Atherothrombosis and Coronary Artery Disease

SECOND EDITION

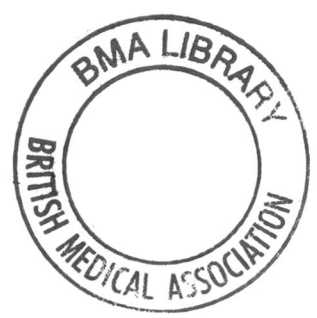

Atherothrombosis and Coronary Artery Disease

SECOND EDITION

Editors

Valentin Fuster, M.D., Ph.D.
Director, The Zena and Michael A. Wiener Cardiovascular Institute
Director, The Marie-Josée and Henry R. Kravis Center for Cardiovascular Health
The Richard Gorlin Professor of Cardiology
President of the World Heart Federation
The Mount Sinai Medical Center
New York, New York

Eric J. Topol, M.D.
Provost and Chief Academic Officer
Chairman, Department of Cardiovascular Medicine
The Cleveland Clinic Foundation
Cleveland, Ohio

Elizabeth G. Nabel, M.D.
Scientific Director, Clinical Research
National Heart, Lung and Blood Institute
National Institutes of Health
Bethesda, Maryland

Acquisitions Editor: Ruth Weinberg
Developmental Editor: Tanya Lazar/Nancy Winter
Project Manager: Alicia Jackson
Senior Manufacturing Manager: Benjamin Rivera
Marketing Manager: Sara Bodison
Designer: Christine Jenny
Production Service: Graphic World Publishing Services
Printer: Courier Kendallville

© 2005 by LIPPINCOTT WILLIAMS & WILKINS
530 Walnut Street
Philadelphia, PA 19106 USA
LWW.com

Printed in the USA

Library of Congress Cataloging-in-Publication Data

Atherothrombosis and coronary artery disease / editors, Valentin Fuster, Eric J. Topol,
  Elizabeth G. Nabel.—2nd ed.
      p. ; cm.
    Rev. ed. of: Atherosclerosis and coronary artery disease / editors, Valentin Fuster,
  Russell Ross, Eric J. Topol. c1996.
    Includes bibliographical references and index.
    ISBN 0-7817-3583-1
      1. Atherosclerosis. 2. Coronary heart disease. I. Fuster, Valentin. II. Topol, Eric J.,
  1954- III. Nabel, Elizabeth G. IV. Atherosclerosis and coronary artery disease.
    [DNLM: 1. Arteriosclerosis. 2. Coronary Disease. 3. Coronary Thrombosis. 4.
  Hypertension. 5. Lipoproteins—metabolism. WG 550 A8699 2005]
  RC692.A7297 2005
  616.1′36—dc22

                                                            2004057755

10 9 8 7 6 5 4 3 2 1

Atherothrombosis and Coronary Artery Disease

Editors
Valentin Fuster, M.D., Ph.D.
Eric J. Topol, M.D.
Elizabeth G. Nabel, M.D.

Hypertension, Cigarette Smoking, Diabetes, Obesity, and Others

II Pathogenesis of Atherothrombosis

General Principles

The Normal Artery

The Lesions of Atherothrombosis

Special Pathogenetic Factors

III Markers and Evolving Imaging of Atherothrombotic Disease

IV Acute Coronary Syndromes

Pathophysiology and Pathogenesis

Clinical Presentation

Management

Contributors

Marios N. Adonis, M.A.
Doctoral Candidate
Ferkauf Graduate School of Psychology
Albert Einstein College of Medicine
Yeshiva University
Bronx, New York;
Intern
Department of Psychiatry
Coler Goldwater Specialty Hospital and Nursing Facility
Roosevelt Island, New York

Jeffrey L. Anderson, M.D., Ph.D.
Professor of Internal Medicine
Department of Internal Medicine
University of Utah;
Associate Chief of Cardiology
Cardiovascular Department
Intermountain Health Care, LDS Hospital
Salt Lake City, Utah

Heidar Arjomand, M.D.
Seacoast Cardiology Associates
Dover, New Hampshire

Doron Aronson, M.D.
Director, Cardiac step-down unit
Division of Cardiology
Rambam Medical Center
Haifa, Israel

Álvaro Avezum, M.D., Ph.D.
Director
Research Division
Dante Pazzanese Institute of Cardiology;
Executive Manager
Clinical Research Center, Teaching and Research Institute
Albert Einstein Hospital
São Paulo, Brazil

Juan Jose Badimon, Ph.D.
Professor of Medicine
Director, Cardiovascular Biology Research Laboratory
Cardiovascular Institute
Mount Sinai School of Medicine
New York, New York

Lina Badimon, Ph.D., F.E.S.C., F.A.H.A.
Director
Cardiovascular Research Center
Hospital de la Santa Creu i Sant Pau
Barcelona, Spain

Donald S. Baim, M.D.
Professor of Medicine
Harvard Medical School;
Director, Center for Integration of Medicine and Innovative
    Technology
Cardiovascular Division, Department of Medicine
Brigham and Women's Hospital
Boston, Massachusetts

**S. Serge Barold, M.D., F.R.A.C.P, F.A.C.C., F.A.C.P.,
    F.E.S.C.**
Professor of Medicine
Department of Cardiology
University of South Florida College of Medicine;
Pacemaker Clinic
USF Cardiology
Harbourside Medical Tower
Tampa General Hospital
Tampa, Florida

George A. Beller, M.D.
Ruth C. Heede Professor of Cardiology
Cardiovascular Division
Department of Medicine
University of Virginia Health System;
Attending Cardiologist
Heart and Vascular Center
University of Virginia Medical Center
Charlottesville, Virginia

Thomas P. Bersot, M.D., Ph.D.
Professor
Department of Medicine
Gladstone Institute of Cardiovascular Disease
University of California San Francisco;
Attending Physician and Chief, Lipid Clinic
Department of Medicine
San Francisco General Hospital
San Francisco, California

Gavin J. Blake, M.D., F.R.C.P.I., M.R.C.P., M.Sc., M.P.H.
Consultant Cardiologist
Mater Misericordiae University Hospital
University College Dublin
Dublin, Ireland

Eugene Braunwald, M.D.
Distinguished Hersey Professor of Medicine
Faculty of Medicine
Harvard Medical School;
Chairman, TIMI Study Group
Department of Medicine
Brigham and Women's Hospital
Boston, Massachusetts

Sorin Brener
Interventional Cardiologist
Director, Angiographic Core Laboratory
Assistant Professor of Medicine
The Cleveland Clinic Foundation
Cleveland, Ohio

H. Bryan Brewer, Jr., M.D.
Chief, Molecular Disease Branch
NHLBI/NIH
Bethesda, Maryland

B. Greg Brown, M.D., Ph.D.
Professor
Department of Medicine/Cardiology
University of Washington School of Medicine;
Cardiologist
Department of Medicine/Cardiology
University of Washington Medical Center
Seattle, Washington

Allen P. Burke, M.D.
Adjunct Professor
Department of Pathology
Georgetown University Hospital;
Associate Chair
Department of Cardiovascular Pathology
Armed Forces Institute of Pathology
Washington, D.C.

Robert M. Califf, M.D., F.A.C.C.
Professor of Medicine
Associate Vice Chancellor for Clinical Research
Department of Medicine
Duke University
Durham, North Carolina

Richard O. Cannon III, M.D.
Clinical Director
National Heart, Lung, and Blood Institute
National Institutes of Health
Bethesda, Maryland

Louis R. Caplan, M.D.
Professor
Department of Neurology
Harvard Medical School;
Chief
Department of Cardiovascular Disease
Beth Israel Deaconess Medical Center
Boston, Massachusetts

Peter Carmeliet, M.D., Ph.D.
Professor of Medicine
Center for Transgene Technology & Gene Therapy
Flanders Institute for Biotechnology (VIB)
University of Leuven, Campus Gasthuisberg
Leuven, Belgium

Alfio Carroccio, M.D.
Assistant Professor of Surgery and Radiology
Mount Sinai School of Medicine
New York, New York

Alexandre Biasi Cavalcanti, M.D.
Medical Researcher
Clinical Research Center
Albert Einstein Education and Research Institute
Albert Einstein Hospital;
Physician
Intensive Care Unit
Albert Einstein Hospital
São Paulo, Brazil

Albert W. Chan, M.D., M.S.C.
Interventional Cardiologist, Department of Cardiology
Royal Columbian Hospital
New Westminster, British Columbia, Canada

Israel F. Charo, M.D., Ph.D.
Department of Medicine
Gladstone Institute of Cardiovascular Disease
University of California
San Francisco, California

Guy M. Chisolm, Ph.D.
Staff Member, Professor
Department of Cell Biology
Cleveland Clinic Foundation
Cleveland, Ohio

Aram V. Chobanian, M.D.
President ad interim
Boston University
Boston, Massachusetts

Robin P. Choudhoury, D.M., M.R.C.P.
Clinical Lecturer
Department of Cardiovascular Medicine
University of Oxford
Oxford, The United Kingdom

Mina K. Chung, M.D.
Staff
Department of Cardiovascular Medicine
Cleveland Clinic Foundation
Cleveland, Ohio

Lynn P. Clemow, Ph.D.
Assistant Professor
Department of Medicine
Columbia University, College of Physicians and Surgeons;
Associate Psychologist
Departments of Medicine & Psychiatry
Columbia University Medical Center
New York, New York

Alexander W. Clowes, M.D.
Professor
Department of Surgery
University of Washington School of Medicine
Seattle, Washington

Marc Cohen, M.D., F.A.C.C.
Professor of Medicine
Department of Internal Medicine
Mount Sinai School of Medicine
New York, New York;
Chief of Cardiology
Department of Internal Medicine
Newark Beth Israel Medical Center
Newark, New Jersey

Peter F. Cohn, M.D.
Professor of Medicine and Vice-Chair for Clinical Affairs
Department of Medicine
State University of New York Health Sciences Center
Stony Brook, New York

Veerle Compernolle
Laboratory for Clinical Biology
Ghent University Hospital
Gent, Belgium

Roberto Corti, M.D.
Assistant Professor
Consultant
Department of Cardiology
University Hospital Zurich
Zurich, Switzerland

Juan Cosín-Sales, M.D.
Consultant in Cardiology
Department of Cardiology
Arnau de Vilanova Hospital
Valencia, Spain

Myron I. Cybulsky, M.D.
Professor
Department of Laboratory Medicine and Pathobiology
University of Toronto;
Senior Scientist
Pathologist
Division of Cell and Molecular Biology
Department of Laboratory Medicine and Pathobiology
Toronto General Research Institute, University Health
  Network
Toronto, Ontario, Canada

Dorota Dajnowiec, H.B.Sc.
Ph.D. Student
Laboratory Medicine and Pathobiology
University of Toronto;
Ph.D. Student
Cellular and Molecular Biology
Toronto General Hospital
Toronto, Ontario, Canada

Karina W. Davidson, Ph.D.
Associate Professor of Behavioral Medicine
Departments of Medicine and Psychiatry
Columbia College of Physicians & Surgeons
Columbia University
New York, New York

Pim J. de Feyter, M.D., Ph.D.
Professor
Department of Cardiology
Erasmus Medical Center
Rotterdam, The Netherlands

Anthony C. De Franco, M.D.
Director, McLaren Heart and Vascular Center
Chief, Division of Cardiology
McLaren Regional Medical Center
Assistant Professor of Medicine
Michigan State University
Flint, Michigan

Louis J. Dell'Italia, M.D.
Professor
Department of Medicine
Division of Cardiovascular Disease
University of Alabama at Birmingham
Center for Heart Failure Research;
Physician/Cardiologist
Department of Cardiovascular Disease
University Hospital
Birmingham, Alabama

Joseph A. Diamond, M.D.
Associate Professor
Department of Medicine
Albert Einstein College of Medicine
Bronx, New York;
Director
Department of Nuclear Cardiology
Division of Cardiology
Long Island Jewish Medical Center
New Hyde Park, New York

Paul E. DiCorleto, Ph.D.
Chairman
Lerner Research Institute
The Cleveland Clinic Foundation
Cleveland, Ohio

Thomas F. Dodson, M.D.
Division of Vascular Surgery
Emory University School of Medicine
Atlanta, Georgia

W. Lane Duvall, M.D.
Instructor of Medicine
Assistant Director of the Cardiac Care Unit
Mount Sinai Medical Center
The Zena and Michael A. Wiener Cardiovascular Institute
New York, New York

Victor J. Dzau, M.D.
Chancellor of Health Affairs
Duke University;
President and Chief Executive Officer
Duke University Health System
Duke University Medical Center
Durham, North Carolina

Simon P. Eggleton, M.B.B.S. (Hons), B.Sc. (med)
Cardiology Registrar
Department of Cardiology
Prince of Wales Hospital
Randwick, Australia

Stephen G. Ellis, M.D.
Professor of Medicine
Department of Cardiovascular Medicine
The Cleveland Clinic Lerner College of Medicine of Case
    Western Reserve University;
Director, Jones Cardia Laboratories
Co-Director, Cardiac Genebank
The Cleveland Clinic Foundation
Cleveland, Ohio

Sharif H. Ellozy, M.D.
Assistant Professor, Department of Surgery
Division of Vascular and Endovascular Surgery
The Mount Sinai Medical Center
New York, New York

Erling Falk, M.D. Ph.D.
Professor of Cardiovascular Pathology
Department of Cardiology
Aarhus University Hospital (Skejby) and Clinical Institute
University of Aarhus
Aarhus, Denmark

John A. Farmer, M.D.
Department of Medicine
Baylor College of Medicine;
Cardiology Service
Ben Taub Hospital
Houston, Texas

Zahi A. Fayad, Ph.D.
Associate Professor
Departments of Radiology and Medicine (Cardiology)
Mount Sinai School of Medicine
New York, New York

James S. Forrester, M.D.
Professor of Medicine
Department of Medicine
UCLA Geffen School of Medicine;
Burns and Allen Professor of Cardiology
Department of Medicine
Cedars Sinai Medical Center
Los Angeles, California

Joan E.B. Fox, Ph.D.
Professor of Medicine
Department of Cardiovascular Medicine
The Cleveland Clinic Foundation;
Director
Center for Integrative Medicine
The Cleveland Clinic Foundation
Cleveland, Ohio

Paul L. Fox, Ph.D.
Department of Cell Biology
Lerner Research Institute
Cleveland Clinic Foundation
Cleveland, Ohio

William H. Frishman, M.D., F.A.C.C.
Professor of Medicine and Pharmacology
Chairman, Department of Medicine
New York Medical College;
Director of Medicine
Westchester Medical Center
Valhalla, New York

Edward D. Frohlich, M.D.
Professor of Medicine and Physiology
Louisiana State University School of Medicine;
Clinical Professor of Medicine and Adjunct Professor
    of Pharmacology
Tulane University School of Medicine;
Alton Ochsner Distinguished Scientist
Ochsner Clinic Foundation
New Orleans, Louisiana

Valentin Fuster, M.D., Ph.D.
Director, The Zena and Michael A. Wiener Cardiovascular
    Institute
Director, The Marie-Josée and Henry R. Kravis Center for
    Cardiovascular Health
The Richard Gorlin Professor of Cardiology
President, World Heart Federation
The Mount Sinai Medical Center
New York, New York

W. Bruce Fye, M.D., M.A.
Professor of Medicine and the History of Medicine
The Mayo Clinic College of Medicine;
Consultant, Cardiology
Mayo Clinic
Rochester, Minnesota

Santhi K. Ganesh, M.D.
Vascular Biology Section, Cardiovascular Branch
National Heart, Lung and Blood Institute
Bethesda, Maryland

William Ganz, M.D., C.Sc.
Professor of Medicine
David Geffen School of Medicine
University of California;
Division of Cardiology
Cedars-Sinai Medical Center
Los Angeles, California

William Gerin, Ph.D.
Associate Professor of Medicine
Department of General Medicine
Columbia University College of Physicians and Surgeons;
Associate Professor of Psychiatry
Department of Psychiatry
New York-Presbyterian Hospital
New York, New York

Henry Gewirtz, M.D.
Associate Professor
Department of Medicine
Harvard Medical School;
Director, Nuclear Cardiology
Department of Medicine
Massachusetts General Hospital
Boston, Massachusetts

Gary H. Gibbons, M.D.
Director, Cardiovascular Research Institute
Professor of Medicine
Cardiovascular Research Institute
Department of Medicine
Morehouse School of Medicine;
Attending Cardiologist
Department of Medicine
Morehouse School of Medicine
Atlanta, Georgia

Robert S. Gibson, M.D.
Lockhart B. McGuire Professor of Medicine
Department of Internal Medicine
University of Virginia
Charlottesville, Virginia

Mladen Golubic, M.D., Ph.D.
Project Scientist
Center for Integrative Medicine and Brain Tumor Institute
Cleveland Clinic Foundation
Cleveland, Ohio

J. Anthony Gomes
The Zena and Michael A. Wiener Cardiovascular Institute
Mount Sinai Medical Center of NYU
New York, New York

Joao A. Gomes, M.D.
Post Doctoral Fellow
Department of Neurology
Division of Neurocritical Care
The Johns Hopkins University Medical School;
Senior Clinical Fellow
Department of Neurology
Division of Neurocritical Care
The Johns Hopkins Hospital
Baltimore, Maryland

David Gordon, M.D.
Department of Pathology
University of Michigan
Ann Arbor, Michigan

Nilesh J. Goswami, M.D.
Clinical Assistant Professor of Medicine
Department of Internal Medicine
Southern Illinois University School of Medicine;
Director, Coronary Care Unit
Prairie Cardiovascular Consultants, Ltd.
Prairie Heart Institute
Springfield, Illinois

Avrum I. Gotlieb, M.D. C.M.
Professor and Chair
Department of Laboratory Medicine and Pathobiology
University of Toronto;
Staff Pathologist
Department of Pathology
University Health Network
Toronto, Ontario, Canada

Antonio M. Gotto, Jr., M.D., D.Phil.
The Stephen and Suzanne Weiss Dean
Professor of Medicine
Weill Medical College of Cornell University
New York, New York

Scott M. Grundy, M.D., Ph.D
Director
Professor
Center for Human Nutrition
Department of Internal Medicine
University of Texas
Southwestern Medical Center at Dallas
Dallas, Texas

Hitinder S. Gurm, M.B.B.S.
Fellow, Interventional Cardiology
Department of Cardiovascular Medicine
Cleveland Clinic Foundation
Cleveland, Ohio

Jonathan L. Halperin, M.D.
Robert and Harriet Heilbrunn Professor of Medicine
The Zena and Michael A. Wiener Cardiovascular Institute
Mount Sinai School of Medicine;
Director, Cardiology Clinical Services
The Zena and Michael A. Wiener Cardiovascular Institute
Mount Sinai Medical Center
New York, New York

Göran K. Hansson, M.D., Ph.D.
Professor and Research Director
Department of Medicine and Center for Molecular
    Medicine
Karolinska Institute;
Professor
Department of Medicine
Karolinska University Hospital
Stockholm, Sweden

Donald C. Harrison, M.D.
Senior Vice President and Provost for Health Affairs
    Emeritus
University of Cincinnati Medical Center
Cincinnati, Ohio

J. Warren Harthorne, M.D., C.M., F.A.C.P., F.A.C.C.
Professor of Medicine
Harvard Medical School
Cardiology Unit
Massachusetts General Hospital
Boston, Massachusetts

H. Coenraad Hemker, M.D., Ph.D.
Senior Professor of Biochemistry
Department of Coagulation Physiology
Cardiovascular Research Institute Maastricht (CARIM);
Director
Synapse bv, Research and Consultation
Maastricht University Holding bv
Maastricht, The Netherlands

Larry H. Hollier, M.D., F.A.C.S., F.A.C.C., F.R.C.S.
Professor of Surgery and Dean
Louisiana Health Sciences Center School of Medicine
New Orleans, Louisiana

William L. Holman, M.D.
Professor in Surgery
Division of Cardiothoracic Surgery
University of Alabama at Birmingham;
Professor in Surgery
Division of Cardiothoracic Surgery
University Hospital
Birmingham, Alabama

David R. Holmes, Jr., M.D.
Professor
Department of Internal Medicine
Division of Cardiovascular Diseases
Mayo Clinic College of Medicine;
Interventional Cardiologist
Department of Internal Medicine
Division of Cardiovascular Diseases
Mayo Clinic, Saint Mary's Hospital
Rochester, Minnesota

Paul N. Hopkins, M.D., M.S.P.H.
Professor of Internal Medicine
Department of Cardiovascular Genetics
University of Utah
Salt Lake City, Utah

Gordon S. Huggins, M.D.
Assistant Professor of Medicine
Division of Cardiology
Tufts University School of Medicine;
Investigator
Molecular Cardiology Research Institute
Tufts-New England Medical Center
Boston, Massachusetts

Steven C. Hunt, Ph.D.
Professor
Cardiovascular Genetics, Department of Internal Medicine
University of Utah
Salt Lake City, Utah

John P. Kane, M.D., Ph.D.
Professor of Medicine, Biochemistry and Biophysics
Director, UCSF Lipid Clinic
Associate Director Cardiovascular Research Institute
Attending Physician
Department of Medicine
University of California, San Francisco
San Francisco, California

William B. Kannel, M.D., M.P.H.
Professor of Medicine
Framingham Heart Study
Boston University School of Medicine
Framingham, Massachusetts

Samir R. Kapadia, M.D.
Staff Cardiologist
Department of Cardiovascular Medicine
The Cleveland Clinic Foundation
Cleveland, Ohio

Norman M. Kaplan, M.D.
Clinical Professor
Department of Internal Medicine
University of Texas Southwestern Medical School
Dallas, Texas

Juan Carlos Kaski, M.D., D.M. (Hons), D.Sc., F.R.C.P.
Professor of Cardiovascular Science and Head
    of Department
Department of Cardiological Sciences
St. George's Hospital Medical School;
Consultant Cardiologist
Department of Cardiology
St. George's Hospital
London, The United Kingdom

Spencer B. King III, M.D.
Clinical Professor of Medicine
Emory University;
Director of Interventional Cardiology
Fuqua Heart Center
Piedmont Hospital
Atlanta, Georgia

Margaret L. Kirby, Ph.D.
Professor
Department of Pediatrics
Duke University
Durham, North Carolina

James K. Kirklin, M.D.
Professor of Surgery
Director of Cardiothoracic Transplantation
Cardiothoracic Department
University of Alabama at Birmingham
Birmingham, Alabama

Larry W. Kraiss, M.D.
Associate Professor & Chief
Division of Vascular Surgery
Department of Surgery
University of Utah School of Medicine;
Attending Surgeon
University of Utah Hospitals & Clinics
Salt Lake City, Utah

Meena S. Kumar, M.D., Ph.D.
Department of Physiology
University of Virginia
Charlottesville, Virginia

B. Lowell Langille, Ph.D.
Professor
Department of Laboratory Medicine and Pathobiology
University of Toronto;
Senior Scientist
Division of Cellular and Molecular Biology
Toronto General Hospital
Toronto, Ontario, Canada

Martin B. Leon, M.D., F.A.C.C.
Associate Director of Cardiovascular Interventional Therapy
Department of Medicine
Columbia University College of Physicians and Surgeons
New York, New York

Peter Libby, M.D.
Mallinckrodt Professor of Medicine
Harvard Medical School;
Chief
Cardiovascular Medicine, Department of Medicine
Brigham and Women's Hospital
Boston, Massachusetts

A. Michael Lincoff, M.D.
Professor of Medicine
Department of Medicine
Cleveland Clinic Lerner College of Medicine of Case
    Western Reserve University;
Staff
Department of Cardiovascular Medicine
The Cleveland Clinic Foundation
Cleveland, Ohio

Theo Lindhout, Ph.D.
Associate Professor
Department of Biochemistry
Maastricht University
Maastricht, The Netherlands

Robert A. Lookstein, M.D.
Department of Surgery
Division of Vascular and Endovascular Surgery
The Mount Sinai Medical Center
New York, New York

Thomas F. Lüscher, M.D.
Professor and Head of Cardiology
University Hospital Zurich
Zurich, Switzerland

Robert W. Mahley, M.D., Ph.D.
Professor of Pathology and Medicine
Director, Gladstone Institute of Cardiovascular Disease
Department of Pathology
University of California, San Francisco
San Francisco, California

John J. Mahmarian, M.D.
Professor of Medicine
Department of Medicine
Section of Cardiology
Baylor College of Medicine
Medical Director
Nuclear Cardiology Laboratory
Methodist DeBakey Heart Center
The Methodist Hospital
Houston, Texas

Joseph F. Malouf, M.D.
Associate Professor
Department of Internal Medicine
Mayo Clinic College of Medicine;
Consultant, Cardiovascular Diseases
Mayo Clinic
Rochester, New York

David Manka
Genome Research Institute
University of Cincinnati
Cincinnati, Ohio

Michael L. Marin, M.D., F.A.C.S.
Professor and Interim Chairman
Henry Kaufmann Professor of Vascular Surgery
Mount Sinai School of Medicine
Attending
Department of Surgery
Mount Sinai Hospital
New York, New York

Daniel B. Mark, M.D., M.P.H.
Professor of Medicine
Department of Medicine
Division of Cardiology
Duke University Medical Center;
Director, Outcomes Research
Duke Clinical Research Institute
Duke University
Durham, North Carolina

David O. Martin, M.D., M.P.H.
Department of Cardiovascular Medicine
The Cleveland Clinic Foundation
Cleveland, Ohio

David C. McGiffin, M.D.
Professor of Surgery
Department of Surgery
University of Alabama at Birmingham;
Professor of Surgery
Department of Surgery
University of Alabama at Birmingham Medical Center
Birmingham, Alabama

Henry C. McGill, Jr., M.D.
Professor Emeritus
Department of Pathology
The University of Texas Health Science Center
  at San Antonio;
Senior Scientist Emeritus
Department of Physiology and Medicine
Southwest Foundation for Biomedical Research
San Antonio, Texas

C. Alex McMahan, Ph.D.
Professor
Department of Pathology
University of Texas Health Science Center at San Antonio
San Antonio, Texas

Murray A. Mittleman, M.D., Dr.P.H.
Associate Professor of Medicine and Epidemiology
Department of Medicine
Harvard Schools of Medicine and Public Health;
Director, Cardiovascular Epidemiology
Department of Medicine/Cardiology
Beth Israel Deaconess Medical Center
Boston, Massachusetts

David J. Moliterno, M.D.
Professor and Vice-Chairman
Department of Internal Medicine
University of Kentucky;
Chief, Cardiovascular Medicine
Gill Heart Institute
University of Kentucky
Lexington, Kentucky

Lori Mosca, M.D., Ph.D.
Associate Professor
Department of Medicine
Columbia University;
Director, Preventive Cardiology
Department of Medicine/Division of Cardiology
New York-Presbyterian Hospital
New York, New York

Andreas Muench, M.D.
Chief Fellow
Division of Cardiology
Instructor in Medicine
Department of Medicine
University of Texas-Houston Medical School at Houston
Houston, Texas

Joseph B. Muhlestein, M.D.
Cardiovascular Department
LDS Hospital
University of Utah School of Medicine
Salt Lake City, Utah

James E. Muller, M.D.
Co-Director, CIMIT Vulnerable Plaque Program
Massachusetts General Hospital
Harvard Medical School
Boston, Massachusetts

Robert J. Myerburg, M.D.
Professor of Medicine
Division of Cardiology
Department of Medicine
University of Miami School of Medicine;
Chief
Division of Cardiology
Department of Medicine
Jackson Memorial Hospital
Miami, Florida

Elizabeth G. Nabel, M.D.
Scientific Director, Clinical Research
National Heart, Lung and Blood Institute
National Institutes of Health
Bethesda, Maryland

Yoshifumi Naka, M.D., Ph.D.
Herbert Irving Assistant Professor of Surgery
Department of Surgery
Columbia University;
Director, Cardiac Transplantation and Mechanical
  Circulatory Support Programs
Department of Surgery
New York Presbyterian Hospital
New York, New York

Konstantin Nikolaou, M.D.
Fellow of Radiology
Department of Radiology
University of Munich
Munich, Germany

Steven E. Nissen, M.D.
Vice-Chairman, Division of Cardiology
Medical Director, Cleveland Clinic Foundation
Professor of Medicine
The Cleveland Clinic Foundation
Cleveland, Ohio

Georg Noll, M.D.
Professor
Cardio Vascular Centre/Cardiology
University Hospital Zurich
Zurich, Switzerland

Patrick T. O'Gara, M.D.
Associate Professor of Medicine
Harvard Medical School;
Director, Clinical Cardiology
Vice-Chairman, Department of Medicine
Cardiovascular Division and Department of Medicine
Brigham and Women's Hospital
Boston, Massachusetts

Jeffrey W. Olin, D.O.
Professor of Medicine
Zena and Michael A. Wiener Cardiovascular Institute
Marie-Josée and Henry R. Kravis Center for Cardiovascular
    Health
Mount Sinai School of Medicine;
Director, Vascular Medicine
Zena and Michael A. Wiener Cardiovascular Institute
Marie-Josée and Henry R. Kravis Center for Cardiovascular
    Health
Mount Sinai Hospital

Robert A. O'Rourke, M.D., F.A.C.C., M.A.C.P.
Charles Conrad Brown Distinguished Professor of
    Medicine
Department of Medicine
University of Texas Health Science Center;
Attending Faculty Cardiologist
Department of Medicine
University Hospital
Audie L. Murphy Veterans' Administration Hospital
San Antonio, Texas

Gary K. Owens, M.D., Ph.D.
Professor of Molecular Physiology and Biological Physics
Cardiovascular Research Center
University of Virginia;
Associate Dean
The School of Medicine
Graduate and Medical Scientist Programs
University of Virginia
Charlottesville, Virginia

Fredric J. Pashkow, M.D.
Professor of Medicine
Department of Medicine
John A. Burns School of Medicine
University of Hawaii
Honolulu, Hawaii;
Director
Department of Medical Affairs
Sanofi~Snthelabo
New York, New York

Richard C. Pasternak, M.D.
Associate Professor of Medicine
Harvard Medical School;
Director of Preventive Cardiology
Cardiology Division
Massachusetts General Hospital
Boston, Massachusetts

Marc S. Penn, M.D., Ph.D.
Adjunct Assistant Professor
Department of Biomedical Engineering
Case Western Reserve University;
Director, Experimental Animal Laboratory
Director, Cardiac Intensive Care Unit
Department of Cardiovascular Medicine and Cell Biology
Cleveland Clinic Foundation
Cleveland, Ohio

Carl J. Pepine, M.D.
Professor and Chief
Division of Cardiovascular Medicine
Department of Medicine
University of Florida
Gainesville, Florida

Marc A. Pfeffer, M.D., Ph.D.
Cardiovascular Division
Brigham and Women's Hospital
Boston, Massachusetts

Robert A. Phillips, M.D., Ph.D.
Professor of Medicine
Department of Medicine
New York University School of Medicine;
Chairman
Department of Medicine
Lenox Hill Hospital
New York, New York

Thomas G. Pickering, M.D., D. Phil.
Director, Behavioral Cardiovascular Health
    and Hypertension Program
Columbia Presbyterian Medical Center
New York, New York

Leopoldo Soares Piegas, M.D., Ph.D.
Associated Professor
Department of Cardioneurolgoy
University of São Paulo School of Medicine;
Technical Director
Dante Pazzanese Institute of Cardiology
São Paulo, Brazil

David J. Pinsky, M.D.
J. Griswold Ruth, M.D. and Margery Hopkins Ruth
  Professor of Internal Medicine
Department of Medicine
University of Michigan;
Chief, Cardiovascular Medicine
Scientific Director, Cardiovascular Center
University of Michigan
Ann Arbor, Michigan

Andrew S. Plump, M.D., Ph.D.
Director
Department of Clinical Molecular Profiling
Merck Research Laboratory
Rahway, New Jersey

Gerald M. Pohost, M.D.
Professor
Department of Medicine
Keck School of Medicine;
Chief
Department of Cardiovascular Medicine
University Hospital
Los Angeles, California

Michael Poon, M.D.
Associate Professor
Department of Medicine (Cardiology)
Mount Sinai School of Medicine;
Chief
Department of Cardiology
Cabrini Medical Center
New York, New York

Eric N. Prystowsky, M.D.
Consulting Professor of Medicine
Department of Medicine
Duke University Medical Center
Durham North Carolina;
Director, Clinical Electrophysiology Laboratory
Department of Cardiology
St. Vincent Hospital
Indianapolis, Indiana

Daniel J. Rader, M.D.
Associate Professor
Departments of Medicine and Pharmacology
University of Pennsylvania School of Medicine;
Director, Preventive Cardiology & Lipid Clinic
Department of Cardiology
University of Pennsylvania Medical Center

Elaine W. Raines, M.S.
Research Professor
Department of Pathology
University of Washington
Harborview Medical Center
Seattle, Washington

Elliot J. Rayfield, M.D.
Clinical Professor
Department of Medicine
Mount Sinai School of Medicine;
Attending Physician
Department of Medicine
Mount Sinai Hospital
New York, New York

Paul M. Ridker, M.D., M.P.H., F.A.C.C.
Eugene Braunwald Professor of Medicine
Department of Medicine
Harvard Medical School;
Director, Center for Cardiovascular Disease Prevention
Division of Preventive Medicine
Brigham and Women's Hospital
Boston, Massachusetts

Thom W. Rooke, M.D., F.A.C.C.
Krehbiel Professor of Vascular Medicine
Department of Vascular Medicine
Mayo Clinic, Gonda Vascular Center;
Head, Section of Vascular Medicine
Department of Vascular Medicine
St. Mary's Hospital
Rochester, Minnesota

Randi Rose, M.D.
Clinical Instructor
Department of Cardiology
Mount Sinai School of Medicine
New York, New York

Michael E. Rosenfeld, Ph.D.
Professor
Department of Pathobiology and Pathology
University of Washington
Seattle, Washington

Gabriella Rothman
Behavioral Cardiovascular Health and Hypertension
  Program
Division of General Medicine
Columbia University, College of Physicians & Surgeons
New York, New York

John D. Rutherford, M.B., Ch.B., F.R.A.C.P.
Vice President for Clinical Operations
Professor of Internal Medicine
Jonsson-Rogers Chair in Cardiology
UT Southwestern Medical Center
Dallas, Texas

Silvia Santamarina-Fojo, M.D., Ph.D.
Chief, Section of Molecular Biology
Molecular Disease Branch
National Heart, Lung and Blood Institute, NIH
Bethesda, Maryland

Javier Sanz, M.D.
Post Doctoral Research Fellow
Cardiovascular Institute
Mount Sinai School of Medicine
New York, New York

Angelo M. Scanu, M.D.
University of Chicago
Chicago, Illinois

Hartzell V. Schaff, M.D.
Stuart W. Harrington Professor of Surgery
Division of Cardiovascular Surgery
Mayo Clinic College of Medicine;
Professor of Surgery
Division of Cardiovascular Surgery
Saint Mary's Hospital
Rochester, Minnesota

Heinrich R. Schelbert, M.D., Ph.D.
George V. Taplin Professor
Department of Molecular and Medical Pharmacology
David Geffen School of Medicine at UCLA
Los Angeles, California

Thomas H. Schindler, M.D.
Research Fellow
Department of Molecular and Medical Pharmacology
David Geffen School of Medicine at UCLA
Los Angeles, California

Paul Schoenhagen, M.D., F.A.H.A.
Department of Radiology and Cardiovascular Medicine
The Cleveland Clinic Foundation
Cleveland, Ohio

Uwe Schönbeck, Ph.D.
Executive Director
Department of Cardiovascular Disease
Boehringer Ingelheim Pharmaceuticals Inc.
Ridgefield, Connecticut

Rafael F. Sequeira, M.D., F.R.C.P., F.A.C.C.
Professor
Department of Medicine
University of Miami Medical Center;
Director, Coronary Care Unit
Department of Cardiology
Jackson Memorial Hospital
Miami, Florida

Patrick W. Serruys, M.D., Ph.D.
Professor of Interventional Cardiology
University Hospital Dijkzigt-Thoraxcenter
Rotterdam, The Netherlands

Prediman K. Shah, M.D.
Professor
Department of Medicine
David Geffen School of Medicine at UCLA;
Shapell and Webb Chair and Director
Cardiology Division
Cedars-Sinai Medical Center
Los Angeles, California

Robert D. Shamburek, M.D.
Molecular Disease Branch
NIH/National Heart, Lung, and Blood Institute
Bethesda, Maryland

Jeffrey D. Simmons, M.D.
Mount Sinai Medical Center
Division of Electrophysiology
Florida

Robert B. Smith III, M.D.
John E. Skandalakis Professor of Surgery, Emeritus
  and Associate Chairman
Department of Surgery
Emory University School of Medicine;
Medical Director
Department of Surgery
Emory University Hospital
Atlanta, Georgia

Lukas Spieker, M.D.
Department of Cardiology
University Hospital
Zurich, Switzerland

Herbert Christian Stary, M.D.
Professor of Pathology
Louisiana State University Health Sciences Center
New Orleans, Louisana

David M. Stern, M.D.
Dean, School of Medicine
Professor of Medicine, Physiology, and Graduate Studies
Medical College of Georgia
Augusta, Georgia

Thoralf M. Sundt, M.D.
Professor of Surgery
Department of Surgery
Mayo College of Medicine;
Consultant
Department of Surgery
Mayo Clinic
Rochester, Minnesota

Geoffrey H. Tofler, M.B., M.D.
Professor of Preventative Cardiology
University of Sydney;
Senior Staff Specialist
Department of Cardiology
Royal North Shore Hospital
Sydney, Australia

Eric J. Topol, M.D.
Provost and Chief Academic Officer
Chairman, Department of Cardiovascular Medicine
The Cleveland Clinic Foundation
Cleveland, Ohio

E. Murat Tuzcu, M.D.
Interventional Cardiologist
Director, Intravascular Ultrasound Laboratory
Professor of Medicine
The Cleveland Clinic Foundation
Cleveland, Ohio

Renu Virmani, M.D.
Chair
Department of Cardiovascular Pathology
Armed Forces Institute of Pathology
Washington D.C.

James A. Vitarius, M.D., Ph.D.
Cardiology Fellow
Zena and Michael A. Wiener Cardiovascular Institute
Marie-Josèe and Henry R. Kravis Center for Cardiovascular
   Health
Mount Sinai School of Medicine
New York, New York

David A. Vorchheimer, M.D.
Assistant Professor
Department of Medicine (Cardiology)
Mount Sinai School of Medicine;
Director, Coronary Care Unit
Cardiovascular Institute
Mount Sinai Medical Center
New York, New York

Brian R. Wamhoff, Ph.D.
Post-doctoral Fellow
Departments of Molecular Physiology and Biological
   Physics
University of Virginia
Charlottesville, Virginia

John C. Wang, M.D., M.Sc.
Interventional Cardiology
Midatlantic Cardiovascular Associates, P.A.
Department of Medicine
St. Joseph Medical Center
Towson, Maryland

Brant M. Weinstein, Ph.D.
Investigator
Laboratory of Molecular Genetics
National Institute of Child Health and Human Development
Bethesda, Maryland

Victor J. Weiss, M.D.
Assistant Clinical Professor of Surgery
University of Mississippi School of Medicine
Cardiovascular Surgical Clinic
Jackson, Mississippi

Paul Wade Wennberg, M.D.
Assistant Professor of Medicine
Department of Cardiovascular Diseases
Mayo Clinic College of Medicine;
Director
Gonda Vascular Laboratory and Vascular Medicine
   Hospital Service
Mayo Clinic
Rochester, Minnesota

Thomas N. Wight, Ph.D.
Affiliate Professor
Department of Pathology
University of Washington School of Medicine;
Member
The Hope Heart Program
Benaroya Research Institute at Virginia Mason
Seattle, Washington

James T. Willerson, M.D.
President
University of Texas, Health Science Center;
Medical Director
Texas Heart Institute
Houston, Texas

Jay S. Yadav, M.D.
The Cleveland Clinic Foundation
Cleveland, Ohio

Phillip C. Yang, M.D.
Assistant Professor
Department of Medicine
Stanford University;
Staff Physician
Department of Medicine
Stanford University Hospital
Stanford, California

Philip T. Zhao
The Zena and Michael A. Wiener Cardiovascular Institute
The Marie-Josée and Henry R. Kravis Cardiovascular
  Health Center
Mount Sinai School of Medicine
New York, New York

Frank J. Zidar, M.D.
Interventional Cardiology Fellow
Adult Cardiac Catheterization Laboratories
Division of Cardiology
Duke University Medical Center
Durham, North Carolina

Pierre Zoldhelyi, M.D.
Associate Professor of Medicine
Divisions of Cardiology & Hematology
University of Texas-Houston Medical School
Houston, Texas

PREFACE

The first edition of *Atherosclerosis and Coronary Artery Disease,* published in 1996, was the first multi-authored, comprehensive textbook to examine this unique and broad discipline of cardiovascular disease. A critical factor leading to its creation was the need for a dialogue on a variety of topics ranging from molecular biology to randomized clinical trials. The text benefitted from the complementary expertise of its three editors and the excellent contributions of about 200 authors. Based on the worldwide response within the first 3 years of its appearance, this first edition was a success. However, those of us who participated in its creation, as well as the medical and scientific community in general, were saddened by the loss of Russell Ross Ph.D., an enthusiastic editor of the first edition and a brilliant and visionary scientist. The editors of this second edition, now including Dr. Elizabeth G. Nabel, dedicate this edition to our former colleague and admired dearest friend, Dr. Russell Ross.

After discussions among the editors, the scientific community, and the staff at Lippincott Williams & Wilkins Publishers, it was concluded that the time was right for a second edition that focuses on the current explosion of research and knowledge at the molecular and cellular levels, and its technological and clinical impact on the diagnosis and therapy of *Atherothrombosis and Coronary Artery Disease.* The title term *Atherothrombosis* has replaced the term *Atherosclerosis* of the former edition, thus reflecting the importance of thrombosis in the cardiovascular discipline approached in the book. This new edition, with 105 chapters written by over 200 outstanding and highly recognized experts in each of the examined fields, has several unique features that distinguish it from the previous edition.

1) At least 60% of the chapters have been modified extensively, particularly in those sections concerned with the most recent advances in the pathogenesis of atherothrombosis, markers and evolving imaging technology, acute coronary syndromes, and primary prevention strategies. Ten new chapters have been added that examine the latest exciting developments concerning the hu-man genome and the genetic basis of atherothrombotic disease, the molecular basis of vasculogenesis, angiogenesis and arteriogenesis, mouse models of lipoprotein metabolism and atherothombosis, the development of "high-" and "low-risk" coronary and noncoronary atherothrombotic plaques, and evolving imaging technology for the assessment of coronary and noncoronary atherosclerotic disease and plaque characterization.

2) Four chapters of this newly revised edition focus on nonsurgical and surgical interventions of peripheral and carotid disease as well as behavioral and alternative medicine in the treatment of atherothrombosis.

3) The second edition of *Atherothombosis and Coronary Artery Disease* includes many new references from the past six months as well as milestone articles that were still in press at the time of publication. The book has been shortened by selectively reducing the number of repetitive references and other unnecessary duplication of information.

The editors are grateful to the outstanding group of authors who participated in the second edition of *Atherothombosis and Coronary Artery Disease* for their extraordinary and timely contributions. As with the previous edition, it took just 20 months from the time the authors agreed to participate to the day of publication. This is a record for a textbook of this size and complexity which deserves the highest tribute and acknowledgment to our authors.

We again gratefully acknowledge the staff at Lippincott Williams & Wilkins Publishers, including Tanya Lazar and Ruth Weinberg, who made production of this endeavor a reality.

Finally, we wish to acknowledge the support of our families and the many sacrifices they have made to make this volume possible.

THE EDITORS
Valentin Fuster, M.D., Ph.D.
Eric J. Topol, M.D.
Elizabeth G. Nabel, M.D.

Introduction

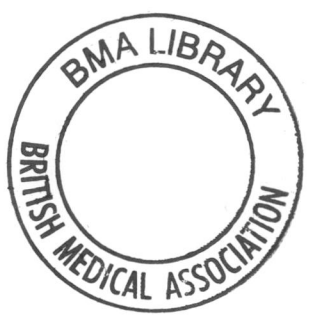

CHAPTER 1

A Historical Perspective on Atherosclerosis and Coronary Artery Disease

W. Bruce Fye

Key Words: Aneurysm; angina pectoris; anticoagulants; arrhythmia; arteriography; atherosclerosis; electrocardiogram; embolism; myocardial infarction; occlusion; reperfusion; thrombosis.

INTRODUCTION

This historical summary focuses on angina pectoris and acute myocardial infarction, the main clinical manifestations of atherothrombosis, a new term that reflects our current understanding of the pathophysiology of a broad range of symptoms, signs, and diseases. It is important to recognize that earlier generations of physicians and scientists did not appreciate the role of thrombosis, and they did not, of course, use the word *atherothrombosis*. In this historical chapter, therefore, I have used the traditional term *atherosclerosis* when it is more appropriate than *atherothrombosis*. This approach avoids the problem of implying that earlier investigators and doctors understood cardiovascular pathophysiology as we do today.

The pathologic features of atherosclerosis were recognized long before the clinical syndromes of angina pectoris and acute myocardial infarction were described in the literature. Even after these clinical conditions were recognized, there was prolonged debate about their pathophysiology. This review provides some insights into the origins of the current understanding of atherosclerosis, angina pectoris, and acute myocardial infarction. It was a challenge to decide which advances to include in this chapter because over the centuries thousands of scientists

W.B. Fye: Mayo Clinic College of Medicine, 200 First Street, SW, Rochester, Minnesota 55905.

and clinicians from around the world have contributed to our current understanding of the pathophysiology, diagnosis, and treatment of coronary artery disease. Inevitably, some well-known names are missing, and some minor individuals are included. Space constraints also made it necessary to exclude several topics and to focus on the period from the mid-eighteenth to the mid-twentieth century.

ANEURYSMS, VASCULAR DISEASE, AND ATHEROSCLEROSIS

Atherosclerosis is a pathologic condition that underlies several important disorders including coronary artery disease, cerebrovascular disease, and diseases of the aorta and peripheral arterial circulation. It is not a new problem. Using sophisticated histologic techniques, paleopathologist A. T. Sandison confirmed that some Egyptian mummies had evidence of atherosclerosis (1). Paleopathologist Roy Moodie concluded that atherosclerosis in ancient Egyptians followed exactly the same course as it does today (2). Galen, the most influential physician of ancient Greece, described vascular aneurysms, but there is no evidence that he recognized other forms of atherosclerotic cardiovascular disease (3). Galen's teachings dominated medical theory and practice, such as they were, until the Renaissance.

Several sixteenth century anatomists, including Andreas Vesalius and Gabriele Falloppio, described aneurysms of the aorta and peripheral arteries (4,5). By the beginning of the seventeenth century, it was recognized that the aorta and other major arteries degenerated with advancing age, but the pathophysiology of this process was unknown. This is not surprising when recalling that William Harvey first proposed that the heart propelled blood through a closed vascular circuit in 1628 (6).

Because aneurysms of the peripheral arteries were visible and could be treated surgically, even before the advent of anesthesia or antisepsis, several articles and books appeared on this subject during the eighteenth century. An 1844 work by British surgeon John Erichsen provides valuable insight into early observations on arterial disease. This book includes nearly two dozen articles on aneurysms from antiquity to the late eighteenth century (7). The authors (and the original publication dates of their works) include Daniel Sennert (1628), Giovanni Maria Lancisi (1728), Alexander Monro (1733), Albrecht von Haller (1749), Pierre Foubert (1753), William Hunter (1757), Donald Monro (1760), Carlo Guattani (1772), John Hunter (1786), and Jacques Louis Dechamps (1799). In his 1628 publication, German chemist and physician Daniel Sennert described two layers in arteries. Sennert's work contained some practical information: He warned practitioners that an aneurysm might result if an artery instead of a vein was accidentally punctured during bloodletting, a popular therapy at the time.

Swiss physiologist Albrecht von Haller made several important observations on the cardiovascular system. In his 1755 monograph, *Opuscula Pathologica,* von Haller described progressive atherosclerotic changes in arteries of the elderly. Six years later, Italian physician and pathologist Giovanni Battista Morgagni published *The Seats and Causes of Disease,* a book that inaugurated the modern era of pathologic anatomy. Morgagni emphasized the value of the microscope as a tool for studying disease processes and stressed the importance of clinicopathologic correlation (Fig. 1–1). Pathologist and historian Esmond Long thought Morgagni's studies of the vascular system were his most significant contribution to special pathology and characterized his observations on aneurysms as "magnificent" (8).

Atherosclerosis was more than an incidental finding at the dissecting table; it sometimes caused diseases that eighteenth century physicians and surgeons tried to treat. Their approaches reflected contemporary medical theories rather than a sophisticated understanding of the pathophysiology of diseases of the heart and vascular system. Although these practitioners did not understand the relation between cerebral atherosclerosis and apoplexy or coronary artery disease and angina pectoris, they surely saw some patients who had these conditions.

Morgagni's pupil Antonio Scarpa, an Italian anatomist and surgeon, extended his mentor's observations on vascular disease. In his 1804 monograph on aneurysms, Scarpa sought to prove that earlier concepts regarding the cause of aneurysms were incorrect. After carefully studying the various layers of arteries, he concluded that the most common and important antecedent to aneurysm formation was an ulcerated atheromatous lesion. Scarpa emphasized that an aneurysm was not simply a dilated portion of normal artery, it was the result of localized disease of the arterial wall (9).

Although interest in vascular disease remained focused on aneurysms throughout much of the nineteenth century,

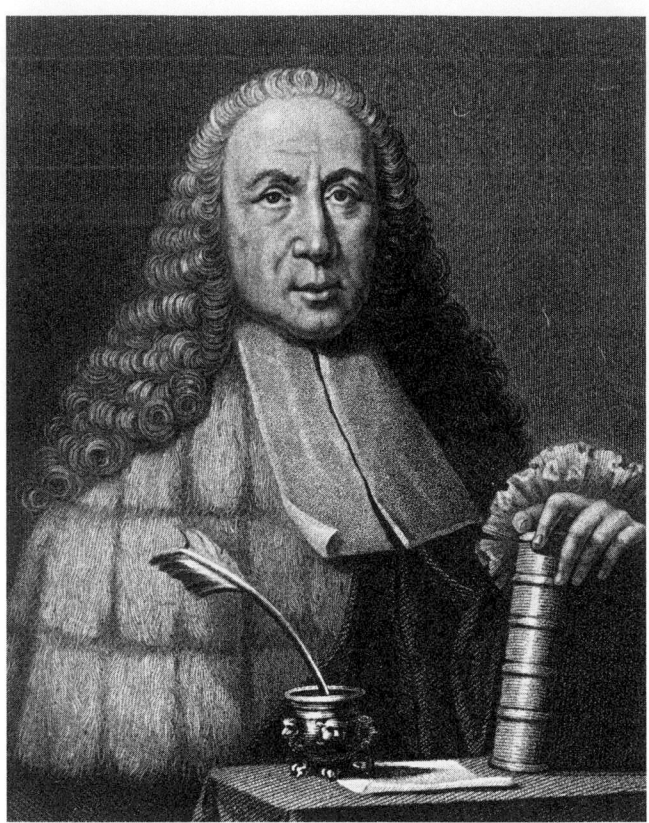

FIG. 1–1. Giovanni Battista Morgagni (1682–1771). The founder of modern pathology, Morgagni emphasized the importance of clinicopathologic correlation. His most significant scientific contributions related to pathology of the vascular system. (From the collection of W. Bruce Fye, Rochester, MN.)

some individuals turned their attention to the pathophysiology of atherosclerosis. London surgeon Joseph Hodgson published an important monograph on vascular disease in 1815. Reflecting contemporary medical theory, Hodgson claimed that inflammation was the underlying cause of atheromatous arteries. By this time, it was known that arteries consisted of three distinct layers. Hodgson identified atheromatous material between the intima and media and proposed that these changes could be traced to an abnormality of the intima. Reflecting a growing appreciation of the value of chemistry in medicine, he also was the first to report the results of chemical analysis of atherosclerotic lesions.

In an 1829 monograph on pathologic anatomy, French pathologist Jean Lobstein introduced the term "arteriosclerosis" and, like Hodgson, published the results of a chemical analysis of calcified arterial plaques. Several atlases of pathologic anatomy were published in Europe during the nineteenth century, and some of them included illustrations of atherosclerotic arteries. Striking engravings of vascular lesions and the cerebral and cardiac complications of atherosclerosis appeared in the spectacular atlas published between 1829 and 1842 by French pathologist Jean Cruveilhier. One hand-colored plate depicted a ventricular aneurysm containing thrombus.

Viennese pathologist Carl Rokitansky's comprehensive monograph on pathologic anatomy (1842–1846) included an extensive section on atherosclerosis. Although much of his theory regarding the cause of atherosclerotic lesions was later proved false, Rokitansky's descriptions of the lesions are striking and accurate. He also recognized that there was a thrombogenic component to the progression of atherosclerosis. In 1852, he published a monograph on arterial diseases that included 61 spectacular illustrations. The book also contained clear descriptions of atheroma and intimal calcification.

It is hard to overestimate German pathologist Rudolf Virchow's significance in the history of medicine (Fig. 1–2). Esmond Long called him "the greatest figure in the history of pathology." Virchow's 1858 book *Cellular Pathology* signaled the end of humoralism and inaugurated a new era in the conceptualization of disease. Reflecting his enthusiasm for microscopy, Virchow used the instrument to study blood vessels. He concluded from his research that atherosclerotic lesions were located within the intimal layer. He believed that these intimal deposits stimulated the proliferation of connective tissue, which triggered further degenerative changes of the vessel wall.

Virchow made pioneering observations on thrombosis and embolism. The first volume of his *Handbuch der Speciellen Pathologie und Therapie,* published in 1854, contained important sections on thrombosis (a term that he also coined),

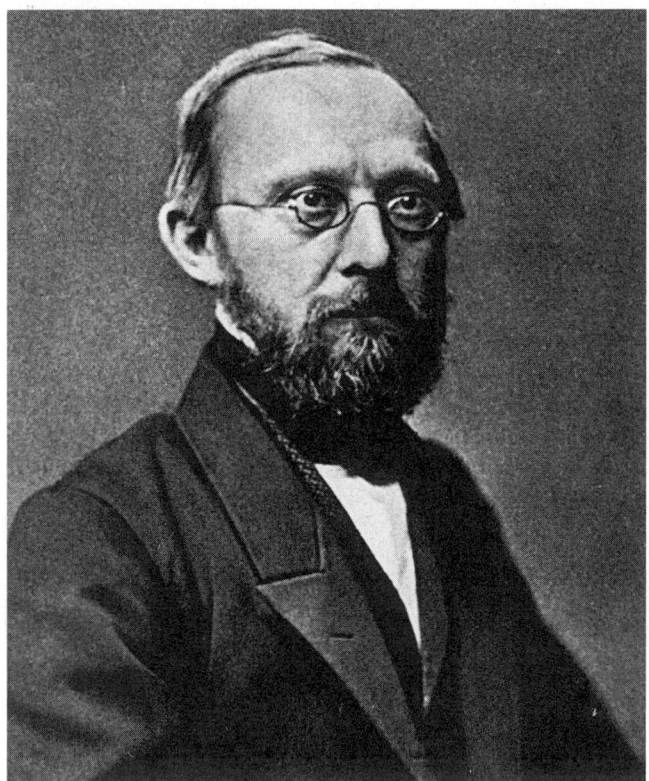

FIG. 1–2. Rudolf Virchow (1821–1902). Virchow's 1858 book on cellular pathology signaled the end of humoralism. He made classic observations on thrombosis (a term that he also coined) and embolism. (From the collection of W. Bruce Fye, Rochester, MN.)

embolism, and vascular obstruction (10). Virchow described the process of thrombosis in this work. He explained,

> The coagulation of blood within vessels takes place in accord with the same laws as outside the vessels, in that the dissolved fibrin, which does not require the access of atmospheric air, alters its state of aggregation and becomes solid....This coagulum we call a blood-clot, a thrombus, and accordingly we suggest for the process the designation clot-formation, thrombosis (11).

During the final decades of the nineteenth century, several theories were advanced to attempt to explain the pathophysiology of the various forms of arterial disease that pathologists had identified. Although attention was initially focused on visible lesions of the aorta, the expanding use of the microscope led to the recognition of vascular disease involving the small blood vessels of the kidneys and other organs. This led to the introduction of the concept of arteriosclerosis. Gradually, pathologists abandoned the view that atherosclerosis was the result of inflammation and adopted the view that it was a degenerative process.

The modern era of atherosclerosis research began in 1908 when Russian scientist Alexander Ignatovski showed that he could experimentally induce atherosclerosis in rabbits by feeding them a diet of milk and egg yolk. Extending these experiments, Nikolai Anitschkov showed that a diet rich in cholesterol caused atherosclerosis in experimental animals. German chemist and Nobel Prize winner Adolf Windaus showed that cholesterol was present in atherosclerotic lesions in humans in 1910. Anitschkov published a valuable summary in English of the early experimental studies of atherosclerosis in 1933 (12).

There was growing interest in the clinical and scientific aspects of atherosclerosis during the early twentieth century (13). This is explained, in part, by the gradually declining morbidity and mortality from infectious diseases that resulted from better nutrition, improved sanitation, and various public health measures. As people lived longer, "degenerative" diseases, such as cancer and disorders of the cardiovascular system, became more important to patients and physicians alike. Some authorities viewed atherosclerosis as inevitable. But German pathologist Ludwig Aschoff did not. In 1933, he claimed, "The widespread belief that arteriosclerosis is merely a manifestation of old age does not tally with the actual facts." Aschoff thought such a fatalistic attitude was inappropriate: "If arteriosclerosis were merely a phenomenon of aging, neither remedies nor prophylactics would be of any avail, for no one can escape age and death" (14). Researchers were motivated to search for clues to the pathophysiology of this disease process because they did not view it as a simple manifestation of aging that could not be modified in some fashion.

Philadelphia pharmacologist Thomas H. F. Smith, claimed in 1960 that "atherosclerosis had emerged by the end of the 1930s from the position of a medical curiosity. It was no longer considered a casual observation at autopsies but was now regarded as a major cause of death" (15). Scientists sought to understand the pathophysiology of atherosclerosis, and patients and their doctors were eager for effective remedies for the many clinical problems that resulted from this process. This growing interest in atherosclerosis was reflected in the publication in 1933 of a 617-page book on the subject (16). Like this volume, that work included contributions by leaders in the field who discussed both the scientific and clinical aspects of atherosclerosis and its complications. Still, effective therapy lagged behind the understanding of the pathology of atherosclerosis and coronary artery disease. This is apparent if one reviews Paul Dudley White's classic book on heart disease, first published in 1931, and other texts from the first half of the twentieth century (17).

Breakthroughs were being made, however, and at an ever-increasing rate. In 1933, the year Cowdry's book appeared, New York bacteriologist William Tillett reported his discovery of the fibrinolytic activity of β-hemolytic streptococci (18). It would be nearly half a century, however, before this observation was translated into the routine use of thrombolytic therapy for acute myocardial infarction. During this time many important discoveries would be made. Initially, these resulted largely from the explosive growth of the biomedical research community in the United States; this expansion was fueled by generous government funding of academic medical centers after World War II. In recent decades workers in many other nations have increasingly contributed to current knowledge (13,19).

ANGINA PECTORIS AND CORONARY ARTERY DISEASE

Renaissance artist Leonardo da Vinci was the first to describe and illustrate the coronary arteries accurately (20). They also were accurately depicted by Belgian anatomist Andreas Vesalius in his monumental work *De Humani Corporis Fabrica* published in 1543. Best known for his discovery of the circulation, reported in 1628 in his monumental book *De Motu Cordis,* English physician and anatomist William Harvey also first described coronary circulation (Fig. 1–3). In a 1649 book he described the anatomy of the coronary arteries and veins and proposed that coronary circulation nourished the heart (21). Using injection techniques, British physician and anatomist Richard Lower described coronary anastomoses two decades later (22). Although other physicians and scientists extended these observations on the anatomy of the coronary circulation, little was known about the functional significance of the coronary arteries until the nineteenth century.

English physician William Heberden first described angina pectoris in a talk presented to members of the College of Physicians of London in July 1768 (Fig. 1–4). His article, published four years later, is still recognized as one of the most classic clinical descriptions in medicine (23,24). Speaking of the condition he called angina pectoris, Heberden claimed,

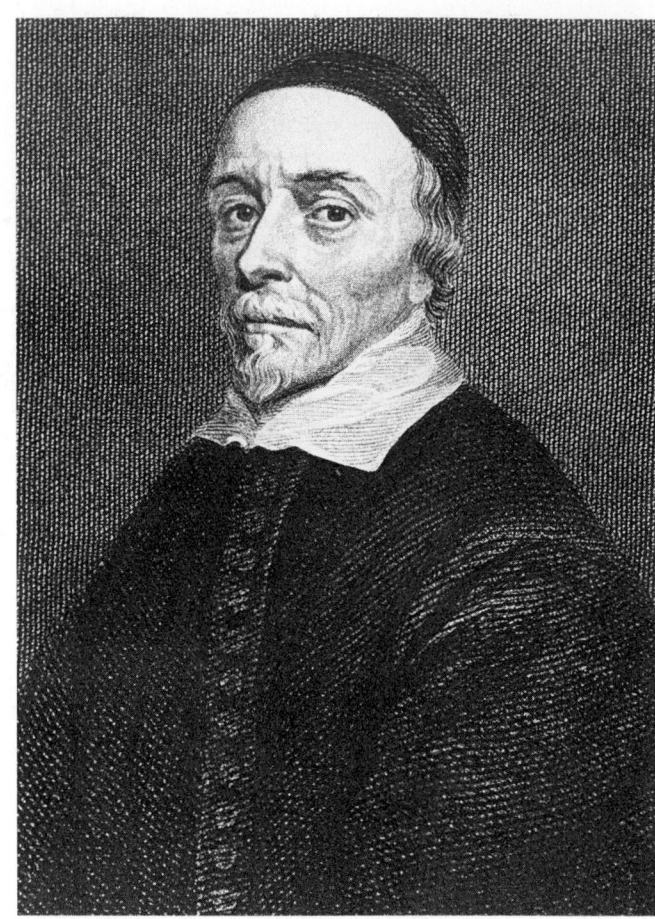

FIG. 1–3. William Harvey (1578–1657). Best known for his discovery of circulation, reported in 1628 in *De Motu Cordis,* Harvey also first described coronary circulation. These observations were published in 1649. (From the collection of W. Bruce Fye, Rochester, MN.)

There is a disorder of the breast, marked with strong and peculiar symptoms, considerable for the kind of danger belonging to it, and not extremely rare, of which I do not recollect any mention among medical authors. The seat of it, and sense of strangling and anxiety with which it is attended, may make it not improperly be called Angina pectoris.

Those, who are afflicted with it, are seized, while they are walking, and more particularly when they walk soon after eating, with a painful and most disagreeable sensation in the breast, which seems as if it would take their life away, if it were to increase or to continue: the moment they stand still, all this uneasiness vanishes. In all other respects the patients are at the beginning of this disorder perfectly well, and in particular have no shortness of breath, from which it is totally different.

After it has continued some months, it will not cease so instantaneously upon standing still; and it will come on, not only when the persons are walking, but when they are lying down and oblige them to rise up out of their beds every night for many months together....When a fit of this sort comes on by walking, its duration is very short, as it goes off almost immediately upon stopping. If it come on in the night, it will last an hour or two....The os sterni is usually pointed to as the seat of this malady, but it seems sometimes as if it was under the lower part of it, and at other times under the middle or

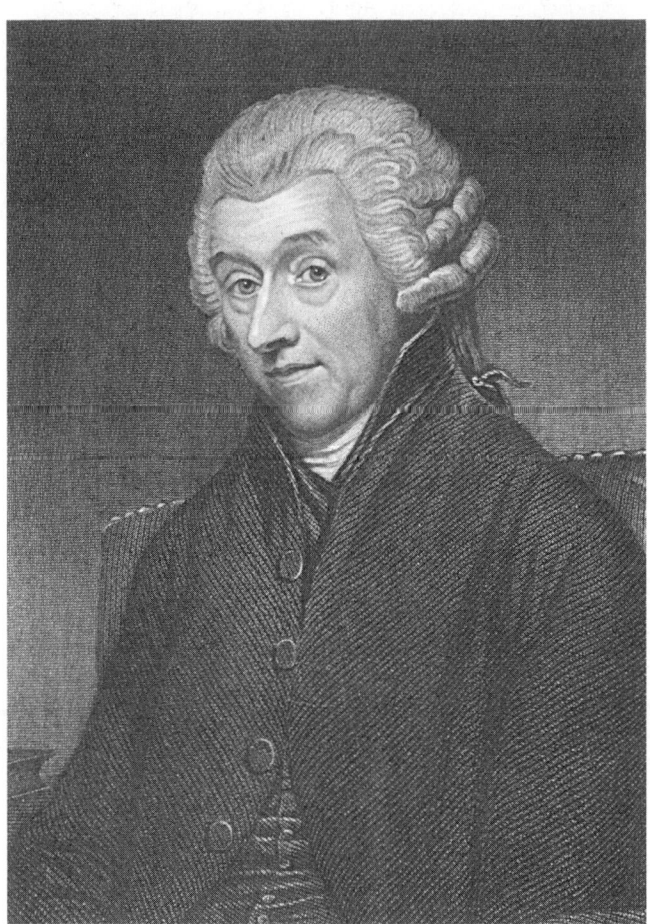

FIG. 1–4. William Heberden (1710–1801). British physician who is remembered eponymically for first describing angina pectoris (1772). (From the collection of W. Bruce Fye, Rochester, MN.)

upper part, but always inclining more to the left side, and sometimes there is joined with it a pain about the middle of the left arm.

By the time Heberden described the syndrome of angina pectoris to his fellow London physicians, he had seen more than 20 patients with the condition. He thought that most people with angina had a poor prognosis and noted that they were prone to sudden death. Still, Heberden recognized that some individuals would survive for many years despite the presence of typical anginal symptoms. Heberden had never seen an autopsy performed on anyone who had had angina and was unsure of the cause of the dramatic clinical picture. His management of angina reflected contemporary thought about the mechanism of disease. Although Heberden found that bleeding and purging did not help his patients, he discovered that opiates seemed to prevent nocturnal episodes of angina. Specific remedies for angina would not be introduced for more than a century.

Heberden remained interested in angina. His book *Commentaries on the History and Cure of Diseases,* published posthumously in 1802, included additional observations on

the malady (25). By the time he finished the manuscript in 1782, Heberden had seen about 100 patients with the disorder. Although Heberden's clinical description of angina pectoris was masterful, he did not speculate on its pathophysiology. Shortly after Heberden published his original observations on angina, he received an anonymous letter from a 52-year-old physician who had the condition. The doctor urged Heberden to perform an autopsy on him in the event of his death, hoping that this might help to clarify the cause of the malady. When "Dr. Anonymous" died three weeks later, Heberden asked surgeon and anatomist John Hunter to perform the autopsy. Edward Jenner, best remembered for his introduction of vaccination a few years later, assisted Hunter in the postmortem examination and later recalled that this was the first case of angina he had seen (Fig. 1–5). Hunter and Jenner found no abnormalities in the heart or other organs to explain the doctor's death, however. Because of Heberden's (as well as Hunter's and Jenner's) lack of recognition that coronary artery disease was the cause of angina, the anonymous doctor's coronary arteries were not examined (26).

After serving as Hunter's assistant for two years, Jenner returned to his hometown of Gloucestershire to begin his career as a country doctor. Once in practice, Jenner saw more patients with angina. His interest in the condition was further stimulated when he realized that his friend John Hunter

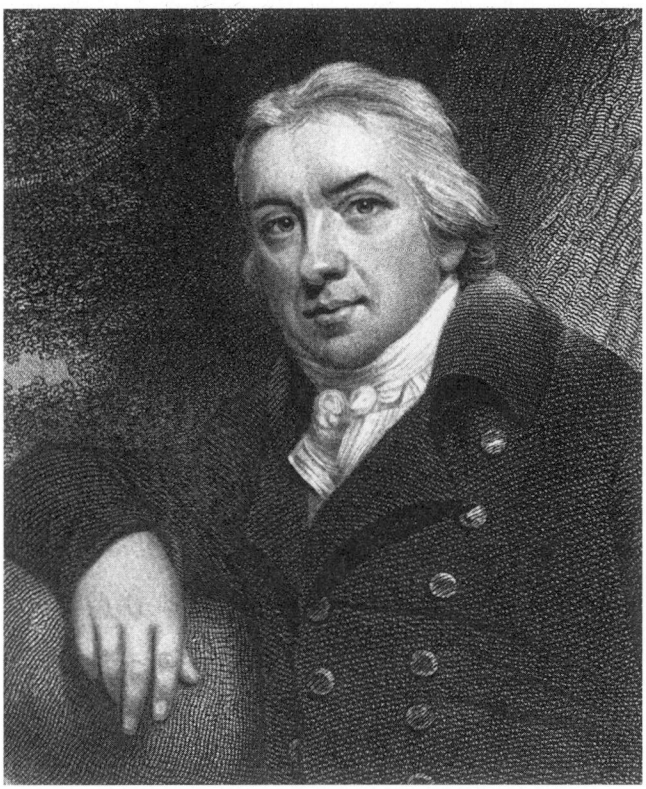

FIG. 1–5. Edward Jenner (1749–1823). Best known for introducing vaccination, this British physician was the first to attribute angina pectoris to coronary artery disease. (From the collection of W. Bruce Fye, Rochester, MN.)

had the disorder. By 1786, Jenner had witnessed three autopsies of patients who had experienced anginal attacks. The postmortem examination on the last of these patients led Jenner to conclude that the symptoms were related to coronary artery disease. He explained in a 1778 letter to William Heberden, that the autopsy revealed "a kind of firm fleshy tube, formed within the [coronary] vessel, with a considerable quantity of ossific matter dispersed irregularly through it." Jenner proposed that this pathologic finding had been overlooked in other patients with angina because the coronary arteries were often covered by epicardial fat (27).

In his letter to Heberden, Jenner explicitly linked coronary artery disease to angina; he was the first to do so. Jenner explained, "the importance of the coronary arteries, and how much the heart must suffer from their not being able to perform their functions, (we cannot be surprised at the painful spasms) is a subject I need not enlarge upon, therefore shall only just remark that it is possible that all the symptoms may arise from this one circumstance." Jenner also told Heberden of his reluctance to share his beliefs with Hunter because "it may deprive him of the hopes of a recovery," as there was no remedy for coronary artery disease (27).

Jenner's friend, Bath physician Caleb Hillier Parry, published the first book on angina pectoris in 1799. Parry credited Jenner with first attributing angina to coronary artery disease. Jenner had told Parry that while carefully dissecting the heart of a patient with angina that he had treated, his "knife struck something so hard and gritty, as to notch it." At first Jenner thought a piece of ceiling plaster had fallen into his dissecting field, but on closer inspection he discovered that the "coronaries were become bony canals." It was this case that led Jenner to conclude that angina was caused by "malorganization of these [coronary] vessels" (28).

Parry accepted Jenner's hypothesis that angina was caused by coronary artery disease. He was surprised, however, that angina had not been described earlier. "Although there can be no reason to doubt," Parry explained, "that mankind must have been subject to this disorder from the remotest antiquity, it is somewhat extraordinary that so many ages should have elapsed without any notice of its existence either as a distinct disease, or as a variety of one commonly known." After a thorough review of the literature, Parry concluded that only ten essays on angina had been published by 1799, and only nine patients with anginal attacks had undergone autopsy.

Parry's case reports were remarkably detailed and, reflecting growing interest in clinicopathologic correlation, included the relevant pathologic findings. He concluded that "there is an important connection between the rigid and obstructed state of these vessels, and the disease in question [angina pectoris]." Parry attributed angina to "induration" and "ossification" of the coronary arteries and proposed that they might be "so obstructed as to intercept the blood, which should be the proper support of the muscular fibres of the heart that [the] organ must become thin and flaccid, and unequal to the task of circulation" (28).

Scottish anatomist and physician Allan Burns published the first English language book on heart disease in 1809. Burns agreed with Parry that angina was caused by "some organic lesions of the nutrient vessels of the heart." He emphasized that because the heart was primarily a muscle, it was "regulated by the same laws which govern other muscles." Burns drew an analogy between coronary artery disease and the ligation of a peripheral artery to support his view of the pathophysiology of angina pectoris (29).

Although the contributions of Jenner, Parry, and Burns seemed to document a relation between coronary artery disease and angina pectoris, other observations made during the nineteenth century undermined the coronary theory of angina. For example, in his 1813 book on dropsy, a condition now known usually to be caused by congestive heart failure, British physician John Blackall described one patient with typical angina who had only trivial coronary artery disease, but whose ascending aorta was severely atherosclerotic. The apparent inconsistent relation between coronary artery disease found at autopsy and symptoms thought to represent angina was an important factor in the long delay between Heberden's description of angina in 1772 and the widespread acceptance of the coronary theory of its cause a century later.

The introduction of mediate auscultation by French physician René Laennec gave physicians a powerful diagnostic tool to help them evaluate diseases of the heart and lungs. But the stethoscope, first described in Laennec's two-volume book on auscultation in 1819, contributed to a shift in emphasis in heart disease. Using a stethoscope, doctors could identify abnormal heart sounds and murmurs. It also helped them correlate their patient's complaints and physical findings with autopsy results. For several decades the literature of heart disease reflected this new orientation toward valvular heart lesions.

Although relatively little progress was made during the nineteenth century with regard to understanding the pathophysiology of angina, an empirical observation led to the use of vasodilators for its treatment. Scottish medical student Thomas Lauder Brunton introduced amyl nitrite for the treatment of angina pectoris in 1867 (30) (Fig. 1–6). Brunton's mentors at the University of Edinburgh had been experimenting with the substance and were impressed by the immediate and profound effects that followed its inhalation. Using a new instrument, the sphygmograph, they found that amyl nitrate predictably decreased the arterial tension in animals and humans.

Brunton found that blood pressure increased and the pulse quickened during anginal attacks. He thought angina was caused by a "derangement of the vaso-motor system," which resulted in increased vascular tone and high arterial tension. This theory eventually proved false, but it was a critical factor in Brunton's decision to administer amyl nitrite in patients with angina. Although the popularity of therapeutic bleeding had declined by the late 1860s, some doctors still used the procedure in angina because it was thought to reduce arterial tension. When Brunton bled patients with

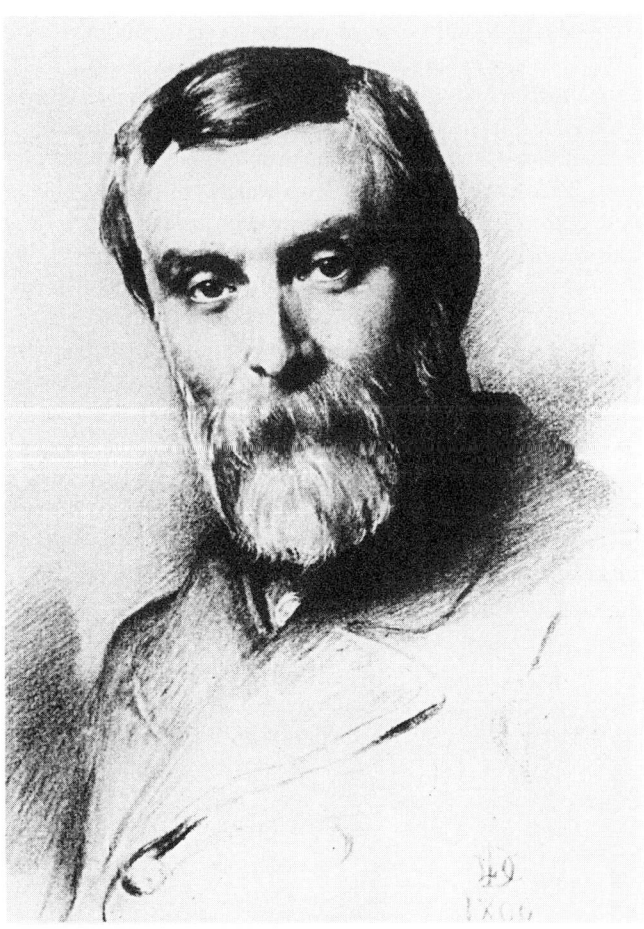

FIG. 1–6. Thomas Lauder Brunton (1844–1916). Scottish physician and pharmacologist who first advocated vasodilator therapy (amyl nitrite) for angina pectoris in 1867. (From the collection of W. Bruce Fye, Rochester, MN.)

angina, some of them seemed to improve. Recognizing that amyl nitrite was a vasodilator, he thought it might be useful in the treatment of the disorder. When Brunton gave amyl nitrite to patients with angina, their chest discomfort often disappeared within a minute.

Twelve years later, British physician and pharmacologist William Murrell reported that nitroglycerin was an effective treatment for angina. Murrell became interested in nitroglycerin, a homeopathic remedy first used by Constantine Hering in the 1840s, because he found that its effect on heart rate and arterial tension was similar to that of amyl nitrite (31). Murrell found that nitroglycerin relieved angina promptly, although its effects came on more slowly and lasted longer than those of amyl nitrite. After Murrell's 1879 report in the *Lancet,* nitroglycerin's value in angina was rapidly and widely acknowledged. This was true, in large part, because its beneficial effects were immediate, dramatic, and reproducible.

By the twentieth century, most physicians and medical scientists interested in heart disease accepted the coronary theory of angina; however, a few did not. T. Clifford Allbutt,

Regius Professor of Medicine at Cambridge and a prolific author, published several articles on angina and, until his death in 1925, held steadfastly to the belief that it was caused by disease of the aortic root. By this time, however, there was growing understanding about the pathophysiology of coronary artery disease and its complications. Much of this new insight about angina pectoris came from pathologic and physiologic research on coronary occlusion and myocardial infarction.

ACUTE MYOCARDIAL INFARCTION

The clinical syndrome currently termed "acute myocardial infarction" was first clearly described in the twentieth century. Several factors contributed to the delay between Heberden's 1772 article on angina pectoris and James Herrick's classic description of acute myocardial infarction in 1912. Probably the most important factor in this delay was the belief that sudden coronary occlusion was invariably fatal. This view predominated until the early twentieth century. Other reasons included the inconsistent relation of symptoms to pathologic findings in ischemic heart disease, the reliance of nineteenth century physicians on auscultation as an indicator of heart disease, the failure to examine the coronary arteries and myocardium routinely at autopsy, the lag between pathologic and physiologic discoveries and their incorporation into medical practice, the preoccupation of late nineteenth century physicians with the new field of bacteriology, and the lack of any diagnostic tool to help physicians identify coronary artery obstruction or its consequences during life (32).

European and American medical scientists and clinicians made several observations during the second half of the nineteenth century that ultimately led to recognition of the clinical and pathologic sequelae of coronary occlusion (33). British surgeon John Erichsen investigated the relation of cardiac arrest and experimental coronary occlusion in the early 1840s. In 1850, British physician Richard Quain described "fatty degeneration" of the myocardium, a process he associated with coronary artery disease. In 1866, French physician Edme Vulpian reported the case of a 75-year-old woman found at autopsy to have cardiac rupture at the site of a dramatically thin left ventricular segment supplied by an occluded coronary artery. Vulpian concluded that a thrombus had formed at the site of an atherosclerotic plaque and occluded the coronary artery, causing the myocardium to become thin and friable. Although Vulpian's interpretation of the pathophysiology of coronary occlusion and its consequences was advanced for the time, he did not address the clinical aspects of the condition or suggest how physicians might recognize coronary occlusion during life (24).

By the end of the nineteenth century, many pathologists had concluded that there was a causal relation between thrombotic coronary occlusion and the degenerative changes of the myocardium that were seen using a microscope and were visible to the naked eye. Despite this, clinicians were either unaware of these conclusions or unimpressed by them. In 1880, Carl Weigert, who worked with German pathologist Julius Cohnheim, published an article that included a clear description of the pathophysiology of thrombotic occlusion of atherosclerotic coronary arteries leading to myocardial necrosis. Weigert differentiated gradual, progressive obstruction of a coronary artery from abrupt occlusion of the vessel. His article is a milestone in the description of the pathologic aspects of coronary thrombosis and myocardial infarction.

Weigert's clinical colleague Karl Huber extended these observations and claimed, in 1882, that angina pectoris and myocardial infarction were both manifestations of coronary artery disease. These important observations on the pathophysiology of occlusive coronary artery disease had essentially no impact on contemporary medical practice, however. In retrospect, some authors described symptoms that are currently recognized as consistent with acute myocardial infarction, but they did not distinguish those episodes from prolonged attacks of angina pectoris.

William Osler, the leading internist of his generation, had studied with Cohnheim and Weigert and appreciated the significance of their observations on coronary artery disease. As early as 1889, Osler observed in an editorial, "The local disturbances of nutrition caused by the blocking of a terminal branch of the coronary artery produces the condition known as infarct of the heart" (34). But Osler was referring to the *pathological* findings of myocardial infarction; he did not comprehend that there was a distinct *clinical* syndrome that accompanied acute coronary occlusion.

American physiologist William Porter performed a series of experiments in the late nineteenth century that were critical for Herrick's formulation of the clinical syndrome of acute myocardial infarction. For more than a decade, Porter studied the effects of experimental occlusion of the coronary arteries. He documented the results of sudden occlusion (produced by ligation or embolization) on the heart rhythm, hemodynamics, and the histology and gross pathology of the organ (35). Porter's assistant Walter Baumgarten studied the effect of myocardial ischemia on contractility, and he raised issues that are currently of great interest in terms of myocardial viability after acute coronary thrombosis and reperfusion therapy. In 1899, Baumgarten found that after acute coronary occlusion, "portions of the mammalian ventricle will resume their contractions if fed with defibrinated blood." On the basis of the experiments he and Porter performed, Baumgarten concluded that the loss of contractility that resulted from experimentally induced ischemia was reversible for up to 11 hours. He also claimed that contractility was most impaired in the central zone of the ischemic area and least affected at the periphery (36).

Gradually, clinicians acknowledged that acute coronary thrombosis was not invariably fatal, but there was no recognition of the clinical syndrome of acute myocardial infarction until Russian physicians W. P. Obrastzow and N. D. Straschesko published the first description of this dramatic event in 1910. They believed that two specific findings were characteristic of acute coronary thrombosis: prolonged chest discomfort ("status anginosus") and persistent dyspnea ("status dyspnoeticus"). After presenting cases with autopsy correlations, Obrastzow and Straschesko concluded that "the differential diagnosis of coronary thrombosis from angina pectoris is made by the presence of status anginosus with coronary thrombosis and its absence with isolated attacks of angina pectoris" (37,38).

Although this article, published in German, attracted little attention, it was known to Chicago internist James Herrick, who eventually convinced the medical community that acute coronary thrombosis could be recognized during life (Fig. 1–7). Herrick's 1912 article, "Certain Clinical Features of Sudden Obstruction of the Coronary Arteries" (39), is a milestone in current understanding of the pathophysiology of coronary artery disease, angina pectoris, and myocardial infarction. It contained the first description in English of the clinical syndrome of acute myocardial infarction.

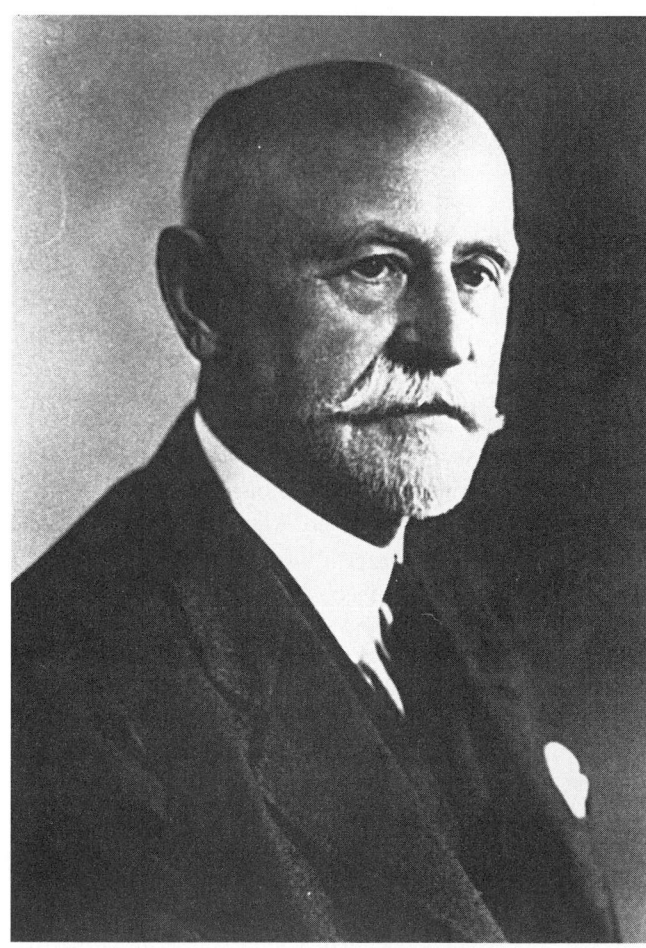

FIG. 1–7. James B. Herrick (1861–1954). Chicago internist who published, in 1912, the first description of the clinical syndrome of acute myocardial infarction in English. He was among the first to advocate using the electrocardiograph to help confirm the diagnosis. (From the National Library of Medicine.)

Herrick had reviewed experimental, clinical, and pathologic reports from Europe and the United States and concluded that acute thrombosis of a major coronary artery did not invariably cause sudden death. He also provided an explanation of the spectrum of symptoms that could accompany coronary thrombosis. "The clinical manifestations of coronary obstruction will evidently vary greatly," Herrick claimed, "depending on the size, location and number of vessels occluded. The symptoms and end-result must also be influenced by blood-pressure, by the condition of the myocardium not immediately affected by the obstruction, and by the ability of the remaining vessels properly to carry on their work, as determined by their health or disease" (39).

Despite his vivid description, Herrick's report on the clinical features of acute coronary thrombosis attracted little attention until doctors had an objective tool to demonstrate that their patients' chest discomfort and associated symptoms were unequivocally cardiac in origin. Electrocardiography, introduced by Dutch physiologist Willem Einthoven in 1902, eventually provided clinicians with a powerful tool to help them recognize acute myocardial infarction and differentiate it from angina pectoris and noncardiac conditions causing chest pain (Fig. 1–8). Initially, the electrocardiogram was used to evaluate cardiac arrhythmias.

Herrick and his assistant Fred Smith were among the first to study the electrocardiographic (ECG) manifestations of experimental coronary occlusion (40). Their findings led Herrick to claim that characteristic ECG changes accompanied acute coronary occlusion and that these typical findings should help physicians to recognize acute coronary thrombosis. Therefore, Herrick provided clinicians with both an intellectual framework for conceptualizing survival after coronary thrombosis and a new diagnostic approach to help them recognize the event. Other investigators extended Herrick's observations during the 1920s and 1930s. The introduction of the precordial leads by Charles Wolferth and Francis Wood in 1932 was a major advance in the ECG diagnosis of myocardial infarction.

In 1929, Boston cardiologist Samuel Levine published the first book in English devoted to coronary thrombosis. He addressed the concept of what is currently termed "cardiac risk factors" and claimed that heredity, male sex, obesity, diabetes, and hypertension predisposed patients to coronary thrombosis. Levine identified a broad spectrum of complications that might result from coronary thrombosis and myocardial infarction. He explained that cardiac arrhythmias, cardiac rupture, and thromboembolic events could follow coronary thrombosis in addition to the well-known complication of sudden death (41).

The routine treatment of myocardial infarction in the 1930s and 1940s consisted mainly of prolonged bed rest, oxygen, and narcotics. Quinidine was used to treat ventricular tachycardia, but arrhythmia was rarely detected because continuous ECG monitoring had not yet been introduced. Prolonged bed rest (up to six weeks) was routinely advocated after acute myocardial infarction. Growing awareness of pulmonary emboli and other complications resulting from prolonged immobilization led to a gradual reduction in the length of hospitalization and strict bed rest after myocardial infarction.

During the 1960s, the treatment of acute myocardial infarction changed dramatically. American cardiologist Mason Sones first performed selective coronary arteriography in 1958 and reported the technique four years later (42) (Fig. 1–9). This procedure, an extension of angiographic techniques that had evolved over three decades, revolutionized the evaluation and management of patients with known or suspected coronary artery disease (22). It provided researchers with a powerful tool to study ischemic heart disease and was critical for the development of coronary bypass surgery, percutaneous transluminal coronary angioplasty, and thrombolytic therapy.

In 1960, William Kouwenhoven and his colleagues published their method of external cardiac massage that inaugurated the modern era of cardiopulmonary resuscitation (43). Around this time pacemakers and defibrillators were introduced into clinical practice, approaches that enabled physicians to effectively treat bradyarrhythmias and tachyarrhythmias. Advances in the pharmacologic treatment of arrhythmias also were reported; lidocaine and procainamide were shown to be effective for ventricular arrhythmias (44).

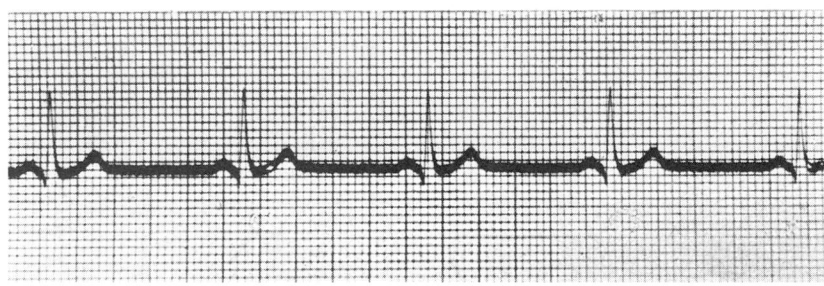

FIG. 1–8. Einthoven's first published electrocardiographic tracing using a string galvanometer. (From Einthoven W. Galvanometrische Registratie van Het Manschelijk Electrocardiogram. In: Rosenstein SS, ed. *Herrineringsbundel.* Leiden: Eduard Ijdo, 1902:107.)

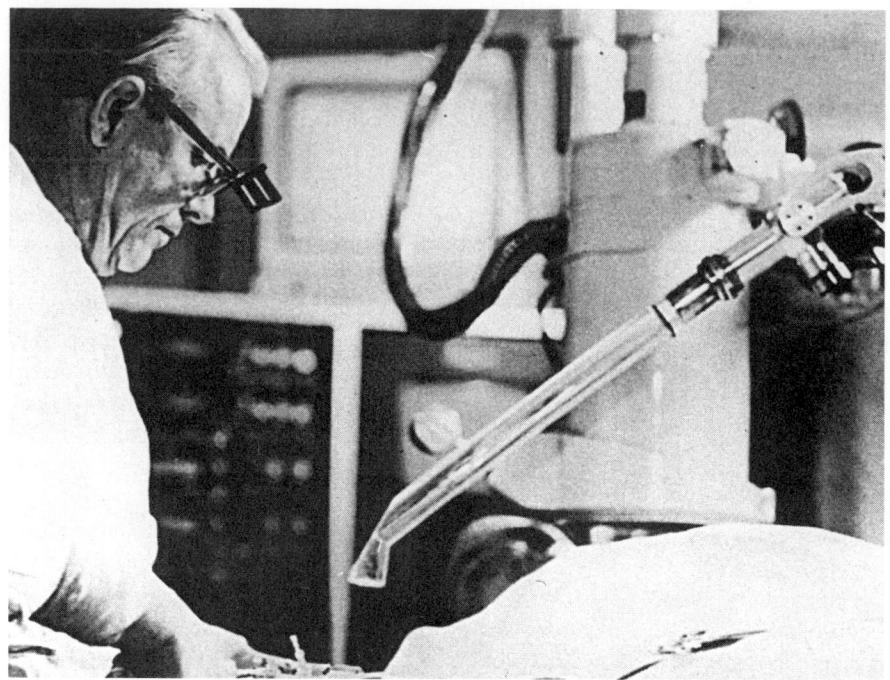

FIG. 1–9. F. Mason Sones, Jr. (1918–1985). American cardiologist who developed the technique of selective coronary arteriography. Reported in 1962, this technique was critical for the future development of coronary bypass surgery, percutaneous transluminal coronary angioplasty, and thrombolytic therapy. (From *Modern Medicine,* with permission.)

In 1962, Kansas cardiologist Hughes Day introduced the concepts of the cardiac arrest team and the coronary care unit (CCU) to the United States. These innovations dramatically changed the management of patients with acute myocardial infarction (45). Continuous ECG monitoring, a critical part of the CCU concept, alerted a specially trained staff to the onset of potentially life-threatening arrhythmias or cardiac arrest. They responded quickly using new mechanical and pharmacologic approaches to treat these problems. Early detection and aggressive management of arrhythmias significantly reduced mortality from acute myocardial infarction, and the CCU concept spread rapidly throughout the nation.

Although early deaths from arrhythmias resulting from acute myocardial infarction were reduced, many patients still died as a result of cardiogenic shock and other less dramatic consequences of extensive myocardial necrosis. The introduction of the flow-directed, balloon-tipped catheter in 1970 facilitated the assessment of the hemodynamic consequences of acute myocardial infarction. This new approach made it possible to evaluate left ventricular filling pressure and cardiac output at the bedside so that the physician could adjust therapy to treat specific hemodynamic abnormalities.

Beginning in the 1950s, various techniques were introduced to estimate infarct size. These approaches included serum enzyme assays, ECG mapping, and evaluation of myocardial performance using radioisotopes, ultrasound, and angiocardiography. They improved the physician's ability to establish a prognosis and helped clinical scientists to evalu-

ate new approaches to myocardial preservation. Although several pharmacologic and mechanical approaches introduced during the 1970s to limit myocardial necrosis failed to show any significant effect on survival, one strategy—thrombolytic therapy—seemed promising.

As noted earlier, some nineteenth century pathologists thought that thrombus played a critical role in causing coronary occlusion, which they believed resulted in the myocardial necrosis identified at autopsy. By 1920, as a result of the observations of Herrick and others, the view that sudden thrombotic occlusion of the diseased coronary artery triggered acute myocardial infarction was widely accepted. Soon after the anticoagulants heparin and bishydroxycoumarin (Dicumarol) were developed in the 1930s, some clinicians and medical scientists thought they might be useful in the treatment of acute myocardial infarction. On the basis of a study of 800 patients reported in 1948, Irving Wright advocated the routine use of anticoagulants after acute myocardial infarction to prevent the extension of coronary thrombosis and the development of mural thrombi (46). Hemorrhagic complications, however, limited the acceptance of this approach. Another factor that contributed to the decline in the routine use of oral anticoagulants was the recognition that venous thrombosis and pulmonary emboli occurred less frequently after myocardial infarction once early ambulation became standard.

Modern thrombolytic therapy can be traced to 1933, when New York bacteriologist William Tillett discovered that β-hemolytic streptococci produced a fibrinolytic substance that he termed "fibrinolysin" (later renamed streptokinase) (47). Extending Tillett's work, Sol Sherry, Anthony Fletcher, and their associates reported on the administration of intravenous streptokinase in 24 patients with acute myocardial infarction in 1958. In this, the first report on thrombolytic therapy for myocardial infarction, they proposed that "the rapid dissolution of a coronary thrombus by enzymatic means could result in reduction of the final area of muscle infarction, reduction of the degree of electrical instability present during the early critical phase of infarction and prevent the appearance of or lyse mural thrombi" (48).

The pyrogenicity of the streptokinase then available retarded further clinical studies using streptokinase. In 1960, Miami cardiologist Robert Boucek and his associates (49) reported administering fibrinolysin, a mixture of human plasmin and streptokinase, to eight patients after acute myocardial infarction. They used a novel approach to deliver the thrombolytic agent: It was administered through a catheter placed in one of the sinuses of Valsalva. Boucek's enthusiasm for the procedure was limited by his recognition that he could not prove that a coronary thrombus was present in any of the patients or whether it was lysed as a result of the administration of fibrinolysin. To understand these concerns, it is important to recognize that Boucek and his associates did not perform coronary arteriograms as part of their study. That procedure was rarely performed in 1960, and when it was used everyone but Mason Sones used a nonselective technique that generally provided inadequate visualization of the coronary circulation.

During the mid-twentieth century, some influential clinicians and pathologists began to question the role of coronary thrombosis in acute myocardial infarction. In 1939, New York cardiologist Charles Friedberg reported that one-third of a series of 37 patients thought to have died of acute myocardial infarction did not have evidence of a fresh coronary thrombus at autopsy (50). A quarter of a century later, San Francisco cardiologist Meyer Friedman, reporting a study of the pathogenesis of coronary thrombus, acknowledged that there was "considerable argument" regarding the relation of thrombus formation and underlying atherosclerosis and "even between thrombosis and infarction." Friedman's findings supported the view held by some, but by no means all, pathologists that "the thrombus lay in direct communication with a preexisting intramural atheromatous process." He concluded that "fracture" of the atheromatous plaque preceded and was "responsible for the formation of thrombus" (51).

Some pathologists questioned the causal role of coronary thrombosis in acute myocardial infarction during the 1960s and 1970s, however. One of them, William Roberts, of the National Institutes of Health, wrote several articles on the subject. In 1972, he explained that a variety of postmortem findings "suggest that coronary thrombi are consequences rather than causes of acute myocardial infarction" (52). Spokane cardiologist Marcus DeWood was aware of this controversy when he published a report on the prevalence of total coronary occlusion during the early hours of myocardial infarction. DeWood performed coronary arteriograms in these patients and found that 87% of those studied within four hours of the onset of symptoms had occlusion of the infarct-related artery (53).

The first report of the intracoronary administration of a thrombolytic agent into a coronary artery was published in 1976 by E. I. Chazov and colleagues from Russia. They reported on two patients in whom coronary angiograms were performed before and after the administration of thrombolytic therapy. Reperfusion was demonstrated in one patient when the lytic therapy was administered four hours after the onset of symptoms. Lytic therapy was unsuccessful in a second case when it was administered ten hours after the onset of symptoms. This article, published in Russian with a brief English summary, was apparently unknown to U.S. workers. This situation is reminiscent of James B. Herrick's original description of acute myocardial infarction, which was preceded by the observations of two Russians a few months earlier (54).

The English-speaking world first learned of the technique of intracoronary thrombolytic therapy in 1979 when German cardiologist Peter Rentrop reported the intracoronary administration of streptokinase in five patients with acute myocardial infarction. He concluded that the infarct was precipitated by thrombus in four of his patients and found that symptoms improved in each of them when the infarct-related artery was reperfused (55). This report, together with DeWood's article (53), inaugurated the modern era of treatment of acute myocardial infarction, which emphasizes prompt reperfusion. Many multicenter clinical trials of thrombolytic therapy have been undertaken since 1971, when the European Working Party reported on a trial they conducted in nine hospitals. They concluded that streptokinase was superior to heparin in reducing mortality and reinfarction after acute myocardial infarction (56).

CONCLUSIONS

The subsequent developments in the dynamic field of thrombolytic therapy are beyond the scope of this historical review. This also is true of immediate or direct percutaneous transluminal coronary angioplasty, an increasingly popular alternative to thrombolytic therapy for achieving reperfusion after acute myocardial infarction. Of necessity, many significant topics have been excluded from this brief review of atherosclerosis and coronary artery disease. The remainder of this book provides a state-of-the-art review of basic and clinical research, diagnostic techniques, and therapeutic approaches in the areas of atherosclerosis and coronary artery disease. While reading this book, I urge you to reflect on the provocative question: Where does the review of the literature end and history begin? The distinction is really quite artificial. History is actually everything that happened before the moment you read this. This historical review emphasizes events that occurred several years to several centuries ago, but my approach has been similar to that used when one prepares a review of the literature. This concept emphasizes the continuity of current knowledge with concepts and practices of earlier generations of physicians and scientists.

REFERENCES

1. Sandison AT. Degenerative vascular disease. In: Brothwell D, Sandison AT, eds. *Diseases in antiquity: a survey of the diseases, injuries and surgery of early populations.* Springfield, IL: Charles C Thomas, 1967:474–488.
2. Moodie RL. *Paleopathology: an introduction to the study of ancient evidences of disease.* Urbana, IL: University of Illinois Press, 1923.
3. Harris CR. *The heart and vascular system in ancient Greek medicine from Alcmaeon to Galen.* Oxford: Clarendon Press, 1973.
4. Bing RJ. Atherosclerosis. In: Bing RJ, ed. *Cardiology: the evolution of the science and the art.* Philadelphia: Harwood Academic Publishers, 1992:127–143.
5. Long ER. Development of our knowledge of arteriosclerosis. In: Blumenthal HT, ed. *Cowdry's atherosclerosis.* Springfield, IL: Charles C Thomas, 1967:5–20.
6. Harvey W. *Exercitatio anatomica. De motu cordis et sanguinis in animalibus.* Springfield, IL: Charles C Thomas, 1928. Leake C, translator.
7. Erichsen JE. *Observations on aneurism selected from the works of the principal writers on that disease from the earliest periods to the close of the last century.* London: Sydenham Society, 1844.
8. Long ER. *A history of pathology.* New York: Dover Publications, 1965.
9. Scarpa A. *A treatise on the anatomy, pathology, and surgical treatment of aneurism, with engravings.* Edinburgh: Mundell, Doig, & Stevenson, 1808. Wishart JH, translator.
10. Virchow R. Örtliche Störungen des Kreislaufes. In: Virchow R, Vogel J, Stiebel SF, eds. *Handbuch der speciellen pathologie und therapie, Vol. 1.* Erlangen: Ferdinand Enke, 1854:95–270.
11. Rather LJ. *A commentary on the medical writings of Rudolf Virchow.* San Francisco: Norman Publishing, 1990.
12. Anitschokov N. Experimental arteriosclerosis in animals. In: Cowdry EV, ed. *Arteriosclerosis: a survey of the problem.* New York: Macmillan, 1933:271–322.
13. Dock W. Research in arteriosclerosis—the first fifty years. *Ann Intern Med* 1958;49:699–705.
14. Aschoff L. Introduction. In: Cowdry EV, ed. *Arteriosclerosis: a survey of the problem.* New York: Macmillan, 1933:1–18.
15. Smith TH. A chronology of atherosclerosis. *Am J Pharm* 1960;132:390–405.
16. Cowdry EV, ed. *Arteriosclerosis: a survey of the problem.* New York: Macmillan, 1933.
17. White PD. *Heart disease.* New York: Macmillan, 1931.
18. Tillett WS, Garner RL. The fibrinolytic activity of hemolytic streptococci. *J Exp Med* 1933;58:485–502.
19. Ahrens EH Jr. *The crisis in clinical research: overcoming institutional obstacles.* New York: Oxford University Press, 1992.
20. Keele KD. *Leonardo da Vinci on the movement of the heart and blood.* London: Harvey and Blythe Ltd, 1952.
21. Bedford DE. Harvey's third circulation. De circulo sanguinis in corde. *Br Med J* 1968;4:273–277.
22. Fye WB. Coronary arteriography: it took a long time. *Circulation* 1984;70:781–787.
23. Heberden W. Some account of a disorder of the breast. *Med Trans Coll Physicians Lond* 1772;2:59–67.
24. Leibowitz JO. *The history of coronary heart disease.* London: Wellcome Institute of the History of Medicine, 1970.
25. Heberden W. *Commentaries on the history and cure of diseases.* London: T. Payne, 1802.
26. Kligfield P. The early pathophysiologic understanding of angina pectoris. *Am J Cardiol* 1982;50:1433–1435.
27. Baron J. *The life of Edward Jenner, M.D.* London: Henry Colburn, 1827.
28. Parry CH. *An inquiry into the symptoms and causes of the syncope anginosa commonly called angina pectoris.* Bath, England: R. Cruttwell, 1799.
29. Burns A. *Observations on some of the most frequent and important diseases of the heart.* Edinburgh: Bryce & Co, 1809.
30. Fye WB. T. Lauder Brunton and amyl nitrite: a Victorian vasodilator. *Circulation* 1986;74:222–229.
31. Fye WB. Nitroglycerin: a homeopathic remedy. *Circulation* 1986;73:21–29.
32. Fye WB. The delayed diagnosis of acute myocardial infarction: it took half a century. *Circulation* 1985;72:262–271.
33. Fye WB, ed. *Classic papers on coronary thrombosis and myocardial infarction.* Birmingham, AL: Classics of Cardiology Library, 1991.
34. [Osler W]. Rupture of the heart. *Med News* 1889;54:129–130.
35. Fye WB. Acute coronary occlusion always results in death, or does it? *Circulation* 1985;71:4–10.
36. Baumgarten W. Infarction in the heart. *Am J Physiol* 1899;2:243–265.
37. Obrastzow WP, Straschesko ND. Zue Kenntnis der Thrombose der Koronararterien des Herzens. *Z Klin Med* 1910;71:116–132.
38. Muller JE. Diagnosis of myocardial infarction: historical notes from the Soviet Union and the United States. *Am J Cardiol* 1977;40:269–271.
39. Herrick JB. Certain clinical features of sudden obstruction of the coronary arteries. *JAMA* 1912;59:2015–2020.
40. Howell JD. Early perceptions of the electrocardiogram: from arrhythmia to infarction. *Bull Hist Med* 1984;58:83–98.
41. Levine SA. *Coronary thrombosis: its various clinical features.* Baltimore: Williams & Wilkins, 1929.
42. Sones FM Jr, Shirey EK. Cine coronary arteriography. *Mod Concepts Cardiovasc Dis* 1962;31:735–738.
43. Fye WB. Ventricular fibrillation and defibrillation: historical perspectives. *Circulation* 1985;71:858–865.
44. Fye WB. Disorders of the heartbeat: a historical overview from antiquity to the mid-20th century. *Am J Cardiol* 1993;72:1055–1070.
45. Day HW. A cardiac resuscitation program. *Lancet* 1962;82:153–156.
46. Wright IS, Marple CD, Beck DF. Report of the committee for the evaluation of anti-coagulants in the treatment of coronary thrombosis with myocardial infarction. *Am Heart J* 1948;36:801–815.
47. Mueller RL, Scheidt S. History of drugs for thrombotic disease: discovery, development, and directions for the future. *Circulation* 1994;89:432–449.
48. Fletcher AP, Alkjaersig N, Smyrniotis F, et al. The treatment of patients suffering from early myocardial infarction with massive and prolonged streptokinase therapy. *Trans Assoc Am Physicians* 1958;71:287–296.
49. Boucek RJ, Murphy WP Jr. Segmental perfusion of the coronary arteries with fibrinolysin in man following a myocardial infarction. *Am J Cardiol* 1960;6:525–533.
50. Friedberg CK, Horn H. Acute myocardial infarction not due to coronary artery occlusion. *JAMA* 1939;112:1675–1679.
51. Friedman M, Van den Bovenkamp GJ. The pathogenesis of a coronary thrombus. *Am J Pathol* 1966;48:19–44.
52. Roberts WC, Buja LM. The frequency and significance of coronary arterial thrombi and other observations in fatal acute myocardial infarction: a study of 107 necropsy patients. *Am J Med* 1972;52:425–443.
53. DeWood MA, Spores J, Notske R, et al. Prevalence of total coronary occlusion during the early hours of transmural myocardial infarction. *N Engl J Med* 1980;303:897–902.
54. Chazov EI, Matveeva LS, Mazaev AV, et al. Intracoronary administration of fibrinolysin in acute myocardial infarction. *Ter Arkh* 1976;48:8–19.
55. Rentrop KP, Blanke H, Karsch KR, et al. Acute myocardial infarction: intracoronary application of nitroglycerin and streptokinase. *Clin Cardiol* 1979;2:354–363.
56. Streptokinase in recent myocardial infarction: a controlled multicentre trial. European working party. *Br Med J* 1971;3:325–331.

CHAPTER 2

Prevalence, Incidence, and Mortality of Coronary Heart Disease

William B. Kannel

Incidence and Prevalence	Secular Trends
The Elderly	Preventive Implications
Prognosis	References
Mortality	

Key Words: Coronary disease; incidence; mortality; risk factors; secular trends.

Life expectancy in the United States is currently at its greatest level, chiefly as a consequence of the 49% age-adjusted decline in cardiovascular mortality during the last 25 years. This indicates the extent to which these leading causes of death are amenable to preventive and therapeutic measures. However, the residual magnitude of the problem is substantial, requiring vigorous preventive measures. Despite major reductions in death rates for the various forms of cardiovascular disease in the United States, it remains the most serious threat to life and health (1,2). Currently in the United States, a major cardiovascular disease develops in one-third of men younger than 60 years; the odds for women are 1 in 10 (3). Coronary heart disease (CHD), in particular, is a major cause of death in men older than 40 years and women older than 64 years (4).

Cardiovascular disease accounts for 44% of mortality and much morbidity in the United States. Its cost to the U.S. economy is by far the largest for any diagnostic group (5). CHD, in particular, kills and disables individuals in the United States in their most productive years. According to National Heart, Lung, and Blood Institute estimates, CHD was associated with $53 billion for medical care and $47 billion in indirect economic costs in 1999 (1). CHD is the third most frequent cause of short-stay hospitalizations and ranks among the greatest costs per hospital admission. It is also the leading cause of premature permanent disability in

W. B. Kannel: Framingham Heart Study, Lung and Blood Institute's Framingham Heart Study, National Institutes of Health, 73 Mt. Wayte Avenue, Framingham, Massachusetts 01702-5827.

the U.S. labor force, accounting for 19% of disability allowances by the Social Security Administration. The five-year medical treatment cost for a myocardial infarction (for diagnostic and therapeutic services) in 1986 was $51,211 (6).

INCIDENCE AND PREVALENCE

Data from the Framingham Study provide reliable estimates of cardiovascular morbidity and mortality on the basis of 44 years of follow-up of a defined population sample of 5,209 men and women aged 35 to 94 years. These data indicate that average annual rates of first major cardiovascular events increase from 7 per 1,000 men at ages 35 to 44 years to 68 per 1,000 at ages 85 to 94 years (7). For women, comparable rates are achieved ten years later in life, with the gap in incidence narrowing with advancing age. CHD comprises al-

TABLE 2–1. *Incidence of atherosclerotic cardiovascular events:44-year follow-up of Framingham Study cohort and 20-year follow-up of offspring by age and sex*

	Average annual incidence per 1,000			
	Aged 35–64 yr		Aged 65–94 yr	
	Men	Women	Men	Women
CVD (all types)	17	9	44	30
Coronary disease	12	5	27	16
Stroke	2	2	13	11
Heart failure	2	1	12	9
Peripheral artery disease	3	2	8	5

Average annual incidence rates are age-adjusted. CVD, cardiovascular disease.

TABLE 2–2. *Percent of first cardiovascular events as coronary heart disease, stroke, and heart failure: 44-year follow-up of Framingham Study cohort and 20-year follow-up of offspring*

Age, yr	CHD		Stroke		CHF	
	Men	Women	Men	Women	Men	Women
35–54	76.1%	60.9%	9.6%	13.8%	5.0%	10.6%
55–64	69.9%	62.2%	11.1%	14.6%	5.2%	8.7%
65–74	57.9%	53.6%	20.8%	24.5%	7.2%	8.4%
75–94	51.0%	39.3%	26.0%	35.0%	13.5%	16.8%

CHD, coronary heart disease; CHF, congestive heart failure.
From Thom TJ, Kannel WB, Silbershatz H, et al. Cardiovascular diseases in the U.S. and preventive approaches. In: Fuster V, Alexander RW, O'Rourke RA, eds. *Hurst's the heart.* New York: McGraw-Hill, 2001:3–17, with permission.

most two-thirds of all cardiovascular disease in men and women. The incidence of CHD in patients younger than 65 years equals that of stroke, heart failure, and peripheral artery disease combined. The male sex predominance is most striking for CHD (Table 2–1). The fraction of cardiovascular events caused by CHD declines with age, whereas the proportions caused by stroke and cardiac failure increase with age. At all ages, a greater proportion of cardiovascular events in men than women are caused by CHD. This is in contrast with the fraction for stroke and heart failure, which predominates in women at all ages (Table 2–2).

The Framingham Study estimated the lifetime risk for development of CHD on the basis of its long-term continuous surveillance of the original and offspring cohorts. The lifetime risk at age 40 years was found to be one in two for men and one in three for women (8). Notably, this risk for women greatly exceeds the one in eight lifetime risk for development of breast cancer, which often is a greater fear for women. Even at age 70 years there is no escaping a high lifetime risk—35% for men and 25% for women (Table 2–3).

It was estimated that in the United States in 1999 12 million people had CHD; half of those individuals had myocardial infarctions (1). Coronary artery disease causes about 800,000 new heart attacks each year and 450,000 recurrent attacks (2). The incidence in women lags behind men by 10 years for total CHD and by 20 years for myocardial infarction and sudden death. The male sex predominance is least pronounced for uncomplicated angina pectoris. The inci-

dence of myocardial infarction increases more sharply with age than angina or sudden death (Table 2–4). The first CHD manifestation in women is more likely to be angina, whereas in men it more often presents as a myocardial infarction. The proportion of CHD events as myocardial infarction increases with age in both men and women reaching 55% to 60% by age 75 to 94 years. The fraction for angina decreases with age, whereas that for sudden death increases sharply with age (Table 2–5). Angina in men occurs more often after a myocardial infarction than before it. Only one in five coronary attacks are preceded by long-standing angina, and even fewer if the infarction is silent or unrecognized. Serious manifestations of CHD, such as myocardial infarction or sudden death, are rare in the premenopausal woman. The incidence and severity of CHD increase with age in both sexes. CHD incidence rates in postmenopausal women are two to three times that of women the same age who remain premenopausal (9), and this applies whether the menopause is natural or surgical. The male predominant sex ratio in incidence narrows progressively with advancing age.

Unrecognized myocardial infarctions are common, numbering about one in every three infarctions (7). Half of the unrecognized infarctions are silent, and the other half are so atypical that neither the patients nor their physicians consider the possibility. Men with diabetes and men and women with hypertension are particularly susceptible to silent or unrecognized infarctions. More than half of these individuals subsequently experience development of overt clinical manifestations of CHD and, hence, eventually come under medical care. Angina less frequently accompanies unrecognized compared with recognized infarctions. Despite the seemingly innocuous effects of unrecognized infarctions, the long-term cardiovascular event and mortality rate experienced by men is nearly the same as for recognized infarctions (Table 2–6).

THE ELDERLY

Cardiovascular disease is an expanding problem in the elderly, causing 70% of all deaths after age 75 years. CHD is the most common and most lethal cardiovascular event in both sexes, causing much disability in old age. Unrecog-

TABLE 2–3. *Lifetime risk for first coronary heart disease events at specified ages: Framingham Study participants*

Age, yr	(95% confidence interval)	
	Men	Women
40	48.6% (45.8–51.3)	31.7% (29.2–34.2)
50	46.9% (44.0–49.8)	31.1% (28.6–33.7)
60	42.7% (39.5–45.8)	29.0% (26.3–31.6)
70	34.9% (31.2–38.7)	24.2% (21.4–27.0)

From Lloyd-Jones DM, Larson MG, Beiser A, et al. Lifetime risk of developing coronary heart disease. *Lancet* 1999;353:89–92, with permission.

TABLE 2–4. *Incidence of specified clinical manifestations of coronary heart disease: 44-year follow-up of Framingham Study cohort and 20-year follow-up of offspring*

| | Average annual age-adjusted incidence rate per 1,000 | | | | | |
| | Angina pectoris | | Myocardial infarction | | Sudden death | |
Age, yr	Men	Women	Men	Women	Men	Women
35–64	8	4	6	2	2	1
65–94	10	8	16	7	3	1

nized myocardial infarctions are especially common in the elderly (10). Women older than 65 years become as vulnerable to cardiovascular mortality as men (11). The predisposing modifiable risk factors for CHD are similar for young and old individuals, as well as for men and women. The relevant risk factors include: hypertension, dyslipidemia, impaired glucose tolerance, physical inactivity, and cigarette smoking. A lower risk ratio for some risk factors in the elderly is offset by a greater absolute risk of CHD in advanced age. As a result, the attributable risk and the potential benefit of treatment increases with age (11). In the elderly, average total and atherogenic LDL-cholesterol often are unacceptable and are greater in women than men. According to National Heart, Lung, and Blood Institute guidelines, about 10 million elderly, with a female-to-male ratio of 2:1, require further investigation and treatment for dyslipidemia. Multivariate risk profiles composed of the major risk factors predict CHD as efficiently in the elderly as in young individuals. This, together with that the decline in cardiovascular mortality has included the elderly, suggests a need for intervention in the elderly. Because of the preponderance of women in the elderly population, trials testing the efficacy of correcting risk factors should focus more on women.

PROGNOSIS

Even after surviving the acute stage of a myocardial infarction, morbidity and mortality are two to nine times that of the general population (12). The incidence of reinfarction, sudden death, angina pectoris, cardiac failure, and stroke are all substantial, and the relative and absolute risks for these oc-

currences are as great in women as in men. After a recognized myocardial infarction, 18% of men and 35% of women will have a recurrent infarction within 6 years, and angina will develop in 27% of men and 14% of women. About 22% of men and 46% of women will be disabled with cardiac failure, and 8% of men and 11% of women will sustain a stroke. Sudden death will occur in 7% of men and 6% of women. The outlook, particularly in men, is not better after an unrecognized infarction (Table 2–6). Although about two-thirds of patients who have had a myocardial infarction do not make a complete recovery, 88% of those patients younger than 65 years are able to return to their usual occupations.

Heart failure often is the end stage of CHD. Once overt indications of failure appear, half of the patients will die within 5 years, despite modern medical management (13). Risk for cardiac failure is increased twofold to sixfold by CHD; the risk for angina is half that of a myocardial infarct. CHD, generally accompanied by hypertension, is responsible for 39% of cases of cardiac failure (14). Sudden death is a common feature of cardiac failure; it occurs at six to nine times the general population rate. Mortality and hospital discharge rates for cardiac failure have not declined substantially since 1970, despite a marked decline in CHD mortality and a marked improvement in hypertension control. This cannot be readily explained. Some postulate that improved survival of cases of angina, myocardial infarction, and hypertensive heart disease may result in an increased prevalence of chronic heart disease and, ultimately, cardiac failure. There also is uncertainty about the prevalence of underlying causes of heart failure, which may have shifted in recent years from predominantly hypertension to CHD (15).

TABLE 2–5. *Percent of first coronary events as myocardial infarction, angina pectoris, or sudden death: 44-year follow-up of Framingham Study cohort and 20-year follow-up of offspring*

| | Percent as specified CHD event | | | | | | | |
| | Myocardial infarction | | Angina pectoris | | Sudden death | | Other CHD | |
Age, yr	Men	Women	Men	Women	Men	Women	Men	Women
35–54	45.3%	29.7%	37.7%	58.2%	8.1%	2.2%	8.9%	9.9%
55–64	42.2%	26.2%	43.3%	59.2%	8.9%	5.6%	5.6%	8.4%
65–74	51.0%	33.3%	34.0%	51.1%	8.3%	7.4%	6.8%	8.2%
75–84	59.4%	54.6%	21.8%	30.3%	14.3%	7.3%	4.5%	7.9%

CHD, coronary heart disease; other CHD, coronary insufficiency and nonsudden CHD death.

TABLE 2–6. *Six-year prognosis after myocardial infarction: 44-year follow-up of Framingham Study cohort and 20-year follow-up of offspring*

| | Percent developing specified event | | | |
| | Recognized MI | | Unrecognized MI | |
Outcome	Men	Women	Men	Women
Death	37%	60%	46%	34%
Sudden death	7%	6%	5%	2%
Myocardial infarct	18%	35%	19%	18%
Angina	27%	14%	11%	17%
Heart failure	22%	46%	27%	21%
Stroke	8%	11%	13%	7%

Excludes deaths within 30 days.
MI, myocardial infarction.
From Thom TJ, Kannel WB, Silbershatz H, et al. Cardiovascular diseases in the U.S. and preventive approaches. In: Fuster V, Alexander RW, O'Rourke RA, eds. *Hurst's the heart.* New York: McGraw-Hill, 2001:3–17, with permission.

MORTALITY

CHD is the leading cause of death for adults in the United States, accounting for more than 25% of deaths in adults older than 35 years (4). In 1998, there were 498,000 deaths attributed to CHD (7). Mortality from this disease increases steeply with age and causes many deaths in adults at the peak of their productive lives. CHD is either the leading cause, or one of the leading causes, of death in men and women of every racial or ethnic group (2). The mortality rate for CHD is 4.5 times greater in men than women 25 to 34 years old, but that ratio declines to 1.5 for the 75 to 84 year age group. The mortality rate for CHD is reported to be greater in black than in white individuals younger than 75 years. Heart disease mortality rates are not quite as great among the Hispanic population as they are among black and white populations (16).

In a substantial proportion of CHD events, the progression from inapparent disease to death is abrupt. Much of the premature CHD mortality surfaces with little warning. Sudden, unexpected, out-of-hospital deaths account for more than half of all coronary fatalities. The fraction of CHD

TABLE 2–7. *Proportion of coronary heart disease deaths as sudden deaths: 44-year follow-up of Framingham Study cohort and 20-year follow-up of offspring*

| | Percent as sudden death | | |
	Aged 35–64 yr	Aged 65–94 yr	Aged 35–94 yr
Men	54%	41%	47%
Women	39%	29%	31%
Total	51%	36%	42%

From Thom TJ, Kannel WB, Silbershatz H, et al. Cardiovascular diseases in the U.S. and preventive approaches. In: Fuster V, Alexander RW, O'Rourke RA, eds. *Hurst's the heart.* New York: McGraw-Hill, 2001:3–17, with permission.

TABLE 2–8. *One-year mortality rate after initial recognized myocardial infarction: 44-year follow-up of Framingham Study cohort and 20-year follow-up of offspring*

| | Percent dead within 1 year | | |
	Aged 35–64 yr	Aged 65–94 yr	Aged 35–94 yr
Men	17%	38%	25%
Women	31%	40%	38%

From Thom TJ, Kannel WB, Silbershatz H, et al. Cardiovascular diseases in the U.S. and preventive approaches. In: Fuster V, Alexander RW, O'Rourke RA, eds. *Hurst's the heart.* New York: McGraw-Hill, 2001:3–17, with permission.

deaths that are sudden deaths is less in women than men and also is less in elderly men (Table 2–7). However, the percentage of sudden coronary deaths that occurs without prior overt CHD is much greater in women than men and also in younger compared with older individuals. Of those individuals who experience sudden death, 50% of the men and 63% of the women did not have prior indication of overt CHD (7). About 80% of CHD deaths of patients younger than 65 years occur at the time of the initial coronary attack (3). Thus, despite a greater death rate after a prior coronary attack, most CHD deaths arise from the segment of the population who are free of symptomatic disease.

After myocardial infarction, sudden deaths occur at four to six times the rate of the general population. The first year after a recognized myocardial infarction is especially dangerous, with 25% of men and 38% of women (including all in- and out-of-hospital deaths) experiencing sudden death (7). The one-year mortality rate increases steeply with age (Table 2–8). Most of these deaths occur within the first 30 days after myocardial infarction. In contrast to initial myocardial infarction incidence rates, where women have lower rates, survival after recognized myocardial infarction in women is not as good compared with men at all ages (Table 2–6). This is because women tend to have a greater burden of risk factors at time of infarction and smaller coronary arteries (17). Long-term survival after unrecognized myocardial infarction is little better than for recognized infarctions, but better for women than men (Table 2–6). After uncomplicated angina pectoris, mortality rates for men younger than 65 years are nearly the same as for patients with recognized myocardial infarctions, but they are much worse than mortality rates for women with angina (7).

SECULAR TRENDS

Mortality from cardiovascular diseases has declined steadily since 1940 (7). After the epidemic increase in the 1940s through the early 1960s, a decline in CHD mortality has continued since the mid-1960s. Since peaking in 1963, the age-adjusted CHD mortality rate declined more than 50% and is currently decreasing 3% to 4% per year. In recent years, the largest absolute decline in cardiovascular mortality has been iin deaths caused by CHD. The decline coincides with reductions in the major cardiovascular risk factors, more effective treatment, and greater efforts at secondary prevention (18). This reduction in CHD mortality in the United States exceeds that observed in most countries.

PREVENTIVE IMPLICATIONS

Epidemiologic perusal of the incidence, prevalence, and mortality of CHD indicates the need for a preventive approach. Further innovations in diagnosis and treatment for CHD undoubtedly will improve the outlook of patients surviving the initial attack. However, this can have only a limited impact because of the unheralded high initial mortality rates. When the heart is infarcted, no therapy can be expected to restore full function. A preventive approach involving detection and correction of predisposing conditions before the advent of overt clinical disease is required for a substantial impact. CHD often emerges without warning, with one in five coronary attacks presenting as a sudden death. In all, two-thirds of CHD fatalities occur too precipitously to be brought under medical attention.

Awaiting overt signs and symptoms of CHD before treatment is no longer justied. In some respects, the occurrence of symptoms may be more properly regarded as a medical failure rather than as the initial indication for treatment. High-risk candidates can be detected for preventive management from a coronary risk profile made up of ingredients easily obtained by office procedures (19).

REFERENCES

1. American Heart Association. 1999 heart and stroke: statistical update. Dallas: American Heart Association, 1999. Available at: http://www.amhrt.org (accessed March 25, 2004).
2. National Heart, Lung and Blood Institute. Morbidity and mortality chartbook on cardiovascular, lung and blood diseases, 1998. Washington: U.S. Department of Health and Human Services, 1998. Available at: http://www.nhlbi.nih.gov/index.htm (accessed March 25, 2004).
3. Gordon T, Kannel WB. Premature mortality from coronary heart disease: the Framingham Study. *JAMA* 1971;215:1617–1625.
4. National Center for Health Statistics. Vital statistics of the United States, 1988, Vol. II, Mortality, Part A, 1991. Hyattsville, MD: Centers for Disease Control and Prevention, 1991.
5. National Heart, Lung and Blood Institute. *NHLBI fact book, fiscal year 1990.* Washington: U.S. Department of Health and Human Services, 1991.
6. Wittels EH, Hay JW, Gotto AM. Medical costs of coronary artery disease in the United States. *Am J Cardiol* 1990;65:432–440.
7. Thom TJ, Kannel WB, Silbershatz H, et al. Cardiovascular diseases in the U.S. and preventive approaches. In: Fuster V, Alexander RW, O'Rourke RA, eds. *Hurst's the heart.* New York: McGraw-Hill, 2001:3–17.
8. Lloyd-Jones DM, Larson MG, Beiser A, et al. Lifetime risk of developing coronary heart disease. *Lancet* 1999;353:89–92.
9. Gordon T, Kannel WB, Hjortland MC, et al. Menopause and coronary heart disease. *Ann Intern Med* 1978;89:157–161.
10. Kannel WB, Cupples LA, Gagnon DR. Incidence precursors and prognosis of unrecognized myocardial infarction. *Adv Cardiol* 1990;37:202–214.
11. Kannel WB, Vokonas PS. Demographics of the prevalence, incidence, and management of coronary heart disease in the elderly and in women. *Ann Epidemiol* 1992;2:5–14.
12. Cupples LA, D'Agostino RB. Survival following initial cardiovascular events: 30-year follow-up. Framingham Heart Study, Section 35. In: Kannel WB, Wolf PA, Garrison RJ, eds. *The Framingham Study: an epidemiological investigation of cardiovascular disease.* Bethesda, MD: National Heart, Lung and Blood Institute, 1988:21; NIH publication no. 88-2969, 1988, 454.
13. Kannel WB, Belanger AJ. Epidemiology of heart failure. *Am Heart J* 1991;121:951–957.
14. Kannel WB. Vital epidemiologic clues in heart failure. *J Clin Epidemiol* 2000;53:229–235.
15. Turlink JR, Goldhaber SJ, Pfeffer MA. An overview of contemporary etiologies of congestive heart failure. *Am Heart J* 1991;121:1852–1853.
16. National Center for Health Statistics. Deaths of Hispanic Origin, 15 Reporting States, 1979-81. Vital and Health Statistics, Series 20, No. 18, DHHS Publication No. (PHS) 91-1855; 1990.
17. Wong ND, Cupples LA, Ostfeld AM, et al. Risk factors for long-term coronary prognosis after initial myocardial infarction. The Framingham Study. *Am J Epidemiol* 1989;130:469–480.
18. Burke GL, Sprafka JM, Folsom AR, et al. Trends in CHD mortality, morbidity and risk factor levels from 1960 to 1986: The Minnesota Heart Survey. *Int J Epidemiol* 1989;18[Suppl 3]:573–581.
19. Grundy SM, Pasternak R, Greenland P. Assessment of cardiovascular risk by use of multiple risk-factor assessment equations: a statement for health care professionals from the American Heart Association and the American College of Cardiology. *Circulation* 1999;34:1348–1359.

PART I

Major Risk Factors and Primary Prevention

CHAPTER 3

Overview

Henry C. McGill, Jr. and C. Alex McMahan

Key Words: Atherothrombosis; atherosclerosis; coronary artery disease; primary prevention; risk factor.

ATHEROTHROMBOSIS AND ITS SEQUELAE AS PREVENTABLE DISEASES

Until the mid-twentieth century, age was considered the major determinant of atherothrombosis and coronary artery disease (CAD). Although it was conventional knowledge that atherosclerotic lesions were rich in cholesterol (1) and that human-like atherothrombosis developed in rabbits that were fed cholesterol (2), it remained difficult to believe that this essential component of human tissues could cause a lethal disease.

H. C. McGill, Jr.: Department of Physiology and Medicine, Southwest Foundation for Biomedical Research, P. O. Box 760549, San Antonio, TX 78245-0549, and The University of Texas Health Science Center at San Antonio, San Antonio, Texas.

C. A. McMahan: The University of Texas Health Science Center at San Antonio, San Antonio, Texas.

A Dutch physician who practiced in Java observed in 1916 that Javanese had lower blood cholesterol levels and also had a lower frequency of atherosclerotic disease than individuals in the Netherlands (3). This report lay without notice in an obscure journal until cited in 1941 in support of an observation that the incidence of atherosclerotic disease in Chinese individuals was low because of their low intake of fat (4).

CAD reached epidemic proportions among the industrialized countries by the mid-twentieth century and commanded the attention of physicians and scientists after World War II. Several observers attributed the decline in frequency of CAD in the Scandinavian countries during the war to reduced availability of butter, eggs, and meat (5,6). These reports stimulated the idea that atherothrombosis and its sequelae might be prevented by modifying dietary fat intake. Wide variations in CAD morbidity and mortality among countries provided further evidence that atherothrombosis might be related to diet and other environmental conditions and, therefore, was not inevitable with aging. Gradually, the idea was accepted that atherothrombosis and the resulting

CAD could be prevented if the environmental causes could be identified and modified.

THE RISK FACTOR CONCEPT

Epidemiologic Studies Identifying the Risk Factors

Between 1930 and 1950, a number of reports indicated that patients with CAD had greater levels of serum cholesterol and greater blood pressures than other patients and were predominantly male (7–9). However, conclusions were limited by the case–control study design because serum cholesterol and blood pressure were measured after myocardial infarction had occurred.

To support a causal relation, it was necessary to measure the suspected variables in healthy persons, to measure the subsequent incidence of CAD, and to relate the occurrence of disease to the previously measured variables (a prospective or longitudinal design). Such a study was initiated by the Division of Chronic Disease of the United States Public Health Service among the residents of Framingham, MA, in 1948; and the project was transferred to the newly established National Heart Institute in 1949 (10). In 1950, The Framingham Study, as it came to be known, enrolled and examined about 5,000 adults 30 to 59 years of age free of cardiovascular disease.

In 1957, when 90% of the subjects had been followed for 4 years, about 1 of 20 subjects had experienced a new episode of CAD (11). The rate of new events in men was about twice that in women. Men with hypertension, obesity, or increased serum cholesterol concentration at the initial examination had from twofold to sixfold greater rates of new CAD events. The effect of obesity was largely accounted for by its association with hypertension. CAD was more frequent in heavy smokers, but the association was not statistically significant. Two years later, a 6-year follow-up report added smoking as a predictor of CAD (12).

During the 1950s and early 1960s, other similar longitudinal epidemiologic studies were started in Albany, NY (13); Tecumseh, MI (14); Chicago (15); and San Francisco (16). Reports from these studies soon confirmed the Framingham results regarding serum cholesterol, hypertension, and smoking. In 1978, data from five major longitudinal studies were pooled for a combined analysis of observations on 8,422 men representing more than 72,011 person-years (17). This comprehensive report firmly established hypertension, increased serum cholesterol concentration, diabetes mellitus, and smoking (in addition to age and male sex) as predictors of the incidence of CAD.

What Is a "Risk Factor"?

The term "risk factor" first appeared in the title of a journal article in 1963 (18). A risk factor is any measurable characteristic of an individual that predicts that individual's probability of experiencing development of a clinically manifest disease. The definition is broad and does not necessarily imply a causal relation. The characteristic may be exposure to an environmental agent (tobacco smoke), an intervening variable (increased serum cholesterol concentration) resulting from an environmental agent (dietary lipids), or a genetic variant (low-density lipoprotein [LDL] receptor defect), another disease (hypertension or diabetes), or an early or preclinical manifestation of CAD (electrocardiographic abnormality). The risk factor concept was widely accepted and the term was extended to traits that predicted stroke, peripheral arterial disease, and other diseases. Research was directed toward the mechanisms of action of the risk factors while the search for new risk factors continued.

This broad definition of a risk factor is most useful in the early stages of investigating a disease, when etiology and pathogenesis are uncertain. However, because the ultimate objective is to prevent the disease, much effort has been devoted to ascertaining whether the risk factors, particularly those that can be modified, are truly causes of CAD, and, by implication, whether modification of the risk factor will reduce the risk for disease. Although a risk factor such as male sex cannot be modified, knowledge of why it predicts the occurrence of CAD may suggest other preventive strategies.

RISK FACTORS: ESTABLISHED, EMERGING, AND CONTROVERSIAL

Serum Lipids and Lipoproteins

Measurement of serum (or plasma) cholesterol became a major concern when its usefulness in predicting CAD risk was established. Methods using automated analyzers and enzymatic assays greatly improved precision and accuracy. The initial observations of cholesterol and risk for CAD were made on the basis of total cholesterol because methods were not available for measuring subclasses of serum lipoproteins in large numbers of persons. Results using the analytic ultracentrifuge (19,20) and, later, paper electrophoresis (21) indicated that the distribution of cholesterol among the lipoproteins improved the prediction of risk (22). The method of heparin-manganese precipitation of the apo-B–containing lipoproteins and measuring high-density lipoprotein (HDL) cholesterol, and then estimating LDL cholesterol (23), facilitated measurement of the lipoprotein profile in large numbers of subjects.

In a longitudinal study using ultracentrifugal analyses, an increased LDL cholesterol concentration was positively associated with CAD (24), and this association has been confirmed in numerous subsequent studies. Recent studies suggest that a simpler and equally effective predictor of CAD risk is non-HDL cholesterol, which contains all of the known and potential atherogenic lipoproteins (25) (see Chapters 6 and 9).

The association of low HDL cholesterol concentration with CAD was initially proposed in 1956 (24), but the finding was ignored until confirmed 20 years later (26). The link of low

HDL to CAD was reinforced by the recognition that the physiologic function of HDL was reverse cholesterol transport (see Chapter 7). Low HDL cholesterol currently is recognized as a common and powerful risk factor for CAD (27).

An immunologically distinctive form of LDL, lipoprotein (a) (Lp[a]), discovered more than 40 years ago (28), was associated with increased incidence of CAD independently of serum LDL cholesterol levels (29). Despite confirmatory reports, Lp(a) received little attention until the structure of the gene for its distinctive protein, apolipoprotein(a), was found to be similar to that for plasminogen (30). This similarity provided a plausible mechanism of action: attenuation of clot lysis by competing with plasminogen for its binding to fibrin (31). Further confirmation of its predictive power, combined with a plausible mechanism, made Lp(a) a promising candidate for risk factor status (32). The role of Lp(a) in CAD continues to be widely studied by measuring Lp(a) directly (33), measuring Lp(a)-cholesterol (34), and measuring apolipoprotein(a) isoforms (35). The results continue to be mixed, sometimes showing Lp(a) or its isoforms to be a risk factor only when other risk factors (particularly increased LDL cholesterol) were present and at other times showing it to be an independent risk factor for clinical CAD. Its role in the pathogenesis of atherosclerotic lesions has not been determined with certainty, and it remains likely that its major role is in the terminal occlusive thrombosis.

The discovery of a chemically modified lipoprotein, oxidized LDL (36), led to extensive investigation of its properties and its putative role in atherogenesis (37). Oxidized LDL is present in human atherosclerotic lesions, but there is no reliable way to measure the rate at which it is formed in lesions (see Chapter 8). Antioxidant agents prevent atherothrombosis in hypercholesterolemic animals, but antioxidant vitamins have failed to prevent disease in humans (38). If a marker of the oxidizing process in tissues can be identified, oxidized LDL may become an important risk factor that can be modified by other antioxidants.

A class of small, dense LDL (39) is associated with risk for CAD (40). The predictive value of this trait has been confirmed in numerous observational studies since it was initially described (41). The role of small, dense LDL is complicated by its association with hypertriglyceridemia, low HDL cholesterol, obesity (particularly central obesity), and insulin resistance—all features of the metabolic syndrome (see Chapter 19). This lipoprotein subclass is influenced both by genetics and diet (42), and by the same interventions that modulate other components of the metabolic syndrome (43). The association is well established, but whether small, dense LDL is the critical agent or simply a marker for the other atherogenic factors remains to be determined (44,45).

Triglycerides

Serum triglyceride concentration as an independent risk factor for CAD was first reported in 1959 (46). Subsequently, both prospective and case–control epidemiologic studies yielded conflicting results. A National Institutes of Health (NIH) Consensus Development Panel in 1993 concluded that although triglyceride-rich lipoproteins were atherogenic, the predictive power of serum triglyceride concentration for CAD often was lost when the analysis included adjustment for other lipid risk factors, particularly low HDL cholesterol (47). A meta-analysis in 1996 concluded that triglycerides were indeed an independent risk factor (48). As the metabolic syndrome was recognized, it became apparent that increased triglyceride concentrations were part of this syndrome with its several atherogenic factors and that its frequent but inconsistent relation with CAD might be because of this association (49) (see Chapter 19).

Blood Pressure

Long before the modern epidemiologic studies of CAD, physicians recognized that individuals with increased blood pressure were more susceptible to CAD (9). The Framingham Study found that systolic blood pressure was as good a predictor of risk as diastolic blood pressure (10). An exhaustive meta-analysis of nine major studies showed a direct, continuous, and independent association between blood pressure and risk for CAD and an even stronger association with stroke (50). Even small increases in blood pressure in young men predicted excess CAD 25 years later (51). Hypertension may produce this effect by several potential mechanisms: cardiac hypertrophy, impairment of endothelial function, or a disordered renin-angiotensin system (52,53) (see Chapter 14). Furthermore, hypertension is associated with insulin resistance and the metabolic syndrome (54) (see Chapter 19), which may affect atherogenesis through other mechanisms. Pharmacologic treatment of hypertension reduces CAD risk, but not as much as it reduces stroke risk.

Smoking

The 1964 Surgeon General's report on the health effects of smoking observed an association of smoking with death rates from CAD, but the evidence for a causal relation was not conclusive (55). By 1971, with access to considerable additional evidence, the Surgeon General concluded that smoking was an independent risk factor for CAD (56). By 1983, the conclusion was clear that smoking was not only causal, but was "the most important of the known modifiable risk factors for CHD" in the United States (57). Subsequently, a massive volume of evidence from around the world has reinforced this conclusion. Smoking accelerates atherogenesis and increases risk for clinically manifest CAD. The mechanism by which tobacco smoke produces these effects is not known, but the effects of thousands of chemicals in tobacco smoke offer many possibilities: vasospasm, endothelial damage, immune responses, inflammatory cytokines, mutagenesis, and thrombosis, to cite only a few (see Chapter 18).

The risk for CAD (as well as other smoking-related diseases) diminishes after cessation of smoking, but it has not been feasible to conduct a controlled clinical trial to demonstrate the benefits of smoking cessation because of ethical considerations. Thus, although the gold standard criterion of efficacy has not been fulfilled, overwhelming observational evidence indicates that smoking cessation is the most effective and least expensive of all the risk factor modifications likely to reduce risk for CAD. Despite all efforts, 23.5% of adults and 27.9% of youths 18 to 24 years old youths were smoking in the United States in 1999, a statistic indicating a substantial opportunity for primary prevention (58).

Male Sex

Male sex is one of the best documented and strongest risk factors for CAD, yet the least understood (59). The sex differential is not explained by differences in the established risk factors. However, the sex differential observed in white populations is not universal and is attenuated in nonwhite populations; also, diabetes abolishes the sex differential (60). The rate of age-related increase in incidence of CAD among men declines after middle age, but continues to increase in women during and after menopause so that the rates become nearly equal in men and women in the older age groups.

For many years, the relative protection of premenopausal women to atherothrombosis and CAD was attributed to the female sex steroid hormones, particularly estrogen; but paradoxically, men treated with estrogen after a myocardial infarct had more frequent recurrent CAD, not less (61). For 30 years, observational studies found lower rates of CAD in postmenopausal women using hormone replacement therapy and these findings continued to support the idea that estrogen was protective (62). This firmly entrenched belief was displaced in 2002 by reports of two major controlled clinical trials of hormone replacement therapy for postmenopausal women. Hormone replacement did not prevent recurrence of CAD (63) and actually increased risk for CAD in healthy women (64) (see Chapter 20). The explanation for the protection of premenopausal women remains unknown.

Family History and Genetic Markers

CAD, particularly when occurring in younger persons, was recognized long ago as clustering in families. The first success in explaining the physiologic basis of familial clustering was the identification of individuals with extremely high serum cholesterol levels (65), a syndrome transmitted as an autosomal-dominant trait known as familial hypercholesterolemia and ultimately traced to a defect in the LDL receptor gene (66) (see Chapter 5).

Subsequently, investigators have found many genes and genetic variants associated with lipid and lipoprotein abnormalities and with risk for CAD. These variants include polymorphisms in genes affecting lipoproteins—apolipoproteins, receptors, enzymes, transport proteins (67); genes affecting hemostasis (68); genes affecting tissues of the arterial wall and the inflammatory response (69); and genes affecting the responses of plasma lipoproteins to diet (70). The application of molecular and population genetic methods combined with progress in mapping the human genome ensure that many more genetic variants contributing to atherothrombosis and CAD will be discovered. The emerging knowledge of the molecular and cellular metabolism of the atherosclerotic lesion will lead to new candidate genes.

Despite this progress, genetic polymorphisms are of limited value in predicting an individual's susceptibility to CAD in everyday clinical practice. Meanwhile, family history of CAD, particularly a history of precocious events, remains a powerful predictor of risk for CAD independent of the other known risk factors (71).

Diabetes Mellitus, Insulin Resistance, and the Metabolic Syndrome

After the use of exogenous insulin began to protect diabetics from diabetic ketoacidosis, surviving patients with diabetes were found to be at high risk for all forms of atherosclerotic disease (72). More recently, insulin resistance, the inability of insulin to stimulate glucose uptake, was recognized as a precursor of type 2 diabetes; and insulin resistance was found to be accompanied by a cluster of disorders, including visceral obesity, glucose intolerance, increased triglyceride and decreased HDL cholesterol concentrations, increased blood pressure, and the presence of small, dense LDL particles in serum (73). This combination of abnormalities, currently called the "metabolic syndrome" (49), affects about one in five adults in the United States (74) and is associated with greatly increased risk for CAD (75). Thus, atherogenesis is probably accelerated in prediabetic individuals long before the onset of clinical diabetes (76) (see Chapter 19). Diabetes and the metabolic syndrome undoubtedly have strong genetic components, but the major modifiable condition predisposing to the metabolic syndrome is obesity, which, in turn, can be controlled by balancing caloric intake with caloric expenditure.

Obesity

The association of obesity with CAD was recognized early in epidemiologic studies, but obesity was closely linked with other risk factors (hypertension, diabetes, and hyperlipidemia) and its effect usually disappeared in multivariate analyses (77). However, when subjects were followed for longer periods (15 years or more), obesity emerged as an independent risk factor (78,79). Furthermore, body fat distribution seemed important because the association of adiposity with CAD was stronger with central (visceral) body fat than with overall body fat, as indicated by the body mass index (80). The pathophysiologic mechanisms by which obesity produces this effect are not clear, but conditions recently found to be associated with obesity suggest several potential intervening variables—for example, C-reactive protein (81), insulin resistance (82), and fibrinogen (83) (see Chapter 19).

Physical Inactivity

An early study comparing the incidence of CAD among London bus drivers (sedentary) and conductors (active) suggested that physical activity protected men from CAD (84). Many reports showing no association with physical activity appeared—for example, the ecologic comparisons of the Seven Countries Study (85); but longitudinal studies found physical activity associated with decreased risk (86). Moderate physical activity favorably affects HDL cholesterol concentration, blood pressure, body weight, and insulin resistance, mechanisms by which it may reduce CAD risk (87). Physical activity may also protect from myocardial infarction by improving the efficiency of cardiac function. Even beginning moderate physical activity in middle age was associated with less risk for CAD (88). Continuing studies have repeatedly confirmed the beneficial effects of physical activity (89). Physical activity, a readily modifiable trait, has emerged with persuasive evidence that it is protective against CAD.

Homocystinemia

The association of increased levels of blood homocysteine with CAD was first suspected because precocious atherothrombosis and thrombosis developed in subjects with a rare genetic disorder of methionine metabolism causing very high levels of plasma homocysteine (90). Subsequent case–control and a few prospective studies indicated that increased plasma homocysteine levels were associated with risk for CAD, and plausible cellular mechanisms involving endothelial damage were proposed. Proposals also were made to fortify foods with folic acid and vitamin B_{12}, which were shown to decrease plasma homocysteine levels (91). Results of additional prospective studies and clinical trials were mixed, however, and reviews of the voluminous literature also have reached mixed conclusions regarding hyperhomocystinemia as an independent and causal risk factor for CAD (92–97).

C-Reactive Protein and Other Inflammatory Biomarkers

Elements of a chronic inflammatory reaction in atherosclerotic lesions led to the discovery that the plasma concentration of C-reactive protein (CRP), a trace plasma protein secreted in response to inflammation, was associated with CAD (98). This association has been confirmed in a number of case–control and prospective studies (99–101). Increased CRP levels also are associated with obesity, but multivariate analyses indicate that the CRP association is independent of obesity and other risk factors (99). There are plausible mechanisms for the association and this relation may suggest rational preventive regimens. Plasma fibrinogen levels (102), leucocyte count (103), interleukin-6 (104), and other markers of inflammation (105) also are associated with risk for CAD. Taken together, these findings suggest that there are many links between inflammation, atherothrombosis, and CAD.

Infections

The suspicion that infections might be involved in atherogenesis and thrombosis led to the observation that periodontitis, an inflammatory reaction to infections of the tooth supporting tissues, was more frequent in patients with unstable angina (106). Similar associations were found in a number of case–control studies, but only weak (107) or no (108) associations were found in large prospective studies. Potential intervening mechanisms involving responses to the chronic inflammation have been suggested (109), but the strong association of periodontitis with smoking often confounds interpretation of its link to CAD. Other infections have been linked to CAD—for example, *Chlamydia pneumoniae, Helicobacter pylori,* and cytomegalovirus—but a meta-analysis concluded that evidence from prospective studies was not sufficient to support strong associations with risk for CAD (110).

Psychologic Characteristics

In the 1970s, several reports linked various psychologic traits—personality type, aggression, hostility, depression, stress—with CAD (111). Both positive (112–114) and negative (115) reports continue to appear. One review (116) concludes that the evidence of an association is convincing, but the mechanism is obscure.

Lesions in the Living: The Ultimate Risk Factor for Coronary Artery Disease?

Because the most proximate cause of clinical CAD is the severity of atherothrombosis in the coronary arteries, the best predictor of risk for imminent clinical disease would be the assessment of these lesions in the living person (117,118). A number of methods to accomplish this end are under development and have been demonstrated in animal models or humans. These include ultrasound (119), electron beam computed tomography (120), and various forms of magnetic resonance imaging (121). As these techniques become more refined, they may be useful in identifying older individuals at risk for a clinical event; in identifying children and young adults with advanced lesions, and therefore at high risk for precocious CAD (122); and in identifying young people with progressing atherothrombosis that if not addressed will ultimately lead to clinical disease.

DO RISK FACTORS AFFECT ATHEROTHROMBOSIS OR CLINICAL DISEASE?

Natural History

Atherothrombosis begins as intimal lipid deposits (fatty streaks) in childhood and adolescence (Fig. 3–1) (123). Fatty streaks in some arterial sites are converted into fibrous plaques by continued accumulation of lipid, smooth muscle, and connective tissue. In middle age, fibrous plaques undergo a variety of changes (hemorrhage, ulceration, thrombosis, or calcification) (see Chapters 30, 31, and 32). Ulceration, or plaque rupture (see Chapter 31), is particularly likely to produce thrombotic occlusion, target organ ischemia, and clinical disease (see Chapter 33). Typically, clinical disease occurs 30 or more years after the process begins as fatty streaks, but it may be accelerated in persons with one or more of the major risk factors.

Risk Factors and Atherothrombosis

The major risk factors were identified on the basis of their ability to estimate risk for clinical CAD and not athero-

sclerotic lesions. This evidence did not permit direct inferences about the association of risk factors with the preclinical stages of atherosclerotic disease described in Figure 3–1. The presence of severe coronary atherothrombosis in many persons dying of other causes and having no symptoms of CAD raised questions about the relation of atherothrombosis to CAD and whether the risk factors for clinical disease influenced the initiation and progression of atherothrombosis or only the terminal occlusive episode. Answers to these questions were important in evaluating the causal relation of the risk factors, in determining which risk factors should be modified, and deciding when the modification should begin.

An international survey of atherothrombosis in autopsy results from 19 geographic and ethnic groups showed a threefold variation in extent of coronary artery raised lesions (fibrous plaques plus complicated lesions) in patients dying because of accidents and cardiovascular and noncardiovascular diseases (124). Individuals with clinical CAD had an average of about 60% of the coronary artery intimal surface covered with raised lesions. CAD became frequent in a population when an average of about 30% of the intimal surface

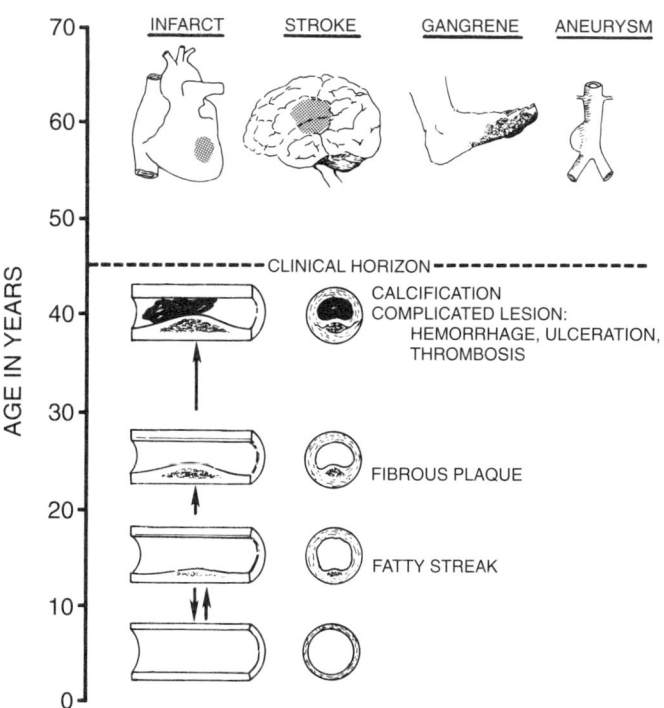

FIG. 3–1. Natural history of human atherothrombosis. The earliest detectable lesion is a deposit of lipid, principally cholesterol and its esters, in the intima and inner media of large muscular and elastic arteries. These appear in the aorta during the first decade of life, in the coronary arteries during the second decade, and in the cerebral arteries during the third decade. The process is similar in molecular and cellular characteristics in all three arterial systems. Continued accumulation of lipid and proliferation of smooth muscle and connective tissue form fibrous plaques, which undergo a variety of changes. The terminal occlusive episode usually results from rupture of a plaque and thrombosis on its intimal surface. Clinical manifestations vary with the artery involved. Risk factors may affect one, several, or all stages of the process. (Redrawn from McGill HC Jr, Geer JC, Strong JP. Natural history of human atherosclerotic lesions. In: Sandler M, Bourne GH, eds. *Atherosclerosis and its origin*. New York: Academic Press, 1963:39–65, with permission.)

was covered with raised lesions. These results were consistent with the idea that the prevalence of advanced atherothrombosis in a population was the major determinant of CAD rates in that population.

Several reports appearing since the mid-1970s have shown associations of risk factors measured during life in longitudinal epidemiologic studies, or estimated after death by indirect methods, with atherosclerotic lesions measured at autopsy (125). It is now well established that high serum cholesterol concentration, increased blood pressure, smoking, diabetes, and male sex are positively associated with atherothrombosis, particularly with raised lesions, in the coronary arteries, aorta, and cerebral arteries of older adults. Many studies using coronary artery angiography and other in vivo quantitative evaluation techniques confirmed the association of coronary atherothrombosis with the same risk factors in living persons, but they did not show how early in life the risk factors began to accelerate atherogenesis.

The risk factors for adult CAD also exist in children (126,127); and although the average values and ranges of most risk factor variables are lower than in adults, there is considerable variability. Both the extent and severity (as measured by histologic characteristics) of atherothrombosis of the abdominal aorta and coronary arteries are associated with high non-HDL cholesterol and low HDL cholesterol concentrations, hypertension, obesity, smoking, and hyperglycemia (128) (see Chapter 32).

Thus, current evidence is strong that lipoproteins, smoking, blood pressure, obesity, and blood glucose influence the early stages of atherothrombosis 20 or more years before clinical CAD appears. This association with the early stages of atherogenesis strengthens the conclusion that the risk factors are causal and encourages the belief that risk factor modification early in life will contribute to primary prevention of CAD.

THE CONCEPT OF PRIMARY PREVENTION

Implications of the Great Decline

In the mid-1960s, a remarkable decline in mortality caused by CAD began in most of the industrialized countries (129). The decline in the United States continued at least until the late 1990s (130,131), and currently approaches a 50% decrease from peak rates. The magnitude and consistency of the declining rates indicate that they were real. Analyses of the changes in risk factors and in treatment of clinical disease indicate that about half of the decline was because of risk factor reductions (serum lipids, blood pressure, and smoking) and about half to improved treatment (emergency medical services, intensive care, medical management, drugs, percutaneous transluminal angioplasty, and bypass surgery) (131). The proportion attributed to treatment was greater during the more recent periods (132,133). The decline gave a powerful stimulus to the belief that primary prevention of CAD was feasible, and the association of decreased mortality with favorable trends in risk factor levels supported the concept that risk factor modification would be beneficial.

Diet and Coronary Artery Disease

Despite the lack of experimental proof that reducing serum cholesterol in humans would prevent atherothrombosis or CAD, in 1957 the American Heart Association recommended that individuals should reduce their total dietary fat intake from the average 40% to 25% or 30% of calories (134). The American Heart Association revised its recommendations periodically thereafter, adding statements that included more specific recommendations about limiting saturated fatty acid and cholesterol intake.

Several small clinical investigations in free-living and metabolic ward subjects and one large trial with 2,000 men indicated that reducing saturated fatty acid and cholesterol intakes decreased serum cholesterol concentrations (135). The effects of fat-modified diets on CAD in varied groups showed predominantly beneficial results (136), but a definitive diet trial to prevent CAD in noninstitutionalized subjects was not feasible.

There has been much progress in defining the effects of different types of fats on lipoproteins (137,138). Dietary intervention was overshadowed in the 1990s by the success of new lipid-lowering drugs, but overwhelming evidence suggests that it should remain the first line of attack for controlling hyperlipidemia in preventive regimens (139).

The Lipid-lowering Drug Era

The Lipid Research Clinics Coronary Primary Prevention Trial tested a bile acid sequestrant in about 4,000 men with high LDL cholesterol levels (140). In 7 years, an 11% reduction in LDL cholesterol was accompanied by a 19% reduction in CAD. The reduction in incidence of CAD was proportional to the reduction in LDL cholesterol. Other clinical trials in Europe with clofibrate (141) and gemfibrozil (142) yielded similar favorable effects of serum cholesterol-decreasing regimens on cardiovascular end points.

The statins, a class of drugs that limited the biosynthesis of cholesterol by inhibiting 3-hydroxy-3-methylglutaryl coenzyme A reductase, revolutionized the physician's ability to modify high serum or LDL cholesterol levels. The change began with a trial of 4,444 men and women with CAD in whom treatment reduced all-cause deaths by 30% (143). This result was soon confirmed in several other similar studies and extended to individuals without CAD but with increased serum cholesterol levels (144), and even to individuals with average serum cholesterol levels (145). These results were achieved with a minimum of adverse effects and with reductions in all-cause and CAD mortality.

Other developments between 1980 and 2000 gave further impetus to the concept of primary prevention. A trial of intervention in men with the three major risk factors—hypercholesterolemia, hypertension, and smoking—showed a reduction in CAD after 16 years (146). Although randomized clinical trials were not feasible with smoking, numerous studies showed that cessation of smoking led to reduction in frequency of CAD (57).

National Campaigns for Primary Prevention

In the United States, Canada, and Europe, many national volunteer health agencies and professional organizations endorsed the recommendations for reducing dietary fat and cholesterol intake to decrease serum cholesterol; controlling increased blood pressure through weight control, physical activity, and drugs; and cessation of smoking to reduce the risk for CAD. The recommendations differed in details and points of emphasis, but all agreed that individuals at high risk—defined by having high serum cholesterol concentration, high blood pressure, and smoking—would benefit from risk factor reduction (see Chapter 11).

Public Health versus Clinical Medicine Strategies

The major difference among the recommended preventive programs was whether risk factor control should be directed toward the entire population, the strategy of public health engineering, or only toward individuals at high risk, the strategy of clinical medicine (147). Because the high-risk individuals are less numerous, they contribute a smaller proportion of the overall disease in the population than the larger groups of individuals at moderate and low risk. Therefore, although risk factor modification may benefit those persons at high risk, it will have a disappointingly small effect in reducing the overall frequency of disease. In contrast, smaller reductions in risk among the larger groups at moderate risk will have a greater effect in reducing disease frequency in the population. The two strategies are not incompatible with one another, but the debate regarding choice of strategies can be confusing and they may compete for scarce resources in conducting preventive campaigns.

THE FUTURE OF RISK FACTORS AND PRIMARY PREVENTION

Criteria by which to judge the causal significance of an association include strength of the association, dose-response relation, temporal sequence, consistency or plausibility, independence, coherence, specificity, and reversibility (55). Many epidemiologic studies from around the world have demonstrated the strength, dose response, temporal sequence, and independence of the major risk factors—serum cholesterol concentration, hypertension, smoking, and diabetes—in varied geographic and ethnic groups. A growing body of knowledge from cellular and molecular biology are fulfilling the requirement of coherence and plausibility by providing mechanisms. The most difficult, but most important, criterion is reversibility, which requires that the disease

risk be reduced when the trait is ameliorated. This final criterion has been met for hypertension and smoking, and overwhelmingly for hyperlipidemia. Persuasive evidence, therefore, indicates that modification of the major risk factors reduces risk for clinical CAD. These conclusions must be communicated to physicians from all medical specialties, including pediatricians; to other health care professionals; and to the public.

New risk factors will be identified, and proposed risk factors will be evaluated by ongoing research. The criteria for a causal relation, which determine their usefulness in primary prevention, remain the same. The most likely new risk factors will be genetic polymorphisms that affect established risk factors or affect atherogenesis directly. Genetic markers of risk will be useful in identifying the high-risk individual for medical care, but will be of little value in the population-based strategy. A simple genetic marker for the individual who is highly sensitive to the lipemic effects of dietary saturated fatty acids or cholesterol would be useful.

Modifying dietary intakes and lifestyles of children older than 2 years to maintain lower serum lipid levels and healthy body weight, preventing smoking among teenagers, and maintaining a healthy lifestyle through young adulthood into middle age offer the greatest long-range potential benefits, at least regarding potential costs, and also offer health benefits other than retarding the onset of CAD. However, experimental proof of effectiveness is lacking, and rigorous proof, such as that gained from a controlled clinical trial, is not likely ever to be available until methods of noninvasive imaging of early lesions are available. As with many medical decisions, action must be taken in the absence of ultimate proof.

The long-term results of all preventive efforts depend on the assumptions that lifetime exposure to the risk factors determine the extent of advanced atherosclerotic lesions, and that reducing the duration or intensity of exposure to the risk factors will substantially delay the age at which coronary atherothrombosis reaches a level of severity sufficient to cause clinical disease. Abundant evidence from more than 50 years of research supports the validity of these conclusions.

REFERENCES

1. Windaus A. Ober den gehalt normaler und atheromatoser aorten an cholesterin und cholesterinestern. *Zeitschr Physiol Chem* 1910;67:174–176.
2. Anitschkow N, Chalatow S. On experimental cholesterin steatosis and its significance in the origin of some pathological processes. *Arteriosclerosis* 1983;3:178–182. Pelias MZ, translator.
3. de Langen CD. Cholesterine-stofwisseling en rassenpathologie. *Geneesk Tijdschr Ned Indie* 1916;56:1–34.
4. Snapper I. *Chinese lessons to Western medicine.* New York: Interscience Publishers, 1941.
5. Vartiainen I, Kanerva K. Arteriosclerosis and wartime. *Ann Med Intern Fenn* 1947;36:748–758.
6. Malmros H. The relation of nutrition to health: a statistical study of the effect of the wartime on arteriosclerosis, cardiosclerosis, tuberculosis and diabetes. *Acta Med Scand Suppl* 1950;246:137–153.

7. Steiner A, Domanski B. Dietary hypercholesterolemia. *Am J Med Sci* 1941;201:820–824.

8. Gertler MM, Garn SM, Lerman J. The interrelationships of serum cholesterol, cholesterol esters and phospholipids in health and in coronary artery disease. *Circulation* 1950;2:205–214.

9. Master AM, Dack S, Jaffe HL. Age, sex and hypertension in myocardial infarction due to coronary occlusion. *Arch Intern Med* 1939;64:767–786.

10. Dawber TR. *The Framingham Study. The epidemiology of atherosclerotic disease.* Cambridge, MA: Harvard University Press, 1980.

11. Dawber TR, Moore FE, Mann GV II. Coronary heart disease in the Framingham Study. *Am J Public Health* 1957;47[April Suppl]:4–23.

12. Dawber TR, Kannel WB, Revotskie N, et al. Some factors associated with the development of coronary heart disease. Six years' follow-up experience in the Framingham Study. *Am J Public Health* 1959;49:1349–1356.

13. Hilleboe HE, James G, Doyle JT. Cardiovascular health center. I. Project design for public health research. *Am J Public Health* 1954;44:851–863.

14. Epstein FH, Ostrander LD Jr, Johnson BC, et al. Epidemiological studies of cardiovascular disease in a total community—Tecumseh, Michigan. *Ann Intern Med* 1965;62:1170–1187.

15. Paul O, Leeper MH, Phelan WH, et al. A longitudinal study of coronary heart disease. *Circulation* 1963;28:20–31.

16. Rosenman RH, Brand RJ, Jenkins CD, et al. Coronary heart disease in the Western Collaborative Group Study. Final follow-up experience of 8 1/2 years. *JAMA* 1975;233:872–877.

17. Pooling Project Research Group. Relationship of blood pressure, serum cholesterol, smoking habit, relative weight and ECG abnormalities to incidence of major coronary events: final report of the Pooling Project. *J Chronic Dis* 1978;31:201–306.

18. Doyle JT. Risk factors in coronary heart disease. *NY State J Med* 1963;63:1317–1320.

19. Lindgren FT, Elliott HA, Gofman JW. The ultracentrifugal characterization and isolation of human blood lipids and lipoproteins, with applications to the study of atherosclerosis. *J Phys Colloid Chem* 1951;55:80–93.

20. Gofman JW, Glazier F, Tamplin A, et al. Lipoproteins, coronary heart disease, and atherosclerosis. *Physiol Rev* 1954;34:589–607.

21. Lees RS, Hatch FT, Sharper separation of lipoprotein species by paper electrophoresis in albumin-containing buffer. *J Lab Clin Med* 1963;61:518–528.

22. Rosenfeld L. Lipoprotein analysis. Early methods in the diagnosis of atherosclerosis. *Arch Pathol Lab Med* 1989;113:1101–1110.

23. Burstein M, Scholnick HR, Morfin R. Rapid method for the isolation of lipoproteins from human serum by precipitation with polyanions. *J Lipid Res* 1970;11:583–595.

24. The Technical Group of the Committee on Lipoproteins and Atherosclerosis. Evaluation of serum lipoprotein and cholesterol measurements as predictors of clinical complications of atherosclerosis. Report of a Cooperative Study of Lipoproteins and Atherosclerosis. *Circulation* 1956;14:691–733.

25. Cui Y, Blumenthal RS, Flaws JA, et al. Non-high-density lipoprotein cholesterol level as a predictor of cardiovascular disease mortality. *Arch Intern Med* 2001;161:1413–1419.

26. Miller GJ, Miller NE. Plasma-high-density-lipoprotein concentration and development of ischaemic heart-disease. *Lancet* 1975;1:16–19.

27. Sharrett AR, Ballantyne CM, Coady SA, et al. Coronary heart disease prediction from lipoprotein cholesterol levels, triglycerides, lipoprotein(a), apolipoproteins A-I and B, and HDL density subfractions: the Atherosclerosis Risk in Communities (ARIC) Study. *Circulation* 2001;104:1108–1113.

28. Berg K. A new serum type system in man—the Lp system. *Acta Pathol Microbiol Scand* 1963;59:369–382.

29. Dahlén G, Berg K, Frick MH. Lp(a) lipoprotein/pre-β_1-lipoprotein, serum lipids and atherosclerotic disease. *Clin Genet* 1976;9:558–566.

30. McLean JW, Tomlinson JE, Kuang WJ, et al. cDNA sequence of human apolipoprotein(a) is homologous to plasminogen. *Nature* 1987;330:132–137.

31. Loscalzo J. Lipoprotein(a): a unique risk factor for atherothrombotic disease. *Arteriosclerosis* 1990;10:672–679.

32. Howard GC, Pizzo SV. Biology of disease. Lipoprotein(a) and its role in atherothrombotic disease. *Lab Invest* 1993;69:373–386.

33. Luc G, Bard JM, Arveiler D, et al. Lipoprotein (a) as a predictor of coronary heart disease: the PRIME Study. *Atherosclerosis* 2002;163:377–384.

34. Seman LJ, DeLuca C, Jenner JL, et al. Lipoprotein(a)-cholesterol and coronary heart disease in the Framingham Heart Study. *Clin Chem* 1999;45:1039–1046.

35. Lundstam U, Herlitz J, Karlsson T, et al. Serum lipids, lipoprotein(a) level, and apolipoprotein(a) isoforms as prognostic markers in patients with coronary heart disease. *J Intern Med* 2002;251:111–118.

36. Henriksen T, Mahoney EM, Steinberg D. Enhanced macrophage degradation of low density lipoprotein previously incubated with cultured endothelial cells: recognition by receptors for acetylated low density lipoproteins. *Proc Natl Acad Sci USA* 1981;78:6499–6503.

37. Steinberg D, Lewis A. Conner Memorial Lecture. Oxidative modification of LDL and atherogenesis. *Circulation* 1997;95:1062–1071.

38. Steinberg D, Witztum JL. Is the oxidative modification hypothesis relevant to human atherosclerosis? Do the antioxidant trials conducted to date refute the hypothesis? *Circulation* 2002;105:2107–2111.

39. Krauss RM, Burke DJ. Identification of multiple subclasses of plasma low density lipoproteins in normal humans. *J Lipid Res* 1982;23:97–104.

40. Austin MA, Breslow JL, Hennekens CH, et al. Low-density lipoprotein subclass patterns and risk of myocardial infarction. *JAMA* 1988;260:1917–1921.

41. Gardner CD, Fortmann SP, Krauss RM. Association of small low-density lipoprotein particles with the incidence of coronary artery disease in men and women. *JAMA* 1996;276:875–881.

42. Krauss RM. Dietary and genetic effects on low-density lipoprotein heterogeneity. *Annu Rev Nutr* 2001;21:283–295.

43. Lamarche B, Lemieus I, Despres JP. The small, dense LDL phenotype and the risk of coronary heart disease: epidemiology, patho-physiology and therapeutic aspects. *Diabetes Metab* 1999;25:199–211.

44. Grundy SM. Small LDL, atherogenic dyslipidemia, and the metabolic syndrome. *Circulation* 1997;95:1–4.

45. Coresh J, Kwiterovich PO Jr. Small, dense low-density lipoprotein particles and coronary heart disease risk. A clear association with uncertain implications. *JAMA* 1996;276:914–915.

46. Albrink MJ, Man EB. Serum triglycerides in coronary artery disease. *Arch Intern Med* 1959;103:4–8.

47. NIH Consensus Development Panel on Triglyceride, High-Density Lipoprotein, and Coronary Heart Disease. *JAMA* 1993;269:505–510.

48. Hokanson JE, Austin MA. Plasma triglyceride level is a risk factor for cardiovascular disease independent of high-density lipoprotein cholesterol level: a meta-analysis of population-based prospective studies. *J Cardiovasc Risk* 1996;3:213–219.

49. Grundy SM. Hypertriglyceridemia, insulin resistance, and the metabolic syndrome. *Am J Cardiol* 1999;83[Suppl]:25F–29F.

50. MacMahon S, Petro R, Cutler J, et al. Blood pressure, stroke, and coronary heart disease. Part 1, Prolonged differences in blood pressure: prospective observational studies corrected for the regression dilution bias. *Lancet* 1990;335:765–774.

51. Miura K, Daviglus ML, Dyer AR, et al. Relationship of blood pressure to 25-year mortality due to coronary heart disease, cardiovascular diseases, and all causes in young adult men. The Chicago Heart Association Detection Project in Industry. *Arch Intern Med* 2001;161:1501–1508.

52. Lembo G, Morisco C, Lanni F, et al. Systemic hypertension and coronary artery disease: the link. *Am J Cardiol* 1998;82:2H–7H.

53. Unger T. The role of the renin-angiotensin system in the development of cardiovascular disease. *Am J Cardiol* 2002;89[Suppl]:3A–9A, discussion 10A.

54. Glasser SP. Hypertension, hypertrophy, hormones, and the heart. *Am Heart J* 1998;135[Suppl]:S16–S20.

55. Department of Health Education and Welfare, Public Health Service (U.S.). Smoking and Health: Report of the Advisory Committee to the Surgeon General of the Public Health Service. Washington: U.S. Government Printing Office, 1964; Public Health Service publication no. 1103.

56. Department of Health Education and Welfare, Public Health Service (U.S.). The Health Consequences of Smoking: A Report of the Surgeon General. Washington: U.S. Government Printing Office, 1971; DHEW publication no. (HSM)71-7513.

57. Department of Health and Human Services, Public Health Service, Office of Smoking and Health (U.S.). The health consequences of smoking: cardiovascular disease: A Report of the Surgeon General.

Rockville, MD: U.S. Department of Health and Human Services, 1983; DHHS publication no. (PHS)84-50204.

58. Centers for Disease Control and Prevention. Cigarette smoking among adults–United States 1999. *Morb Mortal Wkly Rep (MMWR)* 2001;50:869–873.

59. McGill HC Jr, Stern MP. Sex and atherosclerosis. *Atheroscler Rev* 1979;4:157–242.

60. Kannel WB, McGee DL. Diabetes and cardiovascular disease: the Framingham Study. *JAMA* 1979;241:2035–2038.

61. Coronary Drug Project Research Group. The Coronary Drug Project. Initial findings leading to modifications of its research protocol. *JAMA* 1970;214:1303–1313.

62. Barrett-Connor E, Bush TL. Estrogen and coronary heart disease in women. *JAMA* 1991;265:1861–1867.

63. Grady D, Herrington D, Bittner V, et al. Cardiovascular disease outcomes during 6.8 years of hormone therapy. Heart and Estrogen/progestin Replacement Study follow-up (HERS II). *JAMA* 2002;288:49–57.

64. Writing Group for the Women's Health Initiative Investigators. Risks and benefits of estrogen plus progestin in healthy postmenopausal women. Principal results from the Women's Health Initiative randomized controlled trial. *JAMA* 2002;288:321–333.

65. Muller C. Xanthomata, hypercholesterolemia, angina pectoris. *Acta Med Scand Suppl* 1938;89:75–84.

66. Goldstein JL, Brown MS. Familial hypercholesterolemia. A genetic regulatory defect in cholesterol metabolism. *Am J Med* 1975;58:147–150.

67. Breslow JL. Genetics of lipoprotein abnormalities associated with coronary heart disease susceptibility. *Annu Rev Genet* 2000;34:233–254.

68. Franco RF, Reitsma PH. Gene polymorphisms of the haemostatic system and the risk of arterial thrombotic disease. *Br J Haematol* 2001;115:491–506.

69. Buono C, Come EC, Witztum JL, et al. Influence of C3 deficiency on atherosclerosis. *Circulation* 2002;105:3025–3031.

70. Krauss RM. Atherogenic lipoprotein phenotype and diet-gene interactions. *J Nutr* 2001;131:340S–343S.

71. Scheuner MT. Genetic predisposition to coronary artery disease. *Curr Opin Cardiol* 2001;16:251–260.

72. Beckman JA, Creager MA, Libby P. Diabetes and atherosclerosis: epidemiology, pathophysiology, and management. *JAMA* 2002;287:2570–2581.

73. Reaven GM. Pathophysiology of insulin resistance in human disease. *Physiol Rev* 1995;75:473–486.

74. Ford ES, Giles WH, Dietz WH. Prevalence of the metabolic syndrome among US adults: findings from the third National Health and Nutrition Examination Survey. *JAMA* 2002;287:356–359.

75. Pyörälä M, Miettinen H, Halonen P, et al. Insulin resistance syndrome predicts the risk of coronary heart disease and stroke in healthy middle-aged men. The 22-year follow-up results of the Helsinki Policemen Study. *Arterioscler Thromb Vasc Biol* 2000;20:538–544.

76. Haffner SM, Stern MP, Hazuda HP, et al. Cardiovascular risk factors in confirmed prediabetic individuals. Does the clock for coronary heart disease start ticking before the onset of clinical diabetes? *JAMA* 1990;263:2893–2898.

77. Alexander JK. Obesity and coronary heart disease. *Am J Med Sci* 2001;321:215–224.

78. Hubert HB, Feinleib M, McNamara PM, et al. Obesity as an independent risk factor for cardiovascular disease: a 26-year follow-up of participants in the Framingham Heart Study. *Circulation* 1983;67:968–977.

79. Jousilahti P, Tuomilehto J, Vartiainen E, et al. Body weight, cardiovascular risk factors, and coronary mortality: 15-year follow-up of middle-aged men and women in eastern Finland. *Circulation* 1996;93:1372–1379.

80. Stern MP, Haffner SM. Body fat distribution and hyperinsulinemia as risk factors for diabetes and cardiovascular disease. *Arteriosclerosis* 1986;6:123–130.

81. Visser M, Bouter LM, McQuillan GM, et al. Elevated C-reactive protein levels in overweight and obese adults. *JAMA* 1999;282:2131–2135.

82. Abate N, Garg A, Peshock RM, et al. Relationships of generalized and regional adiposity to insulin sensitivity in men. *J Clin Invest* 1995;96:88–98.

83. Cook DG, Whincup PH, Miller G, et al. Fibrinogen and factor VII

levels are related to adiposity but not to fetal growth or social class in children aged 10-11 years. *Am J Epidemiol* 1999;150:727–736.

84. Morris JN, Heady JA, Raffle PA, et al. Coronary heart-disease and physical activity of work. *Lancet* 1953;2:1053–1057.

85. Keys A. *Seven countries: a multivariate analysis of death and coronary heart disease.* Cambridge, MA: Harvard University Press, 1980.

86. Paffenbarger RS Jr, Hale WE. Work activity and coronary heart mortality. *N Engl J Med* 1975;292:545–550.

87. Berlin JA, Colditz GA. A meta-analysis of physical activity in the prevention of coronary heart disease. *Am J Epidemiol* 1990;132:612–628.

88. Paffenbarger RS Jr, Hyde RT, Wing AL, et al. The association of changes in physical-activity level and other lifestyle characteristics with mortality among men. *N Engl J Med* 1993;328:538–545.

89. Kavanagh T. Exercise in the primary prevention of coronary artery disease. *Can J Cardiol* 2001;17:155–161.

90. McCully KS. Vascular pathology of homocystinemia: implications for the pathogenesis of arteriosclerosis. *Am J Pathol* 1969;56:111–128.

91. Boushey CJ, Beresford SA, Omenn GS, et al. A quantitative assessment of plasma homocysteine as a risk factor for vascular disease. Probable benefits of increasing folic acid intakes. *JAMA* 1995;274:1049–1057.

92. Nygård O, Vollset SE, Refsum H, et al. Total homocysteine and cardiovascular disease. *J Intern Med* 1999;246:425–454.

93. Meleady R, Graham I. Plasma homocysteine as a cardiovascular risk factor: causal, consequential, or of no consequence? *Nutr Rev* 1999;57:299–305.

94. Eikelboom JW, Lonn E, Genest J Jr, et al. Homocyst(e)ine and cardiovascular disease: a critical review of the epidemiologic evidence. *Ann Intern Med* 1999;131:363–375.

95. Ueland PM, Refsum H, Bersford SA, et al. The controversy over homocysteine and cardiovascular risk. *Am J Clin Nutr* 2000;72:324–332.

96. Christen WG, Ajani UA, Glynn RJ, et al. Blood levels of homocysteine and increased risks of cardiovascular disease: causal or casual? *Arch Intern Med* 2000;160:422–434.

97. Ford ES, Smith SJ, Stroup DF, et al. Homocyst(e)ine and cardiovascular disease: a systematic review of the evidence with special emphasis on case-control studies and nested case-control studies. *Int J Epidemiol* 2002;31:59–70.

98. Berk BC, Weintraub WS, Alexander RW. Elevation of C-reactive protein in "active" coronary artery disease. *Am J Cardiol* 1990;65:168–172.

99. Albert CM, Ma J, Rifai N, et al. Prospective study of C-reactive protein, homocysteine, and plasma lipid levels as predictors of sudden cardiac death. *Circulation* 2002;105:2595–2599.

100. Pradhan AD, Manson JE, Rossouw JE, et al. Inflammatory biomarkers, hormone replacement therapy, and incident coronary heart disease. Prospective analysis from the Women's Health Initiative observational study. *JAMA* 2002;288:980–987.

101. de Ferranti S, Rifai N. C-reactive protein and cardiovascular disease: a review of risk prediction and interventions. *Clin Chim Acta* 2002;317:1–15.

102. Kannel WB, Wolf PA, Castelli WP, et al. Fibrinogen and risk of cardiovascular disease. The Framingham Study. *JAMA* 1987;258:1183–1186.

103. Ernst E, Hammerschmidt DE, Bagge U, et al. Leukocytes and the risk of ischemic diseases. *JAMA* 1987;257:2318–2324.

104. Lindmark E, Diderholm E, Wallentin L, et al. Relationship between interleukin 6 and mortality in patients with unstable coronary artery disease. Effects of an early invasive or noninvasive strategy. *JAMA* 2001;286:2107–2113.

105. Ridker PM. On evolutionary biology, inflammation, infection, and the causes of atherosclerosis. *Circulation* 2002;105:2–4.

106. Mattila KJ, Nieminen MS, Valtonen VV, et al. Association between dental health and acute myocardial infarction. *Br Med J* 1989;298:779–781.

107. DeStefano F, Anda RF, Kahn HS, et al. Dental disease and risk of coronary heart disease and mortality. *Br Med J* 1993;306:688–691.

108. Hujoel PP, Drangsholt M, Spiekerman C, et al. Periodontal disease and coronary heart disease risk. *JAMA* 2000;284:1406–1410.

109. Beck JD, Offenbacher S, William R, et al. Periodontitis: a risk factor for coronary heart disease? *Ann Periodontol* 1998;3:127–141.

110. Danesh J. Coronary heart disease, *Helicobacter pylori*, dental disease, *Chlamydia pneumoniae*, and cytomegalovirus: meta-analyses of prospective studies. *Am Heart J* 1999;138:S434–S437.

111. Jenkins CD. Recent evidence supporting psychologic and social risk factors for coronary heart disease. *N Engl J Med* 1976;294:987–994, 1033–1038.

112. Ford DE, Mead LA, Chang PP, et al. Depression is a risk factor for coronary artery disease in men. The Precursors Study. *Arch Intern Med* 1998;158:1422–1426.

113. Kawachi I, Sparrow D, Kubzansky LD, et al. Prospective study of a self-report type A scale and risk of coronary heart disease. Test of the MMPI-2 type A scale. *Circulation* 1998;98:405–412.

114. Gullette EC, Blumenthal JA, Babyak M, et al. Effects of mental stress on myocardial ischemia during daily life. *JAMA* 1997;277:1521–1526.

115. O'Malley PG, Jones DL, Feuerstein IM, et al. Lack of correlation between psychological factors and subclinical coronary artery disease. *N Engl J Med* 2000;343:1298–1304.

116. Krantz DS, McCeney MK. Effects of psychological and social factors on organic disease: a critical assessment of research on coronary heart disease. *Annu Rev Psychol* 2002;53:341–369.

117. Greenland P, Abrams J, Aurigemma GP, et al. Prevention Conference V: beyond secondary prevention: identifying the high-risk patient for primary prevention: noninvasive tests of atherosclerotic burden: Writing Group III. *Circulation* 2000;101:e16–e22.

118. Fayad ZA, Fuster V. Clinical imaging of the high-risk or vulnerable atherosclerotic plaque. *Circ Res* 2001;89:305–316.

119. Tobis JM, Mallery J, Mahon D, et al. Intravascular ultrasound imaging of human coronary arteries *in vivo*. Analysis of tissue characterizations with comparison to *in vitro* histological specimens. *Circulation* 1991;83:913–926.

120. Nallamothu BK, Saint S, Bielak LF, et al. Electron-beam computed tomography in the diagnosis of coronary artery disease. A meta-analysis. *Arch Intern Med* 2001;161:833–838.

121. Choudhury RP, Fuster V, Badimon JJ, et al. MRI and characterization of atherosclerotic plaque. Emerging applications and molecular imaging. *Arterioscler Thromb Vasc Biol* 2002;22:1065–1074.

122. Järvisalo MJ, Jartti L, Näntö-Salonen K, et al. Increased aortic intima-media thickness. A marker of preclinical atherosclerosis in high-risk children. *Circulation* 2001;104:2943–2947.

123. McGill HC Jr, Geer JC, Strong JP. Natural history of human atherosclerotic lesions. In: Sandler M, Bourne GH, eds. *Atherosclerosis and its origin*. New York: Academic Press, 1963:39–65.

124. Tejada C, Strong JP, Montenegro MR, et al. Distribution of coronary and aortic atherosclerosis by geographic location, race, and sex. *Lab Invest* 1968;18:509–526.

125. Solberg LA, Strong JP. Risk factors and atherosclerotic lesions. A review of autopsy studies. *Arteriosclerosis* 1983;3:187–198.

126. Frerichs RR, Srinivasan SR, Webber LS, et al. Serum cholesterol and triglyceride levels in 3,446 children from a biracial community. The Bogalusa Heart Study. *Circulation* 1976;54:302–309.

127. Lauer RM, Conner WE, Leaverton PE, et al. Coronary heart disease risk factors in school children: the Muscatine study. *J Pediatr* 1975;86:697–706.

128. McGill HC Jr, McMahan CA, Herderick EE, et al. Origin of atherosclerosis in childhood and adolescence. *Am J Clin Nutr* 2000;72[Suppl]:1307S–1315S.

129. Havlik RJ, Feinlieb M, eds. Proceedings of the Conference on the Decline in Coronary Heart Disease Mortality. Bethesda, MD: National Institutes of Health, 1979; NIH publication no. 79-1610.

130. ARIC Study Investigators. The decline of ischaemic heart disease mortality in the ARIC Study communities. *Int J Epidemiol* 1989;18[Suppl 1]:S88–S98.

131. Hunink MG, Goldman L, Tosteson AN, et al. The recent decline in mortality from coronary heart disease, 1980-1990. The effect of secular trends in risk factors and treatment. *JAMA* 1997;277:535–542.

132. McGovern PG, Pankow JS, Shahar E, et al. Recent trends in acute coronary heart disease. Mortality, morbidity, medical care, and risk factors. *N Engl J Med* 1996;334:884–890.

133. Capewell S, Morrison CE, McMurray JJ. Contribution of modern cardiovascular treatment and risk factor changes to the decline in coronary heart disease mortality in Scotland between 1975 and 1994. *Heart* 1999;81:380–386.

134. Page IH, Stare FJ, Corcoran AC, et al. Atherosclerosis and the fat content of the diet. *Circulation* 1957;16:163–178.

135. National Diet-Heart Study Research Group. The National Diet-Heart Study Final Report. *Circulation* 1968;37[Suppl 1]:I-428–I-428.

136. Dayton S, Pearce ML. Prevention of coronary heart disease and other complications of atherosclerosis by modified diet. *Am J Med* 1969;46:751–762.

137. Hu FB, Manson JE, Willett WC. Types of dietary fat and risk of coronary heart disease: a critical review. *J Am Coll Nutr* 2001;20:5–19.

138. Schaefer EJ. Lipoproteins, nutrition, and heart disease. *Am J Clin Nutr* 2002;75:191–212.

139. Kromhout D, Menotti A, Kesteloot H, et al. Prevention of coronary heart disease by diet and lifestyle. Evidence from prospective cross-cultural, cohort, and intervention studies. *Circulation* 2002;105:893–898.

140. Lipid Research Clinics Program. The Lipid Research Clinics Coronary Primary Prevention Trial Results. I. Reduction in incidence of coronary heart disease. *JAMA* 1984;251:351–364.

141. Geizerova H, Gyarfas I, Green KG, et al. Committee of Principal Investigators. A co-operative trial in the primary prevention of ischaemic heart disease using clofibrate. Report from the Committee of Principal Investigators. *Br Heart J* 1978;40:1069–1118.

142. Frick MH, Elo O, Haapa K, et al. Helsinki Heart Study: primary-prevention trial with gemfibrozil in middle-aged men with dyslipidemia. Safety of treatment, changes in risk factors, and incidence of coronary heart disease. *N Engl J Med* 1987;317:1237–1245.

143. Scandinavian Simvastatin Survival Study Group. Randomised trial of cholesterol lowering in 4,444 patients with coronary heart disease: the Scandinavian Simvastatin Survival Study (4S). *Lancet* 1994;344:1383–1389.

144. West of Scotland Coronary Prevention Group. West of Scotland Coronary Prevention Study: identification of high-risk groups and comparison with other cardiovascular intervention trials. *Lancet* 1996;348:1339–1342.

145. Downs JR, Clearfield M, Weis S, et al. Primary prevention of acute coronary events with lovastatin in men and women with average cholesterol levels. Results of AFCAPS/TexCAPS. *JAMA* 1998;279:1615–1622.

146. The Multiple Risk Factor Intervention Trial Research Group. Mortality after 16 years for participants randomized to the multiple risk factor intervention trial. *Circulation* 1996;94:946–951.

147. Rose G. Strategy of prevention: lessons from cardiovascular disease. *Br Med J* 1981;282:1847–1851.

Lipid Abnormalities

CHAPTER 4

Nutrition, Lipid Disorders, and the Metabolic Syndrome

Scott M. Grundy

Key Words: Cardiovascular disease; lipids; metabolic syndrome; metabolism; nutrition.

Nutrition is the cornerstone of the prevention of coronary heart disease (CHD). This claim primarily is based on a large body of epidemiologic data indicating that the incidence of CHD in various countries correlates closely with the type of diet consumed in these countries (1–4). Although factors other than nutrition undoubtedly affect rates of CHD, a mass of epidemiologic evidence leaves little doubt that nutrition contributes importantly to coronary atherothrombosis and CHD. Several different dietary factors appear to modify atherogenesis. The mechanisms whereby these various factors impart their effects also are becoming better understood. Although nutrition may influence atherogenesis and risk for CHD in ways yet to be discovered, the diet clearly affects several of the known risk factors. This chapter focuses mainly on two major areas of the diet–heart relation—namely, the primacy of increased low density lipoprotein (LDL) and the growing importance of the metabolic syndrome.

S. M. Grundy: The Center for Human Nutrition, Departments of Internal Medicine and Clinical Nutrition, The University of Texas Southwestern Medical Center at Dallas, Dallas, Texas 75390-9052.

INCREASED LOW-DENSITY LIPOPROTEIN CHOLESTEROL LEVELS: PRIMARY TARGET OF DIETARY INTERVENTION

A positive relation exists between serum total cholesterol levels and risk for atherosclerotic CHD (5,6). That a high serum cholesterol level can induce atherothrombosis was demonstrated first when a group of rabbits were fed cholesterol as part of their diet (7). Many studies in experimental animals, including primates, subsequently showed that diet-induced hypercholesterolemia produces arterial lesions resembling human atherothrombosis (8–10). Moreover, a human condition first called familial xanthomatosis was early to be characterized by very high levels of serum cholesterol and premature coronary atherothrombosis. A number of epidemiologic surveys, including those carried out between populations (11), within countries (4,6), and in migrating populations (12), further revealed a positive association between serum total cholesterol and rates of atherosclerotic CHD. In more recent years, several controlled clinical trials have conclusively documented that decreasing serum cholesterol levels will retard risk for CHD and the progression of atherothrombosis (13–19). The sum of accumulated data thus proves that increased serum total cholesterol is a major risk factor for CHD. Although serum *total* cholesterol correlates with risk, serum cholesterol is not homogeneous. Because cholesterol is completely insoluble in aqueous solutions, special mechanisms are needed to keep it in solution. This is accomplished by combining it as a complex with other lipids and proteins. These complexes are called lipoproteins. The categories of lipoproteins are distinguished by their densities. They include LDLs, high-density lipoproteins (HDLs), very low-density lipoproteins (VLDLs), and intermediate-density lipoproteins (IDLs). In healthy individuals, about two-thirds of serum total cholesterol is carried in LDL. This lipoprotein contains mostly cholesterol ester in its lipid core; it has unesterified cholesterol, phospholipids, and protein in its surface coat. The only protein present in LDL is apolipoprotein B-100 (apo B-100). Among the lipoproteins, increased LDL contributes most importantly to CHD in several ways. Genetic forms of high LDL cholesterol predispose to premature CHD (20–24). In epidemiologic studies, LDL has emerged as the major atherogenic lipoprotein. Investigations in experimental animals and *in vitro* systems reveal mechanisms whereby excess LDL promotes atherogenesis. Finally, clinical trials in which LDL levels were therapeutically decreased document a reduction in risk for CHD (13–19). Thus, LDL cholesterol is the major serum cholesterol fraction linked to coronary atherothrombosis. Consequently, the National Cholesterol Education Program (NCEP) (25) has identified LDL cholesterol as the primary target of cholesterol-lowering therapy.

Definitions of Serum Cholesterol Levels

Three categories of serum total cholesterol are defined by the NCEP (25): desirable (<200 mg/dL), borderline high (200–239 mg/dL), and high (>240 mg/dL). For clinical purposes a more refined definition of LDL cholesterol is provided as follows:

- Optimal   <100 mg/dL
- Near optimal   100–129 mg/dL
- Borderline high   130–159 mg/dL
- High   160–189 mg/dL
- Very high   <190 mg/dL

Relation of Low-Density Lipoprotein Cholesterol Levels to Coronary Heart Disease Risk

Epidemiologic studies (1,25) suggest that for every 1% increase in total cholesterol the risk for CHD increases by 2%. This relation has been called the 1%/2% rule. Clinical trials support this relation. In clinical trials of 5 years in duration, a 1% reduction in LDL cholesterol results in a 1% reduction in risk (13–19). It seems likely, however, that over the long term, a 1% reduction in LDL cholesterol will produce a greater risk reduction (e.g., 1.5–2% decrease) (26).

Causes of Increased Serum Low-Density Lipoprotein Cholesterol Levels

Approximately 45% of adults in the United States have LDL-cholesterol levels of 130 mg/dL or greater (25). These greater than desirable levels contribute significantly to the high rates of CHD in the United States. All humans do not have such high LDL levels. For example, a 20-year-old man who is not obese and who consumes a diet low in saturated fatty acids and cholesterol should have an LDL-cholesterol level in the range of 75 to 90 mg/dL (27,28). This level is well below 130 mg/dL, and little clinical CHD develops in those populations that maintain optimal LDL-cholesterol levels (<100 mg/dL) into middle age.

Pathologic and epidemiologic surveys indicate when LDL-cholesterol levels increase to the range of 100 to 129 mg/dL, atherogenesis begins to accelerate. Rates of atherogenesis seemingly are proportional to cholesterol levels over a broad range, from high to low (29). Populations that have the greatest rates of CHD generally have, on average, LDL-cholesterol levels greater than 130 mg/dL. Therefore, the mechanisms for the increase of LDL cholesterol into this range must be of great importance for the pathogenesis of atherothrombosis and CHD. Although genetic factors may help to increase concentrations into this range, other factors common in the general population appear to be mainly responsible. These include diet, obesity, aging, and in postmenopausal women, loss of estrogen. For example, excess cholesterol in the U.S. diet, which is about 200 mg/day greater than optimal, increases the LDL cholesterol level by about 5 mg/dL (30). Moreover, the excess cholesterol-increasing fatty acids (mostly saturated fatty acids), which exceed optimal intakes by approximately 7% of total calories (25), increase LDL cholesterol by another 15 mg/dL (31). The precise contribution of the increase of body weight with age is not known, but probably accounts for another 10- to 20-mg/dL increment in middle-aged adults in the United States compared with 20-year-old individuals (32). A further increase associated with aging appears to be caused by metabolic aging (32). This adds another 15 to 20 mg/dL. Finally, loss of estrogen in women after menopause frequently yields another increment of about 20 mg/dL (25). Because of these factors, middle-aged adults in the United States typically have LDL-cholesterol levels that are 50 to 70 mg/dL above optimal levels.

The probable mechanisms whereby these factors increase cholesterol concentrations are becoming better understood. Most mechanisms apparently are related to expression of LDL receptors. Humans, compared with other species, seemingly have a low activity of LDL receptors, accounting for relatively high baseline levels compared with other species. In addition, excess dietary cholesterol (33–35) and saturated fatty acids (36–38), aging (39–41), and loss of estrogen (in postmenopausal women) (42,43) all seemingly decrease the activity of LDL receptors. Obesity, in contrast, enhances the secretion of VLDL-apo B (44,45), leading to increased formation of LDL (46).

Borderline high LDL cholesterol levels (130–159 mg/dL) are largely because of the previously mentioned factors. Approximately 25% of middle-aged and older adults in the United States have still greater LDL-cholesterol concentrations (≥160 mg/dL). Presumably, these greater concentrations result from the addition of genetic aberrations. Two genetic factors have been mainly implicated: (a) a further reduction in LDL-receptor activity (20,47), and (b) a greater hepatic secretion of apo B-containing lipoproteins beyond that induced by obesity. Two other mechanisms also deserve consideration: (c) a decreased clearance of LDL because of the presence of LDL particles that are poor ligands for LDL receptors (21,22), and (d) an enhanced conversion of VLDL to LDL, leading to an overproduction of LDL particles (47). Mechanisms related to decreased clearance of LDL (i.e., reduced activity of LDL receptors and LDL particles having low affinity for receptors) have been identified with certainty, whereas those responsible for an overproduction of LDL (i.e., increased hepatic secretion of lipoproteins and increased conversion of VLDL to LDL) are less well-documented. Identified genetic causes of reduced LDL clearance involve defects in the gene encoding for LDL receptors (familial hypercholesterolemia) (19) and abnormalities in the apo B molecule imparting poor binding of LDL to receptors (familial defective apo B) (21,22). Specific genetic defects leading to overproduction of LDL have not been identified, but indirect evidence for their existence comes from isotope kinetic studies (48–50).

An important question is whether some people are genetically hyperresponsive to the LDL-increasing effects of diet and obesity. Limited data indicate that some people respond to dietary cholesterol and saturated fatty acids with a greater increase in LDL levels than do others (51). Furthermore, we reported that patients with hypercholesterolemia with a relatively low clearance capacity for LDL tend to be hyperresponsive to saturated fatty acids (52). Although these studies suggest genetic variability in responsiveness, the molecular basis for this variability has not been elucidated.

Role of Diet Composition and Specific Nutrients

As a group, saturated fatty acids undoubtedly increase LDL-cholesterol levels (53); the issue of what is their best replacement in the diet, however, is the subject of ongoing interest but also uncertainty. Because the protein content of the diet must be kept relatively constant, possible replacements include carbohydrates or other types of fats, or both. The issue is broader than just replacement of saturated fatty acids because of the possibility that other nutrients have health benefits or detrimental effects within themselves. For this reason, overall composition of the diet must be taken into consideration.

Dietary Fat

Dietary fat consists largely of triglycerides that are made up of three molecules of fatty acid esterified to glycerol. Different types of dietary fat contain different patterns of fatty acids. These include saturated, monounsaturated, and polyunsaturated fatty acids. Each type contains two or more subtypes (Table 4–1), and each fatty acid seemingly has characteristic effects on lipid and lipoprotein metabolism, and perhaps other unique metabolic actions as well; each fatty acid, therefore, deserves to be considered separately.

Palmitic Acid

The major saturated fatty acid in the U.S. diet is palmitic acid (16:0); it makes up about 60% of total saturated acids. Palmitic acid is abundant in most meats and dairy fats, but it also occurs in large amounts in some plant oils (e.g., palm oil and coconut oil). Many reports indicate that dietary palmitic acid increases the serum total cholesterol level; this effect is observed when palmitic acid replaces unsaturated fatty acids and carbohydrates in the diet. The hypercholesterolemic action of palmitic acid has been documented best in metabolic ward studies (54–57). Increments in total cholesterol occur almost entirely in LDL, with little change in HDL or VLDL. Palmitic acid seemingly suppresses the expression of LDL receptors (36–38).

Some researchers have questioned whether palmitic acid truly increases the serum LDL cholesterol. In fact, in several animal species, including some primates, high intakes of palmitic acid have only a small cholesterol-increasing action, seemingly less than reported for humans. Moreover, when experimental designs for human studies have not been rigorous, cholesterol-increasing by palmitic acid can appear to be small. Conversely, more definitive human studies (56,57) clearly show that this fatty acid increases LDL-

TABLE 4–1. *Dietary fatty acids*

Saturated fatty acids
  Stearic acid (18:0)
  Palmitic acid (16:0)
  Myristic acid (14:0)
  Lauric acid (12:0)
  Medium-chain fatty acids (8:0 and 10:0)
Monounsaturated fatty acids
  Oleic acid (16:cis 1)
  Trans fatty acids (16:trans 1)
Polyunsaturated fatty acids
  N-6 fatty acids
    Linoleic acid (18:2)
  N-3 fatty acids
    Linolenic acid (18:3)
    Eicosapentanoic acid (EPA) (20:5)
    Docosahexanoic acid (DHA) (22:6)

The first number in parentheses indicates the number of carbon atoms; the second number denotes the number of double bonds per molecule.

cholesterol levels compared with unsaturated fatty acids (or carbohydrate). Indeed, palmitic acid is the predominant saturated fatty acid in the U.S. diet; therefore, it is the major cholesterol-increasing fatty acid in the diet.

Myristic Acid

Myristic acid has 14 carbons and no double bonds (14:0). It occurs in appreciable amounts in butter fat and in certain tropical oils (coconut oil and palm kernel oil). Myristic acid increases cholesterol levels at least as much as palmitic acid (54) and perhaps even more (55). Still, it is less influential than palmitic acid because it is ingested in much smaller amounts.

Lauric Acid

Lauric acid has 12 carbons and no double bonds (12:0). Longer chain fatty acids (e.g., myristic and palmitic acids) are absorbed chylomicron triglycerides. Lauric acid, however, is absorbed partly with chylomicron triglycerides and partly into the portal circulation as a free fatty acid. Until recently it was uncertain whether dietary lauric acid increases serum cholesterol levels (58,59). Previous studies (54,55) on different fatty acids failed to provide a solid answer. If lauric acid does not increase cholesterol levels, it could be useful as a substitute for the cholesterol-increasing saturated fatty acids. To resolve this uncertainty, we tested for its effects on cholesterol levels (60). Lauric acid was incorporated into a synthetic triglyceride. Essentially the only fatty acids present in this test fat were lauric and oleic acid. They were present in equal proportions. This lauric acid–enriched fat was compared with palm oil; the latter essentially differed only by having palmitic rather than lauric acid. These two fats also were compared with high-oleic safflower oil, which consists almost entirely of oleic acid. As expected, palm oil strikingly increased LDL-cholesterol levels compared with the safflower oil. The lauric acid–enriched oil also increased LDL-cholesterol levels compared with safflower oil, but only about two-thirds as much as did palm oil. Nonetheless, lauric acid *did* raise the LDL-cholesterol level relative to oleic acid; consequently, lauric acid definitely must be considered a cholesterol-increasing fatty acid; consequently, it would not be an acceptable substitute for palmitic acid in the diet.

Medium-Chain Fatty Acids

Until recently, the actions of medium-chain fatty acids (8:0 and 10:0) on serum cholesterol levels were uncertain. Workers in early studies (61) argued that these fatty acids are hypercholesterolemic because butter fat, which is rich in medium-chain fatty acids, is especially hypercholesterolemic compared with other hard fats. Nonetheless, as already mentioned, at least two studies (58,59) failed to demonstrate a cholesterol-increasing

effect of medium-chain acids. Nonetheless, a detailed metabolic study from our laboratory observed that medium-chain fatty acids do in fact increase LDL-cholesterol levels (62).

Stearic Acid

Early research in humans by Ahrens and coworkers (61), Keys and coworkers (54), and Hegsted and coworkers (55) suggest that stearic acid, contrary to other saturated fatty acids, does not increase serum cholesterol levels. This suggestion was confirmed more recently by our laboratory (57,63). Stearic acid also does not increase LDL-cholesterol levels (57,63). Although one study (64) reports a mild LDL-increasing action, compared with linoleic acid, most data indicate that stearic acid has a "neutral" effect on LDL-cholesterol levels (54,55,57,63). In this regard, stearic acid is similar to oleic acid, the effects of which are discussed later.

The reason stearic acid does not increase LDL levels, whereas other long-chain saturates do, is not completely understood. Contrary to early evidence in laboratory animals, more than 90% of stearic acid in the human diet is absorbed (57). Investigations in both laboratory animals (65, 66) and in humans (57) have noted that much of stearic acid is rapidly transformed into oleic acid. Seemingly, stearic acid does not remain long in the body as a saturated fatty acid, and this could account for its failure to increase LDL levels.

Monounsaturated Fatty Acids

Two types of monounsaturated fatty acids occur in the diet. The major kind is omega-9, *cis* 18:1 (oleic acid). It is present in both animal and vegetable products. In fact, oleic acid is the predominant fatty acid in the U.S. diet. A lesser group of monounsaturates consist of the *trans* 18:1 fatty acids. They are produced by hydrogenation of polyunsaturated oils. The most common acid is elaidic acid (omega-9, *trans* 18:1), but other *trans* isomers are formed during hydrogenation. The actions of these two types of monounsaturates on serum cholesterol levels can be reviewed separately.

Dietary *oleic acid* is considered to be "neutral," neither increasing nor decreasing serum cholesterol levels. As indicated earlier, most saturated fatty acids increase the serum cholesterol relative to oleic acid (54–56). This neutrality extends to all lipoproteins—VLDL, LDL, and HDL. Why oleic acid does not increase serum LDL-cholesterol levels is not fully understood. One reason may be that oleic acid is the favored substrate for acyl cholesterol acyl transferase in the liver (67). A large amount of oleic acid in the liver may promote the esterification of cholesterol by acyl cholesterol acyl transferase; this should decrease unesterified cholesterol in the liver cell, and, if so, the suppressive action of unesterified cholesterol on LDL-receptor transcription could be withdrawn (34). Alternative LDL-decreasing mechanisms for oleic acid have been envisioned. For example, enrichment of cell membranes with oleic acid might promote receptor-mediated uptake of LDL (68). Moreover, the secretion of lipoproteins by the liver could be reduced, although there is not strong evidence to support this mechanism.

Trans Monounsaturated Fatty Acids

Trans monounsaturated fatty acids recently have received considerable attention. For many years there was uncertainty about their effects on cholesterol levels in humans. Until recently, *trans* monounsaturates were assumed to be "neutral," similar to the *cis* counterpart, oleic acid. Recent evidence, however, argues the opposite view (69): *trans* fatty acids actually increase LDL levels relative to oleic acid. This increase in LDL may be somewhat less than that induced by palmitic acid (69). Nonetheless, the *cis* and *trans* forms of monounsaturated fatty acids must be considered separately for their effects on LDL levels.

The reasons *trans* fatty acids increase LDL levels, compared with oleic acid, are not clear. Clearly their *cis* and *trans* configurations are different. Oleic acid molecules do not pack tightly together, which explains why high-oleic oils, like olive oil, are liquids at room temperature. *Trans* monounsaturated fatty acid molecules, in contrast, fit together compactly and impart solidity to their oils. In terms of physical properties, *trans* monounsaturates behave similarly to saturated fatty acids; this similarity might explain why *trans* fatty acids have an LDL-increasing property like saturated acids—that is, they might have a similar effect on cholesterol distribution in the liver.

Polyunsaturated Fatty Acids

Polyunsaturated fatty acids are of two types: omega-6 and omega-3 acids. The major omega-6 fatty acid is linoleic acid (ω-6, 18:2). The predominant omega-3 fatty acid found in plants is linolenic acid (ω-3, 18:3); but longer chain, omega-3 fatty acids, notably eicosapentaenoic acid (EPA; ω-3, 20:5) and docosahexanoic acid (DHA; ω-3, 22:6) occur in fish oils. EPA and DHA comprise about 26% of the total fatty acids of fish oils.

For many years *linoleic acid* was the preferred dietary fatty acid because it was thought to be the best acid for decreasing serum cholesterol. Several early studies (54,55) reported that linoleic acid reduces total cholesterol levels compared with oleic acid. This observation contributed to recommendations for increased use of polyunsaturated vegetable oils in U.S. and European diets. Indeed, during the last 40 years, linoleic acid intakes have increased from about 4% to about 7% of total calories in the U.S. diet. Paradoxically, at the same time, there was a growing reservation about the safety of increased consumption of this fatty acid. First, there was concern on epidemiologic grounds: No large population has ever consumed high amounts of linoleic acid

with proven long-term safety. Moreover, in laboratory animals, diets high in linoleic acid can promote chemical carcinogenesis (70,71) and suppress the immune system (72). In humans, large amounts of linoleic acid in the diet can decrease HDL-cholesterol levels (73–75), and possibly predispose to cholesterol gallstones (76,77). Finally, enrichment of LDL lipids with linoleic acid makes them more likely to be oxidized (78,79); this action might promote atherogenesis. These possible side effects of high intakes of linoleic acid have led to a general recommendation that linoleic acid intake probably should be limited to no more than 7% of total calories.

Moreover, reports in human studies (56,80,81) note that linoleic acid provides little additional decreases in cholesterol compared with oleic acid. In particular, LDL cholesterol appears to be reduced similarly (56,80–82). The total cholesterol lowering of linoleic acid occurs mostly in VLDL and HDL fractions (73–75). Thus, because of possible long-term adverse effects of high intakes of linoleic acid, there is little reason to advocate greater intakes than the current standards.

The other category of polyunsaturated fatty acids—omega-3—also has generated considerable interest. The major focus of this interest has been on EPA and DHA. These fatty acids, found in fish oils, have been claimed to improve the lipoprotein profile, to reduce the danger of thrombosis, and to slow down atherogenesis. The major action of omega-3 fatty acids on plasma lipids is to decrease serum triglyceride levels (83,84). Otherwise, however, EPA and DHA appear to have little beneficial effect on lipoprotein metabolism. In fact, in patients with high triglycerides, when triglycerides are reduced by omega-3 fatty acids, LDL-cholesterol concentrations often increase (84). Also, in the absence of high triglycerides, these fatty acids do not uniquely reduce LDL-cholesterol. When they are exchanged for saturated fatty acids, LDL-cholesterol levels decline, but this effect is no different from that found with other types of unsaturated fatty acids.

Carbohydrates

Although much attention has been paid to dietary cholesterol and fats, the role of carbohydrates must not be overlooked. Carbohydrates are the major source of dietary calories, even in populations consuming high-fat diets. Carbohydrates provide 45% to 60% of the total calories in the diet. Moreover, they occur in several forms. These include simple sugars (monoglycerides and diglycerides), complex digestible carbohydrates (starches), and nondigestible carbohydrate (fiber). Fiber is present in soluble and insoluble forms; being undigestible, fiber does not contribute to total caloric intake. Generally, the complex digestible carbohydrates have been lumped together as a single group. However, it may be useful for practical purposes to divide the sources of complex carbohydrates into (a) starchy foods and (b) fruits and vegetables.

The starchy foods consist of refined starches (breads and pasta) or foods of concentrated carbohydrate content (rice, potatoes, and legumes). Starchy foods contrast to fruits and vegetables in that the latter contain a significant amount of other nutrients other than their complex-carbohydrate content.

As a class, digestible carbohydrates class appear to affect total cholesterol and LDL-cholesterol levels similarly to the effects of oleic acid (54,55,85–88). They neither increase nor decrease the levels; hence, they also are called "neutral." Furthermore, no strong evidence indicates that different types of digestible carbohydrates (simple sugars or complex carbohydrates) affect LDL-cholesterol levels differently from one another. This is not to say that carbohydrates and oleic acid have identical effects on LDL metabolism. Carbohydrates tend to increase serum triglyceride concentrations (86,89), an effect that may reduce LDL particle size and decrease LDL-cholesterol/apo B ratios. For example, Kuusi and coworkers (90) report that high-carbohydrate (low-fat) diets reduce LDL-cholesterol levels more than they decrease LDL-apo B levels, when compared with a diet high in saturated fats. In contrast, a previous study (56) showed that replacement of saturated fatty acids with oleic acid decreases levels of LDL cholesterol without reducing LDL-cholesterol/apo B ratios—that is, LDL-apo B and LDL-cholesterol levels are decreased equally. An important question is whether high-carbohydrate diets produce any decrease of apo B levels relative to saturated fatty acids. Abbott and coworkers (91) report that carbohydrates, compared with saturated fatty acids, modestly reduce LDL-apo B concentrations, but two other reports (92,93) indicate that replacement of saturated fatty acids with carbohydrate produces no reduction in apo B levels despite decreasing LDL-cholesterol concentrations. These latter findings raise questions about the use of carbohydrates as a substitute for saturated fatty acids for decreasing LDL.

Another unresolved issue has to do with the influence of undigestible fiber on cholesterol levels. Several reports suggest that dietary fiber actively decreases serum cholesterol levels (94–98). This action appears to be greater for soluble fiber than for the insoluble form. A review (98) of all available data indicates that increasing intakes of soluble fiber has the potential to decrease total cholesterol levels by about 3% to 5%, or perhaps somewhat less.

Table 4–2 summarizes the influence of the specific nutrients discussed earlier on serum levels of lipids and lipoproteins. It can be seen that each nutrient has a different action, and the net effect of the diet depends on the total amount of each nutrient consumed. Available evidence indicates that each nutrient is relatively independent of the others in this effect.

Obesity and Low-Density Lipoprotein Cholesterol

More attention generally has been given to the composition of the diet than to intake of total calories for their effects on serum cholesterol. A few early reports claimed that obesity per se has little or no effect on cholesterol levels. Most epidemiologic studies, however, have found a positive correlation between body weight and cholesterol levels (99–103). Denke and coworkers (32) examined the link between body weight, expressed as body mass index, and serum cholesterol in both men and women. These results were derived from the large database of the Second National Health and Nutrition Examination Survey (NHANES II). Serum cholesterol levels correlated positively with body mass index for both sexes. The link, however, was more pronounced in younger adults than in older ones. A greater increment in cholesterol levels moreover occurred as body weight increased from lean weight to mild obesity than from the latter to marked obesity.

TABLE 4–2. *Summary of influence of specific nutrients on serum lipid and lipoprotein levels*

Specific nutrient	Total cholesterol	Triglycerides	LDL	HDL
Dietary cholesterol	↑↑	—	↑↑	↑
Saturated fatty acids				
Palmitic acid	↑↑↑	—	↑↑↑	↑
Myristic acid	↑↑↑↑	—	↑↑↑↑	—
Lauric acid	↑↑	—	↑↑	—
Medium-chain fatty acids	↑	↑	↑	↑
Stearic acid	—	—	—	—
Monounsaturated fatty acids				
Oleic acid	—	—	—	—
Trans fatty acids	↑↑	—	↑↑	↑
Polyunsaturated fatty acids				
N-6 (linolenic acid)	↓	↓	↓	↓
N-3 (EPA, DHA)	↓	↓↓↓	—	—
Carbohydrates	—	↑↑	—	↓↓

↑, increase (number = relative increase); ↓, decrease; —, no change; DHA, docosahexanoic acid; EPA, eicosapentanoic acid; HDL, high-density lipoprotein; LDL, low-density lipoprotein.

Only a few investigations have addressed whether weight gain *per se* will increase cholesterol levels. For example, Anderson, Lawler, and Keys (104) report that for young adult men the total cholesterol increases approximately 4 mg/dL for every kilogram of weight gain. This change is consistent with the population data reported by Denke and coworkers (32); both studies suggest that cholesterol concentrations in young adult men are particularly sensitive to weight gain. Although no metabolic ward studies are available in older adults, population evidence suggests a less pronounced effect of weight gain in older age groups (32).

The primary mechanism whereby obesity increases cholesterol levels seemingly is an enhancement of hepatic secretion of lipoproteins. Isotope kinetic studies indicate that the obese state promotes secretion of VLDL (44,45); this, in turn, provides more VLDL for conversion to LDL (46). In many obese people, this effect increases total cholesterol and LDL-cholesterol levels (32). The extent to which the LDL-cholesterol level increases in response to obesity depends on the individual's ability to clear LDL from the circulation. If the LDL-receptor activity is high, LDL particles should be removed efficiently; therefore, LDL-cholesterol levels should not increase to abnormally high levels. Conversely, if LDL-receptor activity is relatively suppressed, onset of obesity seemingly can produce a substantial increase in LDL levels.

Clinical experience suggests that individuals vary in their LDL-cholesterol response to changes in body weight. Some people are highly sensitive to slight increases in weight, and small weight gains induce a substantial increase in LDL levels. Others appear to be more resistant and manifest little if any increase in cholesterol concentrations with weight gain. This difference in responsiveness could have a genetic basis. Two mechanisms can be visualized. First, development of obesity could stimulate the secretion of apo B-containing lipoproteins more in some people than in others. Alternatively, there almost certainly is variability in different individual's inherent LDL-receptor activity; those having a relatively low activity should demonstrate a greater hypercholesterolemic response to the development of obesity than would those with a greater baseline activity. The response in LDL levels to weight reduction may vary in a reverse way.

Although LDL responsiveness to weight reduction may be influenced by genetic factors, it also depends on diet composition. For example, both in the Multiple Risk Factor Intervention Trials (105) and in the National Diet-Heart Study (106) serum cholesterol decreases induced by removing saturated fatty acids from the diet were doubled when patients simultaneously lost weight. In a metabolic ward study, Wolf and Grundy (107) found that weight reduction in obese, normolipidemic patients often did not decrease LDL-cholesterol levels when there was no change in diet composition—that is, no reduction in intake of saturated fatty acids. Thus, to achieve the maximal benefit for LDL decreasing from weight reduction, a simultaneous decrease in intake of saturated fatty acids and cholesterol appears to be necessary.

NUTRITION, NON–LOW-DENSITY LIPOPROTEIN LIPID DISORDERS, AND THE METABOLIC SYNDROME

Definition of Metabolic Syndrome

According to NCEP Adult Treatment Panel III (ATP III) (25), the metabolic syndrome and increased LDLs have become equal partners, together with increased LDL, as major risk factors for CHD. The metabolic syndrome in fact consists of a constellation of cardiovascular disease (CVD) risk factors occurring in one individual. These risk factors are of three types: *underlying risk factors, established major risk factors,* and *emerging risk factors* (Table 4–3). The *underlying risk factors* include the following:

- Abdominal obesity
- Physical inactivity
- Atherogenic diet

The *established major risk factors* and *emerging risk factors* can be listed together and include the following:

- Atherogenic dyslipidemia
- Increased blood pressure
- Insulin resistance and hyperglycemia
- Proinflammatory state
- Prothrombotic state

Atherogenic dyslipidemia is composed of four serum lipid and lipoprotein abnormalities: increased triglyceride, increased apo B, small LDL particles, and reduced HDL-cholesterol levels.

Medical Complications of the Metabolic Syndrome

Cardiovascular Disease

The metabolic syndrome was first recognized as a multiplex risk factor for CVD, particularly CHD. More recently, the increasing prevalence of obesity, together with the decline in cigarette smoking, could make the metabolic syndrome the major cause of CHD in the United States. Reports (108–111) attest to the increased risk for CHD accompanying this syndrome. When patients with the metabolic syndrome develop type 2 diabetes, the risk for CVD is compounded.

Type 2 Diabetes

Most people who experience development of type 2 diabetes have been affected by the metabolic syndrome for several years before diagnosis. Without doubt, patients with the metabolic syndrome are at high risk for development of type 2 diabetes (112). On the basis of relative prevalence rates of dia-

TABLE 4–3. *Risk factor categories*

Underlying risk factors	Major risk factors	Emerging risk factors
• Obesity (especially abdominal obesity) • Physical inactivity • Atherogenic diet	• Cigarette smoking • Hypertension (or on antihypertensive medication) • Low HDL cholesterol • Family history of premature CHD (CHD in male first degree relative <55 years; CHD in female first degree relative <65 years) • Age (men ≥45 years; women ≥55 years)	• Emerging lipid risk factors (elevations in triglyceride, apolipoprotein B, lipoprotein(a) • Emerging nonlipid risk factors (insulin resistance, impaired fasting glucose and impaired glucose tolerance, elevated proinflammatory and prothrombotic factors, elevated homocysteine)

CHD, coronary heart disease; HDL, high-density lipoprotein.

betes and the metabolic syndrome in the general population, it can be estimated that type 2 diabetes eventually will develop in at least one-third of patients with the metabolic syndrome (111). This is because insulin resistance is one important component of the metabolic syndrome (Table 4–3). Type 2 diabetes is defined as categoric hyperglycemia resulting from two defects in glucose metabolism: namely, insulin resistance and reduced insulin secretion. When secretory capacity for insulin declines in a person with the metabolic syndrome, categoric hyperglycemia (fasting plasma glucose ≥ 126 mg/dL) can develop. Thus, type 2 diabetes can be alternatively defined as the metabolic syndrome plus categoric hyperglycemia. The medical complications of type 2 diabetes are manifold; but two of them—macrovascular and microvascular disease—carry particular importance to the cardiovascular field. Moreover, hypertension is extremely common in patients with type 2 diabetes (113). Simultaneous increases of blood pressure and glucose particularly contribute to peripheral vascular disease, chronic renal failure, congestive heart failure, and stroke.

Other Medical Complications

A growing interest in the metabolic syndrome has uncovered associations with other medical conditions of importance. Among them are fatty liver, cholesterol gallstones, polycystic ovary disease, and acanthosis nigricans. The syndrome may be further accompanied by increased risk for certain kinds of cancer (e.g., colon, breast, and prostate cancer).

Underlying Causes of the Metabolic Syndrome

Obesity and Adipose Tissue Disorders

Adipose Tissue Excess (Obesity)

The increasing prevalence of the metabolic syndrome in many countries can be attributed largely to an increasing prevalence of obesity. The most visible effect of obesity is an increase in fat content of adipose tissue. But excess fat hidden in other organs associated with obesity is critical

for the development of the metabolic syndrome. The key target organs of this syndrome are adipose tissue, liver, muscle, and likely, pancreatic β cells. Fat overload in target organs results from excessive intakes of both fats and carbohydrates—that is, if nutrient intakes exceed energy expenditure, fat accumulation in target organs will occur.

Lipid overload in target organs links importantly to all of the metabolic risk factors. Lipid overload in muscle causes insulin resistance, which, in turn, predisposes to hyperglycemia. Lipid overload in liver contributes to atherogenic dyslipidemia (114); it also enhances hepatic glucose output, which adds to insulin resistance and hyperglycemia. Excess lipid in adipose tissue causes secretion of several factors that not only promote insulin resistance but also predispose to a proinflammatory state and a prothrombotic state. Finally, excess lipid in pancreatic β cells appears to promote hyperinsulinemia and, thus, secondary insulin resistance (115), and through lipotoxicity to β cells, a decline in insulin secretory capacity (116).

Adipose Tissue Deficiencies

Another type of adipose tissue abnormality that leads to the metabolic syndrome is a deficiency of this tissue. The most dramatic forms of deficiency are called *lipodystrophy*. The lipodystrophies come in several forms. *Congenital generalized lipodystrophy* results from a defect in the synthesis of triglyceride and phospholipids in adipose tissue (117). Adipose tissue is virtually absent. This defect causes extreme fat accumulation in liver and muscle. *Familial partial lipodystrophy* derives from mutations in either lamin A/C (118,119) or peroxisome proliferator-activated receptor-γ (120). Patients with human immunodeficiency virus infection who are treated with protease inhibitors also commonly manifest partial lipodystrophy (121). In the various forms of partial lipodystrophy, subcutaneous adipose tissue is greatly diminished and fat redistributes to liver and muscle. All forms of lipodystrophy are accompanied by the metabolic syndrome. The lipodystrophies provide a prime example of how organ accumulation of fat can cause the metabolic syndrome.

Adipose Tissue Distribution Disorders

Adipose tissue distribution disorders are probably also related to a partial deficiency of adipose tissue. A condition called *abdominal obesity* is characterized by reduced stores of gluteofemoral fat, distribution of fat into the abdomen, excess liver fat, insulin resistance, and metabolic syndrome (25). This pattern of fat distribution is common in white men (122), in South Asians (123), and in women with polycystic ovary disease (124).

Primary Insulin Resistance of Adipose Tissue

With primary insulin resistance of adipose tissue, normal levels of insulin do not suppress triglyceride lipolysis in the absence of other obvious abnormalities of adipose tissue. Consequently, plasma concentrations of nonesterified fatty acids (NEFA) are high (125). These increased NEFA concentrations produce lipid overload in muscle, liver, and B-cells, which accentuates the metabolic syndrome.

Abnormalities in Adipose Tissue Secretory Products

Important products produced by adipose tissue include leptin, inflammatory cytokines, thrombotic factors (e.g., plasminogen activator inhibitor-1 [PAI-1]), and adiponectin (126). Abnormalities in these secretory products occur in patients with obesity, with adipose tissue deficiencies and distribution disorders, and possibly with primary insulin resistance of adipose tissue. They contribute in one way or another to the increased risk for CVD or type 2 diabetes in patients with the metabolic syndrome.

The development of the metabolic syndrome secondary to disorders of adipose tissue generally requires some degree of overnutrition. If nutrient intake does not exceed energy expenditure, the metabolic syndrome generally will not develop. Only when some excess of nutrient intake is present does fat begin to accumulate in target organs outside of adipose tissue. Thus, to prevent the development of the metabolic syndrome in individuals who are predisposed to it, excessive nutrient intake must be greatly curtailed.

Physical Inactivity

Lack of physical activity is a known risk factor for CVD. Conversely, increased physical activity reduces risk for CVD. The mechanisms underlying this relation are not fully understood. However, a significant portion of the benefit of regular exercise appears to be through reducing metabolic risk factors for CVD: namely, insulin resistance (127), increased triglyceride (128), low HDL cholesterol (129), proinflammatory state (130,131), and possibly prothrombotic state (132,133). Physical inactivity, therefore, must be considered one of the underlying causes of the metabolic syndrome.

High-Carbohydrate Diets

In individuals who already have the features of the metabolic syndrome, a diet high in carbohydrates and low in fat can exacerbate several of the metabolic risk factors. With high-carbohydrate diets, postprandial glucose and insulin levels are greater (134,135), fasting triglycerides are increased (85), and HDL-cholesterol levels are lower (85). There is dispute whether high-carbohydrate diets in patients with the metabolic syndrome or type 2 diabetes actually accentuate the risk for CVD; although this question has not been answered definitively, there is little doubt that several of the metabolic risk factors are worsened.

Genetic Factors

Many lines of evidence indicate that genetic factors can contribute to the metabolic syndrome. Some notable examples include the high prevalence of this syndrome in certain population groups (e.g., South Asians) (136,137) and offspring of parents with type 2 diabetes (138). Genetic factors contributing to the metabolic syndrome can be considered in two areas: upstream factors and downstream factors. The former can be considered to be related to the disorders of adipose tissue that were discussed earlier. These genetic factors will contribute to excessive release of NEFA from adipose tissue; this will lead to tissue overload of lipid. Downstream factors are those that modify the major and emerging risk factors of the syndrome. Each of these risk factors is under complex genetic control, and many possibilities exist for genetic variation that can modify them.

Major and Emerging Risk Factors of the Metabolic Syndrome

Atherogenic Dyslipidemia

The degree of dyslipidemia that develops in subjects with the adipose tissue disorders is variable. Severity is related in part to the degree of lipid overload in the liver. However, the response in lipoprotein levels to hepatic lipid overload also depends on an individual's genetic architecture. Key proteins that regulate lipoprotein metabolism are lipoprotein lipase, hepatic lipase, and likely those affecting fatty acid oxidation. If fatty acid oxidation in the liver is sluggish, more fatty acids will be diverted into triglycerides for secretion with VLDLs. This will accentuate hypertriglyceridemia. The same is true if genetic polymorphism of lipoprotein lipase is present and contributes to impaired lipolysis of VLDL triglyceride. In individuals who have a particular isoform of apolipoprotein E, called apo E_2, the conversion of VLDL into LDL is impaired; this leads to an accumulation of VLDL remnants known as β-VLDL. Patients who have both the metabolic syndrome and apo E_2 often experience a marked accumulation of β-VLDL; this condition is characterized by approximately equal increases in plasma triglycerides and cholesterol and is named *familial dysbetalipoproteinemia* (139).

Other forms of hypertriglyceridemia are common of persons with the metabolic syndrome. *Familial hypertriglyceridemia,* which manifests raised VLDL triglycerides in affected family members, is more likely to become clinically manifest when other risk factors of the metabolic syndrome are present (140). Multiple different and mild genetic defects in triglyceride metabolism likely can elicit this form of hypertriglyceridemia. A more complex genetic architecture is responsible for multiple lipoprotein phenotypes occurring in one family. This familial pattern is called *familial combined hyperlipidemia* (141). The hyperlipidemia also manifests more severely in family members affected by a metabolic syndrome.

Patients having small LDL particles as a component of atherogenic dyslipidemia usually have the metabolic syndrome as well (142). Small LDL particles most commonly are secondary to raised triglycerides. Small particles result from exchange of triglycerides in VLDLs with cholesterol esters in LDLs. Other genetic factors, yet to be discovered, may contribute further to small LDLs (143). This genetic predisposition is revealed in individuals who have a constellation of metabolic risk factors.

Most individuals in affluent societies who have low HDL cholesterol also have insulin resistance and the metabolic syndrome (144). This is because of two factors: increased VLDL triglycerides and increased activity of hepatic lipase (145). Both decreased HDL levels are secondary to hepatic liver overload. Increased VLDL triglyceride reduces HDL cholesterol by exchange of triglyceride in VLDL for cholesterol in HDLs. High activity of hepatic lipase reduces HDL cholesterol by degrading larger HDL particles. Other factors of genetic origin can further contribute to HDL decrease in patients with the metabolic syndrome. These have not been well-defined and are the subject of intensive research. Factors under investigation include gene polymorphisms in hepatic lipase, adenosine triphosphate-binding cassette A1 transporters, and cholesterol-ester transfer protein.

Elevated Blood Pressure. Multiple mechanisms link elevated blood pressure to the metabolic syndrome. One theory holds that insulin resistance and hyperinsulinemia increase blood pressure (146). Another postulated mechanism includes sodium and fluid retention (147). Activation of the renin–angiotensin system may increase tubular reabsorption of sodium; and even small increases in angiotensin II levels can increase blood pressure, especially after volume expansion. Yet another effect may be compression of the kidney from excess adiposity under the kidney capsule. Thus, Hall (148) suggests that increased volume retention in obesity may be related to increases in interstitial fluid hydrostatic pressure. This condition could cause increased resistance to flow through the loop of Henle and, consequently, a reduction in tubular flow rate and increased sodium reabsorption. In a word, the association of increased blood pressure and metabolic syndrome occurs through multiple mechanisms (148).

Insulin Resistance. Many investigators believe that insulin resistance is the primary *cause* of the metabolic syndrome (149,150); this belief is based on their close association. Association and causality, however, are not synonymous; the relation between insulin resistance and metabolic syndrome is complex. Furthermore, insulin resistance may be a risk factor for CVD independent of other metabolic risk factors (151). Thus, the *causes* of insulin resistance are a topic of great interest. Obesity is with little doubt one cause of insulin resistance, as discussed earlier. Physical inactivity also is a contributing factor. But there also appears to be a strong genetic component. The mechanisms of insulin signaling are complicated and multifaceted. Indeed, the possibility that polymorphisms in genes regulating insulin signaling may modify the insulin response is high. Putative dysfunctional polymorphisms in fact have been reported (152,153). Currently, however, no common polymorphisms that alone confer insulin resistance in large populations have been discovered. Current research nonetheless is being carried out in search of such polymorphisms.

Proinflammatory State. Patients with the metabolic syndrome commonly have increased C-reactive protein (CRP) (154). This finding accords with reports that adipose tissue secretes inflammatory cytokines (155). Thus, obesity itself appears to induce a proinflammatory state. If so, cytokine overproduction could be one mechanism whereby obesity predisposes to CVD; and for many obese individuals, an increase of CRP is one marker of the presence of a proinflammatory state.

Prothrombotic State. People with the metabolic syndrome commonly have high levels of PAI-1 and fibrinogen (156). Research indicates that adipose tissue secretes PAI-1 (157). Increases in fat content of adipose tissue, particularly with visceral obesity, are accompanied by high levels of PAI-1. Increased fibrinogen further represents an acute phase response to high levels of cytokines. Both increased PAI-1 and high fibrinogen levels contribute to the prothrombotic state of the metabolic syndrome.

Clinical Diagnosis of the Metabolic Syndrome

The NCEP ATP III (25) has proposed criteria that can be used in the clinical setting for a diagnosis of the metabolic syndrome (Table 4–4). The diagnosis can be made when a patient has three of five of the characteristics listed in Table 4–4. This diagnosis is arbitrary, but it has the advantage of simplicity of application in the clinic. Some reports (108–110) indicate that patients who meet these criteria are at increased risk for CVD. These patients are also at risk for type 2 diabetes. Another set of criteria for the metabolic syndrome have been proposed by the World Health Organization (WHO) (158). These criteria are similar but require the presence of glucose intolerance as one of the components. By WHO criteria, glucose intolerance can be manifest in one of three ways: (a) by impaired fasting glucose (100–125 mg/dL), (b) by impaired glucose tolerance (2-hour postprandial glucose (140 mg/dL), or type 2 diabetes

TABLE 4–4. *Clinical identification of the metabolic syndrome*

Risk factor	Defining level
Abdominal obesity[a]	Waist circumference[b]
Men	>102 cm (>40 in)
Women	>88 cm (>35 in)
Triglycerides	≥150 mg/dL
High-density lipoprotein cholesterol	
Men	<40 mg/dL
Women	<50 mg/dL
Blood pressure	≥130/≥85 mmHg
Fasting glucose	≥100 mg/dL

[a]Being overweight or obese is associated with insulin resistance and the metabolic syndrome. However, the presence of abdominal obesity is more highly correlated with metabolic risk factors than is an increased body mass index. Therefore, the simple measure of waist circumference is recommended to identify the body weight component of the metabolic syndrome.

[b]Some male patients can develop multiple metabolic risk factors when the waist circumference is only marginally increased, for example, 94 to 102 cm (37–39 in.). Such patients may have a strong genetic contribution to insulin resistance. They should benefit from changes in life habits, similarly to men with categoric increases in waist circumference.

(fasting glucose (≥126 mg/dL). Although there is considerable overlap between ATP III and WHO criteria, the former will identify more patients at high risk for CVD, whereas the latter will identify more at high risk for type 2 diabetes.

Prevalence of Metabolic Syndrome

The prevalence of the metabolic syndrome differs in different populations throughout the world. The United States has one of the highest frequencies in the general population in the world. A report (111) highlighted its high prevalence using ATP III criteria for diagnosis. This reflects the high prevalence of obesity in the United States. Table 4–5 shows the age-adjusted prevalence of metabolic risk factors shown in Table 4–4 among 8,814 adults 20 years of age or older in the United States. By ATP III criteria, those subjects with three or more metabolic abnormalities have the metabolic syndrome (Table 4–4). Approximately one-fourth of the whole U.S. population has the metabolic syndrome. Frequency of the metabolic syndrome increases with age, and some ethnic groups are particularly susceptible.

Metabolic Syndrome: Implications for Clinical Intervention

The introduction of the metabolic syndrome in ATP III guidelines (25) has placed new emphasis on an aggregation of CVD risk factors beyond the focus on single risk factors. Often patients with the metabolic syndrome do not have severe, single risk factors; consequently, their greater risk for CVD is overlooked in clinical practice. Moreover, primary management of the metabolic syndrome resides in modifica-

TABLE 4–5. *Age-adjusted prevalence of one or more abnormalities of the metabolic syndrome among 8,814 adults 20 years of age or older in the United States: National Health and Nutrition Examination Survey III, 1988–1994*

	No. of Metabolic Abnormalities, % (SE)				
	≥1	≥2	≥3	≥4	5
Total	71	44	24	10	3
Men	72	45	24	11	2
Women	71	43	23	10	3
Race or ethnicity					
White	70	43	24	11	3
African American	76	45	22	8	2
Mexican American	79	54	32	12	2
Other	71	42	20	7	2
Men					
White	72	46	25	12	3
African American	70	37	16	6	1
Mexican American	75	52	28	9	2
Other	70	43	21	4	1
Women					
White	68	41	23	9	3
African American	80	51	26	10	2
Mexican American	84	58	36	15	3
Other	71	40	20	11	2

Ford ES, Giles WH, Dietz WH. Prevalence of the metabolic syndrome among US adults: findings from the third National Health and Nutrition Examination Survey. *JAMA* 2002;287: 356–359.

tion of the underlying risk factors—that is, obesity, physical inactivity, and atherogenic diet. In the next section, practical suggestions are presented for the nutritional management of increased LDL cholesterol and of the metabolic syndrome.

PRACTICAL APPROACHES TO LIFESTYLE MODIFICATION FOR PREVENTION OF CARDIOVASCULAR DISEASE

The NCEP ATP III (25) has outlined a practical nutritional approach to nutrition prevention of CVD that is called *therapeutic lifestyle change*. The primary thrust of these recommendations is to reduce LDL-cholesterol levels and to reduce the risk factors of the metabolic syndrome. The basic concept of this approach is that multiple dietary and lifestyle changes are required to achieve maximal CVD risk reduction with nondrug therapies. This section discusses practical approaches to *therapeutic lifestyle changes*. These goals are achieved in three ways: (a) by an LDL-decreasing diet, (b) by weight reduction, and (c) by increased physical activity. These therapeutic changes are presented in summary form in Table 4–6.

Low-Density Lipoprotein–Decreasing Dietary Changes

The primary dietary change to achieve a decrease of serum LDL cholesterol is reduction in intake of cholesterol. Other

TABLE 4–6. *Essential components of therapeutic lifestyle changes*

Component	Recommendation
LDL-increasing nutrients	
Saturated fats*	<7% of total calories
Dietary cholesterol	<200 mg/day
Therapeutic options for LDL decrease	
Plant stanol/sterols	2 g/day
Increased viscous (soluble)fiber	10–25 g/day
Total calories (energy)	Adjust total caloric intake to maintain desirable body weight/prevent weight gain
Physical activity	Include enough moderate exercise to expend at least 200 kcal/day

TABLE 4–8. *Adult Treatment Panel IIII macronutrient recommendations*

Component	Recommendation
Saturated fat	<7% of total calories
Trans fatty acids	Reduce as much as practical
Polyunsaturated fat	Up to 10% of total calories
Monounsaturated fat	Up to 20% of total calories
Total fat	25–35% of total calories
Carbohydrate	50–60% of total calories
Dietary fiber	20–30 g/day
Protein	Approximately 15% of total calories

changes, including use of plant stanol/sterols and increased dietary fiber, also will decrease LDL cholesterol. Finally, it is important that the whole diet be modified to improve health. For this reason, the NCEP ATP III tailored its dietary recommendations to be in accord with the latest recommendations of Dietary Guidelines for Americans (159) (Table 4–7).

The ATP III report further focused on aspects of the Dietary Guidelines for Americans that relate more directly to prevention of CVD. Its recommendations for other macronutrient intakes are given in Table 4–8. An important change in this recommendation was that total fat was allowed to range from 25% to 35% of total calories. A greater percentage of total fat is most appropriate for patients with the metabolic syndrome.

To assess intakes of LDL-increasing nutrients, the ATP III panel devised a brief dietary CAGE that may be helpful (Table 4–9). These questions are most appropriate for physicians during patient interviews; they are not a substitute for a

systematic dietary assessment by a nutrition professional. CAGE questions can be used to identify the common food sources of LDL-increasing nutrients—saturated fat and cholesterol—in the patient's diet. Without doubt effective dietary modification will be facilitated by consultation with a registered dietitian or other qualified nutrition professional for *medical nutrition therapy*. Both physicians and nutritional professionals can provide useful information to patients on dietary change to reduce LDL cholesterol. Suggestions for foods to increase and foods to decrease to achieve LDL reduction and to promote health are provided in Table 4–10.

Weight Control and Increased Physical Activity

For individuals who are overweight or obese, weight reduction and increased physical activity will both enhance LDL-cholesterol decline and reduce the severity of the metabolic syndrome. In 1998, the National Heart, Lung, and Blood Institute published *Clinical Guidelines on the Identification, Evaluation, and Treatment of Overweight and Obesity in Adults* from the Obesity Education Initiative (OEI) (160). This is an evidence-based report, and its recommendations for techniques of weight reduction were accepted by ATP III for individuals undergoing management for cholesterol disorders. The major recommendations of the OEI can be summarized as a guide to weight reduction in patients who have increased LDL cholesterol and the metabolic syndrome.

The primary goals of weight-loss therapy are (a) to prevent further weight gain, (b) to reduce excess body weight,

TABLE 4–7. *Dietary guidelines for Americans (2000)*

Aim for fitness
- Aim for a healthy weight.
- Be physically active each day.

Build a healthy base
- Let the pyramid guide your food choices.
- Choose a variety of grains daily, especially whole grains.
- Choose a variety of fruits and vegetables daily.
- Keep foods safe to eat.

Choose sensibly
- Choose a diet that is low in saturated fat and cholesterol and moderate in total fat.
- Choose beverages and foods to moderate your intake of sugars.
- Choose and prepare foods with less salt.
- If you drink alcoholic beverages, do so in moderation.

TABLE 4–9. *Dietary CAGE questions for assessment of intakes of saturated fat and cholesterol*

C—Cheese (and other sources of dairy fats—whole milk, 2% milk, ice cream, cream, whole fat yogurt)
A—Animal fats (hamburger, ground meat, frankfurters, bologna, salami, sausage, fried foods, fatty cuts of meat)
G—Got it away from home (high-fat meals either purchased and brought home or eaten in restaurants)
E—Eat (extra) high-fat commercial products: candy, pastries, pies, doughnuts, cookies

TABLE 4–10. *Practical suggestions for a low-density lipoprotein (LDL)–decreasing diet*

Food Items to Choose More Often	Food Items to Choose Less Often
Breads and cereals ≥6 servings per day, adjusted to caloric needs Breads, cereals, especially whole grain; pasta; rice; potatoes; dry beans and peas; low fat crackers and cookies	Many bakery products, including doughnuts, biscuits, butter rolls, muffins, croissants, sweet rolls, Danish, cakes, pies, coffee cakes, cookies Many grain-based snacks, including chips, cheese puffs, snack mix, regular crackers, buttered popcorn
Vegetables 3–5 servings/day fresh, frozen, or canned, without added fat, sauce, or salt	Vegetables fried or prepared with butter, cheese, or cream sauce
Fruits 2–4 servings per day fresh, frozen, canned, dried	Fruits fried or served with butter or cream
Dairy products 2–3 servings/day fat-free, 0.5%, 1% milk, buttermilk, yogurt, cottage cheese; fat-free and low-fat cheese	Whole milk/2% milk, whole milk yogurt, ice cream, cream, cheese
Eggs ≥2 egg yolks/wk; egg whites or egg substitute	Egg yolks, whole eggs
Meat, poultry, fish ≥5 oz/day lean cuts loin, leg, round; extra-lean hamburger; cold cuts made with lean meat or soy protein; skinless poultry; fish	Higher fat meat cuts: ribs, t-bone steak, regular hamburger, bacon, sausage; cold cuts: salami, bologna, hot dogs; organ meats: liver, brains, sweetbreads; poultry with skin; fried meat; fried poultry; fried fish
Fats and oils Amount adjusted to caloric level: unsaturated oils; soft or liquid margarines and vegetable oil spreads, salad dressings, seeds, and nuts	Butter, shortening, stick margarine, chocolate, coconut
LDL-lowering dietary options Stanol/sterol-containing margarines; viscous fiber food sources: barley, oats, psyllium, apples, bananas, berries, citrus fruits, nectarines, peaches, pears, plums, prunes, broccoli, brussel sprouts, carrots, dry beans, peas, soy products (tofu, meso)	

and (c) to keep a lower body weight in the long term. Increased physical activity should be made an integral part of any weight reduction diet. Furthermore, it should be encouraged for its benefits beyond weight loss. The *initial goal* of weight loss therapy is to reduce body weight by approximately 10% from baseline weight. If this goal is achieved, further weight loss can be attempted, if indicated through further evaluation. A *reasonable time* for a 10% reduction in body weight is 6 months. A decrease of 300 to 500 kcal/day usually will result in weight loss of about 0.5 to 1 lb/wk. For most patients, this loss will translate into a 10% loss in 6 months. However, for more severely obese patients, reductions in energy intakes of up to 500 to 1,000 kcal/day may be necessary; these energy deficits will lead to weight losses of about 1 to 2 lb/week and a 10% weight loss in 6 months. After 6 months, weight loss rates usually decline and weight plateaus because of a lesser energy expenditure at the lower weight.

Any lost weight usually will be regained unless a weight maintenance program consisting of dietary therapy, physical activity, and behavior therapy is continued thereafter. If a pa-

tient loses about 10% of body weight, the risk factors of the metabolic syndrome usually are much improved. However, if more weight reduction is necessary, the process of weight reduction can be continued after 6 months. This will require further adjustment of the diet and physical activity prescriptions. For those patients who are unable to achieve adequate weight reduction, prevention of further weight gain becomes a high priority.

There are several modalities available to achieve weight reduction in patients with the metabolic syndrome. These include dietary therapy; increased physical activity; behavior therapies; combinations of dietary, exercise, and behavior therapies; pharmacotherapies; and surgical therapies. Each of these modalities are reviewed briefly in this chapter.

Dietary Therapy

A diet that is individually planned and takes into account the patient's overweight status to help create a deficit of 300 to 500 kcal/day should be the foundation of weight reduction therapy. Suggestions to promote caloric restriction are provided in Table 4–11. The weight reduction diet should be consistent in composition with that recommended for the LDL-lowering diet. Frequent contact with the practitioner and, if possible, a nutrition professional during dietary therapy helps to promote weight loss and weight maintenance at a lower weight.

Physical Activity

An increase in physical activity per se will not lead to substantially greater weight loss over six months. Most weight loss occurs because of decreased caloric intake. Nonetheless, physical activity will improve the metabolic syndrome independently of weight reduction. Furthermore, sustained physical activity is most helpful in the prevention of regaining weight. Suggestions for a regimen of routine physical activity are provided in Table 4–12. For most obese patients, exercise should be initiated slowly, and the intensity should be increased gradually. It does not matter whether exercise is done all at one time or intermittently during the course of the day. A good plan is to start by walking for 30 minutes 3 days a week, and then building to 45 minutes to 1 hour of more intense walking at least 5 days a week. Depending on amounts of exercise, expenditures of 100 to 300 calories per day can be achieved that will assist in weight reduction. Walking is a particularly attractive exercise because of its safety. Exercise within the home—weight exercise, walking or running in place, treadmill exercise—also are attractive because they can be done in the security of the home, they save time, and they are not affected by weather. Simple daily exercises such as taking the stairs instead of the elevator also are helpful. Competitive sports such as tennis and volleyball are fun, but care must be taken to avoid injury. Reducing sedentary time is another way to increase activity by undertaking frequent, less strenuous activities.

TABLE 4–11. *Practical recommendations for weight reduction through dietary modifications*

Weigh regularly
Record weight, body mass index, and waist circumference
Lose weight gradually
Goal: lose 10% of body weight in 6 months. Lose 0.5–1
  lb/wk
Develop healthy eating patterns
• Choose healthy foods (see Table 4–10)
• Reduce intake of foods that increase low-density lipoprotein cholesterol (see Table 4–10)
• Limit number of eating occasions
• Select sensible portion sizes
• Avoid second helpings
• Identify and reduce hidden fat by reading food labels to choose products lower in saturated fat and calories, and ask about ingredients in ready-to-eat foods prepared away from home
• Identify and reduce sources of excess carbohydrates such as fat-free and regular crackers, cookies and other desserts, snacks, and sugar-containing beverages

---

TABLE 4–12. *Suggestions for regular physical activity*

Make physical activity part of daily routines
• Reduce sedentary time.
• Walk, wheel, or bike-ride more, drive less. Take the stairs instead of an elevator. Get off the bus a few stops early and walk the remaining distance. Mow the lawn with a push mower. Rake leaves. Garden. Push a stroller. Clean the house. Do exercises or pedal a stationary bike while watching television. Play actively with children. Take a brisk ten-minute walk or wheel before work, during your work break, and after dinner.

Make physical activity part of exercise or recreational activities
• Walk, wheel, or jog. Bicycle or use an arm pedal bicycle. Swim or do water aerobics. Play basketball. Join a sports team. Play wheelchair sports. Golf (pull cart or carry clubs). Canoe. Cross-country ski. Dance. Take part in an exercise program at work, home, school, or gym.

Behavior Therapy

Behavior therapy is based on learning principles such as reinforcement, self-monitoring of both eating habits and physical activity, stress management, stimulus control, problem solving, contingency management, cognitive restructuring, and social support. Nutritional professionals are trained in these techniques, and they can be reinforced by physicians in their interactions with patients.

Combined Therapies

A combined intervention of dietary therapy, increased physical activity, and behavior therapy offers the greatest likelihood of success for weight loss and weight maintenance.

Pharmacotherapy

The combined therapies listed earlier should be considered for at least six months before even considering weight reduction drugs. In selected patients who have severe medical consequences from obesity, the possibility of weight reduction drugs can be considered. Unfortunately, Food & Drug Administration–approved weight loss drugs have limited efficacy and often are accompanied by side effects. For example, sibutramine has been reported to modestly enhance weight loss and to help facilitate weight loss maintenance. Even so, increases in blood pressure and heart rate may occur. This drug should not be used in patients with a history of hypertension, CHD, congestive heart failure, arrhythmias, or stroke. Many patients with the metabolic syndrome have increased blood pressure and thus are not good candidates for sibutramine therapy. Another drug, orlistat, partially blocks absorption of dietary fat. With orlistat, fat-soluble vitamins may require replacement. The primary side effect of orlistat is steatorrhea, which many patients find to be unacceptable.

Weight Loss Surgery

Gastrointestinal surgery for the purpose of weight reduction should be reserved for patients in whom efforts at medical therapy have failed and who are experiencing the complications of obesity. Gastrointestinal surgery (gastric restriction [vertical gastric banding] or gastric bypass [Roux-en Y]) is one intervention currently being used (161). Although this approach is used in clinical practice, clinical trial evidence is insufficient to be certain that benefits outweigh the side effects in the long term. Because of a lack of clinical trial evidence, this approach is controversial. Some investigators believe that this approach has weight loss potential for selected patients, whereas others consider it too dangerous to be used except under unusual circumstances.

Other Considerations for Weight Control

Obesity is multifactorial in origin, and approaches to weight reduction must take individual differences into account. No "cookbook" or standardized set of rules to optimize weight reduction for all subjects exists. Physicians and nutrition professionals also should be sensitive to cultural factors that exist for patients. The patient's age also must be considered. Although people older than 65 years may be obese, there are issues that must be considered. The benefits of weight loss must be considered in the context of other medical problems that may exist in older persons.

Although smoking cessation has a high priority in smokers, there is some weight gain in about 80% of individuals after quitting smoking. This weight gain averages about 5 lb, but about 10% of patients can gain 20 to 30 lb. Generally, this side effect is less detrimental than continuing to smoke, but it often requires increased attention to the risk factors of the metabolic syndrome.

REFERENCES

1. Carleton RA, Dwyer J, Finberg L, et al. Report of the expert panel on population strategies for blood cholesterol reduction. A statement from the Nation. Cholesterol Education Program, National Heart, Lung, and Blood Institute, National Institutes of Health. *Circulation* 1991;83:2154–2232.
2. Grundy SM, Bilheimer D, Blackburn H, et al. Rationale of the diet-heart statement of the American Heart Association. Report of Nutrition Committee. *Circulation* 1982;65:839A–854A.
3. National Research Council, Committee on Diet and Health, Food and Nutrition Board, and Commission on Life Science. *Diet and health: implications for reducing chronic disease risk.* Washington, D.C.: National Academy Press, 1989:749.
4. Gordon T, Kannel WB, Castelli WP, et al. Lipoproteins, cardiovascular disease, and death: the Framingham study. *Arch Intern Med* 1981; 141:1128.
5. Stamler J, Wentworth D, Neaton J. Is the relationship between serum cholesterol and risk of death from CHD continuous and graded? *JAMA* 1986;256:2823–2828.
6. Anderson KM, Castelli WP, Levy DL. Cholesterol and mortality: 30 years of follow-up from the Framingham study. *JAMA* 1987;257: 2176–2180.
7. Anitschkow N, Chalatow S. Veber experimentelle cholesterinseatose und ihre bedeutung fur die entstehung einiger pathologisher prozesse. *Zentralbl Allg Pathol Pathol Anat* 1913;24:1–9.
8. Strong JP, McGill HC. Diet and experimental atherosclerosis in baboons. *Am J Pathol* 1967;50:669–690.
9. Strong JP. Atherosclerosis in primates. Introduction and overview. *Primates Med* 1976;9:1–15.
10. McGill HC Jr, McMahan CA, Kruski AW, et al. Relationship of lipoprotein cholesterol concentrations to experimental atherosclerosis in baboons. *Arteriosclerosis* 1981;1:3–12.
11. Keys A. *Seven countries: a multivariate analysis on death and coronary heart disease.* Cambridge, MA: Harvard University Press, 1980:132–133.
12. Kagan A, Harris BR, Winkelstein W Jr, et al. Epidemiologic studies of coronary heart disease and stroke in Japanese men living in Japan, Hawaii and California: demographic physical, dietary and biochemical characteristics. *J Chronic Dis* 1974;27:345–364.
13. Shepherd J, Cobbe SM, Ford I, et al. Prevention of coronary heart disease with pravastatin in men with hypercholesterolemia. West of Scotland Coronary Prevention Study Group. *N Engl J Med* 1995;333: 1301–1307.
14. Sacks FM, Pfeffer MA, Moye LA, et al. The effect of pravastatin on coronary events after myocardial infarction in patients with average cholesterol levels. *N Engl J Med* 1996;335:1001–1009.
15. Prevention of cardiovascular events and death with pravastatin in patients with coronary heart disease and a broad range of initial cholesterol levels. The Long-Term Intervention with Pravastatin in Ischaemic Disease (LIPID) Study Group. *N Engl J Med* 1998;339: 1349–1357.
16. Randomised trial of cholesterol lowering in 4444 patients with coronary heart disease: the Scandinavian Simvastatin Survival Study (4S). *Lancet* 1994;344:1383–1389.
17. Downs JR, Clearfield M, Whitney E, et al. Primary prevention of acute coronary events with lovastatin in men and women with average cholesterol levels. Results of AFCAPS/TexCAPS. *JAMA* 1998;279: 1615–1622.
18. Heart Protection Study Collaborative Group: MRC/BHF Heart Protection Study of cholesterol lowering with simvastatin in 20,536 high-risk individuals: a randomised placebo-controlled trial. *Lancet* 2002; 360:7–22.
19. Brown BG, Zhao XQ, Sacco DE, et al. Lipid lowering and plaque regression. New insights into prevention of plaque disruption and clinical events in coronary disease. *Circulation* 1993;87:1781–1791.
20. Goldstein JL, Brown MS. Familial hypercholesterolemia. In: Scriver CR, Beaudet AL, Sly WS, et al., eds. *The metabolic basis of inherited disease,* 6th ed. New York: McGraw-Hill, 1989:1215–1250.
21. Vega GL, Grundy SM. In vivo evidence for reduced binding of low density lipoproteins to receptors as a cause of primary moderate hypercholesterolemia. *J Clin Invest* 1986;78:1410–1414.
22. Innerarity TL, Mahley RW, Weisgraber KH, et al. Familial defective apolipoprotein B-100: a mutation of apolipoprotein B that causes hyper-cholesterolemia. *J Lipid Res* 1990;31:1337–1349.
23. Rauh G, Keller C, Kormann B, et al. Familial defective apolipoprotein B100: clinical characteristics of 54 cases. *Atherosclerosis* 1992; 92(2–3):233–241.
24. Tybjaerg-Hansen A, Humphries SE. Familial defective apo-lipoprotein B-100: a single mutation that causes hypercholesterolemia and premature coronary artery disease. *Atherosclerosis* 1992;96:91–107.
25. National Cholesterol Education Program (NCEP) Expert Panel on Detection, Evaluation, and Treatment of High Blood Cholesterol in Adults (Adult Treatment Panel III). Third Report of the National Cholesterol Education Program (NCEP) Expert Panel on Detection, Evaluation, and Treatment of High Blood Cholesterol in Adults (Adult Treatment Panel III) final report. *Circulation* 2002;106: 3143–3421.
26. Davis C, Rifkind B, Brenner H, et al. A single cholesterol measurement underestimates the risk of CHD. An empirical example from the Lipid Research Clinics mortality follow-up study. *JAMA* 1990;264: 3044–3046.
27. Kesteloot H, Huang DX, Yang XS, et al. Serum lipids in the People's Republic of China: comparison of western and eastern populations. *Arteriosclerosis* 1985;5:427–433.
28. Knuiman JT, West CE, Katan MB, et al. Total cholesterol and high density lipoprotein cholesterol levels in populations differing in fat and carbohydrate intake. *Arteriosclerosis* 1987;7:612–619.
29. Grundy SM. Cholesterol and coronary heart disease: a new era. *JAMA* 1986;256:2849–2858.

30. Grundy SM, Barrett-Connor E, Rudel LL, et al. Workshop on the impact of dietary cholesterol on plasma lipoproteins and atherogenesis. *Arteriosclerosis* 1988;8:95–101.
31. Mensink RP, Katan MB. Effects of dietary fatty acids on serum lipids and lipoproteins: a meta-analysis of 27 trials. *Arteriosclerosis* 1992;12:911–919.
32. Denke MA, Sempos CT, Grundy SM. Excess body weight: an underrecognized contributor to high blood cholesterol in Caucasian American men. *Arch Intern Med* 1993;153:1093–1103.
33. Goldstein JL, Brown MS. The low density lipoprotein receptor and its relation to atherosclerosis. *Ann Rev Biochem* 1977;46:879–930.
34. Kovanen PT, Brown MS, Basu SK, et al. Saturation and suppression of hepatic lipoprotein receptors: a mechanism for the hypercholesterolemia of cholesterol-fed rabbits. *Proc Natl Acad Sci USA* 1981;78:1396–1400.
35. Sorci-Thomas M, Wilson MD, Johnson FL, et al. Studies on the expression of genes encoding apolipoproteins B100 and B48 and the low density lipoprotein receptor in nonhuman primates. *J Biol Chem* 1989;264:9039–9045.
36. Spady DK, Dietschy JM. Dietary saturated triglycerides suppress hepatic low density lipoprotein receptors in the hamster. *Proc Natl Acad Sci USA* 1985;82:4526–4530.
37. Fox JC, McGill HC Jr, Carey KD, et al. In vivo regulation of hepatic LDL receptor mRNA in the baboon: differential effects of saturated and unsaturated fat. *J Biol Chem* 1987;262:7014–7020.
38. Nicolosi RJ, Stucchi AF, Kowala MC, et al. Effect of dietary fat saturation and cholesterol on LDL composition and metabolism. *Arteriosclerosis* 1990;10:119–128.
39. Miller NE. Why does plasma low density lipoprotein concentration in adults increase with age? *Lancet* 1984;1:263–266.
40. Grundy SM, Vega GL, Bilheimer DW. Kinetic mechanisms determining variability in low density lipoprotein levels and their rise with age. *Arteriosclerosis* 1985;5:623–630.
41. Ericsson S, Eriksson M, Vitols S, et al. Influence of age on the metabolism of plasma low density lipoproteins in healthy males. *J Clin Invest* 1991;87:591–596.
42. Ma PT, Yamamoto T, Goldstein JL, et al. Increased mRNA for low density lipoprotein receptor in livers of rabbits treated with 17 alpha-ethinyl estradiol. *Proc Natl Acad Sci USA* 1986;83:792–796.
43. Eriksson M, Berglund L, Rudling M, et al. Effects of estrogen on low density lipoprotein metabolism in males: short-term and long-term studies during hormonal treatment of prostatic carcinoma. *J Clin Invest* 1989;84:802–810.
44. Kesaniemi YA, Beltz WF, Grundy SM. Comparisons of metabolism of apolipoprotein B in normal subjects, obese patients, and patients with coronary heart disease. *J Clin Invest* 1985;76:586–595.
45. Egusa G, Beltz WF, Grundy SM, et al. Influence of obesity on the metabolism of apolipoprotein B in man. *J Clin Invest* 1985;76:596–603.
46. Kesaniemi YA, Grundy SM. Increased low density lipoprotein production associated with obesity. *Arteriosclerosis* 1983;3:170–177.
47. Grundy SM. Multifactorial etiology of hypercholesterolemia: implications for prevention of coronary heart disease. *Arterioscler Thromb* 1991;11:1619–1635.
48. Janus ED, Nicoll AM, Turner PR, et al. Kinetic basis of the primary hyperlipidaemias: studies of apolipoprotein B turnover in genetically-defined subjects. *Eur J Clin Invest* 1980;10:161–171.
49. Teng B, Sniderman AD, Soutar AK, et al. Metabolic basis of hyperapobetalipoproteinemia: turnover of apolipoprotein B in low density lipoproteins and its precursors and subfractions compared with normal and familial hypercholesterolemia. *J Clin Invest* 1986;77:663.
50. Kissebah AH, Alfarsi S, Evans DJ. Low density lipoprotein metabolism in familial combined hyperlipidemia: mechanism of the multiple lipoprotein phenotypic expression. *Arteriosclerosis* 1984;4:614–624.
51. Grundy SM, Vega GL. Plasma cholesterol responsiveness to saturated fatty acids. *Am J Clin Nutr* 1988;47:822–824.
52. Denke MA, Grundy SM. Individual responses to a cholesterol-lowering diet in fifty men with moderate hypercholesterolemia. *Arch Intern Med* 1994;154:317–325.
53. Grundy SM, Denke MA. Dietary influences on serum lipids and lipoproteins. *J Lipid Res* 1990;31:1149–1172.
54. Keys A, Anderson JT, Grande F. Serum cholesterol response to changes in the diet. IV. Particular saturated fatty acids in the diet. *Metabolism* 1965;14:776–787.
55. Hegsted DM, McGandy RB, Myers ML, et al. Quantitative effects of dietary fat on serum cholesterol in man. *Am J Clin Nutr* 1965;17:281–295.
56. Mattson FH, Grundy SM. Comparison of effects of dietary saturated, monounsaturated, and polyunsaturated fatty acids on plasma lipids and lipoproteins in man. *J Lipid Res* 1985;26:194–202.
57. Bonanome A, Grundy SM. Effect of dietary stearic acid on plasma cholesterol and lipoprotein levels. *N Engl J Med* 1988;318:1244–1248.
58. Grande F. Dog serum lipid responses to dietary fats differing in the chain length of the saturated fatty acids. *J Nutr* 1962;76:255–264.
59. Hashim SA, Arteaga A, van Itallie TB. Effect of a saturated medium-chain triglyceride on serum-lipids in man. *Lancet* 1960;1:1105–1108.
60. Denke MA, Grundy SM. Comparison of effects of lauric acid and palmitic acid on plasma lipids and lipoproteins. *Am J Clin Nutr* 1992;56:895–898.
61. Ahrens EH, Hirsch J, Insull W, et al. The influence of dietary fats on serum-lipid levels in man. *Lancet* 1957;1:943–953.
62. Cater NB, Heller HJ, Denke MA. Comparison of the effects of medium-chain triacylglycerols, palm oil, and high oleic acid sunflower oil on plasma triacylglycerol fatty acids and lipid and lipoprotein concentrations in humans. *Am J Clin Nutr* 1997;65(1):41–45.
63. Denke MA, Grundy SM. Effects of fats high in stearic acid on lipid and lipoprotein concentrations in men. *Am J Clin Nutr* 1991;54:1036–1040.
64. Zock PL, Katan MB. Hydrogenation alternatives: effects of trans fatty acids and stearic acid versus linoleic acid on serum lipids and lipoproteins in humans. *J Lipid Res* 1992;33:399–410.
65. Elovson J. Immediate fate of albumin bound [I-14C] stearic acid following its intraportal injection into carbohydrate refed rats. Early course of desaturation and esterification. *Biochim Biophys Acta* 1965;106:480–494.
66. Bonanome A, Bennett M, Grundy SM. Metabolic effects of dietary stearic acid in mice: changes in the fatty acid composition of triglycerides and phospholipids in various tissues. *Atherosclerosis* 1992;94:119–127.
67. Daumeri CM, Woollett LA, Dietary JM. Fatty acids regulate hepatic low density lipoprotein receptor activity through redistribution of intracellular cholesterol pools. *Proc Natl Acad Sci USA* 1992;89:10797–10801.
68. Loscalzo J, Fredman J, Rudd RM, et al. Unsaturated fatty acids enhance low density lipoprotein uptake and degradation by peripheral blood mononuclear cells. *Arteriosclerosis* 1987;7:450–455.
69. Mensink RP, Katan MB. Effect of dietary trans fatty acids on high-density and low-density lipoprotein cholesterol levels in healthy subjects. *N Engl J Med* 1990;323:439–445.
70. Carroll KK, Khor HT. Effects of level and type of dietary fat on incidence of mammary tumors induced in female Sprague-Dawley rats by 7, 12-dimethylbenz (alpha) anthracene. *Lipids* 1971;6:415–420.
71. Reddy BS. Amount and type of dietary fat and colon cancer: animal model studies. *Prog Clin Biol Res* 1986;222:295–309.
72. Weyman C, Berlin J, Smith AD, et al. Linoleic acid as an immunosuppressive agent. *Lancet* 1975;2:33–34.
73. Vega GL, Groszek E, Wolf R, et al. Influence of polyunsaturated fats on composition of plasma lipoproteins and apolipoproteins. *J Lipid Res* 1982;23:811–822.
74. Shepherd J, Packard CJ, Patsch JR, et al. Effects of dietary polyunsaturated and saturated fat on the properties of high density lipoprotein and the metabolism of apolipoprotein. *J Clin Invest* 1978;60:1582–1592.
75. Jackson RL, Kashyap ML, Barnhart RL, et al. Influence of polyunsaturated and saturated fats on plasma lipids and lipoproteins in man. *Am J Clin Nutr* 1984;39:589–597.
76. Grundy SM. Effects of polyunsaturated fats on lipid metabolism in patients with hypertriglyceridemia. *J Clin Invest* 1975;55:269–282.
77. Sturdevant RA, Pearce ML, Dayton S. Increased prevalence of cholelithiasis in men ingesting a serum cholesterol-lowering diet. *N Engl J Med* 1973;288:24–27.
78. Parthasarathy S, Khoo JC, Miller E, et al. Low density lipoprotein rich in oleic acid is protected against oxidative modification: implications for dietary prevention of atherosclerosis. *Proc Natl Acad Sci USA* 1990;87:3894–3898.
79. Berry E, Kaufmann N, Friedlander Y, et al. The effect of dietary substitution of monounsaturated with polyunsaturated fatty acids on lipoprotein levels, structure, and function in free-living population. *Circulation* 1989;80:II-85.

80. Valsta LM, Jauhiainen M, Mutanen M, et al. Effects of a monounsaturated rapeseed oil and a polyunsaturated sunflower oil diet on lipoprotein levels in humans. *Arterioscler Thromb* 1992;12:50–57.

81. Mensink, RP, Katan MB. Effect of a diet enriched with monounsaturated or polyunsaturated fatty acids on levels of low-density and high-density lipoprotein cholesterol in healthy women and men. *N Engl J Med* 1989;321:436–441.

82. Connor WE. Effects of omega-3 fatty acids in hypertriglyceridemic states. *Semin Thromb Hemost* 1988;14:271–284.

83. Sanders TAB, Sullivan DR, Reeve J, et al. Triglyceride-lowering effect of marine polyunsaturates in patients with hypertriglyceridemia. *Arteriosclerosis* 1985;5:459–465.

84. Sullivan DR, Sanders TAB, Trayner IM, et al. Paradoxical elevation of LDL apoprotein B levels in hypertriglyceridemic patients and normal subjects ingesting fish oil. *Atherosclerosis* 1986;61:129–134.

85. Grundy SM. Comparison of monounsaturated fatty acids and carbohydrates for lowering plasma cholesterol. *N Engl J Med* 1986;314:745–748.

86. Grundy SM, Florentin L, Nix D, et al. Comparison of monounsaturated fatty acids and carbohydrates for reducing raised levels of plasma cholesterol in man. *Am J Clin Nutr* 1988;47:965–969.

87. Mensink RP, Katan MB. Effect of monounsaturated fatty acids versus complex carbohydrates on high-density lipoproteins in healthy men and women. *Lancet* 1987;1:122–125.

88. Mensink RP, de Groot MJM, van den Broeke LT, et al. Effects of monounsaturated fatty acids v complex carbohydrates on serum lipoproteins and apoproteins in healthy men and women. *Metabolism* 1989;38:172–178.

89. Knittle JL, Ahrens EH Jr. Carbohydrate metabolism in two forms of hyperglyceridemia. *J Clin Invest* 1964;43:485–495.

90. Kuusi T, Ehnholm C, Huttunen JK, et al. Concentration and composition of serum lipoproteins during a low-fat diet at two levels of polyunsaturated fat. *J Lipid Res* 1985;26:360–367.

91. Abbott WG, Swinburg B, Routolo G, et al. Effect of a high-carbohydrate, low-saturated-fat diet on apolipoprotein B and triglyceride metabolism in Pima Indians. *J Clin Invest* 1990;150:1313–1319.

92. Dreon DM, Fernstrom HA, Miller B, et al. Low density lipoprotein subclass patterns and lipoprotein response to a reduced-fat diet in men. *FASEB J* 1994;8:121–126.

93. Ginsberg HN, Karmally W, Barr SL, et al. Effects of increasing dietary unsaturated fatty acids within guidelines of the AHA Step I diet on plasma lipid and lipoprotein levels in normal males. *Arterioscler Thromb* 1994;14:892–901.

94. Bell LP, Hectorn KJ, Reynolds H, et al. Cholesterol-lowering effects of soluble-fiber cereals as part of a prudent diet for patients with mild to moderate hypercholesterolemia. *Am J Clin Nutr* 1990;52:1020–1026.

95. Anderson JW, Garrity TF, Wood CL, et al. Prospective, randomized, controlled comparison of the effects of low-fat and low-fat plus high-fiber diets on serum lipid concentrations. *Am J Clin Nutr* 1992;56:887–894.

96. Lepre F, Crane S. Effect of oatbran on mild hyperlipidaemia. *Med J Aust* 1992;157:305–308.

97. Whyte JL, McArthur R, Topping D, et al. Oat bran lowers plasma cholesterol levels in mildly hypercholesterolemic men. *J Am Diet Assoc* 1992;92:446–449.

98. Ripsin CM, Keenan JM, Jacobs DR Jr. Oat products and lipid lowering: a meta-analysis. *JAMA* 1992;267:3317–3325.

99. Ashley FW Jr, Kannel WB. Relation of weight change to changes in atherogenic traits: the Framingham Study. *J Chron Dis* 1974;27:103–114.

100. Kannel WB, Gordon T, Castelli WP. 1979. Obesity, lipids, and glucose intolerance: the Framingham Study. *Am J Clin Nutr* 1979;32:1238–1245.

101. Garrison RJ, Wilson PW, Castelli WP, et al. Obesity and lipoprotein cholesterol in the Framingham offspring study. *Metabolism* 1980;29:1053–1060.

102. Shekelle RB, Shryock AM, Paul O, et al. Diet, serum cholesterol, and death from coronary heart disease: the Western Electric Study. *N Engl J Med* 1981;304:65–70.

103. Stamler J. Overweight, hypertension, hypercholesterolemia and coronary heart disease. In: Mananni M, Lewis B, Contaldo F, eds. *Medical complications of obesity*. New York: Academic Press, 1979:191–216.

104. Anderson JT, Lawler A, Keys A. Weight gain from simple overeating. II. Serum lipids and blood volume. *J Clin Invest* 1957;36:81–88.

105. Caggiula AW, Christakis G, Farrand M, et al. The Multiple Risk Factor Intervention Trial (MRFIT) IV. Intervention blood lipids. *Prev Med* 1981;10:443–475.

106. National Diet-Heart Study Research Group. The National Diet-Heart Study Final Report. *Circulation* 1968(Monograph);18:I-201.

107. Wolf RN, Grundy SM. Influence of weight reduction on plasma lipoproteins in obese patients. *Arteriosclerosis* 1983;3(2):160–169.

108. Lakka HM, Laaksonen DE, Lakka TA, et al. The metabolic syndrome and total and cardiovascular disease mortality in middle-aged men. *JAMA* 2002;288:2709–2716.

109. Onat A, Ceyhan K, Basar O, et al. Metabolic syndrome: major impact on coronary risk in a population with low cholesterol levels-a prospective and cross-sectional evaluation. *Atherosclerosis* 2002;165:285–292.

110. Knopp RH. Risk factors for coronary artery disease in women. *Am J Cardiol* 2002;89[Suppl 12]:28E–34E.

111. Ford ES, Giles WH, Dietz WH. Prevalence of the metabolic syndrome among US adults: findings from the third National Health and Nutrition Examination Survey. *JAMA* 2002;287:356–359.

112. Laaksonen DE, Lakka HM, Niskanen LK, et al. Metabolic syndrome and development of diabetes mellitus: application and validation of recently suggested definitions of the metabolic syndrome in a prospective cohort study. *Am J Epidemiol* 2002;156:1070–1077.

113. Jandeleit-Dahm K, Cooper ME. Hypertension and diabetes. *Curr Opin Nephrol Hypertens* 2002;11:221–228.

114. Grundy SM. Metabolic complications of obesity. *Endocrine* 2000;13:155–165.

115. McGarry JD. Banting lecture 2001. Dysregulation of fatty acid metabolism in the etiology of type 2 diabetes. *Diabetes* 2002;51:7–18.

116. Unger RH, Zhou YT. Lipotoxicity of beta-cells in obesity and in other causes of fatty acid spillover. *Diabetes* 2001;50[Suppl 1]:S118–S121.

117. Agarwal AK, Arioglu E, De Almeida S, et al. AGPAT2 is mutated in congenital generalized lipodystrophy linked to chromosome 9q34. *Nat Genet* 2002;31:21–23.

118. Cao H, Hegele RA. Nuclear lamin A/C R482Q mutation in Canadian kindreds with Dunningan-type familial partial lipodystrophy. *Hum Mol Genet* 2000;9:109–112.

119. Garg A, Vinaitheerthan M, Weatherall PT, et al. Phenotypic heterogeneity in patients with familial partial lipodystrophy (dunningan variety) related to the site of missense mutations in lamin a/c gene. *J Clin Endocrinol Metab* 2001;86:59–65.

120. Agarwal AK, Garg A. A novel heterozygous mutation in peroxisome proliferator-activated receptor-gamma gene in a patient with familial partial lipodystrophy. *J Clin Endocrinol Metab* 2002;87:408–411.

121. Chen D, Misra A, Garg A. Clinical review 153: lipodystrophy in human immunodeficiency virus-infected patients. *J Clin Endocrinol Metab* 2002;87:4845–4856.

122. Abate N, Garg A, Peshock RM, et al. Relationships of generalized and regional adiposity to insulin sensitivity in men. *J Clin Invest* 1995;96:88–98.

123. Chandalia M, Abate N, Garg A, et al. Relationship between generalized and upper body obesity to insulin resistance in Asian Indian men. *J Clin Endocrinol Metab* 1999;84:2329–2335.

124. Gambineri A, Pelusi C, Vicennati V, et al. Obesity and the polycystic ovary syndrome. *Int J Obes Relat Metab Disord* 2002;26:883–896.

125. Mostaza JM, Vega GL, Snell P, et al. Abnormal metabolism of free fatty acids in hypertriglyceridaemic men: apparent insulin resistance of adipose tissue. *J Intern Med* 1998;243:265–274.

126. Prin JB. Adipose tissue as an endocrine organ. *Best Pract Res Clin Endocrinol Metab* 2002;16:639–651.

127. Perseghin G, Price TB, Petersen KF, et al. Increased glucose transport-phosphorylation and muscle glycogen synthesis after exercise training in insulin-resistant subject. *N Engl J Med* 1996;335:1357–1362.

128. Koutsari C, Karpe F, Humphreys SM, et al. Exercise prevents the accumulation of triglyceride-rich lipoproteins and their remnants seen when changing to a high-carbohydrate diet. *Arterioscler Thromb Vasc Biol* 2001;21:1520–1525.

129. Wood PD, Stefanick ML, Williams PT, et al. The effects of plasma lipoproteins of a prudent weight-reducing diet, with or without exercise, in overweight men and women. *N Engl J Med* 1991;325:461–466.

130. Church TS, Barlow CE, Earnest CP, et al. Associations between cardiorespiratory fitness and C-reactive protein in men. *Arterioscler Thromb Vasc Biol* 2002;22:1869–1876.

131. Ford ES. Does exercise reduce inflammation? Physical activity and C-reactive protein among U.S. adults. *Epidemiology* 2002;13:561–568.

132. Gardner AW, Killewich LA. Association between physical activity and endogenous fibrinolysis in peripheral arterial disease: a cross-sectional study. *Angiology* 2002;53:367–374.

133. Koenig W, Ernst N. Exercise and thrombosis. *Coron Artery Dis* 2000;11:123–127.

134. Garg A, Grundy SM, Unger RH. Comparison of effects of high and low carbohydrate diets on plasma lipoproteins and insulin sensitivity in patients with mild NIDDM. *Diabetes* 1992;41:1278–1285.

135. Garg A, Bantel JP, Henry RR, et al. Effects of varying carbohydrate content of diet in patients with noninusulin dependent diabetes mellitus. *JAMA* 1994;271:1421–1428.

136. McKeigue PM, Shah B, Marmot MG. Relation of central obesity and insulin resistance with high diabetes prevalence and cardiovascular risk in South Asians. *Lancet* 1991;337:382–386.

137. Hughes K, Aw TC, Kuperan P, et al. Central obesity, insulin resistance, syndrome X, lipoprotein(a), and cardiovascular risk in Indians, Malays, and Chinese in Singapore. *J Epidem Comm Health* 1997;51:394–399.

138. Perseghin G, Ghosh S, Gerow K, et al. Metabolic defects in lean nondiabetic offspring on NIDDM parents: a cross-sectional study. *Diabetes* 1997;46:1001–1009.

139. Mahley RW, Huang Y, Rall SC Jr. Pathogenesis of type III hyperlipoproteinemia (dysbetalipoproteinemia). Questions, quandaries, and paradoxes. *J Lipid Res* 1999;40:1933–1949.

140. Laws A, Stefanick ML, Reaven GM. Insulin resistance and hypertriglyceridemia in nondiabetic relatives of patients with noninsulin-dependent diabetes mellitus. *J Clin Endocrinol Metab* 1989;69:343–347.

141. van der Kallen CJ, Voors-Pette C, Bouwman FG, et al. Evidence of insulin resistant lipid metabolism in adipose tissue in familial combined hyperlipidemia, but not type 2 diabetes mellitus. *Atherosclerosis* 2002;164:337–346.

142. Kang HS, Gutin B, Barbeau P, et al. Low-density lipoprotein particle size, central obesity, cardiovascular fitness, and insulin resistance syndrome markers in obese youths. *Int J Obes Relat Metab Disord* 2002;26:1030–1035.

143. Austin MA, Krauss RM. Genetic control of low density lipoprotein subclasses. *Lancet* 1986;I:592–595.

144. Karhapaa P, Malkki M, Laakso M. Isolated low HDL cholesterol. An insulin-resistance state. *Diabetes* 1994;43:411–417.

145. Blades B, Vega GL, Grundy SM. Activities of lipoprotein lipase and hepatic triglyceride lipase in postheparin plasma of patients with low concentrations of HDL cholesterol. *Arterioscler Thromb* 1993;13:1227–1235.

146. Lind L, Berne C, Lithell H. Prevalence of insulin resistance in essential hypertension. *J Hypertens* 1995;13(12 Pt 1):1457–1462.

147. Strazzullo P, Barbato A, Vuotto P, et al. Relationships between salt sensitivity of blood pressure and sympathetic nervous system activity: a short review of evidence. *Clin Exp Hypertens* 2001;23(1–2):25–33.

148. Hall JE. Pathophysiology of obesity hypertension. *Curr Hypertens Rep* 2000;2:139–147.

149. Reaven GM. Banting lecture 1988. Role of insulin resistance in human disease. *Diabetes* 1988;37:1595–1607.

150. DeFronzo RA, Ferrannini E. Insulin resistance: a multifaceted syndrome responsible for NIDDM, obesity, hypertension, dyslipidemia and atherosclerotic cardiovascular disease. *Diabetes Care* 1991;14:173–194.

151. Grundy SM. Is insulin resistance an independent risk factor for coronary heart disease? In: Fletcher GF, Grundy SM, Hayman LL, eds. *Obesity: impact on cardiovascular disease.* Armonk, NY: Futura Publishing, 1999:169–188.

152. Goldfine ID, Maddux BA, Youngren JF, et al. Role of PC-1 in the etiology of insulin resistance. *Ann NY Acad Sci* 1999;892:204–222.

153. Le Fur S, Le Stunff C, Bougneres P. Increased insulin resistance in obese children who have both 972 IRS-1 and 1057 IRS-2 polymorphisms. *Diabetes* 2002;51[Suppl 3]:S304–S307.

154. Frohlich M, Imhof A, Berg G, et al. Association between C-reactive protein and features of the metabolic syndrome: a population-based study. *Diabetes Care* 2000;23:1835–1839.

155. Straczkowski M, Dzienis-Straczkowska S, Stepien A, et al. Plasma interleukin-8 concentrations are increased in obese subjects and related to fat mass and tumor necrosis factor-alpha system. *J Clin Endocrinol Metab* 2002;87:4602–4606.

156. Festa A, D'Agostino R Jr, Tracy RP, et al, The Insulin Resistance Atherosclerosis Study. Elevated levels of acute-phase proteins and plasminogen activator inhibitor-1 predict the development of type 2 diabetes: the insulin resistance atherosclerosis study. *Diabetes* 2002;51:1131–1137.

157. Bastelica D, Morange P, Berthet B, et al. Stromal cells are the main plasminogen activator inhibitor-1-producing cells in human fat: evidence of differences between visceral and subcutaneous deposits. *Arterioscler Thromb Vasc Biol* 2002;22:173–178.

158. World Health Organization Department of Noncommunicable Disease Surveillance. *Definition, diagnosis, and classification of diabetes mellitus and its complications: report of a WHO consultation.* Geneva: World Health Organization, 1999.

159. US Department of Agriculture and US Department of Health and Human Services. Nutrition and your health: dietary guidelines for Americans, 5th edition. Home and Garden Bulletin no. 232. Washington: US Department of Agriculture, 2000;44 pages.

160. Clinical Guidelines on the Identification, Evaluation, and Treatment of Overweight and Obesity in Adults—The Evidence Report. National Institutes of Health. *Obes Res* 1998;6[Suppl 2]:51S–209S.

161. Brolin RE. Bariatric surgery and long-term control of morbid obesity. *JAMA* 2002;288:2793–2796.

CHAPTER 5

Genetic Dyslipoproteinemias

H. Bryan Brewer, Jr., Silvia Santamarina-Fojo, and Robert D. Shamburek

Key Words: Apolipoproteins; dysbetalipoproteinemia; dyslipoproteinemia; familial hypercholesterolemia; hepatic lipase; hypoalphalipoproteinemia; lipoprotein lipase; Tangier disease.

INTRODUCTION

Plasma lipids are transported by lipoproteins composed of several classes of lipids and proteins designated apolipoproteins. There are six major classes of human plasma lipoproteins: chylomicrons, very low-density lipoproteins (VLDLs), intermediate-density lipoproteins (IDLs), low-density lipoproteins (LDLs), high-density lipoproteins (HDLs), and lipoprotein(a) [Lp(a)] (1–4). HDLs can be further separated by hydrated density into HDL_2 and HDL_3. Over the last two decades the roles

H. B. Brewer, Jr.: Molecular Disease Branch, National Heart, Lung & Blood Institute, National Institutes of Health, Building 10, Room 7N115, 10 Center Drive MSC 1666, Bethesda, Maryland 20892-1666.
S. Santamarina-Fojo: Molecular Disease Branch, NIH/National Heart, Lung, and Blood Institute, Bethesda, Maryland 20892.
R. D. Shamburek: Molecular Disease Branch, NIH/National Heart, Lung, and Blood Institute, Bethesda, Maryland 20892.

of apolipoproteins, enzymes, lipoprotein receptors, and transfer proteins in lipoprotein metabolism have been elucidated, and this new information provides a conceptual framework for understanding lipid transport in healthy individuals and in patients with the genetic dyslipoproteinemias.

LIPOPROTEIN METABOLISM

On the basis of current information, the metabolism of the human plasma lipoproteins can be conceptually separated into two separate pathways: One pathway is composed of the apolipoprotein B (apoB)-containing lipoproteins (chylomicrons, VLDLs, IDLs, and LDLs), and the second pathway involves HDL. Schematic overviews of the two metabolic pathways for lipoprotein biosynthesis, transport, and catabolism in healthy subjects are illustrated in Figures 5–1 and 5–2.

Apolipoprotein B-Lipoprotein Metabolic Pathways

The metabolism of the plasma lipoproteins containing the B apolipoproteins, apoB-48 and apoB-100, consists of two separate pathways (3–7). The first apoB pathway involves the stepwise delipidation of triglyceride-rich chylomicron parti-

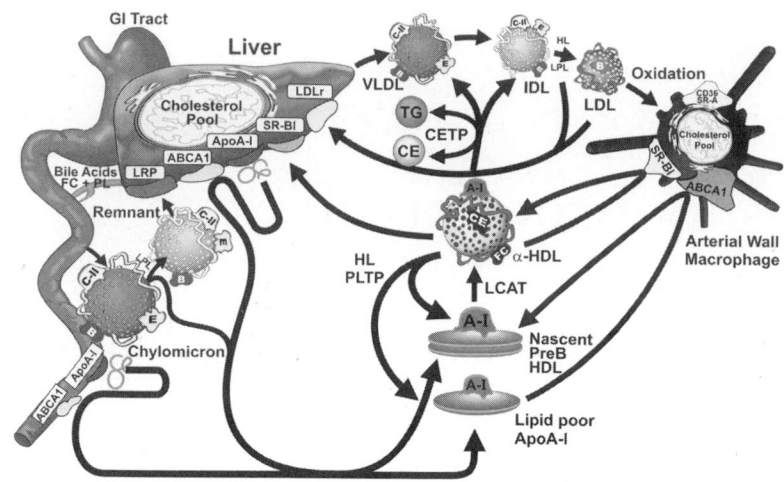

FIG. 5–1. Schematic overview of the metabolic pathways of the apolipoprotein B (apoB)-containing lipoprotein particles including chylomicrons, very low-density lipoproteins (VLDLs), intermediate-density lipoproteins (IDLs), and low-density lipoproteins (LDL). The "intestinal apoB cascade" involves the metabolism of triglyceride-rich chylomicrons secreted from the intestine. Chylomicron triglycerides undergo hydrolysis by lipoprotein lipase and chylomicrons remnant particles are formed that have an initial hydrated density of VLDL and finally IDL. The small chylomicron remnants are removed from the plasma and taken up by the liver through LRP and the LDL receptors. The "hepatic apoB cascade" involves the metabolic conversion of triglyceride rich VLDL secreted by the liver. VLDL triglycerides are also hydrolyzed by lipoprotein lipase and remnants undergo stepwise delipidation with the formation of particles with a hydrated density of IDL and finally LDL. VLDL remnants are cleared from the plasma by interacting with the LDL receptor-related protein (LRP) and LDL receptors. Plasma LDL are catabolized primarily by uptake by the LDL receptor that initiates receptor-mediated endocytosis and LDL degradation. LDL may also undergo oxidation and the modified LDL is taken up by the scavenger receptors, CD36 and SRA, resulting in lipid accumulation in macrophages. Cholesterol is removed by HDL in the process termed reverse cholesterol transport in which nascent HDL containing apoA-I interacts with the adenosine triphosphate-binding cassette transporter A1 (ABCA1) facilitating the removal of excess cellular cholesterol. The hepatic SR-BI receptor selectively removes cholesterol and cholesteryl esters from both HDLs and IDLs/LDLs without intracellular uptake and degradation of the lipoprotein particles. Thus, the ABC1 transporter and SR-BI receptor are key receptors in the reverse cholesterol transport pathway. LCAT, lecithin-cholesterol acyltransferase.

cles containing apoB-48, which transport dietary cholesterol and triglycerides from the intestine to peripheral tissues and finally to the liver. After secretion, chylomicrons acquire two apolipoproteins, apoE and apoC-II, present on HDL. apoC-II activates the lipolytic enzyme lipoprotein lipase (LPL), which is attached to the capillary endothelium. Activation of LPL results in triglyceride hydrolysis and remodeling of the triglyceride-rich lipoprotein particles. Concomitant with the hydrolysis of triglycerides, apolipoproteins and lipid constituents are transferred from chylomicrons to HDL. With lipolysis the chylomicrons are converted to small chylomicron remnants with a hydrated density of initially VLDLs and then IDLs.

The second apoB pathway involves triglyceride-rich VLDLs containing apoB-100 secreted by the liver. apoC-II and apoE dissociate from HDL and reassociate with the hepatogenous triglyceride-rich VLDLs secreted from the liver. apoC-II activates LPL, as outlined earlier, and VLDLs are serially converted to VLDL remnants, IDL, and finally LDL. Hepatic lipase (HL), a second lipolytic enzyme, and apoE have been proposed to be required for

the efficient conversion of IDL to LDL. HL plays an important role in lipoprotein metabolism as both a phospholipase and triacylglycerol hydrolase. During the metabolic conversion of VLDL to LDL, approximately 50% of VLDL remnants and IDL are removed from the plasma by the liver.

Remnants of both the chylomicron and VLDL pathways have been proposed to be removed from the plasma primarily by the interaction of either apoE or apoB-100 with the hepatic remnant or LDL receptors. The LDL receptor has been extensively characterized, and two apolipoproteins on the triglyceride remnants, apoB-100 and apoE, serve as ligands for the LDL receptor (8,9). Several genetic and physiologic studies in mice have confirmed a function of LDL receptor-related protein (LRP), together with the LDL receptor, in hepatic remnant metabolism (10–12). The LRP is a glycosylated 600-kD protein that belongs to an ancient family of endocytic receptors that include the LDL receptor (13–18). LRP binds not only apoE, chylomicrons remnants, and lipases, but also multiple other ligands that include pro-

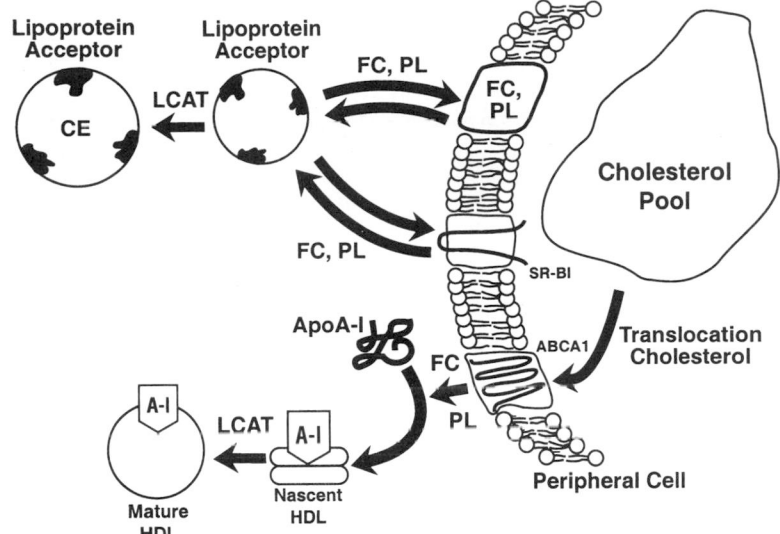

FIG. 5–2. Schematic model of the three primary pathways for the removal of excess cholesterol from peripheral cells. Nascent high-density lipoprotein (HDL)–containing apolipoprotein A-I (apoA-I) facilitates cholesterol efflux from the cell through an interaction with the adenosine triphosphate-binding cassette transporter A1 (ABCA1). Net excess cellular cholesterol also is removed by passive diffusion process to lipoproteins including HDL and low-density lipoprotein (LDL). A third pathway for cholesterol efflux involves the interaction of lipoproteins with SR-BI, which facilitates the removal of free cholesterol from the cell.

teinases, proteinase–inhibitor complexes, extracellular matrix proteins, bacterial toxins, viruses, and various intracellular proteins (13–18). Thus, in addition to serving as a receptor for remnant lipoproteins, LRP may have a major role as a multifunctional scavenger receptor protein.

LDL, the final lipoprotein in the VLDL cascade, contains virtually only apoB-100 and interacts primarily with the LDL receptor present on the plasma membrane of the liver (Fig. 5–1). In addition, LDL interacts with the LDL receptor on peripheral cells, including adrenal, fibroblasts, and smooth muscle cells (8,9,18). The interaction of LDL with the LDL receptor initiates receptor-mediated endocytosis and transport of LDL to intracellular lysosomes, where the protein moiety is degraded and cholesteryl esters are hydrolyzed to free cholesterol, which are then transferred to the intracellular cholesterol pool. An additional pathway for LDL metabolism is the uptake by macrophages with the formation of foam cells in the arterial wall. Native LDL is not readily taken up by macrophages. However, oxidative modification of LDL results in markedly enhanced LDL uptake by the scavenger receptor on macrophages with foam cell formation (19–23). Oxidative modifications of LDL were observed after *in vitro* incubation with endothelial cells, smooth muscle cells, and macrophages, or after modification with malondialdehyde. Studies have indicated that oxidized lipids within LDL may play an important role in the pathophysiology of the atherosclerotic lesion by stimulating the secretion of cytokines and other factors that modulate endothelial cell function and facilitate the recruitment of plasma monocytes into the vessel wall (19–23). On the basis of current data, it has been proposed that oxidative modification of LDL may be a prerequisite for the macrophage uptake of LDL, foam cell formation, and the development of the atherosclerotic lesion.

High-Density-Lipoprotein Metabolism

An important role of HDL in lipoprotein metabolism is to transport cholesterol from peripheral tissues back to the liver, where it is removed from the body after conversion to bile acids or as biliary cholesterol. This hypothetical process is termed reverse cholesterol transport (24,25). Three major pathways for the removal or efflux of cholesterol from peripheral cells are summarized in Figure 5–2. Nascent HDL, composed primarily of apo-A-I phospholipid discs, are secreted from both the human intestine and the liver. Nascent HDLs acquire excess cholesterol from tissues, a process facilitated by the adenosine triphosphate (ATP)-binding cassette transporter A1 (ABCA1) (Fig. 5–3) (26–32), and the enzyme lecithin-cholesterol acyltransferase (LCAT) catalyzes the esterification of plasma lipoprotein cholesterol to cholesteryl esters. With the formation of cholesteryl esters, the nascent HDLs are converted to spherical lipoproteins with a hydrated density of HDL_3. HDL_3 are converted to the larger HDL_2 by the acquisition of apolipoproteins and lipids released during the stepwise delipidation and remodeling of the triglyceride-rich chylomicrons and VLDLs, as well as by the esterification of the cholesterol removed from peripheral tissues. Excess intracellular cholesterol also is removed by passive diffusion to lipoprotein acceptors including mature

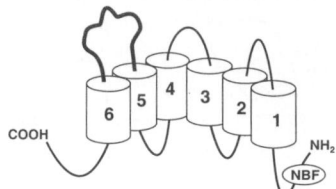 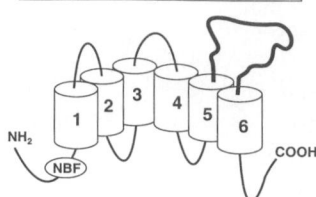

FIG. 5–3. Schematic model of the adenosine triphosphate-binding cassette transporter A1 (ABCA1) transporter that facilitates cholesterol efflux and is defective in Tangier disease.

HDLs and LDLs (33) (Fig. 5–2). The third pathway for cholesterol removal involves the efflux of cholesterol to lipoprotein acceptors facilitated by the SR-BI receptors (34,35). Thus, three separate pathways modulate the efflux of excess cellular cholesterol Fig. 5–2).

Mature HDL transfers the cholesterol removed from the peripheral tissues to the liver. HDL_2 are converted back to HDL_3 by HL through the removal of phospholipids and triglycerides and the generation of nascent apoA-I HDLs (6,7,20,36–38). The cycle of uptake of cholesterol from the peripheral tissues and then transport of cholesterol to the liver is repeated. An additional pathway for transport of cholesterol to the liver is the transfer of cholesteryl esters in HDL to VLDL, IDL, and LDL by the cholesteryl ester transfer protein (CETP), with ultimate transfer of cholesterol to the liver by the apoB-containing lipoproteins (6,7,39,40).

Lipoprotein(a)

Lipoprotein(a), a cholesterol-rich atherogenic lipoprotein that closely resembles LDLs in lipid composition, has a hydrated density intermediate between LDLs and HDLs. The protein moiety of Lp(a) consists of apoB-100 and a unique apolipoprotein, designated apolipoprotein(a) [Apo(a)] (41–44). Apo(a) is linked by a single disulfide bridge to apoB-100 on LDLs to form Lp(a). Apo(a) is a large glycoprotein ranging in size from 400 to 700 kD. The amino acid sequence of Apo(a) is similar to the sequence of plasminogen and contains cysteine-rich domains of 80 to 114 amino acids in length termed kringles (41–44). Apo(a) contains a variable number of copies of kringle IV and a single copy of kringle V, followed by the protease domain of plasminogen (45). In contrast to plasminogen, Apo(a) has no serine protease enzymic activity, and it cannot be converted to an active plasmin-like enzyme by tissue plasminogen activator, streptokinase, or urokinase. Current data suggest that Apo(a) is synthesized and directly secreted into plasma independent of the biosynthetic pathways of the apoB-containing lipoproteins.

Plasma Lp(a) levels range from less than 1 to greater than 100 mg/dL. Of clinical importance is the correlation of the size of the Apo(a) isoprotein and the plasma Lp(a) levels (46). The different molecular weights of Lp(a) in human plasma are because of a variable number of copies of kringle

IV in the amino acid sequence of Apo(a) (47,48). Lp(a) isoproteins of greater and smaller molecular weights are associated with smaller and greater plasma concentrations, respectively. The molecular size and plasma levels of Lp(a) are inheritable. Approximately 20% of the population has

TABLE 5–1. *Known molecular defects in patients with genetic dyslipoproteinemias*

Disease	Genetic defect
Hyperlipoproteinemias	
Familial hypercholesterolemia	LDL receptor
Familial defective apolipoprotein B-100	Apolipoprotein B
Familial combined hyperlipidemia	Unknown
Familial dysbetalipoproteinemia	Apolipoprotein E
Familial autosomal-dominant hypercholesterolemia	PCSK9
ARH	ARH
Hypertriglyceridemia-low-HDL syndrome	Probably polygenic
Familial hyperchylomicronemia	
Apolipoprotein C-II deficiency	Apolipoprotein C-II
Lipoprotein lipase deficiency	Lipoprotein lipase
Hepatic lipase deficiency	Hepatic lipase
Increased lipoprotein(a)	Unknown
Sitosterolemia	ABCG5 and ABCG8
Hypoalphalipoproteinemias	
Tangier disease	ABCA1
Apolipoprotein A-I deficiency	Apolipoprotein A-I
Familial hypoalphalipoproteinemia	Unknown
LCAT deficiency/Fish Eye	LCAT deficiency
Hypobetalipoproteinemias	
Abetalipoproteinemia	Microsomal Transfer Protein
Hypobetalipoproteinemia	Apolipoprotein B
Chylomicron retention disease	SARA2
Hyperalphalipoproteinemias	
CETP deficiency	CETP deficiency

Twenty percent of the population has lipoprotein(a) greater than 30 mg/dL, which is associated with an increased risk for premature cardiovascular disease.

ABCA1, adenosine triphosphate-binding cassette transporter A1; ABCG5, adenosine triphosphate-binding cassette transporter G5; ABCG8, adenosine triphosphate-binding cassette transporter G8; ARH, autosomal-recessive hypercholesterolemia; CETP, cholesteryl ester transfer protein; HDL, high-density lipoprotein; LCAT, lecithin-cholesterol acyltransferase; LDL, low-density lipoprotein.

levels greater than 30 mg/dL, which is associated with a twofold increase in the relative risk for premature cardiovascular disease (41,49–55). The mechanism(s) by which increased plasma levels of Lp(a) increase the risk for premature heart disease has not been definitively ascertained. Lp(a) may be taken up by macrophages resulting in cholesterol deposition and foam cell formation. Alternatively, its atherogenic properties may be related to its role in increasing thrombosis. Lp(a) has been reported to interact with fibrin peptides, inhibit thrombolysis, and be a competitive inhibitor of plasminogen for the plasminogen receptor present on endothelial cells (41,49–55). Individuals with increased plasma Lp(a) levels have no diagnostic clinical features, and subjects with relatively normal total cholesterol levels may have increased plasma levels of Lp(a), which increase the risk for premature heart disease. The precise physiologic function(s) of Lp(a) in lipoprotein metabolism remains to be established.

The rapid expansion of our knowledge of the pathways for lipoprotein metabolism has permitted the classification of the molecular defects in patients with the genetic dyslipoproteinemias into defects in either lipoprotein receptors, apolipoproteins, enzymes, or transfer proteins. The major genetic dyslipoproteinemias currently identified are summarized in Table 5–1. Each of these genetic dyslipoproteinemias has characteristic clinical features and lipoprotein profiles and are summarized in this chapter.

HYPERLIPOPROTEINEMIAS

Familial Hypercholesterolemia

The elucidation of the molecular defect in familial hypercholesterolemia (FH) has provided an understanding of the role of receptor-mediated endocytosis in lipoprotein metabolism, the importance of phenotypic heterogeneity in the expression of genetic diseases, and the development of therapies that can halt the progression of atherothrombosis.

Young adults with homozygous FH have total and LDL cholesterol concentrations fourfold to sevenfold greater than normal and a constellation of physical findings that bring them to medical attention. The raised, yellowish beige, rugous xanthomas on the knuckles and in the interdigital web of the fingers (Fig. 5–4) often are the initial manifestation of the disease. By the ages of 5 to 12 years, the other stigmatas, including arcus cornea, tuberous xanthomas, and planar xanthomas, appear. Histologic analysis reveals that these xanthomas are from cells derived from the deposition of LDL-derived lipid in monocyte-macrophages (18,56). Lipid deposition is a key component of the atherosclerotic lesion in the arterial wall. The lesions in the coronary arteries are readily detectable by coronary angiography. The premature atherothrombosis in FH, as well as lesions not detectable by angiography, can now be detected noninvasively by electron beam tomography. (Electron beam tomography was previously termed ultrafast computed tomography [CT].) In contrast to conventional CT, the x-rays scans are generated by a beam of electrons that are focused by a magnet, analogous to that used in standard television cathode-ray tubes. This permits the acquisition of images within 50 to 100 msec. This fast focusing is then gated to the electrocardiogram, and the heart can be imaged in a freeze-frame, stroboscopic manner. This permits fine resolution of all of the structures of the mediastinum, including the coronary arteries. In addition to the coronary artery lesions observed by angiography, this new method can both detect and quantitate the calcific atherothrombosis in the coronary ostia and the ascending aortic root. The severity of calcific atherothrombosis is highly correlated with both the severity of the hypercholesterolemia and the duration of exposure of the endothelium to the high concentrations of LDL particles (57). This formulation has led to the concept of the cholesterol-year score (58), which parallels the cigarette pack-year score for assessing the risk for pulmonary disease.

The human LDL receptor gene is located on chromosome 1 (59) and is 45.5 kb in length. The gene contains 18 exons ranging in size from 78 to 2,535 nucleotides, which are separated by 17 introns (60). The single-chain nascent protein has a molecular weight of 93 kD, and the glycosylated receptor has an apparent molecular weight of 164 kD by sodium dodecyl sulfate–polyacrylamide gel electrophoresis (61,62). The deduced protein structure of the LDL receptors from several species suggests several functional domains (18,63) (Fig. 5–5). The LDL receptor is an acidic protein (Pi = 4.6) that contain 839 amino acids, and cysteine residues comprise 15% of the 322 amino-terminal residues. In the amino-terminal domain there are seven 40-amino acid, cysteine-rich repeated cassettes (18,63). Deletion of one or more of the seven 40-amino acid, cysteine-rich repeats abolishes binding of LDL to the LDL receptor (64). In addition to the cysteine-rich, ligand-binding domain, the LDL receptor contains four other domains. The second 350-amino acid domain initially resides on the extracellular side of the plasma membrane and contains a high degree of homology with the epidermal growth factor (EGF) precursor (62). The EGF precursor homology domain contains a six-bladed _-propeller region involved in the delivery and intracellular ligand release of LDL (65). In the acidic environment of the endosome, the LDL-receptor ligand releases LDL, allowing recycling of the receptor when the _-propeller of the EGF precursor folds back on itself (63). The third domain is rich in serine and threonine residues, which are glycosylation sites, the fourth domain consists of 22 hydrophobic amino acid residues that span the plasma membrane, and the fifth domain, a 50-amino acid carboxyl-terminus domain, is important for the cellular metabolism of the LDL receptor (Fig. 5–5).

The study of skin fibroblasts from patients with FII provided the first insight into the abnormalities in cellular cholesterol metabolism. In contrast to fibroblasts from normolipidemic control subjects, cells from patients with FH did not down-regulate endogenous cholesterol biosynthesis

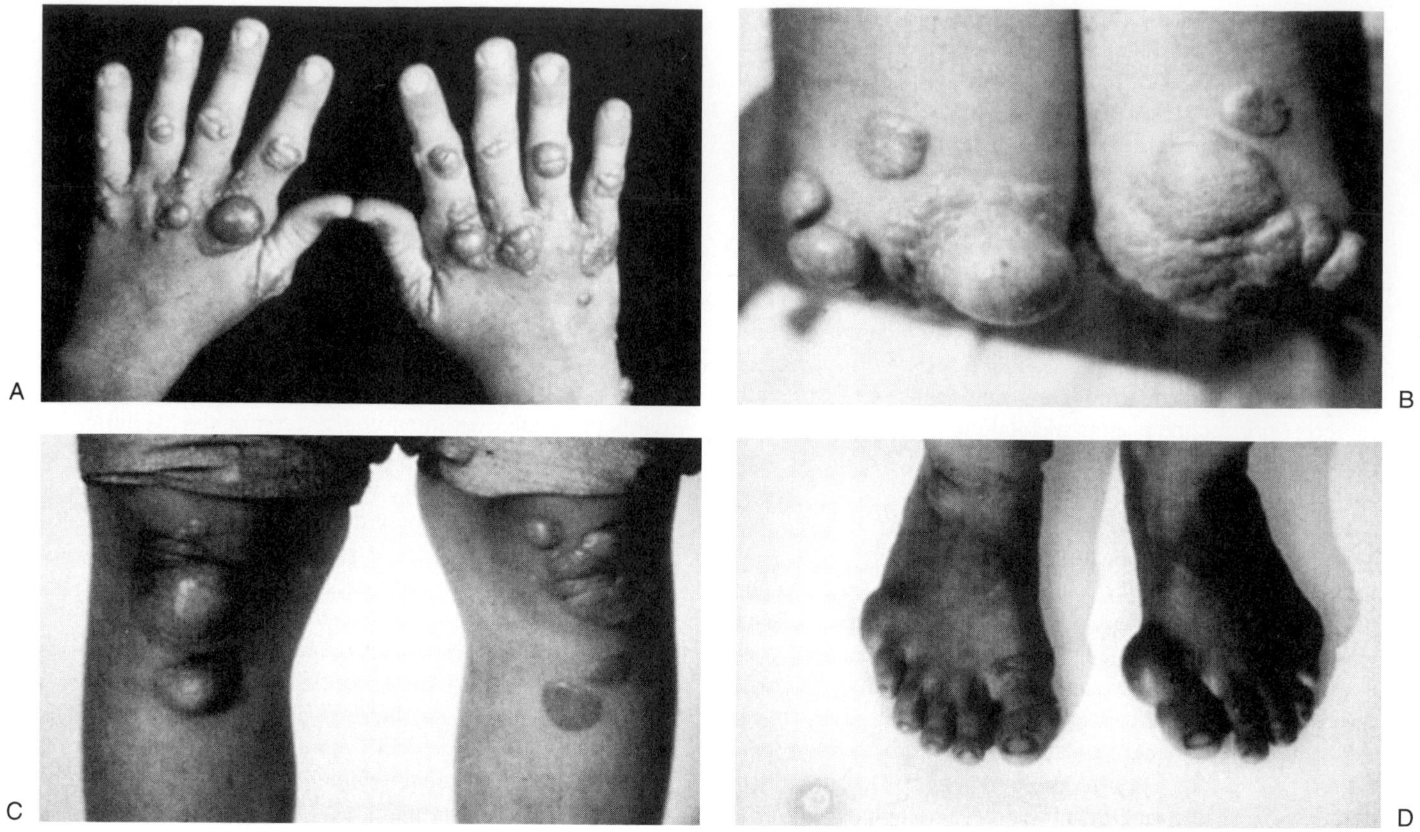

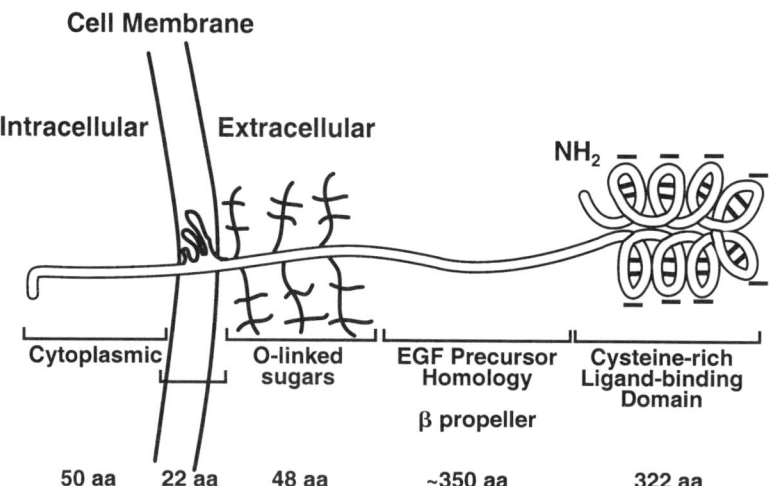

FIG. 5–4. Clinical features of patients with homozygous familial hypercholesterolemia include tendon and cutaneous xanthomas.

in the presence of LDL (66). This cellular defect was shown to be caused by mutations in the gene encoding for cell surface LDL receptors, which resulted in the inability of the LDL-derived cholesterol to enter the cell and undergo lysosomal degradation (67).

Since the initial studies, more than 900 different mutations in the LDL receptor have been characterized that result in FH (18,63,68). Point mutations, as well as insertional and deletional mutations, have been reported, and these mutations can be classified on the basis of the aberrant function

FIG. 5–5. Schematic representation of the structural features of the low-density lipoprotein (LDL) receptor. The proposed protein structural domains were determined by analysis of the amino acid *(aa)* sequence derived from the determination of the LDL receptor complementary DNA structure. EGF, epidermal growth factor.

of the cellular metabolism of the LDL receptor. Class 1 mutations lead to the failure to synthesize the LDL receptor protein, whereas class 2 mutations lead to the synthesis of an LDL receptor that cannot be effectively transported from the endoplasmic reticulum to the cell surface. Class 2a mutations lead to a complete block in transport, whereas class 2b mutations lead to a partial block in transport. In the case of class 3 mutations, the LDL receptor reaches the cell surface but cannot bind normally to LDL. The inability of LDL receptors to cluster into coated pits derives from mutations designated as class 4. Finally, the normal life cycle of LDL receptors involves the uptake of the membrane-bound receptor by endocytosis and the recycling of the internalized LDL receptors back to the plasma membrane. Mutations that lead to receptors that cannot be normally recycled are termed class 5 mutations.

Heterozygotes for FH have increased LDL cholesterol concentrations and a fourfold to sixfold increased risk for premature cardiovascular disease; furthermore, by age 39 years, 90% of patients with heterozygous FH have detectable tendon xanthomas (Fig. 5–6). The heterozygotes have one normal allele, and therapy can be effective in reducing the concentration of LDL by up-regulating the activity of the normal LDL receptors. The hepatocyte is the principal cell type expressing LDL receptors (18,69). Use of bile acid sequestrants and inhibitors of 3-hydroxy-3-methylglutaryl coenzyme A (HMG-CoA) reductase can effectively increase the expression of hepatic LDL receptors. Combined, these drugs are additive in both expressing LDL receptors and in reducing the concentration of plasma LDL cholesterol. Diet plus a combination of niacin, an inhibitor of HMG-CoA reductase, and a bile acid sequestrant can reduce the total and LDL-cholesterol concentrations in heterozygous FH by 35% to 50% (70–72). Ezetimibe, a newly available cholesterol absorption inhibitor, has an additive effect with a HMG-CoA reductase inhibitor in decreasing cholesterol. Ezetimibe is absorbed and binds to the brush border of enterocytes inhibiting a putative intestinal cholesterol transporter (73). Although the majority of patients have a substantial improvement in their plasma lipoprotein concentrations with drugs, a large fraction of these patients do not achieve the goal LDL-cholesterol concentrations outlined by the Adult Treatment Panel of the National Cholesterol Education Program (74). These therapies can retard the progression of atherogenesis and even reduce cardiovascular and all-cause mortality rates, as shown in the initial 4S clinical trial (75); however, even more aggressive measures may be required to halt, as well as reverse, the atherosclerotic process. A variety of techniques have been used to remove atherogenic lipoproteins from patients heterozygous for FH. Plasma exchange, heparin extracorporeal lipoprotein precipitation, and dextran-sulfate LDL adsorption are all effective in reducing LDL-cholesterol con-

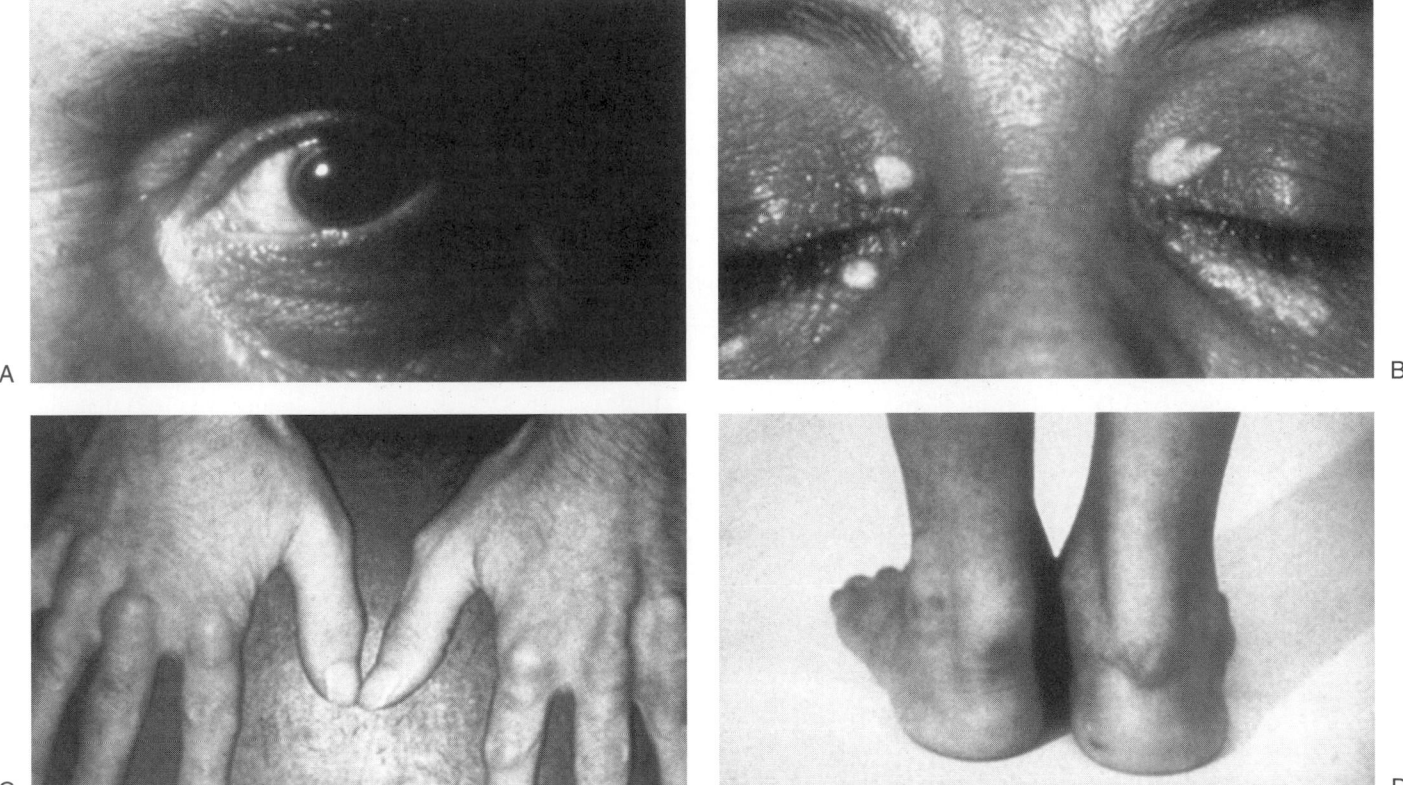

FIG. 5–6. Clinical features of heterozygotes with familial hypercholesterolemia include arcus (A), xanthelasma (B), and tendon xanthomas (C and D).

centrations and affecting the angiographic progression of coronary artery disease (CAD) (76). The use of LDL apheresis is being advocated as a useful adjunct to diet and pharmacologic therapy in treating patients with heterozygous FH with established CAD (76,77).

Individuals inheriting mutant LDL receptor genes in both alleles are either homozygous for the same mutation or are termed compound heterozygotes. A founder effect has been observed in unique populations such as in Quebec, Canada and in South Africa, where virtually all of the patients with FH have the same mutation. In these regions, there is a high likelihood that patients with total cholesterol concentrations greater than 600 mg/dL and classical xanthomas are true homozygotes. In contrast, in more outbred populations and in the absence of consanguinity, there is a greater likelihood that patients with FH are compound heterozygotes. Rather than the specific mutation, the residual activity of the LDL receptors in both true homozygotes and compound heterozygotes is the major determinant of the severity of the atherosclerotic process. Fibroblast LDL-receptor activity correlates with plasma LDL-cholesterol concentration and with the response to dietary and drug therapy (78). A variety of dietary and pharmacologic interventions have been tested in patients with homozygous FH. The addition of ezetimibe to a high-dose HMG-CoA reductase inhibitor further reduces LDL-C by 14% to 20% (73). In addition, more aggressive and experimental therapies such as partial ileal bypass, portacaval shunt, plasma exchange (79,80), or apheresis using dextran-sulfate adsorption (81,82), heparin precipitation (83), or immunosorption (84,85), and liver transplantation (86–88) have all been used to prevent the cardiovascular sequelae of this disease. An additional approach to replacing the hepatic LDL receptors is *ex vivo* gene therapy (89,90). Hepatocytes isolated from homozygous patients with FH have been cultured, transformed by retroviral infection, selected for transformation, and reinfused into the portal circulation. This therapy appears to have been successful in reducing the total and LDL-cholesterol concentrations in the plasma of an animal model for FH, the Watanabe heritable hyperlipidemic rabbit (91,92). Currently, the removal of LDL particles by either plasma exchange or LDL apheresis is the treatment of choice for homozygous FH. LDL apheresis is preferable because it removes only the atherogenic lipoprotein particles. With these apheresis techniques there is not only a profound reduction in LDL-cholesterol concentrations, there also is regression of the skin xanthomas, stabilization of the coronary atherothrombosis, and even regression of substantial, flow-limiting coronary artery lesions (18,81).

Familial Defective Apolipoprotein B-100

In addition to genetic defects in the LDL receptor, structural mutations in the ligand-binding domain of apoB-100 also can lead to hypercholesterolemia and xanthomatosis. Hy-

percholesterolemia occurs in familial defective apoB-100 (FDB) because the abnormal LDL binds poorly to LDL receptors. The metabolic defect in FDB is reduced clearance of autologous LDL compared with LDL from normolipidemic study subjects (93). LDL from one of these probands and from the proband's first-degree relatives had substantially reduced binding to LDL receptors expressed in normal skin fibroblasts (94). Sequence analysis of the two alleles of the *apoB* gene of a subject heterozygous for this disorder revealed a glutamine-for-arginine substitution in the codon for amino acid 3,500 (95). This same mutant allele was found in six unrelated subjects and in eight affected relatives in two of these kindreds. On the basis of these results, this disease has been designated FDB. A monoclonal antibody (96) whose epitope was within residues 3,350 and 3,506 of apoB has been isolated and characterized. This antibody, MB47, bound with a higher affinity to abnormal LDL compared with normal LDL, permitting the development of a useful assay for clinical and epidemiologic studies.

The frequency of the glutamine-for-arginine mutation in hypercholesterolemic individuals suggests a prevalence of 1:500 to 1:700 in central European populations (97,98). The mutation is rare among non-Europeans, suggesting a common ancestor. Other mutations that cause FCH are much less common but appear to alter the conformation of apoB-100 near the receptor binding site (99).

As in patients heterozygous for FH, heterozygotes for FDB also have been observed to have corneal arcus, tendon xanthomas, and premature cardiovascular disease. However, the clinical consequences of FDB tend to be less severe than heterozygotes for FH. LDL is increased in FDB but not to the same extent as in FH. Patients with FDB respond to drug therapy, but their response to specific therapy may differ from heterozygous FH. Patients with FDB appear to be more resistant to lovastatin compared with patients with heterozygous FH. At 40 mg/day lovastatin, patients with heterozygous FH had LDL-cholesterol concentrations decline by 32% compared with only a 22% decrease in patients with FDB (100). In contrast, patients with FDB appeared to respond more favorably to both niacin (FDB vs. FH, 24% vs. 14% LDL reduction) (101) and bile acid sequestrant therapy (FDB vs. FH, 32% vs. 22% LDL reduction) (102) than did patients with heterozygous FH. These data suggest that the specific molecular defect in the LDL receptor ligand pathway may have important therapeutic implications. These combined results now indicate that patients with type II hyperlipoproteinemia may have either a defect in the LDL receptor resulting in FH, or the ligand, apoB-100, for the LDL receptor leading to FDB.

Familial Combined Hyperlipidemia

Familial combined hyperlipidemia (FCHL) was originally described as one of the most common monogenetic disorders in humans, with a gene frequency assuming a single defect as great as 3 to 5 per 1,000 (103–108). FCHL accounts for 10% to 15% of myocardial infarctions in a North American and European population (4,109). The FCHL phenotype occurs in 1% of the general population and the inheritance appears more complex, suggesting both additive effects of several genes and gene–environment interactions. The clinical features of FCHL usually are expressed in the fourth and fifth decades of life. A characteristic feature of FCHL is the presence of multiple lipoprotein profiles in the proband and affected relatives. The lipoproteins that are most frequently increased are VLDLs, LDLs, or LDLs + VLDLs (lipoprotein phenotypes IV, IIa, or IIb, respectively), with small, dense LDL particles and increased apoB levels consistently present (110). Patients with FCHL have two changes in their plasma lipoproteins that can be used to establish the diagnosis of FCHL. The first is a cholesterol-rich plasma LDL containing an abnormal cholesterol-to-apoB ratio (normal, <1.3; FCH, >1.3), which is designated "dense LDL." The second is an LDL-apoB level greater than 130 mg/dL. In addition, HDL levels are frequently reduced, particularly in patients with hypertriglyceridemia. The most important clinical sequela of FCHL is the development of premature coronary heart disease, which is similar in severity and clinical course to the cardiovascular disease present in FH heterozygotes. Patients with FCHL often present with features of insulin resistance such as hyperinsulinemia, impaired glucose tolerance, and abdominal obesity. FCHL has several of the features of the metabolic syndrome and may be included as a subset of such individuals.

A subset of patients with FCHL has been identified having normal LDL cholesterol levels but increased levels of LDL apoB greater than 130 mg/dL. This syndrome, termed hyperapobetalipoproteinemia, is characterized by increased plasma levels of LDL-apoB and the presence of dense LDL in the absence of hyperlipidemia (107,108). Kinetic studies of radiolabeled VLDLs and LDLs revealed an increase in VLDL-apoB synthesis and a relatively normal rate of LDL catabolism (111,112). Of particular clinical importance is the development of premature cardiovascular disease in patients with hyperapobetalipoproteinemia. These patients can mistakenly be considered not to have a dyslipoproteinemia that requires treatment, because they may have "normal LDL-cholesterol levels."

The clinical features of patients with FCHL include arcus cornea and xanthelasma; however, tendon xanthomas are unusual. The lack of tendon xanthomas in a patient with hypercholesterolemia is a useful clinical feature to differentiate FCHL from FH.

The presumptive diagnosis of FCHL can be established only by the identification of a characteristic pattern of dyslipoproteinemia in the propositus and family members. No homozygotes for FCHL have been identified. Affected individuals in a number of kindreds with FCHL may be genetic compounds, containing two defective genes—one for FCHL and the other for another underlying genetic dyslipopro-

teinemia. The discovery of definitive genes has been hampered by the lack of standardized diagnostic inclusion and exclusion criteria, unknown mode of inheritance, and genetic heterogeneity. Both genetic and environmental factors likely affect the FCHL phenotype. Genomic scans on Finnish, Dutch, and their combined populations have identified several chromosomal areas with linkage to FCHL. The Finnish families with FCHL localized the first locus for FCHL on chromosome 1q21 (113). Genomic scans on Dutch families with FCHL detected the short arm of chromosome 11 as a possible locus, but not to the 1q21 locus (114). The combined analysis of genome scans of Finnish and Dutch families identified chromosome 16q24.1 for the low HDL trait in FCHL. Additional chromosomal regions were identified as possible sites (115). The region on chromosome 1q21 has been confirmed in U.S., German, and Chinese populations, and it is likely the strongest candidate for a gene in FCHL (116). No major gene has been identified as causing FCHL, but many genes involved in lipid metabolism have been shown to have some effect as modifiers on the FCHL phenotype. The emerging view of the complex genetic basis of FCHL is that it has a multigenic inheritance with a number of modifying genes and environmental factors influencing the phenotype.

Other Autosomal-Dominant Forms of Hypercholesterolemia

Patients with clinical features indistinguishable from FH and FDB but whose disease does not segregate with either the LDL receptor or apoB have been reported (117,118). Mutations in the PCSK9 gene, which encodes a neural apoptosis-regulated convertase, a member of the proteinase K family of subtilases, have been shown to be responsible for the disorder (119,120). Little is currently known about this protein and its role in LDL metabolism.

Autosomal-Recessive Hypercholesterolemia

The molecular defect responsible for an autosomal-recessive form of hypercholesterolemia (ARH) has been identified (121,122). Patients with ARH have markedly delayed LDL clearance rates, yet have normal LDL receptor function in their cultured fibroblast (123). They present with clinical features similar to homozygous FH, including marked hypercholesterolemia and large tendon xanthomas (124,125), although the plasma levels of LDL-C in patients with ARH tend to be intermediate between those in FH heterozygotes and those in FH homozygotes (125). The onset of clinically significant coronary atherosclerotic disease is later in patients with ARH than in patients with homozygous FH (124,125).

ARH is caused by mutations in the ARH gene, which encodes a novel adaptor protein that may function to link the LDL receptor to the endocytic machinery of the coated pit and facilitate internalization of the LDL receptor–LDL complex (126). ARH contains a phosphotyrosine-binding domain that binds a sequence motif (NPXY) in the cytoplasmic tail of the LDL receptor required for receptor internalization (127–129). This sequence also binds inositol phospholipids, which may anchor the protein to the plasma membrane (130). The C-terminal portion of the protein contains a canonical clathrin box consensus sequence (LL-DLE) and a 27-amino acid sequence that bind structural components of clathrin-coated pits (129). All currently reported mutations in the *ARH* gene interrupt the reading frame and result in the synthesis of a truncated protein (121,131). LDL receptor function, although normal in fibroblasts, is defective in transformed lymphocytes from patients with ARH (132). In these cells, ARH appears to reside primarily on the plasma membrane (132), and although cell surface LDL binding is increased, LDL degradation is markedly reduced.

The therapeutic approach to patients with ARH is similar to that of patients with FH. Increased expression of hepatic LDL receptors induced by bile acid sequestrants and inhibitors of HMG-CoA reductase may compensate for the abnormal LDL receptor function in ARH. Although the cholesterol-decreasing response to drug therapy in patients with ARH is more substantial than patients with homozygous FH, most require LDL apheresis to reach optimal treatment goals (125).

Familial Hyperchylomicronemia

Familial chylomicronemia, a rare genetic syndrome inherited as an autosomal-recessive trait, is characterized by severe fasting hypertriglyceridemia and massive accumulations of chylomicrons in plasma (133–135). Affected individuals often present early in childhood with recurrent episodes of abdominal pain or pancreatitis, or both, frequently precipitated by the ingestion of a fatty meal. In these patients, both serum and urine amylase levels may appear normal because of interference by the plasma lipids, by circulating inhibitors with the amylase assays, or by both (133,136–138). Thus, classic pancreatitis may be difficult to diagnose. The major clinical findings seen in patients with chylomicronemia are illustrated in Figure 5–7. Lipid accumulation in the liver and spleen of some patients leads to hepatosplenomegaly and mild but reversible increase of liver transaminase. Eruptive xanthomas, small yellow papular skin lesions localized primarily over the buttocks and extensor surfaces, appear when plasma triglyceride levels exceed 1,000 to 2,000 mg/dL, and usually regress within a few weeks after triglyceride levels are decreased (139). Simi-

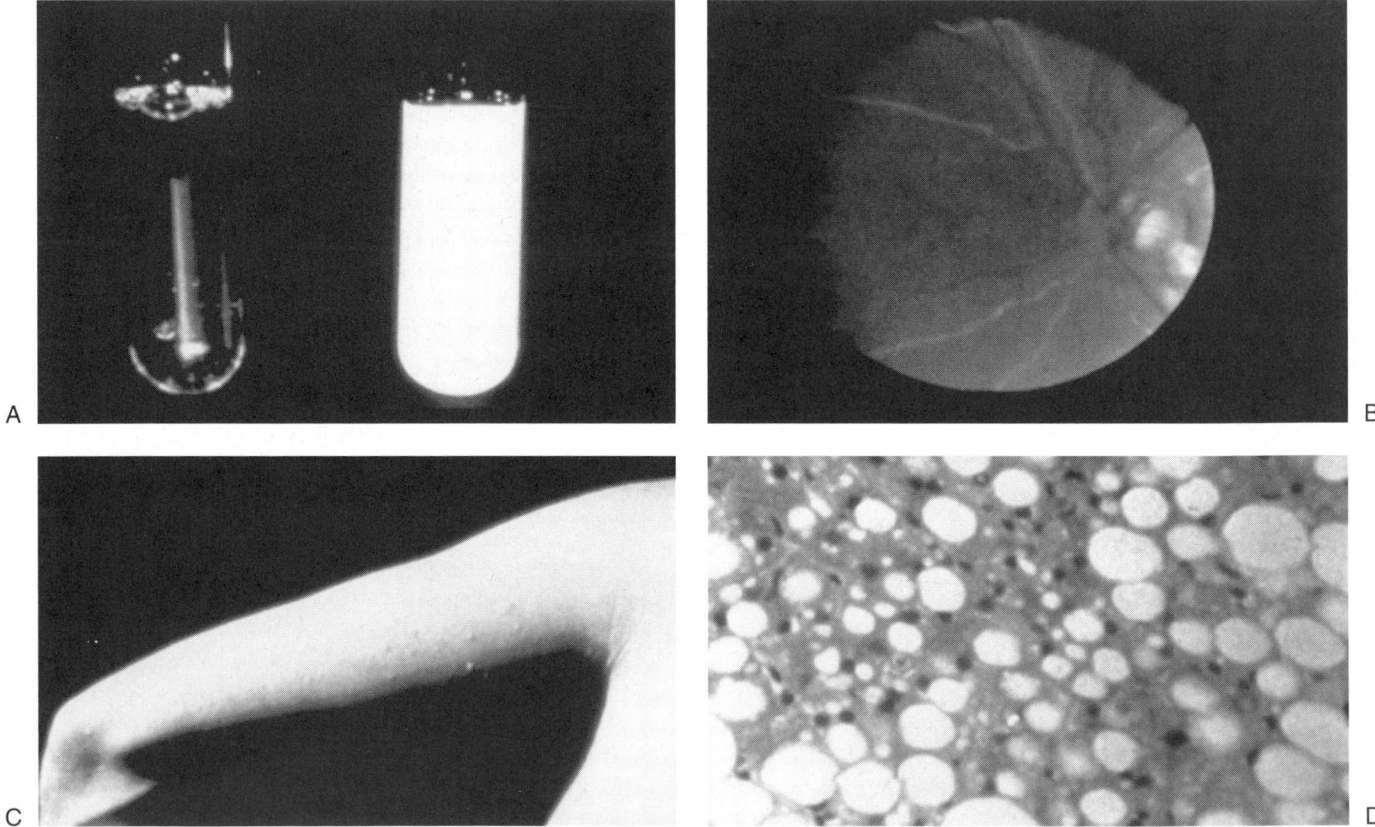

FIG. 5–7. Milky or cream of tomato soap plasma (**A:** control left, patient right), lipemia retinalis (**B**), eruptive xanthomas (**C**), and fatty liver (**D**) characteristic of patients with hyperchylomicronemia.

larly, lipemia retinals may be detected by funduscopic examination when triglyceride values are greater than 2,000 to 3,000 mg/dL. The retinal vessels in these patients appear lipemic, and the fundus has a pale pink appearance because of light scattering by circulating chylomicrons. All of these clinical features are reversible and do not lead to either progressive liver dysfunction or visual impairment. Patients with familial chylomicronemia do not appear to be at risk for development of premature cardiovascular disease. The major morbidity associated with this disorder is recurrent episodes of pancreatitis, which in some affected individuals have resulted in pancreatic insufficiency.

Abnormalities in the lipid profile of patients with familial chylomicronemia include severe fasting hypertriglyceridemia, with levels between 500 and 5,000 mg/dL, and plasma cholesterol concentrations that range from normal to as high as 1,000 mg/dL. Chylomicrons, which are normally rapidly cleared from the circulation, are present in the patient's plasma after a 12-hour fast, and VLDL concentrations also are frequently increased. In addition, LDL- and HDL-cholesterol values are reduced as a result of both decreased synthesis and increased catabolism (135). The two major molecular defects that lead to the familial chylomicronemia are a deficiency of LPL or of its cofactor, apoC-II. These two genetic disorders are summarized in the following sections.

The goal of therapy in all patients with familial chylomicronemia is to reduce plasma triglycerides to levels less than 1000 mg/dL, which will reverse many of the clinical manifestations of the syndrome (133–135). Treatment involves restriction of dietary fat to less than 15% of total calories (10–15 g of fat daily). Both unsaturated and saturated fats should be limited, and agents that can increase plasma triglyceride levels, such as alcohol, estrogens, diuretics, and β-adrenergic drugs should be avoided. Patients requiring additional fat calories can be supplemented with medium-chain triglycerides, which can replace other cooking oils in the diet. Such supplements should be used with caution because of a possible association with hepatic fibrosis (133–135). Patients with recurrent pancreatitis and increased VLDL may respond to therapy with fibric acids or niacin, but response to these agents is highly variable. Transient normalization of plasma triglycerides after plasma infusion has been demonstrated in patients with LPL, but not in those with apoC-II deficiency (133,135).

Apolipoprotein C-II Deficiency

ApoC-II is a small, 8,800-molecular weight protein that is present in plasma associated with chylomicrons, VLDLs, and HDLs. It is synthesized primarily by the liver (139) and serves as a cofactor for the lipolytic enzyme. In the presence of apoC-II, LPL hydrolyses triglycerides present in chylomicrons and VLDL to monoglycerides and diglycerides, as well as free fatty acids that can be used as sources of energy or reesterified for storage in adipose tissue (133,135).

Thus, a deficiency of apoC-II results in marked derangements of both triglyceride and lipoprotein metabolism.

Deficiency of apoC-II is a rare cause of familial chylomicronemia (140). With few exceptions (141,142), this genetic disorder is inherited as an autosomal-recessive trait, and affected homozygous individuals present with many of the classical features of familial chylomicronemia as described previously (133–135). The diagnosis of apoC-II deficiency is made when the plasma of a patient with the chylomicronemia syndrome is unable to activate LPL *in vitro,* suggesting a functional deficiency of apoC-II. In addition, a deficiency of apoC-II or an apoC-II variant can be identified by analysis of the patient's plasma by isoelectric focusing or two-dimensional gel electrophoresis. Postheparin plasma LPL activity in the presence of exogenous apoC-II ranges from normal to increased in these individuals.

The underlying molecular defects that lead to a functional deficiency of apoC-II have been identified in several kindreds by sequence analysis of the *apoC-II* gene of affected family members (133,143). Most of the identified gene defects are single-point mutations that result in decreased expression of the apolipoprotein, and thus lead to markedly reduced concentrations or total absence of plasma apoC-II. These include mutations in the *apoC-II* gene that either introduce a premature termination codon, substitute the initiation codon, or disrupt a donor splice site (133,143). In the case of apoC-II Toronto and apoC-II St. Michael (133,143), frameshift mutations in the proposed LPL binding domain (residues 65–79) of apoC-II result in the synthesis of an altered protein that cannot activate bovine LPL *in vitro.* Unlike the situation in most apoC-II—deficient patients, significant amounts of a nonfunctional apoC-II are detected in the plasma of affected individuals. Characterization of the various kindreds indicates that the underlying molecular defects that lead to apoC-II deficiency are heterogeneous with no evidence of a founder gene effect that would permit rapid screening of affected individuals or identification of carriers for the trait.

Lipoprotein Lipase Deficiency

Human LPL is a glycoprotein of approximately 55,000 daltons (144) that is synthesized primarily by adipocytes, heart and skeletal muscle, macrophages, and mammary gland (145). The active enzyme is a noncovalent homodimer that is anchored to the endothelial cell surface by a membrane-bound heparin sulfate proteoglycan. In the presence of its cofactor, apoC-II, LPL hydrolyses the 1- and 3-ester bonds in triglycerides present in chylomicrons and VLDL to monoglycerides, diglycerides, and free fatty acids. In the process, LPL in combination with apoC-II facilitates the intravascular remodeling of lipoprotein particles and the ultimate clearance of remnant lipoproteins from the circulation. In addition to its role as a lipolytic enzyme, LPL has a separate role in lipoprotein metabolism as a ligand that facilitates the cellular uptake of lipoproteins or lipoprotein lipids by cell surface receptors and proteoglycans (see References 146–151 for reviews of functions of LPL in lipoprotein metabolism).

The majority of patients with the familial chylomicronemia syndrome have a deficiency of LPL. Unlike apoC-II deficiency, LPL deficiency is a relatively common disorder, with a frequency of 1:5,000 to 1:10,000 in some populations (152,153). The carrier state for LPL deficiency is as prevalent as, and in some areas more prevalent (152,154,155) than, the heterozygous state for FH. The diagnosis of LPL deficiency is suspected from the clinical presentation and is established by finding markedly reduced or absent LPL activity in the patient's postheparin plasma. A bolus of 60 U/kg of heparin sulfate will release LPL bound to the endothelial vessel wall into the circulation, where it can be easily quantitated (133). Determination of adipocyte LPL activity obtained from a fat biopsy also can be used to form the diagnosis (133).

Almost 100 naturally occurring mutations in the *LPL* gene that lead to the expression of familial chylomicronemia have been identified (140,148,150,156,157). Several major gene rearrangements that result in markedly reduced levels of *LPL* in the postheparin plasma of affected individuals have been described. Approximately 60 point mutations that lead to the substitution of a single amino acid in *LPL* and to the synthesis of a nonfunctional enzyme also have been reported. Interestingly, most of these mutations are clustered around the highly conserved fourth, fifth, and sixth exons of the *LPL* gene, which encode for amino acids involved in the catalytic function (127). Defects that result in the introduction of a premature stop codon and splicing defects also have been reported. Unlike apoC-II, evidence for a founder gene effect as a cause for *LPL* deficiency has been identified in the French Canadian and other populations that have mutations at positions 188 and 207 of *LPL*.

Although many carriers for the *LPL* deficiency trait appear to have normal plasma lipids, analysis of several extended kindreds with different mutations in the *LPL* gene indicate that the heterozygous state for LPL deficiency may underlie some of the more common hyperlipidemic disorders found in the general population (148,150,156,158–160). Thus, a significant association is present between the carrier state for LPL deficiency and familial hypertriglyceridemia (161), FCHL (136), and postprandial lipemia (162–164). In addition, mutations in the *LPL* gene have been linked to other diseases including Alzheimer's (165), hypertension (166,167), cerebrovascular disease (168), and preeclampsia (169). Given the high frequency of the carrier state for *LPL* deficiency in the general population, mutations in LPL alone or through interactions with either environmental or genetic factors may account for a significant proportion of hyperlipidemias within a given population.

Homozygous individuals with *LPL* deficiency do not appear to be at an increased risk for development of premature cardiovascular disease (156). However, the partial *LPL* deficiency observed in carriers for the trait may result, at least in a subset of patients, in an increased risk for atherothrombosis. In the general population, carriers for the Asp_Asn and Gly188Glu LPL mutations have increased risk for CAD, whereas heterozygosity for the Asn291Ser mutation enhances CAD risk in patients with FCHL (170,171). Recent studies have provided some insights into potential processes by which LPL function may enhance atherothrombosis. The synthesis of LPL by either macrophages or smooth muscle cells present in atherosclerotic lesions has been demonstrated (156). Enhanced lipolysis mediated by LPL may, in turn, increase the accumulation of cholesteryl esters in these cells, and ultimately result in enhanced foam cell formation in the arterial wall. In addition, the presence of LPL in the subendothelial space may promote the binding and retention of LDL (172) and VLDL (173) to the subendothelial matrix, potentially enhancing the conversion of these lipoproteins to more atherogenic forms. LPL also enhances the binding of atherogenic lipoproteins to smooth muscle cells (174) and increases monocyte adhesion to aortic endothelial cells (175). A significant association between high levels of LPL synthesis and secretion in macrophages and susceptibility to atherothrombosis in inbred murine strains (176) has been reported. Compelling data concerning the relation between macrophage LPL and atherothrombosis has come from studies in transgenic mice and bone marrow transplantation experiments (177–180). In these studies, macrophage LPL synthesis promoted foam cell formation and atherothrombosis, providing further evidence for a role of LPL in atherothrombosis.

Characterization of transgenic mice overexpressing LPL primarily in adipose tissue, heart, and skeletal muscle (175,181,182) suggests that expression of LPL in tissues other than those found in the arterial wall may, in fact, be beneficial. Thus, these animals have a markedly improved lipid profile, including increases in total HDL (183) and HDL$_2$-cholesterol (181) and reduction in plasma triglyceride and cholesterol-rich LDL and they appear to be protected against diet-induced hypertriglyceridemia and hypercholesterolemia. In other studies (184), the treatment of rats with the novel compound NO-1886, which increases LPL activity, leads to greater levels of HDL and protection against the development of coronary artery lesions.

Thus, LPL may play a dual role in the development of atherothrombosis. The synthesis of LPL by cells present in the arterial wall may promote the atherosclerotic process, whereas LPL-mediated lipoprotein uptake by the liver may result in enhanced catabolism of atherogenic particles, thereby reducing lesion formation. Ultimately, the role of LPL in the development of or protection against atherothrombosis may be dictated by its site of synthesis and interaction with other genetic and environmental factors.

Hepatic Lipase Deficiency

HL deficiency, a rare genetic disorder first described in 1982 by Breckenridge and coworkers (185), currently has been identified in only four different kindreds (185–190). The frequency of this disorder in the general population, however, may be underestimated because of the difficulty in identifying affected individuals. HL, 64-kD glycoprotein synthesized primarily in hepatocytes, is an important enzyme that mediates the hydrolysis of triglycerides and phospholipids present in plasma lipoproteins (191–193). Its action as both an acylglycerol hydrolase and phospholipase results in the conversion of IDL to LDL and HDL$_2$ to HDL$_3$ (194–196). In addition to its role as a lipolytic enzyme, HL, like LPL, also functions as a ligand that facilitates the cellular uptake of lipoproteins or lipoprotein lipids by cell surface receptors and proteoglycans (146–148). HL plays an important role in the metabolism of remnant lipoproteins and HDL.

The diagnosis of HL deficiency is established by finding markedly reduced or absent HL activity but normal LPL activity in the patient's postheparin plasma. The underlying molecular defects that lead to HL deficiency have been investigated in several independent kindreds (197–201). Individuals with a deficiency of HL may present with features characteristic of type III hyperlipoproteinemia, including hypercholesterolemia, hypertriglyceridemia, accumulation of triglyceride-rich lipoproteins and β-VLDL, palmar xanthomas, and premature cardiovascular disease (185–190). Triglyceride levels can range from normal to 4,000 mg/dL in affected individuals. In addition, pancreatitis has been described in a patient with severe hypertriglyceridemia caused by combined HL deficiency and partial deficiency of LPL (186,187). However, unlike patients with type III hyperlipoproteinemia, patients with a deficiency of HL have triglyceride-enriched lipoproteins and a normal VLDL-cholesterol/total triglyceride ratio of less than 0.3, a finding that is useful in distinguishing the two genetic syndromes (186,187,190). In addition, many patients with HL deficiency have increased plasma apoB concentrations (185,187,202), which appear to be the result of a reduced fractional clearance rate of apoB from VLDL and IDL (202).

Although several patients with HL deficiency have experienced development of premature cardiovascular disease (185,187), the role that deficiency of this enzyme plays in the development of atherothrombosis remains to be established. Human and animal studies support a dual role for HL in atherogenesis (146–148,203–214). HL beneficially alters the plasma lipid profile by reducing the amount of cholesterol present in the proatherogenic apoB-containing lipoproteins. However, HL has been shown to be synthesized by macrophages (214), and bone marrow transplantation studies in HL-deficient mice have shown that macrophage HL synthesis promotes foam cell formation and atherothrombosis (215), providing evidence for a dual role of HL in atherothrombosis.

Familial Dysbetalipoproteinemia: Type III Hyperlipoproteinemia

Individuals with familial dysbetalipoproteinemia have a delayed clearance of remnants of triglyceride-rich lipoproteins, resulting in the accumulation of remnants from both the hepatic VLDL and chylomicron pathways. Several different nomenclatures have been used for the codification of familial dysbetalipoproteinemia (216–221). Patients with this disorder have been classified as having dysbetalipoproteinemia when low or normal plasma lipid values are present and as having type III hyperlipoproteinemia when hyperlipidemia has developed. The remnant lipoproteins have the hydrated density of VLDL and IDL, but have the electrophoretic mobility of β rather than the usual pre-β lipoproteins. These cholesterol-rich, β electrophoretically migrating lipoproteins are present with the density less than 1.006 g/mL. As a result of the change in VLDL electrophoretic mobility, patients with this disease also have been classified as having β-VLDL, floating β lipoproteins (density < 1.006 g/mL), or broad-β disease. Additional important diagnostic features of familial dysbetalipoproteinemia include an increase of cholesterol and triglycerides with a ratio of approximately 1:1 and a VLDL-cholesterol/plasma-triglyceride ratio greater than 0.3 (control subjects < 0.3). Patients with dysbetalipoproteinemia often experience development of hyperlipidemia and other clinical symptomatology in the fourth and fifth decades of life. One of the fascinating clinical features of dysbetalipoproteinemia is the presence of palmar xanthomas (xanthoma striata palmaris), which are virtually pathognomonic of this dyslipoproteinemia (Fig. 5–8). Palmar xanthomas are frequently accompanied by tuberous lesions over the elbows, knees, and buttocks. Occasionally, the patients may develop Achilles tendon xanthomas, characteristic of patients with FH. The important clinical sequelae of this disorder is an increased risk for both premature coronary heart disease and peripheral vascular disease (220,221).

The underlying metabolic defect in familial dysbetalipoproteinemia is the presence of a defective apoE, which plays a key role in the metabolism and cellular uptake of remnants of triglyceride-rich lipoproteins (222). Population studies have indicated that apoE is controlled at a single genetic locus with an unusual degree of polymorphism (223–226). There are three common alleles in the general population, which have been designated ϵ_2, ϵ_3, and ϵ_4. The three E apolipoproteins encoded by these three alleles are separable by isoelectrofocusing and are designated apoE$_2$, apoE$_3$, and apoE$_4$, respectively. Six major apoE phenotypes are present in the population, including homozygotes for apolipoproteins E$_2$, E$_3$, and E$_4$ and heterozygotes for apolipoproteins E$_{2,3}$, E$_{2,4}$, and E$_{3,4}$. The structural differences in the apoE isoproteins have been shown to be caused by one or two amino acid substitutions involving cysteine and arginine exchanges at amino acid residues 112 and 158 (227).

The predominant E isoprotein in the normolipidemic population is apoE$_3$, and it is considered the normal or parent isoprotein. Two different modes of inheritance have been identified in hyperlipidemic patients with familial dysbetalipoproteinemia. The majority of individuals who have hyperlipidemia have the autosomal-recessive form of the disease. An increased fre-

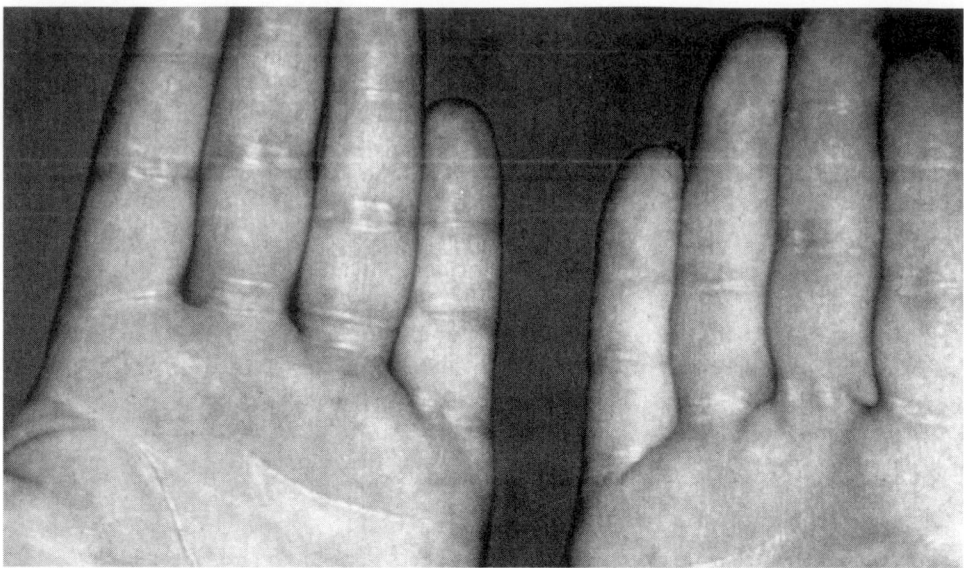

FIG. 5–8. Palmar xanthoma characteristic of the clinical features of patients with type III hyperlipoproteinemia.

quency of the E_2 allele (apoE$_{2,2}$ phenotype) (220,224–227) or E_0 allele (apoE absence) (228–231) has been observed in hyperlipidemic patients with familial dysbetalipoproteinemia. However, the majority of individuals with the apoE$_{2,2}$ phenotype are normocholesterolemic or hypocholesterolemic (220,221,226). Subjects with the apoE$_{2,2}$ phenotype and no hyperlipidemia have been categorized as normolipidemic E_2 dysbetalipoproteinemic homozygotes. The development of hyperlipidemia in the recessive form of familial dysbetalipoproteinemia has been proposed to require the presence of an additional environmental or genetic abnormality such as obesity, hypothyroidism, or a second dyslipoproteinemia, particularly FCHL. Thus, a second genetic defect may be required for the apoE$_{2,2}$ subject to become hyperlipidemic.

Patients with the dominant form of inheritance of familial dysbetalipoproteinemia experience development of hyperlipidemia as heterozygotes. The apoE mutations associated with the dominant form of this dyslipoproteinemia have included mutations at residue 142, residue 146, or a seven-amino acid insertion at residue 121 of apoE (232–236). The hyperlipidemia observed in some cases of the dominant form of the disease often appears at an earlier age and is associated with significant cardiovascular disease.

Individuals with the apoE4 variant have increased plasma levels of total as well as LDL cholesterol when compared with subjects with the apoE$_{3,3}$ phenotype. Kinetic studies using radiolabeled apoE isoproteins have established that apoE$_4$ is catabolized more rapidly than apoE$_3$ (237,238). On the basis of these results, it has been proposed that patients with the apoE$_4$ phenotype have a more rapid clearance of plasma chylomicrons and VLDL remnants by the liver than do apoE$_3$ subjects. The increased rate of hepatic clearance of the remnant particles leads to down-regulation of the LDL receptor, resulting in greater plasma concentrations of cholesterol, LDL, and remnant particles. An increased level of plasma LDL would be expected to increase the risk for premature cardiovascular disease in patients with the apoE$_4$ phenotype. Of major importance is the recent observation that patients with Alzheimer's disease have an increased frequency of the apoE$_4$ allele (239–243). The role of apoE$_4$ in development of Alzheimer's disease is not as yet completely understood and remains an active area of research (239–243).

Hypertriglyceridemia Low High-Density Lipoprotein Syndrome

A common lipoprotein profile present in patients with established coronary heart disease is increased triglycerides and decreased HDL-cholesterol levels (244). There are no characteristic clinical features and the patients have a significantly increased risk for premature heart disease. The lipid and lipoprotein profiles in these patients may vary depending on the diet and lifestyle, as well as the presence of a second genetic dyslipoproteinemia. The mode of inheritance of this syndrome has not been established and there may be several different molecular defects resulting in this lipoprotein phenotype. The increased risk in the development of premature cardiovascular disease may be because of the increase of atherogenic remnants of triglyceride-rich particles or low HDL, or a combination of both.

Sitosterolemia

Sitosterolemia is a rare autosomal-recessive disease characterized by plasma and tissue accumulation of plant sterols, including sitosterol, campesterol, and stigmasterol, as well as other sterols, including shellfish sterols (245,246). In fact this disease can more appropriately be considered a pan sterol defect in which all of the dietary sterols are absorbed by the intestine. The increased plasma concentrations of sterols are frequently accompanied by an increase in cholesterol levels. The clinical manifestations of sitosterolemia begin in childhood or the first and second decades of life. Tendon xanthomas may develop even if the plasma cholesterol concentrations are relatively normal. The disease should be suspected in patients with hypercholesterolemia who have a greater than usual response to dietary cholesterol restriction or to bile acid resins. The presence of tendon xanthomas in a child without hypercholesterolemia may also be a clue to the diagnosis of sitosterolemia. The disease also should be considered in young patients with tendon xanthomas and hypercholesterolemia. In these individuals, LDL-receptor function is normal and some of these patients have been classified as "pseudofamilial hypercholesterolemia."

The diagnosis of sitosterolemia can be definitively ascertained by the determination of the plasma levels of plant sterols (upper limit of normal is 0.5% of total plasma sterols), which are transported primarily within LDL. The fecal bile acid pattern is unusual, with increased levels of deoxycholic and lithocholic acids and fecal bile alcohols. The characteristic clinical features of sitosterolemia in addition to the tendon xanthomas are tuberous xanthomas, arcus cornea, xanthelasma, and premature cardiovascular disease. Hemolytic anemia may also occur in sitosterolemia. Patients with sitosterolemia are unusually responsive to dietary cholesterol restriction and bile acid–binding resins. The addition of ezetimibe to a low-sterol diet has been shown to be particularly effective in decreasing plasma plant sterols and cholesterol in these patients (247).

Sitosterolemia is caused by mutations in either of two adjacent genes that encode ABC half-transporters, ABCG5 and ABCG8 (Fig. 5–9) (248–254). They are members of a superfamily of transmembrane proteins, which translocate a variety of molecules, including proteins, ions, sugars, and lipids, across extracellular and intracellular membranes with energy derived from ATP (253). All patients with sitosterolemia have mutations in either both ABCG5 alleles (Japanese patients) or both ABCG8 alleles (white patients);

currently, no affected individuals with mutations in both transporter genes have been reported (248,249). ABCG5 and ABCG8 are expressed primarily in the liver and small intestine (250,251,254–256), where they limit intestinal cholesterol absorption and enhance biliary cholesterol excretion. Both genes are up-regulated by cholesterol feeding in mice (250), a process that is dependent on liner X receptor α (LXRα), a nuclear hormone receptor that orchestrates the regulation of several genes involved in the trafficking of cholesterol from tissues to the liver (*ABCA1, apoE, CETP,* and others) (257).

The importance of ABCG5 and ABCG8 in regulating excretion of cholesterol and other sterols from the body has been demonstrated in genetically engineered mice with altered expression of ABCG5 and ABCG8. Deficiency of ABCG5 and ABCG8 leads to increased intestinal cholesterol absorption and decreased gall bladder bile cholesterol concentration (258), a phenotype similar to that of patients with sitosterolemia. Conversely, overexpression of human G5/G8 increased the gallbladder cholesterol concentrations by more than fivefold and reduced dietary sterol absorption by 50% in transgenic mice (259). The pivotal role that G5/G8 play in sterol trafficking and promoting sterol excretion from the body identify these genes as potential targets for reducing atherogenesis.

Abetalipoproteinemia

Abetalipoproteinemia is a rare genetic disorder first described in 1950 by Bassen and Kornzweig (260). Abetalipoproteinemia is a rare autosomal-recessive disorder characterized in homozygotes by the absences of all lipoproteins containing apoB-48 and apoB-100, including chylomicrons, VLDLs, IDLs, and LDLs. Heterozygotes with abetalipoproteinemia have no detectible clinical or biochemical abnormalities. The clinical manifestations of abetalipoproteinemia include steatorrhea, retinitis pigmentosa, hemolytic anemia, and neurologic dysfunction (Fig. 5–10) (98,261). The most serious sequelae of abetalipoproteinemia are the progressive blindness and the progressive neurologic. The first symptoms to appear often are related to fat malabsorption during the first years of life. Radi-

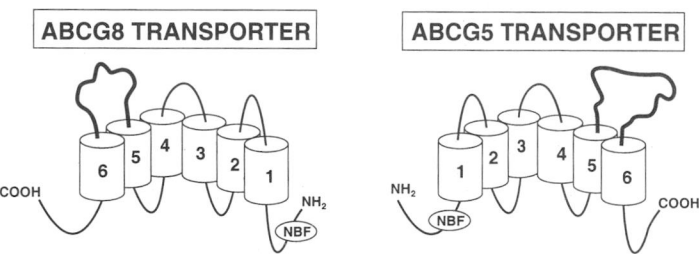

FIG. 5–9. Schematic model of the adenosine triphosphate (ATP)-binding cassette transporter G5 (ABCG5) and ATP-binding cassette transporter G8 (ABCG8) transporters that function as a heterodimer to decrease intestinal absorption of cholesterol. A genetic defect in either ABCG5 or ABCG8 results in sitosterolemia.

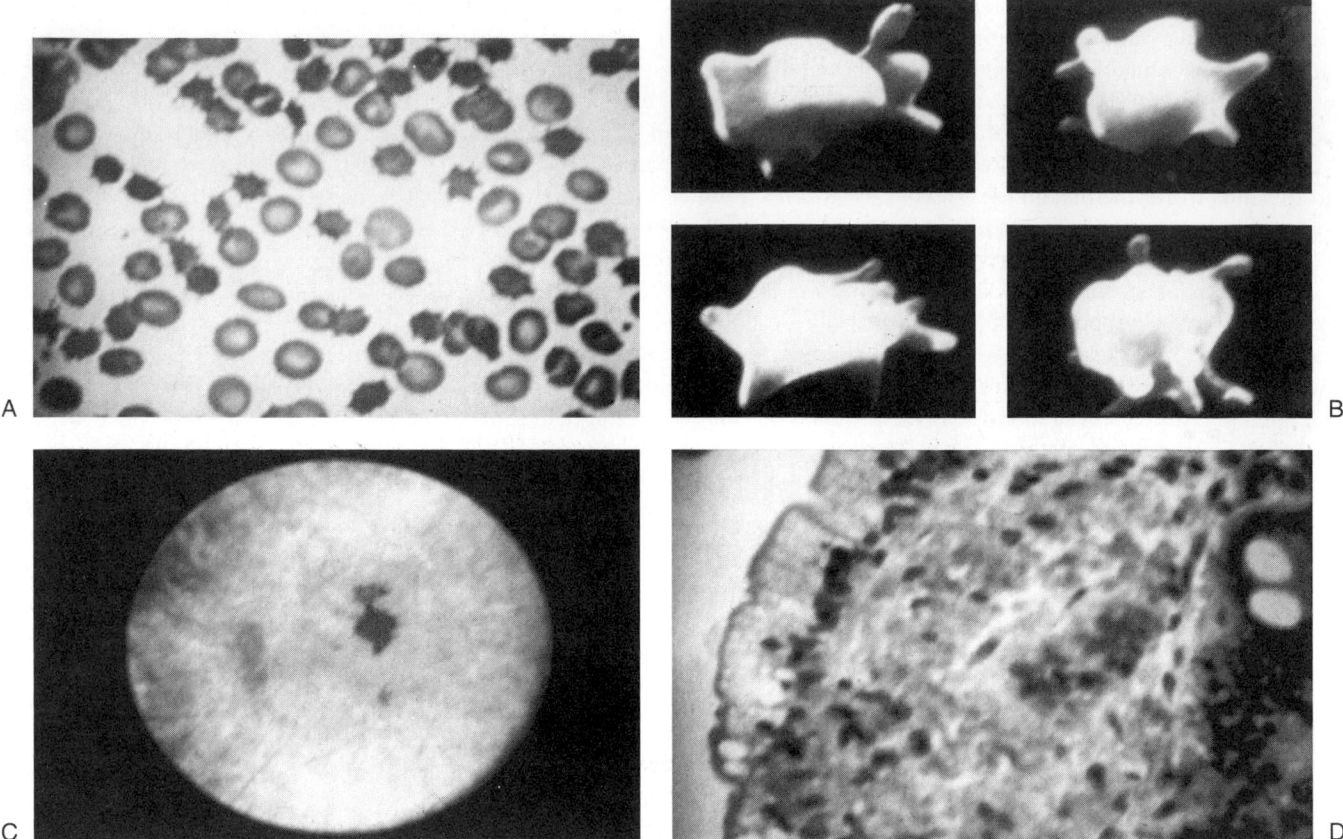

FIG. 5–10. Clinical features of abetalipoproteinemia include lipid-filled enterocytes **(A)**, atypical acanthronigricans **(B)**, and acanthocytes **(C** and **D)**.

ographic findings are not diagnostic and a small intestinal biopsy reveals a snow-white mucosa with unblunted, well-formed villi containing lipid-laden mucosal cells (Fig. 5–10). These mucosal findings are characteristic and distinguish abetalipoproteinemia from celiac disease. Of major clinical importance is the severe malabsorption of fat-soluble vitamins, particularly A and E (262). Acanthocytes with altered cholesterol and phospholipid contents are present, often leading to episodes of hemolysis and anemia. The cardinal ophthalmologic physical findings include nystagmus, retinitis pigmentosa, and decreased visual acuity. Visual symptoms often present as night blindness because of vitamin A deficiency. During the course of the disease nystagmus and progressive retinal degeneration develop. The first neurologic deficient is loss of deep tendon. Abetalipoproteinemia progresses to muscular weakness (kyphoscoliosis, lordosis), loss of proprioception (loss of position and vibratory sense), and cerebellar dysfunction (ataxia) attributed to spinocerebelar degeneration. The neurologic defects have been proposed to be caused by a profound deficiency of vitamin E. Death may occur in the fourth and fifth decade of life and may be related to cardiac arrhythmias.

The plasma concentrations of cholesterol are extremely low (<50 mg/dL) and triglyceride concentrations less than 10 mg/dL is a clue to the diagnosis. Triglyceride concentrations do not increase after a fat-rich meal. All apoB-containing lipoproteins are absent including chylomicrons, VLDLs, IDLs, and LDLs. HDLs are the only lipoproteins detected and their composition is abnormal with increased ratios of free to esterified cholesterol and sphingomyelin to phosphatidylcholine. The characteristic feature of abetalipoproteinemia is the absence of plasma apoB-100 and apoB-48. The cellular defect is characterized by a defect in the assembly or secretion of apoB-containing lipoproteins. The genetic defect was determined to be the absence of microsomal triglyceride transfer protein (MTP) in the intestine and liver (263). The inability to assemble and secrete chylomicrons by the intestine results in malabsorption and a deficiency of fat-soluble vitamins, whereas the absence of hepatic production of VLDL severely diminishes the transport of endogenous triglycerides and abolishes the transport of cholesterol to peripheral cells through the LDL receptor pathway.

MTP is a dimeric lipid transfer protein located on chromosome 4q22 (263). The heterodimer is composed of a 58-kD protein disulfide-isomerase involved in disulfide bond formation and a unique 97-kD subunit that possesses the lipid transfer activity (264,265). MTP is located in the endoplasmic reticulum and accelerates the transport of triglycerides, cholesteryl ester, and phospholipid between membranes. Chylomicron and VLDL are assembled within the endoplasmic reticulum lumen of enterocytes and hepatocytes and are subsequently transported to the Golgi apparatus and then secreted. ApoB is synthesized and translocated through the endoplasmic reticulum membrane where the addition of lipid to apoB begins cotranslationally. MTP plays a primary role in the first step of lipoprotein assembly (261,265). More than 25 mutations have been described in MTP, with all being located in the large 97-kD subunit (261).

Treatment of abetalipoproteinemia with high doses of vitamin A and E ameliorates the progressive retinopathy and neuropathy (262,266–268). There is marked heterogeneity in response to treatment and replacement does not always prevent the appearance of the neurologic and ophthalmologic signs.

Hypobetalipoproteinemia

Homozygous familial hypobetalipoproteinemia is a rare autosomal disease that, like classical abetalipoproteinemia, is characterized by the absence of plasma lipoproteins containing apoB-48 and apoB-100. There are two major differences between the two clinical syndromes. First, the clinical manifestations of homozygous hypobetalipoproteinemia are milder than abetalipoproteinemia. Second, the heterozygous carrier state of familial hypobetalipoproteinemia is associated with reduced concentrations of plasma apoB and LDL. In homozygotes, malabsorption leads to a mild deficiency of fat-soluble vitamins. An intestinal biopsy reveals lipid-laden columnar cells similar to that observed in patients with abetalipoproteinemia. Circulating acanthocytes are present; however, hemolytic anemia is milder than in abetalipoproteinemia. Ocular manifestations include night blindness and the development of progressive retinal degeneration. Of particular importance in the clinical course of patients with homozygous hypobetalipoproteinemia is a relative sparing of the neurologic system. The majority of the patients have minimal ataxia, cerebellar signs, or motor-sensory dysfunction, which is in marked contrast to the severe ataxia and neurologic disease observed in abetalipoproteinemia.

The biochemical defect in many of the patients with familial hypobetalipoproteinemia, unlike abetalipoproteinemia, is caused by a structural mutation in the *apoB* gene leading to decreased biosynthesis of apoB and the inability to effectively secrete chylomicron and hepatogenous VLDL. More than 40 truncations of apoB have been identified in the *apoB* gene on chromosome 2 (98,269, 270). Many mutations result from deletions and substitutions that cause frameshifts leading to premature stop codons. Truncated proteins are named on the basis of percent of amino acid in the mutated *apoB* relative to the full-length apoB-100 and have been described as short as apoB-2 to apoB-89. ApoBs shorter than apoB 27 are usually absent from the plasma (98,270,271). Truncated forms of apoB are poorly lapidated

and are secreted at greatly reduced rates and the size influences the clearances by the LDL receptor (271).

There is evidence that genetic disorders other than truncations can cause hypobetalipoproteinemia. If hypobetalipoproteinemia is defined by less than 5 percentile levels of total cholesterol (150 mg/dL), apoB (50 mg/dL), or LDL (70 mg/dL), then less than 5% of individuals have an apoB truncation–producing mutation (272). This would include most individuals presumed to be heterozygotes for familial hypobetalipoproteinemia. A genomic scan on families with hypobetalipoproteinemia revealed linkage to a susceptibility gene on chromosome 3p21 (273). Another genomic scan found no linkage to chromosome 2 or chromosome 3p21 (270). Factors other than mutations in apoB likely contribute in hypobetalipoproteinemia.

Treatment of hypobetalipoproteinemia with high doses of vitamin A and E is warranted when fat-soluble vitamin levels are reduced. Most heterozygotes for familial hypobetalipoproteinemia are asymptomatic and only have reduced plasma apoB and LDL. Studies have shown that as many as 60% of heterozygotes with mutations in the *apoB* gene have a fivefold increase in percentage of liver fat on the basis of magnetic resonance spectroscopy (270). The clinical significance of the hepatic steatosis is unknown.

Chylomicron Retention Disease

Chylomicron retention disease, or Anderson's disease, is a rare autosomal-recessive disorder first described in 1961 by Anderson (275). Homozygotes for chylomicron retention disease have a selective absence of apoB-48–containing chylomicrons. Heterozygotes have no detectible clinical, lipid, or biochemical abnormalities. The major finding that distinguishes chylomicron retention disease from abetalipoproteinemia and familial hypobetalipoproteinemia is the presence of LDL and apoB-100 in the plasma, and the absence of acanthocytes, retinitis pigmentosa, and ataxia (98,276–278). The liver is capable of synthesizing VLDL, and plasma contains the liver-derived lipoproteins. The major symptoms are related to fat malabsorption during the first year of life. Diarrhea and failure to thrive are common with varying degrees of growth retardation. Radiographic findings are not diagnostic. Endoscopy shows a white stippling-like frosting on the intestinal mucosal surface and a small intestinal biopsy reveals fat-laden enterocytes. Fat-soluble vitamin levels including vitamin A and E are near normal, unlike abetalipoproteinemia and familial hypobetalipoproteinemia, but may be reduced in infancy. Acanthocytes are generally absent. Neurologic findings are mild or absent. Symptoms might include diminished or absent deep tendon reflexes and diminished vibratory sense. Subclinical ophthalmologic findings include mild defects in color vision or retinal electrophysiologic abnormalities (98,277), but atypical retinitis pigmentosa has not been described. The cellular defects by electron microscopy are heterogeneous and range from cytoplasmic fat droplets to an accumulation of chylomicron-like particles in membrane-bound compartments of enterocytes, which contain large cytoplasmic lipid droplets (98,276–278). The distinction between chylomicron retention disease and Anderson's disease has been largely derived in the partitioning of the lipid between cytoplasmic and membrane-bound compartments (276,277). Genetic studies excluded the *apoB* gene (279,280) and MTP levels were normal. The genetic defect was identified through a genome-wide screen, and a mutation in SARA2 was found on chromosome 5q31.1 (281). SARA2 belongs to a family of guanosine triphosphatases involved in the intracellular assembly and disassembly of COPII vesicles in the enterocyte. Sar1a is the gene product of SARA2 and is involved in the binding of guanosine triphosphate with COPII vesicles. Mutations in SARA2 were found in patients with chylomicron retention disease and Anderson's disease and also found in chylomicron retention disease with the neuromuscular disorder Marinesco-Sjögren (281). The inability to secrete apoB-48–containing chylomicrons by the intestine results in malabsorption, whereas the liver is able to produce apoB-100–containing VLDL.

The total cholesterol concentration is usually 50 to 100 mg/dL. HDL, LDL, and apoB levels are half of the normal levels. Triglyceride concentrations are nearly normal and fail to increase in response to a fat-load because of the failure to secrete chylomicrons. Treatment primarily includes restriction of dietary fat. Adherence to the diet is required to prevent a recurrence of symptoms. Vitamins A and E should be supplemented if fat-soluble vitamin levels are reduced or with the appearance of ophthalmologic or neurologic symptoms.

HYPOALPHALIPOPROTEINEMIAS

The genetic dyslipoproteinemias that are characterized by abnormally low concentrations of plasma lipoproteins and an increased risk for early heart disease involve primarily genetic defects in HDL.

Tangier Disease

Tangier disease is a genetic dyslipoproteinemia characterized clinically by orange tonsils, cloudy corneas, hepatosplenomegaly, lymphadenopathy, intermittent peripheral neuropathy, and a mild increase in risk for premature cardiovascular disease (Fig. 5–11) (6,282,283). Tangier disease should be suspected in patients with plasma cholesterol less than 120 mg/dL and normal or slightly increased triglycerides. Marked decreases in the plasma levels of HDL cholesterol, apoA-I, and apoA-II (<2–5% of normal) are the lipoprotein profile hallmark of patients with Tangier disease. Kinetic studies using radiolabeled HDL established that the low plasma HDL levels in Tangier disease are caused by markedly increased HDL catabolism (6,283,284).

The onset of the clinical features of Tangier disease is insidious, presumably reflecting the slow tissue accumulation of cholesteryl esters. The most characteristic site of deposition is the pharyngeal tonsils, and the presence of orange tonsils is virtually pathognomonic and can provide the diagnosis of Tangier disease at a glance. Frequently, however, the tonsils have been removed previously and, therefore, cannot be examined by the physician. Hepatosplenomegaly, caused by lipid accumulation in the reticuloendothelial system, often is present. Hypersplenism is rare; however, removal of the spleen for splenomegaly may lead to hyperplasia of the reticuloendothelial cells in the omentum or other areas of the body. Patients with Tangier disease may present with transient recurrent peripheral neuropathy, which also is caused by an accumulation of lipids within the nerve sheaths. Neurologic symptoms include motor weakness, paresthesia, and dysesthesia, but they often wax and wane. The clinical course of patients with Tangier disease is extremely variable, and the diagnosis may not be made until the third or fourth decade of life. Despite the low plasma HDL levels, the risk for premature cardiovascular disease is moderate (6,282,283). Heterozygotes have plasma HDL, apoA-I, and apoA-II that are approximately 50% of normal levels and triglyceride levels that are mildly increased. Heterozygotes appear to have a mild increased risk for cardiovascular disease. On physical examination, the unique clinical feature of homozygotes with Tangier disease is the presence of lobulated, bright orange—yellow tonsils Fig. 5–10). If the tonsils have been removed, pharyngeal tags of orange—yellow tissue may still be evident on examination. The rectal mucosa may have a similar orange appearance, and the identification of cholesteryl esters in foam cells in the rectal mucosa may be used to establish the diagnosis. Asymptomatic corneal opacities often require slit-lamp examination for identification. Mild hepatosplenomegaly and lymphadenopathy may also be present. The neuropathy in Tangier disease may be detected by decreased deep tendon reflexes and sensory motor abnormalities.

In vitro analysis of HDL-facilitated cholesterol efflux from cholesterol-loaded fibroblasts revealed decreased cholesterol efflux from cells from patients with Tangier disease compared with cells from control subjects, indicating that the molecular defect in Tangier disease is an intracellular defect in cholesterol metabolism (285). This concept was confirmed by the identification of ABCA1 as the gene defect in Tangier disease (26–32). ABCA1 is a 240-kD transmembrane protein that belongs to a superfamily of transmembrane proteins that translocate a variety of molecules, including proteins, ions, sugars, and lipids, across extracellular and intracellular membranes with energy derived from ATP (286,287). ABCA1 is a full transporter containing two ABCs and two transmembrane domains. It is intimately involved in the reverse cholesterol transport process by facilitating intracellular cholesterol and promotes the first step in reverse cholesterol transport (24,25, 288,289)—namely, the efflux of cellular cholesterol and phospholipids to apolipoprotein acceptors (285,290–294). The removal of excess cholesterol is of critical importance in preventing cholesterol accumulation and foam cell formation in

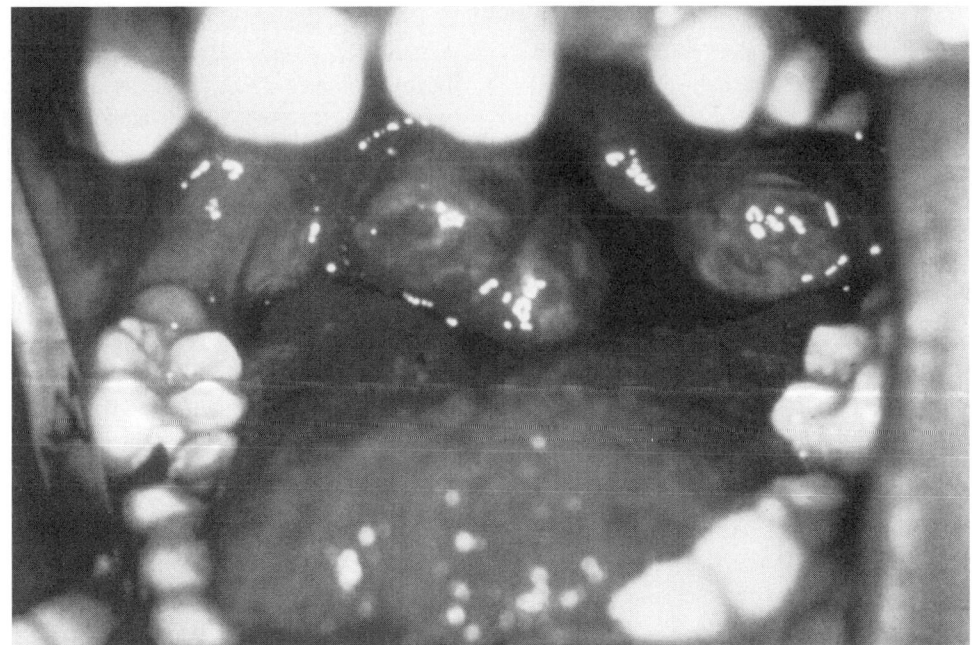

FIG. 5–11. Orange tonsils, the unique feature of Tangiers disease.

macrophages (290,295–298), Studies in humans and mice with ABCA1 deficiency have provided evidence that ABCA1 function is a major determinant of plasma HDL concentrations and may beneficially influence atherogenic risk (292,297–302). Over the past several years, ABCA1 has emerged as a transporter of major importance in lipoprotein metabolism, macrophage cholesterol homeostasis, and atherothrombosis, and it is currently considered a major therapeutic target for the treatment of low HDL syndromes and cardiovascular disease.

Apolipoprotein A-I Deficiency

ApoA-I, a major apolipoprotein of HDL, is of clinical importance because of the inverse association of plasma apoA-I levels and the development of premature coronary heart disease. The majority of structural mutations that have been identified in apoA-I do not affect HDL levels and have apparently little clinical significance. However, identification of structural mutations in apoA-I that lead to decreased plasma HDL levels and premature cardiovascular disease have important clinical implications for the diagnosis and treatment of patients with early heart disease. Two point mutations in the amino acid sequence of apoA-I, the deletion of apoA-I lysine 107 and the substitution of proline 165 for arginine, are associated with reduced levels of HDL cholesterol (303). Mutations in the apoA-I + apoC-III + apoA-IV gene complex on chromosome 11 that lead to the virtual absence of plasma apoA-I and HDL cholesterol are associated with severe premature heart disease. Four illustrative kindreds will be reviewed with premature coronary heart disease, markedly decreased plasma HDL levels, and a deficiency of apoA-I alone or in combination with apoC-III or apoC-III + apoA-IV.

Isolated Apolipoprotein A-I Deficiency

Two representative kindreds with apoA-I deficiency are summarized in this section. In the first kindred, the proband with apoA-I deficiency was a 5-year-old Turkish girl with planar xanthomas and a markedly reduced level of plasma HDL (304). Family history was positive for early heart disease. Clinical features included mild hepatomegaly, but no splenomegaly, neuropathy, or orange tonsils. Plasma apoA-I was absent, apoA-II was reduced to 10% of control subjects, and apoC-III and apoA-IV levels were within the control range. The molecular defect in the proband was identified as a deletion of a base resulting in a frameshift introducing a premature stop codon at residue 27 in apoA-I.

The proband in a second kindred with apoA-I deficiency was a 25-year-old man of Philippine origin with planar xanthomas (305) and established coronary heart disease based on ultrafast CT. The lipoprotein profile included normal plasma triglycerides, reduced total cholesterol, markedly decreased HDL cholesterol (<3 mg/dL) and apoA-II (7–13 mg/dL), and absence of plasma apoA-I. The proband's 62-year-old aunt also had no plasma apoA-I and had coronary artery bypass surgery at age 61 years. The structural defect in the *apoA-I* gene in this kindred has not been reported.

Apolipoprotein A-I + Apolipoprotein C-III Deficiency

The affected individuals in apoA-I + apoC-III kindred are two sisters identified at ages 31 and 32 years with mild corneal opacities and planar xanthomas on the trunk, neck, and eyelids and severe CAD (306,307). Plasma levels of

VLDL were reduced, LDL was normal, and HDL was severely decreased (6 mg/dL). ApoA-I and apoC-III were absent and apoA-II was reduced to less than 5% of normal. The molecular defect in this kindred was a rearrangement in the *apoA-I* and *apoC-III* genes resulting in the failure of synthesis of both *apoA-I* and *apoC-III*.

Apolipoprotein A-I + Apolipoprotein C-III + Apolipoprotein A-IV Deficiency

The proband was a 45-year-old woman with mild corneal opacities and severe premature heart disease (308,309). There were no xanthomas, orange tonsils, or organomegaly. Plasma triglycerides and VLDL were reduced, LDL and plasma apoB were normal, and HDL was markedly decreased. Plasma apolipoproteins A-I, C-III, and A-IV were absent from plasma, and apoA-II was decreased to less than 10% of normal. The genetic defect in this kindred is a 7.5-kb deletion that results in the failure of synthesis of all three apolipoproteins—A-I, C-III, and apoA-IV.

These kindreds with apoA-I deficiency illustrate two clinically important points. First, the close proximity and tandem array of the genes for apolipoproteins A-I, C-III, and A-IV on chromosome 11 permits the loss of the expression of up to three apolipoproteins by a single mutation. Second, the absence of synthesis of plasma apoA-I and markedly decreased HDL-cholesterol levels because of a genetic defect in the *apoA-I* gene alone or in combination with a deficiency of *apoC-III* or *apoC-III* + *apoA-IV* results in the development of severe premature heart disease. Thus, *apoA-I* is necessary for normal plasma levels of HDL, and a defect in the *apoA-I* gene that results in decreased *apoA-I* synthesis dramatically increases the risk for premature cardiovascular disease.

Familial Hypoalphalipoproteinemia

Kindreds with familial hypoalphalipoproteinemia have been identified with normal plasma triglycerides and decreased plasma HDL-cholesterol levels (310,311). A subset of these kindreds has cosegregation of low plasma HDL levels and an increased risk for premature cardiovascular disease. There are no characteristic clinical features and the plasma lipids and lipoproteins often are normal, except for the reduced plasma levels of HDL cholesterol. The genetic defect(s) leading to familial hypoalphalipoproteinemia has not been identified. Patients with CAD with "normal lipids" may be members of kindreds with familial hypoalphalipoproteinemia.

Lecithin-Cholesterol Acyltransferase Deficiency Syndromes

Lecithin-cholesterol acyltransferase (LCAT) deficiency is a genetic dyslipoproteinemia characterized by reduced or absent plasma LCAT activity and marked hypoalphalipoproteinemia. LCAT, the major enzyme responsible for the esterification of free cholesterol present in circulating plasma lipoproteins catalyzes the transfer of an unsaturated fatty acid from the sn-2 position of lecithin to free cholesterol, generating cholesteryl ester and lysolecithin (312–319). The esterification of free cholesterol removed by nascent HDL after interaction with the ABCA1 by LCAT is essential for the maturation of disc-shaped nascent pre-β HDL into spherical α-HDL particles and for facilitating reverse cholesterol transport (315). LCAT-derived cholesteryl ester is transported back to the liver directly by HDL or after transfer to the apoB-containing lipoproteins by CETP.

Mutations in the *LCAT* gene are associated with either a partial or complete absence of plasma LCAT activity, leading to fish eye disease (FED) or familial *LCAT* deficiency, respectively (312,316). Familial *LCAT* deficiency is characterized by hypertriglyceridemia, markedly reduced HDL levels, cloudy corneas, hemolytic anemia, and renal disease. The major clinical manifestations of patients with FED are cloudy corneas and markedly decreased plasma HDL levels (Fig. 5–12) (312,316). Both groups of patients have reduced plasma concentrations of apoA-I and apoA-II. The deficiency in LCAT results in failure of the formation of cholesteryl esters and the maturation of the nascent HDL particles (320). The poorly lipidated HDL particles undergo rapid catabolism resulting in low plasma HDL levels. The apoB-containing lipoproteins, which are increased in concentration, also undergo rapid catabolism. In addition, there is decreased conversion of IDL to LDL resulting in low plasma LDL levels in LCAT deficiency. Abnormal multilaminar lipoprotein particles resembling lipoprotein X (LpX) may also be present in VLDLs, IDLs, and LDLs in LCAT deficiency (316,321–323). Despite decreased HDL, the risk for atherothrombosis in most patients with LCAT deficiency is not increased (316,321–323).

The importance of LCAT in modulating plasma lipoprotein metabolism has been demonstrated in genetically engineered mice with altered expression of the enzyme. Overexpression of LCAT in transgenic rabbits (324) and mice (325–329) increases the plasma concentrations of total cholesterol, cholesteryl ester, HDL-cholesterol, and apoA-I. Similar findings have been reported in nonhuman primates transiently expressing the human enzyme after recombinant adenovirus infusion (330). Deficiency of LCAT leads to markedly reduced plasma HDL-C levels, accumulation of LpX, hemolytic anemia, and glomerulosclerosis in mice (331). Glomset (288) first proposed that by generating a concentration gradient for the diffusion of free cholesterol from peripheral tissues to HDL, LCAT could facilitate the process of reverse cholesterol transport and modulate the development of atherothrombosis. Although there is an increasing body of evidence that supports this concept, the role of LCAT in atherothrombosis remains to be definitively established.

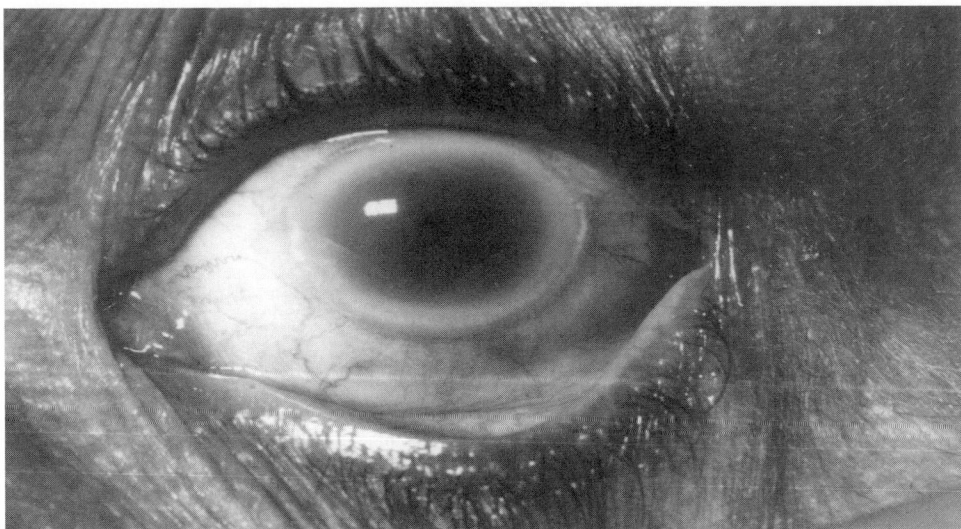

FIG. 5–12. Cloudy cornea observed in patients with fish eye disease or lecithin-cholesterol acyltransferase deficiency.

FAMILIAL HYPERALPHALIPOPROTEINEMIA

Cholesteryl Ester Transfer Protein Deficiency

A number of epidemiologic studies have demonstrated a negative correlation between HDL cholesterol levels and the incidence of coronary heart disease, suggesting a protective role of HDL in cardiovascular disease. A novel cause of familial hyperalphalipoproteinemia, CETP deficiency, has been identified (332). As illustrated in Figure 5–1, CETP catalyzes the exchange of triglycerides and cholesteryl esters between plasma lipoproteins. Kindreds with a deficiency of CETP have a marked increase of plasma HDLs, which are enriched in CE and apoE, as well as decreased levels of LDL, which are polydisperse and poor in CE. The initial patients identified with CETP deficiency had cardiovascular disease and premature corneal opacities. Several mutations have been identified in the *CETP* gene including an intron 14 splicing defect and missense mutation at exon 15 (D442), which are the most frequent molecular causes of CETP deficiency (333). Kinetic studies in patients with CETP established that the increased HDLs was caused by delayed catabolism and the decreased LDLs resulted from increased catabolism (334,335). The relation between CETP deficiency and premature cardiovascular has been controversial. *In vitro* studies have established that the large HDLs have a reduced ability to efflux cholesterol (336) and the polydisperse LDLs have a lower affinity than normal LDL for the LDL receptor on fibroblasts (337). The limited number of homozygous subjects with CETP deficiency has limited the conclusive analysis of cardiovascular disease in these individuals and the majority of the data come from heterozygous subjects. A high frequency of CETP deficiency was found in the Omagari area of Japan. In this area, the prevalence of marked increases in HDLs and the *CETP*

gene mutation decreased with age. In these studies, a U-shaped relation between plasma HDL levels and ischemic changes identified by electrocardiogram was identified. In contrast, in other studies in the Japanese population both moderate and high levels of HDL were reported to be associated with less cardiovascular disease (332). An analysis of the association of CETP gene polymorphisms and the development of cardiovascular disease has been undertaken. A CETP Taq1B gene polymorphism has been associated with increased HDLs and a decreased risk for cardiovascular disease in men (338). In contrast, the I405V polymorphism in women participants of the Copenhagen City Heart study was associated with increased HDL and increased cardiovascular disease (339). In an additional study, carriers of the 451Q/373P mutation had decreased HDL levels and a lower atherothrombosis (340). In animal studies, inhibition of CETP in rabbits by antisense oligodeoxynucleotides (341), anti-CETP antibodies (342,343), or a chemical inhibitor (344) were all associated with decreased aortic atherothrombosis. Further studies will be required to definitively establish if CETP deficiency is associated with increased risk for atherothrombosis. The resolution of this question is of great interest because of the potential development of drugs to increase HDL by inhibition of CETP.

SUMMARY

During the last two decades there has been a progressive increase in our knowledge of the pathways of cholesterol and triglyceride metabolism. The detailed information currently available on the role of the plasma lipoproteins in lipid transport and the specific functions in metabolism of lipoprotein receptors, enzymes, transfer proteins, and apolipoproteins has provided the framework for a detailed understanding of lipid transport. In addition, the role of the plasma lipoproteins, enzymes, and receptors in the development of the atherosclerotic process has been more clearly defined. This new knowledge has markedly facilitated the elucidation of the molecular defects in patients with genetic dyslipoproteinemias. Identification of the specific gene defects and the resulting clinical phenotypes now provides the opportunity to develop improved methods for identification of the individual at risk for development of a dyslipoproteinemia and the potential for more selective and specific treatment programs. The ultimate goal of these studies is to identify and treat effectively the patient with a potential risk for premature cardiovascular disease. The current availability of more effective drugs for the treatment of the dyslipoproteinemias and the ultimate ability to correct gene defects by gene therapy provide an encouraging future for the eventual reduction in atherothrombosis and the prevention of premature cardiovascular disease.

REFERENCES

1. Brewer HB Jr, Gregg RE, Hoeg JM, et al. Apolipoproteins and lipoproteins in human plasma: an overview. *Clin Chem* 1988;34:4–8.
2. Brewer HB Jr, Gregg RE, Hoeg JM. Apolipoproteins, lipoproteins, and atherosclerosis. In: Braunwald E, ed. *Heart disease: a textbook of cardiovascular medicine.* Philadelphia: WB Saunders, 1989:121–144.
3. Schaefer EJ. Diagnosis and management of lipoprotein disorders. In: Rifkind BM, ed. *Drug treatment of hyperlipidemia.* New York: Marcel-Dekker, 1991:17–52.
4. Havel RJ, Kane JP. Introduction: structure and metabolism of plasma lipoprotein. *The metabolic basis of inherited disease.* New York: McGraw-Hill, 2001:2705–2716.
5. Davignon J, Gregg RE, Sing CF. Apolipoprotein E polymorphism and atherosclerosis. *Arteriosclerosis* 1988;8:1–21.
6. Assman G, von Eckardstein A, Brewer HB. Familial analphalipoproteinemia: Tangier disease. *The metabolic basis of inherited disease.* New York: McGraw-Hill, 2001:2937–2980.
7. Brewer HB, Santamarina-Fojo S. Clinical significance of high-density lipoproteins and the development of atherosclerosis: focus on the role of the adenosine triphosphate-binding cassette protein A1 transporter. *Am J Cardiol* 2003;92(4B):10K–16K.
8. Goldstein JL, Brown MS. The LDL receptor locus and the genetics of familial hypercholesterolemia. *Annu Rev Genet* 1979;13:259–289.
9. Goldstein JL, Brown MS, Anderson RG, et al. Receptor-mediated endocytosis: concepts emerging from the LDL receptor system. *Annu Rev Cell Biol* 1985;1:1–39.
10. Willnow TE, Sheng Z, Ishibashi S, et al. Inhibition of hepatic chylomicron remnant uptake by gene transfer of a receptor antagonist. *Science* 1994;264:1471–1474.
11. Willnow TE, Armstrong SA, Hammer RE, et al. Functional expression of low density lipoprotein receptor-related protein is controlled by receptor-associated protein *in vivo. Proc Natl Acad Sci USA* 1995;92:4537–4541.
12. Rohlmann A, Gotthardt M, Hammer RE, et al. Inducible inactivation of hepatic LRP gene by cre-mediated recombination confirms role of LRP in clearance of chylomicron remnants. *J Clin Invest* 1998;101:689–695.
13. Herz J, Hamann U, Rogne S, et al. Surface location and high affinity for a calcium of a 500 kDa liver membrane protein closely related to the LDL receptor suggest a physiological role as a lipoprotein receptor. *EMBO J* 1988;7:4119–4127.
14. Strickland DK, Ashcom JD, Williams S, et al. Sequence identity between alpha2-macroglobulin receptor and low density lipoprotein receptor-related protein suggests that this molecule is a multifunctional receptor. *J Biol Chem* 1990;265:17401–17404.
15. Willnow TE, Nykjaer A, Herz J. Lipoprotein receptors: new roles for ancient proteins. *Nat Cell Biol* 1999;1(6):E157–E162.
16. Strickland DK. LRP: a multifunctional scavenger and signaling receptor. *J Clin Invest* 2001;108:779–784.
17. Herz J, Beffert U. Apolipoprotein E receptors: linking brain development and Alzheimer's disease. *Nat Rev Neurosci* 2000;1(1):51–58.
18. Goldstein JL, Hobbs HH, Brown MS. Familial hypercholesterolemia. In: Scriver CR, Beaudet AL, Sly WS, et al., eds. *The metabolic and molecular bases of inherited disease.* New York: McGraw-Hill, 2001:2863–2914.
19. Steinberg D. Lipoproteins and atherosclerosis. A look back and a look ahead. *Arteriosclerosis* 1983;3:283–301.
20. Steinberg D. Antioxidants and atherosclerosis: a current assessment. *Circulation* 1991;84:1420–1425.
21. Van Lenten BJ, Fogelman AM. Processing of lipoproteins in human monocyte-macrophages. *J Lipid Res* 1990;31:1455–1466.
22. Haberland ME, Fogelman AM. The role of altered lipoproteins in the pathogenesis of atherosclerosis. *Am Heart J* 1987;113:573–557.
23. Navab M, Hama SY, Nguyen TB, et al. Monocyte adhesion and transmigration in atherosclerosis. *Coron Artery Dis* 1994;5:198–204.
24. Glomset JA, Janssen ET, Kennedy R, et al. Role of plasma lecithin:cholesterol acyltransferase in the metabolism of high density lipoproteins. *J Lipid Res* 1966;7:638–648.
25. Glomset JA. The plasma lecithins:cholesterol acyltransferase reaction. *J Lipid Res* 1968;9:155–167.
26. Brooks-Wilson A, Marcil M, Clee SM, et al. Mutations in ABC1 in Tangier disease and familial high-density lipoprotein deficiency. *Nat Genet* 1999;22:336–345.
27. Bodzioch M, Orso E, Klucken J, et al. The gene encoding ATP-binding cassette transporter 1 is mutated in Tangier disease. *Nat Genet* 1999;22:347–351.
28. Rust S, Rosier M, Funke H, et al. Tangier disease is caused by mutations in the gene encoding ATP-binding cassette transporter 1. *Nat Genet* 1999;22:352–355.
29. Remaley AT, Rust S, Rosier M, et al. Human ATP-binding cassette transporter 1 (ABC1): genomic organization and identification of the genetic defect in the original Tangier disease kindred *Proc Natl Acad Sci USA* 1999;96:12685–12690.
30. Santamarina-Fojo S, Peterson K, Knapper C, et al. Complete genomic sequence of the human ABCA1 gene: analysis of the human and mouse ATP-binding cassette A promoter. *Proc Natl Acad Sci USA* 2000;97:7987–7992.
31. Lawn RM, Wade DP, Garvin MR, et al. The Tangier disease gene product ABC1 controls the cellular apolipoprotein-mediated lipid removal pathway. *J Clin Invest* 1999;104:25–31.
32. Brousseau ME, Schaefer EJ, Dupuis J, et al. Novel mutations in the gene encoding ATP-binding cassette 1 in four tangier disease kindreds. *J Lipid Res* 2000;41:433–441.
33. Yancey PG, Bortnick AE, Kellner-Weibel G, et al. Importance of different pathways of cellular cholesterol efflux. *Arterioscler Thromb Vasc Biol* 2003;23:712–719.
34. Williams DL, Connelly MA, Temel RE, et al. Scavenger receptor BI and cholesterol trafficking. *Curr Opin Lipidol* 1999;10:329–339.
35. Trigatti BL, Krieger M, Rigotti A. Influence of the HDL receptor SR-BI on lipoprotein metabolism and atherosclerosis. *Arterioscler Thromb Vasc Biol* 2003;23:1732–1738.
36. Eisenberg S. High density lipoprotein metabolism. *J Lipid Res* 1984;25:1017–1058.
37. Rader DJ, Castro G, Zech LA, et al. *In vivo* metabolism of apolipoprotein A-I on high density lipoprotein particles LpA-I and LpA-I, A-II. *J Lipid Res* 1991;32:1849–1859.
38. Brinton EA, Eisenberg S, Breslow JL. Human HDL cholesterol levels are determined by apoA-I fractional catabolic rate, which correlates inversely with estimates of HDL particle size: effects of gender, hepatic and lipoprotein lipases, triglyceride and insulin levels, and body fat distribution. *Arterioscler Thromb* 1994;14:707–720.
39. Tall AR. Plasma cholesteryl ester transfer protein. *J Lipid Res* 1993;34:1255–1274.
40. Schwartz CC, Zech LA, VandenBroek JM, et al. Cholesterol kinetics in subjects with bile fistula. Positive relationship between size of the bile acid precursor pool and bile acid synthetic rate. *J Clin Invest* 1993;91:923–938.
41. Utermann G, Weber W. Protein composition of Lp(a) lipoprotein from human plasma. *FEBS Lett* 1983;154:357–361.
42. Fless GM, Rolih CA, Scanu AM. Heterogeneity of human plasma

lipoprotein (a). Isolation and charcterization of the lipoprotein subspecies and their apoproteins. *J Biol Chem* 1984;259:11470–11478.

43. Eaton DL, Fless GM, Kohr WJ, et al. Partial amino acid sequence of apolipoprotein(a) shows that it is homologous to plasminogen. *Proc Natl Acad Sci USA* 1987;84:3224–3228.

44. Utermann G. Lipoprotein(a). *The metabolic basis of inherited disease.* New York: McGraw-Hill, 2001:2753–2788.

45. McLean JW, Tomlinson JE, Kuang WJ, et al. cDNA sequence of human apolipoprotein(a) is homologous to plasminogen. *Nature* 1987;330:132–137.

46. Utermann G, Menzel HJ, Kraft HG, et al. Lp(a) glycoprotein phenotypes. Inheritance and relation to Lp(a)-lipoprotein concentrations in plasma. *J Clin Invest* 1987;80:458–465.

47. Koschinsky ML, Beisiegel U, Henne-Bruns D, et al. Apolipoprotein(a) size heterogeneity is related to variable number of repeat sequences in its mRNA. *Biochemistry* 1990;29:640–644.

48. Azrolan N, Gavish D, Breslow JL. Lp(a) levels correlate inversely with apo(a) size and KIV copy number but not with apo(a) mRNA levels in a cynomolgus monkey model. *Circulation* 1990;82:III-90.

49. Kostner GM, Avagaro P, Zazzolato G, et al. Lipoprotein Lp(a) and the risk for myocardial infarction. *Arteriosclerosis* 1981;38:51–61.

50. Armstrong VW, Cremer P, Eberle E, et al. The association between serum Lp(a) concentrations and angiographically assessed coronary atherosclerosis. Dependence on serum LDL levels. *Atherosclerosis* 1986;62:249–257.

51. Utermann G. The mysteries of lipoprotein(a). *Science* 1989;246:904–910.

52. Scanu AM. Genetic basis and pathophysiological implications of high plasma Lp(a) levels. *J Intern Med* 1992;231:679–683.

53. Schaefer EJ, Lamon-Fava S, Jenner JL, et al. Lipoprotein(a) levels and risk of coronary heart disease in men: the Lipid Research Clinics Coronary Primary Prevention Trial. *JAMA* 1994;271:999–1003.

54. Loscalzo J. Lipoprotein(a). A unique risk factor for atherothrombotic disease. *Arteriosclerosis* 1990;10:672–679.

55. Miles LA, Plow EF. Lp(a): an interloper in the fibrinolytic system. *Thromb Haemostasis* 1990;63:331–335.

56. Bulkley BH, Buja LM, Ferrans VJ, et al. Tuberous xanthoma in homozygous type II hyperlipoproteinemia. A histologic, histochemical, and electron microscopical study. *Arch Pathol* 1975;99:293–300.

57. Hoeg JM, Feuerstein IM, Tucker EE. Detection and quantitation of calcific atherosclerosis by ultrafast CT in children and young adults with homozygous familial hypercholesterolemia. *Arterioscler Thromb* 1994;14:1066–1074.

58. Hoeg JM. Familial hypercholesterolemia: what the zebra can teach us about the horse. *JAMA* 1994;271:543–546.

59. Lindgren V, Luskey KL, Russell DW, et al. Human genes involved in cholesterol metabolism: chromosomal mapping of the loci for the low density lipoprotein receptor and 3-hydroxy-3-methylglutaryl coenzyme A reductase with cDNA probes. *Proc Natl Acad Sci USA* 1985;82:8567–8571.

60. Sudhof TC, Goldstein JL, Brown MS, et al. The LDL receptor gene: a mosiac of exons shared with different proteins. *Science* 1985;228:815–822.

61. Schneider WJ, Beisiegel U, Goldstein JL, et al. Purification of the low density lipoprotein receptor, an acidic glycoprotein of 164,000 molecular weight. *J Biol Chem* 1982;257:2664–2673.

62. Cummings RD, Kornfield S, Schneider WJ, et al. Biosynthesis of N- and O-linked oligosaccharides of the low density lipoprotein receptor. *J Biol Chem* 1983;258:15261–15273.

63. Rudenko G, Henry L, Henderson K, et al. Structure of the LDL receptor extracellular domain at endosomal pH. *Science* 2002;298:2353–2358.

64. Hobbs HH, Brown MS, Goldstein JL, et al. Deletion of exon encoding cysteine-rich repeat of low density lipoprotein receptor alters its binding specificity in a subject with familial hypercholesterolemia. *J Biol Chem* 1986;261:13114–13120.

65. Jeon H, Meng W, Takagi J, et al. Implications for familial hypercholesterolemia from the structure of the LDL receptor YWTD-EGF domain pair. *Nat Struct Biol* 2001;8:499–504.

66. Brown MS, Goldstein JL. Familial hypercholesterolemia: defective binding of lipoproteins to cultured fibroblasts associated with impaired regulation of 3-hydroxy-3-methylglutaryl coenzyme A reductase activity. *Proc Natl Acad Sci USA* 1974;71:788–792.

67. Brown MS, Goldstein JL. Analysis of a mutant strain of human fibroblasts with a defect in the internalization of receptor-bound low density lipoprotein. *Cell* 1976;9:663–674.

68. Hobbs HH, Brown MS, Goldstein JL. Molecular genetics of the LDL receptor gene in familial hypercholesterolemia. *Hum Mutat* 1992;1:445–446.

69. Edge SB, Hoeg JM, Triche T, et al. Cultured human hepatocytes. Evidence for metabolism of low density lipoproteins by a pathway independent of the classical low density lipoprotein receptor. *J Biol Chem* 1986;261:3800–3806.

70. Witztum JL, Simmons D, Steinberg D, et al. Intensive combination drug therapy of familial hypercholesterolemia with lovastatin, probucol, and colestipol hydrochloride. *Circulation* 1989;79:16–28.

71. Illingworth DR. Management of hyperlipidemia: goals for the prevention of atherosclerosis. *Clin Invest Med* 1990;13:211–218.

72. Eric B, Philippe G, Tellier P. Perspectives in cholesterol-lowering therapy: the role of ezetimibe, a new selective inhibitor of intestinal cholesterol absorption. *Circulation* 2003;107:3124–3128.

73. Gagne C, Gaudet D, Bruckert E. Efficacy and safety of ezetimibe coadministered with atorvastatin or simvastatin in patients with homozygous familial hypercholesterolemia. *Circulation* 2002;105:2469–2475.

74. Cleeman JI, Grundy SM, Becker D, et al. Executive summary of the Third Report of the National Cholesterol Education Program (NCEP) expert panel on detection, evaluation, and treatment of high blood cholesterol in adults (Adult Treatment Panel III). *JAMA* 2001;285:2486–2497.

75. Scandinavian Simvastatin Survival Study Group. Randomized trial of cholesterol lowering in 4444 patients with coronary heart disease: the Scandinavian Simvastatin Survival Study (4S). *Lancet* 1994;344:1383–1389.

76. Thompson GR. LDL apheresis. *Atherosclerosis* 2003;167:1–13.

77. Gordon BR, Stein E, Jones P, et al. Indications for low-density lipoprotein apheresis. *Am J Cardiol* 1994;74:1109–1112.

78. Sprecher DL, Hoeg JM, Schaefer EJ, et al. The association of LDL receptor activity, LDL cholesterol level, and clinical course in homozygous familial hypercholesterolemia. *Metabolism* 1985;34:294–299.

79. Postiglione A, Thompson GR. Experience with plasma-exchange in homozygous familial hypercholesterolemia. *Prog Clin Biol Res* 1985;188:213–220.

80. Stein EA, Glueck CJ, Wesselman A, et al. Repetitive intermittent flow plasma exchange in patients with severe hypercholesterolemia. *Atherosclerosis* 1981;38:149–164.

81. Tatami R, Inoue N, Itoh H, et al. Regression of coronary atherosclerosis by combined LDL-apheresis and lipid-lowering drug therapy in patients with familial hypercholesterolemia: a multicenter study. *Atherosclerosis* 1992;95:1–13.

82. Gordon BR, Kelsey SF, Bilheimer DW, et al. Treatment of refractory familial hypercholesterolemia by low-density lipoprotein apheresis using an automated dextran sulfate cellulose adsorption system. *Am J Cardiol* 1992;70:1010–1016.

83. Eisenhauer T, Schuff-Werner P, Armstrong VW, et al. Long-term experience with the HELP system for treatment of severe familial hypercholesterolemia. *ASAIO Trans* 1987;33:395–397.

84. Borberg H, Gaczkowski A, Oette K, et al. Immunosorptive apheresis of LDL. *Prog Clin Biol Res* 1990;337:163–167.

85. Borberg H, Gaczkowski A, Hombach V, et al. Regression of atherosclerosis in patients with familial hypercholesterolemia under LDL-apheresis. *Prog Clin Biol Res* 1988;255:317–326.

86. Starzl TE, Bilheimer DW, Bahnson HT, et al. Heart–liver transplantation in a patient with familial hypercholesterolemia. *Lancet* 1984;1:1382–1383.

87. Bilheimer DW, Goldstein JL, Grundy SM, et al. Liver transplantation to provide low-density-lipoprotein receptors and lower plasma cholesterol in a child with homozygous familial hypercholesterolemia. *N Engl J Med* 1984;311:1658–1664.

88. Hoeg JM, Starzl TE, Brewer HB Jr. Liver transplantation for treatment of cardiovascular disease: comparison with medication and plasma exchange in homozygous familial hypercholesterolemia. *Am J Cardiol* 1987;59:705–707.

89. Wilson JM, Chowdhury JR. Prospects for gene therapy of familial hypercholesterolemia. *Mol Biol Med* 1990;7:223–232.

90. Grossman M, Rader DJ, Muller DWM, et al. A pilot study of ex vivo gene therapy for homozygous familial hypercholesterolaemia. *Nat Med* 1995;1:1148–1154.

91. Chowdhury JR, Grossman M, Gupta S, et al. Long-term improvement of hypercholesterolemia after *ex vivo* gene therapy in LDLR-deficient rabbits. *Science* 1991;254:1802–1805.

92. Wilson JM, Grossman M, Wu CH, et al. Hepatocyte-directed gene transfer *in vivo* leads to transient improvement of hypercholesterolemia in low density lipoprotein receptor-deficient rabbits. *J Biol Chem* 1992;267:963–967.

93. Vega GL, Grundy SM. *In vivo* evidence for reduced binding of low density lipoproteins to receptors as a cause of primary moderate hypercholesterolemia. *J Clin Invest* 1986;78:1410–1414.

94. Innerarity TL, Weisgraber KH, Arnold KS, et al. Familial defective apolipoprotein B-100: low density lipoproteins with abnormal receptor binding. *Proc Natl Acad Sci USA* 1987;84:6919–6923.

95. Soria LF, Ludwig EH, Clarke HR, et al. Association between a specific apolipoprotein B mutation and familial defective apolipoprotein B-100. *Proc Natl Acad Sci USA* 1989;86:587–591.

96. Weisgraber KH, Innerarity TL, Newhouse YM, et al. Familial defective apolipoprotein B-100: enhanced binding of monoclonal antibody MB47 to abnormal low density lipoproteins. *Proc Natl Acad Sci USA* 1988;85:9758–9762.

97. Myant NB. Familial defective apolipoprotein B-100: a review, including some comparisons with familial hypercholesterolaemia. *Atherosclerosis* 1993;104:1–18.

98. Kane JP, Havel RJ. Disorders of the biogenesis and secretion of lipoproteins containing the B apolipoproteins. In: Scriver CR, Beaudet AL, Sly WS, et al., eds. *The metabolic and molecular bases of inherited disease.* New York: McGraw-Hill, 2001:2717–2752.

99. Boren J, Ekstrom U, Agren B, et al. The molecular mechanism for the genetic disorder familial defective apolipoprotein B100. *J Biol Chem* 2001;276:9214–9218.

100. Illingworth DR, Vakar F, Mahley RW, et al. Hypocholesterolemia effects of lovastatin in familial defective apolipoproteinemia B-100. *Lancet* 1992;339:598–600.

101. Schmidt EB, Illingworth DR, Bacon S, et al. Hypolipidemic effects of nicotinic acid in patients with familial defective apolipoprotein B-100. *Metabolism* 1993;42:137–139.

102. Schmidt EB, Illingworth DR, Bacon S, et al. Hypocholesterolemia effects of cholestyramine and colestipol in patients with familial defective apolipoprotein B-100. *Atherosclerosis* 1993;98:213–217.

103. Goldstein JL, Schrott HG, Hazzard WR, et al. Hyperlipidemia in coronary heart disease. II. Genetic analysis of lipid levels in 176 families and delineation of a new inherited disorder, combined hyperlipidemia. *J Clin Invest* 1973;52:1544–1568.

104. Rose HG, Kranz P, Weinstock M, et al. Inheritance of combined hyperlipoproteinemia: evidence for a new lipoprotein phenotype. *Am J Med* 1973;54:148–160.

105. Nikkila EA, Aro A. Family study of serum lipids and lipoproteins in coronary heart-disease. *Lancet* 1973;1:954–959.

106. Brunzell JD, Albers JJ, Chait A, et al. Plasma lipoproteins in familial combined hyperlipidemia and monogenic familial hypertriglyceridemia. *J Lipid Res* 1983;24:147–155.

107. Sniderman A, Shapiro S, Marpole D, et al. Association of coronary atherosclerosis with hyperapobetalipoproteinemia [increased protein but normal cholesterol levels in human plasma low density (beta) lipoproteins]. *Proc Natl Acad Sci USA* 1980;77:604–608.

108. Sniderman AD, Wolfson C, Teng B, et al. Association of hyperapolipoproteinemia with endogenous hypertriglyceridemia and atherosclerosis. *Ann Intern Med* 1982;97:833–839.

109. Hopkins PN, Heiss G, Ellison RC, et al. Coronary artery disease risk in familial combined hyperlipidemia and familial hypertriglyceridemia: a case-control comparison from the National Heart, Lung, and Blood Institute Family Heart Study. *Circulation* 2003;108:519–523.

110. Ayyobi AF, McGladdery SH, McNeely MJ, et al. Small, dense LDL and elevated apolipoprotein B are the common characteristics for the three major lipid phenotypes of familial combined hyperlipidemia. *Arterioscler Thromb Vasc Biol* 2003;23:1289–1294.

111. Janus ED, Nicoll AM, Turner PR, et al. Kinetic bases of the primary hyperlipidaemias: studies of apolipoprotein B turnover in genetically defined subjects. *Eur J Clin Invest* 1980;10:161–172.

112. Thompson GR, Teng B, Sniderman AD. Kinetics of LDL subfractions. *Am Heart J* 1987;113:514–557.

113. Pajukanta P, Nuotio I, Terwilliger JD, et al. Linkage of familial com-

114. Aouizerat BE, Allayee H, Cantor RM, et al. A genome scan for familial combined hyperlipidemia reveals evidence of linkage with locus on chromosome 11. *Am J Hum Genet* 1999;65:397–412.

115. Pajukanta P, Allayee H, Krass KL, et al. Combined analysis of genome scans of Dutch and Finnish families reveals a susceptibility locus for high-density lipoprotein cholesterol on chromosome 16q. *Am J Hum Genet* 2003;72:903–917.

116. Eurlings PMH, van der Kallen CJH, Geurts JMW, et al. Genetic dissection of familial combined hyperlipidemia. *Mol Genet Metab* 2001;74:98–104.

117. Haddad L, Day IN, Hunt S, et al. Evidence for a third genetic locus causing familial hypercholesterolemia. A non-LDLR, non-APOB kindred. *J Lipid Res* 1999;40:1113–1122.

118. Varret M, Rabes JP, Saint-Jore B, et al. A third major locus for autosomal dominant hypercholesterolemia maps to 1p34.1-p32. *Am J Hum Genet* 1999;64:1378–1387.

119. Abifadel M, Varret M, Rabes JP, et al. Mutations in PCSK9 cause autosomal dominant hypercholesterolemia. *Nat Genet* 2003;34:154–156.

120. Seidah NG, Benjannet S, Wickham L, et al. The secretory proprotein convertase neural apoptosis-regulated convertase 1 (NARC-1): liver regeneration and neuronal differentiation. *Proc Natl Acad Sci USA* 2003;100:928–933.

121. Cohen JC, Kimmel M, Polanski A, et al. Molecular mechanisms of autosomal recessive hypercholesterolemia. *Curr Opin Lipidol* 2003;14:121–127.

122. Rader DJ, Cohen J, Hobbs HH. Monogenic hypercholesterolemia: new insights in pathogenesis and treatment *J Clin Invest* 2003;111:795–1803.

123. Zuliani G, Vigna GB, Corsini A, et al. Severe hypercholesterolaemia: unusual inheritance in an Italian pedigree. *Eur J Clin Invest* 1995;25:322–331.

124. Khachadurian AK, Uthman SM. Experiences with the homozygous cases of familial hypercholesterolemia. A report of 52 patients. *Nutr Metab* 1973;15:132–140.

125. Arca M, Zuliani G, Wilund K, et al. Autosomal recessive hypercholesterolaemia in Sardinia, Italy, and mutations in ARH: a clinical and molecular genetic analysis. *Lancet* 2002;359:841–847.

126. Garcia CK, Wilund K, Arca M, et al. Autosomal recessive hypercholesterolemia caused by mutations in a putative LDL receptor adaptor protein. *Science* 2001;292:1394–1398.

127. Forman-Kay JD, Pawson T. Diversity in protein recognition by PTB domains. *Curr Opin Struc Biol* 1999;9:690–695.

128. Davis CG, van Driel IR, Russell DW, et al. The low density lipoprotein receptor. Identification of amino acids in cytoplasmic domain required for rapid endocytosis. *J Biol Chem* 1987;262:4075–4082.

129. He G, Gupta S, Michaely P, et al. ARH is a modular adaptor protein that interacts with the LDL receptor, clathrin and AP-2. *J Biol Chem* 2002;277:44044–44049.

130. Mishra SK, Watkins SC, Traub LM. The autosomal recessive hypercholesterolemia (ARH) protein interfaces directly with the clathrin-coat machinery. *Proc Natl Acad Sci USA* 2002;99:16099–16104.

131. Eden ER, Patel DD, Sun XM, et al. Restoration of LDL receptor function in cells from patients with autosomal recessive hypercholesterolemia by retroviral expression of *ARH1*. *J Clin Invest* 2002;110:1695–1702.

132. Norman D, Sun XM, Bourbon M, et al. Characterization of a novel cellular defect in patients with phenotypic homozygous familial hypercholesterolemia. *J Clin Invest* 1999;104:619–628.

133. Fojo SS, Brewer HB Jr. The familial hyperchylomicronemia syndrome. *JAMA* 1991;265:904–908.

134. Santamarina-Fojo S. The familial chylomicronemia syndrome. *Endocrinol Metab Clin North Am* 1998;27:551–567.

135. Brunzell JD, Deeb SS. Familial lipoprotein lipase deficiency, apo c-ii deficiency and hepatic lipase deficiency. *The metabolic basis of inherited disease.* New York: McGraw-Hill, 2001:2789–2816.

136. Fallat RW, Vester JW, Glueck CJ. Suppression of amylase activity by hypertriglyceridemia. *JAMA* 1973;225:1331–1334.

137. Lesser PB, Warshaw AL. Diagnosis of pancreatitis masked by hyperlipemia. *Ann Intern Med* 1975;82:795–798.

138. Warshaw AL, Bellini CA, Lesser PB. Inhibition of serum and urine amylase activity in pancreatitis with hyperlipemia. *Ann Surg* 1975;182:72–75.

bined hyperlipidaemia to chromosme 1q21-23. *Nat Genet* 1998;18:369–373.

139. Austin MA, McKnight B, Edwards KL, et al. Cardiovascular disease mortality in familial forms of hypertriglyceridemia: a 20-year prospective study. *Circulation* 2000;101:2777–2782.

140. Santamarina-Fojo S. Genetic dyslipoproteinemias: role of lipoprotein lipase and apoC-II. *Curr Opin Lipidol* 1992;3:186–195.

141. Brunzell JD, Miller NE, Alaupovic P, et al. Familial chylomicronemia due to a circulating inhibitor of lipoprotein lipase activity. *J Lipid Res* 1983;24:12–19.

142. Kihara S, Matsuzawa Y, Kubo M, et al. Autoimmune hyperchylomicronemia. *N Engl J Med* 1989;320:1255–1259.

143. Fojo SS, Brewer HB Jr. Hypertriglyceridaemia due to genetic defects in lipoprotein lipase and apolipoprotein C-II. *J Intern Med* 1992;231:669–677.

144. Cheng C, Bensadoun A, Bersot T, et al. Purification and characterization of human lipoprotein lipase and hepatic triglyceride lipase. *J Biol Chem* 1985;260:10720–10727.

145. Wion KL, Kirchgessner TG, Lusis AJ, et al. Human lipoprotein lipase complementary DNA sequence. *Science* 1987;235:1638–1641.

146. Thuren T. Hepatic lipase and HDL metabolism. *Curr Opin Lipidol* 2000;11:277–283.

147. Cohen JC, Vega GL, Grundy SM. Hepatic lipase: new insights from genetic and metabolic studies. *Curr Opin Lipidol* 1999;10:259–267.

148. Santamarina-Fojo S, Haudenschild C, Amar M. The role of hepatic lipase in lipoprotein metabolism and atherosclerosis *Curr Opin Lipidol* 1998;9:211–219.

149. Mead JR, Irvine SA, Ramji DP. Lipoprotein lipase: structure, function, regulation, and role in disease. *J Mol Med* 2002;80:753–769.

150. Merkel M, Eckel RH, Goldberg IJ. Lipoprotein lipase: genetics, lipid uptake, and regulation. *J Lipid Res* 2002;43:1997–2006.

151. Beisiegel U, Heeren J. Lipoprotein lipase (EC 3.1.1.34) targeting of lipoproteins to receptors. *Proc Nutr Soc* 1997;56:731–737.

152. Gagne C, Brum LDF, Julien P, et al. Primary lipoprotein lipase activity deficiency: clinical investigation of a French Canadian population. *Can Med Assoc J* 1989;140:405–411.

153. Evans V, Kastelein JJ. Lipoprotein lipase deficiency—rare or common? *Cardiovasc Drug Ther* 2002;16:283–287.

154. Julien P. High frequency of lipoprotein lipase deficiency in the Quebec population. *Can J Cardiol* 1992;8:675–676.

155. Dionne C, Gagne C, Julien P, et al. Geneaology and regional distribution of lipoprotein lipase deficiency in French-Canadians of Quebec. *Hum Biol* 1993;65:29–39.

156. Santamarina-Fojo S, Dugi K. Structure, function and role of lipoprotein lipase in lipoprotein metabolism. *Curr Opin Lipidol* 1994;5:117–125.

157. Santamarina-Fojo S, Brewer HB Jr. Lipoprotein lipase: structure, function and mechanism of action. *Int J Clin Lab Res* 1994;24:143–147.

158. Devlin RH, Deeb S, Brunzell J, et al. Partial gene duplication involving exon-*Alu* interchange results in lipoprotein lipase deficiency. *Am J Hum Genet* 1990;46:112–119.

159. Emmerich J, Beg OU, Peterson J, et al. Human lipoprotein lipase. Analysis of the catalytic triad by site-directed mutagenesis of Ser-132, Asp-156, and His-241. *J Biol Chem* 1992;267:4161–4165.

160. Miesenboeck G, Hoelzl B, Foeger B, et al. Heterozygous lipoprotein lipase deficiency due to a missense mutation as the cause of impaired triglyceride tolerance with multiple lipoprotein abnormalities. *J Clin Invest* 1993;91:448–455.

161. Gagne C, Brun D. Primary lipoprotein lipase deficiency. *Presse Med* 1993;22:212–217.

162. Dionne C, Gagne C, Julien P, et al. Genetic epidemiology of lipoprotein lipase deficiency in Saguenay-Lac-St-Jean. *Ann Genet* 1992;35:89–92.

163. Pimstone SN, Clee SM, Gagne SE, et al. A frequently occurring mutation in the lipoprotein lipase gene (Asn291Ser) results in altered postprandial chylomicron triglyceride and retinyl palmitate response in normolipidemic carriers. *J Lipid Res* 1996;37:1675–1684.

164. Gerdes C, Fisher RM, Nicaud V, et al. Lipoprotein lipase variants D9N and N291S are associated with increased plasma triglyceride and lower high-density lipoprotein cholesterol concentrations: studies in the fasting and postprandial states: the European Atherosclerosis Research Studies. *Circulation* 1997;96:733–740.

165. Baum L, Chen L, Masliah E, et al. Lipoprotein lipase mutations and Alzheimer's disease. *Am J Med Genet* 1999;88:136–139.

166. Wu DA, Bu X, Warden CH, et al. Quantitative trait locus mapping of human blood pressure to a genetic region at or near the lipoprotein lipase gene locus on chromosome 8p22. *J Clin Invest* 1996;97:2111–2118.

167. Sprecher DL, Harris BV, Stein EA, et al. Higher triglycerides, lower high-density lipoprotein cholesterol, and higher systolic blood pressure in lipoprotein lipase-deficient heterozygotes. A preliminary report. *Circulation* 1996;94:3239–3245.

168. Wittrup HH, Nordestgaard BG, Sillesen H, et al. A common mutation in lipoprotein lipase confers a 2-fold increase in risk of ischemic cerebrovascular disease in women but not in men. *Circulation* 2000;101:2393–2397.

169. Hubel CA, Roberts JM, Ferrell RE. Association of pre-eclampsia with common coding sequence variations in the lipoprotein lipase gene. *Clin Genet* 1999;56:289–296.

170. Merkel M, Eckel RH, Goldberg IJ. Lipoprotein lipase: genetics, lipid uptake, and regulation. *J Lipid Res* 2002;43:1997–2006.

171. Hokanson JE. Functional variants in the lipoprotein lipase gene and risk cardiovascular disease. *Curr Opin Lipidol* 1999;10:393–399.

172. Saxena U, Klein MG, Vanni TM, et al. Lipoprotein lipase increases low density lipoprotein retention by subendothelial cell matrix. *J Clin Invest* 1992;89:373–380.

173. Saxena U, Ferguson E, Auerbach BJ, et al. Lipoprotein lipase facilitates very low density lipoprotein binding to the subendothelial cell matrix. *Biochem Biophys Res Commun* 1993;194:769–774.

174. Tabas I, Li Y, Brocia RW, et al. Lipoprotein lipase and sphingomyelinase synergistically enhance the association of atherogenic lipoproteins with smooth muscle cells and extracellular matrix. *J Biol Chem* 1993;268:20419–20432.

175. Saxena U, Kulkarni NM, Ferguson E, et al. Lipoprotein lipase-mediated lipolysis of very low density lipoproteins increase monocyte adhesion to aortic endothelial cells. *Biophys Res Commun* 1992;189:1653–1658.

176. Renier G, Skamene E, DeSanctis JB, et al. High macrophage lipoprotein lipase expression and secretion are associated in inbred murine strains with susceptibility to atherosclerosis. *Arterioscler Thromb* 1993;13:190–196.

177. Semenkovich CF, Coleman T, Daugherty A. Effects of heterozygous lipoprotein lipase deficiency on diet-induced atherosclerosis in mice. *J Lipid Res* 1998;39:1141–1151.

178. Babaev VR, Fazio S, Gleaves LA, et al. Macrophage lipoprotein lipase promotes foam cell formation and atherosclerosis in vivo. *J Clin Invest* 1999;103:1697–1705.

179. Van Eck M, Zimmermann R, Groot PHE, et al. Role of macrophage-derived lipoprotein lipase in lipoprotein metabolism and atherosclerosis. *Arterioscler Thromb Vasc Biol* 2000;20:E53–E62.

180. Babaev VR, Patel MB, Semenkovich CF, et al. Macrophage lipoprotein lipase promotes foam cell formation and atherosclerosis in low density lipoprotein receptor-deficient mice. *J Biol Chem* 2000;275:26293–26299.

181. Shimada M, Shimano H, Gotoda T, et al. Overexpression of human lipoprotein lipase in transgenic mice. *J Biol Chem* 1993;268:17924–17929.

182. Santamarina-Fojo S, Haudenschild C. Role of hepatic and lipoprotein lipase in lipoprotein metabolism and atherosclerosis: studies in transgenic and knockout animal models and somatic gene transfer. *Int J Tissue React* 2000;22:39–47.

183. Hayden MR, Liu MS, Jirik F, et al. Expression of human lipoprotein lipase in transgenic mice. *J Cell Biochem* 1993;17E:242.

184. Tsutsumi K, Inoue Y, Shima A, et al. The novel compound NO-1886 increases lipoprotein lipase activity with resulting elevation of high density lipoprotein cholesterol, and long-term administration inhibits atherogenesis in the coronary arteries of rats with experimental atherosclerosis. *J Clin Invest* 1993;92:411–417.

185. Breckenridge WC, Little JA, Alaupovic P, et al. Lipoprotein abnormalities associated with a familial deficiency of hepatic lipase. *Atherosclerosis* 1982;45:161–179.

186. Carlson LA, Holmquist L, Nilsson-Ehle P. Deficiency of hepatic lipase activity in post-heparin plasma in familial hyper-α-triglyceridemia. *Acta Med Scand* 1986;219:435–447.

187. Auwerx JH, Marzetta CA, Hokanson JE, et al. Large buoyant LDL-like particles in hepatic lipase deficiency. *Arteriosclerosis* 1989;9:319–325.

188. Auwerx JH, Babirak SP, Hokanson JE, et al. Coexistence of abnor-

malities of hepatic lipase and lipoprotein lipase in a large family. *Am J Hum Genet* 1990;46:470–477.

189. Ikeda Y, Takagi A. Hypertriglyceridemia in a deficiency of lipoprotein lipase and hepatic lipase. *Tanpakushitsu Kakusan Koso* 1988;33:783–790.

190. Connelly PW, Maguire GF, Lee M, et al. Plasma lipoproteins in familial hepatic lipase deficiency. *Arteriosclerosis* 1990;10:40–48.

191. Kuusi T, Nikkila EA, Taskinen MR, et al. Human postheparin plasma hepatic lipase activity against triacylglycerol and phospholipid substrates. *Clin Chim Acta* 1982;16:39–45.

192. Jensen GL, Daggy B, Bensadoun A. Triacylglycerol lipase, monoacylglycerol lipase and phospholipase activities of highly purified rat hepatic lipase. *Biochim Biophys Acta* 1982;710:464–470.

193. Laboda HM, Glick JM, Phillips MC. Hydrolysis of lipid monolayers and the substrate specificity of hepatic lipase. *Biochim Biophys Acta* 1986;876:233–242.

194. Kuusi T, Saarinen P, Nikkila EA. Evidence for the role of hepatic endothelial lipase in the metabolism of plasma high density lipoprotein$_2$ in man. *Atherosclerosis* 1980;36:589–593.

195. Rao SN, Cortese C, Miller NE, et al. Effects of heparin infusion on plasma lipoproteins in subjects with lipoprotein lipase deficiency. Evidence for a role of hepatic endothelial lipase in the metabolism of high-density lipoprotein subfractions in man. *FEBS Lett* 1982;150:255–259.

196. Kinnunen PKJ. Hepatic endothelial lipase: isolation, some characteristics, and physiological role. In: Borgstrom B, Brockman HL, eds. *Lipases.* New York: Elsevier, 1984:307–328.

197. Hegele RA, Little JA, Vezina C, et al. Hepatic lipase deficiency: clinical, biochemical, and molecular genetic characteristics. *Arterioscler Thromb* 1993;13:720–728.

198. Hegele RA, Little JA, Connelly PW. Compound heterozygosity for mutant hepatic lipase in familial hepatic lipase deficiency. *Biochim Biophys Res Commun* 1991;179:78–84.

199. Hegele RA, Vezina C, Moorjani S, et al. A hepatic lipase gene mutation associated with heritable lipolytic deficiency. *J Clin Endocrinol* 1991;72:730–732.

200. Durstenfeld A, Ben-Zeev O, Reue K, et al. Molecular characterization of human hepatic lipase deficiency. *In vitro* expression of two naturally occurring mutations. *Arterioscler Thromb* 1994;14:381–385.

201. Brand K, Dugi KA, Brunzell JD, et al. Alternative splicing: a novel mechanism leading to deficiency of hepatic lipase. *Circulation* 1993;88:I-178.

202. Demant T, Carlson LA, Holmquist L, et al. Lipoprotein metabolism in hepatic lipase deficiency: studies on the turnover of apolipoprotein B and on the effect of hepatic lipase on high density lipoprotein UK. *J Lipid Res* 1988;29:1603–1611.

203. Shohet RV, Vega GL, Anwar A, et al. Hepatic lipase (LIPC) promoter polymorphism in men with coronary artery disease. Allele frequency and effects on hepatic lipase activity and plasma HDL-C concentrations. *Arterioscler Thromb Vasc Biol* 1999;19:1975–1978.

204. Santamarina-Fojo S, Haudenschild C, Amar M. The role of hepatic lipase in lipoprotein metabolism and atherosclerosis. *Curr Opin Lipidol* 1998;9:211–219.

205. Dugi KA, Brandauer K, Schmidt N, et al. Low hepatic lipase activity is a novel risk factor for coronary artery disease. *Circulation* 2001;104:3057–3062.

206. Hokanson JE, Cheng S, Snell-Bergeon JK, et al. A common promoter polymorphism in the hepatic lipase gene (LIPC-480C>T) is associated with an increase in coronary calcification in type 1 diabetes. *Diabetes* 2002;51:1208–1213.

207. Katzel LI, Coon PJ, Busby MJ, et al. Reduced HDL2 cholesterol subspecies and elevated postheparin hepatic lipase activity in older men with abdominal obesity and asymptomatic myocardial ischemia. *Arterioscler Thromb* 1992;12:814–823.

208. Zambon A, Deeb SS, Brown BG, et al. Common hepatic lipase gene promoter variant determines clinical response to intensive lipid-lowering treatment. *Circulation* 2001;103:792–798.

209. Zambon A, Deeb SS, Hokanson JE, et al. Common variants in the promoter of the hepatic lipase gene are associated with lower levels of hepatic lipase activity, buoyant LDL, and higher HDL2 cholesterol. *Arterioscler Thromb Vasc Biol* 1998;18:1723–1729.

210. Fan J, Wang J, Bensadoun A, et al. Overexpression of hepatic lipase in transgenic rabbits leads to a marked reduction of plasma high density lipoproteins and intermediate density lipoproteins. *Proc Natl Acad Sci USA* 1994;91:8724–8728.

211. Busch SJ, Barnhart RL, Martin GA, et al. Human hepatic triglyceride lipase expression reduces high density lipoprotein and aortic cholesterol in cholesterol-fed transgenic mice. *J Biol Chem* 1994;269:16376–16382.

212. Mezdour H, Jones R, Dengremont C, et al. Hepatic lipase deficiency increases plasma cholesterol but reduces susceptibility to atherosclerosis in apolipoprotein E–deficient mice. *J Biol Chem* 1997;272:13570–13575.

213. Bergeron N, Kotite L, Verges M, et al. Lamellar lipoproteins uniquely contribute to hyperlipidemia in mice doubly deficient in apolipoprotein E and hepatic lipase. *Proc Natl Acad Sci USA* 1998;95:15647–15652.

214. Nong ZX, Gonzalez-Navarro H, Amar M, et al. Hepatic lipase expression in macrophages contributes to atherosclerosis in apoE-deficient and LCAT-transgenic mice. *J Clin Invest* 2003;112:367–378.

215. Gonzalez-Navarro H, Nong ZX, Freeman L, et al. Identification of mouse and human macrophages as a site of synthesis of hepatic lipase. *J Lipid Res* 2002;43:671–675.

216. Mahley RW. Dietary, fat, cholesterol, and accelerated atherosclerosis. *Atheroscler Rev* 1979;5:1–34.

217. Brewer HB Jr, Zech LA, Gregg RE, et al. Type III hyperlipoproteinemia: diagnosis, molecular defects, pathology, and treatment. *Ann Intern Med* 1983;98:623–640.

218. Havel RJ. Familial dysbetalipoproteinemia. New aspects of pathogenesis and diagnosis. *Med Clin N Am* 1982;66:441–454.

219. Mahley RW, Rall SC. Type III Hyperlipoprotein (Dysbetalipoproteinemia): the role of apolipoprotein E in normal and abnormal lipoprotein metabolism. *The metabolic basis of inherited disease.* New York: McGraw-Hill, 2001:2835–2862.

220. Davignon J, Cohn JS, Mabile L, et al. Apolipoprotein E and atherosclerosis: insight from animal and human studies. *Clin Chim Acta* 1999;286:115–143.

221. Curtiss LK, Boisvert WA. Apolipoprotein E and atherosclerosis. *Curr Opin Lipidol* 2000;11:243–251.

222. Gregg RE, Zech LA, Schaefer EJ, et al. Type III hyperlipoproteinemia: defective metabolism of an abnormal apolipoprotein E. *Science* 1981;211:584–586.

223. Rall SC Jr, Weisgraber KH, Innerarity TL, et al. Structural basis for receptor binding heterogeneity of apolipoprotein E from type III hyperlipoproteinemic subjects. *Proc Natl Acad Sci USA* 1982;79:4696–4700.

224. Utermann G, Vogelberg KH, Steinmetz A, et al. Polymorphism of apolipoprotein E. II. Genetics of hyperlipoproteinemia type III. *Clin Genet* 1979;15:37–62.

225. Zannis VI, Just PW, Breslow JL. Human apolipoprotein E isoprotein subclasses are genetically determined. *Am J Hum Genet* 1981;33:11–24.

226. Mahley RW, Innerarity TL, Rall SC Jr, et al. Plasma lipoproteins: apolipoprotein structure and function. *J Lipid Res* 1984;25:1277–1294.

227. Strittmatter WJ, Bova Hill C. Molecular biology of apolipoprotein E. *Curr Opin Lipidol* 2002;13:119–123.

228. Schaefer EJ, Gregg RE, Ghiselli G, et al. Familial apolipoprotein E deficiency. *J Clin Invest* 1986;78:1206–1219.

229. Lohse P, Brewer HB III, Meng MS, et al. Familial apolipoprotein E deficiency and type III hyperlipoproteinemia due to a premature stop codon in the apolipoprotein E gene. *J Lipid Res* 1992;33:1583–1590.

230. Mabuchi H, Itoh H, Takeda M, et al. A young type III hyperlipoproteinemic patient associated with apolipoprotein E deficiency Medicine, Kanazawa, Japan. *Metabolism* 1989;38:115–119.

231. Kurosaka D, Teramoto T, Matsushima T, et al. Apolipoprotein E deficiency with a depressed mRNA of normal size. *Atherosclerosis* 1991;88:15–20.

232. Mann WA, Gregg RE, Sprecher DL, et al. Apolipoprotein E-1$_{Harrisburg}$: a new variant of apolipoprotein E dominantly associated with type III hyperlipoproteinemia. *Biochim Biophys Acta* 1989;1005:239–244.

233. Rall SC Jr, Newhouse YM, Clarke HR, et al. Type III hyperlipoproteinemia associated with apolipoprotein E phenotype E3/3. Structure and genetics of an apolipoprotein E3 variant. *J Clin Invest* 1989;83:1095–1101.

234. Wardell MR, Weisgraber KH, Havekes LM, et al. Apolipoprotein E3-Leiden contains a seven-amino acid insertion that is a tandem repeat of residues 121-127. *J Biol Chem* 1989;264:21205–21210.

235. Brewer HB Jr, Santamarina-Fojo S, Hoeg JM. Genetic defects in the human plasma apolipoproteins. *Atheroscler Rev* 1991;23:51–61.

236. Lohse P, Mann WA, Stein EA, et al. Apolipoprotein E-4$_{Philadelphia}$ (Glu^{13}_Lys,Arg^{145}_Cys). Homozygosity for two rare point mutations in the apolipoprotein E gene combined with severe type III hyperlipoproteinemia. *J Biol Chem* 1991;266:10479–10484.
237. Gregg RE, Zech LA, Schaefer EJ, et al. Abnormal *in vivo* metabolism of apolipoprotein E4 in humans. *J Clin Invest* 1986;78:815–821.
238. Gregg RE, Brewer HB Jr. The role of apolipoprotein E and lipoprotein receptors in modulating the *in vivo* metabolism of apolipoprotein B-containing lipoproteins in humans. *Clin Chem* 1988;34:28–32.
239. Roses AD. Apolipoprotein E affects the rate of Alzheimer disease expression: beta-amyloid burden is a secondary consequence dependent on APOE genotype and duration of disease. *J Neuropathol Exp Neurol* 1994;53:429–437.
240. Herz J, Beffert U. Apolipoprotein E receptors: linking brain development and Alzheimer's disease. *Nat Rev Neurosci* 2000;1:51–58.
241. Saunders AM. Apolipoprotein E and Alzheimer disease: an update on genetic and functional analyses. *J Neuropathol Exp Neurol* 2000;59:751–758.
242. Strittmatter WJ. Apolipoprotein E and Alzheimer's disease: signal transduction mechanisms. *Biochem Soc Symp* 2001;67:101–109.
243. Irizarry MC, Rebeck GW, Cheung B, et al. Modulation of A beta deposition in APP transgenic mice by an apolipoprotein E null background. *Ann NY Acad Sci* 2000;920:171–178.
244. Schaefer EJ, Genest JJ Jr, Ordovas JM, et al. Familial lipoprotein disorders and premature coronary artery disease. *Atherosclerosis* 1994;108[Suppl]:S41–S54.
245. Salens G, Shefer S, Nguyen L, et al. Sitosterolemia. *J Lipid Res* 1992;33:945–955.
246. Bjorkhem I, Boberg KM Leitersdorj E. Inborn errors in bile acid biosynthesis and storage of sterols other than cholesterol. In: Scriver CR, Beaudet AL, Sly WS, et al., eds. *The metabolic and molecular bases of inherited disease.* New York: McGraw-Hill, 2001:2961–2988.
247. Salen G, von Bergmann K, Kwiterovich P, et al. Ezetimibe is an effective treatment for homozygous sitosterolemia. *Circulation Supp* 2002;106:ll–185.
248. Berge KE, Tian H, Graf GA, et al. Accumulation of dietary cholesterol in sitosterolemia caused by mutations in adjacent ABC transporters. *Science* 2000;290:1771–1775.
249. Lee MH, Lu K, Hazard S, et al. Identification of a gene, ABCG5, important in the regulation of dietary cholesterol absorption. *Nat Genet* 2001;27:79–83.
250. Hubacek JA, Berge KE, Cohen JC, et al. Mutations in ATP-cassette binding proteins G5 (ABCG5) and G8 (ABCG8) causing sitosterolemia. *Hum Mutat* 2001;18:359–360.
251. Heimer S, Langmann T, Moehle C, et al. Mutations in the human ATP-binding cassette transporters ABCG5 and ABCG8 in sitosterolemia. *Hum Mutat* 2002;20:151.
252. Lu K, Lee M, Hazard S, et al. Two genes that map to the *STSL* locus cause sitosterolemia: genomic structure and spectrum of mutations involving Sterolin-1 and Sterolin-2, encoded by ABCG5 and ABCG8, respectively. *Am J Hum Genet* 69:278–290, 2001.
253. Dean M, Rzhetsky A, Allikmets R. The human ATP-binding cassette (ABC) transporter superfamily. *Genome Res* 11:1156–1166, 2001.
254. Dean M, Hamon Y, Chimini G. The human ATP-binding cassette (ABC) transporter superfamily. *J Lipid Res* 2001;42:1007–1017.
255. Turley SD, Dietschy JM. Sterol absorption by the small intestine. *Curr Opin Lipidol* 2003;14:233–240.
256. Lu K, Lee M, Yu H, et al. Molecular cloning, genomic organization, genetic variations, and characterization of murine sterolin genes ABCG5 and ABCG8. *J Lipid Res* 2002;43:565–578.
257. Repa JJ, Berge KE, Pomajzl C, et al. Regulation of ATP-binding cassette sterol transporters ABCG5 and ABCG8 by the liver X receptors alpha and beta. *J Biol Chem* 2002;277:18793–18800.
258. Yu LQ, Hammer RE, Li-Hawkins J, et al. Disruption of Abcg5 and Abcg8 in mice reveals their crucial role in biliary cholesterol secretion. *Proc Natl Acad Sci USA* 2002;99:16237–16242.
259. Yu LQ, Li-Hawkins J, Hammer RE, et al. Overexpression of ABCG5 and ABCG8 promotes biliary cholesterol secretion and reduces fractional absorption of dietary cholesterol. *J Clin Invest* 2002;110:671–680.
260. Bassen FA, Kornzweig AL. Malformation of the erythrocytes in a case of atypical retinitis pigmentosa. *Blood* 1950;5:381–387.
261. Berriot-Varoqueaux N, Aggerbeck LP, Samson-Bouma M-E, et al. The role of the microsomal triglyceride transfer protein in abetalipoproteinemia. *Annu Rev Nutr* 2000;20:663–697.
262. Kayden HJ, Silber R. The role of vitamin E deficiency in the abnormal autohemolysis of acanthocytosis. *Trans Assoc Am Phys* 1965;78:334–342.
263. Wetterau JR, Aggerbeck LP, Bouma ME, et al. Absence of microsomal triglyceride transfer protein in individuals with abetalipoproteinemia, *Science* 1992;258:999–1001.
264. Jamil H, Dickson JK Jr, Chu CH, et al. Microsomal triglyceride transfer protein. Specificity of lipid binding and transport. *J Biol Chem* 1995;270:6549–6554.
265. Gordon DA, Jamil H. Progress towards understanding the role of microsomal triglyceride transfer protein in apolipoprotein-B lipoprotein assembly. *Biochim Biophys Acta* 2000;1486:72–83.
266. Bishar S, Merin S, Cooper M, et al. Combined vitamin A, E therapy prevents retinal electrophysiological deterioration in abetalipoproteinemia. *Br J Ophtalmol* 1982;66:767–770.
267. Dieri JG, Hoeg JM, Scheafer EJ, et al. Vitamin A and vitamin E replacement in abetalipoproteinemia. *Ann Intern Med* 1984;100:238–240.
268. Muller DPR, Lloyd JK. Effect of large oral doses of vitamin E on the neurological sequalae of patients with abetalipoproteinemia. *Ann NY Acad Sci* 1982;393:133–144.
269. Young SG, Bertics SJ, Curtiss LK, et al. Characterization of an abnormal species of apolipoprotein B, apolipoprotein B-37, associated with familial hypobetalipoproteinemia. *J Clin Invest* 1987;79:1831–1841.
270. Schonfeld G. Familial hypobetalipoproteinemia: a review. *J Lipid Res* 2003;44:878–883.
271. Schonfeld G. The hypobetalipoproteinemias. *Annu Rev Nutr* 1995;15:23–34.
272. Wu JS, Kim J, Li Q, et al. Known mutations of apoB account for only a small minority of hypobetalipoproteinemia. *J Lipid Res* 1999;40:955–959.
273. Pulai JI, Neuman RJ, Groenewegen AW, et al. Genetic heterogeneity in familial hypobetalipoproteinemia: linkage and nonlinkage to the apoB gene in Caucasian families. *Am J Hum Genet* 1998;76:79–86.
274. Schonfeld G, Patterson BW, Yablonskiy DA, et al. Fatty liver in familial hypobetalipoproteinemia: triglyceride assembly into VLDL particles is affected by the extent of hepatic steatosis. *J Lipid Res* 2003;44:470–478.
275. Anderson CM, Townley RRW, Freeman M, et al. Unusual causes of steatorrhea in infancy and childhood. *Med J Aust* 1961;2:617–622.
276. Bouma ME, Beucler I, Aggerbeck LP, et al. Hypobetalipoproteinemia with accumulation of an apoprotein B-like protein in intestinal cells. Immunoenzymatic and biochemical characterization of seven cases of Anderson's disease. *J Clin Invest* 1986;78:398–410.
277. Roy CC, Levy E, Green PHR, et al. Malabsorption, hypocholesterolemia, and fat-filled enterocytes with increased intestinal apoprotein B: chylomicron retention disease. *Gastroenterology* 1987;92:390–399.
278. Dannoura AH, Berriot-Varoqueaux N, Amati P, et al. Anderson's disease: exclusion of apolipoprotein and intracellular lipid transport genes. *Arterioscler Thromb Vasc Biol* 1999;19:2494–2508.
279. Pessah M, Benlian P, Beucler I, et al. Anderson's disease: genetic exclusion of the apolipoprotein-B gene in two families. *J Clin Invest* 1991;87:367–370.
280. Strich D, Goldstein R, Phillips A, et al. Anderson's disease: no linkage to the apo B locus. *J Pediatr Gastroenterol Nutr* 1993;16:257–264.
281. Jones B, Jones EL, Bonney SA, et al. Mutations in a Sar1 GTPase of COPII vesicles are associated with lipid absorption disorders. *Nat Genet* 2003;34:29–31.
282. Schaefer EJ, Zech LA, Schwartz DE, et al. Coronary heart disease prevalence and other clinical features in familial high-density lipoprotein deficiency (Tangier disease). *Ann Intern Med* 1980;93:261–266.
283. Serfaty-Lacrosniere C, Civeira F, Lanzberg A, et al. Homozygous Tangier disease and cardiovascular disease. *Atherosclerosis* 1994;107:85–98.
284. Bojanovski D, Gregg RE, Zech LA, et al. *In vivo* metabolism of proapolipoprotein A-I in Tangier disease. *J Clin Invest* 1987;80:1742–1747.
285. Francis GA, Oram JF. Defective excretion of cholesterol from Tangier patients' fibroblasts to apolipoprotein A-I: a potential cause of hypoalphalipoproteinemia. *Circulation* 1994;90:I-241.
286. Dean M, Hamon Y, Chimin G. The human ATP-binding cassette (ABC) transporter superfamily. *J Lipid Res* 2001;42:1007–1017.

287. Dean M, Rzhetsky A, Allikmets R. The human ATP-binding cassette (ABC) trasporter superfamily. *Genome Res* 2001;11:1156–1166.

288. Fielding CJ, Fielding PE. Molecular physiology of reverse cholesterol transport. *J Lipid Res* 1995;36:211–228.

289. Fielding CJ, Fielding PE. Cellular cholesterol efflux. *Biochim Biophys Acta* 2001;1533:175–189.

290. Bortnick AE, Rothblat GH, Stoudt G, et al. The correlation of ATP-binding cassette 1 mRNA levels with cholesterol efflux from various cell lines. *J Biol Chem* 2000;275:28634–28640.

291. Remaley AT, Stonik JA, Demosky SJ, et al. Apolipoprotein specificity for lipid efflux by the human ABCA1 transporter. *Biochem Biophys Res Commun* 2001;280:818–823.

292. Orso E, Broccardo C, Kiminski WE, et al. Transport of lipids from Golgi to plasma membrane is defective in tangier disease patients and Abc1-deficient mice. *Nat Genet* 2000;24:192–196.

293. Wang N, Silver DL, Thiele C, et al. ABCA1 functions as a cholesterol efflux regulatory protein. *J Biol Chem* 2001;276:23742–23747.

294. Yokoyama S. Release of cellular cholesterol: molecular mechanism for cholesterol homeostasis in cells and in the body. *Biochim Biophys Acta Mol Cell Res* 2000;1529:231–244.

295. Oram JF, Lawn RM, Garvin MR, et al. ABCA1 is the cAMP-inducible apolipoprotein receptor that mediates cholesterol secretion from macrophages. *J Biol Chem* 2000;275:34508–34511.

296. Aiello RJ, Brees D, Bourassa PAK, et al. Increased atherosclerosis in hyperlipidemic mice with inactivation of ABCA1 in macrophages. *Arterioscler Thromb Vasc Biol* 2002;22:630–637.

297. van Eck M, Sophie I, Bos T, et al. Leukocyte ABCA1 controls susceptibility to atherosclerosis and macrophage recruitment into tissues. *Proc Natl Acad Sci USA* 2002;99:6298–6303.

298. Attie AD, Kastelein JP, Hayden MR. Pivotal role of ABCA1 in reverse cholesterol transport influencing HDL levels and susceptibility to atherosclerosis. *J Lipid Res* 2001;42:1717–1726.

299. Clee SM, Zwinderman AH, Engert JC, et al. Common genetic variation in ABCA1 is associated with altered lipoprotein levels and a modified risk for coronary artery disease. *Circulation* 2001;103:1198.

300. van Dam MJ, de Groot E, Clee SM, et al. Association between increased aterial-wall thickness and impairment in ABCA1-driven cholesterol efflux: an observational study. *Lancet* 2002;359:37–42.

301. McNeish J, Aiello RJ, Guyot D, et al. High density lipoprotein deficiency and foam cell accumulation in mice with targeted disruption of ATP-binding cassette transporter-1. *Proc Natl Acad Sci USA* 2000;97:4245–4250.

302. Christiansen-Weber TA, Voland JR, Wu Y, et al. Functional loss of ABCA1 in mice causes severe placental malformation, aberrant lipid distribution, and kidney glomerulonephritis as well as high-density lipoprotein cholesterol deficiency. *Am J Pathol* 2000;157:1017–1029.

303. von Eckardstein A, Funke H, Henke A, et al. Apolipoprotein A-I variants. Naturally occurring substitutions of proline residues affect plasma concentration of apolipoprotein A-I. *J Clin Invest* 1989;84:1722–1730.

304. Schmitz G, Lackner K. High density lipoprotein deficiency with xanthomas: a defect in apoA-I synthesis. In: Crepaldi G, Baggio G, eds. *Atherosclerosis VIII.* Rome: Tekno Press, 1989:399–403.

305. Bekaert ED, Alaupovic P, Knight-Gibson CS, et al. Characterization of apoA- and apoB-containing lipoprotein particles in a variant of familial apoA-I deficiency with planar xanthoma: the metabolic significance of LP-A-II particles. *J Lipid Res* 1991;32:1587–1599.

306. Norum RA, Lakier JB, Goldstein S, et al. Familial deficiency of apolipoproteins A-I and C-III and precocious coronary-artery disease. *N Engl J Med* 1982;306:1513–1519.

307. Karathanasis SK, Zannis VI, Breslow JL. A DNA insertion in the apolipoprotein A-I gene of patients with premature atherosclerosis. *Nature* 1983;305:823–825.

308. Schaefer EJ, Ordovas JM, Law SW, et al. Familial apolipoprotein A-I and C-III deficiency, variant II. *J Lipid Res* 1985;26:1089–1101.

309. Ordovas JM, Cassidy DK, Civeira F, et al. Familial apolipoprotein A-I, C-III, and A-IV deficiency and premature atherosclerosis due to deletion of a gene complex on chromosome 11. *J Biol Chem* 1989;264:16339–16342.

310. Third JL, Montag J, Flynn M, et al. Primary and familial hypoalphalipoproteinemia. *Metabolism* 1984;33:136–146.

311. Genest J Jr, Bard JM, Fruchart JC, et al. Familial hypoalphalipoproteinemia in premature coronary artery disease. *Arterioscler Thromb* 1993;13:1728–1737.

312. Santamarina-Fojo S, Hoeg JM, Assmann G, et al. Lecithin cholesterol acyltransferase deficiency and fish eye disease. In: Scriver CR, Beaudet AL, Sly WS, et al., eds. *The metabolic and molecular bases of inherited disease.* New York: McGraw-Hill, 2001:2817–2834.

313. Jonas A. Regulation of lecithin cholesterol acyltransferase activity. *Prog Lipid Res* 1998;37:209–234.

314. Dobiasova M, Frohlich JJ. Advances in understanding of the role of lecithin cholesterol acyltransferase (LCAT) in cholesterol transport. *Clin Chim Acta* 1999;286:257–271.

315. Applebaum-Bowden D. Lipases and lecithin:cholesterol acyltransferase in the control of lipoprotein metabolism. *Curr Opin Lipidol* 1995;6:130–135.

316. Kuivenhoven JA, Pritchard H, Hill J, et al. The molecular pathology of lecithin:cholesterol acyltransferase (LCAT) deficiency syndromes. *J Lipid Res* 1997;38:191–205.

317. Peelman F, Vinaimont N, Verhee A, et al. A proposed architecture for lecithin cholesterol acyl transferase (LCAT): identification of the catalytic triad and molecular modeling. *Protein Sci* 1998;7:587–599.

318. Peelman F, Vandekerckhove J, Rosseneu M. Structure and function of LCAT: new insights from structural predictions and animal models. *Curr Opin Lipidol* 2000;11:155–160.

319. Santamarina-Fojo S, Hoeg JM, Assmann G, et al. Lechitin cholesterol acyltranserase deficiency and fish eye disease. *The metabolic basis of inherited disease.* New York: McGraw-Hill, 2001:2817–2834.

320. Rader DJ, Ikewaki K, Duverger N, et al. Markedly accelerated catabolism of apolipoprotein A-II (ApoA-II) and high density lipoproteins containing ApoA-II in classic lecithin:cholesterol acyltransferase deficiency and fish-eye disease. *J Clin Invest* 1994;93:321–330.

321. Teh EM, Chisholm JW, Dolphin PJ, et al. Classical LCAT deficiency resulting from a novel homozygous dinucleotide deletion in exon 4 of the human lecithin:cholesterol acyltransferase gene causing a frameshift and stop codon at residue 144. *Atherosclerosis* 1999;146:141–151.

322. Yang X-P, Inazu A, Honjo A, et al. Catalytically inactive lecithin:cholesterol acyltransferase (LCAT) caused by a Gly 30 to Ser mutation in a family with LCAT deficiency. *J Lipid Res* 1997;38:585–591.

323. Klein H-G, Lohse P, Duverger N, et al. Two different allelic mutations in the lecithin:cholesterol acyltransferase (LCAT) gene resulting in classic LCAT deficiency: LCAT (tyr83–> stop) and LCAT (tyr156–> asn). *J Lipid Res* 1993;34:49–58.

324. Hoeg JM, Vaisman BL, Demosky SJ Jr, et al. Lecithin:cholesterol acyltransferase overexpression generates hyperalphalipoproteinemia and a nonatherogenic lipoprotein pattern in transgenic rabbits. *J Biol Chem* 1996;271:4396–4402.

325. Vaisman BL, Klein H-G, Rouis M, et al. Overexpression of human lecithin cholesterol acyltransferase leads to hyperalphalipoproteinemia in transgenic mice. *J Biol Chem* 1995;270:12269–12275.

326. Francone OL, Gong EL, Ng DS, et al. Expression of human lecithin-cholesterol acyltransferase in transgenic mice: effect of human apolipoprotein AI and human apolipoprotein AII on plasma lipoprotein cholesterol metabolism. *J Clin Invest* 1995;96:1440–1448.

327. Mehlum A, Staels B, Duverger N, et al. Tissue-specific expression of the human gene for lecithin-cholesterol acyltransferase in transgenic mice alters blood lipids, lipoproteins and lipases towards a less atherogenic profile. *Eur J Biochem* 1995;230:567–575.

328. Amar MJA, Vaisman BL, Koch CA, et al. Expression of murine LCAT in transgenic mice; evaluation of the role of LCAT cholesteryl ester-fatty acid specificity in the development of atherosclerosis. *Circulation* 1999;100:I-401.

329. Berard AM, Remaley AT, Vaisman BL, et al. High plasma HDL concentrations associated with enhanced atherosclerosis in transgenic mice overexpressing lecithin cholesteryl acyltransferase. *Nat Med* 1997;3:744–749.

330. Amar MJA, Shamburek RD, Foger B, et al. Adenovirus-mediated expression of LCAT in non-human primates leads to an antiatherogenic lipoprotein profile with increased HDL and decreased LDL. *Circulation* 1998;98:I-35.

331. Sakai N, Vaisman BL, Koch CA, et al. Analysis of aortic atherosclerosis and glomerulosclerosis in LCAT knockout mice. *Circulation* 1997;96:I-229.

332. Matsuzawa Y, Yamashita S, Kameda K, et al. Marked hyper-HDL2-cholesterolemia associated with premature corneal opacity. A case report. *Atherosclerosis* 1984;53:207–212.

333. Hirano K, Yamashita S, Matsuzawa Y. Pros and cons of inhibiting

cholesteryl ester transfer protein. *Curr Opin Lipidol* 2000;11: 589–596.

334. Ikewaki K, Rader DJ, Sakamoto T, et al. Delayed catabolism of high density lipoprotein apolipoproteins A-I and A-II in human cholesteryl ester transfer protein deficiency. *J Clin Invest* 1993;92:1650–1658.

335. Ikewaki K, Nishiwaki M, Sakamoto T, et al. Increased catabolic rate of low density lipoproteins in humans with cholesteryl ester transfer protein deficiency. *J Clin Invest* 1995;96:1573–1581.

336. Ishigami M, Yamashita S, Sakai N, et al. Large and cholesteryl ester-rich high-density lipoproteins in cholesteryl ester transfer protein (CETP) deficiency can not protect macrophages from cholesterol accumulation induced by acetylated low-density lipoproteins. *J Biochem (Tokyo)* 1994;116:257–262.

337. Sakai N, Yamashita S, Hirano K, et al. Decreased affinity of low density lipoprotein (LDL) particles for LDL receptors in patients with cholesteryl ester transfer protein deficiency. *Eur J Clin Invest* 1995;25.332–339.

338. Ordovas JM, Cupples LA, Corella D, et al. Association of cholesteryl ester transfer protein-TaqIB polymorphism with variations in lipoprotein subclasses and coronary heart disease risk: the Framingham study. *Arterioscler Thromb Vasc Biol* 2000;20:1323–1329.

339. Agerholm-Larsen B, Tybjaerg-Hansen A, Schnohr P, et al. Common cholesteryl ester transfer protein mutations, decreased HDL cholesterol, and possible decreased risk of ischemic heart disease: the Copenhagen City Heart Study. *Circulation* 2000;102:2197–2203.

340. Agerholm-Larsen B, Tybjaerg-Hansen A, Schnohr P, et al. Common cholesteryl ester transfer protein mutations, decreased HDL cholesterol, and possible decreased risk of ischemic heart disease: the Copenhagen City Heart Study. *Circulation* 2000;102:2197–2203.

341. Sugano M, Makino N, Sawada S, et al. Effect of antisense oligonucleotides against cholesteryl ester transfer protein on the development of atherosclerosis in cholesterol-fed rabbits. *J Biol Chem* 1998;273: 5033–5036.

342. Whitlock ME, Swenson TL, Ramakrishnan R, et al. Monoclonal antibody inhibition of cholesteryl ester transfer protein activity in the rabbit. Effects on lipoprotein composition and high density lipoprotein cholesteryl ester metabolism. *J Clin Invest* 1989;84:129–137.

343. Rittershaus CW, Miller DP, Thomas LJ, et al. Vaccine-induced antibodies inhibit CETP activity in vivo and reduce aortic lesions in a rabbit model of atherosclerosis. *Arterioscler Thromb Vasc Biol* 2000;20: 2106–2112.

344. Okamoto H, Yonemori F, Wakitani K, et al. A cholesteryl ester transfer protein inhibitor attenuates atherosclerosis in rabbits. *Nature* 2000;406:203–207.

CHAPTER 6

Structure and Function of the Plasma Lipoproteins and Their Receptors

John P. Kane

Key Words: Apolipoprotein; chylomicrons; high-density lipoproteins, intermediate-density lipoproteins, low-density lipoproteins; lipids; phospholipids; triglycerides; very low-density lipoproteins.

OVERVIEW

It is estimated that as much as 80% of the carbon and hydrogen in energy substrates used by the human body passes through lipid intermediaries at some point before being oxidized to terminal products. Most of that lipid transits the blood in the form of free fatty acids (FFAs) or triglycerides. Furthermore, there is a constant bidirectional movement of the lipid constituents of membranes between cells and the blood. The lipids of plasma are virtually all solubilized and dispersed by association with a highly evolved group of proteins. The simplest association among these is that between unesterified fatty acids and albumin, which has three high-affinity sites (1). The transport of more complex lipids is chiefly accomplished by lipoproteins. These are spherical microemulsion particles, with cores containing hydrophobic cholesteryl esters and triglycerides in variable proportions,

surrounded by a monolayer of phospholipids and unesterified cholesterol. The charged head groups of the phospholipids and the hydroxyl group of cholesterol associate with water dipoles and proteins, whereas the hydrophobic fatty acid chains of phospholipids and the sterol ring structure are in contact with each other and with the core lipids. A number of proteins (apolipoproteins:apoproteins) interact with the lipid microemulsions. Proteins of one family between 6 and 50 kD, containing amphipathic helices, can move among lipoprotein species. In contrast, the B apoproteins have much greater molecular weights, few amphipathic helices, and a large content of β structure (2). They remain with the particles on which they were secreted. Plasma lipoproteins vary greatly in diameter. The principal core constituent of the largest is triglyceride, whereas smaller lipoproteins contain progressively more cholesteryl esters, which become predominant at diameters less than 230 Å [low-density lipoproteins (LDLs)]. The densities of lipoproteins increase as diameters decrease, because protein-to-core lipid ratio increases. Preparative ultracentrifugation is widely used to separate lipoproteins (3). Proteins associated with lipoproteins represent several families. A family of nine small proteins containing amphipathic helices (apolipoproteins A-I, A-II, A-IV, A-V, C-I, C-II, C-III, C-IV, and E) are characterized by tandem repeats of 11 codons (4). Each of these is exchangeable among lipoproteins. A second

J. P. Kane: Cardiovascular Research Institute, University of California, San Francisco, San Francisco, California 94143.

family, the apoL proteins, are phylogenetically distinct (5). The B apoproteins comprise two very large proteins, apoB-100 and apoB-48, products of a single gene. Unlike other apoproteins, they are unexchangeable among lipoprotein particles (2,6). Another group, including apoD, cholesteryl ester transfer protein (CETP), and phospholipid transfer protein (PLTP), function in lipid exchange. Lastly, a number of proteins that are present in molecular dispersion in plasma that have known functions outside of lipid transport partially associate with lipoproteins and may have roles in the lipoprotein context. These include transferrin, ceruloplasmin, haptoglobin-associated protein, paraoxonase, factor VII, complement 4 component-binding protein, lipopolysaccharide-binding protein (LBP), and others (7,8).

Thematic roles for lipoproteins involve transport of exogenous and endogenous triglycerides, delivery of cholesterol to tissues through LDLs, and retrieval of lipids from peripheral sites through high-density lipoproteins (HDLs). Chylomicrons, large triglyceride-rich lipoproteins of enteric origin, carry exogenous triglycerides into plasma (6,9), whereas very low-density lipoproteins (VLDLs) originate in the liver and carry endogenous triglycerides. FFAs for hepatic triglyceride synthesis come chiefly from adipocytes, released by hormone-sensitive lipase. Some FFAs come from hydrolysis of triglycerides in VLDLs and chylomicrons. Lipolysis in adipocytes is stimulated by catecholamines, growth hormone, glucagon, and afferent autonomic stimulation. It is suppressed by insulin. One-third of FFAs that perfuse the liver are removed in each circulatory pass, independent of plasma level. A high rate of lipolysis increases FFA uptake by the liver, providing fatty acids for oxidation, export of triglycerides, or ketogenesis. Uptake of FFA in the liver is facilitated by a fatty acid transfer protein belonging to a family of transfer proteins (10). Chylomicrons and VLDLs marginate in capillaries, where they undergo lipolysis by lipoprotein lipase (LPL), liberating FFAs that are chiefly taken up locally. As a result, the particles decrease in size and the cores become relatively enriched in cholesteryl esters, forming remnant lipoproteins. Chylomicron remnants are removed quantitatively by endocytosis into hepatocytes. About half of VLDL remnants are similarly endocytosed. The remainder undergo further depletion of triglycerides forming LDLs (6). LDLs are endocytosed through the LDL receptor, principally in hepatocytes and degraded within lysosomes.

Nascent VLDLs and chylomicrons contain apoproteins that, together with phospholipids and free cholesterol, migrate from the triglyceride-rich lipoproteins during lipolysis to appear in HDLs. Cholesterol and phospholipids also are effluxed to HDL from peripheral tissues. Free cholesterol is esterified by lecithin-cholesterol acyl transferase (LCAT) (11) to form cholesteryl esters, the chief core constituent of HDL. Cholesteryl esters are then transferred to VLDLs, intermediate-density lipoproteins (IDLs), and LDLs mediated by CETP. Finally, the endocytosis of these acceptor lipoproteins by hepatocytes and direct transfer of cholesteryl esters from HDLs, provide the means for delivery of cholesterol from peripheral tissues to the liver. Modern models of atherogenesis place the apoB-containing lipoproteins in a pro-atherogenic role, whereas HDLs act to countervail this effect by improving the retrieval of cholesterol from peripheral sites and inhibiting oxidation of LDL. Emerging functions of lipoproteins outside of lipid transport suggest broader biological roles than was previously appreciated. For example, apoL-1 in HDLs mediates resistance to trypanosomes (12). Chylomicrons and VLDLs bind and remove endotoxins from plasma through endocytosis into hepatocytes (13). Thus, increases in plasma triglycerides occurring in sepsis and inflammation, reflecting increased VLDL synthesis and decreased lipolysis, may have evolved adaptively to protect against endotoxemia (14). Some determinants of lipoprotein metabolism may emanate from other systems in which they play a role. Emerging functions include involvement in blood clotting (15) and thrombolysis, and in the inhibition of the infectivity of endogenous C viruses.

TRANSPORT OF EXOGENOUS LIPIDS

Secretion of Chylomicrons

Ingested fats are hydrolyzed by pancreatic lipase to form a mixture of β-monoglycerides and unesterified fatty acids, which are absorbed by the enterocyte. Unesterified cholesterol is liberated from ingested cholesteryl esters by a cholesteryl esterase. Enterocytes absorb both cholesterol and phytosterols. Most of the latter are transported back to the lumen by a pair of adenosine triphosphate (ATP) cassette transporters (G5/G8). Mutations in these loci cause primary phytosterolemia (16,17). The intracellular transport of FFA is facilitated by fatty acid–binding proteins. After esterification with coenzyme A (CoA), the fatty acyl groups directly transacylate the β-monoglyceride to triglycerides. Some free cholesterol is esterified, chiefly with oleic and linoleic acids, by an intestinal acyl CoA-cholesterol acyl transferase (ACAT) to yield esters that will appear in the chylomicron. apoB-48, found in chylomicrons, is a product of the same gene that produces apoB-100. ApoB-48, so named because it is completely homologous with the N-terminal 48% of B-100, results from a tissue-specific RNA-editing process that produced a truncated protein (18).

ApoB-48 protein is synthesized in the endoplasmic reticulum of the intestine analogous to secretion of VLDLs by the liver. These processes cannot be completely equated, however. There is a disorder, chylomicron retention disease (Anderson's disease), in which there is selective inability to secrete chylomicrons, although VLDL secretion proceeds normally (6). Partial lipidation of apoB-48 proceeds as it is translocated across the membrane of the endoplasmic reticulum, forming a small spherical precursor of the chylomicron. In a second step, a lipid particle fuses with the partially lipidated apoB. This is mediated by microsomal triglyceride transport protein (MTP), and a protein disulfide isomerase

(19). The particles are then transported to the Golgi apparatus where more phospholipid and apolipoproteins A-I, A-II, and A-IV (apoA-I, apoA-II, and apoA-IV, respectively) are added. Secretion of chylomicrons into the extracellular space occurs when membranes of the *trans*-cisternae of the Golgi fuse with the basolateral membrane. Chylomicrons pass into intestinal lacteals and transit the thoracic duct to the subclavian vein. The capillaries of the intestine are fenestrated such that HDLs can pass into the lymph spaces allowing exchange of phospholipid to HDLs and acquisition of C proteins and apoE by chylomicrons. ApoA-I, apoA-II, and apoA-IV dissociate rapidly on exposure of chylomicrons to lymph and enter the HDL pool. HDLs in intestinal lymph may also facilitate sequestration of endotoxins (8). The intestine accommodates large fluxes of triglyceride by increasing chylomicron size. Synthesis of apoB-48 is increased only minimally with fat feeding, whereas triglyceride transport can increase up to 20-fold.

Intravascular Lipolysis of Chylomicrons

Lipolysis of triglycerides in chylomicrons and VLDLs proceed at the vascular endothelium. They marginate on capillary walls in adipose tissue and in skeletal and cardiac muscle where a complex interaction of lipoproteins, LPLs, and endothelial proteoglycans is involved (20), with the lipase binding both to heparan sulfate and to lipoproteins (21). The active form of LPL is a homodimer. ApoC-II is an obligate activator of the enzyme. LPL is synthesized and secreted most significantly in adipose tissue, striated muscle, and mammary gland. It moves across endothelium to the luminal surface in these tissues. LPL is transcriptionally upregulated by peroxisome proliferate-activated receptor α. Fasting decreases LPL activity in adipose tissue, whereas it increases activity in cardiac and skeletal muscle (22), sparing FFA for skeletal and cardiac muscle when energy substrates are scarce. Insulin deficiency results in very low levels of LPL activity in adipose tissue, contributing to hypertriglyceridemia (23). A number of mutations resulting in impaired function of LPL are recognized. In the homozygous state, they cause severe chylomicronemia. They also can contribute to lipemia in heterozygotes especially if factors such as pregnancy, poorly controlled diabetes, or alcohol use are present. Individuals homozygous for mutations causing deficiency of apoC-II also have severe impairment of lipolysis (20).

Intravascular lipolysis liberates FFA and glycerol. The major fraction of FFA is taken up in the tissue where hydrolysis occurred, and glycerol is removed by tissues that possess glycerokinase activity, principally the liver and intestine. Albumin is a transient ligand for transport to cell membranes. The marked albumin deficiency of severe nephrosis causes significant impairment of lipolysis resulting from product inhibition of LPL by FFA. Depletion of triglycerides leads to the production of smaller particles until about 70% of the triglyceride has been removed. Surface phospholipid and free cholesterol sheds to HDL apace with the decrease in particle size. This is dependent on PLTP (24). PLTP is synthesized in the placenta, pancreas, lung, kidney, liver, and brain. As lipolysis proceeds, the C proteins and a portion of apoE move to HDLs. The small (about 500–800 Å in diameter) triglyceride-depleted products of lipolysis that contain apoB-48 and apoE are termed chylomicron remnants. Lipolysis requires about 15 minutes in healthy individuals (25).

Metabolism of Chylomicron Remnants

Chylomicron remnants are removed from blood rapidly and categorically into hepatocytes, through the LDL receptor-related protein (LRP), and the LDL receptor (6,26). LRP contains a number of structurally distinct regions that exhibit homology with the LDL receptor (27). It recycles through endosomal compartments in a fashion analogous to the LDL receptor. The protein is synthesized as a precursor that undergoes selective proteolysis to yield subunits of 515 and 85 kD that remain noncovalently associated. It binds apoE. Although it binds chylomicron remnants poorly *in vitro*, their ligand property may be enhanced by acquiring apoE from hepatic microvilli. This may occur during interaction with hepatic lipase (HL) and is perhaps facilitated by interaction with heparan sulfate. The presence of HL in endosomal compartments is compatible with this model (28). LPL bound to lipoproteins may also be a ligand for LRP. Unlike the metabolism of VLDL remnants, no circulating daughter particles such as LDL are formed from chylomicrons. Triglycerides and cholesterol of chylomicron remnants are used in secretion of VLDLs by the liver. Tocopherols also enter the hepatocyte in chylomicron remnants, to be sorted on the basis of stereoisomerism and resecreted in VLDLs (29).

A common variant allele of apoE, apoE$_2$, has low affinity for both receptors. In individuals homozygous for apoE$_2$, remnants of chylomicrons and VLDLs accumulate in plasma if factors that potentiate lipemia are present. This disorder is termed familial dysbetalipoproteinemia.

TRANSPORT OF ENDOGENOUS TRIGLYCERIDES

The Hepatic Triglyceride Economy

VLDL secretion provides a pathway for export of triglyceride fatty acids, cholesterol, certain exchangeable apoproteins, and tocopherol (Fig. 6–1). Production rate of VLDL varies greatly, reflecting the supply of disposable energy substrate, and is significantly increased by estrogens and alcohol. Fatty acids used in triglyceride synthesis come from lipolysis in adipose tissue by intracellular lipase, from intravascular lipolysis, and from *de novo* synthesis. The fraction extracted from blood by the liver is about one-third, independent of level. Hence, increased lipolysis in adipocytes will increase FFA uptake. The most potent down-regulator

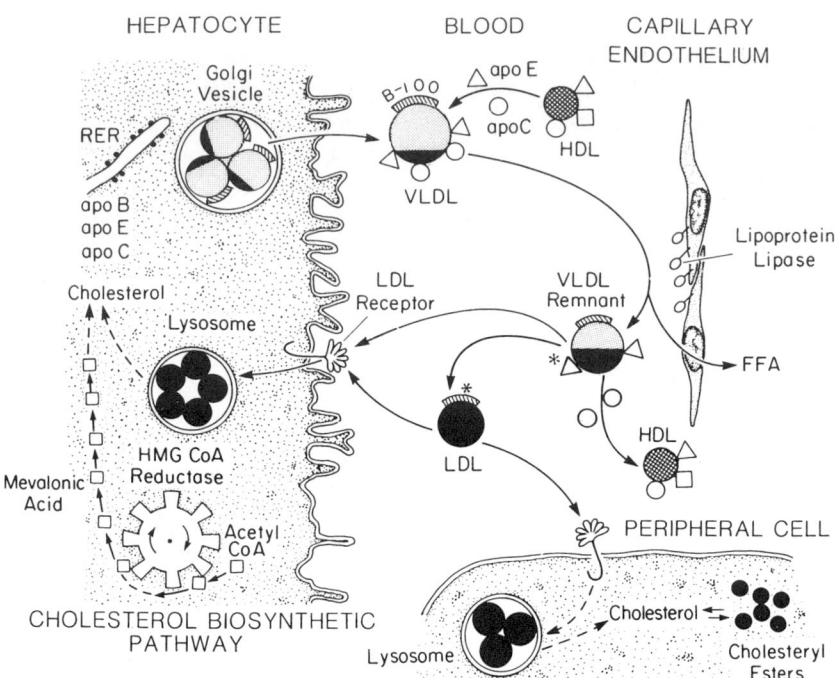

FIG. 6–1. Metabolism of lipoproteins of hepatic origin. Nascent very low-density lipoproteins (VLDLs) are secreted through the Golgi apparatus. They acquire additional C apolipoproteins and apolipoprotein E (apoE) from high-density lipoproteins (HDLs). Lipolysis by lipoprotein lipase produces remnant particles, which yield C apolipoproteins and a portion of their apoE to HDLs. A portion of VLDL remnants is endocytosed in liver after binding of their apoE moieties to receptors. The remaining VLDL remnants are converted to low-density lipoproteins (LDLs) by further loss of triglycerides and loss of apoE. A major pathway for LDL degradation involves the endocytosis of LDLs by LDL receptors, for which B-100 is the ligand. *Black areas,* cholesteryl esters; *stippled areas,* triglycerides; *cross-hatched areas,* HDL particles; *asterisk,* a functional ligand for LDL receptor; *triangles,* apoE; *open circles* and *squares,* C apolipoproteins. FFA, free fatty acid; HMG-CoA, 3-hydroxy-3-methylglutaryl coenzyme A.

of intracellular lipase is insulin. Hepatic biosynthesis of fatty acids proceeds using carbon sources derived from the catabolism of glucose, amino acids, and ethanol. Fatty acid synthesis is enhanced in the fed state and is suppressed during prolonged fasting, when ketogenesis is active.

Assembly and Secretion of Very Low-Density Lipoproteins

ApoB-100 is the sole B protein produced in the human liver. This is supported by the finding that apoB-48 is absent despite normal production of apoB-100, in patients with abetalipoproteinemia who have undergone liver transplant. Each VLDL and LDL particle contains a single copy of apoB-100 (6). The gene for apoB is located on chromosome 2 (30). Both positive and negative transcriptional regulatory sites are present in its promotor. The glycosylated B-100 protein is approximately 549 kD. It contains about 40 lipophilic sequences that allow it to associate with the lipid moieties of VLDL, IDL, and LDL with such high affinity that it remains with a single-lipoprotein particle from secretion to ultimate endocytosis (31). ApoB-100 is synthesized on ribosomes attached to the endoplasmic

reticulum. It is partially lipidated during transfer into the endoplasmic reticulum. The lipids in this stage probably come from the inner leaflet of the endoplasmic membrane (6). A substantial fraction of newly synthesized apoB is degraded without being secreted, suggesting that lipidation may induce conformational changes that allow it to proceed to a second stage of lipidation (32,33). Lipidation of apoB-100 has been postulated to be a two-step process (34). The first phase produces LDL-sized particles and the second involves coalescence of these with triglyceride-rich particles produced in the smooth endoplasmic reticulum. MTP appears to be involved in both steps (6,19). Fully lipidated VLDLs normally are transported to the Golgi vesicles, where glycosylation proceeds, before they are transported to the plasma membrane and released into the space of Disse. Homozygous ablative mutations for MTP result in abetalipoproteinemia in which no VLDLs or chylomicrons are present in plasma.

Nascent Very Low-Density Lipoproteins

Nascent VLDLs isolated from the Golgi apparatus contain newly synthesized apoE and the C apoproteins. They contain more phospholipid and much less unesterified cholesterol than plasma VLDLs (35). On secretion, phospholipid migrates to HDL, possibly nucleating new HDL particles and unesterified cholesterol, and E and C proteins move from HDLs to VLDLs (35). The transfer of phospholipid to HDL is dependent on PLTP (24). Because the human liver has relatively low ACAT activity, VLDLs contain little cholesteryl ester.

Regulation of Very Low-Density Lipoprotein Synthesis

Triglyceride biosynthesis *de novo* in the liver is regulated by the transcriptional regulatory mechanism involving SREBP (sterol response element-binding protein) 1-a and 1-c, which are derived from a single gene through alternative transcription (36). The 1-c product is the principal regulator of fatty acid biosynthesis. Activation is mediated by proteolytic events that release the amino terminal domain from the membrane-bound precursor, when it enters the nucleus, upregulating about 30 genes that code for enzymes of fatty acid synthesis and modification. Another member of the regulatory gene family, SREBP2, chiefly regulates genes involved in cholesterol synthesis. Proteolytic activation is mediated by SREBP cleavage-activating protein that facilitates cleavage of SREBP2 in response to decreasing ambient sterol levels.

Increases of triglyceride secretion in VLDLs are largely accommodated by increases in particle volume, although a modest increment in secretion of apoB-100 can take place when triglyceride secretion is maximal. Because so much apoB-100 is degraded intracellularly, it is probable that increases in secretion may reflect changes in the rate of degradation. That apoB-100 message increases in abetalipoproteinemia suggests that there is significant regulation of expression or degradation (37). Insulin is known to inhibit synthesis and secretion of apoB. The most commonly encountered form of hyperlipidemia in humans, familial combined hyperlipidemia, involves an increased secretion rate for VLDLs (6).

Metabolism of Very Low-Density Lipoproteins

VLDLs are subject to lipolysis by LPL as described for chylomicrons. The circulating half-life of VLDL particles is 30 to 60 minutes in healthy humans (25). The rate of lipolysis of triglycerides is regulated partly by the inhibitory effects of apoC-III, which also inhibit premature binding of VLDLs to the LDL receptor. Progressive lipolysis leads to a cascade of successively smaller particles. Lipids of the surface monolayer and C proteins are transferred to HDLs, a process dependent on PLTP. Loss of apoC-II, a cofactor of LPL, causes lipolysis to become less efficient. The particles have now become IDLs, enriched in cholesteryl esters, and retaining some apoE in addition to one copy of apoB-100. The fate of remnant particles is dichotomous at this point. About half, perhaps those with a larger complement of apoE, are endocytosed in the liver; the remainder become cholesteryl ester–rich LDL. It is possible that a subclass of VLDLs that is devoid of apoE may be converted quantitatively to LDLs. VLDL remnants are endocytosed through the LDL receptor in the liver, with apoE as the ligand (38). The receptors cluster in coated pits, which subsequently are endocytosed as coated vesicles. The receptors are dissociated with the CURL (compartment for uncoupling of receptor and ligand) and return to the cell surface, whereas the remnants are degraded, returning triglycerides and cholesterol to hepatic pools. A related receptor, the VLDL receptor, appears to endocytose VLDL, particularly in adipose tissue (39). ApoE, a protein of about 35 kD, contains a ligand domain for the LDL and LRP receptors (40–42). It is synthesized in a number of tissues including the liver, intestine, central nervous system, and retinal pigment epithelium. Expression is greatest in the liver, where a tissue-specific regulatory domain directs expression of both the *apoE* and *apoC-I* genes (43). Human apoE deficiency leads to the accumulation of remnant lipoproteins in plasma.

Formation of Low-Density Lipoproteins

The loss of C proteins from VLDL remnants relieves inhibition of HL, allowing hydrolysis of most of the remaining triglycerides. Although HL is in the family of lipases with LPL and pancreatic lipase, it has distinct properties that comport with its role in lipolysis of remnants. This protein of 499 amino acids does not require apoC-II as cofactor, but it is activated by apoE (44). It also has more phospholipase activity than does LPL (45). The formation of LDL appears to involve interaction of VLDL remnants with heparan sulfate on hepatocyte membrane, mediated by apoE. ApoE binds poorly to the terminal lipoprotein products of lipolysis by HL, probably accounting for their release from the liver membranes. These mature LDL particles, of approximately 215 Å in diameter with a cholesteryl ester–rich core, have apoB-100 as the sole apoprotein. Both HDLs and IDLs accumulate in the plasma of individuals who lack active HL, indicating a dual role for the enzyme in the metabolism of remnant particles and HDL.

CENTRIFUGAL TRANSPORT OF CHOLESTEROL

Structure of Low-Density Lipoproteins

Because each LDL particle contains one copy of apoB-100, two populations of LDL exist in plasma-containing apoB-100 molecules that are products of different alleles (6). The apoB-100 appears to be disposed circumferentially around the lipid core of LDL (46). In the presence of hypertriglyceridemia, the triglyceride content of LDL is increased, and the particles assume smaller diameters within an array of five quantized states (47). Conformational differences in apoB-100 characterize these states, and the two with the smallest diameters have diminished affinity for the LDL receptor and are either more atherogenic than normal LDL or are markers for increased risk (48).

Metabolism of Low-Density Lipoproteins

The circulating half-life of LDL is approximately 2.5 days in healthy humans. The principal mechanism by which LDL are removed from blood is endocytosis into nucleated cells through the LDL receptor, for which apoB-100 is the ligand. Hepatocytes account for more than half of total uptake. The ligand domain remains latent in VLDLs and IDLs of larger particle diameters but is exposed in LDLs. It is a complex domain including sequence located around an interdomain loop in the carboxyl-terminal region (6). Receptor-mediated endocytosis of LDLs provides a major source of cholesterol to cells for the maintenance of cell membranes. Because LDLs contain tocopherols, this mechanism serves to deliver them to cells as well (29,49). Receptor number is increased during cell division and under other circumstances when an increased supply of cholesterol is required. The greatest levels of receptor expression occur in malignant cells. LDL receptor–mediated endocytosis also delivers cholesterol to steroidogenic tissues. Expression of LDL receptors is regulated transcriptionally by SREBP-1 (36,50,51). The synthesis of cholesterol is controlled by transcriptional regulation of 3-hydroxy-3-methylglutaryl coenzyme A (HMG-CoA) reductase and HMG-CoA synthase (50). HMG-CoA reductase activity also is regulated by degradation of the enzyme, a mechanism activated by both sterol and isoprenoid compounds (52–54).

The LDL receptor gene located on chromosome 19 contains 18 exons. Five exons encode the ligand interactive domain (55). Interaction with the ligands apoB-100 and apoE occur through a domain consisting of seven repeats, rich in negative charges, and rigidly constrained by disulfide bridges. The fate of endocytosed LDL is similar to that described for VLDL remnants. Decreasing pH in endosomes dissociates ligand and receptor. The latter are returned to the cell surface through the CURL compartment, whereas the lipoproteins undergo proteolysis. Cholesteryl esters are hydrolyzed by acid esterase activity, and the cholesterol enters cellular pools. It can then be esterified, largely with oleic acid, by ACAT, providing for storage of cholesterol in the ester form. The principal mechanism for chemical degradation of cholesterol is its oxidative conversion to bile acids in the liver, a process initiated by cholesterol 7-α-hydroxylase. Two pathways then result in the formation of cholic and chenodeoxycholic acids. Defects in cholesterol 7-α-hydroxylase cause the cholesterol content of the liver to increase, down-regulating LDL receptors, and leading to increased levels of LDL in plasma. Resistance to HMG-CoA reductase inhibitors and premature gallstone disease may also occur (56).

More than 400 mutations of the LDL receptor gene have been described that result, variously, in failure to produce the protein, failure of glycosylation or transport of the receptor to the cell surface, failure of the receptor to localize in coated pits or to endocytose, and, most common, failure to bind ligand lipoproteins with normal affinity. Phenotypically, any of these mutations can lead to accumulation of LDL in plasma, even in the heterozygous state, a condition termed familial hypercholesterolemia (FH) (49). Increased levels of LDL in plasma also can result from mutations that impair the ligand properties of apoB-100 for the LDL receptor (57,58). In addition to endocytosis through the LDL receptor, LDL can be taken up in all nucleated cells by nonreceptor-mediated processes that are of low efficiency but that become significant as the LDL concentration in extracellular fluid increases greatly, as in homozygous FH. Genetic defects in a protein that acts in an auxiliary role result in a disorder termed autosomal-recessive hypercholesterolemia (59). Furthermore, macrophages and transformed smooth muscle cells can endocytose LDL that is chemically or physically modified through a pair of structurally interrelated scavenger receptors (60,61). The two receptors, products of a single gene, differ in that one has an additional carboxyl-terminal cysteine-rich domain. Other receptors on macrophages also are capable of endocytosis of oxidized LDL (62–64).

HIGH-DENSITY LIPOPROTEIN METABOLISM

Origins of High-Density Lipoproteins

Protein and lipid constituents that will form HDL originate in both hepatocytes and enterocytes. Precursor complexes of apoA-I, cholesterol, and phospholipids are excellent substrates for LCAT. Esterification of cholesterol generates a hydrophobic phase that accumulates in the interlamellar space, forming spherical microemulsion particles typical of plasma HDL (65). The association of some apoA-I and apoE with nascent VLDLs (35) suggests that some of the proteins of HDLs originate in VLDLs and presumably, by analogy, in chylomicrons. As VLDLs reach the space of Disse and chylomicrons enter the intestinal lymphatics, some phospholipid dissociates from the surface with lipoproteins A-I, A-II, and possibly E, to nucleate new HDL particles or to join existing HDL. Nascent VLDLs are enriched in phosphatidylethanolamine (66), which is selectively depleted during the loss of phospholipids. LCAT then esterifies free cholesterol acquired during dissociation of surface lipids from the nascent triglyceride-rich lipoprotein. A major source of both unesterified cholesterol and phospholipid is efflux from peripheral cells to HDLs. Macrophages secrete particles that contain phospholipid and cholesterol accompanied by apoE (67), which they synthesize. These particles probably contribute lipid substrates for LCAT and merge into the circulating HDLs, although some may be endocytosed directly in the liver through the LDL receptor. The process of secretion of precursors of HDLs from the liver is not dependent on secretion of apoB-containing lipoproteins, however, as the accumulation of apoA-I, phospholipid, and cholesterol is normal in perfusates of the liver in which apoB secretion is completely blocked by orotic acid (68).

High-Density Lipoprotein Structure

ApoA-I is present in nearly all HDL molecular species as a primary structural element. This 28-kD protein is rich in amphipathic helical structure. ApoA-I is synthesized in the liver and intestine and is secreted with a six-amino acid prosequence that is cleaved by proteolysis in plasma to form the mature protein. ApoA-I apparently can assume several conformations in accommodating to different lipid-to-protein ratios. The *apoA I* gene is clustered on the long arm of chromosome 11 with the genes for apoC-III and apoA-IV (69). Overexpression of apoA-I in transgenic mice appears to retard atherogenesis (70). ApoA-II also is a major protein constituent of HDL, but it is not present in all HDL particles. It is a disulfide-bridged homodimer of a monomeric chain of only 77 amino acids. The monomer also forms heterodimers with the E_2 and E_3 isoforms of apoE. Its gene is located on chromosome 1. ApoA-II is secreted as a proprotein that undergoes proteolytic cleavage to form the mature protein. ApoA-IV, a 46-kD protein that has extensive homology with apoA-I, is found in both HDLs and chylomicrons (71). In humans, it is synthesized largely in the intestine and occurs in a number of isoforms. It is capable of activating LCAT with some substrates. All of the C proteins are found in HDLs, which serves as a reservoir of C proteins and apoE for recycling to nascent VLDLs and chylomicrons. ApoC-I is predominantly associated with HDLs. This protein, containing 57 amino acids, is synthesized in the liver. Most HDL particles contain cores of cholesteryl esters and monolayers of phospholipid and unesterified cholesterol with which the helical apoproteins associate. The core domains can contain significant amounts of triglycerides, especially in the presence of hypertriglyceridemia. When plasma triglyceride levels are abnormally increased, triglycerides exchange for a portion of the cholesteryl esters of HDLs, providing the basis for a log-inverse relation between HDL cholesterol levels and total plasma triglycerides (72).

The Centripetal Transport Pathway

Cholesterol is retrieved from peripheral tissues by a transport system that is initiated by the efflux of phospholipid and cholesterol by the ATP-binding cassette transporter A1 (ABCA1) (73–76). This transporter is transcriptionally regulated by LXR-RXR nuclear hormone receptors in response to cholesterol loading of the cell. It is expressed in many tissues and is active in cholesterol-laden macrophages (77). Genetic defects in the ABCA1 transporter result in Tangier disease characterized by low levels of HDLs. Effluxed phospholipid and cholesterol is chiefly acquired by pre-β_1 HDLs, a 70-kD particle containing two copies of apoA-1. As cholesterol in this particle is esterified by LCAT, larger HDL particles of α mobility are formed. Cholesterol reaches the

liver by two processes. Cholesteryl esters transfer to chylomicrons, VLDLs, their remnant particles, and LDLs, mediated by CETP. The uptake of LDL and remnant particles by receptor-mediated endocytosis then delivers the cholesterol to hepatocytes (78). The second process involves transfer of cholesteryl esters to hepatocytes through the scavenger receptor BI (SR-BI) receptor (64). The centripetal transport system is entropically driven: Esterification of cholesterol by LCAT reduces its chemical potential, maintaining a diffusion gradient from the cell membranes. The increase in entropy associated with the transfer of cholesteryl esters into the cores of acceptor lipoproteins provides energy for the transfer process. As cholesteryl esters transfer to acceptor lipoproteins, triglycerides move from VLDLs and chylomicrons to the cores of α species of HDLs (79). As cholesteryl esters and triglycerides are removed from HDLs, 70-kD pre-β_1 HDL is regenerated, contributing the final portion of a newly recognized metabolic cycle (Fig. 6–2) (79). HDL particles with and without apoA-II are both capable of forming pre-β_1 HDL as cholesteryl esters are transferred to lipoprotein acceptors (80). HL is chiefly responsible for the removal of triglycerides from HDLs.

LCAT is a hydrophobic protein composed of 416 amino acids that is secreted by the liver, for which apoA-I is a required cofactor. LCAT catalyzes the transacylation of a fatty acid from the *sn*-2 position of lecithin to cholesterol. Integrated transesterification and centripetal movement of cholesterol appear to involve two additional elements, apoD and CETP. ApoD is a highly glycosylated protein of 33 kD, a product of a gene on chromosome 3 (81), synthesized by many tissues including the placenta, liver, and intestine. CETP with a mass of 53 kD is more hydrophobic than other apoproteins, consistent with its function as a lipid transfer protein. Synthesized in the liver, intestine, adrenals, and probably in macrophages, it catalyzes the transfer of triglycerides and, to a lesser extent, phospholipids and cholesteryl esters. In LCAT deficiency, abnormal lamellar lipoproteins containing unesterified cholesterol and phospholipid accumulate in plasma in place of spherical cholesteryl ester–rich HDLs (11). In CETP deficiency, there is a marked accumulation of cholesteryl ester–rich HDLs in plasma (82).

Speciation of High-Density Lipoproteins

The realization that ultracentrifugation causes the denaturation and loss of some elements of HDL led to the development of the technique of selected affinity immunosorption for isolation of native molecular species (83). Nondenaturing gel electrophoresis after immunosorption demonstrates up to 15 discrete HDL species containing many more proteins than are associated with ultracentrifugally prepared HDL. A number of these proteins exist in molecular dispersion in plasma in addition to a fraction that is bound to HDL (7). These include haptoglobin-associated protein, apoJ (84), fibrinogen, the binding protein for complement component 4 (C4BP), and LBP (8). In addition, an HDL species

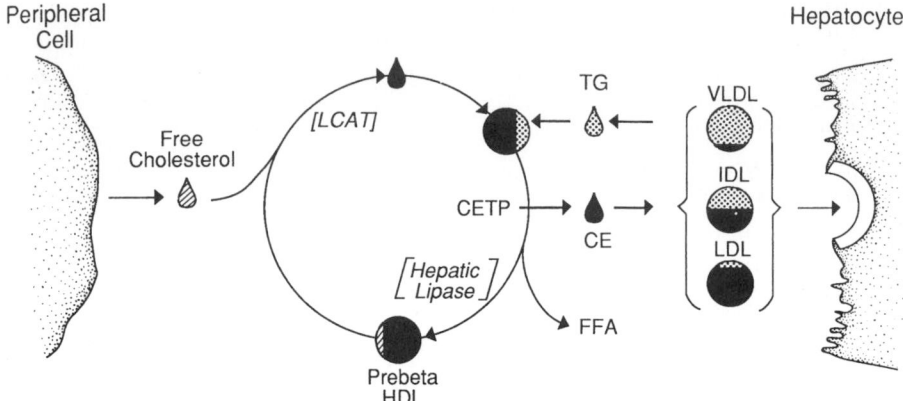

FIG. 6–2. The role of pre-β_1 high-density lipoprotein (HDL) in reverse cholesterol transport. *Black areas,* cholesteryl esters; *stippled areas,* triglycerides; *hatched areas,* free cholesterol. CE, cholesteryl ester; CETP, cholesteryl ester transfer protein; FFA, free fatty acid; IDL, intermediate-density lipoprotein; LCAT, lecithin-cholesterol acyl transferase; LDL, low-density lipoprotein; TG, triglyceride; VLDL, very low-density lipoprotein.

that contains tightly bound transferrin can chelate transition metals and inhibit the oxidation of LDLs (85). Another species contains ceruloplasmin (85). ApoL-1 is found in two species of large α HDL particles (86,87). The best characterized of the newly recognized species of HDL is the 70-kD pre-β_1 HDL (88). This particle contains about 85% protein, representing two copies of apoA-I. The conformation of apoA-I is markedly different from that in other HDL species (89), and its binding affinity for SR-BI is much less (90). Content of this particle in plasma increases monotonically with increasing triglyceride levels and during exercise. Discrete HDL species that contain apoE and apoA-IV also have been characterized (91,92). The distribution of discrete molecular species of HDL is the result of processes involving LCAT, CETP, PLTP, LPL, HL, and also endothelial lipase. The latter primarily modifies the phospholipid content of HDL particles (93,94). It is likely that further understanding of the molecular basis of HDL speciation will lead to insights of importance in the formation and degradation of HDLs.

REFERENCES

1. He XM, Carter DC. Atomic structure and chemistry of human serum albumin. *Nature* 1992;358:209–215.
2. Schumaker VN, Phillips ML, Chatterton JE. Apolipoprotein B and low density lipoprotein structure: implications for biosynthesis of triglyceride-rich lipoproteins. *Adv Protein Chem* 1994;45:205–248.
3. Havel RJ, Eder HA, Bragdon JH. The distribution and chemical composition of ultracentrifugally separated lipoproteins in human serum. *J Clin Invest* 1955;34:1345–1353.
4. Segrest JP, Garber DW, Brouilette CG, et al. The amphipathic alpha-helix: a multifunctional structural motif in plasma apolipoproteins. *Adv Protein Chem* 1994;45:303–369.
5. Duchateau PN, Movsesyan I, Yamashita S, et al. Plasma apolipoprotein L concentrations correlate with plasma triglycerides and cholesterol levels in normolipidemic, hyperlipidemic and diabetic subjects. *J Lipid Res* 2000;41:1231–1236.
6. Kane JP, Havel RJ. Disorders of the biogenesis and secretion of lipoproteins containing the B-apolipoproteins. In: Scriver CR, Beaudet

AL, Sly WS, et al., eds. *The metabolic bases of inherited disease.* New York: McGraw-Hill, 2002:2717–2752.
7. Kunitake ST, Carilli CT, Lau K, et al. Identification of proteins associated with apolipoprotein A-I-containing lipoproteins purified by selected affinity immunosorption. *Biochemistry* 1994;33:1988–1993.
8. Wurfel MM, Kunitake ST, Lichenstein H, et al. Lipopolysaccharide (LPS) binding protein is carried on lipoproteins and acts as a cofactor in the neutralization of LPS. *J Exp Med* 1994;180:1025–1035.
9. Havel RJ, Kane JP. Introduction: structure and metabolism of plasma lipoproteins. In: Scriver CR, Beaudet AL, Sly WS, et al., eds. *The metabolic bases of inherited disease.* New York: McGraw-Hill, 2002:2705–2716.
10. Stahl A, Gimeno RE, Tartaglia LA, et al. Fatty acid transport proteins: a current view of a growing family. *Trends Endocrinol Metab* 2001;12:266–273.
11. Santamarina-Fojo S, Hoeg JM, Assmann G, et al. Lecithin-cholesterol acyltransferase deficiency and fish eye disease. In: Scriver CR, Beaudet AL, Sly WS, et al., eds. *The metabolic and molecular bases of inherited disease.* New York: McGraw-Hill, 2001:2817–2834.
12. Vanhamme L, Paturiaux-Hanocq F, Poelvoorde P, et al. Apolipoprotein L-I is the trypanosomelytic factor of human serum. *Nature* 2003;422:83–87.
13. Read TE, Harris HW, Grunfeld C, et al. Chylomicrons enhance endotoxin excretion in bile. *Infect Immun* 1993;61:3496–3502.
14. Feingold KR, Staprans I, Memon RA, et al. Endotoxin rapidly induces changes in lipid metabolism that produce hypertriglyceridemia: low doses stimulate hepatic triglyceride production while high doses inhibit clearance. *J Lipid Res* 1992;33:1765–1776.
15. Bowie EJ. Lipid-related clotting reactions of clinical significance. *Arch Pathol Lab Med* 1992;116:1345–1349.
16. Berge KE, Tian H, Graf GA, et al. Accumulation of dietary cholesterol in sitosterolemia caused by mutations in adjacent ABC transporters. *Science* 2001;290(5497):1771–1775.
17. Lu K, Lee MH, Hazard S, et al. Two genes that map to the STSL locus cause sitosterolemia: genomic structure and spectrum of mutations involving sterolin-1 and sterolin-2, encoded by ABCG5 and ABCG8, respectively. *Am J Hum Genet* 2001;68:278–290.
18. Powell LM, Wallis SC, Pease RJ, et al. A novel form of tissue-specific RNA processing produces apolipoprotein B-48 in intestine. *Cell* 1987;50:831–840.
19. Wetterau JR, Aggerbeck LP, Bouma ME, et al. Absence of microsomal triglyceride transfer protein in individuals with abetalipoproteinemia. *Science* 1992;258:999–1001.
20. Brunzel JD, Deeb SS. Familial lipoprotein lipase deficiency, Apo C-II deficiency, and hepatic lipase deficiency. In: Scriver CR, Beaudet AL, Sly WS, et al., eds. *The metabolic and molecular bases of inherited disease.* New York: McGraw-Hill, 2001:2789–2816.
21. Eisenberg S, Sehayek E, Olivecrona T, et al. Lipoprotein lipase en-

hances binding of lipoproteins to heparan sulphate on cell surfaces and extracellular matrix. *J Clin Invest* 1992;90:2013–2021.

22. Doolittle MH, Ben-Zeev O, Elovson J, et al. The response of lipoprotein lipase to feeding and fasting. Evidence for posttranslational regulation. *J Biol Chem* 1990;265:4570–4577.

23. Frayn KN. Insulin resistance and lipid metabolism. *Curr Opin Lipidol* 1993;4:197–204.

24. Tollefson JH, Ravnik S, Albers JJ. Isolation and characterization of a phospholipid transfer protein (LTP-II) from human plasma. *J Lipid Res* 1988;15:1593–1602.

25. Stalenhoef AFH, Malloy MJ, Kane JP, et al. Metabolism of apolipoprotein B-48 and B-100 of triglyceride-rich lipoproteins in normal and lipoprotein lipase-deficient humans. *Proc Natl Acad Sci USA* 1984;81: 1839–1843.

26. Havel RJ. Remnant lipoproteins as therapeutic targets. *Curr Opin Lipidol* 2000;11:615–620.

27. Herz J, Kowal RC, Goldstein JL, et al. Proteolytic processing of the 600 kD low density lipoprotein receptor related protein (LRP) occurs in a *trans*-Golgi compartment. *EMBO J* 1990;9:1769–1776.

28. Belcher JD, Hamilton RL, Brady SE, et al. Hepatic endosomes have hepatic lipase. *Circulation* 1988;28:II-145.

29. Kayden HJ, Traber MG. Absorption, lipoprotein transport and regulation of plasma concentrations of vitamin E in humans. *J Lipid Res* 1993;34:343–358.

30. Blackhart BD, Ludwig EH, Pierotti VR, et al. Structure of the human apolipoprotein B gene. *J Biol Chem* 1986;261:15364–15367.

31. Segrest JP, Jones MK, Mishra VK, et al. Apolipoprotein B-100: conservation of lipid-associating amphipathic secondary structural motifs in nine species of vertebrates. *J Lipid Res* 1998;39(1):85–102.

32. Dixon JL, Ginsberg HN. Regulation of hepatic secretion of apolipoprotein B-containing lipoproteins: information obtained from cultured liver cells. *J Lipid Res* 1993;34:167–179.

33. Liang J, Wu X, Jiang H, et al. Translocation efficiency, susceptibility to proteasomal degradation, and lipid responsiveness of apolipoprotein B are determined by the presence of beta sheet domains. *J Biol Chem* 1998;273:35216–35221.

34. Hamilton RL. Apolipoprotein-B-containing plasma lipoproteins in health and in disease. *Trends Cardiovasc Med* 1994;4:131–139.

35. Hamilton RL, Moorehouse A, Havel RJ. Isolation and properties of nascent lipoproteins from highly purified rat hepatocytic Golgi fractions. *J Lipid Res* 1991;32:529–543.

36. Horton JD, Goldstein JL, Brown MS. SREBPs: activators of the complete program of cholesterol and fatty acid synthesis in the liver. *J Clin Invest* 2002;109:1125–1131.

37. Lackner KJ, Monge JC, Gregg RE, et al. Analysis of the apolipoprotein B gene and messenger ribonucleic acid in abetalipoproteinemia. *J Clin Invest* 1986;78:1707–1712.

38. Havel RJ, Hamilton RL. Hepatocytic lipoprotein receptors and intracellular lipoprotein catabolism. *Hepatology* 1988;8:1689–1704.

39. Tacken PJ, Hofker MH, Havekes LM, et al. Living up to a name: the role of the VLDL receptor in lipid metabolism. *Curr Opin Lipidol* 2001;12:275–279.

40. Mahley RW, Rall SC Jr. Type III hyperlipoproteinemia (dysbetalipoproteinemia): the role of apolipoprotein E in normal and abnormal lipoprotein metabolism. In: Scriver CR, Beaudet AL, Sly WS, et al., eds. *The metabolic and molecular bases of inherited disease.* New York: McGraw-Hill, 2001:2835–2862.

41. Weisgraber KH. Apolipoprotein E: structure–function relationships. *Adv Protein Chem* 1994;45:249–302.

42. Wilson C, Wardell MR, Weisgraber KH, et al. Three dimensional structure of the LDL receptor binding domain of human apolipoprotein E. *Science* 1991;252:1817–1822.

43. Simonet WS, Bucay N, Lauer SJ, et al. A far-downstream hepatocyte-specific control region directs expression of the linked human apolipoprotein E and C-I genes in transgenic mice. *J Biol Chem* 1993;268: 8221–8229.

44. Thuren T, Weisgraber KH, Sisson P, et al. Role of apolipoprotein E in hepatic lipase catalyzed hydrolysis of phospholipid in high density lipoproteins. *Biochemistry* 1992;31:2332–2338.

45. Deckelbaum RJ, Ramakrishnan R, Eisenberg S, et al. Triacylglycerol and phospholipid hydrolysis in human plasma lipoproteins. Role of lipoprotein and hepatic lipase. *Biochemistry* 1992;31:8544–8551.

46. Chatterton JE, Phillips ML, Curtiss LK, et al. Mapping apolipoprotein

47. Chen GC, Liu W, Duchateau P, et al. Conformational differences in human apolipoprotein B-100 among subspecies of low density lipoproteins (LDL). *J Biol Chem* 1994;269:29121–29128.

48. Krauss RM. Heterogeneity of plasma low-density lipoproteins and atherosclerosis risk. *Curr Opin Lipidol* 1994;5:339–349.

49. Goldstein JL, Hobbs HH, Brown MS. Familial hypercholesterolemia. In: Scriver CR, Beaudet AL, Sly WS, et al., eds. *The metabolic and molecular bases of inherited disease.* New York: McGraw-Hill, 2001: 2863–2914.

50. Goldstein JL, Brown MS. Regulation of the mevalonate pathway. *Nature* 1990;343:425–430.

51. Wang X, Sato R, Brown MS, et al. SREBP-1 a membrane-bound transcription factor released by sterol-regulated proteolysis. *Cell* 1994;77: 53–62.

52. Inoue S, Simoni RD. 3-Hydroxy-3-methylglutaryl-coenzyme-A reductase and T cell receptor alpha subunit are differentially degraded in the endoplasmic reticulum. *J Biol Chem* 1992;267:9080–9086.

53. Roitelman J, Simoni RD. Distinct sterol and non-sterol signals for the regulated degradation of 3-hydroxy-3-methylglutaryl coenzyme-A reductase. *J Biol Chem* 1992;267:25264–25273.

54. Rudney H, Panini SR. Cholesterol biosynthesis. *Curr Opin Lipidol* 1993;4:230–237.

55. Brown MS, Goldstein JL. A receptor-mediated pathway for cholesterol homeostasis. *Science* 1986;232:34–47.

56. Pullinger CR, Eng G, Salen S, et al. Human cholesterol 7α-hydroxylase (CYP7A1) deficiency has a hypercholesterolemic phenotype. *J Clin Invest* 2002;110:109–117.

57. Soria LF, Ludwig EH, Clarke HR, et al. Association between a specific apolipoprotein B mutation and familial defective B-100. *Proc Natl Acad Sci USA* 1989;86:587–591.

58. Pullinger CR, Hennessy LK, Chatterton JE, et al. Familial ligand-defective apolipoprotein B: identification of a new mutation that decreases LDL receptor binding affinity. *J Clin Invest* 1995;95: 1225–1234.

59. Garcia CK, Wilund K, Arca M, et al. Autosomal recessive hypercholesterolemia caused by mutations in a putative LDL receptor adaptor protein. *Science* 2001;292:1394–1398.

60. Kodama T, Freeman M, Rohrer L, et al. Type I macrophage scavenger receptor contains alpha helical and collagen-like coiled coils. *Nature* 1990;343:531–535.

61. Rohrer L, Freeman M, Kodama T, et al. Coiled-coil fibrous domains mediate ligand binding by macrophage scavenger receptor type II. *Nature* 1990;343:570–572.

62. Endemann G, Stanton LW, Madden KS, et al. CD36 is a receptor for oxidized low density lipoprotein. *J Biol Chem* 1993;268:11811–11816.

63. Stanton LW, White RT, Bryant CM, et al. A macrophage Fc receptor for IgG is also a receptor for oxidized low density lipoprotein. *J Biol Chem* 1992;267:22446–22451.

64. Acton SL, Kozarsky KF, Rigotti A. The HDL receptor SR-BI: a new therapeutic target for atherosclerosis? *Mol Med Today* 1999;5: 518–524.

65. Forte TM, Goth-Goldstein R, Nordhausen RW, et al. Apolipoprotein A-I-cell membrane interaction: extracellular assembly of heterogeneous nascent HDL particles. *J Lipid Res* 1993;34:317–324.

66. Hamilton RL, Fielding PE. Nascent very low density lipoproteins from rat hepatocytic Golgi fractions are enriched in phosphatidylethanolamine. *Biochem Biophys Res Commun* 1989;160:162–167.

67. Basu SK, Goldstein JL, Brown MS. Independent pathways for secretion of cholesterol and apolipoprotein E by macrophages. *Science* 1983;219:871–873.

68. Hamilton RL, Guo LS, Felker TE, et al. Nascent high density lipoproteins from liver perfusates of orotic acid-fed rats. *J Lipid Res* 1986;27: 967–978.

69. Cheung P, Kao FT, Law ML, et al. Localization of the structural gene for human apolipoprotein A-I on the long arm of human chromosome 11. *Proc Natl Acad Sci USA* 1984;81:508–511.

70. Rubin EM, Ishida BY, Clift SM, et al. Expression of human apolipoprotein A-I in transgenic mice results in reduced plasma levels of murine apolipoprotein A-I and the appearance of two new high density lipoprotein size subclasses. *Proc Natl Acad Sci USA* 1991;88: 434–438.

71. Elshourbagy NA, Walker DW, Boguski MS, et al. The nucleotide and

derived amino acid sequence of human apolipoprotein A-IV mRNA and the close linkage of its gene to the genes of apolipoprotein A-I and C-III. *J Biol Chem* 1986;261:1998–2002.

72. Myers LH, Phillips NR, Havel RJ. Mathematical evaluation of methods for estimation of the concentration of the major lipid components of human serum lipoproteins. *J Lab Clin Med* 1976;88:491–505.

73. Brooks-Wilson A, Marcil M, Clee SM, et al. Mutations in ABC1 in Tangier disease and familial high-density lipoprotein deficiency. *Nat Genet* 1999;22:336–345.

74. Bodzioch M, Orso E, Klucken J, et al. The gene encoding ATP-binding cassette transporter 1 is mutated in Tangier disease. *Nat Genet* 1999; 22:347–351.

75. Rust S, Rosier M, Funke H, et al. Tangier disease is caused by mutations in the gene encoding ATP-binding cassette transporter 1. *Nat Genet* 1999;22:352–355.

76. Lawn RM, Wade DP, Garvin MR, et al. The Tangier disease gene product ABC1 controls the cellular apolipoprotein-mediated lipid removal pathway. *J Clin Invest* 1999;104(8):R25–R31.

77. Tall AR, Costet P, Wang N. Regulation and mechanisms of macrophage cholesterol efflux. *J Clin Invest* 2002;110:899–904.

78. Fielding CJ, Fielding PE. Molecular physiology of reverse cholesterol transport. *J Lipid Res* 1995;36:211–228.

79. Kunitake ST, Mendel CM, Hennessy LK. Interconversion between apolipoprotein A-I-containing lipoproteins of prebeta and alpha electrophoretic mobilities. *J Lipid Res* 1992;33:1807–1816.

80. Hennessy LK, Kunitake ST, Kane JP. Apolipoprotein A-I-containing lipoproteins, with or without apolipoprotein A-II, as progenitors of prebeta HDL particles. *Biochemistry* 1993;32:5759–5765.

81. Drayna D, Fielding C, McLean J, et al. Cloning and expression of human apolipoprotein D cDNA. *J Biol Chem* 1986;261:16535–16538.

82. Kurasawa T, Yokoyama S, Miyake Y, et al. Rate of cholesteryl ester transfer between high and low density lipoproteins in human serum and a case with decreased transfer rate in association with hyperalphalipoproteinemia. *J Biochem* 1985;98:1499–1508.

83. McVicar JP, Kunitake ST, Hamilton RL, et al. Characteristics of human lipoproproteins isolated by selected-affinity immunosorption of apolipoprotein A-I (high density lipoproteins). *Proc Natl Acad Sci USA* 1984;81:1356–1360.

84. de Silva HV, Stuart WD, Duvic CR, et al. A 70-kDa apolipoprotein designated apoJ is a marker for subclasses of human plasma high density lipoproteins. *J Biol Chem* 1990;265:13240–13247.

85. Kunitake ST, Jarvis M, Hamilton RL, et al. Binding of transition metals by apolipoprotein A-I-containing plasma lipoproteins: inhibition of oxidation of low density lipoproteins. *Proc Natl Acad Sci USA* 1992; 89:6993–6997.

86. Duchateau PN, Pullinger CR, Orellana RE, et al. Apolipoprotein L, a new human HDL-apolipoprotein expressed by the pancreas. Identification, cloning, characterization, and plasma distribution of apolipoprotein L. *J Biol Chem* 1997;41:25576–25582.

87. Duchateau PN, Pullinger CR, Cho MH, et al. Apolipoprotein-L gene family: tissue-specific expression, splicing, promoter regions; discovery of a new gene. *J Lipid Res* 2001;42:620–630.

88. Kunitake ST, La Sala KJ, Kane JP. Apoprotein A-I-containing lipoproteins with prebeta electrophoretic mobility. *J Lipid Res* 1985;26:549–553.

89. Kunitake ST, Chen GC, Kung SF, et al. Prebeta high density lipoprotein. Unique disposition of apolipoprotein A-I increases susceptibility to proteolysis. *Arteriosclerosis* 1990;10(1):25–30.

90. Liadaki KN, Liu T, Xu S, et al. Binding of high density lipoprotein (HDL) and discoidal reconstituted HDL to the HDL receptor scavenger receptor Class B Type I. *J Biol Chem* 2000;275:21262–21271.

91. Duverger N, Ghalim N, Ailhaud G, et al. Characterization of apo A-IV containing lipoprotein particles isolated from human plasma and intestinal fluid. *Arterioscler Thromb* 1993;13:126–132.

92. Hennessy LK, Kunitake ST, Jarvis M, et al. Isolation of subpopulations of high density lipoproteins: three particle species containing apoE and two species devoid of apoE that have affinity for heparin. *J Lipid Res* 1997;38:1859–1868.

93. Choi SY, Hirata K, Ishida T, et al. Endothelial lipase: a new lipase on the block. *J Lipid Res* 2002;43:1763–1769.

94. Jin W, Millar JS, Broedl U, et al. Inhibition of endothelial lipase causes increased HDL cholesterol levels in vivo. *J Clin Invest* 2003;111:357–362.

CHAPTER 7

Plasma High-Density Lipoproteins and Atherogenesis

Daniel J. Rader

Key Words: Adenosine triphosphate-binding cassette protein A1; apolipoprotein A-I; atherothrombosis; cholesterol; cholesteryl ester transfer protein; high-density lipoproteins; lipases; reverse cholesterol transport; scavenger receptor B-I.

D. J. Rader: University of Pennsylvania School of Medicine, 654 BRB II/III, 421 Curie Blvd, Philadelphia, Pennsylvania 19104.

INTRODUCTION

High-density lipoproteins (HDLs) are a class of lipoproteins characterized by their high density, small size, and specific apolipoprotein composition. There is a strong inverse association between plasma HDL-C levels and incidence of atherosclerotic cardiovascular disease (ASCVD) that is independent of other known risk factors (1). This strong epidemiologic association has focused tremendous attention on the relation between HDL metabolism and atherothrombosis. The National Cholesterol Education Program (NCEP) recommends screening with HDL-C as an independent risk factor in routine cardiovascular risk screening of all adults, and there is substantial interest in the development of new therapeutic approaches for atherothrombosis based on targeting HDL metabolism.

HIGH-DENSITY LIPOPROTEIN COMPOSITION AND STRUCTURE

Like other lipoproteins, HDLs are composed of lipids (including phospholipid, cholesterol, and triglyceride) and apolipoproteins. The major structural apolipoprotein of HDL is apolipoprotein A-I (apoA-I), and the majority of HDLs contain apoA-I. Mature apoA-I is 243 amino acids in length and consists largely of eight 22-amino acid-long amphipathic α helices. ApoA-II is the second most abundant HDL structural protein. The mature apoA-II polypeptide chain contains 77 amino acids with a single cysteine at residue 6 and exists in plasma primarily as a homodimer. In addition, HDL contains small amounts of apoC proteins (apoC-I, apoC-II, and apoC-III), apoE, apoA-IV, apoAV, apoD, apoJ, and apoL. High-density lipoprotein newly formed by secretion or as a byproduct of lipolysis has a distinctive discoidal structure. Nascent discoidal HDLs are excellent substrates for lecithin-cholesterol acyltransferase (LCAT), leading to the generation of cholesteryl esters and the conversion of discoidal particles into spherical structures.

HIGH-DENSITY LIPOPROTEIN HETEROGENEITY

HDL is heterogeneous with regard to its density and the closely related issue of size. The major subclassification of HDL has been based on the separation of HDL_2 (density, 1.063–1.125 g/mL) and HDL_3 (density, 1.125–1.210 g/mL). Whereas HDL_2 contains about 60% lipid and 40% protein, HDL_3 consists of about 45% lipid and 55% protein. The mean diameter of HDL_2 particles is about 10 to 12 nm, and that of HDL_3 is about 8 to 9 nm. Patients with coronary disease generally have smaller HDL particles, leading to the concept that larger HDL particles may be associated with greater protection from coronary heart disease (CHD). However, the data regarding the predictive ability of large (i.e., HDL_2) versus small (i.e., HDL_3) HDL particles for CHD risk is conflicting and there is no concensus regarding the clinical value of assessing HDL subclasses on the basis of density or size.

Another mode of classifying lipoproteins and HDL is according to their electrophoretic mobility in agarose gels. HDL was originally defined as an α migrating particle. However, a significant subfraction of apoA-I is found in particles with pre-β mobility. Pre-β HDL appears to have distinctive structural and metabolic properties and may have particular importance in mediating cellular cholesterol efflux.

Another aspect of HDL heterogeneity relates to apolipoprotein composition, specifically the content of apoA-I and apoA-II. There are two broad categories of HDL particles: those that do not contain apoA-II and therefore contain apoA-I as the major apolipoprotein [these often are referred to as lipoprotein A-I (LpA-I)], and those that contain both apoA-I and apoA-II (these often are referred to as LpA-I:A-II). In general, LpA-I:A-II particles represent approximately two-thirds of the HDL particles and LpA-I particles represent the remaining approximately one-third. Although centrifugally isolated HDL_2 is somewhat enriched in LpA-I compared with LpA-I:A-II, there is no exact correspondence between the subclassification based on size and density and that based on apoprotein composition. When analyzed by native polyacrylamide gradient gel electrophoresis, LpA-I is found to contain particles of both large and small size, as does LpA-I:A-II.

HIGH-DENSITY LIPOPROTEIN METABOLISM

The metabolism of HDL is a dynamic process. A schematic diagram depicting HDL metabolism is shown in Figure 7–1 (see color insert).

Biosynthesis of Apolipoprotein A-I and High-Density Lipoprotein

ApoA-I is synthesized and secreted by both the intestine and the liver, whereas apoA-II is made only in the liver. There are one or more distinct cis-acting DNA elements required for intestinal expression that are distinct from the liver elements. Many of the factors that regulate apoA-I production rates do not influence the level of apoA-I messenger RNA, indicating important regulation of apoA-I production on a posttranscriptional level. Whether apoA-I is secreted as a preformed HDL particle or as a lipid-poor apolipoprotein that quickly acquires lipid after secretion is not yet fully established.

Lipolysis of Tryglyceride-rich Lipoproteins and High-Density Lipoprotein Formation

A portion of the apolipoprotein and phospholipid destined to become HDL is initially secreted on large, triglyceride-transporting VLDLs (derived from the liver) or chylomicrons (derived from the small intestine). During lipolysis of chylomicrons and VLDLs by lipoprotein lipase (LPL), surface lipids (phospholipid and cholesterol) and apolipoproteins (apoA-I, apoA-II, and C apolipoproteins) are shed from the lipoproteins and form nascent discoidal HDL particles. LPL is synthesized in adipocytes, and skeletal as well as in cardiac myocytes, and is transported to the capillary endothelial surface where, bound to heparan sulfate proteoglycans, it hydrolyzes triglycerides in the triglyceride-rich lipoproteins chylomicrons and VLDL. After lipolysis, surface phospholipids and apolipoproteins from these lipoproteins dissociate and are acquired by

HDLs. Transgenic overexpression of LPL in mice results in increased HDL-cholesterol (HDL-C) levels. Conversely, the gene knockout of LPL is associated not only with severe hypertriglyceridemia, but also with very low HDL-C levels in targeted mice. In LPL-deficient mice rescued by crossbreeding with mice expressing LPL in cardiac muscle alone, plasma triglycerides and HDL-C levels were normalized in adult animals. However, although mice expressing LPL only in skeletal muscle have normal triglycerides, they have reduced HDL-C levels compared with wild-type mice.

Lipidation of Apolipoprotein A-I

Lipid-poor apoA-I and nascent HDL particles must acquire lipid to generate mature HDL particles (2). Phospholipids and unesterified cholesterol are acquired by apoA-I from cells as a key step in the formation of HDL. The molecular mechanisms by which apoA-I and HDL mediate lipid efflux have been the subject of intensive investigation. A key observation was that efflux of cellular unesterified cholesterol and phospholipids occurred at a faster rate when apoA-I (or other HDL apolipoproteins) were present in the extracellular environment and that cells from patients with Tangier disease were defective in effluxing cholesterol and phospholipids to apoA-I (3). A major advance in our understanding of the molecular regulation of this process was the discovery in 1999 that the molecular etiology of Tangier disease is genetic deficiency in adenosine triphosphate-binding cassette protein A1 (ABCA1) (4–6). Thus, ABCA1 was established as a major cellular protein that facilitates efflux of cellular phospholipids and cholesterol to lipid-poor apoA-I. The ABCA1 knockout mouse also has markedly reduced HDL-C and apoA-I levels and evidence of cellular lipid accumulation. However, the relation of ABCA1 expression to reverse cholesterol transport (RCT) and atherogenesis remains uncertain (discussed later).

The regulation of ABCA1 expression and activity has become an important area of investigation. ABCA1 is regulated both at the transcriptional and posttranscriptional levels. The transcriptional regulation of ABCA1 is mediated in large part by the nuclear receptor heterodime LXR/RXR (7). LXR is a receptor for oxysterols and when ligated promotes the transcription of ABCA1, thus serving a homeostatic mechanism to protect the cell from cholesterol toxicity. LXR is transcriptionally regulated by peroxisome proliferator-activated receptor (PPAR)-α and PPAR-γ (8).

ABCA1 activity also is regulated at the posttranslational level. The cellular turnover of the ABCA1 protein is rapid. ABCA1 contains a sequence that enhances the degradation of ABCA1 by calpain protease, thereby regulating the cholesterol efflux activity of ABCA1 (9). ApoA-I stabilizes calpain-mediated ABCA1 turnover. Infusion of apoA-I/phospholipid complexes was shown to increase ABCA1 protein, but not messenger RNA, *in vivo*. Therefore, apoA-I not only promotes ABCA1-mediated cholesterol efflux, but stabilizes the ABCA1 protein, thus magnifying its effects.

Scavenger receptor B-I (SR-BI) also can promote net cholesterol efflux from cells (10). In contrast to ABCA1-mediated cholesterol efflux, the optimal acceptors for SR-BI–mediated cholesterol efflux are larger phospholipid-rich HDL particles (2). The importance of SR-BI–mediated cholesterol efflux to the regulation of HDL metabolism and RCT remains to be determined.

Cholesterol Esterification and Maturation of the High-Density Lipoprotein Particle

LCAT transfers a fatty acid from phosphatidylcholine to unesterified cholesterol, thus resulting in the generation of cholesteryl ester (CE). This is thought to provide a driving force for the net movement of unesterified cholesterol from cells into HDL. ApoA-I can activate LCAT, probably by organizing the lipid substrates for optimal presentation to LCAT. Some regions of apoA-I, possibly because of secondary structural features, appear to be more important than other regions. The CE generated by LCAT forms a neutral lipid core required for the generation of mature spherical HDL. Thus, LCAT activity results in the conversion of nascent discoidal HDL particles to HDL_3, and further from smaller HDL_3 to larger HDL_2.

The importance of LCAT in HDL metabolism is clarified by human and animal studies. LCAT deficiency in humans is associated with markedly reduced HDL-C and apoA-I levels (11). LCAT knockout mice also have markedly reduced levels of HDL-C and apoA-I. Conversely, overexpression of LCAT in mice and rabbits causes increased HDL-C and apoA-I levels. The relation of LCAT activity to atherothrombosis is complex (discussed later).

Lipid Transfer Between High-Density Lipoprotein and Apolipoprotein B–containing Lipoproteins

Plasma lipid transfer proteins play an important part in the transfer of phospholipids and neutral lipids between HDLs and other plasma lipoproteins. In humans, much of the CE formed within HDL is transferred into larger triglyceride-rich lipoproteins as a result of cholesteryl ester transfer protein (CETP) activity. CETP mediates transfer of CE from HDL to apoB-containing lipoproteins in exchange for triglycerides, resulting in CE depletion and triglyceride enrichment of HDL. Genetic deficiency of CETP is associated with markedly increased HDL-C levels (12). Increased transfer of CE from HDL to apoB-containing lipoproteins through CETP is probably a major factor in the low HDL-C levels associated with hypertriglyceridemia and type 2 diabetes. Mice naturally lack CETP, and transgenic expression of CETP in mice results in reduction of plasma HDL-C levels. The relation of CETP activity to atherothrombosis is still being debated (discussed later).

The net movement of phospholipids between HDL and other lipoproteins is facilitated by the phospholipid transfer protein (PLTP) (13). PLTP is a member of the same gene family as CETP. Phospholipid exchange is important in replenishing HDL with unsaturated phospholipids which, among other functions, are optimal for the LCAT reaction. Deficiency of PLTP in knockout mice markedly reduced HDL-C levels; levels of apoB-containing lipoproteins and atherothrombosis also were markedly reduced. Transgenic overexpression of PLTP in the liver of human apoA-I transgenic mice was associated with modestly increased HDL-C and apoA-I levels and reduced atherothrombosis.

Lipid Uptake from High-Density Lipoprotein to Cells

Although much HDL CE is transferred to apoB-containing lipoproteins by CETP, there also is a net transfer of cholesterol from tissues to liver directly through HDL, both as CE and as unesterified cholesterol (14). SR-BI mediates selective uptake of HDL CE and unesterified cholesterol by the liver and, therefore, may be important in the regulation of RCT (15). Animal studies have helped to clarify the role of SR-BI in HDL metabolism. SR-BI knockout mice have increased HDL-C levels. Hepatic overexpression of SR-BI in mice results in markedly reduced HDL-C levels. The relation of SR-BI with atherothrombosis is complex (discussed later).

Remodeling of High-Density Lipoproteins by Lipases

Remodeling of HDLs is a critical process that regulates HDL size and density heterogeneity (16). Lipid transfer through CETP and PLTP plays an important role in HDL remodeling. In addition, lipases play a key role in HDL remodeling. Hepatic lipase (HL) is one factor that plays a role in the conversion of the larger HDL_2 particles to the smaller HDL_3 particles through hydrolysis of HDL triglyceride and possibly phospholipids. HL is a member of the same triglyceride lipase gene family as LPL and is found primarily on the endothelial cells of the liver sinusoids. Overexpression of HL in rabbits and mice results in decreased levels of HDL-C and smaller HDL particles. Female HL-deficient mice have modestly increased HDL-C levels. Overexpression of HL reduced atherothrombosis in cholesterol-fed mice; HL deficiency also reduced atherothrombosis in apoE-deficient mice. In humans, high plasma HL activity is associated with reduced HDL-C levels and smaller HDL particles. Both increased (17) and decreased (18) postheparin plasma HL activity levels have been reported in humans with CHD compared with control subjects. Genetic deficiency in HL is associated with modestly increased HDL-C levels and larger HDL particles, but paradoxically it may be associated with increased risk for atherosclerotic vascular disease, possibly because of greater levels of atherogenic lipoproteins (19). Lower levels of HL activity and increased levels of HDL_2 are found in association with

a common single nucleotide polymorphism in the HL promoter (20).

Endothelial lipase (EL) is a member of the same triglyceride lipase gene family as LPL and HL (21). It was cloned independently by two different groups (22,23). EL has triglyceride lipase activity, but relative to LPL and HL has substantially greater phospholipase activity, putting it at the other end of the lipolytic spectrum from LPL. EL is more effective at hydrolyzing lipids in HDL than LPL or HL. Overexpression of human EL in the livers of mice with a recombinant adenoviral vector caused markedly reduced plasma concentrations of HDL-C and apoA-I (22). Overexpression of human EL in mice under the control of its own promoter modestly reduced HDL-C levels (24). Inhibition of EL in mice with antibodies resulted in significantly increased HDL-C and apoA-I levels (25). EL knockout mice have increased levels of HDL-C (24,26). Although EL-deficient humans have not yet been described, some variants in EL may be more common in individuals with increased HDL-C levels (27), and one common polymorphism was shown to be associated with variation in HDL-C levels (26). Therefore, like HL, EL may play a role in converting larger HDL to smaller HDL particles. The effects of EL on atherothrombosis are unknown.

High-Density Lipoprotein Apolipoprotein Catabolism

Studies in animals have indicated that apoA-I is catabolized in both the liver and kidneys (28). Renal catabolism appears to be regulated by the availability of lipid-poor apoA-I, which is filtered by the glomerulus and then catabolized by proximal tubular cells. The molecular mechanism of tubular cell catabolism appears to be binding to cubulin and internalization by megalin/gp330, with subsequent targeting to the lysosome. However, the regulation of this process is glomerular filtration of lipid-poor apoA-I rather than level of expression of cubulin and megalin/gp330 on the apical surface of the tubular cells. Therefore, factors that regulate the concentration of lipid-poor apoA-I, such as HDL remodeling, play an important role in determining the rate of renal catabolism of apoA-I.

The molecular mechanism of the hepatic uptake of apoA-I has been something of a mystery. SR-BI may have the ability to mediate HDL holoparticle uptake and to direct catabolism of some apoA-I, but is unlikely to be the sole mechanism. There have been other cell-surface HDL binding proteins described in hepatocytes (29). A high-affinity receptor for apoA-I recently was shown to be the β-chain of adenosine triphosphate synthase, a principal protein complex of the mitochondrial inner membrane (30). Receptor stimulation of an ectopic plasma membrane localized adenosine triphosphate synthase complex by apoA-I triggers the holoparticle endocytosis of HDL by a mechanism that depends on the generation of adenosine diphosphate. This phenomenon was shown in hepatocytes *in vitro* and perfused rat liver *ex vivo,* but whether this is an important mechanism of hepatic catabolism of apoA-I *in vivo* remains to be determined.

APOLIPOPROTEIN A-I AND ATHEROTHROMBOSIS IN ANIMALS

Although it is still not entirely clear whether the association of HDL-C levels with ASCVD in humans is causal in nature, a wealth of evidence in animals indicates that HDLs and apoA-I are directly antiatherogenic (31). Repeated intravenous injection of human HDLs into cholesterol-fed rabbits resulted in regression of atherosclerotic lesions, and repeated intravenous injection of rabbit apoA-I into cholesterol-fed rabbits resulted in reduced progression of atherosclerotic lesions. Hepatic overexpression of human apoA-I in transgenic mice reduced progression of atherothrombosis in C57BL/6 mice fed a high-fat, high-cholesterol diet, in apoE-deficient mice, and in apolipoprotein (a) transgenic mice. Somatic gene transfer and hepatic expression of human apoA-I induced significant regression of preexisting atherosclerotic lesions in low density lipoprotein receptor (LDLR)-deficient mice (32) and reduced the progression of atherothrombosis in apoE-deficient mice. Transgenic overexpression of human apoA-I in the livers of cholesterol-fed rabbits reduced the development of aortic atherothrombosis (33). Expression of apoA-I in macrophages also was demonstrated to reduce atherothrombosis progression.

Studies of apoA-I deficiency and atherothrombosis in animals have been relatively limited (31). ApoA-I–deficient mice have reduced levels of HDL-C, but when fed a chow diet or even when fed an atherogenic diet, atherothrombosis does not spontaneously develop. ApoA-I–deficient mice crossed with human apoB transgenic mice had a moderate increase in atherothrombosis when fed a cholate-containing atherogenic diet or a western-type diet.

HIGH-DENSITY LIPOPROTEIN FUNCTION AND MECHANISMS OF ANTIATHEROGENESIS

Reverse Cholesterol Transport

ApoA-I and HDLs are thought to protect against atherothrombosis at least in part by promoting efflux of excess cholesterol from macrophages in the arterial wall and returning that cholesterol to the liver for excretion into the bile, a process known as "reverse cholesterol transport" (RCT) (Fig. 7–1). There have been various efforts to determine the effects of modulating apoA-I levels on the rate of RCT *in vivo,* concluding that differences in plasma apoA-I levels had no effect on total peripheral RCT (31). However, none of the methods involved measuring RCT specifically from the macrophage, the most important cholesterol-accumulating cell in atherothrombosis. A recent method involves the loading of macrophages *ex vivo* with labeled cholesterol and then injecting them intraperitoneally in mice

and quantitating the rate of excretion of tracer in the feces. Using this approach, mice overexpressing apoA-I had a significantly greater rate of excretion of labeled cholesterol, establishing that apoA-I overexpression promotes macrophage RCT (34). In addition, four patients with heterozygous familial hypercholesterolemia were injected with a bolus of apoA-I/PC liposomes, and fecal sterol excretion was monitored 9 days before and 9 days after the injection; the fecal excretion of neutral sterols was increased by 39% and of bile acids by 30%, suggesting promotion of RCT (35).

Another approach to addressing the important question of the relation between RCT and atherothrombosis involves gain and loss of function of genes involved in specific steps of the RCT. The ABCA1 knockout mouse has markedly reduced HDL-C levels and evidence of macrophage lipid accumulation. However, when ABCA1 knockout mice were reconstituted with wild-type bone marrow (and thus macrophages), HDL-C and apoA-I levels were only slightly increased; conversely, transplantation of ABCA1-deficient marrow into wild-type mice did not affect HDL-C and apoA-I levels (36). Therefore, although macrophages are the cell type most affected by ABCA1 deficiency with regard to cholesterol accumulation, macrophages themselves contribute little to the bulk lipidation of plasma apoA-I and, therefore, to plasma HDL-C levels. Hepatic overexpression of ABCA1 increased HDL-C levels in mice (37), suggesting that the liver may be a contributor to lipidation of lipid-poor apoA-I through ABCA1. Fecal sterol excretion and biliary cholesterol and bile acid secretion rates in the steady-state condition concluded that there were no differences in rates of RCT from the periphery in ABCA1 knockout mice (38). ABCA1 deficiency was not associated with increased atherothrombosis in LDLR-deficient or apoE-deficient mice (39). However, selective deficiency of ABCA1 in macrophages was found to significantly increase atherothrombosis in apoE-deficient (40) and LDLR-deficient (39) mice. Mice overexpressing ABCA1 in liver and macrophages had reduced atherothrombosis when fed a high-fat cholate diet, but increased atherothrombosis on the background of apoE deficiency and LDLR deficiency (41). Therefore, the relation between ABCA1 expression, RCT, and atherothrombosis remains unclear.

LCAT is thought to play an important role in RCT (42). Overexpression of human LCAT in cholesterol-fed rabbits was associated with increased HDL-C levels and markedly reduced atherothrombosis (43), but this effect required the presence of functional LDL receptors. By contrast, transgenic overexpression of human LCAT in mice either resulted in increased atherothrombosis or afforded no evidence of protection from it. When human LCAT was overexpressed in mice that were also transgenic for human CETP expression, atherothrombosis was significantly reduced (44), suggesting that the antiatherogenic effect of LCAT requires the presence of CETP. The impact of LCAT deficiency on atherothrombosis in mice is uncertain. In one report, aortic atherothrombosis was significantly reduced in three different mouse models with LCAT deficiency. However, in another report, LCAT deficiency was associated with increased atherothrombosis in LDLR knockout and apoE knockout mice. Therefore, the relation between LCAT deficiency and atherothrombosis remains uncertain.

SR-BI initiates a process of selective uptake of cholesterol from HDL into the liver and is thought to play a key role in RCT (15). Transgenic mice overexpressing SR-BI in the liver had reduced HDL-C levels and reduced atherothrombosis, but also had markedly reduced plasma levels of atherogenic apoB-containing lipoproteins. Hepatic overexpression of SR-BI using gene transfer in LDLR-deficient mice significantly reduced HDL-C levels and atherothrombosis but did not reduce plasma levels of apoB-containing lipoproteins (45). Genetic deficiency of SR-BI increased atherothrombosis in apoE-deficient mice despite greater HDL-C levels and is associated with markedly premature death caused by apparent myocardial infarctions (MIs) (46). It is believed, although unproven, that SR-BI deficiency is associated with reduced RCT. It is unknown whether deficiency in macrophage SR-BI, hepatic SR-BI, or both contribute to the increased atherothrombosis.

Transfer of CE from HDL to apoB-containing lipoproteins in exchange for triglycerides through CETP is one potential pathway of RCT (47). Some reports suggest that expression of CETP in mice resulted in increased atherothrombosis. Conversely, another study showed that expression of CETP reduced atherothrombosis in mice with hypertriglyceridemia, suggesting that the effect of CETP expression on atherothrombosis may depend on other aspects of lipoprotein metabolism. Studies of CETP inhibition in rabbits (which have high levels of CETP) have demonstrated significant reduction in atherothrombosis, using antisense approaches, small molecule inhibition, and an anti-CETP immunization strategy (47). The relation between CETP and atherothrombosis in humans is still in question.

Other Potential Mechanisms of Antiatherogenesis of High-Density Lipoprotein

HDL has a variety of other properties that have been demonstrated *in vitro* that, in theory, could contribute to its antiatherogenic effects. HDL is widely considered to have antioxidant properties. HDL was shown to protect LDL from copper-mediated oxidation *ex vivo*. LDL from mice genetically susceptible to fatty streak lesion formation was highly susceptible to oxidation by artery wall cells and was rendered resistant to oxidation after incubation with apoA-I *in vitro*. Treatment of human endothelial cells with HDL or apoA-I rendered the cells unable to oxidize LDL. A single intravenous injection of a large dose of human HDL$_3$ to rabbits with induced hypercholesterolemia led to a decrease in conjugated dienes and trienes by 20% to 30%. Injection of

apoA-I into mice and humans rendered their LDL resistant to oxidation (48).

HDL also is believed to have direct antiinflammatory properties. Pretreatment of endothelial cells with HDL reduced the cytokine-induced up-regulation of adhesion molecules such as intracellular adhesion molecule-1, vascular cell adhesion molecule-1 (VCAM-1), and E-selectin (49). HDL inhibited tumor necrosis factor-alpha (TNF-α)–stimulated sphingosine kinase activity in endothelial cells, resulting in a decrease in sphingosine 1-phosphate production and nuclear factor-κB signaling cascades (50). *In vivo*, reconstituted HDL-containing human apoA-I reduced VCAM-1 expression after carotid injury in apoE-deficient mice. In a porcine model of vascular inflammation, bolus injection of reconstituted discoidal HDL inhibited basal and interleukin (IL)-1α–induced E-selectin expression by porcine microvascular endothelial cells *in vivo* (51). However, not all studies have been consistent with an antiinflammatory effect of HDLs *in vivo*. In an apoA-I transgenic mouse model there were no differences in endothelial VCAM-1 expression in apoA-I transgenic compared with wild-type mice (52). Few data exist that address the relation between HDL and *in vivo* markers of inflammation in humans.

HDL has been shown to have a variety of other properties. HDL stimulated the release of prostacyclin from endothelial cells and prostaglandin E$_2$ from smooth muscle cells, in part by increasing cyclooxygenase-2 expression. In perfused isolated rat hearts, the administration of HDL during the 10 minutes immediately before ischemia improved postischemic functional recovery, caused a dose-dependent reduction of ischemia-induced cardiac TNF-α expression, and enhanced ischemia-induced prostaglandin release. In addition, HDL may also bind and stabilize prostacyclin. HDL has been shown to result in endothelial nitric oxide synthase (eNOS) activation and nitric oxide production (53). SR-BI was shown to be required for this effect, both *in vitro* and in using aortic rings *ex vivo*. HDL stimulates eNOS through Src-mediated signaling, leading to parallel activation of Akt and mitogen-activated protein kinases, which modulate eNOS activity. The ability of HDL to stimulate eNOS may be dependent on its estrogen content (54). HDL also has antiplatelet and anticoagulant effects (55).

REGULATION OF HIGH-DENSITY LIPOPROTEIN METABOLISM IN HUMANS

Levels of HDL-C and apoA-I in humans are influenced both by rates of biosynthesis and rates of catabolism (56). An example of a factor that influences the rate of apoA-I production is a low saturated fat diet, which causes decreases in HDL-C and apo A-I levels as a result of decreased synthesis of apo A-I without any changes in fractional catabolism (57). Variations in HDL-C and apoA-I levels are more generally correlated with differences in the fractional catabolic rate (FCR) of apoA-I and not with variations in its production rate. The catabolic half-lives of apoA-I and apoA-II in healthy humans is about 4 to 5 days and the FCR of apoA-I is slightly faster than that of apo A-II. This may reflect the more rapid catabolism of LpA-I compared with LpA-I/A-II (58). Metabolic turnover studies on a large number of subjects with a wide range of HDL-C values confirmed a strong inverse correlation between HDL-C levels and the FCR of apoA-I; in contrast, there was little or no association between HDL-C levels and the transport rate of apoA-I (59,60).

Thus, a variety of observations indicate that factors influencing the catabolism of apoA-I are important in the modulation of HDL levels in humans. Factors that decrease the size of HDLs appear to promote the dissociation of apoA-I from HDL, leading to their catabolism (60). Reduced HDL-C and apoA-I levels are commonly associated with hypertriglyceridemia in humans. Hypertriglyceridemia from a variety of causes results in accelerated transfer of CE from HDL to triglyceride-rich lipoproteins. The more triglyceride-enriched the HDL particles, the more susceptible they are to reductions in size and apoprotein content as a result of HL action. Thus, it appears that processes regulating the rate of transfer of CE from HDL to other lipoproteins may play a critical role in determining the size of the HDL CE pool, the size of HDL particles, and the catabolic rates of apoA-I. Another important factor determining the size of the HDL core lipid pool may be the activity of HL. Studies have demonstrated that the apoA-I FCR is strongly correlated with HL activity (60).

Studies of HDL and apoA-I metabolism in humans with genetic disorders of HDL metabolism have provided important insights into the role of specific genes in modulating HDL and apoA-I metabolism. The catabolic rates of several apoA-I mutants such as apoA-I Milano (61) and apoA-I Iowa (62) have been investigated in humans and found to be substantially increased compared with wild-type apoA-I. This suggests that apoA-I mutants associated with low HDL-C and apoA-I levels have altered structures that lead to increased catabolism. The catabolism of apoA-I was demonstrated to be markedly increased in Tangier disease well before the genetic etiology of this disorder was known (63). These data establish firmly that ABCA1 activity is a major determinant of apoA-I catabolic rate and that failure to effectively lipidate apoA-I through ABCA1 results in markedly increased catabolism of lipid-poor apoA-I. HDL metabolic studies in LCAT-deficient humans demonstrated dramatically increased catabolic rates of apoA-I and especially apoA-II (64), demonstrating that effective esterification of cholesterol is essential for maintaining normal metabolism of apoA-I and apoA-II. Studies in humans with genetic CETP deficiency demonstrated that apoA-I (and apoA-II) catabolism were significantly delayed, providing direct evidence that CETP-mediated lipid exchange promotes the catabolism of HDL apolipoproteins (65). Studies in patients with primary hypoalphalipoproteinemia indicate that increased catabolism of apoA-I is a general feature of this syndrome (66,67).

ENVIRONMENTAL AND SECONDARY FACTORS INFLUENCING HIGH-DENSITY LIPOPROTEIN METABOLISM IN HUMANS

Smoking is associated with lower levels of HDL-C, but the mechanism is poorly understood. Vegetarians and others who habitually consume high-carbohydrate, low-fat diets with high P/S ratios tend to have low levels of HDL-C, at least in part because of reduced production of apoA-I. Low levels of HDL-C are commonly found in obese individuals. Increased triglyceride levels caused by any etiologic factor are frequently associated with low HDL-C levels. Possibly the most common form of low HDL-C in humans is that seen in association with the metabolic syndrome, which includes visceral obesity and insulin resistance; low HDL-C and apoA-I levels also are common in patients with type 2 diabetes, a disease associated with insulin resistance. Individuals who are insulin resistant exhibit a dyslipidemia characterized by increased triglyceride levels, low HDL-C and apoA-I levels, and an increase in small, dense, low-density lipoprotein cholesterol (LDL-C); this lipid profile is associated with increased risk for cardiovascular disease (68). Most individuals with low HDL-C have an environmental or secondary factor that at least contributes to the low HDL-C phenotype. Several drugs other than those specifically used for treatment of lipid disorders also affect HDL-C levels. Oral estrogens and diphenylhydantoin increase HDL-C levels, and androgens, some progestins, and β-blockers decrease HDL-C. Frequent aerobic exercise and physical activity in general are associated with greater levels of HDL-C, possibly related at least in part to increases in LPL activity. Alcohol intake is an important factor contributing to increased HDL-C. The mechanisms by which alcohol increases HDL levels may involve alterations in triglyceride metabolism and changes in lipase and CETP activity.

GENETIC INFLUENCES ON HIGH-DENSITY LIPOPROTEIN CHOLESTEROL LEVELS

Although environmental influences account for some of the variance of HDL-C levels, genetic factors also are important. For example, twin studies have indicated a high degree of heritability of HDL-C levels. The Lipid Research Clinics Program Family Study determined the genetic heritablility of HDL-C levels to be 0.48 (69). The National Heart, Lung and Blood Institute (NHLBI) Family Heart Study (FHS) observed a correlation of 0.32 for parent-child and 0.29 for sibling-sibling in HDL-C levels, and less than 10% of this was explained by measurable lifestyle habits (70). These studies are highly suggestive of major genetic influences on HDL-C levels.

An assessment of major genetic locus effects on HDL-C levels can be derived by complex segregation analysis. Several studies revealed no major gene for high HDL-C levels, whereas others found evidence for major genes with various modes of transmission. In the San Antonio Family Heart Study, evidence for a major locus with codominant inheritance influencing plasma HDL-C levels was reported (71). Using the same cohort, strong evidence of linkage of a quantitative trait locus for HDL-C levels was mapped to chromosome 9p in Mexican Americans (72). Segregation analysis of the NHLBI FHS showed no evidence for a major gene causing low HDL-C levels, but demonstrated evidence for a recessive allele that was associated with greater HDL-C levels (73). It remains to be determined whether there are a limited number of major gene loci with appreciable effects on HDL-C levels in humans or many loci, each with small effects on HDL-C levels. Relatively few of the genes that impact on variation in HDL-C levels in humans are currently known.

GENETIC CONDITIONS ASSOCIATED WITH LOW HIGH-DENSITY LIPOPROTEIN CHOLESTEROL LEVELS

Apolipoprotein A-I

ApoA-I is required for normal biosynthesis and metabolism of HDL. Complete deletion of the *apoA-I* gene in humans results in very low levels of HDL-C and premature CHD. A Japanese female homozygous for a codon 84 nonsense mutation (Gln:stop) had absent plasma apoA-I and HDL-C, premature CHD, and planar xanthomas. A large Canadian family with an *apoA-I* gene mutation resulting in complete deficiency of apoA-I was described. Two homozygous sisters had xanthomas and premature CHD, whereas other homozygous family members appeared to be healthy. Thus, complete deficiency of apoA-I is a strong predisposing factor to premature atherothrombosis. However, the rate of disease development is variable and may be modified by other factors such as increased LDL-C levels. For example, a homozygous nonsense mutation in codon 32 (Q32X) of the *apoA-I* gene was found to cause apoA-I deficiency in a 31-year-old woman who did not present with clinical signs of atherothrombosis, and a Turkish girl with apoA-I deficiency caused by frameshift mutation resulting in a premature termination codon had planar xanthomas and corneal clouding but no evidence of CHD, presumably because of her young age.

Missense mutations in apoA-I are sometimes associated with low HDL-C levels. The first of these to be described was apoA-I Milano, which is a substitution of cysteine for arginine at position 173. Heterozygotes for this mutation have an average 40% decrease in apoA-I and a 67% decrease in HDL-C. Turnover of the mutant apoA-I Milano protein and of the wild-type apoA-I in the heterozygotes is markely increased (61). Despite the low levels of HDL-C, this mutation is not associated with increased atherothrombosis. A frameshift mutation in apoA-I with introduction of cysteines and premature termination at codon 230 has been described associated with massive corneal opacifications, complete absence of HDL, and half-normal LCAT activity, but no overt coronary artery disease. An in-frame deletion in apoA-I was described with apparent dominant effect causing low HDL-C. Several missense mutations in apoA-I result in familial amyloidosis associated with deposition of amino-terminal fragments of apoA-I in amyloid fibrils in various tissues (74). One of these, apoA-I Iowa, was shown to have markedly increased catabolism in heterozygotes for the mutation (62).

Commonly observed genetic variations in the promoter sequence of the human *apoA-I* gene may be associated with differences in apoA-I production rate (75). In general, genetic variation in the *apoA-I* gene is probably not a common source of variation in HDL-C levels.

Adenosine Triphosphate-Binding Cassette Protein A1

Tangier disease is a rare disorder characterized by cholesterol accumulation in the reticuloendothelial system and markedly reduced HDL-C levels (76). It is caused by genetic deficiency of ABCA1 (4–6). Fibroblasts from patients with Tangier disease have markedly reduced cholesterol and phospholipid efflux to apolipoproteins that is corrected by expression of ABCA1. ABCA1 plays a critical role in the generation and stabilization of the mature HDL particle, and when genetically absent, HDL and apoA-I are rapidly cleared from the circulation. Patients with Tangier disease have plasma HDL-C levels less than 5 mg/dL and extremely low levels of apoA-I. The disease is associated with cholesterol accumulation in the reticuloendothelial system resulting in hepatosplenomegaly and pathognomonic enlarged, grayish yellow or orange tonsils.

Heterozygotes for *ABCA1* mutations have moderately reduced HDL-C levels, suggesting a gene dosage effect of ABCA1 expression on rates of cellular cholesterol efflux. Mutations in *ABCA1* are one cause of primary hypoalphalipoproteinemia (low HDL-C levels) in some families (5,77). Patients with Tangier disease and even obligate heterozygotes are at some increased risk for premature CHD (78,79). Patients with Tangier disease, but not obligate heterozygotes, have low plasma levels of LDL-C, which may attenuate the atherosclerotic risk (76).

Some data suggest that common variation in the *ABCA1* gene may account for variation in HDL-C levels and possibly premature CHD in the general population (80,81). However, this issue has yet to be definitively established.

Lecithin-Cholesterol Acyltransferase Deficiency

LCAT deficiency in humans is associated with markedly reduced HDL-C and apoA-I levels (11). The HDL-C levels are less than 10 mg/dL and apo A-I levels are less than 30% of normal. The HDL consists primarily of disk-shaped particles resembling nascent HDLs. LCAT mediates the esterification of cholesterol, therefore in this disorder the proportion of free cholesterol in circulating lipoproteins is greatly increased (from ~25% to more than 70% of total plasma cholesterol). Lack of normal cholesterol esterification leads to inability to form mature HDL particles and, therefore, to rapid catabolism of circulating apoA-I. HDL apolipoprotein metabolic studies in LCAT-deficient humans demonstrated dramatically increased catabolic rates of apoA-I and especially apoA-II (64). Two genetic forms of LCAT deficiency have been described in humans: complete deficiency (also called classic LCAT deficiency) and partial deficiency (also called fish eye disease). Progressive corneal opacification caused by the deposition of free cholesterol in the lens, very low plasma levels of HDL-C (usually <10 mg/dL), and variable hypertriglyceridemia are characteristic of both types. Complete LCAT deficiency is characterized by a hemolytic anemia and progressive renal insufficiency that eventually leads to end stage renal disease. Despite the extremely low plasma levels of HDL-C and apoA-I, premature coronary disease is not generally a common feature of LCAT deficiency, although some patients have been described with premature CHD. Therefore, although LCAT clearly has important effects on HDL metabolism, its relation to atherothrombosis remains unclear.

The role that genetic variation in LCAT plays in influencing HDL-C levels in the general population is uncertain. Some studies in humans have shown a positive correlation between HDL-C levels and LCAT activity or LCAT mass, but common polymorphisms in LCAT do not appear to have a major association with variation in HDL-C.

Lipoprotein Lipase Deficiency

After lipolysis of triglyceride-rich lipoproteins by LPL, surface phospholipids and apolipoproteins from these lipoproteins dissociate and are acquired by HDLs. In humans, deficiency of LPL is associated with severe hypertriglyceridemia and very low HDL-C levels. Even heterozygosity for LPL deficiency in humans is associated with reduced HDL-C levels. Postheparin plasma LPL activity is directly correlated with plasma HDL-C levels (82). Interestingly, the relatively common LPL variant Ser447Stop is associated with increased LPL activity and increased HDL-C levels.

Primary Hypoalphalipoproteinemia

Primary hypoalphalipoproteinemia is defined as a condition associated with a plasma HDL-C level less than the 10th percentile in the setting of relatively normal cholesterol and triglyceride levels—that is, no apparent secondary or primary monogenic causes of low plasma HDL-C. It is the most common inherited cause of low plasma levels of HDL-C and often follows an autosomal-dominant pattern of inheritance. The metabolic etiology of this disease appears to be

primarily accelerated catabolism of apoA-I. Increased incidence of premature CHD has been reported in association with this condition.

GENETIC CONDITIONS ASSOCIATED WITH HIGH HIGH-DENSITY LIPOPROTEIN CHOLESTEROL LEVELS

Cholesteryl Ester Transfer Protein Deficiency

Genetic deficiency of CETP is associated with markedly increased HDL-C levels (12). CETP deficiency is primarily found in Japan. Four different CETP gene mutations have been described in Japanese subjects. Two of the mutations result in gene-splicing defects at the intron 14 splice donor (83)—one produces a missense change in the coding sequence (aspartate 442:glycine), and the other produces a nonsense mutation at codon 309. All forms of genetic CETP deficiency cause increases in plasma HDL-C and apo A-I levels. The degree of increase of HDL-C is inversely related to the residual CETP activity in plasma. Homozygotes for the intron 14 splicing defect have absent plasma CETP activity and HDL-C levels of 120 to 200 mg/dL, and heterozygotes have modestly increased HDL-C levels. In contrast, heterozygotes for the missense D442G mutation have substantially increased HDL-C, whereas homozygotes have residual plasma CETP activity and HDL-C levels similar or only slightly greater than heterozygotes, suggesting a dominant inhibitory effect of this mutation.

The relation of CETP deficiency with atherothrombosis is unclear (47). One report suggests that homozygous CETP deficiency was protective against CHD, although another suggests it may be associated with increased atherosclerotic disease. Heterozygous CETP deficiency, which is associated with modestly increased HDL-C levels, was shown in one large epidemiologic study to be associated with an increased risk for CHD for those individuals with HDL-C levels in the range of 40 to 60 mg/dL (84).

Two different mutations of the *CETP* gene are sufficiently common to influence the distribution of HDL-C values in the general Japanese population (83). These mutations are present in about 6% of the Japanese population and account for about 10% of the variance of HDL-C values. The intronic Taq1B polymorphism in the *CETP* gene is common outside Japan and is associated with variation in HDL-C levels and CHD risk (85).

Hepatic Lipase Deficiency

Genetic HL deficiency in humans is rare and is associated with modestly increased HDL-C levels and larger HDL particles (19). The phenotype indicates a role of HL in the hydrolysis of HDL triglycerides and phospholipids, resulting in conversion of HDL_2 into HDL_3. Humans who are HL-deficient have been reported to be at increased risk for atherosclerotic vascular disease, but they also have increased levels of atherogenic lipoproteins that may contribute to the risk. Humans with CHD have been reported to have increased or decreased postheparin plasma HL activity levels compared with control subjects in cross-sectional studies. There might be an optimal level of HL activity with regard to atherothrombosis: Whereas low HL could impair remnant clearance and increase cardiovascular risk, increased HL reduces HDL-C levels and increases risk.

A common single nucleotide polymorphism in the HL promoter has been associated with lower levels of HL activity and increased levels of HDL-C, especially HDL$_2$ (20). The relation of this single nucleotide polymorphism with coronary artery disease is unclear.

Familial Hyperalphalipoproteinemia

Familial hyperalphalipoproteinemia is defined as an HDL-C level greater than 90th percentile for age and sex, no secondary or monogenic causes of high HDL-C, and familial evidence of high HDL-C. In general, HDL-C levels are usually greater than 80 mg/dL in women and greater than 70 mg/dL in men. This condition may be associated with decreased risk for CHD and increased longevity. Other than CETP deficiency, the molecular causes of familial hyperalphalipoproteinemia are unknown.

HIGH-DENSITY LIPOPROTEIN AND ATHEROTHROMBOSIS IN HUMANS

Observational Studies

Although several earlier studies suggest a protective effect of HDL in coronary artery disease, the first major population-based, case–control study to document this effect was the Honolulu Heart Program study, which was based on a cohort of about 1,500 men of Japanese ancestry living in Hawaii. Subsequently, numerous prospective epidemiologic investigations in North America and elsewhere have shown a significant and independent inverse relation between HDL-C levels and the incidence of coronary artery disease (1). The change in risk associated with increasing levels of HDL-C can be estimated. A standardized analysis of the incidence of fatal and nonfatal MI in four large U.S. studies showed a decrease of about 2% to 3% in coronary risk for each 1% increase in HDL-C levels (1). Apo A-I levels are highly correlated with HDL-C levels and predict risk equally well.

The association of alcohol intake, HDL-C levels, and CHD risk deserves particular mention. Moderate alcohol intake is associated with a protective effect against coronary artery disease, possibly mediated in part by alcohol-induced increases in HDL-C levels (86). Approximately 50% of the reduction in risk attributable to alcohol consumption is explained by the changes in HDL-C levels. Although the effects of moderate alcohol may be beneficial, heavy alcohol intake increases overall morbidity and mortality from cardiovascular diseases (86) caused by dilated cardiomyopathy, dysrhythmias, and hypertensive heart disease.

Interventional Studies

Lifestyle interventions that are known to increase HDL-C levels, such as smoking cessation, regular aerobic exercise, weight control, and control of diabetes, are associated with reduced cardiovascular risk. However, there are multiple effects of these lifestyle interventions and the specific contribution of the increased HDL-C to reduced cardiovascular risk is unknown. Clinical trials of the effect of drug therapy targeted toward low HDL-C on clinical cardiovascular events are very limited, reflecting in part the paucity of interventions that substantially increase HDL-C levels. Statins are primarily LDL-decreasing drugs that significantly reduce cardiovascular risk. They also increase HDL-C by about 5% to 10%, which could potentially contribute to their benefit. Several of the large statin outcome trials performed subgroup analyses on the basis of baseline HDL-C levels. The AFCAPS/TexCAPS trial was a trial in healthy subjects with a mean LDL-C level of 150 mg/dL who were selected for relatively low HDL-C levels (87). Treatment with lovastatin significantly reduced major coronary events by 36%, and the relative risk reduction was greatest in the group with the lowest tertile of baseline HDL-C levels. In the Heart Protection Study, high-risk patients were randomized to 40 mg simvastatin versus placebo regardless of baseline cholesterol levels (88). Simvastatin treatment was associated with a significant reduction in major coronary events, including those subjects with low HDL-C levels at baseline. Thus, statin therapy in patients with low HDL-C is an effective method of reducing cardiovascular risk.

Fibric acid derivatives, or fibrates, are agonists of PPAR-α, a nuclear hormone receptor involved in energy and lipid metabolism (89). They decrease triglyceride levels and increase HDL-C levels modestly (5–15%). Fibrates are more effective in increasing HDL-C when triglycerides are elevated. Fibrates have multiple mechanisms by which they influence HDL-C. Part of the ability of fibrates to increase HDL-C is related to the reduction of tryglyceride levels, which occurs as the result of up-regulation of LPL and down-regulation of apoC-III. Through activation of PPAR-α, fibrates also increase HDL-C through induction of hepatic apoA-I and apoA-II expression. There is *in vitro* evidence to suggest that fibrates, through PPAR-α, up-regulate the nuclear receptor liver X receptor (LXR), and thus up-regulate the ABCA1 transporter and promote cholesterol efflux.

There have been several large outcome trials with fibrates. The Helsinki Heart Study in healthy men with increased non–HDL-C greater than 200 mg/dL demonstrated a significant 34% reduction in combined fatal and nonfatal MI associated with gemfibrozil therapy, and at least part of the benefit was attributed to the modest increase in HDL-C (90). The Veterans Affairs High-Density

Lipoprotein Cholesterol Intervention Trial (VA-HIT) tested the benefit of gemfibrozil therapy targeted specifically to patients with low HDL-C and low LDL-C levels (91). A total of 2,531 men with CHD, low HDL-C (mean, 32 mg/dL), low LDL-C (mean, 112 mg/dL), and triglycerides less than 300 mg/dL were randomized to treatment with gemfibrozil 1,200 mg daily or placebo and were then followed for an average of 5.1 years. Gemfibrozil therapy was associated with a significant 22% reduction in the primary end point (nonfatal MI and coronary death) compared with placebo. Compared with placebo, gemfibrozil resulted in a 6% increase in HDL-C, 31% decrease in triglycerides, and no change in LDL-C levels. An analysis suggested that the benefit may have been associated more with the modest increase in HDL-C than with the reduction in triglycerides. In contrast, the Bezafibrate Infarction Prevention (BIP) trial tested the effect of another fibrate, bezafibrate, in 3,090 patients with CHD, low HDL-C, and moderately increased LDL-C (mean 150 mg/dL) and found no significant reduction in major coronary events in the bezafibrate group compared with placebo (92). However, a subgroup analysis indicated that those individuals with increased triglyceride levels at baseline did have a significant benefit from bezafibrate therapy.

Nicotinic acid, or niacin, is the most effective method of increasing HDL-C and can result in up to 30% increases in HDL-C (93). The mechanisms by which niacin increases HDL-C remain somewhat unclear. Niacin reduces triglycerides and apoB-containing lipoproteins, and this has a secondary effect of increasing HDL-C. In addition, metabolic studies in humans indicate that niacin also reduces apoA-I catabolism. There also is *in vitro* evidence that niacin selectively decreases uptake of HDL apoA-I by hepatocytes. There are limited clinical outcome data with niacin. The Coronary Drug Project reported that immediate-release niacin decreased the risk for coronary events (CHD death or nonfatal MI) by 15% and nonfatal MI by 26% compared with placebo and was associated with reduced mortality at 15 years of follow-up (94). Several other clinical trials have found niacin to be effective alone or in combination with other drugs in preventing coronary events, slowing atherosclerotic disease progression, and promoting lesion regression (95).

Thiazolidinediones (also known as glitazones) are PPAR-α agonists and insulin-sensitizing medications that improve glycemic control in patients with type 2 diabetes. They have been noted to increase HDL-C from 7% to 13%. Studies reporting the HDL-C effects of glitazones were designed to investigate effects on glycemic control and included only one or several low doses, compared with placebo. There are few published data reporting the effects of the glitazones in the nondiabetic population. The mechanisms of glitazone-mediated increases in HDL-C are uncertain, but may be involved in improving insulin resistance. Another possible mechanism of the HDL-C–increasing effects of glitazones is through promotion of cholesterol efflux by up-regulation of LXR and ABCA1.

Estrogen can increase HDL-C by 5% to 15%. Effects of estrogen on HDL-C may be mediated in part by inhibition of HL and in part by promotion of hepatic apoA-I production. In the Heart and Estrogen/Progestin Replacement Study (HERS), postmenopausal women who had coronary disease were randomized to placebo or conjugated equine estrogen 0.625 mg plus medroxyprogesterone acetate 2.5 mg. No benefit of treatment in reducing CHD events was observed over approximately 4 years, with a pattern of early increased risk with estrogen/progestin treatment being observed. In the Women's Health Initiative trial, 16,608 healthy postmenopausal women with an intact uterus were randomized to either estrogen/progestin or placebo. The trial was stopped at a mean of 5.2 years because increases in the rates of CHD, stroke, pulmonary embolism, and invasive breast cancer outweighed the reductions in the rates of colorectal cancers and hip fractures associated with estrogen/progestin therapy. Therefore, the current consensus is that combined estrogen/progestin therapy, although it increases HDL-C, should not be used for prevention of CHD in postmenopausal women.

MANAGEMENT OF PATIENTS WITH LOW HIGH-DENSITY LIPOPROTEIN CHOLESTEROL

The NCEP Adult Treatment Panel III (ATP III) guidelines (96) recommended that all adults be screened with a full fasting lipid profile including triglycerides, total cholesterol, LDL-C, and HDL-C levels. The ATP III guidelines also increased the threshold for low HDL-C from 35 to 40 mg/dL (96). Furthermore, the ATP III guidelines included low HDL-C as a criterion for diagnosis of the metabolic syndrome, recommending that an HDL-C level of less than 40 mg/dL in men and less than 50 mg/dL in women be considered one marker of the metabolic syndrome (96).

Although there are no formal guidelines for the management of patients with low levels of HDL-C, several reasonable recommendations can be made. The first step in the management of patients with low HDL-C is counseling on therapeutic lifestyle changes. Patients who smoke should be encouraged to quit, which is usually associated with an increase in HDL-C. Regular aerobic exercise can help increase HDL-C levels, but its effects are modest unless accompanied by weight loss (97). Dietary recommendations need to be individually tailored, but in general patients should be advised to reduce caloric intake (if overweight), limit total fat intake to 30% of total calories, replace saturated fat with monounsaturates rather than polyunsaturates, and limit intake of simple carbohydrates. Alcohol use is clearly associated with increased HDL-C levels in a dose-dependent fashion and with reduced cardiovascular risk, but is not recommended as a therapeutic strategy for increasing HDL-C levels or reducing risk. Hormone replacement therapy can increase HDL-C levels, but is not currently recommended for reduction of cardiovascular risk. Diabetes mellitus should be optimally controlled. Thiazolidinediones have modest HDL-C–increasing effects and could be considered.

Drug therapy specifically targeted to patients with low HDL-C should be considered in selected patients. Patients with low HDL-C and increased or borderline LDL-C levels should be treated to reduce the LDL-C, and in most such cases a statin is the appropriate choice. Statins increase HDL-C levels only modestly, but they significantly reduce risk in patients with low HDL-C and should be considered the first line of drug therapy in patients with increased LDL-C levels. For patients with low HDL-C and substantially increased triglycerides, initial treatment with a fibrate should be considered. Fibrates increase HDL-C levels modestly and significantly reduce cardiovascular risk in patients with low HDL-C. If the HDL-C is low, the LDL-C is already well controlled, and the triglycerides are less than 400 mg/dL, a more difficult issue is whether pharmacologic intervention should be targeted specifically toward the HDL-C level. In individuals with established CHD or a CHD risk equivalent, this may be a reasonable approach, especially in light of the VA-HIT study results. In healthy persons, there are no published clinical trials demonstrating benefit of treatment targeted specifically toward a low HDL-C. After therapeutic lifestyle intervention, high-risk individuals, including those with diabetes or the metabolic syndrome and those with strong family histories of premature CHD, are candidates for drug therapy targeted toward low HDL-C. Fibrates have more overall outcome data, whereas niacin is more effective in increasing HDL-C levels; neither have been used in clinical outcome trials in a primary prevention population with isolated low HDL-C.

It is common for patients to achieve their LDL-C goal on initial drug therapy with a statin but have a persistently low HDL-C level. If the triglycerides are greater than 200 mg/dL, the NCEP ATP III guidelines recommend focusing next on the non–HDL-C, targeting it to a goal 30 points greater than the LDL-C goal (i.e., 130 mg/dL for patients with CHD or CHD risk equivalent). However, even with appropriate treatment of the non–HDL-C, the HDL-C levels frequently remain low in such patients. Currrently available data suggest that a persistent low HDL-C in the setting of statin therapy is a predictor of future cardiovascular events. For patients on a statin with persistently low HDL-C, the addition of a fibrate or niacin can help increase HDL-C levels. No outcome trials comparing either combination to statin montherapy have been reported; nevertheless, in patients with CHD or patients at high cardiovascular risk who are receiving statin therapy with a well controlled LDL-C but a low HDL-C, the addition of niacin or a fibrate should be considered. The combination of a statin and a fibrate and the combination of a statin and a niacin can be associated with myopathy and abnormal liver function tests, respectively, both of which must be carefully monitored in patients receiving combination therapy.

NEW APPROACHES TO THERAPEUTIC TARGETING OF HIGH-DENSITY LIPOPROTEIN METABOLISM

New and more effective approaches to increasing HDL-C and RCT are needed (31). As noted earlier, there is a wealth of animal data that increasing apoA-I production reduces progression and even induces regression of atherothrombosis. Therefore, a small molecule that increases apoA-I production, perhaps through increasing gene transcription, in the liver, the intestine, or both would be highly desirable. However, no such small molecules have yet advanced to the point of large clinical trials. Therefore, other approaches to increasing apoA-I are being actively investigated. A particularly interesting approach is the administration of synthetic peptides based on the apoA-I amphipathic helical sequence. Oral adminstration of an apoA-I mimetic D-peptide was shown to significantly reduce atherothrombosis in mice (98). The use of somatic gene transfer to express apoA-I awaits the development of improved gene transfer vectors before it can be considered in humans.

Promotion of cellular cholesterol efflux and RCT is an attractive therapeutic target. Pharmacologic up-regulation of ABCA1 in macrophages could, in theory, promote cellular cholesterol efflux and reduce atherothrombosis. There has been tremendous interest in understanding the transcriptional regulation of ABCA1, which appears to be primarily through the nuclear heterodimer LXR/RXR. Synthetic ligands for either LXR or RXR are being explored as therapeutic approaches. Furthermore, PPAR-α agonists (fibrates) and PPAR-α agonists (thiadolizinediones) have been shown to up-regulate LXR, ABCA1, and cholesterol efflux, and new "dual PPAR agonists" are being developed. Intravenous infusions of large phospholipid liposomes have been shown to promote peripheral cholesterol mobilization and to reduce atherothrombosis in rabbits.

Antoher therapeutic target is CETP (47). Studies of CETP inhibition in rabbits (which have high levels of CETP) have demonstrated significant reduction in atherothrombosis, using antisense inhibition, a small molecule inhibitor, and an anti-CETP immunization strategy. A CETP inhibitor has been shown to increase levels of HDL-C in humans (99). There remains substantial uncertainty about whether CETP inhibition will reduce atherothrombosis in humans, and this question will only be definitely answered through the appropriate clinical trials.

ACKNOWLEDGMENTS

Dr. Rader is a recipient of the Burroughs Wellcome Fund Clinical Scientist Award in Translational Research, is a Doris Duke Charitable Foundation Distinguished Clinical Scientist, and is supported by NIH grants from the NHLBI, NIDDK, and NCRR.

REFERENCES

1. Gordon DJ, Rifkind BM. High-density lipoproteins—the clinical implications of recent studies. *N Engl J Med* 1989;321:1311–1316.
2. Rothblat GH, de la Llera-Moya M, Atger V, et al. Cell cholesterol efflux: integration of old and new observations provides new insights. *J Lipid Res* 1999;40:781–796.
3. Francis GA, Knopp RH, Oram JF. Defective removal of cellular cholesterol and phospholipids by apolipoprotein A-I in Tangier Disease. *J Clin Invest* 1995;96:78–87.
4. Bodzioch M, Orso E, Klucken J, et al. The gene encoding ATP-binding cassette transporter 1 is mutated in Tangier disease. *Nat Genet* 1999; 22:347–351.
5. Wilson AB, Marcil M, Clee SM, et al. Mutations in ABC1 in Tangier disease and familial high-density lipoprotein deficiency. *Nat Genet* 1999;22:336–345.
6. Rust S, Rosier M, Funke H, et al. Tangier disease is caused by mutations in the gene encoding ATP-binding cassette transporter 1. *Nat Genet* 1999;22:352–355.
7. Repa JJ, Mangelsdorf DJ. The liver X receptor gene team: potential new players in atherosclerosis. *Nat Med* 2002;8:1243–1248.
8. Chinetti G, Lestavel S, Bocher V, et al. PPAR-alpha and PPAR-gamma activators induce cholesterol removal from human macrophage foam cells through stimulation of the ABCA1 pathway. *Nat Med* 2001;7: 53–58.
9. Wang N, Chen W, Linsel-Nitschke P, et al. A PEST sequence in ABCA1 regulates degradation by calpain protease and stabilization of ABCA1 by apoA-I. *J Clin Invest* 2003;111:99–107.
10. Oram JF, Yokoyama S. Apolipoprotein-mediated removal of cellular cholesterol and phospholipids. *J Lipid Res* 1996;37:2473–2491.
11. Kuivenhoven JA, Pritchard H, Hill J, et al. The molecular pathology of lecithin:cholesterol acyltransferase (LCAT) deficiency syndromes. *J Lipid Res* 1997;38:191–205.
12. Inazu A, Brown ML, Hesler CB, et al. Increased high-density lipoprotein levels caused by a common cholesteryl-ester transfer protein gene mutation. *N Engl J Med* 1990;323:1234–1238.
13. Lagrost L, Desrumaux C, Masson D, et al. Structure and function of the plasma phospholipid transfer protein. *Curr Opin Lipidol* 1998;9: 203–209.
14. Schwartz CC, Vlahcevic ZR, Berman M, et al. Central role of high density lipoprotein in plasma free cholesterol metabolism. *J Clin Invest* 1982;70:105–116.
15. Rigotti A, Trigatti B, Babitt J, et al. Scavenger receptor BI—a cell surface receptor for high density lipoprotein. *Curr Opin Lipidol* 1997;8: 181–188.
16. Rye KA, Clay MA, Barter PJ. Remodeling of high density lipoproteins by plasma factors. *Atherosclerosis* 1999;145:227–238.
17. Katzel LI, Coon PJ, Busby MJ, et al. Reduced HDL2 cholesterol subspecies and elevated postheparin hepatic lipase activity in older men with abdominal obesity and asymptomatic myocardial ischemia. *Arterioscler Thromb* 1992;12:814–823.
18. Dugi KA, Brandauer K, Schmidt N, et al. Low hepatic lipase activity is a novel risk factor for coronary artery disease. *Circulation* 2001;104: 3057–3062.
19. Hegele R, Little JA, Vezina C, et al. Hepatic lipase deficiency: clinical, biochemical, and molecular genetic characteristics. *Arterioscler Thromb* 1993;13:720–728.
20. Cohen JC, Vega GL, Grundy SM. Hepatic lipase: new insights from genetic and metabolic studies. *Curr Opin Lipidol* 1999;10:259–267.
21. Rader DJ, Jaye M. Endothelial lipase: a new member of the triglyceride lipase gene family. *Curr Opin Lipidol* 2000;11:141–147.
22. Jaye M, Lynch KJ, Krawiec J, et al. A novel endothelial-derived lipase that modulates HDL metabolism. *Nat Genet* 1999;21:424–428.
23. Hirata K, Diechek HL, Cioffi JA, et al. Cloning of a unique lipase from endothelial cells extends the lipase gene family. *J Biol Chem* 1999;274: 14170–14175.
24. Ishida T, Choi S, Kundu RK, et al. Endothelial lipase is a major determinant of HDL level. *J Clin Invest* 2003;111:347–355.
25. Jin W, Millar JS, Broedl U, et al. Inhibition of endothelial lipase causes increased HDL cholesterol levels in vivo. *J Clin Invest* 2003;111: 357–362.
26. Ma K, Cilingiroglu M, Otvos JD, et al. Endothelial lipase is a major genetic determinant for high-density lipoprotein concentration, structure, and metabolism. *Proc Natl Acad Sci USA* 2003;100: 2748–2753.
27. deLemos AS, Wolfe ML, Long CJ, et al. Identification of genetic variants in endothelial lipase in persons with elevated high-density lipoprotein cholesterol. *Circulation* 2002;106:1321–1326.
28. Glass C, Pittman RC, Weinstein DB, et al. Dissociation of tissue uptake of cholesterol ester from that of apoprotein A-I of rat plamsa high density lipoprotein: selective delivery of cholesterol ester to liver, adrenal, and gonad. *Proc Natl Acad Sci USA* 1983;80:5435–5439.
29. Fidge NH. High density lipoprotein receptors, binding proteins, and ligands. *J Lipid Res* 1999;40:187–201.
30. Martinez LO, Jacquet S, Esteve JP, et al. Ectopic beta-chain of ATP synthase is an apolipoprotein A-I receptor in hepatic HDL endocytosis. *Nature* 2003;421:75–79.
31. Rader DJ. High-density lipoproteins and atherosclerosis. *Am J Cardiol* 2002;90:62i–70i.
32. Tangirala RK, Tsukamoto K, Chun SH, et al. Regression of atherosclerosis induced by liver directed gene transfer of apolipoprotein A-I in mice. *Circulation* 1999;100:1816–1822.
33. Duverger N, Kruth H, Emmanuel F, et al. Inhibition of atherosclerosis development in cholesterol-fed human apolipoprotein A-I-Transgenic rabbits. *Circulation* 1996;94:713–717.
34. Zhang Y, Zanotti I, Reilly M, et al. Overexpression of apoA-I promotes reverse transport of cholesterol from macrophages to feces in vivo. *Circulation* 2003;108:661–663.
35. Eriksson M, Carlson LA, Miettinen TA, et al. Stimulation of fecal steroid excretion after infusion of recombinant proapolipoprotein A-I: potential reverse cholesterol transport in humans. *Circulation* 1999; 100:594–598.
36. Haghpassand M, Bourassa PA, Francone OL, et al. Monocyte/macrophage expression of ABCA1 has minimal contribution to plasma HDL levels. *J Clin Invest* 2001;108:1315–1320.
37. Vaisman BL, Lambert G, Amar M, et al. ABCA1 overexpression leads to hyperalphalipoproteinemia and increased biliary cholesterol excretion in transgenic mice. *J Clin Invest* 2001;108:303–309.
38. Groen AK, Bloks VW, Bandsma RH, et al. Hepatobiliary cholesterol transport is not impaired in Abca1-null mice lacking HDL. *J Clin Invest* 2001;108:843–850.
39. van Eck M, Bos IS, Kaminski WE, et al. Leukocyte ABCA1 controls susceptibility to atherosclerosis and macrophage recruitment into tissues. *Proc Natl Acad Sci USA* 2002;99:6298–6303.
40. Aiello RJ, Brees D, Bourassa PA, et al. Increased atherosclerosis in hyperlipidemic mice with inactivation of ABCA1 in macrophages. *Arterioscler Thromb Vasc Biol* 2002;22:630–637.
41. Joyce CW, Amar MJ, Lambert G, et al. The ATP binding cassette transporter A1 (ABCA1) modulates the development of aortic atherosclerosis in C57BL/6 and apoE-knockout mice. *Proc Natl Acad Sci USA* 2002;99:407–412.
42. Santamarina-Fojo S, Lambert G, Hoeg JM, et al. Lecithin-cholesterol acyltransferase: role in lipoprotein metabolism, reverse cholesterol transport and atherosclerosis. *Curr Opin Lipidol* 2000; 11:267–275.
43. Hoeg JM, Santamarina-Fojo S, Berard AM, et al. Overexpression of lecithin:cholesterol acyltransferase in transgenic rabbits prevents diet-induced atherosclerosis. *Proc Natl Acad Sci USA* 1996;93:11448–11453.
44. Foger B, Chase M, Amar MJ, et al. Cholesteryl ester transfer protein corrects dysfunctional high density lipoproteins and reduces aortic atherosclerosis in lecithin cholesterol acyltransferase transgenic mice. *J Biol Chem* 1999;274:36912–36920.
45. Kozarsky KF, Donahee MH, Glick JM, et al. Gene transfer and hepatic overexpression of the HDL receptor SR-BI reduces atherosclerosis in the cholesterol-fed LDL receptor-deficient mouse. *Arterioscler Thromb Vasc Biol* 2000;20:721–727.
46. Braun A, Trigatti BL, Post MJ, et al. Loss of SR-BI expression leads to the early onset of occlusive atherosclerotic coronary artery disease, spontaneous myocardial infarctions, severe cardiac dysfunction, and premature death in apolipoprotein E-deficient mice. *Circ Res* 2002;90: 270–276.
47. Barter PJ, Brewer HB Jr, Chapman MJ, et al. Cholesteryl ester transfer protein: a novel target for raising HDL and inhibiting atherosclerosis. *Arterioscler Thromb Vasc Biol* 2003;23:160–167.
48. Navab M, Hama SY, Cooke CJ, et al. Normal high density lipoprotein

inhibits three steps in the formation of mildly oxidized low density lipoprotein: step 1. *J Lipid Res* 2000;41:1481–1494.

49. Cockerill G, Rye K, Gamble J, et al. High density lipoproteins inhibit cytokine-induced expression of endothelial cell adhesion molecules. *Arterioscler Thromb Vasc Biol* 1995;15:1987–1994.

50. Xia P, Vadas MA, Rye KA, et al. High density lipoproteins (HDL) interrupt the sphingosine kinase signaling pathway. A possible mechanism for protection against atherosclerosis by HDL. *J Biol Chem* 1999;274:33143–33147.

51. Cockerill GW, Huehns TY, Weerasinghe A, et al. Elevation of plasma high-density lipoprotein concentration reduces interleukin-1-induced expression of E-selectin in an in vivo model of acute inflammation. *Circulation* 2001;103:108–112.

52. Dansky HM, Charlton SA, Barlow CB, et al. Apo A-I inhibits foam cell formation in Apo E-deficient mice after monocyte adherence to endothelium. *J Clin Invest* 1999;104:31–39.

53. Yuhanna IS, Zhu Y, Cox BE, et al. High-density lipoprotein binding to scavenger receptor-BI activates endothelial nitric oxide synthase. *Nat Med* 2001;7:853–857.

54. Gong M, Wilson M, Kelly T, et al. HDL-associated estradiol stimulates endothelial NO synthase and vasodilation in an SR-BI-dependent manner. *J Clin Invest* 2003;111:1579–1587.

55. Griffin JH, Kojima K, Banka CL, et al. High-density lipoprotein enhancement of anticoagulant activities of plasma protein S and activated protein C. *J Clin Invest* 1999;103:219–227.

56. Rader DJ, Ikewaki K. Unraveling high density lipoprotein-apolipoprotein metabolism in human mutants and animal models. *Curr Opin Lipidol* 1996;7:117–123.

57. Brinton EA, Eisenberg S, Breslow JL. A low-fat diet decreases high density lipoprotein (HDL) cholesterol levels by decreasing HDL apolipoprotein transport rates. *J Clin Invest* 1990;85:144–151.

58. Rader DJ, Castro G, Zech LA, et al. In vivo metabolism of apolipoprotein A-I on high density lipoprotein particles LpA-I and LpA-I, A-II. *J Lipid Res* 1991;32:1849–1859.

59. Brinton EA, Eisenberg S, Breslow JL. Increased apo A-I and apo A-II fractional catabolic rate in patients with low high density lipoprotein-cholesterol levels with or without hypertriglyceridemia. *J Clin Invest* 1991;87:536–544.

60. De O, Kong M, Han Z, et al. Metabolic and genetic determinants of HDL metabolism and hepatic lipase activity in normolipidemic females. *J Lipid Res* 1999;40:1211–1221.

61. Roma P, Gregg RE, Meng MS, et al. In vivo metabolism of a mutant form of apolipoprotein A-I, apo A-IMilano, associated with familial hypoalphalipoproteinemia. *J Clin Invest* 1993;1445–1452.

62. Rader DJ, Gregg RE, Meng MS, et al. In vivo metabolism of a mutant apolipoprotein, apoA-IIowa, associated with hypoalphalipoproteinemia and hereditary systemic amyloidosis. *J Lipid Res* 1992;33:755–763.

63. Schaefer EJ, Blum CB, Levy RI, et al. Metabolism of high-density lipoprotein apolipoproteins in Tangier disease. *N Engl J Med* 1978;299:905–910.

64. Rader DJ, Ikewaki K, Duverger N, et al. Markedly accelerated catabolism of apolipoprotein A-II (ApoA-II) and high density lipoproteins containing ApoA-II in classic lecithin: cholesterol acyltransferase deficiency and fish-eye disease. *J Clin Invest* 1994;93:321–330.

65. Ikewaki K, Rader DJ, Sakamoto T, et al. Delayed catabolism of high density lipoprotein apolipoproteins A-I and A-II in human cholesteryl ester transfer protein deficiency. *J Clin Invest* 1993;92:1650–1658.

66. Rader DJ, Ikewaki K, Duverger N, et al. Very low high-density lipoproteins without coronary atherosclerosis. *Lancet* 1993;342:1455–1458.

67. Roma P, Gregg RE, Bishop C, et al. Apolipoprotein A-I metabolism in subjects with a PstI restriction fragment length polymorphism of the apoA-I gene and familial hypoalphalipoproteinemia. *J Lipid Res* 1990;31:1753–1760.

68. Ginsberg HN, Huang LS. The insulin resistance syndrome: impact on lipoprotein metabolism and atherothrombosis. *J Cardiovasc Risk* 2000;7:325–331.

69. Heuch I, Namboodiri KK, Green PP, et al. A multivariate analysis of familial associations of lipoprotein levels in the Lipid Research Clinics Collaborative Family Study: I. Familial correlation and regression analyses. *Genet Epidemiol* 1985;2:283–300.

70. Ellison RC, Myers RH, Zhang Y, et al. Effects of similarities in lifestyle habits on familial aggregation of high density lipoprotein and low density lipoprotein cholesterol: the NHLBI Family Heart Study. *Am J Epidemiol* 1999;150:910–918.

71. Mahaney CM, Blangero J, Rainwater LD, et al. A major locus influencing plasma high-density lipoprotein cholesterol levels in the San Antonio family heart study. *Arterioscler Thromb Vasc Biol* 1995;15:1730–1739.

72. Arya R, Duggirala R, Almasy L, et al. Linkage of high-density lipoprotein-cholesterol concentrations to a locus on chromosome 9p in Mexican Americans. *Nat Genet* 2002;30:102–105.

73. Kronenberg F, Coon H, Ellison RC, et al. Segregation analysis of HDL cholesterol in the NHLBI Family Heart Study and in Utah pedigrees. *Eur J Hum Genet* 2002;10:367–374.

74. Benson MD. Apolipoprotein AI and amyloidosis: a genetic model for aging. *Kidney Int* 1998;53:508–509.

75. Smith JD, Brinton EA, Breslow JL. Polymorphism in the human apolipoprotein A-I gene promoter region: association of the minor allele with decreased production rate in vivo and promoter activity in vitro. *J Clin Invest* 1992;89:1796–1800.

76. Hobbs HH, Rader DJ. ABC1: connecting yellow tonsils, neuropathy, and very low HDL. *J Clin Invest* 1999;104:1015–1017.

77. Marcil M, Brooks-Wilson A, Clee SM, et al. Mutations in the ABC1 gene in familial HDL deficiency with defective cholesterol efflux. *Lancet* 1999;354:1341–1346.

78. Schaefer EJ, Zech LA, Schwartz DE, et al. Coronary heart disease prevalence and other clinical features in familial high-density lipoprotein deficiency (Tangier disease). *Ann Intern Med* 1980;93:261–266.

79. Serfaty-Lacrosniere C, Civeira F, Lanzberg A, et al. Homozygous Tangier disease and cardiovascular disease. *Atherosclerosis* 1994;107:85–98.

80. Clee SM, Zwinderman AH, Engert JC, et al. Common genetic variation in ABCA1 is associated with altered lipoprotein levels and a modified risk for coronary artery disease. *Circulation* 2001;103:1198–1205.

81. Brousseau ME, Bodzioch M, Schaefer EJ, et al. Common variants in the gene encoding ATP-binding cassette transporter 1 in men with low HDL cholesterol levels and coronary heart disease. *Atherosclerosis* 2001;154:607–611.

82. Blades B, Vega GL, Grundy SM. Activities of lipoprotein lipase and hepatic triglyceride lipase in postheparin plasma of patients with low concentrations of HDL cholesterol. *Arterioscler Thromb Vasc Biol* 1993;13:1227–1235.

83. Inazu A, Jiang XC, Haraki T, et al. Genetic cholesteryl ester transfer protein deficiency caused by two prevalent mutations as a major determinant of increased levels of high density lipoprotein cholesterol. *J Clin Invest* 1994;94:1872–1882.

84. Zhong S, Sharp DS, Grove JS, et al. Increased coronary heart disease in Japanese-American men with mutations in the cholesteryl ester transfer protein gene despite increased HDL levels. *J Clin Invest* 1996;97:2687–2688.

85. Ordovas JM, Cupples LA, Corella D, et al. Association of cholesteryl ester transfer protein-TaqIB polymorphism with variations in lipoprotein subclasses and coronary heart disease risk: the Framingham study. *Arterioscler Thromb Vasc Biol* 2000;20:1323–1329.

86. Gaziano JM, Buring JE, Breslow JL, et al. Moderate alcohol intake, increased levels of high-density lipoprotein and its subfractions, and decreased risk of myocardial infarction. *N Engl J Med* 1993;329:1829–1834.

87. Downs JR, Clearfield M, Weis S, et al. Primary prevention of acute coronary events with lovastatin in men and women with average cholesterol levels. *JAMA* 1998;279:1615–1622.

88. Heart Protection Study Collaborative Group. MRC/BHF Heart Protection Study of cholesterol lowering with simvastatin in 20,536 high-risk individuals: a randomised placebo-controlled trial. *Lancet* 2002;360:7–22.

89. Fruchart JC, Staels B, Duriez P. The role of fibric acids in atherosclerosis. *Curr Atheroscler Rep* 2001;3:83–92.

90. Frick MH, Elo O, Haapa K, et al. Helsinki Heart Study: primary-prevention trial with gemfibrozil in middle-aged men with dyslipidemia. Safety of treatment, changes in risk factors, and incidence of coronary heart disease. *N Engl J Med* 1987;317:1237–1245.

91. Rubins HB, Robins SJ, Collins D, et al. Gemfibrozil for the secondary prevention of coronary herat disease in men with low levels of high-density lipoprotein cholesterol. *N Engl J Med* 1999;341:410–418.

92. Secondary prevention by raising HDL cholesterol and reducing triglycerides in patients with coronary artery disease: the Bezafibrate Infarction Prevention (BIP) study. *Circulation* 2000;102:21–27.

93. Kamanna VS, Kashyap ML. Mechanism of action of niacin on lipoprotein metabolism. *Curr Atheroscler Rep* 2000;2:36–46.

94. Canner PL, Berge KG, Wenger NK, et al. Fifteen year mortality in Coronary Drug Project patients: long-term benefit with niacin. *J Am Coll Cardiol* 1986;8:1245–1255.

95. Brown BG, Zhao XQ, Chait A, et al. Simvastatin and niacin, antioxidant vitamins, or the combination for the prevention of coronary disease. *N Engl J Med* 2001;345:1583–1592.

96. Executive Summary of the Third Report of The National Cholesterol Education Program (NCEP) Expert Panel on Detection, Evaluation, And Treatment of High Blood Cholesterol In Adults (Adult Treatment Panel III). *JAMA* 2001;285:2486–2497.

97. Thompson PD, Rader DJ. Does exercise increase HDL cholesterol in those who need it the most? *Arterioscler Thromb Vasc Biol* 2001;21: 1097–1098.

98. Navab M, Anantharamaiah GM, Hama S, et al. Oral administration of an Apo A-I mimetic Peptide synthesized from D-amino acids dramatically reduces atherosclerosis in mice independent of plasma cholesterol. *Circulation* 2002;105:290–292.

99. de Grooth GJ, Kuivenhoven JA, Stalenhoef AF, et al. Efficacy and safety of a novel cholesteryl ester transfer protein inhibitor, JTT-705, in humans: a randomized phase II dose-response study. *Circulation* 2002;105:2159–2165.

CHAPTER 8

Lipoprotein Oxidation, Arterial Inflammation, and Atherogenesis

Marc S. Penn and Guy M. Chisolm

Key Words: Antioxidants; atherothrombosis; mouse models; oxidized low-density lipoprotein; vitamin E.

INTRODUCTION

The concept that oxidized lipoproteins are involved in atherothrombosis lesion development was formulated more than two decades ago from reports that (a) low-density lipoprotein (LDL) can injure cells under certain conditions (1,2)—that is, those that facilitated oxidation of the lipoprotein (3,4); (b) LDL modified by malondialdehyde, a product of the oxidation of unsaturated fatty acids, was taken up by monocyte/macrophages through scavenger receptors (5); and (c) macrophages also will take up through scavenger receptors LDL that was modified by cultured endothelial cells (6). Endothelial modification of LDL was later shown to be through oxidation, mediated by reactive oxygen species produced by the cells (7,8). Smooth muscle cells (7,9), stimulated monocytes (10), and macrophages (11)—cell types

M. S. Penn: Departments of Cardiovascular Medicine and Cell Biology, Cleveland Clinic Foundation, 9500 Euclid Avenue, Cleveland, Ohio 44195.
G. M. Chisolm: Department of Cell Biology, Lerner Research Institute, Cleveland Clinic Foundation (NC-10), 9500 Euclid Avenue, Cleveland, Ohio 44195.

present in arterial lesions—also were shown to oxidize LDL *in vitro*. Since these early observations, the research area of lipoprotein oxidation and atherothrombosis has undergone a virtual explosion, leading to revision of the response to injury hypothesis of atherothrombosis to include oxidized lipoproteins and their lipids as the injurious agents *in vivo* (12). The revised hypothesis predicts that the initial and sustaining vascular insult leading to endothelial cell activation and lipoprotein accumulation is caused by oxidized lipoproteins, their altered apolipoproteins, and/or any of the dozens of newly formed lipid byproducts. Further evolution of an oxidation theory draws on new information about the role of inflammatory processes in exacerbating clinically important cardiovascular events (13–15). The following discussion focuses on the current state of knowledge regarding how oxidized lipoproteins could be formed *in vivo;* their potential roles in atherogenesis, lesion progression, and thrombosis; and current promise or failure of treatment strategies focused on inhibiting oxidation and oxidation-mediated pathways.

There are a few dominating reasons underlying the attraction of the oxidation theory of atherothrombosis (16–20). First, oxidized LDL has been shown to exist *in vivo* both in atherothrombosis-susceptible animal models and in humans. "LDL" fractions extracted from lesions show evidence of oxidation. In atherothrombotic lesions, lipids known to be formed as LDL oxidizes also have been shown to accumulate in lesions. Antibodies that recognize oxidized but not native LDL bind lesion epitopes. Radiolabeled antibodies to oxidized LDL have been used to image vulnerable plaque noninvasively in animals (21). In plasma of humans and animals, circulating subpopulations of LDL have been shown to have features of oxidized LDL. Moreover, antibodies to oxidized LDL circulate in the blood of patients with coronary artery disease (CAD) (18). These are increased in patients with clinical evidence of acute coronary syndrome (22). Second, known features of atherothrombosis can be mimicked by introducing oxidized LDL, but not native LDL, to cultures of the cell types present in lesions—that is, smooth muscle cells, endothelial cells, and macrophages. These include effects that can theoretically explain monocyte recruitment, foam cell formation, smooth muscle cell proliferation, cell injury and apoptosis, and procoagulant tendencies, among others (see later). Third, known links exist between inflammatory processes and the effects of oxidized LDL and its lipids, including the induction by oxidized LDL of inflammatory mediators in vascular cells and macrophages. Fourth, animal studies in which events that block or enhance steps in the hypothesized sequence of events evoked by lipoprotein oxidation support the oxidation theory. In addition, some (but certainly not all) antioxidant treatments in animal models show impaired progression of arterial disease.

DEFINING OXIDIZED LIPOPROTEINS

As with many complex biochemical systems, early studies of oxidized lipoproteins introduced ambiguities that have been difficult to resolve. The term "oxidized LDL" does not indicate the degree to which the lipoprotein is oxidatively modified, and it is clear that LDL oxidation can be regarded as a continuum. One can oxidize LDL in vitro to any desired level, stop the progression, and study the attributes of the altered particle. It is possible, therefore, to introduce into an experiment LDL that is oxidized to an infinite number of different levels. These differentially oxidized preparations can evoke different responses in cells and in vivo. This is illustrated by several diverse studies. In one of these, LDL was oxidized to a limited degree, such that it was still recognized by the LDL (B/E) receptor (23). The authors referred to this preparation as "minimally modified" LDL. It induced monocyte adhesion in endothelial cells, whereas native LDL or LDL that was oxidized to a greater extent did not (23).

The term oxidized LDL is used irrespective of the means by which the oxidation was initiated, but the mode of initiation can lead to differences. For example, LDL oxidized by metal ions can have different properties from LDL oxidized by ultraviolet irradiation. Whereas both lead to lipid peroxidation, LDL receptor recognition is more readily destroyed in the former than the latter (24). Furthermore, the same term has been applied to describe LDL-like extracts from vascular lesions identified by antibodies that recognize oxi-

dized LDL but not native LDL. Although this would suggest that the epitope to which the antibody would bind—for example, a lipid peroxidation product linked to a particular amino acid residue (25)—was in common with LDL oxidized in vitro, it does not validate that other similarities exist between LDL oxidized in vitro and oxidized LDL residing in a lesion. Finally, the term oxidized LDL does not distinguish between LDL subjected to free radical–initiated lipid peroxidation and LDL that has incorporated, or gained by exchange, various lipid oxidation products from adjacent cells, tissue sites, or other lipoproteins.

These considerations make generalizations about oxidized LDL difficult with respect to its categorization, biochemical properties, effects on cell functions, and disposition in vivo. Until more is determined about the nature of oxidized LDL in vivo in terms of measurable parameters, one should maintain a balanced skepticism about extrapolating in vitro findings to an in vivo setting. Although the phrase "oxidized LDL" is a general term that is useful to differentiate a preparation from "native LDL," it requires a more precise description to appreciate its limitations in any specific context. We should point out that this text and the field, in general, have focused on LDL oxidation, presumably because of the known association between LDL and atherothrombosis risk; however, consequences of HDL and VLDL oxidation also are profound and are being studied in various contexts.

MECHANISMS OF LOW-DENSITY LIPOPROTEIN OXIDATION *IN VIVO*

Multiple mechanisms for LDL oxidation in vivo have been proposed and characterized in vitro, but the means by which the oxidation occurs in vivo remains unknown. The failure of antioxidant regimens in the treatment of complications of atherothrombotic heart disease in humans (discussed later) has highlighted the necessity to identify the enzymatic systems responsible for lipoprotein oxidation in vivo to develop more precisely targeted treatment paradigms.

Much of the cell culture research on oxidized LDL-induced atherogenic effects has taken advantage of the ease of preparing oxidized LDL by incubating it with cupric or ferrous ion or exposing LDL to cells in culture in metal ion-containing media; however, a role for free metal ions causing LDL oxidation in vivo is doubted (26). Conversely, one proposed mechanism involves the expression and secretion of ceruloplasmin by macrophages. Ceruloplasmin has been shown to be increased in lesions and to oxidize LDL in a reaction involving one of its bound copper atoms (27,28). Many speculate that LDL becomes oxidized after entering the artery wall in a lesion-prone site, suggesting that the cells within that site, smooth muscle cells, endothelial cells, and monocyte-derived macrophages are the effectors of the oxidation. Smooth muscle cells and endothelial cells are capable of oxidizing LDL in vitro in the presence of metal ions in the media; whereas under specific conditions, monocyte-

TABLE 8–1. *Enzyme systems known to oxidize low-density lipoprotein in vitro*

Enzyme system	Cells	Mechanism of oxidation
Nitric oxide synthase (e.g., iNOS)	Macrophages/SMCs/ECs	Nitric oxide, superoxide anion, formation of peroxynitrite
Lipoxygenase (e.g., 15-LO)	Macrophages/ECs	Enzymatic insertion of molecular oxygen
NADPH oxidase	Macrophages/SMCs/ECs	Generation of superoxide anion
Cp	Macrophages	Oxidation catalyzed by Cp-bound copper
MPO	Neutrophils/Macrophages	Chlorination and nitration

Cp, ceruloplasmin; EC, endothelial cell; iNOS, inducible nitric oxide synthase; MPO, Myeloperoxidase; NADPH, nicotinamide adenine dinucleotide phosphate; SMC, smooth muscle cell.

derived macrophages can oxidize LDL without exogenous metal ion (29). This has led many to focus on the macrophage, bathed in LDL-enriched interstitial fluid, as the source of oxidants that modify LDL (29).

A number of enzymatic systems, almost all expressed in macrophages, have been shown capable of participating in lipoprotein oxidation *in vitro*. These include 15-lipoxygenase (15-LO), ceruloplasmin, nicotinamide adenine dinucleotide phosphate (NADPH) oxidase, myeloperoxidase (MPO) and inducible nitric oxide synthase (Table 8–1). There is tantalizing evidence to support each of these (29), and they are not mutually exclusive. A number of studies have tested the effects of genetically altering the expression of these enzyme systems in mouse models of atherothrombosis (Table 8–2). Importantly, some of these *in vivo* studies have demonstrated significant decreases in lesion formation. An example is offered by studies on the *12/15-LO* gene. Mice deficient in the *12/15-LO* gene have been shown to have significantly less atherothrombosis (30,31), whereas mice engineered to overexpress the *15-LO* gene on an endothelial cell-specific promoter had accelerated atherothrombosis (32). Interestingly, the mice null for *12/15-LO* also exhibited decreased evidence of LDL oxidation, as measured by decreased levels of isoprostanes (breakdown products of oxidized LDL) and circulating levels of antibodies to oxidized LDL (18,30). In addition to suggesting a role

for LO, these findings also suggest and begin to validate potential markers that can be used clinically to quantify atherothrombosis burden and response to therapy.

Studies also have addressed the possible role of MPO. Recent studies have demonstrated that circulating leukocyte MPO levels were greater in patients with CAD than in control subjects who had no evidence of CAD by coronary angiography (33,34). Furthermore, clinical populations that lack the *MPO* gene, or have a polymorphism in the promoter of *MPO* leading to less *MPO* expression, have demonstrably less CAD (35). These data are compelling, but deletion of the *MPO* gene did not result in significant changes in atherothrombosis burden in the apolipoprotein $E^{-/-}$ (apoE$^{-/-}$) mouse model of atherothrombosis (36). Perhaps the latter serves to remind us that there are clear differences between mice and men in the pathophysiology of atherothrombosis.

The role of NADPH oxidase also has been tested for its possible link to atherothrombosis with the result that it, too, may play an important role. Mice deficient in one of the essential proteins of the NADPH oxidase complex, p47phox, were used. Measuring atherothrombotic lesion formation in wild-type, p47phox$^{-/-}$, apoE$^{-/-}$, and (apoE$^{-/-}$)(p47phox$^{-/-}$) mice, Barry-Lane et al. (37) showed that (apoE$^{-/-}$)(p47phox$^{-/-}$) mice had less total lesion area than apoE$^{-/-}$ mice, regardless of whether mice were fed standard chow or a high-fat diet.

TABLE 8–2. *Mouse models used to test the oxidation hypothesis of atherothrombosis*

Gene	Genetic manipulation	Atherosclerosis model	Change in lesion area	Effect on LDL oxidation	Reference
LDL oxidation					
MPO	Knockout	apoE$^{-/-}$	↑		36
12/15-LO	Knockout	apoE$^{-/-}$	↓↓	↓ Oxidation	155
12/15-LO	Overexpress	LDLR$^{-/-}$	↑	↑ Oxidation	32
iNOS	Knockout	apoE$^{-/-}$	↓	↓ Oxidation	156
NADPH oxidase gp91phox subunit	Knockout	apoE$^{-/-}$	—	ND	157
NADPH oxidase p47phox subunit	Knockout	apoE$^{-/-}$	↓↓	ND	37
OxLDL Removal					
CD36	Knockout	apoE$^{-/-}$	↓↓	↓ Uptake	73
SR-A	Knockout	apoE$^{-/-}$	↓	↓ Uptake	72
Paraoxonase	Knockout	apoE$^{-/-}$	↑	↓ Clearance	108
Paraoxonase	Overexpress	apoE$^{-/-}$	↓	↓ Clearance ↑ Oxidation	158

apoE, apolipoprotein E; iNOS, inducible nitric oxide synthase; LDL, low-density lipoprotein; LDLR, low density lipoprotein receptor; 12/15-LO, 12-/15-lipoxygenase; MPO, myeloperoxidase; NADPH, nicotinamide adenine dinucleotide phosphate; ND, not determined; SR-A, scavenger receptor A.

Whether the decreased atherothrombosis in these models is because of the role of these enzymes in the oxidation of lipoproteins that enter the artery wall is, of course, uncertain, but the results represent enticing invitations for further testing of hypotheses of atherogenesis suggesting these enzymes as oxidative sources.

The mechanism of LDL oxidation, the cell(s) responsible, and the site of oxidation remain unknown. Determining these could lead to the identity of markers that can be used clinically to quantify atherothrombosis burden and responses to therapy. The ultimate promise of such studies is the development of inhibitors that will blunt the oxidation of lipoproteins and arrest disease progression.

A THEORY OF ATHEROTHROMBOSIS SUGGESTING A ROLE FOR LOW-DENSITY LIPOPROTEIN OXIDATION

Although oxidized LDL is toxic to cells in culture, voluminous studies have shown that sublethal levels of oxidized LDL markedly alter numerous functions in a variety of cells and tissues in ways that are distinct from the effects of native LDL. These functions include the induction or suppression of the expression of multiple genes, changes in cell motility, changes in cell–cell adhesion, changes in growth factor and cytokine production, influences on cellular lipid metabolism, and alterations in enzyme activities. Many, but not all of these findings can be fit into a hypothetical sequence in which oxidized LDL exacerbates atherothrombosis. Endothelial activation and injury, LDL retention in intimal interstitium, monocyte recruitment into intima, engorgement of macrophages with lipoprotein-derived lipid, smooth muscle cell migration and proliferation, accumulation of necrotic cell debris, procoagulant activity and effects favoring vasoconstriction are characteristics of atherothrombosis that can be predicted by oxidized LDL interactions with cultured cells or isolated vascular tissue. Much of the focus of research related to the role of oxidized LDL in atherothrombosis has been *in vitro* attempts to characterize these cell function changes, to identify the oxidized LDL moieties responsible for the effects, to determine the mechanisms by which these components act, and to use those findings to assess *in vivo* relevance.

Oxidized Low-Density Lipoprotein Accumulates in the Arterial Intima

It is known that LDL enters the normal arterial wall interstitium and accumulates in amounts that are regulated by the endothelium and likely the internal elastic lamina (38). Increases in the level of plasma LDL increase proportionately to the rate of LDL entry (39). Thus, high interstitial LDL secondary to high plasma LDL, and the tendency for LDL to bind proteoglycans would increase the residence time for an LDL molecule entering the tissue (40) and would increase the probability of opportunistic LDL oxidation, perhaps by free radical production from adjacent endothelium or smooth muscle cells or an isolated macrophage (7,8,10,11). Small,

dense LDL, shown to signal increased risk for atherothrombosis and to be more readily oxidized than other LDL subfractions (41,42), may be able to pass the endothelium more readily. LDL bound to proteoglycans is more susceptible to oxidation (43). Once oxidized, subtle injury to endothelium by oxidized LDL may lead to local increases in endothelial cell turnover and further enhanced entry of lipoprotein (44). Intravenous infusion of oxidized LDL into otherwise healthy rats has been shown to increase endothelial cell turnover and macromolecular transport into the artery wall significantly (45). Thus, the initiating event for atherothrombosis may be the accumulation of LDL, secondary to increased plasma LDL, in a thickened intima site near a bifurcation, which, because of the increased LDL residence time, is likely to become oxidized.

Monocyte Infiltration Promoted by Oxidized Low-Density Lipoprotein

Early atherothrombotic lesions in animals are characterized by increased monocyte adhesion to the overlying endothelium, diapedesis into the intima, and differentiation into macrophages (46,47). Oxidized LDL may participate in a number of actions that encourage monocyte invasion of intima. Oxidized LDL causes monocyte chemotactic protein-1 (MCP-1) to be produced by endothelium (48), causes expression by endothelium of monocyte-binding proteins (23, 49,50), and acts itself as a monocyte chemoattractant (51). Oxidized LDL has been shown to induce endothelial cell expression of intercellular adhesion molecule-1 (ICAM-1), platelet-endothelial cell adhesion molecule-1 (PECAM-1), P-selectin, and E-selectin with distinct kinetics, and studies with blocking antibodies demonstrated that ICAM-1 and P-selectin mediate more than half of cell adhesion. Blocking PECAM-1 has no effect on adhesion, but significantly reduces transmigration (52). Other studies have demonstrated that the increase in monocyte adhesion in response to oxidized LDL was suppressed by the presence of HDL (53).

The ability of oxidized LDL to induce monocyte adhesion is, at least in part, mediated by lysoPC (54), a product of phospholipase A_2 activity apparent on oxidation of LDL. VCAM-1 and ICAM-1 expression have been shown to be increased on endothelial cells after exposure to lysoPC. In concert with these observations, stimulators of phospholipase A_2, such as interleukin-1β and tumor necrosis factor, also have been shown to increase surface adhesion molecule expression. Inhibitors of phospholipase A_2 block the effects of phospholipase A_2 stimulators, but not lysoPC (54).

Injections of oxidized LDL have been shown to induce binding of leukocytes to the endothelial cell surface, demonstrating that this is at least possible *in vivo* (55). Furthermore, it has been demonstrated that the injection of antibodies to platelet-activating factor (56) and CD11b/CD18 (57) blocked leukocyte adhesion, suggesting a role for these receptor complexes in the binding of leukocytes to the endothelial cell surface.

The chemotactic effects of oxidized LDL are mediated by a direct effect of oxidized LDL on monocytes and by an indirect effect on endothelial cells. The direct chemotactic and chemostatic effects of oxidized LDL have been shown to be contained in the lipid fraction of oxidized LDL, and are thought to be caused by lysoPC. lysoPC was shown to be a chemoattractant for monocytes (58), whereas oxidized LDL was shown to immobilize macrophages in the presence of known chemoattractants (51). Thus, oxidized LDL may attract monocytes to a lesion, and then inhibit the movement of the differentiated macrophages. The chemostatic effect of oxidized LDL on macrophages may initiate a positive feedback loop, in which the presence of more oxidized LDL leads to the immobilization of cells capable of forming additional oxidized LDL.

Oxidized LDL also has been shown to alter monocyte motility indirectly by inducing the increased production and release of MCP-1 by endothelial cells and smooth muscle cells (23,48). That this observation may have relevance *in vivo* is supported by the decreased atherothrombosis observed when the MCP-1–null mouse was crossed with the low density lipoprotein receptor (LDLR)$^{-/-}$ mouse (59) or the apoB transgenic mouse (60) compared with the control animals expressing wild-type MCP-1.

Oxidized LDL also has been shown to have potentially important effects on other vascular cells—for example, it blunts the migration of endothelial cells (61) and enhances that of smooth muscle cells (62).

Foam Cell Formation from Oxidized Low-Density Lipoprotein

As LDL oxidation progresses, the lipoprotein loses its ability to be recognized by the LDL receptor and its affinity increases for other receptors, including the macrophage scavenger receptor A (SR-A) types I and II (6,63) and CD36 (64), which recognize oxidized, but not native, LDL. Once recruited into the intima, the monocyte-derived phagocytes are able to internalize oxidized LDL by expressing select scavenger receptors, including SR-A (65), CD36 (66), and a specific macrophage Fc-γ receptor (67). In addition, Fc-γ receptors could bind oxidized LDL complexed with antibodies. Such antibodies have been demonstrated in plasma and have been shown to bind oxidized, but not native, LDL (68). It was shown that C-reactive protein can bind oxidized LDL (69,70). This opens the further possibility that Fc-γ receptor subclasses that recognize CRP could also be a means for macrophage ingestion of oxidized LDL. The known tendency of LDL to aggregate on oxidation suggests yet another possibility for macrophage uptake potentially independent of scavenger or Fc receptors—that is, particulate oxidized LDL aggregates may be taken up through nonspecific phagocytosis (71). As a result of encountering phagocytic stimuli, resident macrophages may be stimulated to produce more reactive oxidant species contributing to further LDL oxidation (10,11).

The potential importance of receptor-mediated uptake of oxidized LDL on atherogenesis is suggested by the observed decrease in lesion formation in mouse models of atherothrombosis that lack either SR-A (72) or CD36 (73). The moieties of oxidized LDL recognized by CD36 appear to be various species of oxidized phospholipids formed during oxidation (74,75). The roles of Fc receptor subclasses and other scavenger receptors—LOX-1, SR-BI, and macrosialin/CD68--and the consequences of their absences are, like CD36 and SR-A subtypes, under intense investigation (76,77).

Oxidized Low-Density Lipoprotein and Smooth Muscle Cell Migration and Proliferation

The migration of smooth muscle cells into intima from media and the vigorous proliferation of these cells is a known feature of lesion development and growth. Oxidized LDL alteration in growth factor production could play a major role in the pathogenesis of atherothrombosis, because many of the growth factors influenced by oxidized LDL stimulate smooth muscle cell proliferation or migration. Oxidized LDL alters growth factor production and release in a variety of cells and promotes smooth muscle cell proliferation *in vitro* (78). This occurs in part because of the oxidized LDL-mediated release of fibroblast growth factor-2 from smooth muscle cells induced by lysoPC and other structurally related phospholipids borne by oxidized LDL (78–80). Other autocrine growth factor effects also are possible. For example, oxidized LDL also enhances platelet-derived growth factor (PDGF) receptor expression and PDGF AA production in smooth muscle cells (81). Whether these effects that have been demonstrated *in vitro* are what stimulate migration and proliferation *in vivo* is unknown.

Oxidized LDL may further stimulate smooth muscle proliferation by increasing heparin-binding epidermal growth factor (HB-EGF) production in neighboring cells. LysoPC has been shown to increase messenger RNA levels for HB-EGF, as well as its release from human monocytes (82) and endothelial cells (83).

Relatively low concentrations of oxidized LDL increase the production of granulocyte-monocyte colony-stimulating factor (GM-CSF), macrophage CSF (M-CSF), and granulocyte CSF (G-CSF) in aortic endothelial cells from humans and rabbits (84). The importance of this effect of oxidized LDL is highlighted by observations that M-CSF–null mice exhibit significantly less atherothrombosis (85). These experiments suggest further links between lipid oxidation and inflammation.

Cell Injury and Apoptosis Induced by Oxidized Low-Density Lipoprotein

Other atherothrombotic actions of oxidized LDL that may speed lesion development include killing of smooth muscle cells or macrophages forming a necrotic core. Cells can be killed by oxidized LDL at concentrations of oxidized LDL that are less than estimated concentrations of LDL in interstitial space (1–4). This has invited speculation that if LDLs in the intimal interstitium were to become oxidized, it could participate in the dysfunction of endothelium believed to occur in early atherothrombosis (12), the abundance of apoptotic cells throughout lesion development, or the accumulation of dead cell debris known to occur in later stages of lesion development. Injury to endothelium could lead, for example, to increased entry of lipoproteins into the intima from the lumen, or it could impair the important anticoagulant functions of this cell layer. The consequences of injury to endothelial cells may be worsened by the inhibition of endothelial migration (61), and thereby the healing process. LysoPC appears to be responsible for at least a portion of the inhibitory activity (86), and the antimigratory effect of lysoPC appears linked to its influence on plasma membrane viscosity (87).

The capacity of oxidized LDL to injure or kill cells appears to be a general result of oxidation that develops regardless of the mode of oxidation (88). In general, the potency of oxidized LDL to kill cells is related to the degree of oxidation, but even moderately oxidized LDL can kill cells (3,4). Proliferating cells are more susceptible (2), especially during DNA synthesis (89). LDL receptors are not required for toxicity, because receptor negative cells can be killed by oxidized LDL (1,90), and cells are vulnerable to the isolated lipids of oxidized LDL (3). Furthermore, cells without scavenger receptors (e.g., foreskin fibroblasts) are susceptible (4). Conversely, if LDL is oxidized in such a way as to preserve LDL receptor recognition, as has been reported for ultraviolet irradiated LDL, the killing of cells expressing the LDL receptor is enhanced (91). These results suggest that internalization of the entire lipoprotein may not be required for cell injury, but receptor-mediated uptake can increase the delivery of the cytotoxins.

Attempts have been made to identify the cytotoxic lipids that are formed during LDL oxidation. Many of the lipid oxidation products known to be produced during LDL oxidation have been previously demonstrated to kill cells. Several oxysterols, including 7-α-hydroxycholesterol, 7-β-hydroxycholesterol, 7-ketocholesterol, epoxycholesterols (92,93), as well as nonsterol-derived oxidation products, such as lysoPC, oxidized fatty acids, and 4-hydroxynonenal, are among substances formed in oxidized LDL that are known toxins (94–96). Attempts to identify the major cytotoxins of LDL oxidized *in vitro* have variably suggested that 7-β-hydroperoxycholesterol (97) or 7-β-hydroxycholesterol (98) play major roles. It is possible that different toxic lipids dominate under different circumstances, or the vulnerability of various cell types to different oxidized lipids may vary. In addition, the relative amounts of the toxic lipids formed can vary with the degree or the mode of LDL oxidation. Many of the toxic lipids formed on oxidized LDL are known to exist *in vivo*. A critical issue toward understanding which oxidation products are candidates for causing injury or inducing apoptosis to cells *in vivo* is the extent to which they are formed and accumulate to reach bioactive concentrations in the interstitial space of a diseased intima. For example, in

one study, 7-β-hydroperoxycholesterol is shown to be the most potent toxin found on oxidized LDL (97) and to kill cells by inducing lipid peroxidation (99). Although it has been shown to reside in human atherothrombotic lesions (97), Brown and Jessup (100) have measured the accumulation of oxysterols in human lesions and found that 7-ketocholesterol and 7-β-hydroxycholesterol, products of cholesterol hydroperoxides, accumulate to greater levels than the more toxic hydroperoxide, suggesting that the atherogenic effects of these products may be more important *in vivo*.

It has become well recognized that cells of arterial lesions in animals and humans exhibit signs of vigorous ongoing apoptosis (101). Because oxidized LDL accumulates in the interstitium surrounding lesion cells, it is tempting to speculate that some of the lipids of oxidized LDL are candidates for the apoptosis inflicted by oxidized LDL and observed in lesions. Certain oxysterols, 7-β-hydroperoxycholesterol, and 7-ketocholesterol have been studied in this context by many groups because they accumulate in lesions and cause apoptosis in cultured cells (88,102). The identity of the stimuli and the mechanisms for apoptosis and necrosis of cells in plaques and the effects of enhancing or reducing apoptosis on lesion progression are topics of speculation and important subjects for current research (101).

A number of enzymes, distinct from those that catabolize native LDL lipids, have been shown to participate in the catabolism, and potentially the detoxification, of oxidized LDL components. Glutathione peroxidase can degrade fatty acid hydroperoxides after the action of esterases on the hydroperoxides of cholesteryl esters, triglycerides, and phospholipids. In addition, phospholipid hydroperoxide glutathione peroxidase, a selenoperoxidase distinct from glutathione peroxidase, which is capable of directly reducing cholesterol hydroperoxides and hydroperoxides of phospholipids, triglycerides, or cholesteryl esters (103), also may play a role in oxidized LDL lipid metabolism and oxidized LDL detoxification (104). Finally, paraoxonases and esterase/peroxidases, some of which are carried on HDL, can degrade oxidized phospholipids to less toxic phospholipids (105–107). The importance of these enzyme systems was highlighted by the findings that apoE$^{-/-}$ mice lacking paraoxonase exhibited greater degrees of atherosclerosis (108).

Procoagulant Activities of Oxidized Low-Density Lipoproteins

Oxidized LDL has been shown to have a number of effects on the expression of coagulation and fibrinolytic pathways. Tissue factor binding to Factor VIIa is the initiating event for the extrinsic blood coagulation cascade, and it can also participate in the formation of Factor Xa through the intrinsic blood coagulation cascade. There is increased expression of TF in coronary atherectomy specimens from patients with unstable compared with stable angina (109,110), which supports the hypothesis that tissue factor is responsible for thrombosis after atherothrombotic plaque rupture. In addition, tissue factor

might significantly alter disease progression and the clinical consequences of atherothrombosis. These include enzymatic pathways speculated to cause LDL oxidation, such as ceruloplasmin, lipoxygenase, NADPH oxidase components, and MPO, as well as receptors for oxidized LDL forms that could mediate foam cell formation, such as CD36 and SR-A. Other potential targets include oxidized LDL-evoked monocyte chemoattractants, such as MCP-1; specific monocyte adhesion molecules; tissue factor–mediated events; and apoptotic signaling pathways.

REFERENCES

1. Henriksen T, Evensen SA, Carlander B. Injury to human endothelial cells in culture induced by low density lipoproteins. *Scand J Clin Lab Invest* 1979;39:361–368.
2. Hessler JR, Robertson AL Jr, Chisolm GM. LDL-induced cytotoxicity and its inhibition by HDL in human vascular smooth muscle and endothelial cells in culture. *Atherosclerosis* 1979;32:213–229.
3. Hessler JR, Morel DW, Lewis LJ, et al. Lipoprotein oxidation and lipoprotein-induced cytotoxicity. *Arteriosclerosis* 1983;3:215–222.
4. Morel DW, Hessler JR, Chisolm GM. Low density lipoprotein cytotoxicity induced by free radical peroxidation of lipid. *J Lipid Res* 1983;24:1070–1076.
5. Shechter I, Fogelman AM, Haberland ME, et al. The metabolism of native and malondialdehyde altered low density lipoproteins by human monocyte-macrophages. *J Lipid Res* 1981;22:63–71.
6. Henriksen T, Mahoney EM, Steinberg D. Enhanced macrophage degradation of low density lipoprotein previously incubated with cultured endothelial cells: recognition by receptors for acetylated low density lipoproteins. *Proc Natl Acad Sci USA* 1981;78:6499–6503.
7. Morel DW, DiCorleto PE, Chisolm GM. Endothelial and smooth muscle cells alter low density lipoprotein in vitro by free radical oxidation. *Arteriosclerosis* 1984;4:357–364.
8. Steinbrecher UP, Parthasarathy S, Leake DS, et al. Modification of low density lipoprotein by endothelial cells involves lipid peroxidation and degradation of low density lipoprotein phospholipids. *Proc Natl Acad Sci USA* 1984;81:3883–3887.
9. Heinecke JW, Rosen H, Chait A. Iron and copper promote modification of low density lipoprotein by human arterial smooth muscle cells in culture. *J Clin Invest* 1984;74:1890–1894.
10. Cathcart MK, Morel DW, Chisolm GM 3rd. Monocytes and neutrophils oxidize low density lipoprotein making it cytotoxic. *J Leukoc Biol* 1985;38:341–350.
11. Parthasarathy S, Printz DJ, Boyd D, et al. Macrophage oxidation of low density lipoprotein generates a form recognized by the scavenger receptor. *Arteriosclerosis* 1986;6:505–510.
12. Ross R. Atherosclerosis—an inflammatory disease. *N Engl J Med* 1999;340:115–126.
13. Navab M, Hama SY, Ready ST, et al. Oxidized lipids as mediators of coronary heart disease. *Curr Opin Lipidol* 2002;13:363–372.
14. Glass CK, Witztum JL. Atherosclerosis: the road ahead. *Cell* 2001;104:503–516.
15. Libby P, Ridker PM, Maseri A. Inflammation and atherosclerosis. *Circulation* 2002;105:1135–1143.
16. Navab M, Berliner JA, Subbanagounder G, et al. HDL and the inflammatory response induced by LDL-derived oxidized phospholipids. *Arterioscler Thromb Vasc Biol* 2001;21:481–488.
17. Chisolm GM, Steinberg D. The oxidative modification hypothesis of atherogenesis: an overview. *Free Radic Biol Med* 2000;28:1815–1826.
18. Binder CJ, Chang MK, Shaw PX, et al. Innate and acquired immunity in atherogenesis. *Nat Med* 2002;8:1218–1226.
19. Witztum JL, Steinberg D. The oxidative modification hypothesis of atherosclerosis: does it hold for humans? *Trends Cardiovasc Med* 2001;11:93–102.
20. Yla-Herttuala S. Is oxidized low-density lipoprotein present in vivo? *Curr Opin Lipidol* 1998;9:337–344.
21. Tsimikas S. Noninvasive imaging of oxidized low-density lipoprotein in atherosclerotic plaques with tagged oxidation-specific antibodies. *Am J Cardiol* 2002;90:22L–27L.
22. Tsimikas S, Bergmark C, Beyer RW, et al. Temporal increases in plasma markers of oxidized low-density lipoprotein strongly reflect the presence of acute coronary syndromes. *J Am Coll Cardiol* 2003;41:360–370.
23. Berliner JA, Territo MC, Sevanian A, et al. Minimally modified low density lipoprotein stimulates monocyte endothelial interactions. *J Clin Invest* 1990;85:1260–1266.
24. Dousset N, Negre-Salvayre A, Lopez M, et al. Ultraviolet-treated lipoproteins as a model system for the study of the biological effects of lipid peroxides on cultured cell. I. Chemical modifications of ultraviolet-treated low-density lipoproteins. *Biochim Biophys Acta* 1990;1045:219–223.
25. Palinski W, Yla-Herttuala S, Rosenfeld ME, et al. Antisera and monoclonal antibodies specific for epitopes generated during oxidative modification of low density lipoprotein. *Arteriosclerosis* 1990;10:325–335.
26. Dabbagh AJ, Frei B. Human suction blister interstitial fluid prevents metal ion-dependent oxidation of low density lipoprotein by macrophages and in cell-free systems. *J Clin Invest* 1995;96:1958–1966.
27. Ehrenwald E, Chisolm GM, Fox PL. Intact human ceruloplasmin oxidatively modifies low density lipoprotein. *J Clin Invest* 1994;93:1493–1501.
28. Fox PL, Mazumder B, Ehrenwald E, et al. Ceruloplasmin and cardiovascular disease. *Free Radic Biol Med* 2000;28:1735–1744.
29. Chisolm GM 3rd, Hazen SL, Fox PL, et al. The oxidation of lipoproteins by monocytes-macrophages. Biochemical and biological mechanisms. *J Biol Chem* 1999;274:25959–25962.
30. Cyrus T, Witztum JL, Rader DJ, et al. Disruption of the 12/15-lipoxygenase gene diminishes atherosclerosis in apo E-deficient mice. *J Clin Invest* 1999;103:1597–1604.
31. George J, Afek A, Shaish A, et al. 12/15-Lipoxygenase gene disruption attenuates atherogenesis in LDL receptor-deficient mice. *Circulation* 2001;104:1646–1650.
32. Harats D, Shaish A, George J, et al. Overexpression of 15-lipoxygenase in vascular endothelium accelerates early atherosclerosis in LDL receptor-deficient mice. *Arterioscler Thromb Vasc Biol* 2000;20:2100–2105.
33. Zhang R, Brennan ML, Fu X, et al. Association between myeloperoxidase levels and risk of coronary artery disease. *JAMA* 2001;286:2136–2142.
34. Brennan ML, Hazen SL. Emerging role of myeloperoxidase and oxidant stress markers in cardiovascular risk assessment. *Curr Opin Lipidol* 2003;14:353–359.
35. Kutter D, Devaquet P, Vanderstocken G, et al. Consequences of total and subtotal myeloperoxidase deficiency: risk or benefit? *Acta Haematol* 2000;104:10–15.
36. Brennan ML, Anderson MM, Shih DM, et al. Increased atherosclerosis in myeloperoxidase-deficient mice. *J Clin Invest* 2001;107:419–430.
37. Barry-Lane PA, Patterson C, van der Merwe M, et al. p47phox is required for atherosclerotic lesion progression in ApoE(-/-) mice. *J Clin Invest* 2001;108:1513–1522.
38. Penn MS, Saidel GM, Chisolm GM. Relative significance of endothelium and internal elastic lamina in regulating the entry of macromolecules into arteries in vivo. *Circ Res* 1994;74:74–82.
39. Bratzler RL, Chisolm GM, Colton CK, et al. The distribution of labeled low-density lipoprotein across the rabbit thoracic aorta in vivo. *Atherosclerosis* 1977;28:289–307.
40. Schwenke DC, Carew TE. Initiation of atherosclerotic lesions in cholesterol-fed rabbits. II. Selective retention of LDL vs. selective increases in LDL permeability in susceptible sites of arteries. *Arteriosclerosis* 1989;9:908–918.
41. Tribble DL, Holl LG, Wood PD, et al. Variations in oxidative susceptibility among six low density lipoprotein subfractions of differing density and particle size. *Atherosclerosis* 1992;93:189–199.
42. Chait A, Brazg RL, Tribble DL, et al. Susceptibility of small, dense, low-density lipoproteins to oxidative modification in subjects with the atherogenic lipoprotein phenotype, pattern B. *Am J Med* 1993;94:350–356.
43. Hurt-Camejo E, Camejo G, Rosengren B, et al. Effect of arterial proteoglycans and glycosaminoglycans on low density lipoprotein oxida-

tion and its uptake by human macrophages and arterial smooth muscle cells. *Arterioscler Thromb* 1992;12:569–583.
44. Chen YL, Jan KM, Lin HS, et al. Relationship between endothelial cell turnover and permeability to horseradish peroxidase. *Atherosclerosis* 1997;133:7–14.
45. Rangaswamy S, Penn MS, Saidel GM, et al. Exogenous oxidized low-density lipoprotein injures and alters the barrier function of endothelium in rats in vivo. *Circ Res* 1997;80:37–44.
46. Ross R. The pathogenesis of atherosclerosis: an update. *N Engl J Med* 1986;314:488–500.
47. Li AC, Glass CK. The macrophage foam cell as a target for therapeutic intervention. *Nat Med* 2002;8:1235–1242.
48. Cushing SD, Berliner JA, Valente AJ, et al. Minimally modified low density lipoprotein induces monocyte chemotactic protein 1 in human endothelial cells and smooth muscle cells. *Proc Natl Acad Sci USA* 1990;87:5134–5138.
49. Kume N, Cybulsky MI, Gimbrone MA Jr. Lysophosphatidylcholine, a component of atherogenic lipoproteins, induces mononuclear leukocyte adhesion molecules in cultured human and rabbit arterial endothelial cells. *J Clin Invest* 1992;90:1138–1144.
50. Frostegard J, Nilsson J, Haegerstrand A, et al. Oxidized low density lipoprotein induces differentiation and adhesion of human monocytes and the monocytic cell line U937. *Proc Natl Acad Sci USA* 1990;87: 904–908.
51. Quinn MT, Parthasarathy S, Fong LG, et al. Oxidatively modified low density lipoproteins: a potential role in recruitment and retention of monocyte/macrophages during atherogenesis. *Proc Natl Acad Sci USA* 1987;84:2995–2998.
52. Dangerfield J, Larbi KY, Huang MT, et al. PECAM-1 (CD31) homophilic interaction up-regulates alpha6beta1 on transmigrated neutrophils in vivo and plays a functional role in the ability of alpha6 integrins to mediate leukocyte migration through the perivascular basement membrane. *J Exp Med* 2002;196:1201–1211.
53. Maier JA, Barenghi L, Pagani F, et al. The protective role of high-density lipoprotein on oxidized-low-density-lipoprotein-induced U937/endothelial cell interactions. *Eur J Biochem* 1994;221:35–41.
54. Yokote K, Morisaki N, Zenibayashi M, et al. The phospholipase-A2 reaction leads to increased monocyte adhesion of endothelial cells via the expression of adhesion molecules. *Eur J Biochem* 1993;217: 723–729.
55. Lehr HA, Hubner C, Nolte D, et al. Oxidatively modified human low-density lipoprotein stimulates leukocyte adherence to the microvascular endothelium in vivo. *Res Exp Med* 1991;191:85–90.
56. Lehr HA, Seemuller J, Hubner C, et al. Oxidized LDL-induced leukocyte/endothelium interaction in vivo involves the receptor for platelet-activating factor. *Arterioscler Thromb* 1993;13:1013–1018.
57. Lehr HA, Krober M, Hubner C, et al. Stimulation of leukocyte/endothelium interaction by oxidized low density lipoprotein in hairless mice. Involvement of CD11b/CD18 adhesion receptor complex. *Lab Invest* 1993;68:388–395.
58. Quinn MT, Parthasarathy S, Steinberg D. Lysophosphatidylcholine: a chemotactic factor for human monocytes and its potential role in atherogenesis. *Proc Natl Acad Sci USA* 1988;85:2805–2809.
59. Gu L, Okada Y, Clinton SK, et al. Absence of monocyte chemoattractant protein-1 reduces atherosclerosis in low density lipoprotein receptor-deficient mice. *Mol Cell* 1998;2:275–281.
60. Gosling J, Slaymaker S, Gu L, et al. MCP-1 deficiency reduces susceptibility to atherosclerosis in mice that overexpress human apolipoprotein B. *J Clin Invest* 1999;103:773–778.
61. Murugesan G, Chisolm GM, Fox PL. Oxidized low density lipoprotein inhibits the migration of aortic endothelial cells in vitro. *J Cell Biol* 1993;120:1011–1019.
62. Arai M, Imai H, Koumura T, et al. Mitochondrial phospholipid hydroperoxide glutathione peroxidase plays a major role in preventing oxidative injury to cells. *J Biol Chem* 1999;274:4924–4933.
63. Hamik A, Setiadi H, Bu G, et al. Down-regulation of monocyte tissue factor mediated by tissue factor pathway inhibitor and the low density lipoprotein receptor-related protein. *J Biol Chem* 1999;274:4962–4969.
64. Remacle J, Michiels C, Raes M. The importance of antioxidant enzymes in cellular aging and degeneration. *EXS* 1992;62:99–108.
65. Freeman M, Ekkel Y, Rohrer L, et al. Expression of type I and type II bovine scavenger receptors in Chinese hamster ovary cells: lipid droplet accumulation and nonreciprocal cross competition by acetylated and oxidized low density lipoprotein. *Proc Natl Acad Sci USA* 1991;88:4931–4935.
66. Endemann G, Stanton LW, Madden KS, et al. CD36 is a receptor for oxidized low density lipoprotein. *J Biol Chem* 1993;268:11811–11816.
67. Stanton LW, White RT, Bryant CM, et al. A macrophage Fc receptor for IgG is also a receptor for oxidized low density lipoprotein. *J Biol Chem* 1992;267:22446–22451.
68. Salonen JT, Yla-Herttuala S, Yamamoto R, et al. Autoantibody against oxidised LDL and progression of carotid atherosclerosis. *Lancet* 1992;339:883–887.
69. Chang MK, Binder CJ, Torzewski M, et al. C-reactive protein binds to both oxidized LDL and apoptotic cells through recognition of a common ligand: phosphorylcholine of oxidized phospholipids. *Proc Natl Acad Sci USA* 2002;99:13043–13048.
70. Hazen SL, Chisolm GM. Oxidized phosphatidylcholines: pattern recognition ligands for multiple pathways of the innate immune response. *Proc Natl Acad Sci USA* 2002;99:12515–12517.
71. Hoff HF, Whitaker TE, O'Neil J. Oxidation of low density lipoprotein leads to particle aggregation and altered macrophage recognition. *J Biol Chem* 1992;267:602–609.
72. Suzuki H, Kurihara Y, Takeya M, et al. A role for macrophage scavenger receptors in atherosclerosis and susceptibility to infection. *Nature* 1997;386:292–296.
73. Febbraio M, Podrez EA, Smith JD, et al. Targeted disruption of the class B scavenger receptor CD36 protects against atherosclerotic lesion development in mice. *J Clin Invest* 2000;105:1049–1056.
74. Podrez EA, Poliakov E, Shen Z, et al. Identification of a novel family of oxidized phospholipids that serve as ligands for the macrophage scavenger receptor CD36. *J Biol Chem* 2002;277:38503–38516.
75. Gillotte KL, Horkko S, Witztum JL, et al. Oxidized phospholipids, linked to apolipoprotein B of oxidized LDL, are ligands for macrophage scavenger receptors. *J Lipid Res* 2000;41:824–833.
76. Dhaliwal BS, Steinbrecher UP. Scavenger receptors and oxidized low density lipoproteins. *Clin Chim Acta* 1999;286:191–205.
77. Yamada Y, Doi T, Hamakubo T, et al. Scavenger receptor family proteins: roles for atherosclerosis, host defense and disorders of the central nervous system. *Cell Mol Life Sci* 1998;54:628–640.
78. Chisolm GM, Chai Y. Regulation of cell growth by oxidized LDL. *Free Radic Biol Med* 2000;28:1697–1707.
79. Chai YC, Binion DG, Chisolm GM. Relationship of molecular structure to the mechanism of lysophospholipid-induced smooth muscle cell proliferation. *Am J Physiol Heart Circ Physiol* 2000;279: H1830–H1838.
80. Chai YC, Howe PH, DiCorleto PE, et al. Oxidized low density lipoprotein and lysophosphatidylcholine stimulate cell cycle entry in vascular smooth muscle cells: evidence for release of FGF-2. *J Biol Chem* 1996;271:17791–17797.
81. Stiko-Rahm A, Hultgardh-Nilsson A, Regnstrom J, et al. Native and oxidized LDL enhances production of PDGF AA and the surface expression of PDGF receptors in cultured human smooth muscle cells. *Arterioscler Thromb* 1992;12:1099–1109.
82. Nakano T, Raines EW, Abraham JA, et al. Lysophosphatidylcholine upregulates the level of heparin-binding epidermal growth factor-like growth factor mRNA in human monocytes. *Proc Natl Acad Sci USA* 1994;91:1069–1073.
83. Kume N, Gimbrone MA Jr. Lysophosphatidylcholine transcriptionally induces growth factor gene expression in cultured human endothelial cells. *J Clin Invest* 1994;93:907–911.
84. Rajavashisth TB, Andalibi A, Territo MC, et al. Induction of endothelial cell expression of granulocyte and macrophage colony-stimulating factors by modified low-density lipoproteins. *Nature* 1990;344: 254–257.
85. Smith JD, Trogan E, Ginsberg M, et al. Decreased atherosclerosis in mice deficient in both macrophage colony-stimulating factor (*op*) and apolipoprotein E. *Proc Natl Acad Sci USA* 1995;92:8264–8268.
86. Lenaz G, Cavazzoni M, Genova ML, et al. Oxidative stress, antioxidant defenses and aging. *Biofactors* 1998;8:195–204.
87. Ghosh PK, Vasanji A, Murugesan G, et al. Membrane microviscosity regulates endothelial cell motility. *Nat Cell Biol* 2002;4:894–900.
88. Colles SM, Maxson JM, Carlson SG, et al. Oxidized LDL-induced injury and apoptosis in atherosclerosis. Potential roles for oxysterols. *Trends Cardiovasc Med* 2001;11:131–138.
89. Kosugi K, Morel DW, DiCorleto PE, et al. Toxicity of oxidized low-

density lipoprotein to cultured fibroblasts is selective for S phase of the cell cycle. *J Cell Physiol* 1987;130:311–320.

90. Borsum T, Henriksen B, Carlander B, et al. Injury to human cells in culture induced by low density lipoprotein: an effect independent of receptor binding and endocytotic uptake of low density lipoprotein. *Scand J Clin Lab Invest* 1982;42:75–81.

91. Negre-Salvayre A, Lopez M, Levade T, et al. Ultraviolet-treated lipoproteins as a model system for the study of the biological effects of lipid peroxides on cultured cells. II. Uptake and cytotoxicity of ultraviolet-treated LDL on lymphoid cell lines. *Biochim Biophys Acta* 1990;1045:224–232.

92. Zhang H, Basra HJK, Steinbrecher UP. Effects of oxidatively modified LDL on cholesterol esterification in cultured macrophages. *J Lipid Res* 1990;31:1361–1369.

93. Bhadra S, Arshad MAQ, Rymaszewski Z, et al. Oxidation of cholesterol moiety of low density lipoprotein in the presence of human endothelial cells or CU^{+2} ions: identification of major products and their effects. *Biochem Biophys Res Commun* 1991;176:431–440.

94. Colles SM, Irwin KC, Chisolm GM. Roles of multiple oxidized LDL lipids in cellular injury: dominance of 7 beta-hydroperoxycholesterol. *J Lipid Res* 1996;37:2018–2028.

95. Jurgens G, Hoff HF, Chisolm GM, et al. Modification of human serum low density lipoprotein by oxidation—characterization and pathophysiologic implications. *Chem Phys Lipids* 1987;45: 315–336.

96. Chisolm GM. Cytotoxicity of oxidized lipoproteins. *Curr Opin Lipidol* 1991;2:311–316.

97. Chisolm GM, Ma G, Irwin KC, et al. 7 beta-hydroperoxycholest-5-en-3 beta-ol, a component of human atherosclerotic lesions, is the primary cytotoxin of oxidized human low density lipoprotein. *Proc Natl Acad Sci USA* 1994;91:11452–11456.

98. Hughes H, Mathews B, Lenz ML, et al. Cytotoxicity of oxidized LDL to porcine aortic smooth muscle cells is associated with the oxysterols 7-ketocholesterol and 7-hydroxycholesterol. *Arterioscler Thromb* 1994;14:1177–1185.

99. Coffey MD, Cole RA, Colles SM, et al. In vitro cell injury by oxidized low density lipoprotein involves lipid hydroperoxide-induced formation of alkoxyl, lipid, and peroxyl radicals. *J Clin Invest* 1995; 96:1866–1873.

100. Brown AJ, Jessup W. Oxysterols and atherosclerosis. *Atherosclerosis* 1999;142:1–28.

101. Mallat Z, Tedgui A. Current perspective on the role of apoptosis in atherothrombotic disease. *Circ Res* 2001;88:998–1003.

102. Salvayre R, Auge N, Benoist H, et al. Oxidized low-density lipoprotein-induced apoptosis. *Biochim Biophys Acta* 2002;1585:213–221.

103. Thomas JP, Maiorino M, Ursini F, et al. Protective action of phospholipid hydroperoxide glutathione peroxidase against membrane-damaging lipid peroxidation. In situ reduction of phospholipid and cholesterol hydroperoxides. *J Biol Chem* 1990;265:454–461.

104. Thomas JP, Geiger PG, Girotti AW. Lethal damage to endothelial cells by oxidized low density lipoprotein: role of selenoperoxidases in cytoprotection against lipid hydroperoxide- and iron-mediated reactions. *J Lipid Res* 1993;34:479–490.

105. Ng CJ, Wadleigh DJ, Gangopadhyay A, et al. Paraoxonase-2 is a ubiquitously expressed protein with antioxidant properties and is capable of preventing cell-mediated oxidative modification of low density lipoprotein. *J Biol Chem* 2001;276:44444–44449.

106. Reddy ST, Wadleigh DJ, Grijalva V, et al. Human paraoxonase-3 is an HDL-associated enzyme with biological activity similar to paraoxonase-1 protein but is not regulated by oxidized lipids. *Arterioscler Thromb Vasc Biol* 2001;21:542–547.

107. Navab M, Hama SY, Hough GP, et al. High density associated enzymes: their role in vascular biology. *Curr Opin Lipidol* 1998;9: 449–456.

108. Shih DM, Gu L, Xia YR, et al. Mice lacking serum paraoxonase are susceptible to organophosphate toxicity and atherosclerosis. *Nature* 1998;394:284–287.

109. Randi AM, Biguzzi E, Falciani F, et al. Identification of differentially expressed genes in coronary atherosclerotic plaques from patients with stable or unstable angina by cDNA array analysis. *J Thromb Haemost* 2003;1:829–835.

110. Ardissino D, Merlini PA, Bauer KA, et al. Thrombogenic potential of human coronary atherosclerotic plaques. *Blood* 2001;98:2726–2729.

111. Yen MH, Pilkington G, Starling RC, et al. Increased tissue factor expression predicts development of cardiac allograft vasculopathy. *Circulation* 2002;106:1379–1383.

112. Wilcox JN, Smith KM, Schwartz SM, et al. Localization of tissue factor in the normal vessel wall and in the atherosclerotic plaque. *Proc Natl Acad Sci USA* 1989;86:2839–2843.

113. Taubman MB. Tissue factor regulation in vascular smooth muscle: a summary of studies performed using in vivo and in vitro models. *Am J Cardiol* 1993;72:55C–60C.

114. Hamilton JA, Myers D, Jessup W, et al. Oxidized LDL can induce macrophage survival, DNA synthesis, and enhanced proliferative response to CSF-1 and GM-CSF. *Arterioscler Thromb Vasc Biol* 1999;19:98–105.

115. Taubman MB, Marmur JD, Rosenfield CL, et al. Agonist-mediated tissue factor expression in cultured vascular smooth muscle cells: role of Ca^{2+} mobilization and protein kinase C activation. *J Clin Invest* 1993;91:547–552.

116. Drake TA, Hannani K, Fei HH, et al. Minimally oxidized low-density lipoprotein induces tissue factor expression in cultured human endothelial cells. *Am J Pathol* 1991;138:601–607.

117. Weis JR, Pitas RE, Wilson BD, et al. Oxidized low-density lipoprotein increases cultured human endothelial cell tissue factor activity and reduces protein C activation. *FASEB J* 1991;5:2459–2465.

118. Brand K, Banka CL, Mackman N, et al. Oxidized LDL enhances lipopolysaccharide-induced tissue factor expression in human adherent monocytes. *Arterioscler Thromb* 1994;14:790–797.

119. Petit L, Lesnik P, Dachet C, et al. Tissue factor pathway inhibitor is expressed by human monocyte-derived macrophages: relationship to tissue factor induction by cholesterol and oxidized LDL. *Arterioscler Thromb Vasc Biol* 1999;19:309–315.

120. Ohsawa M, Koyama T, Yamamoto K, et al. 1alpha,25-dihydroxyvitamin D(3) and its potent synthetic analogs downregulate tissue factor and upregulate thrombomodulin expression in monocytic cells, counteracting the effects of tumor necrosis factor and oxidized LDL. *Circulation* 2000;102:2867–2872.

121. Lewis JC, Bennett-Cain AL, DeMars CS, et al. Procoagulant activity after exposure of monocyte-derived macrophages to minimally oxidized low density lipoprotein: co-localization of tissue factor antigen and nascent fibrin fibers at the cell surface. *Am J Pathol* 1995;147: 1029–1040.

122. Cui MZ, Penn MS, Chisolm GM. Native and oxidized low density lipoprotein induction of tissue factor gene expression in smooth muscle cells is mediated by both Egr-1 and Sp1. *J Biol Chem* 1999;274: 32795–32802.

123. Penn MS, Cui MZ, Winokur AL, et al. Smooth muscle cell surface tissue factor pathway activation by oxidized low-density lipoprotein requires cellular lipid peroxidation. *Blood* 2000;96:3056–3063.

124. Penn MS, Patel CV, Cui MZ, et al. LDL increases inactive tissue factor on vascular smooth muscle cell surfaces: hydrogen peroxide activates latent cell surface tissue factor. *Circulation* 1999;99:1753–1759.

125. Cui MZ, Zhao G, Winokur AL, et al. Lysophosphatidic acid induction of tissue factor expression in aortic smooth muscle cells. *Arterioscler Thromb Vasc Biol* 2003;23:224–230.

126. Edgington TS, Ruf W, Rehemtulla A, et al. The molecular biology of initiation of coagulation by tissue factor. *Curr Stud Hematol Blood Transfus* 1991;(58):15–21.

127. Kugiyama K, Sakamoto T, Misumi I, et al. Transferable lipids in oxidized low-density lipoprotein stimulate plasminogen activator inhibitor-1 and inhibit tissue-type plasminogen activator release from endothelial cells. *Circ Res* 1993;73:335–343.

128. Morel DW, Chisolm GM. Antioxidant treatment of diabetic rats inhibits lipoprotein oxidation and cytotoxicity. *J Lipid Res* 1989;30: 1827–1834.

129. Carew TE, Schwenke DC, Steinberg D. Antiatherogenic effect of probucol unrelated to its hypocholesterolemic effect: evidence that antioxidants in vivo can selectively inhibit low density lipoprotein degradation in macrophage-rich fatty streaks and slow the progression of atherosclerosis in the Watanabe heritable hyperlipidemic rabbit. *Proc Natl Acad Sci USA* 1987;84:7725–7729.

130. Kita T, Nagano Y, Yokode M, et al. Probucol prevents the progression of atherosclerosis in Watanabe heritable hyperlipidemic rabbit, an animal model for familial hypercholesterolemia. *Proc Natl Acad Sci USA* 1987;84:5928–5931.

131. Steinberg D, Lewis A. Conner memorial lecture. Oxidative modification of LDL and atherogenesis. *Circulation* 1997;95:1062–1071.

132. Brasen JH, Koenig K, Bach H, et al. Comparison of the effects of alpha-tocopherol, ubiquinone-10 and probucol at therapeutic doses on atherosclerosis in WHHL rabbits. *Atherosclerosis* 2002;163:249–259.

133. Tangirala RK, Casanada F, Miller E, et al. Effect of the antioxidant N,N'-diphenyl 1,4-phenylenediamine (DPPD) on atherosclerosis in apoE-deficient mice. *Arterioscler Thromb Vasc Biol* 1995;15:1625–1630.

134. Bird DA, Tangirala RK, Fruebis J, et al. Effect of probucol on LDL oxidation and atherosclerosis in LDL receptor-deficient mice. *J Lipid Res* 1998;39:1079–1090.

135. Pratico D, Tangirala RK, Rader DJ, et al. Vitamin E suppresses isoprostane generation in vivo and reduces atherosclerosis in ApoE-deficient mice. *Nat Med* 1998;4:1189–1192.

136. Cyrus T, Yao Y, Rokach J, et al. Vitamin E reduces progression of atherosclerosis in low-density lipoprotein receptor-deficient mice with established vascular lesions. *Circulation* 2003;107:521–523.

137. Shaish A, George J, Gilburd B, et al. Dietary beta-carotene and alpha-tocopherol combination does not inhibit atherogenesis in an ApoE-deficient mouse model. *Arterioscler Thromb Vasc Biol* 1999;19:1470–1475.

138. Thomas SR, Leichtweis SB, Pettersson K, et al. Dietary cosupplementation with vitamin E and coenzyme Q(10) inhibits atherosclerosis in apolipoprotein E gene knockout mice. *Arterioscler Thromb Vasc Biol* 2001;21:585–593.

139. Gey KF, Puska P. Plasma vitamins E and A inversely correlated to mortality from ischemic heart disease in cross-cultural epidemiology. *Ann NY Acad Sci* 1989;570:268–282.

140. Rimm EB, Stampfer MJ, Ascherio A, et al. Vitamin E consumption and the risk of coronary heart disease in men. *N Engl J Med* 1993;328:1450–1456.

141. Stampfer MJ, Hennekens CH, Manson JE, et al. Vitamin E consumption and the risk of coronary disease in women. *N Engl J Med* 1993;328:1444–1449.

142. Stephens NG, Parsons A, Schofield PM, et al. Randomized controlled trial of vitamin E in patients with coronary disease: Cambridge Heart Antioxidant Study. *Lancet* 1996;347:781–786.

143. de Gaetano G. Low-dose aspirin and vitamin E in people at cardiovascular risk: a randomised trial in general practice. Collaborative Group of the Primary Prevention Project. *Lancet* 2001;357:89–95.

144. MRC/BHF Heart Protection Study of antioxidant vitamin supplementation in 20,536 high-risk individuals: a randomised placebo-controlled trial. *Lancet* 2002;360:23–33.

145. The effect of vitamin E and beta carotene on the incidence of lung cancer and other cancers in male smokers. The Alpha-Tocopherol, Beta Carotene Cancer Prevention Study Group. *N Engl J Med* 1994;330:1029–1035.

146. Yusuf S, Dagenais G, Pogue J, et al. Vitamin E supplementation and cardiovascular events in high-risk patients. The Heart Outcomes Prevention Evaluation Study Investigators. *N Engl J Med* 2000;342:154–160.

147. Dietary supplementation with n-3 polyunsaturated fatty acids and vitamin E after myocardial infarction: results of the GISSI-Prevenzione trial. Gruppo Italiano per lo Studio della Sopravvivenza nell'Infarto miocardico. *Lancet* 1999;354:447–455.

148. Vivekananthan DP, Penn MS, Sapp SK, et al. Use of antioxidant vitamins for the prevention of cardiovascular disease: meta-analysis of randomised trials. *Lancet* 2003;361:2017–2023.

149. Upston JM, Kritharides L, Stocker R. The role of vitamin E in atherosclerosis. *Prog Lipid Res* 2003;42:405–422.

150. Heinecke JW. Is the emperor wearing clothes? Clinical trials of vitamin E and the LDL oxidation hypothesis. *Arterioscler Thromb Vasc Biol* 2001;21:1261–1264.

151. Pratico D. Vitamin E: murine studies versus clinical trials. *Ital Heart J* 2001;2:878–881.

152. Heinecke JW. Clinical trials of vitamin E in coronary artery disease: is it time to reconsider the low-density lipoprotein oxidation hypothesis? *Curr Atheroscler Rep* 2003;5:83–87.

153. Parthasarathy S, Khan-Merchant N, Penumetcha M, et al. Did the antioxidant trials fail to validate the oxidation hypothesis? *Curr Atheroscler Rep* 2001;3:392–398.

154. Heinecke JW. Oxidative stress: new approaches to diagnosis and prognosis in atherosclerosis. *Am J Cardiol* 2003;91:12A–16A.

155. Cyrus T, Pratico D, Zhao L, et al. Absence of 12/15-lipoxygenase expression decreases lipid peroxidation and atherogenesis in apolipoprotein e-deficient mice. *Circulation* 2001;103:2277–2282.

156. Detmers PA, Hernandez M, Mudgett J, et al. Deficiency in inducible nitric oxide synthase results in reduced atherosclerosis in apolipoprotein E-deficient mice. *J Immunol* 2000;165:3430–3435.

157. Kirk EA, Dinauer MC, Rosen H, et al. Impaired superoxide production due to a deficiency in phagocyte NADPH oxidase fails to inhibit atherosclerosis in mice. *Arterioscler Thromb Vasc Biol* 2000;20:1529–1535.

158. Tward A, Xia YR, Wang XP, et al. Decreased atherosclerotic lesion formation in human serum paraoxonase transgenic mice. *Circulation* 2002;106:484–490.

CHAPTER 9

Lipoprotein(a)

Angelo M. Scanu

Key Words: Apolipoprotein(a); apolipoprotein B-100; atherothrombosis; lipoprotein(a).

INTRODUCTION

Lipoprotein(a) (Lp[a]), discovered by Kare Berg more than 40 years ago (1), represents a class of lipoprotein particles having as a protein moiety apolipoprotein B-100 (apoB-100), linked to apolipoprotein(a) (apo[a]), a highly glycosylated multikringle structure exhibiting a marked degree of homology with plasminogen. apo(a) represents a quantitative genetic trait transmitted in an autosomal codominant mode. The biomedical interest in this lipoprotein has emerged from several epidemiologic studies showing an association between its high plasma levels and coronary heart disease, peripheral vascular disease, and stroke. It also has been recognized that this association can be influenced by ethnic background, age, and sex. The plasma levels of Lp(a) vary about 1,000-fold among individuals, but they are rather steady throughout life in the same individual. Complicating this picture of the Lp(a) assays are the lack of standardized methodology, universally accepted primary and secondary standards, and uniformity in the cutoff point between normal and abnormal plasma levels (2).

LIPOPROTEIN(A) STRUCTURE

In a normotriglyceridemic state, the lipoprotein component of Lp(a) is an low-density lipoprotein (LDL)-like structure that may vary in size and density depending on lipid content

and distribution (3). The protein moiety, apoB-100, approximately 500 kD, is linked by a single disulfide bond in a 1:1 molar ratio to apo(a), varying in mass between 300 and 800 kD. Because of this important size polymorphism, the Lp(a) varies markedly in density and molecular weight (3). apoB-100 wraps about the lipid sphere (Fig. 9–1), making multiple contacts within and below the particle surface. Conversely, apo(a) is a highly elongated protein that greatly increases the intrinsic viscosity of Lp(a). The bulk of circulating apo(a) is linked to LDL particles with no apparent preference for their density or size. In hypertriglyceridemic states, a small portion of the apoB:apo(a) complex also is present in triglyceride-rich particles. Usually, there is little free apo(a) in the circulation, probably because once dissociated from parent Lp(a), apo(a), largely fragmented, is rapidly cleared from the plasma through the kidney.

apo(a), although similar to plasminogen (Fig. 9–2), has distinctive features that differ from plasminogen. For example, (i) apo(a) has several exact tandem copies of kringle IV that determine its size; (ii) the kringle IV lidomains contain glycosylation sites (N-glycans) not present in kringle IV of plasminogen; (iii) the interlinkers of apo(a) are highly glycosylated (O-glycans), contributing to a large extent to the high carbohydrate content of apo(a) (about 30% by weight); (iv) kringle IV_{10} contains the lysine-binding site involved in many critical functions of apo(a); and (v) kringle IV_9 contains an "extra" cysteine residue involved in covalent linkage with an unpaired cysteine in the C-terminal region of apoB-100 (3). The protein's size varies largely among individuals. The *apo(a)* gene contains from a 15 to 40 kringle domains—encoding proteins that range in molecular mass from 300 to 800 kD (Fig. 9–3).

A. M. Scanu: University of Chicago, Chicago, Illinois 60637

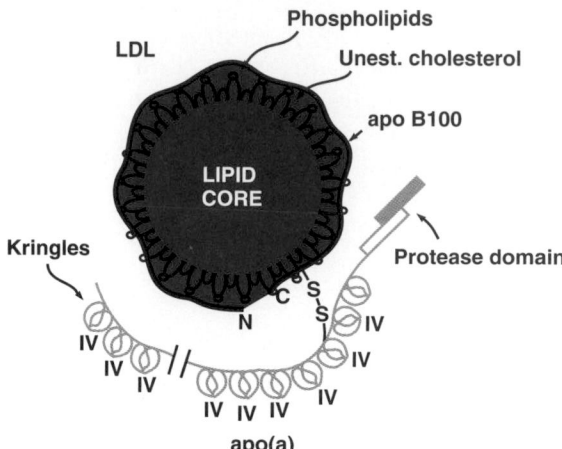

FIG. 9–1. Schematic model of the structure of human Lp(a). Lipoprotein(a) is made up of an LDL-like particle containing cholesterol, phospholipids, and apo B100, to which is covalently linked apo(a), the glycoprotein that is the specific marker of Lp(a). The dominant structural motif of apo(a) is a large domain made up of a number of kringles that resemble the kringle 4 of plasminogen. Individual alleles of apo(a) contain a range of from 13 to 40 kringle 4-like units and a single kringle 5 homolog. Kringles are looped structures stabilized by three disulfide bridges. Kringles are also found in proteins of the coagulation/fibrinolytic system. The homologous protease-like domain of apo(a) appears to be enzymatically inactive, suggesting that apo(a) may share substrates of plasminogen and compete for its binding and activation. (Scanu AM, Fless GM. Lipoprotein(a): Heterogeneity and biological relevance. *J Clin Invest* 1990;85:1709–1715.)

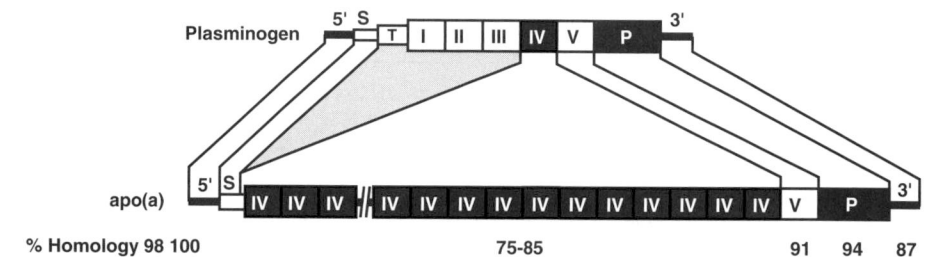

FIG. 9–2. Comparison of the sequence of apo(a) and plasminogin cDNA. Connecting lines indicate regions of homology with the percentage of DNA sequence identity for each domain shown below. Domain symbols refer to the 5′ untranslated, signal sequence, tail (or preactivation peptide), kringles 1–5, protease and 3′ untranslated regions. The apo(a) probably evolved from a duplicated *plasminogen* gene that has subsequently undergone deletion of several exons, multiplication of kringle-encoding domains, and base substitutions. (McLean JW, Tomlinson JE, Kuang WJ, Eaton DL, Chen EY, Fless GM, Scanu AM, Lawn RM. Human apolipoprotein(a): cDNA sequence of an apolipoprotein homologous to plasminogen. *Nature* 1987;330:132–137.)

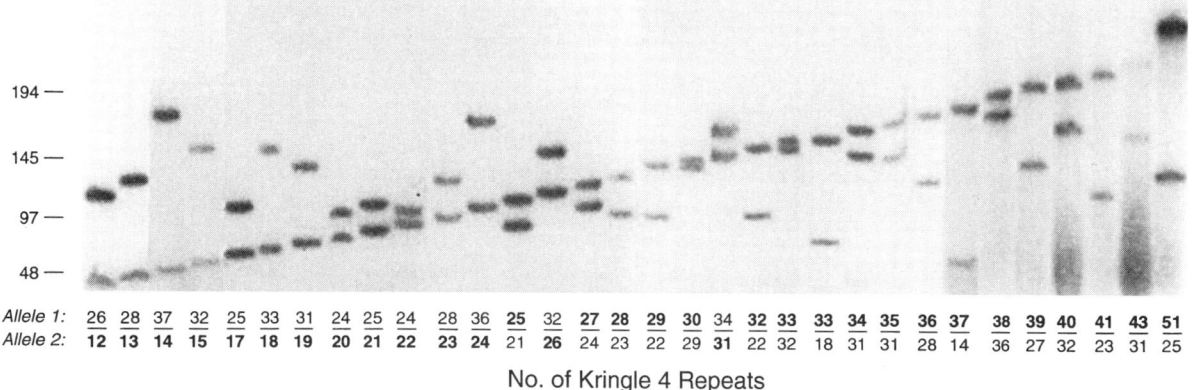

FIG. 9–3. Variation in the number of kringle repeats in the *apo(a)* gene leads to variation in the size of the protein. Genomic blots of the *apo(a)* gene after pulse-field electrophoresis from different human subjects shows that copies of the *apo(a)* gene may contain from about 15 to 40 kringles, encoding proteins with molecular mass ranging from about 300,000 to 800,000. (Lackner C, Cohen JC, Hobbs HH. Molecualr definition of the extreme size polymorphism in apolipoprotein(a). *Hum Mol Genet* 1993;2: 933–940.)

SYNTHESIS AND METABOLISM OF LIPOPROTEIN(A)

The synthesis of circulating apo(a) occurs in the liver (2,3). Currently, it is not established whether the assembly of Lp(a) takes place within or outside the hepatocyte. The most recent studies in primary baboon hepatocytes (4) indicate that apo(a) links to apoB-100 at the cell surface. In contrast, Edelstein and coworkers (5) provided evidence for the intracellular occurrence of the disulfide linkage in long-term primary human hepatocytes. Other studies have shown that much of the maturation of Lp(a) takes place in the circulation after hepatic secretion of apo(a) (6). The latter possibility receives support from human studies showing that in a given individual, the properties of the LDL of Lp(a) reflect those of the circulating apo(a)-free LDL particles (7).

In terms of catabolism, the major routes of plasma clearance of Lp(a) remain unknown, although they do not seem to involve the LDL receptor (see reviews in References 2 and 3). However, two turnover studies in humans have shown that from 10% to 20% of apo(a) can detach from Lp(a) in the circulation, resulting in the generation of Lp(a-) particle candidates for uptake by the LDL receptor (8,9). The site of this thiolytic event was not defined.

Control of Apo(a) Synthesis

Studies in human populations have indicated a general trend toward an inverse relation between apo(a) size and plasma Lp(a) levels (10,11). However, this is not always the case,

because within a given apo(a) size, important variations in plasma Lp(a) levels are observed pointing at the contribution of distinct regulatory elements in the *apo(a)* gene. Multiple factors are probably involved at the level of gene transcription, mRNA stability and translation, rate of apo(a) secretion affected by the efficiency of apo(a) folding and transport out of the endoplasmic reticulum, and degradation by proteasomes. In the Golgi, apo(a) is modified by the addition of N- and O-oligosaccharides before reaching the cell surface. In general, small apo(a) isoforms are secreted more efficiently than the large ones, because the latter tend to be degraded by proteasomes (12).

Although it is generally true that plasma Lp(a) levels remain constant throughout life, transient changes, although modest, have been reported after myocardial infarction and the administration of hormones, particularly estrogen and testosterone. Lp(a) levels also increase after menopause, orchidectomy, and the administration of growth hormone. Disease states that can affect plasma Lp(a) levels are hypothyroidism, acromegaly, nephrotic syndrome, and renal insufficiency (see Reference 12 for a review).

LIPOPROTEIN(A) AS A CARDIOVASCULAR PATHOGEN

Considering the pleiotropic functions of Lp(a), it is likely that several mechanisms contribute to its cardiovascular pathogenicity. Notably, because of sequence differences with plasminogen at the activation site, apo(a) is unable to

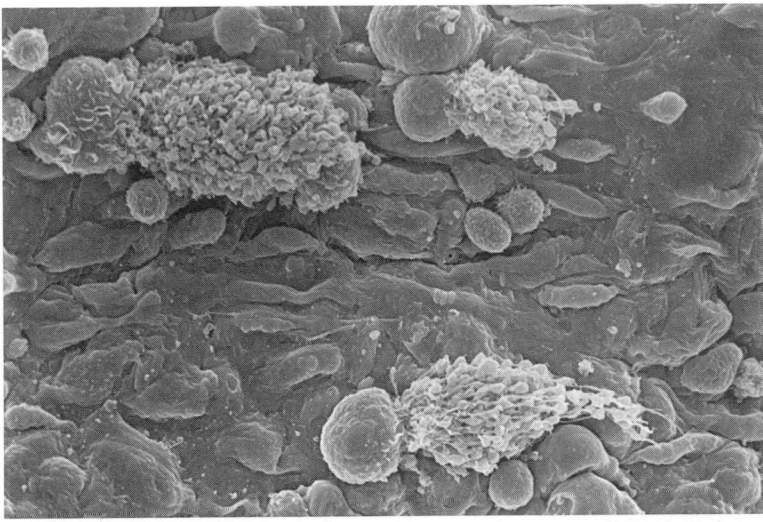

FIG. 9–4: Mural thrombi on the surface of vessel lesions, such as these seen here by scanning electron microscopy, may be a driving force in the growth of atherosclerotic plaque. Such thrombi might persist longer in individuals with elevated levels of Lp(a) because of inhibition of plasminogen activation. (Ross R. The pathogenesis of atherosclerosis: A perspective for the 1990s. *Nature* 1993;362:801–809.)

function as an active plasmin-like protease. apo(a), either free or constitutive of Lp(a), has been shown *in vitro* to act as a competitive inhibitor of the processes of plasminogen–plasmin conversion, clot lysis, the binding of plasminogen to endothelial and monocytoid cells and platelets, all indicative of a prothrombotic function (13,14). However, *in vivo*, no correlation has been found between high plasma Lp(a) levels and fibrinolytic parameters such as euglobulin clot lysis time, fibrin split products, or α_2-antiplasmin. It is possible that the study of plasma parameters are inadequate markers of the prothrombogenic function of Lp(a), because its expression may be more topical than generalized. Thrombi often are present on the surface of coronary vessels and within existing plaque (Fig. 9–4). Supportive evidence for a relation between plasma Lp(a) levels and thrombosis derives from studies on nonhuman primates showing a direct correlation between increased plasma levels of Lp(a) and enhancement of thrombosis in a segment of carotid artery with a clamp-induced injury (15). Thus, under defined settings, Lp(a) can function as a cardiovascular pathogen. It is possible that some of the inconsistencies in the literature may depend on the polymorphism of Lp(a) particles and apo(a) phenotype, with a varying effect on function also influenced by type of experimental models and procedures. A direct effect of Lp(a) on clot lysis *in vivo* recently has been demonstrated using apo(a) transgenic mice. In these animals, the lysis of radiolabeled clots was shown to be significantly retarded in comparison with control animals (16).

OTHER ACTIVITIES OF LIPOPROTEIN(A)

The inhibition of plasminogen activation by Lp(a) may have repercussions beyond clot lysis. Transforming growth factor-β (TGF-β) is a multipotential cytokine that inhibits cell proliferation in a number of cell types. The TGF-β is synthesized as a latent molecule that requires cleavage of its propeptide region by proteases such as plasmin. Grainger and colleagues (17) report that Lp(a) or recombinant apo(a) stimulates proliferation of cultured human vascular smooth cells in a dose-dependent manner, whereas LDL does not. This effect results from inhibition of plasminogen activation and, consequently, activation of plasmin, a latent TGF-β. Similarly, apo(a), in addition to TGF-β activation, increases the motility of smooth muscle cells cocultured with endothelial cells in a wound response model (18). Because smooth muscle proliferation and migration are hallmarks of atherothrombosis and restenosis, these results point to other possible mechanisms for the pathogenic action of Lp(a).

Another property of Lp(a) is to bind to components of the vascular extracellular matrix typically found in atherothrombotic plaques such as glycosaminoglycans, proteoglycans, and fibronectin, accounting for the increased accumulation of Lp(a) as compared with LDL in the atherothrombotic lesions. In addition, bound Lp(a) can either readily aggregate, be readily degraded by oxidative, lipolytic proteolytic events, or undergo thiolysis of the disulfide bond. The aggregated

Lp(a) is readily taken up and internalized by macrophages, leading to the formation of foam cells, an early event in the atherothrombotic process. It also has been suggested that proteolytically-derived apo(a) fragments can be bioactive in terms of perpetuating macrophage activation (2,3).

ANIMAL MODELS

The *apo(a)* gene may have developed from a duplicated *plasminogen* gene during the course of evolution of primates. Currently, Lp(a) has been detected only in humans, some species of the Old World monkeys, apes, and an insectivore, the European hedgehog. The common features in all of these species is the covalent linkage between apo(a) and apoB-100 and the presence of multiple kringle domains (12). However, there are important sequence differences, the most salient among them, the presence of only kringle III and the absence of the protease domain in hedgehog apo(a). Moreover, in rhesus monkey, apo(a) Trp72 is replaced by Arg in the lysine-binding site of kringle IV 10, and thus is a lysine negative species (3).

The transgenic mouse has become a valuable tool in the study of apo(a) and its interactions with other gene products involved in lipid transport and metabolism. The human *apo(a)* gene has been successfully introduced into the mouse, an animal species that normally lacks this protein. In contrast to the human model, the apo(a) circulating in the mouse was almost entirely free of lipid association, because of the lack of affinity of the human recombinant for mouse LDL. These transgenic mice developed extensive fatty streak-type vascular lesions when maintained on a high-fat diet for 3 months (19). However, no lesion development was noted in the animals fed a low-fat diet. The results of these studies suggest that free apo(a) can be atherogenic in addition to another risk factor. These transgenic mice have subsequently been used to study the effects of apo(a) on clot lysis (16) and TGF-β activation (20) *in vivo* and the counteracting effect of the human *apoA-1* gene (21). In addition, a double transgenic mouse expressing both human apo(a) and human apoB-100 has been shown to be capable of forming a complete Lp(a) particle with a disulfide linkage between the two apolipoproteins (22,23).

HUMAN VARIANTS

It is now apparent that single nucleotide substitutions in the *apo(a)* gene can occur. However, because of its large size, the search for these substitutions has to be limited to regions of suspected functional importance. In this respect, the region of the *apo(a)* gene coding for the lysine-binding pocket of kringle IV_{10} can now be readily amplified (24). The technique has been used successfully to identify a mutation in the lymphocyte DNA of human subjects exhibiting an Lp(a) with a functional defect in lysine binding (24). Pfaffinger and coworkers (24) have found an important variation in lysine binding among subjects, and the heterogeneity motif is likely also to apply for other functions of apo(a). As we continue to develop suitable techniques to correlate given apo(a) functions to specific domains in the *apo(a)* gene, we should be in a position to assess the actual frequency of the sequence-dependent functional polymorphism of apo(a) and of its role in atherothrombogenesis. However, it is important to realize that changes in apo(a) function may not all be secondary to mutations at the gene level and may depend, for example, on reductive or oxidative events occurring in the circulation leading to changes in the structural organization and stability of the kringles of apo(a). These events are more likely to occur in disease states or during the administration of pharmacologic agents capable of interacting with kringle structures, or both.

THERAPEUTIC APPROACHES

Thus far, the main goal has been to decrease the plasma levels of Lp(a) on the undocumented premise that its cardiovascular pathogenicity is related to high plasma levels. However, it is now apparent that neither changes in lifestyle commonly used in the treatment of dyslipoproteinemic states nor pharmacologic agents such as 3-hydroxy-3-methylglutaryl coenzyme A reductase inhibitors and fibrates have proven to be effective. An exception is niacin, which, in dosages of 3 to 4 g daily, has been shown to decrease the plasma levels of Lp(a) by about 30% (25,26). However, this experience is not universal and may depend on pretreatment plasma Lp(a) levels, apo(a) phenotype, dosage, and length of treatment. Because of the potential side effects of high doses of niacin, the risk/benefit relations must be carefully evaluated with particular reference to impaired liver function, glucose intolerance, hyperuricemia, and dermatologic changes. Thus, the use of niacin may be confined to those cases with high plasma levels of Lp(a) and a personal or family history of atherosclerotic cardiovascular disease for whom niacin may also act on a frequently present dyslipidemic state. Several reports have shown that hormones, particularly estrogen, may significantly decrease plasma Lp(a) (27–29); however, their safety in a sustained treatment program remains to be established. What obviously is needed are specific agents targeted at apo(a). Some progress in this area has been made using ribozyme oligonucleotides against apo(a) (30) or apo(a) antisense RNA (31). However, the results obtained in either cell cultures or mice, although promising, cannot yet be translated to humans.

While waiting for these and other encouraging developments, an effective way to reduce the plasma levels of Lp(a) in severe cases is by LDL-apheresis. However, this technique is only available in specialized centers and is invasive, costly, and demanding of patient time and commitment.

FUTURE DIRECTIONS

Although epidemiologic studies have provided evidence for the atherothrombotic potential of Lp(a), many unknown factors remain regarding mechanisms likely to be pleiotropic. An emerging notion is that pathogenicity of Lp(a) may not just be related to total particle concentration, but also to the properties and heterogeneity of its constituents. It also is becoming apparent that Lp(a), like LDL, is subject to modifications by oxidative, lipolytic, and proteolytic events, inviting a close examination of the potential pathogenic function of the resulting products. At the same time, there is also a need to develop animal models that can meaningfully be applied to human pathology and also address therapies not only on the basis of reducing plasma levels of Lp(a), but also on pathogenetic mechanisms. Not of lesser importance is to shed light on the physiologic role of Lp(a), which is currently surrounded by a total mystery

REFERENCES

1. Berg K. A new serum type system in man: the Lp system. *Acta Pathol Microbiol Scand* 1963;59:369–382.
2. Scanu AM. The role of lipoprotein(a) in the pathogenesis of atherosclerotic cardiovascular disease and its utility as predictor of coronary heart disease events. *Curr Cardiol Reports* 2001;3:385–390.
3. Scanu AM, Nakajima K, Edelstein C. Apolipoprotein(a): structure and biology. *Front Biosci* 2001;6:546–554.
4. White AL, Lanford RE. Cell surface assembly of lipoprotein(a) in primary cultures of baboon hepatocytes. *J Biol Chem* 1994;269:28716–28723.
5. Edelstein C, Davidson NO, Scanu AM. Oleates stimulates the formation of triglyceride-rich particles containing apoB100-apo(a) in long-term primary cultures of human hepatocytes. *Chem Phys Lipids* 1994;67/68:135–143.
6. Chiesa G, Hobbs HH, Koschinsky ML, et al. Reconstitution of lipoprotein(a) by infusion of human LDL into transgenic mice expressing human apolipoprotein(a). *J Biol Chem* 1992;267:24369–24374.
7. Nakajima K, Hinman J, Pfaffinger D, et al. Changes in plasma triglyceride levels shift lipoprotein (a) density in parallel with that of LDL independently of apolipoprotein(a) size. *Arterioscler Thromb Vasc Biol* 2001;21:1238–1243.
8. Knight BL, Perombelon YF, Soutar AK, et al. Catabolism of lipoprotein (a) in familial hypercholesterolaemic subjects. *Atherosclerosis* 1991;87:227–237.
9. Rader DJ, Mann WA, Cain W, et al. The low density lipoprotein receptor is not required for normal catabolism of Lp(a) in humans. *J Clin Invest* 1985;95:1403–1408.
10. Utermann G, Duba C, Menzel HJ. Genetics of the quantitative Lp(a) lipoprotein trait. II. Inheritance of Lp(a) glycoprotein phenotypes. *Hum Genet* 1988;78:47–50.
11. Gaubatz JW, Ghanem KI, Guevara J Jr, et al. Polymorphic forms of human apolipoprotein(a) inheritance and relationship of their molecular weight to plasma levels of lipoprotein(a). *J Lipid Res* 1990;31:603–613.
12. Hobbs HH, White AL. Lipoprotein(a): intrigues and insights. *Curr Opin Lipidol* 1999;10:225–236.
13. Miles LA, Plow EF. Lp(a): an interloper into the fibrinolytic system? *Thromb Haemost* 1990;63:331–335.
14. Hajjar KA, Nachman RL. The role of lipoprotein(a) on atherogenesis and thrombosis. *Annu Rev Med* 1996;47:423–442.
15. Williams JK, Bellinger DA, Nichols TC, et al. Occlusive arterial thrombosis in cynomolgus monkeys with varying plasma concentrations of lipoprotein(a). *Arterioscler Thromb* 1993;13:548–554.
16. Palabrica TM, Liu AC, Aronovitz MJ, et al. Antifibrinolytic activity of apolipoprotein(a) in vivo: human apolipoprotein(a) transgenic mice are resistant to tissue plasminogen activator-mediated thrombolysis. *Nat Med* 1995;1:256–259.
17. Grainger DJ, Kirschenlohr HL, Metcalfe JC, et al. The proliferation of human smooth muscle cells is promoted by lipoprotein(a). *Science* 1993;260:1655–1658.
18. Kojima S, Harpel PC, Rifkin DB. Lipoprotein(a) inhibits the genera-

tion of transforming growth factor beta: an endogenous inhibitor of smooth muscle cell migration. *J Cell Biol* 1991;113:1439–1445.

19. Lawn RM, Wade DP, Hammer RE, et al. Atherogenesis in transgenic mice expressing human apolipoprotein(a). *Nature* 1992;360:670–672.

20. Grainger DJ, Kemp PR, Liu AC, et al. Activation of transforming growth factor-β is inhibited in apolipoprotein(a) transgenic mice. *Nature* 1994;370:460–462.

21. Liu AC, Lawn RM, Verstuyft JG, et al. Human apolipoprotein A-I prevents atherosclerosis associated with apolipoprotein(a) in transgenic mice. *J Lipid Res* 1994;35:2263–2267.

22. Callow M, Stoltzfus L, Lawn RM, et al. Expression of human apolipoprotein B and assembly of lipoprotein (a) in transgenic mice. *Proc Natl Acad Sci USA* 1994;91:2130–2134.

23. Linton MF, Farese RV, Chiesa G, et al. Transgenic mice expressing high plasma concentrations of human apolipoprotein B100 and lipoprotein(a). *J Clin Invest* 1993;92:3029–3037.

24. Pfaffinger D, McLean J, Scanu AM. Amplification of human apo(a) kringle 4-37 from blood lymphocyte DNA. *Biochim Biophys Acta* 1993;1225:107–109.

25. Gurakar A, Hoeg JM, Kostner G, et al. Levels of lipoprotein Lp(a) decline with neomycin and niacin treatment. *Atherosclerosis* 1985;57: 293–301.

26. Carlson LA, Hamsten A, Asplund A. Pronounced lowering of serum levels of lipoprotein Lp(a) in hyperlipidaemic subjects treated with nicotinic acid. *J Int Med Res* 1989;226:271–276.

27. Henriksson P, Angelin B, Berglund L. Hormonal regulation of serum Lp(a) levels: opposite effects after estrogen treatment and orchidectomy in males with prostatic carcinoma. *J Clin Invest* 1992;89: 1166–1171.

28. Soma MR, Osnago-Gadda I, Paoletti R, et al. The lowering of lipoprotein(a) induced by estrogen plus progesterone replacement therapy in postmenopausal women. *Arch Intern Med* 1993;153:1462–1468.

29. Crook D, Sidhu M, Seed M, et al. Lipoprotein Lp(a) levels are reduced by danazol, an anabolic steroid. *Atherosclerosis* 1992;92:41–47.

30. Morishita R, Yamada S, Yamamoto K, et al. Novel therapeutic strategies for atherosclerosis ribozyme oligonucleotides against apolipoprotein(a) selectively inhibit apolipoprotein(a) but not plasminogen gene expression *Circulation* 1998;98:1898–1904.

31. Frank S, Gauster M, Strauss J, et al. Adenovirus-mediated apo(a) antisense RNA expression efficiently inhibits apo(a) synthesis in vitro and in vivo. *Gene Ther* 2001;8:425–430.

CHAPTER 10

Clinical Classifications of Lipid Abnormalities

Thomas P. Bersot and Robert W. Mahley

Key Words: Dyslipidemia; lipoprotein phenotyping; atherogenic dyslipidemia; remnant lipoproteins; xanthoma.

INTRODUCTION

In the last 10 to 15 years, remarkable advances have been made in our understanding of the molecular pathophysiology and genetics of dyslipidemia and atherothrombosis (1–4). A host of clinical trials have been completed that validated the benefits of lipid-lowering therapy in adult patients with various degrees of risk for coronary heart disease (CHD) (5–11). A variety of novel (or nontraditional) risk assessment tests and technologies are being touted to better evaluate the extent of disease risk so that the intensity of treatment of risk factors is more appropriately matched to the degree of CHD risk (see Part III of this textbook). In support of this approach, the National Cholesterol Education Program (NCEP) has published an updated dyslipidemia treatment paradigm: the Adult Treatment Panel (ATP) III guidelines (12). These guidelines match the intensity of treatment of dyslipidemia to the degree of risk on the basis of assessment of traditional risk factors identified by the Framingham Study (13). For the

T. P. Bersot: Gladstone Institute of Cardiovascular Disease, Clinical Professor of Medicine, University of California, San Francisco, P.O. Box 419100, San Francisco, California 94141-9100.

R. W. Mahley: Gladstone Institute of Cardiovascular Disease, Professor of Pathology and Medicine, University of California, San Francisco, P.O. Box 419100, San Francisco, California 94141-9100.

primary providers of healthcare and the lay public, the volume of new information, the uncertainty about how to optimally assess risk factors, and concerns about the safety of hypolipidemic drugs have led to confusion about the management of dyslipidemia and undertreatment of patients with dyslipidemia (14,15).

It is important for everyone to realize that the major risk factors—smoking, hypertension (blood pressure > 120/180 mm Hg), and hypercholesterolemia (total cholesterol > 160 mg/dL)—identified years previously explain about 85% of excess CHD risk in the United States (16,17). Consequently, primary caregivers and public health policy makers should focus on detecting and managing the traditional risk factors and the lifestyle factors (diet and exercise) that modulate their severity. Lifestyle factors have become particularly important in view of the epidemic of overweight and obesity affecting adults and children in the United States (18,19).

Because insulin resistance is a consequence of being obese or overweight, the accompanying atherogenic dyslipidemia, which is characterized by low levels of high-density lipoprotein cholesterol (HDL-C) and hypertriglyceridemia, has become common (20). The ATP III guidelines proposed diagnostic criteria, including low HDL-C levels and hypertriglyceridemia, that define the high-CHD risk, insulin-resistant state under the rubric "metabolic syndrome" (12). When these criteria were applied to population-based data collected between 1988 and 1994, more than 40% of adults older than 60 years were found to have the metabolic syndrome (21). The metabolic syndrome is certain to be more prevalent now, given the increases in the rates of overweight and obese individuals during the last decade (18,19).

EVOLUTION OF THE CLASSIFICATION OF LIPID DISORDERS

Xanthomas Associated with Hyperlipidemia

The classification of clinical syndromes associated with hyperlipidemia began with descriptions of xanthomas, which are still useful in categorizing dyslipidemia (Table 10–1; Fig. 10–1). In the nineteenth century, planar xanthomas (those within the plane of the skin; Fig. 10–1, A and B) were described in association with biliary tract disease, and eruptive xanthomas (Fig. 10–1, J and K) were described in association with diabetes mellitus (22). Subsequently, tuberous xanthomas (Fig. 10–1, E–G) were recognized in siblings who died suddenly in childhood, which established the familial basis of this type of xanthoma and its serious medical consequences. It is likely that these children had homozygous familial hypercholesterolemia (FH) (22). Analysis of tuberous xanthomas revealed a high cholesterol content, which ultimately led to the correlation between this xanthoma type and severe hypercholesterolemia (22). Rare patients with severe hyperlipidemia and eruptive xanthomas in the absence of diabetes mellitus also were discovered, prompting the suggestion that hypertriglyceridemia might also play a role in the formation of certain types of xanthomas. However, real progress in the classification of lipid disorders began with application of techniques for measuring concentrations of blood lipids and the recognition that the metabolism of blood lipids is governed by the metabolism of the plasma lipoproteins.

Lipoprotein Identification and Hyperlipoproteinemia Phenotyping

The four major lipoprotein classes are chylomicrons, very low-density lipoproteins (VLDLs), low-density lipoproteins (LDLs), and HDLs (for a review see Reference 23). As the HDLs were studied further, two major subfractions were defined: HDL_2 and HDL_3. Almost immediately, the LDLs (for

a review see Reference 24) were found to have a direct relation with atherothrombosis, whereas the HDLs had an inverse relation (25).

In 1967, a diagnostic and treatment classification system was proposed on the basis of the identification of the specific lipoprotein abnormalities causing hyperlipidemia in patients (26). The plasma lipoprotein abnormalities were identified by fat staining of electrophoretically separated plasma and estimation of the cholesterol concentrations of VLDLs, LDLs, and HDLs (27). This approach identified six common phenotypes (I, IIa, IIb, III, IV, and V) that became quite useful as a shorthand method of describing the lipoprotein abnormalities of patients with hyperlipidemia. For each phenotype, disorders causing secondary phenocopies were identified, and it was suggested that one or more genetic disorders might produce the same lipoprotein phenotype.

GENETIC DIVERSITY OF LIPOPROTEIN PHENOTYPES

Studies of the lipid and lipoprotein abnormalities in survivors of myocardial infarction and their family members provide evidence that persons affected with different lipoprotein phenotypes could exist in the same kindred (28,29). Later it was found that mutations of separate genes produce phenocopies of each of the six phenotypes (24,30–37). These observations proved that lipoprotein phenotyping was not useful for identifying specific genetic disorders that cause hyperlipidemia.

Single-Gene Mutations for Lipid Disorders

In the last decade, mutations have been detected in most of the genes' encoding proteins involved in plasma lipid metabolism (for a review see Reference 23). These include the apolipoproteins (38,39), the LDL receptor (40), lipoprotein lipase and hepatic lipase (41,42), lecithin:cholesterol acyltransferase (43), cholesterol ester transfer protein (44), microsomal triglyceride transfer protein (45), and the adenosine triphosphate–binding cassette proteins (46). Despite the vast number of mutations that have been discovered, the clinically relevant single-gene mutations that promote atherothrombosis are those causing increased concentrations of LDLs or of remnant lipoproteins. It remains to be

TABLE 10–1. *Classification of xanthomas associated with primary and secondary dyslipidemia*

Xanthoma	Location	Associated conditions
Planar	Palmar and intertriginous creases of the extremities	*Primary dyslipidemia:* type III hyperlipoproteinemia; *Secondary dyslipidemia:* obstructive liver disease, multiple myeloma, hypothyroidism
Tuberous or tuberoeruptive	Elbow, dorsum of hand, knee, buttocks	Type III hyperlipoproteinemia, homozygous familial hypercholesterolemia
Tendon	Extensor tendons of hands, Achilles tendon	Familial hypercholesterolemia, autosomal-recessive hypercholesterolemia, familial defective apolipoprotein B-100, type III hyperlipoproteinemia (rare), β-sitosterolemia
Eruptive	Arm and thigh (posterolateral surface), back, buttocks	*Primary dyslipidemia:* lipoprotein lipase deficiency, apolipoprotein C-II deficiency; *Secondary dyslipidemia:* diabetes mellitus, pancreatitis, dysproteinemia (myeloma, lupus)

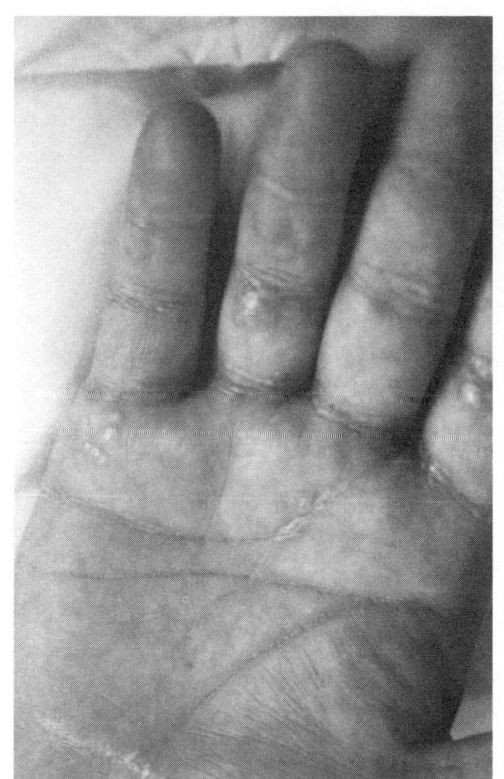

A

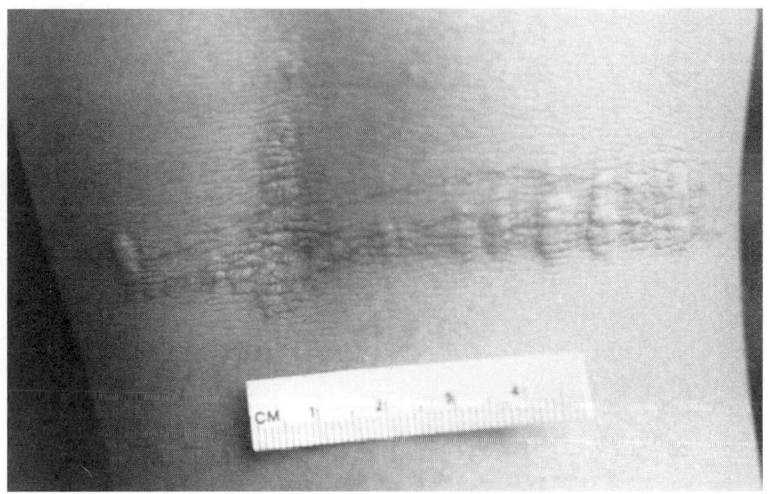

B

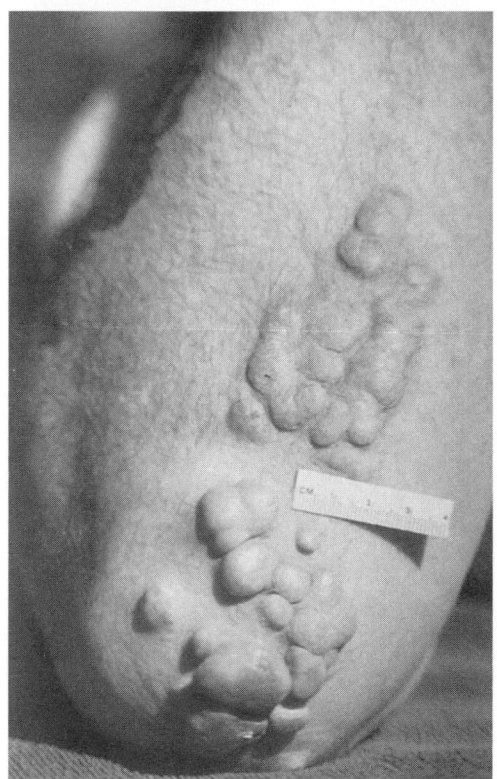

C

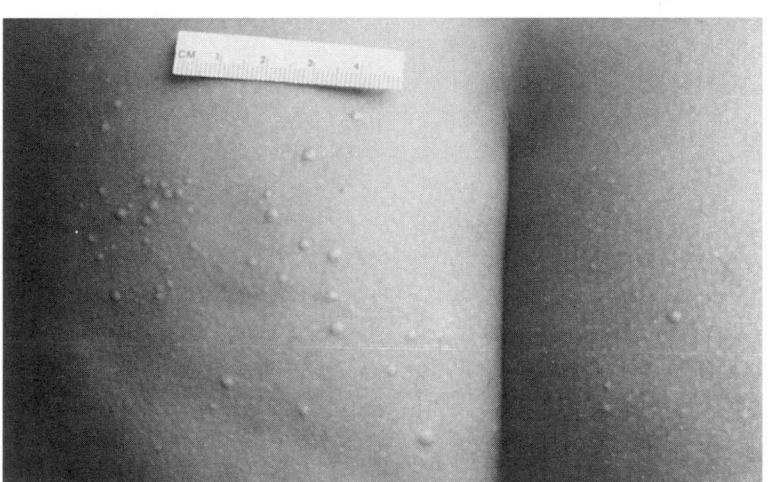

D

FIG. 10–1. Xanthomas associated with hyperlipidemia. Xanthomas **(A–H)** are associated with disorders predominantly causing hypercholesterolemia, whereas xanthomas **J** and **K** are found in patients with severe hypertriglyceridemia. Shown are planar xanthomas of the creases of the palm **(A)** and of the popliteal fossa **(B)** of untreated patients with type III hyperlipoproteinemia. Also apparent are tuberous xanthomas **(A)** (raised above the surface of the skin) of the digits. Planar xanthomas also may be caused by biliary obstruction, hypothyroidism, or paraproteinemia. Shown are tuberoeruptive xanthomas of the forearm **(C)** and buttocks **(D)** of patients with type III hyperlipoproteinemia. Tuberous xanthomas of the hands
continued

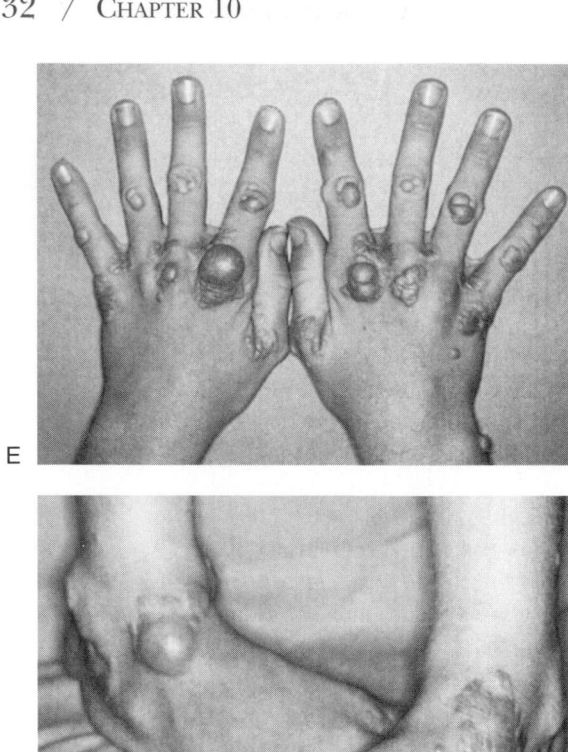

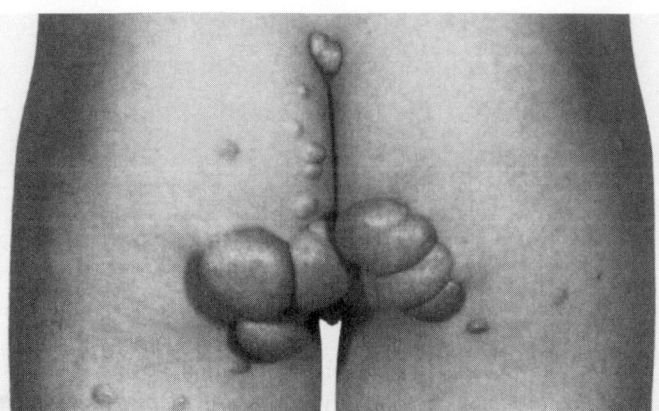

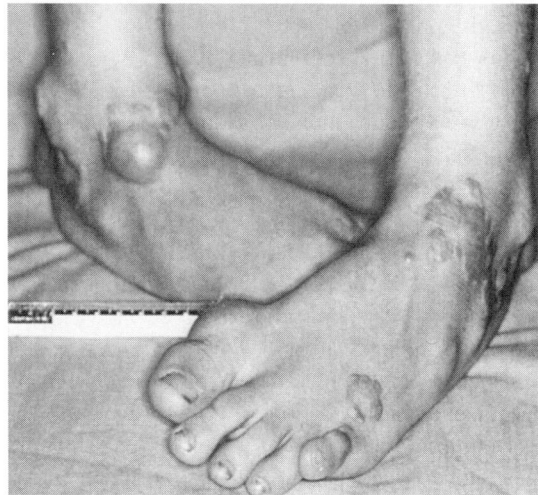

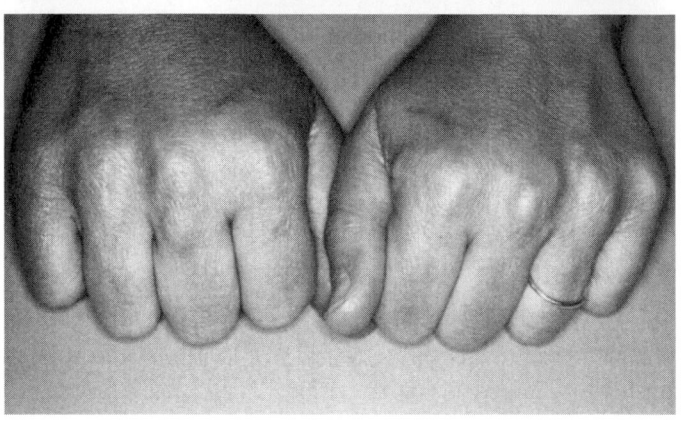

FIG. 10–1. *Continued.* **(E),** buttocks **(F),** and feet **(G)** of a patient with homozygous familial hypercholesterolemia are shown. Xanthomas of the extensor tendons of the hands **(H)** and the Achilles tendon **(I)** of a patient with heterozygous familial hypercholesterolemia. Tendon xanthomas are also present occasionally in patients with type III hyperlipoproteinemia. Eruptive xanthomas associated with severe hypertriglyceridemia are shown.

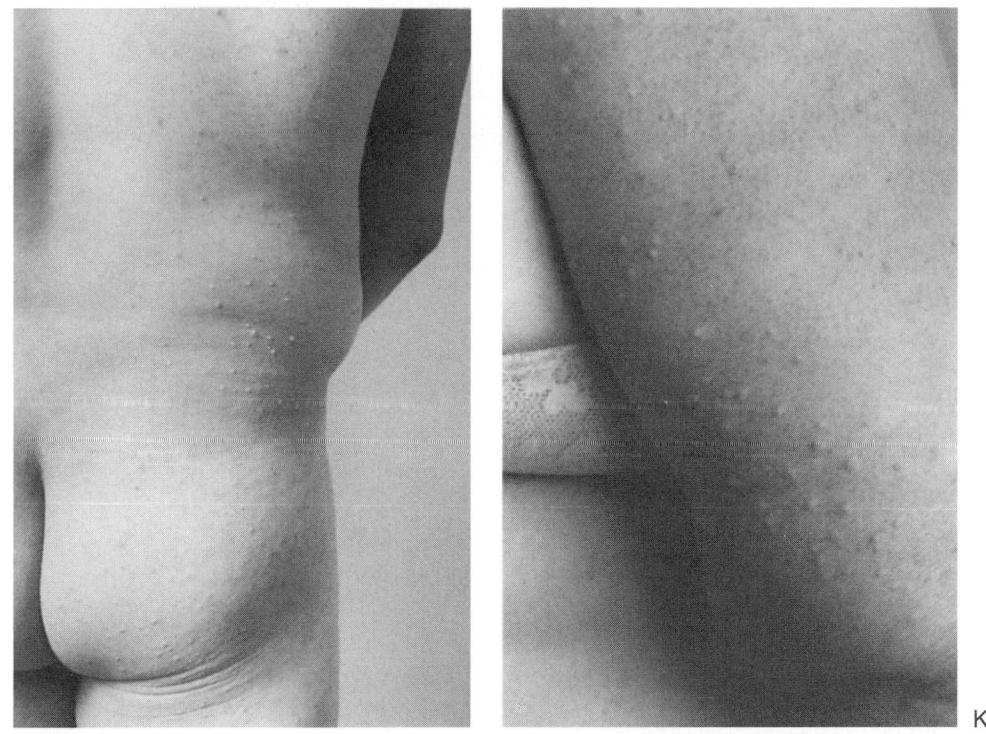

FIG. 10–1. *Continued.* Back and buttocks **(J)** and posterolateral arm **(K)** of patients with severe chylomicronemia (triglyceride levels > 3,000 mg/dL).

determined if moderate hypertriglyceridemia and the associated low HDL levels are caused by single-gene mutations or by the interaction among polymorphisms of multiple genes.

FH and type III hyperlipoproteinemia are both caused by single-gene mutations that have provided many insights into the pathophysiology of plasma lipid metabolism (33,40). The discovery of the LDL receptor and the finding that mutations of the LDL receptor gene are responsible for increased LDL concentrations in FH provided powerful insights into the regulation of plasma LDL levels and intracellular cholesterol metabolism. These insights include the recognition that plasma LDL levels are inversely related to the number of LDL receptors expressed on the cell surfaces within the body, the finding that depletion of intracellular cholesterol and inhibition of cholesterol biosynthesis enhance LDL receptor expression by cells, the discovery of cholesterol biosynthesis inhibitors (the statins) that are the most potent and clinically useful cholesterol-lowering drugs, the recognition of the liver as the organ with most (>50%) of the body's complement of LDL receptors, and the determination that dietary saturated fatty acids of 12-, 14-, and 16-carbon chain lengths and dietary cholesterol influence plasma cholesterol levels by reducing the hepatic expression of the LDL receptor (24,47,48).

Type III hyperlipoproteinemia was found to be associated with mutations of the apolipoprotein E (apoE) gene (33). The accumulation of remnant lipoproteins in type III patients with apoE gene mutations suggested that apoE plays a role in the clearance of these lipoproteins. It also was observed that apoE binds to the LDL receptor, but the lack of substantial remnant accumulation in patients with homozygous FH with few, if any, functional LDL receptors suggests that apoE-enriched remnant lipoproteins are not removed from the blood exclusively by apoE–LDL receptor interactions. Ultimately, a remnant receptor, the LDL receptor–related protein, was identified, and apoE was found to be the ligand that binds remnant lipoproteins to this receptor (49,50).

ATHEROGENIC LIPOPROTEINS

Accumulated remnant lipoproteins and LDLs, associated with type III hyperlipoproteinemia and FH, respectively, are two of four currently recognized dyslipidemic states associated with accelerated atherogenesis. The other two are low HDL concentrations, which occur most commonly with hypertriglyceridemia in conjunction with insulin resistance and increased concentrations of lipoprotein(a) [Lp(a)].

Remnant lipoproteins initiate atheroma formation through their uptake by macrophages in the arterial wall (51,52), resulting in the delivery of remnant cholesterol and the accumulation of excessive intracellular cholesterol. This excessive cholesterol content transforms the macrophage into the conductor of the symphony of events that lead to atheroma formation (53–56).

Unlike remnants, plasma LDLs were noted to be incapable of binding to macrophages, precluding their involvement in cholesterol accumulation and initiation of atherogenesis. Subsequently, investigators found that modifications of LDLs *in vitro* produced LDLs that are bound by specific receptors on macrophages and internalized (57). How LDLs are modified *in vivo* is still under active investigation (58). Oxidation of LDL constituents is the modification that has been most thoroughly investigated. In clinical trials, two antioxidants, β-carotene and vitamin E, were not effective in reducing risk for CHD (11,59).

The causes of reduced HDL concentrations and the role of low HDL levels in atherogenesis remain relatively obscure. Studies of families with low HDL levels and population studies (60–64) have clearly shown that low HDL concentrations, especially of the HDL_2 subfraction, are associated with accelerated coronary atherothrombosis. Investigations of the HDL of patients from low-HDL kindreds suggest that the reduction in HDL_2 levels is specifically caused by low concentrations of HDL particles containing only apolipoprotein A-I (apoA-I) (65).

Although much has been learned about the structure of Lp(a) in recent years, its precise role in atherogenesis is unclear (66). Studies of Lp(a) concentrations and the risk for CHD have shown a clear association. However, the difficulty of measuring Lp(a) levels reliably has led to recommendations against routine screening (12). The risk associated with Lp(a) also is modulated by the degree of increase of LDL cholesterol levels. High Lp(a) levels confer no additional risk if hypercholesterolemia is managed aggressively (67).

TREATMENT-ORIENTED CLASSIFICATION OF DYSLIPIDEMIA: A CONTEMPORARY APPROACH

Currently, the clinical classification of dyslipidemia for management purposes does not require establishing a precise genetic diagnosis, although it may be helpful for genetic counseling and will assume great importance when gene-transfer therapy becomes possible. The classification of dyslipidemia depends on measurement of the concentrations of plasma triglycerides, total cholesterol, and HDL-C (Table 10–2). If the cholesterol concentration is increased to a greater extent than the triglyceride concentration, the patient's hypercholesterolemia is caused by an increased LDL level, usually as a result of one of the cholesterol disorders listed in Table 10–3. Conversely, the fasting triglyceride concentration exceeds the cholesterol level in patients with any of the genetic disorders causing predominant hypertriglyceridemia (Table 10–3). (See Reference 68 for a detailed discussion of the classification and treatment of dyslipidemia.)

Effective treatment can be prescribed based on both assignment of each patient to the cholesterol disorders group, the triglyceride disorders group, or the low-HDL group, and subsequent use of the NCEP ATP III guidelines for initiating therapy and establishing treatment goals

TABLE 10–2. *Classification of dyslipidemia according to triglyceride, total cholesterol, and high-density lipoprotein cholesterol concentrations*

Cholesterol disorders[a]	Cholesterol level is increased and exceeds triglyceride concentration
Triglyceride disorders[b]	Triglyceride level is increased and exceeds cholesterol concentration
HDL-C concentration reduced	Men: <40 mg/dL; women: <50 mg/dL

[a]Total cholesterol: desirable, <200 mg/dL; borderline high, 200–239 mg/dL; high, ≥240 mg/dL. Low-density lipoprotein cholesterol: optimal, <100 mg/dL; near optimal, 100–129 mg/dL; borderline high, 130–159 mg/dL; high, 160–189 mg/dL; very high, ≥190 mg/dL.
[b]Triglyceride: normal, <150 mg/dL; borderline high, 150–199 mg/dL; high, 200–499 mg/dL; very high, ≥500 mg/dL.
HDL-C, high-density lipoprotein cholesterol.

(12). All patients should be managed with reductions in total dietary fat, saturated fat, and cholesterol. Patients with increased triglyceride concentrations and low HDL-C levels should also lose weight, if indicated, and restrict their alcohol intake. Lipid-lowering drugs for patients with cholesterol disorders include statins as the preferred drugs (68). Niacin, resins, and ezetimibe may be used in combination with statins in patients with very high LDL levels. For patients with triglyceride problems, niacin and the fibrates are the drugs of choice, although maximal dosages (80 mg daily) of atorvastatin or simvastatin reduce triglyceride levels almost as much as niacin and fibrates (12,69,70).

Patients with low HDL-C concentrations deserve further consideration. Often these patients have normal total cholesterol concentrations, triglyceride levels greater than 150 mg/dL, and normal or only slightly increased LDL cholesterol levels, and they are frequently insulin resistant (20). Their LDL levels may not be increased enough to meet the NCEP ATP III guidelines to initiate hypolipidemic drug therapy, even though these patients are at increased risk for

TABLE 10–3. *Genetic lipid disorders*

Genetic causes of cholesterol disorders
Familial hypercholesterolemia (40)
Autosomal recessive hypercholesterolemia (32)
Familial defective apolipoprotein B-100 (37)
Familial combined hyperlipidemia (29)
Polygenic hypercholesterolemia (28)

Genetic causes of triglyceride disorders
Familial hypertriglyceridemia (81)
Familial combined hyperlipidemia (29)
Familial type III hyperlipoproteinemia (33)
Chylomicronemia syndrome (41)
• Apolipoprotein C-II mutations
• Lipoprotein lipase mutations

CHD (71,72). To guide effective treatment of patients with low HDL-C levels, it is useful to compute the ratio of the total cholesterol level to the HDL-C concentration. Several studies indicate that this ratio is the most sensitive indicator of lipid-related cardiovascular disease risk (73–76). In the Framingham Study, ratios greater than 4.5 were associated with increased CHD risk, and the optimal ratio was less than 3.5 (77).

Some caveats apply in using the total cholesterol:HDL-C ratio. First is the difficulty of obtaining accurate, reproducible HDL-C determinations. Careful attention is required in the laboratory to reliably measure HDL-C levels. Errors can drastically affect the ratio. Another important concern is that no clinical trials have been designed solely to determine the benefit of reducing the total cholesterol:HDL-C ratio of patients with low HDL concentrations as their only dyslipidemia. However, it is clear that high-risk patients with low HDL-C levels benefit from lipid-lowering therapy even if their baseline LDL cholesterol level is less than the threshold value for initiating drug therapy as defined by the NCEP ATP III guidelines (8,10,11).

Aggressive treatment of high-risk patients with established atherothrombotic vascular disease or multiple risk factors has been recommended (12,68). This includes reducing the LDL cholesterol concentration to well below 100 mg/dL for patients with established vascular disease. All patients with vascular disease should be strongly considered for treatment with statins, including those with baseline LDL cholesterol levels less than 130 mg/dL. Clinical trial data support vigorous cholesterol lowering (11).

SECONDARY CAUSES OF HYPERLIPIDEMIA

Secondary causes of hyperlipidemia should be sought and excluded immediately when dyslipidemia is first identified. The causes of secondary hyperlipidemia are listed in Table 10–4.

TABLE 10–4. *Secondary causes of dyslipidemia*

Associated with hypercholesterolemia	Associated with hypertriglyceridemia
Nephrotic syndrome	Diabetes mellitus
Dysglobulinemia	Renal transplantation
Hepatoma	Nephrotic syndrome
Multiple myeloma	Alcohol
Hypothyroidism	Cushing syndrome
Acute intermittent porphyria	Uremia
Obstructive jaundice	Chronic dialysis
	Contraceptive steroids
	Dysglobulinemia
	Protease inhibitor therapy of patients infected with human immunodeficiency virus

See References 23 and 68 for a detailed discussion of secondary causes of dyslipidemia.

TABLE 10–5. *Causes of hypolipidemia*

Genetic
Hypobetalipoproteinemia: truncations of apolipoprotein B-100 (78)
Abetalipoproteinemia: mutations of microsomal triglyceride transfer protein gene (45)
Hypoalphalipoproteinemia: Tangier disease (46)
Mutations of the apolipoprotein A-I gene (38)

Nutritional
Low-fat diets

LOW BLOOD LIPID LEVEL— A HEALTH HAZARD?

Hypolipidemia, unusually low concentrations of cholesterol or cholesterol and triglycerides, occurs as a result of genetic disorders affecting certain apolipoproteins (apoB-100 and apoA-I) and the microsomal triglyceride transfer protein (Table 10–5) (36,78). These disorders are relatively rare. In the general population, hypocholesterolemia is much more common in individuals consuming low-fat diets. It has been speculated that low total cholesterol levels may be associated with excess mortality from a variety of causes (79). However, a comprehensive meta-analysis of pertinent studies suggests that only hemorrhagic stroke appears to be increased in persons with low total cholesterol levels and hypertension (80). Although of concern, the enhanced risk for stroke is more than compensated for by a 90% reduction in CHD events relative to the increase in the incidence of stroke in hypertensive patients with low total cholesterol levels. Excess total mortality or cause-specific excess mortality has not occurred in any of the clinical trials of lipid-lowering therapy with statins or the fibrates gemfibrozil and fenofibrate.

UNCERTAINTIES OF TREATMENT

The classification of dyslipidemia is most important for making rational treatment choices for patients with dyslipidemia. Brewer and coworkers (see Chapter 5) provide the details needed to evaluate patients for specific genetic disorders, and Farmer and Gotto (see Chapter 11) describe the detailed use of appropriate therapeutic strategies (see also References 23 and 68). It is important to keep in mind that clinical trials provide evidence that coronary disease events can be prevented by appropriate lipid-lowering therapies (5–11). The clinical trials have proven the value of cholesterol-lowering therapy in patients with increased LDL levels, in patients with low concentrations of HDL irrespective of LDL level, in patients older than 65 years with lipid abnormalities, and in patients with diabetes mellitus who have increased triglyceride and reduced HDL concentrations. In patients with low HDL concentrations, treatment guidelines that focus solely on reducing LDL cholesterol concentrations may not be adequate. Treatment of these patients should focus on reducing

LDL concentrations to correct the total cholesterol:HDL-C ratio rather than increasing the HDL-C concentration.

FUTURE DEVELOPMENT OF CLINICAL CLASSIFICATIONS OF LIPID DISORDERS

The clinical classification of lipid disorders is advancing on two fronts. First, scientists are attempting to identify the mutations, monogenic and polygenic, that underlie familial lipid disorders. The value of this approach is that therapeutic efforts can be targeted with a greater chance of efficacy when the metabolic bases of the disorders are understood. Second, our knowledge of the complexities of genetic regulation of plasma lipid levels and the role of lipoproteins in atherogenesis is expanding, especially in the area of HDL metabolism. Discoveries likely to be made regarding obesity and lipoprotein metabolism will enhance our understanding of this increasingly prevalent high-risk condition. The ability to identify patients for treatment by using novel risk assessment techniques and the availability of new lipid-lowering agents also will shape diagnostic and treatment paradigms of the future.

ACKNOWLEDGMENTS

The authors thank Sylvia Richmond for manuscript preparation, Gary Howard and Stephen Ordway for editorial assistance, John C.W. Carroll and Jack Hull for graphics, and Stephen Gonzales and Chris Goodfellow for photography. This work was supported in part by Program Project Grant HL47660 from the National Institutes of Health.

REFERENCES

1. Doevendans PA, Jukema W, Spiering W, et al. Molecular genetics and gene expression in atherosclerosis. *Int J Cardiol* 2001;80:161–172.
2. Lopes N, Vasudevan SS, Alvarez RJ, et al. Pathophysiology of plaque instability: insights at the genomic level. *Prog Cardiovasc Dis* 2002; 44:323–338.
3. Horton JD, Goldstein JL, Brown MS. SREBPs: activators of the complete program of cholesterol and fatty acid synthesis in the liver. *J Clin Invest* 2002;109:1125–1131.
4. Hegele RA. Monogenic dyslipidemias: window on determinants of plasma lipoprotein metabolism. *Am J Hum Genet* 2001;69:1161–1177.
5. Randomised trial of cholesterol lowering in 4444 patients with coronary heart disease: the Scandinavian Simvastatin Survival Study (4S). *Lancet* 1994;344:1383–1389.
6. Sacks FM, Pfeffer MA, Moye LA, et al. The effect of pravastatin on coronary events after myocardial infarction in patients with average cholesterol levels. *N Engl J Med* 1996;335:1001–1009.
7. Shepherd J, Cobbe SM, Ford I, et al. Prevention of coronary heart disease with pravastatin in men with hypercholesterolemia. *N Engl J Med* 1995;333:1301–1307.
8. Rubins HB, Robins SJ, Collins D, et al. Gemfibrozil for the secondary prevention of coronary heart disease in men with low levels of high-density lipoprotein cholesterol. *N Engl J Med* 1999;341:410–418.
9. Prevention of cardiovascular events and death with pravastatin in patients with coronary heart disease and a broad range of initial cholesterol levels. The Long-Term Intervention with Pravastatin in Ischaemic Disease (LIPID) Study Group. *N Engl J Med* 1998;339: 1349–1357.
10. Downs JR, Clearfield M, Weis S, et al. Primary prevention of acute coronary events with lovastatin in men and women with average cholesterol levels. Results of AFCAPS/TexCAPS. *JAMA* 1998;279:1615–1622.
11. Heart Protection Study Collaborative Group. MRC/BHF Heart Protection Study of cholesterol lowering with simvastatin in 20 536 high-risk individuals: a randomised placebo-controlled trial. *Lancet* 2002;360:7–22.
12. The Expert Panel. Third Report of the National Cholesterol Education Program (NCEP) Expert Panel on Detection, Evaluation, and Treatment of High Blood Cholesterol in Adults (Adult Treatment Panel III). Final Report. Bethesda, MD: U.S. Department of Health & Human Services, 2002; NIH publication no. 02-5215.
13. Wilson PW, D'Agostino RB, Levy D, et al. Prediction of coronary heart disease using risk factor categories. *Circulation* 1998;97:1837–1847.
14. Pearson TA, Laurora I, Chu H, et al. The Lipid Treatment Assessment Project (L-TAP). A multicenter survey to evaluate the percentages of dyslipidemic patients receiving lipid-lowering therapy and achieving low-density lipoprotein cholesterol goals. *Arch Intern Med* 2000;160: 459–467.
15. Fonarow GC, French WJ, Parsons LS, et al. Use of lipid-lowering medications at discharge in patients with acute myocardial infarction. Data from the National Registry of Myocardial Infarction 3. *Circulation* 2001;103:38–44.
16. Grundy SM, Balady GJ, Criqui MH, et al. Primary prevention of coronary heart disease: guidance from Framingham. A statement for healthcare professionals from the AHA Task Force on Risk Reduction. *Circulation* 1998;97:1876–1887.
17. Stamler J, Wentworth D, Neaton JD. Is relationship between serum cholesterol and risk of premature death from coronary heart disease continuous and graded? Findings in 356 222 primary screenees of the Multiple Risk Factor Intervention Trial (MRFIT). *JAMA* 1986;256: 2823–2828.
18. Flegal KM, Carroll MD, Ogden CL, et al. Prevalence and trends in obesity among US adults, 1999–2000. *JAMA* 2002;288:1723–1727.
19. Ogden CL, Flegal KM, Carroll MD, et al. Prevalence and trends in overweight among US children and adolescents, 1999–2000. *JAMA* 2002;288:1728–1732.
20. Grundy SM. Hypertriglyceridemia, insulin resistance, and the metabolic syndrome. *Am J Cardiol* 1999;83:25F–29F.
21. Ford ES, Giles WH, Dietz WH. Prevalence of the metabolic syndrome among US adults. Findings from the Third National Health and Nutrition Examination Survey. *JAMA* 2002;287:356–359.
22. Fredrickson DS, Goldstein JL, Brown MS. The familial hyperlipoproteinemias. In: Stanbury JB, Wyngaarden JB, Fredrickson DS, eds. *The metabolic basis of inherited disease,* 4th ed. New York: McGraw-Hill, 1978:604–655.
23. Mahley RW, Weisgraber KH, Farese RV Jr. Disorders of lipid metabolism. In: Larsen PR, Kronenberg HM, Melmed S, et al., eds. *Williams textbook of endocrinology,* 10th ed., Philadelphia: WB Saunders, 2003:1642–1705.
24. Brown MS, Goldstein JL. A receptor-mediated pathway for cholesterol homeostasis. *Science* 1986;232:34–47.
25. Barr DP, Russ EM, Eder HA. Protein-lipid relationships in human plasma. II. In atherosclerosis and related conditions. *Am J Med* 1951;11:480–493.
26. Fredrickson DS, Levy RI, Lees RS. Fat transport in lipoproteins—an integrated approach to mechanisms and disorders. *N Engl J Med* 1967;276:34–44, 94–103, 148–156, 215–225, 273–281.
27. Friedewald WT, Levy RI, Fredrickson DS. Estimation of the concentration of low-density lipoprotein cholesterol in plasma, without use of the preparative ultracentrifuge. *Clin Chem* 1972;18:499–502.
28. Goldstein JL, Hazzard WR, Schrott HG, et al. Hyperlipidemia in coronary heart disease. I. Lipid levels in 500 survivors of myocardial infarction. *J Clin Invest* 1973;52:1533–1543.
29. Goldstein JL, Schrott HG, Hazzard WR, et al. Hyperlipidemia in coronary heart disease. II. Genetic analysis of lipid levels in 176 families and delineation of a new inherited disorder, combined hyperlipidemia. *J Clin Invest* 1973;52:1544–1568.
30. Breckenridge WC, Little JA, Steiner G, et al. Hypertriglyceridemia associated with deficiency of apolipoprotein C-II. *N Engl J Med* 1978;298:1265–1273.
31. Pullinger CR, Hennessy LK, Chatterton JE, et al. Familial ligand-defective apolipoprotein B. Identification of a new mutation that decreases LDL receptor binding affinity. *J Clin Invest* 1995;95:1225–1234.

32. Wilund KR, Yi M, Campagna F, et al. Molecular mechanisms of autosomal recessive hypercholesterolemia. *Hum Mol Genet* 2002;11:3019–3030.
33. Mahley RW, Rall SC Jr. Type III hyperlipoproteinemia (dysbetalipoproteinemia): the role of apolipoprotein E in normal and abnormal lipoprotein metabolism. In: Scriver CR, Beaudet AL, Sly WS, et al., eds. *The metabolic and molecular bases of inherited disease, Vol 2*, 8th ed. New York: McGraw-Hill, 2001:2835–2862.
34. Rall SC Jr, Newhouse YM, Clarke HR, et al. Type III hyperlipoproteinemia associated with apolipoprotein E phenotype E3/3. Structure and genetics of an apolipoprotein E3 variant. *J Clin Invest* 1989;83:1095–1101.
35. Minnich A, Kessling A, Roy M, et al. Prevalence of alleles encoding defective lipoprotein lipase in hypertriglyceridemic patients of French Canadian descent. *J Lipid Res* 1995;36:117–124.
36. Santamarina-Fojo S. The familial chylomicronemia syndrome. *Endocrinol Metab Clin North Am* 1998;27:551–567.
37. Innerarity TL, Mahley RW, Weisgraber KH, et al. Familial defective apolipoprotein B100: a mutation of apolipoprotein B that causes hypercholesterolemia. *J Lipid Res* 1990;31:1337–1349.
38. Tall AR, Breslow JL, Rubin EM. Genetic disorders affecting plasma high-density lipoproteins. In: Scriver CR, Beaudet AL, Sly WS, et al., eds. *The metabolic and molecular bases of inherited disease, Vol 2*, 8th ed. New York: McGraw-Hill, 2001:2915–2936.
39. Dammerman M, Breslow JL. Genetic basis of lipoprotein disorders. *Circulation* 1995;91:505–512.
40. Goldstein JL, Hobbs HH, Brown MS. Familial hypercholesterolemia. In: Scriver CR, Beaudet AL, Sly WS, et al., eds. *The metabolic and molecular bases of inherited disease, Vol 2*, 8th ed. New York: McGraw-Hill, 2001:2863–2913.
41. Brunzell JD, Deeb SS. Familial lipoprotein lipase deficiency, apo C-II deficiency, and hepatic lipase deficiency. In: Scriver CR, Beaudet AL, Sly WS, et al., eds. *The metabolic and molecular bases of inherited disease, Vol 2*, 8th ed. New York: McGraw-Hill, 2001:2789–2816.
42. Cohen JC, Vega GL, Grundy SM. Hepatic lipase: new insights from genetic and metabolic studies. *Curr Opin Lipidol* 1999;10:259–267.
43. Santamarina-Fojo S, Hoeg JM, Assmann G, et al. Lecithin cholesterol acyltransferase deficiency and fish eye disease. In: Scriver CR, Beaudet AL, Sly WS, et al., eds. *The metabolic and molecular bases of inherited disease, Vol 2*, 8th ed. New York: McGraw-Hill, 2001:2817–2833.
44. Barter PJ, Brewer HB Jr, Chapman MJ, et al. Cholesteryl ester transfer protein. A novel target for raising HDL and inhibiting atherosclerosis. *Arterioscler Thromb Vasc Biol* 2003;23:160–167.
45. Berriot-Varoqueaux N, Aggerbeck LP, Samson-Bouma M, et al. The role of the microsomal triglyceride transfer protein in abetalipoproteinemia. *Annu Rev Nutr* 2000;20:663–697.
46. Assmann G, von Eckardstein A, Brewer HB Jr. Familial analphalipoproteinemia: Tangier disease. In: Scriver CR, Beaudet AL, Sly WS, et al., eds. *The metabolic and molecular bases of inherited disease, Vol 2*, 8th ed. New York: McGraw-Hill, 2001:2937–2960.
47. Grundy SM, Vega GL. Influence of mevinolin on metabolism of low density lipoproteins in primary moderate hypercholesterolemia. *J Lipid Res* 1985;26:1464–1475.
48. Dietschy JM. Dietary fatty acids and the regulation of plasma low density lipoprotein cholesterol concentrations. *J Nutr* 1998;128:444S–448S.
49. Herz J, Strickland DK. LRP: a multifunctional scavenger and signaling receptor. *J Clin Invest* 2001;108:779–784.
50. Mahley RW, Ji Z-S. Remnant lipoprotein metabolism: key pathways involving cell-surface heparan sulfate proteoglycans and apolipoprotein E. *J Lipid Res* 1999;40:1–16.
51. Innerarity TL, Arnold KS, Weisgraber KH, et al. Apolipoprotein E is the determinant that mediates the receptor uptake of β-very low density lipoproteins by mouse macrophages. *Arteriosclerosis* 1986;6:114–122.
52. Koo C, Wernette-Hammond ME, Garcia Z, et al. Uptake of cholesterol-rich remnant lipoproteins by human monocyte-derived macrophages is mediated by low density lipoprotein receptors. *J Clin Invest* 1988;81:1332–1340.
53. Mahley RW, Weisgraber KH, Innerarity TL, et al. Genetic defects in lipoprotein metabolism. Elevation of atherogenic lipoproteins caused by impaired catabolism. *JAMA* 1991;265:78–83.
54. Ross R. Atherosclerosis—an inflammatory disease. *N Engl J Med* 1999;340:115–126.
55. Libby P. Changing concepts of atherogenesis. *J Intern Med* 2000;247:349–358.
56. Peters W, Charo IF. Involvement of chemokine receptor 2 and its ligand, monocyte chemoattractant protein-1, in the development of atherosclerosis: lessons from knockout mice. *Curr Opin Lipidol* 2001;12:175–180.
57. Steinberg D, Parthasarathy S, Carew TE, et al. Beyond cholesterol. Modifications of low-density lipoprotein that increase its atherogenicity. *N Engl J Med* 1989;320:915–924.
58. Witztum JL, Steinberg D. The oxidative modification hypothesis of atherosclerosis: does it hold for humans? *Trends Cardiovasc Med* 2001;11:93–102.
59. Chisolm GM, Steinberg D. The oxidative modification hypothesis of atherogenesis: an overview. *Free Radic Biol Med* 2000;28:1815–1826.
60. Miller GJ, Miller NE. Plasma-high-density-lipoprotein concentration and development of ischæmic heart-disease. *Lancet* 1975;1:16–19.
61. Third JL, Montag J, Flynn M, et al. Primary and familial hypoalphalipoproteinemia. *Metabolism* 1984;33:136–146.
62. Gordon DJ, Probstfield JL, Garrison RJ, et al. High-density lipoprotein cholesterol and cardiovascular disease. Four prospective American studies. *Circulation* 1989;79:8–15.
63. Assmann G, Funke H. HDL metabolism and atherosclerosis. *J Cardiovasc Pharmacol* 1990;16[Suppl 9]:S15–S20.
64. Miller NE. Associations of high-density lipoprotein subclasses and apolipoproteins with ischemic heart disease and coronary atherosclerosis. *Am Heart J* 1987;113:589–597.
65. Duriez P, Fruchart JC. High-density lipoprotein subclasses and apolipoprotein A-I. *Clin Chim Acta* 1999;286:97–114.
66. Utermann G. Lipoprotein(a). In: Scriver CR, Beaudet AL, Sly WS, et al., eds. *The metabolic and molecular bases of inherited disease, Vol 2*, 8th ed. New York: McGraw-Hill, 2001:2753–2787.
67. Maher VM, Brown BG, Marcovina SM, et al. Effects of lowering elevated LDL cholesterol on the cardiovascular risk of lipoprotein(a). *JAMA* 1995;274:1771–1774.
68. Mahley RW, Bersot TP. Drug therapy for hypercholesterolemia and dyslipidemia. In: Hardman JG, Limbird LE, eds. *Goodman & Gilman's the pharmacological basis of therapeutics,* 10th ed. New York: McGraw-Hill, 2001:971–1002.
69. Bakker-Arkema RG, Davidson MH, Goldstein RJ, et al. Efficacy and safety of a new HMG-CoA reductase inhibitor, atorvastatin, in patients with hypertriglyceridemia. *JAMA* 1996;275:128–133.
70. Ose L, Davidson MH, Stein EA, et al. Lipid-altering efficacy and safety of simvastatin 80 mg/day: long-term experience in a large group of patients with hypercholesterolemia. *Clin Cardiol* 2000;23:39–46.
71. Castelli WP, Garrison RJ, Wilson PW, et al. Incidence of coronary heart disease and lipoprotein cholesterol levels. The Framingham Study. *JAMA* 1986;256:2835–2838.
72. Rubins HB, Robins SJ, Collins D, et al. Distribution of lipids in 8,500 men with coronary artery disease. *Am J Cardiol* 1995;75:1196–1201.
73. Kinosian B, Glick H, Garland G. Cholesterol and coronary heart disease: predicting risks by levels and ratios. *Ann Intern Med* 1994;121:641–647.
74. Lemieux I, Lamarche B, Couillard C, et al. Total cholesterol/HDL cholesterol ratio vs LDL cholesterol/HDL cholesterol ratio as indices of ischemic heart disease risk in men. The Quebec Cardiovascular Study. *Arch Intern Med* 2001;161:2685–2692.
75. Ridker PM, Glynn RJ, Hennekens CH. C-reactive protein adds to the predictive value of total and HDL cholesterol in determining risk of first myocardial infarction. *Circulation* 1998;97:2007–2011.
76. Gotto AM Jr, Whitney E, Stein EA, et al. Relation between baseline and on-treatment lipid parameters and first acute major coronary events in the Air Force/Texas Coronary Atherosclerosis Prevention Study (AFCAPS/TexCAPS). *Circulation* 2000;101:477–484.
77. Castelli WP. The folly of questioning the benefits of cholesterol reduction. *Am Fam Physician* 1994;49:567–574.
78. Young SG. Recent progress in understanding apolipoprotein B. *Circulation* 1990;82:1574–1594.
79. Jacobs D, Blackburn H, Higgins M, et al. Report of the Conference on Low Blood Cholesterol: mortality associations. *Circulation* 1992;86:1046–1060.
80. Law MR, Thompson SG, Wald NJ. Assessing possible hazards of reducing serum cholesterol. *Br Med J* 1994;308:373–379.
81. Schaefer EJ. Familial lipoprotein disorders and premature coronary artery disease. *Med Clin North Am* 1994;78:21–39.

CHAPTER 11

Management and Adult Treatment Panel III Guidelines

Antonio M. Gotto, Jr. and John A. Farmer

Key Words: Drug therapy; global risk; guidelines; lipids; prevention.

INTRODUCTION

Age-adjusted mortality rates for cardiovascular disease have significantly declined over the last three decades in the United States (1). The improvement in prognosis after an atherothrombotic event represents a complex interplay among increased diagnostic capabilities, risk factor modification, and refinements in revascularization techniques. Because dyslipidemia is central to atherogenesis, modification of lipid abnormalities represents a fundamental component of coronary heart disease (CHD) risk reduction programs (2–4).

The U.S. National Cholesterol Education Program (NCEP) Adult Treatment Panel (ATP) publishes guidelines for CHD risk stratification by lipid levels combined with recommendations for therapeutic options with dietary or pharmacologic therapy. The ATP III, published in 2001, reflects both advances in basic science and the results of five major trials of the 3-hydroxy-3-methylglutaryl coenzyme A (HMG-CoA) reductase inhibitors (also known as statins) that demonstrate clinical cardiovascular benefits across a wide spectrum of lipid ranges

A. M. Gotto, Jr.: Department of Medicine, Weill Medical College of Cornell University, 445 E. 69th St., New York, New York 10021.
J. A. Farmer: Department of Medicine, Baylor College of Medicine, and Cardiology Service, Ben Taub Hospital, One Baylor Plaza, Houston, Texas 77030.

encompassing both primary and secondary prevention (5). This chapter reviews the diagnostic and therapeutic guidelines promulgated by the ATP III and briefly examines lifestyle and pharmacologic strategies for lipid modification.

RISK ASSESSMENT AND ADULT TREATMENT PANEL III

The most recent revision of U.S. guidelines contains several new features. Among these, the ATP III describes the use of global risk calculation, emphasizes the metabolic syndrome as a secondary target of therapy, revises definitions for high-density lipoprotein cholesterol (HDL-C), and introduces the concept of CHD risk equivalence in primary prevention risk assessment. The ATP III guidelines establish an optimal low-density lipoprotein cholesterol (LDL-C) level as less than 100 mg/dL in both primary and secondary prevention (Table 11–1), on the basis of epidemiologic studies that showed a log linear relation between LDL-C levels and heart disease, suggesting individuals whose LDL-C levels were less than 100 mg/dL had an extremely low lifetime CHD risk (6). The definition of low HDL-C was also increased from 35 mg/dL in ATP II to 40 mg/dL in ATP III, to represent depressed levels of this antiatherogenic particle more accurately. Triglyceride guidelines also were altered because of the increasing evidence supporting the epidemiologic relation between serum triglycerides and CHD (Table 11–1) (7).

The guidelines prefer that physicians perform a full fasting lipoprotein analysis that includes total cholesterol, LDL-C,

TABLE 11-1. *Adult Treatment
Panel III classification of lipid levels*

Total cholesterol level, mg/dL	
<200	Desirable
200–239	Borderline high
≥240	High
LDL-C level, mg/dL	
<100	Optimal
100–129	Near optimal/above optimal
130–159	Borderline high
160–189	High
≥190	Very high
HDL-C level, mg/dL	
<40	Low
≥60	High
Triglycerides level, mg/dL	
<150	Normal
150–199	Borderline high
200–499	High
≥500	Very high

HDL-C, high-density lipoprotein cholesterol; LDL-C, low-density lipoprotein cholesterol.

Adapted from Expert Panel on Detection, Evaluation and Treatment of High Blood Cholesterol in Adults. Executive Summary of the Third Report of the National Cholesterol Education Program (NCEP) Expert Panel on the Detection, Evaluation and Treatment of High Blood Cholesterol in Adults (Adult Treatment Panel III). *JAMA* 2001;285:2486–2497.

HDL-C, and triglycerides as the initial lipid screening in all patients. Increased LDL-C remains the primary guide for treatment decisions and target for therapy (Table 11–2). The ATP III uses an algorithm derived from the Framingham Heart Study to project a patient's absolute 10-year risk for development of CHD (Fig. 11–1) on the basis of multiple CHD risk factors. Calculating this global risk may identify individuals who would benefit from more intensive therapy (8).

Primary Prevention

The goal of primary prevention is to reduce the risk for the first clinical coronary event. However, this traditional definition of primary prevention is arbitrary because the atherothrombotic process begins early in life and progresses slowly over a period of decades in vascular sites besides the coronary arteries. Thus, patients who have never had an ischemic event may nevertheless have substantial vessel disease that warrants intervention. Physicians must implement appropriate primary prevention in patients who qualify for such treatment.

In ATP III, the intensity of lipid decreasing should be tailored to the overall risk for the individual patient (Table 11–2). Global risk assessment begins by assessing the risk factor profile. The major coronary risk factors included in ATP III are described in Table 11–3. Individual patients are divided into three categories according to their potential for the development of an acute coronary event over the subsequent 10-year period according to Framingham risk scoring: (i) low risk is considered to be less than 10% over 10 years, (ii) intermediate risk levels are between 10% and 20% over 10 years, (iii) whereas an individual whose 10-year risk calculates to be greater than 20% is considered to be at high risk.

Subjects in primary prevention at low risk (0–1 risk factors and <10% projected ischemic event rate over the next decade) should be treated to decrease the LDL-C level to less than 160 mg/dL. Therapeutic lifestyle changes (TLC) also should be the first line of treatment in primary prevention when the LDL-C level is in the range of 130 to 159 mg/dL. When LDL-C levels are between 160 and 189 mg/dL even after TLC, the physician should use clinical judgment in deciding whether to initiate drugs. The presence of genetic hyperlipidemias (e.g., familial hypercholesterolemia) frequently accounts for severely increased LDL-C levels in excess of 190 mg/dL. Patients in these

TABLE 11-2. *Adult Treatment Panel III treatment decisions based on low-density lipoprotein cholesterol level*

Risk category	LDL-C goal	TLC initiation level	Drug treatment initiation level
0–1 other risk factor[a]	<160 mg/dL	≥160 mg/dL	≥190 mg/dL (160–189; LDL-C–decreasing drug optional)
2+ other risk factors (10-year risk ≤20%)	<130 mg/dL	≥130 mg/dL	10-year risk 10–20%: ≥130 mg/dL; 10-year risk <10%: ≥160 mg/dL
CHD or CHD Risk equivalents (10-year risk > 20%)	<100 mg/dL	≥100 mg/dL	≥130 mg/dL (100–129; drug optional)[b]

[a]Almost all people with 0 to 1 other risk factor have a 10-year risk less than 10%; thus, 10-year risk assessment in people with 0 to 1 risk factor is not necessary.

[b]Some authorities recommend use of LDL-C–decreasing drugs in this category if an LDL-C level of less than 100 mg/dL cannot be achieved by TLC alone. Others prefer use of drugs that primarily modify triglyceride and HDL levels, for example, nicotinic acid or fibrate. Clinical judgment also may call for deferring drug therapy in this subcategory.

CHD, coronary heart disease; LDL-C, low-density lipoprotein cholesterol; TLC, therapeutic lifestyle changes.

Adapted from Expert Panel on Detection, Evaluation and Treatment of High Blood Cholesterol in Adults. Executive Summary of the Third Report of the National Cholesterol Education Program (NCEP) Expert Panel on the Detection, Evaluation and Treatment of High Blood Cholesterol in Adults (Adult Treatment Panel III). *JAMA* 2001;285:2486–2497.

1. Add Up Points by Age and Sex

Age (years)	Points Men	Points Women
20-34	-9	-7
35-39	-4	-3
40-44	0	0
45-49	3	3
50-54	6	6
55-59	8	8
60-64	10	10
65-69	11	12
70-74	12	14
75-79	13	16

TC (mg/dL)	20-39 M	20-39 W	40-49 M	40-49 W	50-59 M	50-59 W	60-69 M	60-69 W	70-79 M	70-79 W
<160	0	0	0	0	0	0	0	0	0	0
160-199	4	4	3	3	2	2	1	1	0	1
200-239	7	8	5	6	3	4	1	2	0	1
240-279	9	11	6	8	4	5	2	3	1	2
≥280	11	13	8	10	5	7	3	4	1	2

Points by Age (years)

	20-39 M	20-39 W	40-49 M	40-49 W	50-59 M	50-59 W	60-69 M	60-69 W	70-79 M	70-79 W
Nonsmoker	0	0	0	0	0	0	0	0	0	0
Smoker	8	9	5	7	3	4	1	2	1	1

Systolic BP (mmHg)	If untreated M	If untreated W	If treated M	If treated W
<120	0	0	0	0
120-129	0	1	1	3
130-139	1	2	2	4
140-159	1	3	2	5
≥160	2	4	3	6

HDL-C (mg/dL)	Points Men	Points Women
≥60	-1	-1
50-59	0	0
40-49	1	1
<40	2	2

2. Estimate Risk

MEN Point Total	MEN 10-year Risk, %	WOMEN Point Total	WOMEN 10-year Risk, %
<0	<1	<9	<1
0	1	9	1
1	1	10	1
2	1	11	1
3	1	12	1
4	1	13	2
5	2	14	2
6	2	15	3
7	3	16	4
8	4	17	5
9	5	18	6
10	6	19	8
11	8	20	11
12	10	21	14
13	12	22	17
14	16	23	22
15	20	24	27
16	25	≥25	≥30
≥17	≥30		

FIG. 11–1. Adult Treatment Panel III Framingham Risk Scoring. Risk estimates were derived from the experience of the Framingham Heart Study, a predominantly white population in Framingham, MA. BP, blood pressure; HDL-C, high-density lipoprotein cholesterol; M, men; TC, total cholesterol; W, women. (Adapted from Expert Panel on Detection, Evaluation and Treatment of High Blood Cholesterol in Adults. Executive Summary of the Third Report of the National Cholesterol Education Program (NCEP) Expert Panel on the Detection, Evaluation and Treatment of High Blood Cholesterol in Adults (Adult Treatment Panel III). *JAMA* 2001;285:2486–2497, with permission.)

TABLE 11–3. *Major risk factors in Adult Treatment Panel III*

Increases risk for CHD
Cigarette smoking	
Hypertension	The standard definition for hypertension is blood pressure 140/90 mm Hg or greater. The use of antihypertensive medication also counts toward this risk factor.
Low HDL-C	ATP III defines a low HDL-C as less than 40 mg/dL.
Family history of premature CHD	Premature CHD is defined CHD in a male first degree relative younger than 55 years or CHD in a female relative younger than 65 years.
Age	Age more than 45 years for men or more than 55 years for women increases the risk for CHD.

Decreases risk for CHD
High HDL-C	The ATP III considers HDL-C greater than 60 mg/dL to be a negative risk factor and allows the subtraction of one factor from the calculated total.

ATP, Adult Treatment Panel; CHD, coronary heart disease; HDL-C, high-density lipoprotein cholesterol.

cases (even if this is the only risk factor) are at a significant long-term risk for CHD and are candidates for pharmacologic therapy.

Patients who have multiple risk factors that are associated with a less than 10% cardiovascular risk over the next decade generally should not receive lipid-lowering agents when the LDL-C level is in the borderline high (130–159 mg/dL) range. However, drugs are an option when the patient has an increased LDL-C level (≥160 mg/dL) and the 10-year risk is between 10% and 20%.

Individuals in the highest risk category (10-year risk >20%) should attain a treatment goal of LDL-C level less than 100 mg/dL, and TLC may be begun in concert with concomitant pharmacologic therapy if the initial baseline LDL-C levels are greater than 130 mg/dL.

Secondary Prevention

Patients who have survived a coronary event are considered to be in the highest risk category. The ATP III affirms the use of a target level of LDL-C less than 100 mg/dL as an optimal goal of therapy in secondary prevention and emphasizes that individuals with established coronary disease should receive intensive decreasing of LDL-C. Secondary prevention patients with increased baseline LDL-C level (≥130 mg/dL) may benefit from the simultaneous institution of TLC and pharmacologic therapy.

Special Considerations

Metabolic Syndrome

The ATP identifies the clustering of coronary risk factors known collectively as the metabolic syndrome as an important secondary target of therapy. The presence of atherogenic dyslipidemia is common in individuals with the metabolic syndrome. Atherogenic dyslipidemia is characterized by increased triglycerides, an increased LDL-C level (with a small, dense phenotype of LDL particles), and a reduced HDL-C level. Although the perturbations of the lipid profile may be only mild by standard criteria, this so-called lipid triad may increase the risk for premature atherothrombosis. Even though LDL-C levels may appear normal, the lipoprotein may exist in the proatherogenic form of small dense LDL (9). These particles express their atherogenic potential through increased penetrance across the endothelial barrier, cytotoxicity, and enhanced susceptibility to oxidative modification. In addition to the lipid abnormalities, risk factors that may be present in this syndrome include truncal obesity, hypercoagulability, and hypertension, all of which may share a common pathophysiology through insulin resistance (10). The increased risk is substantial; in an analysis from Finland, men with metabolic syndrome as defined by the ATP III were 2.9 times more likely to die of CHD, even in the absence of baseline diabetes or cardiovascular disease (11).

In ATP III, a diagnosis of metabolic syndrome may be made when any three of the five risk factors in Table 11–4 are present. The ATP III emphasizes TLC with weight loss and increased physical activity as the first line of treatment to address the metabolic abnormalities in this syndrome. Such approaches may beneficially alter the lipid triad by reducing triglycerides and increasing the HDL-C level. Physicians should also address other lipid and nonlipid risk factors that may be present.

Coronary Heart Disease Risk Equivalents

Atherothrombosis is a generalized macrovascular disease, and pathologic studies have demonstrated that the presence of peripheral vascular disease, carotid artery disease, or abdominal aneurysms increases the risk for overall development of CHD (12–14). Because individuals with noncoronary cardiovascular disease may have a similar 10-year risk for the development of CHD (i.e., >20%), the ATP III classifies such individuals as having a CHD risk equivalent that requires primary prevention, but with the same LDL-C goal (<100 mg/dL) as individuals with established CHD. The major CHD risk equivalents include:

- Other clinical forms of cardiovascular disease (peripheral arterial disease, abdominal aortic aneurysm, and symptomatic carotid artery disease)
- Diabetes
- Multiple risk factors that confer a 10-year risk for CHD of greater than 20%

Non–High-Density Lipoprotein Cholesterol

As a secondary target of therapy, non–HDL-C may be a clinically useful measurement in patients with high triglycerides (200–499 mg/dL). This parameter is believed to capture not only LDL-C, but also the cholesterol in triglyceride-rich very low-density lipoprotein (VLDL)—that is, LDL-C + VLDL-C. It may be calculated simply by subtracting HDL-C from the total cholesterol value. Treatment goals for non–HDL-C are 30 points greater than the LDL-C goals (Table 11–2). Therefore, the non–HDL-C goal in low-risk patients is less than 190 mg/dL; in intermediate-risk patients it is less than 160 mg/dL; and in high-risk patients it is less than 130 mg/dL. Although weight reduction and physical activity are the first lines of treatment, intensifying LDL-C decreasing drug, with the possible—and cautious—addition of fibrates or nicotinic acid, will reduce the non–HDL-C level. In patients with triglycerides 500 mg/dL or greater, the

TABLE 11–4. General features of the metabolic syndrome

Risk factor	Defining level
Abdominal obesity[a] (waist circumference)[b]	
Men	>102 cm (>40 in.)
Women	>88 cm (>35 in.)
Increased triglycerides level	≥150 mg/dL
Low HDL-C	
Men	<40 mg/dL
Women	<50 mg/dL
Increased blood pressure	≥130/≥85 mm Hg
Fasting glucose	≥110 mg/dL

[a]Overweight and obesity are associated with insulin resistance and the metabolic syndrome. However, the presence of abdominal obesity is more highly correlated with the metabolic risk factors than is an increased body mass index. Therefore, the simple measure of waist circumference is recommended to identify the body weight component of the metabolic syndrome.

[b]Some male patients can experience development of multiple metabolic risk factors when the waist circumference is only marginally increased (e.g., 94–102 cm [37–40 in.]). Such patients may have a strong genetic contribution to insulin resistance and they should benefit from changes in life habits similarly to men with categoric increases in waist circumference.

Adapted from Expert Panel on Detection, Evaluation and Treatment of High Blood Cholesterol in Adults. Executive Summary of the Third Report of the National Cholesterol Education Program (NCEP) Expert Panel on the Detection, Evaluation and Treatment of High Blood Cholesterol in Adults (Adult Treatment Panel III). *JAMA* 2001;285:2486–2497.

initial goal must be to decrease triglycerides to reduce the risk for pancreatitis before addressing LDL-C.

Novel Risk Markers

In the last decade, a number of new risk markers have emerged that may assist the optimal evaluation of cardiovascular risk. These markers include lipoprotein (a), homocysteine, prothrombotic and proinflammatory markers (e.g., fibrinogen or C-reactive protein), impaired fasting glucose, and evidence of subclinical atherothrombosis as assessed by various modalities (e.g., carotid ultrasound, coronary calcium score, ankle brachial index, vascular magnetic resonance imaging, or intravascular ultrasound). The ATP III does not use these emerging factors to modify the LDL-C goal. However, the guidelines do acknowledge that they may be of use for clinical judgment, especially in patients who appear to be at borderline risk on the basis of traditional risk factors alone. For example, an increased C-reactive protein in a seemingly intermediate-risk patient may justify the intensification of lipid therapy.

THERAPY

Therapeutic Lifestyle Changes

The NCEP advocates both individual patient- and population-based interventions to reduce the risk for CHD. The ATP III recommends TLC that include a dietary reduction of saturated fat and cholesterol intake combined with enhancing the reduction of LDL-C through the consumption of plant stanol/sterols and increased soluble fiber. In addition, strategies for weight reduction and regular physical activity were recommended.

Saturated Fat and Cholesterol

Reduction of intake of saturated fat and cholesterol represents the basic approach recommended in the TLC diet (Table 11–5). Serum cholesterol will roughly increase 2% for each 1% of increase in calories derived from saturated fatty acid intake (15). A trial that reduced saturated fatty acids from 15% to 6% of total caloric intake yielded an LDL-C reduction of 11% (16). A metaanalysis that included 6,356 subjects in six large-scale dietary trials demonstrated that the reduction of saturated fatty acid intake decreased the incidence of coronary events by 24% without an increase in noncardiovascular mortality (17). The NCEP recommends that the intake of fatty acids should be reduced to less than 7% of total caloric intake to achieve maximal reduction of LDL-C levels.

Trans fatty acids are produced by the hydrogenation of vegetable oils and are also found in animal fats. Epidemiologic data suggest that a high intake of trans fatty acids is associated with increased risk for CHD (18). Trans fatty acids currently account for approximately 2.6% of total caloric

TABLE 11–5. *Components of the therapeutic lifestyle changes diet*

Nutrient	Recommended intake
Saturated fat	Less than 7% of total calories
Polyunsaturated fat	Up to 10% of total calories
Monounsaturated fat	Up to 20% of total calories
Total fat	25–35% of total calories
Carbohydrate	50–60% of total calories
Fiber	20–30 g/day
Protein	Approximately 15% of total calories
Cholesterol	Less than 200 mg/day
Total calories (energy)	Balance energy intake and expenditure to maintain desirable body weight and prevent weight gain

energy consumed in the United States. Trans fatty acid intake can be altered by reducing the intake of products that are rich in partially hydrogenated oils frequently used in baked products, butter, and some margarines. However, definitive prospective clinical trial data that demonstrate a reduction in coronary events by modifying dietary composition of trans fatty acid are currently lacking.

Dietary Cholesterol

A high intake of cholesterol may adversely affect the ratio of total cholesterol to HDL-C, despite the lack of a significant impact on circulating cholesterol levels (19). A general consensus is that dietary cholesterol may alter atherothrombotic risk independently of an effect on LDL-C, and the NCEP recommends that the total intake per day of cholesterol be less than 200 mg to maximize clinical benefits on the lipid profile.

Monounsaturated Fats

Oleic acid is the most common monounsaturated fat and an increased proportional intake may reduce LDL-C levels and cardiac risk (20). However, extensive controlled prospective clinical trial evidence comparing the effects of monounsaturated versus saturated fatty acid consumption on CHD end points is lacking. The Lyon Heart Study reported that after a myocardial infarction (MI) a Mediterranean-type diet, which is relatively rich in monounsaturated fats, reduced recurrent coronary event rates, with a 72% relative risk reduction ($p = 0.0001$) compared with a prudent "Western"-type diet (21). Monounsaturated fat consumption generally does not have an adverse effect on HDL-C and may decrease LDL-C relative to saturated fat intake.

Polyunsaturated Fatty Acids

Polyunsaturated acids reduce LDL-C levels when substituted for saturated fatty acids and have been demonstrated in a metaanalysis to reduce the risk for coronary disease, which supports experimental work previously performed in nonhuman primates (22,23). Linoleic acid is an N-6 polyunsaturated fatty acid that also may produce a reduction in HDL-C and triglycerides, although individual responses are variable. However, high intake of polyunsaturated fatty acids have not been proven safe in large population studies because of the lack of adequate statistical and epidemiologic data (24). The NCEP recommends that polyunsaturated fatty acids could optimally range up to 10% of total calories.

Total Fat

The ATP II recommended that the total amount of fat be reduced to less than 30% of total caloric intake (3). However, severely restricted total fat intake may lead to a substitution of carbohydrates as percent of total calories and may increase overall body weight. Carbohydrate intake that exceeds 60% of total calories may aggravate the metabolic syndrome and result in glucose intolerance, insulin resistance, and weight gain (25). It is not necessary to reduce total fat intake as a primary means to reduce LDL-C if reduction of saturated fatty acids are reduced to goal levels (<7% of total calories).

Additional Dietary Options for Decreasing Low-Density Lipoprotein Cholesterol

Reduction in LDL-C may also be achieved by increasing the intake of soluble fiber and plant stanol/sterols (26). The addition of viscous fiber (5–10 g/day) to the diet is associated with approximately a 5% reduction in LDL-C. The ATP III recommends the intake of soluble fiber (rich in oats, barley, pectin, and beans) be increased to at least 5 to 10 g per day on the basis of a large-scale metaanalysis of 67 trials (27). In addition, plant sterols isolated from a variety of dietary sources including soybeans and margarine products have been demonstrated to decrease LDL-C. Plant-derived stanol or sterol esters consumed at a level of 2 to 3 g per day may decrease LDL-C by up to 15% without an adverse effect on HDL-C or triglyceride levels (28). However, gastrointestinal absorption of certain nutrients such as carotenoids may be altered by a diet rich in plant sterols.

Weight Reduction

The adult population of the United States has a 60% prevalence of being either overweight or frankly obese. The trends in obesity have a potentially adverse impact on vascular morbidity and mortality (29). For example, the incidence of congestive heart failure is directly related to body mass index in the Framingham Study (30). The ATP III guidelines emphasize weight reduction as a primary intervention that should be delayed until other dietary measures (reduction of saturated fat and cholesterol) have been implemented. Weight reduction has beneficial effects beyond alteration of circulating lipid levels and may improve blood pressure and

insulin sensitivity (31). Achievement of ideal body weight is a therapeutic goal.

Drug Therapy to Achieve Low-Density Lipoprotein Cholesterol Goals

Pharmacologic therapy generally should be reserved for individuals who do not reach established lipid goals after an adequate trial of TLC. The NCEP has presented a mechanism to allow the orderly progression of the initiation and assessment of efficacy of drug therapy. In individuals who are considered to be at relatively low risk, a trial of TLC may be used for approximately 3 months before the consideration of pharmacologic intervention. However, in individuals at high risk, a more aggressive approach to pharmacologic therapy may be advisable, especially in subjects with dyslipidemia after an acute coronary syndrome. The initiation and evaluation of pharmacologic efficacy is a stepwise process (Fig. 11–2). Because of space limitations, we refer physicians to the package inserts for dosing and detailed safety information on the various agents discussed later in this chapter.

Pharmacologic Agents

Predominant Low-Density Lipoprotein Cholesterol-Lowering Agents

3-Hydroxy-3-methylglutaryl Coenzyme A Reductase Inhibitors (Statins)

The currently available HMG CoA reductase inhibitors are lovastatin, pravastatin, simvastatin, fluvastatin, atorvastatin, and rosuvastatin (Table 11–6). In 2001, cerivastatin was removed from the worldwide marketplace because of an increase of fatal cases of rhabdomyolysis that occurred both in monotherapy or in combination with gemfibrozil.

Mechanism of Action. The mechanism of action of the statins is complex and multifactorial. The HMG CoA reductase enzyme is the rate-limiting step in cholesterol biosynthesis, and its activity is partially inhibited by statins. Cholesterol synthesis occurs primarily in the liver and a statin-mediated reduction in intrahepatic cholesterol pools results in a secondary up-regulation of the LDL receptor with increased clearance from the circulation of lipoproteins containing apolipoprotein B (apoB) or apolipoprotein E (apoE). Statins with increased tissue penetrance may also affect the endogenous cholesterol pathway by inhibition of lipoprotein assembly because of apoB fragmentation and reduced incorporation into VLDL (32). In addition, statins have a number of nonlipid or pleiotropic effects that may impact clinical benefit, but they have not been conclusively demonstrated to represent major mechanisms of action of these agents (33,34).

The statins reduce LDL-C reduction in the range of 18% to 55%, depending on the agent and dosage used. The statin dose response usually follows the rule of sixes where a dou-

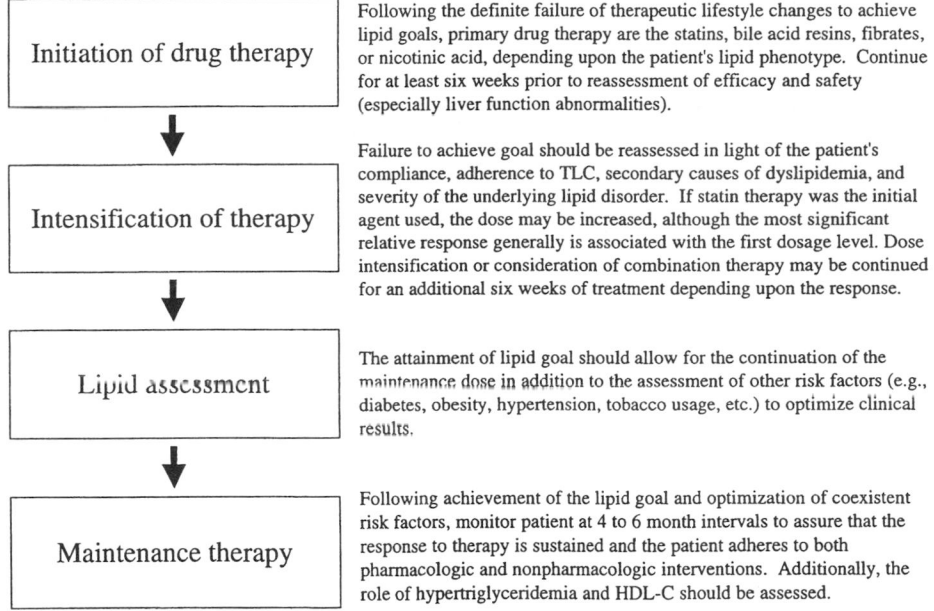

| Initiation of drug therapy | Following the definite failure of therapeutic lifestyle changes to achieve lipid goals, primary drug therapy are the statins, bile acid resins, fibrates, or nicotinic acid, depending upon the patient's lipid phenotype. Continue for at least six weeks prior to reassessment of efficacy and safety (especially liver function abnormalities). |

| Intensification of therapy | Failure to achieve goal should be reassessed in light of the patient's compliance, adherence to TLC, secondary causes of dyslipidemia, and severity of the underlying lipid disorder. If statin therapy was the initial agent used, the dose may be increased, although the most significant relative response generally is associated with the first dosage level. Dose intensification or consideration of combination therapy may be continued for an additional six weeks of treatment depending upon the response. |

| Lipid assessment | The attainment of lipid goal should allow for the continuation of the maintenance dose in addition to the assessment of other risk factors (e.g., diabetes, obesity, hypertension, tobacco usage, etc.) to optimize clinical results. |

| Maintenance therapy | Following achievement of the lipid goal and optimization of coexistent risk factors, monitor patient at 4 to 6 month intervals to assure that the response to therapy is sustained and the patient adheres to both pharmacologic and nonpharmacologic interventions. Additionally, the role of hypertriglyceridemia and HDL-C should be assessed. |

FIG. 11–2. Implementation of drug therapy. HDL-C, high-density lipoprotein cholesterol; TLC, therapeutic lifestyle changes.

bling of the dose results in an additive 6% reduction in LDL-C for each progressive increment. Statin therapy generally increases HDL-C, although the achieved change may be modest and ranges from 5% to 15%. Triglyceride reduction is a function of pretreatment triglycerides and underlying metabolic abnormalities, but generally ranges from 7% to 30%.

Side Effects. The majority of data suggest statins have an acceptable risk factor profile. The major side effects of statin therapy relate to hepatic or muscle toxicity. Increased hepatic transaminases occur in approximately 0.5 to 2% of individuals and generally relate with dosing intensity (35). Increases of transaminase levels occur in about 1 per 1,000 patients who receive 20 mg lovastatin per day, which increases to approximately 2% if the dose is increased to 80 mg per day. However, in large clinical trials, the risks for sustained increases of circulating transaminase levels (two to three times the upper limit of normal) were essentially equal for statin-treated and placebo-treated arms. Fatal cases of hepatic failure with statin monotherapy are extremely rare, and liver function generally returns to normal after drug discontinuation. However, active or significant chronic liver disease is considered to be an absolute contraindication for statin use.

Myotoxicity is less common than hepatic toxicity, but it has been associated with fatal rhabdomyolysis and associated renal failure (36). The spectrum of muscle symptoms associated with statin therapy ranges from nonspecific myalgia with normal creatine kinase levels to clinical myositis with borderline increases of creatine kinase to frank rhabdomyolysis. The failure to recognize the clinical manifestations of significant muscle involvement and discontinue

therapy may lead to diffuse muscle breakdown and acute renal failure caused by myoglobinuria. The risk for muscle toxicity is increased in combination therapy, especially with cyclosporine, fibric acid derivatives, erythromycin, and nicotinic acid. The risk for interaction with the fibrates is especially increased in renal insufficiency because fibrates are primarily cleared by the kidney. The mechanism by which statins cause myotoxicity is more complicated than simple interactions with the cytochrome P450-3A4 enzyme system (37). However, the coadministration of statins with agents that are also metabolized by this pathway potentially increase the risk for muscle toxicity. Pravastatin does not use the 3A4 pathway and, therefore, may have hypothetical advantages in combination therapy.

Clinical Trial Evidence. Statin therapy has a robust trial database that includes angiographic regression studies, monotherapy trials, and combination therapy trials. The most compelling evidence of clinical efficacy has been derived from the large-scale primary and secondary trials that used statin therapy in a wide spectrum of patients (36–43). In both primary and secondary prevention, statins have reduced the risk for coronary events and the need for revascularization procedures. In secondary prevention and other high-risk prevention, statins have also reduced the risk for stroke and all-cause mortality rates.

Bile Acid Sequestrants

Bile acid sequestrants (or resins) were among the initial hypolipidemic agents used to treat increased LDL-C levels. Available agents include cholestyramine and colestipol, with the recent addition of colesevelam (44).

TABLE 11–6. *Summary of major classes of lipid-modifying drugs*

Drug class	Statins	Fibrates	Resins	Nicotinic acid
Available in United States	Lovastatin, pravastatin, simvastatin, fluvastatin, atorvastatin, rosuvastatin	Gemfibrozil, clofibrate, fenofibrate	Cholestyramine, colestipol, colesevelam	Various preparations
Lipid/lipoprotein effects	LDL-C: ↓ 18–55% HDL-C: ↑ 5–15% TG: ↓ 7–30%	LDL-C: variable HDL-C: 10–20% TG: 20–50%	LDL-C: 15–30% HDL-C: 3–5% TG: no change or increase	LDL-C: 5–25% HDL-C: 15–35% TG: 20–50%
Major use	To decrease LDL-C level	To decrease TG level, increase HDL-C level	To decrease LDL-C level	To decrease LDL-C and TG levels, increase HDL-C level
Contraindications				
Absolute	Active or chronic liver disease	Severe renal or hepatic disease	Dysbetalipoproteinemia, TG > 400 mg/dL	Chronic liver disease, severe gout
Relative	Concomitant use of cyclosporine, gemfibrozil, niacin, macrolide antibiotics, various antifungal agents, and cytochrome P-450 inhibitors		TG > 200 mg/dL	Diabetes, hyperuricemia, peptic ulcer disease
Efficacy	Reduce angiographic progression of atherothrombosis Reduce risk for CHD in primary prevention Reduce risk for CHD, all-cause death, and stroke in secondary prevention	Reduce risk for angiographic progression of atherothrombosis Reduce risk for CHD in primary and secondary prevention	Reduce risk for angiographic progression of atherothrombosis Reduce risk for CHD in primary prevention	Reduce risk for CHD and possibly all-cause mortality
Safety	Side effects minimal in clinical trials; infrequent myopathy with rare cases of rhabdomyolysis; increased liver enzymes	Dyspepsia, gallstones, myopathy; unexplained increase in non-CHD deaths in WHO study	Gastrointestinal distress; constipation; decreased absorption of other drugs	Flushing, hyperglycemia, hyperuricemia (or gout), upper gastrointestinal distress, hepatotoxicity
Usual starting dose/ maximum FDA-approved dose	Lovastatin: 20 mg/80 mg Pravastatin: 20 mg/80 mg Simvastatin: 20 mg/80 mg Fluvastatin: 20 mg/80 mg Atorvastatin: 10 mg/80 mg Rosuvastatin: 10 mg/40 mg	Gemfibrozil: 600 mg twice daily/1200 mg Fenofibrate: 200 mg daily/200 mg Clofibrate: 1000 mg twice daily/2000 mg	Cholestyramine: 4–16 g/24 g Colestipol: 5–20g/30 g Colesevelam: 2.6–3.8g/4.4 g	Crystalline: 1.5–3 g/ 4.5 g Sustained-release: 1–2 g/2 g Extended-release: 1–2 g/2 g

CHD, coronary heart disease; FDA, Food and Drug Administration; HDL-C, high-density lipoprotein cholesterol; LDL-C, low-density lipoprotein cholesterol; TG, triglyceride; WHO, World Health Organization.

Mechanism of Action. The bile acid sequestrants interfere with the enterohepatic circulation of the cholesterol-rich bile acid pool. Normally, the bile acid pool is nearly completely (97%) reabsorbed at the ileal level. By binding with bile acids, resins reduce the normal reabsorption in the ileum and increase fecal bile acid removal. The increased fecal loss stimulates the conversion of cholesterol into bile acids by stimulating 7-α-dehydrogenase. Hepatic cholesterol levels are decreased and a secondary up-regulation of the apoB/E receptor results in increased LDL removal from the circulation. However, the reduction in intrahepatic cholesterol level results in a secondary stimulation of cholesterol synthesis by HMG CoA reductase induction, which may diminish the long-term reduction of LDL-C as a new steady state is reached. For this reason, statins may be prescribed in combination with resins to exploit their complementary modes of action.

The bile acid sequestrants are generally pure LDL-C decreasing agents and may achieve a reduction of 15% to 30% depending on maximum dose achieved. The resins do not decrease triglycerides and may slightly increase circulating levels if the patient is predisposed to hypertriglyceridemia because of the presence of diabetes or obesity. The effect of resins on HDL-C is minimal and increases of 3% to 5% may be achieved, although the mechanism is unclear.

Side Effects. The resins are not absorbed by the gastrointestinal tract and thus lack direct systemic effects, but they are associated with significant gastrointestinal symptomatology including bloating, constipation, and nausea. In addition, the bile acid sequestrants are nonspecific binders and will interfere with the absorption of a number of anionic drugs including Coumadin, digoxin, β-blockers, and other cardiac medications. Therefore, concomitant medications should be taken at least 1 hour before the administration of resins. Resins may exacerbate hypertriglyceridemia in susceptible individuals (e.g., in obese, diabetic, or insulin-resistant subjects).

Clinical Trial Evidence. Resins have been used in both monotherapy and combination regimen trials. In clinical trials, cholestyramine has reduced the risk for nonfatal MI and CHD death, as well as slowed angiographic progression of atherothrombosis (45,46).

Cholesterol Absorption Inhibitors

Recently, a novel type of LDL-C decreasing agent has been introduced known as a cholesterol absorption inhibitor. The first of these is ezetimibe.

Mechanism of Action. Ezetimibe reduces blood cholesterol by inhibiting the absorption of cholesterol in the small intestine, leading to a decrease in the delivery of intestinal cholesterol to the liver. The decrease in intrahepatic cholesterol increases clearance of cholesterol from the circulation, thereby reducing total cholesterol. Ezetimibe (10 mg/day) may reduce total cholesterol by about 13%, LDL-C by 19%, apoB by 14%, and triglycerides by 8%. Ezetimibe increases HDL-C by 3%. It may be administered as monotherapy or in combination with statins.

Side Effects. Because of its novelty, there is limited clinical experience with ezetimibe. It appears to have no activity with the cytochrome P450 isozymes and, therefore, is unlikely to affect the metabolism of drugs metabolized by this pathway. When used in combination with statins, ezetimibe may increase the risk for liver enzyme elevations three times greater than the upper limit of normal, but it does not seem to increase the risk for skeletal muscle toxicity.

Clinical Trial Evidence. There are no data evaluating the clinical effects of ezetimibe as monotherapy or combination therapy on the risk for coronary and other cardiovascular events.

Predominant Triglyceride-decreasing Agents

Fibrates

The fibric acid derivatives have a long history of clinical use, and the currently available agents in the United States are gemfibrozil, fenofibrate, and clofibrate.

Mechanism of Action. The mechanisms of action of the fibrates are complex and involve the peroxisome proliferator-activated receptor-alpha (PPAR-α) (47). The PPAR-α system is a family of nuclear transcription factors that when activated by agonists results in an increase in HDL-C and reduction in triglyceride levels. Fibrates down-regulate the ex-

pression of apolipoprotein C-III, which is an inhibitor of lipoprotein lipase (48). Gemfibrozil increases catabolism of VLDL and chylomicron remnant lipoproteins and will reduce postprandial lipemia. Fibric acid derivatives may alter the phenotype of small, dense LDL to a larger, more buoyant, and presumably less atherogenic form.

The fibric acid derivatives have modest effects on LDL-C that are a function of pretreatment triglyceride levels and efficiency of apoB/E receptor activity. In general, LDL-C decreases between 5% and 20% after administration of fibrates, but may be increased in individuals with significant hypertriglyceridemia before the administration of the agents. Depending on baseline triglyceride levels, HDL-C level generally will increase between 10% and 35%. Triglyceride level decreases between 20% and 50% may be achieved with administration of fibric acid derivatives.

Side Effects. The fibric acid derivatives are generally well tolerated and free of serious side effects. However, early clinical trials suggested a potential increase in noncardiac mortality with the use of clofibrate (49). The fibrates appear to be associated with increased risk for cholelithiasis because of an increased incidence of cholesterol gallstones. The fibrates are protein-bound and thus may alter circulating levels of coadministered drugs that also demonstrate binding to albumin. The prothrombin time may need to be adjusted in individuals who are receiving combined Coumadin and fibrate therapy. The fibric acid derivatives are mainly excreted by renal mechanisms, and dosage levels may be altered in the presence of renal insufficiency. A major concern for combination therapy has been the interaction between fibric acid derivatives and statins, increasing the risk for myotoxicity. Some data have suggested that gemfibrozil may inhibit glucuronidation of statins, thereby increasing exposure to the active form of the statin, especially cerivastatin, and increasing the risk for rhabdomyolysis (50).

Clinical Trial Evidence. Clinical trials with other fibrates have not demonstrated the same safety concerns as clofibrate. Gemfibrozil has reduced primary and recurrent CHD and slowed atherothrombotic progression in at-risk men with a low HDL-C level (51–53). Fenofibrate has slowed progression in a cohort of patients with diabetes (54).

Nicotinic Acid

Nicotinic acid is an essential B vitamin associated with the deficiency state pellagra. Pellagra, which is a systemic disorder, may be prevented by 5 mg per day of nicotinic acid. However, doses of this essential B vitamin that exceed those needed to prevent deficiency will improve the lipid profile. Nicotinic acid is converted into nicotinamide, which is the substrate for nicotinamide adenine dinucleotide. However, a significant hypolipidemic effect requires the presence of the parent molecule.

Mechanism of Action. Nicotinic acid has a complex mechanism of action involving both hepatic and peripheral effects. Nicotinic acid is associated with a reduction in the release and flux of free fatty acids from peripheral adipocytes to the liver, resulting in a decrease in available substrate for VLDL synthesis. Therefore, the niacin-mediated reduction in hepatic secretion of VLDL decreases catabolic generation of intermediate-density lipoprotein and LDL. Nicotinic acid has been demonstrated to increase total HDL-C and both major circulating subfractions (HDL-2 and HDL-3). Nicotinic acid also increases the HDL-associated and cardioprotective lipoprotein A-I. Nicotinic acid may inhibit hepatic removal of HDL-apoprotein A-I without interfering with the removal of cholesterol by HDL, and thus may increase the efficiency of reverse cholesterol transport (55).

Nicotinic acid is the only hypolipidemic agent that demonstrates beneficial effects on all circulating lipid subfractions. Nicotinic acid therapy will reduce LDL-C levels by 5% to 25%, increase HDL-C levels by 15% to 35%, and reduce triglyceride levels by up to 50%. Nicotinic acid is the only standard hypolipidemic agent that reduces lipoprotein (a), an emerging CHD risk factor (56).

Side Effects. The most common side effect of nicotinic acid is diffuse flushing and pruritus secondary to prostaglandin-mediated vasodilatation. The cutaneous complications of niacin may be minimized by premedication with aspirin, initial low dose with gradual subsequent uptitration, and the ingestion of nicotinic acid with meals. The flushing is most marked with crystalline niacin and is less prominent when long-acting preparations are used. Nicotinic acid is associated with a variety of gastrointestinal disorders and peptic ulcer disease may be activated with the potential for hemorrhagic complications.

Nicotinic acid may worsen glucose control. However, meticulous administration of niacin with monitoring of metabolic parameters has been safely used in patients with diabetes (57). Niacin may be considered as an alternative therapy in subjects with diabetes who do not tolerate fibric acid derivatives or statins (58).

Hyperuricemia may be associated with nicotinic acid use, and clinical exacerbations of gout may occur. The most serious complication of nicotinic acid is fulminant acute hepatic failure. The incidence of hepatic failure is idiosyncratic and should be suspected when a sudden precipitous decline in circulating lipid levels occurs. However, increased liver enzymes greater than three times the upper limit of normal occurs in 0.5% of individuals, even with the combination of nicotinic acid and a statin (59). Nicotinic acid may also be associated with acanthosis nigricans, toxic amblyopia, and conjunctivitis.

Clinical Indications. Nicotinic acid therapy reduces the risk for coronary events and may be associated with reduced all-cause mortality (60). In combination with a statin, it may slow atherothrombotic progression (61).

Omega-3 Polyunsaturated Fatty Acids

Diets rich in omega-3 polyunsaturated fatty acids may be associated with a reduced incidence of CHD (62). Dietary sources of omega-3 fatty acids include fish oils that are rich in eicosapentaenoic acid and docosahexaenoic acid. In addition, vegetables rich in α-linolenic acid are also a dietary source of omega-3 fatty acids. Omega-3 fatty acids may also be obtained in fish oil capsules at a dosage range of 3 to 12 g per day.

Mechanism of Action. High-dose omega-3 fatty acids have major effects on the reduction of the hepatic production of triglyceride-rich lipoproteins and may be used in individuals who are intolerant of fibric acid derivatives or nicotinic acid. In addition, chylomicronemia may also be decreased by omega-3 fatty acids (63). The effect of fish oils may transcend lipid effects, and antithrombotic properties have been attributed to fish oils (64). Eicosapentaenoic acid has been demonstrated to reduce the synthesis of thromboxane A_2, which is a powerful agonist for platelet activation and vasoconstriction (65). Endothelial function also is improved by the ingestion of omega-3 fatty acids. Omega-3 fatty acids may also demonstrate an antiarrhythmic effect, which occurs from stabilization of the electrical activity of cardiac myocytes by a prolongation of the relative refractory period (66). The administration of fish oil may also have beneficial effects on lipid peroxidation and antioxidant activity (67).

Side Effects. The side effects of nondietary fish oil administration are generally mild and consist of an unpleasant aftertaste when administered as fish oil capsules. The role of fish oil supplementation has been controversial in individuals with diabetes or impaired glucose tolerance. However, a metaanalysis of 18 trials that analyzed the effects of fish oil on serum lipids and glucose tolerance demonstrated no significant changes in hemoglobin A_{1C} in patients with diabetes treated with fish oil (68). A trend toward increased fasting blood glucose levels was determined but did not reach statistical significance.

Clinical Trial Evidence. The ATP III guidelines analyzed the clinical trial evidence for omega-3 fatty acids and determined the strength of definite benefit to be moderate. Fish oil treatment has been shown to reduce the risk for cardiovascular events by 10% in secondary prevention (69). Although the data are promising, more definitive clinical trials are needed before recommending an increase in omega-3 fatty acid intake (69–71).

Combination Therapy

Some patients will require combination therapy to reach ATP III goals. Common combinations include a statin plus a resin, which increases LDL-C decreasing potency; a statin plus a fibrate, which addresses the combined hyperlipidemia of increased LDL-C and triglycerides; a statin plus nicotinic acid, which favorably affects all lipid fractions; and a fibrate plus nicotinic acid, which is attractive for atherogenic dyslipidemia. Although combination therapy may increase lipid-modifying efficacy, certain combinations also may increase the risk for side effects, such as the interaction of statins with fibrates or nicotinic acid that may increase the risk for myopathy. Although several trials have examined the effect of combination therapies on lipid parameters and only a handful of trials have explored their effect on clinical end points, these latter trials generally report beneficial effects on such measures as atherothrombotic progression (61).

Special Considerations

Diabetes

Diabetic dyslipidemia is characterized by relatively normal total cholesterol levels associated with small, dense LDL particles, low HDL-C levels, and increased triglyceride-rich lipoproteins (72). In addition, the metabolic syndrome, which is characterized by insulin resistance, has this lipid phenotype as one of its major features. Diabetes is clearly associated with increased risk for cardiovascular disease and its complications (73). Regulation of blood sugar reduces microvascular complications of diabetes, such as retinopathy and peripheral neuropathy. However, macrovascular complications are more clearly related to the prevalence of dyslipidemia and hypertension (74). Patients with type 2 diabetes have an increased risk for mortality after unstable angina and non-ST elevation MI (75). Patients with diabetes who survive the initial coronary event have an adverse long-term survival rate because of increased rates of congestive heart failure and fatal and nonfatal MIs. The ATP III panel considers diabetes to be a CHD risk equivalent, on the basis of epidemiologic studies that demonstrate that morbidity and mortality rates in nondiabetic individuals in secondary prevention are similar to those in subjects with diabetes who would qualify for primary prevention (76). Subgroup analyses from the major statin trials in high-risk patients suggest a statistically significant decrease in major coronary events with statin therapy compared with placebo (77,78).

The ATP III developed therapeutic recommendations on the basis of lipid levels in subjects with diabetes. Because of diabetes' CHD risk equivalency, the LDL-C goal would be less than 100 mg/dL.

1. LDL-C levels greater than 130 mg/dL: Individuals whose LDL-C level exceeds 130 mg/dL are candidates for TLC. In addition, statins would be the first choice for LDL-C decreasing drugs. If the triglycerides exceed 200 mg/dL, non–HDL-C should be less than 130 mg/dL. Fibric acid derivatives or nicotinic acid may be used as alternative therapy to statins or in combination to achieve the goal for non–HDL-C.
2. LDL-C levels 120 to 129 mg/dL: Individuals with borderline LDL-C level increase should have intensive treatment of nonlipid risk factors and TLC. The lipid profile should focus on a non–HDL-C goal of less than 130 mg/dL, if baseline triglycerides are in excess of 200 mg/dL. Fibrates and nicotinic acid may be used as alternatives to statin therapy. Nicotinic acid may worsen glu-

cose tolerance; therefore, at all LDL-C levels, the dose should not exceed 3,000 mg per day. An LDL-C level of 100 to 129 mg/dL even with therapy should result in intensification of therapy.
3. LDL-C levels less than 100 mg/dL: Individuals with diabetes whose LDL-C levels already are within the ATP III goals should have intense treatment of nonlipid risk factors including hypertension control, weight reduction, smoking cessation and exercise, and other TLC.

Elderly

Although the relative relation between cholesterol and coronary events weakens with age, the absolute attributable risk, which may be defined as the difference in coronary event rates between the highest and lowest quintiles of cholesterol, actually increases with advancing age, because of the high prevalence of atherothrombosis in the elderly population. Hypertension, obesity, and diabetes are also more prevalent in the older age group and increase overall risk (79). Metaanalysis of the statin trials indicate comparable benefits of treatment in older versus younger participants (80). The Prospective Evaluation of Pravastatin in the Elderly (PROSPER) trial assessed the effect of pravastatin versus placebo in a cohort of high-risk patients, 72 to 80 years of age, treated for 3.2 years. This study reported a 15% reduction in the risk for cardiovascular events ($p = 0.014$), largely because of a reduction in the risk for CHD death or nonfatal MI (81).

The ATP III argues that chronologic age alone should not exclude patients who may benefit from lipid treatment. Similar action limits may be used for older and younger patients (Table 11–2). However, in the older subgroup, because of the decreased predictability of cholesterol, clinical judgment may be needed. The use of noninvasive screening modalities, such as carotid ultrasonography, ankle brachial index, or coronary calcium score, may help identify elderly patients with subclinical atherothrombosis. Management of associated risk factors including hypertension, diabetes, and smoking are of paramount importance in this subgroup. Treatment must also consider quality of life issues that are especially germane to the elderly, such as cost, impact on quality of life, and the patient's level of functionality.

Low High-Density Lipoprotein Cholesterol

The ATP III defines a low HDL-C level as less than 40 mg/dL. An HDL-C level in excess of 60 mg/dL is a negative risk factor and allows subtraction of one risk factor from the total risk factor profile. A low HDL-C level is frequently associated with physical inactivity, obesity, the metabolic syndrome, and diabetes (82). Dietary composition may alter HDL-C levels and a very high carbohydrate intake that accounts for more than 60% of total energy is associated with low HDL-C. Cigarette smoking may decrease HDL-C by up to 5 mg/dL and should be discontinued (83). Genetic conditions may also be associated with HDL-C reduction caused by either reduced production or increased catabolism.

The ATP III does not identify a goal for HDL-C levels, but does recommend the management of individuals with low HDL-C. The target for lipid intervention in these individuals is LDL-C. After achieving the LDL-C goal, the next step should emphasize increased physical activity and optimization of body weight. When low HDL-C occurs with triglycerides of 200 mg/dL or more, a secondary priority goes to achieving the non–HDL-C goal. Pharmacologic therapy of low HDL-C levels in primary prevention using traditional HDL-C increasing drugs (fibric acid derivatives or nicotinic acid) does not have a robust clinical trial database; however, isolated increasing of HDL-C levels may be considered in patients with CHD or CHD risk equivalent (84).

Estrogen

In women, CHD develops approximately 10 years later than in men and is relatively rare in the premenopausal years, unless a genetic hyperlipidemia (e.g., familial hypercholesterolemia) is present. The epidemiologic pattern of coronary atherothrombosis suggests a protective role for endogenous estrogen in women who are premenopausal (85). However, the role of hormone replacement therapy as a means to prevent CHD has been controversial. Oral estrogens reduce the LDL-C level, presumably by increasing LDL receptor activity. In addition, the HDL-C level is increased by exogenous estrogen therapy when administered through the oral route. In contrast, estrogen therapy may increase triglycerides and increase the potential for coagulation by increasing fibrinogen (86). In addition, inflammatory markers (hsCRP) have been increased by hormone replacement therapy (87).

The Heart Estrogen/Progestin Replacement Study (HERS) was a randomized, double-blinded, placebo-controlled trial that evaluated the role of 0.625 mg of conjugated estrogen plus 2.5 mg of medroxyprogesterone in 2,763 postmenopausal women with documented CHD (88). Despite a large body of observational data that suggested a benefit to women who used hormone replacement therapy, the combination therapy used in the HERS did not demonstrate a significant difference between hormone and placebo groups in the primary outcome, which was fatal and nonfatal CHD. Extended follow-up of the original HERS reported no benefit over a total of 6.8 years of hormone replacement therapy (89). Along the same line, in the Estrogen Replacement Atherosclerosis (ERA) study, hormone replacement therapy did not slow atherothrombotic progression in postmenopausal women with angiographic evidence of CHD (90).

The primary prevention Women's Health Initiative (WHI) of 16,608 postmenopausal women likewise showed no coronary benefits in the 5.2-year trial period with conjugated equine estrogen 0.625 mg per day plus medroxyprogesterone 2.5 mg per day in one tablet form (91). The composite results of the WHI, ERA, and HERS do not support the use of hormone replacement therapy in postmenopausal women as CHD prevention.

CONCLUSION

The most recent guidelines of the U.S. NCEP reflect a major step forward for the management of cardiovascular risk. First, they embrace the concept of global risk assessment in prevention, recognizing that the composite effect of dyslipidemia with other major risk factors is the primary determinant of the patient's overall risk and should guide treatment intensity. Second, these guidelines keep pace with important clinical and basic scientific advances, putting forth a diagnostic and treatment strategy for the metabolic syndrome, an important constellation of cardiovascular risk factors that should be a secondary target of therapy. Third, as a whole, they present a useful algorithm for the clinician that simplifies a body of knowledge that has grown increasingly sophisticated.

REFERENCES

1. American Heart Association. *Heart and Stroke Facts Update 2004.* Dallas, TX: AHA, 2003.
2. Report of the National Cholesterol Education Program Expert Panel on Detection, Evaluation, and Treatment of High Blood Cholesterol in Adults. The Expert Panel. *Arch Intern Med* 1988;148:36–69.
3. National Cholesterol Education Program. Second Report of the Expert Panel on Detection, Evaluation and Treatment of High Blood Cholesterol in Adults (Adult Treatment Panel II). *Circulation* 1994;89: 1333–1445.
4. Rossouw JE, Lewis B, Rifkind BM. The value of lowering cholesterol after myocardial infarction. *N Engl J Med* 1990;323:1112–1119.
5. Expert Panel on Detection, Evaluation and Treatment of High Blood Cholesterol in Adults. Executive Summary of the Third Report of the National Cholesterol Education Program (NCEP) Expert Panel on the Detection, Evaluation and Treatment of High Blood Cholesterol in Adults (Adult Treatment Panel III). *JAMA* 2001;285:2486–2497.
6. Law MR. Lowering heart disease risk with cholesterol reduction: evidence from observational studies in clinical trials. *Eur Heart J Suppl* 1999;[Suppl 1]:S3–S8.
7. Assmann G. Pro and con: high density lipoprotein, triglycerides and other lipid subfractions of the future of lipid management. *Am J Cardiol* 2001;87(5A):2B–7B.
8. Wilson TWF, D'Agostino RB, Levy D, et al. Prediction of coronary heart disease using risk factor categories. *Circulation* 1998;97: 1837–1847.
9. Superko HR. Small dense low density lipoprotein and atherosclerosis. *Curr Atheroscler Rep* 2000;2:226–231.
10. Reaven G. Metabolic syndrome: pathophysiology and implications for management of cardiovascular disease. *Circulation* 2002;106: 286–288.
11. Lakka HM, Laaksonen DE, Lakka TA, et al. The metabolic syndrome and total and cardiovascular disease mortality in middle-aged men. *JAMA* 2002;288:2709–2716.
12. Leng GC, Papacosta O, Whincup P, et al. Femoral atherosclerosis in an older British population: prevalence and risk factors. *Atherosclerosis* 2000;152:167–174.
13. Ferguson GC, Eliasziw M, Barr HW, et al. The North American Symptomatic Carotid Endarterectomy Trial surgical results in 1,415 patients. *Stroke* 1999;30:1751–1758.
14. Norman PE, Semmens JB, Lawrence-Brown MM. Long-term survival following surgery for abdominal aortic aneurysm: a review. *Cardiovasc Surg* 2001;9:219–224.
15. Muller H, Kirkhus B, Pedersen JI. Serum cholesterol predictive equa-

tions with special emphasis on trans and saturated fatty acids. An analysis from designed controlled trials. *Lipids* 2001;36:783–791.

16. Ginsberg HN, Kris-Etherton P, Dennis D, et al. Effects of reducing dietary saturated fatty acids on plasma lipids and lipoproteins in healthy subjects. *Arterioscler Thromb Vasc Biol* 1998;18:441–449.

17. Gordon DJ. Cholesterol lowering and total mortality. In: Rifkind BM, ed. *Contemporary issues in cholesterol lowering: clinical and population aspects.* New York: Marcel-Dekker, 1994:33–48.

18. Oomen CM, Ocke MC, Feskens EJ, et al. Association between trans fatty acid intake and 10-year risk of coronary artery disease in the Zutphen Elderly Study: a prospective population based study. *Lancet* 2001;357:746–751.

19. Weggemans RM, Zock PL, Katan MB. Dietary cholesterol from eggs increases the ratio of total cholesterol to high density lipoprotein cholesterol in humans: a meta-analysis. *Am J Clin Nutr* 2001;73:885–891.

20. Kris-Etherton PM, Pearson TA, Wan Y, et al. High monounsaturated fatty acid diets lower both plasma cholesterol and triacyglycerol con centrations. *Am J Clin Nutr* 1999;70:1009–1015.

21. de Lorgeril M, Salen P, Martin JL, et al. Mediterranean diet, traditional risk factors and the risk of cardiovascular complications after myocardial infarction: final report of the Lyon Diet Heart Study. *Circulation* 1999;99:779–785.

22. Olson RE. The key to an enigma: how the dietary polyunsaturated fatty acids lower serum cholesterol. *J Nutr* 2002;132:134–135.

23. Rudel LL, Parks JS, Sawyer JK. Compared with dietary monounsaturated and saturated fat, polyunsaturated fat protects African Green monkeys from coronary artery atherosclerosis. *Arterioscler Thromb Vasc Biol* 1995;15:2101–2110.

24. Kris-Etherton P, Daniels SR, Eckel RH, et al. Summary of the scientific conference on dietary fatty acids and cardiovascular health: conference summary from the Nutrition Committee of the American Heart Association. *Circulation* 2001;103:1034–1039.

25. Howard BV, Wylie-Rosett J. Sugar and cardiovascular disease. A statement for healthcare professionals from the Committee on Nutrition of the Council on Nutrition, Physical Activity and Metabolism of the American Heart Association. *Circulation* 2000;106:523–527.

26. Kris-Etherton PM, Etherton TD, Carlson J, et al. Recent discoveries in inclusive food based approaches and dietary patterns for reduction in risk for cardiovascular disease. *Curr Opin Lipidol* 2002;13:397–407.

27. Brown L, Rosner B, Willett WW, et al. Cholesterol lowering effects of dietary fiber: a meta-analysis. *Am J Clin Nutr* 1999;69:30–42.

28. Lichtenstein AH. Plant sterols and blood lipid levels. *Curr Opin Clin Nutr Metab Care* 2002;5:147–152.

29. Eckel RH, Barouch WW, Ershow AG. Report of the NHLBI and NIKKD Working Group on the pathophysiology of obesity associated heart disease. *Circulation* 2002;105:2923–2928.

30. Kenchaiah S, Evans JC, Levy D, et al. Obesity and the risk of heart failure. *N Engl J Med* 2002;347:305–313.

31. The Obesity Evidence Report. NIH publication no. 98-4083; September 1998.

32. Burnett JR, Wilcox LJ, Telford DE, et al. The magnitude of decrease in hepatic very low density lipoprotein apo B secretion is determined by the extent of 3-hydroxy-3-methylglutaryl coenzyme A reductase inhibition. *Endocrinology* 1999;140:5293–5302.

33. Rifai N, Ridker VM. Inflammatory markers and coronary heart disease. *Curr Opin Lipidol* 2002;13:383–389.

34. Farmer JA, Gotto AM. Dyslipidemia and the vulnerable plaque. *Prog Cardiovasc Dis* 2002;44:415–428.

35. Tolman KG. The liver and lovastatin. *Am J Cardiol* 2002;89:1374–1380.

36. Evans M, Rees A. Effects of HMG Co A reductase inhibitors on skeletal muscle: are all statins the same? *Drug Saf* 2002;25:649–663.

37. Farmer JA. Learning from the cerivastatin experience. *Lancet* 2001; 358:1383–1385.

38. Downs JR, Clearfield M, Weis S, et al. Primary prevention of acute coronary events with lovastatin in men and women with average cholesterol levels: results of the AFCAPS/TexCAPS Air Force/Texas Coronary Atherosclerosis Prevention Study. *JAMA* 1998;279:1615–1622.

39. Shepherd J, Cobbe SM, Ford I, et al. Prevention of coronary heart disease with pravastatin in men with hypercholesterolemia. West of Scotland Coronary Prevention Study Group. *N Engl J Med* 1995;333:1301–1307.

40. Randomized trial of cholesterol lowering in 4444 patients with coronary heart disease: the Scandinavian Simvastatin Survival Study (4S). *Lancet* 1994;344:1383–1389.

41. Sacks FM, Pfeffer MA, Moye LA, et al. The effect of pravastatin on coronary events after myocardial infarction in patients with average cholesterol levels. Cholesterol and Recurrent Events Trial Investigators. *N Engl J Med* 1996;335:1001–1009.

42. Prevention of cardiovascular events and death with pravastatin in patients with coronary heart disease and a broad range of initial cholesterol levels. The Long-Term Intervention with Pravastatin in Ischemic Disease (LIPID) Study Group. *N Engl J Med* 1998;339:1349–1357.

43. Heart Protection Study Collaborative Group. MRC/BHF Heart Protection Study of cholesterol lowering with simvastatin in 20,536 high risk individuals: a randomized, placebo-controlled trial. *Lancet* 2002;360:7–22.

44. Wong NN. Colesevelam: a new bile acid sequestrant. *Heart Dis* 2001; 3:63–70.

45. The Lipid Research Clinics Coronary Primary Prevention Trial results. I. Reduction in incidence of coronary artery disease. *JAMA* 1984;251: 351–364.

46. Watts GF, Lewis D, Brunt JN, et al. Effects on coronary artery disease of lipid lowering diet or diet plus cholestyramine in the Saint Thomas Atherosclerosis Regression Study (STARS). *Lancet* 1992;339:563–569.

47. Vosper H, Khoudoli G, Grahm T, et al. Peroxisome proliferator activated receptor agonists, hyperlipidemia and atherosclerosis. *Pharmacol Ther* 2002;95:47–62.

48. Fredenrich A. Role of apolipoprotein C-III in triglyceride rich lipoprotein metabolism. *Diabetes Metab* 1998;24:490–495.

49. WHO cooperative trial on primary prevention of ischemic heart disease with clofibrate to lower serum cholesterol: final mortality follow-up. Report of the Committee of Principal Investigators. *Lancet* 1984;2:600–604.

50. Prueksaritanont T, Tang C, Qiu Y, et al. Effects of fibrates on metabolism of statins in human hepatocytes. *Drug Metab Dispos* 2002;30:1280–1287.

51. Manninen D, Tenkanen L, Koskinen P, et al. Joint effects of serum triglyceride, LDL cholesterol and HDL cholesterol concentrations on coronary heart disease risk in the Helsinki Heart Study. *Circulation* 1992;85:37–45.

52. Frick MH, Syvanne M, Nieminen MS, et al. Prevention of the angiographic progression of coronary artery and vein graft atherosclerosis by gemfibrozil after coronary artery bypass surgery in men with low levels of HDL-C. Lopid Coronary Angiography Trial (LOCAT) Study Group. *Circulation* 1997;96:2137–2143.

53. Rubins HB, Robins SJ, Collins D, et al. Gemfibrozil for the secondary prevention of coronary heart disease in men with low levels of HDL cholesterol. Veterans Affairs High Density Lipoprotein Cholesterol Intervention Trial Study Group. *N Engl J Med* 1999;341:410–418.

54. Effect of fenofibrate on progression of coronary artery disease in type 2 diabetes: the Diabetes Atherosclerosis Intervention Study, a randomised study. *Lancet* 2001;357:905–910.

55. Kamanna VS, Kashyap ML. Mechanism of action of niacin on lipoprotein metabolism. *Curr Atheroscler Rep* 2000;2:36–46.

56. Morrisett JD. The role of lipoprotein (a) in atherosclerosis. *Curr Atheroscler Rep* 2002;243–250.

57. Elam MB, Hunninghake DD, Davis KD, et al. Effect of niacin on lipid and lipoprotein levels and glycemic control in patients with diabetes and peripheral vascular disease. *JAMA* 2000;284:1263–1270.

58. Grundy SM, Vega GL, McGovern NE, et al. Efficacy, safety and tolerability of once daily niacin for the treatment of dyslipidemia associated with type 2 diabetes. *Arch Intern Med* 2002;162:1568–1576.

59. Kashyap ML, McGovern ME, Berra K, et al. Long-term safety and efficacy of a once daily niacin/lovastatin formulation for patients with dyslipidemia. *Am J Cardiol* 2002;89:672–678.

60. Kanner PL, Berge KG, Wenger NK, et al. Fifteen year mortality in Coronary Drug Project patients: long-term benefit with niacin. *J Am Coll Cardiol* 1986;8:1245–1255.

61. Brown BG, Zhao XQ, Chait A, et al. Simvastatin and niacin, antioxidant vitamins or the combination for the prevention of coronary disease. *N Engl J Med* 2001;345:1583–1592.

62. Harper CR, Jacobson TA. The fats of life: the role of omega-3 fatty acids in the prevention of coronary heart disease. *Arch Intern Med* 2001;161:2185–2192.

63. Malloy MJ, Kane JP. A risk factor for atherosclerosis: triglyceride rich lipoproteins. *Adv Intern Med* 2001;47:111–136.

64. Kristensen SD, Iversen AM, Schmidt EB. n-3 polyunsaturated fatty acids and coronary thrombosis. *Lipids* 2001;36[Suppl]:S79–S82.

65. Di Minno G, Piemontino U, Cerbone AM. Nutrition and thrombogenic factors. *Nutr Metab Cardiovasc Dis* 1999;9[Suppl 4]:16–20.

66. Leaf A, Kang JX. Omega-3 fatty acids and cardiovascular disease. *World Rev Nutr Diet* 2001;89:161–172.

67. Kesabulu MN, Kameswararao B, Apparao CH, et al. Effect of omega-3 fatty acids on lipid peroxidation and antioxidant enzyme status in type 2 diabetic patients. *Diabetes Metab* 2002;28:20–26.

68. Montori DM, Farmer A, Wollan PC, et al. Fish oil supplementation in type 2 diabetes. A quantitative systematic review. *Diabetes Care* 2000; 23:1407–1415.

69. Marchioli R, Schweiger C, Tavazzi L, et al. Efficacy of N3 polyunsaturated fatty acids after myocardial infarction. Results of the GISSI-Prevenzione. *Lipids* 2001;36[Suppl]:S119–S126.

70. de Lorgeril M, Salen P. Fish and N3 fatty acids for the prevention and treatment of coronary heart disease. Nutrition is not pharmacology. *Am J Med* 2002;112:316–319.

71. Iso H, Rexrode KM, Stampfer MJ, et al. Intake of fish and omega-3 fatty acids and the risk of stroke in women. *JAMA* 2001;285:304–312.

72. Beckman JA, Creager MA, Libby P. Diabetes and atherosclerosis: epidemiology, pathophysiology and management. *JAMA* 2002;287:2570–2581.

73. Resnick HE, Howard EV. Diabetes and cardiovascular disease. *Ann Rev Med* 2002;53:245–267.

74. Grundy SM, Howard B, Smith S, et al. Prevention Conference VI: Diabetes and Cardiovascular Disease: Executive Summary: Conference Proceeding for Health Care Professionals from a special writing group of the American Heart Association. *Circulation* 2002;105:2231–2239.

75. Kjaergaard SC, Hansen HH, Fog L, et al. In hospital outcome for diabetic patients with acute myocardial infarction in the thrombolytic area. *Scand Cardiovasc J* 1999;33:166–170.

76. Haffner SM. Coronary heart disease in patients with diabetes. *N Engl J Med* 2000;342:1040–1042.

77. Haffner SM, Alexander CM, Cook TJ, et al. Reduced coronary events in simvastatin treated patients with coronary heart disease and diabetes or impaired fasting glucose levels: subgroup analysis in the Scandinavian Simvastatin Survival Study. *Arch Intern Med* 1999;159:2661–2667.

78. Sacks FM, Tonkin AM, Craven T, et al. Coronary heart disease in patients with low LDL cholesterol: benefit of pravastatin in diabetics and enhanced role for HDL-C and triglycerides as risk factors. *Circulation* 2002;105:1424–1428.

79. Wilson PW, Kannel WD. Obesity, diabetes and risk of cardiovascular disease in the elderly. *Am J Geriatr Cardiol* 2002;11:119–123.

80. LaRosa JC, He J, Vupputuri S. Effect of statins on risk of coronary disease: a meta-analysis of randomized controlled trials. *JAMA* 1999;282:2340–2346.

81. Shepherd J, Blauw GJ, Murphy MB, et al. Pravastatin in elderly individuals at risk of vascular disease (PROSPER): a randomised controlled trial. *Lancet* 2002;360:1623–1630.

82. Grundy SM. Obesity, metabolic syndrome and coronary atherosclerosis. *Circulation* 2002;105:2696–2698.

83. Rogotti NA, Pasternack RC. Cigarette smoking and coronary heart disease: risks and management. *Cardiol Clin* 1996;14:51–68.

84. Robins SJ, Collins D, Wittes JT, et al. Relation of gemfibrozil treatment and lipid levels with major coronary events: VA-HIT: a randomized controlled trial. *JAMA* 2001;285:1585–1591.

85. Denke MA. Primary prevention of heart disease in women. *Curr Atheroscler Rep* 2001;3:136–138.

86. Cushman M. Effects of hormone replacement therapy and estrogen receptor modulators on markers of inflammation and coagulation. *Am J Cardiol* 2002;90(1A):7F–10F.

87. Skouby SO, Gram H, Andersen LF, et al. Hormone replacement therapy: estrogen and progestin effects on plasma C-reactive protein concentrations. *Am J Obstet Gynecol* 2002;186:969–977.

88. Hulley S, Grady D, Bush T, et al. Randomized trial of estrogen plus progestin for secondary prevention of coronary heart disease in postmenopausal women. Heart and Estrogen/Progestin Replacement Study (HERS) Research Group. *JAMA* 1998;280:605–613.

89. Grady D, Herrington D, Bittner D, et al. Cardiovascular disease outcomes during 6.8 years of hormone therapy: Heart and Estrogen/Progestin Replacement Study Follow-up (HERS II). *JAMA* 2002;288:49–57.

90. Herrington DM, Reboussin DM, Brosnihan KB, et al. Effect of estrogen replacement on the progression of coronary artery atherosclerosis. *N Engl J Med* 2000;343:522–529.

91. Risks and benefits of estrogen plus progestin in healthy postmenopausal women: principal results from the Women's Health Initiative randomized controlled trial. *JAMA* 2002;288:321–333.

CHAPTER 12

Impact of Management on Stabilization of Plaque and Reduction of Cardiovascular Events

B. Greg Brown and Antonio M. Gotto, Jr.

Key Words Core lipids; fibrous cap; foam cells; plaque disruption; plaque stability; quantitative arteriography; regression trials.

INTRODUCTION

The past two decades have witnessed important advances in the understanding of the vascular biology of atherogenesis and the dynamic interplay among atherothrombotic plaque size, vasomotor tone, blood flow, thrombosis, and, most recently, the pathologic processes that lead to plaque disruption and clinical ischemic events. This chapter reviews a series of angiographic "regression" trials and interprets these studies from the perspective of the underlying pathologic processes that promote coronary atherothrombosis regression and retard its progression. This chapter presents the evidence supporting the unifying hypothesis that lipid depletion from two important plaque pools results in plaque stability and thereby reduces clinical events.

B. G. Brown: Department of Medicine, Cardiology Division, University of Washington School of Medicine, 1959 NE Pacific Street, Seattle, Washington 98195.

A. M. Gotto, Jr.: Office of the Dean, Weill Medical College of Cornell University, New York, New York, 10021.

MANAGEMENT OBJECTIVES FOR PATIENTS WITH CORONARY ARTERY DISEASE

Comprehensive management of coronary artery disease (CAD) has two fundamental objectives. The first objective is to reduce the severity of ischemic symptoms that occur when myocardial perfusion is impaired by one or more of the following mechanisms: a fixed flow-limiting coronary stenosis (1,2), abnormal epicardial vessel tone (3,4), intermittent arterial vasospasm (5), microvascular dysfunction (6,7), and/or incomplete collateral development.

A variety of medical approaches are currently used to relieve symptoms by favorably altering the O_2 supply–demand imbalance. Alternatively, more direct structural or physiologic changes that favorably affect the above mechanisms of diminished vascular flow capacity may provide symptom relief. Regression has been questioned as a possible mechanism for symptom relief. In this chapter, the evidence for the occurrence of regression and its mechanisms are reviewed, with a focus on lipid therapy.

The second fundamental management objective in CAD is to prevent the anticipated worsening of symptoms, or progression to a *clinical event* such as cardiac death, myocardial infarction (MI), or worsening angina requiring bypass surgery or angioplasty. In this chapter, the mechanisms of gradually progressive arterial obstruction are briefly reviewed, together with the mechanism of plaque disruption resulting in abrupt worsening of arterial obstruction. Evidence is presented that indicates a linkage between lipid reduction and stabilization of the plaque structure. This set of observations supports the idea that lipid-lowering therapy prevents clinical events by selectively lipid-depleting or "regressing" a relatively small subgroup of lipid-rich plaques that are at high risk for plaque disruption, ulceration, and hemorrhage, and which account for most clinical events.

EVIDENCE FOR REGRESSION

The basic term *regression* means something quite different to the experimental pathologist than to the clinician, both of whom have contributed to our understanding. To the research pathologist, regression means shrinkage of intimal plaque through a reduction in its major components: smooth muscle, macrophages, connective tissues, calcium, and lipid. To the physician interpreting human disease from its arteriographic appearance, regression is defined as an enlargement in the caliber of the narrowed arterial lumen. Such improvement occurs infrequently in the natural course of the disease (8). It may occur by a variety of mechanisms including plaque shrinkage, lysis of occlusive or of mural thrombi, healing of a disrupted plaque (9–11), remodeling of the underlying arterial architecture, and/or relaxation of arterial vasomotor tone (3,4). The endothelium and the relation(s) of therapy to its function contribute to many of these processes (4,7,13–19). Arteriographic images do not distinguish among the various processes of regression, thus our understanding of its principal mechanisms in patients is limited.

Thus, the key question is not: "Does regression occur in patients?" (it does), but rather: "Can such regression be induced by a therapeutic strategy?" Important related questions are "What are its mechanisms?," "Does regression provide clinical benefits?," and "If so, how?" Although there is not yet a consensus, the emerging evidence is encouraging.

Evidence in Experimental Models

Atherothrombosis has been shown convincingly to regress with lipid reduction in the nonhuman primate studies (20–23). In the typical regression experiment, the amount and composition of intimal growth is assessed among cholesterol-fed animals at specified times, using group-averaged chemical and histologic end points. During a sustained exposure to an "atherogenic" diet, plasma cholesterol may increase to more than 600 mg/dL, and there are substantial increases in coronary artery content of collagen (threefold), elastin (fourfold), and cholesterol (sevenfold, mostly esterified). On return to a native vegetarian "regression" diet, plasma cholesterol decreases quickly to normal

(140 mg/dL), and the arterial lipid and connective tissue accumulates partially regress over 20 to 40 months. Collagen content does not decline much from its peak value (~20%), but elastin (~50%) and cholesterol (~60%) do (21,23); and there is a fibrous transformation that thins the myointimal cellular response (24). Not all forms of cholesterol are readily depleted from these lipid-rich intimal deposits. The more mobile forms, including cholesteryl esters in foam cells, lipoproteins, and cholesteryl ester droplets, are known to diminish in response to decreased plasma cholesterol (22), but the cholesterol monohydrate crystals of the core lipid region are relatively resistant to mobilization (22,24). Histologic morphometry shows that plaque mass is reduced during regression therapy (20,22).

Evidence in the Human

As late as 1987, there was only anecdotal evidence that the observations of regression in animals could be extended to patients with atherothrombotic disease (26–30). In general, these pioneering studies concluded that lipid-lowering therapy reduced the frequency of disease progression, but regression was rarely observed and was not increased by the therapies tested. A more recent series of randomized clinical arteriographic trials has provided a perspective on the magnitude, frequency, and conditions under which regression can occur in patients. The more recent trials have incorporated more powerful therapeutic combinations to modify lipids and more objective methods for analysis of the arteriogram. These trials (25,29–48) and their lipid response data are summarized in Table 12–1. Their results, based on arteriographic and clinical outcomes, are summarized in Table 12–2.

More recently, a series of trials (40,42–48) has examined the effect of monotherapy with one of the 3-hydroxy-3-methylglutaryl coenzyme A reductase inhibitors, also known as statins, on atherothrombosis, as assessed quantitatively from the coronary arteriogram or from percutaneous B-mode ultrasound of the carotid bifurcation.

In all studies except the National Heart, Lung, and Blood Institute Type II (NHLBI II) study, the Cholesterol Lowering and Atherosclerosis studies (CLAS I and CLAS II), and the Program on the Surgical Control of the Hyperlipidemias (POSCH; in which change in disease severity was assessed visually, using panels of experts blinded to patient identity, treatment, and film sequence), the similarly blinded analysis incorporated techniques of computer-assisted quantitative arteriography (47). Despite the diversity among these trials in clinical presentation, lipid entry requirements, treatment regimens, and methods for arteriographic analysis, the outcomes (summary in Table 12–2) are surprisingly consistent. Each study demonstrated a benefit from treatment, whether by diet or by diet supplemented by other lifestyle changes or by lipid-lowering drugs. As a generalization of the composite of results (not a metaanalysis), 8% of the control group patients were considered to have improvement in arterial ob-

TABLE 12–1. *Summary descriptions for 15 reported arteriographic lipid-lowering trials: lipid response to treatments*

Study[a]	N	Entry requirements	Control regimen[b]	Treatment regimen	Treatment response		Years
					LDL	HDL	
Combination therapy studies							
CLAS	188	CABG	D (−)	D + R + N	−43%	+37%	2
POSCH	838	MI, chol	D	D + PIB ± R	−42%	+5%	9.7
Lifestyle	48	CAD	U	V + M + E	−37%	−3%	1
FATS (N + C)	146	CAD, apoB	D ± R	D + R + N	−32%	+43%	2.5
FATS (N + C)	146	CAD, apoB	D ± R	D + R + L	−46%	+15%	2.5
CLAS II	138	CABG	D	D + R + N	−40%	+37%	4
UC-SCOR	97	FH	U	D + R + N ± L	−39%	+25%	2
STARS (D + R)	90	CAD, chol	U	D + R	−36%	−4%	3
SCRIP	300	CAD	U	D + (R/N/LF) + E, BP	−22%	+12%	4
Heidelberg	113	CAD	U	D + Ex	−8%	+3%	1
HARP	91	CAD "NL" lipids	D ± R	P ± N ± R ± F	−41%	+13%	2.5
Monotherapy studies							
NHLBI	143	CAD, LDL	D	D + R	−31%	+8%	5
STARS (D)	90	CAD, chol	U	D	−16%	0%	3
MARS	270	CAD	D	D + L	−38%	+9%	2
CCAIT	331	CAD, chol	D	D + L	−29%	+7%	2
PLAC I	408	CAD, LDL	D	D + P	−28%	+9%	3
MAAS	381	CAD	D	D + S	−31%	+9%	4
REGRESS	885	CAD	D	D + P	−29%	+10%	2

apoB, apolipoprotein B ≤ 125 mg/dL; BP, blood pressure therapy; C, colestipol; CABG, coronary artery bypass graft surgery; CAD, coronary artery disease; chol, cholesterol > 200 mg/dL; CCAIT, Canadian Coronary Atherosclerosis Intervention Trial; CLAS; Cholesterol Lowering and Atherosclerosis studies; D, diet; Ex, exercise program; F, fibrate-type drugs; FATS, Familial Atherosclerosis Treatment Study; FH, familial hypercholesterolemia; HARP, Harvard Atherosclerosis Regression Project; HDL, high-density lipoprotein >90th percentile; L, lovastatin; LDL, low-density lipoprotein; M, relaxation techniques; MAAS, Multicenter Anti-Atheroma Study; MARS, Monitored Atherosclerosis Regression Study; MI, myocardial infarction; N, nicotinic acid; NHLBI, National Heart, Lung, and Blood Institute; NL, normal; PIB, partial ileal bypass; PLAC, Pravastatin Limitation of Atherosclerosis in the Coronary Arteries; POSCH, Program on the Surgical Control of the Hyperlipidemias; R, resin (colestipol or cholestyramine); REGRESS, Regression Growth Evaluation Statin Study; S, simvastin; SCRIP, Stanford Coronary Risk Intervention Project; STARS, St. Thomas' Atherosclerosis Regression Study; U, usual care; UC-SCOR, University of California Specialized Center of Research; V, vegetarian diet < 10% fat.
[a]See text for details of these studies.
[b]Mean LDL cholesterol response to control regimen, −7%; mean HDL cholesterol response, 0%.

struction ("regression"), and more than half had worsening ("progression") during the study period. By contrast, about one fourth of treated patients regressed and one fourth progressed.

As a generalization from Table 12–2, averaged estimates of disease severity, per patient, worsened (progressed) by about 3% stenosis among the control subjects while improving (regressing) by 1% to 2% stenosis among intensively treated patients. The "monotherapy" studies with somewhat less pronounced low-density lipoprotein (LDL) cholesterol or high-density lipoprotein (HDL) cholesterol changes, or both, did not achieve net regression among treated patients; instead, progression was significantly slowed in each. In nearly every study, the frequency of clinical cardiovascular events was reduced substantially, although the reductions achieved statistical significance in only 40% of the studies. This was because these trials were powered to demonstrate arteriographic benefits, with marginal power to detect clinical effects.

Multivariate statistical analysis has been used to identify those factors correlated with change in disease severity. Such change was usually characterized, per patient, as the mean difference (final to baseline) in percentage stenosis among all lesions assessed. In the NHLBI II study, changes in the ratios HDL cholesterol/total cholesterol or HDL cholesterol/LDL cholesterol were the only significant negative correlates of disease change among the study cohorts (49). In CLAS, non-HDL cholesterol best correlated with global change among placebo patients, as did the level of apolipoprotein (apo) C-III in HDL among treated patients (50). In the Lifestyle Heart Study, an index of adherence to all aspects of the program best correlated with arteriographic outcome. In the Familial Atherosclerosis Treatment Study (FATS), the multivariate expression including the treatment-induced change in apoB (or LDL cholesterol), HDL cholesterol, systolic blood pressure, and baseline ischemia on the exercise

TABLE 12-2. *Summary of arteriographic outcomes, treatment lipid response, and frequencies of reported clinical events in 15 lipid-lowering coronary arteriographic trials*

Study[a]	Control patients				Changes among treated patients				"Event"[d] reduction (%)
	Progression	Regression	Δ%S[b]	ΔMLD (mm)	Progression	Regression	Δ%S(P)[c]	ΔMLD (mm) (P)	
Combination therapy studies									
CLAS	61%	2%	—	—	39%	16%	—	—	25%
POSCH, 10 yr	65%	6%	—	—	37%	14%	—	—	35% (62%)[e,f]
Lifestyle	32%	32%	+3.4%	—	14%	41%	−2.2 (0.001)[g]	—	0 vs. 1 (↑)
FATS (N + C)	46%	11%	+2.1%	−0.05	25%	39%	−0.9 (0.005)	+0.035 (0.005)	80%§
FATS (L + C)	46%	11%	+2.1%	−0.05	22%	32%	−0.7 (0.02)	+0.012 (0.06)	70%
CLAS II	83%	6%	—	—	30%	18%	—	—	43%
UC-SCOR	41%	13%	+0.8%	—	20%	33%	−1.5 (0.04)	—	1 vs. 0
STARS (D + R)	46%	4%	+5.8%	−0.23	12%	33%	−1.9 (0.01)	+0.12 (0.001)	89%[f]
SCRIP	50%	10%	+3.2%	−0.20	50%	20%	+1.2 (0.02)	−0.08 (0.003)	50%
Heidelberg	42%	4%	+3.0%	−0.13	20%	30%	−1.0 (0.05)[g]	0.00 (0.05)	−27% (↑)[h]
HARP	38%	15%	+2.4%	−0.17	33%	13%	+2.1 (NS)	−1.2 (NS)	33%
Monotherapy studies									
NHLBI	49%	7%	—	—	32%	7%	—	—	33%
STARS (D)	46%	4%	+5.8%	−0.23	15%	38%	−1.1 (NS)	+0.03 (0.05)	69%
MARS	41%	12%	+2.2%	−0.06	29%	23%	+1.6% (0.2)	−0.03 (0.2)	29%
CCAIT	50%	7%	+2.9%	−0.09	33%	10%	+1.7% (0.04)	−0.05 (0.01)	22%
PLAC I	38%	14%	+3.4%	−0.15	26%	14%	+2.1% (0.13)	−0.09 (0.04)	13% (54%)[i]
MAAS	32%	12%	3.6%	−0.13	23%	19%	1.0	−0.04 (0.007)	22%[f]
REGRESS	NA	NA	NA	−0.09	NA	NA	NA	−0.03 (0.001)	39%[f]

See Table 1 for explanation of abbreviations.

[a]See text for details of these studies. Progression and regression are variably defined, per patient, in each study.

[b]Δ(%S) is usually reported as the average change in percent stenosis over all the lesions measured per patient. A positive (+) value represents "progression"; (−), "regression."

[c]p = Value for comparison of Δ%S or ΔMLD in control versus treated groups.

[d]Events are variably defined in these studies; in general, the frequency of cardiovascular events (death, myocardial infarction [MI], unstable ischemia requiring revascularization or hospitalization, or both) in control and treated groups are compared using the sometimes sketchy details and definitions provided.

[e]A 62% reduction in coronary bypass surgery.

[f]Studies for which the reduction in cardiovascular clinical events was statistically significant.

[g]Statistical comparison in Lifestyle uses a lesion-based method.

[h]An increase of −27% reduction means 27% increase (NS).

[i]A 54% reduction in coronary heart disease death and nonfatal MI.

§: p < 0.01.

MLD, minimum lumen diameter.

treadmill test, predicting the change in mean proximal percent stenosis ($\Delta\%S_{prox}$), correlated well with the observed change ($r = 0.51$; $p < 0.001$). In these men with CAD and increased LDL cholesterol, lipoprotein (a) [Lp(a)] levels were dominant correlates of baseline disease severity, its progression, and event rate over 2.5 years. However, among patients with substantial treatment-induced LDL cholesterol reductions and HDL cholesterol increases, persistent increases of Lp(a) were no longer atherogenic or clinically threatening (51). In the University of California Specialized Center of Research (UC-SCOR) trial of patients with heterozygous familial hypocholesterolemia, only in-treatment LDL cholesterol correlated with arteriographic outcome, perhaps because the presence of extreme increases of LDL cholesterol mitigated the predictivity of other lipid and nonlipid risk factors. In the St. Thomas' Atherosclerosis Regression Study (STARS), changes in LDL cholesterol/HDL cholesterol ratio and mean BP change during therapy were significant independent correlates of disease change. In the HDL Atherosclerosis Treatment Study (HATS) (41), in-treatment apoC-III and small HDL particle size joined apoB as key determinants of disease progression. In the NHLBI-II, FATS, UC-SCOR, the Lifestyle Heart Study, and STARS, the insertion of these predictive variables in the analysis abolished the association of benefit with treatment group, implying that the therapy effect was mediated by its effect on these variable(s).

In summary, reduction of LDL cholesterol, apoB, and the LDL cholesterol/HDL cholesterol ratio have frequently correlated with arterial benefit. Blood pressure reduction, apoC-III distribution, Lp(a) levels, and compliance with lifestyle changes also have emerged in one or more studies. The differences in variables that correlated with treatment effects in these trials may reflect differences both in the population being treated and in the mechanisms of action of the therapeutic strategies used. The more recent "monotherapy" studies suggest that the arterial and clinical benefits are less striking when LDL cholesterol, HDL cholesterol, or both are less intensively altered. When women are included in these studies (37,39), the arterial treatment benefits appear comparable with those in men.

Figure 12–1 illustrates cases of lesion regression seen in intensively treated FATS patients over a 2.5-year period. Regression may occur in mild, moderate, and severe lesions. Although a few lesions (about 5%) "naturally" regress by 10% or more, and more (about 12%) regress with lipid therapy, most stenoses do not improve even with "intensive" regimens that result in marked alterations in the lipid and lipoprotein profile. Yet, these regimens are commonly associated with much more substantial reductions in clinical

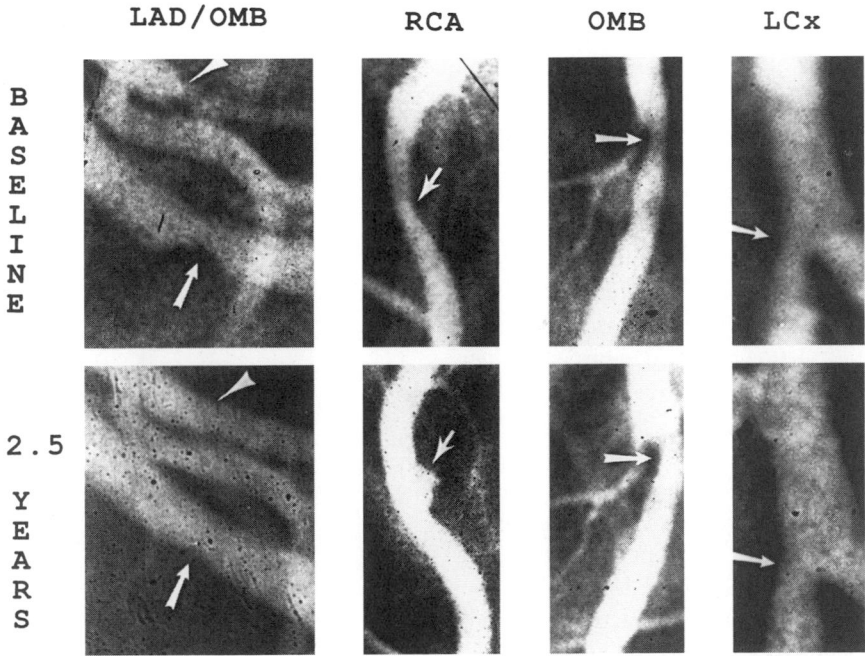

FIG. 12–1. Examples of definite regression in intensively treated patients in the Familial Atherosclerosis Treatment Study (FATS). **Top row:** Baseline. **Bottom row:** 2.5 years later. LAD *(top arrow),* left anterior descending artery (100 → 20%S); OMB *(bottom arrow),* obtuse marginal branch (39 → 18%S); RCA, right coronary artery (48 → 30%S) (note plaque ulcer at 2.5 years); OMB (69% → 37%); LCx, left circumflex artery (44 → 30%S). (Modified from Brown BG, Albers JJ, Fisher LD, et al. Regression of coronary artery disease as a result of intensive lipid-lowering therapy in men with high levels of apolipoprotein B. *N Engl J Med* 1990;323:1289–1298, with permission.)

event rate (Table 12–2). This apparent paradox is detailed later in this chapter.

PREVENTING PROGRESSION

Pathologic Processes

This section focuses briefly on several clinically important aspects of plaque biology: lipid accumulation in the foam cells and core region, disruption of plaques and their healing, and variation in vasoconstrictor tone.

Arterial Lipid Accumulation

LDL and, more recently, Lp(a) have been localized in the intimal extracellular space, the cholesterol content of which is thought to derive from plasma LDL cholesterol (52–55). Intimal lipid also accumulates in subendothelial monocyte-derived macrophages (56,57). Such "foam cell" formation is thought to occur by unregulated scavenger receptor uptake of oxidized LDL (58,59) and possibly of Lp(a) (60,61) by macrophages. Foam cells are abundant in precursor fatty streak lesions (62), in the cap of early fibrous plaques, and in the shoulders, cap, and basilar neovascular complex of advanced plaques (63). Lipid may enter the core region of the fibrous plaque by transmural flux (64) of its more mobile forms (lipoprotein particles, droplets, and vesicles) (65,66), or it may be deposited there as a result of foam cell necrosis (62,67). There, lipids coalesce into lower-energy phases dictated by the local cholesterol, phospholipid, and cholesteryl ester concentrations (22). Cholesteryl ester droplets and vesicles and cholesterol monohydrate crystals are the dominant core lipids (22,63). The flux of small perifibrous lipid droplets through the endothelium has been thought to initiate core lipid accumulation in the earliest human aortic lesions (65,68). The subsequent contribution of foam cell necrosis to its continued accumulation in the larger mature fibrous plaques remains to be determined. This last question is a key one because of the proposed therapeutic role of antioxidants (58), which, by preventing LDL oxidation, may act to prevent foam cell formation and, ultimately, core lipid accumulation.

Arterial Lipid Content

It is unclear why certain patients or certain arterial segments develop lipid-rich plaques whereas adjacent segments have the more stable fibrous intimal involvement. Using quantitative morphometry of the histologic section, Roberts and coworkers (69–72) have determined the proportion of intimal area that is contributed by each of the principal plaque components: (a) dense fibrous tissue, (b) cellular fibrous tissue, (c) calcific deposits, (d) inflammatory infiltrates, (e) extracellular core lipid (as "pultaceous debris"), and (f) foam cell lipid (69). They separated serially sampled arterial sections into four ranges of lumen area reduction. They found,

on average, that early intimal involvement is almost entirely fibrocellular, but at the stage of severe arterial obstruction, the cellular contribution has declined to about 25% of total intimal area, whereas dense fibrous tissue occupies about 50%. Foam cells appear in some numbers when intimal involvement is moderate; their fraction increases to 10% of the area in the more severe stages and then declines in the most severe stage. Calcific deposits and extracellular lipid become relatively abundant in the more severe stages; each increases progressively to contribute about 10% of intimal area in the most severe stage.

Plaque Disruption

As described later, the structural disruption of plaques is currently recognized as the critical event triggering abrupt arterial occlusion and ischemia. Also, "silent" disruption can occur in the absence of ischemic symptoms (11,73,74), possibly defining another mechanism of plaque growth, in which mural or intramural thrombus can undergo mesenchymal organization, thus expanding the plaque connective tissue mass (11,74,75).

Vasoconstrictor Tone

Increased vasoconstrictor tone may contribute to progressive luminal narrowing. Atherothrombosis affects vascular tone by interfering with the endothelial production and normal release of the endogenous vasodilator, endothelium-derived relaxing factor (nitric oxide [NO]), or an analog (15–18,76–78). Endothelial NO dysfunction appears to account for the apparently paradoxic epicardial coronary vasoconstrictor effects of isometric and aerobic exercise in patients with CAD (79,80). The mechanism of impairment is unknown, but LDL cholesterol, HDL cholesterol, and LDL oxidation have been implicated (81–84).

Evidence in Humans

Randomized trial evidence that lipid-lowering therapy can effectively retard arterial obstruction is surprisingly consistent (Table 12–2 provides a summary of evidence). Approximately one-half of the control group patients were judged to have worsening arterial obstruction during the study period; by contrast, about one-fourth of the treated patients (a 50% reduction from control) experienced worsening of their condition.

PREVENTING PLAQUE DISRUPTION AND CLINICAL EVENTS

Prevention of Clinical Events

The landmark Lipid Research Clinics Coronary Primary Prevention Trial (85) demonstrated that clinical coronary events, but not cardiac or total mortality, were significantly reduced (~19%) in association with a 9% reduction, relative to the dietary control, in total cholesterol and a 13% reduction in LDL cholesterol, accomplished with diet and cholestyramine. Importantly, the magnitude of cardiovascular benefit correlated with the degree of both total and LDL cholesterol reduction (86). The Helsinki Heart Trial (87) also achieved a significant reduction in total cardiac events but not in mortality. The 15-year follow-up of the Coronary Drug Project showed a significant 11% reduction in all-cause mortality in the group that received niacin therapy 9 years earlier (88).

The statin era introduced a series of secondary prevention trials, including the Scandinavian Simvastatin Survival Study (4S) (89), the Cholesterol and Recurrent Events (CARE) trial (90), and the Long-term Intervention with Pravastatin in Ischaemic Disease (LIPID) trial (91), in which reduction of clinical coronary event rates (23–34%) were largely related to percent LDL-lowering (25–35%). A surprising finding, the event and survival curves for placebo treatment versus statin treatment generally began to diverge after the first or second year of the trial, in favor of statins. This divergence does not seem to coincide with the theoretic timeline for plaque regression, and therefore, significant diminution of plaque burden may not explain the benefits observed.

Under the premise that the distinction between primary and secondary prevention may be somewhat arbitrary (that is, someone who has never had a clinical coronary event may nevertheless bear a substantial amount of atherothrombotic vessel disease), examining clinical trials on the basis of their cohort's global risk for CAD provides additional insight (see Chapter 11 for a discussion of the concept of global risk). The Air Force/Texas Coronary Atherosclerosis Prevention Study (AFCAPS/TexCAPS) randomized the lowest risk cohort of any of the large statin clinical trials; the annual event rate was just greater than 1% per year in the placebo group (92). Treatment with lovastatin in this study reduced the relative risk for the first acute coronary event by 37% over a 5-year period. The statin-treated group was also at lower risk for unstable angina, with the benefit beginning to emerge after 1 year into the trial, suggesting a major effect of intervention was near-term stabilization of atherothrombosis rather than frank regression.

The angiographic trials are also congruent with this hypothesis (Table 12–2). For each trial, when reported, we have classified as clinical events cardiac death, confirmed MI, and progressive or unstable ischemia requiring revascularization. Thus, clinical cardiovascular events are clearly reduced by lipid-lowering therapy. The amount of risk reduction seems out of proportion to the small average regression in lesion severity (1–2% stenosis) and with the fact that only about 12% of all intensively treated lesions actually regress. To understand how regression of a small number of lesions can result in a substantial clinical benefit, one must understand the series of events in the plaque that turn a stable quiescent lesion into an unstable culprit lesion triggering a clinical event.

Determinants of Plaque Disruption

Acute ischemic syndromes are most commonly precipitated when sites of mild or moderate atherothrombotic narrowing become disruptively transformed into severely obstructive culprit lesions. As seen in Figure 12–2B, such a transformation usually involves avulsion of the fibrous cap of the atheroma, often with intramural hemorrhage and mural or occlusive thrombus. The plaque at high risk for such fissuring and subsequent hemorrhage or thrombosis usually has a large core lipid pool and a structurally weakened fibrous cap. The cap can be weakened by the migration or death of its smooth muscle cells, by an accumulation of lipid-laden macrophages, or by proteolytic or mechanical damage to its collagen. Evolving insights into three clinically important aspects of atherothrombosis have greatly altered our understanding of the precipitation of plaque events leading to acute clinical events.

First, mild and moderate coronary lesions (<70% stenosis) may progress abruptly to severe obstruction, with resulting unstable angina, MI, or death. In fact, a majority of clinical events occur under these circumstances (9,89–92). Although a given severe (≥70%) lesion is more likely to progress or totally occlude than those of the less severe variety, clinical events are more frequently triggered by lesions that are initially mild or moderate, because (a) these are much more numerous in the patient's anatomy (93), and (b) because the majority of occlusions of severe stenoses occur without an event (94).

A second insight was originally brought into focus by Constantinides (98) but has received renewed attention (11,73,74,95–101). It is that, for the great majority of ischemic coronary events, a "culprit" lesion can be identified with variations of the following morphologic features at histologic examination (Figure 12–2B): (a) a fissure, tear, or vent in the fibrous cap overlying the core lipid pool; (b) a thrombus adherent at the site of the fissure; (c) bleeding into the core lipid region; and (d) severe arterial obstruction by the composite mass of expanded plaque and thrombus.

A third insight is that there are features of plaque structure and lipid composition that predict the risk for disruption, which virtually never occurs in the absence of atheroma. Among patients dying of noncardiac causes, new nonobstructive cap rupture can be found in 9% to 17%, suggesting that not all such episodes progress to severe obstruction (74). The greater the core lipid content, the greater the likelihood of cap rupture. In a detailed histologic assessment of 86 infarct lesions, an intimal fissure extended from the lumen into an unstructured pool of extracellular lipid in 83% of cases (98,100) (Fig. 12–2B). Yet, in any given patient, only a small subgroup of all plaques (about one in eight) has a substantial core lipid accumulation. Certain aspects of fibrous cap composition also heighten the risk for fissuring. The macrophage density in disrupted caps is greater than that in intact caps (96,97). It occurs most commonly at the shoulder of an eccentric lipid-rich plaque (Fig. 12–2B), a location of high macrophage density (100) and also of high

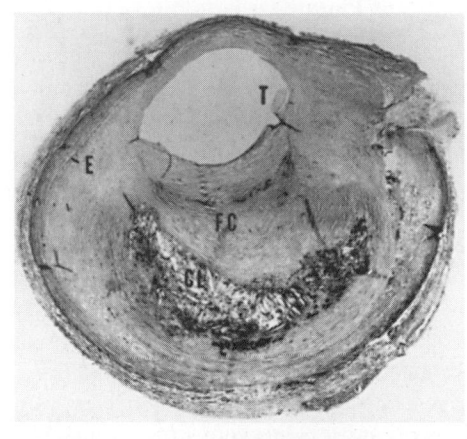

A

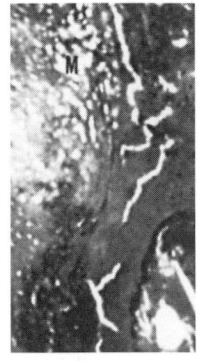

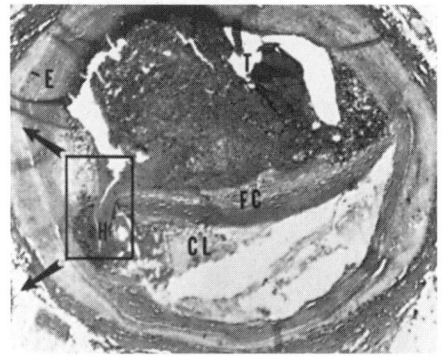

B

FIG. 12–2. A: Histologic section through a structurally stable coronary plaque in a patient with vasospastic angina. Morphologic features include: internal elastic lamina *(E);* a thick fibrous cap *(FC)* composed largely of collagen and smooth muscle cells (SMCs); core lipid *(CL),* here largely crystalline; and a small tag of thrombus *(T).* **B:** Section through a structurally unstable coronary plaque in a patient dying of myocardial infarction. The lumen, only moderately narrowed by the plaque, is acutely occluded by thrombus *(T).* There are many features in common with the section in **A.** In the unstable plaque, core lipid (some dislodged by sectioning artifact) comprises a much larger fraction of the plaque. The fibrous cap is much thinner than in **A,** and is fissured (or vented) at its left shoulder, permitting a small pocket of hemorrhage *(H)* in the plaque. This fissure, the associated hemorrhagic pocket, and the plaque shoulder, here rich in lipid-laden macrophages *(M; round, bright spots),* are shown at increased magnification in the *inset.* Also at greater magnification (not shown), the fibrous cap has few SMCs but many Ms. **(B:** Reproduced from Brown BG, Zhao XQ, Sacco DE, et al. Lipid lowering and plaque regression. New insights into prevention of plaque disruption and clinical events in coronary disease. *Circulation* 1993;87:1781–1791, with permission.)

circumferential stress when there is significant core lipid, according to computer models (101,102). Finally, the fibrous cap is thinned and weakened by the disappearance of smooth muscle cells and by lysis of collagen. Cytotoxic agents, including T-cell interferon-γ, macrophage secretory products, and oxidatively modified LDL (103–107), can transform a viable and structurally intact cap (Fig. 12–2A) into one that is thinned and acellular, and thus much more susceptible to disruption (Fig. 12–2B). Oxidation or acetyla-

tion of LDL produces a modified species of LDL more susceptible to uptake by macrophages. The macrophage and monocyte scavenger receptor CD36 is a major pathway for transport of oxidized LDL, leading to increased inflammatory activity (108). Statin therapy may reduce CD36 activity (109), thus a reduction in CD36 and therefore a decrease in the uptake of oxidized LDL by macrophages in the arterial wall may be one mechanism contributing to plaque stabilization.

This perception of plaque disruption as a "passive" process related to the softness and size of the core lipid pool and the strength of the fibrous cap is being refined as our understanding of the "active" macrophage inflammatory mechanisms evolves (110,111). Atherectomy specimens from culprit lesions for unstable angina have a significantly greater macrophage content than those from stable angina lesions (112). Macrophages release metalloproteinases such as interstitial collagenase, gelatinase, and stromelysin, all of which have been identified in atherothrombotic plaques (113) and in cultured macrophages (114). The inflammatory aspect of macrophages and T cells is emphasized by Van der Wal and coworkers (111), who found intimal rupture into a large core lipid pool in only 12 (60%) of 20 infarct lesions, but uniformly identified increased macrophage density at focal sites of plaque erosion or disruption and also demonstrated focal expression of HLA-DR inflammatory antigens. This emphasis is supported by the seminal studies of Davies

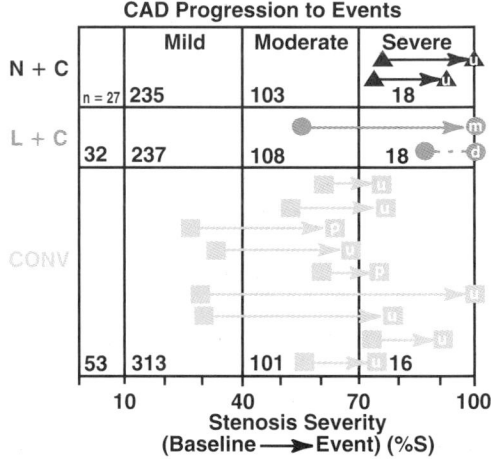

FIG. 12–3. Lesion changes associated with the 13 coronary events as measured from 1,316 lesions in 120 patients of the Familial Atherosclerosis Treatment Study (FATS). Among lesions exposed to intensive lipid-lowering therapy, only 1 of 683 mild or moderate lesions, at baseline, among 74 such patients progressed to a clinical event, whereas 8 of 414 such lesions among 46 conventionally treated patients did (per patient or per lesion, *p* < 0.004). By this standard, severe lesions did not appear to benefit from therapy. C, colestipol; CONV, conventional therapy; D, death; L, lovastatin; MI, myocardial infarction; N, niacin; P, progressive angina; %S, percentage diameter stenosis; U, unstable angina event. The number in each panel represents the number of lesions at risk, at baseline, in each subgroup.

and coworkers (103) and by Fuster and coworkers (11). The extent to which these inflammatory changes occur after the rupture remains to be determined. A growing body of evidence demonstrated the association of the inflammatory marker C-reactive protein with atherothrombosis (115,116) and especially with acute coronary syndromes. Its plasma levels are reduced with lipid therapy (115).

Prevention of Plaque Disruption

As described earlier, plaque disruption is predicted by certain lipid-related plaque features including macrophage foam cell density, core lipid pool size, and possible cytotoxicity from oxidized LDL. Reduction of plasma LDL would be expected to reduce the likelihood of fissuring because of the experimentally documented favorable effects of LDL reduction on these predictors. As a clinical consequence, LDL-lowering therapy should decrease the frequency of abrupt progression to clinical events. Indeed, this was the case in 13 coronary events among 146 patients in the FATS trial (32,33) (Fig. 12–3).

UNIFYING HYPOTHESIS

The above series of observations can be used to support the hypothesis that angiographic coronary stenosis regression, seen in 12% of all coronary lesions during intensive lipid-lowering therapy, reflects depletion of cholesteryl esters selectively from the "vulnerable" subgroup of lipid-rich and foam cell–rich lesions, which comprise about 15% of all visible coronary lesions. Such lipid depletion typically reduces stenosis severity by 10% to 20%, but, more importantly, it stabilizes the plaque in terms of its mechanical strength and endothelial functional integrity. The plaque fibrous cap is strengthened by favorable geometric changes and a marked reduction in the number of intimal inflammatory cells (macrophages and T lymphocytes) that secrete proinflammatory cytokines and proteolytic enzymes. Plaque stabilization by these mechanisms appears to explain the substantial reduction of clinical events associated with intensive lipid reduction.

SUMMARY

The consensus of evidence from angiographic trials demonstrates both coronary artery and clinical benefits from lipid decreasing, using any of a variety of treatment regimens. The findings of decreased arterial disease progression and increased regression have been convincing but, at best, modest in their magnitude. In view of these modest arterial benefits, the associated reductions in cardiovascular events have been surprisingly great. For example, coronary events were reduced 75% with intensive lipid therapy in FATS (34,35); this was entirely explained by a 93% reduction with therapy in the likelihood that a mildly or moderately diseased arterial segment would experience substantial pro-

gression to become the severe lesion that triggered the clinical event. We believe the magnitude of the clinical benefit is best explained in terms of this observation, using the following lines of reasoning. Clinical events most commonly spring from lesions that are initially of mild or moderate severity and that abruptly undergo a disruptive transformation to a severe "culprit" lesion. The process of plaque fissuring leading to plaque disruption and thrombosis triggers most clinical coronary events. Fissuring is predicted by a large accumulation of core lipid in the plaque and by a high density of lipid-laden inflammatory cells, T-lymphocytes, and macrophages in its thinned fibrous cap. Lesions with these characteristics comprise only 10% to 20% of the overall lesion population but account for 80% to 90% of the acute clinical events. In the experimental setting, normalization of an atherogenic lipid profile substantially decreases the number of lipid-laden intimal macrophages (foam cells) and gradually depletes cholesterol from the core lipid pool. In the clinical setting, intensive lipid decreasing virtually halts the abrupt progression of mild and moderate lesions to severe obstructions precipitating clinical events.

Briefly stated, the composite of data presented in this chapter supports the hypothesis that lipid-lowering therapy selectively lipid-depletes (regresses) that relatively small, but dangerous, subgroup of lipid-rich and foam cell–rich lesions containing a large lipid core and dense clusters of intimal macrophages. These lesions are thereby effectively stabilized, and clinical event rate is accordingly decreased.

FUTURE DIRECTIONS

The concept that abrupt disruption of the atherothrombotic plaque, with associated thrombosis, precipitates cardiovascular events is now firmly embedded in our understanding of the pathogenesis of clinical coronary disease. Several current lines of investigation relate to mechanisms of plaque instability. These include studies of (a) histocytochemistry and *in situ* hybridization to identify biochemical or cellular markers of plaque vulnerability; (b) plaque structure and connective tissue strength as determinants of plaque instability; (c) the role of endothelial functional vasorelaxation and resistance to thrombosis; (d) the role of the various plaque lipid pools in relation to plaque vulnerability; (e) the role of circulating lipid levels (LDL cholesterol, Lp(a), HDL cholesterol, and their subfractions) and their molecular, genetic, and pharmacologic regulation in the dynamics of plaque lipid accumulation or depletion; (f) the role of antioxidants in the process(es) of plaque lipid accumulation in these pools; and (g) the role of arterial remodeling as a means of adapting to these pathologic processes. Newly emerging tools will be used to probe these procedures, including intravascular ultrasound, magnetic resonance imaging (117), catheter-based segmental therapy including gene transfer techniques, and gene chip technology.

ACKNOWLEDGMENTS

The authors greatly appreciate the efforts of Heather Bruggman in preparing the manuscript for this chapter, which was extensively modified from a previous publication (35). This work was supported in part by National Institutes of Health (NIH) grants R01 HL 19451, P01 HL 30086, and R01 HL 42419 from the National Heart, Lung, and Blood Institute, in part by the University of Washington Clinical Research Center (NIH #RR37), by a grant (NIH DK 35816) to the Clinical Nutrition Research Unit, and in part by a grant from the John L. Locke, Jr. Charitable Trust, Seattle, Washington.

REFERENCES

1. Demer LL, Gould KL, Goldstein RA, et al. Assessment of coronary artery disease severity by positron emission tomography. Comparison with quantitative arteriography in 193 patients. *Circulation* 1989;79: 825–835.
2. Klocke FJ. Measurements of coronary flow reserve: defining pathophysiology versus making decisions about patient care. *Circulation* 1987;76:1183–1189.
3. Ludmer PL, Selwyn AP, Shook TL, et al. Paradoxical vasoconstriction induced by acetylcholine in atherosclerotic coronary arteries. *N Engl J Med* 1986;315:1046–1051.
4. Nabel EG, Selwyn AP, Ganz P. Large coronary arteries in humans are responsive to changing blood flow: an endothelium-dependent mechanism that fails in patients with atherosclerosis. *J Am Coll Cardiol* 1990;16:349–356.
5. Kaski JC, Crea F, Meran DO, et al. Local coronary supersensitivity to diverse vasoconstrictive stimuli in patients with variant angina. *Circulation* 1986;74:1255–1265.
6. Cannon RO, Camici PG, Epstein SE. Pathophysiological dilemma of syndrome X. *Circulation* 1992;85:883–892.
7. Loscalzo J, Dzau VJ. Flow activates an endothelium potassium channel to release an endogenous nitrovasodilator. *J Clin Invest* 1991;88: 1663–1671.
8. Brown BG, Bolson EL, Pierce CD, et al. Regression of atherosclerosis in man: current data and their methodological limitations. In: Malinkow MR, Blaton VH, eds. *Regression of atherosclerotic lesions.* New York: Plenum Press, 1984:289–310.
9. Brown BG, Gallery CA, Badger RS, et al. Incomplete lysis of thrombus in the moderate underlying atherosclerotic lesion during intracoronary infusion of streptokinase for acute myocardial infarction: quantitative angiographic observations. *Circulation* 1986;73:653–661.
10. Early effects of tissue-type plasminogen activator added to conventional therapy on the culprit coronary lesion in patients presenting with ischemic cardiac pain at rest. Results of the Thrombolysis in Myocardial Ischemia (TIMI IIIA) Trial. *Circulation* 1993;87:38–52.
11. Fuster V, Badimon L, Badimon JJ, et al. The pathogenesis of coronary artery disease and the acute coronary syndromes. *N Engl J Med* 1992;326:310–318.
12. Glasgov S, Weisenberg E, Zarins CK, et al. Compensatory enlargement of human atherosclerotic coronary arteries. *N Engl J Med* 1987;316:1371–1375.
13. Langille BL, O'Donnell F. Reductions in arterial diameter produced by chronic decreases in blood flow are endothelium-dependent. *Science* 1986;231:405–407.
14. Jaffe RB, Glancy DC, Epstein SE, et al. Coronary arterial-right heart fistulae: long-term observations in seven patients. *Circulation* 1973; 47:133–143.
15. McLenachan JM, Williams JK, Fish RD, et al. Loss of flow-mediated endothelium-dependent dilation occurs early in the development of atherosclerosis. *Circulation* 1991;84:1273–1278.
16. Furchgott RF, Zawadzki JV. The obligatory role of endothelial cells in the relaxation of arterial smooth muscle by acetylcholine. *Nature* 1980;299:373–376.

17. Furchgott RF, Vanhoutte PM. Endothelium-derived relaxing and contracting factors. *FASEB J* 1989;3:2007–2018.
18. Selke FW, Armstrong ML, Harrison DG. Endothelium-dependent vascular relaxation is abnormal in the coronary microcirculation of atherosclerotic primates. *Circulation* 1990;81:1568–1593.
19. Armstrong ML, Megan MB. Lipid depletion in atheromatous coronary arteries in rhesus monkeys after regression diets. *Circ Res* 1972;30:675–680.
20. Clarkson TB, Bond MG, Bullock BC, et al. A study of atherosclerosis regression in *Macaca mulatta.* IV. Changes in coronary arteries from animals with atherosclerosis induced for 19 months and then regressed for 24 or 48 months at plasma cholesterol concentrations of 300 or 200 mg/dl. *Exp Mol Pathol* 1981;34:345–368.
21. Small DM, Bond MG, Waugh D, et al. Physiochemical and histological changes in the arterial wall of nonhuman primates during progression and regression of atherosclerosis. *J Clin Invest* 1984;73: 1590–1605.
22. Armstrong MC, Megan MB. Arterial fibrous protein in cynomolgus monkeys after atherogenic and regression diets. *Circ Res* 1975;36: 256–261.
23. Brown BG, Fry DL. The fate and fibrogenic potential of subintimal implants of crystalline lipid in the canine aorta. Quantitative histological and autoradiographic studies. *Circ Res* 1978;43:261–273.
24. Kuo PT, Hayase K, Kostic JB, et al. Use of combined diet and colestipol in long-term (7–7.5 years) treatment of patients with type II hyperlipoproteinemia. *Circulation* 1979;59:199–214.
25. Brensike JF, Levy RI, Kelsey SF, et al. Effects of therapy with cholestyramine on progression of coronary atherosclerosis: results of the NHLBI Type II coronary intervention study. *Circulation* 1984;69:313–324.
26. Duffield RG, Lewis B, Miller NE, et al. Treatment of hyperlipidemia retards progression of symptomatic femoral atherosclerosis. *Lancet* 1983;ii:639–642.
27. Nash DT, Gensini G, Esente P. Effect of lipid lowering therapy on the progression of coronary atherosclerosis assessed by scheduled repetitive coronary arteriography. *Int J Cardiol* 1982;2:43–55.
28. Nikkila EA, Viikinkoski P, Valle M, et al. Prevention of progression of coronary atherosclerosis by treatment of hyperlipidemia: a seven-year prospective angiographic study. *Br Med J* 1984;289:220–223.
29. Blankenhorn DH, Nessim SA, Johnson RL, et al. Beneficial effects of colestipol niacin therapy on coronary atherosclerosis and coronary venous bypass grafts. *JAMA* 1987;257:3233–3240.
30. Buchwald H, Matts JP, Ritch LL, et al. Effect of partial ileal bypass on mortality and morbidity from coronary heart disease in patients with hypercholesterolemia. Report of the Program on Surgical Control of the Hyperlipidemias (POSCH). *N Engl J Med* 1990;323:946.
31. Ornish D, Brown SE, Scherwitz LW, et al. Can lifestyle changes reverse coronary heart disease? *Lancet* 1990;336:129–133.
32. Brown BG, Albers JJ, Fisher LD, et al. Regression of coronary artery disease as a result of intensive lipid-lowering therapy in men with high levels of apolipoprotein B. *N Engl J Med* 1990;323:1289–1298.
33. Brown BG, Zhao XQ, Sacco DE, et al. Lipid lowering and plaque regression. New insights into prevention of plaque disruption and clinical events in coronary disease. *Circulation* 1993;87:1781–1791.
34. Cashin-Hemphill L, Mack WJ, Pogoda JM, et al. Beneficial effects of colestipol-niacin on coronary atherosclerosis. *JAMA* 1990;264:3013–3017.
35. Kane JP, Malloy MJ, Ports TA, et al. Regression of coronary atherosclerosis during treatment of familial hypercholesterolemia with combined drug regimens. *JAMA* 1990;264:3007.
36. Watts GF, Lewis B, Brunt JN, et al. Effects on coronary artery disease of lipid-lowering diet, or diet plus cholestyramine, in the St. Thomas' Atherosclerosis Regression Study (STARS). *Lancet* 1992;339:563–569.
37. Alderman E, Haskell WL, Fain JM, et al. Beneficial angiographic and clinical response to multifactor modification in the Stanford Coronary Risk Intervention Project (SCRIP). *Circulation* 1991;84[Suppl II]:II-140(abst).
38. Schuler G, Hambrecht R, Schlierf G, et al. Regular physical exercise and low-fat diet. Effects on progression of coronary artery disease. *Circulation* 1992;86:1–11.
39. Sacks F, Pasternak RC, Gibson CM, et al. Effect on coronary atherosclerosis of decrease in plasma cholesterol concentrations in normocholesterolemic patients. *Lancet* 1994;344:1182–1186.

40. Herd JA, Ballantyne CM, Farmer JA, et al. Effects of fluvastatin on coronary atherosclerosis in patients with mild to moderate cholesterol elevations (Lipoprotein and Coronary Atherosclerosis Study [LCAS]). *Am J Cardiol* 1997;80:278–286.

41. Brown BG, Zhao XQ, Chait A, et al. Simvastatin and niacin, antioxidant vitamins, or the combination for the prevention of coronary disease. *N Engl J Med* 2001;345:1583–1592.

42. Effect of fenofibrate on progression of coronary-artery disease in type 2 diabetes: the Diabetes Atherosclerosis Intervention Study, a randomised study. *Lancet* 2001;357:905–910.

43. Ericsson CG, Hamsten A, Nilsson J, et al. Angiographic assessment of effects of bezafibrate on progression of coronary artery disease in young male postinfarction patients. *Lancet* 1996;347:849–853.

44. Blankenhorn DH, Azen SP, Kramsch DM, et al. Coronary angiographic changes with lovastatin therapy: the Monitored Atherosclerosis Regression Study (MARS). *Ann Intern Med* 1993;119:967–976.

45. Waters D, Higginson L, Gladstone P, et al. Effect of monotherapy with an HMG-CoA reductase inhibitor on the progression of coronary atherosclerosis as assessed by serial quantitative arteriography: the Canadian Coronary Atherosclerosis Intervention Trial. *Circulation* 1994;89:959–968.

46. Pitt B, Mancini GB, Ellis SG, et al. Pravastatin Limitation of Atherosclerosis in the Coronary Arteries (PLAC I). *J Am Coll Cardiol* 1994;23[Suppl]:131A(abst).

47. Effect of simvastatin on coronary atheroma: the Multicentre Anti-Atheroma Study (MAAS). *Lancet* 1994;344:633–638.

48. Jukema JW, Bruschke AV, van Boven AJ, et al. Effects of lipid lowering by pravastatin on progression and regression of coronary artery disease in symptomatic men with normal to moderately elevated serum cholesterol levels. The Regression Growth Evaluation Statin Study (REGRESS). *Circulation* 1995;91:2528–2540.

49. Brown BG, Bolson EL, Dodge HT. Quantitative computer techniques for analyzing coronary arteriograms. *Prog Cardiovasc Dis* 1986;28:403–418.

50. Levy RI, Brensike JF, Epstein SE, et al. The influence of changes in endothelial values induced by cholestyramine and diet on progression of coronary artery disease: results of the NHLBI Type II Coronary Intervention Study. *Circulation* 1984;69:325–337.

51. Blankenhorn DH, Alaupovic P, Wickham E, et al. Prediction of angiographic change in native human coronary arteries and aortocoronary bypass grafts. Lipid and non-lipid factors. *Circulation* 1990;81:470–476.

52. Maher VM, Brown BG, Marcovina SM, et al. Effects of lowering elevated LDL cholesterol on the cardiovascular risk of lipoprotein(a). *JAMA* 1995;274:1771–1774.

53. Smith EB. The relationship between plasma and tissue lipids in human atherosclerosis. *Adv Lipid Res* 1974;12:1–49.

54. Walton KW, Williamson N. Histological and immunofluorescent studies on the evolution of the human atheromatous plaque. *J Atheroscler Res* 1968;8:599–624.

55. Rath M, Niendorf A, Reblin T, et al. Detection and quantification of lipoprotein (a) in the arterial wall of 107 coronary bypass patients. *Arteriosclerosis* 1989;9:579–592.

56. Cushing GL, Gaubatz JW, Nava ML, et al. Quantitation and localization of apolipoproteins (a) and B in coronary artery bypass vein grafts resected at operation. *Arteriosclerosis* 1989;9:593–603.

57. Gerrity RG. The role of monocyte in atherogenesis. I. Transition of blood-borne monocytes into foam cells in fatty lesions. *Am J Pathol* 1981;103:181–190.

58. Ross R. Atherosclerosis—an inflammatory disease. *N Engl J Med* 1999;340:115–126.

59. Steinberg D, Parthasarathy S, Carew TE, et al. Beyond cholesterol: modifications of low-density lipoprotein that increase its atherogenicity. *N Engl J Med* 1989;320:915–924.

60. Berliner JA, Territo MC, Sevanian A, et al. Minimally modified LDL stimulates monocyte endothelial interactions. *J Clin Invest* 1990;85:1260–1266.

61. Yamaguchi J, Hoff MF. Apolipoprotein B accumulation and development of foam cell lesions in coronary arteries of hypercholesterolemic swine. *Lab Invest* 1984;51:325–332.

62. Krempler F, Kostner GM, Roscher A, et al. The interaction of human apoB containing lipoproteins with mouse peritoneal macrophages: a comparison of Lp(a) with LDL. *J Lipid Res* 1984;25:283–287.

63. Stary HC. Changes in the cells of atherosclerotic lesions as advanced lesions evolve in coronary arteries of children and young adults. In: Glagou S, Newman WP, Schaffer SA, eds. *Pathobiology of the human atherosclerotic plaque.* New York: Springer-Verlag, 1989:93–106.

64. Guyton JR, Klemp KF. The lipid-rich core region of human atherosclerotic fibrous plaques. *Am J Pathol* 1989;1343:705–717.

65. Fry DL. Mass transport, atherogenesis, and risk. *Arteriosclerosis* 1987;7:88–100.

66. Guyton JR, Bocan TM. Human aortic fibrolipid lesions. Progenitor lesions for fibrous plaques, exhibiting early formation of the cholesterol-rich core. *Am J Pathol* 1985;120:193–206.

67. Smith EB, Evans PH, Pownham MD. Lipid in the aorta intima: the correlation of morphological and chemical characteristics. *J Atheroscler Res* 1967;7:171–186.

68. Haust MD. The morphogenesis and fate of potential and early atherosclerotic lesions in man. *Hum Pathol* 1971;2:1–29.

69. Guyton JR, Klemp KF. Development of the atherosclerotic core region. Chemical and ultrastructural analysis of microdissected atherosclerotic lesions from human aorta. *Arterioscler Thromb* 1994;14:1305–1314.

70. Kragel AH, Reddy SG, Wittes JT, et al. Morphometric analysis of the composition of atherosclerotic plaques in the four major epicardial coronary arteries in acute myocardial infarction and in sudden coronary death. *Circulation* 1989;80:1747–1756.

71. Dollar AL, Kragel AH, Fernicola DJ, et al. Composition of atherosclerotic plaques in coronary arteries in women less than 40 years of age with fatal coronary artery disease and implications for plaque reversibility. *Am J Cardiol* 1991;67:1223–1227.

72. Gertz SD, Malezadah S, Dollar MA, et al. Composition of atherosclerotic plaques in the four major epicardial coronary arteries in patients greater than or equal to 90 years of age. *Am J Cardiol* 1991;67:1228–1233.

73. Kragel AH, Roberts WC. Composition of atherosclerotic plaques in the coronary arteries in homozygous familial hypercholesterolemia. *Am Heart J* 1991;121:210–211.

74. Tracey RE, Devaney K, Kissling G. Characteristics of the plaque under a coronary thrombus. *Virchows Arch Pathol Anat* 1985;405:411–427.

75. Davies MJ, Krikler DM, Katz D. Atherosclerosis: inhibition or regression as therapeutic possibilities. *Br Heart J* 1991;65:302–310.

76. Duguid JB. Thrombosis as a factor in the pathogenesis of aortic atherosclerosis. *J Pathol Bacteriol* 1948;60:57–69.

77. Moncada S, Palmer RM, Higgs EA. Nitric oxide physiology, pathophysiology, and pharmacology. *Pharmacol Rev* 1991;43:109–142.

78. Stamler JS, Simon DI, Osborne JA, et al. S-Nitrosylation of proteins with nitric oxide-synthesis and characterization of novel biologically active compounds. *Proc Natl Acad Sci USA* 1992;89:444–448.

79. Chilian WM, Dellsperger KC, Layne SM, et al. Effects of atherosclerosis on the coronary micro-circulation. *Am J Physiol* 1990;258:H529–H539.

80. Brown BG, Lee AB, Bolson EL, et al. Reflex constriction of significant coronary stenosis as a mechanism contributing to ischemic ventricular dysfunction during isometric exercise. *Circulation* 1984;70:18–24.

81. Hess OM, Bortone A, Eid K, et al. Coronary vasomotor tone during static and dynamic exercise. *Eur Heart J* 1989;10[Suppl F]:105–110.

82. Harrison DG, Armstrong ML, Freeman PC, et al. Restoration of endothelium-dependent relaxation by dietary treatment of atherosclerosis. *J Clin Invest* 1987;80:808–811.

83. Vita JA, Treasure CB, Nabel EG, et al. Coronary vasomotor response to acetylcholine relates to risk factors for coronary artery disease. *Circulation* 1990;81:491–497.

84. Muegge A, Edwell JH, Peterson TE, et al. Chronic treatment with polyethylene-glycolated superoxide dismutase partially restores endothelium-dependent vascular relaxations in cholesterol-fed rabbits. *Circ Res* 1991;69:1293–1300.

85. The Lipid Research Clinics Coronary Primary Prevention Trial results. I. Reduction in incidence of coronary heart disease. *JAMA* 1984;251:351–364.

86. The Lipid Research Clinics Coronary Primary Prevention Trial results. II. The relationship of reduction in incidence of coronary heart disease to cholesterol lowering. *JAMA* 1984;251:365–374.

87. Manninen V, Elo MO, Frick MH, et al. Lipid alterations and decline

in the incidence of coronary heart disease in the Helsinki Heart Study. *JAMA* 1988;260:641–651.

88. Canner PL, Berge KG, Wenger NK, et al. Fifteen year mortality in Coronary Drug Project patients: long-term benefit with niacin. *J Am Coll Cardiol* 1986;8:1245–1255.

89. Randomized trial of cholesterol lowering in 4444 patients with coronary heart disease: the Scandinavian Simvastatin Survival Study (4S). *Lancet* 1994;344:1383–1389.

90. Sacks FM, Pfeffer MA, Moye LA, et al. The effect of pravastatin on coronary events after myocardial infarction in patients with average cholesterol levels. Cholesterol and Recurrent Events Trial investigators. *N Engl J Med* 1996;335:1001–1009.

91. Prevention of cardiovascular events and death with pravastatin in patients with coronary heart disease and a broad range of initial cholesterol levels. The Long-Term Intervention with Pravastatin in Ischaemic Disease (LIPID) Study Group. *N Engl J Med* 1998;339: 1349–1357.

92. Downs JR, Clearfield M, Weis S, et al. Primary prevention of acute coronary events with lovastatin in men and women with average cholesterol levels: results of the AFCAPS/TexCAPS Air Force/Texas Coronary Atherosclerosis Prevention Study. *JAMA* 1998;279:1615–1622.

93. Ambrose JA, Tannenbaum MA, Alexopoulos D, et al. Angiographic progression of coronary artery disease and the development of myocardial infarction. *J Am Coll Cardiol* 1988;12:56–62.

94. Little WC, Constantinescu M, Applegate RM, et al. Can coronary angiography predict the site of a subsequent myocardial infarction in patients with mild-to-moderate coronary artery disease? *Circulation* 1988;78:1157–1166.

95. Little WC. Angiographic assessment of the culprit coronary artery lesion before acute myocardial infarction. *Am J Cardiol* 1990;66: 44G–47G.

96. Brown BG, Lin JT, Kelsey S, et al. Progression of coronary atherosclerosis in patients with probable familial hypercholesterolemia. Quantitative arteriographic assessment of patients in NHLBI Type II Study. *Arteriosclerosis* 1989;9[Suppl I]:I-81–I-90.

97. Webster MWI, Chesebro JH, Smith HC, et al. Myocardial infarction and coronary artery occlusion: a prospective 5-year angiographic study. *J Am Coll Cardiol* 1990;15[Suppl A]:218A(abst).

98. Constantinides P. Plaque fissures in human coronary thrombosis. *J Atheroscler Res* 1966;6I:1–17.

99. Constantinides P. Plaque hemorrhages, their genesis and their role in supraplaque thrombosis and atherogenesis. In: Glagov S, Newman W, Schaffer SA, eds. *Pathobiology of the human atherosclerotic plaque.* New York: Springer-Verlag, 1990:393–411.

100. Lendon CL, Davies MJ, Born GVR, et al. Atherosclerotic plaque caps are locally weakened when macrophage density is increased. *Atherosclerosis* 1991;87:87–90.

101. Richardson PD, Davies MJ, Born GV. Influence of plaque configuration and stress distribution on fissuring of coronary atherosclerotic plaques. *Lancet* 1989;334:941–944.

102. Loree HM, Kamm RD, Strongfellow RG, et al. Effects of fibrous cap thickness on peak circumferential stress in model atherosclerotic vessels. *Circ Res* 1992;71:850–858.

103. Davies MJ, Richardson PD, Woolf N, et al. Risk of thrombosis in human atherosclerotic plaques: role of extracellular lipid, macrophages, and smooth muscle cell content. *Br Heart J* 1993;69:377–381.

104. Hessler JR, Morel DW, Lewis LJ, et al. Lipoprotein oxidation and lipoprotein-induced cytotoxicity. *Arteriosclerosis* 1983;3:215–222.

105. Kugiyama K, Kerns SA, Morrisett JD, et al. Impairment of endothelium-dependent arterial relaxation by lysolecithin in modified low-density lipoproteins. *Nature* 1990;344:160–162.

106. Yla-Herttuala S, Palinski W, Rosenfeld ME, et al. Evidence for the presence of oxidatively modified low density lipoprotein in atherosclerotic lesions of rabbit and man. *J Clin Invest* 1989;84:1086–1095.

107. Haberland M, Fong D, Cheng L. Malondialdehyde-altered protein occurs in atheroma of Watanabe heritable hyperlipidemic rabbits. *Science* 1988;24:215–218.

108. Kunjathoor VV, Febbraio M, Podrez EA, et al. Scavenger receptors class A-I/II and CD36 are the principal receptors responsible for the uptake of modified low density lipoprotein leading to lipid loading in macrophages. *J Biol Chem* 2002;277:49982–49988.

109. Fuhrman B, Koren L, Volkova N, et al. Atorvastatin therapy in hypercholesterolemic patients suppresses cellular uptake of oxidized-LDL by differentiating monocytes. *Atherosclerosis* 2002;164:179–185.

110. Davies MJ. A macro and micro view of coronary vascular insult in ischemic heart disease. *Circulation* 1990;82[Suppl II]:II38–II46.

111. Van der Wal AC, Becker AE, Van der Loos CM, et al. Site of intimal rupture or erosion of thrombosed coronary atherosclerotic plaques is characterized by an inflammatory process irrespective of the dominant plaque morphology. *Circulation* 1994;89:36–44.

112. Moreno PR, Falk E, Palacios IF, et al. Macrophage infiltration in acute coronary syndromes: implications for plaque rupture. *Circulation* 1994;90:775–778.

113. Shah PK, Falk E, Badimon JJ, et al. Human monocyte-derived macrophages express collagenase and induce collagen breakdown in atherosclerotic fibrous caps: implication for plaque rupture. *Circulation* 1993;88[Suppl I]:I-254(abst).

114. Henney AM, Wakeley PR, Davies MJ, et al. Location of stromelysin gene in atherosclerotic plaques using in-site hybridization. *Proc Natl Acad Sci USA* 1991;88:8154–8158.

115. Ridker PM, Rifai N, Clearfield M, et al. Measurement of C-reactive protein for the targeting of statin therapy in the primary prevention of acute coronary events. *N Engl J Med* 2001;344:1959–1965.

116. Libby P. Current concepts of the pathogenesis of the acute coronary syndromes. *Circulation* 2001;104:365–372.

117. Zhao XQ, Yuan C, Hatsukami TS, et al. Effects of prolonged intensive lipid-lowering therapy on the characteristics of carotid atherosclerotic plaques in vivo by MRI: a case-control study. *Arterioscler Thromb Vasc Biol* 2001;21:1623–1629.

Hypertension, Cigarette Smoking, Diabetes, Obesity, and Others

CHAPTER 13

Hypertension Genetics and Mechanisms

Steven C. Hunt and Paul N. Hopkins

Key Words: Adducin; angiotensinogen; genetic association; genetic linkage; genetic marker; metabolic syndrome; Na-Li countertransport; Na-K-ATPase transport.

INTRODUCTION

Blood pressure is controlled by multiple physiologic systems, each with many components that are highly interrelated (1). Part of the difficulty in studying the causes of hypertension is that unless specific variables can be studied in isolation from other variables, their characteristics will be confounded by those other variables. At the same time, hypertension may result from defective interactions among variables, so that isolating a single variable may make it impossible to identify any defect. By studying the genetic mechanisms related to specific components of blood pressure control, more specific abnormalities might be identified that can then be studied in combination with modifying factors.

Hypertension clearly has multiple causes and is heterogeneous even within defined populations (2). Perhaps the

most important finding resulting from the substantial number of genome searches for hypertension or blood pressure genes is that there are probably no common mutations in genes that explain a large proportion of hypertension or blood pressure variation (3–8). Genetic control, therefore, is probably a result of small to moderate effects from many genes. Heterogeneity masks the effects of any particular gene being studied because of the variation in a phenotype that is independent of the genetic mechanism of interest. However, progress has been made in identifying specific variables associated with hypertension that seem to be genetically controlled. Some of these variables are also risk factors for cardiovascular disease. Whether these common factors lead directly to both hypertension and cardiovascular disease or whether they lead to hypertension that increases risk for cardiovascular disease is still being determined.

Cardiovascular disease may develop from the direct effects of hypertension independent of the effects of atherothrombosis. Chronic increase of blood pressure is known to induce structural alterations in the vasculature and in other organs. Thus, increasing levels of blood pressure or greater duration of hypertension can lead progressively to arteriosclerosis with increased stress on the myocardium caused by lack of aortic compliance, thereby promoting congestive heart failure. Arteriolosclerosis, and more severe arteriolar damage such as fibrinoid change and fibrinoid necrosis, can directly cause end-organ damage such as hem-

S. C. Hunt: Cardiovascular Genetics Division, Department of Internal Medicine, University of Utah School of Medicine, Salt Lake City, Utah 84108.

P. N. Hopkins: Cardiovascular Genetics Division, Department of Internal Medicine, University of Utah School of Medicine, Salt Lake City, Utah 84108.

orrhagic and lacunar stroke, malignant hypertension, renal failure, and retinal damage. Hypertension may also cause associated physiologic systems to respond to the greater pressures, thereby changing other components related to increased risk for coronary disease. There may also be factors that lead to the development of both hypertension and coronary heart disease (CHD) independently, not requiring a direct relation to exist between increased pressure and coronary disease.

It is not the purpose of this chapter to review the basic physiology of each system that controls blood pressure; however, major components that could be altered by a genetic abnormality are described. The hypotheses relating high blood pressure to atherothrombosis and cardiovascular end points also are briefly discussed.

BLOOD PRESSURE AS A MAJOR CARDIOVASCULAR RISK FACTOR

Both coronary artery disease (CAD) and stroke are strongly and positively associated with blood pressure in a graded, independent, and consistent fashion, as shown in a meta-analysis of nine major prospective studies (9). Moreover, treatment of hypertension markedly decreased risk for stroke and modestly reduced CAD end points in multiple studies (10–13). Considering these trials together, treatment resulted in a significant reduction of CAD end points by

17% (95% confidence interval [CI], 10–23%), whereas stroke incidence declined 38% (95% CI, 30–44%) (14). The Antihypertensive and Lipid-Lowering Treatment to Prevent Heart Attack Trial (ALLHAT) study clearly showed the benefits of antihypertensive treatment in subjects with hypertension with other CHD risk factors (15). These results establish hypertension as a major, causal risk factor for cardiovascular disease. Systolic blood pressure is at least as predictive a risk factor as diastolic blood pressure (Fig. 13–1), as shown in numerous prospective studies (16–18) and by the positive benefits realized by treating isolated systolic hypertension (12). In fact, CAD risk increases progressively with systolic pressure independent of diastolic pressure (19). Systolic blood pressure is now included in the staging scheme for severity of hypertension in the report of the Joint National Committee on Detection, Evaluation, and Treatment of High Blood Pressure (20) as amply justified by epidemiologic observations.

In the Multiple Risk Factor Intervention Trial (MRFIT), a 6-year follow-up of 356,222 middle-aged men, ideal ranges for systolic and diastolic blood pressures were less than 120 and 80 mm Hg, respectively (16) (Figs. 13–1 and 13–2). Only 25% of the men had systolic blood pressures in this ideal range. Importantly, the blood pressure strata where the attributable risk for CHD was greatest (a function of both prevalence and relative risk) was in the high normal range (85–89 mm Hg) of diastolic blood pressure and in the low

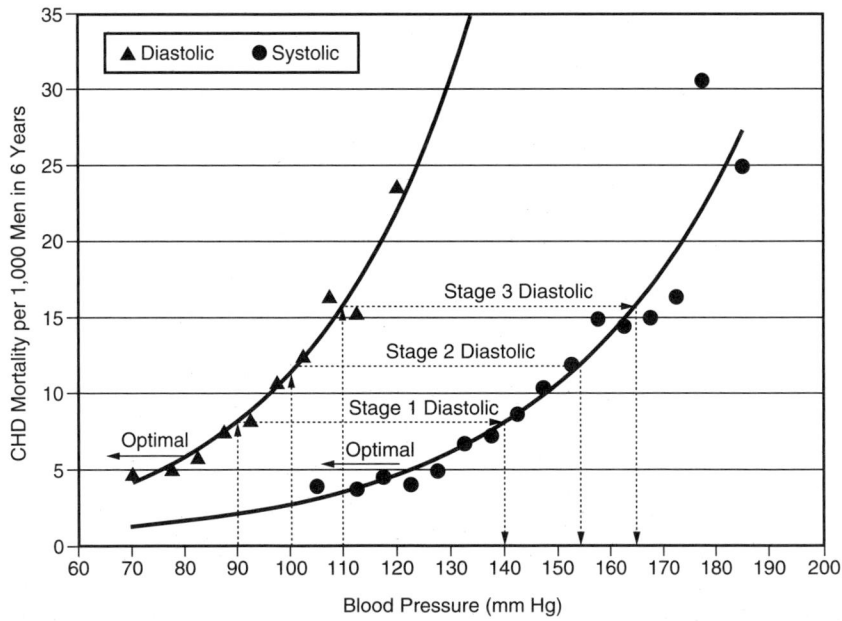

FIG. 13–1. Age-adjusted coronary heart disease (CHD) mortality in 6 years (per 1,000 individuals) as a function of systolic and diastolic blood pressure among the 356,222 men 35 to 57 years of age screened and free of myocardial infarction in the Multiple Risk Factor Intervention Trial. Equivalent risk is shown for systolic blood pressure using the current diastolic blood pressure guidelines. (Data from Stamler J. Epidemiology, established major risk factors, and the primary prevention of coronary heart disease. In: Parmley WW, Chatterjee K, eds. *Cardiology.* Philadelphia: JB Lippincott, 1987:1:1–1:41.)

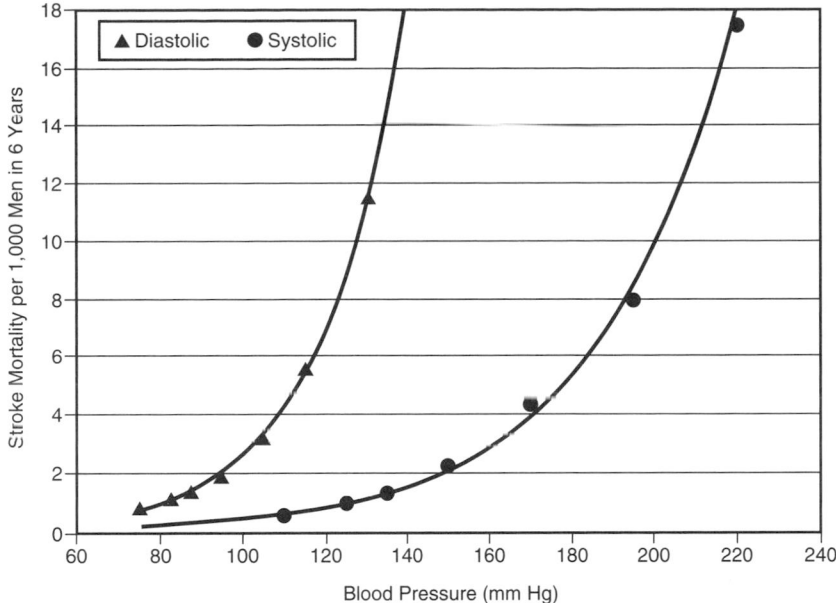

FIG. 13–2. Age-adjusted stroke mortality in 6 years (per 1,000 individuals) as a function of systolic and diastolic blood pressure among the 356,222 men 35 to 57 years of age screened and free of myocardial infarction in the Multiple Risk Factor Intervention Trial. (Data from Stamler J. Epidemiology, established major risk factors, and the primary prevention of coronary heart disease. In: Parmley WW, Chatterjee K, eds. *Cardiology.* Philadelphia: JB Lippincott, 1987:1:1–1:41.)

hypertensive range for systolic blood pressure (140–144 mm Hg). On the basis of these MRFIT data, 32% of all CHD deaths could be attributed to diastolic blood pressure greater than 80 mm Hg and 42% could be attributed to systolic blood pressure greater than 120 mm Hg (16).

Relative risks associated with hypertension are typically greater for stroke than for CHD (9). This also appears to be true of atherothrombotic stroke and other forms of stroke. However, atherothrombosis in individuals with hypertension is not more extensive in carotid or intracerebral vessels than in coronary arteries. Rather, hypertension largely reverses the relative protection against atherothrombosis that the carotid and intracerebral vessels normally enjoy (21,22). This is graphically illustrated in Figure 13–3. The increased relative risk is therefore caused by a low baseline risk for cerebral atherothrombosis in normotensive individuals rather than markedly increased absolute risks in hypertensive individuals. In patients with familial hypercholesterolemia who generally are not hypertensive (23), the cerebral vessels are relatively spared compared with coronary arteries (24).

Some international studies have reported no association between clinically defined CHD end points and high blood pressure in which serum cholesterol is consistently low (25–27). Possibly, there were too few CHD events to detect the effect of blood pressure in these studies. In autopsy, hypertension was associated with more raised coronary lesions even in countries with a very low incidence of clinical disease (21). High-resolution carotid ultrasound revealed an excess of plaques in patients with hypertension (28,29). However, if these raised lesions did not progress sufficiently fast because of low plasma cholesterol, they may not lead to a statistically significant excess of clinically detectable disease. Alternatively, blood pressure may only foster atherothrombosis when serum cholesterol levels are sufficiently high (30–32).

FAMILIAL AGGREGATION OF CARDIOVASCULAR END POINTS

CHD, hypertension, and stroke all aggregate within families, suggesting that genetic factors, shared common environmental factors, or both, make significant contributions to each of these end points. A family history of hypertension is an independent predictor of the development of hypertension (33–37). A positive family history of either hypertension or CHD increases the risk for future disease onset in unaffected family members (Table 13–1) (33). Family history is more predictive when multiple family members are affected or if they are affected at young ages. A majority of cases of both early stroke and early CHD occur in a small percentage of families in the population, demonstrating the marked aggregation of early disease (38). Family history as a prediction variable also has advantages over biochemical, anthropometric, or other risk factors in the sense that its relation to hypertension is not confounded by heterogeneity between families (39). Two families may have completely

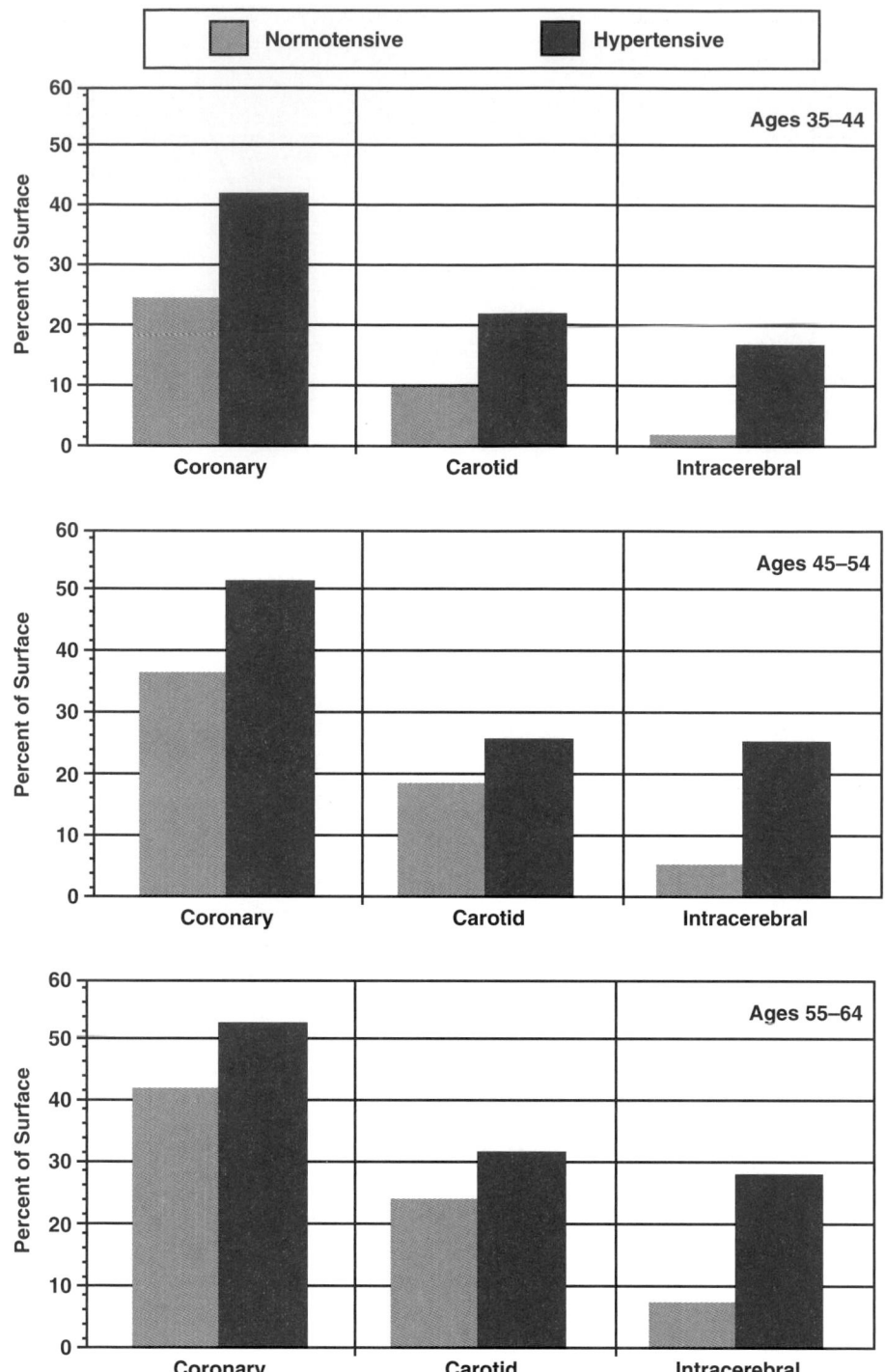

FIG. 13–3. Percent of surface involved in raised atherothrombotic lesions in an autopsy among men from Oslo, Norway, with and without diagnosed hypertension in the International Atherosclerosis Project. (Data from Robertson WB, Strong JP. Atherosclerosis in persons with hypertension and diabetes mellitus. *Lab Invest* 1968;18:539–551; and Solberg LA, McGarry PA. Cerebral atherosclerosis in persons with selected diseases. *Lab Invest* 1968;18:613–619.)

different causes of their positive family history, but each cause will increase the probability that other family members will become hypertensive at early ages. Not only does the same disease aggregate within a family, but a positive family history of one disease increases the likelihood of a positive family history of another disease. The prevalence of a positive family history of CHD (two or more affected members) is increased threefold if the family has a positive family history of hypertension, stroke, or diabetes and suggests that there are probably genetic components that are common to the development of both hypertension and CHD in the same family (40).

TABLE 13–1. *Relative risks for coronary heart disease and hypertension after 13 years of follow-up for individuals in families with a positive family history of coronary heart disease or hypertension*

Age group, yr	CHD		HBP	
	≥2 Early events	≥1 Event	≥2 Early events	≥1 Event
Men				
20–39	12.7[a]	2.9[a]	4.1[a]	2.5[a]
50–59	2.9[a]	1.3[a]	2.4[a]	1.7[a]
≥70	0.7	1.3[a]	0.8	0.9
Women				
20–39	8.0[a]	1.4	5.0[a]	2.8[a]
50–59	3.7	1.2	1.5	1.5[a]
≥70	1.5	1.1	0.8	1.0
% of population	1.7%	38.1%	11.4%	53.1%

Relative risks of a positive family history compared with families with no events.
CHD, coronary heart disease; HBP, high blood pressure.
[a]$P < 0.05$.
Adapted from Hunt SC, Williams RR, Barlow GK. A comparison of positive family history definitions for defining risk of future disease. *J Chron Dis* 1986;39:809–821.

HEMODYNAMIC FACTORS AND ATHEROGENESIS

Blood pressure in the arterial range appears to be an essential requirement for the development of atherothrombosis. Venous atherothrombosis does not develop even in patients with homozygous familial hypercholesterolemia (41). The relatively rapid progression of atherothrombosis in saphenous veins used in coronary artery bypass suggests there is nothing uniquely resistant about veins themselves. The normal pulmonary arterial circulation with its systolic pressures of 12 to 22 mm Hg is another protected site. Nevertheless, with pulmonary hypertension, atherothrombotic plaques are commonly seen (42).

Studies have provided further insights into the roles of blood pressure and hemodynamics in atherogenesis. In one study, rabbit aorta was isolated *in vitro* and pressurized to either 70 or 160 mm Hg. The penetration of radiolabeled low-density lipoprotein (LDL) into layers of the artery wall was determined at the two pressures. LDL concentration in the intima and inner media was increased 44-fold at the greater pressure. LDL concentration decreased rapidly in more peripheral layers until, in the adventitia, LDL concentrations at the two pressures were nearly equal. In contrast, albumin concentration was increased tenfold at the high pressure, but was distributed evenly throughout the arterial wall layers. The investigators suggest that at greater pressures, the subintimal tissues are compacted and thereby retard the movement of the relatively large LDL particles through the wall. Thus, trapping of LDL at the internal elastic lamina together with pressure-driven convection of LDL into the artery wall appear to be the major mechanisms underlying the relation between blood pressure and atherothrombosis (43).

Sites of atherothrombosis predilection can largely be explained by hemodynamic models. Plaques are much more frequent in areas *opposite* flow dividers—in areas of slow flow (low shear) or eddy currents (Fig. 13–4). Turbulence is not a feature of flow in these sites. In fact, essentially no turbulence is seen in most of the normal cardiovascular system (44). At the flow divider, the pattern of flow is laminar and fast (45). The shearing forces along the vessel wall in such areas are relatively high. Although intimal thickening is stimulated early at arterial sites exposed to high shear stress (primarily from smooth muscle cell accumulation), the process does not proceed on to atherothrombosis (46). Release of growth factors may mediate this early proliferation of smooth muscle cells (47,48).

In a mathematical model with parameters fit to human autopsy findings, intimal thickening increased gradually with age to a point when macrophages became trapped at a critical intimal thickness, at which time intimal thickness increased rapidly as macrophages accumulated (49). Increased residence time near the artery wall in slow-flow areas might promote penetration by blood components such as LDL, monocytes, and platelets into the intima (50). Intimal plaques accumulated exclusively in areas of low shear created experimentally by aortic stenoses placed in hypercholesterolemic beagles (51). Finally, low-shear stress, calculated by anatomic features in 20 arterial segments, was strongly correlated with greater progression of coronary atherothrombosis over 3 years among patients in the Harvard Atherosclerosis Reversibility Project (52). The unique hemodynamics of the coronary circulation, with near cessation of flow during systole, together with the high pressures generated at the aortic root may explain the predilection of coronary arteries to atherothrombosis. As heart rate increases, relatively more time is spent in systole with proportionately more time for penetration of blood elements into the arterial wall. This may help to explain the fourfold increase in risk for CAD as resting heart rate increased from less than 60 to more than 100 beats per minute (53).

METABOLIC SYNDROME AND HYPERTENSION

Epidemiologic studies have clearly shown consistent associations among hypertension, diabetes, and dyslipidemia, as have been reported from Framingham (54), the Lipid Re-

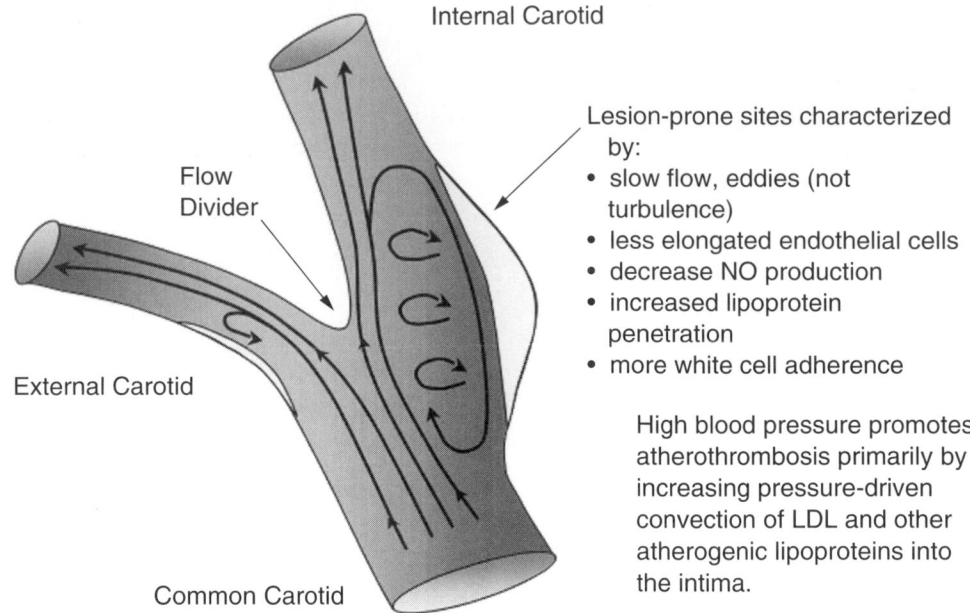

Internal Carotid

Flow
Divider

External Carotid

Common Carotid

Lesion-prone sites characterized
by:
• slow flow, eddies (not
turbulence)
• less elongated endothelial cells
• decrease NO production
• increased lipoprotein
penetration
• more white cell adherence

High blood pressure promotes
atherothrombosis primarily by
increasing pressure-driven
convection of LDL and other
atherogenic lipoproteins into
the intima.

FIG. 13–4. Hemodynamic factors favoring development of atherothrombosis. Lesion-prone sites are characterized by slow flow, eddy currents, prolonged residence time for formed blood elements, potentially higher side pressures, and increased adhesion of monocytes mediated in part by lower rates of production of nitric oxide (NO) and prostacyclin. *Arrows:* Streamlines and flow patterns of bubbles injected into glass casts of human arteries. LDL, low-density lipoprotein.

search Clinic (LRC) population (55), and Stanford subjects (56–58). Abnormalities associated with hypertension have included increased levels of cholesterol, LDL cholesterol (LDL-C), apolipoprotein B, triglycerides, and very low-density lipoprotein (VLDL) cholesterol, as well as decreased levels of high-density lipoprotein cholesterol (HDL-C) and apolipoprotein A-I. Insulin resistance, obesity, and diabetes are other common occurrences in what has been termed the metabolic syndrome.

Twin and family studies suggest that genetic factors play an important role in the coaggregation of lipid abnormalities and hypertension, as shown from the National Heart, Lung, and Blood Institute (NHLBI) twin cohort (58) and studies of Utah families (59,60). In Utah sibling pairs ascertained only for the diagnosis of hypertension before age 60 years in both siblings, high triglycerides and low HDL-C levels were found three times more often than expected ($p < 0.0001$). These abnormalities occurred in individuals with normal weight and in obese individuals. This syndrome was descriptively labeled "familial dyslipidemic hypertension" and occurs in about 12% of individuals with essential hypertension and in 1% to 2% of the general population (Table 13–2). Occurrence of CHD after 16 years of follow-up was much greater in individuals with both hypertension and dyslipidemia than in individuals with only hypertension or dyslipidemia (58).

Familial combined hyperlipidemia (FCHL) is one of the most common lipid syndromes associated with CHD (60, 61). A 6-year prospective study has shown that although only 4.3% of the study participants had increased baseline triglycerides and a baseline LDL-C/HDL-C ratio greater

than 5, a total of 25% of all definite myocardial infarctions occurred in this subgroup (62). More recently, the NHLBI Family Heart Study has shown that CHD risk in families with familial hypertriglyceridemia is the same as in families with FCHL, and the phenotypic expression of the syndromes are much more similar than previously thought (63).

TABLE 13–2. *Familial dyslipidemic hypertension in the National Heart, Lung, and Blood Institute twins versus Utah siblings*

Characteristic tabulated	NHLBI	Utah
Study subjects	Twins	Siblings
Number of hypertensives tested	185	131
Frequency of FDH		
In general population (%)	2	1.5
In all hypertensives (%)	10	12
Frequency of lipid abnormalities		
HDL-C <10th percentile (%)	83	62
Triglyceride >90th percentile (%)	33	45
LDL-C >90th percentile (%)	22	22

National Heart, Lung, and Blood Institute (NHLBI) Twin Concordance for Familial Dyslipidemic Hypertension (FDH): monozygotes three times dizygotes ($p = 0.06$).

HDL-C, high-density lipoprotein cholesterol; LDL-C, low-density lipoprotein cholesterol.

Adapted from Selby JV, Newman B, Quiroga J, et al. Concordance for dyslipidemic hypertension in male twins. *JAMA* 1991;265:2079–2084; and Williams RR, Hunt SC, Hopkins PN, et al. Familial dyslipidemic hypertension: evidence from 58 Utah families for a syndrome present in approximately 12% of patients with essential hypertension. *JAMA* 1988; 259:3579–3586.

FCHL and familial dyslipidemic hypertension, which usually appear by young adulthood, may influence the development of hypertension through various pathways, such as alteration of ion transport systems, structural changes in the vasculature, or increasing responsiveness of vascular smooth muscle to hormonal or other factors in addition to shared associations with obesity. For example, a randomized treatment trial using pravastatin found that it had a significant blood pressure–decreasing effect in addition to its lipid-decreasing effect (64). Normotensive individuals with familial hypercholesterolemia showed greater Na-Li countertransport and intracellular sodium than normolipidemic control subjects, both of which were reduced by fluvastatin treatment of the increased lipids (65). Three studies have shown that increased lipids increase the blood pressure response to an angiotensin II infusion (66–68), and this response can be partially reduced by statin treatment (67). The lipid modification of blood pressure responsiveness may be partly caused by up-regulation of the angiotensin type 1 (AT-1) receptor by LDL-C (69). AT-1 receptor density or regulation also can arise from changes in salt, estrogens, insulin, and insulin resistance (70–73).

Insulin resistance is closely related to several metabolic and clinical conditions, including hyperinsulinemia, CHD, diabetes, and obesity (57,74–76). At least three prospective studies have shown plasma insulin associated with CHD (77–79). The metabolic syndrome, defined by National Cholesterol Education Program (NCEP) criteria (80), predicted CHD, cardiovascular disease, and total mortality in men (81) and CHD risk factors in the Third National Health and Nutrition Examination Survey (NHANES III) study (82).

The causal relation of insulin or insulin resistance with hypertension is somewhat more controversial than with CHD. Prospective studies have shown insulin or postglucose 1-hour insulin level is related to the development of hypertension (83–86). Insulin resistance is hypothesized to promote hypertension in various ways, including (a) stimulation of cation transport and sodium reabsorption in the distal and proximal tubule causing renal sodium retention and hypertension (87,88); (b) stimulation of norepinephrine and increased blood pressure (89) (this is likely because of insulin-related peripheral vasodilation with reflex stimulation of the sympathetic nervous system); (c) stimulation of smooth muscle cells to hypertrophy, increasing peripheral vascular resistance and blood pressure (i.e., growth factor–like effect of insulin) (90); (d) stimulation of intracellular calcium and increased smooth muscle contractility (91); and (e) obesity-related angiotensinogen production in adipose tissue leading to insulin resistance (92).

Many studies have shown that individuals with untreated hypertension have greater insulin levels than do normotensive control subjects (74,93,94). Furthermore, treatment of hypertension does not necessarily normalize the insulin levels (94), suggesting that the increased levels are not caused by hypertension. There is evidence that abnormalities in glucose and insulin metabolism precede and may play a role in the causes of hypertension.

Increased dietary intake of calories increases insulin levels and sympathetic response (95). This sympathetic response increases thermogenesis to burn off the excess calories, preventing further weight gain. However, increased norepinephrine also increases vasoconstriction and sodium retention, which further increases blood pressure. Catecholamines also buffer the insulin effects on glucose metabolism (96), which increases insulin resistance (97). Body fat distribution as measured by waist-to-hip ratio also plays an important role relating sympathetic response to systolic and diastolic blood pressure (98). The amount of intraabdominal fat correlates with the insulin response to a glucose load (99), indicating that upper or central obesity may aggravate preexisting insulin resistance or be responsible for part of the initiation of that resistance. Euglycemic clamp studies have shown increases in blood pressure and sympathetic stimulation as the insulin levels increased in nonobese subjects (89), indicating that insulin resistance also occurs in the absence of obesity.

Studies suggest that high plasma triglycerides or fatty acids, or both, promote insulin resistance (100–102). Patients with type V hyperlipoproteinemia have high triglycerides from both increased chylomicrons and high VLDL and also experience insulin resistance. Increased insulin levels increase the synthesis and secretion of VLDL-triglyceride by the liver, possibly explaining some of the observed hypertriglyceridemia commonly seen in patients with hypertension (103). After weight loss, which increases the effectiveness of insulin, VLDL-triglyceride secretion and plasma triglyceride concentrations decrease (104). It has been shown that blood pressure in obese individuals could be decreased by physical training without a loss of weight, but only in those who were hyperinsulinemic and hypertriglyceridemic at baseline (105). Insulin sensitivity defects appear to occur in skeletal muscle of subjects with hypertension, even in those of normal weight (93).

Insulin resistance and hyperinsulinemia are not always synonymous. For example, patients with pheochromocytoma have insulin resistance and hypertension without hyperinsulinemia (106). Neither rats nor humans with renal vascular hypertension have hyperinsulinemia (107,108). Hypertensive and normotensive rats with acutely increased insulin levels do not experience an increase in sodium reabsorption (109). Chronic insulin infusion (28 days) in healthy dogs does not increase blood pressure or sympathetic stimulation (110,111). Therefore, some researchers believe that hypertension is related more to an underlying cause of insulin resistance than to hyperinsulinemia. Obesity is likely a major cause of insulin resistance, because adjustment for adiposity and controlling for background polygenes and environment by using a sib-pair study design removed most of the insulin differences seen between hypertensive and normotensive subjects (112). Subjects with isolated systolic hypertension showed no insulin differences.

An *in vivo* study on humans showed that insulin infusion with a glucose clamp decreased sodium excretion even though there was decreased sodium reabsorption in the proximal tubule of the kidney (113). The decreased net sodium excretion occurred because there was increased distal tubule reabsorption of sodium that more than counterbalanced the decreased reabsorption in the proximal tubule. Further studies on hypertension incidence are needed to clarify the role of insulin levels as an independent risk factor in both men and women of all ages. However, whatever the causes of insulin resistance, dyslipidemia, and hyperinsulinemia, these phenotypes are clearly associated with coronary heart disease and are highly familial (40,114).

ENDOTHELIAL FACTORS

The effects of a number of vasoactive substances in both hypertension and atherogenesis have been the subject of much recent research.

Endothelin

Endothelin is a potent vasoconstricting peptide and is mitogenic for smooth muscle cells. It occurs in at least three forms: endothelin-1, -2, and -3. Endothelial cells produce only endothelin-1 (115). Endothelin-converting enzyme inhibitors and endothelin antagonists have shown some efficacy in reducing blood pressure in certain genetic animal models of hypertension (116,117). Plasma levels of endothelin (which are variably increased or normal in human hypertension) do not necessarily reflect endothelial production rates, because most endothelin is probably not secreted luminally. Nevertheless, several interesting observations suggest potential roles in promoting hypertension, hyperlipidemia, and atherothrombosis through inflammatory mechanisms (118,119). Endothelin production by cultured endothelial cells and intact aorta is stimulated by oxidized LDL (120,121). Endothelin can also induce oxidative stress (122). Whether increased endothelin production may be involved in the hypertension associated with dyslipidemia is unknown, but it is an attractive hypothesis. At least in salt-sensitive hypertension using the Sabra rat model, left ventricular hypertrophy is prevented when the endothelin-A receptor is blocked (123). Serum and vascular concentrations of endothelin were increased in patients with atherothrombosis (124). Endothelin may thus promote excess vasoconstriction known to occur at diseased vascular sites, especially if unopposed by nitric oxide (NO; discussed later).

Endothelin infusion causes renal afferent vasoconstriction, decreased glomerular filtration rate, salt retention, and hypertension (125,126). This salt-sensitive hypertension, which develops after endothelin infusion in animals, is prevented by captopril, implicating the renin-angiotensin system as a mediator of the hypertensive effects of endothelin (127).

At least three studies have shown a genetic association between endothelin-1 and blood pressure (128,129), although another study did not find an association (130).

Nitric Oxide and Nitric Oxide Synthase

Decreased endothelial NO production has been consistently associated with atherothrombosis in the coronary arteries and other vascular beds. Furthermore, impaired endothelial NO production or availability has been associated with virtually every risk factor for atherothrombosis including hypertension, diabetes, cigarette smoking, hypercholesterolemia, hypertriglyceridemia, low HDL, increased lipoprotein (a), increased homocysteine, and high C-reactive protein (131–137).

NO is produced by several isozymes, among them two constitutively synthesized and calmodulin-dependent, noninducible NO synthases (one cytosolic, *NOS1* or neuronal NOS, and another membrane-bound obtained from endothelial cells and producing picomolar quantities of NO, *NOS3*, or endothelial NOS) and two inducible enzymes that predominate in smooth muscle cells (138). The inducible enzymes *(NOS2)* can produce sufficient NO (nanomolar quantities of NO) to cause shock when production is sufficiently stimulated by lipopolysaccharide, endotoxin, or several cytokines including tumor necrosis factor and interleukin-1.

The constitutive endothelial NOS *(NOS3)* is calcium- and calmodulin-dependent and is stimulated by a variety of hormones (acetylcholine, bradykinin, serotonin, norepinephrine, histamine, and adenosine diphosphate), peptides (endothelin, vasopressin, and substance P), and mechanical factors such as flow or shear stress, all of which mediate increased intracellular calcium concentrations. NO diffuses across cell membranes and binds to soluble guanylate cyclase resulting in increased production of cyclic guanosine monophosphate (cGMP). In smooth muscle cells, increased cGMP activates cGMP kinase, which can increase permeability of potassium channels, increase calcium ATPase, decrease phospholipase C activity with reduced concentration of inositol phosphatides, and decrease phosphorylation of myosin light chain. In smooth muscle these effects lead directly and indirectly to relaxation. Interestingly, in endothelial and smooth muscle cells, increased cGMP inhibits endothelin production, resulting in a negative feedback loop (because endothelin increases activity of the constitutive NOS in endothelial cells).

In general, the endothelium provides a buffer to many potentially vasoconstricting agents by producing NO in response to the same intracellular signal (increasing calcium concentration) that causes vasoconstriction in smooth muscle cells. Hence, for example, acetylcholine or serotonin causes vasodilatation in an intact artery, but causes constriction if the endothelium is removed or impaired. Although NO can cause hyperpolarization of the smooth muscle cells leading to vasodilatation (139), an endothelium-derived hyperpolarizing factor (EDHF or C-type natriuretic peptide) also exists that results in vasodilatation even when the NO and prostaglandin I_2 actions are blocked (140).

NO may be unique among vasoactive substances in that tonic production appears to be involved in maintenance of normal blood pressure in animals (141,142) and humans (143), because infusion of NOS inhibitors increases blood pressure and vascular resistance even in normal individuals. There is impaired NO production in hypertensive individuals (144,145). At least part of the impaired NO production appears to be caused by the high blood pressure itself, being in part reversible with decreased pressure (146). Yet, sustained hypertension in normal rats was induced by prolonged administration of an NOS inhibitor (147,148). The vasodilatation of muscle vascular beds by insulin has been reported to be mediated by NO release (149,150).

In kidneys, several mechanisms may contribute to antihypertensive effects of NO. Renal blood flow appears to be controlled by the balance between angiotensin II and NO. A 3-day infusion of N^G-nitro-L-arginine methyl ester in conscious dogs at doses below the threshold to acutely affect blood pressure led to a 35% decrease in glomerular filtration rate, a 32% decrease in urinary sodium excretion, a sustained reduction in urine flow rate, and a 45% increase in plasma renin activity. These effects were reversible with administration of L-arginine (151). Part of the increase in sodium excretion induced by volume loading was shown to be mediated by NO in dogs (152). NO also is produced by *NOS1* in macula densa cells and is induced by a high-salt diet and stimulated by increasing tubular sodium chloride concentration (153). The long-term effects on renin release, however, may be small (154).

The genes regulating NO have been suggested as candidate genes involved with the development of hypertension with varying results (155–165). A variant of the gene coding *NOS3* has been related to basal NO production levels (156). *NOS1* variants may affect susceptibility to end-stage renal disease in black individuals (166). A G894T polymorphism in the endothelial NOS gene *(NOS3)* was associated with blood pressure, and this association was stronger in subjects with greater insulin resistance (167). Insulin increases *NOS3* expression (168), and polymorphisms that interfere with that expression could lead to decreased NO and increased blood pressure. Functional and clinical studies of the known genetic variants will be required to validate the importance of the various polymorphisms. One such study did not find any functional differences for the Glu298Asp variant of *NOS3* (169).

RENIN-ANGIOTENSIN-KALLIKREIN SYSTEMS

The renin-angiotensin system plays an important role in salt and water homeostasis and the maintenance of vascular tone. Each component of this system represents a potential candidate in the etiology of hypertension. Accordingly, ge-

netic investigations of renin activity, angiotensin-converting enzyme (ACE) activity, angiotensinogen, and angiotensin II have been done. Briefly, linkage of the renin and *ACE* genes to hypertension were initially rejected (170,171). Although the renin gene has not been linked to hypertension, renin levels are important in the pathophysiology of hypertension, because they are modulated by genetic and phenotypic variations of other, related variables. A newly identified polymorphism in the renin gene enhancer region at −5,312 base pair has been shown to affect gene transcription and may have more relevance to blood pressure (172). The association of the *ACE* gene with hypertension seems to be easier to detect in men than women, because two studies found significant results when stratifying by sex (173,174). Additional polymorphisms in *ACE* have been identified that explain greater amounts of variation in plasma ACE levels and also show association with blood pressure (175). Previous studies that yielded negative results using the *ACE* I/D polymorphism should be repeated using these more informative polymorphisms.

Plasma Angiotensinogen and Angiotensin II

Angiotensin II is formed after cleavage of angiotensinogen by renin and cleavage of angiotensin I by ACE. Renin conversion of angiotensinogen to angiotensin I decreases the amount of angiotensinogen. Increased angiotensin II levels stimulate hepatic angiotensinogen production and release, returning angiotensinogen levels to normal. Angiotensin II–stimulated angiotensinogen production seems to occur by stabilization of the messenger RNA (mRNA) for angiotensinogen, not by activation of transcription by any known DNA sequence (176). Renin release is normally stimulated by reduced perfusion pressure and inhibited by increased sodium loads sensed by the macula densa in the juxtaglomerular apparatus in the kidney. In the presence of decreased pressure or sodium loads, plasma renin is increased, producing more angiotensin II (177). Vasoconstriction occurs reducing the renin levels and replenishing the angiotensinogen levels through the angiotensin II positive feedback loop. Any genetic abnormality resulting in increased angiotensinogen production appears to increase angiotensinogen levels, resulting in greater amounts converted to angiotensin II (178). The greater angiotensinogen levels also would be maintained through higher feedback by angiotensin II. Increased angiotensin II increases blood pressure by stimulating vasoconstriction, proximal tubular sodium reabsorption, and aldosterone release, which further increases sodium and water retention.

Long-term administration of angiotensin II at subpressor doses has been shown to increase blood pressure (179). Increased blood pressure resulting from chronic angiotensinogen elevation would tend to reduce the renin released in the kidney. Greater angiotensin II levels also have a negative feedback on renin, decreasing renin levels (180). Because it has been shown that increased amounts of angiotensinogen are associated with higher blood pressure, this implies that if renin activity is reduced, it is still sufficient to maintain the increased conversion of angiotensinogen to angiotensin I. However, angiotensin II does not seem to be increased in subjects with hypertension. Preliminary results from a rat study suggest that if plasma renin activity remains low, there is no relation between blood pressure and angiotensinogen; whereas for rats with high renin, there was a strong relation (181): High renin led to angiotensinogen depletion.

Plasma angiotensinogen was greater in subjects with hypertension and in the offspring of hypertensive parents than in normotensive control subjects (182–184). The correlation between angiotensinogen levels and blood pressure in another study was $r = 0.39$ (185). Therefore, the *angiotensinogen (AGT)* gene appears to have functional significance and at least one of the variants (A-6G) explains 10% to 30% of circulating angiotensinogen levels (186,187).

However, it appears that the effect of the *AGT* gene on angiotensinogen levels in the collecting duct of the kidney is more important than on circulating angiotensinogen levels, because the collecting duct is where the final determination of sodium handling is made and where there is a local renin-angiotensin system (188–190). Therefore, urinary angiotensinogen may be a better indicator of sodium homeostasis than plasma levels.

An infusion of angiotensinogen increases blood pressure (191), whereas if angiotensinogen antibodies are administered, blood pressure is decreased (192). Blood pressure is increased in transgenic animals that are overexpressing angiotensinogen (193). Vascular injury induces angiotensinogen gene expression (194). In another study, an association of the *AGT* gene with blood pressure was found in subjects younger than 50 years and an association with left ventricular mass was found in the whole group (195).

Obesity is an important promoter of hypertension. In a rat feeding experiment, it was shown that fasted rats decreased the production of mRNA for angiotensinogen in adipose cells, decreased the cellular release of angiotensinogen into the local circulation, and decreased central blood pressure (92). It was hypothesized that decreased local angiotensinogen led to local vasodilatation and increased tissue perfusion allowing (a) free fatty acids to be removed from the tissue into the general circulation for fuel use, (b) increased insulin-stimulated glucose uptake by the adipose tissue, and (c) decreased blood pressure from the decreased vasoconstriction of vessels surrounded by adipose tissue. When the rats were overfed, angiotensinogen mRNA increased 16-fold from fasted levels and more than 2-fold greater than control levels, with increased cellular release of angiotensinogen. This results in local vasoconstriction, increased systemic blood pressure, reduced fatty acid removal from the tissues (even though cellular release was increased), and decreased glucose uptake by adipose tissue because of the local vasoconstriction preventing glucose deliv-

ery to the adipose tissue. These changes would result in insulin resistance and hyperinsulinemia. Despite the increased local release of angiotensinogen and increased blood pressure, there was no increase in systemic circulating levels of angiotensinogen.

Therefore, an environmental response to overfeeding had similar responses on adipocyte angiotensinogen control that a gene for high angiotensinogen levels would have—a chronically overstimulated local angiotensinogen system that increased blood pressure and resulted in insulin resistance and decreased central utilization of free fatty acids. A functional polymorphism in the *AGT* gene might have greater effects, because it appears that hepatic release of angiotensinogen is also increased in those with a gene variant, resulting in increased circulating levels of angiotensinogen, whereas circulating levels were not increased by overfeeding. In addition, differentiation of preadipocytes to adipocytes is related to the activation of the angiotensinogen promoter (196), suggesting that the greater the accrual of adipocytes, the greater the activation of the *AGT* gene. Increased body weight has been correlated with increased angiotensinogen levels in humans (197–199).

Linkage of hypertension to angiotensinogen levels has been demonstrated in multiple populations (200–203). Association of hypertension with the M235T variant or the G-6A variant, which is in nearly total disequilibrium with M235T, within the *AGT* gene also has been found in some studies (187,200–202,204), but not in others (195,205,206). Some of these discrepancies may be because of differences in statistical power arising from varying allele frequencies across racial and ethnic groups or from small sample size. Additional problems could be different background genetic or environmental influences on gene expression across studies. For example, haplotypes of the *AGT* gene interact with *ACE* (207), and the A-20C angiotensinogen variant appears to alter the body mass index relations with blood pressure in black individuals (208). Genetic or background influences on detecting significant associations are well illustrated in a study of the α-*adducin* gene in two Italian populations, Milan and Sardinia (209). Association of α-*adducin* with hypertension was only significant in Milan. However, the same functional abnormalities and clinical responses were identified in both populations, indicating that this gene is functional even though association was not found in Sardinia. The α-*adducin* example probably also applies to angiotensinogen. Further evidence of direct effects of angiotensinogen on renal function comes from a study of high and low salt intake and angiotensin infusions to determine changes in renal blood flow and adrenal responses. These responses were significantly related to the G-6A angiotensinogen polymorphism, with the A allele, which is associated with hypertension, being related to decreased renal and adrenal responses to angiotensin II infusions (210). To form a conclusion whether this gene or any other gene has functional significance, one must look beyond association studies and examine function and clinical expression of the gene.

Three clinical trials investigating blood pressure–decreasing effects of specific interventions have confirmed the clinical use of the angiotensinogen polymorphisms. The Trials of Hypertension Prevention study found that either sodium reduction or weight loss intervention compared with usual care had significantly greater blood pressure–decreasing effects in subjects with the "at risk" angiotensinogen alleles (211). A second intervention of reduced sodium and increased potassium, calcium, and magnesium also showed a greater blood pressure–decreasing response in subjects with the hypertension-associated alleles (212). Finally, the Dietary Approaches to Stop Hypertension (DASH) study, which held sodium constant but reduced fat and increased fruit and vegetable intake, confirmed the previous findings (213), suggesting that there are multiple pathways downstream from the *AGT* gene that can be modified to induce lower blood pressures or to protect against blood pressure increases.

Kallikrein System and Angiotensin-converting Enzyme

ACE has a dual effect in controlling blood pressure: It can convert angiotensin I to angiotensin II, and it can inactivate bradykinin. ACE is a more potent factor in the kallikrein-kinin system than in the renin-angiotensin system because bradykinin has a very low K_m (214). Bradykinin is a powerful vasodilator formed by the action of kallikrein on kininogen and stimulates prostaglandin formation. Greater ACE levels and the *ACE* D allele of the I/D polymorphism increase inactivation of bradykinin while increasing angiotensin II formation (215). ACE blockers decrease angiotensin II formation and increase the total bradykinin activity. Decreased kallikrein levels have been associated with hypertension (216–221). A major gene has been shown in segregation analyses to be responsible for a large portion of the phenotypic variability of urinary kallikrein excretion (222). It was found that inheritance followed a codominant pattern after the interactive effects of dietary potassium (as measured by urinary potassium excretion) were modeled. In individuals inferred to be heterozygous at the kallikrein locus, urinary kallikrein excretion had a strong relation with dietary potassium. Increased intake of potassium was related to increased kallikrein excretion, and theoretically could protect the heterozygotes if there is a direct cause and effect relation.

There are multiple polymorphisms in the promoter region of the kallikrein gene that appear to have significant effects on kallikrein excretion, hypertension, and end-stage renal disease (223,224). A polymorphism causing an amino acid change in the *kallikrein* gene, R53H, has been identified and has been associated with a more than 50% reduction in urinary kallikrein excretion (225). However, this polymorphism was not related to blood pressure. A promoter poly-

morphism in the *bradykinin B_2* gene was associated with hypertension in black individuals, (226) and a polymorphism in the *kininogen* gene had significant effects on kininogen levels (227).

Susceptibility loci alone presumably do not account for hypertension in the absence of other risk factors. Defects in the renin-angiotensin vasoconstricting system and the kallikrein-kinin vasodilating system may act synergistically or may not be in balance with each other, thereby promoting hypertension (228). Long-term blockade of bradykinin B_2 receptors by Hoe-140 in Wistar-Kyoto normotensive rats did not cause an increase in blood pressure (229). However, blockade of the B_2 receptors during a normally nonpressor infusion of A-II caused significant blood pressure increase. Infusion of low A-II doses into Brown Norway normotensive rats with normal kallikrein levels does not increase blood pressure. If the same dose of A-II is given to Brown Norway Katholiek rats, which have a complete lack of kallikrein, blood pressure increases faster than in control rats (230). Factors leading to hypertension may also change as hypertension develops. However, contrary to these earlier experiments, a series of experiments in rats has suggested that there is little blood pressure control by the kallikrein-kinin system even though there were significant strain differences in kallikrein and kininogen concentrations (231). Blockade of the bradykinin B_2 receptor did not affect blood pressure in the rats even when angiotensin II or high salt were administered. However, the kinin system appeared to be involved in the antihypertensive effects of ACE inhibitors. These series of conflicting experiments suggest that additional physiologic studies should be done to get a consensus regarding the effects of the kallikrein-kinin system on blood pressure control.

CELLULAR ION TRANSPORT SYSTEMS

Ion transport across cell membranes has been the focus of a great deal of research on blood pressure control because of the inferred relation of the activity of these systems to cellular sodium and calcium homeostasis and vascular smooth muscle contractility. Some of these systems include Na-Li countertransport, Na-K cotransport, Na-K-ATPase transport, Na-H antiporter, Na-Ca exchange, Ca-ATPase, Cl-HCO_3 transport, and the associated intracellular and extracellular levels of the ions these systems exchange. There are multiple mechanisms that control the activity of these cellular transport systems and intracellular ion content, including genetic control of baseline activity, ion concentration, and the number of transporters, cellular pH, cellular membrane lipid composition, and local or systemic circulating factors.

Table 13–3 shows that there appears to be considerable genetic involvement in the activity or concentration of many of the ionic variables involved with hypertension. These genetic factors combine to give hypertension the appearance of a polygenic trait. The h^2 term is an estimate of polygenic

TABLE 13–3. *Heritability, common household, and shared screening date effects of biochemical measurements on 2,500 members of 98 Utah pedigrees*

Variables	h^2	c^2	d^2
Cell cation tests			
Na-Li countertransport	0.58	0.02	0.08
Intraerythrocytic Na	0.58	0.14	0.20
Ouabain binding sites	0.56	0.16	0.12
Na-K-ATPase pump activity	0.22	0.03	0.35
Li-K cotransport	0.30	0.00	0.26
Lithium leak	0.43	0.00	0.40
Intraerythrocytic Mg	0.29	0.00	0.56
Blood tests			
Mg concentration	0.57	0.24	0.00
Na concentration	0.14	0.01	0.52
K concentration	0.23	0.07	0.18
Total Ca concentration	0.14	0.13	0.17
Phosphate concentration	0.30	0.08	0.04
Renin activity	0.07	0.00	0.74
Uric acid concentration	0.31	0.08	0.04
Fasting blood glucose	0.15	0.00	0.09
Total cholesterol	0.42	0.08	0.00

c^2, Common household effect (chronic shared environment); d^2, same-day screening effect (immediate shared environment or same-day measurement effects); h^2, polygenic heritability.

Adapted from Williams RR, Hasstedt SJ, Hunt SC, et al. Genetic traits related to hypertension and electrolyte metabolism. *Hypertension* 1991;17[Suppl 1]:I69–I73.

heritability and low estimates do not mean that there is no major gene effect.

Adducin, Na-K-2Cl Cotransport, and Na-K-ATPase Transport

Investigations of the genetic causes of hypertension in the salt-sensitive Milan hypertensive rat resulted in significant associations with the α-*adducin* gene (232). Mutations in either the α or β subunits of this gene affect the cytoskeleton of the cell membrane, influencing the rates of sodium reabsorption by the Na-K-ATPase pump (233–235). Similar findings were found in humans, and studies showed that either acute or chronic volume depletion had differential blood pressure–decreasing effects depending on the adducin genotype (236,237). *Adducin* also has been directly associated with Na-K-2Cl cotransport, Na-Li countertransport, and Na-K-ATPase transport (238). The effects of the α-*adducin* Gly460Trp polymorphism on blood pressure response to a saline load or to diuretic therapy also appear to depend on the *ACE* genotype, because there was a significant additive effect of the two genes on diuretic response of blood pressure (239) or a significant interaction between the two genes on a sodium load response of blood pressure (240). Although some large studies have found smaller or nonsignificant effects of the *adducin* gene on hypertension status or blood pressure (241–244), a prospective study found significant associa-

tions and interactions of α-*adducin, ACE,* and *aldosterone synthase* on the incidence of hypertension (245). In addition, the physiologic, biochemical, and structural analyses of this gene appear to substantiate its importance in hypertension and blood pressure control despite some association studies that reported negative results (209).

Studies have identified the presence of natriuretic substances that inhibit the sodium/potassium pump. At least four such inhibitory substances have been identified: ouabain (246), linoleic and oleic acids (247), and lysophosphatidylcholine (248). The last three substances have a common precursor, phosphatidylcholine, which is a phospholipid in the cell membrane. Population genetic analyses have not shown strong evidence for major gene determination of the Na-K-ATPase pump, but a study in rats suggested that a mutation in the transporter was associated with hypertension (249). This study was later confirmed in humans and showed a significant interaction between the Na-K-ATPase transporter and the Na-K-2Cl cotransporter on hypertension (250). The thiazide-sensitive sodium channel located in the distal renal tubule and involved in the hypotensive Gitelman syndrome was shown not to be associated with hypertension or to interact with either the Na-K-ATPase transporter or the Na-K-2Cl cotransporter (251).

Na-Li Countertransport and the Na-H Antiporter

Na-Li countertransport is clearly familial and increased in hypertensive versus normotensive subjects. Na-Li countertransport has been related to hypertension and blood pressure increases in two prospective studies (252–254). Segregation analysis suggests that a recessive gene can account for high Na-Li countertransport in about 5% of the population (255,256). This system is thought to represent some form of Na-H exchange (257) but has its own unique properties (258). More recent evidence suggests that the transporters for the two systems are different (259).

Two important genetic studies have been published on Na-Li countertransport. The first was a genome-wide linkage analysis of the trait in the Tecumseh population (260). Suggestive linkage was found on the q arm of chromosome 15. Despite the high heritability and the likelihood that fewer genes control this hypertension intermediate phenotype, strong linkage was not found after correcting for the number of statistical tests in the genome search. An impressive study was a genome-wide association analysis of Na-Li countertransport in lymphoblast cell lines from centre d' Etude du Polymorphisme Humain (CEPH) families. More than 7,000 markers were analyzed, with significant association and linkage being found near the *AGT* gene and near families of antioxidant genes, primarily glutathione-related genes (261).

Despite the attractive hypotheses surrounding Na-Li countertransport, a linkage study of the gene *NHE1* controlling the ubiquitous expression of Na-H exchange to Na-Li countertransport, blood pressure, or hypertension failed to show linkage (262). Other isoforms exist for expression of the antiporter specifically in the kidney and remain as candidate genes for hypertension and ion transport.

Na-H exchange is an important cellular control system to maintain pH within an optimal range for proper cellular function (263). Na-H antiporter units are found in many cells and tissues, including skeletal muscle and the brush border of the kidney proximal tubule. Increased cellular functions that cause greater acidity and decrease pH invoke an otherwise silent Na-H antiport system to extrude H, thereby increasing pH. A metabolic shift toward use of fats rather than carbohydrates may produce more acid products, promoting more acid intracellular pH. Increased stimulation of Na-H exchange increases sodium reabsorption, perhaps leading to volume-related blood pressure increases. This may be followed by compensating increased Na-Ca exchange and increased intracellular calcium, fostering increased smooth muscle contractility and hypertension (264). Intracellular calcium may be a mediating factor between transport system abnormalities and vasoconstriction. Increased intracellular free calcium stimulates Na-H exchange across the plasma membrane, whereas increased cellular calcium in the juxtaglomerular cells in the kidney also has direct effects on renin release and enzyme activity (265).

Insulin increases activation of the antiporter, as it does with other transport systems (266). Resnick and coworkers (267,268) proposed that intracellular cation imbalances may be responsible for an underlying insulin resistance, specifically decreased cellular pH and magnesium and increased calcium. Metabolic cellular abnormalities reflected by cation and pH imbalances may stimulate insulin production to activate the Na-H exchange system to compensate for these abnormalities. In addition, catecholamines, which reduce the effectiveness of insulin on glucose uptake, increase intracellular levels of calcium (97,269) and may be synergistic with the above mechanisms.

Membrane Fluidity and Lipids

Multiple factors influence membrane fluidity, such as lipids, calcium, NO, estrogens, and insulin (270,271). Lipids and lipoproteins influence the level of most ion transport systems, with triglycerides or VLDL cholesterol having the strongest correlations (272,273). Triglyceride and VLDL-C levels also are greater in individuals inferred to have the high Na-Li countertransport genotype (255). If triglyceride levels alter ion transport in a causal pathway leading to hypertension, this may be one link between dyslipidemic hypertension and CHD. The hypothesized mechanism is through alterations in membrane lipid content, changing the membrane fluidity and capability of individual transport units to operate normally. There are mixed findings supporting the relation among dyslipidemia, ion transport, and hypertension. Changes in membrane fluidity have been associated with increased countertransport levels (274,275). Membrane fluidity is decreased by cellular calcium loading (276), and this decrease is greater in hy-

pertensive than in normotensive patients (277). Low dietary salt intake increases membrane fluidity (278), providing another pathway for the prevention of hypertension. However, a cholesterol-decreasing intervention study did not show an important effect of cholesterol levels per se on countertransport, even though membrane cholesterol is reduced (279).

Systems Analysis Approach to Ion Transport

No one gene involved with cellular ionic homeostasis acts independently of other controls of cellular function. For example, a gene with large effects on the number of Na-K-ATPase exchange sites may also affect cellular concentrations of sodium, potassium, or calcium or changed activity of other associated transport systems. In addition to multiple effects of a single gene, each transport system likely reflects influences of multiple genetic variants. To separate multiple genetic influences on a single variable and allow for correlated secondary effects of other variables, a segregation analysis of statistically derived principal components created from relations among multiple ion transport concentrations and transporters showed that there was evidence for five common and three rare major genes among these components (280). These components were related to (a) familial dyslipidemic hypertension or the multiple metabolic syndrome, with the expected moderate increase in Na-Li countertransport levels; (b) a smaller number of ouabain-binding sites and increased intracellular sodium; (c and d) two genes affecting Na-Li countertransport levels, one dominant and one recessive; and (e) moderate obesity, but with normal triglyceride levels. Therefore, this methodology appeared to extract subsets of variables into different genetically influenced pathways.

OTHER CANDIDATE GENES

Although not discussed as extensively in this review, there are other important candidate genes that have been associated with hypertension or blood pressure. Two genes in the renin-angiotensin-aldosterone pathway are the *angiotensin receptor type 1* and *aldosterone synthase*, both of which have some evidence for association with blood pressure–related phenotypes, although weaker than for *AGT* (281–284). *Aldosterone synthase*, even though related to hypertension (285), was not related to salt sensitivity in a subsequent study (286).

Another potentially important gene is the β_3 *subunit* of a G protein that has variably been associated with blood pressure, insulin resistance, or obesity (287–294). Physiologic alterations led to the investigation of this gene rather than genetics. A pertussis toxin that poisons the G protein suppressed the greater calcium transients, suppressed Na-H exchange, and decreased the cell proliferation seen in lymphocytes from patients with hypertension compared with those who were normotensive (287,295). Increased renal perfusion also was related to this gene (296). A pharmacogenetic study of blood pressure reductions by diuretics according to G protein genotypes has shown a 6-mm Hg difference between the two groups of subjects homozygous for the hypertension-associated polymorphism (297).

Adrenergic genes and catecholamine levels have been implicated in the development of hypertension. The most consistent of the genetic findings occur for the β_2-*adrenergic receptor*. This gene became a strong candidate from a genome scan by one of the four networks of the NHLBI Family Blood Pressure Program, because it and a few other important genes were under the linkage peak on chromosome 5 (298,299). Another network in this program replicated these results (300), although as with most genes there have been negative studies (301). The β_1-*adrenergic receptor* gene has been associated with heart rate (302), hypertension (303), and obesity (fat mass) (304). The β_3-*adrenergic receptor* gene has been more widely associated with obesity, diabetes, and insulin resistance (305–309). An interaction with a gene regulating thyroid hormone, *deiodinase type 2,* with the β_3-*adrenergic* gene on insulin resistance also has been reported (310). No association of the α_{2B} gene was found with hypertension (311).

A variant in a G protein–coupled *receptor kinase 4* gene has been associated with salt sensitivity and hypertension (312,313). This polymorphism increases G protein–coupled receptor kinase activity and uncouples the dopamine D_1 receptor from its G protein in the renal proximal tubule. Dopamine is increased by a high sodium diet and down-regulates sodium transport by the Na-H exchange isoform in the kidney *(NHE3).* The polymorphism thereby decreases sodium excretion and is expected to be related to hypertension. The dopamine D_1 receptor itself also has shown association with hypertension (314).

GENOME SCANS FOR BLOOD PRESSURE AND HYPERTENSION

A number of genome scans for blood pressure and related phenotypes have been published (Table 13–4). As more are published, one would expect significant results for specific regions to overlap by chance. However, there are clearly some areas that have greater support for an underlying gene contributing to blood pressure abnormalities. In addition, there are interesting overlaps of linkage with published regions for both lipid disorders and diabetes, perhaps explaining the close association of these three conditions.

Chromosome 1 between 170 and 192 cM on the Marshfield map appears to contain an important quantitative trait locus (QTL) related to blood pressure (Table 13–4), dyslipidemia (315–318), obesity (319), and diabetes (320–324), although there could be separate genes for each disorder. Although a mouse gene has been identified in this region and has been related to fatty acid metabolism and the cellular redox state (325), studies in humans have not been published. A strong signal for linkage to preeclampsia also has been found in this region (326).

The multiple linkage signals on chromosome 7 for blood pressure overlap a linkage region that included fasting insulin (327) and one for pulse pressure (328). These linkages are also not far away from obesity linkages near the leptin gene (329). Chromosome 6 has a linkage region that includes putative genes for both blood pressure and FCHL (330,331).

The most concordant chromosome of linkage of blood pressure from multiple studies is chromosome 2. Although there are linkage signals on both the p and q arms of the chromosome, the majority of the results appear to center around 100 cM. There are a number of attractive candidate genes in the area that are currently being pursued.

A genome scan for postural systolic blood pressure change found linkage to chromosome 18 (logarithm of odds [LOD] = 2.6) (332) near a region found significantly linked to hypertension (Iceland; LOD = 4.6) (333). A candidate gene under this peak, *NEDD4L,* has been shown to bind with the epithelial sodium channel more strongly than the originally identified *NEDD4* on chromosome 15 (334), and it could result in increased sodium reabsorption if defective binding occurs. Pulse pressure has shown linkage to chromosomes 7, 8, 18, and 21 (328). Blood pressure during exercise showed suggestive linkage to chromosomes 8, 10, 11, and 18 (335).

CAUSAL GENETIC MUTATIONS

Rare mutations in multiple genes lead either to hypertension or to hypotension. A review of the hypotension genes can be found in Scheinman and coworkers (336). These syndromes include Bartter syndrome involving the Na-K-2Cl cotransporter in the thick ascending limb of the loop of Henle, a chloride channel, or a potassium channel (337,338); Gitelman syndrome involving the thiazide-sensitive sodium channel in the distal convoluted tubule (339); and pseudohypoaldosteronism type I with both dominant and recessive mutations in the epithelial sodium channel (340–342).

The first hypertension-related gene mutations were found for glucocorticoid-remediable aldosteronism, which has been shown to be determined by a single, dominantly inherited genetic defect on chromosome 8 (343). There is an unequal crossing over between the paired chromosomes containing the gene for 11-β-*hydroxylase* with a homologous (95% identical) gene for *aldosterone synthase* resulting in hypertension. This occurrence can completely explain the observed pathophysiology of this disorder, which causes severe hypertension in youths, very early strokes, and mortality. Diagnosis of this condition is important because it is unresponsive to usual antihypertensive therapies (e.g., diuretics), which greatly decrease serum potassium in this disorder, but it is responsive to glucocorticoid therapy.

Liddle syndrome is caused by defects in the β and γ subunits of the sodium channel of the kidney epithelium (344,345). It also is dominantly inherited, increases the activity of the epithelial sodium channels, and results in early

TABLE 13–4. Genome-wide scans reporting suggestive (LOD 1.9) or greater evidence for blood pressure–related traits

Reference no.	Trait	Sample	Chromosome and location (cM) of linkage																						
			1	2	3	4	5	6	7	8	9	10	11	12	13	14	15	16	17	18	19	20	21	22	X
299	SBP	W, S					190	144[a]									97								
350	SBP	C, S		58	6								58						24			39			
	DBP	C, S										46					105	64				39	25		
351	SBP	W, F				73													67[a] 94 74						
352	DBP	W, F		97 103 210[a]																7					
	SBP	W, F					32		135	87											4				
353	DBP	W, F		185																					
354	HTN	W, S		161																					
355	HTN	W, S			166[a]																				
356	HTN	C, S																						39	67
357	SBP	W, F		99[a]																					
357	DBP	MA, F							114	165										116	37				
	PP	MA, F							128	154										116	37				
327	SBP	W, F	4																						
	MAP	W, F	4																						
331	HTN	W, F	192						58 127					83			103								
330	SBP	W, F				90[a]		89[a]																	
	SBP	W, F						89																	
	DBP	W, F																			10				
358	HTN	W, F	76	12[a]		117					43				115		79		15		54[a]				42
359	SBP	W, S											105					49							
360	SBP	W, F												95							49				
361	SBP	B, F		104	16																				
	DBP	B, F							81 109			76													
	SBP	B, F																			47 78				
	DBP	B, F																		89[a]					
333	HTN	W, F														100									
4	HTN	C, S										30													
5	DBP	W, F			119																				
3	HTN	B, S	170	63																					

Totally negative scan (6).

B, black subject; C, Chinese subject; DBP, diastolic blood pressure; HTN, hypertension; MA, Mexican-American subject; PP, pulse pressure; SBP, systolic blood pressure; W, white subject.

[a]Logarithm of odds (LOD) scores ≥3.0.

age at onset of hypertension and usually hypokalemia. Plasma renin activity and aldosterone are low even when dietary sodium is low. Pseudohypoaldosteronism type II has been shown to result from genes on either chromosomes 1 or 17 (346). The responsible gene on chromosome 17 is the *WNK4* gene, which again involves a Na-Cl co-transporter (347).

SUMMARY OF THE FUTURE OF HYPERTENSION GENETICS

Over the last few years, large family collections have been examined, genotyped, and analyzed. The resulting linkage analyses, together with the large number of association studies, have begun to identify genes or regions likely to be involved with the development of hypertension. As candidate genes under the linkage peaks are identified, sequenced, and tested for association, further advances are expected in the next few years. Validation of these gene targets with multiple association studies, functional studies, and clinical studies may take longer.

The angiotensinogen and adducin genes are representative of the class of genes that increase susceptibility to hypertension. These types of genes will facilitate division of patients into risk or diagnostic groups so that effects of other identified genes or environmental factors may be determined within more homogeneous groups. True gene–environment and gene–gene interactions will be able to be more consistently observed and described, allowing better pharmacologic investigation of how to effectively treat hypertension. Controlling one of the major risk factors for cardiovascular disease by treating hypertension without aggravating other risk factors, such as lipid or glucose metabolism, should reduce morbidity and mortality.

REFERENCES

1. Guyton AC. *Textbook of medical physiology,* 5th ed. Philadelphia: WB Saunders, 1976.
2. Hunt SC, Hopkins PN, Lalouel JM. Hypertension. In: King RA, Rotter JI, Motulsky AG, eds. *The genetic basis of common diseases.* New York: Oxford University Press, 2002:127–154.
3. Rao DC, Province MA, Leppert MF, et al. A genome-wide affected sibpair linkage analysis of hypertension: the HyperGEN network. *Am J Hypertens* 2003;16:148–150.
4. Ranade K, Hinds D, Hsiung CA, et al. A genome scan for hypertension susceptibility loci in populations of Chinese and Japanese origins. *Am J Hypertens* 2003;16:158–162.
5. Thiel BA, Chakravarti A, Cooper RS, et al. A genome-wide linkage analysis investigating the determinants of blood pressure in whites and African Americans. *Am J Hypertens* 2003;16:151–153.
6. Kardia SL, Rozek LS, Krushkal J, et al. Genome-wide linkage analyses for hypertension genes in two ethnically and geographically diverse populations. *Am J Hypertens* 2003;16:154–157.
7. Province MA, Kardia SL, Ranade K, et al. A meta-analysis of genome-wide linkage scans for hypertension: the National Heart, Lung and Blood Institute Family Blood Pressure Program. *Am J Hypertens* 2003;16:144–147.
8. Turner ST, Boerwinkle E. Genetics of blood pressure, hypertensive complications, and antihypertensive drug responses. *Pharmacogenomics* 2003;4:53–65.
9. MacMahon S, Peto R, Cutler J, et al. Blood pressure, stroke, and coronary heart disease. Part 1. Prolonged differences in blood pressure: prospective observational studies corrected for the regression dilution bias. *Lancet* 1990;335:765–774.
10. Medical Research Council Working Party. MRC trial of treatment of mild hypertension: principal results. *BMJ* 1985;291:97–104.
11. Collins R, Peto R, MacMahon S, et al. Blood pressure, stroke, and coronary heart disease. Part 2. short-term reductions in blood pressure: overview of randomised drug trials in their epidemiological context. *Lancet* 1990;335:827–838.
12. Prevention of stroke by antihypertensive drug treatment in older persons with isolated systolic hypertension. Final results of the Systolic Hypertension in the Elderly Program (SHEP). SHEP Cooperative Research Group. *JAMA* 1991;265:3255–3264.
13. Dahlöf B, Lindholm LH, Hansson L, et al. Morbidity and mortality in the Swedish Trial in Old Patients with Hypertension (STOP-Hypertension). *Lancet* 1991;338:1281–1285.
14. Yusuf S, Lessem J, Jha P, et al. Primary and secondary prevention of myocardial infarction and strokes: an update of randomly allocated, controlled trials. *J Hypertens* 1993;11[Suppl 4]:S61–S73.
15. Major outcomes in high-risk hypertensive patients randomized to angiotensin-converting enzyme inhibitor or calcium channel blocker vs diuretic: the Antihypertensive and Lipid-Lowering Treatment to Prevent Heart Attack Trial (ALLHAT). *JAMA* 2002;288:2981–2997.
16. Stamler J. Epidemiology, established major risk factors, and the primary prevention of coronary heart disease. In: Parmley WW, Chatterjee K, eds. *Cardiology.* Philadelphia: JB Lippincott, 1987:1:1–1:41.
17. Neaton JD, Wentworth D. Serum cholesterol, blood pressure, cigarette smoking, and death from coronary heart disease. *Arch Intern Med* 1992;152:56–64.
18. Strandberg TE, Pitkala K. What is the most important component of blood pressure: systolic, diastolic or pulse pressure? *Curr Opin Nephrol Hypertens* 2003;12:293–297.
19. Neaton JD, Kuller LH, Wentworth D, et al. Total and cardiovascular mortality in relation to cigarette smoking, serum cholesterol concentration, and diastolic blood pressure among black and white males followed up for five years. *Am Heart J* 1984;108:759–769.
20. The sixth report of the Joint National Committee on prevention, detection, evaluation, and treatment of high blood pressure. *Arch Intern Med* 1997;157:2413–2446.
21. Robertson WB, Strong JP. Atherosclerosis in persons with hypertension and diabetes mellitus. *Lab Invest* 1968;18:539–551.
22. Solberg LA, McGarry PA. Cerebral atherosclerosis in persons with selected diseases. *Lab Invest* 1968;18:613–619.
23. Stephens T, Craig CL, Ferris BF. Adult physical fitness and hypertension in Canada: findings from the Canada Fitness Survey II. *Can J Pub Health* 1986;77:291–298.
24. Sprecher DL, Schaefer EJ, Kent KM, et al. Cardiovascular features of homozygous familial hypercholesterolemia: analysis of 16 patients. *Am J Cardiol* 1984;54:20–30.
25. Gordon T, Garcia-Palmieri MR, Kapan A. Differences in coronary heart disease in Framingham, Honolulu and Puerto Rico. *J Chron Dis* 1974;27:329–344.
26. Kozarevic D, Pirc B, Racic Z. The Yugoslavia cardiovascular disease study. II. Factors in the incidence of coronary heart disease. *Am J Epidemiol* 1976;104:133–140.
27. Keys A, Menotti A, Aravanis C, et al. The Seven Countries Study: 2,289 Deaths in 15 Years. *Prev Med* 1984;13:141–154.
28. Ferrara LA, Mancini M, Celentano A, et al. Early changes of the arterial carotid wall in uncomplicated primary hypertensive patients. Study by ultrasound high-resolution B-mode imaging. *Arterioscler Thromb* 1994;14:1290–1296.
29. Suurkula M, Agewall S, Fagerberg B, et al. Ultrasound evaluation of atherosclerotic manifestations in the carotid artery in high-risk hypertensive patients. Risk Intervention Study (RIS) Group. *Arterioscler Thromb* 1994;14:1297–1304.
30. Hopkins PN, Williams RR. A survey of 246 suggested coronary risk factors. *Atherosclerosis* 1981;40:1–52.
31. Chobanian AV, Lichtenstein AH, Nilakhe V, et al. Influence of hypertension on aortic atherosclerosis in the Watanabe rabbit. *Hypertension* 1989;14:203–209.
32. Xu C, Glagov S, Zatina MA, et al. Hypertension sustains plaque progresson despite reduction of hypercholesterolemia. *Hypertension* 1991;18:123–129.

33. Hunt SC, Williams RR, Barlow GK. A comparison of positive family history definitions for defining risk of future disease. *J Chron Dis* 1986;39:809–821.
34. Hunt SC, Stephenson SH, Hopkins PN, et al. Predictors of an increased risk of future hypertension in Utah pedigrees: a screening analysis. *Hypertension* 1991;17:969–976.
35. Hunt KJ, Heiss G, Sholinsky PD, et al. Familial history of metabolic disorders and the multiple metabolic syndrome: the NHLBI family heart study. *Genet Epidemiol* 2000;19:395–409.
36. van der Sande MA, Walraven GE, Milligan PJ, et al. Family history: an opportunity for early interventions and improved control of hypertension, obesity and diabetes. *Bull World Health Organ* 2001;79:321–328.
37. Tozawa M, Oshiro S, Iseki C, et al. Family history of hypertension and blood pressure in a screened cohort. *Hypertens Res* 2001;24:93–98.
38. Williams RR, Hunt SC, Heiss G, et al. Usefulness of cardiovascular family history data for population-based preventive medicine and medical research (the Health Family Tree Study and the NHLBI Family Heart Study). *Am J Cardiol* 2001;87:129–135.
39. Hunt SC, Gwinn M, Adams TD. Family history assessment. Strategies for prevention of cardiovascular disease. *Am J Prev Med* 2003;24:136–142.
40. Carmelli D, Cardon LR, Fabsitz R. Clustering of hypertension, diabetes, and obesity in adult male twins: same genes or same environments? *Am J Hum Genet* 1994;55:566–573.
41. Buja LM, Kovanen PT, Bilheimer DW. Cellular pathology of homozygous familial hypercholesterolemia. *Am J Pathol* 1979;97:327–357.
42. Glagov S, Ozoa AK. Significance of the relatively low incidence of atherosclerosis in the pumonary, renal and mesenteric arteries. *Ann NY Acad Sci* 1968;149:940–955.
43. Curmi PA, Juan L, Tedgui A. Effect of transmural pressure on low density lipoprotein and albumin transport and distribution across the intact arterial wall. *Circ Res* 1990;66:1692–1702.
44. Friedman MH. How hemodynamic forces in the human affect the topography and development of atherosclerosis. In: Glagov S, Newman WP III, Schaffer SA, eds. *Pathobiology of the human atherosclerotic plaque.* New York: Springer-Verlag, 1990:303–315.
45. Ku DN, Giddens DP. Pulsatile flow in a model carotid bifurcation. *Arteriosclerosis* 1983;3:31–39.
46. Malek AM, Alper SL, Izumo S. Hemodynamic shear stress and its role in atherosclerosis. *JAMA* 1999;282:2035–2042.
47. Haudenschild CC, Grunwald J, Chobanian AV. Effects of hypertension on migration and proliferation of smooth muscle in culture. *Hypertension* 1985;7[Suppl I]:I-101–I-104.
48. Scannapieco G, Pauletto P, Pagnan A, et al. Lipoprotein binding to cultured aortic smooth muscle cells from normotensive and hypertensive rats. *J Hypertens* 1988;6:S269–S271.
49. Friedman MH. A biologically plausible model of thickening of arterial intima under shear. *Arteriosclerosis* 1989;9:511–522.
50. Glagov S, Zarins C, Giddens DP, et al. Hemodynamics and atherosclerosis. Insights and perspectives gained from studies of human arteries. *Arch Pathol Lab Med* 1988;112:1018–1031.
51. Uematsu M, Kitabatake A, Tanouchi J, et al. Reduction of endothelial microfilament bundles in the low-shear region of the canine aorta. Association with intimal plaque formation in hypercholesterolemia. *Arterioscler Thromb* 1991;11:107–115.
52. Gibson CM, Diaz L, Kandarpa K, et al. Relation of vessel wall shear stress to atherosclerosis progression in human coronary arteries. *Arterioscler Thromb* 1993;13:310–315.
53. Berkson DM, Stamler J, Lindberg HA, et al. Heart rate: an important risk factor for coronary mortality. Ten-year experience of the Peoples Gas Co. Epidemiologic Study (1958-68). In: Jones RJ, ed. *Atherosclerosis Proceedings of the 2nd International Symposium on Atherosclerosis.* New York: Springer-Verlag, 1970:382–389.
54. Castelli WP, Garrison RJ, Wilson PWF, et al. Incidence of coronary heart disease and lipoprotein cholesterol levels. The Framingham Study. *JAMA* 1986;256:2835–2838.
55. Criqui MH, Cowan LD, Heiss G, et al. Frequency and clustering of nonlipid coronary risk factors in dyslipoproteinemia: the Lipid Research Clinic's program prevalence study. *Circulation* 1986;73[Suppl1]:140–150.
56. Williams PT, Fortmann SP, Terry RB, et al. Associations of dietary fat, regional adiposity, and blood pressure in men. *JAMA* 1987;257:3251–3256.
57. Reaven GM, Hoffman BB. A role for insulin in the aetiology and course of hypertension? *Lancet* 1987;2:435–436.
58. Selby JV, Newman B, Quiroga J, et al. Concordance for dyslipidemic hypertension in male twins. *JAMA* 1991;265:2079–2084.
59. Williams RR, Hunt SC, Hopkins PN, et al. Familial dyslipidemic hypertension: evidence from 58 Utah families for a syndrome present in approximately 12% of patients with essential hypertension. *JAMA* 1988;259:3579–3586.
60. Williams RR, Hopkins PN, Hunt SC, et al. Population-based frequency of dyslipidemia syndromes in coronary prone families in Utah. *Arch Intern Med* 1990;150:582–588.
61. Genest JJ, Martin-Munley SS, McNamara JR, et al. Familial lipoprotein disorders in patients with premature coronary artery disease. *Circulation* 1992;85:2025–2033.
62. Assmann G, Schulte H. Relation of high-density lipoprotein cholesterol and triglycerides to incidence of atherosclcerotic coronary artery disease (the PROCAM experience) *Am J Cardiol* 1992;70;733–737.
63. Hopkins PN, Heiss G, Ellison RC, et al. Coronary artery disease risk in familial combined hyperlipidemia and familial hypertriglyceridemia: a case-control comparison from the National Heart, Lung, and Blood Institute Family Heart Study. *Circulation* 2003;108:519–523.
64. Glorioso N, Troffa C, Filigheddu F, et al. Effect of the HMG-CoA reductase inhibitors on blood pressure in patients with essential hypertension and primary hypercholesterolemia. *Hypertension* 1999;34:1281–1286.
65. Saitta A, Castaldo M, Sardo A, et al. Effects of fluvastatin treatment on red blood cell Na$^+$ transport systems in hypercholesterolemic subjects. *J Cardiovasc Pharmacol* 2000;35:376–382.
66. John S, Delles C, Klingbeil AU, et al. Low-density lipoprotein-cholesterol determines vascular responsiveness to angiotensin II in normocholesterolaemic humans. *J Hypertens* 1999;17:1933–1939.
67. Nickenig G, Baumer AT, Temur Y, et al. Statin-sensitive dysregulated AT1 receptor function and density in hypercholesterolemic men. *Circulation* 1999;100:2131–2134.
68. Vuagnat A, Giacche M, Hopkins PN, et al. Blood pressure response to angiotensin II, low-density lipoprotein cholesterol and polymorphisms of the angiotensin II type 1 receptor gene in hypertensive sibling pairs. *J Mol Med* 2001;79:175–183.
69. Nickenig G, Sachinidis A, Michaelsen F, et al. Upregulation of vascular angiotensin II receptor gene expression by low-density lipoprotein in vascular smooth muscle cells. *Circulation* 1997;95:473–478.
70. Gaboury CL, Simonson DC, Seely EW, et al. Relation of pressor responsiveness to angiotensin II and insulin resistance in hypertension. *J Clin Invest* 1994;94:2295–2300.
71. Nickenig G, Strehlow K, Roeling J, et al. Salt induces vascular AT1 receptor overexpression in vitro and in vivo. *Hypertension* 1998;31:1272–1277.
72. Nickenig G, Baumer AT, Grohe C, et al. Estrogen modulates AT1 receptor gene expression in vitro and in vivo. *Circulation* 1998;97:2197–2201.
73. Nickenig G, Roling J, Strehlow K, et al. Insulin induces upregulation of vascular AT1 receptor gene expression by posttranscriptional mechanisms. *Circulation* 1998;98:2453–2460.
74. Fuh MM, Shieh SM, Wu DA, et al. Abnormalities of carbohydrate and lipid metabolism in patients with hypertension. *Arch Intern Med* 1987;147:1035–1038.
75. Reaven G. Role of insulin resistance in human disease. *Diabetes* 1988;37:1595–1607.
76. Kaplan NM. Upper-body obesity, glucose intolerance, hypertriglyceridemia, and hypertension. *Arch Intern Med* 1989;149:1514–1520.
77. Welborn TA, Wearne K. Coronary heart disease incidence and cardiovascular mortality in Busselton with reference to glucose and insulin concentrations. *Diabetes Care* 1979;2:154–160.
78. Pyörälä K. Relationship of glucose tolerance and plasma insulin to the incidence of coronary heart disease: results from two population studies in Finland. *Diabetes Care* 1979;2:131–141.
79. Ducimetiere P, Eschwege L, Papoz JL, et al. Relationship of plasma insulin levels to the incidence of myocardial infarction and coronary heart disease mortality in a middle-aged population. *Diabetologia* 1980;19:205–210.

80. Expert Panel on Detection, Evaluation, and Treatment of High Blood Cholesterol in Adults. Executive Summary of the Third Report of the National Cholesterol Education Program (NCEP) Expert Panel on Detection, Evaluation, and Treatment of High Blood Cholesterol in Adults (Adult Treatment Panel III). *JAMA* 2001;285:2486–2497.

81. Lakka HM, Laaksonen DE, Lakka TA, et al. The metabolic syndrome and total and cardiovascular disease mortality in middle-aged men. *JAMA* 2002;288:2709–2716.

82. Park YW, Zhu S, Palaniappan L, et al. The metabolic syndrome: prevalence and associated risk factor findings in the US population from the Third National Health and Nutrition Examination Survey, 1988-1994. *Arch Intern Med* 2003;163:427–436.

83. Skarfors ET, Lithell HO, Selinus I. Risk factors for the development of hypertension: a 10-year longitudinal study in middle-aged men. *J Hypertens* 1991;9:217–223.

84. Niskanen LK, Uusitupa MI, Pyorala K. The relationship of hyperinsulinemia to the development of hypertension in type 2 diabetic patients and in non-diabetic subjects. *J Hum Hypertens* 1991;5:155–159.

85. Haffner SM, Valdez RA, Hazuda HP, et al. Prospective analysis of the insulin-resistance syndrome (syndrome X). *Diabetes* 1992;41:715–722.

86. Lissner L, Bengtsson C, Lapidus L, et al. Fasting insulin in relation to subsequent blood pressure changes and hypertension in women. *Hypertension* 1992;20:797–801.

87. DeFronzo RA, Cooke CR, Andres R, et al. The effect of insulin on renal handling of sodium, potassium, calcium, and phosphate in man. *J Clin Invest* 1975;55:845–855.

88. Klisic J, Hu MC, Nief V, et al. Insulin activates Na(+)/H(+) exchanger 3: biphasic response and glucocorticoid dependence. *Am J Physiol Renal Physiol* 2002;283:F532–F539.

89. Rowe JW, Young JB, Minaker KL, et al. Effect of insulin and glucose infusions on sympathetic nervous system activity in normal man. *Diabetes* 1981;30:219–225.

90. King GL, Goodman AD, Buzney S, et al. Receptors and growth-promoting effects of insulin and insulinlike growth factors on cells from bovine retinal capillaries and aorta. *J Clin Invest* 1985;75:1028–1036.

91. Draznin B, Kao M, Sussman KE. Insulin and glyburide increase cytosolic free-Ca^{2+} concentration in isolated rat adipocytes. *Diabetes* 1987;36:174–178.

92. Frederich RC Jr, Kahn BB, Peach MJ, et al. Tissue-specific nutritional regulation of angiotensinogen in adipose tissue. *Hypertension* 1992;19:339–344.

93. Ferrannini E, Buzzigoli G, Bonadonna R, et al. Insulin resistance in essential hypertension. *N Engl J Med* 1987;317:350–356.

94. Reaven GM. Insulin resistance, hyperinsulinemia, and hypertriglyceridemia in the etiology and clinical course of hypertension. *Am J Med* 1991;90[Suppl 2A]:7S–12S.

95. Daly PA, Landsberg L. Hypertension in obesity and NIDDM: role of insulin and sympathetic nervous system. *Diabetes Care* 1991;14:240–248.

96. Cryer PE. Physiology and pathophysiology of the human sympathoadrenal neuroendocrine system. *N Engl J Med* 1980;303:436–444.

97. Roth J, Grunfeld C. Mechanism of action of peptide hormones and catecholamines. In: Wilson JD, Foster DW, eds. *Williams textbook of endocrinology,* 7th ed. Philadelphia: WB Saunders, 1985:76–122.

98. Troisi RJ, Weiss ST, Segal MR, et al. The relationship of body fat distribution to blood pressure in normotensive men: the normative aging study. *Int J Obes* 1990;14:515–525.

99. Peiris AN, Sothmann MS, Hoffmann RG, et al. Adiposity, fat distribution, and cardiovascular risk. *Ann Intern Med* 1989;110:867–872.

100. Kissebah AH, Adams PW, Wynn V. Interrelationship between insulin secretion and plasma free fatty acid and triglyceride transport kinetics in maturity onset diabetes and the effect of phenethylbiguanide (Phenformin). *Diabetologia* 1974;10:119–130.

101. Ferrannini E, Barrett EJ, Bevilacqua S, et al. Effect of fatty acids on glucose production and utilization in man. *J Clin Invest* 1983;72:1737–1747.

102. Berliner JA, Territo M, Almada L, et al. Lipoprotein-induced insulin resistance in aortic endothelium. *Diabetes* 1984;33:1039–1044.

103. Reaven GM. Insulin resistance, hyperinsulinemia, hypertriglyceridemia, and hypertension: parallels between human disease and rodent models. *Diabetes Care* 1991;14:195–202.

104. Olefsky J, Reaven GM, Farquhar HW. Effects of weight reduction on obesity. *J Clin Invest* 1974;53:64–76.

105. Krotkiewski M, Mandroukas K, Sjostrom L, et al. Effects of long-term physical training on body fat, metabolism, and blood pressure in obesity. *Metabolism* 1979;28:650–658.

106. Izzo JL, Swislocki AL. Workshop III—insulin resistance: is it truly the link? *Am J Med* 1991;90[Suppl 2A]:2A-26S–2A-31S.

107. Marigliano A, Tedde R, Sechi LA, et al. Insulinemia and blood pressure: relationships in patients with primary and secondary hypertension, and with or without glucose metabolism impairment. *Am J Hypertens* 1990;3:512–526.

108. Reaven GM, Ho H. Renal vascular hypertension does not lead to hyperinsulinemia in Sprague-Dawley rats. *Am J Hypertens* 1992;5:314–317.

109. Finch D, Davis G, Bower J, et al. Effect of insulin on renal sodium handling in hypertensive rats. *Hypertension* 1990;14:514–518.

110. Hall JE, Coleman TG, Mizelle HL. Does chronic hyperinsulinemia cause hypertension? *Am J Hypertens* 1989;2:171–173.

111. Hall JE, Brands MW, Kivlighn SD, et al. Chronic hyperinsulinemia and blood pressure. Interaction with catecholamines? *Hypertension* 1990;15:519–527.

112. Kronenberg F, Rich SS, Sholinsky P, et al. Insulin and hypertension in the NHLBI Family Heart Study: a sibpair approach to a controversial issue. *Am J Hypertens* 2000;13:240–250.

113. Kageyama S, Yamamoto J, Isogai Y, et al. Effect of insulin on sodium reabsorption in hypertensive patients. *Am J Hypertens* 1994;7:409–415.

114. Schumacher MC, Hasstedt SJ, Hunt SC, et al. Major gene effect for insulin levels in familial NIDDM pedigrees. *Diabetes* 1992;41:416–423.

115. Lüscher TF, Boulanger CM, Dohi Y, et al. Endothelium-derived contracting factors. *Hypertension* 1992;19:117–130.

116. Nishikibe M, Tsuchida S, Okada M, et al. Antihypertensive effect of a newly synthesized endothelin antagonist, BQ-123, in a genetic hypertensive model. *Life Sci* 1993;52:717–724.

117. McMahon EG, Palomo MA, Brown MA, et al. Effect of phosphoramidon (endothelin converting enzyme inhibitor) and BQ-123 (endothelin receptor subtype A antagonist) on blood pressure in hypertensive rats. *Am J Hypertens* 1993;6:667–673.

118. Rossi GP, Colonna S, Pavan E, et al. Endothelin-1 and its mRNA in the wall layers of human arteries ex vivo. *Circulation* 1999;99:1147–1155.

119. Virdis A, Schiffrin EL. Vascular inflammation: a role in vascular disease in hypertension? *Curr Opin Nephrol Hypertens* 2003;12:181–187.

120. Boulanger CM, Tanner FC, Hahn AW, et al. Oxidized low-density lipoproteins induce mRNA expression and release of endothelin from human and porcine endothelium. *Circ Res* 1992;70:1191–1197.

121. He Y, Kwan WC, Steinbrecher UP. Effects of oxidized low density lipoprotein on endothelin secretion by cultured endothelial cells and macrophages. *Atherosclerosis* 1996;119:107–118.

122. Browatzki M, Schmidt J, Kubler W, et al. Endothelin-1 induces interleukin-6 release via activation of the transcription factor NF-kappaB in human vascular smooth muscle cells. *Basic Res Cardiol* 2000;95:98–105.

123. Rothermund L, Vetter R, Dieterich M, et al. Endothelin-A receptor blockade prevents left ventricular hypertrophy and dysfunction in salt-sensitive experimental hypertension. *Circulation* 2002;106:2305–2308.

124. Lerman A, Edwards BS, Hallet JW, et al. Circulating and tissue endothelin immunoreactivity in advanced atherosclerosis. *N Engl J Med* 1991;325:997–1001.

125. Bunchman TE, Brookshire CA. Cyclosporine-induced synthesis of endothelin by cultured human endothelial cells. *J Clin Invest* 1991;88:310–314.

126. Kon V, Badr KF. Biological actions and pathophysiologic significance of endothelin in the kidney. *Kidney Int* 1991;40:1–12.

127. Mortensen LH, Fink GD. Captopril prevents chronic hypertension produced by infusion of endothelin-1 in rats. *Hypertension* 1992;19:676–680.

128. Asai T, Ohkubo T, Katsuya T, et al. Endothelin-1 gene variant associates with blood pressure in obese Japanese subjects: the Ohasama Study. *Hypertension* 2001;38:1321–1324.

129. Jin JJ, Nakura J, Wu Z, et al. Association of endothelin-1 gene variant with hypertension. *Hypertension* 2003;41:163–167.

130. Berge KE, Berg K. No effect of a Taq1 polymorphism in DNA at the

endothelin I (EDN1) locus on normal blood pressure level or variability. *Clin Genet* 1992;41:90–95.

131. Vita JA, Treasure CB, Nabel EG, et al. Coronary vasomotor response to acetylcholine relates to risk factors for coronary artery disease. *Circulation* 1990;81:491–497.

132. Kuhn FE, Mohler ER, Satler LF, et al. Effects of high-density lipoprotein on acetylcholine-induced coronary vasoreactivity. *Am J Cardiol* 1991;68:1425–1430.

133. Egashira K, Inou T, Kirooka Y, et al. Impaired coronary blood flow response to acetylcholine in patients with coronary risk factors and proximal atherosclerotic lesions. *J Clin Invest* 1993;91:29–37.

134. Sorensen KE, Celermajer DS, Georgakopoulos D, et al. Impairment of endothelium-dependent dilation is an early event in children with familial hypercholesterolemia and is related to the lipoprotein(a) level. *J Clin Invest* 1994;93:50–55.

135. Reddy KG, Nair RN, Sheehan HM, et al. Evidence that selective endothelial dysfunction may occur in the absence of angiographic or ultrasound atherosclerosis in patients with risk factors for atherosclerosis. *J Am Coll Cardiol* 1994,23.833–843.

136. Dandona P. Endothelium, inflammation, and diabetes. *Curr Diab Rep* 2002;2:311–315.

137. Ikeda U, Maeda Y, Yamamoto K, et al. C-Reactive protein augments inducible nitric oxide synthase expression in cytokine-stimulated cardiac myocytes. *Cardiovasc Res* 2002;56:86–92.

138. Chen PY, Sanders PW. Role of nitric oxide synthesis in salt-sensitive hypertension in Dahl/Rapp rats. *Hypertension* 1993;22:812–818.

139. Chauhan S, Rahman A, Nilsson H, et al. NO contributes to EDHF-like responses in rat small arteries: a role for NO stores. *Cardiovasc Res* 2003;57:207–216.

140. Chauhan SD, Nilsson H, Ahluwalia A, et al. Release of C-type natriuretic peptide accounts for the biological activity of endothelium-derived hyperpolarizing factor. *Proc Natl Acad Sci USA* 2003;100: 1426–1431.

141. Rees DD, Palmer RM, Moncada S. Role of endothelium-derived nitric oxide in the regulation of blood pressure. *Proc Natl Acad Sci USA* 1989;86:3375–3378.

142. Lacolley PJ, Lewis SJ, Brody MJ. Role of sympathetic nerve activity in the generation of vascular nitric oxide in urethane-anesthetized rats. *Hypertension* 1991;17:881–887.

143. Vallance P, Collier J, Moncada S. Effects of endothelium-derived nitric oxide on peripheral arteriolar tone in man. *Lancet* 1989:997–1000.

144. Linder L, Kiowski W, Buhler FR, et al. Indirect evidence for release of endothelium-derived relaxing factor in human forearm circulation in vivo. Blunted response in essential hypertension. *Circulation* 1990;81:1762–1767.

145. Panza JA. Endothelial dysfunction in essential hypertension. *Clin Cardiol* 1997;20:II-26–II-33.

146. Lüscher TF, Vanhoutte PM, Raij L. Antihypertensive treatment normalizes decreased endothelium-dependent relaxations in rats with salt-induced hypertension. *Hypertension* 1987;9:III193–III197.

147. Baylis C, Mitruka B, Deng A. Chronic blockade of nitric oxide synthesis in the rat produces systemic hypertension and glomerular damage. *J Clin Invest* 1992;90:278–281.

148. Dananberg J, Sider RS, Grekin RJ. Sustained hypertension induced by orally administered nitro-L-arginine. *Hypertension* 1993;21:359–363.

149. Steinberg HO, Brechtel G, Johnson A, et al. Insulin-mediated skeletal muscle vasodilation is nitric oxide dependent. A novel action of insulin to increase nitric oxide release. *J Clin Invest* 1994;94: 1172–1179.

150. Zeng G, Quon MJ. Insulin-stimulated production of nitric oxide is inhibited by wortmannin. Direct measurement in vascular endothelial cells. *J Clin Invest* 1996;98:894–898.

151. Salazar FJ, Pinilla JM, Lopez F, et al. Renal effects of prolonged synthesis inhibition of endothelium-derived nitric oxide. *Hypertension* 1992;20:113–117.

152. Alberola A, Pinilla JM, Quesada T, et al. Role of nitric oxice in mediating renal response to volume expansion. *Hypertension* 1992;19: 780–784.

153. Liu R, Pittner J, Persson AE. Changes of cell volume and nitric oxide concentration in macula densa cells caused by changes in luminal NaCl concentration. *J Am Soc Nephrol* 2002;13:2688–2696.

154. Ollerstam A, Persson AE. Macula densa neuronal nitric oxide synthase. *Cardiovasc Res* 2002;56:189–196.

155. Friend LR, Morris BJ, Gaffney PT, et al. Examination of the role of

156. Wang XL, Mahaney MC, Sim AS, et al. Genetic contribution of the endothelial constitutive nitric oxide synthase gene to plasma nitric oxide levels. *Arterioscler Thromb Vasc Biol* 1997;17:3147–3153.

157. Miyamoto Y, Saito Y, Kajiyama N, et al. Endothelial nitric oxide synthase gene is positively associated with essential hypertension. *Hypertension* 1998;32:3–8.

158. Lacolley P, Gautier S, Poirier O, et al. Nitric oxide synthase gene polymorphisms, blood pressure and aortic stiffness in normotensive and hypertensive subjects. *J Hypertens* 1998;16:31–35.

159. Uwabo J, Soma M, Nakayama T, et al. Association of a variable number of tandem repeats in the endothelial constitutive nitric oxide synthase gene with essential hypertension in Japanese. *Am J Hypertens* 1998;11:125–128.

160. Kato N, Sugiyama T, Morita H, et al. Lack of evidence for association between the endothelial nitric oxide synthase gene and hypertension. *Hypertension* 1999;33:933–936.

161. Glenn CL, Wang WY, Morris BJ. Different frequencies of inducible nitric oxide synthase genotypes in older hypertensives. *Hypertension* 1999;33:927–932.

162. Kajiyama N, Saito Y, Miyamoto Y, et al. Lack of association between T-786→C mutation in the 5'-flanking region of the endothelial nitric oxide synthase gene and essential hypertension. *Hypertens Res* 2000;23:561–565.

163. Benjafield AV, Morris BJ. Association analyses of endothelial nitric oxide synthase gene polymorphisms in essential hypertension. *Am J Hypertens* 2000;13:994–998.

164. Rutherford S, Johnson MP, Curtain RP, et al. Chromosome 17 and the inducible nitric oxide synthase gene in human essential hypertension. *Hum Genet* 2001;109:408–415.

165. Hyndman ME, Parsons HG, Verma S, et al. The T-786→C mutation in endothelial nitric oxide synthase is associated with hypertension. *Hypertension* 2002;39:919–922.

166. Freedman BI, Yu H, Anderson PJ, et al. Genetic analysis of nitric oxide and endothelin in end-stage renal disease. *Nephrol Dial Transplant* 2000;15:1794–1800.

167. Achenbach S, Giesler T, Ropers D, et al. Detection of coronary artery stenoses by contrast-enhanced, retrospectively electrocardiographically-gated, multislice spiral computed tomography. *Circulation* 2001;103:2535–2538.

168. Kuboki K, Jiang ZY, Takahara N, et al. Regulation of endothelial constitutive nitric oxide synthase gene expression in endothelial cells and in vivo: a specific vascular action of insulin. *Circulation* 2000;101: 676–681.

169. Schneider MP, Erdmann J, Delles C, et al. Functional gene testing of the Glu298Asp polymorphism of the endothelial NO synthase. *J Hypertens* 2000;18:1767–1773.

170. Jeunemaitre X, Lifton RP, Hunt SC, et al. Absence of linkage between the angiotensin converting enzyme locus and human essential hypertension. *Nat Genet* 1992;1:72–75.

171. Jeunemaitre X, Rigat B, Charru A, et al. Sib pair linkage analysis of renin gene haplotypes in human essential hypertension. *Hum Genet* 1992;88:301–306.

172. Fuchs S, Philippe J, Germain S, et al. Functionality of two new polymorphisms in the human renin gene enhancer region. *J Hypertens* 2002;20:2391–2398.

173. O'Donnell CJ, Lindpaintner K, Larson MG, et al. Evidence for association and genetic linkage of the angiotensin-converting enzyme locus with hypertension and blood pressure in men but not women in the Framingham Heart Study. *Circulation* 1998;97: 1766–1772.

174. Fornage M, Amos CI, Kardia S, et al. Variation in the region of the angiotensin-converting enzyme gene influences interindividual differences in blood pressure levels in young white males. *Circulation* 1998;97:1773–1779.

175. Zhu X, Bouzekri N, Southam L, et al. Linkage and association analysis of angiotensin I-converting enzyme (ACE)-gene polymorphisms with ACE concentration and blood pressure. *Am J Hum Genet* 2001;68:1139–1148.

176. Klett C, Bader M, Ganten D, et al. Mechanism by which angiotensin II stabilizes messenger RNA for angiotensinogen. *Hypertension* 1994;23:I-120–I-125.

177. Blaine EH, Davis JO, Harris PD. A steady-state control analysis of the

renin-angiotensin-aldosterone system. *Circulation Res* 1972;30:713–730.

178. Smithies O, Kim HS, Takahashi N, et al. Importance of quantitative genetic variations in the etiology of hypertension. *Kidney Int* 2000;58:2265–2280.

179. Brown AJ, Casals-Stenzel J, Gofford S, et al. Comparison of fast and slow pressor effects of angiotensin II in the conscious rat. *Am J Physiol* 1981;241:H381–H388.

180. Sealey JE, Blumenfeld JD, Bell GM, et al. On the renal basis for essential hypertension: nephron heterogeneity with discordant renin secretion and sodium excretion causing a hypertensive vasoconstriction-volume relationship. In: Laragh JH, Brenner BM, eds. *Hypertension: pathophysiology, diagnosis and management.* New York: Raven Press, 1990:1089–1103.

181. Gahnem F, von Lutterotti N, Camargo MJ, et al. Angiotensinogen dependency of blood pressure in two high-renin hypertensive rat models. *Am J Hypertens* 1994;7:899–904.

182. Fasola AF, Martz BL, Helmer OM. Plasma renin activity during supine exercise in offspring of hypertensive parents. *J Appl Physiol* 1968;25:410–415.

183. Watt GC, Harrap SB, Foy CJ, et al. Abnormalities of glucocorticoid metabolism and the renin-angiotensin system: a four-corners approach to the identification of genetic determinants of blood pressure. *J Hypertens* 1992;10:473–482.

184. Jeunemaitre X, Gimenez-Roqueplo AP, Celerier J, et al. Angiotensinogen variants and human hypertension. *Curr Hypertens Rep* 1999;1:31–41.

185. Walker WG, Whelton PK, Saito H, et al. Relation between blood pressure and renin, renin substrate, angiotensin II, aldosterone and urinary sodium and potassium in 574 ambulatory subjects. *Hypertension* 1979;1:287–291.

186. Jeunemaitre X, Soubrier F, Kotelevtsev Y, et al. Molecular basis of human hypertension: role of angiotensinogen. *Cell* 1992;71:169–180.

187. Staessen JA, Kuznetsova T, Wang JG, et al. M235T angiotensinogen gene polymorphism and cardiovascular renal risk. *J Hypertens* 1999;17:9–17.

188. Lantelme P, Rohrwasser A, Gociman B, et al. Effects of dietary sodium and genetic background on angiotensinogen and Renin in mouse. *Hypertension* 2002;39:1007–1014.

189. Kobori H, Nishiyama A, Abe Y, et al. Enhancement of intrarenal angiotensinogen in Dahl salt-sensitive rats on high salt diet. *Hypertension* 2003;41:592–597.

190. Kobori H, Nishiyama A, Harrison-Bernard LM, et al. Urinary angiotensinogen as an indicator of intrarenal Angiotensin status in hypertension. *Hypertension* 2003;41:42–49.

191. Ménard J, El Amrani AI, Savoie F, et al. Angiotensinogen: an attractive and underrated participant in hypertension and inflammation. *Hypertension* 1991;18:705–706.

192. Gardes J, Bouhnik J, Clauser E, et al. Role of angiotensinogen in blood pressure homeostasis. *Hypertension* 1982;4:185–189.

193. Kimura S, Mullins JJ, Bunnemann B, et al. High blood pressure in transgenic mice carrying the rat angiotensinogen gene. *EMBO J* 1992;11:821–827.

194. Rakugi H, Jacob HJ, Krieger JE, et al. Vascular injury induces angiotensinogen gene expression in the media and neointima. *Circulation* 1993;87:283–290.

195. Iwai N, Shimoike H, Ohmichi N, et al. Angiotensinogen gene and blood pressure in the Japanese population. *Hypertension* 1995;25:688–693.

196. Tamura K, Umemura S, Iwamoto T, et al. Molecular mechanism of adipogenic activation of the angiotensinogen gene. *Hypertension* 1994;23:364–368.

197. Bloem LJ, Manatunga AK, Tewksbury DA, et al. The serum angiotensinogen concentration and variants of the angiotensinogen gene in white and black children. *J Clin Invest* 1995;95:948–953.

198. Schorr U, Blaschke K, Turan S, et al. Relationship between angiotensinogen, leptin and blood pressure levels in young normotensive men. *J Hypertens* 1998;16:1475–1480.

199. Cooper R, Forrester T, Ogunbiyi O, et al. Angiotensinogen levels and obesity in four population samples. *J Hypertens* 1998;16:571–576.

200. Jeunemaitre X, Soubrier F, Kotelevtsev YV, et al. Molecular basis of human hypertension: role of angiotensinogen. *Cell* 1992;71:169–180.

201. Jeunemaitre X, Charru A, Chatellier G, et al. M235T variant of the human angiotensinogen gene in unselected hypertensive patients. *J Hypertens* 1993;11[Suppl 5]:S80–S81.

202. Hata A, Namikawa C, Sasaki M, et al. Angiotensinogen as a risk factor for essential hypertension in Japan. *J Clin Invest* 1994;93:1285–1287.

203. Caulfield M, Lavender P, Farrall M, et al. Linkage of the angiotensinogen gene to essential hypertension. *N Engl J Med* 1994;330:1629–1633.

204. Sethi AA, Nordestgaard BG, Agerholm-Larsen B, et al. Angiotensinogen polymorphisms and elevated blood pressure in the general population: the Copenhagen City Heart Study. *Hypertension* 2001;37:875–881.

205. Rotimi C, Morrison L, Cooper R, et al. Angiotensinogen gene in human hypertension. Lack of an association of the 235T allele among African Americans. *Hypertension* 1994;24:591–594.

206. Province MA, Boerwinkle E, Chakravarti A, et al. Lack of association of the angiotensinogen-6 polymorphism with blood pressure levels in the comprehensive NHLBI Family Blood Pressure Program. National Heart, Lung and Blood Institute. *J Hypertens* 2000;18:867–876.

207. Tsai CT, Fallin D, Chiang FT, et al. Angiotensinogen gene haplotype and hypertension: interaction with ACE gene I allele. *Hypertension* 2003;41:9–15.

208. Tiago AD, Samani NJ, Candy GP, et al. Angiotensinogen gene promoter region variant modifies body size-ambulatory blood pressure relations in hypertension. *Circulation* 2002;106:1483–1487.

209. Glorioso N, Manunta P, Filigheddu F, et al. The role of alpha-adducin polymorphism in blood pressure and sodium handling regulation may not be excluded by a negative association study. *Hypertension* 1999;34:649–654.

210. Hopkins PN, Hunt SC, Jeunemaitre X, et al. Angiotensinogen genotype affects renal and adrenal responses to angiotensin II in essential hypertension. *Circulation* 2002;105:1921–1927.

211. Hunt SC, Cook NR, Oberman A, et al. Angiotensinogen genotype, sodium reduction, weight loss, and prevention of hypertension: trials of hypertension prevention, phase II. *Hypertension* 1998;32:393–401.

212. Hunt SC, Geleijnse JM, Wu LL, et al. Enhanced blood pressure response to mild sodium reduction in subjects with the 235T variant of the angiotensinogen gene. *Am J Hypertens* 1999;12:460–466.

213. Svetkey LP, Moore TJ, Simons-Morton DG, et al. Angiotensinogen genotype and blood pressure response in the Dietary Approaches to Stop Hypertension (DASH) study. *J Hypertens* 2001;19:1949–1956.

214. Skidgel RA, Erdös EG. Angiotensin I-converting enzyme. In: Izzo JL Jr, Black HR, eds. *Hypertension primer.* Dallas: American Heart Association, 1999:19–20.

215. Murphey LJ, Gainer JV, Vaughan DE, et al. Angiotensin-converting enzyme insertion/deletion polymorphism modulates the human in vivo metabolism of bradykinin. *Circulation* 2000;102:829–832.

216. Margolius HS, Horwitz D, Pisano JJ, et al. Urinary kallikrein excretion in hypertensive man: relationships to sodium intake and sodium-retaining steroids. *Circ Res* 1974;35:820–825.

217. Carretero OA, Oza NB, Schork A. Renal tissue kallikrein, plasma renin, and plasma aldosterone in renal hypertension. *Acta Physiol Lat Am* 1974;24:448–452.

218. Mersey JH, Williams GH, Emanuel R, et al. Plasma bradykinin levels and urinary kallikrein excretion in normal renin essential hypertension. *J Clin Endocrinol Metab* 1979;48:642–647.

219. Keiser HR. The kallikrein-kinin system in essential hypertension. *Clin Exp Hypertens* 1980;2:675–691.

220. Ura N, Shimamoto K, Nakao T, et al. The excretion of human urinary kallikrein quantity and activity in normal and low renin subgroups of essential hypertension. *Clin Exp Hypertens A* 1983;A5(3):329–337.

221. Katori M, Majima M. The renal kallikrein-kinin system: its role as a safety valve for excess sodium intake, and its attenuation as a possible etiologic factor in salt-sensitive hypertension. *Crit Rev Clin Lab Sci* 2003;40:43–115.

222. Hunt SC, Hasstedt SJ, Wu LL, et al. A gene-environment interaction between inferred kallikrein genotype and potassium. *Hypertension* 1993;22:161–168.

223. Song Q, Chao J, Chao L. DNA polymorphisms in the 5'-flanking region of the human tissue kallikrein gene. *Hum Genet* 1997;99:727–734.

224. Yu H, Song Q, Freedman BI, et al. Association of the tissue kallikrein gene promoter with ESRD and hypertension. *Kidney Int* 2002;61:1030–1039.

225. Slim R, Torremocha F, Moreau T, et al. Loss-of-function polymorphism of the human kallikrein gene with reduced urinary kallikrein activity. *J Am Soc Nephrol* 2002;13:968–976.

226. Gainer JV, Brown NJ, Bachvarova M, et al. Altered frequency of a

promoter polymorphism of the kinin B2 receptor gene in hypertensive African-Americans. *Am J Hypertens* 2000;13:1268–1273.

227. Hayashi I, Oh-ishi S, Kato H, et al. Identification of T-kininogen in high and low molecular weight kininogens deficient rat (brown Norway Katholiek strain). *Thromb Res* 1985;39:313–321.

228. Sanchez R, Nolly H, Giannone C, et al. Reduced activity of the kallikrein-kinin system predominates over renin-angiotensin system overactivity in all conditions of sodium balance in essential hypertensives and family-related hypertension. *J Hypertens* 2003;21:411–417.

229. Madeddu P, Parpaglia PP, Demontis MP, et al. Chronic inhibition of bradykinin B2-receptors enhances the slow vasopressor response to angiotensin II. *Hypertension* 1994;23:646–652.

230. Majima M, Mizogami S, Kuribayashi Y, et al. Hypertension induced by a nonpressor dose of angiotensin II in kininogen-deficient rats. *Hypertension* 1994;24:111–119.

231. Rhaleb NE, Yang XP, Nanba M, et al. Effect of chronic blockade of the kallikrein-kinin system on the development of hypertension in rats. *Hypertension* 2001;37:121–128.

232. Bianchi G, Tripodi G, Casari G, et al. Two point mutations within the adducin genes are involved in blood pressure variation. *Proc Natl Acad Sci USA* 1994;91:3999–4003.

233. Tripodi G, Valtorta F, Torielli L, et al. Hypertension-associated point mutations in the adducin alpha and beta subunits affect actin cytoskeleton and ion transport. *J Clin Invest* 1996;97:2815–2822.

234. Manunta P, Burnier M, D'Amico M, et al. Adducin polymorphism affects renal proximal tubule reabsorption in hypertension. *Hypertension* 1999;33:694–697.

235. Ferrandi M, Salardi S, Tripodi G, et al. Evidence for an interaction between adducin and Na(+)-K(+)-ATPase: relation to genetic hypertension. *Am J Physiol* 1999;277:H1338–H1349.

236. Cusi D, Barlassina C, Glorioso N, et al. a-adducin G460W variant is associated with salt-sensitive hypertension. *Hypertension* 1996;28:694.

237. Cusi D, Barlassina C, Azzani T, et al. Polymorphisms of alpha-adducin and salt sensitivity in patients with essential hypertension. *Lancet* 1997;349:1353–1357.

238. Glorioso N, Filigheddu F, Cusi D, et al. alpha-Adducin 460Trp allele is associated with erythrocyte Na transport rate in North Sardinian primary hypertensives. *Hypertension* 2002;39:357–362.

239. Sciarrone MT, Stella P, Barlassina C, et al. ACE and alpha-adducin polymorphism as markers of individual response to diuretic therapy. *Hypertension* 2003;41:398–403.

240. Barlassina C, Schork NJ, Manunta P, et al. Synergistic effect of alpha-adducin and ACE genes causes blood pressure changes with body sodium and volume expansion. *Kidney Int* 2000;57:1083–1090.

241. Province MA, Arnett DK, Hunt SC, et al. Association between the alpha-adducin gene and hypertension in the HyperGEN Study. *Am J Hypertens* 2000;13:710–718.

242. Ranade K, Hsuing AC, Wu KD, et al. Lack of evidence for an association between alpha-adducin and blood pressure regulation in Asian populations. *Am J Hypertens* 2000;13:704–709.

243. Bray MS, Li L, Turner ST, et al. Association and linkage analysis of the alpha-adducin gene and blood pressure. *Am J Hypertens* 2000;13:699–703.

244. Schork NJ, Chakravarti A, Thiel B, et al. Lack of association between a biallelic polymorphism in the adducin gene and blood pressure in whites and African Americans. *Am J Hypertens* 2000;13:693–698.

245. Staessen JA, Wang JG, Brand E, et al. Effects of three candidate genes on prevalence and incidence of hypertension in a Caucasian population. *J Hypertens* 2001;19:1349–1358.

246. Hamlyn JM, Harris DW, Clark MA, et al. Isolation and characterization of a sodium pump inhibitor from human plasma. *Hypertension* 1989;13:681–689.

247. Tamura M, Kuwano H, Kinoshita T, et al. Identification of linoleic and oleic acids as endogenous Na+,K+,-ATPase inhibitors from acute volume-expanded hog plasma. *J Biol Chem* 1985;260:9672–9677.

248. Tamura M, Inagami T, Kinoshita T, et al. A search for endogenous Na+,K+-ATPase inhibitor in acutely volume-expanded hog plasma led to lysophosphatidylcholine g-stearoyl. *J Hypertens* 1987;5:219–225.

249. Ruiz-Opazo N, Barany F, Hirayama K, et al. Confirmation of mutant alpha 1 Na,K-ATPase gene and transcript in Dahl salt-sensitive/JR rats. *Hypertension* 1994;24:260–270.

250. Glorioso N, Filigheddu F, Troffa C, et al. Interaction of alpha(1)-Na,K-ATPase and Na,K,2Cl-cotransporter genes in human essential hypertension. *Hypertension* 2001;38:204–209.

251. Song Y, Herrera VL, Filigheddu F, et al. Non-association of the thiazide-sensitive Na,Cl-cotransporter gene with polygenic hypertension in both rats and humans. *J Hypertens* 2001;19:1547–1551.

252. Laurenzi M, Cirillo M, Panarelli W, et al. Baseline sodium-lithium countertransport and 6-year incidence of hypertension. The Gubbio Population Study. *Circulation* 1997;95:581–587.

253. Strazzullo P, Siani A, Cappuccio FP, et al. Red blood cell sodium-lithium countertransport and risk of future hypertension: the Olivetti Prospective Heart Study. *Hypertension* 1998;31:1284–1289.

254. Cirillo M, Laurenzi M, Panarelli W, et al. Prospective analysis of traits related to 6-year change in sodium-lithium countertransport. Gubbio Population Study Research Group. *Hypertension* 1999;33:887–893.

255. Hasstedt SJ, Wu LL, Ash KO, et al. Hypertension and sodium-lithium countertransport in Utah pedigrees: evidence for major locus inheritance. *Am J Hum Genet* 1988;43:14–22.

256. Rebbeck TR, Turner ST, Sing CF. Sodium-lithium countertransport genotype and the probability of hypertension in adults. *Hypertension* 1993;22:560–568.

257. Canessa ML, Morgan K, Semplicini A. Genetic differences in lithium-sodium exchange and regulation of the sodium-hydrogen exchanger in essential hypertension. *J Cardiovasc Pharmacol* 1988;12[Suppl 3]:S92–S98.

258. Semplicini A. The Li+/Na+ countertransport in hypertension. In: Coca A, Garay RP, eds. *Ionic transport in hypertension: new perspectives*. Boca Raton: CRC Press, 1994:89–117.

259. Orlov SN, Kuznetsov SR, Pokudin NI, et al. Can we use erythrocytes for the study of the activity of the ubiquitous Na+/H+ exchanger (NHE-1) in essential hypertension? *Am J Hypertens* 1998;11:774–783.

260. Weder AB, Delgado MC, Zhu X, et al. Erythrocyte sodium-lithium countertransport and blood pressure: a genome-wide linkage study. *Hypertension* 2003;41:842–846.

261. Knoll R, Hoshijima M, Hoffman HM, et al. The cardiac mechanical stretch sensor machinery involves a Z disc complex that is defective in a subset of human dilated cardiomyopathy. *Cell* 2002;111:943–955.

262. Lifton RP, Hunt SC, Williams RR, et al. Exclusion of the Na+/H+ antiporter as a candidate gene in human essential hypertension by genetic linkage analysis. *Hypertension* 1991;17:8–14.

263. Aviv A, Lasker N. Proposed defects in membrane transport and intracellular ions as pathogenic factors in essential hypertension. In: Laragh JH, Brenner BM, eds. *Hypertension: pathophysiology, diagnosis, and management*. New York: Raven Press, 1990:923–937.

264. Blaustein MP, Hamlyn JM. Sodium transport inhibition, cell calcium, and hypertension. The natriuretic hormone/Na+ -Ca2+ exchange/hypertension hypothesis. *Am J Med* 1984:45–59.

265. Fray JC, Park CS, Valentine AN. Calcium and control of renin secretion. *Endocrine Rev* 1987;8:53–93.

266. Moore RD. Effects of insulin upon ion transport. *Biochim Biophys Acta* 1983;737:1–49.

267. Resnick LM, Gupta RK, Soza RE, et al. Intracellular pH in human and experimental hypertension. *Proc Natl Acad Sci USA* 1987;84:7663–7667.

268. Resnick LM, Gupta RK, Gruenspan H, et al. Hypertension and peripheral insulin resistance: possible mediating role of intracellular free magnesium. *Am J Hypertens* 1990;3:373–379.

269. Landsberg L, Young JB. Catecholamines and the adrenal medulla. In: Wilson JD, Foster DW, eds. *Williams textbook of endocrinology*, 7th ed. Philadelphia: WB Saunders, 1985:891–965.

270. Zicha J, Kunes J, Devynck MA. Abnormalities of membrane function and lipid metabolism in hypertension: a review. *Am J Hypertens* 1999;12:315–331.

271. Tsuda K, Nishio I. Membrane fluidity and hypertension. *Am J Hypertens* 2003;16:259–261.

272. Hunt SC, Williams RR, Smith JB, et al. Associations of three erythrocyte cation transport systems with plasma lipids in Utah subjects. *Hypertension* 1986;8:30–36.

273. Hunt SC, Williams RR, Ash KO. Changes in sodium-lithium countertransport correlate with changes in triglyceride levels and body mass index over two and one-half years of followup in Utah. *Cardiovasc Drugs Ther* 1990;4:357–362.

274. Levy R, Paran E, Keynan A, et al. Essential hypertension: improved

differentiation by the temperature dependence of Li efflux in erythrocytes. *Hypertension* 1983;5:821–827.

275. Engelmann B, Op den Kamp JA, Roelofsen B. Replacement of molecular species of phosphatidylcholine: influence on erythrocyte Na transport. *Am J Physiol* 1990;258[4 Pt 1]:C682–C691.

276. Sauerheber RD, Lewis UJ, Esgate JA, et al. Effect of calcium, insulin and growth hormones on membrane fluidity: a spin label study of rat adipocytes and human erythrocyte ghosts. *Biochim Biophys Acta* 1980;597:292–304.

277. Tsuda K, Masuyama Y. Age-related changes in membrane fluidity of erythrocytes in essential hypertension. *Am J Hypertens* 1990;3:714–716.

278. Masuyama Y, Tsuda K, Shima H, et al. Membrane abnormality of erythrocytes is highly dependent on salt intake and renin profile in essential hypertension: an electron spin resonance study. *J Hypertens* 1988;6[Suppl 4]:S266–S268.

279. Lijnen P, Celis H, Fagard R, et al. Influence of cholesterol lowering on plasma membrane lipids and cationic transport systems. *J Hypertens* 1994;12:59–64.

280. Hasstedt SJ, Hunt SC, Wu LL, et al. Evidence for multiple genes determining sodium transport. *Genet Epidemiol* 1994;11:553–568.

281. Hautanena A, Lankinen L, Kupari M, et al. Associations between aldosterone synthase gene polymorphism and the adrenocortical function in males. *J Intern Med* 1998;244:11–18.

282. Kainulainen K, Perola M, Terwilliger J, et al. Evidence for involvement of the type 1 angiotensin II receptor locus in essential hypertension. *Hypertension* 1999;33:844–849.

283. Davies E, Holloway CD, Ingram MC, et al. Aldosterone excretion rate and blood pressure in essential hypertension are related to polymorphic differences in the aldosterone synthase gene CYP11B2. *Hypertension* 1999;33:703–707.

284. Duncan JA, Scholey JW, Miller JA. Angiotensin II type 1 receptor gene polymorphisms in humans: physiology and pathophysiology of the genotypes. *Curr Opin Nephrol Hypertens* 2001;10:111–116.

285. Brand E, Chatelain N, Mulatero P, et al. Structural analysis and evaluation of the aldosterone synthase gene in hypertension. *Hypertension* 1998;32:198–204.

286. Brand E, Schorr U, Ringel J, et al. Aldosterone synthase gene (CYP11B2) C-344T polymorphism in Caucasians from the Berlin Salt-Sensitivity Trial (BeSST). *J Hypertens* 1999;17:1563–1567.

287. Siffert W, Rosskopf D, Siffert G, et al. Association of a human G-protein beta3 subunit variant with hypertension. *Nat Genet* 1998;18:45–48.

288. Schunkert H, Hense HW, Doring A, et al. Association between a polymorphism in the G protein beta3 subunit gene and lower renin and elevated diastolic blood pressure levels. *Hypertension* 1998;32:510–513.

289. Siffert W, Forster P, Jockel KH, et al. Worldwide ethnic distribution of the G protein beta3 subunit 825T allele and its association with obesity in Caucasian, Chinese, and Black African individuals. *J Am Soc Nephrol* 1999;10:1921–1930.

290. Beige J, Hohenbleicher H, Distler A, et al. G-Protein beta3 subunit C825T variant and ambulatory blood pressure in essential hypertension. *Hypertension* 1999;33:1049–1051.

291. Brand E, Herrmann SM, Nicaud V, et al. The 825C/T polymorphism of the G-protein subunit beta3 is not related to hypertension. *Hypertension* 1999;33:1175–1178.

292. Benjafield AV, Lin RC, Dalziel B, et al. G-protein beta3 subunit gene splice variant in obesity and overweight. *Int J Obes Relat Metab Disord* 2001;25:777–780.

293. Poston WS, Haddock CK, Spertus J, et al. Physical activity does not mitigate G-protein-related genetic risk for obesity in individuals of African descent. *Eat Weight Disord* 2002;7:68–71.

294. Wascher TC, Paulweber B, Malaimare L, et al. Associations of a human G protein beta3 subunit dimorphism with insulin resistance and carotid atherosclerosis. *Stroke* 2003;34:605–609.

295. Siffert W, Rosskopf D, Moritz A, et al. Enhanced G protein activation in immortalized lymphoblasts from patients with essential hypertension. *J Clin Invest* 1995;96:759–766.

296. Zeltner R, Delles C, Schneider M, et al. G-protein beta(3) subunit gene (GNB3) 825T allele is associated with enhanced renal perfusion in early hypertension. *Hypertension* 2001;37:882–886.

297. Turner ST, Schwartz GL, Chapman AB, et al. C825T polymorphism of the G protein beta(3)-subunit and antihypertensive response to a thiazide diuretic. *Hypertension* 2001;37:739–743.

298. Krushkal J, Xiong M, Ferrell R, et al. Linkage and association of adrenergic and dopamine receptor genes in the distal portion of the long arm of chromosome 5 with systolic blood pressure variation. *Hum Mol Genet* 1998;7:1379–1383.

299. Krushkal J, Ferrell R, Mockrin SC, et al. Genome-wide linkage analyses of systolic blood pressure using highly discordant siblings. *Circulation* 1999;99:1407–1410.

300. Ranade K, Shue WH, Hung YJ, et al. The glycine allele of a glycine/arginine polymorphism in the beta2-adrenergic receptor gene is associated with essential hypertension in a population of Chinese origin. *Am J Hypertens* 2001;14:1196–1200.

301. Jia H, Sharma P, Hopper R, et al. beta2-adrenoceptor gene polymorphisms and blood pressure variations in East Anglian Caucasians. *J Hypertens* 2000;18:687–693.

302. Ranade K, Jorgenson E, Sheu WH, et al. A polymorphism in the beta1 adrenergic receptor is associated with resting heart rate. *Am J Hum Genet* 2002;70:935–942.

303. Bengtsson K, Melander O, Orho-Melander M, et al. Polymorphism in the beta(1)-adrenergic receptor gene and hypertension. *Circulation* 2001;104:187–190.

304. Dionne IJ, Garant MJ, Nolan AA, et al. Association between obesity and a polymorphism in the beta(1)-adrenoceptor gene (Gly389Arg ADRB1) in Caucasian women. *Int J Obes Relat Metab Disord* 2002;26:633–639.

305. Shuldiner AR, Silver K, Roth J, et al. Beta 3-adrenoceptor gene variant in obesity and insulin resistance. *Lancet* 1996;348:1584–1585.

306. Silver K, Mitchell BD, Walston J, et al. TRP64ARG beta 3-adrenergic receptor and obesity in Mexican Americans. *Hum Genet* 1997;101:306–311.

307. Kim-Motoyama H, Yasuda K, Yamaguchi T, et al. A mutation of the beta 3-adrenergic receptor is associated with visceral obesity but decreased serum triglyceride. *Diabetologia* 1997;40:469–472.

308. Mitchell BD, Blangero J, Comuzzie AG, et al. A paired sibling analysis of the beta-3 adrenergic receptor and obesity in Mexican Americans. *J Clin Invest* 1998;101:584–587.

309. Walston J, Silver K, Hilfiker H, et al. Insulin response to glucose is lower in individuals homozygous for the Arg 64 variant of the beta-3-adrenergic receptor. *J Clin Endocrinol Metab* 2000;85:4019–4022.

310. Mentuccia D, Proietti-Pannunzi L, Tanner K, et al. Association between a novel variant of the human type 2 deiodinase gene Thr92Ala and insulin resistance: evidence of interaction with the Trp64Arg variant of the beta-3-adrenergic receptor. *Diabetes* 2002;51:880–883.

311. Baldwin CT, Schwartz F, Baima J, et al. Identification of a polymorphic glutamic acid stretch in the alpha2B-adrenergic receptor and lack of linkage with essential hypertension. *Am J Hypertens* 1999;12:853–857.

312. Felder RA, Sanada H, Xu J, et al. G protein-coupled receptor kinase 4 gene variants in human essential hypertension. *Proc Natl Acad Sci USA* 2002;99:3872–3877.

313. Jose PA, Eisner GM, Felder RA. Dopamine and the kidney: a role in hypertension? *Curr Opin Nephrol Hypertens* 2003;12:189–194.

314. Sato M, Soma M, Nakayama T, et al. Dopamine D1 receptor gene polymorphism is associated with essential hypertension. *Hypertension* 2000;36:183–186.

315. Pajukanta P, Nuotio I, Terwilliger JD, et al. Linkage of familial combined hyperlipidaemia to chromosome 1q21-q23. *Nat Genet* 1998;18:369–373.

316. Pei W, Baron H, Muller-Myhsok B, et al. Support for linkage of familial combined hyperlipidemia to chromosome 1q21-q23 in Chinese and German families. *Clin Genet* 2000;57:29–34.

317. Coon H, Myers RH, Borecki IB, et al. Replication of linkage of familial combined hyperlipidemia to chromosome 1q with additional heterogeneous effect of apolipoprotein A-I/C-III/A-IV locus. The NHLBI Family Heart Study. *Arterioscler Thromb Vasc Biol* 2000;20:2275–2280.

318. Coon H, Leppert MF, Eckfeldt JH, et al. Genome-wide linkage analysis of lipids in the hypertension genetic epidemiology network (HyperGEN) blood pressure study. *Arterioscler Thromb Vasc Biol* 2001;21:1969–1976.

319. Kotchen TA, Broeckel U, Grim CE, et al. Identification of hypertension-related QTLs in African American sib pairs. *Hypertension* 2002;40:634–639.

320. Hanson RL, Ehm MG, Pettitt DJ, et al. An autosomal genomic scan

for loci linked to type II diabetes mellitus and body-mass index in Pima Indians. *Am J Hum Genet* 1998;63:1130–1138.

321. Elbein SC, Hoffman MD, Teng K, et al. A genome-wide search for type 2 diabetes susceptibility genes in Utah Caucasians. *Diabetes* 1999;48:1175–1182.

322. Vionnet N, Hani El H, Dupont S, et al. Genomewide search for type 2 diabetes-susceptibility genes in French whites: evidence for a novel susceptibility locus for early-onset diabetes on chromosome 3q27-qter and independent replication of a type 2-diabetes locus on chromosome 1q21-q24. *Am J Hum Genet* 2000;67:1470–1480.

323. Wiltshire S, Hattersley AT, Hitman GA, et al. A genomewide scan for loci predisposing to type 2 diabetes in a U.K. population (the Diabetes UK Warren 2 Repository): analysis of 573 pedigrees provides independent replication of a susceptibility locus on chromosome 1q. *Am J Hum Genet* 2001;69:553–569.

324. Hsueh WC, St Jean PL, Mitchell BD, et al. Genome-wide and fine-mapping linkage studies of type 2 diabetes and glucose traits in the Old Order Amish: evidence for a new diabetes locus on chromosome 14q11 and confirmation of a locus on chromosome 1q21-q24. *Diabetes* 2003;52:550–557.

325. Bodnar JS, Chatterjee A, Castellani LW, et al. Positional cloning of the combined hyperlipidemia gene Hyplip1. *Nat Genet* 2002;30:110–116.

326. Arngrimsson R, Sigurard ttir S, Frigge ML, et al. A genome-wide scan reveals a maternal susceptibility locus for pre-eclampsia on chromosome 2p13. *Hum Mol Genet* 1999;8:1799–1805.

327. Cheng LS, Davis RC, Raffel LJ, et al. Coincident linkage of fasting plasma insulin and blood pressure to chromosome 7q in hypertensive Hispanic families. *Circulation* 2001;104:1255–1260.

328. Atwood LD, Samollow PB, Hixson JE, et al. Genome-wide linkage analysis of pulse pressure in Mexican Americans. *Hypertension* 2001;37:425–428.

329. Feitosa MF, Borecki IB, Rich SS, et al. Quantitative-trait loci influencing body-mass index reside on chromosomes 7 and 13: the National Heart, Lung, and Blood Institute Family Heart Study. *Am J Hum Genet* 2002;70:72–82.

330. Allayee H, de Bruin TW, Michelle Dominguez K, et al. Genome scan for blood pressure in Dutch dyslipidemic families reveals linkage to a locus on chromosome 4p. *Hypertension* 2001;38:773–778.

331. Hunt SC, Ellison RC, Atwood LD, et al. Genome scans for blood pressure and hypertension: the National Heart, Lung, and Blood Institute Family Heart Study. *Hypertension* 2002;40:1–6.

332. Pankow JS, Rose KM, Oberman A, et al. Possible locus on chromosome 18q influencing postural systolic blood pressure changes. *Hypertension* 2000;36:471–476.

333. Kristjansson K, Manolescu A, Kristinsson A, et al. Linkage of essential hypertension to chromosome 18q. *Hypertension* 2002;39:1044–1049.

334. Dunn DM, Ishigami T, Pankow J, et al. Common variant of human NEDD4L activates a cryptic splice site to form a frameshifted transcript. *J Hum Genet* 2002;47:665–676.

335. Rankinen T, An P, Rice T, et al. Genomic scan for exercise blood pressure in the Health, Risk Factors, Exercise Training and Genetics (HERITAGE) Family Study. *Hypertension* 2001;38:30–37.

336. Scheinman SJ, Guay-Woodford LM, Thakker RV, et al. Genetic disorders of renal electrolyte transport. *N Engl J Med* 1999;340:1177–1187.

337. Simon DB, Karet FE, Hamdan JM, et al. Bartter's syndrome, hypokalaemic alkalosis with hypercalciuria, is caused by mutations in the Na-K-2Cl cotransporter NKCC2. *Nat Genet* 1996;13:183–188.

338. Simon DB, Karet FE, Rodriguez-Soriano J, et al. Genetic heterogeneity of Bartter's syndrome revealed by mutations in the K^+ channel, ROMK. *Nat Genet* 1996;14:152–156.

339. Simon DB, Nelson-Williams C, Bia MJ, et al. Gitelman's variant of Bartter's syndrome, inherited hypokalaemic alkalosis, is caused by mutations in the thiazide-sensitive Na-Cl cotransporter. *Nat Genet* 1996;12:24–30.

340. Chang SS, Grunder S, Hanukoglu A, et al. Mutations in subunits of the epithelial sodium channel cause salt wasting with hyperkalaemic acidosis, pseudohypoaldosteronism type 1. *Nat Genet* 1996;12:248–253.

341. Strautnieks SS, Thompson RJ, Gardiner RM, et al. A novel splice-site mutation in the g subunit of the epithelial sodium channel gene in three pseudohypoaldosteronism type 1 families. *Nat Genet* 1996;13:248–250.

342. Geller DS, Rodriguez-Soriano J, Vallo Boado A, et al. Mutations in the mineralocorticoid receptor gene cause autosomal dominant pseudohypoaldosteronism type I. *Nat Genet* 1998;19:279–281.

343. Lifton RP, Dluhy RG, Powers M, et al. A chimaeric 11ß-hydroxylase/aldosterone synthase gene causes glucocorticoid-remediable aldosteronism and human hypertension. *Nature* 1992;355:262–265.

344. Shimkets RA, Warnock DG, Bositis CM, et al. Liddle's syndrome: heritable human hypertension caused by mutations in the b subunit of the epithelial sodium channel. *Cell* 1994;79:407–414.

345. Schild L, Lu Y, Gautschi I, et al. Identification of a PY motif in the epithelial Na channel subunits as a target sequence for mutations causing channel activation found in Liddle syndrome. *EMBO J* 1996;15:2381–2387.

346. Mansfield TA, Simon DB, Farfel Z, et al. Multilocus linkage of familial hyperkalaemia and hypertension, pseudohypoaldosteronism type II, to chromosomes 1q31-42 and 17p11-q21. *Nat Genet* 1997;16:202–205.

347. Wilson FH, Disse-Nicodeme S, Choate KA, et al. Human hypertension caused by mutations in WNK kinases. *Science* 2001;293:1107–1112.

CHAPTER 14

Role of Angiotensin in the Pathobiology of Cardiovascular Disease

Victor J. Dzau and Aram V. Chobanian

Introduction	Integrated Model of Tissue Angiotensin and Vascular
Endothelium, Oxidative Stress, and Vascular Disease	Pathobiology
Direct Vascular Effects of Angiotensin II	Tissue Angiotensin-converting Enzyme and Angiotensin
Evidence for Increased Tissue Production of	as Therapeutic Targets
Angiotensin II: A Vicious Cycle	References

Key Words: Cardiovascular diseases; endothelium-derived factors; molecular biology; risk factors; vasculature.

INTRODUCTION

Evidence is increasing that direct pathobiologic events of the vessel wall play an important role in vascular disease. An important mechanism involves the perturbation of the homeostatic balance between nitric oxide (NO) and reactive oxygen species (ROS). Increased ROS can inactivate NO and produce peroxynitrite. Angiotensin II (Ang II) is a potent mediator of oxidative stress and stimulates the release of cytokines and the expression of leukocyte adhesion molecules that mediate vessel wall inflammation. Inflammatory cells release enzymes, including angiotensin-converting enzyme (ACE) that generate Ang II. Thus, a local positive feedback mechanism could be established in the vessel wall for oxidative stress, inflammation, and endothelial dysfunction. Ang II also acts as a direct growth factor for vascular smooth muscle cells and can stimulate the local production of metalloproteinases and plaminogen activator inhibitor. Taken together, Ang II can promote vasoconstriction, inflammation, thrombosis, and vascular remodeling. In this chapter, we propose a model that unifies the interrelation among cardiovascular risk factors, Ang II, and the pathobio-

logic mechanisms contributing to cardiovascular disease. This model may also explain the beneficial effects of ACE inhibitors and angiotensin II type 1 (AT-1) receptor blockade on cardiovascular events beyond blood pressure reduction.

Since its discovery a century ago, the role of the renin-angiotensin system as an endocrine system involved in blood pressure and fluid electrolyte regulation has been well established (1). Disorders of this system contribute importantly to the pathophysiology of hypertension, renal disease, and congestive heart failure. The recent discoveries of the tissue actions of Ang II have revolutionized the perception of the role of this peptide in cardiovascular disease. Evidence indicates that Ang II is more than a hormone that exerts hemodynamic and renal actions; it is also a local, biologically active mediator that has direct effects on endothelial and smooth muscle cells (2). It plays a key role in the initiation and amplification of pathobiologic events that lead to vascular disease. Indeed, clinical trials of ACE inhibitors have consistently documented the salutary effects of this class of agents in treating and preventing cardiovascular disease with impressive reductions in coronary and cerebral vascular events (3–5). Initial studies also suggest that AT-1 receptor blockade also may have a favorable effect in reducing cardiovascular events (6,7). These data suggest that ACE and angiotensin inhibition may also exert direct actions on the blood vessel beyond their hemodynamic effects. This chapter reviews the evidence for the direct tissue actions of Ang II, the cellular signaling pathways, and the interactions of Ang II with other local mediators. It is hypothesized that these tissue effects are important in the process of vascular disease and may mediate the additional

V. J. Dzau: Brigham and Women's Hospital, Department of Medicine, 75 Francis Street, Tower 1, Suite 210, Boston, Massachusetts 02115.

A. V. Chobanian: Boston University School of Medicine, 715 Albany Street, L-103, Boston, Massachusetts 02118-2394.

nonhemodynamic actions of ACE inhibitors and AT-1 receptor blockers in treating cardiovascular conditions such as coronary artery disease (CAD).

ENDOTHELIUM, OXIDATIVE STRESS, AND VASCULAR DISEASE

To understand the effect of Ang II on vascular pathobiology, the role of the endothelium must first be examined. Ang II is synthesized by and has a key action on the endothelium: It exerts direct influence on endothelial function. The endothelium is well recognized as having a pivotal role in maintaining normal vascular function and structure (8). The endothelium presents a thromboresistant surface to blood and forms a macromolecular barrier between blood and the vessel wall. Endothelial cells produce factors that regulate vessel tone, coagulation, cell growth and death, and leukocyte migration. Vascular tone is maintained by a balance between vasodilators such as NO and vasoconstrictors such as Ang II. Under the influence of the endothelium and other factors, vascular smooth muscle cells are also capable of releasing cytokines and growth regulatory factors that can influence vascular cellular phenotype and growth.

The association between endothelial dysfunction and vascular disease is well established. Endothelial dysfunction may result in increased vasoconstrictor activity. It may induce alterations in local mediators (e.g., cytokines, chemokines, and adhesion molecules) such that they favor inflammation. Endothelial dysfunction may also create an imbalance between tissue plasminogen activator (tPA) and plasminogen activator inhibitor type 1 (PAI-1) that can predispose to thrombosis.

A key determinant of endothelial biology is the cell redox state (9), and a key molecule that mediates endothelial function is NO. Evidence indicates that a homeostatic balance between NO and ROS such as superoxide anion and hydrogen peroxide regulates cell redox and is necessary for normal endothelial function. The impairment in the capacity of the vessel to dilate in the presence of endothelial dysfunction reflects, at least in part, increased oxidative stress due to an enhanced catabolism of NO caused by increased generation of superoxide anion. In addition to being a vasodilator, NO is an endogenous inhibitor of vascular smooth muscle cell growth and migration (10), activity of the transcription factor nuclear factor-kappaB (NF-κB), and expression of proinflammatory molecules (11,12). With an imbalance between NO and ROS, there is a propensity for vasospasm, smooth muscle cell proliferation, prothrombosis, and proinflammatory and prooxidant states.

The well established cardiovascular risk factors such as dyslipidemia, increased blood pressure, diabetes, and smoking can initiate endothelial dysfunction by altering the cell redox state (oxidative stress) in the vessel wall (13–18). Dyslipidemia is associated with increased generation of superoxide anions and enhanced oxidation of low-density lipoprotein (LDL) cholesterol within the vessel wall (14,15). In patients with diabetes, potentiation of atherogenesis may be related to induction of oxidative stress by advanced glycation end products (13). Cigarette smoking also induces endothelial dysfunction, as documented by an impairment of endothelium-dependent vasodilation (16,17). It has been shown that these risk factors act synergistically, worsening endothelial dysfunction (18). Indeed, an amplified effect of smoking-induced impairment of endothelial-dependent vasodilatation occurs in association with increased oxidized LDL (17).

Oxidative stress induces the expression of redox-sensitive genes for chemoattractant proteins (e.g., monocyte chemotactic protein-1 [MCP-1]) and leukocyte adhesion molecules (e.g., vascular cell and intracellular adhesion molecules). Superoxide anion may function as a signaling molecule, mediating increased activity of NF-κB that coordinates the upregulation of these proinflammatory genes (19,20). These gene products stimulate leukocyte interaction with the vessel wall and subsequent transmigration into the subintimal layer of the cell wall. Once in the vessel wall, monocytes are transformed to macrophages capable of taking up modified and oxidized LDL, thereby becoming foam cells, which constitute fatty streaks and contribute importantly to the atherothrombotic process.

DIRECT VASCULAR EFFECTS OF ANGIOTENSIN II

Ang II exerts multiple actions on the blood vessel (Table 14–1). It is a major mediator of oxidative stress and reduced NO activity. Ang II activates a powerful membrane oxidase (nicotinamide adenine dinucleotide/nicotinamide adenine dinucleotide phosphate oxidase) that results in the production of superoxide anion and, subsequently, hydrogen peroxide (21). Accordingly, Ang II induces MCP-1 messenger RNA expression in monocytes and vascular smooth muscle cells, an effect that is inhibited by coadministration of an intracellular antioxidant (22). Ang II induces endothelial dysfunction and activates the expression of proinflammatory phenotype of human vascular smooth muscle cells (23). It activates NF-κB and stimulates the expression of vascular cell adhesion molecule and the release of the cytokines interleukin-6 (24) and tumor necrosis factor-α (25). This proinflammatory action of Ang II on the vessel wall interacts synergistically with those of other cardiovascular risk factors such as dyslipidemia and diabetes.

Ang II also is involved in vascular remodeling, acting as a bifunctional growth factor that induces increased expression of autocrine growth factors (e.g., platelet-derived growth factor, basic fibroblast growth factor, insulin-like growth factor, and transforming growth factor-β_1) in vascular smooth muscle cells (26,27). Other mechanisms whereby Ang II may promote vascular remodeling and formation of vascular lesions are the modulation of vascular cell migration, decreased vascular smooth muscle apoptosis (28), and altered extracellular matrix composition (29,30). Indeed, Ang II can stimulate the synthesis and release of matrix glycoproteins and metalloproteinases. Ang II is, therefore, a

TABLE 14-1. *Direct vascular effects of angiotensin*

I. Vasoconstriction
- Directs AT-1 receptor stimulation
- Releases endothelin and norepinephrine
- Reduces nitric oxide bioactivity and produces peroxynitrite

II. Inflammation
- Activates NADH/NADPH oxidase and produces superoxide anion
- Induces expression of MCP-1, VCAM, TNF-α, and IL-6
- Activates monocytes/macrophages

III. Remodeling
- Stimulates smooth muscle migration, hypertrophy, and replication
- Induces PDGF, bFGF, IGF-1, and TGF-β expression
- Stimulates production of matrix glycoproteins and metalloproteinases

IV. Thrombosis
- Stimulates PAI-1 synthesis and alters tPA/PAI-1 ratio
- Activates platelets with increased aggregation and adhesion

AT-1, angiotensin II type 1; bFGF, basic fibroblast growth factor; IGF-1, insulin-like growth factor 1; IL-6, interleukin-6; MCP-1, monocyte chemoattractant protein-1; NADH, nicotinamide adenine dinucleotide (reduced form); NADPH, nicotinamide adenine dinucleotide phosphate; PAI-1, plasminogen activator inhibitor type 1; PDGF, platelet-derived growth factor; TGF-β, transforming growth factor-beta; TNF-α, tumor necrosis factor-alpha; tPA, tissue plasminogen activator; VCAM, vascular cell adhesion molecule.

pleiotropic local mediator of vascular remodeling and lesion formation.

Ang II also can upset the balance between the fibrinolytic and coagulation systems through its effect on the endothelium. Ang II induces formation of PAI-1 (31–34), an effect that is mediated by specific angiotensin receptors on en-dothelial cells (33). Independent of its stimulation of PAI-1 synthesis through Ang II production, tissue ACE also down-regulates tPA production through degradation of bradykinin, which is a potent stimulator of tPA production in the endothelium (35). These actions of tissue ACE(Ang II on the fibrinolytic system can enhance the development of a pro-thrombotic state.

EVIDENCE FOR INCREASED TISSUE PRODUCTION OF ANGIOTENSIN II: A VICIOUS CYCLE

High levels of ACE expression and Ang II have been shown in experimental and human vascular lesions (36–38). Indeed, ACE, Ang II, and its receptor colocalize in areas of inflammation in human atherothrombotic lesions (38). Recent data indicate that inflammatory cells can release enzymes that generate Ang II, including ACE from monocytes/macrophages (38,39), cathepsin G from neutrophils (40), and chymase from mast cells (41). Furthermore, we have reported that as macrophages become activated with modified LDL, its ACE expression increases significantly (38). This creates a positive feedback mechanism (Fig. 14–1) for local Ang II formation. Tissue ACE and Ang II produced within an atherothrombotic lesion contribute to high local levels of Ang II, which when activating Ang II receptors on different cell types, lead to progressive lesion formation through proliferation of smooth muscle cells, formation of foam cells, and facilitation of thrombosis. Notably, we have reported a marked accumulation of tissue ACE and Ang II in the inflamed shoulder regions of vulnerable plaques that are prone to rupture (38). It is attractive to hypothesize that the increased production of ACE and Ang II contributes to this process of acute ischemic complication. In addition to its effects on inflammation and vascu-

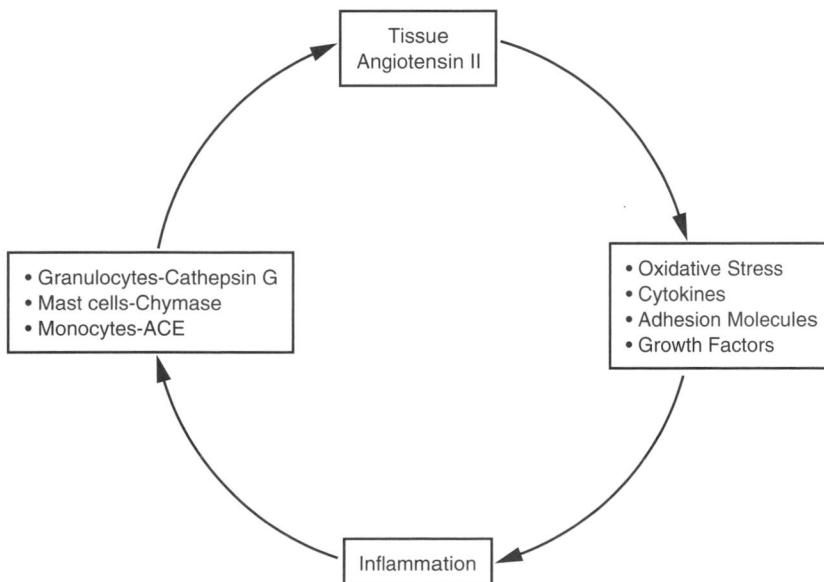

FIG. 14-1. Activation of tissue angiotensin-converting enzyme (ACE) creates a positive feedback mechanism for tissue angiotensin II formation with subsequent induction of oxidative stress and inflammation. Activation of tissue ACE promotes release of cytokines and growth factors that increase vessel wall inflammation. Inflammatory cells, in turn, release enzymes and other substances that generate angiotensin II. (Reproduced with permission from V. J. Dzau.)

lar contraction, local Ang II stimulates metalloproteinases (29,42) that can break down extracellular matrix, weakening this vulnerable region that is subject to increased circumferential stress (43), and thus enhancing the probability of rupture.

INTEGRATED MODEL OF TISSUE ANGIOTENSIN AND VASCULAR PATHOBIOLOGY

The effects of many of the biologically active mediators produced in the vessel wall are long-term, reflecting the progressive nature of vascular disease. In this chapter, we propose a model that integrates the complex interrelation of tissue ACE and Ang II with the various biologically active mediators, cardiovascular risk factors, and pathobiologic mechanisms that contribute to the vascular disease process (Fig. 14–2). In this paradigm, a common mechanism by which cardiovascular risk factors initiate the disease process is oxidative stress leading to endothelial dysfunction and vascular inflammation. The latter pathways increase local ACE and Ang II production. Thus, a positive feedback mechanism involving increased tissue Ang II and decreased NO production exists in vascular pathology, in which Ang II acts as a direct mediator and an amplifier. Through its acti-

vation of oxidative stress, local Ang II magnifies endothelial dysfunction and smooth muscle phenotypic alterations induced by cardiovascular risk factors and serves as a vicious positive amplification mechanism for decreased NO, increased ROS, and the activation of other biologically active mediators for vascular disease. Thus, through its direct tissue effects, increased tissue Ang II activates various pathobiologic processes that lead to vascular complications.

In addition, other potentially important interactions may occur between angiotensin and LDL, which may amplify their adverse effects. Incubation of cultured rat aortic smooth muscle cells with human LDL has been reported to cause a marker increase in AT-1 receptor expression (44), and aortic rings from hypercholesterolemic rabbits demonstrated exaggerated contractile responses to Ang II (45). In addition, in a double transgenic model of malignant hypertension in which human renin and angiotensinogen genes are overexpressed, the cholesterol decreasing drug, cervastatin, surprisingly reduced blood pressure, decreased cardiac and renal injury, and markedly improved life span, suggesting diminishment in the adverse effects of Ang II (46). Furthermore, patients with hypercholesterolemia appear to have increased blood pressure responses to infused Ang II

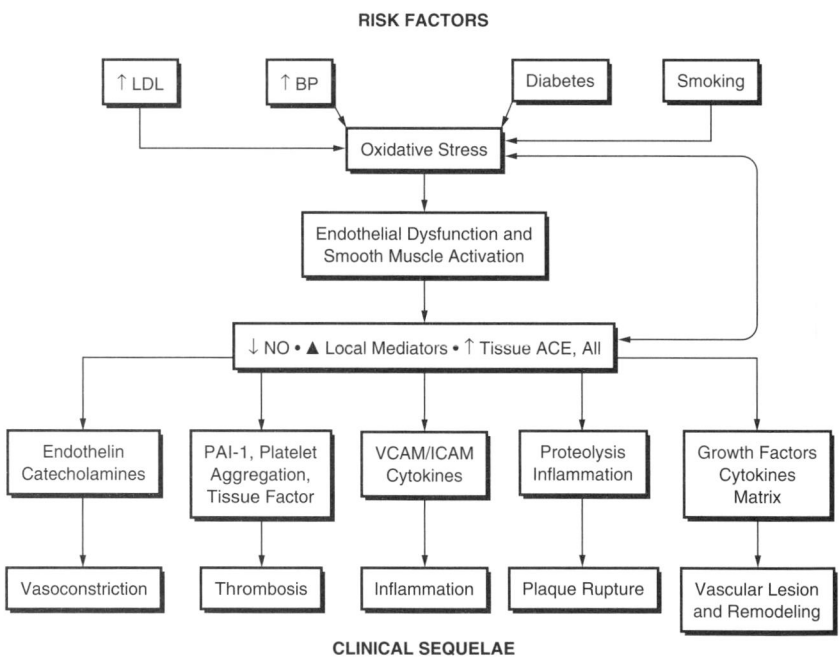

FIG. 14-2. Proposed model that integrates the role of angiotensin II in the complex pathobiologic processes that occur in the development and progression of vascular disease. Central to the pathogenesis of cardiovascular disease is oxidative stress and endothelial dysfunction, which alters the normal homeostatic balance maintained by the endothelium. ACE, angiotensin-converting enzyme; BP, blood pressure; ICAM, intracellular adhesion molecule; LDL, low-density lipoprotein; NO, nitric oxide; PAI-1, platelet activator inhibitor type 1; VCAM, vascular cell adhesion molecule.(Reproduced with permission from V. J. Dzau.)

and increased platelet AT-1 receptor expression when compared with normocholesterolemic subjects (47), and treatment of the patients with hypercholesterolemia with statin drugs reduced both the angiotensin pressor responses and AT-1 receptor expression to control levels.

TISSUE ANGIOTENSIN-CONVERTING ENZYME AND ANGIOTENSIN AS THERAPEUTIC TARGETS

Therapeutic strategies for cardiovascular disease would include antioxidants, antiinflammatory agents, agents that enhance NO activity, and agents that reduce Ang II. In this context, an important therapeutic target is tissue ACE, which has multiple actions. Inhibition of tissue ACE not only reduces Ang II, oxidative stress, and Ang II–induced inflammatory states, but it also increases bradykinin formation; this increases NO and prostacylin, which also exert antiinflammatory, antithrombotic, and vasorelaxant actions.

Evidence from experimental (48) and clinical (49–51) trials supports the role of direct vascular effects of tissue ACE and angiotensin inhibition. ACE inhibitors have been shown to reduce the development of atherosclerosis in several hypercholesterolemic animal models (52–56). More recently, AT-1 receptor antagonists have been reported to inhibit atherogenesis (57–60). In the Watanabe heritable hyperlipidemic rabbit, the effects were almost identical (58) when the ACE inhibitor, trandolapril, was compared with the AT-1 antagonist, irbesartan. A direct vascular effect of angiotensin inhibition also has been suggested in clinical studies. The Trial on Reversing Endothelial Dysfunction (TREND study) demonstrated that 6 months of treatment with the tissue ACE inhibitor quinapril normalized endothelial function in patients with CAD, as evidenced by a reversal of the paradoxic vasoconstriction caused by intracoronary administration of acetylcholine (49). In another study, improvement in forearm vasodilation was noted after 6 months of treatment with lisinopril in patients with hyperlipidemia (50). Enalaprilat also has been shown to improve acetylcholine- and bradykinin-mediated epicardial and microvascular dilation in patients with CAD or its risk factors, or both (51).

ACE inhibition has emerged as an important therapeutic modality for cardiovascular disease. In addition to hypertension and congestive heart failure, ACE inhibitors are now shown to be effective for treatment of coronary heart disease. Studies of ACE inhibitor administration in patients with left ventricular dysfunction after myocardial infarction (MI) demonstrated that ACE inhibitor treatment was associated with significant reductions in risk for recurrent MI. The risk reduction was approximately 24% in the Studies of Left Ventricular Dysfunction (SOLVD) (4,61,62) and Survival and Ventricular Enlargement (SAVE) (3) trials and approximately 37% in the Survival of Myocardial Infarction Long-term Evaluation (SMILE) study (63), as well as with a 25% reduction in sudden death in the Trandolapril Cardiac Evaluation (TRACE) (64). Several long-term clinical trials were

initiated to evaluate the potential clinical benefits of ACE inhibition in patients with CAD *without* left ventricular dysfunction: the Quinapril Ischemic Events Trial (QUIET) (65,66), Heart Outcomes Prevention Evaluation (HOPE) (3), Antihypertensive and Lipid-Lowering Treatment to Prevent Heart Attack Trial (ALLHAT) (67), Prevention of Events with Angiotensin-Converting Enzyme Inhibition (PEACE) (68), and the European Trial on Reduction of Cardiac Events with Perindopril in Stable Coronary Artery Disease (EUROPA) (69). Of these, the QUIET and HOPE studies have been completed. Results of QUIET were neutral with respect to the effect on cardiac ischemic end points of ACE inhibition initiated within 72 hours of revascularization (66). This outcome may have been due, in part, to its being a small study (1,750 patients) of relatively brief duration (3 years) with an enrollment of a relatively lower risk patient population (i.e., normal LDL cholesterol and normal body mass index).

The HOPE study, which evaluated ramipril, provides compelling data regarding the beneficial effects of ACE inhibition on cardiovascular morbidity and mortality (3). The study followed 9,297 high-risk patients who had evidence of vascular disease or diabetes plus one other cardiovascular risk factor but who did not have a low ejection fraction or heart failure. The planned 5-year treatment period was terminated early because of the significant, and much greater than anticipated, effect of ACE inhibition on the composite primary outcome of MI, stroke, or death from cardiovascular causes (22% greater reduction with ramipril compared with placebo), as well as significantly greater reductions in the individual end points (MI, 20%; stroke, 31%; death from cardiovascular causes, 25%). In addition, significant reductions in all-cause mortality (relative risk [RR], 0.84), need for revascularization procedures (RR, 0.84), cardiac arrest (RR, 0.63), heart failure (RR, 0.77), worsening angina (RR, 0.89), and new diagnosis of diabetes (RR, 0.68) or complications related to diabetes (RR, 0.84) were observed. ACE inhibitor treatment demonstrated beneficial effects within 1 year, which were significant at 2 years. The favorable effects of treatment were noted in all subgroups, including those with/without diabetes, hypertension, microalbuminuria, CAD, or history of MI; men and women; and those older/younger than 65 years. The findings from the HOPE study indicate that a broad spectrum of patients potentially can derive additional benefit from ACE inhibitor treatment. The blood pressure reduction effect of ACE inhibition was modest and could not account completely for the risk reductions observed in HOPE. As the investigators noted, "it is likely that angiotensin-converting-enzyme inhibitors exert additional direct mechanisms on the heart or the vasculature that are important" (3).

Another trial of patients with hypertension at high risk for cardiovascular complications was the LIFE study, which compared the long-term effects of losartan and atenolol in 9,173 individuals with blood pressure in the 160 to 200/95 to 115 mm Hg range and electrocardiogram-documented left ventricular hypertrophy (6). Despite comparable degrees of blood pressure reduction in the two treatment groups, the subjects treated with losartan had significantly lower rates in total primary outcomes of death, MI, and stroke (risk ration 0.87) as compared with the atenolol-treated group. The findings again indicate that the beneficial effects of angiotensin blockade are at least in part independent of blood pressure reduction. In subjects with diabetes, the rate of primary outcomes with losartan was 24% less in the lasartan than in the atenolol group (7). In addition, the incidence of new-onset diabetes was 25% less with losartan, which is somewhat similar to the reduction observed in the HOPE study with ramipril.

The studies assessing the effect of ACE inhibitors and AT-1 receptor antagonists on clinical outcomes in patients with CAD support the body of experimental evidence indicating that locally generated vasoactive mediator substances like NO and Ang II are important determinants in the progression of vascular disease and that restoring the local balance of these mediators is an important therapeutic goal. As therapeutic strategy, inhibiting ACE and angiotensin appears to be an effective target for preventing premature death, MI, and stroke in patients at high risk for vascular disease. In summary, advances in renin angiotensin research have improved our understanding of the role of this system in cardiovascular pathobiology and have validated its importance as a target for pharmacologic inhibition.

REFERENCES

1. Oparil S, Haber E. The renin-angiotensin system. *N Engl J Med* 1974;291:381–401,446–457.
2. Reference deleted in proofs.
3. Yusuf S, Sleight P, Pogue J, et al. Effects of an angiotensin-converting enzyme inhibitor, ramipril, on cardiovascular events in high-risk patients. The Heart Outcomes Prevention Evaluation Study Investigators. *N Engl J Med* 2000;342:145–153.
4. Yusuf S, Pepine CJ, Garces C, et al. Effect of enalapril on myocardial infarction and unstable angina in patients with low ejection fractions. *Lancet* 1992;430:1173–1178.
5. Pfeffer MA, Braunwald E, Moyé LA, et al., on behalf of the SAVE Investigators. Effect of captopril on mortality and morbidity in patients with left ventricular dysfunction after myocardial infarction: results of the Survival and Ventricular Enlargement Trial. *N Engl J Med* 1992;327:669–677.
6. Dahlof B, Devereux RB, Kjeldsen SE, et al. Cardiovascular morbidity and mortality in the Losartan Intervention for Endpoint Reduction in hypertension study (LIFE): a randomized trial against atenolol. *Lancet* 2002;359:995–1003.
7. Lindholm LH, Ibsen H, Daholf B, et al. Cardiovascular morbidity and mortality in patients with diabetes in the Losartan Intervention for Endpoint Reduction in hypertension study (LIFE): a randomized trial against atenolol. *Lancet* 2002;359:1004–1110.
8. Gibbons GH, Dzau VJ. The emerging concept of vascular remodeling. *N Engl J Med* 1992;327:669–677.
9. Alexander RW. Oxidative stress and the mediation of arterial inflammatory response: a new perspective. *Hypertension* 1995;25:155–161.
10. Dubey RK, Jackson EK, Lüscher TF. Nitric oxide inhibits angiotensin II-induced migration of rat aortic smooth muscle cell: role of cyclic-nucleotides and angiotensin 1 receptors. *J Clin Invest* 1995;96:141–149.
11. Peng HB, Libby P, Liao JK. Induction and stabilization of 1 kappa B alpha by nitric oxide mediates inhibition of NF-kappa B. *J Biol Chem* 1995;270:14214–14219.
12. De Caterina R, Libby P, Peng HB, et al. Nitric oxide decreases cytokine-induced endothelial activation. Nitric oxide selectively reduces endothelial expression of adhesion molecules and proinflammatory cytokines. *J Clin Invest* 1995;96:60–68.
13. Schmidt AM, Hori O, Chen JX, et al. Advanced glycation endproducts interacting with their endothelial receptor induce expression of vascular cell adhesion molecule-1 (VCAM-1) in cultured human endothelial cells and in mice: a potential mechanism for the accelerated vasculopathy of diabetes. *J Clin Invest* 1995;95:1395–1403.
14. Ohara Y, Peterson TE, Sayegh HS, et al. Dietary correction of hypercholesterolemia in the rabbit normalized endothelial superoxide anion production. *Circulation* 1995;92:898–903.
15. Steinberg D. Role of oxidized LDL and antioxidants in atherosclerosis. *Adv Exp Med Biol* 1995;369:39–48.
16. Celermajer DS, Sorensen KE, Georgakopoulos D, et al. Cigarette smoking is associated with dose-related and potentially reversible impairment of endothelium-dependent dilation in healthy young adults. *Circulation* 1993;88:2149–2155.
17. Heitzer T, Ylä-Herttuala S, Luoma J, et al. Cigarette smoking potentiates endothelial dysfunction of forearm resistance vessels in patients with hypercholesterolemia: role of oxidized LDL. *Circulation* 1996;93:1346–1353.
18. Vita JA, Treasure CB, Nabel EG, et al. Coronary vasomotor response to acetylcholine relates to risk factors for coronary artery disease. *Circulation* 1990;81:491–497.
19. Marui N, Offermann MK, Swerlick R, et al. Vascular cell adhesion molecule-1 (VCAM-1) gene transcription and expression are regulated through an antioxidant-sensitive mechanism in human vascular endothelial cells. *J Clin Invest* 1993;92:1866–1874.
20. Collins T, Read MA, Neish AS, et al. Transcriptional regulation of endothelial cell adhesion molecules: NF-kappa B and cytokine-inducible enhancers. *FASEB J* 1995;9:899–909.
21. Griendling KK, Minieri CA, Ollerenshaw JD, et al. Angiotensin II stimulates NADH and NADPH oxidase activity in cultured vascular smooth muscle cells. *Circ Res* 1994;74:1141–1148.
22. Hernández-Presa M, Bustos C, Ortego M, et al. Angiotensin-converting enzyme inhibition prevents arterial nuclear factor-kB activation, monocyte chemoattractant protein-1 expression, and macrophage infiltration in a rabbit model of early accelerated atherosclerosis. *Circulation* 1997;95:1532–1541.
23. Kranzhöfer R, Schmidt J, Pfeiffer CAH, et al. Angiotensin induces inflammatory activation of human vascular smooth muscle cells. *Arterioscler Thromb Vasc Biol* 1999;19:1623–1629.
24. Han Y, Runge MS, Brasier AR. Angiotensin II induces interleuken-6 transcription in vascular smooth muscle cells through pleiotropic activation of nuclear factor-kappa B transcription factors. *Circ Res* 1999;84:695–703.
25. Hahn AW, Jonas U, Buhler FR, et al. Activation of human peripheral monocytes by angiotensin II. *FEBS Lett* 1994;347:178–180.
26. Naftilan AJ, Pratt RE, Dzau VJ. Induction of PDGF A-chain and c-myc gene expression by angiotensin II in vascular smooth muscle cells. *J Clin Invest* 1989;83:1419–1424.
27. Itoh H, Mukoyama M, Pratt RE, et al. Multiple autocrine growth factors modulate vascular smooth muscle cell growth response to angiotensin II. *J Clin Invest* 1993;91:2268–2274.
28. Pollman MJ, Yamada T, Horiuchi M, et al. Vasoactive substances regulate vascular smooth muscle cell apoptosis: countervailing influences of nitric oxide and angiotensin II. *Circ Res* 1996;79:748–756.
29. Takagishi T, Murahashi N, Azagami S, et al. Effect of angiotensin II and thromboxane A2 on the production of matrix metalloproteinase by human aortic smooth muscle cells. *Biochem Mol Biol Int* 1995;35:265–273.
30. Scott-Burden ST, Mackie EJ, Buhler FR. Angiotensin II induction of smooth muscle matrix synthesis in culture. *J Vasc Med Biol* 1991;3:271–276.
31. Vaughan DE, Lazos SA, Tong K. Angiotensin II regulates the expression of plasminogen activator inhibitor-1 in cultured endothelial cells. *J Clin Invest* 1995;95:995–1001.
32. Ridker PM, Gaboury CL, Conlin PR, et al. Stimulation of plasminogen activator inhibitor in vivo by infusion of angiotensin II: evidence of a potential interaction between the renin-angiotensin system and fibrinolytic function. *Circulation* 1993;87:1969–1973.
33. Kerins DM, Hao Q, Vaughan DE. Angiotensin induction of PAI-1 expression in endothelial cells is mediated by the hexapeptide angiotensin IV. *J Clin Invest* 1995;96:2515–2520.

34. Van Leeuwen RT, Kol A, Andreotti F, et al. Angiotensin II increases plasminogen activator inhibitor type 1 and tissue-type plasminogen activator messenger RNA in cultured rat aortic smooth muscle cells. *Circulation* 1994;90:362–368.

35. Oikawa T, Freeman M, Lo W, et al. Modulation of plasminogen activator inhibitor-1 in vivo: a new mechanism for the anti-fibrotic effect of renin-angiotensin inhibition. *Kidney Int* 1997;51:164–172.

36. Rakugi H, Kim DK, Krieger JE, et al. Induction of angiotensin converting enzyme in the neointima after vascular injury. Possible role in restenosis. *J Clin Invest* 1994;90:449–455.

37. Rakugi H, Wang D, Dzau VJ, et al. Potential importance of tissue angiotensin converting enzyme inhibition in preventing neointima formation. *Circulation* 1994;90:449–455.

38. Diet F, Pratt RE, Berry GJ, et al. Increased accumulation of tissue ACE in human atherosclerotic coronary artery disease. *Circulation* 1996;94:2756–2767.

39. Kitazono T, Padgett RC, Armstrong ML, et al. Evidence that angiotensin II is present in human monocytes. *Circulation* 1995;91:1129–1134.

40. Snyder RA, Kaempfer CE, Wintroub BU. Chemistry of a human monocyte-derived cell line (U937): identification of the angiotensin 1-converting activity as leukocyte cathepsin G. *Blood* 1985;65:176–182.

41. Kinoshita A, Urata H, Bumpus M, et al. Multiple determinants for the high substrate specificity of an angiotensin II-forming chymase from the human heart. *J Biol Chem* 1991;266:19192–19197.

42. Rouet-Benzineb P, Gontero B, Dreyfus P, et al. Angiotensin II induces nuclear factor-kappa B activation in cultured neonatal rat cardiomyocytes through protein kinase C signaling pathway. *J Mol Cell Cardiol* 2000;32:1767–1778.

43. Lee RT, Schoen FJ, Loree HM, et al. Circumferential stress and matrix metalloproteinase 1 in human coronary atherosclerosis: implications for plaque rupture. *Arterioscler Thromb Vasc Biol* 1996;16:1070–1073.

44. Nickenig G, Sachinidis A, Michaelson F, et al. Upregulation of vascular angiotensin II receptor gene expression by low density lipoprotein in vascular smooth muscle cells. *Circulation* 1997;95:473–478.

45. Yang BC, Phillips I, Mohuczy D, et al. Increased angiotensin II type 1 receptor expression in hypercholesterolemic atherosclerosis in rabbits. *Arteriocler Thromb Vasc Biol* 1998;18:1433–1439.

46. Dechend R, Fiebler A, Lindschau C, et al. Modulating angiotensin II-induced inflammation by HMG-CoA reductase inhibition. *Am J Hypertens* 2001;14:55S–61S.

47. Nickenig G, Baumer AT, Temur Y, et al. Statin-sensitive dysregulated AT-I receptor function and density in hypercholesterolemic men. *Circulation* 1999;100:2131–2134.

48. Finta KM, Fischer MJ, Lee L, et al. Ramipril prevents endothelium-dependent relaxation in arteries from rabbits fed an atherogenic diet. *Atherosclerosis* 1993;100:149–156.

49. Mancini GB, Henry GC, Macaya C, et al. Angiotensin-converting enzyme inhibition with quinapril improves endothelial vasomotor dysfunction in patients with coronary artery disease: the TREND (Trial on Reversing Endothelial Dysfunction) Study. *Circulation* 1996;94:258–265.

50. Lee AF, Dick JB, Struthers AD. Can lisinopril improve endothelial function in hyperlipidaemics? *J Am Coll Cardiol* 1997;29:46A(abst).

51. Prasad A, Husain S, Mincemoyer R, et al. Coronary endothelial dysfunction in humans improves with angiotensin converting enzyme inhibition. *Circulation* 1996;94[Suppl I]:I-61(abst).

52. Chobanian AV, Haudenchild CC, Nickerson C, et al. Anti-atherogenic effect of captopril in the Watanabe Heritable Hyperlipidemic Rabbit. *Hypertension* 1990;15:327–331.

53. Hernandez A, Barberi L, Ballerio R, et al. Delapril slows the progression of atherosclerosis and maintains endothelial function in cholesterol-fed rabbits. *Atherosclerosis* 1998;137:71–76.

54. Aberg G, Ferrer P. Effects of captopril on atherosclerosis in cynomolgus monkeys. *J Cardiovasc Pharmacol* 1990;15:S65–S72.

55. Kowala MC, Grove RI, Aberg G. Inhibitors of angiotensin-converting enzyme decrease early atherosclerosis in hyperlipidemic hamsters. Fosinopril reduces plasma cholesterol and captopril inhibits macrophage-foam cell accumulation, independently of blood pressure and plasma lipids. *Atherosclerosis* 1994;108:61–72.

56. Charpiot P, Rolland PH, Friggi A, et al. ACE inhibition with perindopril and atherogenesis-induced structural and functional changes in minipig arteries. *Arteriocler Thromb* 1993;13:1125–1138.

57. Keider S, Attias J, Smith J, et al. The angiotensin-II receptor antagonist, losartan, inhibits LDL lipid peroxidation and atherosclerosis in apolipoprotein E-deficient mice. *Biochem Biophys Res Comm* 1997;236.622–625.

58. Hope S, Brecher P, Chobanian AV. Comparison of the effects of AT-I receptor blockade and angiotensin converting enzyme inhibition on atherosclerosis. *Am J Hypertens* 1999;12:28–34.

59. Makaritsis KP, Gavras H, Du Y, et al. Alpha 1-adrenergic receptor blockade reduces atherosclerosis in apolipoprotein E-deficient mice. *Hypertension* 1998;32:1044–1048.

60. Strawn WB, Chappell MC, Dean RH, et al. Inhibition of early atherogenesis by losartan in monkeys with diet-induced hypercholesterolemia. *Circulation* 2000;101:1586–1593.

61. Effect of enalapril on survival in patients with reduced left ventricular ejection fractions and congestive heart failure. The SOLVD Investigators. *N Engl J Med* 1991;325:293–301.

62. Effect of enalapril on mortality and the development of heart failure in asymptomatic patients with reduced left ventricular ejection fractions. The SOLVD Investigators. *N Engl J Med* 1992;327:685–691.

63. Ambrosioni E, Borghi C, Magnani B. The effect of the angiotensin-converting enzyme inhibitor zofenopril on mortality and morbidity after anterior myocardial infarction: the Survival of Myocardial Infarction Long-term Evaluation (SMILE) Study. *N Engl J Med* 1995;332:80–85.

64. Køber L, Torp-Pederson C, Carlsen J, et al., for the Trandolapril Cardiac Evaluation (TRACE) Study Group. A clinical trial of the angiotensin-converting-enzyme inhibitor trandolapril in patients with left ventricular dysfunction after myocardial infarction. *N Engl J Med* 1995;333:1670–1676.

65. Texter M, Lees RS, Pitt B, et al. The QUinapril Ischemic Event Trial (QUIET) design and methods: evaluation of chronic ACE inhibitor therapy after coronary artery intervention. *Cardiovasc Drugs Ther* 1993;7:273–282.

66. Cashin-Hemphill L, Holmvang G, Chan RC, et al., for the QUIET Investigators. Angiotensin-converting enzyme inhibition as antiatherosclerotic therapy: no answer yet. *Am J Cardiol* 1999;83:43–47.

67. Davis BR, Cutler JA, Gordon DJ, et al., for the ALLHAT Research Group. Rationale and design for the Antihypertensive and Lipid Lowering Treatment to Prevent Heart Attack Trial (ALLHAT). *Am J Hypertens* 1996;9:342–360.

68. Pfeffer MA, Domanski M, Rosenberg Y, et al. Prevention of events with angiotensin-converting enzyme inhibition (the PEACE study design). *Am J Cardiol* 1998;82[Suppl 3A]:25H–30H.

69. Fox KM, Henderson JR, Bertrand ME, et al. The European trial on reduction of cardiac events with perindopril in stable coronary artery disease (EUROPA). *Eur Heart J* 1998;29[Suppl J]:J52–J55.

CHAPTER 15

Clinical Classifications of Hypertensive Diseases

Edward D. Frohlich

Key Words: α-Adrenergic receptor blockers; angiotensin-converting enzyme inhibitors; antihypertensive therapy; β-adrenergic receptor blockers; calcium antagonists; diuretics; essential hypertension; hypertension, diagnostic evaluation; hypertension, pathophysiology; hypertension, target organ involvement; left ventricular hypertrophy; pressor mechanisms.

INTRODUCTION

Systemic arterial hypertension is one of the most common cardiovascular diseases in industrialized societies. More than 43 million individuals in the United States have systemic arterial hypertension, and it occurs with increasing prevalence with aging. Furthermore, the disease is a major risk factor underlying coronary heart disease, it exacerbates the atherothrombotic disease process, and it frequently is associated with obesity or diabetes mellitus.

In this chapter, several hypertensive diseases are discussed in terms of a series of classifications. The large number of pressor and depressor mechanisms that maintain arterial pressure in the healthy individual are discussed. This concept is then extended to an etiologic classification of the various primary and secondary forms of hypertensive disease by indicating the interrelations of these factors that participate multifactorially and pathophysiologically in these diseases and how they are also brought into play with anti-

hypertensive treatment. The discussion continues by considering the classification of hypertensive disease according to severity of arterial pressure increase, as well as with respect to suppressing intraorgan mechanisms as related to target organ involvement of the diseases.

The final aspect of this chapter considers a classification of antihypertensive therapy and how this is related to the recent recommendations for antihypertensive therapy by the sixth report of the Joint National Committee (JNC-VI). This discussion is not restricted to a single algorithm for therapy; it also considers how treatment can be modified when complicating factors of disease (including comorbidity) are considered through a rational approach to individualization of drug therapy.

HYPERTENSION: A MULTIFACTORIAL DISEASE

As presented in this discussion of the classifications of hypertensive disease, the fundamental considerations underlying the hypertensive diseases continue to expand dramatically. Specific genetic mechanisms are being elucidated in experimental forms of naturally developing hypertension. Notably, the first reports of the specific genes involved in clinical hypertension are currently beginning to be identified. In addition to these fundamental factors, experimental and clinical studies have identified new biologic mechanisms that participate importantly in the various expressions of the hypertensive diseases. These mechanisms involve local growth factors, hormones, and peptides in vessels, heart, kidney, and brain and their roles in controlling or increasing arterial pressure, in producing arteriolar thickening and ventricular hypertrophy, and in promot-

E. D. Frohlich: Departments of Medicine and Physiology, Louisiana State University; Departments of Medicine and Pharmacology, Tulane University; and Alton Ochsner Medical Foundation, New Orleans, Louisiana 70121.

ing glomerular hyperfiltration and possibly hypertensive renal disease. Of particular importance is that these local mechanisms participate in organ dysfunction, even independently of the height of arterial pressure. In addition, some of these local growth factors also have been implicated in the atherogenic process and, hence, may open a way to a clearer understanding of the interrelation between hypertension and atherothrombosis, as one disease exacerbates the other. Finally, these new considerations no doubt will make possible the consideration of innovative modes of therapy involving some of the new local factors (e.g., endothelin, atrial natriuretic factor, peptides, and their antagonists), agonists and antagonists of membrane channel receptors, intracellular regulators, and even gene therapy in hypertension.

Over the years, new concepts of the pathogenesis and treatment of hypertension have provided mind-boggling extrapolations to other cardiovascular diseases. Consider, for example, the concepts of "unloading" the heart with ganglion-blocking therapy, vasodilators and angiotensin-converting enzyme (ACE) inhibitors, control of intravascular (i.e., plasma) volume, adrenergic receptor blockade, inhibition of the renin-angiotensin system, development and reversal of ventricular hypertrophy, and prevention of further deterioration of renal function in diabetes mellitus. With this record of successes and the anticipated innovations suggested earlier, the future for further understanding of hypertension and its relations with other cardiovascular diseases is truly exciting.

REGULATION OF BLOOD PRESSURE AND HYPERTENSION

Most workers in the field of hypertension have come to appreciate the concept that the control of arterial pressure is multifactorial (1,2). Thus, increase of arterial pressure, even when specific causes can be identified, is amplified through the interaction of physiologic pressor and depressor factors (Fig. 15–1) (3,4). This concept is most clearly evidenced in patients with the most common clinical expression of systemic arterial hypertension: essential hypertension. This primary form of hypertension occurs in more than 90% of patients with abnormally increased arterial pressure. Thus, despite the more obvious or apparent participation of perhaps only a few specific pressor mechanisms in certain patients, the interrelation that exists among those pressor mechanisms means that other possibilities exist whereby the increased pressure may be expressed clinically in those affected patients. This becomes most evident and important clinically when antihypertensive therapy is prescribed, because reduction of the increased pressure brings into play a variety of additional physiologically adaptive systemic homeostatic responses, even though pressure was abnormally increased at the outset.

This "mosaic" concept, introduced by Page (1) more than 50 years ago, emphasizes the multifactorial causation of increased arterial pressure in hypertension and has been supported clinically by observations that the disease is frequently associated with familial (i.e., hereditable) predispositions that may be associated with other abnormalities that also have a familial or genetic predisposition. Among these other comorbid conditions are exogenous obesity, enhanced sodium sensitivity, carbohydrate intolerance and diabetes mellitus, hyperuricemia and gout, hypercholesterolemia and other hyperlipidemias, and, of course, accelerated atherosclerogenesis with occlusive coronary artery disease, stroke, sudden death, and renal functional impairment (5). More recently, this pathophysiologic multifactorial concept has been reinforced by the

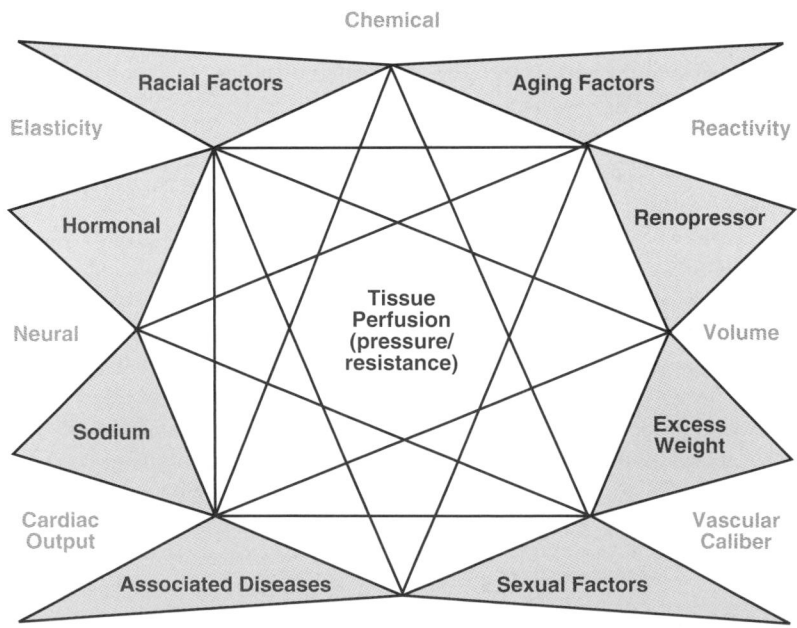

FIG. 15–1. Mosaic. (From Frohlich ED. The first Irvine H. Page lecture: the mosaic of hypertension; past, present, and future. *J Hypertens* 1988;6[Suppl 4]:2–11, with permission.)

demonstration of a number of genetic alterations that also have been associated with hypertension (6). Thus, hypertension does not seem to be based solely on one or even two genetic abnormalities, but rather is considered to be polygenetic in basis with facilitated expression of certain alterations of gene function by environmental factors (e.g., excess sodium intake). Moreover, some of these genetic alterations have been associated with specific pressor and depressor mechanisms, so that there is great likelihood of interrelations between altered genotype and phenotype in patients with hypertension. For example, one report relates development of left ventricular hypertrophy to the DD genotype of the ACE or angiotensinogen genes in middle-aged men (7).

PATHOPHYSIOLOGIC MECHANISMS

Because of the foregoing concept concerning the pathogenesis of hypertensive diseases, in this chapter hypertension is considered from a pathophysiologic viewpoint and then by a more traditional etiologic means of disease. This is followed by a more recent approach of staging the severity of hypertensive disease, then by a more pragmatic clinical functional approach, and, finally, with a therapeutic classification taking into consideration the "wedding" of pathophysiologic mechanisms with mechanisms of drug action.

Control of arterial pressure is subserved through a large number of pressor and depressor mechanisms in normotensive and hypertensive individuals (Table 15–1) (8,9). As has been indicated, these were initially termed by Page as a "mosaic" of factors that interrelate with each other in a more or less kaleidoscopic fashion to maintain normal tissue perfusion in response to systemic arteriolar constriction, but at the "expense" of the abnormally increased pressure (1,4). In any individual with hypertension, the seeming participation of any single factor naturally impacts on the participation of and, hence, interaction with many others. For example, in what might appear to be a straightforward mechanism for increasing arterial pressure by means of a mechanical obstruction to the forward flow of blood by a coarctation of the aorta, a variety of other factors also can participate in the pathophysiologic problem. Thus, if the coarctation is above the renal arteries, renal ischemic changes might result so that the intrarenal angiotensin system is secondarily stimulated through the release of renin from the juxtaglomerular apparatus. Should this be severe enough, secondary hyperaldosteronism may also result through the generation of angiotensin II, which, in turn, stimulates aldosterone release from the adrenal cortex. This, in turn, would result in the development of hypokalemic alkalosis and additional associated electrolytic and metabolic changes. In addition, experimental work suggests that the increased aldosterone may promote intraorgan fibrosis (*vide infra*). Furthermore, even when the coarctation is repaired surgically, during the immediate postoperative period there may be a precipitous increase in arterial pressure, which frequently is controlled by sympathetic

TABLE 15–1. *Pressor and depressor mechanisms involved in hypertension*

1. Mechanical
2. Neural
   a. Adrenergic, parasympathetic
   b. Central, peripheral
3. Catecholamines
   a. Norepinephrine
   b. Epinephrine
   c. Dopamine
4. Renopressor (i.e., renin-angiotensin) system
5. Renal
   a. Sodium
   b. Other ions (e.g., potassium, magnesium, calcium, chloride)
   c. Water and fluid balance
6. Hormonal
   a. Thyroid
   b. Parathyroid
   c. Growth
   d. Adrenal cortical (e.g., cortisol, aldosterone)
   e. Vasopressin
   f. "Third factor" (i.e., ouabain)
   g. Erythropoietin
7. Peptides and growth factors
   a. Atrial natriuretic factor
   b. Endothelin
   c. Insulin
   d. Vasoactive intestinal polypeptide
   e. Protooncogenes
   f. Growth factors (e.g., platelet-derived growth factor, β-transforming growth factor, insulin-derived growth factors)
   g. Endothelial-derived relaxing (nitric oxide) and constriction factors
   h. Many others
8. Volume
   a. Renal factors
   b. Electrolytic (e.g., sodium)
   c. Humoral control (e.g., antidiuretic hormone, atrial natriuretic factor, "third factor")
9. Serotonin
10. Depressor factors
    a. Histamine
    b. Kinins
    c. Prostaglandins
    d. Renal neutral medullary phospholipid

From Frohlich ED. Current approaches in the treatment of hypertension. *Curr Prob Cardiol* 1994;19:399–469; and Frohlich ED. *Hypertension: evaluation and treatment.* Philadelphia: Lippincott Williams & Wilkins, 1998, with permission.

blockade. This suggests the possible provocation of an augmented sympathetic discharge as the baroreceptors sense the sudden reduction of arterial pressure that is associated with the repair of the coarctation.

As another example of the participation of a multiplicity of pressor mechanisms in causation of hypertension, consider the patient with occlusive renal arterial disease. In this patient, arterial pressure is increased by the release of renin from the renal juxtaglomerular apparatus as a consequence of the reduced renal blood flow, renal baroreceptor stimulation, and other intrarenal factors. In addition, consequences of the increased circulating level of angiotensin II include release of aldosterone from the adrenal cortex, possibly an initial release of catecholamines from the adrenal medulla, secondary enhanced adrenergic outflow from specific cardiovascular medullary centers in the brain, stimulation of specific central thirst-promoting centers, and a contracted plasma volume as a result of postcapillary venoconstriction and a pressure natriuresis by the kidney. Accompanying this secondary hyperaldosteronism are hypokalemic alkalosis, hypomagnesemia, hypercalcemia and, perhaps, intraorgan fibrosis. Not only does each of these mechanisms interact in the patient with hypertension and with hemodynamically significant renal arterial disease, local autocrine/paracrine mechanisms (involving the kinin, prostaglandin, endothelin, and perhaps other systems) come into play within the kidney and elsewhere. These latter factors are extremely important when one considers the management of the patient with bilateral renal arterial disease who had been treated with an ACE inhibitor and who subsequently developed an acceleration of the hypertensive disease process with malignant hypertension and, perhaps, further renal functional impairment (8).

The foregoing clinical examples were selected to demonstrate the importance of the multiplicity of pathophysiologic factors that participate in patients with what might otherwise be considered straightforward forms of secondary hypertension from a mechanistic point of view. These very same interrelations occur, but perhaps more subtly, in patients with primary or essential hypertension. However, in these patients, the underlying disease mechanisms are related to inborn genetic alterations, which, in turn, impact on their clinical expressions in primary hypertension (6,10,11). Thus, this ubiquitous disease, essential hypertension, is considered to result from genetic alterations involving abnormal gene expression that may be facilitated through specific environmental factors (e.g., sodium). Even the role of sodium is highly complex and may also promote intraorgan fibrosis over and above sodium's classically accepted mechanism of volume expansion. Among these genetic alterations are functional expressions of the renin-angiotensin system (e.g., angiotensinogen, renin, ACE), the autonomic nervous system (e.g., through catecholamine biosynthesis), endocrine systems (e.g., expression of altered enzymes of steroid hormone biosynthesis), sodium metabolism (e.g., through enzymes that control sodium ionic channel and exchange mechanisms), and control of other humoral and peptide agents. Thus, each of the genetic factors that participate in normal blood pressure regulation may be altered in hypertensive diseases. Furthermore, these factors frequently come into play when arterial pressure is reduced therapeutically. In that regard, when arterial pressure is reduced by certain antihypertensive agents (e.g., antiadrenergic agents or direct-acting vascular smooth muscle relaxants), there is an ingress of extravascular water into the circulation that offsets the therapeutic reduction in pressure (12,13). This phenomenon leads to the state of pseudotolerance and may be counteracted by the addition of small doses of diuretics

if not already prescribed or by greater doses of diuretics if smaller doses have been used (14). These factors may explain the finding in the Antihypertensive and Lipid-Lowering Treatment to Prevent Heart Attack Trial (ALLHAT) study of the production of cardiac failure by doxycycline, which mandated the withdrawal of this drug from the study.

ETIOLOGIC CLASSIFICATION

From a clinical viewpoint, the various hypertensive diseases have been classified according to whether they result from a known factor or disease (i.e., secondary forms of hypertension) or whether no known specific clinical cause of the hypertension can be identified (i.e., primary or essential hypertension). Actually, 90% to 95% of all patients with hypertension have essential hypertension; and only 5% to 10% of patients with persistently increased arterial pressures have hypertension of a known cause (Table 15–2).

Following the concept presented earlier concerning the mechanisms that participate in increasing arterial pressure, it is logical to relate the various secondary forms of hypertensive disease to specific pressor and depressor mechanism(s) that can be identified clinically (Tables 15–1 and 15–2). Thus, a mechanical factor impairing the forward flow of blood in the aorta (e.g., aortic coarctation, mechanical obstruction of the aorta by tumor) will increase pressure proximal to that aortic obstruction. A number of neurologic diseases are complicated by hypertension. They may be central (e.g., brain tumors or trauma, porphyria, diencephalic syndrome) or peripheral (e.g., pheochromocytoma). In either case, the final common pathway explaining the increased arterial pressure is based on increased adrenergic outflow from the brain, catecholamine release from nerve endings, or abnormal adrenergic receptor stimulation (e.g., hyperdynamic β-adrenergic circulatory state). Increased participation of the renin-angiotensin system is classically demonstrated by occlusive renal arterial lesions (e.g., by fibrosis or atherothrombosis) (15), although not all patients with these lesions have an increased arterial pressure (16). This latter concept is exceedingly important considering clinical reports of placing renal arterial stents coincident with coronary arterial catheterization procedures (the practice of so-called driveby angiography). Hemodynamically significant occlusive renal arterial lesions may also be produced by emboli to the kidney, renal cysts or tumors, radiation fibrosis of the kidney, or compression of the renal artery by tumor, and hypertension can be caused by renin-producing tumors within the kidney.

Many, but not all, patients with parenchymal disease of the kidney will have hypertension. In those patients who do have parenchymal renal disease and hypertension, the increased arterial pressure is related primarily to an inability of the kidney to maintain fluid and electrolyte balance and especially to excrete sodium and water, even if renal function is normal clinically. In other patients, there may be an

TABLE 15–2. *Primary and secondary hypertension*

Primary (essential) hypertension (hypertension of
   undetermined cause)
Borderline (labile) essential hypertension
Essential hypertension (sustained arterial hypertension)
   Diastolic hypertension
   Isolated systolic hypertension
Secondary hypertensions
Coarctation of the aorta
Renal arterial diseases (renal vascular disease with
   hypertension)
   Nonatherothrombotic (fibrosing) renal arterial disease
   Atherothrombotic renal arterial disease
   Aneurysm(s) of renal artery
   Embolic renal arterial disease
   Extravascular compression (of renal artery): tumor,
     fibrosis
   Perinephric hull (Page kidney)
Renal parenchymal diseases
   Chronic pyelonephritis
   Acute glomerulonephritis
   Chronic glomerulonephritis
   Polycystic renal disease
   Diabetic nephropathy
   Others: amyloidosis, ureteral obstruction, etc.
Hormonal disease
   Thyroid
     Hyperthyroidism
     Hypothyroidism
     Hashimoto's thyroiditis
   Adrenal
     Cushing disease or Cushing syndrome
     Primary hyperaldosteronism
       Adenoma
       Bilateral hyperplasia
     Adrenal enzyme deficiencies
     Pheochromocytoma
   Others
     Ectopic production of pressor hormones
     Growth hormone excess
     Hypercalcemic disease states (including
       hyperparathyroidism)
Drugs, chemicals, and foods
   Excessive alcohol intake
   Excessive dietary sodium intake
   Exogenously administered adrenal steroids: birth control
     pills; adrenal steroids for asthma and malignancies;
     anabolic steroids
   Licorice excess (imported)
   Over-the-counter preparations (e.g.,
     phenylpropanolamine, nasal decongestants)
   Milk-alkali syndrome; hypervitaminosis D
   Snuff
   Complications from specific therapy
     Antidepressant therapy (tricyclics, monoamine oxidase
       inhibitors)
     Chronic steroid administration
     Cyclosporine (transplantation and certain diseases
       requiring immunosuppressive therapy)
     β-Adrenergic receptor agonists (e.g., for asthma)
     Radiation nephritis, arteritis

From Frohlich ED. Pathophysiology of systemic arterial hypertension. In: Schlant RC, Alexander RW, O'Rourke RA, et al., eds. *Hurst's the heart,* 8th ed. New York: McGraw-Hill, 1993:1391–1401, with permission.

additional participation of the renin-angiotensin system (17). In the former group, the arterial pressure is directly related to the expansion of intravascular (plasma) volume (17). The impaired renal excretory component of the hypertension has been termed by some workers in the field to be a "renoprival" factor, which may be demonstrated best by the patient with severe renal functional impairment who is able to achieve optimal control of increased arterial pressure before hemodialysis by increasing the filtration pressures during dialysis (18). A number of hormonal substances, when produced in excess, may increase arterial pressure—including thyroid, parathyroid, growth hormone, and several adrenal steroidal hormones (produced by tumor, hyperplasia, or enzymatic deficiencies).

In addition to these better known clinical entities, hypertension may be produced by an excessive amount of circulating humoral substances. This might be exemplified by the patient with metastatic carcinoid, who produces excessive amounts of serotonin that are inadequately metabolized by metastatic liver disease, or in porphyria, in which participation of the central nervous system occurs in those patients with essential hypertension who may have impaired endothelial-dependent vasodilating or constricting factors (19–21). It also is possible that arterial pressure might be increased in the patient with deficient amounts of vasodilating agents (8,19). Finally, secondary hypertension might be produced by any of a variety of ingested over-the-counter medications (e.g., nose drops, oral contraceptives, aspirin, steroidal and nonsteroidal antiinflammatory agents, and tricyclic antidepressants with guanethidine or guanabenz), foodstuffs (e.g., licorice, tyramine-containing foods, and beverages), or diets with excessive amounts of sodium in the patient who is more sensitive to dietary sodium excess (e.g., patients with renal or cardiac failure) (22).

Primary (or essential) hypertension is, by far, the most common hypertension, occurring in approximately 90% to 95% of all patients with hypertension. In 1993, The Third National Health and Nutrition Survey estimated that there were approximately 50 million individuals with essential hypertension in the United States (23). This reduction of approximately 17% from the prior survey (which estimated 59 million people with essential hypertension in the United States) has been attributed to the broad acceptance of several lifestyle modifications by the general public. These nonpharmacologic modifications of personal lifestyle include weight control, sodium restriction, alcohol moderation, adoption of a regular isotonic exercise program, and smoking cessation (23,24). Thus, this decrease of 10 million patients with essential hypertension has been attributed to an unanticipated practice of primary prevention measures that would otherwise predispose the involved individuals to an abnormally increased arterial pressure.

With the publication of the Seventh Report of the Joint National Committee (JNC-VII) in 2003, a new classification of essential hypertension was introduced (Table 15–3) (24). For the first time this report took into consideration in-

TABLE 15–3. *Classification of blood pressure for adults 18 years of age and older*

Category	Systolic (mm Hg)		Diastolic (mm Hg)
Optimal	<120	and	<80
Normal	<130	and	<85
High-normal	130–139	or	85–89
Hypertension			
Stage 1	140–159		90–99
Stage 2	160–179		100–109
Stage 3	≥180	or	≥110–119

Modified from The sixth report of the Joint National Committee on detection, evaluation, and treatment of high blood pressure. *Arch Intern Med* 1997;157:2413–2446, with permission.

creased systolic and diastolic pressure. The patient's baseline (or pretreatment) blood pressure should be established after at least three indirect pressure measurements are obtained on at least three separate occasions. The measurements should be obtained under well prescribed resting conditions not influenced by prior smoking, restrictive clothing, and other factors (24). However, if the physician believes that the height of arterial pressure is of sufficient concern to warrant immediate treatment, subsequent pressure measurements on other occasions obviously are not warranted.

Increased systolic and diastolic pressures are defined in JNC report as 140 and 90 mm Hg or greater, respectively (24). Patients with systolic and diastolic pressures less than 120 and 80, less than 130 and 85, or ranging from 130 through 139 and 85 through 89 mm Hg, respectively, are considered to have optimal, normal, and high normal pressures, respectively. Moreover, the heights of the systolic and diastolic pressures are classified according to stages of increasing severity of pressure elevation (Stages 1 through 3). Most importantly, the pressure (i.e., systolic or diastolic) that is greatest permits rating of the stage severity (24). This classification, then, accomplishes three major points: (a) it clearly defines normal, optimal, and high-normal systolic and diastolic pressures; (b) it underscores the concept that the increase of systolic pressure is at least as important as the diastolic pressure increase, and (c) no longer is any increase of arterial pressure to be considered "mild," because

all levels of severity confer a significantly amplified risk for increased (and premature) cardiovascular morbidity and mortality (24). The concept of "borderline" hypertension is not considered and, hence, this ambiguous term was excluded (24). This term relating to whether the physician should institute pharmacologic treatment for those patients whose systolic and diastolic pressures range from 140 through 159 and 90 through 94 mm Hg, respectively, is now clarified. These patients are currently included in a presently existing group (or Stage 1 hypertension) that includes the pressure range 140 through 159 mm Hg systolic and 90 through 99 mm Hg, which should be treated depending on risk group (*vide infra*).

Functional Classification

Hypertension as a disease is manifested clinically by its effects on its major target organs (i.e., heart, brain, and kidneys). These effects are assessable by means of clinical and laboratory studies. As already indicated, not all patients having hypertension may warrant pharmacologic therapy. However, all patients with hypertension should come under close medical management, even if this means that the patient is instructed to institute the various nonpharmacologic lifestyle modifications with instructions to return for further follow-up consultations at regularly prescribed intervals. To arrive at an appropriate plan for subsequent management, the patient should be evaluated comprehensively. Thus, to assess target organ involvement, the initial evaluation should include a careful medical history, physical examination, and certain laboratory studies (24). To emphasize this point a new concept of risk stratification was introduced in JNC-VI in which target organ involvement, clinical evidence of clinical cardiovascular disease, and coexisting cardiovascular risk factors and diabetes mellitus are considered (Table 15–4) (24).

Inherent in this evaluation is a careful search for a family history of cardiovascular illnesses and premature death, as well as for other major risk factors predisposing the patient to hypertension, coronary heart disease, stroke, and renal failure. This clinical evaluation should include a number of laboratory studies that will be of value in detecting those comorbid risk factors, clinical evidence of target organ involvement resulting from hypertensive vascular disease,

TABLE 15–4. *Risk stratification and treatment*

BP Classification	Systolic BP, mm HG		Diastolic BP, mm Hg	
Normal	<120	and	<80	
Prehypertension	120–139	or	80–89	Lifestyle modification
Stage 1 hypertension	140–159	or	90–99	Lifestyle modification and encourage drug therapy
Stage 2 hypertension	≥160	or	≥100	Drug therapy

BP, blood pressure.

TABLE 15–5. *Laboratory studies that may be of value in the diagnostic evaluation of the patient with hypertension*

Complete blood count
  White blood cell count (and differential)
  Hemoglobin concentration[a]
  Hematocrit[a]
  Adequacy of platelets
Blood chemistries
  Sugar (fasting, 2-hr postprandial, or tolerance test)[a]
  Uric acid[a]
  Cholesterol and triglyceride concentrations[a]
  Low- and high-density cholesterol concentrations[a]
  Renal function (blood urea and/or serum creatinine)[a]
  Serum electrolytes (Na,[a] K, Cl, CO2) concentrations
  Calcium and phosphate concentrations
  Total protein and albumin concentration
  Hepatic function (alkaline phosphatase, bilirubin, serum enzymes)
Urine studies
  Urinalysis[a]
  Urine culture
  24-hr collection (protein, Na, K, creatinine)
  Electrocardiogram (12-lead)[a]

[a]These tests are currently recommended in the Fifth Report of the Joint National Committee (22).

and methods for the detection of secondary causes of hypertensive disease (Tables 15–5 and 15–6). In this regard, it is also extremely important to evaluate the patient for hypertensive retinopathy (Table 15–7) (25,26) and history of transient ischemic attacks or more severe sensory or motor neurologic deficit. Cardiac involvement can be ascertained using electrocardiographic criteria for left atrial abnormality and left ventricular hypertrophy (Table 15–8) (27–32), which have been confirmed by echocardiographic criteria of increased left atrial size, left ventricular mass or wall thicknesses, and ventricular function (33,34). (See Chapter 17 for a complete discussion of the criteria for calculating left ventricular mass, wall thicknesses, and indices of ventricular function.) Renal functional impairment is assessed by quantitative measurement of proteinuria and increase of serum creatinine or blood urea nitrogen concentration. Clinical evaluation is extremely valuable and includes ascertaining evidence of secondary forms of hypertension (e.g., renal arterial bruits, facial and body habitus and characteristics of Cushing syndrome or disease, reduction or delay of femoral pulsations for aortic coarctation, hypokalemic alkalosis for indication of primary or secondary hyperaldosteronism, and symptoms presented in the patient's history suggesting pheochromocytoma or ingestion

TABLE 15–6. *Classification of known hypertensive diseases according to pressor mechanisms*

Primary pressor mechanisms	Clinical diagnosis	Other implicated pressor mechanisms	Specific tests
Mechanical	Coarctation of aorta	Renopressor	Chest radiograph, angiography
Catecholamines	Pheochromocytoma	Volume, renopressor, neural	Plasma catecholamines, CAT scan
Renopressor	Renal arterial disease	Aldosterone, volume, neural	Renal arteriography; plasma renin activity or angiotensin I level
Hormonal	Thyrotoxicosis	Thyroid, neural	Thyroid function studies
	Hyperparathyroidism	Calcium on vascular smooth muscle	Serum calcium; parathormone level
	Oral contraceptives	Renopressor	Plasma renin activity
	Acromegaly, gigantism	Growth hormone and factors	Growth hormone
	Cushing syndrome or disease	Compounds D, F	17-OH steroids
	Primary hyperaldosteronism	Volume, electrolytes	Aldosterone, rennin
	Adrenal virilism	Volume, electrolytes	Ketosteroids
	Hydroxylase deficiencies	Volume, electrolytes	Corticosteroids
	DOC-tumors	Volume, electrolytes	17-OH steroids
Volume	Renal parenchymal disease	Electrolytes, renopressor	IVP, urine culture, renal biopsy, renal function studies, measurement of body fluid volumes
Neural	Essential hypertension; borderline hypertension	Catecholamines, volume, renopressor	Hemodynamics; plasma renin activity; measurement of fluid volumes; assessment
	β-Adrenergic hypercirculatory state	Adenylate cyclase, cAMP	Hemodynamics; isoproterenol infusion
	Porphyria	Catecholamines	
	Diencephalic syndrome	Renopressor	Porphobilinogen
	Brain tumor		CAT scan, MRI

cAMP, cyclic adenosine monophosphate; CAT, computed axial tomography; DOC, deoxycorticosterone; IVP, intravenous pyelography; MRI, magnetic resonance imaging.

TABLE 15–7. *Classification of hypertensive retinopathy*

A. Keith-Wagener-Barker Classification (23)
  Group I: tortuosity, minimal constriction
  Group II: above + arteriovenous nicking
  Group III: above + hemorrhages and exudates
  Group IV: papilledema
B. American Ophthalmological Society Committee
  Classification (Wagener-Clay-Gipner) (24)
  1. Generalized arteriolar constriction
    Grade 1: arterioles 3/4 normal caliber; A/V ratio of 1:2
    Grade 2: arterioles 1/2 normal caliber; A/V ratio of 1:3
    Grade 3: arterioles 1/3 normal caliber; A/V ratio of 1:4
    Grade 4: arterioles thread-like or invisible
  2. Focal arteriolar constriction or sclerosis
    Grade 1: localized arteriolar narrowing to 2/3 caliber of proximal segment
    Grade 2: localized arteriolar narrowing to 1/2 caliber of proximal segment
    Grade 3: localized arteriolar narrowing to 1/3 caliber of proximal segment
    Grade 4: arterioles invisible beyond focal constriction
  3. Generalized sclerosis
    Grade 1: increased light striping; mild AV nicking
    Grade 2: coppery arteriolar color; moderate AV nicking; veins almost completely invisible below arteriolar crossing
    Grade 3: silver arteriolar color; severe AV nicking
    Grade 4: arterioles visible only as fibrous cords without bloodstreams
  4. Hemorrhage and exudates: grades 1 to 4 (based on number of affected quadrants divided by 2)
  5. Papilledema: grades 1 to 4 (based on diopters of elevation)

A/V, arteriolar/venular.

TABLE 15–8. *Diagnostic electrocardiographic cardiac criteria*

1. Left atrial abnormality (ECG): two of four (25)
  a. P wave in lead II $\geq$ 0.3 mV and $\geq$ 0.12 second (26)
  b. Bipeak interval in notched P wave $\geq$ 0.04 second (27)
  c. Ratio of P wave duration to PR segment $\geq$ 1.6 (lead II) (28)
  d. Terminal atrial forces (in V_1) $\geq$ 0.04 second
2. Left ventricular hypertrophy (25)
  a. Ungerleider index $\geq$ +15% (chest radiograph alone)
  b. Ungerleider index $\geq$ +10% (chest radiograph + two of the following ECG criteria):
    1. Sum of tallest R and deepest S waves $\geq$ 4.5 mV (precordial) (29)
    2. LV "strain"—i.e., QRS and T wave vectors 180° apart (30)
    3. QRS frontal axis < 0°
  c. All three ECG criteria (above)

ECG, electrocardiogram; LV, left ventricular.

of certain drugs or foods). Each of these considerations, including the patient's age, race, and sex, should provide information that suggests the need for immediacy and intensity of medical treatment.

Therapeutic Classification

It is clear from the foregoing discussions concerning these various classifications of hypertension that a consideration of therapeutic classifications naturally should follow. Treatment may be selected on the basis of etiologic factors, functional mechanisms, severity of pressure increase, target organ involvement, and comorbid diseases.

High Normal

Patients with "high normal" levels of arterial pressure (i.e., 130–139/85–89 mm Hg) are more likely to be predisposed to development of increased pressure at some subsequent time. These patients should return for repeated blood pressure measurements at more frequent intervals. This may be facilitated with the use of sphygmomanometers that can be calibrated and are suitable for home use. The likelihood of subsequent development of hyperten-

sion is enhanced particularly if there is a family history of hypertension and premature death. If blood pressure increases to the lower levels of Stage I blood pressure levels (i.e., 140–150/90–95 mm Hg), earlier pharmacologic therapy may be indicated, particularly if there is evidence of target organ (i.e., heart, kidneys, and brain) involvement from hypertensive disease. In any event, it is of particular value to instruct these patients who are more predisposed to development of hypertension about the value and feasibility of lifestyle modifications, including tobacco cessation, weight control (to within 15% of ideal body weight), dietary sodium restriction (<100 mEq or 2.3 g sodium daily), alcohol moderation ($\leq$1 oz ethanol intake daily), and a regular isotonic exercise program (Table 15–9). This program not only has been shown to be of value in the primary prevention of hypertension (23), but it will significantly reduce the number of antihypertensive drugs and their dosages if and when they are ultimately prescribed (24).

TABLE 15–9. *Lifestyle modifications for hypertension control or overall cardiovascular risk, or both*

- Lose weight if overweight.
- Limit alcohol intake to no more than 1 oz ethanol per day (24 oz beer, 8 oz wine, or 2 oz 100-proof whiskey).
- Exercise (aerobic) regularly.
- Reduce sodium intake to less than 100 mmol per day (<2.3 g sodium or <6 g sodium chloride).
- Maintain adequate dietary potassium (approximately 90 mmol/day), calcium, and magnesium intake.
- Stop smoking and reduce dietary saturated fat and cholesterol intake for overall cardiovascular health. Reducing fat intake also helps to reduce caloric intake, which is important for control of weight and type II diabetes.

From Oren S, Grossman E, Messerli FH, et al. High blood pressure: side effects of drugs, poisons, and food. *Cardiol Clin North Am* 1988;6:467–474.

Stage I Hypertension

Currently, patients with lower levels of diastolic pressure elevation (i.e., 90–94 mm Hg) are at definite risk for premature cardiovascular morbidity and mortality (24) and certainly should be considered as potential beneficiaries of an antihypertensive treatment program. This might be instituted initially, as described earlier, with lifestyle modification measures. Each of these measures (with the exception of stopping smoking) has been shown to reduce arterial pressure significantly in a population of patients with hypertension. However, with respect to the smoking issue, several multicenter studies have shown that when smokers who receive propranolol for antihypertensive therapy are treated, and their outcomes are compared with those of a similar group of patients with hypertension who smoke but are treated with a thiazide diuretic, they achieve similar reductions in arterial pressure, but myocardial infarction (MI) and stroke are not prevented (35,36). Patients with Stage I isolated systolic hypertension (i.e., 140–159 mm Hg) also are

at a greater risk for subsequent development of cardiovascular events. In general, however, the JNC-VI recommends that antihypertensive drug therapy be initiated with Stage I hypertension, especially if target organ involvement and family history suggesting high risk are present (24).

Stage I and II Hypertension

If blood pressure is not controlled within a reasonable time (1–3 months) in patients with levels of 140 to 159/90 to 95 mm Hg, institution of antihypertensive drug therapy is a wise option. In these individuals, therapy may be initiated with low doses of a diuretic, β-adrenergic receptor blocking agent, ACE inhibitor, angiotensin (type 1) receptor blocker, calcium antagonist, or α_1- or α/β-adrenergic receptor blocking agent (Fig. 15–2). The most recent JNC-VI report indicated that the diuretic and β-blocker may be considered "preferred" choices, because in multicenter, controlled, clinical trials these agents have been shown to reduce cardiovas-

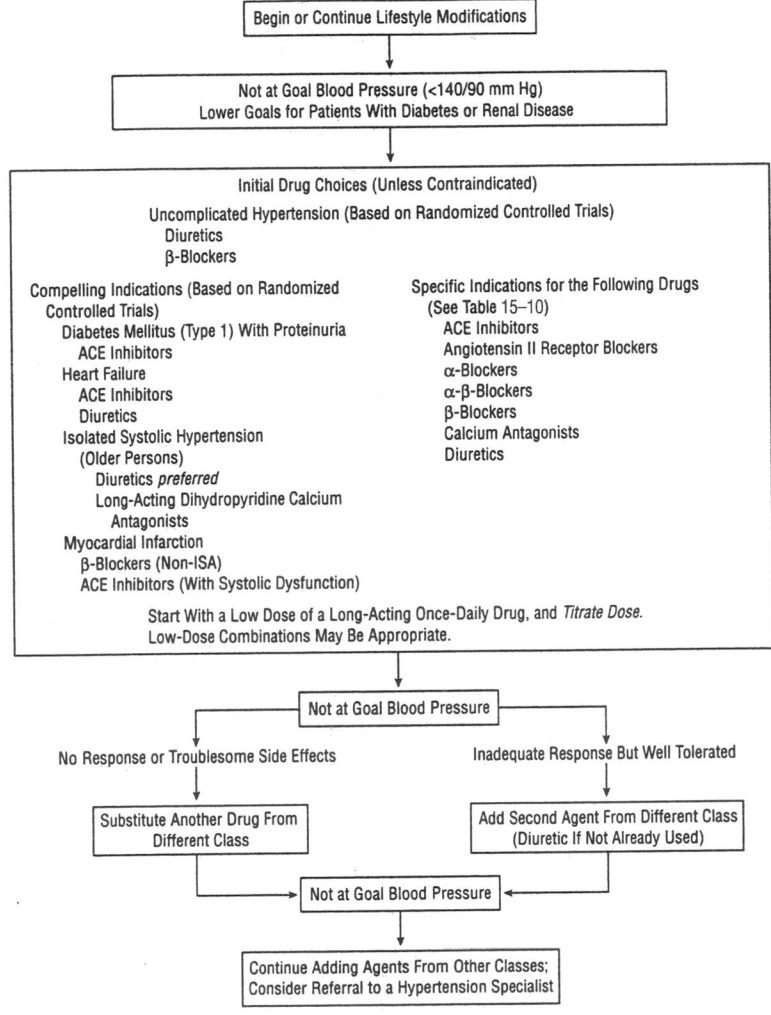

FIG. 15–2. Treatment algorithm. ACE, angiotensin-converting enzyme; ISA, intrinsic sympathomimetic activity. (Modified from The sixth report of the Joint National Committee on detection, evaluation, and treatment of high blood pressure. *Arch Intern Med* 1997;157:2413–2446.)

TABLE 15–10. *Antihypertensive agent*

Drug	Usual dosage range (mg/day)[a]	Frequency (qd unless otherwise noted)	Mechanisms of antihypertensive drug action	Comments
Initial choices				
I. Diuretics Thiazides and related agents			Decreased plasma volume, decreased extracellular fluid volume, and decreased cardiac output initially, followed by decreased total peripheral resistance with normalization of cardiac output. Chronic effects include a slight decrease in extracellular fluid volume.	• For thiazide and loop diuretics, lower doses and dietary counseling should be used to avoid metabolic changes.
• Bendroflumethiazide	2.5–5.0			• Thiazides and related agents are more effective antihypertensives than loop diuretics, except in patients with serum creatinine ≥221 μmol/liter (2.5 mg/dL).
• Benzthiazide	12.5–50.0			
• Chlorothiazide	125–500	bid		
• Chlorthalidone	12.5–50.0			• Hydrochlorothiazide and chlorthalidone are generally the preferred thiazides. They were the most often used thiazides in clinical trials.
• Cyclothiazide	1–2			
• Hydrochlorothiazide	12.5–50.0			
• Hydroflumethiazide	12.5–50.0			
• Indapamide	2.5–5.0			
• Methyclothiazide	2.5–5.0			
• Metolazone	0.5–5.0			
• Polythiazide	1–4			
• Quinethazone	25–100			
• Trichlormethiazide	1–4			
Loop diuretics			See thiazides.	• Greater doses of loop diuretics may be needed for patients with renal impairment or congestive heart failure.
• Bumetanide	0.5–5.0	bid		• Ethacrynic acid is the only alternative for patients with allergy to thiazide and sulfur-containing diuretics.
• Ethacrynic acid	25–100	bid		
• Furosemide	20–320	bid		• Weak diuretics.
Potassium-sparing			Increased potassium reabsorption.	• Used mainly in combination with other diuretics to avoid or reverse hypokalemia from other diuretics.
• Amiloride HCl	5–10	qd or bid		
• Spironolactone	25–100	qd or bid	Aldosterone antagonist.	• Avoid when serum creatinine ≥221 μmol/L (2.5 mg/dL).
• Triamterene	50–150	qd or bid		• May cause hyperkalemia, and this may be exaggerated when combined with ACE inhibitors or potassium supplements.
• Eplerinone (not yet released)				
II. Adrenergic Inhibitors				
β-blockers			Decreased cardiac output and increased total peripheral resistance. Decreased plasma renin activity. Atenolol, betaxolol, and metoprolol are cardioselective.	• Selective agents will also inhibit β-receptors in greater doses; all may aggravate asthma.
• Atenolol	25–100[b]			
• Betaxolol HCl	5–40			
• Bisoprolol fumarate	5–20			
• Metoprolol tartrate	50–200			
• Metoprolol (extended release)	50–200	qd or bid		
• Nadolol	20–240[b]			
• Propranolol HCl	40–240	bid		
• Propranolol (long acting)	60–240			
• Timolol maleate	20–40	bid		

Continued

TABLE 15–10. *Antihypertensive agent*

Drug	Usual dosage range (mg/day)[a]	Frequency (qd unless otherwise noted)	Mechanisms of antihypertensive drug action	Comments
β-blockers with ISA			Acebutolol is cardioselective.	No clear advantage for agents with ISA except in patients with bradycardia who must receive β-blocker; these drugs produce fewer or no metabolic side effects.
• Acebutolol HCl	200–1,200[b]	bid		
• Carteolol HCl	2.5–10.0[b]			
• Penbutolol sulfate	20–80[b]			
• Pindolol	10–60[b]	bid		
α/β-blocker			Same as β-blockers plus α₁-blockade.	• Possibly more effective in blacks than other β-blockers. • May cause postural effects, and titration should be based on standing blood pressure.
• Labetalol HCl	200–1,200	bid		
α₁-receptor blockers			Block postsynaptic α₁-receptors and cause vasodilation.	All may cause postural effects, and titration should be based on standing blood pressure.
• Doxazosin mesylate	1–16			
• Prazosin HCl	1–20	bid or tid		
• Terazosin	1–20			
III. ACE inhibitors			Block formation of angiotensin II, promoting vasodilation and decreased aldosterone. Also increase bradykinin and vasodilatory prostaglandins.	• Contraindicated in pregnant women and those with history of angioneurotic edema or prior reactions to ACE inhibitors. • Diuretic doses should be reduced or discontinued before starting ACE inhibitors whenever possible to prevent excessive hypotension. • Reduce dose of those drugs marked with a superscript [b] in patients with serum creatinine ≥221 μmol/L (2.5 mg/dL). • May cause hyperkalemia in patients with renal impairment or in those receiving potassium-sparing agents. • Can cause acute renal failure in patients with severe bilateral renal artery stenosis or severe stenosis in an artery to a solitary kidney.
Benazepril HCl	10–40[b]	qd or bid		
Captopril	12.5–150.0[b]	bid		
Cilazapril	2.5–5.0	qd or bid		
Enalapril maleate	2.5–40.0[b]	qd or bid		
Fosinopril sodium	10–40	qd or bid		
Moexipril	7.5–30	qd or bid		
Lisinopril	5–40[b]	qd or bid		
Perindopril[c]	1–16[b]	qd or bid		
Quinapril HCl	5–80	qd or bid		
Ramipril	1.25–20.0[b]	qd or bid		
Spirapril[c]	12.5–50.0	qd or bid		
Trandolapril	2–4	qd		
IV. Calcium antagonists Diltiazem HCl/verapamil HCl			Block the inward movement of calcium ions across cell membranes and cause smooth muscle relaxation.	Diltiazem and verapamil also block the slow channels in the heart and may reduce the sinus rate and produce heart block.
• Diltiazem	90–360	tid		
• Diltiazem (sustained release)	120–360	bid		
• Diltiazem (extended release)	180–360			
• Verapamil	80–480	bid		
• Verapamil (long acting)	120–480	qd or bid		
Dihydropyridines				Dihydropyridines are more potent peripheral vasodilators than diltiazem and verapamil and may cause more dizziness, headache, flushing, peripheral edema, and tachycardia.
• Amlodipine besylate	2.5–10.0	bid		
• Felodipine	5–20	tid		
Isradipine	2.5–10.0	tid		
Nicardipine HCl	60–120			
Nifedipine	30–120			
Nifedipine (GITS)	30–90			
Nisoldipine	10–20			

Continued

TABLE 15–10. *Antihypertensive agent*

Drug	Usual dosage range (mg/day)[a]	Frequency (qd unless otherwise noted)	Mechanisms of antihypertensive drug action	Comments
Supplemental choices				
I. Centrally acting α₂-agonists			Stimulate central α_2-receptors that inhibit efferent sympathetic activity.	Clonidine patch is replaced once a week. None of these agents should be withdrawn abruptly. Avoid in nonadherent patients.
• Clonidine HCl	0.1–1.2	bid		
• Clonidine TTS (patch)[d]	0.1–0.3	qw		
• Guanabenz acetate	4–64	bid		
• Guanfacine HCl	1–3			
• Methyldopa	250–2,000	bid		
II. Peripheral-acting adrenergic antagonist			Inhibit catecholamine release from neuronal storage sites.	May cause serious orthostatic and exercise-induced hypotension.
Guanadrel sulfate	10–75	bid		
Guanethidine monosulfate	10–100		Deplete tissue stores of catecholamines.	
Rauwolfia alkaloids				
• Rauwolfia root	50–200			
• Reserpine	0.05[e]–0.25			
III. Direct vasodilators			Direct smooth muscle vasodilation (primarily arteriolar).	Hydralazine is subject to phenotypically determined metabolism (acetylation). With each agent, the patient should be given a diuretic and a β-blocker for fluid retention and reflex tachycardia.
Hydralazine HCl	50–300	bid to qid		
Minoxidil	2.5–80.0	qd or bid		

In all patients, lifestyle modifications are also advised.

ACE, angiotensin-converting enzyme.

[a]The lower dose indicated is the preferred initial dose, and the greater dose is the maximum per day. Most agents require 2 to 4 weeks for complete efficacy; more frequent dosage adjustments are not advised except for severe hypertension. The dosage range may differ slightly from what is recommended on the package insert.

[b]These drugs are excreted by the kidney and require dosage reduction in the presence of renal impairment (serum creatinine $\geq$221 μmol/L [2.5 mg/dL]).

[c]This drug is not approved by the Food and Drug Administration.

[d]Weekly patch is 1,2,3 equivalent to 0.1 to 0.3 mg/day, respectively.

[e]A 0.1-mg dose may be given qod to achieve this dosage.

From The sixth report of the Joint National Committee on detection, evaluation, and treatment of high blood pressure. *Arch Intern Med* 1997;157:2413–2446, with permission.

cular morbidity and mortality. This is in contrast to the ACE inhibitors, calcium antagonists, α_1-adrenergic and α/β-adrenergic receptor blockers, which have been shown to be equally efficacious in controlling arterial pressure but have not yet been demonstrated to reduce cardiovascular morbidity and mortality in controlled trials involving patients with hypertension (24). Controlled trials have shown such benefit with ACE inhibitors in patients with coronary heart disease who have had prior MI or cardiac failure, but these trials did not involve patients with hypertension (24). Should arterial pressure not be controlled with low doses of these various classes of antihypertensive drugs, full doses may then be administered. Alternatively, it may be wise to change to another class of drugs or to add a second antihypertensive agent from the six classes of drugs. A listing of all currently available antihypertensive agents, their usual dosage range, and mechanism(s) of action (6) is presented in Table 15–10.

Some individuals have interpreted the JNC-V and JNC-VI to state that only the diuretics and β-blockers are recommended for the initial treatment of patients with hypertension. To the contrary, each of the foregoing six classes of antihypertensive agents (diuretics, β-blockers, calcium antagonists, ACE inhibitors, α_1-blockers, and α/β-blockers) is recommended for initial therapy. To this end, certain classes (not necessarily diuretics or β-blockers) of agents are particularly recommended for individualized therapy (Table 15–11). The reports specifically detail distinct and "compelling" cardiovascular, renal, and other clinical conditions in which certain drug classes (or even specific agents) are particularly preferred, when special monitoring of therapy is required, and which of these agents are relatively or absolutely contraindicated.

Hypertension with Compelling Indications

As indicated earlier, the JNC-VI indicates that patients with uncomplicated hypertension may be best treated with a diuretic (e.g., 12.5 or 25 mg daily of hydrochlorothiazide initially, with an increase in dosage to 50 mg, as necessary) or a β-adrenergic receptor blocking agent (e.g., 25 mg daily of atenolol initially, with an increase in dose to 100 mg, as necessary). However, certain compelling factors may suggest reevaluation of the initial selection of antihypertensive agent over and above the height of arterial pressure. For example, if a patient has diabetes mellitus (insulin-dependent or not), it is wise to control arterial pressure levels to less than 130 mm Hg systolic pressure and less than 80 mm Hg diastolic pressure. (Some other guidelines have suggested <120 and <70 mm Hg systolic and diastolic pressure, respectively.) These levels have been shown to markedly and significantly retard the development of end-stage renal disease in patients with diabetes (37,38). Moreover, the agents that were recommended in JNC-VI for patients with hypertension and diabetes were the ACE inhibitors (24). However, since publication of JNC-6 in 1997, several controlled multicenter trials have demonstrated that certain angiotensin II (type 1)

receptor–blocking agents also will retard the progression of end-stage renal disease (39–41). One such agent, losartan, has received approval for marketing for that specific indication (41).

Another compelling indication identified in JNC-VI is that of cardiac failure, for which the diuretics and ACE inhibitors were recommended. The best prevention of cardiac failure with systolic dysfunction is the excellent control of arterial pressure; however, diastolic dysfunction is usually characterized by being more common in elderly patients or those with ischemic heart disease. Diastolic dysfunction, especially, is characterized by ventricular ischemia and fibrosis (in extracellular matrix and around the myocardial arterioles). Several reports have appeared in recent years demonstrating the improvement of ventricular ischemia with the ACE inhibitors and the calcium antagonists; these drugs, as well as the angiotensin II (type 1) receptor antagonists, also have been shown experimentally and clinically to reverse the fibrotic process within the ventricular wall (42,43). Thus, the best compelling therapy in these situations include excellent control of arterial pressure and the judicious use of the ACE inhibitors or type 1 receptor antagonists, or both. Moreover, if angina pectoris is coexistent with hypertension (and this not infrequently occurs even in the absence of occlusive atherothrombotic epicardial coronary arterial disease), the use of β-blockers are indicated. If chest pain is not controlled with the β-blocker, it is important to prescribe the calcium antagonist together with the foregoing agents.

In addition to cardiac failure as a complication of hypertension, it is also important to consider MI as another compelling indication of specific antihypertensive therapy. In this regard, those β-adrenergic receptors blocking agents, which do not possess intrinsic sympathomimetic activity, have been demonstrated in repeated multicenter trials with a number of these agents to prevent the reoccurrence of a second infarction. It also should be emphasized that β-blockers continue to be underused in the foregoing group of patients. In addition, to this consideration, it also is important to recognize that a number of ACE inhibitors have been shown to be exceedingly important in preventing cardiac failure, a recurrent MI, and death in the patient with a prior MI. These findings were well documented first in the Survival and Ventricular Enlargement Trial study with captopril; since this first documentation, they have been repeated with several other drugs of this therapeutic group (44–46).

Hence, there are a number of clinical situations in which agents other than the diuretic and β-blocker may be selected for the initial therapy of hypertension; and these compelling indications may be independent of the height of arterial pressure.

Stage III Hypertension

Therapy should be initiated with any one of the six classes of antihypertensive agents in less than full doses. Patients with stage III hypertension should return for follow-up examina-

TABLE 15–11. *Guideline for selecting initial antihypertensive drug therapy in the presence of special considerations*

Clinical situation	Preferred	Requires special monitoring	Relatively or absolutely contraindicated
I. Cardiovascular			
Angina pectoris	β-Blockers, calcium antagonists		Direct vasodilators
Bradycardia/heart block, sick sinus syndrome			β-Blockers, labetalol HCl, diltiazem HCl, verapamil HCl
Cardiac failure	Diuretics, ACE inhibitors		β-Blockers, calcium antagonist, labetalol
Hypertrophic cardio-myopathy with severe diastolic dysfunction	β-Blockers, diltiazem, verapamil		Diuretics, ACE inhibitors, α_1-blockers, hydralazine HCl, minoxidil
Hyperdynamic circulation	β-Blockers		Direct vasodilators
Peripheral vascular oc-clusive disease		β-Blockers	
Postmyocardial infarction	Nonintrinsic sympathomimetically active β-blockers		
II. Renal			
Bilateral renal arterial disease or severe stenosis in artery to solitary kidney			ACE inhibitors
Renal insufficiency			
• Early (serum creatinine 130–221 μmol/L, 1.5–2.5 mg/dL)			Potassium-sparing agents, potassium supplements
• Advanced (serum cre-atinine ≥221 μmol/L [2.5 mg/dL])	Loop diuretics	ACE inhibitors	Potassium-sparing agents, potassium supplements
III. Other			
Asthma/chronic obstruc-tive pulmonary disease			β-Blocker, labetalol
Cyclosporine-associated hypertension	Nifedipine, labetalol	Verapamil, diltiazem, nicardipine HCl	
Depression		α_2-Agonists	Reserpine
Diabetes mellitus			
• Type I (insulin-dependent)		β-Blockers	
• Type II		β-Blockers: diuretics	
Dyslipidemia		β-Blockers: diuretics	
Liver disease		Labetalol	Methyldopa
Vascular headache			
Pregnancy			
• Preeclampsia	Methyldopa; hydralazine		Diuretics; ACE inhibitors
• Chronic hypertension	Methyldopa		ACE inhibitors

ACE, angiotensin-converting enzyme.

From The sixth report of the Joint National Committee on detection, evaluation, and treatment of high blood pressure. *Arch Intern Med* 1997;157:2413–2446, with permission.

tion more frequently (perhaps in 2 weeks or earlier), and, if pressure is not optimally controlled, the same alternatives as depicted in Figure 15–2 might be pursued. Thus, the dose of the initially prescribed agent might be increased to its full amount, or an alternative agent might be prescribed, or a second agent may be added to the agent that was prescribed initially. In selecting the second agent to be added to the one initially prescribed, it is wise to choose one that will at least add to or potentiate the antihypertensive effectiveness of the first compound. In this regard, the diuretic (in less than full doses, perhaps 12.5 or 25 mg hydrochlorothiazide or its equiva-

lents) has been found to be particularly effective without significantly exacerbating its intrinsic potential to produce metabolic side effects. This consideration is of particular relevance if the diuretic was not selected initially because of preexisting carbohydrate intolerance, hyperlipidemia, hyperuricemia, or the concern for development of hypokalemia (particularly in those patients with left ventricular hypertrophy or a history of cardiac failure. In selecting an initial agent for antihypertensive therapy, it might be especially worthwhile to consider comorbid diseases, other prescribed drug therapy, or preexisting metabolic alterations. In this regard, a

TABLE 15–12. *Adverse antihypertensive drug effects*

Drug	Selected side effects	Precautions and special considerations
I. Diuretics		
Thiazides and related diuretics	Hypokalemia, hypomagnesemia, hyponatremia, hyperuricemia, hypercholesterolemia, hypertriglyceridemia, dysfunction, weakness	Except for metolazone and indapamide, ineffective in renal failure (serum creatine ≥221 μmol/L (2.5 mg/dL); hypokalemia increases digitalis toxicity; may precipitate acute gout.
Loop diuretics	Same as for thiazides except loop diuretics do not cause hypercalcemia.	Effective in chronic renal failure.
Potassium-sparing agents	This group is associated with hyperkalemia. Spironolactone can cause gynecomastia, mastodynia, menstrual irregularities, diminished libido in male individuals.	Danger of hyperkalemia in patients with renal failure, in patients treated with ACE inhibitors or with nonsteroidal antiinflammatory agents. Triamterene is associated with the danger of renal calculi.
II. Adrenergic inhibitors		
β-Blockers	Bronchospasm, may aggravate peripheral arterial insufficiency, fatigue, insomnia, exacerbation of CHF, masking of symptoms of hypoglycemia. Also, hypertriglyceridemia, decreased high-density lipoprotein cholesterol (except for those drugs with intrinsic sympathomimetic activity). Reduced exercise tolerance.	Should not be used in patients with asthma, COPD, CHF with systolic dysfunction, heart block (greater than first degree), and sick sinus syndrome; use with caution in patients with insulin-treated diabetes and patients with peripheral vascular disease; should not be discontinued abruptly in patients with ischemic heart disease.
α/β-Blocker	Bronchospasm, may aggravate peripheral vascular insufficiency, orthostatic hypotension.	Should not be used in patients with asthma, COPD, CHF, heart block (greater than first degree), and sick sinus syndrome; use with caution in patients with insulin-treated diabetes and patients with peripheral vascular disease.
α-Receptor blockers	Orthostatic hypotension, syncope, weakness, palpitations, headache	
III. ACE inhibitors	Cough, rash, angioneurotic edema, hyperkalemia, dysgeusia	Hyperkalemia can develop, particularly in patients with renal insufficiency; hypotension has been observed with initiation of ACE inhibitors, especially in patients with high plasma renin activity or in those receiving diuretic therapy; can cause reversible, acute renal failure in patients with bilateral renal artery stenosis or unilateral stenosis in a solitary kidney and in patients with cardiac failure and with volume depletion; rarely can induce neutropenia or proteinuria; absolutely contraindicated in the second and third trimesters of pregnancy.
IV. Calcium antagonists Dihydropyridines • Amlodipine besylate • Felodipine • Isradipine • Nicardipine HCl • Nifedipine • Nisoldipine	Headache, dizziness, peripheral edema, tachycardia, gingival hyperplasia	Use with caution in patients with CHF; may aggravate angina and myocardial ischemia.

ACE, angiotensin-converting enzyme; CHF, congestive heart failure; COPD, chronic obstructive pulmonary disease.
From The sixth report of the Joint National Committee on detection, evaluation, and treatment of high blood pressure. *Arch Intern Med* 1997;157:2413–2446, with permission.

TABLE 15–13. *Selected drug interactions with antihypertensive therapy*

Diuretics

Possible situations for decreased antihypertensive effects
- Cholestyramine and colestipol HCl decrease absorption.
- NSAIDs, including aspirin and OTC ibuprofen, may antagonize diuretic effectiveness.

Possible situations for increased antihypertensive effects
- Combinations of thiazides—especially metolazone—with furosemide can produce profound diuresis, natriuresis, and kaliuresis in renal impairment.

Effects of diuretics on other drugs
- Diuretics can increase serum lithium levels and increase toxicity by enhancing proximal tubular reabsorption of lithium.
- Diuretics may make it more difficult to control dyslipidemia and diabetes.

β-Blockers

Possible situations for decreased antihypertensive effects
- NSAIDs may decrease the effects of β-blockers.
- Rifampin, smoking, and phenobarbital decrease serum levels of agents primarily metabolized by the liver through enzyme induction.

Possible situations for increased antihypertensive effects
- Cimetidine may increase serum levels of β-blockers that are primarily metabolized by the liver through enzyme inhibition.
- Quinidine may increase the risk for hypotension.

Effects of β-blockers on other drugs
- Combinations of diltiazem HCl or verapamil HCl with β-blockers may have additive sinoatrial and atrioventricular node depressant effects and may also promote negative inotropic effects on the failing myocardium.
- The combination of β-blockers and reserpine may cause marked bradycardia and syncope.
- β-Blockers may increase serum levels of theophylline, lidocaine HCl, and chlorpromazine through reduced hepatic clearance.
- Nonselective β-blockers prolong insulin-induced hypoglycemia and promote rebound hypertension by unopposed α stimulation. All β-blockers mask the adrenergically mediated symptoms of hypoglycemia and have the potential to aggravate diabetes.
- β-Blockers may make it more difficult to control dyslipidemia.
- Phenylpropanolamine, which can be obtained OTC in cold and diet preparations, pseudoephedrine, ephedrine, and epinephrine can cause increases in blood pressure by unopposed α-receptor–induced vasoconstriction.

ACE inhibitors

Possible situations for decreased antihypertensive effects
- NSAIDs, including aspirin and OTC ibuprofen, may decrease blood pressure control.
- Antacids may decrease the bioavailability of ACE inhibitors.

Possible situations for increased antihypertensive effects
- Diuretics may lead to excessive hypotensive effects (hypovolemia).

Effects of ACE inhibitors on other drugs
- Hypokalemia may occur with potassium supplements, potassium-sparing agents, and NSAIDs.
- ACE inhibitors may increase serum lithium levels.

Calcium antagonists

Possible situations for decreased antihypertensive effects
- Serum levels and antihypertensive effects of calcium antagonists may be diminished by these interactions—rifampin/verapamil; carbamazepine/diltiazem and verapamil; phenobarbital and phenytoin/verapamil.

Possible situations for increased antihypertensive effects
- Cimetidine may increase pharmacologic effects of all calcium antagonists by inhibition of hepatic metabolizing enzymes resulting in increased serum levels.

Effects of calcium antagonists on other drugs
- Digoxin and carbamazepine serum levels and toxicity may be increased by verapamil and possibly diltiazem.
- Serum levels of prazosin HCl, quinidine, and theophylline may be increased by verapamil.
- Serum levels of cyclosporine may be increased by diltiazem, nicardipine HCl, and verapamil. The cyclosporine dose may need to be decreased.

α-Blockers

Possible situations for increased antihypertensive effects
- Concomitant antihypertensive drug therapy, especially diuretics, may increase chance of postural hypotension.

Sympatholytics

Possible situations for decreased antihypertensive effects
- Tricyclic antidepressants may decrease the effects of centrally acting and peripheral norepinephrine depleters.
- Sympathomimetics, including OTC cold and diet preparations, amphetamines, phenothiazine, and cocaine, may interfere with the antihypertensive effects of guanethidine monosulfate and guanadrel sulfate.
- The severity of clonidine HCl withdrawal reaction can be increased with β-blockers.
- Monoamine oxidase inhibitors may prevent degradation and metabolism of norepinephrine released by tyramine-containing foods and may cause hypertension. They may also cause hypertensive reactions when combined with reserpine or guanethidine.

Effects of sympatholytics on other drugs
- Methyldopa may increase lithium levels.

This table does not include all potential drug interactions with antihypertensive drugs.

ACE, angiotensin-converting enzyme; NSAIDs, nonsteroidal antiinflammatory drugs; OTC, over-the-counter.

From The sixth report of the Joint National Committee on detection, evaluation, and treatment of high blood pressure. *Arch Intern Med* 1997;157:2413–2446, with permission.

TABLE 15–14. *Effects of therapy in older patients with hypertension*

Characteristics	Clinical trial						
	Australian (50)	EWPHE (51)	Coope and Warrender (52)	STOP-Hypertension (49)	MRC (48)	SHEP (47)	HDFP (36)
Patients, n	582	840	884	1,627	4,396	4,736	2,374
Age range, yr	60–69	>60	60–79	70–84	65–74	60 to ≥80[b]	60–69
Mean BP at entry, mm Hg	165/101	182/101	197/100	195/102	185/91	170/77	170/101
Relative risk of event (treated vs. control)							
Stroke	0.67	0.64	0.58[b]	0.53[b]	0.75[b]	0.67[b]	0.56[b]
CAD	0.82	0.80	1.03	0.87[c]	0.81	0.73[b]	0.85[b]
CHF	—	0.78	0.68	0.49[b]	—	0.45[b]	—
All CVD	0.69	0.71[b]	0.76[b]	0.60[b]	0.83[b]	0.68[b]	0.84[b]

BP, blood pressure; CAD, coronary artery disease; CHF, congestive heart failure; CVD, cardiovascular disease; EWPHE, European Working Party on High Blood Pressure in the Elderly; HDFP, Hypertension Detection and Follow-Up Program; MRC, Medical Research Council; SHEP, Systolic Hypertension in the Elderly Program; STOP, Swedish Trial in Old Patients.
[b]Statistically significant.
[c]Myocardial infarction only; sudden deaths decreased from 13 to 4.

series of additional tables were included in the JNC-VI report that may be of particular value to the physician with particular interest in cardiovascular medicine. In addition to those cited earlier (Tables 15–10 and 15–11), Table 15–12 concerns adverse effects of particular relevance, and Table 15–13 details important drug interactions. Space does not permit further discussion of those urgent or emergent complications of hypertensive disease, but these are also summarized well and succinctly in the JNC-VI (24).

Isolated Systolic Hypertension

Until relatively recently, although it was well known that isolated systolic pressure increase was associated with increased risk, information was not available to indicate whether therapeutic reduction of that pressure increase would be associated with a reduction in those risks. At least three independent national studies (the Systolic Hypertension in the Elderly Program in the United States [47], the Medical Research Council Trial in Great Britain [48], and the STOP-Hypertension Trial in Sweden [49]) demonstrated that pressure reduction was associated with a significant reduction in risk. Each of these studies used the diuretic alone or in combination with a β-blocker. Other earlier reports emphasized the efficacy and importance of treating diastolic hypertension in the elderly (50–52) (Table 15–14). Subsequent to these studies, the dihydropyridine calcium antagonist nitrendipine demonstrated reduction of deaths in elderly patients with isolated systolic hypertension (53). Moreover, other studies in patients with systolic and diastolic pressure increase also have shown reduction in fatal and nonfatal strokes with ACE inhibitors and angiotensin II (type 1) receptor blockers (54–56).

SUMMARY

The various hypertensive diseases, with particular emphasis on essential hypertension, have been discussed presenting a sequence of clinically relevant classifications. By initially discussing the means by which arterial pressure is normally controlled through a mechanistic classification, an etiologic classification of the variety of hypertensive diseases seemed reasonable. With these concepts taken into consideration, it followed that a classification of disease by severity of arterial pressure increase and target organ involvement was offered. This approach was followed by a classification of therapeutic alternatives that took into consideration the severity of pressure increase, target organ involvement, comorbid diseases, and coexisting therapy for other conditions.

REFERENCES

1. Page IH. Pathogenesis of arterial hypertension. *JAMA* 1949;140: 451–458.
2. Frohlich ED. Pathophysiology of systemic arterial hypertension. In: Schlant RC, Alexander RW, O'Rourke RA, et al., eds. *Hurst's the heart,* 8th ed. New York: McGraw-Hill, 1993:1391–1401.
3. Frohlich ED. The first Irvine H. Page lecture: the mosaic of hypertension; past, present, and future. *J Hypertens* 1988;6[Suppl 4]:2–11.
4. Frohlich ED. Pathophysiology: disease mechanisms. In: Frohlich ED, ed. *Pathophysiology: disease mechanisms.* Philadelphia: Lippincott Williams & Wilkins, 1998:1–21.
5. Stokes J III. Cardiovascular risk factors. In: Frohlich ED, ed. *Preventive aspects of coronary heart disease.* Philadelphia: FA Davis, 1990:3–20.
6. Kurtz TW, Spence MA. Genetics of essential hypertension. *Am J Med* 1993;94:77–84.
7. Schunkert H, Hense HW, Holmer SR, et al. Association between a deletion polymorphism of the angiotensin-converting-enzyme gene and left ventricular hypertrophy. *N Engl J Med* 1994;330:1634–1638.
8. Frohlich ED. Current approaches in the treatment of hypertension. *Curr Prob Cardiol* 1994;19:399–469.
9. Frohlich ED. *Hypertension: evaluation and treatment.* Philadelphia: Lippincott Williams & Wilkins, 1998.

10. Ward R. Familial aggregation and genetic epidemiology of blood pressure. In: Laragh JH, Brenner BM, eds. *Hypertension: pathophysiology, diagnosis, and management, Vol. 1.* New York: Raven Press, 1990: 81–100.

11. Morris BJ. Identification of essential hypertension genes. *J Hypertens* 1993;11:115–120.

12. Tarazi RC, Dustan HP, Frohlich ED. Relation of plasma to interstitial fluid volume in essential hypertension. *Circulation* 1969;40:357–365.

13. Weil JV, Chidsey CA. Plasma volume expansion resulting from interference with adrenergic functions in normal man. *Circulation* 1968;37:54–61.

14. Dustan HP, Tarazi RC, Bravo EL. Dependence of arterial pressure on intravascular volume in treated hypertensive patients. *N Engl J Med* 1972;286:861–866.

15. McCormack LJ, Poutasse EF, Meaney TF, et al. A pathologic-arteriographic correlation of renal arterial disease. *Am Heart J* 1966;72:188–198.

16. Dustan HP, Humphries AW, DeWolfe VG, et al. Normal arterial pressure in patients with renal arterial stenosis. *JAMA* 1964;187: 1028–1029.

17. Frohlich ED, Tarazi RC, Dustan HP. Hemodynamic and functional mechanisms in two renal hypertension: arterial and pyelonephritis. *Am J Med Sci* 1971;261:189–195.

18. Dustan HP, Page IH. Some factors in renal and renoprival hypertension. *J Lab Clin Med* 1964;64:948–959.

19. Panza JA, Casino PR, Kilcoyne CM, et al. Impaired endothelium-dependent vasodilation in patients with essential hypertension: evidence that the abnormality is not at the muscarinic receptor level. *J Am Coll Cardiol* 1994;23:1610–1616.

20. Yanagisawa M, Kurihara H, Kimura S, et al. A novel potent vasoconstrictor peptide produced by vascular endothelial cells. *Nature* 1988;332:411–415.

21. Sadoshima J, Xu Y, Slayter HS, et al. Autocrine release of angiotensin II mediates stretch-induced hypertrophy of cardiac myocytes *in vitro*. *Cell* 1993;75:977–984.

22. Oren S, Grossman E, Messerli FH, et al. High blood pressure: side effects of drugs, poisons, and food. *Cardiol Clin North Am* 1988;6: 467–474.

23. Whelton PK, He J, Appel LJ, et al. Primary prevention of hypertension: clinical and public health advisory from The National High Blood Pressure Education Program Working Group. *Arch Intern Med* 1993;153:186–208.

24. The seventh report of the Joint National Committee on detection, evaluation, and treatment of high blood pressure. *JAMA* 2003;289:2560–2572.

25. Keith HM, Wagener HP, Barker NN. Some different types of essential hypertension: their course and prognosis. *Am J Med Sci* 1939;197: 332–343.

26. Wagener HP, Clay GE, Gipner JF. Classification of retinal lesions in presence of vascular hypertension: report submitted by committee. *Trans Am Ophthalmol Soc* 1947;45:57–73.

27. Frohlich ED, Tarazi RC, Dustan HP. Clinical-physiological correlations in the development of hypertensive heart disease. *Circulation* 1971;44:446–455.

28. Thomas P, DeJong D. The P-wave in the electrocardiogram in the diagnosis of heart disease. *Br Heart J* 1967;16:241.

29. Macruz R, Perloff JK, Case RB. Method for the ECG recognition of atrial enlargement. *Circulation* 1958;17:882–889.

30. Morris JJ Jr, Estes HR Jr, Whalen RE, et al. P-wave analysis in valvular heart disease. *Circulation* 1964;29:242–252.

31. McPhie J. Left ventricular hypertrophy: electrocardiographic diagnosis. *Australas Ann Med* 1958;7:317–327.

32. Grant RP, ed. *The spatial vector approach: clinical electrocardiography.* New York: McGraw-Hill, 1957.

33. Dunn FG, Chandraratna PN, de Carvalho JG, et al. Pathophysiologic assessment of hypertensive heart disease by echocardiography. *Am J Cardiol* 1977;39:789–795.

34. Dreslinski GR, Frohlich ED, Dunn FG, et al. Echocardiographic diastolic ventricular abnormality in hypertensive heart disease: atrial emptying index. *Am J Cardiol* 1981;47:1087–1090.

35. Greenberg G, Thompson SG, Brennan PJ. The relationship between smoking and the response to antihypertensive treatment in mild hypertensives in the Medical Research Council's Trial of Treatment. *Int J Epidemiol* 1987;16:25–30.

36. Langford HG, Stamler J, Wassertheil-Smoller S, et al. All-cause mortality in the Hypertension Detection and Follow-Up Program: findings in the whole cohort and for persons with less severe hypertension, with and without other traits related to risk of mortality. *Prog Cardiovasc Dis* 1986;29[Suppl 1]:29–54.

37. Tight blood pressure control and risk of macrovascular and microvascular complications in type 2 diabetes: UKPDS 38. UK Prospective Diabetes Study Group. *BMJ* 1998;317:703–713.

38. Efficacy of atenolol and captopril in reducing risk of macrovascular and microvascular complications in type 2 diabetes: UKPDS39. UK Prospective Diabetes Study Group. *BMJ* 1998;317:713–720.

39. Parving HH, Lehnert H, Bröchner-Mortensen J, et al. The effect of irbesartan on the development of diabetic nephropathy in patients with type 2 diabetes. *N Engl J Med* 2001;345:870–878.

40. Lewis EJ, Hunsicker LG, Clarke WR, et al. Renoprotective effect of the angiotensin-receptor antagonist irbesartan in patients with nephropathy due to type 2 diabetes. *N Engl J Med* 2001;345:851–860.

41. Brennen BM, Cooper ME, de Zeeuw D, et al. Effects of losartan on renal and cardiovascular outcomes in patients with type 2 diabetes and nephropathy. *N Engl J Med* 2001;345:861–869.

42. Frohlich ED. Risk mechanisms in hypertensive heart disease. *Hypertension* 1999;34:782–789.

43. Frohlich ED. Promise of prevention and reversal of target organ involvement in hypertension. *J Renin Angiotensin Aldosterone Syst* 2001;2[Suppl 1]:S4–S9.

44. Pfeffer MA, Braunwald E, Moyé LA, et al. Effect of captopril on mortality and morbidity in patients with left ventricular dysfunction after myocardial infarction. Results of the Survival and Ventricular Enlargement Trial. *N Engl J Med* 1992;327:669–677.

45. Swedberg K, Held P, Kjekshus J, et al. Effects of the early administration of enalapril on mortality in patients with acute myocardial infarction. Results of the Cooperative New Scandinavian Enalapril Survival Study II (CONSENSUS II). *N Engl J Med* 1992;327: 678–684.

46. Køber L, Torp-Pedersen C, Carlsen JE, et al. A clinical trial of the angiotensin-converting-enzyme inhibitor trandolapril in patients with left ventricular dysfunction after myocardial infarction. *N Engl J Med* 1995;333:1670–1676.

47. Prevention of stroke by antihypertensive drug treatment in older persons with isolated systolic hypertension. Final results of the Systolic Hypertension in the Elderly Program (SHEP). SHEP Cooperative Research Group. *JAMA* 1991;265:3255–3264.

48. Medical Research Council trial of treatment of hypertension in older adults: principal results. MRC Working Party. *Br Med J* 1992;304: 405–412.

49. Dahlöf B, Lindholm LH, Hansson L, et al. Morbidity and mortality in the Swedish Trial in Old Patients with Hypertension (STOP-Hypertension). *Lancet* 1991;338:1281–1285.

50. Treatment of mild hypertension in the elderly. A study initiated and administered by the National Heart Foundation or Australia. *Med J Aust* 1981;2:398–402.

51. Amery A, Birkenhäger W, Brixko P, et al. Mortality and morbidity results from the European Working Party on High Blood Pressure in the Elderly trial. *Lancet* 1985;1:1349–1354.

52. Coope J, Warrender TS. Randomized trial of treatment of hypertension in elderly patients in primary care. *Br Med J* 1986;293:1145–1151.

53. Staessen JA, Fagard R, Thijs L, et al., Randomised double-blind comparison of placebo and active treatment for older patients with isolated systolic hypertension. The Systolic Hypertension-Europe (Syst-Eur) Trial Investigators. *Lancet* 1997;360:757–764.

54. Effects of ramipril on cardiovascular and microvascular outcomes in people with diabetes: results of the HOPE study and MICRO-HOPE substudy. Heart Outcomes Prevention Evaluation (HOPE) Study Investigators. *Lancet* 2000;355:253–259.

55. Dahlöf B, Devereux RB, Kjeldsen SE, et al. Cardiovascular morbidity and mortality in the Losartan Intervention For Endpoint and reduction in hypertension study (LIFE): a randomized trial against atenolol. *Lancet* 2002;359:995–1003.

56. Lindholm LH, Ibsen H, Dahlöf B, et al. Cardiovascular morbidity and mortality in patients with diabetes in the Losartan Intervention For Endpoint reduction in hypertension study (LIFE): a randomized trial against atenolol. *Lancet* 2002;359:1004–1010.

CHAPTER 16

Management of Hypertension

Norman M. Kaplan

Key Words: Antihypertensive drugs; lifestyle modification; hypertension; treatment.

Hypertension is easy to treat but often difficult to control. As the most common of the major risk factors for atherothrombotic vascular diseases, the number of patients being treated has markedly increased over the last few decades, but still only about one-fourth of all patients with hypertension have their condition adequately managed (1).

PROBLEMS OF DIAGNOSIS AND ADHERENCE

Such poor management reflects the basic nature of hypertension. On the one hand, blood pressure (BP) fluctuates constantly and usually is considerably greater in the offices and clinics where it is usually measured, giving rise to a 20% to 30% likelihood that the increased pressure is "isolated office hypertension" or "white-coat hypertension." Although the natural history of such office-only hypertension remains incompletely ascertained, the limited data currently available support a benign course, little different than normotension (2). Therefore, a considerable number of people are being diagnosed and treated either prematurely or unnecessarily. On the other hand, documented hypertension typically has characteristics that make it difficult to treat: a lifelong, incurable condi-

tion that is asymptomatic and whose treatment provides benefits that show up only after many years while causing immediate burdens of costs and side effects.

One maneuver has surfaced as a complete solution to the overdiagnosis of office-only hypertension and a major stimulus for the continuance of antihypertensive therapy: the measurement of BP outside of the physician's office, either by self-taken readings with an electronic device or by ambulatory automatic recorders. Multiple readings with home devices not only can document the initial nature of the BP, but it also can monitor the long-term response to therapy, thereby providing feedback to the patient that encourages adherence to therapy. Ambulatory monitoring more rapidly establishes the nature of the BP and, by assessing the nocturnal pattern, provides additional prognostic information (3).

THE DECISION TO TREAT

At the same time that out-of-office measurements have provided greater certainty of the initial nature of the BP and more assurance about the effectiveness of therapy, major changes have occurred in the perceptions about the criteria for institution of treatment. Not long ago, the criteria were based almost entirely on the level of BP. During the past few years, the criteria have been considerably broadened to take into account other factors that determine overall risk for premature cardiovascular disease (4) (Table 16–1). Using either the looser classifications of risk advocated in guidelines of expert committees (4,5) or the more

N. M. Kaplan: University of Texas Southwestern Medical Center, 5323 Harry Hines Blvd., Dallas, Texas 75390-8899.

TABLE 16–1. *Factors influencing prognosis*

Risk factors for cardiovascular disease used for risk stratification	Target-organ damage	Associated clinical conditions
• Levels of systolic and diastolic blood pressure (grades 1–3) • Men > 55 years • Women > 65 years • Smoking • Total cholesterol > 5.1 mmol/L (200 mg/dL) • Increased LDL cholesterol > 2.5 mmol/L (100 mg/dL) • Reduced HDL cholesterol: M < 1.0 mmol/L (<40 mg/dL), F < 1.2 mmol/L (<45 mg/dL) • Family history of premature cardiovascular disease	• Left ventricular hypertrophy (electrocardiogram or echocardiogram) • Microalbuminuria (30–300 mg/day) • Ultrasound or radiologic evidence of atherothrombotic plaque (carotid, iliac and femoral arteries, aorta) • Generalized or focal narrowing of the retinal arteries	Cerebrovascular disease • Ischemic stroke • Cerebral hemorrhage • Transient ischemic attack Heart disease • Myocardial infarction • Angina • Coronary revascularization • Congestive heart failure Renal disease • Renal impairment (plasma creatinine concentration: F > 1.4 mg/dL, M > 1.5 mg/dL) • Albuminuria > 300 mg/day Peripheral vascular disease Diabetes

F, female; HDL, high-density lipoprotein; LDL, low-density lipoprotein; M, male.

exact ascertainments provided by application of the Framingham study data to each patient (6), the relative risk for a cardiovascular event in the next 10 years is being taken as the best criterion for the decision to institute antihypertensive therapy.

This shift in criteria has been coupled with the positive results of several randomized, controlled, therapeutic trials to bring about two major changes in clinical practice: (i) the recognition that millions of elderly patients with isolated systolic hypertension need to be given antihypertensive therapy; and (ii) the establishment of lower thresholds for the institution of therapy and lower goals for the intensiveness of therapy for patients with concomitant diabetes, renal damage, coronary disease, congestive failure, or cerebrovascular disease who are at high risk for hypertension.

LIFESTYLE MODIFICATIONS

Together with the acceptance of more frequent and more intensive antihypertensive therapy has come a greater awareness of the contributions of multiple adverse lifestyle habits to the development of hypertension and to overall cardiovascular risk. Table 16–2 lists those modifications known to be useful in both prevention and management.

TABLE 16–2. *Lifestyle modifications*

- Lose weight if overweight
- Increase aerobic physical activity (30–60 minutes most days of the week)
- Reduce sodium intake to no more than 100 mmol/day (2.4 g sodium or 6 g sodium chloride)
- Limit alcohol intake
- Increase intake of potassium-rich foods
- Stop smoking

Weight Loss

Almost everywhere people are gaining weight, no place more so than in the United States, where more than half of the population is overweight (7). With weight gain even within the limits of presumably normal body size, particularly if it is predominantly deposited in the upper body (i.e., visceral or abdominal), the prevalence of hypertension increases together with other elements of the metabolic syndrome (6). Weight loss, regardless of the method, decreases BP. Rather than waiting until obesity is obvious and almost impossible to overcome, small gains in weight and abdominal circumference should be vigorously attacked by diet and physical activity. In addition, the contribution of obstructive sleep apnea, usually occurring in obese individuals, should be recognized and intensively treated (8).

Physical Activity

The need for increased levels of physical activity has been clearly documented. Physical inactivity contributes greatly to weight gain and afflicts not only middle-aged "couch potatoes" but also adolescents (9). Fortunately, activity as easy as brisk walking will reduce the incidence of cardiovascular events (10), an effect that likely involves a reduction in BP (11) and glucose intolerance (12).

Sodium Reduction

A moderate reduction in dietary sodium intake (e.g., a decline to 100–120 mmol/day from the usual intake of 150–175 mmol/day, which is the average level in the U.S. population) will decrease BP. In the Dietary Approaches to Stop Hypertension (DASH) trial, a reduction in sodium intake added to the antihypertensive effect of a diet with increased potassium, fiber, and calcium and decreased saturated fat (13). The desired reduction in sodium intake should be easy to accomplish, simply by avoiding processed foods with more than 400 mg sodium per portion as identified on the label.

Moderation of Alcohol

Too much alcohol—more than 3 portions a day—will increase BP. Reduction of intake to 1 portion per day will decrease the BP of individuals who drink too much alcohol (14). Regular consumption of 1 to 2 portions (one portion = 12 ounces of beer, 5 ounces of wine, 1.5 ounces of whiskey) of alcohol per day provides significant protection against cardiovascular diseases and dementia (15); therefore, in the absence of liver dysfunction, such healthful drinking need not be curtailed.

Potassium Intake

The antihypertensive effects of the DASH diet (13) may reflect the increased intake of potassium from fresh fruits and vegetables. Greater intake of dietary potassium is protective against stroke (16), likely as an effect on BP.

Smoking

Beyond all of the nefarious effects of cigarette smoking, nicotine increases BP (17). Unfortunately, the transitory pressor effect of smoking each cigarette, lasting 20 to 30 minutes, is usually not recognized when BP is measured in a setting where smoking is prohibited. If the measurement cannot be taken while the patient is smoking, BP can be assumed to be at least 10 mm Hg greater and should be treated accordingly.

Other Factors

Numerous other dietary components, including fiber and fish oil (18), but not calcium, magnesium, or antioxidants, may decrease BP (19).

ANTIHYPERTENSIVE DRUGS

If lifestyle changes are not adequate to decrease BP to the appropriate goal of therapy, as will be true in the majority of patients with hypertension with one or more additional risk factors, antihypertensive drugs are indicated. During the last decade, major changes have occurred in the relative usage of the various classes of agents (Fig. 16–1).

These major changes are largely the result of the intensive promotion by their pharmaceutical marketers and the natural desire of hypertension specialists and practitioners to be on the cutting edge of clinical practice. The choice of drug often is based on perceived differences in efficacy in decreasing BP and the likelihood of side effects. In fact, overall antihypertensive efficacy varies little among the various available drugs. To gain approval from regulatory agencies in various countries, the drug must be effective in reducing BP in a large portion of the 1,500 or more patients given the drug during its preapproval clinical trials. Moreover, the dosage and formulation of drug are chosen so as not to de-

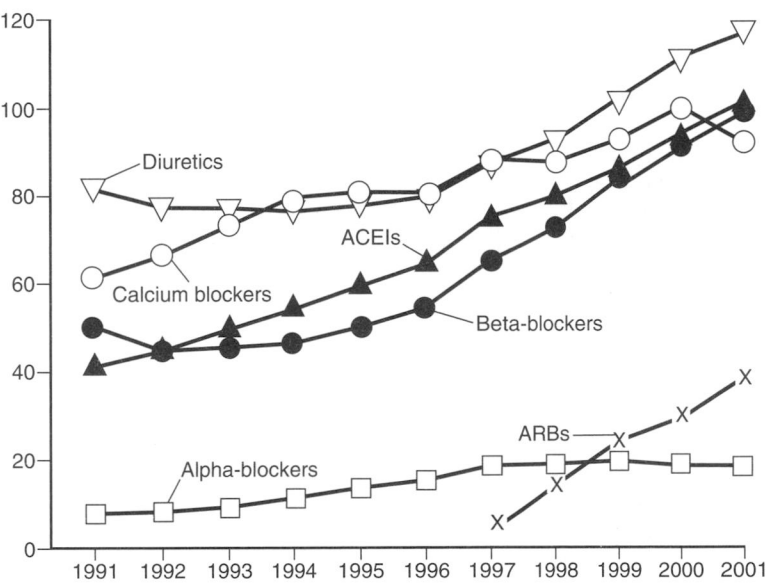

FIG. 16–1. Number of prescriptions in millions for antihypertensive drugs dispensed in retail channels in the United States from 1991 to 2000. ACEI, angiotensin-converting enzyme inhibitor; ARB, angiotensin II-receptor blocker. (Reprinted from National Prescription Audit. Ambler, PA: IMS, 2000, with permission.)

crease BP too much or too fast to avoid hypotensive side effects. Virtually all oral drugs are designed to do the same thing: decrease BP at least 10% in the majority of patients with mild to moderate hypertension.

Comparisons of Efficacy

Each new drug must be shown to be effective in a large percentage of patients with hypertension and must be tested against currently available agents to show at least equal efficacy. When comparisons among various drugs have been made, they almost always come out close to one another in antihypertensive efficacy. The best such comparison was the Treatment of Mild Hypertension Study (TOMHS) (20). The TOMHS study involved random allocation of five drugs: the diuretic chlorthalidone, the β-blocker acebutolol, the α-blocker doxazosin, the calcium channel blocker (CCB) amlodipine, or the angiotensin-converting enzyme inhibitor (ACEI) enalapril. Each drug was given to almost 200 subjects with mild hypertension, whereas another group took a placebo; all subjects remained on a nutritional-hygienic program. The overall antihypertensive efficacy of the five drugs over 4 years was virtually equal.

Nonetheless, individual patients may vary considerably in their response to different drugs. Some of this variability can be accounted for by patient characteristics, including age and race. This was shown in a Veterans Administration (VA) cooperative 1-year trial in which 1,292 men were randomly given one of six drugs from each major class. Overall and in the black patients, the CCB was most effective, but the ACEI was best in younger white patients, and the β-blocker was best in older white patients (21). In a randomized crossover trial of younger patients with combined systolic and diastolic hypertension who were given a representative drug from four classes (ACEI, β-blocker, CCB, and diuretic) the ACEI and β-blocker were more effective than the CCB or diuretic (22). In a similar randomized crossover trial of elderly patients with isolated systolic hypertension, diuretic and CCB were more effective than the β-blocker or ACEI (23).

These different effects on decreasing BP are of interest, but the critical issue is effectiveness in reducing morbidity and mortality. All major classes of antihypertensive drugs, except α-blockers, have been shown to reduce mortality and morbidity in large randomized controlled trials and there are few differences among them (24,25).

In all of the 18 randomized controlled trials completed before 1995, diuretics or β-blockers were used (24) (Table 16–3). The major conclusion of the metaanalysis of the data from these 18 randomized controlled trials is that low-dose diuretic therapy (12.5 to 25 mg hydrochlorothiazide or its equivalent) provided excellent protection against coronary disease, whereas high doses of diuretic and β-blocker–based therapies did not, although all provided protection against stroke and congestive heart failure (CHF).

TABLE 16–3. *Randomized controlled trials before 1995: first drug therapy*

	Relative risk vs. placebo			
	Stroke	CHD	CHF	CV mortality
High dose diuretic (50–100 mg)	0.49	0.99	0.17	0.78
Low dose diuretic (12.5–25 mg)	0.66	0.72	0.58	0.76
β-Blocker	0.71	0.93	0.58	0.89

CHD, coronary heart disease; CHF, congestive heart failure; CV, cardiovascular.

Adapted from Psaty BM, Smith NL, Siscovick DS, et al. Health outcomes associated with antihypertensive therapies used as first-line agents. *JAMA* 1997;277:739–745, with permission.

After 1995, randomized controlled trials compared either ACEIs or CCBs against a diuretic with or without β-blocker or against one another (25). As seen in Table 16–4, one conclusion from these more recent trials seems obvious: Neither ACEI-based nor CCB-based therapies are better than therapies based on diuretics with or without β-blocker. CCB therapy protected better against stroke and less well against coronary heart disease and CHF, but ACEIs and CCBs provided identical effects on overall morbidity and mortality.

The results of the eight comparative trials completed since 1995 are by no means definitive. Fortunately, a large number of trials are currently in progress; therefore, more definitive data should soon be available to guide choices in therapy. In particular, data from the Antihypertensive and Lipid Lowering (ALLHAT) trial has provided a great deal of important comparative data.

In a sense, the process of determining which one drug is best is irrelevant. As the need to achieve lower goals of therapy has become obvious, the need to use more than one drug in the majority of hypertensives has also become obvious. This is nowhere better seen than among patients with diabetes who have hypertension. Therefore, the best combination of agents, which almost always is likely to include a low dose of diuretic, will be a more pertinent goal of future trials.

Putative Serious Adverse Effects

The various antihypertensive agents vary significantly, both in the frequency of adverse effects and, to an even greater degree, in their nature. The only currently available comparisons of a representative drug from all major classes given as monotherapy to sizable numbers of patients are TOMHS (20) and the VA Cooperative Study (21). Side effects differed among the drugs, but no one drug was markedly more or less acceptable than the others.

More serious problems have been blamed on various classes of antihypertensive drugs. Virtually all of these claims have come from noncontrolled, often retrospective,

TABLE 16–4. *Prospective overview of randomized trials for hypertension*

	Stroke	CHD	CHF	Major CV event	CV death	Total mortality
ACEI vs. placebo	0.70	0.80	0.84	0.79	0.74	0.84
(4 trials; 12,124 pts)	(0.57–0.85)	(0.72–0.89)	(0.68–1.04)	(0.73–0.86)	(0.64–0.85)	(0.76–0.94)
CCB vs. placebo	0.61	0.79	0.72	0.72	0.72	0.87
(2 trials; 5,520 pts)	(0.44–0.85)	(0.59–1.06)	(0.48–1.07)	(0.59–0.87)	(0.52–0.98)	(0.70–1.09)
ACEI vs. D/βB	1.05	1.00	0.92	1.00	1.00	1.03
(3 trials; 16,161 pts)	(0.92–1.19)	(0.88–1.14)	(0.77–1.09)	(0.93–1.08)	(0.87–1.15)	(0.93–1.14)
CCB vs. D/βB	0.87	1.12	1.12	1.02	1.05	1.01
(5 trials; 23,454 pts)	(0.77–0.98)	(1.0–1.26)	(0.95–1.33)	(0.95–1.10)	(0.92–1.2)	(0.92–1.11)
ACEI vs. CCB	1.02	0.81	0.82	0.92	1.04	1.03
(2 trials; 4,871 pts)	(0.85–1.21)	(0.68–0.97)	(0.67–1.0)	(0.83–1.01)	(0.87–1.24)	(0.91–1.18)

ACEI, angiotensin-converting enzyme inhibitor; CCB, calcium channel blocker; CHD, coronary heart disease; CHF, congestive heart failure; CV, cardiovascular; D/βB, diuretics/beta-blockers; pts, patients.

Adapted from Neal B, MacMahon S, Chapman N. Effects of ACE inhibitors, calcium antagonists, and other blood-pressure-lowering drugs: results of prospectively designed overviews of randomised trials. Blood Pressure Lowering Treatment Trialists' Collaboration. *Lancet* 2000;356:1955–1964.

observational case–control studies, and most of these claims subsequently have been disproved.

Cancer

The first erroneous claim was that the use of reserpine was associated with a twofold to fourfold increased risk for breast cancer in women, a claim made in three simultaneously published articles from outstanding investigators. As subsequently shown, these studies were all contaminated by the bias of excluding women at high risk for cancer from the control groups. Multiple subsequently published prospective studies have shown no association (26).

More recently, Pahor and coworkers (27) reported a twofold greater risk for cancer in elderly patients taking short-acting CCBs compared with users of β-blockers. Because they made no ascertainment of drug use after the original observation that the subjects had the respective drugs in their possession, the actual intake of drugs is totally unknown. Multiple subsequent reports of much larger populations in which drug use was appropriately ascertained have found *no increase* in cancer among users of CCBs. In their review of 14 case–control and cohort studies, Kizer and Kimmel (28) concluded that "the ensuing clinical evidence has failed to substantiate an elevation in cancer risk, overall or site specific."

Coronary Disease

A few years ago, Psaty and coworkers (29) reported a 60% increase in the risk for acute myocardial infarction (MI) among patients taking short-acting CCBs. This report coincided with republication of a metaanalysis of the adverse effects of high doses of short-acting CCBs in the immediate post-MI period (30). The two publications received tremendous press coverage claiming that CCBs could endanger more than 6 million patients with hypertension in the United

States alone, which led to major disruptions in the management of patients with both angina and hypertension who were receiving these agents.

Both Psaty and coworkers (29) and Furberg and coworkers (30) strongly suggested that their claims against short-acting CCBs (which had never been approved for the treatment of hypertension) also carried over to the longer acting agents (which are approved for the treatment of hypertension). There are significant differences in the hemodynamic and hormonal responses to short-acting versus long-acting CCBs, so that the faults of the former should not be assumed to apply to the latter.

Whereas some additional cohort observational studies have shown a greater mortality rate among CCB users than other drugs (31), no such increased mortality risk for CCB users was found among the 3,539 subjects in the Framingham Heart Study (32). As Michels and coworkers (31) concluded: "Whether the observed elevated risk [in CCB users] is real, or a result of residual confounding by indication, or chance, or a combination of the above cannot be evaluated with certainty on the basis of these observational data." The probability that confounding was a major factor in these associations is supported by the finding that, among 77,000 patients, the likelihood of being prescribed a CCB rather than other antihypertensives was significantly greater for patients with coexisting coronary disease (7.8-fold) or diabetes (1.5-fold) (33). As reviewed by Kizer and Kimmel (28), prospective, controlled data show no increase in coronary disease among users of long-acting CCBs.

As seen in Table 16–4, in the comparative trials of CCBs versus diuretic/β-blocker therapy, the slight increase in coronary events seen with CCBs was balanced by a smaller risk for strokes in the CCB-treated patients, with no differences in mortality between different classes (25). As previously noted, data from additional large comparative trials will resolve this issue.

The Individualized Approach

Increasingly, the treatment of hypertension is being individualized. The individualized approach is predicated on four major principles. The first choice may be one of a variety of antihypertensives from any of the major classes of drugs. Second, the choice can be logically based on the characteristics of the patients, in particular, the presence of concomitant diseases. Third, rather than proceeding with a second drug if the first is not effective or if side effects ensue, a substitution approach is used (stop the first drug and try another from a different class). Fourth, to reach the appropriate goal of therapy, multiple drugs, usually two and sometimes three or more, will be needed. In fact, additional drugs often were needed to achieve the goal of therapy in every randomized controlled trial comparing initial monotherapy against either placebo or another active drug.

Characteristics of the Drugs

Each class of drugs has different features that make its members more or less attractive.

Diuretics

In the past, diuretics were almost always chosen first, particularly because reactive fluid retention with other drugs used without a diuretic often blunted their effect. However, recognition of the electrolyte and metabolic side effects of diuretics, together with the lesser protection from coronary mortality in the initial trials where they were used in high doses shown in Table 16–3, caused many clinicians to doubt the wisdom of the routine use of diuretics. At the least, these factors have led to the more widespread use of lower doses of diuretics and their combinations with potassium-sparing agents. Low-dose, diuretic-based therapy is clearly protective and, as seen in Table 16–4, has now been shown to be as protective as either ACEI- or CCB-based therapies.

β-*Blockers*

In the 1970s and 1980s, β-blockers became increasingly popular. However, contraindications to their use and recognition of their potential for altering lipids and glucose tolerance adversely dampened their popularity. The failure to find primary protection against coronary disease in trials with a β-blocker, particularly in the elderly, further weakened the argument for their use. However, their ability to provide secondary cardioprotection and to treat heart failure has recently embellished their status.

Vasodilators

Drugs that act primarily as indirect vasodilators (α-blockers, ACEIs, angiotensin II-receptor blockers [ARBs], and CCBs) are being more widely advocated for initial therapy. There seems to be an inherent logic in using drugs that induce vasodilation, because an increased peripheral resistance is the hemodynamic fault of established hypertension, and these drugs have been shown to reverse the structural abnormalities of the disease (34).

Characteristics of the Patient

Demographic Features

Individual patient's characteristics may affect the likelihood of a good response to various classes of drugs. As shown in crossover rotations of the four major classes (22,23), younger and white patients will usually respond better to either an ACEI or a β-blocker, perhaps because they tend to have greater renin levels, whereas older and black patients will respond better to diuretics and CCBs, perhaps because they have lower renin levels and their hypertension is more "volume" mediated. These differences apply to monotherapy; with a low-dose of a diuretic as part of the regimen, responses to all other agents are largely equalized. Moreover, for each individual patient, any drug may work well or poorly, and there is no set formula that can be used to predict certain success without side effects.

Compelling Indications

Patients with hypertension, particularly the elderly, often have other medical problems, some related to their hypertension, some coincidental. Current guidelines list specific choices of drug for a variety of "compelling" indications (Table 16–5). There is evidence, mostly from controlled trials, of additional benefits to the use of these choices in various subgroups of hypertensives. Thus, a patient with hypertension with angina would logically be given a β-blocker or a CCB; a patient with CHF would be given an ACEI and diuretic. In an elderly man with hypertension

TABLE 16–5. *Compelling indications for antihypertensive drugs*

Indication	Drug
Elderly with ISH	Diuretic, CCB-DHP
Black	Diuretic, CCB
Heart Disease	
Post-MI	ACEI, β-blocker
LV dysfunction	ACEI
CHF	ACEI, β-blocker, spironolactone
Cerebrovascular disease	Diuretic ± ACEI
Nephropathy	
Type I DM	ACEI
Type 2 DM	ARB
Nondiabetic	ACEI
Prostatism	α-Blocker

ACEI, angiotensin-converting enzyme inhibitor; ARB, angiotensin II-receptor blocker; CCB, calcium channel blocker; CHF, congestive heart failure; DHP, dihydropyridine; DM, diabetes mellitus; ISH, isolated systolic hypertension; LV, left ventricular; MI, myocardial infarction.

with benign prostatic hypertrophy, an α-blocker would be the logical choice. In view of the benefits of addition of the ACEI ramipril to the therapy of high-risk patients shown in the Heart Outcomes Prevention Evaluation trial (35), it may be appropriate to use an ACEI in all suitable patients at high risk for atherothrombotic cardiovascular events. However, the assumption that the ACEI provided benefits beyond its antihypertensive effect has been questioned (36); therefore, perhaps other classes of drugs may also have provided additional protection as they further decreased BP.

At the same time, claims of special benefits of one class or another must be tempered when they are not placebo-controlled or based only on limited comparisons. For example, the claim that an ARB is preferred for patients with hypertension with left ventricular hypertrophy (LVH) is based only on its greater benefit when compared with a β-blocker (37), a class of drug long known to be less effective for LVH regression than other classes (38).

The same caveat applies to the evidence favoring the use of ARBs in the treatment of patients with type 2 diabetes with nephropathy. In the three trials showing benefit of an ARB (39–41), the ARB was compared with placebo but not with an ACEI, the class of drug clearly known to be renoprotective in other nephropathies (42).

An Overall Algorithm

Taking all of the preceding into account, the most appropriate individualized approach to therapy should almost always be based on a foundation of a low-dose of a diuretic except for the few who are intolerant to diuretic because of allergy, gout, or other conditions (Fig. 16–2). For most patients with hypertension, a combination of 12.5 mg hydrochlorothiazide or its equivalent plus a potassium-sparing agent should be used. In view of evidence that aldosterone antagonists provide protection against cardiac and renal fibrosis (43), spironolactone or, now that it has become available, eplerenone, is the logical choice as the potassium-sparing component. In those patients with hypertension with renal insufficiency, a more potent diuretic will be needed. Although furosemide has usually been chosen, the need for 2 or 3 doses per day make it an unattractive choice. A once daily dose of metolazone works as well and is more likely to be taken.

Even if the low-dose diuretic decreases BP to the goal of therapy, a second drug often will be indicated for those with the compelling indications shown in Figure 16–2. It could be argued that these other drugs should be given first and the diuretic added only for those whose BP is not adequately controlled with the first drug. This approach may be appropriate for those patients with hypertension with minimally increased BPs who resist the reactive sodium retention that frequently accompanies a reduction in BP with nondiuretic agents and who are able to maintain a diet that is moderately restricted of sodium. Nonetheless, I believe that the majority of patients with hypertension will need a combination of a low-dose diuretic together with whatever else they require because of the compelling indications shown in Table 16–5.

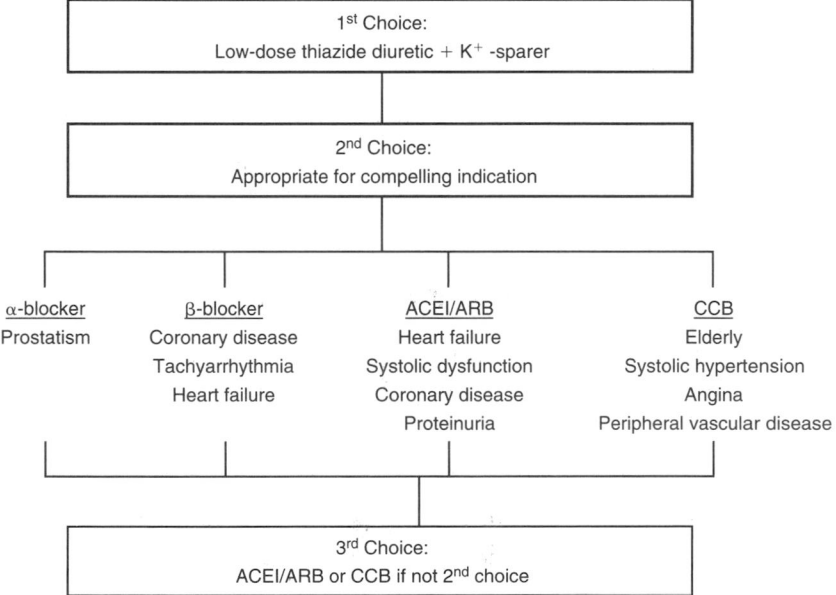

FIG. 16–2. An individualized approach to the treatment of hypertension that begins in most patients with a low dose diuretic and proceeds to those drugs for which there is a compelling indication. ACEI, angiotensin-converting enzyme inhibitor; ARB, angiotensin II-receptor blocker; CCB, calcium channel blocker.

TABLE 16–6. *Goals of therapy for patients with hypertension*

Group	Goal
Combined systolic and diastolic; low to medium overall risk	<140/90 mm Hg
Isolated systolic in the elderly	140–150 mm Hg
Diabetics and other high-risk patients	<130/80 mm Hg
Renal insufficiency	<125/75 mm Hg

GOALS OF THERAPY

A growing consensus has established different goals of therapy for different groups of patients with hypertension (Table 16–6). For most middle-aged patients at low to medium overall risk, a level less than 140/90 mm Hg is desirable. Therapy may need to be started in "high-normal" patients (i.e., with levels of pressure 130–139/85–89), because they clearly are at increased risk when compared with individuals with 120/80 mm Hg BP (44). However, in the absence of trial data documenting benefits beyond costs, most physicians would wait to begin therapy until the usual level is greater than 140/90 mm Hg.

In the elderly with isolated systolic hypertension, currently available data have all come from trials with initial systolic levels of 160 mm Hg or greater wherein treatment decreased the levels to 140 to 145 mm Hg. Those who are at high overall risk should probably have their levels reduced further, but that may be exceedingly difficult to accomplish.

The need for earlier and more intensive therapy in diabetics and other patients at high risk for hypertension has been well documented (45). The appropriate goal for those with renal insufficiency, accepted to be as low as 125/75 mm Hg, is based on rather limited data (46).

As desirable as these goals may be, they have rarely been reached, even in carefully controlled trials in which impediments to successful therapy have been removed (47). In typical clinical practice, the goals of therapy may be even harder to reach. Nonetheless, in general, the lower the better (48) so that efforts to achieve adequate control should be intensified to better protect vulnerable hypertensive patients.

REFERENCES

1. Kaplan NM. Hypertension in the population at large. In: Kaplan NM, ed. *Kaplan's clinical hypertension,* 8th ed. Philadelphia: Lippincott Williams & Wilkins, 2002.
2. Verdecchia P. Prognostic value of ambulatory blood pressure. *Hypertension* 2000;35:844–851.
3. Lurbe E, Redon J, Kesani A, et al. Increase in nocturnal blood pressure and progression to microalbuminuria in type 1 diabetes. *N Engl J Med* 2002;347:797–805.
4. Chobanian AV, Bakris GL, Black HR, et al. The seventh report of the Joint National Committee on prevention, detection, evaluation, and treatment of high blood pressure: the JNC 7 report. *JAMA* 2003;289:2560–2572.
5. 2003 World Health Organization (WHO)/International Society of Hypertension (ISH) statement on management of hypertension. *J Hypertens* 2003;21:1983–1992.
6. Expert Panel on Detection, Evaluation, and Treatment of High Blood Cholesterol in Adults. Executive Summary of the Third Report of the National Cholesterol Education Program (NCEP) Expert Panel on Detection, Evaluation, and Treatment of High Blood Cholesterol in Adults (Adult Treatment Panel III). *JAMA* 2001;285:2486–2497.
7. Hedley AA, Ogden CL, Johnson CL, et al. Prevalence of overweight and obesity among US children, adolescents, and adults, 1999–2002. *JAMA* 2004;291:2847–2850.
8. Pepperell JC, Ramdassingh-Dow S, Crosthwaite N, et al. Ambulatory blood pressure after therapeutic and subtherapeutic nasal continuous positive airway pressure for obstructive sleep apnoea: a randomised parallel trial. *Lancet* 2002;359:204–210.
9. Kimm SY, Glynn NW, Kriska AM, et al. Decline in physical activity in black girls and white girls during adolescence. *N Engl J Med* 2002;347:709–715.
10. Manson JE, Greenland P, LaCroix AZ, et al. Walking compared with vigorous exercise for the prevention of cardiovascular events in women. *N Engl J Med* 2002;347:716–725.
11. Whelton SP, Chin A, Xin X, et al. Effects of aerobic exercise on blood pressure: a meta-analysis of randomized, controlled trials. *Ann Intern Med* 2002:136:493–503.
12. Knowler WC, Barrett-Connor E, Fowler SE, et al. Reduction in the incidence of type 2 diabetes with lifestyle intervention or metformin. *N Engl J Med* 2002;346:393–403.
13. Sacks FM, Svetkey LP, Vollmer WM, et al. Effects of blood pressure on reduced dietary sodium and the Dietary Approaches to Stop Hypertension (DASH) diet. *N Engl J Med* 2001;344:3–10.
14. Xin X, He J, Frontini MG, et al. Effects of alcohol reduction on blood pressure. A meta-analysis of randomized controlled trials. *Hypertension* 2001;38:1112–1117.
15. Ruitenberg A, van Swieten JC, Witteman JC, et al. Alcohol consumption and risk of dementia: the Rotterdam study. *Lancet* 2002;359:281–286.
16. Green DM, Ropper AH, Kronmal RA, et al. Serum potassium level and dietary potassium intake as risk factors for stroke. *Neurology* 2002;59:314–320.
17. Benowitz NL, Hansson A, Jacob P. Cardiovascular effects of nasal and transdermal nicotine and cigarette smoking. *Hypertension* 2002;39:1107–1112.
18. Geleijnse JM, Giltay EJ, Grobbee DE, et al. Blood pressure response to fish oil supplementation: metaregression analysis of randomized trials. *J Hypertens* 2002;20:1493–1499.
19. Kaplan NM. Treatment of hypertension: drug therapy. In: Kaplan NM, ed. *Kaplan's clinical hypertension,* 8th ed. Philadelphia: Lippincott Williams & Wilkins, 2002.
20. Neaton JD, Grimm RH Jr, Prineas RJ, et al. Treatment of mild hypertension study (TOMHS). *JAMA* 1993;270:713–724.
21. Materson BJ, Reda DJ, Cushman WC. Department of Veterans Affairs single-drug therapy of hypertension study. *Am J Hypertens* 1995;8:189–192.
22. Dickerson JE, Hingorani AD, Ashby MJ, et al. Optimisation of antihypertensive treatment by crossover rotation of four major classes. *Lancet* 1999;353:2008–2013.
23. Morgan TO, Anderson AI, MacInnis RJ. ACE inhibitors, beta-blockers, calcium blockers, and diuretics for the control of systolic hypertension. *Am J Hypertens* 2001;14:241–247.
24. Psaty BM, Smith NL, Siscovick DS, et al. Health outcomes associated with antihypertensive therapies used as first-line agents. *JAMA* 1997;277:739–745.
25. Neal B, MacMahon S, Chapman N. Effects of ACE inhibitors, calcium antagonists, and other blood-pressure-lowering drugs: results of prospectively designed overviews of randomised trials. Blood Pressure Lowering Treatment Trialists' Collaboration. *Lancet* 2000;356:1955–1964.
26. Mayes LC, Horwitz R, Feinstein AR. A collection of 56 topics with contradictory results in case-control research. *Int J Epidemiol* 1988;17:680–685.
27. Pahor M, Guralnik JM, Ferrucci L, et al. Calcium-channel blockade and incidence of cancer in aged populations. *Lancet* 1996;348:493–497.
28. Kizer JR, Kimmel SE. Epidemiologic review of the calcium channel blocker drugs: an up-to-date perspective on the proposed hazards. *Arch Intern Med* 2001;161:1145–1158.
29. Psaty BM, Heckbert SR, Koepsell TD, et al. The risk of myocardial infarction associated with antihypertensive drug therapies. *JAMA* 1995;274:620–625.

30. Furberg CD, Psaty BM, Meyer JV. Nifedipine. Dose-related increase in mortality in patients with coronary heart disease. *Circulation* 1995;92: 1326–1331.
31. Michels KB, Rosner BA, Manson JE, et al. Prospective study of calcium channel blocker use, cardiovascular disease, and total mortality among hypertensive women. *Circulation* 1998;97:1540–1548.
32. Abascal VM, Larson MG, Evans JC, et al. Calcium antagonists and mortality risk in men and women with hypertension in the Framingham Heart Study. *Arch Intern Med* 1998;158:1882–1886.
33. Leader S, Mallick R, Roht L. Using medication history to measure confounding by indication in assessing calcium channel blockers and other antihypertensive therapy. *J Hum Hypertens* 2001;15:153–159.
34. Christensen KL, Mulvany MJ. Vasodilatation, not hypotension, improves resistance vessel design during treatment of essential hypertension: a literary survey. *J Hypertens* 2001;19:1001–1006.
35. Yusuf S, Sleight P, Pogue J, et al. Effects of an angiotensin-converting-enzyme inhibitor, ramipril, on cardiovascular events in high-risk patients. The Heart Outcomes Prevention Evaluation Study Investigators. *N Engl J Med* 2000;342:145–153.
36. Yudkin JS. Superiority of particular class of antihypertensive agent remains to be shown [Letter]. *BMJ* 2002;325:439.
37. Dalhöf B, Devereux RB, Kjeldsen SE, et al. Cardiovascular morbidity and mortality in the Losartan Intervention for Endpoint reduction in hypertension study (LIFE): a randomised trial against atenolol. *Lancet* 2002;359:995–1003.
38. Van Zwieten PA. The influence of antihypertensive drug treatment on the prevention and regression of left ventricular hypertrophy. *Cardiovasc Res* 2000;45:82–91.
39. Brenner BM, Cooper ME, De Zeeuw D, et al. Effects of losartan on renal and cardiovascular outcomes in patients with type 2 diabetes and nephropathy. *N Engl J Med* 2001;345:861–869.
40. Lewis EJ, Hunsicker LG, Clarke WR, et al. Renoprotective effect of the angiotensin-receptor antagonist irbesartan in patients with nephropathy due to type 2 diabetes. *N Engl J Med* 2001;345:51–60.
41. Parving HH, Lehnert H, Bröchner-Mortensen J, et al. The effect of irbesartan on the development of diabetic nephropathy in patients with type 2 diabetes. *N Engl J Med* 2001;345:870–878.
42. Jaffar TH, Schmid CH, Landa M, et al. Angiotensin converting enzyme inhibitors and progression of nondiabetic renal disease: a meta-analysis of patient-level data. *Ann Intern Med* 2001;135:73–87.
43. Young MJ, Funder JW. Mineralocorticoid receptors and pathophysiological roles for aldosterone in the cardiovascular system. *J Hypertens* 2002;20:1465–1468.
44. Vasan RS, Larson MG, Leip EP, et al. Impact of high-normal blood pressure on the risk of cardiovascular disease. *N Engl J Med* 2001;345: 1291–1297.
45. Kaplan NM. What is goal blood pressure for the treatment of hypertension? *Arch Intern Med* 2001;161:1480–1482.
46. Bakris GL, Williams M, Dworkin L, et al. Preserving renal function in adults with hypertension and diabetes. *Am J Kidney Dis* 2000;36: 646–661.
47. Mancia G, Grassi G. Systolic and diastolic blood pressure control in antihypertensive drug trials. *J Hypertens* 2002;20:1461–1464.
48. Staessen JA, Wang JG, Thijs L. Cardiovascular protection and blood pressure reduction: a meta-analysis. *Lancet* 2001;358:1305–1315.

CHAPTER 17

Hypertensive Heart Disease

Robert A. Phillips and Joseph A. Diamond

Key Words: Coronary flow reserve; left ventricular diastolic function; left ventricular hypertrophy; techniques; treatment.

INTRODUCTION

Hypertensive heart disease is a common disorder associated with a markedly increased risk for cardiovascular morbidity and mortality. It is a result of a complex interaction of genetic and hemodynamic factors that lead to increased left ventricular (LV) mass, diastolic dysfunction, congestive heart failure (CHF), arrhythmias, and abnormalities of blood flow caused by microvascular disease. The purpose of this chapter is to review (a) the epidemiologic evidence for left ventricular hypertrophy (LVH) as a risk factor for cardiovascular disease, (b) the genetic and structural changes in the hypertensive heart that provide the substrate for increased risk, (c) the cause of LVH, (d) the identification and treatment of LVH in clinical practice, and (e) the abnormalities of diastolic function and coronary microcirculation that accompany LVH.

R. A. Phillips: Department of Medicine, Lenox Hill Hospital, New York, New York 10021.

J. A. Diamond: Division of Cardiology, Long Island Jewish Medical Center, New Hyde Park, New York 10040.

Definition of Hypertensive Heart Disease and Epidemiology of Left Ventricular Mass

Manifestations of hypertensive heart disease include diastolic dysfunction, increased LV mass, and microvascular changes that cause coronary blood flow abnormalities. Echocardiographically determined LVH is defined as LV mass in the upper 2.5% to 5% of the adult population. It occurs in 15% to 20% of patients with hypertension (1). Considered as a discrete, categorical variable, LVH significantly increases the risk for coronary artery disease (CAD), CHF, cerebrovascular accidents, ventricular arrhythmia, and sudden death (2,3). LVH increases the relative risk for mortality by twofold in subjects with CAD and by fourfold in those with normal epicardial coronary arteries (4,5). In addition, when LV mass is considered as a continuous variable, a direct and progressive relation exists between cardiovascular risk and the absolute amount of LV mass (3).

Etiology of Left Ventricular Hypertrophy

Genetic Factors in the Development of Left Ventricular Hypertrophy

It is estimated that up to 60% of the variance of LV mass may be caused by genetic factors independent of blood pressure (BP) (6). Epidemiologic evidence for genetic influence on LV mass includes offspring studies that generally demonstrate that LV mass in children of hypertensive parents is increased independently of BP and other known determinants of LVH (7,8). Additional evidence for a genetic influence on LV mass is that race appears to be a determinant of ventricular structure. Studies during the last three decades suggest that for equal levels of BP, black individuals have increased relative wall thickness and LV mass for equivalent degrees of hypertension compared with white individuals. In the Trial of Mild Hypertension Study (TOMHS), even though BP and LV mass were the same, black subjects had greater wall thickness than white subjects (9). Similarly, a study from London showed that for equal levels of previously untreated BP, black subjects had greater LV mass and relative wall thickness than white subjects (10).

One of the first and most studied genetic factors in the development of LVH in hypertension in humans is an insertion/deletion polymorphism of a 287-base pair marker in intron 16 (noncoding region) of the gene for angiotensin-converting enzyme (ACE). It is estimated from population studies that the ACE gene contributes 3% to 4% to the variation of BP in the general population. The homozygous genotype for the deletion (DD) is associated with electrocardiographic (ECG) evidence of LVH (11). The association was strongest in men who were normotensive, supporting the concept that this association is independent of hemodynamic factors. However, the Framingham study did not find a relation between echocardiographically measured LV mass and ACE genotype (11). An Italian study showed that the DD genotype was a risk factor for increased echocardiographically determined LV mass (12). Furthermore, a study in an ethnically diverse New York City population found that the DD genotype was associated with concentric remodeling of the left ventricle, a geometric pattern associated with increased cardiovascular risk (13).

In addition to the angiotensin gene, there is strong evidence that another gene on chromosome 1, the angiotensinogen gene, contributes to the development of LVH in individuals with hypertension. In the Hypertension Genetic Epidemiology Network (HyperGEN) study, two polymorphisms of the angiotensinogen gene have been associated with LVH. The M235T polymorphism on exon 2 of the angiotensinogen gene appears to be a marker for a functional variant, the G-6A polymorphism, which is tightly linked to the marker (e.g., 6 base pairs away) and affects the transcriptional rate of this gene (14). Additional studies applying the principles of physiologic genomics are assessing the effect of the ACE and angiotensinogen genes on hypertensive heart disease. This is accomplished by altering expression levels through transgenics, knockouts, and gene targeting in animal models (15). In spontaneously hypertensive rats, antisense targeted to angiotensinogen messenger RNA delivered by an adeno-associated virus produced sustained reduction in BP and reduction in LVH (16). This suggests a potential future gene therapy approach for the treatment of hypertension and regression of LVH.

In addition to the ACE and angiotensinogen genes, more recent studies are focusing on other genes with different physiologic mechanisms that could contribute to hypertensive heart disease. Table 17–1 summarizes current genes, which appear to contribute to LVH.

Hemodynamic and Nonhemodynamic Factors and Left Ventricular Hypertrophy

The effect of BP, as well as virtually every factor known to influence BP, has been investigated for its independent effect on LV mass (Table 17–2).

The sequence of events that leads from increased wall stress to cellular hypertrophy is only beginning to be elucidated (70). Because failure to hypertrophy in response to increased wall stress would result in a mechanical disadvantage and decreased LV function, it is likely that there are redundant systems that translate wall stress into cardiac myocyte hypertrophy. It is likely that increased wall stress activates a stretch receptor, which, through a series of cellular and subcellular events, activates fetal cardiac and growth genes, such as c-*myc* and c-*jun*, to up-regulate myocardial cell protein synthesis. Shear stress has been shown to activate these growth genes in endothelial cells by stimulating the production of several mitogen-activated protein kinases (Fig. 17–1) (71). The underlying molecular mechanisms that couple hypertrophic signals at the cell membrane to the reprogramming of cardiomyocyte gene expression are begin-

TABLE 17–1. *Genes implicated in the development of left ventricular hypertrophy in essential hypertension*

Gene	Location	Physiologic role
Angiotensin-converting enzyme gene (11,13,17)	Insertion/deletion polymorphism of 287-base pair marker intron 16 on chromosome 17	Production of angiotensinII
Angiotensinogen gene (18)	G-6A polymorphism in exon 2 on chromosome 1	Production of angiotensinogen
G protein β$_3$ subunit gene (19,20)	Single base substitution at position 825 of exon 9 in the short arm of chromosome 12	Enhanced Na$^+$-H$^+$ exchange because of enhanced G protein activation
Type A human natriuretic peptide receptor gene (21)	Deletion mutation of the 5′ flanking region in chromosome 1	Increased brain natriuretic peptide because of decreased natriuretic peptide receptors

TABLE 17–2. *Association between left ventricular mass and hemodynamic and nonhemodynamic factors*

Factor	Strength of evidence supporting a causal role in LV mass (references)
Blood pressure/wall stress	Very strong (22,23–29)
Stroke volume	Very strong (27,30)
Obesity	Very strong (31,32,33–35)
Growth hormone and IGF-1	Strong (36,37)
Sex	Strong (38,39–41)
Race	Strong (9,10,42,43)
Age	Strong (women only?) (44,45,31,46,47)
Intracellular [Ca^{2+}]	Strong (48,49)
Insulin resistance	Strong (35,50,51)
Angiotensin II	Strong (52,53)
Alcohol	Needs confirmation (54)
Intrinsic myocardial contractility	Needs confirmation (27)
Blood viscosity	Needs confirmation (55)
Parathyroid hormone	Needs confirmation (56)
Aldosterone (collagen synthesis)	Needs confirmation (53,57,58)
Sodium intake	Needs confirmation (59)
Na$^+$-H$^+$ exchanger and Na$^+$-K$^+$-Cl$^-$ cotransport system	Needs confirmation (60)
Polymorphism of the ACE gene	Controversial (11,12)
Plasma renin activity	Controversial (56, 61,62)
Norepinephrine	Controversial (61,63–66)
Na$^+$-Li$^+$ exchanger	Controversial (60,67)
βARK	Controversial (68,69)

ACE, angiotensin-converting enzyme; βARK, β-adrenergic receptor kinase; IGF-1, insulin-like growth factor-1; LV, left ventricular.

ning to be elucidated. Intracellular calcium release may be an early response to myocyte stretch and other humoral stimuli, including angiotensin II, phenylephrine, and endothelin. The increase in intracellular calcium results in activation of the phosphatase calcineurin, which then dephosphorylates transcription factor NF-AT3, resulting in its translocation to the nucleus. In the nucleus, AT3 interacts with another transcription factor, GATA4, to initiate transcription of genes that lead to myocyte hypertrophy (48) such as β-myosin heavy chain, β-skeletal actin (Fig. 17–2). In the hypertrophic response, other genes are also upregulated, such as those for atrial natriuretic peptide and phospholamban (72).

Calcineurin appears to be both necessary and sufficient to induce hypertrophy; pharmacologic inhibition of calcineurin activity with cyclosporine blocks development of hypertrophy in several circumstances: (i) mice prone to LVH because they are genetically engineered to produce high levels of calcineurin (48), (ii) mice genetically predisposed to development of hypertrophic cardiomyopathy (73); and (iii) rats with an aorta that was banded so as to produce a pressure stimulus for hypertrophy (73). Although cyclosporine will not be clinically useful in the nontransplant population, it is

likely that new classes of calcineurin inhibitors (e.g., FK 506) that regulate transcription will become available to modulate responses such as hypertrophy (74). It is likely the ACE inhibitors and angiotensin II type I (AT-1) receptor blockers also attenuate the development of cardiac hypertrophy by inhibiting angiotensin from up-regulating the production of factors that stimulate fetal-type genes, particularly calcineurin. Nonantihypertensive doses of the AT-1 receptor blocker, candesartan, suppresses calcineurin production and subsequent LVH and fibrosis in salt-sensitive, hypertensive, Dahl rats (74).

Sex, age, obesity, and dietary factors affect LV mass. Aging is associated with increased LV mass, but this effect may be more pronounced in women than in men (44,45). Women have less LV mass for the same level of office-determined BP (38), but whether this difference is biologic or an artifact of the method of BP measurement or indexing of LV mass is controversial. For example, for similar levels of clinic BP, women often have lower ambulatory BPs than men. This results in less hypertrophy in women for the same level of clinic pressure (75). In the Framingham study, obesity increased LV mass in elderly men and women (31). These changes are reversible with weight loss (32). Excessive alcohol intake is directly related to increased LV mass (54), and excess sodium intake may be a signal for hypertrophy (59).

Several hormones have been related to the hypertrophic process. The plasma renin-angiotensin-aldosterone axis in hypertensive end organ pathophysiology has been the most extensively explored. Experimental and human studies (56,61) have linked plasma renin activity to degree of LVH, but this is not universally accepted (62). The product of renin activity, angiotensin I, is the substrate for ACE. Expression and regulation of the ACE gene and, thus, angiotensin II levels, may modulate development of LVH. This is supported by *in vitro* studies in which local release of angiotensin II in response to the mechanical stretch is a necessary permissive factor for induction of the hypertrophic growth response (52). Although there is ample evidence that angiotensin II is involved in the hypertrophic response, it is apparently not a necessary factor for the response to occur. This was shown in a study in which LVH developed in mice in response to pressure overload despite "knockout" of the AT-1 receptor (87). Aldosterone, the synthesis of which is partially controlled by angiotensin II levels, appears to regulate cardiac fibroblast metabolism and growth (57). These observations may explain why increased plasma renin levels confer a greater risk for myocardial infarction (MI) in patients with hypertension.

Left Ventricular Mass Regression

Regression of LV mass with effective BP reduction has been demonstrated in more than 400 clinical studies, but less than 10% have been double-blind, placebo-controlled studies (88). Data indicate that LV mass regression improves survival in patients with hypertension. Verdecchia and coworkers showed decreased risk for cardiac events with LV mass

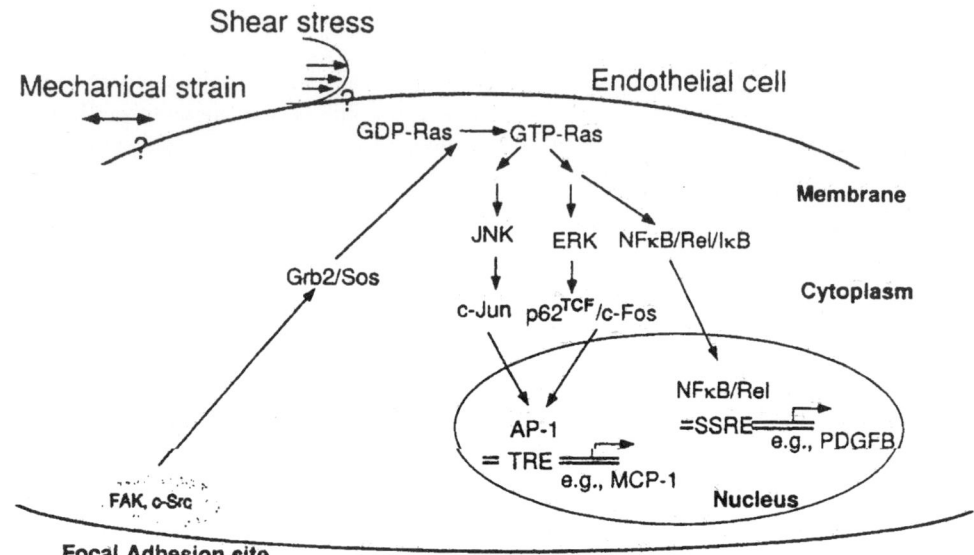

FIG. 17–1. The sequential events of signaling and gene expression in endothelial cells in response to shear stress or mechanical strain. Tyrosine kinases in the focal adhesion site of endothelial cells such as FAK and c-SRC are involved in the mechanochemical transduction. Through the Src homology 2–containing adaptor Grbe, the small guanosine triphosphatase (GTPase) Ras is activated by Sos, a guanine nucleotide exchange factor that converts the inactive guanosine diphosphate (GDP)-Ras to the activated GTP-Ras. As a result, JNK and ERK in the cytoplasm are activated to phosphorylate, c-Jun and p62^{TCF}/c-Fos, respectively, which are components of the transcription factor AP-1. In the nucleus, the action of the activated AP-1 on its target sequence (e.g., the TRE site in the promoter of the monocyte chemotactic protein-1 [*MCP-1*] gene) causes an up-regulation of gene expression. Concurrently, nuclear factor-kappa B (NF-κB)/Rel is activated by eliminating its inhibitor IκB so that genes with a shear stress-responsive element or κB site (e.g., platelet-derived growth factor-β [PDGF-β]) can be activated. AP-1, (mitogen) activating protein-1; c-Src, nonreceptor protein tyrosine kinase; ERK, extracellular signal-regulated kinase; FAK, focal adhesion kinase; JNK, c-Jun N-terminal kinase; TRE, phorbol ester tissue 12-0-tetradecanoylphorbol 13-acetate-responsive element. (Reproduced from Chien S, Li S, Shyy YJ. Effects of mechanical forces on signal transduction and gene expression in endothelial cells. *Hypertension* 1998;31[1 Pt 2]:162–169, with permission.)

regression independent of the baseline LV mass, baseline clinic and ambulatory BP, and the degree of BP reduction (89). Similar findings were reported in a more recent prospective study of 172 patients with essential hypertension, in which the absence or presence of LV hypertrophy on the follow-up echocardiogram was the strongest predictor of subsequent morbid events (90). Total cardiovascular events also were reduced in TOMHS, in which there was LV mass regression (91). A mechanism that might explain these findings is that midwall fractional shortening, a sensitive measure of intrinsic myocardial systolic performance, appears to improve with LV mass regression, as does Doppler-assessed stroke volume (92,93).

BP reduction with all classes of antihypertensive agents reduces LV mass, with the possible exception of pure vasodilators such as minoxidil and hydralazine (61). A meta-analysis of more than 100 studies yielded a moderately strong relation between BP reduction and LV mass regression (94). This confirms the hemodynamic contribution to LV mass and demonstrates that greater BP reduction is associated with greater mass regression.

It is not clear, however, whether antihypertensive agents can regress LV mass independent of their effect on BP. In animal studies, ACE inhibitors reduce LV mass without decreasing BP (95). The Losartan Intervention for Endpoint Reduction (LIFE) study showed a significant and continued decrease in LV mass over a 2-year treatment period, despite only a small decrease in BP after the first year of blinded therapy with either atenolol or Losartan (93). However, one metaanalysis of human studies suggested that for equal levels of BP reduction, β-blockers, ACE inhibitors, and calcium channel blockers cause the same degree of LVH regression, whereas diuretics reduce chamber dimension but do not lead to regression of hypertrophied muscle. This conclusion, however, has been challenged in two randomized trials that suggest that diuretics are as effective as, if not more effective than, other drug classes for reducing LV mass. In TOMHS, BP was reduced by a combination of weight loss plus either placebo or one of five antihypertensive drug classes (β-blocker, α-blocker, calcium channel blocker, ACE inhibitor, and diuretic) (91). At 1 and 4 years, all groups showed LV mass regression, confirming that

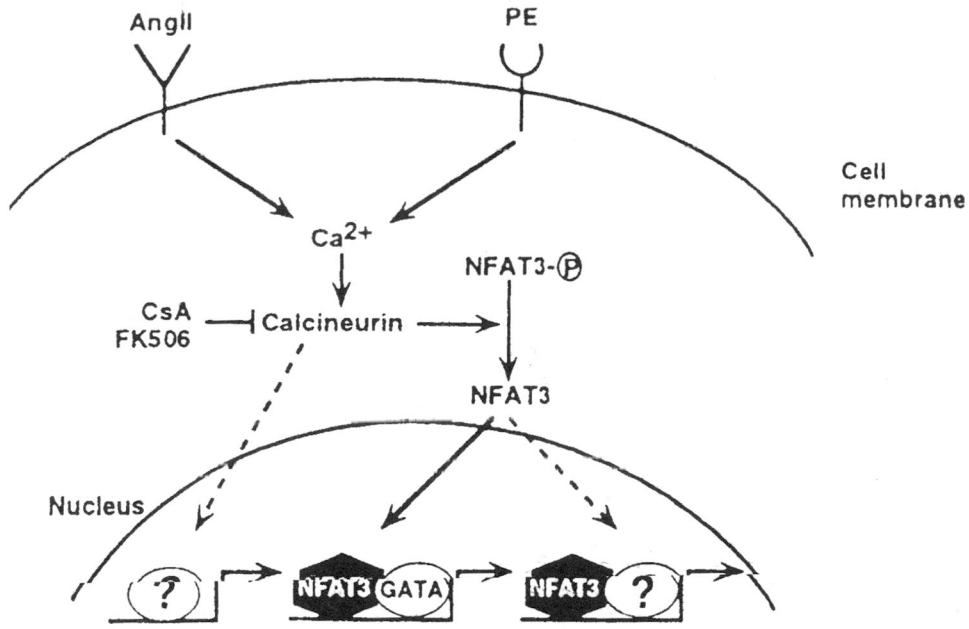

Hypertrophic response genes

FIG. 17–2. A model for the calcineurin-dependent transcriptional pathway in cardiac hypertrophy. Angiotensin II (Ang II), phenylephrine (PE), and possibly other hypertrophic stimuli acting at the cell membrane lead to increase of intracellular Ca^{2+} and activation of calcineurin in the cytoplasm. Calcineurin dephosphorylates NFAT3, resulting in its translocation to the nucleus, where it interacts with GATA4 to synergistically activate transcription. Whether all actions of NF-AT3 are mediated by its interaction with GATA4 or whether there are GATA4-independent pathways for activation of certain hypertrophic responses remains to be determined. *Solid arrows* denote pathways that are known. *Dotted lines* denote possible pathways that have not been demonstrated. (Reproduced from Molkentin JD, Lu JR, Antos CL, et al. A calcineurin-dependent transcriptional pathway for cardiac hypertrophy. *Cell* 1998;93:215–228, with permission, ©Cell Press.)

weight loss in conjunction with BP reduction reduces LV mass. Surprisingly, only subjects receiving chlorthalidone had greater LV mass regression than those undergoing weight loss and receiving placebo. Reduced internal dimension and reduced wall thickness accounted for this. The Veterans Affairs (VA) Cooperative Study Group reported similar results: For equal levels of BP reduction, hydrochlorothiazide had a greater effect on LV mass regression than other antihypertensive agents (96). In this trial of 493 patients who completed 1 year of antihypertensive maintenance therapy, LV mass was not reduced despite hemodynamic improvement in patients taking prazosin, clonidine, or diltiazem. In the VA trial, ACE inhibition was nearly as beneficial as diuretic-based therapy.

DIASTOLIC FUNCTION IN HYPERTENSION

Clinical Presentation, Etiologic Factors, and Prognosis

The clinical presentation of diastolic dysfunction in hypertensive heart disease is variable, ranging from asymptomatic findings on noninvasive testing to overt CHF, despite normal systolic function (97–100). The prevalence of asymptomatic

LV filling abnormalities in adults without hypertrophy and with ambulatory awake BP greater than 130/85 mm Hg may be as high as 33% (22). An estimated 30% to 45% of patients with CHF have normal systolic function but abnormal diastolic function (CHF-D) (100). In a large community-based study of CHF, the prognosis for patients with diastolic heart failure was poor. Survival rate at 3 months, 1 year, and 5 years was 86%, 76%, and 48%, respectively (Fig. 17–3) (101). In a cohort of patients with diastolic dysfunction and underlying CAD, 7-year cardiovascular mortality approaches 50%. Many of these patients also were hypertensive (102). Symptoms in the presence of diastolic dysfunction are accounted for by prolonged LV relaxation or decreased compliance, which causes shifts in the diastolic LV pressure–volume relation that result in increased left atrial and LV filling pressures (103).

Factors Affecting Diastolic Function

Genetic structural, metabolic, and hemodynamic factors can affect diastolic function under resting conditions and during states of increased demand or ischemia (Fig. 17–4).

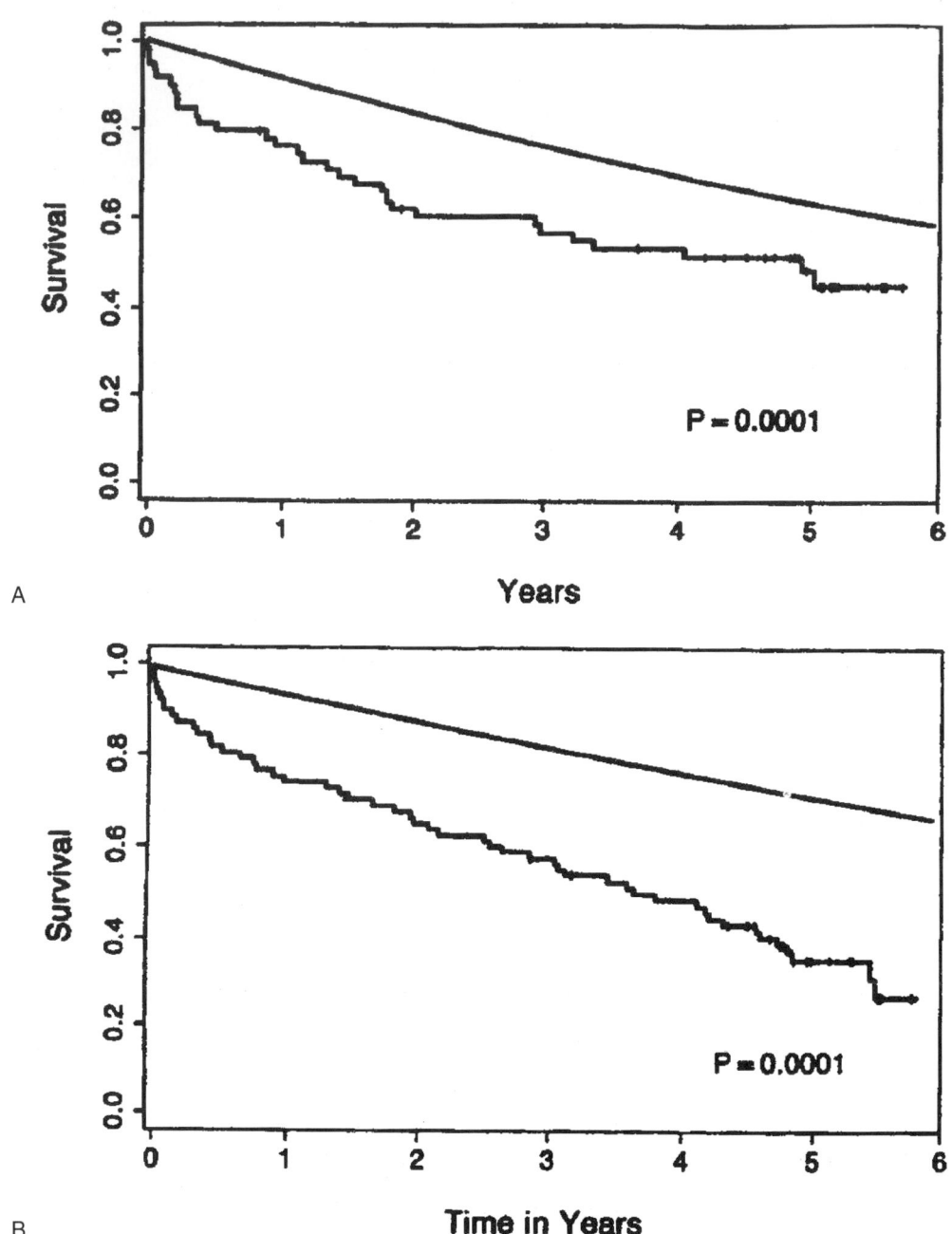

FIG. 17–3. Survival of patients with ejection fraction of ≥50% **(A)** and <50% **(B)** compared with that for age- and sex-matched population. (Reproduced from Senni M, Tribouilloy CM, Rodeheffer RJ, et al. Congestive heart failure in the community: a study of all incident cases in Olmsted County, Minnesota, in 1991. *Circulation* 1998;98:2282–2289, with permission.)

Genetic Factors

Using E and A Doppler mitral inflow velocities as a phenotype for diastolic filling, the Hypertension Genetic Epidemiology Network study performed linkage analyses that identified two potentially significant genes on chromosome 5 that contribute to diastolic dysfunction in hypertension (104). One is a calcium-modulating cyclophilin ligand, which is an integral membrane protein involved in the regulation of calcium ion signaling. This protein is expressed in multiple tissues and may play a role in calcium transport in myocardial contraction/relaxation. The other is α-1B–adrenergic receptor (*ADRA1B*) gene, which is expressed in myocardium and may indirectly stimulate intracellular calcium release and protein kinase C activation. Other genes are likely involved in diastolic dysfunction. SR-Ca^{2+} adenosine triphosphatase pump is up-regulated in CHF. Phospholamban is overexpressed in rats with prolonged isovolumic relaxation and increased LV end-diastolic pressure. In addition, abnormal diastolic filling

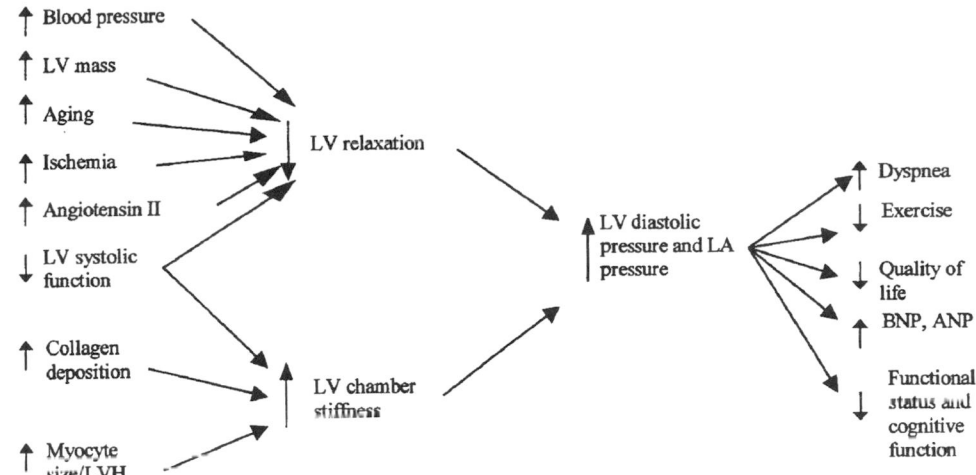

FIG. 17–4. Causes of left ventricular (LV) diastolic dysfunction and its clinical consequences. ANP, atrial natriuretic peptide; BNP, brain natriuretic peptide; LA, left atrial; LVH, LV hypertrophy.

parameters have been associated with ACE I/D and G protein β_3 subunit *C825T* gene polymorphisms.

Structural Factors

Reports in the late 1980s and early 1990s suggest that diastolic abnormalities occur early in the course of hypertension and precede detectable hypertrophy (22,105–108). More recent studies challenge the notion that diastolic abnormalities are the first sign of hypertensive heart disease; they suggest that diastolic abnormalities do not precede structural changes, but rather occur simultaneously. In general, diastolic function is inversely related to LV mass in patients with hypertension (97,106,109–111), and regression of LV mass with calcium channel blockers, β-blockers, and ACE inhibitors is often (112–117), but not always (118), associated with improved LV diastolic function.

Ischemia

Ischemia has pronounced effects on diastolic function, and this is exacerbated even in the minimally hypertrophied heart (119). Several metabolic/biochemical factors, which are not fully elucidated, that slow inactivation of the actin-myosin complex and delay relaxation are probably involved. Baseline adenosine triphosphate levels in the pressure overload hypertrophied heart are similar to or slightly less than those in control hearts (120,121). Although it may be normal in the resting state (122), the rate of sarcoplasmic uptake of calcium, an energy-dependent and adenosine triphosphate–requiring step, is markedly reduced by hypoxia (123).

Hemodynamic Load

Increased hemodynamic load affects diastolic performance. In isolated hearts, increases in afterload early in systole im-

pair relaxation (124). Wall stress in untreated individuals with hypertension is inversely related to diastolic function (111). When studied with ambulatory monitoring, previously untreated patients with borderline or mild hypertension demonstrate a linear relation between BP and abnormal LV filling (22,125). The degree to which an acute reduction in BP per se improves LV diastolic performance is not known, and studies are difficult to interpret because the agents used can themselves affect performance (126,127).

Systolic Function

Systolic function, as measured by ejection fraction, does not appear to decrease during episodes of severe hypertension with pulmonary edema (128). However, systolic and diastolic dysfunction are closely linked. Midwall fractional shortening, a more sensitive measure of intrinsic myocardial systolic function than endocardial fractional shortening, is abnormal in a substantial portion of individuals with asymptomatic hypertension (129,130). Schussheim and coworkers (131) found that depressed midwall fractional shortening and diastolic dysfunction occur simultaneously in individuals with asymptomatic hypertension with normal endocardial fractional shortening. Conversely, those with normal midwall fractional shortening tend to have normal Doppler indices of mitral inflow. In the Hypertension Genetic Epidemiology Network Study, impaired LV relaxation, as measured by prolonged isovolumic relaxation time, was associated with lower midwall fractional shortening, but not with lower fractional shortening (104). The prognostic implications of these findings were illustrated in the Cardiovascular Health Study, a population-based study of 5,201 men and women 65 years or age and older. Those with the greatest risk for development of CHF had the greatest LV mass index and the lowest stress-corrected, midwall, fractional shortening (132).

Enhanced systolic performance, such as during exercise, is associated with improved diastolic function (111,133). Systolic function directly affects the efficiency of elastic recoil (133). Increased recoil, in turn, augments the ability of the heart to generate negative pressure during early diastole, a "suction" phenomenon that increases LV filling. Catecholamines enhance diastolic function and improve LV filling through enhancement of myocardial restoring forces and recoil during isovolumetric relaxation (134).

Aging

Aging has profound effects on diastolic function, which is reflected in a reduced rate of LV relaxation and increased diastolic stiffness. This effect has been confirmed by various noninvasive measurements of diastolic function (22,135–137). Among healthy subjects in the Framingham Heart Study, age was the predominant factor affecting Doppler indices of diastolic function, with a Pearson correlation coefficient of -0.80 between age and the E/A ratio (138).

Hormones and Paracrine Factors

As noted earlier, catecholamines are believed to favorably affect diastolic performance by improving systolic performance. Several other studies suggest that angiotensin II adversely affects diastolic function by impairing LV relaxation and stimulating aldosterone-mediated myocardial fibrosis (57).

Noninvasive Measurement of Diastolic Function

Diastolic function may be evaluated by several methods. The rate of isovolumic pressure decay (tau), early and late LV filling, and pressure–volume relations can be derived from cardiac catheterization (139–141). Although these measurements are the most accurate indices of diastolic function, they require an invasive procedure. Inferences regarding the diastolic properties of the ventricle can be obtained noninvasively with radionuclide angiography (142) and M-mode (143) or Doppler echocardiography (144) and acoustic quantification (145). These techniques (Table 17–3) yield information on all phases of diastole, including isovolumetric relaxation, early and late LV filling (22,107,146), and temporal differences in regional filling (regional nonuniformity) (147).

Doppler echocardiographic evaluation of LV inflow is the most widely used noninvasive measure of diastolic function (148). The LV diastolic flow velocity profile obtained with Doppler echocardiography correlates well with radionuclide angiographic variables in the evaluation of LV diastolic function (142). However, Doppler echocardiographic assessment is easy and convenient and does not add much time to study acquisition. Furthermore,

significant prognostic information may be obtained from Doppler-determined mitral inflow. The Strong Heart Study evaluated the prognostic significance of abnormal mitral inflow as a measure of diastolic dysfunction in a population-based sample of middle aged and elderly American Indians. In this population, a restrictive pattern of inflow with mitral E/A ratio greater than 1.5 was associated with a threefold increase in cardiac mortality independent of other covariates (149). A low E/A ratio (e.g., < 0.6), indicative of delayed LV relaxation, was also associated with increased cardiovascular mortality, but not as an independent variable. A younger Italian population was evaluated in the Progretto Ipertensione Umbria Monitoraggio Ambulatoriale (PIUMA) study. The investigators did not observe a J-shaped pattern as noted in the Strong Heart study. There was, however, significantly increased cardiovascular mortality associated with a low E/A ratio and a 21% greater risk for cardiovascular events for each 0.3-decrease in age-adjusted E/A ratio below the median value for this group (0.98) (150). There are several new and emerging Doppler techniques that may allow for serial noninvasive interpretation of LV end-diastolic pressure (Table 17–3).

Effect of Treatment on Congestive Heart Failure with Abnormal Diastolic Function

Treatment of patients with hypertension with symptoms of CHF-D is guided by relatively few studies. Topol and coworkers (99), in a landmark study, analyzed the effect of treatment on morbidity and mortality in 21 elderly patients with hypertension with marked concentric hypertrophy, supernormal LV systolic function, and depressed LV diastolic function. These patients were treated with a variety of antihypertensive and cardioactive agents because of heart failure, angina, stoke, or syncope (99). Of the 12 patients who received vasodilators (nitrates, hydralazine, prazosin, or captopril), 6 had a severe hypotensive reaction and 1 patient died. In contrast, all nine patients who received β-blockers or calcium antagonists improved, and four subjects had less dyspnea after discontinuation of digoxin and furosemide. In a more recent study of 144 patients with CHF and Doppler evidence of restrictive LV diastolic filling, as measured by a shortened deceleration time of early mitral filling, cardiac mortality was assessed after 2 years of unblinded oral therapy. Various combinations of digoxin, diuretics, ACE inhibitors, nitrates, and β-blockers were used. Survival was significantly better in patients with prolongation of the deceleration time over the treatment period compared with patients with no change in deceleration time (151). The latter group used more digoxin. No other significant difference in medication use was noted. Thus, although reversing diastolic dysfunction may relieve symptoms and prolong survival, the optimal regimen remains unclear.

The few systematic studies of various agents on CHF-D are reviewed in this chapter. The paucity of data that form the basis for conflicting recommendations by authorities on the optimal treatment of CHF-D suggests a need for a randomized trial using drug classes with an efficacy in treatment of CHF-D that has not been proved in a clinical trial.

Angiotensin-converting Enzyme Inhibitors

Three studies have evaluated the efficacy of ACE inhibitors in CHF-D. In one study, 10 subjects with hypertension, LVH, and CHF-D were treated in a nonrandomized, uncontrolled study with the ACE inhibitor enalapril and a low-sodium diet (116). After an average of 9 months of treatment, heart failure symptoms resolved in all subjects, without use of diuretics. Diastolic function as measured by Doppler echocardiography did not change after initial decrease in BP, but did significantly improve (decreased A/E ratio and deceleration time) after LV mass regression. Another study compared treatment with enalapril to standard therapy without enalapril in 21 elderly patients with CHF-D, prior non–Q-wave MI, and normal ejection fraction (152). In the enalapril group, BP and LV mass were significantly reduced with treatment, and this was accompanied by a significant improvement in New York Heart Association functional score (decrease from 3.0 to 2.4, $p < 0.01$), an increase in exercise time on a treadmill, and an improvement in diastolic function, as measured by Doppler echocardiography. In the third study, 35 patients with hypertension and LVH underwent endocardial biopsy after 6 months of treatment with lisinopril (153). There was evidence of significant regression of myocardial fibrosis, as evidenced by collagen volume fraction and myocardial hydroxyproline concentration, irrespective of the degree of LVH regression. Echocardiographic signs of improved LV diastolic function, including increased E/A and decreased isovolumic relaxation time, accompanied these findings.

Calcium Channel Blockers

Two small, short-term studies have been reported in which calcium channel blockers were the mainstay of therapy in CHF. In a prospective study of 20 patients (15 of whom had hypertension), verapamil and placebo were compared in a 5-week crossover design. Compared with baseline, verapamil significantly improved LV filling, decreased symptoms, and improved exercise time (154), whereas placebo had no significant effect. However, possibly because of a "carryover" effect of verapamil-induced improvement into the placebo phase of the crossover design, there was no difference between verapamil and placebo in LV filling. In six patients with severe hypertension who were managed for 4 months, of whom four received a concomitant diuretic, treatment with nifedipine was associated with symptomatic improvement (155).

β-Blockade

To our knowledge, no study has evaluated the role of β-blockade in isolated CHF-D. A study in patients with idiopathic dilated cardiomyopathy (ejection fraction <25%) evaluated the effect of metoprolol, up to 50 mg three time daily, on diastolic dysfunction (156). Not only did diastolic function improve within 3 months of treatment, but the investigators suggested that better diastolic performance may have allowed for the subsequent observed boost in systolic function.

Diuretics

Although no clinical trial data are available, several investigators recommend cautious use of diuretics to reduce the congested state in CHF-D (98,157). Diuretics reduce congestion by decreasing LV preload and reducing right ventricular filling pressure, thereby relieving pericardial restraint on the LV (158). However, use of diuretics remains controversial because of the lack of clinical trial evaluation of this strategy and the concern that preload may be inappropriately reduced with "overdiuresis." In fact, the Fifth Report of the Joint National Committee on the Detection and Treatment of Hypertension considers diuretic therapy in diastolic dysfunction as "relatively or absolutely contraindicated" in patients with hypertensive hypertrophic cardiomyopathy with diastolic dysfunction (159). Diuretic-based therapy effectively prevents development of CHF in patients with hypertension.

Digoxin and Inotropes

Although digoxin may improve LV filling by decreasing heart rate, its ability to increase intracellular calcium may increase LV stiffness (160). In the recent National Institutes of Health–sponsored Digitalis Investigation Group trial of almost 8,000 patients (161), digoxin did not appear to be deleterious in those patients with CHF with abnormal systolic function (CHF-S) and it might have improved functional status.

CORONARY MICROCIRCULATION ABNORMALITIES IN PATIENTS WITH HYPERTENSION

In patients with hypertension with LVH, structural and functional alterations in the small coronary vessels, increasing ventricular wall stress, and alterations in the rheologic properties of blood (e.g., increased viscosity) inhibit the ability of the coronary microcirculation to regulate overall coronary blood flow (162). These abnormalities result in diminished coronary flow reserve, which is the increase in total coronary blood flow that occurs with maximal vasodilatation (Fig. 17–5). A better (although less frequently used) term

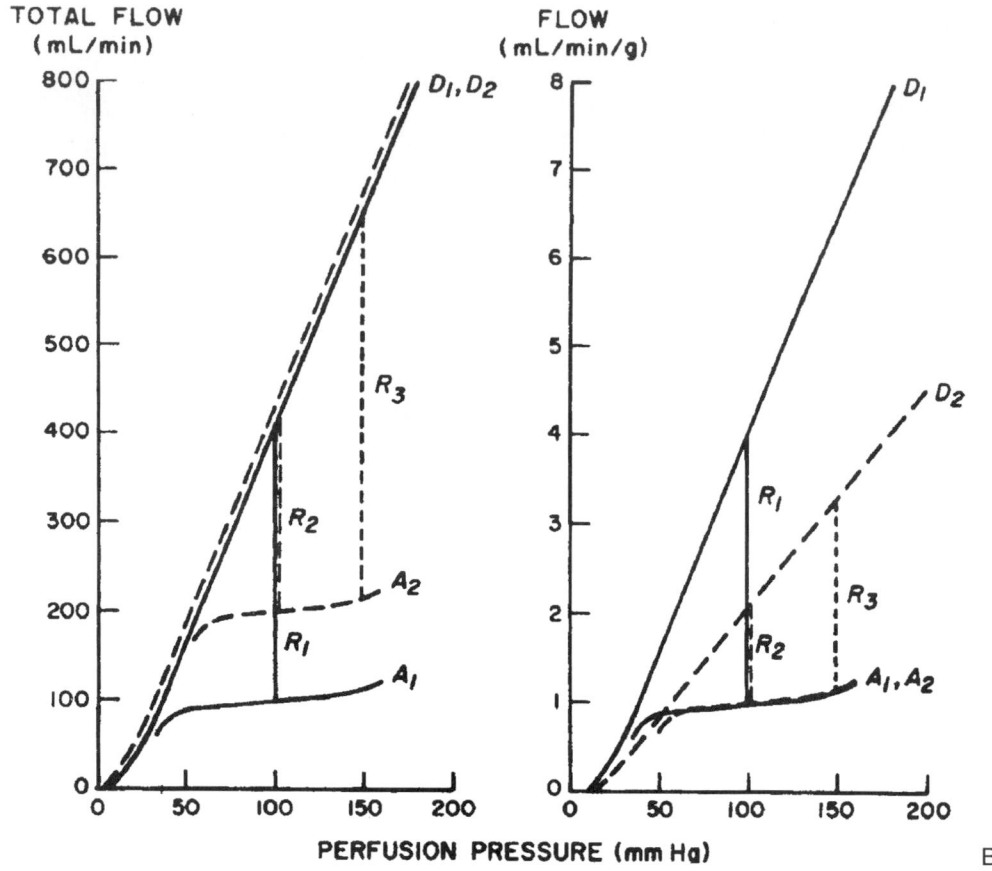

FIG. 17–5. Diagram of coronary flow reserve in the presence of hypertrophy. **A:** Absolute flow is measured (mL/min). **B:** Flow per unit mass (mL/min/g) is measured. *A,* autoregulated flows; *D,* pressure flow line during maximal vasodilatation; *R,* flow reserve. Normal are A_1, D_1, R_1, and *solid lines.* Hypertrophied are A_2, D_2, R_2, R_3, and *dashed lines.* In both scenarios, coronary flow reserve is diminished. R_3 represents coronary flow reserve when perfusion pressures are increased. (Reproduced from Hoffman JI. A critical view of coronary reserve. *Circulation* 1987;75[Suppl I]:I-6–I-11, with permission.)

may be myocardial perfusion reserve, because this indicates the total circulation of the myocardium rather than just the epicardial coronary arteries. Abnormal coronary flow reserve may predispose the patient with hypertension to ischemic syndromes, which lead to heart failure, MI, and sudden death.

Coronary Vessel Pathology in Left Ventricular Hypertrophy

Various vascular abnormalities result in a reduction in the total maximal cross-sectional area of the coronary microvasculature. These include inadequate vascular growth in response to increasing muscle mass, changes in vessel wall composition, vascular remodeling, and vascular endothelial dysfunction.

Increased wall stress (which is one factor initiating the development of LVH in patients with hypertension) may directly moderate coronary flow reserve by causing physical compression of blood vessels. Increased wall stress may stimulate the release of vasoactive substances that alter vascular function and growth (162). Patients with nonhyper-

tensive LVH without ventricular dilatation and increased wall tension (i.e., some cases of aortic stenosis, hypertrophic obstructive and hypertrophic nonobstructive cardiomyopathy with no ventricular dilatation) do not have decreased coronary flow reserve. Those with hypertension with similar degrees of LVH, or aortic stenosis with ventricular dilation and increased LV end-diastolic pressures, however, show abnormally decreased flow reserve (163,164). This effect also is seen in patients with dilated cardiomyopathy (165) and dilated ventricles caused by aortic regurgitation (166,167).

Alterations of Coronary Autoregulation and Flow Reserve with Left Ventricular Hypertrophy

The coronary circulation is able to maintain a relatively stable blood flow supply over a wide range of perfusion pressures (168–171). This range varies in different experiments but is generally between 70 and 130 mm Hg in humans (172). Coronary flow decreases markedly when perfusion pressure decreases to less than the lower limit of autoregulation.

Relationship Between Autoregulated Coronary Flow and Maximal Coronary Flow

Coronary flow reserve is, for any given perfusion pressure, the decrease in coronary resistance over the resting state that occurs after maximal coronary vasodilatation. A healthy human heart can increase coronary flow by a factor of 4 to 5 times over the resting state (163). Coronary flow increases above resting autoregulated levels after transient coronary arterial occlusion (reactive hyperemia), exercise, pacing, or injection of agents like dipyridamole, adenosine, papaverine, or hyperosmolar iodinated contrast media (173). Loss of autoregulation occurs during these events. Coronary flow reserve is a dynamic value that is dependent on coronary perfusion pressure. Because there is no autoregulation during states that produce maximal coronary flow, the relation between coronary flow and coronary perfusion pressure is linear. Relatively small changes in perfusion pressure produce large changes in coronary flow reserve.

Effect of Hypertension and Left Ventricular Hypertrophy on Coronary Flow Reserve

Coronary flow reserve can be measured as absolute flow (mL/min) or flow per unit muscle mass (mL/min/g; Fig. 17–5) (172). Although resting absolute coronary blood flow of the entire left ventricle increases with LVH, resting coronary blood flow per gram myocardium is unchanged. Total maximal ventricular flow does not significantly change with acquired LVH, whereas total flow per gram of myocardium decreases. This is because of the lack of vascular growth in response to increasing muscle mass. Thus, when absolute flow is measured, resting flow is high and maximal flow is normal (Fig. 17–5, A). If flow per gram is measured, resting flow per gram myocardium is normal, but maximal flow per gram myocardium is reduced (Fig. 17–5, B). Consequently, coronary flow reserve is less than normal whether measured as absolute flow (mL/min) or flow per gram (mL/min/gm) myocardium.

In the presence of hypertension, absolute coronary flow reserve may theoretically be normal or increased, despite greater resting absolute coronary blood flow. This is because of the greater coronary perfusion pressure (shift to the right side of the curve, as shown by R_3 in Fig. 17–5, A). Nevertheless, in most cases of hypertensive heart disease, vascular abnormalities and increased LV end-diastolic pressure result in reduced maximal flow, and thus a decrease in coronary flow reserve (164,174–176). Most (166,175,177), but not all (178,179), studies show an inverse linear relation between the extent of LVH and vascular endothelial function as noted by either forearm blood flow or coronary blood flow reserve (Fig. 17–6).

Hypertension may alter coronary flow reserve before the development of LVH. This was suggested by a cross-sectional analysis of patients with and without hypertension. Although coronary flow reserve was lowest in patients with untreated hypertension with increased LV mass, patients with hypertension and normal LV mass had lower coronary flow reserve than normotensive patients (180). This must be viewed with caution, however, because cross-sectional studies do not allow for analysis of other factors that may influence coronary blood flow such as duration of hypertension and prior antihypertensive therapies. Whether related linearly, most studies suggest that LVH is strongly associated with reduced coronary flow reserve. Thus, abnormalities of coronary flow reserve may partially explain why patients with hypertension and LVH are at increased risk for myocardial ischemia and infarction (3).

Effect of Blood Pressure Reduction on Autoregulated Blood Flow and Coronary Flow Reserve

Experimental and clinical studies demonstrate that BP reduction in patients with hypertension with LVH may result in increased myocardial ischemia. Resting absolute coronary flow is high in these patients, and loss of autoregulated flow occurs at greater perfusion pressures (the autoregulatory curve is shifted upward and to the right). In experimentally induced LVH, although marked reductions in coronary perfusion pressure from 100 to 40 mm Hg have minimal effect on autoregulation in the subepicardium, the ability of the subendocardium to autoregulate is reduced by greater than 50% (181). This may account for the increased size of MI associated with experimentally induced coronary ligation in hypertrophied hearts (182,183). Recovery of stunned myocardium (systolic thickening and regional myocardial blood flow) in the period immediately after transient coronary occlusion is delayed in the presence of LVH, and even more so when BP is decreased during this early reperfusion period (184).

BP reduction in hypertensive human subjects without LVH does not significantly change resting coronary blood flow when perfusion pressure is acutely decreased with nitroprusside from 120 to 70 mm Hg. However, when hypertrophy is present with hypertension, there is a marked decline in flow as perfusion pressure decreases from 90 to 70 mm Hg (Fig. 17–7) (185). This suggests that a reduction of BP to less than 90 mm Hg in patients with LVH could cause ischemia. This observation may, in part, explain the limited impact that BP reduction has on reducing mortality from CAD compared with reducing the incidence of nonfatal and fatal stroke in studies in which patients had both systolic and diastolic hypertension. Analysis of several large, prospective, observational studies suggests that a 5- to 6-mm Hg decrease in diastolic BP would cause a 20% to 25% reduction in coronary events. However, this degree of reduction in BP has resulted in only a 14% decrease in coronary events (186,187).

A J-curve may describe the relation between mortality rate from MI and treated diastolic BP (188). The J-curve implies that patients with hypertension without coronary disease may benefit from decreasing BP as much as possible; however, those patients with ischemic disease and a treated

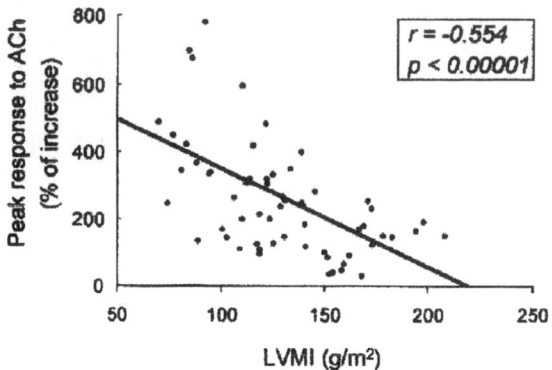

A

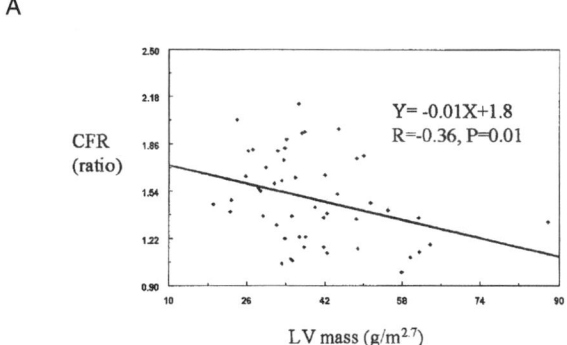

B

FIG. 17–6. Inverse relation between left ventricular (LV) mass and vascular endothelial function. **A:** Increase in left ventricular mass index (LVMI) is associated with a decrease in the increase in forearm blood flow in response to acetylcholine (Ach) infusion. **B:** The same relation is shown when comparing LVMI to coronary flow reserve (CFR), as determined by "split-dose" Tl-201 single photon emission tomography in subjects with moderate to severe hypertension (Reproduced from Diamond JA, Krakoff LR, Goldman A, et al. Comparison of two calcium blockers on hemodynamics, left ventricular mass, and coronary vasodilatory in advanced hypertension. *Am J Hypertens* 2001;14:231–240; Perticone F, Maio R, Ceravolo R, et al. Relationship between left ventricular mass and endothelium-dependent vasodilation in never-treated hypertensive patients. *Circulation* 1999;99:1991–1996, with permission).

diastolic BP less than 85 to 95 mm Hg may have an upturn in coronary events. This is presumably a result of inadequate perfusion of coronary arteries. Support for and against this relation is based on differing interpretations and results of retrospective analyses of several large treatment trials or programs (189–193). For example, in one retrospective analysis, men with LVH or ischemic patterns on ECG had increased incidence of MI when treated diastolic BPs were less than 95 mm Hg (194). By contrast, in the Systolic Hypertension in the Elderly (SHEP) trial, coronary events were decreased in subjects with evidence of LVH by ECG criteria and low treatment diastolic BP (195). Although this may argue against a J-curve, it is important to realize that these patients had low diastolic pressures before treatment, and, hence, their autoregulatory curve was already adjusted to lower pressure.

Recommendations for the safest level of BP reduction in patients with LVH can be only speculative at this point. In patients with isolated systolic hypertension, in which the pretreatment diastolic BP is already low, SHEP trial data indicate that further reduction of diastolic BP is safe. Conversely, patients with diastolic hypertension and LVH (without renal disease) may experience complications of reduced coronary blood flow when BP is decreased to less than 85 to 90 mm Hg, particularly in the presence of CAD. Whether decreasing BP to less than 85 to 90 mm Hg is warranted in the presence of renal disease and LVH requires further study. The presence of systolic dysfunction, particularly in the presence of CAD, adds more controversial variables to this dilemma and also requires further investigation.

Prognostic Implications of Abnormal Coronary Microvascular Function

Patients with hypertension with LVH have increased cardiac morbidity and mortality even in the absence of epicardial CAD. Only recently has this been attributed to abnormal coronary microvasculature function. A positive

TABLE 17–3. *New Doppler techniques that may allow for serial noninvasive interpretation of left ventricular diastolic function*

Doppler technique	Measure	References
Pulmonary venous inflow	Increase in the "reverse flow" wave caused by high LV end-diastolic pressure	76–78
A–Ar interval	Diastolic flow first directed toward apex of LV, then to LV outflow tract. This interval shortens with stiffening LV	79,80
Color M-mode	Interval from color M-mode peak velocity at the mitral leaflet tips to peak velocity in the apex of the LV	81
Doppler tissue imaging	Quantification of intramural myocardial velocities by detection of consecutive phase shifts of the ultrasound signal reflected from contracting myocardium	82–85
Ultrasonic backscatter	Quantitative characterization of myocardial texture obtained by analysis of ultrasonic reflectivity; amount of backscatter produced when ultrasound interacts with components of tissue correlates with the degree of myocardial fibrillar collagens	86

LV, left ventricle.

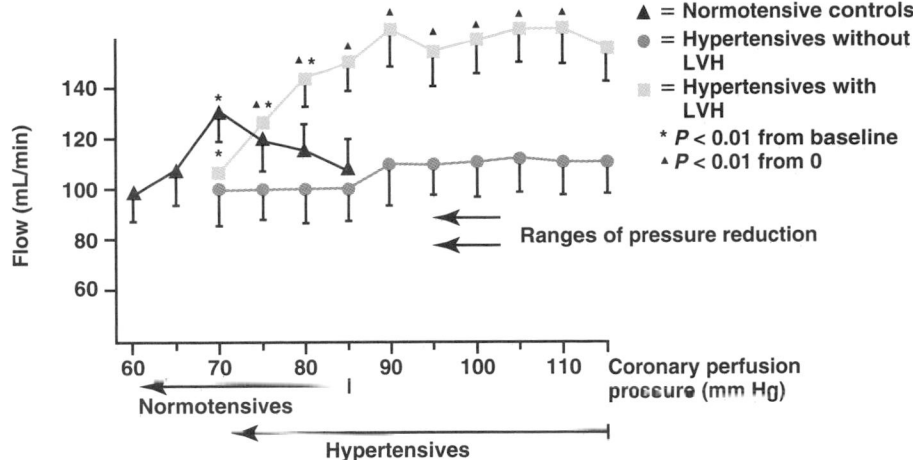

FIG. 17–7. Effect of acute reduction in coronary perfusion pressure on coronary autoregulation in control subjects with normotension, patients with hypertension without left ventricular hypertrophy (LVH), and patients with hypertension and LVH. The autoregulatory curve for hypertension with LVH is shifted upward and to the right. At coronary perfusion pressure less than 90 mm Hg, patients with hypertension and LVH have marked loss of coronary autoregulation. (Modified from Polese A, DeCesare N, Montorsi P, et al. Upward shift of the lower range of coronary flow autoregulation in hypertensive patients with hypertrophy of the left ventricle. *Circulation* 1991;83:845–853.)

family history of premature CAD has been associated with a genetic predisposition to abnormal endothelium-dependent vasodilatation, as demonstrated by response to acetylcholine (197). Although the genetic cause is not known, there may be an association with abnormal homocysteine metabolism. Suwaidi and coworkers (198) showed increased overall cardiovascular morbidity in individuals with an abnormal forearm blood flow response to acetylcholine. However, this study was limited by the small total number of cardiac events (6 events in 42 subjects with abnormal endothelial function). Halcox and coworkers (199) demonstrated increased cardiovascular morbidity and mortality in individuals with endothelial dysfunction. In individuals with mild CAD or no CAD, a blunted decrease in coronary arterial resistance and an increase in epicardial coronary artery diameter in response to intracoronary acetylcholine infusion was independently associated with an increased incidence of future vascular events (199).

Effect of Antihypertensive Treatment on Coronary Flow Reserve

To reduce the risk for coronary events in arterial hypertension, therapy should be geared at reversing the chief cardiac manifestations: LVH and coronary microcirculatory abnormalities.

Studies in hypertensive rodent and canine models show that reduction of wall stress results in regression of LVH, reversal of coronary vascular abnormalities, and improved overall coronary blood flow (200–204). The effects of antihypertensive therapy on vascular pathology in humans,

however, are not well understood. Heagerty and coworkers (205) obtained serial skin biopsies of subcutaneous resistance arterioles in patients with hypertension. After long-term treatment with various combinations of β-blockers, calcium channel blockers, diuretics, and ACE inhibitors, they demonstrated partial regression of the medial layer of these vessels (205). It is not known if parallel changes occur in coronary vessels.

Angiotensin-converting Enzyme Inhibitors and Angiotensin II Receptor Blockers

There are few human studies on the effects of antihypertensive therapy on coronary blood flow reserve. Preliminary data using the gas chromatographic Argon method of quantifying coronary flow reserve showed improved flow reserve in patients with hypertension after 12 months of therapy with enalapril (206). By blocking the production of angiotensin II, ACE inhibitors may be effective in improving coronary flow reserve. This may be because of reduction in perivascular and interstitial fibrosis (207). Akinboboye and coworkers (208) used ^{15}O-water positron emission tomography to quantify myocardial perfusion reserve in a small population of predominantly African American subjects with hypertension. This study demonstrated improved myocardial perfusion reserve after treatment with lisinopril for a mean of 11 months (208). Using a modification of traditional Tl-201 myocardial perfusion imaging to permit quantification of myocardial perfusion reserve, Diamond and coworkers (209) showed a modest improvement in myocardial perfusion reserve after 6 months of antihypertensive treatment with the angiotensin receptor blocker eprosartan. In this study, however, there was no significant change in MPR with the ACE inhibitor enalapril. However, this may be because of the short follow-up period. The Brachial Artery Normalization of Forearm Function (BANFF) study was a randomized, crossover trial examining the effects of quinapril, enalapril, losartan, and amlodipine on flow-mediated vasodilatation of the brachial artery in 80 subjects with CAD (210). Significant improvement was observed only with quinapril and only in subjects with either the ID or II (insertion) ACE genotype. This study suggests that ACE inhibitors with significant tissue affinity may be important in improving vascular endothelial function. However, the observations of this study may be, in part, because of the dosage of drugs administered and the duration of therapy. The maximal dosage of enalapril and losartan used were 10 and 50 mg daily, respectively, and the treatment duration was only 8 weeks.

Calcium Channel Blockers

The effect of calcium channel blockers on coronary flow reserve is even less clear. Although they produce favorable hemodynamic effects with reversal of pressure overload and regression of LVH, several studies suggest that certain calcium channel blockers do not significantly change, or may even reduce coronary flow reserve (211–213). Theoretically, calcium channel blockers may reduce coronary flow reserve by blocking the effect of endogenous vasodilators such as adenosine (214).

β-Blockers

Using positron emission tomography quantification of myocardial perfusion, β-blockers have been shown to augment coronary flow reserve in healthy volunteer subjects (215). Billinger and coworkers (216) showed in patients with CAD that postischemic coronary flow reserve (hyperemic flow), is significantly augmented in those patients taking the β-blocker, metoprolol. By augmenting coronary flow reserve, oxygen supply to the heart is enhanced. This may explain, in part, the benefit of β-blockers in patients with CAD.

REFERENCES

1. Levy D, Anderson KM, Savage D, et al. Echocardiographically detected left ventricular hypertrophy: prevalence and risk factors. The Framingham Heart Study. Ann Intern Med 1988;108:7–13.
2. Bikkina M, Larson MG, Levy D. Asymptomatic ventricular arrhythmias and mortality risk in subjects with left ventricular hypertrophy. J Am Coll Cardiol 1993;22:1111–1116.
3. Levy D, Garrison RJ, Savage DD, et al. Prognostic implications of echocardiographically determined left ventricular mass in the Framingham Heart Study. N Engl J Med 1990;322:1561–1566.
4. Cooper RS, Simmons BE, Castaner A, et al. Left ventricular hypertrophy is associated with worse survival independent of ventricular function and number of coronary arteries severely narrowed. Am J Cardiol 1990;65:441–445.
5. Ghali JK, Liao Y, Simmons B, et al. The prognostic role of left ventricular hypertrophy in patients with or without coronary artery disease. Ann Intern Med 1992;117:831–836.
6. Deschepper CF, Boutin-Ganache I, Zahabi A, et al. In search of cardiovascular candidate genes: interactions between phenotypes and genotypes. Hypertension 2002;39[2 Pt 2]:332–336.
7. Himmelmann A, Svensson A, Hansson L. Blood pressure and left ventricular mass in children with different maternal histories of hypertension: the Hypertension in Pregnancy Offspring Study. J Hypertens 1993;11:263–268.
8. van Hooft IM, Grobbee DE, Waal-Manning HJ, et al. Hemodynamic characteristics of the early phase of primary hypertension: the Dutch Hypertension and Offspring study. Circulation 1993;87:1100–1106.
9. Liebson PR, Grandits G, Prineas R, et al. Echocardiographic correlates of left ventricular structure among 844 mildly hypertensive men and women in the treatment of mild hypertension study (TOMHS). Circulation 1993;87;476–486
10. Mayet J, Shahi M, Foale RA, et al. Racial differences in cardiac structure and function in essential hypertension. Br Med J 1994;308:1011–1014.
11. Schunkert H, Hense HW, Holmer SR, et al. Association between a deletion polymorphism of the angiotensin converting-enzyme gene and left ventricular hypertrophy. N Engl J Med 1994;330:1634–1638.
12. Perticone F, Ceravolo R, Cosco C, et al. Deletion polymorphism of angiotensin-converting enzyme gene and left ventricular hypertrophy in southern Italian patients. J Am Coll Cardiol 1997;29:365–369.
13. Gharavi AG, Lipkowitz MS, Diamond JA, et al. Deletion polymorphism of the angiotensin-converting enzyme gene is independently associated with left ventricular mass and geometric remodeling in systemic hypertension. Am J Cardiol 1996;77:1315–1319.
14. Lifton RP, Gharavi AG, Geller DS. Molecular mechanisms of human hypertension. Cell 2001;104:545–556.
15. Glueck SB, Dzau VJ. Physiological genomics: implications in hypertension research. Hypertension 2002;39[2 Pt 2]:310–315.
16. Kimura B, Mohuczy D, Tang X, et al. Attenuation of hypertension and heart hypertrophy by adeno-associated virus delivering angiotensinogen antisense. Hypertension 2001;37[2 Pt 2]:376–380.
17. Perticone F, Ceravolo R, Cosco C, et al. Deletion polymorphism of angiotensin-converting enzyme gene and left ventricular hypertrophy in southern Italian patients. J Am Coll Cardiol 1997;29:365–369.
18. Tang W, Devereux RB, Rao DC, et al. Associations between angiotensinogen gene variants and left ventricular mass and function in the HyperGEN study. Am Heart J 2002;143:854–860.
19. Poch E, Gonzalez D, Gomez-Angelats E, et al. G-Protein beta(3) subunit gene variant and left ventricular hypertrophy in essential hypertension. Hypertension 2000;35[1 Pt 2]:214–218.
20. Obineche EN, Frossard PM, Bokhari AM. An association study of five genetic loci and left ventricular hypertrophy amongst Gulf Arabs. Hypertens Res 2001;24:635–639.
21. Nakayama T, Soma M, Takahashi Y, et al. Functional deletion mutation of the 5'-flanking region of type A human natriuretic peptide receptor gene and its association with essential hypertension and left ventricular hypertrophy in the Japanese. Circ Res 2000;86:841–845.
22. Phillips RA, Goldman ME, Ardeljan M, et al. Determinants of abnormal left ventricular filling in early hypertension. J Am Coll Cardiol 1989;14:979–985.
23. Chantin A, Barksdale EE. Experimental renal insufficiency produced by partial nephrectomy. II. Relationship of left ventricular hypertrophy, the width of the cardiac muscle fiber and hypertension in the rat. Arch Intern Med 1933;52:739.
24. Rowlands DB, Glover DR, Ireland MA, et al. Assessment of left-ventricular mass and its response to antihypertensive treatment. Lancet 1982;1:467–470.
25. Devereux RB, Pickering TG, Harshfield GA, et al. Left ventricular hypertrophy in patients with hypertension: importance of blood pressure response to regular recurring stress. Circulation 1983;68:470–476.
26. Lauer MS, Anderson KM, Levy D. Influence of contemporary versus 30-year blood pressure levels on left ventricular mass and geometry: the Framingham Heart Study. J Am Coll Cardiol 1991;18:1287–1294.
27. Ganau A, Devereux RB, Pickering TG, et al. Relation of left ventricular hemodynamic load and contractile performance to left ventricular mass in hypertension. Circulation 1990;81:25–36.
28. Guerrier M, Schillaci G, Verdecchia P, et al. Circadian blood pressure changes and left ventricular hypertrophy in essential hypertension. Circulation 1990;81:528–536.
29. Fagard R, Staessen J, Thijs L, et al. Relation of left ventricular mass

and filling to exercise blood pressure and rest blood pressure. *Am J Cardiol* 1995;75(1):53–57.

30. Ramakrishna G, Schechter CB, Phillips RA. Diagnosis and treatment of isolated systolic hypertension (ISH) in the elderly. Results of a survey four years post-SHEP. *Am J Geriatr Cardiol* 1997;6(4):20–36.
31. Levy D, Garrison RJ, Savage DD, et al. Left ventricular mass and incidence of coronary heart disease in an elderly cohort: the Framingham Heart Study. *Ann Intern Med* 1989;110:101–107.
32. MacMahon SW, Wilcken DE, MacDonald GJ. The effect of weight reduction on left ventricular mass. *N Engl J Med* 1986;314:334–339.
33. Lauer MS, Anderson KM, Levy D. Separate and joint influences of obesity and mild hypertension on left ventricular mass and geometry: the Framingham Heart Study. *J Am Coll Cardiol* 1992;19:130–134.
34. de Simone G, Devereux RB, Roman MJ, et al. Relation of obesity and gender to left ventricular hypertrophy in normotensive and hypertensive adults. *Hypertension* 1994;23:600–606.
35. Marcus R, Krause L, Weder AB, et al. Sex specific determinants of increased left ventricular mass in the Tecumseh blood pressure study. *Circulation* 1994;90:928–936.
36. Lim MJ, Barkan AL, Buda AJ. Rapid reduction of left ventricular hypertrophy in acromegaly after suppression of growth hormone hypersecretion. *Ann Intern Med* 1992;117:719–726.
37. Andronico G, Mangano MT, Nardi E, et al. Insulin-like growth factor 1 and sodium-lithium countertransport in essential hypertension and in hypertensive left ventricular hypertrophy. *J Hypertens* 1993;11:1097–1101.
38. Hinderliter AL, Light KC, Willis PW 4th. Gender differences in left ventricular structure and function in young adults with normal or marginally elevated blood pressure. *Am J Hypertens* 1992;5:33–36.
39. Devereux RB, Lutas EM, Casale PN, et al. Standardization of M-mode echocardiographic left ventricular anatomic measurements. *J Am Coll Cardiol* 1984;4:1222–1230.
40. Cabral AM, Vasquez EC, Moyses MR, et al. Sex hormone modulation of ventricular hypertrophy in sino-aortic denervated rats. *Hypertension* 1988;11[Suppl 1]:93–97.
41. Douglas PS, Katz SE, Weinberg EO, et al. Hypertrophic remodeling: gender differences in the early response to left ventricular pressure overload. *J Am Coll Cardiol* 1998;32:1118–1125.
42. Beaglehole R, Tyroler HA, Cassel JC, et al. An epidemiological study of left ventricular hypertrophy in the biracial population of Evans County, Georgia. *J Chronic Dis* 1974;28:549–559.
43. Hinderliter AL, Light KC, Willis PW. Racial differences in left ventricular structure in healthy young adults. *Am J Cardiol* 1992;69:1196–1199.
44. Shub C, Klein AL, Zachariah PK, et al. Determination of left ventricular mass by echocardiography in a normal population: effect of age and sex in addition to body size. *Mayo Clin Proc* 1994;69:205–211.
45. de Simone G, Devereux RB, Roman MJ, et al. Gender differences in left ventricular anatomy, blood viscosity and volume regulatory hormones in normal adults. *Am J Cardiol* 1991;68:1704–1708.
46. Savage DD, Drayer JI, Henry WL, et al. Echocardiographic assessment of cardiac anatomy and function in hypertensive patients. *Circulation* 1979;59:623–632.
47. Gerstenblith G, Frederiksen J, Yin FC, et al. Echocardiographic assessment of a normal adult aging population. *Circulation* 1977;56:273–278.
48. Molkentin JD, Lu JR, Antos CL, et al. A calcineurin-dependent transcriptional pathway for cardiac hypertrophy. *Cell* 1998;93:215–228.
49. Marban E, Koretsune Y. Cell calcium, oncogenes, and hypertrophy. *Hypertension* 1990;15:652–658.
50. Phillips RA, Krakoff LR, Ardeljan M, et al. Relation of left ventricular mass to insulin resistance and blood pressure in non-obese subjects. *J Am Coll Cardiol* 1994;23:48A(abst).
51. Phillips RA, Krakoff LR, Dunaif A, et al. Relation among left ventricular mass, insulin resistance, and blood pressure in nonobese subjects. *J Clin Endocrinol Metab* 1998;83:4284–4288.
52. Sadoshima J, Xu Y, Slayter HS, et al. Autocrine release of angiotensin II mediates stretch-induced hypertrophy of cardiac myocytes in vitro. *Cell* 1993;75:977–984.
53. Schmieder RE, Langenfeld MR, Friedrich A, et al. Angiotensin II related to sodium excretion modulates left ventricular structure in human essential hypertension. *Circulation* 1996;94:1304–1309.
54. Manolio TA, Levy D, Garrison RJ, et al. Relation of alcohol intake to left ventricular mass: the Framingham study. *J Am Coll Cardiol* 1991;17,3:717–721.

55. Devereux RB, Drayer JI, Chien S, et al. Whole blood viscosity as a determinant of cardiac hypertrophy in systemic hypertension. *Am J Cardiol* 1986;54:592–595.
56. Bauwens FR, Duprez DA, de Buyzere ML, et al. Influence of the arterial blood pressure and nonhemodynamic factors on left ventricular hypertrophy in moderate essential hypertension. *Am J Cardiol* 1991;68:925–929.
57. Weber KT, Brilla CG. Pathological hypertrophy and cardiac interstitium. Fibrosis and renin-angiotensin-aldosterone system pathological hypertrophy and cardiac interstitium. Fibrosis and renin-angiotensin-aldosterone system. *Circulation* 1991;83:1849–1865.
58. Rossi GP, Sacchetto A, Visentin P, et al. Changes in left ventricular anatomy and function in hypertension and primary aldosteronism. *Hypertension* 1996;27:1039–1045.
59. Schmieder RE, Messerli FH, Garavaglia GE, et al. Dietary salt intake: a determinant of cardiac involvement in essential hypertension. *Circulation* 1988;78:951–956.
60. de la Sierra A, Coca A, Paré JC, et al. Erythrocyte ion fluxes in essential hypertensive patients with left ventricular hypertrophy. *Circulation* 1993;88:1628–1633.
61. Sen S, Tarazi RC, Khairallah PA, et al. Cardiac hypertrophy in spontaneously hypertensive rats. *Circ Res* 1974;35:775–781.
62. Devereux RB, Pickering TG, Cody RJ, et al. Relation of renin-angiotensin system activity to left ventricular hypertrophy and function in experimental and human hypertension. *J Clin Hypertens* 1987;3:87–103.
63. Adams TD, Yanowitz FG, Fisher AG, et al. Heritability of cardiac size: an echocardiographic and electrocardiographic study of monozygotic and dizygotic twins. *Circulation* 1985;71:39–44.
64. Trimarco B, Ricciardelli B, de Luca N, et al. Participation of endogenous catecholamines in the regulation of left ventricular mass in progeny of hypertensive parents. *Circulation* 1985;72:38–46.
65. Simpson P. Role of proto-oncogenes in myocardial hypertrophy. *Am J Cardiol* 1988;62:13G–19G.
66. Shub C, Cueto-Garcia L, Sheps S, et al. Echocardiographic findings in pheochromocytoma. *Am J Cardiol* 1986;57:971–975.
67. Nosadini R, Semplicini A, Fioretto P, et al. Sodium-lithium countertransport and cardiorenal abnormalities in essential hypertension. *Hypertension* 1991;18:191–198.
68. Akhter SA, Milano CA, Shotwell KF, et al. Transgenic mice with cardiac overexpression of alpha1B-adrenergic receptors. In vivo alpha1-adrenergic receptor-mediated regulation of beta-adrenergic signaling. *J Biol Chem* 1997;272:21253–21259.
69. Choi DJ, Koch WJ, Hunter JJ, et al. Mechanism of beta-adrenergic receptor desensitization in cardiac hypertrophy is increased beta-adrenergic receptor kinase. *J Biol Chem* 1997;272:17223–17229.
70. Morgan HE, Baker KM. Cardiac hypertrophy. Mechanical, neural and endocrine dependence. *Circulation* 1991;83:13–25.
71. Schunkert H, Jahn L, Izumo S, et al. Localization and regulation of c-fos and c-jun protooncogene induction by systolic wall stress in normal and hypertrophied rat hearts. *Proc Natl Acad Sci USA* 1991;88:11480–11484.
72. Hsueh WA, Law RE, Do YS. Integrins, adhesion, and cardiac remodeling. *Hypertension* 1998;31[1 Pt 2]:176–180.
73. Sussman MA, Lim HW, Gude N, et al. Prevention of cardiac hypertrophy in mice by calcineurin inhibition. *Science* 1998;281:1690–1693.
74. Nagata K, Somura F, Obata K, et al. AT1 receptor blockade reduces cardiac calcineurin activity in hypertensive rats. *Hypertension* 2002;40:168–174.
75. Diamond JA, Krakoff LR, Martin K, et al. Comparison of ambulatory blood pressure and amounts of left ventricular hypertrophy in men versus women with similar levels of hypertensive clinic blood pressures. *Am J Cardiol* 1997;79:505–508.
76. Matsuda Y, Toma Y, Matsuzaki M, et al. Change of left atrial systolic pressure waveform in relation to left ventricular end-diastolic pressure. *Circulation* 1990;82:1659–1667.
77. Rossvoll O, Hatle LK. Pulmonary venous flow velocities recorded by transthoracic Doppler ultrasound: relation to left ventricular diastolic pressures. *J Am Coll Cardiol* 1993;21:1687–1696.
78. Appleton CP, Galloway JM, Gonzales MS, et al. Estimation of left ventricular filling pressures using two-dimensional and Doppler echocardiography in adult patients with cardiac disease. Additional value of analyzing left atrial size, left atrial ejection fraction and the

difference in duration of pulmonary venous and mitral flow velocity at atrial contraction. *J Am Coll Cardiol* 1993;22:1972–1982.

79. Pai RG, Suzuki M, Heywood JT, et al. Mitral A velocity wave transit time to the outflow tract as a measure of left ventricular diastolic stiffness: hemodynamic correlations in patients with coronary artery disease. *Circulation* 1994;89:553–557.

80. Pai RG, Shakudo M, Yoganathan AP, et al. Clinical correlates of the rate of transmission of transmitral "A" wave to the left ventricular outflow tract in left ventricular hypertrophy secondary to system hypertension, hypertrophic cardiomyopathy or aortic valve stenosis. *Am J Cardiol* 1994;73:831–834.

81. Garcia MJ, Thomas JD, Klein AL. New Doppler echocardiographic applications for the study of diastolic function. *J Am Coll Cardiol* 1998;32:865–875.

82. Derumeaux G, Ovize M, Loufoua J, et al. Doppler tissue imaging quantitates regional wall motion during myocardial ischemia and reperfusion. *Circulation* 1998;97:1970–1977.

83. Galiuto L, Ignone G, DeMaria AN. Contraction and relaxation velocities of the normal left ventricle using pulsed-wave tissue Doppler echocardiography. *Am J Cardiol* 1998;81:609–614.

84. Stewart RE, Miller DD, Bowers TR, et al. PET perfusion and vasodilator function after angioplasty for acute myocardial infarction. *J Nucl Med* 1997;38:770–777.

85. Stoylen A, Slordahl S, Skjelvan GK, et al. Strain rate imaging in normal and reduced diastolic function: comparison with pulsed Doppler tissue imaging of the mitral annulus. *J Am Soc Echocardiogr* 2001;14:264–274.

86. Maceira AM, Barba J, Beloqui O, et al. Ultrasonic backscatter and diastolic function in hypertensive patients. *Hypertension* 2002;40:239–243.

87. Harada K, Komuro I, Shiojima I, et al. Pressure overload induces cardiac hypertrophy in angiotensin II type 1A receptor knockout mice. *Circulation* 1998;97:1952–1959.

88. Schmieder RE. Reversal of left ventricular hypertrophy: analysis of 412 published studies. *Am J Hypertens* 1994;7[4 Pt 2]:25a(abst).

89. Verdecchia P, Schillaci G, Borgioni C, et al. Prognostic significance of serial changes in left ventricular mass in essential hypertension. *Circulation* 1998;97:48–54.

90. Koren MJ, Ulin RJ, Koren AT, et al. Left ventricular mass change during treatment and outcome in patients with essential hypertension. *Am J Hypertens* 2002;15:1021–1028.

91. Neaton JD, Grimm RH Jr, Prineas RJ, et al. Treatment of mild hypertension study: final results. *JAMA* 1993;270:713–724.

92. Schussheim AE, Diamond JA, Phillips RA. Left ventricular midwall function improves with antihypertensive therapy and regression of left ventricular hypertrophy in patients with asymptomatic hypertension. *Am J Cardiol* 2001;87:61–65.

93. Wachtell K, Palmieri V, Olsen MH, et al. Change in systolic left ventricular performance after 3 years of antihypertensive treatment: the Losartan Intervention for Endpoint (LIFE) Study. *Circulation* 2002;106:227–232.

94. Dahlof B, Pennert K, Hansson L. Reversal of left ventricular hypertrophy in hypertensive patients. A metaanalysis of 109 treatment studies. *Am J Hypertens* 1992;5:95–110.

95. Linz W, Schaper J, Wiemer G, et al. Ramipril prevents left ventricular hypertrophy with myocardial fibrosis without blood pressure reduction: a one year study in rats. *Br J Pharmacol* 1992;107:970–975.

96. Gottdiener JS, Reda DJ, Massie BM, et al. Effect of single-drug therapy on reduction of left ventricular mass in mild to moderate hypertension: comparison of six antihypertensive agents. The Department of Veterans Affairs Cooperative Study Group on Antihypertensive Agents. *Circulation* 1997;95:2007–2014.

97. Inouye I, Massie B, Loge D, et al. Abnormal left ventricular filling: an early finding in mild to moderate systemic hypertension. *Am J Cardiol* 1984;53:120–126.

98. Bonow RO, Udelson JE. Left ventricular diastolic dysfunction as a cause of congestive heart failure: mechanisms and management. *Ann Intern Med* 1992;117:502–510.

99. Topol EJ, Traill GV, Fortuin NJ. Hypertensive cardiomyopathy of the elderly. *N Engl J Med* 1985;312:277–282.

100. Soufer R, Wohlgelernter D, Vita N, et al. Intact systolic left ventricular function in clinical congestive heart failure. *Am J Cardiol* 1985;55:1032–1036.

101. Senni M, Tribouilloy CM, Rodeheffer RJ, et al. Congestive heart failure in the community: a study of all incident cases in Olmsted County, Minnesota, in 1991. *Circulation* 1998;98:2282–2289.

102. Setaro JF, Soufer R, Remetz MS, et al. Long-term outcome in patients with congestive heart failure and intact systolic left ventricular performance. *Am J Cardiol* 1992;69:1212–1216.

103. Carroll JD, Lang RM, Neumann AL, et al. The differential effects of positive inotropic and vasodilator therapy on diastolic properties in patients with congestive cardiomyopathy. *Circulation* 1986;74:815–825.

104. Tang W, Arnett DK, Devereux RB, et al. Linkage of left ventricular early diastolic peak filling velocity to chromosome 5 in hypertensive African Americans: the HyperGEN echocardiography study. *Am J Hypertens* 2002;15[7 Pt 1]:621–627.

105. Snider AR, Gidding SS, Rocchini AP, et al. Doppler evaluation of left ventricular diastolic filling in children with systemic hypertension. *Am J Cardiol* 1985;56:921–926.

106. Smith VE, Schulman P, Karimeddini M, et al. Rapid ventricular filling in left ventricular hypertrophy II. Pathological hypertrophy. *J Am Coll Cardiol* 1985;5:869–874.

107. Phillips RA, Coplan NL, Krakoff LR, et al. Doppler echocardiographic analysis of left ventricular filling in treated hypertensive patients. *J Am Coll Cardiol* 1987;9:317–322.

108. Dianzumba SB, DiPette DJ, Cornman C, et al. Left ventricular filling characteristics in mild untreated hypertension. *Hypertension* 1986;8[Suppl I]:I-156–I-160.

109. Shapiro LM, McKenna WJ. Left ventricular hypertrophy: relationship of structure to diastolic function in hypertension. *Br Heart J* 1984;51:637–642.

110. Hartford M, Wikstrand J, Wallentin I, et al. Diastolic function of the heart in untreated primary hypertension. *Hypertension* 1984;6:329–338.

111. Fouad FM, Slominski JM, Tarazi RC. Left ventricular diastolic function in hypertension: relation to left ventricular mass and systolic function. *J Am Coll Cardiol* 1984;3:1500–1506.

112. Smith VE, White WB, Meeran MK, et al. Improved left ventricular filling accompanies reduced left ventricular mass during therapy of essential hypertension. *J Am Coll Cardiol* 1986;8:1449–1454.

113. White WB, Schulman P, Karimeddini MK, et al. Regression of left ventricular mass is accompanied by improvement in rapid left ventricular filling following antihypertensive therapy with metoprolol. *Am Heart J* 1989;117:145–150.

114. Trimarco B, DeLuca N, Rosiello G. Improvement of diastolic function after reversal of left ventricular hypertrophy induced long-term antihypertensive treatment with tertatolol. *Am J Cardiol* 1989;64:745–751.

115. Schulman SP, Weiss JL, Becher LC, et al. The effects of antihypertensive therapy on left ventricular mass in elderly patients. *N Engl J Med* 1990;322:1350–1356.

116. Gonzalez-Fernandez RB, Altieri PI, Diaz LM, et al. Effects of enalapril on heart failure in hypertensive patients with diastolic dysfunction. *Am J Hypertens* 1992;5:480–483.

117. Phillips RA, Ardeljan M, Shimabukuro S, et al. Normalization of left ventricular mass and associated changes in neurohormones and atrial natriuretic peptide after one year of sustained nifedipine therapy for severe hypertension. *J Am Coll Cardiol* 1991;17:1595–1602.

118. Shahi M, Thorn S, Poulter N, et al. Regression of hypertensive left ventricular hypertrophy and left ventricular diastolic dysfunction. *Lancet* 1990;336:458–461.

119. Lorell BH, Grice WN, Apstein CS. Influence of hypertension with minimal hypertrophy on diastolic function during demand ischemia. *Hypertension* 1989;13:361–370.

120. Wexler LF, Lorell BH, Momomura S, et al. Enhanced sensitivity to hypoxia-induced diastolic dysfunction in pressure-overload left ventricular hypertrophy in the rat: role of high-energy phosphate depletion. *Circ Res* 1988;62:766–775.

121. Osbakken M, Douglas PS, Ivanics T, et al. Creatinine kinase kinetics studied by phosphorus-31 nuclear magnetic resonance in a canine model of chronic hypertension-induced cardiac hypertrophy. *J Am Coll Cardiol* 1992;19:223–228.

122. Ito Y, Suko J, Chidsey CA. Intracalcium and myocardial contractility. V. Calcium uptake of sarcoplasmic reticulum fractions in hypertrophied and failing rabbit hearts. *J Mol Cell Cardiol* 1974;6:237–247.

123. Harding DP, Poole-Wilson PA. Calcium exchange in rabbit myocardium during and after hypoxia: effect of temperature and substrate. *Cardiovasc Res* 1980;14:435–445.

124. Brutsaert DL, Rademakers FE, Sys SU, et al. Analysis of relaxation in the evaluation of ventricular function of the heart. *Prog Cardiovasc Dis* 1985;28:143–163.

125. White WB, Schulman P, Dey HM, et al. Effects of age and 24-hour ambulatory blood pressure on rapid left ventricular filling. *Am J Cardiol* 1989;63:1343–1347.

126. Franchi F, Fabbri G, Monopoli A, et al. Left ventricular diastolic filling improvement obtained by intravenous verapamil in mild to moderate essential hypertension: a complex effect. *Cardiology* 1989;76:32–41.

127. Betocchi S, Cuocolo A, Pace L, et al. Effect of intravenous verapamil administration of left ventricular diastolic function in systemic hypertension. *Am J Cardiol* 1987;59:624–629.

128. Gandhi SK, Powers JC, Nomeir AM, et al. The pathogenesis of acute pulmonary edema associated with hypertension. *N Engl J Med* 2001;344:17–22.

129. de Simone G, Devereux RB, Koren MJ, et al. Midwall left ventricular mechanics. An independent predictor of cardiovascular risk in arterial hypertension. *Circulation* 1996;93:259–265.

130. de Simone G, Devereux RB, Roman MJ, et al. Assessment of left ventricular function by the midwall fractional shortening/end-systolic stress relation in human hypertension [published erratum appears in J Am Coll Cardiol 1994;24:844]. *J Am Coll Cardiol* 1994;23:1444–1451.

131. Schussheim AE, Diamond JA, Jhang JS, et al. Midwall fractional shortening is an independent predictor of left ventricular diastolic dysfunction in asymptomatic patients with systemic hypertension. *Am J Cardiol* 1998;82:1056–1059.

132. Aurigemma GP, Gottdiener JS, Shemanski L, et al. Predictive value of systolic and diastolic function for incident congestive heart failure in the elderly: the cardiovascular health study. *J Am Coll Cardiol* 2001;37:1042–1048.

133. Udelson JE, Bacharach SL, Cannon RO, et al. Minimum left ventricular pressure during b-adrenergic stimulation in human subjects. Evidence for elastic recoil and diastolic "suction" in the normal heart. *Circulation* 1990;82:1174–1182.

134. Rademakers FE, Buchalter MB, Rogers WJ, et al. Dissociation between left ventricular untwisting and filling. Accentuation by catecholamines. *Circulation* 1992;85:1572–1581.

135. Harrison TR, Dixon K, Russell RO, et al. The relation of age to the duration of contraction, ejection, and relaxation of the normal human heart. *Am Heart J* 1964;67:189–199.

136. Spirito P, Maron BJ. Influence of aging on Doppler echocardiographic indices of left ventricular diastolic function. *Br Heart J* 1988;59:672–679.

137. Arora RR, Machac J, Goldman ME, et al. Atrial kinetics and left ventricular diastolic filling in the healthy elderly. *J Am Coll Cardiol* 1987;9:1255–1260.

138. Benjamin EJ, Plehn JF, D'Agostino RB, et al. Mitral annular calcification and the risk of stroke in an elderly cohort. *N Engl J Med* 1992;327:374–379.

139. Weiss JL, Frederiksen JW, Weisfeldt ML. Hemodynamic determinants of the time-course of fall in canine left ventricular pressure. *J Clin Invest* 1976;58:751–760.

140. Grossman W, McLaurin LP. Diastolic properties of the left ventricle. *Ann Intern Med* 1976;84:316–326.

141. Hess OM, Ritter M, Schneider J, et al. Diastolic stiffness and myocardial structure in aortic valve disease before and after valve replacement. *Circulation* 1984;69:855–865.

142. Spirito P, Maron BJ, Bonow RO. Noninvasive assessment of left ventricular diastolic function: comparative analysis of Doppler echocardiographic and radionuclide angiographic techniques. *J Am Coll Cardiol* 1986;7:518–526.

143. Shapiro LM, Mackinnon J, Beevers DG. Echocardiographic features of malignant hypertension. *Br Heart J* 1981;46:374–379.

144. Kitabatake A, Inoue M, Asao M, et al. Transmitral blood flow reflecting diastolic behavior of the left ventricle in health and disease: a study by pulsed Doppler technique. *Jpn Circ J* 1982;46:92–102.

145. Chenzbraun A, Pinto FJ, Popylisen S, et al. Filling patterns in left ventricular hypertrophy: a combined acoustic quantification and Doppler study. *J Am Coll Cardiol* 1994;23:1179–1185.

146. Hanrath P, Mathey DG, Siegert R, et al. Left ventricular relaxation and filling pattern in different forms of left ventricular hypertrophy: an echocardiographic study. *Am J Cardiol* 1980;45:15–23.

147. Nakashima Y, Nii T, Ikeda M, et al. Role of left ventricular regional nonuniformity in hypertensive diastolic dysfunction. *J Am Coll Cardiol* 1993;22:790–795.

148. Spirito P, Maron BJ. Doppler echocardiography for assessing left ventricular diastolic function. *Ann Intern Med* 1988;109:122–126.

149. Bella JN, Palmieri V, Roman MJ, et al. Mitral ratio of peak early to late diastolic filling velocity as a predictor of mortality in middle-aged and elderly adults: the Strong Heart Study. *Circulation* 2002;105:1928–1933.

150. Schillaci G, Pasqualini L, Verdecchia P, et al. Prognostic significance of left ventricular diastolic dysfunction in essential hypertension. *J Am Coll Cardiol* 2002;39:2005–2011.

151. Temporelli PL, Corra U, Imparato A, et al. Reversible restrictive left ventricular diastolic filling with optimized oral therapy predicts a more favorable prognosis in patients with chronic heart failure. *J Am Coll Cardiol* 1998;31:1591–1597.

152. Aronow WS, Kronzon I. Effect of enalapril on congestive heart failure treated with diuretics in elderly patients with prior myocardial infarction and normal left ventricular ejection fraction. *Am J Cardiol* 1993;71:602–604.

153. Brilla CG, Funck RC, Rupp H. Lisinopril-mediated regression of myocardial fibrosis in patients with hypertensive heart disease. *Circulation* 2000;102:1388–1393.

154. Setaro JF, Zaret BL, Schulman DS, et al. Usefulness of verapamil for congestive heart failure associated with abnormal left ventricular diastolic filling and normal left ventricular systolic performance. *Am J Cardiol* 1990;66:981–986.

155. Given BD, Lee TH, Stone PH, et al. Nifedipine in severely hypertensive patients with congestive heart failure and preserved ventricular systolic function. *Arch Intern Med* 1985;145:281–285.

156. Andersson B, Caidahl K, di Lenarda A, et al. Changes in early and late diastolic filling patterns induced by long-term adrenergic beta-blockade in patients with idiopathic dilated cardiomyopathy. *Circulation* 1996;94:673–682.

157. Gaasch WH. Diagnosis and treatment of heart failure based on left ventricular systolic or diastolic dysfunction. *JAMA* 1994;271:1276–1280.

158. Packer M. Abnormalities of diastolic function as a potential cause of exercise intolerance in chronic heart failure. *Circulation* 1990;81[2 Suppl]:III78–III86.

159. The fifth report of the Joint National Committee on Detection, Evaluation, and Treatment of High Blood Pressure (JNC V). *Arch Intern Med* 1993;153:154–183.

160. Lorell BH, Isoyama S, Grice WN, et al. Effects of ouabain and isoproterenol on left ventricular diastolic function during low-flow ischemia in isolated, blood-perfused rabbit hearts. *Circ Res* 1988;63:457–467.

161. The effect of digoxin on mortality and morbidity in patients with heart failure. The Digitalis Investigation Group. *N Engl J Med* 1997;336:525–533.

162. Strauer BE. The concept of coronary flow reserve. *J Cardiovasc Pharmacol* 1992;19[Suppl 5]:S67–S80.

163. Strauer BE. Coronary hemodynamics in hypertensive heart disease. Basic concepts, clinical consequences, and experimental analysis of regression of hypertensive microangiopathy. *Am J Med* 1988;84[Suppl 3A]:45–54.

164. Strauer BE. Ventricular function and coronary hemodynamics in hypertensive heart disease. *Am J Cardiol* 1979;44:999–1006.

165. Cannon RO III. Dynamic limitation of coronary vasodilator reserve in patients with dilated cardiomyopathy and chest pain. *J Am Coll Cardiol* 1987;10:1190–1200.

166. Prichard AD, Smith H, Holt J, et al. Coronary vascular reserve in left ventricular hypertrophy secondary to chronic aortic regurgitation. *Am J Cardiol* 1983;51:315–320.

167. Villari B, Hess OM, Moccetti D, et al. Effect of progression of left ventricular hypertrophy on coronary artery dimensions in aortic valve disease. *J Am Coll Cardiol* 1992;20:1073–1079.

168. Rouleau J, Boerboom LE, Surjadhana A, et al. The role of autoregulation and tissue diastolic pressures in the transmural distribution of left ventricular blood flow in anesthetized dogs. *Circ Res* 1979;45:804–815.

169. Guyton RA, McClenathan JH, Michaelis LL. Evolution of regional ischemia distal to a proximal coronary stenosis: self propagation of ischemia. *Am J Cardiol* 1977;40:381–392.

170. Mosher P, Ross J, McFate PA, et al. Control of coronary blood flow by an autoregulatory mechanism. *Circ Res* 1964;14:250.

171. Driscol TE, Moir TW, Eckstein RW. Autoregulation of coronary blood flow: effect of intraarterial pressure gradients. *Circ Res* 1964; 15:103–111.

172. Hoffman JI. A critical view of coronary reserve. *Circulation* 1987;75[Suppl I]:I-6–I-11.

173. Hoffman JI. Maximal coronary flow and the concept of coronary vascular reserve. *Circulation* 1984;70:153–159.

174. Opherk D, Mall G, Zebe H, et al. Reduction of coronary reserve: a mechanism for angina pectoris in patients with arterial hypertension and normal coronary arteries. *Circulation* 1984;69:1–7.

175. Prichard AD, Gorlin R, Smith H, et al. Coronary flow studies in patients with left ventricular hypertrophy of the hypertensive type: evidence for an impaired coronary vascular reserve. *Am J Cardiol* 1981;47:547–554.

176. Goldstein RA, Haynie M. Limited myocardial perfusion reserve in patients with left ventricular hypertrophy. *J Nucl Med* 1990;31: 255–258.

177. Diamond JA, Machac J, Vallabhajosula S, et al. Validation in the canine model of a new non-invasive method of measuring coronary blood flow reserve: split dose thallium-201 rest / stress imaging. *Int J Card Imaging* 2001;17:145–152.

178. Houghton JL, Frank MJ, Carr AA, et al. Relations among impaired coronary flow reserve, left ventricular hypertrophy and thallium perfusion defects in hypertensive patients without obstructive coronary artery disease. *J Am Coll Cardiol* 1990;15:43–51.

179. Marcus ML, White CW. Coronary flow reserve in patients with normal coronary angiograms. *J Am Coll Cardiol* 1990;15:43–51.

180. Antony I, Nitenberg A, Foult JM, et al. Coronary vasodilator reserve in untreated and treated hypertensive patients with and without left ventricular hypertrophy. *J Am Coll Cardiol* 1993;22:514–520.

181. Harrison DG, Florentine MS, Brooks LA, et al. The effect of hypertension and left ventricular hypertrophy on the lower range of coronary autoregulation. *Circulation* 1988;77:1108–1115.

182. Koyanagi S, Eastham CL, Harrison DG, et al. Increased size of myocardial infarction in dogs with chronic hypertension and left ventricular hypertrophy. *Circ Res* 1982;50:55.

183. Dellsperger KC, Clothier JL, Hartnett JA, et al. Acceleration of the wavefront of myocardial necrosis by chronic hypertension and left ventricular hypertrophy in dogs. *Circ Res* 1988;63:87–96.

184. Taylor AL, Murphree S, Buja LM, et al. Segmental systolic responses to brief ischemia and reperfusion in the hypertrophied canine left ventricle. *J Am Coll Cardiol* 1992;20:994–1002.

185. Polese A, DeCesare N, Montorsi P, et al. Upward shift of the lower range of coronary flow autoregulation in hypertensive patients with hypertrophy of the left ventricle. *Circulation* 1991;83:845–853.

186. MacMahon S, Peto R, Cutler J, et al. Blood pressure, stroke, and coronary heart disease. Part 1, prolonged differences in blood pressure: prospective observational studies corrected for the regression dilution bias. *Lancet* 1990;335:765–774.

187. Collins R, Peto R, MacMahon S, et al. Blood pressure, stroke, and coronary heart disease. Part 2, short-term reductions in blood pressure: overview of randomized drug trials in their epidemiological context. *Lancet* 1990;335:827–838.

188. Cruickshank JM, Thorp JM, Zacharias FJ. Benefits and potential harm of lowering high blood pressure. *Lancet* 1987;1:581–584.

189. Alderman MH, Ooi WL, Madhavan S, et al. Treatment-induced blood pressure reduction and the risk of myocardial infarction. *JAMA* 1989;262:920–924.

190. Farnett L, Mulrow CD, Linn WD, et al. The J-curve phenomenon and the treatment of hypertension. Is there a point beyond which pressure reduction is dangerous? *JAMA* 1991;265:489–495.

191. Fletcher AE, Bulpitt CJ. How far should blood pressure be lowered? *N Engl J Med* 1992;326:251–254.

192. McCloskey LW, Psaty BM, Koepsell TD, et al. Level of blood pressure and risk of myocardial infarction among treated hypertensive patients. *Arch Intern Med* 1992;152:513–520.

193. Weinberger MH. Do No Harm. Antihypertensive therapy and the "J" curve. *Arch Intern Med* 1992;152:473–476.

194. Lindblad U, Rastam L, Ryden L, et al. Control of blood pressure and risk of first acute myocardial infarction: Skaraborg hypertension project. *BMJ* 1994;308:681–686.

195. Hansson L. Future goals for the treatment of hypertension in the elderly with reference to STOP-hypertension, SHEP, and the MRC trial in older adults. *Am J Hypertens* 1993;6[Suppl]:40S–43S.

196. Walker WG, Neaton JD, Cutler JA, et al. Renal function change in hypertensive members of the Multiple Risk Factor Intervention Trial: racial and treatment effects. *JAMA* 1992;268:3085–3091.

197. Schachinger V, Britten MB, Elsner M, et al. A positive family history of premature coronary artery disease is associated with impaired endothelium-dependent coronary blood flow regulation. *Circulation* 1999;100:1502–1508.

198. Suwaidi JA, Hamasaki S, Higano ST, et al. Long-term follow-up of patients with mild coronary artery disease and endothelial dysfunction. *Circulation* 2000;101:948–954.

199. Halcox JP, Schenke WH, Zalos G, et al. Prognostic value of coronary vascular endothelial dysfunction. *Circulation* 2002;106:653–658.

200. Isoyama S, Ito J, Sato K, et al. Collagen deposition and the reversal of coronary reserve in cardiac hypertrophy. *Hypertension* 1992;20: 491–500.

201. Anderson PG, Bishop SP, Digerness SB. Vascular remodeling and improvement of coronary reserve after hydralazine treatment in spontaneously hypertensive rats. *Circ Res* 1989;64:1127–1136.

202. Canby CA, Tomanek RJ. Role of lowering arterial pressure on maximal coronary flow with and without regression of cardiac hypertrophy. *Am J Physiol* 1989;257:H1110–H1118.

203. Ishihara K, Zile MR, Nagatsu M, et al. Coronary blood flow after the regression of pressure-overload left ventricular hypertrophy. *Circ Res* 1992;71:1472–1481.

204. Sato F, Isoyama S, Takishima T. Normalization of impaired coronary circulation in hypertrophied rat hearts. *Hypertension* 1990;16:26–34.

205. Heagerty AM, Bund SJ, Aalkjaer C. Effects of drug treatment on human resistance arteriole morphology in essential hypertension: direct evidence for structural remodelling of resistance vessels. *Lancet* 1988;2:1209–1212.

206. Vogt M, Motz WH, Schwartzkopf B, et al. Pathophysiology and clinical aspects of hypertensive hypertrophy. *Eur Heart J* 1993; 14[Suppl D]:2–7.

207. Yamada H, Fabris B, Allen AM, et al. Localization of angiotensin converting enzyme in the rat heart. *Circ Res* 1991;68:141–149.

208. Akinboboye OO, Chou RL, Bergmann SR. Augmentation of myocardial blood flow in hypertensive heart disease by angiotensin antagonists: a comparison of lisinopril and losartan. *J Am Coll Cardiol* 2002;40:703–709.

209. Diamond JA, Gharavi AG, Roychoudhury D, et al. Effect of long-term eprosartan versus enalapril antihypertensive therapy on left ventricular mass and coronary flow reserve in stage I-II hypertension. *Curr Med Res Opin* 1999;15(1):1–8.

210. Anderson TJ, Elstein E, Haber H, et al. Comparative study of ACE-inhibition, angiotensin II antagonism, and calcium channel blockade on flow-mediated vasodilation in patients with coronary disease (BANFF study). *J Am Coll Cardiol* 2000;35:60–66.

211. Rossen JD, Simonetti I, Marcus ML, et al. The effect of diltiazem on coronary flow reserve in humans. *Circulation* 1989;80:1240–1246.

212. Vrolix MC, Sionis D, Piessens J, et al. Changes in human coronary flow reserve after administration of intracoronary diltiazem. *J Cardiovasc Pharmacol* 1991;18[Suppl 9]:S64–S67.

213. Diamond JA, Krakoff LR, Goldman A, et al. Comparison of two calcium blockers on hemodynamics, left ventricular mass, and coronary vasodilatory in advanced hypertension. *Am J Hypertens* 2001;14: 231–240.

214. Merrill G, Young M, Dorell S, et al. Coronary interactions between nifedipine and adenosine in the intact dog heart. *Eur J Pharmacol* 1982;81:543–550.

215. Bottcher M, Czernin J, Sun K, et al. Effect of beta 1 adrenergic receptor blockade on myocardial blood flow and vasodilatory capacity. *J Nucl Med* 1997;38:442–446.

216. Billinger M, Seiler C, Fleisch M, et al. Do beta-adrenergic blocking agents increase coronary flow reserve? *J Am Coll Cardiol* 2001;38: 1866–1871.

CHAPTER 18

Smoking and Atherothrombosis

Lynn P. Clemow, Thomas G. Pickering, Marios N. Adonis, and Gabriella Rothman

Key Words: Addiction; endothelium; leukocytes; neurotransmitter; nicotine; plaque; thrombosis.

INTRODUCTION

Cigarette smoking is a powerful risk factor for atherothrombosis and cardiovascular events. As a contributor to almost 150,000 annual smoking-related cardiovascular deaths in

L. P. Clemow: Behavioral Cardiovascular Health and Hypertension Program, Columbia University, College of Physicians and Surgeons, 622 W. 168th St., PH-9, Room 942, New York, New York 10032.

T. G. Pickering: Behavioral Cardiovascular Health and Hypertension Program, Columbia University, College of Physicians and Surgeons, 622 W. 168th St., PH-9, Room 942, New York, New York 10032.

M. N. Adonis: Behavioral Cardiovascular Health and Hypertension Program, Columbia University, College of Physicians and Surgeons, 622 W. 168th St., PH-9, Room 942, New York, New York 10032.

G. Rothman: Behavioral Cardiovascular Health and Hypertension Program, Columbia University, College of Physicians and Surgeons, 622 W. 168th St., PH-9, Room 942, New York, New York 10032.

the United States (1), cigarette smoking is a critical public health problem with a national and international scope. Although smoking rates in the United States have decreased, worldwide smoking-related mortality is expected to increase from 3 to 10 million deaths annually by 2030 (70% of those deaths occurring in developing countries) (2).

Tobacco smoke is a complex mixture of chemicals with a broad range of biologic activities. In interaction with other risk factors, smoking contributes to atherothrombosis through a number of biologic pathways involving the central and peripheral nervous systems, the walls of blood vessels, the coagulation system, and the immune system. Over the last 30 years, the more than 50% reduction in cardiovascular mortality has followed reductions in cigarette smoking (3). Despite these trends, approximately 25% of adults in the United States continue to smoke cigarettes (1). Clinical interventions that focus on smoking cessation are a key strategy in the treatment and prevention of cardiovascular disease (CVD). Using a simple, systematic approach that focuses on treating nicotine addiction and engaging in problem-solving, physicians can effectively assist patients in altering the smoking-related biologic mechanisms that lead to atherothrombosis and its complications.

245

The purpose of this chapter is to describe the relation of tobacco consumption to the pathogenesis of CVD and its complications, briefly review the various mechanisms that may be involved in this relation, review the beneficial effects of smoking cessation, explore the barriers to smoking cessation and the characteristics of current smokers, and review in detail the strategies of smoking cessation and overcoming addiction to nicotine in the prevention and treatment of CVD in the clinical setting.

TRENDS IN TOBACCO USE AND ATHEROTHROMBOSIS

CVD is the major cause of disability and death in the United States. It is estimated that between 1995 and 1999 approximately 500,000 people died annually of various CVDs. Of these deaths, about 150,000 per year were directly related to smoking cigarettes (1). The contribution to CVD deaths in younger smokers is particularly high, with 40% of CVD deaths in adults younger than 65 years related to smoking (1). A dose–response relation has been established between smoking and the severity of atherothrombosis in coronary and cerebral arteries and the aorta, particularly in men (4), and also between smoking status and the progression of carotid atherothrombosis (Fig. 18–1). There has been a decrease in deaths from CVD of more than 50% over the last 30 years (3). The decline in CVD mortality has been attributed to improvements in primary and secondary prevention and improved medical care, although the exact impact of each factor is a topic of ongoing debate (5). It is estimated that as much as 24% of this decrease is related to reductions in cigarette smoking.

Despite improving trends in smoking cessation in the United States in recent years, approximately 25% of adults continue to smoke (1), and much remains to be done at the primary and secondary prevention level to reduce smoking-related morbidity and mortality.

Individual Differences in the Impact of Smoking

Although no one appears to be protected from the negative effects of smoking on the cardiovascular system, some populations appear to be particularly vulnerable to the toxic effects of smoking. Smoking plays a major role in increasing the relative risk of women for cardiovascular events, although their absolute risk for CVD for age is, of course, less than for men (6) (Fig. 18–2). The mechanisms related to the disproportionately increased risk in women have not been extensively studied, but they seem to include that smoking reduces estrogen levels and alters estradiol levels in women (7).

It appears that levels of serum cotinine (a major metabolite of nicotine) are greater in black than in white smokers who smoke equivalent amounts, implying differences in rate of metabolism (8). These differences may help account for, beyond the increased incidence of hypertension, the more rapid rate of progression of atherothrombosis observed in black compared with white smokers.

Genetic research regarding CVD susceptibility suggested that the effect of smoking on CVD is strongly affected by apolipoprotein E (*apoE*) ε2/ε3/ε4 genotype, such that individuals with the ε4 allele who smoke are at particularly high risk (9,10). However, a large-scale study has found the inter-

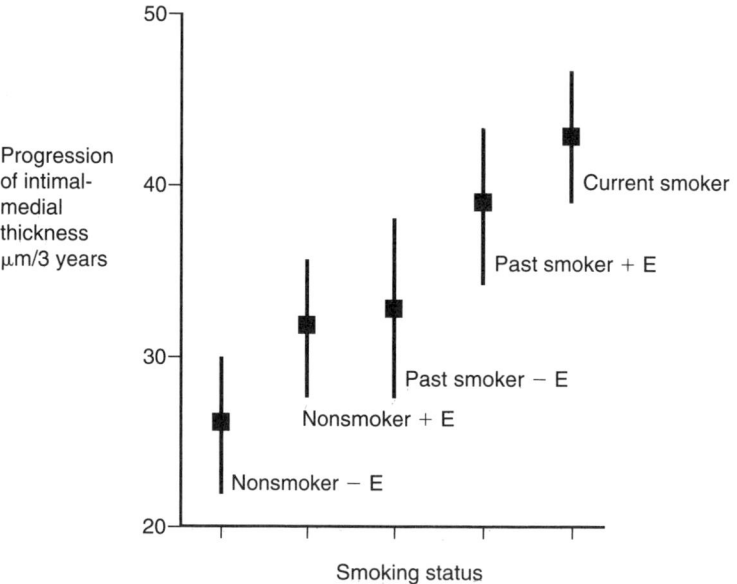

FIG. 18–1. Smoking status (with or without environmental exposure to smokers *[E]*) correlates closely with the progression of atherothrombosis of the carotid artery over a 3-year period. (Redrawn from Howard G, Wagenknecht LE, Burke GL, et al. Cigarette smoking and progression of atherosclerosis: The Atherosclerosis Risk in Communities (ARIC) Study. *JAMA* 1998;279:119–124, with permission.)

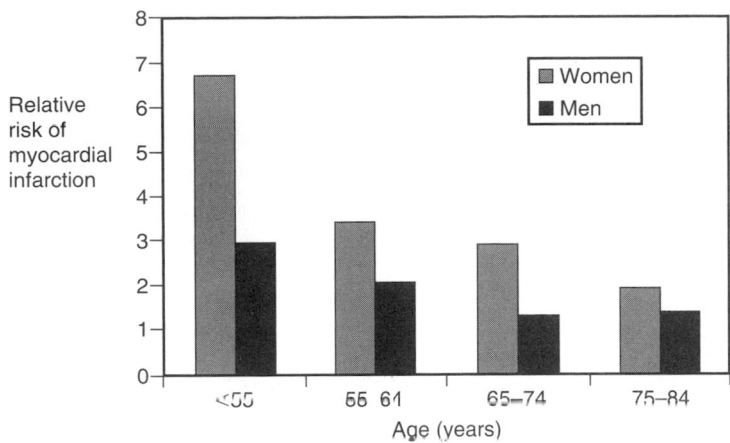

FIG. 18–2. Women are at proportionally greater risk than men for myocardial infarction as a consequence of smoking. (From Prescott E, Hippe M, Schnohr P, et al. Smoking and risk of myocardial infarction in women and men: longitudinal population study. *BMJ* 1998;316:1043–1047, with permission.)

action of smoking with the *apoE ε2/ε3/ε4* genotype to be nonsignificant (11).

Individuals who begin smoking at a younger age appear to have an enduring increased risk for CVD. For example, those who start smoking at age 16 years or younger have more than double the risk for future symptomatic peripheral arterial occlusive disease, regardless of the total amount of exposure to cigarette smoking (12).

Tobacco

The cigarette has a highly efficient drug delivery system. Mainstream smoke, which is inhaled through the cigarette, contains approximately 500 compounds in the gas phase including nitrogen (58%), oxygen (12%), carbon dioxide (13%), and carbon monoxide (3.5%). The vapor also includes hydrogen, methane and other hydrocarbons, aldehydes and ketones, hydrogen cyanide, nitrogen oxides, and several hundred other chemicals in smaller amounts (13). The particulates in cigarette smoke contain the majority of carcinogenic substances, polyphenols and their phenolic and catechol derivatives, and, in most cases, nicotine (14). The particulate phase of smoke also contains free radicals, which may be important in inducing tissue injury through effects on proteins or on lipid peroxidation, or in modifying other constituents of smoke (15). In addition, the particulates contain a variety of insecticides, as well as aluminum, cadmium, lead, mercury, and other metals (13,16). Sidestream smoke, which is typically produced at a lower burning temperature between puffs, contains compounds generated by reduction reactions, including ammonia, aromatic amines, and volatile carcinogenic amines (13).

PATHWAYS BY WHICH SMOKING CONTRIBUTES TO THE DEVELOPMENT OF CARDIOVASCULAR DISEASE

Many of the highly chemically reactive substances in either mainstream or sidestream smoke may participate in the initiation of atherothrombosis and its complications. The biologic effects of many of these substances have not been thoroughly studied; therefore, our understanding of the mechanisms is almost certainly incomplete. Many of the effects of smoking on the cardiovascular system may be related to the lung as an entry point for smoke. The pulmonary epithelium allows the passage of even relatively large molecules, which can then react with the cellular components of blood. In addition, the lung is rich in macrophages, mast cells, and lymphocytes, which, stimulated by components of cigarette smoke, can release a number of biologically active substances including cytokines. The products of these reactions are rapidly delivered into the systemic arterial circulation. The effects of the substances contained in cigarette smoke appear to occur in interaction with each other and with the biologic characteristics of the smoker, including cardiac risk factors independent of smoking (e.g., cholesterol and hypertension), immunologic sensitization, and the rate at which the body forms metabolites. This chapter briefly reviews several of the mechanisms that have been described to date.

Nicotine, Neurotransmitter Release, and Endothelial Damage

Nicotine has powerful effects on central and peripheral nervous system function. In the central nervous system (CNS), it appears to act presynaptically, leading to the release of acetylcholine, norepinephrine, dopamine, serotonin, vasopressin, growth hormone, adrenocorticotropic hormone, β-endorphin, prolactin, and cortisol. Nicotine also excites nicotinic receptors in the spinal cord, autonomic ganglia, and adrenal medulla, leading to release of epinephrine. The sympathetic activation induced by smoking depends on an increased release and/or a reduced clearance of catecholamines at the neuroeffector junctions, and it facilitates the release of neurotransmitters from sympathetic nerves in blood vessels (17). Release of these catecholamines contributes to the acute increase in heart rate and blood pressure associated with smoking. With chronic exposure, circulating catecholamines have direct and indirect effects on platelets and the cells of blood vessel walls, which may contribute to atherogenesis.

Interestingly, whereas peripheral sympathetic activity is increased by nicotine, central sympathetic activity is inhibited by smoking. This inhibition is presumably caused by a baroreceptor stimulation triggered by the smoking-related pressor response (18). The baroreflex is impaired by chronic smoking (19), which raises the possibility that smoking contributes to dysregulation of autonomic input into the cardiovascular system.

Nicotine also has been reported to be directly toxic to vascular endothelial cells *in vitro*. Metabolites of nicotine have proven to be carcinogenic (20), and nicotine may also enhance tumor growth by inhibiting apoptosis or programmed cell death (21). To the extent that nicotine inhibits apoptosis, it may also permit plaque growth.

Many investigators have reported that exposure to tobacco smoke results in endothelial injury or perturbation. This toxicity has been attributed to nicotine, carbon monoxide, or both (although the effects of carbon monoxide recently have come into question) (22). More recently, however, attention has focused on the multiple roles of oxidants in cigarette smoke in contributing to atherogenesis, including the induction of endothelial dysfunction. In addition to the endothelial injury caused by the free radicals present in smoke, it also has been hypothesized that the oxidative damage to endothelial cells, which results in a nitric oxide (NO) shortage, is an important cause of the adverse effects of smoking. Smoking a single cigarette temporarily decreases nitrate and serum antioxidant concentrations in the plasma. These transient changes may partially contribute to coronary vasoconstriction (23).

Smoking and Blood Pressure

Does smoking increase blood pressure? As mentioned earlier, the effects of nicotine on sympathetic arousal and blood pressure are complex, and different ways of studying the effects of smoking on blood pressure have yielded conflicting results. Laboratory studies have clearly demonstrated that smoking a cigarette increases blood pressure; however, epidemiologic studies have shown smokers to have lower rather than higher blood pressure than nonsmokers.

On closer examination, these findings can be reconciled (24). Although smoking acutely increases blood pressure and heart rate (25), presumably by an effect on the peripheral sympathetic nerves, tolerance develops over time (26)

so that the effects are not sustained. Studies with ambulatory recording, which include periods when people are actually smoking, suggest that any effect is small and may be manifest as a slightly increased difference between daytime and nighttime pressures that is more pronounced in older people (27). Finally, epidemiologic studies, in which blood pressure was recorded when participants were not smoking, have generally shown no significant effect of smoking on blood pressure, particularly when controlling for weight and alcohol intake (25,28).

A related issue is the effect of nicotine replacement on blood pressure and the safety of the use of these products in patients with hypertension. Two studies have directly assessed the physiologic effects of nicotine replacement (22,29) and found that no nicotine patch that was tested had any effect on heart rate or blood pressure, although urine epinephrine was increased. The explanation for the lack of sustained cardiovascular effect of nicotine was that when it is given in a sustained dosing, as with the patch, tolerance to its cardiovascular effects develops within about 35 minutes (22). In summary, nicotine patches seem to have little adverse effect on the cardiovascular system and, therefore, can be safely recommended to patients with hypertension.

Cigarette Smoke and Lipoproteins

Cigarette smoking is associated with significant changes in the blood level of lipoproteins and lipids and in the structure of lipoproteins that may contribute to the development of atherothrombosis. Smokers had significantly greater serum concentrations of cholesterol, triglycerides, very low-density lipoprotein (VLDL) cholesterol, and low-density lipoprotein (LDL) cholesterol and also lower serum concentrations of high-density lipoprotein (HDL) cholesterol and apolipoprotein A-I compared with nonsmokers, and these changes were greater in heavy smokers (30). The effect of oxidants in cigarette smoke on plasma LDL may be particularly important in the relation between smoking and the development of atherothrombosis. It has been demonstrated that cigarette smoking renders LDL more susceptible to peroxidative modification by cellular elements such as macrophages and vascular smooth muscle cells (31).

Smoking may also affect other aspects of lipid metabolism. Treatment of plasma *in vitro* with the vapor phase of cigarette smoke was found to dramatically inhibit lecithin-cholesterol acyltransferase activity and both increase the negative charge on HDL and cross-linking with apolipoproteins A-I and A-II (32). Overviews of the multiple roles that oxidized LDL may have in the pathogenesis of atherothrombosis can be found in Chapter 8 of this textbook.

Cigarette Smoke, Leukocytes, and the Immune System

Some elements of cigarette smoke may affect different aspects of immune reactions. One process that may affect the development of atherothrombosis is the activation of components of the classical complement cascade, which may act to increase the adhesion of leukocytes to the vascular endothelium, both by effects on the leukocytes and the sensitization of the cells of the blood vessels (33).

Another set of processes may involve the effects of nicotine on immune function, the conflicting findings of which remain a topic of controversy in the literature. Some investigators have presented evidence that nicotine promotes inflammation (34), whereas others indicate that nicotine may have immunosuppressive effects, particularly at high doses (35). In addition to affecting CNS sites, nicotine activates nicotinic acetylcholine receptors on cells such as monocytes, endothelial cells, and epithelial cells. Nicotine was shown to promote progression of advanced atherothrombotic plaques (36), and there are indications that both innate and adaptive immune responses play an important role in the growth and instability of these plaques. One recently discovered immune-activating mechanism involves the detection of dendritic cells in the arterial wall (37), which occur in greater numbers in atherothrombotic lesions (38). Dendritic cells are potent antigen-presenting cells that are required for the initiation of adaptive immune responses. Nicotine induces a sevenfold increase in the secretion of the proinflammatory cytokine interleukin (IL)-12 and also increases T-cell proliferation (39). Nicotine also profoundly enhances the recruitment of dendritic cells to atherothrombotic lesions *in vivo* (39). Taken together, these immune system effects of nicotine may contribute to its influence on the progression of atherothrombotic lesions. Smoking also has been reported to be associated with increased C-reactive protein (40).

In addition, immune responses to tobacco constituents may greatly amplify their pathogenic potential. Tobacco glycoprotein is a complex of glycoprotein, iron, and polyphenols or their derivatives that can be isolated from flue-cured tobacco leaves and from cigarette smoke (41) and has been shown to stimulate release of cytokines such as IL-1α, IL-1β, and IL-6 (42) and selective expression of immunoglobulin E (IgE) in animal studies (43,44). Smokers have greater serum levels of IgE than nonsmokers (42,45), with levels of IgE correlating better with a history of smoking than with allergy. Moreover, IgE level does not decrease with age in smokers as it does in nonsmokers, and increased levels have been positively associated with myocardial infarction (MI), stroke, and large-vessel peripheral arterial disease in men (46). It also has been reported that increased numbers of mast cells were present in the adventitia, outer media, and intima in raised arteriosclerotic lesions in the aortas and coronary arteries of young individuals (45).

Cigarette Smoke Constituents and Thrombosis

As noted in the section previous, inflammatory reactions in the walls of arteries help convert the endothelial surface from antithrombotic to prothrombotic (47). In addition, certain chemicals in tobacco smoke tend to activate factor XII and favor thrombus formation on a surface with diminished

TABLE 18–1. *Cardiovascular risk factors affected by smoking*

↑ Blood pressure
↑ Low-density lipoprotein cholesterol
↓ High-density lipoprotein cholesterol
↑ Triglycerides
↑ Insulin resistance
↑ Fibrinogen
↑ C-reactive protein

capacity to dissolve thrombi (48) or after a plaque erosion or rupture. Tobacco glycoprotein, described in the previous section, can also stimulate proliferation of bovine aortic smooth muscle cells (49) and activate factor XII of the intrinsic pathway of coagulation.

Both fibrinogen and platelet function are key elements in thrombus formation and are affected by smoking. Higher fibrinogen is a risk factor for atherothrombosis (50), and significantly increased fibrinogen levels are found in chronic smokers (51). Platelet function also is significantly altered in smokers. Decreased platelet survival time, increased numbers of aggregated platelets in the circulation, and release of platelet proteins have been described in smokers (52). Long-term smoking also diminishes the inhibition of platelet aggregation in response to nitroglycerin (53).

Other conditions may also contribute to the process of atherothrombosis. For example, chronic smokers have been reported to be insulin resistant and hyperinsulinemic and to have increased VLDL cholesterol and triglycerides and lower HDL cholesterol than nonsmokers (54). Indeed, smokers have been found to have a sixfold increase in the prevalence of the metabolic syndrome (55). A summary of the major cardiovascular risk factors that are associated with smoking are listed in Table 18–1.

BENEFICIAL EFFECTS OF SMOKING CESSATION

Having enumerated the various pathways by which smoking may contribute to CVD, it seems important to emphasize the benefits of smoking cessation. Overall, the negative cardiovascular effects of smoking are almost all reversible (56). By quitting smoking a person reduces his or her risk for a CVD-related event by half almost immediately (57).

In the first week of smoking cessation, increases in HDL cholesterol levels and decreases in serum lipoprotein levels and plasma plasminogen activator inhibitor-1 levels are seen (58). In addition, there are significant decreases in ambulatory blood pressure during the daytime, heart rate, and plasma norepinephrine and epinephrine (59). Evidence for reductions in the oxidation caused by cigarette smoke also can be found in the first week of cessation (60). Two weeks after cessation there are significant decreases in the rate of fibrinogen synthesis by the liver, with concomitant reductions in plasma fibrinogen concentration (51). Much of the oxidation stress is reversed by 4 weeks after cessation (60).

Eight weeks of abstinence results in further improvements in HDL and LDL levels and further reductions in the mean white blood cell counts (61).

After an MI, smokers are at increased risk for recurrent coronary events, but for those who quit smoking after MI, the risk declines to that of nonsmokers after approximately 3 years, with the relative risk for recurrence decreasing as the duration of smoking abstinence increases (62).

Although quitting smoking entirely is quickly and powerfully effective in reducing cardiovascular risk, simply reducing the amount smoked is much less effective in reducing mortality and morbidity (63). It is clear that even limited cigarette consumption (as little as 3–5 cigarettes per day) has negative effects on health (64).The increased homocysteine levels seen in smokers (65) are reduced when these individuals stop smoking, but they do not decline in people who reduce smoking or continue to smoke (66). However, some improvements have been noted in fibrinogen, white blood cell counts, and HDL/LDL ratio after reduction of smoking (e.g., 20 cigarettes per day reduced to approximately 10) (61). There appears to be no safe level of smoking; therefore, promoting complete cessation remains the eventual goal of intervention efforts, although reducing the number of cigarettes smoked may be an initial step for some patients and an interim harm-reduction measure for smokers unwilling or unable to quit (67).

CHARACTERISTICS OF CURRENT SMOKERS

In 2000, 23.2% of adults in the United States were current smokers (Centers for Disease Control and Prevention, Behavioral Risk Factors Survey website: http://apps.nccd.cdc.gov/brfss/). Although the overall trend indicates a gradual decrease in smoking over the last 40 years, there are troubling disparities among demographic groups in the U.S. population, with the strongest effects reflected in the high rates of smoking among those groups with lower levels of education and socioeconomic status (68).

Because many of the patients seen in the cardiac care setting are 50 years and older, more detailed description of the smokers in this age group is warranted. Approximately 20% of adults 50 years and older smoke cigarettes (69), and as the baby boomers continue to age, the overall number of older smokers is likely to increase (although the rates have decreased). The "young old" (age 65–75 years) smoke at twice the rate of older people (age >75) (70). Interest in quitting smoking among senior citizens also appears to be increasing; in 1999, 42% of senior citizens reported having made an attempt to quit in the past year (70). More than half of a large sample of smokers aged 50 years or older reported that they welcomed physician advice to quit, approximately half said such advice greatly influenced their quitting decision, and a third said it increased their confidence in their ability to quit (71). The older smoker is likely to have more contact with health care providers and also is more likely to be already experiencing health consequences of smoking,

making the health care setting an obvious important point of contact for smoking interventions

BARRIERS TO SMOKING CESSATION

Barriers to smoking cessation include nicotine addiction, behavioral dependency on nicotine and other aspects of smoking, and beliefs and attitudes that lead people to minimize their personal risk or otherwise diminish their motivation to quit smoking.

Nicotine Addiction

Nicotine addiction is the main reason patients have difficulty quitting smoking. Nicotine is extremely addictive, a fact clearly reflected by the extremely high proportion (approximately 90%) of casual users who become addicted daily users (72). Nicotine interacts with specific membrane receptors in the nervous system known as neuronal nicotinic acetylcholine receptors. Nicotine acts primarily as a psychostimulant drug, increasing the outflow of dopamine in the nucleus accumbens (73). Although addiction generally involves the interactions of many CNS effects, the importance of the dopamine system in nicotine addiction has been a primary area of study (74). There is strong evidence linking nucleus accumbens dopamine levels and reward/pleasure, although the effects of dopamine may be more complex and may signal novelty or reward expectation rather than reward itself (75). Over time in the addiction process, the molecular actions that alter the activity and metabolism of the nicotine-sensitive neurons eventually alter the properties of the individual neurons and circuits, which leads to complex behaviors such as dependence, tolerance, sensitization, and craving (76).

Central Nervous System Effects of Nicotine

There is considerable evidence that nicotine has a number of beneficial effects on CNS functioning that may contribute to tobacco dependence. Nicotine has properties that enhance cognition, improve attention, increase alertness, alleviate stress, and regulate weight (77). Imaging studies have confirmed that nicotine has a biphasic effect on arousal that is dose-dependent, with low doses having a stimulant effect and greater doses a sedative effect (78). Blood flow in the right hemisphere reticular system showed a dose-related effect of nicotine and also correlated highly with subjective ratings of cravings for cigarettes (78). In addition, increases in metabolism are seen during cravings in heavy smokers in limbic and cortical areas related to arousal, compulsive repetitive behaviors, sensory integration, and episodic memory (79). There also is a dose-related decrease in blood flow to the left hemisphere amygdala, possibly accounting for some of the anxiety-reducing and antiaggressive effects of cigarette smoking (78). Frontal regions also appear to be affected, with activation in the left hemisphere being greater than right hemisphere arousal (78) and with activation in areas associated with visual attention, arousal, and motor activation (80).

SMOKING CESSATION INTERVENTIONS

Methods to encourage people to quit or never to begin smoking have been developed and intensively researched over the last 30 years. As a public health problem with many different faces, a wide variety of approaches have been proposed and tested. The focus of this section is to review clinical approaches to smoking cessation, including the assessment of smoking, brief interventions tested in the medical practice setting, and more intensive specialized clinical interventions for smoking cessation.

Overview of Treatment Recommendations: Agency for Healthcare Research and Quality Guidelines

The effectiveness of smoking cessation programs has been reviewed by the Agency for Healthcare Research and Quality (AHRQ) (81) and has led to the suggestion of clinical settings such as cardiology practices as ideal for the provision of such treatments. The metaanalytic approach of this panel weighed the results and strength of evidence for various aspects of smoking cessation treatment. Their *key recommendations* are summarized as follows:

1. Tobacco dependence is a chronic condition that may require repeated interventions to be effective. However, effective treatments do exist to assist patients in achieving long-term abstinence.
2. Because effective treatments are available, every smoker should be offered: (a) one of the effective treatments, if willing to make a quit attempt; or (b) a brief counseling intervention to help increase their motivation, if unwilling to try to quit.
3. Clinicians and health care systems need to build systems to support the identification and treatment of every tobacco user seen in the health care setting.
4. Every patient seen in the medical setting should be offered at least brief treatment.
5. There is a strong dose–response relation between the intensity of smoking interventions and their effectiveness—that is, more is better.
6. Three types of counseling and behavioral therapies have shown consistently good results and should be included in all interventions: (a) offering practical counseling such as problem-solving, goal setting, training in self-management skills; (b) providing social support as part of treatment; and (c) helping patients develop support for their efforts outside of treatment.
7. Numerous effective pharmacotherapies for smoking cessation are available, including nicotine replacement (currently available as over-the-counter [OTC] drugs) and Bupropion SR (Zyban), and their use should be encouraged.
8. Treatment for tobacco dependence is both clinically effective and cost-effective compared with other medical interventions, and clinicians should be reimbursed for delivering these services (81).

This chapter will be referring to the AHRQ Guidelines throughout the descriptions of the treatment modalities and will note specific recommendations contained in this document. Notably, as with any methodology, there are limitations to metaanalysis. One of the areas in which problems have been noted (68) is the specific components of behavioral/psychosocial interventions, which are not always specified in studies and are somewhat arbitrarily classified in the metaanalyses on which the AHRQ Guidelines are based.

Assessment of Smokers

The AHRQ Guidelines suggest that physicians in practice have a unique opportunity to intervene successfully with patients regarding tobacco use. The often cited statistic is that 70% of smokers see a physician each year (82) and that as many as 70% of smokers report that they would like to quit (83). Importantly, smokers report that physicians are a credible source of personalized information about their health risks and that a physician's advice to quit is an important motivator for them (84).

Basic Assessment: Current Smoking Status

It is recommended that patients be asked about their smoking status regularly and have it documented in the medical record. There is excellent evidence that gathering the information alone increases the likelihood that an intervention will occur (81). Although this may seem like an obvious step, it should be noted that as many as 30% of current smokers report never having been asked by a physician if they smoke (85).

Further Assessment

Further assessment beyond current smoking status is strongly recommended. If patients are currently smoking, it is most important to ask if they are interested in trying to quit at this time. If they are currently nonsmokers, it may be helpful to know their smoking history, primarily to identify recent smoking cessation efforts so as to support them appropriately, or to know to check in from time to time with those who have had occasional relapses. The AHRQ Guidelines outline approaches to counseling smokers primarily on their current smoking status, readiness to change, and smoking history (Fig. 18–1).

Readiness to Change

Although the basic information noted earlier will be adequate for many smokers, more detail on the barriers seen in current smokers not interested in quitting may be useful. Several models of health behavior (86,87) have identified distinct stages through which most people pass when dealing with a health risk, from their initial awareness of a health risk through making a change in that behavior to reduce their risk. Current smokers who are not ready to quit may fall into either of the following stages:

1. *Not thinking about quitting (Precontemplative):* This encompasses at least two sets of patients: (a) those who are unaware that smoking is a risk factor; and (b) those who may accept the risk for others, but do not acknowledge their personal risk. Clinicians frequently encounter people in the second group, because there is a widespread tendency for people to minimize their personal risk, particularly in areas over which they perceive themselves to have considerable control, such as smoking. People in this stage frequently have beliefs about their health that reduce their personal sense of risk for harm from smoking. This may include the beliefs that they do not smoke very much compared with others or that no smoking-related diseases run in their families, therefore they are not vulnerable. Physicians are in a uniquely powerful position to give specific, personalized risk information to their patients in the form of advice, perhaps coupled with printed literature and a plan to discuss smoking in the future. Such a discussion could act as a potent cue to action for the patient.

2. *Thinking about quitting (Contemplative):* Patients in this stage report having given some thought to quitting smoking and seem to appreciate their personal risk, but feel unable or unwilling to act. In many cases, barriers to change are emotional in nature and may relate to fears about negative effects of quitting smoking. The fears may include concerns about nicotine withdrawal symptoms, possible weight gain, worsening of emotional or stress-related symptoms, or an inability to concentrate or work effectively. Helping patients work around these issues is an important step in helping them move toward another quit attempt. Two areas deserve particular mention. First, if the patient has a psychiatric comorbidity (particularly depression, anxiety, schizophrenia, or attention-deficit hyperactivity disorder [ADHD]), he or she may have special needs (discussed later in this chapter). In the clinical setting, some of these patients have a history of multiple attempts to quit smoking, only to relapse relatively quickly. Second, some patients who are in recovery from alcohol or drugs through 12-step programs may fear that giving up smoking could compromise their sobriety.

Nicotine Dependence

One dimension on which matching patient characteristics to smoking interventions has been shown to be important is the extent of the smoker's nicotine dependence. Patients who show evidence of a greater level of nicotine dependence have been shown to be more successful at maintaining abstinence if using greater doses of nicotine replacement.

To determine the extent of nicotine dependence, a few simple indicators are useful. Patients who are more dependent on nicotine tend (a) to be heavy smokers (>20 cigarettes per day); (b) to have suffered severe withdrawal symptoms during previous attempts to quit; and (c) to have their first cigarette of the day within 30 minutes of awakening (88).

Other Specialized Assessment Approaches

The following indices for further assessment of smokers and smoking behavior are presented with the following caveat: There is no consistent evidence that matching patients to particular treatments improves outcomes. Indeed, except for nicotine dosing recommendations noted earlier, few studies have attempted to match patient characteristics to elements of treatment and none has shown strong and consistent results. However, it must be noted that a considerable amount of tailoring to patient characteristics and needs is embedded in the cognitive–behavioral and pharmacologic approaches with strong empirical support.

Further assessment from the psychosocial side might include the following: (a) patient's level of motivation to quit; (b) willingness to quit within the next month; (c) level of confidence in his or her ability to quit (self-efficacy); (d) degree to which the smoker's living and work environment is smoke-free; and (e) smoking behavior of others in their household and social network. These issues are generally measured with self-ratings on a 0 to 10 scale (or 0–100 scale).

One other relevant issue is the current or anticipated level of life stress, particularly the existence of major life events such as divorce or health problems in the family. Again, the presence or absence of these factors should not argue against making an attempt to quit, but rather help the patient anticipate potential problem areas and formulate ways of coping with likely barriers in advance. It also is useful to inquire about previous attempts to quit, and to seek specific information about the nature of "failed" attempts to help identify problem areas in future attempts. In addition, previous attempts may have been extremely successful initially, but then ended in a relapse. These experiences can be mined for both examples of strategies or treatments that worked (or at least seemed to help) and those that may have led to relapse.

Brief Clinical Interventions

Brief interventions for smoking cessation are defined as interventions taking 3 to 5 minutes or less in the medical care setting; these interventions are recommended for all patients identified as smokers in clinical settings (81). There is excellent evidence that even minimal interventions consisting primarily of physician advice to quit significantly increase the smoking abstinence rate. Although the magnitude of the change may seem small (the difference between the 7.9% yearly spontaneous quit rate and the 10.7% seen with advice only), each smoker who quits will add an additional 13 to 15 years to his or her life. With the addition of a brief patient-centered counseling intervention plus nicotine replacement, 6-month cessation rates may be as high as 20% (89). Follow-up visits (particularly four or more) apparently further increase the rate of successful cessation in patients (81).

Smokers Who Express an Interest in Quitting at This Time

The components of a brief clinical smoking intervention have been summarized as the "5 As" in the treatment guidelines (derived from the National Cancer Institute's model [90]) (Table 18–2). The strategies (81) are as follows:

1. *ASK* about tobacco use. Ask every patient at every visit. The assessment issues discussed previously describe this step in greater detail.
2. *ADVISE* to quit: In a clear, strong, and personalized manner, urge every cigarette smoker to quit.
3. *ASSESS* willingness to try to make a quit attempt: Determine whether the smoker is prepared to make a quit attempt at this time.
4. *ASSIST* in quit attempt: For the patient who is willing to make an attempt to quit, use pharmacotherapy and counseling to help him or her quit. This may include offering support, setting specific goals, reviewing options for pharmacotherapy and other approaches, and setting a quit date.
5. *ARRANGE* follow-up: Schedule a follow-up appointment, ideally within a week of the decided quit date.

Pharmacotherapy

The treatment guidelines recommend that all smokers should receive pharmacotherapy unless special circumstances (e.g., pregnancy, adolescence) exist that contraindicate the use of these agents. Each modality has been shown to approximately double the rate of success at abstaining from smoking; for this reason, they are strongly recommended.

Nicotine Replacement Therapy. Nicotine replacement comes in five U.S. Food and Drug Administration (FDA)-approved forms: (a) nicotine gum; (b) nicotine inhaler; (c) nicotine nasal spray; (d) nicotine patch; and (e) nicotine lozenges. All have been proven to increase smoking cessa-

TABLE 18–2. *The five As for smoking cessation*

1. ASK about use
2. ADVISE to quit
3. ASSESS willingness
4. ASSIST to quit
5. ARRANGE follow-up

tion rates. Doses and recommendations for use from the Guidelines are outlined in Table 18–3.

Nicotine replacement therapy (NRT) in patients with CVD merits specific comment. A possible link between the use of NRT and cardiovascular problems has received considerable study, and three separate analyses documented a lack of association between the nicotine patch and acute cardiovascular events, even in patients who continued to smoke occasionally while on the nicotine patch (91). However, because of the negative media coverage, patients may need some reassurance that NRT does not increase cardiovascular event risk. There are warnings on the package inserts for NRT products that NRT should be used with caution in patients during the 2 weeks immediately after an MI, in those with serious arrhythmias, and in patients with serious and worsening angina.

Beyond the basic dosing recommendations for use of a single NRT agent, there is evidence that patients who are unsuccessful with a single modality of the approved NRT methods may benefit from supplementing nicotine patches with either nicotine gum or nicotine nasal spray on an as needed basis. These methods allow the patient to more precisely manage nicotine levels by quickly delivering greater nicotine doses in response to urges to smoke or withdrawal symptoms. Abstinence rates increase from approximately 17% with a single NRT agent to 28.6 % using combination therapy (81), and nicotine withdrawal symptoms are also better controlled (92). Because of limited safety data on combined therapies and the possibility of overdosing on nicotine, combination NRT is recommended only if the patient has been unsuccessful with single-modality treatment (81).

Bupropion SR (Zyban or Wellbutrin SR). Bupropion SR has been approved as a first-line pharmacotherapy for smoking cessation, and it approximately doubles the rate of success versus placebo (81). Bupropion is an atypical antidepressant that affects both dopamine and noradrenergic activity (93). One of the mechanisms by which Bupropion appears to help is in reducing withdrawal symptoms and negative effect (94). Unlike NRT, smokers should begin Bupropion 1 to 2 weeks before the planned quit date. The recommended dosage should begin at 150 mg per day, and can be increased after 3 days to 300 mg per day. One study suggests that the combination of NRT and Bupropion produces greater quit rates than either treatment alone (95). Treatment should be continued for at least 7 to 12 weeks, and it may be extended if there are concerns about depression or weight gain (which is not prevented, but can be delayed) (96). Improved maintenance of tobacco abstinence has been seen in patients treated with 150 mg per day over a 6-month period (81). The drug is generally well tolerated in patients with CVD, although there have been infrequent reports of hypertension.

With more widespread use of NRT (particularly because patches and gum have become OTC items), physicians are more likely to encounter smokers who have previously tried NRT without success. It is important to inform patients that

TABLE 18–3. *Nicotine prescription recommendations from Clinical Practice Guidelines*

NRT modality	Dosage recommended	Comments
Nicotine gum	2 mg (per piece) gum for those smoking <20 cig/day 4 mg gum for >20 cig/day; up to 24 pieces/day Chew slowly then hold between cheek and gum for 30 min.	OTC only Dosage and duration tailored to patient individual needs Patients often do not use enough; instruct to use on fixed schedule every 1–2 hours × 1–3 months.

Nicotine patch	Dose determined by amount smoked, use lower dose in smokers of <10 cig/day.
	Stepped doses:
	  21 mg for 4 weeks
	  14 mg for 2 weeks
	  7 mg for 2 weeks
	Single dose:
	  15 mg for 8 weeks
		OTC and prescription
		Local skin irritation common, usually mild and self-limiting, 0.5% hydrocortisone cream helps
		Insomnia a common side effect, may decide to remove at bedtime
		24-h and 16-h patches equally effective
		May consider extended use beyond 8 weeks as needed

Nicotine spray	Dose is 0.5-mg delivery to each nostril; initial dose 1–2 doses/h, increase as needed for symptom relief Minimum recommended is 8 doses/day up to maximum of 40 Duration: 3–6 months	Prescription only Each bottle contains 100 doses; 94% report nasal irritation in first 2 days of use, milder thereafter Dependency potential relatively greater than other NRT; 15–20% report using 6–12 mo, 5% used greater doses than recommended
Nicotine inhaler	A dose is a puff or inhalation, each cartridge = 4 mg nicotine per 80 puffs; recommend 6–16 cartridges/day; duration up Duration 3–6 mo, should taper last 9–12 weeks Frequent puffing works best	Prescription only Local irritation in throat and nose common (40%), usually mild, may be cough Not effective at <40°F, keep warm in cold weather Acidic beverages reduce absorption, avoid 15 min before and during use

Overall Guidelines: Pregnant smokers encouraged to quit first without pharmacologic treatment. Nicotine replacement therapy (NRT) should be used only if increased likelihood of abstinence and its benefits outweigh risks associated with NRT or continued smoking.

cig, cigarettes; OTC, over-the-counter.

From Fiore M, Bailey W, Cohen S, et al. Treating tobacco use and dependence; Clinical Practice Guideline. Rockville, MD: U.S. Department of Health and Human Services, 2000.

most smokers make more than five attempts to quit before they are successful. In addition, it may be useful to add or change medications (either another NRT or Bupropion), because there is little evidence of success with re-treatment with the same NRT method. Notably, successful quit attempts that last several weeks or months but end in a relapse are different from an unsuccessful attempt. In the case of a relapse, reinstituting a previously successful NRT method may be effective.

Second-Line Drugs. Two other medications, clonidine and nortriptyline, have been approved as second-line treatments for smoking cessation—that is, their use is only recommended if patients either did not respond to the first-line treatments or have contraindications that rule out their use. Unfortunately, the role of second-line drugs in treating patients with CVD is extremely limited because of side effect profiles and interactions with other drugs used in these patients. Although they are not approved by the FDA for smoking cessation, there is considerable evidence of efficacy. Clonidine is an antihypertensive drug that has approximately doubled cessation rates in trials versus placebo (81), although no dose–response relation was seen. The dose range in clinical trials ranged from 0.1 to 0.75 mg, either orally or with transdermal patch, and no clear dosing recommendations have been established for smoking cessation.

The clinician obviously must consider potential drug interactions in patients taking other antihypertensive drugs, and, in any case, patients should be cautioned not to abruptly discontinue treatment with clonidine because of the risk for acutely increased blood pressure. The tricyclic antidepressant, nortriptyline, also has been shown to significantly improve smoking cessation rates, but its use is strongly cautioned in patients with CVD because of the cardiotoxicity of this class of drugs.

Smokers Who Do Not Express an Interest in Attempting to Quit

For smokers who do not express an interest in making a quit attempt, the following outline is offered ("5 *R*s") for a brief intervention intended to increase their motivation to eventually quit (Table 18–4). The major points are summarized as follows:

1. *RELEVANCE:* Encourage the patient to consider why quitting smoking might be personally relevant to them. The most powerful information is likely to be that which relates to their personal health problems, family situation, and other personal concerns. It is important to note that the individual's reasons for quitting always

TABLE 18–4. *The five Rs for reluctant quitters*

1. RELEVANCE of quitting
2. RISKS of continuing
3. REWARDS of quitting
4. ROADBLOCKS to quitting
5. REPETITION of motivation

have more impact than those we might propose as clinicians, however scientifically accurate and cogently argued.

2. *RISKS:* The clinician should ask the patient to identify any potentially negative consequences for continuing to smoke. These risks may include short-term risks, such as shortness of breath, increased vulnerability to respiratory infections, and exacerbation of asthma or angina symptoms. There are also long-term risks, including increased risk for acute cardiovascular events, chronic lung disease, accelerated aging, and other health risks. Additional risks include environmental issues, such as second-hand smoke exposure for family members.

3. *REWARDS:* The clinician should ask the patient to identify benefits that might accrue if he or she quits smoking. The most important rewards are, again, those that are most personally relevant to that patient; these may include improved health, saving money, feeling better, setting good example for children/grandchildren, and other rewards.

4. *ROADBLOCKS:* The patients should be encouraged to identify potential barriers to successful quitting, which might include issues like withdrawal symptoms, fear of failure, weight gain, lack of support, depression, and other concerns. The clinician can advise strategies to ameliorate the potential barriers, such as medication, adjunctive treatments, and others.

5. *REPETITION:* The motivational intervention should be repeated on every appropriate occasion when the patient visits the clinical setting.

Motivational Interviewing

Motivational interviewing (97) is an alternative counseling format that incorporates these five elements. The model was developed for working with patients with addiction, and it has been widely applied in the area of health behavior change. The basic approach attempts to draw on the patient's own beliefs and engage him or her in a conversation about reasons to change his or her behavior, while avoiding a struggle with the patient by being on the opposite side of an argument. By identifying the person's own reasons in favor of behavior change, the conflict between his or her behavior and basic beliefs and values is heightened. For example, the clinician initially queries the patient on how *important* he or she believes it is to quit smoking (on a scale of 0–10). If the patient's rating is greater than zero, the clinician asks why it is not zero, thus eliciting the patient's rea-

sons for quitting. The next question is what might increase that importance rating by several points. The second dimension the patient is asked to rate is, if he or she believed it were important to quit smoking, how *confident* is he or she about his or her ability to quit (again, on a 0–10 scale). Again, if the rating is not zero, the patient is asked to explain why it is not zero, eliciting any sources of confidence the patient may have in his or her ability to change. The follow-up questions include asking what it would take to increase the confidence rating by several points and what the physician could do to assist the patient in increasing that rating. The patient also is asked to enumerate the costs and benefits of changing versus not changing his or her behavior. This approach has considerable empirical support and has been widely disseminated in the primary care setting.

The Patient Who Has Recently Quit Smoking

The final brief intervention recommendation in the clinical guidelines is to assist patients who are in the early days of a smoking cessation attempt, with the goal of supporting the effort and preventing relapse. Because most relapses occur within the first 3 months of cessation, patients deserve particularly close attention during this time (98). The recommended interventions are divided into two forms: (a) Minimal Intervention—that is, congratulating the patient on progress to date, continuing to check in with the patient, and offering assistance for any problems that arise; and (b) Prescriptive Intervention, which is based on a more active, detailed assessment of the patient's quit attempt and barriers that have arisen. The more intensive relapse prevention interventions may be done in person in medical follow-up, by telephone, or through a specialized smoking cessation program (81).

Intensive Tobacco Dependence Interventions

A wide variety of program formats using a range of providers have been tested and have been proven effective in promoting smoking cessation in patients willing to participate in them (68,81). Detailed description of such specialized services is beyond the scope of this chapter, but it is important to know that such programs exist and can be effective in patients who have failed or relapsed with brief interventions or those with psychiatric comorbidities that are likely to complicate the cessation process.

Services for Hospitalized Smokers

The assessment and treatment algorithms outlined earlier, although most often tested in the outpatient medical setting, are applicable to smokers who are hospitalized. Admission for cardiovascular problems is often an excellent opportunity for smoking cessation intervention. The patient has a heightened sense of vulnerability to the ill effects of smoking, may be very motivated to quit, and has not been smoking for several days, which has reduced his or her nicotine dependence (99). A number of bedside interventions with cardiac patients have proven effective (100–103), even at 5-year follow-up examination (104). As with outpatient interventions, the rule of thumb seems to be that more treatment is better. The most robust effects are seen in more intensive interventions (approximately 1-hour inpatient counseling plus telephone follow-up contacts) (101,104). Briefer interventions (15–30 minute nurse-delivered counseling, physician advice and prescription of pharmacotherapy, and self-help literature) have shown mixed results (105), most often showing small but significant improvements in cessation rates (106).

Barriers to Physician Intervention in Smokers

Although every recent consensus on cardiac care and prevention (107) advocates smoking cessation interventions for patients with CVD, much remains to be done to implement these recommendations. Although cardiologists usually advise their patients to stop smoking (85,108), only a few actually support patients through the cessation process (99, 109–112).

Why do so few physicians pay attention to smoking cessation? First, many physicians are not trained in behavioral techniques such as counseling, even though this is an activity to which they devote substantial time. They believe that their patients already know that smoking is harmful and are not interested in hearing about smoking, and that counseling is unlikely to have any significant effect (113). Second, physicians often are pressed for time and smoking counseling is poorly reimbursed by health insurance, which give it a low priority (114). However, the reason most often cited in recent surveys is that physicians do not think their patients will follow through with taking their advice (109–114). This is particularly unfortunate in that even a low rate of success in encouraging smoking cessation would yield substantial health benefits in a population of patients. It has been established that brief (approximately 3 minutes) counseling from a physician can double the spontaneous quit rate of smokers, which is about 2.5% per year. If a physician counsels 100 patients per year, 95% will continue to smoke, a despairingly large number. But of the 2.5 smokers who quit—above the further 2.5 smokers who will quit spontaneously—1 ex-smoker will avoid a premature smoking-related death, and another ex-smoker will gain up to 15 years of life expectancy. The cost of this benefit would have been 3 hours and 20 minutes of the physician's time.

Psychologic and Psychiatric Comorbidities and Smoking Cessation

The strong relation between smoking and psychiatric comorbidities has become increasingly clear. More patients with mood disorders, alcohol and other substance abuse, attention deficit disorder, and schizophrenia tend to be smok-

ers than in the general population (overall, 41% vs. the average of 23%) (115). A self-medication model has been advanced to explain the high rate of nicotine dependence among these individuals (116) and may provide some understanding of why psychiatric comorbidity (either current or by history) appears to predict greater difficulty in quitting smoking successfully (117). Although the literature for treating smoking and psychiatric comorbidity is not always consistent, the greater prevalence and relapse rate among patients with these disorders nonetheless warrants particular clinical attention.

Depression

Tailoring treatment for depression has been addressed to a limited extent. Depressed smokers are more responsive to NRT (118) and to treatment with antidepressants (119,120). In patients with chronic low-level depressive symptoms, selective serotonin reuptake inhibitors have improved cessation rates (fluoxetine) (121,122); and in patients with a history of major depression, they have reduced withdrawal symptoms, anxiety, and cravings (sertraline) (121). Regarding psychosocial treatments, there is some evidence that cognitive–behavioral therapy for depression (rather than treatment focused on smoking cessation alone) improved smoking cessation rates in smokers with major depression (122) or with a history of depression (123), and there is evidence of benefit from combined cognitive–behavioral therapy and smoking cessation interventions (124).

Attention-Deficit Hyperactivity Disorder

ADHD is a prevalent disorder that may not have been diagnosed in the older adult population, although they may have children or grandchildren with ADHD. Patients may report using smoking to improve their ability to concentrate on their work. Although there is relatively little definitive research concerning smoking cessation treatment of these patients, Bupropion SR may have some beneficial effects on symptoms of adult ADHD (93). Beyond this recommendation, the best treatment approach would include a psychiatric consultation and specialty smoking cessation clinic referral.

Smoking cessation treatment of patients with severe psychiatric disorders (e.g., schizophrenia or severe bipolar disorder) is a particular challenge, because nicotine appears to relieve both some of the psychiatric symptoms and the side effects of antipsychotic medication. Addressing the needs of these patients clearly requires a specialty referral with strong psychiatric services.

Harm Reduction and Alternative Strategies

The patient's physical dependence on nicotine may be too great to realistically implement a plan of immediate and complete cessation. Moreover, the psychologic factors noted earlier place the patient at greater risk for treatment failure when full abstinence is required. In such cases, the tapering of nicotine use as an alternative treatment strategy may be necessary. The addictions literature suggests the alternative "warm turkey" approach in which treatment for patients identified as high risk for smoking relapse and/or high levels of emotional distress follows a set of progressive stages, with full cessation defined as the optimal and ultimate goal state (124). Together with the clinician, high-risk patients select one of the following options to begin treatment: (a) a negotiated period of trial abstinence, (b) a process of gradual tapering down toward abstinence; or (c) a period of trial moderation. The validity of these approaches is recognized in the treatment outcome literature (125) where matching patients to treatment strategy has been demonstrated as most effective for successful treatment adherence and long-term abstinence from nicotine use.

Having discussed the challenges facing people with psychologic comorbidities, it is important to note that it is often possible for these individuals to quit smoking successfully. Coordinated specialty care, with referrals for psychiatric consultation, is likely to be extremely important. When the comorbid condition is effectively treated or managed, smoking cessation in these patients may be much more successful.

SUMMARY

Quitting smoking is the single most powerful action a person can take to reduce his or her cardiovascular risk. Our increasing knowledge of the mechanisms by which tobacco use acts to initiate or promote the development of atherothrombosis highlights the importance of assisting our patients in moving toward successful smoking cessation. At the same time, the increasing knowledge of the biology of addiction and the complex actions of nicotine makes clear the great difficulties faced by patients attempting to quit smoking. Fortunately, a variety of treatment modalities have been proven to be effective tools in assisting patients in this process, including nicotine replacement products, antidepressant medications, and behavioral and supportive counseling approaches. Physicians and other health care professionals in the practice of cardiology are in a uniquely influential position to advise and assist their patients in the process of quitting smoking. The investment of a modest amount of time and effort can yield highly significant results over the process of continuing care, making brief counseling for smoking cessation the most cost-effective intervention a physician can perform (126). Our goal has been to provide an overview of brief treatment models, practice guidelines, and aspects of treatment with strong empirical support to assist physicians in this important process.

ACKNOWLEDGMENTS

The authors are indebted to Randall S. Stafford and Carl G. Becker, authors of the chapter "Cigarette Smoking and Atherosclerosis" in the previous edition of this book, for the structure of the chapter and the background information on the physiologic mechanisms in the pathogenesis of atherothrombosis.

REFERENCES

1. Annual smoking-attributable mortality, years of potential life lost, and economic costs: United States, 1995-1999. *MMWR Morb Mortal Wkly Rep* 2002;51(14):300–303.
2. Fagerstrom K. The epidemiology of smoking: health consequences and benefits of cessation. *Drugs* 2002;62[Suppl 2]:1–9.
3. Stein Y, Harats D, Stein O. Why is smoking a major risk factor for hyperlipidemic subjects? *Ann NY Acad Sci* 1993;686:66–69.
4. Gariepy J, Denarie N, Chironi G, et al. Gender difference in the influence of smoking on arterial wall thickness. *Atherosclerosis* 2000;153: 139–145.
5. Kuulasmaa K, Tunstall-Pedoe H, Dobson A. Estimation of contribution of changes in classic risk factors to trends in coronary event rates across the WHO MONICA Project. *Lancet* 2000;355:675–687.
6. Bolego C, Poli A, Paoletti R. Smoking and gender. *Cardiovasc Res* 2002;53:568–576.
7. Meek M, Finch G. Diluted mainstream cigarette smoke condensates activate estrogen receptor and aryl hydrocarbon receptor-mediated gene transcriptase. *Environ Res* 1999;80:9–17.
8. Benowitz NL, Perez-Stable EJ, Fong I, et al. Ethnic differences in N-glucuronidation of nicotine and cotinine. *J Pharmacol Exp Ther* 1999;291:1196–1203.
9. Stengard J, Kardia S, Tervahauta M, et al. Utility of the predictors of coronary heart disease mortality in a longitudinal study of elderly Finnish men aged 65 to 84 years is dependent on context defined by APOE genotype and area of residence. *Clin Genet* 1999;56:367–377.
10. Humphries S, Talmud P, Hawe E, et al. Aplipoprotein E4 and coronary heart disease in middle-aged men who smoke: a prospective study. *Lancet* 2001;358:115–119.
11. Keavney B, Parish S, Palmer A, et al. Large-scale evidence that the cardiotoxicity of smoking is not significantly modified by the apolipoprotein E e2/e3/e4 genotype. *Lancet* 2003;361:398.
12. Planas A, Clara A, Marrugat J, et al. Age at onset of smoking is an independent risk factor in peripheral artery disease development. *J Vasc Surg* 2002;35:506–509.
13. Hoffmann D, Wynder E. Chemical constituents and bioactivity of tobacco smoke. *IARC Sci Publ* 1986;74:145–165.
14. Hoffmann D, Rivenson A, Hecht SS, et al. Model studies in tobacco carcinogenesis with the Syrian golden hamster. *Prog Exp Tumor Res* 1979;24:370–390.
15. Park E, Park Y, Gwak Y. Oxidative damage in the tissues of rats exposed to cigarette smoke. *Free Radic Biol Med* 1998;25(1):79–86.
16. Chiba M, Masironi R. Toxic and trace elements in tobacco and tobacco smoke. *Bull WHO* 1992;70:269–275.
17. Benowitz N. Pharmacologic aspects of cigarette smoking and nicotine addiction. *N Engl J Med* 1988;319:1318–1330.
18. Grassi G, Seravalle G, Calhoun D, et al. Mechanisms responsible for sympathetic activation by cigarette smoking in humans. *Circulation* 1994;90:248–253.
19. Gerhardt U, Vorneweg P, Riedasch M, et al. Acute and persistent effects of smoking on the baroreceptor function. *J Auton Pharmacol* 1999;19:105–108.
20. Hoffmann D, Hecht S. Perspectives in cancer research. Nicotine-derived N-nitrosamines and tobacco related cancer: current status and future directions. *Cancer Res* 1985;45:944.
21. Wright S. Nicotine inhibition of apoptosis suggests a role in tumor progression. *FASEB J* 1993;7:1045–1051.
22. Zevin S, Saunders S, Gourlay S, et al. Cardiovascular effects of carbon monoxide and cigarette smoking. *J Am Coll Cardiol* 2001;38: 1633–1638.
23. Tsuchiya M, Asada A, Kasahara E, et al. Smoking a single cigarette rapidly reduces combined concentrations of nitrate and nitrite and concentrations of antioxidants in plasma. *Circulation* 1998;105: 1155–1157.
24. Pickering T. Effects of stress and behavioral interventions in hypertension—the effects of smoking and nicotine replacement therapy on blood pressure. *J Clin Hypertens (Greenwich)* 2001;3:319–321.

25. Omvik P. How smoking affects blood pressure. *Blood Press* 1996;5: 71–77.
26. Perkins K, Gerlach D, Broge M, et al. Dissociation of nicotine tolerance from tobacco dependence in humans. *J Pharmacol Exp Ther* 2001;296:849–856.
27. Mann S, James G, Wang R, et al. Elevation of ambulatory systolic blood pressure in hypertensive smokers. A case-control study. *JAMA* 1991;265:2226–2228.
28. Primatesta P, Falaschetti E, Gupta S, et al. Association between smoking and blood pressure: evidence from the health survey for England. *Hypertension* 2001;37:187–193.
29. Tanus-Santos J, Toledo J, Cittadino M, et al. Cardiovascular effects of transdermal nicotine in mildly hypertensive smokers. *Am J Hypertens* 2001;14[7 Pt 1]:610–614.
30. Craig W, Palomaki G, Haddow J. Cigarette smoking and serum lipid and lipoprotein concentrations: an analysis of published data. *BMJ* 1989;298:784–788.
31. Harats D, Ben-Naim M, Dabach Y, et al. Cigarette smoking renders LDL susceptible to peroxidative modification and enhanced metabolism by macrophages. *Atherosclerosis* 1989;79:245–252.
32. Wilztum J. Role of oxidized low-density lipoprotein in atherogenesis. *Br Heart J* 1993;69[Suppl]:S12–S18.
33. Collins T. Endothelial nuclear factor-kB and the initiation of the atherosclerotic lesion. *Lab Invest* 1993;68:499–508.
34. Furie M, Raffanello J, Gergel E, et al. Extracts of smokeless tobacco induce pro-inflammatory. *Immunopharmacology* 2000;47:13–23.
35. Matsunaga K, Klein T, Friedman H, et al. Involvement of nicotinic acetylcholine receptors in suppression of antimicrobial activity and cytokine responses of alveolar macrophages to Legionella pneumophila infection by nicotine. *J Immunol* 2001;167:6518–6524.
36. Hansson G. Regulation of immune mechanisms in atherosclerosis. *Ann NY Acad Sci* 2001;947:157–165.
37. Millonig G, Niederegger H, Rabl W, et al. Network of vascular-associated dendritic cells in intima of healthy young individuals. *Arterioscler Thromb Vasc Biol* 2001;21:503–508.
38. Lord R, Bobryshev Y. Clustering of dendritic cells in athero-prone areas of the aorta. *Atherosclerosis* 1999;146:197–198.
39. Aicher A, Heeschen C, Mohaupt M, et al. Nicotine strongly activates dendritic cell-mediated adaptive immunity. *Circulation* 2003;107: 604–611.
40. Saito M, Ishimitsu T, Minami J, et al. Relations of plasma high-sensitivity C-reactive protein to traditional cardiovascular risk factors. *Atherosclerosis* 2003;167(1):73–79.
41. Becker C, Dubin T. Activation of factor XII by tobacco glycoprotein. *J Exp Med* 1977;146:1712–1716.
42. Criqui M, Lee ER, Hamburger RN, et al. IgE and cardiovascular disease. *Am J Med* 1987;82:964–968.
43. Francus T, Siskind G, Becker C. The role of antigen structure in the regulation of IgE isotype expression. *Proc Natl Acad Sci USA* 1983; 80:3430–3434.
44. Becker C, Levi R, Zavecz J. Induction of IgE antibodies to antigen isolated from tobacco leaves and from cigarette smoke condensate. *Am J Pathol* 1979;96:249–255.
45. Atkinson JB, Harlan CW, Harlan GC, et al. The association of mast cells and atherosclerosis: a morphologic study of early atherosclerotic lesions in young people. *Hum Pathol* 1994;25:154–159.
46. Criqui MH, Seibles JA, Hamburger RN, et al. Epidemiology of immunoglobulin E levels in a defined population. *Ann Allergy* 1990;64: 308–313.
47. Pober J, Cotran R. Cytokines and endothelial biology. *Physiol Rev* 1990;70:427–451.
48. Nachman R. Thrombosis and atherogenesis: molecular connections. *Blood* 1992;79:1897–1906.
49. Becker C, Hajjar D, Hefton J. Tobacco constituents are mitogenic for arterial smooth muscle cells. *Am J Pathol* 1985;120:1–5.
50. Heinrich J, Balleisen L, Schulte H, et al. Fibrinogen and factor VII in the prediction of coronary risk: results from the PROCAM study in healthy men. *Arterioscler Thromb* 1994;14:54–59.
51. Hunter K, Garlick P, Broom I, et al. Effects of smoking and abstention from smoking on fibrinogen synthesis in humans. *Clin Sci (London)* 2001;100:459–465.
52. Schmidt K, Rasmussen J. Acute platelet activation induced by smoking. *Thromb Haemostasis* 1984;51:279–282.
53. Haramake N, Ikeda H, Takajo Y, et al. Long-term smoking causes ni-

troglycerin resistance in platelets by depletions of intraplatelet glutathione. *Arterioscler Thromb Vasc Biol* 2001;21:1852–1856.
54. Wallenfeldt K, Hulthe J, Bokemark L, et al. Carotid and femoral atherosclerosis, cardiovascular risk factors and C-reactive protein in relation to smokeless tobacco use or smoking in 58-year-old men. *J Intern Med* 2001;250:492–501.
55. Tahtinen T, Vanhala M, Oikarinen J, et al. Effect of smoking on the prevalence of insulin resistance-associated cardiovascular risk factors among Finnish men in military service. *J Cardiovasc Risk* 1998; 5:319–323.
56. Rosenberg L, Kaufman D, Helmrich S, et al. The risk of myocardial infarction after quitting smoking in men under 55 years of age. *N Engl J Med* 1985;313:1511–1514.
57. Mehta R, Eagle K. Secondary prevention in acute myocardial infarction. *BMJ* 1998;316:838–842.
58. Minami J, Todoroki M, Yoshii M, et al. Effects of smoking cessation or alcohol restriction on metabolic and fibrinolytic variables in Japanese men. *Clin Sci (London)* 2002;103:117–122.
59. Oncken C, White W, Cooney J, et al. Impact of smoking cessation on ambulatory blood pressure and heart rate in postmenopausal women. *Am J Hypertens* 2001;14:942–949.
60. Pilz H, Oguogho A, Chehne F, et al. Quitting cigarette smoking results in a fast improvement of in vivo oxidation injury (determined via plasma, serum, and urinary isoprostanes). *Thromb Res* 2000;99:209–221.
61. Eliasson B, Hjalmarson A, Kruse E, et al. Effect of smoking reduction and cessation on cardiovascular risk factors. *Nicotine Tob Res* 2001;3:249–255.
62. Rea T, Heckbert S, Kaplan R, et al. Smoking status and risk for recurrent coronary events after myocardial infarction. *Ann Intern Med* 2002;137:494–500.
63. Godtfredsen N, Holst D, Prescott E, et al. Smoking reduction, smoking cessation, and mortality: a 16-year follow-up of 19,732 men and women from the Copenhagen Centre for Prospective Population Studies. *Am J Psychiatry* 2002;156:994–1001.
64. Prescott E, Scharling H, Osler M, et al. Importance of light smoking and inhalation habits on risk of myocardial infarction and all-cause mortality: a 22-year follow-up of 12,149 men and women in the Copenhagen City Heart Study. *J Epidemiol Community Health* 2002;56:702–706.
65. O'Callaghan P, Meleady R, Fitzgerald T, et al. Smoking and plasma homocysteine. *Eur Heart J* 2002;23:1580–1586.
66. Stein J, Bushara M, Bushara K, et al. Smoking cessation, but not reduction, reduces plasma homocysteine levels. *Clin Cardiol* 2002;25: 23–26.
67. *Clearing the smoke: assessing the science base for harm reduction.* Washington, DC: Institute of Medicine, National Academy Press, 2001.
68. Niaura R, Abrams D. Smoking cessation: progress, priorities, and prospectus. *J Consult Clin Psychol* 2002;70:494–509.
69. Rimer B, Orleans C, Fleisher L, et al. Does tailoring matter? The impact of a tailored guide on ratings and short-term smoking-related outcomes for older smokers. *Health Educ Res* 1994;9(1): 69–84.
70. Arday D, Lapin P, Chin J, et al. Smoking patterns among seniors and the Medicare Stop Smoking Program. *J Am Geriatr Soc* 2002;50: 1689–1697.
71. Ossip-Klein D, McIntosh S, Utman D, et al. Smokers ages 50+: who gets physician advice to quit? *Prev Med* 2000;31:364–369.
72. Henningfield J, Fant R. Tobacco use as drug addiction: the scientific foundation. *Nicotine Tob Res* 1999;1[Suppl 2]:S31–S35.
73. Dani J, DeBiasi M. Cellular mechanisms of nicotine addiction. *Pharmacol Biochem Behav* 2001;70:439–446.
74. Mansvelder H, McGehee D. Cellular and synaptic mechanisms of nicotine addiction. *J Neurobiol* 2002;53:606–617.
75. DiChiara G. Role of dopamine in the behavioural actions of nicotine related to addiction. *Eur J Pharmacol* 2000;393:295–314.
76. Nestler E, Aghajanian G. Molecular and cellular basis of addiction. *Science* 1997;278:58–63.
77. Parrott A, Garnham N, Wesnes K, et al. Cigarette smoke and abstinence: comparative effects upon cognitive task performance and mood state over 24 hours. *Hum Psychopharmacol* 1996;11:391–400.
78. Rose J, Behm F, Westman E, et al. PET studies of the influences of nicotine on neural systems in cigarette smokers. *Am J Psychiatry* 2003;160:323–333.

79. Brody A, Mandelkern M, London E, et al. Brain metabolic changes during cigarette craving. *Arch Gen Psychiatry* 2002;59:1162–1172.

80. Lawrence N, Ross T, Stein E. Cognitive mechanisms of nicotine on visual attention. *Neuron* 2002;36:539–548.

81. Fiore M, Bailey W, Cohen S, et al. Treating tobacco use and dependence; Clinical Practice Guideline. Rockville, MD: U.S. Department of Health and Human Services, 2000.

82. Davis R. Uniting physicians against smoking: the need for a coordinated national strategy [editorial]. *JAMA* 1988;259:2900–2901.

83. Cigarette smoking among adults—United States, 1993. *MMWR Morb Mortal Wkly Rep* 1994;43(50):925–930.

84. National Cancer Institute. Tobacco and the clinician: interventions for medical and dental practice. *Monographs of the National Cancer Institute* 1994;5:1–22.

85. Thorndike A, Rigotti N, Stafford R, et al. National patterns in the treatment of smokers by physicians. *JAMA* 1998;279:604–608.

86. Prochaska J, DiClemente C. The transtheoretical approach: crossing traditional boundaries of change. Homewood, IL: Irwin, 1984.

87. Weinstein N. The precaution adoption process. *Health Psychol* 1988; 7:355–386.

88. Heatherton R, Kozlowski L, Frecker R, et al. The Fagerstrom Test for Nicotine Dependence: A revision of the Fagerstrom Tolerance Questionnaire. *Br J Addict* 1991;86:1119–1127.

89. Ockene J, Kristeller J, Pbert L, et al. The physician-delivered smoking intervention project: can short-term interventions produce long-term effects for a general outpatient population? *Health Psychol* 1994;13: 278–281.

90. Manley M, Epps R, Husten C, et al. Clinical interventions in tobacco control: a National Cancer Institute training program for physicians. *JAMA* 1991;266:3172–3173.

91. Nicotine replacement therapy for patients with coronary artery disease. Working Group for the Study of Transdermal Nicotine in Patients with Coronary artery disease. *Arch Intern Med* 1994;154:989–995.

92. Fagerstrom KO. The combined use of nicotine replacement products. *Health Values* 1994;18(3):15–20.

93. Ascher J, Cole J, Colin J. Buproprion: a review of its mechanism of antidepressant activity. *J Clin Psychiatry* 1995;56:395–401.

94. Lerman C, Roth D, Kaufmann V, et al. Mediating mechanisms for the impact of buproprion in smoking cessation treatment. *Drug Alcohol Depend* 2002;67:219–223.

95. Jorenby D, Leischow S, Nides M, et al. A controlled trial of sustained release buproprion, a nicotine patch, or both for smoking cessation. *N Engl J Med* 1999;340:685–691.

96. Hughes J, Goldstein M, Hurt R, et al. Recent advances in the pharmacotherapy of smoking. *JAMA* 1999;281:72–76.

97. Rollnick S, Butler C, Stott N. Helping smokers make decisions: the enhancement of brief intervention for general medical practice. *Patient Educ Couns* 1997;31:191–203.

98. Carroll K. Relapse prevention as a psychosocial treatment: a review of controlled clinical trials. *Exp Clin Psychopharmacol* 1996;4(1):46–52.

99. Emmons K, Goldstein M. Smokers who are hospitalized: a window of opportunity for cessation interventions. *Prev Med* 1992;21:262–269.

100. Houston-Miller N, Smith P, DeBusk R, et al. Smoking cessation in hospitalized patients. Results of a randomized trial. *Arch Intern Med* 1997;157:409–415.

101. Ockene J, Kristeller J, Goldberg R, et al. Smoking cessation and severity of disease: the Coronary Artery Smoking Intervention Study. *Health Psychol* 1992;11:119–126.

102. Taylor C, Miller N, Herman S, et al. A nurse-managed smoking cessation program for hospitalized smokers. *Am J Public Health* 1996; 86:1557–1560.

103. Rigotti N, McKool K, Shiffman S. Predictors of smoking cessation af-

104. Rosal M, Ockene J, Ma Y, et al. Coronary artery smoking intervention study (CASIS): 5-year follow-up. *Health Psychol* 1998;17:476–478.

105. Hajak P, Taylor T, Mills P. Brief intervention during hospital admission to help patients to give up smoking after myocardial infarction and bypass surgery: randomised controlled trial. *BMJ* 2002;324:1–6.

106. Bolman C, deVries H, van Breukelen G. Evaluation of a nurse-managed minimal-contact smoking cessation intervention for cardiac inpatients. *Health Educ Res* 2002;17(1):99–116.

107. Smith S Jr, Blair S, Bonow R, et al. AHA/ACC guidelines for preventing heart attack and death in patients with atherosclerotic cardiovascular disease: 2001 Update. *J Am Coll Cardiol* 2001;38;1581–1583.

108. van Berkel T, Boersma H, Roos-Hesselink J, et al. Impact of smoking cessation and smoking interventions in patients with coronary heart disease. *Eur Heart J* 1999;20:1773–1782.

109. Goldstein M, DePue J, Monroe A, et al. A population-based survey of physician smoking cessation counseling practices. *Prev Med* 1998; 27(5 Pt 1):720–729.

110. Emmons K, Goldstein M. Smokers who are hospitalized: a window of opportunity for cessation interventions. *Prev Med* 1992;21:262–269.

111. Tessier J, Thomas D, Nejjari C, et al. Attitudes and opinions of French cardiologists towards smoking. *Eur J Epidemiol* 1995;11:615–620.

112. Frank E, Winkleby M, Altman D, et al. Predictors of physician's smoking cessation advice. *JAMA* 1991;266:3139–3144.

113. McIlvain H, Backer E, Crabtree B, et al. Physician attitudes and the use of office-based activities for tobacco control. *Fam Med* 2002; 34(2):114–119.

114. O'Loughlin J, Makni H, Tremblay M, et al. Smoking cessation counseling practices of general practitioners in Montreal. *Prev Med* 2001; 33:627–638.

115. Lasser K, Boyd J, Woolhandler S, et al. Smoking and mental illness: a population-based prevalence study. *JAMA* 2000;284:2606–2610.

116. Carmody T. Affect regulation, nicotine addiction, and smoking cessation. *J Psychoactive Drugs* 1989;21:331–342.

117. Hughes J, Fiester S, Goldstein M, et al. American Psychiatric Association practice guidelines for the treatment of patients with nicotine dependence. *Am J Psychiatry* 1996;153[Suppl 1]:1–31.

118. Kinnunen T, Doherty K, Militello F, et al. Depression and smoking cessation: characteristics of depressed smokers and effects of nicotine replacement. *J Consult Clin Psychol* 1996;64:791–798.

119. Hitsman B, Pingitore R, Spring B, et al. Antidepressant pharmacotherapy helps some cigarette smokers more than others. *J Consult Clin Psychol* 1999;67:751–760.

120. Niaura R, Goldstein M, DePue J, et al. Fluoxetine, symptoms of depression, and smoking cessation. *Ann Behav Med* 1995;17[Suppl]:61.

121. Covey L, Glassman A, Stetner F, et al. A randomized clinical trial of sertraline as a cessation aid for smokers with a history of major depression. *Am J Psychiatry* 2002;159:1731–1737.

122. Brown R, Kahler C, Niaura R, et al. Cognitive-behavioral treatment for depression in smoking cessation. *J Consult Clin Psychol* 2001;69: 471–480.

123. Hall S, Munoz R, Reus V. Cognitive-behavioral intervention increases abstinence rates for depressive-history smokers. *J Consult Clin Psychol* 1994;62:141–146.

124. Miller W, Page A. Warm turkey: other routes to abstinence. *J Subst Abuse Treat* 1991;8:227–232.

125. Brown T, Seraganian P, Tremblay J, et al. Matching substance abuse aftercare treatments to client characteristics. *Addict Behav* 2002;27: 585–604.

126. Tengs T, Adams M, Pilskin J, et al. Five hundred life saving interventions and their cost-effectiveness. *Risk Anal* 1995;15:360–390.

CHAPTER 19

Diabetes, Obesity, and the Metabolic Syndrome

Doron Aronson and Elliot J. Rayfield

Key Words: Diabetes; dyslipidemia; endothelium; glycosylation; insulin resistance; obesity; thrombosis.

EPIDEMIOLOGY OF DIABETES

In the last two decades, there has been an explosive worldwide increase in the number of people diagnosed with diabetes. The diabetes epidemic relates particularly to type 2 diabetes and is taking place both in developed and developing countries. The World Health Organization (WHO) estimates that the global number of people with diabetes will increase from the current estimate of 150 million to 220 million in 2010, and to 300 million in 2025 (1,2).

D. Aronson: Division of Cardiology, Rambam Medical Center, Bat Galim, Haifa 31096, Israel.

E. J. Rayfield: Division of Endocrinology, Diabetes, and Bone Disease, Mount Sinai School of Medicine, One Gustave Levy Place, New York, New York 10029.

In the United States, almost 8% of the adult population and 19% of the population older than 65 years have diabetes (3); and 800,000 new cases of diabetes are being diagnosed each year. Approximately 90% of patients with diabetes have type 2, which is now being diagnosed in young people, including adolescents (4). On the basis of fasting plasma glucose levels, one third to one half of cases of type 2 diabetes are undiagnosed and untreated (3,5,6).

Impaired glucose tolerance (IGT) is defined as hyperglycemia with glucose values intermediate between normal and diabetes; it affects at least 200 million people worldwide. Approximately 40% of individuals with IGT experience progression to diabetes within 5 to 10 years (1).

Whereas the mortality rates for other major multifactorial diseases (e.g., heart disease, stroke, and many cancers) have declined or remained stable, the age-adjusted death rate for diabetes in the United States has increased 30% since 1980 (7). The decline in heart disease mortality in the general

U.S. population has been attributed to the reduction in cardiovascular risk factors and to improvement in treatment of heart disease. However, patients with diabetes have not experienced the reduction in age-adjusted heart disease mortality that has been observed in the nondiabetic population, and an increase in age-adjusted heart disease mortality has been reported in women with diabetes (8).

Both type 1 and type 2 diabetes are powerful and independent risk factors for coronary artery disease (CAD), stroke, and peripheral arterial disease (9–11). Atherothrombosis accounts for 65% to 80% of all deaths among North American patients with diabetes, compared with about 33% of all deaths in the general North American population (12). More than 75% of all hospitalizations for diabetic complications are attributable to cardiovascular disease (12). A history of diabetes is equivalent in risk for death to a history of myocardial infarction (MI), and the combination compounds the risk (13).

In patients with type 1 diabetes, the earliest manifestations of CAD occur late in the third decade or in the fourth decade of life regardless of whether diabetes developed early in childhood or in late adolescence (14). The risk increases rapidly after 40 years of age, and by 55 years of age, 35% of patients type 1 diabetes die of CAD. The protection from CAD observed in women without diabetes is lost in women with type 1 diabetes (14,15).

The risk for CAD increases dramatically in the subset of patients with type 1 diabetes in whom diabetic nephropathy develops (this complication develops in only 30–40% of patients with type 1 diabetes) (14,16,17). In a case–control study of patients with type 1 diabetes who were followed from the onset of microalbuminuria (a urinary albumin excretion rate >20 μg/min but less than 200 μg/min or 30–300 mg/24 hours), coronary heart disease developed eight times more frequently than in a diabetic population of similar age, sex, and diabetes duration (17).

When nephropathy is superimposed on diabetes, some of the atherogenic mechanisms present in diabetes are accentuated. An aggregation of cardiovascular risk factors for cardiovascular disease, including hypertension, lipid abnormalities, and a hypercoagulable state, are detectable in the early stages of diabetic nephropathy, when renal function is still normal (18). Hypertension is frequently present in diabetic nephropathy even when the creatinine concentrations remain normal and can intensify CAD in patients with type 1 diabetes. In the WHO Multinational Study on Vascular Disease in Diabetes, patients with both hypertension and proteinuria experienced 11-fold and 18-fold increased mortality for men and women, respectively (19). Microalbuminuria is associated with an atherogenic lipoprotein profile that includes increased low-density lipoprotein (LDL) and chylomicron remnants levels and decreased high-density lipoprotein (HDL) levels (20). In addition, plasminogen activator inhibitor-1 (PAI-1) activity, factor VII, and plasma fibrinogen are significantly greater in patients with microalbuminuria with type 1 diabetes (21). Finally, nephropathy

results in accelerated accumulation of advanced glycosylation end products (AGEs) in the circulation and tissue that parallels the severity of renal functional impairment (22). The accumulation of AGEs improves markedly with successful renal transplantation (23).

Coronary heart disease is the leading cause of death among patients with type 2 diabetes regardless of duration of diabetes. Several population-based studies have shown that the relative risk for cardiovascular disease in type 2 diabetes compared with the general population is increased twofold to fourfold (10). The increased cardiovascular risk is particularly striking in women. A number of studies reported a disproportionate impact of CAD in women with diabetes compared with men with diabetes (24). Indeed, the usual protection that premenopausal women have against atherothrombosis is almost completely lost when diabetes is present.

THE METABOLIC SYNDROME

In individuals who are genetically prone to development of type 2 diabetes, insulin resistance is the earliest detectable metabolic defect and can occur 15 to 25 years or more before the clinical onset of overt diabetes (25). Although there is some uncertainty regarding the primary lesion and the relative importance of the different tissues, metabolic defects in the liver and peripheral tissues such as fat, muscle, and pancreatic β-cells all contribute to the syndrome. Initially, despite the presence of insulin resistance, compensatory increases in pancreatic insulin secretion are able to maintain glucose concentrations within the normal range. However, as the diseases progresses, insulin production gradually diminishes with the progressive development of hyperglycemia.

The term *insulin resistance* usually connotes resistance to the effects of insulin on glucose uptake and metabolism in adipocytes and skeletal muscle, and impaired suppression of hepatic glucose output (26). Insulin resistance is a common condition, associated with genetic predisposition, sedentary lifestyle, obesity, and aging. Even in the absence of diabetes, insulin resistance is a major risk factor for CAD (27) because insulin resistance clusters with a number of proatherogenic abnormalities referred to as the insulin resistance syndrome, the metabolic syndrome, or the cardiovascular dysmetabolic syndrome (Table 19-1). The nature of the associations in the cluster has not been fully elucidated. For some of them, such as dyslipidemia or increased PAI-1, the underlying physiology is sufficiently clear (see "Obesity and Atherothrombosis"); for others (e.g., hypertension), the mechanism is incompletely understood. The primary importance of the metabolic syndrome is that each of its components is an established risk factor for CAD. Alone, each component of the cluster conveys increased CAD risk; but as a combination, they become even more powerful (28).

Insulin resistance and its associated proatherogenic risk factors are present many years before the development of

TABLE 19–1. *Cardiovascular risk factors associated with the metabolic syndrome*

Hypertension
Abdominal obesity
Dyslipidemia
   Increased very low-density lipoprotein triglyceride
   Decreased high-density lipoprotein
   Small, dense atherogenic low-density lipoprotein particles
   Postprandial lipemia
Prothrombotic state: increased plasminogen activator
   inhibitor-1
Endothelial dysfunction
Chronic subclinical inflammation

overt diabetes (29). In addition, the proatherogenic metabolic risk factors associated with the metabolic syndrome appear to worsen over time and across the spectrum of glucose tolerance. In the Framingham Offspring Study, the deterioration of insulin resistance (and glucose tolerance) over time was associated with a continuous increasing gradient of metabolic atherogenic risk factors (30). Therefore, in subjects with the metabolic syndrome who eventually experience development of diabetes, the risk for CAD is increased years before the clinical diagnosis of diabetes. In the Nurses' Health Study, the risk for MI and stroke began to increase at least 15 years before diagnosis of diabetes (31).

Several prospective studies reported the association between fasting or postprandial hyperinsulinemia and CAD (32). Other studies reported inverse correlations between insulin sensitivity and atherothrombosis (33). In addition, it has been suggested that chronic hyperinsulinemia exerts a direct deleterious effect on the arterial wall (34). However, the clinical relevance of these observations is disputed, and the association between hyperinsulinemia and atherothrombosis remains controversial.

The inconsistent association between plasma insulin levels and CAD may stem from that hyperinsulinemia is only a compensatory response of pancreatic β cells to the peripheral insulin resistance. Prospective studies have shown that type 2 diabetes progresses over a continuum of worsening insulin action, beginning with peripheral insulin resistance and ending with a loss of insulin secretion. Thus, plasma insulin levels reflect not only the degree of insulin resistance but also the ability of β cells to compensate. In fact, the natural course of type 2 diabetes is characterized by gradual loss of insulin secretion. The failure of the β cell to continue to hypersecrete insulin underlies the transition from insulin resistance with compensatory hyperinsulinemia to IGT and, subsequently, to overt diabetes. Whereas hyperinsulinemia is characteristic in patients with IGT and mild type 2 diabetes, increased glucose levels seen in patients with moderate to severe type 2 diabetes are associated with a progressive decline in both fasting and postprandial insulin concentrations as a result of pancreatic β cell failure (26). Cross-sectional (30) and prospective (35) studies have shown that fasting and glucose-stimulated insulin concentrations have an inverted U-shaped curve when plotted against plasma glucose concentrations. This pattern has been termed the *Starling curve of the pancreas* (26). Thus, the insulin resistance state itself (not the accompanying compensatory hyperinsulinemia) is more important than hyperinsulinemia as a risk factor for atherothrombosis (33).

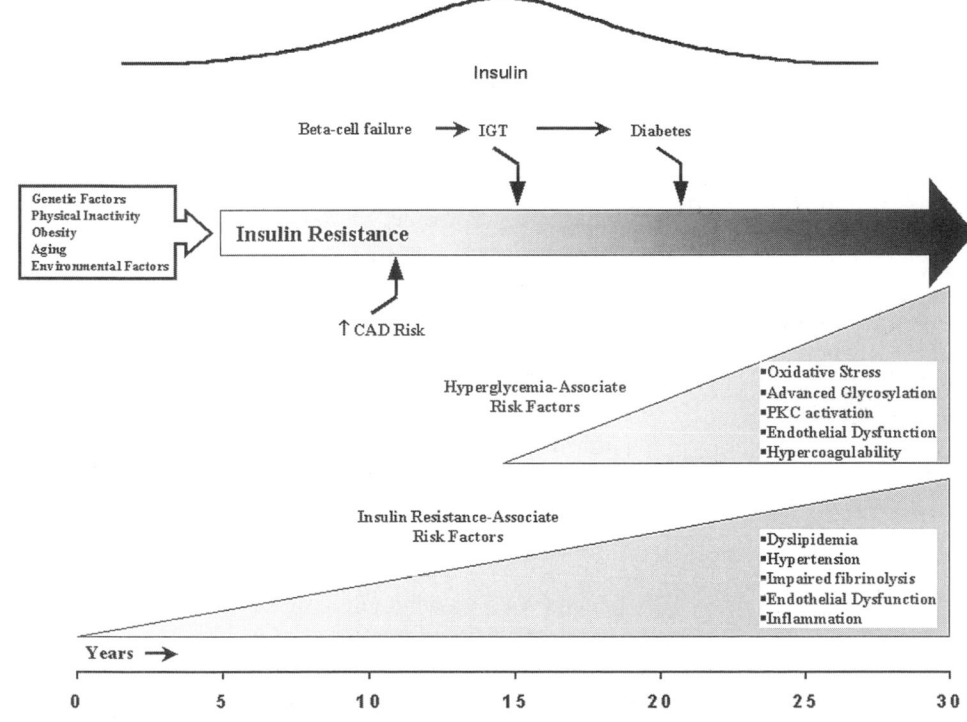

FIG. 19–1. Scheme of cardiovascular risk factor in patients with the metabolic syndrome and type 2 diabetes. Patients are exposed to proatherogenic factors associated with the metabolic syndrome many years before the development of frank hyperglycemia. Patients with the metabolic syndrome who go on to develop type 2 diabetes become exposed to the proatherogenic effects of hyperglycemia. CAD, coronary artery disease; IGT, impaired glucose tolerance; PKC, protein kinase C.

Insulin-resistant individuals who go on to experience development of type 2 diabetes become exposed to the atherogenic effects of hyperglycemia (Fig. 19–1). Indeed, the atherogenic risk factor profile observed in patients with insulin resistance accounts for only a portion of the excess risk for CAD in patients with type 2 diabetes, indicating that hyperglycemia itself plays a central role in accelerating atherothrombosis in these patients. Because many years of asymptomatic hyperglycemia may precede the clinical diagnosis of type 2 diabetes, the duration of diabetes is frequently underestimated. However, population-based studies in patients with type 2 diabetes have shown a positive association between the degree of glycemic control and CAD morbidity and mortality in middle-aged and elderly patients with type 2 diabetes (36,37).

It is important to emphasize that the threshold above which hyperglycemia becomes atherogenic is unknown (38). Glucose cutoffs that define diabetes (fasting and 2-hour postglucose load values of 7.0 and 11.1 mmol/L, respectively) were chosen to identify people at risk for diabetic retinopathy and nephropathy (39). Thus, there is no reason for this threshold to represent a meaningful value with respect to the risk for cardiovascular disease. In fact, a progressive relation between glucose levels and the risk for cardiovascular events exists throughout the whole range of concentrations, including glucose concentrations below the threshold for diabetes and IGT (40–43).

The prevalence of the metabolic syndrome has varied markedly among studies, mostly because of the lack of accepted criteria for the definition of the syndrome. The WHO (44) and the National Cholesterol Education Program Adult Treatment Panel III (NCEP/ATP III) (Table 19–2) proposed unifying definitions for the syndrome. When applying the latter criteria to the National Health and Nutrition Examination Survey III (NHANES III) population, it is estimated that 1 of 4 adults living in the United States merits the diagnosis (45). The prevalence of CAD, MI, and stroke are nearly threefold greater in subjects with the metabolic syndrome than in those without the syndrome (28).

TABLE 19–2. *Adult Treatment Panel III criteria for identification of the metabolic syndrome*

Abdominal obesity (waist circumference)	
Men	>102 cm (40 in.)
Women	>88 cm (35 in.)
Triglycerides	≥150 mg/dL
High-density lipoprotein cholesterol	
Men	<40 mg/dL
Women	<50 mg/dL
Blood pressure	≥130/(85 mm Hg
Fasting glucose	≥110 mg/dL

From the Executive Summary of the Third Report of The National Cholesterol Education Program (NCEP) Expert Panel on Detection, Evaluation, and Treatment of High Blood Cholesterol in Adults (Adult Treatment Panel III). *JAMA* 2001;285:2486–2497.

HYPERGLYCEMIA AS AN ATHEROGENIC FACTOR

Prolonged exposure to hyperglycemia is currently recognized as the primary causal factor in the pathogenesis of diabetic complications (6,37,46). Hyperglycemia induces a large number of alterations in vascular tissue that potentially promote accelerated atherothrombosis. Several major mechanisms have emerged that encompass most of the pathologic alterations observed in the vasculature of animals and humans with diabetes, including: (a) nonenzymatic glycosylation of proteins and lipids, (b) protein kinase C (PKC) activation, (c) increased flux through the hexosamine pathway, and (d) increased oxidative stress.

Advanced Glycosylation End Products

The effects of hyperglycemia often are irreversible and lead to progressive cell dysfunction (47). For example, in patients with diabetes with functioning pancreatic transplants, renal pathology continues to progress for at least 5 years after diabetes has been cured (47). The mechanism for these observations is unclear, but it suggests that cellular perturbations may persist despite the return of normoglycemia (the so-called memory effect) (48). Thus, persistent, rather than transient, acute metabolic changes are of pivotal importance in the pathogenesis of diabetic complications.

One of the important mechanisms responsible for the accelerated atherothrombosis in diabetes is the nonenzymatic reaction between glucose and proteins or lipoproteins in arterial walls, collectively known as Maillard, or browning reaction (49,50) (Fig. 19–2). In 1912, Maillard (50) first incubated glucose with amino acids and observed the formation of yellow–brown pigments that resulted from a nonenzymatic glycosylation reaction of glucose with protein. Glucose forms chemically reversible early glycosylation products with reactive amino groups of proteins (Schiff bases). Formation of the Schiff base from glucose and amine is relatively fast and highly reversible (49), and it represents an equilibrium reaction in which the amount of Schiff base formed is dictated by glucose concentration. When glucose is removed or decreased, the unstable Schiff base reverses within minutes.

Over a period of days, the unstable Schiff base subsequently rearranges to form the more stable Amadori-type early glycosylation products. Formation of Amadori product from the Schiff base is slow, but much faster than the reverse reaction, and therefore tends to accumulate on proteins. Equilibrium levels of Amadori products are reached within weeks (Fig. 19–2). As with the formation of the Schiff base, the amount of Amadori product formed is related to the glucose concentration (49). The best known Amadori product is hemoglobin A_{1C}, which is an adduct of glucose with the N-terminal valine amino group of the β chain of hemoglobin. Thus, measurement of hemoglobin A_{1C} allows assessment of the degree of glucose control integrated over several weeks.

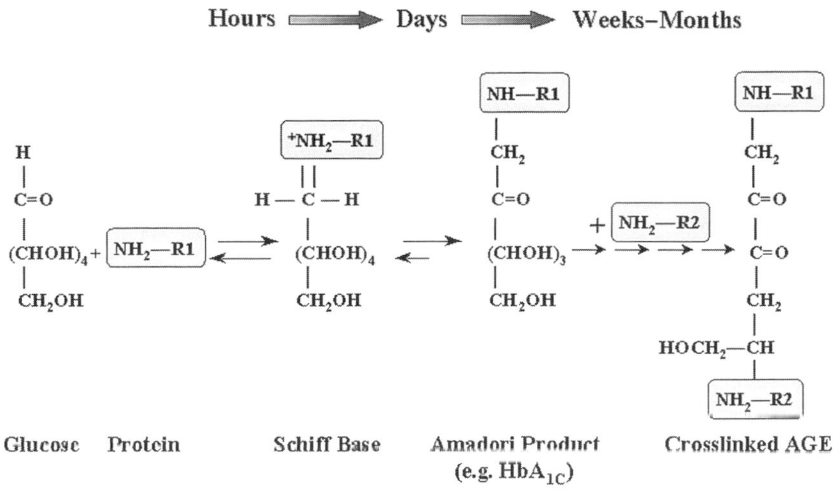

Hours ⟹ Days ⟹ Weeks–Months

FIG. 19–2. Formation of advanced glycosylation end products (AGEs). The process can be inhibited by aminoguanidine, which reacts with Amadori products and prevents the development of more advanced products. AGE cross-link breakers bind to a fully formed AGE and create a ring prone to a sequence of spontaneous break. The result is a severing of AGE cross-bridges between collagen and other macromolecules. HbA$_{1C}$, Glycosylated hemoglobin.

Proteins bearing Amadori products are referred to as glycated proteins (distinguishing them from enzymatically glycosylated proteins), and the process of Amadori product formation is called glycation (49). Some of the early glycosylation products on long-lived proteins (e.g., vessel wall collagen) continue to undergo complex series of chemical rearrangements in vivo to form complex compounds and cross-links known as AGEs (49,51) (Fig. 19–2). An important distinction of AGEs compared with the Amadori products is that once formed, AGE-protein adducts are stable and virtually irreversible. The degree of nonenzymatic glycation is determined mainly by the glucose concentration and time of exposure. Therefore, AGEs accumulate continuously on long-lived vessel wall proteins with aging and at an accelerated rate in diabetes (51). However, another critical factor to the formation of AGEs is the tissue microenvironment redox potential. Thus, in situations in which the local redox potential has been shifted to favor oxidant stress, AGEs formation increases substantially (52,53).

AGEs can accelerate the atherothrombotic process by diverse mechanisms. Glycosylation of proteins and lipoproteins can interfere with their normal function by disrupting molecular conformation, alter enzymatic activity, reduce degradative capacity, and interfere with receptor recognition. Thus, changes in the normal physiology of proteins that are relevant to atherogenesis may promote atherothrombosis in individuals with diabetes. A notable example is interference of the normal physiology of LDL cholesterol described earlier (Fig. 19–9).

On the most important consequences of AGE formation is its ability to cross-link adjacent proteins. Collagen can become cross-linked because AGEs form covalent heat-stable intermolecular bonds (54). The amount of cross-linked collagen peptides formed increase as a function of both time and glucose concentration (54,55). In contrast to normal cross-links within normal collagen, which occur only at two discrete sites at the N-terminal and C-terminal ends of the molecule, AGEs form cross-links throughout the collagen molecule (51). Studies have demonstrated that collagen cross-linking plays an important role in changing the mechanical properties of tissues, leading to the increased vascular rigidity and the reduced left ventricular compliance in patients with diabetes. Collagen cross-linking plays a major role in the pathogenesis of isolated systolic hypertension and diastolic heart failure (see "Arterial Stiffness and Diastolic Dysfunction in Diabetes").

Interruption of AGE formation has been shown to ameliorate microvascular and macrovascular complications of diabetes. Aminoguanidine (an analogue of the side chain of arginine), a small nucleophilic compound, is a potent inhibitor of AGE formation and protein-to-protein cross-linking (54). The terminal amino group of the compound reacts with glucose-derived reactive α-carbonyl intermediates at the post-Amadori stage (Fig. 19–2). Aminoguanidine has been proven to be effective in inhibiting AGE formation in vivo in a variety of animal models and clinical studies (49,56).

Vasan and coworkers (57) developed a new class of anti-AGE agents that contained a thiazolium structure, which could break α-carbonyl compounds by cleaving the carbon–carbon bond between the carbonyls. The thiazolium agent 3-phenacylthiazolium bromide (PTB) was found to cleave a major proportion of AGE cross-links formed under physiologic conditions. Subsequently, a more stable and more active derivative, 4,5-dimethyl-3-phenacylthiazolium chloride (DPTC or ALT-711) was developed for preclinical studies (49). This agent has been shown to ameliorate arterial stiffness and diastolic dysfunction in both animal and human studies (see "Arterial Stiffness and Diastolic Dysfunction in Diabetes").

The Advanced Glycosylation End Product Receptor Mediates Inflammation

The pathophysiologic significance of AGEs stems not only from their ability to modify the functional properties of proteins, but also their ability to interact with AGE-binding proteins or AGE receptors, through which AGEs elicit several biologic phenomena. The cellular interactions of AGEs are mediated through a specific receptor for AGE determinants on cell surfaces (52). The presence of the AGE receptor (RAGE), a member of the immunoglobulin superfamily of receptors (58), has been demonstrated in all cells relevant to the atherothrombotic process including monocyte-derived macrophages, endothelial cells (ECs), and smooth muscle cells (52,58) (Table 19–3).

In mature animals, RAGE expression on these cells is low. However, under certain pathologic circumstances, sustained up-regulation of RAGE occurs. In pathologic lesions, abundance of RAGE-expressing cells is usually associated with sites of accumulated RAGE ligands. In diabetic vasculature, cells expressing high levels of RAGE are often proximal to areas in which AGEs are abundant (52,67).

AGE interaction with RAGE on ECs results in the induction of oxidative stress and consequently of the transcription factor nuclear factor-kappaB (NF-κB) (61,62) and increases the expression of adhesion molecules including vascular cell adhesion molecule-1 (VCAM-1), intracellular adhesion molecule (ICAM-1), and E-selectin (65,66). In addition, engagement of AGEs with their specific receptors results in reduced endothelial barrier function (63,65), with increased permeability of EC monolayers (63,64). Thus, the interaction of AGEs with RAGE-bearing ECs can promote initiating events in atherogenesis such as increased lipid entry into the subendothelium and adhesive interactions of monocytes with the endothelial surface with subsequent transendothelial migration.

Binding of soluble AGEs to RAGE-bearing monocytes induces chemotaxis (68), followed by mononuclear infiltration

TABLE 19–3. *Atherothrombosis promoting effects of receptor for advanced glycosylation end products activation*

Promoting inflammation
  Secretion of cytokines such as TNF-α, IL-1 (54)
  Chemotactic stimulus for monocyte/macrophages (56,59)
Induction of cellular proliferation
  Stimulation of PDGF from monocytes (59)
  Stimulation of IGF-1 secretion from monocytes (60)
Endothelial dysfunction
  Stimulation of transcription factor NF-κB (61,62)
  Increased permeability of EC monolayers (63,64)
  Increased procoagulant activity (e.g., tissue factor expression) (64)
  Increased expression of adhesion molecules (65,66)
  Increased intracellular oxidative stress (61,63)

EC, endothelial cell; IGF-I, insulin-like growth factor I; IL-1, interleukin-1; NF-κB, nuclear factor-kappaB PDGF, platelet-derived growth factor; TNF-α, tumor necrosis factor-α.

through an intact endothelial monolayer (56,59). Monocyte/macrophage interaction with AGEs also results in the production of mediators such as interleukin (IL)-1, tumor necrosis factor-α (TNF-α), platelet-derived growth factor, and insulin growth factor-I (59,60,69), which have a pivotal role in the pathogenesis of atherothrombosis (70). Thus, under conditions of enhanced tissue AGE deposition, receptor-mediated interaction of AGE proteins with vascular wall cells facilitate the migration of inflammatory cells into the lesion with the subsequent release of growth-promoting cytokines.

Schmidt and coworkers (52,58) proposed the following *two–hit model* for RAGE-mediated perturbations in diabetic vasculature. In the setting of hyperglycemia, formation and deposition of AGEs in tissues and vasculature is accelerated. The presence of AGEs (RAGE ligands) in the vasculature results in a basal state of increased RAGE expression and activation (first hit). The superimposition of another stimulus, such as deposition of oxidized lipoproteins or inflammation, results in an exaggerated, chronic inflammation and promotes accelerated atherothrombosis (second hit). In contrast to other inflammatory processes, in which a negative feedback loop terminates cellular activation, RAGE activation appears to result in a smoldering degree of cellular stimulation (52,58,66).

The potential role of RAGE in the atherogenic process in diabetes has been demonstrated by Park and associates (71). In the model of atherothrombosis-prone mice due to homozygous deletion of apolipoprotein E (*apoE*) gene, the induction of diabetes using streptozotocin resulted in atherothrombosis of increased severity compared with euglycemic *apoE* control mice. The development of vascular disease was more rapid with the formation of more complex lesions (fibrous caps, extensive monocyte infiltration, and others) and atherothrombosis extending distally in the aorta and major arteries. Increased expression of RAGE and the presence of AGEs in the vessel wall, especially at sites of vascular lesions, were also evident. Blockade of AGE-RAGE interaction using a truncated soluble extracellular domain of RAGE resulted in a striking suppression of lesions in diabetic mice, with lesions largely arrested at the fatty streak stage and a large reduction in complex lesions (Fig. 19–3). These effects were independent of glucose and lipid levels (71). Activation of RAGE-dependent mechanisms contributes not only to lesion formation but also to lesion progression in the same mouse model of atherothrombosis. When established atherothrombosis is already present, RAGE blockade halts the progression of vascular inflammation (72).

RAGE is not the only receptor for AGE-modified proteins that is relevant to atherothrombosis. The macrophage scavenger receptor class A mediates endocytic uptake of AGE bearing proteins by macrophages (73). Similarly, CD36, a member of the class B scavenger receptor family, also recognizes and endocytoses AGE proteins (74). That foam cells in the early phase of atherothrombosis are driven from

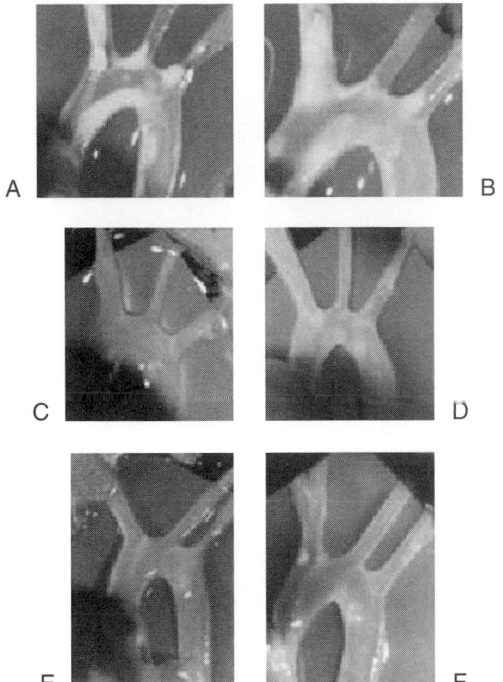

FIG. 19–3. Effect of blockade of interaction of advanced glycosylation end products and its receptor (AGE-RAGE) using a truncated soluble extracellular domain of RAGE (sRAGE) on the development of atherothrombotic lesions in diabetic apolipoprotein E (apoE)-null mice. Diabetic mice without treatment **(A** and **B)**; diabetic mice treated with sRAGE at 20 mg/day **(C)** or 40 mg/day **(D)**; control euglycemic apoE-null mice without treatment **(E)** or sRAGE at 20 mg/day **(F)**. Also, note that diabetic apoE-null mice **(A** and **B)** develop atherothrombosis of increased severity compared with euglycemic control mice **(E** and **F)**. (Modified from Park L, Raman KG, Lee KJ, et al. Suppression of accelerated diabetic atherosclerosis by the soluble receptor for advanced glycation endproducts. *Nat Med* 1998;4:1025–1031, with permission.)

monocyte/macrophages, in which these scavenger receptors are highly expressed (serving as major oxidized LDL receptors), raises the possibility that scavenger receptors also are involved in AGE-mediated diabetic macrovascular complications.

Protein Kinase C

The metabolic consequences of hyperglycemia can be expressed in cells in which glucose transport is largely independent of insulin. The resulting intracellular hyperglycemia has been implicated in the pathogenesis of diabetic complications through the activation of the PKC system (34,75,76).

High ambient glucose concentrations activate PKC by increasing the formation of diacylglycerol (DAG), the major endogenous cellular cofactor for PKC activation, from glycolytic intermediates such as dihydroxy-acetone phosphate and glyceraldehyde-3-phosphate. The increase of DAG and

subsequent activation of PKC in the vasculature can be maintained chronically (76).

PKC is a family of at least 12 isoforms of serine and threonine kinases. Although several PKC isoforms are expressed in vascular tissue, in the rat model of diabetes there is a preferential activation of PKC β_2 in the aorta, heart, and retina, and PKC β_1 in the glomeruli (76,77).

The PKC system is ubiquitously distributed in cells and is involved in the transcription of several growth factors and in signal transduction in response to growth factors (78,79), nitric oxide (NO) (80), and endothelin production (81). In vascular smooth muscle cells, PKC activation has been shown to modulate growth rate, DNA synthesis, and growth factor receptor turnover (76). For example, hyperglycemia-induced PKC activation also results in increased platelet-derived growth factor-β receptor expression on smooth muscle cells and other vascular wall cells (e.g., ECs, monocyte/macrophages) (82).

PKC activation increases the expression of transforming growth factor-β (TGF-β), which is one of the most important growth factors regulating extracellular matrix (ECM) production by activating gene expression of proteoglycans and collagen and decreasing the synthesis of proteolytic enzymes that degrade matrix proteins. Increased expression of TGF-β is thought to lead to thickening of capillary basement membrane—one of the early structural abnormalities observed in almost all tissues in diabetes. PKC β-selective inhibitor (LY333531) attenuates glomerular expression of TGF-β and ECM proteins such as fibronectin and type IV collagen (77,78).

PKC activation also appears to be involved in the increased permeability of ECs in diabetes (83), and it contributes to endothelial dysfunction by increasing oxidative stress and decreasing NO bioavailability (11,48).

The Hexosamine Pathway

Shunting of excess intracellular glucose into the hexosamine pathway may contribute to diabetic macrovascular disease. In this pathway, fructose-6–phosphate derived from glycolysis provides substrate to reactions that require UDP-*N*-acetylglucosamine, such as proteoglycan synthesis and the formation of *O*-linked glycoproteins (48,84) (Fig. 19–4).

O-glycosylation typically involves the addition of a single sugar, usually *N*-acetylglucosamine (GlcNAc) to the protein's serine and threonine residues. Serine/threonine phosphorylation is a critical step in the regulation of various enzymes, raising the possibility that *O*-glycosylation might result in perturbations in normal enzyme function.

Many transcription factors and other nuclear and cytoplasmic proteins are dynamically modified by *O*-linked GlcNAc and show reciprocal modification by phosphorylation (48,85) (Fig. 19–4). For example, hyperglycemia increases endothelial nitric oxide synthase (eNOS)–associated *O*-GlcNAc, resulting in a parallel decrease in eNOS serine phosphorylation (which results in enzyme activation) and, therefore, a decrease in eNOS activity (86). This pathway also is involved in

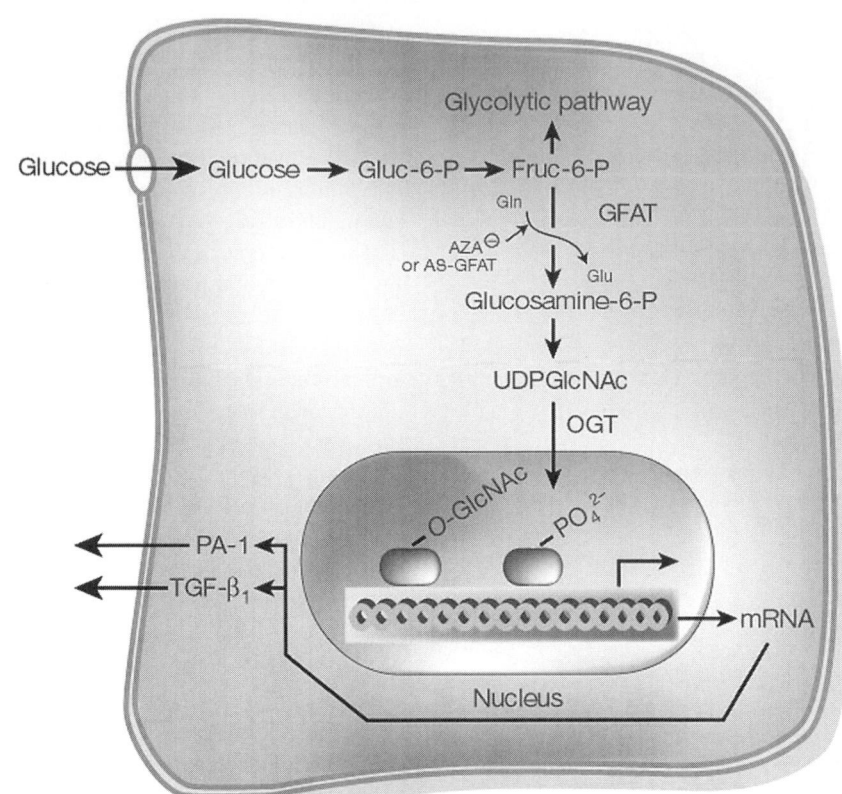

FIG. 19–4. The hexosamine pathway. The glycolytic intermediate fructose-6-phosphate (Fruc-6-P) is converted to glucosamine-6-phosphate by the enzyme glutamine:fructose-6-phosphate amidotransferase (GFAT). Intracellular glycosylation by the addition of *N*-acetylglucosamine (GlcNAc) to serine and threonine is catalyzed by the enzyme *O*-GlcNAc transferase (OGT). Increased donation of GlcNAc moieties to serine and threonine residues of transcription factors such as Sp1, often at phosphorylation sites, increases the production of factors as plasminogen activator inhibitor type 1 (PAI-1) and transforming growth factor (TGF)-β_1. AZA, azaserine; AS-GFAT, antisense to GFAT.

hyperglycemia-induced increase in the transcription of TGF-β and PAI-1. Inhibition of glutamine:fructose-6-phosphate amidotransferase (GFAT), the rate-limiting enzyme in the conversion of glucose to glucosamine (Fig. 19–4), blocks the increase of TGF-β (84) and PAI-1 (87) transcription.

Oxidative Stress

Oxidative stress is widely invoked as a pathogenic mechanism for atherothrombosis. Oxidative damage to arterial wall proteins occurs even with short-term exposure to hyperglycemia in the diabetic range (88). Among the sequelae of hyperglycemia, oxidative stress has been suggested as a potential mechanism for accelerated atherothrombosis (53, 89). Importantly, there appears to be a tight pathogenic link between hyperglycemia-induced oxidant stress and other hyperglycemia-dependent mechanisms of vascular damage described earlier, namely AGE formation, PKC activation, and increased flux through the hexosamine pathway (Fig. 19–5).

Hyperglycemia can increase oxidative stress through several pathways. A major mechanism appears to be the overproduction of the superoxide anion (O_2^-) by the mitochondrial electron transport chain (53). Physiologic generation of O_2 species (particularly the superoxide radical) occurs during normal electron shuttling by cytochromes within the electron transport chain. Hyperglycemia leads to an increased production of electron donors (reduced nicotinamide adenine dinucleotide [NADH] and reduced flavin adenine dinucleotide [FADH$_2$]) by the tricarboxylic cycle. This generates a high mitochondrial membrane potential by pumping protons across the mitochondrial inner membrane. The resulting inhibition of electron transport at complex III increases the half-life of free radical intermediates of coenzyme Q (ubiquinone), which reduces O_2 to superoxide, and markedly increases the production of superoxide (48,53,86,87).

An additional mechanism involves the transition metal-catalyzed autoxidation of protein-bound Amadori products, which yields superoxide and hydroxyl radicals and highly reactive dicarbonyl compounds (89). Some of the individual advanced glycosylation products such as N$^\epsilon$-(carboxymethyl)lysine and pentosidine are formed in reactions of protein with glucose only under oxidative conditions (90, 91). Thus, some AGEs are produced by combined processes of glycation and oxidation and have been termed glycoxida-

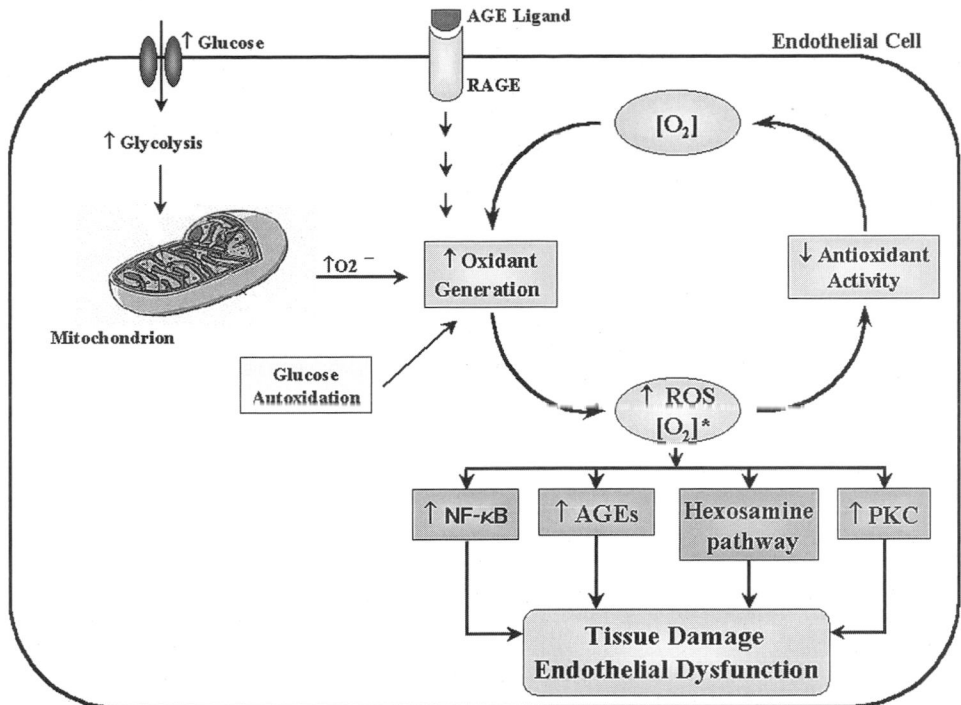

FIG. 19–5. Relation between rates of oxidant generation, antioxidant activity, oxidative stress, and oxidative damage in diabetes. $[O_2]^*$ represents various forms of reactive oxygen species (ROS). The overall rate of formation of oxidative products leading to oxidative tissue damage is dependent on ambient levels of both $[O_2]^*$ and substrate. Increased generation of $[O_2]^*$ depends on several sources including glucose autoxidation, increased mitochondrial superoxide production, and as a result of the receptor for advanced glycosylation end product (RAGE) activation. $[O_2]^*$ deactivation is reduced because antioxidant defenses are compromised in diabetes. Note that oxidative stress also promotes other hyperglycemia-induced mechanisms of tissue damage. Oxidative stress activates protein kinase C (PKC) and accelerates the formation of advanced glycosylation end products (AGEs). NF-κB, Nuclear factor-kappaB.

tion products. Each AGE structure has its own formation mechanism, and thus its own dependence on oxidative stress. However, because glycoxidation products on proteins are irreversible, it has been suggested that they may be an integrative biomarker for the accumulated oxidative stress to which the respective tissue has been exposed (89). Indeed, there are strong correlations between levels of glycoxidation products in skin collagen and the severity of diabetic retinal, renal, and vascular disease (92,93).

Another potential mechanism contributing to oxidative stress involves the transition metal-catalyzed autoxidation of free glucose, as described in cell-free systems. Through this mechanism, glucose itself initiates an autoxidative reaction and free radical production yielding superoxide anion (O_2^-) and hydrogen peroxide (H_2O_2) (94–96). This reaction often is catalyzed by transition metals, but even with the catalyst, the reaction is very slow.

Finally, as previously discussed, the interaction between AGE epitopes and the cell surface AGE receptor up-regulate oxidative stress response genes (61) and release oxygen radicals (97). Thus, hyperglycemia simultaneously enhances both AGE formation and oxidative stress, and the interaction between glycation and oxidation chemistry can augment

each of these processes. Furthermore, oxidative stress generated in the setting of hyperglycemia can lead to the activation of DAG-PKC in vascular tissue (53,98).

Importantly, all mechanisms of hyperglycemia-induced cellular dysfunction appear to be interrelated and augmented by increased oxidative stress (53) (Fig. 19–5). Nishikawa and coworkers (53) have shown that hyperglycemia-induced overproduction of mitochondrial superoxide promotes the formation of AGEs, PKC activation, and hexosamine pathway activity. Inhibition of superoxide production by overexpression of manganese dismutase (which rapidly converts superoxide to H_2O_2) or of uncoupling protein-1 (which collapses the proton electromechanical gradients) prevents hyperglycemia-induced superoxide overproduction. Concomitantly, increased intracellular AGE formation, PKC activation, and increased hexosamine formation are prevented (48,53).

ENDOTHELIAL CELL DYSFUNCTION IN DIABETES

ECs situated at the vessel wall–blood interface participate in a number of important homeostatic and cellular functions that protect against atherothrombosis and intraluminal thrombosis. Endothelial cell dysfunction (ECD) can promote both the formation of atherothrombotic plaques and the occurrence of acute events. One of the hallmarks of vascular disease in diabetes is ECD, which contributes to the initiation, progression, and clinical presentation of the atherothrombotic process in these patients.

Impaired Endothelium-dependent Vasodilation

Impaired endothelium-dependent relaxation, mediated through the release of NO, is a consistent finding in animal models and in humans with diabetes (99,100), and it occurs in a variety of vascular beds including the coronary arteries (100). Impaired endothelium-dependent relaxation has been demonstrated in both type 1 and type 2 diabetes in the absence of clinical complications (99–101), whereas endothelium-independent vasodilation is preserved (100).

The alterations in the NO regulation in diabetes are complex and involve increased reactive oxygen species (ROS) (53), quenching of bioactive NO by glucose (102), changes in eNOS levels or its cofactors (103,104), and perturbations in eNOS activation (86,105) (Fig. 19–6).

The loss of normal endothelial function exerts a profound effect on the arterial wall because NO protects against the development of vasculature by inhibiting platelets aggregation and adhesion, circulating monocyte adhesion to ECs, and vascular smooth muscle proliferation

(see Chapter 27). Consequently, multiple abnormalities in EC function have been described in association with diabetes (Table 19–4).

Hyperglycemia Impairs Endothelium-dependent Vasodilation

Hyperglycemia appears to be the primary mediator of endothelial dysfunction in diabetes. Endothelium-dependent vasodilatation is impaired during acute hyperglycemia in both healthy subjects (99) and patients with diabetes (110). A short exposure (several hours) to high glucose concentrations is sufficient to induce impaired endothelium-dependent relaxation (99).

Hyperglycemia decreases bioavailability of NO in a progressive and concentration-dependent manner (111). Moreover, diminished capacity of eNOS has been demonstrated experimentally when ECs are exposed to hyperglycemia (86). There is abundant evidence supporting the importance of ROS in inducing and maintaining ECD in diabetes (86,107,112,113). Furthermore, experimental and clinical data suggest that scavengers of oxygen radicals and antioxidants such as vitamins E and C improve endothelium-dependent relaxation in diabetic arteries (101,107,114).

EC overproduction of superoxide (53,86,105) reduces NO bioactivity because superoxide reacts rapidly with NO, producing the oxidative peroxynitrite radical. In addition to

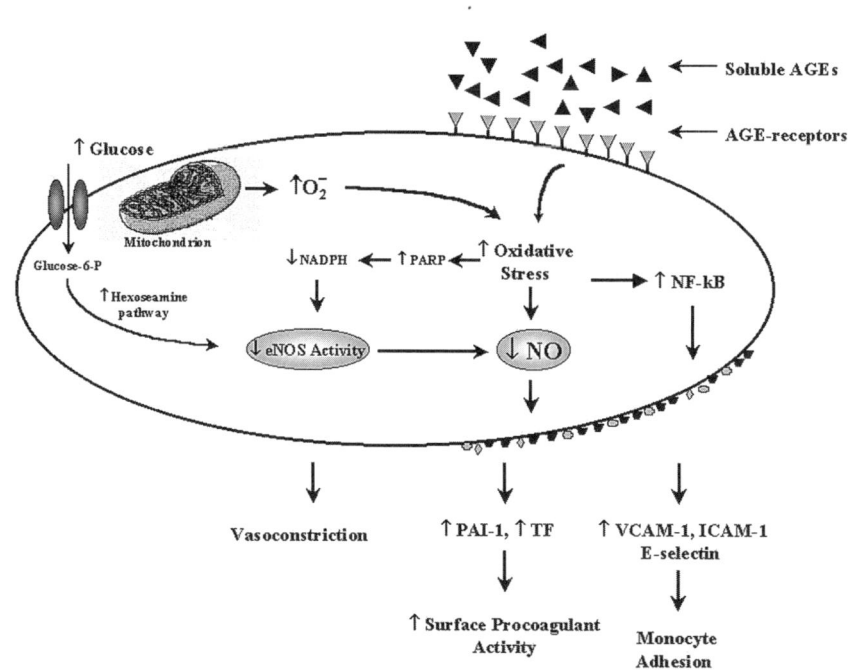

FIG. 19–6. Potential mechanisms of endothelial dysfunction in diabetes. Diabetes leads to reduced nitric oxide (NO) bioavailability and nuclear factor-kappaB (NF-κB) activation, resulting in perturbations in vascular tone, increased procoagulant activity, and increased expression of adhesion molecules on endothelial cells. AGE, advanced glycosylation end product; eNOS, endothelial nitric oxide synthase; ICAM, intracellular adhesion molecule; NADPH, nicotinamide adenine dinucleotide phosphate; PAI-1, plasminogen activator inhibitor type 1; PARP, poly(ADP-ribose) polymerase; TF, tissue factor; VCAM, vascular cell adhesion molecule.

TABLE 19–4. *Diabetes-induced alterations in endothelial cell functional properties*

Endothelial function	Effectors	Diabetes-induced perturbations	Atherothrombosis/Events promoting effects
Selective permeability barrier	Continuous endothelium with tight junctions in the lateral borders	Increased permeability Delayed regeneration (63,65)	Allow LDL or bloodborne mitogens to reach the subendothelial space
Provides a nonthrombogenic surface	NO, PGI$_2$ t-PA, HS; thrombo-modulin; TF	Reduced antithrombotic and fibrinolytic phenotype ($\downarrow$NO, $\downarrow$PGI$_2$, $\uparrow$PAI-1, $\uparrow$TF) (106)	Promote thrombosis and inhibit fibrinolysis
Provides a nonadherent surface for circulating leukocytes	NO	Induction of adhesion molecules (e.g., VCAM-1, E-selectin) (61,62,65)	Recruit macrophages into the vascular wall
Regulation of vascular tone	NO, PGI$_2$, ET-1	Reduced vasodilator function ($\downarrow$NO, $\downarrow$PGI$_2$, $\uparrow$ET-1) (107)	Failure of vasodilation
Secrete growth inhibitors	NO, HS	Inactivation of NO (108); reduced NO production (109)	Reduced antiproliferative activity of NO on vascular smooth muscle cells

AGE, advanced glycosylation end product; ET-1, endothelin-1; HS, heparan sulfate; LDL, low-density lipoprotein; NO, nitric oxide; PAI-1, plasminogen activator inhibitor; PGI$_2$, prostacyclin; TF, tissue factor; t-PA, tissue plasminogen activator; VCAM, vascular cell adhesion molecule.

NO scavenging, superoxide overproduction may alter the activity and regulation of eNOS through activation of the hexosamine pathway (86,105), leading to reduced eNOS activity (86) (Fig. 19–6).

Diabetes-related oxidative stress also induces DNA single-strand breakage leading to the activation of the nuclear enzyme poly(adenosine diphosphate-ribose) polymerase (PARP). The result of this process is rapid depletion of endothelial energy sources, including nicotinamide adenine dinucleotide phosphate (NADPH). Because eNOS is an NADPH-dependent enzyme, its activity is suppressed (103,104). A PARP inhibitor can maintain normal vascular responsiveness, despite the persistence of severe hyperglycemia (104).

Insulin-resistant Subjects Exhibit Impaired Endothelium-dependent Vasodilation

ECD occurs concomitantly with insulin resistance and antedates overt hyperglycemia in patients with type 2 diabetes. Insulin is a physiologic vasodilator of skeletal muscle vasculature in humans and exhibits a dose- and time-dependent induction of vasodilation, which is partially NO-mediated (115). Under normal conditions, insulin induces vasodilation by modulating eNOS activity and expression (80,116) and, therefore, NO bioavailability.

However, the vasodilatory effect of insulin is blunted in insulin-resistant subjects. Thus, impaired endothelium-dependent relaxation is present in insulin-resistant *normoglycemic* subjects (117), including first-degree relatives of subjects with type 2 diabetes (118), subjects at risk for type 2 diabetes (119), and in other insulin resistance states (120).

The mechanism by which insulin resistance impairs endothelium-dependent vasodilation is not well understood. Absolute or relative deficiency of insulin action on the vessel wall may reduce insulin-mediated vasodilation. For example, a positive correlation has been reported between endothelial NO production and insulin sensitivity in healthy subjects (109).

Alternatively, the compensatory hyperinsulinemia associated with insulin resistance states can also induce ECD in large conduit arteries (121). In addition, metabolic abnormalities that accompany insulin resistance, and especially increased circulating free fatty acids (FFAs) (122,123), can contribute to ECD in insulin-resistant subjects.

Endothelial Permeability

The endothelial lining of the large arteries is of the continuous type characterized by tight junctions in the lateral borders, which restrict the movement of macromolecules from reaching the subendothelial space. Human vascular ECs cultured in glucose concentrations comparable to those of uncontrolled diabetes exhibit delay in reaching confluence and in the rate of replication (124). EC regeneration after deendothelialization (e.g., after balloon angioplasty) is slower (125). ECs in diabetic animals also exhibit morphologic abnormalities that include the presence of craters resulting from weakened intercellular junctions (126). Furthermore, AGEs with their specific receptor diminishes endothelial barrier function (63,65). These abnormalities may explain the increased vascular permeability and transendothelial macromolecular transport (124).

Leukocyte Adhesion to the Vascular Endothelium

Binding of monocytes to the endothelium represents one of the earliest events in atherogenesis. The process is mediated through the expression of inducible adhesion molecules on the EC surface and allows subsequent monocyte entry into the vessel wall.

High glucose concentrations potently promote leukocyte adhesion to ECs under flow conditions through glucose-induced up-regulation of the adhesion molecules E-selectin, ICAM-1, and VCAM-1 (127). This phenomenon may be mediated through PKC-induced NF-κB activation (127) or through AGE interaction with the AGE receptor, which results in the induction of oxidative stress, NF-κB activation (61,62), and up-regulation of adhesion molecules (65,66) (Fig. 19–6). Thus, early events in the atherothrombosis process in diabetes may be mediated through enhanced adhesive interactions of monocytes with the endothelial surface.

LIPOPROTEIN DISORDERS IN DIABETES

The metabolic abnormalities associated with type I and type II diabetes result in changes in the transport, composition, and metabolism of lipoproteins. Lipoprotein metabolism is influenced by several factors including type of diabetes, glycemic control, obesity, insulin resistance, the presence of diabetic nephropathy, and genetic background (128). Abnormalities in plasma lipoprotein concentrations are commonly observed in individuals with diabetes, and they have a profound impact on the atherothrombotic process. Today, Elliot P. Joslin's presentation to the American College of Physicians in 1927 seems appropriate:

> I believe the chief cause of premature development of arteriosclerosis in diabetes, save for advancing age, is due to an excess of fat, an excess of fat in the body, obesity, an excess of fat in the diet, and an excess of fat in the blood. With an excess of fat diabetes begins and from an excess of fat diabetics die, formerly of coma, recently from arteriosclerosis.[128a]

Lipoprotein Profile in Type 1 Diabetes

Glycemic control is the chief determinant of lipoprotein profile levels in patients with type 1 diabetes (129). In well to moderately controlled diabetes, lipoprotein levels are usually within the normal range (130). In poorly controlled patients, triglycerides are markedly increased, LDL is modesty increased (usually when glycosylated hemoglobin [HbA$_{1C}$] is >11%), and HDL levels are decreased (130) (Table 19–5). Hypertriglyceridemia and hypercholesterolemia are readily reversible with intensive insulin therapy (130), and HDL levels may be greater than in healthy control subjects (20). When high LDL levels exist in a well controlled individual with type 1 diabetes, diabetic nephropathy or a separately inherited lipid disorder should be suspected (129).

Lipoprotein Profile in Type 2 Diabetes

The dyslipidemia in type 2 diabetes results from a complex interaction among an insulin resistance state, obesity, and hyperglycemia (128), and is often present for years before the development of fasting hyperglycemia and the diagnosis of type 2 diabetes (29). The typical lipoprotein profile associated with type 2 diabetes includes high triglycerides, low HDL and normal LDL levels (Table 19–5). However, the composition of LDL particles is altered, resulting in a preponderance of small, triglyceride-enriched and cholesterol-depleted particles (small, dense LDL). This lipoprotein profile has been termed *atherogenic lipoprotein phenotype* (131), and it is also characteristic of the metabolic syndrome and obesity (132–134).

The most consistent change is an increase in VLDL-triglyceride levels (135,136). Population studies, including of the Pima Indians, who have virtually no forms of genetic hyperlipidemia, indicate that type II diabetes generally produces only a 50% to 100% increase in total triglyceride levels (137). Thus, patients with type II diabetes with total triglyceride levels greater than 350 to 400 mg/dL probably have other genetic disorders in lipoprotein metabolism, which may be exacerbated by diabetes. HDL levels are typically 25% to 30% less than in nondiabetics and are commonly associated with other lipid and lipoprotein abnormalities, particularly high triglyceride levels.

TABLE 19–5. *Lipoprotein abnormalities in diabetes*

	Type 1 diabetes		Type 2 diabetes		
Lipoprotein	Conventional therapy	Intensive therapy	Poor control	Good control	Atherogenic modifications
VLDL-TG	Normal or increased	Decreased	Increased	Normal or increased	Cholesteryl ester–rich VLDL
LDL	Normal or increased	Normal or decreased	Normal	Normal	Glycosylation of LDL apoB increases uptake through the scavenger receptor; LDL susceptible to oxidative modification; high proportion of small, dense LDL
HDL	Normal	Increased	Decreased	Normal or decreased	Decreased HDL; increased CETP activity

apoB, apolipoprotein B; CETP, cholesteryl ester transfer protein; HDL, high-density lipoprotein; LDL, low-density lipoprotein; TG, triglyceride; VLDL, very low-density lipoprotein.

Very Low-Density Lipoprotein Metabolism in Diabetes

Hypertriglyceridemia in type 2 diabetes results from high fasting and postprandial triglyceride-rich lipoproteins, especially VLDL (135), which is the consequence of both overproduction and impaired catabolism of VLDL (128,136). Increased VLDL production is almost uniformly present in patients with type 2 diabetes and hypertriglyceridemia because of an increase in FFA flux to the liver (136). Because maintenance of stored fat in adipose tissue depends on the suppression of hormone-sensitive lipase by insulin, insulin deficiency or resistance results in increased hormone-sensitive lipase activity and excessive release of FFA from adipocytes. As FFA availability is a major determinant of VLDL production by the liver, VLDL overproduction and hypertriglyceridemia ensues (136) (Fig. 19–7). Increased delivery of glucose to the liver may also contribute to the secretion of triglyceride-enriched VLDL particles by the liver.

In patients with type 2 diabetes with more severe hypertriglyceridemia, VLDL clearance by lipoprotein lipase (LPL), the rate-limiting enzyme responsible for the removal of plasma triglyceride-rich lipoproteins, also is impaired (135). LPL requires insulin for maintenance of normal tissue levels (138), and its activity is low in patients with poorly controlled type II diabetes (135). The result is enzymatic activity insufficient to match the overproduction rate, with further accumulation of VLDL triglyceride.

Increased fatty acid flux to the liver also results in the production of large triglyceride-rich VLDL particles because the size of VLDL is also mainly determined by the amount of triglycerides available. VLDL size is an important determinant of its metabolic fate. Large triglyceride-rich VLDL particles may be less efficiently converted to LDL (139), thereby increasing direct removal from the circulation by non-LDL pathways. In addition, overproduction of large triglyceride-rich VLDL is associated with the atherogenic small, dense LDL subclass (discussed later).

The rest of the dyslipidemic phenotype that characterizes insulin resistance and type 2 diabetes (low HDL and small, dense LDL) follows once VLDL plasma concentrations increase, mainly through the action of cholesteryl ester transfer protein (CETP) and lipoprotein compositional changes that occur in plasma (140).

High-Density Lipoprotein Metabolism in Diabetes

Decreased HDL levels in diabetes are closely related to the abnormal metabolism of triglyceride-rich lipoproteins (135,136) (Fig. 19–8). During lipolysis of chylomicrons and VLDL, surface components (free cholesterol, redundant phospholipids, and apolipoproteins) are transferred into the HDL fraction. These components may enter nascent discoid HDL particles secreted by the liver. The free cholesterol is esterified by lecithin cholesterol acyl transferase to generate mature spherical HDLs (see Chapter 7). Alternatively, these surface components may be incorporated into preexisting HDL particles. The latter process results in an increase in size and

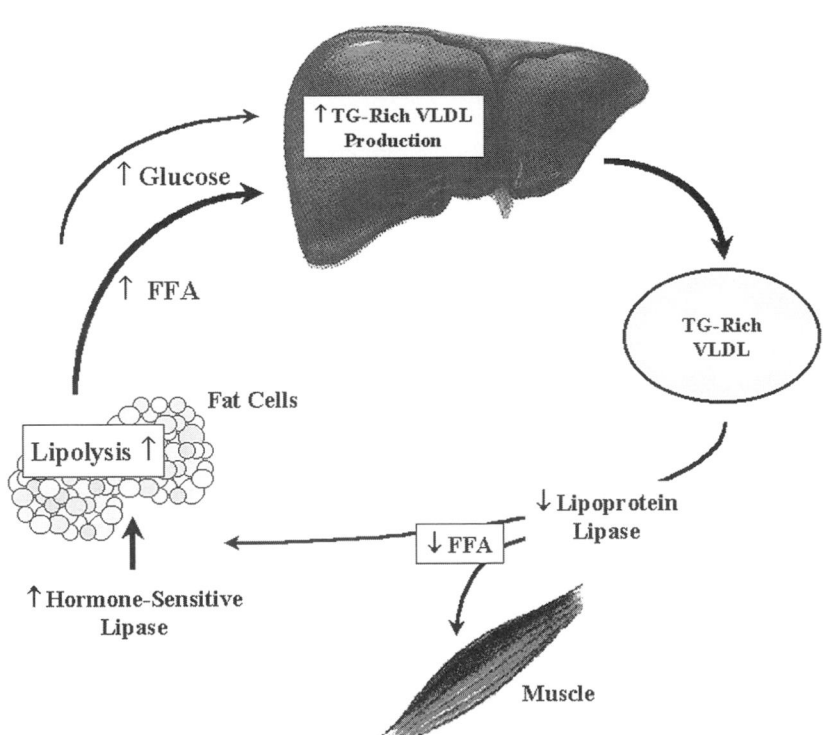

FIG. 19–7. Mechanism of increased very low-density lipoprotein (VLDL)-triglyceride in diabetes: in the setting of insulin deficiency or insulin resistance, greater rates of glucose and free fatty acids (FFAs) flux to the liver lead to enhanced VLDL production and secretion. Decreased lipoprotein lipase activity contributes to the accumulation of these particles in the plasma.

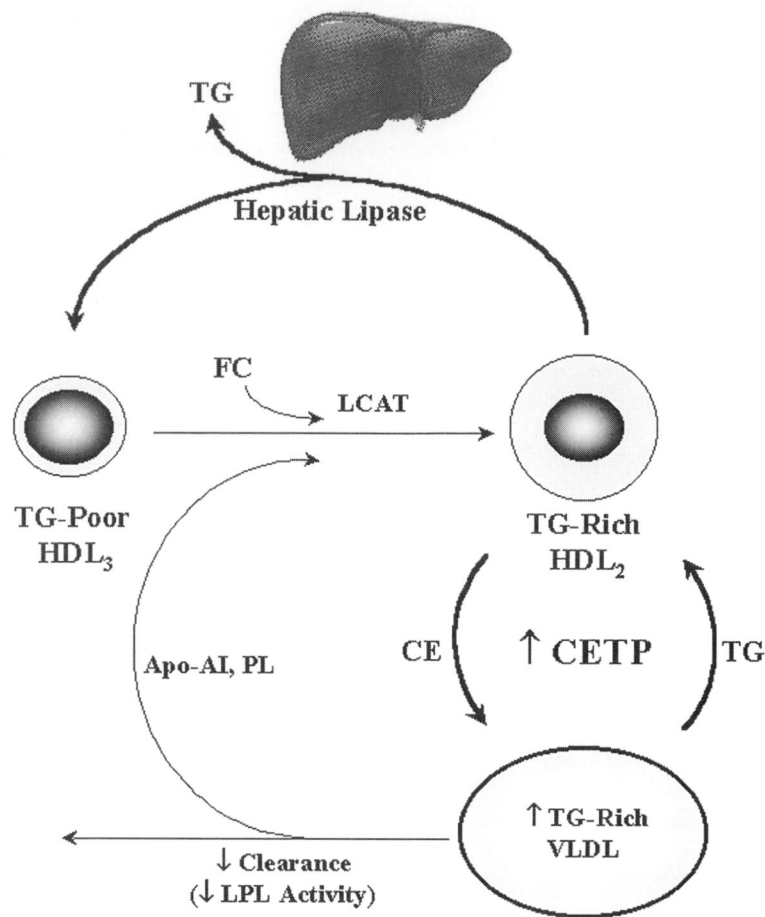

FIG. 19–8. Mechanism of decreased high-density lipoprotein (HDL) in diabetes: the rate of HDL_2 formation is dependent on the rate of flux of surface components from lipolysis of triglyceride (TG)-rich lipoproteins. Inefficient lipoprotein lipase (LPL)–mediated triglyceride-rich lipoprotein catabolism reduces the rate of HDL_2 formation. Excess of triglyceride-rich lipoproteins enhances cholesteryl ester transfer protein (CETP), resulting in the formation of HDL_2, which is a triglyceride-rich particle that efficiently interacts with hepatic lipase. The result is the predominance of the small and dense HDL_3 in patients with diabetes. A similar mechanism governs the predominance of small, dense species of low-density lipoprotein (LDL). Apo-AI, apolipoprotein A-I; CE, cholesteryl ester; FC, free cholesterol; LCAT, lecithin cholesterol acyltransferase; PL, phospholipids.

decrease in density of HDL particles, leading to the conversion of preexisting HDL_3 (triglyceride depleted) to HDL_2.

In diabetes, decreased HDL synthesis is related to the decreased LPL activity because the rate of HDL_2 formation is dependent on the rate of flux of surface components from lipolysis of triglyceride-rich lipoprotein (Fig. 19–8). When LPL-mediated VLDL catabolism is inefficient, less surface material is transferred to HDL, impairing HDL formation.

Increased catabolism of HDL in diabetes also occurs because increased secretion of VLDL into plasma promotes the transfer of triglycerides from these lipoproteins to HDLs in exchange for cholesteryl ester. This exchange occurs in plasma and is facilitated by CETP, generating a triglyceride-enriched (and cholesteryl ester–depleted) HDL_2. This particle is highly susceptible to catabolism by hepatic triglyceride lipase (HTGL), an enzyme found primarily on ECs of hepatic sinusoids (136,141). HTGL has both triglyceride hydrolase and phospholipase activity, and generates smaller

HDL_3 particles, which are depleted in triglycerides and phospholipids (Fig. 19–8).

Low-Density Lipoprotein Metabolism in Diabetes

In diabetes, although the absolute number of LDL particles is normal, alterations in LDL clearance and susceptibility to oxidative modification result in an increase in LDL atherogenic potential. The composition of LDL particles is altered, resulting in a preponderance of small, triglyceride-enriched and cholesterol-depleted particles (132–134). The formation of small, dense LDLs in diabetes occurs in a similar fashion to the increased formation of small and dense HDL_3, as described earlier. CETP mediates the exchange of triglyceride from VLDL for cholesteryl ester in LDL. If sufficient LDL cholesteryl ester is replaced by triglyceride from VLDL, then when the particle comes into contact with hepatic lipase, hydrolysis of newly acquired triglyceride in LDL and HDL by HTGL in turn decreases the size of LDL particles (142). The symmetry of the mechanisms for the formation of small, dense species of LDL and HDL (Fig. 19–8) helps to explain why low HDL levels and a preponderance of small, dense LDLs are associated with diabetes and the metabolic syndrome and why HDL cholesterol level is strongly correlated with LDL size (142).

Small, dense LDL has been associated with CHD risk independent of the absolute concentrations of LDL cholesterol or other CHD risk factors (131). These particles are more susceptible to oxidative modification, are particularly prone to induce endothelial dysfunction, and easily penetrate the arterial wall (see Chapter 8).

Low-Density Lipoprotein Glycosylation

The glycosylation process (see "Advanced Glycosylation End Products") occurs both on the apoprotein B (143) and phospholipid (144) components of LDL. Clinical studies have shown an increased level of AGEs on LDL obtained from diabetics as compared with normal individuals (144,145). Glycosylation of LDL apoB occurs mainly on a positively charged lysine residue within the putative LDL receptor–binding domain, which is essential for the recognition of LDL by the LDL receptor (145). LDL glycosylation increases with glucose levels and impairs LDL receptor–mediated LDL clearance (Fig. 19–9).

Another atherogenic effect of glycation is to increase LDL susceptibility to oxidative modification. Advanced glycosylation of an amine-containing phospholipids component of LDL is accompanied by progressive oxidative modification of unsaturated fatty acid residues (144) (Fig. 19–9). Thus, glycation confers increased susceptibility of LDL to oxidative modification (146,147), which is considered a critical step in its atherogenicity.

DIABETES AS A PROTHROMBOTIC STATE

The coagulation and fibrinolytic systems are especially important in atherothrombosis because thrombotic occlusion plays a vital role in the development of clinical events. In most cases, the fundamental mechanism in the development of potentially life-threatening events such as unstable angina or MI is thrombosis arising at sites of plaque disruption (148). Not all disruptions of atherothrombotic plaques result in clinically apparent or symptomatic events. Thus, both local and systemic *thrombogenic risk factors* at the time of plaque disruption may determine the degree of thrombus formation and, hence, the clinical outcome. Diabetes is characterized by a variety of individual alterations in the coagulation and fibrinolytic systems that combine to produce a prothrombotic state (Table 19–6). Although it remains possible that some of the hemostatic abnormalities in diabetes are partly markers of underlying vascular disease rather than primary abnormalities, the clotting and fibrinolytic profile of patients with diabetes bears a striking similarity to that of patients at high risk for a cardiovascular event (158) (Table 19–6).

Platelet Aggregation

Platelets from patients with diabetes exhibit enhanced adhesiveness and hyperaggregability in response to both strong (e.g., thrombin and thromboxane A$_2$) and weak (e.g., adenosine diphosphate [ADP], epinephrine, and collagen) agonists (149). Shear-induced platelet adhesion and aggregation is increased in patients with diabetes (159). Platelet hypersensitivity is more evident in patients with diabetes with vascular complications. However, it is also observed in patients with newly diagnosed diabetes, sug-

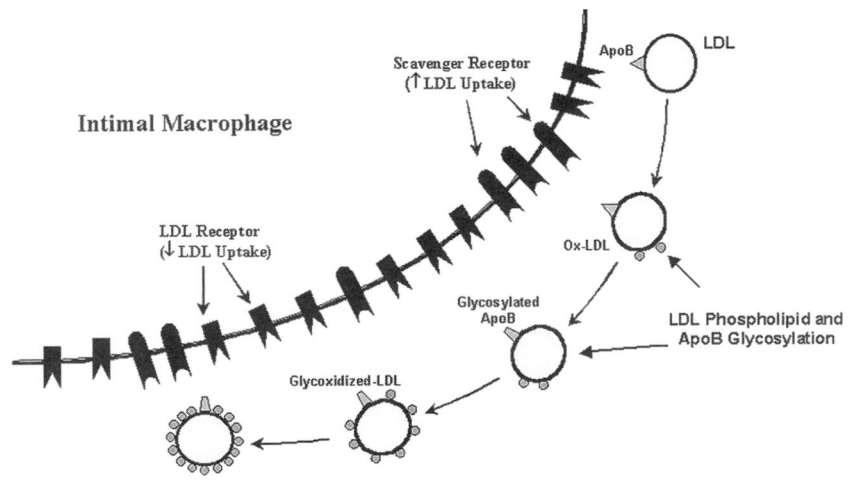

FIG. 19–9. Potential mechanisms by which low-density lipoprotein (LDL) glycosylation increases its atherogenicity. Advanced glycosylation of the phospholipid component of LDL is accompanied by the progressive oxidative modification of unsaturated fatty acid residues. Glycosylation of LDL apolipoprotein B (apoB) reduces its recognition by the LDL receptor.

TABLE 19–6. *Coagulation and fibrinolytic abnormalities of prognostic significance in diabetes*

Factor	Prognostic significance	Diabetes effect
Platelet hyper-activity	Spontaneous platelet aggregation *in vitro* predicts coronary events and mortality in patients surviving MI	Platelet hyperaggregability in response to agonists (149) and increased fractions of circulating activated platelets (150)
vWF	Increased concentrations of endothelium-derived vWF reflect endothelial perturbation (21,151) and is associated with subsequent MI (151)	Increased vWF levels, especially in the presence of vascular complications and endothelial dysfunction (21) or insulin resistance; confers a high risk for cardiovascular events
Fibrinogen	High fibrinogen levels associated with increased risk for reinfarction and death (151)	Increased in patients with diabetes
Factor VII	High levels of factor VII coagulant activity is associated with increased risk for coronary events	Increased and correlates with glycemic control and microalbuminuria
PAI-1	Reduced fibrinolytic capacity caused by increased plasma PAI-1 levels is predisposed to MI in patients after infarction or in patients with angina (151,152)	Increased PAI-1 levels occur as a result of obesity (153,154,155,156) or hyperglycemia (87)
Tissue factor	Expressed in coronary atherothrombotic plaques and may account for the magnitude of the thrombotic responses to rupture of coronary atherothrombotic plaques	AGE-RAGE interaction induces cell surface expression of tissue factor (106,157)

AGE, advanced glycosylation end products; MI, myocardial infarction; PAI-1, plasminogen activator inhibitor 1; RAGE, receptor for advanced glycosylation end products; vWF, von Willebrand factor.

gesting that altered platelet function may be a consequence of metabolic changes secondary to the diabetic state (160). Increased numbers of GPIb (the von Willebrand receptor, to which platelets are exposed at injury sites) and GPIIb/IIIa (the fibrinogen receptor) have been found in patients with diabetes (161). Increased fractions of CD62$^+$/CD63$^+$ (activated) platelets circulate in patients with diabetes in the absence of clinically detectable vascular lesions (150,162).

The mechanism for these abnormalities is not well understood. There is a significant correlation between glucose levels and platelet-dependent thrombosis (163). Increased oxidant stress might lead to enhanced generation of certain isoprostanes, which induce platelet activation (164). In addition, hyperglycemia increases mitochondrial ROS generation in human platelets, leading to increased platelet aggregation through the activation of intracellular signaling systems (165).

Alterations in Coagulation Factors

The von Willebrand factor (vWF) is synthesized and secreted by ECs, and high circulating levels of vWF are considered a marker of endothelial dysfunction. In patients with diabetes plasma concentrations of vWF are increased and are closely associated with the presence of vascular complications and endothelial dysfunction (21). Epidemiologic data demonstrated a relation between plasma vWF and the insulin resistance syndrome (166).

Fibrinogen levels are often increased in diabetes, and this increase is associated with poor glycemic control (167). However, the association between diabetes and increased fibrinogen may be partly related to the presence of vascular disease at the clinical or preclinical stage (168). Fibrinogen levels may decrease with intensive insulin therapy (169), although this finding is not consistent, and transient increase of fibrinogen with intensive insulin therapy has been reported (170).

Plasma factor VII levels have been shown to increase in healthy subjects after a meal (171). Plasma levels of factor VII increase in healthy subjects in response to moderate hyperglycemia, but not during hyperinsulinemia with euglycemia (172). Plasma factor VII levels decrease with improved glycemic control (169).

Altered Fibrinolysis in Diabetes

The intensity of endogenous fibrinolysis depends on a dynamic equilibrium involving plasminogen activators, primarily tissue-type plasminogen activator (t-PA), and inhibitors. The principal physiologic inhibitor of t-PA is PAI-1. Attenuated fibrinolysis caused by increased PAI-1 activity has been associated with increased risk for MI in patients with established CAD (152).

Reduced plasma fibrinolytic activity caused by increased PAI-1 levels is a characteristic feature of insulin resistance and strongly correlates with body mass index (BMI) and visceral accumulation of body fat, rather than with diabetes per se. This association probably represents production of PAI-1 by adipocytes (see "Obesity and Atherothrombosis"). Interventions that lower insulin resistance, such as weight loss, are invariably accompanied with a reduction in plasma PAI-1 concentrations (173). Hyperglycemia can also increase PAI-1 levels because it stimulates transcription of

PAI-1 gene caused by activation of the hexosamine pathway (87) (Fig. 19–4).

ARTERIAL STIFFNESS AND DIASTOLIC DYSFUNCTION IN DIABETES

Part of the normal aging process of humans and other long-lived species is the gradual decrease in the elasticity of the cardiovascular system, which leads to increased arterial and left ventricular stiffness and, consequently, to systolic hypertension and diastolic dysfunction. Arterial stiffness increases systolic pressure, decreases diastolic pressure, and increases pulse pressure at any given mean pressure, and it is considered necessary for the development of isolated systolic hypertension. The normal aging process is known to depress left ventricular diastolic performance, and heart failure caused by diastolic dysfunction increases dramatically with age.

Patients with diabetes manifest increased arterial stiffness at a relatively young age compared with individuals without diabetes (174). Many studies have shown that patients with diabetes manifest diminished left ventricular compliance in the presence of normal left ventricular systolic function (175–177). Although most of these patients are asymptomatic, subclinical diastolic dysfunction becomes clinically important in the presence of myocardial ischemia (158,178), and contributes to the fourfold to eightfold increase in risk for congestive heart failure (CHF) in patients with diabetes (179). Thus, compared with individuals who do not have diabetes, patients with diabetes manifest premature development of both arterial stiffness and diminished left ventricular compliance. These observations suggest that the mechanism underling the loss of vascular and myocardial compliance with normal aging is accelerated in the presence of diabetes.

The ability of advanced glycosylation to form protein–protein cross-links on collagen *in vivo* is a key determinant in the pathogenesis of the reduced vascular and myocardial compliance observed with aging and diabetes (Fig. 19–10). The amount of cross-linked collagen peptides formed increase as a function of both time and glucose concentration (54). In contrast to normal cross-links within normal collagen, which occur only at two discrete sites at the N-terminal and C-terminal ends of the molecule, AGEs form cross-links throughout the collagen molecule (54). The result is loss of elasticity and flexibility and increased brittleness. In addition, AGE-mediated crosslinks may confer a high resistance to enzymatic proteolysis and a decrease in degradation rate. The balance between synthesis and hydrolysis of collagen would thus be shifted in favor of larger amounts of collagen in tissues such as the arterial wall and myocardium.

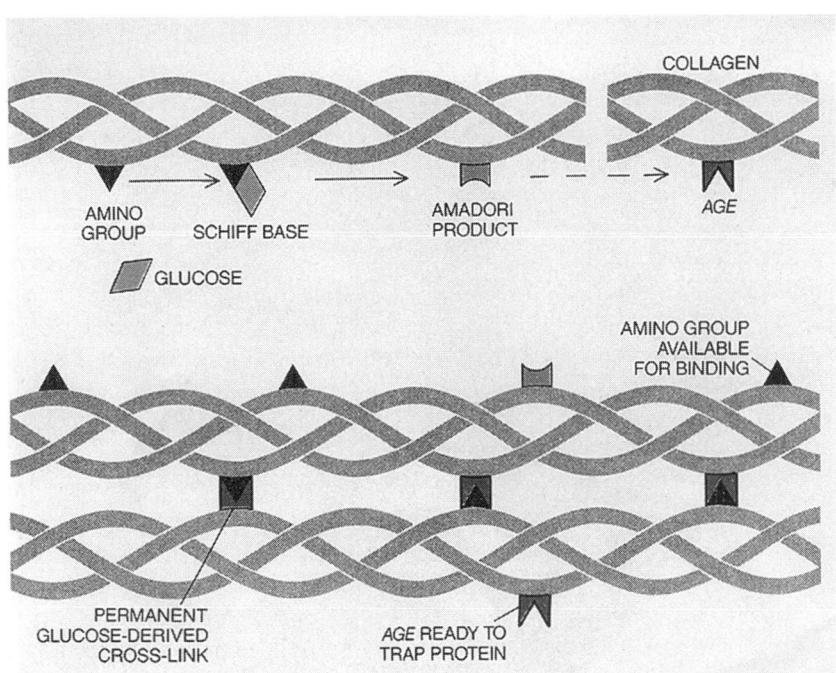

FIG. 19–10. Schematic description of the formation of collagen cross-links. Glucose attaches to an amino group (NH$_2$) of a protein (*top*), such as collagen to form a Schiff base, which subsequently transforms itself into an Amadori product (see Fig. 19–1 for chemical structure). The latter can pass through several incompletely understood steps (*broken arrows*) to become an advanced glycosylation end product (AGE). AGEs can react with free amino groups on an adjacent protein to form cross-links (*bottom*). Cross-linking can lead to decreased compliance of large vessels and of the myocardium. (Reproduced from Cerami A, Vlassara H, Brownlee M. Glucose and aging. *Sci Am* 1987;256:90–96, with permission.)

Aminoguanidine, an inhibitor of AGE formation, prevents age-related decrease in arterial compliance in rats (180). In addition, aminoguanidine retards or prevents the development of diabetes-related decline in arterial (181) and myocardial (182) compliance. Experiments using aminoguanidine provided important evidence supporting the AGE hypothesis with regard to vascular and myocardial stiffness in diabetes and aging. However, the limitation of aminoguanidine and other AGE formation inhibitors is that they cannot affect preexisting AGE cross-linking. In contrast, studies have used the newly developed AGE "breaker" compound (ALT-711) to demonstrate that such agents have the potential to improve existing vascular and myocardial stiffness. In animals with preexisting age- and diabetes-related abnormalities in vascular tissue mechanical properties, ALT-711 improved large vessel (183,184) and myocardial (185) compliance. Preliminary studies have shown the efficacy of ALT-711 in humans (186).

THE PATIENT WITH DIABETES WITH AN ACUTE ISCHEMIC EVENT

Acute coronary syndromes (ACSs) represent a major cause of death in patients with diabetes. Whether presenting with unstable angina (187,188), acute MI (158), or cardiogenic shock (189), patients with diabetes have a greater mortality in the acute phase and worse long-term outcome.

The fundamental mechanism in the development of acute coronary events such as unstable angina or MI is thrombosis arising at sites of unstable plaque disruption (see Chapter 31). Diabetes is associated with multiple alterations that promote vascular inflammation, potentially leading to plaque instability and disruption. Furthermore, the prothrombotic state associated with diabetes increases the likelihood that plaque disruption will result in a clinically apparent or symptomatic event. Indeed, greater proportions of ulcerated plaque (94% vs. 60%) and intracoronary thrombi (94% vs. 55%) are observed by angioscopy in patients with diabetes presenting with unstable angina (190). Coronary tissue obtained from culprit lesions of patients with diabetes and unstable angina or MI exhibit a larger content of lipid-rich atheroma and macrophage infiltration and a greater incidence of coronary thrombus, which occupies a larger area (191).

Unstable Angina in Patients with Diabetes

Of all patients presenting with non–ST-segment elevation ACS, 20% to 25% have diabetes (187,192). Diabetes is an important risk factor for an adverse outcome in this setting, with greater 30-day (188,193) and 1-year mortality rates, as well as greater readmissions with unstable angina (194). In a metaanalysis of six large-scale ACS trials, patients with diabetes had a twofold greater mortality rate (188). Studies suggest that therapy with platelet glycoprotein IIb/IIIa inhibitors may improve the outcome of patients with diabetes

and ACS, particularly in those undergoing percutaneous coronary intervention (188,195,196).

Acute Myocardial Infarction

The in-hospital mortality rate from MI in patients with diabetes is 1.5-to 2-fold greater than in patients without diabetes (158,178,197–200). In the Global Utilization of Streptokinase and t-PA for Occluded Coronary Arteries (GUSTO)-I trial, the 30-day mortality rate was greatest among patients with diabetes treated with insulin (12.5%) compared with noninsulin-treated diabetic (9.7%) and nondiabetic (6.2%) patients (197). Women with diabetes have a particularly poor prognosis, with an almost twofold increase in mortality compared with men with diabetes (178,199).

The excess in-hospital mortality rate associated with diabetes correlates primarily with an increased incidence of CHF (158,178,199), although increased reinfarction, infarct extension, and recurrent ischemia also are more common among patients with diabetes (178,199). Diabetes also is a risk factor for cardiogenic shock in the setting of acute ischemic syndromes (201).

CHF and cardiogenic shock are more common and more severe in patients with diabetes than would be predicted from the size of the index infarction (158,198). Indeed, although CHF develops at twice the rate in patients with than in patients without diabetes, there is no evidence that diabetes is associated with larger infarctions, and systolic function is similar in patients with and without diabetes (158,202). These observations led to the suggestion that preexisting diastolic dysfunction (see "Arterial Stiffness and Diastolic Dysfunction in Diabetes") is a major culprit of the congestive symptoms (178,202). Interestingly, patients with diabetes may develop CHF in the post-MI period with less ventricular enlargement than patients without diabetes. This decreased ability for ventricular remodeling may result in increased filling pressures with the same degree of contractile loss (202).

Other contributing mechanisms to the worse clinical outcome of patients with diabetes in the acute phase of infarction include: (a) the diffuse nature of coronary atherothrombosis in diabetes, (b) reduced ability to develop collateral blood vessels in the presence of CAD (203), and (c) an abnormal pattern of exogenous substrate use in the setting of ischemia and in the postreperfusion period leading to increased oxygen consumption by the myocardium, reduced contractility, and reduced myocardial preservation.

Patients with diabetes who survive the acute phase of MI have high late mortality rates, which are mainly related to recurrent MI and the development of new CHF (158,198,204).

Medical Therapy in Patients with Diabetes with Myocardial Infarction

Patients with diabetes treated with fibrinolytic agents benefit by the same reduction in mortality rate as patients without diabetes (158,199,205). Importantly, no increase in serious

The protective effects of CABG are probably related to the increased restenosis rates after angioplasty in diabetes and incomplete revascularization associated with multivessel angioplasty (223,243). Complete revascularization is accomplished almost exclusively through CABG. In the BARI study population, 3.1 grafts were placed per patient undergoing CABG, whereas the mean number of successfully treated lesions in the PTCA group was 2.0 (215). Together with the high restenosis rate, it is likely that a greater proportion of the myocardium remains unrevascularized in patients with diabetes. The impact of incomplete revascularization may be even more severe in view of the more diffuse and distal CAD (213,215), poor collateral development (203), and microcirculatory dysfunction in diabetes.

THERAPY

Prevention of cardiovascular disease in patients with diabetes requires intensified multifactorial intervention comprising behavioral modification and pharmacologic therapies aimed at several modifiable risk factors (244).

Dyslipidemia

Nonpharmacologic strategies to treat dyslipidemia in patients with diabetes include dietary modification (similar to those recommended by the NCEP), weight loss, physical exercise, and improved glycemic control (245). In patients with type 1 diabetes, optimal glycemic control should result in normal or less than normal lipoprotein levels and should prevent the atherogenic state associated with lipoprotein glycosylation. Improved diabetic control in type 2 diabetes is beneficial, but it is not always associated with reversal of lipoprotein abnormalities. Improved glycemic control using sulfonylurea, insulin (20), metformin (246), or thiazolidinediones (e.g., Pioglitazone, Rosiglitazone) (247) therapy often causes a substantial reduction (20–50%) in VLDL triglyceride levels. The magnitude of improvement in triglycerides generally correlates with the change in glucose levels rather than the mode of therapy. However, agents that improve insulin sensitivity such as metformin (246) and thiazolidinediones (247) lead to greater decline of triglyceride compared with sulfonylurea. The effect of improved glycemic control on HDL is more variable and often results in only a small increase (3–4 mg/dL) in HDL levels (20). During therapy with thiazolidinediones, LDL cholesterol usually increases (~10%), without an increase in apoB and with an increase in LDL particle size and a decrease in the propensity to oxidative modifications, indicating a possible antiatherogenic effect (248).

Antihyperlipidemic drug therapy in patients with diabetes is similar to patients who do not have diabetes (see Chapter 11) with several specific considerations. Some publications have argued against the relevance of the traditional classification to primary and secondary CHD prevention in the setting of diabetes (13,20). The rationale for this approach stems from both the high event rates in patients with dia-

betes without clinical evidence of CAD (presumably because of the high rates of subclinical atherothrombosis) (20), as well as the worse prognosis in patients with diabetes who have had a clinical event compared with subjects without diabetes (158). These considerations led to the recommendation that LDL cholesterol should be decreased to less than 100 mg/dL in patients with diabetes who do not have prior CAD (13,20,249,250).

The first priority of pharmacologic therapy is to decrease LDL cholesterol to a target goal of less than 100 mg/dL, followed by an emphasis on HDL cholesterol, and lastly on triglyceride levels (251) (Table 19–7). 3-Hydroxy-3-methylglutaryl coenzyme A (HMG-CoA) reductase inhibitors are highly effective in decreasing cholesterol levels in patients with type 2 diabetes in whom the principal finding is increased LDL cholesterol levels. In three secondary prevention studies using HMG-CoA reductase inhibitors, patients with diabetes achieved significant reductions in coronary and cerebrovascular events (204,252,253). A primary prevention study using statins showed a similar trend of reduced events (253).

The fibric acid derivatives are effective in the treatment of hypertriglyceridemia in patients with diabetes. These agents decrease VLDL levels, increase HDL, and can increase LDL particle size in patients with hypertriglyceridemia with small, dense LDL particles. Fenofibrate has been shown to reduce the angiographic progression of CAD in type 2 diabetes (254). The Veterans Affairs High-Density Lipoprotein Cholesterol Intervention Trial randomized 2,531 patients with CHD (25% of whom had diabetes) with low HDL cholesterol to gemfibrozil or placebo (255). Treatment with gemfibrozil over 5 years increased HDL 6% and reduced 22% of major coronary artery events, without decreasing LDL cholesterol.

Fibric acid derivatives do not adversely affect glucose metabolism. In patients with normal triglyceride levels, these drugs decrease LDL cholesterol by 5% to 15%. However, in patients with hypertriglyceridemia, the decrease in triglyceride levels is frequently accompanied by an increase in LDL cholesterol levels (256). This increase probably reflects the elimination of small, dense LDL particles characteristic of the hypertriglyceridemic patients, resulting in less atherogenic LDL cholesterol.

Fibric acid derivatives such as gemfibrozil should not be initiated alone in patients with diabetes who have undesirable levels of both triglyceride and LDL cholesterol. Fenofibrate, a recently approved fibric acid derivative, may have greater LDL-decreasing effects and may be useful in patients with combined hyperlipidemia. This agent can be used in a patients with HDL level less than 40 mg/dL and LDL level between 100 and 129 mg/dL (251).

Nicotinic acid is the most effective drug in increasing HDL levels in patients with hypertriglyceridemia, and it can increase particle size in patients with small, dense LDL particles. The use of nicotinic acid has been discouraged in patients with diabetes because of possible deterioration in

TABLE 19–7. *Standards of medical care in patients with diabetes*

Indications for initial treatment and goals for adult patients with diabetes with hypertension

	Systolic	Diastolic
Goal (mm Hg)	<130	<80
Behavioral therapy alone (maximum 3 months), then add pharmacologic treatment	130–139	80–89
Behavioral therapy and pharmacologic treatment	≥140	≥90

Target lipid levels and treatment priorities for adult patients with diabetes[a]

Order of priorities
I. LDL cholesterol decreasing
II. HDL cholesterol increasing
III. Triglyceride decreasing

Target lipid levels	
LDL cholesterol	<100 mg/dL (2.6 mmol/L)
LDL cholesterol	Men: >45 mg/dL (1.15 mmol/L) Women: >55 mg/dL (1.40 mmol/L)
Triglycerides	<150 mg/dL (1.7 mmol/L)

Glycemic control for nonpregnant individuals with diabetes[b]

	Normal	Goal	Additional action suggested[c]
Average preprandial glucose (mg/dL)	<110	90–130	<90/>150
Average bedtime glucose (mg/dL)	<120	10–150	<110/<180
HbA$_{1C}$ (%)	<6	<7	>8

[a]The recent National Cholesterol Education Program Adult Treatment Panel III guidelines suggest that in patients with triglycerides 200 mg/dL or greater the "non-HDL cholesterol" be calculated with a goal being less than 130 mg/dL.

[b]Values calibrated to plasma glucose. Whole blood values are 10 mg/dL lower.

[c]Values greater than or less than these levels are not "goals" nor are they "acceptable" in most patients; they are an indication for a significant change in the treatment plan. A$_{1C}$ is referenced to a nondiabetic range 4.0% to 6.0% (mean 5.0%, SD 0.5%).

Data from Grundy SM, Benjamin IJ, Burke GL, et al. Diabetes and cardiovascular disease: a statement for healthcare professionals from the American Heart Association. *Circulation* 1999;100:1134–1146; Standards of medical care for patients with diabetes mellitus. *Diabetes Care* 2002;25:213–229; Executive Summary of the Third Report of The National Cholesterol Education Program (NCEP) Expert Panel on Detection, Evaluation, and Treatment of High Blood Cholesterol in Adults (Adult Treatment Panel III). *JAMA* 2001;285:2486–2497; and Arauz-Pacheco C, Parrott MA, Raskin P. The treatment of hypertension in adult patients with diabetes. *Diabetes Care* 2002; 25:134–147.

glycemic control (20) secondary to the induction of insulin resistance. However, at dosages of 3.0 or less g per day niacin produced a 8% reduction in LDL, 23% reduction in triglycerides, and 29% increase in HDL level, whereas increasing HbA$_{1C}$ by only 0.3% (257). Similar results have been shown for low doses (1,000 or 1,500 mg/day) of ex-

tended-release niacin (258). Therefore, niacin therapy may be considered as an alternative to statin drugs or fibrates in patients with diabetes in whom these agents are not tolerated or in whom they fail to sufficiently correct hypertriglyceridemia or low HDL (257). The combination of statins with nicotinic acid is extremely effective in modifying diabetic dyslipidemia, but may significantly worsen hyperglycemia. Therefore, low doses of nicotinic acid (≤2 g/day) should be used in this situation, with frequent glucose monitoring (251).

Hypertension

The prevalence of hypertension in the diabetic population is 1.5 to 3 times greater than that of the nondiabetic age-matched group (259). The combined presence of hypertension and diabetes considerably accelerates the development of both macrovascular and microvascular diabetic complications. However, the most significant manifestation of this combination of diseases is that they confer a greater risk for ischemic heart disease, stroke, and peripheral vascular disease in affected individuals. Serious cardiovascular events are more than twice as likely in patients with both diabetes and hypertension than in patients with either disease alone (10). The high cardiovascular risk associated with the coexistence of hypertension and diabetes led the Joint National Committee on Prevention, Detection, Evaluation, and Treatment of High Blood Pressure to include hypertensive patients with diabetes in the same risk group as hypertensive patients who have clinically manifest cardiovascular disease (260). In addition, because of the high cardiovascular risk associated with blood pressure 130/80 mm Hg or greater in patients with diabetes, this value is considered to be the cutoff point for defining hypertension, rather than 140/90 mm Hg, as in the general population.

Randomized controlled trials have shown impressive benefits of reducing blood pressure to less than 130/80 mm Hg (261,262). The United Kingdom Prospective Diabetes Study (UKPDS) indicated that among patients with hypertension and type 2 diabetes, aggressive reduction of blood pressure (mean 144/82 vs. 154/87 mmHg) either with ACE inhibitors or a β-blocker provides greater protection against death from cardiovascular causes and major nonfatal events than did less aggressive therapy (261). A similar benefit was observed in the Hypertension Optimal Treatment (HOT) study among patients with hypertension with diabetes (n = 1,501, representing the largest calcium antagonist trial in patients with diabetes), who were randomly assigned to achieve diastolic pressures of 80, 85, or 90 mm Hg. A difference of only 4.1 mm Hg in diastolic pressure was associated with significant reductions of 60%, 43%, and 77% in coronary events, stroke, and mortality, respectively (262).

The American Diabetes Association has incorporated these principles for the treatment of hypertension in the presence of diabetes and have included a more aggressive program of blood pressure reduction, aiming for a target of less than 130/80 mm Hg in patients with diabetes (249,259) (Table 19–7). In addition, a target of 125/75 mm Hg is recommended in patients with greater than 1 g per day proteinuria (260). In attempting to achieve this goal, it is important to emphasize that hypertension control usually requires two or three antihypertensive agents in patients with diabetes (261,263,264).

Pharmacologic Therapy of Hypertension in Patients with Diabetes

Current evidence suggests that, for the prevention of cardiovascular events, ACE inhibitors (263,265), diuretics (266), β-adrenergic blockers (264), and calcium antagonists (267) effectively reduce mortality and morbidity in patients with diabetes with hypertension. However, there is no clear proof that one class of drugs is better than another (259,268,269). Because of the large number of studies in patients with diabetes demonstrating improvement in both microvascular and macrovascular outcomes, it is now an established practice to begin antihypertensive drug therapy in patients with diabetes with an ACE inhibitor even in the absence of microalbuminuria (259). Data also indicate that angiotensin II receptor blockers (ARBs) can be considered equal to ACE inhibitors in patients with type 2 diabetes (270).

Thiazides are often effective antihypertensive agents in diabetes, in which the total body sodium is increased and the extracellular volume is expanded. These agents are considered an appropriate choice for a second or third drug (259). Because in the UKPDS no difference was found between atenolol and captopril in improving multiple diabetes-related end points (264), β-blockers are also an appropriate choice for a second drug.

Although some studies suggest that calcium channel blockers (CCBs) are inferior to ACE inhibitors (263), these agents contribute to improvements in outcomes when combined with ACE inhibitors to achieve low-targeted blood pressure (265) and even as monotherapy (262,267). Therefore, CCBs can be used when ACE inhibitors, ARBs, or β-blockers are not tolerated or are contraindicated or when a second or third drug is required (259). It is important to emphasize that aggressive blood pressure reduction may be more important than the specific drug regimen being used (259).

Glycemic Control

Glycemic control is fundamental to the management of diabetes. Prospective, randomized, controlled studies have shown that achieving glycemic control is associated with decreased rate of retinopathy, nephropathy, and neuropathy (271). The effects of improved glycemic control on cardiovascular outcomes are less impressive.

In the Diabetes Control and Complications Trial (DCCT) the number of combined major macrovascular events was almost twice as high in the conventionally treated group as in the intensive treatment group. However, the differences were not statistically significant ($p = 0.08$) because patients participating in this study were young and were early in the course of their disease (46). Data from the Stockholm Diabetes Intervention Study indicate that tight control retards the development of atherothrombosis in patients with type 1 diabetes as measured by the development of carotid intima media thickening (272).

The UKPDS was a prospective, randomized, intervention trial aimed at determining whether patients with noninsulin-dependent diabetes mellitus (NIDDM) can obtain clinical benefit from intensive glycemic control. In this study, 3,867 patients with newly diagnosed NIDDM were randomly assigned to intensive treatment policy or to a conventional treatment policy. Compared with the conventional treatment group, the intensive treatment group demonstrated a 16% risk reduction ($p = 0.052$) for fatal and nonfatal MI (271). However, epidemiologic analysis of the UKPDS cohort showed a statistically significant effect of HbA_{1C} decline with an approximate 14% reduction in all-cause mortality and MI for every 1% reduction in HbA_{1C} (273). The current recommendations of the American Diabetes Association for glycemic control are summarized in Table 19–7.

Current approaches to achieve glycemic control are beyond the scope of this chapter and are discussed in detail elsewhere (274,275). However, the insulin-sensitizing thiazolidinediones are agonists of the nuclear receptor peroxisome proliferator-activated receptor-γ (PPAR-γ) that in vitro can decrease proinflammatory functions of macrophages and smooth muscle cells (276). Thus, these agent may have direct effects on key processes in atherothrombosis.

Prevention of Type 2 Diabetes

Several randomized controlled trials have shown that the onset of type 2 diabetes can be prevented or delayed with lifestyle modifications or pharmacologic interventions (277–279). During an average follow-up of approximately 3 years, a 25% to 58% relative reduction in the incidence of diabetes has been demonstrated with lifestyle changes (278, 279), the biguanide metformin (278), and the α-glucosidase inhibitor acarbose (277). Although not designed to determine directly whether there was also cardiovascular benefit, a reduction in the magnitude of some cardiovascular risk factors was observed (279).

In the Diabetes Prevention Program, metformin was about half as effective as diet and exercise in delaying the onset of diabetes. This effect was obtained with modest weight loss (5–10% of body weight) and modest physical activity (30 min daily). The greater benefit of weight loss and physical inactivity strongly suggests that lifestyle modification should be the first choice to prevent or delay diabetes (280). Currently, there is insufficient evidence to support the use of drug therapy as a substitute for, or routinely used in addition to, lifestyle modifications to prevent diabetes (280).

Clinical trials suggest that blockade of the renin-angiotensin system (281,282), either by inhibiting the ACE or by blocking the angiotensin type 1 receptor (283), may substantially reduce the risk for type 2 diabetes. In the Heart Outcomes Prevention Evaluation (HOPE) trial, there was a 34% reduction in relative risk for the development of type 2 diabetes in the ramipril group (282). Currently, several large studies are underway to further explore the relation between renin-angiotensin system (RAS) blockade and the development of type 2 diabetes.

In the West of Scotland Coronary Prevention Study, assignment to pravastatin therapy resulted in a 30% reduction in the risk for development of diabetes (284). The mechanisms for the beneficial effects of RAS inhibition and statins on glucose tolerance are unknown, but they may be related to antiinflammatory effects or improved endothelial function.

OBESITY AND ATHEROTHROMBOSIS

The proportion of overweight adults in the United States has been steadily increasing in the past several decades. Currently, most adults in the United States are overweight (>56%), and approximately 1 in 5 are obese (BMI $\geq$ 30 kg/m^2) (285). Each year, an estimated 300,000 adults in the United States die of causes related to obesity (286). Twin studies, analyses of familial aggregation and adoption studies, both indicate that genetic factors have a major role in obesity (287). However, the marked increase in the prevalence of obesity is best explained by behavioral and environmental contributions, and especially diets high in fat and calories and a reduced expenditure of energy in the form of physical activity (288). Importantly, changes in adult prevalence of obesity are reflected by a striking increase in childhood and adolescent weight in both industrialized and developing countries (288–290). The early onset of obesity leads to increased likelihood of obesity in later life (291), as well as an increased prevalence of obesity-related disorders.

The relation between BMI and the incidence of common conditions associated with excess body fat is presented in Figure 19–11. The relation between BMI and risk appears approximately linear for BMI of 30 or less, but increases greatly above this cutoff point. In particular, obesity is associated with the development of type 2 diabetes and CHD (Fig. 19–11). BMI is one of the strongest predictors of diabetes. For every 1-kg increase in body weight, the risk for diabetes increases by 4.5% to 9.0% (285,292). Conversely, a modest weight loss (5%) results in a dramatic reduction in the incidence of diabetes (279).

There is a strong link between obesity and the metabolic syndrome. Therefore, the relation between obesity and CHD is partly indirect and mediated through covariates related to both obesity and CAD. However, obesity independently predicts coronary atherothrombosis (293), coronary events, and coronary mortality (294–296).

Definition of Overweight and Obesity

Body fat is most commonly estimated by using a formula that combines weight and height, because most variation in weight for persons of the same height is because of fat mass (288). A graded classification of overweight and obesity that applies to both men and woman has been proposed by a WHO expert committee (Table 19–8).

Visceral Obesity

The cardiovascular risk factors associated with obesity are closely related to the pattern of distribution of adipose tissue throughout the body. A predominantly abdominal or visceral distribution of body fat is closely associated with insulin resistance and the presence of one or more components of the metabolic syndrome. Upper body obesity correlates better with cardiovascular morbidity and mortality than total adipose tissue mass. In contrast, individuals with comparable amounts of fat distributed in the femoral or gluteal depots (lower body obesity) have a much lower risk for metabolic disturbances and CAD morbidity (297).

Upper body fat includes both the intraabdominal (visceral) and abdominal subcutaneous adipose depots. The visceral fat depot is contained within the body cavity, surrounding the internal organs, and is composed of the mesenteric and the greater and lesser omental depots. Visceral depots represent ~20% and 6% of total body fat in men and women,

TABLE 19–8. *World Health Organization classification of overweight*

Body mass index (kg/m^2)	
Overweight	25.0–29.9
Class I obese	30.0–34.9
Class II obese	35.0–39.9
Class III obese	$\geq$40.0
Waist circumference (cm)[a,b]	
Increased risk	$\geq$102 cm for men and $\geq$89 cm for women
Substantially increased risk	$\geq$94 cm for men and $\geq$88 cm for women

[a]Sex-specific cutoff points for waist circumference may be of guidance in interpreting values in adults with respect to metabolic complications associated with obesity in white individuals. Level 1 (increased risk) is being intended to alert clinicians to potential risk, and level 2 (substantially increased risk) should initiate therapeutic action.
[b]Waist circumference and the ratio of waist circumference to hip circumference are similarly correlated with measures of risk factors for CHD, and neither method has been consistently superior in predicting risk for disease. Thus, because of its greater simplicity, waist circumferences may be the most useful in clinical practice (291).
From World Health Organization Expert Committee. Physical status: the use and interpretation of anthropometry. Geneva: World Health Organization; 1995; WHO Tech Rep serial no. 854; and Clinical Guidelines on the Identification, Evaluation, and Treatment of Overweight and Obesity in Adults—The Evidence Report. National Institutes of Health. *Obes Res* 1998;6[Suppl 2]:51S–209S.

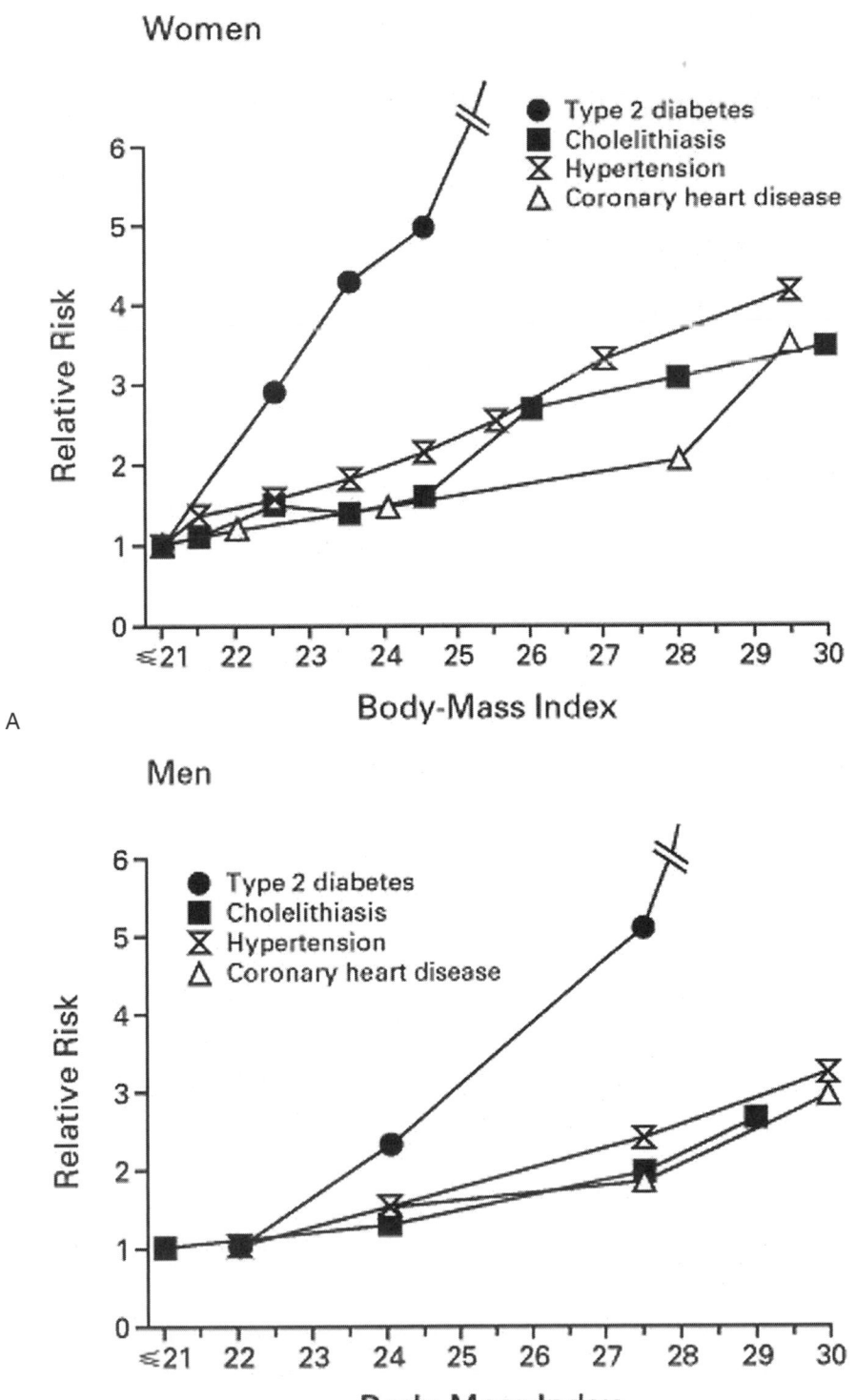

FIG. 19–11. The relation between body mass index up to 30 and the relative risk for type 2 diabetes, hypertension, coronary heart disease, and cholelithiasis. **A:** These relations for women in the Nurses' health study, initially 30 to 55 years of age, who were followed up to 18 years. **B:** The same relations for men in the Health Professionals Follow-up Study, initially 40 to 65 years of age, who were followed up to 10 years. (Reproduced from Willett WC, Dietz WH, Colditz GA. Guidelines for healthy weight. *N Engl J Med* 1999;341:427–434, with permission.)

respectively, and are most closely linked to adverse outcome. The abdominal subcutaneous fat depot is situated immediately below the skin in the abdominal region. In the lower body, all adipose depots are subcutaneous, and the two largest sites of storage are in the gluteal and femoral regions (297).

Waist circumference and waist-to-hip circumference ratio are the most widely used indices of regional adipose tissue distribution and are similarly correlated with risk factors for CHD (298). Waist-to-hip circumference ratio is obtained by measuring the circumference of the abdomen at the smallest part below the rib cage and above the umbilicus, and the gluteal region or hip at the largest circumference at the posterior extension of the buttocks, and taking the ratio. Because neither method has been consistently superior in predicting the risk for disease, waist circumference may be most useful in clinical practice because of its greater simplicity (299).

Sex is the most important determinant of fat distribution. Men tend to have more abdominal fat, giving them the central or "apple" pattern of fat distribution. Women manifest a peripheral fat distribution, with greater amounts of gluteal fat, and thus have larger hip circumferences, giving them the "pear" pattern of fat distribution. Although a predominant abdominal fat distribution is more common in men, both men and women show an increased risk for heart disease when their abdominal fat is increased. Because body fat distribution is more important then obesity per se with regard to its effect on cardiovascular risk, methods of accurate measurement of the amount and distribution of body fat have become an important clinical consideration.

Diabetes

BMI is a dominant predictor of diabetes after adjustment for age. For example, the risk for diabetes increases 5-fold for women with a BMI of 25 kg/m^2, 28-fold for those with a BMI of 30 Kg/m^2, and 93-fold for those with a BMI of 35 kg/m^2 or greater (300). The distribution of fat depots provides additional information on the risk for diabetes: A waist circumference greater than 102 cm (>40 inches) increases the risk for diabetes 3.5-fold after adjusting for BMI (301).

Hypertension

The risk for hypertension appears to parallel the degree of increased body weight. The hypertension associated with obesity is reversible by weight loss and exercise (302). Modest weight losses (i.e., 10% of body weight) improve blood pressure, and in many patients decrease arterial pressure to normal. Blood pressure reduction in response to chronic physical conditioning in obese individuals is greatest in patients with the greatest circulating insulin levels. The mechanisms by which insulin resistance and hyperinsulinemia has been most frequently postulated to increased blood pressure have been discussed earlier in this chapter. Obstructive sleep apnea, which frequently occurs in obesity, may be an important secondary cause of hypertension. This disorder causes increased sympathetic activity that persists even through the waking hours and is associated with altered vascular responses that include increased blood pressure (289).

Dyslipidemia

Obesity often is associated with an atherogenic lipid profile, which is similar to that observed in subjects with the metabolic syndrome, and is more prominent in individuals with abdominal obesity. The most common lipid alteration in obese individuals is the reduction of HDL (289,303). This abnormality is partly dependent on the presence of hypertriglyceridemia and its associated compositional changes in HDL and LDL cholesterol (see "High-Density Lipoprotein Metabolism in Diabetes"). However, reduced HDL cholesterol often is seen in obese subjects with normal triglyceride levels.

In summary, in abdominal obesity, an insulin-resistant state is consistently observed and is a central component of the relation among body fat distribution, plasma lipid abnormalities, hypertension, and CAD. The metabolic alterations observed in abdominal obesity are analogous to those observed in the metabolic syndrome. Assessment of visceral adiposity is more relevant than obesity alone in the evaluation of cardiovascular risk.

Heart Failure in Obesity

There is a progressive increase in the risk for heart failure as BMI increases from the normal range (18.5–24.9 kg/m^2) to values indicating overweight (25.0–29.9 kg/m^2) and obesity ($\geq$30 kg/m^2). In obese subjects, the risk for development of heart failure is approximately twice that in subjects with normal BMI (304). Total blood volume increases with obesity and leads to an increase in left ventricular preload and an increase in resting cardiac output. Volume expansion and increased cardiac output result in increased left ventricular cavity radius, whereas wall thickness remains preserved (eccentric hypertrophy). Left ventricular mass increases in proportion to BMI or the degree that the individual is overweight (288,305). In obese subjects with concomitant hypertension, concentric hypertrophy may also develop. Systolic dysfunction occurs when the left ventricle can no longer adapt to volume overload. Excess of fatty acids can directly damage cardiac myocytes by increasing triglyceride content and the rate of apoptosis (306).

Metabolic Activities of Adipose Tissue

Adipocytes not only have a role in energy storage, but also actively participate in physiologic homeostasis through the secretion hormones, cytokines, and procoagulant factors that are linked to insulin resistance and to the cardiovascular complications of obesity (153,154,307–309) (Fig. 19–12).

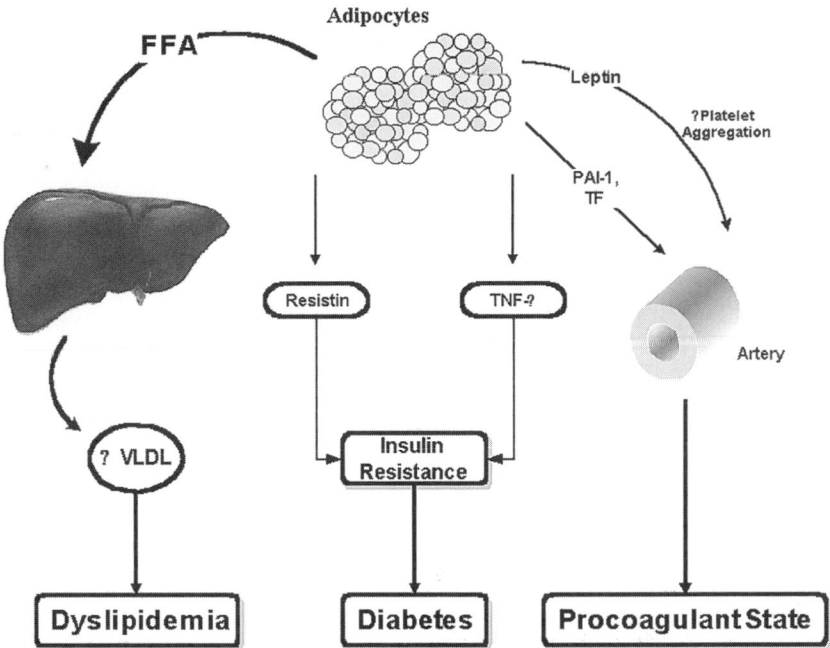

FIG. 19–12. Adipose tissue actively participates in physiologic homeostasis through the secretion hormones, cytokines, and procoagulant factors that contribute to insulin resistance and to the cardiovascular complications of obesity. FFA, free fatty acids; PAI-1, plasminogen activator inhibitor type 1; TF, tissue factor; TNF-α, tumor necrosis factor-α; VLDL, very low-density lipoprotein.

Adipose tissue is functionally heterogeneous and marked regional differences can be found in cell number and size, LPL activity, and basal and catecholamine-stimulated lipolytic (hormone-sensitive lipase) activities. Specifically, the intraabdominal adipose tissue has some metabolic characteristics that are unique in comparison with other adipose tissue. These special features seem to be most pronounced in the regions that are drained by the portal circulation (omental and mesenteric adipose tissue).

Thus, portal adipose tissue has an exceedingly sensitive system for the mobilization of FFA caused by a preponderance of β-adrenergic receptors, little α-adrenergic inhibition, and a low density of insulin receptors. Human adipocytes contain catecholamine receptors able to stimulate (β) and inhibit (α_2) the hormone-sensitive lipase through their effects on adenylate cyclase. The higher lipolytic response to catecholamines in omental compared with subcutaneous or femoral adipose cells is, in part, because of reduced α_2- and increased β-adrenergic receptor density in the former. In addition, subcutaneous abdominal adipocytes are more sensitive then omental adipocytes to the inhibitory action of insulin on the lipolytic process. The high lipolytic activity of omental adipocytes results in a greater flux of FFAs to the liver through the portal circulation. Increased portal FFA concentrations stimulate hepatic triglyceride production and VLDL secretion. In addition, FFAs reduce hepatic extraction of insulin, contributing to increased hepatic gluconeogenesis and systemic hyperinsulinemia (288,297).

Visceral and subcutaneous fat exhibit profound differences in the regulation of the enzyme 11β-hydroxysteroid dehydrogenase type 1, which regulates intracellular conversion of inactive cortisone to hormonally active cortisol and serves as a tissue-specific amplifier of glucocorticoid action. Enzyme activity is greater in omental than in subcutaneous fat, leading to the production of greater local concentrations of cortisol in visceral fat depots (310). Transgenic mice overexpressing 11β-hydroxysteroid dehydrogenase selectively in adipose tissue to an extent similar to that found in adipose tissue from obese humans develop visceral obesity, hyperlipidemia, and insulin-resistant diabetes (309). This suggests that increased adipocyte 11β-hydroxysteroid dehydrogenase activity may contribute to the metabolic alteration observed in subjects with the metabolic syndrome.

Tumor Necrosis Factor-α

TNF-α is expressed in normal adipocytes and is overexpressed in adipocytes from obese individuals (307,311). TNF-α has a direct role in the development of insulin resistance in obesity through its effect on insulin-mediated intracellular signaling pathways. TNF-α impairs insulin-stimulated glucose uptake in muscle and adipose cells, and it suppresses the expression of the insulin-responsive glucose transporter (GLUT-4) that mediates insulin-dependent glucose uptake in these cells (307,311). In addition to its deleterious effects on insulin sensitivity, TNF-α contributes to the hypercoagulable state associated with obesity and the metabolic syndrome.

The increased expression of PAI-1 in adipocytes appears to be partly mediated by chronically increased TNF-α levels (154).

Resistin

A new adipocyte hormone—resistin—has been identified (308). In mice, resistin is expressed predominantly in white adipose tissue and is detectable in serum. In obese mice, serum resistin levels are markedly increased. Neutralization of resistin activity decreases blood glucose level and improves insulin sensitivity in obese, insulin-resistant mice, and the injection of resistin into mice worsens glucose tolerance and induces insulin resistance (308). Interestingly, the thiazolidinedione class of antidiabetic drugs (e.g., Pioglitazone, Rosiglitazone) that reduce insulin resistance by acting through the nuclear receptor protein PPAR-γ down-regulate resistin in mature adipocytes.

Plasminogen Activator Inhibitor-1 and Tissue Factor

As previously mentioned, increased PAI-1 level is a characteristic feature of the metabolic syndrome and type 2 diabetes (152,155), and it correlates with BMI and visceral accumulation of body fat, rather than with diabetes per se (155,156). In addition, increased tissue factor (TF) levels and TF-mediated coagulation has been demonstrated in obese and insulin-resistant subjects (312,313). Adipocytes synthesize and secrete increased amounts of PAI-1 and TF, under the influence of TNF-α, TGF-β, and insulin (153,154, 314).

Leptin, the most well known adipocyte hormone, is positively correlated with BMI and percentage of body fat. Leptin receptors are present on platelets, and high leptin concentrations (in the range that can be found in obese individuals) potentiate agonist-induced (e.g., ADP, thrombin) platelet aggregation and may contribute to the risk for atherothrombotic in obese individuals (315,316).

Obesity and Inflammation

The presence of the metabolic syndrome, and especially obesity, was found to cluster with increase of inflammatory markers such as C-reactive protein (CRP) and proinflammatory cytokines (307,317–320). Both TNF-α and IL-6 are expressed in and released by adipose tissue (307,321). There is a close relation between circulating CRP and cytokine concentrations (321) and between CRP concentrations and anthropometric measures of obesity (320,321). Because the synthesis of CRP by the liver is predominantly regulated by IL-6, it is believed that IL-6 originating from adipose tissue contributes to the increased CRP concentrations in obese insulin-resistant subjects. TNF-α does not induce CRP directly, but can potentiate the induction of CRP by IL-6. This hypothesis is consistent with the strong relation of BMI with CRP levels observed in virtually all studies (317–322).

Treatment of Obesity

There is overwhelming evidence that a modest loss (5–10%) of body weight is associated with substantial improvement in obesity-related conditions such as diabetes (279), hypertension (302), and dyslipidemia. However, only limited data support the notion that interventional weight loss will reduce total mortality rates.

Obese adults can lose 0.5 kg per week by decreasing their daily intake by 500 to 1,000 kcal less than the caloric intake required for maintenance of their current weight. Adding exercise to caloric restriction minimally increases weight loss during the acute phase, but promotes long-term maintenance of reduced weight. Unfortunately, weight loss is frequently followed by a slow increase to the preintervention body weight, or even higher (323). Approximately two thirds of individuals who loose weight will regain it within 1 year, and almost all individuals who loose weight will regain it within 5 years.

National Institute of Health Guidelines recommend that pharmacotherapy should be initiated only in patients with BMI of at least 30 kg/m^2 in the absence of obesity-related medical conditions, or BMI of at least 27 kg/m^2 in the presence of such conditions (303). Drug therapy should be considered only if nonpharmacologic therapies were attempted for 6 months with unsatisfactory results. Available pharmacologic agents include appetite suppressants (e.g., sibutramine) and drugs that reduce nutrient absorption (e.g., orlistat) (323). Surgical therapies such as gastric bypass can improve long-term weight loss but are appropriate only for selected patients with BMI 40 kg/m^2 or greater, or BMI 35 kg/m^2 or greater in the presence of obesity-related medical conditions (303).

REFERENCES

1. Zimmet P, Alberti KG, Shaw J. Global and societal implications of the diabetes epidemic. *Nature* 2001;414:782–787.
2. King H, Aubert RE, Herman WH. Global burden of diabetes, 1995-2025: prevalence, numerical estimates, and projections. *Diabetes Care* 1998;21:1414–1431.
3. Harris MI. Diabetes in America: epidemiology and scope of the problem. *Diabetes Care* 1998;21[Suppl 3]:C11–C14.
4. Sinha R, Fisch G, Teague B, et al. Prevalence of impaired glucose tolerance among children and adolescents with marked obesity. *N Engl J Med* 2002;346:802–810.
5. Howard BV, Rodriguez BL, Bennett PH, et al. Prevention Conference VI: Diabetes and Cardiovascular disease: Writing Group I: epidemiology. *Circulation* 2002;105:e132–e137.
6. Grundy SM, Benjamin IJ, Burke GL, et al. Diabetes and cardiovascular disease: a statement for healthcare professionals from the American Heart Association. *Circulation* 1999;100:1134–1146.
7. McKinlay J, Marceau L. US public health and the 21st century: diabetes mellitus. *Lancet* 2000;356:757–761.
8. Gu K, Cowie CC, Harris MI. Diabetes and decline in heart disease mortality in US adults. *JAMA* 1999;281:1291–1297.
9. Schwartz CJ, Valente AJ, Sprague EA, et al. Pathogenesis of the atherosclerotic lesion. Implications for diabetes mellitus. *Diabetes Care* 1992;15:1156–1167.
10. Stamler J, Vaccaro O, Neaton JD, et al. Diabetes, other risk factors, and 12-yr cardiovascular mortality for men screened in the Multiple Risk Factor Intervention Trial. *Diabetes Care* 1993;16:434–444.

11. Beckman JA, Creager MA, Libby P. Diabetes and atherosclerosis: epidemiology, pathophysiology, and management. *JAMA* 2002;287: 2570–2581.

12. American Diabetes Association. Consensus Statement: role of cardiovascular risk factors in prevention and treatment of macrovascular disease in diabetes. *Diabetes Care* 1993;16:72–78.

13. Haffner SM, Lehto S, Ronnemaa T, et al. Mortality from coronary heart disease in subjects with type 2 diabetes and in nondiabetic subjects with and without prior myocardial infarction. *N Engl J Med* 1998;339:229–234.

14. Krolewski AS, Kosinski EJ, Warram JH, et al. Magnitude and determinants of coronary artery disease in juvenile-onset, insulin-dependent diabetes mellitus. *Am J Cardiol* 1987;59:750–755.

15. Donahue RP, Orchard TJ. Diabetes mellitus and macrovascular complications. An epidemiological perspective. *Diabetes Care* 1992;15: 1141–1155.

16. Borch-Johnsen K, Kreiner S. Proteinuria: value as predictor of cardiovascular mortality in insulin dependent diabetes mellitus. *Br Med J* (Clin Res Ed) 1987;294:1651–1654.

17. Jensen T, Borch-Johnsen K, Kofoed-Enevoldsen A, et al. Coronary heart disease in young type 1 (insulin-dependent) diabetic patients with and without diabetic nephropathy: incidence and risk factors. *Diabetologia* 1987;30:144–148.

18. Deckert T, Kofoed-Enevoldsen A, Norgaard K, et al. Microalbuminuria. Implications for micro- and macrovascular disease. *Diabetes Care* 1992;15:1181–1191.

19. Wang SL, Head J, Stevens L, et al. Excess mortality and its relation to hypertension and proteinuria in diabetic patients. The World Health Organization multinational study of vascular disease in diabetes. *Diabetes Care* 1996;19:305–312.

20. Haffner SM. Management of dyslipidemia in adults with diabetes. *Diabetes Care* 1998;21:160–178.

21. Stehouwer CD, Nauta JJ, Zeldenrust GC, et al. Urinary albumin excretion, cardiovascular disease, and endothelial dysfunction in non-insulin-dependent diabetes mellitus. *Lancet* 1992;340:319–323.

22. Makita Z, Radoff S, Rayfield EJ, et al. Advanced glycosylation end products in patients with diabetic nephropathy. *N Engl J Med* 1991;325:836–842.

23. Makita Z, Bucala R, Rayfield EJ, et al. Reactive glycosylation endproducts in diabetic uraemia and treatment of renal failure. *Lancet* 1994;343:1519–1522.

24. Barrett-Connor EL, Cohn BA, Wingard DL, et al. Why is diabetes mellitus a stronger risk factor for fatal ischemic heart disease in women than in men? The Rancho Bernardo Study [published erratum appears in JAMA 1991;265:3249]. *JAMA* 1991;265:627–631.

25. Kahn CR. Banting Lecture. Insulin action, diabetogenes, and the cause of type II diabetes. *Diabetes* 1994;43:1066–1084.

26. DeFronzo RA. Lilly lecture 1987. The triumvirate: beta-cell, muscle, liver. A collusion responsible for NIDDM. *Diabetes* 1988;37:667–687.

27. Lempiainen P, Mykkanen L, Pyorala K, et al. Insulin resistance syndrome predicts coronary heart disease events in elderly nondiabetic men. *Circulation* 1999;100:123–128.

28. Isomaa B, Almgren P, Tuomi T, et al. Cardiovascular morbidity and mortality associated with the metabolic syndrome. *Diabetes Care* 2001;24:683–689.

29. Haffner SM, Stern MP, Hazuda HP, et al. Cardiovascular risk factors in confirmed prediabetic individuals. Does the clock for coronary heart disease start ticking before the onset of clinical diabetes? *JAMA* 1990;263:2893–2898.

30. Meigs JB, Nathan DM, Wilson PW, et al. Metabolic risk factors worsen continuously across the spectrum of nondiabetic glucose tolerance. The Framingham Offspring Study. *Ann Intern Med* 1998;128: 524–533.

31. Hu FB, Stampfer MJ, Haffner SM, et al. Elevated risk of cardiovascular disease prior to clinical diagnosis of type 2 diabetes. *Diabetes Care* 2002;25:1129–1134.

32. Despres JP, Lamarche B, Mauriege P, et al. Hyperinsulinemia as an independent risk factor for ischemic heart disease. *N Engl J Med* 1996;334:952–957.

33. Howard G, O'Leary DH, Zaccaro D, et al. Insulin sensitivity and atherosclerosis. The Insulin Resistance Atherosclerosis Study (IRAS) Investigators. *Circulation* 1996;93:1809–1817.

34. Feener EP, King GL. Vascular dysfunction in diabetes mellitus. *Lancet* 1997;350[Suppl 1]:SI9–SI13.

35. Saad MF, Knowler WC, Pettitt DJ, et al. Sequential changes in serum insulin concentration during development of non-insulin-dependent diabetes. *Lancet* 1989;1:1356–1359.

36. Turner RC, Millns H, Neil HA, et al. Risk factors for coronary artery disease in non-insulin dependent diabetes mellitus: United Kingdom Prospective Diabetes Study (UKPDS: 23). *BMJ* 1998;316:823–828.

37. Laakso M. Hyperglycemia and cardiovascular disease in type 2 diabetes. *Diabetes* 1999;48:937–942.

38. Gerstein HC, Yusuf S. Dysglycaemia and risk of cardiovascular disease. *Lancet* 1996;347:949–950.

39. Report of the Expert Committee on the Diagnosis and Classification of Diabetes Mellitus. *Diabetes Care* 1997;20:1183–1197.

40. Khaw KT, Wareham N, Luben R, et al. Glycated haemoglobin, diabetes, and mortality in men in Norfolk cohort of european prospective investigation of cancer and nutrition (EPIC-Norfolk). *BMJ* 2001;322: 15–18.

41. Coutinho M, Gerstein HC, Wang Y, et al. The relationship between glucose and incident cardiovascular events. A metaregression analysis of published data from 20 studies of 95,783 individuals followed for 12.4 years. *Diabetes Care* 1999;22:233–240.

42. Pais P, Pogue J, Gerstein H, et al. Risk factors for acute myocardial infarction in Indians: a case-control study. *Lancet* 1996;348:358–363.

43. Lowe LP, Liu K, Greenland P, et al. Diabetes, asymptomatic hyperglycemia, and 22-year mortality in black and white men. The Chicago Heart Association Detection Project in Industry Study. *Diabetes Care* 1997;20:163–169.

44. Alberti KG, Zimmet PZ. Definition, diagnosis and classification of diabetes mellitus and its complications. Part 1: diagnosis and classification of diabetes mellitus provisional report of a WHO consultation. *Diabet Med* 1998;15:539–553.

45. Ford ES, Giles WH, Dietz WH. Prevalence of the metabolic syndrome among US adults: findings from the third National Health and Nutrition Examination Survey. *JAMA* 2002;287:356–359.

46. The effect of intensive treatment of diabetes on the development and progression of long-term complications in insulin-dependent diabetes mellitus. The Diabetes Control and Complications Trial Research Group. *N Engl J Med* 1993;329:977–986.

47. Fioretto P, Steffes MW, Sutherland DE, et al. Reversal of lesions of diabetic nephropathy after pancreas transplantation. *N Engl J Med* 1998;339:69–75.

48. Brownlee M. Biochemistry and molecular cell biology of diabetic complications. *Nature* 2001;414:813–820.

49. Ulrich P, Cerami A. Protein glycation, diabetes, and aging. *Recent Prog Horm Res* 2001;56:1–21.

50. Maillard L. Action des acides amines sur les sucres: formation des melanoidines par voie methodique. *C R Hebd Seances Acad Sci* 1912;154:66–68.

51. Brownlee M, Cerami A, Vlassara H. Advanced glycosylation end products in tissue and the biochemical basis of diabetic complications. *N Engl J Med* 1988;318:1315–1321.

52. Schmidt AM, Yan SD, Wautier JL, et al. Activation of receptor for advanced glycation end products: a mechanism for chronic vascular dysfunction in diabetic vasculopathy and atherosclerosis. *Circ Res* 1999;84:489–497.

53. Nishikawa T, Edelstein D, Du XL, et al. Normalizing mitochondrial superoxide production blocks three pathways of hyperglycaemic damage. *Nature* 2000;404:787–790.

54. Brownlee M, Vlassara H, Kooney A, et al. Aminoguanidine prevents diabetes-induced arterial wall protein cross-linking. *Science* 1986; 232:1629–1632.

55. Monnier VM, Bautista O, Kenny D, et al. Skin collagen glycation, glycoxidation, and crosslinking are lower in subjects with long-term intensive versus conventional therapy of type 1 diabetes: relevance of glycated collagen products versus HbA1c as markers of diabetic complications. DCCT Skin Collagen Ancillary Study Group. Diabetes Control and Complications Trial. *Diabetes* 1999; 48:870–880.

56. Vlassara H, Fuh H, Makita Z, et al. Exogenous advanced glycosylation end products induce complex vascular dysfunction in normal animals: a model for diabetic and aging complications. *Proc Natl Acad Sci USA* 1992;89:12043–12047.

57. Vasan S, Zhang X, Zhang X, et al. An agent cleaving glucose-derived protein crosslinks in vitro and in vivo. *Nature* 1996;382:275–278.

58. Schmidt AM, Yan SD, Yan SF, et al. The multiligand receptor RAGE

as a progression factor amplifying immune and inflammatory responses. *J Clin Invest* 2001;108:949–955.

59. Kirstein M, Brett J, Radoff S, et al. Advanced protein glycosylation induces transendothelial human monocyte chemotaxis and secretion of platelet-derived growth factor: role in vascular disease of diabetes and aging. *Proc Natl Acad Sci USA* 1990;87:9010–9014.

60. Kirstein M, Aston C, Hintz R, et al. Receptor-specific induction of insulin-like growth factor I in human monocytes by advanced glycosylation end product-modified proteins. *J Clin Invest* 1992;90:439–446.

61. Yan SD, Schmidt AM, Anderson GM, et al. Enhanced cellular oxidant stress by the interaction of advanced glycation end products with their receptors/binding proteins. *J Biol Chem* 1994;269:9889–9897.

62. Wautier JL, Wautier MP, Schmidt AM, et al. Advanced glycation end products (AGEs) on the surface of diabetic erythrocytes bind to the vessel wall via a specific receptor inducing oxidant stress in the vasculature: a link between surface-associated AGEs and diabetic complications. *Proc Natl Acad Sci USA* 1994;91:7742–7746.

63. Wautier JL, Zoukourian C, Chappey O, et al. Receptor-mediated endothelial cell dysfunction in diabetic vasculopathy. Soluble receptor for advanced glycation end products blocks hyperpermeability in diabetic rats. *J Clin Invest* 1996;97:238–243.

64. Esposito C, Gerlach H, Brett J, et al. Endothelial receptor-mediated binding of glucose-modified albumin is associated with increased monolayer permeability and modulation of cell surface coagulant properties. *J Exp Med* 1989;170:1387–1407.

65. Schmidt AM, Hori O, Chen JX, et al. Advanced glycation endproducts interacting with their endothelial receptor induce expression of vascular cell adhesion molecule-1 (VCAM-1) in cultured human endothelial cells and in mice. A potential mechanism for the accelerated vasculopathy of diabetes. *J Clin Invest* 1995;96:1395–1403.

66. Basta G, Lazzerini G, Massaro M, et al. Advanced glycation end products activate endothelium through signal-transduction receptor RAGE: a mechanism for amplification of inflammatory responses. *Circulation* 2002;105:816–822.

67. Ritthaler U, Deng Y, Zhang Y, et al. Expression of receptors for advanced glycation end products in peripheral occlusive vascular disease. *Am J Pathol* 1995;146:688–694.

68. Schmidt AM, Yan SD, Brett J, et al. Regulation of human mononuclear phagocyte migration by cell surface-binding proteins for advanced glycation end products. *J Clin Invest* 1993;91:2155–2168.

69. Vlassara H, Brownlee M, Manogue KR, et al. Cachectin/TNF and IL-1 induced by glucose-modified proteins: role in normal tissue remodeling. *Science* 1988;240:1546–1548.

70. Ross R. Atherosclerosis—an inflammatory disease. *N Engl J Med* 1999;340:115–126.

71. Park L, Raman KG, Lee KJ, et al. Suppression of accelerated diabetic atherosclerosis by the soluble receptor for advanced glycation endproducts. *Nat Med* 1998;4:1025–1031.

72. Bucciarelli LG, Wendt T, Qu W, et al. RAGE blockade stabilizes established atherosclerosis in diabetic apolipoprotein E-null mice. *Circulation* 2002;106:2827–2835.

73. Suzuki H, Kurihara Y, Takeya M, et al. A role for macrophage scavenger receptors in atherosclerosis and susceptibility to infection. *Nature* 1997;386:292–296.

74. Ohgami N, Nagai R, Ikemoto M, et al. Cd36, a member of the class b scavenger receptor family, as a receptor for advanced glycation end products. *J Biol Chem* 2001;276:3195–3202.

75. Ishii H, Jirousek MR, Koya D, et al. Amelioration of vascular dysfunctions in diabetic rats by an oral PKC beta inhibitor. *Science* 1996;272:728–731.

76. Koya D, King GL. Protein kinase C activation and the development of diabetic complications. *Diabetes* 1998;47:859–866.

77. Koya D, Jirousek MR, Lin YW, et al. Characterization of protein kinase C beta isoform activation on the gene expression of transforming growth factor-beta, extracellular matrix components, and prostanoids in the glomeruli of diabetic rats. *J Clin Invest* 1997;100:115–126.

78. Koya D, Haneda M, Nakagawa H, et al. Amelioration of accelerated diabetic mesangial expansion by treatment with a PKC beta inhibitor in diabetic db/db mice, a rodent model for type 2 diabetes. *FASEB J* 2000;14:439–447.

79. Inoguchi T, Battan R, Handler E, et al. Preferential elevation of protein kinase C isoform beta II and diacylglycerol levels in the aorta and heart of diabetic rats: differential reversibility to glycemic control by islet cell transplantation. *Proc Natl Acad Sci USA* 1992;89:11059–11063.

80. Kuboki K, Jiang ZY, Takahara N, et al. Regulation of endothelial constitutive nitric oxide synthase gene expression in endothelial cells and in vivo: a specific vascular action of insulin. *Circulation* 2000;101:676–681.

81. Park JY, Takahara N, Gabriele A, et al. Induction of endothelin-1 expression by glucose: an effect of protein kinase C activation. *Diabetes* 2000;49:1239–1248.

82. Inaba T, Ishibashi S, Gotoda T, et al. Enhanced expression of platelet-derived growth factor-beta receptor by high glucose. Involvement of platelet-derived growth factor in diabetic angiopathy. *Diabetes* 1996;45:507–512.

83. Yuan SY, Ustinova EE, Wu MH, et al. Protein kinase C activation contributes to microvascular barrier dysfunction in the heart at early stages of diabetes. *Circ Res* 2000;87:412–417.

84. Kolm-Litty V, Sauer U, Nerlich A, et al. High glucose-induced transforming growth factor beta1 production is mediated by the hexosamine pathway in porcine glomerular mesangial cells. *J Clin Invest* 1998;101:160–169.

85. Wells L, Vosseller K, Hart GW. Glycosylation of nucleocytoplasmic proteins: signal transduction and O-GlcNAc. *Science* 2001;291:2376–2378.

86. Du XL, Edelstein D, Dimmeler S, et al. Hyperglycemia inhibits endothelial nitric oxide synthase activity by posttranslational modification at the Akt site. *J Clin Invest* 2001;108:1341–1348.

87. Du XL, Edelstein D, Rossetti L, et al. Hyperglycemia-induced mitochondrial superoxide overproduction activates the hexosamine pathway and induces plasminogen activator inhibitor-1 expression by increasing Sp1 glycosylation. *Proc Natl Acad Sci USA* 2000;97:12222–12226.

88. Pennathur S, Wagner JD, Leeuwenburgh C, et al. A hydroxyl radical-like species oxidizes cynomolgus monkey artery wall proteins in early diabetic vascular disease. *J Clin Invest* 2001;107:853–860.

89. Baynes JW, Thorpe SR. Role of oxidative stress in diabetic complications: a new perspective on an old paradigm. *Diabetes* 1999;48:1–9.

90. Wells-Knecht MC, Thorpe SR, Baynes JW. Pathways of formation of glycoxidation products during glycation of collagen. *Biochemistry* 1995;34:15134–15141.

91. Wells-Knecht KJ, Zyzak DV, Litchfield JE, et al. Mechanism of autoxidative glycosylation: identification of glyoxal and arabinose as intermediates in the autoxidative modification of proteins by glucose. *Biochemistry* 1995;34:3702–3709.

92. Beisswenger PJ, Moore LL, Brinck-Johnsen T, et al. Increased collagen-linked pentosidine levels and advanced glycosylation end products in early diabetic nephropathy. *J Clin Invest* 1993;92:212–217.

93. McCance DR, Dyer DG, Dunn JA, et al. Maillard reaction products and their relation to complications in insulin-dependent diabetes mellitus. *J Clin Invest* 1993;91:2470–2478.

94. Hunt JV, Smith CC, Wolff SP. Autoxidative glycosylation and possible involvement of peroxides and free radicals in LDL modification by glucose. *Diabetes* 1990;39:1420–1424.

95. Hunt JV, Dean RT, Wolff SP. Hydroxyl radical production and autoxidative glycosylation. Glucose autoxidation as the cause of protein damage in the experimental glycation model of diabetes mellitus and ageing. *Biochem J* 1988;256:205–212.

96. Wolff SP. Diabetes mellitus and free radicals. Free radicals, transition metals and oxidative stress in the aetiology of diabetes mellitus and complications. *Br Med Bull* 1993;49:642–652.

97. Yan SD, Chen X, Schmidt AM, et al. Glycated tau protein in Alzheimer disease: a mechanism for induction of oxidant stress. *Proc Natl Acad Sci USA* 1994;91:7787–7791.

98. Konishi H, Tanaka M, Takemura Y, et al. Activation of protein kinase C by tyrosine phosphorylation in response to H2O2. *Proc Natl Acad Sci USA* 1997;94:11233–11237.

99. Williams SB, Goldfine AB, Timimi FK, et al. Acute hyperglycemia attenuates endothelium-dependent vasodilation in humans in vivo. *Circulation* 1998;97:1695–1701.

100. De Vriese AS, Verbeuren TJ, Van de Voorde J, et al. Endothelial dysfunction in diabetes. *Br J Pharmacol* 2000;130:963–974.

101. Calles-Escandon J, Cipolla M. Diabetes and endothelial dysfunction: a clinical perspective. *Endocr Rev* 2001;22:36–52.

102. Brodsky SV, Morrishow AM, Dharia N, et al. Glucose scavenging of nitric oxide. *Am J Physiol Renal Physiol* 2001;280:F480–F486.

103. Garcia Soriano F, Virag L, Jagtap P, et al. Diabetic endothelial dysfunction: the role of poly(ADP-ribose) polymerase activation. *Nat Med* 2001;7:108–113.

104. Soriano FG, Pacher P, Mabley J, et al. Rapid reversal of the diabetic endothelial dysfunction by pharmacological inhibition of poly(ADP-ribose) polymerase. *Circ Res* 2001;89:684–691.
105. Guzik TJ, Mussa S, Gastaldi D, et al. Mechanisms of increased vascular superoxide production in human diabetes mellitus: role of NAD(P)H oxidase and endothelial nitric oxide synthase. *Circulation* 2002;105:1656–1662.
106. Bierhaus A, Illmer T, Kasper M, et al. Advanced glycation end product (AGE)-mediated induction of tissue factor in cultured endothelial cells is dependent on RAGE. *Circulation* 1997;96:2262–2271.
107. Ting HH, Timimi FK, Boles KS, et al. Vitamin C improves endothelium-dependent vasodilation in patients with non-insulin-dependent diabetes mellitus. *J Clin Invest* 1996;97:22–28.
108. Bucala R, Tracey KJ, Cerami A. Advanced glycosylation products quench nitric oxide and mediate defective endothelium-dependent vasodilatation in experimental diabetes. *J Clin Invest* 1991;87:432–438.
109. Petrie JR, Ueda S, Webb DJ, et al. Endothelial nitric oxide production and insulin sensitivity. A physiological link with implications for pathogenesis of cardiovascular disease. *Circulation* 1996;93:1331–1333.
110. Makimattila S, Virkamaki A, Groop PH, et al. Chronic hyperglycemia impairs endothelial function and insulin sensitivity via different mechanisms in insulin-dependent diabetes mellitus. *Circulation* 1996;94:1276–1282.
111. Giugliano D, Marfella R, Coppola L, et al. Vascular effects of acute hyperglycemia in humans are reversed by L-arginine. Evidence for reduced availability of nitric oxide during hyperglycemia. *Circulation* 1997;95:1783–1790.
112. Cosentino F, Hishikawa K, Katusic ZS, et al. High glucose increases nitric oxide synthase expression and superoxide anion generation in human aortic endothelial cells. *Circulation* 1997;96:25–28.
113. Rosen P, Nawroth PP, King G, et al. The role of oxidative stress in the onset and progression of diabetes and its complications: a summary of a Congress Series sponsored by UNESCO-MCBN, the American Diabetes Association and the German Diabetes Society. *Diabetes Metab Res Rev* 2001;17:189–212.
114. Zanetti M, Sato J, Katusic ZS, et al. Gene transfer of superoxide dismutase isoforms reverses endothelial dysfunction in diabetic rabbit aorta. *Am J Physiol Heart Circ Physiol* 2001;280:H2516–H2523.
115. Steinberg HO, Brechtel G, Johnson A, et al. Insulin-mediated skeletal muscle vasodilation is nitric oxide dependent. A novel action of insulin to increase nitric oxide release. *J Clin Invest* 1994;94:1172–1179.
116. Zeng G, Nystrom FH, Ravichandran LV, et al. Roles for insulin receptor, PI3-kinase, and Akt in insulin-signaling pathways related to production of nitric oxide in human vascular endothelial cells. *Circulation* 2000;101:1539–1545.
117. Steinberg HO, Chaker H, Leaming R, et al. Obesity/insulin resistance is associated with endothelial dysfunction. Implications for the syndrome of insulin resistance. *J Clin Invest* 1996;97:2601–2610.
118. Balletshofer BM, Rittig K, Enderle MD, et al. Endothelial dysfunction is detectable in young normotensive first-degree relatives of subjects with type 2 diabetes in association with insulin resistance. *Circulation* 2000;101:1780–1784.
119. Caballero AE, Arora S, Saouaf R, et al. Microvascular and macrovascular reactivity is reduced in subjects at risk for type 2 diabetes. *Diabetes* 1999;48:1856–1862.
120. Paradisi G, Steinberg HO, Hempfling A, et al. Polycystic ovary syndrome is associated with endothelial dysfunction. *Circulation* 2001;103:1410–1415.
121. Arcaro G, Cretti A, Balzano S, et al. Insulin causes endothelial dysfunction in humans: sites and mechanisms. *Circulation* 2002;105:576–582.
122. Steinberg HO, Tarshoby M, Monestel R, et al. Elevated circulating free fatty acid levels impair endothelium-dependent vasodilation. *J Clin Invest* 1997;100:1230–1239.
123. Steinberg HO, Paradisi G, Hook G, et al. Free fatty acid elevation impairs insulin-mediated vasodilation and nitric oxide production. *Diabetes* 2000;49:1231–1238.
124. Lin SJ, Hong CY, Chang MS, et al. Increased aortic endothelial death and enhanced transendothelial macromolecular transport in streptozotocin-diabetic rats. *Diabetologia* 1993;36:926–930.
125. Winocour PD, Richardson M, Kinlough-Rathbone RL. Continued platelet interaction with de-endothelialized aortae associated with slower re-endothelialization and more extensive intimal hyperplasia in spontaneously diabetic BB Wistar rats. *Int J Exp Pathol* 1993;74:603–613.
126. Dolgov VV, Zaikina OE, Bondarenko MF, et al. Aortic endothelium of alloxan diabetic rabbits: a quantitative study using scanning electron microscopy. *Diabetologia* 1982;22:338–343.
127. Morigi M, Angioletti S, Imberti B, et al. Leukocyte-endothelial interaction is augmented by high glucose concentrations and hyperglycemia in a NF-kB-dependent fashion. *J Clin Invest* 1998;101:1905–1915.
128. Ginsberg HN. Lipoprotein physiology in nondiabetic and diabetic states. Relationship to atherogenesis. *Diabetes Care* 1991;14:839–855.
128a. Joslin EP. Arteriosclerosis and diabetes. *Ann Clin Med* 1927;5:1061–1079.
129. Garg A. Management of dyslipidemia in IDDM patients [published erratum appears in Diabetes Care 1994;17:349]. *Diabetes Care* 1994;17:224–234.
130. Sosenko JM, Breslow JL, Miettinen OS, et al. Hyperglycemia and plasma lipid levels: a prospective study of young insulin-dependent diabetic patients. *N Engl J Med* 1980;302:650–654.
131. Austin MA, King MC, Vranizan KM, et al. Atherogenic lipoprotein phenotype. A proposed genetic marker for coronary heart disease risk. *Circulation* 1990;82:495–506.
132. Selby JV, Austin MA, Newman B, et al. LDL subclass phenotypes and the insulin resistance syndrome in women. *Circulation* 1993;88:381–387.
133. Reaven GM, Chen YD, Jeppesen J, et al. Insulin resistance and hyperinsulinemia in individuals with small, dense low density lipoprotein particles. *J Clin Invest* 1993;92:141–146.
134. Haffner SM, D'Agostino R Jr, Goff D, et al. LDL size in African Americans, Hispanics, and non-Hispanic whites: the insulin resistance atherosclerosis study. *Arterioscler Thromb Vasc Biol* 1999;19:2234–2240.
135. Syvanne M, Taskinen MR. Lipids and lipoproteins as coronary risk factors in non-insulin-dependent diabetes mellitus. *Lancet* 1997;350:SI20–SI23.
136. Ginsberg HN. Diabetic dyslipidemia: basic mechanisms underlying the common hypertriglyceridemia and low HDL cholesterol levels. *Diabetes* 1996;45[Suppl 3]:S27–S30.
137. Howard BV, Knowler WC, Vasquez B, et al. Plasma and lipoprotein cholesterol and triglyceride in the Pima Indian population. Comparison of diabetics and nondiabetics. *Arteriosclerosis* 1984;4:462–471.
138. Eckel RH. Lipoprotein lipase. A multifunctional enzyme relevant to common metabolic diseases [published erratum appears in N Engl J Med 1990;322:477]. *N Engl J Med* 1989;320:1060–1068.
139. Packard CJ, Munro A, Lorimer AR, et al. Metabolism of apolipoprotein B in large triglyceride-rich very low density lipoproteins of normal and hypertriglyceridemic subjects. *J Clin Invest* 1984;74:2178–2192.
140. Ginsberg HN. Insulin resistance and cardiovascular disease. *J Clin Invest* 2000;106:453–458.
141. Patsch JR, Prasad S, Gotto AM Jr, et al. Postprandial lipemia. A key for the conversion of high density lipoprotein2 into high density lipoprotein3 by hepatic lipase. *J Clin Invest* 1984;74:2017–2023.
142. Packard CJ, Shepherd J. Lipoprotein heterogeneity and apolipoprotein B metabolism. *Arterioscler Thromb Vasc Biol* 1997;17:3542–3556.
143. Bucala R, Mitchell R, Arnold K, et al. Identification of the major site of apolipoprotein B modification by advanced glycosylation end products blocking uptake by the low density lipoprotein receptor. *J Biol Chem* 1995;270:10828–10832.
144. Bucala R, Makita Z, Koschinsky T, et al. Lipid advanced glycosylation: pathway for lipid oxidation in vivo. *Proc Natl Acad Sci USA* 1993;90:6434–6438.
145. Bucala R, Makita Z, Vega G, et al. Modification of low density lipoprotein by advanced glycation end products contributes to the dyslipidemia of diabetes and renal insufficiency. *Proc Natl Acad Sci USA* 1994;91:9441–9445.
146. Lyons TJ. Glycation and oxidation: a role in the pathogenesis of atherosclerosis. *Am J Cardiol* 1993;71:26B–31B.
147. Bowie A, Owens D, Collins P, et al. Glycosylated low density lipoprotein is more sensitive to oxidation: implications for the diabetic patient? *Atherosclerosis* 1993;102:63–67.
148. Libby P. Current concepts of the pathogenesis of the acute coronary syndromes. *Circulation* 2001;104:365–372.
149. Vinik AI, Erbas T, Park TS, et al. Platelet dysfunction in type 2 diabetes. *Diabetes Care* 2001;24:1476–1485.
150. Tschoepe D, Driesch E, Schwippert B, et al. Exposure of adhesion molecules on activated platelets in patients with newly diagnosed

IDDM is not normalized by near-normoglycemia. *Diabetes* 1995;44:890–894.

151. Thompson SG, Kienast J, Pyke SD, et al. Hemostatic factors and the risk of myocardial infarction or sudden death in patients with angina pectoris. European Concerted Action on Thrombosis and Disabilities Angina Pectoris Study Group. *N Engl J Med* 1995;332:635–641.

152. Kohler HP, Grant PJ. Plasminogen-activator inhibitor type 1 and coronary artery disease. *N Engl J Med* 2000;342:1792–1801.

153. Samad F, Pandey M, Loskutoff DJ. Tissue factor gene expression in the adipose tissues of obese mice. *Proc Natl Acad Sci USA* 1998;95:7591–7596.

154. Samad F, Uysal KT, Wiesbrock SM, et al. Tumor necrosis factor alpha is a key component in the obesity-linked elevation of plasminogen activator inhibitor 1. *Proc Natl Acad Sci USA* 1999;96:6902–6907.

155. Juhan-Vague I, Alessi MC. PAI-1, obesity, insulin resistance and risk of cardiovascular events. *Thromb Haemost* 1997;78:656–660.

156. Alessi MC, Peiretti F, Morange P, et al. Production of plasminogen activator inhibitor 1 by human adipose tissue: possible link between visceral fat accumulation and vascular disease. *Diabetes* 1997;46:860–867.

157. Kislinger T, Tanji N, Wendt T, et al. Receptor for advanced glycation end products mediates inflammation and enhanced expression of tissue factor in vasculature of diabetic apolipoprotein E-null mice. *Arterioscler Thromb Vasc Biol* 2001;21:905–910.

158. Aronson D, Rayfield EJ, Chesebro JH. Mechanisms determining course and outcome of diabetic patients who have had acute myocardial infarction. *Ann Intern Med* 1997;126:296–306.

159. Knobler H, Savion N, Shenkman B, et al. Shear-induced platelet adhesion and aggregation on subendothelium are increased in diabetic patients. *Thromb Res* 1998;90:181–190.

160. Davi G, Gresele P, Violi F, et al. Diabetes mellitus, hypercholesterolemia, and hypertension but not vascular disease per se are associated with persistent platelet activation in vivo. Evidence derived from the study of peripheral arterial disease. *Circulation* 1997;96:69–75.

161. Tschoepe D, Roesen P, Kaufmann L, et al. Evidence for abnormal platelet glycoprotein expression in diabetes mellitus. *Eur J Clin Invest* 1990;20:166–170.

162. Tschoepe D, Roesen P, Schwippert B, et al. Platelets in diabetes: the role in the hemostatic regulation in atherosclerosis. *Semin Thromb Hemost* 1993;19:122–128.

163. Shechter M, Merz CN, Paul-Labrador MJ, et al. Blood glucose and platelet-dependent thrombosis in patients with coronary artery disease. *J Am Coll Cardiol* 2000;35:300–307.

164. Davi G, Ciabattoni G, Consoli A, et al. In vivo formation of 8-iso-prostaglandin f2alpha and platelet activation in diabetes mellitus: effects of improved metabolic control and vitamin E supplementation. *Circulation* 1999;99:224–229.

165. Yamagishi SI, Edelstein D, Du XL, et al. Hyperglycemia potentiates collagen-induced platelet activation through mitochondrial superoxide overproduction. *Diabetes* 2001;50:1491–1494.

166. Conlan MG, Folsom AR, Finch A, et al. Associations of factor VIII and von Willebrand factor with age, race, sex, and risk factors for atherosclerosis. The Atherosclerosis Risk in Communities (ARIC) Study. *Thromb Haemost* 1993;70:380–385.

167. Kannel WB, D'Agostino RB, Wilson PW, et al. Diabetes, fibrinogen, and risk of cardiovascular disease: the Framingham experience. *Am Heart J* 1990;120:672–676.

168. Vague P, Juhan-Vague I. Fibrinogen, fibrinolysis and diabetes mellitus: a comment. *Diabetologia* 1997;40:738–740.

169. D'Elia JA, Weinrauch LA, Gleason RE, et al. Fibrinogen and factor VII levels improve with glycemic control in patients with type 1 diabetes mellitus who have microvascular complications. *Arch Intern Med* 2001;161:98–101.

170. Emanuele N, Azad N, Abraira C, et al. Effect of intensive glycemic control on fibrinogen, lipids, and lipoproteins: Veterans Affairs Cooperative Study in Type II Diabetes Mellitus. *Arch Intern Med* 1998;158:2485–2490.

171. Kapur R, Hoffman CJ, Bhushan V, et al. Postprandial elevation of activated factor VII in young adults. *Arterioscler Thromb Vasc Biol* 1996;16:1327–1332.

172. Rao AK, Chouhan V, Chen X, et al. Activation of the tissue factor pathway of blood coagulation during prolonged hyperglycemia in young healthy men. *Diabetes* 1999;48:1156–1161.

173. Svendsen OL, Hassager C, Christiansen C, et al. Plasminogen activator inhibitor-1, tissue-type plasminogen activator, and fibrinogen: effect of dieting with or without exercise in overweight postmenopausal women. *Arterioscler Thromb Vasc Biol* 1996;16:381–385.

174. Lehmann ED, Riley WA, Clarkson P, et al. Non-invasive assessment of cardiovascular disease in diabetes mellitus. *Lancet* 1997;350:SI14–SI19.

175. Poirier P, Bogaty P, Garneau C, et al. Diastolic dysfunction in normotensive men with well-controlled type 2 diabetes: importance of maneuvers in echocardiographic screening for preclinical diabetic cardiomyopathy. *Diabetes Care* 2001;24:5–10.

176. Albanna, II, Eichelberger SM, Khoury PR, et al. Diastolic dysfunction in young patients with insulin-dependent diabetes mellitus as determined by automated border detection. *J Am Soc Echocardiogr* 1998;11:349–355.

177. Annonu AK, Fattah AA, Mokhtar MS, et al. Left ventricular systolic and diastolic functional abnormalities in asymptomatic patients with non-insulin-dependent diabetes mellitus. *J Am Soc Echocardiogr* 2001;14:885–891.

178. Stone PH, Muller JE, Hartwell T, et al. The effect of diabetes mellitus on prognosis and serial left ventricular function after acute myocardial infarction: contribution of both coronary disease and diastolic left ventricular dysfunction to the adverse prognosis. The MILIS Study Group. *J Am Coll Cardiol* 1989;14:49–57.

179. Ho KK, Pinsky JL, Kannel WB, et al. The epidemiology of heart failure: the Framingham Study. *J Am Coll Cardiol* 1993;22:6A–13A.

180. Corman B, Duriez M, Poitevin P, et al. Aminoguanidine prevents age-related arterial stiffening and cardiac hypertrophy. *Proc Natl Acad Sci USA* 1998;95:1301–1306.

181. Huijberts MS, Wolffenbuttel BH, Boudier HA, et al. Aminoguanidine treatment increases elasticity and decreases fluid filtration of large arteries from diabetic rats. *J Clin Invest* 1993;92:1407–1411.

182. Norton GR, Candy G, Woodiwiss AJ. Aminoguanidine prevents the decreased myocardial compliance produced by streptozotocin-induced diabetes mellitus in rats. *Circulation* 1996;93:1905–1912.

183. Wolffenbuttel BH, Boulanger CM, Crijns FR, et al. Breakers of advanced glycation end products restore large artery properties in experimental diabetes. *Proc Natl Acad Sci USA* 1998;95:4630–4634.

184. Vaitkevicius PV, Lane M, Spurgeon H, et al. A cross-link breaker has sustained effects on arterial and ventricular properties in older rhesus monkeys. *Proc Natl Acad Sci USA* 2001;98:1171–1175.

185. Asif M, Egan J, Vasan S, et al. An advanced glycation endproduct cross-link breaker can reverse age-related increases in myocardial stiffness [published erratum appears in Proc Natl Acad Sci USA 2000;97:5679]. *Proc Natl Acad Sci USA* 2000;97:2809–2813.

186. Kass DA, Shapiro EP, Kawaguchi M, et al. Improved arterial compliance by a novel advanced glycation end-product crosslink breaker. *Circulation* 2001;104:1464–1470.

187. Malmberg K, Yusuf S, Gerstein HC, et al. Impact of diabetes on long-term prognosis in patients with unstable angina and non-Q-wave myocardial infarction: results of the OASIS (Organization to Assess Strategies for Ischemic Syndromes) Registry. *Circulation* 2000;102:1014–1019.

188. Roffi M, Chew DP, Mukherjee D, et al. Platelet glycoprotein IIb/IIIa inhibitors reduce mortality in diabetic patients with non-ST-segment-elevation acute coronary syndromes. *Circulation* 2001;104:2767–2771.

189. Shindler DM, Palmeri ST, Antonelli TA, et al. Diabetes mellitus in cardiogenic shock complicating acute myocardial infarction: a report from the SHOCK Trial Registry. SHould we emergently revascularize Occluded Coronaries for cardiogenic shocK? *J Am Coll Cardiol* 2000;36:1097–1103.

190. Silva JA, Escobar A, Collins TJ, et al. Unstable angina. A comparison of angioscopic findings between diabetic and nondiabetic patients. *Circulation* 1995;92:1731–1736.

191. Moreno PR, Murcia AM, Palacios IF, et al. Coronary composition and macrophage infiltration in atherectomy specimens from patients with diabetes mellitus. *Circulation* 2000;102:2180–2184.

192. Braunwald E, Antman EM, Beasley JW, et al. ACC/AHA guidelines for the management of patients with unstable angina and non-ST-segment elevation myocardial infarction: executive summary and recommendations. A report of the American College of Cardiology/American Heart Association task force on practice guidelines (committee on the management of patients with unstable angina). *Circulation* 2000;102:1193–1209.

193. McGuire DK, Emanuelsson H, Granger CB, et al. Influence of diabetes mellitus on clinical outcomes across the spectrum of acute coro-

nary syndromes. Findings from the GUSTO-IIb study. GUSTO IIb Investigators. *Eur Heart J* 2000;21:1750–1758.

194. Calvin JE, Klein LW, VandenBerg BJ, et al. Risk stratification in unstable angina. Prospective validation of the Braunwald classification. *JAMA* 1995;273:136–141.

195. Bhatt DL, Marso SP, Lincoff AM, et al. Abciximab reduces mortality in diabetics following percutaneous coronary intervention. *J Am Coll Cardiol* 2000;35:922–928.

196. Theroux P, Alexander J Jr, Pharand C, et al. Glycoprotein IIb/IIIa receptor blockade improves outcomes in diabetic patients presenting with unstable angina/non-ST-elevation myocardial infarction: results from the platelet receptor inhibition in ischemic syndrome management in patients limited by unstable signs and symptoms (PRISM-PLUS) study. *Circulation* 2000;102:2466–2472.

197. Mak KH, Moliterno DJ, Granger CB, et al. Influence of diabetes mellitus on clinical outcome in the thrombolytic era of acute myocardial infarction. GUSTO-I Investigators. Global Utilization of Streptokinase and Tissue Plasminogen Activator for Occluded Coronary Arteries. *J Am Coll Cardiol* 1997;30:171–179.

198. Zuanetti G, Latini R, Maggioni AP, et al. Influence of diabetes on mortality in acute myocardial infarction: data from the GISSI-2 study. *J Am Coll Cardiol* 1993;22:1788–1794.

199. Granger CB, Califf RM, Young S, et al. Outcome of patients with diabetes mellitus and acute myocardial infarction treated with thrombolytic agents. The Thrombolysis and Angioplasty in Myocardial Infarction (TAMI) Study Group. *J Am Coll Cardiol* 1993;21:920–925.

200. Woodfield SL, Lundergan CF, Reiner JS, et al. Angiographic findings and outcome in diabetic patients treated with thrombolytic therapy for acute myocardial infarction: the GUSTO-I experience. *J Am Coll Cardiol* 1996;28:1661–1669.

201. Holmes DR Jr, Berger PB, Hochman JS, et al. Cardiogenic shock in patients with acute ischemic syndromes with and without ST-segment elevation. *Circulation* 1999;100:2067–2073.

202. Solomon SD, St John Sutton M, Lamas GA, et al. Ventricular remodeling does not accompany the development of heart failure in diabetic patients after myocardial infarction. *Circulation* 2002;106:1251–1255.

203. Abaci A, Oguzhan A, Kahraman S, et al. Effect of diabetes mellitus on formation of coronary collateral vessels. *Circulation* 1999;99:2239–2242.

204. Goldberg RB, Mellies MJ, Sacks FM, et al. Cardiovascular events and their reduction with pravastatin in diabetic and glucose-intolerant myocardial infarction survivors with average cholesterol levels: subgroup analyses in the cholesterol and recurrent events (CARE) trial. The Care Investigators. *Circulation* 1998;98:2513–2519.

205. Indications for fibrinolytic therapy in suspected acute myocardial infarction: collaborative overview of early mortality and major morbidity results from all randomized trials of more then 1000 patients. Fibrinolytic Therapy Trialists' (FTT) Collaborative Group. *Lancet* 1994;343:311–322.

206. Mahaffey KW, Granger CB, Toth CA, et al. Diabetic retinopathy should not be a contraindication to thrombolytic. *J Am Coll Cardiol* 1997;30:1606–1610.

207. Hasdai D, Granger CB, Srivatsa SS, et al. Diabetes mellitus and outcome after primary coronary angioplasty for acute myocardial infarction: lessons from the GUSTO-IIb Angioplasty Substudy. Global Use of Strategies to Open Occluded Arteries in Acute Coronary Syndromes. *J Am Coll Cardiol* 2000;35:1502–1512.

208. Hsu LF, Mak KH, Lau KW, et al. Clinical outcomes of patients with diabetes mellitus and acute myocardial infarction treated with primary angioplasty or fibrinolysis. *Heart* 2002;88:260–265.

209. Collaborative overview of randomized trials of antiplatelet therapy. I. Prevention of death, myocardial infarction, and stroke by prolonged antiplatelet therapy in various categories of patients. Antiplatelet Trialist' Collaboration. *BMJ* 1994;308:81–106.

210. Kendall MJ, Lynch KP, Hjalmarson A, et al. Beta-blockers and sudden cardiac death. *Ann Intern Med* 1995;123:358–367.

211. Zuanetti G, Latini R, Maggioni AP, et al. Effect of the ACE inhibitor lisinopril on mortality in diabetic patients with acute myocardial infarction: data from the GISSI-3 study. *Circulation* 1997;96:4239–4245.

212. Gustafsson I, Torp-Pedersen C, Kober L, et al. Effect of the angiotensin-converting enzyme inhibitor trandolapril on mortality and morbidity in diabetic patients with left ventricular dysfunction after

acute myocardial infarction. Trace Study Group. *J Am Coll Cardiol* 1999;34:83–89.

213. Kip KE, Faxon DP, Detre KM, et al. Coronary angioplasty in diabetic patients. The National Heart, Lung, and Blood Institute Percutaneous Transluminal Coronary Angioplasty Registry. *Circulation* 1996;94:1818–1825.

214. Levine GN, Jacobs AK, Keeler GP, et al. Impact of diabetes mellitus on percutaneous revascularization (CAVEAT-I). CAVEAT-I Investigators. Coronary Angioplasty Versus Excisional Atherectomy Trial. *Am J Cardiol* 1997;79:748–755.

215. Influence of diabetes on 5-year mortality and morbidity in a randomized trial comparing CABG and PTCA in patients with multivessel disease. The Bypass Angioplasty Revascularization Investigation (BARI). *Circulation* 1997;96:1761–1769.

216. Abizaid A, Mintz GS, Pichard AD, et al. Clinical, intravascular ultrasound, and quantitative angiographic determinants of the coronary flow reserve before and after percutaneous transluminal coronary angioplasty. *Am J Cardiol* 1998;82:423–428.

217. Elezi S, Kastrati A, Neumann F, et al. Vessel size and long-term outcome after coronary stent placement. *Circulation* 1998;98:1875–1880.

218. Kleiman NS, Lincoff AM, Kereiakes DJ, et al. Diabetes mellitus, glycoprotein IIb/IIIa blockade, and heparin: evidence for a complex interaction in a multicenter trial. EPILOG Investigators. *Circulation* 1998;97:1912–1920.

219. Goldberg S, Savage MP, Fischman DL. The interventional cardiologist and the diabetic patient. Have we pushed the envelope too far or not far enough? [editorial]. *Circulation* 1996;94:1804–1806.

220. Kastrati A, Schomig A, Elezi S, et al. Predictive factors of restenosis after coronary stent placement. *J Am Coll Cardiol* 1997;30:1428–1436.

221. Carrozza JP Jr, Kuntz RE, Fishman RF, et al. Restenosis after arterial injury caused by coronary stenting in patients with diabetes mellitus. *Ann Intern Med* 1993;118:344–349.

222. Elezi S, Kastrati A, Pache J, et al. Diabetes mellitus and the clinical and angiographic outcome after coronary stent placement. *J Am Coll Cardiol* 1998;32:1866–1873.

223. Gum P, O'Keefe JJ, Borkon A, et al. Bypass surgery versus coronary angioplasty for revascularization of treated diabetic patients. *Circulation* 1997;96:II-7–II-10.

224. Abizaid A, Kornowski R, Mintz GS, et al. The influence of diabetes mellitus on acute and late clinical outcomes following coronary stent implantation. *J Am Coll Cardiol* 1998;32:584–589.

225. Kornowski R, Mintz GS, Kent KM, et al. Increased restenosis in diabetes mellitus after coronary interventions is due to exaggerated intimal hyperplasia. A serial intravascular ultrasound study. *Circulation* 1997;95:1366–1369.

226. Aronson D, Bloomgarden Z, Rayfield EJ. Potential mechanisms promoting restenosis in diabetic patients. *J Am Coll Cardiol* 1996;27:528–535.

227. Aronson D. Potential role of advanced glycosylation end products in promoting restenosis in diabetes and renal failure. *Med Hypotheses* 2002;59:297–301.

228. Park SH, Marso SP, Zhou Z, et al. Neointimal hyperplasia after arterial injury is increased in a rat model of non-insulin-dependent diabetes mellitus. *Circulation* 2001;104:815–819.

229. Indolfi C, Torella D, Cavuto L, et al. Effects of balloon injury on neointimal hyperplasia in streptozotocin-induced diabetes and in hyperinsulinemic nondiabetic pancreatic islet-transplanted rats. *Circulation* 2001;103:2980–2986.

230. Sakaguchi T, Yan SF, Yan SD, et al. Central role of RAGE-dependent neointimal expansion in arterial restenosis. *J Clin Invest* 2003;111:959–972.

231. Van Belle E, Abolmaali K, Bauters C, et al. Restenosis, late vessel occlusion and left ventricular function six months after balloon angioplasty in diabetic patients. *J Am Coll Cardiol* 1999;34:476–485.

232. Van Belle E, Ketelers R, Bauters C, et al. Patency of percutaneous transluminal coronary angioplasty sites at 6-month angiographic follow-up: a key determinant of survival in diabetics after coronary balloon angioplasty. *Circulation* 2001;103:1218–1224.

233. Thourani VH, Weintraub WS, Stein B, et al. Influence of diabetes mellitus on early and late outcome after coronary artery bypass grafting. *Ann Thorac Surg* 1999;67:1045–1052.

234. Eagle KA, Guyton RA, Davidoff R, et al. ACC/AHA guidelines for coronary artery bypass graft surgery: executive summary and recommendations: a report of the American College of Cardiology/Ameri-

can Heart Association Task Force on Practice Guidelines (Committee to revise the 1991 guidelines for coronary artery bypass graft surgery). *Circulation* 1999;100:1464–1480.

235. Zerr KJ, Furnary AP, Grunkemeier GL, et al. Glucose control lowers the risk of wound infection in diabetics after open heart operations. *Ann Thorac Surg* 1997;63:356–361.

236. Hoogwerf BJ, Waness A, Cressman M, et al. Effects of aggressive cholesterol lowering and low-dose anticoagulation on clinical and angiographic outcomes in patients with diabetes: the Post Coronary Artery Bypass Graft Trial. *Diabetes* 1999;48:1289–1294.

237. Schwartz L, Kip KE, Frye RL, et al. Coronary bypass graft patency in patients with diabetes in the Bypass Angioplasty Revascularization Investigation (BARI). *Circulation* 2002;106:2652–2658.

238. Barsness GW, Peterson ED, Ohman EM, et al. Relationship between diabetes mellitus and long-term survival after coronary bypass and angioplasty. *Circulation* 1997;96:2551–2556.

239. The Bypass Angioplasty Revascularization Investigation (BARI) Investigators. Comparison of coronary bypass surgery with angioplasty in patients with multivessel disease. *N Engl J Med* 1996;335:217–225.

240. King SB 3rd, Kosinski AS, Guyton RA, et al. Eight-year mortality in the Emory Angioplasty versus Surgery Trial (EAST). *J Am Coll Cardiol* 2000;35:1116–1121.

241. Abizaid A, Costa MA, Centemero M, et al. Clinical and economic impact of diabetes mellitus on percutaneous and surgical treatment of multivessel coronary disease patients: insights from the Arterial Revascularization Therapy Study (ARTS) trial. *Circulation* 2001;104:533–538.

242. The BARI Investigators. Seven-year outcome in the Bypass Angioplasty Revascularization Investigation (BARI) by treatment and diabetic status. *J Am Coll Cardiol* 2000;35:1122–1129.

243. Detre KM, Lombardero MS, Brooks MM, et al. The effect of previous coronary-artery bypass surgery on the prognosis of patients with diabetes who have acute myocardial infarction. Bypass Angioplasty Revascularization Investigation Investigators. *N Engl J Med* 2000;342:989–997.

244. Gaede P, Vedel P, Larsen N, et al. Multifactorial intervention and cardiovascular disease in patients with type 2 diabetes. *N Engl J Med* 2003;348:383–393.

245. American diabetes association. Position statement. Management of dyslipidemia in adults with diabetes. *Diabetes Care* 1998;21:179–182.

246. DeFronzo RA, Goodman AM. Efficacy of metformin in patients with non-insulin-dependent diabetes mellitus. The Multicenter Metformin Study Group. *N Engl J Med* 1995;333:541–549.

247. Ghazzi MN, Perez JE, Antonucci TK, et al. Cardiac and glycemic benefits of troglitazone treatment in NIDDM. The Troglitazone Study Group. *Diabetes* 1997;46:433–439.

248. Tack CJ, Smits P, Demacker PN, et al. Troglitazone decreases the proportion of small, dense LDL and increases the resistance of LDL to oxidation in obese subjects. *Diabetes Care* 1998;21:796–799.

249. Standards of medical care for patients with diabetes mellitus. *Diabetes Care* 2002;25:213–229.

250. Executive Summary of the Third Report of The National Cholesterol Education Program (NCEP) Expert Panel on Detection, Evaluation, and Treatment of High Blood Cholesterol in Adults (Adult Treatment Panel III). *JAMA* 2001;285:2486–2497.

251. American Diabetes Association. Consensus statement: management of dyslipidemia in adults with diabetes. *Diabetes Care* 2002;25[Suppl]:S74–S77.

252. Pyorala K, Pedersen TR, Kjekshus J, et al. Cholesterol lowering with simvastatin improves prognosis of diabetic patients with coronary heart disease. A subgroup analysis of the Scandinavian Simvastatin Survival Study (4S). *Diabetes Care* 1997;20:614–620.

253. Prevention of cardiovascular events and death with pravastatin in patients with coronary heart disease and a broad range of initial cholesterol levels. The Long-Term Intervention with Pravastatin in Ischaemic Disease (LIPID) Study Group. *N Engl J Med* 1998;339:1349–1357.

254. Effect of fenofibrate on progression of coronary-artery disease in type 2 diabetes: the Diabetes Atherosclerosis Intervention Study, a randomised study. *Lancet* 2001;357:905–910.

255. Rubins HB, Robins SJ, Collins D, et al. Gemfibrozil for the secondary prevention of coronary heart disease in men with low levels of high-density lipoprotein cholesterol. Veterans Affairs High-Density Lipoprotein Cholesterol Intervention Trial Study Group. *N Engl J Med* 1999;341:410–418.

256. Vega GL, Grundy SM. Gemfibrozil therapy in primary hypertriglyceridemia associated with coronary heart disease. Effects on metabolism of low-density lipoproteins. *JAMA* 1985;253:2398–2403.

257. Elam MB, Hunninghake DB, Davis KB, et al. Effect of niacin on lipid and lipoprotein levels and glycemic control in patients with diabetes and peripheral arterial disease: the ADMIT study: a randomized trial. Arterial Disease Multiple Intervention Trial. *JAMA* 2000;284:1263–1270.

258. Grundy SM, Vega GL, McGovern ME, et al. Efficacy, safety, and tolerability of once-daily niacin for the treatment of dyslipidemia associated with type 2 diabetes: results of the assessment of diabetes control and evaluation of the efficacy of niaspan trial. *Arch Intern Med* 2002;162:1568–1576.

259. Arauz-Pacheco C, Parrott MA, Raskin P. The treatment of hypertension in adult patients with diabetes. *Diabetes Care* 2002;25:134–147.

260. The Sixth Report of the Joint National Committee on prevention, evaluation, and treatment of high blood pressure. *Arch Intern Med* 1997;157:2413–2446.

261. Tight blood pressure control and risk of macrovascular and microvascular complications in type 2 diabetes: UKPDS 38. *BMJ* 1998;317:703–713.

262. Hansson L, Zanchetti A, Carruthers SG, et al. Effects of intensive blood-pressure lowering and low-dose aspirin in patients with hypertension: principal results of the Hypertension Optimal Treatment (HOT) randomised trial. HOT Study Group. *Lancet* 1998;351:1755–1762.

263. Estacio RO, Jeffers BW, Hiatt WR, et al. The effect of nisoldipine as compared with enalapril on cardiovascular outcomes in patients with non-insulin-dependent diabetes and hypertension. *N Engl J Med* 1998;338:645–652.

264. Efficacy of atenolol and captopril in reducing risk of macrovascular and microvascular complications in type 2 diabetes: UKPDS 39. *BMJ* 1998;317:713–720.

265. Tatti P, Pahor M, Byington RP, et al. Outcome results of the Fosinopril versus Amlodipine Cardiovascular Events Randomized Trial (FACET) in patients with hypertension and NIDDM. *Diabetes Care* 1998;21:597–603.

266. Curb JD, Pressel SL, Cutler JA, et al. Effect of diuretic-based antihypertensive treatment on cardiovascular disease risk in older diabetic patients with isolated systolic hypertension. Systolic Hypertension in the Elderly Program Cooperative Research Group [published erratum appears in JAMA 1997;277:1356]. *JAMA* 1996;276:1886–1892.

267. Tuomilehto J, Rastenyte D, Birkenhager WH, et al. Effects of calcium-channel blockade in older patients with diabetes and systolic hypertension. Systolic Hypertension in Europe Trial Investigators. *N Engl J Med* 1999;340:677–684.

268. Kaplan NM. Management of hypertension in patients with type 2 diabetes mellitus: guidelines based on current evidence. *Ann Intern Med* 2001;135:1079–1083.

269. Grossman E, Messerli FH, Goldbourt U. High blood pressure and diabetes mellitus: are all antihypertensive drugs created equal? *Arch Intern Med* 2000;160:2447–2452.

270. Brenner BM, Cooper ME, de Zeeuw D, et al. Effects of losartan on renal and cardiovascular outcomes in patients with type 2 diabetes and nephropathy. *N Engl J Med* 2001;345:861–869.

271. Intensive blood-glucose control with sulphonylureas or insulin compared with conventional treatment and risk of complications in patients with type 2 diabetes (UKPDS 33). UK Prospective Diabetes Study (UKPDS) Group. *Lancet* 1998;352:837–853.

272. Jensen-Urstad KJ, Reichard PG, Rosfors JS, et al. Early atherosclerosis is retarded by improved long-term blood glucose control in patients with IDDM. *Diabetes* 1996;45:1253–1258.

273. Stratton IM, Adler AI, Neil HA, et al. Association of glycaemia with macrovascular and microvascular complications of type 2 diabetes (UKPDS 35): prospective observational study. *BMJ* 2000;321:405–412.

274. Inzucchi SE. Oral antihyperglycemic therapy for type 2 diabetes: scientific review. *JAMA* 2002;287:360–372.

275. Nathan DM. Clinical practice. Initial management of glycemia in type 2 diabetes mellitus. *N Engl J Med* 2002;347:1342–1349.

276. Jiang C, Ting AT, Seed B. PPAR-gamma agonists inhibit production of monocyte inflammatory cytokines. *Nature* 1998;391:82–86.

277. Chiasson JL, Josse RG, Gomis R, et al. Acarbose for prevention of type 2 diabetes mellitus: the STOP-NIDDM randomised trial. *Lancet* 2002;359:2072–2077.

278. Knowler WC, Barrett-Connor E, Fowler SE, et al. Reduction in the

incidence of type 2 diabetes with lifestyle intervention or metformin. *N Engl J Med* 2002;346:393–403.

279. Tuomilehto J, Lindstrom J, Eriksson JG, et al. Prevention of type 2 diabetes mellitus by changes in lifestyle among subjects with impaired glucose tolerance. *N Engl J Med* 2001;344:1343–1350.

280. The prevention or delay of type 2 diabetes. *Diabetes Care* 2002;25:742–749.

281. Hansson L, Lindholm LH, Niskanen L, et al. Effect of angiotensin-converting-enzyme inhibition compared with conventional therapy on cardiovascular morbidity and mortality in hypertension: the Captopril Prevention Project (CAPPP) randomised trial. *Lancet* 1999;353:611–616.

282. Yusuf S, Gerstein H, Hoogwerf B, et al. Ramipril and the development of diabetes. *JAMA* 2001;286:1882–1885.

283. Lindholm LH, Ibsen H, Borch-Johnsen K, et al. Risk of new-onset diabetes in the Losartan Intervention For Endpoint reduction in hypertension study. *J Hypertens* 2002;20:1879–1886.

284. Freeman DJ, Norrie J, Sattar N, et al. Pravastatin and the development of diabetes mellitus: evidence for a protective treatment effect in the West of Scotland Coronary Prevention Study. *Circulation* 2001;103:357–362.

285. Mokdad AH, Bowman BA, Ford ES, et al. The continuing epidemics of obesity and diabetes in the United States. *JAMA* 2001;286:1195–1200.

286. Allison DB, Fontaine KR, Manson JE, et al. Annual deaths attributable to obesity in the United States. *JAMA* 1999;282:1530–1538.

287. Barsh GS, Farooqi IS, O'Rahilly S. Genetics of body-weight regulation. *Nature* 2000;404:644–651.

288. Kopelman PG. Obesity as a medical problem. *Nature* 2000;404:635–643.

289. Eckel RH, Barouch WW, Ershow AG. Report of the National Heart, Lung, and Blood Institute-National Institute of Diabetes and Digestive and Kidney Diseases Working Group on the pathophysiology of obesity-associated cardiovascular disease. *Circulation* 2002;105:2923–2928.

290. Troiano RP, Flegal KM. Overweight children and adolescents: description, epidemiology, and demographics. *Pediatrics* 1998;101:497–504.

291. Whitaker RC, Wright JA, Pepe MS, et al. Predicting obesity in young adulthood from childhood and parental obesity. *N Engl J Med* 1997;337:869–873.

292. Ford ES, Williamson DF, Liu S. Weight change and diabetes incidence: findings from a national cohort of US adults. *Am J Epidemiol* 1997;146:214–222.

293. McGill HC Jr, McMahan CA, Herderick EE, et al. Obesity accelerates the progression of coronary atherosclerosis in young men. *Circulation* 2002;105:2712–2718.

294. Manson JE, Willett WC, Stampfer MJ, et al. Body weight and mortality among women. *N Engl J Med* 1995;333:677–685.

295. Calle EE, Thun MJ, Petrelli JM, et al. Body-mass index and mortality in a prospective cohort of U.S. adults. *N Engl J Med* 1999;341:1097–1105.

296. Rimm EB, Stampfer MJ, Giovannucci E, et al. Body size and fat distribution as predictors of coronary heart disease among middle-aged and older US men. *Am J Epidemiol* 1995;141:1117–1127.

297. Montague CT, O'Rahilly S. The perils of portliness: causes and consequences of visceral adiposity. *Diabetes* 2000;49:883–888.

298. Han TS, van Leer EM, Seidell JC, et al. Waist circumference action levels in the identification of cardiovascular risk factors: prevalence study in a random sample. *BMJ* 1995;311:1401–1405.

299. Willett WC, Dietz WH, Colditz GA. Guidelines for healthy weight. *N Engl J Med* 1999;341:427–434.

300. Colditz GA, Willett WC, Rotnitzky A, et al. Weight gain as a risk factor for clinical diabetes mellitus in women. *Ann Intern Med* 1995;122:481–486.

301. Lean ME, Han TS, Seidell JC. Impairment of health and quality of life in people with large waist circumference. *Lancet* 1998;351:853–856.

302. Huang Z, Willett WC, Manson JE, et al. Body weight, weight change, and risk for hypertension in women. *Ann Intern Med* 1998;128:81–88.

303. Clinical Guidelines on the Identification, Evaluation, and Treatment of Overweight and Obesity in Adults—The Evidence Report. National Institutes of Health. *Obes Res* 1998;6[Suppl 2]:51S–209S.

304. Kenchaiah S, Evans JC, Levy D, et al. Obesity and the risk of heart failure. *N Engl J Med* 2002;347:305–313.

305. Alpert MA. Obesity cardiomyopathy: pathophysiology and evolution of the clinical syndrome. *Am J Med Sci* 2001;321:225–236.

306. Zhou YT, Grayburn P, Karim A, et al. Lipotoxic heart disease in obese rats: implications for human obesity. *Proc Natl Acad Sci USA* 2000;97:1784–1789.

307. Hotamisligil GS, Arner P, Caro JF, et al. Increased adipose tissue expression of tumor necrosis factor-alpha in human obesity and insulin resistance. *J Clin Invest* 1995;95:2409–2415.

308. Steppan CM, Bailey ST, Bhat S, et al. The hormone resistin links obesity to diabetes. *Nature* 2001;409:307–312.

309. Masuzaki H, Paterson J, Shinyama H, et al. A transgenic model of visceral obesity and the metabolic syndrome. *Science* 2001;294:2166–2170.

310. Bujalska IJ, Kumar S, Stewart PM. Does central obesity reflect "Cushing's disease of the omentum"? *Lancet* 1997;349:1210–1213.

311. Hotamisligil GS, Shargill NS, Spiegelman BM. Adipose expression of tumor necrosis factor-alpha: direct role in obesity-linked insulin resistance. *Science* 1993;259:87–91.

312. Matsuda T, Morishita E, Jokaji H, et al. Mechanism on disorders of coagulation and fibrinolysis in diabetes. *Diabetes* 1996;45[Suppl 3]:S109–S110.

313. Mansfield MW, Heywood DM, Grant PJ. Sex differences in coagulation and fibrinolysis in white subjects with non-insulin-dependent diabetes mellitus. *Arterioscler Thromb Vasc Biol* 1996;16:160–164.

314. Shimomura I, Funahashi T, Takahashi M, et al. Enhanced expression of PAI-1 in visceral fat: possible contributor to vascular disease in obesity. *Nat Med* 1996;2:800–803.

315. Konstantinides S, Schafer K, Koschnick S, et al. Leptin-dependent platelet aggregation and arterial thrombosis suggests a mechanism for atherothrombotic disease in obesity. *J Clin Invest* 2001;108:1533–1540.

316. Nakata M, Yada T, Soejima N, et al. Leptin promotes aggregation of human platelets via the long form of its receptor. *Diabetes* 1999;48:426–429.

317. Frohlich M, Imhof A, Berg G, et al. Association between C-reactive protein and features of the metabolic syndrome: a population-based study. *Diabetes Care* 2000;23:1835–1839.

318. Ford ES. Body mass index, diabetes, and C-reactive protein among U.S. adults. *Diabetes Care* 1999;22:1971–1977.

319. Hak AE, Stehouwer CD, Bots ML, et al. Associations of C-reactive protein with measures of obesity, insulin resistance, and subclinical atherosclerosis in healthy, middle-aged women. *Arterioscler Thromb Vasc Biol* 1999;19:1986–1991.

320. Lemieux I, Pascot A, Prud'homme D, et al. Elevated C-reactive protein: another component of the atherothrombotic profile of abdominal obesity. *Arterioscler Thromb Vasc Biol* 2001;21:961–967.

321. Yudkin JS, Stehouwer CD, Emeis JJ, et al. C-reactive protein in healthy subjects: associations with obesity, insulin resistance, and endothelial dysfunction: a potential role for cytokines originating from adipose tissue? *Arterioscler Thromb Vasc Biol* 1999;19:972–978.

322. Festa A, D'Agostino R Jr, Howard G, et al. Chronic subclinical inflammation as part of the insulin resistance syndrome: the Insulin Resistance Atherosclerosis Study (IRAS). *Circulation* 2000;102:42–47.

323. Yanovski SZ, Yanovski JA. Obesity. *N Engl J Med* 2002;346:591–602.

CHAPTER **20**

Estrogen and Atherothrombosis

Lori Mosca

INTRODUCTION

Coronary heart disease (CHD) is the leading cause of death in both men and women in the United States and most other industrialized countries. However, women experience initial manifestations of CHD about 10 years later than men (1), and compared with premenopausal women, postmenopausal women experience a threefold increase in risk for CHD (2). This observation of a delayed onset of CHD in women, coupled with a greater rate of disease in men, has contributed to the hypothesis that there is something about being female, most likely endogenous estrogen, that is good for cardiovascular health (3).

Postmenopausal hormone therapy has been used for more than 50 years for the alleviation of menopausal symptoms, and in more recent decades for the prevention of several chronic diseases, including cardiovascular disease (CVD). However, in the past several years, data from randomized,

L. Mosca: Preventive Cardiology, New York Presbyterian Hospital; and Department of Medicine, Columbia University College of Physicians and Surgeons, ICCR PH 10-203D, 622 West 168th St., New York, New York 10032.

placebo-controlled trials challenged the conventional wisdom that hormone replacement therapy (HRT) would prevent postmenopausal women from succumbing to CVD. Clinical trials and other studies suggest that estrogen therapy may be associated with some deleterious cardiovascular effects, especially in the period early after initiation of treatment.

Estrogen produces varied effects in different tissues in the body. Functional estrogen receptors (ERs) are present in the smooth muscle, endothelial cells, and myocardium of men and women. When activated, these steroid hormone receptors serve as transcription factors that bind estrogen response elements on target genes, and then alter their expression. Nonhormone therapy with selective estrogen receptor modulators (SERMs) may take advantage of the beneficial effects of ER activation and altered gene expression in specific target organs, while avoiding untoward effects by blocking estrogen action in certain other tissues. A current limitation of SERMs is that they do not treat menopausal symptoms. Therefore, the role of traditional and newer sex receptor–targeted therapy for postmenopausal women and the impact on CVD is discussed.

POTENTIAL MECHANISMS FOR CARDIOPROTECTIVE AND ADVERSE CARDIOVASCULAR EFFECTS OF HORMONE THERAPY

The effects of estrogen on the cardiovascular system fall into two broad categories: (a) systemic effects on circulating factors, including lipids, coagulation and fibrinolysis, and inflammation; and (b) direct effects on the heart and vasculature, including the rapid effects of an increase in nitric oxide and vasodilation, and longer-term effects related to gene expression. Among the genomic effects are a decrease in atherothrombosis, vascular injury, and smooth muscle cell growth, and an increase in endothelial cell growth (4,5).

Estrogen Receptors and Signaling Pathways

Our understanding of the effects of estrogen on the cardiovascular system has changed significantly during the last decade, particularly with regard to the pathways for ER action.

Estrogen acts by binding to intracellular steroid hormone receptors that are present in cardiovascular cells, reproductive tissue, mammary gland, bone, liver, and brain (6,7). Two types of ERs have been identified: ER-α and ER-β. Both types are found in smooth muscle and endothelial cells of the vasculature. Cell-specific effects of estrogen are mediated by the differential expression of proteins that interact with the ERs, either as coactivators or corepressors, and modulate downstream effects (8).

Research suggests that estrogen and its receptors may play a direct and functional role in vascular protection. For example, diminished ER expression in vascular smooth muscle was found in premenopausal women who had premature atherothrombosis (9).

The cardiovascular effects of estrogen involve multiple signaling pathways that result in cell-specific responses in both vascular and nonvascular cells. Estrogen has been shown to up-regulate the transcription of inducible nitric oxide synthase (iNOS) and attenuate vasoconstriction in animals through an ER-β–mediated genomic pathway (10). Estrogen also produces rapid vasodilatory effects on endothelial cells by directly activating endothelial nitric oxide synthase (eNOS) through ER-α (8). Unlike the classic signaling pathway, this rapid response requires no change in gene expression and is often referred to as the nongenomic effect of estrogen. Rapid signal transduction and activation of eNOS has been shown to involve the phosphatidylinositol-3-kinase Akt pathway (5, 11,12).

Slower transcriptional related effects include inhibition of intimal hyperplasia through increased endothelial cell renewal and decreased smooth muscle cell proliferation; promotion of angiogenesis; decreased oxidation of low-density lipoprotein (LDL) and, therefore, decreased macrophage foam cell maturation.

Beneficial Effects by Estrogen on Intermediate Endpoints

Estrogen has both systemic and direct effects on the cardiovascular system (Table 20–1). Systemic effects include changes in lipoprotein metabolism, inflammatory coagulation, and fibrinolysis pathways. The direct effects of estrogen include vasodilation and a decrease in the vascular injury response.

Lipoprotein Metabolism

Initial studies indicated that cardioprotection derives from the beneficial effects of estrogen on lipoproteins. These lipid effects are mainly caused by the altered hepatic expression of apolipoprotein (*apo*) genes and LDL receptors. However, the Post-menopausal Estrogen/Progesterone Intervention (PEPI) study also revealed other factors (13). In healthy, postmenopausal women, estrogen alone or in combination with a progestin significantly improved lipoproteins and decreased fibrinogen levels. LDL cholesterol levels were decreased by 10% to 12%; high-density lipoprotein (HDL) cholesterol levels showed a similar increase; and lipoprotein(a), an independent risk factor for CHD and stroke (13), was reduced by 25%. Although the study was not powered for clinical end points, rates of cardiovascular events and mortality were found to be equivalent between treated groups and a comparison placebo group (14).

Estrogen replacement therapy (ERT) also has been shown to increase apoA-1 levels, decrease apoB-100 levels, and inhibit the oxidation of LDL cholesterol (15–17). Studies have demonstrated that alterations in lipoprotein metabolism account for approximately one-third of the cardiovascular benefit seen in observational studies of estrogen (11).

Vasodilation

Estrogen promotes vasodilation by increasing prostacyclin levels and decreasing endothelin-1 levels, angiotensin-converting enzyme activation, renin levels, and angiotensin II receptor levels (18). Estrogen directly activates NOS through nongenomic effects. The increase in nitric oxide facilitates endothelium-dependent vasodilation and reverses the paradoxic coronary vasoconstriction seen in diseased endothelium (8). Estrogen also has been shown to have direct effects on calcium-activated potassium channels in vascular smooth muscle cells, which further promotes vasodilation (19).

Coagulation

Estrogen alters hemostasis and can inhibit coagulation by decreasing levels of fibrinogen and factor XII. It also has been shown to promote fibrinolysis by decreasing levels of

ESTROGEN AND ATHEROTHROMBOSIS / 299

TABLE 20–1. *Qualitative comparison of cardiovascular effects with hormone replacement therapy, selective estrogen receptor modulators, and tibolone in postmenopausal women*

	HRT	Raloxifene	Tamoxifen	Tibolone
Serum lipids				
Total-C	↓	↓	↓	NC
LDL-C	↓	↓	↓	NC
HDL-C	↑	NC	NC	↓
HDL$_2$-C	↑↑	↑	NC	↓
Non–HDL-C	↓	↓	a	a
Triglycerides	↑	NC	NC	↓
Apolipoprotein B	↓	↓	↓	NC
Apolipoprotein A1	↑↑	↑	↑	↓
Lipoprotein(a)	↓↓	↓	↓↓	↓↓
Homocysteine	↓	↓	↓	a
Endothelial function				
Endothelium-dependent relaxation	↑	↑	↑ to NC	a
Plasma nitrates	↑	↑	↑	a
Endothelin-1	↓	↓	↓	a
Vascular inflammation/plaque stability				
HsCRP	↑	NC	↓	↑
MMP-9	↑	NC	a	a
TNF-α	↓	↓	a	a
Fibrinogen	↓ to NC	↓↓	↓↓	↓
E-selectin	↓	↓	a	a
ICAM-1	↓↓	↓	a	a
VCAM-1	↓	NC	a	a
MCP-1	↓	a	a	a

[a]Data not available.

HDL-C, high-density lipoprotein cholesterol; hsCRP, high-sensitivity C-reactive protein; ICAM-1, intercellular adhesion molecule-1; LDL, low-density lipoprotein cholesterol; MCP-1, monocyte chemotactic protein-1; MMP-9, matrix metalloproteinase-9; NC, no significant change; PAI-1, plasminogen activator inhibitor-1; TNF-α, tumor necrosis factor-α; VCAM-1, vascular cell adhesion molecule-1.

plasminogen activator inhibitor-1 and increasing levels of tissue plasminogen activator (18).

Antiinflammatory Action

The impact of estrogen on measures of inflammation is mixed. That atherothrombosis increases after menopause indicates that endogenous estrogen may have antiinflammatory effects. The antiinflammatory effects of estrogen on the endothelium are mediated by decreased levels of circulating adhesion molecules, which are responsible for leukocyte/endothelial attachment, such as E-selectin, vascular cell adhesion molecule-1 (VCAM-1), intercellular adhesion molecule-1 (ICAM-1), and several chemokines (20,21). By decreasing leukocyte adhesion, and therefore migration, these effects may result in a decrease in the inflammatory response to vascular injury, a process that is pivotal in the pathogenesis of atherothrombosis.

Vascular Injury Response

There are several mechanisms by which estrogen may decrease the vascular response to injury and maintain endothelial integrity by several mechanisms. The migration and proliferation of vascular smooth muscle cells in inhibited by decreased levels of transforming growth factor-β, epidermal growth factor receptor, platelet-derived growth factor, and flt4 tyrosine kinase (11). In addition, research shows that estrogen can up-regulate expression of vascular endothelial growth factor (22).

Insulin Resistance

Estrogen also appears to decrease insulin resistance. However, there is currently no clear evidence that HRT can modify insulin sensitivity and carbohydrate metabolism (23).

Homocysteine

Another systemic effect of estrogen is a decrease in levels of plasma homocysteine, an independent risk factor for CVD (24). Studies suggest that homocysteine-derived free radicals damage the endothelial lining of vessels. Decreasing serum levels of homocysteine may diminish the damage, such that endothelial injury will not progress to more advanced atherothrombosis (24). Homocysteine is a product of the transsulfuration and demethylation of methionine. This conversion of methionine to homocysteine is associated with production of methyl group that is donated to DNA, RNA, proteins, and hormones. Estrogen appears to reduce the level of homocysteine either indirectly by its effect on gene expression, or directly by effects on homocysteine synthesis. This effect on methionine/homocysteine metabolism may play a role in the antiatherothrombotic action of estrogen (25).

As the previously mentioned evidence shows, estrogen has both systemic and direct vascular actions that affect lipoprotein metabolism, vasodilation, and inflammatory and coagulation pathways, all of which may confer vasoprotection.

Biologic Basis for Adverse Cardiovascular Effects of Estrogen/Progestin

In contrast to numerous potentially cardioprotective biologic effects of estrogen, some of its other biologic actions may have adverse cardiovascular consequences in postmenopausal women (Table 20–1). Several mechanisms may explain these adverse effects of estrogen, including (a) prothrombic, (b) proinflammatory, (c) proarrhythmic, and (d) adverse lipid profile changes.

Prothrombic Effect

Despite some anticoagulant effects, estrogen can adversely affect the cardiovascular system by promoting thrombosis. Clinically, ERT has been shown to increase the risk for deep venous thromboembolism by threefold (26). The procoagulant effect of estrogen is mediated in part by increased levels of prothrombin fragments 1 and 2 and fibrinopeptide A, and decreased levels of antithrombin III and protein S (18,27). Increased levels of factor VII and factor VIII antigen may also contribute; however, data are inconsistent. Estrogen can also lead to increased activated protein C resistance that, when superimposed on the inherited factor V Leiden mutation, may increase atherothrombosis risk in hyperlipidemic women treated with ERT (28,29). Here, too, data on the association between factor V Leiden and CHD appear to be conflicting (30).

Research also suggests an increased risk for atherothrombosis with ERT in postmenopausal women carrying the prothrombin mutation G20210A, compared with the wild-type genotype (31). Although larger studies are needed to confirm these findings, they suggest that the assessment of thrombotic risk may be important in decisions on use of ERT.

Proinflammatory Effect

In addition to previously mentioned antiinflammatory effects at the endothelial levels, estrogen also has been shown to alter proinflammatory cytokine gene expression in monocytes. Although *in vitro* data have not been consistent, some *in vivo* studies suggest that estrogen treatment may be associated with increases in proinflammatory cytokines such as interleukin (IL)-6 and tumor necrosis factor-α, which may play a role in the evolution of atherogenic plaques (32).

Estrogen also has been shown to increase levels of C-reactive protein (CRP), a nonspecific marker of inflamma-

tion that activates the complement cascade (33), stimulates the release of inflammatory cytokines (34), and induces tissue factor expression from macrophage foam cells (35). CRP may also act as a primary inflammatory instigator of coronary instability (34), and it has been independently associated with increased CVD in women (21,36). Research also shows that increased levels of CRP induce VCAM-1, ICAM-1, and E-selectin (37). The resulting increase in leukocyte adhesion may negate the potential antiinflammatory effects of estrogen. Matrix metalloproteinase-9, an enzyme capable of digesting matrix proteins and leaving atherothrombotic plaques vulnerable to rupture or fissure, also increases with estrogen treatment (38).

Findings of a prospective study from the Women's Health Initiative Observational Study showed that CRP and IL-6 independently predicted future cardiovascular events in apparently healthy postmenopausal women and that HRT increases CRP (39). Research indicates that statin administration may attenuate the increase in CRP during estrogen therapy (40).

Proarrhythmic Effect

In the Heart and Estrogen/progestin Replacement Study (HERS) (41) and its follow-up HERS II (42), women who were assigned to hormone therapy had a greater rate of nonfatal ventricular arrhythmia compared with those assigned to placebo. Although this increase was not associated with an increased risk for sudden death, most of these events required resuscitation.

Adverse Lipid Profile Changes

Increased triglyceride levels are strongly correlated with increased CHD risk (43). Estrogen therapy has been shown to cause a 20% increase in triglyceride levels by increasing hepatic apoB and very low-density lipoprotein (VLDL) expression (44,45). However, it is important to note that hepatic first-pass metabolism is responsible for this effect. Natural and transdermal ERTs do not result in significant lipid alterations, because they enter the systemic circulatory system, rather than the portal.

Because of the combined favorable and unfavorable effects of estrogen on markers of coagulation, inflammation, and lipid metabolism, laboratory measurements may not predict the predominant effect (3). Clinical studies are needed to determine net cardiovascular outcomes.

HORMONE THERAPY FOR SECONDARY PREVENTION OF CARDIOVASCULAR DISEASE

Observational Data

More than 30 observational studies have examined the role of postmenopausal ERT in the prevention of CVD in women without CHD. Results consistently showed a reduction in cardiovascular risk with treatment. In several metaanalyses, aggregate relative risks for CHD mortality were between 0.50 and 0.65 for comparisons of women who had once used ERT or combined HRT versus women who had never used ERT/HRT (46–49). The Nurses' Health Study, the largest of the observational studies, noted a 40% decrease in CHD in current users versus never-users of HRT after adjustment for CHD risk factors, and it also showed a greater benefit among women at high-risk for CHD (50).

Epidemiologic studies examining the role of ERT in women with established CVD are limited in number, but they also have shown cardiovascular benefits such as decreased angiographic disease and increased long term survival in users of ERT, compared with never-users (51,52).

Although the overwhelming body of observational evidence indicates a cardiovascular benefit with estrogen therapy in primary prevention, several studies have shown a possible early adverse effect among estrogen users. An examination of data from the Nurses' Health Study showed that short-term users of HRT (<1 year) had a 25% increased risk for recurrent CHD events compared with never-users, whereas long-term users had lower event rates relative to never-users (53). Several other observational studies in women with established CHD also suggest an early increased risk associated with estrogen therapy (54–56). In the Coumadin Aspirin Reinfarction Study (CARS), postmenopausal women who initiated HRT after a recent myocardial infarction (MI) had a greater incidence of unstable angina, compared with women who had never used HRT or had been taking HRT before their index event (55).

Despite the observational data that support a cardioprotective role of ERT in primary prevention, there are many limitations of observational studies that may overestimate or account for the apparent beneficial effect of ERT. One important confounding factor is the healthy women selection bias, because women who use ERT tend to be healthier, more educated, and of higher socioeconomic status (57). Similarly, physicians may tend to provide better preventive care and monitoring for women on hormone therapy (preventional bias). Other biases include prevalence/incidence bias, compliance bias, and survivor bias (58). These limitations of the observational data emphasize the importance of clinical trials, because double-blinded, randomized, controlled study designs are able to minimize bias.

Heart and Estrogen/Progestin Replacement Study (HERS I and II)

No benefit for secondary prevention of CHD has yet been demonstrated with HRT in postmenopausal women. HERS, the first prospective, randomized, placebo-controlled trial to examine HRT in women with preexisting coronary artery disease, found no overall benefit for women assigned to conjugated equine estrogen (CEE) 0.625 mg per day and medroxyprogesterone acetate (MPA) 2.5 mg per day, compared with placebo (41). At the completion of the trial (4.1 years), there was no difference between the treatment and placebo arms of the study in the primary outcome of CHD events (nonfatal MI plus CHD-related death) or in any secondary cardiovascular outcomes. Surprisingly, a 52% increase in risk for CHD events for hormone-assigned study patients was detected in Year 1 of HERS (42.5/1,000 person-years vs. 28.0/1,000 person-years), although a protective effect was seen during Years 3 to 5. Patients in the treatment group were also found to be more vulnerable to gallbladder disease and venous thromboembolism while receiving HRT.

The HERS II trial provided data on an additional 2.7 years of observation in 93% of the original HERS subjects (42). The HERS investigators found that lower rates of CHD events in the HRT group did not persist during the additional years of follow-up. After 6.8 years, there was no evidence that HRT reduces the risk for cardiovascular events in women with established disease (Fig. 20–1).

Angiographic Trials

Lack of benefit also was reported in the Papworth HRT Atherosclerosis Study Enquiry (PHASE), which randomized women with established CHD to HRT (transdermal 17-β estradiol plus cyclic norethisterone) or placebo (59). Patients were followed for more than 3 years. In the first 2 years of the study, there were more thromboembolic events in the treatment arm than in the placebo arm, although the difference was not statistically significant.

The Estrogen Replacement and Atherosclerosis (ERA) trial showed no difference in progression of coronary atherothrombosis in women randomized to CEE 0.625 mg per day plus progesterone, CEE alone, or placebo (60)

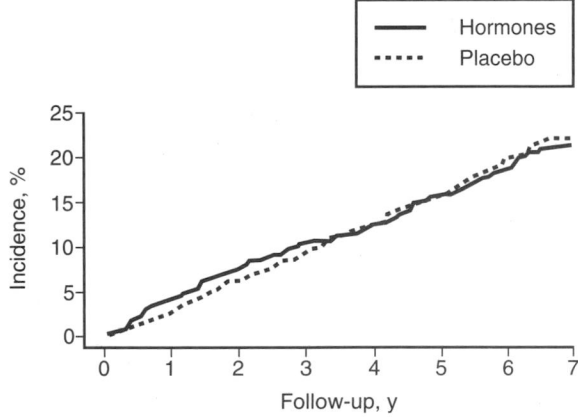

No. at Risk
Hormones	1380	1303	1247	1196	1133	1043	984	354
Placebo	1383	1334	1269	1209	1122	1039	976	336

FIG. 20–1. Cumulative incidence of coronary heart disease events in postmenopausal women in Heart and Estrogen/progestin Replacement Study II. (From Grady D, Herrington D, Bittner V, et al. Cardiovascular disease outcomes during 6.8 years of hormone therapy: Heart and Estrogen/Progestin Replacement Study follow-up (HERS II). *JAMA* 2002;288: 49–57.)

Women included in this study, as in HERS, were elderly (mean age, 65.8 years), and had undergone menopause an average of 23.1 years earlier. This prolonged time interval may be relevant because of diminished numbers or activity of ERs in aging or diseased vessels. Post and coworkers (61) found that inactivation of the ER-α by a process of methylation occurred in cardiovascular tissue with aging. In studies by Losordo and coworkers (9), ERs were less prevalent in atherothrombotic vessels of premenopausal women versus normal arteries. Although this relation no longer held true in atherothrombotic vessels of postmenopausal women, the authors postulated that the estrogen-deficient state of women after menopause obviated any potentially protective effect of the ER (9).

The possibility of an increase in cardiovascular events early after HRT use was explored in an analysis of the CARS (Coumadin Aspirin Reinfarction Study) database, which followed post-MI patients randomized to two possible doses each of aspirin or Coumadin (55). The authors found that postmenopausal women who began taking HRT during the study had a greater incidence of unstable angina during follow-up than those women who had never used HRT, as well as those who had been taking HRT before their index event. Women who were current users of HRT had a significantly decreased risk for death when compared with women who had never taken HRT.

Several reported trials also deserve mention. Schulman and coworkers (62) randomized postmenopausal women with unstable angina either to placebo or acute hormone therapy (using intravenous followed by oral conjugated estrogen, with or without MPA) for 21 days. They found no difference among the three study arms in the primary end point of ambulatory electrocardiographic ischemic events over 48 hours, and no difference in clinical outcomes. In the Women's Estrogen for Stroke Trial (WEST), women with established cerebrovascular disease were randomized to treatment with 17-β estradiol or placebo (63). After a mean follow-up of 2.7 years, there was no difference between treatment and placebo arms in the incidence of recurrent cerebral ischemia or all-cause mortality, although there was a trend toward increased incidence of fatal stroke. These data are consistent with an angiographic trial of 226 postmenopausal women with CHD showing no significant effect of 17-β estradiol alone or with MPA on the progression of artherosclerosis (64).

Multiple explanations for the lack of benefit have been postulated, including negative effects of the progestational agent used, bidirectional estrogen effects (early harm and late benefit), an elderly study population that could no longer benefit from therapy, and the possibility that HRT is simply not effective in preventing recurrent events in women with established coronary artery disease (65). One hypothesis for explaining the early increased risk with HRT suggests a potential interaction of HRT with coagulation and/or inflammation mechanisms in a subset of women with vulnerable plaques. It may be that certain women have a susceptibility factor in the form of an increased blood or tissue level, or an augmented response to HRT caused by a genetic mutation, which could result in plaque destabilization and thrombosis (29).

HORMONE THERAPY FOR PRIMARY PREVENTION OF CARDIOVASCULAR DISEASE

Epidemiologic Studies

Observational studies have consistently demonstrated a reduced CHD risk among postmenopausal women currently using HRT compared with nonusers. A 35% decrease in risk for CHD was documented in a metaanalysis (66). However, as mentioned earlier, women taking HRT are generally better educated and of higher socioeconomic status than nonusers, and this may account for some, or all, of the observed benefit (57). HRT users have healthier lifestyles and are more likely to have preventive evaluations, which also may bias results in favor of HRT (65).

Women's Health Initiative

The Women's Health Initiative (WHI), sponsored by the National Heart, Lung, and Blood Institute, was a large multicenter trial designed to test the effects of several interventions on the development of CHD, breast and colorectal cancers, and fractures (67). WHI investigators randomized healthy postmenopausal women to estrogen plus progestin (n = 8,506), estrogen alone in women who had a hysterectomy (n = 10,739), or placebo (n = 8,102). The WHI data and safety monitoring board stopped the conjugated estrogen/MPA arm of the trial after 5.2 years, because health risks were found to outweigh benefits (67). Although a significant benefit was seen in the prevention of hip fractures and colorectal cancer, the HRT group showed an increase in breast cancer, CHD, stroke, and pulmonary embolism (Fig. 20–2).

The findings of the estrogen alone arm were recently published and showed no CHD benefit of CEE 0.25 mg daily compared to placebo among postmenopausal women with hysterectomy (68). Although CEE decreased hip fractures and did not effect CHD incidence, the risk of stroke was increased (OR = 1.39, 95% CI 1.10–1.77). The consistent increase in stroke risk in the HERS trial and both arms of the WHI suggest this adverse effect and is attributable to the estrogen component.

Hormone Therapy and Progression of Subclinical Atherothrombosis

The Estrogen in the Prevention of Atherosclerosis Trial (EPAT) looked at healthy postmenopausal women without preexisting CVD whose high LDL levels ((130 mg/dL) indicated that they were at high risk for development of CHD (68). Participants were randomized to receive 17-β estradiol or placebo. Progression of atherothrombosis was measured by carotid artery ultrasonography. There also was a planned subgroup of patients with LDL levels of 160 mg/dL or greater who received lipid-lowering medications (primarily statins).

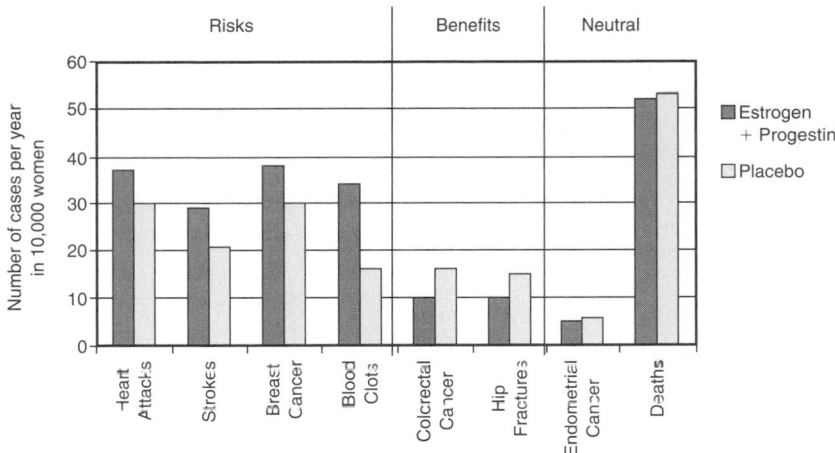

FIG. 20–2. Disease Rates for Postmenopausal Women on CEE/MPA versus Placebo in the Women's Health Initiative. (From the National Heart, Lung, and Blood Institute/National Institutes of Health (NHLBI/NIH) Women's Health Initiative Participant website. Available at: http://www.whi.org/update/2002update.asp)

Results from EPAT showed a significantly slower progression of atherothrombosis in women who were treated with 17-β estradiol, although the protective effect was not significant in women who were receiving lipid decreasing therapy.

In another primary prevention trial, Angerer and coworkers (69) studied healthy postmenopausal women with increased risk for CHD, as shown by increased intima-media thickness in one or more segments of the carotid arteries. During 1 year of treatment, women received 17-β estradiol plus standard progestin or low-dose progestin, or no HRT. Results showed that HRT was not effective in slowing the progression of subclinical atherothrombosis.

These results suggest that ERT might be useful only for primary prevention of CHD during the earliest stages of atherothrombosis, and not in women with more damaged epithelium and more advanced atherothrombotic lesions. However, the WHI, which evaluated women in the age range from 50 to 70 years, found that age did not modify the association between HRT and CHD (67). These data may or may not be generalizable to women with premature menopause or to symptomatic postmenopausal women.

POTENTIAL ROLE OF OTHER SEX RECEPTOR–TARGETED THERAPEUTICS IN CARDIOVASCULAR DISEASE PREVENTION

SERMs are nonhormonal agents that bind with high affinity to ERs. SERMs may exhibit either estrogen agonist or estrogen antagonist effects, depending on the end organ affected. Examples of clinically used compounds with the SERM profile include tamoxifen (Nolvadex), toremifene (Fareston), and raloxifene (Evista).

Tamoxifen and toremifene are triphenylethylene compounds used for the prevention and treatment, respectively, of breast cancer in postmenopausal women. Raloxifene is a benzothiophene compound used for the prevention and treatment of postmenopausal osteoporosis. Tibolone (Livial), al-

though not a SERM, is a synthetic steroid with tissue-selective estrogenic, progestational, and androgenic effects. Outside of the United States, tibolone is used in the treatment of climacteric symptoms and for the prevention of osteoporosis in postmenopausal women.

Cardiovascular Effects of Selective Estrogen Receptor Modulators and Tibolone

In addition to the effects related to their primary indications, all of these compounds have effects on the cardiovascular system that may influence the risk for CHD in postmenopausal women. SERMs have not been associated with the early increased risk for cardiovascular events seen in clinical trials using ERT/HRT. However, clinical studies of SERMs in postmenopausal women have focused primarily on biomarkers for cardiovascular risk (serum lipids and lipoproteins, homocysteine, and markers of vascular inflammation) and on vascular endothelial function (Table 20–1). Unlike HRT, SERMs do not increase HDL cholesterol or triglycerides levels and do not appear to increase CRP, a proinflammatory marker (24).

Raloxifene

Raloxifene has estrogen-like effects in preventing bone loss and decreases cholesterol levels in a similar fashion to estrogen, although to a lesser degree (71). At the same time, raloxifene produces estrogen-antagonist effects on breast and endometrial tissue, and it has been shown to decrease the risk for breast cancer (72). In small studies of healthy postmenopausal women, raloxifene showed favorable effects on vascular reactivity. Saitta and coworkers (73) demonstrated improved flow-mediated, endothelium-dependent vasodilation of the brachial artery equal to HRT, in a placebo-controlled trial involving 90 postmenopausal women randomized to 6 months of treatment with either raloxifene 60 mg daily, 17-β estradiol 1 mg daily plus norethisterone acetate 0.5 mg daily, or control (73). The study also demonstrated that raloxifene led to increases in nitric oxide products in the bloodstream.

Raloxifene may also reduce markers of vascular inflammation in an estrogen-like fashion, with consequent antiatherogenic properties. A raloxifene analogue has been shown to inhibit VCAM expression and adhesion of monocytes *in vitro,* similar to estrogen (74). Studies indicate that raloxifene also decreases plasma homocysteine (24,75,76) and does not increase CRP levels (24,77).

Tamoxifen

Tamoxifen is prescribed for the primary and secondary prevention of breast cancer. In large trials undertaken to examine its effects as adjuvant therapy for breast cancer treatment, tamoxifen has been reported to substantially decrease both fatal MI and hospitalization for acute coronary syndromes (78–80). However, the Breast Cancer Prevention Trial, which studied women who did not have a diagnosis of breast cancer, showed no differences in ischemic heart disease rates between women receiving tamoxifen versus those receiving a placebo (81). Notably, these trials reported CHD events as secondary, not primary, end points and had wide confidence intervals.

The cardiovascular effects of tamoxifen also have been specifically studied. Clarke and coworkers (82) reported that tamoxifen improved flow-mediated, endothelium-dependent vasodilation in men with angiographically proven coronary atherothrombosis, as well as those with normal coronary arteries. Tamoxifen also had beneficial effects on levels of total cholesterol, lipoprotein(a), and fibrinogen. Furthermore, in a 6-month substudy of women participating in a breast cancer primary prevention trial, 20 mg per day tamoxifen led to significant reductions in the levels of CRP, fibrinogen, and cholesterol in comparison with placebo (83).

Toremifene

Toremifene shows similar hypocholesterolemic effects to tamoxifen and, like tamoxifen, does not generally affect serum triglycerides in postmenopausal women (84). Both tamoxifen and toremifene also inhibit the oxidation of human LDL or lipid peroxidation in cell membranes *in vitro* (85). The antioxidant effects of these SERMs are generally 10- to 15-fold more potent than that of estrogen (85,86). Similar to HRT, toremifene, tamoxifen, and raloxifene all increase levels of plasma nitrate, a systemic metabolite of nitric oxide, and decrease plasma endothelin-1 levels, a potent endothelium-derived vasoconstrictor. These effects are consistent with an improvement in endothelium function *in vivo* (87).

Tibolone

Tibolone differs from both SERMs and estrogen in its effect on serum lipids, most likely because of its mixed estrogen/progesterone/androgenic profile. In randomized trials in postmenopausal women, tibolone decreased total cholesterol, triglycerides, and lipoprotein(a) levels, but, unlike estrogen and most SERMs, did not affect LDL cholesterol or apoB levels (88–91). Tibolone also consistently decreased HDL cholesterol and apo-A1 levels in postmenopausal women, whereas estrogen increases and SERMs generally have minimal effects on HDL and apo-A1 levels (88–91). Tibolone and raloxifene also have been shown to increase coronary and uterine artery blood flow *in vivo* through an ER-dependent mechanism at least partially dependent on nitric oxide (92–95). In another study, tibolone was found to induce endothelium-dependent venous vasodilation in the hand in postmenopausal women (96).

Clinical End Point Studies

The Multiple Outcomes of Raloxifene Evaluation (MORE) trial is the largest study of raloxifene completed to date (97,98). It was designed to test the effects of raloxifene on bone mineral density and vertebral fractures in more than 7,000 postmenopausal women with osteoporosis. Cardiovascular events and mortality were monitored as safety end points and were subsequently adjudicated by a cardiologist. Results of MORE showed no evidence that raloxifene was associated with an early increase in the risk for cardiovascular events, either overall or in subsets of women at high risk for or with a history of CHD (99). At the 4-year point, the risk for cardiovascular events (coronary and cerebrovascular events combined) was not significantly different in the placebo versus the raloxifene groups in the total study cohort, but was significantly reduced by 40% among women at high risk for cardiovascular events who were taking raloxifene (99).

Raloxifene was also associated with a significant 62% decrease in the likelihood of any stroke among women at increased cardiovascular risk. In addition, the MORE study showed that 4 years of treatment with raloxifene resulted in significant reductions of total cholesterol and LDL cholesterol levels, without a significant effect on HDL cholesterol or triglycerides levels (99).

Raloxifene Use for the Heart Trial

These data on surrogate end points are promising, but additional research is needed to demonstrate whether SERMs are a useful alternative to estrogen therapy for the prevention of CVD. More definitive evidence is expected from the ongoing Raloxifene Use for the Heart (RUTH) study, an international, placebo-controlled, long-term investigation evaluating the effects of raloxifene on cardiovascular and breast cancer morbidity and mortality in more than 10,000 women at increased risk for CVD or with documented coronary artery disease (100). Co-primary end points include (i) hospitalization for acute coronary syndrome other than MI, nonfatal MI, or coronary death and (ii) invasive breast cancer. Results should shed further light on the usefulness of this class of medications as a preventive strategy for postmenopausal women.

CURRENT CLINICAL RECOMMENDATIONS

Results from trials do not lend support for a role of hormone therapy in the prevention of CHD and suggest stroke risk is increased. Therefore, a recent expert panel of the American Heart Association that developed evidence-based guidelines for the prevention of CVD in women recommend hormone therapy as a class III intervention that should not be used to prevent CVD (101).

According to these latest guidelines, lifestyle approaches, including smoking avoidance, proper nutrition, and regular exercise, are indicated in all women. Blood pressure control with pharmacotherapy is indicated in women who do not meet blood pressure levels with lifestyle interventions. For high-risk women, statin therapy antiplatelet agents or (when indicated) anticoagulants, β-blockers, and angiotensin-converting enzyme inhibitors also should be used, unless there are contraindications to therapy. Lipid management with drug therapy is also indicated in some intermediate and lower risk women.

CHD is a significant cause of morbidity and mortality for millions of women worldwide. Efforts to decrease the number of women affected must focus on these proven risk reduction strategies.

REFERENCES

1. American Heart Association. *2002 Heart and stroke statistical update.* Dallas, TX: American Heart Association, 2001.
2. Kannel WB, Wilson PW. Risk factors that attenuate the female coronary disease advantage. *Arch Intern Med* 1995;155:57–61.
3. Rossouw JE. Hormones, genetic factors, and gender differences in cardiovascular disease. *Cardiovasc Res* 2002;53:550–557.
4. Karas RH, Mosca L. Introduction. A symposium: hormone replacement therapy and the pathophysiology of cardiovascular disease. *Am J Cardiol* 2002;90[Suppl]:1F–2F.
5. Chen Z, Yuhanna IS, Galcheva-Gargova Z, et al. Estrogen receptor α mediates the nongenomic activation of endothelial nitric oxide synthase by estrogen. *J Clin Invest* 1999;103:401–406.
6. Mendelsohn ME. Protective effects of estrogen on the cardiovascular system. *Am J Cardiol* 2002;89[Suppl]:12E–18E.
7. Mendelsohn ME. Genomic and nongenomic effects of estrogen in the vasculature. *Am J Cardiol* 2002;90[Suppl]:3F–6F.
8. Mendelsohn ME, Karas RH. The protective effects of estrogen on the cardiovascular system. *N Engl J Med* 1999;340:1801–1811.
9. Losordo DW, Kearney M, Kim EA, et al. Variable expression of the estrogen receptor in normal and atherosclerotic coronary arteries of premenopausal women. *Circulation* 1994;89:1501–1510.
10. Zhu Y, Bian Z, Lu P, et al. Abnormal vascular function and hypertension in mice deficient in estrogen receptor beta. *Science* 2002;295:505–508.
11. Haynes MP, Sinha D, Russell KS, et al. Membrane estrogen receptor engagement activates endothelial nitric oxide synthase via the P13-kinase Akt pathway in human endothelial cells. *Circ Res* 2000;87:677–682.
12. Simoncini T, Hafezi-Moghadam A, Brazil DP, et al. Interaction of oestrogen receptor with the regulatory subunit of phosphatidylinositol-3-OH kinase. *Nature* 2000;407:538–541.
13. Espeland MA, Marcovina SM, Miller V, et al. Effect of postmenopausal hormone therapy on lipoprotein(a) concentration. PEPI investigators. Postmenopausal Estrogen/Progestin Interventions. *Circulation* 1998;97:979–986.
14. Effects of estrogen or estrogen/progestin regimens on heart disease risk factors in postmenopausal women. The Postmenopausal Estrogen/Progestin Interventions (PEPI) Trial. *JAMA* 1995;273:199–208.
15. Brinton EA. Oral estrogen replacement therapy in postmenopausal women selectively raises levels and production rates of lipoprotein A-1 and lowers hepatic lipase activity without lowering the fractional catabolic rate. *Arterioscler Thromb Vasc Biol* 1996;16:431–440.
16. Nabulsi AA, Folsom AR, White A, et al. Association of hormone-replacement therapy with various cardiovascular risk factors in postmenopausal women. The Atherosclerosis Risk in Communities Study Investigators. *N Engl J Med* 1993;328:1069–1075.
17. Sack MN, Rader DJ, Cannon RO 3rd. Oestrogen and inhibition of oxidation of low-density lipoproteins in postmenopausal women. *Lancet* 1994;343:269–270.
18. Mendelsohn ME, Karas RH. Estrogen and the blood vessel wall. *Curr Opin Cardiol* 1994;9:619–626.
19. White RE, Darkow DJ, Lang JL. Estrogen relaxes coronary arteries by opening BKCa channels through a cGMP-dependent mechanism. *Circ Res* 1995;77:938–942.
20. Koh KK, Horne MK 3rd, Cannon RO 3rd. Effects of hormone replacement therapy on coagulation, fibrinolysis, and thrombosis risk in postmenopausal women. *Thromb Haemost* 1999;82:626–633.
21. Cushman M, Legault C, Barrett-Connor E, et al. Effect of postmenopausal hormones on inflammation-sensitive proteins: the Postmenopausal Estrogen/Progestin Interventions (PEPI) Study. *Circulation* 1999;100:717–722.
22. Agarwal R, Prelevic G, Conway GS, et al. Serum vascular endothelial growth factor concentrations in postmenopausal women: the effect of hormone replacement therapy. *Fertil Steril* 2000;73:56–60.
23. Vehkavaara S, Westerbacks J, Hakala-Ala-Pietila T, et al. Effect of estrogen replacement therapy on insulin sensitivity of glucose metabolism and preresistance and resistance vessel function in healthy postmenopausal women. *J Clin Endocrinol Metab* 2000;85:4663–4670.
24. Walsh BW, Paul S, Wild RA, et al. The effects of hormone replacement therapy and raloxifene on C-reactive protein and homocysteine in healthy postmenopausal women: a randomized, controlled trial. *J Clin Endocrinol Metab* 2000;85:214–218.
25. Dimitrova KR, DeGroot K, Myers AK, et al. Review: estrogen and homocysteine. *Cardiovasc Res* 2002;53:577–588.
26. Grady D, Wenger NK, Herrington D, et al. Postmenopausal hormone therapy increases risk for venous thromboembolic disease. The Heart and Estrogen/progestin Replacement Study. *Ann Intern Med* 2000;132:689–696.
27. Braunstein JB, Kershner DW, Bray P, et al. Interaction of hemostatic genetics with hormone therapy: new insights to explain arterial thrombosis in postmenopausal women. *Chest* 2002;121:906–920.
28. Clueck CJ, Wang P, Fontaine RN, et al. Effect of exogenous estrogen on atherothrombotic vascular disease risk related to the presence or absence of the factor V Leiden mutation (resistance to activated protein C). *Am J Cardiol* 1999;84:549–559.
29. Herrington DM, Vittinghoff E, Howard TD, et al. Factor V Leiden, hormone replacement therapy, and risk of venous thromboembolic events in women with coronary disease. *Arterioscler Thromb Vasc Biol* 2002;22:1012–1017.
30. Rossouw JE. Hormones, genetic factors, and gender differences in cardiovascular disease. *Cardiovasc Res* 2002;53:550–557.
31. Psaty BM, Smith NL, Lemaitre RN, et al. Hormone replacement therapy, prothrombotic mutations, and the risk of incident nonfatal myocardial infarction in postmenopausal women. *JAMA* 2001;285:906–913.
32. Herrington DM, Brosnihan KB, Pusser BE, et al. Differential effects of E and droloxifene on C-reactive protein and other markers of inflammation in healthy postmenopausal women. *J Clin Endocrinol Metab* 2001;86:4216–4222.
33. Wolbink GJ, Brouwer MC, Buysmann S, et al. CRP-mediated activa-

tion of complement in vivo: assessment by measuring circulating complement-C-reactive protein complexes. *J Immunol* 1996;157:473–479.

34. Galve-de Rochemonteix B, Wiktorowicz K, Kushner I, et al. C-reactive protein increases production of IL-1α, IL-1β, and TNF-α, and expression of mRNA by human alveolar macrophages. *J Leukoc Biol* 1993;53:439–445.

35. Nakagoma A, Freedman SB, Geczy CL. Interferon-γ and lipopolysaccharide potentiate monocyte tissue factor induction by C-reactive protein: relationship with age, sex, and hormone replacement treatment. *Circulation* 2000;101:1785–1791.

36. Ridker PM, Hennekens CH, Rifai N, et al. Hormone replacement therapy and increased plasma concentration of C-reactive protein. *Circulation* 1999;100:713–716.

37. Pasceri V, Willerson JT, Yeh ET. Direct proinflammatory effect of C-reactive protein on human endothelial cells. *Circulation* 2000;102: 2165–2168.

38. van Baal WM, Emes JJ, Kenemans P, et al. Short-term hormone replacement therapy reduced plasma levels of soluble adhesion molecules. *Eur J Clin Invest* 1999;29:913–921.

39. Pradhan AD, Manson JE, Rossouw JE, et al. Inflammatory biomarkers, hormone replacement therapy, and incident coronary heart disease. Prospective analysis from the Women's Health Initiative Observational Study. *JAMA* 2002;288:980–987.

40. Koh KK, Schenke WH, Waclawiw MA, et al. Statin attenuates increase in C-reactive protein during estrogen replacement therapy in postmenopausal women. *Circulation* 2002;105:1531–1533.

41. Hulley SH, Grady D, Bush T, et al. Randomized trial of estrogen plus progestin for secondary prevention of coronary heart disease in postmenopausal women. *JAMA* 1998;280:605–613.

42. Grady D, Herrington D, Bittner V, et al. Cardiovascular disease outcomes during 6.8 years of hormone therapy: Heart and Estrogen/progestin Replacement Study follow-up (HERS II). *JAMA* 2002;288:49–57.

43. LaRosa J. Triglycerides and coronary risk in women and elderly. *Arch Intern Med* 1997;157:961–968.

44. Bush TL, Barrett-Connor E, Cowan LD, et al. Cardiovascular mortality and noncontraceptive use of estrogen in women: results from the Lipid Research Clinics Program follow-up study. *Circulation* 1987;75:1102–1109.

45. Walsh BW, Schiff I, Rosner B, et al. Effects of postmenopausal estrogen replacement on the concentrations and metabolism of plasma lipoproteins. *N Engl J Med* 1991;325:1196–1204.

46. Col NF, Pauker SG, Goldberg RJ, et al. Individualizing therapy to prevent long-term consequences of estrogen deficiency in postmenopausal women. *Arch Intern Med* 1999;159:1458–1466.

47. Stampfer MJ, Colditz GA. Estrogen replacement therapy and coronary heart disease: a quantitative assessment of the epidemiologic evidence. *Prev Med* 1991;20:47–63.

48. Grady D, Rubin SM, Petitti DB, et al. Hormone therapy to prevent disease and prolong life in postmenopausal women. *Ann Intern Med* 1992;117:1016–1037.

49. Grodstein F, Stampfer M. The epidemiology of coronary heart disease and estrogen replacement in postmenopausal women. *Prog Cardiovasc Dis* 1995;38:199–210.

50. Grodstein F, Manson JE, Colditz GA, et al. A prospective, observational study of postmenopausal hormone therapy and primary prevention of cardiovascular disease. *Ann Intern Med* 2000;133:933–941.

51. Sullivan JM, Vander Zwaag R, Lemp GF, et al. Postmenopausal estrogen use and coronary atherosclerosis. *Ann Intern Med* 1988;108:358–363.

52. Sullivan JM. Coronary arteriography in estrogen-treated postmenopausal women. *Prog Cardiovasc Dis* 1995;38:211–222.

53. Grodstein F, Manson JE, Stampfer MJ. Postmenopausal hormone use and secondary prevention of coronary events in the Nurses' Health Study: a prospective observational study. *Ann Intern Med* 2001;135:1–8.

54. Wenger NK, Knatterud GL, Canner PL. Early risks of hormone therapy in patients with coronary heart disease. *JAMA* 2000;284:41–43.

55. Alexander KP, Newby LK, Hellkamp AS, et al. Initiation of hormone replacement therapy after acute myocardial infarction is associated with more cardiac events during follow-up. *J Am Coll Cardiol* 2001;38:1–7.

56. Heckbert SR, Kaplan RC, Weiss NS, et al. Risk of recurrent coronary events in relation to use and recent initiation of postmenopausal hormone therapy. *Arch Intern Med* 2001;161:1709–1713.

57. Humphrey LL, Chan BKS, Sox HC. Postmenopausal hormone replacement therapy and the primary prevention of cardiovascular disease. *Ann Intern Med* 2002;137:273–284.

58. Mosca L. Estrogen and atherosclerosis. *J Invest Med* 1998;46:381–386.

59. Clarke S, Kelleher J, Lloyd-Jones H, et al. A study of hormone replacement therapy in postmenopausal women with ischaemic heart disease: the Papworth HRT Atherosclerosis Study. *Br J Obstet Gynaecol* 2002;109:1056–1062.

60. Herrington DM, Reboussin DM, Brosnihan KB, et al. Effects of estrogen replacement on the progression of coronary-artery atherosclerosis. *N Engl J Med* 2000;343:522–529.

61. Post WS, Goldschmidt-Clermont PJ, Wilhide CC, et al. Methylation of the estrogen receptor gene is associated with aging and atherosclerosis in the cardiovascular system. *Cardiovasc Res* 1999;43:985–991.

62. Schulman S, Thiemann D, Ouyang P, et al. Effects of acute hormone therapy on recurrent ischemia in postmenopausal women with unstable angina. *J Am Coll Cardiol* 2001;37:648A.

63. Viscoli CM, Brass LM, Kernan WN, et al. A clinical trial of estrogen-replacement therapy after ischemic stroke. *N Engl J Med* 2001;345: 1243–1249.

64. Hodis HN, Mack WJ, Azen SP. Hormone therapy and the progression of coronary-artery artherosclerosis in postmenopausal women. *N Engl J Med* 2003;349:535–545.

65. Petitti DB. Hormone replacement therapy and heart disease prevention: experimentation trumps observation. *JAMA* 1998;280:650–652.

66. Barrett-Connor E, Grady D. Hormone replacement therapy, heart disease, and other considerations. *Ann Rev Public Health* 1998;19:55–72.

67. Risks and benefits of estrogen plus progestin in healthy postmenopausal women: principal results from the Women's Health Initiative randomized controlled trial. *JAMA* 2002;288:321–333.

68. Women's Health Initiative Steering Committee. Effects of conjugated equine estrogen in postmenopausal women with hysterectomy. The Women's Health Initiative Randomized Controlled Trial. *JAMA* 2004;291:1701–1712.

69. Hodis HN, Mack WJ, Lobo RA, et al. Estrogen in the prevention of atherosclerosis. *Ann Intern Med* 2001;125:939–953.

70. Angerer P, Störk S, Kothny W, et al. Effect of oral postmenopausal hormone replacement on progression of atherosclerosis: a randomized, controlled trial. *Arterioscler Thromb Vasc Biol* 2001;21:262–268.

71. Delmas P, Bjarnason N, Mitlak B, et al. Effects of raloxifene on bone mineral density, serum cholesterol concentrations, and uterine endometrium in postmenopausal women. *N Engl J Med* 1997;337: 1641–1647.

72. Cummings SR, Eckert S, Krueger KA, et al. The effect of raloxifene on risk of breast cancer in postmenopausal women: results from the MORE randomized trial. Multiple Outcomes of Raloxifene Evaluation. *JAMA* 1999;281:2189–2197.

73. Saitta A, Altavilla D, Cucinotta D, et al. Randomized, double-blind, placebo-controlled study on effects of raloxifene and hormone replacement therapy on plasma nitric oxide concentrations, endothelin-1 levels, and endothelium-dependent vasodilation in postmenopausal women. *Arterioscler Thromb Vasc Biol* 2001;21:1512–1519.

74. Simoncini T, De Caterina R, Genazzani AR. Selective estrogen receptor modulators: different actions on vascular cell adhesion molecule-1 (VCAM-1) expression in human endothelial cells. *J Clin Endocrinol Metab* 1999;84:815–818.

75. Mijatovic V, Netelenbos C, van der Mooren MJ, et al. Randomized, double-blind, placebo-controlled study of the effects of raloxifene and conjugated equine estrogen on plasma homocystein levels in healthy postmenopausal women. *Fertil Steril* 1998;70:1085–1090.

76. De Leo V, la Marca A, Morgante G, et al. Randomized control study of the effects of raloxifene on serum lipids and homocysteine in older women. *Am J Obstet Gynecol* 2001;184:350–353.

77. de Valk-de Roo GW, Stehouwer CD, Meijer P, et al. Both raloxifene and estrogen reduce major cardiovascular risk factors in healthy postmenopausal women: a 2-year placebo-controlled study. *Arterioscler Thromb Vasc Biol* 1999;19:2993–3000.

78. Rutqvist LE, Mattsson A. Cardiac and thromboembolic morbidity among postmenopausal women with early-stage breast cancer in a randomized trial of adjuvant tamoxifen. The Stockholm Breast Cancer Study Group. *J Natl Cancer Inst* 1993;85:1398–1406.

79. McDonald CC, Alexander FE, Whyte BW, et al. Cardiac and vascular morbidity in women receiving adjuvant tamoxifen for breast cancer in a randomised trial. The Scottish Cancer Trials Breast Group. *BMJ* 1995;311:977–980.

80. McDonald CC, Stewart HJ. Fatal myocardial infarction in the Scottish adjuvant tamoxifen trial. The Scottish Breast Cancer Committee. *BMJ* 1991;303:435–437.

81. Fisher B, Constantino JP, Wickerham DL, et al. Tamoxifen for prevention of breast cancer: Report of the National Surgical Adjuvant Breast and Bowel Project P-1 Study. *J Natl Cancer Inst* 1998;90:1371–1388.

82. Clarke SC, Schofield PM, Grace AA, et al. Tamoxifen effects on endothelial function and cardiovascular risk factors in men with advanced atherosclerosis. *Circulation* 2001;103:1497–1502.

83. Cushman M, Constantino JP, Tracy RP, et al. Tamoxifen and cardiac risk factors in healthy women: suggestion of an anti-inflammatory effect. *Arterioscler Thromb Vasc Biol* 2001;21:255–261.

84. Gylling H, Pyrhonen S, Mantyla E, et al. Tamoxifen and toremifene lower serum cholesterol by inhibition of delta 8-cholesterol conversion to lathosterol in women with breast cancer. *J Clin Oncol* 1995;13:2900–2905.

85. Ahotupa M, Mantyla E, Kangas L. Antioxidant properties of the triphenylethylene antiestrogen drug toremifene. *Naunyn Schmiedebergs Arch Pharmacol* 1997;356:297–302.

86. Rattan AK, Arad Y. Inhibition of LDL oxidation by a new estradiol receptor compound LY-139478, comparative with other steroids. *Atherosclerosis* 1998;136:305–314.

87. Marttunen MB, Hietanen P, Tiitinen A, et al. Antiestrogens reduce plasma levels of endothelin-1 without affecting nitrate levels in breast cancer patients. *Gynecol Endocrinol* 2000;14:55–59.

88. Farish E, Barnes JF, Fletcher CD, et al. Effects of tibolone on serum lipoprotein and apolipoprotein levels compared with a cyclical estrogen/progestogen regimen. *Menopause* 1999;6:98–104.

89. Hanggi W, Lippuner K, Riesen W, et al. Long-term influence of different postmenopausal hormone replacement regimens on serum lipids and lipoprotein(a): a randomised study. *Br J Obstet Gynaecol* 1997;104:708–717.

90. Bjarnason NH, Bjarnason K, Haarbo J, et al. Tibolone: influence on markers of cardiovascular disease. *J Clin Endocrinol Metab* 1997;82:1752–1756.

91. Farish E, Barnes JF, Rolton HA, et al. Effects of tibolone on lipoprotein(a) and HDL subfractions. *Maturitas* 1994;20:215–219.

92. Zoma WD, Baker RS, Clark KE. Coronary and uterine vascular responses to raloxifene in the sheep. *Am J Obstet Gynecol* 2000;182:521–528.

93. Zoma WD, Baker RS, Lang U, et al. Hemodynamic response to tibolone in reproductive and nonreproductive tissues in the sheep. *Am J Obstet Gynecol* 2001;184:544–551.

94. Clark KE, Zoma WD, Baker RS, et al. Effect of chronic raloxifene on cardiovascular responses. *J Soc Gynecol Invest* 2000;7:187A.

95. Zoma WE, Baker RS, Friedman A, et al. Inhibition of raloxifene induced hemodynamic changes by the anti-estrogen ICI 182,780. *J Soc Gynecol Invest* 2000;7:226A.

96. Ceballos C, Ribes C, Amado JA, et al. Venous endothelial function in postmenopausal women after six months of tibolone therapy. *Maturitas* 2001;39:63–70.

97. Cummings S, Eckert S, Krueger K, et al. The effect of raloxifene on risk of breast cancer in postmenopausal women. *JAMA* 1999;281:2189–2197.

98. Cauley JA, Norton L, Lippman ME, et al. Continued breast cancer risk reduction in postmenopausal women treated with raloxifene: 4-year results from the MORE Trial. *Breast Cancer Res Treat* 2001;65:125–134.

99. Barrett-Connor E, Grady D, Sashegyi A, et al. Raloxifene and cardiovascular events in osteoporosis postmenopausal women: four-year results from the MORE (Multiple Outcomes of Raloxifene Evaluation) randomized trial. *JAMA* 2002;287:847–857.

100. Mosca L, Barrett-Connor E, Wenger KN, et al. Design and methods of the Raloxifene Use for The Heart (RUTH study). *Am J Cardiol* 2001;88:392–395.

101. Mosca L, Appel LJ, Benjamin EJ, et al. Evidence-based guidelines for cardiovascular disease prevention in women. *Circulation* 2004;109:672–693.

CHAPTER 21

Vitamins in Coronary Artery Disease

Mladen Golubic and Joan E.B. Fox

Key Words: Antioxidant; cardiovascular disease; coronary artery disease; inflammation; nutrition; supplement; vitamin.

INTRODUCTION

People who consume diets high in fruits and vegetables have a lower risk for cardiovascular disease (CVD), most cancer types, diabetes, and all-cause mortality (1,2). It is often assumed that vitamins in fruits and vegetables are responsible for the protective effects of these foods, hence, the considerable interest in the potential for vitamin supplementation in disease prevention. As part of a $30 billion a year alternative medicine industry (3), the public is bombarded with claims for benefits of commercial vitamin supplements; an estimated 40% of the U.S. population uses these products (4). Many physicians support this practice, suggesting that all adults take a daily vitamin supplement (5). This recommendation is based on several assumptions. First, it is assumed that benefits of diets rich in fruits and vegetables derive from vitamins in these foods. Second, it is assumed that benefits of dietary vitamins will still occur when a vitamin is taken as an individual supplement. Third, it is assumed that the use of high doses of vitamin supple-

ments is safe. With the exception of folic acid supplementation in the first trimester of pregnancy, there is, however, little evidence from clinical trials that supports the claims that vitamin supplementation improves health. Moreover, vitamin supplementation is not always safe. Vitamin A levels in the range readily attained with a normal diet and a multivitamin supplement are associated with an increased risk for fracture and birth defects (5). In two trials, high-dose β-carotene increased the risk for death in individuals who smoked (6,7). The interaction between vitamins and prescription drugs also is a concern. For example, adverse interactions between antioxidant vitamins and lipid-lowering medications have been reported (8).

In the case of CVD, two groups of vitamins have drawn considerable attention. First, supplementation with vitamin B$_6$, vitamin B$_{12}$, and folic acid decreases elevated homocysteine levels. Because increased homocysteine is a risk factor for CVD, these vitamins might be expected to have beneficial effects; clinical trials to evaluate this are underway. Second, there is interest in the potential benefits of the antioxidant vitamins, vitamin E, vitamin C, and β-carotene. Evidence for a role for oxidative stress in the development of CVD is compelling (9), and antioxidants inhibit development of coronary artery disease in animal models (10). Several prospective cohort studies have provided evidence for decreased cardiovascular events and deaths in healthy individuals taking antioxidant vitamins. Large clinical trials, however, have failed to provide evidence for benefits of vitamin supplements (11–13). Most importantly, several trials have demonstrated the potential for harm (6–8,14). In contrast, trials addressing the effects of diets rich in fruits and vegetables have continued to show clear benefits.

M. Golubic: Brain Tumor Institute, Center for Integrative Medicine, The Cleveland Clinic Foundation, 9500 Euclid Avenue, Cleveland, Ohio 44195.

J. E. B. Fox: Center for Integrative Medicine, Joseph J. Jacobs Center for Thrombosis and Vascular Biology, Department of Molecular Cardiology, The Cleveland Clinic Foundation, 9500 Euclid Avenue, Cleveland, Ohio 44195; and Department of Physiology and Biophysics, School of Medicine, Case Western Reserve University, Cleveland, Ohio 44106.

The purpose of this chapter is to summarize recent clinical trials of vitamin supplements and dietary interventions in CVD, to discuss reasons for the inconclusive findings from the vitamin trials, and to suggest directions for future research and clinical practice.

DEVELOPMENT OF CORONARY ARTERY DISEASE

Some of the pathways involved in initiation and development of coronary artery disease are shown in Figure 21–1 (see color insert). Endothelial cells serve as sensors of the environment. Under healthy conditions, they produce nitric oxide (NO), which stimulates soluble guanyl cyclase and maintains the cells in an unstimulated state. Stimuli such as thrombin, cytokines, or angiotensin II activate signaling pathways that decrease the bioavailability of NO and increase expression of proteins such as vascular cell adhesion molecule-1, tumor necrosis factor-alpha (TNF-α), interleukin-8, and monocyte chemoattractant protein 1 that induce binding of monocytes to activated endothelial cells and migration of monocytes into the intima. As indicated in the insert in Figure 21–1, the genes encoding these proinflammatory proteins are under the control of the transcription factor nuclear factor-kappaB (NF-κB) (15). This factor is maintained in an inactive state by interaction with a family of inhibitory proteins. Phosphorylation of these inhibitory proteins causes them to dissociate from NF-κB, which can then migrate into the nucleus, where it binds to specific regions in the promotor of target genes. Studies have shown that reactive oxygen species (ROS) are important second messengers in the signaling pathways leading to activation of NF-κB (15). Nicotinamide adenine dinucleotide phosphate (NADPH) oxidase is thought to be responsible for agonist-induced production of ROS in endothelial cells (16). Although the initial ROS targets in the signaling pathways are not known, changes in cytosolic calcium concentrations and altered activity of protein kinase C, tyrosine kinases, and protein phosphatases have been implicated as ROS-induced events occurring upstream of NF-κB activation (15).

Under normal conditions, the production of low amounts of ROS is an important component of physiologic intracellular signaling pathways and is balanced by the presence of endogenous antioxidant mechanisms. However, the presence of continuing endothelial cell activation shifts the equilibrium between NO and ROS-induced pathways, leading to an inflammatory response, lipid peroxidation, the formation of foam cells, and tissue damage (9). All of the common risk factors for CVD, including inflammatory cytokines, angiotensin II, oxidized low-density lipoprotein (LDL), TNF-α, interferon γ, mechanical forces, homocysteine, and diabetes-induced hyperglycemia are associated with activation of signaling pathways in endothelial cells. Many of these risk factors have been shown to stimulate production of ROS and the resulting expression of proinflammatory genes in endothelial cells (15,16). ROS are also emerging as important second messengers in signaling pathways in leukocytes, platelets, smooth muscle cells, and fibroblasts (15,17). As endothelial cell activation, the inflammatory response, and development of the atherothrombotic lesion continue, the oxidative stress increases and ROS-induced events such as metalloproteinase activation and endothelial cell–induced apoptosis contribute to the development and complications of the disease (9).

Factors present in a diet rich in fruits and vegetables could potentially modulate the development of CVD by neutralizing risk factors or by inhibiting pathways involved in the development or the complications of CVD. One of the risk factors is homocysteine, which can be decreased by folate supplementation; hence, the interest in the use of the B vitamins in the prevention of CVD. Interest in the use of antioxidant vitamins originated from the elucidation of the critical role of oxidation of LDL in the formation of foam cells. However, consideration of potential benefits of antioxidant vitamins must now include the myriad of steps in which oxidation reactions regulate physiologic and pathologic events in the vasculature.

FOLIC ACID, VITAMIN B₆, AND VITAMIN B₁₂

Although the association between homocysteine levels and coronary disease is less substantial in healthy populations than originally thought, increased homocysteine is still considered to be a risk factor for CVD (18). Increasing evidence suggests that the primary mechanism by which homocysteine exerts its effects is through stimulation of endothelial cells. Flow-mediated dilatation of the brachial artery is impaired in individuals with hyperhomocystinemia and in experimental hyperhomocystinemia, induced by methionine loading in healthy subjects. Increased homocysteine induces production of ROS, decreases NO bioavailability, and is associated with lipid peroxidation and oxidative damage (19,20).

Vitamin B₆, vitamin B₁₂, and folic acid are required for the normal metabolism of homocysteine to methionine, and one cause of increased homocysteine is decreased B vitamin intake (19). Several studies have shown that daily supplementation with folate, vitamin B₆, and vitamin B₁₂ can decrease elevated homocysteine levels (21,22). A metaanalysis of 12 randomized trials (23) found that folic acid is the most effective in restoring homocysteine concentrations to normal levels, vitamin B₁₂ induces only a small additional effect, and addition of vitamin B₆ to folic acid has no effect over folate alone. The effects of folate supplementation are greatest in individuals with the greatest homocysteine or lowest folate levels before treatment (23).

Given the association between increased homocysteine and CVD, decreasing homocysteine might be expected to provide beneficial effects. Many small studies have shown that folate supplementation can improve endothelial function in healthy adults and in subjects with increased homocysteine (19–22). Such studies have identified the concentrations of homocysteine that induce endothelial dysfunction and forms and concentrations of B vitamins that can inhibit this. Thus, information required for the rational design of clinical trials is now available. Several small randomized trials have evaluated the effects of B vitamins on intermediate clinical outcomes. One trial involved 158 siblings of patients with premature atherothrombotic disease who showed post-methionine hyperhomocystinemia (24). Fewer abnormal exercise electrocardiography tests were observed in those treated with folate and vitamin B$_6$ for 2 years compared with placebo. In another trial (25), patients received a daily combination of folic acid, vitamin B$_{12}$, and vitamin B$_6$ for 6 months before angioplasty. The rate of restenosis in 105 patients receiving supplements was less than in 100 patients receiving placebo. In a follow-up trial involving 533 patients and using a protocol in which supplements were stopped at 6 months, decreased restenosis was observed 1 year after angioplasty (26).

Although the results from large clinical trials are not yet available, nine such trials are currently underway (22). They involve more than 50,000 participants, all of whom have vascular disease or risk factors for CVD. They are all evaluating end points such as fatal and nonfatal CVD, strokes, and other coronary events. The results will become available in about 2 to 4 years. Three of the trials are taking place in North America. These trials were designed before the instigation of the program to fortify cereal grain flour products with folic acid. This program has had marked effects on folate levels, and concern has been expressed that because of this only 20% to 25% of the planned effects will be achieved, leaving the studies inadequately powered (27). Because of the food fortification program, there seems to be little rational for recommending the use of folate supplementation for the prevention of CVD except in individuals such as those taking methotrexate, the elderly with decreased vitamin B$_{12}$ absorption, or vegans who may be consuming inadequate B vitamins in their diet.

ANTIOXIDANT VITAMINS AND CORONARY DISEASE

Given the compelling evidence that ROS are intimately involved in the development and progression of CVD, antioxidants might be expected to be beneficial. In support of this concept, considerable *in vitro* data have shown that antioxidants can inhibit oxidation of LDL, activation of NF-κB, or induction of adhesion receptors on endothelial cells stimulated *in vitro* by agonists such as angiotensin II, TNF-α, or oxidized LDL (15). Studies in animal models have shown that antioxidants inhibit development of coronary artery disease (10). Epidemiologic studies have shown that diets rich in fruits and vegetables are associated with decreased death from CVD and associations between β-carotene, vitamin C, and vitamin E content and health benefits have been noted (28). Several prospective cohort studies have shown vitamin E intake in the form of supplements is associated with a reduction in cardiovascular events (29,30) or death from CVD (31) in healthy individuals. The Nurses Health Study (29) followed 87,245 female nurses and found that those who reported using vitamin E supplements for a period of 8 years

had a 34% decreased risk for having a cardiac event. Similar findings were reported in the Health Professionals Follow-up study (30), which followed 39,910 male health professionals for 4 years. In the Established Populations for Epidemiologic Studies of the Elderly (EPESE) study (31), long-term use of vitamin E and vitamin C supplements in a healthy population was associated with a 63% decrease in risk for death from CVD. In contrast to the prospective studies, however, randomized clinical trials have generated inconclusive results.

β-Carotene

Five major trials evaluating the effects of β-carotene supplements have been completed, and all have failed to show a reduction of all-cause death or death from CVD (Table 21–1). Three of the trials followed individuals without risk factors for CVD. In the Skin Cancer Prevention (SCP) study (32), 1,188 men and 532 women were followed for 8.2 years. The Physicians Health Study (PHS) (33) involved 22,071 healthy male physicians who were followed for a 12-year period. In the Women's Health Study (WHS) (34), 39,876 women were followed for 2.1 years. Two other studies evaluated individuals who were smokers and both of these found not only that were no benefits of β-carotene supplementation, but also that there was a significantly increased risk for death. In the Alpha-Tocopherol, Beta-Carotene Cancer Prevention (ATBC) study (6) 29,133 male Finnish smokers received β-carotene or placebo for a 5- to 8-year period. There were more deaths caused by ischemic heart disease and ischemic and hemorrhagic stroke among men who received β-carotene than among those who did not. In addition, a significantly greater incidence (18% increase) of lung cancer and overall mortality (8%) was observed in recipients of β-carotene. When a subgroup of participants who not only smoked but also had a previous myocardial infarction (MI) was analyzed, there were significantly more deaths from fatal coronary heart disease in the β-carotene group than in the placebo group (35). The Beta-Carotene and Retinol Efficacy Trial (CARET) (7) randomized 18,314 people with risk factors for lung cancer to receive a combination of β-carotene and retinyl palmitate or placebo for a 4-year period. The study was terminated 21 months before scheduled completion because the treatment group had a 26% greater incidence of death from cardiovascular causes, 17% greater overall mortality, and 28% greater incidence of lung cancer than the placebo. Taken together, the results from these five primary prevention trials do not provide any evidence for a protective effect of β-carotene on cardiovascular mortality. In fact, taking β-carotene supplements may be hazardous for smokers.

Vitamin E

The results of five major clinical trials evaluating the use of vitamin E, administered as an individual supplement, have

TABLE 21–1. *Summary of trials using antioxidant vitamins*

Trial name (reference)	Publication date	Population characteristics	Trial size, n	Daily dose/ plasma concentration	Duration, yr	Adverse effects	Outcomes
β-Carotene							
ATBC (6)	1994	Male smokers	29,133	20 mg[a]	6.1	↑ in lung cancer (18%)	↑ deaths from ischemic heart disease and stroke ↑ overall mortality (8%)
CARET (7)	1996	Smokers, former smokers, people exposed to asbestos	18,314	30 mg 25,000 IU vitamin A[a]	4.0	↑ in lung cancer (28%)	↑ death from CVD (26%) ↑ overall mortality (17%)
SCP (32)	1996	Biopsy results showed skin cancer	1,720	50 mg[a]	4.3	None reported	No effect on all cause or CVD deaths
PHS (33)	1996	Healthy male physicians	22,071	50 mg qod[a]	12.0	Yellow skin	No effect on all cause or CVD deaths
WHS (34)	1999	Healthy female health professionals	39,876	50 mg qod[b]	2.1	Yellow skin	No effect on MI, stroke, or CVD deaths
Vitamin E							
ATBC (6)	1994	Male smokers	29,133	50 mg (s)[a]	6.1	↑ cancer deaths (other than lung cancer)	↑ in CVD death (8%) No effect on nonfatal cardiovascular events
CHAOS (37)	1996	CVD	2,002	400 or 800 IU (n)[a]	1.4	None	↑ CVD, nonfatal MI and CVD death No effect on CVD deaths
GISSI (38)	1999	Previous MI	11,324	300 mg (s)[b]	3.5	None	No effect on combined end points of CVD, death, all-cause death, nonfatal MI, and strokes
HOPE (39)	2000	CVD risk factors	9,541	400 IU (n)[b]	4.5	None	No effect on CVD or all-cause deaths
PPP (40)	2001	CVD risk factors	4,495	300 mg (s)[b]	3.6	None	No effect on prespecified CVD end points
Combination							
AREDS (41)	2001	High risk for age-related eye diseases	4,757	β-Carotene 15 mg Vitamin E 400 IU Vitamin C 500 mg[a]	6.3	Yellow skin	No effect on mortality or ophthalmologic end points
HPS (42)	2002	CVD, diabetes, or other vascular disease	20,536	β-Carotene 20 mg Vitamin E 600 mg Vitamin C 250 mg[a]	5	None	No effect on CVD death, nonfatal vascular events, or cancer

AREDS, Age-Related Eye Disease Study; ATBC, Alpha-Tocopherol, Beta-Carotene Cancer Prevention; CARET, Beta-Carotene and Retinol Efficacy Trial; CHAOS, Cambridge Heart Antioxidant Study; CVD, cardiovascular disease; GISSI, Gruppo Italiano per lo Studio della Sopravvivenza nell 'Infarto Miocardico; HOPE, Health Outcomes Prevention Evaluation; HPS, Heart Protection Study; MI, myocardial infarction; n, natural; PHS, Physicians Health Study; PPP, Primary Prevention Project; s, synthetic; SCP, Skin Cancer Prevention; WHS, Women's Health Study.

[a]Plasma vitamin concentration was measured.
[b]Plasma vitamin concentration was not measured.

produced inconsistent findings (Table 21–1). Four of the trials (ATBC, Cambridge Heart Antioxidant Study [CHAOS], Gruppo Italiano per lo Studio della Sopravvivenza nell 'Infarto Miocardico [GISSI], and Health Outcomes Prevention Evaluation [HOPE]) have involved secondary prevention; only one (Primary Prevention Project [PPP]) has been on a healthy population. In the ATBC study (6), deaths from CVD were reduced by 8% in those receiving vitamin E (36). The total number of nonfatal coronary events, however, was not reduced. Moreover, analysis of outcomes of a subset of 1,862 men who had experienced a previous MI at the time of enrollment showed that they received no benefits from vitamin use (35). In the CHAOS (37), 2,002 patients with angiographic evidence of coronary artery disease were assigned to treatment groups receiving vitamin E or placebo for 1.4 years. Vitamin E had no effect on cardiovascular mortality. However, major cardiovascular events were reduced by 47%. The difference was largely attributable to a 77% reduction in the number of nonfatal MIs. In the GISSI-Prevenzione Trial (38), 11,324 patients with a recent MI were given a daily dose of vitamin E alone or in combination with v-3 polyunsaturated fatty acids for 3.5 years. In contrast to v-3 polyunsaturated fatty acids, vitamin E did not yield any beneficial effect on the preselected end point of combined all-cause deaths, cardiovascular deaths, nonfatal MI, and nonfatal strokes. However, if individual variables were considered as end points, 20% reduction in deaths from CVD and 35% in sudden death were observed (38).

Despite some promising findings from these first three trials, findings from subsequent major trials have been negative. In the HOPEβ-carotene, vitamin E, vitamin C, and selenium or simvastatin plus niacin, either alone or in combination. This trial differed from most others in that it included measurement of oxidative stress and showed that this was decreased in the experimental group: The resistance of LDL to oxidation increased by 35%. Despite the demonstration of efficacy of the vitamin therapy, no beneficial effects of vitamin therapy on major cardiovascular outcomes were detected. In fact, the simvastatin and niacin-induced increase in HDL_2 cholesterol was decreased: HDL_2 levels increased by 65% with simvastatin alone and only 28% when antioxidant vitamins were added. The statin-induced angiographic benefits also were significantly decreased in the group receiving vitamins: Stenosis regressed by 0.4% with simvastatin-niacin alone and progressed by 0.7% with simvastatin-niacin plus vitamin. The frequency of clinical end point (change in stenosis and incidence of a first coronary event) was 24% in the placebo group, 3% in the simvastatin-niacin alone group, 21% with vitamins alone, and 14% with simvastatin-niacin plus vitamins. The Women's Angiographic Vitamin and Estrogen (WAVE) trial (14) involved 423 postmenopausal women with at least one angiographically demonstrated coronary stenosis. Patients in seven clinical sites in North America were randomly assigned to receive either hormone replacement therapy or placebo or vitamin E plus vitamin C or placebo. The main

outcome measure was the change in minimum lumen diameter from baseline to concluding angiogram of all qualifying coronary lesions. Neither hormone replacement therapy nor the antioxidant vitamins provided any cardiovascular benefit. In fact, both treatments had negative effects: All-cause mortality was significantly greater in women assigned to vitamins compared with vitamin placebo. Death, nonfatal MI, or stroke occurred in 26 of the patients receiving vitamins compared with 18 patients in the vitamin placebo group.

Summary of Clinical Trials of Antioxidant Vitamin Supplements

Five major clinical trials on the use of β-carotene have failed to provide evidence for benefits in primary prevention, five major trials using vitamin E have produced inconsistent findings, whereas two trials using combinations of vitamins have failed to show benefits. Although metaanalysis of the existing data demonstrates that there is no evidence for benefits of antioxidant vitamins (11,12), we find it difficult to compare the data from the trials and impossible to evaluate the reliability of the information from many. The U.S. Preventive Services Task Force (USPSTF) reached a similar conclusion, reporting that the existing data are conflicting, inadequate, or impossible to evaluate because confounding variables cannot be assessed (13). The USPSTF concluded that there is insufficient evidence to recommend for or against the use of vitamins for prevention of CVD (13). None of the existing trials have reported benefits from the use of β-carotene, and in two trials the use of this vitamin was associated with increased death in smokers. One outcome that is uniformly recommended is that β-carotene supplements, either alone or in combination with other vitamins, should be avoided (11–13).

Initiation of trials with vitamin C, vitamin E, and β-carotene was based on the recommendations of the National Institutes of Health (NIH) panel of experts that convened in 1991 (44). At that time, there was evidence from animal studies that antioxidants could inhibit coronary artery disease. However, the studies had used primarily probucol. There were no studies showing that vitamin E, vitamin C, or β-carotene had beneficial effects. Thus, the clinical trials were initiated without data on concentration and efficacy or preclinical evidence that would normally be available. In the absence of such information, protocols have varied widely, making outcomes difficult to compare. The choice of vitamin and dosage for each trial was made on the basis of little scientific evidence, therefore it is possible that the vitamins used did not affect the critical oxidation-induced modifications. In some trials, the vitamin levels were not measured (Table 21–1), therefore it is not known whether these levels increased as a result of supplementation. Even in those trials in which increases were demonstrated, it is not known whether these increases were sufficient to inhibit oxidation-induced pathways. This makes it difficult to evaluate the reliability of the trials or to assess reasons for differing outcomes.

Before initiating future trials it will be critical to determine optimal vitamins and concentrations. Antioxidant vitamins work in different ways (45). For example, vitamin E can repair ROS directly, and in this way it functions as a chain-breaking antioxidant. β-Carotene traps singlet oxygen, but it is less effective in terminating free radical chain reactions. Natural vitamin E, produced by plants, includes eight forms of related fat-soluble compounds (α-, β-, γ-, and δ-tocopherol and α-, β-, γ-, and δ-tocotrienol) (45). Although the antioxidant property is similar, the bioavailability of the forms is different and distinct biologic effects can be distinguished at the molecular level. Thus, a reason for the failure of trials using synthetic α-tocopherol may be that this is not the ideal form of the vitamin. However, even in studies (HOPE and CHAOS trials) in which natural vitamin E was used, no benefits were observed (Table 21–1).

One problem with deciding which vitamin to use is that we do not know what we want it to inhibit. At the time that the NIH panel recommended clinical trials, it was assumed that ROS-induced oxidation of LDL was the mechanism by which oxidative stress exerted its effects on the vasculature. However, our increasing knowledge about the role of ROS in signaling pathways and modifying proteins involved in numerous steps of the atherothrombotic process makes it critical that an antioxidant is chosen carefully. It is now clear that signaling pathways in many different cell types are dependent on ROS, and a redox imbalance favors the development of coronary artery disease because it accelerates many different pathways, including those that regulate the expression of proinflammatory genes, monocyte signaling, smooth muscle cell proliferation, leukocyte activation, apoptosis, and lipid peroxidation (Fig. 21–1). Investigation of mechanisms by which ROS are produced is beginning to identify enzymes such as NADPH oxidase as an enzyme responsible for ROS production by risk factor stimulation of endothelial cells (16) and myeloperoxidase, secreted by monocytes, as an enzyme involved in ROS-induced lipid peroxidation (46). Investigation of specific targets suggests that the activity of intracellular signaling molecules such as protein kinase C, tyrosine kinases, protein phosphatases, and NF-κB activity are affected by the actions of ROS (15,16), but it is not currently known which of these molecules are directly modified. Without this information, it is difficult to know which antioxidants might be beneficial. If more information was available on ways in which ROS induce their harmful effects and cellular locations at which they act, we would be in a better position to know whether to expect a specific vitamin to inhibit these effects.

Once a vitamin is selected, a marker is needed to ensure that the vitamin has reduced the oxidative stress and inhibited pathways of interest. None of the major trials reported to date has determined whether oxidative stress was increased at baseline or shown that the intervention was effective in decreasing oxidative stress. For these reasons, the results of the trials are not able to be interpreted. As pointed out by Steinberg and Witztum (10), "it is as if a cholesterol-lowering drug was being tested for efficacy in preventing coronary heart disease but without measurements of plasma cholesterol as part of the protocol." Assays available to determine whether a vitamin inhibits ROS-induced pathways include protection of plasma LDL from oxidation *ex vivo*, inhibition of platelet aggregation, and inhibition of H_2O_2-induced lipid peroxidation in erythrocytes. However, it is not clear whether these assays would predict the ability of an antioxidant to protect against ROS-induced damage related to the progression of CVD *in vivo*. Unless it is known which are the critical pathways affected by ROS and which of these would be expected to be modified by antioxidant vitamins, it cannot be known which assays to use to reliably determine whether the vitamin has inhibited oxidation reactions of interest.

Another reason that it is difficult to draw conclusions from the existing clinical trials is that they have been performed on populations with varying characteristics. One important variable in trials that evaluate benefits of vitamins is the nutritional intake of the participants. If subjects were consuming antioxidants from dietary sources, supplements might not provide further benefits. Similarly, those who were nutritionally deficient might benefit most. The use of Italian subjects, who were presumably consuming a Mediterranean diet rich in plant foods, may have been responsible for the lack of benefits of vitamin E supplementation in the GISSI trial (38). In the absence of measurements of vitamin E and oxidative stress, at baseline and during the supplementation, it is impossible to interpret the results of this trial. One study that used a nutritionally deficient population was the Nutrition Intervention in Linxian Trial (47). The population of the Linxian province of China, where this trial was performed, is deficient in micronutrients. In this trial, 29,584 subjects were randomly assigned to placebo or intervention groups receiving four different combinations of nutrients, including a group that was receiving β-carotene, vitamin E, and selenium for 5.2 years. Although there was no reduction in mortality from CVD, cancer mortality was reduced by 13% and mortality from cerebrovascular disease by 10% in the group taking vitamins compared with placebo. Other high-risk populations that might benefit are those known to have high oxidative stress, such as those with diabetes, undergoing cardiac transplantation, or on hemodialysis. One such trial was the Secondary Prevention with Antioxidants of Cardiovascular disease in Endstage renal disease (SPACE) study (48), in which 196 subjects with CVD and undergoing hemodialysis received vitamin E for 1.4 years. The intervention caused a 54% reduction in cardiovascular events and a 70% reduction of MI (36).

Another major difference in the participants in the various trials is that they varied from healthy individuals to those with advanced CVD, obesity, diabetes, and increased lipids. Because of the different locations of ROS production and different cells and targets involved, an antioxidant would not be expected to be equally effective at all stages of CVD. Oxidation reactions are essential in the normal intracellular signaling of many cell types. Cells have their own sensitive mechanisms for regulating the redox equilibrium; as with other cellular processes, problems arise when the equilibrium between ROS-induced and antioxidant-induced pathways is shifted. In the presence of excess ROS, events leading to coronary artery disease are activated. By the same logic, problems can presumably arise in the presence of excess antioxidants, particularly if the system is flooded with one antioxidant that may act at a specific location in the cell or reduce oxidation of a specific target. It seems likely, therefore, that supplementation with an antioxidant could be beneficial or harmful depending on the balance of antioxidants and ROS that exist at any particular time or cellular location. Primary outcomes in most trials have been death or cardiovascular events. These outcomes involve disruption of the fibrous cap, an event that involves release and activation of metalloproteinases, tissue damage, and endothelial cell apoptosis. Transition metals bound to metalloproteinases can exert prooxidant activities when they are in the reduced state. Because antioxidants reduce transition metals, they could conceivably promote, rather than inhibit, events involved in disruption of fibrous caps (45).

On the basis of current knowledge of actions of ROS, antioxidants might be expected to be more beneficial in primary prevention than in preventing the complications of more advanced disease. The initial prospective studies showing benefits of antioxidant vitamins were performed on healthy individuals (29–31). The animal studies that showed benefits all involved administering antioxidants before the start of lesion development (10). In evaluating primary prevention, outcomes such as endothelial dysfunction or intimal thickening would be more appropriate than death or cardiovascular events. In support of the potential benefit of antioxidants in early stages of coronary artery disease, numerous studies have shown that α-tocopherol and other antioxidants inhibit early steps of the disease process such as endothelial cell activation, monocyte adhesion, cytokine production, platelet aggregation, and signaling pathways in monocytes (15,45,49). One small trial (50) evaluated the effect of antioxidant vitamins on intimal thickening in transplant-associated coronary artery disease, a situation in which the progression of new lesions could be followed. One year after cardiac transplantation, those subjects receiving a combination of vitamins C and E showed no change in intimal index compared with an 8% increase in the placebo group. In another study, decreases in the rate of intimal thickening were observed in healthy individuals with hypercholesterolemia. In this Antioxidant Supplementation in Atherosclerosis Prevention (ASAP) study (51), the average annual increase of the mean common carotid artery intima-media thickness was reduced by 25% in individuals who received vitamin E plus vitamin C for 6 years compared with those receiving placebo.

Antioxidant Capacity of Fruits and Vegetables

Although the epidemiologic evidence showing an association between diets rich in fruit and vegetables and decreased risk for CVD is strong, there is little scientific basis for the assumption that it is the antioxidant vitamins in these foods that are responsible for the protective effects. Several prospective cohort studies have shown an inverse relation between the incidence of CVD and intake of vitamin E, vitamin C, or β-carotene, either from dietary sources or supplements (28–30). However, accumulating evidence suggests that nutrients other than the antioxidant vitamins may provide the major benefits. The Iowa Women's Health Study followed 34,486 postmenopausal women for 7 years and found that vitamin E intake from foods, but not supplements, was inversely associated with the risk for death from CHD (52). Although an increased incidence of death in subjects taking the β-carotene supplements caused the CARET to be stopped in 1996, active follow up of all participants continued until September 2003. Analysis of the follow-up data has demonstrated an association between fruit and vegetable intake and decreased cancer risk in subjects in the placebo group; no such association has been demonstrated in those who received the β-carotene supplement (53). This finding suggests that β-carotene supplements may interfere with the beneficial effects of the bioactive components in fruits and vegetables. It is currently known that fruits and vegetables contain thousands of unique phytochemicals, and that more than 80% of the antioxidant capacity of most fruits and vegetables comes from phytochemicals other than vitamins (54–56). Many phytochemicals have synergistic, additive, or inhibitory effects on each other (57).

Flavonoids have been identified as the most abundant plant antioxidants, particularly in foods such as soy, the onion family of vegetables, apples, berries, green and black tea, and red wine (58). Flavonoids exert antiinflammatory and antithrombogenic effects that could be important in the development and progression of coronary artery disease and other chronic diseases such as cancer and diabetes (59,60). Measurement of the total antioxidant capacity of plasma after ingestion of foods that are rich sources of flavonoids shows that these foods significantly increase the antioxidant capacity and decrease oxidative stress (58,61–65).

Whole Diet Studies

Randomized trials of dietary interventions in prevention of CVD have demonstrated impressive benefits. Several studies suggest that a reduction of 70% to 80% of CVD can be achieved by combining a low-fat, plant-based diet with other lifestyle modifications (28,66,67). The Mediterranean diet has been associated with a low incidence of CVD and other chronic diseases. This diet is rich in plant foods such as fruits, vegetables, whole grain cereal, nuts, and legumes. Olive oil is the major source of fat; fish and poultry are consumed in low to moderate amounts, and there is low consumption of red meat and dairy products. There is moderate consumption of wine. In a population-based study involving 22,043 healthy adults in Greece, adherence to the Mediterranean diet was associated with decreased death from CVD (2). Several large, randomized, secondary prevention trials have provided evidence of benefits of the Mediterranean diet. In the Lyon Diet Heart Study, 605 patients were randomly assigned to a Mediterranean style diet or a control diet resembling the American Heart Association (AHA) step 1 diet. After 46 months, individuals consuming the Mediterranean-style diet showed a 77% reduction in an end point that combined CVD deaths and nonfatal MI compared with those in the AHA diet group (67). In the Indian Heart Study, consumption of a low-fat diet enriched with fruits and vegetables, whole grains, and nuts was associated with a 40% reduction in cardiac events and a 45% reduction in mortality (68). In the Indo-Mediterranean Diet Heart Study (69), patients ate step I diet recommended by the National Cholesterol Education Program for 2 years. Patients in the intervention group, however, were advised to consume at least 250 to 300 g fruit, 125 to 150 g vegetables, and 25 to 50 g walnuts or almonds per day, as well as whole grains and variety of legumes. The intervention group had a significant reduction in risk for nonfatal MI (51%), sudden cardiac death (62%), and total cardiac end points (49%) compared with the control group.

In another, nonrandomized trial, 18 patients who had experienced 49 coronary events in the 8 years before entering the study ate a plant-based diet in which less than 10% of calories were derived from fats, in combination with lipid-decreasing medication. During a 12-year follow-up, none of the patients experienced further coronary events, and the CAD was arrested and/or reversed, as demonstrated by angiography (70). In contrast, 6 noncompliant patients who were under standard care sustained 13 new cardiac events. A study of 409 patients with stable CVD adds strong support for the idea that a combination of a low-fat, plant-based diet with cholesterol-decreasing drugs is a highly effective approach to decreasing CVD (71). Over 5 years, coronary events occurred in only 6.6% of patients on a strict low-fat diet with lipid-decreasing drugs, compared with 30.6% of patients with a standard diet and no lipid-decreasing drugs, and 20.3% in a combined group who were consuming either an AHA diet and lipid-decreasing drugs or a strict low-fat diet with no lipid-decreasing drugs. Finally, the Lifestyle Heart Study (72) showed that a combination of a low-fat, plant-based diet with exercise, yoga, and stress management significantly reduced coronary artery disease even without lipid decreasing medication in patients with moderate to severe CAD.

Taken together, the information from clinical trials on plant-based diets provides clear evidence for the dramatic benefits that can be attained by dietary intervention. Accumulating evidence suggests that antioxidant vitamins are probably not the critical nutrients. Although associations be-

tween flavonoid content of foods and decreased incidence of CVD have been documented, there is no evidence that these antioxidants are responsible for the beneficial effects of the plant-based diets either. In a report of 22,043 adults eating a Mediterranean diet (2), associations between intake of any one food group and decreased CVD were not observed, supporting findings from other studies that many different nutrients and phytochemicals have overlapping mechanisms of action and synergistic, additive, or inhibitory effects on each other, and that a combination of nutrients is more powerful than a single factor alone (28,57).

SUMMARY AND RECOMMENDATIONS

The only group of vitamins for which there is good evidence that supplementation is beneficial are those of vitamin B. Intake of folic acid is sufficient to maintain homocysteine levels at normal baselines in most individuals. Supplementation is advisable only for those with increased homocysteine levels such as may occur in the elderly who can show malabsorption of vitamin B_{12}, individuals who consume one or two alcoholic drinks a day, or vegans who may have decreased vitamin B_{12} intake.

Diets rich in fruits and vegetables and low in saturated fats have a powerful protective effect, both in primary and secondary prevention. Studies suggest that 70% to 80% of CVD could be prevented by combining such a diet with other healthy lifestyle practices (66). Although it is often assumed that antioxidant vitamins are the beneficial ingredient of plant-based diets, there is no good evidence for this. Clinical trials on the use of antioxidant vitamins have produced inconclusive results, at least in part because the studies have been performed without the necessary scientific rationale and background information and did not provide information needed to evaluate the reliability of the outcomes. The absence of evidence for benefits of antioxidant vitamins from clinical trials argues against recommendation of vitamin supplementation. A few trials have suggested that antioxidant use may be appropriate in specific groups of patients (48,50,51), but further studies are needed to confirm the observed benefits. Most importantly, trials that show that vitamin use is not always safe makes it difficult to rationalize the use of population-wide recommendations for supplementation with antioxidant vitamins. Adverse effects of vitamin A supplementation such as increased risk for fractures and birth defects if used during pregnancy have been reported. Clinical trials on the use of β-carotene in smokers have demonstrated an increased risk for lung cancer and cardiovascular death. Thus, the use of this vitamin by smokers should be discouraged. The interaction between vitamins and prescription drugs such as statins is another cause for concern. Before additional trials are initiated, it will be important to obtain more information on mechanisms by which oxidative stress is involved in CVD. Elucidation of ROS-induced pathways and sites of action of different antioxidants will be essential so that choices of antioxidants, concentrations, and populations that might benefit can be based on scientific rationale.

The idea that vitamins are the most appropriate antioxidants to investigate needs to be reconsidered. Our current knowledge suggests that plant-derived molecules other than vitamins provide greater benefits than antioxidant vitamins. Plants contain thousands of antioxidant flavonoids and other phytochemicals that provide more than 80% of the antioxidant capacity of many fruits and vegetables. Most importantly, the idea that antioxidant vitamins could be used as a "magic bullet" in the treatment of CVD is overly simplistic and needs to be reevaluated. There is no evidence that any antioxidants will have protective effects when removed from the plant source and administered as separate supplements. Given the multitude of potential sites at which ROS may be involved in the development of coronary artery disease, it appears likely that a mixture of antioxidants, such as is obtained in protective diets, will be more effective than a single one or a combination of a few. The lack of association between any individual nutrient or food type and protective effects in the diet trials (2) supports this idea, as does the accumulating evidence of synergism and interactions between individual phytochemicals (28,57). Given the clear evidence of benefits of consumption of plant foods that contain thousands of biologically active compounds, including hundreds of natural antioxidants, flavonoids, and carotenoids, efforts to elucidate the most beneficial foods and diets would be a wiser and more effective strategy than attempting to identify the "magic bullet."

Although it is easier to recommend a supplement than to suggest that patients change their diets, the evidence that CVD could be almost completely prevented and even reversed by dietary and other lifestyle changes can no longer be ignored. A key factor in the success of dietary interventions is adherence. Epidemiologic data and intervention studies with diets rich in plant foods show that clinical benefits can be obtained by consumption of vegetables and fruits within a range that is behaviorally possible and culturally normative. In contrast to current opinion, patients are able to readily adopt new dietary habits when given detailed instructions, their adherence is closely monitored, and families and support groups are engaged in following the new dietary or other lifestyle changes, or both (67,73). There is a growing awareness by the public about the benefits of fruits, vegetables, and low-fat diets, and many of those using vitamin supplements are doing so because of their interest in prevention and empowerment. In the absence of support from the medical profession, many people resort to the Internet and media for their information about prevention and diet, and in this way they are susceptible to claims by supplement manufacturers about the benefits of these products. Thus, there is an urgent need for medical professionals to recognize the importance of dietary and lifestyle intervention programs that will educate and support those patients who are ready to take an active role in prevention or in managing their disease.

ACKNOWLEDGMENTS

This work was supported by research grants HL30657, HL56264, and HL00903 (to J.E.B.F.) from the National Institutes of Health and the "Finding Cures for Glioblastoma Award" (to M.G.).

REFERENCES

1. Bazzano LA, He J, Ogden LG, et al. Fruit and vegetable intake and risk of cardiovascular disease in US adults: the First National Health and Nutrition Examination Survey Epidemiologic Follow-up Study. *Am J Clin Nutr* 2002;76(1):93–99.
2. Trichopoulou A, Costacou T, Bamia C, et al. Adherence to a Mediterranean diet and survival in a Greek population. *N Engl J Med* 2003;348:2599–2608.
3. Eisenberg DM, Davis RB, Ettner SL, et al. Trends in alternative medicine use in the United States, 1990-1997: results of a follow-up national survey. *JAMA* 1998;280:1569–1575.
4. Kaufman DW, Kelly JP, Rosenberg L, et al. Recent patterns of medication use in the ambulatory adult population of the United States: the Slone Survey. *JAMA* 2002;287:337–344.
5. Fletcher RH, Fairfield KM. Vitamins for chronic disease prevention in adults: clinical applications. *JAMA* 2002;287:3127–3129.
6. The effect of vitamin E and beta-carotene on the incidence of lung cancer and other cancers in male smokers. The Alpha-Tocopherol, Beta-Carotene Cancer Prevention Study Group. *N Engl J Med* 1994; 330:1029–1035.
7. Omenn GS, Goodman GE, Thornquist MD, et al. Effects of a combination of beta carotene and vitamin A on lung cancer and cardiovascular disease. *N Engl J Med* 1996;334:1150–1155.
8. Brown BG, Zhao XQ, Chait A, et al. Simvastatin and niacin, antioxidant vitamins, or the combination for the prevention of coronary disease. *N Engl J Med* 2001;345:1583–1592.
9. Libby P. Vascular biology of atherosclerosis: overview and state of the art. *Am J Cardiol* 2003;91[Suppl]:3A–6A.
10. Steinberg D, Witztum JL. Is the oxidative modification hypothesis relevant to human atherosclerosis? Do the antioxidant trials conducted to date refute the hypothesis? *Circulation* 2002;105:2107–2111.
11. Vivekananthan DP, Penn MS, Sapp SK, et al. Use of antioxidant vitamins for the prevention of cardiovascular disease: meta-analysis of randomized trials. *Lancet* 2003;361:2017–2023.
12. Morris CD, Carson S. Routine vitamin supplementation to prevent cardiovascular disease: a summary of the evidence for the U.S. Preventive Services Task Force. *Ann Intern Med* 2003;139:56–70.
13. Routine vitamin supplementation to prevent cancer and cardiovascular disease: recommendations and rationale: U.S. Preventive Services Task Force. *Ann Intern Med* 2003;139:51–55.
14. Waters DD, Alderman EL, Hsia J, et al. Effects of hormone replacement therapy and antioxidant vitamin supplements on coronary atherosclerosis in postmenopausal women: a randomized controlled trial. *JAMA* 2002;288:2432–2440.
15. Kunsch C, Medford RM. Oxidative stress as a regulator of gene expression in the vasculature. *Circ Res* 1999;85:753–766.
16. Harrison D, Griendling KK, Landmesser U, et al. Role of oxidative stress in atherosclerosis. *Am J Cardiol* 2003;91[Suppl]:7A–11A.
17. Chakraborti T, Ghosh SK, Michael JR, et al. Targets of oxidative stress in cardiovascular system. *Mol Cell Biochem* 1998;187:1–10.
18. Homocysteine Studies Collaboration. Homocytsteine and risk of ischemic heart disease and stroke: a meta-analysis. *JAMA* 2002; 288:2015–2022.
19. De Bree A, Verschuren WM, Kromhout A, et al. Homocysteine determinants and the evidence to what extent homocysteine determines the risk of coronary heart disease. *Pharmacol Rev* 2002;54:599–618.
20. Haynes GH. Hyperhomocysteinemia, vascular function, and atherosclerosis: effects of vitamins. *Cardiovasc Drugs Ther* 2003;16: 391–399.
21. Clarke R, Armitage J. Vitamin supplements and cardiovascular risk: review of the randomized trials of homocysteine-lowering vitamin supplements. *Semin Thromb Hemost* 2000;26:341–348.
22. Graham IM, O'Callaghan P. Vitamins, homocysteine and cardiovascular risk. *Cardiovasc Drugs Ther* 2002;16:383–389.

23. Lowering blood homocysteine with folic acid based supplements: meta-analysis of randomised trials. Homocysteine Lowering Trialists' Collaboration. *BMJ* 1998;316:894–898.

24. Vermeulen EG, Stehouwer CD, Twisk JW, et al. Effect of homocysteine-lowering treatment with folic acid plus vitamin B6 on progression of subclinical atherosclerosis: a randomized, placebo-controlled trial. *Lancet* 2000;355:517–522.

25. Schnyder G, Roffi M, Pin R, et al. Decreased rate of coronary restenosis after lowering of plasma homocysteine levels. *N Engl J Med* 2001;345:1593–1600.

26. Schnyder G, Roffi M, Flammer Y, et al. Effect of homocysteine-lowering therapy with folic acid, vitamin B12, and vitamin B6 on clinical outcome after percutaneous coronary intervention: the Swiss Heart Study: a randomized controlled trial. *JAMA* 2002;288:973–979.

27. Bostom AG, Selhub J, Jacques PF, et al. Power shortage: clinical trials testing the homocysteine hypothesis against a background of folic acid-fortified cereal grain flour. *Ann Intern Med* 2001;135:133–137.

28. Hu FB, Willett WC. Optimal diets for prevention of coronary heart disease. *JAMA* 2002;288:2569–2578.

29. Stampfer MJ, Hennekens CH, Manson JE, et al. Vitamin E consumption and the risk of coronary disease in women. *N Engl J Med* 1993;328:1444–1449.

30. Rimm EB, Stampfer MJ, Ascherio A, et al. Vitamin E consumption and the risk of coronary heart disease in men. *N Engl J Med* 1993;328:1450–1456.

31. Losonczy KG, Harris TB, Havlik RJ. Vitamin E and vitamin C supplement use and risk of all-cause and coronary heart disease mortality in older persons: the Established Populations for Epidemiologic Studies of the Elderly. *Am J Clin Nutr* 1996;64:190–196.

32. Greenberg ER, Baron JA, Karagas MR, et al. Mortality associated with low plasma concentration of beta carotene and the effect of oral supplementation. *JAMA* 1996;275:699–703.

33. Hennekens CH, Buring JE, Manson JE, et al. Lack of effect of long-term supplementation with beta carotene on the incidence of malignant neoplasms and cardiovascular disease. *N Engl J Med* 1996;334:1145–1149.

34. Lee IM, Cook NR, Manson JE, et al. Beta-carotene supplementation and incidence of cancer and cardiovascular disease: the Women's Health Study. *J Natl Cancer Inst* 1999;91:2102–2106.

35. Rapola JM, Virtamo J, Ripatti S, et al. Randomized trial of alpha-tocopherol and beta-carotene supplements on incidence of major coronary events in men with previous myocardial infarction. *Lancet* 1997;349:1715–1720.

36. Virtamo J, Rapola JM, Ripatti S, et al. Effect of vitamin E and beta carotene on the incidence of primary nonfatal myocardial infarction and fatal coronary heart disease. *Arch Intern Med* 1998;158:668–675.

37. Stephens NG, Parsons A, Schofield PM, et al. Randomised controlled trial of vitamin E in patients with coronary disease: Cambridge Heart Antioxidant Study (CHAOS). *Lancet* 1996;347:781–786.

38. Dietary supplementation with n-3 polyunsaturated fatty acids and vitamin E after myocardial infarction: results of the GISSI-Prevenzione trial. Gruppo Italiano per lo Studio della Sopravvivenza nell'Infarto miocardico. *Lancet* 1999;354:447–455.

39. Vitamin E supplementation and cardiovascular events in high-risk patients. *N Engl J Med* 2000;342:154–160.

40. Low-dose aspirin and vitamin E in people at cardiovascular risk: a randomized trial in general practice. *Lancet* 2001;357:89–95.

41. A randomized, placebo-controlled, clinical trial of high-dose supplementation with vitamins C and E and beta carotene for age-related cataract and vision loss: AREDS report no. 9. *Arch Ophthalmol* 2001;119:1439–1452.

42. MRC/BHF Heart Protection Study of antioxidant vitamin supplementation in 20,536 high-risk individuals: a randomised placebo-controlled trial. *Lancet* 2002;360:23–33.

43. Cheung MC, Zhao XQ, Chait A, et al. Antioxidant supplements block the response of HDL to simvastatin-niacin therapy in patients with coronary artery disease and low HDL. *Arterioscler Thromb Vasc Biol* 2001;21:1320–1326.

44. Steinberg D. Antioxidants in the prevention of human atherosclerosis. Summary of the proceedings of a National Heart, Lung, and Blood Institute workshop: September 5-6, 1991, Bethesda, Maryland. *Circulation* 1992;85:2337–2344.

45. Brigelius-Flohe R, Kelly FJ, Salonen JT, et al. The European per-

spective on vitamin E: current knowledge and future research. *Am J Clin Nutr* 2002;76:703–716.

46. Zhang R, Brennan ML, Shen Z, et al. Myeloperoxidase functions as a major enzymatic catalyst for initiation of lipid peroxidation at sites of inflammation. *J Biol Chem* 2002;277:46116–46122.

47. Blot WJ, Li JY, Taylor PR, et al. Nutrition intervention trials in Linxian, China: supplementation with specific vitamin/mineral combinations, cancer incidence, and disease-specific mortality in the general population. *J Natl Cancer Inst* 1993;85:1483–1492.

48. Boaz M, Smetana S, Weinstein T, et al. Secondary Prevention with Antioxidants of Cardiovascular disease in Endstage renal disease (SPACE): randomised placebo-controlled trial. *Lancet* 2000;356:1213–1218.

49. Cai H, Harrison DG. Endothelial dysfunction in cardiovascular diseases: the role of oxidant stress. *Circ Res* 2000;87:840–844.

50. Fang JC, Kinlay S, Beltrame J, et al. Effect of vitamins C and E on progression of transplant-associated arteriosclerosis: a randomised trial. *Lancet* 2002;359:1108–1113.

51. Salonen RM, Nyyssonen K, Kaikkonen J, et al. Six-year effect of combined vitamin C and E supplementation on atherosclerotic progression: the Antioxidant Supplementation in Atherosclerosis Prevention (ASAP) study. *Circulation* 2003;107:947–953.

52. Kushi LH, Folsom AR, Prineas RJ, et al. Dietary antioxidant vitamins and death from coronary heart disease in postmenopausal women. *N Engl J Med* 1996;334:1156–1162.

53. Neuhouser ML, Patterson RE, Thornquist MD, et al. Fruits and vegetables are associated with lower lung cancer risk only in the placebo arm of the beta-Carotene And Retinol Efficacy Trial (CARET). *Cancer Epidemiol Biomarkers Prev* 2003;12:350–358.

54. Cao G, Sofic E, Prior R. Antioxidant capacity of tea and common vegetables. *J Agric Food Chem* 1996;44:3426–3431.

55. Sun J, Chu YF, Wu X, et al. Antioxidant and antiproliferative activities of common fruits. *J Agric Food Chem* 2002;50:7449–7454.

56. Chu YF, Sun J, Wu X, et al. Antioxidant and antiproliferative activities of common vegetables. *J Agric Food Chem* 2002;50:6910–6916.

57. Lampe JW. Health effects of vegetables and fruit: assessing mechanisms of action in human experimental studies. *Am J Clin Nutr* 1999;70[3 Suppl]:475S–490S.

58. Tapiero H, Tew KD, Ba GN, et al. Polyphenols: do they play a role in the prevention of human pathologies? *Biomed Pharmacother* 2002;56:200–207.

59. Nijveldt RJ, van Nood E, van Hoorn DE, et al. Flavonoids: a review of probable mechanisms of action and potential applications. *Am J Clin Nutr* 2001;74:418–425.

60. Knekt P, Kumpulainen J, Jarvinen R, et al. Flavonoid intake and risk of chronic diseases. *Am J Clin Nutr* 2002;76:560–568.

61. Cao G, Booth SL, Sadowski JA, et al. Increases in human plasma antioxidant capacity after consumption of controlled diets high in fruit and vegetables. *Am J Clin Nutr* 1998;68:1081–1087.

62. Bub A, Watzl B, Abrahamse L, et al. Moderate intervention with carotenoid-rich vegetable products reduces lipid peroxidation in men. *J Nutr* 2000;130:2200–2206.

63. Freedman JE, Parker C 3rd, Li L, et al. Select flavonoids and whole juice from purple grapes inhibit platelet function and enhance nitric oxide release. *Circulation* 2001;103:2792–2798.

64. O'Byrne DJ, Devaraj S, Grundy SM, et al. Comparison of the antioxidant effects of Concord grape juice flavonoids and alpha-tocopherol on markers of oxidative stress in healthy adults. *Am J Clin Nutr* 2002;76:1367–1374.

65. Lu SC, Wu WH, Lee CA, et al. LDL of Taiwanese vegetarians are less oxidizable than those of omnivores. *J Nutr* 2000;130:1591–1596.

66. Willett WC. Balancing life-style and genomics research for disease prevention. *Science* 2002;296:695–698.

67. de Lorgeril M, Salen P, Martin JL, et al. Mediterranean diet, traditional risk factors, and the rate of cardiovascular complications after myocardial infarction: final report of the Lyon diet heart study. *Circulation* 1999;99:779–785.

68. Singh RB, Niaz MA, Ghosh S, et al. Effect on mortality and reinfarction of adding fruits and vegetables to a prudent diet in the Indian Experiment of Infarct Survival (IEIS). *J Am Coll Nutr* 1993;12:255–261.

69. Singh RB, Dubnov G, Niaz MA, et al. Effect of an Indo-Mediterranean diet on progression of coronary artery disease in high

risk patients (Indo-Mediterranean diet heart study): a randomized single-blind trial. *Lancet* 2002;360:1455–1461.

70. Esselstyn CB Jr. Updating a 12-year experience with arrest and reversal therapy for coronary heart disease (an overdue requiem for palliative cardiology). *Am J Cardiol* 1999;84:339–341, A8.

71. Sdringola S, Nakagawa K, Nakagawa Y, et al. Combined intense lifestyle and pharmacologic lipid treatment further reduce coronary events and myocardial perfusion abnormalities compared with usual-care cholesterol-lowering drugs in coronary artery disease. *J Am Coll Cardiol* 2003;41:263–272.

72. Ornish D, Scherwitz LW, Billings JH, et al. Intensive lifestyle changes for reversal of coronary heart disease. *JAMA* 1998;280:2001–2007.

73. Barnard ND, Akhtar A, Nicholson A. Factors that facilitate compliance to lower fat intake. *Arch Fam Med* 1995;4:153–158.

PART II

Pathogenesis of Atherothrombosis

General Principles

CHAPTER 22

Developmental Biology of the Vasculature

Margaret L. Kirby

Key Words: Angiogenesis; early vascular development; patterning; signaling; vasculogenesis.

INTRODUCTION

The two major processes that generate blood vessels are vasculogenesis and angiogenesis. During vasculogenesis, vesicles of angioblasts form *de novo* and coalesce to form tubes or sinusoids. Angiogenesis, by contrast, is the formation of vessels by growth or *sprouting from preexisting vessels.* All of the earliest vascular development is by vasculogenesis, which lays down a primary capillary plexus that prefigures, with remodeling and growth, the adult vascular system. The capillary network is remodeled into a hierarchical system of large to small blood vessels by sprouting, or angiogenesis, of new vessels from preexisting vessels and regression of existing channels. These vessels are stabilized by perivascular cells attracted during the period of remodeling. The vessels recruit investing cells that will be organized into the tunics of the mature vessels or pericytes of capillaries.

The earliest vascular development is found in the yolk sac, but is soon thereafter initiated intraembryonically. Intraembryonic blood vessels arise from intraembryonic angioblasts. Precursors for angioblasts are thought to be born as early as gastrulation, although little is known about their developmental history before the expression of definitive markers. From their birth, these cells are migratory, invasive, and quickly distributed widely throughout the intraembryonic and extraembryonic mesenchyme.

M. L. Kirby: Department of Pediatrics and Cell Biology, Neonatal-Perinatal Research Institute, Duke University Medical Center, Durham, North Carolina 27710.

Although there are considerable variations on vascular patterning, especially in the venous system, arteries and veins are identifiable by their location from individual to individual, indicating that the basic vertebrate plan of the vasculature is remarkably stable even among widely varying species. The earliest embryonic vascular pattern is bilaterally symmetric, but the central vessels undergo extensive remodeling during organogenesis and the pattern of both veins and arteries in the trunk becomes asymmetric (Fig. 22–1).

The driving force for vascular developmental is multifactorial, but surely oxygen need plays a major role in growth of the vasculature. During early development, metabolic needs are satisfied by diffusion and so the prepattern for the vasculature is formed by strands of angioblasts that are guided by molecular patterning cues involving cell–cell interaction; it is only later that growth of the vasculature is driven by metabolic requirements.

PATTERNING THE VASCULATURE: THE PRIMARY CAPILLARY PLEXUS

Little is known about how vascular patterns are generated in the embryo. Because the endothelial cells seem to adhere to a prepattern at least reminiscent of the pattern they will have after circulation begins, it is likely that they follow a pattern established by other cells in a situation reminiscent of neural crest migration, which follows paths laid down by nonneural crest cells (1). Endothelial cells interact with their surrounding matrix and with each other to migrate and to form vesicles and finally tubes (Fig. 22–2). Integrin-mediated cell adhesion is necessary for normal endothelial tube formation. Endothelial cells express the α_5 integrin subunit in addition

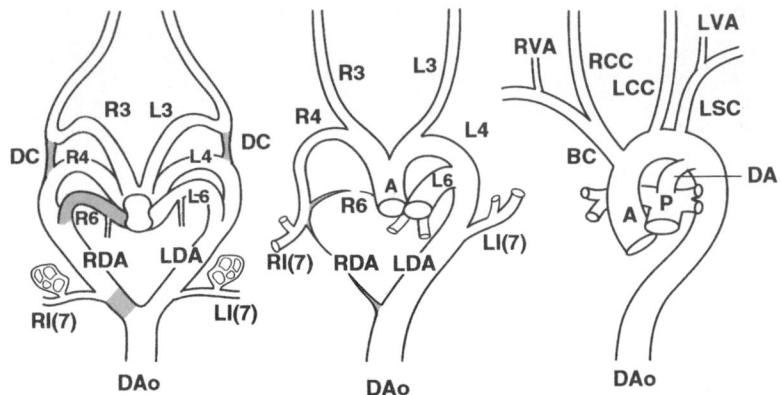

FIG. 22–1. Diagram of the bilaterally symmetric aortic arch arteries that carry the early cardiac output to the dorsal aorta, which then distributes blood to the embryo. The early symmetry is lost when these vessels are remodeled to be the adult great arteries of the thorax. A, aorta; BC, brachiocephalic; DA, ductus arteriosus; DAo, dorsal aorta; DC, ductus caroticus; LCC, left common carotid; LDA, left dorsal aorta; LI(7), left seventh intercostal; LSC, left subclavian artery; P, pulmonary trunk; R3/L3, right or left aortic arch 3; R4/L4, right or left aortic arch 4; R6/L6, right or left aortic arch 6; RCC, right common carotid; RDA, right dorsal aorta; RI(7), right seventh intercostal.

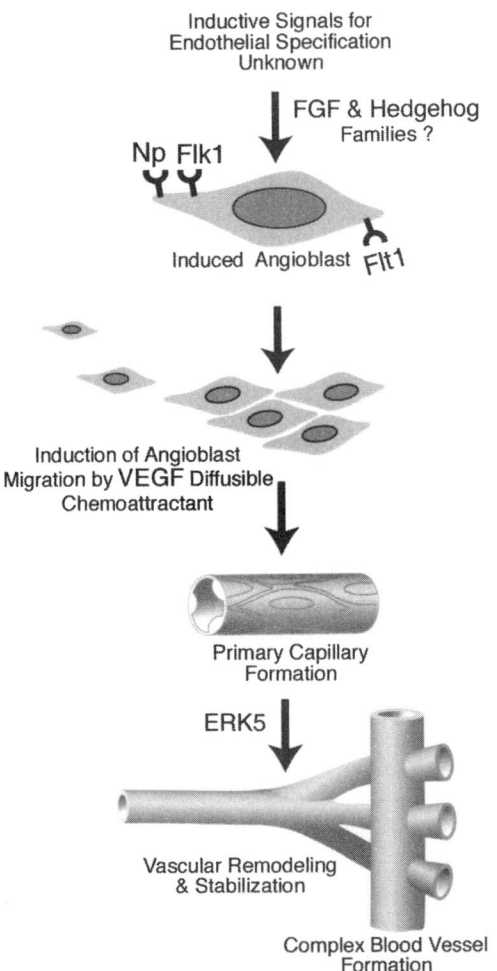

FIG. 22–2. Diagram showing the steps in conversion of angioblasts to blood vessels. The early steps are dependent on a variety of signals, but vascular endothelial growth factor (VEGF) signaling is critical for the process. FGF, fibroblast growth factor; Np, neuropilin.

to other integrin subunits to interact with fibronectin for vasculogenesis and angiogenesis (2). After tube formation, interendothelial tight junctions regulate paracellular permeability and maintain endothelial cell polarity (3).

The first endothelial cells to differentiate are seen in the yolk sac in clusters of hemangioblasts. The early hemangioblast is capable of differentiation into both hematoblasts, which will give rise to hematopoietic stem cells and angioblasts, which will give rise to the endothelial cell line. Vascular endothelial growth factor (VEGF) signaling is essential for the specification, proliferation, and migration of angioblasts. On the basis of the localization of VEGF receptors in cells of the gastrulating embryo and on clonal culture experiments, two types of intraembryonic endothelial precursor cells can be distinguished: posterior mesodermal hemangioblasts, which can differentiate into either endothelial or hemopoietic cells, and anterior angioblasts, which are restricted to an endothelial cell lineage (4).

The initial blood vessels form from coalescence of vesicles composed of angioblasts. The angioblasts, vesicles, or both appear to be laid down in a pattern corresponding roughly to the vascular pattern of the earliest vascularized embryos. This early pattern is highly symmetric (Fig. 22–1). The first recognizable vessels are the bilaterally paired dorsal aortae, which form by fusion of small vesicles of angioblasts. Many organs also contain their own endothelial precursors (i.e., lung, pancreas, spleen, and stomach), which self-assemble by vasculogenesis, whereas other organs (i.e., the brain, kidney, thymus and limb bud) are vascularized by angiogenic ingrowth from preexisting vessels (5–7). The vasculature of the heart develops by a mixture of vasculogenesis followed by angiogenesis. The endothelial precursors for the coronary circulation are generated from the epicardium by epithelial-to-mesenchymal transformation. The endothelial cells then self-assemble—that is, vasculogenesis—and then grow to provide circulation on a one-to-one basis with myocardial cells by angiogenesis. The last step in coronary angiogenesis is ingrowth of the vessels into the base of the aorta where, with remodeling and growth, they form the coronary stems (8). Many other organs acquire their vasculature through vasculogenesis followed by angiogenesis and only later contact their blood supply in a similar fashion (9).

The bilateral aortic arch arteries, which will form the definitive great arteries of the thorax, form from endothelial strands that are located roughly segmentally along the ventral pharynx in a pattern reminiscent of the arch arteries. As the pharyngeal arches form, the endothelial strands are lifted away from the ventral pharyngeal endoderm and begin to open at their ventral and dorsal extremities, adjacent to the aortic sac and dorsal aorta, respectively. The central portion of the aortic arch artery is the last to become patent. The cranial two aortic arch arteries regress into capillary beds, whereas the caudal three are remodeled to form the great arteries (Fig. 22–1). Part of the remodeling process involves a transition from bilateral symmetry to a distinctly asymmetric pattern that adheres to strict left-right axis instructions. The venous system in the trunk behaves in a similar manner in that a bilaterally symmetric venous vasculature is laid down and then extensively remodeled into an asymmetric venous system.

Some of the bilaterally symmetric patterns that are established early are maintained as bilaterally symmetric. The vasculature of the zebrafish trunk has an extremely regular pattern. The intersegmental vessels that originate from the dorsal aorta run between each pair of somites and connect to the dorsal longitudinal anastomotic vessel (10). The same type of intersegmental vessels develop in mammalian embryos and are maintained symmetrically.

SIGNALING AND EARLY VASCULAR DEVELOPMENT: VASCULAR ENDOTHELIAL GROWTH FACTOR

Understanding signaling networks is essential to understanding vasculogenesis and angiogenesis. The inductive signals for endothelial specification are not known and possibly include members of the fibroblast growth factor and hedgehog families. The immediate response of the induced endothelial cell is the expression VEGF of receptors, Flk1 (VEGFR2) followed later by Flt1 (VEGFR1) (Fig. 22–2) (11,12). VEGF regulates endothelial cell protrusive activity necessary for the establishment of a primary vascular pattern, and thus acts as a vascular morphogen. It is secreted by cells in four isoforms that have somewhat different functions. Localized sources of VEGF play a role in patterning the primary capillary plexus. A diffusible form of VEGF released by the hypochord acts as a chemoattractant for angioblasts that migrate from the lateral plate mesoderm to the midline, where they form a single dorsal aorta (13). Stimulation of embryonic endothelial cells with exogenous VEGF results in a massive "fusion" of vessels (14). When embryos are injected with VEGF antibody before the onset of circula-

tion, endothelial cells fail to form the elongated processes necessary for vessel morphogenesis.

Null mutation of the VEGF-A ligand is one of the few null mutations with a haploinsufficiency phenotype, suggesting that the availability of VEGF ligand is critical for vascular development (15,16). Heterozygous embryos die early in gestation with a reduction in the size and diameter of blood vessels.

Loss of Flk1 leads to absent development of angioblasts and failure to form any of the primary capillary plexus (17). Flt1 may be a negative regulator of VEGF signaling, and embryos that have null mutation of Flt1 have disorganized primary blood vessels with an overgrowth in endothelial cells (18,19). VEGF continues to play a role in promoting growth of blood vessels in later development and support vascularization of developing organs. The different isoforms of VEFG are important because an isoform-specific knockout causes abnormal myocardial angiogenesis with a loss of blood vessel growth in other organs (20).

Neuropilins (Np), which are transmembrane proteins associated with axon guidance, act as coreceptors for Flk1-mediated VEGF signaling. Np1 and Np2 are critical for vasculogenesis and angiogenesis as double mutation leads to failure of vasculature to develop (21,22). The binding of VEGF ligand to its receptors is enhanced by complexing with heparin-bound Np. Np is found to enhance VEGF-Flk1–dependent migration. Using transgenic zebrafish embryos in which an endothelial cell-specific promoter drives expression of enhanced green fluorescent protein in all blood vessels throughout embryogenesis, Lawson and Weinstein (23) have shown that blood vessels undergoing angiogenesis display extensive filopodia activity and pathfinding behavior similar to neuronal growth cones that also use Np.

ERK5 is a mitogen-activated protein (MAP) kinase, which plays a specific role in early vessel development (Fig. 22–2). Embryos deficient for the ERK5 MAP kinase die between E10.5 and E11.5 because they are unable to form a complex vasculature. This is thought to be because ERK5 deficiency leads to increased expression of VEGF, which impedes vascular remodeling and stabilization (24). Vasculogenesis occurs, but extraembryonic and embryonic blood vessels are disorganized and fail to mature. Furthermore, the investment of embryonic blood vessels with smooth muscle cells is attenuated (25).

ANGIOGENESIS AND REMODELING: TIE AND EPHRIN

The primary capillary network prefigures the adult vasculature but does not represent it perfectly, and extensive remodeling and growth occur. Remodeling of blood vessels involves branching, fusion of endothelial tubes to form larger vessels, and elimination of excess branches. Endothelial cells must interact with associated cells to organize a smooth muscle tunic. Several growth factor families are prominently involved in these steps. Angiopoietin and its receptors Tie1 and Tie2 (Tek) (26–29) are major contributors to vascular

328 / CHAPTER 22

remodeling and vessel stabilization. Little is known about angiopoietin signaling through the Tie1 receptor. More is known about the Tie2 receptor, which is a receptor tyrosine kinase that forms autophosphorylated homodimers on ligand binding (30). Null mutation of Tie2 or angiopoietin 1 causes embryonic death in midgestation because of the inability of blood vessels to remodel and stabilize (31,32). Angiopoietin 2 overexpression leads to a phenotype similar to the null phenotype of Tie2 or angiopoietin 1, indicating that it acts as an antagonist of angiopoietin 1/Tie2 signaling (33). Because angiopoietin 2 is expressed at sites of remodeling and branching, it is thought to act locally to block angiopoietin 1 signaling, which leads to vessel destabilization. Destabilization is an important step in remodeling (33). If VEGF is present, the vessel remodels at sites of destabilization. In the absence of VEGF the destabilized endothelial cells undergo apoptosis and the vessel regresses (34).

As mentioned previously, the primary capillary plexus is symmetric, and during remodeling it becomes asymmetric. The presence of left-right axis asymmetry is indicated molecularly in the primary capillary plexus. Tie1 is expressed symmetrically in the sinus venosus, whereas angiopoietin 1 is expressed only in the right side before the time when the vasculature shows any morphologic asymmetry, suggesting that there is a distinct genetic program for the establishment of the right-hand side and left-hand side vascular networks well before the network asymmetry becomes morphologically discernible (34). Null mutation indicates that angiopoietin 1/Tie1 signaling are necessary for the development of the right-sided venous system, but they are dispensable for the left-sided venous system.

Unlike VEGF, the angiopoietin/Tie2 signaling system does not appear to function until circulation begins. Injection of angiopoietin 2, a naturally occurring inhibitor of Tie2-mediated signaling, results in endocardial and aortic anomalies. Injected embryos display malformed endocardial tubes, which appear perforated and discontinuous. Instead of large vessels with a single lumen, angiopoietin 2–treated aortic primordia resemble a small plexus of microvessels. Because angiopoietin 2 is an inhibitory ligand, it may compete with angiopoietin 1 for Tie2 binding (35).

Ephrin signaling also is required for vessel remodeling. As for the Nps, ephrin signaling was first characterized in the nervous system and neural crest cell migration, where it is needed for pathfinding and bundling of nerves. Eph receptors are tyrosine kinases that bind several ephrin ligands. The ephrin ligands can be soluble, but the most numerous class is membrane-attached cell-surface molecules (36). Membrane-bound ephrin ligands are themselves active in signaling, in addition to serving as ligands for Eph receptors, resulting in bidirectional signaling (37). EphrinA ligands are chemoattractant for migrating endothelial cells (38) and are found at sites of remodeling (39,40).

Mesenchymal cells adjacent to some vessels express EphB2 receptors where they could interact with ephrinB ligands expressed by endothelial cells (41). Disrupted interactions between EphB4 on intersomatic vessels and ephrinB ligands on somites lead to disrupted patterning of the segmental vessels that are unable to recognize boundaries in the absence of normal ephrin signaling (42). This type of cell-to-cell repellent effect is caused by bidirectional EphB/ephrin-B2 signaling and is similar to the mechanism described for neuronal development (43).

STABILIZATION AND DEVELOPMENT OF THE VESSEL WALL: TRANSFORMING GROWTH FACTOR-β AND PLATELET-DERIVED GROWTH FACTOR

Embryogenesis of the primary capillary plexus does not seem to depend on the perivascular cells, but subsequent vessel remodeling relies on mesenchymal–endothelial short-range signaling for assembly of the vessel wall (44). Vascular mural cells are derived from mesoderm, neural crest, or epicardium (Fig. 22–3). These cells migrate to associate with endothelial cells and form the vessel wall. There is some evidence that endothelial cells have the potential to give rise to vascular smooth muscle cells in that Flk1-positive cells derived from embryonic stem cells can differentiate into both endothelial and mural cell types. The Flk1-positive angioblasts can organize into vessel-like structures consisting of endothelial tubes supported by mural cells in three-dimensional culture. Injected Flk1-positive embryonic stem cells in chick embryos incorporate as endothelial and mural cells in vivo (45).

The proper recruitment of vascular smooth muscle cells to the endothelium is a critical event in blood vessel development (Fig. 22–4). The first mesodermally derived cells to as-

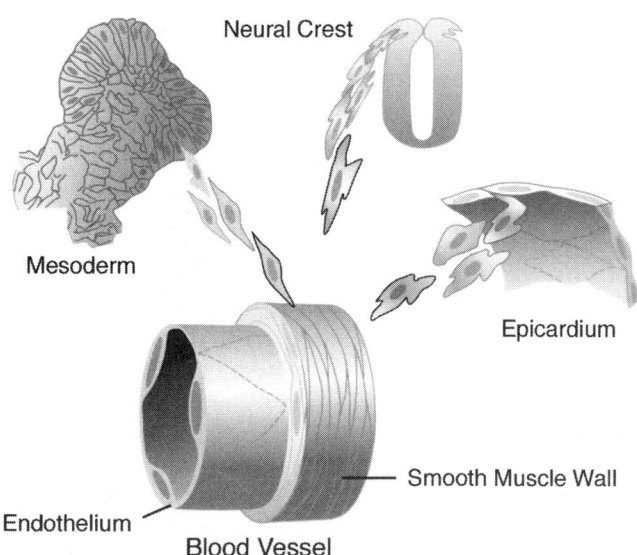

FIG. 22–3. Diagram showing the three sources of vascular smooth muscle from embryonic mesenchyme. The cells from two of the sources, neural crest and epicardium, must undergo the additional step of epithelial-to-mesenchymal transformation.

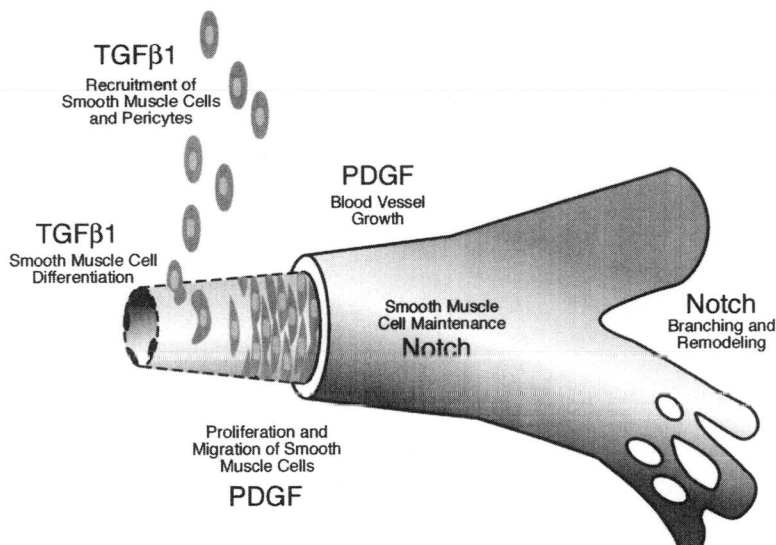

FIG. 22–4. Diagram showing the factors that are involved in recruitment of vascular smooth muscle cells and pericytes to stabilize blood vessels after remodeling and branching. PDGF, platelet-derived growth factor; TGF-β_1, transforming growth factor-β_1.

sociate with the aortic endothelium do so at the ventral surface. Recruitment of these cells proceeds in a ventral to dorsal direction along the aorta and in a radial direction from the endothelium. Differential expression of fibulin-1 by the initial population of vascular smooth muscle cells before elastin is expressed suggests that there may be early diversity among embryonic vascular smooth muscle cells (46,47). Vascular smooth muscle cells can be thought of as existing along a continuum of phenotypes. This spectrum varies from mainly matrix-producing cells to primarily contractile cells; thus, no one cell type typifies vascular smooth muscle (14).

Platelet-derived growth factor (PDGF)-B, PDGF receptor-β (PDGFR-β), angiopoietin 1, and tie2 knockout mice all show deficient development of perivascular cells. PDGF signaling is critical for proliferation and migration of smooth muscle cells and pericytes to support the endothelial cell wall (44). This process involves reciprocal interactions of endothelial and smooth muscle cells (14). Endothelial cells express the PDGF ligand, whereas smooth muscle cells express the PDGFR-β (48). Mutation of PDGF-B results in failure of recruitment of pericytes (44). Smooth muscle cells and pericytes initially form around endothelial vessels, but cells lacking PDGF signaling cannot proliferate and migrate as the vessels sprout and enlarge (49).

Notch1-deficient embryos have defects in remodeling with vascular degeneration (50). Mutants of Jagged1 form endothelial cells but fail to remodel to form large veins and show poor branching (51). Notch signaling is needed to support branching and vascular maintenance, which includes maintaining a smooth muscle coat. Because there may be a common endothelial/smooth muscle lineage, it is possible that Notch signaling could play a role in determining the ratio of endothelial/smooth muscle cells (45).

TGF-β_1 signaling is needed for vascular smooth muscle cell differentiation and recruitment (52,53). TGF-β_1 binds to the TGF-β type II receptor (TβRII). In endothelial cells, the TβRII recruits and phosphorylates type I receptors (Alk) (54). The heterodimer then complexes with Smads 1 and 5, and finally with Smad 4, which is translocated to the nucleus where it activates the transcription of target genes (55). Endothelial cells express a type II receptor called endoglin, which reduces the TGF signaling response (56,57). Embryos deficient for Alk5 die at E10.5 to E11.5, with vascular defects similar to TGF-β_1 and TβRII mutants (53)—that is, reduced smooth muscle walls.

ESTABLISHING THE IDENTITY OF ARTERIES AND VEINS: EPHRIN AND NOTCH SIGNALING

Artery versus vein identity is programmed developmentally rather than developing as a functional characteristic (Fig. 22–5). A signaling cascade has been recognized in establishing artery and vein identity. VEGF signaling may be involved in establishing artery and vein identity. Although Flk1 is expressed in both arteries and veins, Np1 is artery-specific, whereas Np2 is restricted to the venous endothelium (58). TGF-β activation of Alk1 signaling also is involved in establishing artery versus vein identity (59). Alk1 null mutation in mice leads to formation of abnormal shunting between the dorsal aorta and cardinal veins. Mutations in the human *alk1* and *endoglin* genes are associated with hereditary hemorrhagic telangiectasia (60), a disorder that results in arteriovenous shunts (59).

Notch and ephrin are expressed on established arteries and veins. Alk1 may activate both ephrin and Notch signaling, which, in turn, suppresses venous fate. In mice with Alk1 null mutation, the dorsal aorta and arteries fail to express

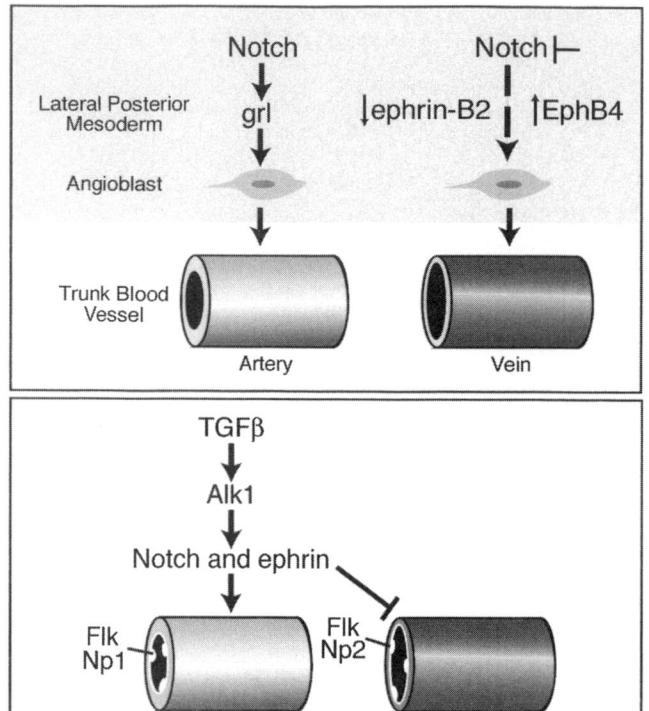

FIG. 22–5. Factors that establish and maintain artery versus vein identity. grl, gridlock; TGF-β, transforming growth factor-β; VEGF, vascular endothelial growth factor.

ephrinB2, which is specific for arterial endothelium (59). The cognate receptor for ephrinB2, EphB4, is expressed in venous endothelial cells (61). An ephrinB2/EphB4 interaction is probably necessary to establish the arterial–venous boundary (36). Venous endothelial cells coexpress EphB3 and EphB4 receptors with the ephrinB1 ligand (41). EphrinB1 and B2 are found with low levels of EphB3 and B4 expressed by arterial endothelium (41,62). However, other factors must be involved, because loss of ephrin signaling does not lead to mixing of arterial and venous endothelial cells (61,62).

Notch is a receptor that binds with a variety of identified ligands. Ligand binding causes proteolytic cleavage of the intracellular domain of the Notch cytoplasmic tail (63,64). The cytoplasmic tail then binds to the transcription factor recombination signal-binding protein J kappa (RBPj-κ) (65), and the complex enters the nucleus where it activates gene transcription (66). Targets of Notch signaling include the *Hes* (Hairy/Enhancer of Split) gene, which is a basic helix-loop-helix (bHLH) transcription factor. *Hes* represses transcription to suppress specific cell fates in the signaled cell (67).

Many Notch ligands and receptors are expressed in the developing vasculature. Notch1, Notch4, Delta4, Jagged1, and Jagged2 are expressed in the arterial endothelium. Notch3 is localized to smooth muscle cells surrounding arteries (68–70). Notch4 and Delta4 are the only Notch family members with expression confined to the endothelium. Mutations in Jagged1 and Notch3 are associated with human diseases that have significant vascular malformations called Alagille syndrome and CADASIL.

Jag1, a Notch ligand, and Notch2 are colocalized and required for glomerular differentiation and patterning. Notch2 null homozygotes also display myocardial hypoplasia, edema, and hyperplasia of cells associated with the hyaloid vasculature of the eye (71). Angioblast precursors for the trunk artery and vein are spatially mixed in the lateral posterior mesoderm. Progeny of each angioblast, however, are restricted to one of the vessels. This arterial–venous decision is guided by gridlock (*grl*), an artery-restricted gene that is expressed in the lateroposterior mesoderm. Graded reduction of *grl* expression, by mutation or morpholino antisense, progressively ablates regions of the artery and expands contiguous regions of the vein, preceded by an increase in expression of the venous marker EphB4 receptor and diminution of expression of the arterial marker ephrinB2. *grl* is downstream of Notch. Interference with Notch signaling, by blocking Suppressor of Hairless (SuH), a cofactor needed for Notch transcriptional activity, similarly reduces the artery and increases the vein. Thus, a Notch-grl pathway controls assembly of the first embryonic artery, apparently by adjudicating an arterial versus venous cell fate decision (72). Dilated vessels and missing major veins are reported in loss and gain of function in Notch mutants. Inhibition of Notch signaling in zebrafish resulted in decreased arterial expression of ephrinB2 and Notch3, both markers of arterial endothelial cells (72,73). The embryos had circulatory shunts between the dorsal aorta and posterior cardinal vein with progressive loss of sections of the dorsal aorta and expansion of the posterior cardinal vein (72,73).

CONCLUSION

Significant advances in understanding the molecular and cell biology of the developing vascular system have allowed major insights in the understanding of vascular development and its exciting cell types. However, many questions remain. How and when are endothelial lineages specified? What patterns the vascular system? What drives growth and remodeling of the blood vessels? What factors are involved in recruitment of the perivascular tissues? We have made some of the initial steps in answering these questions, but we remain a long way from a comprehensive understanding of this dynamic system.

ACKNOWLEDGMENTS

The author thanks Karen Waldo, who produced the illustrations for this chapter, and Mary Hutson, for critical comments and continuing lively discussions of cardiovascular development. This chapter was supported by National Institutes of Health grants HL36059, HD17065, and HD39946.

REFERENCES

1. LeDouarin NM, Kalcheim C. *The neural crest, 2nd ed. Developmental and cell biology series.* Cambridge, UK: Cambridge University Press, 2001.
2. Francis SE, Goh KL, Hodivala-Dilke K, et al. Central roles of alpha5beta1 integrin and fibronectin in vascular development in mouse embryos and embryoid bodies. *Arterioscler Thromb Vasc Biol* 2002;22: 927–933.
3. Bazzoni G, Martinez Estrada O, Dejana E. Molecular structure and functional role of vascular tight junctions. *Trends Cardiovasc Med* 1999;9:147–152.
4. Eichmann A, Corbel C, Le Douarin NM. Segregation of the embryonic vascular and hemopoietic systems. *Biochem Cell Biol* 1998;76:939–946.
5. Stewart PA, Wiley MJ. Developing nervous tissue induces formation of blood-brain barrier characteristics in invading endothelial cells: a study using quail-chick transplantation chimeras. *Dev Biol* 1981;84:183–192.
6. Risau W. Developing brain produces an angiogenesis factor. *Proc Natl Acad Sci USA* 1986;83:3855–3859.
7. Sariola H, Ekblom P, Lehtonen E, et al. Differentiation and vascularization of the metanephric kidney grafted on the chorioallantoic membrane. *Dev Biol* 1983;96:427–435.
8. Waldo KL, Willner W, Kirby ML. Origin of the proximal coronary artery stems and a review of ventricular vascularization in the chick embryo. *Am J Anat* 1990;188:109–120.
9. Robert B, St. John PL, Abrahamson DR. Direct visualization of renal vascular morphogenesis in Flk1 heterozygous mutant mice. *Am J Physiol* 1998;275:F164–F172.
10. Childs S, Chen JN, Garrity DM, et al. Patterning of angiogenesis in the zebrafish embryo. *Development* 2002;129:973–982.
11. Millauer B, Wizigmann-Voos S, Schnurch H, et al. High affinity VEGF binding and developmental expression suggest Flk-1 as a major regulator of vasculogenesis and angiogenesis. *Cell* 1993;72:835–846.
12. Yamaguchi TP, Dumont DJ, Conlon RA, et al. flk-1, an flt-related receptor tyrosine kinase is an early marker for endothelial cell precursors. *Development* 1993;118:489–498.
13. Cleaver O, Krieg PA.VEGF mediates angioblast migration during development of the dorsal aorta in Xenopus. *Development* 1998;125: 3905–3914.
14. Drake CJ, Hungerford JE, Little CD. Morphogenesis of the first blood vessels. *Ann NY Acad Sci* 1998;857:155–179.
15. Carmeliet P, Ferreira V, Breier G, et al. Abnormal blood vessel development and lethality in embryos lacking a single VEGF allele. *Nature* 1996;380:435–439.
16. Ferrara N, Carver-Moore K, Chen H, et al. Heterozygous embryonic lethality induced by targeted inactivation of the VEGF gene. *Nature* 1996;380:439–442.
17. Shalaby F, Rossant J, Yamaguchi TP, et al. Failure of blood-island formation and vasculogenesis in Flk-1-deficient mice. *Nature* 1995;376:62–66.
18. Fong GH, Rossant J, Gertsenstein M, et al. Role of the Flt-1 receptor tyrosine kinase in regulating the assembly of vascular endothelium. *Nature* 1995;376:66–70.
19. Fong TA, Shawver LK, Sun L, et al. SU5416 is a potent and selective inhibitor of the vascular endothelial growth factor receptor (Flk-1/KDR) that inhibits tyrosine kinase catalysis, tumor vascularization, and growth of multiple tumor types. *Cancer Res* 1999;59:99–106.
20. Carmeliet P. Basic concepts of (myocardial) angiogenesis: role of vascular endothelial growth factor and angiopoietin. *Curr Interv Cardiol Rep* 1999;1:322–335.
21. Neufeld G, Cohen T, Shraga N, et al. The neuropilins: multifunctional semaphorin and VEGF receptors that modulate axon guidance and angiogenesis. *Trends Cardiovasc Med* 2002;12:13–19.
22. Takashima S, Kitakaze M, Asakura M, et al. Targeting of both mouse neuropilin-1 and neuropilin-2 genes severely impairs developmental yolk sac and embryonic angiogenesis. *Proc Natl Acad Sci USA* 2002;99: 3657–3662.
23. Lawson N, Weinstein B. In vivo imaging of embryonic vascular development using transgenic zebrafish. *Dev Biol* 2002;248:307–318.
24. Sohn SJ, Sarvis BK, Cado D, et al. ERK5 MAPK regulates embryonic angiogenesis and acts as a hypoxia-sensitive repressor of vascular endothelial growth factor expression. *J Biol Chem* 2002;277:43344–43351.
25. Regan CP, Li W, Boucher DM, et al. Erk5 null mice display multiple extraembryonic vascular and embryonic cardiovascular defects. *Proc Natl Acad Sci USA* 2002;99:9248–9253.
26. Dumont DJ, Yamaguchi TP, Conlon RA, et al. tek, a novel tyrosine kinase gene located on mouse chromosome 4, is expressed in endothelial cells and their presumptive precursors. *Oncogene* 1992;7:1471–1480.
27. Korhonen J, Polvi A, Partanen J, et al. The mouse tie receptor tyrosine kinase gene: expression during embryonic angiogenesis. *Oncogene* 1994;9:395–403.
28. Sato TN, Qin Y, Kozak CA, et al. Tie-1 and tie-2 define another class of putative receptor tyrosine kinase genes expressed in early embryonic vascular system. *Proc Natl Acad Sci USA* 1993;90:9355–9358.
29. Schnurch H, Risau W. Expression of tie-2, a member of a novel family of receptor tyrosine kinases, in the endothelial cell lineage. *Development* 1993;119:957–968.
30. Jones N, Master Z, Jones J, et al. Identification of Tek/Tie2 binding partners. Binding to a multifunctional docking site mediates cell survival and migration. *J Biol Chem* 1999;274:30896–30905.
31. Dumont DJ, Gradwohl G, Fong GH, et al. Dominant-negative and targeted null mutations in the endothelial receptor tyrosine kinase, tek, reveal a critical role in vasculogenesis of the embryo. *Genes Dev* 1994;8:1897–1909.
32. Sato TN, Tozawa Y, Deutsch U, et al. Distinct roles of the receptor tyrosine kinases Tie-1 and Tie-2 in blood vessel formation. *Nature* 1995;376:70–74.
33. Maisonpierre PC, Suri C, Jones PF, et al. Angiopoietin-2, a natural antagonist for Tie2 that disrupts in vivo angiogenesis. *Science* 1997;277: 55–60.
34. Loughna S, Sato TN. Angiopoietin and Tie signaling pathways in vascular development. *Matrix Biol* 2001;20:319–325.
35. Drake CJ, Little CD. The de novo formation of blood vessels. *J Histochem Cytochem* 1999;47:1643–1643.
36. Adams RH, Klein R. Eph receptors and ephrin ligands. Essential mediators of vascular development. *Trends Cardiovasc Med* 2000;10:183–188.
37. Bruckner K, Klein R. Signaling by Eph receptors and their ephrin ligands. *Curr Opin Neurobiol* 1998;8:375–382.
38. Daniel TO, Stein E, Cerretti DP, et al. ELK and LERK-2 in developing kidney and microvascular endothelial assembly. *Kidney Int Suppl* 1996;57:S73–S81.
39. Flenniken AM, Gale NW, Yancopoulos GD, et al. Distinct and overlapping expression patterns of ligands for Eph-related receptor tyrosine kinases during mouse embryogenesis. *Dev Biol* 1996;179:382–401.
40. McBride JL, Ruiz JC. Ephrin-A1 is expressed at sites of vascular development in the mouse. *Mech Dev* 1998;77:201–204.
41. Adams RH, Wilkinson GA, Weiss C, et al. Roles of ephrinB ligands and EphB receptors in cardiovascular development: demarcation of arterial/venous domains, vascular morphogenesis, and sprouting angiogenesis. *Genes Dev* 1999;13:295–306.
42. Helbling PM, Saulnier DM, Robinson V, et al. Comparative analysis of embryonic gene expression defines potential interaction sites for Xenopus EphB4 receptors with ephrin-B ligands. *Dev Dyn* 1999;216:361–373.
43. Oike Y, Ito Y, Hamada K, et al. Regulation of vasculogenesis and angiogenesis by EphB/ephrin-B2 signaling between endothelial cells and surrounding mesenchymal cells. *Blood* 2002;100:1326–1333.
44. Lindahl P, Hellstrom M, Kalen M, et al. Endothelial-perivascular cell signaling in vascular development: lessons from knockout mice. *Curr Opin Lipidol* 1998;9:407–411.
45. Yamashita J, Itoh H, Hirashima M, et al. Flk1-positive cells derived from embryonic stem cells serve as vascular progenitors. *Nature* 2000;408:92–96.
46. Wunsch AM, Little CD, Markwald RR. Cardiac endothelial heterogeneity defines valvular development as demonstrated by the diverse expression of JB3, an antigen of the endocardial cushion tissue. *Dev Biol* 1994;165:585–601.
47. Hungerford JE, Owens GK, Argraves WS, et al. Development of the aortic vessel wall as defined by vascular smooth muscle and extracellular matrix markers. *Dev Biol* 1996;178:375–392.
48. Betsholtz C, Karlsson L, Lindahl P. Developmental roles of platelet-derived growth factors. *Bioessays* 2001;23:494–507.
49. Hellstrom M, Kal NM, Lindahl P, et al. Role of PDGF-B and PDGFR-beta in recruitment of vascular smooth muscle cells and pericytes dur-

ing embryonic blood vessel formation in the mouse. *Development* 1999;126:3047–3055.

50. Krebs LT, Xue Y, Norton CR, et al. Notch signaling is essential for vascular morphogenesis in mice. *Genes Dev* 2000;14:1343–1352.

51. Xue Y, Gao X, Lindsell CE, et al. Embryonic lethality and vascular defects in mice lacking the Notch ligand Jagged1. *Hum Mol Genet* 1999;8:723–730.

52. Pepper MS. Transforming growth factor-beta: vasculogenesis, angiogenesis, and vessel wall integrity. *Cytokine Growth Factor Rev* 1997;8:21–43.

53. Larsson J, Goumans MJ, Sjostrand LJ, et al. Abnormal angiogenesis but intact hematopoietic potential in TGF-beta type I receptor-deficient mice. *EMBO J* 2001;20:1663–1673.

54. Hoodless PA, Wrana JL. Mechanism and function of signaling by the TGF beta superfamily. *Curr Top Microbiol Immunol* 1998;228:235–272.

55. Oh SP, Seki T, Goss KA, et al. Activin receptor-like kinase 1 modulates transforming growth factor-beta 1 signaling in the regulation of angiogenesis. *Proc Natl Acad Sci USA* 2000;97:2626–2631.

56. Barbara NP, Wrana JL, Letarte M. Endoglin is an accessory protein that interacts with the signaling receptor complex of multiple members of the transforming growth factor-beta superfamily. *J Biol Chem* 1999;274:584–594.

57. Letamendia A, Lastres P, Botella LM, et al. Role of endoglin in cellular responses to transforming growth factor-beta. A comparative study with betaglycan. *J Biol Chem* 1998;273:33011–33019.

58. Herzog Y, Kalcheim C, Kahane N, et al. Differential expression of neuropilin-1 and neuropilin-2 in arteries and veins. *Mech Dev* 2001;109: 115–119.

59. Urness LD, Sorensen LK, Li DY. Arteriovenous malformations in mice lacking activin receptor-like kinase-1. *Nat Genet* 2000;26:328–331.

60. Azuma H. Genetic and molecular pathogenesis of hereditary hemorrhagic telangiectasia. *J Med Invest* 2000;47:81–90.

61. Wang HU, Chen ZF, Anderson DJ. Molecular distinction and angio-

62. Gerety SS, Wang HU, Chen ZF, et al. Symmetrical mutant phenotypes of the receptor EphB4 and its specific transmembrane ligand ephrin-B2 in cardiovascular development. *Mol Cell* 1999;4:403–414.

63. Schroeter EH, Kisslinger JA, Kopan R. Notch-1 signalling requires ligand-induced proteolytic release of intracellular domain. *Nature* 1998;393:382–386.

64. Struhl G, Adachi A. Nuclear access and action of notch in vivo. *Cell* 1998;93:649–660.

65. Fortini ME, Artavanis-Tsakonas S. The suppressor of hairless protein participates in notch receptor signaling. *Cell* 1994;79:273–282.

66. Artavanis-Tsakonas S, Rand MD, Lake RJ. Notch signaling: cell fate control and signal integration in development. *Science* 1999;284:770–776.

67. Cau E, Gradwohl G, Casarosa S, et al. Hes genes regulate sequential stages of neurogenesis in the olfactory epithelium. *Development* 2000; 127:2323–2332.

68. Shirayoshi Y, Yuasa Y, Suzuki T, et al. Proto-oncogene of int-3, a mouse Notch homologue, is expressed in endothelial cells during early embryogenesis. *Genes Cells* 1997;2:213–224.

69. Shutter JR, Scully S, Fan W, et al. Dll4, a novel Notch ligand expressed in arterial endothelium. *Genes Dev* 2000;14:1313–1318.

70. Uyttendaele H, Marazzi G, Wu G, et al. Notch4/int-3, a mammary proto-oncogene, is an endothelial cell-specific mammalian Notch gene. *Development* 1996;122:2251–2259.

71. McCright B, Gao X, Shen L, et al. Defects in development of the kidney, heart and eye vasculature in mice homozygous for a hypomorphic Notch2 mutation. *Development* 2001;128:491–502.

72. Zhong TP, Childs S, Leu JP, et al. Gridlock signalling pathway fashions the first embryonic artery. *Nature* 2001;414:216–220.

73. Lawson ND, Scheer N, Pham VN, et al. Notch signaling is required for arterial-venous differentiation during embryonic vascular development. *Development* 2001;128:3675–3683.

genic interaction between embryonic arteries and veins revealed by ephrin-B2 and its receptor Eph-B4. *Cell* 1998;93:741–753.

CHAPTER **23**

Molecular Basis of Vasculogenesis, Angiogenesis, and Arteriogenesis

David Manka, Veerle Compernolle, and Peter Carmeliet

Key Words: Angiogenesis; collateral growth; placental growth factor; stem cell; vascular endothelial growth factor.

The purpose of this review is to provide an overview of vessel growth, its cellular and molecular mechanisms, and emerging therapeutic targets for cardiovascular disease.

The growth of new blood vessels begins during embryonic development and is subsequently integral to homeostatic maintenance and adaptation of the adult vasculature. Dysfunctional blood vessel formation is likewise associated with a rich gamut of pathologies and genetic defects. Angiogenesis is commonly used as a comprehensive term when referring to the appearance of new blood vessels, large and small, healthy and diseased, embryonic and adult. To be more precise, though, the formation of new vessels is segregated according to three classic paradigms: *vasculogenesis, angiogenesis,* and *arteriogenesis.* Vasculogenesis is the *in situ* formation of vessels from angioblasts during embryonic development. Later in development, smaller capillaries sprout from the primary vessels, and this is referred to as angiogenesis. Arteriogenesis is

the maturation of a preexisting thin-walled vessels into a muscular vessel through recruitment of mural cells, resulting in a more robust and durable vessel. In the adult, vessels are normally quiescent, but they can start to grow rapidly and extensively in response to stress conditions such as malignancy, inflammation, or ischemia—a process coined the *angiogenic switch.* As in the embryo, vessel growth in the adult also is mediated by vasculogenesis (with bloodborne circulating vascular progenitors), angiogenesis, and arteriogenesis (Fig. 23–1). In addition, preexisting collateral vessels can enlarge and salvage ischemic tissues by supplying them bulk flow (Fig. 23–1). The field of angiogenesis is converging with diverse fields such as stem cell biology and neurobiology to yield novel and provocative avenues of research. For example, recent experimental evidence suggests significant crosstalk between the vascular and nervous systems during differentiation, growth, patterning, and maintenance of blood vessels and nerves with important implications for neurovascular disorders such as neurodegeneration (1). These topics, as well as a reference to therapeutic strategies aimed at increasing or inhibiting new vessel growth, are discussed in this chapter.

VASCULOGENESIS IN THE EMBRYO AND ADULT

Hematopoietic and (at least some) endothelial cells share a common progenitor in the embryo: the hemangioblast (Fig. 23–2). In the yolk sac, for example, hemangioblasts form aggregates in which the inner cells develop into hematopoietic precursors and the outer population into endothelial

D. Manka: Genome Research Institute, University of Cincinnati, 2180 East Galbraith Road, Building 44, Cincinnati, Ohio 45237.

V. Compernolle: Laboratory for Clinical Biology, Ghent University Hospital, De Pintelaan 185, B-9000 Gent, Belgium.

P. Carmeliet: Center for Transgene Technology and Gene Therapy, Flanders Interuniversity Institute for Biotechnology, KU Leuven, Campus Gasthuisberg, Herestraat 49, B-3000 Leuven, Belgium.

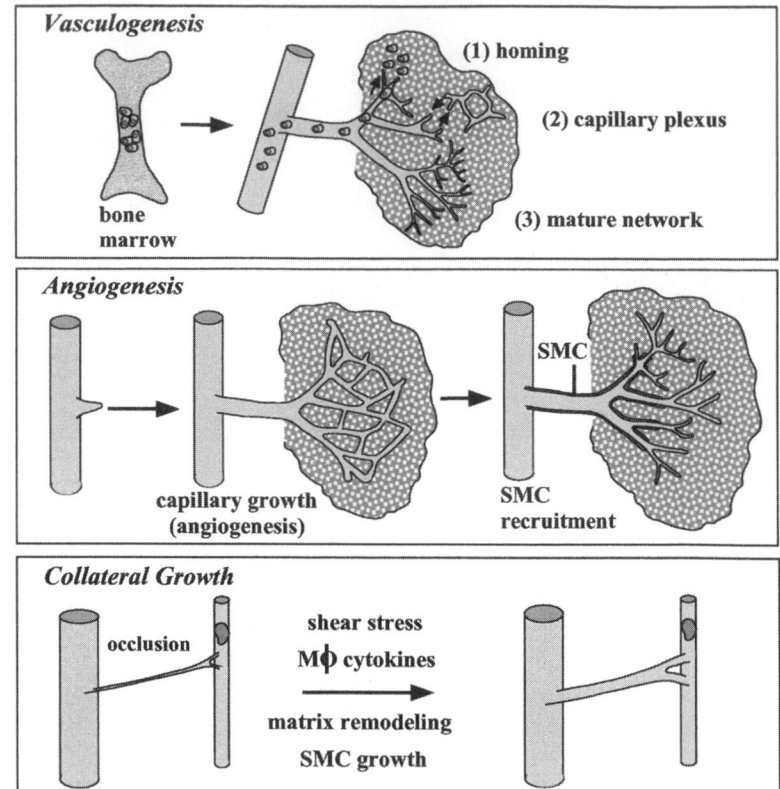

FIG. 23–1. Vessel growth in the adult. **Top:** Vasculogenesis, or the recruitment of endothelial progenitors to sites of active vessel growth. **Middle:** Angiogenesis, or the sprouting of vessel branches from preexisting vessels, which then become covered by mural cells (arteriogenesis). **Bottom:** Collateral vessel growth, or the enlargement of a preexisting collateral vessel after occlusion of a feeder supply artery. SMC, smooth muscle cells. (Reprinted from Carmeliet P. Mechanisms of angiogenesis and arteriogenesis. *Nat Med* 2000;6:389–395, with permission.)

cells. Hemangioblasts express VEGFR2 (also fetal liver kinase-1 [Flk1], a receptor of vascular endothelial growth factor [VEGF]) and the helix-loop-helix transcription factor Tal1 (or Scl) (2–4). VEGF promotes hemangioblast differentiation into endothelium, but it is not a prerequisite, because endothelial cells develop in the absence of VEGF (5,6). VEGFR1 (also fms-like tyrosine kinase-1 or Flt1), another VEGF receptor, also has been implicated in hemangioblast commitment to endothelial cells (7,8) and endothelial cell division (9). Tal1 in combination with VEGFR2 determines hemangioblast formation and differentiation (10). Several additional genes are expressed and/or regulate hematopoietic and endothelial cell lineage development—for example, Tie1 and Tie2, VE-cadherin, basic fibroblast growth factor (bFGF), CD34, podocalyxin-like protein 1, cloche, Hex, Vezf, hedgehog, and members of the GATA,

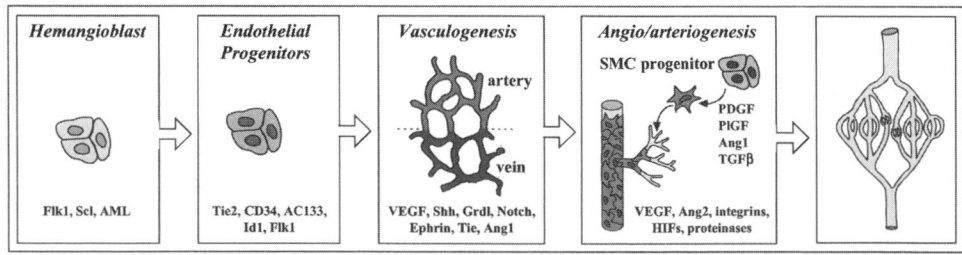

FIG. 23–2. Endothelial progenitors differentiate to arterial and venous endothelial cells (EC), which assemble in a primitive capillary plexus. Vessels then sprout and become stabilized by smooth muscle cells (SMC), differentiating from their progenitors. A partial list of molecules is indicated. AML, acute myeloid leukemia; Ang, angiopoietin; HIF, hypoxia-inducible transcription factor; Id1, inhibitor of differentiation 1; PDGF, platelet-derived growth factor; PlGF, placental growth factor; shh, sonic hedgehog; TGF, transforming growth factor; VEGF, vascular endothelial growth factor. (Reprinted from Carmeliet P. Angiogenesis in health and disease. *Nat Med* 2003;9:653–660, with permission.)

Hox, Ets, and inhibitor of differentiation (Id) protein families (11–13).

Angioblasts may migrate extensively before *in situ* differentiation and plexus formation. For example, the myocardium of the early embryo is initially avascular, receiving diffusing oxygen from the ventricular cavity (14). As the myocardial wall thickens, a vascular network develops to supply oxygen to the cardiomyocytes. The vascular precursors that establish this network are derived from outside the heart. Mesothelial cells located on the right side of the sinus venosus, the proepicardial organ, invade the embryonic epicardium and differentiate *in situ* into endothelial precursor cells, or angioblasts (15). Their derivative endothelial cells subsequently assemble into a primitive, unorganized labyrinth of capillaries. In aggregate, these steps constitute vasculogenesis (16). Myocardial vessels subsequently branch and sprout into smaller terminal vessels (angiogenesis). Coronary vascular smooth muscle cells, recruited from a subpopulation of epicardial cells, the epicardium-derived cells, migrate alongside the preexisting endothelial channels and later invest the walls with one or more muscular layers (arteriogenesis) (17).

The prevailing dogma had been that vessels in the embryo develop from endothelial progenitors, whereas angiogenic sprouting of capillaries was the result of division and migration of neighboring differentiated endothelial cells (Fig. 23–1). It is becoming more clear, however, that endothelial progenitor cells (EPCs) contribute to angiogenesis in both the embryo and in ischemic, malignant, or inflamed tissues in the adult (Fig. 23–1); this process can be amplified and harnessed during ischemia (18–22), a process that has been termed *therapeutic vasculogenesis* (23–25). EPCs are not only present in the embryo, they also have been identified in the peripheral blood in the adult (26). These circulating bone marrow–derived progenitors express CD34, VEGFR2 and VE-cadherin (26), and AC133 (27) and can be distinguished from mature endothelial cells by their high proliferation potential and late outgrowth *ex vivo* (28). Endothelial cells may also differentiate from additional cell types such as mesoangioblasts (29), multipotent adult progenitor cells (30), or side-population cells (31). EPCs are recruited to sites of neoangiogenesis by the increased availability of angiogenic growth factors or chemokines such as VEGF, angiopoietin, and stromal cell–derived factor-1α (32–35). Ischemic conditions increase the circulating levels of EPCs up to 1000-fold (21,36), and these levels may be used as a prognostic marker for determination of cardiovascular risk (37–39). Once arrived at the site of neovascularization, EPCs may recruit additional EPCs by releasing growth factors such as VEGF, hepatocyte growth factor, granulocyte colony-stimulating factor, and granulocyte-macrophage colony-stimulating factor (40,41). The VEGF homologue placental growth factor (PlGF) also is involved in this process, because bone marrow–derived cells (including EPCs) restored impaired VEGF-driven angiogenesis in mice lacking PlGF (42). EPCs might thus contribute in two ways to vessel growth: for example, by differentiating to mature endothelial cells,

which then become incorporated as building blocks in nascent vessels; and, secondly, by creating a proangiogenic microenvironment through the release of cytokines and growth factors. Reports on the numeric contribution of EPCs to vessel growth in ischemia, tumor growth, and wound healing are variable, ranging from less than 0.1% to as high as 50% (43,44). In some cases, neovascularization even seemed to be almost exclusively dependent on the contribution of bone marrow–derived precursor cells, such as in tumor vascularization in Id-mutant mice (45). The growing interest in circulating EPCs in adults has challenged traditional tenets of angiogenesis in healthy tissue and disease and offers new therapeutic opportunities for regenerative vascular medicine.

VASCULAR IDENTITY

Traditionally, arteries and veins have been defined by the direction of blood flow in relation to the heart. The largest arteries efficiently transport energy developed from the contracting heart throughout the vascular tree. Pressure drives flow from the arterial to the venous system, and arteries, therefore, experience the highest hydrodynamic pressures. Arterioles are smaller, more muscular, and regulate their resistance to blood flow, and thus perfusion of distal capillary beds. Veins return blood to the heart and are relatively thin-walled and of a larger diameter than their arterial counterparts, and they are characterized by low blood velocities and pressures. It had been thought that characteristic physical forces were transduced by mechanosensors in the vessel wall into structural differences that are apparent between the arterial and venous circulation (46). For example, coronary veins develop before arteries, but the arteries are the first to be invested with muscular wall of smooth muscle cells (47,48). Presumably, increased pressure and flow, as well as differences in oxygen content after connection to the aorta, triggers smooth muscle cell differentiation in arteries, whereas it is delayed in the low-pressure veins (49,50).

Recently, however, genetic differences between the endothelium of arteries and veins in the developing embryo have been uncovered (Fig. 23–2). That these differences arise very early in embryonic angiogenesis before blood flow is established is proof of arterial or venous lineage-specific genetic divergence. Cell transplantation and genetic studies further revealed that endothelial cells remain plastic and can differentiate into both arterial and venous endothelial cells until late in embryonic development, and that growth of arterial endothelial cells can be induced by VEGF in the adult heart (51) and neonatal retina (52). Several molecules such as bone marrow tyrosine kinase, neuropilin-1 (Np-1, a VEGF$_{164}$-specific receptor), and VEGF, derived from peripheral nerves, influence arterial specification (52–54). A family that also seems to play a critical role in arterial cell fate decision is the Notch pathway, comprising ligands (Delta-like-4, Jagged1, and Jagged2) and receptors (Notch1, 3, and 4). Loss of Notch signaling abolishes arterial specification, whereas ectopic activation represses venous cell fate, indicating that Notch represses venous differentiation within developing arteries (55,56). Sonic hedgehog (shh) and VEGF (which is induced by shh and up-regulates Notch1 and Delta-like-4) act upstream, whereas Gridlock acts downstream of Notch to determine arterial fate, even before the onset of flow (56,57). It remains to be determined whether Notch signals also determine the fate of a quiescent versus branching endothelial cell—that is, whether lateral inhibition by Notch signaling permits one endothelial cell to sprout but restrains its neighbors from sprouting. Such a mechanism would provide a mechanistic basis of the stereotyped branching of vessels at predestined positions along the vascular tree, similar as it occurs in the trachea in the fruit fly (58). Notch signaling also is critical for arterial maintenance. Mutations of the smooth muscle cell–specific Notch3 receptor, which disrupt smooth muscle cell anchorage to extracellular matrix (ECM) and impair smooth muscle cell survival, cause progressive degeneration of cerebral arterioles, leading to cerebral autosomal dominant arteriopathy with subcortical infarcts and leukoencephalopathy (CADASIL) (59).

An important requirement for multicellular organisms to function properly is that various cell types acquire distinct identity so that each of them can exert specialized functions. However, this identity must remain established, and for cells to perform many tasks, cells of the same identity should stick together and be prevented from intermixing with cells of another identity. These processes thus require signals specifying cellular identity and boundaries. Endothelial cells are not a uniform class of identical cell types. Instead, there are multiple different subtypes of endothelial cells, exerting specialized functions in different tissues (60–62). A remarkable finding is that endothelial cells in a single vessel may even have distinct cell fates. Three types of endothelial cells, for example, each with a distinct cell fate, build the intersegmental vessels (ISVs) in the zebrafish embryo (63). Vessels in different regions also arise from distinct angioblasts (64). The transcriptional code determining endothelial cell fate involves basic helix-loop-helix transcriptional activators (hypoxia-inducible factor-2α, stem cell leukemia factor, Tfeb) (13,65–67), as well as Id repressors—as exemplified by the perturbed developmental and tumor angiogenesis in mice lacking Id1/3 (68). VEGF and platelet-derived growth factor (PDGF)-BB influence endothelial and smooth muscle cell fate, respectively (69). The blood–brain barrier endothelial cell phenotype is codetermined by glial-derived neurotrophic factor and other glial cell-derived factors (70), or the selective stimulation of endocrine gland endothelial cells by EG-VEGF (71). Malignant cells induce endothelial cells in tumor vessels to acquire a distinct fate and express unique "vascular zip codes," which are absent in other vessels (72).

The ephrins, ligands for the large family of receptor tyrosine kinase (RTK) ephrin (eph) receptors, are involved in arterial–venous identity and boundary formation (73,74). The ephrins and their receptors were first described in the context of neural cell guidance and the demarcation of distinct cellular compartments, and they can mediate repulsive events between ligand-bearing cell types and those expressing the cognate receptor (75). The ephrins and their receptors are unlike other ligand-RTK pairs in that the membrane-bound ephrinB ligands can themselves be tryosine phosphorylated on activation, so-called reverse signaling. For example, ephrinB1 (arterial and venous) reverse signaling resulting after binding with its receptor EphB2 in the surrounding mesenchyme leads to local actin cytoskeletal deconstruction, suggesting a role for the ephrin–receptor system in neuronal and vascular guidance and inhibition of reciprocal cell mixing (76). This likely results in bidirectional signaling between the two juxtaposed cell types expressing complementing ephrin ligand–receptor pairs. *EphrinB2,* present in arterial endothelial cells, binds the RTK *EphB4,* which is restricted to the venous endothelium. Null mutations of either gene are embryonically lethal because of dysfunctional vascular remodeling and a failure of correct interconnection between the arterial and venous plexus in the yolk sac (77–79). *EphrinB2* must be membrane-bound to activate its receptor *EphB4,* which means they are paired at the interface between the venous and arterial circulations (80). They meet approximately halfway between terminal arterioles and postcapillary venules in the capillary bed, suggesting that the smallest sprouting microvessels have arterial or venous identity (80). *EphrinB2/Eph4* interaction enables bidirectional signaling that may also provide vital navigational cues for angiogenic endothelial cells (81,82). In the adult, the respective expression patterns of *ephrinB2* and *EphB4* continue to be restricted to the arterial or venous endothelium, respectively, and persist in healthy and pathologic angiogenesis (80,83). It is noteworthy that *ephrinB2* expression extends to periendothelial smooth muscle cells with time, first appearing in those closest to the lumen and then spreading outward to encompass the entire wall (80). This is reminiscent in the developing embryo of the first layers of smooth muscle cells in the dorsal aorta, which transdifferentiate from the endothelium (46,84). Expression of *ephrinB2* also is found in the arterial side of vas vasorum perfusing the walls of the largest veins (83). Other ephrin–ephrin receptor interactions are not repulsive but seem to be directly linked to endothelial cell migration. *EphrinB1* activation by *EphB1* stimulates endothelial cell migration and $\alpha_v\beta_3$ and $\alpha_5\beta_1$ integrin–mediated attachment. These effects were not caused by an increase in integrin expression, providing evidence that ephrin activation and integrin function are coupled (85).

VASCULAR BRANCHING AND PATTERNING

Vascular branching can occur in various ways: through sprouting, splitting, or intussusception (16). Endothelial cells can sprout toward a cluster of cells that produce an appropriate angiogenic stimulus. The lack of oxygen is a strong attractant for vessel sprouts. In cells farther than the oxygen diffusion limit from a vessel, hypoxia activates hypoxia-inducible transcription factor-1α and -2α, which turn on the expression of angiogenic genes such as VEGF, induc-

are similarly associated with low VEGF levels and increased risk for ALS (114). The SNPs in the at-risk genotypes impaired transcription and translation of the normally secreted VEGF isoforms, providing a molecular explanation for lower *Vegf* expression by cells or subjects carrying these polymorphisms (114). Interestingly, numerous smaller studies suggest that the inverse polymorphisms that result in a relatively greater level of *Vegf* expression may be associated with acute renal allograft rejection (112), diabetic retinopathy (115), and increased tumor thickness and decreased survival of cutaneous malignant melanoma (116).

Numerous studies also established VEGF as a key angiogenic player in cancer and almost any other inflammatory or ischemic disorder (61,102). VEGF is expressed in most tumors; its expression is induced by hypoxia, hypoglycemia, growth factors, and oncogenes—all present in tumors—and correlates with tumor progression. Plasma VEGF levels often are increased in patients with cancer and are a marker of poor clinical outcome (117–119). Forced overexpression of VEGF in tumors increases tumor vascularization and growth, whereas capturing VEGF or blocking VEGFR2 by VEGF receptor tyrosine kinase inhibitors, antisense oligonucleotides, vaccination, or neutralizing antibodies reduced tumor angiogenesis and growth in preclinical studies (120–132). Several clinical efforts are currently underway to evaluate the therapeutic potential of VEGF or VEGFR2 inhibitors (see the National Cancer Institute website for more information at: www.cancer.gov/clinicaltrials/). Over the past several years, promising clinical results were obtained using VEGF inhibitors (102), and the anti-VEGF Avastatin antibody prolonged the survival of patients with colorectal cancer for longer periods than expected (see the Genentech website for more information at: www.gene.com/gene/news/press-releases; see also comment in McCarthy [133]). This landmark study provides a milestone in the field and underlines the overall feasibility of angiogenesis inhibition strategies, in particular those targeting VEGF receptor signaling.

PLACENTAL GROWTH FACTOR: A KEY MEDIATOR OF PATHOLOGIC BUT NOT PHYSIOLOGIC ANGIOGENESIS

Several homologues of the *Vegf* gene have been discovered: VEGF-B, -C, -D, -E, and PlGF, although much less is known about their functions. Due to alternative splicing, three isoforms of PlGF exist in humans: PlGF-1, -2, and -3, which vary in amino acid length from 131, 152, and 203, respectively. Only PlGF-2 is present in mice, and it specifically binds VEGFR1. The role of both PlGF and VEGFR1 have remained enigmatic for more than a decade, but genetic and pharmacologic studies have unraveled their important role in the angiogenic switch (for review see Autiero and coworkers [134]). PlGF in absence or excess seems to have no effect on vascular development. PlGF knockout mice do not exhibit a vascular phenotype until stressed with ischemia or a strong angiogenic stimulus, such as a growing tumor

(42). Blocking VEGFR1 reduced angiogenesis and/or inflammation during angiogenic and inflammatory disorders (135). These findings, together with the evidence that deletion of the tyrosine kinase domain of VEGFR1 or inhibition of VEGFR1 by antagonists impaired pathologic angiogenesis (136,137) and that PlGF stimulates angiogenesis in a variety of conditions *in vivo* (138–143) (also discussed later in this chapter) indicate that PlGF and VEGFR1 are key molecules in regulating the angiogenic switch during pathologic conditions (Fig. 23–3).

VEGF/VEGFR2-mediated endothelial cell survival, migration, and proliferation is blunted in the absence of PlGF and amplified in its presence (42) and, conversely, PlGF activation of VEGFR1 amplifies VEGF-mediated effects on endothelial cells (42,135,144). VEGFR1 has low tyrosine kinase activity, and until recently the mechanism by which VEGFR1 signaling affected angiogenesis was unknown. In earlier mouse experiments, VEGFR1 deletion was found to be embryonically lethal because of a vascular defect in which excess endothelial cells block the lumens of blood vessels, indicating the loss of a negative feedback mechanism for endothelial cell growth (7). Subsequent studies revealed that deletion of the tyrosine kinase domain of VEGFR1 did not impair vascular development (145), but pathologic angiogenesis in the adult was attenuated (137). The suggested mechanism based on these results was that VEGFR1 acted as an inert sink for VEGF, which could be displaced in pathologic conditions to increase the availability of VEGF for binding to VEGFR2 and to modulate endothelial cell biology (42).

The role of VEGFR-1 is, however, more complex than simply serving as a sink. In cultured PlGF-deficient endothelial cells, anti-Flt1 antibodies, which would displace VEGF from Flt1 in the sink model, *decrease* VEGF/VEGFR2-mediated endothelial cell survival (42). If VEGFR1 were only a reservoir that reversibly sequestered VEGF, inhibition of VEGFR1 would have enhanced endothelial cell survival. In fact, PlGF enhances VEGF-induced VEGFR2 tyrosine phosphorylation (including tyrosine residue 1175) and intermolecular transphosphorylation of VEGFR2 by VEGFR1 (144). Because activated endothelial cells up-regulate their PlGF levels, they therefore can regulate their own responsiveness to VEGF during the angiogenic switch. Interestingly, while PlGF enhances, VEGF suppresses VEGFR2 transphosphorylation by VEGFR1 (144), which is consistent with previous findings that VEGF/VEGFR1 suppresses VEGF/VEGFR2 activity (146–148). Moreover, the two ligands stimulate phosphorylation of distinct tyrosine residues on VEGFR1 (144). This suggests that VEGF and PlGF, although highly homologous ligands, transmit distinct signals through their common receptor VEGFR1. Besides inducing an intermolecular crosstalk between VEGFR1 and VEGFR2 with consequent enhancement of the response to VEGF-A, PlGF also activates an intramolecular crosstalk between the two receptors when in complex with VEGF-A; PlGF also initiates its own signaling cascade through VEGFR1, independently of VEGFR2 (144). PlGF further contributes to the angiogenic switch in pathologic conditions through additional mechanisms—that is, by affecting smooth muscle cells and stimulating vessel maturation and stabilization, by recruiting inflammatory cells, which play a critical role in growth of collateral vessels (discussed later), and by mobilizing vascular and hematopoietic stem cells/progenitors from the bone marrow, which contribute to adult vasculogenesis (Figs. 23–1 and 23–3). Because it affects all known modes of vessel growth in the adult, PlGF is an attractive candidate for therapeutic stimulation of revascularization of ischemic tissues, and PlGF antagonists are candidates for therapeutic inhibition of angiogenesis in malignant and inflamed tissues.

VESSEL MATURATION THROUGH ARTERIOGENESIS

When endothelial cells establish vessels, they initially assemble as stringlike cords and, subsequently, become perfused as channels. These nascent vessels, however, are fragile, easily break, are prone to regression, and lack any vasoregulation. For these growing vessels to become functional and durable, they must first mature and become stabilized. This is achieved through several mechanisms, including the deposition of ECM and the recruitment of mural cells, pericytes and smooth muscle cells in small and larger vessels, respectively (Fig. 23–3). The latter process is called *arteriogenesis,* and it is of utmost importance for the building of a stable vascular network both in normal health and on treatment of ischemic disease. Indeed, when this process fails, vessels become fragile, nonperfused, and are doomed to regress (Fig. 23–3). Numerous disorders are attributable to an imbalance in vessel maturation and regression (61). Genetic and other studies have provided key insights into this process over the last decade, which is reviewed in this section.

In the decade after the discovery of the VEGF family of vascular growth factors and their receptors, a second family, the angiopoietins (angiopoietin-1, -2), was discovered (75). The angiopoietins bind Tie2, which like the VEGF receptors is a receptor tyrosine kinase expressed on the vascular endothelium. Lack of angiopoietin-1 or Tie2 is embryonically lethal because of vascular defects, although at a later stage than in VEGF/VEGFR knockout embryos (149,150). Vasculogenesis remains unaffected, but the primitive vessels are unable to sprout and permit the vasculature to invade avascular embryonic tissue, preventing organogenesis. Angiopoietin-1 is widely expressed by periendothelial smooth muscle cells and pericytes in the embryo and adult, and stabilizes appropriate endothelial cell interactions with the subendothelial matrix and mural cells through Tie2 activation (151) (Fig. 23–3). Angiopoietin-1 promotes the interaction between endothelial and mural cells by serving as an adhesive ECM-associated and α_5-binding protein, and it recruits pericytes (152,153). Angiopoietin-1 is capable of stabilizing vessels also without mural cell recruitment (154). Because of these properties, angiopoietin-1 also blocks vascular leakage in sepsis, lung injury, stroke, local inflamma-

tion, and cancer (155,156). The role of angiopoietin-1 is, however, pleiotropic and context-dependent. For example, angiopoietin-1 promotes angiogenesis in the skin, ischemic limb, gastric ulcers (157–159), and in some tumors (160). This proangiogenic effect is attributable to the ability of angiopoietin-1 to stimulate endothelial cell survival and growth, capillary tube formation, and EPC mobilization (34). But, angiopoietin-1 also suppresses angiogenesis in tumors (161,162) and the heart (51), presumably because it tightens vessels too much, and thereby impedes vessel sprouting (155,163). Angiopoietin-2 is an antagonist of Tie2 activation by angiopoietin-1, and its expression is restricted to sites of vascular remodeling (151). In a quiescent vessel, there exists a stable interaction between endothelial and mural cells. Angiopoietin-2 is thought to disrupt this interaction by interfering with angiopoietin-1, loosening up the endothelial layer, and priming it for action (161,164,165). In the absence of VEGF, the angiopoietin-2–perturbed endothelial cells die and the vessel regresses (166) (such as the hyaloid vessel network [167]), whereas in its presence, angiogenic sprouting results (51) (Fig. 23–3). Thus, the proangiogenic or antiangiogenic effects of angiopoietin-2 are modulated by VEGF and its survival and mitogenic effects on activated endothelial cells.

There is another growth factor family of PDGF that plays a critical role in vessel stabilization—in particular by recruiting mural cells around nascent vessels. There are four family members (e.g., PDGF-A to -D) that bind, with distinct selectivity, the receptor tyrosine kinases PDGFRα and PDGFRβ expressed on endothelial and smooth muscle cells. PDGF-CC promotes vascular development in the embryo and in healing wounds and angiogenesis in avascular tissues (168), whereas PDGF-D stimulates tumor neovascularization (169). Sprouting endothelial cells express PDFGβ, which attracts neighboring adventitial mural cell progenitors that on arrival stabilize the nascent vessel (170,171) (Fig. 23–3). Blockade of the receptor for PDGF-β (PDGFRβ) results in leaky, immature vessels that lack periendothelial support cells (172). Absence of pericytes in embryos lacking PDGF-B or PDGFRβ increases endothelial cell growth, permeability, and deformity, enlarges the vessel size, and enhances fragility, resulting in bleeding, impaired perfusion, and hypoxia (170). Consequently, VEGF levels increase, which further aggravate vascular permeability and edema and promote hemangioma formation. Individuals with diabetic retinopathy also suffer similar neovascularization when their pericytes are killed by toxic metabolites. PDGF-BB has a therapeutic potential, as dual delivery of VEGF and PDGF-BB results in the formation of a more mature vascular network than when each factor was given alone (173).

Individuals with hereditary hemorrhagic telangiectasia (HHT) have lesions characterized by mucocutaneous telangiectasias and arteriovenous malformations. Genetic studies revealed that HHT-1 and -2 were attributable to loss of function mutations of endoglin and activin receptor-like kinase-1 (ALK-1), respectively (174). These molecules belong to signaling cascades of the transforming growth factor (TGF)-β superfamily ligands of the TGF-β, activin, and bone morphogenetic protein families; these ligands stimulate type II receptors, which phosphorylate type I receptors (e.g., activin receptor-like kinase or ALK-1 to -7) and, in turn, activate the downstream signaling Smads. Endoglin is a type III receptor, which facilitates binding of TGF-β$_1$ to the type II receptors. TGF-β$_1$ has both proangiogenic and antiangiogenic properties; some of these effects are caused by direct effects on endothelial cells, but this growth factor also regulates angiogenesis indirectly by affecting other cell types. At low doses, TGF-β$_1$ stimulates vessel growth by increasing the expression of angiogenic factors (e.g., VEGF) and proteinases urokinase-type plasminogen activator (uPA). Conversely, at high doses, TGF-β$_1$ suppresses endothelial cell proliferation and migration and induces the basement membrane to reform. TGF-β$_1$ further contributes to the resolution of angiogenesis by stimulating the recruitment of mesenchymal cells and their differentiation to smooth muscle cell (Fig. 23–3). It remains, however, unclear how endoglin and ALK-1 mutations cause excessive fusion of capillary plexuses into cavernous vessels and hyperdilation of large vessels in the vascular lesions in patients with HHT, but they are likely because of an imbalance between vessel growth and maturation (175,176). The confusion about ALK-1 stems from that ALK-1 increases the expression of Id1, which would switch on angiogenesis, whereas ALK-1 also directly inhibits endothelial migration, and thus also could be involved in vessel stabilization (175,177–179). Whatever the mechanism, the severity of the clinical HHT syndrome indicates that this growth factor family plays a significant role in vessel growth and stabilization.

EXTRACELLULAR MATRIX AND ANGIOGENESIS

Molecules mediating interactions between endothelial cells and the ECM also affect vasculogenesis. Integrins, the cell surface receptors that anchor cells to ECM proteins, are the two-way transducers that allow for communication between the intracellular and extracellular environments (180,181). More than 24 different heterodimers, with at least 18 α and 9 β subunits interacting noncovalently, constitute the integrin family. Although endothelial cells express many different integrins, with distinct and often overlapping specificity for ECM proteins, α$_v$β$_3$ is especially important. It is minimally expressed on resting vessels, but it is up-regulated on endothelial precursors in embryos and on vascular cells in tumors and ischemic tissues (182,183). α$_v$β$_3$ antagonists disrupt vascular development in the embryo and block pathologic angiogenesis in animal models with few side effects on established blood vessels, which has made this integrin an attractive target for therapeutic intervention (182,183). Pharmacologic blockade of the integrins α$_v$β$_3$ and α$_v$β$_5$ with antagonists inhibits angiogenesis in cancer, arthritis, and ischemic retinopathy (182,183). In addition, extensive crosstalk occurs between VEGF and the α$_v$ integrins. VEGF up-regulates and increases the activity of α$_v$β$_3$ and α$_v$β$_5$, stimulating endothelial migration. Likewise, α$_v$β$_3$ associates with VEGFR2 and amplifies VEGF-mediated effects on endothelial cell survival and proliferation. The unexpected finding that mice lacking β$_3$ or β$_5$ integrins, or both, show increased pathologic angiogenesis (184), however, is a note of caution that our understanding of the role of integrins in angiogenesis is incomplete, which may serve a dual proangiogenic and antiangiogenic function (185).V

Proteolytic degradation of the ECM also is an integral part of neovascularization and in tumors. By degrading the thicket of the ECM around vascular cells, proteinases such as the plasminogen activators (e.g., uPA and its inhibitor plasminogen activator inhibitor-1), matrix metalloproteinases (e.g., MMPs and their tissue inhibitor of metalloproteinase (TIMP) inhibitors), heparinases, chymases, tryptases, cathepsins, and kallikreins (and their inhibitor kallistatin) clear a path for migrating vascular cells (186–194). But, their action is much broader and proteinases can switch on angiogenesis by liberating matrix-bound angiogenic activators (e.g., bFGF, VEGF, TGF-β, tumor necrosis factor [TNF]-α, hepatocyte growth factor, and others) and proteolytically activating angiogenic chemokines (e.g., interleukin [IL]-1β) (195). The role of proteinases in angiogenesis is, however, pleiotropic and dependent of the context and concentration. This is further illustrated by that proteinases turn the angiogenic switch off, by liberating matrix-bound inhibitors (TSP-1; canstatin; Arrestin; tumstatin; angiostatin; endostatin; and cleaved antithrombin III, PF4) and inactivating angiogenic cytokines (e.g., stromal cell–derived factor-1). In addition, it is crucial that the activity of proteinases is somehow controlled. Indeed, when excessive, proteolysis may suppress angiogenesis by removing all structural ECM support for the nascent vessels such that the nascent vessel falls apart. This explains why increased levels of proteinase inhibitors in patients with cancer are often associated with a poor clinical outcome (196,197).

COLLATERAL VESSEL GROWTH

For vascularization to be successful in improving tissue perfusion, not only capillary angiogenesis but also the growth of the conducting supply arteries should be stimulated, as the former distributes flows distally, whereas the latter provides bulk flow to the tissue. When such a feeder artery becomes occluded by, for instance, a thrombus, the tissue in the vascular territory of this occluded artery becomes ischemic. Often, however, the tissue also is nourished by preexisting collateral vessels, which are interconnected with the primary arterial systems. These collaterals may salvage the ischemic tissue, at least when they remodel and enlarge in size (198) (Fig. 23–1). This process of *collateral vessel growth* is cellularly and molecularly quite distinct from the mechanisms governing vasculogenesis and angiogenesis. VEGF, for example, is well known to stimulate capillary angiogenesis, but its effects on collateral vessel growth remain controversial (159,198,199). The reason VEGF, which is especially active in stimulating vessel growth in ischemic tissues, is less effective or even ineffective relates to that ischemia is not the driving force for collateral vessel enlargement. Instead, the increased shear stress, resulting from the large pressure differences between the perfusion territories, activates endothelial cells, which then express monokines (monocyte chemotactic protein-1 [MCP-1]), the leukocyte adhesion molecules vascular cell adhesion molecule-1 and intercellular adhesion molecule-1. Monocytes adhere to these activated endothelial cells and subsequently infiltrate the vessel wall and perforate the basement membrane and media, using proteinases (uPA and MMPs) and death factors (TNF-α). Local production of bFGF, PDGF-B, and TGF-β$_1$ stimulates endothelial and smooth muscle cell growth. Delivery of acidic FGF, FGF-4, or bFGF (together with PDGF-BB) stimulates collateral growth, in part through upregulation of PDGFR expression (200). The importance of monocytes is illustrated by the fact that depletion of monocytes impairs, whereas delivery of monocytes enhances collateral growth (201,202). Cytokines that attract monocytes or prolong their lifespan (MCP-1, granulocyte-macrophage colony-stimulating factor, TGF-β$_1$, TNF-α, and TNF-α/Rp55) enhance collateral growth (203–206), whereas anti-inflammatory cytokines (e.g., IL-10) are inhibitory. PlGF also enhances collateral growth, not only because it recruits monocytes, but also because it stimulates endothelial and smooth muscle cell growth (141,207).

CONCLUSION

Blood vessels have a vital function in health and play important roles in numerous disorders. In fact, studies over the past decade have revealed that many more disorders are *angiogenic* in nature. This important realization, together with the emerging molecular insights in how blood vessels grow, now permits proposal of rational designs to therapeutically stimulate vessel growth is ischemic tissues or to block excessive vessel growth in malignant or inflamed tissues. The recent success obtained with an anti-VEGF antibody in prolonging the survival of patients with colorectal cancer provides the long awaited first proof of the concept that inhibiting angiogenesis is a feasible strategy to combat cancer. Building new blood vessels to revascularize ischemic tissues is perhaps more challenging than originally anticipated, but not less rewarding. With the rapidly advancing pace of science in this field, this goal might be achieved in the near future.

ACKNOWLEDGMENTS

The authors express their gratitude to all internal and external collaborators who have contributed to these studies and to A. Vandenhoeck for artwork.

REFERENCES

1. Carmeliet P. Blood vessels and nerves: common signals, pathways and diseases. *Nat Rev Genet* 2003;4:710–720.
2. Drake CJ, Fleming PA. Vasculogenesis in the day 6.5 to 9.5 mouse embryo. *Blood* 2000;95:1671–1679.
3. Gering M, Rodaway AR, Gottgens B, et al. The SCL gene specifies haemangioblast development from early mesoderm. *EMBO J* 1998;17:4029–4045.
4. Shalaby F, Rossant J, Yamaguchi TP, et al. Failure of blood-island formation and vasculogenesis in Flk-1-deficient mice. *Nature* 1995;376:62–66.
5. Carmeliet P, Ferreira V, Breier G, et al. Abnormal blood vessel development and lethality in embryos lacking a single VEGF allele. *Nature* 1996;380:435–439.
6. Ferrara N, Carver-Moore K, Chen H, et al. Heterozygous embryonic lethality induced by targeted inactivation of the VEGF gene. *Nature* 1996;380:439–442.
7. Fong GH, Rossant J, Gertsenstein M, et al. Role of the Flt-1 receptor tyrosine kinase in regulating the assembly of vascular endothelium. *Nature* 1995;376:66–70.
8. Fong GH, Zhang L, Bryce DM, et al. Increased hemangioblast commitment, not vascular disorganization, is the primary defect in flt-1 knock-out mice. *Development* 1999;126:3015–3025.
9. Kearney JB, Ambler CA, Monaco KA, et al. Vascular endothelial growth factor receptor Flt-1 negatively regulates developmental blood vessel formation by modulating endothelial cell division. *Blood* 2002;99:2397–2407.
10. Ema M, Faloon P, Zhang WJ, et al. Combinatorial effects of Flk1 and Tal1 on vascular and hematopoietic development in the mouse. *Genes Dev* 2003;17:380–393.
11. Choi K. The hemangioblast: a common progenitor of hematopoietic and endothelial cells. *J Hematother Stem Cell Res* 2002;11:91–101.
12. Ribatti D, Vacca A, Nico B, et al. Cross-talk between hematopoiesis and angiogenesis signaling pathways. *Curr Mol Med* 2002;2:537–543.
13. Mikkola HK, Orkin SH. The search for the hemangioblast. *J Hematother Stem Cell Res* 2002;11:9–17.
14. Tomanek RJ. Formation of the coronary vasculature: a brief review. *Cardiovasc Res* 1996;31:E46–E51.
15. Poelmann RE, Lie-Venema H, Gittenberger-de Groot AC. The role of the epicardium and neural crest as extracardiac contributors to coronary vascular development. *Tex Heart Inst J* 2002;29:255–261.
16. Carmeliet P. Mechanisms of angiogenesis and arteriogenesis. *Nat Med* 2000;6:389–395.
17. Vrancken Peeters MP, Gittenberger-de Groot AC, Mentink MM, et al. Smooth muscle cells and fibroblasts of the coronary arteries derive from epithelial-mesenchymal transformation of the epicardium. *Anat Embryol (Berl)* 1999;199:367–378.
18. Asahara T, Masuda H, Takahashi T, et al. Bone marrow origin of endothelial progenitor cells responsible for postnatal vasculogenesis in physiological and pathological neovascularization. *Circ Res* 1999;85:221–228.
19. Gehling UM, Ergun S, Schumacher U, et al. In vitro differentiation of endothelial cells from AC133-positive progenitor cells. *Blood* 2000;95:3106–3112.
20. Kalka C, Masuda H, Takahashi T, et al. Transplantation of ex vivo expanded endothelial progenitor cells for therapeutic neovascularization. *Proc Natl Acad Sci USA* 2000;97:3422–3427.
21. Takahashi T, Kalka C, Masuda H, et al. Ischemia- and cytokine-induced mobilization of bone marrow-derived endothelial progenitor cells for neovascularization. *Nat Med* 1999;5:434–438.
22. Schatteman GC, Hanlon HD, Jiao C, et al. Blood-derived angioblasts accelerate blood-flow restoration in diabetic mice. *J Clin Invest* 2000;106:571–578.
23. Luttun A, Carmeliet G, Carmeliet P. Vascular progenitors: from biology to treatment. *Trends Cardiovasc Med* 2002;12:88–96.
24. Asahara T, Isner JM. Endothelial progenitor cells for vascular regeneration. *J Hematother Stem Cell Res* 2002;11:171–178.
25. Rafii S, Lyden D, Benezra R, et al. Vascular and haematopoietic stem cells: novel targets for anti-angiogenesis therapy? *Nat Rev Cancer* 2002;2:826–835.
26. Asahara T, Murohara T, Sullivan A, et al. Isolation of putative progenitor endothelial cells for angiogenesis. *Science* 1997;275:Z964–967.
27. Peichev M, Naiyer AJ, Pereira D, et al. Expression of VEGFR-2 and AC133 by circulating human CD34(+) cells identifies a population of functional endothelial precursors. *Blood* 2000;95:952–958.

28. Lin Y, Weisdorf DJ, Solovey A, et al. Origins of circulating endothelial cells and endothelial outgrowth from blood. *J Clin Invest* 2000; 105:71–77.

29. Minasi MG, Riminucci M, De Angelis L, et al. The meso-angioblast: a multipotent, self-renewing cell that originates from the dorsal aorta and differentiates into most mesodermal tissues. *Development* 2002; 129:2773–2783.

30. Reyes M, Dudek A, Jahagirdar B, et al. Origin of endothelial progenitors in human postnatal bone marrow. *J Clin Invest* 2002;109:337–346.

31. Hirschi K, Goodell M. Common origins of blood and blood vessels in adults? *Differentiation* 2001;68:186–192.

32. Yamaguchi J, Kusano K, Masuo O, et al. Stromal cell-derived factor-1 effects on ex vivo expanded endothelial progenitor cell recruitment for ischemic neovascularization. *Circulation* 2003;107:1322–1328.

33. Iwaguro H, Yamaguchi J, Kalka C, et al. Endothelial progenitor cell vascular endothelial growth factor gene transfer for vascular regeneration. *Circulation* 2002;105:732–738.

34. Hattori K, Dias S, Heissig B, et al. Vascular endothelial growth factor and angiopoietin-1 stimulate postnatal hematopoiesis by recruitment of vasculogenic and hematopoietic stem cells. *J Exp Med* 2001; 193:1005–1014.

35. Asahara T, Takahashi T, Masuda H, et al. VEGF contributes to postnatal neovascularization by mobilizing bone marrow-derived endothelial progenitor cells. *EMBO J* 1999;18:3964–3972.

36. Gill M, Dias M, Hattori K, et al. Vascular trauma induces rapid but transient mobilization of VEGFR2(+)AC133(+) endothelial precursor cells. *Circ Res* 2001;88:167–174.

37. Vasa M, Fichtlscherer S, Aicher A, et al. Number and migratory activity of circulating endothelial progenitor cells inversely correlate with risk factors for coronary artery disease. *Circ Res* 2001;89:E1–E7.

38. Shintani S, Murohara T, Ikeda H, et al. Mobilization of endothelial progenitor cells in patients with acute myocardial infarction. *Circulation* 2001;103:2776–2779.

39. Hill JM, Zalos G, Halcox JP, et al. Circulating endothelial progenitor cells, vascular function, and cardiovascular risk. *N Engl J Med* 2003;348:593–600.

40. Rehman J, Li J, Orschell CM, et al. Peripheral blood "endothelial progenitor cells" are derived from monocyte/macrophages and secrete angiogenic growth factors. *Circulation* 2003;107:1164–1169.

41. Carmeliet P, Luttun A. The emerging role of the bone marrow-derived stem cells in (therapeutic) angiogenesis. *Thromb Haemost* 2001;86: 289–297.

42. Carmeliet P, Moons L, Luttan A, et al. Synergism between vascular endothelial growth factor and placental growth factor contributes to angiogenesis and plasma extravasation in pathological conditions. *Nat Med* 2001;7:575–583.

43. De Palma M, Venneri MA, Roca C, et al. Targeting exogenous genes to tumor angiogenesis by transplantation of genetically modified hematopoietic stem cells. *Nat Med* 2003;9:789–795.

44. Orlic D, Kajstura J, Chimenti S, et al. Bone marrow cells regenerate infarcted myocardium. *Nature* 2001;410:701–705.

45. Lyden D, Hattori K, Dias S, et al. Impaired recruitment of bone-marrow-derived endothelial and hematopoietic precursor cells blocks tumor angiogenesis and growth. *Nat Med* 2001;7:1194–1201.

46. Gittenberger-de Groot AC, DeRuiter MC, Bergwerff M, et al. Smooth muscle cell origin and its relation to heterogeneity in development and disease. *Arterioscler Thromb Vasc Biol* 1999;19:1589–1594.

47. Reese DE, Mikawa T, Bader DM. Development of the coronary vessel system. *Circ Res* 2002;91:761–768.

48. Vrancken Peeters MP, Gittenberger-de Groot AC, Mentink MM, et al. Differences in development of coronary arteries and veins. *Cardiovasc Res* 1997;36:101–110.

49. Cowan DB, Langille BL. Cellular and molecular biology of vascular remodeling. *Curr Opin Lipidol* 1996;7:94–100.

50. Hungerford JE, Little CD. Developmental biology of the vascular smooth muscle cell: building a multilayered vessel wall. *J Vasc Res* 1999;36:2–27.

51. Visconti RP, Richardson CD, Sato TN. Orchestration of angiogenesis and arteriovenous contribution by angiopoietins and vascular endothelial growth factor (VEGF). *Proc Natl Acad Sci USA* 2002; 99:8219–8224.

52. Stalmans I, Ng YS, Rohan R, et al. Arteriolar and venular patterning in retinas of mice selectively expressing VEGF isoforms. *J Clin Invest* 2002;109:327–336.

53. Moyon D, Pardanaud L, Yuan L, et al. Plasticity of endothelial cells during arterial-venous differentiation in the avian embryo. *Development* 2001;128:3359–3370.

54. Mukouyama YS, Shin D, Britsch S, et al. Sensory nerves determine the pattern of arterial differentiation and blood vessel branching in the skin. *Cell* 2002;109:693–705.

55. Lawson ND, Scheer N, Pham VN, et al. Notch signaling is required for arterial-venous differentiation during embryonic vascular development. *Development* 2001;128:3675–3683.

56. Zhong TP, Childs S, Leu JP, et al. Gridlock signalling pathway fashions the first embryonic artery. *Nature* 2001;414:216–220.

57. Lawson ND, Vogel AM, Weinstein BM. Sonic hedgehog and vascular endothelial growth factor act upstream of the Notch pathway during arterial endothelial differentiation. *Dev Cell* 2002;3:127–136.

58. Metzger RJ, Krasnow MA. Genetic control of branching morphogenesis. *Science* 1999;284:1635–1639.

59. Kalimo H, Ruchoux MM, Viitanen M, et al. CADASIL: a common form of hereditary arteriopathy causing brain infarcts and dementia. *Brain Pathol* 2002;12:371–384.

60. Carmeliet P. Developmental biology. One cell, two fates. *Nature* 2000;408:43–45.

61. Carmeliet P. Angiogenesis in health and disease. *Nat Med* 2003;9:653–660.

62. Cleaver O, Melton DA. Endothelial signaling during development. *Nat Med* 2003;9:661–668.

63. Childs S, Chen JN, Garrity DM, et al. Patterning of angiogenesis in the zebrafish embryo. *Development* 2002;129:973–982.

64. Rovainen CM. Labeling of developing vascular endothelium after injections of rhodamine-dextran into blastomeres of Xenopus laevis. *J Exp Zool* 1991;259:209–221.

65. Liao W, Ho CY, Yan YL, et al. Hhex and scl function in parallel to regulate early endothelial and blood differentiation in zebrafish. *Development* 2000;127:4303–4313.

66. Brown LA, Rodaway AR, Schilling TF, et al. Insights into early vasculogenesis revealed by expression of the ETS-domain transcription factor Fli-1 in wild-type and mutant zebrafish embryos. *Mech Dev* 2000;90:237–252.

67. Carmeliet P. Developmental biology. Controlling the cellular brakes. *Nature* 1999;401:657–658.

68. Neufeld G, Cohen T, Shraga N, et al. The neuropilins: multifunctional semaphorin and VEGF receptors that modulate axon guidance and angiogenesis. *Trends Cardiovasc Med* 2002;12:13–19.

69. Yamashita J, Itoh H, Hirashima M, et al. Flk1-positive cells derived from embryonic stem cells serve as vascular progenitors. *Nature* 2000;408:92–96.

70. Abbot NJ. Glial-endothelial communication in physiology and pathology. *J Neurochem* 2003;85[Suppl 2]:2.

71. LeCouter J, Lin R, Ferrara N. Endocrine gland-derived VEGF and the emerging hypothesis of organ-specific regulation of angiogenesis. *Nat Med* 2002;8:913–917.

72. Ruoslahti E. Specialization of tumour vasculature. *Nat Rev Cancer* 2002;2:83–90.

73. Cheng N, Brantley DM, Chen J. The ephrins and Eph receptors in angiogenesis. *Cytokine Growth Factor Rev* 2002;13:75–85.

74. Himanen JP, Nikolov DB. Eph receptors and ephrins. *Int J Biochem Cell Biol* 2003;35:130–134.

75. Gale NW, Yancopoulos GD. Growth factors acting via endothelial cell-specific receptor tyrosine kinases: VEGFs, angiopoietins, and ephrins in vascular development. *Genes Dev* 1999;13:1055–1066.

76. Cowan CA, Henkemeyer M. The SH2/SH3 adaptor Grb4 transduces B-ephrin reverse signals. *Nature* 2001;413:174–179.

77. Gerety SS, Wang HU, Chen ZF, et al. Symmetrical mutant phenotypes of the receptor EphB4 and its specific transmembrane ligand ephrin-B2 in cardiovascular development. *Mol Cell* 1999;4:403–414.

78. Wang HU, Chen ZF, Anderson DJ. Molecular distinction and angiogenic interaction between embryonic arteries and veins revealed by ephrin-B2 and its receptor Eph-B4. *Cell* 1998;93:741–753.

79. Adams RH, Wilkinson GA, Weiss C, et al. Roles of ephrinB ligands and EphB receptors in cardiovascular development: demarcation of arterial/venous domains, vascular morphogenesis, and sprouting angiogenesis. *Genes Dev* 1999;13:295–306.

80. Shin D, Garcia-Cardena G, Hayashi S, et al. Expression of ephrinB2 identifies a stable genetic difference between arterial and venous vascular smooth muscle as well as endothelial cells, and marks subsets of

microvessels at sites of adult neovascularization. *Dev Biol* 2001; 230:139–150.

81. Mellitzer G, Xu Q, Wilkinson DG. Eph receptors and ephrins restrict cell intermingling and communication. *Nature* 1999;400:77–81.

82. Xu Q, Mellitzer G, Robinson V, et al. In vivo cell sorting in complementary segmental domains mediated by Eph receptors and ephrins. *Nature* 1999;399:267–271.

83. Gale NW, Baluk P, Pan L, et al. Ephrin-B2 selectively marks arterial vessels and neovascularization sites in the adult, with expression in both endothelial and smooth-muscle cells. *Dev Biol* 2001;230:151–160.

84. DeRuiter MC, Poelmann RE, VanMunsteren JC, et al. Embryonic endothelial cells transdifferentiate into mesenchymal cells expressing smooth muscle actins in vivo and in vitro. *Circ Res* 1997;80:444–451.

85. Huynh-Do U, Vindis C, Liu H, et al. Ephrin-B1 transduces signals to activate integrin-mediated migration, attachment and angiogenesis. *J Cell Biol* 2002;115:3073–3081.

86. Pugh CW, Ratcliffe PJ. Regulation of angiogenesis by hypoxia: role of the HIF system. *Nat Med* 2003;9:677–684.

87. Isogai S, Horiguchi M, Weinstein BM. The vascular anatomy of the developing zebrafish: an atlas of embryonic and early larval development. *Dev Biol* 2001;230:278–301.

88. Carmeliet P. Fibroblast growth factor-1 stimulates branching and survival of myocardial arteries: a goal for therapeutic angiogenesis? *Circ Res* 2000;87:176–178.

89. Hilgers KF, Norwood VF, Gomez RA. Angiotensin's role in renal development. *Semin Nephrol* 1997;17:492–501.

90. Miao HQ, Soker S, Feiner L, et al. Neuropilin-1 mediates collapsin-1/semaphorin III inhibition of endothelial cell motility: functional competition of collapsin-1 and vascular endothelial growth factor-165. *J Cell Biol* 1999;146:233–242.

91. Lee SH, Schloss DJ, Jarvis L, et al. Inhibition of angiogenesis by a mouse sprouty protein. *J Biol Chem* 2001;276:4128–4133.

92. Helbling PM, Saulnier DM, Brandli AW. The receptor tyrosine kinase EphB4 and ephrin-B ligands restrict angiogenic growth of embryonic veins in Xenopus laevis. *Development* 2000;127:269–278.

93. Ruhrberg C, Gerhardt H, Golding M, et al. Spatially restricted patterning cues provided by heparin-binding VEGF-A control blood vessel branching morphogenesis. *Genes Dev* 2002;16:2684–2698.

94. Carmeliet P, Ng YS, Nuyens D, et al. Impaired myocardial angiogenesis and ischemic cardiomyopathy in mice lacking the vascular endothelial growth factor isoforms VEGF164 and VEGF188. *Nat Med* 1999;5:495–502.

95. Mattot V, Moons L, Lupu F, et al. Loss of the VEGF(164) and VEGF(188) isoforms impairs postnatal glomerular angiogenesis and renal arteriogenesis in mice. *J Am Soc Nephrol* 2002;13:1548–1560.

96. Stalmans I, Lambrechts D, De Smet F, et al. VEGF: a modifier of the del22q11 (DiGeorge) syndrome? *Nat Med* 2003;9:173–182.

97. Gerhardt H, Golding M, Fruttiger M, et al. VEGF guides angiogenic sprouting utilizing endothelial tip cell filopodia. *J Cell Biol* 2003; 161:1163–1177.

98. Djonov VG, Kurz H, Burri PH. Optimality in the developing vascular system: branching remodeling by means of intussusception as an efficient adaptation mechanism. *Dev Dyn* 2002;224:391–402.

99. Egginton S, Zhou AL, Brown MD, et al. Unorthodox angiogenesis in skeletal muscle. *Cardiovasc Res* 2001;49:634–646.

100. Carmeliet P, Jain RK. Angiogenesis in cancer and other diseases. *Nature* 2000;407:249–257.

101. Hanahan D, Folkman J. Patterns and emerging mechanisms of the angiogenic switch during tumorigenesis. *Cell* 1996;86:353–364.

102. Ferrara N, Gerber HP, LeCouter J. The biology of VEGF and its receptors. *Nat Med* 2003;9:669–676.

103. Claesson-Welsh L. Signal transduction by vascular endothelial growth factor receptors. *Biochem Soc Trans* 2003;31:20–24.

104. Senger DR, Galli SJ, Dvorak AM, et al. Tumor cells secrete a vascular permeability factor that promotes accumulation of ascites fluid. *Science* 1983;219:983–985.

105. Neufeld G, Kessler O, Herzog Y. The interaction of Neuropilin-1 and Neuropilin-2 with tyrosine-kinase receptors for VEGF. *Adv Exp Med Biol* 2002;515:81–90.

106. Cleaver O, Krieg PA. VEGF mediates angioblast migration during development of the dorsal aorta in Xenopus. *Development* 1998;125: 3905–3914.

107. Nasevicius A, Larson J, Ekker SC. Distinct requirements for zebrafish angiogenesis revealed by a VEGF-A morphant. *Yeast* 2000;17: 294–301.

108. Carmeliet P, Ng YS, Nuyens D, et al. Impaired myocardial angiogenesis and ischemic cardiomyopathy in mice lacking the vascular endothelial growth factor isoforms VEGF164 and VEGF188. *Nat Med* 1999;5:495–502.

109. Eremina V, Sood M, Haigh J, et al. Glomerular-specific alterations of VEGF-A expression lead to distinct congenital and acquired renal diseases. *J Clin Invest* 2003;111:707–716.

110. Maes C, Carmeliet P, Moermans K, et al. Impaired angiogenesis and endochondral bone formation in mice lacking the vascular endothelial growth factor isoforms VEGF164 and VEGF188. *Mech Dev* 2002; 111:61–73.

111. Stalmans I, Lambrechts D, De Smet F, et al. VEGF: a modifier of the del22q11 (DiGeorge) syndrome? *Nat Med* 2003;9:173–182.

112. Shahbazi M, Fryer AA, Pravica V, et al. Vascular endothelial growth factor gene polymorphisms are associated with acute renal allograft rejection. *J Am Soc Nephrol* 2002;13:260–264.

113. Oosthuyse B, Moons L, Storkebaum E, et al. Deletion of the hypoxia-response element in the vascular endothelial growth factor promoter causes motor neuron degeneration. *Nat Genet* 2001;28:131–138.

114. Lambrechts D, Storkebaum E, Morimoto M, et al. VEGF is a modifier of amyotrophic lateral sclerosis in mice and humans and protects motoneurons against ischemic death. *Nat Genet* 2003;34:383–394.

115. Awata T, Inoue K, Kurihara S, et al. A common polymorphism in the 5'-untranslated region of the VEGF gene is associated with diabetic retinopathy in type 2 diabetes. *Diabetes* 2002;51:1635–1639.

116. Howell WM, Bateman AC, Turner SJ, et al. Influence of vascular endothelial growth factor single nucleotide polymorphisms on tumour development in cutaneous malignant melanoma. *Genes Immun* 2002;3:229–232.

117. Dvorak HF. Vascular permeability factor/vascular endothelial growth factor: a critical cytokine in tumor angiogenesis and a potential target for diagnosis and therapy. *J Clin Oncol* 2002;20:4368–4380.

118. Ferrara N. VEGF and the quest for tumour angiogenesis factors. *Nat Rev Cancer* 2002;2:795–803.

119. Bellamy WT. Vascular endothelial growth factor as a target opportunity in hematological malignancies. *Curr Opin Oncol* 2002;14:649–656.

120. Carmeliet P, Jain RK. Angiogenesis in cancer and other diseases. *Nature* 2000;407:249–257.

121. Jain RK, Carmeliet P. Vessels of death or life. *Sci Am* 2001;285: 38–45.

122. Rafii S. Vaccination against tumor neovascularization: promise and reality. *Cancer Cell* 2002;2:429–431.

123. Kendall RL, Thomas KA. Inhibition of vascular endothelial cell growth factor activity by an endogenously encoded soluble receptor. *Proc Natl Acad Sci USA* 1993;90:10705–10709.

124. Aiello LP, Pierce EA, Foley ED, et al. Suppression of retinal neovascularization in vivo by inhibition of vascular endothelial growth factor (VEGF) using soluble VEGF-receptor chimeric proteins. *Proc Natl Acad Sci USA* 1995;92:10457–10461.

125. Kim KJ, Li B, Winer J, et al. Inhibition of vascular endothelial growth factor-induced angiogenesis suppresses tumour growth in vivo. *Nature* 1993;362:841–844.

126. Presta LG, Chen H, O'Connor SJ, et al. Humanization of an anti-vascular endothelial growth factor monoclonal antibody for the therapy of solid tumors and other disorders. *Cancer Res* 1997;57: 4593–4599.

127. Lee CG, Heijn M, di Tomaso E, et al. Anti-Vascular endothelial growth factor treatment augments tumor radiation response under normoxic or hypoxic conditions. *Cancer Res* 2000;60:5565–5570.

128. Benjamin LE, Golijanin D, Itin A, et al. Selective ablation of immature blood vessels in established human tumors follows vascular endothelial growth factor withdrawal. *J Clin Invest* 1999;103:159–165.

129. Prewett M, Huber J, Li Y, et al. Antivascular endothelial growth factor receptor (fetal liver kinase 1) monoclonal antibody inhibits tumor angiogenesis and growth of several mouse and human tumors. *Cancer Res* 1999;59:5209–5218.

130. Strawn LM, McMahon G, App H, et al. Flk-1 as a target for tumor growth inhibition. *Cancer Res* 1996;56:3540–3545.

131. Dias S, Hattori K, Heissig B, et al. Inhibition of both paracrine and autocrine VEGF/VEGFR-2 signaling pathways is essential to induce

long-term remission of xenotransplanted human leukemias. *Proc Natl Acad Sci USA* 2001;98:10857–10862.

132. Fong TA, Shawver LK, Sun L, et al. SU5416 is a potent and selective inhibitor of the vascular endothelial growth factor receptor (Flk-1/KDR) that inhibits tyrosine kinase catalysis, tumor vascularization, and growth of multiple tumor types. *Cancer Res* 1999;59:99–106.

133. McCarthy M. Antiangiogenesis drug promising for metastatic colorectal cancer. *Lancet* 2003;361:1959.

134. Autiero M, Luttun A, Tjwa M, et al. Placental growth factor and its receptor, vascular endothelial growth factor receptor-1: novel targets for stimulation of ischemic tissue revascularization and inhibition of angiogenic and inflammatory disorders. *J Thromb Haemost* 2003;1:1356–1370.

135. Luttun A, Tjwa M, Moons L, et al. Revascularization of ischemic tissues by PlGF treatment, and inhibition of tumor angiogenesis, arthritis and atherosclerosis by anti-Flt1. *Nat Med* 2002;8:831–840.

136. Weng DE, Usman N. Angiozyme: a novel angiogenesis inhibitor. *Curr Oncol Rep* 2001;3:141–146.

137. Hiratsuka S, Maru Y, Okada A, et al. Involvement of Flt-1 tyrosine kinase (vascular endothelial growth factor receptor-1) in pathological angiogenesis. *Cancer Res* 2001;61:1207–1213.

138. Ziche M, Maglione D, Ribatti D, et al. Placenta growth factor-1 is chemotactic, mitogenic, and angiogenic. *Lab Invest* 1997;76:517–531.

139. Carmeliet P, Moons L, Luttun A, et al. Synergism between vascular endothelial growth factor and placental growth factor contributes to angiogenesis and plasma extravasation in pathological conditions. *Nat Med* 2001;7:575–583.

140. Odorisio T, Schietroma C, Zaccaria ML, et al. Mice overexpressing placenta growth factor exhibit increased vascularization and vessel permeability. *J Cell Sci* 2002;115:2559–2567.

141. Luttun A, Tjwa M, Moons L, et al. Revascularization of ischemic tissues by PlGF treatment, and inhibition of tumor angiogenesis, arthritis and atherosclerosis by anti-Flt1. *Nat Med* 2002;8:831–840.

142. Parenti A, Brogelli L, Filippi S, et al. Effect of hypoxia and endothelial loss on vascular smooth muscle cell responsiveness to VEGF-A: role of flt-1/VEGF-receptor-1. *Cardiovasc Res* 2002;55:201–212.

143. Oura H, Bertoncini J, Velasco P, et al. A critical role of placental growth factor in the induction of inflammation and edema formation. *Blood* 2003;101:560–567.

144. Autiero M, Waltenberger J, Communi D, et al. Role of PlGF in the intra- and intermolecular cross talk between the VEGF receptors Flt1 and Flk1. *Nat Med* 2003;9:936–943.

145. Hiratsuka S, Minowa O, Kuno J, et al. Flt-1 lacking the tyrosine kinase domain is sufficient for normal development and angiogenesis in mice. *Proc Natl Acad Sci USA* 1998;95:9349–9354.

146. Zeng H, Zhao D, Mukhopadhyay D. Flt-1-mediated down-regulation of endothelial cell proliferation through pertussis toxin-sensitive G proteins, beta gamma subunits, small GTPase CDC42, and partly by Rac-1. *J Biol Chem* 2002;277:4003–4009.

147. Rahimi N, Dayanir V, Lashkari K. Receptor chimeras indicate that the vascular endothelial growth factor receptor-1 (VEGFR-1) modulates mitogenic activity of VEGFR-2 in endothelial cells. *J Biol Chem* 2000;275:16986–16992.

148. Gille H, Kowalski J, Yu L, et al. A repressor sequence in the juxtamembrane domain of Flt-1 (VEGFR-1) constitutively inhibits vascular endothelial growth factor-dependent phosphatidylinositol 3′-kinase activation and endothelial cell migration. *EMBO J* 2000;19:4064–4073.

149. Patan S. TIE1 and TIE2 receptor tyrosine kinases inversely regulate embryonic angiogenesis by the mechanism of intussusceptive microvascular growth. *Microvasc Res* 1998;56:1–21.

150. Suri C, Jones PF, Patan S, et al. Requisite role of angiopoietin-1, a ligand for the TIE2 receptor, during embryonic angiogenesis. *Cell* 1996;87:1171–1180.

151. Loughna S, Sato TN. Angiopoietin and Tie signaling pathways in vascular development. *Matrix Biol* 2001;20:319–325.

152. Xu Y, Yu Q. Angiopoietin-1, unlike angiopoietin-2, is incorporated into the extracellular matrix via its linker peptide region. *J Biol Chem* 2001;276:34990–34998.

153. Carlson TR, Feng Y, Maisonpierre PC, et al. Direct cell adhesion to the angiopoietins mediated by integrins. *J Biol Chem* 2001;276:26516–26525.

154. Oh H, Takagi H, Otani A, et al. Selective induction of neuropilin-1 by

155. Thurston G, Rudge JS, Ioffe E, et al. Angiopoietin-1 protects the adult vasculature against plasma leakage. *Nat Med* 2000;6:460–463.

156. Zhang Z, Chopp M. Vascular endothelial growth factor and angiopoietins in focal cerebral ischemia. *Trends Cardiovasc Med* 2002;12:62–66.

157. Suri C, McClain J, Thurston G, et al. Increased vascularization in mice overexpressing angiopoietin-1. *Science* 1998;282:468–471.

158. Shyu KG, Manor O, Magner M, et al. Direct intramuscular injection of plasmid DNA encoding angiopoietin-1 but not angiopoietin-2 augments revascularization in the rabbit ischemic hindlimb. *Circulation* 1998;98:2081–2087.

159. Chae JK, Kim I, Lim ST, et al. Coadministration of angiopoietin-1 and vascular endothelial growth factor enhances collateral vascularization. *Arterioscler Thromb Vasc Biol* 2000;20:2573–2578.

160. Shim WS, Teh M, Bapna A, et al. Angiopoietin 1 promotes tumor angiogenesis and tumor vessel plasticity of human cervical cancer in mice. *Exp Cell Res* 2002;279:299–309.

161. Ahmad SA, Liu W, Jung WD, et al. The effects of angiopoietin-1 and -2 on tumor growth and angiogenesis in human colon cancer. *Cancer Res* 2001;61:1255–1259.

162. Tian S, Hayes AJ, Metheny-Barlow LJ, et al. Stabilization of breast cancer xenograft tumour neovasculature by angiopoietin-1. *Br J Cancer* 2002;86:645–651.

163. Gamble JR, Drew J, Trezise L, et al. Angiopoietin-1 is an antipermeability and anti-inflammatory agent in vitro and targets cell junctions. *Circ Res* 2000;87:603–607.

164. Etoh T, Inoue H, Tanaka S, et al. Angiopoietin-2 is related to tumor angiogenesis in gastric carcinoma: possible in vivo regulation via induction of proteases. *Cancer Res* 2001;61:2145–2153.

165. Gale NW, Thurston G, Hackett SF, et al. Angiopoietin-2 is required for postnatal angiogenesis and lymphatic patterning, and only the latter role is rescued by Angiopoietin-1. *Dev Cell* 2002;3:411–423.

166. Maisonpierre PC, Suri C, Jones PF, et al. Angiopoietin-2, a natural antagonist for Tie2 that disrupts in vivo angiogenesis. *Science* 1997;277:55–60.

167. Hackett SF, Wiegand S, Yancopoulos G, et al. Angiopoietin-2 plays an important role in retinal angiogenesis. *J Cell Physiol* 2002;192:182–187.

168. Cao R, Brakenhielm E, et al. Angiogenesis stimulated by PDGF-CC, a novel member in the PDGF family, involves activation of PDGFR-alphaalpha and -alphabeta receptors. *FASEB J* 2002;16:1575–1583.

169. Li H, Fredriksson L, Li X, et al. PDGF-D is a potent transforming and angiogenic growth factor. *Oncogene* 2003;22:1501–1510.

170. Hellstrom M, Gerhardt H, Kalen M, et al. Lack of pericytes leads to endothelial hyperplasia and abnormal vascular morphogenesis. *J Cell Biol* 2001;153:543–553.

171. Hellstrom M, Kalen M, Lindahl P, et al. Role of PDGF-B and PDGFR-beta in recruitment of vascular smooth muscle cells and pericytes during embryonic blood vessel formation in the mouse. *Development* 1999;126:3047–3055.

172. Uemura A, Ogawa M, Hirashima M, et al. Recombinant angiopoietin-1 restores higher-order architecture of growing blood vessels in mice in the absence of mural cells. *J Clin Invest* 2002;110:1619–1628.

173. Richardson TP, Peters MC, Ennett AB, et al. Polymeric system for dual growth factor delivery. *Nat Biotechnol* 2001;19:1029–1034.

174. Begbie ME, Wallace GM, Shovlin CL. Hereditary haemorrhagic telangiectasia (Osler-Weber-Rendu syndrome): a view from the 21st century. *Postgrad Med J* 2003;79:18–24.

175. Oh SP, Seki T, Goss KA, et al. Activin receptor-like kinase 1 modulates transforming growth factor-beta 1 signaling in the regulation of angiogenesis. *Proc Natl Acad Sci USA* 2000;97:2626–2631.

176. Srinivasan S, Hanes MA, Dickens T, et al. A mouse model for hereditary hemorrhagic telangiectasia (HHT) type 2. *Hum Mol Genet* 2003;12:473–482.

177. Lamouille S, Mallet C, Feige JJ, et al. Activin receptor-like kinase 1 is implicated in the maturation phase of angiogenesis. *Blood* 2002;100:4495–4501.

178. Ota T, Fujii M, Sugizaki T, et al. Targets of transcriptional regulation by two distinct type I receptors for transforming growth factor-beta in human umbilical vein endothelial cells. *J Cell Physiol* 2002;193:299–318.

179. Goumans MJ, Valdimarsdottir G, Itoh S, et al. Balancing the activa-

tion state of the endothelium via two distinct TGF-beta type I receptors. *EMBO J* 2002;21:1743–1753.

180. Hynes RO. Cell adhesion: old and new questions. *Trends Cell Biol* 1999;9:M33–M37.
181. Giancotti FG, Ruoslahti E. Integrin signaling. *Science* 1999;285: 1028–1032.
182. Eliceiri BP, Cheresh DA. Adhesion events in angiogenesis. *Curr Opin Cell Biol* 2001;13:563–568.
183. Rupp PA, Little CD. Integrins in vascular development. *Circ Res* 2001;89:566–572.
184. Reynolds LE, Wyder L, Lively JC, et al. Enhanced pathological angiogenesis in mice lacking beta3 integrin or beta3 and beta5 integrins. *Nat Med* 2002;8:27–34.
185. Carmeliet P. Integrin indecision. *Nat Med* 2002;8:14–16.
186. Pepper MS. Extracellular proteolysis and angiogenesis. *Thromb Haemost* 2001;86:346–355.
187. Jackson C. Matrix metalloproteinases and angiogenesis. *Curr Opin Nephrol Hypertens* 2002;11:295–299.
188. Luttun A, Dewerchin M, Collen D, et al. The role of proteinases in angiogenesis, heart development, restenosis, atherosclerosis, myocardial ischemia, and stroke: insights from genetic studies. *Curr Atheroscler Rep* 2000;2:407–416.
189. Berchem G, Glondu M, Gleizes M, et al. Cathepsin-D affects multiple tumor progression steps in vivo: proliferation, angiogenesis and apoptosis. *Oncogene* 2002;21:5951–5955.
190. Kostoulas G, Lang A, Nagase H, et al. Stimulation of angiogenesis through cathepsin B inactivation of the tissue inhibitors of matrix metalloproteinases. *FEBS Lett* 1999;455:286–290.
191. Yousef GM, Diamandis EP. Expanded human tissue kallikrein family—a novel panel of cancer biomarkers. *Tumour Biol* 2002;23:185–192.
192. Miao RQ, Agata J, Chao L, et al. Kallistatin is a new inhibitor of angiogenesis and tumor growth. *Blood* 2002;100:3245–3252.
193. Overall CM, Lopez-Otin C. Strategies for MMP inhibition in cancer: innovations for the post-trial era. *Nat Rev Cancer* 2002;2:657–672.
194. Egeblad M, Werb Z. New functions for the matrix metalloproteinases in cancer progression. *Nat Rev Cancer* 2002;2:161–174.
195. Bergers G, Brekken R, McMahon G, et al. Matrix metalloproteinase-9 triggers the angiogenic switch during carcinogenesis. *Nat Cell Biol* 2000;2:737–744.
196. Bajou K, Noel A, Gerard RD, et al. Absence of host plasminogen activator inhibitor 1 prevents cancer invasion and vascularization. *Nat Med* 1998;4:923–928.
197. Luttun A, Dewerchin M, Collen D, et al. The role of proteinases in angiogenesis, heart development, restenosis, atherosclerosis, myocardial ischemia, and stroke: insights from genetic studies. *Curr Atheroscler Rep* 2000;2:407–416.
198. Helisch A, Schaper W. Arteriogenesis: the development and growth of collateral arteries. *Microcirculation* 2003;10:83–97.
199. Isner JM. Myocardial gene therapy. *Nature* 2002;415:234–239.
200. Cao R, Brakenhielm E, Pawliuk R, et al. Angiogenic synergism, vascular stability and improvement of hind-limb ischemia by a combination of PDGF-BB and FGF-2. *Nat Med* 2003;9:604–613.
201. Kamihata H, Matsubara H, Nishiue T, et al. Improvement of collateral perfusion and regional function by implantation of peripheral blood mononuclear cells into ischemic hibernating myocardium. *Arterioscler Thromb Vasc Biol* 2002;22:1804–1810.
202. Heil M, Ziegelhoeffer T, Pipp F, et al. Blood monocyte concentration is critical for enhancement of collateral artery growth. *Am J Physiol Heart Circ Physiol* 2002;283:H2411–H2419.
203. van Royen N, Hoefer I, Buschmann I, et al. Exogenous application of transforming growth factor beta 1 stimulates arteriogenesis in the peripheral circulation. *FASEB J* 2002;16:432–434.
204. Buschmann IR, Hoefer IE, van Royen N, et al. GM-CSF: a strong arteriogenic factor acting by amplification of monocyte function. *Atherosclerosis* 2001;159:343–356.
205. Voskuil M, van Royen N, Hoefer IE, et al. Modulation of collateral artery growth in a porcine hindlimb ligation model using MCP-1. *Am J Physiol Heart Circ Physiol* 2003;284:H1422–1428.
206. Hoefer IE, van Royen N, Rectenwald JE, et al. Direct evidence for tumor necrosis factor-alpha signaling in arteriogenesis. *Circulation* 2002;105:1639–1641.
207. Pipp F, Heil M, Issbrucker K, et al. VEGFR-1-selective VEGF homologue PlGF is arteriogenic: evidence for a monocyte-mediated mechanism. *Circ Res* 2003;92:378–385.

CHAPTER 24

Embryogenesis of the Vascular System

Brant M. Weinstein

Key Words: Arteries; Flk1; hedgehog; hemangioblast; lymphatics; Notch, Prox1; SCL/Tal1; vascular endothelial growth factor; veins.

INTRODUCTION

The growth of new blood and lymphatic vessels is a complex process that, as might be expected, is exquisitely controlled in adults by the adjacent tissues that these vessels serve. However, the patterning of major blood and lymphatic vessels during development and, in particular, the specification and differentiation of the cells that comprise these vessels are under the control of defined genetic programs during embryogenesis. This chapter reviews recent discoveries on the origins of the cellular building blocks of blood and lymphatic vessels.

BASIC CONCEPTS

Blood vessels are composed of two basic cell types: vascular endothelial cells (VECs) and vascular smooth muscle cells (VSMCs). The inner epithelial lining of blood vessels, adjacent to the lumen, is a single layer of endothelial cells, whereas smooth muscle cells or pericytes surround the endothelial tube. Arteries and veins are the two fundamental types of blood vessels, carrying blood away from and toward the heart, respectively. Higher pressure arteries generally have thicker, medial, smooth muscle–containing layers, whereas larger veins have thinner, more elastic walls and valves to prevent backflow. In addition to blood vessels, an additional important but often overlooked component of the

circulatory system is the lymphatic vasculature. Lymphatics are a separate vascular network important for tissue fluid homeostasis, waste removal, and immune functions that is lined by lymphatic endothelial cells (LECs), which are most likely derived from venous VECs (discussed later). As described later in this chapter, the endothelial cells contributing to arteries, veins, and lymphatic vessels have distinct molecular and functional identities that are established early during development.

EMBRYONIC ORIGINS OF THE VASCULATURE

The first, major embryonic vessels form by coalescence of individual endothelial progenitor cells or "angioblasts" that arise from lateral mesoderm (1). These progenitors migrate medially to form cords of attached VECs, which undergo morphogenesis to form epithelial tubes. This process, called *vasculogenesis,* was thought to be restricted to early vascular development, but evidence has shown that vasculogenesis also occurs later during development and even postnatally. Most later developmental and postnatal blood vessel formation, however, occurs by sprouting and elongation of new vessels from preexisting vessels or remodeling of preexisting vessels, collectively known as *angiogenesis.* A variety of evidence suggests that angioblasts also emerge *de novo* at later stages of development from other mesodermal tissues such as the paraxial/somitic mesoderm, mesodermal mesenchyme, and even, as recently described, during adult life from hematopoietic stem cells.

Vessels generally form initially as unlined endothelial tubes but soon become associated with supporting pericytes or VSMCs. A large number of studies have shown that the acquisition of these supporting cells is critical for proper morphogenesis, stability, and survival of nascent blood vessels (for comprehensive review of vascular smooth muscle

B. M. Weinstein: Laboratory of Molecular Genetics, NICHD, NIH, Bethesda, Maryland 20892.

development see Majesky and coworkers [2]). The origins of pericytes or VSMCs is in many if not most cases unclear. Cranial neural crest contributes to the VSMCs of the aortic arches, whereas the epicardium gives rise to that of the coronary vasculature. Most other VSMCs are believed to be of mesodermal origin, but more specific information on their ontogeny has been largely lacking. Recent work suggests that VSMCs may in at least some cases share common origins with cells contributing to the endothelial and hematopoietic lineages and that there may be a multipotent common progenitor for these lineages at least transiently during development (discussed later).

There has been controversy over the origins of the LECs that line lymphatic vessels (reviewed in Oliver and Detmar [3]). Ink injection studies performed by Florence Sabin around the turn of the twentieth century (4,5) and other more recent studies suggested that the LECs in the earliest primitive lymph sacs originate from endothelial cells that lined veins earlier in development, in particular larger veins including the subclavian and anterior cardinal veins. The peripheral lymphatic system then forms by endothelial sprouting from these primitive sacs into surrounding tissues and organs. This *centrifugal* model has received support from recent characterization of molecular markers of LECs that have revealed budding of LECs from veins to form primitive lymph sacs exactly as described by Sabin (discussed later). The centrifugal model, however, was challenged by an alternative model (6) proposing that LECs comprising the primary lymph sacs originate from mesenchyme, independently from veins, and secondarily establish venous connections to vessels such as the cardinal and subclavian veins. This *centripetal* model for lymphatic vessel formation also has received some support from studies on the origin of LECs of the avian wing bud that have suggested these cells are derived from somitic or paraxial mesoderm (7,8). The two models for LEC genesis are, of course, not mutually exclusive, and it seems likely that although the primitive lymph sacs and central lymphatic vessels arise largely by budding from veins, some progenitors for LECs in distal lymphatic vessels and capillaries may arise *de novo* from mesenchyme in a manner analogous to that proposed for the emergence of additional VEC progenitors.

Although most of the larger blood vessels form early during development with a pattern of interconnections that is relatively stable thereafter, significant growth and remodeling of blood vessels does continue throughout adult life—for example, during uterine cycling or in conjunction with gain or loss of fat or muscle mass. Postnatal vessel growth also occurs in pathologic contexts, notably cancer. Tumors recruit new blood vessels (and lymphatic vessels) from their hosts to provide themselves with access to the host circulation and obtain oxygen and nutrients. Acquisition of a host vascular blood supply is an essential step in tumor progression and tumor survival, and antiangiogenic therapies targeting these tumor blood vessels are currently a subject of intensive investigation as one of the most promising new methods for combating cancer.

THE HEMANGIOBLAST

The existence of a progenitor for both vascular and hematopoietic lineages has been debated for many years. The idea was first proposed by Florence Sabin (9) on the basis of the observed common origin of these cell types in blood islands, but until recently there was little definitive evidence for the existence of such a common progenitor cell. In recent years, however, a variety of reports have demonstrated that a common hemangioblast progenitor is at least a transient intermediate in the development of some but probably not all endothelial and hematopoietic cells (for review see Forrai and Robb [10]), and the possible lineage relations have been expanded further to include smooth muscle and possibly other cell types (discussed later in this chapter and see also Ema and Rossant [11]).

With the advent of molecular biology and characterization of genes expressed in hematopoietic and endothelial cells, it became apparent that during their early development these cell types share expression of many genes, including *Flk1, Flt1, SCL/Tal1, Tie1, Tie2,* and *Runx1.* Targeted disruption of some of these genes in mice has revealed their functional importance for both lineages as well. Mice homozygous for knockouts of *Flk1*/vascular endothelial growth factor receptor 2 *(VEGFR2)* (12) or *Flt1*/VEGFR1 (13,14) have severe defects in both blood and vascular development. The *SCL* gene is expressed in vascular, hematopoietic, and neural tissues (15). The *SCL* knockout lacks both primitive and definitive hematopoietic lineages, but endothelium is still present (16–19). However, $SCL^{-/-}$ mice in which hematopoietic expression of *SCL* is "rescued" by expression of an *SCL* transgene display defective angiogenic remodeling of yolk sac vessels (20) and ectopic expression of *SCL* in zebrafish embryos results in an increase in the number of hematopoietic and vascular cells (21), suggesting that *SCL* promotes the specification of both lineages. The zebrafish *cloche* mutant (22) also has provided suggestive genetic evidence in support of the existence of a hemangioblast. *Cloche* mutants lack virtually all endothelial and blood cells and are deficient in an as yet unidentified gene functioning early in both lineages, or in a common progenitor (22–24). Experimental studies suggest that *cloche* acts upstream of *flk* (23) and downstream of or in parallel to *hhex* (25) and *fli1* (26). Transplantation experiments indicate that *cloche* is required cell-autonomously for both the formation of vascular endothelium (22) and for the differentiation and/or survival of red blood cells (27), although there is evidence it also plays a cell-nonautonomous role in hematopoietic development, perhaps as a result of a requirement for interaction with endothelium to generate blood cells (27).

While the data on shared expression and function of vascular and hematopoietic genes are highly suggestive, *in vitro* experiments using cultured embryonic stem (ES) cell differentiation have provided the best evidence to date for the existence of an hemangioblast. ES cells differentiated into embryoid bodies give rise to clonal *blast colonies* containing both hematopoietic and endothelial cells *in vitro* (28). These "BL-CFC" cells are or are derived from cells coexpressing both *VEGFR2* and *SCL* (29,30), and additional studies (31–34) have led to a proposed model in which multipotential *VEGFR2*-positive mesodermal precursors are directed into hematopoietic, endothelial, and smooth muscle lineages on the basis of their expression of additional factors including *SCL/Tal1* and *Runx1* (Fig. 24–1; also reviewed in more detail in Ema and Rossant [11]). The existence of common multipotential progenitor for all three lineages including smooth muscle is a particularly interesting possibility that has gained support from a number of *in vitro* and *in vivo* findings. Flk1$^+$ cells derived from embryonic stem cells can differentiate into both endothelial and mural (VSMC) cells and form organized vascular networks *in vitro* (31). Interestingly, this fate choice can be modulated by *SCL/Tal1* levels: ES cells with increased *Tal1* expression show reduced smooth muscle differentiation, whereas loss of *Tal1* promotes smooth muscle formation (34). Mice with cre recombinase "knocked in" to the *Flk* locus crossed to a cre reporter line have shown that Flk$^+$ cells can give rise to various muscle cell types in addi-

tion to vascular and hematopoietic cells (32), suggesting a common progenitor may also be present during normal development *in vivo*. A variety of additional evidence has arisen to suggest that adults also possess multipotential mesodermal progenitors, cells transdifferentiating from one lineage to another, or both, including reports that adult human or hematopoietic stem cells can contribute to both blood and vascular cell types (35,36) and a number of different studies that suggest VECs can transdifferentiate into vascular smooth muscle cells, at least under certain circumstances (see review in Majesky and coworkers [2]).

ARTERIAL–VENOUS FATE DETERMINATION

Blood vessels are most fundamentally divided into two types: arteries and veins. Although the classical view of arterial–venous (A-V) identity is that it follows from physiologic parameters such as differences in blood flow and pressure, some work has shown that in the early embryo, genetic programs specify arterial and venous endothelial cell types (Fig. 24–1, reviewed in References 37 through 39). Initial evidence that arterial and venous endothelial cells possess dis-

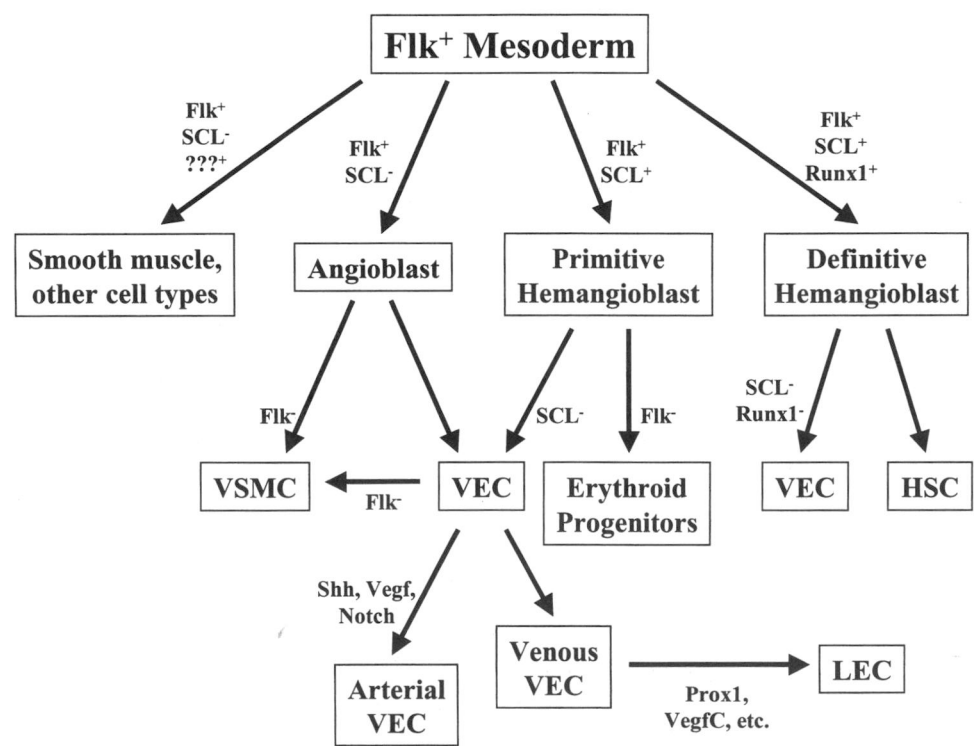

FIG. 24–1. A proposed model for specification of various cell lineages from Flk1$^+$ mesodermal precursors. The presence or absence of SCL/Tal1, Runx1, and as yet undetermined transcription factor expression determines whether Flk11 cells produce vascular endothelial cells (VECs), primitive or definitive hematopoietic precursors, or other cell types including smooth muscle cells (SMCs). VECs differentiate into arterial VECs under the direction of a molecular pathway including sonic hedgehog (shh), vascular endothelial growth factor (VEGF), and Notch signaling. Venous differentiation is likely the default identity of VECs. Venous VECs also can differentiate into lymphatic endothelial cells (LECs) under the direction of Prox1 and other factors. Transdifferentiation of VECs to smooth muscle also may occur. HSC, hematopoietic stem cell; VSMC, vascular smooth muscle cell. (Modified from Ema M, Rossant J. Cell fate decisions in early blood vessel formation. *Trends Cardiovasc Med* 2003;13:254–259.)

tinct molecular identities came from work with *ephrin* and *Eph* genes in mice (40). Wang and coworkers (40) described the expression of ephrinB2, a member of the ephrin family of membrane ligands. Before the onset of flow, ephrinB2, a member of the ephrin family of membrane ligands, is expressed specifically in arterial endothelial cells and is absent in venous endothelial cells, whereas the ephrinB2 receptor EphB4 is preferentially expressed in veins. Targeted gene deletion of each member of this ligand receptor pair resulted in similar cardiovascular abnormalities, demonstrating that they are necessary for normal vascular development and likely directly interact (40,41). The *ephrinB2* mutant mice were generated with the *LacZ* "knocked in" to the *ephrinB2* locus, and homozygotes continued to express *LacZ* appropriately in the arterial compartment, indicating that initial specification of arterial or venous fate involves additional factors upstream of *ephrinB2* (40).

Zebrafish studies have been critical in uncovering and dissecting the functional roles of these upstream factors, resulting in the identification of a signaling cascade for arterial fate determination consisting of sequential hedgehog, vascular endothelial growth factor, and Notch signaling (Fig. 24–2). A variety of studies in mammals and other vertebrates have revealed the specific expression of Notch signaling genes (e.g., *Notch, Delta,* and *Jagged*) in arterial but not in venous endothelial cells, and murine knockout studies showed that these molecules play an important functional role in the vasculature (reviewed comprehensively in References 37, 38, and 42). Although the nature of this functional role was not determined in the murine studies, the arterial-specific expression of these genes suggested that they might be playing a role in artery formation. Studies in the zebrafish (43–45) have now shown that Notch signaling promotes arterial differentiation at the expense of venous differentiation during vascular development. Repression of Notch signaling in zebrafish embryos using either the neurogenic *mindbomb* (*mib*) mutant or injection of mRNA encoding a dominant-negative DNA binding mutant of Xenopus suppressor of hairless protein (45) resulted in loss of *ephrinB2a* expression from arteries and ectopic expansion of normally venous-restricted markers such as *ephb4* and *flt-4* into the arterial domain. Conversely, activation of Notch signaling using either ubiquitous or endothelial-specific expression of the activated Notch intracellular domain suppressed expression of vein-restricted markers and promoted ectopic expression of *ephrinB2a* and other arterial markers in venous vessels.

Lawson and colleagues (44) further dissected the A-V differentiation signaling hierarchy by demonstrating that *sonic hedgehog (shh)* and *VEGF* act upstream of Notch during arterial differentiation. Embryos lacking *shh* or *VEGF* also fail

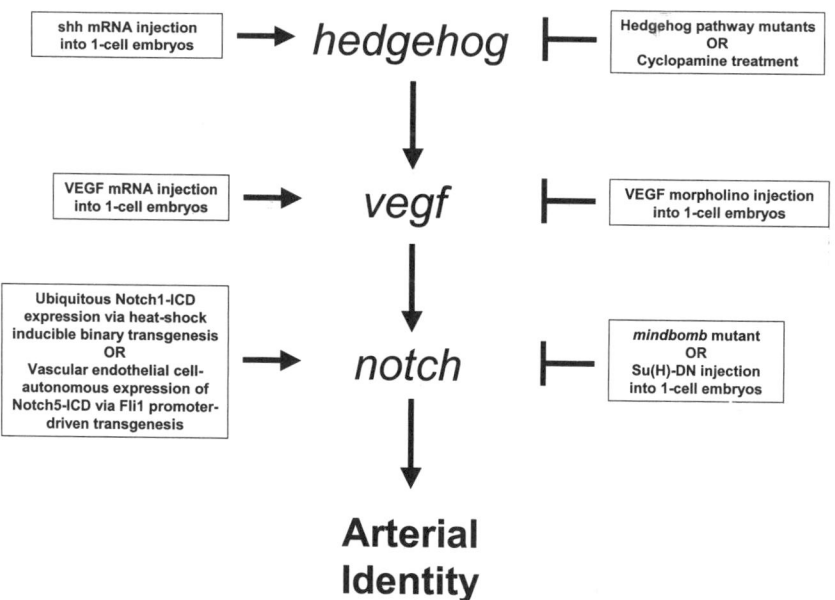

Arterial Identity

FIG. 24–2. A molecular pathway for arterial–venous fate determination. Studies in the zebrafish have shown that vascular endothelial growth factor (VEGF) acts downstream of sonic hedgehog (shh) and upstream of the Notch pathway to determine arterial cell fate. A variety of different methods were used to either increase *(left)* or decrease *(right)* the levels, activities, or both of each of these signaling pathways. Loss of Notch, VEGF, or shh signaling results in loss of arterial identity, whereas exogenous activation or overexpression of these factors causes ectopic expression of arterial markers. *Molecular epistasis* experiments were performed by combining different methods to assemble these components into an ordered pathway. For example, microinjection of VEGF mRNA into embryos homozygous mutant for hedgehog pathway genes can rescue their arterial differentiation defect. Likewise, inducible transgenic activation of the Notch pathway in zebrafish embryos rescues the loss of arterial marker gene expression caused by "knock-down" of VEGF signaling. (For further information on the zebrafish studies used to derive this pathway see Lawson et al. [44,45].) (See color insert for Fig. 24–3.)

to express *ephrinB2a* within their blood vessels, like embryos deficient in Notch signaling. Overexpression of *shh* promotes ectopic arterial vessel formation in the trunk, whereas overexpression of *VEGF* through injection of VEGF mRNA suppresses expression of vein-restricted markers and results in expression of *ephrinB2a* and other arterial markers in venous vessels. *Molecular epistasis* experiments were used to show that shh activity induces expression of VEGF in the somites, and that VEGF then activates Notch signaling in the endothelial cells of the developing dorsal aorta, promoting arterial differentiation. Genetic screening methods were used to identify a zebrafish mutant deficient in both angiogenesis and arterial differentiation as a result of a defect in *phospholipase C gamma-1 (plcg1)* (46). Phospholipase Cγ genes are known effectors of signaling through receptor tyrosine kinases such as the VEGF receptor Flk1. The vascular expression of *plcg1* and vascular-specific phenotype of the mutant in this gene suggested that it might be functioning downstream of VEGF signaling. Indeed, it was found that *plcg1* mutants are insensitive to both angiogenic and arterial differentiation responses to VEGF overexpression, demonstrating that this gene plays a major role in signaling downstream from VEGF *in vivo*.

Studies in mice have also implicated shh and VEGF signaling in regulating blood vessel growth and arterial differentiation. shh induces expression of all three VEGF-1 isoforms, angiopoietin 1, and angiopoietin 2 in ischemic limbs, and it induces new blood vessel growth without affecting endothelial cell migration or proliferation (47). Mukouyama and coworkers (48) evaluated the influence of the nervous system on blood vessel development and found that peripheral nerves express VEGF and influence vascular patterning and arteriogenesis in embryonic skin. They demonstrated that VEGF-expressing neurons and Schwann cells induced ephrinB2 expression in endothelial cells when cocultured and that exogenously added VEGF had a similar effect. They also demonstrated that a VEGF-blocking antibody could abrogate this response. Two additional studies performed in adult animals suggest that VEGF also plays a role in postnatal arterial differentiation. Visconti and coworkers (49) showed myosin heavy chain alpha (αMHC)::VEGF transgenic mice expressing VEGF-A in the heart had an increased percentage of arterial (ephrinB2$^+$) vessels in adult cardiac tissue compared with wild type mice. In another study, Springer and coworkers (50) demonstrated an increase in arterial concentration in adult skeletal muscle in response to VEGF-A expression. Transplantation of myoblasts expressing VEGF-A into nonischemic skeletal muscle resulted in an increased capillary density in the region of the implanted cells and a region of arteriogenic growth immediately adjacent to the implanted cells. The authors noted that this type of arteriogenic growth is distinct from that typically seen as a result of collateral arteriole formation because of its proximity to the site of VEGF delivery in a region of tissue that has few if any preexisting arteriolar vessels. Some of the links in the pathway shown in Figure 24–2 have been further confirmed by other *in vitro* experiments. *Notch4* activation by

Delta4 (vascular expression of both of these genes is restricted to arteries) in cultured primary human dermal microvascular endothelial cells (HMVECd) up-regulates expression of ephrinB2 and hairy-related factors HES1, HERP1, and HERP2 (51). VEGFs (but not fibroblast growth factors) induces *Notch4* and *Delta4* expression in cultured arterial endothelial cells (52). This induction requires functional VEGF receptors VEGFR1 and VEGFR2, as well as PI3-kinase pathway. Constitutive activation of Notch in these cells inhibits proliferation and promotes survival and network formation, whereas Notch blockade may partially inhibit network formation.

Although the results above indicate that the A-V identity of early blood vessels precedes circulatory flow or even angioblast assembly, other work suggests that this fate choice is not irreversible and that maintenance of differentiated A-V identity might require components of the vascular wall. Two separate groups performed quail–chick grafting experiments to examine the plasticity of A-V endothelial cell fate (53,54). Portions of embryonic arteries or veins were grafted from quail donors at various stages of development into chick hosts, and the A-V identity of donor cells contributing to different host vessels was assessed using artery- or vein-specific molecular markers. Up until approximately E7 donor cells populate both types of vessels and assume the appropriate molecular identity, but after E7 this plasticity is progressively lost. However, isolated endothelial cells or isolated dissected endothelia were still plastic even in older vessels, suggesting that components of the vascular wall are necessary to maintain, or are sufficient to redirect, the A-V identity of adjacent endothelial cells.

LYMPHATIC FATE DETERMINATION

As noted earlier, a separate but interconnected network of lymphatic vessels composed of LECs rather than VECs parallels the blood vascular network. Molecular characterization of LEC and VEC has shown that these cell types share most of their genes in common, a fact that has also made isolation and functional characterization of LEC difficult. In the past few years, however, a number of reasonably specific or at least diagnostic markers of LEC have been uncovered that have helped us begin to understand the specification and differentiation of these cells. These include the lymphatic endothelial hyaluronan receptor LYVE-1 (55, 56), podoplanin (57), VEGFR3, a receptor for VEGF-C and VEGF-D (58,59), and Prox-1 (60). Interestingly, many LEC markers are also transiently expressed in developing VECs, particularly in the venous blood vessels. This might be expected if, as proposed by Florence Sabin, LECs are derived from venous VECs (Fig. 24–1). Immunohistochemical studies using LEC markers to examine successive stages of development have shown that the primitive lymphatic sacs, at least, form by budding off from the cardinal veins and other major venous vessels, validating Sabin's *centrifugal* model for formation of the lymphatic vasculature (discussed earlier).

Many of the genes used as markers for LECs also have been shown to have important functional roles in these cells, and analysis of their null phenotypes has led to a model for specification and differentiation of these cells from venous VECs (Fig. 24–3 [see color insert]; see Oliver and Detmar [3] for a recent comprehensive review of lymphatic development and LEC specification). The homeobox gene *Prox-1* appears to be a critical "master regulator" of LECs specification from VECs. *Prox-1* is a very early marker of prospective LEC progenitors in veins such as the cardinal and subclavian veins. It localizes to a subpopulation of the venous VECs that subsequently sprout and bud off to give rise to lymphatic vessels. In Prox1-null mice this sprouting and budding becomes arrested (60) and the cells that do bud off have a VEC rather than LEC phenotype as determined by expression of various marker genes (61). Ectopic expression of *Prox-1* in cultured endothelial cells induces genes specific for LEC such as VEGFR3 and suppresses expression of VEC-specific genes (62,63). The VEGFR3 (Flt1) receptor is another important regulator of lymphangiogenesis, together with its ligands VEGF-C and VEGF-D. Like most lymphatic-specific genes, *VEGFR3* is initially expressed in VECs early in development, but later becomes restricted to LEC (58,59). VEGFR3 null mice die of cardiovascular failure at E9.5 because of defects in blood vessel formation and morphogenesis (58), precluding assessment of the lymphatic phenotype of loss of *VEGFR3* function. However, some patients with hereditary lymphedema have nonsense mutations in *VEGFR3* (64) and transgenic expression of soluble *VEGFR3* in the skin of adult mice causes extensive loss of lymphatic vessels, whereas the rest of the circulatory system is normal (65). Furthermore, transgenic overexpression of the VEGFR3 ligands VEGF-C or VEGF-D in skin results in lymphatic hyperplasia (66,67).

A number of other genes also have been shown to be important for proper development and function of the lymphatic vasculature. Podoplanin is not required for specification of the lymphatic vasculature (its expression also is regulated by *Prox-1*), but rather for the proper morphogenesis and/or function of lymphatic vessels. Podoplanin null mice have lymphatic vessels, but there is diminished lymphatic transport, congenital lymphedema, and dilation of lymphatic vessels (57). Angiopoietin 2 signaling through Tie2 is required for lymphangiogenesis and for proper angiogenic remodeling of blood vessels (68). This ligand is dispensable for embryonic vascular development despite its proposed important role as an antagonist of angiopoietin 1 signaling in VECs (69). Interestingly, the lymphatic but not vascular defects in angiopoietin 2 knockout mice can be rescued by angiopoietin 1, suggesting that in the lymphatic system, at least, angiopoietin 2 is functioning as a Tie2 agonist rather than an antagonist (68). The *Neuropilin-1* and *Neuropuilin-2* genes are believed to act as VEGFR cofactors in the vasculature. *Neuropilin-2* null mice display loss of smaller lymphatic vessels and capillaries, although larger vessels and lymph sacs still form,

suggesting a specific role in branching morphogenesis of smaller lymphatics (70).

CONCLUSION

Lymphatic, arterial, and venous vessels respond to the needs of local tissues and hemodynamic changes during adult life by remodeling or initiating new vessel growth. However, it has become clear that genetic programs during early development direct the specification of the endothelial progenitors for these vessels. A number of critical molecular regulators of A-V and lymphatic fate determination have now been identified, but our understanding of how these factors work together in defined molecular pathways is still limited.

REFERENCES

1. Risau W, Flamme I. Vasculogenesis. *Annu Rev Cell Dev Biol* 1995;11: 73–91.
2. Majesky MW, Dong X-R, Lu J. In: Tomanek RJ, ed. *Assembly of the vasculature and its regulation.* Boston: Birkhauser, 2002:111–131.
3. Oliver G, Detmar M. The rediscovery of the lymphatic system: old and new insights into the development and biological function of the lymphatic vasculature. *Genes Dev* 2002;16:773–783.
4. Sabin FR. On the origin of the lymphatic system from the veins, and the development of the lymph hearts and thoracic duct in the pig. *Am J Anat* 1902;1:367–389.
5. Sabin FR. On the development of the superficial lymphatics in the skin of the pig. *Am J Anat* 1904;3:183–195.
6. Huntington GS, McClure CF. The anatomy and development of the jugular lymphatic sac in the domestic cat *(Felis domestica). Am J Anat* 1910;10:177–311.
7. Wilting J, Papoutsi M, Schneider M, et al. The lymphatic endothelium of the avian wing is of somitic origin. *Dev Dyn* 2000;217:271–278.
8. Schneider M, Othman-Hassan K, Christ B, et al. Lymphangioblasts in the avian wing bud. *Dev Dyn* 1999;216:311–319.
9. Sabin FR. Studies on the origin of blood vessels and of red corpuscles as seen in the living blastoderm of the chick during the second day of incubation. *Contrib Embryol* 1920;9:213–262.
10. Forrai A, Robb L. The hemangioblast—between blood and vessels. *Cell Cycle* 2003;2:86–90.
11. Ema M, Rossant J. Cell fate decisions in early blood vessel formation. *Trends Cardiovasc Med* 2003;13:254–259.
12. Shalaby F, Rossant J, Yamaguchi TP, et al. Failure of blood-island formation and vasculogenesis in Flk-1-deficient mice. *Nature* 1995;376: 62–66.
13. Fong GH, Rossant J, Gertsenstein M, et al. Role of the Flt-1 receptor tyrosine kinase in regulating the assembly of vascular endothelium. *Nature* 1995;376:66–70.
14. Fong GH, Zhang L, Bryce DM, et al. Increased hemangioblast commitment, not vascular disorganization, is the primary defect in flt-1 knock-out mice. *Development* 1999;126:3015–3025.
15. Elefanty AG, Begley CG, Hartley L, et al. SCL expression in the mouse embryo detected with a targeted lacZ reporter gene demonstrates its localization to hematopoietic, vascular, and neural tissues. *Blood* 1999; 94:3754–3763.
16. Robb L, Elwood NJ, Elefanty AG, et al. The scl gene product is required for the generation of all hematopoietic lineages in the adult mouse. *EMBO J* 1996;15:4123–4129.
17. Robb L, Lyons I, Li R, et al. Absence of yolk sac hematopoiesis from mice with a targeted disruption of the scl gene. *Proc Natl Acad Sci USA* 1995;92:7075–7079.
18. Shivdasani RA, Mayer EL, Orkin SH. Absence of blood formation in mice lacking the T-cell leukaemia oncoprotein tal-1/SCL. *Nature* 1995;373:432–434.
19. Porcher C, Swat W, Rockwell K, et al. The T cell leukemia oncoprotein SCL/tal-1 is essential for development of all hematopoietic lineages. *Cell* 1996;86:47–57.

20. Visvader JE, Fujiwara Y, Orkin SH. Unsuspected role for the T-cell leukemia protein SCL/tal-1 in vascular development. *Genes Dev* 1998;12:473–479.

21. Gering M, Rodaway AR, Gottgens B, et al. The SCL gene specifies haemangioblast development from early mesoderm. *EMBO J* 1998;17:4029–4045.

22. Stainier DY, Weinstein BM, Detrich HW 3rd, et al. Cloche, an early acting zebrafish gene, is required by both the endothelial and hematopoietic lineages. *Development* 1995;121:3141–3150.

23. Liao W, Bisgrove BW, Sawyer H, et al. The zebrafish gene cloche acts upstream of a flk-1 homologue to regulate endothelial cell differentiation. *Development* 1997;124:381–389.

24. Thompson MA, Ransom DG, Pratt SJ, et al. The cloche and spadetail genes differentially affect hematopoiesis and vasculogenesis. *Dev Biol* 1998;197:248–269.

25. Liao W, Ho CY, Yan YL, et al. Hhex and scl function in parallel to regulate early endothelial and blood differentiation in zebrafish. *Development* 2000;127:4303–4313.

26. Brown LA, Rodaway AR, Schilling TF, et al. Insights into early vasculogenesis revealed by expression of the ETS domain transcription factor Fli-1 in wild-type and mutant zebrafish embryos. *Mech Dev* 2000;90:237–252.

27. Parker L, Stainier DY. Cell-autonomous and non-autonomous requirements for the zebrafish gene cloche in hematopoiesis. *Development* 1999;126:2643–2651.

28. Choi K, Kennedy M, Kazarov A, et al. A common precursor for hematopoietic and endothelial cells. *Development* 1998;125:725–732.

29. Chung YS, Zhang WJ, Arentson E, et al. Lineage analysis of the hemangioblast as defined by FLK1 and SCL expression. *Development* 2002;129:5511–5520.

30. Faloon P, Arentson E, Kazarov A, et al. Basic fibroblast growth factor positively regulates hematopoietic development. *Development* 2000;127:1931–1941.

31. Yamashita J, Itoh H, Hirashima M, et al. Flk1-positive cells derived from embryonic stem cells serve as vascular progenitors. *Nature* 2000;408:92–96.

32. Motoike T, Markham DW, Rossant J, et al. Evidence for novel fate of Flk1+ progenitor: contribution to muscle lineage. *Genesis* 2003;35:153–159.

33. Fehling HJ, Lacaud G, Kubo A, et al. Tracking mesoderm induction and its specification to the hemangioblast during embryonic stem cell differentiation. *Development* 2003;130:4217–4227.

34. Ema M, Faloon P, Zhang WJ, et al. Combinatorial effects of Flk1 and Tal1 on vascular and hematopoietic development in the mouse. *Genes Dev* 2003;17:380–393.

35. Cogle CR, Wainman DA, Jorgensen ML, et al. Adult human hematopoietic cells provide functional hemangioblast activity. *Blood* 2004;103:133–135.

36. Bailey AS, Jiang S, Afentoulis M, et al. Transplanted adult hematopoietic stem cells differentiate into functional endothelial cells. *Blood* 2004;103:13–19.

37. Lawson ND, Weinstein BM. Arteries and veins: making a difference with zebrafish. *Nat Rev Genet* 2002;3:674–682.

38. Weinstein BM, Lawson ND. Arteries, veins, notch, and VEGF. *Cold Spring Harb Symp Quant Biol* 2002;67:155–162.

39. D'Amore PA, Ng YS. Won't you be my neighbor? Local induction of arteriogenesis. *Cell* 2002;110:289–292.

40. Wang HU, Chen ZF, Anderson DJ. Molecular distinction and angiogenic interaction between embryonic arteries and veins revealed by ephrin-B2 and its receptor Eph-B4. *Cell* 1998;93:741–753.

41. Gerety SS, Anderson DJ. Cardiovascular ephrinB2 function is essential for embryonic angiogenesis. *Development* 2002;129:1397–1410.

42. Torres-Vazquez J, Kamei M, Weinstein BM. Molecular distinction between arteries and veins. *Cell Tissue Res* 2003;314:43–59.

43. Zhong TP, Childs S, Leu JP, et al. Gridlock signalling pathway fashions the first embryonic artery. *Nature* 2001;414:216–220.

44. Lawson ND, Vogel AM, Weinstein BM. Sonic hedgehog and vascular endothelial growth factor act upstream of the Notch pathway during arterial endothelial differentiation. *Dev Cell* 2002;3:127–136.

45. Lawson ND, Scheer N, Pham VN, et al. Notch signaling is required for arterial-venous differentiation during embryonic vascular development. *Development* 2001;128:3675–3683.

46. Lawson ND, Mugford JW, Diamond BA, et al. phospholipase C gamma-1 is required downstream of vascular endothelial growth factor during arterial development. *Genes Dev* 2003;17:1346–1351.

47. Pola R, Ling LE, Silver M, et al. The morphogen Sonic hedgehog is an indirect angiogenic agent upregulating two families of angiogenic growth factors. *Nat Med* 2001;7:706–711.

48. Mukouyama YS, Shin D, Britsch S, et al. Sensory nerves determine the pattern of arterial differentiation and blood vessel branching in the skin. *Cell* 2002;109:693–705.

49. Visconti RP, Richardson CD, Sato TN. Orchestration of angiogenesis and arteriovenous contribution by angiopoietins and vascular endothelial growth factor (VEGF). *Proc Natl Acad Sci USA* 2002;99:8219–8224.

50. Springer ML, Ozawa CR, Banfi A, et al. Localized arteriole formation directly adjacent to the site of VEGF-Induced angiogenesis in muscle. *Mol Ther* 2003;7:441–449.

51. Shawber CJ, Das I, Francisco E, et al. Notch signaling in primary endothelial cells. *Ann NY Acad Sci* 2003;995:162–170.

52. Liu ZJ, Shirakawa T, Li Y, et al. Regulation of Notch1 and Dll4 by vascular endothelial growth factor in arterial endothelial cells: implications for modulating arteriogenesis and angiogenesis. *Mol Cell Biol* 2003;23:14–25.

53. Othman-Hassan K, Patel K, Papoutsi M, et al. Arterial identity of endothelial cells is controlled by local cues. *Dev Biol* 2001;237:398–409.

54. Moyon D, Pardanaud L, Yuan L, et al. Plasticity of endothelial cells during arterial-venous differentiation in the avian embryo. *Development* 2001;128:3359–3370.

55. Prevo R, Banerji S, Ferguson DJ, et al. Mouse LYVE-1 is an endocytic receptor for hyaluronan in lymphatic endothelium. *J Biol Chem* 2001;276:19420–19430.

56. Jackson DG. The lymphatics revisited: new perspectives from the hyaluronan receptor LYVE-1. *Trends Cardiovasc Med* 2003;13:1–7.

57. Schacht V, Ramirez MI, Hong YK, et al. T1alpha/podoplanin deficiency disrupts normal lymphatic vasculature formation and causes lymphedema. *EMBO J* 2003;22:3546–3556.

58. Dumont DJ, Jussila L, Taipale J, et al. Cardiovascular failure in mouse embryos deficient in VEGF receptor-3. *Science* 1998;282:946–949.

59. Kaipainen A, Korhonen J, Mustonen T, et al. Expression of the fms-like tyrosine kinase 4 gene becomes restricted to lymphatic endothelium during development. *Proc Natl Acad Sci USA* 1995;92:3566–3570.

60. Wigle JT, Oliver G. Prox1 function is required for the development of the murine lymphatic system. *Cell* 1999;98:769–778.

61. Wigle JT, Harvey N, Detmar M, et al. An essential role for Prox1 in the induction of the lymphatic endothelial cell phenotype. *EMBO J* 2002;21:1505–1513.

62. Petrova TV, Makinen T, Makela TP, et al. Lymphatic endothelial reprogramming of vascular endothelial cells by the Prox-1 homeobox transcription factor. *EMBO J* 2002;21:4593–4599.

63. Hong YK, Harvey N, Noh YH, et al. Prox1 is a master control gene in the program specifying lymphatic endothelial cell fate. *Dev Dyn* 2002;225:351–357.

64. Karkkainen MJ, Ferrell RE, Lawrence EC, et al. Missense mutations interfere with VEGFR-3 signalling in primary lymphoedema. *Nat Genet* 2000;25:153–159.

65. Makinen T, Jussila L, Veikkola T, et al. Inhibition of lymphangiogenesis with resulting lymphedema in transgenic mice expressing soluble VEGF receptor-3. *Nat Med* 2001;7:199–205.

66. Veikkola T, Jussila L, Makinen T, et al. Signalling via vascular endothelial growth factor receptor-3 is sufficient for lymphangiogenesis in transgenic mice. *EMBO J* 2001;20:1223–1231.

67. Jeltsch M, Kaipainen A, Joukov V, et al. Hyperplasia of lymphatic vessels in VEGF-C transgenic mice. *Science* 1997;276:1423–1425.

68. Gale NW, Thurston G, Hackett SF, et al. Angiopoietin-2 is required for postnatal angiogenesis and lymphatic patterning, and only the latter role is rescued by Angiopoietin-1. *Dev Cell* 2002;3:411–423.

69. Maisonpierre PC, Suri C, Jones PF, et al. Angiopoietin-2, a natural antagonist for Tie2 that disrupts in vivo angiogenesis. *Science* 1997;277:55–60.

70. Yuan L, Moyon D, Pardanaud L, et al. Abnormal lymphatic vessel development in neuropilin 2 mutant mice. *Development* 2002;129:4797–4806.

CHAPTER **25**

Mouse Models of Lipoprotein Disorders and Atherosclerosis

Andrew S. Plump

Key Words: Atherosclerosis; knockout; lipoproteins; mouse; transgenic.

A complex set of environmental and genetic determinants define a human's susceptibility to atherosclerosis. A continuum of genetic susceptibility exists in the general population. At one extreme, individuals with monogenic disorders such as low-density lipoprotein (LDL) receptor deficiency (familial hypercholesterolemia [FH]) will experience uniform development of clinically relevant atherosclerosis, regardless of environmental influences. At the other extreme, certain individuals with a genetic tendency toward very high levels of high-density lipoprotein cholesterol (HDL-C) will almost never experience development of clinically relevant atherosclerosis. For most, though, a mixture of underlying

genetic predisposition and environmental influences will determine susceptibility.

Despite a substantial knowledge of the genes that determine susceptibility in patients with monogenic disorders, little is known of the interplay of polygenetic factors in the general population. To dissect atherosclerosis susceptibility, scientists rely on a combination of mouse and human genetics. This chapter highlights the former model organism, focusing specifically on genes involved in lipoprotein metabolism. By assessing the role of genes individually and in combination, the mouse offers a powerful system for understanding the biology of lipoprotein metabolism and atherosclerosis. The use of modern genomic technology in combination with mouse genetics will eventually result in a thorough understanding of atherosclerosis susceptibility and streamline therapies.

Monogenic causes of atherosclerosis have long been studied. In recent years, a series of novel atherosclerosis-related genes involved in human monogenic disorders have been identified. For many of these human genetic diseases, phe-

A. S. Plump: Clinical Molecular Profiling, Merck Research Laboratory, 126 East Lincoln Avenue, Rahway, New Jersey 07065.

notypically the pathology has been apparent for quite some time, but the genetic etiology has been elusive. The genomics era has heralded the discovery of several of these genes, including those for hereditary sitosterolemia (1), Tangier disease (2,3), Niemann Pick Type C (4), and additional genes for FH (5). The recent cloning of these genes and the identification of a handful of additional lipid metabolism genes, such as apolipoprotein A-V (6) and endothelial lipase (EL) (7), has provided lipoprotein biologists with a new set of factors that influence the complex set of events that determine lipid profiles and atherosclerosis susceptibility and pathogenesis. Although genetic deficiency of each of these genes is rare, they clearly are key players in the regulation of physiologically relevant lipid trafficking and lipoprotein metabolism, and the potential exists (and requires further study) that common genetic variation in these genes contributes to atherosclerosis susceptibility in the general population. The mouse has been a critical tool for understanding the function that each of these genes plays in lipid metabolism and atherosclerosis susceptibility.

Although the mouse is inadequate at times in terms of its relevance to human lipid and atherosclerosis biology, it offers a tremendously powerful substrate to study physiology and pathogenesis. Long argued as a poor model for human atherogenesis, the mouse has become the front-line model for studying genetic, environmental, and pharmacologic influences on lipid metabolism and atherogenesis. The generation of apolipoprotein E (apoE)–deficient (8,9) and LDL receptor–deficient mice (10,11) has led to nearly a decade of studies with publications numbering in the thousands, and an unprecedented understanding of this complex biologic process and fatal disease.

This chapter reviews the history of the mouse as a model organism, focusing initially and extensively on efforts to model the various lipoprotein abnormalities most commonly associated with human coronary artery disease (CAD). Then it centers on the existence and relative use of various mouse models (Fig. 25–1), and finally highlights a number of recent studies defining the role of newly recognized atherosclerosis susceptibility genes (such as the Tangier disease gene and adenosine triphosphate–binding cassette transporter A1 [ABCA1]), biological processes (such as lipoxygenase-mediated lipid modification), and drugs (such as the glucose decreasing peroxisome proliferator-activated receptor γ [PPAR-γ] agonists known as thiazolidinediones or glitazones). The literature is massive

with respect to mouse studies of lipid metabolism and atherosclerosis, and a complete review is beyond the scope of this chapter. This overview has been designed to identify some of the critical studies and provide examples of where the mouse has been particularly useful in either proving existing dogma or in uncovering new biology.

HUMAN LIPOPROTEIN PATTERNS AND ATHEROSCLEROSIS

In humans, lipoprotein disorders are strongly associated with CAD susceptibility. Several types of abnormal lipoprotein patterns are commonly observed in heart attack victims, including: (a) increased LDL-C; (b) decreased HDL-C, usually with increased triglycerides (commonly seen in the metabolic syndrome, in which this lipoprotein pattern is associated with hypertension, obesity, and insulin resistance); (c) increased chylomicron remnant and intermediate density lipoprotein cholesterol (IDL-C) levels; and (d) increased levels of lipoprotein(a) [Lp(a)]. These patterns are caused by an interplay of environmental or genetic factors, or both, that alter the synthesis, processing, or catabolism of lipoprotein particles. The genes encoding lipoprotein transport proteins, including apolipoproteins that coat lipoprotein particles, lipoprotein-processing enzymes, and lipoprotein receptors, have been used as candidates to identify mutations underlying lipoprotein phenotypes associated with CAD susceptibility (12). Their role in lipoprotein transport is described in Figure 25–2, and the existence of mouse models for each of these patterns is outlined in Table 25–1.

INCREASED LOW-DENSITY LIPOPROTEIN CHOLESTEROL LEVELS

Increased levels of LDL-C are a significant risk factor for CAD in humans. There is a 2% to 3% increased risk for heart disease for each 1 mg/dL change in LDL-C levels. LDL particles are a constituent of the endogenous (nondietary) fat transport pathway (Fig. 25–2). Dietary carbohydrate or fat reaching the liver not required for energy or synthetic purposes is converted into triglycerides, packaged with apolipoproteins, and secreted as very low-density lipoprotein (VLDL) particles. Lipoprotein lipase (LPL) present on the capillary endothelium, mainly in adipose tissue and skeletal muscle, hydrolyzes VLDL core triglyc-

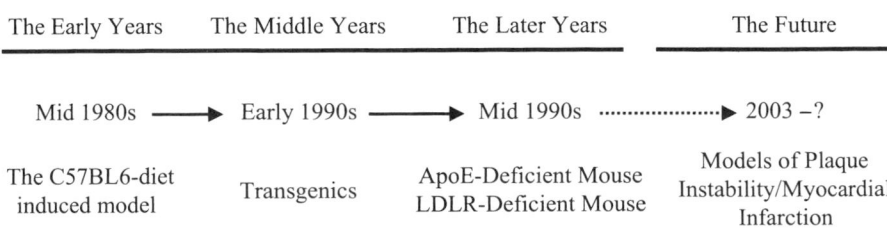

FIG. 25–1. The mouse as an atherosclerosis model: two decades of experience.

A   EXOGENOUS FAT TRANSPORT

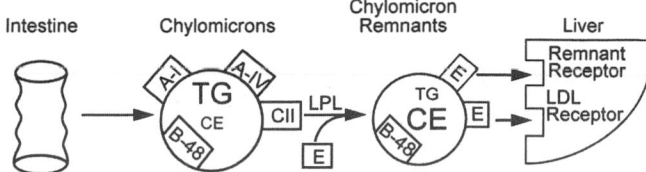

B   ENDOGENOUS FAT TRANSPORT

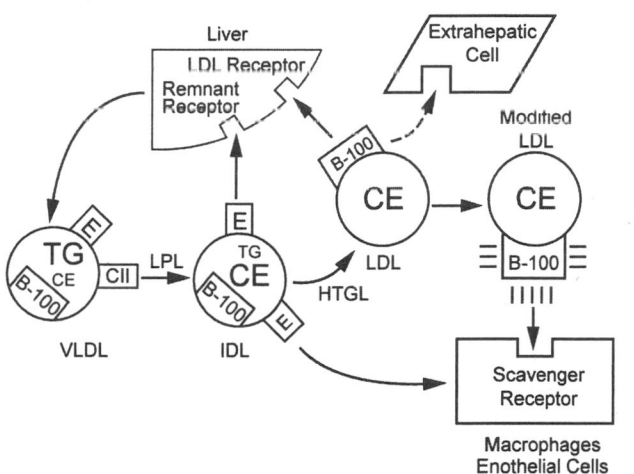

C   REVERSE CHOLESTEROL TRANSPORT

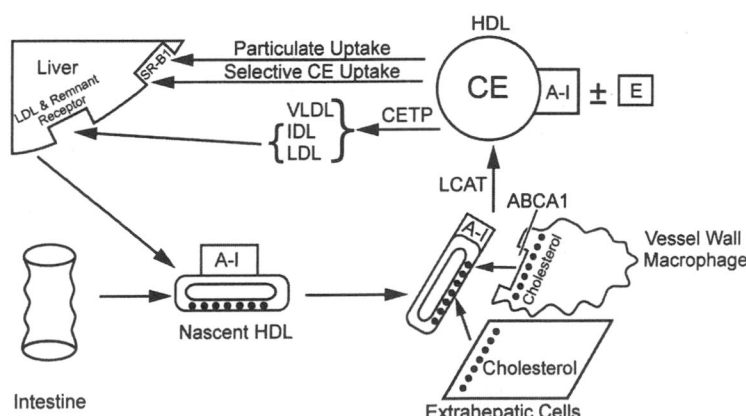

FIG. 25–2. The major lipoprotein metabolic pathways. ABCA1, adenosine triphosphate–binding cassette transporter A1; CE, cholesterol ester; CETP, cholesteryl ester transfer protein; HDL, high-density lipoprotein; HTGL, hepatic triglyceride lipase; IDL, intermediate density lipoprotein; LCAT, lecithin cholesterol acyltransferase; LDL, low-density lipoprotein; LPL, lipoprotein lipase; SR, scavenger receptor; TG, triglyceride; VLDL, very low-density lipoprotein.

erides, resulting in the conversion of VLDL to IDL. The liberated fatty acids are reesterified to form triglycerides in adipose tissue or are oxidized to generate energy in muscle. IDL is cleared from plasma by the LDL receptor, which binds apoE on the IDL surface. IDL particles that escape clearance by this route are subject to further triglyceride hydrolysis by hepatic lipase (HL) to form cholesterol ester–enriched LDL particles. The LDL surface contains a single molecule of apoB, which is recognized by LDL receptors. Approximately 70% of LDL is cleared by the LDL receptor (primarily in the liver).

Mouse lipoprotein metabolism differs from that in humans (Table 25–2). The mouse is a poor model for increased

LDL-C levels. On a chow diet, mouse LDL-C levels are less than 10 mg/dL, and on a Western-type diet, levels are less than 20 mg/dL. This contrasts with average human LDL-C levels of ~140 mg/dL. Several inherited disorders are recognized in humans that cause high levels of LDL-C, and these disorders have suggested genetic manipulations in the mouse that could be used to produce animals with increased LDL-C levels.

The first of these conditions is FH, an autosomal-dominant disorder caused by a defective LDL receptor gene and characterized by increased plasma LDL. Two phenomena contribute to increased LDL levels: decreased degradation and increased synthesis. Reduction in functional cell

TABLE 25–1. *Examples of mouse models of human lipoprotein disorders associated with enhanced coronary artery disease susceptibility*

Lipoprotein pattern	Mouse	Reference
↑ LDL-C	LDL receptor–deficient	10
	apoB transgenic	18–20
↓ HDL-C and ↑ VLDL triglyceride	apoA-I–deficient	37–39
	apoC-III transgenic	66,67
	apoC-I transgenic	68
	apoC-II transgenic	69
	CETP transgenic	70,73,57,103
	apoA-I, CETP transgenic	95
	apoA-I, apoC-III, CETP transgenic	72
↑ IDL and chylomicron remnant cholesterol	apoE-deficient	8,9,94
	apoE$_{3\text{-Leiden}}$	92
	apoE$_4$-Arg^{142}Cys transgenic	93
↑ Lp(a)	Apo(a) transgenic	97
	Apo(a), apoB transgenic	19,20

apo, apolipoprotein; CETP, cholesterol ester transfer protein; HDL-C, high-density lipoprotein cholesterol; IDL, intermediate-density lipoprotein; LDL-C, low-density lipoprotein cholesterol; Lp(a), lipoprotein(a); VLDL, very low-density lipoprotein.

surface LDL receptor molecules impairs LDL catabolism, and failure to carry out receptor-mediated IDL uptake results in enhanced conversion of IDL to LDL, increasing LDL synthesis. FH heterozygotes have LDL-C levels approximately double those in unaffected family members. They have premature CAD and premature mortality. FH homozygotes have LDL-C levels in the 600 to 1,000 mg/dL range. CAD often is apparent before age 10 years, and most untreated homozygotes experience fatal myocardial infarction before age 20 years. In addition to tendon xanthomas, planar cutaneous xanthomas develop in homozygotes.

Low-Density Lipoprotein Receptor Transgenic Mice

Two lines of LDL receptor transgenic mice have been created: First, a human LDL receptor cDNA driven by an inducible metallothionein-I promoter (13), and the second, a human LDL receptor minigene driven by the constitutively expressed transferrin receptor promoter (14). Mice with the LDL receptor under control of the inducible promoter express low levels of hepatic LDL receptor in the uninduced state, but increase expression twofold when induced with the metallothionein promotor-sensitive element: cad-

TABLE 25–2. *Critical differences in lipoprotein profiles and atherosclerosis sensitivity in humans and mice*

Parameter	Human	Mouse
HDL	~50 mg/dL	~50 mg/dL
LDL	~140 mg/dL	~10 mg/dL
CETP	Present	Absent
Lp(a)	Present	Absent
apoB editing	Intestine	Liver, intestine
Atherosclerosis	Susceptible	Resistant

apoB, apolipoprotein B; CETP, cholesterol ester transfer protein; HDL, high-density lipoprotein; LDL, low-density lipoprotein; Lp(a), lipoprotein(a).

mium. After cadmium induction, transgenic mice clear injected radiolabeled LDL 8 to 10 times faster than control mice, and the plasma concentrations of LDL receptor ligands, apoB and apoE, decline by more than 90%. Unfortunately, when administered over extended periods, cadmium has significant hepatotoxicity, thus precluding long-term studies. In the transferrin receptor-driven LDL receptor transgenic mice, high levels of hepatic LDL receptor activity could be achieved without toxicity. After a high cholesterol–containing diet, a diet that normally leads to substantial increases in IDL and LDL in mice, IDL and LDL levels were unaffected in these mice. Unregulated expression of LDL receptors thus can affect the dietary responsiveness of plasma IDL and LDL levels. By extension, variability in LDL receptor expression in humans may help to explain the differences in diet-induced IDL and LDL levels seen from person to person.

Low-Density Lipoprotein Receptor–Deficient Mice

LDL receptor knockout mice experience an eightfold increase in IDL- and LDL-C levels as a result of decreased lipoprotein clearance (10). The LDL receptor typically acts to remove lipoproteins that contain the largest apolipoprotein, apoB, using either apoB or apoE as a ligand (15). Studies in these mice further support a role for LDL receptor variation in determining the response of plasma cholesterol to dietary fat and cholesterol intake. When fed a high-fat, 0.2% cholesterol, 10% coconut oil diet, the LDL receptor–deficient mice have an additional threefold increase in the IDL plus LDL-C level, whereas this diet does not affect these lipoproteins in control mice.

The LDL receptor knockout mice also have been used as a model for gene replacement therapy. Intravenous administration of an adenovirus vector containing a human LDL receptor cDNA driven by the cytomegalovirus promoter causes high levels of hepatic LDL receptor expression, increased clearance of apoB-containing lipoproteins, and reduced IDL and LDL lipoproteins. These data support similar experiments in LDL receptor–deficient humans (familial hypercholesterolemics) (16) and LDL receptor–deficient rabbits (Watanabe heritable hyperlipidemic rabbits) (17) in which various viral delivery systems have been used to ameliorate, at least temporarily, the hypercholesterolemia found in the LDL receptor–deficient state.

Apolipoprotein B Transgenic Mice

There are two other inherited conditions in humans characterized by increased LDL-C. The first condition is familial defective apoB, in which an amino acid substitution leads to disrupted apoB binding to the LDL receptor and impaired LDL uptake. Heterozygosity for this disorder increases LDL-C levels by at least 50%. The second condition is familial combined hyperlipidemia (FCHL), a complex but common disorder of unknown cause. This disorder is characterized by varying degrees of increases of VLDL-C, LDL-C, and VLDL triglycerides, as well as VLDL overproduction. Familial defective apoB and FCHL suggest that production of a receptor-binding defective form of apoB or overproduction of apoB in mouse liver would increase mouse LDL-C levels. Because human apoB is recognized poorly by mouse LDL receptors, both strategies can be realized by creating transgenic mice that overproduce human apoB in the liver.

In humans, full-length apoB, B-100, is produced in the liver, whereas truncated apoB, B-48, is produced in the intestine by a messenger RNA (mRNA) editing mechanism. In rodent liver, apoB mRNA editing also occurs, so mouse liver produces both B-48 and B-100. Transgenic mice expressing a human apoB minigene have very low levels of human apoB in plasma (<1% of normal), but the human apoB mRNA transcripts produced in the transgenic mouse liver undergo editing at an efficiency comparable to endogenous mouse apoB mRNA (18). This indicates that the apoB mRNA editing process can occur across species. Human apoB transgenic mice also have been made with the entire 43-kb gene and 15 to 20 kb of 5′ and 3′ flanking sequence (19,20). Human apoB mRNA was found only in the liver, and mRNA editing occurred. High expressing human apoB transgenic mice have increased total cholesterol with an increase in LDL-C. A major difference between mouse and human lipoprotein patterns is the low LDL-C level in the mouse. The human apoB transgenic mice are more similar to humans in this respect, although the absolute levels of LDL-C are still low compared with those in individuals with hypercholesterolemia. The apoB editing–deficient mouse (apoBEC$^{-/-}$), when crossed with an LDL receptor–deficient mouse, is another example of a high LDL model (21).

Gene targeting has been used to alter the endogenous mouse apoB gene (22–24), and a mouse was created that expressed a truncated protein that is 70% of the wild-type size. This mimics human hypobetalipoproteinemia, a disorder associated with a variety of truncated apoB mutations and characterized by low plasma cholesterol and triglyceride levels. Mice homozygous for the mutant apoB-70 allele have reduced VLDL-C, IDL-C, LDL-C, and triglyceride levels. These mice are an excellent model of hypobetalipoproteinemia; however, they also display findings not associated with human hypobetalipoproteinemia such as low HDL-C levels and central nervous system abnormalities, exencephalus and hydrocephalus, for reasons that are not known.

REDUCED HIGH-DENSITY LIPOPROTEIN CHOLESTEROL AND INCREASED TRIGLYCERIDE LEVELS

Reduced HDL-C is the most common lipoprotein abnormality associated with CAD. Each 1 mg/dL decrease in HDL-C is associated with a 4% increase in CAD risk. Low HDL-C often is found along with other lipoprotein abnormalities, including high levels of triglycerides in VLDL and increased levels of IDL and small, dense LDL. Nascent HDL particles produced by the liver and small intestine consist primarily of complexes of phospholipid and apoA-I, and remodeling of these particles occurs as they circulate in plasma. The HDL particles attract excess free cholesterol from extrahepatic tissues and from other types of lipoprotein particles. The cholesterol is esterified by the enzyme lecithin cholesterol acyl transferase (LCAT) using apoA-I and, to a lesser extent, other apolipoproteins as cofactors, and the resulting cholesterol ester enters the HDL core, enlarging the particle. The HDL particles may become smaller as a result of the action of cholesteryl ester transfer protein (CETP), which exchanges the cholesterol ester in HDLs for triglyceride in VLDLs and IDLs. HL can then hydrolyze HDL triglycerides, reducing HDL size. Excess cholesterol in peripheral tissues thus can be transferred from HDL to other lipoprotein particles, which are cleared from plasma primarily by hepatic receptors. This process, termed *reverse cholesterol transport,* may account in part for the protective effect of HDL on atherosclerosis susceptibility (Fig. 25–2).

Apolipoprotein A-I Transgenic Mice

Levels of HDL-C are strongly correlated with the levels of its major apolipoprotein, apoA-I. Transgenic animals have been made with the human apoA-I gene (25–27). The apoA-I gene is in a gene cluster consisting in order of apoA-I, apoC-III, and apoA-IV, and it is expressed primarily in the liver and intestine. Experiments in transgenic mice have revealed a region approximately 6 kb 3′ to the apoA-I gene, required for apoA-I intestinal expression. A hormone-responsive element in this region has been shown to direct intestinal apoA-I expression and also influence hepatic expression (28).

ApoA-I overexpression in mice selectively increases HDL-C levels. Human apoA-I expression in the mouse also results in decreased levels of mouse apoA-I (27,29,30), as well as changes in the physical properties of HDL. Mouse HDL normally consists of a single major size distribution of particles approximately 10 nM in diameter. In human apoA-I transgenic mice, there are two major size distributions of particles, with diameters of approximately 10.3 and 8.8 nM. This corresponds to the two major size distributions of HDL particles in human plasma, HDL$_{2b}$ and HDL$_{3a}$, respectively. The transgenic mouse studies show that the structure of apoA-I is an important determinant of HDL particle size distribution and suggest an explanation for HDL subspeciation in humans.

Human apoA-I transgenic mice have served as a model system to examine the mechanisms whereby diet and drugs alter HDL-C and apoA-I levels. A high-fat Western-type diet increases HDL-C and apoA-I levels in humans, and this effect has been mimicked in transgenic mice (31). Following a high-cholesterol diet there is an increase in HDL cholesterol ester and apoA-I synthetic rates without an increase in apoA-I mRNA levels (31). Transgenic CETP models also have been used to define mechanisms whereby diet and endogenous changes in cholesterol can affect CETP expression, again suggesting a transcriptional regulation of cholesterol homeostasis. Transgenic studies have shown that CETP contains natural flanking sequences that are bound and activated by the nuclear hormone receptor, LXR, a transcription factor critical for the regulation of many lipid-responsive genes that mediate up-regulation in response to dietary or endogenous cholesterol (32–35). The identification of apoA-I and CETP promotor elements that mediate cholesterol responsiveness highlights the use of transgenic models in understanding diet–gene relations.

In addition to use as a model organism for assessing the mechanism of dietary responsiveness, transgenic mice have been useful in elucidating drug effects. The lipid-lowering and antioxidant drug probucol decreases HDL-C and apoA-I levels, an effect that is reproducible in transgenic mice (36). In probucol-treated mice, HDL cholesterol ester fractional catabolic rate increased and apoA-I synthetic rate decreased, although there was no change in apoA-I mRNA levels.

When considered together, the diet and drug studies suggest a pattern of biologic responses. Over the wide range of apoA-I levels observed in the high-fat feeding and probucol experiments, there were no changes observed in apoA-I fractional catabolic rates or in apoA-I mRNA levels. Two interesting implications can be drawn from these studies. The first implication is that over the physiologic range of apoA-I levels there is no saturable apoA-I or HDL receptor. The second implication is that previously unrecognized, potent, post-mRNA levels of regulation exist that regulate apoA-I production in relevant clinical situations.

Apolipoprotein A-I–Deficient Mice

Although it is clear that low HDL-C levels are an important risk factor for CAD in the general population, there is little understanding of mechanism. Several theories have been proposed: Low HDL reflects decreased reverse cholesterol transport from peripheral tissues including the artery wall to the liver, where it can be excreted; low HDL results in decreased direct protection of the blood vessel wall; HDL acts as an antioxidant; HDL can alter expression of adhesion molecules, such as vascular cell adhesion molecule-1, necessary for inflammatory cell infiltration into the vessel wall; and low HDL is merely reflective of increased levels of atherogenic lipoproteins such as VLDL, IDL, and small, dense LDL.

The physiological consequences of low HDL have been modeled in mice. ApoA-I knockout mice have been created by gene targeting in embryonic stem cells (37,38). ApoA-I–deficient mice maintained on a chow diet have a 75% reduction in total and HDL-C levels. These mice have been used to study reverse cholesterol transport. The amount of cholesterol ester flux through HDL is diminished by more than sevenfold in apoA-I–deficient mice, a decrease consistent with the ~10-fold decrease in HDL cholesterol ester levels. Despite this large decrease in cholesterol flux, peripheral tissues do not accumulate cholesterol or cholesterol ester, and these mice do not experience development of atherosclerosis (38,39).

These observations suggest that either the amount of non–HDL-C in the apoA-I–deficient mice is not sufficient to induce cholesterol loading in peripheral tissues and macrophages of the arterial intima, or that homeostatic mechanisms are being invoked in peripheral tissues to compensate for the diminished flux (e.g., decreased LDL receptor and 3-hydroxy-3-methylglutaryl coenzyme A [HMG-CoA] reductase activity). In all likelihood, a combination of decreased loading, reduced LDL receptor activity, and decreased peripheral biosynthesis contributes to the absence of peripheral cholesterol accumulation. To test the former hypothesis, apoA-I–deficient mice were bred onto a line of mice with high levels of LDL (apoB transgenic) and fed a high-fat diet (40). The apoA-I null, apoB-expressing transgenic mice developed significantly more lesion area than control mice.

Reverse cholesterol transport involves the delivery of peripheral cholesterol stores (such as those from deposits in atherosclerotic lesions) to the liver. In apoA-I–deficient mice, the liver was found to have normal cholesterol and cholesterol ester stores (38). Although levels of hepatic LDL receptor and HMG-CoA reductase mRNA was normal, 7α-hydroxylase mRNA was decreased by more than 60%. These data suggest that in response to diminished HDL-C flux to the liver, apoA-I–deficient mice are regulating intrahepatic cholesterol levels by decreasing cholesterol excretion in the form of bile acids. The study of reverse cholesterol transport cannot be done directly because cholesterol easily diffuses across lipid surfaces, making labeling studies challenging to interpret; therefore the effect of apoA-I deficiency and the resulting decrease in HDL-C on reverse cholesterol transport has been challenging to assess, and that it results in increased atherosclerosis in an atherosensitive animal does not speak to mechanism (i.e., a loss of direct protective effects of HDL vs. decreased reverse cholesterol transport). Follow-up studies, however, suggest that the apoA-I–deficient HDL has less ability to accept cholesterol from cultured fibroblasts and from an *in vivo* tissue depot than control HDL, lending support to a defect in the reverse cholesterol transport cascade (41,42).

In summary, apoA-I deficiency leads to significant reductions in HDL-C levels and HDL cholesterol ester flux, and it likely leads to diminished reverse cholesterol transport, although definitive demonstration of the latter is still needed.

Apolipoprotein A-II Transgenic Mice

The second most abundant HDL protein is apoA-II, and transgenic mice expressing human apoA-II have been produced (43–45). ApoA-II transgenic mice develop hypertriglyceridemia and low HDL-C (44,45), phenomena related to multiple factors including functional deficits in LCAT and HL activity, leading to both decreased production and increased clearance of HDL-C (46,47). The clinical relevance of these findings is not clear, but the inability of excess apoA-II production to increase HDL-C is compatible with clinical studies that fail to show a correlation between plasma apoA-II and HDL-C levels and the relatively normal HDL-C levels reported in an apoA-II–deficient patient (48). The human apoA-II transgenics did show an alteration of HDL particle size with the appearance of a population of 8.0 n*M*-diameter particles, consisting almost entirely of human apoA-II. The larger, endogenous particles consisted of mouse apoA-I and either mouse or human apoA-II. Thus, human apoA-II appears to affect the quality of HDL particles.

A transgenic mouse line expressing mouse apoA-II was derived with a twofold to threefold increase of apoA-II levels (49). These animals have a twofold increase in HDL-C levels, larger HDL particles, and a twofold to threefold increase in non–HDL-C and triglyceride levels. The marked differences in the lipoprotein profiles between mouse and human apoA-II transgenics may be caused by the different physical properties of the two proteins. Mouse apoA-II is monomeric, whereas human apoA-II is homodimeric. In addition, the two proteins are only about 60% identical in their amino acid sequences. As with apoA-I, apoA-II provides another example of how species differences can affect apolipoprotein behavior *in vivo* and offers a unique perspective on apolipoprotein function.

Lipase Transgenic Mice

Four lipases are critical for proper lipoprotein metabolism in humans: LPL, HL, EL, and hormone-sensitive lipase (HSL). Each has different specificity for lipoproteins, and whereas LPL, HSL, and HL preferentially act on triglycerides, EL has greater specificity for phospholipids. The lipases have distinct functions with respect to modulating lipoprotein and

lipid trafficking. Low HDL-C levels often are associated with high triglycerides. The principal triglyceride-rich lipoproteins are VLDL and chylomicrons. The initial step in the metabolism of these particles is triglyceride hydrolysis, carried out by LPL, a molecule that resides on endothelial surfaces, principally in muscle and adipose tissue. LPL is known to require apoC-II as a cofactor.

Transgenic and knockout mice have been made that overexpress or underexpress each of the lipases. LPL overexpression leads to reduced serum triglycerides, increased HDL levels, accelerated clearance of VLDLs, rapid clearance of dietary fat, suppression of diet-induced hypercholesterolemia following a high-cholesterol diet, and reduced atherogenesis (50,51). In addition, muscle-specific expression of LPL leads to accumulation of intramuscular fatty acids and subsequent insulin resistance (52,53). Interestingly, catalytically inactive LPL transgenics have been constructed and have demonstrated that LPL can act as a bridging factor allowing for receptor-mediated uptake of circulating VLDL, suggesting that its role in lipoprotein metabolism extends beyond its enzymatic function (54). Mice deficient in LPL die in the perinatal period because of overwhelming hypertriglyceridemia and stasis of blood flow in the pulmonary vasculature (55). The LPL transgenic mice confirm that LPL has a strong influence on triglyceride levels *in vivo* and suggest that LPL genetic variation may influence responsiveness to dietary cholesterol in humans.

HL (56–61), HSL (62–64), and EL (7,65) also have been studied in transgenic and knockout mice. EL was the most recent of the lipases to be cloned, and its preferential phospholipase activity (and its expression in cultured endothelial cells) distinguish it. Despite its limited triglyceride hydrolytic activity, animals that overexpress EL have decreased HDL-C levels (7) and knockout mice have increased HDL-C levels (65), demonstrating a pivotal role for this novel lipase in lipoprotein metabolism, and perhaps atherosclerosis susceptibility.

Apolipoprotein C Transgenic Mice

The apoC genes have LPL modulatory ability. Prior to transgenic studies in mice, apoC-II was recognized in humans to be a critical LPL cofactor. The ability of the apoC-I and apoC-III to modulate LPL activity was uncovered by transgenic mice studies. The apoC-III story is particularly intriguing, because its role in triglyceride metabolism was accidentally uncovered in a "genetic accident." In the course of making transgenic mice to study the *cis*-acting regions responsible for the tissue-specific expression of the apoA-I gene, a DNA construction was used that contained the apoA-I gene plus the neighboring apoC-III gene, which codes for a protein found in VLDL and HDL (14). These mice were found to have massive hypertriglyceridemia, whereas mice made with the apoA-I gene alone had normal triglyceride levels. To determine the physiologic relevance of these findings, several transgenic mouse lines were subsequently made with only the apoC-III gene, and triglyceride levels were found to be proportional to apoC-III gene expression and human apoC-III plasma concentrations (66).

The human apoC-III transgenic mice were the first animal model of primary hypertriglyceridemia. The mechanism of primary hypertriglyceridemia has been extensively studied in apoC-III transgenic mice (67). These animals accumulate large, triglyceride-rich VLDLs, with an increased apoC-III/apoE ratio. The increased VLDL triglyceride level results from decreased VLDL fractional catabolic rate with a small increase in the VLDL triglyceride (but not apoB) production rate. *In vitro*, the transgenic VLDL has decreased LDL receptor–mediated uptake by tissue culture cells but normal lipolysis by purified LPL. Thus, the hypertriglyceridemia appears to result from a prolonged VLDL residence time because of a combination of slightly increased production and delayed clearance, a process that, interestingly, does not lead to the accumulation of cholesterol ester–enriched remnant particles. This implies decreased *in vivo* lipolysis and tissue uptake, presumably secondary to altered surface apolipoprotein composition.

Transgenic mouse models of hypertriglyceridemia also have been made with apoC-I and apoC-II. Human apoC-I transgenics are mildly hypertriglyceridemic (68). The human apoC-II transgenic mice are as hypertriglyceridemic as the apoC-III transgenics, a surprising result considering that apoC-II is an activator of LPL (69). As with the human apoC-III transgenics, the human apoC-II transgenic mice accumulate VLDL of almost normal size but with an increased apoC/apoE ratio. These mice also have delayed VLDL clearance but not increased production. The human apoC-II transgenic mouse VLDL had markedly decreased binding to heparin-Sepharose, suggesting that apoC-II–rich, apoE–poor VLDL may be less accessible to cell surface lipases or receptors within capillary-associated glycosaminoglycan matrices. The human apoC-II transgenic mice are a model of primary hypertriglyceridemia and suggest a more complex role for apoC-II in the metabolism of triglycerides than previously thought. apoC-II deficiency is known to cause hypertriglyceridemia by decreasing LPL activity. Overproduction of apoC-II might do this as well, probably by preventing association of VLDL with matrix-bound LPL.

Cholesterol Ester Transfer Protein Transgenic Mice

The mouse lacks CETP activity. In humans, it is thought that hypertriglyceridemia actually causes low HDL-C levels through the CETP-mediated exchange of HDL cholesterol esters for triglycerides with subsequent HDL triglyceride hydrolysis by HL. CETP deficiency has been described in humans and causes increased HDL-C levels and reduced levels of non–HDL-C. CETP mutations occur frequently among Japanese individuals, and in this population they are a common cause of high HDL-C levels.

Mice with human CETP transgenes (70) have 35% and 24% lower levels of HDL-C and apoA-I, respectively, and smaller HDL particles. These effects of CETP were less than expected based on studies comparing healthy and CETP-deficient humans. One possibility for this difference is that mouse and human HDLs are significantly different. To create mice with a more human-like HDL, the CETP transgenics were crossed with human apoA-I transgenic mice. CETP was found to be more potent at reducing HDL levels in the setting of human apoA-I expression (71). Compared with the human apoA-I transgenic mice, the doubly transgenic mice had a more pronounced reduction in HDL-C and apo A-I levels—66% and 42%, respectively—with smaller HDL particles (mean particle diameter of 10.4, 8.8, and 7.4 n*M* as compared with 9.7, 8.5, and 7.3 n*M*). In the doubly transgenic mice, it was also found that 100% of the CETP was associated with HDL, compared with 22% in the singly transgenic animals. Thus, CETP overexpression can reduce HDL-C levels and particle size—an effect that is more dramatic in the setting of human apoA-I–containing HDL, implying a specific interaction of human CETP with human apoA-I or the particles it produces.

CETP-mediated exchange of triglycerides for HDL cholesterol ester is driven by the level of VLDL triglyceride, which is quite low in the mouse. To study the relation between high triglycerides and low HDL-C, a CETP transgene was introduced into the hypertriglyceridemic human apoC-III mice that coexpressed human apoA-I (72). In these mice, human CETP gene expression reduced HDL-C and apoA-I to very low levels with a dramatic reduction in HDL particle size. This mimics the high triglyceride/low HDL-C phenotype in humans (a component of the metabolic syndrome). The human apoA-I, apoC-III, CETP transgenic mice are the first animal model of this disorder.

A cynomolgus monkey CETP transgenic mouse also has been generated (73). The monkey CETP transgenic mice showed a strong inverse correlation of CETP activity with HDL-C levels, apoA-I levels, and HDL size, and a positive correlation of CETP activity with apoB levels and the size of apoB-containing lipoproteins. These mice also were more diet responsive than control animals. Human CETP transgenic mice also were found to show a gene dosage-dependent effect on apoB levels (32). Despite its anticipated negative effect on HDL, studies with CETP in mice suggest variable results with respect to atherosclerosis susceptibility (74–77), a phenomenon likely related to genetic background. From these data it is clear that the knee-jerk association between high HDL-C and atheroprotection is not correct, and that this association, although in general true, is often dependent on other dynamic factors. That CETP overexpression in mice does not influence the flux of cholesterol from the periphery to the liver (78) would further suggest that genetic background and an individual's underlying lipoprotein profile dictate whether CETP is proatherogenic or antiatherogenic. The dynamic role that CETP plays in lipoprotein metabolism, its relation to atherosclerosis, and the therapeutic potential of CETP inhibition remain unclear.

Adenosine Triphosphate–binding Cassette Transporter A1 and Scavenger Receptor B-I Models

The recent discovery of the HDL-forming factor, ABCA1 (2,3), and the HDL-binding protein, scavenger receptor B-I (SR-BI) (79), and their study in transgenic mice have shed considerable light on the reverse cholesterol transport process. These two factors play a substantial role in determining HDL levels and turnover in the plasma. SR-BI aids in the delivery of cholesterol and phospholipid from cells to HDL, moving lipid bidirectionally. ABCA1 actions are more one-sided, moving cholesterol from cells to HDL. The two factors differ in their relative specificity for HDL. SR-B1 appears to require a phosphatidyl choline–rich particle and will interface not only with HDL but with multiple lipoprotein particles. ABCA1 interacts with HDL more specifically (although all small, relatively lipid-poor lipoproteins are potential acceptors of ABCA1-mediated cholesterol flux) and does so through a combination of lipid and apolipoprotein cofactors.

The role of SR-BI in reverse cholesterol transport and the net transport of cholesterol from the periphery to the liver is not clear. That SR-BI can effect bidirectional lipid transport suggests that its role could be to act both in the centrifugal and reverse cholesterol transport processes. In the liver, SR-BI appears to act to "receive" HDL-C, and many believe that low HDL-C levels caused by increased hepatic SR-BI activity could be beneficial (i.e., low HDL-C levels caused by enhanced reverse cholesterol transport). Conversely, the role of SR-BI in the periphery and specifically in the vessel wall is less clear, depending on a host of factors including net cholesterol content in the vessel, the presence of lipid-poor, apolipoprotein-rich nascent HDL, and other factors that will help to determine the net direction of cholesterol flux. Given the difficulty in quantifying reverse cholesterol transport experimentally, only indirect evidence supports a more precise role for SR-BI in atherosclerosis susceptibility. Transgenic mice studies, however, have shown that SR-BI is antiatherogenic. Hepatic overexpression of SR-BI reduces atherosclerosis in LDL receptor knockout mice (80), whereas SR-BI/LDL receptor double knockout mice have increased atherosclerosis (81). The mechanism for this apparent atheroprotection remains speculative.

Several mouse studies have been done with ABCA1 confirming human and in vitro data showing that ABCA1 is clearly linked to HDL production and that, as expected, it serves an antiatherogenic function; however, as with most factors that affect HDL-C, the mechanism is dynamic, depending on a number of concurrent genetic and environmental influences. Increased liver and macrophage expression of ABCA1 leads to increased HDL-C level (82). These studies have led to a novel concept that the liver perhaps acts as a source of HDL-C in plasma, questioning the mantra that HDL-C is derived primarily from peripheral tissues and further confusing the understanding of reverse cholesterol transport. One hypothesis is that liver-derived HDL is a cholesterol source for certain peripheral tissues, such as the adrenal gland and ovary, that rely on HDL-mediated uptake to meet requirements for steroidogenic hormone synthesis. Liver-derived HDL-C could further act to modulate intrahepatic cholesterol concentrations and to promote hepatic cholesterol uptake through other pathways (such as through SR-BI or the LDL receptor), or it could act to increase the circulating pool of HDL providing greater substrate for reverse cholesterol transport or oxidative protection of peripheral tissues such as the vascular wall.

The role of ABCA1 in atherosclerosis has been at least partially clarified by animal models (82–87). When transferred to the atherosclerosis-susceptible LDL receptor– or apoE-deficient mice, macrophages deficient in ABCA1 cause increased atherosclerosis as compared with animals receiving wild-type macrophages, supporting an atheroprotective role for ABCA1. Less clear have been the results from overexpression studies. On a C57Bl6 diet-induced background, ABCA1 overexpression causes decreased atherosclerosis; however, in apoE-deficient mice, conflicting results have been obtained. In one study in which no appreciable change in plasma lipoproteins were observed, atherosclerosis actually increased, whereas in a second strain in which the predicted beneficial changes in plasma lipoproteins were observed, atherosclerosis decreased. Clearly, the biology is complicated, and overexpression studies suggest that the effects of ABCA1 may, in part, depend on apoE-mediated lipoprotein metabolism or direct effects on the vessel wall.

INCREASED CHYLOMICRON REMNANTS AND INTERMEDIATE-DENSITY LIPOPROTEIN CHOLESTEROL

Chylomicron remnant and IDL are atherogenic cholesterol ester–rich particles, normally cleared from plasma by hepatic remnant and LDL receptors that recognize surface apoE. There are three common apoE alleles: E_3 (frequency in white population, 77%), E_4 (15%), and E_2 (8%), specifying six common apoE phenotypes: $E_{3/3}$ (frequency, 59%), $E_{4/4}$ (2%), $E_{2/2}$ (1%), $E_{4/3}$ (23%), $E_{3/2}$ (12%), and $E_{4/2}$ (2%). $apoE_2$ is defective in receptor binding, whereas $apoE_3$ and $apoE_4$ bind receptors normally. Individuals with type III hyperlipoproteinemia, who have increased plasma levels of chylomicron remnants and IDL particles as a result of impaired catabolism, generally have the $E_{2/2}$ phenotype. These patients are susceptible to premature CAD, strokes, and peripheral vascular disease. Type III hyperlipoproteinemia also can be caused by heterozygosity for other rare mutations of apoE. In addition to type III hyperlipoproteinemia, the apoE phenotype can affect LDL-C levels, atherosclerosis susceptibility, longevity, and predisposition to Alzheimer's disease.

Apolipoprotein E Transgenic Mice

Human apoE transgenic mice have been made (88,89). The apoE gene is in a cluster with two other apolipoprotein genes consisting of apoE, apoC-I, and apoC-II. apoE is expressed primarily in the liver, with lower expression in most body tissues. Early human apoE transgenic mice were made with constructions that lacked a liver control element and, as a result, had relatively poor apoE expression with no significant lipoprotein alterations. apoE transgenic mice have been made with heterologous promotors (90,91) that have a four-fold increase in apoE levels and significantly decreased VLDL-C and LDL-C. Metabolic studies indicate a several-fold increase in the clearance rate of radiolabeled VLDL and LDL, consistent with the established role for apoE in mediating lipoprotein uptake through the LDL receptor. In addition, these animals are resistant to diet-induced hypercholesterolemia, indicating that apoE overexpression decreases fasting levels of atherogenic lipoproteins and can decrease the response of these lipoprotein fractions to a high-cholesterol diet.

Transgenic mice also have been made with mutant forms of apoE associated with dominantly inherited type III hyperlipoproteinemia, including $E_{3\text{-Leiden}}$ (tandem duplication of apoE amino acids 120 to 126) (92) and $E_4Arg^{142}Cys$ (93). In both cases, there were increased levels of cholesterol and triglyceride in the VLDL and IDL lipoprotein fractions. The $E_{3\text{-Leiden}}$ mice were shown to be extremely responsive to dietary cholesterol. The $E_{3\text{-Leiden}}$ and the $E_4Arg^{142}Cys$ mice appear to be reasonable phenocopies of human type III hyperlipoproteinemia and are useful models for the study of genetic and environmental influences on the manifestation of this disease.

Apolipoprotein E–Deficient Mice

apoE-deficient mice have been created (8,9,94). Homozygous-deficient animals are viable and fertile. On a chow diet (low in cholesterol, 0.01%, and fat, 4.5%) they have serum cholesterol levels of 400 to 500 mg/dL (Table 25–3). Most

of this is in the VLDL plus IDL lipoprotein fractions. When the homozygous apoE knockout mice are fed a Western-type diet (moderate amounts of cholesterol, 0.15%, and fat, 20%), they develop cholesterol levels of approximately 1,800 mg/dL (9). The lipoprotein particles that accumulate in the apoE-deficient mice are similar in size to normal VLDL, but are cholesterol ester enriched, similar to β-VLDL (95). Metabolic studies indicate a severe defect in lipoprotein clearance from plasma, as predicted from the known function of apoE as a ligand for lipoprotein receptors. The β-VLDL in the apoE-deficient mice are probably remnants of intestinally derived lipoproteins. Heterozygous apoE knockout mice have diminished plasma apoE levels, normal fasting lipoprotein levels, and slightly delayed postprandial lipoprotein clearance. Thus, half-normal apoE expression in the mouse is nearly sufficient for normal lipoprotein metabolism. The accumulation of atherogenic β-VLDL in the apoE knockout mice is sufficient to produce human-like atherosclerotic lesions. The creation of the apoE-deficient mouse has generated substantial new data with regard to apoE and lipoprotein metabolism and has led to the development of a widely used and well validated model of atherosclerosis (see later; see also review by Callow and coworkers [96]).

INCREASED LIPOPROTEIN(a)

Increased levels of Lp(a) have been found to be an independent risk factor for CAD. In humans, genetic variation at the apolipoprotein(a) [Apo(a)] locus leads to variable Lp(a) levels in the general population. Lp(a) consists of a large glycoprotein, Apo(a), disulfide bonded to the apoB moiety of LDL. Apo(a) resembles plasminogen, containing domains of plasminogen-like kringle IV in multiple copies and of plasminogen-like kringle V and protease in single copies. Apo(a) alleles specify proteins that differ in size because of variation in the number of kringle IV–like domains. The larger Apo(a) size forms are associated with lower plasma Lp(a) levels and vice versa. Lp(a) is a tightly bound constituent of the atherosclerotic plaque. In addition, through its plasminogen-like properties, Lp(a) may also participate in thrombogenic processes. The physiologic function of Lp(a) is unknown.

TABLE 25–3. *Approximate plasma lipoprotein levels in apolipoprotein E–deficient mice and humans*

	TC, mg/dL	VLDL-C, mg/dL	HDL, mg/dL
Mouse			
$apoE^{+/+}$	100	20	65
$apoE^{-/-}$	600	400	50
$apoE^{-/-}$, apoA-I	600	400	100
Human			
$apoE^{+/+}$	200	15	50
$apoE^{-/-}$	500	250	50

Values represent approximate total plasma cholesterol (TC), very low-density lipoprotein cholesterol (VLDL-C), and high-density lipoprotein cholesterol (HDL-C) levels in control, apolipoprotein E (apoE)–deficient, and apoE-deficient mice that overexpress a human apoA-I transgene (data from Plump and coworkers [107]). For comparison, approximate plasma cholesterol and lipoprotein levels are given for normal and apoE-deficient humans (data from Haemerle and coworkers [64]).

Apolipoprotein(a) Transgenic Mice

Lp(a) has a limited phylogenetic distribution and is found only in humans, Old World primates, and hedgehogs. Mice do not express Apo(a), but transgenic animals have been made with a human Apo(a) gene (97). Mean plasma levels equivalent to 9 mg/dL Lp(a) are observed (human range, 0.1–200 mg/dL), but, in contrast to humans, Apo(a) is found in the lipoprotein-free fraction. Infusion of human LDL into these transgenic mice results in the formation of Lp(a). In addition, when Apo(a) transgenic mice were cross-bred with human apoB transgenic mice, Lp(a) was also formed

(19,20). These experiments suggest that human Apo(a) can bind to human apoB but not mouse apoB, perhaps because of the lack of conservation of a crucial cysteine in the mouse protein. Mice that overexpress Apo(a) have slightly increased atherosclerosis as compared with wild-type mice, and when coexpressed with human apoB, susceptibility increases (98,99).

MOUSE MODELS OF ATHEROSCLEROSIS

The mouse is highly resistant to atherosclerosis (Table 25–2). The benefits of the mouse as a genetic tool have prompted substantial efforts directed at altering environment and genes to create an atherosclerosis-sensitive species. To date, these efforts have focused on altering the mouse's lipoprotein profile to create more atherogenic lipoprotein patterns (Table 25–1).

The C57BL/6 Mouse Model of Atherosclerosis

The first attempts at creating an atherosclerosis-sensitive mouse involved dietary interventions. Mice have been fed an unphysiological diet consisting of 1.25% cholesterol, 15% fat, and 0.5% cholic acid. This diet contains 10 to 20 times the amount of cholesterol of a human diet and an unnatural dietary constituent, cholic acid. Although toxic to mice when fed over a long time period, this diet leads to cholesterol levels of 200 to 300 mg/dL with increased non-HDL lipoproteins. This is in contrast to a standard chow diet, which produces cholesterol levels of 60 to 80 mg/dL, mostly in HDL. Although the majority of mouse strains do not experience development of atherosclerosis in response to the high-cholesterol diet, a handful of inbred mouse strains will experience development of foam cell lesions at the base of the aorta in the region of the aortic valves after chronic administration.

Transgenic Mouse Models of Atherosclerosis

Initial studies examining the genetics of atherosclerosis in mice used transgenic manipulation in diet-induced athero-susceptible mouse strains. In a pioneering study examining susceptibility to diet-induced fatty streaks, human apoA-I gene expression was found to reduce dramatically aortic sinus foam cell lesion area (100), suggesting that apoA-I expression with its attendant increase in HDL-C levels can protect against early events in atherogenesis. In a related study, human apoA-I and human apoA-II transgenic mice were crossed, and substantially less protection was seen when both genes were expressed than when only human apoA-I was expressed (101). In this study, apoA-I only and apoA-I/apoA-II transgenic mice had similarly increased levels of HDL-C; however, human apoA-II expression led to a decrease in the subpopulation of HDL that contained only apoA-I and an increase in the HDL population that contained both apoA-I and apoA-II. Because human apoA-II

gene expression did not decrease HDL-C levels but rather altered the composition of the existing HDL, this experiment suggests that not all HDL particles are equally antiatherogenic. Studies have likewise demonstrated that over-expression of mouse apoA-II leads to similar conclusions concerning the role of HDL protein composition in determining atherosclerosis susceptibility (102). Mice that express mouse apoA-II at twofold to threefold greater levels than control mice have increased HDL-C levels. On a chow diet, small, but detectable, fatty streak lesions develop in these mice at the base of the aorta. The results question whether HDL levels alone are sufficient to predict risk for atherosclerotic heart disease.

In addition to HDL levels and protein composition, other factors can determine the ability of HDL to influence atherosclerosis susceptibility. The ratio of non-HDL to HDL-C in humans is an excellent predictor of CAD and suggests that the combination of increased non–HDL-C and decreased HDL-C may create an atherogenic environment. This profile was created in a line of CETP transgenic mice (103). CETP activity was ~20-fold greater in these mice than in humans. With this high level of CETP activity, a reciprocal increase in non-HDL and decrease in HDL-C was observed. When challenged with the atherogenic high-cholesterol diet, these mice developed slightly more fatty streaks than control animals. The degree of atherosclerosis could be correlated with the ratio of non-HDL to HDL-C.

That HDL levels alone are not sufficient to determine susceptibility to atherosclerosis was further demonstrated in apoA-I–deficient mice. These mice have an 80% reduction in HDL-C level, but atherosclerosis does not develop in mice on a chow, high-fat, or high-cholesterol diet (38,39). Increased non–HDL-C level appears necessary to create a susceptible environment with HDL-C acting as a modifier.

The use of a high-cholesterol diet to induce fatty streaks has offered insight into the mechanism by which Apo(a) is atherogenic. When fed the high-cholesterol diet, mice expressing a human Apo(a) transgene experience development of fatty streak lesions at the base of the aorta (104). This result is striking in light of the observation that the majority of Apo(a) in the plasma of these mice is not lipid associated. The conclusion from this study is that the atherogenicity of Lp(a) does not rely fully on the association of Apo(a) with the lipoprotein particle.

The Low-Density Lipoprotein Receptor– and Apolipoprotein E–Deficient Mouse Models of Atherosclerosis

The apoE knockout mouse was the first model of human atherosclerosis to experience development of disease on a chow diet (8,9). Although these animals are outbred on a typically atheroresistant genetic background, widespread fibroproliferative atherosclerotic lesions develop when they are fed a low-fat diet (Fig. 25–3) (see also color insert) (105–107). In the apoE-deficient mice, lesions are widespread, developing

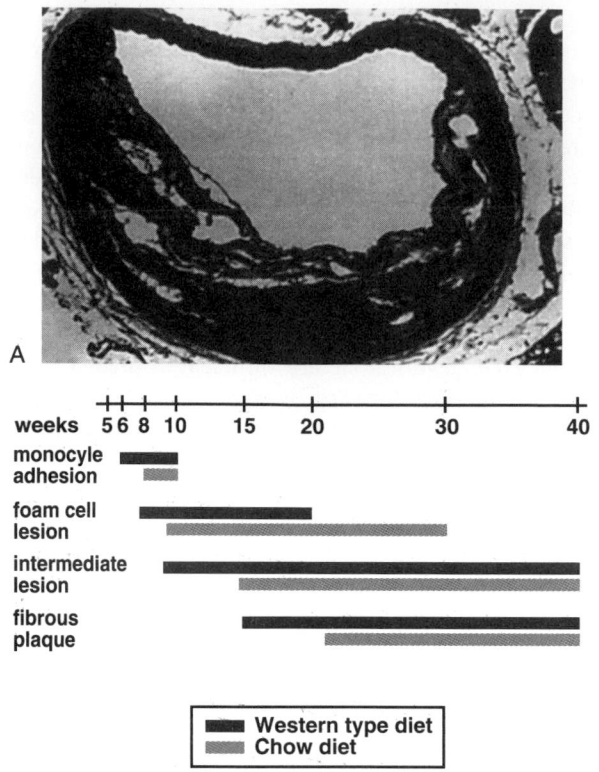

weeks 5 6 8 10   15   20   30   40

monocyle
adhesion

foam cell
lesion

intermediate
lesion

fibrous
plaque

```
■■■■ Western type diet
■■■■ Chow diet
```

B

FIG. 25–3. Atherosclerosis in the apolipoprotein E (apoE)–deficient mouse. **A:** An advanced atherosclerotic fibrous plaque from the carotid artery of an apoE-deficient mouse. **B:** The progression of lesion formation in apoE-deficient mice fed chow and Western-type diets. **C:** An aorta from an apoE-deficient mouse stained for lipid with oil red O. (**A** and **B:** Reproduced from Nakashima Y, Plump AS, Raines EW, et al. Apo E-deficient mice develop lesions of all phases of atherosclerosis throughout the arterial tree. *Arterioscler Thromb* 1994;14:133–140, with permission; **C:** reproduced from Palinski W, Ord VA, Plump AS, et al. Apolipoprotein E-deficient mice are a model of lipoprotein oxidation in atherogenesis: demonstration of oxidation-specific epitopes in lesions and high titers of autoantibodies to malondialdehydelysine in serum. *Arterioscler Thromb* 1994;14:606–616, with permission.) (See color insert for Fig. 25–3C.)

mation of the potent effect that apoA-I can have in modulating atherosclerosis (108). Overexpression of human apoA-I can increase HDL-C levels, which can reduce the size and delay the onset of atherosclerotic lesions in the apoE-deficient mouse. The decrease in lesion size in the apoE-deficient, apoA-I transgenic mouse was inversely proportional to the increase in HDL. Variability in HDL could explain more than 75% of the variability of lesion size in the apoE-deficient mouse (Fig. 25–4).

The single genetic lesion causing apoE absence and severe hypercholesterolemia is sufficient to convert the mouse from a species that is highly resistant to one that is highly susceptible to atherosclerosis. After the establishment of the apoE-deficient mouse as an atherosclerosis model, two subsequent, potent genetic mouse models have been developed, the LDL receptor– and the LDL receptor/apoBEC-deficient mice (81,84). Mice in both models experience development of extensive atherosclerosis on Western-type diets, not requiring the toxic cholic acid–containing diet. Both have emerged as accepted models of human atherosclerosis. The LDL receptor– and the apoE-

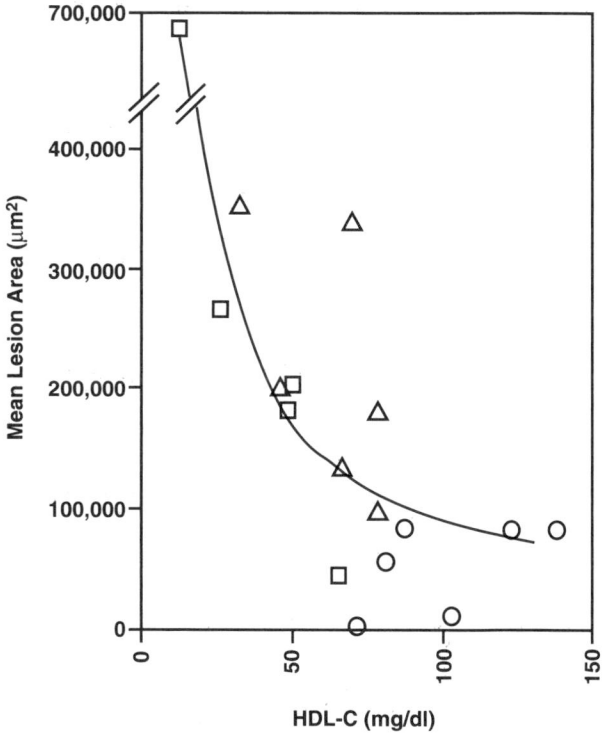

FIG. 25–4. Correlation of mean lesion area and high-density lipoprotein (HDL) cholesterol levels in apolipoprotein E (apoE)–deficient and apoE-deficient, human apoA-I transgenic mice. *Squares,* apoE$^{-/-}$ mice; *triangles,* apoE$^{-/-}$, low-expressing human apoA-I mice; *circles,* apoE$^{-/-}$, high-expressing human apoA-I mice. (Reproduced from Plump AS, Scott CJ, Breslow JL. Human apolipoprotein A-I gene expression increases high density lipoproteins and suppresses atherosclerosis in the apolipoprotein E-deficient mouse. *Proc Natl Acad Sci USA* 1994;91:9607–9611, with permission.)

at multiple points along the arterial tree including the base of the aorta, the proximal coronaries, branch points of the major vessels coming off the aorta, and within the carotid, intercostal, mesenteric, renal, and femoral arteries (105). Electron microscopy has demonstrated that these lesions probably begin by endothelial cell–monocyte adhesions that progress to fatty streaks composed of subintimal foam cells at 6 to 10 weeks of age. Unlike the other mouse models, these lesions rapidly progress to advanced lesions that contain muscular fibrous caps with extracellular matrix deposition and necrotic cores by 15 to 20 weeks of age (Fig. 25–3). Some lesions show fibrous plaques flanked by foam cells at the shoulder areas. Other lesions have medial necrosis with occasional aneurysm formation.

A particularly dramatic and one of the first demonstrations of the use of the apoE-deficient mouse came on confir-

deficient mice have been widely used to test diet, therapeutic, genetic, and environmental modifiers of atherosclerosis. Over the last decade literally thousands of studies have been published in abstract and article form in which these animals have been used to assess modifiers of atherosclerosis.

New Mouse Models of Atherosclerosis

The LDL receptor– and apoE-deficient mouse models of atherosclerosis have become gold standards. They are routinely used to assess the effects of genetics, environment, and pharmacotherapy on atherosclerosis. Although imperfect, they provide rapid screening tools for the assessment of atherosusceptibility. In recent years, dozens of additional genetic models have been created in mice to study atherosclerosis. Table 25–4 highlights some key models published in a 2-year span between 2000 and 2001, with many of the models based on the susceptible LDL receptor– or apoE-deficient background. Although initial focus had been on quantifying the atherogenicity of factors directly involved in lipoprotein metabolism, such as apolipoproteins and lipoprotein-modifying enzymes, more recent efforts have been focused on deciphering the role of genes involved in

TABLE 25–4. *Mouse models*

Model	Background[a]	Phenotype	Reference
apoB-100/100	LDLR$^{-/-}$	↑ Lesions, ↑ VLDL-C	138
apoB-100/100	apoE$^{-/-}$	↑ Lesions, ↑ LDL-C	138
Pltp$^{-/-}$	apoB Tg	↓ Lesions, ↓ secretion and levels of apoB lipoproteins	139
Pltp$^{-/-}$	apoE$^{-/-}$	↓ Lesions, ↓ production and levels of apoB lipoproteins	139
ABCA1$^{-/-}$	DBA/1	No change hepatic cholesterol, phospholipids, biliary secretion	140
Hnf-1$\alpha^{-/-}$	C57BL/6	↑ HDL-C, ↓ bile acid transport, type 2 diabetes	141
Induction of HO-1	LDLR$^{-/-}$	↓ Lesions, ↓ lipid hydroperoxides	142
MPO$^{-/-}$	LDLR$^{-/-}$	↑ Lesions, neutrophils fail to kill *Candida albicans*	143
Ttpa$^{-/-}$	apoE$^{-/-}$	↑ Lesions, ↑ levels of isoprostanes	144
12/15-LO$^{-/-}$	apoE$^{-/-}$	↓ Lesions, ↓ levels of isoprostanes, ↓ levels of IgG MDA-LDL autoantibodies	108
15-LO Tg	LDLR$^{-/-}$	↑ Lesions, LDL more susceptible to oxidation, Mø/T-cell density unchanged	110
ACAT1$^{-/-}$ (Mᵠ)	LDLR$^{-/-}$	↑ Lesions, ↓ Mø	145
Ap2$^{-/-}$ (Mᵠ)	apoE$^{-/-}$	↓ Lesions, ↓ Mø cholesterol uptake, ↓ inflammatory cytokines	146
Rag1$^{-/-}$	LDLR$^{-/-}$	↓ Lesions in early stages (8 weeks)	147
Rag2$^{-/-}$	apoE$^{-/-}$	↓ Lesions, ↓ cholesterol and triglyceride	148
CD18$^{-/-}$ (Mᵠ)	C57BL/6 x 129/SvEv	↓ ROS production by Mø stimulates by oxidized-LDL	149
eNOS$^{-/-}$	apoE$^{-/-}$	↑ Lesions, ↑ blood pressure, ↑ aneurysms	150
iNOS$^{-/-}$	C57BL/6 x 129/SvEv	↑ Lesions, ↑ serum cholesterol	151
iNOS$^{-/-}$	apoE$^{-/-}$	↓ Lesions, ↓ lipoperoxides	152
iNOS$^{-/-}$	C57BL/6 x 129/SvEv	No difference lesion size, plasma lipids, cellular density ↑ Collagen content	153
MMP-3$^{-/-}$	apoE$^{-/-}$ ↓ Mᵠ in lesions	↑ Lesions, ↑ fibrillar collagen, ↓ aneurysms	154
HuMMP-1 Tg (Mᵠ)	apoE$^{-/-}$	↓ Lesions, ↓ fibrillar collagen content	155
PPAR-$\alpha^{-/-}$	apoE$^{-/-}$	↓ Lesions, ↓ insulin resistance	156
VCAM-1$^{-/-}$	LDLR$^{-/-}$	↓ Lesions	157
Fld$^{-/-}$ (lipin)	LDLR$^{-/-}$	Adipose tissue deficiency, glucose intolerance	158
apoA-V$^{-/-}$	C57BL/6 x 129/SvEv	↑ Triglycerides	6
Diet1$^{-/-}$	C57BL/6By	↑ Bile acid excretion, resistance to diet-induced hypercholesterolemia	159
Txnip	C3H/DisnA	↑ Triglycerides, ketone bodies, and cholesterol	160

apo, apolipoprotein; eNOS, endothelial nitric oxide synthase; HDL, high-density lipoprotein; HO-1, heme oxygenase-1; Hu, human; iNOS, inducible nitric oxide synthase; LDL-C, low-density lipoprotein cholesterol; LDLR, low-density lipoprotein receptor; LO, lipoxygenase; Mø, macrophage; MDA-LDL, malondialdehyde-LDL; MMP, matrix metalloproteinase; MPO, myeloperoxidase; Pltp, phospholipid transfer protein; PPAR, peroxisome proliferator-activated receptor; ROS, reactive oxygen species; Tg, transgenic; Ttpa, α-tocopherol transfer protein; VLDL, very low-density lipoprotein.
[a]LDLR$^{-/-}$ and apoE$^{-/-}$ are on the background of the C57BL/6 strain.

lipid oxidation, adhesion molecules, immunoregulatory modifiers, transcription factors, and vessel wall components. Although the scope of this chapter is too limited to permit a discussion of each of these studies, some key studies deserve mention.

The role of lipid oxidation in atherosclerosis susceptibility has long been speculated. Studies in mice deficient in 12/15-lipoxygenase (LO), an intracellular enzyme known to oxidize lipid, have shown that when crossed into an athero-susceptible background, lesions are significantly decreased (109,110); conversely, overexpression of 12/15-LO leads to increased atherosclerosis (111). In both cases, strong direct correlations were made between the magnitude of athero-sclerosis and the amount of lipid peroxidation. The studies with 12/15-LO are supported by a host of additional athero-sclerosis studies examining other antioxidants, such as vitamin E and probucol (112–116). Antioxidants could have therapeutic benefit in decreasing atherosclerosis risk; however, both clinical and mouse data suggest conflicting conclusions. For example, the first probucol clinical efficacy trial, PQRST, showed no effect of probucol on femoral artery lesions (117), but more recent studies in different patient populations with other anatomic end points have suggested that probucol administration to humans is atheroprotective (118–121). Assuming that these studies are all appropriately designed, the suggestion is that the mechanism of atherogenesis may vary between individuals and at different anatomic locations. Mouse studies would support this claim. As with humans, increased lesions develop in probucol-treated atherosusceptible mice in certain parts of the arterial tree and decreased lesions develop elsewhere (116).

Mouse studies have been useful in understanding effects of the insulin-sensitizing thiazolidinedione (TZD) drugs on atherosclerosis. The TZDs are agonists of the transcription factor PPAR-γ and are often prescribed to patients with the metabolic syndrome. Two of these TZD drugs, rosiglitazone and troglitazone, have been shown to decrease atherosclerosis in susceptible mouse strains (122,123). This pharmacologic observation is consistent with genetic data. PPAR-γ–deficient mice die during embryogenesis, but PPAR-γ–deficient macrophages, which can be derived from cultured PPAR-γ–deficient embryonic stem cells or from mice with conditional disruptions of macrophage PPAR-γ, have diminished expression of ABCA1 (124,125). Diminished ABCA1 expression leads to an inability to fully export cellular cholesterol, hence impeding the reverse cholesterol transport process. Conversely, bone marrow transplantation studies in which LDL receptor–deficient mice transplanted with PPAR-γ–deficient bone marrow have less atherosclerosis than those transplanted with wild-type cells (124). The long-term benefit of the marketed PPAR-γ agonists with regard to atherosclerosis has yet to be established in humans, but these overlapping lines of evidence in mice suggest the strong likelihood of protective effects.

One area in which the mouse has been inadequate as a model has been in replicating advanced aspects of human atherosclerosis, plaque instability, and subsequent clinical events such as myocardial infarction and stroke. Although lesions in both the LDL receptor– and apoE-deficient mouse can become quite large, they tend not to rupture. Studies suggest that in older apoE-deficient mice (42–54 weeks), the brachiocephalic artery might serve as a nidus for studying spontaneous plaque rupture. Feeding diets high in fat to these animals results in increased death rates (126) and ruptured thrombotic plaques in the brachiocephalic artery (127). These spontaneous models are perhaps impractical for hypothesis testing, given the timelines required; however, several physical approaches have been developed to induce rupture (128). Although artificial, these induced methods open portals for studying complex atherogenesis and perhaps will provide a means for assessing the next wave of more advanced therapeutic modalities. Clearly, the development of a genetic model that develops reproducible unstable lesions will mark a major advance in the field.

GENOMICS AND MOUSE ATHEROSCLEROSIS

The genomics era has heralded new fronts for the study of mouse atherosclerosis. Although several studies have emerged recently highlighting the importance of new genetic technologies, three are noted here as clever examples of the different approaches one might take with genomic tools. One study used cross-species comparative sequence analysis to identify a new apolipoprotein gene, apoA-V (6); another study used more traditional positional cloning (but in a genomics era accelerated fashion) (129–131), with transgenic confirmation of a new atherosclerosis susceptibility locus; and the third study used a combination of molecular profiling and positional cloning in humans to identify the gene for hereditary sitosterolemia (1,132). The identification of each of these genes has been followed by critical proof of concept experiments in mice.

Apolipoprotein A-V Mice

Using cross-species sequence comparisons of the apoA-I–C-III–A-IV gene cluster to search for regulatory regions, a stretch of several kilobytes of highly conserved residues was identified approximately 30 kb from the cluster (6). This region was found to contain an open reading frame that encoded a gene highly homologous to apoA-IV, and was hence named apoA-V. The discovery of this new gene so many years after the initial sequencing of this locus was remarkable, considering its high homology to apoA-IV and that this was and remains an intensely studied region of the genome. Overexpression of apoA-V in mice led to a significant decrease in serum triglycerides and gene knockout led to hypertriglyceridemia (6). In the same study as the genetic identification, the overexpression, and the mouse knockout, the authors went on the demonstrate that haplotypes across the human apoA-V locus were associated with hypertriglyceridemia in two separate association studies (6), an observation that has since been made even more robust by independent association studies in distinct ethnic populations (133,134). The role of apoA-V in terms of atherosclerosis susceptibility has yet to be firmly established, but clearly apoA-V is a key determinant of human lipoprotein metabolism.

5-Lipoxygenase

Genetics provide a powerful unbiased tool into the dissection of complex traits. Quantitative trait locus mapping in mice fed an atherogenic diet was used to identify a locus on chromosome 6 that was highly linked to atherosclerosis susceptibility (129,130). When crossed onto the LDL receptor–deficient mouse background, this locus led to near complete resistance to atherosclerosis. Interestingly, when initially identified, the prime candidate in the locus was the PPAR-γ gene. Although subsequent studies failed to confirm PPAR-γ as the causative gene, a second candidate, 5-LO, emerged as the likely effector. 5-LO is a key enzyme in leukotriene biosynthesis, catalyzing the production of chemokines thought necessary for recruitment of inflammatory cells into atherosclerotic lesions. 5-LO mRNA levels were reduced fivefold in congenic mice harboring the chromosome 6 susceptibility locus, and significant sequence differences were detected between wild-type and susceptible 5-LO mouse DNA. The proof of concept experiments came when macrophages from knockout 5-LO mice were transplanted into LDL receptor–deficient animals and when heterozygous 5-LO–deficient mice were bred onto an LDL receptor–deficient background (131). In both cases, animals with either 5-LO–deficient macrophages or 5-LO deficiency had significantly less atherosclerosis than LDL receptor–deficient mice with wild-type 5-LO.

Hereditary Sitosterolemia (Adenosine Triphosphate–binding Cassette Transporters G5 and G8)

Hereditary sitosterolemia is a rare autosomal recessive disease characterized by increased dietary absorption of the plant sterol, sitosterol, and of cholesterol, with associated decreased biliary cholesterol excretion, hypercholesterolemia, and premature atherosclerosis. The genes for this disease have been identified through a clever sequence of experiments (1,132). Gene microarray data from mice treated with an LXR agonist (known to decrease intestinal cholesterol absorption) led to the identification of an upregulated adenosine triphosphate–binding cassette (ABC) transporter that was named ABCG5. Since an ABC had been previously linked to cholesterol absorption and that a human homologue of ABCG5 existed on a portion of chromosome 2 for which hereditary sitosterolemia had previously been mapped, it became a likely candidate. ABCG5 is a half-transporter with a closely linked gene, ABCG8, the other functional half of this transporter. Mutations in both have been implicated as causative for hereditary sitosterolemia. Studies in transgenic mice have subsequently confirmed the

crucial role that this complex plays in cholesterol uptake and atherosclerosis susceptibility (135–137). Whether common genetic variation in these genes can influence cholesterol uptake, lipoprotein metabolism, and atherosclerosis susceptibility in the general population remains unknown.

SUMMARY

In humans, lipoprotein disorders are found in the majority of individuals with atherosclerotic heart disease. Four lipoprotein patterns are commonly recognized, including increased LDL-C levels, reduced HDL-C levels in association with increased triglycerides, increased levels of IDL-C and chylomicrons, and increased Lp(a). Conversely, increased levels of HDL-C, low LDL-C, IDL-C, and chylomicron remnants, and absent or diminished Lp(a) are associated with resistance to atherosclerosis. Each of the protective profiles and each of the aberrant lipoprotein profiles either exists naturally or has been created in transgenic mice by overexpressing one or a combination of human lipoprotein transport genes or by disrupting endogenous mouse genes. These studies have provided vast insight into the mechanisms of a variety of genetic factors and lipoprotein metabolism. The use of quantitative assays of fatty streak formation in the C57BL/6 diet-induced mouse model and of atherosclerosis in the LDL receptor– and apoE-deficient mouse models has provided additional concrete evidence for involvement of several lipoprotein transport genes in the determination of atherosclerosis susceptibility. These latter studies have considerably expedited the evaluation of genes, environment, and pharmacotherapy on atherosclerosis susceptibility. More recent and hopefully future studies will lay the groundwork for more advanced mouse models of human atherosclerosis in which processes such as plaque instability and clinical sequelae can be more faithfully studied.

REFERENCES

1. Berge KE, Tian H, Graf GA, et al. Accumulation of dietary cholesterol in sitosterolemia caused by mutations in adjacent ABC transporters. *Science* 2000;290:1709–1711.
2. Brooks-Wilson A, Marcil M, Clee SM, et al. Mutations in ABC1 Tangier disease and familial high-density lipoprotein deficiency. *Nat Genet* 1999;22:336–345.
3. Marcil M, Brooks-Wilson A, Clee SM, et al. Mutations in the ABC1 gene in familial HDL deficiency with defective cholesterol efflux. *Lancet* 1999;354:1341–1346.
4. Carstea ED, Morris JA, Coleman KG, et al. Niemann-Pick C1 disease gene: homology to mediators of cholesterol homeostasis. *Science* 1997;277:228–231.
5. Garcia CK, Wilund K, Arca M, et al. Autosomal recessive hypercholesterolemia caused by mutations in a putative LDL receptor adaptor protein. *Science* 2001;292:1394–1398.
6. Pennacchio LA, Oliver M, Hubacek JA, et al. An apolipoprotein influencing triglycerides in humans and mice revealed by comparative sequencing. *Science* 2001;294:169–173.
7. Jaye M, Lynch KJ, Kraweic J, et al. A novel endothelial-derived lipase that modulates HDL metabolism. *Nat Genet* 1999;21:424–428.
8. Zhang SH, Reddick RL, Piedrahita JA, et al. Spontaneous hypercholesterolemia and arterial lesions in mice lacking apolipoprotein E. *Science* 1992;258:468–471.
9. Plump AS, Smith JD, Hayek T, et al. Severe hypercholesterolemia

and atherosclerosis in apolipoprotein E-deficient mice created by homologous recombination in ES cells. *Cell* 1992;71:343–353.

10. Ishibashi S, Brown MS, Goldstein JL, et al. Hypercholesterolemia in
    low density lipoprotein receptor knockout mice and its reversal by
    adenovirus-mediated gene delivery. *J Clin Invest* 1993;92:883–893.

11. Ishibashi S, Goldstein JL, Brown MS, et al. Massive xanthomatosis
    and atherosclerosis in cholesterol-fed low density lipoprotein recep-
    tor-negative mice. *J Clin Invest* 1994;93:1885–1893.

12. Breslow JL. Lipoprotein metabolism and atherosclerosis susceptibil-
    ity in transgenic mice. *Curr Opin Lipidol* 1994;5:175–184.

13. Hofmann SL, Russell DW, Brown MS, et al. Overexpression of low
    density lipoprotein (LDL) receptor eliminates LDL from plasma in
    transgenic mice. *Science* 1988;239:1277–1281.

14. Yokode M, Hammer RE, Ishibashi S, et al. Diet-induced hypercholes-
    terolemia in mice: prevention by overexpression of LDL receptors.
    Science 1990;250:1273–1275.

15. Myant N. *Cholesterol metabolism, LDL, and the LDL receptor.* San
    Diego: Academic Press, 1990.

16. Grossman M, Raper SE, Kozarsky K, et al. Successful *ex vivo* gene
    therapy directed to liver in a patient with familial hypercholes-
    terolemia. *Nat Genet* 1994;6:335–341.

17. Chowdhury JR, Grossman M, Gupta S, et al. Long-term improvement
    of hypercholesterolemia after *ex vivo* gene therapy in LDLR-deficient
    rabbits. *Science* 1991;254:1802–1805.

18. Chiesa G, Johnson DF, Yao Z, et al. Expression of human apolipopro-
    tein B100 in transgenic mice. *J Biol Chem* 1993;268:23747–23750.

19. Linton MF, Farese RV Jr, Chiesa G, et al. Transgenic mice expressing
    high plasma concentrations of human apolipoprotein B100 and
    lipoprotein(a). *J Clin Invest* 1993;92:3029–3037.

20. Callow MJ, Stoltzfus LJ, Lawn RM, et al. Expression of human
    apolipoprotein B and assembly of lipoprotein(a) in transgenic mice.
    Proc Natl Acad Sci USA 1994;91:2130–2134.

21. Powell-Braxton L, Veniant M, Latvala RD, et al. A mouse model of
    human familial hypercholesterolemia: markedly elevated low density
    lipoprotein cholesterol levels and severe atherosclerosis on a low-fat
    chow diet. *Nat Med* 1998;4:934–938.

22. Homanics GE, Smith TJ, Zhang SH, et al. Targeted modification of
    the apolipoprotein B gene results in hypobetalipoproteinemia and de-
    velopmental abnormalities in mice. *Proc Natl Acad Sci USA*
    1993;90:2389–2393.

23. Homanics GE, Maeda N, Traber MG, et al. Exencephaly and hydro-
    cephaly in mice with targeted modification of the apolipoprotein B
    (ApoB) gene. *Teratology* 1995;51(1):1–10.

24. Huang LS, Voyiaziakis E, Markenson DF, et al. Apo B gene knockout
    in mice results in embryonic lethality in homozygotes and neural tube
    defects, male infertility, and reduced HDL cholesterol ester and apo
    A-I transport rates in heterozygotes. *J Clin Invest* 1995;96:2152–2161.

25. Walsh A, Ito Y, Breslow JL. High levels of human apolipoprotein A-I
    in transgenic mice result in increased plasma levels of small high den-
    sity lipoprotein (HDL) particles comparable to human HDL3. *J Biol
    Chem* 1989;264:6488–6494.

26. Walsh A, Azrolan N, Wang K, et al. Intestinal expression of the hu-
    man apo A-I gene in transgenic mice is controlled by a DNA region 3′
    to the gene in the promoter of the adjacent convergently transcribed
    apo C-III gene. *J Lipid Res* 1993;34:617–623.

27. Rubin EM, Ishida BY, Clift SM, et al. Expression of human
    apolipoprotein A-I in transgenic mice results in reduced plasma levels
    of murine apolipoprotein A-I and the appearance of two new high
    density lipoprotein size subclasses. *Proc Natl Acad Sci USA* 1991;88:
    434–438.

28. Kan HY, Georgopoulous S, Zannis V. A hormone response element in
    the human apolipoprotein CIII (ApoCIII) enhancer is essential for in-
    testinal expression of the ApoA-I and ApoCIII genes and contributes
    to the hepatic expression of the two linked genes in transgenic mice. *J
    Biol Chem* 2000;275:30423–30431.

29. Swanson ME, Hughes TE, Denny IS, et al. High level expression of
    human apolipoprotein A-I in transgenic rats raises total serum high
    density lipoprotein cholesterol and lowers rat apolipoprotein A-I.
    Transgenic Res 1992;1:142–147.

30. Chajek-Shaul T, Hayek T, Walsh A, et al. Expression of the human
    apolipoprotein A-I gene in transgenic mice alters high density lipopro-
    tein (HDL) particle size distribution and diminishes selective uptake of
    HDL cholesteryl esters. *Proc Natl Acad Sci USA* 1991;88:6731–6735.

31. Hayek T, Ito Y, Azrolan N, et al. Dietary fat increases high density

lipoprotein (HDL) levels both by increasing the transport rates and
decreasing the fractional catabolic rates of HDL cholesterol ester and
apolipoprotein (apo) A-I. *J Clin Invest* 1993;91:1665–1671.

32. Jiang XC, Masucci-Magoulas L, Ma J, et al. Down regulation of LDL
    receptor mRNA in CETP transgenic mice: mechanism to explain ac-
    cumulation of lipoprotein B particle. *Circulation* 1993;88:I-421.

33. Masucci-Magoulas L, Plump A, Jiang XC, et al. Profound induction
    of hepatic cholesteryl ester transfer protein transgene expression in
    apolipoprotein E and low density lipoprotein receptor gene knockout
    mice. A novel mechanism signals changes in plasma cholesterol lev-
    els. *J Clin Invest* 1996;97:154–161.

34. Olivera HC, Chouinard RA, Agellon LB, et al. Human cholesteryl es-
    ter transfer protein gene proximal promoter contains dietary choles-
    terol positive responsive elements and mediates expression in small
    intestine and periphery while predominant liver and spleen expression
    is controlled by 5′-distal sequences. Cis-acting elements mapped in
    transgenic mice. *J Biol Chem* 1996;271:31831–31838.

35. Luo Y, Tall AR. Sterol upregulation of human CETP expression in
    vitro and transgenic mice by an LXR element. *J Clin Invest* 2000;
    105:513–520.

36. Hayek T, Chajek-Shaul T, Walsh A, et al. Probucol decreases apo-
    lipoprotein A-I transport rate in control and human apolipoprotein A-I
    transgenic mice. *Arterioscler Thromb* 1991;11:1295–1302.

37. Williamson R, Lee D, Hagaman J, et al. Marked reduction of high
    density lipoprotein cholesterol in mice genetically modified to lack
    apolipoprotein A-I. *Proc Natl Acad Sci USA* 1992;89:7134–7138.

38. Plump AS, Azrolan N, Odaka H, et al. ApoA-I knockout mice: char-
    acterization of HDL metabolism in homozygotes and identification of
    a post-RNA mechanism of apoA-I up-regulation in heterozygotes. *J
    Lipid Res* 1997;38:1033–1047.

39. Li H, Reddick RL, Maeda N. Lack of apo A-I is not associated with
    increased susceptibility to atherosclerosis in mice. *Arterioscler
    Thromb* 1993;13:1814–1821.

40. Voyiaziakis E, Goldberg IJ, Plump AS, et al. ApoA-I deficiency
    causes both hypertriglyceridemia and increased atherosclerosis in hu-
    man apoB transgenic mice. *J Lipid Res* 1998;39:313–321.

41. Huang Y, Zhu Y, Langer C, et al. Effects of genotype and diet on cho-
    lesterol efflux into plasma and lipoproteins of normal, apolipoprotein
    A-I-, and apolipoprotein E-deficient mice. *Arterioscler Thromb Vasc
    Biol* 1997;17:2010–2019.

42. Stein O, Dabach Y, Hollander G, et al. Delayed loss of cholesterol
    from a localized lipoprotein depot in apolipoprotein A-I-deficient
    mice. *Proc Natl Acad Sci USA* 1997;94:9820–9824.

43. Schultz JR, Gong EL, McCall MR, et al. Expression of human
    apolipoprotein A-II and its effect on high density lipoproteins in
    transgenic mice. *J Biol Chem* 1993;267:21630–21636.

44. Marzal-Casscubertam A, Blanco-Vaca F, Ishida BY, et al. Functional
    lecithin:cholesterol acyltransferase deficiency and HDL deficiency in
    transgenic mice overexpressing human apolipoprotein A-II. *J Biol
    Chem* 1996;271:6720–6728.

45. Pastier D, Dugue S, Boisfer E, et al. Apolipoprotein A-I/A-II ration is a
    key determinant in vivo of HDL concentration and formation of pre-β
    containing apolipoprotein A-II. *Biochemistry* 2001;40:12243–12253.

46. Julve-Gil J, Ruiz-Perez E, Casaroli-Marano R, et al. Free cholesterol
    deposition in corneas of human apoA-II transgenic mice with func-
    tional LCAT deficiency. *Metabolism* 1999;48:415–421.

47. Julve J, Escolà-Gil JC, Ribas V, et al. Mechanisms of HDL deficiency
    in mice overexpressing human apoA-II. *J Lipid Res* 2002;43:1734–
    1742.

48. Deeb SS, Takata K, Peng RL, et al. A splice-junction mutation re-
    sponsible for familial apolipoprotein A-II deficiency. *Am J Hum
    Genet* 1990;46:822–827.

49. Hedrick CC, Castellani LW, Warden CH, et al. Influence of mouse
    apolipoprotein A-II on plasma lipoproteins in transgenic mice. *J Biol
    Chem* 1993;268:20676–20682.

50. Shimada M, Shimano H, Gotoda T, et al. Overexpression of human
    lipoprotein lipase in transgenic mice. *J Biol Chem* 1993;268:17924–
    17929.

51. Yagyu H, Ishibashi S, Chen Z, et al. Overexpressed lipoprotein lipase
    protects against atherosclerosis in apolipoprotein E knockout mice. *J
    Lipid Res* 1999;40:1677–1685.

52. Kim JK, Filmore JJ, Chen Y, et al. Tissue-specific overexpression of
    lipoprotein lipase causes tissue-specific insulin resistance. *Proc Natl
    Acad Sci USA* 2001;98:7522–7527.

53. Ferreira LD, Pulawa LK, Jensen DR, et al. Overexpressing human lipoprotein lipase in mouse skeletal muscle is associated with insulin resistance. *Diabetes* 2001;50:1064–1068.

54. Merkel M, Kako Y, Radner H, et al. Catalytically inactive lipoprotein lipase expression in muscle of transgenic mice increases very low density lipoprotein uptake: direct evidence that lipoprotein lipase bridging occurs in vivo. *Proc Natl Acad Sci USA* 1998;98:13841–13846.

55. Weinstock PH, Bisgaier CLK Aalto-Setälä, et al. Severe hypertriglyceridemia, reduced high density lipoprotein, and neonatal death in lipoprotein lipase knockout mice. Mild hypertriglyceridemia with impaired very low density lipoprotein clearance in heterozygotes. *J Clin Invest* 1995;96:2555–2568.

56. Dichek HL, Brecht W, Fan J, et al. Overexpression of hepatic lipase in transgenic mice decreases apolipoprotein B-containing and high density lipoproteins. Evidence that hepatic lipase acts as a ligand for lipoprotein uptake. *J Biol Chem* 1998:273:1896–1903.

57. Dichek HL, Johnson SM, Akeefe H, et al. Hepatic lipase overexpression lowers remnant and LDL levels by a noncatalytic mechanism in LDL receptor-deficient mice. *J Lipid Res* 2001;42:201–210.

58. Qiu S, Bergeron N, Kotite L, et al. Metabolism of lipoproteins containing apolipoprotein B in hepatic lipase-deficient mice. *J Lipid Res* 1998;39:1661–1668.

59. Mezdour H, Jones R, Dengreomnt C, et al. Hepatic lipase deficiency increases plasma cholesterol but reduces susceptibility to atherosclerosis in apolipoprotein E-deficient mice. *J Biol Chem* 1997;272:13570–13575.

60. Lambert G, Amar MJ, Martin P, et al. Hepatic lipase deficiency decreases the selective uptake of HDL-cholesteryl esters in vivo. *J Lipid Res* 2000;41:667–672.

61. Homanics GE, de Silva HV, Osada J, et al. Mild dyslipidemia in mice following targeted inactivation of the hepatic lipase gene. *J Biol Chem* 1995;270:2974–2980.

62. Escary JL, Choy HA, Reue K, et al. Paradoxical effect on atherosclerosis of hormone-sensitive lipase overexpression in macrophages. *J Lipid Res* 1999;40:397–404.

63. Lucas S, Tavernier G, Triaby C, et al. Expression of human hormone-sensitive lipase in white adipose tissue of transgenic mice increases lipase activity but does not enhance in vitro lipolysis. *J Lipid Res* 2003;44:154–163.

64. Haemmerle G, Zimmermann R, Strauss JG, et al. Hormone-sensitive lipase deficiency in mice changes the plasma lipid profile by affecting the tissue-specific expression pattern of lipoprotein lipase in adipose tissue and muscle. *J Biol Chem* 2002;277:12946–12952.

65. Ishida T, Choi S, Ramendra K, et al. Endothelial lipase is a major determinant of HDL level. *J Clin Invest* 2003;111:347–355.

66. Ito Y, Azrolan N, O'Connell A, et al. Hypertriglyceridemia as a result of human apolipoprotein CIII gene expression in transgenic mice. *Science* 1990;249:790–793.

67. Aalto-Setälä K, Fisher EA, Chen X, et al. Mechanism of hypertriglyceridemia in human apo CIII transgenic mice: diminished VLDL fractional catabolic rate associated with increased apo CIII and reduced apo E on the particles. *J Clin Invest* 1992;90:1889–1900.

68. Simonet WS, Bucay N, Pitas RE, et al. Multiple tissue-specific elements control the apolipoprotein E/C-I gene locus in transgenic mice. *J Biol Chem* 1991;265:8651–8654.

69. Shachter NS, Hayek T, Leff T, et al. Overexpression of apolipoprotein CII causes hypertriglyceridemia in transgenic mice. *J Clin Invest* 1994;93:1683–1690.

70. Agellon LB, Walsh A, Hayek T, et al. Reduced high density lipoprotein cholesterol in human cholesteryl ester transfer protein transgenic mice. *J Biol Chem* 1991;266:10796–10801.

71. Hayek T, Chajek-Shaul T, Walsh A, et al. An interaction between the human cholesteryl ester transfer protein (CETP) and apolipoprotein A-I genes in transgenic mice results in a profound CETP-mediated depression of high density lipoprotein cholesterol levels. *J Clin Invest* 1992;90:505–510.

72. Hayek T, Azrolan N, Verdery RB, et al. Hypertriglyceridemia and cholesteryl ester transfer protein interact to dramatically alter high density lipoprotein levels, particle sizes, and metabolism. *J Clin Invest* 1993;92:1143–1152.

73. Marotti KR, Castle CK, Murray RW, et al. The role of cholesteryl ester transfer protein in primate apolipoprotein A-I metabolism. Insights from studies with transgenic mice. *Arterioscler Thromb* 1992;12:736–744.

74. Plump AS, Masucci-Magoulas L, Bruce C, et al. Increased atherosclerosis in ApoE and LDL receptor gene knock-out mice as a result of human cholesteryl ester transfer protein transgene expression. *Arterioscler Thromb Vasc Biol* 1999;19:1105–1110.

75. Cazita PM, Berti JA, Aoki C, et al. Cholesteryl ester transfer protein expression attenuates atherosclerosis in ovariectomized mice. *J Lipid Res* 2003;44:33–40.

76. Hayek T, Masucci-Magoulas L, Jiang X, et al. Decreased early atherosclerotic lesions in hypertriglyceridemic mice expressing cholesteryl ester transfer protein transgene. *J Clin Invest* 1995;96:2071–2074.

77. Foger B, Chase M, Amar MJ, et al. Cholesteryl ester transfer protein corrects dysfunctional high density lipoproteins and reduces aortic atherosclerosis in lecithin cholesterol acyltransferase transgenic mice. *J Biol Chem* 1999;274:36912–36920.

78. Stein O, Dabach Y, Hollander G, et al. Reverse cholesterol transport in mice expressing simian cholesteryl ester transfer protein. *Atherosclerosis* 2002;164:73–78.

79. Acton S, Rigotti A, Landschulz KT, et al. Identification of scavenger receptor SR-BI as a high density lipoprotein receptor. *Science* 1996;27:518–520.

80. Kozarsky KF, Donahee MH, Glick JM, et al. Gene transfer and hepatic overexpression of the HDL receptor SR-BI reduces atherosclerosis in the cholesterol-fed LDL receptor-deficient mouse. *Arterioscler Thromb Vasc Biol* 2000;20:721–727.

81. Huszar D, Varban ML, Rinninger F, et al. Increased LDL cholesterol and atherosclerosis in LDL receptor-deficient mice with attenuated expression of scavenger receptor B1. *Arterioscler Thromb Vasc Biol* 2000;20:1068–1073.

82. Joyce C, Freeman L, Brewer HB Jr, et al. Study of ABCA1 function in transgenic mice. *Arterioscler Thromb Vasc Biol* 2003;23:1–6.

83. Attiem AD, Kastelein JP, Hayden MR. Pivotal role of ABCA1 in reverse cholesterol transport influencing HDL levels and susceptibility to atherosclerosis. *J Lipid Res* 2001;42:1717–1726.

84. van Eck M, Bos IS, Kaminski WE, et al. Leukocyte ABCA1 controls susceptibility to atherosclerosis and macrophage recruitment into tissues. *Proc Natl Acad Sci USA* 2002;99:6298–6303.

85. Aiello RJ, Brees D, Bourassa PA, et al. Increased atherosclerosis in hyperlipidemic mice with inactivation of ABCA1 in macrophages. *Arterioscler Thromb Vasc Biol* 2002;22:630–637.

86. Joyce CW, Amar MJ, Lambert G, et al. The ATP binding cassette transporter A1 (ABCA1) modulates the development of aortic atherosclerosis in C57BL/6 and apoE-knockout mice. *Proc Natl Acad Sci USA* 2002;99:407–412.

87. Singaraja RR, Fivete C, Castro G, et al. Increased ABCA1 activity protects against atherosclerosis. *J Clin Invest* 2002;110:35–42.

88. Simonet WS, Bucay N, Lauer SJ, et al. In the absence of a downstream element, the apolipoprotein E gene is expressed at high levels in kidneys of transgenic mice. *J Biol Chem* 1990;265:10809–10812.

89. Smith JD, Plump AS, Hayek T, et al. Accumulation of human apolipoprotein E in the plasma of transgenic mice. *J Biol Chem* 1990;265:14709–14712.

90. Shimano H, Yamada N, Katsuki M, et al. Overexpression of apolipoprotein E in transgenic mice: marked reduction in plasma lipoproteins except high density lipoprotein and resistance against diet-induced hypercholesterolemia. *Proc Natl Acad Sci USA* 1992;89:1750–1754.

91. Shimano H, Yamada N, Katsuki M, et al. Plasma lipoprotein metabolism in transgenic mice overexpressing apolipoprotein E. *J Clin Invest* 1992;90:2084–2091.

92. van den Maagdenberg AM, Hofker MH, Krimpenfort PJ, et al. Transgenic mice carrying the apolipoprotein E3-Leiden gene exhibit hypercholesterolemia. *J Biol Chem* 1993;268:10540–10545.

93. Fazio S, Lee Y, Ji ZS, et al. Type III hyperlipoproteinemic phenotype in transgenic mice expressing dysfunctional apolipoprotein E. *J Clin Invest* 1993;92:1497–1503.

94. Piedrahita JA, Zhu ZS, Hagaman JR, et al. Generation of mice carrying a mutant apolipoprotein E gene inactivated by gene targeting in embryonic stem cells. *Proc Natl Acad Sci USA* 1992;89:4471–4475.

95. Plump AS, Forte TM, Eisenberg S, et al. Atherogenic β-VLDL in the apo E-deficient mouse: composition, origin, and fate. *Circulation* 1993;88:I-2.

96. Plump AS, Breslow JL. Apolipoprotein E and the apolipoprotein E-deficient mouse. *Annu Rev* 1995;15:495–518.

97. Chiesa G, Hobbs HH, Koschinsky ML, et al. Reconstitution of lipoprotein(a) by infusion of human low density lipoprotein into transgenic mice expressing human apolipoprotein(a). *J Biol Chem* 1992;267:24369–24374.

98. Callow MJ, Verstuyft J, Tangirala R, et al. Atherosclerosis in transgenic mice with human apolipoprotein B and lipoprotein (a). *J Clin Invest* 1995;96:1639–1646.

99. Mancini FP, Newland DL, Mooser V, et al. Relative contributions of apolipoprotein (a) and apolipoprotein-B to the development of fatty lesions in the proximal aorta of mice. *Arterioscler Thromb Vasc Biol* 1995;15:1911–1916.

100. Rubin EM, Krauss RM, Spangler EA, et al. Inhibition of early atherogenesis in transgenic mice by human apolipoprotein AI. *Nature* 1991;353:265–267.

101. Schultz JR, Verstuyft JG, Gong EL, et al. Protein composition determines the anti-atherogenic properties of HDL in transgenic mice. *Nature* 1993;365:762–764.

102. Warden CH, Hedrick CC, Qiao JH, et al. Atherosclerosis in transgenic mice overexpressing apolipoprotein A-II. *Science* 1993;261:469–472.

103. Marotti KR, Castle CK, Boyle TP, et al. Severe atherosclerosis in transgenic mice expressing simian cholesteryl ester transfer protein. *Nature* 1993;364:73–74.

104. Lawn RM, Wade DP, Hammer RE, et al. Atherogenesis in transgenic mice expressing human apolipoprotein(a). *Nature* 1992;360:670–671.

105. Nakashima Y, Plump AS, Raines EW, et al. Apo E-deficient mice develop lesions of all phases of atherosclerosis throughout the arterial tree. *Arterioscler Thromb* 1994;14:133–140.

106. Ishibashi S, Goldstein JL, Brown MS, et al. Massive xanthomatosis and atherosclerosis in cholesterol-fed low density receptor-negative mice. *J Clin Invest* 1994;93:1885–1893.

107. Reddick RL, Zhang SH, Maeda N. Atherosclerosis in mice lacking ApoE. *Arterioscler Thromb* 1994;14:141–147.

108. Plump AS, Scott CJ, Breslow JL. Human apolipoprotein A-I gene expression increases high density lipoproteins and suppresses atherosclerosis in the apolipoprotein E-deficient mouse. *Proc Natl Acad Sci USA* 1994;91:9607–9611.

109. Cyrus T, Pratico D, Zaho L, et al. Absence of 12/15-lipoxygenase expression decreases lipid peroxidation and atherogenesis in apolipoprotein E-deficient mice. *Circulation* 2001;103:2277–2282.

110. Georgem J, Afekm A, Shaish A, et al. 12/15 Lipoxygenase gene disruption attenuates atherogenesis in LDL receptor-deficient mice. *Circulation* 2001;104:1646–1650.

111. Harats D, Shaish A, George J, et al. Overexpression of 15-lipoxygenase in vascular endothelium accelerates early atherosclerosis in LDL receptor-deficient mice. *Arterioscler Thromb Vasc Biol* 2000;20: 2100–2105.

112. Crawford RS, Kirk EA, Rosenfeld ME, et al. Dietary antioxidants inhibit development of fatty streak lesions in the LDL receptor-deficient mouse. *Arterioscler Thromb Vasc Biol* 1998;18:1506–1513.

113. Pratico D, Tangirala RK, Rader DJ, et al. Vitamin E suppresses isoprostane generation in vivo and reduces atherosclerosis in ApoE-deficient mice. *Nat Med* 1998;4:1189–1192.

114. Terasawa Y, Ladha Z, Leonard SW, et al. Increased atherosclerosis in hyperlipidemic mice deficient in α-tocopherol transfer protein and vitamin E. *Proc Natl Acad Sci USA* 2000;97:13830–13834.

115. Zhang SH, Reddick RL, Avdievich E, et al. Paradoxical enhancement of atherosclerosis by probucol treatment in apolipoprotein E-deficient mice. *J Clin Invest* 1997;99:2858–2866.

116. Witting PK, Pettersson K, Ostlund-Lindqvist AM, et al. Inhibition by a coantioxidant of aortic lipoprotein lipid peroxidation and atherosclerosis in apolipoprotein E and low density lipoprotein receptor gene double knockout mice. *FASEB J* 1999;13:667–675.

117. Walldius G, Erikson U, Olsson AG, et al. The effect of probucol on femoral atherosclerosis: the Probucol Quantitative Regression Swedish Trial (PQRST). *Am J Cardiol* 1994;74:875–883.

118. Sawayama Y, Shimizu C, Maeda N, et al. Effects of probucol and pravastatin on common carotid atherosclerosis in patients with asymptomatic hypercholesterolemia. *J Am Coll Cardiol* 2002;39:610–616.

119. Sekiya M, Funada J, Watanabe K, et al. Effects of probucol and cilostazol alone and in combination on frequency of poststenting restenosis. *Am J Cardiol* 1998;82:144–147.

120. Rodes J, Cote G, Lesperance J, et al. Prevention of restenosis after angioplasty in small coronary arteries with probucol. *Circulation* 1998; 97:429–436.

121. Tardif J, Gregorie J, Schwartz L, et al. Effects of AGI-1067 and probucol after percutaneous coronary interventions. *Circulation* 2003;107: 552–558.

122. Levi Z, Shaish A, Yacov N, et al. Rosiglitazone (PPARgamma-agonist) attenuates atherogenesis with no effect on hyperglycemia in a combined diabetes-arteriosclerosis mouse model. *Diabetes Obes Metab* 2003;5:45–50.

123. Chen Z, Ishibashi S, Perrey S, et al. Troglitazone inhibits atherosclerosis in apolipoprotein E-knockout mice. Pleiotropic effects on CD36 expression and HDL. *Arterioscler Thromb Vasc Biol* 2001;21:372–377.

124. Chawla WA, Boisvert M, Lee CH, et al. A PPAR gamma-LXR-ABCA1 pathway in macrophages is involved in cholesterol efflux and atherogenesis. *Mol Cell* 2001;7:161–171.

125. Akiyama TE, Sakai S, Lambert G, et al. Conditional disruption of the peroxisome proliferator-activated receptor gamma gene in mice results in lowered expression of ABCA1, ABCG1, and apoE in macrophages and reduced cholesterol efflux. *Mol Cell Biol* 2002;22:2607–2619.

126. Johnson JL, Jackson CL. Atherosclerotic plaque rupture in the apolipoprotein E knockout mouse. *Atherosclerosis* 2001;154:399–406.

127. Rosenfeld MA, Polinsky P, Virmani R, et al. Advanced atherosclerotic lesions in the innominate artery of the ApoE knockout mice. *Arterioscler Thromb Vasc Biol* 2000;20:2587–2592.

128. Reddick RL, Zhang SH, Maeda N. Aortic atherosclerotic plaque injury in apolipoprotein E deficient mice. *Atherosclerosis* 1998;140:297–305.

129. Mehrabian M, Wong J, Wang X, et al. Genetic locus in mice that blocks development of atherosclerosis despite extreme hyperlipidemia. *Circ Res* 2001;89:125–130.

130. Welch CL, Bretschger S, Latib N, et al. Localization of atherosclerosis susceptibility loci to chromosomes 4 and 6 using the Ldlr knockout mouse model. *Proc Natl Acad Sci USA* 2001;98:7946–7951.

131. Mehrabian M, Allayee H, Wong J, et al. Identification of 5-lipoxygenase as a major gene contributing to atherosclerosis susceptibility in mice. *Circ Res* 2002;91:120–126.

132. Lee MH, Lu K, Hazard S, et al. Identification of a gene, ABCG5, important in the regulation of dietary cholesterol absorption. *Nat Genet* 2001;27:79–83.

133. Nabika T, Nasreen S, Kobayashi S, et al. The genetic effect of the apoprotein AV gene on the serum triglyceride level in Japanese. *Atherosclerosis* 2002;165:201–204.

134. Aouizerat BE, Kulkarni M, Heilbron D, et al. Genetic analysis of a polymorphism in the human apoA-V gene: effect on plasma lipids. *J Lipid Res* 2003;44:1167–1173.

135. Yu L, York J, Von Bergmann K, et al. Stimulation of cholesterol excretion by the liver X receptor agonist requires ATP-binding cassette transporters G5 and G8. *J Biol Chem* 2003;278:15565–15570.

136. Yu L, Hammer RE, Li-Hawkins J, et al. Disruption of Abcg5 and Abcg8 in mice reveals their crucial role in biliary cholesterol secretion. *Proc Natl Acad Sci USA* 2002;99:16237–16242.

137. Yu L, Li-Hawkins J, Hammer RE, et al. Overexpression of ABCG5 and ABCG8 promotes biliary cholesterol secretion and reduced fractional absorption of dietary cholesterol. *J Clin Invest* 2002;110:671–680.

138. Veniant MM, Suillvan MA, Kim SK, et al. Defining the atherogenicity of large and small lipoproteins containing apolipoprotein B100. *J Clin Invest* 2000;106:1501–1510.

139. Jiang XC, Quin S, Qiao C, et al. Apolipoprotein B secretion and atherosclerosis are decreased in mice with phospholipid-transfer protein deficiency. *Nat Med* 2001;7:847–852.

140. Groen AK, Bloks VW, Bandsma RH, et al. Hepatobiliary cholesterol transport is not impaired in Abca 1-null mice lacking HDL. *J Clin Invest* 2001;108:843–850.

141. Shih DQ, Bussen M, Sehayek E, et al. Hepatocyte nuclear factor-1 alpha is an essential regulator of bile acid and plasma cholesterol metabolism. *Nat Genet* 2001;27:375–382.

142. Ishikawa K, Sugawara D, Wang X, et al. Heme oxygenase-1 inhibits atherosclerotic lesion formation in ldl-receptor knockout mice. *Circ Res* 2001;88:506–512.

143. Brennan ML, Anderson MM, Shih DM, et al. Increased atherosclerosis in myeloperoxidase-deficient mice. *J Clin Invest* 2001;107:419–430.

144. Terasawa Y, Ladha Z, Leonard SW, et al. Increased atherosclerosis in hyperlipidemic mice deficient in alpha-tocopherol transfer protein and vitamin E. *Proc Natl Acad Sci USA* 2000;97:13830–13834.

145. Fazio S, Major AS, Swift LL, et al. Increased atherosclerosis in LDL receptor-null mice lacking ACAT1 in macrophages. *J Clin Invest* 2001;106:163–171.

146. Makowski L, Boord JB, Maeda K, et al. Lack of macrophage fatty-acid-binding protein aP2 protects mice deficient in apolipoprotein E against atherosclerosis. *Nat Med* 2001;7:699–705.

147. Song L, Leung C, Schindler C. Lymphocytes are important in early atherosclerosis. *J Clin Invest* 2001;108:251–259.

148. Reardon CA, Blachowicz L, White T, et al. Effect of immune deficiency in lipoproteins and atherosclerosis in male apolipoprotein E-deficient mice. *Arterioscler Thromb Vasc Biol* 2001;21:1011–1016.

149. Husemann J, Obstfeld A, Fennraio M, et al. CD11b/CD18 mediates production of reactive oxygen species by mouse and human macrophages adherent to matrixes containing oxidized LDL. *Arterioscler Thromb Vasc Biol* 2001;21:1301–1305.

150. Kuhlencordt PJ, Gyurko R, Han F, et al. Accelerated atherosclerosis, aortic aneurysm formation, and ischemic heart disease in apolipoprotein E/endothelial nitric oxide synthase double-knockout mice. *Circulation* 2001;104:448–454.

151. Ihrig M, Dangler CA, Fox JG. Mice lacking inducible nitric oxide synthase develop spontaneous hypercholesterolemia and aortic atheromas. *Atherosclerosis* 2001;56:103–107.

152. Kuhlencordt PJ, Chen J, Han F, et al. Genetic deficiency of inducible nitric oxide synthases reduces atherosclerosis and lowers plasma lipids peroxides in apolipoprotein E-knockout mice. *Circulation* 2001;103:3099–3104.

153. Niu XL, Yang X, Hoshiai K, et al. Inducible nitric oxide synthase deficiency does not affect the susceptibility of mice to atherosclerosis but increases collagen content in lesions. *Circulation* 2001;103:1115–1120.

154. Silence J, Lupu F, Collen D, et al. Persistence of atherosclerotic plaque but reduced aneurysm formation in mice with stromelysin-1 (MMP-3) gene inactivation. *Arterioscler Thromb Vasc Biol* 2001;21:1440–1445.

155. Lemaitre V, O'Byrne TK, Borczuk AC, et al. ApoE knockout mice expressing human matrix metalloproteinase-1 in macrophages have less advanced atherosclerosis. *J Clin Invest* 2001;107:1227–1234.

156. Tordjman K, Bernal-Mizrachi C, Zemany L, et al. PPARalpha deficiency reduces insulin resistance and atherosclerosis in apoE-null mice. *J Clin Invest* 2001;107:1025–1034.

157. Cybulsky MI, Iiyama K, Li L, et al. A major role for VCAM-1, but not ICAM-1, in early atherosclerosis. *J Clin Invest* 2001;107:1255–1262.

158. Reue K, Xu P, Wang XP, et al. Adipose tissue deficiency, glucose intolerance, and increased atherosclerosis result from mutation in the mouse fatty liver dystrophy (FLD) gene. *J Lipid Res* 2000;41:1067–1076.

159. Phan J, Pesaran T, Davis RC, et al. The diet1 locus confers protection against hypercholesterolemia through enhanced bile acid metabolism. *J Biol Chem* 2002;277:469–477.

160. Bodnar JS, Chatterjee A, Castellani LW, et al. Positional cloning of the combined hyperlipidemia gene Hyplip1. *Nat Genet* 2001;30:110–116.

CHAPTER **26**

Genetics of Atherothrombotic Disease

Andreas Muench and Pierre Zoldhelyi

Key Words: Acute coronary syndromes; atherosclerosis; coronary artery disease; genetics; population studies; risk factors; thrombosis.

INTRODUCTION

Atherothrombosis of coronary, carotid, and peripheral arteries is the leading cause of death and disability in the industrialized world. Acute ischemic exacerbations, such as myocardial infarction (MI), are caused in general by plaque rupture and superimposed thrombosis (1). The term *athero-*

A. Muench: Division of Cardiology, Department of Medicine, University of Texas Health Science Center at Houston, 64311 Fannin, Room 1.246, Houston, Texas 77030.
P. Zoldhelyi: Department of Internal Medicine, Division of Cardiology, Wafic Said Molecular Cardiology and Gene Therapy Research Laboratories, Texas Heart Institute at St. Luke's Episcopal Hospital, Houston, Texas.

thrombosis has been coined to describe the intimately connected phenomena of slowly developing atherothrombosis and intermittent thrombosis.

As in other complex disorders, genotype, penetrance (the degree to which a genotype is phenotypically expressed), and environment determine to varying degree the incidence and severity of atherothrombotic disorders. Goals of genetic research related to these disorders are the identification of specific genes or gene variants involved in the individuals' susceptibility to these diseases and the dissection of the underlying molecular pathways. In addition to the complex pathophysiology of the atherothrombotic disorders (involving a multitude of genes and proteins), this task is further complicated by that the function of more than half of the estimated 35,000 to 40,000 genes of the human genome is unknown (2,3), which undoubtedly include unknown determinants of atherothrombosis and thrombosis. The delineation of the genetic basis of common complex disorders is challenging and involves integration of such different types of information as DNA sequence data from the Human Genome Project, genotype associations, gene expression profiling data, structural and functional genomics data, protenomic studies, results of clinical studies, and other information.

For most patients with an acute coronary or cerebrovascular event, the practical implications of the genetically determined risk are still few because the "genetic inquiry" is usually limited to obtaining a family history of premature coronary artery disease (CAD). The emphasis in the prevention of further events usually focuses exclusively on modification of environmental rather than genetic factors. Clinical trials in *gene therapy* are limited to a relatively small number of studies of local somatic gene transfer, but they have not yet advanced to modify the underlying genetic risk for atherothrombotic disorders.

Despite these limitations in the clinical application of genetics, the understanding of the genetic basis of atherothrombotic disorders has grown substantially as witnessed by a rapidly growing list of genes and proteins involved in the pathogenesis of these disorders. This review illustrates concepts and methods of genetic research related to atherothrombotic disease and points out relevant examples and studies.

PRINCIPLES AND METHODS OF GENE DISCOVERY IN ATHEROTHROMBOTIC DISEASE

A variety of methods is used to study the heritability of common complex disorders and to discover novel disease genes, gene variants, or factors altering gene expression. Heritability of atherothrombotic vascular disease may exceed 50% in the general population (4,5).

Linkage Analysis

Linkage analysis allows the identification of genes underlying a specific disease or phenotype on the basis of their recombination frequencies with markers in related chromosomal regions. Linkage disequilibrium refers to a close allelic association of two or more loci that is preserved over many generations. Analysis of linkage and linkage disequilibrium is made on the basis of genomic location and distance and does not require any prior knowledge about biologic or functional pathways. Strategies of linkage analysis include genome scans, with markers interspersed throughout the genome, or the screening of single candidate genes that are believed to play a role in the phenotype of interest. Linkage analysis has been successfully applied to many relatively rare monogenic (Mendelian) diseases but is far more challenging when applied to complex common disorders such as atherothrombosis, where disease expression is determined by the cooperation of a multitude of genes with various environmental modifiers (6). Other problems in linkage analysis of atherothrombotic disorders are phenotype variability, long generation time intervals, and the generally late onset

of clinical manifestations. A German study completed total genome scans in 513 families having at least two members with acute MI or severe CAD before age 60 years; this study uncovered a new "MI locus" on chromosome 14 (14q32) in addition to genetically mapping known risk factors including increased plasma levels of lipoprotein(a) [Lp(a)], low-density lipoprotein (LDL), and triglycerides (TGs) (7). Another study in Finish families with angiographically defined premature CAD provided evidence for linkage to two chromosomal regions: 2q21.1-22 and Xq23-26 (8).

Genetic Polymorphisms and Genotype Association Studies

Variation in the DNA sequence of the genome forms the genetic basis of our individuality. Specific sequence variants that are found in more than 1% of the population are referred to as *polymorphisms*. The term *mutation* is generally applied to sequence alterations that produce overt disease. *Single nucleotide polymorphisms* (SNPs) are used to discriminate different alleles by restriction enzyme digestion (restriction fragment length polymorphism), polymerase chain reaction (PCR), or DNA-microarray. More than 1.4 million SNPs were identified in the initial sequencing of the human genome, most of which in noncoding DNA regions without phenotypic consequences (9). Short elements of repetitive DNA sequences such as microsatellites (dinucleotide repeats) or minisatellites (repetitive DNA sequences of greater complexity) have a greater degree of variability (i.e., more alleles) than the SNPs. Polymorphisms are the basis for genotyping, linkage analysis, DNA fingerprinting, paternity testing, and so on.

Genotype association studies investigate potential differences in the frequency of polymorphisms or gene variants when compared between control and disease populations. The number of known associations of allelic variance with risk factors or overt manifestations of atherothrombotic disorders is rapidly increasing. Automation of genotyping procedures enables large-scale association studies that examine many polymorphisms simultaneously. A Japanese study examined 112 polymorphisms of 71 candidate genes in 2,819 unrelated individuals with MI and 2,242 control subjects (10). The study found a significant association of MI in men with the C1019 polymorphism in the *connexin 37* gene (gene map locus *1p35.1*), an endothelial cell gap junction protein. In women, there was a significant link with the 4G-668/5G polymorphism within the promoter region of the plasminogen-activator inhibitor type 1 *(PAI-1)* gene (gene map locus *7q21.3-q22*) and with the 5A-117/6A polymorphism of the *stromelysin* (matrix metalloproteinase 3 [MMP-3]; *11q23*) gene.

A number of genotype association studies have reported links between the increased incidence of atherothrombotic disorders and gene polymorphisms associated with qualitative and quantitative alteration proteins involved in coagulation, fibrinolysis, platelet function, and more recently inflammation. However, many of the reported findings are inconsistent, if not conflicting, especially with regard to establishing a direct correlation of a genotype with thrombotic disease. Thus, the results of most genotype association studies remain controversial with no consensus on their practical implications (some examples are discussed later in this chapter).

Potential inconsistencies may be because of phenotype complexity, small effects of individual allelic variants, limited size of the study populations, improper population mix, and interfering environmental factors (11). Furthermore, linkage disequilibrium may falsely indicate an effect of a gene variant that is actually caused by another nearby locus. Finally, even a statistically significant association may not translate into a clinical consequence. Despite all these limitations, genotype association studies have contributed significantly to our understanding of the genetic basis and the molecular mechanisms of many complex diseases, including atherothrombotic disorders.

Gene Expression Profiling

Several recently developed technologies allow large-scale gene expression profiling in diseased and healthy tissue or during different stages of disease progression. For example, *DNA-microarrays* permit simultaneous profiling of expression patterns of thousands of genes during a single experiment (12). *Serial analysis of gene expression* (SAGE) is another technique to analyze a large number of transcripts simultaneously (13). A third approach is *differential display of randomly primed messenger RNA (mRNA) by reverse transcription (RT)-PCR* (DD/RT-PCR), where mRNA are targeted in random fashion by oligonucleotide primers, then amplified after RT and finally analyzed on DNA sequencing gels (14). These different methods of large-scale gene expression profiling produce a wealth of data, which in most cases still await confirmation of specificity and determination of the biologic significance.

De Waard and coworkers (15) used SAGE to investigate differential gene expression of human arterial endothelial cells in the quiescent stage and after activation with a strong atherogenic and inflammatory stimulus (oxidized LDL). Transcripts derived from 14 unknown and 42 known genes were differentially expressed. Among the latter were endothelial cell activation marker, growth factor, and fibrinolysis factor genes. Stanton and coworkers (16) studied temporal and spatial gene expression in a rat model of acute MI using DNA microarrays. More than 200 of 4,000 examined genes were found to be differentially expressed in response to MI (16).

Animal Models

As discussed in Chapter 25, the mouse is the most used animal model to study the genetic basis of atherothrombosis and its complications. The ability to manipulate the mouse genome, specifically to silence ("knockout") or overexpress genes, has made it possible to study the *in vivo* function of single genes. Currently, the most widely used mouse strain in atherothrombosis research is the apolipoprotein E (apoE)-knockout mouse, in which spontaneous hypercholesterolemia is accompanied by the development of extensive atherothrombosis. Mice models also are used for linkage analysis, genome wide expression studies, evaluation of new pharmacologic agents, and gene therapy. The transgenic work is likely to continue to shift from the purely hyperlipidemic (apoE$^{-/-}$ or LDL receptor–null mice) strains to those with additional mutations of genes involved in inflammation, plaque stability, and thrombosis (17).

Other examples of transgenic atherothrombosis models are the Watanabe heritable hyperlipidemic rabbit, a model of human familial hypercholesterolemia (FH) (18), and a new genetic variant of the Dahl salt-sensitive hypertensive rats overexpressing the human cholesteryl ester transfer protein, which was reported to have atherothrombotic lesions resulting in spontaneous MI and decreased survival (19).

EXAMPLES FOR ATHEROTHROMBOSIS SUSCEPTIBILITY GENE VARIANTS

Lipoproteins

In most individuals, the genetic basis of a high-risk lipoprotein profile is complex and polygenic. However, monogenic traits are responsible in some families. Examples are FH caused by mutations in the LDL receptor gene *(19p13.2)* or Tangier disease. The latter is a rare condition characterized by the virtual absence of circulating high-density lipoprotein (HDL) caused by mutations in the adenosine triphosphate–binding cassette (ABC) transporter A1 *(ABCA1; 9q22-q31)* gene (20). Although genetic dyslipoproteinemias are reviewed in Chapter 5, two examples stand out for the well known role in atherothrombotic disease: Lp(a) and apoE.

Lipoprotein(a)

High levels of serum Lp(a) are an independent risk factor for MI and stroke (21,22). Plasma Lp(a) concentrations vary widely among individuals, remain relatively constant over time, and have defied most drug and dietary intervention. Variants of the apolipoprotein(a) [*Apo(a); 6q27*] gene account for more than 90% of the observed interindividual variation of Lp(a) plasma levels (23). The extensive polymorphism of the *Apo(a)* gene is caused by a varying number of the tandemly-repeated (VNTR) kringle structure encoding the sequence element kringle 4. In general, there is an inverse relation between the number of kringle repeats and Lp(a) levels (23). Other polymorphisms in the coding and regulatory regions of the gene have been described, and numerous genotype associations studies have attempted to correlate the risk for coronary events with *Apo(a)* gene variants with mixed results. Five Apo(a) polymorphisms lacked any association with MI in the Etude Cas-Temoins de l'Infarctus du Myocarde (ECTIM) study (24).

Apolipoprotein E

ApoE gene variants and their relation to different diseases are among the most extensively studied loci in the apolipoprotein gene family. The *apoE* gene *(19q13.2)* is polymorphic with three common alleles (ε_2, ε_3, and ε_4) distinguished by single amino acid substitutions at two different sites (cys or arg at residues 112 and 158) (25). A metaanalysis on *apoE* alleles and risk for CAD in 1996 showed only a weak association of the ε_4 allele with CAD (odds ratio [OR], 1.26; 95% confidence interval [CI], 1.13–1.41) (26). Results of the international Monitoring of Trends and Determinants in Cardiovascular Disease (MONICA) study suggested a stronger association with fatal CAD, showing an increase in the CAD mortality rate by 24.5 per 100,000 for an increase of 0.01 in the relative frequency of the ε_4 allele (27). A subanalysis of the Scandinavian Simvastatin Survival Study (4S) trial concluded that MI survivors carrying the ε_4 allele had a nearly twofold risk for death during 5.5-year follow-up period compared with noncarriers that was abolished by treatment with simvastatin (28).

Homocysteine

The suggestion that increased serum homocysteine levels are linked to atherothrombotic disease stems from early observations that genetic defects of cystathionine β-synthase and methylenetetrahydrofolate reductase (MTHFR) lead to increased plasma homocysteine associated with premature vascular disease and the demonstration that high concentrations of homocysteine produce severe endothelial dysfunction. Numerous studies evaluated the association of increased plasma homocysteine levels with coronary and cerebrovascular disease. A metaanalysis of prospective studies showed a modest link, whereas a 25% below average homocysteine level (about 3 μM [0.41 mg/L]) was associated with an 11% reduction in the risk for ischemic heart disease (OR, 0.89; 95% CI, 0.83–0.96) and a 19% reduction in stroke risk (OR, 0.81; 95% CI, 0.69–0.95) (29).

An extensively studied MTHFR (1p36.3) polymorphism is an SNP where a C/T substitution (TT-genotype) at base 677 results in an alanine/valine exchange in the mature protein and reduced MTHFR activity resulting in increased serum homocysteine concentrations (30). A metaanalysis of 40 studies on the association of the MTHFR-TT genotype with CAD demonstrated a small (16% higher odds; OR, 1.16; 95% CI, 1.05–1.28) increase in the risk for CAD when compared with individuals with the CC genotype (30). Nonetheless, these findings may be of clinical importance, especially because folic acid supplementation alleviates these adverse effects of the MTHFR-TT genotype (30).

Angiotensin-converting Enzyme

The angiotensin-converting enzyme *(ACE; 17q23)* gene exhibits polymorphism with regard to the insertion of a 287 base pair (bp) alu-repeat within intron 16, resulting in three possible genotypes based on the presence (insertion = I) or absence (deletion = D) of the alu-sequence element (DD, DI, and II) (31). The *D* allele is strongly associated with an increased level of circulating *ACE*. The role of *ACE* gene variants has been investigated in diverse disorders including MI, heart failure, left ventricular hypertrophy, hypertension, nephropathy, and restenosis after percutaneous coronary intervention.

Cambien and coworkers (32) were the first to report an increased frequency of the *DD* genotype in patients with MI, which was followed by a number of studies with conflicting results (33). A metaanalysis in 1996 combining 3,394 MI cases and 5,479 control subjects supported a weak association of the *ACE-DD* genotype with the risk for MI (mean OR for MI of *DD* vs. *ID/II* genotypes was 1.26; 95% CI, 1.15–1.39; $p < 0.0001$) with an increased relative risk in the Japanese population (33). Whether allelic variation of *ACE* influences the risk for MI by direct effects on plaque stability or thrombosis, or through interactions with various other metabolic or prothrombotic factors is debated.

EXAMPLES OF GENETIC FACTORS ASSOCIATED WITH RESISTANCE TO ATHEROTHROMBOTIC DISEASE

Resistance to atherothrombosis is exemplified by individuals without apparent clinical manifestations in the presence of a high-risk profile or by those with extensive atherothrombosis but relatively few thrombotic complications.

High-Density Lipoprotein

The best recognized factor associated with a reduced risk for CAD is HDL-cholesterol, which is routinely included in the screening test for cardiovascular risk assessment. Key atheroprotective mechanisms of HDL involve lipid clearance from the circulation and the vascular wall by reverse cholesterol transport and also antiinflammatory effects.

HDL plasma levels have a strong genetic determination. The principal apolipoprotein in HDL is apoA-I, a cofactor for the enzyme lecithin cholesterol acyltransferase. Overexpression of apoA-I in a variety of transgenic animal models inhibits progression of atherothrombosis and promotes regression of existing atherothrombotic lesions (34). The *apoA_1* gene is located within a cluster of closely related apolipoprotein genes on the long arm of chromosome 7 (APO A1-C3-A4). Multiple variants of *apoA_1* and its adjacent loci are described. These account for a large part of the familial hypoalphalipoproteinemia (low HDL) cases and are generally associated with high TG levels and accelerated atherothrombosis (35).

previous MI, compared with those without MI. The odds ratio for MI was even greater in the youngest individuals of the study sample (<49 years; n = 223; OR, 2.61; 95% CI, 1.26–5.41; $p = 0.009$) (80). In contrast, there was no association with MI in studies in the United Kingdom or Japan or with MI and cerebrovascular events in a study in Spain (81–83).

Glycoprotein Ib/IX/V Receptor Complex

The *trans*-membrane GP Ib/IX/V complex is present with approximately 25,000 copies per platelet and is the major receptor for von Willebrand factor, mediating initial platelet adhesion to injured arterial wall. GP 1b is composed of two polypeptide chains: GP 1bα and GP 1bβ. The α subunit, the functional dominant part of the complex, is encoded by a relatively small gene (6 kb, 1 exon) located on chromosome 17-p12. The rare bleeding diathesis Bernard-Soulier syndrome (type A) is caused by a mutation in the *GP Ibα* gene (84). The relation of atherothrombosis to two closely linked and common polymorphisms (Thr145Met or HPA-2 and VNTR-A,B,C,D) within the coding region of the *GP Ibα* gene has been studied. The Ibα HPA-2/VNTR-B haplotype was associated with fatal MI and sudden cardiac death in middle-aged Finnish men in the Helsinki Sudden Death Study (85). The *B* allele of the VNTR polymorphisms also was associated with an increased risk for acute coronary syndromes and acute cerebral vascular disease in middle-aged patients (86). Several other studies on this subject exist from Japan and Europe with inconsistent results (77).

In summary, epidemiologic evidence to date does not support an important influence of gene variants related to platelet function on the atherothrombotic risk, which is similar to the genotype association studies involving the coagulation factor genes. However, genetic and molecular research of platelet function has just begun. Because platelets can be easily removed during stages activation, such as acute coronary syndromes, they are good subjects for genetic analysis. Future large-scale studies of gene expression and the proteome of activated platelets are likely to reveal new insights into the pathogenesis of atherothrombotic disease.

GENES AND GENE VARIANTS INVOLVED IN INFLAMMATION, CELL SIGNALING, AND PLAQUE DESTABILIZATION

Interest in the role of inflammation in atherothrombotic disease has recently surged. Genes of mediators of inflammation direct cell–cell interactions during initiation and progression of atherothrombotic lesions, mediate the turnover of the lipid core and of the fibrous cap matrix of the atherothrombotic plaque, and alter the thrombogenicity of plaque constituents (87). The four cell types that are mainly involved in these processes are vascular endothelial cells, smooth muscle cells, leukocytes, and platelets. An array of cell signaling factors and cytokines regulate interactions between these different cells during atherogenesis and arterial thrombosis. Genetically determined variation in these complex pathways may account for a part of the variation in the risk for atherothrombotic disease between individuals or populations. A growing number of studies evaluate the association of gene variants of inflammatory mediators with atherothrombotic disease. A few examples of these studies are mentioned in this chapter and also some biochemical mechanisms are discussed.

C-Reactive Protein

C-Reactive protein (CRP) is an indicator of low-grade systemic inflammation and has been recognized to be a powerful risk marker for vascular disease, including acute coronary disorders and stroke (88). There also is a possible active involvement of the CRP protein in the pathogenesis of atherothrombotic disease (89). A polymorphism in the *CRP* gene (1059G/C within exon 2) and its relation to future vascular events was examined in 726 case–control pairs out of the large Physician Health Study. The C variant (GC or CC as compared with GG) of the polymorphism was associated with reduced CRP levels, but there was no significant association with risk for arterial thrombosis (nonfatal MI, nonfatal stroke, or cardiovascular death) with either variant (90).

Cell Adhesion Molecules

Endothelial activation represents an early stage of atheroma development and is characterized by decreased vasoreactivity, alteration of endothelial interface–integrity, and leucocyte adhesion. Activated endothelial cells express chemoattractant and adhesion molecules, mediating leukocyte adhesion and transmigration. Examples are vascular cell adhesion molecule-1 (VCAM-1), intercellular adhesion molecule-1 (ICAM-1), and proteins of the selectin family (selectin E and P).

Intercellular Adhesion Molecule-1

Gene variants of the *ICAM-1* gene *(19p13.3-p13.2)* have been studied in disorders as diverse as dementia, different types of arthritis, inflammatory bowel disease, type-1 diabetes, and atherothrombosis. Smaller studies have linked ICAM-1 polymorphism to CAD, MI, and peripheral arterial occlusive disease (Table 26–1).

E-Selectin and P-Selectin

The gene for endothelial leukocyte adhesion molecule-1 (E-selectin, 1q23-q25) has several polymorphisms (128Ser/Arg, 554-Leu/Phe, and 98G/T). Genotype association studies relating to CAD and MI had conflicting results (Table 26–1).

The P-selectin gene (map locus *1q23-q25*) is highly polymorphic. Among several polymorphisms the variant 715-Pro has a possible protective role from MI (lower frequency in cases than in control subjects) (Table 26–1).

TABLE 26–1. *Association studies of gene polymorphisms of factors involved in inflammation and cell signaling with coronary artery disease and myocardial infarction*

Gene	Polymorphism	Author (reference)	n (cases/control subjects)	Suggested results
CRP	1059G/C	Zee et al. (90)	726/726	No significant association with non-fatal MI, stroke, or cardiovascular death
ICAM-1	Lys-469-Glu	Jiang et al. (100)	349/213	Association to MI and CAD
E-selectin	Ser-128-Arg	Wenzel et al. (101)	97 patients <50 years	Associated with angiographic severe CAD in patients <50 years
	Ser-128-Arg, Leu-554-Phe, G98T	Wenzel et al. (102)	40 patients <40 years	Associated with angiographic severe CAD in younger patients
	Ser-128-Arg	Herrmann et al. (103)	99/100	No association with MI
	G98T	Zheng et al. (104)	647/758 (all male)	*T* allele more common in younger patients with angiographic CAD
P-selectin	Ser-128-Arg	Ye et al. (105)	82/71	Association with early-onset CAD
	Pro715	Herrmann et al. (103)	647/758 (all male)	Possible protective from MI
	Pro715	Kee et al. (106)	696/561	Possible protective from MI
	S290N, N562D, V599L, T715P, T741T	Tregouet et al. (107)	582/630	Protective effect of the P715; S290N and N562D associated with MI, when carried by certain haplotype
	C-2123G, A-1969G, Thr715Pro	Barbaux et al. (108)	869/334	Polymorphisms associated with P-selectin levels but not with MI
TNF-α and β	-863C/A, -308G/A (TNF-α), 252G/A (TNF-β)	Koch et al. (109)	998 (CAD); 793 (MI)/340	No association of TNF or IL-10 polymorphisms with MI or CAD
TNF-α	Five polymorphisms	Herrmann et al. (110)	641/710	No association to MI or CAD
TNF-α and β	TNF-α 308 G/A, TNF-β 252 A/G	Padovani et al. (111)	148/148	No association to MI
TNF-α and β	TNF-β 308 G/A, TNF-β 252 A/G	Keso et al. (112)	700 men (autopsy)	No association to old MI by autopsy or CAD
TNF-α	308 G/A	Francis et al. (113)	674/232	No association to angiographic CAD
IL-1 cluster	IL-1A(−889), IL-1B(−511), IL-1B(+3953), IL-1RA intron 2 VNTR	Francis et al. (113)	674/232	IL-1RA VNTR allele 2 associated with single-vessel CAD
IL-1-RA	IL-1RA intron 2 VNTR	Manzoli et al. (114)	115/80	No clearcut association to CAD or MI
IL-1 cluster	IL-1b 511 C/T, IL-1RA intron 2 VNTR	Vohnout et al. (115)	355/205	No association to angiographic CAD with either polymorphism
IL-1-RA	IL1RN-VNTR	Zee et al. (116)	385/385 (prospective)	No association with risk for future MI
IL-1β, IL-RA	IL-1b 511 C/T, IL-1RA intron 2 VNTR	Momiyama et al. (117)	188/104	IL-1b (−511) C/C and IL-1Ra (intron 2) 2- or 3-repeat allele both associated with CAD, association with MI only in patients who are seropositive for *Chlamydia pneumoniae*

Gene	Polymorphism	Reference	Sample (cases/controls)	Association
IL-6	IL-6 G(−174)C promoter polymorphism	Nauck et al. (118)	2559/729	No association with the risk for CAD or MI
	−174 (G/C), −572 (G/C), −596 (G/A) +528 I/D	Georges et al. (119)	640/719	−174 C associated with MI (OR, 1.34); −174 C more frequent in patients with two or fewer stenosed vessels than in patients with three-vessel lesions
IL-10	3 IL-10 promoter polymorphisms (1082G/A, −819C/T and −592C/A)	Koch et al. (109)	998 (CAD); 793 (MI)/340	No association with MI or CAD
TGF-β₁	7 polymorphisms	Donger et al. (120)	1107/1082	No association with risk for MI
	29 T/C	Yokota et al. (92)	315/591	T allele is a risk factor for MI in middle-aged Japanese men
	−509T	Wang et al. (121)	371 cases	No association with CAD
	7 polymorphisms	Cambien et al. (122)	563/629	No association with the degree of angiographic CAD, Pro25 allele associated with MI in some regions
Stromelysin (MMP-3)	5 polymorphisms	Syrris et al. (123)	655/244	No association of either polymorphism with CAD
	5A-1171/6A promoter polymorphism (5A/6A)	Schwarz et al. (124)	1848 (coronary angiography)/515 healthy control subjects	No association with risk for MI, 6A allele marker for progression of CAD
	5A/6A	Terashima et al. (125)	330 (AMI)/330	5A allele associated with risk for MI
	5A/6A	Kim et al. et al. (126)	131 (stable angina)/117	5A allele associated with stable angina
	5A/6A	Humphries et al. (127)	125/375 (prospective study)	6A genotypes at greater risk for CAD related events in nonsmokers 5A/5A genotype amplifies risk in smokers
PECAM-1 (CD31)	5A/6A	Ye et al. (128)	72/354	Homozygosis for 6A associated with greater progression of angiographic CAD
	Val125Leu, Asn563Ser, and Gly670Arg	Sasaoka et al. (129)	136 Japanese patients with MI/235	563Ser/Ser and 670Arg/Arg genotypes associated with MI
	Val125Leu, Asn563Ser	Wenzel et al. (130)	98 German patients with early CAD/103	125Val and 563Asn associated with early CAD (<50 years)
	Leu125Val, Ser563Asn	Song et al. (131)	156/75	125Val and 563Asn associated with CAD
	Val125Leu	Gardemann et al. (132)	2,500	No association with MI; weak association of Val125 with CAD in low-risk patients without HTN or DM (OR, 1.54; 95% CI, 1.03–2.3)

Examples are given; not a complete list. Studies evaluating acute events were not separated from those assessing risk for coronary artery disease (CAD; angina, angiographic disease). Not listed are studies on restenosis or cerebrovascular disease.

CI, confidence interval; CRP, C-reactive protein; DM, diabetes mellitus; HTN, hypertension; ICAM, intercellular adhesion molecule; IL, interleukin; MI, myocardial infarction; MMP, matrix metalloproteinase; OR, odds ratio; PECAM, platelet endothelial cell adhesion molecule; TGF, transforming growth factor; TNF, tumor necrosis factor; VNTR, variable number of tandem repeats.

Cytokines and Growth Factors

The involvement of cytokines and growth factors (and their genes) in atherothrombotic disease is multifaceted with numerous effects on endothelial function, lipid metabolism, and blood coagulation. Cytokines such as interferon-γ and tumor necrosis factor-β (TNF-β) stimulate endothelial cells, vascular smooth muscle cells, and macrophages during initiation and progression of atherothrombotic lesions. Interferon-γ can halt collagen synthesis by vascular smooth muscle cells leading to plaque instability (87). Growth factor proteins are implemented in cell proliferation leading to plaque stabilization, lesion progression, or in-stent restenosis.

Tumor Necrosis Factor

The *TNF-α* and *β* genes are located in close proximity on 6p21.3. A Japanese large-scale case–control association study, analyzing 92,788 SNP markers, showed an association of TNF-β markers with MI (91). Genotype association studies of several functionally relevant polymorphisms of the TNF-α and β with risk for CAD or MI genes have been largely negative however (Table 26–1).

Transforming Growth Factor-β (gene map locus 19q13.1)

Of special interest are the effects of transforming growth factor-β (TGF-β) on vascular remodeling and its possible role as an inhibiting factor in atherothrombosis progression. Japanese investigators showed an association of a *TGF-β* gene SNP (29 T→C transition, resulting in Leu-10-Pro substitution) with MI in middle-aged Japanese men (n = 234, *TT* + *TC* vs. *CC; p* < 0.0001; OR, 3.5; 95% CI, 2.0–6.3) (92). In contrast, there was no association with MI in women. In both men and women serum concentrations of *TGF-β* were significantly greater in individuals with the *CC* genotype than in subjects with the *TT* or *TC* genotype. Other *TGF-β* genotype association studies with CAD or MI are listed in Table 26–1; the table also summarizes studies involving genes of other cytokines, such as the interleukin-1 cluster.

Matrix Metalloproteinases

An important mechanism of plaque erosion is degradation of the fibrous cap by MMPs. The family of MMPs includes interstitial collagenases, gelatinases and stromelysin (MMP-3). Initial research on the MMPs has focused on their role in connective tissue disorders, cancer, arthritis, and rupture of aortic aneurysms. More recently, interest in their involvement, especially of MMP-2, 9, and 3 (stromelysin), in atherothrombotic plaque rupture has emerged. For example, stromelysin is abundant in atherothrombotic plaques, can cleave different substrates, and can activate other MMPs. Interestingly, a significant association of increased risk for MI with the *6A* allele of the *stromelysin 5A-1171-6A* gene poly-

morphism was found in women in the large study by Yamada (10) discussed earlier in this chapter. Results of smaller genotype association studies have been mixed and are also listed in Table 26–1.

PHARMACOGENOMICS AND ATHEROTHROMBOTIC DISEASE

The effectiveness of cardiovascular pharmacotherapy and the occurrence of unwanted side effects or toxicities varies among individuals and populations. Although many nongenetic factors such as age, patient's compliance, nature and stage of the disease, concomitant therapy, and others all play a role, genetic determinants account for a substantial part of the individual differences in the response to pharmacologic therapy. Virtually every pathway of drug metabolism and action is likely to have some genetic variation (93). The following sections highlight two examples of commonly prescribed agents: aspirin and statins.

Aspirin

Aspirin, one of the most widely used drugs worldwide, reduces the risk for cardiovascular events by inhibiting platelet aggregation. The drug inhibits platelet thromboxane A_2 synthesis by means of irreversible acetylation of a serine residue at position 529 of the platelet cyclooxygenase-1 (COX-1). A subset of individuals has limited benefit from aspirin, also termed *aspirin resistance.* In an analysis of Canadian patients enrolled in the Heart Outcomes Prevention Evaluation (HOPE) study, concentrations of urinary 11-dehydro-thromboxane B_2, an indicator of incomplete suppression of thromboxane generation, were measured. The odds for the composite study end points (first MI, stroke, or cardiovascular death) increased with greater urinary concentrations of the metabolite (OR, 1.8; 95% CI, 1.2–2.7; p = 0.009 for patients in the upper quartile of urinary 11-dehydro-thromboxane B_2 concentration) (94). These results raise the question whether allelic variation of the *COX-1* gene or other genes involved in prostaglandin biosynthesis may account for aspirin resistance in acute coronary disorders. There are more than 100 SNPs located within the genes involved in thromboxane A_2 synthesis (95). The previously mentioned PLA_1/PLA_2 gene variant of the platelet *GP IIIa* gene also been implicated in aspirin insensitivity. Individuals with the PLA_2 allele showed decreased response to the antithrombotic action of aspirin (96).

3-Hydroxy-3-methylglutaryl Coenzyme A Reductase Inhibitors ("Statins")

Large landmark trials have established the benefit of cholesterol-lowering therapy with statins in the primary and secondary prevention of cardiovascular events. These data are impressive, but represent average risk reductions and do not take into account the genetic variability of the response to these drugs or the individual susceptibility to side effects. Several gene variants and their influence on the effects of statins have been investigated. Among others, these include polymorphisms in the genes for cholesteryl ester transfer protein (Taq1B), stromelysin-1 (5A/6A polymorphism in promoter region), β-fibrinogen ((455G/A), apoE$_4$, lipoprotein lipase (Asp-9-Asn), hepatic lipase (-514 CT) and the ACE deletion type polymorphism (97).

This chapter mentioned few examples of genetic influences on effects of commonly used drugs. Most inherited factors of the response to pharmacologic therapy are polygenic. There are also numerous drug gene and gene–gene interactions. The strategies to dissect these polygenic determinants of varying effects of pharmacotherapy are akin to the ones discussed earlier in the genetics of common complex disorders. They may involve genetic mapping of factors associated with drug effects by genome-wide and candidate gene approaches, gene expression profiling, and protenomic approaches (98,99).

Genetic-based research will bring a large number of novel targets for pharmacologic therapy. Expectations in the future impact of pharmacogenomics are raising the possibility of a pharmacotherapy tailored to the individuals' genetic background to identify the right drug and dose for each patient. With the rapid evolution of automated genotyping methods, simultaneous screening of thousands of polymorphisms relevant to pharmacotherapy will be possible. Whether broad and extensive genetic screening of large populations in cardiovascular pharmacology and medicine is beneficial is uncertain. Before the wide application of this approach a number of questions, including clinical significance, molecular mechanisms of gene variants and cost considerations, need to be addressed. Genetic research will bring about new powerful therapeutic options that will continue to transform the clinical practice. One must, however, realize that the currently available pharmacologic tools for prevention of atherothrombotic events are quite powerful and are widely underused.

CONCLUSION

This chapter reviewed some of the methods to delineate the genetic basis of atherothrombotic diseases and highlighted a few examples of studies. The elucidation of the genetics of such common complex disorders remains a formidable challenge for molecular research in the twenty-first century.

ACKNOWLEDGMENTS

The authors have no conflict of interest to disclose.

1. 5R01 HL073346-02 (NHLBI)
2. Texas State Grant, Subsection "Gene Therapy"
3. Introgen Therapeutics, Inc., Houston, TX 77030
4. Rodney MacDonald Fund, St. Luke's Episcopal Health Systems, Dallas, TX.

REFERENCES

1. Fuster V, Badimon L, Badimon JJ, et al. The pathogenesis of coronary artery disease and the acute coronary syndromes. *N Engl J Med* 1992;326:242–250.
2. Lander ES, Linton LM, Birren B, et al. Initial sequencing and analysis of the human genome. *Nature* 2001;409:860–921.
3. Venter JC, Adams MD, Myers EW, et al. The sequence of the human genome. *Science* 2001;291:1304–1351.
4. Nora JJ, Lortscher RH, Spangler RD, et al. Genetic-epidemiologic study of early-onset ischemic heart disease. *Circulation* 1980;61:503–508.
5. Schildkraut JM, Myers RH, Cupples LA, et al. Coronary risk associated with age and sex of parental heart disease in the Framingham Study. *Am J Cardiol* 1989;64:555–559.
6. Menzel S. Genetic and molecular analyses of complex metabolic disorders. genetic linkage. *Ann NY Acad Sci* 2002;967:249–257.
7. Broeckel U, Hengstenberg C, Mayer B, et al. A comprehensive linkage analysis for myocardial infarction and its related risk factors. *Nat Genet* 2002;30:210–214.
8. Pajukanta P, Cargill M, Viitanen L, et al. Two loci on chromosomes 2 and X for premature coronary heart disease identified in early- and late-settlement populations of Finland. *Am J Hum Genet* 2000;67:1481–1493.
9. Sachidanandam R, Weissman D, Schmidt SC, et al. A map of human genome sequence variation containing 1.42 million single nucleotide polymorphisms. *Nature* 2001;409:928–933.
10. Yamada Y, Izawa H, Ichihara S, et al. Prediction of the risk of myocardial infarction from polymorphisms in candidate genes. *N Engl J Med* 2002;347:1916–1923.
11. Altshuler D, Kruglyak L, Lander E. Genetic polymorphisms and disease. *N Engl J Med* 1998;338:1626.
12. Duggan DJ, Bittner M, Chen Y, et al. Expression profiling using cDNA microarrays. *Nat Genet* 1999;21[1 Suppl]:10–14.
13. Velculescu VE, Zhang L, Vogelstein B, et al. Serial analysis of gene expression. *Science* 1995;270:484–487.
14. Liang P, Pardee AB. Differential display of eukaryotic messenger RNA by means of the polymerase chain reaction. *Science* 1992;257:967–971.
15. de Waard V, van den Berg BM, Veken J, et al. Serial analysis of gene expression to assess the endothelial cell response to an atherogenic stimulus. *Gene* 1999;226:1–8.
16. Stanton LW, Garrard LJ, Damm D, et al. Altered patterns of gene expression in response to myocardial infarction. *Circ Res* 2000;86:939–945.
17. Reardon CA, Getz GS. Mouse models of atherosclerosis. *Curr Opin Lipidol* 2001;12:167–173.
18. Buja LM, Kita T, Goldstein JL, et al. Cellular pathology of progressive atherosclerosis in the WHHL rabbit. An animal model of familial hypercholesterolemia. *Arteriosclerosis* 1983;3:87–101.
19. Herrera VL, Makrides SC, Xie HX, et al. Spontaneous combined hyperlipidemia, coronary heart disease and decreased survival in Dahl salt-sensitive hypertensive rats transgenic for human cholesteryl ester transfer protein. *Nat Med* 1999;5:1383–1389.
20. Orso E, Broccardo C, Kaminski WE, et al. Transport of lipids from Golgi to plasma membrane is defective in Tangier disease patients and ABC1-deficient mice. *Nat Genet* 2000;24:192–196.
21. Rhoads GG, Dahlen G, Berg K, et al. Lp(a) lipoprotein as a risk factor for myocardial infarction. *JAMA* 1986;256:2540–2544.
22. Zenker G, Koltringer P, Bone G, et al. Lipoprotein (a) as a strong indicator for cerebrovascular disease. *Stroke* 1986;17:942–945.
23. Boerwinkle E, Leffert CC, Lin J, et al. Apolipoprotein(a) gene accounts for greater than 90% of the variation in plasma lipoprotein(a) concentrations. *J Clin Invest* 1992;90:52–60.
24. Brazier L, Tiret L, Luc G, et al. Sequence polymorphisms in the apolipoprotein(a) gene and their association with lipoprotein(a) levels and myocardial infarction. The ECTIM Study. *Atherosclerosis* 1999;144:323–333.
25. Weisgraber KH, Rall SC, Mahlcy RW. Human E apoprotein heterogeneity: cysteine-arginine interchanges in the amino acid sequence of the apo E isoforms. *Biol Chem* 1981;256:9077–9083.
26. Wilson PW, Schaefer EJ, Larson MG, et al. Apolipoprotein E alleles and risk of coronary disease. A meta-analysis. *Arterioscler Thromb Vasc Biol* 1996;16:1250–1255.
27. Stengard JH, Weiss KM, Sing CF. An ecological study of association

between coronary heart disease mortality rates in men and the relative frequencies of common allelic variations in the gene coding for apolipoprotein E. *Hum Genet* 1998;103:234–241.

28. Gerdes LU, Gerdes C, Kervinen K, et al. The apolipoprotein ε allele determines prognosis and the effect on prognosis of simvastatin in survivors of myocardial infarction. A substudy of the Scandinavian Simvastatin Survival Study. *Circulation* 2000;101:1366–1371.

29. Homocysteine Studies Collaboration. Homocysteine and risk of ischemic heart disease and stroke: a meta-analysis. *JAMA* 2002;288:2015–2022.

30. Klerk M, Verhoef P, Clarke R, et al. MTHFR Studies Collaboration Group. MTHFR 677C→T polymorphism and risk of coronary heart disease: a meta-analysis. *JAMA* 2002;288:2023–2031.

31. Rigat B, Hubert C, Alhenc-Gelas F, et al. An insertion/deletion polymorphism in the angiotensin I-converting enzyme gene accounting for half the variance of serum enzyme levels. *J Clin Invest* 1990;86:1343–1346.

32. Cambien F, Poirier O, Lecerf L, et al. Deletion polymorphism in the gene for angiotensin-converting enzyme is a potent risk factor for myocardial infarction. *Nature* 1992;359:641–643.

33. Samani NJ, Thompson JR, O'Toole L, et al. A meta-analysis of the association of the deletion allele of the angiotensin-converting enzyme gene with myocardial infarction. *Circulation* 199615;94:708–712.

34. Rader JD. High-density lipoproteins and atherosclerosis. *Am J Cardiol* 2002;90:62i–70i.

35. Calabresi L, Franceschini G. High density lipoprotein and coronary heart disease: insights from mutations leading to low high density lipoprotein. *Curr Opin Lipidol* 1997;8:219–224.

36. Sirtori CR, Calabresi L, Franceschini G, et al. Cardiovascular status of carriers of the apolipoprotein A-I(Milano) mutant: the Limone sul Garda study. *Circulation* 2001;103:1949–1954.

37. Weisgraber KH, Rall SC Jr, Bersot TP, et al. Apolipoprotein A-I (Milano): detection of normal A-I in affected subjects and evidence for a cysteine for arginine substitution in the variant A-I. *J Biol Chem* 1983;258:2508–2513.

38. Kern F Jr. Normal plasma cholesterol in an 88-year-old man who eats 25 eggs a day. Mechanisms of adaptation. *N Engl J Med* 1991;324:896–899.

39. Gylling H, Miettinen TA. Cholesterol absorption and synthesis related to low density lipoprotein metabolism during varying cholesterol intake in men with different apoE phenotypes. *J Lipid Res* 1992;33:1361–1371.

40. Ordovas JM, Schaefer EJ. Genetic determinants of plasma lipid response to dietary intervention: the role of the APOA1/C3/A4 gene cluster and the APOE gene. *Br J Nutr* 2000;83[Suppl 1]:S127–S136.

41. Buhman KK, Accad M, Novak S, et al. Resistance to diet-induced hypercholesterolemia and gallstone formation in ACAT2-deficient mice. *Nat Med* 2000;6:1341–1347.

42. Stein O, Thiery J, Stein Y. Is there a genetic basis for resistance to atherosclerosis? *Atherosclerosis* 2002;160:1–10.

43. Wilhelmsen L, Svardsudd K, Korsan-Bengtsen K, et al. Fibrinogen as a risk factor for stroke and myocardial infarction. *N Engl J Med* 1984;311:501–505.

44. Humphries SE, Cook M, Dubowitz M, et al. Role of genetic variation at the fibrinogen locus in determination of fibrinogen concentrations. *Lancet* 1987;1:1452–1455.

45. Lane DA, Grant PJ. Role of hemostatic gene polymorphisms in venous and arterial thrombotic disease. *Blood* 2000:95:1517–1532.

46. Tybjaerg-Hansen A, Agerholm-Larsen B, Humphries SE, et al. A common mutation (G-455-A) in the b-fibrinogen promoter is an independent predictor of plasma fibrinogen, but not of ischemic heart disease: a study of 9,127 individuals based on the Copenhagen City Heart Study. *J Clin Invest* 1997;99:3034–3039.

47. Gardemann A, Schwartz O, Haberbosch W, et al. Positive association of the b fibrinogen H1/H2 gene variation to basal fibrinogen levels and to increase in fibrinogen concentration during acute phase reaction but not to coronary artery disease and myocardial infarction. *Thromb Haemost* 1997;77:1120–1126.

48. Wang XL, Wang J, McCredie RM, et al. Polymorphisms of factor V, factor VII, and fibrinogen genes: relevance to severity of coronary artery disease. *Arterioscler Thromb Vasc Biol* 1997;17:246–251.

49. Folsom AR, Aleksic N, Ahn C, et al. Beta-fibrinogen gene -455G/A polymorphism and coronary heart disease incidence: the Atheroscle-

rosis Risk in Communities (ARIC) Study. *Ann Epidemiol* 2001;11:166–170.

50. Soejima H, Ogawa H, Yasue H, et al. Heightened tissue factor associated with tissue factor pathway inhibitor and prognosis in patients with unstable angina. *Circulation* 1999;99:2908–2913.

51. Arnaud E, Barbalat V, Nicaud V, et al. Polymorphisms in the 5′ regulatory region of the tissue factor gene and the risk of myocardial infarction and venous thromboembolism: the ECTIM and PATHROS studies. Etude Cas-Temoins de l'Infarctus du Myocarde. Paris Thrombosis case-control Study. *Arterioscler Thromb Vasc Biol* 2000;20:892–898.

52. Badimon JJ, Lettino M, Toschi V, et al. Local inhibition of tissue factor reduces the thrombogenicity of disrupted human atherosclerotic plaques: effects of tissue factor pathway inhibitor on plaque thrombogenicity under flow conditions. *Circulation* 1999;99:1780–1787.

53. Zoldhelyi P, McNatt J, Shelat HS, et al. Thromboresistance of balloon-injured porcine carotid arteries after local gene transfer of human tissue factor pathway inhibitor. *Circulation* 2000;101:289–295.

54. Zoldhelyi P, Chen ZQ, Shelat HS, et al. Local gene transfer of tissue factor pathway inhibitor regulates intimal hyperplasia in atherosclerotic arteries. *Proc Natl Acad Sci USA* 2001;98:4078–4083.

55. Nishida T, Ueno H, Atsuchi N, et al. Adenovirus-mediated local expression of human tissue factor pathway inhibitor eliminates shear stress-induced recurrent thrombosis in the injured carotid artery of the rabbit. *Circ Res* 1999;84:1446–1452.

56. Moatti D, Seknadji P, Galand C, et al. Polymorphisms of the tissue factor pathway inhibitor (TFPI) gene in patients with acute coronary syndromes and in healthy subjects: impact of the V264M substitution on plasma levels of TFPI. *Arterioscler Thromb Vasc Biol* 1999;19:862–869.

57. Meade TW, Mellows S, Brozovic M, et al. Haemostatic function and ischaemic heart disease: principal results of the Northwick Park Heart Study. *Lancet* 1986;2:533–537.

58. Heinrich J, Balleisen L, Schulte H, et al. Fibrinogen and factor VII in the prediction of coronary risk: results from the PROCAM study in healthy men. *Arterioscler Thromb* 1994;14:54–59.

59. Smith FB, Lee AJ, Fowkes FG, et al. Hemostatic factors as predictors of ischemic heart disease and stroke in the Edinburgh Artery Study. *Arterioscler Thromb Vasc Biol* 1997;17:3321–3325.

60. Girelli D, Russo C, Ferraresi P, et al. Polymorphisms in the factor VII gene and the risk of myocardial infarction in patients with coronary artery disease. *N Engl J Med* 2000;343:774–780.

61. Bertina RM, Koeleman BP, Koster T, et al. Mutation in blood coagulation factor V associated with resistance to activated protein C. *Nature* 1994;369:64–67.

62. Ridker PM, Hennekens CH, Lindpaintner K, et al. Mutation in the gene coding for coagulation factor V and the risk of myocardial infarction. *N Engl J Med* 1995;332:912–917.

63. Doggen CJ, Cats VM, Bertina RM, et al. Interaction of coagulation defects and cardiovascular risk factors: increased risk of myocardial infarction associated with factor V Leiden or prothrombin 20210A. *Circulation* 1998;97:1037–1041.

64. Van der Bom, JG, de Knijff P, Haverkate F, et al. Tissue plasminogen activator and risk of myocardial infarction. The Rotterdam study. *Circulation* 1997;95:2623–2627.

65. Ridker PM, Baker MT, Hennekens CH, et al. Alu-repeat polymorphism in the gene coding for tissue-type plasminogen activator (t-PA) and risks of myocardial infarction among middle-aged men. *Arterioscler Thromb Vasc Biol* 1997;17:1687–1690.

66. Steeds R, Adams M, Smith P, et al. Distribution of tissue plasminogen activation insertion/deletion polymorphism in myocardial infarction and control subjects. *Thromb Haemost* 1998;79:980–984.

67. Kohler HP, Grant PJ. Plasminogen-activator inhibitor type 1 and coronary artery disease. *N Engl J Med* 2000;342:1792–1801.

68. Iacoviello L, Burzotta F, Di Castelnuovo A, et al. The 4G/5G polymorphism of PAI-1 promoter gene and the risk of myocardial infarction: a meta-analysis. *Thromb Haemost* 1998;80:1029–1030.

69. Kottke-Marchant K. Genetic polymorphisms associated with venous and arterial thrombosis: an overview. *Arch Pathol Lab Med* 2002;126:295–304.

70. Franco RF, Reitsma PH. Gene polymorphisms of the haemostatic system and the risk of arterial thrombotic disease. *Br J Haematol* 2001;115:491–506.

71. Atherosclerosis, Thrombosis, and Vascular Biology Italian Study Group. No evidence of association between prothrombotic gene poly-

morphisms and the development of acute myocardial infarction at a young age. *Circulation* 2003;107:1117–1122.

72. Newman PJ, Derbes RS, Aster RH. The human platelet alloantigens, PlA1 and PlA2, are associated with a leucine33/proline33 amino acid polymorphism in membrane glycoprotein IIIa, and are distinguishable by DNA typing. *J Clin Invest* 1989;83:1778–1781.

73. Ridker PM, Hennekens CH, Schmitz C, et al. PlA1/A2 polymorphism of platelet glycoprotein IIIa and risks of myocardial infarction, stroke and venous thrombosis. *Lancet* 1997;349:385–388.

74. Herrmann SM, Poirier O, Marques-Vidal P, et al. The Leu 33/Pro polymorphism (PlA1/PlA2) of the glycoprotein IIIa (GPIIIa) receptor is not related to myocardial infarction in the ECTIM Study. *Thomb Haemost* 1997;77:1179–1181.

75. Aleksic N, Juneja H, Folsom AR, et al. Platelet Pl(A2) allele and incidence of coronary heart disease: results from the Atherosclerosis Risk In Communities (ARIC) Study. *Circulation* 2000;102:1901–1905.

76. Zhu MM, Weedon J, Clark LT. Meta-analysis of the association of platelet glycoprotein IIIa PlA1/A2 polymorphism with myocardial infarction. *Am J Cardiol* 2000;86:1000–1005.

77. Reiner AP, Siscovick DS, Rosendaal FR. Platelet glycoprotein gene polymorphisms and risk of thrombosis: facts and fancies. *Rev Clin Exp Hematol* 2001;5:262–287.

78. Nieuwenhuis HK, Akkerman JW, Houdijk WP, et al. Human blood platelets showing no response to collagen fail to express surface glycoprotein Ia. *Nature* 1985;318:470–472.

79. Kunicki TJ, Kritzik M, Annis DS, et al. Hereditary variation in platelet integrin α2 β1 density is associated with two silent polymorphisms in the α2 gene coding sequence. *Blood* 1997;89:1939–1943.

80. Santoso S, Kunicki TJ, Kroll H, et al. Association of the platelet glycoprotein Ia $C_{807}T$ gene polymorphism with nonfatal myocardial infarction in younger patients. *Blood* 1999;93:2449–2453.

81. Croft SA, Hampton KK, Sorrell JA, et al. The GPIa C807T dimorphism associated with platelet collagen receptor density is not a risk factor for myocardial infarction. *Br J Haematol* 1999;106:771–776.

82. Morita H, Kurihara H, Imai Y, et al. Lack of association between the platelet glycoprotein Ia C807T gene polymorphism and myocardial infarction in Japanese. *Thromb Haemost* 2001;85:226–230.

83. Corral J, Gonzalez-Conejero R, Rivera J, et al. Role of the 807 C/T polymorphism of the (2 gene in platelet GP Ia collagen receptor expression and function. Effect in thromboembolic diseases. *Thromb Haemost* 1999;81:951–956.

84. Ware J, Russell SR, Vicente V, et al. Nonsense mutation in the glycoprotein Ib alpha coding sequence associated with Bernard-Soulier syndrome. *Proc Natl Acad Sci USA* 1990;87:2026–2030.

85. Mikkelsson J, Perola M, Penttilä A, et al. Platelet glycoprotein Ibα HPA-2 Met/VNTR B haplotype as a genetic predictor of myocardial infarction and sudden cardiac death. *Circulation* 2001;104:876–880.

86. Gonzalez-Conejero R, Lozano ML, Rivera J, et al. Polymorphisms of platelet membrane glycoprotein Ib alpha associated with arterial thrombotic disease. *Blood* 1998;92:2771–2776.

87. Libby P, Ridger PM, Maseri A. Inflammation and atherosclerosis. *Circulation* 2002;105:1135–1143.

88. Blake GJ, Ridker PM. C-reactive protein, subclinical atherosclerosis, and risk of cardiovascular events. *Arterioscler Thromb Vasc Biol* 2002;22:1512–1513.

89. Pasceri V, Willerson JT, Yeh ET. Direct proinflammatory effect of C-reactive protein on human endothelial cells. *Circulation* 2000;102:2165–2168.

90. Zee RY, Ridker PM. Polymorphism in the human C-reactive protein (CRP) gene, plasma concentrations of CRP, and the risk of future arterial thrombosis. *Atherosclerosis* 2002;162:217–219.

91. Ozaki K, Ohnishi Y, Iida A, et al. Functional SNPs in the lymphotoxin-alpha gene that are associated with susceptibility to myocardial infarction. *Nat Genet* 2002;32:650–654.

92. Yokota M, Ichihara S, Lin TL, et al. Association of a T29→C polymorphism of the transforming growth factor-beta1 gene with genetic susceptibility to myocardial infarction in Japanese. *Circulation* 2000; 101:2783–2787.

93. Evans WE, McLeod HL. Pharmacogenomics—drug disposition, drug targets, and side effects. *N Engl J Med* 2003;348:538–549.

94. Eikelboom JW, Hirsh J, Weitz JI, et al. Aspirin-resistant thromboxane biosynthesis and the risk of myocardial infarction, stroke, or cardiovascular death in patients at high risk for cardiovascular events. *Circulation* 2002;105:1650–1655.

95. Halushka MK, Halushka PV. Why are some individuals resistant to the cardioprotective effects of aspirin? Could it be tromboxane A_2? *Circulation* 2002;105:1620–1622.

96. Undas A, Brummel K, Musial J, et al. Pl(A2) polymorphism of beta(3) integrins is associated with enhanced thrombin generation and impaired antithrombotic action of aspirin at the site of microvascular injury. *Circulation* 2001;104:2666–2672.

97. Maitland-van der Zee AH, Klungel OH, Stricker BH, et al. Genetic polymorphisms: importance for response to HMG-CoA reductase inhibitors. *Atherosclerosis* 2002;163:213–222.

98. Staunton JE, Slonim DK, Coller HA, et al. Chemosensitivity prediction by transcriptional profiling. *Proc Natl Acad Sci USA* 2001;98:10787–10792.

99. Liotta LA, Kohn EC, Petricoin EF. Clinical proteomics: personalized molecular medicine. *JAMA* 2001;286:2211–2214.

100. Jiang H, Klein RM, Niederacher D, et al. C/T polymorphism of the intercellular adhesion molecule-1 gene (exon 6, codon 469). A risk factor for coronary heart disease and myocardial infarction. *Int J Cardiol* 2002;84(2-3):171–177.

101. Wenzel K, Felix S, Kleber FX, et al. E-selectin polymorphism and atherosclerosis: an association study. *Hum Mol Genet* 1994;3:1935–1937.

102. Wenzel K, Ernst M, Rohde K, et al. DNA polymorphisms in adhesion molecule genes—a new risk factor for early atherosclerosis. *Hum Genet* 1996;97:15–20.

103. Herrmann SM, Ricard S, Nicaud V, et al. The P-selectin gene is highly polymorphic: reduced frequency of the Pro715 allele carriers in patients with myocardial infarction. *Hum Mol Genet* 1998;7:1277–1284.

104. Zheng F, Chevalier JA, Zhang LQ, et al. HphI polymorphism in the E-selectin gene is associated with premature coronary artery disease. *Clin Genet* 2001;59:58–64.

105. Ye SQ, Usher D, Virgil D, et al. PstI polymorphism detects the mutation of serine128 to arginine in CD 62E gene—a risk factor for coronary artery disease. *J Biomed Sci* 1999;6:18–21.

106. Kee F, Morrison C, Evans AE, et al. Polymorphisms of the P-selectin gene and risk of myocardial infarction in men and women in the ECTIM extension study. Etude cas-temoin de l'infarctus myocarde. *Heart* 2000;84:548–552.

107. Tregouet DA, Barbaux S, Escolano S, et al. Specific haplotypes of the P-selectin gene are associated with myocardial infarction. *Hum Mol Genet* 2002;11:2015–2023.

108. Barbaux SC, Blankenberg S, Rupprecht HJ, et al. Association between P-selectin gene polymorphisms and soluble P-selectin levels and their relation to coronary artery disease. *Arterioscler Thromb Vasc Biol* 2001;21:1668–1673.

109. Koch W, Kastrati A, Bottiger C, et al. Interleukin-10 and tumor necrosis factor gene polymorphisms and risk of coronary artery disease and myocardial infarction. *Atherosclerosis* 2001;159:137–144.

110. Herrmann SM, Ricard S, Nicaud V, et al. Polymorphisms of the tumour necrosis factor-alpha gene, coronary heart disease and obesity. *Eur J Clin Invest* 1998;28:59–66.

111. Padovani JC, Pazin-Filho A, Simoes MV, et al. Gene polymorphisms in the TNF locus and the risk of myocardial infarction. *Thromb Res* 2000;100:263–269.

112. Keso T, Perola M, Laippala P, et al. Polymorphisms within the tumor necrosis factor locus and prevalence of coronary artery disease in middle-aged men. *Atherosclerosis* 2001;154:691–697.

113. Francis SE, Camp NJ, Dewberry RM, et al. Interleukin-1 receptor antagonist gene polymorphism and coronary artery disease. *Circulation* 1999;99:861–866.

114. Manzoli A, Andreotti F, Varlotta C, et al. Allelic polymorphism of the interleukin-1 receptor antagonist gene in patients with acute or stable presentation of ischemic heart disease. *Cardiologia* 1999;44:825–830.

115. Vohnout B, Di Castelnuovo A, Trotta R, et al. Interleukin-1 gene cluster polymorphisms and risk of coronary artery disease. *Haematologica* 2003;88:54–60.

116. Zee RY, Lunze K, Lindpaintner K, et al. A prospective evaluation of the interleukin-1 receptor antagonist intron 2 gene polymorphism and the risk of myocardial infarction. *Thromb Haemost* 2001;86:1141–1143.

117. Momiyama Y, Hirano R, Taniguchi H, et al. Effects of interleukin-1 gene polymorphisms on the development of coronary artery disease associated with Chlamydia pneumoniae infection. *J Am Coll Cardiol* 2001;38:712–717.

118. Nauck M, Winkelmann BR, Hoffmann MM, et al. The interleukin-6 G(−174)C promoter polymorphism in the LURIC cohort: no associa-

tion with plasma interleukin-6, coronary artery disease, and myocardial infarction. *J Mol Med* 2002;80:507–513.

119. Georges JL, Loukaci V, Poirier O, et al. Interleukin-6 gene polymorphisms and susceptibility to myocardial infarction: the EC-TIM study. Etude Cas-Temoin de l'Infarctus du Myocarde. *J Mol Med* 2001;79(5-6):300–305.

120. Donger C, Georges JL, Nicaud V, et al. New polymorphisms in the interleukin-10 gene—relationships to myocardial infarction. *Eur J Clin Invest* 2001;31:9–14.

121. Wang XL, Sim AS, Wilcken DE. A common polymorphism of the transforming growth factor-beta1 gene and coronary artery disease. *Clin Sci (Lond)* 1998;95:745–746.

122. Cambien F, Ricard S, Troesch A, et al. Polymorphisms of the transforming growth factor-beta 1 gene in relation to myocardial infarction and blood pressure. The Etude Cas-Temoin de l'Infarctus du Myocarde (ECTIM) Study. *Hypertension* 1996;28:881–887.

123. Syrris P, Carter ND, Metcalfe JC, et al. Transforming growth factor-beta1 gene polymorphisms and coronary artery disease. *Clin Sci (Lond)* 1998;95:659–667.

124. Schwarz A, Haberbosch W, Tillmanns H, et al. The stromelysin-1 5A/6A promoter polymorphism is a disease marker for the extent of coronary heart disease. *Dis Markers* 2002;18:121–128.

125. Terashima M, Akita H, Kanazawa K, et al. Stromelysin promoter 5A/6A polymorphism is associated with acute myocardial infarction. *Circulation* 1999;99:2717–2719.

126. Kim JS, Park HY, Kwon JH, et al. The roles of stromelysin-1 and the gelatinase B gene polymorphism in stable angina. *Yonsei Med J* 2002;43:473–481.

127. Humphries SE, Martin S, Cooper J, et al. Interaction between smoking and the stromelysin-1 (MMP3) gene 5A/6A promoter polymorphism and risk of coronary heart disease in healthy men. *Ann Hum Genet* 2002;66[Pt 6]:343–352.

128. Ye S, Watts GF, Mandalia S, et al. Preliminary report: genetic variation in the human stromelysin promoter is associated with progression of coronary atherosclerosis. *Br Heart J* 1995;73:209–215.

129. Sasaoka T, Kimura A, Hohta SA, et al. Polymorphisms in the platelet-endothelial cell adhesion molecule-1 (PECAM-1) gene, Asn563Ser and Gly670Arg, associated with myocardial infarction in the Japanese. *Ann NY Acad Sci* 2001;947:259–270.

130. Wenzel K, Baumann G, Felix SB. The homozygous combination of Leu125Val and Ser563Asn polymorphisms in the PECAM1 gene (CD31) is associated with early severe coronary heart disease. *Hum Mutat* 1999;14:545.

131. Song FC, Chen AH, Tang XM, et al. Association of platelet endothelial cell adhesion molecule-1 gene polymorphism with coronary heart disease. *Di Yi Jun Yi Da Xue Xue Bao* 2003;23:156–158.

132. Gardemann A, Knapp A, Katz N, et al. No evidence for the CD31 C/G gene polymorphism as an independent risk factor of coronary heart disease. *Thromb Haemost* 2000;83:629.

The Normal Artery

CHAPTER 27

Vascular Endothelium

Paul E. DiCorleto and Paul L. Fox

Key Words: Adhesion molecules; cytokines; endothelial dysfunction; endothelium-derived relaxing factor; platelet-derived growth factor; transforming growth factor-β; vascular endothelium.

INTRODUCTION

The entire circulatory system is lined by a continuous, single cell–thick layer: the vascular endothelium. In the aorta and its main branches (e.g., the coronary arteries), this transparent tissue, together with a modest amount of extracellular matrix, constitutes the normal tunica intima. It is this inner concentric layer of the artery wall that is the primary locus of the atherothrombotic disease process. More than a century ago, anatomic pathologists began to catalog the gross and microscopic changes involving the intima that mark the progression from the early fatty streak lesion to the clinically important complicated plaque (1). However, an understanding of the pathogenic mechanisms underlying these changes has developed in the last three decades, largely through the application of modern cellular and molecular biologic techniques (2,3). During the course of these studies, the working concept of the role of vascular endothelium in health and disease has undergone a dramatic evolution. Originally viewed simply as a passive barrier or insulation,

P. E. DiCorleto: Department of Cell Biology-NB21, Lerner Research Institute, Cleveland Clinic Foundation, Cleveland, Ohio 44195.
P. L. Fox: Department of Cell Biology-NC10, Lerner Research Institute, Cleveland Clinic Foundation, Cleveland, Ohio 44195.

the endothelial lining is now considered to be a multifunctional organ, the health of which is essential to normal vascular physiology, and the dysfunction of which leads to multiple diseases (4,5).

In health, vascular endothelium comprises a "container" for blood and forms the biologic interface between circulating blood components and all of the tissues of the body. It is strategically situated to monitor systemic, as well as locally generated, stimuli and to alter its functional state. This adaptive process typically proceeds without notice, contributing to normal homeostasis. However, nonadaptive changes in endothelial structure and function, provoked by pathophysiologic stimuli, can result in localized, acute and chronic, alterations in the interactions of endothelium with the cellular and macromolecular components of circulating blood and of the blood vessel wall. These alterations include enhanced permeability to (and subsequent oxidative modification of) plasma lipoproteins, hyperadhesiveness for blood leukocytes, and functional imbalances in local prothrombotic and antithrombotic factors, growth stimulators and inhibitors, and vasoactive (dilator and constrictor) substances. These manifestations, collectively termed *endothelial dysfunction,* play an important role in the initiation, progression, and clinical complications of various forms of inflammatory and degenerative vascular diseases.

This chapter briefly summarizes our current understanding of normal endothelial biology, thus providing a background for discussion of its role in the pathogenesis of atherothrombotic lesions and their thrombotic, inflammatory, and vasospastic complications.

NORMAL VASCULAR ENDOTHELIUM

Anatomic and Functional Organization

By virtue of its *anatomic location,* vascular endothelium is a biologically significant interface: It defines intravascular and extravascular compartments, serves as a selectively permeable barrier, and provides a continuous nonthrombogenic lining for the cardiovascular system. Its location is also a key factor in its dynamic, reciprocal interactions with other cells, both in the circulating blood and within the vessel wall proper. Endothelial cells send signals both outward to blood cells and inward to smooth muscle cells and infiltrated leukocytes. The molecules that send these signals may be subject to modulating influences exerted by extracellular matrix and blood factors in the vicinity. Another functionally important consequence of endothelium's location is its ability to monitor, integrate, and transduce bloodborne signals and mechanical forces, thus making it a type of "sensory organ."

A second important aspect of the structural organization of endothelium is its large luminal *surface area.* The endothelium is the body's most extensive simple epithelium; its aggregate area has been estimated to be several thousand square meters (6). This essentially continuous expanse of living cells can function as a vast solid-phase reactor, a highly selective affinity chromatography "sieve," or a relatively nonspecific adsorptive "sponge." These surface-related activities are especially enhanced in the microcirculation, where the ratio of the surface of the endothelial container to the volume of contained blood reaches a maximum. The realization that the walls of this *in vivo* blood container actively participate in the biochemical reactions of blood constituents represented a significant conceptual advance (7). Equally important from the pathophysiologic standpoint is that key surface-related functions of vascular endothelium can be dynamically modulated, thus making the luminal endothelial surface a locus of physiologic regulation and pathologic alteration (8).

Another relevant aspect of endothelial organization is its *regional specialization.* Despite its apparent morphologic simplicity and relative homogeneity, there is increasing evidence that the vascular endothelial lining does exhibit site-to-site variations that may have important physiologic and pathophysiologic implications. These differences are manifested in properties such as permeability to macromolecules, secretion of biosynthetic products, and responsiveness to various exogenous mediators (9). Regional specialization may in fact extend down to the level of the individual endothelial cell (10). In addition, despite its thin configuration, each vascular endothelial cell has a clearly definable "apical" or luminal surface, which faces the bloodstream, and a "basal" or abluminal surface, which is in contact with the subendothelial connective tissues; each is outfitted with its own distinct complement of intrinsic proteins (11).

Taken together, these basic principles of endothelial organization—its interface location, dynamic surface properties, and regional specialization—have important implications for the vital functions of this tissue in health and disease.

Vital Functions of Endothelium

Selective Permeability Barrier

Endothelium is the primary anatomic site for restriction of macromolecular flux between the blood and the extravascular space. When viewed with the electron microscope, the endothelial lining of the heart and large arteries is of the continuous type, characterized by tight junctions at the lateral borders of each cell, which restrict the movement of macromolecules, and a complex microvesicular system, which has been implicated in macromolecular transport. The latter consists of simple vesicles or caveolae, branched surface–connected canaliculi, and beaded transcellular channels (12). In addition, the endothelial surface–associated glycocalyx contains sulfated glycosaminoglycans and other charged species that can selectively adsorb macromolecules, such as growth factors and cytokines.

Dramatic changes can occur in endothelial permeability to bloodborne molecules, acutely and chronically, in response to various physiologic and pathophysiologic stimuli. For example, histamine and other acute inflammatory mediators can act directly on microvascular (primarily postcapillary venular) endothelial cells to stimulate opening of their intercellular junctions. It has been suggested that macrovascular endothelium (arterial and venous) can respond acutely to certain soluble mediators with a similar type of permeability change, and that transient gap formation may contribute to the trapping of the relatively large lipoprotein particles in the subendothelial space. The vascular endothelial growth factor (VEGF) family increases the permeability of the endothelium by multiple mechanisms including gap formation and vesiculovacuolar organelle formation (13).

Detailed studies of atherothrombosis lesion-prone areas in hypercholesterolemic rabbits and other animal models have documented enhanced lipoprotein permeability, manifested by the accumulation of plasma-derived low-density lipoprotein (LDL) and β-very low-density lipoprotein Ω(β-VLDL), primarily through the transcytotic route (14). Normal LDL particles also can enter endothelial cells through the LDL receptor–mediated endocytic route and are then subject to hydrolysis and reesterification of their cholesterol contents, analogous to the process in other cell types. However, in response to increased plasma levels of lipoproteins, this receptor-mediated pathway usually is down-regulated. Lipoproteins delivered to the subendothelial space in hypercholesterolemic animals appear to undergo a complex process of oxidative and physicochemical modification and can accumulate in relatively large quantities extracellularly in association with newly synthesized, proteoglycan-rich matrix material (15). Endothelial cells, as well as other cells in developing atherothrombotic plaques, can contribute to the superoxide-dependent oxidative modification of LDL (16), which results in its endocytic uptake through so-called scavenger receptors, as discussed elsewhere in this textbook. In addition, components of oxidized lipoproteins, such as lysophospholipids, can act on endothelial cells to modify their function (e.g., motility) (17) and their expression of growth factors, cytokines, and adhesion molecules (18–20). The multiple potential interactions of lipoproteins with endothelium and other cellular components of developing atherothrombotic lesions are considered in more detail later in this chapter and in Chapters 6–9.

The Hemostatic/Thrombotic Balance

Blood normally does not clot inside of its endothelial "container." This failure of endothelium to activate the coagulation cascade or to promote platelet adhesion has been termed *nonthrombogenicity*. For many years, this vital function was considered simply as a passive form of insulation, attributable to ill-defined physicochemical properties of the luminal endothelial surface. With the discovery that the vascular wall and, in particular, endothelial cells (21) synthesize the unique arachidonate metabolite prostacyclin (PGI$_2$), which proved to be an extraordinarily potent inhibitor of platelet aggregation, a more active *antithrombotic* role for endothelium became apparent. In addition to its major influence on platelet function, the endothelium plays a pivotal role in the coagulation and fibrinolytic system (22). Many of these functions appear to be antithrombotic in nature. For example, several of the body's natural anticoagulant mechanisms (23), including the heparin–antithrombin mechanism, the protein C–thrombomodulin mechanism, and the tissue plasminogen activator mechanism, are endothelial-associated. The molecular components of several of these antithrombotic mechanisms are considered in detail in Chapters 41 and 42.

In contrast to these antithrombotic functions, the endothelial cell also appears capable of active *prothrombotic* behavior (22). It synthesizes adhesive cofactors for platelets, such as von Willebrand factor, fibronectin, and thrombospondin; procoagulant components, such as factor V; and, as discussed later, it can be activated by various pathophysiologic stimuli to express tissue factor, a trigger for the fibrin-generating coagulation cascade (24). Endothelium also generates an inhibitor of the fibrinolytic pathway (plasminogen activator inhibitor-1 [PAI-1]), which can reduce the rate of fibrin breakdown. Thus, the endothelial cell appears capable of playing a number of roles, both *pro-* and *anti-* hemostatic/thrombotic, that are relevant to maintaining normal blood fluidity, stopping hemorrhage at sites of vascular injury, and affecting pathologic thrombosis. These endothelial-dependent mechanisms contribute to a dynamic physiologic antagonism or "balance," which can significantly influence the status of local hemostatic/thrombotic activity (Fig. 27–1).

The Vasoconstrictor/Vasodilator Balance

The maintenance of cardiovascular tone traditionally has been viewed as a function of the vascular smooth muscle

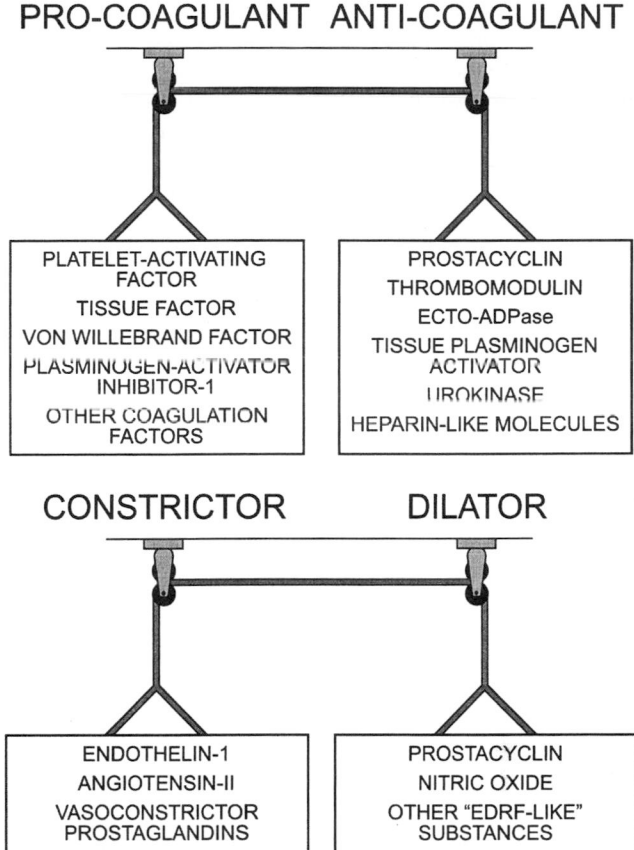

FIG. 27–1. The vascular endothelial hemostatic/thrombotic balance and vasoconstrictor/vasodilator balance. Various endothelial-associated factors and functions contribute to a dynamic physiologic antagonism or "balance," which determines the status of local hemostatic versus thrombotic activity, as well as the local regulation of vascular tone. EDRF, Endothelium-derived relaxation factor.

cell, responding primarily to sympathetic/parasympathetic nerve stimulation or circulating hormones (e.g., products of the renin-angiotensin system). In 1980, the discovery by Furchgott and Zawadzki (25) of a potent endothelium-derived relaxing factor (EDRF) pointed to a significant role for the vascular endothelial cell in the *local* regulation of vascular tone. The elucidation of the chemical nature of EDRF as endogenous nitric oxide, its metabolic pathway of generation through (one or more) nitric oxide synthases, and the cellular mechanisms of its action that result in vasodilatation has added a new dimension to our understanding of the role of cell–cell interactions in the regulation of vascular functions (26). Together with prostacyclin, which also has a potent vasorelaxor effect (through different mechanisms of generation and target cell action), nitric oxide and related compounds thus constitute a class of "natural" endothelial-derived antihypertensives.

Balancing the action of these endothelial-derived vasorelaxors are a number of endothelium-derived substances that have vasoconstrictor activity (Fig. 27–1). These include angiotensin II, generated at the luminal endothelial surface by angiotensin-converting enzyme; platelet-derived growth factor (PDGF), which is secreted by endothelial cells and can act as a smooth muscle contractile agonist; and the vasoconstrictor substance endothelin-1 (27). The latter 18–amino acid peptide is generated by the proteolytic cleavage of a larger precursor, "big endothelin," and resembles the lethal toxin in the venom of certain snakes whose bite can induce coronary vasospasm. Endothelin-1 is reported to be the most potent known vasoconstrictor. Understanding the production of these endothelial-derived vasoconstrictor substances and their mechanisms of target cell action may help provide valuable insights into the normal regulation of vascular tone, as well as new strategies for antihypertensive therapies.

Cytokines and Growth Regulatory Molecules

The vascular endothelial lining also is the source of a wide variety of cytokines, growth factors, and growth inhibitors that can act locally, within a given segment of the circulatory tree, to influence the behavior of adjacent vascular cells and interacting blood elements. This makes the endothelium a special kind of endocrine organ that can secrete its hormones in a paracrine (acting on neighbors) or even autocrine (acting on self) fashion. Analogous to the physiologic antagonism of prothrombotic and antithrombotic agents and vasoconstrictor/vasodilators described earlier, a similar balance also is evident in certain of the endothelial-derived cytokines and growth regulatory molecules with regard to their effects on vascular smooth muscle migration and proliferation. Further details concerning the regulation of the production of these endothelial products, their primary cellular targets, and the pathophysiologic implications of their actions are discussed later, in the context of endothelial dysfunction, and also in Chapters 28 and 39.

Transducer of Biomechanical Forces

By virtue of its unique position, in direct contact with flowing blood, the endothelium is constantly exposed to a variety of biomechanical stimuli. These stimuli take the form of specialized types of mechanical forces generated by pulsatile blood flow (e.g., fluid shear stresses, wall tension, and intraluminal pressure). Some of these forces appear to be passively transduced across the endothelial layer to other components—cells and extracellular matrix—of the vessel wall, whereas other forces act directly on the endothelial cell to modify its metabolic state and even regulate (positively or negatively) gene expression (28). Certain of these biomechanically induced effects, which include changes in growth factors, vasoconstrictors, vasodilators, and fibrinolytic components, appear to involve transcriptional modulation (29). Shear stress–response elements have now been identified in the promoters of multiple endothelial cell–expressed genes (30,31). Experimental analysis of the transduction mechanisms that link externally applied forces to genetic regula-

tory events within the nucleus may provide new insights into the endothelial activation process (32).

In addition to its intrinsic cell biologic interest, the question of the role of the endothelium as a transducer of biomechanical forces is of particular interest in the context of atherogenesis. It has long been appreciated that the early lesions of atherothrombosis arise in a nonrandom pattern, showing a predilection for branch points and regions of curvature, areas characterized by disturbed blood flow (33); more recently, it has been suggested that laminar flow induces the endothelium to exert atheroprotective effects (34). The topic of hemodynamics and atherogenesis is considered in greater detail in Chapter 40.

DYSFUNCTIONAL OR ACTIVATED ENDOTHELIUM

Endothelial Cell Activation: Stimuli and Consequences

As discussed in detail in Chapters 1 and 31, a proposed mechanism for the development of the atherothrombotic plaque, referred to as the "response-to-injury" hypothesis, has had a marked influence during the last three decades on atherothrombosis research. A basic tenet of the original model was that the initiating event in blood vessel disease was an undefined injury to the endothelium that led to endothelial cell loss and exposure of the underlying thrombogenic basement membrane (35). Platelet adherence to this surface and subsequent degranulation would result in the release of multiple bioactive molecules, including PDGF, a potent mitogen and chemoattractant for vascular smooth muscle cells and monocytes. Intimal proliferation of smooth muscle cells, lipid accumulation, and monocyte infiltration then generated the early atherothrombotic plaque. In this model, the sole *function* of the endothelial cell in the disease process was its susceptibility to injury leading to cell death and sloughing. However, frank denudation of endothelium does not occur as an early event in atherogenesis; only in advanced atherothrombotic plaques have regions of vessel wall lacking intact endothelium been verified morphologically.

The presence of an intact endothelium over lesion-prone areas of artery raises the possibility that the endothelial cell may play an active role in atherogenesis (4,5). Injury to, or activation of, the endothelium may lead to the induction of genes that are suppressed under physiologic, rather than pathologic conditions, or to the halting of expression of "beneficial" genes, or both. As depicted in Figure 27–2, specific endothelial cell functions that may be directly relevant to atherothrombosis and its clinical sequelae include the expression of leukocyte binding sites on the endothelial cell surface; the altered production of paracrine growth factors, chemoattractants, and vasoreactive molecules; the ability to oxidize LDL and to respond to oxidized lipids and lipoproteins; the ability to express procoagulant rather than anticoagulant activities; and the modulation of plasma component levels within the vessel wall through changes in permeability function (36,37).

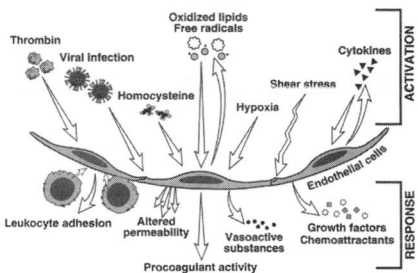

FIG. 27–2. Generation of a dysfunctional endothelium. A variety of stimulatory or "injury-provoking" agents have been implicated in the process of endothelial cell activation. Many of the responses of the endothelium are associated with the progression of vascular disease.

An important question that remains unanswered is the source of injury—that is, causative factor—that leads to altered endothelial cell gene expression during atherogenesis. Multiple candidates for the atherogenic agent have been proposed; however, rigorous identification of the molecule(s) responsible for the initial changes in endothelial cell function that potentially lead to vascular disease has not been achieved. Candidates include local cytokines or proteases, infection, variations in shear, free radicals and oxidized lipids, and homocysteine (Fig. 27–2). These various injury agents may act through common transcriptional factors, such as nuclear factor-kappaB (38) or Egr-1 (39), leading to dysfunction that is most readily quantified clinically by measuring endothelium-dependent vasorelaxation (40).

Expression of Leukocyte Adhesion Molecules

Molecular interactions between bloodborne leukocytes and the endothelium are of great interest to atherothrombosis researchers because of the well recognized involvement of both monocytes and T-lymphocytes in the developing lesion. The monocyte-derived macrophage has been implicated in multiple aspects of atherothrombotic plaque development (41). These cells contribute to the formation of fatty streak lesions by ingesting massive amounts of lipid and thus developing into foam cells. They also produce growth factors for vascular smooth muscle cells, generate cytotoxic factors for neighboring cells, and emigrate as foam cells from the vessel wall leading to physical damage to the endothelium.

The first step in monocyte recruitment into the subendothelial space is the attachment of this bloodborne cell to the endothelium. The focal adherence of mononuclear cells to lesion-prone regions of large vessels is one of the earliest readily detectable events that occurs in experimentally induced atherothrombosis in various animal models. Topics that remain under investigation in multiple laboratories include the nature of the underlying mechanisms regulating the expression of leukocyte adhesion proteins on the endothelial cell surface after cellular activation, the mechanism underlying the induction of adhesion by hypercholes-

terolemia, the specificity of this monocyte adhesion with little, if any, involvement of neutrophils, and finally the reason monocytes adhere only to specific regions of the vasculature. A currently well accepted model to describe the process of leukocyte attachment to the endothelium and subsequent diapedesis involves the sequential involvement of various adhesion molecules and chemokines (42,43). Both cell types play an active role in the process, which includes an initial rolling or tethering event (selectins), a signaling process (chemokines), and a strong attachment step (the immunoglobulin family members). It must be kept in mind that *in vivo* data supporting this model have been limited to the microvasculature, and that leukocyte adhesion to larger arteries that develop atherothrombosis may not occur by the same mechanism.

Many studies have implicated lipoproteins and their components in inducing leukocyte adhesion to endothelial cells. Minimally modified (oxidized) LDL and native LDL at atherogenic concentrations have been shown to specifically increase monocyte adhesion to cultured endothelial cells (44,45). As discussed earlier, lysophosphatidylcholine, as well as other lysophospholipids and oxidized phospholipids, present in oxidized LDL, increase mononuclear cell adhesion to cultured endothelial cells (18–20,46). These lipids appear to induce the adhesion molecules vascular cell adhesion molecule-1 (VCAM-1) and intercellular adhesion molecule-1 (ICAM-1), but not E-selectin, on the endothelial cell surface, thus distinguishing this stimulus from many other agonists of leukocyte adhesion. The primary candidate for the *atherogenic* leukocyte adhesion molecule is VCAM-1 (47). The kinetics of expression of this cytokine-inducible leukocyte adhesion molecule is consistent with its involvement in monocyte adhesion to rabbit aorta after the feeding of a high-cholesterol diet (48). Other adhesion molecules for which some evidence exists, albeit mostly *in vitro,* for their involvement in monocyte adhesion include E-selectin, ICAM-1, and P-selectin (41).

A second class of molecules whose action is required for leukocyte emigration is the chemokines (49). These cytokine-like proteins act as cell-specific chemoattractants for leukocytes; thus, when present in the subendothelial space they lead to the transmigration of the adherent leukocyte from the endothelial cell surface into the intima. These chemokines can be expressed by endothelial cells, smooth muscle cells, and leukocytes in response to various "activating" agents.

Prothrombotic Properties of the Activated Endothelium

As discussed earlier, a healthy physiologic endothelium presents a nonthrombogenic surface to blood cells; however, multiple pathways may be induced in dysfunctional endothelial cells that render these cells thrombogenic. The anticoagulant properties of the endothelium include the production of prostaglandin derivatives and other lipids that inhibit platelet aggregation and the elaboration of antithrombotic proteoglycans and proteins, such as thrombomodulin. Mechanisms by which the procoagulant state develops in large-vessel endothelial cells have been studied principally *in vitro*. Activated endothelial cells express tissue factor, which initiates blood coagulation through the extrinsic pathway. Tissue factor activity has been shown to be induced in endothelial cells in response to various agonists, such as endotoxin, interleukin-1 (IL-1), tumor necrosis factor, and thrombin, and altered flow conditions (24,50–52). The tissue factor expressed by cultured endothelial cells in response to IL-1β is localized principally at the luminal or apical surface of the cell (50).

In both native and activated states, the endothelium participates actively in the process of fibrinolysis as it relates to both clot dissolution and tissue repair (36). Activated endothelial cells can inhibit fibrin degradation by reducing the expression of plasminogen activators whereas increasing expression of PAI-1. Oxidized lipoproteins, as well as native lipoproteins, cause increased synthesis of PAI-1 by cultured human endothelial cells (53). Multiple proteases, including cathepsin G, play a role in the fibrinolytic system by regulating the release of PAI-1 and plasminogen activator from the endothelial cell surface (54). Finally, a link exists between vasoreactivity and the fibrinolytic activity of endothelial cells, because endothelin (discussed later) augments release of both tissue plasminogen activator and PAI-1 from cultured endothelial cells (55).

Vasospasm and the Activated Endothelium

The ability of blood vessels to contract in response to humoral and paracrine vasoactive substances is affected by the diseased state of the vessel under study (36,37,56). Understanding the regulation of endothelial cell production of vasoreactive molecules is therefore of direct relevance to clinical situations and end points, such as occlusion of blood flow. A key paracrine modulator of vascular reactivity is endothelin-1, a highly potent vasoconstrictive agent, which is regulated both by oxidized lipoproteins (57) and by shear stress (58). Endothelin-1 is secreted by endothelial cells into the basolateral compartment (59), and its production is modulated by lysophosphatidylcholine, interferon-γ, IL-1β, and thrombin (60,61).

The endothelium also controls vascular tone, depending on the physiologic state of the blood vessel, by secreting vasorelaxants, such as nitric oxide, which act reciprocally to endothelin-1 and angiotensin (62,63). Multiple studies from a decade ago in both animal models and in humans have established the interrelations between endothelium-dependent relaxation and hypercholesterolemia (64–66). An inverse relation between atherothrombotic plaque development and vasorelaxation has been well documented (67–70). Impaired endothelium-dependent vasodilatation of forearm resistance vessels has been shown in patients with hypercholesterolemia (64). Also, patients with coronary risk factors and proximal atherothrombotic lesions exhibit impaired responsiveness of their coronary vessels to acetylcholine (71). These studies have been reinforced by those in patients with hypercholesterolemia in which cholesterol reduction therapy improved coronary endothelium-dependent relaxation (72,73).

Growth Factor Production by the Activated Endothelium

As discussed earlier, the endothelium is a potential source of the growth factor(s) responsible for smooth muscle cell migration and proliferation that is a hallmark of the atherothrombotic lesion. The production of PDGF, a mitogen that has been implicated in atherothrombotic plaque development, by endothelial cells has been shown to correlate with endothelial dysfunction and vascular disease (74). The most efficacious inducer of PDGF production by endothelial cells remains the coagulation system protease α-thrombin, which acts both transcriptionally and posttranscriptionally to cause release of PDGF (75–77). Thrombin would be expected to be present at sites of vascular injury, and it is known to have multiple effects on the vessel wall (78). The promoter of the PDGF B-chain gene also contains elements that confer both shear stress and cyclic strain responsiveness to this gene (79,80). As discussed earlier in this chapter, this observation, as well as previous studies reporting modulation of PDGF production by mechanical/physical activation, support a potential mechanistic link between regions of altered shear stress and susceptibility to atherothrombotic plaque development.

The endothelium also is known to produce other growth factors in addition to PDGF, for example, insulin-like growth factor-1 (IGF-1), which can modulate gene expression and augment proliferation of neighboring smooth muscle cells (81). The endothelium also expresses several IGF-binding proteins that can modulate the activity of this growth factor (82). Basic fibroblast growth factor (bFGF), a ubiquitous mitogen, also exhibits regulated expression by the endothelium. Thrombin releases active bFGF from glycosaminoglycans in the subendothelial matrix (83). The endothelium also is a well recognized source of the pluripotent growth factor/growth inhibitor transforming growth factor-β (TGF-β). bFGF induces activation of latent TGF-β in endothelial cell cultures by increasing plasminogen activator activity (84). Endothelial cells also respond to TGF-β as a growth inhibitor and it has been suggested that this protein may alter the differentiated state of endothelium, causing expression of genes by endothelial cells in culture previously thought to be smooth muscle cell–specific (85). Endothelial cells are unique in their ability to distinguish between the isoforms of TGF-β. Specifically, the ability of TGF-β to suppress endothelial cell migration is highly specific for the type-1 but not the type-2 isoform (86).

Regenerated Endothelium and Collateral Circulation

A continuous endothelial monolayer is required for the maintenance and control of normal vessel wall properties. This continuity may be challenged by pathologic damage induced by one or more of the agents depicted in Figure 27–2 or by physical damage caused by, for example, a passing catheter or an angioplasty procedure. Much of what is known about the regeneration of endothelium derives from studies of gross denudation, mostly in animal models of vessel wall hyperplasia. A strong correlation between the duration of denudation and the degree of intimal thickening has been shown (87), and injured regions that are covered by regenerated endothelium within 7 days after injury are completely spared from intimal thickening (88). Rat carotid arteries that are entirely, but gently, denuded are capable of complete endothelial regrowth (89). In contrast to balloon denudation, this method does not cause significant medial damage. These results suggest that the intensity of the vessel trauma also is a critical determinant of endothelial regeneration. The mechanism(s) by which confluent endothelium reduces or prevents intimal thickening has not been resolved. It may be because of the secretion of growth inhibitory substances or limiting the exposure of the subendothelial tissue to stimulatory elements in the blood.

Endothelial regeneration proceeds from the uninjured luminal surface and from the intercostal arteries at approximately 0.1–0.4 mm/day (88). Endothelial regeneration after balloon catheter injury is limited in duration and extent in most animal species. Total axial ingrowth in the rabbit and rat is limited to approximately 3 and 10 mm, respectively (90). The minimal ingrowth of endothelial cells from vessel anastomoses onto impermeable synthetic vascular grafts suggests that a similar limitation exists in humans. The cause of the incomplete regeneration of endothelium remains unknown; however, growth factors are likely to have a role in endothelial regeneration, because several, including TGFs, angiogenin, VEGF, and acidic and basic FGF, influence endothelial cell migration and proliferation *in vitro* (91). In addition to stimulatory molecules, endogenous inhibitors of endothelial cell migration have been identified; TGF-β_1, thrombospondin-1, tissue inhibitors of metalloproteinases, and fibronectin are particularly potent and may regulate repair *in vivo* (92).

The development of collateral circulation, a form of angiogenesis, is another process that requires the migration and proliferation of endothelial cells. The formation of new vessels involves multiple steps, including (a) receipt of angiogenic signals by large-vessel endothelial cells, (b) degradation of the extracellular matrix surrounding the existing vascular bed by secretion of proteases, (c) formation of a capillary "bud" by migrating endothelial cells, (d) capillary extension by proliferation of endothelial cells at the distal tip of the vessel, and (e) anastomosis of newly formed tubes to form a continuous microvessel (92). Migration, rather than proliferation, appears to be the controlling step in capillary growth, because angiogenic factors have been identified

that stimulate endothelial cell migration but not proliferation *in vitro,* and because irradiation of tumors grafted into corneal tissues completely blocks endothelial cell proliferation without altering rates of angiogenesis (93). Both VEGF and bFGF may be important physiologic regulators of angiogenesis (94). Continuous delivery of bFGF in solid-phase pellets increases both collateral circulation (95) and formation of vasa vasorum (96) after arterial injury. VEGF is thought to be particularly important in regulating endothelial cell motility during development of the vasculature and in tumor angiogenesis (92,97).

SUMMARY

The endothelium, although only a single layer thick at any vascular site, is now understood to be a massive, regionally specific, multifunctional organ, the health of which is essential to normal vascular physiology, and whose dysfunction can be a critical factor in the pathogenesis of multiple vascular diseases. The vascular endothelium is strategically situated to monitor systemic and locally generated stimuli and to alter its functional state. This adaptive process typically proceeds without notice, contributing to normal homeostasis. However, nonadaptive changes in endothelial structure and function, provoked by pathophysiologic stimuli, can result in localized, acute and chronic, alterations in the interactions of endothelium with the cellular and macromolecular components of circulating blood and of the blood vessel wall. These alterations include enhanced permeability to (and subsequent oxidative modification of) plasma lipoproteins, hyperadhesiveness for blood leukocytes, and functional imbalances in local prothrombotic and antithrombotic factors, growth stimulators and inhibitors, and vasoactive (dilator, constrictor) substances. These manifestations, collectively termed *endothelial dysfunction,* play an important role in the initiation, progression, and clinical complications of various forms of inflammatory and degenerative vascular diseases. Further challenges include identification of the triggering agents responsible for endothelial dysfunction in specific vascular diseases, and the design of therapeutic regimens that will serve to either prevent the genesis of the dysfunctional endothelium or cause such endothelium to revert to a more physiologic phenotype.

ACKNOWLEDGMENTS

Original research in the authors' laboratories was supported by grants from the National Heart, Lung and Blood Institute, National Institutes of Health (P01-HL29582 to P.E.D. and P.L.F., and R01 HL64357 to P.L.F.).

REFERENCES

1. Virchow R. Der ateromatose Prozess der Arterien. *Wien Med Wochenschr* 1856;6:825–841.

2. Ross R. Atherosclerosis: an inflammatory disease. *N Engl J Med* 1999;340:115–126.
3. Glass CK, Witztum JL. Atherosclerosis. The road ahead. *Cell* 2001; 104:503–516.
4. DiCorleto PE, Chisolm GM. Participation of the endothelium in the development of the atherosclerotic plaque. *Prog Lipid Res* 1986;25: 365–374.
5. Gimbrone MA Jr. Endothelial dysfunction and atherosclerosis. *J Card Surg* 1989;4:180–183.
6. Krogh A. *The anatomy and physiology of capillaries*. New Haven, CT: Yale University Press, 1929:22.
7. Gimbrone MA Jr, Bevilacqua MP. Vascular endothelium: functional modulation at the blood interface. In: Simionescu N, Simionescu M, eds. *Endothelial cell biology in health and disease*. New York: Plenum Press, 1988;255–273.
8. Middleton J, Patterson AM, Gardner L, et al. Leukocyte extravasation: chemokine transport and presentation by the endothelium. *Blood* 2002;100:3853–3860.
9. Fishman AP. Endothelium: a distributed organ of diverse capabilities. *Ann NY Acad Sci* 1982;401:1–8.
10. Davies PF, Polacek DC, Shi C, et al. The convergence of haemodynamics, genomics, and endothelial structure in studies of the focal origin of atherosclerosis. *Biorheology* 2002;39:299–306.
11. Muller WA, Gimbrone MA Jr. Plasmalemmal proteins of cultured vascular endothelial cells exhibit apical-basal polarity: analysis by surface-selective iodination. *J Cell Biol* 1986;103:2389–2402.
12. Wagner R, Chen SC. Transcapillary transport of solute by the endothelial vesicular system: evidence from thin serial section analysis. *Microvasc Res* 1991;42:139–150.
13. Bates DO, Hillman NJ, Williams B, et al. Regulation of microvascular permeability by vascular endothelial growth factors. *J Anat* 2002;200: 581–597.
14. Simionescu N, Simionescu M. Cellular interactions of lipoproteins with the vascular endothelium: endocytosis and transcytosis. In: Shaw JM, ed. *Lipoproteins as carriers of pharmacological agents*. New York: Marcel-Dekker, 1991:45–95.
15. Chisolm GM, Hazen SL, Fox PL, et al. The oxidation of lipoproteins by monocytes-macrophages. Biochemical and biological mechanisms. *J Biol Chem* 1999;274:25959–25962.
16. Fang X, Weintraub NL, Rios CD, et al. Overexpression of human superoxide dismutase inhibits oxidation of low-density lipoprotein by endothelial cells. *Circ Res* 1998;82:1289–1297.
17. Ghosh PK, Vasanji A, Murugesan G, et al. Membrane microviscosity regulates endothelial cell motility. *Nat Cell Biol* 2002;4:894–900.
18. Kume N, Gimbrone MA Jr. Lysophosphatidylcholine transcriptionally induces growth factor gene expression in cultured human endothelial cells. *J Clin Invest* 1994;93:907–911.
19. Zimmerman GA, McIntyre TM, Prescott SM. Adhesion and signaling in vascular cell-cell interactions. *J Clin Invest* 1997;100:S3–S5.
20. Leitinger N, Watson AD, Hama SY, et al. Role of group II secretory phospholipase A2 in atherosclerosis: 2. Potential involvement of biologically active oxidized phospholipids. *Arterioscler Thromb Vasc Biol* 1999;19:1291–1298.
21. Weksler BB, Marcus AJ, Jaffe EA. Synthesis of prostaglandin I2 (prostacyclin) by cultured human and bovine endothelial cells. *Proc Natl Acad Sci USA* 1977;74:3922–3928.
22. Edelberg JM, Christie PD, Rosenberg RD. Regulation of vascular bed-specific prothrombotic potential. *Circ Res* 2001;89:117–124.
23. Esmon CT. The regulation of natural anticoagulant pathways. *Science* 1987;235:1348–1352.
24. Rauch U, Nemerson Y. Tissue factor, the blood, and the arterial wall. *Trends Cardiovasc Med* 2000;10:139–143.
25. Furchgott RF, Zawadzki JV. The obligatory role of endothelial cells in the relaxation of arterial smooth muscle by acetylcholine. *Nature* 1980; 288:373–379.
26. Dinerman JL, Lowenstein CJ, Snyder SH. Molecular mechanisms of nitric oxide regulation: potential relevance to cardiovascular disease. *Circ Res* 1993;73:217.
27. Masaki T, Kimura S, Yanagisawa M, et al. Molecular and cellular mechanism of endothelin regulation. Implications for vascular function. *Circulation* 1991;84:1457–1468.
28. Shyy JY, Chien S. Role of integrins in endothelial mechanosensing of shear stress. *Circ Res* 2002;91:769–775.
29. Fisher AB, Chien S, Barakat AI, et al. Endothelial cellular response to altered shear stress. *Am J Physiol* 2001;281:L529–L533.
30. Resnick N, Collins T, Atkinson W, et al. Platelet-derived growth factor B chain promoter contains a cis-acting fluid shear-stress-responsive element. *Proc Natl Acad Sci USA* 1993;90:4591–4595.
31. Gimbrone MA Jr, Topper JN, Nagel T, et al. Endothelial dysfunction, hemodynamic forces, and atherogenesis. *Ann NY Acad Sci* 2000;902: 230–239.
32. Davies PF. Multiple signaling pathways in flow-mediated endothelial mechanotransduction: PYK-ing the right location. *Arterioscler Thromb Vasc Biol* 2002;22:1755–1757.
33. Glagov S, Zarins C, Giddens DP, et al. Hemodynamics and atherosclerosis, insights and perspectives gained from studies of human arteries. *Arch Pathol Lab Med* 1988;112:1018–1031.
34. Traub O, Berk BC. Laminar shear stress: mechanisms by which endothelial cells transduce an atheroprotective force. *Arterioscler Thromb Vasc Biol* 1998;18:677–685.
35. Ross R, Glomset JA. The pathogenesis of atherosclerosis. *N Engl J Med* 1976;295:369–377,420–425.
36. Cines DB, Pollak ES, Buck CA, et al. Endothelial cells in physiology and in the pathophysiology of vascular disorders. *Blood* 1998;91:3527–3561.
37. Cai H, Harrison DG. Endothelial dysfunction in cardiovascular diseases: the role of oxidant stress. *Circ Res* 2000;87:840–844.
38. Collins T. Endothelial nuclear factor-kappa B and the initiation of the atherosclerotic lesion. *Lab Invest* 1993;68:499–508.
39. Yan SF, Fujita T, Lu J, et al. Egr-1, a master switch coordinating upregulation of divergent gene families underlying ischemic stress. *Nat Med* 2000;6:1355–1361.
40. Celermajer DS, Sorensen KE, Gooch VM, et al. Non-invasive detection of endothelial dysfunction in children and adults at risk of atherosclerosis. *Lancet* 1992;340:1111–1115.
41. Faruqi RM, DiCorleto PE. Mechanisms of monocyte recruitment and accumulation. *Br Heart J* 1993;69:S19–S29.
42. Springer TA. Traffic signals for lymphocytes recirculation and leukocyte emigration: the multistep paradigm. *Cell* 1994;76:301–314.
43. Butcher EC. Leukocyte-endothelial cell recognition: three (or more) steps to specificity and diversity. *Cell* 1991;67:1033–1036.
44. Berliner JA, Territo MC, Sevanian A, et al. Minimally modified low density lipoprotein stimulates monocyte endothelial interactions. *J Clin Invest* 1990;85:1260–1266.
45. Smalley DM, Lin JH, Curtis ML, et al. Native LDL increases endothelial cell adhesiveness by inducing intercellular adhesion molecule-1. *Arterioscler Thromb Vasc Biol* 1996;16:585–590.
46. Berliner JA, Subbanagounder G, Leitinger N, et al. Evidence for a role of phospholipid oxidation products in atherogenesis. *Trends Cardiovasc Med* 2001;11:142–147.
47. Cybulsky MI, Gimbrone MA Jr. Endothelial expression of a mononuclear leukocyte adhesion molecule during atherogenesis. *Science* 1991;251:788–791.
48. Li H, Cybulsky MI, Gimbrone MA Jr, et al. An atherogenic diet rapidly induces VCAM-1, a cytokine-regulatable mononuclear leukocyte adhesion molecule, in rabbit aortic endothelium. *Arterioscler Thromb* 1993;13:197–204.
49. Mackay CR. Chemokines: immunology's high impact factors. *Nat Immunol* 2001;2:95–101.
50. Narahara N, Enden T, Wiiger M, et al. Polar expression of tissue factor in human umbilical vein endothelial cells. *Arterioscler Thromb* 1994;14:1815–1820.
51. Ishii H, Horie S, Kizaki K, et al. Retinoic acid counteracts both the downregulation of thrombomodulin and the induction of tissue factor in cultured human endothelial cells exposed to tumor necrosis factor. *Blood* 1992;80:2556–2562.
52. Herbert JM, Savi P, Laplace MC, et al. IL-4 inhibits LPS-, IL-1β- and TNFα-induced expression of tissue factor in endothelial cells and monocytes. *FEBS Lett* 1992;310:31–33.
53. Tremoli E, Camera M, Maderna P, et al. Increased synthesis of plasminogen activator inhibitor-1 by cultured human endothelial cells exposed to native and modified LDL: an LDL receptor-independent phenomenon. *Arterioscler Thromb* 1993;13:338–346.
54. Pintucci G, Iacoviello L, Amore C, et al. Cathepsin G, a polymorphonuclear cell protease, affects the fibrinolytic system by releasing PAI-1 from endothelial cells and platelets. *Ann NY Acad Sci* 1992;667: 286–288.

55. Yamamoto C, Kaji T, Sakamoto M, et al. Effect of endothelin on the release of tissue plasminogen activator and plasminogen activator inhibitor-1 from cultured human endothelial cells and interaction with thrombin. *Thromb Res* 1992;67:619–624.

56. Kisanuki A, Asada Y, Hatakeyama K, et al. Contribution of the endothelium to intimal thickening in normocholesterolemic and hypercholesterolemic rabbits. *Arterioscler Thromb* 1992;12:1198–1205.

57. Jougasaki M, Kugiyama K, Saito Y, et al. Suppression of endothelin-1 secretion by lysophosphatidylcholine in oxidized low density lipoprotein in cultured vascular endothelial cells. *Circ Res* 1992;71:614–619.

58. Kuchan MI, Frangos JA. Shear stress regulates endothelin-1 release via protein kinase C and cGMP in cultured endothelial cells. *Am J Physiol* 1993;264:H150–H156.

59. Wagner OF, Christ G, Wojta J, et al. Polar secretion of endothelin-1 by cultured endothelial cells. *J Biol Chem* 1992;267:16066–16068.

60. Mawji IA, Marsden PA. Perturbations in paracrine control of the circulation: role of the endothelial-derived vasomediators, endothelin 1 and nitric oxide. *Microsc Res Tech* 2003;60:46–58

61. Schiffrin EL. Role of endothelin-1 in hypertension and vascular disease. *Am J Hypertens* 2001;14:83S–89S.

62. Rossi GP, Seccia TM, Nussdorfer GG. Reciprocal regulation of endothelin-1 and nitric oxide: relevance in the physiology and pathology of the cardiovascular system. *Int Rev Cytol* 2001;209:241–272.

63. Calo L, Semplicini A. Physiological relevance of nitric oxide-angiotensin II interplay in the cardiovascular system. *J Hypertens* 2000;18:351–352.

64. Chowienczyk PJ, Watts GF, Cockcroft JR, et al. Impaired endothelium-dependent vasodilation of forearm resistance vessels in hypercholesterolaemia. *Lancet* 1992;340:1430–1432.

65. Lefer AM, Ma X. Decreased basal nitric oxide release in hypercholesterolemia increases neutrophil adherence to rabbit coronary artery endothelium. *Arterioscler Thromb* 1993;13:771–776.

66. Matsuda Y, Hirata K, Inoue N, et al. High density lipoprotein reverses inhibitory effect of oxidized low density lipoprotein on endothelium-dependent arterial relaxation. *Circ Res* 1993;72:1103–1109.

67. Cooke JP, Dzau VJ. Derangements of the nitric oxide synthase pathway, L-arginine, and cardiovascular diseases. *Circulation* 1997;96:379–382.

68. Ignarro LJ, Napoli C, Loscalzo J. Nitric oxide donors and cardiovascular agents modulating the bioactivity of nitric oxide: an overview. *Circ Res* 2002;90:21–28.

69. Papapetropoulos A, Rudic RD, Sessa WC. Molecular control of nitric oxide synthases in the cardiovascular system. *Cardiovasc Res* 1999;43:509–520.

70. Shah AM. Inducible nitric oxide synthase and cardiovascular disease. *Cardiovasc Res* 2000;45:148–155.

71. Egashira K, Inou T, Hirooka Y, et al. Impaired coronary blood flow response to acetylcholine in patients with coronary risk factors and proximal atherosclerotic lesions. *J Clin Invest* 1993;91:29–37.

72. Leung WH, Lau CP, Wong CK. Beneficial effect of cholesterol-lowering therapy on coronary endothelium-dependent relaxation in hypercholesterolaemic patients. *Lancet* 1993;341:1496–1500.

73. Puddu P, Puddu GM, Muscari A. HMG-CoA reductase inhibitors: is the endothelium the main target? *Cardiology* 2001;95:9–13.

74. DiCorleto PE, Fox PL. Growth factor production by endothelial cells. In: Ryan U, ed. *Endothelial cells, vol II.* Boca Raton, FL: CRC Press, 1988:51–61.

75. Soyombo AA, DiCorleto PE. Stable expression of human platelet-derived growth factor B chain by bovine aortic endothelial cells: cell-association and selective proteolytic cleavage by thrombin. *J Biol Chem* 1994;269:17734–17740.

76. Stenina OI, Poptic EJ, DiCorleto PE. Thrombin activates a Y box-binding protein (DNA-binding protein B) in endothelial cells. *J Clin Invest* 2000;106:579–587.

77. Stenina OI, Shaneyfelt K, DiCorleto PE. Thrombin induces the release of the Y-box protein dpbB from mRNA: a new mode of transcription factor activation. *Proc Natl Acad Sci USA* 2001;98:7277–7282.

78. Patterson C, Stouffer GA, Madamanchi N, et al. New tricks for old dogs: nonthrombotic effects of thrombin in vessel wall biology. *Circ Res* 2001;88:987–997.

79. Resnick N, Collins T, Atkinson W, et al. Platelet-derived growth factor B chain promoter contains a cis-acting fluid shear-stress-responsive element. *Proc Natl Acad Sci USA* 1993;90:4591–4595.

80. Sumpio BE, Du W, Galagher G, et al. Regulation of PDGF-B in endothelial cells exposed to cyclic strain. *Arterioscler Thromb Vasc Biol* 1998;18:349–355.

81. Taylor WR, Nerem RM, Alexander RW. Polarized secretion of IGF-I and IGF-I binding protein activity by cultured aortic endothelial cells. *J Cell Physiol* 1993;154:139–142.

82. Dahlfors G, Arnqvist HJ. Vascular endothelial growth factor and transforming growth factor-beta1 regulate the expression of insulin-like growth factor-binding protein-3, -4, and -5 in large vessel endothelial cells. *Endocrinology* 2000;141:2062–2067.

83. Benezra M, Vlodavsky I, Ishai-Michaeli R, et al. Thrombin-induced release of active basic fibroblast growth factor-heparan sulfate complexes from subendothelial extracellular matrix. *Blood* 1993;83:3324–3331.

84. Flaumenhaft R, Abe M, Mignatti P, et al. Basic fibroblast growth factor-induced activation of latent transforming growth factor-β in endothelial cells: regulation of plasminogen activator activity. *J Cell Biol* 1992;118:901–909.

85. Arciniegas E, Sutton AB, Allen TD, et al. Transforming growth factor beta-1 promotes the differentiation of endothelial cells into smooth muscle-like cells. *J Cell Sci* 1992;103:521–529.

86. Qian SW, Burmester JK, Merwin JR, et al. Identification of a structural domain that distinguishes the actions of the type 1 and 2 isoforms of transforming growth factor-β on endothelial cells. *Proc Natl Acad Sci USA* 1992;89:6290–6294.

87. Fishman JA, Ryan GB, Karnovsky MJ. Endothelial regeneration in the rat carotid artery and the significance of endothelial denudation in the pathogenesis of myointimal thickening. *Lab Invest* 1975;32:339–351.

88. Haudenschild CC, Schwartz SM. Endothelial regeneration. II. Restitution of endothelial continuity. *Lab Invest* 1979;41:407–418.

89. Lindner V, Reidy MA, Fingerle J. Regrowth of arterial endothelium. Denudation with minimal trauma leads to complete endothelial cell regrowth. *Lab Invest* 1989;61:556–563.

90. Reidy MA, Clowes AW, Schwartz SM. Endothelial regeneration. V. Inhibition of endothelial regrowth in arteries of rat and rabbit. *Lab Invest* 1983;49:569–575.

91. Yancopoulos GD, Klagsbrun M, Folkman J. Vasculogenesis, angiogenesis, and growth factors: ephrins enter the fray at the border. *Cell* 1998;93:661–664.

92. Anand-Apte B, Fox, PL. Tumor angiogenesis. In: Borden EC, ed. *Melanoma: biologically targeted therapeutics.* Totowa, NJ: Humana Press, 2002.

93. Folkman J, Klagsbrun M. Angiogenic factors. *Science* 1987;235:442–447.

94. Cross MJ, Claesson-Welsh L. FGF and VEGF function in angiogenesis: signalling pathways, biological responses and therapeutic inhibition. *Trends Pharmacol Sci* 2001;22:201–207.

95. Chleboun JO, Martins RN, Mitchell CA, et al. bFGF enhances the development of the collateral circulation after acute arterial occlusion. *Biochem Biophys Res Commun* 1992;185:510–516.

96. Edelman ER, Nugent MA, et al. Basic fibroblast growth factor enhances the coupling of intimal hyperplasia and proliferation of vasa vasorum in injured rat arteries. *J Clin Invest* 1992;89:465–473.

97. Traver D, Zon LI. Walking the walk: migration and other common themes in blood and vascular development. *Cell* 2002;108:731–734.

CHAPTER 28

Role of Alterations in the Differentiated State of the Smooth Muscle Cell in Athcrothrombogenesis

Brian R. Wamhoff, Meena S. Kumar, and Gary K. Owens

Key Words: Atherosclerosis; bone marrow; differentiation; smooth muscle; transgenic mice.

B. R. Wamhoff: Department of Molecular Physiology and Biological Physics, The Cardiovascular Research Center, University of Virginia, Charlottesville, Virginia 22903.

M. S. Kumar: Department of Molecular Physiology and Biological Physics, The Cardiovascular Research Center, University of Virginia, Charlottesville, Virginia 22903.

G. K. Owens: Department of Molecular Physiology and Biological Physics, The Cardiovascular Research Center, University of Virginia, Charlottesville, Virginia 22903.

PHENOTYPIC MODULATION OF THE SMOOTH MUSCLE CELL PLAYS A KEY ROLE IN THE DEVELOPMENT, PROGRESSION, AND CLINICAL CONSEQUENCES OF ATHEROTHROMBOTIC DISEASE

As is evident from the material presented in this textbook, atherothrombosis is an extremely complex disease involving many cell types including macrophages, lymphocytes, neutrophils, endothelial cells, and vascular smooth muscle cells (SMCs) (1). In addition, relatively recent evidence has implicated possible involvement of circulating multipotential stem cells derived from bone marrow that may give rise to a variety of lesion cells including SMCs (2–4), although the contribution of these cells in human disease remains quite controversial (5,6) (see "Origin of the Intimal Smooth Muscle Cell in Atherothrombotic Lesions"). Of interest, the role of the SMC appears to vary depending on the stage of the disease, with it playing a maladaptive role in lesion development and progression (1,7), but likely playing a beneficial adaptive role in stabilizing plaques before activation of protease cascades that may contribute to end-stage disease events such as plaque rupture (8,9). What has also become clear is that the contributions of the SMC are not a simple function of alterations in its growth state, but rather they are a function of very complex changes in the differentiated state of the SMC including increased matrix production (10–12), production of various proteases (9), participation in chronic inflammatory responses including production of inflammatory cytokines and expression of at least some inflammatory cell markers (13–15), altered contractility and expression of contractile proteins (16,17), and a variety of other changes that have collectively been referred to as *phenotypic modulation* (see review by Owens [7]), a useful descriptive term originally coined by Julie Chamley-Campbell and coworkers almost 30 years ago (18) (see "Origin, Characteristics, and Role of Phenotypic Modulation of the Smooth Muscle Cell in the Development, Progression, and End-Stage Clinical Sequelae Of Atherothrombosis").

The focus of this chapter is to consider the role of the vascular SMCs in development and progression of atherothrombotic lesions, as well as in end-stage clinical events. Vascular development is not reviewed because this topic has been well summarized in recent years by others (19,20); a comprehensive review of the function of various SMC differentiation marker genes also is not provided, although information from the previous edition of this book has been extensively updated. Rather, this chapter focuses on consideration of those properties of the normal SMC that are altered in atherothrombotic disease and postulated to play a key role in its etiology and on examination of possible mechanisms responsible for these changes. The nature of phenotypic switching of the SMC in the lesion is likely to be a key factor in determining whether the lesion is benign or has catastrophic clinical consequences such as plaque rupture with resulting thrombosis and myocardial infarction. In the end, although this research is at its infancy, a goal of this chapter is to convince the reader that an understanding of molecular mechanisms that normally control the differentiated state of the vascular SMCs *in vivo* is critical to understanding the molecular mechanisms that control phenotypic modulation of the SMC associated with the complex pathophysiology of atherothrombosis.

SMOOTH MUSCLE CELL DIFFERENTIATION AND MATURATION

Vascular Smooth Muscle Cell Functions Vary During Different Stages of Vascular Development

Before considering how dysregulation of SMC differentiation or phenotypic modulation contributes to the pathogenesis of atherothrombosis, it is important to first briefly review some general principals of regulation of normal cellular differentiation, as well as some unique aspects of control of differentiation of vascular SMCs.

Cellular differentiation is simply the process by which multipotential cells in the developing organism acquire those cell-specific characteristics that distinguish them from other cell types. Although the process of cellular differentiation is quite complex, in the final analysis it can be subdivided into the following three major regulatory components:

1. Selective activation of the subset of genes required for the cell's differentiated function or functions
2. Coordinate control of expression of cell-selective/specific genes at precise times and stoichiometries
3. Continuous regulation of gene expression through effects of local environmental cues on the genetic program that determines cell lineage

A major challenge in understanding differentiation of the SMC is that it can exhibit a wide range of different phenotypes at different stages of development, and even in adult organisms the cell is not terminally differentiated and is capable of major changes in its phenotype in response to changes in its local environment (see reviews by Owens [7] and Schwartz and coworkers [21]) (Fig. 28–1). For example, during early stages of vasculogenesis, SMCs are highly migratory and undergo rapid cell proliferation. Indeed, recent live videos of vascular development, the SMC investment process, and vascular remodeling in zebrafish (22) and avian systems (23) indicate that there is a remarkable amount of movement of SMCs and SM progenitor cells as part of the complex morphogenic events that result in formation of the cardiovascular system. During vascular development, SMCs also exhibit high rates of synthesis of extracellular matrix components including collagen, elastin, proteoglycans, cadherins, and integrins that comprise a major portion of the blood vessel mass. At this stage of development, SMCs form abundant gap junctions with endothelial cells, and the process of investment of endothelial tubes with SMCs or pericytes is critical for vascular maturation and vessel remodeling. In contrast, in adult blood vessels, the SMC shows an exceedingly low rate of proliferation/turnover, is largely nonmigratory, shows a low rate of synthesis of extracellular matrix components, and is a cell virtually completely committed to carrying out its contractile function. The mature fully differentiated SMC expresses a repertoire of appropriate receptors, ion channels, signal transduction molecules, calcium regulatory proteins, and contractile proteins necessary for the unique contractile properties of the SMC (7). However, on vascular injury, *contractile* SMCs are capable of undergoing transient modification of their phenotype to a highly synthetic phenotype (see "Origin, Characteristics, and Role of Phenotypic Modulation of the Smooth Muscle Cell in the Development, Progression, and End-Stage Clinical Sequelae Of Atherothrombosis"), and they play a critical role in repair of the vascular injury. On resolution of the injury, the local environmental cues within the vessel return to normal, and SMCs reacquire their contractile phenotype/properties. Taken together, the model that has emerged is that SMCs within adult mammals are highly plastic cells that are capable of rather profound alterations in their phenotype in response to changes in local environmental cues important for their differentiation (Fig. 28–1). Thus, the key questions are: (a) What genes and gene products serve as appropriate markers with which to study SMC differentiation/maturation?; and (b) What are the key environmental cues or signals that control the expression of these SMC-specific/selective marker genes?

Smooth Muscle Cell Differentiation and Maturation: No Single Marker Exclusively Identifies a Smooth Muscle Cell to the Exclusion of All Other Cell Types

The initial step in studying cellular differentiation is to identify a set of cell-specific/selective target genes that contribute to the differentiated function or functions of the cell.

This task has proved particularly challenging for the SMC field because of the diverse functions of the SMC, and because most (if not all) SMC markers, although *selective* for SMCs in adult animals, are expressed, at least transiently, in other cell types. Nevertheless, a variety of SMC-selective or specific genes and gene products have been identified that serve as useful markers of the relative state of differentiation/maturation of the fully mature contractile state SMC. These include the smooth muscle isoforms of contractile apparatus proteins: SM α-actin (24–26), SM myosin heavy chain (SM MHC) (27–31), h_1-calponin (32,33), SM22α (32,34,35), aortic carboxypeptidase-like protein (ACLP) (36), desmin (37,38), h-caldesmon (39–41), metavinculin (42), telokin (43), and smoothelin (44). A detailed description of these proteins and other potentially useful SMC differentiation markers and their expression patterns have been reviewed previously (7; see also the first edition of this book) and are not repeated in this chapter. The goals of this section include briefly summarizing the various SMC markers that are useful for assessing SMC differentiation/maturation with a particular focus on identifying issues of impor-

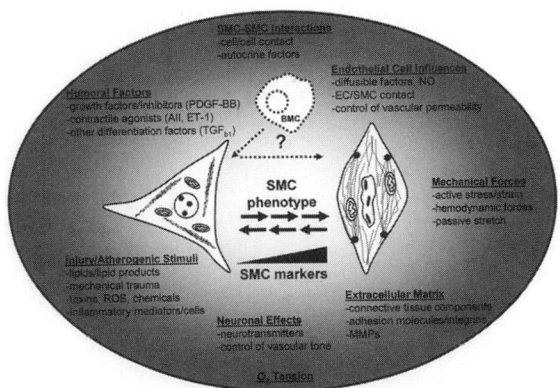

FIG. 28–1. The differentiation state of the vascular smooth muscle cell (SMC) is highly plastic and dependent on integration of multiple local environmental cues. Depicted is a summary of some of the extrinsic factors or local environmental cues that are either known or believed to be important in influencing the differentiation/maturation of the vascular SMC. This schematic emphasizes the point that SMC phenotypic modulation is dependent on the complex interaction of a multitude of local environmental cues, not any single factor, and that a change in any one of these may lead to alterations in the phenotypic state of the SMC (i.e., phenotypic switching). This includes a spectrum of phenotypes ranging from the highly synthetic/proliferative SMC **(left)** to the highly contractile fully differentiated/mature SMC **(right).** The *multiple arrows* connecting the two cell types are meant to illustrate the complexity of steps involved in transitions between the different phenotypes and that changes appear to be reversible. Two separate pathways are depicted rather than a single reversible pathway because it is not at all clear that transitions in phenotype follow the same pathway. The gradient scale **(middle)** depicts increasing expression of the repertoire of SMC-selective markers that typify a fully differentiated mature SMC, although it should not be implied that the "synthetic state" SMC **(left)** does not necessarily express any SMC differentiation marker genes. In fact, it is well known that "synthetic" SMCs often express at least some early SMC differentiation marker genes such as SM α-actin but not SM myosin heavy chain (MHC). Finally, this figure has been updated from the previous edition of this textbook to indicate that there is considerable controversy as to whether bone marrow–derived progenitor cells (BMC, *dashed cell*) give rise to immature SMCs in the developing neointima or if these cells invest as SM-like cells (i.e., SM α-actin positive), with the potential to become fully differentiated SMCs (as indicated by the *question mark* and *dashed arrows*). EC, endothelial cell; ET-1, endothelin-1; MMP, matrix metalloproteinase; NO, nitric oxide; PDGF, platelet-derived growth factor; ROS, reactive oxygen species; TGF, transforming growth factor.

tance for assessing phenotypic modulation of SMC in atherothrombosis and vascular injury.

One of the major deficiencies in studies of the role of the SMC in atherogenesis has been the failure of most studies to adequately distinguish *differentiation markers* that serve as indices of the relative state of differentiation of the SMC versus *lineage markers* that can serve to identify SMCs to the exclusion of all other cell types. Consequently, many cells may have been misidentified as SMCs because of assessment of the wrong or more often an inadequate number of markers (see discussion in "Origin of the Intimal Smooth Muscle Cells in Atherothrombotic Lesions"). Alternatively, many SMCs may not have been identified as such, because of the inability to recognize phenotypically modified SMCs caused by loss of expression of SMC markers as part of the disease process. The problem is further confounded by that virtually all known SMC differentiation markers, with the possible exception of SM MHC, have been shown to be expressed, at least transiently, in other cell types either during development or in response to pathophysiologic stimuli (see review by Owens [7]). For example, the most widely used SMC marker by far is SM α-actin, in part because of the commercial availability of a number of high-affinity and highly selective antibodies for this protein. Indeed, SM α-actin is an excellent SMC differentiation marker in that it is the first known protein expressed during differentiation of the SMC during development (26,39), and it is highly selective for SMC or SMC-like cells in adult animals under normal circumstances. Moreover, it is required for the high force development properties of fully differentiated SMCs, and it is the single most abundant protein in differentiated SMCs, making up to 40% of total cell protein (45). However, by no means is it a definitive SMC lineage marker in that it is known to be expressed in a wide variety of non-SMC cell types under certain circumstances including: (a) skeletal and cardiac muscle during normal development (46); (b) in adult cardiomyocytes in association with various cardiomyopathies (47); (c) in fibroblasts (or so-called myofibroblasts) in a wide range of circumstances including wound repair (see review in Sartore and coworkers [48]); (d) in endothelial cells during vascular remodeling or response to transforming growth factor-β (TGF-β), or both (49,50); and (e) in numerous tumor cells (51,52). Despite this fact, there are literally hundreds of articles in the literature in some of the highest quality journals that have inappropriately equated expression of SM α-actin as sufficient evidence for identification of SMC lineage.

Similarly, virtually all the remaining SMC differentiation marker genes are expressed in a variety of circumstances in other cell types. SM22α, a calponin-like protein of unknown function, exhibits an expression pattern similar to SM α-actin being expressed in skeletal and cardiac muscle during development and within activated fibroblasts under a variety of conditions (32,34,35,48). h_1-calponin, a calcium regulatory protein, is expressed in cardiac myocytes, myofibroblasts, and a variety of tumor cells (53–56). Metavinculin

is an intracellular protein localized at sites of insertion of microfilament bundles into cell membranes and is expressed in cardiac muscle and myofibroblasts in addition to SMCs (57–59). ACLP is widely expressed in many tissues (60). Telokin appears to be relatively specific for SMCs (43), but unfortunately is expressed at low levels in many vascular SMCs of interest in terms of atherogenesis including the aorta and coronary arteries. Smoothelin appears to be selectively expressed in differentiated SMCs as two known isoforms: a 55-kD (or type A) and 120-kD (type B) isoform that are expressed selectively in visceral SMC and vascular SMC, respectively (44,61). However, as acknowledged in the initial articles identifying smoothelin (44,61), this gene is expressed at relatively high levels in a variety of organs and tissues including heart, kidney, and brain (e.g., see Fig. 4 of Rensen and coworkers [61]).

Expression of SM MHC has been extensively scrutinized by a large number of different laboratories (28,29,62–64). Notably, Miano and coworkers (29) carried out very detailed *in situ* hybridization analyses of expression of SM MHC throughout development and maturation of whole mouse embryos and found no evidence for expression of this marker in cell types other than SMCs. Consistent with these results, we found complete SMC specificity of expression of a −4.2 to 11.7 SM MHC promoter enhancer reporter gene in transgenic mice either using direct measurement of a LacZ reporter transgene (28) or a highly sensitive cre recombinase inducible system (62). Importantly, the latter involved crossing mice containing a SM MHC promoter enhancer cre recombinase gene to an indicator mouse strain that shows cre inducible (permanent) activation of a *LacZ* gene in any cell that has ever expressed this promoter-enhancer throughout development and maturation. Results showed complete specificity of expression in SMCs with the exception of a small population of cells within the right atrium at E8.5 that may represent a population of epicardial cells that may have been derived from the proepicardial organ, which gives rise to the coronary circulation. Moreover, we found no evidence of activation of this gene in myofibroblasts in a dermal wound healing model (Owens, Raines, and Tomasek, unpublished observations). As such, expression of SM MHC seems to be highly restricted to SMCs. There are, however, a number of reports of expression of SM MHC within myofibroblasts, endothelial cells, and tumor cells (65,66). However, we have found that the antibody used in these studies cross-reacts with a nonmuscle isoform of MHC—that is, SMemb or NM-B MHC—in a number of species, thus raising some uncertainty regarding reports of expression of SM MHC outside of SMCs (67). In summary, whereas we cannot rule out that SM MHC may be expressed, at least transiently or under certain circumstances, in cells other than SMCs *in vivo*, to our knowledge, conclusive evidence of SM MHC expression in a non-SMC *in vivo* does not exist, and currently it is the most discriminating marker for SMCs identified. However, we would not be surprised if SM MHC is found in non-SMCs, and as such it is recommended that identification of vascular SMCs use SM MHC and several other markers such as SM α-actin, smoothelin, SM22α, and h$_1$-calponin.

Rather than focusing on markers that decline during transition of contractile SMC to an alternative state, a number of workers have focused on identifying genes that serve as markers of these states and investigating mechanisms that regulate their expression. In our opinion, some of the most exciting work in this area has been carried out by Nagai and coworkers who have shown that one of the most useful definitive *positive* markers of the phenotypically modulated SMC is the nonmuscle MHC isoform designated SMemb, or NM-B MHC (68–70). Interestingly, this marker appears to be relatively specific for phenotypically modified or embryonic SMC, although it is expressed in neuronal lines as well (71). Its expression also seems to be induced in association with vascular injury and within intimal SMCs within atherothrombotic lesions (see "Characterization of the Smooth Muscle Cell Within Atherothrombotic Lesions"). These authors also have extensively characterized mechanisms that control transcription of this gene (69,70), and, interestingly, there appear to be some reciprocal control processes as compared with genes indicative of contractile state SMCs.

Environmental Cues Important in Control of Smooth Muscle Cell Differentiation

Despite extensive evidence indicating that phenotypic modulation of the SMC plays a key role in the cause of atherothrombosis and injury repair, little is known regarding the specific environmental cues and mechanisms that regulate SMC differentiation/maturation *in vivo*. Results of gene knockout studies in mice have implicated a number of factors/pathways, but results are equivocal because of uncertainties regarding whether loss of the gene in question had a direct or indirect effect on SMC differentiation. For example, knockout of the type I TGF-β receptor alk-1 (72), the TGF-β receptor II (73), the TGF-β signaling molecule Smad5 (74), TGF-β$_1$ (75), or the thrombin receptor PAR1 (76) are all associated with early embryonic lethality caused by, at least in part, defective vascular maturation, SMC investment/differentiation, or both, although in some cases there is incomplete penetrance in some individual animals. However, in no case has it been shown that the primary defect was the result of a direct effect on the SMC (see details regarding atherothrombosis in "Examples of Environmental Factors Thought to Be Important").

Whereas little direct evidence exists regarding factors that regulate SMC differentiation *in vivo,* results of studies in cultured SMCs have implicated a large number of factors including mechanical forces (77), contractile agonists (78–80), extracellular matrix components such as laminin and type I and IV collagens (81–84), neuronal factors (85), reactive oxygen species (86), endothelial-SMC interactions (87), thrombin (88), and TGF-β$_1$ (89–92) (see reviews by Owens

[7] and Chamley-Campbell and coworkers [18]), all which have been shown to promote expression of at least some SMC marker genes in cultured cell systems (Fig. 28–1). However, these results, including the studies from our own laboratory, need to be interpreted with caution, because there is unequivocal evidence showing that the cultured SMC systems used fail to adequately recapitulate regulatory pathways that are critical *in vivo* (see the first edition of this textbook for a detailed discussion). Perhaps most telling are studies in our own laboratory showing that regions of the SM α-actin promoter or *SM MHC* genes that are sufficient to drive cell-specific expression in cultured SMCS were completely inactive *in vivo* in transgenic mice (25,28). For example, we found that 547 base pair (bp) of the 5' region of the SM α-actin promoter had more than 50-fold greater activity than control constructs in multiple independent lines of cultured SMCs but was inactive in endothelial cells, 10T1/2 cells, 3T3 fibroblasts, adventitial fibroblasts, and rat2 fibroblasts in culture (93), suggesting that we had defined sufficient regions of the promoter to control cell-specific expression of this gene. However, this same 547 bp promoter construct was completely inactive in SMCs *in vivo* in more than 12 independent founder lines, although it was sufficient to drive high expression in cardiac and skeletal muscle during development in a manner similar to the endogenous SM α-actin gene (25). Our conclusion from these studies is that cultured SMCs, although they express high levels of their endogenous SM α-actin gene, do not fully recapitulate cell-specific gene regulatory pathways critical *in vivo*.

Surprisingly, despite that cultured SMC lines are highly modulated and that phenotypic modulation is a critical process in atherogenesis and vascular injury repair, few factors/pathways have been identified that selectively and directly promote phenotypic modulation of SMCs with the exception of platelet-derived growth factor (PDGF)-BB (94–97). The reason for the paucity of studies in this area is likely because of two factors: (a) the incorrect belief that SMC phenotypic modulation is simply secondary to growth stimulation—that is, the old and incorrect adage that differentiation and proliferation are mutually exclusive processes in all cell types; and (b) the untested assumption by many that phenotypic modulation of SMCs is a passive rather than active process and is simply because of loss of positive SMC differentiation factors.

It is now well established that differentiation and proliferation are not necessarily mutually exclusive processes and that many factors other than the SMC proliferation status influences its differentiation state. This topic has been reviewed extensively (7); thus, only a briefly summary of several relevant observations that substantiate this point is provided. First, during late embryogenesis and postnatal development, SMCs are known to have an extremely high rate of proliferation, yet at this time they undergo the most rapid rate of induction of expression of multiple SMC differentiation marker genes (98). Indeed, we showed convincing evidence that proliferating SMCs within the aorta of newborn rats expressed the early SMC marker SM α-actin. Second, SMCs within advanced atherothrombotic lesions show a low rate of proliferation that approaches that of fully differentiated SMCs, yet they are highly phenotypically modulated as evidenced by marked reductions in expression of SMC marker genes (99,100). The latter results indicate that cessation of proliferation alone is not sufficient to promote SMC differentiation and suggest that other SMC differentiation cues are absent, there are active repressors of SMC differentiation present, or both.

Consistent with the hypothesis that phenotypic modulation of the SMC may be controlled actively and not simply by loss of positive differentiation signals, we (94,96,97) and others (95,101,102) have shown that treatment of postconfluent cultures of rat aortic SMCs with PDGF-BB is associated with rapid down-regulation of expression of multiple SMC differentiation marker genes. Of particular significance, under the conditions of our experiments, we found that PDGF-BB elicited only a transient mitogenic effect with cell proliferation returning to control values within 36 hours despite repeated pulsing with PDGF-BB (94). Moreover, suppression of SMC marker gene expression, including SM α-actin and SM MHC, persisted as long as PDGF-BB was present, and on removal of PDGF-BB, SMC marker genes were rapidly reinduced. Of further interest, we also showed that the concentration of PDGF-BB required for inducing SMC phenotypic modulation was 10-fold less than that required to elicit a growth response—that is, we could induce down-regulation of SM α-actin expression in the absence of cell cycle entry. In contrast, we found that bFGF and fetal bovine serum (FBS) had little or no effect on SMC differentiation marker gene expression in postconfluent cultures despite eliciting nearly identical proliferative responses, and thrombin-induced proliferation was associated with increased not decreased expression of SMC marker genes (94,96). Taken together, these results indicate that PDGF-BB is a highly efficacious and selective negative regulator of SMC differentiation, and its effects on differentiation are not secondary to growth stimulation. Whereas the results of these culture studies are interesting, currently there is no definitive evidence that PDGF-BB is a potent negative regulator of SMC differentiation in vivo, although conventional PDGF-β receptor knockout mice do show reduced investment of arterioles with SMC (103) (see "Examples of Environmental Factors Thought to Be Important").

In summary, although there is extensive evidence showing that SMCs are highly plastic and can respond to changes in environmental cues by changing their phenotype, the precise factors and mechanisms that regulate both normal and abnormal differentiation of SMCs in vivo are poorly understood. However, the model that has evolved is that differentiation/maturation of vascular SMC is dependent on constant integration of a large number of local environment cues, which in aggregate determine the pattern of gene expression appropriate for that circumstance (Fig. 28–1). Importantly, this model is probably applicable irrespective of the origins of the SMC in question (e.g., preexisting SMC or bone marrow–derived SM progenitor cells; see the following section and "Mechanisms That Contribute to Phenotypic Modulation of Smooth Muscle Cells Associated with Vascular Injury and Experimental Atherothrombosis").

ORIGIN, CHARACTERISTICS, AND ROLE OF PHENOTYPIC MODULATION OF THE SMOOTH MUSCLE CELL IN THE DEVELOPMENT, PROGRESSION, AND END-STAGE CLINICAL SEQUELAE OF ATHEROTHROMBOSIS

Chapters 30 through 33 provide a detailed and elegant description of the various morphologic characteristics of the human atherothrombotic lesion at various stages of disease progression. The focus in this section is to briefly summarize specific changes that occur in SMCs within atherothrombotic lesions with a particular focus on consideration of the possible contributions of phenotypic modulation of SMC to lesion development, progression, and clinical sequelae including plaque rupture. The key points conveyed in this section are the following: (a) a broad range of changes in the phenotype of the SMC have been described that vary as a function of disease stage and location within the atherothrombotic lesion (e.g., cells within the fibrous cap differ from those in the base of the lesion or the necrotic core); (b) the phenotypically modified SMC itself is likely to contribute to alterations in the extracellular milieu within the intima through production of extracellular matrix components and other secreted products that, in turn, influence the state of differentiation of the SMC; (c) the repertoire of environmental cues that exist within atherothrombotic lesions are no doubt very different than those that exist within a normal healthy blood vessel or cell culture models; and (d) it is often difficult to identify whether lesion cells were derived from SMCs, because phenotypically modified SMCs no longer express most of the markers that allow for their identification. Before considering these issues, evidence that has challenged the dogma for the last three decades that intimal SMCs are derived primarily from preexisting medial SMCs is first considered (104).

Origin of the Intimal Smooth Muscle Cell in Atherothrombotic Lesions

Several lines of evidence have evolved that challenge the dogma that repair of vascular injury is carried out principally (or exclusively) by reversible phenotypic modulation of preexisting SMCs. Two alternative mechanisms have been proposed, although neither is mutually exclusive with the model presented earlier. First, SMC populations within blood vessels are extremely heterogeneous with resident stable populations of preexisting SMCs that are phenotypically distinct from the classical definition of a contractile SMC (105,106), and these cells carry out injury repair. Second, circulating bone marrow–derived SM progenitor cells *may* play a major role in normal vascular injury repair (2–4) (Fig. 28–1).

There are several reports in the literature suggesting that there are heterogeneities among SMCs within a given blood vessel with retention of a resident stable population of cells that have a "synthetic phenotype" (105–107). For example, Frid and coworkers (105) used a panel of antibodies specific for different markers of SMC differentiation including SM α-actin, SM MHC, calponin, desmin, and metavinculin to perform immunofluorescence labeling studies on cryosections of adult and fetal bovine main pulmonary arteries. They reported the presence of what they categorized as four distinct populations or clusters of SMCs on the basis of (a) morphology, (b) cell orientation, (c) pattern of elastic laminae, and (d) immunostaining patterns, speculating that these distinct populations may represent unique lineages that may serve different functions with the arterial media and respond differently to pathophysiologic stimuli. Similarly, studies by Benditt and Benditt (107) also reported that human atherothrombotic lesions may be derived from a monoclonal origin. Whereas there is without question overwhelming evidence for the existence of heterogeneous populations of SMCs *in vivo,* no study has shown that these represent *distinct stable SMC lineages that play a preferential role in carrying out repair of vascular injury.* Indeed, the classic studies of Clowes and coworkers (108–111) would seem to be incompatible with such a possibility in that they showed SMC growth fractions (i.e., the fraction of medial SMCs at time zero that leaves G_0 and reenters the cell cycle) of up to 60% after balloon injury of the rat carotid artery, indicating that most, if not all, SMCs within the media retain the capacity to reenter the cell cycle and contribute to vessel repair in adult animals, although the response to balloon injury in the rat is very different from that of the developing atherothrombotic lesion in humans. In addition, no study has clearly demonstrated that the SMC subtypes observed by Frid and coworkers (105) and Benditt and Benditt (107) represent distinct SMC lineages using classic and well established methodologies for studying cell lineages—that is, demonstration that a putative distinct SMC lineage retains its unique identity after transplantation to the locus of another putative lineage. Until such studies are done, it cannot be ruled out that the different properties observed are a function of differences in local environmental cues as opposed to genetically distinct stable SMC lineages with fixed developmental potential.

There is compelling evidence that cells resident in the circulating blood invest in the neointima and give rise to cells that express at least some properties of vascular SMCs (112,113). For example, Sata and coworkers (3) lethally irradiated wild-type mice and reconstituted with bone marrow cells from a ROSA26 mouse that expressed a *β-galactosidase* gene, thus allowing lineage tracing. They then injured the femoral artery with a large wire that caused severe damage of the vessel including complete loss of endothelium and medial

SMC apoptosis/necrosis and examined for investment by LacZ$^+$ cells at 1 and 4 weeks, as well as expression of the SMC differentiation marker gene *SM α-actin* by immunostaining. Interestingly, at 4 weeks, a significant amount of neointimal (63.0 ± 9.3%) and medial cells (45.9 ± 6.9%) were LacZ$^+$, as determined by X-gal staining, whereas no LacZ$^+$ cells were present in uninjured femoral arteries. Moreover, at least some of the LacZ$^+$ cells also expressed either SM α-actin (a marker for SMC and myofibroblasts, see "Smooth Muscle Cell Differentiation and Maturation: No Single Marker Exclusively Identifies a Smooth Muscle Cell to the Exclusion of All Other Cell Types") or CD31 (a marker for endothelial cells). They interpreted these studies as evidence that bone marrow–derived cells can give rise to vascular cells after mechanical injury and contribute to vessel repair (3). Consistent with the preceding results, Han and coworkers (2) had previously conducted similar experiments in which they lethally irradiated female C57Bl/6 mice and reconstituted with bone marrow cells from congenic (Ly5.1) male donors and characterized the contributions of the bone marrow cells to neointima formation and medial repair by *in situ* hybridization with a Y chromosome–specific probe. Of particular significance, they examined a scratch injury, or silk suture models of vascular injury that evoked varying severity of medial injury. Results demonstrated the presence of abundant bone marrow cells within the media and intima in cases of severe injury, whereas no bone marrow cells was present in cases where there was denudation of endothelial cells but minimal damage to the media (2). These results suggest that bone marrow cells are recruited in vascular healing to complement resident SMC. However, of critical importance, Han and coworkers (2) found that the relative proportion of these cells that contributed varied as a function of the severity of medial damage, and only in cases of severe medial damage, when few resident SMCs are available to affect repair, was the bone marrow contribution extensive. Therefore, the high frequency of investment by circulating bone marrow cells observed in some studies may be artificial and not reflective of normal vascular repair processes. In addition, a major general limitation in studies thus far that have explored the possible contribution of bone marrow cells to neointimal SMCs is the failure to provide compelling evidence regarding expression of definitive markers of SMC lineage such as SM MHC (see "Smooth Muscle Cell Differentiation and Maturation: No Single Marker Exclusively Identifies a Smooth Muscle Cell to the Exclusion of All Other Cell Types"). As stated clearly by Han and coworkers (2), the use of SM α-actin to further characterize bone marrow–derived neointimal cells shows that "these marrow-derived cells resemble fetal/immature vascular SMC or myofibroblasts" at best.

There also have been a number of studies showing that bone marrow cells contribute to intimal lesion formation in mouse models of transplant atherothrombosis (3–5). Blood vessel allograft atherothrombosis typically results in the accumulation of mononuclear cell types and enhanced SMC proliferation that ultimately culminates in vascular stenosis and ischemic graft failure. Until recently, the source of SMC investment in allograft blood vessel stenosis was unknown. In two separate studies involving lethal irradiation followed by reconstitution with bone marrow cells from mice expressing LacZ, Sata and coworkers (3) and Shimizu and coworkers (4) found that ~10% to 20% of SM α-actin–positive cells in the neointimal lesions of aortic allografts were colocalized or in close proximity with LacZ⁺ stained cells. The authors concluded that bone marrow–derived cells gave rise to SMC-like cells within the neointima, although again studies lacked presentation of compelling evidence of expression of definitive SMC markers like SM MHC and failed to clearly resolve whether SM α-actin/LacZ⁺ cells were in fact one cell or merely two adjacent cells. To overcome this limitation, Hu and coworkers (5) carried out a clever series of studies using bone marrow cells derived from a SM22α-LacZ transgenic mouse to allow simultaneous lineage tracing and characterization of expression of this SMC differentiation marker within the same cell. These workers found that there were no LacZ⁺ cells in the neointima of mice that received bone marrow from the SM22α-LacZ mice 6 weeks after allograft implantation. Although consistent with other studies, they did see investment of bone marrow cells from ROSA LacZ mice within the neointima. To confirm that the SM22α-LacZ promoter can be potentially active at 6 weeks in the allograft neointima, a BALB/c to SM22α-LacZ aortic transplant was performed. SM22α-LacZ⁺ cells were identified in the allograft neointima, indicating that SM22α-LacZ⁺ cells migrated from the host vessel to the neointima and that the SM22α-LacZ promoter is active in the neointima at 6 weeks in this model (5). Taken together, these studies seem to refute earlier studies in that although bone marrow–derived cells clearly invest the neointima, these cells failed to express even the early SMC differentiation marker SM22α as detected by LacZ staining. One way to reconcile these results is that SM α-actin staining may have been more sensitive than detection of the SM22α LacZ. However, in any case, the lack of demonstration of expression of multiple definitive markers of SMC lineage raises doubts as to whether bone marrow cells can undergo differentiation into mature SMCs.

The most important question is whether there is evidence that "SMC or SMC-like cells" within *human* atherothrombotic lesions are derived from bone marrow, although relatively few studies have been published in this area because of inherent limitations underlying the use of human subjects. However, of interest, three studies have analyzed the contribution of host versus recipient contributions to intimal lesions (6,114,115). In each study, Y chromosome labeling was done to ascertain the possibility of investment of recipient cells into lesions in male cardiac transplantation patients who received a female donor heart. As such, Y-chromosome–positive cells within blood vessels of the transplanted heart may have come through the systemic circulation from undifferentiated cells in the male recipient's bone marrow, from cells that entered the

circulation from non–bone marrow sources, or because of its proximity from the cardiac remnant. Results from two of these studies (6,115) differed greatly from the third (114), and none of the studies provides definitive insight into the investment of blood-derived cells in the developing lesion. Quaini and coworkers (115) estimated that as many as 60% of cells investing in newly developed arterioles in the collateral circulation were Y-chromosome/SM α-actin–positive. In contrast, Glaser and coworkers (6) showed that at most 6% (the observed frequency was actually 2.7%, but authors appropriately allowed for possible false negatives) of the cells were Y chromosome/SM α-actin–positive in medium and small arteries, whereas collateral arterioles were not examined. Consistent with the latter findings, Hruban and coworkers (114) found no evidence of bone marrow–derived SMCs within coronary lesions. Regardless of these discrepancies, it appears that at least some recipient-derived cells can give rise to a SMC-like/myofibroblast cell in newly developed arterioles of the collateral circulation and medium and small coronary arteries. However, insight into the investment of blood-derived cells into the developing atherothrombotic lesion was not evident, and vessels with advanced neointimal SMC proliferation did not have markedly increased or decreased numbers of Y chromosome/SM α-actin–positive cells (6). *Thus, whether blood-derived cells can give rise to SMCs that play a functional role in the developing atherothrombotic lesions in humans is still uncertain* (Fig. 28–1). Irrespective of whether this is true, studies showing that bone marrow–derived cells have the capacity to invest injured blood vessels raise the exciting possibility of exploiting this process for possible stem cell–based gene therapies.

In summary, whereas there appears to be clear evidence that blood-derived cells can give rise to SMC-like or myofibroblast-like cells in the developing neointima in models of allograft rejection, severe vessel injury, or both, it remains to be determined if these cells are capable of full differentiation into SMCs (Fig. 28–1) or whether bone marrow–derived SMCs play a significant role in development of atherothrombosis in humans, or both. Thus, it is important that future studies in this area address a number of limitations in previous studies including the following: (a) the persistent use of SM α-actin expression as the sole marker for identification of SMC lineage; (b) the use of animal models that result in severe medial damage/necrosis, thus resulting in possible gross overestimation of the contribution of bone marrow–derived cells in normal vascular repair processes; (c) the failure to adequately resolve whether there is truly coexpression of bone marrow lineage tracer markers and SMC markers within an individual cell and to rule out the possibility of fusion of circulating stem cells and resident SMCs, as suggested may be the case by studies showing a high frequency of such an event in hepatocytes (116,117); and (d) a lack of long-term studies in animal models that undergo spontaneous/naturally occurring atherothrombosis.

Characterization of the Smooth Muscle Cell Within Atherothrombotic Lesions

The terms *contractile* and *synthetic* phenotype have been used extensively in the literature to describe the many phenotypic states of the vascular SMC. Indeed, these terms have proven to be useful (if for no other reason than economy of language) for describing distinct generic spectrums of phenotypes available to the SMC. However, it is now recognized that a simple two state model is inadequate to explain the diverse range of phenotypes that can be exhibited by the SMC under different physiologic and pathologic circumstances (Fig. 28–1) (see review by Owens [7]). Not surprisingly, as the repertoire of SMC markers has expanded, the picture that has emerged is that there is likely a continuous spectrum of possible SMC phenotypes that might exist such that it may be artificial to assign cells to distinct subcategories. If this logic is extended to consider quantitative measures of large numbers of markers that represent the *contractile* and *synthetic* state of the SMC, the distinctions between these subtypes become difficult to distinguish, as in the case of vascular development when SMCs are first acquiring their contractile properties yet also simultaneously must participate in vessel growth and remodeling. In the case of SMCs within atherothrombotic lesions, there is clear evidence that the morphologic, biochemical, and molecular properties of SMCs vary at different stages of atherothrombosis, within different lesion types, and among SMCs located in different regions within a given lesion. With this in mind, this chapter does not attempt to review the literally thousands of articles that have been published on this topic and unequivocally establish that intimal SMCs are altered with respect to normal medial SMCs after vascular injury or in association with experimental or human atherothrombosis (see review by Ross [1]). Rather, just a few representative examples of SMC phenotypes that appear to exist within atherothrombotic lesions are briefly described, beginning with what we believe were several seminal studies by Aikawa and coworkers (63,118,119) that focused on analysis of the definitive SMC differentiation marker SM MHC, as well as nonmuscle-type myosin heavy chain (NM-B MHC or SMemb) in human and rabbit lesions ("Smooth Muscle Cell Differentiation and Maturation: No Single Marker Exclusively Identifies a Smooth Muscle Cell to the Exclusion of All Other Cell Types").

Aikawa and colleagues (63,118) found evidence for altered expression of SM MHC isoforms (SM-1 an SM-2) and SM α-actin in tissue samples obtained from autopsied patients and atherectomy specimens from patients undergoing percutaneous transluminal coronary angioplasty (PTCA). Medial SMCs were positive for SM-1, SM-2, and SM α-actin; however, 16 to 20 days after PTCA, neointimal cells contained SM α-actin but little or no SM-1 or SM-2, indicating partial SMC phenotypic modulation to an immature state. In contrast, 6 months after PTCA, SMCs sequentially recovered SM-1 and then SM-2 expression and conse-

quently a more mature phenotype. Increased expression of SMemb, a marker of fetal SMCs or immature adult SMCs (118), was found throughout the intima with no apparent relation to the time after PTCA. These findings were extended in a separate experimentally controlled study in a rabbit hypercholesterolemic angioplasty model of atherothrombosis (119). Whereas expression of SM-1 and SM-2 were significantly reduced in the media and outermost edge of the atheroma, animals undergoing the same treatment followed by extensive lipid reduction for 16 months showed a time-dependent increase in SM-1 and SM-2 expression in the media and neointima, indicating that SMCs exhibit a more mature phenotype after lipid reduction. Perhaps of even greater interest, the authors observed that intimal SMCs in the group undergoing lipid decreasing showed marked reductions in expression of matrix metalloproteinase (MMP)-2 and 9, reduced expression of PDGF-B, and acquired the morphologic appearance of a mature/contractile SMC, similar to the "contractile" phenotype (119).

Intimal SMCs have been shown to exhibit many additional changes including: (a) increased DNA synthesis and expression of proliferation markers and cyclins such as proliferating cell nuclear antigen (120); (b) decreased expression of proteins that typify differentiated SMCs including SM MHCs (SM-1, SM-2), SM α-actin, SM22α, smoothelin, h-caldesmon, desmin, calponin, and vinculin and increased ACLP and SMemb (16,17,60,118,121,122); (c) alterations in calcium handling and contractility (123–125); and (d) alterations in cell ultrastructure, including a general loss of myofilaments, which is replaced largely by synthetic organelles such as Golgi and rough endoplasmic reticulum, rounding of the cell from its typical elongated contractile morphology, and alterations in basement membrane (16,17,122). These latter changes in SMC ultrastructure are illustrated in Figure 28–2, which shows transmission electron micrographs (micrographs by the late Dr. Russel Ross) clearly depicting the morphologic and cytoskeletal changes in SMCs in the normal artery compared with SMCs localized to the neointimal human atherothrombotic lesion. These studies have been extended to the extreme by Geary and coworkers (126), who carried out microarray-based profiling of gene expression patterns of SMCs in the neointima formed 4 weeks after aortic grafting compared with those from the normal aorta in primates. A total of 147 genes were differentially expressed in neointimal SMCs versus normal aorta SMCs, most genes underscoring the importance of matrix production during neointimal formation. However, as informative as these studies are, we feel they fail to capture the dynamic aspects of SMC phenotypic modulation in the naturally occurring lesion, and clearly represent an oversimplification. For example, although the rate of SMC proliferation may be increased during early stages of lesion formation, or after balloon injury of an advanced lesion as part of an angioplasty procedure, the proliferation index of SMCs within mature advanced lesions is not increased (120). Sim-

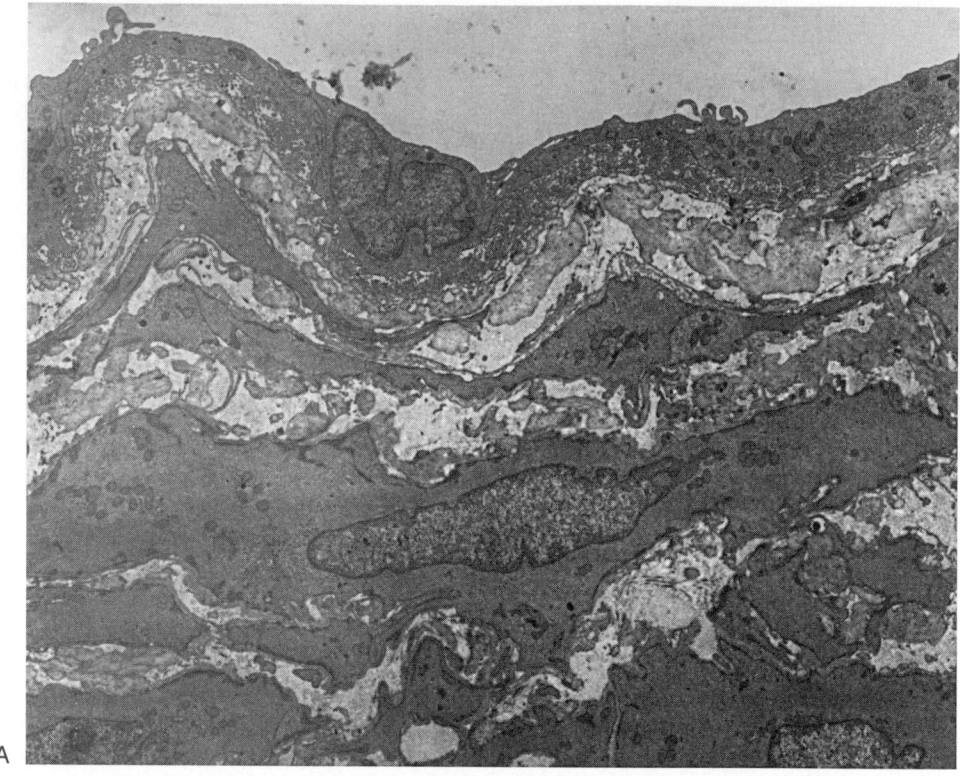

A

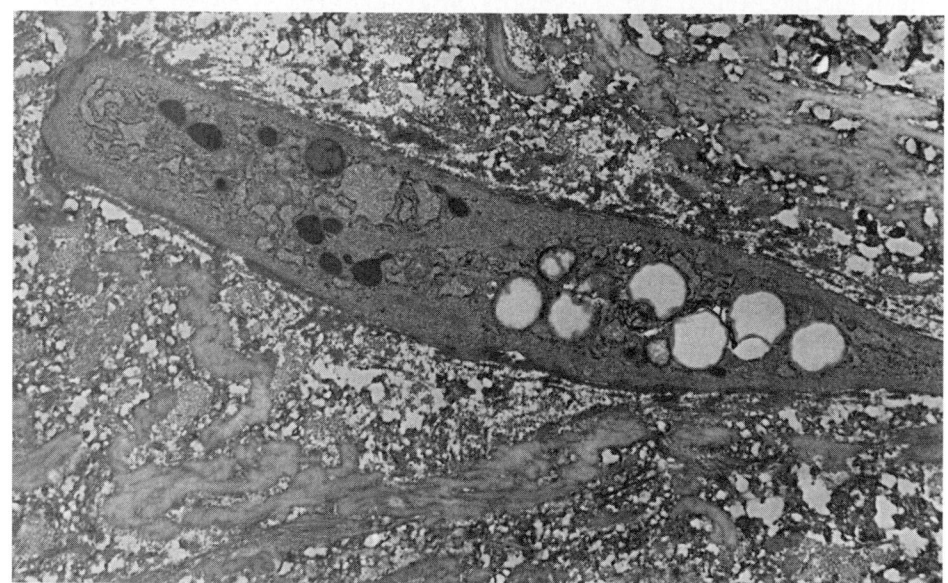

B

FIG. 28–2. Intimal smooth muscle cell (SMC) within human atherothrombotic lesions show a multitude of phenotypic alterations. Figure shows transmission electron micrographs from human coronary arteries. **A:** A SMC from a normal coronary artery (the top of this micrograph is the lumen). The endothelial cells lie in proximity to the internal elastic lamina, beneath which are seen several smooth muscle cells. These cells contain a large complement of myofilaments that surrounds the nucleus and few cellular organelles. It is characteristic of the "contractile" phenotype depicted in the schematic diagram in Figure 28–1. **B:** A SMC within the intima of an atherothrombotic lesion. This cell is surrounded by large amounts of connective tissue matrix, including collagen fibrils, an irregular basement membrane, and elastic fibers and proteoglycans. Within the cell can be seen numerous cisternae of rough endoplasmic reticulum and numerous forms of lipid. Mitochondria and some myofilaments are visible. This cell is typical of the "synthetic state" SMC usually seen in atherothrombotic lesions deep within the intima. (Courtesy of the late Dr. Russell Ross, University of Washington, Seattle, WA.) (See color insert for Fig. 28–3.)

ilarly, depending on the nature of the lesion, intimal SMCs may or may not show loss of many SMC marker genes (100). Finally, aortic grafting and vessel injury in healthy animals develop a predominantly SMC-rich neointima over a relatively short time period compared with the naturally occurring multicellular atherothrombotic lesion, which takes decades to develop.

Taken together, the preceding studies support a model in which the SMC can exhibit a wide range of different phenotypes depending on the stage of lesion development (or regression), the location of the SMC within a specific region of the atherothrombotic lesion, or both. Therefore, the functional role of phenotypic modulation of the SMC likewise must also vary depending on the stage of the disease. For example, it presumably plays a maladaptive role in early lesion development and progression (1,127), but it may have a beneficial adaptive role in stabilizing plaques in mature eccentric atherothrombotic lesions. However, it may later contribute to plaque destabilization through apoptosis or activation of various protease cascades, or both (8,9). In any case, these few examples illustrate that understanding the regulation of transitions in the phenotypic state of the SMC, and the functional consequences of these transitions, is likely to be extremely complex—a topic the following section attempts to address.

MECHANISMS THAT CONTRIBUTE TO PHENOTYPIC MODULATION OF SMOOTH MUSCLE CELLS ASSOCIATED WITH VASCULAR INJURY AND EXPERIMENTAL ATHEROTHROMBOSIS

Examples of Environmental Factors Thought to Be Important

It is not possible to consider all environmental factors thought to be important in SMC phenotypic modulation—that is, many factors have been implicated on the basis of morphologic and biochemical characteristics of human lesions, as well as numerous studies in cultured cell systems and animal models. However, our synopsis of many studies is that phenotypic modulation of SMCs within lesions is complex and likely to involve many factors including growth factors and cytokines, inflammatory cell mediators, lipids, lipid peroxidation products, reactive oxygen species, and others (see reviews by Ross [1] and Lusis [128]). Rather than trying to do justice to these studies, this section focuses on several selected examples in which we feel there is sufficient evidence implicating possible involvement of that factor in phenotypic modulation of SMCs associated with the natural progression of atherothrombosis *in vivo* including: (a) PDGF ("Environmental Cues Important in Control of Smooth Muscle Cell Differentiation"); (b) TGF-β; (c) endothelial nitric oxide synthase (eNOS); and (d) MMPs. The goal is to convince the reader that although gain and loss of function studies involving each factor provide new insight

into the role of the SMCs at a particular stage of atherothrombosis—that is, SMC investment of the fibrotic cap—considerable efforts must still be taken to identify the complex interactions of single and multiple factors throughout the many stages of atherothrombosis lesion development and not simply the end stage of advanced lesion formation. This distinction is important because loss or gain of function studies may not yield differences in the end-stage lesion, but they provide novel insight into the role of the SMC and SMC phenotypic modulation during early lesion formation (discussed later).

Although the rat model of vascular injury was initially used by investigators to characterize the complex interaction between potential growth factors involved in phenotypic SMC modulation associated with neointimal hyperplasia, this model more closely mimics vascular repair or at best restenosis in humans and not the natural progression of atherothrombosis, which occurs over decades (129). However, the initial observations regarding growth factor expression that were made in the rat (109,110,130) were important in guiding subsequent studies in mice and, ultimately, were the foundation of many human clinical restenosis trials. Here, the focus is on reviewing studies in genetically modified mouse models of atherothrombosis that we believe illustrate general paradigms that may be operative in atherothrombotic lesion formation in humans, although recognizing there are likely to be many important differences. In mice, a detailed analysis of lesion development throughout the arterial tree by Nakashima and coworkers (131) and Zhang and coworkers (132) showed that atherothrombotic lesions in the apoE-deficient mouse (apoE$^{-/-}$) contained a spectrum of lesions similar to those observed during atherogenesis in humans, including: (a) monocyte attachment to endothelial cells and subendothelial infiltration and macrophage investment, (b) foam cell lesion formation and fatty streaks, and (c) complex fibrous plaque formation including recruitment of SMCs to the cap—processes that are enhanced by a high-fat/cholesterol–enriched diet as in humans (see Chapter 25 for a more detailed discussion).

Platelet-derived Growth Factor

PDGF is a potent SMC chemoattractant produced by activated platelets and lesion macrophages (133) that rapidly down-regulates SM-selective markers in cell culture (94, 96,97) and stimulates SMC proliferation and migration in arterial injury models (134,135). PDGF exists as a disulfide-linked dimer and is composed of two chains: A and B (136). There are two PDGF receptors, PDGFR-α and PDGFR-β, whose intrinsic tyrosine kinase activity is activated by PDGF-A alone, or PDGF-A and PDGF-B, respectively (137). The role of PDGF receptors have been described in several postinjury models (138), and it is reported that both PDGF chains and their receptors are detected in human coronary arteries after balloon angioplasty (139,140). Conventional knockout of PDGF-A (141), PDGF-B (142), PDGFR-α (143), and PDGFR-β (144) has been shown to result in early embryonic or perinatal lethality, thereby prohibiting use of these mice to investigate the role of PDGF signaling in vascular injury responses or experimental atherogenesis. However, in apoE$^{-/-}$ mice fed a Western diet for 12 to 18 weeks, Sano and coworkers (145) showed a 67% reduction in atherothrombotic lesion size and an 80% reduction in SMC cell investment of the neointima (as identified by SM α-actin–positive cells) after injection of rat monoclonal antibodies directed against both the PDGF α and β receptors compared with IgG injected control mice. Blockade of PDGFR-α alone had no effect on lesion size or smooth muscle investment compared with control mice. Thus, regulating signal transduction through the PDGFR-β receptor in SMCs may play a critical role in SMC migration and proliferation. Elegant work by Kozaki and coworkers (146) tested a similar hypothesis but extended the length of atherothrombosis development up to 50 weeks on a Western diet. PDGF-B–deficient embryonic liver cells were used to reconstitute circulating blood cells in lethally irradiated apoE$^{-/-}$ mice, where no PDGF-B was detected in circulating platelets and macrophages. At 35 weeks, lesions in the PDGF-B$^{-/-}$ mice contained mostly macrophages, appeared less mature, and had a reduced frequency of a fibrous cap. However, after 45 weeks, SMC accumulation in the fibrous cap was indistinguishable from control mice. The delayed onset of SMC proliferation and migration also was observed in the same study by dosing apoE$^{-/-}$ mice with a PDGFR-α/β antagonist, CT52923. Thus, results show that inhibition of PDGF signaling or elimination of PDGF-B from circulating cells does not appear sufficient to prevent SMC accumulation in advanced lesions, and these results suggest that PDGF-BB is not required for lesion formation at this stage, or that other growth factor signaling pathways mediate these effects when PDGF signaling is blocked. However, it also is possible that non–blood cell-derived PDGF-BB is important—that is, endothelial cell and SMC PDGF production (133)—or that PDGF receptor blockade was incomplete, or both. In addition, it is not possible to deduce from the preceding studies which effects were the result of PDGF-dependent signaling in SMCs, nor whether any of the observed effects were secondary to alterations in SMC phenotype per se. Indeed, resolution of these many possibilities will be extremely difficult and likely will be dependent on development of SMC-specific or conditional gene knockout mice, or both, that show selective abrogation of PDGF-dependent signaling pathways in SMCs (discussed at the end of this section).

Transforming Growth Factor-β

TGF-β was first identified as an antiinflammatory cytokine and shown to promote SMC differentiation in cell culture by coordinately up-regulating SM-selective markers such as SM α-actin and SM MHC (89,90,147). Thus far, knockout gene studies in mice for type I TGF-β receptor (72), TGF-β receptor II (73), TGF-β$_1$ (75), TGF-β signaling molecules

(74), and cardiovascular overexpression of TGF-β$_1$ under control of the SM22α promoter are embryonic lethal (148). TGF-β levels are rapidly increased within 6 to 24 hours in experimental balloon injury models (149). Neointimal formation, matrix deposition, and smooth muscle proliferation are increased by overexpression of TGF-β and the reciprocal occurs by selective inhibition of endogenous TGF-β (150,151). However, there also exists a paucity of in vivo data implicating a protective role of TGF-β in the "natural" progression of atherothrombosis. Of interest, McCaffrey and coworkers (152) showed that advanced human plaque SMCs contain mutations in the TGF-β type II receptor that decrease the sensitivity of these cells to TGF-β, and patients with unstable angina typically have decreased plasma levels of TGF-β (153). The most convincing evidence for a protective role of TGF-β comes from two studies in the apoE$^{-/-}$ mouse that suggest that TGF-β may be critical for SMC matrix production and development of a stable fibrotic plaque (154,155). Neutralizing antibodies to TGF-β$_1$, TGF-β$_2$, and TGF-β$_3$ were shown to accelerate the development of atherothrombosis at 15 weeks, and the lesions displayed increased inflammatory cells and decreased collagen content (155). The latter findings suggested that TGF-β may mediate a critical balance between inflammation and fibrosis, presumably by SMC matrix production, during atherothrombotic plaque development. To test this hypothesis, a similar study was performed by Lutgens and coworkers (154), whereby 12-week treatment with a soluble TGF-β receptor II protein, which inhibits TGF-β signaling, increased CD3$^+$ and CD45$^+$ cells in the atherothrombotic lesion at 17 weeks. More profound effects were found when the 12-week treatment was started 17 weeks into the development of atherothrombosis. In these mice, lipid cores were 65% larger, the inflammatory cell content had increased 2.7-fold, fibrosis decreased 50%, and intraplaque hemorrhages were observed frequently. Thus, although not directly addressed in either study, these results strongly imply that TGF-β may be essential for SMC matrix production and fibrotic stabilization of the developing atherothrombotic plaque.

Endothelial Nitric Oxide Synthase

Nitric oxide (NO), constitutively produced by NOS in the endothelium, is a potent vasodilator and possesses various cardioprotective attributes such as inhibition of platelet aggregation (156), suppression of leukocyte/monocyte adhesion to vascular endothelial cells, and inhibition of SMC proliferation and migration, as identified at the level of SM differentiation marker genes (157). Chronic administration of L-arginine to increase NO levels or adenoviral-mediated administration of eNOS inhibited neointimal hyperplasia in several balloon injury models (158,159). However, these beneficial effects were only examined in the short time frame of experimental injury models, and insight into long-term gain and loss of function studies in the apoE$^{-/-}$ mouse have revealed a novel paradox regarding the *protective* effects of eNOS. In the apoE/eNOS double knockout mouse, atherothrombosis is accelerated, as predicted, and further complications include aortic aneurysms, coronary stenosis, and ischemic heart disease, which are not common to the wild-type apoE$^{-/-}$ mouse. Paradoxically, crossing eNOS overexpressing transgenic mice to apoE$^{-/-}$ mice resulted in increased, not decreased, acceleration of atherothrombosis. Excess NO production ultimately resulted in increased superoxide anion (O_2^-) production, a strong oxidant implicated as a proliferative stimulus for the SMC *in vitro* and *in vivo* (160,161). Moreover, in wild-type apoE$^{-/-}$ mice, production of superoxide anion is increased in SMCs throughout the artery wall causing two detrimental effects: (a) decreased NO bioavailability and (b) concomitant impaired endothelial-dependent vasodilation. Of particular interest, the expression of the transcription factor Id3 (inhibitor of differentiation 3), which is increased with vascular injury (162) and suppresses SM α-actin expression *in vitro* (163), also is increased by superoxide anion (164). Thus, there is presumably a tightly regulated balance between the production of eNOS that provides an antiatherothrombotic effect and the role of excess superoxide anion in promoting SMC phenotypic modulation, proliferation, and migration in the developing lesion, although this mechanism has not been directly addressed.

Matrix Metalloproteinases

MMPs are endopeptidases produced by SMCs and macrophages that are believed to contribute significantly to the degradation and remodeling of the plaque extracellular matrix. Although MMPs are not environmental cues that regulate SMC phenotypic modulation per se, they appear to be a functional marker of the phenotypically modulated SMC in the developing lesion whose expression is effected by environmental cues discussed earlier: PDGF (165), TGF-β (166), NO (167), and reactive oxygen species (168). In nondiseased human and experimental animal arteries, MMP-2 (72 kD gelatinase) and TIMP-1 and TIMP-2 (tissue inhibitor of metalloproteinase) are constitutively expressed at levels providing a stable balance between endogenous matrix production and matrix degradation, a healthy MMP:TIMP ratio (8). This ratio is tipped toward MMPs in the developing lesion as described in part by an increase in MMP-3 (stromelysin) and MMP-9 (92 kD gelatinase) increased MMP:TIMP ratio (8). Presumably, MMP overexpression would be required for SMC migration and formation of a SMC-rich fibrous plaque and subsequent plaque stabilization. However, and elegant study by Galis and coworkers (9) showed that SMCs in the shoulder region of human atherothrombotic plaques also can express MMP-3 and MMP-9, possibly leading to plaque destabilization and rupture. Furthermore, as discussed in great detail in "Characterization of the Smooth Muscle Cell Within Atherothrombotic Lesions," Aikawa and coworkers (119) showed

that decreased SM-1 and SM-2 marker expression correlated with increased PDGF and MMP-3/9 expression in the rabbit neointima. Thus far, knockout genes studies for MMP-9 have shown decreased intimal SMC hyperplasia and reduced late lumen loss in the mouse carotid artery flow cessation model (169) and similar results in the carotid wire injury model (170). To our knowledge, there are no studies in the MMP-9/apoE–deficient mouse; however, in wild-type apoE$^{-/-}$ mice, differential expression of MMP-9 increases with time in lesional areas versus nonlesion areas during the natural progression of atherothrombosis (171). Thus, a critical unresolved question is: What environmental cues within the lesion differentially regulate SMC MMP production, as well as production of various TIMPs, thereby influencing plaque formation or stability, or both? (See Galis and Khatri [8] for an excellent review of this critically important topic.)

In summary, although the preceding studies have implicated a possible role of these factors in atherothrombogenesis, few studies have directly examined if or how these factors alter the phenotypic state of the SMC *in vivo*. Given the dynamic nature of SMC phenotypic switching, further detailed analyses of the expression pattern of various environmental cues—that is, PDGF and TGF-β—are needed throughout the time course of the natural lesion development in mouse atherothrombotic models (109,110,130). Although such studies would only provide correlative evidence regarding the large plethora of signals present within an atherothrombotic lesion, such studies should help to identify candidate regulatory pathways that could be directly tested by various loss of function approaches. In any case, much additional work is needed to address a fundamentally important question in the field: What factors in the lesion are responsible for inducing phenotypic switching of SMCs at various stages of vascular injury or lesion development/progression? In the next section, we will briefly describe an experimental approach that we have used to begin to address this question.

Molecular Mechanisms of Decreased Smooth Muscle Cell Differentiation Marker Expression Associated with Atherothrombosis: A Novel Experimental Approach to Studying Smooth Muscle Cell Phenotypic Modulation *In Vivo*

Tremendous progress has been made in the last decade in identifying mechanisms that contribute to transcriptional regulation of SMC marker genes (see reviews by Owens and coworkers [88,172], Firulli and Olson [173], Miano [174]). For example, a review article by our group summarizes the complex interaction of cis regulatory elements and trans acting factors involved in regulating expression of SM α-actin (172). Given the focus of this chapter on the role of SMC phenotypic switching in atherogenesis, we do not attempt to review this complex topic, but rather the focus is on consideration of regulatory pathways that may act to repress expression of SMC marker genes in response to vascular injury or atherothrombosis.

As an alternative to attempting to individually dissect which of the wide plethora of altered environmental cues associated with vascular injury, or atherogenesis, directly contribute to phenotypic modulation of SMC phenotype *in vivo,* we developed what we refer to as the "inside-out" approach (175). That is, because we know that a signature feature of the phenotypically modified SMC is reduced expression of SMC marker genes such as SM α-actin and SM MHC, we first asked two simple questions: (a) Is injury-induced down-regulation of SMC marker genes mediated at the transcriptional level? (b) If so, what specific cis elements and trans factors are required for this effect?

Whereas it may seem intuitive that repression of SMC marker expression in lesions would be transcriptionally mediated, this had never been directly tested despite that the knowledge that phenotypic modulation occurs has been available for more than 30 years (176). Moreover, results of our studies in cultured SMCs showed that PDGF-BB–induced transcriptional repression was mediated in large part by selective destabilization of transcripts for SMC marker genes (94–97), thus raising the possibility that phenotypic modulation *in vivo* might not include a transcriptional component. To directly address this question, we carried out a series of vascular injury experiments in SM α-actin, SM MHC, and SM22α LacZ transgenic mice (175). As shown in Figure 28–3 (see color insert), A through L, the SM α-actin, SM MHC, and SM22α LacZ transgenes were highly expressed throughout the media of the uninjured mouse carotid artery (175). However, after vascular injury, we observed nearly complete loss of expression of all three transgenes, thus demonstrating for the first time that SMC phenotypic modulation *in vivo* was mediated at least in part by transcriptional repression (175). However, of interest, we also observed that after 14 days of injury, subpopulations of cells began to show redifferentiation as evidenced by increased expression of SM α-actin and SM MHC, further documenting the very dynamic nature of SMC phenotypic switching *in vivo* as emphasized in the previous section and in Figure 28–1.

Studies from our laboratory had identified a G/C-rich cis regulatory element positioned between two CArG elements in the SM MHC promoter that functioned as a repressor *in vitro* and was shown to bind the transcription factors Sp1 and Sp3, both of which are increased in vascular models of injury (177,178). The presence of the CArG cis regulatory elements and CArG:SRF interaction are required for both *in vivo* and *in vitro* expression of SM MHC (175,177–179). Of major significance, we showed that mutation of a similar G/C-rich cis regulatory element in the SM22α promoter (also positioned between both CArGs) had no effect on the normal pattern of expression of this transgene during development, but completely abrogated injury-induced down-regulation (175) (Fig. 28–3, compare panels I through P). These results thus indicate that the G/C repressor element is dispensable for normal developmental regulation of this gene but is *required* for injury-induced down-regulation. Moreover, we showed that expression of the G/C repressor element-binding factor Sp1 was dramatically up-regulated

by vascular injury (177). Because G/C repressor elements are found between CArG elements of many SMC marker gene promoters, results support the hypothesis that phenotypic modulation of the SMC (or at least repression of SMC marker genes) may be regulated at least in part by injury-induced increases in expression of Sp1 or other Kruppel-like (KLF) transcription factors that bind to the G/C repressor element and disrupt interactions between CArG elements, thereby inhibiting SMC gene expression (see Black and coworkers [180] for review of Sp1 and KLF transcription factors). For example, KLF5, a KLF factor also known as BTEB2 or IKLF, is similarly up-regulated in the neointima of developing lesions. Homozygous knockout of KLF5 is embryonic lethal, but mice heterozygous for KLF5 showed decreased neointimal and medial thickening and SMC proliferation (181). Although KLF5 has not been directly linked to SMC gene regulation *in vivo,* these results do support the general paradigm presented earlier involving the role of Sp1-like or KLF factors in *SMC* gene regulation. Of further interest, there is evidence that Sp1-dependent mechanisms may also be responsible for activation of genes characteristic of the phenotypically modulated SMC such as the constitutive expression of PDGF-BB (182,183), SMemb (70), and ACLP (60)—that is, there may be common factors/pathways that turn off certain subsets of genes whereas simultaneously turning on others. Whereas much additional work needs to be done to thoroughly test this hypothesis, this work clearly provides a foundation of information with which to identify specific environmental cues that control phenotypic switching of SMC—that is, one can simply identify which of the plethora of factors present in the lesion activate transcriptional control pathways directly linked to the end-stage markers of phenotypic modulation.

We feel that this field is in its infancy and that similar "inside-out" approaches (175) need to be applied to elucidate mechanisms that activate expression of many of the genes that exemplify the many phenotypic states of the SMC in atherothrombotic lesions including, for example, switching the balance of production of gene products that stabilize the fibrous cap versus those that result in destabilization.

Finally, we would like to emphasize two last points in this section. First, on the basis of studies conducted to date, it has not been possible to distinguish whether phenotypic switching of the SMC is an initial *cause* or an *effect* of atherothrombosis. We would argue that in terms of the long-term consequences of atherothrombosis, it probably does not matter. That is, whether phenotypic modulation of the SMC plays a role in initial development of atherothrombosis, or whether atherothrombosis develops and leads to SMC modulation, in the final analysis, this process is a key part of the progression and final clinical sequelae of the disease. Second, although several studies have shown that deletion of a particular candidate gene results in atheroprotection, the underlying atheroprotective mechanisms are seldom resolved or understood. A major rate-limiting factor in conventional gene knockout studies is that the gene of interest is absent from all cells throughout the entire developmental history of the animal such that there are likely to be a wide range of secondary compensatory changes in these mice that confound data interpretation. For example, knockout of intracellular adhesion molecule-1 (ICAM-1) resulted in the attenuation of atherothrombosis when crossed to the apoE$^{-/-}$ mouse (184). However, an unpredicted result in the ICAM-1$^{-/-}$ knockout mouse was the development of severe obesity as compared with control mice, suggesting that there are a large number of undefined secondary metabolic changes in these mice, and that any observed phenotypic differences with wild-type mice cannot be simply ascribed simply to the absence of the ICAM-1 receptor on leucocytes or endothelial cells, as has often been assumed (185). Likewise, many candidate pathways that may play a role in regulating SMC phenotypic switching are also involved in regulating responses in many different cell types during development and maturation, and when knocked out may result in embryonic lethality (e.g., as was the case with PDGF-BB and TGF-β above). Therefore, further progress in this area is likely to be highly dependent on development of both SMC-specific and conditional gene knockout mice that permit selective abrogation of candidate pathways of interest. One of the most powerful approaches is to make use of cre-recombinase gene targeting systems such as the SM MHC cre mouse developed by our laboratory (62). However, currently, these approaches are only beginning to be used to investigate SMC phenotypic modulation.

In summary, because of inherent limitations in human studies, further progress in this field will likely be dependent on use of animal models, albeit ones that are unlikely to completely recapitulate many of the regulatory processes involved in humans. Nevertheless, studies of these simple animal models have already yielded and will continue to yield some interesting potential insights into SMC phenotypic modulation and particularly mechanisms that regulate this process during the natural development of the atherothrombotic lesion.

SUMMARY, CONCLUSIONS, AND FUTURE DIRECTIONS AND CHALLENGES

The model that has evolved is that regulation of SMC differentiation is extremely complex and involves constant interplay between environmental cues and the genetic program that controls the coordinate expression of genes characteristic of the SMC lineage (Fig. 28–1). Whereas studies in animal models have clearly demonstrated that circulating bone marrow–derived cells can contribute to formation of the intimal lesions under some circumstances involving extensive medial necrosis or transplant rejection, the role of these circulating cells in formation of human atherothrombotic lesions is unclear. Indeed, preliminary studies suggest they do not play a major role in most human lesions. Rather, the majority of SMCs within lesions appear to be derived from phenotypic switching/modulation of preexisting SMCs in response to the plethora of alterations in environmental cues present within the atherothrombotic lesion or site of vascular injury, or both. Indeed, it is likely that our susceptibility to

development of atherothrombosis may be, at least in part, a consequence of the necessity of the fully differentiated SMC to retain extensive plasticity—a property that is essential for vascular wound repair and survival, but which unfortunately makes us susceptible to a plethora of atherogenic stimuli prevalent in modern society.

Despite compelling evidence that phenotypic modulation of SMCs plays a key role in development, progression, or both of atherothrombosis, relatively little is known about how this process is regulated. In fact, we are just beginning to understand some of the molecular mechanisms and factors that control transitions in the phenotypic state of SMCs associated with vascular injury, and almost nothing is known regarding what controls these transitions during different stages of development of atherothrombosis in humans. Key unresolved questions include: (a) What are the key environmental cues/factors that induce phenotypic modulation of the SMC within atherothrombotic lesions? (b) What are the molecular mechanisms by which these environmental cues/factors induce phenotypic modulation of the SMC? (c) What factors and mechanisms convert a SMC to a phenotype that promotes plaque stabilization versus plaque destabilization? (d) Can the phenotypic state of the SMC within lesions be manipulated for therapeutic purposes?

Clearly there has been much exciting progress in our understanding of molecular mechanisms that regulate SMC differentiation in recent years, but much additional work is needed. Given that many of the factors that appear to play an important role in control of SMC differentiation are also involved in regulating many other cellular processes, it is likely that major progress in this area is going to be dependent on development of sophisticated loss of function approaches including SMC-specific conditional gene knockout models, local inhibition of candidate regulatory factors/pathways specifically at sites of lesion formation, or both. Finally, much additional work also is needed to identify the precise origins of intimal SMCs and to clearly define the specific contributions of SMCs versus other cell types within the lesion, such as macrophages and endothelial cells, to the end-stage clinical sequelae of atherothrombosis including plaque rupture, thrombosis, infarction, vasospasm, myocardial ischemia, and death.

ACKNOWLEDGMENTS

This work was supported by grants RO1 HL38854, R37 HL57353, and PO1 HL19242 from the National Institutes of Health to Gary K. Owens and a Post-doctoral Fellowship in Physiological Genomics from the American Physiological Society to Brian R. Wamhoff.

REFERENCES

1. Ross R. The pathogenesis of atherosclerosis: a perspective for the 1990s. *Nature* 1993;362:801–809.
2. Han CI, Campbell G, Campbell JH. Circulating bone marrow cells can contribute to neointimal formation. *J Vasc Res* 2001;38:113–119.
3. Sata M, Saiura A, Kunisato A, et al. Hematopoietic stem cells differ-

entiate into vascular cells that participate in the pathogenesis of atherosclerosis. *Nat Med* 2002;8:403–409.

4. Shimizu K, Sugiyama S, Aikawa M, et al. Host bone-marrow cells are a source of donor intimal smooth muscle-like cells in murine aortic transplant arteriopathy. *Nat Med* 2001;7:738–741.

5. Hu Y, Davison F, Ludewig B, et al. Smooth muscle cells in transplant atherosclerotic lesions are originated from recipients, but not bone marrow progenitor cells. *Circulation* 2002;106:1834–1839.

6. Glaser R, Lu MM, Narula N, et al. Smooth muscle cells, but not myocytes, of host origin in transplanted human hearts. *Circulation* 2002;106:17–19.

7. Owens GK. Regulation of differentiation of vascular smooth muscle cells. *Physiol Rev* 1995;75:487–517.

8. Galis ZS, Khatri JJ. Matrix metalloproteinases in vascular remodeling and atherogenesis: the good, the bad, and the ugly. *Circ Res* 2002;90:251–262.

9. Galis ZS, Sukhova GK, Lark MW, et al. Increased expression of matrix metalloproteinases and matrix degrading activity in vulnerable regions in human atherosclerotic plaques. *J Clin Invest* 1994;94:2493–2503.

10. Liau G, Winkles JA, Cannon MS, et al. Dietary-induced atherosclerotic lesions have increased levels of acidic FGF mRNA and altered cytoskeletal and extracellular matrix mRNA expression. *J Vasc Res* 1993;30:327–332.

11. Tan EM, Galssberg E, Olsen DR, et al. Extracellular matrix gene expression by human endothelial and smooth muscle cells. *Matrix* 1991;11:380–387.

12. Turley EA. Extracellular matrix remodeling: multiple paradigms in vascular disease. *Circ Res* 2001;88:2–4.

13. Hansson GK, Jonasson L, Holm J, et al. Class II MHC antigen expression in the atherosclerotic plaque: smooth muscle cells express HLA-DR, HLA-DQ and the invariant gamma chain. *Clin Exp Immunol* 1986;64:261–268.

14. Rong JX, Berman JW, Taubman MB, et al. Lysophosphatidylcholine stimulates monocyte chemoattractant protein-1 gene expression in rat aortic smooth muscle cells. *Arterioscler Thromb Vasc Biol* 2002;22:1617–1623.

15. Roque M, Kim WJ, Gazdoin M, et al. CCR2 deficiency decreases intimal hyperplasia after arterial injury. *Arterioscler Thromb Vasc Biol* 2002;22:554–559.

16. Kocher O, Gabbiani F, Gabbiani G, et al. Phenotypic features of smooth muscle cells during the evolution of experimental carotid artery intimal thickening. Biochemical and morphologic studies. *Lab Invest* 1991;65:459–470.

17. Kocher O, Gabbiani G. Cytoskeletal features of normal and atheromatous human arterial smooth muscle cells. *Hum Pathol* 1986;17:875–880.

18. Chamley-Campbell J, Campbell GR, Ross R. The smooth muscle cell in culture. *Physiol Rev* 1979;59:1–6.

19. Drake CJ, Hungerford JE, Little CD. Morphogenesis of the first blood vessels. *Ann NY Acad Sci* 1998;857:155–179.

20. Hungerford JE, Little CD. Developmental biology of the vascular smooth muscle cell: building a multilayered vessel wall. *J Vasc Res* 1999;36:2–27.

21. Schwartz SM, Heimark RL, Majesky MW. Developmental mechanisms underlying pathology of arteries. *Physiol Rev* 1990;70:1177–1209.

22. Isogai S, Horiguchi M, Weinstein BM. The vascular anatomy of the developing zebrafish: an atlas of embryonic and early larval development. *Dev Biol* 2001;230:278–301.

23. Czirok A, Rupp PA, Rongish BJ, et al. Multi-field 3D scanning light microscopy of early embryogenesis. *J Microsc* 2002;206:209–217.

24. Gabbiani G, Schmid E, Winter S, et al. Vascular smooth muscle cells differ from other smooth muscle cells: predominance of vimentin filaments and a specific-type actin. *Proc Natl Acad Sci USA* 1981;78:298–300.

25. Mack CP, Owens GK. Regulation of SM alpha-actin expression in vivo is dependent upon CArG elements within the 5′ and first intron promoter regions. *Circ Res* 1999;84:852–861.

26. Hungerford JE, Owens GK, Argraves WS, et al. Development of the aortic vessel wall as defined by vascular smooth muscle and extracellular matrix markers. *Dev Biol* 1996;178:375–392.

27. Arimura C, Suzuki T, Yanagisawa M, et al. Primary structure of chicken skeletal muscle and fibroblast alpha-actinins deduced from cDNA sequences. *Eur J Biochem* 1988;177:649–655.

28. Madsen CS, Regan CP, Hungerford JE, et al. Smooth muscle-specific expression of the smooth muscle myosin heavy chain gene in trans-

genic mice requires 5″-flanking and first intronic DNA sequence. *Circ Res* 1998;82:908–917.

29. Miano JM, Cserjesi P, Ligon K, et al. Smooth muscle myosin heavy chain marks exclusively the smooth muscle lineage during mouse embryogenesis. *Circ Res* 1994;75:803–812.

30. Babij P, Kelly C, Periasamy M. Characterization of a mammalian smooth muscle myosin heavy-chain gene: complete nucleotide and protein coding sequence and analysis of the 5″ end of the gene. *Proc Natl Acad Sci USA* 1991;88:10676–10681.

31. Frid MG, Printesva OY, Chiavegato A, et al. Myosin heavy-chain isoform composition and distribution in developing and adult human aortic smooth muscle. *J Vasc Res* 1993;30:279–292.

32. Duband JL, Gimona M, Scatena M, et al. Calponin and SM 22 as differentiation markers of smooth muscle: spatiotemporal distribution during avian embryonic development. *Differentiation* 1993;55:1–11.

33. Strasser P, Gimona M, Moessler H, et al. Mammalian calponin: identification and expression of genetic variants. *FEBS Lett* 1993;330:13–18.

34. Li L, Miano JM, Cserjesi P, et al. SM22 alpha, a marker of adult smooth muscle, is expressed in multiple myogenic lineages during embryogenesis. *Circ Res* 1996;78:188–195.

35. Kim S, Ip HS, Lu MM, et al. A serum response factor-dependent transcriptional regulatory program identifies distinct smooth muscle cell sublineages. *Mol Cell Biol* 1997;17:2266–2278.

36. Watanabe M, Layne MD, Hsieh CM, et al. Regulation of smooth muscle cell differentiation by AT-rich interaction domain transcription factors Mrf2alpha and Mrf2beta. *Circ Res* 2002;91:382–389.

37. Bolmont C, Lilienbaum A, Paulin D, et al. Expression of the desmin gene in skeletal and smooth muscle by in situ hybridization using a human desmin gene probe. *J Submicrosc Cytol Pathol* 1990;22:117–122.

38. Mericskay M, Parlakian A, Porteu A, et al. An overlapping CArG/Octamer element is required for regulation of desmin gene transcription in arterial smooth muscle. *Dev Biol* 2000;226:192–208.

39. Frid MG, Shekhonin BV, Koteliansky VE, et al. Phenotypic changes of human smooth muscle cells during development: late expression of heavy caldesmon and calponin. *Dev Biol* 1992;153:185–193.

40. Sobue K, Sellers JR. Caldesmon, a novel regulatory protein in smooth muscle and nonmuscle actomyosin systems. *J Biol Chem* 1991;266:12115–12118.

41. Yano H, Hayashi K, Momiyama T, et al. Transcriptional regulation of the chicken caldesmon gene. Activation of gizzard-type caldesmon promoter requires a CArG box-like motif. *J Biol Chem* 1995;270:23661–23666.

42. Gimona M, Furst DO, Small JV. Metavinculin and vinculin from mammalian smooth muscle: bulk isolation and characterization. *J Muscle Res Cell Motil* 1987;8:329–341.

43. Herring BP, Lyons GE, Hoggatt AM, et al. Telokin expression is restricted to smooth muscle tissues during mouse development. *Am J Physiol Cell Physiol* 2001;280:C12–C21.

44. van der Loop FT, Schaart G, Timmer ED, et al. Smoothelin, a novel cytoskeletal protein specific for smooth muscle cells. *J Cell Biol* 1996;134:401–411.

45. Fatigati V, Murphy RA. Actin and tropomyosin variants in smooth muscles. Dependence on tissue type. *J Biol Chem* 1984;259:14383–14388.

46. Woodcock-Mitchell J, Mitchell JJ, Low RB, et al. Alpha-smooth muscle actin is transiently expressed in embryonic rat cardiac and skeletal muscles. *Differentiation* 1988;39:161–166.

47. Adachi S, Ito H, Tamamori M, et al. Skeletal and smooth muscle alpha-actin mRNA in endomyocardial biopsy samples of dilated cardiomyopathy patients. *Life Sci* 1998;63:1779–1791.

48. Sartore S, Chiavegato A, Faggin E, et al. Contribution of adventitial fibroblasts to neointima formation and vascular remodeling: from innocent bystander to active participant. *Circ Res* 2001;89:1111–1121.

49. Arciniegas E, Sutton AB, Allen TD, et al. Transforming growth factor beta 1 promotes the differentiation of endothelial cells into smooth muscle-like cells in vitro. *J Cell Sci* 1992;103:521–529.

50. Basson CT, Kocher O, Basson MD, et al. Differential modulation of vascular cell integrin and extracellular matrix expression in vitro by TGF-beta 1 correlates with reciprocal effects on cell migration. *J Cell Physiol* 1992;153:118–128.

51. Cintorino M, Vindigni C, Del Vecchio MT, et al. Expression of actin isoforms and intermediate filament proteins in childhood orbital rhabdomyosarcomas. *J Submicrosc Cytol Pathol* 1989;21:409–419.

52. Cintorino M, Bellizzi de Marco E, Leoncini P, et al. Expression of al-

pha-smooth-muscle actin in stromal cells of the uterine cervix during epithelial neoplastic changes. *Int J Cancer* 1991;47:843–846.

53. Miano JM, Olson EN. Expression of the smooth muscle cell calponin gene marks the early cardiac and smooth muscle cell lineages during mouse embryogenesis. *J Biol Chem* 1996;271:7095–7103.

54. Werling RW, Hwang H, Yaziji H, et al. Immunohistochemical distinction of invasive from noninvasive breast lesions: a comparative study of p63 versus calponin and smooth muscle myosin heavy chain. *Am J Surg Pathol* 2003;27:82–90.

55. Sakamoto A, Oda Y, Yamamoto H, et al. Calponin and h-caldesmon expression in atypical fibroxanthoma and superficial leiomyosarcoma. *Virchows Arch* 2002;440:404–409.

56. Samaha FF, Ip HS, Morrisey EE, et al. Developmental pattern of expression and genomic organization of the calponin-h1 gene. A contractile smooth muscle cell marker. *J Biol Chem* 1996;271: 395–403.

57. Geiger B, Tokuyasu KT, Dutton AH, et al. Vinculin, an intracellular protein localized at specialized sites where microfilament bundles terminate at cell membranes. *Proc Natl Acad Sci USA* 1980;77:4127–4131.

58. Ehler E, Babiychuk E, Draeger A. Human foetal lung (IMR-90) cells: myofibroblasts with smooth muscle-like contractile properties. *Cell Motil Cytoskeleton* 1996;34:288–298.

59. Belkin AM, Ornatsky OI, Kabakov AE, et al. Diversity of vinculin/meta-vinculin in human tissues and cultivated cells. Expression of muscle specific variants of vinculin in human aorta smooth muscle cells. *J Biol Chem* 1988;263:6631–6635.

60. Layne MD, Yet SF, Maemura K, et al. Characterization of the mouse aortic carboxypeptidase-like protein promoter reveals activity in differentiated and dedifferentiated vascular smooth muscle cells. *Circ Res* 2002;90:728–736.

61. Rensen S, Merkx G, Doevendans P, et al. Structure and chromosome location of Smtn, the mouse smoothelin gene. *Cytogenet Cell Genet* 2000;89:225–229.

62. Regan CP, Manabe I, Owens GK. Development of a smooth muscle-targeted cre recombinase mouse reveals novel insights regarding smooth muscle myosin heavy chain promoter regulation. *Circ Res* 2000;87:363–369.

63. Aikawa M, Sivam PN, Kuro-o M, et al. Human smooth muscle myosin heavy chain isoforms as molecular markers for vascular development and atherosclerosis. *Circ Res* 1993;73:1000–1012.

64. Sartore S, Scatena M, Chiavegato A, et al. Myosin isoform expression in smooth muscle cells during physiological and pathological vascular remodeling. *J Vasc Res* 1994;31:61–81.

65. Lazard D, Sastre X, Frid MG, et al. Expression of smooth muscle-specific proteins in myoepithelium and stromal myofibroblasts of normal and malignant human breast tissue. *Proc Natl Acad Sci USA* 1994;90:999–1003.

66. Borrione AC, Zanellato AM, Giuriato L, et al. Nonmuscle and smooth muscle myosin isoforms in bovine endothelial cells. *Exp Cell Res* 1990;190:1–10.

67. Rovner AS, Murphy RA, Owens GK. Expression of smooth muscle and nonmuscle myosin heavy chains in cultured vascular smooth muscle cells. *J Biol Chem* 1986;261:14740–14745.

68. Manabe I, Kurabayashi M, Shimomura Y, et al. Isolation of the embryonic form of smooth muscle myosin heavy chain (SMemb/NMHC-B) gene and characterization of its 5′-flanking region. *Biochem Biophys Res Commun* 1997;239:598–605.

69. Sekiguchi K, Kurabayashi M, Oyama Y, et al. Homeobox protein hex induces SMemb/nonmuscle myosin heavy chain-B gene expression through the cAMP-responsive element. *Circ Res* 2001;88:52–58.

70. Watanabe N, Kurabayashi M, Shimomura Y, et al. BTEB2, a Kruppel-like transcription factor, regulates expression of the SMemb/Nonmuscle myosin heavy chain B (SMemb/NMHC-B) gene. *Circ Res* 1999; 85:182–191.

71. Itoh T, Adelstein RS. Neuronal cell expression of inserted isoforms of vertebrate nonmuscle myosin heavy chain II-B. *J Biol Chem* 1995;270:14533–14540.

72. Oh SP, Seki T, Goss KA, et al. Activin receptor-like kinase 1 modulates transforming growth factor-beta 1 signaling in the regulation of angiogenesis. *Proc Natl Acad Sci USA* 2000;97:2626–2631.

73. Oshima M, Oshima H, Taketo MM. TGF-beta receptor type II deficiency results in defects of yolk sac hematopoiesis and vasculogenesis. *Dev Biol* 1996;179:297–302.

74. Yang X, Castilla LH, Xu X, et al. Angiogenesis defects and mes-

75. Dickson MC, Martin JS, Cousins FM, et al. Defective haematopoiesis and vasculogenesis in transforming growth factor-beta 1 knock out mice. *Development* 1995;121:1845–1854.

76. Griffin CT, Srinivasan Y, Zheng YW, et al. A role for thrombin receptor signaling in endothelial cells during embryonic development. *Science* 2001;293:1666–1670.

77. Reusch P, Wagdy H, Reusch R, et al. Mechanical strain increases smooth muscle and decreases nonmuscle myosin expression in rat vascular smooth muscle cells. *Circ Res* 1996;79:1046–1053.

78. Hautmann M, Thompson MM, Swartz EA, et al. Angiotensin II-induced stimulation of smooth muscle alpha-actin expression by serum response factor and the homeodomain transcription factor MHox. *Circ Res* 1997;81:600–610.

79. Higashita R, Li L, Van Putten V, et al. Galpha16 mimics vasoconstrictor action to induce smooth muscle alpha-actin in vascular smooth muscle cells through a Jun-NH2-terminal kinase-dependent pathway. *J Biol Chem* 1997;272:25845–25850.

80. Garat C, Van Putten V, Refaat ZA, et al. Induction of smooth muscle alpha-actin in vascular smooth muscle cells by arginine vasopressin is mediated by c-Jun amino-terminal kinases and p38 mitogen-activated protein kinase. *J Biol Chem* 2000;275:22537–22543.

81. Thyberg J, Hultgardh-Nilsson A. Fibronectin and the basement membrane components laminin and collagen type IV influence the phenotypic properties of subcultured rat aortic smooth muscle cells differently. *Cell Tissue Res* 1994;276:263–271.

82. Hedin U, Bottger BA, Luthman J, et al. A substrate of the cell-attachment sequence of fibronectin (Arg-Gly-Asp-Ser) is sufficient to promote transition of arterial smooth muscle cells from a contractile to a synthetic phenotype. *Dev Biol* 1989;133:489–501.

83. Drake CJ, Davis LA, Walters L, et al. Avian vasculogenesis and the distribution of collagens I, IV, laminin, and fibronectin in the heart primordia. *J Exp Zool* 1990;255:418–421.

84. Carey DJ. Control of growth and differentiation of vascular cells by extracellular matrix proteins. *Annu Rev Physiol* 1991;53:161–177.

85. Chamley JH, Campbell GR, Burnstock G. Dedifferentiation, redifferentiation and bundle formation of smooth muscle cells in tissue culture: the influence of cell number and nerve fibres. *J Embryol Exp Morphol* 1974;32:297–323.

86. Su B, Mitra S, Gregg H, et al. Redox regulation of vascular smooth muscle cell differentiation. *Circ Res* 2001;89:39–46.

87. Hess H. Significance of blood platelets and coagulation for development, progression and regression of arteriosclerosis [Ger]. *Vasa Suppl* 1987;20:56–61.

88. Owens GK, Vernon SM, Madsen CS. Molecular regulation of smooth muscle cell differentiation. *J Hypertens* 1996;14:S55–S64.

89. Hautmann M, Madsen CS, Owens GK. A transforming growth factor beta (TGF) control element drives TGF-induced stimulation of SM alpha-actin gene expression in concert with two CArG elements. *J Biol Chem* 1997;272:10948–10956.

90. Adam PJ, Regan CR, Hautmann MB, et al. Positive and negative acting krupple-like transcription factors bind a transforming growth factor beta control element required for expression of the smooth muscle differentiation marker SM22alpha in vivo. *J Biol Chem* 2000;275:37798–37806.

91. Shah NM, Groves AK, Anderson DJ. Alternative neural crest cell fates are instructively promoted by TGFbeta superfamily members. *Cell* 1996;85:331–343.

92. Jain MK, Layne MD, Watanabe M, et al. In vitro system for differentiating pluripotent neural crest cells into smooth muscle cells. *J Biol Chem* 1998;273:5993–5996.

93. Shimizu RT, Blank RS, Jervis R, et al. The smooth muscle a-actin gene promoter is differentially regulated in smooth muscle versus non-smooth muscle cells. *J Biol Chem* 1995;270:7631–7643.

94. Blank RS, Owens GK. Platelet-derived growth factor regulates actin isoform expression and growth state in cultured rat aortic smooth muscle cells. *J Cell Physiol* 1990;142:635–642.

95. Li X, Van Putten V, Zarinetchi F, et al. Suppression of smooth muscle alpha-actin expression by platelet-derived growth factor in vascular smooth-muscle cells involves Ras and cytosolic phospholipase A2. *Biochemistry* 1997;327:709–716.

96. Corjay MH, Thompson MM, Lynch KR, et al. Differential effect of platelet-derived growth factor versus serum-induced growth on smooth muscle alpha-actin and nonmuscle beta-actin mRNA expres-

sion in cultured rat aortic smooth muscle cells. *J Biol Chem* 1989; 264:10501–10506.

97. Holycross BJ, Blank RS, Thompson MM, et al. Platelet-derived growth factor-BB-induced suppression of smooth muscle cell differentiation. *Circ Res* 1992;71:1525–1532.

98. Owens GK, Thompson MM. Developmental changes in isoactin expression in rat aortic smooth muscle cells in vivo. Relationship between growth and cytodifferentiation. *J Biol Chem* 1986;261:13373–13380.

99. O'Brien ER, Alpers CE, Stewart DK, et al. Proliferation in primary and restenotic coronary atherectomy tissue. Implications for antiproliferative therapy. *Circ Res* 1993;73:223–231.

100. Wilcox JN. Analysis of local gene expression in human atherosclerotic plaques. *J Vasc Surg* 1992;15:913–916.

101. Thyberg J, Palmberg L, Nilsson J, et al. Phenotypic modulation in primary cultures of arterial smooth muscle cells: on the role of platelet-derived growth factor. *Differentiation* 1983;25:156–167.

102. Somasundaram C, Kallmeier RC, Babij P. Regulation of smooth muscle myosin heavy chain gene expression in cultured vascular smooth muscle cells by growth factors and contractile agonists. *Basic and Applied Mycology* 1995;6:31–36.

103. Lindahl P, Johansson BR, Leveen P, et al. Pericyte loss and microaneurysm formation in PDGF-B-deficient mice. *Science* 1997;277: 242–245.

104. Ross R, Glomset JA. The pathogenesis of atherosclerosis. *N Engl J Med* 1976;295:369–377,420–425.

105. Frid MG, Moiseeva EP, Stenmark KR. Multiple phenotypically distinct smooth muscle cell populations exist in the adult and developing bovine pulmonary arterial media in vivo. *Circ Res* 1994;75:669–681.

106. Hao H, Ropraz P, Verin V, et al. Heterogeneity of smooth muscle cell populations cultured from pig coronary artery. *Arterioscler Thromb Vasc Biol* 2002;22:1093–1099.

107. Benditt EP, Benditt JM. Evidence for the monoclonal origin of human atherosclerotic plaques. *Proc Natl Acad Sci USA* 1973;70:1753–1756.

108. Clowes AW, Reidy MA, Clowes MM. Mechanisms of stenosis after arterial injury. *Lab Invest* 1983;49:208–215.

109. Clowes AW, Reidy MA, Clowes MM. Kinetics of cellular proliferation after arterial injury. I. Smooth muscle growth in the absence of endothelium. *Lab Invest* 1983;49:327–333.

110. Clowes AW, Clowes MM, Reidy MA. Kinetics of cellular proliferation after arterial injury. III. Endothelial and smooth muscle growth in chronically denuded vessels. *Lab Invest* 1986;54:295–303.

111. Clowes AW, Clowes MM, Fingerle J, et al. Kinetics of cellular proliferation after arterial injury. V. Role of acute distension in the induction of smooth muscle proliferation. *Lab Invest* 1989;60:360–364.

112. Simper D, Stalboerger PG, Panetta CJ, et al. Smooth muscle progenitor cells in human blood. *Circulation* 2002;106:1199–1204.

113. Remy-Martin JP, Marandin A, Challie B, et al. Vascular smooth muscle differentiation of murine stroma: a sequential model. *Exp Hematol* 1999;27:1782–1795.

114. Hruban RH, Long PP, Perlman EJ, et al. Fluorescence in situ hybridization for the Y-chromosome can be used to detect cells of recipient origin in allografted hearts following cardiac transplantation. *Am J Pathol* 1993;142:975–980.

115. Quaini F, Urbanek K, Beltrami AP, et al. Chimerism of the transplanted heart. *N Engl J Med* 2002;346:5–15.

116. Wang X, Willenbring H, Akkari Y, et al. Cell fusion is the principal source of bone-marrow-derived hepatocytes. *Nature* 2003;422:897–901.

117. Vassilopoulos G, Wang PR, Russell DW. Transplanted bone marrow regenerates liver by cell fusion. *Nature* 2003;422:901–904.

118. Aikawa M, Sakomura Y, Ueda M, et al. Redifferentiation of smooth muscle cells after coronary angioplasty determined via myosin heavy chain expression. *Circulation* 1997;96:82–90.

119. Aikawa M, Rabkin E, Voglic SJ, et al. Lipid lowering promotes accumulation of mature smooth muscle cells expressing smooth muscle myosin heavy chain isoforms in rabbit atheroma. *Circ Res* 1998;83: 1015–1026.

120. Gordon D, Reidy MA, Benditt EP, et al. Cell proliferation in human coronary arteries. *Proc Natl Acad Sci USA* 1990;87:4600–4604.

121. van der Loop FT, Gabbiani G, Kohnen G, et al. Differentiation of smooth muscle cells in human blood vessels as defined by smoothelin, a novel marker for the contractile phenotype. *Arterioscler Thromb Vasc Biol* 1997;17:665–671.

122. Mosse PR, Campbell GR, Campbell JH. Smooth muscle phenotypic expression in human carotid arteries. II. Atherosclerosis-free diffuse in-

123. Wamhoff BR, Dixon JL, Sturek M. Atorvastatin treatment prevents alterations in coronary smooth muscle nuclear Ca2+ signaling in diabetic dyslipidemia. *J Vasc Res* 2002;39:208–220.

124. Hill BJ, Wamhoff BR, Sturek M. Functional nucleotide receptor expression and sarcoplasmic reticulum morphology in dedifferentiated porcine coronary smooth muscle cells. *J Vasc Res* 2001;38:432–443.

125. Dixon JL, Stoops JD, Parker JL, et al. Dyslipidemia and vascular dysfunction in diabetic pigs fed an atherogenic diet. *Arterioscler Thromb Vasc Biol* 1999;19:2981–2992.

126. Geary RL, Wong JM, Rossini A, et al. Expression profiling identifies 147 genes contributing to a unique primate neointimal smooth muscle cell phenotype. *Arterioscler Thromb Vasc Biol* 2002;22:2010–2016.

127. Ross R. The pathogenesis of atherosclerosis—an update. *N Engl J Med* 1986;314:488–500.

128. Lusis AJ. Atherosclerosis. *Nature* 2000;407:233–241.

129. Schwartz SM, deBlois D, O'Brien ER. The intima. Soil for atherosclerosis and restenosis. *Circ Res* 1995;77:445–465.

130. Clowes AW, Clowes MM, Fingerle J, et al. Kinetics of cellular proliferation after arterial injury. V. Role of acute distension in the induction of smooth muscle proliferation. *Lab Invest* 1989;60:360–364.

131. Nakashima Y, Plump AS, Raines EW, et al. ApoE-deficient mice develop lesions of all phases of atherosclerosis throughout the arterial tree. *Arterioscler Thromb* 1994;14:133–140.

132. Zhang SH, Reddick RL, Piedrahita JA, et al. Spontaneous hypercholesterolemia and arterial lesions in mice lacking apolipoprotein E. *Science* 1992;258:468–471.

133. Heldin CH, Ostman A, Ronnstrand L. Signal transduction via platelet-derived growth factor receptors. *Biochim Biophys Acta* 1998;1378: F79–F113.

134. Ferns GA, Raines EW, Sprugel KH, et al. Inhibition of neointimal smooth muscle accumulation after angioplasty by an antibody to PDGF. *Science* 1991;253:1129–1132.

135. Jawien A, Bowen Pope DF, Lindner V, et al. Platelet-derived growth factor promotes smooth muscle migration and intimal thickening in a rat model of balloon angioplasty. *J Clin Invest* 1992;89:507–511.

136. Heldin CH, Westermark B. Platelet-derived growth factor: mechanism of action and possible in vivo function. *Cell Regul* 1990;1:555–566.

137. Claesson Welsh L, Heldin CH. Platelet-derived growth factor. Three isoforms that bind to two distinct cell surface receptors. *Acta Oncol* 1989;28:331–334.

138. Davies MG, Owens EL, Mason DP, et al. Effect of platelet-derived growth factor receptor-a and -b blockage on flow-induced neointimal formation in endothelialized baboon vascular grafts. *Circ Res* 2000; 86:779–786.

139. Tanizawa S, Ueda M, van der Loos CM, et al. Expression of platelet derived growth factor B chain and beta receptor in human coronary arteries after percutaneous transluminal coronary angioplasty: an immunohistochemical study. *Heart* 1996;75:549–556.

140. Ueda M, Becker AE, Kasayuki N, et al. In situ detection of platelet-derived growth factor-A and -B chain mRNA in human coronary arteries after percutaneous transluminal coronary angioplasty. *Am J Pathol* 1996;149:831–843.

141. Bostrom H, Willetts K, Pekny M, et al. PDGF-A signaling is a critical event in lung alveolar myofibroblast development and alveogenesis. *Cell* 1996;85:863–873.

142. Leveen P, Pekny M, Gebre-Medhin SG, et al. Mice deficient for PDGF B show renal, cardiovascular, and hematological abnormalities. *Genes Dev* 1994;8:1875–1887.

143. Soriano P. The PDGF alpha receptor is required for neural crest cell development and for normal patterning of the somites. *Development* 1997;124:2691–2700.

144. Soriano P. Abnormal kidney development and hematological disorders in PDGF beta-receptor knockout mice. *Genes Dev* 1994;8:1888–1896.

145. Sano H, Sudo T, Yokode M, et al. Functional blockade of platelet-derived growth factor receptor-beta but not of receptor-alpha prevents vascular smooth muscle cell accumulation in fibrous cap lesions in apolipoprotein E-deficient mice. *Circulation* 2001;103:2955–2960.

146. Kozaki K, Kaminski WE, Tang J, et al. Blockade of platelet-derived growth factor or its receptors transiently delays but does not prevent fibrous cap formation in ApoE null mice. *Am J Pathol* 2002;161: 1395–1407.

147. Owens GK, Geisterfer AA, Yang YW, et al. Transforming growth fac-

timal thickenings compared with the media. *Arteriosclerosis* 1986;6: 664–669.

tor-beta-induced growth inhibition and cellular hypertrophy in cultured vascular smooth muscle cells. *J Cell Biol* 1988;107:771–780.

148. Agah R, Prasad KS, Linnemann R, et al. Cardiovascular overexpression of transforming growth factor-beta(1) causes abnormal yolk sac vasculogenesis and early embryonic death. *Circ Res* 2000;86:1024–1030.

149. Majesky MW, Lindner V, Twardzik DR, et al. Production of transforming growth factor beta 1 during repair of arterial injury. *J Clin Invest* 1991;88:904–910.

150. Schulick AH, Taylor AJ, Zuo W, et al. Overexpression of transforming growth beta1 in arterial endothelium causes hyperplasia, apoptosis, and cartilaginous metaplasia. *Proc Natl Acad Sci USA* 1998;95:6983–6988.

151. Smith JD, Bryant SR, Couper LL, et al. Soluble transforming growth factor beta type II receptor inhibits negative remodeling, fibroblast transdifferentiation, and intimal lesion formation but not endothelial growth. *Circ Res* 1999;84:1212–1222.

152. McCaffrey TA, Du B, Consigli S, et al. Genomic instability in the Type II TGF-beta I receptor gene in atherosclerotic and restenotic vascular cells. *J Clin Invest* 1997;100:2182–2188.

153. Grainger DJ, Kemp PR, Metcalfe JC, et al. The serum concentration of active transforming growth factor-beta is severely depressed in advanced atherosclerosis. *Nat Med* 1995;1:74–79.

154. Lutgens E, Gijbels M, Smook M, et al. Transforming growth factor-beta mediates balance between inflammation and fibrosis during plaque progression. *Arterioscler Thromb Vasc Biol* 2002;22:975–982.

155. Mallat Z, Gojova A, Marchiol-Fournigault C, et al. Inhibition of transforming growth factor-beta signaling accelerates atherosclerosis and induces an unstable plaque phenotype in mice. *Circ Res* 2001;89:930–934.

156. De Caterina R, Libby P, Peng HB, et al. Nitric oxide decreases cytokine-induced endothelial activation. Nitric oxide selectively reduces endothelial expression of adhesion molecules and proinflammatory cytokines. *J Clin Invest* 1995;96:60–68.

157. Itoh S, Katoh Y, Konishi H, et al. Nitric oxide regulates smooth-muscle-specific myosin heavy chain gene expression at the transcriptional level—possible role of SRF and YY1 through CArG element. *J Mol Cell Cardiol* 2001;33:95–107.

158. Hamon M, Vallet B, Bauters C, et al. Long-term oral administration of L-arginine reduces intimal thickening and enhances neoendothelium-dependent acetylcholine-induced relaxation after arterial injury. *Circulation* 1994;90:1357–1362.

159. Channon KM, Qian H, Neplioueva V, et al. In vivo gene transfer of nitric oxide synthase enhances vasomotor function in carotid arteries from normal and cholesterol-fed rabbits. *Circulation* 1998;98:1905–1911.

160. Li PF, Dietz R, von Harsdorf R. Differential effect of hydrogen peroxide and superoxide anion on apoptosis and proliferation of vascular smooth muscle cells. *Circulation* 1997;96:3602–3609.

161. Laukkanen MO, Kivela A, Rissanen T, et al. Adenovirus-mediated extracellular superoxide dismutase gene therapy reduces neointima formation in balloon-denuded rabbit aorta. *Circulation* 2002;106:1999–2003.

162. Matsumura ME, Li F, Berthoux L, et al. Vascular injury induces post-transcriptional regulation of the Id3 gene: cloning of a novel Id3 isoform expressed during vascular lesion formation in rat and human atherosclerosis. *Arterioscler Thromb Vasc Biol* 2001;21:752–758.

163. Kumar MS, Hendrix J, Johnson AD, et al. Smooth muscle alpha-actin gene requires two E-boxes for proper expression in vivo and is a target of class I basic helix-loop-helix proteins. *Circ Res* 2003;92:840–847.

164. Nickenig G, Baudler S, Muller C, et al. Redox-sensitive vascular smooth muscle cell proliferation is mediated by GKLF and Id3 in vitro and in vivo. *FASEB Lett* 2002;16:1077–1086.

165. Cho A, Graves J, Reidy MA. Mitogen-activated protein kinases mediate matrix metalloproteinase-9 expression in vascular smooth muscle cells. *Arterioscler Thromb Vasc Biol* 2000;20:2527–2532.

166. Ma C, Chegini N. Regulation of matrix metalloproteinases (MMPs) and their tissue inhibitors in human myometrial smooth muscle cells by TGF-β1. *Mol Hum Reprod* 1999;5:950–954.

167. Gurjar MV, DeLeon J, Sharma RV, et al. Mechanism of inhibition of matrix metalloproteinase-9 induction by NO in vascular smooth muscle cells. *J Appl Physiol* 2001;91:1380–1386.

168. Gurjar MV, DeLeon J, Sharma RV, et al. Role of reactive oxygen species in IL-1beta–stimulated sustained ERK activation and MMP-9 induction. *Am J Physiol Heart Circ Physiol* 2001;281:H2568–H2574.

169. Galis ZS, Johnson C, Godin D, et al. Targeted disruption of the matrix metalloproteinase-9 gene impairs smooth muscle cell migration and geometrical arterial remodeling. *Circ Res* 2002;91:852–859.

170. Cho A, Reidy MA. Matrix metalloproteinase-9 is necessary for the regulation of smooth muscle cell replication and migration after arterial injury. *Circ Res* 2002;91:845–851.

171. Jormsjo S, Wuttge DM, Sirsjo A, et al. Differential expression of cysteine and aspartic proteases during progression of atherosclerosis in apolipoprotein E-deficient mice. *Am J Pathol* 2002;161:939–945.

172. Kumar MS, Owens GK. Combinatorial control of smooth muscle-specific gene expression. *Arterioscler Thromb Vasc Biol* 2003;23:737–747.

173. Firulli AB, Olson EN. Modular regulation of muscle gene transcription: a mechanism for muscle cell diversity. *Trends Genet* 1997;13:364–369.

174. Miano JM. Cardiac-specific gene expression: a HANDful of factors. *J Mol Cell Cardiol* 2002;34:1287–1291.

175. Regan CP, Adam PJ, Madsen CS, et al. Identification of molecular mechanisms that contribute to vascular injury-induced decreases in expression of smooth muscle differentiation marker genes in vivo. *J Clin Invest* 2000;106:1139–1147.

176. Schwartz SM, Campbell GR, Campbell JH. Replication of smooth muscle cells in vascular disease. *Circ Res* 1986;58:427–444.

177. Madsen CS, Hershey JC, Hautmann MB, et al. Expression of the smooth muscle myosin heavy chain gene is regulated by a negative-acting GC-rich element located between two positive-acting serum response factor-binding elements. *J Biol Chem* 1997;272:6332–6340.

178. Madsen CS, Regan CP, Owens GK. Interaction of CArG elements and a GC-repressor element in transcriptional regulation of the smooth muscle myosin heavy chain gene in vascular smooth muscle. *J Biol Chem* 1997;272:29842–29851.

179. Manabe I, Owens GK. CArG elements control smooth muscle subtype-specific expression of smooth muscle myosin in vivo. *J Clin Invest* 2001;107:823–834.

180. Black AR, Black JD, Azizkhan-Clifford J. Sp1 and kruppel-like factor family of transcription factors in cell growth regulation and cancer. *J Cell Physiol* 2001;188:143–160.

181. Shindo T, Manabe I, Fukushima Y, et al. Kruppel-like zinc-finger transcription factor KLF5/BTEB2 is a target for angiotensin II signaling and an essential regulator of cardiovascular remodeling. *Nat Med* 2002;8:856–863.

182. Rafty LA, Khachigian LM. Sp1 phosphorylation regulates inducible expression of platelet-derived growth factor B-chain gene via atypical protein kinase C-zeta. *Nucleic Acids Res* 2001;29:1027–1033.

183. Rafty LA, Khachigian LM. Zinc finger transcription factors mediate high constitutive platelet-derived growth factor-B expression in smooth muscle cells derived from aortae of newborn rats. *J Biol Chem* 1998;273:5758–5764.

184. Kitagawa K, Matsumoto M, Sasaki T, et al. Involvement of ICAM-1 in the progression of atherosclerosis in APOE-knockout mice. *Atherosclerosis* 2002;160:305–310.

185. Dong ZM, Gutierrez-Ramos JC, Coxon A, et al. A new class of obesity genes encodes leukocyte adhesion receptors. *Proc Natl Acad Sci USA* 1997;94:7526–7530.

CHAPTER 29

The Vascular Extracellular Matrix

Thomas N. Wight

Key Words: Collagen; elastic fibers; extracellular matrix; glycoproteins; glycosaminoglycans; hyaluronan; low-density lipoproteins; proteoglycans.

INTRODUCTION

The vascular extracellular matrix (ECM) is a reinforced composite of collagen and elastic fibers embedded in a viscoelastic gel consisting of proteoglycans, hyaluronan, glycoproteins, and water. These components interact through entanglement and cross-linking to form a biomechanically active polymer network that imparts tensile strength, elastic recoil, compressibility, and viscoelasticity to the vascular wall. In addition, this network interacts with vascular cells and participates in the regulation of cell adhesion, migration, and proliferation during vascular development and disease. This regulation involves molecular interactions that govern the attachment of vascular cells to specific ECM components, detachment of cells from these components, and molecular rearrangements in the ECM that allow cells to change their shape during division and migration. Furthermore, components of the ECM bind plasma proteins, growth factors, cytokines, and enzymes, and these interactions modulate arterial wall metabolism. Thus, the vascular ECM not only maintains vascular wall structure, it also regulates key events in vascular physiology.

T. N. Wight: The Hope Heart Program, Benaroya Institute at Virginia Mason, 1124 Columbia Street, Seattle, Washington 98104 and the University of Washington School of Medicine.

The composition of the ECM is controlled by the coordinate and differential regulation of synthesis and turnover of each of the components. Such differential regulation creates differences in the composition of the vascular ECM during vascular development, between different vascular beds, and in different forms of vascular disease. For example, each layer of the vessel wall (i.e., intima, media, and adventitia) has a different ECM composition. An ECM rich in fibrillar collagen, as is found in the adventitia, will impart stiffness and rigidity, whereas a layer enriched in proteoglycans and hyaluronan, as found in the intima, is more viscoelastic and compressible. Maintaining the appropriate balance of the components in each layer is critical for maintaining vascular wall integrity and resisting rupture and hemorrhage. In addition, an ECM composition that forms a "loose" and hydrated network enriched in attachment proteins promotes vascular cell adhesion, proliferation, and migration in developmental and early stages of vascular disease, whereas a "dense" and fibrous ECM typifies more differentiated vascular tissue and advanced vascular lesions. This review covers the major components of the vascular ECM and discusses the role these molecules play in the normal physiology and pathology of the vascular wall.

COLLAGENS

Collagens are proteins that consist of a triple helix of polypeptide chains, in which each chain contains at least one stretch of the repeating amino acid sequence, Gly-X-Y. Collagens comprise a family of proteins of at least 19 genetically distinct types, classified by differences in their amino acid composition and the proportion of the molecule forming the triple helix. Common collagen types that have been identified in normal and diseased blood vessels are types I, III, IV, V, VI, and VIII (see reviews by Barnes [1] and Rauterberg and coworkers [2]). The predominant vascular collagens are type I and III, which comprise up to 80% to 90% of the total blood vessel wall collagens. These collagens are assembled into crossbanded fibrils and are prominent throughout the ECM of all vascular layers (Figs. 29–1 and 29–2). In the normal arterial wall, types I and III collagens are organized into distinct fibrillar bundles, either wedged between elastic fibers in elastic arteries or organized into "nests" surrounding medial arterial smooth muscle cells in muscular arteries (3,4). It is unclear whether these fibrillar collagens align to form a distinct network in vascular tissue, because most images demonstrate a wavy fiber random orientation. Wavy collagen fibers are generally found in "soft" tissues and align during loading or pressure changes to prevent tissue failure (5). These collagens provide tensile strength to the vascular wall. Less abundant collagens such as type VIII are present in association with different types of vascular cells (6).

Types and Distribution

The principal source of collagens in the arterial intima and media is the smooth muscle cell. Modulation of collagen synthesis by these cells frequently accompanies phenotypic changes associated with altered cellular behavior. For example, as arterial smooth muscle cells modulate from a quiescent or "contractile state" typical of the normal vessel phenotype to a proliferative or "synthetic state" characteristic of the atherothrombotic phenotype, type I collagen synthesis increases (7). A number of factors regulate collagen synthesis by arterial smooth muscle cells (see review by Rekhter [8]). For example, the growth state of the cells, different growth factors and cytokines, and the nature of the ECM substrate influence collagen synthesis by these cells. Cytokines and growth factors generally enhance the synthesis of types I, III, and V collagen, with transforming growth factor (TGF)-β_1 exhibiting the most potent effect. However, TGF-β_1–induced type I and III collagen synthesis by human arterial smooth muscle cells is inhibited by interferon-γ.

Vascular smooth muscle cells normally reside in the media of the vessel wall surrounded by abundant collagen molecules. Thus, collagens serve as attachment proteins for arterial smooth muscle cells and influence cell behavior. For example, inhibiting collagen synthesis in vascular smooth muscle cells inhibits their proliferative and migratory behavior (9–12). Smooth muscle cells interact with collagen through integrin and nonintegrin receptors. For example, cultured arterial smooth muscle cells express $\alpha_2\beta_1$ receptors when stimulated to migrate on type I collagen substrates (13). Such an interaction regulates intracellular signaling pathways that control cell proliferation and migration and cell survival (see reviews by Raines and coworkers [14] and Pickering [15]). Vascular smooth muscle cells also interact with type I and VIII collagens through the discoidin family of ECM receptors (see review by Hou and coworkers [16]). These nonintegrin receptors are a novel class of receptor tyrosine kinases that bind several collagens and stimulate matrix metalloproteinase activity and control vascular smooth

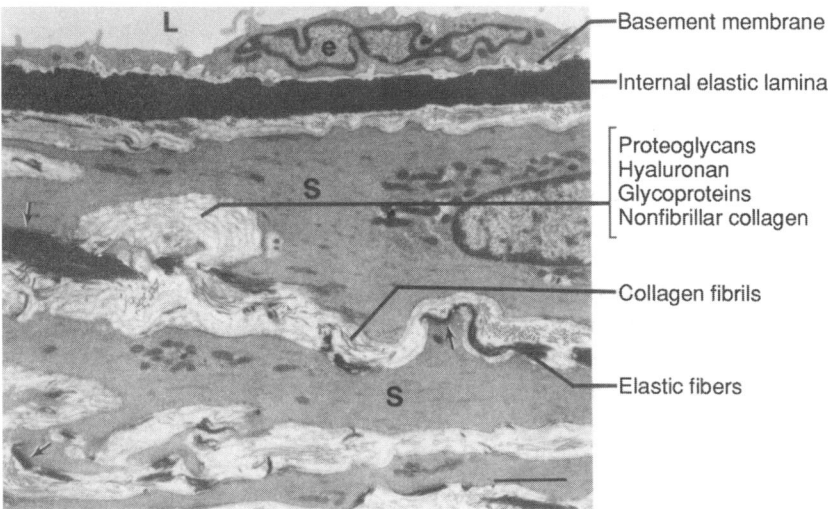

FIG. 29–1. An electron micrograph of a cross section of a rat superior mesenteric artery. This low-power view demonstrates location of specific extracellular matrix (ECM) components in relation to vascular cells. e, Endothelial cell; L, lumen; S, smooth muscle cell. *Arrows* point to areas of the cell that are closely apposed to elastic fibers. Scale bar = 2 μm. (From Walker-Caprioglio HM, Trotter JA, Little SA, et al. Organization of cells and extracellular matrix in mesenteric arteries of spontaneously hypertensive rats. *Cell Tissue Res* 1992;269:141–149, with permission.)

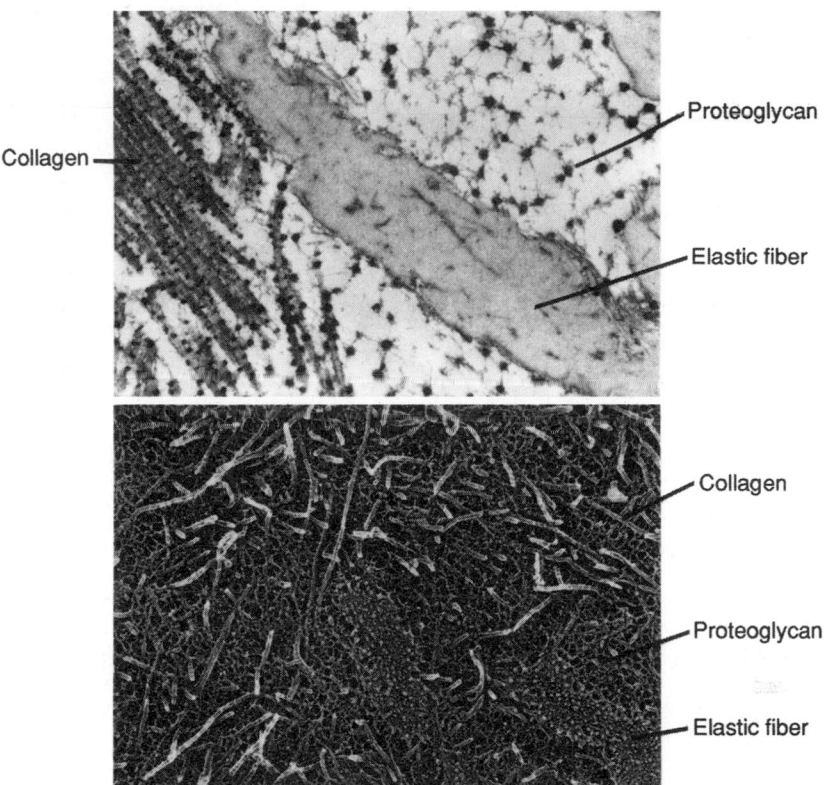

FIG. 29–2. Top: Electron micrograph of vascular extracellular matrix (ECM) demonstrating organization of collagen, elastic fiber, and proteoglycans. The proteoglycans have been preserved with ruthenium red and can be visualized as large granules filling the extracellular space and small granules attached to collagen fibrils. Original magnification ×86,000. **Bottom:** Electron micrograph of a similar ECM prepared using a quick-freeze/deep-etch procedure without chemical fixation. The ECM consists of a finely woven meshwork of proteoglycan-containing elastic fibers and collagen fibrils. Scale bar = 0.2 μm. (From Mecham, RP, Geuser JE. In: Hay E, ed. *Cell biology of extracellular matrix.* New York: Plenum Press, 1991, with permission.)

muscle cell proliferation and migration. Such results indicate that collagens can regulate vascular smooth muscle cell phenotype through specific cell–ECM interactions.

Endothelial cells also express genes that code for types I, III, IV, and VIII collagens, which influence endothelial cell behavior (see review by Vernon and Sage [17]). Collagens are known to play a role in the formation of new blood vessels (i.e., angiogenesis). For example, a substrate of type I collagen induces endothelial cells to form capillary tubes *in vitro,* and expression of type I collagen by endothelial cells is characteristic of neovascularization *in vivo.* When endothelial cells "sprout" and form capillary tubes *in vitro,* type I collagen synthesis is induced. Although the role that type I collagen plays in this process is not fully understood, collagen fibrils may serve as a template or cable onto which endothelial cells wrap themselves through tractive restructuring.

Vascular Disease

Vascular collagens are critical to vascular wall integrity. Defects in the synthesis and deposition of either type I or type III vascular collagen, such as occurs in lethal mutations of the type I collagen gene and in some forms of Ehlers–Danlos syndrome, result in aneurysms and rupture of both elastic and muscular arteries (18,19). Vascular collagens also change in amount and location in different forms of vascular disease. For example, there is topographic variation in the location of collagen types in human atherothrombotic plaques (20–22) and changes in the amount of collagens in the development of restenotic lesions (23,24). Type I collagen expression occurs principally in the fibrous caps and vascularized regions of primary plaques, with less type I collagen in the plaque center where lipid is highest (Fig. 29–3). However, both normal and oxidized low-density lipoproteins interact with type I and III collagen, suggesting a role for collagen in lipoprotein retention during the development of atherothrombosis. Yet, other studies suggest that molecules associated with collagen, such as the proteoglycan decorin, may be partially responsible for lipoprotein interaction (25).

Variations in distribution of fibrillar collagen throughout vascular lesions may create regions within the plaque that differ in tensile strength and stiffness. These variations can

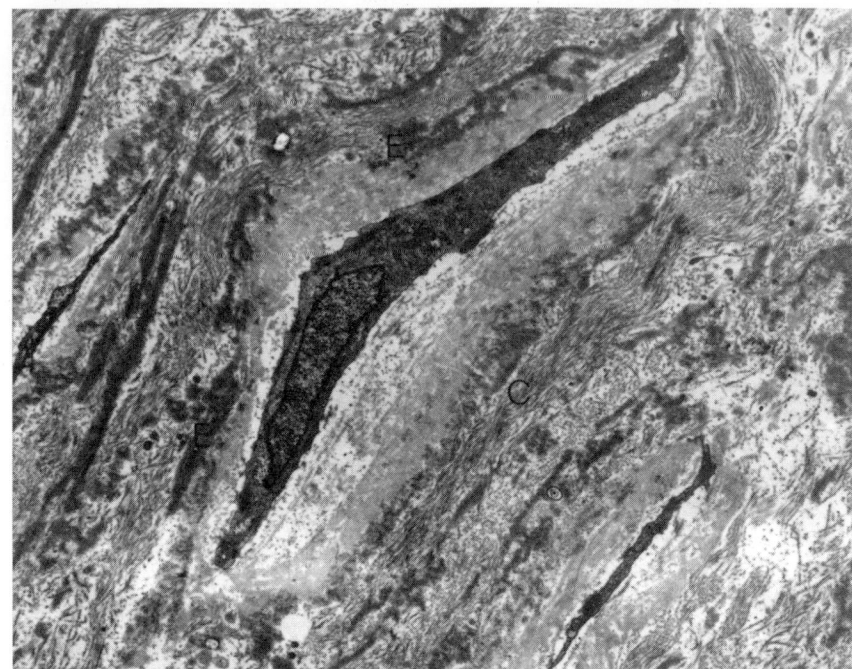

FIG. 29–3. Electron micrograph of an area of the fibrous cap of a human atherothrombotic lesion demonstrating a smooth muscle cell surrounded by extensive collagen *(C)* fibrils. E, elastin. Original magnification ×10,000. (From Ross R, Wight TN, Strandness E, et al. Human atherosclerosis. I. Cell constitution and characteristics of advanced lesions of the superficial femoral artery. *Am J Pathol* 1984;114:79–93, with permission.)

lead to differences in susceptibility to plaque rupture reviewed by Libby (26). For example, plaque fissuring and subsequent thrombosis often occur at boundaries between collagen-rich and collagen-poor zones, such as at the base of thin fibrous caps or near collagen-poor and lipid-rich regions of plaque, or both. Exposure of collagen fibrils during vascular tearing results in platelet activation and thrombosis. Thrombosis associated with plaque fissures is the most common cause of acute myocardial infarction, sudden cardiac death, and unstable angina. Thus, although fibrillar collagens provide blood vessels with tensile strength essential for plaque stability, they also provide a potential substrate for initiating the events that lead to occlusive arterial disease. Considerable attention has focused on the possible protective role of collagen in stabilizing the fibrous cap and possibly preventing plaque rupture (27). It is of interest that agents such as statins not only reduce serum cholesterol but appear to have an additional beneficial effect on the vascular wall by preventing proteolytic activity and enhancing collagen content in the developing atherothrombotic lesion (28,29). Absence of vitamin C, a cross-linking catalyst for collagens, produces vulnerable plaques in experimental animals (30). Another way to manipulate the collagen content and organization of atherothrombotic plaques is to introduce genes whose products associate with collagen and regulate collagen organization and structure. One such gene is decorin. Introducing smooth muscle cells that overexpress decorin into injured vessels leads to a marked enrichment in collagen accumulation and reduces intimal thickening (31).

ELASTIC FIBERS

Another major structural component of blood vessels is the elastic fiber. Together with collagens, elastic fibers provide mechanical strength and elasticity needed to accommodate pressure changes arising from the pulsatile nature of blood flow, as well as the hemodynamic changes created on the wall by the rheology of blood. Whereas the collagen fibers bear load in the circumferential direction, elastic fibers provide longitudinal and circumferential support (32).

Properties and Distribution

Elastic fibers are complex structures that include a hydrophobic 72-kD tropoelastin subunit associated with hydrophilic glycoproteins and enzymes responsible for the internal cross-linking of elastin peptides (33,34). Cross-linking is controlled by lysyl oxidase, an enzyme that catalyzes the oxidative deamination and condensation of lysyl side chains in the elastin molecule. This is the same enzyme that catalyzes the cross-linking of collagen fibrils. Elastin has an unusual amino acid composition in that it is low in acidic and basic amino acids but rich in hydrophobic amino acids such as valine. Such cross-links impart "rubber-like" recoil properties to this protein and render it highly insoluble. Aortic elastin turns over very slowly, if at all, and, therefore, synthesis of elastin occurs principally during perinatal and early growth and decreases to insignificant levels in the adult. In the absence of arterial pathology, arterial elastin is highly stable and long-lasting.

Like the fibrillar collagens, elastic fibers form discrete structures within the ECM that can readily be visualized at the light and electron microscopic level (3,4) (Figs. 29–1, 29–2, and 29–4). Elastic fibers are arranged into concentric sheets or lamellae that separate different vascular layers. A thick layer of elastic tissue separates the intima from the media (internal elastic lamina) and the media from the adventitia (external elastic lamella). In addition, elastic lamellae form boundaries between successive concentric layers of smooth muscle (Fig. 29–4). Frequently, the elastic lamellae are interconnected by radially oriented elastic fibers that facilitate the transfer of stress throughout the vessel wall (3,4).

The concentration of elastin varies throughout the vascular system. Elastic lamellae are prominent in the larger vessels such as the thoracic aorta, which receives high-pressure pulses of blood from the left ventricle. Elastin concentration decreases in the smaller, more muscular arteries such as the smaller mesenteric arteries (3,4). In large vessels, such as the aorta of adult mammals, the number of lamellar units and the radius of the vessel are nearly proportional (35). This allows for tension carried by each lamella to be nearly constant, regardless of the animal's weight, the aortic diameter, or the medial thickness. Thus, elastin acts as a dampening chamber to smooth the pressure wave as it is transmitted down the vessel.

The principal source of elastic fibers in blood vessels is the arterial smooth muscle cell, which supports elastic fibrillogenesis in vitro (36,37). A number of factors stimulate the synthesis of tropoelastin (see reviews by Rosenbloom and coworkers [33] and Davidson [38]) and proteins that associate with elastin such as lysyl oxidase (see review by Bank and van Hinsbergh [39]). Elastic fibers consist of two morphologically distinct components: an amorphous core of elastin and a peripheral mantle of 10- to 12-nanaometer microfibrils that contain the protein fibrillin. Elastic fiber formation takes place close to the cell membrane, generally within infoldings of the cell surface. Microfibrils are the first components to appear, followed by discrete foci of elastin that associates with the microfibrils. Accessory proteins at the cell surface help target elastic fiber assembly along the smooth muscle cell surface. For example, a 67-kD protein binds tropoelastin at the cell surface and regulates elastic fiber assembly (40,41). The 67-kD protein is a galactoside lectin and its affinity for the cell surface is greatly diminished by interaction with molecules that contain galactose sugars such as proteoglycans (42). Such an interaction interrupts elastic fiber fibrillogenesis and impairs elastic fiber assembly (41). Other cell surface–associated proteins may play similar roles in elastic fiber assembly. For example, fibulin 5, an ECM protein that contains binding sites for integrins, is required for proper vascular elastic fiber formation in mice (43–45).

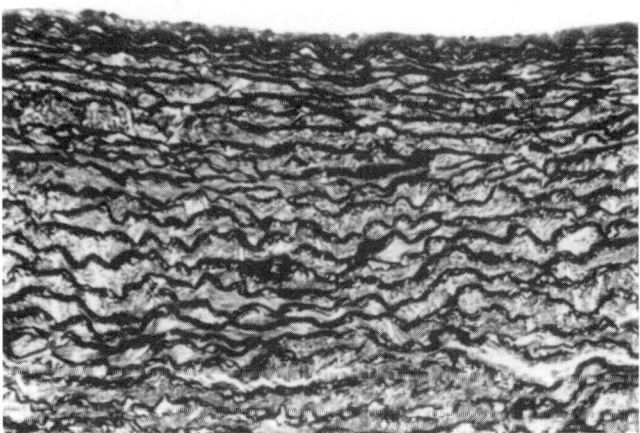
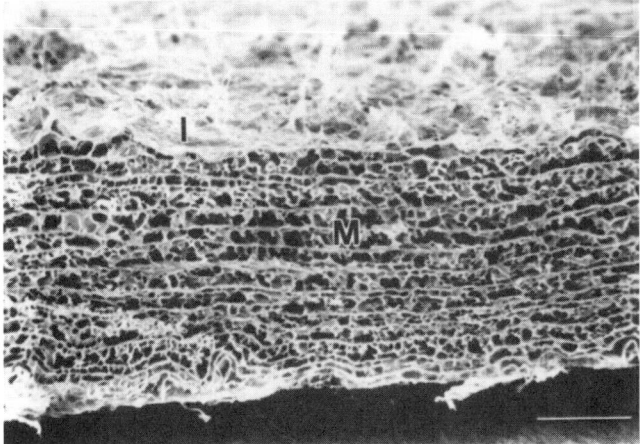

FIG. 29–4. Organization of elastin in bovine pulmonary artery. **Top:** Cross section of the artery stained with Verheff–Van Gieson elastic stain to demonstrate multiple layers of elastin. Original magnification ×80. **Bottom:** Scanning electron micrograph of adult rat aorta after removal of nonelastin components. Scale bar = 50 μm. (From Mecham RP, Geuser JE. In: Hay E, ed. *Cell biology of extracellular matrix.* New York: Plenum Press, 1991, with permission.)

Maintenance of structural integrity of the elastic fibers in blood vessels is an important factor in regulating the phenotype of vascular cells. For example, elastin fragments or peptides and reduced elastic fiber formation stimulate migration and proliferation of arterial smooth muscle cells (46). Furthermore, elastin peptides are chemotactic for monocytes, which may promote the inflammatory response characteristic of vascular disease. The importance of elastic fiber integrity in controlling the proliferative and migratory phenotype of arterial smooth muscle cells is exemplified by the elastin knockout mouse, which dies of occlusive arterial disease shortly after birth because of excessive vascular smooth muscle cell proliferation and migration (47).

Vascular Disease

Vascular diseases involving elastic fibers are caused by genetic mutations in elastin or elastin-associated genes or are secondary to other metabolic problems (48). The genetic causes involve either mutations in the elastin gene leading to supravalvular aortic stenosis or mutations in elastin-associated proteins such as fibrillin, which lead to aneurysms as found in Marfan syndrome (see review by Ramirez and coworkers [49]). Marfan syndrome is characterized by changes in large artery stiffness, pulse pressures, dilatation and defective elastic fiber formation, and/or elastic fiber fragmentation leading to "weakening" of the vascular wall and aneurysms. Furthermore, alterations in the fibrillin 1 genotype are associated with aortic stiffness and disease severity in patients with coronary artery disease (50).

Fragmentation or loss of elastic fibers also is frequently seen during atherothrombosis (51,52) and in arteriovenous fistulas (53). The cause of elastic fiber tears in these conditions is not entirely clear, it but may relate to vascular wall tension brought on by the turbulent flow of blood and to the release of proteases from a variety of cell types including smooth muscle cells (54) and infiltrating inflammatory cells. A variety of proteases are found in atherothrombotic plaques that are capable of degrading elastin including matrix metalloproteinases (55,56), and cysteine proteases (57). In addition, serine proteases capable of degrading elastin are found in pulmonary vessels in experimental hypertension in rats

(58). In fact, a complete reversal of hypertension in this animal model has been accomplished by using an inhibitor of serine protease activity (59).

Although elastin turns over very slowly in normal vessels, active elastin synthesis takes place during vascular matrix remodeling associated with vascular injury (Fig. 29–5). Vascular injury can result from conditions such as hypertension or from physical insults to the blood vessels such as occur during balloon angioplasty or suturing in vascular grafting. It is of interest that, although tropoelastin synthesis is increased in response to vascular injury, elastic fibers do not form during this remodeling phase. Therefore, the presence of excessive amounts of nonassembled elastin coupled to a lack of elastic fibers may promote the proliferative and migratory response seen in the early phases of atherothrombosis. In addition, expressing an isoform of versican, V3, in arterial smooth muscle cells promotes elastic fiber assembly *in vitro* and *in vivo* after vascular injury (60). Such results indicate that elastic fiber assembly must rely on a number of interacting components.

Modification of elastic fibers occurs in vascular disease, which can cause loss of normal elastic fiber function. For example, normal aortic elastin appears to consist of a protein–lipid complex with lipids presumably bound by hy-

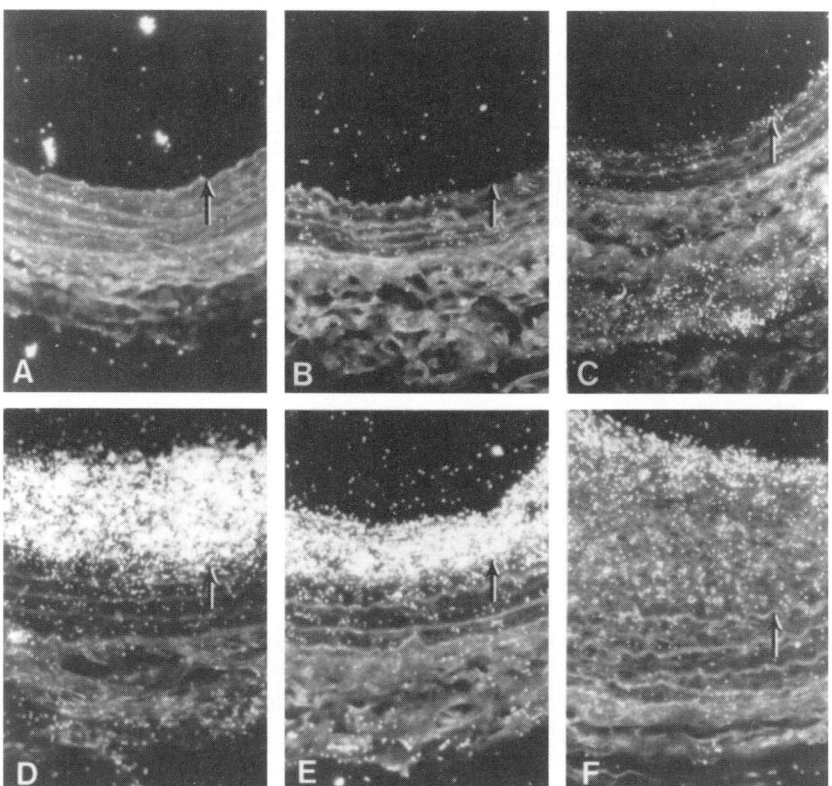

FIG. 29–5. Dark-field photomicrographs showing time course of tropoelastin transcript induction after rat carotid artery injury by *in situ* hybridization. **A:** Uninjured. **B:** Two days after injury. **C:** One week after injury. **D:** Two weeks after injury plus heparin treatment. **F:** Four weeks after injury. (From Nikkari ST, Järveläinen HT, Wight TN, et al. Smooth muscle cell expression of extracellular matrix genes after arterial injury. *Am J Pathol* 1994;144:1348–1356, with permission.)

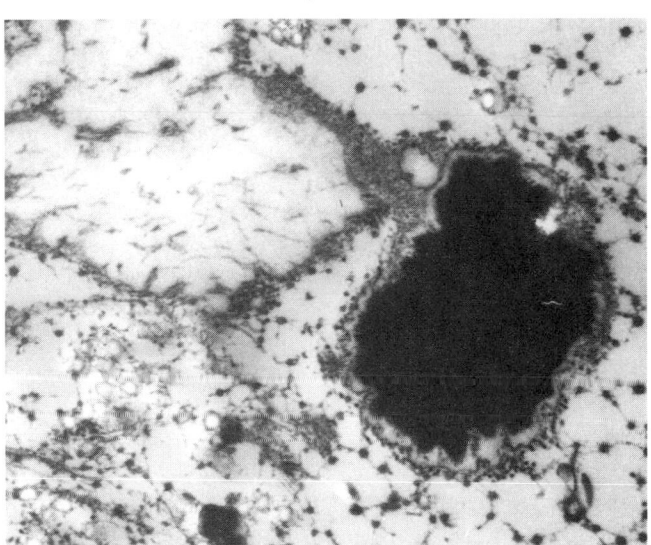

FIG. 29–6. An electron micrograph of a section of vascular extracellular matrix (ECM) from a patient with idiopathic infantile arterial calcinosis (68). The elastic fiber on the right is extensively calcified, whereas the elastic fiber on the left appears normal. Original magnification ×43,000.

drophobic stacking to hydrophobic sites in elastin molecules (51,61). Although the lipid moiety of normal elastin is small, it is greater in elastin from atherothrombotic arteries (62, 63). Morphologic studies show lipid deposited adjacent to and within elastic fibers (64) and lipid–elastin complexes have been isolated from human atherothrombotic vessels (65). Such binding or trapping of lipid in elastin could interfere with normal elastic fiber formation by preventing proper alignment of peptide monomers during the cross-linking reaction. Lipid associated with elastic fibers may also interfere with elastic recoil because recoil is somewhat dependent on the exposure of lipophilic groups of the native elastin molecule (51). Lipids may also facilitate the breakdown of the elastic fiber because free fatty acids bound to elastin increase the binding of elastolytic enzymes (66,67).

Elastic fibers may also form a depot for accumulation of calcium in vascular disease (68–70) (Fig. 29–6). For example, calcium is a cofactor for several of the elastolytic enzymes, such as the matrix metalloproteinases and inhibition of matrix metalloproteinases significantly inhibits calcification of elastin implants in an animal model of calcification (71). Conformational changes induced by organic solvents in elastin promote calcium binding to elastic fibers (72). Thus, elastin–lipid complexes may promote deposits of calcium in advancing atherothrombosis and facilitate elastic fiber destruction.

PROTEOGLYCANS/HYALURONAN

Proteoglycans and hyaluronan are hydrophilic molecules that interact with a variety of other ECM molecules in the interstitial space to create tissue turgor and viscoelasticity.

In addition, these macromolecules interact with components in a number of vascular events and participate in the regulation of vascular permeability, lipid metabolism, hemostasis, and thrombosis (see reviews by Camejo [73], Radhakrishnamurthy and coworkers [74], Williams and Tabas [75], and Rosenberg and coworkers [76]). In addition, proteoglycans and hyaluronan interact with vascular cells and with growth factors and cytokines to modify vascular cell adhesion, migration, and proliferation (see reviews by Wight [77] and Toole and coworkers [78]).

Types and Distribution

Proteoglycans are protein polysaccharides that share the common structural feature of one or more glycosaminoglycan (GAG) chains covalently attached to a core glycoprotein backbone (79). The GAG chains are linear polymers of repeating disaccharides that contain a hexosamine and either a carboxylate or a sulfate ester or both. As a rule, GAGs do not exist "free" in tissue but are attached to core glycoproteins to form distinct families of proteoglycans. However, the GAG hyaluronan, formerly termed hyaluronic acid, is an exception in that it is not covalently linked to a core glycoprotein and exists in the ECM as a high molecular weight random-coiled polysaccharide occupying large hydrodynamic domains. Hyaluronan polymers self-associate and form regions of ordered helical structures creating continuous networks of pronounced viscoelasticity.

Traditionally, proteoglycans have been classified on the basis of the predominant type of GAG attached to a specific core glycoprotein, for example, chondroitin sulfate (CSPG), dermatan sulfate (DSPG), heparan sulfate (HSPG), and keratan sulfate (KSPG). However, more recent comparisons of proteoglycan core protein structure by immunochemical and cloning methods have shown that proteoglycans exist as multigenic families of related core proteins that share common functions within their respective families (80). A number of different core proteins with variable numbers of GAG chains of different length and composition exist, creating enormous structural diversity in these proteoglycans. Vascular proteoglycans can be found in four locations: (a) in the interstitial ECM; (b) as part of specialized ECM structures such as basement membranes; (c) as part of cell membranes; and (d) intracellularly. Proteoglycans found in each of these locations tend to share common structural features that in part determine their role in these tissue compartments.

More than 30 different proteoglycans have been shown to exist in vascular tissue or to be synthesized by vascular cells (81). However, the major types of proteoglycans found in the interstitial space include large (~1,000 kD) CSPGs such as versican (82), small (~120–300 kD) leucine-rich DSPGs such as decorin and biglycan (83,84), KSPGs such as lumican (85), and HSPGs such as perlecan, syndecans, and glypicans (86). All of these proteoglycans associate with different components of the vascular ECM (Fig. 29–2) and influence the properties of these components. For example, decorin is located along collagen fibrils and is known to regulate collagen fiber diameter and organization (87). Perlecan interacts with components of basement membranes and contributes to the permeability characteristics of this structure, serves as substrate for vascular cells, and retains growth factors involved in vascular remodeling and new blood vessel formation (see review by Dunlevy and Hassell [88]). Versican is present throughout the interstitial space of the vascular ECM (89) and interacts with hyaluronan and link proteins (90) to fill the ECM space not occupied by the fibrous components of the ECM. These complexes create a reversibly compressible compartment in the vascular ECM and provide a swelling pressure within the ECM that is offset by the collagen fibrils, reviewed in Comper and Laurent (91).

The distribution of proteoglycans throughout the blood vessel wall is variable. For example, the intima is particularly enriched in proteoglycans with lower amounts in the media and adventitia (Fig. 29–7). Versican/hyaluronan complexes and biglycan are prominent in the intima and media, and decorin is concentrated in the collagen-containing adventitia. Perlecan is present in basement membranes throughout both the intimal and medial layers. Lumican appears to be associated with collagen fibers within the arterial wall. Not only are there differences in the types of proteoglycans between the different layers of the blood vessel wall, but differences exist between different vascular beds (89).

The arterial smooth muscle cell is a principal source for vascular proteoglycans and hyaluronan, although virtually every cell that is present in the vascular wall, with the exception of red blood cells, synthesize proteoglycans. A number of studies indicate that the synthesis of these molecules is differentially regulated by growth factors and cytokines such as platelet-derived growth factor (PDGF) and TGF-β_1 (92–95). PDGF stimulation leads to an increase in the pericellular matrix that surrounds the smooth muscle cells, which is required for their proliferation and migration (95,96). Whereas versican and hyaluronan appear to promote arterial smooth muscle cell proliferation, HSPGs such as perlecan inhibit proliferation in some situations (97–100). The mechanism for this inhibitory effect is unknown.

Endothelial cells also synthesize a variety of proteoglycans and hyaluronan and modulate their synthesis in different phenotypic states. For example, decorin is not synthesized by confluent cultures of endothelial cells (101) and is absent from the endothelial lining of adult arteries (102). However, when endothelial cells sprout to a migratory phe-

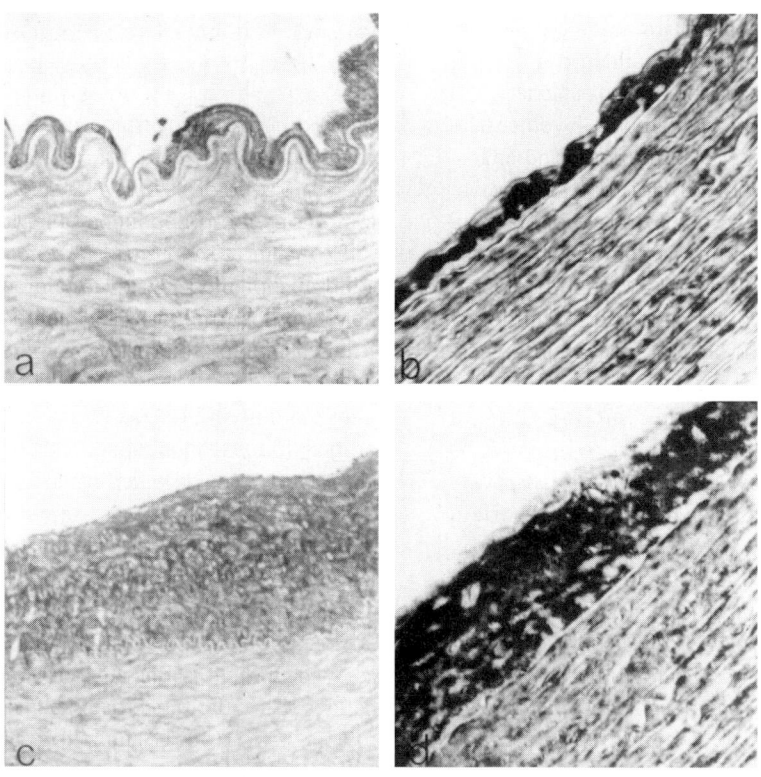

FIG. 29–7. Light micrographs illustrating that the narrow intima of a normal blood vessel stains more intensely with **(A)** Alcian blue and **(B)** a monoclonal antibody to chondroitin sulfate proteoglycan (CSPG) than the underlying medial layer. Intimal thickening after injury exhibits intense staining for proteoglycan **(C)** Alcian blue; **(D)** monoclonal antibody to CSPG. Scale bar = 50 μm. (From Wight TN, Lark MW, Kinsell MG. In: Wight T, Mecham R, eds. *Biology of proteoglycans.* Orlando, FL: Academic Press, 1987:267–300, with permission.)

notype and form tubes *in vitro,* they express decorin and type I collagen (103). In addition, decorin-positive microvessels are found in vascular tissue undergoing remodeling (104). These two ECM molecules may thus provide the appropriate substrate for endothelial cell rearrangement during new vessel formation.

Vascular Disease

The content and distribution of vascular proteoglycans and hyaluronan change as the ECM is remodeled in hypertension (4), diabetes (105–108), atherothrombosis, and restenosis (see reviews by Toole and coworkers [78] and Wight [109]). Overall, proteoglycans and hyaluronan increase in the early and middle phases of vascular disease and decrease as the lesions become more advanced and fibrotic. However, with the development of more precise probes to examine regional deposits and expression of these molecules, it is clear that there are topographic variations in the distribution of different classes of proteoglycans and hyaluronan as lesions develop. For example, versican is prominent in the ECM of human diffuse intimal thickenings during early stages of human vascular disease (110,111) and is located at the edge of the necrotic core in more advanced late-stage disease (112,113). Interestingly, versican, together with hyaluronan, is present at the plaque thrombus interface, suggesting a role in thrombosis in late-stage disease (114). Conversely, biglycan colocalizes with apoB- and apoE-containing lipoproteins (115), suggesting a role in lipoprotein accumulation in vascular disease. *In vitro* binding assays show that biglycan interacts with LDL with saturable kinetics and with an association constant of 1.7×10^{-7} M (116). Lumican is another proteoglycan that associates with collagen, is expressed by vascular smooth muscle cells (117), and is present in human atherothrombotic lesions (118). The role of lumican in developing atherothrombosis is not clear but is likely to involve effects on collagen organization and accumulation in the developing lesion.

Proteoglycans and hyaluronan also form a significant part of the ECM as the human vascular wall thickens during restenosis after angioplasty. For example, the fibroproliferative tissue typical of human restenosis contains vascular smooth muscle cells embedded in a loose ECM containing mostly proteoglycan (i.e., versican and biglycan) and hyaluronan (Fig. 29–8). Experimental injury models of restenosis confirm that balloon angioplasty leads to increased expression and deposition of proteoglycans and hyaluronan during the early vascular remodeling phase (119–122). These changes accompany increases in arterial smooth muscle cell proliferation and migration and raise the possibility that proteoglycans or hyaluronan, or both, contribute to events leading to arterial wall thickening in vascular disease. For example, antibodies or antisense to TGF-β_1 reduces versican accumulation and significantly retards balloon injury–induced neointimal expansion in experimental animals (123,124). Such findings indicate the potential importance of targeting these ECM molecules in the prevention of injury-induced restenosis.

Changes in the proteoglycan and hyaluronan content of the ECM in vascular disease dramatically affect the permeability of the vascular wall. For example, increases in proteoglycan and hyaluronan lead to an expansion of the ECM and a network of highly charged and interactive macromolecules. This arrangement creates an ECM that regulates the movement of small and large molecules as they enter the vascular wall from the plasma (125). Macromolecules that encounter this network may be retained through ionic interaction or excluded by steric hindrance. An important example is the retention of plasma lipoproteins by proteoglycans (see reviews by Williams and Tabas [75,126]). The interaction is ionic, either directly between two macromolecules (127–129) or through bridging molecules such as apoE or lipoprotein lipase (75,130,131). Lipoproteins interact with a number of different proteoglycans through positively charged amino acids in the apoprotein and negatively charged residues in the GAG chains. The proteoglycan binding site has been mapped to residue 3363 in apoprotein B in human LDL, because replacing this charged residue with a neutral amino acid by site-directed mutagenesis eliminates proteoglycan binding to LDL in an *in vitro* assay (132). These *in vitro* results have been extended *in vivo* by showing that transgenic mice expressing the defective proteoglycan binding form of LDL do not develop atherothrombosis when fed a high-fat diet, whereas control mice expressing normal LDL develop severe atherothrombosis under the same conditions (133). Other proteoglycans such as those containing heparan sulfate influence lipoprotein metabolism by regulating uptake and processing of lipoproteins at nonvascular sites such as the liver (see review by Conde-Knape [134]).

Although most studies implicate proteoglycans and their associated GAGs in the promotion of arterial disease, a subset of these molecules are protective against atherothrombosis and thrombosis. For example, some forms of heparin, heparan sulfate, and dermatan sulfate are powerful anticoagulants and are therefore useful in preventing the generation of fibrin and subsequent thrombosis (see reviews by Rosenberg and coworkers [76] and Bourin and Lindahl [135]). The basis for this activity lies in the ability of these GAGs to interact with serine protease inhibitors (serpins) such as antithrombin III and heparin cofactor II to potentiate the inactivation of clotting enzymes such as factor Xa and thrombin. Heparin and heparan sulfate principally target the inactivation of thrombin through antithrombin III, whereas dermatan sulfate, in addition to heparin and heparan sulfate, accelerates the inactivation of thrombin by heparin cofactor II. Interestingly, genetic manipulation of perlecan expression can inhibit thrombosis after deep vascular injury in experimental animals (100). Decorin and biglycan also influence the coagulation cascade and the generation of fibrin by thrombin during thrombosis. Both of these proteoglycans interact with heparin cofactor II and potentiate the inactivation of thrombin (136). Because decorin and biglycan inter-

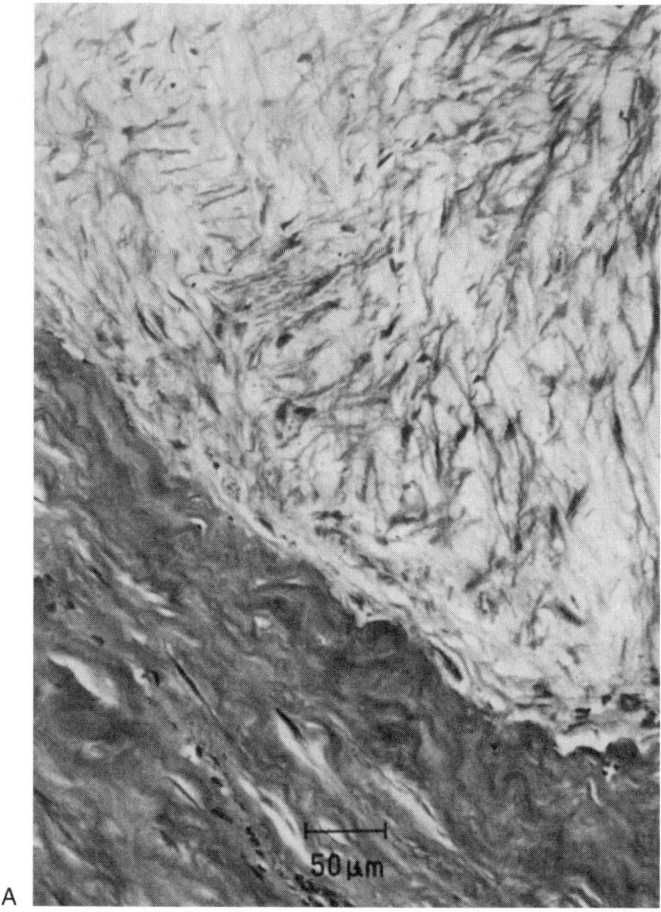

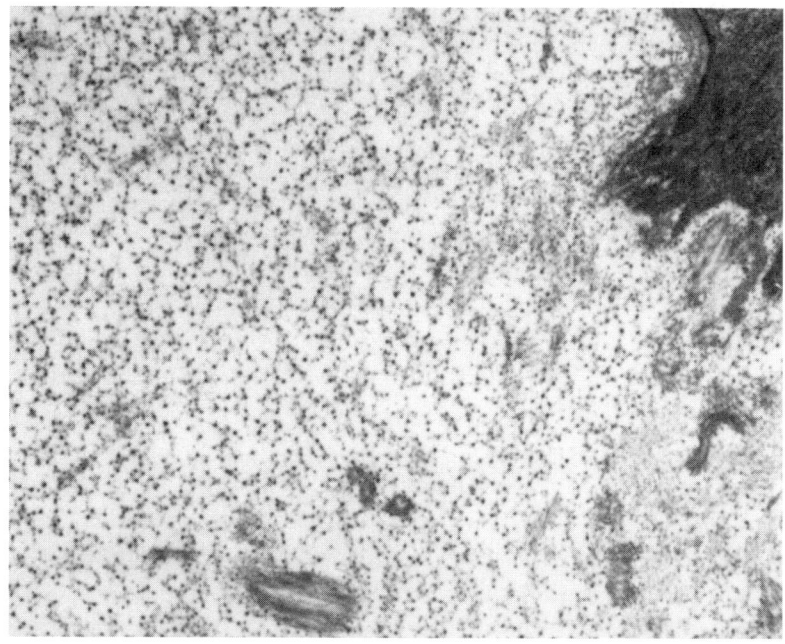

FIG. 29–8. A: A light microscopic view of typical restenotic tissue exhibiting a loose connective tissue zone and a dense connective zone. Original magnification ×50. **B:** An electron micrograph of a section of the loose connective tissue zone demonstrating abundant proteoglycan granules. **C:** Section from the dense connective tissue zone demonstrating abundant collagen fibrils. Original magnification ×50,000.

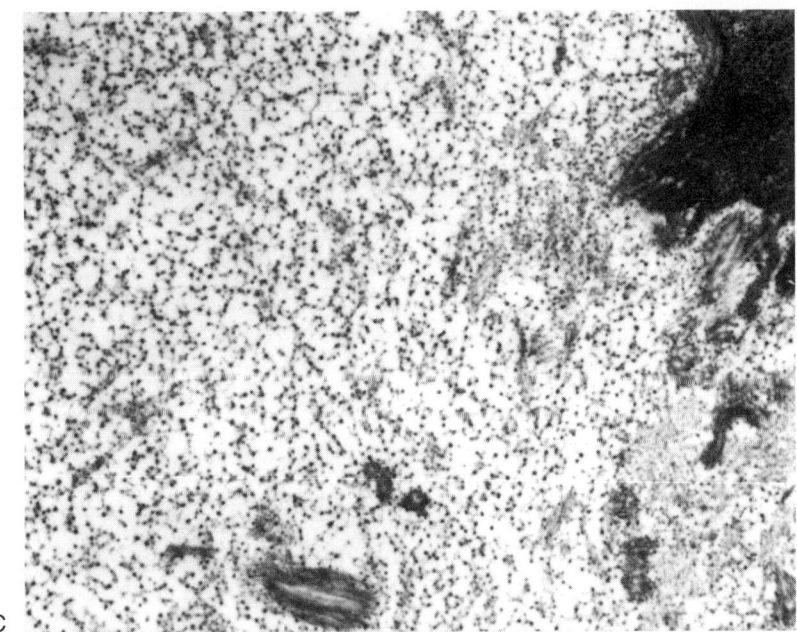

FIG. 29–8. *Continued.*

act with a number of other ECM molecules throughout the atherothrombotic plaque, focal accumulation of these proteoglycans may, in part, contribute a thromboresistance to the ECM portion of the lesion. Furthermore, biglycan and decorin extracted from human atherothrombotic plaques exhibit reduced inactivation of thrombin when mixed with heparin cofactor II compared with similar extracts from normal vessels. Consistent with this observation, both decorin and biglycan are missing from human atherothrombotic plaque/thrombus boundaries (114).

GLYCOPROTEINS

The principal glycoproteins in vascular tissue and synthesized by vascular cells include fibronectin, laminin, thrombospondin (TSP), tenascin, and osteopontin. These proteins have similar modular structures and contain sequences that allow them to self-associate, interact with other ECM components, and bind to cells through specific cell surface receptors. Through multiple interactions, these macromolecules regulate vascular ECM integrity and provide a variety of substrates for vascular cells.

Fibronectins

Fibronectins are a family of glycoproteins that are present in blood plasma and the ECM of most tissues. This glycoprotein consists of two similar peptide chains of ~220 kD held together at one end by disulfide bonds (137). Each chain consists of repeated copies of three distinct types of polypeptide domains (types I, II, and III). There are 12 type I repeats, 2 type II repeats, and 15 to 17 type III repeats in human fibronectin. Approximately 20 different fibronectin chains have been identified in humans, all of which are generated by alternative splicing of the RNA transcript of a single fibronectin gene. Many of these variants are expressed in vascular tissue during development and remodeling (138,139).

Fibronectin is present throughout all layers of the vascular ECM and in increased amounts during development and in the neointima in response to injury and hypertension (140–142). In addition, fibronectin synthesis is increased as smooth muscle cells proliferate and migrate in the intima during closure of the ductus arteriosus during fetal development (143). This glycoprotein also accumulates in intimal thickenings associated with postcardiac transplant coronary arteriopathy and vascular restenosis (144–146). Deposits of this glycoprotein in altered vascular tissue may influence the retention of lipoproteins in the vascular ECM because fibronectin interacts with lipoproteins, possibly through its heparin-binding domain (147). Fibronectin is a principal attachment protein for vascular cells and serves as a substrate for the migration of vascular cells during development and remodeling and is mediated primarily by the $\alpha_5\beta_1$ integrin (see review by Casscells [148]).

Laminin

Laminin is an ~800-kD trimeric glycoprotein present in vascular basement membranes of endothelial and smooth muscle cells. Like fibronectin, this molecule consists of subunits of polypeptides that contain multiple binding sites for cell surface receptors and other ECM molecules (149). Laminin also exists as multiple isoforms. These isoforms belong to a family of proteins containing several genetically distinct subunit chains.

Laminin interacts with key basement membrane components such as type IV collagen, nidogen, and HSPG to form the fabric of the basement membrane during embryonic vasculogenesis and vascular wall maturation. Because laminin peptides contain multiple cell-binding sites, this glycoprotein serves as a substrate for vascular cells. For example, the A chain of laminin contains RGD sequences, which can be recognized by multiple integrin receptors, of which $\alpha_6\beta_1$ appears to be the most specific. The B chain of laminin contains the YIGSR sequence, which also serves as a ligand for some cells. Vascular endothelial cells attach to laminin through both β_1 and β_3 integrins and use multiple laminin binding sites, including SIKVAV sequences, to form endothelial tubes *in vitro* (150,151).

Laminin also interacts with arterial smooth muscle cells through more than one receptor (152,153). This interaction in part maintains these cells in a nonproliferative and contractile phenotype, unlike fibronectin, which promotes modulation of arterial smooth muscle cells to a proliferative and secretory phenotype. The potential importance of laminin in vascular disease is highlighted by studies that demonstrate that the synthetic peptide YIGSR inhibits new blood vessel formation (151).

Thrombospondin

TSP is a 450-kD trimeric glycoprotein that consists of three identical 150-kD chains joined together by disulfide linkages. The glycoprotein exists in more than one form and may constitute a family of related proteins generated by alternative splicing, although more than one TSP gene exists (see review by Bornstein [154]). TSP was first identified in platelet α granules where on release it promotes platelet aggregation. TSP interacts with a number of plasma proteins such as fibrinogen, plasminogen, and histidine-rich glycoprotein and copolymerizes with fibrin in clot formation. However, as is true for many of the other platelet proteins, TSP is synthesized by a variety of cells including vascular endothelial and smooth muscle cells. TSP possesses multiple binding sites and interacts with a variety of ECM components such as fibronectin, a number of different collagens, laminin, and HSPGs. Interestingly, TSP also binds to growth factors such as TGF-β_1 and may be involved in the activation of this cytokine within the vascular ECM (155). Unlike fibronectin and laminin, which promote cell adhesion, TSP exerts antiadhesive effects that lead to cell rounding and cell detachment (156).

TSP is present in different vascular layers but is increased in the thickened intima in human vascular disease (157) and in the neointima after experimental balloon angioplasty (158). Increased expression of TSP appears to be linked to a vascular cell growth response (158–160). Antibodies to TSP inhibit PDGF-induced proliferation of arterial smooth muscle cells. Although TSP appears necessary for arterial smooth muscle cell proliferation, this glycoprotein inhibits endothelial cell proliferation *in vitro* (161) and angiogenesis

in vivo (162). Such opposing actions on two different vascular cell types indicate that this glycoprotein plays a key and somewhat complicated role in regulating vascular cell growth.

Tenascin

Tenascin is a glycoprotein that is transiently present in the vascular ECM. This glycoprotein is a large hexameric protein with disulfide-linked multidomain subunits of 190 to 240 kD organized into a six-armed structure. Tenascin is composed of several distinct domains and resembles fibronectin in that a large part of the molecule is composed of fibronectin type III repeats. As is true of other ECM glycoproteins, more than one form of tenascin exists, generated by alternative splicing involving various exons that code for the type III repeats in the molecule (163).

Tenascin is an ECM glycoprotein with a spatially and temporally restricted distribution. It is present in the vascular ECM at early stages of embryonic vasculogenesis (164,165) and, like TSP, is present in increased levels in the neointima after experimental balloon angioplasty in animals (166,167) and in neointimal lesions of human coronary arteries after percutaneous transluminal coronary angioplasty (168). Furthermore, tenascin expression is increased in the arterialization of human vein grafts (169) and in hypertension (170).

Tenascin is synthesized by both vascular smooth muscle and endothelial cells and is regulated in part by factors such as PDGF, TGF-β_1, and angiotensin II (170,171). Tenascin influences vascular cell adhesion (172,173). For example, there is an RGD cell-binding domain in one of the fibronectin type III repeats within tenascin to which endothelial cells attach by $\alpha_2\beta_1$ and $\alpha_2\beta_3$ integrin receptors. However, tenascin also interferes with endothelial cell adhesion by causing disruption of focal adhesion sites and destabilizing endothelial cell attachment. Destabilization of cell contact is accompanied by the expression of tenascin splice variants lacking some of the type III fibronectin repeats, suggesting that different tenascin isoforms may differentially regulate cell attachment. Thus, the expression of vascular tenascin appears to be confined to cellular events associated with embryonic development and remodeling in vascular disease.

Osteopontin

Osteopontin is an acidic, highly phosphorylated glycoprotein first identified in bone but subsequently found in a variety of tissues including blood vessels (see review by Giachelli and coworkers [174]). Osteopontin is small compared to most ECM molecules and has an average molecular mass ranging from 44 to 85 kD. The protein contains an RGD cell-binding domain, two potential Ca^{2+} binding sites, and an HSPG binding domain as well. Osteopontin is encoded by a single gene, but alternatively spliced variants exist. Currently, functions associated with different splice variants of osteopontin are unknown.

Osteopontin is not present in the ECM of normal blood vessels, but it appears in the neointima after experimental balloon angioplasty and is present in human atherothrombotic plaques (175–178). There is a spatial and temporal expression of osteopontin that is coincident with the proliferation and migration of arterial smooth muscle cells during the invasion of the intima after vascular injury and in remodeling (179). The synthesis of osteopontin by arterial smooth muscle cells is partially regulated by cytokines such as basic fibroblast growth factor, TGF-β_1, and angiotensin II (see review by Giachelli and coworkers [174]). Osteopontin also is synthesized by macrophages, which may be an important source of this glycoprotein in the reaction to tissue injury (177). These observations suggest a role for osteopontin in the early events associated with vascular disease. Because it contains an RGD cell-binding motif, osteopontin could serve as an adhesive ligand for vascular cells during the early phases of vascular remodeling. In fact, osteopontin supports the adhesion of arterial smooth muscle and endothelial cells through the $\alpha_v\beta_3$ integrin, which is an integrin implicated in smooth muscle cell and endothelial migration (180,181). In addition, osteopontin is chemotactic for arterial smooth muscle cells.

The finding of osteopontin in advanced atherothrombotic lesions also suggests a role for this molecule in late events of vascular disease. Osteopontin tends to localize around areas of calcification in advanced human atherothrombotic plaques (see reviews by Giachelli and coworkers [174] and Shanahan and coworkers [182]). These findings, coupled with that osteopontin contains specific domains for Ca^{2+} binding, suggest a role for osteopontin in the calcification process involved in human disease. Whether this protein regulates arterial calcification remains to be determined.

Vitronectin

Vitronectin is a glycoprotein present in plasma and serum (183). Like several other glycoproteins, vitronectin serves as an attachment protein for vascular cells, interacting with these cells through the $\alpha_v\beta_3$ and $\alpha_v\beta_5$ integrin receptors (184). Vitronectin induces migration of smooth muscle cells in a Boyden chamber assay in an $\alpha_v\beta_3$-dependent manner. Vitronectin is up-regulated after vascular injury, as well as the $\alpha_v\beta_3$ and $\alpha_v\beta_5$ integrins (185). Blocking antibodies to vitronectin and the vitronectin integrins decreased intimal thickening after vascular injury, suggesting a critical role for vitronectin in the vascular injury response. Vitronectin is found in human atherothrombotic plaques (186).

SUMMARY

The vascular ECM is a collection of vastly different macromolecules organized into a highly ordered network in close association with the vascular cells that produce them. Each component of the ECM possesses unique structural properties that form the basis for their separate functions within vascular tissue. Together these molecules form the architectural framework of vascular tissue and the milieu for vascular cells. Considerable progress has been made within the past few years identifying specific ECM components that regulate key events in vascular wall physiology and pathology. Thus, it is now clear that the vascular ECM not only serves as a biomechanically active scaffold for blood vessel function, but it also plays a more complex role in regulating the behavior of vascular cells. Furthermore, because virtually all vascular pathology involves significant and specific changes in the vascular ECM, a more thorough understanding of the properties of this matrix and the factors that regulate synthesis and turnover of individual components of the ECM should hasten a cure for cardiovascular disease—the leading cause of death in the United States and Europe.

ACKNOWLEDGMENTS

This review was prepared with grant support from the National Institutes of Health (HL 18645-26 and DK02456-42). The author thanks Kathleen Braun for preparation of the figures, Anna Lewak Wight for careful editing, Dr. Susan Potter-Perigo for helpful discussions, and Ellen Briggs for assisting with the preparation of the manuscript.

REFERENCES

1. Barnes MJ. Collagens in atherosclerosis. *Coll Relat Res* 1985;5:65–97.
2. Rauterberg J, Jaeger E, Althaus M. Collagens in atherosclerotic vessel wall lesions. *Curr Top Pathol* 1993;87:163–192.
3. Clark JM, Glagov S. Transmural organization of the arterial media. The lamellar unit revisited. *Arteriosclerosis* 1985;5:19–34.
4. Walker-Caprioglio HM, Trotter JA, Little SA, et al. Organization of cells and extracellular matrix in mesenteric arteries of spontaneously hypertensive rats. *Cell Tissue Res* 1992;269:141–149.
5. Birk D, Silver F, Trelstad R. Matrix assembly. In: Hay E, ed. *Cell biology of the extracellular matrix.* New York: Plenum Press, 1991:221–254.
6. Kittelberger R, Davis PF, Greenhill NS. Immunolocalization of type VIII collagen in vascular tissue. *Biochem Biophys Res Commun* 1989;159:414–419.
7. Ang AH, Tachas G, Campbell JH, et al. Collagen synthesis by cultured rabbit aortic smooth-muscle cells. Alteration with phenotype. *Biochem J* 1990;265:461–469.
8. Rekhter MD. Collagen synthesis in atherosclerosis: too much and not enough. *Cardiovasc Res* 1999;41:376–384.
9. Miyazawa K, Kikuchi S, Fukuyama J, et al. Inhibition of PDGF- and TGF-beta 1-induced collagen synthesis, migration and proliferation by tranilast in vascular smooth muscle cells from spontaneously hypertensive rats. *Atherosclerosis* 1995;118:213–221.
10. McCaffrey TA, Pomerantz KB, Sanborn TA, et al. Specific inhibition of eIF-5A and collagen hydroxylation by a single agent. Antiproliferative and fibrosuppressive effects on smooth muscle cells from human coronary arteries. *J Clin Invest* 1995;95:446–455.
11. Nagler A, Miao HQ, Aingorn H, et al. Inhibition of collagen synthesis, smooth muscle cell proliferation, and injury-induced intimal hyperplasia by halofuginone. *Arterioscler Thromb Vasc Biol* 1997;17:194–202.
12. Rocnik EF, Chan BM, Pickering JG. Evidence for a role of collagen synthesis in arterial smooth muscle cell migration. *J Clin Invest* 1998;101:1889–1898.

13. Skinner MP, Raines EW, Ross R. Dynamic expression of alpha 1 beta 1 and alpha 2 beta 1 integrin receptors by human vascular smooth muscle cells. Alpha 2 beta 1 integrin is required for chemotaxis across type I collagen-coated membranes. *Am J Pathol* 1994;145:1070–1081.

14. Raines EW, Koyama H, Carragher NO. The extracellular matrix dynamically regulates smooth muscle cell responsiveness to PDGF. *Ann NY Acad Sci* 2000;902:39–52.

15. Pickering JG. Regulation of vascular cell behavior by collagen: form is function. *Circ Res* 2001;88:458–459.

16. Hou G, Vogel WF, Bendeck MP. Tyrosine kinase activity of discoidin domain receptor 1 is necessary for smooth muscle cell migration and matrix metalloproteinase expression. *Circ Res* 2002;90:1147–1149.

17. Vernon RB, Sage EH. Between molecules and morphology. Extracellular matrix and creation of vascular form. *Am J Pathol* 1995;147:873–883.

18. Lohler J, Timpl R, Jaenisch R. Embryonic lethal mutation in mouse collagen I gene causes rupture of blood vessels and is associated with erythropoietic and mesenchymal cell death. *Cell* 1984;38:597–607.

19. Pyeritz RE, Stolle CA, Parfrey NA, et al. Ehlers-Danlos syndrome IV due to a novel defect in type III procollagen. *Am J Med Genet* 1984;19:607–622.

20. Katsuda S, Okada Y, Minamoto T, et al. Collagens in human atherosclerosis. Immunohistochemical analysis using collagen type-specific antibodies. *Arterioscler Thromb* 1992;12:494–502.

21. Rekhter MD, Zhang K, Narayanan AS, et al. Type I collagen gene expression in human atherosclerosis. Localization to specific plaque regions. *Am J Pathol* 1993;143:1634–1648.

22. Bode MK, Mosorin M, Satta J, et al. Complete processing of type III collagen in atherosclerotic plaques. *Arterioscler Thromb Vasc Biol* 1999;19:1506–1511.

23. Coats WD Jr, Whittaker P, Cheung DT, et al. Collagen content is significantly lower in restenotic versus nonrestenotic vessels after balloon angioplasty in the atherosclerotic rabbit model. *Circulation* 1997;95:1293–1300.

24. Wight TN, Lara S, Reissen R, et al. Selective deposits of versican in the extracellular matrix of restenotic lesions from human peripheral arteries. *Am J Pathol* 1997;151:963–973.

25. Kovanen PT, Pentikainen MO. Decorin links low-density lipoproteins (LDL) to collagen: a novel mechanism for retention of LDL in the atherosclerotic plaque. *Trends Cardiovasc Med* 1999;9:86–91.

26. Libby P. Changing concepts of atherogenesis. *J Intern Med* 2000;247:349–358.

27. Rekhter MD, Hicks GW, Brammer DW, et al. Hypercholesterolemia causes mechanical weakening of rabbit atheroma: local collagen loss as a prerequisite of plaque rupture. *Circ Res* 2000;86:101–108.

28. Aikawa M, Rabkin E, Okada Y, et al. Lipid lowering by diet reduces matrix metalloproteinase activity and increases collagen content of rabbit atheroma: a potential mechanism of lesion stabilization. *Circulation* 1998;97:2433–2444.

29. Fukumoto Y, Libby P, Rabkin E, et al. Statins alter smooth muscle cell accumulation and collagen content in established atheroma of Watanabe heritable hyperlipidemic rabbits. *Circulation* 2001;103:993–999.

30. Nakata Y, Maeda N. Vulnerable atherosclerotic plaque morphology in apolipoprotein E-deficient mice unable to make ascorbic acid. *Circulation* 2002;105:1485–1490.

31. Fischer JW, Kinsella MG, Clowes MM, et al. Local expression of bovine decorin by cell-mediated gene transfer reduces neointimal formation after balloon injury in rats. *Circ Res* 2000;86:676–683.

32. Silver FH, Horvath I, Foran DJ. Viscoelasticity of the vessel wall: the role of collagen and elastic fibers. *Crit Rev Biomed Eng* 2001;29:279–301.

33. Rosenbloom J, Abrams WR, Mecham R. Extracellular matrix 4: the elastic fiber. *FASEB J* 1993;7:1208–1218.

34. Cleary E, Gibson M: Elastic tissue, elastin, and elastin associated proteins. In: Comper W, ed. *Extracellular matrix.* Amsterdam: Harwood Academic Publishers, 1996:95–140.

35. Wolinsky H, Glagov S. A lamellar unit of aortic medial structure and function in mammals. *Circ Res* 1967;20:99–111.

36. Ross R. The smooth muscle cell. II. Growth of smooth muscle in culture and formation of elastic fibers. *J Cell Biol* 1971;50:172–186.

37. Martin BM, Ritchie AR, Toselli P, et al. Elastin synthesis and accumulation in irradiated smooth muscle cell cultures. *Connect Tissue Res* 1992;28:181–189.

38. Davidson JM. Smad about elastin regulation. *Am J Respir Cell Mol Biol* 2002;26:164–166.

39. Bank RA, van Hinsbergh VW. Lysyl oxidase: new looks on LOX. *Arterioscler Thromb Vasc Biol* 2002;22:1365–1366.

40. Hinek A, Wrenn DS, Mecham RP, et al. The elastin receptor: a galactoside-binding protein. *Science* 1988;239:1539–1541.

41. Hinek A, Mecham RP, Keeley F, et al. Impaired elastin fiber assembly related to reduced 67-kD elastin-binding protein in fetal lamb ductus arteriosus and in cultured aortic smooth muscle cells treated with chondroitin sulfate. *J Clin Invest* 1991;88:2083–2094.

42. Hinek A, Boyle J, Rabinovitch M. Vascular smooth muscle cell detachment from elastin and migration through elastic laminae is promoted by chondroitin sulfate-induced "shedding" of the 67-kDa cell surface elastin binding protein. *Exp Cell Res* 1992;203:344–353.

43. Yanagisawa H, Davis EC, Starcher BC, et al. Fibulin-5 is an elastin-binding protein essential for elastic fibre development in vivo. *Nature* 2002;415:168–171.

44. Nakamura T, Lozano PR, Ikeda Y, et al. Fibulin-5/DANCE is essential for elastogenesis in vivo. *Nature* 2002;415:171–175.

45. Midwood KS, Schwarzbauer JE. Elastic fibers: building bridges between cells and their matrix. *Curr Biol* 2002;12:R279–R281.

46. Mochizuki S, Brassart B, Hinek A. Signaling pathways transduced through the elastin receptor facilitate proliferation of arterial smooth muscle cells. *J Biol Chem* 2002;277:44854–44863.

47. Li DY, Brooke B, Davis EC, et al. Elastin is an essential determinant of arterial morphogenesis. *Nature* 1998;393:276–280.

48. Milewicz DM, Urban Z, Boyd C. Genetic disorders of the elastic fiber system. *Matrix Biol* 2000;19:471–480.

49. Ramirez F, Pereira L, Zhang H, et al. The fibrillin-Marfan syndrome connection. *Bioessays* 1993;15:589–594.

50. Medley TL, Cole TJ, Gatzka CD, et al. Fibrillin-1 genotype is associated with aortic stiffness and disease severity in patients with coronary artery disease. *Circulation* 2002;105:810–815.

51. Sandberg LB, Soskel NT, Leslie JG. Elastin structure, biosynthesis, and relation to disease states. *N Engl J Med* 1981;304:566–579.

52. Robert L, Jacob MP, Frances C, et al. Interaction between elastin and elastases and its role in the aging of the arterial wall, skin and other connective tissues. A review. *Mech Ageing Dev* 1984;28:155–166.

53. Davis PF, Ryan PA, Osipowicz J, et al. The biochemical composition of hemodynamically stressed vascular tissue: the insoluble elastin of experimental arteriovenous fistulae. *Exp Mol Pathol* 1989;51:103–110.

54. Cohen JR, Sarfati I, Danna D, et al. Smooth muscle cell elastase, atherosclerosis, and abdominal aortic aneurysms. *Ann Surg* 1992;216:327–332.

55. Brown DL, Hibbs MS, Kearney M, et al. Identification of 92-kD gelatinase in human coronary atherosclerotic lesions. Association of active enzyme synthesis with unstable angina. *Circulation* 1995;91:2125–2131.

56. Galis ZS, Sukhova GK, Lark MW, et al. Increased expression of matrix metalloproteinases and matrix degrading activity in vulnerable regions of human atherosclerotic plaques. *J Clin Invest* 1994;94:2493–2503.

57. Sukhova GK, Shi GP, Simon DI, et al. Expression of the elastolytic cathepsins S and K in human atheroma and regulation of their production in smooth muscle cells. *J Clin Invest* 1998;102:576–583.

58. Todorovich-Hunter L, Dodo H, Ye C, et al. Increased pulmonary artery elastolytic activity in adult rats with monocrotaline-induced progressive hypertensive pulmonary vascular disease compared with infant rats with nonprogressive disease. *Am Rev Respir Dis* 1992;146:213–223.

59. Cowan KN, Heilbut A, Humpl T, et al. Complete reversal of fatal pulmonary hypertension in rats by a serine elastase inhibitor. *Nat Med* 2000;6:698–702.

60. Merrilees MJ, Lemire JM, Fischer JW, et al. Retrovirally mediated overexpression of versican v3 by arterial smooth muscle cells induces tropoelastin synthesis and elastic fiber formation in vitro and in neointima after vascular injury. *Circ Res* 2002;90:481–487.

61. Winlove CP, Parker KH, Ewins AR. Some factors influencing the interactions of plasma lipoproteins with arterial elastin. *Artery* 1988;15:292–303.

62. Kramsch DM, Hollander W. The interaction of serum and arterial lipoproteins with elastin of the arterial intima and its role in the lipid accumulation in atherosclerotic plaques. *J Clin Invest* 1973;52:236–247.

63. Saulnier JM, Hauck M, Fulop T Jr, et al. Human aortic elastin from normal individuals and atherosclerotic patients: lipid and cation contents; susceptibility to elastolysis. *Clin Chim Acta* 1991;200:129–136.

64. Guyton JR, Bocan TM, Schifani TA. Quantitative ultrastructural analysis of perifibrous lipid and its association with elastin in nonatherosclerotic human aorta. *Arteriosclerosis* 1985;5:644–652.

65. Srinivasan SR, Yost C, Radhakrishnamurthy B, et al. Lipoprotein-elastin interactions in human aorta fibrous plaque lesions. *Atherosclerosis* 1981;38:137–147.

66. Jordan RE, Hewitt N, Lewis W, et al. Regulation of elastase-catalyzed hydrolysis of insoluble elastin by synthetic and naturally occurring hydrophobic ligands. *Biochemistry* 1974;13:3497–3503.

67. Kagan HM, Milbury PE Jr, Kramsch DM. A possible role for elastin ligands in the proteolytic degradation of arterial elastic lamellae in the rabbit. *Circ Res* 1979;44:95–103.

68. Juul S, Ledbetter D, Wight TN, et al. New insights into idiopathic infantile arterial calcinosis. Three patient reports. *Am J Dis Child* 1990;144:229–233.

69. Dobryshev YV, Lord RS, Warren BA. Calcified deposit formation in intimal thickenings of the human aorta. *Atherosclerosis* 1995;118:9–21.

70. Niederhoffer N, Lartaud-Idjouadiene I, Giummelly P, et al. Calcification of medial elastic fibers and aortic elasticity. *Hypertension* 1997;29:999–1006.

71. Vyavahare N, Jones PL, Tallapragada S, et al. Inhibition of matrix metalloproteinase activity attenuates tenascin-C production and calcification of implanted purified elastin in rats. *Am J Pathol* 2000;157: 885–893.

72. Rucker RB, Ford D, Riemann WG, et al. Additional evidence for the binding of calcium ions to elastin at neutral sites. *Calcif Tissue Res* 1974;14:317–325.

73. Camejo G. The interaction of lipids and lipoproteins with the intercellular matrix of arterial tissue: its possible role in atherogenesis. *Adv Lipid Res* 1982;19:1–53.

74. Radhakrishnamurthy B, Srinivasan SR, Vijayagopal P, et al. Arterial wall proteoglycans—biological properties related to pathogenesis of atherosclerosis. *Eur Heart J* 1990;11:148–157.

75. Williams KJ, Tabas I. The response-to-retention hypothesis of atherogenesis reinforced. *Curr Opin Lipidol* 1998;9:471–474.

76. Rosenberg RD, Shworak NW, Liu J, et al. Heparan sulfate proteoglycans of the cardiovascular system. Specific structures emerge but how is synthesis regulated? *J Clin Invest* 1997;100:S67–S75.

77. Wight TN. Cell biology of arterial proteoglycans. *Arteriosclerosis* 1989;9:1–20.

78. Toole BP, Wight TN, Tammi MI. Hyaluronan-cell interactions in cancer and vascular disease. *J Biol Chem* 2002;277:4593–4596.

79. Wight T, Heinegard D, Hascall V. Proteoglycans: structure and function. In Hay E, ed. *Cell biology of extracellular matrix*. New York, Plenum Press, 1991.

80. Iozzo R, ed. *Proteoglycans: stucture, biology, and molecular interactions*. New York: Marcel Dekker, 2000.

81. Jarvelainen H, Wight T. Vascular proteoglycans. In: Garg H, Roughly P, Hales P, eds. *Proteoglycans in lung disease*. New York: Marcel Dekker, 2002.

82. Yao LY, Moody C, Schönherr E, et al. Identification of the proteoglycan versican in aorta and smooth muscle cells by DNA sequence analysis, in situ hybridization and immunohistochemistry. *Matrix Biol* 1994;14:213–225.

83. Dreher KL, Asundi V, Matzura D, et al. Vascular smooth muscle biglycan represents a highly conserved proteoglycan within the arterial wall. *Eur J Cell Biol* 1990;53:296–304.

84. Stocker G, Meyer HE, Wagener C, et al. Purification and N-terminal amino acid sequence of a chondroitin sulfate/dermatan sulfate proteoglycan isolated from intima/media preparations of human aorta. *Biochem J* 1991;274:415–420.

85. Funderburgh JL, Funderburgh ML, Mann MM, et al. Arterial lumican. Properties of a corneal-type keratan sulfate proteoglycan from bovine aorta. *J Biol Chem* 1991;266:24773–24777.

86. Clowes AW, Clowes MM, Gown AM, et al. Localization of proteoheparan sulfate in rat aorta. *Histochemistry* 1984;80:379–384.

87. Danielson KG, Baribault H, Holmes DF, et al. Targeted disruption of decorin leads to abnormal collagen fibril morphology and skin fragility. *J Cell Biol* 1997;136:729–743.

88. Dunlevy J, Hassell J. Heparan sulfate proteoglycans in basement membranes. In: Iozzo R, ed. *Proteoglycans: structure, biology and molecular interactions*. New York: Marcel Dekker, 2000:275–326.

89. Merrilees MJ, Beaumont B, Scott LJ. Comparison of deposits of versican, biglycan and decorin in saphenous vein and internal thoracic,

90. Binette F, Cravens J, Kahoussi B, et al. Link protein is ubiquitously expressed in non-cartilaginous tissues where it enhances and stabilizes the interaction of proteoglycans with hyaluronic acid. *J Biol Chem* 1994;269:19116–19122.

91. Comper WD, Laurent TC. Physiological function of connective tissue polysaccharides. *Physiol Rev* 1978;58:255–315.

92. Schönherr E, Järveläinen HT, Sandell LJ, et al. Effects of platelet-derived growth factor and transforming growth factor-beta 1 on the synthesis of a large versican-like chondroitin sulfate proteoglycan by arterial smooth muscle cells. *J Biol Chem* 1991;266:17640–17647.

93. Schönherr E, Järveläinen HT, Kinsella MG, et al. Platelet-derived growth factor and transforming growth factor-β1 differentially affect the synthesis of biglycan and decorin by monkey arterial smooth muscle cells. *Arterioscler Thromb* 1993;13:1026–1036.

94. Schönherr E, Kinsella MG, Wight TN. Genistein selectively inhibits platelet-derived growth factor stimulated versican biosynthesis in monkey arterial smooth muscle cells. *Arch Biochem Biophys* 1997;339: 353–361.

95. Evanko SP, Johnson PY, Braun KR, et al. Platelet-derived growth factor stimulates the formation of versican-hyaluronan aggregates and pericellular matrix expansion in arterial smooth muscle cells. *Arch Biochem Biophys* 2001;394:29–38.

96. Evanko SP, Angello JC, Wight TN. Formation of hyaluronan and versican-rich pericellular matrix is required for proliferation and migration of vascular smooth muscle cells. *Arterioscler Thromb Vasc Biol* 1999;19:1004–1013.

97. Weiser MC, Grieshaber NA, Schwartz PE, et al. Perlecan regulates Oct-1 gene expression in vascular smooth muscle cells. *Mol Biol Cell* 1997;8:999–1011.

98. Bingley JA, Campbell JH, Hayward IP, et al. Inhibition of neointimal formation by natural heparan sulfate proteoglycans of the arterial wall. *Ann NY Acad Sci* 1997;811:238–244.

99. Paka L, Goldberg IJ, Obunike JC, et al. Perlecan mediates the antiproliferative effect of apolipoprotein E on smooth muscle cells. An underlying mechanism for the modulation of smooth muscle cell growth? *J Biol Chem* 1999;274:36403–36408.

100. Nugent MA, Nugent HM, Iozzo RV, et al. Perlecan is required to inhibit thrombosis after deep vascular injury and contributes to endothelial cell-mediated inhibition of intimal hyperplasia. *Proc Natl Acad Sci USA* 2000;97:6722–6727.

101. Järveläinen HT, Kinsella MG, Wight TN, et al. Differential expression of small chondroitin/dermatan sulfate proteoglycans, PG-I/biglycan and PG-II/decorin, by vascular smooth muscle and endothelial cells in culture. *J Biol Chem* 1991;266:23274–23281.

102. Bosse A, Schwarz K, Vollmer E, et al. Divergent and co-localization of the two small proteoglycans decorin and proteoglycan-100 in human skeletal tissues and tumors. *J Histochem Cytochem* 1993;41:13–19.

103. Järveläinen HT, Iruela-Arispe ML, Kinsella MG, et al. Expression of decorin by sprouting bovine aortic endothelial cells exhibiting angiogenesis in vitro. *Exp Cell Res* 1992;203:395–401.

104. Nelimarkka L, Salminen H, Kuopio T, et al. Decorin is produced by capillary endothelial cells in inflammation-associated angiogenesis. *Am J Pathol* 2001;158:345–353.

105. Wasty F, Alavi MZ, Moore S. Distribution of glycosaminoglycans in the intima of human aortas: changes in atherosclerosis and diabetes mellitus. *Diabetologia* 1993;36:316–322.

106. Heickendorff L, Ledet T, Rasmussen LM. Glycosaminoglycans in the human aorta in diabetes mellitus: a study of tunica media from areas with and without atherosclerotic plaque. *Diabetologia* 1994;37:286–292.

107. Chajara A, Raoudi M, Delpech B, et al. Effects of diabetes and insulin treatment of diabetic rats on hyaluronan and hyaluronectin production in injured aorta. *J Vasc Res* 1999;36:209–221.

108. Camejo G, Olsson U, Hurt-Camejo E, et al. The extracellular matrix on atherogenesis and diabetes-associated vascular disease. *Atheroscler Suppl* 2002;3:3–9.

109. Wight TN. Proteoglycans and hyaluronan in vascular disease. In: Ernst B, Hart G, Sinay P. *Oligosaccharides in chemistry and biology*. Weinheim, Germany: Wiley VCH, 1999.

110. Gutierrez PS, Reis MM, Higuchi ML, et al. Distribution of hyaluronan and dermatan/chondroitin sulfate proteoglycans in human aortic dissection. *Connect Tissue Res* 1998;37:151–161.

111. Lin H, Wilson JE, Roberts CR, et al. Biglycan, decorin and versican protein expression patterns in coronary arteriopathy of human cardiac allograft: distinctness as compared to native atherosclerosis. *J Heart Lung Transplant* 1996;15:1233–1247.

112. Halpert I, Sires U, Potter-Perigo S, et al. Matrilysin is expressed by lipid-laden macrophages at sites of potential rupture in atherosclerotic lesions and localized to areas of versican deposits. *Proc Natl Acad Sci USA* 1996;93:9748–9753.

113. Evanko S, Raines EW, Ross R, et al. Proteoglycan distribution in lesions of atherosclerosis depends on lesion severity, structural characteristics and the proximity of PDGF and TGF-β1. *Am J Pathol* 1998;152:533–546.

114. Kolodgie F, Burke A, Farb A, et al. Differential accumulation of proteoglycans and hyaluronan in culprit lesions: insights into plaque erosion. *Arterioscler Thromb Vasc Biol* 2002;22:1642–1648.

115. O'Brien KD, Olin KL, Alpers CE, et al. A comparison of apolipoprotein and proteoglycan deposits in human coronary atherosclerotic plaques: co-localization of biglycan with apolipoproteins. *Circulation* 1998;98:519–527.

116. Olin KL, Potter-Perigo S, Barrett PH, et al. Lipoprotein lipase enhances the binding of native and oxidized low density lipoproteins to versican and biglycan synthesized by cultured arterial smooth muscle cells. *J Biol Chem* 1999;274:34629–34636.

117. Qin H, Ishiwata T, Asano G. Effects of the extracellular matrix on lumican expression in rat aortic smooth muscle cells in vitro. *J Pathol* 2001;195:604–608.

118. Onda M, Ishiwata T, Kawahara K, et al. Expression of lumican in thickened intima and smooth muscle cells in human coronary atherosclerosis. *Exp Mol Pathol* 2002;72:142–149.

119. Richardson M, Ihnatowycz, I, Moore S. Glycosaminoglycan distribution in rabbit aortic wall following balloon catheter deendothelialization. An ultrastructural study. *Lab Invest* 1980;43:509–516.

120. Nikkari ST, Järveläinen HT, Wight TN, et al. Smooth muscle cell expression of extracellular matrix genes after arterial injury. *Am J Pathol* 1994;144:1348–1356.

121. Chajara A, Levesque H, Courel MN, et al. Hyaluronan and hyaluronectin production in injured rat thoracic aorta. *Atherosclerosis* 1996;125:193–207.

122. Riessen R, Wight TN, Pastore C, et al. Distribution of hyaluronan during extracellular matrix remodeling in human restenotic arteries and balloon-injured rat carotid arteries. *Circulation* 1996;93:1141–1147.

123. Merrilees MJ, Scott L. Antisense S-oligonucleotide against transforming growth factor-beta 1 inhibits proteoglycan synthesis in arterial wall. *J Vasc Res* 1994;31:322–329.

124. Wolf YG, Rasmussen LM, Ruoslahti E. Antibodies against transforming growth factor-β1 suppress intimal hyperplasia in a rat model. *J Clin Invest* 1994;93:1172–1178.

125. Weinbaum S, Chien S. Lipid transport aspects of atherogenesis. *J Biomech Eng* 1993;115:602–610.

126. Williams KJ, Tabas I. The response-to-retention hypothesis of early atherogenesis. *Arterioscler Thromb Vasc Biol* 1995;15:551–561.

127. Jackson RL, Busch SJ, Cardin AD. Glycosaminoglycans: molecular properties, protein interactions and role in physiological processes. *Physiol Rev* 1991;71:481–539.

128. Camejo G, Hurt-Camejo E, Wiklund O, et al. Association of apo B lipoproteins with arterial proteoglycans: pathological significance and molecular basis. *Atherosclerosis* 1998;139:205–222.

129. Chait A, Wight TN. Interaction of native and modified low-density lipoproteins with extracellular matrix. *Curr Opin Lipidol* 2000;11:457–463.

130. Goldberg IJ. Lipoprotein lipase and lipolysis: central roles in lipoprotein metabolism and atherogenesis. *J Lipid Res* 1996;37:693–707.

131. Pentikainen MO, Oksjoki R, Oorni K, et al. Lipoprotein lipase in the arterial wall: linking LDL to the arterial extracellular matrix and much more. *Arterioscler Thromb Vasc Biol* 2002;22:211–217.

132. Borén J, Olin K, Lee I, et al. Identification of a principal proteoglycan binding site in LDL: a single point mutation in apo B-100 severely affects proteoglycan interaction without affecting LDL receptor binding. *J Clin Invest* 1998;101:2658–2664.

133. Skalen K, Gustafsson M, Rydberg EK, et al. Subendothelial retention of atherogenic lipoproteins in early atherosclerosis. *Nature* 2002;417:750–754.

134. Conde-Knape K. Heparan sulfate proteoglycans in experimental models of diabetes: a role for perlecan in diabetes complications. *Diabetes Metab Res Rev* 2001;17:412–421.

135. Bourin MC, Lindahl U. Glycosaminoglycans and the regulation of blood coagulation. *Biochem J* 1993;289:313–330.

136. Whinna HC, Choi HU, Rosenberg LC, et al. Interaction of heparin cofactor II with biglycan and decorin. *J Biol Chem* 1993;268:3920–3924.

137. Schwarzbauer JE. Alternative splicing of fibronectin—three variants, three functions. *Bioessays* 1991;13:527–533.

138. Saouaf R, Takasaki I, Eastman E, et al. Fibronectin biosynthesis in the rat aorta in vivo: changes due to experimental hypertension. *J Clin Invest* 1991;88:1182–1189.

139. Takasaki I, Chobanian AV, Mamuya WS, et al. Hypertension induces alternatively spliced forms of fibronectin in rat aorta. *Hypertension* 1992;20:20–25.

140. Stenman S, Vaheri A. Distribution of a major connective tissue protein, fibronectin, in normal human tissues. *J Exp Med* 1978;147:1054–1064.

141. Smith EB, Ashall C. Fibronectin distribution in human aortic intima and atherosclerotic lesions: concentration of soluble and collagenase-releasable fractions. *Biochim Biophys Acta* 1986;880:10–15.

142. Rasmussen LH, Garbarsch C, Chemnitz J, et al. Injury and repair of smaller muscular and elastic arteries. *Virchows Arch A Pathol Anat Histopathol* 1989;415:579–585.

143. Boudreau N, Turley E, Rabinovitch M. Fibronectin, hyaluronan and a hyaluronan binding protein contribute to increased ductus arteriosus smooth muscle cell migration. *Dev Biol* 1991;143:235–247.

144. Molossi S, Clausell N, Rabinovitch M. Coronary artery endothelial interleukin-1 beta mediates enhanced fibronectin production related to post-cardiac transplant arteriopathy in piglets. *Circulation* 1993;88:II248–II256.

145. Clausell N, Rabinovitch M. Upregulation of fibronectin synthesis by interleukin-1 beta in coronary artery smooth muscle cells is associated with the development of the post-cardiac transplant arteriopathy in piglets. *J Clin Invest* 1993;92:1850–1858.

146. Clausell N, de Lima VC, Molossi S, et al. Expression of tumour necrosis factor α and accumulation of fibronectin in coronary artery restenotic lesions retrieved by atherectomy. *Br Heart J* 1995;73:534–539.

147. van der Hoek YY, Sangrar W, Cote GP, et al. Binding of recombinant apolipoprotein(a) to extracellular matrix proteins. *Arterioscler Thromb* 1994;14:1792–1798.

148. Casscells W. Migration of smooth muscle and endothelial cells. Critical events in restenosis. *Circulation* 1992;86:723–729.

149. Tryggvasson K. The laminin family. *Curr Opin Cell Biol* 1993;5:877–882.

150. Grant DS, Tashiro KI, Segui-Real B, et al. Two different laminin domains mediate the differentiation of human endothelial cells into capillary-like structures in vitro. *Cell* 1989;58:933–943.

151. Schnaper HW, Kleinman HK, Grant DS. Role of laminin in endothelial cell recognition and differentiation. *Kidney Int* 1993;43:20–25.

152. Hedin U, Bottger BA, Forsberg E, et al. Diverse effects of fibronectin and laminin on phenotypic properties of cultured arterial smooth muscle cells. *J Cell Biol* 1988;107:307–319.

153. Thyberg J, Hultgardh-Nilsson A. Fibronectin and the basement membrane components laminin and collagen type IV influence the phenotypic properties of subcultured rat aortic smooth muscle cells differently. *Cell Tissue Res* 1994;276:263–271.

154. Bornstein P. Thrombospondins: structure and regulation of expression. *FASEB J* 1992;6:3290–3299.

155. Schultz-Cherry S, Chen H, Mosher DF, et al. Regulation of transforming growth factor-β activation by discrete sequences of thrombospondin 1. *J Biol Chem* 1995;270:7304–7310.

156. Sage EH, Bornstein P. Extracellular proteins that modulate cell-matrix interactions. *J Biol Chem* 1991;266:14831–14834.

157. Wight T, Raugi GJ, Mumby SM, et al. Light microscopic immunolocalization of thrombospondin secretion in human tissues. *J Histochem Cytochem* 1984;33:280–288.

158. Miano JM, Vlasic N, Tota RR, et al. Smooth muscle cell immediate-early gene and growth factor activation follows vascular injury. A putative in vivo mechanism for autocrine growth. *Arterioscler Thromb* 1993;13:211–219.

159. Majack RA, Goodman LV, Dixit VM. Cell surface thrombospondin is functionally essential for vascular smooth muscle proliferation. *J Cell Biol* 1988;106:415–422.

160. Scott-Burden T, Resink TJ, Hahn AW, et al. Induction of throm-

bospondin expression in vascular smooth muscle cells by angiotensin II. *J Cardiovasc Pharmacol* 1990;16[Suppl 7]:S17–S20.

161. Taraboletti G, Roberts D, Liotta LA, et al. Platelet thrombospondin modulates endothelial cell adhesion, motility, and growth: a potential angiogenesis regulatory factor. *J Cell Biol* 1990;111:765–772.

162. Good DJ, Polverini PJ, Rastinejad F, et al. A tumor suppressor-dependent inhibitor of angiogenesis is immunologically and functionally indistinguishable from a fragment of thrombospondin. *Proc Natl Acad Sci USA* 1990;87:6624–6628.

163. Erickson HP. Tenascin-C, tenascin-R and tenascin-X: a family of talented proteins in search of functions. *Curr Opin Cell Biol* 1993;5: 869–876.

164. Hurle JM, Garcia-Martinez V, Ros MA. Immunofluorescent localization of tenascin during the morphogenesis of the outflow tract of the chick embryo heart. *Anat Embryol* 1990;181:149–155.

165. Riou JF, Umbhauer M, Shi DL, et al. Tenascin: a potential modulator of cell-extracellular matrix interactions during vertebrate embryogenesis. *Biol Cell* 1992;75:1–9.

166. Hedin U, Holm J, Hansson GK. Induction of tenascin in rat arterial injury. *Am J Pathol* 1991;139:649–656.

167. Wallner K, Shah PK, Sharifi BG. Balloon catheterization induces arterial expression of new Tenascin-C isoform. *Atherosclerosis* 2002; 161:75–83.

168. Imanaka-Yoshida K, Matsuura R, Isaka N, et al. Serial extracellular matrix changes in neointimal lesions of human coronary artery after percutaneous transluminal coronary angioplasty: clinical significance of early tenascin-C expression. *Virchows Arch* 2001;439:185–190.

169. Wallner K, Li C, Fishbein MC, et al. Arterialization of human vein grafts is associated with tenascin-C expression. *J Am Coll Cardiol* 1999;34:871–875.

170. Mackie EJ, Scott-Burden T, Hahn AW, et al. Expression of tenascin by vascular smooth muscle cells. Alterations in hypertensive rats and stimulation by angiotensin II. *Am J Pathol* 1992;141:377–388.

171. LaFleur DW, Fagin JA, Forrester JS, et al. Cloning and characterization of alternatively spliced isoforms of tenascin. Platelet-derived growth factor-BB markedly stimulates expression of spliced variants of tenascin mRNA in arterial smooth muscle cells. *J Biol Chem* 1994;269:20757–20763.

172. Murphy-Ullrich JE, Lightner VA, Aukhil I, et al. Focal adhesion integrity is downregulated by the alternatively spliced domain of human tenascin. *J Cell Biol* 1991;115:1127–1136.

173. Sriramarao P, Mendler M, Bourdon MA. Endothelial cell attachment and spreading on human tenascin is mediated by alpha 2 beta 1 and alpha v beta 3 integrins. *J Cell Sci* 1993;105:1001–1012.

174. Giachelli CM, Liaw L, Murry CE, et al. Osteopontin expression in cardiovascular disease. *Ann NY Acad Sci* 1995;760:109–126.

175. Hirota S, Imakita M, Kohri K, et al. Expression of osteopontin messenger RNA by macrophages in atherosclerotic plaques. *Am J Pathol* 1993;143:1003–1008.

176. Ikeda T, Shiraswa T, Esaki Y, et al. Osteopontin mRNA is expressed by smooth muscle derived foam cells in human atherosclerotic lesions of the aorta. *J Clin Invest* 1993;92:2814–2820.

177. O'Brien ER, Garvin MR, Stewart DK, et al. Osteopontin is synthesized by macrophage, smooth muscle, and endothelial cells in primary and restenotic human coronary atherosclerotic plaques. *Arterioscler Thromb* 1994;14:1648–1656.

178. Gadeau AP, Campan M, Millet D, et al. Osteopontin overexpression is associated with arterial smooth muscle cell proliferation in vitro. *Arterioscler Thromb* 1993;13.120–125.

179. Isoda K, Nishikawa K, Kamezawa Y, et al. Osteopontin plays an important role in the development of medial thickening and neointimal formation. *Circ Res* 2002;91:77–82.

180. Choi ET, Engel L, Callow AD, et al. Inhibition of neointimal hyperplasia by blocking alpha V beta 3 integrin with a small peptide antagonist GpenGRGDSPCA. *J Vasc Surg* 1994;19:125–134.

181. Brooks PC, Montgomery AM, Rosenfeld M, et al. Integrin alpha 3 beta v antagonists promote tumor regression by inducing apoptosis of angiogenic blood vessels. *Cell* 1994;79:1157–1164.

182. Shanahan CM, Cary NR, Metcalfe JC, et al. High expression of genes for calcification-regulating proteins in human atherosclerotic plaques. *J Clin Invest* 1994;93:2393–2402.

183. Preissner KT, Jenne D. Vitronectin: a new molecular connection in haemostasis. *Thromb Haemost* 1991;66:189–194.

184. Stefansson S, Lawrence DA. The serpin PAI-1 inhibits cell migration by blocking integrin alpha V beta 3 binding to vitronectin. *Nature* 1996;383:441–443.

185. Dufourcq P, Couffinhal T, Alzieu P, et al. Vitronectin is up-regulated after vascular injury and vitronectin blockade prevents neointima formation. *Cardiovasc Res* 2002;53:952–962.

186. Dufourcq P, Louis H, Moreau C, et al. Vitronectin expression and interaction with receptors in smooth muscle cells from human atheromatous plaque. *Arterioscler Thromb Vasc Biol* 1998;18:168–176.

The Lesions of Atherothrombosis

CHAPTER **30**

Histologic Classification of Human Atherosclerotic Lesions

Herbert Christian Stary

Key Words: Aorta; atherosclerotic lesion development; atherosclerotic lesion regression; calcification; coronary arteries; pathology; thrombosis.

INTRODUCTION

This chapter describes the successive morphologic steps in the development of atherosclerotic disease—from the initial, only microscopically visible, lipid-filled macrophages in susceptible locations of arteries to lesions that produce clinical symptoms. Also described is the effect of drastic therapeutic reduction of high blood cholesterol levels on the components of the various types of lesion. The information on lesion development and progression relies in large part on an autopsy study of a large human population extending in age from childhood to middle age (1,2), whereas the data on lesion regression come from a series of studies in rhesus monkeys (3).

In all studies, coronary arteries and aortas were sectioned at close intervals along the length of standard segments highly susceptible to the formation of advanced (clinically important) atherosclerotic lesions. Evaluation of plastic-embedded, only 1-μm-thick sections by light microscopy al-

lowed three-dimensional reconstruction of the structure and composition of the susceptible segments and of the lesions contained therein. Because of the extreme thinness of the large sections superior detail of structure and components was obtained. Additional detail of smaller areas or cells was obtained through the use of electron microscopy. The coronary arteries and their lesions had been restored to their *in vivo* dimensions and configurations through fixation by perfusion with glutaraldehyde at approximately physiologic pressures.

The sequence in the evolution of human lesions was deduced by comparing the lesions at different ages. The approach was to characterize the intima in the susceptible segments of infants and children and then to study the same locations in adolescents and adults. The contiguous nature of the changes and the time of life at which characteristic types of lesions occurred and predominated provide strong evidence that each type represents a gradation or stage in a temporal sequence.

CLASSIFICATION OF ATHEROSCLEROTIC LESIONS ACCORDING TO THEIR PATHWAYS OF DEVELOPMENT

Currently, various classifications of human atherosclerotic lesions, many specialized and with focused objectives, are in use. How lesions are described and classified depends on the objectives and on whether the lesions are imaged in living

H. C. Stary: Department of Pathology, Louisiana State University Health Sciences Center, 1901 Perdido Street, New Orleans, Louisiana 70112.

persons or examined at autopsy or after resection in the course of a therapeutic procedure. How closely the true nature of lesions is reflected in a classification depends on the sensitivity of the techniques used in each instance.

In pathology, two classifications developed through the study of vessels and lesions obtained at autopsy are used. The older one is a gross classification that is primarily based on examination of vessels and lesions with the unaided eye, consisting of a sequence of four lesion types (fatty streak, fibrous plaque, complicated lesion, and calcified plaque). A far more precise classification emerged when standard highly susceptible vessel segments were studied using state-of-the-art histologic methods, with eight types of lesion being identified (Fig. 30–1) (3).

The roman numerals assigned to lesion types in the histologic classification indicate the sequence in which characteristic components appear or are added. At least this statement applies to the first half of the classification which covers the steps in the evolution to atheroma (type IV lesion). Once this stage is reached, the mechanisms of further progression are less predictable and the higher numerals indicate possible morphologic outcomes rather than predicting a set chronologic sequence. The *arrows* in Figure 30–1 indicate the diversity of pathways that commonly take place.

Most children have some lipid-filled macrophages in the intima in susceptible locations of the arterial system. Minimal accumulations of such cells (lesion types I and II) do not

disorganize or deform the arterial wall, and most stabilize at that level and do not progress. Yet, after puberty, some people have, at a predictable subset of susceptible points, lesions with an additional feature (type III, preatheroma) that histologically renders them the link between the minimal changes and the first clinically important lesion type (type IV, atheroma).

After type IV has formed, mechanisms of progression include the development of various types of surface defect, thrombotic deposits, and hematoma. Lesions with these additional features are labeled type VI. Other features predominate in lesions labeled type V, VII, or VIII.

Lesion types IV to VIII are collectively regarded as clinically important because histologically they include tissue destruction to a degree that makes them susceptible to thrombus formation and because some degree of arterial wall thickening is present. Although clinically important by histologic criteria, some of these lesions (particularly many type IV) cause little narrowing of the arterial lumen and are not visible on angiography. Many potentially clinical lesions remain silent for a lifetime.

The sequence of changes in lesions that are regressing has been determined in experiments with rhesus monkeys (see "Sequence of Histologic Changes During Lesion Regression ") and extrapolation to the human situation is possible. When high blood cholesterol is drastically reduced, lesion types I to III can disappear completely and lesion

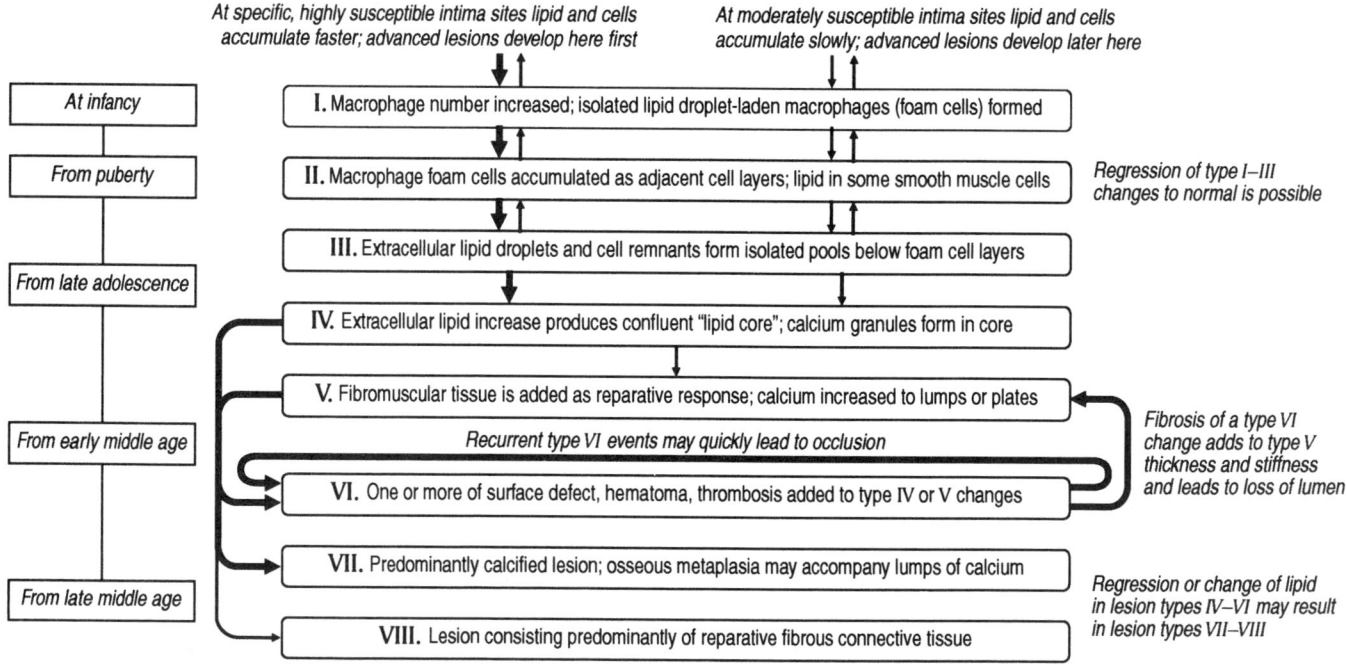

FIG. 30–1. Pathways of atherosclerosis progression and regression. The order in which distinct lesion types usually develop is designated with the numerals I to VIII. Diagram lists the main histologic characteristics of each sequential step (lesion type). *Thick* or *thin arrows* differentiate between the relative ease with which lesions develop in specific locations, or they indicate the relative frequency and importance of a specific pathway section.

types IV to VI may decrease in size and assume the compositions of types VII and VIII.

Working with the histologic classification, we found the same sequence of lesion types in coronary arteries and aortas and, except for size, no fundamental differences between lesions in the two vascular beds. Nevertheless, some authors have described differences between the clinically important lesions of specific vascular beds: less lipid and more hematoma in carotid than coronary arteries, and longer lesions with more calcium and thrombus in leg arteries (besides the involvement also of small arteries in the legs of patients with diabetes).

In this chapter the term *atherosclerosis* is used for the entire disease process, including the minimal changes, even though, in many people, minimal lesions will not proceed and develop into clinically important ones. It also is understood that atherosclerosis includes lesions with thrombus, as well as other components besides lipid and reparative fibrous tissue (sclerosis).

Subsequent sections of this chapter describe the characteristic types (i.e., the developmental stages) of lesions. But to understand lesions, the nature of vascular sites at which clinically important lesions mostly develop must first be understood.

NORMAL ASYMMETRIES IN ARTERIAL WALL THICKNESS, FLOW MECHANICAL FORCES, AND ARTERIAL SITES SUSCEPTIBLE TO LIPID ACCUMULATION

An artery responds to normal asymmetries in flow along its course and around its circumference by adjusting its contour, wall thickness, and lumen size. Arteries thus have both thin and thick regions, and their contour ranges between oval and round. Thicker intima segments that are focal and eccentric occur inevitably at and near bifurcations of arteries and at the mouths of even the smallest branch vessels. The thick segments are called *adaptive intimal thickening,* although many other terms also have been used (4).

In microscopic sections of properly distended arteries, adaptive thickenings appear as crescent-shaped increases in the thickness of the half of the arterial wall circumference opposite flow dividers of bifurcations. They measure as much as twice the thickness of the media from the time of birth, but, in the coronary arteries of young children, considerable individual variation in degree has been found (5).

From the initial appearance of minimal lipid and macrophage foam cell accumulations, the accumulations are more prominent in a subset of locations that also contain adaptive intimal thickening. These are sites at which clinically important lesions develop first and foremost. The explanation for the preferred accumulation of lipid and macrophage foam cells in specific locations is the nature of flow mechanical forces in these regions. These forces give rise to adaptive thickening, but, independently, they also enhance the influx of plasma proteins including lipoprotein. A distinct force acting at such locations is low shear stress (6,7).

The significance of adaptive intimal thickening has been disputed. Some authors view it as the first stage of atherosclerosis mainly because atheroma, when present, is found superimposed on some of the same locations. Other authors have speculated that adaptive thickening, although not a lesion itself, is a prerequisite for retention and accumulation of lipid and, thus, for lesion formation. Neither assumption is likely, because when blood lipoprotein levels are very high (as in familial hypercholesterolemia homozygotes), macrophage foam cells and extracellular lipid do accumulate, and clinically important lesions develop readily also at sites without adaptive intimal thickening.

PHASE OF MINIMAL LESIONS

The changes that represent minimal atherosclerosis have been subdivided into lesion types I and II. The most minimal change (type I lesion) that is detectable by high-resolution light microscopy at highly susceptible intima points consists of isolated groups of a few macrophages loaded with and enlarged by lipid droplets (macrophage foam cells) and isolated monocyte/macrophages without droplets. Lymphocytes may not be present. In the first 8 months of life, 45% of infants have type I changes in their coronary arteries (5).

After a temporary decline following infancy, macrophage foam cells, now more numerous, emerge at the highly susceptible and additional susceptible locations in children at puberty (type II lesion). The foam cells, accompanied by monocyte/macrophages, are generally stratified into layers rather than occurring as isolated groups of only a few cells. A variable number of intimal smooth muscle cells at the involved sites also contain lipid droplets. T lymphocytes have been identified (8,9), but they are less numerous than macrophages. Type II lesions vary greatly in the overall number of foam cells, number of other cell types, and their proportions to each other. Neither the media adjacent to the lesions nor the adventitia is affected. Such minimal changes never obstruct the flow of blood and, thus, never produce clinical manifestations. Of children aged 12 to 15 years, 69% have mostly type II lesions (few have only type I, and even fewer have lesions advanced beyond type II) in coronary arteries.

Although generally the only lesions in infants and children, lesion types I and II also are present in adults in addition to more advanced lesions. Most of the minimal changes do not develop further. In themselves, they are harmless, and the term *lesion* when applied to them should not be taken to indicate mandatory treatment. Lesion types I and II are included in the natural history of atherosclerosis because the sequence of histologic changes (see type III lesion) indicates that, when clinically important lesions are present, they have developed from initially minimal changes.

Type II lesions resemble type I in that almost the entire microscopically visible lipid within a region of the intima is within cells. Chemical and immunochemical data indicate that the presence of intracellular lipid droplets is a consequence and a marker of excess atherogenic lipoproteins in those regions of the intima. Minimal extracellular lipid particles may be present in type II lesions, but extracellular accumulations that disrupt the intimal architecture (characteristic of subsequent lesion types) are absent. Extracellular lipid accumulation (defined in the next section) must not be confused with excess intimal lipoprotein. The latter does not disrupt intima structure. Indeed, without immunostaining, neither high-resolution light nor electron microscopy reveals the plasma-derived lipoprotein in the intimal intercellular space.

Type II lesions are usually (but not always) visible with the unaided eye as flat yellow (fatty) streaks, dots, or patches on the intimal surface. Because the number of foam cells is so small in type I lesions, these may not be visible even when Sudan staining is used.

Many authors had rejected (and some still do [10]) the evidence that clinically important lesions derive from the minimal ones, considering the minimal changes (referred to by most authors by the gross term *fatty streak*) as unrelated to the pathogenesis of atherosclerosis. The manner in which minimal, fatty streak–type lesions change into clinically important ones is explained in the next section.

LINK BETWEEN MINIMAL AND CLINICALLY IMPORTANT LESIONS

The histologic feature that follows intracellular accumulation of lipid is the accumulation of extracellular lipid. Thus, the emergence of small, only microscopically visible, pools of lipid particles and droplets below the layers of lipid-laden cells (the type III lesion) constitutes the initiation of progression from minimal to clinically important lesions. The pools of packed particles and droplets widen the spaces between the normally closely adjoining resident smooth muscle cells of the deep intima. This disruption of deep intimal structure constitutes the precursor of the lipid core—the hallmark of the first clinically important lesion type (type IV).

Extracellular lipid represents the remnants of lipid-laden cells (primarily macrophages) that have died. The component particles and droplets are of variable size and morphology, much larger than plasma-derived LDLs. The extracellular accumulations are not phagocytosed and broken down by macrophages or other cells. Instead, very slow degradation, perhaps partly by mechanical means, takes place in the intercellular space. Electron microscopic studies of the sequence in which lesion components regress (see "Sequence of Histologic Changes During Lesion Regression ") support this observation. When high blood cholesterol levels were drastically decreased in monkeys, monocytes, macrophages, and macrophage foam cells were the first lesion components to disappear; only subsequently did extracellular lipid accumulations decrease.

The existence of a histologically contiguous step (the type III lesion) between minimal and clinically important lesions is evidence that clinical lesions develop from minimal ones, although, clearly, not every minimal change develops further. Past skepticism about a connection between minimal and clinical lesions was based on the view that the two differ too sharply from each other both histologically and grossly, and that a precise topographic correspondence between the two is lacking. The seeming lack of conformity between locations with only foam cell accumulations and those with clinical lesions is, in part, the consequence of relying on the unaided eye to evaluate blood vessels. This popular means of studying atherosclerosis often is unable to discover foam cell accumulations at the highly susceptible (i.e., progression-prone) intima sites nor that more foam cells are present here than at other locations. Because intima has greater depth at the highly susceptible sites, foam cells come to rest some distance below the endothelial cell layer and may not be visible from the surface. Conversely, the smaller number of foam cells in thin (less progression-prone) segments of intima are easily visible as fatty streaks because they are forced to lie close to the endothelial surface. With the use of high-resolution light microscopy, a strong correlation between the locations containing more foam cells in children and the preferred sites of the clinically important lesions of adults is found (1–3).

Furthermore, there is no insurmountable difference between the morphologies of minimal and clinically important lesions considering that layers of smooth muscle cells are not just a hallmark of clinically important lesions but also a normal component of the susceptible intima sites. The observation that, at such smooth muscle–rich locations, small pools of extracellular lipid may follow foam cell accumulation and that pools may enlarge and merge to form a lipid core provide the link between minimal and clinically important lesions.

GENERAL COMMENTS ON CLINICALLY IMPORTANT LESIONS

Clinically important lesions have a range of characteristic compositions designated lesion types IV, V, VI, VII, and VIII. Although any of these may produce symptoms, those that do not obstruct blood flow much may be silent. Type VI is the histology that produces symptoms most often and is mostly found in fatal cases.

The common histologic hallmark of these lesion types is complete structural disorganization and thickening of the intima. An accumulation of extracellular lipid entirely replacing a central part (core) of the arterial wall is a feature of lesion types IV to VI and to a lesser extent type VII. The lipid core constitutes a region of arterial wall that has lost all structure, strength, and resilience. In type IV lesions, a lipid core is the dominant lesion component. In type V lesions, lipid cores are comparable to those of type IV, but constitute a smaller proportion of the overall lesion volume as newly added (reparative) fibromuscular layers constitute an equal or greater mass. Intimal changes, including the lipid core, may extend into the adjacent media and as far as the adventitia. Lesion types IV and V that have a thrombotic deposit (usually associated with disruption of the lesion surface and often with a hematoma) are designated type VI. Thrombotic deposits and hematoma contribute to wall thickness and lumen reduction. Unless fatal, they convert to fibromuscular tissue.

At older ages, lesions often are heterogeneous in composition. Thus, a type VII lesion (characteristic for a predominantly mineral content) might, somewhere along its extent, contain a lipid core, layers of reparative fibrous tissue, and an eroded surface with a thrombotic deposit. A lesion like that might be classified as type V/VI/VII. In practice, I would classify it as type VI because knowing about the thrombus would be more important than knowing that it was predominantly mineralized.

The numbers of monocyte/macrophages, macrophage foam cells, and lymphocytes vary in lesions of the same type, as do the proportions of these cell types to each other. Generally, macrophage foam cells outnumber monocyte/macrophages and these outnumber lymphocytes. In some lesion types IV to VII, monocyte/macrophages and lymphocytes equal foam cells in the intimal part of lesions, where they tend to predominate in the upper and peripheral regions. In lesions extending to the media/adventitia border, nests or even sheets of monocyte/macrophages and lymphocytes, outnumbering all leukocytes in the intima, may colonize particularly the region around the vasa vasorum (11). The deep media is also the preferred location for multinucleated giant cells (often containing cholesterol crystals) when these are present. According to Moreno and coworkers (12), inflammatory cell infiltrates occur in the media in 35% and in the adventitia in 79% of lesions with a disrupted intimal surface (type VI lesions), more often than in any other lesion type.

Mast cells, always occurring as single cells, are rare in the intimal part and more numerous in the adventitial part of lesions. Plasma cells are rarer still than mast cells. Acute inflammatory cells (neutrophil granulocytes) are not a feature of atherosclerotic lesions.

When macrophage foam cells predominate in lesions, macrophage function is clearly phagocytic in response to excess atherogenic lipoprotein in the tissue. When large numbers of lymphocytes are present, there may be additional reasons for the presence of leukocytes.

LESIONS WITH A LIPID CORE AS THE MAIN FEATURE

The first clinically important lesion type (type IV or atheroma) is found at the highly susceptible arterial locations in some individuals at the end of the second decade of life, and it remains the predominant clinical lesion type for the following decade. It consists of all the components of type II lesions plus a lipid core, the latter accounting for arterial wall thickness now increased over what is normal for the arterial site involved. The lipid core is a well delineated region of intima where structural elements normally present (proteoglycan matrix, fibers, and smooth muscle cells) have been replaced with packed particles and droplets of lipid. This large mass of extracellular material forms through the increase and coalescence of the small, separate pools of the same material that are the hallmark of type III lesions (Fig. 30–2).

In contrast to the small pools of type III lesions, lipid cores almost always also contain cholesterol crystals and calcium particles. The quantity of cholesterol crystals varies, but is usually less than 10% of the lipid core volume in young adults. Rarely, a lipid core will consist entirely of cholesterol crystals. Smooth muscle cells normally resident in the region now occupied by the lipid core are decreased in number or are absent. The packed extracellular material presumably hinders the function and existence of the cells. Any remaining smooth muscle cells become widely dispersed and have developed attenuated and elongated cell bodies and often unusually thick basement membranes. Some cell organelles are calcified and calcium particles of variable size and extent are also found among the extracellular lipid of a core.

At this developmental stage, the thickness of the intima layer overlying the lipid core (the cap of the core) does not much exceed the usual thickness of that location. The cap consists of proteoglycan-rich intercellular matrix, smooth muscle cells with and without lipid-droplet inclusions, monocytes, macrophages, macrophage foam cells, and lymphocytes. Reparative fibrous connective tissue layers are not part of the cap at this stage. Those who use the gross classification of lesions include type IV lesions under the term *fibrous plaque*. Use of this term is responsible for the misconception that pathologic fibrous tissue layers are present from the start.

Although lipid cores, and thus type IV lesions, clearly thicken the arterial wall, the vascular lumen often is only slightly reduced, partly because the vessel wall may give somewhat to the outside. Some clinical angiographic studies indicate that lesions that narrow the arterial lumen only mildly can suddenly progress to critical obstructions (13,14). The clinical terms *high risk* or *vulnerable* or *culprit* lesion have been applied to them. By histopathology, type IV lesions are vulnerable because when a lipid core is present, lesion rupture and thrombosis are facilitated (discussed later).

Although the first type IV lesions arise at the highly susceptible sites of arteries, with advancing age, additional type IV lesions may develop in locations of lesser susceptibility. In subjects with genetic lipoprotein abnormalities causing high levels of blood cholesterol, type IV lesions develop at both highly susceptible and at additional locations before adulthood.

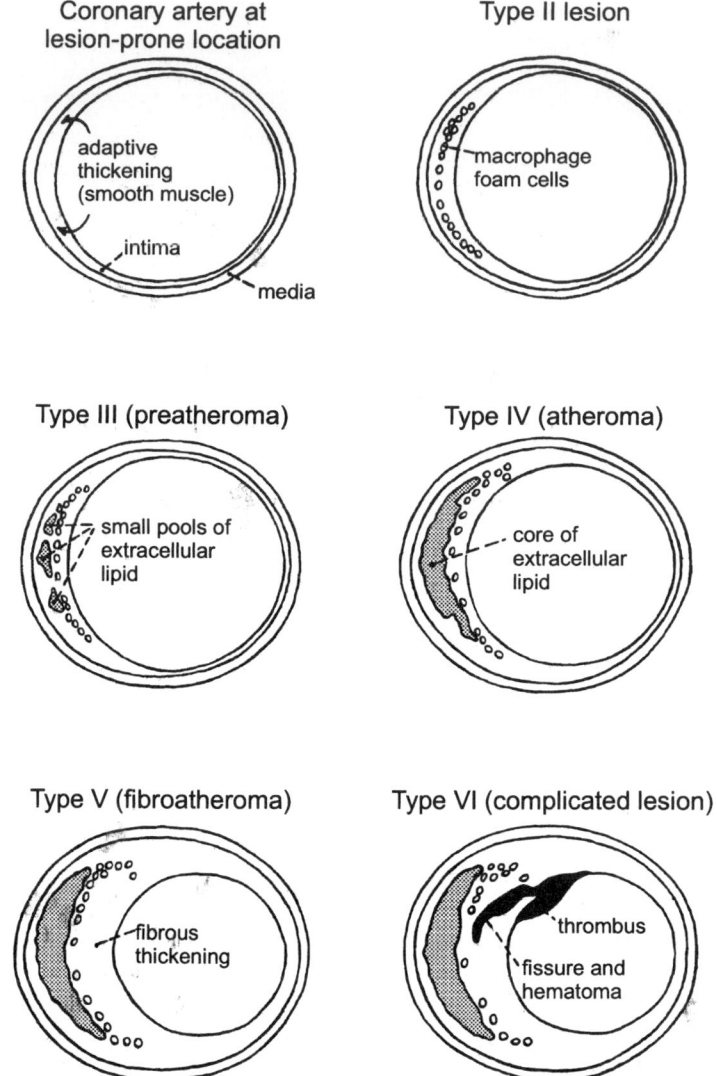

FIG. 30–2. Drawings of cross sections of the anterior descending coronary artery taken at an identical, proximal point from six individuals of different ages to illustrate the usual sequence in the development of atherosclerosis. The morphology of the intima in this location ranges from adaptive intimal thickening that is always present in this location to a type VI lesion in a person with clinically important atherosclerosis.

ADDITION OF REPARATIVE FIBROMUSCULAR TISSUE

Lesions in which layers of reparative fibrous connective tissue and often an increased number of smooth muscle cells are present in addition to the components of type IV lesions are designated type V or fibroatheroma. Tissue death and thrombosis are the two stimuli that account for the reparative response. Reparative tissue produced in response to disruption of arterial wall by the accumulated extracellular lipid is gradual and moderate, whereas rapid and substantial production follows thrombotic deposits. The larger amounts of reparative tissue are found in the *cap* region—that is, between lipid core and endothelial surface. Smooth muscle cells residing in the cap region respond to thrombotic deposits by increasing in number and producing fibrous tissue.

Type V lesions may consist of two or more lipid cores of unequal size, separated by unequal layers of reparative fibromuscular tissue, stacked one on top of the other. Some multilayered type V lesions may be a consequence of modification of flow mechanical forces because of the development of a vascular stenosis causing a slight shifting of the site of continuing lipid accumulation (15). Other lesions may be a consequence of separate episodes of surface fissure and thrombus formation, each such episode being followed by a reparative phase and renewed lipid accumulation.

It has been argued that reparative fibromuscular tissue in the cap region protects lesions from fissuring and thrombosis. However, histologic evidence indicates that type V is no less susceptible than type IV. The susceptibility of type V lesions to such complications lies in their uneven composition and contour. Regions between fibromuscular layers are still occupied by nests of macrophage foam cells and extracellular lipid. The tissue at the shoulders of type V lesions often is rich in monocyte/macrophages, lymphocytes, and proteoglycan matrix, similar to the peripheries of type IV lesions.

THROMBOSIS

When thrombotic deposits develop on lesions, the lesions are designated as type VI. Often the deposit is secondary to a fissure, erosion, or ulceration of the lesion surface. Hematoma may also be present. Such complicating features usually are superimposed on lesions with an underlying type IV or V composition. Occasionally, a thrombotic deposit with or without a surface defect occurs in association with a lesion that does not contain a lipid core. Histologic evidence indicates that a type VI event may be followed by months or longer without additional damage to the surface or thrombus enlargement. However, additional layers of thrombus often are superimposed at short intervals, sometimes to the point where the lumen of a medium-sized artery becomes occluded within hours, days, or weeks. When not fatal, a thrombotic deposit is colonized by intimal smooth muscle cells and changed into a layer of fibromuscular tissue. The changes result in a lesion of type V morphology, larger and with greater obstruction of the arterial lumen than before the complicating episode.

In an autopsy study of a population aged 30 to 59 years, the amount of thrombotic material on or within atherosclerotic lesions was variable (in most cases it was small), whereas the incidence was high. Of subjects having lesions type IV or greater in the aorta, 38% had thrombotic deposits on these lesions. Immunohistochemistry revealed that an additional 29% of the lesions contained products related to fibrin that might also represent remnants of thrombi (16).

The susceptibility of a lesion's surface to fissure or erosion cannot be predicted precisely, although an abundance of macrophages, macrophage foam cells and lymphocytes in lesions, and the release of toxic substances and proteolytic enzymes have been proposed as the factors that predispose to intima weakness (17,18). More likely, it is the packed extracellular lipidic material that leads mechanically to disruption and loss of tissue, structural weakness, and loss of surface integrity.

In our studies, we have occasionally found occlusive or near-occlusive thrombi of identical histologic age superimposed on separate lesions in more than one branch of an individual's coronary arteries. It is unlikely that fissures would develop in separate lesions at quite the same time, at least not on the basis of the lesion's morphology.

In view of the finding of multiple simultaneous occlusive thrombi and the observed individual variability in thrombus amount, it may be more feasible and rewarding to identify and treat persons with a systemic thrombogenic propensity before attempting to predict and then reduce a particular lesion's susceptibility to fissure.

CALCIFICATION

From the fifth decade of life onward, lesions often have a predominantly mineral character. When about half or more of a lesion consists of mineral, it may be called a type VII or calcific lesion. In addition, such lesions generally contain an abundance of lipid and reparative fibrous connective tissue.

We have used electron microscopy to follow the formation of calcium deposits in atherosclerotic lesions. Calcium granules emerge in the lipid cores of type IV lesions of young adults. At that early stage, mineralization is in the organelles of intimal smooth muscle cells trapped among the extracellular material that constitutes lipid cores. When the cells die and disintegrate, mineralized organelles become a part of the extracellular accumulation. The extracellular remnants of other dead cells may also serve as sites for calcium granule formation. In most lipid cores, extracellular calcium granules outnumber intracellular ones from the beginning of their formation. Granules are scattered throughout a lipid core in a pepper and salt–like manner, although their density often is greater in deep parts of the core (parts facing the media).

In the type IV lesions of individuals 20 to 29 years old, mineral granules might account for up to 10% of the volume of the lesions' lipid cores. The amount varies greatly in different individuals even when the lesions and lipid cores look similar otherwise.

With age, calcium granules increase in size and merge to form ever larger aggregates. From middle age, large clumps or sheets of mineral may dominate the core of a lesion by replacing the extracellular lipid at the base or (less often) throughout the lesion core (type VII lesion). Lamellar bone formation tends to occur when sheetlike calcifications are present (19).

A focal calcium deposit identified in arterial intima by clinical imaging generally represents at least a type IV lesion. Although it is not necessarily a marker of clinically significant obstruction of the lumen (20), it is a marker of disease advanced at least to the point where surface disruption and thrombosis may develop. There may be exceptions, however. Animal experiments indicate that focal mineral deposits persist in locations of arteries in which lesions of types IV and V have changed or regressed to lesion types VII or VIII after therapeutic reduction of high blood cholesterol. Furthermore, diffuse mineralization of the media of arteries (Mönckeberg's medial calcification) must be distinguished from the irregularly focal calcifications of atherosclerotic lesions that extend into media from intima.

FIBROUS THICKENING WITHOUT THE PRESENCE OF LIPID

Some intimal lesions consist mainly of reparative fibrous connective tissue that may be partly hyalinized. Lipid cores are absent, other accumulated lipid is minimal and, sometimes, there is apparently no lipid at all; some mineralization may be present. Such lesions may be designated type VIII (fibrotic) lesions.

Fibrotic lesions may be the result of one or more processes, including organization of thrombus, extension of the fibrous component of an adjacent fibroatheroma, or resorption (regression) of a lipid core and replacement with fibrous tissue.

Type VIII lesions must not be confused with focal and eccentric adaptive thickening of the intima. The smooth muscle cells and fibrous connective tissue matrix of type VIII lesions have the characteristics of reparative reactions, whereas adaptive intimal thickening has a predictably harmonious structure with smooth muscle cells and intercellular matrix present in normal proportions.

SEQUENCE OF HISTOLOGIC CHANGES DURING LESION REGRESSION

The feasibility of atherosclerosis regression has been examined by many investigators in various animal species (21–25). The primary aim of the animal experiments was to demonstrate that, through manipulation of the diet, lesions could be made to decrease in thickness, thereby enlarging the lumina of obstructed arteries. In our series of regression studies in rhesus monkeys, we investigated the degree and sequence in which particular cell and matrix components of lesions changed, decreased, and disappeared in the belief that the same happens in human lesions and that this information could guide therapy. We studied the same susceptible segments of coronary arteries and aortas in monkeys as in humans and we used the same histologic techniques and methods. Lesions comparable to human types I to V were first produced by feeding the monkeys atherogenic diets for periods from 12 weeks to 5.5 years (see details in Reference 3). To determine the compositions of these baseline lesions, a group of monkeys was killed in each experiment at the point at which the atherogenic diet was changed to a low-cholesterol regression diet in the remaining monkeys. Mon-

keys fed the regression diets were killed in small groups at intervals from 3 weeks to 3.5 years after switching from the atherogenic food.

Monkeys killed after 12 weeks of atherogenic food had lesions resembling human types I to III. Feeding the atherogenic diet for 2 or 5.5 years produced lesions similar to type IV or V.

Characteristic sequential changes occurred in the cells and tissues of lesions after serum total cholesterol concentrations (range, 300–500 mg/dL) were decreased to less than 180 mg/dL. The sequence can be divided into an early phase (the 6-month period after total cholesterol decreased to <180 mg/dL) and a subsequent late phase, which lasted for several years when existing lesions were type IV or V (Fig. 30–3).

Changes became visible by electron microscopy in the macrophage and macrophage foam cell populations within 3 months of reducing high serum total cholesterol to less than 180 mg/dL. Typical was the marked increase in lysosomal reduction of lipid droplets in macrophage foam cells. Shrinkage of lipid droplets to small residual bodies resulted in smaller overall cell size. Concomitantly, these and other leukocytes were progressively declining in number. Dead cells were identifiable by electron microscopy. Six months after cholesterol had decreased to less than 180 mg/dL, macrophages, macrophage foam cells, and other leukocyte types were absent or found as rare isolated cells (3,26).

Processes that constituted the late phase were those that occurred in lesions comparable to human types IV and V after completion of the characteristic early changes. Most of the longer lasting processes began in the early phase of regression and continued beyond it. They included the slow reduction of lipid droplets in the cytoplasm of smooth muscle cells (3,27) (in contrast to the rapid reduction in macrophages completed in the early phase), reduction of extracellular lipid pools and cores, and production of fibrous connective tissue to repair regions of the arterial wall as lipid cleared.

	Lesion types I–III	Lesion types IV–V
Early phase of regression (3–6 months after reduction of high s. cholesterol to below 180 mg/dl)	• rapid degradation of lipid droplets in macrophage foam cells • slow degradation of lipid droplets in smooth muscle cells • cessation of macrophage foam cell mitosis in lesions • death of macrophage foam cells in lesions • slow reduction of extracellular lipid	
Late phase of regression (6 months to several years after reduction of high s. cholesterol to below 180 mg/dl)	mostly back to normal	• macrophages and macrophage foam cells absent or rare • other WBC types absent • continued degradation of lipid droplets in smooth muscle cells • progressive reduction of extracellular lipid
Final outcome		conversion to fibrocalcific lesions (types VII and VIII) containing minimal or no lipid

FIG. 30–3. Changes in lesion composition during atherosclerosis regression. s., serum; WBC, white blood cell.

Aggregates of calcium occurred in the larger type IV and type V lesions of monkeys killed after 2 or 5.5 years of hypercholesterolemia. After 3.5 years of continuously low cholesterol levels, large calcium aggregates were still present in the larger residual lesions (3,28). The amount about equaled that found in the baseline lesions. Monkeys that had been on the low-cholesterol diet for 3.5 years had lesions that, judging from the cholesterol level during the hypercholesterolemic phase had been types IV and V, resembled human lesion types VII and VIII.

Although normal arterial wall composition, structure, thickness, and elasticity were not reestablished, the loss of macrophages and lymphocytes, the massive reduction in lipid content, and the replacement of disrupted regions with reparative fibrous tissue must be regarded as a therapeutic success. In humans, the same changes might improve structural stability and reduce susceptibility to surface disruption and thrombosis. The persistence of calcium may not be detrimental. Calcium in comparably deep locations in the arterial wall is seen in some older individuals as so-called Mönckeberg's medial calcification (medial calcinosis) and does not predispose to vascular complications. Furthermore, patients with stenosing calcified lesions have fewer ischemic events than those with stenosing lesions lacking calcium (19).

There is no reason to doubt that the changes of lesion composition in the monkeys would occur in human lesions if high blood cholesterol levels were similarly reduced.

ACKNOWLEDGMENTS

The chapter is based, for the most part, on studies by the author that have been supported by the National Institutes of Health (grants HL-22739 and HL-08974).

REFERENCES

1. Stary HC. Evolution and progression of atherosclerotic lesions in coronary arteries of children and young adults. *Arteriosclerosis* 1989;9[Suppl I]:19–32.
2. Stary HC. The sequence of cell and matrix changes in atherosclerotic lesions of coronary arteries in the first forty years of life. *Eur Heart J* 1990;11[Suppl E]:3–19.
3. Stary HC. *Atlas of atherosclerosis progression and regression,* 2nd ed. New York: Parthenon Publishing, 2003.
4. Stary HC, Blankenhorn DH, Chandler AB, et al. A definition of the intima of human arteries and of its atherosclerosis-prone regions. *Circulation* 1992;85:391–405.
5. Stary HC. Macrophages, macrophage foam cells, and eccentric intimal thickening in the coronary arteries of young children. *Atherosclerosis* 1987;64:91–108.
6. Zarins CK, Giddens DP, Bharadvaj BK, et al. Carotid bifurcation atherosclerosis. Quantitative correlation of plaque localization with flow velocity profiles and wall shear stress. *Circ Res* 1983;53:502–514.
7. Caro CG, Parker KH, Fish PJ, et al. Blood flow near the arterial wall and arterial disease. *Clin Hemor* 1985;5:849–871.
8. Jonasson L, Holm J, Skalli O, et al. Regional accumulations of T cells, macrophages, and smooth muscle cells in the human atherosclerotic plaque. *Arteriosclerosis* 1986;6:131–138.
9. Katsuda S, Boyd HC, Fligner C, et al. Human atherosclerosis. III. Immunocytochemical analysis of the cell composition of lesions of young adults. *Am J Pathol* 1992;140:907–914.
10. Stehbens WE. Integrated vascular pathology. In: Lanzer P, Topol EJ, eds. *Pan vascular medicine.* Berlin: Springer-Verlag, 2002:76–113.
11. Mitchell JR, Schwartz CJ. *Arterial disease.* Philadelphia: FA Davis, 1965.
12. Moreno PR, Purushothaman KR, Fuster V, et al. Intimomedial interface damage and adventitial inflammation is increased beneath disrupted atherosclerosis in the aorta: implications for plaque vulnerability. *Circulation* 2002;105:2504–2511.
13. Little WC, Constantinescu M, Applegate RJ, et al. Can coronary angiography predict the site of a subsequent myocardial infarction in patients with mild-to-moderate coronary artery disease? *Circulation* 1988;78:1157–1166.
14. Fuster V. Mechanisms leading to myocardial infarction: insights from studies of vascular biology. *Circulation* 1994;90:2126–2146.
15. Glagov S, Zarins C, Giddens DP, et al. Hemodynamics and atherosclerosis: insights and perspectives gained from studies of human arteries. *Arch Pathol Lab Med* 1988;112:1018–1031.
16. Yin J, Stary HC. Differences in thrombosis and composition of advanced atherosclerotic lesions between natives and non-natives of Alaska. *FASEB J* 1994;8:A268.
17. Davies MJ. The concept of the vulnerable plaque in coronary heart disease. In: Jacotot B, Mathe D, Fruchart JC, eds. *Atherosclerosis XI.* Amsterdam: Elsevier, 1998:57–62.
18. Libby P, Mach F, Schonbeck U, et al. Regulation of the thrombotic potential of atheroma. *Thromb Haemost* 1999;82:736–741.
19. Hunt JL, Fairman R, Mitchell ME, et al. Bone formation in carotid plaques: a clinicopathological study. *Stroke* 2002;33:1214–1219.
20. Wexler L, Brundage B, Crouse J, et al. Coronary artery calcification: pathophysiology, epidemiology, imaging methods, and clinical implications. *Circulation* 1996;94:1175–1192.
21. Armstrong ML, Warner ED, Connor WE. Regression of coronary atheromatosis in rhesus monkeys. *Circ Res* 1970;27:59–67.
22. Armstrong ML. Connective tissue in regression. In: Paoletti R, Gotto AM, eds. *Atherosclerosis reviews 3.* New York: Raven Press, 1978:147–168.
23. Stary HC. Regression of atherosclerosis in primates. *Virchows Arch* 1979;383:117–134.
24. Clarkson TB, Bond MG, Bullock BC, et al. A study of atherosclerosis regression in Macaca mulatta. IV. Changes in coronary arteries from animals with atherosclerosis induced for 19 months and then regressed for 24 or 48 months at plasma cholesterol concentrations of 300 or 200 mg/dl. *Exp Mol Pathol* 1981;34:345–368.
25. Clarkson TB, Bond MG, Bullock BC, et al. A study of atherosclerosis regression in Macaca mulatta. V. Changes in abdominal aorta and carotid and coronary arteries from animals with atherosclerosis induced for 38 months and then regressed for 24 or 48 months at plasma cholesterol concentrations of 300 or 200 mg/dl. *Exp Mol Pathol* 1984;41:96–118.
26. Stary HC. Arterial cell injury and cell death in hypercholesterolemia and after reduction of high serum cholesterol levels. *Prog Biochem Pharmacol* 1977;13:241–247.
27. Stary HC, Strong JP, Eggen DA. Differences in the degradation-rate of intercellular lipid droplets in the intimal smooth muscle cells and macrophages of regressing atherosclerotic lesions of primates. In: Gotto AM, Smith LC, Allen B, eds. *Atherosclerosis V.* New York: Springer-Verlag, 1980:753–756.
28. Strong JP, Bhattacharyya AK, Eggen DA, et al. Long-term induction and regression of diet-induced atherosclerotic lesions in rhesus monkeys. II. Morphometric evaluation of lesions by light microscopy in coronary and carotid arteries. *Arterioscler Thromb* 1994;14:2007–2016.

CHAPTER 31

Pathogenesis of Atherothrombosis

Role of Vulnerable, Ruptured, and Eroded Plaques

Erling Falk and Prediman K. Shah

Key Words: Atherosclerosis; atherothrombosis; plaque erosion; plaque rupture; thrombosis; vulnerable plaque.

INTRODUCTION

Atherosclerosis is the underlying cause of nearly all cases of coronary artery disease and peripheral arterial disease and many cases of stroke. Superimposed thrombosis is the proximate cause of most of the acute and potentially lethal

   E. Falk: Coronary Pathology Research, and Department of Cardiology, Aarhus University Hospital (Skejby), DK-8200 Aarhus N, Denmark.
   P. K. Shah: Cardiology and Atherosclerosis Research Center, Cedars Sinai Medical Center; Department of Medicine, David Geffen School of Medicine at UCLA, Los Angeles, California 90048.

manifestations of atherosclerosis, including the acute coronary syndromes (unstable angina, myocardial infarction [MI], and sudden death), acute peripheral ischemia, and ischemic stroke. Thus, atherosclerosis with superimposed thrombosis, *atherothrombosis,* is the leading cause of death and severe disability in the affluent countries, and it will soon be so worldwide because of the pandemic growth of obesity, insulin resistance, and type 2 diabetes (1,2).

Symptomatic coronary lesions (culprit lesions) contain a variable mix of chronic atherosclerosis and acute thrombosis, but because the exact nature of the mix is unknown in the individual patient, the term *atherothrombosis* is indeed appropriate. Generally, atherosclerosis predominates in lesions responsible for chronic stable angina, whereas a component of thrombosis is usually present in culprit lesions responsible for acute coronary syndromes (3).

DEFINITIONS AND TERMINOLOGY

To avoid confusion, the terms that have been and are used to describe the characteristic features of atherothrombotic plaques will first be reviewed.

Atherosclerosis is a multifocal smoldering inflammatory disease that primarily affects the intima of medium-sized and large arteries, resulting in intimal thickening that may lead to luminal narrowing and inadequate blood supply. As the name implies, mature atherosclerosis plaques consist typically of two main components: One is lipid-rich and soft (*athére* is Greek for gruel or porridge) and the other is collagen-rich and hard (*skleros* is Greek for hard). The flow-limiting potential of an intimal plaque may be modified by reactive changes in the underlying media and adventitia that may attenuate (positive remodeling) or accentuate (negative remodeling) luminal compromise and consequent hemodynamic impact of the plaque.

Plaque rupture, but not plaque disruption, is a well defined term. It is a deep plaque injury that involves much more than just a missing or "disrupted" endothelium (3–5). In plaque rupture, there is a real defect—a gap—in the fibrous cap that separates a lipid-rich atheromatous core from the flowing blood (Fig. 31-1) (see color insert). The thrombogenic core is exposed (risk for thrombosis) and blood may enter the soft core through the gap in the cap (rupture-related plaque hemorrhage). The size of the gaps varies greatly in width, length, and depth (6).

In contrast to plaque rupture, *plaque disruption* is not a well defined term. It has been used synonymously with plaque rupture (3,7,8), but also for all other kinds of plaque injuries found beneath thrombi, including superficial injuries in which only the endothelium is missing or *disrupted* (so-called plaque erosion) (9–11). Muller probably had this broad meaning in mind when he originally used (12), and still uses (10,13), the term *disruption.* Virmani and coworkers (5) used the expression *fibrous cap disruption* when they introduced a rare nonrupture type of plaque injury: the calcified nodule. Therefore, to avoid confusion, the term *disruption* should be used with great caution.

Davies and Thomas (14,15) used the term *plaque fissuring* in the mid-1980s, when they suggested a common pathogenetic basis for the acute coronary syndromes. They probably used the term synonymously with plaque rupture (3), but *fissuring* also has been used for superficial intimal tearing in the absence of a lipid-rich core (16). Thus, *fissuring* is not an unambiguous term. Terms like *plaque ulceration, breaks, rents, and tears* also are poorly defined and should be avoided (15).

The term *unstable plaque* usually refers to culprit lesions in unstable angina and the other acute coronary syndromes (17,18). Pathoanatomically, the term has been used for plaques assumed to be *vulnerable,* rupture-prone, and/or thrombosis-prone and for plaques that already have a thrombus superimposed (17–19). Thus, *unstable plaque* also is an ambiguous term.

Plaque erosion is an old nonspecific term with a new meaning. The term was revived by van der Wal and coworkers (20) and (re)defined by Virmani and coworkers (5) in the following way: "'Plaque erosion' is identified when serial sectioning of a thrombosed arterial segment fails to reveal fibrous cap rupture. Typically, the endothelium is absent at the erosion site." Thus, it is the lack of plaque rupture rather than any specific pathoanatomic feature that "characterizes" these lesions. According to this definition, rupture and erosion will together account for all plaque changes found at the plaque–thrombus interface (20–23).

The term *vulnerable* has been used for about two decades to describe coronary lesions assumed to be dangerous, but confusion exists on its use. In 1985, Muller and coworkers (12) introduced the term *vulnerable* in a seminal article dealing with the circadian onset of acute MI (12). A sentence in the abstract reads as follows: "If coronary arteries become vulnerable to occlusion when the intima covering an atherosclerotic plaque is disrupted, the circadian timing of MI may result from a variation in the tendency to thrombosis." The focus was soon concentrated on rupture-prone plaques, characterized by a large lipid-rich core covered by a thin fibrous cap that was inflamed and depleted of smooth muscle cells (6). Outward (positive) remodeling was later added as another characteristic feature (24–26). A kind of consensus developed during the 1990s, and the term *vulnerable* was generally used only for rupture-prone plaques (6–8,21,24,25,27–29). Virmani and coworkers (17) introduced the purely descriptive term *thin-cap fibroatheroma* for rupture-prone plaques and preferred to reserve the term *vulnerable* for thrombosis-prone plaques. Thus, *vulnerable* has historically been used for occlusion-prone, rupture-prone, and thrombosis-prone plaques and also could be used for culprit-prone plaques (plaques at high risk for causing a heart attack) and for plaques at high risk for rapid progression. These different definitions focus on different aspects of plaques assumed to be dangerous. Regarding atherothrombosis and coronary artery disease, *vulnerable* is an ambiguous term that currently needs to be specified when used.

A *thrombus* is defined as any solid mass that arises in the bloodstream during life from components of the blood (30). Thus, a thrombus may not only form within the heart and vessels, it may form where blood is streaming, for example, in a false channel within the vessel wall (e.g., aortic dissection) or through a large gap in the surface of a ruptured plaque. Extravasation of blood is usually called a hemorrhage or bleeding, but Davies and Thomas (14,15,21) introduced the term *intraintimal thrombi* for rupture-related hemorrhages into plaques because of their composition (often relatively rich in platelets and fibrin) and location (often next to a luminal thrombus). However, many defects in ruptured caps are small without significant potential for to-and-fro flow and, consequently, the accumulated blood often looks more like a hemorrhage than a thrombus.

EARLY ATHEROSCLEROTIC LESIONS

The earliest lesions of atherosclerosis, *fatty streaks,* are present in the aorta from early childhood and may, in fact, begin to develop already during fetal life, particularly in fetuses of mothers with hypercholesterolemia (31). They are highly cellular inflammatory lesions consisting of macrophage foam cells (intracellular lipid) and T lymphocytes (immune reaction). Extracellular lipid is hardly identifiable microscopically, and B lymphocytes and neutrophils are not seen. Fatty streaks do not protrude into the lumen; therefore, they are asymptomatic.

Fatty streaks develop under an intact but activated and dysfunctioning endothelium, particularly in atherosclerosis-prone areas with preexisting intimal thickening. Inflammation and immune responses play an important role in atherogenesis from its beginning (32–36). Hypercholesterolemia is associated with increased endothelial permeability, increased transcytosis and intimal retention of lipoproteins, and endothelial activation with focal expression of vascular cell adhesion molecule-1 (VCAM-1), leading to monocyte and T lymphocyte adhesion. It is generally believed that inflammatory cells are recruited by adhesion molecules and chemokines such as monocyte chemoattractant protein-1 (MCP-1) and activated in the intima by factors such as oxidized lipids and cytokines such as macrophage-colony stimulating factor (M-CSF). Within intima, the monocyte-derived macrophages engulf the blood-derived low-density lipoprotein (LDL), probably through their scavenger receptors after oxidative modification, and become lipid-filled foam cells. These inflammatory cells constitute by far the major part of the early fatty streak lesion, with a ratio of approximately 1:10 to 1:50 between T cells and macrophages (35), and they probably play a significant role in the progression of fatty streaks to mature atherothrombotic plaques. The presence of activated macrophages and T cells strongly suggest that an immunologic reaction is taken place in the atherosclerotic plaque. The antigens that elicit this response are unknown but there are many candidates, including exogenous microorganisms (e.g., *Chlamydia pneumoniae*) and endogenous proteins such as heat shock proteins, β_2-glyco-protein-1, and modified LDL (34). The most extensive data obtained so far support the idea that oxidized LDL is important as a neoantigen (34,35).

Although immunoglobulins are found in abundance in lesions, B cells are noticeably absent from human plaques. Similarly, whereas plasma cells have been noted in inflammatory infiltrates in the adventitia surrounding atherosclerotic arteries, few, if any, such cells have been seen in the plaque itself (36).

Fate of Fatty Streaks

The fate of fatty streaks remains controversial. It is generally assumed that fatty streaks can progress to more advanced lesions because they occur at the same anatomic sites and because transitional stages have been observed (37). A smaller subgroup of fatty streaks, those superimposed on preexisting intimal thickenings, appears to be particularly prone to progress to advanced symptomatic lesions, but the mode of progression and the factors controlling it are not clear (37). Aortic fatty streaks are universally present in all populations around the world early in life, even in populations at low risk for symptomatic atherothrombosis later in life such as the South African Bantu (38). Female individuals have more aortic fatty streaks than males early in life, despite that male individuals develop more advanced lesions than females later in life (38,39). Black individuals have more aortic fatty streaks than white individuals early in life, but the latter have more advanced lesions than the former later in life (38,39). The thoracic aorta has more fatty streaks than the abdominal aorta early in life, but the opposite applies for advanced lesions later in life (38). These contrasting relations seen in the human aorta between asymptomatic fatty streaks in young persons and advanced and potentially symptomatic lesions in adults may question the relevance of results obtained in short-term animal experiments in which only the development of foam cell lesions (fatty streaks) in aorta are studied.

ADVANCED ATHEROSCLEROTIC PLAQUES

Advanced lesions (plaques) may cause luminal narrowing and give rise to ischemic symptoms. In contrast to most laboratory animals, smooth muscle cells are already present within the human intima early during atherogenesis, beneath developing fatty streaks (37). When lipids begin to accumulate extracellularly, then atherogenesis has passed beyond the fatty streak stage. Oxidized LDL is present in atherosclerotic plaques but not in the normal intima (32,36). Two different processes are responsible for the extracellular accumulation of lipids: Blood-derived atherogenic lipoprotein particles may be trapped and retained directly within the proteoglycan-rich extracellular matrix and/or lipid may be released from macrophage foam cells after their death (40). Macrophages both proliferate and die within atherosclerotic plaques, and the balance probably depends on whether the lesion is progressing, quiescent, or regressing. Later, when a lipid-rich core has formed, erythrocytes and their lipid-rich membranes may contribute to the expansion of the core (plaque rupture and hemorrhages; see later).

Progression beyond the fatty streak stage is not only associated with lipid accumulation, but connective tissue, produced by smooth muscle cells, accumulates, giving rise to heterogenous atherosclerotic plaques. Some plaques are lipid-rich, whereas others are lipid-poor, and morphologically dissimilar plaques may evolve next to each other. The endothelium is intact early during atherogenesis, but denuded areas (often related to superficial foam cell infiltration) with adherent platelets are later seen over mature plaques (41,42). Then, growth factors released from adherent platelets and microthrombi may stimulate the smooth muscle cells within the plaque to produce more connective tissue matrix (32,43). Because of a leaky endothelium, not only lipoproteins but also many other blood-derived components, including albumin and fibrinogen, are present in evolving lesions (44).

Endothelial cells and vascular smooth muscle cells are, according to conventional wisdom, presumed to be resident arterial cells. A series of investigations have, however, suggested a new paradigm in which smooth muscle cells and endothelial cells in atherothrombosis and neointimal lesions after vascular injury may derive, at least in part, from bone marrow or circulating blood cells (45).

Neovascularization and Low-Pressure Plaque Hemorrhages

Neovascularization, often expressing leukocyte adhesion molecules such as VCAM-1 and intercellular adhesion molecule-1 (ICAM-1) and associated with inflammatory cell infiltration, is frequently present at the base of advanced plaques, and it has been suggested that these vasa vasorum–derived new vessels could play an active role in the recruitment of leukocytes into plaques, and thus contribute to the progression of the disease (46,47). Regardless of the integrity of the plaque surface, small low-pressure hemorrhages (extravasated erythrocytes) are also common in these neovascularized areas (14). There is no convincing evidence that such low-pressure bleedings may precipitate rupture of the plaque surface, luminal thrombosis, or both. Leaky microvessels in plaques may, however, contribute to plaque growth (47).

Coronary Calcification

Focal calcification in atherosclerotic plaques is common and increases with age, both in men and women. Both lipid-rich and collagen-rich components may calcify, and the process may be active and controlled, resembling calcification in bone, rather than being passive and "dystrophic" (48,49). Coronary calcification in adults is almost always caused by atherosclerosis (50). Medial calcification (Mönckeberg's calcinosis) is rare in coronary arteries, even in patients with diabetes, in whom it frequently occurs in other arteries, particularly the muscular arteries of the legs (51). Both autopsy and clinical data indicate that coronary calcification is a marker for, and correlates closely with, the overall atherosclerotic plaque burden (52–54), but calcification of a plaque does not correlate with its flow-limiting capacity (degree of stenosis) (52,53) or its risk for sudden occlusion (vulnerability). If anything, heavily calcified plaques appear to be more stable than noncalcified plaques (53,55–58). Vascular remodeling is a likely explanation for the poor correlation of plaque calcification with lumen narrowing, stenosis severity, or both (52).

Noninvasive detection of coronary calcification may identify patients, rather than plaques, at increased risk for a heart attack. The greater the number of plaques, the greater the likelihood of one of them being vulnerable to rupture and thrombosis.

RUPTURE-PRONE AND RUPTURED PLAQUES

A subset of advanced, but not necessarily stenotic, plaques is particularly dangerous because of their high risk for becoming complicated by superimposed thrombosis. Pathoanatomic studies have revealed that rupture of the plaque surface with superimposed thrombosis is the most frequent proximate cause of acute heart attacks (3,4,29). Although not all thrombi are precipitated by plaque rupture (discussed later), atherosclerosis would undoubtedly be a much more benign disease if plaque rupture could be prevented.

The precise mechanisms responsible for plaque rupture are unknown, but detailed microscopic studies of ruptured plaques indicate that plaque type (composition) rather than plaque size (or stenosis severity) plays the major role (7). Plaques that have ruptured and, by inference, plaques at risk for rupturing (vulnerable plaques) are usually characterized by a relatively large lipid-rich core that is covered by a thin, inflamed, and smooth muscle–depleted fibrous cap (7,29) (Table 31–1). After rupturing, the exposed lipid-rich core appears to be highly thrombogenic because of a high content of tissue factor (59–62). Such plaques tend to grow outward rather than inward, preserving the lumen (positive remodeling), which may explain why vulnerable plaques are easily missed by angiography and stress testing (24–26,63).

Lipid-rich Core

The lipid-rich core of a plaque is avascular, hypocellular, softlike gruel and is totally devoid of supporting collagen (7,21). It contains free cholesterol, cholesterol crystals, and esterified cholesterol assumed to originate both from lipids

---

TABLE 31–1. *Features associated with plaque rupture*

Structural
- Large and soft lipid-rich core
- Thin and collagen-poor fibrous cap

Cellular
- Lack of smooth muscle cells at rupture site
- Accumulation of macrophages at rupture site

Function
- Impaired matrix synthesis (smooth muscle cell–related)
- Increased matrix breakdown (macrophage-derived matrix metalloproteinases)

Remodeling
- Outward (positive) vascular remodeling

Others
- Adventitial inflammation and neovascularization

that have infiltrated into the arterial wall from circulating blood and lipids derived from death of foam cells by apoptosis and necrosis, primarily of macrophage origin (7,40, 64–66). The latter explains why the lipid-rich core has been referred to as the "graveyard of dead macrophages" to emphasize its inflammatory origin (64–66). A large lipid-rich core is associated with a preferential distribution of circumferential stress to the shoulder regions of an eccentric plaque, where 60% of plaque ruptures tend to occur.

The size and consistency of the lipid-rich core are, of course, critical for the stability of a plaque. At autopsy, Gertz and Roberts (57) found that coronary plaques with ruptured (vs. intact) surface contained much larger lipid-rich cores, and Davies and coworkers (67) found a strong relation between core size and plaque rupture in aorta; in ruptured plaques, the lipid-rich core often occupied 30% to 40% or more of the plaque (67,68).

The lipid-rich core not only destabilizes plaques, it also is highly thrombogenic when exposed to circulating blood (59), caused by a high level of functionally active tissue factor most likely derived from the death of macrophages inside the plaque (60–62).

Fibrous Cap

The fibrous cap that separates the lipid-rich core from the arterial lumen varies considerably in thickness and often is thinned out in the vicinity of rupture (7,29). The fibrous cap contains extracellular matrix components that include collagen, elastin, and proteoglycans derived from smooth muscle cells. Thinning of the fibrous cap is generally considered a prelude to rupture and is therefore considered a feature of vulnerability. Fibrous caps from ruptured plaques contain less extracellular matrix (collagen and proteoglycans) and fewer smooth muscle cells than fibrous caps from intact plaques (7,29).

Plaque rupture results probably from an imbalance between synthesis and breakdown of extracellular matrix in the fibrous cap resulting in depletion of collagen and other matrix components, which, in turn, leads to thinning of the cap, predisposing the cap to spontaneous rupture or rupture in response to a variety of triggers (3,7,8,29).

Smooth Muscle Cells and Matrix Synthesis

Because vascular smooth muscle cells are responsible for secretion of extracellular matrix, reduced synthetic function or reduced smooth muscle cell numbers may play an important role in depleting matrix from the fibrous cap, which eventually may lead to plaque rupture (7,29). On the basis of *in vitro* experiments, Libby (47) has shown that interferon γ inhibits collagen gene expression in smooth muscle cells, suggesting the possibility that activated T cells in the plaque may inhibit matrix synthesis by producing interferon γ. Increased death of smooth muscle cells by apoptosis also has been demonstrated by several investigators in human atherothrombosis, and several key players of the apoptotic pathway have been demonstrated in atherothrombotic lesions (65,66, 69–80). The precise signals that induce smooth muscle cell death are unknown, but some of the putative culprits include oxidized lipids and cytokines (75,81). We have observed evidence of *in vivo* cleavage of macrophage-derived Tenascin-c in some human atherothrombotic plaques and demonstrated that epidermal growth factor–like domain of cleaved Tenascin-c is a potent inducer of apoptosis in vascular smooth muscle cells (81a). Because it is known that matrix metalloproteinases (MMPs) can cleave Tenascin-c, we have hypothesized that macrophages in atherothrombotic lesions may contribute to smooth muscle cell death, at least in part, through this mechanism.

Inflammation and Matrix Breakdown

Increased breakdown of extracellular matrix may also contribute to matrix depletion, thinning, and eventual rupture of the fibrous cap. Pathoanatomic studies have shown that compared with intact plaques, ruptured plaques and, by inference, intact but rupture-prone plaques have increased numbers of inflammatory cells, mostly macrophages but also including, to a less extent, T cells and mast cells (7,29). The fibrous cap is usually thinnest and most inflamed at the shoulder regions where the cap tends to rupture (~60% of cases) (16,82–85). Inflammatory cells may also be seen at the base of the lipid-rich core, around areas of neovascularization, and in the adjacent adventitia (20,68,86–90). These inflammatory cells often show evidence of heightened activity (20,87). It is generally believed that inflammatory cells are recruited into the atherosclerotic plaques by adhesion molecules such as VCAM-1 and chemokines such as MCP-1 and activated in the vessel wall by factors such as oxidized lipids and cytokines such as M-CSF. However, it also has been postulated that adventitial neovasculature, enhanced in atherosclerosis, provides another potential avenue for the entry and recruitment of inflammatory cells inside the atherosclerotic lesion. Factors that may contribute to recruitment of inflammatory cells and their activation in atherothrombosis include oxidized lipids, increased angiotensin II activity, increased arterial pressure, diabetes, chronic infections remote from the arterial wall creating a heightened systemic proinflammatory state, potential infectious organisms in the vessel wall (e.g., *Chlamydia pneumoniae*, cytomegalovirus), and activation of the immune system (29). Macrolide antibiotics (against Chlamydia) have been tested in the secondary prevention of cardiovascular disease, including patients with acute coronary syndromes (e.g., the AZithromycin in Acute Coronary Syndromes Trial by Cercek and coworkers.) (91). No clearcut benefit has emerged from these trials (92). A recent case–control study by Naghavi and coworkers (93) and an influenza vaccine pilot study by Gurfinkel and coworkers. (FLU Vaccination Acute Coronary Syndromes [FLUVACS] Study) (94) indicated, however, that influenza infection might play a role in triggering acute coronary events.

Increased matrix breakdown has been primarily attributed to a number of matrix-degrading metalloproteinases that are expressed in atherothrombotic plaques by inflammatory cells (macrophages, foam cells, and, to a lesser extent, smooth muscle cells and endothelial cells) (95–103). This family of enzymes collectively is capable of degrading all components of the extracellular matrix and has been shown to be catalytically active both *in vitro* and *in vivo* (96,104–106). The activity of these enzymes is tightly regulated at the level of gene transcription and by their secretion in an inactive zymogen form requiring extracellular activation and cosecretion of their tissue inhibitors (tissue inhibitor of metalloproteinases [TIMPS]) (105). Thus, increased gene transcription or enhanced activation of MMPs or reduced activity of TIMPS can create a milieu for increased matrix proteolysis. Activation of latent MMPs can be induced by plasmin generated by the activity of urokinase type plasminogen activator from plasminogen, trypsin, and chymase (derived from degranulating mast cells). Increased MMP production can be induced by oxidized lipids, reactive oxygen species, thrombin, chlamydial heat shock proteins, T cell interaction involving CD-40 ligation, inflammatory cytokines, and hemodynamic stress (89,101,103,105,107–111). We have shown that Tenascin-c, a complex matrix protein expressed in atherothrombotic plaques, also can increase MMP-9 production by monocyte-derived macrophages (112). Thus, all components necessary for the activation of the MMP pathway exist in the atherothrombotic plaques. In addition to MMPs, increased expression of elastolytic cysteine protease cathepsin-S and K and reduced expression of their inhibitor cystatin-c in human atherothrombotic lesions also have been demonstrated (113, 114). Despite the attractiveness of the MMP hypothesis, several limitations must be pointed out. Although MMPs are expressed in experimental animal models of atherosclerosis, convincing demonstration of human-like plaque rupture with superimposed thrombosis has proven elusive in such models (10,115–122). Even overexpression of human MMP-1 (interstitial collagenase) has failed to induce plaque rupture in murine models (123).

Thus, according to the current hypothesis, inflammatory cells play a critical role in plaque rupture by contributing to depletion of extracellular matrix in the fibrous cap through increased proteolysis or reduced matrix synthesis. Furthermore, data indicate that, contrary to conventional wisdom, neutrophils also are present in culprit lesions responsible for acute coronary syndromes (124).

Remodeling

Vascular remodeling is the ability of the vessel wall to reorganize its cellular and extracellular components in response to a chronic stimulus (125). Remodeling is a bidirectional process (126). Vulnerable plaques (large lipid-rich core, thin cap, and ongoing inflammation) and those responsible for the acute coronary syndromes are usually relatively large and are associated with compensatory enlargement (positive remodeling), which tends to preserve a normal lumen despite the presence of significant, and potentially dangerous, vessel wall disease (24–26,63). In contrast, plaques responsible for stable angina are usually smaller but, nevertheless, often cause more severe luminal narrowing because of concomitant local shrinkage of the artery (negative remodeling) (127). The reason for these different modes of remodeling is unknown, but processes in adventitia could play a critical role.

Potential Triggers for Plaque Rupture

Sudden rupture of a thin and inflamed fibrous cap may occur spontaneously, but triggering could also play a role, and thus help explain the nonrandom onset of acute coronary syndromes (12,13). Potential triggers may include extreme physical activity, especially in someone unaccustomed to regular physical activity; severe emotional trauma; sexual activity; exposure to illicit drugs such as cocaine, marijuana, or amphetamines; cold exposure; and acute infections—or just normal daily activities (12,13).

THROMBOSIS CAUSED BY PLAQUE RUPTURE

Plaque rupture was first reported as a fatal coronary event in 1844 in a Danish medical journal (128). The famous Danish sculptor Bertel Thorvaldsen suddenly died during the overture in the Royal Theater in Copenhagen, and a "plugged coronary" (Herrick's wording many years later [129]) caused by a rupture plaque was found at autopsy (6). In 1926, Benson (130) described that plaques beneath coronary thrombi often were physically broken, and Leary (131) stressed a few years later that plaque rupture is the standard terminal lesion in older individuals. But not until the mid-1960s was the critical role of plaque rupture in the pathogenesis of coronary thrombosis convincingly documented by detailed pathoanatomic studies performed in Europe by Sinapius (132) and in the United States by Chapman (133), Constantinides (134), and Friedman and van den Bovenkamp (135). It took, however, another 15 to 20 years before the significance of these observations were realized, when clinical studies revived the primary role of thrombosis in MI (136–140).

Cause, Consequence, or Epiphenomenon?

When a ruptured plaque is found beneath a thrombus, the question arises, of course, which came first? The frequent finding of components from the lipid-rich core within the thrombus or downstream of the rupture site clearly indicates the sequence of events: Plaque rupture precedes thrombus formation (4,20,133–135). Furthermore, this sequence, rather than the opposite, makes sense; the lipid-rich core contains active tissue factor and is, thus, thrombogenic. Therefore, if a ruptured plaque is found beneath a thrombus, it is generally considered a plausible precipitating cause.

However, plaque rupture does not inevitably lead to significant luminal thrombosis (21,141). The two other components of the triad of Virchow (blood and flow) are also decisive for the magnitude of the thrombotic response to plaque rupture (141).

Plaque Rupture Worldwide

A worldwide search revealed 18 autopsy studies in which 1,460 coronary thrombi were identified and studied carefully with the purpose to characterize the surface of the underlying atherothrombotic plaque (Table 31–2). Overall, a ruptured plaque was identified beneath 1,114 (76%) of the 1,460 coronary thrombi. The youngest mean age (48 years) and lowest frequency of plaque rupture (59%) were found in the medical examiner cases reported by Virmani and coworkers (5), and an even lower frequency of plaque rupture in coronary thrombosis (40–55%) was more recently reported by the same group (17).

Stratification for where the autopsies were performed revealed no major difference in the frequency of plaque rupture in coronary thrombosis (hospital: 79%, n = 935; coroner/medical examiner: 71%, n = 525). Thus, plaque rupture plays a major role in fatal coronary thrombosis, regardless of clinical presentation (MI or sudden death).

Risk Factors for Rupture-mediated Thrombosis

Many risk factors for atherothrombosis and ischemic heart disease have been identified, and it is generally assumed that these risk factors influence the speed of atherogenesis (plaque burden) (152). They could, however, also influence the composition of plaques and their risk for rupture and

thrombosis. On the basis of the data from our worldwide search, the possibility of a more specific role for cardiovascular risk factors in rupture-mediated coronary thrombosis was evaluated.

Age

Stratification for age revealed no major differences in the percentage of thrombi precipitated by plaque rupture (age > 60 years: 78%, n = 837; age < 60 years: 73%, n = 217; age unknown: 74%, n = 406).

Sex

Sex-specific data were reported in five studies (4,5,23,149, 151). The consistent message was that plaque rupture is a more frequent cause of coronary thrombosis in male (81%, n = 523) than in female individuals (59%, n = 203).

Menopause

Only one study contained a relatively large number of young female individuals (n = 16), and plaque rupture was a rare cause of coronary thrombosis in this series (6% vs. 70% in female individuals > 50 years of age) (153).

Ethnicity and Race

Stratified for geographic location, no major differences emerged in the frequency of rupture-mediated coronary thrombosis (Asia: 81%, n = 320; United States: 77%, n = 253; Europe: 75%, n = 887). Plaque rupture is the major cause of coronary thrombosis in China (92%, n = 61),

TABLE 31–2. *Worldwide 1,114 (76%) of 1,460 fatal coronary thrombi were precipitated by plaque rupture*

Patients	Age, years[a]	n	Rupture	Study, year (reference)
Hospital	—	19	19 = 100%	Chapman, 1965 (133)
Hospital	—	17	17 = 100%	Constantinides, 1966 (134)
Hospital, AMI+SCD	58	40	39 = 98%	Friedman and van den Bovenkamp, 1966 (135)
Hospital, AMI	62	88	71 = 81%	Bouch and Montgomery, 1970 (142)
Hospital, AMI	66	91	68 = 75%	Sinapius, 1972 (143)
Coroner, SCD	53	20	19 = 95%	Friedman et al., 1973 (144)
Hospital, AMI	67	76	69 = 91%	Horie et al., 1978 (145)
Hospital, AMI	67	49	40 = 82%	Falk, 1983 (4)
Coroner, SCD	<65	32	26 = 81%	Tracy et al., 1985 (146)
Medical examiner, SCD	<70	61	39 = 64%	el Fawal et al., 1987 (147)
Hospital, AMI	—	83	52 = 63%	Yutani et al., 1987 (148)
Coroner	—	85	71 = 84%	Richardson et al., 1989 (16)
Hospital, AMI	63	20	12 = 60%	van der Wal et al., 1994 (20)
Coroner, SCD	—	202	143 = 71%	Davies, 1997 (149)
Hospital, AMI	69	291	218 = 75%	Arbustini et al., 1999 (23)
Hospital, AMI	61	61	56 = 92%	Shi et al., 1999 (150)
Hospital, AMI	69	100	81 = 81%	Kojima et al., 2000 (151)
Medical examiner, SCD	48	125	74 = 59%	Virmani et al., 2000 (5)
AMI+SCD, overall		1,460	1,114 = 76%	Worldwide

Davies (149) and Virmani and coworkers (5) are updated summaries, including previously published data.
[a]Mean: —, not reported; AMI, acute myocardial infarction; SCD, sudden coronary death.

which is a population with a low average plasma cholesterol level (150).

Regarding black compared with white individuals in the United States, Burke and coworkers (28) concluded that "Race was not significantly associated with plaque rupture in men." No data on women alone has been reported, and the combined data (both sexes) is difficult to interpret because of relatively more and younger female individuals among the black compared with the white population (154).

Hypercholesterolemia

Burke and coworkers (28,153) found a positive association between plasma cholesterol (total and total:HDL ratio) and rupture-mediated coronary thrombosis, but the association was not strong and was not confirmed by Kojima and coworkers (151). As mentioned earlier, plaque rupture is the major cause of coronary thrombosis in China, where the average plasma cholesterol level is low (150).

Smoking

Only sparse and conflicting information is available on the role of smoking in rupture-mediated coronary thrombosis. Kojima and coworkers (151) found that smoking favored rupture-mediated coronary thrombosis, whereas Burke and coworkers (28,153) found a nonsignificant trend going in the opposite direction. Considering all evidence, smoking appears to be thrombogenic rather than atherogenic (155), and the increased risk for thrombus-mediated ischemic events in smokers might be explained by smoking-induced tissue factor expression in atherosclerotic plaques (156).

Diabetes

Contrasting results have been reported on the role of diabetes (predominantly type 2) in rupture-mediated coronary thrombosis. In our autopsy series, diabetes was less frequent in thrombosis caused by plaque rupture than in thrombosis without plaque rupture (13% vs. 33%, n = 8 thrombi in patients with diabetes) (4), and this trend was later confirmed in a larger series (11% vs. 64%, n = 41) (157). However, the opposite trend also has been reported (61% vs. 42%, not significant, n = 57) (151). On the basis of postmortem measurement of glycohemoglobin, Burke and coworkers (28, 153) found no significant association between impaired glucose metabolism and rupture-mediated coronary thrombosis. Therefore, type 2 diabetes does not appear to favor any particular type of coronary thrombosis.

Hypertension

Data on a possible relation between hypertension and rupture-mediated coronary thrombosis are available from four studies (4,28,151,153). Hypertension did not favor any particular type of coronary thrombosis.

Inflammation and C-Reactive Protein

Acute-phase reactants can usually be identified in advanced plaques, including fibrinogen, C-reactive protein (CRP), and serum amyloid A (152), but only one study has tried to evaluated their role in rupture-mediated coronary thrombosis (158). In this study, the CRP level determined postmortem did not correlate with the presence or mechanism of coronary thrombosis (55 ruptures and 18 erosions) in 144 persons who had died suddenly of coronary artery disease (158).

Infection

Microbial agents and their products have been identified in atherothrombotic plaques, but no published evidence suggests that plaques containing infectious agent–related products differ histologically from those without signs of plaque infection (159).

Exercise

Burke and coworkers (160) examined coronary thrombi in sudden coronary deaths and found that among those who died during acute exertion (n = 19), 89% of the thrombi were precipitated by plaque rupture. Among those who did not exercise immediately before sudden death (n = 51), "only" 53% had a ruptured plaque beneath the thrombus. These data suggest that severe exertion may trigger rupture-mediated coronary thrombosis (13,161). It should be remembered, however, that most heart attacks do not occur during strenuous exercise and that exercise appears to confer protection in the long run (13).

Stenosis and Local Shear

Contrasting results have been reported in the five studies in which the role of preexisting atherosclerotic stenosis (a major determinant of local flow and shear) in rupture-mediated coronary thrombosis has been evaluated (4,22,151,153, 157). Three studies found a positive association between stenosis severity and rupture-mediated coronary thrombosis (22,151,153), whereas two studies found the opposite (4,157).

Calcification

Ruptured plaques have been reported to be calcified more frequently than nonruptured plaques (69% vs. 23%) (22). It does not indicate, however, that calcification destabilizes plaques (17). Clinical observations suggest that culprit lesions responsible for acute coronary syndromes generally are less calcified than plaques responsible for stable angina, indicating that calcium confers stability to plaques rather than the opposite (53,55–58). The total amount of calcification—the calcium score—is a marker of plaque burden (and thus a marker of cardiovascular risk) rather than a marker of risk conferred by the individual calcified plaque (17).

Thus, regarding rupture-mediated thrombosis, plaque rupture is the major cause of coronary thrombosis, being responsible for approximately 76% of the fatal thrombotic events worldwide. Plaque rupture is a more frequent cause of coronary thrombosis in male (81%) than in female individuals (59%). It is rare in one extremely small subgroup of patients, namely premenopausal female individuals, who constitutes less than 1% of heart attack victims in the United States (162). Except for sex and menopause, no particular risk factors have consistently been connected with a particular type of coronary plaque or mechanism of thrombosis.

THROMBOSIS NOT CAUSED BY PLAQUE RUPTURE

The term plaque erosion has gained popularity for the minority of thrombi not precipitated by plaque rupture (~20% in male and ~40% in female individuals) (Fig. 31–2) (see color insert). Virmani and coworkers (5) have published extensively on the role of these lesions in sudden coronary death, and they introduced the term *calcified nodule* for a rare subtype of plaque erosion. It is a heterogenous group of atherothrombotic plaques where no deep injury is present to explain the overlying thrombus, only the endothelium is missing at the plaque–thrombus interface. The pathogenetic role of inflammation is controversial (5,17,20,21), and although tissue factor immunoreactivity has been identified in some of these lesions (163), its functional role is unknown.

The precise mechanisms of thrombosis over eroded plaques are unknown but probably reflect the heterogeneity of these plaques. It is conceivable that systemic thrombogenic factors such as platelet hyperaggregability, hypercoagulability, circulating tissue factor, and/or depressed fibrinolysis play a major role in thrombosis over plaques that are only eroded (vs. ruptured) (17,29). Studies have suggested that activated circulating leukocytes may transfer active tissue factor by shedding microparticles and transferring them onto adherent platelets (164,165). It is possible that such circulating sources of tissue factor rather than plaque-derived tissue factor can contribute to thrombosis at sites of endothelial denudation such as in plaque erosion.

THROMBOTIC RESPONSE TO PLAQUE RUPTURE

The three major determinants of the thrombotic response to plaque rupture (or the amount of thrombosis formed on top of an eroded plaque) are (a) local thrombogenic substrate, (b) local flow disturbances, and (c) systemic thrombotic propensity.

Local Thrombogenic Substrate

Ongoing inflammation, particularly macrophage infiltration and activation, and lipid accumulation not only destabilize plaques making them vulnerable to rupture, these plaque components also appear to be highly thrombogenic when exposed to the flowing blood after plaque rupture. Activated macrophages express tissue factor, and the lipid-rich atheromatous core contains a lot of active tissue factor, probably originating from dead macrophages (60–62). Culprit lesions responsible for the acute coronary syndromes contain more tissue factor than plaques responsible for stable angina (166). Oxidized lipids in the lipid-rich core may also directly stimulate platelet aggregation (167).

Local Flow Disturbances

In contrast to venous thrombosis, rapid flow and high shear forces promote arterial thrombosis, probably through shear-induced platelet activation (141). A platelet-rich thrombus may indeed form and grow within a severe stenosis, where the blood velocity and shear forces are greatest. Irregularities of the exposed surface also increase platelet-mediated thrombus formation (59).

Systemic Thrombotic Propensity

The state (activation) of platelets, coagulation, and fibrinolysis is critical for the outcome of plaque rupture, documented by the protective effect of antiplatelet agents and anticoagulants in patients at risk for coronary thrombosis. Tissue factor probably plays an important prothrombotic role both locally (expressed by macrophages in the culprit lesion) and systemically (expressed by activated leukocytes in the peripheral blood) (164,165,168).

Platelets and Fibrin

In coronary thrombosis, the initial flow obstruction is usually caused by platelet aggregation, but fibrin is important for the subsequent stabilization of the early and fragile platelet thrombus (141). Thus, both platelets and fibrin are involved in the evolution of a stable and persisting coronary thrombus.

Dynamic Thrombosis and Microembolization

The thrombotic response to plaque rupture is dynamic; thrombosis and thrombolysis, often associated with vasospasm (169), tend to occur simultaneously, causing intermittent flow obstruction and distal embolization. The latter leads to microvascular obstruction, which may prevent myocardial reperfusion despite a "successfully" recanalized infarct-related artery (170).

Clinical Manifestations

Atherosclerosis with ruptured and eroded coronary plaques is common and clinically silent for long periods. However, acute thrombosis (with or without vasospasm) may cause sudden flow obstruction, giving rise to an acute coronary syndrome (3,47,171). The culprit lesion is frequently "dynamic," causing intermittent flow obstruction, and the clinical presentation and the outcome depend on the location of the obstruction and the severity and duration of myocardial ischemia. A nonocclusive or transiently occlusive thrombus most frequently underlies acute coronary syndromes without ST-segment elevation, whereas a more stable and occlusive thrombus prevails in ST-segment elevation MI—overall modified by vascular tone and collateral flow. A critical thrombotic component also is frequent in culprit lesions responsible for out-of-hospital cardiac arrest and sudden coronary death.

MULTIPLE "ACTIVE" PLAQUES IN ACUTE CORONARY SYNDROMES

The risk for a recurrent event is particularly high during the first month after an acute coronary syndrome, and it has generally been assumed that the same atherothrombotic plaque, the culprit lesion, is responsible not only for the initial but also for the recurrent event. Recent observations indicate, however, that not just one but multiple "active," complex, and rapidly progressing coronary lesions frequently are present in patients who have had an acute heart attack (172–174).

Pathoanatomic Observations

Plaque rupture is not a rare event. It is followed by a variable amount of hemorrhage into the plaque and luminal thrombosis (often small and nonobstructive), causing sudden and rapid, but often clinically silent, growth of the lesion. It is probably the most important mechanism underlying the episodic (vs. linear) progression of some coronary lesions observed by serial angiography (175,176). Davies and coworkers (177) found ruptured coronary plaques without luminal thrombosis in 9% of persons who died suddenly of noncardiac causes, increasing to 22% (including 5% with nonocclusive thrombosis) if an atheroma-related disease such as diabetes or hypertension was present (177). And many more ruptured plaques are found in patients dying of rather than with coronary atherothrombosis (4,14,178). In 47 of such patients, we identified 103 ruptured coronary plaques (an average of 2.2 per patient) of which only 40 had obstructive, and probably fatal, luminal thrombosis superimposed, whereas the remaining 63 ruptures were without luminal thrombosis or covered only by a small nonobstructive, and thus probably asymptomatic, thrombus (4). None of these ruptured plaques were healed, suggesting they had developed within a relatively short period before death, although not necessarily simultaneously. Frink (178) identified 211 ulcerated plaques, of which many were judged to be chronic, in 83 cases of acute coronary death and concluded that ulcerated plaques without thrombosis are ubiquitous and multiple in such patients. Finally, a special nonuniform pattern of dense (older) and loosely arranged (younger) collagen, judged to represent the healed stage of subclinical

plaque disruption, has been identified in many coronary plaques, particularly in those causing chronic high-grade stenosis (175,176). Therefore, plaque rupture, causing episodic plaque growth, is not a rare event in the spontaneous progression of coronary atherosclerosis, and more than one ruptured plaque, with or without thrombosis superimposed, are usually present in individuals dying of the disease. The temporal relation among multiple ruptured plaques, particularly whether they occurred simultaneously or not, remains, however, elusive because exact dating of acute coronary lesions is difficult if not impossible.

Not only multiple ruptured plaques but even multiple thrombi are relatively frequent in those who die of an acute heart attack. We identified 51 recent coronary thrombi (and 29 old coronary occlusions) in 44 patients who died of coronary atherosclerosis (4). In the landmark study by Davies and Thomas (14) of sudden coronary death (n = 100), coronary thrombosis was present in 74 cases of which 28 (38%) had more than one discontinuous segment with thrombosis. In all, 115 separate thrombi were found, and major coronary thrombosis, occluding more than 50% of the lumen, was present in 44 of the 74 cases (14). That is, many of the thrombi identified in this thorough autopsy study were small and nonobstructive and thus probably asymptomatic. Arbustini and coworkers (23) reported their experience in a large autopsy series of 298 patients with acute MI; they found multiple coronary thrombi in 29 (10%) of the cases, apparently unrelated to the integrity of the underlying plaque surface (whether it was ruptured or just eroded). Therefore, multiple ruptured plaques, of which many are unhealed and probably ruptured recently, are frequently present in patients with an acute coronary syndrome, and multiple coronary thrombosis is found in more than 10% of autopsied cases. It seems likely that multiple coronary thrombosis often has a rapid and fatal course, which may explain why it is rarely recognized clinically (179).

Clinical Observations

Some years ago cardiologists were puzzled by that the number and severity of coronary stenoses were similar in patients with stable and unstable angina, despite the worse short-term prognosis of the latter (180). Ambrose and coworkers (181) were the first to draw attention to the different angiographic morphology of culprit lesions, and it was soon realized that the behavior of culprit lesions also differed in the two syndromes. In unstable angina, a typical culprit lesion is angiographically complex (ruptured plaque), intraluminal filling defects (nonocclusive thrombosis) and vasospasm are frequent in the acute phase, and rapid progression to total occlusion (occlusive thrombosis) is impending (180). Later it was realized, primarily thanks to a series of provocative angiographic observations by Kaski's group (182,183), that unstable patients often harbor multiple complex coronary lesions (an average of 2.6 per patient) (184) of which only one is usually pointed out as the main culprit. And, importantly, the more complex the plaques, the worse the prognosis (180). Supportive evidence for the presence of multiple "active" lesions in unstable angina was provided by the demonstration of widespread (i.e., involvement of more than one major coronary artery) activation of neutrophils across the coronary vascular bed, regardless of the location of the culprit stenosis (185). These findings have been extended to patients with MI (26,179,186–188). Goldstein and coworkers (187) identified multiple complex coronary plaques in as many as 40% of infarct patients undergoing angiographic examination, and the presence of multiple (vs. single) complex plaques was associated with adverse clinical outcomes. This finding suggests multifocal disease activity with rapid progression of nonculprit lesions after MI. Patients with single and multiple complex plaques did not differ significantly in age, sex ratio, or the frequency of coronary risk factors, including current smoking, diabetes mellitus, and hypercholesterolemia (187). In non–Q-wave infarction, 423 complex lesions were identified in 274 patients (189). Although these figures for complex lesions are impressive, it should be remembered that angiography is able to identify only major plaque events, and thus underestimates the real number of "active" coronary lesions. Overall, not only culprit lesions but also other complex, but not considered culprit, lesions progress rapidly during and shortly after an acute heart attack, indicating that multiple plaque ruptures or thrombosis, or both, occur simultaneously or within a relatively short period in the coronary arteries of clinically unstable patients.

CONCLUSIONS

Atherothrombosis is a systemic inflammatory disease, and inflammation is particularly frequent and intense in ruptured plaques beneath coronary thrombi. The role of inflammation in plaque erosion is more questionable. Similar to other chronic inflammatory diseases such as rheumatoid arthritis, a stable phase may suddenly be punctuated by an acute crisis in atherosclerosis, probably caused by activation of the disease. The chronic atherogenic stimuli are better, although not exhaustively, characterized than those leading to or "precipitating" acute crises, but some candidates are emerging. Indeed, the frequent finding of more than one "active" coronary lesion of which one is the main but not the only culprit in unstable patients suggests that more generalized pathogenetic processes may precipitate an acute crisis. An invasive approach may be needed to obtain rapid, complete, and sustained reperfusion of infarct-related arteries (primary angioplasty) or to "passivate" one or a few complex lesions that pose a particularly high short-term risk in unstable angina, but a target lesion-based approach alone will not eliminate the threat posed by all the other existing coronary plaques, and their overall risk determines the long-term prognosis. Atherosclerosis is a systemic disease and needs (also) systemic treatment.

REFERENCES

1. Murray CJ, Lopez AD. Mortality by cause for eight regions of the world: Global Burden of Disease Study. *Lancet* 1997;349:1269–1276.
2. Fuster V. Epidemic of cardiovascular disease and stroke: the three main challenges. Presented at the 71st scientific sessions of the American Heart Association. Dallas, Texas. *Circulation* 1999;99:1132–1137.
3. Davies MJ. The pathophysiology of acute coronary syndromes. *Heart* 2000;83:361–366.
4. Falk E. Plaque rupture with severe pre-existing stenosis precipitating coronary thrombosis. Characteristics of coronary atherosclerotic plaques underlying fatal occlusive thrombi. *Br Heart J* 1983;50:127–134.
5. Virmani R, Kolodgie FD, Burke AP, et al. Lessons from sudden coronary death: a comprehensive morphological classification scheme for atherosclerotic lesions. *Arterioscler Thromb Vasc Biol* 2000;20:1262–1275.
6. Falk E. Why do plaques rupture? *Circulation* 1992,86[Suppl]:III30–III42.
7. Falk E, Shah PK, Fuster V. Coronary plaque disruption. *Circulation* 1995;92:657–671.
8. Libby P. Molecular bases of the acute coronary syndromes. *Circulation* 1995;91:2844–2850.
9. Stary HC, Chandler AB, Dinsmore RE, et al. A definition of advanced types of atherosclerotic lesions and a histological classification of atherosclerosis. A report from the Committee on Vascular Lesions of the Council on Arteriosclerosis, American Heart Association. *Circulation* 1995;92:1355–1374.
10. Abela GS, Picon PD, Friedl SE, et al. Triggering of plaque disruption and arterial thrombosis in an atherosclerotic rabbit model. *Circulation* 1995;91:776–784.
11. Clubb FJ, Cerny JL, Deferrari DA, et al. Development of atherosclerotic plaque with endothelial disruption in Watanabe heritable hyperlipidemic rabbit aortas. *Cardiovasc Pathol* 2001;10:1–11.
12. Muller JE, Stone PH, Turi ZG, et al. Circadian variation in the frequency of onset of acute myocardial infarction. *N Engl J Med* 1985;313:1315–1322.
13. Servoss SJ, Januzzi JL, Muller JE. Triggers of acute coronary syndromes. *Prog Cardiovasc Dis* 2002;44:369–380.
14. Davies MJ, Thomas A. Thrombosis and acute coronary-artery lesions in sudden cardiac ischemic death. *N Engl J Med* 1984;310:1137–1140.
15. Davies MJ, Thomas AC. Plaque fissuring—the cause of acute myocardial infarction, sudden ischaemic death, and crescendo angina. *Br Heart J* 1985;53:363–373.
16. Richardson PD, Davies MJ, Born GV. Influence of plaque configuration and stress distribution on fissuring of coronary atherosclerotic plaques. *Lancet* 1989;2:941–944.
17. Virmani R, Burke AP, Farb A, et al. Pathology of the unstable plaque. *Prog Cardiovasc Dis* 2002;44:349–356.
18. Falk E. Morphologic features of unstable atherothrombotic plaques underlying acute coronary syndromes. *Am J Cardiol* 1989;63:114E–120E.
19. Willerson JT. Systemic and local inflammation in patients with unstable atherosclerotic plaques. *Prog Cardiovasc Dis* 2002;44:469–478.
20. van der Wal AC, Becker AE, van der Loos CM, et al. Site of intimal rupture or erosion of thrombosed coronary atherosclerotic plaques is characterized by an inflammatory process irrespective of the dominant plaque morphology. *Circulation* 1994;89:36–44.
21. Davies MJ. Going from immutable to mutable atherosclerotic plaques. *Am J Cardiol* 2001;88[Suppl]:2F–9F.
22. Farb A, Burke AP, Tang AL, et al. Coronary plaque erosion without rupture into a lipid core. A frequent cause of coronary thrombosis in sudden coronary death. *Circulation* 1996;93:1354–1363.
23. Arbustini E, Dal Bello B, Morbini P, et al. Plaque erosion is a major substrate for coronary thrombosis in acute myocardial infarction. *Heart* 1999;82:269–272.
24. Pasterkamp G, Schoneveld AH, van der Wal AC, et al. Relation of arterial geometry to luminal narrowing and histologic markers for plaque vulnerability: the remodeling paradox. *J Am Coll Cardiol* 1998;32:655–662.
25. Varnava AM, Mills PG, Davies MJ. Relationship between coronary artery remodeling and plaque vulnerability. *Circulation* 2002;105:939–943.
26. Rioufol G, Finet G, Ginon I, et al. Multiple atherosclerotic plaque

rupture in acute coronary syndrome: a three-vessel intravascular ultrasound study. *Circulation* 2002;106:804–808.

27. Mann JM, Davies MJ. Vulnerable plaque. Relation of characteristics to degree of stenosis in human coronary arteries. *Circulation* 1996; 94:928–931.

28. Burke AP, Farb A, Malcom GT, et al. Coronary risk factors and plaque morphology in men with coronary disease who died suddenly. *N Engl J Med* 1997;336:1276–1282.

29. Shah PK. Pathophysiology of coronary thrombosis: role of plaque rupture and plaque erosion. *Prog Cardiovasc Dis* 2002;44:357–368.

30. Majno G, Joris I. *Cells, tissues, and disease. Principles of general pathology.* Malden, MA: Blackwell Science, 1996:646.

31. Napoli C, Glass CK, Witztum JL, et al. Influence of maternal hypercholesterolaemia during pregnancy on progression of early atherosclerotic lesions in childhood: Fate of Early Lesions in Children (FELIC) study. *Lancet* 1999;354:1234–1241.

32. Ross R. Atherosclerosis—an inflammatory disease. *N Engl J Med* 1999;340:115–126.

33. Hansson GK, Libby P, Schonbeck U, et al. Innate and adaptive immunity in the pathogenesis of atherosclerosis. *Circ Res* 2002;91:281–291.

34. Binder CJ, Chang MK, Shaw PX, et al. Innate and acquired immunity in atherogenesis. *Nat Med* 2002;8:1218–1226.

35. Hansson GK. Immune responses in atherosclerosis. In: Hansson GK, Libby P, eds. *Immune functions of the vessel wall.* Amsterdam: Harwood Academic Publishers, 1996.

36. Witztum JL, Palinski W. Are immunological mechanisms relevant for the development of atherosclerosis? *Clin Immun* 1999;90:153–156.

37. Stary HC, Chandler AB, Glagov S, et al. A definition of initial, fatty streak, and intermediate lesions of atherosclerosis. A report from the Committee on Vascular Lesions of the Council on Arteriosclerosis, American Heart Association. *Circulation* 1994;89:246–278.

38. McGill HC Jr. George Lyman Duff memorial lecture. Persistent problems in the pathogenesis of atherosclerosis. *Arteriosclerosis* 1984;4: 443–451.

39. McGill HC Jr, McMahan CA, Malcom GT, et al. Effects of serum lipoproteins and smoking on atherosclerosis in young men and women. The PDAY Research Group. Pathobiological Determinants of Atherosclerosis in Youth. *Arterioscler Thromb Vasc Biol* 1997;17: 95–106.

40. Guyton JR. Phospholipid hydrolytic enzymes in a 'cesspool' of arterial intimal lipoproteins: a mechanism for atherogenic lipid accumulation. *Arterioscler Thromb Vasc Biol* 2001;21:884–886.

41. Davies MJ, Woolf N. Atherosclerosis: what is it and why does it occur? *Br Heart J* 1993;69[Suppl]:S3–S11.

42. Burrig KF. The endothelium of advanced arteriosclerotic plaques in humans. *Arterioscler Thromb* 1991;11:1678–1689.

43. Ruggeri ZM. Platelets in atherothrombosis. *Nat Med* 2002;8: 1227–1234.

44. Falk E, Fernández-Ortiz A. Role of thrombosis in atherosclerosis and its complications. *Am J Cardiol* 1995;75:5B–11B.

45. Doherty TM, Shah PK, Rajavashisth TB. Cellular origins of atherosclerosis: towards ontogenetic endgame? *FASEB J* 2003;17:592–597.

46. O'Brien KD, McDonald TO, Chait A, et al. Neovascular expression of E-selectin, intercellular adhesion molecule-1, and vascular cell adhesion molecule-1 in human atherosclerosis and their relation to intimal leukocyte content. *Circulation* 1996;93:672–682.

47. Libby P. Current concepts of the pathogenesis of the acute coronary syndromes. *Circulation* 2001;104:365–372.

48. Donley GE, Fitzpatrick LA. Noncollagenous matrix proteins controlling mineralization; possible role in pathologic calcification of vascular tissue. *Trends Cardiovasc Med* 1998;8:199–206.

49. Wexler L, Brundage B, Crouse J, et al. Coronary artery calcification: pathophysiology, epidemiology, imaging methods, and clinical implications. A statement for health professionals from the American Heart Association. Writing Group. *Circulation* 1996;94:1175–1192.

50. Blankenhorn DH. Coronary arterial calcification: a review. *Am J Med Sci* 1961;242:41–49.

51. Lachman AS, Spray TL, Kerwin DM, et al. Medial calcinosis of Monckeberg. A review of the problem and a description of a patient with involvement of peripheral, visceral and coronary arteries. *Am J Med* 1977;63:615–622.

52. Sangiorgi G, Rumberger JA, Severson A, et al. Arterial calcification and not lumen stenosis is highly correlated with atherosclerotic plaque burden in humans: a histologic study of 723 coronary artery

segments using nondecalcifying methodology. *J Am Coll Cardiol* 1998;31:126–133.

53. Mintz GS, Pichard AD, Popma JJ, et al. Determinants and correlates of target lesion calcium in coronary artery disease: a clinical, angiographic and intravascular ultrasound study. *J Am Coll Cardiol* 1997;29:268–274.

54. Baumgart D, Schmermund A, Goerge G, et al. Comparison of electron beam computed tomography with intracoronary ultrasound and coronary angiography for detection of coronary atherosclerosis. *J Am Coll Cardiol* 1997;30:57–64.

55. Hodgson JM, Reddy KG, Suneja R, et al. Intracoronary ultrasound imaging: correlation of plaque morphology with angiography, clinical syndrome and procedural results in patients undergoing coronary angioplasty. *J Am Coll Cardiol* 1993;21:35–44.

56. Rasheed Q, Nair R, Sheehan H, et al. Correlation of intracoronary ultrasound plaque characteristics in atherosclerotic coronary artery disease patients with clinical variables. *Am J Cardiol* 1994;73: 753–758.

57. Gertz SD, Roberts WC. Hemodynamic shear force in rupture of coronary arterial atherosclerotic plaques. *Am J Cardiol* 1990;66:1368–1372.

58. Beckman JA, Ganz J, Creager MA, et al. Relationship of clinical presentation and calcification of culprit coronary artery stenoses. *Arterioscler Thromb Vasc Biol* 2001;21:1618–1622.

59. Fernandez-Ortiz A, Babimon JJ, Falk E, et al. Characterization of the relative thrombogenicity of atherosclerotic plaque components: implications for consequences of plaque rupture. *J Am Coll Cardiol* 1994;23:1562–1569.

60. Toschi V, Gallo R, Lettino M, et al. Tissue factor modulates the thrombogenicity of human atherosclerotic plaques. *Circulation* 1997; 95:594–599.

61. Badimon JJ, Lettino M, Toschi V, et al. Local inhibition of tissue factor reduces the thrombogenicity of disrupted human atherosclerotic plaques: effects of tissue factor pathway inhibitor on plaque thrombogenicity under flow conditions. *Circulation* 1999;99:1780–1787.

62. Mallat Z, Hugel B, Ohan J, et al. Shed membrane microparticles with procoagulant potential in human atherosclerotic plaques: a role for apoptosis in plaque thrombogenicity. *Circulation* 1999;99:348–353.

63. Schoenhagen P, Ziada KM, Kapadia SR, et al. Extent and direction of arterial remodeling in stable versus unstable coronary syndromes: an intravascular ultrasound study. *Circulation* 2000;101:598–603.

64. Ball RY, Stowers EC, Burton JH, et al. Evidence that the death of macrophage foam cells contributes to the lipid core of atheroma. *Atherosclerosis* 1995;114:45–54.

65. Björkerud S, Björkerud B. Apoptosis is abundant in human atherosclerotic lesions, especially in inflammatory cells (macrophages and T cells), and may contribute to the accumulation of gruel and plaque instability. *Am J Pathol* 1996;149:367–380.

66. Geng YJ, Libby P. Evidence for apoptosis in advanced human atheroma. *Am J Pathol* 1995;147:251–266.

67. Davies MJ, Richardson PD, Woolf N, et al. Risk of thrombosis in human atherosclerotic plaques: role of extracellular lipid, macrophage, and smooth muscle cell content. *Br Heart J* 1993;69:377–381.

68. Felton CV, Crook D, Davies MJ, et al. Relation of plaque lipid composition and morphology to the stability of human aortic plaques. *Arterioscler Thromb Vasc Biol* 1997;17:1337–1345.

69. Bennett MR, Evan GI, Schwartz SM. Apoptosis of human vascular smooth muscle cells derived from normal vessels and coronary atherosclerotic plaques. *J Clin Invest* 1995;95:2266–2274.

70. Kockx, MM, DeMeyer GR, Muhring J, et al. Distribution of cell replication and apoptosis in atherosclerotic plaques of cholesterol-fed rabbits. *Atherosclerosis* 1996;120:115–124.

71. Crisby M, Nordin-Fredriksson G, Shah PK, et al. Cell death in human atherosclerotic plaques involves both oncosis and apoptosis. *Atherosclerosis* 1997;130:17–27.

72. Ihling C, Haendeler J, Menzel G, et al. Co-expression of p53 and MDM2 in human atherosclerosis: implications for the regulation of cellularity of atherosclerotic lesions. *J Pathol* 1998;185:303–312.

73. Bennett MR. Apoptosis of vascular smooth muscle cells in vascular remodelling and atherosclerotic plaque rupture. *Cardiovasc Res* 1999; 41:361–368.

74. Galle J, Heermeier K, Wanner C. Atherogenic lipoproteins, oxidative stress, and cell death. *Kidney Int* 1999;[Suppl 71]:S62–S65.

75. Vieira O, Escargueil-Blanc I, Jurgens G, et al. Oxidized LDLs alter the activity of the ubiquitin-proteasome pathway: potential role in oxidized LDL-induced apoptosis. *FASEB J* 2000;14:532–542.

76. Rossig L, Dimmeler S, Zeiher AM. Apoptosis in the vascular wall and atherosclerosis. *Basic Res Cardiol* 2001;96:11–22.

77. Geng YJ, Henderson LE, Levesque EB, et al. Fas is expressed in human atherosclerotic intima and promotes apoptosis of cytokine-primed human vascular smooth muscle cells. *Arterioscler Thromb Vasc Biol* 1997;17:2200–2208.

78. Kockx MM, Herman AG. Apoptosis in atherosclerosis: beneficial or detrimental? *Cardiovasc Res* 2000;45:736–746.

79. Kockx MM, Knaapen MW. The role of apoptosis in vascular disease. *J Pathol* 2000;190:267–280.

80. Mallat Z, Tedgui A. Apoptosis in the vasculature: mechanisms and functional importance. *Br J Pharmacol* 2000;130:947–962.

81. Geng YJ, Wu Q, Muszynski M, et al. Apoptosis of vascular smooth muscle cells induced by in vitro stimulation with interferon-gamma, tumor necrosis factor-alpha, and interleukin-1 beta. *Arterioscler Thromb Vasc Biol* 1996;16:19–27.

81a. Wallner K, Li C, Shah PK, et al. FGF-like domain of tenascin-C is proapoptotic for cultured smooth muscle cells. *Arterioscler Thromb Vasc Biol* 2004;24:1416–1421.

82. Loree HM, Kamm RD, Stringfellow RG, et al. Effects of fibrous cap thickness on peak circumferential stress in model atherosclerotic vessels. *Circ Res* 1992;71:850–858.

83. Cheng GC, Loree HM, Kamm RD, et al. Distribution of circumferential stress in ruptured and stable atherosclerotic lesions. A structural analysis with histopathological correlation. *Circulation* 1993;87:1179–1187.

84. Loree HM, Tobias BJ, Gibson LJ, et al. Mechanical properties of model atherosclerotic lesion lipid pools. *Arterioscler Thromb* 1994;14:230–234.

85. Huang H, Virmani R, Younis H, et al. The impact of calcification on the biomechanical stability of atherosclerotic plaques. *Circulation* 2001;103:1051–1056.

86. Kovanen PT. The mast cell—a potential link between inflammation and cellular cholesterol deposition in atherogenesis. *Eur Heart J* 1993;14[Suppl K]:105–117.

87. Kovanen PT, Kaartinen M, Paavonen T. Infiltrates of activated mast cells at the site of coronary atheromatous erosion or rupture in myocardial infarction. *Circulation* 1995;92:1084–1088.

88. Kovanen PT. Chymase-containing mast cells in human arterial intima: implications for atherosclerotic disease. *Heart Vessels* 1997;[Suppl 12]:125–127.

89. Kaartinen M, van der Wal AC, van der Loos CM, et al. Mast cell infiltration in acute coronary syndromes: implications for plaque rupture. *J Am Coll Cardiol* 1998;32:606–612.

90. Laine P, Kaartinen M, Penttila A, et al. Association between myocardial infarction and the mast cells in the adventitia of the infarct-related coronary artery. *Circulation* 1999;99:361–369.

91. Cercek B, Shah PK, Noc M, et al. Effect of short-term treatment with azithromycin on recurrent ischaemic events in patients with acute coronary syndrome in the Azithromycin in Acute Coronary Syndrome (AZACS) trial: a randomised controlled trial. *Lancet* 2003;361:809–813.

92. Neumann FJ. Chlamydia pneumoniae-atherosclerosis link: a sound concept in search for clinical relevance. *Circulation* 2002;106:2414–2416.

93. Naghavi M, Barlas Z, Siadaty S, et al. Association of influenza vaccination and reduced risk of recurrent myocardial infarction. *Circulation* 2000;102:3039–3045.

94. Gurfinkel EP, de la Fuente RL, Mendiz O, et al. Influenza vaccine pilot study in acute coronary syndromes and planned percutaneous coronary interventions: the FLU Vaccination Acute Coronary Syndromes (FLUVACS) Study. *Circulation* 2002;105:2143–2147.

95. Henney AM, Wakeley PR, Davies MJ, et al. Localization of stromelysin gene expression in atherosclerotic plaques by in situ hybridization. *Proc Natl Acad Sci USA* 1991;88:8154–8158.

96. Galis ZS, Sukhova GK, Lark MW, et al. Increased expression of matrix metalloproteinases and matrix degrading activity in vulnerable regions of human atherosclerotic plaques. *J Clin Invest* 1994;94:2493–2503.

97. Brown DL, Hibbs MS, Kearney M, et al. Identification of 92-kD gelatinase in human coronary atherosclerotic lesions. Association of active enzyme synthesis with unstable angina. *Circulation* 1995;91:2125–2131.

98. Nikkari ST, O'Brien KD, Ferguson M, et al. Interstitial collagenase (MMP-1) expression in human carotid atherosclerosis. *Circulation* 1995;92:1393–1398.

99. Li Z, Li L, Zielke HR, et al. Increased expression of 72-kd type IV collagenase (MMP-2) in human aortic atherosclerotic lesions. *Am J Pathol* 1996;148:121–128.

100. Galis ZS, Sukhova GK, Kranzhofer R, et al. Macrophage foam cells from experimental atheroma constitutively produce matrix-degrading proteinases. *Proc Natl Acad Sci USA* 1995;92:402–406.

101. Xu XP, Meisel SR, Ong JM, et al. Oxidized low-density lipoprotein regulates matrix metalloproteinase-9 and its tissue inhibitor in human monocyte-derived macrophages. *Circulation* 1999;99:993–998.

102. Rajavashisth TB, Xu XP, Jovinge S, et al. Membrane type 1 matrix metalloproteinase expression in human atherosclerotic plaques: evidence for activation by proinflammatory mediators. *Circulation* 1999;99:3103–3109.

103. Rajavashisth TB, Liao JK, Galis ZS, et al. Inflammatory cytokines and oxidized low density lipoproteins increase endothelial cell expression of membrane type 1-matrix metalloproteinase. *J Biol Chem* 1999;274:11924–11929.

104. Shah PK, Falk E, Badimon JJ, et al. Human monocyte-derived macrophages induce collagen breakdown in fibrous caps of atherosclerotic plaques. Potential role of matrix-degrading metalloproteinases and implications for plaque rupture. *Circulation* 1995;92:1565–1569.

105. Shah PK. Role of inflammation and metalloproteinases in plaque disruption and thrombosis. *Vasc Med* 1998;3:199–206.

106. Sukhova GK, Schonbeck U, Rabkin E, et al. Evidence for increased collagenolysis by interstitial collagenases-1 and -3 in vulnerable human atheromatous plaques. *Circulation* 1999;99:2503–2509.

107. Lee RT, Schoen FJ, Loree HM, et al. Circumferential stress and matrix metalloproteinase 1 in human coronary atherosclerosis. Implications for plaque rupture. *Arterioscler Thromb Vasc Biol* 1996;16:1070–1073.

108. Galis ZS, Muszynski M, Sukhova GK, et al. Enhanced expression of vascular matrix metalloproteinases induced in vitro by cytokines and in regions of human atherosclerotic lesions. *Ann NY Acad Sci* 1995;748:501–507.

109. Kol A, Sukhova GK, Lichtman AH, et al. Chlamydial heat shock protein 60 localizes in human atheroma and regulates macrophage tumor necrosis factor-alpha and matrix metalloproteinase expression. *Circulation* 1998;98:300–307.

110. Mach F, Schonbeck U, Fabunmi RP, et al. T lymphocytes induce endothelial cell matrix metalloproteinase expression by a CD40L-dependent mechanism: implications for tubule formation. *Am J Pathol* 1999;154:229–238.

111. Schonbeck U, Mach F, Sukhova GK, et al. Regulation of matrix metalloproteinase expression in human vascular smooth muscle cells by T lymphocytes: a role for CD40 signaling in plaque rupture? *Circ Res* 1997;81:448–454.

112. Wallner K, Li C, Shah PK, et al. Tenascin-C is expressed in macrophage-rich human coronary atherosclerotic plaque. *Circulation* 1999;99:1284–1289.

113. Sukhova GK, Shi GP, Simon DI, et al. Expression of the elastolytic cathepsins S and K in human atheroma and regulation of their production in smooth muscle cells. *J Clin Invest* 1998;102:576–583.

114. Shi GP, Sukhova GK, Grubb A, et al. Cystatin C deficiency in human atherosclerosis and aortic aneurysms. *J Clin Invest* 1999;104:1191–1197.

115. Rekhter MD, Hicks GW, Brammer DW, et al. Animal model that mimics atherosclerotic plaque rupture. *Circ Res* 1998;83:705–713.

116. Rosenfeld ME, Polinsky P, Virmani R, et al. Advanced atherosclerotic lesions in the innominate artery of the ApoE knockout mouse. *Arterioscler Thromb Vasc Biol* 2000;20:2587–2592.

117. Johnson JL, Jackson CL. Atherosclerotic plaque rupture in the apolipoprotein E knockout mouse. *Atherosclerosis* 2001;154:399–406.

118. Zhou J, Moller J, Danielsen CC, et al. Dietary supplementation with methionine and homocysteine promotes early atherosclerosis but not plaque rupture in ApoE-deficient mice. *Arterioscler Thromb Vasc Biol* 2001;21:1470–1476.

119. Calara F, Silvestre M, Casanada F, et al. Spontaneous plaque rupture and secondary thrombosis in apolipoprotein E-deficient and LDL receptor-deficient mice. *J Pathol* 2001;195:257–263.

120. Williams H, Johnson JL, Carson KG, et al. Characteristics of intact and ruptured atherosclerotic plaques in brachiocephalic arteries of apolipoprotein E knockout mice. *Arterioscler Thromb Vasc Biol* 2002;22:788–792.

121. von der Thüsen JH, van Vlijmen BJ, Hoeben RC, et al. Induction of

atherosclerotic plaque rupture in apolipoprotein E-/- mice after adenovirus-mediated transfer of p53. *Circulation* 2002;105:2064–2070.

122. Napoli C, Palinski W. Unraveling the mechanisms of plaque rupture in murine models. *Circulation* 2002;106:e186.

123. Lemaitre V, O'Byrne TK, Borczuk AC, et al. ApoE knockout mice expressing human matrix metalloproteinase-1 in macrophages have less advanced atherosclerosis. *J Clin Invest* 2001;107:1227–1234.

124. Naruko T, Ueda M, Haze K, et al. Neutrophil infiltration of culprit lesions in acute coronary syndromes. *Circulation* 2002;106:2894–2900.

125. Gibbons GH, Dzau VJ. The emerging concept of vascular remodeling. *N Engl J Med* 1994;330:1431–1438.

126. Mintz GS, Kent KM, Pichard AD, et al. Contribution of inadequate arterial remodeling to the development of focal coronary artery stenoses. An intravascular ultrasound study. *Circulation* 1997;95: 1791–1798.

127. Smits PC, Pasterkamp G, Quarles van Ufford MA, et al. Coronary artery disease: arterial remodelling and clinical presentation. *Heart* 1999;82:461–464.

128. Mødet den 26de Marts. *Ugeskr Læg* 1844;10:214–218.

129. Herrick JB. Clinical features of sudden obstruction of the coronary arteries. *JAMA* 1912;59:2015–2020.

130. Benson RL. The present status of coronary arterial disease. *Arch Pathol* 1926;2:876–916.

131. Leary T. Coronary spasm as a possible factor in producing sudden death. *Am Heart J* 1934;10:338–344.

132. Sinapius D. Über Wandveränderungen bei Coronarthrombose: Bemerkungen zur Häufigkeit, Entstehung und Bedeutung. *Klin Wschr* 1965;43:875–880.

133. Chapman I. Morphogenesis of occluding coronary artery thrombosis. *Arch Pathol* 1965;80:256–261.

134. Constantinides P. Plaque fissures in human coronary thrombosis. *J Atheroscler Res* 1966;6:1–17.

135. Friedman M, van den Bovenkamp GJ. The pathogenesis of a coronary thrombus. *Am J Pathol* 1966;48:19–44.

136. DeWood MA, Spores J, Notski R, et al. Prevalence of total coronary occlusion during the early hours of transmural myocardial infarction. *N Engl J Med* 1980;303:897–902.

137. DeWood MA, Spores J, Hensley GR, et al. Coronary arteriographic findings in acute transmural myocardial infarction. *Circulation* 1983;68[2 Pt 2]:139–149.

138. DeWood MA, Stifter WS, Simpson CS, et al. Coronary arteriographic findings soon after non-Q-wave myocardial infarction. *N Engl J Med* 1986;315:417–423.

139. Rentrop P, Blanke H, Karsch KR, et al. Selective intracoronary thrombolysis in acute myocardial infarction and unstable angina pectoris. *Circulation* 1981;63:307–317.

140. Ganz W, Ninomiya K, Hashida J, et al. Intracoronary thrombolysis in acute myocardial infarction: experimental background and clinical experience. *Am Heart J* 1981;102:1145–1149.

141. Falk E. Coronary thrombosis: pathogenesis and clinical manifestations. *Am J Cardiol* 1991;68:28B–35B.

142. Bouch DC, Montgomery GL. Cardiac lesions in fatal cases of recent myocardial ischaemia from a coronary care unit. *Br Heart J* 1970;32:795–803.

143. Sinapius D. Beziehungen zwischen Koronarthrombosen und Myokardinfarkten. *Dtsch Med Wochenschr* 1972;97:443–448.

144. Friedman M, Manwaring JH, Rosenman RH, et al. Instantaneous and sudden deaths. Clinical and pathological differentiation in coronary artery disease. *JAMA* 1973;225:1319–1328.

145. Horie T, Sekiguchi M, Hirosawa K. Coronary thrombosis in pathogenesis of acute myocardial infarction. Histopathological study of coronary arteries in 108 necropsied cases using serial section. *Br Heart J* 1978;40:153–161.

146. Tracy RE, Devaney K, Kissling G. Characteristics of the plaque under a coronary thrombus. *Virchows Arch A Pathol Anat Histopathol* 1985;405:411–427.

147. el Fawal MA, Berg GA, Wheatley DJ, et al. Sudden coronary death in Glasgow: nature and frequency of acute coronary lesions. *Br Heart J* 1987;57:329–335.

148. Yutani C, Ishibashi-Ueda H, Konishi M, et al. Histopathological study of acute myocardial infarction and pathoetiology of coronary thrombosis: a comparative study in four districts in Japan. *Jpn Circ J* 1987;51:352–361.

149. Davies MJ. The composition of coronary-artery plaques. *N Engl J Med* 1997;336:1312–1314.

150. Shi H, Wei L, Yang T, et al. Morphometric and histological study of coronary plaques in stable angina and acute myocardial infarctions. *Chin Med J* 1999;112:1040–1043.

151. Kojima S, Nonogi H, Miyao Y, et al. Is preinfarction angina related to the presence or absence of coronary plaque rupture? *Heart* 2000;83:64–68.

152. Falk E, Fuster V. Atherogenesis and its determinants. In: Fuster V, Alexander RW, O'Rourke RA, et al., eds. *Hurst's the heart,* 10th ed. New York: McGraw-Hill, 2001.

153. Burke AP, Farb A, Malcom GT, et al. Effect of risk factors on the mechanism of acute thrombosis and sudden coronary death in women. *Circulation* 1998;97:2110–2116.

154. Burke AP, Farb A, Pestaner J, et al. Traditional risk factors and the incidence of sudden coronary death with and without coronary thrombosis in blacks. *Circulation* 2002;105:419–424.

155. Bottcher M, Falk E. Pathology of the coronary arteries in smokers and non-smokers. *J Cardiovasc Risk* 1999;6:299–302.

156. Matetzky S, Tani S, Kangavari S, et al. Smoking increases tissue factor expression in atherosclerotic plaques: implications for plaque thrombogenicity. *Circulation* 2000;102:602–604.

157. Davies MJ. Stability and instability: two faces of coronary atherosclerosis. The Paul Dudley White Lecture 1995. *Circulation* 1996;94: 2013–2020.

158. Burke AP, Tracy RP, Kolodgie F, et al. Elevated C-reactive protein values and atherosclerosis in sudden coronary death: association with different pathologies. *Circulation* 2002;105:2019–2023.

159. Kol A, Libby P. The mechanisms by which infectious agents may contribute to atherosclerosis and its clinical manifestations. *Trends Cardiovasc Med* 1998;8:191–199.

160. Burke AP, Farb A, Malcom GT, et al. Plaque rupture and sudden death related to exertion in men with coronary artery disease. *JAMA* 1999;281:921–926.

161. Ciampricotti R, elGamal M. Exercise-induced plaque rupture producing myocardial infarction. *Int J Cardiol* 1986;12:102–108.

162. American Heart Association. *2002 heart and stroke statistical update.* Dallas, TX: American Heart Association, 2001:12.

163. Schonbeck U, Mach F, Sukhova GK, et al. CD40 ligation induces tissue factor expression in human vascular smooth muscle cells. *Am J Pathol* 2000;156:7–14.

164. Rauch U, Nemerson Y. Circulating tissue factor and thrombosis. *Curr Opin Hematol* 2000;7:273–277.

165. Mallat Z, Benamer H, Hugel B, et al. Elevated levels of shed membrane microparticles with procoagulant potential in the peripheral circulating blood of patients with acute coronary syndromes. *Circulation* 2000;101:841–843.

166. Ardissino D, Merlini PA, Ariens R, et al. Tissue-factor antigen and activity in human coronary atherosclerotic plaques. *Lancet* 1997;349: 769–771.

167. Essler M, Retzer M, Bauer M, et al. Stimulation of platelets and endothelial cells by mildly oxidized LDL proceeds through activation of lysophosphatidic acid receptors and the Rho/Rho-kinase pathway. Inhibition by lovastatin. *Ann NY Acad Sci* 2000;905:282–286.

168. Jude B, Agraou B, McFadden EP, et al. Evidence for time-dependent activation of monocytes in the systemic circulation in unstable angina, but not in acute myocardial infarction or in stable angina. *Circulation* 1994;90:1662–1668.

169. Bogaty P, Hackett D, Davies G, et al. Vasoreactivity of the culprit lesion in unstable angina. *Circulation* 1994;90:5–11.

170. Topol EJ, Yadav JS. Recognition of the importance of embolization in atherosclerotic vascular disease. *Circulation* 2000;101:570–580.

171. Fuster V, Badimon L, Badimon J, et al. The pathogenesis of coronary artery disease and the acute coronary syndromes. *N Engl J Med* 1992;326:242–250,310–318.

172. Falk E. Multiple culprits in acute coronary syndromes: systemic disease calling for systemic treatment [editorial]. *Ital Heart J* 2000;1:835–838.

173. Goldstein JA. Angiographic plaque complexity: the tip of the unstable plaque iceberg [editorial]. *J Am Coll Cardiol* 2002;39:1464–1467.

174. Schoenhagen P, Tuzcu EM, Ellis SG. Plaque vulnerability, plaque rupture, and acute coronary syndromes: (multi)-focal manifestation of a systemic disease process [editorial]. *Circulation* 2002;106:760–762.

175. Mann J, Davies MJ. Mechanisms of progression in native coronary artery disease: role of healed plaque disruption. *Heart* 1999;82:265–268.

176. Burke AP, Kolodgie FD, Farb A, et al. Healed plaque ruptures and

sudden coronary death: evidence that subclinical rupture has a role in plaque progression. *Circulation* 2001;103:934–940.

177. Davies MJ, Bland JM, Hangartner JR, et al. Factors influencing the presence or absence of acute coronary artery thrombi in sudden ischaemic death. *Eur Heart J* 1989;10:203–208.

178. Frink RJ. Chronic ulcerated plaques: new insights into the pathogenesis of acute coronary disease. *J Invasive Cardiol* 1994;6:173–185.

179. Asakura M, Ueda Y, Yamaguchi O, et al. Extensive development of vulnerable plaques as a pan-coronary process in patients with myocardial infarction: an angioscopic study. *J Am Coll Cardiol* 2001;37: 1284–1288.

180. Falk E, Fuster V. Angina pectoris and disease progression [editorial]. *Circulation* 1995;92:2033–2035.

181. Ambrose JA, Winters SL, Stern A, et al. Angiographic morphology and the pathogenesis of unstable angina pectoris. *J Am Coll Cardiol* 1985;5:609–616.

182. Chen L, Chester MR, Redwood S, et al. Angiographic stenosis progression and coronary events in patients with 'stabilized' unstable angina. *Circulation* 1995;91:2319–2324.

183. Kaski JC, Chester MR, Chen L, et al. Rapid angiographic progression of coronary artery disease in patients with angina pectoris. The role of complex stenosis morphology. *Circulation* 1995;92:2058–2065.

184. Garcia-Moll X, Coccolo F, Cole D, et al. Serum neopterin and complex stenosis morphology in patients with unstable angina. *J Am Coll Cardiol* 2000;35:956–962.

185. Buffon A, Biasucci LM, Liuzzo G, et al. Widespread coronary inflammation in unstable angina. *N Engl J Med* 2002;347:5–12.

186. Guazzi MD, Bussotti M, Grancini L, et al. Evidence of multifocal activity of coronary disease in patients with acute myocardial infarction. *Circulation* 1997;96:1145–1151.

187. Goldstein JA, Demetriou D, Grines CL, et al. Multiple complex coronary plaques in patients with acute myocardial infarction. *N Engl J Med* 2000;343:915–922.

188. Kerensky RA, Wade M, Deedwania P, et al. Revisiting the culprit lesion in non-Q-wave myocardial infarction. Results from the VANQWISH trial angiographic core laboratory. *J Am Coll Cardiol* 2002;39:1456–1463.

189. Boden WE, Kerensky RA, Bertolet BD, et al. Coronary angiographic findings after non-Q-wave myocardial infarction: an analysis from the VANQWISH trial. *Eur Heart J* 1997;18[Suppl]:123(abst).

CHAPTER 32

Atherothrombosis in Youth

Henry C. McGill, Jr. and C. Alex McMahan, for the Pathobiological Determinants of Atherosclerosis in Youth (PDAY) Research Group

Key Words: Atherosclerosis; atherothrombosis; coronary artery disease; primary prevention; risk factor; youth.

ORIGIN OF ATHEROTHROMBOSIS IN CHILDHOOD AND ADOLESCENCE

The origin of atherosclerosis in childhood and its progression through adolescence and young adulthood to atherothrombosis, the lesion directly causing coronary artery disease (CAD), have been inferred from observations on the arteries of individuals dying at various ages. The study of autopsy material was necessary because atherothrombotic lesions, particularly the early lesions before they produced luminal obstruction or became calcified, could not be assessed in living persons. It was even more difficult to relate suspected causative agents and intervening variables—the conditions commonly known as risk factors—to the rate of progression of these early stages of atherogenesis.

When atherothrombosis and CAD became recognized as preventable diseases shortly after the middle of the twentieth century, attention was focused initially on the advanced stages of disease leading directly to the clinical manifestations of angina pectoris, myocardial infarction, and sudden cardiac death. The concept of risk factors in longitudinal

H. C. McGill, Jr.: Department of Physiology and Medicine, Southwest Foundation for Biomedical Research, P.O. Box 760549, San Antonio, Texas 78245-0549; and the University of Texas Health Sciences Center at San Antonio, San Antonio, Texas.

C. A. McMahan: University of Texas Health Science Center at San Antonio, San Antonio, Texas.

epidemiologic studies was based on the ability of those traits to predict the probability of occurrence of clinical disease. Forty years of clinical trials have demonstrated the effectiveness of risk factor control in reducing the risk for clinical disease.

A number of clinical and autopsy studies have shown the association of the same risk factors with the extent and severity of atherothrombosis in adults (see Chapter 3). They also have shown by various imaging methods that risk factor control leads to regression of advanced lesions in living persons. However, the age at which the risk factors began to influence the process was not known. The need to answer this question was first appreciated in 1953 when it was found that 77% of young Korean War battle casualties, average age 22.1 years, had atherothrombotic lesions in their coronary arteries, and 15% had plaques producing 50% or greater stenosis (1). Subsequent studies of coronary arteries of young persons in the industrialized counties confirmed and extended this observation by quantifying different types of atherothrombotic lesions in successive age groups (2,3) and tracing the progression of lesions from uncomplicated fatty streaks to raised fibrous plaques, and thereafter to ruptured plaques and occlusive thrombosis (4,5).

RISK FACTORS IN YOUTH

As knowledge about the preclinical stages of atherogenesis developed, evidence accumulated that the risk factors for adult CAD also were present in children and adolescents. In the 1970s, several centers in the United States and Europe surveyed children and adolescents for levels of serum lipids and lipoproteins, blood pressure, obesity, and smoking (6–8). Although the average values and ranges of most risk factor variables were less than in adults, there was considerable variability. Furthermore, these variables tracked: children with high values tended to stay high, and children with low values remained low (9). The risk factors also tracked from childhood into young adulthood (10). Serum lipid and lipoprotein levels were greater in children of parents who had experienced precocious CAD (11), an observation consistent with the identification of family history as a risk factor. However, the only direct evidence that any of the risk factors affected atherothrombosis in children came from rare cases of homozygous familial hypercholesterolemia (12).

A few of the school-age children whose risk factors had been measured during life subsequently died of external causes and their arteries were examined at autopsy. Body mass index (BMI), systolic and diastolic blood pressure, and serum concentrations of cholesterol, low density-lipoprotein (LDL) cholesterol, and high-density lipoprotein (HDL) cholesterol were associated with coronary artery lesions (13,14). These observations supported the suspicion that the adult risk factors not only existed among children at modified levels, but might be important in determining the rate of progression of atherothrombosis in youth.

PATHOBIOLOGICAL DETERMINANTS OF ATHEROSCLEROSIS IN YOUTH STUDY

A multicenter cooperative study of atherothrombosis (Pathobiological Determinants of Atherosclerosis in Youth [PDAY]) (15) in autopsied young individuals dying of external causes was organized in 1985 to examine the relation of risk factors to early atherothrombosis. Participating investigators collected coronary arteries, aortas, blood, and other tissues from nearly 3,000 individuals aged 15 to 34 years who died of accidents, homicide, or suicide and were autopsied in medical examiners' laboratories. The collection took place between 1987 and 1994 in seven participating centers in the United States. The tissues and resulting data were analyzed in central laboratories. Methods of grading atherothrombosis, measuring risk factors, and analyzing data are described in detail in related publications (16–20) and are summarized briefly later in this chapter.

The right coronary artery (RCA) was opened longitudinally, fixed in the flattened state, and stained grossly with Sudan IV. Pathologists estimated the percent of intimal surface involved by Sudan-stained fatty streaks and by raised lesions, which included fibrous plaques and complicated lesions. The grading team also divided fatty streaks into flat fatty streaks and raised fatty streaks (the latter also known as intermediate lesions, transitional lesions, or raised fatty plaques). Raised fatty streaks represented lesions in transition from fatty streaks to fibrous plaques (21). To supplement the visual estimates of surface involvement by lesions, photographs of the stained RCAs were digitized and converted to standard formats, and composite images of specified groups were produced that showed the prevalence of fatty streaks and raised lesions at each pixel location (22). The aorta was bisected longitudinally and was fixed, stained, and graded in the same manner as the RCA.

The left anterior descending coronary artery (LADCA) was fixed under pressure, and microscopic sections stained for smooth muscle, connective tissue, and fat were prepared from a standard site just distal to the origin of the left circumflex artery. These sections were graded by the American Heart Association (AHA) system from 0 to 5 (23) (see Chapter 30) as follows:

0 = a normal arterial intima
1 = an early fatty streak with scattered macrophage foam cells
2 = a more advanced fatty streak with clusters of macrophage foam cells
3 = an intermediate lesion with many macrophage foam cells and small pools of extracellular lipid, corresponding to the grossly defined raised fatty streak (21)
4 = a fibrous plaque with one or more large pools of extracellular lipid and a thin fibromuscular cap
5 = a fibrous plaque with large pools of extracellular lipid and a thick fibromuscular cap

Grade 4 and 5 lesions had characteristics that indicated vulnerability to rupture and thrombosis (see Chapter 30). Atherothrombotic stenosis of 40% or greater was assessed by computerized morphometry of the same microscopic sections.

Central laboratories measured total serum cholesterol and HDL cholesterol concentrations and obtained the non-HDL cholesterol concentration by subtraction. The non-HDL cholesterol concentration was considered elevated if it was 160 mg/dL or greater (≥ 4.14 mM); and HDL cholesterol was considered low if it was less than 35 mg/dL (<0.91 mM). Smoking was judged present if the serum thiocyanate concentration was 90 µM or greater. Hypertension was present if the thickness of the intima of small renal arteries indicated a mean arterial pressure of 110 mm Hg or greater. Adiposity was evaluated by the BMI, computed as weight (kg) divided by height (m) squared; a BMI greater than 30 indicated the subject was obese. A red blood cell glycohemoglobin concentration of 8% or greater indicated a blood glucose concentration of approximately 150 mg/dL or greater (≥ 8.33 mM) during the previous 2 to 3 months.

NATURAL HISTORY OF ATHEROTHROMBOSIS IN YOUTH

The progression of atherothrombosis with age is shown in Figure 32–1 as the percent intimal surface involvement with fatty streaks and raised lesions in the RCA of men and women by 5-year age groups. The extent of fatty streaks in women was similar to that in men at all ages, but raised lesions were less extensive, becoming about half the extent in men at ages 30 to 34 years. This difference in raised lesions

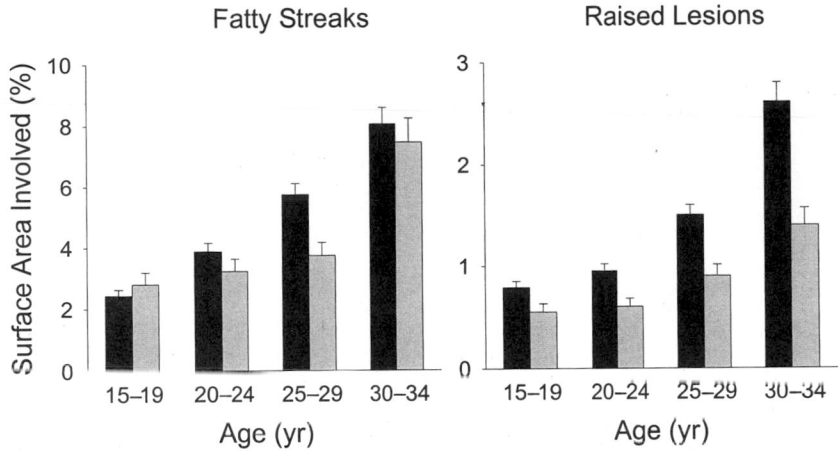

FIG. 32–1. Mean (+SE) extent involvement with fatty streaks **(left)** and raised lesions **(right)** in the right coronary artery by 5-year age groups of men *(black bars)* and women *(gray bars)*. (See color insert for Fig. 32–2.)

between men and women precedes by two decades the well known difference in clinical disease between the sexes during the premenopausal years. The sex difference was not explained by differences in risk factors.

The distribution of both fatty streaks and raised lesions in the RCA is shown in topographic prevalence maps for men and women by 5-year age groups in Figure 32–2 (see color insert). Fatty streaks increased with age in a characteristic anatomic pattern, and raised lesions followed a similar pattern, an observation consistent with the idea of progression from fatty streaks to raised lesions.

The prevalence of microscopically advanced lesions of the LADCA also increased with age and was greater in men than in women (Fig. 32–3). Less than 5% of subjects younger than 30 years of age had Grade 4 or 5 lesions, but by age 30 to 34 years, the prevalence in men approached

20%. Likewise, the prevalence of stenotic lesions increased slowly in the late teens and 20s, but became nearly as frequent as Grade 4 or 5 lesions in the early 30s. By both measures, as with gross extent of raised lesions in the RCA, the prevalence was twice as great for men than for women.

RISK FACTOR EFFECTS ON GROSS LESIONS

The effects of the risk factors measured in this study are summarized in Table 32–1, which shows the ratio of the extent of each type of lesion—flat fatty streaks, raised fatty streaks, and raised lesions—in subjects with the risk factor (as defined earlier) to the extent in subjects without the risk factor. Table 32–1 also includes ratios for the abdominal aorta and for the RCA to show both similarities and differences between the two arteries.

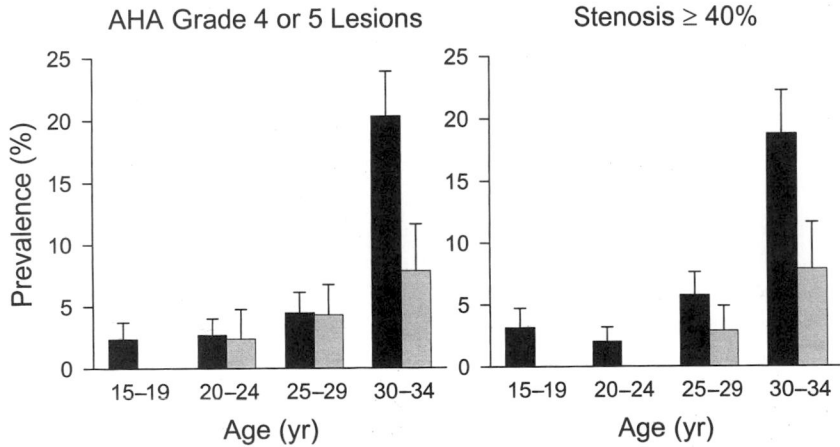

FIG. 32–3. Prevalence (%; +SE) of American Heart Association (AHA) Grade 4 or 5 lesions **(left)** and prevalence of stenosis 40% or greater **(right)** in the left anterior descending coronary artery by 5-year age groups of men *(black bars)* and women *(gray bars)*. (Reproduced from McGill HC Jr, McMahan CA, Zieske AW, et al. Association of coronary heart disease risk factors with microscopic qualities of coronary atherosclerosis in youth. *Circulation* 2000;102:374–379, with permission.) (See color insert for Fig. 32–4.)

TABLE 32–1. *Ratio of percent intimal surface area involved for high level of a risk factor to involvement for low level of the risk factor by age*

Risk factor and group	Lesion	Abdominal aorta		Right coronary artery	
		15–24 yr	25–34 yr	15–24 yr	25–34 yr
High non-HDL cholesterol[a]					
All	Flat fatty streaks	1.24 ± 0.06^{bc}	1.25 ± 0.04^b	1.33 ± 0.18^b	1.72 ± 0.18^b
	Raised fatty streaks	1.93 ± 0.26^b	2.39 ± 0.24^b	1.39 ± 0.17^b	1.91 ± 0.18^b
	Raised lesions	0.96 ± 0.15	1.44 ± 0.14^b	1.30 ± 0.18	1.79 ± 0.19^b
Low HDL cholesterol[a]					
All	Flat fatty streaks	1.09 ± 0.06	1.22 ± 0.05^b	1.19 ± 0.17	1.27 ± 0.17
	Raised fatty streaks	1.27 ± 0.17	1.63 ± 0.20^b	1.10 ± 0.14	1.56 ± 0.19^b
	Raised lesions	0.89 ± 0.15	1.05 ± 0.14	1.02 ± 0.15	1.20 ± 0.16
Smoking[a]					
All	Flat fatty streaks	1.16 ± 0.05^b	1.08 ± 0.04^b	1.15 ± 0.14	1.01 ± 0.11
	Raised fatty streaks	1.00 ± 0.12	1.27 ± 0.11^b	1.08 ± 0.12	0.93 ± 0.10
	Raised lesions	1.11 ± 0.14	2.92 ± 0.25^b	1.02 ± 0.13	1.12 ± 0.11
Hypertension[d]					
Whites	Flat fatty streaks	0.94 ± 0.07	1.00 ± 0.06	0.79 ± 0.15	0.96 ± 0.15
	Raised fatty streaks	1.00 ± 0.16	1.33 ± 0.20	0.86 ± 0.13	0.92 ± 0.14
	Raised lesions	0.66 ± 0.15^b	1.07 ± 0.16	0.96 ± 0.16	1.58 ± 0.23^b
Blacks	Flat fatty streaks	0.98 ± 0.06	1.03 ± 0.04	0.79 ± 0.13	0.96 ± 0.12
	Raised fatty streaks	0.90 ± 0.13	1.21 ± 0.14	1.03 ± 0.13	1.10 ± 0.12
	Raised lesions	1.29 ± 0.19	1.90 ± 0.21^b	1.27 ± 0.18	2.07 ± 0.25^b
Obesity[e]					
Men	Flat fatty streaks	1.02 ± 0.07	1.13 ± 0.06^b	1.53 ± 0.21^b	1.44 ± 0.17^b
	Raised fatty streaks	1.49 ± 0.21^b	1.29 ± 0.15^b	1.95 ± 0.25^b	1.58 ± 0.18^b
	Raised lesions	1.02 ± 0.16	1.01 ± 0.13	1.88 ± 0.26^b	2.22 ± 0.26^b
Women	Flat fatty streaks	0.92 ± 0.10	1.02 ± 0.07	1.23 ± 0.29	1.17 ± 0.23
	Raised fatty streaks	1.09 ± 0.26	0.95 ± 0.20	1.17 ± 0.25	0.95 ± 0.18
	Raised lesions	0.88 ± 0.25	0.88 ± 0.20	1.15 ± 0.28	1.43 ± 0.27
Elevated glycohemoglobin[a]					
All	Flat fatty streaks	0.92 ± 0.09	0.91 ± 0.07	1.33 ± 0.29	1.32 ± 0.26
	Raised fatty streaks	1.18 ± 0.26	1.00 ± 0.20	1.36 ± 0.27	1.34 ± 0.24
	Raised lesions	0.90 ± 0.22	1.36 ± 0.25	1.18 ± 0.27	2.43 ± 0.46^b

[a]Results adjusted for sex and race.
[b]Ratios significantly different from 1.00 ($P < 0.05$).
[c]Standard error.
[d]Results adjusted for sex.
[e]Results adjusted for race.
Reproduced from McGill HC Jr, McMahan C, Zieske A, et al. Associations of coronary heart disease risk factors with the intermediate lesion of atherosclerosis in youth. *Arterioscler Thromb Vasc Biol* 2000; 20:1998–2004, with permission.

High non-HDL cholesterol had a substantial and significant effect on all types of lesions beginning in the decade of life from 15 to 24 years of age and becoming even greater in the decade of life from 25 to 34 years of age. Low HDL cholesterol had a smaller effect on lesions, being significant only for raised fatty streaks in the decade of life from 25 to 34 years. These effects are consistent with the overwhelming data showing dyslipidemia as a major contributor to adult atherothrombosis and to clinically manifest CAD, with the early results from the Bogalusa Heart Project (13) and with the results of long-term follow-up of men whose serum cholesterol levels had been measured in youth (24). The conclusion is that dyslipidemia accelerates the progression of atherothrombosis at all ages beginning at least in adolescence.

Smoking increased the extent of fatty streaks in the abdominal aortas of 15- to 24-year-old subjects and increased both raised fatty streaks and raised lesions in the abdominal aortas of 25- to 34-year-old subjects, but it did not affect the extent of RCA lesions (17). Smoking was associated with a nearly threefold increase in raised lesions of the abdominal aorta of the older group. The smoking effect on the abdominal aorta began in the teenage years and was substantial by the fourth decade of life, an observation consistent with the high prevalence of aortic aneurysm among adult smokers (25). Smoking was previously shown to be associated with advanced coronary atherothrombosis in individuals older than 35 years (26).

Hypertension was associated with more extensive raised lesions almost exclusively, and the effect was greater in the aortas of black than in white individuals (18). Hypertension was the only risk factor measured in this study that was associated with more extensive raised lesions but not with flat fatty streaks or raised fatty streaks. The greater effect in black individuals is probably because of the well established greater severity of hypertension in the black population (18). The observed effect of hypertension is consistent with the observa-

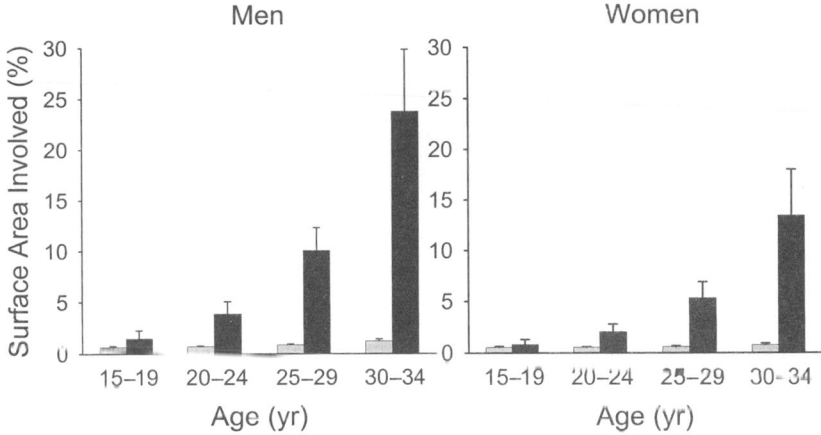

FIG. 32–5. Mean (+SE) extent involvement with raised lesions in the right coronary artery by sex, 5-year age groups, and risk status, adjusted for race. Low-risk subjects *(gray bars)* have non–high-density lipoprotein (HDL) cholesterol less than 160 mg/dL, HDL cholesterol 35 mg/dL or greater, body mass index (BMI) 30 k/m² or greater, glycohemoglobin less than 8%, and are normotensive and non-smokers. High-risk subjects *(black bars)* have non-HDL cholesterol 160 mg/dL or greater, HDL cholesterol less than 35 mg/dL, BMI greater than 30 k/m², glycohemoglobin 8% or greater, and are hypertensive and smokers. (See color insert for Fig. 32–6.)

tions from the Bogalusa Heart Study (13) and with the results of long-term follow-up of men whose blood pressure was measured in youth (27). As with dyslipidemia, hypertension begins to affect atherogenesis early in life and does so by accelerating the conversion of fatty streaks to raised lesions.

Obesity was associated strongly with all types of lesions in the RCAs of men, but not of women, although there was a trend toward such an association in women with a thick panniculus adiposus (central obesity pattern) (28). The effect was independent of the other risk factors measured in this study. Finding an association with obesity despite the negative results of many previous studies that found no association may be because of the prevalence and severity of obesity, which were increasing in the population from which these cases were drawn in the early 1990s. The explanation for the sex difference in the effects of obesity is not apparent, but may be because of the slower progression of atherothrombosis in premenopausal women. Obesity was the only risk factor measured in this study that affected the sexes differently.

Hyperglycemia, as indicated by increased glycohemoglobin, was associated with substantially greater extent of raised lesions of the RCA (29). This result is consistent with the reported evidence that blood glucose levels are associated with cardiovascular disease risk in a continuous and progressive relation, even below the diabetic threshold (30).

These risk factor effects are illustrated graphically in Figure 32–4 (see color insert) by topographic prevalence maps comparing the distribution of raised lesions in the RCAs of men in two age groups with high and low non-HDL cholesterol, low and high HDL cholesterol, hypertension, and obesity. The additive effects of these risk factors are illustrated in Figure 32–5, which compares the mean extent of raised lesions in the RCAs of men and women by 5-year age

groups with and without the six major risk factors. The additive risk factor effects are even more dramatically illustrated in Figure 32–6 (see color insert), which shows topographic prevalence maps of raised lesions in men in two age groups with zero, one, two, and three or more of the risk factors.

RISK FACTOR EFFECTS ON LESION QUALITIES

The risk factors also were associated with advanced lesions (AHA Grades 4 and 5 and stenosis ≥ 40%) in the LADCA (Table 32–2) (19). Although not all of the odds ratios were statistically significant, all were in the same direction as

TABLE 32–2. *Odds ratios for risk factor effects adjusted for other risk factors and 5-year age group*

Risk factor	AHA Grade (4–5 vs. 0–1)		Atherothrombotic stenosis ≥ 40%	
	OR	95% CI	OR	95% CI
Male sex	2.47	1.00–6.10[a]	2.80	1.11–7.03[a]
High non-HDL cholesterol	2.59	1.32–5.09[a]	2.95	1.53–5.70[a]
Low HDL cholesterol	1.81	0.84–3.91	1.32	0.61–2.88
Smoking	1.12	0.53–2.38	0.87	0.45–1.66
Hypertension	2.18	0.96–4.93	1.29	0.56–2.96
Obesity	2.66	1.18–6.03[a]	2.27	1.08–4.74[a]
Impaired glucose tolerance	2.33	0.53–10.33	1.33	0.35–5.12

CI, confidence interval; HDL, high-density lipoprotein; OR, odds ratio.
[a]95% CIs that do not include 1.00.
Adapted from McGill HC Jr, McMahan CA, Zieske AW, et al. Association of coronary heart disease risk factors with microscopic qualities of coronary atherosclerosis in youth. *Circulation* 2000;102:374–379.

seen in the effects of the risk factors on gross lesions. Thus, the risk factors were associated with the severity of coronary atherothrombosis and with the gross extent of involvement. The qualities of AHA Grades 4 and 5 are those associated with the vulnerability of plaques to rupture and to occlusive thrombosis.

IMPLICATIONS FOR PATHOGENESIS

The results of this intensive examination of atherothrombotic lesions in young individuals in the United States are consistent with the prevailing concept of pathogenesis that begins with intimal lipid deposition to form a lesion termed the fatty streak (AHA Grade 1 or 2); progresses with continued lipid deposition to produce the raised fatty streak (variously termed the intermediate or transitional lesion, or fatty plaque, AHA Grade 3); and proceeds with additional lipid deposition and reactive fibrosis to form the raised lesion also called the fibrous plaque (AHA Grade 4 or 5). Certain characteristics of the raised lesion render it susceptible to rupture and thrombosis, which commonly occur only after age 35 years (see Chapter 31).

Clearly, lipid deposition begins in childhood in the aorta (31) and in the coronary arteries during the second decade of life (2). However, not all fatty streaks are equally disposed to progression: Those in the thoracic aorta and in the proximal half of the abdominal aorta rarely are converted to raised lesions, whereas those in the dorsolateral intimal surface of the distal half are highly susceptible, particularly in the presence of smoking (22). In contrast to the pattern of distribution in the aorta, the pattern of distribution of fatty streaks in the coronary arteries is similar to that of raised lesions. However, there is another incongruity in the behavior of fatty streaks of the coronary arteries: Although young women and men have approximately equal involvement with fatty streaks, men develop more extensive raised lesions than women having a similar risk factor status. We interpret this observation to indicate that the fatty streak is a labile lesion, and its fate is determined by its anatomic location and the presence of identified risk factors and also by as yet unidentified risk factors. The anatomic location may involve either the tissue structure of the artery wall or local physiologic conditions, such as lateral pressure or flow factors, or both.

IMPLICATIONS FOR ETIOLOGY

The strength and consistency of the associations of the risk factors with one or more of the stages of evolution of atherothrombosis leave little doubt that they are involved in the chain of causation, either as external agents acting through unknown intervening variables (for example, smoking); as external agents interacting with genetically programmed metabolic systems to produce atherogenic conditions (for example, genotype and diet causing dyslipidemia); or as other diseases acting through known and unknown

mechanisms (for example, hypertension, impaired glucose tolerance, and obesity).

Dyslipidemia has long been thought to be the primary proximate cause of atherothrombosis, and the other risk factors only augment the effects of dyslipidemia. In these young persons, however, the nonlipid risk factors are associated with greater extent and severity of coronary atherothrombosis even in the presence of a favorable lipoprotein profile (non-HDL cholesterol < 160 mg/dL, HDL cholesterol > 35 mg/dL) (32). This result may mean that the currently designated "desirable" lipoprotein profile is actually not an "ideal" profile—that is, that the non-HDL cholesterol concentration should be much less to ensure protection from atherogenesis.

Although the effects of hypertension, hyperglycemia, and obesity are strong and independent of other risk factors, these results do not indicate the molecular, cellular, or physiologic mechanisms by which they produce their effects. Many possibilities can be suggested for each association; for example, obesity in children is associated with increased C-reactive protein (33), increased fibrinogen (34), and insulin resistance (35). Other types of evidence must be sought to explain these relations.

IMPLICATIONS FOR PREVENTION

No matter how strong or consistent, we must acknowledge that the associations of the risk factors with atherothrombosis in youth are based exclusively on observational evidence in a sample of convenience. A controlled clinical trial is the gold standard for evidence-based medicine. However, it is not feasible to conduct a clinical trial when the end point can be determined only at autopsy or 20 to 30 years later when clinically manifest CAD begins to appear. When noninvasive imaging methods become sufficiently sensitive to assess coronary artery lesions in young persons, it will be possible to conduct a clinical trial of regression following risk factor control. In the meantime, preventive regimens must depend on the best available data derived from observational studies. The results of the PDAY study suggest that, for long-range effective prevention of CAD, risk factor control must start in youth (36).

ACKNOWLEDGMENTS

The following lists the institutions cooperating in the PDAY study and the supporting grants from the National Heart Lung and Blood Institute: University of Alabama (HL-33733, HL-33728), Albany Medical College (HL-33765), Baylor College of Medicine (HL-33750), University of Chicago (HL-33740, HL-45715), The University of Illinois (HL-33758), Louisiana State University Health Science Center (HL-33746, HL-45720), University of Maryland (HL-33752, HL-45693), Medical College of Georgia (HL-33772), University of Nebraska Medical Center (HL-33778), The Ohio State University (HL-33760, HL-45694),

Southwest Foundation for Biomedical Research (HL-39913), The University of Texas Health Science Center at San Antonio (HL-33749, HL-45719), Vanderbilt University (HL-33770, HL-45718), and West Virginia University Health Sciences Center (HL-33748).

REFERENCES

1. Enos WF, Holmes RH, Beyer J. Coronary disease among United States soldiers killed in action in Korea: preliminary report. *JAMA* 1953;152:1090–1093.
2. Strong JP, McGill HC Jr. The natural history of coronary atherosclerosis. *Am J Pathol* 1962;40:37–49.
3. Tejada C, Strong JP, Montenegro MR, et al. Distribution of coronary and aortic atherosclerosis by geographic location, race, and sex. *Lab Invest* 1968;18:509–526.
4. Stary HC, Chandler AB, Glagov S, et al. A definition of initial, fatty streak, and intermediate lesions of atherosclerosis: a report from the Committee on Vascular Lesions of the Council on Arteriosclerosis, American Heart Association. *Circulation* 1994;89:2462–2478.
5. Stary HC, Chandler AB, Dinsmore RE, et al. A definition of advanced types of atherosclerotic lesions and a histological classification of atherosclerosis: a report from the Committee on Vascular Lesions of the Council on Arteriosclerosis, American Heart Association. *Arterioscler Thromb Vasc Biol* 1995;15:1512–1531.
6. Frerichs RR, Srinivasan SR, Webber LS, et al. Serum cholesterol and triglyceride levels in 3,446 children from a biracial community. The Bogalusa Heart Study. *Circulation* 1976;54:302–309.
7. Lauer RM, Connor WE, Leaverton PE, et al. Coronary heart disease risk factors in school children: the Muscatine Study. *J Pediatr* 1975;86:697–706.
8. Vartiainen E, Puska P, Salonen JT. Serum total cholesterol, HDL cholesterol and blood pressure levels in 13-year-old children in eastern Finland. The North Karelia Project. *Acta Med Scand* 1982;211:95–103.
9. Clarke WR, Schrott HG, Leaverton PE, et al. Tracking of blood lipids and blood pressures in school age children: the Muscatine Study. *Circulation* 1978;58:626–634.
10. Orchard TJ, Donahue RP, Kuller LH, et al. Cholesterol screening in childhood: does it predict adult hypercholesterolemia? The Beaver County experience. *J Pediatr* 1983;103:687–691.
11. Tamir I, Bojanower Y, Levtow O, et al. Serum lipids and lipoproteins in children from families with early coronary heart disease. *Arch Dis Child* 1972;47:808–810.
12. Sprecher DL, Schaefer EJ, Kent KM, et al. Cardiovascular features of homozygous familial hypercholesterolemia: analysis of 16 patients. *Am J Cardiol* 1984;54:20–30.
13. Newman WP III, Freedman DS, Voors AW, et al. Relation of serum lipoprotein levels and systolic blood pressure to early atherosclerosis. The Bogalusa Heart Study. *N Engl J Med* 1986;314:138–144.
14. Berenson GS, Srinivasan SR, Bao W, et al. Association between multiple cardiovascular risk factors and atherosclerosis in children and young adults. The Bogalusa Heart Study. *N Engl J Med* 1998;338:1650–1656.
15. Wissler RW. USA Multicenter Study of the pathobiology of atherosclerosis in youth. *Ann NY Acad Sci* 1991;623:26–39.
16. McGill HC Jr, Strong JP, Tracy RE, et al. Relation of a postmortem renal index of hypertension to atherosclerosis in youth. *Arterioscler Thromb Vasc Biol* 1995;15:2222–2228.
17. McGill HC Jr, McMahan CA, Malcom GT, et al. Effects of serum lipoproteins and smoking on atherosclerosis in young men and women. *Arterioscler Thromb Vasc Biol* 1997;17:95–106.
18. McGill HC Jr, McMahan CA, Tracy RE, et al. Relation of a postmortem renal index of hypertension to atherosclerosis and coronary artery size in young men and women. *Arterioscler Thromb Vasc Biol* 1998;18:1108–1118.
19. McGill HC Jr, McMahan CA, Zieske AW, et al. Association of coronary heart disease risk factors with microscopic qualities of coronary atherosclerosis in youth. *Circulation* 2000;102:374–379.
20. McGill HC Jr, McMahan C, Zieske A, et al. Associations of coronary heart disease risk factors with the intermediate lesion of atherosclerosis in youth. *Arterioscler Thromb Vasc Biol* 2000;20:1998–2004.
21. Wissler RW, Hiltscher L, Oinuma T, et al. The lesions of atherosclerosis in the young. From fatty streaks to intermediate lesions. In: Fuster V, Ross R, Topol EJ, eds. *Atherosclerosis and coronary artery disease, Vol 1.* Philadelphia: Lippincott-Raven Publishers, 1996:475–489.
22. McGill HC Jr, McMahan CA, Herderick EE, et al. Effects of coronary heart disease risk factors on atherosclerosis of selected regions of the aorta and right coronary artery. *Arterioscler Thromb Vasc Biol* 2000;20:836–845.
23. Stary HC. The histological classification of atherosclerotic lesions in human coronary arteries. In: Fuster V, Ross RR, Topol EJ, eds. *Atherosclerosis and coronary artery disease, Vol 1.* Philadelphia: Lippincott-Raven Publishers, 1996:463–474.
24. Stamler J, Daviglus ML, Garside DB, et al. Relationship of baseline serum cholesterol levels in 3 large cohorts of younger men to long-term coronary, cardiovascular, and all-cause mortality and to longevity. *JAMA* 2000;284:311–318.
25. Auerbach O, Hammond EC, Garfinkel L. Smoking in relation to atherosclerosis of the coronary arteries. *N Engl J Med* 1965;273:775–779.
26. Strong JP, Richards ML. Cigarette smoking and atherosclerosis in autopsied men. *Atherosclerosis* 1976;23:451–476.
27. Miura K, Daviglus ML, Dyer AR, et al. Relationship of blood pressure to 25-year mortality due to coronary heart disease, cardiovascular diseases, and all causes in young adult men. The Chicago Heart Association Detection Project in Industry. *Arch Intern Med* 2001;161:1501–1508.
28. McGill HC Jr, McMahan CA, Herderick EE, et al. Obesity accelerates the progression of coronary atherosclerosis in young men. *Circulation* 2002;105:2712–2718.
29. McGill HC Jr, McMahan CA, Malcom GT, et al. Relation of glycohemoglobin and adiposity to atherosclerosis in youth. *Arterioscler Thromb Vasc Biol* 1995;15:431–440.
30. Coutinho M, Gerstein HC, Wang Y, et al. The relationship between glucose and incident cardiovascular events. A metaregression analysis of published data from 20 studies of 95,783 individuals followed for 12.4 years. *Diabetes Care* 1999;22:233–240.
31. Holman RL, McGill HC Jr, Strong JP, et al. The natural history of atherosclerosis: the early aortic lesions as seen in New Orleans in the middle of the 20th century. *Am J Pathol* 1958;34:209–235.
32. McGill HC Jr, McMahan CA, Zieske AW, et al. Effects of nonlipid risk factors on atherosclerosis in youth with a favorable lipoprotein profile. *Circulation* 2001;103:1546–1550.
33. Cook DG, Mendall MA, Whincup PH, et al. C-reactive protein concentration in children: relationship to adiposity and other cardiovascular risk factors. *Atherosclerosis* 2000;149:139–150.
34. Cook DG, Whincup PH, Miller G, et al. Fibrinogen and factor VII levels are related to adiposity but not to fetal growth or social class in children aged 10-11 years. *Am J Epidemiol* 1999;150:727–736.
35. Steinberger J, Moran A, Hong CP, et al. Adiposity in childhood predicts obesity and insulin resistance in young adulthood. *J Pediatr* 2001;138:469–473.
36. Van Horn L, Greenland P. Prevention of coronary artery disease is a pediatric problem. *JAMA* 1997;278:1779–1780.

CHAPTER 33

Coronary Thrombosis

Local and Systemic Factors

Roberto Corti, Lina Badimon, Valentin Fuster, and Juan Jose Badimon

Introduction	Shear Stress, Vascular Remodeling, and Neointima
Endothelium and Atherogenesis	Formation
Blood Flow and Shear Stress	Effect of Blood Flow on Thrombus Formation
Vessel Wall–Platelet Interaction	and Growth
Thrombus Formation and Thrombus Growth	Conclusion
Endothelium and Rheology	References

Key Words: Atherothrombosis; blood flow; endothelium; platelet.

INTRODUCTION

Pulsatile blood flow through coronary, carotid, and peripheral arteries is an important regulator of the structure and function of these arteries and has been implicated in the pathogenesis of atherothrombosis (1–3). Several risk factors (such as diabetes, hypercholesterolemia, hypertension, and smoking) have been implicated in the initiation and progression of atherothrombosis. Although these risk factors are systemic in nature, atherothrombotic plaques are not randomly distributed, but occur with preference to specific locations in the arterial tree. Atherothrombotic lesions colocalize with regions of low shear stress throughout the arterial tree, such as the carotid artery bifurcation (4,5), the coronary arteries (1), the infrarenal aorta, and the femoral artery (2). The vascular or arterial wall and particularly its endothelial surface are constantly exposed

R. Corti: Department of Cardiology, University Hospital Zurich, CH-8091 Zurich, Switzerland.

L. Badimon: Cardiovascular Research Center, CSIC-HSCSP-UAB, Barcelona, Spain.

V. Fuster: Cardiovascular Institute, The Mount Sinai School of Medicine, New York, New York 10029.

J. J. Badimon: The Cardiovascular Research Laboratory, Zena and Michael A. Wiener Cardiovascular Institute, The Mount Sinai School of Medicine, New York, New York 10029.

to the mechanical forces exerted by the flowing blood: the hemodynamic shear stress. The interaction between rheology and the functional phenotype of endothelium plays a critical role in the atherothrombotic process. It has been shown that sudden changes in flow induce rapid adaptive changes in the endothelial phenotype, expression, and production of endothelial-derived substances responsible for vascular homeostasis and hemostasis. Acute changes in rheologic conditions induce regulation or reorganization of preexisting proteins or structures, whereas chronic flow changes involve *de novo* protein synthesis, which, in turn, reflects regulation at the level of gene expression. The activation of specific transcriptional regulatory elements termed shear stress response elements (SSREs) in the promoters of shear-responsive genes is responsible for the changes in gene expression (6–8).

ENDOTHELIUM AND ATHEROGENESIS

The endothelium plays a pivotal role in preserving vascular homeostasis and hemostasis (Fig. 33–1). The endothelium, the inner layer of blood vessels, is a dynamic autocrine and paracrine organ that regulates contractile, secretory, and mitogenic activities in the vessel wall and hemostatic process within the vessel lumen by producing several local active substances (Table 33–1). The vascular homeostasis is guaranteed by the balanced production of potent vasodilator (such as nitric oxide [NO]) and vasoconstrictor (such as endothelin-1 [ET-1]) agents (Fig. 33–2). Vascular hemostasis,

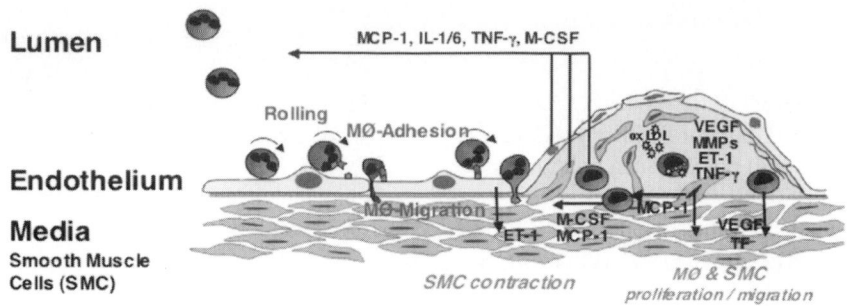

FIG. 33–1. Pathogenesis of plaque development. The endothelium plays a pivotal role in vascular homeostasis and hemostasis. Normal functioning endothelium **(left)** produces several substances aimed at maintaining normal shear conditions by balancing the production of vasodilator (nitric oxide) and vasoconstrictor (ET-1) and avoiding excessive platelet aggregation (nitric oxide and prostacyclin). Dysfunctional endothelium **(right)** favors macrophages adhesion and migration (MCP-1) and plaque growth and induces vasoconstriction. Dashed line means inhibition; arrow represents inducement or promotion. ET, endothelin; MCP-1, monocyte chemotactic protein-1; M-CSF, macrophage colony-stimulating factor; IL, interleukin; M(, macrophage; MMP, matrix metalloproteinase; ox LDL, oxidized low-density lipoprotein; SMC, smooth muscle cells; TF, tissue factor; TNF, tumor necrosis factor; VEGF, vascular endothelial growth factor.

defined as the ability of the vascular system to maintain blood fluidity and vascular integrity, is achieved by the interaction between the endothelium and blood cells (Figs. 33–1 and 33–2). In physiologic conditions, the normal endothelium actively supports the fluid state of flowing blood and prevents activation of circulating cells. Endothelial dysfunction, as well as a breach of the endothelial integrity, triggers a series of biochemical and molecular reactions such as vasoconstriction, platelet adhesion, and fibrin formation. Endothelial dysfunction is considered a precursor of the

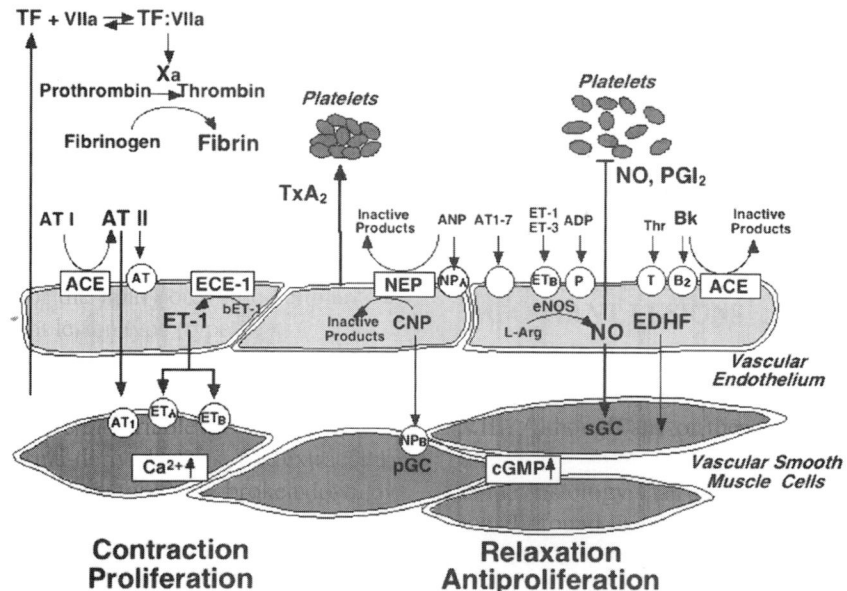

FIG. 33–2. The endothelium is a source of paracrine mediators that act as vasodilators such as nitric oxide (NO), endothelial-derived hyperpolarizing factor (EDHF), or potent vasoconstrictor such as endothelin (ET). In addition, several substances that act as chemoattractant for bloodborne cells or proliferative substances are produced and are responsible for the initiation and progression of atherothrombotic lesions. ACE, angiotensin-converting enzyme; AT, angiotensin; CNP, natriuretic peptide type C; cGMP, cyclic guanosine monophosphate; ECE, endothelin converting enzyme; eNOS, endothelial nitric oxide synthase; NEP, neutral endo-peptidase; NP, natrium peptide; pGC, particulate guanylyl cyclase; PGI2, prostacyclin; sGC, soluable guanylyl cyclase; TF, tissue factor; TxA2, thromboxane A2.

TABLE 33–1. *Function of normal endothelium*

- Permeability barrier
- Production of thrombogenic and nonthrombogenic products
- Metabolism of vasoactive substances
- Production of cytokines and growth factor
- Synthesis of leukocyte adhesion molecules
- Synthesis of basement membrane constituents
- Lipid metabolism

atherothrombotic process and is characterized by the increased expression of adhesion molecules (e.g., selectins, vascular cell adhesion molecules, and intercellular adhesion moleculars) that participate in "homing" and infiltration of monocytes (Fig. 33–1) (9,10). The monocytes migrate into the subendothelium, where they transform into macrophages.

This differentiation process includes the up-regulation of different receptors including CD36 and the scavenger receptor A, which are responsible for the oxidized low-density lipoprotein (LDL) internalization. On lipid enrichment, macrophages transform into foam cells leading to the formation of fatty streaks. These activated macrophages release mitogens and chemoattractants that perpetuate the process by recruiting additional macrophages and vascular smooth muscle cells from the media into the injured media, which may eventually compromise the vascular lumen. The recruited smooth muscle cells and macrophages will significantly contribute to plaque growth, not only by increasing their number, but also by synthesizing extracellular matrix components. The ratio between smooth muscle cells and macrophages plays an important role in the plaque vulnerability because of their lytic activity. Macrophages are able to elaborate matrix metalloproteinases, and those enzymes, by digesting the extracellular matrix, will facilitate plaque disruption and thrombus formation (11).

Studies have confirmed the importance of hemodynamic shear stress in endothelial dysfunction, atherogenesis, remodeling, and restenosis after angioplasty and thrombus formation. The endothelium, by virtue of its location interfacing between the blood and the vascular wall, responds rapidly and sensitively to biochemical and biomechanical stimuli to maintain constant rheologic conditions.

BLOOD FLOW AND SHEAR STRESS

The vascular or arterial wall and particularly its endothelial surface are constantly exposed to the mechanical forces exerted by the flowing blood: the hemodynamic shear stress. The magnitude of the shear stress can be estimated in most of the vasculature by Poiseuille's law ($\tau = [4 v Q]/[\pi R^3]$; where v is viscosity, Q is volumetric flow, and R is the vessel radius), which states that shear stress is proportional to blood flow viscosity and is inversely proportional to the third power of the internal radius. This ratio is important

within the context of atherothrombosis because it is defined by thickening of the arterial wall and subsequent lumen reduction. Therefore, a small reduction in lumen diameter will be associated with a significant increase in local shear rate conditions (Fig. 33–3). Shear rate decreases with increasing vessel diameter for constant flow. Measurements using different modalities show that shear stress ranges from 1 to 6 dyne/cm^2 in the venous system and between 10 and 70 dyne/cm^2 in the arterial vascular network (12). In numerous experiments, shear stress has been shown to actively influence vessel wall remodeling. Specifically, chronic increases in blood flow, and consequently shear stress, lead to expansion of the luminal radius such that mean shear stress is returned to its baseline level. Conversely, decreased shear stress resulting from lower flow or blood viscosity induces a decrease in internal vessel radius. The net effect of these endothelial-mediated compensatory responses is the maintenance of mean arterial hemodynamic shear stress magnitude at approximately 15 to 20 dyne/cm^2. This shear stress–stabilizing process is dependent on intact endothelial function and is abolished by prior selective destruction of the endothelial monolayer.

Interestingly, two contradictory hypotheses were advanced more than 30 years ago to explain the typical distribution of atherothrombotic lesions at the vessel bifurcation. The first hypothesis implicated high shear stress through endothelial injury and denudation. The second hypothesis proposed low shear stress as an atherogenic factor (13). Similarly, in the complex process of thrombus formation, the rate of platelet adhesion was shown to increase with increasing shear rates up to approximately 800 per second, whereas fibrin formation (the end product of coagulation) has been ob-

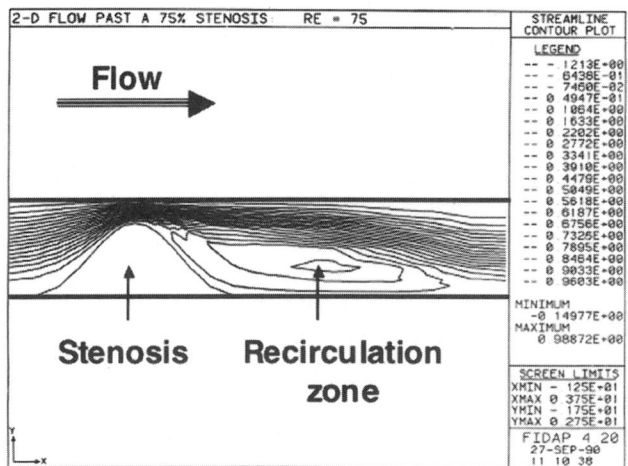

FIG. 33–3. Computer-generated two-dimensional plot of the rheologic conditions developed in a 75% stenotic vessel. Shear stress progressively increases up to the maximum achieved at the top of the stenosis. Distal from the stenosis the shear stress consequently decreases as the lumen increases. Note the area of recirculation immediately distal from the stenosis.

served to decrease with increasing wall shear stress (14). More conclusive evidence for the direct effect of hemodynamic forces on endothelial structure and function derives from *in vitro* studies with cultured monolayers subjected to various rheologic conditions (6). Importantly, recognition of the modulator effect of the changes of shear stress on cultured cell monolayers and on gene modulation led to further research under more complex flow conditions. Several endothelial targets have been suggested to act as shear stress responsive elements (6,15,16), which may be activated by changes in shear stress conditions leading to the various signaling cascades, resulting in highly coordinated and orchestrated mechanotransduction messages with the ultimate goal to restore physiologic conditions.

VESSEL WALL–PLATELET INTERACTION

The inherent capacity of platelets to aggregate is regulated by the physiologic systems that inhibit platelet activation. The endothelium is a major contributor to the inhibitor system that controls platelet activation (Fig. 33–2). Endothelial cells are able to synthesize several potent inhibitors of platelet aggregation such as prostacyclin (PGI_2) and NO. Both compounds act as paracrine inhibitors of platelet activation and exhibit potent vasodilator properties (17). Interestingly, NO was found to cause disaggregation of preformed platelet aggregates, in addition to its inhibitory effect on platelet adhesion and aggregation. Shear stress and pulsatile flow are major stimuli that induce endothelial release of NO under basal condition (18); however, long-lasting disturbances of blood flow condition result in rearrangement of the endothelial phenotype (15) ending in its dysfunction with consequent reduction in NO production. The physical forces exerted by pulsatile and turbulent flow also are responsible for the rheologic arrangement of platelets in the flowing blood close to the surface of endothelial cells, allowing interaction between platelets and the endothelial paracrine-released substances.

The platelet hemostasis is warranted by efficient balance between activator and inhibitor substances, which demonstrate a synergistic behavior within their group. In fact, synergistic enhancement of aggregation has been described during interactions involving adenosine diphosphate (ADP) and thromboxane (19). In contrast, subthreshold amounts of NO strengthen the platelet inhibitory effects of PGI_2 (20). Therefore, it is not surprising that proatherothrombotic conditions characterized by hypercholesterolemia, hypertension, smoking, diabetes, aging, and inflammation may promote an endothelial dysfunction generating a prothrombotic condition, which may trigger acute cardiovascular events.

THROMBUS FORMATION AND THROMBUS GROWTH

Endothelial dysfunction is considered the earliest stage of atherothrombosis. It initiates atherothrombosis by favoring the accumulation of LDL-cholesterol and macrophages, as well as the migration of smooth muscle cells in the subendothelial space, by increasing the endothelial permeability, up-regulating adhesion molecules, and chemoattracting factors (9,10). In addition, endothelial dysfunction may end in a prothrombotic and procoagulant stage favoring thrombotic obstruction (21). On plaque disruption, platelets and the coagulation cascade are rapidly activated as a consequence of the interaction between vascular tissue factor (TF) and flowing blood. Abrupt episodic disruption or erosion of atherothrombotic plaques leading to thrombus formation has been associated with the onset of acute cardiovascular events (11,22–25). The balance between platelet activator and inhibitor substances is moved toward the agonist, such as thromboxane A_2, inducing rapid platelet aggregation (26). Thromboxane A_2 is released from the platelet membrane by the stimulatory effect of collagen, thrombin, ADP, and serotonin. Platelet-released ADP and serotonin stimulate adjacent platelets, further enhancing the process of platelets activation, leading to thrombus growth. Platelet function depends on adhesive interactions modulated by surface receptors. Several receptors, whose modulating genes and ligands have been recognized and served as targets for therapeutic approaches aiming to decrease platelet adhesion have been developed and are currently in clinical use. The more abundant platelet receptor families and their ligands are presented in Table 33–2. The effectiveness of the platelet IIb/IIIa receptors' antagonist has been demonstrated in several large clinical trials. Despite the clinical benefit of this class of agent, the bleeding complication rate is still not negligible and is probably dose-related. We described a new bedside method to test platelet activation with a shear-dependent platelet function test for monitoring long-term glycoprotein (GP) IIb/IIIa inhibition that does not require a baseline reference (27). Such a test may prove to be a valuable tool in monitoring GP IIb/IIIa dose/response and finding the adequate dose for long-term GP IIb/IIIa inhibition.

TABLE 33–2. *Platelet receptors*

Ligand	Receptor	Other names
Collagen	GPIa/IIa	VLA-2, $\alpha_2\beta_1$
	GPIIb/IIIa	$\alpha IIb\beta_3$
	GPIV	GPIIIb
Fibrinogen	GPIIb/IIIa	$\alpha IIb\beta_3$
Fibronectin	GPIc/IIa	VLA-5, $\alpha_5\beta_1$
	GPIIb/IIIa	$\alpha IIb\beta_3$
Thrombospondin	Vn-R	$\alpha_v\beta_3$
	GPIV	GPIIIb
Vitronectin	Vn-R	$\alpha_v\beta_3$
	GPIIb/IIIa	$\alpha IIb\beta_3$
vWF	GPIb/IX	—
	GPIIb/IIIa	$\alpha IIb\beta_3$
Laminin	GPIc/IIa region	VLA-6, $\alpha_6\beta_1$

GP, glycoprotein; VLA, very late antigen; Vn-R, vitronectin receptor; vWF, von Willebrand Factor

Disrupted lipid-rich plaques are highly thrombogenic by triggering the coagulation cascade and enhancing platelet aggregation. Disruption of the plaques facilitates the interaction between the flowing blood and the deeper components of lipid-rich lesions such as TF (28,29). TF is a cell surface protein that is expressed by endothelial cells, monocytes, and smooth muscle cells in response to a variety of stimuli including oxidized LDL. TF, a small-molecular-weight GP, binds to coagulation factor VII, leading to the activation of factors IX and X and, therefore, to both the intrinsic and extrinsic blood coagulation cascade (30). Colocalization analysis of coronary atherectomy specimens of culprit lesions from patients with unstable angina showed a strong relation between TF and macrophages, suggesting a cell-mediated thrombogenicity in patients with acute coronary syndromes (31). Our group showed that the thrombogenicity of disrupted atherothrombotic plaques is modulated by their TF content and, furthermore, specific inhibition of the TF pathway (by using tissue factor pathway inhibitor [TFPI]) significantly reduces their thrombogenicity (32). TFPI is expressed in the adventitial layer of large arteries, and, in atherothrombotic vessels, TFPI is expressed by macrophages in focal areas throughout the plaque. Local production of TFPI may regulate procoagulant activity and thrombotic events within atherothrombotic plaques (33).

TF expression was found in a variety of cells in culture after growth factor or cytokine stimulation (34). Data have suggested that the majority of cell-associated TF is either encrypted on the cell surface or present in an intracellular pool. Arterial injury may, therefore, involve the deencryption of surface TF or the release of intracellular TF (35). TF was reported in the extracellular matrix, whereas latent TF was found on the outside of unbroken smooth muscle cells, and TF activity was found in native whole blood and in plasma. In addition, inhibition of this circulating TF was shown to prevent formation of thrombi on collagen-coated glass slides in an *ex vivo* perfusion system (36). Therefore, bloodborne TF may play a major role in thrombosis. Encryption of TF present in the circulation could be a mechanism that prevents thrombosis. Alternatively, circulating TF may be active but below the threshold required for the initiation of blood coagulation.

It has been demonstrated that high cell death caused by apoptosis and necrosis is a basic *in situ* feature found in advanced coronary primary lesions associated with unstable angina, possibly explaining their low density of (viable) smooth muscle cells (37). Apoptotic cells have been postulated as a source for TF. We investigated the relation between TF expression and apoptosis after percutaneous transluminal coronary angioplasty in a porcine model. Arterial injury leads to a high simultaneous expression of TF and caspase-3 (a marker for apoptotic cells) in the media. Immunofluorescence double labeling showed almost complete colocalization of TF and caspase-3 (38). There is increasing evidence for apoptosis as a major determinant of the thrombogenicity of the plaque lipid core and a potential contributor to plaque erosion and associated thrombosis. Apoptosis may directly affect blood thrombogenicity through the release of apoptotic cells and microparticles into the bloodstream (39).

All this evidence has highlighted a possible link between inflammation, apoptosis, and TF-mediated thrombosis (40). Therefore, interventions aiming to decrease TF expression may be helpful in preventing atherothrombotic complications.

ENDOTHELIUM AND RHEOLOGY

Despite the systemic nature of the major cardiovascular risk factors, atherothrombosis is a geometric focal disease preferentially affecting the outer edges of vessel bifurcation (41) and is characterized by low and oscillatory shear stress as observed by Caro and coworkers (13) in the early 1970s. Atherothrombotic lesions colocalize with regions of low shear stress throughout the arterial tree, from the carotid artery bifurcation (4,5) to the coronary (1) infrarenal, and femoral artery vasculatures (2). The rate of atherothrombosis progression in patients with coronary artery disease was found, by serial quantitative coronary angiography, to correlate inversely with shear stress magnitude, even when corrected for other cardiovascular risk factors such as lipoproteins levels (42).

The interaction between rheology and the functional phenotype of endothelium plays a critical role in the atherothrombotic process. The early stage of atherothrombosis is characterized by an increased permeability of the vessel wall to bloodborne cells and proteins (macrophages, lymphocytes, LDL-lipoprotein, and others). Caro and coworkers (43) first proposed a shear stress–dependent transfer of lipids into the vessel wall. Interestingly, cultured endothelial cells exposed to physiologic laminar shear stress elongate and align in the direction of blood flow, whereas those exposed to low shear stress (or cultured in static condition) do not change their shape or orientation (Fig. 33–4).

The endothelium promptly reacts to increased shear stress by increasing the production of NO. The nitric oxide synthase (NOS) messenger RNA protein and activity are stimulated in high shear stress conditions, leading to vasodilation aiming to normalize the shear condition. In contrast, low shear stress induces endothelial cell loss and desquamation probably consequent to a proapoptotic situation (44), alters the morphology with decreased elongation, decreases actin fibers, stimulates monocyte attachment to and migration across the endothelial layer (45), and increases endothelial surface expression of vascular cell adhesion molecules (Fig. 33–4) (46). Two different mechanisms appear to be responsible for the endothelial molecular responses to shear stress (15). The first mechanism is the regulation or reorganization of preexisting proteins or structures by sudden changes in flow. Many of these effects are rapid and occur in just seconds, involving regulatory system at the level of rate-limiting enzymes or substrate availability. One of the most

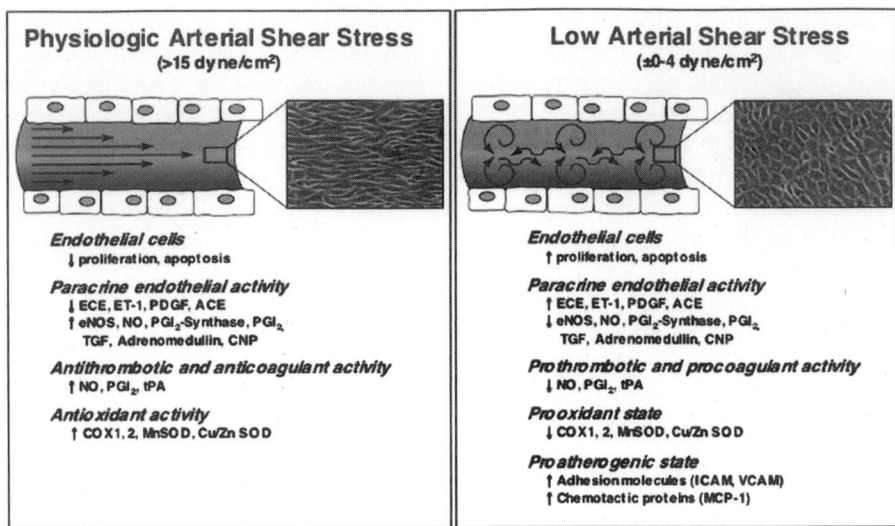

FIG. 33–4. Effect of shear stress on endothelial phenotype and activity. In physiologic shear stress conditions **(left)**, endothelial cells are elongated and align in the direction of blood flow and their function is mainly characterized by the production of vasodilators and substances with antithrombotic, anticoagulant, and antioxidant properties. In low flow conditions (such as turbulent flow, **right**), cultured endothelial cells show a random pattern and produce substances favoring cell apoptosis and proliferation, inflammation, vasoconstriction, thrombosis, and atherogenesis. ACE, angiotensin-converting enzyme; CNP, natriuretic peptide type C; COX, cyclooxygenase; ECE, endothelin converting enzyme; eNOS, endothelial nitric oxide synthase; ET-1, endothelin-1; ICAM, intercellular adhesion molecular; MCP-1, monocyte chemotactic protein-1; MnSOD, manganese superoxide dismutase; NO, nitric oxide; PDGF, platelet-derived growth factor; PGI_2, prostacyclin; TGF, transforming growth factor; tPA, tissue plasminogen activator; VCAM, vascular cell adhesion molecule.

studied enzymes that shows a rapid response to an increase in shear stress is the NOS. This enzyme catalyzes the production of NO in a potent and rapid response to shear stress, within milliseconds of the onset of flow. The second mechanism mediates the endothelial response to chronic flow changes. The delayed or chronic shear-mediated effects involve *de novo* protein synthesis, which, in turn, reflects regulation at the level of gene expression. The activation of specific transcriptional regulatory elements, SSREs, in the promoters of shear-responsive genes is responsible for the changes in gene expression (6). Several endothelial genes are influenced by shear stress (7,8). For example, shear stress influences the expression of genes involved in vascular homeostasis, activating the expression NOS-encoding gene and cyclooxygenase-2–encoding gene (responsible for the production of PGI_2) and down-regulating the expression of the gene encoding preproendothelin-1 (the precursor of ET-1) (15). In addition, a number of genes involved in thrombosis (such as thrombomodulin and tissue plasminogen activator) and in inflammation, such as the adhesion molecules (vascular cell adhesion molecule-1 and intercellular adhesion molecular-1) and macrophage chemotactic protein-1, are modulated by shear stress (6,8,15,47).

In addition to the effective paracrine and endocrine endothelial production of a multitude of vasoactive substances with the ultimate goal to maintain shear stress condition in a physiologic range, the shear stress–dependent changes in endothelial function may play a central role in vascular remodeling and neointima formation.

SHEAR STRESS, VASCULAR REMODELING, AND NEOINTIMA FORMATION

The vessel wall reacts to a sustained increment in flow with a structural increase in vessel diameter (positive remodeling) mediated by the activation of several genes. The magnitude of the vascular remodeling induced by chronic rheologic changes is surpassingly more important than that induced by acute changes in flow (48). A negative feedback loop between shear stress and vessel lumen was postulated in the 1980s and suggested that increased shear stress induces vasodilatation aimed to renormalize the shear stress (49). Glagov and coworkers (50) demonstrated in 1987 that a compensatory enlargement of human atherothrombotic coronary already exists before compromising the arterial lumen. Thereafter, compensation is lost and lumen narrowing occurs. These postmortem observations have been confirmed *in vivo* using intravascular ultrasound (51,52) and magnetic resonance imaging (53). New understanding of the cellular and molecular mechanisms of endothelium-mediated vascular remodeling may have important implications in the pathogenesis and treatment of atherothrombotic disease. TF (54), ET-1 (55), and other growth factors are involved in vascular remodeling and may serve as targets for specific intervention.

Neointima formation in aortoiliacal graft

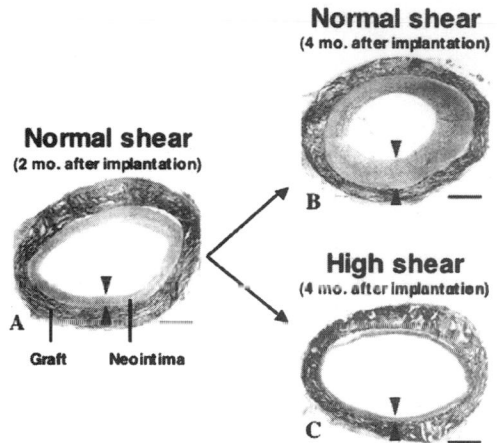

FIG. 33–5. Shear stress and neointima formation. High shear stress condition reduces preformed intima hyperplasia in aortoiliac polytetrafluoroethylene graft implanted in primates. Progressive neointima formation is described in normal shear condition in this model in the first 2 to 4 months **(A and B),** whereas significant reduction of neointimal thickening is seen after increasing shear stress condition **(C).** (Adapted from Mattsson EJ, Kohler TR, Vergel SM, et al. Increased blood flow induces regression of intimal hyperplasia. *Arterioscler Thromb Vasc Biol* 1997;17:2245–2249.)

Several studies performed in the last decade have clarified the importance of shear stress in neointima formation after percutaneous coronary intervention. Increased shear stress has been shown to prevent neointima formation and even to reduce previously established neointima in different experimental settings (Fig. 33–5) (56) In addition, shear-related neointima formation has been reported at the edges of anastomosis (57,58), where a disturbance in the flow and low shear stress was present. Low blood flow seems to promote restenosis after angioplasty through its adverse effect on vessel remodeling, associated with the augmented expression of multiple genes central to cell migration and restenosis (59).

EFFECT OF BLOOD FLOW ON THROMBUS FORMATION AND GROWTH

Platelet–vessel wall interaction and thrombus formation *in vivo* takes place under flow conditions. The process of thrombosis, especially in the vicinity of advanced atherothrombotic lesions, is complex, involving platelets, coagulation proteins, the condition of the vessel wall, and local blood flow condition. Both physical and chemical factors can influence the activity of platelets and coagulation factors responsible for the formation of thrombotic and hemostatic masses in the vicinity of injured vessel wall. Thrombus growth is seen in cases of major plaque disruption, lipid extrusion, vasospasm and slow flow, low fibrinolytic activity,

procoagulant states and high tissue factor activity, high levels of fibrinogen, and reactive platelets.

Several *in vitro* systems capable of modeling the different flow conditions developing in the blood vessels have been developed to investigate the mechanisms by which mechanical forces affect platelet–thrombus formation. To investigate the dynamics of platelet deposition and thrombus formation after vascular damage and to study the influence of various biochemical and physical factors, our group developed a tubular perfusion chamber that retains the cylindrical shape of the vascular system and permits *ex vivo* exposure of thrombogenic substrate to blood under characteristic rheologic conditions (Fig. 33–6) (60). Dual radioactive labeling allowed us to establish the contribution of both platelet and fibrinogen on thrombus formation and to validate the method in animal experiments.

Exposure of deendothelialized vessel wall (thus mimicking mild vascular injury) to flowing blood demonstrated the shear-dependent platelet deposition. At low shear rates, platelet deposition reaches the maximum within 5 to 10 minutes of exposure, after which platelet deposition remains constant. At high wall shear rate (1,690/s), initial platelet deposition is greater than at the lower shear stress. Maximum platelet deposition also is reached at 5 to 10 minutes of perfusion; however, the thrombi appear fragile and may be dislodged from the substrate. Exposure of fibrillar collagen (thus mimicking a deeper vessel wall injury) to blood produced platelet deposition of more than two orders of magnitude greater than on subendothelium (60). Even at high shear rate, platelet thrombus formed was not dislodged but remained adherent to the surface (Fig. 33–7). Thus, this extracorporal flow chamber can be used to test the effect of interventions (such as antithrombotic agents) in humans at different shear rate conditions.

These observations emphasize the importance not only of the shear rate, but also the influence of the degree of injury on platelet deposition and thrombus formation. Overall, it is likely that in mild injury the thrombogenic stimulus is relatively limited, the thrombus relatively fragile, and the resulting thrombotic occlusion may be transient, as occurs in unstable angina. Conversely, deep vessel injury secondary to plaque disruption results in the exposure of highly thrombogenic substrate leading to larger and more stable thrombi ending in relatively persistent thrombotic occlusion. The proximity of stenotic regions could result in a synergistic production of platelets and fibrin-rich thrombi, as it is well established that platelets are activated by high shear stress and coagulation tends to proceed more rapidly in low shear stress areas.

Disruption of atherothrombotic plaque is believed to be the major trigger of thrombus formation *in vivo*. The localization of these thrombotic masses is modulated by local flow conditions. The high shear rate areas, typical of flow at the apex of stenotic lesions, are the preferred sites for platelet thrombus formation on injured vessel wall; in fact, platelet deposition increases with increasing stenosis (61). Thus, the

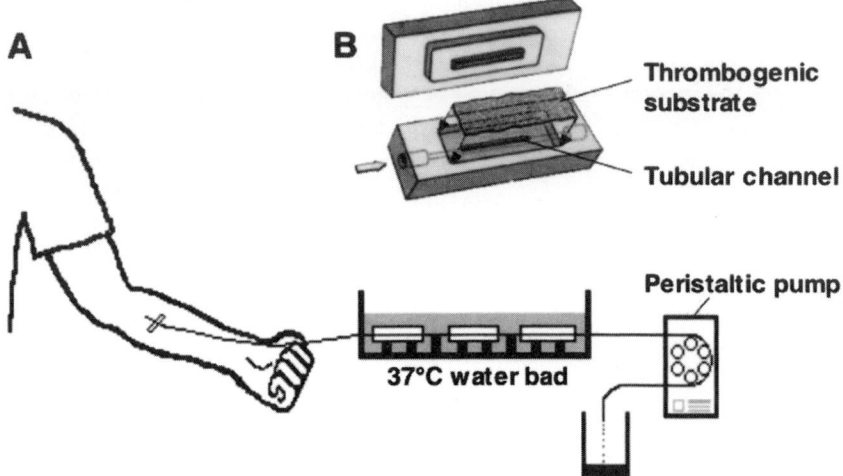

FIG. 33–6. The study of thrombus formation. Schematic of experimental setting with the use of the Badimon chamber **(A).** The blood from the studied subject flows to serial chambers with specific shear rate (defined by the size of the tubular channel) where it flows over the thrombogenic substrate **(B).** The contact of the flowing blood with the surface of the thrombogenic substrate (mainly deendothelialized pig aorta) induces platelet activation and fibrin deposition, forming a surface thrombus. The amount of the thrombus formed on the surface of the thrombogenic substrate can be quantified by morphometric analysis of the histologic section.

degree of vascular damage and local flow condition are important parameters for the study of clinically relevant thrombosis. Platelet deposition depends on shear rate, thrombogenic substrate, and platelet activity. Thrombus formation on atheromatous core has been demonstrated to be up to sixfold greater than on other substrates, including collagen-rich matrix (62). The lipid-rich core is the most thrombogenic component of human atherothrombotic plaques and, therefore, plaques with large atheromatous core contents are at high

risk to lead to thrombosis after spontaneous or mechanically induced rupture, because of the increased thrombogenicity of their content (62). Disruption of atherothrombotic plaques facilitates the interaction between the flowing blood and the deeper components of lipid-rich lesions such as TF, which was shown to modulate the thrombogenicity of human atherothrombotic plaques (28).

Systemic factors such as dyslipoproteinemia, hypertension, diabetes, cigarette smoking, and aging, which were rec-

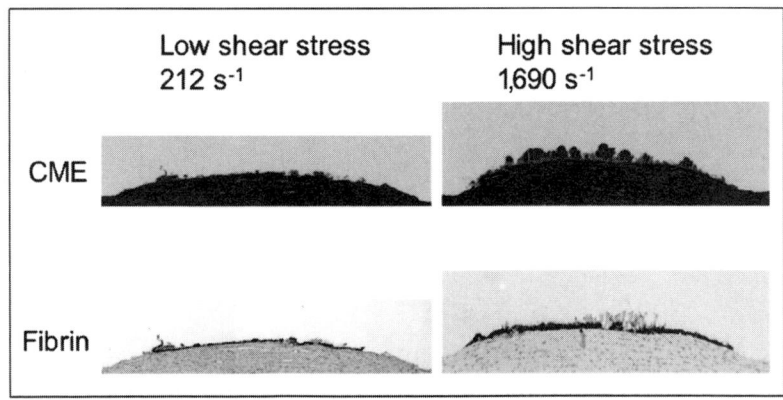

FIG. 33–7. The effect of shear stress on thrombus formation. Representative histologic sections of thrombus formed on the thrombogenic surface (in this case, the media of porcine aorta) at low and high shear stress conditions. The rheologic conditions in the first chamber **(left)** simulated those of patent coronary arteries (medium caliber arteries; shear rate, 212/s), whereas those in the second chambers **(right)** simulated those of mildly stenosed coronary arteries (shear rate, 1,690/s). Thrombus formation on the tunica media surface and the fibrin/fibrinogen (collectively referred to as fibrin) contribution to the content of the thrombus can be quantified using microscopic morphometry. The perfused substrates are formalin-fixed, paraffin-embedded, sectioned, and stained for the presence of either total thrombus, using a combined Masson's trichrome-elastin (CME) stain, or fibrin, using a fibrin-specific antibody.

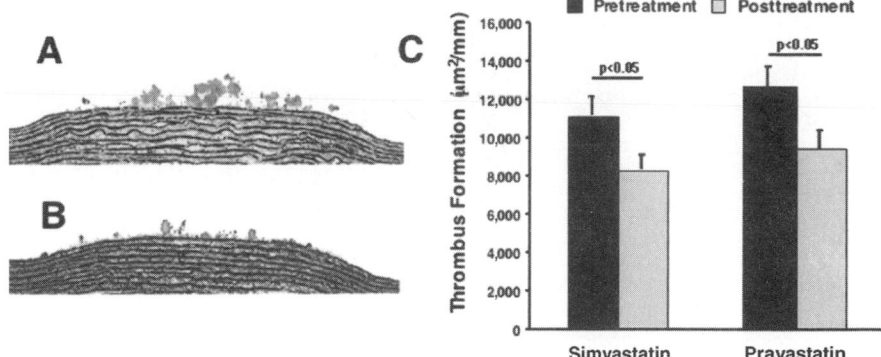

FIG. 33–8. Effect of lipid reduction on thrombus formation. Representative histologic sections of thrombus formed on the surface of the thrombogenic surface (in this case, the media of porcine aorta) before **(A)** and after **(B)** cholesterol reduction therapy. Similar reduction of thrombus formation has been reported used lipophilic and hydrophilic statins. (Adapted from Rauch U, Osende JI, Chesebro JH, et al. Statins and cardiovascular diseases: the multiple effects of lipid-lowering therapy by statins. *Atherosclerosis* 2000;153:181–189.)

ognized to induce endothelial dysfunction (63) and increase sympathetic nerve activity (64) (both positively correlated with atherogenesis, morbidity, and mortality for coronary heart disease), may induce a hypercoagulable or thrombogenic state, favoring progression or recurrence of thrombi (65). Cigarette smokers (66–68), patients with hypertension (69) and hypercholesterolemia (70,71), and patients with all of the other classic cardiovascular risk factors show enhanced platelet reactivity. More importantly, discontinuation of smoking (72) and lipid-decreasing interventions (in primary and secondary prevention trials) reduce vascular events most often associated with thrombosis. Lipid-lowering therapy with statins normalizes the hypercholesterolemia-induced platelet thrombogenicity (71) and improves endothelial function. In this context, we demonstrated a significant decrease in thrombus formation using the Badimon chamber in patients with hypercholesterolemia after lipid reduction (70,73). Interestingly, all the statins tested showed a similar reduction in thrombus formation (Fig. 33–8) (70).

CONCLUSION

Considering the important role of endothelium in maintaining vascular homeostasis and hemostasis—with its strategic localization interfacing between vessel wall and the flowing blood, its magnitude, and the efficient production of potent vasoactive agents—and the pivotal role of TF in the initiation of the thrombosis, both the endothelium and TF should be considered major pharmaceutical targets for the prevention of atherothrombotic disease. In addition, because of the cross-linking effects among platelets, coagulation and fibrinolytic system, endothelial function, and rheologic factors and the positive effect of influencing each single factor on the clinical outcome, all of these effects should be considered in the evaluation of new treatment strategies.

REFERENCES

1. Asakura T, Karino T. Flow patterns and spatial distribution of atherosclerotic lesions in human coronary arteries. *Circ Res* 1990;66:1045–1066.
2. Pedersen EM, Agerbaek M, Kristensen IB, et al. Wall shear stress and early atherosclerotic lesions in the abdominal aorta in young adults. *Eur J Vasc Endovasc Surg* 1997;13:443–451.
3. Gimbrone MA Jr, Cybulsky MI, Kume N, et al. Vascular endothelium. An integrator of pathophysiological stimuli in atherogenesis. *Ann NY Acad Sci* 1995;748:122–132.
4. Gnasso A, Irace C, Carallo C, et al. In vivo association between low wall shear stress and plaque in subjects with asymmetrical carotid atherosclerosis. *Stroke* 1997;28:993–998.
5. Motomiya M, Karino T. Flow patterns in the human carotid artery bifurcation. *Stroke* 1984;15:50–56.
6. Resnick N, Yahav H, Schubert S, et al. Signalling pathways in vascular endothelium activated by shear stress: relevance to atherosclerosis. *Curr Opin Lipidol* 2000;11:167–177.
7. Nagel T, Resnick N, Dewey CF Jr, et al. Vascular endothelial cells respond to spatial gradients in fluid shear stress by enhanced activation of transcription factors. *Arterioscler Thromb Vasc Biol* 1999;19:1825–1834.
8. Chien S, Li S, Shyy JY. Effects of mechanical forces on signal transduction and gene expression in endothelial cells. *Hypertension* 1998;31:162–169.
9. Luscher TF, Tanner FC, Noll G. Lipids and endothelial function: effects of lipid-lowering and other therapeutic interventions. *Curr Opin Lipidol* 1996;7:234–240.
10. Ross R. Atherosclerosis—an inflammatory disease. *N Engl J Med* 1999;340:115–126.
11. Libby P. Current concepts of the pathogenesis of the acute coronary syndromes. *Circulation* 2001;104:365–372.
12. Malek AM, Alper SL, Izumo S. Hemodynamic shear stress and its role in atherosclerosis. *JAMA* 1999;282:2035–2042.
13. Caro CG, Fitz-Gerald JM, Schroter RC. Atheroma and arterial wall shear. Observation, correlation and proposal of a shear dependent mass transfer mechanism for atherogenesis. *Proc R Soc Lond B Biol Sci* 1971;177:109–159.
14. Turitto VT, Hall CL. Mechanical factors affecting hemostasis and thrombosis. *Thromb Res* 1998;92:S25–S31.
15. Topper JN, Gimbrone MA Jr. Blood flow and vascular gene expression: fluid shear stress as a modulator of endothelial phenotype. *Mol Med Today* 1999;5:40–46.
16. Traub O, Berk BC. Laminar shear stress: mechanisms by which endothelial cells transduce an atheroprotective force. *Arterioscler Thromb Vasc Biol* 1998;18:677–685.
17. Radomski MW, Palmer RM, Moncada S. Comparative pharmacology of endothelium-derived relaxing factor, nitric oxide and prostacyclin in platelets. *Br J Pharmacol* 1987;92:181–187.

18. Cooke JP, Rossitch E Jr, Andon NA, et al. Flow activates an endothelial potassium channel to release an endogenous nitrovasodilator. *J Clin Invest* 1991;88:1663–1671.

19. Grant JA, Scrutton MC. Positive interaction between agonists in the aggregation response of human blood platelets: interaction between ADP, adrenaline and vasopressin. *Br J Haematol* 1980;44:109–125.

20. Radomski MW, Palmer RM, Moncada S. The anti-aggregating properties of vascular endothelium: interactions between prostacyclin and nitric oxide. *Br J Pharmacol* 1987;92:639–646.

21. Corti R, Badimon JJ. Biologic aspects of vulnerable plaque. *Curr Opin Cardiol* 2002;17:616–625.

22. Virmani R, Kolodgie FD, Burke AP, et al. Lessons from sudden coronary death: a comprehensive morphological classification scheme for atherosclerotic lesions. *Arterioscler Thromb Vasc Biol* 2000;20:1262–1275.

23. Corti R, Fuster V, Badimon JJ. Pathogenetic concepts of acute coronary syndromes. *J Am Coll Cardiol* 2003;41:S7–S14.

24. Fuster V, Badimon L, Badimon JJ, et al. The pathogenesis of coronary artery disease and the acute coronary syndromes (2). *N Engl J Med* 1992;326:310–318.

25. Zaman AG, Helft G, Worthley SG, et al. The role of plaque rupture and thrombosis in coronary artery disease. *Atherosclerosis* 2000;149:251–266.

26. Corti R, Farkouh ME, Badimon JJ. The vulnerable plaque and acute coronary syndromes. *Am J Med* 2002;113:668–680.

27. Osende JI, Fuster V, Lev EI, et al. Testing platelet activation with a shear-dependent platelet function test versus aggregation-based tests: relevance for monitoring long-term glycoprotein IIb/IIIa inhibition. *Circulation* 2001;103:1488–1491.

28. Toschi V, Gallo R, Lettino M, et al. Tissue factor modulates the thrombogenicity of human atherosclerotic plaques. *Circulation* 1997;95:594–599.

29. Kaikita K, Ogawa H, Yasue H, et al. Tissue factor expression on macrophages in coronary plaques in patients with unstable angina. *Arterioscler Thromb Vasc Biol* 1997;17:2232–2237.

30. Rosenberg RD, Aird WC. Vascular-bed—specific hemostasis and hypercoagulable states. *N Engl J Med* 1999;340:1555–1564.

31. Moreno PR, Bernardi VH, Lopez-Cuellar J, et al. Macrophages, smooth muscle cells, and tissue factor in unstable angina. Implications for cell-mediated thrombogenicity in acute coronary syndromes. *Circulation* 1996;94:3090–3097.

32. Badimon JJ, Lettino M, Toschi V, et al. Local inhibition of tissue factor reduces the thrombogenicity of disrupted human atherosclerotic plaques: effects of tissue factor pathway inhibitor on plaque thrombogenicity under flow conditions. *Circulation* 1999;99:1780–1787.

33. Drew AF, Davenport P, Apostolopoulos J, et al. Tissue factor pathway inhibitor expression in atherosclerosis. *Lab Invest* 1997;77:291–298.

34. Giesen PL, Nemerson Y. Tissue factor on the loose. *Semin Thromb Hemost* 2000;26:379–384.

35. Taubman MB, Giesen PL, Schecter AD, et al. Regulation of the procoagulant response to arterial injury. *Thromb Haemost* 1999;82:801–805.

36. Giesen PL, Rauch U, Bohrmann B, et al. Blood-borne tissue factor: another view of thrombosis. *Proc Natl Acad Sci USA* 1999;96:2311–2315.

37. Bauriedel G, Hutter R, Welsch U, et al. Role of smooth muscle cell death in advanced coronary primary lesions: implications for plaque instability. *Cardiovasc Res* 1999;41:480–488.

38. Hutter R, Sauter B, Fallon JT, et al. Pig coronary angioplasty is followed by the coordinated upregulation of tissue-factor and caspase-3. *J Am Coll Cardiol* 2001;37:36A.

39. Mallat Z, Tedgui A. Current perspective on the role of apoptosis in atherothrombotic disease. *Circ Res* 2001;88:998–1003.

40. Penn MS, Topol EJ. Tissue factor, the emerging link between inflammation, thrombosis, and vascular remodeling. *Circ Res* 2001;89:1–2.

41. Zarins CK, Giddens DP, Bharadvaj BK, et al. Carotid bifurcation atherosclerosis. Quantitative correlation of plaque localization with flow velocity profiles and wall shear stress. *Circ Res* 1983;53:502–514.

42. Gibson CM, Diaz L, Kandarpa K, et al. Relation of vessel wall shear stress to atherosclerosis progression in human coronary arteries. *Arterioscler Thromb* 1993;13:310–315.

43. Caro CG, Fitz-Gerald JM, Schroter RC. Atheroma: a new hypothesis. *Br Med J* 1971;2:651.

44. Cho A, Mitchell L, Koopmans D, et al. Effects of changes in blood flow rate on cell death and cell proliferation in carotid arteries of immature rabbits. *Circ Res* 1997;81:328–337.

45. Walpola PL, Gotlieb AI, Langille BL. Monocyte adhesion and changes in endothelial cell number, morphology, and F-actin distribution elicited by low shear stress in vivo. *Am J Pathol* 1993;142:1392–1400.

46. Walpola PL, Gotlieb AI, Cybulsky MI, et al. Expression of ICAM-1 and VCAM-1 and monocyte adherence in arteries exposed to altered shear stress. *Arterioscler Thromb Vasc Biol* 1995;15:2–10.

47. Malek AM, Zhang J, Jiang J, et al. Endothelin-1 gene suppression by shear stress: pharmacological evaluation of the role of tyrosine kinase, intracellular calcium, cytoskeleton, and mechanosensitive channels. *J Mol Cell Cardiol* 1999;31:387–399.

48. Tronc F, Wassef M, Esposito B, et al. Role of NO in flow-induced remodeling of the rabbit common carotid artery. *Arterioscler Thromb Vasc Biol* 1996;16:1256–1262.

49. Kamiya A, Togawa T. Adaptive regulation of wall shear stress to flow change in the canine carotid artery. *Am J Physiol* 1980;239:H14–H21.

50. Glagov S, Weisenberg E, Zarins CK, et al. Compensatory enlargement of human atherosclerotic coronary arteries. *N Engl J Med* 1987;316:1371–1375.

51. Mintz GS, Popma JJ, Pichard AD, et al. Arterial remodeling after coronary angioplasty: a serial intravascular ultrasound study. *Circulation* 1996;94:35–43.

52. Wentzel JJ, Kloet J, Andhyiswara I, et al. Shear-stress and wall-stress regulation of vascular remodeling after balloon angioplasty: effect of matrix metalloproteinase inhibition. *Circulation* 2001;104:91–96.

53. Worthley SG, Helft G, Fuster V, et al. Serial in vivo MRI documents arterial remodeling in experimental atherosclerosis. *Circulation* 2000;101:586–589.

54. Singh R, Pan S, Mueske CS, et al. Role for tissue factor pathway in murine model of vascular remodeling. *Circ Res* 2001;89:71–76.

55. Dzau VJ, Gibbons GH. Endothelium and growth factors in vascular remodeling of hypertension. *Hypertension* 1991;18:III115–III121.

56. Mattsson EJ, Kohler TR, Vergel SM, et al. Increased blood flow induces regression of intimal hyperplasia. *Arterioscler Thromb Vasc Biol* 1997;17:2245–2249.

57. Ethier CR, Steinman DA, Zhang X, et al. Flow waveform effects on end-to-side anastomotic flow patterns. *J Biomech* 1998;31:609–617.

58. Steinman DA, Frayne R, Zhang XD, et al. MR measurement and numerical simulation of steady flow in an end-to-side anastomosis model. *J Biomech* 1996;29:537–542.

59. Ward MR, Tsao PS, Agrotis A, et al. Low blood flow after angioplasty augments mechanisms of restenosis: inward vessel remodeling, cell migration, and activity of genes regulating migration. *Arterioscler Thromb Vasc Biol* 2001;21:208–213.

60. Mailhac A, Badimon JJ, Fallon JT, et al. Effect of an eccentric severe stenosis on fibrin(ogen) deposition on severely damaged vessel wall in arterial thrombosis. Relative contribution of fibrin(ogen) and platelets. *Circulation* 1994;90:988–996.

61. Badimon L, Badimon JJ. Mechanisms of arterial thrombosis in nonparallel streamlines: platelet thrombi grow on the apex of stenotic severely injured vessel wall. Experimental study in the pig model. *J Clin Invest* 1989;84:1134–1144.

62. Fernandez-Ortiz A, Badimon JJ, Falk E, et al. Characterization of the relative thrombogenicity of atherosclerotic plaque components: implications for consequences of plaque rupture. *J Am Coll Cardiol* 1994;23:1562–1569.

63. Luscher TF, Tanner FC, Tschudi MR, et al. Endothelial dysfunction in coronary artery disease. *Annu Rev Med* 1993;44:395–418.

64. Corti R, Binggeli C, Sudano I, et al. The beauty and the beast: aspects of the autonomic nervous system. *News Physiol Sci* 2000;15:125–129.

65. Rauch U, Osende JI, Fuster V, et al. Thrombus formation on atherosclerotic plaques: pathogenesis and clinical consequences. *Ann Intern Med* 2001;134:224–238.

66. Fuster V, Chesebro JH, Frye RL, et al. Platelet survival and the development of coronary artery disease in the young adult: effects of cigarette smoking, strong family history and medical therapy. *Circulation* 1981;63:546–551.

67. Rangemark C, Benthin G, Granstrom EF, et al. Tobacco use and urinary excretion of thromboxane A2 and prostacyclin metabolites in women stratified by age. *Circulation* 1992;86:1495–1500.

68. Yasuda K, Takashima M, Sawaragi I. Influence of a cigarette smoke ex-

CHAPTER 34

Leukocytes, Adhesion Molecules, and Chemokines in Atherothrombosis

Myron I. Cybulsky and Israel F. Charo

Key Words: CCL2 (monocyte chemoattractant protein-1); CCR2; CX3CL1 (fractalkine); CX3CR1; CXCL8 (interleukin-8); CXCR2; hypercholesterolemia; intercellular adhesion molecule-1; integrin; knockout mice; lymphocytes; monocytes; mononuclear leukocytes; mouse models; selectin; vascular cell adhesion molecule-1.

INTRODUCTION

Although the major risk factors for atherothrombosis have been identified, the cellular and molecular mechanisms of atherothrombotic lesion initiation and progression are still not understood. The recruitment of blood monocytes and lymphocytes to the arterial intima is a key feature of early and advanced atherothrombotic lesions (1–3). Adherent monocytes transmigrate into the intima, transform into macrophages, engulf lipids, and become foam cells. Monocyte recruitment contributes to the growth and expansion of

early lesions, and, in advanced lesions, recruited monocytes may directly participate in plaque destabilization, resulting in thrombotic complications that are associated with significant morbidity and mortality. In humans, atherothrombosis develops indolently for decades before the onset of complications and clinical manifestations. Understanding the pathogenesis of early atherothrombotic lesions may lead to appropriate interventions in populations at risk, which may prevent or delay future complications.

A critical feature of an inflammatory disease process, including atherothrombosis, is the recruitment of leukocytes to the site of inflammation. This process involves the emigration of leukocytes from blood into the extravascular tissues, where leukocytes migrate along chemotactic gradients and can cause tissue damage by releasing enzymes, chemical mediators, and toxic oxygen free radicals. Leukocyte-induced injury occurs in many acute and chronic inflammatory diseases and may be subject to therapeutic intervention.

The nature of the inflammatory response and the type of leukocyte subpopulations that are recruited are regulated by the repertoire of cytokines and chemokines that are produced locally by the inflammatory stimulus. Cytokines modulate the biologic properties of endothelial cells that form the interface between blood and tissues and have important homeostatic functions, including maintenance of a nonadhesive and an-

M. I. Cybulsky: Department of Laboratory Medicine and Pathobiology, University of Toronto, Toronto General Research Institute, UHN, 200 Elizabeth Street, Eaton-4, Toronto, Ontario, M5G 2C4 Canada.
    I. F. Charo: Department of Medicine, 365 Vermont Street, Gladstone Institute of Cardiovascular Disease, University of California, San Francisco, California 94103.

tithrombotic surface and regulation of protein and lipoprotein permeability (4). Endothelial cells can respond to stimuli derived from the vessel wall and blood. Examples include inflammatory cytokines, oxidized lipoproteins trapped in the subendothelium, and even hemodynamic forces of flowing blood. Many of these stimuli can induce a phenotypic change in endothelial cells. For example, in response to the inflammatory cytokines interleukin-1 (IL-1) or tumor necrosis factor-α (TNF-α), endothelial cells synthesize and express on their surface adhesion molecules, which are transmembrane proteins, and present chemokines, which are bound to cell surface proteoglycans. Adhesion molecules and chemokines promote the recruitment of leukocytes from blood into the artery wall.

ROLE OF LEUKOCYTES IN THE FORMATION OF ATHEROTHROMBOTIC LESIONS

The recruitment of blood monocytes and lymphocytes to the arterial intima is one of the earliest events in the formation of an atherothrombotic lesion and persists even in advanced lesions (1,3,5–8). Adherent monocytes transmigrate into the intima, transform into macrophages, engulf lipids, and become foam cells. Monocyte recruitment, particularly at the periphery of lesions (9), may contribute to their lateral growth. Monocytes and macrophage foam cells may also contribute to the progression of atherothrombotic lesions by producing cytokines and growth factors. These, in turn, may amplify mononuclear leukocyte recruitment, induce migration of smooth muscle cells into the intima, and stimulate cell replication. Because early fatty streaks are composed almost entirely of macrophage foam cells, recruitment of monocytes to the intima may be a critical event in lesion initiation and expansion.

The importance of leukocytes in atherogenesis was illustrated in osteopetrotic (op/op) mice. These mice are deficient in macrophage-colony stimulating factor (M-CSF or CSF-1) because of a point mutation in the *M-CSF* gene. Through binding to its receptor, c-fms, M-CSF functions as a monocyte chemotactic factor and regulates the growth, survival, and expression of genes in macrophages, including the class A scavenger receptor. Op/op mice have impaired production of blood monocytes and deficiency of peritoneal and tissue macrophages. A lack of osteoclasts accounts for osteopetrosis, and an inability for teeth to erupt impairs consumption of solid food and requires feeding of a special liquid diet. When bred into an atherothrombosis-susceptible background, op/op mice have markedly reduced atherothrombotic lesions formation (10–12). Even heterozygous (op/+) mice have dramatically reduced lesion size, despite only a 20% reduction in circulating monocytes and absence of osteopetrosis (13). Mice deficient in macrophage class A scavenger receptors also have reduced lesion formation (14), which highlights the importance of monocyte/macrophages in atherothrombotic lesion formation.

Lymphocytes also participate in atherogenesis. CD4$^+$ T helper 1 cells (Th1) are the predominant T-cell subtype in

atherothrombotic lesions and respond to antigenic challenge by releasing proinflammatory cytokines, including interferon-γ (IFN-γ), TNF-α, and lymphotoxin (15). Apolipoprotein E$^{-/-}$ (apoE$^{-/-}$) mice deficient in the recombinase activating gene-1 (Rag-1$^{-/-}$) lack adaptive immunity and develop twofold less atherothrombosis when fed standard chow, but had lesions comparable to immunocompetent apoE$^{-/-}$ mice when fed a Western-type diet (16). In the low-density lipoprotein receptor–deficient (LDLR$^{-/-}$) background, lesion development in Rag-1$^{-/-}$ mice was reduced by 54% after 8 weeks of consuming a Western-type diet; however, significant differences in lesion area gradually subsided as the diet was continued for 12 and 16 weeks (17). apoE$^{-/-}$ mice with severe combined immunodeficiency experienced development of 75% less atherothrombosis, and reconstitution of these mice with CD4$^+$ T cells increased atherothrombosis (18). This proatherogenic activity may be exerted at least partly through secretion of the cytokine IFN-γ, because smaller atherothrombotic lesions develop in mice deficient in IFN-γ or IFN-γ receptor (19–22).

MECHANISMS OF LEUKOCYTE EMIGRATION FROM BLOOD INTO TISSUES

Leukocyte Emigration: A Multistep Process

Intravital microscopy experiments and *in vitro* modeling have determined that leukocyte emigration in postcapillary venules and arteries involves several distinct interactions between leukocytes and endothelial cells (Fig. 34–1). These include tethering and rolling, arrest, firm or stable adhesion, and transendothelial migration (diapedesis). Each of these sequential steps is mediated by binding and detachment of adhesion molecules expressed on leukocytes and endothelium. Endothelial cell adhesion molecules and their respective leukocyte ligands or counter-receptors belong to several families, including selectin, selectin carbohydrate ligands on mucins, immunoglobulin gene superfamily, and integrin (Table 34–1). The adhesive interactions between leukocytes and endothelium initiate signaling in both cells that are critical for emigration. For example, during rolling, chemokines presented on the surface of inflamed endothelial cells activate leukocyte integrins, which up-regulates their adhesive function and enables them to bind efficiently to their endothelial ligands. This chapter reviews key features and concepts of inflammatory adhesion molecule and chemokine biology. Primary references are too numerous to be cited comprehensively; however, reviews of this area with abundant citations are available (23–26).

Endothelial Cell Activation and Identification of Adhesion Molecules

The discovery in the 1980s and early 1990s of endothelial cell adhesion molecules relevant to leukocyte emigration was largely dependent on the development of efficient and

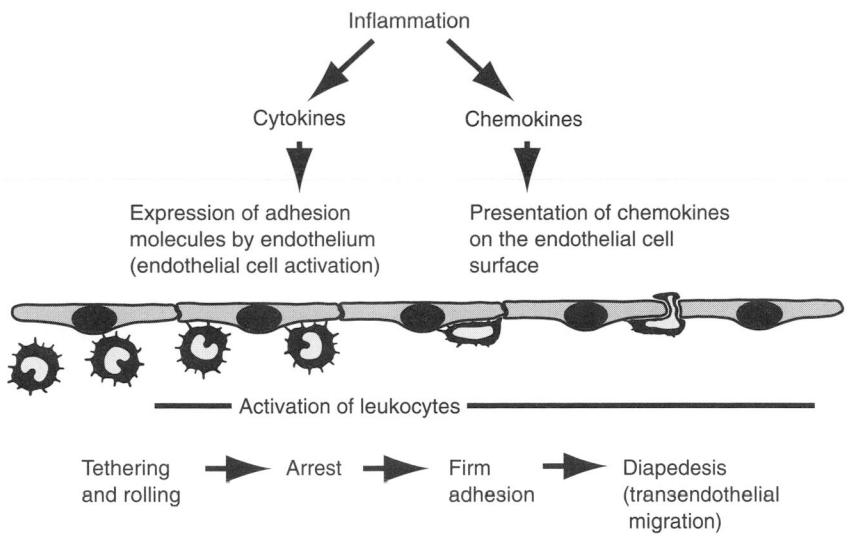

FIG. 34–1. Stages of leukocyte emigration.

TABLE 34–1. *Endothelial and leukocyte adhesion molecules relevant to inflammation*

Adhesion molecule (alternative designation)	Cell expression	Ligands
Selectins		
E-selectin (CD62E, ELAM-1)	Endothelium	CD15s (on ESL-1?)
P-selectin (CD62P, GMP-140, PADGEM)	Endothelium, platelets	CD15s on PSGL-1
L-selectin (CD62L, LAM-1)	Leukocytes	GlyCAM-1, CD34, podocallixin, gp200, MadCAM-1, PSGL-1, (inducible endothelial ligand?)
Immunoglobulin gene superfamily		
ICAM-1 (CD54)	Endothelium	LFA-1, Mac-1
ICAM-2 (CD102)	Endothelium	LFA-1
ICAM-3 (CD50)	Leukocytes	LFA-1
VCAM-1 (CD106)	Endothelium	$\alpha_4\beta_1$, $(\alpha_4\beta_7)$
MadCAM-1	Endothelium	$\alpha_4\beta_7$, L-selectin
PECAM-1 (CD31)	Endothelium, leukocytes	PECAM-1, heterotypic
Integrins		
$\alpha_L\beta_2$ (LFA-1, CD11a/CD18)	Leukocytes	ICAM-1, 2, 3
$\alpha_M\beta_2$ (Mac-1, CD11b/CD18)	Granulocytes, monocytes	ICAM-1, iC3b, fibrinogen, factor X
$\alpha_X\beta_2$ (p150/95, CD11c/CD18)	Granulocytes, monocytes	iC3b, fibrinogen
$\alpha_d\beta_2$ (CD11d/CD18)	Leukocytes (myeloid > lymphoid)	ICAM-3, (VCAM-1)
$\alpha_4\beta_1$ (VLA-4, CD49d/CD29)	Leukocytes (not neutrophils)	VCAM-1, fibronectin CS-1
$\alpha_4\beta_7$ (LPAM-1)	Lymphocytes	MadCAM-1, fibronectin CS-1, (VCAM-1)

ELAM, endothelial–leukocyte adhesion molecule-1; ESL-1, E-selectin ligand-1; GMP, α-granule membrane protein; ICAM-1, intercellular adhesion molecule-1; LAM-1, leukocyte adhesion molecule-1; LFA-1, leukocyte function-associated antigen-1; LPAM-1, lymphocyte Peyer's patch adhesion molecule-1; Mac-1, macrophage-1; MadCAM-1, mucosal addressin cell adhesion molecule-1; PADGEM, platelet activation-dependent granule-external membrane; PECAM-1, platelet–endothelial cell adhesion molecule-1; PSGL-1, P-selectin glycoprotein ligand; VCAM-1, vascular cell adhesion molecular-1; VLA-4, very late antigen-4.

reproducible techniques for culturing of human umbilical vein endothelial cells. Early experiments showed that IL-1 treatment of cultured endothelial cells elicited a protein synthesis–dependent phenotype change, resulting in prothrombotic and hyperadhesive cell surface properties, which was one of the first examples of endothelial cell activation *in vitro*. Subsequent studies involved production of monoclonal antibodies to IL-1–inducible endothelial cell antigens and antibody adhesion blocking assays to determine which of the activation antigens were leukocyte adhesion molecules. This approach identified a neutrophil adhesion molecule designated endothelial-leukocyte adhesion molecule-1, and subsequently renamed E-selectin. Monoclonal antibodies to E-selectin also were used to characterize its biochemical properties, expression patterns in human and experimental tissues, and in expression cloning of the cDNA (27). Vascular cell adhesion molecule-1 (VCAM-1) was discovered using a novel expression cloning strategy, in which a cDNA library from cytokine-activated endothelial cells was expressed in COS cells and plasmids were extracted from transfected cells that supported leukocyte adhesion (28). Other endothelial cell adhesion molecules were initially identified in other cell types. These include P-selectin, identified in platelets, and intercellular adhesion molecule-1 (ICAM-1), in leukocytes (see review by Springer [23]).

Leukocyte adhesion molecules expressed by endothelial cells can be classified into three general categories on the basis of their expression pattern (Table 34–2). Adhesion molecules, such as ICAM-2 and platelet–endothelial cell adhesion molecule-1 (PECAM-1), are expressed constitutively on the endothelial cell surface, and their expression levels are not up-regulated by treatment with inflammatory cytokines. PECAM-1 is unique in that it is localized to endothelial junctions, a feature that may contribute to its role in leukocyte transendothelial migration. Expression of E-selectin, VCAM-1, and ICAM-1 is up-regulated by inflammatory cytokines or lipopolysaccharide (LPS) through induction of transcription, although the kinetics and duration of induced expression of each molecule is different. P-selectin was originally described in α granules of platelets. In endothelium it is present constitutively on the membrane of Weibel-Palade granules and can be rapidly translocated to the plasma membrane on exposure of cells to thrombin, histamine, platelet-activating factor, oxidants, and

hypoxia. This occurs within minutes, does not require protein synthesis, and depends on increased concentrations of cytosolic calcium. P-selectin molecules can be recycled back to the cytoplasmic storage pool. Activation of endothelium by inflammatory cytokines induces P-selectin transcription and increases its expression on the cell surface.

Selectins and Selectin Ligands

Selectins are highly homologous type 1 transmembrane glycoproteins that share structurally related domains, which include an N-terminal calcium-dependent lectin, endothelial growth factor–like, variable number of complement regulatory repeats, transmembrane, and C-terminal cytoplasmic domain (23,29). Selectins are designated as E (endothelial), P (platelet), or L (leukocyte) on the basis of their expression, and the genes are clustered on the long arm of chromosome 1. E-selectin expression is restricted to activated endothelial cells, and L-selectin is restricted to leukocytes. Although L-selectin is expressed constitutively, stimulation of leukocytes by chemoattractants induces its proteolytic cleavage and shedding. P-selectin is expressed by platelets and endothelium. The cytoplasmic domain of each selectin is distinct. This domain targets P-selectin molecules to α granules in platelets and Weibel-Palade bodies in endothelium, and L-selectin to the tips of lymphocyte microvilli and ruffles on myeloid cells. Selectins bind ligands via the N-terminal lectin domain. Their ligands are sialylated carbohydrate determinants closely related to sialyl-Lewis^x (sialyl-CD15) and its isomer sialyl-Lewis^a, which are linked to mucin-like molecules, such as P-selectin glycoprotein ligand-1 (PSGL-1). PSGL-1 is a 120-kD disulfide-linked dimer expressed on leukocytes and is the preferential ligand for P-selectin, although it can bind other selectins. E-selectin ligand-1 (ESL-1) has been identified; however, it is not clear if it is expressed on the leukocyte surface, and thus whether it is relevant to leukocyte emigration. L-selectin recognizes sulfated and sialylated CD15 on several mucin-like molecules expressed by lymph node high endothelial venules. Several have been identified, including glycosylation-dependent cell adhesion molecule-1, which is secreted, and CD34 and podocalyxin, which are on the cell surface (30,31).

Immunoglobulin Gene Superfamily and Integrins

VCAM-1, the ICAMs, and PECAM-1 are members of the immunoglobulin gene superfamily. They are type 1 transmembrane proteins that contain multiple domains homologous to variable and constant domains of the immunoglobulin genes. These domains are composed of a sandwich of two β-sheets stabilized by a conserved disulfide bond. VCAM-1, ICAM-1, and ICAM-2 bind leukocyte integrins, whereas PECAM-1 supports homotypic adhesive interactions (23). The biologic function of immunoglobulin gene superfamily members is regulated primarily by their expression patterns.

TABLE 34–2. *Expression patterns of leukocyte adhesion molecules on endothelial cells*

Inducible, cell surface	Constitutive, cell surface	Constitutive, cytoplasmic granules
E-selectin	ICAM-2	P-selectin
VCAM-1	PECAM-1	
ICAM-1	ICAM-1	
P-selectin		

ICAM, intercellular adhesion molecule; PECAM-1, platelet–endothelial cell adhesion molecule-1; VCAM-1, vascular cell adhesion molecule-1.

Leukocyte integrins are heterodimeric transmembrane proteins composed of noncovalently associated α and β chains. More than 20 different integrins have been identified; however, 2 groups of integrins are relevant to leukocyte emigration. These include β_2 integrins, which are exclusively expressed by leukocytes and α_4 integrins. Four types of β_2 integrins have been identified. Of these, $\alpha_L\beta_2$ (LFA-1) and $\alpha_M\beta_2$ (Mac-1) have been studied most extensively. Integrins are expressed on the cell surface of leukocytes and also are stored in cytoplasmic granules of granulocytes and monocytes. LFA-1 and $\alpha_d\beta_2$ are expressed by all leukocyte types, whereas Mac-1 and $\alpha_X\beta_2$ are expressed by myeloid cells. α_4 integrins include $\alpha_4\beta_1$ and $\alpha_4\beta_7$. They are expressed on the cell surface of all circulating leukocytes except mature human neutrophils and like L-selectin are localized to the tips of microvilli of lymphoid and ruffles of myeloid cells.

Integrins are highly dynamic molecules. Their activation state determines binding of ligands (32). Modulation of integrin function provides a regulatory mechanism by which leukocyte adhesion to endothelium is strengthened or weakened at different stages of emigration. Integrins have low ligand-binding activity on circulating leukocytes; however, they are "activated" in a highly regulated manner while undergoing emigration during inflammation or physiologic trafficking. The process by which extracellular stimuli modulate integrin adhesive function has been referred to as inside-out signaling. Inside-out signals are produced by stimulation of a wide array of leukocyte receptors. During leukocyte emigration, potential mechanisms of integrin activation include signaling by chemokine or chemoattractant receptors (Fig. 34–2), binding of L-selectin to endothelial ligands, and outside-in signaling by other integrins. Integrin ligand-binding capacity can be up-regulated in two ways: by increasing integrin affinity or avidity, or both.

The affinity of an integrin is determined by its molecular conformation, because this influences the nature of the bond between each integrin molecule and its ligand (Fig. 34–3). A number of advances have provided insights to the structural basis for integrin conformational changes. High-affinity integrins form persistent bonds with ligands, whereas low-affinity bonds are transient. Therefore, high, but not low, affinity integrins can be detected by binding of soluble ligands or peptides (see review by Chan and coworkers [33]).

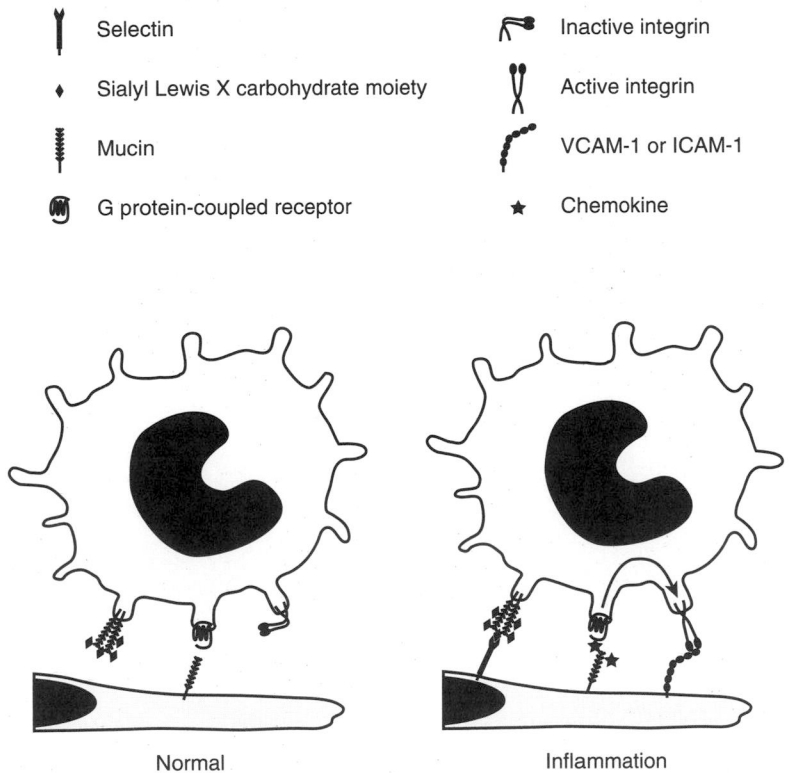

ⵉ Selectin	⌐ Inactive integrin
♦ Sialyl Lewis X carbohydrate moiety	ⵋ Active integrin
ⵊ Mucin	⌐ VCAM-1 or ICAM-1
ⓦ G protein-coupled receptor	★ Chemokine

Normal   Inflammation

FIG. 34–2. Integrin activation during leukocyte emigration. **A:** Integrins on circulating leukocytes are inactive and incapable of firm or prolonged binding of ligands. Furthermore, adhesion molecules, including selectins vascular cell adhesion molecule-1 (VCAM-1) and intercellular adhesion molecular-1 (ICAM-1), are not expressed on the endothelial surface in the absence of an inflammatory stimulus. **B:** At a site of inflammation, endothelial cells are activated by cytokines to express adhesion molecules and present chemoattractants and chemokines on their surface, which activate leukocyte integrins. Only active integrins are capable of mediating firm/persistent adhesion, resulting in leukocyte arrest, stable adhesion, and diapedesis.

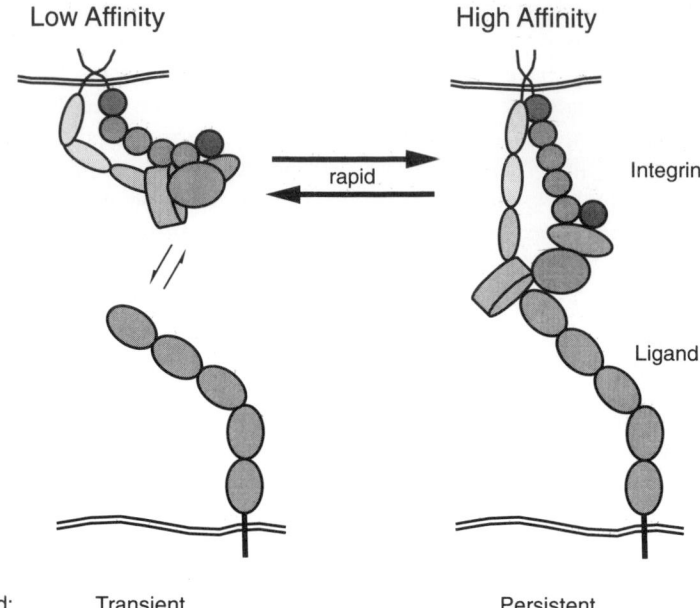

FIG. 34–3. Integrin affinity modulation. Integrins are thought to exist in low- and high-affinity conformations. A low-affinity integrin binds ligand transiently, whereas binding of a ligand to a high-affinity integrin is persistent. Therefore, binding of soluble ligand can be used to detect high-affinity integrins. Manganese binds directly to the extracellular domains of integrins and locks them in the high-affinity conformation.

Conformation changes and ligand binding by integrins result in exposure of previously masked epitopes that can be detected with monoclonal antibodies.

Integrin avidity refers to the number of simultaneous bonds that integrins on a cell can form with ligand. Multiple simultaneous bonds strengthen cell adhesion irrespective of whether each bond is transient or persistent (low or high affinity). Relatively few-high affinity bonds can mediate persistent cell adhesion, whereas alignment of many receptor–ligand pairs is necessary for adhesive interactions mediated solely by increased integrin avidity (32). Multivalent ligand binding can be enhanced by the release of integrins from the cytoskeleton resulting in rapid diffusion in the cell membrane, by active clustering of integrins, by increased cell spreading and contact area, and by a high density of ligand (Fig. 34–4).

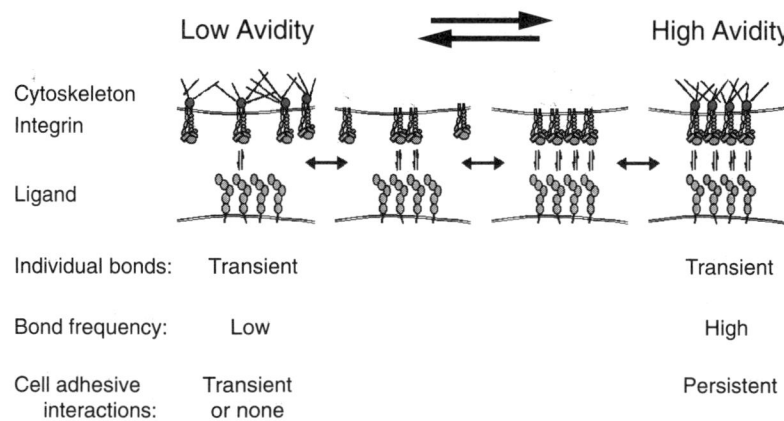

FIG. 34–4. Integrin avidity modulation. Release of integrins from cytoskeletal restraint increases their mobility in the plasma membrane, and adhesive interactions with ligands results in diffusion trapping and formation of multiple simultaneous bonds. Attachment to the cytoskeleton is subsequently reestablished. Depending on the activation stimulus, avidity modulation can occur with or without changes in integrin affinity.

TABLE 34–3. *Stages of leukocyte emigration and key adhesion molecules*

Stage	Key endothelial molecules	Key leukocyte molecules
Tethering and rolling	E-selectin, P-selectin ? VCAM-1	Selectin ligands (PSGL-1) L-selectin α_4 integrins
Arrest, firm (stable) adhesion	VCAM-1, ICAM-1	Integrins: α_4, LFA-1, Mac-1
Transendothelial migration (diapedesis)	VCAM-1, ICAM-1 PECAM-1 CD99	Integrins PECAM-1

ICAM, intercellular adhesion molecule; LFA-1, lymphocyte function-associated antigen-1; PECAM-1, platelet–endothelial cell adhesion molecule-1; PSGL-1, P-selectin glycoprotein ligand; VCAM-1, vascular cell adhesion molecule-1.

Adhesion Molecules and Leukocyte Emigration

Different adhesion molecules mediate each stage of leukocyte emigration (Table 34–3). This knowledge is based on intravital microscopy experiments, in which function-blocking antibodies or genetically engineered mice lacking specific adhesion molecules were used, as well as *in vitro* studies in which interactions between leukocytes and purified adhesion molecules immobilized on a surface were observed. Interactions of selectins with sialyl-Lewis[x,a] and VCAM-1 with α_4 integrins mediate leukocyte tethering and rolling (23–26). L-selectin, PSGL-1, and α_4 integrins are localized on the tips of leukocyte ruffles or microvilli; thus, they are strategically positioned to mediate the initial interactions with endothelium. The transition from rolling to arrest, firm (stable) adhesion, and transendothelial migration is mediated by leukocyte integrin binding to members of the immunoglobulin gene superfamily. At these stages, leuko-

cyte activation and modulation of integrin ligand binding activity plays a key role. PECAM-1 and CD99 contribute to leukocyte transendothelial migration.

Chemokines

Chemokines are small heparin-binding proteins that direct the migration of circulating leukocytes to sites of inflammation or injury (see reviews in References 34 through 37). There are 40 to 50 human chemokines, and these can be divided into four families on the basis of differences in their structure and function (Table 34–4). The largest family is known as the CC chemokines, because the first two of the four conserved cysteines residues that are characteristic of chemokines are adjacent to each other. CC chemokines tend to attract mononuclear cells and are found at sites of chronic inflammation. The most thoroughly characterized CC chemokine is monocyte chemoattractant protein-1 (MCP-1), which is a potent agonist for monocytes, memory T cells, and basophils. As discussed later in this chapter, MCP-1 has been implicated as a key player in the recruitment of monocytes from the blood into early atherothrombotic lesions. Other members of the CC family include RANTES (regulated on activation, normal T expressed and secreted), monocyte inflammatory protein-1α (MIP-1α), and MIP-1β. The CXC family of chemokines, of which IL-8 is the prototypic member, mediates acute inflammation and attracts polymorphonuclear leukocytes. CXC chemokines have a single amino acid residue interposed between the first two canonical cysteines. Lymphotactin is the sole member of the C family of chemokines, and it attracts lymphocytes. The fourth family is the CX3C family, of which fractalkine is the only known member. In fractalkine, a soluble chemokine domain similar in structure to other chemokines is fused to a mucin-like stalk and a transmembrane domain. Thus, unlike other chemokines, fractalkine is a type 1 transmembrane

TABLE 34–4. *Partial list of chemokine receptors, ligands, and receptor expression patterns*

Receptor	Chemokine ligands	Receptor expression on: Leukocytes
CCR1	CCL3 (MIP-1α), CCL5 (RANTES), CCL7 (MCP-3), CCL8 (MCP-2)	Eo, M, T, NK, D
CCR2	CCL2 (MCP-1), CCL7, CCL8, CCL13 (MCP-4)	M, T, NK, D
CCR3	CCL11 (Eotaxin-1), CCL24 (Eotaxin-2), CCL26 (Eotaxin-3) CCL5, CCL7, CCL8, CCL13	Eo, Ba, T
CCR4	CCL17 (TARC), CCL22 (MDC)	Ba, T, D
CCR5	CCL3, CCL4, (MIP-1β) CCL5, CCL8,	M, T, NK, D
CCR6	CCL20, (MIP-3α)	M, T, D
CCR7	CCL21 (SLC), CCL19 (MIP-3β)	T
CXCR1	CXCL8 (IL-8)	N, T, NK, D
CXCR2	CXCL8, CXCL1 (Gro-α), CXCL2 (Gro-β), CXCL3 Gro-γ), CXCL7 (NAP-2), CXCL5 (ENA-78), CXCL6 (GCP-2)	N, M, T, B, NK, D
CXCR3	CXCL9 (MIG), CXCL10 (IP-10), CXCL11 (I-TAC)	T
CXCR4	CXCL12 (SDF-1α)	N, T, B (pre and pro), M, NK, D
CXCR6	CXCL16	T
CX3CR1	CX3CL1 (Fractalkine)	M, T (human), NK (mouse)

B, B lymphocytes; Ba, basophils; D, dendritic cells; Eo, eosinophils; M, monocytes/macrophages; N, neutrophils; NK, natural killer cells; T, T lymphocytes.

protein. Fractalkine can be cleaved from the cell membrane to release a soluble protein that is a potent chemoattractant for monocytes and T cells. Finally, CXCL16 a second chemokine with an architecture similar to fractalkine, has been identified.

Many of the chemokines are rapidly inducible, early response genes—for example, MCP-1 and IL-8. These chemokines have little or no constitutive expression, but they are rapidly up-regulated in response to cytokines such as TNF-α or LPS. These chemokines have been referred to as "inflammatory chemokines," in part because they are often present at sites of inflammation. Virtually any parenchymal cell can synthesize and secrete these chemokines if activated by the appropriate cytokines. Fractalkine is expressed on activated endothelial cells and smooth muscle cells and, as discussed later in this chapter, is also likely to be involved in monocyte recruitment to the vessel wall in atherothrombosis. Other chemokines are produced constitutively to regulate normal homeostatic processes. Examples of these are the CC chemokines SLC and ELC, which are made in secondary lymphoid tissues and direct the trafficking of naive T cells in the lymph nodes and the spleen.

Chemokines exert their effects on cells through activation of seven transmembrane domain G protein–coupled receptors. Whether a leukocyte responds to a particular chemokine is determined by its complement of chemokine receptors. Chemokine binding activates a signal transduction cascade that results in activation of phosphatidylinositol 3 (PI3)-kinase to increase levels of inositol 1,4,5, triphosphate (IP$_3$), elevation of intracellular calcium, activation of Rho and mitogen-activated protein kinases, and eventually leads to actin rearrangement, shape change, and cell movement. The precise signaling pathways that lead to chemotaxis are not yet fully understood, but they rely on activation of the G$_{\alpha i}$ protein as the initial link to the activated receptor and appear to be dependent on activation of one or more isoforms of PI3-kinase. Treatment of cells with pertussis toxin, which prevents receptor coupling to G$_{\alpha i}$, blocks chemotaxis.

As discussed earlier in this chapter, the movement of leukocytes from the blood to the subendothelial space can be envisioned to be a four-step process. Chemokines can facilitate at least two steps of this process. First, certain chemokines can directly capture cells rolling along the blood vessel wall, and thus complement the function of the selectins. Fractalkine does this particularly well, in part because its unique architecture serves to position the chemokine domain above the glycocalyx of the cell and in good position to interact with its cognate receptor on monocytes and T cells. Cell capture by fractalkine is not dependent on receptor activation and is not blocked by pertussis toxin. IL-8 also is efficient at capturing cells under flow conditions. How IL-8 and other typical soluble chemokines are presented to circulating cells is not firmly established, but they may be transported by endothelial cells from the extravascular space to the luminal surface, where they can associate with heparin sulfate proteoglycans (38,39).

Chemokines also contribute to cell capture by activating integrins on the leukocyte. Integrin activation results in the firm adherence of leukocytes to the endothelium, and chemokine receptor–activated signaling pathways result in inside-out integrin activation. Unlike direct cell capture, chemokine-dependent activation of integrins is dependent on receptor activation and is blocked by pertussis toxin. An example of this is the activation of Mac-1 (α_M/β_2, CD11b/CD18) for ICAM-1 binding by the chemokine RANTES. In addition to increasing integrin affinity, chemokines can facilitate cell capture by inducing clustering of integrins on the leukocyte surface, without direct effects of integrin–ligand affinities. Microclustering of α_4/β_1 integrins also is dependent on G$_{\alpha i}$ signaling.

Specificity of Leukocyte Emigration

A combination of factors determines which leukocyte subtypes are recruited in different inflammatory responses. Neutrophils are the predominant leukocytes recruited in acute inflammation, whereas it is lymphocytes and monocytes in chronic inflammation, and it is eosinophils in allergic reactions and parasitic infections. The specificity of leukocyte recruitment is regulated by the inflammatory stimulus, repertoire cytokines and chemokines that are produced, the expression pattern of endothelial cell adhesion molecules, and the type of vascular bed that is involved. Chemokines orchestrate the movement of virtually all types of leukocytes throughout the body. Specificity of emigration is achieved through a combination of the chemokines produced in response to the inflammatory stimulus, the expression pattern of receptors on different leukocytes, and the particular selectins and integrins present on endothelium. This paradigm applies equally well to normal homeostatic processes, such as the recirculation of lymphocytes through lymph nodes and spleen; to classic inflammatory settings, such as acute and chronic infection; and, as discussed later, to diseases in which leukocyte recruitment contributes to pathogenesis, such as atherothrombosis.

The anatomic features and hemodynamic conditions of the blood vessel involved by inflammation can influence the functions of adhesion molecules at different stages of leukocyte emigration. Rolling is an essential step for leukocyte recruitment when blood flow is laminar, as in postcapillary venules. Selectins mediate leukocyte tethering and rolling under these conditions, but are only minimally functional if blood flow decreases to near-static conditions. In contrast, LFA-1 usually does not contribute to early leukocyte–endothelial interactions, but it can mediate rolling when stress is low. During acute inflammation in lungs, a significant component of neutrophil emigration occurs through the capillary plexus. Because the diameter of capillaries is slightly smaller than that of neutrophils, these leukocytes must deform during passage through this vascular bed, and rolling is not an important feature of emigration. In arteries, hemodynamic conditions, such as high shear forces and regions of disturbed flow, may also influence early stages of leukocyte emigration. Finally, adhesion inhibitors, such as nitric oxide, transforming growth factor-β, and lipoxin, participate in regulating leukocyte emigration.

FUNCTIONS OF ADHESION MOLECULES AND CHEMOKINES IN ATHEROTHROMBOSIS

During atherogenesis, the trapping and oxidation of low-density lipoproteins (LDLs) in the arterial intima (40) initiates an inflammatory response leading to the emigration of mononuclear leukocytes from the blood, which is a key feature of initiation and progression of atherothrombotic plaques. The paradigms for leukocyte recruitment to the arterial wall during atherogenesis are likely similar to those proposed for a variety of inflammatory and immune processes in postcapillary venules; however, there may be important differences in the contribution of individual adhesion molecules and chemokines. In the last decade, research has progressed from descriptive studies on the expression patterns of adhesion molecules and chemokines in atherothrombotic lesions to functional studies predominantly using mice with an engineered molecular overexpression or deficiency. Because experimental atherothrombotic lesions develop over a period of weeks to months, genetic approaches were used for evaluating functions of molecules. However, leukocyte recruitment has not been directly evaluated in mouse models of atherothrombosis. Instead, atherothrombotic lesion size, area, cellular composition, and histologic features are assessed and an assumption is made that lesion size directly correlates with the magnitude of leukocyte recruitment. In many instances, this reasoning is probably correct; however, adhesion molecules and chemokines are expressed by cells within plaques in addition to endothelium and may influence the biology of leukocytes within lesions. The recruitment of leukocytes versus their survival and proliferation in atherothrombotic lesions has not been addressed. Despite this limitation, important insights have been gained into the role of different adhesion molecules and chemokines, and these data are reviewed in the next section.

Expression of Adhesion Molecules and Chemokines in Atherothrombosis

The formation of foam cell–rich lesions during hypercholesterolemia appears to be a highly regulated process during which the vascular endothelium remains intact and regulates leukocyte recruitment into the intima. Studies in the early 1990s identified up-regulated expression of VCAM-1 on endothelial cells overlying early atherothrombotic lesions in rabbits and provided the first molecular evidence of endothelial cell activation during atherothrombosis (41). Subsequent studies characterized the expression patterns of VCAM-1 and other adhesion molecules in rabbit and mouse models of atherothrombosis. In aortas of normal chow-fed rabbits and wild-type mice, VCAM-1 and ICAM-1, but not E-selectin,

were expressed by endothelial cells in regions predisposed to atherothrombotic lesion formation, such as the lesser curvature of the aortic arch and downstream of artery ostia (42). In the setting of hypercholesterolemia, VCAM-1 and ICAM-1 protein expression is increased in endothelial cells (42–44), and increased steady-state mRNA levels of VCAM-1 and ICAM-1, but not E-selectin, were detected in the aorta (42). Increased VCAM-1 expression in endothelium is an early event in atherogenesis, occurring within 1 week after the initiation of a hypercholesterolemic diet in rabbits and preceding detectable intimal monocyte/macrophage accumulation (45a). Endothelial cell expression of VCAM-1 and ICAM-1 is prominent at and adjacent to lesion borders and is variable over the surface of lesions. ICAM-1 staining extended into the uninvolved aorta, in contrast to VCAM-1, which was generally restricted to lesions.

In early lesions, VCAM-1 and ICAM-1 are expressed predominantly by endothelium, whereas in more advanced lesions, abundant expression is found in intimal cells (42). Neointimal smooth muscle cells near the surface and base of intimal lesions and in the medial smooth muscle cells adjacent to the internal elastic lamina express VCAM-1, as do cultured rabbit and human arterial vascular smooth muscle cells when treated with appropriate cytokines (45b). The pathophysiologic function of VCAM-1 in smooth muscle cells remains unknown. Possibilities include retention of mononuclear leukocytes within lesions, signaling through α_4 integrins on leukocytes to activate cytokine and protease production, or simply it may be a marker of smooth muscle cell migration, activation, or differentiation.

Several studies used immunohistochemistry to examine the expression patterns of leukocyte adhesion molecules in human atherothrombotic plaques obtained at autopsy or from hearts of transplant recipients. Unlike the rabbit models, in which early lesions were examined, the human atherothrombotic plaques were generally advanced. In all cases, ICAM-1 expression was found in endothelial cells over plaques and in intimal smooth muscle cells and macrophages (46–50). In advanced human coronary artery plaques, VCAM-1 was expressed focally by luminal endothelial cells, usually in association with inflammatory infiltrates (50,51). Focal endothelial VCAM-1 expression also was found in uninvolved vessels with diffuse intimal thickening. Within plaques, VCAM-1 was expressed by subsets of smooth muscle cells and macrophages and by endothelial cells of neovasculature. The variability of VCAM-1 expression in human atherothrombotic lesions, apart from possible technical difficulties with detection, may reflect states of plaque activity or quiescence with regard to leukocyte recruitment. In contrast to rabbit models, in which relatively high levels of hypercholesterolemia are maintained by an atherogenic diet and intimal lesion growth is progressive, humans with atherothrombosis generally have low levels of hypercholesterolemia, and human plaque expansion, as a result of leukocyte recruitment, may develop at intervals.

In rabbit models, increased expression of P-selectin by endothelium precedes lesion formation and is sustained (44). In contrast, E-selectin expression was found in only occasional cells overlying lesions (42,44), but may be more prominent in an alloxan diabetic model (52). E-selectin expression was variable in human atherothrombosis (48–50). Caution should be applied to the interpretation of these data, because one of the antibodies to human E-selectin used in these studies (BBA 1) was subsequently found to cross-react with P-selectin.

Mononuclear leukocytes can respond chemotactically to numerous substances including peptides, lipids, and modified plasma components. Monocyte chemotactic activities have been isolated from atherothrombotic lesions in hypercholesterolemic swine and pigeons (53,54). These activities may result from modification of plasma lipoproteins and from chemokines produced locally in the arterial wall by endothelium, smooth muscle, and infiltrating leukocytes. MCP-1 is a key mediator of monocyte chemotaxis and its expression has been detected in human and experimental atherothrombotic plaques (55,56). Many other chemokines and chemoattractants have been found in human and experimental atherothrombotic lesions, including IL-8 and RANTES, fractalkine and M-CSF (57–63). In addition to acting locally, M-CSF may stimulate increased monocyte production by the bone marrow and account for the monocytosis in hypercholesterolemic animals (64).

Mouse Models of Atherothrombosis

Mouse models are currently at the forefront in the study of atherothrombosis because of the availability of multiple genetic approaches to overexpress or suppress the expression of genes in mice in a global or tissue-specific manner. These include conventional and conditional tissue-specific transgenesis, conventional and tissue-specific (Cre-lox) gene inactivation through homologous recombination in embryonic stem cells, and bone marrow transplantation. Normal mice are resistant to development of diet-induced hypercholesterolemia. Some strains, such as C57BL/6, develop foam cell lesions only in the aortic root when placed on a hypercholesterolemic diet containing cholate. In contrast, LDLR$^{-/-}$ (65) and apoE$^{-/-}$ mice (66,67) develop marked hypercholesterolemia and atherothrombotic lesions throughout the aorta. Their lesions have morphologic features that closely resemble human atherothrombosis (68–70), suggesting that pathogenic mechanisms similar to human atherothrombosis may be involved. LDLR$^{-/-}$ mice fed a normal chow diet have only a twofold increase in plasma cholesterol (primarily intermediate density lipoprotein [IDL]/LDL fraction) and do not develop lesions (65). When fed a cholesterol-enriched diet these mice experience development of marked hypercholesterolemia, with increased very low-density lipoprotein (VLDL), IDL, and LDL and decreased high-density lipoprotein, and readily experience development of lesions throughout the aorta (71,72). Therefore, cholesterol feeding in the LDLR$^{-/-}$ model enables

precise timing of lesion initiation. ApoE$^{-/-}$ mice experience spontaneous development of hypercholesterolemia (400–500 mg/dL, predominantly VLDL) and atherothrombotic lesions when fed a normal chow diet; however, on a Western-type diet (0.15% cholesterol, 21% fat), the hypercholesterolemia is pronounced (>1,500 mg/dL) and lesions develop more rapidly (66).

Adhesion Molecules in Atherothrombosis

During the 1990s, many lines of mice with an endothelial cell or leukocyte adhesion molecule deficiency have been developed (see reviewed by Bullard [73]), and the contribution of these adhesion molecules in atherogenesis has been investigated. Mice were backcrossed into the apoE$^{-/-}$ or LDLR$^{-/-}$ background, and the extent of atherothrombotic lesion formation was assessed by estimating the volume of lesions in the aortic root or determining the surface area of the aorta occupied by lesions. The histologic features of lesions and their cellular composition also were determined.

P-selectin deficiency in the LDLR$^{-/-}$ background had a modest effect in male but not female mice (74), and the effect was greater in the apoE$^{-/-}$ background (75–77). For example, at 4 months of age in the apoE$^{-/-}$ background, the P-selectin–deficient group had 3.5-fold smaller aortic sinus lesions than the P-selectin wild-type group. In the P-selectin–deficient group, lesions were limited to fatty streaks and contained less macrophages (76). By 15 months, progression to fibrous plaques was observed throughout the aorta in both groups, although lesions in the aortic sinus were smaller and less calcified in the P-selectin–deficient group. E-selectin deficiency had a relatively small effect on lesion formation (75). Mice with combined P- and E-selectin deficiency had less lesion formation than P-selectin$^{-/-}$ alone (78). Platelets may also contribute to atherogenesis (77,79–81). P-selectin is involved in mediating the adhesion of activated platelets to endothelial cells and leukocytes (81) and the deposition of platelet chemokines onto endothelium (82). Soluble P-selectin, derived primarily from endothelial cells, induces the formation of procoagulant microparticles (77).

Deficiency of VCAM-1 or α_4 integrin results in embryonic lethality (83–85). During embryogenesis, these molecules mediate the fusion of the allantois to the chorion. This is because VCAM-1 is normally expressed on the tip of the allantois, which subsequently forms the umbilical cord and the fetal vasculature of the placenta, whereas α_4 integrin is expressed on the chorion. The embryonic lethality of VCAM-1 null mice was circumvented by generating mice that express a mutant form of VCAM-1 at markedly reduced levels. Approximately 25% of these VCAM-1 domain 4–deficient (VCAM-1 D4D) mice were viable, which was sufficient for breeding them into the LDLR$^{-/-}$ background. Mice were fed a 1.25% cholesterol-enriched diet for 8 weeks and en face analysis of oil red O–stained aortas revealed reduced lesion area compared with VCAM-1$^{+/+}$ mice (86). VCAM-1 D4D mice also were bred into the apoE$^{-/-}$ background, and lesion formation in the aortic root was quantified. These studies revealed a *VCAM-1* gene dosage effect on aortic root atherothrombotic lesions at 16 weeks of age. The aortic root lesion area was reduced by 84% and 56% in VCAM-1$^{D4D/D4D}$ and VCAM-1$^{+/D4D}$ mice, respectively, and lesions in VCAM-1$^{D4D/D4D}$ mice were limited to small nascent fatty streaks (87). Together these studies suggest that VCAM-1 has a critical role in atherogenesis. Similarly its ligand, the α_4 integrin, should have an important function in atherothrombosis. This has been difficult to test, because mice deficient in α_4 integrin are not viable. However, data supporting this have been generated using infusion of α_4 integrin blocking peptide, which reduced lesion formation in mice (88). VCAM-1 and α_4 integrin also were key mediators of U937 cell rolling and adhesion in an *ex vivo* perfusion model of the carotid artery bifurcation harvested from apoE$^{-/-}$ mice (89).

In contrast to VCAM-1, ICAM-1 appears to have a minor role in the formation of early atherothrombotic lesions. In experiments carried out in parallel with VCAM-1 D4D mice, ICAM-1–deficient mice in the LDLR$^{-/-}$ background had lesion formation in the aorta comparable to wild-type littermate control mice (86). In the apoE$^{-/-}$ background, deficiency of ICAM-1 reduced the extent of aortic lesions, but to a lesser degree than P-selectin (75). Leukocyte CD11b expression was not essential for the development of atherothrombosis (90).

Chemokines in Atherothrombosis

Fatty streaks, the hallmark of early atherothrombotic lesions, are composed of lipid-laden macrophages, or foam cells. Studies in swine, nonhuman primates, and mice indicate that circulating blood monocytes are the precursors of these foam cells (91–93). Recent work has revealed that several members of the chemokine family play important roles in recruiting monocytes from the blood to the vessel wall. Insights into the mechanism governing monocyte migration into the blood vessel wall initially came from studies in which MCP-1 was found in macrophage-rich atherothrombotic plaques (94,95). Oxidized lipids have long been implicated as important mediators of atherothrombosis and foam cell formation (96), and minimally oxidized LDL, but not native LDL, induces MCP-1 production in vascular wall cells such as endothelial and smooth muscle cells (97). Chemokines thus emerged as a possible molecular link between oxidized lipoproteins and foam cell recruitment to the vessel wall.

Studies in transgenic mice overexpressing MCP-1 and mice in which either MCP-1 or CCR2 have been genetically deleted have provided strong evidence in support of this hypothesis. In bone marrow transplantation studies in mice, overexpression of MCP-1 in the blood vessel wall macrophages leads to increased foam cell formation and increased atherothrombosis (98). Similarly, deletion of MCP-1 in mice blocked the progression of dietary-induced atherothrombosis (99–101). CCR2 is the only known receptor for MCP-1, and deletion of CCR2 in mice afforded significant protection from both macrophage accumulation and atherothrombotic lesion formation in response to a high-fat diet (102,103). Finally, studies have shown that treatment of mice with an MCP-1 antagonist resulted in a reduction in dietary-induced atherothrombosis (104). Collectively, these studies provide strong evidence that activation of CCR2 by MCP-1 plays an important role in monocyte recruitment into early atherothrombotic lesions and suggest that interruption of the MCP-1/CCR2 axis can reduce lesion formation.

The degree to which monocytes respond to MCP-1 is influenced by the number of CCR2 receptors on their surface, and studies indicate that lipoproteins contribute to the regulation of CCR2 expression. Individuals with hypercholesterolemia have greater levels of CCR2 on their monocytes; CCR2 expression correlates positively with plasma LDL cholesterol levels and negatively with plasma high-density plasma lipoprotein levels (105,106). These findings suggest that high cholesterol levels lead to increased sensitivity of monocyte/macrophages to MCP-1, thereby increasing the movement of blood monocytes into early atherothrombotic lesions. The subsequent down-regulation of CCR2, as monocytes differentiate into macrophages, might then serve to keep the monocyte/macrophages in the lesion.

Oxidized lipids, which accumulate in early atherothrombotic lesions and induce production of MCP-1, also influence the level of CCR2 expression on monocytes. Unlike native LDL, which up-regulates CCR2, oxidized lipids down-regulate CCR2 (105). The mechanism for this down-regulation may involve the binding and internalization of oxidized lipids by CD36, a scavenger receptor, and subsequent activation of the peroxisome proliferator-activated receptor (PPAR)-γ, a member of the nuclear hormone receptor family. Indeed, purified components of oxidized lipids, such as 9-hydroxyoctadecadienoic acid (9-HODE) and 13-HODE are known to activate PPAR-γ Furthermore, rosiglitazone, a synthetic ligand that activates PPAR-γ, decreases CCR2 expression on monocytes (107). Systemic administration of rosiglitazone inhibits the development of atherothrombosis in mice, consistent with its effects on CCR2 expression (108). Further evidence for the importance of MCP-1/CCR2 in atherothrombosis comes from the observation that individuals who are homozygous for the *–2518 G/G* allele in the MCP-1 regulator region, a change that leads to increased levels of MCP-1 mRNA, have a greater incidence of coronary artery disease (109). Although provocative, this study included relatively small groups of patients, and the clinical relevance of this polymorphism will have to be verified in larger studies.

At least two other chemokines—IL-8 and fractalkine—have been directly linked to the development of early atherothrombotic lesions. IL-8 is perhaps the best characterized of the neutrophil chemoattractants, but studies have demonstrated that it is also a monocyte agonist and is present in macrophage-rich atherothrombotic plaques. Bone marrow transplantation has been used to repopulate LDLR$^{-/-}$ mice with cells that either lacked or overexpressed CXCR2, the murine IL-8 receptor (110). After feeding mice an atherogenic diet, the investigators noted a decrease in both macrophage accumulation and atherothrombotic lesion size in mice that lacked CXCR2. In addition to its role as a chemoattractant, IL-8 was shown to trigger the arrest of monocytes under flow conditions (111). This effect did not correlate with either chemotaxis or the induction of an intracellular calcium flux, and thus may be mediated by novel signaling pathways. Taken together, these data provide strong evidence that IL-8 plays a pivotal role in monocyte capture and in the initiation of atherothrombotic lesions.

Fractalkine is a novel chemokine composed of a chemokine-like domain fused to a mucin stalk (112). Fractalkine has a transmembrane domain and exists both as a full-length immobilized protein and, after cleavage at a site(s) near the plasma membrane, as a soluble protein. Full-length transmembrane fractalkine is an efficient cell adhesion molecule and can capture cells expressing its cognate receptor (CX3CR1) under physiologically relevant flow conditions (113,114). Fractalkine is present in atherothrombotic lesions, and the M280 polymorphism of its receptor CX3CR1 has been linked to a decrease in the incidence of coronary artery disease in humans and exhibits lower fractalkine binding (115,116). Mice with genetic deficiency of CX3CR1 have been created and crossed into the apoE$^{-/-}$ background, and like the CCR2 and IL-8 receptor null mice, show substantially smaller lesions throughout the aorta in diet-induced atherothrombosis (117,118). Thus, in addition to MCP-1 and IL-8, fractalkine appears to be the third member of the chemokine family intimately involved in fatty streak formation.

Currently, it is unclear whether each of these chemokines is acting independently or in concert with each other, and this remains an area of intense investigation. For example, it is possible that MCP-1 and IL-8 are acting primarily as chemoattractants, and that full-length, membrane-bound fractalkine is acting as a cell adhesion molecule. This is only one of many possible scenarios, however. Other chemokines may also participate in atherogenesis. For example, the chemokine KC (mouse GRO-α or CXCL2), but not MCP-1, triggers α$_4$ integrin-dependent monocyte arrest on atherothrombotic endothelium (119). It should be emphasized that the effects of chemokines in atherothrombosis are not exerted through changes in the cholesterol level or the lipoprotein profile. Although it is clear that lipids are a major factor in the pathogenesis of atherothrombosis, these findings suggest that one of the effects of hyperlipidemia may be to cause monocyte/macrophage recruitment through up-regulation of chemokines.

A thorough understanding of mechanisms of leukocyte recruitment to atherothrombotic plaques will provide the basis for effective therapeutic interventions in patients, with the goal of inhibiting lesion formation, reducing the risk for thrombotic complications, and diminishing the morbidity and mortality associated with this disease process.

ACKNOWLEDGMENTS

Supported by the Heart and Stroke Foundation of Ontario grant T 4608 (to M. I. Cybulsky), the Canadian Institutes of Health Research grant MOP-14151 (to M. I. Cybulsky), and the National Institutes of Health, National Heart, Lung, and Blood Institute grants HL52773 and HL63894 (to I. F. Charo). Dr. Cybulsky is a recipient of a Career Investigator Award from the Heart and Stroke Foundation of Ontario.

REFERENCES

1. Munro JM, Cotran RS. The pathogenesis of atherosclerosis: atherogenesis and inflammation. *Lab Invest* 1988;58:249–261.
2. Ross R. The pathogenesis of atherosclerosis—an update. *N Engl J Med* 1986;314:488–500.
3. Ross R. Atherosclerosis—an inflammatory disease. *N Engl J Med* 1999;340:115–126.
4. Gimbrone MA Jr, Cybulsky MI, Kume N, et al. Vascular endothelium. An integrator of pathophysiological stimuli in atherogenesis. *Ann NY Acad Sci* 1995;748:122–132.
5. Lusis AJ. Atherosclerosis. *Nature* 2000;407:233–241.
6. Glass CK, Witztum JL. Atherosclerosis: the road ahead. *Cell* 2001; 104:503–516.
7. Steinberg D. Atherogenesis in perspective: hypercholesterolemia and inflammation as partners in crime. *Nat Med* 2002;8:1211–1217.
8. Libby P. Inflammation in atherosclerosis. *Nature* 2002;420:868–874.
9. Walker LN, Reidy MA, Bowyer DE. Morphology and cell kinetics of fatty streak lesion formation in the hypercholesterolemic rabbit. *Am J Pathol* 1986;125:450–459.
10. Smith JD, Trogan E, Ginsberg M, et al. Decreased atherosclerosis in mice deficient in both macrophage colony-stimulating factor (op) and apolipoprotein E. *Proc Natl Acad Sci USA* 1995;92:8264–8268.
11. Qiao JH, Tripathi J, Mishra NK, et al. Role of macrophage colony-stimulating factor in atherosclerosis: studies of osteopetrotic mice. *Am J Pathol* 1997;150:1687–1699.
12. de Villiers WJ, Smith JD, Miyata M, et al. Macrophage phenotype in mice deficient in both macrophage-colony-stimulating factor (op) and apolipoprotein E. *Arterioscler Thromb Vasc Biol* 1998;18: 631–640.
13. Rajavashisth T, Qiao JH, Tripathi S, et al. Heterozygous osteopetrotic (op) mutation reduces atherosclerosis in LDL receptor-deficient mice. *J Clin Invest* 1998;101:2702–2710.
14. Suzuki H, Kurihara Y, Takeya M, et al. A role for macrophage scavenger receptors in atherosclerosis and susceptibility to infection. *Nature* 1997;386:292–296.
15. Hansson GK. Immune mechanisms in atherosclerosis. *Arterioscler Thromb Vasc Biol* 2001;21:1876–1890.
16. Dansky HM, Charlton SA, Harper MM, et al. T and B lymphocytes play a minor role in atherosclerotic plaque formation in the apolipoprotein E-deficient mouse. *Proc Natl Acad Sci USA* 1997;94:4642–4646.
17. Song L, Leung C, Schindler C. Lymphocytes are important in early atherosclerosis. *J Clin Invest* 2001;108:251–259.
18. Zhou X, Nicoletti A, Elhage R, et al. Transfer of CD4(+) T cells aggravates atherosclerosis in immunodeficient apolipoprotein E knockout mice. *Circulation* 2000;102:2919–2922.
19. Gupta S, Pablo AM, Jiang X, et al. IFN-gamma potentiates atherosclerosis in ApoE knock-out mice. *J Clin Invest* 1997;99:2752–2761.
20. Whitman SC, Ravisankar P, Elam H, et al. Exogenous interferon-gamma enhances atherosclerosis in apolipoprotein E-/- mice. *Am J Pathol* 2000;157:1819–1824.

21. Whitman SC, Ravisankar P, Daugherty A. IFN-gamma deficiency exerts gender-specific effects on atherogenesis in apolipoprotein E-/- mice. *J Interferon Cytokine Res* 2002;22:661–670.

22. Buono C, Come CE, Stavrakis G, et al. Influence of interferon-gamma on the extent and phenotype of diet-induced atherosclerosis in the LDLR-deficient mouse. *Arterioscler Thromb Vasc Biol* 2003;23: 454–460.

23. Springer TA. Traffic signals for lymphocyte recirculation and leukocyte emigration: the multistep paradigm. *Cell* 1994;76:301–314.

24. Butcher EC, Picker LJ. Lymphocyte homing and homeostasis. *Science* 1996;272:60–66.

25. Campbell JJ, Butcher EC. Chemokines in tissue-specific and microenvironment-specific lymphocyte homing. *Curr Opin Immunol* 2000;12:336–341.

26. Ley K. Pathways and bottlenecks in the web of inflammatory adhesion molecules and chemoattractants. *Immunol Res* 2001;24:87–95.

27. Bevilacqua MP, Stengelin S, Gimbrone MA Jr, et al. Endothelial leukocyte adhesion molecule 1: an inducible receptor for neutrophils related to complement regulatory proteins and lectins. *Science* 1989;243:1160–1165.

28. Osborn L, Hession C, Tizard R, et al. Direct expression cloning of vascular cell adhesion molecule 1, a cytokine-induced endothelial protein that binds to lymphocytes. *Cell* 1989;59:1203–1211.

29. Patel KD, Cuvelier SL, Wiehler S. Selectins: critical mediators of leukocyte recruitment. *Semin Immunol* 2002;14:73–81.

30. Rosen SD, Hwang ST, Giblin PA, et al. High-endothelial-venule ligands for L-selectin: identification and functions. *Biochem Soc Trans* 1997;25:428–433.

31. Sassetti C, Tangemann K, Singer MS, et al. Identification of podocalyxin-like protein as a high endothelial venule ligand for L-selectin: parallels to CD34. *J Exp Med* 1998;187:1965–1975.

32. Hughes PE, Pfaff M. Integrin affinity modulation. *Trends Cell Biol* 1998;8:359–364.

33. Chan JR, Hyduk SJ, Cybulsky MI. Detecting rapid and transient upregulation of leukocyte integrin affinity induced by chemokines and chemoattractants. *J Immunol Methods* 2003;273:43–52.

34. Baggiolini M. Chemokines and leukocyte traffic. *Nature* 1998;392: 565–568.

35. Rollins BJ. Chemokines. *Blood* 1997;90:909–928.

36. Zlotnik A, Morales J, Hedrick JA. Recent advances in chemokines and chemokine receptors. *Crit Rev Immunol* 1999;19:1–47.

37. Gerard C, Rollins BJ. Chemokines and disease. *Nat Immunol* 2001;2: 108–115.

38. Tanaka Y, Adams DH, Hubscher S, et al. T-cell adhesion induced by proteoglycan-immobilized cytokine MIP-1 beta. *Nature* 1993;361: 79–82.

39. Middleton J, Neil S, Wintle J, et al. Transcytosis and surface presentation of IL-8 by venular endothelial cells. *Cell* 1997;91:385–395.

40. Skalen K, Gustafsson M, Rydberg EK, et al. Subendothelial retention of atherogenic lipoproteins in early atherosclerosis. *Nature* 2002;417: 750–754.

41. Cybulsky MI, Gimbrone MA Jr. Endothelial expression of a mononuclear leukocyte adhesion molecule during atherogenesis. *Science* 1991;251:788–791.

42. Iiyama K, Hajra L, Iiyama M, et al. Patterns of vascular cell adhesion molecule-1 and intercellular adhesion molecule-1 expression in rabbit and mouse atherosclerotic lesions and at sites predisposed to lesion formation. *Circ Res* 1999;85:199–207.

43. Nakashima Y, Raines EW, Plump AS, et al. Upregulation of VCAM-1 and ICAM-1 at atherosclerosis-prone sites on the endothelium in the ApoE-deficient mouse. *Arterioscler Thromb Vasc Biol* 1998;18: 842–851.

44. Sakai A, Kume N, Nishi E, et al. P-selectin and vascular cell adhesion molecule-1 are focally expressed in aortas of hypercholesterolemic rabbits before intimal accumulation of macrophages and T lymphocytes. *Arterioscler Thromb Vasc Biol* 1997;17:310–316.

45a. Li H, Cybulsky MI, Gimbrone Ma Jr, et al. An atherogenic diet rapidly induces VCAM-1, a cytokine-regulatable mononuclear leukocyte adhesion molecule, in rabbit aortic endothelium. *Arterioscler Thromb* 1993;13:197–204.

45b. Li H, Cybulsky MI, Gimbrone MA Jr, et al. Inducible expression of vascular cell adhesion molecule-1 by vascular smooth muscle cells in vitro and within rabbit atheroma. *Am J Pathol* 1993;143:1551–1559.

46. Poston RN, Haskard DO, Coucher JR, et al. Expression of intercellular adhesion molecule-1 in atherosclerotic plaques. *Am J Pathol* 1992;140:665–673.

47. Printseva O, Peclo MM, Gown AM. Various cell types in human atherosclerotic lesions express ICAM-1. Further immunocytochemical and immunochemical studies employing monoclonal antibody 10F3. *Am J Pathol* 1992;140:889–896.

48. Wood KM, Cadogan MD, Ramshaw AL, et al. The distribution of adhesion molecules in human atherosclerosis. *Histopathology* 1993;22: 437–444.

49. van der Wal AC, Das PK, Tigges AJ, et al. Adhesion molecules on the endothelium and mononuclear cells in human atherosclerotic lesions. *Am J Pathol* 1992;141:1427–1433.

50. Davies MJ, Gordon JL, Gearing AJ, et al. The expression of the adhesion molecules ICAM-1, VCAM-1, PECAM, and E-selectin in human atherosclerosis. *J Pathol* 1993;171:223–229.

51. O'Brien KD, Allen MD, McDonald TO, et al. Vascular cell adhesion molecule-1 is expressed in human coronary atherosclerotic plaques. Implications for the mode of progression of advanced coronary atherosclerosis. *J Clin Invest* 1993;92:945–951.

52. Richardson M, Hadcock SJ, DeReske M, et al. Increased expression in vivo of VCAM-1 and E-selectin by the aortic endothelium of normolipemic and hyperlipemic diabetic rabbits. *Arterioscler Thromb* 1994;14:760–769.

53. Gerrity RG, Goss JA, Soby L. Control of monocyte recruitment by chemotactic factor(s) in lesion-prone areas of swine aorta. *Arteriosclerosis* 1985;5:55–66.

54. Denholm EM, Lewis JC. Monocyte chemoattractants in pigeon aortic atherosclerosis. *Am J Pathol* 1987;126:464–475.

55. Yla-Herttuala S, Lipton BA, Rosenfeld ME, et al. Expression of monocyte chemoattractant protein 1 in macrophage-rich areas of human and rabbit atherosclerotic lesions. *Proc Natl Acad Sci USA* 1991;88:5252–5256.

56. Kowala MC, Recce R, Beyer S, et al. Characterization of atherosclerosis in LDL receptor knockout mice: macrophage accumulation correlates with rapid and sustained expression of aortic MCP-1/JE. *Atherosclerosis* 2000;149:323–330.

57. Reape TJ, Groot PH. Chemokines and atherosclerosis. *Atherosclerosis* 1999;147:213–225.

58. Reape TJ, Rayner K, Manning CD, et al. Expression and cellular localization of the CC chemokines PARC and ELC in human atherosclerotic plaques. *Am J Pathol* 1999;154:365–374.

59. Wong BW, Wong D, McManus BM. Characterization of fractalkine (CX3CL1) and CX3CR1 in human coronary arteries with native atherosclerosis, diabetes mellitus, and transplant vascular disease. *Cardiovasc Pathol* 2002;11:332–338.

60. Greaves DR, Hakkinen T, Lucas AD, et al. Linked chromosome 16q13 chemokines, macrophage-derived chemokine, fractalkine, and thymus- and activation-regulated chemokine, are expressed in human atherosclerotic lesions. *Arterioscler Thromb Vasc Biol* 2001;21: 923–929.

61. Rosenfeld ME, Yla-Herttuala S, Lipton BA, et al. Macrophage colony-stimulating factor mRNA and protein in atherosclerotic lesions of rabbits and humans. *Am J Pathol* 1992;140:291–300.

62. Clinton SK, Underwood R, Hayes L, et al. Macrophage colony-stimulating factor gene expression in vascular cells and in experimental and human atherosclerosis. *Am J Pathol* 1992;140:301–316.

63. Wang J, Wang S, Lu Y, et al. GM-CSF and M-CSF expression is associated with macrophage proliferation in progressing and regressing rabbit atheromatous lesions. *Exp Mol Pathol* 1994;61:109–118.

64. Averill LE, Meagher RC, Gerrity RG. Enhanced monocyte progenitor cell proliferation in bone marrow of hyperlipemic swine. *Am J Pathol* 1989;135:369–377.

65. Ishibashi S, Brown MS, Goldstein JL, et al. Hypercholesterolemia in low density lipoprotein receptor knockout mice and its reversal by adenovirus-mediated gene delivery. *J Clin Invest* 1993;92:883–893.

66. Plump AS, Smith JD, Hayek T, et al. Severe hypercholesterolemia and atherosclerosis in apolipoprotein E-deficient mice created by homologous recombination in ES cells. *Cell* 1992;71:343–353.

67. Zhang SH, Reddick RL, Piedrahita JA, et al. Spontaneous hypercholesterolemia and arterial lesions in mice lacking apolipoprotein E. *Science* 1992;258:468–471.

68. Nakashima Y, Plump AS, Raines EW, et al. ApoE-deficient mice de-

velop lesions of all phases of atherosclerosis throughout the arterial tree. *Arterioscler Thromb* 1994;14:133–140.

69. Reddick RL, Zhang SH, Maeda N. Atherosclerosis in mice lacking apo E. Evaluation of lesional development and progression. *Arterioscler Thromb* 1994;14:141–147.

70. Ishibashi S, Goldstein JL, Brown MS, et al. Massive xanthomatosis and atherosclerosis in cholesterol-fed low density lipoprotein receptor-negative mice. *J Clin Invest* 1994;93:1885–1893.

71. Lichtman AH, Clinton SK, Iiyama K, et al. Hyperlipidemia and atherosclerotic lesion development in LDL receptor-deficient mice fed defined semipurified diets with and without cholate. *Arterioscler Thromb Vasc Biol* 1999;19:1938–1944.

72. Tangirala RK, Rubin EM, Palinski W. Quantitation of atherosclerosis in murine models: correlation between lesions in the aortic origin and in the entire aorta, and differences in the extent of lesions between sexes in LDL receptor-deficient and apolipoprotein E-deficient mice. *J Lipid Res* 1995;36:2320–2328.

73. Bullard DC. Adhesion molecules in inflammatory diseases: insights from knockout mice. *Immunol Res* 2002;26:27–33.

74. Johnson RC, Chapman SM, Dong ZM, et al. Absence of P-selectin delays fatty streak formation in mice. *J Clin Invest* 1997;99:1037–1043.

75. Collins RG, Velji R, Guevara NV, et al. P-Selectin or intercellular adhesion molecule (ICAM)-1 deficiency substantially protects against atherosclerosis in apolipoprotein E-deficient mice. *J Exp Med* 2000;191: 189–194.

76. Dong ZM, Brown AA, Wagner DD. Prominent role of P-selectin in the development of advanced atherosclerosis in ApoE-deficient mice. *Circulation* 2000;101:2290–2295.

77. Burger PC, Wagner DD. Platelet P-selectin facilitates atherosclerotic lesion development. *Blood* 2003;101:2661–2666.

78. Dong ZM, Chapman SM, Brown AA, et al. The combined role of P- and E-selectins in atherosclerosis. *J Clin Invest* 1998;102:145–152.

79. Methia N, Andre P, Denis CV, et al. Localized reduction of atherosclerosis in von Willebrand factor-deficient mice. *Blood* 2001;98:1424–1428.

80. Massberg S, Brand K, Gruner S, et al. A critical role of platelet adhesion in the initiation of atherosclerotic lesion formation. *J Exp Med* 2002;196:887–896.

81. Huo Y, Schober A, Forlow SB, et al. Circulating activated platelets exacerbate atherosclerosis in mice deficient in apolipoprotein E. *Nat Med* 2003;9:61–67.

82. Schober A, Manka D, von Hundelshausen P, et al. Deposition of platelet RANTES triggering monocyte recruitment requires P-selectin and is involved in neointima formation after arterial injury. *Circulation* 2002;106:1523–1529.

83. Gurtner GC, Davis V, Li H, et al. Targeted disruption of the murine VCAM1 gene: essential role of VCAM-1 in chorioallantoic fusion and placentation. *Genes Dev* 1995;9:1–14.

84. Kwee L, Baldwin HS, Shen HM, et al. Defective development of the embryonic and extraembryonic circulatory systems in vascular cell adhesion molecule (VCAM-1) deficient mice. *Development* 1995; 121:489–503.

85. Yang JT, Rayburn H, Hynes RO. Cell adhesion events mediated by alpha 4 integrins are essential in placental and cardiac development. *Development* 1995;121:549–560.

86. Cybulsky MI, Iiyama K, Li H, et al. A major role for VCAM-1, but not ICAM-1, in early atherosclerosis. *J Clin Invest* 2001;107:1255–1262.

87. Dansky HM, Barlow CB, Lominska C, et al. Adhesion of monocytes to arterial endothelium and initiation of atherosclerosis are critically dependent on vascular cell adhesion molecule-1 gene dosage. *Arterioscler Thromb Vasc Biol* 2001;21:1662–1667.

88. Shih PT, Brennan ML, Vora DK, et al. Blocking very late antigen-4 integrin decreases leukocyte entry and fatty streak formation in mice fed an atherogenic diet. *Circ Res* 1999;84:345–351.

89. Huo Y, Hafezi-Moghadam A, Ley K. Role of vascular cell adhesion molecule-1 and fibronectin connecting segment-1 in monocyte rolling and adhesion on early atherosclerotic lesions. *Circ Res* 2000;87: 153–159.

90. Kubo N, Boisvert WA, Ballantyne CM, et al. Leukocyte CD11b expression is not essential for the development of atherosclerosis in mice. *J Lipid Res* 2000;41:1060–1066.

91. Gerrity RG. The role of the monocyte in atherogenesis: I. Transition of blood-borne monocytes into foam cells in fatty lesions. *Am J Pathol* 1981;103:181–190.

92. Faggiotto A, Ross R, Harker L. Studies of hypercholesterolemia in the nonhuman primate. I. Changes that lead to fatty streak formation. *Arteriosclerosis* 1984;4:323–340.

93. Lessner SM, Prado HL, Waller EK, et al. Atherosclerotic lesions grow through recruitment and proliferation of circulating monocytes in a murine model. *Am J Pathol* 2002;160:2145–2155.

94. Nelken NA, Coughlin SR, Gordon D, et al. Monocyte chemoattractant protein-1 in human atheromatous plaques. *J Clin Invest* 1991;88: 1121–1127.

95. Yu X, Dluz S, Graves DT, et al. Elevated expression of monocyte chemoattractant protein 1 by vascular smooth muscle cells in hypercholesterolemic primates. *Proc Natl Acad Sci USA* 1992;89:6953–6957.

96. Steinberg D, Lewis A. Conner Memorial Lecture. Oxidative modification of LDL and atherogenesis. *Circulation* 1997;95:1062–1071.

97. Cushing SD, Berliner JA, Valente AJ, et al. Minimally modified low density lipoprotein induces monocyte chemotactic protein 1 in human endothelial cells and smooth muscle cells. *Proc Natl Acad Sci USA* 1990;87:5134–5138.

98. Aiello RJ, Bourassa PA, Lindsey S, et al. Monocyte chemoattractant protein-1 accelerates atherosclerosis in apolipoprotein E-deficient mice. *Arterioscler Thromb Vasc Biol* 1999;19:1518–1525.

99. Gosling J, Slaymaker S, Gu L, et al. MCP-1 deficiency reduces susceptibility to atherosclerosis in mice that overexpress human apolipoprotein B. *J Clin Invest* 1999;103:773–778.

100. Gu L, Okada Y, Clinton SK, et al. Absence of monocyte chemoattractant protein-1 reduces atherosclerosis in low density lipoprotein receptor-deficient mice. *Mol Cell* 1998;2:275–281.

101. Gosling J, Slaymaker S, Gu L, et al. MCP-1 deficiency reduces susceptibility to atherosclerosis in mice that overexpress human apolipoprotein B. *J Clin Invest* 1999;103:773–778.

102. Boring L, Gosling J, Cleary M, et al. Decreased lesion formation in CCR2-/- mice reveals a role for chemokines in the initiation of atherosclerosis. *Nature* 1998;394:894–897.

103. Dawson TC, Kuziel WA, Osahar TA, et al. Absence of CC chemokine receptor-2 reduces atherosclerosis in apolipoprotein E-deficient mice. *Atherosclerosis* 1999;143:205–211.

104. Egashira K, Koyanagi M, Kitamoto S, et al. Anti-monocyte chemoattractant protein-1 gene therapy inhibits vascular remodeling in rats: blockade of MCP-1 activity after intramuscular transfer of a mutant gene inhibits vascular remodeling induced by chronic blockade of NO synthesis. *FASEB J* 2000;14:1974–1978.

105. Han KH, Tangirala RK, Green SR, et al. Chemokine receptor CCR2 expression and monocyte chemoattractant protein-1–mediated chemotaxis in human monocytes. A regulatory role for plasma LDL. *Arterioscler Thromb Vasc Biol* 1998;18:1983–1991.

106. Han KH, Han KO, Green SR, et al. Expression of the monocyte chemoattractant protein-1 receptor CCR2 is increased in hypercholesterolemia. Differential effects of plasma lipoproteins on monocyte function. *J Lipid Res* 1999;40:1053–1063.

107. Han KH, Chang MK, Boullier A, et al. Oxidized LDL reduces monocyte CCR2 expression through pathways involving peroxisome proliferator–activated receptor γ. *J Clin Invest* 2000;106:793–802.

108. Li AC, Brown KK, Silvestre MJ, et al. Peroxisome proliferator–activated receptor γ ligands inhibit development of atherosclerosis in LDL receptor–deficient mice. *J Clin Invest* 2000;106:523–531.

109. Szalai C, Duba J, Prohászka Z, et al. Involvement of polymorphisms in the chemokine system in the susceptibility for coronary artery disease (CAD). Coincidence of elevated Lp(a) and MCP-1 −2518 G/G genotype in CAD patients. *Atherosclerosis* 2001;158:233–239.

110. Boisvert WA, Santiago R, Curtiss LK, et al. A leukocyte homologue of the IL-8 receptor CXCR-2 mediates the accumulation of macrophages in atherosclerotic lesions of LDL receptor- deficient mice. *J Clin Invest* 1998;101:353–363.

111. Gersten RE, Garcia-Zepeda EA, Lim Y-C, et al. MCP-1 and IL-8 trigger firm adhesion of monocytes to vascular endothelium under flow conditions. *Nature* 1999;398:718–723.

112. Bazan JF, Bacon KB, Hardiman G, et al. A new class of membrane-bound chemokine with a CX₃C motif. *Nature* 1997;385:640–644.

113. Fong AM, Robinson LA, Steeber DA, et al. Fractalkine and CX₃CR1 mediate a novel mechanism of leukocyte capture, firm adhesion, and activation under physiologic flow. *J Exp Med* 1998;188:1413–1419.

114. Haskell CA, Cleary MD, Charo IF. Molecular uncoupling of

fractalkine-mediated cell adhesion and signal transduction. Rapid flow arrest of CX$_3$CR1-expressing cells is independent of G-protein activation. *J Biol Chem* 1999;274:10053–10058.

115. Moatti D, Faure S, Fumeron F, et al. Polymorphism in the fractalkine receptor CX3CR1 as a genetic risk factor for coronary artery disease. *Blood* 2001;97:1925–1928.

116. McDermott DH, Fong AM, Yang Q, et al. Chemokine receptor mutant CX3CR1-M280 has impaired adhesive function and correlates with protection from cardiovascular disease in humans. *J Clin Invest* 2003;111:1241–1250.

117. Lesnik P, Haskell CA, Charo IF. Decreased atherosclerosis in CX3CR1-/- mice reveals a role for fractalkine in atherogenesis. *J Clin Invest* 2003;111:333–340.

118. Combadiere C, Potteaux S, Gao JL, et al. Decreased atherosclerotic lesion formation in CX3CR1/apolipoprotein E double knockout mice. *Circulation* 2003;107:1009–1016.

119. Huo Y, Weber C, Forlow SB, et al. The chemokine KC, but not monocyte chemoattractant protein-1, triggers monocyte arrest on early atherosclerotic endothelium. *J Clin Invest* 2001;108:1307–1314.

CHAPTER 35

The Role of Macrophages

Elaine W. Raines, Peter Libby, and Michael E. Rosenfeld

Key Words: Atherothrombosis; lipid; macrophage; monocyte; phagocyte.

INTRODUCTION

A common feature of lesions of atherothrombosis at all stages of development is the presence of monocytes/macrophages (1). In addition to their ability to accumulate large amounts of lipid, some of the specific products of these cells while they are resident in the artery wall are beginning to be understood. However, it is less clear how the multiple capabilities of these pluripotent cells are balanced within lesions. Lesion macrophages express a number of mediators that may stimulate lesion progression, whereas their ability to take up foreign material is part of the innate protective response that may, particularly early in lesion development, prevent lesion expansion. However, with chronic inflammation and continued monocyte influx, a failure of that protective response may contribute to lesion progression and, ulti-mately, to the clinical sequelae associated with coronary heart disease.

This chapter summarizes current knowledge of some of the general properties of the monocyte/macrophage with a particular focus on the properties of macrophages in developing lesions of atherothrombosis. We discuss how these and other capabilities of the monocyte/macrophage may affect cells in the artery wall and alter lesion development and progression.

THE MONOCYTE/MACROPHAGE: GENERAL PROPERTIES OF A MULTIPOTENT EFFECTOR CELL

Mononuclear phagocytes are an important part of normal host defenses, principally through their capacity as scavenger cells, as antigen-presenting cells, and as secretory cells. The presence of numerous macrophages together with variable numbers of lymphocytes constitutes a hallmark of any chronic inflammatory response (1). In most inflammatory situations, the macrophage contributes to the resolution by scavenging debris from interstitial tissues and then migrating from the site of injury, thereby removing tissue debris (Fig. 35–1). However, animal studies have shown that reducing macrophage numbers or monocyte recruitment can markedly decrease lesion development, suggesting that macrophages contribute to atherogenesis (2–5).

E. W. Raines: Department of Pathology, University of Washington, Harborview Medical Center, Box 359675, 325 9th Avenue, Seattle, Washington 98104.
P. Libby: Brigham and Women's Hospital, Harvard Medical School, Eugene Braunwald Research Center 307, 221 Longwood Avenue, Boston, Massachusetts 02115.
M. E. Rosenfeld: Department of Pathobiology, University of Washington, Box 353410, 324D Raitt Hall, Seattle, Washington 98195.

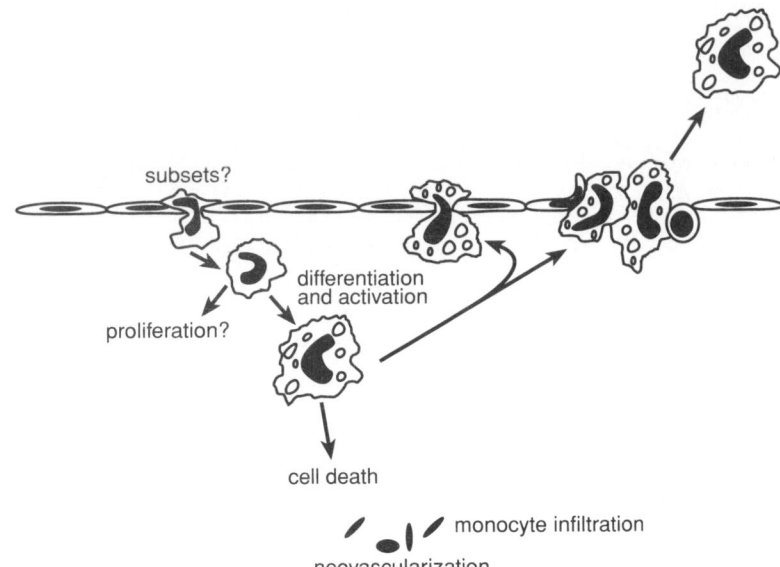

FIG. 35–1. Monocyte/macrophage influx and turnover in lesions of atherothrombosis. Monocytes adhere to the endothelium at lesion-prone sites (Fig. 35–2), crawl between the endothelial cells, and localize within the forming intima. Many of these monocytes/macrophages display proliferating cell nuclear antigen, consistent with cell replication. Uptake of lipid with subsequent "foam cell" formation is observed at all stages of lesion development. This uptake may depend on monocyte differentiation and may be involved in monocyte/macrophage activation. Lipid-filled macrophages can be observed squeezing between endothelial cells in an apparent exit from the intima (Fig. 35–3). These foam cells are also seen in areas of endothelial cell denudation and may contribute to endothelial cell dysfunction associated with endothelial cell loss and thrombosis. Macrophages in the core of the lesion die, but they leave cellular antigens that can be detected (Fig. 35–6). Within more advanced lesions, areas of neovascularization serve as an additional avenue for monocyte infiltration.

Monocytes and recently immigrated macrophages are not fully mature cells and can develop further functional competence, as well as undergo further divisions, after they have entered the tissue (6). The transformation into tissue macrophages depends on both developmental and tissue-specific stimuli. In the bone marrow, for example, the presence of colony-stimulating factors (CSFs) such as granulocyte-monocyte colony-stimulating factor (GM-CSF) and monocyte colony-stimulating factor (M-CSF) help determine different macrophage phenotypes after migration of the committed bone marrow progenitors (monocytes) into specific tissues (7). Furthermore, tissue macrophages exhibit extensive functional and antigenic variations that may reflect stages of differentiation or activation of the macrophages (8), or both, in response to tissue-specific stimuli. These variations exist both among different tissues and in different areas of the same tissue (9).

Circulating monocytes spontaneously undergo programmed cell death (apoptosis) in the absence of M-CSF or other survival factors (10). As circulating monocytes differentiate into mature macrophages, this requirement is lost and tissue macrophages can even resist apoptotic stimuli (11). However, differentiated macrophages retain a novel pathway that initiates apoptosis after activation with specific stimuli, such as zymosan (12). Sensitivity to activation-induced apoptosis appears to be determined in part by previous exposure to particular cytokines. M-CSF exposure prevents apoptosis, whereas even transient exposure to the proinflammatory cytokine interferon-γ (IFN-γ) increases this apoptotic pathway (13).

The process of monocyte/macrophage activation is also complex, as the effect of the activating signals depends on the state of differentiation of the cell and on the other signals it has met (8,14). Among leukocytes, the monocyte/macrophage secretes the most diverse selection of substances in response to stimuli, and these substances have myriad effects on surrounding tissues and adjacent cells (15). Table 35–1 lists the different categories of molecules secreted by macrophages, many with potential relevance to the process of atherogenesis. Macrophages taken from sites of active inflammation have greatly increased properties for endocytosis, digestion, and secretion of a number of proteins, including a factor increasing monocytopoiesis (16). Interestingly, terminally differentiated macrophages containing endocytosed material appear to be the most inhibited in terms of phagocytic and adherent functions (17). In contrast, when macrophages enter their terminal stage of maturation, evidence exists for a 20- to 30-fold increase in their production of reactive oxygen species in response to zymosan and for down-regulation of c-*fms,* the M-CSF receptor (18). All of these elements may limit the extent of an inflammatory response.

TABLE 35–1. *Multipotent molecules secreted by monocytes/macrophages*

Cyclic nucleotides
Cytokines and immune-modulating factors
Cytotoxic substances
Enzymes and enzyme inhibitors involved in:
   Coagulation
   Hydrolysis of connective tissue
   Lipoprotein metabolism
Extracellular matrix proteins
Factors regulating vascular tone
Prostaglandins and leukotrienes
Reactive oxygen intermediates
Regulators of lipoprotein metabolism
Substances regulating the migration and growth of other
   cells

PROPERTIES OF THE MONOCYTE/ MACROPHAGE IN DEVELOPING LESIONS OF ATHEROTHROMBOSIS

Early Attraction and Retention in Lesion-prone Areas

Monocyte adherence to the endothelium in nonrandom clusters at lesion-prone sites (19,20) occurs early in atherogenesis in animal models that mimic the cellular changes observed in human disease (Fig. 35–2). As described by Cybulsky and Charo (see Chapter 34), this process depends on regulated expression of specific adherence molecules on endothelial cells, especially vascular cell adhesion molecule-1 (VCAM-1), specific for monocytes and lymphocytes. Expression of VCAM-1 on the surface of the endothelial cells of hypercholesterolemic rabbits precedes detectable intimal monocyte/macrophage accumulation by approximately 1 week (21), and aortic endothelial cells in normocholesterolemic rabbits do not express VCAM-1 except at lesion-prone sites that presumably reflect flow-induced expression (22). Studies of mouse models of atherothrombosis have established a critical role of VCAM-1 in monocyte accumulation. Reduction of VCAM-1 protein levels to 2% to 8% of the wild-type allele levels by mutation of the extracellular domain of VCAM-1 resulted in a 40% reduction in the total lesion area in early-stage lesions (23).

Although the regulation of endothelial cell adhesion molecules appears to be at the level of quantitative differences in expression, qualitative changes in adhesion receptor avidity stimulated by chemokines appear to be the major determinant of monocyte adhesion (24). Integrin receptors on circulating monocytes are normally in an inactive or low-avidity state. Chemokine signaling through G protein–coupled receptors triggers leukocyte arrest through β_2 and α_4 integrin binding to intercellular adhesion moelcule-1 (ICAM-1) and VCAM-1, respectively (24). The transient nature of avidity changes provides a potential mechanism for rapid deadhesion during cell migration.

Although adhesion molecule expression appears essential for the accumulation of monocytes at particular sites in the artery wall, many lines of evidence indicate that a key event in early attraction of monocytes to these sites is the subendothelial retention of cholesterol-rich, atherogenic lipoproteins. Before subendothelial accumulation of monocytes occurs, hypercholesterolemia induces enhanced transport of plasma lipoproteins across the endothelial layer followed by intimal accumulation of modified and reassembled lipoproteins (25). Substantial evidence has been obtained for interactions between lipoproteins and proteoglycans, and for

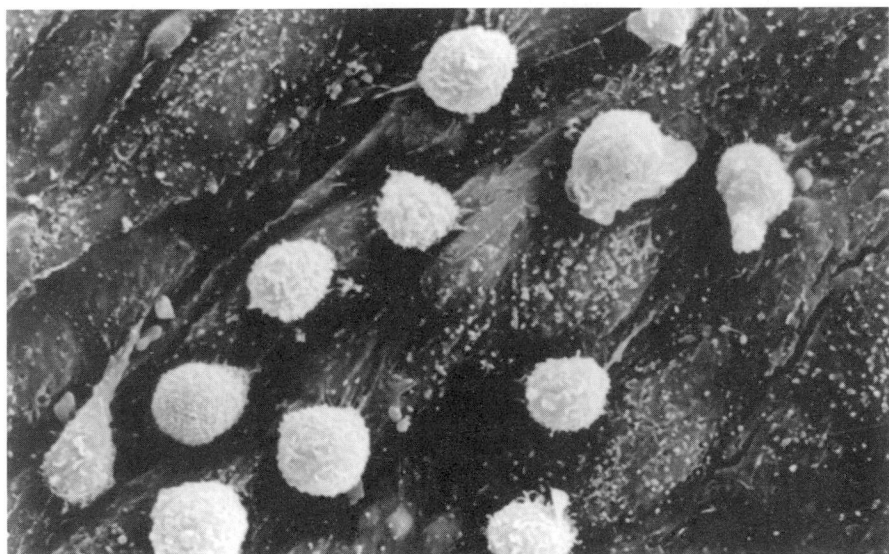

FIG. 35–2. Monocyte adherence to lesion-prone sites is among the earliest changes seen in developing lesions and persists throughout development of lesions of atherothrombosis. This scanning electron micrograph shows adherent leukocytes attached to the intact endothelium in the thoracic aorta of a hypercholesterolemic nonhuman primate.

proteoglycans mediating the retention of the modified lipoproteins (26,27). In a mouse model of atherothrombosis, mutation of the proteoglycan binding site in atherogenic apolipoprotein B-100 resulted in an approximately 60% reduction in total aortic lesion area at early stages of lesion development (28). Retained lipoproteins can stimulate local synthesis of proteoglycans and, directly and indirectly, accelerate further retention and aggregation of lipoproteins and monocyte accumulation (26,29).

After adherence of monocytes to the endothelium, they spread on the endothelium, crawl between the endothelial cells, and localize in the intima where they become foam cells (19,20). These data from animal models of atherothrombosis suggest that the monocytes squeeze between the endothelial cells and migrate into the intima in response to a gradient of chemoattractants situated within the subendothelial space. Expression and production of monocyte-specific chemoattractants monocyte chemotactic protein-1 (MCP-1) (30), tumor necrosis factor-α (TNF-α) (31), interleukin-1 (IL-1) (32), and M-CSF (33) appear to be increased in atherothrombotic lesions of both humans and experimental animals. However, on the basis of immunocytochemistry and *in situ* hybridization results at the light microscopic level, it appears that the expression of these factors by smooth muscle cells and monocytes/macrophages already resident within developing lesions may be the primary source of chemoattractants within developing lesions. In mouse models of atherothrombosis, targeted deletion of the leukocyte chemoattractant MCP-1 or its receptor CC chemokine receptor 2 (CCR2) significantly delays lesion formation (2–4).

Although morphologic studies suggest that macrophages filled with lipid can push their way out between endothelial cells (Fig. 35–3) and egress back into the circulation with their ingested material (34), many monocytes/macrophages appear to remain in the lesions until they die. Macrophages express a variety of integrins that interact with several different matrix proteins and may prevent egress and movement within the plaque. For example, the β$_2$ integrin (very late-activation antigen-4) expressed by monocytes not only interacts with VCAM-1 but also with the matrix protein fibronectin (35). *In vitro,* the chemoattractants MCP-1, macrophage inhibitory protein-1α (MIP-1α), and RANTES (regulated on activation, normal T expressed and secreted) increase expression of the β$_2$ integrins (36), which could enhance both endothelial cell binding and retention of the macrophages within the lesion. Freezing the integrins in the activated state, as has been observed with α$_5$β$_1$ integrin in the human monocyte cell line THP-1 after differentiation (37), also could prevent cell migration out of the lesion. Smooth muscle cell expression of VCAM-1 and ICAM-1 in atherothrombotic, but not normal vessels (21,38), may further contribute to monocyte/macrophage retention. Interestingly, scavenger receptors abundant in macrophages in lesions of atherothrombosis can serve as adhesion receptors in addition to taking up modified lipoproteins (39).

States of Differentiation and Activation

Are All Stages of Macrophage Differentiation Observed in Lesions?

The activation state of monocytes/macrophages within a developing lesion likely depends on both the differentiation state of the cell and the local environment, as suggested by

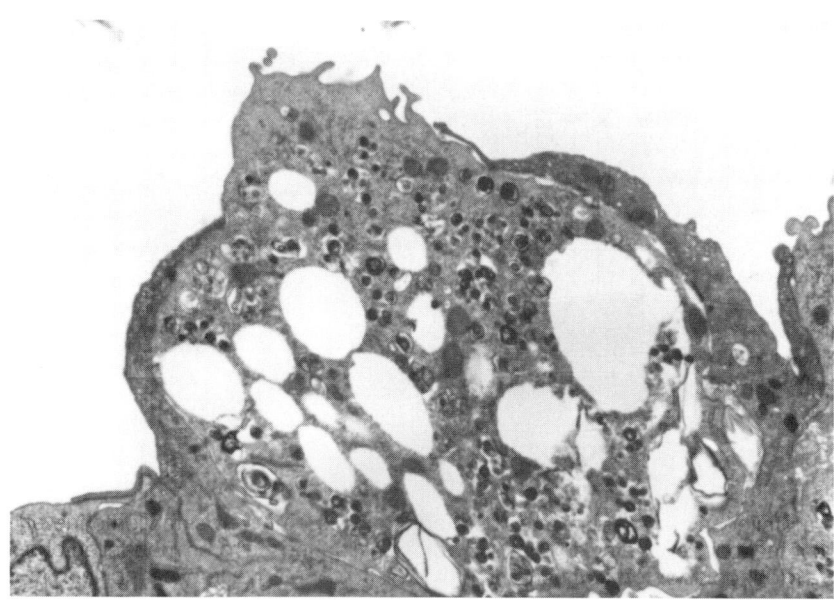

FIG. 35–3. A lipid-filled foam cell protruding between two endothelial cells. This transmission electron micrograph demonstrates a lipid-filled macrophage that is exposed to the lumen in a transitional lesion from the thoracic aorta of a 9-month-old homozygous Watanabe heritable hyperlipidemic (WHHL) rabbit. Original magnification ×40,000.

an immunohistochemical study of human aorta and coronary and carotid arteries that evaluated the differentiation state of monocytes in diffuse intimal thickening, fatty streaks, and atheromatous plaques (40). Cells that stained for major histocompatibility complex Class II antigens and CD14 were abundant in diffuse intimal thickening and also localized in subendothelial layers in fatty streaks and more advanced plaques. Many of these cells closely apposed T cells that also stained for major histocompatibility complex Class II antigens. CD1 molecules, a family of cell surface proteins that present lipid antigens to T cells, are observed in foam cell lesions, but not in normal vessels, and colocalize in areas of the arterial wall that also contain abundant T lymphocytes (41). Plaques may also contain specialized antigen-presenting cells, or dendritic cells (42). These observations suggest that macrophages serve as antigen-presenting cells in local immune response (see Chapter 36).

Most monocytic phagocytes in fatty streaks and the outer layers of more advanced lesions stain for the complement C3bi receptor (OKM1) together with acid phosphatase and lipid (oil red O) (40). In the case of more advanced lesions, large monocytic cells filled with lipid and acid phosphatase bear the thrombospondin receptor but express little of the C3bi receptor (40). These observations indicate a gradual shift toward a more differentiated phenotype as residence time within the lesion increases. Binding by cells in fatty streaks of antibodies more specific to circulating monocytes that do not recognize tissue macrophages or foam cells in lesions also supports this interpretation (43). The presence of macrophage differentiation-stimulating cytokine, GM-CSF, in plaque tissues has been suggested to provide a microenvironment that promotes monocyte macrophage survival and differentiation (44). Several proteins overexpressed in atherothrombosis may have considerable functional significance within developing lesions (Table 35–2), including scavenger receptors, the low-density lipoprotein receptor–related protein (LRP), and extracellular matrix metalloproteinase inducer (EMMPRIN), which are also increased during monocyte/macrophage differentiation and foam cell formation *in vitro* (45–47).

What is the State of Activation of Circulating Cells and Cells within Developing Lesions?

Given the long list of products expressed by the monocyte/macrophage (Table 35–1), what do we know about their secretory activity in developing lesions of atherothrombosis (Table 35–2)? Selective activation may depend on the stage of lesion development. For example, platelet-derived growth factor (PDGF)-B chain localizes to only a subset of the macrophages in advanced human lesions (Fig. 35–4) (48). In contrast, PDGF-B chain staining is observed in macrophages throughout an early-stage fatty streak from a hypercholesterolemic nonhuman primate (Fig. 35–4). Similarly, not all macrophages in the lesions are simultaneously induced to express 15-lipoxygenase (15-LO) (49), MCP-1

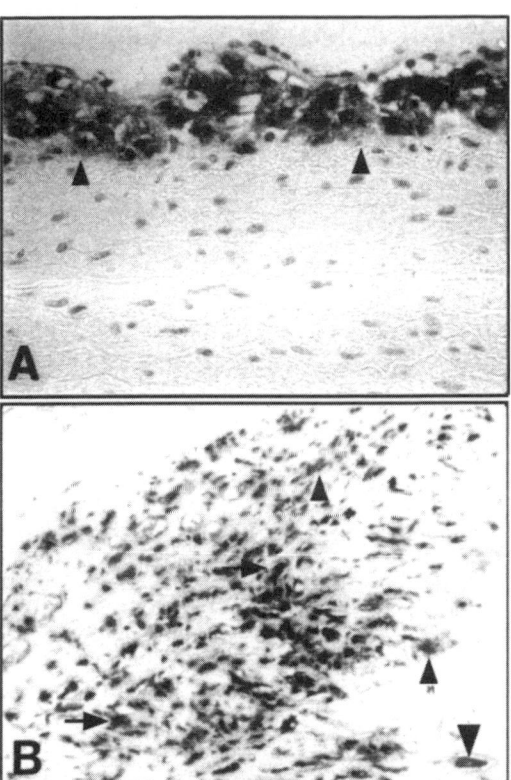

FIG. 35–4. Varying numbers of monocyte/macrophages contain platelet-derived growth factor (PDGF)-B chain in lesions of atherothrombosis. Both the fatty streak from a nonhuman primate with hypercholesterolemia **(A)** and the advanced human lesion **(B)** contain cells that stain with an antibody specific for the B-chain of PDGF. **A:** The anti-PDGF antibody stained almost all of the intimal macrophages *(gray)*, whereas only a subset of the macrophages *(gray, arrowheads)* in **B** stained with the anti-PDGF antibody *(black, arrows)*. **A:** *Arrowheads* indicate the location of the internal elastic lamina.

(30), tissue factor (50,51), and M-CSF (33). These and other studies indicate heterogeneity of monocytes in developing lesions.

Under some circumstances, activation of circulating monocytes may occur before entry into the lesions. Monocytes from homozygous familial hypercholesterolemic patients show abnormalities in eicosanoid metabolism (consequently, in the formation of leukotrienes), decreased superoxide anion generation, and increased adhesion (52). Examination of 26 patients with unstable angina demonstrated increased tissue factor expression in isolated monocytes, with and without stimulation, and increased plasma levels of fibrinogen (53). However, the increase in tissue factor expression does not appear to be related to hypercholesterolemia (53). Monocytes from patients with acute myocardial infarction show increased levels of urokinase receptor and activation of β_2 integrins lymphocyte function-associated antigen-1 (LFA-1) and macrophage antigen-1 (54). Patients with ischemic heart disease also have increased secretion of TNF-α in isolated monocytes (55). The

TABLE 35–2. *Molecules expressed by monocytes/macrophages in atherothrombosis*

Molecule	Possible role	Reference
Secreted proteins		
Cytokines and immune-modulating factors		
CD40 Ligand	Proinflammatory stimulation	145
Fractalkine	Leukocyte chemoattractant	150
IL-1	Increase adhesion molecule expression, SMC migration and proliferation, immune modulation, secondary gene induction	32
IL-6	Activation of coagulation, SMC secondary gene induction	151
IL-8	Recruitment of lymphocytes and endothelial cells	152
IL-10	Antiinflammatory cytokine	153
IL-12	T-cell growth factor and induces Th1 cytokines	153
IL-15	Proinflammatory cytokine that is growth factor and chemoattractant for T cells	154
IL-18	Inducer of interferon-γ and promotes Th1 response	155
Leukemia inhibitory factor	Differentiation and proliferation of T cells	156
Macrophage inhibitory protein-1α and 1β	Monocyte chemoattractant	157
Monocyte chemoattractant protein-1	Monocyte chemoattractant, activation of α_2 integrins	30
Monocyte colony-stimulating factor	Monocyte chemoattraction, proliferation, and survival	33
RANTES	Monocyte chemoattractant	157
TNF-α	Increase endothelial cell adhesion molecule expression, monocyte chemoattractant and activator, SMC proliferation	31
Enzymes and inhibitors		
Cathepsin K and S	Matrix degradation, regulation of immune function	158
Collagenases (MMP-1,-8,-13)	Matrix degradation, cell migration, possible plaque rupture, and plaque expansion	141, 159, 160
Complement C3b	Prothrombotic and promoter of lipoprotein uptake	161
EMMPRIN	Induction of MMPs	47
Factor XIIIa	Prothrombotic	162
Gelatinase (MMP-2,-9)	Matrix degradation, cell migration, possible plaque rupture and expansion	141
Lipoprotein lipase	Alteration of lipoprotein metabolism and hydrolysis of core triglycerides of lipoproteins	163, 164
5-lipoxygenase	Promote leukotriene production and inflammatory response	165
15-Lipoxygenase	LDL oxidation and foam cell formation	49, 165
Lipoprotein-associated PLA(2)	Enzyme capable of hydrolyzing PAF and phospholipids	166
Matrilysin (MMP-7)	Matrix degradation, cell migration, possible plaque rupture and expansion	167
Membrane type MMP-1,-3	MMP activation	168, 169
Myeloperoxidase	Formation of cytotoxins and reactive oxygen intermediates that oxidize lipoproteins	126
Plasminogen activator-1	Mediates plasmin generation involved in fibrinolysis and MMP activation	147
Plasminogen-activator inhibitor (PAI-1)	Antifibrinolytic	148
Stromelysin (MMP-3)	Connective tissue degradation, cell migration, and possible plaque rupture and expansion	140, 141
TIMP-1,-2,-3	Prevention of matrix degradation by blocking proteolytic processing of zymogens or blocking substrate binding and contributions to complex formation and activation	141, 170
Urokinase	Mediates plasmin generation involved in fibrinolysis and MMP activation	147
Extracellular proteins		
Collagen type VIII	Areas of tissue remodeling	171
Matrix Gla protein	Cell adhesion, regulation of calcification	172
Osteopontin	Cell adhesion and migration, neovessel formation, and calcification	173
SPARC, osteonectin	Cell migration, proliferation, and neovessel formation	174
Thrombospondin	Cell migration, neovessel formation	175

TABLE 35–2. *Continued*

Molecule	Possible role	Reference
Regulators of lipoprotein metabolism		
Apolipoprotein E	Modulation of lipoprotein uptake	176
27-Hydroxycholesterol	Side-chain degradation in the formation of bile acids from cholesterol	177
Serum amyloid A	Acute phase reactant associated with high-density lipoprotein alteration of lipoprotein metabolism, immune response and platelet function, monocyte chemoattractant	178
Substances regulating the migration and growth of other cells		
Acidic fibroblast growth factor	Endothelial cell chemoattractant and mitogen	179
Basic fibroblast growth factor	SMC chemoattractant and mitogen	180
Activin A	Promotes differentiation of SMCs	181
Betacellulin	SMC proliferation	182
Endothelin-1	Vasoconstriction	183
Fas ligand	Monocyte apoptosis and macrophage activation	184
Heparin-binding epidermal growth factor	SMC chemoattraction and proliferation	185
Insulin-like growth factor I	SMC chemoattraction and survival	186
Platelet-derived growth factor	SMC chemoattraction and proliferation	48
Transforming growth factor-β_1 and β_3	Promote or inhibit SMC proliferation depending on concentration	187
Cell-associated proteins		
Adhesion molecules		
Very late-activation antigen-4	Monocyte counter-receptor for VCAM-1	188
VCAM-1	Monocyte/macrophage activation and retention	134
ICAM-1	Monocyte/macrophage activation and retention	134
Connexin 37	Gap junctional communication	189
Connexin 43	Gap junctional communication	190
SIGN	C-type lectin that mediates adhesion to T lymphocytes and endocytosis	42
Receptors		
Adenosine triphosphate (ATP)–binding cassette transporter A1 (ABCA1)	Reverse cholesterol transport	191
For advanced glycation end products	Monocyte activation and induction of oxidant stress	192
CC Chemokine-3	Monocyte chemoattraction	193
For complement C3bi	Thrombosis and lipoprotein uptake	161
CXCR2	IL-8 receptor	194
FGF receptors	SMC and endothelial cell migration and proliferation	[195]
α_2-Macroglobulin/LDL receptor-related clearance including–PAI complexes	Foam cell formation, uptake of cytokine α_2-M complexes, protease protein (LDL receptor-related protein)	[106]
For modified LDL (scavenger receptor)	Foam cell formation, monocyte recruitment and adhesion	91–94
For thrombin	Monocyte/macrophage activation	196
Toll-like receptors 1, 2, 4	Regulators of innate immunity	128
TNFRSF14	Receptor for TNF superfamily 14 (LIGHT) that induces MMPs	197
TGF-βII	SMC growth inhibition	187
For urokinase	Pericellular proteolysis facilitate migration	198
Other cell-associated proteins		
60-kD heat shock protein	Cytoprotective to stress and lethal stimuli and inducers of immune response	199
70-kD heat shock protein	Cytoprotective to stress and lethal stimuli	200
Tissue factor	Coagulation and thrombosis	51

EMMPRIN, extracellular matrix metalloproteinase inducer; ICAM-1, intercellular adhesion molecular-1; IL, interleukin; LDL, low-density lipoprotein; MMP, matrix metalloproteinase; PAF, platelet activating factor; PLA, phospholipase A; RANTES, regulated on activation, normal T expressed and secreted; SMC, smooth muscle cell; TGF, transforming growth factor; TIMP, tissue inhibitor of metalloproteinase; TNF, tumor necrosis factor; VCAM-1, vascular cell adhesion molecule-1.

adhesion process itself may suffice to induce activation and the expression of particular monocyte products. Blocking ICAM-1–mediated interaction with endothelial cells can inhibit production of the mononuclear chemoattractant protein, MIP-1α (56). Both TNF-α and IL-1 release from monocytes *in vitro* can also be induced *in vitro* by engagement of monocyte proteoglycans (LFA-3, CD44, and CD45) known to be involved in cell–cell adhesion (57).

Evidence for the Presence of Macrophage-activating Agents in Atherothrombotic Lesion

The presence of T cells and expression of major histocompatibility Class II antigens indicate an ongoing immune response to foreign antigens in developing lesions (see Chapter 36). The high prevalence and early onset of cardiovascular disease in patients with diabetes mellitus have focused attention on the potential role of advanced glycosylation end products (AGEs) that accumulate on long-lived extracellular matrix proteins in individuals with diabetes (58). *In vitro* studies suggest that AGEs within the vascular wall can trap lipoproteins (59), modify lipoproteins (60), inactivate nitric oxide activity (61), and interact with specific cell surface receptors to induce cytokine and growth factor release from monocytes (62). AGEs accumulate in lesions in coronary vessels of patients with type II diabetes, but not in lesions from individuals without diabetes (63). As detailed later in this chapter and elsewhere in this textbook, there is also evidence for viral (cytomegalovirus, herpes simplex, and Epstein-Barr) and infectious (*Chlamydia pneumoniae* and *Helicobacter pylori*) antigens and nucleic acid in atherothrombotic lesions (64). For *C. pneumoniae,* one of the most extensively investigated infectious agents, the current body of evidence establishes it as a plausible and potentially modifiable risk factor in cardiovascular disease (65). However, currently, no rigorous clinical trial evidence indicates a role for antibiotics in secondary prevention of myocardial infarction. Thus, a number of examples exist for the presence of potential monocyte-activating agents such as AGEs and viral antigens in atherothrombotic lesions.

Macrophage Proliferation

As in other inflammatory responses, monocytes/macrophages in lesions of atherothrombosis can proliferate. Early morphologic studies by McMillan and Duff (66) demonstrated the presence of mitotic spindles in foam cells within rabbit lesions. Up to 40% of the cells that take up thymidine in atherothrombotic lesions of rabbits are monocytes/macrophages (67). Studies with antibodies to proliferating cell nuclear antigen have provided evidence for proliferating monocytes/macrophages in human coronary and carotid atherothrombotic lesions (68).

It is still unclear what stimulates DNA synthesis in macrophages within atherothrombotic lesions, and whether the proliferating cells are monocytes or promonocytes. Many proliferating monocytes/macrophages are foam cells

suggesting at least partial differentiation. Several cell types within lesions including macrophages within both human and animal lesions express hematopoietic growth factors M-CSF and GM-CSF (33,69,70). Mice lacking M-CSF have few macrophages and resist the development of atherothrombosis despite an increase in circulating cholesterol levels (5,71,72). Similarly, blockade of the M-CSF receptor (c-*fms*) inhibits development of early lesions in apolipoprotein E (apoE)–deficient mice (73).

Macrophages and Lipid Accumulation

Presence of "Foam Cells" in Atherothrombotic Lesions

Macrophages in most tissues function as "scavenger" cells—that is, they phagocytose necrotic cell debris and sometimes appear to engulf whole cells (Fig. 35–5). Early morphologic studies of human lesions demonstrated the presence of phagocytic cells containing large numbers of vacuoles and nonmembrane-bound lipid droplets in both human and experimental atherothrombotic lesions (74). The presence of a large number of lipid droplets gives the cells a "foamy" appearance by light and electron microscopy. Thus, the cells are generally referred to as "foam cells." Immunocytochemical analyses identify many of these foam cells as monocytes/macrophages (75) and show that macrophage-derived foam cells populate atherothrombotic plaques at all stages of lesion development (76). Biochemical studies of atherothrombotic tissue have demonstrated that lipids deposited in the artery wall during the atherogenic process are predominantly cholesteryl esters derived from the direct deposition of lipoproteins in the artery wall (77,78). In particular, studies using ^{125}I-tyramine-cellobiose–labeled low-density lipoprotein (LDL) (a nondegradable LDL probe) demonstrate preferential trapping and retention of lipoproteins before the appearance of monocytes in arteries of cholesterol-fed animals (79). Once the monocytes have entered the intima, they appear to rapidly become foam cells (80).

Mechanisms of Lipid Accumulation in Macrophages

The quest for pathways that enable macrophages to accumulate large amounts of lipoprotein-derived cholesteryl esters led to the discovery that rapid lipid loading depended on lipoprotein modification and the expression of specific receptors on the macrophage surface that bind and internalize the modified lipoproteins (81–85). Murine peritoneal macrophages showed that these cells take up nonmodified LDL at slow rates that do not lead to foam cell formation. However, LDL particles modified by being made more cationic or by acetylation undergo rapid uptake and form intracellular lipid droplets. The process is saturable and mediated by a receptor termed the *acetyl-LDL* receptor, or the *scavenger* receptor (86,87). A variety of different types of lipoprotein modifications facilitate foam cell formation *in vitro,* including acetylation, oxidation, aggregation, immune or matrix

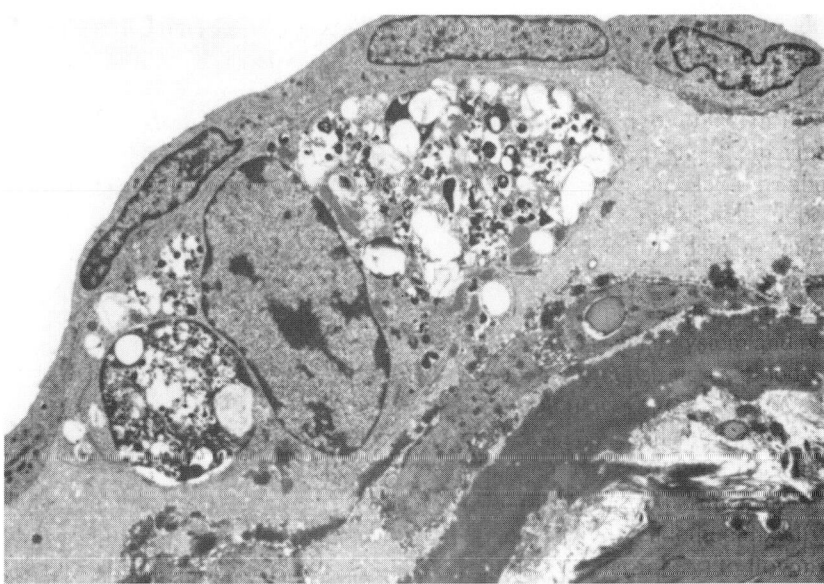

FIG. 35–5. The monocyte/macrophage is a phagocytic effector cell. This transmission electron micrograph shows a lipid-filled macrophage that appears to have engulfed another cell in an early atherothrombotic lesion from the thoracic aorta of a 6-week-old homozygous Watanabe heritable hyperlipidemic (WHHL) rabbit. Original magnification ×24,000.

protein complex formation, and glycation (88). Immunocytochemical studies suggest that oxidized and glycated lipoproteins and lipoprotein–antibody complexes exist in atherothrombotic lesions (63,89,90).

Human atherothrombotic lesions contain at least three families of broad specificity macrophage scavenger receptors that are expressed within. These include the type A family (subtypes I–III and the macrophage receptor with collagenous structure, or MARCO); type B receptors that include CD36, scavenger receptor B-I (SR-BI)/CD36 and LIMPII analog 1 (CLA-1) and the splice variant SR-BII, and an additional group of receptors such as the mucin-like receptor macrosalin/CD68 and lactin-like oxidized LDL receptor 1 (LOX-1) (49,91–94). All of these receptors bind oxidized LDL, but CD36 now appears to be the major receptor on macrophages responsible for accumulation of oxidized LDL (95). Studies of hyperlipidemic mice with targeted deletions of SR-AI/II or CD36 have established that both types of receptors play a fundamental role in foam cell formation and lesion initiation *in vivo* (96,97).

Unlike LDL receptors, increased cellular content of cholesterol does not suppress the expression of macrophage scavenger receptors (98). On the contrary, increasing uptake of modified lipoproteins appears to stimulate both type A and B receptor expression (99). Levels of the type A receptors also increase during differentiation of monocytes to macrophages (45). Uptake of modified lipoproteins and polyunsaturated fatty acids induces the expression of the type B receptors CD36 and SR-BI through activation of the nuclear receptor peroxisome proliferator-activated receptor-γ (93,100,101), whereas CD36 expression is inhibited by vitamin E (102) and IL-6 (103), and SR-BI expression is reduced

by inflammatory mediators such as lipopolysaccharide (LPS) (104). Transforming growth factor-β treatment of macrophages inhibits the expression of both type A and B scavenger receptors, but it increases expression of the LOX-1 receptor (105).

Macrophages within human lesions also express specific receptors that recognize AGE proteins, the LDL receptor, very low-density lipoprotein receptor, and the LRP/α_2-macroglobulin receptor, a receptor with a very high affinity for lipoproteins containing apoprotein E (106) that increases with macrophage differentiation (46). Macrophages in human and rabbit atherothrombotic lesions produce and secrete apoE (107,108), and the simultaneous expression of both apoE and the LRP may facilitate further lipid accumulation.

Why Do Foam Cells Form?

Accumulation of large amounts of lipid within macrophages may represent a protective phagocytic response to the accumulated and modified lipid. The large lipid content may result from unrestricted uptake of modified lipoproteins, because lipid accumulation does not suppress expression of scavenger receptors (98). Trapping of cholesteryl ester in lesional cells may be caused by a deficit in hydrolysis of free cholesterol from stored cholesteryl esters, as only free cholesterol can diffuse out of a cell (109), and/or because of reduced expression of the cholesterol transporter ABCA1, a member of the adenosine triphosphate (ATP)–binding cassette transporter family. Insufficient availability of extracellular acceptors of free cholesterol, such as apoprotein A1, could also lead to lipid retention. Macrophages within atherothrombotic lesions express ABCA1 (110), a transporter that mediates the movement of free cholesterol to the cell surface for egress and binding to apoprotein A1 (111). Targeted deletion of ABCA1 in macrophages increases atherothrombosis in hyperlipidemic mice (112).

Macrophage Cell Death and Formation of the "Necrotic Core"

The lipid core characterizes advanced atherothrombotic lesions, generally localized at the base of the plaque, filled with cell debris, and sometimes calcified. The presence of a necrotic core can radically alter the structural and mechanical properties of the artery (113). However, it remains unclear how the necrotic core arises. Immunocytochemical and biochemical studies of advanced lesions in humans and hypercholesterolemic animals strongly implicate macrophages in the formation of the necrotic core. These studies have demonstrated that, despite the paucity of intact cells within the core, macrophage-specific antigens persist throughout the core region (114) (Fig. 35–6). Macrophage-derived foam cells may become trapped within the lesion by formation of the overlying fibrous cap. These cells must eventually die, either from apoptosis or possibly from hypoxia or the cytotoxic effects of oxidized lipids or cytokines secreted by other cells within the lesions. If the macrophages become necrotic, they would be expected to release their stored lipid and proteolytic enzymes into the extracellular space, which could lead to the formation of a large pool of lipid and cell debris. Consistent with this possibility, levels of heat shock protein-60 (HSP-60) and HSP-70, proteins expressed by cells under metabolic stress, increase in lesions of atherothrombosis (115,116), particularly around sites of necrosis and lipid accumulation (117).

Numerous studies have reported apoptosis of cells in human atherothrombotic lesions as demonstrated by terminal deoxynucleotide transferase-mediated dUTP nick-end labeling (TUNEL) staining (118,119). Although the TUNEL as-

say for apoptosis has pitfalls (120), many macrophages undergo apoptosis in lesions (121). Caspase 2, a survival factor, has been observed in macrophage-derived foam cells around the necrotic core of advanced human atherothrombotic plaques, and it may increase in response to DNA damage (115). *In vitro* studies demonstrate apoptosis in macrophages, especially after treatment with cytokines or oxidized LDLs present in developing lesions (121). Abundant evidence supports the presence of oxidized derivatives of cholesterol within atherothrombotic lesions, especially in lesions rich in macrophage-derived foam cells (122). High concentrations of oxidized LDLs can kill many types of cells *in vitro,* including macrophages (123). Death of macrophage in atheromata probably occurs by both apoptosis and necrosis. It is unknown if the balance between these processes shifts with particular risk factors or with other characteristics of the lesions.

POTENTIAL ROLES OF MACROPHAGES IN LESION DEVELOPMENT AND PROGRESSION

The Macrophage as a Phagocytic Effector Cell

The early attraction and retention of monocytes in lesion-prone sites most likely represents the normal inflammatory response to clear the area of foreign or noxious materials that have accumulated locally. Thus, the scavenging of cytotoxic lipids resulting in foam cell formation appears to be a normal protective mechanism with pathologic consequences. Immunocytochemical and biochemical evidence shows that lipid hydroperoxides, oxysterols, and other oxidation-specific epitopes characteristic of oxidized LDL exist in atherothrombotic lesions in association with macrophages of both humans and hypercholesterolemic animals (89,90, 122,124). However, macrophages can themselves induce lipid hydroperoxide formation and the resultant cytotoxic products (123,125), for example, as a byproduct of the production of reactive oxygen species formed during the respiratory burst or through other cellular mechanisms including the production and secretion of 15-LO or myeloperoxidase. The presence of both 15-LO and myeloperoxidase associated predominantly with macrophages has been demonstrated in human atherothrombotic plaques (49,126). The spectrum of oxidant species generated during phagocytic stimulation varies considerably depending on the extracellular environment (125).

Macrophages play a fundamental role in host innate and acquired immunity through their capacity to recognize, phagocytose, and kill infectious organisms and as antigen-presenting cells. It is becoming increasingly clear that infectious organisms may contribute to the atherogenic process. As discussed earlier in this chapter, viruses and bacteria are found in human atherothrombotic plaques. Macrophages within atherothrombotic plaques express cell surface receptors that bind bacterial factors such as LPS and HSPs and that facilitate phagocytosis of the bacteria.

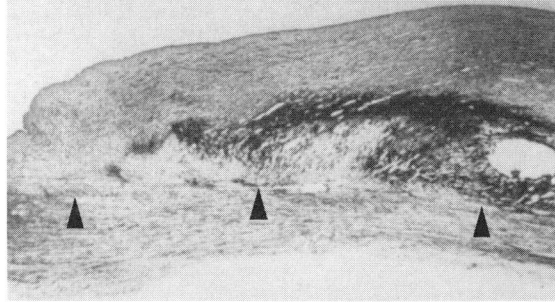

FIG. 35–6. Cell debris within the core of fibrous plaques contains antigens recognized by anti-macrophage antibodies. This advanced human lesion was stained with antibodies to monocytes/macrophages, and macrophage-specific antigens *(black)* were detected within the necrotic core of the lesion. *Arrowheads* indicate the location of the internal elastic lamina. Original magnification ×50.

These include CD14 and several members of the toll-like receptor family (43,127–129). Binding of LPS or HSPs, or both, to the toll-like receptors activates the cells to produce superoxide and hydrogen peroxide (130) and to express and secrete a large number of cytokines (131). These include both proinflammatory cytokines such as TNF-α, IL-1β, IL-12, and IFN-γ and antiinflammatory cytokines such as IL-10 and IL-6. Binding of LPS to the toll-like receptors also increases the capacity of macrophages to present antigen to T cells (132). Toll-like receptor expression is induced during macrophage differentiation (133) and by treatment with oxidized LDL (127). The induction of cytokine secretion and the respiratory burst by infectious organisms could exacerbate inflammatory mechanisms already ongoing within athcrothrombotic lesions and contribute to lesion progression.

In the normal cycle of the inflammatory response, cells take up foreign substances and reenter the circulation. Although some lipid-filled macrophages may reenter the circulation in experimental models of hypercholesterolemia (38) (Fig. 35–3), numerous macrophages remain within the atherothrombotic lesions. As discussed earlier in this chapter, many of the macrophages that remain within the lesions die, through either apoptosis or necrosis. However, recruitment of monocytes into lesions continues throughout lesion development, primarily at shoulders or within neovascularized areas (Fig. 35–1). As a result of this ongoing recruitment of monocytes, a gradient of macrophage differentiation will occur. The least mature cells are at the periphery, and the most differentiated are within the core (134). Because the activation of monocytes/macrophages varies with the state of differentiation and the local stimulants, a gradient of activation and response of adjacent cells to released activation products could be predicted.

Effects of Macrophages on Other Cells Within the Artery Wall

Macrophages produce a myriad of mediators within human lesions (Table 35–2) that may significantly alter the function of adjacent vascular cells. Reactive oxygen species such as superoxide anion can annihilate nitric oxide radical, an endothelial-dependent vasodilator, and thus can impair the control of arterial tone in affected vessels. The resultant peroxynitrite ion found within human lesions (135) can further promote oxidant stress (136). Myeloperoxidase release from a subset of plaque macrophages can sensitize endothelial and smooth muscle cells to apoptosis, and Fas ligand produced by macrophages can promote the death of smooth muscle cells (137). The macrophage may also function as an antigen-presenting cell, thus locally regulating the immune responses within lesions (138). Macrophages can present antigens such as modified lipoproteins through major histocompatibility Class II antigens (40) and certain lipid antigens through lesion macrophage expression of CD1 (41).

It also could be predicted that the capacity of the activated macrophage as an effector cell would depend on its proximity to smooth muscle cells, lymphocytes, endothelial cells, or other macrophages. Electron microscopic evaluation of contacts between macrophages and lymphocytes, as well as other macrophages in lesions of atherothrombosis, has shown frequent close contacts (139). In contrast, there is an absence of contacts between smooth muscle cells and macrophages, implying more of a paracrine response to macrophage products.

Just as the monocyte/macrophage depends on other cells within the artery wall for the provision of M-CSF for survival, it can secrete a number of substances that affect the migration, proliferation, adherence, and metabolic state of other adjacent cells. Effects of macrophage products (Table 35–2) will be limited locally by other factors. For stimulation by growth, migration, and survival factors, the expression of the specific receptor on the target cell is required. Matrix degradation induced by metalloproteinases and other matrix-degrading enzymes (140–142) may be required to enhance migration of smooth muscle cells stimulated by chemoattractants. However, the enzyme activation depends on removal of inhibitory prodomains, and the active enzyme can be blocked by the presence of natural inhibitors. Other macrophage products, such as apoE and lipoprotein lipase, may modulate lipoprotein modification and uptake by surrounding macrophages and endothelial and smooth muscle cell expression of other growth and metabolic mediators. Although numerous macrophage products that associate with human lesions have been identified in this chapter, their roles have been difficult to test, particularly in lesion progression and late-stage lesion rupture.

Macrophages and the Fibrinolytic Process

Macrophages can play a major role in regulating the thrombogenicity of atherothrombotic plaques. A subset of foam cells in established atherothrombotic plaques expresses a potent procoagulant, tissue factor (50,51). Tissue factor accelerates thrombosis by increasing several fold the enzymatic activity of activated factors VII and X (143). Normal human monocytes/macrophages do not express appreciable tissue factor on their surface, and the usual soluble cytokines long implicated in atherogenesis such as IL-1 and TNF-α do not substantially induce tissue factor gene expression by mononuclear phagocytes. However, a cell surface–associated TNF-α homologue, CD40 ligand or CD154, can robustly induce tissue factor expression by human monocytes/macrophages (144). CD40 ligand and its receptor colocalize with tissue factor–bearing macrophages in human lesions (145), consistent with the probable regulation of macrophage tissue factor expression by CD40 ligand.

Once blood clots form, endogenous fibrinolytic mechanisms can limit clot stability (146). Human monocytes/macrophages can express two forms of plasminogen activator, enzymes that cause the production of the fibrinolytic enzyme plasmin from its precursor plasminogen. Urokinase and tissue-type plasminogen activator colocalize with macrophages in human and experimental models of atherothrombosis (147). Many cells, including mononuclear phagocytes, also can express the endogenous inhibitor of these enzymes, plasminogen activator inhibitor-1 (148). Plasminogen activators may have functions beyond participation in fibrinolysis. They may help mononuclear phagocytes to transverse extracellular matrix barriers during their trafficking into and out of lesions.

UNRESOLVED QUESTIONS

Determination of the molecular mechanisms required for lesion initiation has progressed substantially, particularly with advances in gene targeting in mice. Targeted deletion or depletion of lipoprotein retention sequences, the monocyte/lymphocyte adhesion molecule VCAM-1, or the monocyte chemoattractant MCP-1 (or its receptor CCR2) significantly delay lesion formation (2,3,23,28). However, the role of the macrophage and specific macrophage products is less clear, especially with regard to the progression of preexisting lesions. As outlined in this chapter, the monocyte/macrophage is an important component of the normal host defense mechanism and, within lesions of atherothrombosis, expresses many of the proteins associated with this function (Table 35–2). However, persistence of the macrophage inflammatory response in the artery may promote lesion progression and, ultimately, may be responsible for clinical manifestations. Understanding the role of the macrophage and specific macrophage products in lesion progression and plaque rupture has clinical relevance because even young adults have preexisting lesions of atherothrombosis. The development of macrophage-specific retroviral expression vectors (149) should allow this topic to be addressed using the combination of gene transduction of bone marrow stem cells and their transplantation into animals with advanced, preexisting lesions of atherothrombosis.

Would enhanced survival of macrophages in lesions promote lesion expansion and chronicity of the inflammatory response? Is dysregulation of macrophage apoptosis a contributor to lesion expansion? Does the prolonged retention of macrophages within the lesion further amplify the inflammatory response? What are the critical macrophage products involved in plaque rupture? Answers to these and other questions related to the regulation of the macrophage inflammatory response will allow for better definition, and possibly modulation, of the role of macrophages in the progression of lesions of atherothrombosis.

ACKNOWLEDGMENT

This research was supported by grants from the National Heart, Lung, and Blood Institute (grants HL-18645 and HL-67267 to E. W. Raines; HL-34636, HL-56985, and HL-48743 to P. Libby; HL-66115 to M. E. Rosenfeld), National Institutes of Health grant RR-00166 to the Northwest Primate Center, and a grant from Fondation Leducq to P. Libby.

REFERENCES

1. Ross R. Atherosclerosis—an inflammatory disease. *N Engl J Med* 1999;340:115–126.
2. Boring L, Gosling J, Cleary M, et al. Decreased lesion formation in CCR2-/- mice reveals a role for chemokines in the initiation of atherosclerosis. *Nature* 1998;394:894–897.
3. Gosling J, Slaymaker S, Gu L, et al. MCP-1 deficiency reduces susceptibility to atherosclerosis in mice that overexpress human apolipoprotein B. *J Clin Invest* 1999;103:773–778.
4. Ni W, Egashira K, Kitamoto S, et al. New anti-monocyte chemoattractant protein-1 gene therapy attenuates atherosclerosis in apolipoprotein E-knockout mice. *Circulation* 2001;103:2096–2101.
5. Smith JD, Trogan E, Ginsberg M, et al. Decreased atherosclerosis in mice deficient in both macrophage colony-stimulating factor (op) and apolipoprotein E. *Proc Natl Acad Sci USA* 1995;92:8264–8268.
6. van Furth R. Origin and turnover of monocytes and macrophages. *Curr Top Pathol* 1989;79:125–150.
7. Wijffels JF, de Rover Z, Kraal G, et al. Macrophage phenotype regulation by colony-stimulating factors at bone marrow level. *J Leukoc Biol* 1993;53:249–255.
8. Adams DO, Hamilton TA. The cell biology of macrophage activation. *Annu Rev Immunol* 1984;2:283–318.
9. Buckley PJ, Smith MR, Braverman MF, et al. Human spleen contains phenotypic subsets of macrophages and dendritic cells that occupy discrete microanatomic locations. *Am J Pathol* 1987;128:505–520.
10. Mangan DF, Wahl SM. Differential regulation of human monocyte programmed cell death (apoptosis) by chemotactic factors and proinflammatory cytokines. *J Immunol* 1991;147:3408–3412.
11. van Furth R. Phagocytic cells: development and distribution of mononuclear phagocytes in normal steady state and inflammation. In: Galilin JI, Snyderman R, eds. *Inflammation: basic principles and clinical correlates.* New York: Raven Press, 1988:218–295.
12. Munn DH, Beall AC, Song D, et al. Activation-induced apoptosis in human macrophages: developmental regulation of a novel cell death pathway by macrophage colony-stimulating factor and interferon gamma. *J Exp Med* 1995;181:127–136.
13. Bingisser R, Stey C, Weller M, et al. Apoptosis in human alveolar macrophages is induced by endotoxin and is modulated by cytokines. *Am J Respir Cell Mol Biol* 1996;15:64–70.
14. Adams DO, Hamilton TA. Molecular transductional mechanisms by which IFN gamma and other signals regulate macrophage development. *Immunol Rev* 1987;97:5–27.
15. Nathan CF. Secretory products of macrophages. *J Clin Invest* 1987;79:319–326.
16. Sluiter W, Hulsing-Hesselink E, Elzenga-Claasen I, et al. Macrophages as origin of factor increasing monocytopoiesis. *J Exp Med* 1987;166:909–922.
17. Elliott DE, Righthand VF, Boros DL. Characterization of regulatory (interferon-alpha/beta) and accessory (LAF/IL 1) monokine activities from liver granuloma macrophages of Schistosoma mansoni-infected mice. *J Immunol* 1987;138:2653–2662.
18. Kreipe H, Radzun HJ, Rudolph P, et al. Multinucleated giant cells generated in vitro. Terminally differentiated macrophages with down-regulated c-fms expression. *Am J Pathol* 1988;130:232–243.
19. Gerrity RG. The role of the monocyte in atherogenesis: I. Transition of blood-borne monocytes into foam cells in fatty lesions. *Am J Pathol* 1981;103:181–190.
20. Faggiotto A, Ross R, Harker L. Studies of hypercholesterolemia in the nonhuman primate. I. Changes that lead to fatty streak formation. *Arteriosclerosis* 1984;4:323–340.
21. Li H, Cybulsky MI, Gimbrone MA Jr, et al. An atherogenic diet rapidly induces VCAM-1, a cytokine-regulatable mononuclear leukocyte adhesion molecule, in rabbit aortic endothelium. *Arterioscler Thromb* 1993;13:197–204.
22. Nagel T, Resnick N, Atkinson WJ, et al. Shear stress selectively up-regulates intercellular adhesion molecule-1 expression in cultured human vascular endothelial cells. *J Clin Invest* 1994;94:885–891.

23. Cybulsky MI, Iiyama K, Li H, et al. A major role for VCAM-1, but not ICAM-1, in early atherosclerosis. *J Clin Invest* 2001;107:1255–1262.

24. Gerszten RE, Garcia-Zepeda EA, Lim YC, et al. MCP-1 and IL-8 trigger firm adhesion of monocytes to vascular endothelium under flow conditions. *Nature* 1999;398:718–723.

25. Simionescu M, Simionescu N. Proatherosclerotic events: pathobiochemical changes occurring in the arterial wall before monocyte migration. *FASEB J* 1993;7:1359–1366.

26. Williams KJ, Tabas I. The response-to-retention hypothesis of early atherogenesis. *Arterioscler Thromb Vasc Biol* 1995;15:551–561.

27. Chait A, Wight TN. Interaction of native and modified low-density lipoproteins with extracellular matrix. *Curr Opin Lipidol* 2000;11:457–463.

28. Skalen K, Gustafsson M, Rydberg EK, et al. Subendothelial retention of atherogenic lipoproteins in early atherosclerosis. *Nature* 2002;417:750–754.

29. Williams KJ, Tabas I. The response-to-retention hypothesis of atherogenesis reinforced. *Curr Opin Lipidol* 1998;9:471–474.

30. Yla-Herttuala S, Lipton BA, Rosenfeld ME, et al. Expression of monocyte chemoattractant protein 1 in macrophage-rich areas of human and rabbit atherosclerotic lesions. *Proc Natl Acad Sci USA* 1991;88:5252–5256.

31. Barath P, Fishbein MC, Cao J, et al. Detection and localization of tumor necrosis factor in human atheroma. *Am J Cardiol* 1990;65:297–302.

32. Moyer CF, Sajuthi D, Tulli H, et al. Synthesis of IL-1 alpha and IL-1 beta by arterial cells in atherosclerosis. *Am J Pathol* 1991;138:951–960.

33. Clinton SK, Underwood R, Hayes L, et al. Macrophage colony-stimulating factor gene expression in vascular cells and in experimental and human atherosclerosis. *Am J Pathol* 1992;140:301–316.

34. Faggiotto A, Ross R. Studies of hypercholesterolemia in the nonhuman primate. II. Fatty streak conversion to fibrous plaque. *Arteriosclerosis* 1984;4:341–356.

35. Mosesson MW. The role of fibronectin in monocyte/macrophage function. *Prog Clin Biol Res* 1984;154:155–175.

36. Vaddi K, Newton RC. Regulation of monocyte integrin expression by beta-family chemokines. *J Immunol* 1994;153:4721–4732.

37. Faull RJ, Kovach NL, Harlan JM, et al. Stimulation of integrin-mediated adhesion of T lymphocytes and monocytes: two mechanisms with divergent biological consequences. *J Exp Med* 1994;179:1307–1316.

38. O'Brien KD, McDonald TO, Chait A, et al. Neovascular expression of E-selectin, intercellular adhesion molecule-1, and vascular cell adhesion molecule-1 in human atherosclerosis and their relation to intimal leukocyte content. *Circulation* 1996;93:672–682.

39. Fraser I, Hughes D, Gordon S. Divalent cation-independent macrophage adhesion inhibited by monoclonal antibody to murine scavenger receptor. *Nature* 1993;364:343–346.

40. van der Wal AC, Das PK, Tigges AJ, et al. Macrophage differentiation in atherosclerosis. An in situ immunohistochemical analysis in humans. *Am J Pathol* 1992;141:161–168.

41. Melian A, Geng YJ, Sukhova GK, et al. CD1 expression in human atherosclerosis. A potential mechanism for T cell activation by foam cells. *Am J Pathol* 1999;155:775–786.

42. Soilleux EJ, Morris LS, Trowsdale J, et al. Human atherosclerotic plaques express DC-SIGN, a novel protein found on dendritic cells and macrophages. *J Pathol* 2002;198:511–516.

43. Poston RN, Hussain IF. The immunohistochemical heterogeneity of atheroma macrophages: comparison with lymphoid tissues suggests that recently blood-derived macrophages can be distinguished from longer-resident cells. *J Histochem Cytochem* 1993;41:1503–1512.

44. Frostegard J, Ulfgren AK, Nyberg P, et al. Cytokine expression in advanced human atherosclerotic plaques: dominance of pro-inflammatory (Th1) and macrophage-stimulating cytokines. *Atherosclerosis* 1999;145:33–43.

45. Geng Y, Kodama T, Hansson GK. Differential expression of scavenger receptor isoforms during monocyte-macrophage differentiation and foam cell formation. *Arterioscler Thromb* 1994;14:798–806.

46. Watanabe Y, Inaba T, Shimano H, et al. Induction of LDL receptor-related protein during the differentiation of monocyte-macrophages. Possible involvement in the atherosclerotic process. *Arterioscler Thromb* 1994;14:1000–1006.

47. Major TC, Liang L, Lu X, et al. Extracellular matrix metalloproteinase inducer (EMMPRIN) is induced upon monocyte differentiation and is expressed in human atheroma. *Arterioscler Thromb Vasc Biol* 2002;22:1200–1207.

48. Ross R, Masuda J, Raines EW, et al. Localization of PDGF-B protein in macrophages in all phases of atherogenesis. *Science* 1990;248:1009–1012.

49. Yla-Herttuala S, Rosenfeld ME, Parthasarathy S, et al. Gene expression in macrophage-rich human atherosclerotic lesions. 15-lipoxygenase and acetyl low density lipoprotein receptor messenger RNA colocalize with oxidation specific lipid-protein adducts. *J Clin Invest* 1991;87:1146–1152.

50. Wilcox JN, Smith KM, Schwartz SM, et al. Localization of tissue factor in the normal vessel wall and in the atherosclerotic plaque. *Proc Natl Acad Sci USA* 1989;86:2839–2843.

51. Landers SC, Gupta M, Lewis JC. Ultrastructural localization of tissue factor on monocyte-derived macrophages and macrophage foam cells associated with atherosclerotic lesions. *Virchows Arch* 1994;425:49–54.

52. Stragliotto E, Camera M, Postiglione A, et al. Functionally abnormal monocytes in hypercholesterolemia. *Arterioscler Thromb* 1993;13:944–950.

53. Jude B, Agraou B, McFadden EP, et al. Evidence for time-dependent activation of monocytes in the systemic circulation in unstable angina but not in acute myocardial infarction or in stable angina. *Circulation* 1994;90:1662–1668.

54. May AE, Schmidt R, Kanse SM, et al. Urokinase receptor surface expression regulates monocyte adhesion in acute myocardial infarction. *Blood* 2002;100:3611–3617.

55. Vaddi K, Nicolini FA, Mehta P, et al. Increased secretion of tumor necrosis factor-alpha and interferon-gamma by mononuclear leukocytes in patients with ischemic heart disease. Relevance in superoxide anion generation. *Circulation* 1994;90:694–699.

56. Lukacs NW, Strieter RM, Elner VM, et al. Intercellular adhesion molecule-1 mediates the expression of monocyte-derived MIP-1 alpha during monocyte-endothelial cell interactions. *Blood* 1994;83:1174–1178.

57. Webb DS, Shimizu Y, Van Seventer GA, et al. LFA-3, CD44, and CD45: physiologic triggers of human monocyte TNF and IL-1 release. *Science* 1990;249:1295–1297.

58. Vlassara H, Bucala R, Striker L. Pathogenic effects of advanced glycosylation: biochemical, biologic, and clinical implications for diabetes and aging. *Lab Invest* 1994;70:138–151.

59. Brownlee M, Vlassara H, Cerami A. Nonenzymatic glycosylation products on collagen covalently trap low-density lipoprotein. *Diabetes* 1985;34:938–941.

60. Bucala R, Makita Z, Koschinsky T, et al. Lipid advanced glycosylation: pathway for lipid oxidation in vivo. *Proc Natl Acad Sci USA* 1993;90:6434–6438.

61. Bucala R, Tracey KJ, Cerami A. Advanced glycosylation products quench nitric oxide and mediate defective endothelium-dependent vasodilatation in experimental diabetes. *J Clin Invest* 1991;87:432–438.

62. Kirstein M, Brett J, Radoff S, et al. Advanced protein glycosylation induces transendothelial human monocyte chemotaxis and secretion of platelet-derived growth factor: role in vascular disease of diabetes and aging. *Proc Natl Acad Sci USA* 1990;87:9010–9014.

63. Nakamura Y, Horii Y, Nishino T, et al. Immunohistochemical localization of advanced glycosylation end products in coronary atheroma and cardiac tissue in diabetes mellitus. *Am J Pathol* 1993;143:1649–1656.

64. Epstein SE, Zhu J, Burnett MS, et al. Infection and atherosclerosis: potential roles of pathogen burden and molecular mimicry. *Arterioscler Thromb Vasc Biol* 2000;20:1417–1420.

65. Kalayoglu MV, Libby P, Byrne GI. Chlamydia pneumoniae as an emerging risk factor in cardiovascular disease. *JAMA* 2002;288:2724–2731.

66. McMillan GC, Duff G. Mitotic activity in the aortic lesions of experimental atherosclerosis in rabbits. *Arch Pathol* 1948;46:179–182.

67. Rosenfeld ME, Ross R. Macrophage and smooth muscle cell proliferation in atherosclerotic lesions of WHHL and comparably hypercholesterolemic fat-fed rabbits. *Arteriosclerosis* 1990;10:680–687.

68. Gordon D, Reidy MA, Benditt EP, et al. Cell proliferation in human coronary arteries. *Proc Natl Acad Sci USA* 1990;87:4600–4604.

69. Rosenfeld ME, Yla-Herttuala S, Lipton BA, et al. Macrophage colony-stimulating factor mRNA and protein in atherosclerotic lesions of rabbits and humans. *Am J Pathol* 1992;140:291–300.

70. Wang J, Wang S, Lu Y, et al. GM-CSF and M-CSF expression is associated with macrophage proliferation in progressing and regressing rabbit atheromatous lesions. *Exp Mol Pathol* 1994;61:109–118.

71. Qiao JH, Tripathi J, Mishra NK, et al. Role of macrophage colony-stimulating factor in atherosclerosis: studies of osteopetrotic mice. *Am J Pathol* 1997;150:1687–1699.

72. Rajavashisth T, Qiao JH, Tripathi S, et al. Heterozygous osteopetrotic (op) mutation reduces atherosclerosis in LDL receptor-deficient mice. *J Clin Invest* 1998;101:2702–2710.

73. Murayamá T, Yokode M, Kataoka H, et al. Intraperitoneal administration of anti-c-fms monoclonal antibody prevents initial events of atherogenesis but does not reduce the size of advanced lesions in apolipoprotein E-deficient mice. *Circulation* 1999;99:1740–1746.

74. Still WJ, Marriott PR. Comparative morphology of the early atherosclerotic lesion in man and cholesterol-atherosclerosis in the rabbit: an electron microscopic study. *J Atheroscler Res* 1964;4:373–386.

75. Gown AM, Tsukada T, Ross R. Human atherosclerosis. II. Immunocytochemical analysis of the cellular composition of human atherosclerotic lesions. *Am J Pathol* 1986;125:191–207.

76. Rosenfeld ME, Pestel E. Cellularity of atherosclerotic lesions. *Coron Artery Dis* 1994;5:189–197.

77. Smith EB. The influence of age and atherosclerosis on the chemistry of aortic intima, part 1: the lipids. *J Atheroscler Res* 1965;5:224–240.

78. Katz SS, Shipley GG, Small DM. Physical chemistry of the lipids of human atherosclerotic lesions. Demonstration of a lesion intermediate between fatty streaks and advanced plaques. *J Clin Invest* 1976;58:200–211.

79. Schwenke DC, Carew TE. Initiation of atherosclerotic lesions in cholesterol-fed rabbits. II. Selective retention of LDL vs. selective increases in LDL permeability in susceptible sites of arteries. *Arteriosclerosis* 1989;9:908–918.

80. Rosenfeld ME, Tsukada T, Gown AM, et al. Fatty streak initiation in Watanabe Heritable Hyperlipemic and comparably hypercholesterolemic fat-fed rabbits. *Arteriosclerosis* 1987;7:9–23.

81. Krieger M, Stern DM. Series introduction: multiligand receptors and human disease. *J Clin Invest* 2001;108:645–647.

82. Platt N, Gordon S. Is the class A macrophage scavenger receptor (SR-A) multifunctional? The mouse's tale. *J Clin Invest* 2001;108:649–654.

83. Herz J, Strickland DK. LRP: a multifunctional scavenger and signaling receptor. *J Clin Invest* 2001;108:779–784.

84. Febbraio M, Hajjar DP, Silverstein RL. CD36: a class B scavenger receptor involved in angiogenesis, atherosclerosis, inflammation, and lipid metabolism. *J Clin Invest* 2001;108:785–791.

85. Krieger M. Scavenger receptor class B type I is a multiligand HDL receptor that influences diverse physiologic systems. *J Clin Invest* 2001;108:793–797.

86. Brown MS, Basu SK, Falck JR, et al. The scavenger cell pathway for lipoprotein degradation: specificity of the binding site that mediates the uptake of negatively-charged LDL by macrophages. *J Supramol Struct* 1980;13:67–81.

87. Goldstein JL, Ho YK, Basu SK, et al. Binding site on macrophages that mediates uptake and degradation of acetylated low density lipoprotein, producing massive cholesterol deposition. *Proc Natl Acad Sci USA* 1979;76:333–337.

88. Steinberg D, Parthasarathy S, Carew TE, et al. Beyond cholesterol. Modifications of low-density lipoprotein that increase its atherogenicity. *N Engl J Med* 1989;320:915–924.

89. Palinski W, Rosenfeld ME, Yla-Herttuala S, et al. Low density lipoprotein undergoes oxidative modification in vivo. *Proc Natl Acad Sci USA* 1989;86:1372–1376.

90. Yla-Herttuala S, Palinski W, Rosenfeld ME, et al. Evidence for the presence of oxidatively modified low density lipoprotein in atherosclerotic lesions of rabbit and man. *J Clin Invest* 1989;84:1086–1095.

91. Matsumoto A, Naito M, Itakura H, et al. Human macrophage scavenger receptors: primary structure, expression, and localization in atherosclerotic lesions. *Proc Natl Acad Sci USA* 1990;87:9133–9137.

92. Nakata A, Nakagawa Y, Nishida M, et al. CD36, a novel receptor for oxidized low-density lipoproteins, is highly expressed on lipid-laden macrophages in human atherosclerotic aorta. *Arterioscler Thromb Vasc Biol* 1999;19:1333–1339.

93. Chinetti G, Gbaguidi FG, Griglio S, et al. CLA-1/SR-BI is expressed in atherosclerotic lesion macrophages and regulated by activators of peroxisome proliferator-activated receptors. *Circulation* 2000;101:2411–2417.

94. Kume N, Kita T. Roles of lectin-like oxidized LDL receptor-1 and its soluble forms in atherogenesis. *Curr Opin Lipidol* 2001;12:419–423.

95. Lougheed M, Lum CM, Ling W, et al. High affinity saturable uptake of oxidized low density lipoprotein by macrophages from mice lacking the scavenger receptor class A type I/II. *J Biol Chem* 1997;272:12938–12944.

96. Suzuki H, Kurihara Y, Takeya M, et al. A role for macrophage scavenger receptors in atherosclerosis and susceptibility to infection. *Nature* 1997;386:292–296.

97. Febbraio M, Podrez EA, Smith JD, et al. Targeted disruption of the class B scavenger receptor CD36 protects against atherosclerotic lesion development in mice. *J Clin Invest* 2000;105:1049–1056.

98. Fogelman AM, Haberland ME, Seager J, et al. Factors regulating the activities of the low density lipoprotein receptor and the scavenger receptor on human monocyte-macrophages. *J Lipid Res* 1981;22:1131–1141.

99. Han J, Hajjar DP, Tauras JM, et al. Cellular cholesterol regulates expression of the macrophage type B scavenger receptor, CD36. *J Lipid Res* 1999;40:830–838.

100. Han J, Hajjar DP, Febbraio M, et al. Native and modified low density lipoproteins increase the functional expression of the macrophage class B scavenger receptor, CD36. *J Biol Chem* 1997;272:21654–21659.

101. Tontonoz P, Nagy L, Alvarez JG, et al. PPARgamma promotes monocyte/macrophage differentiation and uptake of oxidized LDL. *Cell* 1998;93:241–252.

102. Fuhrman B, Volkova N, Aviram M. Oxidative stress increases the expression of the CD36 scavenger receptor and the cellular uptake of oxidized low-density lipoprotein in macrophages from atherosclerotic mice: protective role of antioxidants and of paraoxonase. *Atherosclerosis* 2002;161:307–316.

103. Keidar S, Heinrich R, Kaplan M, et al. Angiotensin II administration to atherosclerotic mice increases macrophage uptake of oxidized ldl: a possible role for interleukin-6. *Arterioscler Thromb Vasc Biol* 2001;21:1464–1469.

104. Hullinger TG, Panek RL, Xu X, et al. p21-activated kinase-1 (PAK1) inhibition of the human scavenger receptor class B, type I promoter in macrophages is independent of PAK1 kinase activity, but requires the GTPase-binding domain. *J Biol Chem* 2001;276:46807–46814.

105. Minami M, Kume N, Kataoka H, et al. Transforming growth factor-beta(1) increases the expression of lectin-like oxidized low-density lipoprotein receptor-1. *Biochem Biophys Res Commun* 2000;272:357–361.

106. Luoma J, Hiltunen T, Sarkioja T, et al. Expression of alpha 2-macroglobulin receptor/low density lipoprotein receptor-related protein and scavenger receptor in human atherosclerotic lesions. *J Clin Invest* 1994;93:2014–2021.

107. Rosenfeld ME, Butler S, Ord VA, et al. Abundant expression of apoprotein E by macrophages in human and rabbit atherosclerotic lesions. *Arterioscler Thromb* 1993;13:1382–1389.

108. Salomon RN, Underwood R, Doyle MV, et al. Increased apolipoprotein E and c-fms gene expression without elevated interleukin 1 or 6 mRNA levels indicates selective activation of macrophage functions in advanced human atheroma. *Proc Natl Acad Sci USA* 1992;89:2814–2818.

109. Harte RA, et al. Low level expression of hormone-sensitive lipase in arterial microphage-derived foam cells: potential explanation for low rates of cholesteryl ester hydrolysis. *Atherosclerosis* 2000;149:343–350.

110. Schmitz G, Kaminski WE, Porsch-Ozcurumez M, et al. ATP-binding cassette transporter A1 (ABCA1) in macrophages: a dual function in inflammation and lipid metabolism? *Pathobiology* 1999;67(5-6):236–240.

111. Oram JF, Lawn RM. ABCA1. The gatekeeper for eliminating excess tissue cholesterol. *J Lipid Res* 2001;42:1173–1179.

112. Aiello RJ, Brees D, Bourassa PA, et al. Increased atherosclerosis in hyperlipidemic mice with inactivation of ABCA1 in macrophages. *Arterioscler Thromb Vasc Biol* 2002;22:630–637.

113. Falk E. Why do plaques rupture? *Circulation* 1992;86[6 Suppl]: III30–III42.

114. Tsukada T, Rosenfeld M, Ross R, et al. Immunocytochemical analysis of cellular components in atherosclerotic lesions. Use of monoclonal antibodies with the Watanabe and fat-fed rabbit. *Arteriosclerosis* 1986;6:601–613.

115. Berberian PA, Myers W, Tytell M, et al. Immunohistochemical localization of heat shock protein-70 in normal-appearing and atherosclerotic specimens of human arteries. *Am J Pathol* 1990;136:71–80.

116. Kleindienst R, Xu Q, Willeit J, et al. Immunology of atherosclerosis. Demonstration of heat shock protein 60 expression and T lymphocytes bearing alpha/beta or gamma/delta receptor in human atherosclerotic lesions. *Am J Pathol* 1993;142:1927–1937.

117. Johnson AD, Berberian PA, Tytell M, et al. Differential distribution of 70-kD heat shock protein in atherosclerosis. Its potential role in arterial SMC survival. *Arterioscler Thromb Vasc Biol* 1995;15:27–36.

118. Geng YJ, Libby P. Evidence for apoptosis in advanced human atheroma. Colocalization with interleukin-1 beta-converting enzyme. *Am J Pathol* 1995;147:251–266.
119. Han DK, Haudenschild CC, Hong MK, et al. Evidence for apoptosis in human atherogenesis and in a rat vascular injury model. *Am J Pathol* 1995;147:267–277.
120. Kockx MM. Apoptosis in the atherosclerotic plaque: quantitative and qualitative aspects. *Arterioscler Thromb Vasc Biol* 1998;18:1519–1522.
121. Martinet W, Kockx MM. Apoptosis in atherosclerosis: focus on oxidized lipids and inflammation. *Curr Opin Lipidol* 2001;12:535–541.
122. Garcia-Cruset S, Carpenter KL, Guardiola F, et al. Oxysterol profiles of normal human arteries, fatty streaks and advanced lesions. *Free Radic Res* 2001;35:31–41.
123. Cathcart MK, Morel DW, Chisolm GM III. Monocytes and neutrophils oxidized low density lipoproteins making it cytotoxic. *J Leukocyte Biol* 1985;38:341–350.
124. Coffey MD, Cole RA, Colles SM, et al. In vitro cell injury by oxidized low density lipoprotein involves lipid hydroperoxide-induced formation of alkoxyl, lipid, and peroxyl radicals. *J Clin Invest* 1995;96:1866–1873.
125. Rosen GM, Pou S, Ramos CL, et al. Free radicals and phagocytic cells. *FASEB J* 1995;9:200–209.
126. Daugherty A, Dunn JL, Rateri DL, et al. Myeloperoxidase, a catalyst for lipoprotein oxidation, is expressed in human atherosclerotic lesions. *J Clin Invest* 1994;94:437–444.
127. Xu XH, Shah PK, Faure E, et al. Toll-like receptor-4 is expressed by macrophages in murine and human lipid-rich atherosclerotic plaques and upregulated by oxidized LDL. *Circulation* 2001;104:3103–3108.
128. Edfeldt K, Swedenborg J, Hansson GK, et al. Expression of toll-like receptors in human atherosclerotic lesions: a possible pathway for plaque activation. *Circulation* 2002;105:1158–1161.
129. Bulut Y, Faure E, Thomas L, et al. Chlamydial heat shock protein 60 activates macrophages and endothelial cells through Toll-like receptor 4 and MD2 in a MyD88-dependent pathway. *J Immunol* 2002;168:1435–1440.
130. Remer KA, Brcic M, Jungi TW. Toll-like receptor-4 is involved in eliciting an LPS-induced oxidative burst in neutrophils. *Immunol Lett* 2003;85:75–80.
131. Netea MG, Kullberg BJ, Galama JM, et al. Non-LPS components of Chlamydia pneumoniae stimulate cytokine production through Toll-like receptor 2-dependent pathways. *Eur J Immunol* 2002;32:1188–1195.
132. Ozato K, Tsujimura H, Tamura T. Toll-like receptor signaling and regulation of cytokine gene expression in the immune system. *Biotechniques* 2002;[Suppl]:66–68,70,72.
133. Li C, Wang Y, Gao L, et al. Expression of toll-like receptors 2 and 4 and CD14 during differentiation of HL-60 cells induced by phorbol 12-myristate 13-acetate and 1 alpha, 25-dihydroxy-vitamin D(3). *Cell Growth Differ* 2002;13:27–38.
134. van der Wal AC, Das PK, Tigges AK, et al. Adhesion molecules on the endothelium and mononuclear cells in human atherosclerotic lesions. *Am J Pathol* 1992;141:1427–1433.
135. Sugiyama S, Okada Y, Sukhova GK, et al. Macrophage myeloperoxidase regulation by granulocyte macrophage colony-stimulating factor in human atherosclerosis and implications in acute coronary syndromes. *Am J Pathol* 2001;158:879–891.
136. Heinecke JW. Mechanisms of oxidative damage by myeloperoxidase in atherosclerosis and other inflammatory disorders [Review]. *J Lab Clin Med* 1999;133:321–325.
137. Geng YJ, Henderson LE, Levesque EB, et al. Fas is expressed in human atherosclerotic intima and promotes apoptosis of cytokine-primed human vascular smooth muscle cells. *Arterioscler Thromb Vasc Biol* 1997;17:2200–2208.
138. Hansson GK. Immune mechanisms in atherosclerosis. *Arterioscler Thromb Vasc Biol* 2001;21:1876–1890.
139. van der Wal AC, Dingemans KP, van den Bergh W, et al. Specialized membrane contacts between immunocompetent cells in human atherosclerotic plaques. *Cardiovasc Pathol* 1994;3:81–85.
140. Henney AM, Wakeley PR, Davies MJ, et al. Localization of stromelysin gene expression in atherosclerotic plaques by in situ hybridization. *Proc Natl Acad Sci USA* 1991;88:8154–8158.
141. Galis ZS, Sukhova GK, Lark MW, et al. Increased expression of matrix metalloproteinases and matrix degrading activity in vulnerable regions of human atherosclerotic plaques. *J Clin Invest* 1994;94:2493–2503.
142. Galis ZS, Sukhova GK, Kranzhofer R, et al. Macrophage foam cells from experimental atheroma constitutively produce matrix-degrading proteinases. *Proc Natl Acad Sci USA* 1995;92:402–406.
143. Toschi V, Gallo R, Lettino M, et al. Tissue factor modulates the thrombogenicity of human atherosclerotic plaques. *Circulation* 1997;95:594–599.
144. Mach F, Schonbeck U, Bonnefoy JY, et al. Activation of monocyte/macrophage functions related to acute atheroma complication by ligation of CD40. Induction of collagenase, stromelysin, and tissue factor. *Circulation* 1997;96:396–399.
145. Mach F, Schonbeck U, Sukhova GK, et al. Functional CD40 ligand is expressed on human vascular endothelial cells, smooth muscle cells, and macrophages: implications for CD40-CD40 ligand signaling in atherosclerosis. *Proc Natl Acad Sci USA* 1997;94:1931–1936.
146. Robbie LA, Booth NA, Brown AJ, et al. Inhibitors of fibrinolysis are elevated in atherosclerotic plaque. *Arterioscler Thromb Vasc Biol* 1996;16:539–545.
147. Lupu F, Heim DA, Bachmann F, et al. Plasminogen activator expression in human atherosclerotic lesions. *Arterioscler Thromb Vasc Biol* 1995;15:1444–1455.
148. Lupu F, Bergonzelli GE, Heim DA, et al. Localization and production of plasminogen activator inhibitor-1 in human healthy and atherosclerotic arteries. *Arterioscler Thromb* 1993;13:1090–1100.
149. Gough PJ, Raines EW. Gene therapy of apolipoprotein E-deficient mice using a novel macrophage-specific retroviral vector. *Blood* 2003;101:485–491.
150. Greaves DR, Hakkinen T, Lucas AD, et al. Linked chromosome 16q13 chemokines, macrophage-derived chemokine, fractalkine, and thymus- and activation-regulated chemokine, are expressed in human atherosclerotic lesions. *Arterioscler Thromb Vasc Biol* 2001;21:923–929.
151. Seino Y, Ikeda U, Ikeda M, et al. Interleukin 6 gene transcripts are expressed in human atherosclerotic lesions. *Cytokine* 1994;6:87–91.
152. Wang N, Tabas I, Winchester R, et al. Interleukin 8 is induced by cholesterol loading of macrophages and expressed by macrophage foam cells in human atheroma. *J Biol Chem* 1996;271:8837–8842.
153. Uyemura K, Demer LL, Castle SC, et al. Cross-regulatory roles of interleukin (IL)-12 and IL-10 in atherosclerosis. *J Clin Invest* 1996;97:2130–2138.
154. Wuttge DM, Eriksson P, Sirsjo A, et al. Expression of interleukin-15 in mouse and human atherosclerotic lesions. *Am J Pathol* 2001;159:417–423.
155. Mallat Z, Corbaz A, Scoazec A, et al. Expression of interleukin-18 in human atherosclerotic plaques and relation to plaque instability. *Circulation* 2001;104:1598–1603.
156. Gillett NA, Lowe D, Lu L, et al. Leukemia inhibitory factor expression in human carotid plaques: possible mechanism for inhibition of large vessel endothelial regrowth. *Growth Factors* 1993;9:301–305.
157. Wilcox JN, Nelken NA, Coughlin SR, et al. Local expression of inflammatory cytokines in human atherosclerotic plaques. *J Atheroscler Thromb* 1994;1[Suppl 1]:S10–S13.
158. Sukhova GK, Shi GP, Simon DI, et al. Expression of the elastolytic cathepsins S and K in human atheroma and regulation of their production in smooth muscle cells. *J Clin Invest* 1998;102:576–583.
159. Herman MP, Sukhova GK, Libby P, et al. Expression of neutrophil collagenase (matrix metalloproteinase-8) in human atheroma: a novel collagenolytic pathway suggested by transcriptional profiling. *Circulation* 2001;104:1899–1904.
160. Sukhova GK, Schonbeck U, Rabkin E, et al. Evidence for increased collagenolysis by interstitial collagenases-1 and -3 in vulnerable human atheromatous plaques. *Circulation* 1999;99:2503–2509.
161. Saito E, Fujioka T, Kanno H, et al. Complement receptors in atherosclerotic lesions. *Artery* 1992;19:47–62.
162. Hansson GK, Seifert PS, Olsson G, et al. Immunohistochemical detection of macrophages and T lymphocytes in atherosclerotic lesions of cholesterol-fed rabbits. *Arterioscler Thromb* 1991;11:745–750.
163. Yla-Herttuala S, Lipton BA, Rosenfeld ME, et al. Macrophages and smooth muscle cells express lipoprotein lipase in human and rabbit atherosclerotic lesions. *Proc Natl Acad Sci USA* 1991;88:10143–10147.
164. O'Brien KD, Gordon D, Deeb S, et al. Lipoprotein lipase is synthesized by macrophage-derived foam cells in human coronary atherosclerotic plaques. *J Clin Invest* 1992;89:1544–1550.
165. Spanbroek R, Grabner R, Lotzer K, et al. Expanding expression of the 5-lipoxygenase pathway within the arterial wall during human atherogenesis. *Proc Natl Acad Sci USA* 2003;100:1238–1243.
166. Hakkinen T, Luoma JS, Hiltunen MO, et al. Lipoprotein-associated

phospholipase A(2), platelet-activating factor acetylhydrolase, is expressed by macrophages in human and rabbit atherosclerotic lesions. *Arterioscler Thromb Vasc Biol* 1999;19:2909–2917.

167. Halpert I, Sires UI, Roby JD, et al. Matrilysin is expressed by lipid-laden macrophages at sites of potential rupture in atherosclerotic lesions and localizes to areas of versican deposition, a proteoglycan substrate for the enzyme. *Proc Natl Acad Sci USA* 1996;93:9748–9753.

168. Uzui H, Harpf A, Liu M, et al. Increased expression of membrane type 3-matrix metalloproteinase in human atherosclerotic plaque: role of activated macrophages and inflammatory cytokines. *Circulation* 2002;106:3024–3030.

169. Rajavashisth TB, Xu XP, Jovinge S, et al. Membrane type 1 matrix metalloproteinase expression in human atherosclerotic plaques: evidence for activation by proinflammatory mediators. *Circulation* 1999;99:3103–3109.

170. Fabunmi RP, Sukhova GK, Sugiyama S, et al. Expression of tissue inhibitor of metalloproteinases-3 in human atheroma and regulation in lesion-associated cells: a potential protective mechanism in plaque stability. *Circ Res* 1998;83:270–278.

171. Weitkamp B, Cullen P, Plenz G, et al. Human macrophages synthesize type VIII collagen in vitro and in the atherosclerotic plaque. *FASEB J* 1999;13:1445–1457.

172. Shanahan CM, Cary NR, Metcalfe JC, et al. High expression of genes for calcification-regulating proteins in human atherosclerotic plaques. *J Clin Invest* 1994;93:2393–2402.

173. Giachelli CM, Bae N, Almeida M, et al. Osteopontin is elevated during neointima formation in rat arteries and is a novel component of human atherosclerotic plaques. *J Clin Invest* 1993;92:1686–1696.

174. Raines EW, Lane TF, Iruela-Arispe ML, et al. The extracellular glycoprotein SPARC interacts with platelet-derived growth factor (PDGF)-AB and -BB and inhibits the binding of PDGF to its receptors. *Proc Natl Acad Sci USA* 1992;89:1281–1285.

175. Botney MD, Kaiser LR, Cooper JD, et al. Extracellular matrix protein gene expression in atherosclerotic hypertensive pulmonary arteries. *Am J Pathol* 1992;140:357–364.

176. Babaev VR, Dergunov AD, Chenchik AA, et al. Localization of apolipoprotein E in normal and atherosclerotic human aorta. *Atherosclerosis* 1990;85(2-3):239–247.

177. Bjorkhem I, Andersson O, Diczfalusy U, et al. Atherosclerosis and sterol 27-hydroxylase: evidence for a role of this enzyme in elimination of cholesterol from human macrophages. *Proc Natl Acad Sci USA* 1994;91:8592–8596.

178. Meek RL, Urieli-Shoval S, Benditt EP. Expression of apolipoprotein serum amyloid A mRNA in human atherosclerotic lesions and cultured vascular cells: implications for serum amyloid A function. *Proc Natl Acad Sci USA* 1994;91:3186–3190.

179. Brogi E, Winkles JA, Underwood R, et al. Distinct patterns of expression of fibroblast growth factors and their receptors in human atheroma and nonatherosclerotic arteries. Association of acidic FGF with plaque microvessels and macrophages. *J Clin Invest* 1993;92:2408–2418.

180. Hughes SE, Crossman D, Hall PA. Expression of basic and acidic fibroblast growth factors and their receptor in normal and atherosclerotic human arteries. *Cardiovasc Res* 1993;27:1214–1219.

181. Engelse MA, Neele JM, van Achterberg TA, et al. Human activin-A is expressed in the atherosclerotic lesion and promotes the contractile phenotype of smooth muscle cells. *Circ Res* 1999;85:931–939.

182. Tamura R, Miyagawa J, Nishida M, et al. Immunohistochemical localization of Betacellulin, a member of epidermal growth factor family, in atherosclerotic plaques of human aorta. *Atherosclerosis* 2001;155:413–423.

183. Zeiher AM, Goebel H, Schachinger V, et al. Tissue endothelin-1 immunoreactivity in the active coronary atherosclerotic plaque. A clue to the mechanism of increased vasoreactivity of the culprit lesion in unstable angina. *Circulation* 1995;91:941–947.

184. Imanishi T, Han DK, Hofstra L, et al. Apoptosis of vascular smooth muscle cells is induced by Fas ligand derived from monocytes/macrophage. *Atherosclerosis* 2002;161:143–151.

185. Miyagawa J, Higashiyama S, Kawata S, et al. Localization of heparin-binding EGF-like growth factor in the smooth muscle cells and macrophages of human atherosclerotic plaques. *J Clin Invest* 1995;95:404–411.

186. Okura Y, Brink M, Zahid AA, et al. Decreased expression of insulin-like growth factor-1 and apoptosis of vascular smooth muscle cells in human atherosclerotic plaque. *J Mol Cell Cardiol* 2001;33:1777–1789.

187. Bobik A, Agrotis A, Kanellakis P, et al. Distinct patterns of transforming growth factor-beta isoform and receptor expression in human atherosclerotic lesions. Colocalization implicates TGF-beta in fibrofatty lesion development. *Circulation* 1999;99:2883–2891.

188. Hemler ME. VLA proteins in the integrin family: structures, functions, and their role on leukocytes. *Annu Rev Immunol* 1990;8:365–400.

189. Kwak BR, Mulhaupt F, Veillard N, et al. Altered pattern of vascular connexin expression in atherosclerotic plaques. *Arterioscler Thromb Vasc Biol* 2002;22:225–230.

190. Polacek D, Lal R, Volin MV, et al. Gap junctional communication between vascular cells. Induction of connexin43 messenger RNA in macrophage foam cells of atherosclerotic lesions. *Am J Pathol* 1993;142:593–606.

191. Lawn RM, Wade DP, Couse TL, et al. Localization of human ATP-binding cassette transporter 1 (ABC1) in normal and atherosclerotic tissues. *Arterioscler Thromb Vasc Biol* 2001;21:378–385.

192. Brett J, Schmidt AM, Yan SD, et al. Survey of the distribution of a newly characterized receptor for advanced glycation end products in tissues. *Am J Pathol* 1993;143:1699–1712.

193. Haley KJ, Lilly CM, Yang JH, et al. Overexpression of eotaxin and the CCR3 receptor in human atherosclerosis: using genomic technology to identify a potential novel pathway of vascular inflammation. *Circulation* 2000;102:2185–2189.

194. Boisvert WA, Curtiss LK, Terkeltaub RA. Interleukin-8 and its receptor CXCR2 in atherosclerosis. *Immunol Res* 2000;21(2-3):129–137.

195. Hughes SE. Localisation and differential expression of the fibroblast growth factor receptor (FGFR) multigene family in normal and atherosclerotic human arteries. *Cardiovasc Res* 1996;32:557–569.

196. Nelken NA, Soifer SJ, O'Keefe J, et al. Thrombin receptor expression in normal and atherosclerotic human arteries. *J Clin Invest* 1992;90:1614–1621.

197. Lee WH, Kim SH, Lee Y, et al. Tumor necrosis factor receptor superfamily 14 is involved in atherogenesis by inducing proinflammatory cytokines and matrix metalloproteinases. *Arterioscler Thromb Vasc Biol* 2001;21:2004–2010.

198. Noda-Heiny H, Daugherty A, Sobel BE. Augmented urokinase receptor expression in atheroma. *Arterioscler Thromb Vasc Biol* 1995;15:37–43.

199. Kol A, Lichtman AH, Finberg RW, et al. Cutting edge: heat shock protein (HSP) 60 activates the innate immune response: CD14 is an essential receptor for HSP60 activation of mononuclear cells. *J Immunol* 2000;164:13–17.

200. Xu Q, Luef G, Weimann S, et al. Staining of endothelial cells and macrophages in atherosclerotic lesions with human heat-shock protein-reactive antisera. *Arterioscler Thromb* 1993;13:1763–1769.

CHAPTER 36

The Role of Lymphocyte

Göran K. Hansson and Peter Libby

Key Words: Antigens; autoimmunity; cytokines; immunity; inflammation.

INTRODUCTION

Atherothrombosis starts when mononuclear cells of the blood infiltrate the arterial intima. These cells, largely monocytes and T lymphocytes, play key roles in the immune system. Hence, the finding of such cells in atherothrombotic plaques led to the hypothesis that immune mechanisms participate in atherothrombosis. Clinical and experimental research has furnished new evidence to support an important role of such mechanisms in the pathogenesis of this disease. This chapter considers the role of adaptive immune responses in atherothrombosis, describes the putative triggering antigens, and evaluates the effector mechanisms in the context of the atherothrombotic arterial wall, beginning with a brief overview of some basic immunologic principles.

INNATE AND ADAPTIVE IMMUNITY

To provide optimal protection against invading pathogens, the vertebrate organism has developed two different strategies: innate and adaptive immunity (1). The former constitutes a rapid first line of defense that responds to pathogen-associated molecular patterns by producing a set of toxic

G. K. Hansson: Center for Molecular Medicine, Department of Medicine, Karolinska Institute, Karolinska Hospital, SE-17176 Stockholm, Sweden.

P. Libby: Vascular Medicine and Atherosclerosis Unit, Harvard Medical School, Brigham & Women's Hospital, 221 Longwood Avenue, Boston, Massachusetts 02115.

molecules, such as antibacterial peptides, oxygen radicals, and lytic enzymes. Adaptive immunity also uses toxic molecules as effectors but requires recognition by highly specific receptors—that is, antibodies and T-cell receptors—which are amplified on first encounter of a specific microorganism. This permits adaptive immunity to develop exceptionally selective and efficient responses against those microbes that the individual has encountered in the past, without affecting components of the normal microbial flora.

An adaptive immune response normally starts when a T lymphocyte recognizes a foreign antigen. Once activated, T cells can kill target cells, initiate antibody production by B cells, and activate macrophages. The activation of the T cell is the key to most immune reactions, because activation of other immunocompetent cells requires T cell help. Therefore, it is not surprising that the activation of T cells is strictly regulated. It depends on processing of protein antigens into short peptides, which associate intracellularly with major histocompatibility complex molecules (human major histocompatibility complex molecules are denominated HLAs) and are transported to the cell surface.

Peptide:major histocompatibility Class I complexes may be derived from viral proteins produced in the antigen-presenting cell. They are recognized by T cells carrying CD8 proteins and often lead to cytolytic attack of the antigen-presenting cell by the CD8$^+$ cytotoxic T cell. Peptide:major histocompatibility Class II complexes are usually derived from endocytosed antigens such as bacteria, appear on professional antigen-presenting cells, and are recognized by CD4$^+$ T cells. *De novo* activation of naive CD4$^+$ T cells usually requires antigen presentation by dendritic cells, which are highly specialized antigen-presenting cells derived from mononuclear hematopoietic cells. The activated CD4$^+$ T cell typically exerts its effector functions by secreting cytokines and displaying surface molecules, both of which induce activation of macrophages, B cells, and other cells. These "T helper" functions can result in cell-mediated immune reactions with activated macrophages and sometimes granuloma formation (Th1 responses), or in allergic reactions with IgE antibodies, eosinophils, and other cells (Th2 responses).

Although host defense was previously thought to rely almost entirely on specific antibodies and immune cells, it is now understood that innate immune responses elicited by ligation of pattern recognition receptors provides an equally important, early defense against invading pathogens (2). Pattern recognition receptors can be divided into endocytosing receptors, among which the scavenger receptors prevail, and signaling receptors called toll-like receptors (TLR). Both types of pattern recognition receptors ligate macromolecules carrying pathogen-associated molecular patterns, including modified lipoproteins, endotoxins, and microbial DNA. A broad variety of cells serve as effectors of innate immunity, including epithelial cells, macrophages, and others. Research has revealed that the vascular endothelium constitutively expresses pattern recognition receptors. As the endothelial layer occupies a strategic location at the interface of the circulation and tissues, these cells may constitute important components of the innate immune system.

IMMUNOCOMPETENT CELLS IN ATHEROTHROMBOTIC PLAQUES

The cellular events in atherogenesis have been described by studies using a spectrum of morphologic techniques, including light and electron microscopy, histochemistry, immunohistochemistry, and *in situ* hybridization. Together, these studies form the basis for the hypothesis that cellular immune reactions take place in the atherothrombotic plaque.

Several early studies showed that monocyte-like cells enter the intima of hypercholesterolemic animals and develop into foam cells (3–5). Immunohistochemical analysis of human atherothrombotic lesions showed that foam cells express surface antigens specific for the monocyte/macrophage lineage (6–9). A plausible sequence of events in early atherogenesis starts with monocyte adhesion to an intact endothelium, followed by infiltration of these leukocytes into the subendothelial intima, accumulation of cholesterol, and transition into lipid-laden foam cells (10–13). The existence of scavenger receptors for modified lipoproteins such as oxidized low-density lipoprotein (oxLDL) on cells of the monocyte/macrophage lineage (14) explains why such a large proportion of foam cells originate from these cells.

The detection of T cells in the atherothrombotic plaque, in contrast to the finding of monocytes, required monoclonal antibody technology, because these cells were fairly inconspicuous by morphologic criteria. The use of monoclonal

antibodies in an immunohistochemical mapping of gene expression in human atheromas (9,15) revealed that many smooth muscle cells express the HLA Class II gene *HLA-DR,* although these cells do not normally express this gene. Because *HLA-DR* is induced by the T-cell cytokine interferon-γ, it appeared likely that T cells present in the lesion induced *HLA-DR* expression on smooth muscle cells by release of this cytokine. About 10% to 20% of all cells in such lesions express T-cell–specific antigens such as CD3, with approximately two-thirds of the T cells expressing CD4 and one-third expressing the CD8 antigen (9). More recent studies have shown that other cells, in addition to T cells, may express interferon-γ in lesions (16); this suggests a scenario in which professional and nonprofessional immune cells interact in an inflammatory signal cascade (17).

The presence of T cells and monocyte-derived macrophages suggests that antigen presentation and immune activation occur in atherothrombotic plaques. One might, however, argue that both cell types accumulate by nonspecific trapping and may have no functional importance. However, immunophenotyping and mRNA analysis indicate to the contrary by demonstrating activation of the T cells. Many T cells in atheroma bear interleukin-2 (IL-2) receptors and *HLA-DR* (18). Flow cytometric analysis of T cells isolated from plaques revealed a total dominance of the memory T-cell phenotype and expression of the very late activation (VLA)-1 antigen (19).

Cytokines characteristic of activated T cells have been found in plaques by immunohistochemistry and polymerase chain reaction (20) and the "aberrant" expression of HLA-DR in the plaque (15) provides indirect evidence for a local interferon-γ secretion, as discussed earlier. Interestingly, Th1 cytokines predominate in lesions (20) and in T-cell clones derived from them (21,22). This supports the notion that atherothrombosis is a "Th1 disease" in which proinflammatory and macrophage-activating cytokines, particularly interferon-γ, play a key role.

MECHANISMS OF LYMPHOCYTE RECRUITMENT

Analysis of human lesions and experimental models support the following scenario for the development of the immunopathologic aspect of the disease (Fig. 36–1) (see color insert). The T lymphocytes enter the arterial wall at a very early stage of lesion formation and are found in fatty streaks together with macrophages (23,24). The latter, however, always outnumber the T cells, with a ratio of T cells to macrophages of approximately 1:10 to 1:50.

Studies in cholesterol-fed rabbits shed light on the recruitment of T lymphocytes and monocytes to the arterial wall during atherogenesis. The two earliest detectable vascular events after initiation of cholesterol feeding are expression of endothelial adhesion molecules and intimal complement deposition. Focal expression of vascular cell adhesion molecule-1 (VCAM-1) occurs as early as 1 week after the start of the atherogenic diet (25,26) and is followed by the entry of monocytes/macrophages and other leukocytes during the ensuing weeks. VCAM-1 is a ligand for VLA-4, a cell surface protein expressed by lymphocytes and monocytes (27). Granulocytes do not bear VLA-4, providing a possible explanation for the dominance of mononuclear cells to the forming atherothrombotic lesion.

VCAM-1 is not expressed constitutively by endothelial cells, but it is inducible by proinflammatory cytokines, including IL-1, tumor necrosis factor (TNF), and interferon-γ (28). The production of such cytokines in the underlying atheroma likely contributes to the continued expression of VCAM-1 on the surface of the forming plaque. It is uncertain whether nascent lesions contain sufficient local concentrations of IL-1, TNF, or interferon-γ to induce VCAM-1. Surprisingly, VCAM-1 expression also is induced by lysophosphatidylcholine and 1-palmitoyl-2-glutaroyl-sn-glycero-3-phosphorylcholine (PGPC), whereas 1-palmitoyl-2-(5-oxovaleroyl)-sn-glycero-3-phosphorylcholine (POVPC) induces surface expression of another VLA-4 ligand—the CS-1 fragment of fibronectin (29). These phospholipids are generated during lipoprotein oxidation and cell membrane injury, which may thereby initiate recruitment of inflammatory cells (30). In the hypercholesterolemic state, lysophosphatidylcholine might therefore induce VCAM-1 expression on the endothelium.

The focal expression of VCAM-1 in lesion-prone areas of hypercholesterolemic animals may result from a combination of local flow alterations that promote influx or retention of lipoproteins and the action of a component of modified lipoprotein, either directly or by inducing a secondary cytokine. Notably, in the context of T-cell activation during atherogenesis (discussed later), VCAM-1 not only serves as a leukocyte adhesion molecule, but by engaging VLA-4 on T cells can function as a costimulator or accessory molecule in the T-cell activation pathway. Although other adhesion molecules may contribute to T-cell recruitment to atheroma, studies in atherothrombosis-prone mice with defective VCAM-1 have established an important role for this molecule in lesion formation (31).

Adhesion is a necessary but not a sufficient stimulus for recruitment of leukocytes to the vessel wall. This process also requires a stimulus for the migration of the bloodborne cells from the endothelial surface into the lesion. Such stimulation is accomplished by chemotaxis, which can be elicited by chemokines (i.e., chemotactic cytokines), by chemotactic fragments of complement, or by certain bacterial peptides.

Several chemokines are produced by endothelial cells, smooth muscle cells, and intimal macrophages during lesion formation. The best characterized of them is the monocyte chemotactic protein-1 (MCP-1), which can be induced by complement activation or cytokines. MCP-1 promotes recruitment of monocytes and T cells, which express the MCP-1 receptor, CCR2. MCP-1 is expressed in significant amounts in all stages of atherothrombosis (32) and has im-

portant effects on disease development in gene-targeted mouse models (33,34). Similarly, the chemokine fractalkine, which exists in a transmembrane and a shedded form and ligates the receptor CX3CR1, plays a significant role in atherothrombosis in gene-targeted mice (35). In addition, other chemokines are expressed, including RANTES, fractalkine, and CXCL16. The latter molecule, which is expressed by macrophages, has the remarkable dual capacity of acting either as a chemokine (in processed soluble form) or a scavenger receptor (in its native transmembrane form) (36–38). A trio of interferon-γ–inducible chemokines—IP10, ITAC, and MIG—also exist in atheroma and may participate in T-cell recruitment (39).

INNATE IMMUNITY IN THE PLAQUE

Pattern recognition receptors abound in the atherothrombotic plaque. Scavenger receptors of several types are expressed by macrophages, endothelial cells, and smooth muscle cells. Although they are certainly mediating foam cell formation through binding and internalization of modified lipoproteins, these receptors also could be involved in degradation of local microbial components.

TLRs, which constitute a family of activating receptors in innate immunity, are also expressed in lesions. The human atheroma contains TLR1, 2, 4, 5, and 9 expressed largely by macrophages and endothelial cells (40). Similarly, TLRs can be detected in the lesions of apolipoprotein E–knockout (apoE-KO) mice (41). These receptors, when expressed in atherothrombosis, may transduce signals that lead to macrophage activation, including the nuclear factor-kappaB (NF-κB) and mitogen-activated protein kinase pathways. TLR2$^+$ and TLR4$^+$ macrophages were found to display the p65 subunit or NF-κB in their nuclei, suggesting that receptor ligation had caused translocation of p65 from cytosol to nucleus (40). Once translocated, NF-κB can induce transcription of a large set of genes involved in inflammatory activation. It is, therefore, likely that TLR ligation is one of several pathways for inflammatory activation in the atherothrombotic plaque.

Several TLR ligands may be important in atherothrombosis. Lipopolysaccharides of gram-negative bacteria are well known ligands for TLR4, whereas peptidoglycans of gram-positive bacteria bind to TLR2. In addition, heat shock protein 60 (HSP-60) can ligate TLR4 and possibly also TLR2. This protein is conserved in evolution and displays a high degree of homology between microbes such as *Chlamydia pneumoniae* and humans. It is, therefore, possible that autologous and microbial HSP-60 can activate TLR signaling in plaques (42). A third group of microbial TLR ligands that may be generated in lesions contain unmethylated CpG motifs found in bacterial DNA; they are well known ligands for TLR9. Interestingly, human oxLDL has been reported to upregulate TLR expression in macrophages (41). Therefore, LDL accumulation in the plaque may lead to increased TLR expression and, in the presence of microbial TLR ligands, promote inflammatory signal transduction and plaque activation. These speculations obviously require testing in experimental models.

ANTIGENS AND ADAPTIVE IMMUNITY IN ATHEROTHROMBOSIS

The presence of activated T cells and macrophages strongly suggests an ongoing immunologic reaction in the atherothrombotic plaque. Although the antigens that elicit this response remain uncertain, candidates include both microorganisms and autoantigens (Table 36–1).

In early lesions, the presence of T cells of the CD8 phenotype suggests an immune response to HLA Class I–restricted, endogenously synthesized antigens. The best known HLA Class I–restricted antigens are *viral proteins,* which are synthesized by the virus-infected cell. It is, therefore, possible that (at least some of) the CD8$^+$ cells respond to viral antigens in plaque. Antigens of herpes simplex virus type 1 and cytomegalovirus are present in cells of the arterial wall during atherothrombosis (43,44). These members of the herpesvirus family are, however, among the most ubiquitous viruses that infect humans, and the mere presence of components of such viruses does not prove that they play any pathogenetic role. However, studies have identified virally encoded gene products that can activate vascular cells and elicit reactions that may contribute to atherogenesis (45). Chapter 37 provides a discussion concerning the role of viruses in atherothrombosis.

Nonviral microorganisms such as *Chlamydia* spp. are other conceivable microbial stimuli for a local immune response during atherogenesis. Seroepidemiologic association of *C. pneumoniae* with myocardial infarction has been reported in several case–control studies, but remains controversial (46). There is no evidence for an etiologic role for *Chlamydia* in atherothrombosis (47,48). However, these microbes or immune responses may lead to ischemic heart disease by aggravating or activating atherothrombotic lesions (49).

The mature atherothrombotic plaque contains a large number of CD4$^+$ T cells. These cells respond to HLA Class II–restricted, exogenous antigens that are taken up from the environment by macrophages, endothelial cells, and other antigen-presenting cells. The ensuing T-cell responses include cytokine secretion and T-cell help for antibody-producing B cells. Analysis of antibody responses to plaque components could, therefore, shed light on the reactivity of the CD4$^+$ T cells.

Autoantibodies to *oxLDLs* are common in humans; their titer appears to correlate with the progression of atherothrombosis (50). Antibodies raised against model antigens such as malondialdehyde (MDA)-conjugated lysine recognize oxidatively modified LDL (51). Plaques contain considerable amounts of MDA-lysine cross-reactive material (52). It is likely that the B-cell response depends on T-cell help; therefore, it has been proposed that CD4$^+$ cells in the plaque may initiate an autoimmune response to oxLDLs. The observation that CD4$^+$ T cells cloned from human plaques respond to oxLDLs in an HLA Class II–restricted fashion (53) supports this hypothesis. In addition, circulating, oxLDL-reactive T cells have been detected in patients with unstable angina, pointing to a disease-related, systemic, cellular, immune response to this antigen (54).

Immunization with oxLDL or MDA-modified LDL reduces atherothrombosis in several animal models (55–58). This underlines the pathobiologic significance of immune reactions to modified LDL and suggests that it may be possible to develop immunoprophylaxis against atherothrombosis.

Many inflammatory and autoimmune diseases, including atherothrombosis, are associated with antibody production against *HSPs*. These are intracellular chaperones that stabilize the conformation of other proteins. They are synthesized in increased amounts during cell injury and induce T-cell–dependent antibody production (59). Several HSPs localize in atherothrombotic lesions (60) and the titer of autoantibodies to HSP-60 correlates with the extent of carotid atherothrombosis (61). Mucosal immunization with HSP-60 (by feeding or by spraying antigen through the nose) protects against disease (62,63), whereas parenteral immunization aggravates atherothrombosis (64–66). Cell-mediated immunity and antibodies are involved in these responses, but the relative importance of specific antigenic epitopes and of adjuvant molecules remains to be determined.

HSPs are exceptionally well conserved during evolution, and antibodies to HSP-60, therefore, react with microbial and human HSP of 60- to 65-kD size. The immune response to HSP-60 associated with cardiovascular disease may reflect an antimicrobial response that cross-reacts with its hu-

---

TABLE 36–1. *Candidate antigens for stimulating cellular immunity in atheroma*

Group of antigens	Antigen	Dominating lymphocyte response
Modified lipoprotein constituents	apoB adducts and modified lipids	B cells, antibody production
	apoB fragments	CD4$^+$ T cells, proinflammatory and immune-regulating cytokines
HSPs	HSP-60	CD4$^+$ T cells with TCRαβ and TCRγδ; B cells
Chlamydia antigens	HSP-60; OMA; others	CD4$^+$ T cells; B cells
Viral antigens	Proteins encoded by CMV and other herpes viruses	CD4$^+$ T, CD8$^+$ T; B cells

apoE, apolipoprotein E; CMV, cytomegalovirus; HSP, heat shock protein; OMA, outer membrane antigen; TCR, T-cell receptor.

man counterpart (42,67). Such molecular mimicry could possibly play a pathogenic role in human disease.

Few B cells are found in the plaque; therefore, it is likely that B-cell activation and antibody production occur in regional lymph nodes. T cells might enter the plaque, respond to antigen, and then migrate through the lymph circulation to regional lymph nodes, where B cells are activated to produce antibodies to the antigen recognized by the T cell. Such a patrolling role of the T cell is known to occur in many other situations (68) and would fit with the phenotypic characteristics of T cells isolated from plaques (53). It probably requires that antigen also is present in the lymph node; this is likely to be the case for oxLDL.

Molecular mimicry may also play a role for the immune responses to LDLs. Phosphorylcholine, an immunogenic epitope in the cell wall of *Streptococcus pneumoniae,* also is present in oxLDL and on the surface of apoptotic cells (69). At least some of the antibodies to oxLDL that are detected in patients may arise in response to infections. Whether such antibodies affect cardiovascular disease remains controversial. However, experiments in apoE$^{-/-}$ mice suggest that this may be the case. Spleen B cells were found to play an atheroprotective role in this model (70); they are known to produce antibodies reactive with pneumococci and oxLDL. Indeed, immunization with *S. pneumoniae* reduced atherothrombosis in mice in parallel with formation of antibodies that blocked oxLDL uptake (71).

Periadventitial inflammation often occurs in advanced cases of atherothrombosis and huge inflammatory infiltrates can be produced around aortic atherothrombotic lesions. Microscopically, B lymphocytes and macrophages dominate the periaortic lesion together with oxidized lipid components and antibodies to oxLDL (72). Hence, the periarterial lesion may represent an autoimmune response to oxLDL (73). Therefore, although the initial B-cell response probably occurs in lymph nodes, B cells may at later stages localize to and be activated in the periarteritic inflammatory infiltrate.

IMMUNE EFFECTOR MECHANISMS IN THE PATHOGENESIS OF ATHEROTHROMBOSIS

It is likely that a local immune reaction occurs in the atherothrombotic plaque, but its pathophysiologic consequences remain largely speculative. Humoral immune mechanisms could be involved in elimination of antigenic compounds, but also initiate complement- and macrophage-dependent cytotoxic mechanisms. Cellular immune responses may initiate inflammatory reactions, cell-mediated cytotoxicity, and cytokine-dependent regulatory loops in the atherothrombotic plaque.

Antibodies to plaque antigens such as oxLDL could represent a mechanism for antigen elimination. Immune complexes consisting of LDL and anti-LDL antibodies are avidly taken up by Fc receptor–bearing macrophages. These

phagocytes can become engorged with lipid in this manner, forming foam cells (74). Antibody binding to cell surfaces may initiate cytotoxic activity. Both the complement cascade and Fc receptor–bearing macrophages and cytotoxic lymphocytes would attack antibody-coated target cells. The presence of membrane-bound C5b-9 complexes in experimental plaques (75) indicates that complement-mediated lysis takes place. It is not clear, however, whether this occurs as the result of antibody binding to specific antigens on the surface of cells or is because of an "innocent bystander" attack after alternative complement activation on the extracellular cholesterol deposits (76). Surprisingly, experimental research suggests that complement activation may play a protective, rather than a harmful, role in early phases of atherothrombosis (77). Further studies will be needed to clarify this issue.

Cellular immune reactions require T-cell activation, and the presence of activated CD4$^+$ and CD8$^+$ T cells suggests that both cytotoxic and immune-regulatory, T-cell-dependent reactions could occur in the plaque. There is little direct evidence for cytotoxic reactions in atherothrombosis. In contrast, several reports demonstrate the presence of immune-regulatory cytokines in the atherothrombotic plaque. Proinflammatory cytokines, including IL-1, TNF, IL-6, and interferon-γ, are secreted in the plaque (78), probably by T lymphocytes, macrophages, endothelial cells, and smooth muscle cells.

The pathogenetic consequences of such paracrine cytokine secretion could include activation of macrophages and endothelial cells, stimulation of immune responses, modulation of cholesterol uptake, and regulation of vascular hemostatic properties. The mechanical and hemodynamic properties of the atherothrombotic arterial wall would be affected by cytokines that inhibit vascular contractility (by stimulating nitric oxide synthesis and inhibiting production of contractile proteins), inhibit cell proliferation, and induce matrix-degrading metalloproteinases (79–83). Most of these mechanisms have been identified and characterized in cell culture studies. There is *in vivo* evidence in experimental animals for cytokine control of endothelial activation and inhibition of smooth muscle proliferation (84) and for an important role of the proinflammatory cytokine interferon-γ in atherothrombosis (85,86). Chapter 38 provides further information regarding cytokine effects on the vessel wall.

DEDUCING THE ROLE OF LYMPHOCYTES IN EXPERIMENTAL MODELS

The development of gene-targeting technology and its application to atherothrombosis research has offered important new insights into the immunopathogenesis of atherothrombosis. Using the atherothrombosis-prone apoE-KO and LDL receptor-knockout (LDLR-KO) mouse strains, investigators have been able to test the role of specific cell types or signaling molecules in genetic and cell transfer experiments. When apoE-KO mice were crossed with immunodeficient recombinase activated gene (RAG) and severe combined immunodeficiency (SCID) mice, atherothrombosis was reduced to approximately 50% of that seen in regular, immunocompetent apoE-KO animals (87–89). However, the effect was substantially reduced if the mice were fed a high-cholesterol diet, increasing serum cholesterol levels to the grams per deciliter range. These results show that T and B cells, which are absent in RAG and SCID mice, exert a substantial modulating influence on atherothrombosis; however, this effect is not strictly necessary and can be overcome under extreme experimental conditions. Reconstitution of SCIDxapoE-KO mice with CD4$^+$ T cells from immunocompetent apoE-KO mice led to a significant increase in lesion formation; this indicates that the CD4$^+$ T cell is a proatherogenic subset (88).

Reduced atherothrombosis also has been reported under conditions of abrogated immune signaling. The effect of defective interferon-γ or interferon-γ receptor genes is striking and leads to a prominent reduction of lesions (85,90). Similarly, atherothrombosis is reduced when the Th1/interferon-γ–inducing cytokines, IL-18, and IL-12 are targeted (91). Injections of these cytokines aggravate disease (92), whereas administration of soluble-binding proteins or drugs that inhibit expression of these cytokines reduce disease in mice (93,94).

Gene targeting of CD40 ligand and administration of blocking antibodies to this cell surface protein can inhibit atherothrombosis (95,96). Antiatherothrombotic effects also are observed after immune modulation with polyclonal immunoglobulins (97) and when immune cell recruitment is inhibited by targeting genes for adhesion molecules or chemokines (discussed earlier).

Atheroprotective and proatherogenic immune effectors affect lesions in mice. IL-10 deficiency increased fatty streak formation on a fatty diet (98,99), IL-10 KO mice on an apoE-KO background develop larger lesions than IL-10–competent ones (100), and transplantation of IL-10–deficient bone marrow into LDLR-KO mice enhances disease progression more than an IL-10–competent marrow transfer (101). Similar sets of data point to transforming growth factor-β (TGF-β) as an antiatherogenic cytokine (102). IL-10 is likely to act by inhibiting the secretion of proinflammatory cytokines including interferon-γ, whereas TGF-β may inhibit atherothrombosis because of its antiinflammatory action. Because different subsets of CD4$^+$ T cells produce cytokines with different actions, it has been suggested that the interferon-γ–producing Th1 cells are proatherogenic and the IL-10–producing Th1 cells may be antiatherogenic. However, the Th1/Th2 dichotomy is less clearcut in humans than in rodents.

The balance of current evidence indicates that proinflammatory immune activity and signaling through proinflammatory cytokines augment atherothrombosis in experimental models and that antiatherogenic immune signals may also exist and may oppose the proatherogenic ones. Our understanding of the human disease is obviously more limited. However, immune responses to oxLDL, HSP-60, and certain microbes occur in patients with atherothrombosis, and

inflammatory markers, such as C-reactive protein and IL-6, have prognostic value in prospective studies of coronary heart disease. These findings encourage further studies on the role of immune mechanisms in atherothrombosis.

REFERENCES

1. Janeway CA Jr, Travers P, Walport M, et al. *Immunbiology,* 5th ed. New York: Garland Science, 2001.
2. Medzhitov R, Janeway C Jr. Innate immunity. *N Engl J Med* 2000; 343:338–344.
3. Poole JC, Florey HW. Changes in the endothelium of the aorta and the behaviour of macrophages in experimental atheroma of rabbits. *J Path Bact* 1958;75:245–252.
4. Fowler S, Shio H, Haley NJ. Characterization of lipid-laden aortic cells from cholesterol-fed rabbits. IV. Investigation of macrophage-like properties of aortic cell populations. *Lab Invest* 1979;41: 372–378.
5. Gerrity RG. The role of the monocyte in atherogenesis. I. Transition of blood-borne monocytes into foam cells in fatty lesions. *Am J Pathol* 1981;103:181–190.
6. Vedeler CA, Nyland H, Matre R. In situ characterization of the foam cells in early human atherosclerotic lesions. *Acta Pathol Microbiol Immunol Scand* 1984.
7. Aqel NM, Ball RY, Waldmann H, et al. Monocytic origin of foam cells in human atherosclerotic plaques. *Atherosclerosis* 1984;53:265–271.
8. Klurfeld DM. Identification of foam cells in human atherosclerotic lesions as macrophages using monoclonal antibodies. *Arch Pathol Lab Med* 1985;109:445–449.
9. Jonasson L, Holm J, Skalli O, et al. Regional accumulations of T cells, macrophages, and smooth muscle cells in the human atherosclerotic plaque. *Arteriosclerosis* 1986;6:131–138.
10. Faggiotto A, Ross R. Studies of hypercholesterolemia in the nonhuman primate. I. Changes that lead to fatty streak formation. *Arteriosclerosis* 1984;4:323–340.
11. Faggiotto A, Ross R. Studies of hypercholesterolemia in the nonhuman primate. II. Fatty streak conversion to fibrous plaque. *Arteriosclerosis* 1984;4:341–356.
12. Rosenfeld ME, Tsukada T, Gown AM, et al. Fatty streak initiation in Watanabe heritable hyperlipemic and comparably hypercholesterolemic fat-fed rabbits. *Arteriosclerosis* 1987;7:9–23.
13. Rosenfeld ME, Tsukada T, Chait A, et al. Fatty streak expansion and maturation in Watanabe heritable hyperlipemic and comparably hypercholesterolemic fat-fed rabbits. *Arteriosclerosis* 1987;7:24–34.
14. Brown MS, Goldstein JL. Lipoprotein metabolism in the macrophage: implications for cholesterol deposition in atherosclerosis. *Annu Rev Biochem* 1983;52:223–261.
15. Jonasson L, Holm J, Skalli O, et al. Expression of class II transplantation antigen on vascular smooth muscle cells in human atherosclerosis. *J Clin Invest* 1985;76:125–131.
16. Gerdes N, Sukhova G, Libby P, et al. Expression of interleukin (IL)-18 and functional IL-18 receptor on human vascular endothelial cells, smooth muscle cells, and macrophages: implications for atherogenesis. *J Exp Med* 2002;195:1–14.
17. Tellides G, Tereb DA, Kirkiles-Smith NC, et al. Interferon-gamma elicits arteriosclerosis in the absence of leukocytes. *Nature* 2000;403: 207–211.
18. Hansson GK, Holm J, Jonasson L. Detection of activated T lymphocytes in the human atherosclerotic plaque. *Am J Pathol* 1989;135:169–175.
19. Stemme S, Holm J, Hansson GK. T lymphocytes in human atherosclerotic plaques are memory cells expressing CD45RO and the integrin VLA-1. *Arterioscl Thromb* 1992;12:206–211.
20. Frostegard J, Ulfgren AK, Nyberg P, et al. Cytokine expression in advanced human atherosclerotic plaques: dominance of pro-inflammatory (Th1) and macrophage-stimulating cytokines. *Atherosclerosis* 1999; 145:33–43.
21. Stemme S, Faber B, Holm J, et al. T lymphocytes from human atherosclerotic plaques recognize oxidized LDL. *Proc Natl Acad Sci USA* 1995;92:3893–3897.
22. Benagiano M, Azzurri A, Ciervo A, et al. T helper type 1 lymphocytes drive inflammation in human atherosclerotic lesions. *Proc Natl Acad Sci USA* 2003;100:6658–6663.

23. Munro JM, van der Walt JD, Munro CS, et al. An immunohistochemical analysis of human aortic fatty streaks. *Hum Pathol* 1987;18:375–380.

24. Hansson GK, Jonasson L, Lojsthed B, et al. Localization of T lymphocytes and macrophages in fibrous and complicated human atherosclerotic plaques. *Atherosclerosis* 1988;72:135–141.

25. Cybulsky MI, Gimbrone MA. Endothelial expression of a mononuclear leukocyte adhesion molecule during atherosclerosis. *Science* 1991;251:788–791.

26. Li H, Cybulsky MI, Gimbrone MA, et al. An atherogenic diet rapidly induces VCAM-1, a cytokine-regulatable mononuclear leukocyte adhesion molecule, in rabbit aortic endothelium. *Arterioscler Thromb* 1993;13:197–204.

27. Elices MJ, Osborn L, Takada Y, et al. VCAM-1 on activated endothelium interacts with the leukocyte integrin VLA-4 at a site distinct from the VLA-4/fibronectin binding site. *Cell* 1990;60:577–584.

28. Bevilacqua MP, Pober JS, Mendrick DL, et al. Identification of an inducible endothelial-leukocyte adhesion molecule. *Proc Natl Acad Sci USA* 1987;84.9238–9242.

29. Leitinger N, Tyner TR, Oslund L, et al. Structurally similar oxidized phospholipids differentially regulate endothelial binding of monocytes and neutrophils. *Proc Natl Acad Sci USA* 1999;96:12010–12015.

30. Kume N, Cybulsky MI, Gimbrone MA. Lysophosphatidylcholine, a component of atherogenic lipoproteins, induces mononuclear leukocyte adhesion molecules in cultured human and rabbit arterial endothelial cells. *J Clin Invest* 1992;90:1138–1144.

31. Cybulsky MI, Iiyama K, Li H, et al. A major role for VCAM-1, but not ICAM-1, in early atherosclerosis. *J Clin Invest* 2001;107:1255–1262.

32. Ylä-Herttuala S, Lipton BA, Rosenfeld ME, et al. Expression of monocyte chemoattractant protein 1 in macrophage-rich areas of human and rabbit atherosclerotic lesions. *Proc Natl Acad Sci USA* 1991;88:5252–5256.

33. Boring L, Gosling J, Cleary M, et al. Decreased lesion formation in CCR2-/- mice reveals a role for chemokines in the initiation of atherosclerosis. *Nature* 1998;394:894–897.

34. Gu L, Okada Y, Clinton SK, et al. Absence of monocyte chemoattractant protein-1 reduces atherosclerosis in low density lipoprotein receptor-deficient mice. *Mol Cell* 1998;2:275–281.

35. Lesnik P, Haskell CA, Charo IF. Decreased atherosclerosis in CX3CR1-/- mice reveals a role for fractalkine in atherogenesis. *J Clin Invest* 2003;111:333–340.

36. Matloubian M, David A, Engel S, et al. A transmembrane CXC chemokine is a ligand for HIV-coreceptor Bonzo. *Nat Immunol* 2000;1:298–304.

37. Shimaoka T, Kume N, Minami M, et al. Molecular cloning of a novel scavenger receptor for oxidized low density lipoprotein, SR-PSOX, on macrophages. *J Biol Chem* 2000;275:40663–40666.

38. Minami M, Kume N, Shimaoka T, et al. Expression of SR-PSOX, a novel cell-surface scavenger receptor for phosphatidylserine and oxidized LDL in human atherosclerotic lesions. *Arterioscler Thromb Vasc Biol* 2001;21:1796–1800.

39. Mach F, Sauty A, Iarossi AS, et al. Differential expression of three T lymphocyte-activating CXC chemokines by human atheroma-associated cells. *J Clin Invest* 1999;104:1041–1050.

40. Edfeldt K, Swedenborg J, Hansson GK, et al. Expression of toll-like receptors in human atherosclerotic lesions: a possible pathway for plaque activation. *Circulation* 2002;105:1158–1161.

41. Xu XH, Shah PK, Faure E, et al. Toll-like receptor-4 is expressed by macrophages in murine and human lipid-rich atherosclerotic plaques and upregulated by oxidized LDL. *Circulation* 2001;104:3103–3108.

42. Kol A, Bourcier T, Lichtman AH, et al. Chlamydial and human heat shock protein 60s activate human vascular endothelium, smooth muscle cells, and macrophages. *J Clin Invest* 1999;103:571–577.

43. Fish KN, Soderberg-Naucler C, Mills LK, et al. Human cytomegalovirus persistently infects aortic endothelial cells. *J Virol* 1998;72:5661–5668.

44. Nicholson AC, Hajjar DP. Herpesviruses in atherosclerosis and thrombosis. Etiologic agents or ubiquitous bystanders? *Arterioscler Thromb Vasc Biol* 1998;18:339–348.

45. Streblow DN, Soderberg-Naucler C, Vieira J, et al. The human cytomegalovirus chemokine receptor US28 mediates vascular smooth muscle cell migration. *Cell* 1999;99:511–520.

46. Danesh J, Collins R, Peto R. Chronic infections and coronary heart disease: is there a link? *Lancet* 1997;350:430–436.

47. Wright SD, Burton C, Hernandez M, et al. Infectious agents are not necessary for murine atherogenesis. *J Exp Med* 2000;191:1437–1442.

48. Caligiuri G, Rottenberg M, Nicoletti A, et al. Chlamydia pneumoniae infection does not induce or modify atherosclerosis in mice. *Circulation* 2001;103:2834–2838.

49. Kalayoglu MV, Libby P, Byrne GI. Chlamydia pneumoniae as an emerging risk factor in cardiovascular disease. *JAMA* 2002;288:2724–2731.

50. Salonen JT, Ylä-Herttuala S, Yamamoto R, et al. Autoantibody against oxidised LDL and progression of carotid atherosclerosis. *Lancet* 1992;339:883–887.

51. Palinski W, Ylä-Herttuala S, Rosenfeld ME, et al. Antisera and monoclonal antibodies specific for epitopes generated during oxidative modification of low density lipoprotein. *Arteriosclerosis* 1990;10:325–335.

52. Ylä-Herttuala S, Palinski W, Rosenfeld ME, et al. Evidence for the presence of oxidatively modified low density lipoprotein in atherosclerotic lesions of rabbit and man. *J Clin Invest* 1989;84:1086–1095.

53. Stemme S, Faber B, Holm J, et al. T lymphocytes from human atherosclerotic plaques recognize oxidized low density lipoprotein. *Proc Natl Acad Sci USA* 1995;92:3893–3897.

54. Caligiuri G, Paulsson G, Nicoletti A, et al. Evidence for antigen-driven T cell response in unstable angina. *Circulation* 2000;102:1114–1119.

55. Palinski W, Miller E, Witztum JL. Immunization of low density lipoprotein (LDL) receptor-deficient rabbits with homologous malondialdehyde-modified LDL reduces atherogenesis. *Proc Natl Acad Sci USA* 1995;92:821–825.

56. Ameli S, Hultgårdh-Nilsson A, Regnström J, et al. Effect of immunization with homologous LDL and oxidized LDL on early atherosclerosis in hypercholesterolemic rabbits. *Arterioscler Thromb Vasc Biol* 1996;16:1074–1079.

57. George J, Afek A, Gilburd B, et al. Hyperimmunization of apo-E-deficient mice with homologous malondialdehyde low-density lipoprotein suppresses early atherogenesis. *Atherosclerosis* 1998;138:147–152.

58. Zhou X, Caligiuri G, Hamsten A, et al. LDL immunization induces T-cell-dependent antibody formation and protection against atherosclerosis. *Arterioscler Thromb Vasc Biol* 2001;21:108–114.

59. Kiessling R, Grînberg A, Ivanyi J, et al. Role of hsp60 during autoimmune and bacterial inflammation. *Immunol Rev* 1991;121:91–111.

60. Xu Q, Kleindienst R, Waitz W, et al. Increased expression of heat shock protein 65 coincides with a population of infiltrating T lymphocytes in atherosclerotic lesions of rabbits specifically responding to heat shock protein 65. *J Clin Invest* 1993;91:2693–2702.

61. Xu Q, Willeit J, Marosi M, et al. Association of serum antibodies to heat-shock protein 65 with carotid atherosclerosis. *Lancet* 1993;341:255–259.

62. Maron R, Sukhova G, Faria AM, et al. Mucosal administration of heat shock protein-65 decreases atherosclerosis and inflammation in aortic arch of low-density lipoprotein receptor-deficient mice. *Circulation* 2002;106:1708–1715.

63. Harats D, Yacov N, Gilburd B, et al. Oral tolerance with heat shock protein 65 attenuates Mycobacterium tuberculosis-induced and high-fat-diet-driven atherosclerotic lesions. *J Am Coll Cardiol* 2002;40:1333–1338.

64. Kleindienst R, Xu Q, Willeit J, et al. Immunology of atherosclerosis. Demonstration of heat shock protein 60 expression and T lymphocytes bearing alpha/beta or gamma/delta receptor in human atherosclerotic lesions. *Am J Pathol* 1993;142:1927–1937.

65. George J, Shoenfeld Y, Afek A, et al. Enhanced fatty streak formation in C57BL/6J mice by immunization with heat shock protein-65. *Arterioscler Thromb Vasc Biol* 1999;19:505–510.

66. Afek A, George J, Gilburd B, et al. Immunization of low-density lipoprotein receptor deficient (LDL-RD) mice with heat shock protein 65 (HSP-65) promotes early atherosclerosis. *J Autoimmun* 2000;14:115–121.

67. Perschinka H, Mayr M, Millonig G, et al. Cross-reactive B-cell epitopes of microbial and human heat shock protein 60/65 in atherosclerosis. *Arterioscler Thromb Vasc Biol* 2003.

68. Mackay CR, Marston WL, Dudler L. Naive and memory T cells show distinct pathways of lymphocyte recirculation. *J Exp Med* 1990;171:801–817.

69. Shaw PX, Horkko S, Chang MK, et al. Natural antibodies with the T15 idiotype may act in atherosclerosis, apoptotic clearance, and protective immunity. *J Clin Invest* 2000;105:1731–1740.

70. Caligiuri G, Nicoletti A, Poirier B, et al. Protective immunity against atherosclerosis carried by B cells of hypercholesterolemic mice. *J Clin Invest* 2002;109:745–753.

71. Binder CJ, Horkko S, Dewan A, et al. Pneumococcal vaccination decreases atherosclerotic lesion formation: molecular mimicry between Streptococcus pneumoniae and oxidized LDL. *Nat Med* 2003;9:736–743.

72. Parums D, Mitchinson MJ. Demonstration of immunoglobulin in the neighbourhood of advanced atherosclerotic plaques. *Atherosclerosis* 1981;38(1-2):211–216.

73. Parums DV, Brown DL, Mitchinson MJ. Serum antibodies to oxidized low-density lipoprotein and ceroid in chronic periaortitis. *Arch Pathol Lab Med* 1990;114:383–387.

74. Griffith RL, Virella GT, Stevenson HC, et al. Low density lipoprotein metabolism by human macrophages activated with low density lipoprotein immune complexes. A possible mechanism of foam cell formation. *J Exp Med* 1988;168:1041–1059.

75. Seifert PS, Hugo F, Hansson GK, et al. Prelesional complement activation in experimental atherosclerosis. Terminal C5b-9 complement deposition coincides with cholesterol accumulation in the aortic intima of hypercholesterolemic rabbits. *Lab Invest* 1989;60:747–754.

76. Seifert PS, Hugo F, Tranum JJ, et al. Isolation and characterization of a complement-activating lipid extracted from human atherosclerotic lesions. *J Exp Med* 1990;172:547–557.

77. Buono C, Come CE, Witztum JL, et al. Influence of C3 deficiency on atherosclerosis. *Circulation* 2002;105:3025–3031.

78. Hansson GK. Immune mechanisms in atherosclerosis. *Arterioscler Thromb Vasc Biol* 2001;21:1876–1890.

79. Friesel R, Komoriya A, Maciag T. Inhibition of endothelial cell proliferation by gamma-interferon. *J Cell Biol* 1987;104:689–696.

80. Hansson GK, Hellstrand M, Rymo L, et al. Interferon-γ inhibits both proliferation and expression of differentiation-specific α-smooth muscle actin in arterial smooth muscle cells. *J Exp Med* 1989;170:1595–1608.

81. Geng YJ, Hansson GK, Holme E. Interferon-γ and tumor necrosis factor synergize to induce nitric oxide production and inhibit mitochondrial respiration in vascular smooth muscle cells. *Circ Res* 1992;71:1268–1276.

82. Galis ZS, Muszynski M, Sukhova GK, et al. Cytokine-stimulated human vascular smooth muscle cells synthesize a complement of enzymes required for extracellular matrix digestion. *Circ Res* 1994;75:181–189.

83. Wang JM, Sica A, Peri G, et al. Expression of monocyte chemotactic protein and interleukin-8 by cytokine-activated human vascular smooth muscle cells. *Arterioscler Thromb* 1991;11:1166–1174.

84. Hansson GK, Holm J, Holm S, et al. T lymphocytes inhibit the vascular response to injury. *Proc Natl Acad Sci USA* 1991;88:10530–10534.

85. Gupta S, Pablo AM, Jiang X-C, et al. IFN-γ potentiates atherosclerosis in apoE knock-out mice. *J Clin Invest* 1997;99:2752–2761.

86. Whitman SC, Ravisankar P, Elam H, et al. Exogenous interferon-gamma enhances atherosclerosis in apolipoprotein E-/- mice. *Am J Pathol* 2000;157:1819–1824.

87. Dansky HM, Charlton SA, Harper MM, et al. T and B lymphocytes play a minor role in atherosclerotic plaque formation in the apolipoprotein E-deficient mouse. *Proc Natl Acad Sci USA* 1997;94:4642–4646.

88. Zhou X, Nicoletti A, Elhage R, et al. Transfer of CD4(+) T cells aggravates atherosclerosis in immunodeficient apolipoprotein E knockout mice. *Circulation* 2000;102:2919–2922.

89. Daugherty A, Puré E, Delfel-Butteiger D, et al. The effects of total lymphocyte deficiency on the extent of atherosclerosis in apolipoprotein E-/- mice. *J Clin Invest* 1997;100:1575–1580.

90. Whitman SC, Ravisankar P, Daugherty A. IFN-gamma deficiency exerts gender-specific effects on atherogenesis in apolipoprotein E-/- mice. *J Interferon Cytokine Res* 2002;22:661–670.

91. Elhage R, Jawien J, Rudling M, et al. Reduced atherosclerosis in interleukin-18 deficient apolipoprotein E-knockout mice. *Cardiovasc Res* 2003; in press.

92. Whitman SC, Ravisankar P, Daugherty A. Interleukin-18 enhances atherosclerosis in apolipoprotein E(-/-) mice through release of interferon-gamma. *Circ Res* 2002;90:E34–E38.

93. Laurat E, Poirier B, Tupin E, et al. In vivo downregulation of T helper cell 1 immune responses reduces atherogenesis in apolipoprotein E-knockout mice. *Circulation* 2001;104:197–202.

94. Mallat Z, Corbaz A, Scoazec A, et al. Interleukin-18/interleukin-18 binding protein signaling modulates atherosclerotic lesion development and stability. *Circ Res* 2001;89:E41–E45.

95. Mach F, Schönbeck U, Sukhova GK, et al. Reduction of atherosclerosis in mice by inhibition of CD40 signalling. *Nature* 1998;394:200–203.

96. Lutgens E, Gorelik L, Daemen MJ, et al. Requirement for CD154 in the progression of atherosclerosis. *Nat Med* 1999;5:1313–1316.

97. Nicoletti A, Kaveri S, Caligiuri G, et al. Immunoglobulin treatment reduces atherosclerosis in apo E knockout mice. *J Clin Invest* 1998;102:910–918.

98. Mallat Z, Besnard S, Duriez M, et al. Protective role of interleukin-10 in atherosclerosis. *Circ Res* 1999;85:e17–e24.

99. Pinderski Oslund LJ, Hedrick CC, Olvera T, et al. Interleukin-10 blocks atherosclerotic events in vitro and in vivo. *Arterioscler Thromb Vasc Biol* 1999;19:2847–2853.

100. Caligiuri G, Rudling M, Olivier V, et al. Interleukin-10 deficiency increases atherosclerosis, thrombosis, and low-density lipoproteins in apolipoprotein E knockout mice. *Mol Med* 2003;9:10–17.

101. Pinderski LJ, Fischbein MP, Subbanagounder G, et al. Overexpression of interleukin-10 by activated T lymphocytes inhibits atherosclerosis in LDL receptor-deficient mice by altering lymphocyte and macrophage phenotypes. *Circ Res* 2002;90:1064–1071.

102. Tedgui A, Mallat Z. Anti-inflammatory mechanisms in the vascular wall. *Circ Res* 2001;88:877–887.

CHAPTER 37

Viral Activation and Causation of Atherothrombosis and Thrombosis

Jeffrey L. Anderson and Joseph B. Muhlestein

Key Words: Atherothrombosis; infection; inflammation; pathogen; virus.

INFLAMMATION IN THE PATHOPHYSIOLOGY OF ATHEROSCLEROSIS AND ATHEROTHROMBOSIS

Epidemiology of Coronary Heart Disease

Despite substantial progress over three decades, cardiovascular (CV) disease remains the leading cause of death at the

J. L. Anderson: Cardiovascular Department, LDS Hospital, and University of Utah School of Medicine, 8th Avenue and C Street, Salt Lake City, Utah 84143.

J. B. Muhlestein: Cardiovascular Department, LDS Hospital, and University of Utah School of Medicine, 8th Avenue and C Street, Salt Lake City, Utah 84143.

beginning of the twenty-first century (1). CV disease claimed 950,000 lives in the United States in 1998, accounting for more than 40% of all deaths. Coronary heart disease (CHD) is the leading cause of CV death (460,000 CHD deaths annually; 220,000 occur suddenly [out-of-hospital deaths]). More than 12,400,000 individuals in the United States are living with clinical CHD.

Much of Coronary Heart Disease Risk Is Unexplained

Several CHD risk factors have been long known (dyslipidemia, hypertension, smoking, diabetes, family history), yet traditional risk factors fail to account for about one-half of residual risk beyond that explained by chance alone (2). Additional environmental and genetic risk factors must be discovered to accurately predict CHD risk at a population level and especially for individuals.

Atherothrombosis Is an Inflammatory Process

Our paradigm of atherothrombosis has shifted from the perception that it is a passive, infiltrative process to the realization that it is active, inflammatory, and thrombotic (3,4). Acute coronary syndromes, the common precipitant of clinical CHD events, result from erosion or rupture of atheromatous plaques (5–8). Disruption often occurs at the intersection of plaque with more normal wall. This shoulder region is rich in T lymphocytes and macrophages, which actively secrete inflammatory cytokines, chemokines, thrombogenic tissue factors, and matrix-degrading metalloproteinases (9,10). Disruption of the thin plaque cap results in hemorrhage within plaque, expanding its volume, and a partially or fully occlusive thrombus in the vessel lumen, triggered by contact of blood elements (platelets, fibrinogen, leukocytes, and others) with collagen, tissue factor, and other thrombogenic substances. If atherothrombosis is inflammatory, what are the inflammatory triggers?

TRIGGERS OF VASCULAR INFLAMMATION: NONINFECTIOUS AND INFECTIOUS

Studies of both plaque and circulating vascular elements have provided ample and growing evidence for an inflammatory process in atherothrombosis/thrombosis (3,4,9). Histologic studies show accumulation of activated inflammatory cells (macrophages, T lymphocytes, mast cells) in atherothrombotic plaque (especially unstable and disrupted plaques). At the same time, increases in circulating markers of inflammation (e.g., C-reactive protein [CRP], interleukins) are present. The specific triggers for the vascular inflammatory responses observed in atherothrombosis are uncertain; noninfectious and possibly infectious stimuli have been implicated.

Noninfectious Factors

A number of noninfectious factors, many related to standard risk factors, lead to circulatory oxidative stress and stimulate vascular inflammation (4,11,12). These include oxidized low-density lipoprotein (LDL) and other modified lipoproteins, hypertension, diabetes, cigarette smoking, hyperhomocystinemia, and activation of the renin-angiotensin and sympathetic nervous systems in association with physical or emotional distress (Table 37–1).

Infectious Factors

Infection is the classic stimulus for inflammation, which is directed at eradication or containment of the offending organism. Whether infection also is an inflammatory stimulus of chronic diseases, such as atherothrombosis or rheumatoid

TABLE 37–1. *Proposed inflammatory triggers of atherothrombosis and acute coronary syndromes*

Noninfectious
- Modified lipoproteins (e.g., oxidized LDL)
- Diabetes (e.g., glycosylated products)
- Hypertension (mechanical stress)
- Products of cigarette smoke
- Hyperhomocystinemia
- Sympathoadrenal activation (physical, emotional stress)
- Neuroendocrine factors (e.g., angiotensin II)
- Renal insufficiency, uremic factors (e.g., ADMA)
- Other inflammatory mediators, cytokines, oxidants
Infectious (Table 37–2)

ADMA, asymmetric dimethyl arginine; LDL, low density lipoprotein.

arthritis, is uncertain, but the concept is gaining support (4,13–16). It has been clearly demonstrated experimentally that infection can trigger the very string of molecular and cellular events involved in vascular inflammation and atherothrombosis (4,13–15). What remains to be established is whether, when, and to what extent infection plays a role in human disease (17). A partial list of the growing number of infectious agents that directly or indirectly have been proposed to play a role in atherogenesis is provided in Table 37–2. This chapter focuses on potential viral atherogens.

The possibility that infection might explain chronic, inflammatory, degenerative diseases previously regarded as noninfectious is well exemplified by the discovery in recent years that *Helicobacter pylori (Hpyl)* is an etiologic factor in human peptic ulcer disease. Takayasu's arteritis, which causes arterial stenosis/obstruction with thrombosis or dilatation with aneurysm formation, is a specific human model of atherothrombotic disease characterized by early inflammatory and late fibrotic changes that is believed to be caused by autoimmune processes stimulated by a viral infection (18).

TABLE 37–2. *Candidate proatherogenic infectious organisms*

Viruses
- Cytomegalovirus
- Herpes simplex viruses (HSV-1, HSV-2)
- Epstein-Barr virus
- Hepatitis A virus
- Human immunodeficiency virus
- Influenza viruses
- Enterovirus (Coxsackie)? Adenovirus? Others?
Bacteria
- *Chlamydia pneumoniae*
- Chronic bacterial respiratory, urinary, dental, other infections
- Periodontal disease (e.g., *Porphyromonas gingivalis, Streptococcus sanguis, Streptococcus viridans*)
- *Mycoplasma pneumoniae*
- *Haemophilus influenzae*
- *Helicobacter pylori*

THE "INFECTION THEORY": HISTORICAL NOTES ON VIRAL ATHEROGENESIS

Speculation on an association between infectious agents and atherothrombosis dates to the late nineteenth century (19). Huchard (1891) followed by Weisel and Klotz (1906) proposed a relation between early atherothrombosis in animals and humans and various common infections of the time, such as typhoid fever, scarlet fever, measles, and general sepsis. Osler, in his classic textbook of medicine (1908), wrote of a potential link between infection and atherothrombosis (20).

A "proof of principle" of viral pathogenesis was provided by the mid-twentieth century with the discovery that Marek disease virus (MDV) in chickens was associated with marked, accelerated atherothrombosis (21). MDV is a DNA virus of the herpes family that causes avian T-cell lymphomatosis. Subsequent work with this avian model by Fabricant, Minick, Hajjar, and others (22–26) established that MDV infection caused vascular wall injury and altered cellular lipid metabolism. Infection stimulated LDL-cholesterol uptake and reduced cholesteryl ester hydrolytic activity. Accumulation of aortic cholesterol, cholesteryl ester, triglyceride, and phospholipid was observed, resulting in marked atherothrombosis.

The report of Melnick and colleagues in 1983 (27) of the presence of antigen from the herpes family cytomegalovirus (CMV) in smooth muscle cells (SMCs) from carotid and aortic plaques of patients undergoing vascular surgery raised interest in the possibility of viral pathogenesis in human disease. Subsequently, the possibility of associations of atherothrombosis with bacterial vectors (i.e., *Chlamydia pneumoniae [Cpn]*) was raised.

Of further historical interest is epidemiologic evidence linking episodes of acute respiratory illness with atherothrombotic events. In 1981, Pesonen and Siitonen (28) noted the interesting finding that a flulike syndrome resembling respiratory infection often precedes myocardial infarction (MI). Then, in 1984, Spodick and coworkers (29) reported that among 150 prospectively investigated patients with acute MI and 150 control patients matched for age, sex, and admission date, those with acute MI had a greater prevalence of upper respiratory tract infection during the 2 weeks preceding clinical infarction (odds ratio [OR] 2.2; $p < 0.02$) (29). The authors surmised (but did not prove) that the respiratory symptoms were virally induced. Finally, in 1989, Mattila and colleagues (30,31) reported associations between both viral and bacterial infections and MI in two case–control studies from Finland. The first series consisted of 40 consecutive male patients with acute MI who were younger than 50 years of age. The other series included 60 patients of both sexes younger than 65 years. In these studies, a preceding flulike syndrome was more common among patients with acute MI than control subjects. Although these early studies did not define the specific infectious agents involved, they did demonstrate temporal correlations between infection and acute coronary syndromes.

CANDIDATE VIRAL PATHOGENS

Cytomegalovirus

CMV is a member of the herpes family of DNA viruses and is a common human pathogen worldwide (19). Serologic exposure rates roughly approximate age: 15% of adolescents, 50% of adults, and 70% or more of the elderly are seropositive (32). CMV causes a wide range of human disorders spanning infancy to old age. Congenital infection can cause devastating encephalitis and hepatitis. In youth and adults, CMV can produce an illness lasting 3 to 6 weeks and clinically indistinguishable from infectious mononucleosis with fever, lymphocytosis, headache, backache, abdominal pain, and fatigue.

CMV produces large, intranuclear inclusions (hence, "cytomegalic inclusion body disease") and inconspicuous cytoplasmic inclusions in infected cells. CMV is excreted in saliva ("salivary gland virus disease") and urine even in the presence of antibody. As with other herpes viruses, CMV persists indefinitely in the host. Unlike herpes simplex and varicella zoster, which develop latent infections at specific sites, CMV has sites of latency that are less certain and specific. CMV may reside in a variety of normal and neoplastic tissues and cell types, including bone marrow, mononuclear cells, and vascular cells (19).

In adults, CMV infection is generally latent, but reactivation can occur in the setting of chronic illness with impaired resistance and other states of immunosuppression. In adults, localized CMV often presents as pneumonitis or gastrointestinal ulcers, but many tissues may be affected, including nasal mucosa, salivary glands, liver, adrenals, and importantly, eye. The central nervous system is usually spared, except in immunosuppressed patients. Disseminated CMV infection often is fatal.

Of relevance to this chapter, cells of the arterial wall are known to be susceptible to CMV (33), including SMCs, endothelial cells, and macrophages, and CMV has been proposed to enhance cardiac allograft atherothrombosis, coronary restenosis, and native atherothrombosis. Evidence for these conjectures includes serologic associations, the presence of viral products at sites of vascular pathology, and animal models (discussed later).

Other Herpesviridae

Other herpes viruses that establish chronic latent infections include herpes simplex virus type 1 (HSV-1), HSV-2, varicella zoster, Epstein-Barr virus (EBV), and human herpesvirus type 6 (HHV-6). HSV-1 and HSV-2 are known to infect endothelial and SMCs (33). These viruses also may have the potential to promote atherothrombosis alone or in aggregate (34,35).

Hepatitis Viruses

Hepatitis viruses are not known to be harbored in vascular lesions, but they can establish chronic infection, induce autoimmune disease (e.g., through molecular mimicry), and perhaps provoke atherogenesis indirectly (35). A possible role for hepatitis A virus (HAV) in human coronary artery disease (CAD) has been suggested by Zhu and coworkers (36).

Human Immunodeficiency Virus

Human immunodeficiency virus (HIV) has increasing worldwide impact and should be considered a candidate pathogen for atherothrombosis. Coronary vasculopathy without other obvious risk factors has been reported with HIV infection (37). HIV-related immune dysfunction, as well as HIV therapy (with protease inhibitors) and its associated dyslipidemia, also may contribute to CV pathogenesis.

ASSOCIATIONS OF VIRAL SEROLOGY WITH ATHEROTHROMBOSIS

Serologic Associations of Cytomegalovirus with Coronary Heart Disease

The prevalence of seropositivity to CMV increases with age and often is greater than 70% to 80% in subjects in the age range that predisposes to coronary events. An initial surgical case–control study suggested an association between seroexposure to CMV and atherothrombosis (38), which spurred additional studies. However, a differential association of CMV seropositivity with clinical CHD or angiographic CAD has been inconsistent or negative in several of these other studies. In an overview of 11 case–control studies, 4 showed a strong association of CMV antibody seropositivity with CHD/CAD, whereas the other 7 showed little or no association (39). Also, the correlation of CMV with age and socioeconomic class was cited as a frequent confounder when apparent associations were reported.

CMV seropositivity was not found to be predictive of primary CAD risk in our database (40). CMV seropositivity also was not predictive of primary risk in several other and larger studies (39,41–43). Similarly, a metaanalysis of three *prospective* prevention studies found an OR not significantly different from unity (OR 0.91, 95% confidence interval [CI] 0.69–1.19) (44). In the Atherosclerosis Risk in Communities (ARIC) study, CMV seropositivity predicted carotid artery thickening in an unadjusted analysis (OR 1.55; $p = 0.03$) of 340 case–control pairs, but significance was lost after adjustment for potential confounders (OR 1.36; $p = 0.24$) (45).

In contrast to the absence of predictive value for primary coronary risk, CMV seropositivity did predict secondary outcomes in those in our database with angiographic CAD (46). A total of 935 consecutive patients with severe, angiographically demonstrated CAD were studied. After controlling for potentially confounding factors, the mortality hazard ratio for seropositivity to CMV was 1.9 ($p < 0.05$). The risk for mortality was primarily carried by the combined presence of increased CRP and CMV serology (Fig. 37–1) ($p < 0.0001$) (46). As part of a study of pathogen burden (discussed later) in an overlapping population of 980 patients with angiographic CAD, the risk for death or nonfatal MI was 2.0 (95% CI 1.3–3.2) (35). Consistent with this finding, CMV seropositivity was a univariate (mortality 8.9% vs. 5.0%; $p = 0.01$) (47) but not multivariate risk predictor

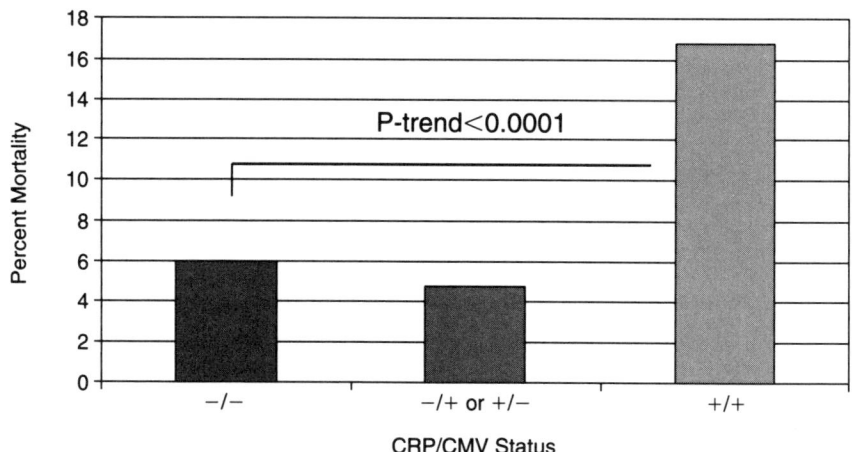

FIG. 37–1. Risk interactions between seropositivity to cytomegalovirus (CMV) and inflammation (C-reactive protein [CRP]). Mortality among 985 patients with angiographic coronary artery disease after a mean of 2.7 years based on relative increase of CRP (second and third tertiles) or seropositivity to CMV, or both. CMV seropositivity and CRP have independent and combined predictive value for mortality in patients with angiographically demonstrated coronary artery disease. (Modified from Muhlestein JB, Horne BD, Carlquist JF, et al. Cytomegalovirus seropositivity and C-reactive protein have independent and combined predictive value for mortality in patients with angiographically demonstrated coronary artery disease. *Circulation* 2000;102:1917–1923.)

(hazard ratio [HR] 1.2–1.4; p = not significant) in the European AtheroGene study (34,47). However, in those patients with an increase of the inflammatory cytokine interleukin-6 (IL-6), CMV seropositivity marked a 3.2-fold ($p < 0.01$) increased risk for death, suggesting that atherogenic effects of CMV are mediated through an associated inflammatory response (47). Most recently, Smieja and coworkers (48) evaluated CMV serology among 3,168 Canadian patients with or at high risk for CHD followed for 4.5 years in the Heart Outcomes Prevention Evaluation (HOPE) study. Over 4.5 years, 494 CV events occurred (MI, stroke, or CV death). Positive CMV serostatus was associated with an increase in CV hazard (adjusted HR 1.24, 95% CI 1.01–1.53). Seropositivity to bacterial candidates (Cpn, Hpyl) and to hepatitis A was not predictive.

To explain the variability of CMV serologic associations with CHD in their database, Zhu and coworkers (49) postulated that CMV elicits a subclinical inflammatory response (marked by increased CRP), but only in certain individuals, and that only those individuals with an inflammatory response are susceptible to atherogenic effects of CMV. In a subsequent study from the same group, sex and individual patterns of inflammatory response to CMV were evaluated for their influence on the CMV-associated risk for atherothrombosis (50). Among 238 subjects evaluated for CAD, increase of CRP was a strong risk predictor for men, and CMV seropositivity was associated with increased CRP. In contrast, for women, CMV seropositivity was independently predictive of CAD, and CRP was less predictive. In addition, CAD prevalence was greater in women with a serologic or mixed, but not cellular only (T cell), response to CMV. Thus, these authors proposed that sex- and host-specific immune responses could determine the etiologic role of CMV in individual patients. Given these observations, young patients (≤50 years or age) with increased inflammatory markers (CRP, IL-6) appear to represent a population subgroup particularly worthy of further investigation of CMV serology as a risk marker for incident MI (51).

Restenosis after coronary angioplasty, usually occurring within 6 months of the procedure, is common (15–50%) and often requires reintervention but is poorly understood. A role for CMV in restenosis after coronary intervention has been proposed. CMV antibody is associated with increased CRP (49),which has been reported to be predictive of restenosis in some but not other studies, including our own (52–54). In one clinical report, patients undergoing atherectomy/angioplasty who were CMV seropositive had a greater rate of angiographic restenosis (55). Before coronary angioplasty and atherectomy in 75 consecutive patients, blood levels for anti-CMV immunoglobulin G (IgG) were measured. After 6 months, seropositive patients had greater reduction in luminal diameter, resulting in a greater rate of angiographic restenosis (43% vs. 8%; $p = 0.002$). In contrast, in our database, we were unable to associate *clinical* restenosis after coronary angioplasty or stenting with CMV seropositivity alone (56), but

greater restenosis risk was predicted by a combined index of infectious serologies ("pathogen burden") (53).

Serologic Associations for Herpes Simplex and Other Viruses

Antibodies to HSV have been measured in several studies. Among patients in the Helsinki Heart Study, seropositivity to HSV-1 showed the strongest association with primary CHD risk (OR 2.1 for the highest quartile) of six serologies tested (HSV-1, adenovirus, enterovirus, CMV, *Cpn,* and *Hpyl*) (42). Risk increased further in those patients with both HSV-1 antibody and increased CRP. In contrast, HSV-1 antibodies were not predictive of primary risk in the U.S. Physician's Health, Women's Health, and ARIC studies (39,43,45).

Hepatitis A serology was studied for associations with CAD in a Washington Heart Center study of 391 patients undergoing angiography (36). CAD prevalence was found to be 74% in HAV seropositive and 52% in seronegative patients. In addition, CRP levels were greater with HAV seropositivity. Predictive value persisted in multivariable analyses.

In two secondary prevention studies, however, herpes viruses contributed to risk both individually and as part of an aggregate score ("pathogen burden"; discussed later) (34,35). Potential risk associations with HSV-2, EBV, and HAV serologies also were raised by these studies. In our U.S. study of 890 patients with angiographic CAD, the HR for death or nonfatal MI associated with HSV-1 seropositivity was 1.57 (95% CI 0.88–2.8) and with HSV-2 seropositivity was 1.51 (1.02–2.23). HAV exposure also predicted an increase in incident events (HR 1.61, 95% CI 1.14–2.2). In contrast, no association with HAV was found in the large HOPE study of more than 3,000 patients (HR 1.01) (57). In the European AtheroGene study (34), the adjusted relative hazard of CV death among 795 patients with angiographic CAD was 3.0 (0.4–22) for HSV-1 and 2.0 (1.0–4.0; $p < 0.05$) for HSV-2. Antibodies to EBV also were tested for predictive value: EBV IgG was not predictive, but EBV IgA seropositivity was significantly predictive (adjusted HR 2.8, 95% CI 1.5–5.0; $p < 0.001$).

PATHOGEN BURDEN: AN INTEGRATED INFECTIOUS MARKER OF CORONARY RISK

Epstein introduced the concept of *total pathogen burden* as a CHD risk factor (14). Exposure to a single atherogenic infectious agent might increase risk modestly, but multiple infectious exposures could combine to substantially increase the aggregate risk for CHD. An initial study evaluated the relation of the presence or absence of angiographic CAD with total pathogen burden, represented by the aggregate number of a panel of five pathogens to which patients showed serologic exposure (58). The study group consisted of 233 patients, and 68% were found to have angiographic

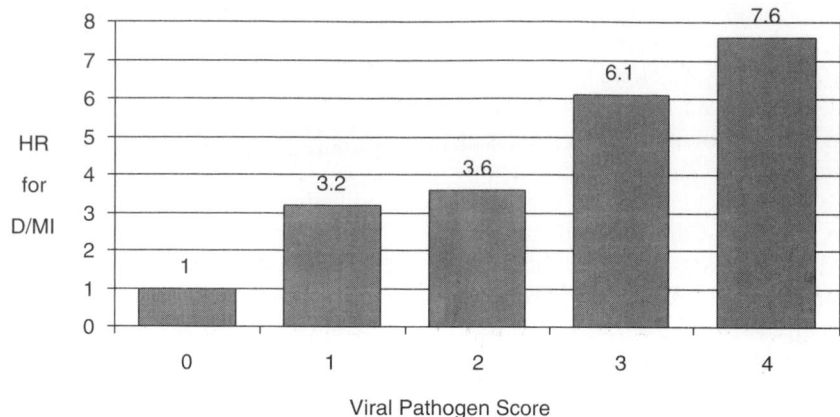

FIG. 37–2. Viral pathogen burden and secondary risk for myocardial infarction (MI) or death (D). Relative hazard rates for MI or D by number of positive IgG antibodies to the four viruses (HSV-1, HSV-2, CMV, hepatitis A). Hazard ratios (HR) are adjusted for age, sex, number of affected vessels, presentation (stable angina, unstable angina, MI), diabetes, smoking, hyperlipidemia, hypertension, family history, and renal failure. (Data from Zhu J, Nieto FJ, Horne BD, et al. Prospective study of pathogen burden and risk of myocardial infarction or death. *Circulation* 2001;103:45–51.)

CAD. The pathogens tested included *Cpn,* CMV, HAV, HSV-1, and HSV-2. The prevalence of CAD was found to be 48%, 69%, and 85% in subjects with antibodies to two or less, three to four, or all five pathogens, respectively. The adjusted OR for CAD was 6.1 for those subjects with five antibodies compared with those with 2 or less antibodies.

The pathogen burden hypothesis was prospectively tested and extended in a subsequent study of patients at secondary CV risk. An independent patient cohort (n = 890) with angiographically documented CAD was tested for antibodies to six vectors—CMV, HSV-1, HSV-2, HAV, *Cpn,* and *Hpyl*—and followed for up to 5 years for the outcomes of death or MI (35). In comparison to having 0 to 1 antibody

positive, those patients with 2, 3, 4, 5, or 6 antibodies positive had fully adjusted relative hazard rates for incident MI or death of 2.4, 3.0, 4.9, 6.5, and 6.3, respectively ($p = 0.0005$).Individually, CMV, HSV-1, HSV-2, and HAV were significantly associated with risk (HR 1.5–2.0) after adjustment for traditional risk factors, whereas *Cpn* and *Hpyl* seropositivities alone were not. Thus, secondary coronary risk essentially was carried entirely by viral pathogen burden (Fig. 37–2).

The European AtheroGene study also found an association between the number of infectious pathogen exposures and prognosis in patients with documented CAD (34). AtheroGene enrolled 1,018 patients with angiographically demon-

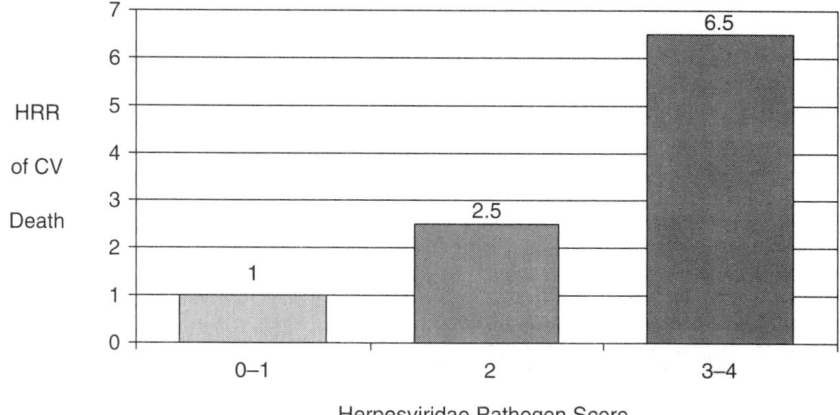

FIG. 37–3. Viral pathogen burden and secondary risk for cardiovascular death. Relative hazard rates (HRR) for cardiovascular (CV) death of Herpesviridae pathogen score (herpes simplex virus type 1 [HSV-1], HSV-2, cytomegalovirus, Epstein-Barr virus). Hazard rate ratios are adjusted for age, sex, diabetes, smoking, high-density lipoprotein cholesterol, ejection fraction (<30%), and C-reactive protein. (Data from Rupprecht HJ, Blankenberg S, Bickel C, et al. Impact of viral and bacterial infectious burden on long-term prognosis in patients with coronary artery disease. *Circulation* 2001;104:25–31.)

strated CAD; measured IgG and IgA antibodies to HSV-1, HSV-2, CMV, EBV, *Haemophilus influenzae, Cpn, Mycoplasma pneumoniae,* and *Hpyl;* and followed the patients for survival outcomes over a mean of 3.1 years. Increasing pathogen burden was highly predictive of long-term prognosis ($p < 0.0001$): CV mortality increased progressively from 3.7% to 12.6% as the number of seropositivities increased from 0 to 3 to a range of 6 to 8. As with our study (35), the AtheroGene result was primarily driven by seropositivity to the Herpesviridae (CMV, HSV-1, HSV-2, EBV) (adjusted HR 5.6; $p < 0.0001$) (Fig. 37–3) (34). Risk (adjusted for clinical and angiographic features) increased incrementally to 2.5, 6.1, and 8.7 for two, three, or four viral serologies when compared with zero to one ($p < 0.0001$ for trend). Risk prediction was retained after further adjusting for left ventricular ejection fraction and CRP (2.5 for two, 6.4 for three to four positive viral serologies; $p = 0.001$). Risk predictions were independent of CRP, which also predicted mortality.

Most recently, the large HOPE study (n = 3,168 patients) assessed the predictive value for CV events (MI, stroke, CV death) of a pathogen burden score among four pathogens (CMV, HAV, *Cpn, Hpyl*) (48). A total score of 4 versus 0 or 1 was associated with an adjusted HR of 1.51 (95% CI 1.02–1.96). The score was driven primarily by CMV serostatus, whereas *Cpn* and *Hpyl* contributed negligibly to the total score and individually were not predictive. The testing of further viral serologies in the HOPE database would be of interest; perhaps greater predictive value could be achieved with a total pathogen score against a panel of several common Herpesviridae (59).

Thus, across a few studies, a greater prevalence of serologic exposures to selected infectious pathogens, particularly viral pathogens, leads to an increased probability of the presence of CAD and of a major incident CV event.

INFECTIOUS PATHOGENS AND PRODUCTS IN VASCULAR TISSUES

DNA Viruses in Native Vessel Atherothrombosis

CMV and other herpes viruses or viral antigens have been found in atherothrombotic arteries (27,60,61), although the database is less robust and consistent than for *Cpn*. Initial reports of herpes family viruses within arterial tissue appeared in 1983–1984. Gyorkey and coworkers (62) reported the detection of herpes-like virions in electron microscopic sections from the aortas of 10 of 60 patients with atherothrombosis undergoing surgery. Benditt and coworkers (63) found HSV nucleic acids by *in situ* hybridization in 11 of 160 aortic tissue samples from patients undergoing coronary bypass surgery. Melnick and coworkers (27) detected CMV antigen in cells cultured from surgically removed arterial tissue from patients with severe atherothrombosis, and Petrie and coworkers (64) later showed superiority of *in situ* hybridization over immunohistochemical tests for detecting CMV in SMCs from atherothrombotic plaque.

More recently, Yamashiroya (61) used DNA hybridization and immunoperoxidase methods and found HSV or CMV, but not EBV, at autopsy in the aorta in 7 and coronary arteries in 8 of 20 young trauma patients. Their presence was observed at sites overlying endothelial cells, SMCs, and early atheroma laden with macrophages. No infectious virus was detected, suggesting the likelihood of abortive infection.

In another small series, Hendrix and coworkers (65) examined samples of aorta and other arteries from patients who had undergone vascular surgery. CMV nucleic acid was found by dot hybridization in one-half of samples from patients with atherothrombosis compared with 22% of samples from CMV seropositive patients without atherothrombotic disease (65). This difference was not significant, however. In a follow-up study using more sensitive polymerase chain reaction (PCR) techniques, CMV nucleic acid sequences were detected in 90% of patients with atherothrombosis compared with 53% without significant atherothrombosis ($p = 0.001$) (66). A greater prevalence of CMV by PCR in arterial samples from patients with compared with those without atherothrombosis (about 85% vs. 7%) also was reported in a Chinese study (67). In contrast, in a third study by Hendrix and coworkers (68), CMV viral nucleic acid was present in seropositive patients independent of the degree of local atherothrombotic change and was found in low levels throughout all major arteries (68).

A Czech study assessed viral DNA to CMV, EBV, and HHV-6 in arterial and venous wall samples and peripheral blood from 244 patients with CAD and 87 angiographically normal control subjects (69). Genomic DNA to CMV was found in 76% and 59%, to EBV in 59% and 50%, and to HHV-6 in 0.1% and 0% of arterial wall samples of patients with CAD and nonischemic control subjects, respectively ($p < 0.01$). No viral DNA was found in venous samples. Thus, a high but differential prevalence of virus occurred by disease status.

These findings suggest widespread vascular presence of CMV nucleic acid after systemic infection, providing a source for reactivation of latent infection, a potential infectious trigger for inflammation, or a cofactor acting with other risk factors for atherothrombosis. However, CMV residence may not be always selective to atherothrombotic arterial segments in exposed subjects.

Cytomegalovirus and Cardiac Allograft Atherothrombosis

Several lines of evidence, including histologic, argue for a role of CMV in allograft atherothrombosis. Both CMV infection and accelerated allograft CAD are common after cardiac transplantation (70). In a Stanford University experience (n = 387), one-third of transplanted patients showed evidence of CMV infection, and graft atherothrombosis developed earlier and more frequently than in uninfected patients and was associated with a greater death rate related to graft CAD (30% vs. 10% at 10 years) (71). Observations from the University of Minnesota program have supported the same conclusion (72). CMV within spindle cells and lymphocytes has been found more commonly (67% vs. 30%) in allografts with than without atherothrombosis (73). Finally, antiviral therapy has been reported to favorably reduce allograft atherothrombosis in an animal model (74), suggesting the potential for prevention (e.g., with ganciclovir) in human transplant recipients.

Cytomegalovirus and Coronary Restenosis

Coronary angioplasty causes vessel wall injury, and "response to injury" leads to vascular SMC proliferation and, frequently, to clinical restenosis. Reactivation of latent CMV might modulate (amplify) this process. Speir and coworkers (75) noted increased prevalence of CMV nucleic acids, of tumor suppression protein p53, and of early viral gene expression (which inhibits p53) in restenotic compared with control tissue. In a subsequent clinical study, restenosis was found to be more common in CMV seropositive patients (43% vs. 8%) (76). The hypothesis that activation of latent CMV at the time angioplasty is a mechanism for restenosis is mechanistically attractive, but the association of CMV with restenosis has been inconsistent and requires further confirmation (discussed earlier) (56).

Cytomegalovirus and Complex Carotid Plaque

Hunter and coworkers (77) analyzed carotid plaque from 51 patients undergoing endarterectomy. CMV by PCR was found in only 2 of 23 (9%) samples, whereas inducible nitric oxide and nitrotyrosine immunoreactivity were found in all complex plaques. These findings led the authors to conclude that free radical oxidative damage not linked to local CMV infection generally was responsible for carotid plaque instability.

POTENTIAL CELLULAR AND MOLECULAR MECHANISMS OF VIRAL ATHEROTHROMBOSIS

General Cellular Mechanisms in Vascular Tissues and Atheroma

CMV and other Herpesviridae-infecting vascular wall cells may provoke or accelerate atherothrombosis by a variety of cellular and molecular mechanisms (14,78,79). During CMV infection, virus is believed to infect monocyte precursors in bone marrow with the viral genome persisting there after clinical infection has resolved (14,80,81). It is further postulated, but not clearly proven, that circulating monocytes, derived from this myelomonocytic precursor cell reservoir, then deliver CMV to the arterial wall (14). These carrier monocytes mature to tissue macrophages in the vascular subintimal space (82). These tissue macrophages, which hone to growing atheromas, provide the local source

from which CMV genes may reactivate and induce their atherogenic effects (83). Vascular SMCs have specifically been shown to support abortive CMV infection, leading to SMC proliferation and accumulation (84,85). Endothelial cells also have been shown to harbor latent CMV, support abortive CMV infection (in which only the immediate early [IE] viral genes are expressed), and, under certain conditions, support productive infection (33,86,87).

Molecular Mechanisms of Viral Atherogenesis

Herpes family viruses (e.g., HSV-1, HSV-2, CMV) are capable of infecting cells of the vascular wall, including human endothelial cells, SMCs, and macrophages (88–91). Infection of cells *in vitro* with herpes viruses results in an inhibition of host cellular protein synthesis, which occurs in early and late stages (33,92). "Early shutoff," mediated by a virion-associated protein, causes dissociation of host cell mRNA from polysomes (92). Delayed shutoff of host cell protein synthesis has been attributed to newly synthesized IE viral gene products that degrade cellular mRNA (33). Among other effects, activation of viral genes (e.g., through abortive [re]infection) and their products could initiate or facilitate atherothrombosis through a number of mechanisms. Epstein and coworkers (14) have summarized several cellular and molecular mechanisms by which infectious agents may directly affect vascular atherothrombosis and thrombosis. Selected proposed mechanisms are summarized in Table 37–3.

TABLE 37–3. *Molecular and cellular mechanisms by which infectious agents may promote atherothrombosis*

Stimulate inflammation
- ↑ Local and circulating inflammatory mediators
  - ↑ Chemokines, cytokines, adhesion molecules
  - ↑ Matrix-degrading proteinases
- ↑ Immune responses directed at pathogen (or pathogen products)
- ↑ Host-directed (autoimmune) responses (molecular mimicry)

Promote lipid accumulation
- ↑ Scavenger receptor activity
- ↑ Cholesteryl esterase activity

Provoke endothelial dysfunction and promote thrombosis
- Impair vasodilator function
- ↓ Anticoagulant activity
- ↑ Procoagulant activity

Promote smooth muscle cell accumulation
- ↑ SMC proliferation
  - Inhibit p53
  - ↑ Growth factor/receptor expression
  - Viral transformation of SMCs
- ↑ SMC migration
- ↓ SMC apoptosis
  - Inhibit p53

SMC, smooth muscle cell.
Modified from Epstein SE, Zhou YF, Zhu J. Infection and atherosclerosis: emerging mechanistic paradigms. *Circulation* 1999;100:e20–e28.

Infection Stimulates Inflammation

Inciting an inflammatory response is a major mechanism by which infection might promote atherothrombosis. Inflammation is triggered by vascular injury caused by a variety of oxidative and mechanical stressors (3).

Noninfectious stressors include hyperlipidemia, increased homocysteine, circulating and tissue cytokines, oxygen free radicals, circulating products of smoke, and biomechanical stressors such as hypertension (Table 37–1). The endothelium reacts to these noninfectious stressors by producing reactive oxygen species (ROS), cytokines, chemokines, and cellular adhesion molecules. ROS lead to oxidative modification of LDLs. Chemokines attract mononuclear and other leukocytes, and adhesion molecules secure their attachment to the vessel wall. After migration to the subintimal space, circulating monocytes transform into macrophages and begin to secrete proinflammatory, prothrombotic, and matrix-degrading molecules, facilitating and amplifying the atherothrombotic process.

Systemic infection similarly promotes generation of ROS and other oxidation- and inflammation-related molecules (93–96). Intracellular ROS activate nuclear factor-kappaB (NF-κB), which mediates transcription of genes involved in inflammatory responses and expression of the CMV promoter (97). CMV induces ROS at least in part through a cyclooxygenase-2 (COX-2)–dependent pathway. IE72 and IE84 gene products transactivate the COX-2 promoter. Aspirin and indomethacin, both COX inhibitors as well as ROS scavengers, can reduce CMV-induced ROS, probably through both of these activities (96). By inhibiting ROS, NF-κB and CMV activation and replication also are inhibited.

Viral infection can up-regulate cytokine gene expression and cytokine release by infected cells (33). CMV infection of macrophages increases expression of IL-1β and tumor necrosis factor-α (TNF-α) (98,99), and HSV-1 strongly up-regulates TNF-α release by monocytes (100). CMV infection of human vascular cells (human umbilical cord vein endothelial cells, [SMCs]) also induces or augments expression of proinflammatory adhesion molecules (e.g., intercellular adhesion molecule-1, vascular cell adhesion molecule-1, E-selectin) (101). Neighboring, uninfected cells show up-regulation of surface molecules caused by the paracrine actions of secreted IL-1β. CMV infection also is associated with increased expression of major histocompatibility complex Class II molecules on multiple cell types.

Differences in host inflammatory response to infection comprise another potentially important but poorly studied factor modifying the inflammatory response to infection that is ripe for further research (14,34,35,42,46,47,49,102–104).

Delayed-type Hypersensitivity, Autoimmunity, and Molecular Mimicry

The atherothrombotic process shows features of a delayed-type hypersensitivity immune response (Th1), which has been compared with that seen in rheumatoid arthritis (9,13,14,105). An important role for specific T-cell sub-groups in directing this response (including natural killer cell-type responses) has been proposed and deserves further consideration and elucidation (13,16). Induction of specific immune responses by infectious pathogens might be directed initially at infectious antigens and subsequently at target host peptides through molecular mimicry (106–108).

Induction of Heat Shock Proteins

Heat shock proteins (HSPs) are important to cellular physiology by acting as chaperones for newly synthesized proteins (109). The importance of their role is emphasized by their high degree of conservation across species, including bacteria, and their substantial homology. HSPs also are induced in response to cellular stresses (heat, biomechanical stress, oxidants) and act to prevent protein denaturation. However, HSPs also might play an atherogenic role either as a target antigen for an (auto)immune response or as an inflammatory stimulus. Infections and common risk factors for atherothrombosis, such as oxidized LDL and hypertension, cause overexpression of HSPs by endothelial cells, SMCs, and macrophages. Soluble HSPs bind to the toll-like receptor 4/CD14 complex, initiating an innate immune response.

Growing evidence points to a central role for HSPs in the pathogenesis of atherothrombosis (109–116). Indeed, HSPs might be a critical link between infection and atherothrombosis (109). Through induction of host or bacterial (e.g., Cpn) HSPs, or both, infection could induce autoreactive or alloreactive cells against HSPs. In addition, HSPs may induce adhesion molecule expression by endothelial cells, SMC proliferation, and proinflammatory cytokine secretion by macrophages (109).

Markers of Inflammation and Immune Stimulation

Several studies support the concept that markers of inflammation (e.g., CRP, IL-6) are complementary to, but are not a surrogate for, markers of infection (e.g., serology, evidence for active infection) (34,35,40,47,49,102). Although increasing infectious exposure often is associated with greater CRP levels, the degree of correlation is low. Only a variable part of risk carried by infectious markers has been explained by adjusting for inflammatory markers. The sum of serologic exposures to eight organisms (five viral) was an independent and additive risk factor on top of CRP in the AtheroGene study (34). Among 985 patients with angiographic CAD, we found that both increased CRP and seropositivity to CMV were independent risk factors (46). However, risk in both studies was greatest and was concentrated among those with both increased CRP and CMV antibody positivity (Fig. 37–1) (46,47). These observations suggest that infection might promote atherothrombosis by inciting an inflammatory response (35). Neither CRP (and IL-6 or other inflammatory markers) nor infectious markers alone fully capture this risk, whereas the presence of both is associated with greatest risk. Similarly, in the setting of chronic bacterial infection, the Bruneck study found independent and additive risk of increased CRP and active infection (102).

Infection May Promote Lipid Accumulation

Marek's disease of chicken, the classic animal infectious model of atherothrombosis, caused by an avian herpes virus, is characterized by marked vascular accumulation of lipids (22,23,25,26,117). The likely mechanism for this effect, also demonstrated in human SMCs infected with HSV, is decreased cellular cholesteryl ester hydrolytic activity with accumulation of saturated cholesteryl esters and triacylglycerols (26). (This topic is discussed in greater detail in an earlier version of this chapter in the previous edition of this textbook [33].)

Enhanced scavenger receptor activity of SMCs and macrophages is another mechanism by which pathogens may increase lipid accumulation. Zhou and coworkers (76) demonstrated this mechanism in human SMCs infected with CMV. An IE gene product appeared to be responsible. We found that CMV also up-regulates scavenger receptor activity in macrophages (86).

Infection Causes Endothelial Dysfunction and Promotes Thrombosis

The healthy endothelium produces a number of vasodilatory and antithrombotic substances, including nitric oxide, prostacyclin, plasminogen activator, thrombomodulin, and heparin sulfate. Several laboratories have shown the ability of infectious agents, including HSV and CMV (as well as *Cpn*), to change this phenotype from anticoagulant to procoagulant (26,118–122). Guetta and coworkers (87) reported that CMV IE gene expression resulted in increased monocyte adhesion to endothelial cells. Furthermore, the major viral IE gene promoter was regulated in endothelial cells by thrombin and by the IE gene products.

Modulation of vascular tone by endothelial cells, which is critical to normal vascular function, is impaired by prior CMV infection and may occur by both nitric oxide–dependent and independent pathways (123).

A clinical correlation of endothelial dysfunction with infectious exposure was provided by Prasad and coworkers (124). Serologic status was assessed to five pathogens (CMV, HSV-1, HAV, *Cpn*, *Hpyl*) among 218 patients who underwent angiography and had endothelium-dependent (with intracoronary acetylcholine) and endothelium-independent function assessed (with nitroprusside and adenosine). Pathogen burden, the number of positive serologies, was associated with CAD presence and extent. Of particular interest, pathogen burden predicted endothelium-dependent ($p = 0.009$), but not endothelium-independent, dysfunction. Pathogen burden also was an independent predictor of en-

dothelial dysfunction in the subgroup with angiographically normal coronary arteries. The authors concluded that endothelial dysfunction might represent a critical mechanism through which pathogens contribute to atherogenesis in humans.

Dysfunctional endothelium is prothrombotic. Laboratory evidence supports the hypothesis that herpes family viruses (HSV, CMV) act as prothrombotic agents, activating the coagulation cascade on endothelium (33,119,121,122,125). HSV infection of endothelium promotes prothrombinase assembly, resulting in more efficient thrombin generation (118,119). Platelet and leukocyte binding increase (119,126). Matrix protein synthesis is inhibited, further destabilizing plaque (89). Viral infection also induces endothelial cell production of tissue factor, a potent procoagulant, and inhibition of anticoagulant production (thrombomodulin, prostacyclin, tissue plasminogen activator) (118,119).

Infection Promotes Smooth Muscle Cell Accumulation

SMC accumulation, with consequent increase in plaque size, may occur through proliferation, migration, and inhibition of apoptosis of SMCs. A further mechanism may be viral transformation of vascular SMCs (33,127). Abortive CMV infection has been shown to lead to SMC proliferation (84,85). An intriguing molecular mechanism for this effect is through the binding and inhibition of the tumor suppressor gene *p53* by an IE CMV gene product (IE2-84) allowing proliferation to proceed unchecked (75,128–130). Another mechanism associated with CMV infection is increased expression of growth factors (i.e., fibroblast growth factors, e.g., basic fibroblast growth factor and acidic fibroblast growth factor, and platelet-derived growth factors [PDGFs], e.g., PDGF-BB) and growth factor receptors (e.g., for PDGF) (84,85,131,132). CMV (and chlamydia) further promote SMC accumulation by inhibiting apoptosis of infected cells (79,133,134). Early viral gene products (i.e., IE2-84) have been found to be involved in the CMV-related inhibition of apoptosis in human SMCs, endothelial cells, and HeLa cells (75,79,128,130,134,135). SMC accumulation also is promoted by migration of SMCs from media and adventitia to neointima. Migration is enhanced by CMV infection of SMCs (84).

Synergistic Effects of Coinfection

Both CMV and *Cpn* have been associated with atherothrombosis. A National Institutes of Health (NIH) study tested whether latent CMV infection could be transactivated by superinfection of HeLa cells with *Cpn* (136). *Cpn* increased the CMV major immediate early promoter (MIEP) essential for viral gene expression in a dose–response fashion by more than twofold. The results suggest that if CMV and *Cpn* are indeed etiologic factors, their copresence might promote atherothrombosis synergistically.

CIRCULATING MEDIATORS PROMOTING ATHEROTHROMBOSIS AT A DISTANCE

Circulating factors might promote atherothrombosis at a distance from the site of infection. That is, infection might cause or amplify vascular dysfunction or injury and facilitate atherothrombosis in the absence of resident pathogens in the vessel wall at the site of plaque formation. Indeed, Zhou and coworkers (137) found that rats infected with CMV showed increased neointimal proliferation in response to vascular injury despite the absence of recoverable virus at the site of arterial injury. CMV was isolated instead from salivary gland and spleen. The responsible circulating factors were not determined, but they could include acute-phase reactants, cytokines, procoagulants, leukocytes, and cross-reactive antibodies. Similar mechanisms might be operative in humans who show increased vascular risk associated with chronic nonvascular infections (102) or with viral (or bacterial) organisms contributing to "pathogen burden" but not causing vascular infection (34,35). A number of procoagulant and proinflammatory factors that act at a distance to enhance progression of atherothrombosis and the initiation of acute ischemic syndromes have been proposed (14); however, these factors will not be further reviewed in this chapter.

It should be noted that although infection can promote atherothrombosis at a distance, systemic infection alone is insufficient to enhance atherogenesis. For example, in an apoE-deficient murine model, both HSV-1 and murine herpes virus 68 (MHV-68) infection induced a systemic immune response (138). However, only MHV-68 message was found in aortic tissue and only MHV-68 accelerated atherothrombosis. Thus, additional cofactors must be present for viral infection not directly involving the arterial wall to promote atherothrombosis.

ANIMAL MODELS OF VIRAL ATHEROTHROMBOSIS

Animal models may be useful for determining the potential for infectious agents to cause or to promote atherothrombosis and for assessing the role of antibiotic or antiviral therapy. The association of MDV infection and atherothrombosis in chickens, first discovered more than 50 years ago, provided the first experimental "proof-of-principle" for a viral cause of atherothrombosis and has remained an important animal model of infection-related atherothrombosis (117,139). These early studies demonstrated conclusively that in a normocholesterolemic animal model, a herpes virus can be an etiologic vector in inducing vascular lesions pathologically and biochemically resembling atherothrombosis, and specifically it can alter arterial wall lipid metabolism, leading to cholesterol deposition (22,24,25).

Additional animal models subsequently have emerged. These have helped greatly in sorting out potential mechanisms of atherogenesis, as noted earlier in this chapter. For example, CMV infection of rats has allowed the discovery of a number of potential atherogenic mechanisms, including induction of growth factor expression, atherogenesis at a distance, and allograft atherothrombosis (85,137).

Murine models of CMV infection have contributed significantly to research advances in recent years. BALB/c mice inoculated with murine cytomegalovirus (MCMV) express viral antigens in aortic endothelial and SMCs and accumulate inflammatory cells at sites of viral antigen expression (140). Immunosuppression increased antigen expression and the size of early atherothrombotic plaques. In apoE knockout mice, atherothrombotic lesion area was increased (by 84%; $p < 0.001$) by infection with MCMV and was not further increased by coinfection with Cpn (141). A concurrent report from NIH confirmed CMV promotion of atherothrombosis in the apoE knockout model and found that augmented atherogenesis at 16 weeks was preceded by measurable levels of circulating interferon-γ (IFN-γ) at 4 weeks. A subsequent study in this model by the NIH group found that serum from CMV-infected mice induced monocyte chemoattractant protein-1 expression by endothelial cells (142). Monocyte chemoattractant protein-1 expression was found to be due, at least in part, to the presence in the serum of INF-γ.

Some work also has been done with HSV infections of mice. Alber and coworkers (143) assessed the effect of MHV-68 infection in apoE knockout mice. Atheroma formation was found to be accelerated over a 24-week period in infected compared with control mice. Acceleration was reduced by antiviral drug administration. Viral mRNA was present in aortic tissue before lesion development. These results suggested a causal rather than "bystander" role for MHV. In a subsequent study in this model, the effects of HSV-1 and MHV-68 were compared (138). Both viruses induced cell and humoral immune responses. However, in contrast to MHV-68 infection, neither viral message in aorta nor accelerated atherothrombosis followed HSV-1 infection. Thus, systemic herpes virus infection alone is not sufficient to enhance atherogenesis; specific vascular infection–induced mechanisms are required in apoE-deficient mice.

Despite the elegant contributions of these models, it should be stressed that no animal model of atherothrombosis exactly mimics or can reliably predict human disease. Therefore, these and many other studies, although generally supportive of the infectious hypothesis of atherothrombosis, do not by themselves prove that vascular infection with CMV, HSV, or other viruses plays a causal role in human disease.

THERAPEUTIC INITIATIVES TARGETING VIRUSES AND RELATED RISK FACTORS

Antiviral Agents and Therapeutic Trials

No antiviral drug trials for prevention of CHD have been conducted for native CAD. However, in the special circumstance of cardiac allograft atherothrombosis, antiviral therapy has shown favorable effects in an animal model (74), suggesting clinical therapeutic potential (e.g., with ganciclovir). In clinical experience, however, CMV disease is unaltered by 4 weeks of ganciclovir prophylaxis in seronegative recipients of hearts from seropositive donors (D^+/R^-). However, a historically controlled experience at Stanford has suggested benefit from a combination of ganciclovir plus CMV hyperimmune globulin (CMVIG) (144). A study population receiving CMVIG (n = 80; 27 heart transplant [D^+/R^-] and 53 heart–lung and lung transplant recipients [R^+ and/or D^+]) were matched with historical control subjects transplanted within the preceding 2 to 3 years. CMVIG-treated patients showed lower rejection rates and greater CMV-free and total survival rates compared with control subjects treated with ganciclovir alone. Important to this discussion, coronary artery intimal thickness (by intravascular ultrasound) was less in the patients receiving CMVIG. These observations suggest a role for CMV-associated immune activation as a cause of transplant-related atherothrombosis; they also support an aggressive preventive approach with anti-CMV therapy, which should be confirmed by a prospective, randomized trial.

Limitations of existing antiviral therapies has spurred the development of new human CMV inhibitors (145). Several of these novel, effective compounds are undergoing preclinical and early clinical evaluation, and some of these might be considered for future trials of atherothrombosis prevention and treatment.

Vaccine Studies

Of recent interest, vaccination against influenza has been reported to reduce the risk for recurrent MI (146). A case–control study was performed on 218 patients with CHD in a single center during the influenza season. The relative risk for MI, adjusted for multiple baseline variables, was found to be 0.33 (95% CI 0.13–0.82; p = 0.02). The mechanism of benefit was not determined, but nine potential antiinflammatory and antiinfectious effects, both viral-specific and nonspecific, were proposed.

Another study compared vaccination histories between 342 subjects who experienced sudden cardiac death in King County, WA, with 549 randomly selected control subjects (147). Those who had received vaccination against influenza within the previous year were 51% less likely to experience primary cardiac arrest. Because sudden cardiac death is commonly precipitated by an acute ischemic event, this study seems to support a protective effect of vaccination against acute coronary syndromes.

However, a more recent study from the same geographic area came to a different conclusion (148). This study cohort consisted of 1,378 Group Health Cooperative enrollees who survived a first MI between 1992 and 1996. Recurrent coronary events, influenza vaccinations, and other covariates were identified from hospital charts and health data systems.

A total of 127 recurrent coronary events were identified during a median of 2.3-years follow-up. Influenza vaccination was not associated with the risk for recurrent coronary events overall (adjusted HR 1.18, 95% CI 0.79–1.75) or during the periods of expected influenza activity (November through April; HR 1.06, 95% CI 0.63–1.78).

In contrast, a smaller but prospective, randomized pilot study from South America reported a beneficial outcome of vaccination after acute coronary syndromes or angioplasty (149). The study enrolled 200 patients with recent MI and 101 elective angioplasty/stent patients and randomized them to single blind influenza vaccination or a control group. After 6 months, CV death had occurred in 2% of the vaccine group compared with 8% of the control group (relative risk, 0.25; 95% CI 0.07–0.86; p = 0.01). The composite end point of death, reinfarction, and rehospitalization for ischemia occurred in 11% of the vaccine group compared with 23% in the control group (p = 0.009).

Others also have proposed vaccination as a therapeutic strategy to prevent atherothrombosis progression and acute coronary syndromes (150), and future vaccine trials against purported viral (and bacterial) pathogens can be expected. Currently, the role of influenza vaccination to prevent acute ischemic events is uncertain and cannot be viewed as clinically established, but it is a worthy topic for research efforts (including adequately powered, double-blind, clinical trials).

Risk Reduction with Standard Coronary Heart Disease Preventive Therapy

Given the absence of proven antiinfective or vaccine therapies for viral-associated CHD risk, we asked whether standard preventive strategies—for example, lipid reduction using a statin (3-hydroxy-3-methylglutaryl coenzyme A reductase inhibitor)—might impact this risk. Because statins have well established antiinflammatory effects, which may be in part "lipid-independent," and CMV may impart risk by stimulating an inflammatory response, we postulated that statin therapy might reduce this associated risk. We studied 2,315 patients with CAD who had plasma drawn at baseline angiography, anti-CMV IgG antibody, and CRP levels and were followed for an average of 2.4 years (151). In untreated patients, mortality increased progressively with the presence of either high CRP or seropositivity to the presence of both. In contrast, those patients prescribed statin therapy at baseline showed "normalization" of risk, similar to those without a positive marker (Fig. 37–4). Although observational, these results support aggressive application of standard preventive therapy, at least with statins, in the setting of CAD with CMV seropositivity. Whether other standard preventive therapies (e.g., β-blockers, angiotensin-converting enzyme inhibitors, smoking cessation) also have greater therapeutic potential in the same setting is uncertain but should be explored. Aspirin attenuates CMV infectivity and gene expression in SMCs by COX-2 inhibition and, hence, might be

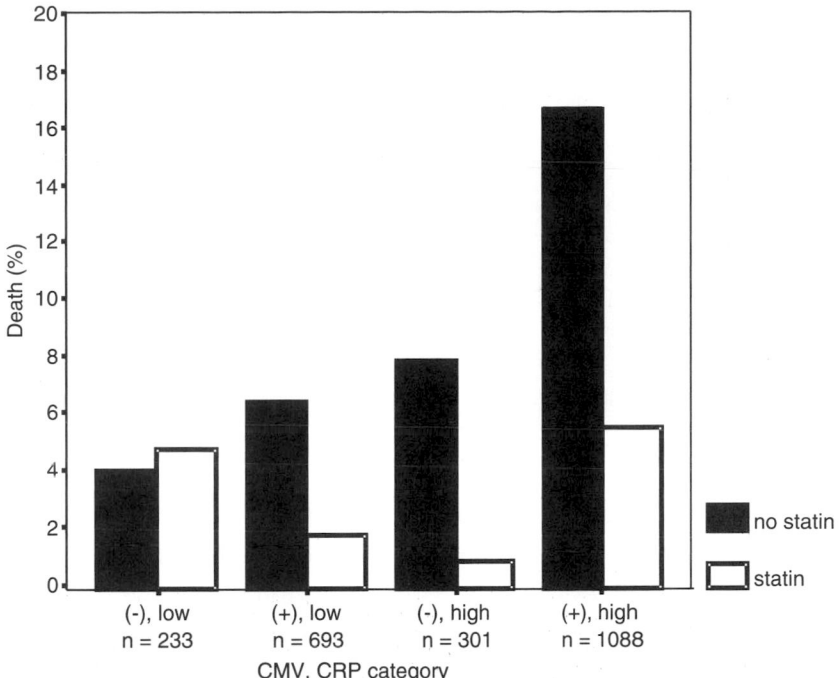

FIG. 37–4. Interaction of statin therapy with cytomegalovirus (CMV) seropositivity and C-reactive protein (CRP) for mortality reductions in patients with coronary artery disease (CAD). Death rates for patients with CAD with or without prescribed statin therapy by categories of CMV and CRP are shown. (Reprinted with permission from Horne BD, Muhlestein JB, Carlquist JF, et al. Statin therapy interacts with cytomegalovirus seropositivity and high C-reactive protein in reducing mortality among patients with angiographically significant coronary disease. *Circulation* 2003;107:258–263.)

postulated to be of particular value for suppressing CMV-related atherogenesis (96).

CURRENT STATE OF KNOWLEDGE AND FUTURE EXPECTATIONS

Expectations of Antiinfective Trials

Enthusiastic expectations of antiviral and antibiotic trials for proving the infection hypothesis of atherothrombosis and establishing therapy must be tempered by a number of limitations and uncertainties (Table 37–4). Negative outcomes might be explained not only by an incorrect hypothesis (infection does not cause CHD) and an inadequate study size or design, but also by an ineffective or inappropriately timed antiinfective regimen. Prevention or elimination of vascular infection with antiinfectives also could be problematic if organisms residing in circulating monocytes, which can carry and disseminate them to the vessel wall, are treatment resistant. Negative studies also might be explained if reactivation of agents from a persistent state, production of proinflammatory mediators, and promotion of atherothrombosis can occur despite an "effective" course of antiinfectives.

However, if studies are positive, the hypothesis also is not entirely proved: a nonspecific antiinflammatory effect, or an antiinfective action against another causal or cocausal or-

ganism, might be operative. This uncertainty already has arisen in attempts to explain the benefits of minocycline therapy for rheumatoid arthritis (152).

In summary, the infectious theory of atherothrombosis does not lend itself well to proof using Koch's classical pos-

TABLE 37–4. *Potential implications and limitations of antiinfective trials*

Negative trial
• Infection hypothesis false?
• False negative; study underpowered
• Treatment incorrect: too short, dose inadequate, drug ineffective
• Treatment-resistant organism (e.g., agent in persistent state) or resistant reservoir (e.g., monocytes/macrophages)
• Wrong organism targeted; multiple organisms involved
• Wrong stage of disease targeted (late vs. early, acute vs. chronic)
• Wrong population tested (what markers predict active/latent atherogenic infection?)
Positive trial
• Infection hypothesis true?
• False positive (small study, chance result)
• Nonspecific antiinflammatory effect
• Nonspecific antiinfective effect

tulates. Thus, new and innovative experimental approaches will be required to gain adequate insight into the role of infection in atherothrombosis and its therapy.

SUMMARY AND CONCLUSIONS

The recognition that atherothrombosis is inflammatory has raised the intriguing question of the inflammatory triggers. Indeed, inflammation underlies atherothrombosis at each stage, including initiation, progression, and advanced disease where plaque instability and disruption lead to acute coronary syndromes. Although noninfectious factors (e.g., oxidized LDL) clearly play a proinflammatory role, interest has been renewed regarding the possibility that infection might be among these triggers.

The finding of Cpn, CMV, and other herpes viruses within human atherothrombotic tissue has raised this issue of infection for human atherothrombotic disease and has begged the question of "innocent bystander versus dangerous pathogen." Certainly, cellular and molecular studies have demonstrated that infectious agents *can* activate the major pathways involved in atherothrombosis and vascular thrombosis. Animal models, beginning with Marek's disease, also show the potential for infection to accelerate and antiinfective treatment to suppress atherothrombosis. CMV and other herpes viruses can stimulate inflammation, facilitate lipid accumulation and matrix degradation, provoke endothelial dysfunction, promote thrombosis, and promote smooth muscle accumulation—all well recognized atherogenic mechanisms. How viral infection impacts common varieties of clinical atherothrombosis remains uncertain, although current evidence is supportive of a role for CMV in cardiac allograft vasculopathy.

Serologic studies have shown high antibody prevalence for several agents (e.g., CMV, HSV) among those with coronary and other vascular diseases. Nevertheless, seropositivity indicates past exposure, not active infection; prevalence is high among the general population; associations have been variable; and confounding has been a concern. Aggregate exposure to many candidate infectious agents ("pathogen burden") appears to be a stronger, more consistent risk marker. Indeed, viral serologies have more consistently contributed to risk prediction than bacterial markers (34,35). However, better markers than serology of active or latent, as opposed to past, resolved infection are clearly needed. HSPs and anti-HSP antibodies are promising possibilities.

Although CMV (a viral atherogen candidate) and Cpn (as a bacterial atherogen candidate) have received the most attention as infectious risk factors, others are likely involved, including common nonvascular infections acting at a distance through proinflammatory and prothrombotic factors.

In the next few years, antiinfective and vaccine trials targeted against viruses will be added to adequately powered antibiotic trials to better assess the therapeutic potential against several potentially atherogenic infective agents.

These will provide additional insight into the role of infection in atherothrombosis and its therapy. However, these trials also will have limitations (Table 37–4). Meanwhile, standard preventive therapies (i.e., lipid reduction with statins, aspirin) should be encouraged and may have particular value for reducing infection (CMV)-related risk (151). Currently, specific antiinfective therapies directed at prevention of coronary heart disease and acute coronary syndromes are unproven and inappropriate. In contrast, innovative research efforts are to be encouraged (153).

REFERENCES

1. American Heart Association. *2002 Heart and stroke statistical update.* Dallas, TX: American Heart Association, 2001.
2. Wilson PW, D'Agostino RB, Levy D, et al. Prediction of coronary heart disease using risk factor categories. *Circulation* 1998;97:1837–1847.
3. Ross R. Atherosclerosis—an inflammatory disease. *N Engl J Med* 1999;340:115–126.
4. Morrow DA, Ridker PM. Inflammation in cardiovascular disease. In: Topol EJ, ed. *Textbook of cardiovascular medicine, Vol 2.* Cedar Knolls, NJ: Lippincott Williams & Wilkins, 1999:1–12.
5. Davies MJ, Thomas AC. Plaque fissuring—the cause of acute myocardial infarction, sudden ischaemic death, and crescendo angina. *Br Heart J* 1985;53:363–373.
6. van der Wal AC, Becker AE, van der Loos CM, et al. Site of intimal rupture or erosion of thrombosed coronary atherosclerotic plaques is characterized by an inflammatory process irrespective of the dominant plaque morphology. *Circulation* 1994;89:36–44.
7. Fuster V, Lewis A. Conner Memorial Lecture. Mechanisms leading to myocardial infarction: insights from studies of vascular biology. *Circulation* 1994;90:2126–2146.
8. Shah PK. Plaque disruption and coronary thrombosis: new insight into pathogenesis and prevention. *Clin Cardiol* 1997;20:II-38–II-44.
9. Libby P. Molecular bases of the acute coronary syndromes. *Circulation* 1995;91:2844–2850.
10. Shah PK, Galis ZS. Matrix metalloproteinase hypothesis of plaque rupture: players keep piling up but questions remain. *Circulation* 2001;104:1878–1880.
11. Chyu KY, Shah PK. The role of inflammation in plaque disruption and thrombosis. *Rev Cardiovasc Med* 2001;2:82–91.
12. Libby P, Ridker PM, Maseri A. Inflammation and atherosclerosis. *Circulation* 2002;105:1135–1143.
13. Libby P, Egan D, Skarlatos S. Roles of infectious agents in atherosclerosis and restenosis: an assessment of the evidence and need for future research. *Circulation* 1997;96:4095–4103.
14. Epstein SE, Zhou YF, Zhu J. Infection and atherosclerosis: emerging mechanistic paradigms. *Circulation* 1999;100:e20–e28.
15. Shah PK. Plaque disruption and thrombosis: potential role of inflammation and infection. *Cardiol Clin* 2000;17:271–281.
16. Weyand CM, Goronzy JJ, Liuzzo G, et al. T-cell immunity in acute coronary syndromes. *Mayo Clin Proc* 2001;76:1011–1020.
17. Shah PK. Link between infection and atherosclerosis: who are the culprits: viruses, bacteria, both, or neither? *Circulation* 2001;103:5–6.
18. Numano F, Kishi Y, Tanaka A, et al. Inflammation and atherosclerosis. Atherosclerotic lesions in Takayasu arteritis. *Ann NY Acad Sci* 2000;902:65–76.
19. Kuvin JT, Kimmelstiel CD. Infectious causes of atherosclerosis. *Am Heart J* 1999;137:216–226.
20. Osler W. Diseases of the arteries. In: Osler W, ed. *Modern medicine: its practice and theory.* Philadelphia: Lea and Febiger, 1908:429–447.
21. Paterson JC, Cottral GE. Experimental coronary sclerosis: lymphomatosis as a cause of coronary sclerosis in chickens. *Arch Pathol* 1950;49:699–709.
22. Fabricant CG, Fabricant J, Litrenta MM, et al. Virus-induced atherosclerosis. *J Exp Med* 1978;148:335–340.
23. Minick CR, Fabricant CG, Fabricant J, et al. Atheroarteriosclerosis induced by infection with a herpesvirus. *Am J Pathol* 1979;96:673–706.
24. Fabricant CG, Hajjar DP, Minick CR, et al. Herpesvirus infection en-

hances cholesterol and cholesteryl ester accumulation in cultured arterial smooth muscle cells. *Am J Pathol* 1981;105:176–184.

25. Hajjar DP, Fabricant CG, Minick CR, et al. Virus-induced atherosclerosis. Herpesvirus infection alters aortic cholesterol metabolism and accumulation. *Am J Pathol* 1986;122:62–70.

26. Hajjar DP, Pomerantz KB, et al. Herpes simplex virus infection in human arterial cells. Implications in arteriosclerosis. *J Clin Invest* 1987;80:1317–1321.

27. Melnick JL, Petrie BL, Dreesman GR, et al. Cytomegalovirus antigen within human arterial smooth muscle cells. *Lancet* 1983;2:644–647.

28. Pesonen E, Siitonen O. Acute myocardial infarction precipitated by infectious disease. *Am Heart J* 1981;101:512–513.

29. Spodick DH, Flessas AP, Johnson MM. Association of acute respiratory symptoms with onset of acute myocardial infarction: prospective investigation of 150 consecutive patients and matched control patients. *Am J Cardiol* 1984;53:481–482.

30. Mattila KJ. Viral and bacterial infections in patients with acute myocardial infarction. *J Intern Med* 1989;225:293–296.

31. Mattila KJ, Valtonen VV, Rasi RP, et al. Association between dental health and acute myocardial infarction. *BMJ* 1989;298:779–781.

32. Melnick JL, Adam E, DeBakey ME. Possible role of cytomegalovirus in atherogenesis. *JAMA* 1990;263:2204–2207.

33. Kaner RJ, Hajjar DP. Viral activation of thrombo-atherosclerosis. In: Fuster V, Topol EJ, eds. *Atherosclerosis and coronary artery disease.* New York: Raven Press, 1996:569–583.

34. Rupprecht HJ, Blankenberg S, Bickel C, et al. Impact of viral and bacterial infectious burden on long-term prognosis in patients with coronary artery disease. *Circulation* 2001;104:25–31.

35. Zhu J, Nieto FJ, Horne BD, et al. Prospective study of pathogen burden and risk of myocardial infarction or death. *Circulation* 2001;103:45–51.

36. Zhu J, Quyyumi AA, Norman JE, et al. The possible role of hepatitis A virus in the pathogenesis of atherosclerosis. *J Infect Dis* 2000;182: 1583–1587.

37. Krishnaswamy G, Chi DS, Kelley JL, et al. The cardiovascular and metabolic complications of HIV infection. *Cardiol Rev* 2000;8: 260–268.

38. Adam E, Melnick JL, Probesfield JL, et al. High levels of cytomegalovirus antibody in patients requiring vascular surgery for atherosclerosis. *Lancet* 1987;2:291–293.

39. Ridker PM, Hennekens CH, Stampfer MJ, et al. Prospective study of herpes simplex virus, cytomegalovirus, and the risk of future myocardial infarction and stroke. *Circulation* 1998;98:2796–2799.

40. Anderson JL, Carlquist JF, Muhlestein JB, et al. Evaluation of C-reactive protein, an inflammatory marker, and infectious serology as risk factors for coronary artery disease and myocardial infarction. *J Am Coll Cardiol* 1998;32:35–41.

41. Strachan DP, Carrington D, Mendall MA, et al. Cytomegalovirus seropositivity and incident ischaemic heart disease in the Caerphilly prospective heart disease study. *Heart* 1999;81:248–251.

42. Roivainen M, Viik-Kajander M, Palosuo T, et al. Infections, inflammation, and the risk of coronary heart disease. *Circulation* 2000; 101:252–257.

43. Ridker PM, Hennekens CH, Buring JE, et al. Baseline IgG antibody titers to Chlamydia pneumoniae, Helicobacter pylori, herpes simplex virus, and cytomegalovirus and the risk for cardiovascular disease in women. *Ann Intern Med* 1999;131:573–577.

44. Danesh J. Coronary heart disease, Helicobacter pylori, dental disease, Chlamydia pneumoniae, and cytomegalovirus: meta-analyses of prospective studies. *Am Heart J* 1999;138:S434–S437.

45. Sorlie PD, Adam E, Melnick SL, et al. Cytomegalovirus/herpesvirus and carotid atherosclerosis: the ARIC Study. *J Med Virol* 1994;42:33–37.

46. Muhlestein JB, Horne BD, Carlquist JF, et al. Cytomegalovirus seropositivity and C-reactive protein have independent and combined predictive value for mortality in patients with angiographically demonstrated coronary artery disease. *Circulation* 2000;102:1917–1923.

47. Blankenberg S, Rupprecht HJ, Bickel C, et al. Cytomegalovirus infection with interleukin-6 response predicts cardiac mortality in patients with coronary artery disease. *Circulation* 2001;103:2915–2921.

48. Smieja M, Gnarpe H, Lonn E, et al. Multiple infections and subsequent cardiovascular events in the Heart Outcomes Prevention Evaluation (HOPE) study. *Circulation* 2003;107:251–257.

49. Zhu J, Quyyumi AA, Norman JE, et al. Cytomegalovirus in the pathogenesis of atherosclerosis: the role of inflammation as reflected by elevated C-reactive protein levels. *J Am Coll Cardiol* 1999;34:1738–1743.

50. Zhu J, Shearer GM, Norman JE, et al. Host response to cytomegalovirus infection as a determinant of susceptibility to coronary artery disease: sex-based differences in inflammation and type of immune response. *Circulation* 2000;102:2491–2496.

51. Danesh J, Wong Y, Ward M, et al. Chronic infection with Helicobacter pylori, Chlamydia pneumoniae, or cytomegalovirus: population based study of coronary heart disease. *Heart* 1999;81:245–247.

52. Buffon A, Liuzzo G, Biasucci LM, et al. Preprocedural serum levels of C-reactive protein predict early complications and late restenosis after coronary angioplasty. *J Am Coll Cardiol* 1999;34:1512–1521.

53. Horne BD, Muhlestein JB, Stroebel GG, et al. Greater pathogen burden but not elevated C-reactive protein increases the risk of clinical restenosis following percutaneous coronary intervention. *Am Heart J* 2002;144:491–500.

54. Zhou YF, Csako G, Grayston JT, et al. Lack of association of restenosis following coronary angioplasty with elevated C-reactive protein levels or seropositivity to Chlamydia pneumoniae. *Am J Cardiol* 1999;84:595–598,A8.

55. Zhou YF, Leon MB, Waclawiw MA, et al. Association between prior cytomegalovirus infection and the risk of restenosis after coronary atherectomy. *N Engl J Med* 1996;335:624–630.

56. Muhlestein JB, Carlquist JF, Horne BD, et al. No association between prior cytomegalovirus infection and the risk of clinical restenosis after percutaneous coronary interventions. *Circulation* 1997;96:I-650.

57. Smieja M, Chong S, Natarajan M, et al. Circulating nucleic acids of Chlamydia pneumoniae and cytomegalovirus in patients undergoing coronary angiography. *J Clin Microbiol* 2001;39:596–600.

58. Zhu J, Quyyumi AA, Norman JE, et al. Effects of total pathogen burden on coronary artery disease risk and C-reactive protein levels. *Am J Cardiol* 2000;85:140–146.

59. Muhlestein JB, Anderson JL. Infectious serology and atherosclerosis: how burdensome is the risk. *Circulation* 2003;107:220–222.

60. Chiu B, Viira E, Tucker W, et al. Chlamydia pneumoniae, cytomegalovirus, and herpes simplex virus in atherosclerosis of the carotid artery. *Circulation* 1997;96:2144–2148.

61. Yamashiroya HM, Ghosh L, Yang R, et al. Herpesviridae in the coronary arteries and aorta of young trauma victims. *Am J Pathol* 1988;130:71–79.

62. Gyorkey F, Melnick JL, Guinn GA, et al. Herpes viridae in the endothelial and smooth muscle cells of the proximal aorta of atherosclerotic patients. *Exp Mol Pathol* 1984;40:328–329.

63. Benditt EP, Barrett T, MacDougal JK. Viruses in the etiology of atherosclerosis. *Proc Natl Acad Sci USA* 1983;80:6386–6389.

64. Petrie BL, Melnick JL, Adam E, et al. Nucleic acid sequences of cytomegalovirus in cells cultured from human arterial tissue. *J Infect Dis* 1987;155:158–159.

65. Hendrix MG, Dormans PH, Kitslaar P, et al. The presence of cytomegalovirus nucleic acids in arterial walls of atherosclerotic and nonatherosclerotic patients. *Am J Pathol* 1989;134:1151–1157.

66. Hendrix MG, Salimans MM, van Boven CP, et al. High prevalence of latently present cytomegalovirus in arterial walls of patients suffering from grade III atherosclerosis. *Am J Pathol* 1990;136:23–28.

67. Hu W, Liu J, Niu S, et al. Prevalence of CMV in arterial walls and leukocytes in patients with atherosclerosis. *Chin Med J* 2001;114:1208–1210.

68. Hendrix MG, Daemen M, Bruggeman CA. Cytomegalovirus nucleic acid distribution within the human vascular tree. *Am J Pathol* 1991;138:563–567.

69. Horvath R, Cerny J, Benedik JJ, et al. The possible role of human cytomegalovirus (HCMV) in the origin of atherosclerosis. *J Clin Virol* 2000;16:17–24.

70. Gao SZ, Alderman EL, Schroeder JS, et al. Accelerated coronary vascular disease in the heart transplant patient: coronary arteriographic findings. *J Am Coll Cardiol* 1988;12:334–340.

71. Grattan M. Accelerated graft atherosclerosis following cardiac transplantation: clinical perspectives. *Clin Cardiol* 1991;14:16–20.

72. McDonald K, Rector TS, Braulin EA, et al. Association of coronary artery disease in cardiac transplant recipients with cytomegalovirus infection. *Am J Cardiol* 1989;64:359–362.

73. Hruban RH, Wu TC, Beschorner WE, et al. Cytomegalovirus nucleic acids in allografted hearts. *Hum Pathol* 1990;21:981–982.

74. Lemstrom K, Sihvola R, Bruggeman C, et al. Cytomegalovirus infection-enhanced cardiac allograft vasculopathy is abolished by DHPG prophylaxis in the rat. *Circulation* 1997;95:2614–2616.

75. Speir E, Modali R, Huang ES, et al. Potential role of human cy-

tomegalovirus and p53 interaction in coronary restenosis. *Science* 1994;265:391–394.

76. Zhou YF, Guetta E, Yu ZX, et al. Human cytomegalovirus increases modified low density lipoprotein uptake and scavenger receptor mRNA expression in vascular smooth muscle cells. *J Clin Invest* 1996;98:2129–2138.

77. Hunter GC, Henderson AM, Westerband A, et al. The contribution of inducible nitric oxide and cytomegalovirus to the stability of complex carotid plaque. *J Vasc Surg* 1999;30:36–49.

78. Muhlestein JB. Chronic infection and coronary artery disease. *Med Clin North Am* 2000;84:123–148.

79. Kovacs A, Weber ML, Burns LJ, et al. Cytoplasmic sequestration of p53 in cytomegalovirus-infected human endothelial cells. *Am J Pathol* 1996;149:1531–1539.

80. Minton EJ, Tysoe C, Sinclair JH, et al. Human cytomegalovirus infection of the monocyte/macrophage lineage in bone marrow. *J Virol* 1994;68:4017–4021.

81. Kondo K, Kaneshima H, Mocarski ES. Human cytomegalovirus latent infection of granulocyte-macrophage progenitors. *Proc Natl Acad Sci USA* 1994;91:11879–11883.

82. Ibanez CE, Schrier R, Ghazal P, et al. Human cytomegalovirus productively infects primary differentiated macrophages. *J Virol* 1991;65:6581–6588.

83. Guetta E, Guetta V, Shibutani T, et al. Monocytes harboring cytomegalovirus: interactions with endothelial cells, smooth muscle cells, and oxidized low-density lipoprotein. Possible mechanisms for activating virus delivered by monocytes to sites of vascular injury. *Circ Res* 1997;81:8–16.

84. Zhou YF, Yu ZX, Wanishsawad C, et al. The immediate early gene products of human cytomegalovirus increase vascular smooth muscle cell migration, proliferation, and expression of PDGF beta-receptor. *Biochem Biophys Res Commun* 1999;256:608–613.

85. Lemstrom KB, Aho PT, Bruggeman CA, et al. Cytomegalovirus infection enhances mRNA expression of platelet-derived growth factor-BB and transforming growth factor-beta 1 in rat aortic allografts. Possible mechanism for cytomegalovirus-enhanced graft arteriosclerosis. *Arterioscler Thromb* 1994;14:2043–2052.

86. Horne BD, Carlquist JF, Habashi J, et al. Cytomegalovirus infection of human macrophages induces increased expression of scavenger receptor CD36 gene and cell surface glycoprotein. *J Am Coll Cardiol* 2000;35:268A(abst).

87. Guetta E, Scarpati EM, DiCorleto PE. Effect of cytomegalovirus immediate early gene products on endothelial cell gene activity. *Cardiovasc Res* 2001;50:538–546.

88. Friedman HM, Macarak EJ, MacGregor RR, et al. Virus infection of endothelial cells. *J Infect Dis* 1981;143:266–273.

89. Lashgari JS, Friedman HM, Kefalides NA. Suppression of matrix protein synthesis by herpes simplex virus in bovine smooth muscle cells. *Biochem Biophys Res Commun* 1987;143:145–151.

90. Ho DD, Rota TR, Anderews CA, et al. Replication of human cytomegalovirus in endothelial cells. *J Infect Dis* 1984;150:956–957.

91. Tumilowicz JJ, Gawlik ME, Powell BB, et al. Replication of cytomegalovirus in human arterial smooth muscle cells. *J Virol* 1985;56:839–845.

92. Fenwick ML, Clark J. Early and delayed shut off of host protein synthesis in cells infected with herpes simplex virus. *J Gen Virol* 1982;61:121–125.

93. Grundy JE, Downes KL. Up-regulation of LFA-3 and ICAM-1 on the surface of fibroblasts infected with cytomegalovirus. *Immunology* 1993;78:405–412.

94. Span AH, Mullers W, Miltenburg AM, et al. Cytomegalovirus induced PMN adherence in relation to an ELAM-1 antigen present on infected endothelial cell monolayers. *Immunology* 1991;72:355–360.

95. Burns LJ, Pooley JC, Walsh DJ, et al. Intercellular adhesion molecule-1 expression in endothelial cells is activated by cytomegalovirus immediate early proteins. *Transplantation* 1999;67:137–144.

96. Speir E, Yu ZX, Ferrans VJ, et al. Aspirin attenuates cytomegalovirus infectivity and gene expression mediated by cyclooxygenase-2 in coronary artery smooth muscle cells. *Circ Res* 1998;83:210–216.

97. Speir E. Cytomegalovirus gene regulation by reactive oxygen species. Agents in atherosclerosis. *Ann NY Acad Sci* 2000;899:363–374.

98. Dudding L, Haskel S, Clark BD, et al. Cytomegalovirus infection stimulates expression of monocyte associated mediator genes. *J Immunol* 1989;143:3343–3352.

99. Smith PD, Saini SS, Raffeld M, et al. Cytomegalovirus induction of tumor necrosis factor-alpha by human monocytes and mucosal macrophages. *J Clin Invest* 1992;90:1642–1648.

100. Gosselin J, Flamand L, D'Addario M, et al. Infection of peripheral blood mononuclear cells by herpes simplex and Epstein-Barr viruses. Differential induction of interleukin 6 and tumor necrosis factor-alpha. *J Clin Invest* 1992;89:1849–1856.

101. Dengler TJ, Raftery MJ, Werle M, et al. Cytomegalovirus infection of vascular cells induces expression of pro-inflammatory adhesion molecules by paracrine action of secreted interleukin-1 beta. *Transplantation* 2000;69:1160–1168.

102. Kiechl S, Egger G, Mayr M, et al. Chronic infections and the risk of carotid atherosclerosis: prospective results from a large population study. *Circulation* 2001;103:1064–1070.

103. Chandra HR, Choudhary N, O'Neill C, et al. Chlamydia pneumoniae exposure and inflammatory markers in acute coronary syndrome (CIMACS). *Am J Cardiol* 2001;88:214–218.

104. Kiechl S, Lorenz E, Reindl M, et al. Toll-like receptor 4 polymorphisms and atherogenesis. *N Engl J Med* 2002;347:185–192.

105. Dechend R, Maass M, Gieffers J, et al. Chlamydia pneumoniae infection of vascular smooth muscle and endothelial cells activates NF-kappa B and induces tissue factor and PAI-1 expression: a potential link to accelerated arteriosclerosis. *Circulation* 1999;100:1369–1373.

106. Oldstone MB. Molecular mimicry and autoimmune disease. *Cell* 1987;50:819–820.

107. Bachmaier K, Neu N, de la Maza LM, et al. Chlamydia infections and heart disease linked through antigenic mimicry. *Science* 1999;283:1335–1339.

108. Epstein SE, Zhu J, Burnett MS, et al. Infection and atherosclerosis: potential roles of pathogen burden and molecular mimicry. *Arterioscler Thromb Vasc Biol* 2000;20:1417–1420.

109. Xu Q. Role of heat shock proteins in atherosclerosis. *Arterioscler Thromb Vasc Biol* 2002;22:1547–1559.

110. Burian K, Kis Z, Virok D, et al. Independent and joint effects of antibodies to human heat-shock protein 60 and Chlamydia pneumoniae infection in the development of coronary atherosclerosis. *Circulation* 2001;103:1503–1508.

111. Mayr M, Metzler B, Kiechl S, et al. Endothelial cytotoxicity mediated by serum antibodies to heat shock proteins of Escherichia coli and Chlamydia pneumoniae: immune reactions to heat shock proteins as a possible link between infection and atherosclerosis. *Circulation* 1999;99:1560–1566.

112. Schett G, Xu Q, Amberger A, et al. Autoantibodies against heat shock protein 60 mediate endothelial cytotoxicity. *J Clin Invest* 1995;96:2569–2577.

113. Xu Q, Willeit J, Marosi M, et al. Association of serum antibodies to heat-shock protein 65 with carotid atherosclerosis. *Lancet* 1993;341:255–259.

114. Xu Q, Kleindienst R, Schett G, et al. Regression of arteriosclerotic lesions induced by immunization with heat shock protein 65-containing material in normocholesterolemic, but not hypercholesterolemic, rabbits. *Atherosclerosis* 1996;123:145–155.

115. Birnie DH, Holme ER, McKay IC, et al. Association between antibodies to heat shock protein 65 and coronary atherosclerosis. Possible mechanism of action of Helicobacter pylori and other bacterial infections in increasing cardiovascular risk. *Eur Heart J* 1998;19:387–394.

116. George J, Shoenfeld Y, Afek A, et al. Enhanced fatty streak formation in C57BL/6J mice by immunization with heat shock protein-65. *Arterioscler Thromb Vasc Biol* 1999;19:505–510.

117. Fabricant CG, Fabricant J. Atherosclerosis induced by infection with Marek's disease herpesvirus in chickens. *Am Heart J* 1999;138:S465–S468.

118. Vercellotti GM. Effects of viral activation of the vessel wall on inflammation and thrombosis. *Blood Coagul Fibrinolysis* 1998;9:S3–S6.

119. Visser MR, Tracy PB, Vercellotti GM, et al. Enhanced thrombin generation and platelet binding on herpes simplex virus-infected endothelium. *Proc Natl Acad Sci USA* 1988;85:8227–8230.

120. Key NS, Vercellotti GM, Winkelmann JC, et al. Infection of vascular endothelial cells with herpes simplex virus enhances tissue factor activity and reduces thrombomodulin expression. *Proc Natl Acad Sci USA* 1990;87:7095–7099.

121. Etingin OR, Silverstein RL, Friedman HM, et al. Viral activation of the coagulation cascade: molecular interactions at the surface of infected endothelial cells. *Cell* 1990;61:657–662.

122. van Dam-Mieras MC, Muller AD, van Hinsbergh VW, et al. The procoagulant response of cytomegalovirus infected endothelial cells.
Thromb Haemost 1992;68:364–370.

123. Prasad A, Zhu J, Mincemoyer R, et al. Cytomegalovirus infection is a
determinant of endothelial dysfunction and coronary flow reserve.
Circulation 1998;98:I-244(abst).

124. Prasad A, Zhu J, Halcox JP, et al. Predisposition to atherosclerosis by
infections: role of endothelial dysfunction. *Circulation* 2002;106:
184–190.

125. Nicholson AC, Hajjar DP. Herpesviruses and thrombosis: activation
of coagulation on the endothelium. *Clin Chim Acta* 1999;286:23–29.

126. Span AH, Van Boven CP, Bruggeman CA. The effect of cytomegalovirus infection on the adherence of polymorphonuclear
leukocytes to endothelial cells. *Eur J Clin Invest* 1989;19:542–548.

127. Benditt EP, Benditt JM. Evidence for a monoclonal origin of human
atherosclerotic plaques. *Proc Natl Acad Sci USA* 1973;70:1753–1756.

128. Levine AJ. p53, the cellular gatekeeper for growth and division. *Cell*
1997;88:323–331.

129. Yonemitsu Y, Kaneda Y, Tanaka S, et al. Transfer of wild-type p53
gene effectively inhibits vascular smooth muscle cell proliferation in
vitro and in vivo. *Circ Res* 1998;82:147–156.

130. Tsai HL, Kou GH, Chen SC, et al. Human cytomegalovirus immediate-early protein IE2 tethers a transcriptional repression domain to
p53. *J Biol Chem* 1996;271:3534–3540.

131. Gonczol E, Plotkin SA. Cells infected with human cytomegalovirus
release a factor(s) that stimulates cell DNA synthesis. *J Gen Virol*
1984;65:1833–1837.

132. Alcami J, Barzu T, Michelson S. Induction of an endothelial cell
growth factor by human cytomegalovirus infection of fibroblasts. *J
Gen Virol* 1991;72:2765–2770.

133. Fan T, Lu H, Hu H, et al. Inhibition of apoptosis in chlamydia-
infected cells: blockade of mitochondrial cytochrome c release and
caspase activation. *J Exp Med* 1998;187:487–496.

134. Tanaka K, Zou JP, Takeda K, et al. Effects of human cytomegalovirus
immediate-early proteins on p53-mediated apoptosis in coronary artery smooth muscle cells. *Circulation* 1999;99:1656–1659.

135. Zhu H, Shen Y, Shenk T. Human cytomegalovirus IE1 and IE2 proteins block apoptosis. *J Virol* 1995;69:7960–7970.

136. Wanishsawad C, Zhou YF, Epstein SE. Chlamydia pneumoniae-
induced transactivation of the major immediate early promoter of cytomegalovirus: potential synergy of infectious agents in the pathogenesis of atherosclerosis. *J Infect Dis* 2000;181:787–790.

137. Zhou YF, Shou M, Guetta E, et al. Cytomegalovirus infection of rats
increases the neointimal response to vascular injury without consistent evidence of direct infection of the vascular wall. *Circulation*
1999;100:1569–1575.

138. Alber DG, Vallance P, Powell KL. Enhanced atherogenesis is not an
obligatory response to systemic herpesvirus infection in the apoE-
deficient mouse: comparison of murine gamma-herpesvirus-68 and

139. Paterson DL, Hall J, Rasmussen SJ, et al. Failure to detect Chlamydia
pneumoniae in atherosclerotic plaques of Australian patients. *Pathology* 1998;30:169–172.

140. Berencsi K, Endresz V, Klurfeld D, et al. Early atherosclerotic
plaques in the aorta following cytomegalovirus infection of mice. *Cell
Adhes Commun* 1998;5:39–47.

141. Burnett MS, Gaydos CA, Madico GE, et al. Atherosclerosis in apoE
knockout mice infected with multiple pathogens. *J Infect Dis*
2001;183:226–231.

142. Rott D, Zhu J, Burnett MS, et al. Serum of cytomegalovirus-infected
mice induces monocyte chemoattractant protein-1 expression by endothelial cells. *J Infect Dis* 2001;184:1109–1113.

143. Alber DG, Powell KL, Vallance P, et al. Herpesvirus infection accelerates atherosclerosis in the apolipoprotein E-deficient mouse. *Circulation* 2000;102:779–785.

144. Valantine HA, Luikart H, Doyle R, et al. Impact of cytomegalovirus
hyperimmune globulin on outcome after cardiothoracic transplantation: a comparative study of combined prophylaxis with CMV hyperimmune globulin plus ganciclovir versus ganciclovir alone. *Transplantation* 2001;72:1647–1652.

145. Martinez A, Castro A, Gil C, et al. Recent strategies in the development of new human cytomegalovirus inhibitors. *Med Res Rev* 2001;
21:227–244.

146. Naghavi M, Barlas Z, Siadaty S, et al. Association of influenza vaccination and reduced risk of recurrent myocardial infarction. *Circulation* 2000;102:3039–3045.

147. Siscovick DS, Raghunathan TE, Lin D, et al. Influenza vaccination
and the risk of primary cardiac arrest. *Am J Epidemiol* 2000;152:
674–677.

148. Jackson LA, Yu O, Heckbert SR, et al. Influenza vaccination is not associated with a reduction in the risk of recurrent coronary events. *Am
J Epidemiol* 2002;156:634–640.

149. Gurfinkel EP, de la Fuente RL, Mendiz O, et al. Influenza vaccine pilot study in acute coronary syndromes and planned percutaneous
coronary interventions: the FLU Vaccination Acute Coronary Syndromes (FLUVACS) Study. *Circulation* 2002;105:2143–2147.

150. Capron L. How to design vaccination trials to prevent atherosclerosis.
Am Heart J 1999;138:S558–S559.

151. Horne BD, Muhlestein JB, Carlquist JF, et al. Statin therapy interacts
with cytomegalovirus seropositivity and high C-reactive protein in reducing mortality among patients with angiographically significant
coronary disease. *Circulation* 2003;107:258–263.

152. Tilley BC, Alarcon GS, Heyse SP, et al. Minocycline in rheumatoid
arthritis. A 48-week, double-blind, placebo-controlled trial. MIRA
Trial Group. *Ann Intern Med* 1995;122:81–89.

153. Hodinka RL. Designing studies to confirm a link between viral infection and atherosclerosis. *Am Heart J* 1999;138:S554–S555.

herpes simplex virus-1. *Arterioscler Thromb Vasc Biol* 2002;22:
793–798.

CHAPTER 38

Cytokines and Growth Regulatory Molecules

Uwe Schönbeck and Peter Libby

Key Words: Cytokines; endothelium; growth factors; macrophages; predictive markers; receptors; smooth muscle cells; T lymphocytes.

INTRODUCTION

An important theme of contemporary atherothrombosis research concerns the proteins that signal changes in cellular functions in the course of lesion formation and its clinical complications. The elucidation of signals that stimulate smooth muscle cell mitogenesis probably provided the initial stimulus for this line of research (1,2). The scope has broadened to include virtually every cell type and function beyond cell division, including adhesion and directed migration, synthesis and breakdown of constituents of the vascular extracellular matrix, apoptosis, modulation of the plaques' thrombogenicity, and control of vasomotor functions of blood vessels, to name just a few.

Originally, the study of growth regulatory molecules, pioneered in the 1950s by Levi-Montalcini (3) and Cohen (4), concentrated on positive regulation of growth control. Accordingly, the proteins mediating cell proliferation were termed *growth factors*. Regulation of the growth of smooth muscle cells provided the basis of early interest in growth factors in the context of atherogenesis. The proliferation of

U. Schönbeck: Boehring Ingelheim, 900 Ridgebury Road, Ridgefied, Connecticut 06877.

P. Libby: Brigham and Women's Hospital, Harvard Medical School, 77 Avenue Louis Pasteur, NRB 741, Boston, Massachusetts 02115.

smooth muscle cells during atherogenesis may occur in waves or cycles (5,6). Indeed, angiographic studies of atherothrombotic lesion progression support such a discontinuous course for the evolution of occlusive epicardial coronary atheroma (7). Waves of proliferation of smooth muscle cells could arise during crises in the progression of the lesion. For example, rupture of a microvessel within a plaque might lead to local thrombin activation with the ensuing direct and evoked mitogenic responses elicited by this molecule. Accordingly, measurement of the rate of proliferation of smooth muscle cells in end-stage lesions does not negate the importance of smooth muscle cell replication at various times even during the phases of lesion progression and complication. In addition to smooth muscle cells, we recognize that replication of other cell types also figures prominently in various phases of atherothrombosis. For example, endothelial repair and neoangiogenesis during plaque evolution require migration or proliferation of endothelial cells, or both (8,9). Moreover, studies measuring replicative rates of the various cell types indicated that macrophages and T lymphocytes divide as often as, if not more frequently than, smooth muscle cells in experimental and human atherothrombotic lesions (10,11). A variety of growth factors can promote proliferation of these distinct cell types, often acting on a broad rather than restricted range of cell types. Thus, the role of growth factors extends to processes beyond cell proliferation such as chemotaxis and the modulation of the plaques' procoagulant activity (discussed later).

Cytokines were first described during the early 1960s in studies originally unrelated to those on growth factors. Workers in the field of inflammation and immunology discovered that nonimmunoglobulin proteins mediate many important aspects of immune and inflammatory responses. Interferons (IFNs) and interleukins (ILs) (identified by their mitogenic functions) were among the first of such nonimmunoglobulin proteins recognized in inflammation or immunity (12–26). Relating to newly discovered functions, as well as in an attempt to separate them from growth factors, the ever growing number of these mediators of inflammation and immunity were denoted *cytokines,* a term derived from the Greek roots for "the cell" (cyto-) and "to move" (-kinein). Even today, appreciation of the complexity of the cytokine network probably remains incomplete, as suggested by the continued discovery not only of new individual members but complete subfamilies of cytokines. The IL, tumor necrosis factor (TNF), and IFN subfamilies have attracted particular interest in the field of atherothrombotic research, whereby distinctions among them are primarily made on the basis of gene sequences and structural features rather than functional criteria. Furthermore, the cytokine family encompasses proteins with predominantly chemotactic function, accordingly designated as *chemokines.*

Although it appears certain that the number of growth factors and cytokines implicated in the different stages of atherogenesis will continue to increase as analysis of the data from the Human Genome Project progresses and will probably be surpassed only by the variety of their proinflammatory and antiinflammatory functions, there is cur-

rently a broad appreciation of the role of these immunomodulators in atherogenesis (Table 38–1). As more has been learned about the molecular structure of cytokines and growth factors and, in particular, their functions, the distinction between these two groups seems increasingly arbitrary. Indeed, the regulation and functions of cytokines and growth factors overlap considerably, such that strict distinction between these families has become less useful. Hence, the joint consideration in this chapter is for both families.

GROWTH FACTORS AND CYTOKINES ARE PRODUCED BY A WIDE RANGE OF CELL TYPES

Growth Factors

One of the principles encountered in the study of growth factors involves their cells of origin, as well as the cells responding to them. The first point to bear in mind is that the original names of growth factors, although convenient, often have proven misleading as knowledge of a particular growth regulatory molecule has increased. For example, platelet-derived growth factor (PDGF) was first described as a serum constituent derived from platelets that stimulated the proliferation of mesenchymal cells *in vitro* (27,28). However, many cells involved in atherogenesis can actually produce

TABLE 38–1. *Examples of growth factor, cytokine, and chemokine families implicated in atherothrombosis*

Nomenclature	Forms	Function
Growth Factors		
FGF	1-23 (aFGF, bFGF)	Mitogen, angiogenesis
PDGF	AA, BB, AB, CC, DD	Mitogen, chemotaxis, angiogenesis
TGF	TGF-α, TGF-β_1, TGF-β_2, TGF-β_3	Cytosis, apoptosis
VEGF	VEGF-A, VEGF-B, VEGF-C, VEGF-D, VEGF-E, PlGF	Angiogenesis, differentiation, chemotaxis
CSF	GM-CSF, M-CSF	Mitogen, differentiation
Cytokines		
IL	IL-1 through IL-29 (IL-1α, IL-1β, IL-4, IL-6, IL-8, IL-10, IL-12, IL-15, IL-18, IL-23)	Proinflammatory/antiinflammatory modulation of adhesion, chemotaxis, cell proliferation and differentiation, matrix turnover, procoagulation status, and others
TNF	TNF-α, TNF-β, CD27L, CD30L, CD40L, CD95 (Fas Ligand), Ox40L	Proinflammatory mediators (promoting adhesion, chemotaxis, apoptosis, cell proliferation and differentiation, matrix turnover, procoagulant status, and others)
IFN	IFN-α, IFN-β, IFN-γ	Cytostasis, proinflammatory/antiinflammatory mediators
Chemokines		
C-Chemokines	Lymphotactin	Chemotaxis (T cells)
CC-Chemokine	CCL1-28 (e.g., MCP-1 to 5, MIP-1 to 4, RANTES, eotaxin-1 to 3, ABCD-1)	Chemotaxis (eosinophils, Mø, T cells, NK cells)
CXC-Chemokine	CXCL1 to 16 (e.g., IL-8, IP-10, MIG, PF-4)	Chemotaxis (PMN, T cells, NK cells)
CX3C-Chemokine	Fractalkine	Chemotaxis (Mø, T cells, NK cells), adhesion

aFGF, acidic fibroblast growth factor; bFGF, basic fibroblast growth factor; CSF, colony-stimulating factor; FGF, fibroblast growth factor; GM-CSF, granulocyte-monocyte colony-stimulating factor; IFN, interferon; IL-interleukin; IP-10, interferon inducible protein-10; MCP, monocyte chemotactic protein; M-CSF, monocyte colony-stimulating factor; MIG, monocyte induced by interferon-gamma; MIP-1, monocyte chemotactic factor-1; Mø, macrophage; NK, natural killer; PDGF, platelet-derived growth factor; PlGF, placental growth factor; RANTES, regulated upon activation, normal T cell expressed and secreted; TGF, transforming growth factor; TNF, tumor necrosis factor; VEGF, vascular endothelial growth factor.

this molecule, including endothelial cells, smooth muscle cells, and mononuclear phagocytes (29–34). In addition to the source, nomenclature has proven misleading regarding the function of growth factors. For example, the function of PDGF was originally considered restricted to mitogenesis, whereas current data strongly support a role for PDGF as a chemoattractant for smooth muscle cells in response to arterial injury (35,36). Moreover, research has implicated PDGF in processes of angiogenesis through induction of the vascular endothelial growth factor (VEGF)/VEGF receptor system (37,38). These points illustrate how PDGF, originally isolated from platelets by virtue of its mitogenic effect, may derive from endothelium, smooth muscle cells, and macrophages as well as platelets, and may be involved in growth stimulation, cell migration, angiogenesis, and protein formation in the context of atherothrombosis.

Although much of the attention focused on PDGF as one of the first and thus probably best characterized growth factor families implicated in vascular diseases, research during the last two decades has generated a continuously growing list of novel growth factor families implicated in atherothrombosis and hypertension. Notably, growth factors of different families often interact, whereby synergistic and antagonistic functions can be observed. For example, members of the transforming growth factor-beta (TGF-β) family, another prototypical class of growth factors, promote autocrine PDGF loops in smooth muscle cells. In addition, however, TGF-β also is expressed by other atheroma-associated cell types, and, when cocultured, endothelial cells and smooth muscle cells can produce activated forms of TGF-β that inhibit smooth muscle cell proliferation (39,40).

More recently, growth factor families such as fibroblast growth factors (FGFs) or VEGFs attracted attention for their potential pathophysiologic roles not only in tumor biology but also in atherothrombosis by promoting neovascularization. As outlined earlier for members of the PDGF and TGF family, the original nomenclature can be deceiving with respect to origin and function. Although VEGFs appear to act selectively on endothelial cells, FGFs are also potent growth factors for cell types other than fibroblasts, for example, endothelial and smooth muscle cells (41,42).

Other growth factors associated with vascular diseases include members of the colony-stimulating factor (CSF) family. Originally named with respect to their requirement for the survival and differentiation of distinct cultured cells such as granulocytes and macrophages (resulting in the terms GM-CSF and M-CSF, respectively), function and expression of these growth factors extend to a range of cell types, including endothelial and smooth muscle cells (43–46). Introducing further complexity, cytokines also can act as stimulatory (e.g., IL-1) or inhibitory (e.g., IFN-γ) growth regulatory molecules.

In summary, research during the past decades revealed that expression and function of a specific growth factor rarely is restricted to a single cell type and process, respectively. Accordingly, the broad expression pattern of growth factors is accompanied by the expression of the respective signal-mediating receptors on a similar range of cell types, although different cells may vary in the number of relevant receptors they display, as previously demonstrated, for example, for PDGF (47).

Cytokines

Similar caveats with respect to nomenclature pertain to the cytokines, as illustrated by the subfamily of ILs, a name derived from the original concept that these proteins mediate signals exclusively "between leukocytes," namely lymphocytes and mononuclear phagocytes. As for PDGF and other growth factors, markedly expanding knowledge about their cellular sources reveals that ILs, although originally conceived as messengers between leukocytes, can derive from most if not all cell types involved in atherothrombosis, including fibroblasts, endothelial cells, and smooth muscle cells, as well as lymphocytes and mononuclear phagocytes, the traditional sources (48–50). Like their range of origin, the number of ILs also has increased, currently encompassing IL-1 to IL-29. The prototype, IL-1, is expressed in two separately encoded isoforms, IL-1α and IL-1β, both of which can occur in all major cell types implicated in atherothrombosis (49–52). *In vitro* and *in vivo* studies revealed the proatherogenic role of the IL-1s and, similarly, of IL-6, IL-12, IL-15, and IL-18 (26). Interestingly, other members of the IL family can exert antiatherogenic properties, as suggested by their ability to mediate antiinflammatory functions *in vitro* or the finding that deficiency/overexpression of the respective molecule worsened/benefited atherothrombosis in experimental models, respectively. Among these antiatherogenic cytokines, expression and function of IL-4 and IL-10 on monocytes and T lymphocytes probably figure most prominently (53–56).

Besides ILs, the TNF (including TNF-α, TNF-β, CD27 ligand, CD30 ligand, CD40 ligand [CD154]), Fas ligand (CD95), lymphotoxin (Ox40 ligand), and the IFN (including IFN-α, IFN-β, and IFN-γ) families encompass cytokines associated with vascular diseases. Within the first family, particular interest focused on the role of TNF-α and CD40L in atherogenesis. Both of these atherogenic cytokines can exist either as cell surface or soluble proteins by atheroma-associated cell types, including endothelial and smooth muscle cells, mononuclear phagocytes, T lymphocytes, and platelets—cell types that also respond to ligation of the respective receptor (57,58). Within the IFN family, the role of IFN-γ in atherogenesis received particular interest. Expression of this proatherogenic cytokine was originally considered restricted to T lymphocytes, but in accord with recognition of broader patterns of expression of growth factors and cytokines, other cell types, including macrophages and smooth muscle cells, can express IFN-γ (59).

Within the group of chemokines, previous *in vitro* and *in vivo* studies provided evidence for atherogenic functions of IL-8, monocyte chemotactic protein-1 (MCP-1), IFN-inducible protein 10 (IP-10), monokine induced by IFN-γ

(MIG), IFN-inducible T-cell α chemoattractant (I-TAC), and RANTES (regulated upon activation, normal T cell expressed and secreted) (60–63). Notably, the expression of these chemokines appears more restricted than that of other cytokines. Although IL-8 is expressed by most cell types implicated in atherogenesis, the expression of and response to chemokines such as MCP-1, RANTES, or IP-10 appears restricted to leukocytes such as T cells and mononuclear phagocytes. According to the location of conserved cysteines within their amino acid sequence, chemokines are divided into the C-Chemokines (lymphotactin), CC-Chemokines (β subfamily; e.g., MCP, MIP-1, RANTES), CXC-Chemokines (α subfamily; e.g., IL-8, IP-10, MIG), and CX₃C-Chemokines (fractalkines), which bind to their respective receptors (termed CCR1-10, CXCR1-6, or CX₃CR1, respectively). Although originally named for their function as chemoattractants, these designations also proved too narrow in this family. The more recently identified fractalkine, expressed on monocytes and endothelial cells, is an unusual chemokine, because it can act both as a soluble chemotactic mediator and as a transmembrane-anchored adhesion receptor for leukocytes (64,65). Notably, deficiency of its receptor CX₃CR1 yields diminished atherothrombosis (66–68), as also observed for other chemokine receptors such as CCR2, demonstrating a central role for chemokines in atherogenesis.

In summary, the expression of growth factors and cytokines, originally considered restricted to distinct cell types, extends from the classical sources such as platelets and leukocytes to cells of the vascular bed such as the endothelium, smooth muscle cells, and fibroblasts. In addition to a broadened expression pattern, research also has expanded our understanding of the range of responding cell types and the type of responses induced. Accordingly, the atheroma-associated functions mediated by growth factors or cytokines extend beyond that of mere promotion of cell growth and differentiation and encompass a range of general inflammatory processes, such as those implicated in adhesion, migration, matrix degradation, coagulation, or vascular tone.

STRINGENT REGULATION OF THE BIOLOGIC FUNCTION OF GROWTH FACTORS AND CYTOKINES

Growth factors and cytokines in general act as upstream triggers of effector mechanisms and processes implicated in most, if not all, pathogenic pathways involved in atherothrombosis and other vascular diseases. As expected for such multipotent modulators of physiologic and pathologic pathways, biologic function of growth factors and cytokines requires stringent control. Control mechanisms include transcriptional regulation, often resulting in the expression of different (iso)forms with distinct functions, and the requirement for processing latent into active forms and for forming homomultimers/heteromultimers to acquire biologic activity. The biologic activities of growth factors and cytokines also undergo regulation by their synergistic or antagonistic interaction with other proteins. In addition, the overall activation status of a certain cell type determines its response to a growth factor or cytokine. For example, both IL-1 and TGF-β can induce programmed cell death in cultures of vascular cells. However, when applied to cultures previously induced to undergo apoptosis, both mediators can prevent cell death, providing yet another level of the complex regulatory mechanisms applying to the biologic function of growth factors and cytokines, depending on the preexisting activation status of a certain cell type. Finally, the induction of proinflammatory or antiinflammatory processes through growth factors and cytokines depends on the presence and density of the respective cognate receptor(s), which often requires accessory molecules to transmit signaling, thus providing additional levels of regulation. Because one may easily become mired in the complexity of these interactive regulatory pathways, this chapter does not aim to provide an exhaustive compendium or catalog of all of the various mediators that may bear relevance to atherogenesis. Instead, certain principles of the biology of cytokines and growth factors are outlines, and general principles are visualized through particular mediators. For more extensive studies, reference is made to the respective original articles and reviews.

Transcriptional Regulation

Transcription of the respective gene commonly embodies the first level of regulation, because the expression of most growth factors or cytokines is not constitutive, but rather requires cell activation (Fig. 38–1) (see color insert). Notably, their own peers can induce synthesis of most, if not all, growth factors and cytokines. The autocrine/paracrine regulation of IL-1 expression was among the first to reveal this potent enhancer mechanism of inflammatory responses (69,70). The range of peers induced by cytokines or growth factors is broad rather than restricted. IL-1, for example, not only induces its own gene expression but also that of other cytokines implicated in atherothrombosis such as IL-6, IL-8, IL-12, and IL-18, as well as a series of chemokines including members of the MCP-1, eotaxin, or MIP-1 families and growth factors such as members of the PDGF, EGF, VEGF, or CSF families (24).

Growth factors and cytokines frequently exist in multiple (iso)forms (derived from different genes or alternative splicing) with distinct biologic functions. As in the case of the prototypic vascular growth factor PDGF, four genes encode the precursors of distinct proteins for the A, B, C, and D chains (71). To function, PDGF must form a covalent dimeric molecule consisting of any of the following possible assortments: PDGF-AA, BB, AB, CC, or DD (Fig. 38–1). The receptors for PDGF, PDGFRα, and PDGFRβ also form different noncovalent dimers that interact differentially with the dimeric forms of PDGF: PDGF-AA, AB, BB and CC induce αα receptor homodimers, whereas PDGF-BB and DD induce the dimerization of ββ receptor subunits, and PDGF-

AB, BB, CC, and DD induce that of αβ heterodimeric receptor. Consequently, these growth factors exert different biologic actions. For example, PDGF-AA stimulates smooth muscle mitogenesis less potent than the BB or CC form (72,73), probably a result of the decreased number of PDGF β receptors compared with α receptors on smooth muscle cells. Moreover, the PDGF-A chain can undergo differential splicing to yield at least two different translation products. Some biologic functions of these splice variant forms of PDGF appear to be significant. For example, PDGF-A can form a truncated version of the A chain, splicing out an amino acid sequence encoded by the sixth exon of the *PDGF-A* gene. This sequence specifically binds to the proteoglycan heparin sulfate. Thus, the ability to bind cell surface–associated proteoglycans or to adhere to extracellular proteoglycans may depend on such sequences contained in one isoform but not in others. The same is true for the precursor form of the PDGF-B chain. PDGF-CC and DD, however, require processing at specific N-terminal domains to achieve biologic activity. Therefore, heterogeneity of PDGF activity exists at the level of the gene and in the assembly of functional dimers, illustrating the imprecision of referring merely to "PDGF" without taking into account its multiple (iso)forms of varying biologic potential.

Similar considerations pertain to other growth factor subfamilies, such as TGF (summarizing term for TGF-α, TGF-β_1, TGF-β_2, TGF-β_3) or FGF (the general term for FGF-1 to 23). The VEGF family provides yet another example for heterogeneity within a growth factor gene family. Currently composed of VEGF-A, B, C, D, E, and the placenta growth factor, several of these family members exist in different isoforms, each mediating unique biologic functions and binding to different receptors (74), including VEGFR-1, 2, and 3, or the proteoglycan neuropilin. Although originally associated with tumor biology, the angiogenic functions triggered by the ligation of VEGF receptors, such as the migration, survival, and differentiation of endothelial cells, provided implications for atherothrombotic disease. Indeed, VEGFs and their receptors are expressed in human and experimental atheroma (75), and therapeutic strategies involving VEGFs have been developed to assist revascularization of ischemic vascular tissue (76,77), although such approaches should be interpreted with the appropriate care (78).

Likewise, IL-1, a monomeric cytokine, can also arise from two different genes that encode the α or β isoforms of this mediator. In contrast to the isoforms of PDGF, which reflect distinct biologic activities, both IL-1 isoforms signal through the same receptor. Although one might, therefore, presume that the biologic responses triggered by both isoforms are identical, they differ in an important aspect of their cell biology. IL-1α, active in its full-length precursor form, is the isoform associated with the cell surface, whereas IL-1β is commonly released, a process requiring maturation of the latent precursor by proteolytic cleavage, as outlined later in this chapter. Because of the different distribution patterns, IL-1α is commonly associated with local effects of this cytokine requiring cell contact, whereas the IL-1β isoform can mediate contact independent of local and systemic functions.

The heterogeneity observed in the examples outlined earlier (PDGF, TGFs, VEGFs, and IL-1) applies to most other cytokines and growth factors and is expandable in mechanisms. For example, heparin-binding EGF and M-CSF, as well as the cytokines TNF-α and CD40L, exist in membrane-associated and soluble forms (79–81). The latter cytokines also require trimerization for optimal signaling capabilities, further adding to the complex regulatory network for biologic functions of cytokines and growth factors, using not only mere gene activation but also the expression of isoforms and differential multimerization thereof.

Posttranslational Regulation

Besides the requirement to form homomultimers/heteromultimers, processing of latent precursors as well as interaction with synergistic or antagonistic counterparts comprise further posttranscriptional mechanisms that modulate the biologic consequences of growth factors and cytokines.

Processing of an inactive, latent precursor into the biologically functional form is probably characterized best for the prototypical cytokine IL-1 (Fig. 38–1). Its isoform IL-1β is expressed as a 33-kD latent form, which is converted into the mature 17-kD form via processing through a specific IL-1β–converting enzyme termed caspase-1. This processing not only equips the protein with biologic function, but it also results in the generation of the soluble IL-1 isoform, markedly extending the reach of this locally expressed cytokine. Activation or release, or both, through conversion of latent precursors is not unique to IL-1β but applies to other cytokines, for example, IL-18, TNF-α, or CD40L, as well as growth factors. The case of TGF-β furnishes an example pertinent to the latter group. Almost all cell types can express the *TGF* gene and synthesize the precursor of this multipotent mediator. However, the precursor of TGF-β lacks biologic activity, and the control of TGF-β activation is complex, requiring interplay among various cell types such as endothelial and smooth muscle cells (39,40). Subtilisin-like proprotein convertases such as furin are thought to mediate TGF-β processing (82). Moreover, enzymatic mechanisms relevant to the regulation of TGF-β activity include cell-associated plasmin. The activity of plasmin further depends on regulation by plasminogen activators (e.g., urokinase-type plasminogen activator, tissue-type plasminogen activator) and plasminogen activator inhibitors (e.g., PAI-1, PAI-2) also expressed by vascular cells, providing yet another example for the complex posttranslational modulation of the biologic activity of growth factors and cytokines.

Interestingly, after passing the abundant transcriptional regulatory mechanisms and posttranslational modifications outlined earlier, expression of mature growth factors or cytokines may still not exert their biologic activities. Typically, interaction with other proteins definitively determines the activity of a certain growth factor or cytokine. Such proteins include other growth factors and/or cytokines, but also specific endogenous inhibitors. With respect to other growth factors and cytokines, the interaction can be synergistic or antagonistic. The examples are numerous and include the synergistic interaction of members of the angiogenic FGF and VEGF families (83,84) or the IFN-γ–inducing cytokines IL-12 and IL-18 (59), as well as the antagonist interactions between T$_H$2 cytokines, such as IL-4 or IL-10, and proinflammatory T$_H$1 cytokines, such as IL-1, TNF-α, or CD40L (26,85), as outlined later in this chapter. With respect to the interaction with specific endogenous inhibitors, several classes of proteins can provide the antagonistic function. Solubilization of the receptors for growth factors or cytokines commonly yields a "trap" for the respective functional ligand, because binding of the ligand to the receptor will constrain the availability of functional ligand through interactions with a detached receptor incapable of signal transduction. Examples for this pathway include the different soluble TGF-β (86,87) and TNF receptor forms (sTNF-RII) (88,89). Receptor antagonists or binding proteins provide another form of receptor-associated inhibitory modulation. Receptor antagonists have distinct structural features that allow them to bind the receptor without triggering signal transduction. Furthermore, the antagonist can effectively block the receptor from accepting functional ligand because of prolonged turnover/dissociation rates. A prototypical example is the IL-1 receptor antagonist (90,91) (Fig. 38–1). Finally, specific binding proteins can interact with the ligand directly, thus preventing its binding to the receptor, as demonstrated for the IL-18 binding protein (92,93).

Commonly, the biologic consequences of growth factors or cytokines depend on the balance between a certain functional ligand and its endogenous inhibitor(s), as well as the responsiveness of a given cell type, frequently dependent on the expression of the respective receptor and associated signal transducers, as discussed in the following section.

Signaling Through Receptor-dependent Mechanisms

Growth factors act primarily through two superfamilies of cell surface receptors that transduce their effects. The first family of receptors has extracellular regions with homology to the immunoglobulin gene, whereas their cytoplasmic portions encode autocatalytic tyrosine kinases. Ligand binding through the extracellular domain of the receptor can cause not only the respective cytoplasmic tyrosine kinase to autophosphorylate the receptor, but it also can yield phosphorylation of other substrates involved in distal intracellular signaling events. The prototypical example of a tyrosine kinase growth factor receptor implicated in vascular biology is the PDGF receptors (94). Other growth factors that use tyrosine kinases for signal transduction include the heparin-binding growth factor family, which includes members of the FGF, VEGF, or insulin-like growth factor family.

Another major category of receptors for growth regulatory molecules spans the cell membrane seven times and interacts with G proteins for intracellular signaling, belonging to the seven transmembrane G protein–coupled receptor superfamily (95,96). For example, products of the arachidonic acid metabolism and angiotensin II, a transducer of smooth muscle contraction, also indirectly stimulate smooth muscle cell growth and act through such seven membrane-spanning receptors (97,98). Reports regarding tethering of the two receptor types suggest integrative signaling for growth factors such as PDGF, EGF, or VEGF, producing more efficient and/or distinct stimulation by activating kinase pathways and G protein–coupled signaling (99–102).

Intracellular signaling mechanisms for the various cytokines, although diverse, can be grouped by structural criteria into those involving one or more members of four major families of receptor proteins: the Class I (e.g., the IL-4, IL-6, IL-12, and IL-15 receptor) or Class II (e.g., the IL-10 and IFN-γ receptor) cytokine receptors; the immunoglobulin superfamily receptors (also termed the "IL-1 receptor family," with the functional form IL-1RI and the antagonistic IL-1RII); and the TNF receptor family (e.g., TNF-RI, CD40, Fas). Most of these receptor families do not exhibit intrinsic tyrosine or seronine/threonine kinase activity, but rather initiate signaling through the recruitment of kinases and cytosolic proteins to the receptor (103,104).

The Class I and II receptors are commonly characterized as heteromers sharing a common receptor chain. For example, IL-4 shares the γ-chain with IL-2, IL-9, and IL-15, whereas IL-6 and IL-12 share a receptor chain with IL-11 and IL-23, respectively. Signaling through Class I or II receptors commonly induces gene transcription through the activation of cytosolic kinase cascades, such as the Jak/STAT (Janus kinase/signal transducers and activators of transcription) pathway, mitogen-activated protein kinases, or extracellular signal-regulated kinases.

A common feature of the molecular mechanisms underlying signaling of members of the TNF family, such as TNF-α and CD40L, is the formation of multiprotein signaling complexes at the cytoplasmic domain of the receptor (26,80,81). Binding of TNF-α to its two receptors, TNFR1 and TNFR2, as well as binding of CD40L to its receptor CD40 results in recruitment of cytoplasmic adapter proteins such as the TNF receptor–associated factors (namely TRAF1, TRAF2, and TRAF3). These factors, through complex signaling cascades and networks, lead to the activation of downstream effectors such as the transcription factors activating protein-1, early growth response, and nuclear factor-kappaB (NF-κB) (26).

The signal transduction pathways activated by IL-1 also can result in the activation of the transcription factor NF-κB, although through a different pathway (Fig. 38–1). Binding of IL-1 results in the recruitment of the IL-1 receptor–associated protein to the functional receptor, IL-1RI, triggering the binding of the IL-1 receptor–associated kinase, which eventually causes activation of the kinase TGF-beta-activated kinase-1 (through MyD88). Activation of this kinase eventually induces association with TRAF-6, which activates the NF-κB inducing kinase, a kinase capable of activating NF-κB through the degradation of inhibitor of NF-kappa B (I-κB) by the I-κB kinase (85). A member of the immunoglobulin superfamily of receptors, IL-1R shares distinct sequence similarities in its cytosolic regions with other family members including the Drosophila melanogaster protein Toll, the IL-18 receptor (IL-18R), and the Toll-like receptors TLR-2 and TLR-4. Accordingly, the signaling proteins activated during signaling by IL-1RI resemble those participating in signaling by IL-18R and TLR-4 (104).

In general, the experimental evidence that surfaced during the last decade suggests that biologic consequences of both growth factors and cytokines result from a stringent regulatory network guarding the intricate balance of proinflammatory and antiinflammatory responses. Such complex control mechanisms appear appropriate with respect to the range and impact of the pathophysiologic pathways initiated by growth factors and cytokines. Disturbance of their equilibriums probably participates in the progression of chronic inflammatory diseases.

GROWTH FACTORS AND CYTOKINES: AGONISTS BUT ALSO ANTAGONISTS OF ATHEROTHROMBOSIS

In accord with the nature of atherothrombosis as a chronic inflammatory disease, proinflammatory growth factors and cytokines are commonly considered proatherogenic and antiinflammatory members are considered antiatherogenic, an admittedly oversimplified view. Interestingly, the distinction between proatherogenic and antiatherogenic cytokines conforms to a large extent with that between the immunoregulatory mediators released by the T_H1 and T_H2 lymphocyte subset, respectively. Indeed, T lymphocytes, and within these the T_H1 predominant immune response, figure centrally in atherogenesis (105–108). Notably, the T-cell subgroups are dichotomized through their growth factor/cytokine release and response pattern rather than by cell type–specific surface markers. Prototypical T_H1 mediators include IL-2, IL-3, IL-12, IL-15, IL-18, and IL-23 (109–113), cytokines expressed by antigen–presenting cells such as mononuclear phagocytes but also vascular endothelial and smooth muscle cells. In addition, T cells can express IL-2 and IFN-γ, cytokines promoting T_H1 polarization in an autocrine loop. This loop includes the suppression of factors promoting a T_H2 predominant immune response such as IL-4, IL-5, IL-10, and IL-13 (114). However, exemptions from this simplified T-cell subset dichotomization pattern exist. The case of CD40L comprises one example. This cytokine promotes not only T_H1 but also T_H2 development, depending on the inflammatory environment (115–117). Indeed, expression of CD40 on antigen-presenting cells is a prerequisite for the initiation of T_H2 but not T_H1 development in response to certain antigens (118–120). However, despite such T_H2-promoting pathways, abrogation of CD40 signaling definitively diminishes atherogenesis in vivo (121–124), probably because of the complex interactions triggered between various growth factors and cytokines (Fig. 38–2). Ligation of CD40 on mononuclear phagocytes induces the expression of IL-12, IL-15, and IL-18, which can reenforce and sustain the expression of CD40L (117,125–130). In addition, IL-15 promotes IL-12 expression, which can, in turn, increase levels of the IL-18 receptor. Ligation of this receptor induces IFN-γ, particularly in combination with IL-12 (131). IFN-γ, however, prominently induces IL-15, as well as CD40 and CD40L (57,111). Moreover, IFN-γ probably

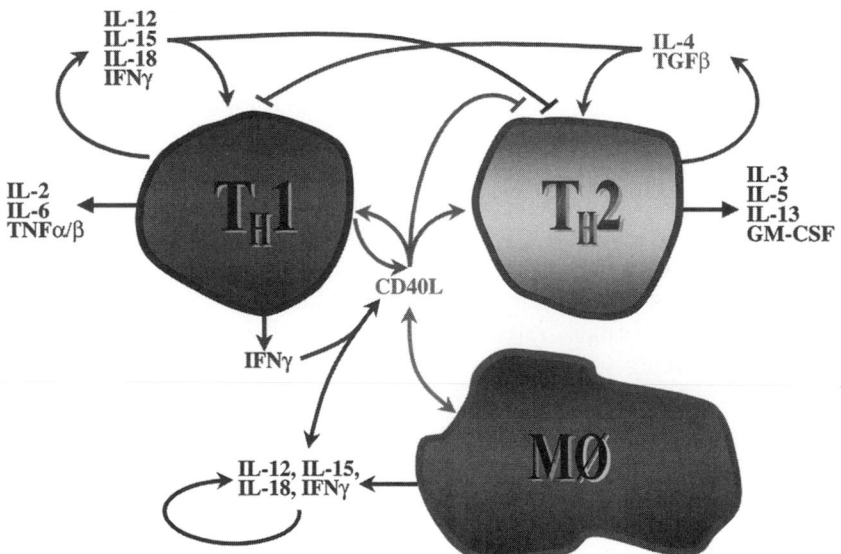

FIG. 38–2. Schema of T_H1/T_H2 balance in atherothrombosis. GM-CSF, granulocyte-monocyte colony-stimulating factor; IFN, interferon; IL, interleukin; Mø, macrophage; TGF, transforming growth factor; TNF, tumor necrosis factor.

further supports CD40-mediated functions by directly impairing IL-4/IL-10–mediated T_H2 immune responses (132), which repress the expression of CD40L (117). CD40L also diminishes the expression of TGF-β in atherothrombotic lesions, a growth factor family that constrains the development of T_H1 immune responses, thus providing yet another example of T_H1-promoting feedback loops that operate in the atherothrombotic plaque.

Ultimately, growth factors and cytokines affect atherothrombosis not only by promoting the development of a certain T cell type, but directly or indirectly by modulation of the underlying pathogenic processes such as cell migration, proliferation and apoptosis, matrix turnover, and the balance of the coagulation and fibrinolytic pathways. These processes depend on the (im)balance of effectors that regulate: (i) cell motility and replication, (ii) programmed cell death, (iii) synthesis and degradation of extracellular matrix, or (iv) the procoagulant status of the plaque. As discussed earlier, current data support the view that T_H1 cytokines modulate these functions in a proatherogenic fashion in most cases. In contrast, T_H2 cytokines may not only oppose the proatherogenic functions induced by T_H1 cytokines, but furthermore can directly promote antiatherogenic processes, such as diminishing the expression of inducible nitric oxide synthase and decreasing rates of apoptosis.

As noted earlier, the field of growth control has traditionally accorded great importance to positive growth control, or stimulation of mitogenesis. Growth factors such as PDGFs and VEGFs, as well as cytokines such as IL-1, figure prominently in lesional cell proliferation. These mitogens, probably in concert with chemokines induced by growth factors, cytokines, or both might contribute to the buildup of the smooth muscle cell–enriched fibrous cap overlaying the developing procoagulant lipid core and to the accumulation of the inflammatory infiltrate. Indeed, PDGF-B derived from bone marrow–derived cells figures centrally in the regulation of lesional smooth muscle cell and fibrous tissue content (but not plaque size per se) in experimental atheroma, as determined by bone marrow reconstitution studies in genetically altered mice (133,134).

Traditionally, growth control was considered synonymous with growth stimulation and, as described earlier, vascular and inflammatory cells, when appropriately activated, can elaborate growth stimulatory molecules that can act on these cells in an autocrine manner or on neighboring cells in a paracrine fashion. These observations raise the specter of untrammeled growth resulting from an initial stimulus, a view that appears incompatible with the apparently indolent nature of replication within atheroma. This conundrum highlights the potential importance of both positive and negative growth control during atherogenesis. Among those negative modulators in atherogenesis, TGF-β has attracted considerable interest. TGF-β was originally isolated by Todaro and colleagues (135,136) as a stimulator of growth of cells in soft agar. At the same time, Holley's group (137) sought the biochemical nature of a growth in-

hibitor present in cultured epithelial cells and converged on the same molecule. Thus, the schizophrenic properties of TGF-β—sometimes a growth stimulator, sometimes an inhibitor—were evident in the earliest studies, illustrating yet again that the original name of a growth factor seldom accounts for the spectrum of actions that emerge from subsequent studies. TGF-β neither transforms nor is it a growth factor either in general or in the context of atherogenesis. *In vitro,* TGF-β appears to inhibit smooth muscle replication rather than stimulate it. The dual designation of TGF-β as a growth stimulator or growth inhibitor may derive from its function as a regulator of both PDGF and PDGF receptor expression (47). To add further complexity to the role of TGF-β, this protein potently stimulates interstitial collagen expression by smooth muscle cells even though it inhibits replication of this major cellular source of the vascular extracellular matrix (138). The dual ability of TGF-β to inhibit smooth muscle growth and enhance production of collagen, the major load-bearing molecule of the plaque, may contribute to the appearance of the dense, cell-depleted fibrous cap of connective tissue that forms in the late stages of plaque development and separates the procoagulant lipid core from the bloodstream. Supporting the role for this growth factor in plaque stability, interruption of TGF-β signaling in hyperlipidemic mice, either by administration of anti–TGF-$β_{1/2/3}$ antibodies or recombinant, soluble TGF-β receptor II, yielded lesions diminished in size and collagen content and demonstrated enhanced lesional accumulation of the inflammatory infiltrate (139,140).

The plaque's structure, however, depends not only on growth factors such as TGF-β, but also on positive and negative regulation by cytokines such as IFN-γ. This cytokine has long been known to exert cytostatic effects on mesenchymal cells. Studies from two laboratories in the 1980s affirmed that this lymphokine limits serum- or growth factor–induced proliferation of vascular smooth muscle cells (141,142). Thus, one function of T cells, a major source of IFN-γ, within atherothrombotic lesions may be inhibition of smooth muscle cell proliferation. Indeed, in the context of experimental vascular injury, Hansson and Holm (143) have provided elegant evidence that IFN-γ acts *in vivo* as an inhibitor of smooth muscle cell replication after injury. In addition to restraining the source of fibrillar collagen, IFN-γ also can abrogate synthesis of this major load-bearing molecule (144–147). Thus, the *in vitro* studies remained controversial regarding the proatherogenic or antiatherogenic function of this cytokine. This controversy was definitively addressed in a dual fashion in experimental models. Mice deficient in IFN-γ exhibited diminished atherogenesis, whereas application of exogenous IFN-γ in wild-type mice promoted the disease, rendering IFN-γ a proatherogenic cytokine (148–150). Notably, IFN-γ also promotes atherothrombosis in the absence of T lymphocytes or mononuclear phagocytes, the traditional sources of this cytokine, by acting on vascular smooth muscle cells (151). The observation that smooth muscle cells themselves can express IFN-γ further supports the importance of nonleukocytic cell types in the inflammatory process of the atherothrombotic vessel wall (59).

Loss of fibrillar collagen, the extracellular matrix component lending tensile strength to the fibrous cap of atherothrombotic lesions (152,153), results from the imbalance in the ratio of synthesis and breakdown. Growth factors and cytokines can modulate collagen expression in a dual fashion, as outlined earlier. However, these proteins control another level of regulation, the breakdown, through specific matrix-degrading enzymes such as matrix metalloproteinases (MMPs). Members of the MMP subfamily of interstitial collagenases, namely MMP-1, MMP-8, and MMP-13, catalyze the initial step in the degradation of interstitial collagen (154–157). Areas of overexpression of these enzymes within human and experimental atherothrombotic lesions colocalize with sites of collagenolysis (158–161), which is consistent with a crucial role of these enzymes as determinants of plaque stability. Indeed, *in vitro,* proatherogenic cytokines such as CD40L shift the balance of synthesis and breakdown toward diminished accumulation of *de novo* synthesized interstitial collagen, probably by increasing breakdown rates through enhanced MMP activity rather than by affecting rates of synthesis (162). In accord with this proatherogenic function of CD40L, *in vivo* studies supported a key role for this cytokine in plaque stability. Inhibition of CD40 signaling either by administration of CD40L antibodies or genetic deficiency of the ligand diminished atherogenesis (121,124). Probably even more clinically relevant, interruption of CD40/CD40L interaction in mice prevented progression of established atherothrombotic lesions and modulated the plaques' structure toward lesions considered less prone to rupture, with enhanced collagen content (122,123). Notably, atherothrombotic lesions in CD40L-deficient mice had increased expression of the collagen-inducing growth factor TGF-β, illustrating again the complex interactions between growth factors and cytokines.

Mechanisms of negative growth control during atherogenesis include the extreme of programmed cell death in addition to cytostasis. Apoptosis of vascular smooth muscle cells and (smooth muscle cell–derived or macrophage-derived) foam cells may contribute considerably to atherogenesis (163–167). This genetically encoded cell death program involves the activation of endonucleases, enzymes that cleave cellular DNA at the nucleosome/linker regions, and thus generate small double-stranded fragments (approximately 200 base pair in length) that, when applied to agarose gel-electrophoresis, yield the so-called oligosomal DNA ladder. Multiple molecular mechanisms may promote programmed cell death in atheroma. However, inflammatory cells such as T lymphocytes that express death ligands on their cell surface or secrete apoptotic mediators may promote vascular cell apoptosis. Ligation of membrane-bound death receptors of the tumor necrosis receptor family, such as Fas (CD95) or death receptors 3 through 6, triggers the recruitment of signal transducers such as Fas-FADD, which eventually can activate caspases such as caspase-8 (FLICE) or caspase-2 by oligomerization. Such functional complexes (termed death-inducing signaling complex) ultimately activate the effector caspase-3, 6, 7, or 9, which can cleave their nuclear substrates, and thus cause death of a cell. As with other pathways outlined in this chapter, apoptosis also is characterized by the intricate balance of proapoptotic pathways such as those outlined earlier and mediators inhibiting cell death. Members of the bcl family of proteins recently received attention in the latter regard. Although both proapoptotic and antiapoptotic processes occur in atherothrombosis (168–170), future studies will have to decipher the molecular mechanisms of their (apparent) imbalance (166).

Although apoptosis might contribute crucially to the formation of the lipid core, the procoagulant activity in this region of the plaque triggers thrombosis after rupture of the overlying fibrous cap and the consequent exposure to blood. Tissue factor accounts for much of the thrombogenic potential of the lipid core. Interestingly, a gamut of mediators modulate the expression of this protein, including growth factors such as PDGF, cytokines such as IL-1, TNF, or CD40L, and chemokines such as MCP-1 or leukotactin (171,172). Similar to patterns outlined earlier for other atherogenic effectors modulated by growth factors and cytokines, the balance between this protein and endogenous inhibitors, principally tissue factor pathway inhibitor 1 (TFPI-1), regulates the procoagulant activity of tissue factor. This Kunitz-type inhibitor antagonizes the initiation of coagulation by the TF/VIIa complex by forming a stable quaternary complex with tissue factor, as well as the coagulation factors Va and Xa. Indeed, hypercholesterolemic mice with a TFPI-1 deficiency exhibited a greater atherothrombotic burden and revealed significantly decreased time to occlusive thrombosis after carotid plaque injury (173). This finding suggests that TFPI protects from atherothrombosis and regulates the thrombosis that occurs in the setting of atherothrombosis. In accord, overexpression of TFPI-1 in rabbit atherothrombotic arteries diminishes the hyperplastic response to injury in the absence of changes in the hemostatic system (174).

SUMMARY

This chapter highlights certain salient features of the biology of growth factors and cytokines in relation to atherothrombosis and does not attempt to catalog exhaustively the entire canon of known members of either family. Rather, we have aimed to emphasize certain principles that apply to growth factor and cytokine biology in general.

Although the functions of growth factors and cytokines are relatively easy to define *in vitro,* definition of their integrated actions *in vivo* and assigning to them a distinct role in the pathogenesis of atherothrombosis have proven more challenging. Indeed, ready extrapolation of the results of *in vitro* experiments to the *in vivo* situation has considerable hazards. Cell culture studies have aided immeasurably the advancement of the growth factor and cytokine field. Nonetheless, investigators must bear in mind that the three-dimensional, multicellular environment within the artery wall differs substantially from the simple single cell type most often studied in monolayer cultures surrounded by unphysiologic fluids on an unnatural substrate. Fortunately, the application of molecular genetic technologies have aided in this task. For example, the ability to perform genetic manipulations that inactivate specific genes permits the design of experiments that test the specific role of the distinct growth factors or cytokines in inflammation and immunity. Furthermore, the availability of mice genetically modified to produce lesions of atherothrombosis when fed appropriate diets, namely apolipoprotein E or low-density-lipoprotein receptor–deficient mice, greatly facilitated the analysis of the actions of growth factors and cytokines in this chronic inflammatory disease through the creation of compound mutant mice. The (still developing) ability to locally alter the expression of growth factor and cytokine genes by vascular gene transfer techniques, as well as the generation of conditional gene deficiencies (in which expression of a certain molecule of interest can be abrogated within a certain cell type or in a time-restricted fashion, or both), will shed further light on the *in vivo* action of these factors. We nonetheless need to bear in mind that important differences may pertain between mice and humans. Also, the exaggerated levels of lipoproteins required to produce atheromata in a practical time scale may render mouse models of atherothrombosis more of a caricature than portrait of human atherothrombosis.

Although the complexities of the actions of growth factors and cytokines might appear daunting and discouraging, viewing this complexity as an opportunity to unravel the signaling pathways at play during atherogenesis, and thus to truly understand the pathogenesis of this chronic inflammatory disease, will allow us to simplify this picture and eventually conquer atherothrombosis. Among the more major hurdles on this future path is the intimidating challenge of controlling a process that contains so many seemingly redundant and overlapping pathways, rendering research on the role of growth factor and cytokines in atherogenesis very exciting today.

ACKNOWLEDGMENT

The late Russell Ross coauthored this chapter with Dr. Libby in the first edition of this book. In gratitude for his many contributions in atherothrombosis research, his inspiration, and his friendship, we respectfully dedicate this updated work to his memory.

REFERENCES

1. Ross R, Glomset JA. The pathogenesis of atherosclerosis I. *N Engl J Med* 1976;295:369–377.
2. Ross R, Glomset JA. The pathogenesis of atherosclerosis II. *N Engl J Med* 1976;295:420–425.
3. Levi-Montalcini R. The nerve growth factor: thirty five years later. In: *Les Prix Nobel–1986.* Stockholm, Sweden: Almquist & Wiksell Intl., 1987:279–299.
4. Cohen S. Epidermal growth factor. In: *Les Prix Nobel–1986.* Stockholm, Sweden: Almquist & Wiksell Intl., 1987:263–275.
5. Libby P, Fleet J, Salomon R, et al. Possible roles of cytokines in atherogenesis. In: Stein O, Eisenberg S, Stein Y, eds. *Atherosclerosis IX.* Tel Aviv, Israel: R&L Creative Communications, 1992:339–350.
6. Libby P. Atherosclerosis: the new view. *Sci Am* 2002;286:46–55.
7. Bruschke AV, Kramer J Jr, Bal ET, et al. The dynamics of progression of coronary atherosclerosis studied in 168 medically treated patients who underwent coronary arteriography three times. *Am Heart J* 1989;117:296–305.
8. Brogi E, Winkles J, Underwood R, et al. Distinct patterns of expression of fibroblast growth factors and their receptors in human atheroma and non-atherosclerotic arteries: association of acidic FGF with plaque microvessels and macrophages. *J Clin Invest* 1993;92:2408–2418.
9. O'Brien ER, Garvin MR, Dev R, et al. Angiogenesis in human coronary atherosclerotic plaques. *Am J Pathol* 1994;145:883–894.
10. Gordon D, Reidy MA, Benditt EP, et al. Cell proliferation in human coronary arteries. *Proc Natl Acad Sci USA* 1990;87:4600–4604.
11. Rosenfeld ME, Ross R. Macrophage and smooth muscle cell proliferation in atherosclerotic lesions of WHHL and comparably hypercholesterolemic fat-fed rabbits. *Arteriosclerosis* 1990;10:680–687.
12. Mazzur SR, Ellsworth B, Paucker K. Studies on the effect of interferon on the formation of antibody in mouse spleen cells. I. Survival of spleen cells in culture and preservation of cellular function. *J Immunol* 1967;98:683–688.
13. Carver DH, Seto DS, Migeon BR. Interferon production and action in mouse, hamster and somatic hybrid mouse-hamster cells. *Science* 1968;160:558–559.
14. Koltai M, Meos E. Inhibition of the acute inflammatory response by interferon inducers. *Nature* 1973;242:525–526.
15. Kuo PT, Wilson AC, Goldstein RC, et al. Suppression of experimental atherosclerosis in rabbits by interferon-inducing agents. *J Am Coll Cardiol* 1984;3:129–134.
16. Kaser A, Tilg H. Interferon-alpha in inflammation and immunity. *Cell Mol Biol (Noisy-le-grand)* 2001;47:609–617.
17. Akbar AN, Lord JM, Salmon M. IFN-alpha and IFN-beta: a link between immune memory and chronic inflammation. *Immunol Today* 2000;21:337–342.
18. Billiau A, Heremans H, Vermeire K, et al. Immunomodulatory properties of interferon-gamma. An update. *Ann NY Acad Sci* 1998;856:22–32.
19. Blyden G, Handschumacher RE. Purification and properties of human lymphocyte activating factor (LAF). *J Immunol* 1977;118:1631–1638.
20. Lachman LB, Moore JO, Metzgar RS. Preparation and characterization of lymphocyte-activating factor (LAF) from acute monocytic and myelomonocytic leukemia cells. *Cell Immunol* 1978;41:199–206.
21. Mizel SB, Oppenheim JJ, Rosenstreich DL. Characterization of lymphocyte-activating factor (LAF) produced by the macrophage cell line, P388D1. I. Enhancement of LAF production by activated T lymphocytes. *J Immunol* 1978;120:1497–1503.
22. Mizel SB. Studies on the purification and structure-functional relationships of murine lymphocyte activating factor (Interleukin 1). *Mol Immunol* 1980;17:571–577.
23. Dinarello CA. Interleukin-1 and the pathogenesis of the acute-phase response. *N Engl J Med* 1984;311:1413–1418.
24. Dinarello CA. Biologic basis for interleukin-1 in disease. *Blood* 1996;87:2095–2147.
25. Dinarello CA. Interleukin-1 beta, interleukin-18, and the interleukin-1 beta converting enzyme. *Ann NY Acad Sci* 1998;856:1–11.
26. Young JL, Libby P, Schönbeck U. Cytokines in the pathogenesis of atherosclerosis. *Thromb Haemost* 2002;88:554–567.
27. Ross R, Glomset JA, Kariya B, et al. A platelet-dependent serum factor that stimulates the proliferation of arterial smooth muscle cells in vitro. *Proc Natl Acad Sci USA* 1974;71:1207–1210.
28. Kohler N, Lipton A. Platelets as a source of fibroblast growth-promoting activity. *Exp Cell Res* 1974;87:297–301.
29. Barrett TB, Gajdusek CM, Schwartz SM, et al. Expression of the sis gene by endothelial cells in culture and in vivo. *Proc Natl Acad Sci USA* 1984;81:6772–6774.
30. Collins T, Pober JS, Gimbrone MA Jr, et al. Cultured human endothelial cells express platelet-derived growth factor A chain. *Am J Pathol* 1987;127:7–12.
31. Shimokado K, Raines EW, Madtes DK, et al. A significant part of macrophage-derived growth factor consists of at least two forms of PDGF. *Cell* 1985;43:277–286.

32. Martinet Y, Bitterman PB, Mornex JF, et al. Activated human monocytes express the c-sis proto-oncogene and release a mediator showing PDGF-like activity. *Nature* 1986;319:158–160.
33. Sjölund M, Hedin U, Sejersen T, et al. Arterial smooth muscle cells express platelet-derived growth factor (PDGF) A chain mRNA, secrete a PDGF-like mitogen, and bind exogenous PDGF in a phenotype- and growth state-dependent manner. *J Cell Biol* 1988;106:403–413.
34. Libby P, Warner SJ, Salomon RN, et al. Production of platelet-derived growth factor-like mitogen by smooth-muscle cells from human atheromata. *N Engl J Med* 1988;318:1493–1498.
35. Fingerle J, Johnson R, Clowes AW, et al. Role of platelets in smooth muscle cell proliferation and migration after vascular injury in rat carotid artery. *Proc Natl Acad Sci USA* 1989;86:8412–8416.
36. Ferns G, Raines E, Sprugel K, et al. Inhibition of neointimal smooth muscle accumulation after angioplasty by an antibody to PDGF. *Science* 1991;253:1129–1132.
37. Edelberg JM, Aird WC, Wu W, et al. PDGF mediates cardiac microvascular communication. *J Clin Invest* 1998;102:837–843.
38. Heldin CH, Westermark B. Mechanism of action and in vivo role of platelet-derived growth factor. *Physiol Rev* 1999;79:1283–1316.
39. Antonelli-Orlidge A, Saunders KB, Smith SR, et al. An activated form of transforming growth factor beta is produced by cocultures of endothelial cells and pericytes. *Proc Natl Acad Sci USA* 1989;86:4544–4548.
40. Sato Y, Rifkin DB. Inhibition of endothelial cell movement by pericytes and smooth muscle cells: activation of a latent transforming growth factor-beta 1-like molecule by plasmin during co-culture. *J Cell Biol* 1989;109:309–315.
41. Gospodarowicz D, Moran JS, Braun DL. Control of proliferation of bovine vascular endothelial cells. *J Cell Physiol* 1977;91:377–385.
42. Gospodarowicz D, Ferrara N, Haaparanta T, et al. Basic fibroblast growth factor: expression in cultured bovine vascular smooth muscle cells. *Eur J Cell Biol* 1988;46:144–151.
43. Broudy VC, Kaushansky K, Harlan JM, et al. Interleukin 1 stimulates human endothelial cells to produce granulocyte- macrophage colony-stimulating factor and granulocyte colony-stimulating factor. *J Immunol* 1987;139:464–468.
44. Sigounas G, Steiner M, Anagnostou A. Synergism of hemopoietic growth factors on endothelial cell proliferation. *Angiology* 1997;48:141–147.
45. Plenz G, Reichenberg S, Koenig C, et al. Granulocyte-macrophage colony-stimulating factor (GM-CSF) modulates the expression of type VIII collagen mRNA in vascular smooth muscle cells and both are codistributed during atherogenesis. *Arterioscler Thromb Vasc Biol* 1999;19:1658–1668.
46. Chen G, Grotendorst G, Eichholtz T, et al. GM-CSF increases airway smooth muscle cell connective tissue expression by inducing TGF-β receptors. *Am J Physiol Lung Cell Mol Physiol* 2002;6:6.
47. Battegay EJ, Raines EW, Seifert RA, et al. TGF-beta induces bimodal proliferation of connective tissue cells via complex control of an autocrine PDGF loop. *Cell* 1990;63:515–524.
48. Libby P, Ordovas JM, Auger KR, et al. Endotoxin and tumor necrosis factor induce interleukin-1 gene expression in adult human vascular endothelial cells. *Am J Pathol* 1986;124:179–185.
49. Libby P, Ordovas JM, Birinyi LK, et al. Inducible interleukin-1 expression in human vascular smooth muscle cells. *J Clin Invest* 1986;78:1432–1438.
50. Hawrylowicz CM, Santoro SA, Platt FM, et al. Activated platelets express IL-1 activity. *J Immunol* 1989;143:4015–4018.
51. Kurt-Jones EA, Fiers W, Pober JS. Membrane IL-1 induction on human endothelial cells and dermal fibroblasts. *J Immunol* 1987;139:2317–2324.
52. Loppnow H, Flad HD, Dürrbaum I, et al. Detection of IL-1 with human dermal fibroblasts. *Immunobiology* 1989;179:283–291.
53. Mallat Z, Besnard S, Duriez M, et al. Protective role of interleukin-10 in atherosclerosis. *Circ Res* 1999;85:e17–e24.
54. Mallat Z, Heymes C, Ohan J, et al. Expression of interleukin-10 in advanced human atherosclerotic plaques: relation to inducible nitric oxide synthase expression and cell death. *Arterioscler Thromb Vasc Biol* 1999;19:611–616.
55. Pinderski Oslund LJ, Hedrick CC, Olvera T, et al. Interleukin-10 blocks atherosclerotic events in vitro and in vivo. *Arterioscler Thromb Vasc Biol* 1999;19:2847–2853.
56. Pinderski LJ, Fischbein MP, Subbanagounder G, et al. Overexpression of interleukin-10 by activated T lymphocytes inhibits atherosclerosis in LDL receptor-deficient Mice by altering lymphocyte and macrophage phenotypes. *Circ Res* 2002;90:1064–1071.
57. Mach F, Schönbeck U, Sukhova GK, et al. Functional CD40 ligand is expressed on human vascular endothelial cells, smooth muscle cells, and macrophages: implications for CD40-CD40 ligand signaling in atherosclerosis. *Proc Natl Acad Sci USA* 1997;94:1931–1936.
58. Henn V, Slupsky JR, Grafe M, et al. CD40 ligand on activated platelets triggers an inflammatory reaction of endothelial cells. *Nature* 1998;391:591–594.
59. Gerdes N, Sukhova GK, Libby P, et al. Expression of interleukin (IL)-18 and functional IL-18 receptor on human vascular endothelial cells, smooth muscle cells, and macrophages: implications for atherogenesis. *J Exp Med* 2002;195:245–257.
60. Nelken N, Coughlin S, Gordon D, et al. Monocyte chemoattractant protein-1 in human atheromatous plaques. *J Clin Invest* 1991;88:1121–1127.
61. Wilcox JN, Nelken NA, Coughlin SR, et al. Local expression of inflammatory cytokines in human atherosclerotic plaques. *J Atheroscler Thromb* 1994;1:310–313.
62. Gu L, Okada Y, Clinton SK, et al. Absence of monocyte chemoattractant protein-1 reduces atherosclerosis in low density lipoprotein receptor-deficient mice. *Mol Cell* 1998;2:275–281.
63. Mach F, Sauty A, Iarossi AS, et al. Differential expression of three T lymphocyte-activating CXC chemokines by human atheroma-associated cells. *J Clin Invest* 1999;104:1041–1050.
64. Greaves DR, Hakkinen T, Lucas AD, et al. Linked chromosome 16q13 chemokines, macrophage-derived chemokine, fractalkine, and thymus- and activation-regulated chemokine, are expressed in human atherosclerotic lesions. *Arterioscler Thromb Vasc Biol* 2001;21:923–929.
65. Harrison JK, Jiang Y, Wees EA, et al. Inflammatory agents regulate in vivo expression of fractalkine in endothelial cells of the rat heart. *J Leukoc Biol* 1999;66:937–944.
66. Boring L, Gosling J, Cleary M, et al. Decreased lesion formation in CCR2-/- mice reveals a role for chemokines in the initiation of atherosclerosis. *Nature* 1998;394:894–897.
67. Dawson TC, Kuziel WA, Osahar TA, et al. Absence of CC chemokine receptor-2 reduces atherosclerosis in apolipoprotein E-deficient mice. *Atherosclerosis* 1999;143:205–211.
68. Lesnik P, Haskell C, Charo I. Decreased atherosclerosis in CXCR1-/- mice reveals a role for fractalkine in atherogenesis. *J Clin Invest* 2003;111:333–340.
69. Warner SJ, Auger KR, Libby P. Interleukin-1 induces interleukin-1. Recombinant human interleukin-1 induces interleukin-1 production by adult human vascular endothelial cells. *J Immunol* 1987;139:1911–1917.
70. Ghezzi P, Dinarello CA. IL-1 induces IL-1. *J Immunol* 1988;140:4238–4244.
71. Heldin CH, Eriksson U, Ostman A. New members of the platelet-derived growth factor family of mitogens. *Arch Biochem Biophys* 2002;398:284–290.
72. Li X, Ponten A, Aase K, et al. PDGF-C is a new protease-activated ligand for the PDGF alpha-receptor. *Nat Cell Biol* 2000;2:302–309.
73. Gilbertson DG, Duff ME, West JW, et al. Platelet-derived growth factor C (PDGF-C), a novel growth factor that binds to PDGF alpha and beta receptor. *J Biol Chem* 2001;276:27406–27414.
74. Matsumoto T, Claesson-Welsh L. VEGF receptor signal transduction. *Sci STKE* 2001;(112):RE21.
75. Couffinhal T, Kearney M, Witzenbichler B, et al. Vascular endothelial growth factor/vascular permeability factor (VEGF/VPF) in normal and atherosclerotic human arteries. *Am J Pathol* 1997;150:1673–1685.
76. Couffinhal T, Silver M, Kearney M, et al. Impaired collateral vessel development associated with reduced expression of vascular endothelial growth factor in ApoE-/- mice. *Circulation* 1999;99:3188–3198.
77. Freedman SB, Isner JM. Therapeutic angiogenesis for coronary artery disease. *Ann Intern Med* 2002;136:54–71.
78. Luttun A, Carmeliet P. Soluble VEGF receptor Flt1: the elusive preeclampsia factor discovered? *J Clin Invest* 2003;111:600–602.
79. Higashiyama S, Lau K, Besner GE, et al. Structure of heparin-binding EGF-like growth factor. Multiple forms, primary structure, and glycosylation of the mature protein. *J Biol Chem* 1992;267:6205–6212.
80. Schönbeck U, Libby P. The CD40/CD154 receptor/ligand dyad. *Cell Mol Life Sci* 2001;58:4–43.
81. Schönbeck U, Libby P. CD40 signaling and plaque instability. *Circ Res* 2001;89:1092–1103.

82. Leitlein J, Aulwurm S, Waltereit R, et al. Processing of immunosuppressive pro-TGF-beta 1,2 by human glioblastoma cells involves cytoplasmic and secreted furin-like proteases. *J Immunol* 2001;166:7238–7243.

83. Xue L, Greisler HP. Angiogenic effect of fibroblast growth factor-1 and vascular endothelial growth factor and their synergism in a novel in vitro quantitative fibrin-based 3-dimensional angiogenesis system. *Surgery* 2002;132:259–267.

84. Yoshiji H, Kuriyama S, Yoshii J, et al. Synergistic effect of basic fibroblast growth factor and vascular endothelial growth factor in murine hepatocellular carcinoma. *Hepatology* 2002;35:834–842.

85. Hanada T, Yoshimura A. Regulation of cytokine signaling and inflammation. *Cytokine Growth Factor Rev* 2002;13:413–421.

86. Zhao W, Kobayashi M, Ding W, et al. Suppression of in vivo tumorigenicity of rat hepatoma cell line KDH-8 cells by soluble TGF-beta receptor type II. *Cancer Immunol Immunother* 2002;51:381–388.

87. Bandyopadhyay A, Zhu Y, Malik SN, et al. Extracellular domain of TGFbeta type III receptor inhibits angiogenesis and tumor growth in human cancer cells. *Oncogene* 2002;21:3541–3551.

88. Higuchi M, Aggarwal BB. Modulation of two forms of tumor necrosis factor receptors and their cellular response by soluble receptors and their monoclonal antibodies. *J Biol Chem* 1992;267:20892–20899.

89. McDermott MF. TNF and TNFR biology in health and disease. *Cell Mol Biol (Noisy-le-grand)* 2001;47:619–635.

90. Seckinger P, Williamson K, Balavoine JF, et al. A urine inhibitor of interleukin 1 activity affects both interleukin 1 alpha and 1 beta but not tumor necrosis factor alpha. *J Immunol* 1987;139:1541–1545.

91. Carter DB, Deibel MR Jr, Dunn CJ, et al. Purification, cloning, expression and biological characterization of an interleukin-1 receptor antagonist protein. *Nature* 1990;344:633–638.

92. Novick D, Kim SH, Fantuzzi G, et al. Interleukin-18 binding protein: a novel modulator of the Th1 cytokine response. *Immunity* 1999;10:127–136.

93. Aizawa Y, Akita K, Taniai M, et al. Cloning and expression of interleukin-18 binding protein. *FEBS Lett* 1999;445:338–342.

94. DeMali KA, Godwin SL, Soltoff SP, et al. Multiple roles for Src in a PDGF-stimulated cell. *Exp Cell Res* 1999;253:271–279.

95. Ye RD. Regulation of nuclear factor kappaB activation by G-protein-coupled receptors. *J Leukoc Biol* 2001;70:839–848.

96. Luttrell LM. Activation and targeting of mitogen-activated protein kinases by G-protein-coupled receptors. *Can J Physiol Pharmacol* 2002;80:375–382.

97. Berk BC, Vekshtein V, Gordon HM, et al. Angiotensin II-stimulated protein synthesis in cultured vascular smooth muscle cells. *Hypertension* 1989;13:305–314.

98. Gibbons GH, Pratt RE, Dzau VJ. Vascular smooth muscle cell hypertrophy vs. hyperplasia. Autocrine transforming growth factor-beta 1 expression determines growth response to angiotensin II. *J Clin Invest* 1992;90:456–461.

99. Paris S, Pouyssegur J. Mitogenic effects of fibroblast growth factors in cultured fibroblasts. Interaction with the G-protein-mediated signaling pathways. *Ann NY Acad Sci* 1991;638:139–148.

100. Asahara T, Bauters C, Zheng LP, et al. Synergistic effect of vascular endothelial growth factor and basic fibroblast growth factor on angiogenesis in vivo. *Circulation* 1995;92:II365–II371.

101. Pepper MS, Mandriota SJ, Jeltsch M, et al. Vascular endothelial growth factor (VEGF)-C synergizes with basic fibroblast growth factor and VEGF in the induction of angiogenesis in vitro and alters endothelial cell extracellular proteolytic activity. *J Cell Physiol* 1998;177:439–452.

102. Ronnstrand L, Heldin CH. Mechanisms of platelet-derived growth factor-induced chemotaxis. *Int J Cancer* 2001;91:757–762.

103. Haddad JJ. Cytokines and related receptor-mediated signaling pathways. *Biochem Biophys Res Commun* 2002;297:700–713.

104. Martin MU, Wesche H. Summary and comparison of the signaling mechanisms of the Toll/interleukin-1 receptor family. *Biochim Biophys Acta* 2002;1592:265–280.

105. Jonasson L, Holm J, Skalli O, et al. Regional accumulations of T cells, macrophages, and smooth muscle cells in the human atherosclerotic plaque. *Arteriosclerosis* 1986;6:131–138.

106. Tsukada T, Rosenfeld M, Ross R, et al. Immunocytochemical analysis of cellular components in lesions of atherosclerosis in the Watanabe and fat-fed rabbit using monoclonal antibodies. *Arteriosclerosis* 1986;6:601–613.

107. Dansky HM, Charlton SA, Harper MM, et al. T and B lymphocytes play a minor role in atherosclerotic plaque formation in the apolipoprotein E-deficient mouse. *Proc Natl Acad Sci USA* 1997;94:4642–4646.

108. Zhou X, Nicoletti A, Elhage R, et al. Transfer of CD4(+) T cells aggravates atherosclerosis in immunodeficient apolipoprotein E knockout mice. *Circulation* 2000;102:2919–2922.

109. O'Garra A, Arai N. The molecular basis of T helper 1 and T helper 2 cell differentiation. *Trends Cell Biol* 2000;10:542–550.

110. Stobie L, Gurunathan S, Prussin C, et al. The role of antigen and IL-12 in sustaining Th1 memory cells in vivo: IL-12 is required to maintain memory/effector Th1 cells sufficient to mediate protection to an infectious parasite challenge. *Proc Natl Acad Sci USA* 2000;97:8427–8432.

111. Avice MN, Demeure CE, Delespesse G, et al. IL-15 promotes IL-12 production by human monocytes via T cell-dependent contact and may contribute to IL-12-mediated IFN-gamma secretion by CD4+ T cells in the absence of TCR ligation. *J Immunol* 1998;161:3408–3415.

112. Akira S. The role of IL-18 in innate immunity. *Curr Opin Immunol* 2000;12:59–63.

113. Lankford CS, Frucht DM. A unique role for IL-23 in promoting cellular immunity. *J Leukoc Biol* 2003;73:49–56.

114. Coffman RL, von der Weid T. Multiple pathways for the initiation of T helper 2 (Th2) responses. *J Exp Med* 1997;185:373–375.

115. De Vita L, Accapezzato D, Mangino G, et al. Defective Th1 and Th2 cytokine synthesis in the T-T cell presentation model for lack of CD40/CD40 ligand interaction. *Eur J Immunol* 1998;28:3552–3563.

116. Ribbens C, Dayer JM, Chizzolini C. CD40-CD40 ligand (CD154) engagement is required but may not be sufficient for human T helper 1 cell induction of interleukin-2- or interleukin-15-driven, contact-dependent, interleukin-1beta production by monocytes. *Immunology* 2000;99:279–286.

117. Lee BO, Haynes L, Eaton SM, et al. The biological outcome of CD40 signaling is dependent on the duration of CD40 ligand expression: reciprocal regulation by interleukin (IL)-4 and IL-12. *J Exp Med* 2002;196:693–704.

118. Poudrier J, van Essen D, Morales-Alcelay S, et al. CD40 ligand signals optimize T helper cell cytokine production: role in Th2 development and induction of germinal centers. *Eur J Immunol* 1998;28:3371–3383.

119. Mackey MF, Barth RJ Jr, Noelle RJ. The role of CD40/CD154 interactions in the priming, differentiation, and effector function of helper and cytotoxic T cells. *J Leukoc Biol* 1998;63:418–428.

120. MacDonald AS, Straw AD, Dalton NM, et al. Cutting edge: Th2 response induction by dendritic cells: a role for CD40. *J Immunol* 2002;168:537–540.

121. Mach F, Schönbeck U, Sukhova GK, et al. Reduction of atherosclerosis in mice by inhibition of CD40 signalling. *Nature* 1998;394:200–203.

122. Schönbeck U, Sukhova GK, Shimizu K, et al. Inhibition of CD40 signaling limits evolution of established atherosclerosis in mice. *Proc Natl Acad Sci USA* 2000;97:7458–7463.

123. Lutgens E, Cleutjens KB, Heeneman S, et al. Both early and delayed anti-CD40L antibody treatment induces a stable plaque phenotype. *Proc Natl Acad Sci USA* 2000;97:7464–7469.

124. Lutgens E, Gorelik L, Daemen MJ, et al. Requirement for CD154 in the progression of atherosclerosis. *Nat Med* 1999;5:1313–1316.

125. Weiler M, Kachko L, Chaimovitz C, et al. CD40 ligation enhances IL-15 production by tubular epithelial cells. *J Am Soc Nephrol* 2001;12:80–87.

126. Mottonen M, Isomaki P, Luukkainen R, et al. Interleukin-15 upregulates the expression of CD154 on synovial fluid T cells. *Immunology* 2000;100:238–244.

127. Skov S, Bonyhadi M, Odum N, et al. IL-2 and IL-15 regulate CD154 expression on activated CD4 T cells. *J Immunol* 2000;164:3500–3505.

128. Zanussi S, D'Andrea M, Simonelli C, et al. The effects of CD40 ligation on peripheral blood mononuclear cell interleukin-12 and interleukin-15 production and on monocyte CD14 surface antigen expression in human immunodeficiency virus-positive patients. *Scand J Immunol* 1999;49:286–292.

129. Kuniyoshi JS, Kuniyoshi CJ, Lim AM, et al. Dendritic cell secretion of IL-15 is induced by recombinant huCD40LT and augments the stimulation of antigen-specific cytolytic T cells. *Cell Immunol* 1999;193:48–58.

130. Sugiura T, Kawaguchi Y, Harigai M, et al. Increased CD40 expression on muscle cells of polymyositis and dermatomyositis: role of CD40-CD40 ligand interaction in IL-6, IL-8, IL-15, and monocyte chemoattractant protein-1 production. *J Immunol* 2000;164:6593–6600.

131. Robinson D, Shibuya K, Mui A, et al. IGIF does not drive Th1 devel-

opment but synergizes with IL-12 for interferon-gamma production and activates IRAK and NFkappaB. *Immunity* 1997;7:571–581.

132. Brossart P, Zobywalski A, Grunebach F, et al. Tumor necrosis factor alpha and CD40 ligand antagonize the inhibitory effects of interleukin 10 on T-cell stimulatory capacity of dendritic cells. *Cancer Res* 2000;60:4485–4492.

133. Sano H, Sudo T, Yokode M, et al. Functional blockade of platelet-derived growth factor receptor-beta but not of receptor-alpha prevents vascular smooth muscle cell accumulation in fibrous cap lesions in apolipoprotein E-deficient mice. *Circulation* 2001;103:2955–2960.

134. Kozaki K, Kaminski WE, Tang J, et al. Blockade of platelet-derived growth factor or its receptors transiently delays but does not prevent fibrous cap formation in ApoE null mice. *Am J Pathol* 2002;161:1395–1407.

135. Sporn MB, Todaro GJ. Autocrine secretion and malignant transformation of cells. *N Engl J Med* 1980;303:878–880.

136. Todaro GJ, De LJ, Fryling C, et al. Transforming growth factors (TGFs): properties and possible mechanisms of action. *J Supramol Struct Cell Biochem* 1981;15:287–301.

137. Tucker RF, Shipley GD, Moses HL, et al. Growth inhibitor from BSC-1 cells closely related to platelet type beta transforming growth factor. *Science* 1984;226:705–707.

138. Liau G, Chan LM. Regulation of extracellular matrix RNA levels in cultured smooth muscle cells. Relationship to cellular quiescence. *J Biol Chem* 1989;264:10315–10320.

139. Mallat Z, Gojova A, Marchiol-Forunigault C, et al. Inhibition of TGF-beta signaling accelerates atherosclerosis and induces an unstable plaque phenotype in mice. *Circ Res* 2001;89:930–934.

140. Lutgens E, Gijbels M, Smook M, et al. Transforming growth factor-beta mediates balance between inflammation and fibrosis during plaque progression. *Arterioscler Thromb Vasc Biol* 2002;22:975–982.

141. Hansson GK, Jonasson L, Holm J, et al. Gamma interferon regulates vascular smooth muscle proliferation and Ia expression in vivo and in vitro. *Circ Res* 1988;63:712–719.

142. Warner SJ, Friedman GB, Libby P. Immune interferon inhibits proliferation and induces 2'-5'-oligoadenylate synthetase gene expression in human vascular smooth muscle cells. *J Clin Invest* 1989;83:1174–1182.

143. Hansson GK, Holm J. Interferon-gamma inhibits arterial stenosis after injury. *Circulation* 1991;84:1266–1272.

144. Granstein RD, Murphy GF, Margolis RJ, et al. Gamma-interferon inhibits collagen synthesis in vivo in the mouse. *J Clin Invest* 1987;79:1254–1258.

145. Jimenez SA, Freundlich B, Rosenbloom J. Selective inhibition of human diploid fibroblast collagen synthesis by interferons. *J Clin Invest* 1984;74:1112–1116.

146. Stephenson ML, Krane SM, Amento EP, et al. Immune interferon inhibits collagen synthesis by rheumatoid synovial cells associated with decreased levels of the procollagen mRNAs. *FEBS Lett* 1985;180:43–50.

147. Amento EP, Ehsani N, Palmer H, et al. Cytokines and growth factors positively and negatively regulate interstitial collagen gene expression in human vascular smooth muscle cells. *Arterioscler Thromb* 1991;11:1223–1230.

148. Nagano H, Mitchell RN, Taylor MK, et al. Interferon-gamma deficiency prevents coronary arteriosclerosis but not myocardial rejection in transplanted mouse hearts. *J Clin Invest* 1997;100:550–557.

149. Gupta S, Pablo AM, Jiang X, et al. IFN-gamma potentiates atherosclerosis in ApoE knock-out mice. *J Clin Invest* 1997;99:2752–2761.

150. Whitman SC, Ravisankar P, Elam H, et al. Exogenous interferon-gamma enhances atherosclerosis in apolipoprotein E-/- mice. *Am J Pathol* 2000;157:1819–1824.

151. Tellides G, Tereb DA, Kirkiles-Smith NC, et al. Interferon-gamma elicits arteriosclerosis in the absence of leukocytes. *Nature* 2000;403:207–211.

152. Smith E. The influence of age and atherosclerosis on the chemistry of aortic intima. *J Atheroscler Res* 1965;5:241–248.

153. Rekhter M, Zhang K, Narayanan A, et al. Type I collagen gene expression in human atherosclerosis. Localization to specific plaque regions. *Am J Pathol* 1993;143:1634–1648.

154. Horwitz AL, Hance AJ, Crystal RG. Granulocyte collagenase: selective digestion of type I relative to type III collagen. *Proc Natl Acad Sci USA* 1977;74:897–901.

155. Welgus HG, Jeffrey JJ, Eisen AZ. The collagen substrate specificity of human skin fibroblast collagenase. *J Biol Chem* 1981;256:9511–9515.

156. Hasty KA, Jeffrey JJ, Hibbs MS, et al. The collagen substrate specificity of human neutrophil collagenase. *J Biol Chem* 1987;262:10048–10052.

157. Knauper V, Lopez-Otin C, Smith B, et al. Biochemical characterization of human collagenase-3. *J Biol Chem* 1996;271:1544–1550.

158. Galis Z, Sukhova G, Lark M, et al. Increased expression of matrix metalloproteinases and matrix degrading activity in vulnerable regions of human atherosclerotic plaques. *J Clin Invest* 1994;94:2493–2503.

159. Nikkari ST, Geary RL, Hatsukami T, et al. Expression of collagen, interstitial collagenase, and tissue inhibitor of metalloproteinases-1 in restenosis after carotid endarterectomy. *Am J Pathol* 1996;148:777–783.

160. Sukhova GK, Schönbeck U, Rabkin E, et al. Evidence for increased collagenolysis by interstitial collagenases-1 and -3 in vulnerable human atheromatous plaques. *Circulation* 1999;99:2503–2509.

161. Herman MP, Sukhova GK, Libby P, et al. Expression of neutrophil collagenase (matrix metalloproteinase-8) in human atheroma: a novel collagenolytic pathway suggested by transcriptional profiling. *Circulation* 2001;104:1899–1904.

162. Horton DB, Libby P, Schönbeck U. Ligation of CD40 on vascular smooth muscle cells mediates loss of interstitial collagen via matrix metalloproteinase activity. *Ann NY Acad Sci* 2001;947:329–336.

163. Libby P, Clinton SK. Cytokines as mediators of vascular pathology. *Nouv Rev Fr Hematol* 1992;34:S47–S53.

164. Geng YJ, Libby P. Evidence for apoptosis in advanced human atheroma. Colocalization with interleukin-1 beta-converting enzyme. *Am J Pathol* 1995;147:251–266.

165. Geng YJ, Henderson LE, Levesque EB, et al. Fas is expressed in human atherosclerotic intima and promotes apoptosis of cytokine-primed human vascular smooth muscle cells. *Arterioscler Thromb Vasc Biol* 1997;17:2200–2208.

166. Geng YJ, Libby P. Progression of atheroma: a struggle between death and procreation. *Arterioscler Thromb Vasc Biol* 2002;22:1370–1380.

167. Bennet MR. Apoptosis in the vascular system. *Heart* 2002;87:480–487.

168. Cai W, Devaux B, Schaper W, et al. The role of Fas/APO 1 and apoptosis in the development of human atherosclerotic lesions. *Atherosclerosis* 1997;131:177–186.

169. Wang A, Bobryshev Y, Cherian S, et al. Expression of apoptosis-related proteins and structural features of cell death in explanted aortocoronary saphenous vein bypass grafts. *Cardiovasc Surg* 2001;9:319–328.

170. Choy J, Granville D, Hunt D, et al. Endothelial cell apoptosis: biochemical characteristics and potential implications for atherosclerosis. *J Mol Cell Cardiol* 2001;33:1673–1690.

171. Ernofsson M, Siegbahn A. Platelet-derived growth factor-BB and monocyte chemotactic protein-1 induce human peripheral blood monocytes to express tissue factor. *Thromb Res* 1996;83:307–320.

172. Lee WH, Kim SH, Jeong EM, et al. A novel chemokine, Leukotactin-1, induces chemotaxis, pro-atherogenic cytokines, and tissue factor expression in atherosclerosis. *Atherosclerosis* 2002;161:255–260.

173. Westrick RJ, Bodary PF, Xu Z, et al. Deficiency of tissue factor pathway inhibitor promotes atherosclerosis and thrombosis in mice. *Circulation* 2001;103:3044–3046.

174. Zoldhelyi P, Chen ZQ, Shelat HS, et al. Local gene transfer of tissue factor pathway inhibitor regulates intimal hyperplasia in atherosclerotic arteries. *Proc Natl Acad Sci USA* 2001;98:4078–4083.

CHAPTER 39

The Role of Rheology in Atherothrombotic Coronary Artery Disease

B. Lowell Langille, Dorota Dajnowiec, and Avrum I. Gotlieb

Key Words: Endothelium; mechanotransduction; remodeling; shear stress.

INTRODUCTION

Pulsatile blood flow through coronary arteries is an important regulator of the structure and function of these vessels and has been implicated in the pathogenesis of atherothrombosis. In the large epicardial coronary arteries, atherothrombosis localizes to the outer wall of one or both daughter vessels at major bifurcations, and compelling evidence implicates hemodynamic forces in this localization (1). In particular, mechanical stresses of flowing blood on the vessel wall are important stimuli that influence atherogenesis by regulating endothelial function, smooth muscle cell behavior, and the interaction of endothelial cells with leukocytes and other blood constituents. This chapter presents information, within the context of atherogenesis, on the nature of the mechanical stresses to which the vessel wall is exposed. These forces

B. L. Langille: Department of Laboratory Medicine and Pathobiology, University of Toronto; and Toronto General Hospital, 200 Elizabeth Street, NU1-121a, Toronto, Ontario M5G 2C4, Canada.

D. Dajnowiec: Toronto General Hospital, 200 Elizabeth Street, NU1-121a, Toronto, Ontario M5G 2C4, Canada.

A. I. Gotlieb: Toronto General Hospital, 200 Elizabeth Street, NU1-119a, Toronto, Ontario M5G 2C4, Canada.

include compression caused by blood pressure, tensile stresses caused by the transmural pressure gradient and by attachments to contiguous myocardium, and shear stresses caused by blood flow and transmural fluid flux, all of which display large spatial and temporal variation. Most evidence points to a predominant role for shear forces, the primary focus of this chapter, although other loads are probably important.

NATURE OF BLOOD FLOW IN ARTERIES

Despite the emphasis that has been placed on shear stress and early atherogenesis, misconceptions persist concerning the distribution of these forces in arteries and its possible implication for atherogenesis. We begin, therefore, with an overview of local blood flow conditions that prevail in coronary and other conduit arteries.

Shear stresses are frictional forces that are derived from blood flow and are imposed directly on vascular endothelium. These stresses depend on local blood flow conditions that, like all fluid flow phenomena, fall into three regimes (Fig. 39–1). At very low flow rates in small vessels, frictional (viscous) forces dominate over forces related to fluid momentum (inertial forces), and flows simply follow the geometry of flow channels *(Stokes flow)*. These conditions are approximated in larger venules and arterioles, but they never occur in coronary arteries except when perfusion is greatly compromised. At very high flow rates in large arteries, inertial forces dominate, blood flows become unstable,

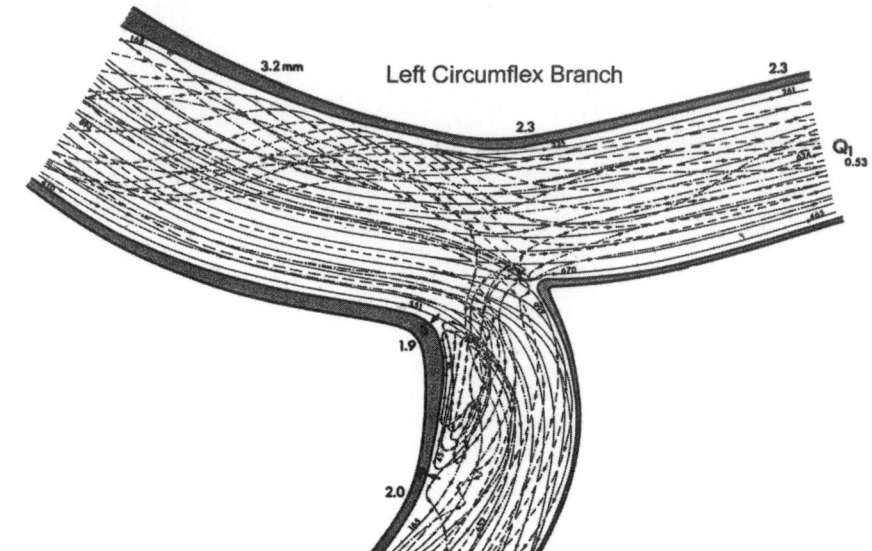

FIG. 39–1. Complex secondary flows arise in large- and medium-sized arteries. Flow streamlines based on perfusion of tracers in a human left circumflex artery are shown. At very low flow rates or in very small vessels, flow trajectories (streamlines) simply follow the geometry of the vessel. High flow rates produce turbulence, which is characterized by random lateral deviations of flow trajectories that are superimposed on net downstream flow. (From Asakura T, Karino T. Flow patterns and spatial distribution of atherosclerotic lesions in human coronary arteries. *Circ Res* 1990;66:1045–1066, with permission.) (See color insert for Fig. 39–2.)

and *turbulence* results—that is, lateral motion of the blood becomes fully randomized. Transient turbulence occurs at peak systole in the human aorta but not at other sites in the healthy arterial system at rest. However, turbulence likely propagates through much of the central arterial system, including coronary arteries, during heavy dynamic exercise. Also, turbulence is promoted by surface irregularities, therefore it can occur distal to arterial stenoses and aneurysms.

When inertial and viscous forces are comparable, *secondary flows* (vortices and other nonaxial flow phenomena) occur at bends and branch sites (Fig. 39–1). Secondary flows are not turbulence because lateral motions are not randomized; instead, instantaneous local flow vectors are reproduced with each cardiac cycle. In most arteries of interest, secondary flows develop at arterial bends and bifurcations and the latter can extend into daughter branches for substantial distances (2,3). Care must therefore be taken when estimating shear stress using formulas that presume fully developed flow. For example, fully developed flows are rarely achieved between branch sites in the superficial coronary arteries.

Flow conditions in arteries are specified by the Reynolds number, which represents the ratio of inertial to viscous forces:

$$Re = 4\rho Q/\pi\mu D$$

where ρ is density of blood (1.03 g/cm^3), D is vessel diameter (cm), μ is blood viscosity (approximately 0.038 P for normal hematocrit), and Q is flow rate (mL/s). Stokes flow prevails when the Reynolds number is well below 1, second-

ary flows arise at greater Reynolds numbers, and the transition to turbulence occurs at Re of 500 to 1,500, depending on flow pulsatility, vascular geometries, and the presence/absence of stenoses (4).

Temporal Variations in Shear Stress

In vivo, arterial endothelium is exposed to large variations in shear stress. Mean shear stresses are typically 10 to 20 dynes/cm^2 in human arteries, but shears may remain close to zero at lateral aspects of some branch sites, and they can exceed 100 dynes/cm^2 adjacent to flow dividers of arterial branch sites at peak systole even at rest (5). Several fold increases occur during heavy exercise.

Temporal gradients in shear stress are large and occur over a great range of time scales. The cardiac cycle imposes oscillations that vary from approximately 1 to 20 Hz when exercise responses and greater harmonics of shear oscillations (6) are considered. Temporal variations in shear stress are particularly important at arterial bends and branches where they cause secondary flows to extend and retract with each cardiac cycle. Consequently, endothelium at these sites is continually exposed to shears that oscillate in both magnitude and direction. Slower variations in mean shear stress accompany the onset of exercise, circadian rhythms, and long-term cardiovascular adaptations to training, reproductive cycles, and pregnancy. Variations that occur over more than approximately 12 hours are particularly germane because they can elicit structural adaptations, first from the endothelium and then from the entire vessel wall (discussed later in this chapter). Finally, at the microscopic level, the passage of blood cells over the endothelium causes extremely rapid local variations in shear stress. At normal hematocrits and arterial shear stresses (15 dynes/cm^2), the frequency of shear fluctuations produced by erythrocytes is typically 200 Hz. The magnitude of these shear fluctuations is difficult to estimate and depends on the tendency for these cells to rotate, deform, and aggregate/disaggregate in shear fields (7,8). The effects of shear fluctuations due to blood cells on arterial endothelium have received little investigation.

Spatial Variations in Shear Stress

Arterial shear stresses can be readily computed only far from bends and branch sites; otherwise, complex numeric analyses or physical models are required. It is generally safe to infer that shear stresses just downstream from branch sites are increased by up to several fold over adjacent regions because high velocity flow is divided at the apices of branches. (In contrast, the apex of the flow divider itself may be subjected to very low shears because blood velocities are perpendicular to the endothelial surface at these sites.) Shears at other areas near branch sites are harder to predict and intuition often is misleading even to the expert, although low fluctuating shears have frequently been reported at lateral aspects of branches (1,9–11).

In the coronary vasculature, flexing of the vessels because of cardiac contraction introduces a complication, but its effects on shear appear to be minor (12). More problematic are the effects of curvature of these vessels as they cross the surface of the heart, because curvature can introduce substantial and unforeseeable effects on shear even in the absence of branches (13). More work is needed on the rheology of the coronary bed if lesion distribution is to be accurately compared with local blood flow.

Local Blood Flow Conditions and Animal Models

Elucidation of cardiovascular development, structure, function, and disease has benefited greatly from exploitation of diverse animal models, including mice, zebrafish, chick, quail, and *Xenopus*. However, important constraints apply to extrapolating flow conditions across species. Small homeotherms (e.g., mice) exhibit relatively high metabolic rates and, therefore, relatively high cardiac outputs that reflect the heat loss implicit in a large body surface area/weight ratio (14). Furthermore, shear stress varies as the inverse cube of vessel diameter. These two factors conspire to produce high shear stresses in smaller species or in juvenile animals. For example, we used very high frequency ultrasound and pulsed Doppler techniques to measure carotid artery size and blood flow rates, respectively, in anesthetized C57Bl6 mice (B.L. Langille and S.L. Adamson, unpublished data). These measurements indicated mean wall shear stresses of 90 dynes/cm^2, which was tenfold greater than those in hu-

man carotid arteries (11). Body size also affects the flow regimens that are encountered in arteries. Although turbulence can occur in large human arteries when flow is increased or the vessel is stenosed, it probably does not occur in mouse arteries, except perhaps in the aorta during maximal exercise. In general, flows are less prone to disturbances that could impact on the distribution of lesions in mouse models of atherothrombosis.

ARTERIAL RESPONSES TO ALTERED SHEAR STRESS

There is now compelling evidence that atherothrombotic lesions, including those in coronary arteries, most often originate near arterial bends and branch sites, where secondary flows occur. This finding, together with observations that experimental perturbations in flow can initiate or redistribute lesions (15,16), strongly implicates local hemodynamics in atherogenesis. Exhaustive study of selected arterial sites (e.g., the carotid bifurcation) has provided clear evidence that low or fluctuating shear stresses, or both, are proatherogenic, and most current work accepts this inference. Nonetheless, generalizations still need to be made cautiously. Flow conditions in arteries are complex, and arterial tissue responses to them are diverse; therefore, other proatherogenic conditions may arise at less well studied locations. Notably, some lesions in mouse models (Fig. 39–2) (see color insert) of atherothrombosis occur at high shear zones, whereas others may be at low shear zones. Indeed, diverse animal models of atherothrombosis confirm both predilection of bends and branch sites for lesions and flow sensitivity of lesion development; however, the evidence from these studies implicating any one manifestation of fluid flow in atherogenesis is weak. Finally, the roles of mechanical stresses other than shear remain unresolved but potentially important (discussed at the end of this chapter).

SHEAR STRESS AND THE ARTERIAL ENDOTHELIUM

Shear stresses are small forces that typically cause bulk deformations (strains) of artery walls that are well below 1% (17), strains that are usually much smaller than those caused by tensile (stretching) forces that are imposed on arterial tissues. However, the endothelial lining of arteries is directly exposed to flowing blood, and these cells have proven to be exquisitely sensitive to shear. This sensitivity impacts on atherogenesis through both modulation of classic functions of endothelium—that is, its role as a nonthrombogenic transport barrier that regulates inflammatory responses—and regulation of growth and contractile functions of smooth muscle.

The ultimate goal of studies of shear sensitivity of endothelial cells, as for mechanosensitivity of other cells, is to define the molecules or structures that sense shear force, the signaling pathways that are regulated by these sensors, the genetic and epigenetic targets of these pathways, and the mechanisms by which these target responses are integrated to produce coherent cellular responses. Understanding shear transduction has proven to be a daunting task and perhaps not surprisingly. Many structures that are not floating freely in the cytoplasm undergo deformation when forces are applied to the surfaces of cells. These structures include the plasma membrane, the cell cytoskeleton, and the adhesion complexes and organelles to which the cytoskeleton attaches. Conformational changes to these structures in response to mechanical loading likely activate many signaling pathways, with evolution culling those signals that are disadvantageous and amplifying or inducing those that are beneficial. It is not surprising, therefore, that multiple signaling cascades are activated by mechanical forces. Figure 39–3 highlights some key pathways that are believed to activate endothelial responses to shear stress.

As do many cell types, endothelium expresses mechanosensitive ion channels (18–21) that may regulate short-term physiologic function of these cells (21), as well as long-term regulators of arterial structure (e.g., transforming growth factor-β) (19). Also, forces are directly transmitted to cells through cell matrix or cell–cell adhesion complexes. Integrin activation, perhaps through formation of new matrix integrin interactions (22), has been widely examined and appears to activate downstream pathways, including the extracellular signal-regulated kinase-1/2 (ERK-1/2), mitogen-activated protein kinases (MAPKs), and phosphatidylinositol 3 kinase (PI3K). Although less well studied, the 67-kD laminin-binding protein also may contribute to sensing shear at the cell matrix interface (23). In addition, there

is evidence that endothelial cell–cell adhesion complexes sense shear stress. VE-cadherin, the primary adhesion molecule at endothelial adherens junctions, activates PI3K and p38 MAPK, and it recruits and signals through vascular endothelial growth factor (VEGF) receptor 2 in response to shear stress (24), a molecule that also can act downstream of integrin activation by shear (25). VEGF receptor 2 or integrin signaling may contribute to the activation of PI3K, which is important in regulating shear-dependent cell survival signals. There also is evidence that an additional endothelial cell–cell adhesion molecule and mediator of endothelial leukocyte interactions, platelet–endothelial cell adhesion molecule-1, acts as a shear transducer that can activate ERK signaling (26). Finally, there is evidence that deformation of endothelial caveolae provides an intriguing level of shear sensing that appears important in activation of endothelial nitric oxide synthase (NOSIII) (27,28).

Alternative pathways to ERK or PI3K activation also include heterotrimeric G proteins, perhaps without activation of G protein–coupled receptors (29,30). These signaling pathways are multifunctional. The ERK-1/2, MAPKs, and PI3Ks are important regulators of cell growth and survival, whereas these pathways and p38 modulate reorganization of adhesion complexes and the actin cytoskeleton (31–33) and, therefore, may also control cell morphologic responses to shear stress. Unsurprisingly, modulation of Rho guanosine triphosphatase activities, and their effect on the cell cytoskeleton, appears to be critical to shear-induced changes in cell morphology (22,34,35).

Atherothrombosis is an inflammatory disease; therefore, the nuclear factor-kappaB (NF-κB) pathway, which regu-

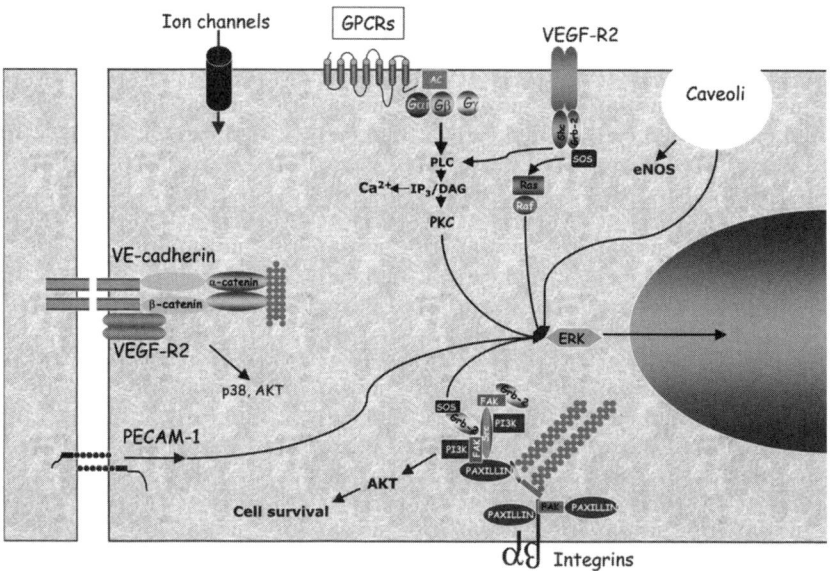

FIG. 39–3. Endothelial cell sensors of shear stress and the signaling pathways they activate. eNOS, endothelial nitric oxide synthase; ERK, extracellular signal-regulated kinase; GPCR, G protein–coupled receptor; PECAM-1, platelet–endothelial cell adhesion molecule-1; PI3K, phosphatidylinositol 3 kinase; PRC, protein kinase C; VEGF-R2, vascular endothelial growth factor receptor 2. (See color insert for Fig. 39–4.)

lates transcription during inflammatory responses and shear-induced growth factor (platelet-derived growth factor [PDGF]-B) expression (36), is relevant to this disease process. NF-κB normally remains cytoplasmic because of association with inhibitory proteins: the inhibitory-kappaBs (I-κBs); however, NF-κB can be activated and translocate to the nucleus by shear, probably through phosphorylation of I-κBs by an I-κB kinase complex that targets the proteins for proteasomal degradation (37). NF-κB is activated by low levels of shear and particularly by the presence of flow disturbances. There is now clear evidence that NF-kB is upregulated and primed for activation at the inner curvature of the mouse aortic arch, a site that is prone to atherogenesis, so that (proatherogenic) inflammatory stimuli lead quickly to nuclear translocation (38). Although hemodynamics in the mouse aorta has not been adequately studied, endothelial morphology at this site is characteristic of low or inconsistent shear stresses (38). These findings are potentially of great importance and they underscore the need to fully characterize flow conditions in this important model.

Endothelial Cellular Responses to Shear Stress

The sensitivity of endothelium to shear forces is most obviously manifested through changes in cell morphology: The cells elongate, the cell outline and its cytoskeleton become highly oriented in the direction of shear stress, and the profile of the cells becomes substantially more flattened when they are exposed to shear stress for more than 8 to 24 hours (39). Morphologic responses also include partial disassembly and then reassembly of adherens junctions, the primary sites of mechanical coupling between endothelial cells (39). Consequently, long-term alterations in secondary flow patterns near branch sites—for example, because of circadian fluctuations in tissue perfusion—may contribute to the high endothelial permeability and low-density lipoprotein (LDL) uptake at atherothrombosis-prone regions near arterial bends and branch sites (40). Shear stress often up-regulates antithrombotic properties of endothelium—for example, by regulating production of cyclooxygenase, prostacyclin, nitric oxide (NO), and tissue plasminogen activator.

Examination of candidate genes has revealed that many atherothrombosis-related genes display shear-sensitive expression by endothelium. Well studied examples include up-regulation at low or disturbed shears of vascular cell adhesion molecule-1 (VCAM-1) both *in vitro* (41) and in arteries (Fig. 39–4) (see color insert) (42), and shear sensitivity of expression of inflammatory regulators such as monocyte chemotactic protein-1 (43), intercellular adhesion molecule-1 (42,44), and modulators of cell proliferation and matrix production, including PDGFs, transforming growth factor-β_1, and endothelin (19,36,43,45,46). VCAM-1, a target of NF-κB signaling, may be a critical mediator of atherogenesis because a mutation that down-regulates both its expression and affinity for counter-receptor, very late activation antigen 4, strongly suppresses atherogenesis in a mouse

model (47) (Fig. 39–4). More recent, microarray-based studies have demonstrated that expression of hundreds of genes displaying sensitivity to both the duration and nature (e.g., laminar vs. turbulent) of shear impose on endothelial cells (48). Indeed, a major challenge, currently, for vascular biologists is appropriately integrating the surfeit of data concerning shear-dependent endothelial gene expression.

Blood Flow, Shear Stress, and Regulation of Arterial Diameter

Increases and decreases in arterial blood flow rates regulate vasomotor tone that rapidly adjusts vessel diameter. Physiologically, these responses amplify vasodilation/vasoconstriction that arise at the tissue level and cause them to propagate upstream to feed vessels that are not directly exposed to tissue metabolites. NO production driven by NOSIII appears to participate in this response, but recent data indicate a role for neuronal NOS, endothelium-derived prostanoids, and endothelium-derived hyperpolarizing factor, at least when NOSIII is suppressed (49–51).

If flow perturbations persist, diameter changes are amplified and entrenched by medial tissue remodeling (17,52). These remodeling responses, like most acute vasomotor responses to altered flow, are endothelium-dependent (17). Current evidence indicates that early, NO-dependent, vasoregulation also is critical for the long-term remodeling in response to altered flow (53,54). Rudic and coworkers (54) found that the capacity of arteries to remodel to a smaller diameter in response to reduced blood flow rate was lost in mice with null mutation of the endothelial NOS (*NOSIII*) gene; instead, these mice displayed a paradoxical wall thickening. More recent data indicate that the story may be more complex than these data suggest. We have found that endothelin-mediated vessel constriction contributes at least as much as NO withdrawal to remodeling in response to reduced blood flow (Pszczolko and Langille, unpublished observations). It also is important that flow-induced remodeling is a critical regulator of arterial development (55,56). That null mutation of NOSIII abolishes remodeling in adult mice that develop normally without the gene suggests that redundant regulators may be lost on maturation. Indeed, there must be multiple regulators and effectors of the complex processes related to flow-induced arterial growth control and remodeling. For example, matrix degradation through production of matrix metalloproteinases (57), and possibly other enzymes, participates in reorganizing matrix, and these likely contribute to the unequivocal changes to elastic lamellae during flow-induced remodeling (58) and during development (59). Arterial narrowing in response to decreased flow goes to completion rapidly, within 2 weeks in rabbit carotid arteries (60), whereas it may take months for diameters to stabilize after flow increases (52). The slower response to increased flow probably occurs because early vasodilator responses to increased flow are limited by the modest tone exhibited by most large arteries; thus, structural remodeling is required to affect substantial diameter increases. In contrast, vasoconstriction in response to decreased blood flow rate usually can accomplish diameter reductions, and then structural modifications simply serve to entrench these reductions and reset the working range of the artery.

PATHOLOGIC ARTERIAL REMODELING

The clinical consequences of arterial disease are most often caused by compromised blood flow. Subsequent flow-induced diameter adjustments of arteries may significantly affect the progression of these diseases, as well as the efficacy of therapeutic interventions. The nature of these adaptations in a pathologic setting remains uncertain, although new data are available in some cases.

Atherogenesis is affected by flow-induced vascular remodeling, and these effects may occur at several levels. Initially, atherothrombotic lesions narrow the vessel lumen and the resulting acceleration of blood flow through the lesion site increases shear stress. Glagov and coworkers (61) demonstrated "compensatory enlargement" in which the media subsequently expand to restore lumen diameter, presumably as a response to the increased shear associated with these accelerated flows. Thus, flow-induced adaptations appear to limit encroachment on the vessel lumen early in lesion development. Ultimately, however, growth of the lesion compromises blood flow, and adjacent healthy segments of the vessel wall experience reduced shear. If these segments respond normally, they will remodel to a smaller diameter, a response that would exacerbate hypoperfusion. Consequently, "adaptive" remodeling may be advantageous during early atherogenesis but disadvantageous in later stages.

Normal, flow-induced remodeling can also affect the development of collateral supply in obstructive arterial disease. In the absence of arterial disease, collateral vessels carry little flow because there is little pressure gradient between the arteries they link; however, obstruction of one of these arteries upstream of the collateral vessel will depressurize that end of the collateral and initiate or enhance flow through it, thereby stimulating collateral growth (62,63). There is also evidence that monocyte/macrophage can participate in flow-induced collateral growth (64). Notably, bypass graft implantation should compromise flow through collaterals and through any residual lumen in the bypassed vessel segment by delivering central arterial pressure downstream of the obstruction, thereby eliminating the pressure gradient driving flow through the stenosis. If collaterals and the obstructed vessel segment narrow in response to this flow reduction, then tissues perfusion may become more vulnerable to acute occlusion of the graft.

The above considerations implicitly assume that arteries will respond normally to changes in shear stress in the setting of vascular disease; however, quite novel responses can sometimes occur. Some well controlled and important experiments have demonstrated the influence of changes in shear stress on intimal proliferative responses. Intimal proliferation after balloon injury of rat carotid arteries is greater under low flow conditions than when flow rates are high (65). In addition, high blood flow rates inhibit intimal proliferation in endothelialized polytetrafluoroethylene grafts in baboons (66,67) and can even effect its reversal (68). PDGF may contribute to these responses (69).

ATHEROGENESIS AND FORCES OTHER THAN LUMINAL SHEAR STRESS

Why does atherothrombosis afflict only large- and medium-sized systemic arteries? It is possible that veins are spared because converging flows (e.g., through venous branch sites) are inherently stable, whereas diverging flows (arterial branch flows) promote flow instability (70,71). However, this consideration cannot explain sparing of the pulmonary arterial system. Sparing of pulmonary arteries suggests a role for arterial pressures. Transmural pressures induce tensile stresses that are very complex near arterial branch sites and bends, and these may be proatherogenic (72,73). It is important, however, that low pulmonary pressures due not imply low wall stress: The stresses are similar because of the thinner walls of the pulmonary vessels (74). High pressures in systemic arteries also enhance transmural fluid transport and, therefore, convection of proatherogenic substances (e.g., mitogens, cytokines, or LDL) to the intima/media. High-pressure gradients may conspire with compromised endothelial permeability barriers at atherothrombosis-prone sites to promote transport (75).

Finally, coronary arteries constantly stretch and shorten longitudinally with the cardiac cycle, and the mean level of such stretch can change as underlying myocardium infarcts or remodels in response to infarction elsewhere. Recent work demonstrates that arteries remodel in response to altered longitudinal forces (76) and these responses may modulate the progression of atherogenesis. It is clear that much work remains to be done on the diverse mechanical loads that are imposed on coronary vessels.

REFERENCES

1. Asakura T, Karino T. Flow patterns and spatial distribution of atherosclerotic lesions in human coronary arteries. *Circ Res* 1990;66:1045–1066.
2. Houle S, Roach MR. Flow studies in a rigid model of an aorto-renal junction: a case for high shear as a cause of the localization of sudanophilic lesions in rabbits. *Atherosclerosis* 1981;40:231–244.
3. Langille BL, Adamson SL. Relationship between blood flow direction and endothelial cell orientation at arterial branch sites in rabbits and mice. *Circ Res* 1981;48:481–488.
4. Nichols WW, O'Rourke MF. *McDonald's blood flow in arteries.* Philadelphia: Lea and Febiger, 1990.
5. Flaherty JT, Pierce JE, Ferrans VJ, et al. Endothelial nuclear patterns in the canine arterial tree with particular reference to hemodynamic events. *Circ Res* 1972;30:23–33.
6. Ling SC, Atabek HB, Letzing WG, et al. Nonlinear analysis of aortic flow in living dogs. *Circ Res* 1973;33:198–212.
7. Schmid-Schonbein H, Wells R. Fluid drop-like transition of erythrocytes under shear. *Science* 1969;165:288–291.

8. Chien S. Shear dependence of effective cell volume as a determinant of blood viscosity. *Science* 1970;168:977–979.

9. Friedman MH, Hutchins GM, Bargeron CB, et al. Correlation between intimal thickness and fluid shear in human arteries. *Atherosclerosis* 1981;39:425–436.

10. Friedman MH, Deters OJ, Mark FF, et al. Arterial geometry affects hemodynamics: a potential risk factor for atherosclerosis. *Atherosclerosis* 1983;46:225–231.

11. Ku DN, Giddens DP, Zarins CK, et al. Pulsatile flow and atherosclerosis in the human carotid bifurcation. Positive correlation between plaque location and low and oscillating shear stress. *Arteriosclerosis* 1985;5:293–302.

12. Zeng D, Ding Z, Friedman MH, et al. Effects of cardiac motion on right coronary artery hemodynamics. *Ann Biomed Eng* 2003;31:420–429.

13. Myers JG, Moore JA, Ojha M, et al. Factors influencing blood flow patterns in the human right coronary artery. *Ann Biomed Eng* 2001;29:109–120.

14. Schmidt-Neilsen K. *Scaling: why is animal size so important?* Cambridge: Cambridge University Press, 1984.

15. Roach MR, Fletcher J. Effect of unilateral nephrectomy of the localization of aortic sudanophilic lesions in cholesterol-fed rabbits. *Atherosclerosis* 1977;24:327–333.

16. Zand T, Hoffman AH, Savilonis BJ, et al. Lipid deposition in rat aortas with intraluminal hemispherical plug stenosis. *Am J Pathol* 1999;155:85–92.

17. Langille BL, O'Donnell F. Reductions in arterial diameter produced by chronic decreases in blood flow are endothelium-dependent. *Science* 1986;231:405–407.

18. Olesen SP, Clapham DE, Davies PF. Haemodynamic shear stress activates a K+ current in vascular endothelial cells. *Nature* 1988;331:168–170.

19. Ohno M, Cooke JP, Dzau VJ, et al. Fluid shear stress induces endothelial transforming growth factor beta-1 transcription and production. Modulation by potassium channel blockade. *J Clin Invest* 1995;95:1363–1369.

20. Forsyth SE, Hoger A, Hoger JH. Molecular cloning and expression of a bovine endothelial inward rectifier potassium channel. *FEBS Lett* 1997;409:277–282.

21. Suvatne J, Barakat AI, O'Donnell ME. Flow-induced expression of endothelial Na-K-Cl cotransport: dependence on K^+ and Cl^- channels. *Am J Physiol Cell Physiol* 2001;280:C216–C227.

22. Tzima E, del Pozo A, Shattil SJ, et al. Activation of integrins in endothelial cells by fluid shear stress mediates Rho-dependent cytoskeletal alignment. *EMBO J* 2001;20:4639–4647.

23. Gloe T, Riedmayr S, Sohn HY, et al. The 67-kDa laminin-binding protein is involved in shear stress-dependent endothelial nitric-oxide synthase expression. *J Biol Chem* 1999;274:15996–16002.

24. Shay-Salit A, Shushy M, Wolfovitz E, et al. VEGF receptor 2 and the adherens junction as a mechanical transducer in vascular endothelial cells. *Proc Natl Acad Sci USA* 2002;99:9462–9467.

25. Chen KD, Li YS, Kim M, et al. Mechanotransduction in response to shear stress. Roles of receptor tyrosine kinases, integrins and Shc. *J Biol Chem* 1999;274:18393–18400.

26. Osawa M, Masuda M, Kusano KI, et al. Evidence for a role of platelet endothelial cell adhesion molecule-1 in endothelial cell mechanosignal transduction: is it a mechanoresponsive molecule? *J Cell Biol* 2002;158:773–785.

27. Rizzo V, McIntosh DP, Schnitzer JE, et al. *In situ* flow activates endothelial nitric oxide synthase in luminal caveolae of endothelium with rapid caveolin dissociation and calmodulin association. *J Biol Chem* 1998;273:34724–34729.

28. Rizzo V, Sung A, Oh P, et al. Rapid mechanotransduction in situ at the luminal cell surface of vascular endothelium and its caveolae. *J Biol Chem* 1998;273:26323–26329.

29. Berthiaume F, Frangos JA. Flow-induced prostacyclin production is mediated by a pertussis toxin-sensitive G protein. *FEBS Lett* 1992;308:277–279.

30. Gudi SR, Clark CB, Frangos JA. Fluid flow rapidly activates G proteins in human endothelial cells: involvement of G proteins in mechanochemical signal transduction. *Circ Res* 1996;79:834–839.

31. Greenwood JA, Theibert AB, Prestwich GD, et al. Restructuring of focal adhesion plaques by PI 3-kinase: regulation by PtdIns (3,4,5)-P_3 binding to a-actinin. *J Cell Biol* 2000;150:627–641.

32. Potempa S, Ridley AJ. Activation of both MAP kinase and phosphatidylinositide 3-kinase by Ras is required for hepatocyte growth factor/scatter factor-induced adherens junction disassembly. *Mol Biol Cell* 1998;9:2185–2200.

33. Azuma N, Akasaka N, Ikeda M, et al. Role of p38 MAP kinase in endothelial cell alignment induced by fluid shear stress. *Am J Physiol* 2001;280:H189–H197.

34. Wojciak-Stothard B, Ridley AJ. Shear stress-induced endothelial cell polarization is mediated by Rho and Rac but not Cdc42 or PI 3-kinases. *J Cell Biol* 2003;161:429–439.

35. Tzima E, Del Pozo MA, Kiosses WB, et al. Activation of Rac1 by shear stress in endothelial cells mediates both cytoskeletal reorganization and effects on gene expression. *EMBO J* 2002;21:6791–6800.

36. Khachigian LM, Resnick N, Gimbrone MA Jr, et al. Nuclear factor-kappaB interacts functionally with the platelet-derived growth factor B-chain shear-stress response element in vascular endothelial cells exposed to fluid shear stress. *J Clin Invest* 1995;96:1169–1175.

37. Collins T, Cybulsky MI. NF-kappaB: pivotal mediator or innocent bystander in atherogenesis? *J Clin Invest* 2001;107:255–264.

38. Hajra L, Evans AI, Chen M, et al. The NF-kB signal transduction pathway in aortic endothelial cells is primed for activation in regions predisposed to atherosclerotic lesion formation. *Proc Natl Acad Sci USA* 2000;97.9052–9057.

39. Noria S, Cowan DB, Gotlieb AI, et al. Transient and steady-state effects of shear stress on endothelial cell adherens junctions. *Circ Res* 1999;85:504–514.

40. Caplan BA, Schwartz CJ. Increased endothelial cell turnover in areas of Evans blue uptake in the pig aorta. *Atherosclerosis* 1973;17:401–417.

41. Ando J, Tsuboi H, Korenaga R, et al. Shear stress inhibits adhesion of cultured mouse endothelial cells to lymphocytes by downregulating VCAM-1 expression. *Am J Physiol Cell Physiol* 1994;267:C679–C687.

42. Walpola PL, Gotlieb AI, Cybulsky MI, et al. Expression of ICAM-1 and VCAM-1 and monocyte adherence in arteries exposed to altered shear stress. *Arterioscler Thromb Vasc Biol* 1995;15:2–10.

43. Bao X, Lu C, Frangos JA. Temporal gradient in shear but not steady shear stress induces PDGF-A and MCP-1 expression in endothelial cells: role of NO, NFkB, and *erg*-1. *Arterioscler Thromb Vasc Biol* 1999;19:996–1003.

44. Nagel T, Resnick N, Atkinson WJ, et al. Shear stress selectively upregulates intercellular adhesion molecule-1 expression in cultured human vascular endothelial cells. *J Clin Invest* 1994;94:885–891.

45. Sharefkin JB, Diamond SL, Eskin SG, et al. Fluid flow decreases preproendothelin mRNA levels and suppresses endothelin-1 peptide release in cultured human endothelial cells. *J Vasc Surg* 1991;14:1–9.

46. Hsieh HJ, Li NQ, Frangos JA. Shear stress increases endothelial platelet-derived growth factor mRNA levels. *Am J Physiol* 1991;260:H642–H646.

47. Cybulsky MI, Iiyama K, Li H, et al. A major role for VCAM-1, but not ICAM-1, in early atherosclerosis. *J Clin Invest* 2001;107:1255–1262.

48. Garcia-Cardena G, Comander J, Anderson KR, et al. Biomechanical activation of vascular endothelium as a determinant of its functional phenotype. *Proc Nat Acad Sci USA* 2001;98:4478–4485.

49. Sun D, Huang A, Smith CJ, et al. Enhanced release of prostaglandins contributes to flow-induced arteriolar dilation in eNOS knockout mice. *Circ Res* 1999;85:288–293.

50. Huang A, Sun D, Shesely EG, et al. Neuronal NOS-dependent dilation to flow in coronary arteries of male eNOS-KO mice. *Am J Physiol Heart Circ Physiol* 2002;282:H429–H436.

51. Huang A, Sun D, Carroll MA, et al. EDHF mediates flow-induced dilation in skeletal muscle arterioles of female eNOS-KO mice. *Am J Physiol Heart Circ Physiol* 2003;280:H2462–H2469.

52. Kamiya A, Togawa T. Adaptive regulation of wall shear stress to flow change in the canine carotid artery. *Am J Physiol* 1980;239:H14–H21.

53. Tronc F, Wassef M, Esposito B, et al. Role of NO in flow-induced remodeling of the rabbit common carotid artery. *Arterioscler Thromb Vasc Biol* 1996;16:1256–1262.

54. Rudic RD, Shesely EG, Maeda N, et al. Direct evidence for the importance of endothelium-derived nitric oxide in vascular remodeling. *J Clin Invest* 1998;101:731–736.

55. Langille BL. Mechanical forces in vascular growth and development. In: Weir E, Archer SL, Reeves JT, eds. *The fetal and neonatal pulmonary circulations.* Armonk, NY: Futura, 2000:201–212.

56. Langille BL. Remodelling of developing and mature arteries: endothelium, smooth muscle and matrix. *J Cardiovasc Pharmacol* 1993;21:S11–S17.

57. Tronc F, Mallat Z, Lehoux S, et al. Role of matrix metalloproteinases

in blood flow-induced arterial enlargement—interaction with NO. *Arterioscler Thromb Vasc Biol* 2000;20:E120–E126.

58. Masuda H, Zhuang YJ, Singh TM, et al. Adaptive remodeling of internal elastic lamina and endothelial lining during flow-induced arterial enlargement. *Arterioscler Thromb Vasc Biol* 1999;19:2298–2307.

59. Wong LC, Langille BL. Developmental remodeling of the internal elastic lamina of rabbit arteries. Effect of blood flow. *Circ Res* 1996;78:799–805.

60. Langille BL, Bendeck MP, Keeley FW. Adaptations of carotid arteries of young and mature rabbits to reduced carotid blood flow. *Am J Physiol* 1989;256:H931–H939.

61. Glagov S, Weisenberg E, Zarins CK, et al. Compensatory enlargement of human atherosclerotic coronary arteries. *N Engl J Med* 1987;316:1371–1375.

62. Schaper W, Ito WD. Molecular mechanisms of coronary collateral vessel growth. *Circ Res* 1996;79:911–919.

63. Langille BL, Gotlieb AI, Kim DW. In vivo responses of endothelial cells to hemodynamic stress. In: Yoshida Y, Yamaguchi T, Caro CG, et al, eds. *Role of blood flow in atherogenesis.* Tokyo: Springer-Verlag, 1988:157–161.

64. Schaper W, Scholz D. Factors regulating arteriogenesis. *Arterioscler Thromb Vasc Biol* 2003;23:1143–1151.

65. Kohler TR, Jawien A. Flow affects development of intimal hyperplasia after arterial injury in rats. *Circ Res* 1992;12:963–971.

66. Kohler TR, Kirkman TR, Kraiss LW, et al. Increased blood flow inhibits neointimal hyperplasia in endothelialized vascular grafts. *Circ Res* 1991;69:1557–1565.

67. Geary RL, Kohler TR, Vergel S, et al. Time course of flow-induced smooth muscle cell proliferation and intimal thickening in endothelialized baboon vascular grafts. *Circ Res* 1994;74:14–23.

68. Mattsson EJ, Kohler TR, Vergel SM, et al. Increased blood flow induces regression of intimal hyperplasia. *Arterioscler Thromb Vasc Biol* 1997;17:2245–2249.

69. Kraiss LW, Geary RL, Mattsson EJ, et al. Acute reductions in blood flow and shear stress induce platelet-derived growth factor-A expression in baboon prosthetic grafts. *Circ Res* 1996;79:45–53.

70. Strong AB, Absolom DR, Zingg W, et al. A new flow cell for platelet adhesion studies. *Ann Biomed Eng* 1982;10:71–82.

71. Batchelor GK. *An introduction to fluid mechanics,* 2nd ed. Cambridge: Cambridge University Press, 1999.

72. Thubrikar MJ, Baker JW, Nolan SP. Inhibition of atherosclerosis associated with reduction of arterial intraluminal stress in rabbits. *Arteriosclerosis* 1988;8:410–420.

73. Thubrikar MJ, Robicsek F. Pressure-induced arterial wall stress and atherosclerosis. *Ann Thorac Surg* 1995;59:1594–1603.

74. Leung DY, Glagov S, Mathews MB. Elastin and collagen accumulation in rabbit ascending aorta and pulmonary trunk during postnatal growth. Correlation of cellular synthetic response with medial tension. *Circ Res* 1977;41:316–323.

75. Tarbell JM. Mass transport in arteries and the localization of atherosclerosis. *Ann Rev Biomed Eng* 2003;5:79–118.

76. Jackson ZS, Gotlieb AI, Langille BL. Wall tissue remodeling regulates longitudinal tension in arteries. *Circ Res* 2002;90:918–925.

CHAPTER 40

Interaction of Platelet Activation and Coagulation

H. Coenraad Hemker and Theo Lindhout

Key Words: Coagulation factors; platelet receptors; platelets; procoagulant activity; thrombin generation; thrombus formation.

The classical paradigm has it that hemostasis is a two-step process: Primary hemostasis, probed by the bleeding time and a result of platelet function, is followed by secondary hemostasis reflected in the clotting time and for which the plasmatic clotting system was held responsible. The interaction between platelets and coagulation, although a central topic until about the mid-twentieth century (1–6), became a relatively neglected area of research that only recently is regaining interest.

For several decades, the main aim of research in platelet physiology has been the understanding of aggregation and adhesion and of the intracellular processes that govern these phenomena. It is not unlikely that this came about through the introduction, by Gustav Born, of the optical aggregometer technique (7) that so much facilitated the study of this aspect of platelet function. Aggregometry is commonly carried out in anticoagulated plasma so that the results necessarily pertain to that part of the hemostatic mechanism in which thrombin

does not play a role. In contrast, blood coagulation—that is, the interaction of clotting factors (furthermore indicated as "factor" plus a roman numeral)—was usually studied in (fractions and preparations from) platelet-poor plasma (PPP), therefore the interactions between the two systems easily escaped attention.

In hemostasis, platelet function and coagulation are closely intertwined and are mutually reinforcing processes. A seminal observation was made in 1982 when Bevers and coworkers (8) showed that activated platelets lose the natural asymmetry of their plasma membrane ("scrambling"), so that the outside of the platelet enriches in phosphatidyl serine (PS) and phosphatidyl ethanolamine (PE) and, consequently, can facilitate the formation of the prothrombinase and tenase complex (discussed later). This prompted further studies on the role of phospholipids in the reaction mechanism of blood coagulation and on the intracellular and intramembrane mechanisms behind membrane scrambling (e.g., see Bevers and coworkers [9]), but not so much on the function of platelet-rich plasma (PRP) as an integrated system.

Experiments that did allow studying interactions between platelets and plasma invariably showed evidence for early participation of thrombin generation in hemostasis. Products of thrombin action (activated F-V and VIII, fibrinopeptide A, and β-thromboglobulin) appear in a wound before clotting can be observed (10,11), and it was reported that thrombin formation can precede platelet activation (12). Also, fibrin is seen in the immediate vicinity of a adhering/aggregating platelets in early stages of plug formation (13).

H. C. Hemker: Department of Biochemistry, Cardiovascular Research Institute Maastricht, P. O. Box 616, 6200 MD Maastricht, The Netherlands.

T. Lindhout: Department of Biochemistry, Cardiovascular Research Institute Maastricht, P. O. Box 616, 6200 MD Maastricht, The Netherlands.

Therefore, although platelet plug formation apparently precedes the bulk of thrombin formation, the interplay between the two systems starts right from the beginning.

The classical key observations at the basis of the concept of primary and secondary hemostasis is that bleeding time is normal in hemophiliacs but clotting time is not, and that in thrombopenia bleeding time is prolonged but clotting time is normal. However, such traces of thrombin as can be formed in hemophilia may suffice in the early stages of hemostasis. Bleeding time is known to be prolonged if thrombin generation is as profoundly affected as in severe overdosage of oral anticoagulants or heparin (14–16). Also, the observation that anticoagulation, by either oral anticoagulants or heparin, is effective in preventing arterial thrombosis (17,18) suggests a role for thrombin in the formation of the arterial "platelet" thrombus. Conversely, aspirin, the antiplatelet drug par excellence, has been reported to prevent venous thrombosis (19).

The picture emerges of thrombin, at very low concentrations, playing a role right from the beginning of the hemostatic–thrombotic reaction. However, studies on thrombin generation (discussed later) show that the role of the platelet is not finished with the forming of an aggregate adhering to a lesion because their role in propagating thrombin formation remains to be played. Coagulation—that is, the conversion of fibrinogen in fibrin—also does not mark the end of the activity of the plasmatic clotting system. When clotting is activated in blood or plasma, a dynamic situation builds up in which prothrombin is converted into thrombin and thrombin disappears by its interaction with antithrombins. Clotting occurs at the very beginning of the process, as soon as 5 to 10 nM thrombin are formed. All fibrinogen is converted into fibrin in a matter of seconds at a moment that ~95% prothrombin remains to be activated and the peak of thrombin concentration is seen minutes after clotting. The velocity of thrombin generation and the amount formed depend on platelet activity and many other variables, such as the concentrations of the about 20 plasma proteins involved, the availability of tissue factor (TF), and procoagulant phospholipid surfaces (PPSs) from circulating microparticles and/or wounded cells, exposed "gruel" from rupturing plaques.

In this review, current insights in the relation of thrombin generation and platelet procoagulant function are discussed that might be relevant for a better understanding of the process of thrombus growth. Currently, the subject is becoming a focus of research and no consensus view has as yet been obtained. Consequently, no uniform picture can emerge. It appears that the development of platelet procoagulant activity can be triggered by a variety of platelet receptor–ligand interactions. In addition, some ligands, like thrombin, interact with a number of different platelet receptors, for example, glycoprotein (GPIb)-V-IX and protease-activated receptors (PARs). In contrast, receptors like integrin $\alpha_{IIb}\beta_3$ can interact with different ligands (e.g., fibrinogen and von Willebrand factor [vWF]). The complexity that arises from the many possible reaction sequences involved in signaling procoagulant response is generally recognized and is poorly understood. It is possible that the actual mechanism is strongly dependent on the experimental or *in vivo* circumstances such as flow, availability of TF, and extracellular matrix proteins.

This chapter first provides a brief outline of the experimental approaches to and mechanism of thrombin generation. Then the following topics will be discussed in more detail: (a) release of clotting factors from platelets; (b) appearance of procoagulant phospholipids in the platelet membrane; (c) role of established clotting factor receptors in rendering the platelet procoagulant; (d) putative clotting factor receptors on the platelet; and the (e) role of circulating TF and interaction between platelets and white blood cells.

METHODS OF STUDYING THE PROCOAGULANT FUNCTION OF PLATELETS: THE IMPORTANCE OF THROMBIN GENERATION

All the tools of chemical physiology can serve in the search for the procoagulant role of platelets, but there are two tests, close to physiologic function, that are of special importance: flow reactors that enable dynamic and kinetic studies on cell adhesion and activation and thrombin generation during both static and flow conditions.

The flow chamber, as developed by Baumgartner (20,21), Sakariassen (22), and Badimon (23) and modified and adapted by numerous others, is especially useful for investigation of platelets at an interface. In combination with fluorescence, confocal microscopy, or both, it also is a powerful tool to study procoagulant properties of platelets. From the earliest applications on, information on the role of thrombin was obtained from the comparison of the behavior of anticoagulated and nonanticoagulated blood. Anticoagulated blood will allow platelets to stick to different surfaces without allowing the platelets to become overtly procoagulant and form a thrombus, showing the importance of early interaction between platelets and the clotting system (20). The use of fluorescent-labeled annexin V, for example, allows visualization of the appearance of the type of phospholipid surface that also supports the binding of clotting factors, both in flow chamber and flow cytometry experiments (24,25).

Flow chambers also can be used to monitor reactants (e.g., thrombin) that are formed during the interaction of the fluid with the adherent cells. Technically, chemical reactions at the fluid–solid interface are more easily investigated using a rotating disk immersed in a limited amount of fluid (26,27), which has the advantage of a uniform accessibility of the surface to the reactants from the fluid and the possibility to follow the build up of reactants in time.

In the late 1980s, Béguin and coworkers (28) reintroduced a technique that had practically disappeared with the advent of adhesion and aggregation studies and that is eminently suited to investigate platelet–plasma interactions, to wit thrombin generation in PRP (28) or whole blood (29,30).

Mann and colleagues (31,32) and Monroe and coworkers (33) developed synthetic plasma models using platelets or membranes, with or without the addition of other cells. Also, the analysis of reactants in clotting whole blood can yield important information on the function of platelet–plasma interactions (30,34–36). Finally, studies on blood flowing from a microvascular wound have yielded important information on thrombin generation under physiologic circumstances (10,11,37,38).

The interaction between platelets and thrombin generation can thus be studied at different levels. The more the experimental design mimics *in vivo* physiologic conditions, the more our analytic understanding decreases. In that order we can distinguish: (a) the interaction between the platelet and isolated single clotting factors; (b) platelets in media reconstituted with isolated clotting factors and inhibitors; (c) PRP; (d) clotting whole blood; and (e) blood emerging from a wound.

Most of these approaches are dependent on measuring the development of reactants in time, which involves labor-intensive subsampling and analysis. Thrombin generation in PRP can now be monitored in real time in up to 48 samples in parallel, however, by measuring the splitting of a fluorescent thrombin substrate and comparing it online to the signal from a calibrator with fixed activity (39). This is as near as the current state of the technique allows measurement of the function of the "isolated organ" PRP.

A thrombin generation curve in PRP (Fig. 40–1) is characterized by a lag (or initiation) phase, in which traces of thrombin and platelets interact so as to prepare the scene for explosive thrombin generation. The importance of thrombin can be judged from the effect of hirudin, which binds tightly, immediately, and irreversibly to thrombin. Already at a low concentration (10 nM), it prolongs the lag time because it scavenges traces of thrombin that form during the initiation phase. Thrombin can engage in the positive feedback reactions (platelets, factors V and VIII) that start explo-sive thrombin formation only after the emerging thrombin has neutralized all hirudin. Virtually the total amount of thrombin is then formed, with only 10 nM thrombin being neutralized. Heparin, which acts as a catalyst of natural antithrombin, is a slow but much more potent inhibitor. Being slow, it allows some thrombin to persist during the initiation phase, so that the lag time is somewhat prolonged but less than with hirudin. The peak of thrombin and the area under the curve are eventually inhibited more than with hirudin because the natural concentration of antithrombin (3 μM) is greater than that of prothrombin (2 μM).

This example shows that long clotting times can accompany almost normal thrombin formation and that low thrombin formation can occur after an almost normal clotting time. There is no single parameter that contains all the information, rather the whole concentration course of thrombin should be considered.

The amount of active thrombin formed can be quantified as the area under the thrombin generation curve, or endogenous thrombin potential (40). It represents the number of "molecule-minutes" (analogous to "man-hours") and determines how much enzymatic work thrombin can do during its short life in plasma. Platelets in the clot play an important role in determining the velocity of thrombin formation and the endogenous thrombin potential (Fig. 40–1). It is not really clear "what all this thrombin is for" (41), but it is evident that it does serve a purpose. Speculating about the function of thrombin formed after the formation of fibrin is complete, one must consider that the amount and the velocity of thrombin formed after coagulation per se has occurred determines the structure of the fibrin clot and its resistance to lysis (42–45). Also, the concentration of thrombin attained at a focus where thrombin generation is triggered determines the concentration gradient of thrombin that develops around that focus. Furthermore, clotting is far from being the only function of thrombin (46). Concentrations of thrombin less than 1 nM suffice to bring about platelet activation and a host of reactions in other cells as well (47–50); the greater the concentration of thrombin formed at the focus, the farther from the focus this threshold can be attained—that is, the larger the size of the thrombotic area.

The amount of thrombin formed depends on the size and the properties of the trigger (wound, ruptured arterial plaque, or venous minitrauma) and the potential of the blood to form thrombin. The importance of the former is generally recognized, the importance of the latter becomes apparent from clinical observation. Resistance to activated protein C (APC) or heparin administration hardly influences the start of the hemostatic/thrombotic reaction triggered by TF, but nevertheless it has an important influence on thrombotic tendency. The lupus anticoagulant brings about a prolongation of the clotting time but an increase of thrombin formation and causes a thrombotic tendency (51,52). Inversely, clinical bleeding in congenital clotting factor deficiencies correlates better with the amount of thrombin formed than with the

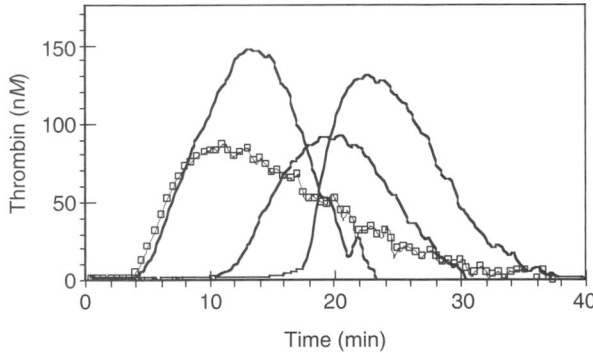

FIG. 40–1. Thrombin generation in platelet-rich plasma (PRP). Calibrated automated thrombinography was used (39). Drawn lines (from left to right): normal PRP, PRP with 0.2 U/mL (~20 nM) unfractionated heparin, and PRP with 20 nM hirudin. *Open circles* represent 20 μg/mL of a monoclonal antibody against GPIIb/IIIa (7e3).

clotting time or with the level of the deficient factor (53). Several antithrombotics (low molecular weight heparins, dermatan sulfate, pentasaccharide) will not significantly influence any form of clotting time, but they do diminish the amount of thrombin formed. In fact, all known antithrombotics, platelet antagonists, and anticoagulants alike cause diminution of thrombin formation and have variable effects on clotting times and/or platelet aggregation and adherence (see Hemker and Béguin [54] for further discussion).

AN OUTLINE OF THE MECHANISM OF THROMBIN GENERATION

In a wound or ruptured plaque, three elements are exposed to blood that activate hemostasis: (a) TF, an integral membrane protein of perivascular connective tissue; (b) collagen; and (c) procoagulant, damaged cell membranes, which are instrumental in bringing about thrombin generation. This not being a review on the blood coagulation mechanism per se, we refrain from exhaustive referencing and refer to a number of review articles for that purpose (54–59).

The clotting mechanism is started by the binding of the plasma protein factor VII(a) to TF. TF functions as an essential cofactor of factor VIIa in the conversion of factors IX and X into the serine proteases factors IXa and Xa. Factor Xa develops into a strong inhibitor of its own formation by binding to TF pathway inhibitor, which two proteins then bind to and prevent further activity of the TF-VIIa complex. Factors Xa and IXa assemble together with their cofactors VIIIa and Va, respectively, on cell membranes containing anionic phospholipids to convert factors X into Xa and prothrombin into thrombin.

The chain of sequential proteolytic activations VII(a) $\Rightarrow$ (IXa) $\Rightarrow$ Xa $\Rightarrow$ (pro)thrombin* has an amplifying effect that ensures an explosive generation of thrombin. Each enzyme in itself is hardly active; however, the helper protein enhances its turnover by 1,000-fold and the membrane surface allows saturation with the substrate, which again can enhance reaction rates 1,000-fold (60). Because of this dependence, thrombin generation can be limited to the site and the moment of injury.

The helper proteins arise from inactive plasma proteins (factors V and VIII) through the action of thrombin itself. Thrombin, however, also reacts with endothelial cell–associated thrombomodulin, and this complex activates protein C. APC degrades factors Va and VIIIa. The product of the coagulation cascade (i.e., thrombin) thus directly promotes its own formation through activation of factors V and VIII, but indirectly limits it by providing APC that removes the helper proteins. This creates a window in time that limits explosive thrombin formation to the minutes after the process is triggered.

Anionic, procoagulant phospholipids are practically restricted to the cytoplasm (inner) side of (blood) cell mem-

branes and, therefore, are not normally exposed to the surrounding plasma or interstitial fluid. Cell damage in a wound will make them appear to a limited extent, and thus the first traces of thrombin may be formed. In the wound platelets will encounter collagen and these traces of thrombin, which induces scrambling of their cell membranes and consequently the appearance of a PPS. The bulk of thrombin formation thus occurs at the surface of activated platelets sticking in a wound and in this way is confined to the wound area.

Not only the composition but also the size of the available surface influences the kinetic properties of the enzymes. A prothrombinase complex on a large surface of procoagulant phospholipid is more efficient than that on a small vesicle because the surface around the complex acts as a "funnel" that guides prothrombin from free solution to the enzyme through lateral diffusion (61). For the interpretation of experiments on clotting factor–platelet interaction, it is essential to realize that mere changes in lipid availability and composition, as they occur during platelet activation, may profoundly change the binding and kinetic characteristics of the platelet membrane. This may be one of the reasons that a number of so far elusive clotting factor receptors have been postulated (discussed later).

TF does not normally occur on circulating platelets, but it is deposited on adherent platelets by leukocytes (discussed later). It can thus be imagined that on damaged cells and platelets provided with TF, the complete thrombin generation process can occur on the same surface. This is probably not the rule, however, otherwise the antithrombin–pentasaccharide complex, which acts on free factor Xa only, would not have an antithrombotic effect (62).

A relatively new insight is that the amount of thrombin formed in a clot also determines the degree of activation of a thrombolysis inhibitor and, therefore, indirectly also determines the resistance of the clot against fibrinolysis (13,43,63–69). This may well explain the clinical observation that in deficiencies of factors VII, IX and XI, where little thrombin is formed, loose clots form that readily lyse. This may explain the common clinical observation in, for example, tooth extraction in hemophiliacs in whom bleeding starts hours after the event. Sometimes this is called a defect in secondary hemostasis, but it is not because the consolidation of a platelet plug, which is the original definition of secondary hemostasis, takes place in the half hour after trauma.

RELEASE OF CLOTTING FACTORS BY PLATELETS

Platelet α-granules contain the clotting protein factor V and the adhesive proteins vWF, fibrinogen, fibronectin, and thrombospondin (13,66–69). Factor V is shed in nonactivated form and activated by thrombin afterward (70). The physiologic function of factor V release is difficult to understand in terms of thrombin generation in plasma because, as is already known from the earliest studies on factor V to-

---

*$\Rightarrow$ is used to indicate "activates."

gether with recent confirmation, 5% or less of the normal plasma concentration of this factor is required for nearly normal thrombin generation (71). Observations on patients suggest that absence of, or inhibitors against, plasmatic factor V do not cause a bleeding syndrome unless platelet factor V also is absent or inhibited (72, and references therein). This in itself is a strong argument in favor of the concept that for the physiologic hemostatic function, thrombin generation in the vicinity of platelets is of prime importance (73).

One can surmise that release of factor V from platelets serves a purpose for thrombin generation within a platelet aggregate that adheres within a wound. It is rarely realized that the circulation time of the blood through the body (~35 s) is smaller than the whole blood clotting time (>60 s). As circulation means mixing, thrombin generation in circulating blood will never reach the limits that allow clotting. Only when very high concentrations of TF reach the bloodstream, as in sepsis or massive brain or lung damage, thrombin generation in circulating blood will ever reach the threshold limits that allow a thrombin burst. This holds *a fortiori* under the high shear conditions—that is, during primary plug formation and in arterial thrombi. There thrombin generation is dependent on the limited amount of plasma factors entrapped in the interstices of the aggregate. In plasma, factor X is in sixfold to eightfold excess to factor V. Extra factor V, supplied from the platelets, will shift this ratio toward unity; hence, allowing the formation of more prothrombinase, and thus more adequate thrombin formation. Results have shown that among washed platelets—that is, under conditions that only intraplatelet factor V counts—a population of platelets (COAT-platelets) can be distinguished that on stimulation by thrombin and collagen together preferably binds released factor V(a) (72). Now thrombin and collagen bring about the exposure of procoagulant phospholipids (PS and PE) in the platelet membrane (see the following section) and factor V(a) binds to such surfaces. One, therefore, can presume that the binding of factor Va to thrombin- and collagen-stimulated platelets is the binding to a PPS as such. It became clear, however, that the retention of procoagulant proteins on COAT-platelets also involves a more specific interaction. Serotonin (abundantly shed by stimulated platelets) binds to procoagulant and adhesive proteins through the action of a transglutaminase. If so modified, these factors bind to the platelet surface, possibly to an as yet unidentified serotonin receptor (74,75).

Also, factor IX, in plasma, is in excess over factor VIII (more than 50-fold). There is no compelling evidence that factor VIII is released from platelets. This factor, however, is carried by vWF, the binding of which to GPIb and activated $\alpha_{IIb}\beta_3$ on the surface of platelets is well documented. Binding of vWF therefore concentrates factor VIII near the platelet surface. As soon as some thrombin is generated on the platelet surface, this factor VIII will be activated and will preferably bind to procoagulant phospholipid rather than to vWF. By making elegant use of that human factor VIII binds to mouse vWF but human vWF hardly to mouse platelets, it could be shown that binding of factor VIII to a platelet aggregate indeed has a prothrombotic effect (76). This also may contribute to the defect in prothrombin consumption in patients with a congenital lack of GPIb (77). The main mechanism behind this observation, however, is probably a direct role of the binding of (activated) vWF to the GPIb receptor (discussed later).

PRESENTATION OF PROCOAGULANT LIPIDS BY PLATELETS

As discussed earlier, the anionic phospholipids PS and PE are essential to thrombin generation because several key reactions in the process occur only at the interface of the solute and a negatively charged phospholipid membrane surface containing these molecules. The virtual absence of PS and PE in the outer layer of the membranes of normal cells, including blood and endothelial cells, may explain the low tendency to thrombin generation in normal blood. If, in drepanocytosis, the asymmetry of the sickling red cell membrane is disturbed by hemoglobin crystals, thrombosis is readily provoked (78).

The phospholipid components of the cell membrane are not evenly distributed between the inner and the outer leaflet. The negatively charged PS and PE, which are essential for the procoagulant function, are to be found at the inside (79–82). Therefore, a cell membrane is not procoagulant unless damaged, apoptotic, or otherwise disturbed. Platelets are the only known cells in which this disturbance ("flip-flop") is a part of their physiologic function, because it brings about their power to facilitate blood coagulation (8,83).

Platelet membranes scramble as a last stage in their activation, after shape change, release, and aggregation. Thrombin alone, for example, will bring about only limited scrambling in washed platelets, whereas it does cause full shape change and release. Full scrambling is brought about by thrombin in combination with collagen and with fibrin and vWF (discussed later). Epinephrine, adenosine diphosphate (ADP), prostanoids, and others may enhance the procoagulant response of platelets but will not by themselves bring it about.

Loss of phospholipid asymmetry is attributed to three putative mechanisms: (a) an inward-directed translocation ("flippase") for PS and PE; (b) an outward-directed translocation ("floppase"); and (c) a scramblase, which facilitates bidirectional migration across the bilayer of all phospholipid classes (9). These activities await further description and definition in terms of protein entities. The precise intracellular events that activate the intramembrane mechanism remain largely obscure. It is clear that an increase in intracellular Ca^{2+} is required: Any Ca^{2+}-ionophore is a potent inducer of scrambling (see Heemskerk and coworkers [84] for more information). The next section describes which platelet receptors and ligands may be involved in inducing the process.

Platelet activation goes hand in hand with extensive rearrangement of the cytoskeleton. In this process patches of the membrane bulge outward and pinch off ("blebbing") (85). This causes minute vesicles (microparticles) to appear, the procoagulant nature of which can be demonstrated (e.g., by annexin V binding) and the platelet origin of which is clear from their containing integral platelet membrane proteins such as GPIb $\alpha_{IIb}\beta_3$ and P-selectin (86,87). Such microparticles bind to fibrin (88), so at least part of them must remain in an emerging thrombus. Probably they are also shed in the bloodstream, because they have been found in the peripheral circulation in various pathologic conditions (88–95).

Calpain inhibitors that inhibit cytoskeleton degradation also inhibit blebbing and microparticle formation but not the generation of procoagulant platelet surfaces (96) (discussed later). They also partially inhibit thrombin generation in PRP (unpublished results), presumably by limiting the contribution of microparticles to the total procoagulant surface. The microparticles can be demonstrated in the serum remaining after a thrombin generation experiment, and their appearance is inhibited by antibodies against vWF and $\alpha_{IIb}\beta_3$. In the presence of fibrin, antibodies against GPIb/IX also inhibit thrombin generation and microparticle formation (97).

PLATELET RECEPTORS INVOLVED IN THE PRESENTATION OF A PROCOAGULANT MEMBRANE SURFACE

There can be no doubt that the platelet receptors GPIb-V-IX, $\alpha_{IIb}\beta_3$, and GPVI, as well as PARs, play a role in the development of a procoagulant membrane surface. There is no consensus, however, on the precise role of each of these receptors or on that of the main ligands: thrombin, vWF, fibrin(ogen), and collagen. The situation is complicated by that different ligands that are released by platelets (ADP, serotonin) modulate the procoagulant response.

It may be illusory to try and find one unifying mechanism that explains the process because, like for other aspects of platelet activation, parallel mechanisms may exist of which the quantitative role differs with the (experimental) circumstances. This is doubtlessly the case with platelets that adhere to collagen through GPVI, because in a wound the majority of platelets will never be in contact with collagen.

Platelets adherent to collagen show important morphologic changes that are accompanied by the exposure of PS (98). The morphologic changes are not essential to PS exposure, however, because they can be inhibited by inhibiting calpain, which has no influence on PS exposure (96). In contrast, of platelets adhering to fibrinogen, only a small fraction (~10%) shows PS. Moreover, they bind less factor Va and consequently convert prothrombin about half as fast as collagen adherent platelets do (99). Further activation by thrombin (as may well be generated by the 10% subpopulation) causes PS exposure in virtually all platelets in a process that is further dependent on vWF and that is activated either by shear or botrocetin (100). Therefore, in adherent platelets, thrombin is not necessarily the sole mediator of platelet procoagulant activity.

After recalcification of PRP, the burst of thrombin generation is invariably preceded by the appearance of subnanomolar amounts (<0.1 U/mL) of thrombin. It probably originates on circulating procoagulant microvesicles or a small subpopulation of procoagulant platelets and may be triggered by minute amounts of circulating TF or minimal contact activation. As already observed by Biggs and Macfarlane (101), adding such amounts of thrombin at zero time to clotting blood dramatically shortens the lag time of the thrombin burst. Similar concentrations of a tight binding thrombin inhibitor like hirudin prolong the lag time (Fig. 40–1) (102,103). The lag phase also can be shortened by addition of synthetic procoagulant phospholipids, by the induction of membrane scrambling through a Ca^{2+} ionophore, or by disrupting cells (freeze thawing, sonication [52]). Conversely, adding factor VIIIa or Va does not abolish the lag phase unless procoagulant phospholipid is available first. Thrombin generation in PRP is completely inhibited by annexin V (103a), which further stresses the pivotal role of exposed procoagulant phospholipid in thrombin generation in PRP. From these and similar observations we conclude that, in PRP, the availability of procoagulant phospholipids is the rate-limiting component for thrombin generation and that thrombin or a thrombin product causes the platelets to produce it.

How thrombin induces platelet procoagulant activity remains uncertain. Jamieson and coworkers (104,105) and Ruggeri and colleagues (106,107) show evidence that GPIb functions directly as the high-affinity receptor for α-thrombin and that this interaction initiates platelet procoagulant activity. However, Liu and coworkers (108) claim that "GPIb plays no role in either thrombin binding or thrombin induced platelet activation" and relate the development of platelet procoagulant activity to the binding of vWF to GPIb. Dicker and coworkers (109) discovered an important role for α-thrombin–GP1b interaction in washed platelets and reported that the PAR-1 activating peptide SFLLRN causes only a low procoagulant reaction as compared with α-thrombin itself; they also saw no effect of PAR-1 antibodies. This in agreement with the absence of an effect of the peptide on the clotting of whole blood (110) and with the observation that SFLLRN, although causing aggregation, does not provoke procoagulant phospholipids (111). Dörmann and coworkers (112), however, concluded that, apart from a key role for GPIb, PAR-1 also is important, and vWF does not play a role at all. It should be kept in mind, however, that these conclusions pertain to washed platelets in the presence of a polymerization inhibitor (discussed later). It also has been reported that in washed platelets by blocking PAR-1 with a peptide (YFLLRNP), with bradykinin, or with an antibody, the appearance of procoagulant phospholipids also is blocked. Some authors believe PAR-1 to be the prime activator involved (113). Probably, GPIb is important in the beginning of thrombin generation at concentrations of thrombin less than 0.5 n*M,* whereas PAR-dependent activation needs greater concentrations. PAR-4 is reported not to be important in this process (113). In summary, these observations suggest that the first trace amounts of thrombin bring about platelet procoagulant activity through GPIb and that PAR-1/-4 plays a role at a later stage.

It may be questioned, however, whether the effect of thrombin on GPIb is necessarily caused by direct ligand–receptor interaction. In PRP of patients with congenital hypofibrinemia, thrombin generation is diminished; and, in fact, in all conditions where no fibrin(-ogen) is present, antibodies against GPIb will not inhibit thrombin generation (114–116). This cannot be explained if direct binding of thrombin to GPIb would be the only, or even the main, mechanism involved. An indirect role of thrombin can be envisaged in two ways.

The first way is through thrombin-mediated activation of the $\alpha_{IIb}\beta_3$ complex in the platelet membrane. Indeed, adding an antibody (abciximab) or another $\alpha_{IIb}\beta_3$ antagonist (MK383) to PRP inhibits the amount of thrombin formed (117–120). Therefore, $\alpha_{IIb}\beta_3$ is part of a loop consisting of the sequence: thrombin $\rightarrow$ GPIb and/or PAR $\rightarrow$ $\alpha_{IIb}\beta_3$ $\rightarrow$ procoagulant phospholipids $\rightarrow$ prothrombinase $\rightarrow$ thrombin (116). Inhibition through blocking $\alpha_{IIb}\beta_3$ does not exceed 50%, therefore this loop is not likely to be the only pathway. Also, the inhibitory effect on the amount of thrombin formed is more important than the effect on the moment of start of thrombin formation, which suggests that another mechanism is the *primum movens*.

Second, thrombin can act through the formation of fibrin. The addition of a fibrin clot (without any adsorbed active thrombin) after recalcification of PRP considerably shortens the lag phase of thrombin formation (114,115) in a vWF- and GPIb-dependent process. Fibrin formation that is provoked during the lag time by adding Agihal, a snake venom enzyme that releases fibrinopeptide A but has no other actions either on the plasmatic clotting factors or on the platelet, provokes immediate thrombin generation (97), which is inhibited by antibodies against GPIb and vWF. Absence of fibrinogen, as in hypofibrinemia or afibrinogenemia, or inhibition of fibrin polymerization inhibits thrombin generation in PRP. Thrombin-independent activation by fibrin also can be observed by electron microscopy (116). However, platelets immobilized on fibrin(ogen) become procoagulant in the presence of vWF and shear stress or botrocetin only after treatment with thrombin (100). For binding of vWF to GPIb, a conformational change of this protein, brought about by shear, by adsorption to a surface or to ristocetin seems a prerequisite condition (121). Goto and coworkers (122) demonstrate that vWF interacts with GPIb in the presence of ristocetin; but after stimulation with thrombin vWF, it binds to GPIIb/IIIa. Together these results do not exclude a role for thrombin binding to GPIb, but strongly suggest also a mediating role of thrombin through

the formation of fibrin and subsequent vWF–GPIb interaction. That Dörmann and coworkers (112) cannot confirm such a role may be because of the virtual absence of fibrinogen and the presence of a polymerization inhibitor in their experiments. In addition, these rather conflicting findings underscore the notion that the mechanisms of generation of platelet procoagulant activity might be quite different for platelets in suspension and adherent platelets.

In the literature, vWF has been reported to be solely important at high shear (e.g., see References 123–125). In our thrombin generation experiments, shear stress is virtually absent. We hypothesize that the interaction of vWF with fibrin monomers in the state of polymerization unfolds the von Willebrand molecule in the same manner as high shear stress, botrocetin, ristocetin, or adsorption on a surface, thus leading to conformational transitions in the von Willebrand molecule that allow interaction with GPIb. The observation that polymerization intermediates of fibrin induce binding of platelet vWF to the glycocalicin portion of GPIb (126) fits well with this hypothesis. This would answer the classical question of what constitutes the natural ristocetin: polymerizing fibrin. We thus postulate the feedback activation loop (thrombin $\rightarrow$ fibrin $\rightarrow$ fibrin-vWF $\rightarrow$ GPIb $\rightarrow$ procoagulant phospholipids $\rightarrow$ prothrombinase $\rightarrow$ thrombin), but do not rule out that it contains a loop within a loop (i.e., thrombin $\rightarrow$ GPIb $\rightarrow$ procoagulant phospholipids $\rightarrow$ prothrombinase $\rightarrow$ thrombin).

In PRP it is impossible to obtain full inhibition of thrombin formation by blocking $\alpha_{IIb}\beta_3$ (117), and the $\alpha_{IIb}\beta_3$ pathway remains active when GPIb is blocked (109) or in the absence of polymerized fibrin. The two receptors therefore seem to function on parallel pathways. Thrombin generation can be blocked more than 75% with antibodies against vWF, and such antibodies have an additional inhibitory power in the presence of antibodies against either GPIB or GPIIb/IIIa but not in the presence of both; therefore, vWF must play a role in both the $\alpha_{IIb}\beta_3$- and the GPIb-dependent pathway (97).

In von Willebrand disease, thrombin generation in PRP is severely diminished (127). This is not caused by a lack of factor VIII, because the defect is not corrected by addition of factor VIII, but it is by procoagulant phospholipid—that is, in contact-activated PPP with added procoagulant phospholipids or in PRP where the platelet membrane is scrambled with a Ca^{2+}-ionophore. In the more severe cases (factor VIII $< \sim$10%), the correction by phospholipid is not complete because factor VIII becomes rate limiting. Half-normal thrombin generation in PRP is seen at a vWF level of ~40% (with factor VIII at 100%) and a factor VIII level of ~5% (with vWF at 100%) (117). In fact, vWF, in PRP, is a clotting factor in the sense that its presence is required for the generation of thrombin.

In agreement with this proposed mechanism, decreased thrombin generation in PRP is not only observed in von Willebrand disease but also in Glanzmann's (117) thrombopathy, as well as afibrinogenemia and hypofibrinemia (115). In all these cases it is normal in PPP with added phospholipids at least as long as, in von Willebrand disease, the level of factor VIII is not less than ~10%.

The literature is not in agreement regarding Bernard-Soulier syndrome (BSS). The original authors (128) as well as others (e.g., Caen and Bellucci [129]) have found defective prothrombin consumption in BSS blood. Bevers and coworkers (130) found normal or slightly increased procoagulant activity in isolated BSS platelets, whereas Dicker and coworkers reported decreased activity (109). In accordance, we found no defect in thrombin generation using the subsampling technique. Aberrant anatomy (128) and lipid composition of the BSS platelet (131) is well recognized. Therefore, it was not a surprise that it proved to be easily damaged, and hence generates a procoagulant surface aspecifically (97). The defect is seen in isolated platelets only when they are handled with utmost care (109). It can be readily observed in native plasma (97) in the presence of an undisturbed clot using the conversion of a fluorogenic substrate (39).

In PRP, the interaction between the plasmatic coagulation system and the platelet is close and mutually reinforcing. A minimal hypothesis requires two parallel, receptor-dependent pathways for the appearance of procoagulant phospholipids that both need vWF: (a) through the $\alpha_{IIb}\beta_3$ heterodimer that originates on the appearance of subnanomolar traces of thrombin (possibly reinforced by thrombin-induced release reactions of, for example, ADP and serotonin); and (b) through GPIb that interacts with vWF adsorbed onto formed fibrin. The primary receptor of subnanomolar traces of thrombin is likely to be GPIb in another role. In the presence of collagen, a third pathway involving GPVI and $\alpha_2\beta_1$ plays a role (see Heemskerk and coworkers [132] for more information).

PUTATIVE PLATELET RECEPTORS FOR OTHER CLOTTING FACTORS?

Procoagulant phospholipids bind clotting factors, and various established platelet receptors such as GPIb-V-IX, $\alpha_{IIb}\beta_3$, GPVI, and others are instrumental in making these binding sites available. Confusingly, the high-affinity binding sites for clotting factors (e.g., prothrombin and factor Xa) that arise from the exposure of procoagulant phospholipids and the adsorption of plasmatic cofactor (e.g., factor Va) are sometimes called receptors (133,134). If we restrict the term receptor to integral membrane proteins that bind specifically to a given plasmatic clotting factor, then are there clotting factor receptors other than those for thrombin and vWF?

Specific receptors, on the platelet membrane, with no other function than binding one or more clotting factors have been described for almost all factors but have been rigorously proven for none (e.g., factor VIII [135] and factor IX [136]). The evidence produced for their existence in our opinion remains open for alternative interpretation. The observations might, for example, be brought about by changes in the lipid composition of the outer face of the platelet membrane. During platelet activation, the composition and the size of the available PPS increases; therefore, the kinetic characteristics of clotting factor binding and conversion increase considerably (61). This can mimic the effect of specific receptors. It may be extremely difficult to distinguish between a protein receptor for a clotting factor and a receptor that is instrumental in producing a phospholipid surface with high affinity for a clotting factor. Also, binding to the serotonin receptor through covalently bound serotonin (74,75) may readily suggest the existence of a specific receptor. In order not to multiply hypotheses beyond necessity, we will disregard postulated specific receptors until more convincing proof is available. A different case can be made for well defined receptors that are shown to bind clotting factors and presumed to play a role in their activation.

Byzova and Plow have described that $\alpha_{IIb}\beta_3$ can act as a receptor for prothrombin (137). If this interaction were of direct importance for thrombin generation, then part of the thrombin generation in PRP would have to be lipid-independent. This has not been demonstrated. We have not been able to find residual thrombin generation in the presence of an excess of annexin V, which also pleads against this possibility.

Effector cell Protease Receptor-1 (EPR-1) has been assigned a regulating role in factor Xa binding and procoagulant activity of platelets (138,139), as well as leukocytes (140), endothelial cells (141), and smooth muscle cells (142), Again, in our opinion, a functional role in normal hemostasis remains to be demonstrated.

GPIb, by virtue of its binding vWF to which factor VIII is bound, may bring factor VIII in the vicinity of the platelet membrane (129). It has indeed been demonstrated that vWF binds to fibrin (143) and to platelet surfaces in a thrombus and that this process leads to enrichment in factor VIII (76).

Walsh and colleagues have convincingly shown that, through its apple 3 domain, factor XI binds to GPIb on activated platelets in a kininogen- and prothrombin-enhanced process (144–146), and that this binding facilitates factor XI activation by thrombin (147). The (patho-)physiologic significance is not yet clear and may, again, depend on the circumstances. The role of factor XII in the platelets may on good grounds be doubted. In fresh plasma from severely factor XI–deficient patients (type 2-2), we found an essentially identical relation between the concentration of added factor XI and thrombin generation in PRP, in PPP supplemented with normal platelets, and in PPP supplemented with 1 μM synthetic procoagulant phospholipid (148). That is, we found no evidence for a facilitating role of platelets in thrombin generation under conditions in which factor XI is rate limiting. A physiologic role for factor XI is suggested by the observation that (arterial) thrombus growth can be inhibited by anti–factor XIa, and it is contradicted by that factor XI deficiency does not protect against coronary infarction (149) and that factor XI is not a risk factor for thrombosis (150).

There is no compelling reason to postulate specific clotting factor receptors. Binding of some clotting factors to known receptors has been demonstrated. A physiologic role of such interactions, with the exception of factor XI-GPIb, remains unclear at this moment.

CIRCULATING TISSUE FACTOR

When blood is led directly from a vein through a flow chamber in which collagen is exposed (either arterial media or purified collagen on glass), platelets adhere to the collagen. Such platelets pick up biologically active TF from leukocytes that roll over the surface of the aggregate. In the free platelet, no TF can be demonstrated. On the surface of the free leukocytes, there also is no active TF; therefore, TF is "decrypted" in the process. The specific leukocyte membrane marker CD15, absent in circulating platelets, is present in adherent platelets that have been exposed to leukocytes, which shows that the leukocyte–platelet contact involves the carryover of pieces of leukocyte membrane ("rafts"). This process, together with the flip-flop induced by fibrin and by fibrin-bound thrombin, makes it possible that a plug or thrombus grows even though the collagen and perivascular TF-carrying cells are shielded from contact with flowing blood by the emerging thrombus/plug (151,152).

Which type of leukocyte is involved in these processes is still a matter of debate. Giesen and coworkers (151) suggest that polymorphonuclears and monocytes contribute. Osterud (153), in experiments in which TF synthesis is induced by lipopolysaccharides, concludes that only monocytes are capable of synthesizing TF, but that platelets and granulocytes play a supporting role. Camera and coworkers (154) reported that activation of platelets by various activators (ADP, epinephrine, TRAP) induces TF expression, which is counteracted by platelet antagonists, and ascribe this to TF carried by platelets per se.

SUMMARY: WHAT MAKES A THROMBUS?

As always when specialists do not agree, the detailed reading of the argument is confusing for the nonspecialist. We therefore end with a summary of our own current understanding. We surmise that about half of it may prove to be incorrect; unfortunately, we do not know which half.

Normally, during the clotting process, all fibrin is formed before 2% to 4% of prothrombin is converted, but almost the totality of prothrombin available is converted into thrombin after clotting. In this process, platelets play an important role and "aggregation" inhibitors or congenital platelet function disorders impair thrombin generation in PRP. The "excess" amount of thrombin formed after clotting is an important determinant of the extent of the thrombotic/hemostatic reaction. Thrombin diffuses in the surroundings where it begets more thrombin and has many other actions that on the whole are prothrombotic and hemostatic. The extent of the thrombin gradient will determine the extent of the thrombotic reaction. Hence, the first law of hemostasis and thrombosis: *The more thrombin the less bleeding; but, the more*

thrombosis the less thrombin, and the less thrombosis the more bleeding. The prime medical importance of measuring and understanding thrombin generation lies in its being a precept that we need to navigate through the therapeutic gap diminishing thrombosis on the one hand and preventing bleeding on the other hand.

Activated platelets foster thrombin generation through release of factor V, through presenting procoagulant phospholipids in their membrane, and through interaction with leukocytes that transfer TF activity to their surface. Activation of platelets may be brought about by collagen, by thrombin, and by vWF adsorbed onto collagen or onto fibrin. *In vivo,* when a hemostatic plug or a thrombus forms, collagen is on the demarcation line with fluid blood for a short time only. As soon as a minimal hemostatic plug or thrombus covers the collagen, the interface is between flowing blood on the one side and polymerizing fibrin and activated platelets on the other side. Further growth occurs at the interface of blood and the preexisting thrombus (hemostatic plug).

Thrombin generated within a focus (clot, hemostatic plug, or thrombus) will diffuse into the surroundings. The gradient is determined by the thrombin generation power (endogenous thrombin potential) within the clot and by hemodynamic conditions. Under low flow (venous thrombosis), the thrombin generated in a platelet aggregate make the surrounding blood clot. At the fibrin–blood interface of that new clot more platelets will adhere and become procoagulant, which starts the process again and makes the thrombus grow. The alternation of blood clot and platelet aggregates explains the striated aspect often observed in venous thrombi. Free platelets in the surroundings of the clot are activated by thrombin (through GPIb and PAR receptors) and are caught in the clot through $\alpha_{IIb}\beta_3$–mediated platelet–platelet interaction and by interaction of GPIb with vWF that has undergone a conformational change through interaction with nascent fibrin. Both receptors in this action trigger intraplatelet processes that make the platelet membrane present procoagulant phospholipids, and thus foster further thrombin formation.

Under high-flow conditions (wound or arterial thrombus), the reactions will be qualitatively the same but quantitatively different. More TF, for example, will be present in a wound or ruptured plaque than in the "head" of a venous thrombus. Thrombin that diffuses out of the aggregate/clot will be strongly diluted by high flow and an appreciable concentration of thrombin will appear only in a thin boundary layer. Platelets may be additionally activated through the high shear conditions. Few fibrin will form in high flow, and no erythrocytes will be entrapped. Any fibrin formed will contain a certain amount of bound thrombin that is able to activate platelets and other clotting factors. Also, several activated clotting factors (e.g., factor Xa) may be incorporated in a natural clot. Thrombin generation at the surface of any clot also is enhanced because, through the interaction of leukocytes and platelets, circulating TF is transferred to the adhering platelets. All together, the picture that emerges stresses the tight interaction between platelets and the plasmatic clotting system under any flow condition, in primary hemostasis, and in arterial and venous thrombi. This explains why anticoagulant drugs can prevent arterial thrombosis (17,18) and why aspirin may be beneficial in venous thrombosis (19), and it challenges previous views in which platelet function was thought to be primarily in adhesion and aggregation and the role of thrombin was restricted to reinforcing a formed platelet aggregate through the clotting of fibrinogen.

REFERENCES

1. Van Creveld S, Paulssen MM. Significance of clotting factors in blood platelets, in normal and pathological conditions. *Lancet* 1951;ii: 242–244.
2. Van Creveld S, Paulssen MM. Isolation and properties of the third clotting factor in blood platelets. *Lancet* 1952;i:23–25.
3. Alkjaersig N, Abe T, Seegers WH. Purification and quantitative determination of platelet factor 3. *Am J Physiol* 1955;181:304–308.
4. Fantl PA, Seegers WH. The thromboplastic component of intact blood platelets is present in masked form. *Austr J Exp Biol Med Sci* 1958;36:499–504.
5. Hardisty RM, Hutton RA. The kaolin clotting time of platelet rich plasma: a test of platelet factor 3 availability. *Br J Haematol* 1965;11:269–275.
6. Spaet TH, Cintron J. Studies on platelet factor-3 availability. *Br J Haematol* 1965;11:269–275.
7. Born GV. The aggregation of blood platelets by adenosine diphosphate and its reversal. *Nature* 1962;194:927.
8. Bevers EM, Comfurius P, van Rijn JL, et al. Generation of prothrombin-converting activity and the exposure of phosphatidylserine at the outer surface of platelets. *Eur J Biochem* 1982;122:429–436.
9. Bevers EM, Comfurius P, Dekkers DW, et al. Lipid translocation across the plasma membrane of mammalian cells. *Biochim Biophys Acta* 1999;1439:317–330.
10. Kyrle PA, Westwick J, Scully MF, et al. Investigation of the interaction of blood platelets with the coagulation system at the site of plug formation in vivo in man—effect of low-dose aspirin. *Thromb Haemost* 1987;57:62–66.
11. Jensen AH, Béguin S, Josso F. Factor V and VIII activation "in vivo" during bleeding. Evidence of thrombin formation at the early stage of hemostasis. *Pathol Biol (Paris)* 1976;[24 Suppl]:6–10.
12. Tindall H, Menys VC, Davies JA. Thrombin generation precedes platelet activation in native blood taken from the hand during multiple blood sampling following cold challenge. *Thromb Res* 1987;46:613–616.
13. Sixma JJ, Kater L, Bouma BN, et al. Immunofluorescent localization of factor VIII-related antigen, fibrinogen, and several other plasma proteins in hemostatic plugs in humans. *J Lab Clin Med* 1976;87:112–119.
14. Marongiu F, Biondi G, Sorano GG, et al. Bleeding time is prolonged during oral anticoagulant therapy. *Thromb Res* 1990;59:905–912.
15. Sato K, Kawasaki T, Taniuchi Y, et al. YM-60828, a novel factor Xa inhibitor: separation of its antithrombotic effects from its prolongation of bleeding time. *Eur J Pharmacol* 1997;339:141–146.
16. Lavelle SM, MacIomhair M. Bleeding times and the antithrombotic effects of high-dose aspirin, hirudin and heparins in the rat. *Ir J Med Sci* 1998;167:216–220.
17. Neri Serneri GG, Rovelli F, Gensini GF, et al. Effectiveness of low-dose heparin in prevention of myocardial reinfarction. *Lancet* 1987;1:937–942.
18. A double-blind trial to assess long-term oral anticoagulant therapy in elderly patients after myocardial infarction. Report of the Sixty Plus Reinfarction Study Research Group. *Lancet* 1980;2:989–994.
19. Prevention of pulmonary embolism and deep vein thrombosis with low dose aspirin: Pulmonary Embolism Prevention (PEP) trial. *Lancet* 2000;355:1295–1302.
20. Baumgartner HR. Effects of anticoagulation on the interaction of hu-
21. Baumgartner HR, Muggli R, Tschopp TB, et al. Platelet adhesion, release and aggregation in flowing blood: effects of surface properties and platelet function. *Thromb Haemost* 1976;35:124–138.
22. Sakariassen KS, Aarts PA, de Groot PG, et al. A perfusion chamber developed to investigate platelet interaction in flowing blood with human vessel wall cells, their extracellular matrix, and purified components. *J Lab Clin Med* 1983;102:522–535.
23. Badimon L, Turitto V, Rosemark JA, et al. Characterization of a tubular flow chamber for studying platelet interaction with biologic and prosthetic materials: deposition of indium 111-labeled platelets on collagen, subendothelium, and expanded polytetrafluoroethylene. *J Lab Clin Med* 1987;110:706–718.
24. Koopman G, Reutelingsperger CP, Kuijten GA, et al. Annexin V for flow cytometric detection of phosphatidylserine expression on B cells undergoing apoptosis. *Blood* 1994;84:1415–1420.
25. van Engeland M, Nieland LJ, Ramaekers FC, et al. Annexin V-affinity assay: a review on an apoptosis detection system based on phosphatidylserine exposure. *Cytometry* 1998;31:1–9.
26. Willems GM, Giesen PL, Hermens WT. Adsorption and conversion of prothrombin on a rotating disc. *Blood* 1993;82:497–504.
27. Salemink I, Franssen J, Willems GM, et al. Inhibition of tissue factor-factor VIIa-catalyzed factor X activation by factor Xa-tissue factor pathway inhibitor. A rotating disc study on the effect of phospholipid membrane composition. *J Biol Chem* 1999;274:28225–28232.
28. Béguin S, Lindhout T, Hemker HC. The effect of trace amounts of tissue factor on thrombin generation in platelet rich plasma, its inhibition by heparin. *Thromb Haemost* 1989;61:25–29.
29. Kessels H, Béguin S, Andree H, et al. Measurement of thrombin generation in whole blood—the effect of heparin and aspirin. *Thromb Haemost* 1994;72:78–83.
30. Rand MD, Lock JB, van't Veer C, et al. Blood clotting in minimally altered whole blood. *Blood* 1996;88:3432–3445.
31. Butenas S, van't Veer C, Mann KG. "Normal" thrombin generation. *Blood* 1999;94:2169–2178.
32. van't Veer C, Mann KG. The regulation of the factor VII-dependent coagulation pathway: rationale for the effectiveness of recombinant factor VIIa in refractory bleeding disorders. *Semin Thromb Hemost* 2000;26:367–372.
33. Monroe DM, Roberts HR, Hoffman M. Platelet procoagulant complex assembly in a tissue factor-initiated system. *Br J Haematol* 1994;88:364–371.
34. Peyrou V, Lormeau JC, Herault JP, et al. Contribution of erythrocytes to thrombin generation in whole blood. *Thromb Haemost* 1999;81:400–406.
35. Cawthern KM, van 't Veer C, Lock JB, et al. Blood coagulation in hemophilia A and hemophilia C. *Blood* 1998;91:4581–4592.
36. Brummel KE, Paradis SG, Butenas S, et al. Thrombin functions during tissue factor-induced blood coagulation. *Blood* 2002;100:148–152.
37. Szczeklik A, Krzanowski M, Gora P, et al. Antiplatelet drugs and generation of thrombin in clotting blood. *Blood* 1992;80:2006–2011.
38. Undas A, Brummel K, Musial J, et al. Blood coagulation at the site of microvascular injury: effects of low-dose aspirin. *Blood* 2001;98:2423–2431.
39. Hemker HC, Giesen P, Al Dieri R, et al. Calibrated automated thrombin generation measurement in clotting plasma. *Pathophysiol Haemost Thromb* 2003;33:4–15.
40. Hemker HC. The endogenous thrombin potential, a new laboratory parameter to indicate the risk of thrombosis and its diminuation by treatment. In: Siegenthaler W, Haas R, eds. *Challenges in medicine.* Stuttgart, Germany: Thieme Verlag, 1996:104–109.
41. Mann KG, Brummel K, Butenas S. What is all that thrombin for? *J Thromb Haemost* 2003;1:1504–1514.
42. Antovic JP, Antovic A, He S, et al. Overall haemostatic potential can be used for estimation of thrombin-activatable fibrinolysis inhibitor-dependent fibrinolysis in vivo and for possible follow-up of recombinant factor VIIa treatment in patients with inhibitors to factor VIII. *Haemophilia* 2002;8:781–786.
43. Von dem Borne PA, Bajzar L, Meijers JC, et al. Thrombin-mediated activation of factor XI results in a thrombin-activatable fibrinolysis inhibitor-dependent inhibition of fibrinolysis. *J Clin Invest* 1997;99:2323–2327.
44. Von dem Borne PA, Meijers JC, Bouma BN. Feedback activation of

factor XI by thrombin in plasma results in additional formation of thrombin that protects fibrin clots from fibrinolysis. *Blood* 1995;86: 3035–3042.

45. Torbet J. The thrombin activation pathway modulates the assembly, structure and lysis of human plasma clots in vitro. *Thromb Haemost* 1995;73:785–792.

46. Narayanan S. Multifunctional roles of thrombin. *Ann Clin Lab Sci* 1999;29:275–280.

47. Major CD, Santulli RJ, Derian CK, et al. Extracellular mediators in atherosclerosis and thrombosis: lessons from thrombin receptor knockout mice. *Arterioscler Thromb Vasc Biol* 2003;23:931–939.

48. Chong AJ, Pohlman TH, Hampton CR, et al. Tissue factor and thrombin mediate myocardial ischemia-reperfusion injury. *Ann Thorac Surg* 2003;75:S649–S655.

49. Cottrell GS, Coelho AM, Bunnett NW. Protease-activated receptors: the role of cell-surface proteolysis in signalling. *Essays Biochem* 2002;38:169–183.

50. Chambers RC, Laurent GJ. Coagulation cascade proteases and tissue fibrosis. *Biochem Soc Trans* 2002;30:194–200.

51. Regnault V, Béguin S, Wahl D, et al. Thrombinography shows acquired resistance to activated protein C in patients with lupus anticoagulants. *Thromb Haemost* 2003;89:208–212.

52. Regnault V, Béguin S, Lecompte T. Calibrated automated thrombin generation in frozen-thawed platelet-rich plasma to detect hypercoagulability. *Pathophysiol Haemost Thromb* 2003;33:23–29.

53. Al Dieri R, Peyvandi F, Santagostino E, et al. The thrombogram in rare inherited coagulation disorders: its relation to clinical bleeding. *Thromb Haemost* 2002;88:576–582.

54. Hemker HC, Béguin S. Phenotyping the clotting system. *Thromb Haemost* 2000;84:747–751.

55. Zwaal RF, Comfurius P, Bevers EM. Lipid-protein interactions in blood coagulation. *Biochim Biophys Acta* 1998;1376:433–453.

56. Dahlback B. Blood coagulation. *Lancet* 2000;355:1627–1632.

57. Esmon CT. Regulation of blood coagulation. *Biochim Biophys Acta* 2000;1477:349–360.

58. Mann KG. Biochemistry and physiology of blood coagulation. *Thromb Haemost* 1999;82:165–174.

59. Bajaj SP, Joist JH. New insights into how blood clots: implications for the use of APTT and PT as coagulation screening tests and in monitoring of anticoagulant therapy. *Semin Thromb Hemost* 1999;25:407–418.

60. Rosing J, Tans G, Govers-Riemslag JW, et al. The role of phospholipids and factor Va in the prothrombinase complex. *J Biol Chem* 1980;255:274–283.

61. Giesen PL, Willems GM, Hemker HC, et al. Membrane-mediated assembly of the prothrombinase complex. *J Biol Chem* 1991;266: 18720–18725.

62. Hemker HC, Choay J, Béguin S. Free factor Xa is on the main pathway of thrombin generation in clotting plasma. *Biochim Biophys Acta* 1989;992:409–411.

63. Bajzar L, Manuel R, Nesheim ME. Purification and characterization of TAFI, a thrombin-activable fibrinolysis inhibitor. *J Biol Chem* 1995;270:14477–14484.

64. Broze GJ Jr, Higuchi DA. Coagulation-dependent inhibition of fibrinolysis: role of carboxypeptidase-U and the premature lysis of clots from hemophilic plasma. *Blood* 1996;88:3815–3823.

65. Nesheim M, Wang W, Boffa M, et al. Thrombin, thrombomodulin and TAFI in the molecular link between coagulation and fibrinolysis. *Thromb Haemost* 1997;78:386–391.

66. Sultan Y, Maisonneuve P, Angles-Cano E. Release of VIII R:Ag and VIII R:WF during thrombin and collagen induced aggregation. *Thromb Res* 1979;15:415–425.

67. Koutts J, Walsh PN, Plow EF, et al. Active release of human platelet factor VIII-related antigen by adenosine diphosphate, collagen, and thrombin. *J Clin Invest* 1978;62:1255–1263.

68. Sixma JJ, Akkerman JW, van Oost B, et al. Intracellular localization of fibrinogen in human blood platelets. *Bibl Haematol* 1977;44:129–133.

69. Osterud B, Rapaport SI, Lavine KK. Factor V activity of platelets: evidence for an activated factor V molecule and for a platelet activator. *Blood* 1977;49:819–834.

70. Baruch D, Hemker HC, Lindhout T. Kinetics of thrombin-induced release and activation of platelet factor V. *Eur J Biochem* 1986;154: 213–218.

71. Mann KG. How much factor V is enough? *Thromb Haemost* 2000; 83:3–4.

72. Alberio L, Safa O, Clemetson KJ, et al. Surface expression and functional characterization of alpha-granule factor V in human platelets: effects of ionophore A23187, thrombin, collagen, and convulxin. *Blood* 2000;95:1694–1702.

73. Monroe DM, Hoffman M, Roberts HR. Platelets and thrombin generation. *Arterioscler Thromb Vasc Biol* 2002;22:1381–1389.

74. Szasz R, Dale GL. Thrombospondin and fibrinogen bind serotonin-derivatized proteins on COAT-platelets. *Blood* 2002;100:2827–2831.

75. Dale GL, Friese P, Batar P, et al. Stimulated platelets use serotonin to enhance their retention of procoagulant proteins on the cell surface. *Nature* 2002;415:175–179.

76. Kawasaki T, Kaida T, Arnout J, et al. A new animal model of thrombophilia confirms that high plasma factor VIII levels are thrombogenic. *Thromb Haemost* 1999;81:306–311.

77. Bellucci S, Girma JP, Lozano M, et al. Impaired prothrombin consumption in Bernard-Soulier syndrome is corrected in vitro by human factor VIII. *Thromb Haemost* 1997;77:383–386.

78. Franck PF, Bevers EM, Lubin BH, et al. Uncoupling of the membrane skeleton from the lipid bilayer. The cause of accelerated phospholipid flip-flop leading to an enhanced procoagulant activity of sickled cells. *J Clin Invest* 1985;75.183–190.

79. Zwaal RF, Roelofsen B, Comfurius P, et al. Organization of phospholipids in human red cell membranes as detected by the action of various purified phospholipases. *Biochim Biophys Acta* 1975;406:83–96.

80. Renooij W, Van Golde LM, Zwaal RF, et al. Topological asymmetry of phospholipid metabolism in rat erythrocyte membranes. Evidence for flip-flop of lecithin. *Eur J Biochem* 1976;61:53–58.

81. Zwaal RF, Comfurius P, van Deenen LL. Membrane asymmetry and blood coagulation. *Nature* 1977;268:358–360.

82. Chap HJ, Zwaal RF, van Deenen LL. Action of highly purified phospholipases on blood platelets. Evidence for an asymmetric distribution of phospholipids in the surface membrane. *Biochim Biophys Acta* 1977;467:146–164.

83. Bevers EM, Comfurius P, Hemker HC, et al. On the clot-promoting activity of human platelets in a one-stage prothrombinase assay. *Haemostasis* 1982;12:268–274.

84. Heemskerk JW, Siljander P, Vuist WM, et al. Function of glycoprotein VI and integrin alpha2beta1 in the procoagulant response of single, collagen-adherent platelets. *Thromb Haemost* 1999;81:782–792.

85. Sims PJ, Wiedmer T, Esmon CT, et al. Assembly of the platelet prothrombinase complex is linked to vesiculation of the platelet plasma membrane. Studies in Scott syndrome: an isolated defect in platelet procoagulant activity. *J Biol Chem* 1989;264:17049–17057.

86. Dachary-Prigent J, Freyssinet JM, Pasquet JM, et al. Annexin V as a probe of aminophospholipid exposure and platelet membrane vesiculation: a flow cytometry study showing a role for free sulfhydryl groups. *Blood* 1993;81:2554–2565.

87. Dachary-Prigent J, Toti F, Satta N, et al. Physiopathological significance of catalytic phospholipids in the generation of thrombin. *Semin Thromb Hemost* 1996;22:157–164.

88. Siljander P, Carpen O, Lassila R. Platelet-derived microparticles associate with fibrin during thrombosis. *Blood* 1996;87:4651–4663.

89. Nomura S, Shouzu A, Nishikawa M, et al. Significance of platelet-derived microparticles in uremia. *Nephron* 1993;63:485.

90. Nomura S, Yasunaga K. Influence of platelet-derived microparticles on coagulation in a lung cancer patient receiving chemotherapy. *Chest* 1993;103:979–980.

91. Lundahl TH, Lindahl TL, Fagerberg IH, et al. Activated platelets and impaired platelet function in intensive care patients analyzed by flow cytometry. *Blood Coagul Fibrinolysis* 1996;7:218–220.

92. Hugel B, Socie G, Vu T, et al. Elevated levels of circulating procoagulant microparticles in patients with paroxysmal nocturnal hemoglobinuria and aplastic anemia. *Blood* 1999;93:3451–3456.

93. Nomura S, Kagawa H, Ozaki Y, et al. Relationship between platelet activation and cytokines in systemic inflammatory response syndrome patients with hematological malignancies. *Thromb Res* 1999;95:205–213.

94. Omoto S, Nomura S, Shouzu A, et al. Significance of platelet-derived microparticles and activated platelets in diabetic nephropathy. *Nephron* 1999;81:271–277.

95. Nieuwland R, Berckmans RJ, McGregor S, et al. Cellular origin and procoagulant properties of microparticles in meningococcal sepsis. *Blood* 2000;95:930–935.

96. Briede JJ, Heemskerk JW, Hemker HC, et al. Heterogeneity in microparticle formation and exposure of anionic phospholipids at the

plasma membrane of single adherent platelets. *Biochim Biophys Acta* 1999;1451:163–172.

97. Béguin S, Keularts I, Al Dieri R, et al. Fibrin polymerization is crucial for thrombin generation in platelet-rich plasma in a vWF-GPIb dependent process, defective in Bernard-Soulier Syndrome. *J Thromb Haemost* 2004;2:170–176.

98. Heemskerk JW, Vuist WM, Feijge MA, et al. Collagen but not fibrinogen surfaces induce bleb formation, exposure of phosphatidylserine, and procoagulant activity of adherent platelets: evidence for regulation by protein tyrosine kinase-dependent Ca2+ responses. *Blood* 1997;90:2615–2625.

99. Briede JJ, Heemskerk JW, van't Veer C, et al. Contribution of platelet-derived factor Va to thrombin generation on immobilized collagen- and fibrinogen-adherent platelets. *Thromb Haemost* 2001;85:509–513.

100. Briede JJ, Wielders SJ, Heemskerk JW, et al. von Willebrand factor stimulates thrombin-induced exposure of procoagulant phospholipids on the surface of fibrin-adherent platelets. *J Thromb Haemost* 2003;1:559–565.

101. Biggs R, Macfarlane RG. Human blood coagulation and its disorders. 1953; Blackwell Scientific Publications, Oxford.

102. Lindhout T, Blezer R, Hemker HC. The anticoagulant mechanism of action of recombinant hirudin (CGP 39393) in plasma. *Thromb Haemost* 1990;64:464–468.

103. Adams TE, Everse SJ, Mann KG. Predicting the pharmacology of thrombin inhibitors. *J Thromb Haemost* 2003;1:1024–1027.

103a. Vanschoonbeek K, Feijge MA, Van Kampen RJ, et al. Initiating and potentiating role of platelets in tissue factor-induced thrombin generation in the presence of plasma: subject-dependent variation in thrombogram characteristics. *J Thromb Haemost* 2004;2:476–484.

104. Jamieson GA. Pathophysiology of platelet thrombin receptors. *Thromb Haemost* 1997;78:242–246.

105. Jamieson GA, Okumura T. Reduced thrombin binding and aggregation in Bernard-Soulier platelets. *J Clin Invest* 1978;61:861–864.

106. De Marco L, Mazzucato M, Masotti A, et al. Function of glycoprotein Ib alpha in platelet activation induced by alpha-thrombin. *J Biol Chem* 1991;266:23776–23783.

107. Soslau G, Class R, Morgan DA, et al. Unique pathway of thrombin-induced platelet aggregation mediated by glycoprotein Ib. *J Biol Chem* 2001;276:21173–21183.

108. Liu L, Freedman J, Hornstein A, et al. Binding of thrombin to the G-protein-linked receptor, and not to glycoprotein Ib, precedes thrombin-mediated platelet activation. *J Biol Chem* 1997;272:1997–2004.

109. Dicker IB, Pedicord DL, Seiffert DA, et al. Both the high affinity thrombin receptor (GPIb-IX-V) and GPIIb/IIIa are implicated in expression of thrombin-induced platelet procoagulant activity. *Thromb Haemost* 2001;86:1065–1069.

110. Butenas S, Cawthern KM, van't Veer C, et al. Antiplatelet agents in tissue factor-induced blood coagulation. *Blood* 2001;97:2314–2322.

111. Ramstrom S, Ranby M, Lindahl TL. Platelet phosphatidylserine exposure and procoagulant activity in clotting whole blood—different effects of collagen, TRAP and calcium ionophore A23187. *Thromb Haemost* 2003;89:132–141.

112. Dörmann D, Clemetson KJ, Kehrel BE. The GPIb thrombin-binding site is essential for thrombin-induced platelet procoagulant activity. *Blood* 2000;96:2469–2478.

113. Andersen H, Greenberg DL, Fujikawa K, et al. Protease-activated receptor 1 is the primary mediator of thrombin-stimulated platelet procoagulant activity. *Proc Natl Acad Sci USA* 1999;96:11189–11193.

114. Kumar R, Beguin S, Hemker HC. The influence of fibrinogen and fibrin on thrombin generation—evidence for feedback activation of the clotting system by clot bound thrombin. *Thromb Haemost* 1994;72:713–721.

115. Kumar R, Béguin S, Hemker HC. The effect of fibrin clots and clot-bound thrombin on the development of platelet procoagulant activity. *Thromb Haemost* 1995;74:962–968.

116. Béguin S, Kumar R. Thrombin, fibrin and platelets, a resonance loop in which von Willebrand factor is a necessary link. *Thromb Haemostas* 1997;78:590–594.

117. Reverter JC, Beguin S, Kessels H, et al. Inhibition of platelet-mediated, tissue factor-induced thrombin generation by the mouse/human chimeric 7E3 antibody. Potential implications for the effect of c7E3 Fab treatment on acute thrombosis and "clinical restenosis." *J Clin Invest* 1996;98:863–874.

118. Herault JP, Peyrou V, Savi P, et al. Effect of SR121566A, a potent GP IIb-IIIa antagonist on platelet-mediated thrombin generation in vitro and in vivo. *Thromb Haemost* 1998;79:383–388.

119. Herault JP, Lale A, Savi P, et al. In vitro inhibition of heparin-induced platelet aggregation in plasma from patients with HIT by SR 121566, a newly developed Gp IIb/IIIa antagonist. *Blood Coagul Fibrinolysis* 1997;8:206–207.

120. Keularts IM, Hamulyak K, Hemker HC, et al. The effect of DDAVP infusion on thrombin generation in platelet-rich plasma of von Willebrand type 1 and in mild haemophilia A patients. *Thromb Haemost* 2000;84:638–642.

121. Miyata S, Goto S, Federici AB, et al. Conformational changes in the A1 domain of von Willebrand factor modulating the interaction with platelet glycoprotein Ibalpha. *J Biol Chem* 1996;271:9046–9053.

122. Goto S, Salomon DR, Ikeda Y, et al. Characterization of the unique mechanism mediating the shear-dependent binding of soluble von Willebrand factor to platelets. *J Biol Chem* 1995;270:23352–23361.

123. Matsui H, Sugimoto M, Mizuno T, et al. Distinct and concerted functions of von Willebrand factor and fibrinogen in mural thrombus growth under high shear flow. *Blood* 2002;100:3604–3610.

124. Houdijk WP, Sakariassen KS, Nievelstein PF, et al. Role of factor VIII-von Willebrand factor and fibronectin in the interaction of platelets in flowing blood with monomeric and fibrillar human collagen types I and III. *J Clin Invest* 1985;75:531–540.

125. Endenburg SC, Hantgan RR, Lindeboom-Blokzijl L, et al. On the role of von Willebrand factor in promoting platelet adhesion to fibrin in flowing blood. *Blood* 1995;86:4158–4165.

126. Parker RI, Gralnick HR. Fibrin monomer induces binding of endogenous platelet von Willebrand factor to the glycocalicin portion of platelet glycoprotein IB. *Blood* 1987;70:1589–1594.

127. Keularts IM, Hamulyak K, Hemker HC, et al. The effect of DDAVP infusion on thrombin generation in platelet-rich plasma of von Willebrand type 1 and in mild haemophilia A patients. *Thromb Haemost* 2000;84:638–642.

128. Bernard J, Soulier JP. Sur une nouvelle variété de dystrophie thrombocitaire hémorrhagipare congénitale. *Semin Hop Paris* 1948;24:321–327.

129. Caen J, Bellucci S. The defective prothrombin consumption in Bernard-Soulier syndrome. Hypotheses from 1948 to 1982. *Blood Cells* 1983;9:389–399.

130. Bevers EM, Comfurius P, Nieuwenhuis HK, et al. Platelet prothrombin converting activity in hereditary disorders of platelet function. *Br J Haematol* 1986;63:335–345.

131. Perret B, Levy-Toledano S, Plantavid M, et al. Abnormal phospholipid organisation in Bernard-Soulier platelets. *Thromb Res* 1983;31:529–537.

132. Heemskerk JW, Bevers EM, Lindhout T. Platelet activation and blood coagulation. *Thromb Haemost* 2002;88:186–193.

133. Scandura JM, Ahmad SS, Walsh PN. A binding site expressed on the surface of activated human platelets is shared by factor X and prothrombin. *Biochemistry* 1996;35:8890–8902.

134. Ahmad SS, Rawala-Sheikh R, Walsh PN. Comparative interactions of factor IX and factor IXa with human platelets. *J Biol Chem* 1989;264:3244–3251.

135. Ahmad SS, Scandura JM, Walsh PN. Structural and functional characterization of platelet receptor-mediated factor VIII binding. *J Biol Chem* 2000;275:13071–13081.

136. Ahmad SS, Wong MY, Rawala R, et al. Coagulation factor IX residues G4-Q11 mediate its interaction with a shared factor IX/IXa binding site on activated platelets but not the assembly of the functional factor X activating complex. *Biochemistry* 1998;37:1671–1679.

137. Byzova TV, Plow EF. Networking in the hemostatic system: integrin alphaIIbbeta3 binds prothrombin and influences its activation. *J Biol Chem* 1997;272:27183–27188.

138. Bouchard BA, Silveira JR, Tracy PB. On the role of EPR-1 or an EPR-1-like molecule in regulating factor Xa incorporation into platelet prothrombinase. *Thromb Haemost* 2001;86:1133–1135.

139. Bouchard BA, Catcher CS, Thrash BR, et al. Effector cell protease receptor-1, a platelet activation-dependent membrane protein, regulates prothrombinase-catalyzed thrombin generation. *J Biol Chem* 1997;272:9244–9251.

140. Altieri DC. Xa receptor EPR-1. *FASEB J* 1995;9:860–865.

141. Bono F, Herault JP, Avril C, et al. Human umbilical vein endothelial cells express high affinity receptors for factor Xa. *J Cell Physiol* 1997;172:36–43.

142. Herbert J, Bono F, Herault J, et al. Effector protease receptor 1 mediates the mitogenic activity of factor Xa for vascular smooth muscle cells in vitro and in vivo. *J Clin Invest* 1998;101:993–1000.

143. Loscalzo J, Inbal A, Handin RI. von Willebrand protein facilitates platelet incorporation in polymerizing fibrin. *J Clin Invest* 1986;78: 1112–1119.

144. Greengard JS, Heeb MJ, Ersdal E, et al. Binding of coagulation factor XI to washed human platelets. *Biochemistry* 1986;25:3884–3890.

145. Baglia FA, Walsh PN. Prothrombin is a cofactor for the binding of factor XI to the platelet surface and for platelet-mediated factor XI activation by thrombin. *Biochemistry* 1998;37:2271–2281.

146. Ho DH, Badellino K, Baglia FA, et al. The role of high molecular weight kininogen and prothrombin as cofactors in the binding of factor XI A3 domain to the platelet surface. *J Biol Chem* 2000;275:25139–25145.

147. Baglia FA, Walsh PN. Thrombin-mediated feedback activation of factor XI on the activated platelet surface is preferred over contact activation by factor XIIa or factor XIa. *J Biol Chem* 2000;275:20514–20519.

148. Keulaïts IM, Zivelin A, Seligsohn U, et al. The role of factor XI in thrombin generation induced by low concentrations of tissue factor. *Thromb Haemost* 2001;85:1060–1065.

149. Salomon O, Steinberg DM, Dardik R, et al. Inherited factor XI deficiency confers no protection against acute myocardial infarction. *J Thromb Haemost* 2003;1:658–661.

150. Rosendaal FR. Clotting and myocardial infarction: a cycle of insights. *J Thromb Haemost* 2003;1:640–642.

151. Giesen PL, Rauch U, Bohrmann B, et al. Blood-borne tissue factor: another view of thrombosis. *Proc Natl Acad Sci USA* 1999;96:2311–2315.

152. Balasubramanian V, Grabowski E, Bini A, et al. Platelets, circulating tissue factor, and fibrin colocalize in ex vivo thrombi: real-time fluorescence images of thrombus formation and propagation under defined flow conditions. *Blood* 2002;100:2787–2792.

153. Osterud B. The role of platelets in decrypting monocyte tissue factor. *Dis Mon* 2003;49:7–13.

154. Camera M, Frigerio M, Toschi V, et al. Platelet activation induces cell-surface immunoreactive tissue factor expression, which is modulated differently by antiplatelet drugs. *Arterioscler Thromb Vasc Biol* 2003;23:1690–1696.

CHAPTER 41

Interaction of Platelet Activation and Thrombosis

Lina Badimon, Valentin Fuster, and Juan Jose Badimon

Key Words: Blood flow; coagulation; fibrin(ogen); platelets; platelet receptors; stenosis; thrombosis; thrombin; vessel wall.

INTRODUCTION

Numerous pathologic and angiographic and several angioscopic and intravascular ultrasound reports have documented the presence of intraluminal thrombi both in unstable angina and in acute myocardial infarction (AMI). In contrast, with the very high incidence of thrombi in AMI, the incidence in unstable angina varied significantly among different studies, related in part to the interval between the onset of symptoms and the angiographic study. Accordingly, when cardiac catheterization was delayed for weeks, the incidence of thrombi was low; in contrast, angiography early after the onset of symptoms revealed the presence of thrombi in approximately two-thirds of cases. Presumably, the thrombus is occlusive at the time of anginal pain and later may become subocclusive and slowly lysed or digested. Local and systemic "thrombogenic risk factors" at the time of coronary plaque disruption may influence the degree and duration of thrombus deposition, and hence the dif-

ferent pathologic and clinical syndromes. This chapter describes some of the local and systemic factors that contribute to the degree of thrombogenicity at a molecular level after plaque rupture.

The concept of vascular injury and local geometry as triggers and modulators of a thrombotic event is relevant to the pathogenesis of different cardiovascular disorders, including the initiation and progression of atherothrombosis, acute coronary syndromes, vein graft disease, and restenosis after coronary angioplasty. The unveiling of the molecular interactions prevalent in thrombosis will serve the development of more accurate strategies of pharmacologic intervention.

PATHOGENESIS OF ARTERIAL THROMBOSIS

The last two decades have highlighted the pivotal role of the endothelium in preserving vascular homeostasis and hemostasis. The endothelium, the inner layer of blood vessels, is a dynamic autocrine and paracrine organ that regulates contractile, secretory, and mitogenic activities in the vessel wall and the hemostatic process within the vessel lumen by producing several local active substances. Vascular hemostasis, defined as the ability of the vascular system to maintain blood fluidity and vascular integrity, is achieved by the interaction between the endothelium and blood cells. In physiologic conditions, the normal endothelium actively supports the fluid state of flowing blood and prevents activation of circulating cells (Fig. 41–1). In this context, of all the endothelial-borne agents, nitric oxide (NO) and prostacyclin (PGI_2) are the most known platelet inhibitors. Endothelial dysfunction, as well as a breach of the endothelial integrity,

L. Badimon: Cardiovascular Research Center, CSIC-ICCC, Hospital de la Santa Creu i Sant Pau, Av. S. Antoni M. Claret, 167 08025 Barcelona, Spain.

V. Fuster: Cardiovascular Institute, Mount Sinai School of Medicine, Annemberg Building 24-201, One Gustave L. Levy Place, New York, New York 10538.

J. J. Badimon: Cardiovascular Institute, Mount Sinai School of Medicine, Annemberg Building 24-201, One Gustave L. Levy Place, New York, New York 10538.

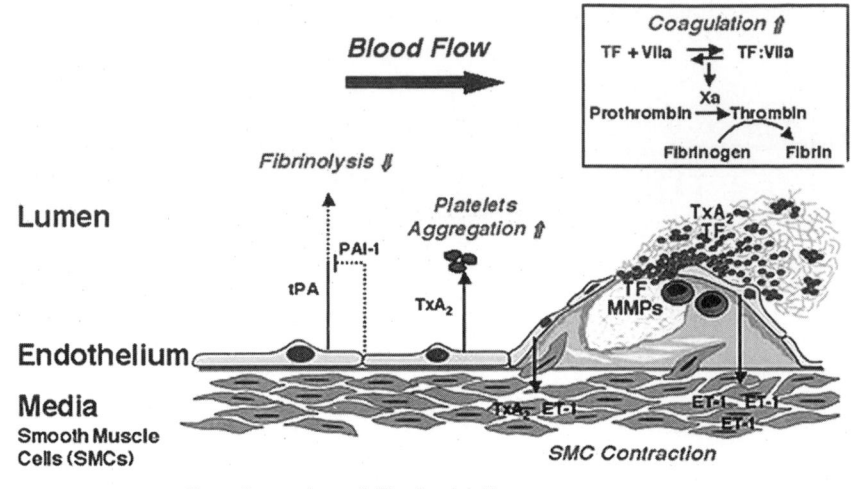

FIG. 41–1. Diagram of dysfunctional endothelium and complicated lesion with thrombosis. ET-1, endothelin; MMP, matrix metalloproteinase; PAI-1, plasminogen activator inhibitor type 1; TF, tissue factor; tPA, tissue plasminogen activator; TxA$_2$, thromboxane A$_2$.

triggers a series of biochemical and molecular reactions aimed at blood arresting and vessel wall repair. Vasoconstriction, platelet adhesion, and fibrin formation at the place of injury aimed to form a hemostatic aggregate are the first steps of the vessel wall repair and prevent excessive loss of blood. A few scattered platelets may interact with subtly injured, dysfunctional endothelium and contribute, by the release of growth factors, to mild intimal hyperplasia. In contrast, with endothelial denudation and mild intimal injury, from a monolayer to a few layers of platelets may deposit on the lesion, with or without mural thrombus formation. The release of platelet growth factors may contribute significantly to an accelerated intimal hyperplasia, as it occurs in the coronary vein graft within the first postoperative year. In severe injury, with exposure of components of deeper layers of the vessel, as in spontaneous plaque rupture or in angioplasty, marked platelet aggregation with mural thrombus formation follows. Vascular injury of this magnitude also stimulates thrombin formation through both the intrinsic (surface-activated) and extrinsic (tissue factor [TF]–dependent) coagulation pathways, in which the platelet membrane facilitates interactions between clotting factors (Fig. 41–1). This concept of vascular injury as a trigger of the platelet coagulation response is important in understanding the pathogenesis of various vascular diseases associated with atherothrombosis and coronary artery disease.

Growing thrombi may locally occlude the lumen or embolize and be washed away by the blood flow to occlude distal vessels. However, thrombi may be physiologically and spontaneously lysed by mechanisms that block thrombus propagation. Thrombus size, location, and composition are regulated by hemodynamic forces (mechanical effects), thrombogenicity of exposed substrate (local molecular effects), relative concentration of fluid phase and cellular

blood components (local cellular effects), and the efficiency of the physiologic mechanisms of control of the system, mainly fibrinolysis (1–4).

Platelets

After plaque rupture, the exposed vessel structures induce platelet aggregation and thrombosis by mechanisms in some instances different from those prevalent in hemostatic plug formation (Fig. 41–1). The ulcerated atherothrombotic plaque may contain a disrupted fibrous cap, a lipid-rich core, abundant extracellular matrix, and inflammatory cells. Such structures exhibit a potent activating effect on platelets and coagulation. The understanding of the biochemical events involved in platelet activation has progressed significantly (5–7). Most platelet aggregation agonists seem to act through the hydrolysis of platelet membrane phosphatidylinositol by phospholipase C, which results in the mobilization of free calcium from the platelet-dense tubular system (8,9). Exposed matrix from the vessel wall and thrombin generated by the activation of the coagulation cascade, as well as circulating epinephrine, are powerful platelet agonists. Adenosine diphosphate (ADP) is a platelet agonist that may be released from hemolyzed red cells in the area of vessel injury. Each agonist stimulates the discharge of calcium from the platelet-dense tubular system and promotes the contraction of the platelet, with the subsequent release of its granule contents. Platelet-related ADP and serotonin stimulate adjacent platelets, further enhancing the process of platelet activation. Arachidonate, which is released from the platelet membrane by the stimulatory effect of collagen, thrombin, ADP, and serotonin, is another platelet agonist. Arachidonate is converted to thromboxane A$_2$ (TxA$_2$) by the sequential effects of cyclooxygenase and thromboxane synthetase. TxA_2 not only promotes further platelet aggregation, but it is also a potent vasoconstrictor (2,3) (Fig. 41–2).

Signal transduction mechanisms initiated on binding of agonists to membrane-spanning receptors on the platelet surface have been partially elucidated (5) (Fig. 41–2). Agonist binding triggers cascades of intracellular second messengers, including inositol 1,4,5-triphosphate (IP_3) and diacylglycerol. IP_3 releases Ca^{2+} from the platelet-dense tubular system, increasing the cytosolic free Ca^{2+} concentration. Diacylglycerol activates the serine/threonine kinase, protein kinase C, translocating it to the plasma membrane and triggering granule secretion and fibrinogen receptor exposure (glycoprotein [GP] IIb/IIIa complex). At the same time, the increasing cytosolic free Ca^{2+} concentration facilitates arachidonate acid release from phospholipids by phospholipase A_2, a process that may occur at both the plasma membrane and the dense tubular system membrane. Arachidonate is metabolized to TxA_2, which diffuses out of the cell, interacts with receptors on the platelet surface, and causes further platelet activation. At some point during this process, tyrosine kinases, including members of the src family, are activated in platelets and cause the phosphorylation on tyrosine of multiple platelet proteins, most of which have not been identified. Tyrosine kinase activation in platelets appears to occur predominantly as a consequence of fibrinogen receptor expression and platelet aggregation, but it also can occur as an early step in platelet activation. In many cases, the interactions between agonists and the enzymes responsible for second messenger generation are mediated by a guanine nucleotide–binding regulatory protein (G protein). In platelets, G proteins have been shown to regulate phosphoinositide hydrolysis and cyclic adenosine monophosphate formation and are probably involved in the activation of phospholipase A_2. Phospholipase C is activated in a pertussis toxin–sensitive manner by the still unidentified G protein, G_p, and in a pertussis toxin–resistant manner by the G protein, G_q. Adenylyl cyclase is stimulated by the G protein, G_s, and is inhibited by the G protein, G_i. The G protein that regulates phospholipase A_2 activity remains to be characterized. Platelet receptors for thrombin, epinephrine, TxA_2, and platelet-activating factor have been cloned and shown to resemble other G protein–coupled receptors with a characteristic structure composed of a single polypeptide with seven transmembrane domains. The low–molecular weight, guanosine triphosphate (GTP)–binding protein, Rap1B, has been shown to form a complex with phospholipase $C\gamma$ and Ras-GTPase activating protein, supplying a potential mechanism for regulating phospholipase $C\gamma$ activity. Other low–molecular weight, GTP-binding proteins may be involved in the regulation of vesicular transport and granule secretion in platelets (5,7).

The initial recognition of damaged vessel wall by platelets involves (a) adhesion, activation, and adherence to recognition sites on the thromboactive substrate (extracellular matrix proteins; e.g., von Willebrand factor [vWF], collagen, fibronectin, vitronectin, and laminin); (b) spreading of the platelet on the surface; and (c) aggregation of platelets with each other to form a platelet plug or white thrombus. The efficiency of the platelet recruitment will depend on the

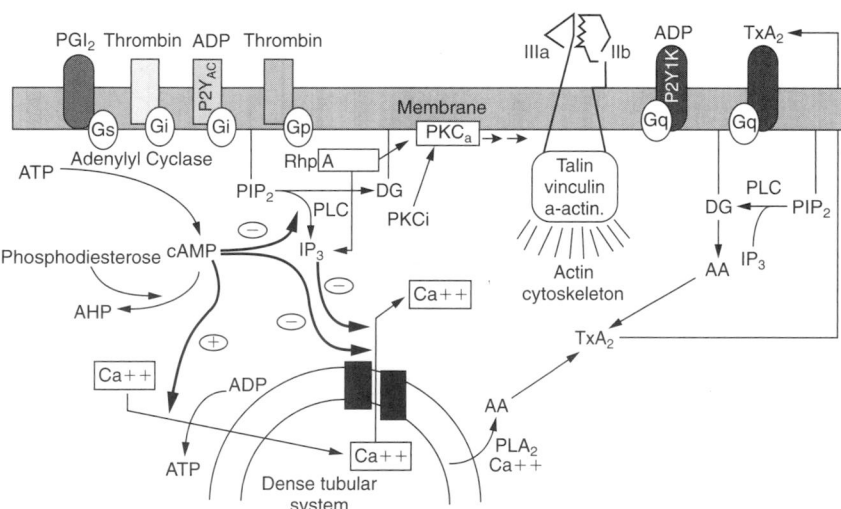

FIG. 41–2. Signal transduction mechanisms initiated on binding of agonists to platelet membrane receptors. Binding activates G proteins and triggers intracellular second messengers such as inositol 1,4,5-triphosphate (IP_3) and diacylglycerol (DG). The final outcome is the activation of the platelet with secretion, further fibrinogen receptor exposure, and aggregation. AA, arachidonic acid; ADP, adenosine diphosphate; AMP, adenosine monophosphate; ATP, adenosine triphosphate; cAMP, cyclic adenosine monophosphate; DG, diacylglycerol; G_s, G_i, G_p, G_q, guanine nucleotide-binding regulatory proteins; IIb/IIIa, receptor glycoprotein for adhesive protein ligands (mainly fibrinogen and von Willebrand factor), which supports platelet aggregation (receptor occupancy triggers tyrosine kinase activation); PGI_2, prostacyclin; PIP_2, phosphoinositol diphosphate; PKC_i and PKC_a, protein kinase C inactivated and activated; PLA_2, phospholipase A_2; PLC, phospholipase C; TxA_2, thromboxane A_2.

underlying substrate and local geometry. A final step of recruitment of other blood cells also occurs; erythrocytes, neutrophils, and occasionally monocytes are found on evolving mixed thrombus (Fig. 41–3).

Platelet function depends on adhesive interactions, and most of the GPs on the platelet membrane surface are receptors for adhesive proteins. Many of these receptors have been identified, cloned, sequenced, and classified within large gene families that mediate a variety of cellular interactions (10,11) (Table 41–1). The most abundant is the integrin family, which includes GPIIb–IIIa, GPIa–IIa, GPIc–IIa, the fibronectin receptor, and the vitronectin receptor, in decreasing order of magnitude. Another gene family present in the platelet membrane glycocalyx is the leucine-rich GP family represented by the GPIb–IX complex, receptor for vWF on unstimulated platelets that mediates adhesion to subendothelium, and GPV. Other gene families include the selectins (such as GMP-140) and the immunoglobulin domain protein (human leukocyte Class I antigen and platelet/endothelial cell adhesion molecule-1). Unrelated to any other gene family is GPIV(IIIa) (10) (Table 41–1).

The GPIb–IX complex consist of two disulfide-linked subunits (GPIbα and GPIbβ) tightly (not covalently) complexed with GPIX in a 1:1 heterodimer. GPIbβ and GPIX are transmembrane GPs and form the larger globular domain. The elongated, protruding part of the receptor corresponds to GPIbα. The major role of GPIb–IX is to bind immobilized vWF on the exposed vascular subendothelium and initiate adhesion of platelets. GPIb does not bind soluble vWF in plasma; apparently, it undergoes a conformation

change on binding to the extracellular matrix and then exposes a recognition sequence for GPIb–IX. The vWF binding domain of GPIb–IX has been narrowed to amino acids 251 through 279 on GPIbα (12). The GPIbα-binding domain of vWF resides in a tryptic fragment extending from residue 449 to 728 of the subunit that does not contain an Arg–Gly–Asp (RGD) sequence (13). The cytoplasmic domain of GPIb–IX has a major function in linking the plasma membrane to the intracellular actin filaments of the cytoskeleton and functions to stabilize the membrane and to maintain the platelet shape (14,15).

TABLE 41–1. *Platelet membrane glycoprotein receptors*

GP receptor	Ligand	Function
GPIIb–IIIa	Fg, vWF, Fn, Ts, Vn	Aggregation, adhesion at high shear rate
Receptor Vn	Vn, vWF, Fn, Fg, Ts	Adhesion
GPIa–IIa	C	Adhesion
GPIc–IIa	Fn	Adhesion
GPIc′–IIa	Ln	Adhesion
GPIb–IX	vWF, T	Adhesion
GPV	Substrate T	Unknown
GPIV (GPIIIb)	Ts, C	Adhesion
GMP-140 (PADGEM)	Unknown	Interaction with leucocytes
PECAM-1 (GPIIa)	Unknown	Unknown

C, collagen; Fg, fibrinogen; Fn, fibronectin; GP, glycoprotein; Ln, laminin; PECAM-1, platelet/endothelial cell adhesion molecule 1; T, thrombin; Ts, thrombospondin; Vn, vitronectin; vWF, von Willebrand factor.

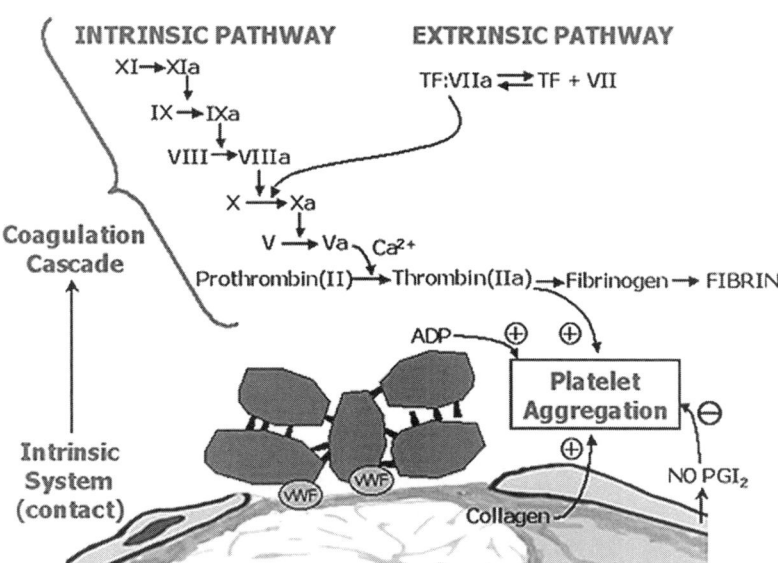

FIG. 41–3. Simplified diagram of platelet–vessel wall interaction and coagulation enzymes. Platelet adhesion to recognition sites occurs in lesioned areas of the endothelium. Adhesion, spreading, and aggregation of new platelets contribute to mural thrombus formation. Platelet aggregation is enhanced by agonists present in the microenvironment *(arrows with plus signs),* whereas there are spontaneous pathways of inhibition *(arrows with minus signs)* derived from neighboring normal endothelium. ADP, adenosine diphosphate; NO, nitric oxide; PGI$_2$, prostacyclin; TF, tissue factor; vWF, von Willebrand factor.

Randomly distributed on the surface of resting platelets are about 50,000 molecules of GPIIb/IIIa. The complex is composed of one molecule of GPIIb (disulfide-linked large and light chains) and one of GPIIIa (single polypeptide chain); it is a Ca^{2+}-dependent heterodimer, noncovalently associated on the platelet membrane (16). Calcium is required for maintenance of the complex and for binding of adhesive proteins (17,18). On activated platelets, the GPIIb/IIIa is a receptor for fibrinogen, fibronectin, vWF, vitronectin, and thrombospondin (19). The receptor recognition sequences are localized to small peptide sequences (RGD) in the adhesive proteins (20). Fibrinogen contains two RGD sequences in its α chain: one near the N-terminus (residues 95–97) and a second near the C-terminus (residues 572–574) (21). Fibrinogen has a second site of recognition for GPIIb/IIIa: the 12-amino acid sequence located at the carboxyl-terminus of the γ chain of the molecule (22). This dodecapeptide is specific for fibrinogen and does not contain the RGD sequence, but it does compete with RGD-containing peptides for binding to GPIIb/IIIa (10,23,24).

Thrombin plays an important role in the pathogenesis of arterial thrombosis (Fig. 41–4). It is one of the most potent known agonists for platelet activation and recruitment. The thrombin receptor has 425 amino acids with seven transmembrane domains and a large NH_2-terminal extracellular extension that is cleaved by thrombin to produce a "tethered" ligand that activates the receptor to initiate signal transduction (25,26). Thrombin is a critical enzyme in early thrombus formation, cleaving fibrinopeptides A and B from fibrinogen to yield insoluble fibrin, which effectively anchors the evolving thrombus. Both free and fibrin-bound fibrin thrombin are able to convert fibrinogen to fibrin, allowing propagation of thrombus at the site of injury.

Therefore, platelet activation triggers intracellular signaling and expression of platelet membrane receptors for adhesion and initiation of cell contractile processes that induce shape change and secretion of the granular contents. The expression of the integrin IIb/IIIa ($\alpha_{IIb}\beta_3$) receptors for adhesive GP ligands (mainly fibrinogen and vWF) in the circulation initiates platelet–platelet interaction. The process becomes perpetuated by the arrival of platelets brought by the circulation. Most of the GPs in the platelet membrane surface are receptors for adhesive proteins or mediate cellular interactions.

The receptor-mediated mechanisms related to platelet interaction in the thrombotic process around stenosis have not been studied directly; however, in laminar parallel flow conditions, platelet GPIb is necessary for normal platelet adhesion to subendothelium at high shear rates (27,28) through its interaction with vWF (29,30). vWF has been shown to bind to platelet membrane GPs in both adhesion (platelet–substrate interaction) and aggregation (platelet–platelet interaction), leading to thrombus formation in perfusion studies conducted at high shear rates (27,31–36). The current consensus is that, at high shear rate conditions, platelet GPIb and GPIIb/IIIa both appear to be involved in the events of platelet adhesion,

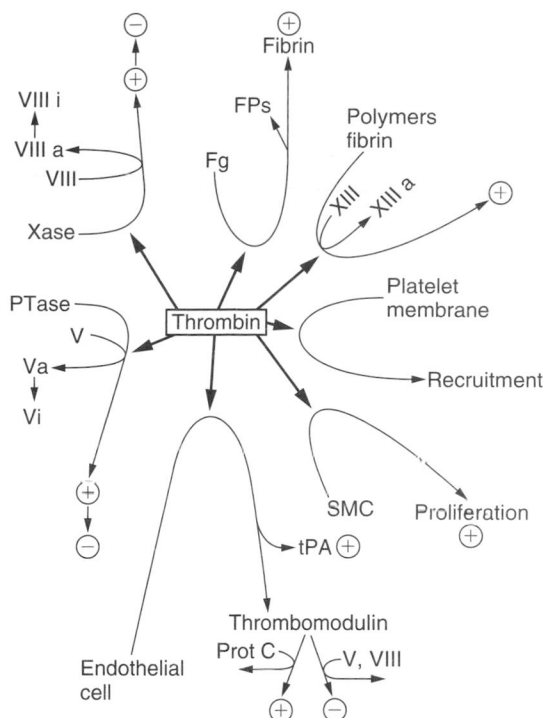

FIG. 41–4. Role of thrombin in the pathogenesis of arterial thrombosis. Positive signs (+) indicate reactions stimulated by thrombin, whereas negative signs (−) indicate reactions inhibited by thrombin. In addition to its effects on the activation of coagulation factors and fibrin formation and stabilization, thrombin activates platelets, induces proliferation of smooth muscle cells (SMCs), and contributes to the activation of the spontaneous anticoagulant pathway of normal endothelium. Fg, fibrinogen; FPs, fibrinopeptides; SMC, smooth muscle cells; tPA, tissue plasminogen activator.

whereas GPIIb/IIIa may be involved predominantly in platelet–platelet interaction. These mechanisms have not been evaluated with respect to events in the vicinity of stenosis.

The specific plasma proteins, which are predominantly involved in platelet–platelet interactions under various shear conditions and triggering atherothrombotic substrates remain to be determined. The absence of platelet aggregation in thrombasthenia (observed using low-shear and nonflow systems) has been ascribed to the inability of platelets to bind fibrinogen, because platelets are known to require fibrinogen for aggregation in plasma or buffer; however, this requirement is not absolute (37,38). In perfusion studies, platelet attachment or aggregate buildup (thrombus formation) on subendothelium was shown to be normal in afibrinogenemia under a wide variety of shear conditions (28, 39,40). Antibodies to fibrinogen, even when added to afibrinogenemic blood to remove any small trace of residual fibrinogen, did not inhibit platelet interaction with the vessel wall (41), although they did reduce aggregation with ADP and collagen when tested in an aggregometer.

Blocking the GPIIb/IIIa receptor site on platelets with either an antibody (LJ-CP8), which blocks the general binding

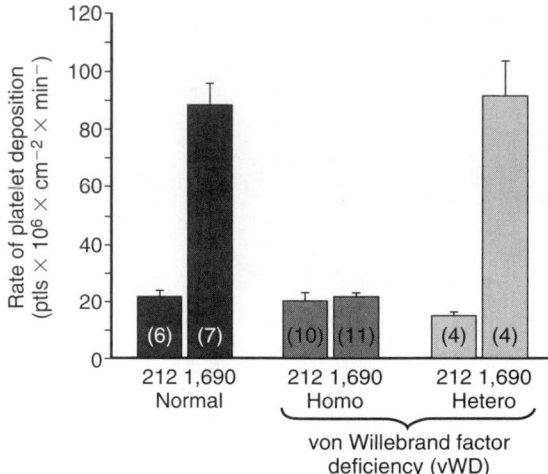

FIG. 41–5. Rate of platelet deposition on native fibrillar collagen type I bundles (model of severe injury to the vessel wall). Results are expressed as millions of platelets deposited per surface area and per unit time. Nonanticoagulated blood derived from a catheterized carotid artery of normal, homozygous von Willebrand factor deficiency (vWD) and heterozygous vWD pigs was perfused at low (212 s^{-1}) and high (1,690 s^{-1}) local shear rates through the Badimon perfusion chamber containing the collagen substrate. Platelet deposition at high shear rate was significantly increased in normal and heterozygous vWD, but not in homozygous vWD (devoid of von Willebrand factor [vWF]). Values in parentheses indicate the numbers of experiments. Heterozygous vWD with intermediate levels of plasma vWF showed normal platelet deposition at high shear rate. The three genotypes showed normal fibrinogen levels; therefore, *in vivo* vWF has an important function in binding glycoprotein IIb/IIIa, mainly at areas with high shear, and supports thrombus formation. (Modified from Badimon L, Badimon JJ, Turitto VT, et al. Platelet thrombus formation on collagen type I. Influence of blood rheology, von Willebrand factor and blood coagulation. *Circulation* 1988;78:1431–1442, with permission.)

of adhesive proteins, or with various peptides, which simulate the RGD sequence, inhibits both platelet adhesion and thrombus formation in flowing blood at high shear rates. These findings reinforce the importance of the GPIIb/IIIa site in platelet–vessel wall interaction and suggest that fibrinogen is not always a necessary component for such interactions. Moreover, the results also are consistent with previous perfusion studies that demonstrated the relatively low importance of fibrinogen in favor of vWF in both platelet–platelet and platelet–vessel wall interactions at certain rheologic conditions in an *in vivo* ^{111}In-platelet thrombosis porcine system (27,28,32–34,42). Additional direct support for the ability of adhesive proteins other than fibrinogen to participate in platelet–platelet interactions has been obtained from studies conducted with a monoclonal antibody (LJ-P5) to GPIIb/IIIa that blocks the binding of vWF and other adhesive proteins, but not of fibrinogen, to platelets (43). In the presence of this antibody, levels of both platelet–vessel wall and platelet–platelet interaction on subendothelium were reduced, suggesting that vWF participates in the thrombotic events occurring in flowing blood.

A peptide-specific monoclonal antibody that inhibits vWF binding to GPIIb/IIIa (152-6) without affecting the binding of other RGD-dependent GPs also has been shown to inhibit significantly platelet deposition to human atherothrombotic vessel wall (44). Pigs that have normal fibrinogen levels but are congenitally deficient in vWF showed a significantly reduced ability to deposit platelets in subendothelium, severely damaged vessel wall, and collagen type I bundles using a variety of *in vivo* and *in vitro* perfusion conditions at high and low local shear rates in native (nonanticoagulated) and anticoagulated blood (45) (Fig. 41–5).

In Figure 41–6, a simplified diagram shows different platelet membrane receptors involved in platelet activation.

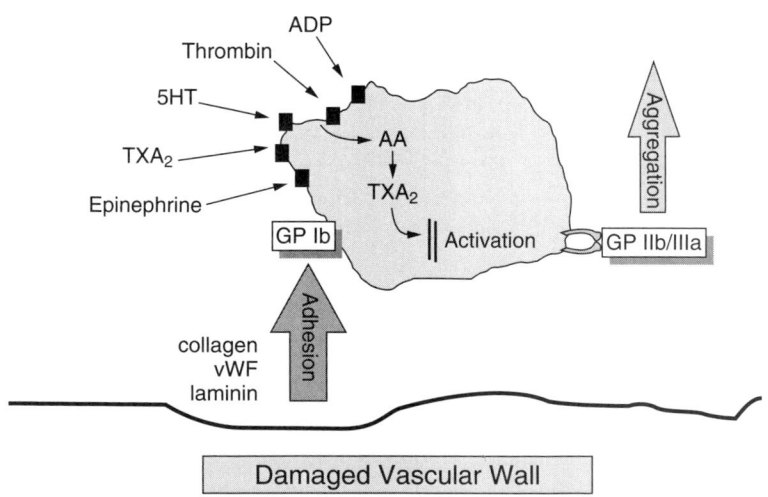

FIG. 41–6. Simplified diagram showing receptors in platelet membrane involved in platelet activation. 5HT, serotonin; ADP, adenosine diphosphate; AA, arachidonate acid; GP, glycoprotein; TxA$_2$, thromboxane A$_2$.

Ligand binding to the different membrane receptors triggers platelet activation with different relative potencies. A lot of interest has been recently generated among the platelet ADP receptors (P2Y$_{AC}$, P2y1R, P2X$_{1R}$) because of available pharmacologic inhibitors.

Activation of the Coagulation System

During plaque rupture, in addition to platelet deposition in the injured area, the clotting mechanism is activated by the exposure of the deendothelialized vascular surface. Blocking TF by a monoclonal antibody has reduced thrombus formation in a rabbit model of angioplasty, and thus TF may be exposed on vessel injury and contribute to thrombosis (46). The activation of the coagulation cascade leads to the generation of thrombin, which, as mentioned earlier, is a powerful platelet agonist that contributes to platelet recruitment in addition to catalyzing the formation and polymerization of fibrin. Fibrin is essential in the stabilization of the platelet thrombus and its withstanding removal forces by flow, shear, and high intravascular pressure. These basic concepts have clinical relevance in the context of the acute coronary syndromes where plaque rupture exposes vessel wall matrix and plaque core materials, which by activating platelets and the coagulation system results in the formation of a fixed and occlusive platelet-fibrin thrombus (Fig. 41–7).

The efficacy of fibrinolytic agents pointedly demonstrates the importance of fibrin-related material in the thrombosis associated with myocardial infarction (MI). However, few studies have considered the influence of flow on procoagulant activity either in laminar or nonparallel streamline conditions. The observation that fibrin formation seems to be diminished at increasing shear rates (30) is currently unexplained and needs to be confirmed. Although dilution of procoagulant moieties has generally been proposed as the mechanism by which flow minimizes clotting events at surfaces, such a mechanism has never been verified experimentally and, in fact, there are theoretical grounds to suspect the validity of such a hypothesis. The proteins that compose the clotting enzymes do not collide and interact on a random basis in the plasma, but interact in complexes in a highly efficient manner on platelet and endothelial surfaces. The major regulatory events in the coagulation (activation, inhibition, generation of anticoagulant proteins) occur on membrane surfaces.

Flow also regulates several endothelial targets that have been suggested to act as shear stress–responsive elements (47–49), which are activated by changes in shear stress conditions leading to the various signaling cascades, resulting in highly coordinated and orchestrated mechanotransduction messages with the ultimate goal to restore physiologic conditions. Two different mechanisms appear to be responsible for the endothelial molecular responses to shear stress. The first is the regulation or reorganization of preexisting proteins or structures by sudden changes in flow. Many of these effects are rapid and occur in just seconds, involving regulatory system at the level of rate-limiting enzymes or substrate

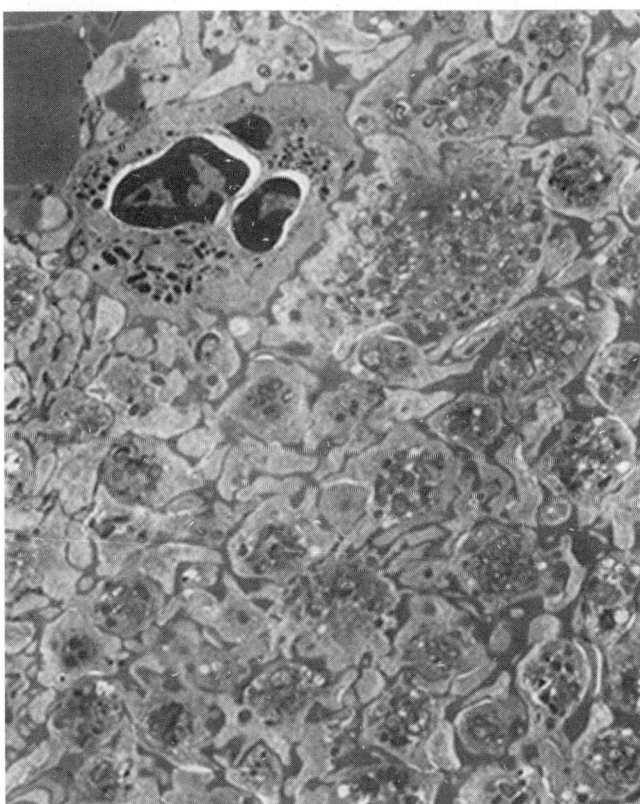

FIG. 41–7. Transmission electron microscopy microphotograph of a thrombus showing a platelet aggregate with completely degranulated platelets, red blood cells, and a leucocyte.

availability. One of the most studied enzymes that shows a rapid response to an increase in shear stress is the nitric oxide synthase (NOS). This enzyme catalyzes the production of NO in a potent and rapid response to shear stress, within milliseconds of the onset of flow. The second mechanism mediates the endothelial response to chronic flow changes. The delayed or chronic shear-mediated effects involve *de novo* protein synthesis, which, in turn, reflects regulation at the level of gene expression. The activation of specific transcriptional regulatory elements termed shear stress response elements in the promoters of shear-responsive genes is responsible for the changes in gene expression (47). Several endothelial genes are influenced by shear stress (50,51). For example, shear stress influences the expression of genes involved in vascular homeostasis, activating the expression of NOS-encoding gene and cyclooxygenase-2–encoding gene (responsible for the production of PGI$_2$), and downregulating the expression of the gene encoding preproendothelin-1 (the precursor of endothelin-1, a potent vasoconstrictor and platelet activator) (48).

Interestingly, venous thrombosis, which is predominantly constituted by fibrin clots, occurs in areas of stasis and low shear rate conditions typical of the venous system. Therefore, the low local shear rate conditions and flow recirculation developing in the poststenotic areas may explain fibrin

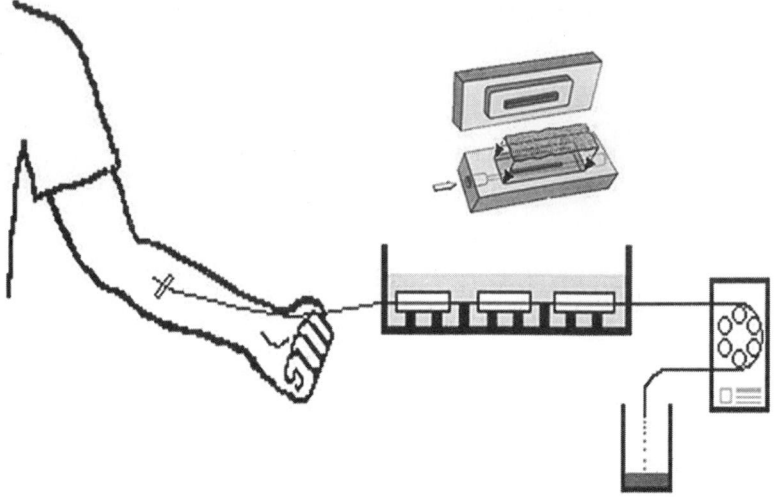

FIG. 41–8. General external view of the Badimon perfusion system.

accumulation. Vascular subendothelium (mildly injured vessel wall), which is completely devoid of endothelial cells, is able to clot whole plasma and more specifically activate factor X in the presence of factor VII (52). This activity results in the deposition of fibrin on the subendothelium at low shear conditions that can be blocked by monoclonal antibody to TF (52). Thus, TF appears to be a major procoagulant factor in the vascular space immediately underlying the endothelial lining of arteries, a site which might be readily accessible on local injury or on rupture of an atherothrombotic plaque.

Using an original stenotic perfusion chamber (Fig. 41–8), local fibrin formation on damaged vessel wall was shown to be dependent on the severity of the lesion and on shear rate conditions. Fibrin deposited in areas under high shear rate conditions (Fig. 41–9). The exposure of deep layers of the

vessel wall to blood will stimulate local fibrin formation also at the apex of stenotic narrowing even in the presence of a systemic heparin (53,54). In eccentric stenosis, fibrin(ogen) and platelet deposition were both significantly greater at the apex of the stenosis than at either the prestenotic or poststenotic area. However, fibrin(ogen) deposition demonstrated a significantly smaller degree of increase from the prestenotic area to the apex, as well as a smaller degree of decrease from the latter to the poststenotic region, compared with platelet deposition. Although both fibrin(ogen) and platelet deposition increased over time, the ratio of fibrin(ogen) to platelet showed a progressive decrease that became significant from 5 to 10 minutes at either low or high shear rate. On severely damaged vessel wall, fibrin(ogen) and platelet deposition is maximal at the apex of the stenosis where shear rate is extremely high and parallel streamlines are deformed. Therefore, fibrin(ogen) deposition is significantly less dependent on high shear rate than platelets, and the pattern is not influenced by time. Fibrin(ogen) deposition seems to be predominant in the thrombus layers adjacent to a severely damaged vessel wall regardless of the local shear stress levels and flow conditions (54).

The blood coagulation system involves a sequence of reactions integrating zymogens (proteins susceptible to be activated to enzymes through limited proteolysis) and cofactors (nonproteolytic enzyme activators) in three groups: (a) the contact activation (generation of factor XIa through the Hageman factor); (b) the conversion of factor X to factor Xa in a complex reaction requiring the participation of factors IX and VIII; and (c) the conversion of prothrombin to thrombin and fibrin formation (55) (Fig 41–10).

The triggering surfaces for *in vivo* initiation of contact activation have been suggested to be sulfatides and glycosaminoglycans of the vessel wall. The physiologic role of this system is unclear, however, because the absence of Hageman factor, prekallikrein, or high–molecular weight kininogen does not induce a clinically apparent pathology. Factor XI deficiency is associated with abnormal bleeding.

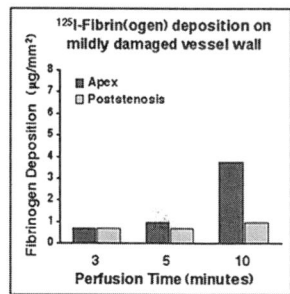
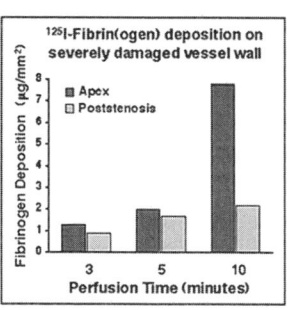

FIG. 41–9. Deposition of ^{125}I-fibrin(ogen) on mildly damaged and severely damaged vessel wall analyzed by perfusing heparinized blood derived from a catheterized carotid artery of a normal pig through the Badimon stenotic perfusion chamber. Fibrin(ogen) depositions on the apex of the stenosis (80%) and on the neighboring poststenotic zone where flow recirculation develops were compared. Fibrinogen deposition is substrate dependent, because it is always greater in severely damaged vessel wall (SDVW) than in mildly damaged vessel wall (MDVW), is flow dependent, and is also greater in the apex of the stenosis than in the recirculation zone (lower shear rate). (Badimon L., et al. unpublished data.)

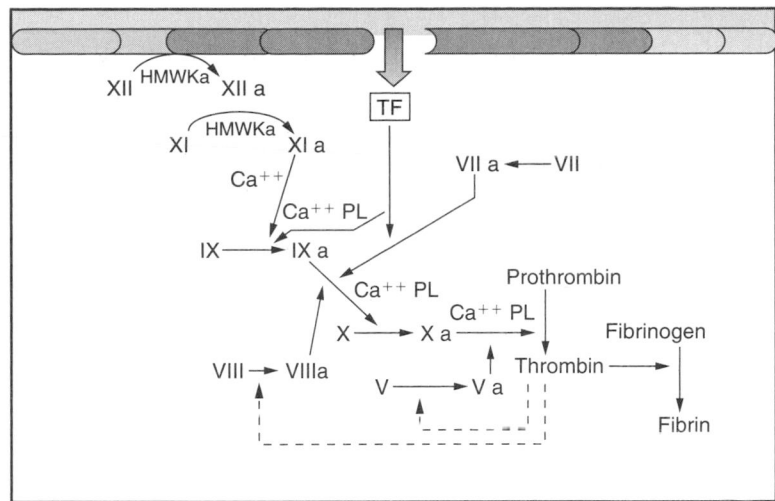

FIG. 41–10. Simplified diagram of the blood coagulation system integrating the contact activation or generation of factor XIa through Hageman factor, the conversion of factor X to Xa with the participation of factors IX and VIII, and the conversion of prothrombin into thrombin and fibrin formation. a, activated factor; BK, bradykinin; HMWK, high–molecular weight kininogen; K, kallikrein; PK, prekallikrein; PL, phospholipids; TF, tissue factor.

Activated factor XI induces the activation of factor IX in the presence of Ca^{2+}. Factor IXa forms a catalytic complex with factor VIII on a membrane surface and efficiently activates factor X in the presence of Ca^{2+}. Factor IX is a vitamin K–dependent enzyme, as are factor VII, factor X, prothrombin, and protein C (Table 41–2).

In citrated plasma, an anticoagulant often used in studies on platelet vessel wall interaction, the coagulation reactions do not proceed further than the activation of factor XI because of their dependence on Ca^{2+}. Platelets may provide the membrane requirements for the activation of factor X, although the participation of other cells of the vessel wall (in exposed injured vessels) has not been excluded (55). As such, endothelial cells in culture have been shown to support the activation of factor X (56). Factor VIII forms a noncovalent complex with vWF in plasma, and its function in coagulation is the acceleration of the effects of IXa on the activation of X to Xa. Absence of factor VIII or IX produces the hemophilic syndromes (57) (Fig. 41–10).

The TF pathway, previously known as extrinsic coagulation pathway, through the TF–factor VII complex in the presence of Ca^{2+} induces the formation of Xa. A second TF-dependent reaction catalyzes the transformation of IX into IXa. TF is an integral membrane protein that serves to initiate the activation of factors IX and X and to localize the reaction to cells on which TF is expressed. Other cofactors include factor VIIIa, which binds to platelets and forms the binding site for IXa, thereby forming the machinery for the activation of X, and factor Va, which binds to platelets and provides a binding site for Xa (Table 41–2). The human genes for these cofactors have been cloned and sequenced. In physiologic conditions, no cells in contact with blood contain active TF, although cells such as monocytes and polymorphonuclear leukocytes can be induced to synthesize and express TF (55).

Activated Xa converts prothrombin into thrombin. The complex that catalyzes the formation of thrombin consists of factors Xa and Va in a 1:1 complex. The activation results in the cleavage of fragment 1.2 and formation of thrombin from fragment 2. The interaction of the four components of the "prothrombinase complex" (Xa, Va, phospholipid, and Ca^{2+}) yield a more efficient reaction (58).

Activated platelets provide procoagulant surface for the assembly and expression of both intrinsic Xase and prothrombinase enzymatic complexes (59–63). These complexes respectively catalyze the activation of factor X to factor Xa and prothrombin to thrombin. The expression of activity is associated with the binding of both the proteases, factors IXa and Xa, and the cofactors, VIIIa and Va, to procoagulant surfaces. The binding of IXa and Xa is promoted by VIIIa and Va, respectively, such that Va and likely VIIIa provide the equivalent of receptors for the proteolytic enzymes (64–66). The surface of the platelet expresses the procoagulant phospholipids that bind coagulation factors and contribute to the procoagulant activity of the cell (64).

Blood clotting is blocked at the level of the prothrombinase complex by the physiologic anticoagulant-activated

TABLE 41–2. *Coagulation system*

Cofactor	Enzyme	Zymogen	Product
Tissue factor	VIIa	IX	IXa
Tissue factor	VIIa	X	Xa
VIIIa	IXa	X	Xa
Va	Xa	Prothrombin	Thrombin

protein C and oral anticoagulants (Fig. 41–11). Oral anticoagulants prevent posttranslational synthesis of γ-carboxyglutamic acid groups on the vitamin K–dependent clotting factors, preventing binding of prothrombin and Xa to the membrane surface. Activated protein C cleaves factor Va to render it functionally inactive. Loss of Va decreases the role of thrombin formation to negligible levels (67).

Thrombin acts on multiple substrates, including fibrinogen, factors XIII, V, and VIII, and protein C, in addition to its effects on platelets (Fig. 41–3). It plays a central role in hemostasis and thrombosis. The catalytic transformation of fibrinogen into fibrin is essential in the formation of the hemostatic plug and in the formation of arterial thrombi. It binds to the fibrinogen central domain and cleaves fibrinopeptides A and B, resulting in fibrin monomer and polymer formation (68). The fibrin mesh holds the platelets together and contributes to the attachment of the thrombus to the vessel wall.

The control of the coagulation reactions occurs by diverse mechanisms, such as hemodilution and flow effects, proteolytic feedback by thrombin, inhibition by plasma proteins (such as antithrombin III) and endothelial cell–localized activation of an inhibitory enzyme (protein C), and fibrinolysis (Fig. 41–11). Although antithrombin III readily inactivates thrombin in solution, its catalytic site is inaccessible while bound to fibrin, and it may still cleave fibrinopeptides even in the presence of heparin. Thrombin has a specific receptor in endothelial cell surfaces, thrombomodulin, that triggers a physiologic anticoagulative system (69). The thrombin-

thrombomodulin complex serves as a receptor for the vitamin K–dependent protein C, which is activated and released from the endothelial cell surface. Activated protein C blocks the effects of factors V and VIII and limits thrombin effects (Fig. 41–11). Endogenous fibrinolysis represents a repair mechanism, such as endothelial cell regrowth and vessel recanalization. Fibrinolysis involves catalytic activation of zymogens, positive and negative feedback control, and inhibitor blockade (70,71).

EFFECTS OF THE SEVERITY OF VESSEL WALL DAMAGE AND LOCAL GEOMETRY ON THE THROMBOTIC RESPONSE TO ATHEROTHROMBOSIS

The dynamics of platelet deposition and thrombus formation after vascular damage are modulated by the type of injury and the local geometry at the damage site (degree of stenosis) (33,72–74). Exposure of deendothelialized vessel wall (mimicking mild vascular injury) to blood at high shear rate (mimicking a stenosed artery) induced significant platelet deposition to the exposed vessel (72). The deposition of platelet reached a maximum within 5 to 10 minutes of exposure; however, the evolving aggregates could be dislodged from the substrate by the flowing blood. Exposure of native fibrillar collagen type I bundles with a rough surface (mimicking type III injury) to blood produced platelet deposition of more than two orders of magnitude greater than on subendothelium (33). Even at high shear rate, the thrombus was not dis-

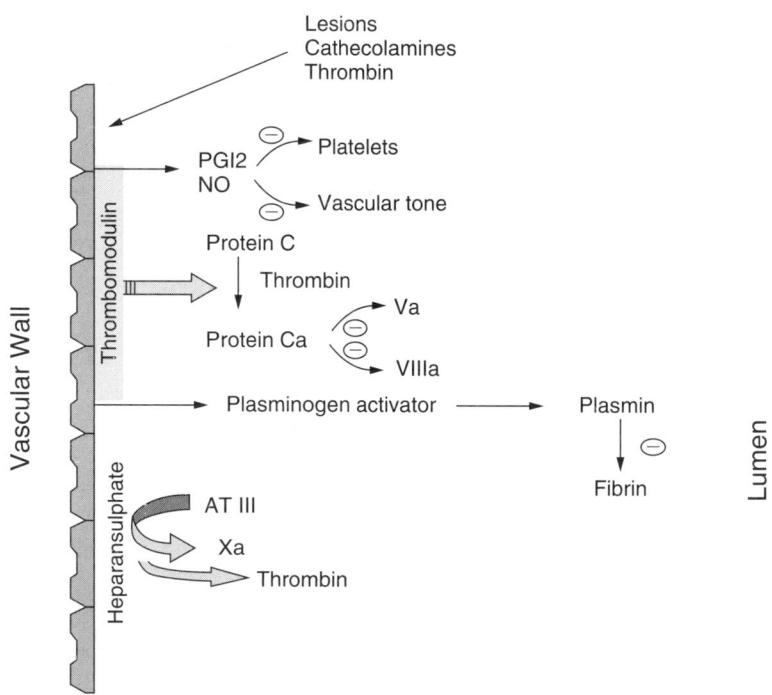

FIG. 41–11. Simplified diagram of the endothelium physiologic anticoagulant system. The thrombomodulin and heparan sulfate systems work as controllers of the coagulation reaction. Endothelial release of prostacyclin (PGI$_2$) and nitric oxide (NO) also inhibit platelet activation and reduce the vascular tone.

lodged, but remained adherent to the surface. Similar experimental quantitative information on the importance of the degree of vascular damage on the degree and stability of thrombus formation has now been documented by varying degrees of stenosis and with severely damaged vessel wall (exposing medial matrix structures to blood) (73,74). Importantly, besides fibrillar collagen (33), exposed thromboplastin or TF (75,76) also seems to contribute to the high thrombogenicity when deep or severe injury to the vessel wall occurs. Overall, it is likely that when injury to the vessel wall is mild, the thrombogenic stimulus is relatively limited, and the resulting thrombotic occlusion is transient, as occurs in unstable angina. However, deep vessel injury secondary to plaque rupture or ulceration (Fig. 41–12) results in exposure of collagen, TF, and other elements of the vessel matrix, leading to relatively persistent thrombotic occlusion and MI (77).

It is likely that the nature of the substrate exposed after spontaneous or angioplasty-induced plaque rupture is one factor determining whether an unstable plaque proceeds rapidly to an occlusive thrombus or persists as nonocclusive mural thrombus. The analysis of the relative contribution of different components of human atherothrombotic plaques (fatty streaks, sclerotic plaques, fibrolipid plaques, atheromatous plaques, hyperplasic cellular plaque and normal intima) to acute thrombus formation showed that the atheromatous core was up to sixfold more active than the other substrates in triggering thrombosis (78). Although the atheromatous core had a more irregular exposed surface and thrombus formation tended to increase with increasing roughness, the atheromatous core remained the most thrombogenic substrate when the substrates were normalized by the degree of irregularity as defined by the roughness index. The atheromatous core is the most thrombogenic component of human atherothrombotic plaques; therefore, plaques with a large atheromatous core content are at high risk for acute coronary syndromes after spontaneous or mechanically induced rupture because of the increased thrombogenicity of their contents (78). The plaque TF content is directly related to its thrombogenicity (Fig. 41–13) (79). As proof of concept, we showed that local tissue blockade of TF, by treatment with TFPI, significantly reduces thrombosis (80). The use of active site inhibited recombinant factor VIIa (FF-rFVIIa) has shown to significantly reduce thrombus growth on severely damaged vessels (81).

Platelet deposition is directly related to the degree of stenosis in the presence of the same degree of injury, indi-

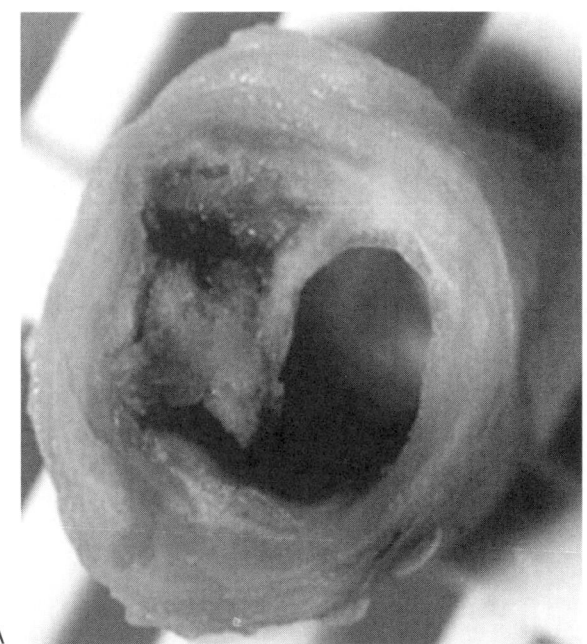
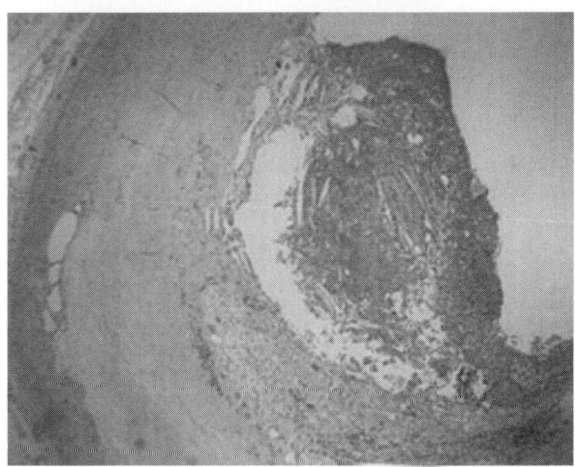

FIG. 41–12. Atherothrombosis. Thrombosis on a ruptured high-risk plaque that resulted in a sudden death episode of an individual. (Courtesy of Badimon L., Juan O. et al., 2003.)

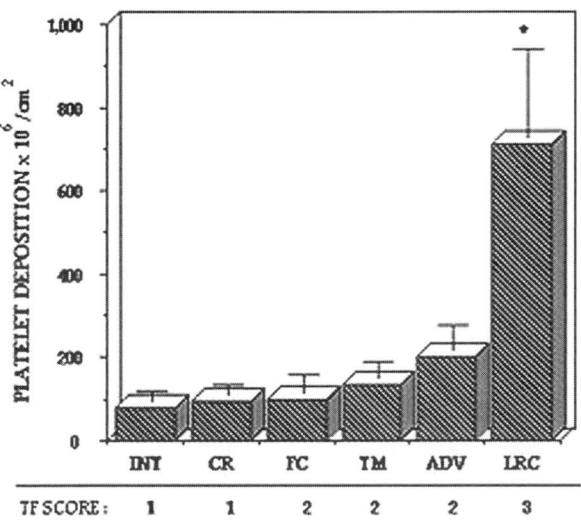

FIG. 41–13. Platelet deposition on atherothrombotic substrates evaluated by perfusing blood with ^{111}In-labeled platelets. The atheromatous core triggers significantly greater thrombosis than other plaque components when perfused at the same hemodynamic conditions. The effect is associated with the content of tissue factor (TF). ADV, adventitia; CR, collagen-rich; FC, fibrous cap; INT, intima; LRC, lipid-rich core; TM, tunica media. (For a more detailed discussion, see Fernández-Ortiz A., et al. [78] and Toschi V., et al. [79].)

cating a shear-induced platelet activation (73,74). In addition, analysis of the axial distribution of platelet deposition indicates that the apex, not the flow recirculation zone distal to the apex, is the segment of greatest platelet accumulation. These data suggest that the severity of the acute platelet response to plaque disruption depends in part on the sudden changes in geometry after rupture (3). Interestingly, hemodynamic effects play a role in the regulation of the thrombotic response in different arteries. In the absence of atherothrombotic changes, in the porcine normolipemic model, the dilatation of carotid and coronary arteries in the same animal rendered a significantly different platelet deposition in both arterial beds, with the coronaries triggering a significantly greater deposition than the carotids (82).

Spontaneous lysis of thrombus does occur, not only in unstable angina (77), but also in AMI. In these patients, as well as in those undergoing thrombolysis for acute infarction, the presence of a residual mural thrombus predisposes to recurrent thrombotic vessel occlusion (83–86). Two main contributing factors for the development of rethrombosis have been identified. First, a residual mural thrombus may encroach into the vessel lumen resulting in increased shear rate, which facilitates the activation and deposition of platelets on the lesion. As mentioned previously, using an experimental animal model of *ex vivo* perfusion, it has been shown that platelet deposition is greater with increasing degrees of vessel stenosis (73,74). Second, the presence of a fragmented thrombus appears to be one of the most powerful thrombogenic surfaces. This was also evaluated in the *ex vivo* Badimon perfusion chamber model, where platelet deposition was assessed by continuous scintigraphic imaging of ^{111}In-labeled platelets. A gradual increase in platelet deposition in the area of maximal stenosis was observed, followed by an abrupt decrease, probably because of the spontaneous thrombus embolization or platelet deaggregation. This was immediately followed by a rapid increase in platelet deposition, suggesting that the remaining thrombus was markedly thrombogenic. In fact, platelet deposition is increased two to four times on residual thrombus compared with deeply injured arterial wall; and thrombus continues to grow during heparin therapy, but is inhibited by specific antithrombin treatment (87).

r-Hirudin, a recombinant molecule that blocks both the catalytic site and the anion-exosite of the thrombin molecule, inhibited significantly the secondary growth (87). Thus, after lysis, thrombin becomes exposed to the circulating blood, leading to activation of the platelets and coagulation, further enhancing thrombosis. The antithrombin activity of heparin is limited for three main reasons. First, a residual thrombus contains active thrombin bound to fibrin, which is thus poorly accessible to the large heparin–antithrombin III complexes; second, a platelet-rich arterial thrombus releases large amounts of platelet factor 4, which may inhibit heparin; third, fibrin II monomer, formed by the action of thrombin on fibrinogen, may also inhibit heparin. Conversely, molecules of hirudin and other specific an-

tithrombins are at least ten times smaller than the heparin–antithrombin III complex, have no natural inhibitors, and therefore have greater accessibility to thrombin bound to fibrin. These experimental results clarify the clinical observations in patients with AMI undergoing thrombolysis, which have shown that residual stenosis is in part related to residual nonlysed thrombus (88). The effects of different antithrombotic treatment regimens on thrombus formation triggered by a residual mural thrombus have been evaluated, and specific thrombin inhibition has been shown to be the most effective regimen in inhibiting the progression of thrombus growth when compared with aspirin, heparin, or both (89,90).

As mentioned earlier, in addition to these prothrombotic effects, thrombin generates a series of reactions that activate the endogenous anticoagulant system (Fig. 41–11). Thrombin generated at the site of injury binds to thrombomodulin, an endothelial surface membrane protein, initiating activation of protein C, which, in turn (in the presence of protein S), inactivates factors Va and VIIIa. Thrombin stimulates successive release of both tissue plasminogen activator (t-PA) and plasminogen activator inhibitor type 1 from endothelial cells, thus initiating endogenous lysis through plasmin generation from plasminogen by t-PA with subsequent modulation through plasminogen activator inhibitor type 1. Thrombin therefore plays a pivotal role in maintaining the complex balance of initial prothrombotic reparative events and subsequent endogenous anticoagulant and thrombolytic pathways (69,91) (Fig. 41–4).

The importance of thrombin lies not just in acute thrombus formation after arterial injury, but also in its contribution to smooth muscle cell (SMC) proliferation by stimulating platelet secretion of growth factors (especially platelet-derived growth factor) and directly acting on SMCs (Fig. 41–4). Thus, thrombin has direct effects on cell proliferation and influences the cellular synthetic mechanisms responsible for matrix protein and collagen production (92). The role of thrombin as a possible mitogen for vascular cells has gained support with the identification of the cellular thrombin receptor (64) and with the detection of messenger RNA for this receptor in human atherothrombotic plaques (93). When thrombin is neutralized by complex formation with antithrombin III, thrombin-induced DNA synthesis and cell proliferation in human arterial SMCs are completely inhibited (94). Because mural thrombosis is usually associated with rescue coronary revascularization procedures, we studied how platelet activation with different agonists may affect SMC proliferation. Among platelet activation agonists ADP, collagen, and thrombin, thrombin was the only one that showed direct proliferative effects on SMC and the release of platelets activated with thrombin also induced significantly greater proliferative effects than the other platelet agonists when coincubated with SMC. Therefore, in severe wall injury, when there is significant *in situ* thrombin generation, platelets will generate a more significant proliferative stimulus for the subjacent SMC than when other agonists for platelet monolayer formation are prevalent (95). Specific thrombin inhibition or blockade of the thrombin generation pathway may also have a potential impact on the relative proliferative response of SMCs after arterial injury (96). It has been reported that thrombin induces expression of neuron-derived orphan receptor-1 (NOR-1) in vascular SMCs (97). Nor-1 is a transcription factor within the nerve growth factor-induced clone B (NGFI-B) subfamily of nuclear receptors that is overexpressed in human coronary atherothrombotic vessels and in balloon-dilated normal vessels (97).

SUMMARY

Arterial thrombus formation seems to be an important factor in the conversion of chronic to acute atherothrombotic coronary events after plaque rupture, in the progression of coronary disease, and in the acute phase of revascularization interventions. The knowledge gained (and studies now in progress) on the mechanisms of platelet activation, signal transduction, receptor binding, zymogen activation and function, substrate recognition, and adhesive events will help to design promising approaches for intervention. Receptors originally thought to be involved only in anchoring functions also are important factors in the transduction of information from the extracellular compartment to the inner cell, and they are involved in governing cell function, shape, proliferation, and differentiation. The availability of monoclonal antibodies and molecular biology techniques applied to the field of thrombosis and blood cell–vessel wall interaction will provide tools to explore specific pathways of cell activation and cell–cell interaction. These studies, together with those to find the most prevalent agonist and substrate to trigger and perpetuate a thrombotic event in every clinical situation, will help to establish strategies of prevention of clinical events and to reduce their associated morbidity and mortality.

ACKNOWLEDGMENTS

Part of the original contributions mentioned in this chapter were generated in a long-standing collaboration with Dr. V. Fuster from the Cardiovascular Institute, Mount Sinai Medical Center. Dr. L. Badimon is supported by grants from FIS, PNS (McyT), and Cardiovascular Research Foundation-Catalana Occidente, Spain. Dr. R. Corti is supported by the Swiss National Research Foundation. Dr. J.J. Badimon is supported by the National Institutes of Health and American Heart Association.

REFERENCES

1. Fuster V, Badimon L, Badimon JJ, et al. The pathogenesis of coronary artery disease and the acute coronary syndromes (1). *N Engl J Med* 1992;326:242–250.
2. Fuster V, Badimon L, Badimon JJ, et al. The pathogenesis of coronary artery disease and the acute coronary syndromes (2). *N Engl J Med* 1992;326:310–318.
3. Badimon L, Chesebro JH, Badimon JJ. Thrombus formation on ruptured atherosclerotic plaques and rethrombosis on evolving thrombi. *Circulation* 1992;86[Suppl III]:III-74–III-85.
4. Badimon JJ, Fuster V, Chesebro JH, et al. Coronary atherosclerosis. *Circulation* 1993;87[Suppl II]:II-3–II-16.
5. Marcus A, Safier LB. Thromboregulation: multicellular modulation of platelet reactivity in hemostasis and thrombosis. *FASEB J* 1993;7:516–522.
6. Kroll MH, Schafer AI. Biochemical mechanisms of platelet activation. *Blood* 1989;74:1181–1195.
7. Brass LF. The biochemistry of platelet activation. In: Hoffman R, Benz EJ Jr, Shattil SJ, et al., eds. *Hematology: basic principles and practice.* New York: Churchill Livingstone, 1991;1176–1197.
8. Colman RW, Walsh PN. Mechanisms of platelet aggregation. In: Colman RW, Hirsh J, Marder VJ, et al., eds. *Hemostasis and thrombosis: basic principles and clinical practice,* 2nd ed. Philadelphia: JB Lippincott, 1987:594–605.
9. Huang EM, Detwiler TC. Stimulus–response coupling mechanisms. In: Philips DR, Shuman MC, eds. *Biochemistry of platelets.* New York: Academic Press, 1986:1–68.
10. Kieffer N, Phillips DR. Platelet membrane glycoproteins: functions in cellular interactions. *Annu Rev Biol* 1990;6:329–357.
11. Kunicki TJ. Organization of glycoproteins within the platelet plasma membrane. In: George JN, Nurden AT, Philips DR, eds. *Platelet membrane glycoproteins.* New York: Plenum Press, 1985:87–101.
12. Vicente V, Houghten RA, Ruggeri ZM. Identification of a site in the α chain of platelet glycoprotein Ib that participates in von Willebrand factor binding. *J Biol Chem* 1990;265:274–280.
13. Fujimura Y, Titani K, Holland LZ, et al. von Willebrand factor. A reduced and alkylated 52/48-kDa fragment beginning at amino acid residue 449 contains the domain interacting with platelet glycoprotein Ib. *J Biol Chem* 1986;261:381–385.
14. Fox JE, Boyles JK, Berndt MC, et al. Identification of a membrane skeleton in platelets. *J Cell Biol* 1988;106:1525–1538.
15. Meyer D, Girma JP. Von Willebrand factor: structure and function. *Thromb Haemostasis* 1993;70:99–104.
16. Fitzgerald LA, Phillips DR. Calcium regulation of the platelet membrane glycoprotein IIb–IIIa complex. *J Biol Chem* 1985;260:11366–11376.
17. Calvete JJ, Henschen A, Gonzalez-Rodriguez J. Complete localization of the intrachain disulphide bonds and the N-glycosylation points in the α subunit of human platelet glycoprotein IIb. *Biochem J* 1989;261:561–568.
18. Beer J, Coller BS. Evidence that platelet glycoprotein IIIa has a large disulfide bonded loop that is susceptible to proteolytic cleavage. *J Biol Chem* 1989;264:17564–17573.
19. Plow EF, Ginsberg MH, Marguerie GA. Expression and function of adhesive proteins on the platelet surface. In: Phillips DR, Shuman MA, eds. *Biochemistry of Platelets.* New York: Academic Press; 1986:225–256.
20. Ruoslahti E, Pierschbacher MD. New perspectives in cell adhesion: RGD and integrins. *Science* 1987;238:491–497.
21. Doolittle RF, Watt KW, Cottrell BA, et al. The amino acid sequence of the α-chain of human fibrinogen. *Nature* 1979;280:464–467.
22. Kloczewiak M, Timmons S, Lukas TJ, et al. Platelet receptor recognition site on human fibrinogen. Synthesis and structure–function relationship of peptides corresponding to the carboxyterminal segment of the γ chain. *Biochemistry* 1984;23:1767–1774.
23. Ginsberg MH, Xiaoping D, O'Toole TE, et al. Platelet integrins. *Thromb Haemostasis* 1993;70:87–93.
24. Shattil SJ. Regulation of platelet anchorage and signaling by integrin αIIbβ₃. *Thromb Haemostasis* 1993;70:224–228.
25. Vu TH, Hung DT, Wheaton VI, et al. Molecular cloning of a functional thrombin receptor reveals a novel proteolytic mechanism of receptor activation. *Cell* 1991;64:1057–1068.
26. Coughlin SR. Thrombin receptor structure and function. *Thromb Haemostasis* 1993;70:184–187.
27. Sakariassen KS, Nievelstein PF, Coller BS, et al. The role of platelet membrane glycoproteins Ib and IIb/IIIa in platelet adherence to human artery subendothelium. *Br J Haematol* 1986;63:681–691.
28. Weiss HJ, Turitto VT, Baumgartner HR. Effect of shear rate on platelet interaction with subendothelium in citrated and native blood. I. Shear rate-dependent decrease of adhesion in von Willebrand's disease and the Bernard–Soulier syndrome. *J Lab Clin Med* 1978;92:750–754.
29. Sixma JJ, Sakariassen KS, Beeser-Vesser NH, et al. Adhesion of platelets

to human artery subendothelium: effects of factor VIII–von Willebrand factor of various multimeric composition. *Blood* 1984;63:128.

30. Turitto VT, Baumgartner HR. Platelet–surface interactions. In: Colman R, Hirsh J, Marder V, et al., eds. *Hemostasis and thrombosis: basic principles and clinical practice,* 2nd ed. Philadelphia: JB Lippincott, 1987:555–571.
31. Sakariassen K, Bolhuis PA, Sixma J. Human blood platelet adhesion to artery subendothelium is mediated by factor VIII–von Willebrand factor bound to the subendothelium. *Nature* 1979;279:636–638.
32. Badimon L, Badimon JJ, Turitto VT, et al. Platelet deposition in von Willebrand factor deficient vessel wall. *J Lab Clin Med* 1987;110:634–647.
33. Badimon L, Badimon JJ, Turitto VT, et al. Platelet thrombus formation on collagen type I. Influence of blood rheology, von Willebrand factor and blood coagulation. *Circulation* 1988;78:1431–1442.
34. Badimon L, Badimon JJ, Chesebro JH, et al. Inhibition of thrombus formation: blockage of adhesive glycoprotein mechanism versus blockage of the cyclooxygenase pathway. *J Am Coll Cardiol* 1988;11:30A.
35. Badimon L, Badimon JJ, Turitto VT, et al. Platelet interaction to vessel wall and collagen. Study in homozygous von Willebrand's disease associated with abnormal collagen aggregation in swine. *Thromb Haemostasis* 1989;61:57–64.
36. Badimon L, Badimon JJ, Turitto VT, et al. Role of von Willebrand factor in mediating platelet–vessel wall interaction at low shear rate; the importance of perfusion conditions. *Blood* 1989;73:961–967.
37. Cattaneo M, Kinlough-Rathbone R, Lecchi A, et al. Fibrinogen-independent aggregation and deaggregation of human platelets: studies in two afibrinogenemic patients. *Blood* 1987;70:221–226.
38. Soria J, Soria C, Borg JY, et al. Platelet aggregation occurs in congenital afibrinogenaemia despite the absence of fibrinogen or its fragments in plasma and platelets, as demonstrated by immunoenzymology. *Br J Haematol* 1985;60:503–510.
39. Turitto VT, Weiss JH, Baumgartner HR. Platelet interaction with rabbit subendothelium in von Willebrand's disease: altered thrombus formation distinct from defective platelet adhesion. *J Clin Invest* 1984;74:1730–1741.
40. Weiss HJ, Turitto VT, Vicic WJ, et al. Fibrin formation, fibrinopeptide A release, and platelet thrombus dimensions on subendothelium exposed to flowing native blood: greater in factor XII and XI than in factor VIII and IX deficiency. *Blood* 1984;63:1004–1014.
41. Weiss HJ, Hawiger J, Ruggeri ZM, et al. Fibrinogen-independent interaction of platelets with subendothelium mediated by glycoprotein IIb–IIIa complex at high shear rate. *J Clin Invest* 1989;83:288–297.
42. Badimon L, Badimon JJ, Cohen M, et al. Thrombosis in stenotic and laminar flow conditions: Effect of an antiplatelet GPIIb/IIIa monoclonal antibody fragment (7E3F(ab′)$_2$). *Circulation* 1989;80[Suppl]:II-422(abst).
43. Lombardo VT, Hodson E, Roberts JR, et al. Independent modulation of von Willebrand factor and fibrinogen binding to the platelet membrane glycoprotein IIb/IIIa complex as demonstrated by monoclonal antibody. *J Clin Invest* 1985;76:1950–1958.
44. Badimon L, Badimon JJ, Ruggeri Z, et al. A peptide-specific monoclonal antibody that inhibits von Willebrand factor binding to GPIIb/IIia (152B6) inhibits platelet deposition to human atherosclerotic vessel wall. *Circulation* 1990;82(4):III-370(abst).
45. Badimon L, Badimon JJ, Chesebro JH, et al. von Willebrand factor and cardiovascular disease. *Thromb Haemostasis* 1993;70:111–118.
46. Pawashe A, Guth BD, Muller TH, et al. Inhibition of experimental thrombosis with monoclonal antibody against rabbit tissue factor. *J Am Coll Cardiol* 1993;21(2):466A.
47. Resnick N, Yahav H, Schubert S, et al. Signalling pathways in vascular endothelium activated by shear stress: relevance to atherosclerosis. *Curr Opin Lipidol* 2000;11:167–177.
48. Topper JN, Gimbrone MA Jr. Blood flow and vascular gene expression: fluid shear stress as a modulator of endothelial phenotype. *Mol Med Today* 1999;5:40–46.
49. Traub O, Berk BC. Laminar shear stress: mechanisms by which endothelial cells transduce an atheroprotective force. *Arterioscler Thromb Vasc Biol* 1998;18:677–685.
50. Nagel T, Resnick N, Dewey CF Jr, et al. Vascular endothelial cells respond to spatial gradients in fluid shear stress by enhanced activation of transcription factors. *Arterioscler Thromb Vasc Biol* 1999;19:1825–1834.
51. Chien S, Li S, Shyy YJ. Effects of mechanical forces on signal transduction and gene expression in endothelial cells. *Hypertension* 1998;31:162–169.

52. Weiss HJ, Turitto VT, Baumgartner HR, et al. Evidence for the presence of tissue-factor activity on subendothelium. *Blood* 1989;73:968–975.
53. Badimon L, Badimon JJ, Lassila R, et al. Thrombin regulation of platelet interaction with damaged vessel wall and isolated collagen type I at arterial flow conditions in a porcine model. Effects of hirudins, heparin and calcium chelation. *Blood* 1991;78:423–434.
54. Mailhac A, Badimon JJ, Fallon JT, et al. Effect of an eccentric severe stenosis on fibrin(ogen) deposition on severely damaged vessel wall in arterial thrombosis. Relative contribution of fibrin(ogen) and platelets. *Circulation* 1994;90:988–996.
55. Nemerson Y. Mechanism of coagulation. In: Williams WJ, Beutler E, Erslev AJ, et al., eds. *Hematology.* New York: McGraw-Hill, 1990:1295–1304.
56. Rimon S, Melamed R, Savion N, et al. Identification of a factor IX/IXa binding protein on the endothelial cell surface. *J Biol Chem* 1987;262:6023–6031.
57. Colman RW, Marder VJ, Salzman EW, et al. Overview of hemostasis. In: Colman RW, Hirsh J, Marder VJ, et al., eds. *Hemostasis and thrombosis: basic principles and clinical practice.* Philadelphia: JB Lippincott, 1987:3–17.
58. Mann KG. Membrane-bound enzyme complexes in blood coagulation. In: Spaet TH, ed. *Progress in hemostasis and thrombosis.* New York: Grune & Stratton, 1984:1–23.
59. Tracy PB. Regulation of thrombin generation at cell surfaces. *Semin Thromb Haemostasis* 1988;14:227–233.
60. Mann KG, Nesheim ME, Church WR, et al. Surface dependent reactions of the vitamin K dependent enzyme complexes. *Blood* 1990;76:1–16.
61. Rawala-Sheikh R, Ahmad SS, Ashby B, et al. Kinetics of coagulation factor X activation by platelet bound factor IXa. *Biochemistry* 1990;29:2606–2611.
62. Tracy PB, Eide LL, Mann KG. Human prothrombinase complex assembly and function on isolated peripheral blood cell populations. *J Biol Chem* 1985;260:2119–2124.
63. Rosing J, van Rijn JL, Bevers EM, et al. The role of activated human platelets in prothrombin and factor X activation. *Blood* 1985;65:319–332.
64. Nesheim ME, Furmaniak-Kazmierczak E, Henin C, et al. On the existence of platelet receptors for factor Va and factor VIIIa. *Thromb Haemostasis* 1993;70:80–86.
65. Tracy PB, Nesheim ME, Mann KG. Coordinate binding of factor Va and factor Xa to the unstimulated platelet. *J Biol Chem* 1981;256:743–751.
66. Ahmad SS, Rawala-Sheikh R, Monroe DM, et al. Comparative platelet binding and kinetic studies with normal and variant factor IXa molecules. *J Biol Chem* 1990;265:20907–20911.
67. Comp PC. Kinetics of plasma coagulation factors. In: Williams WJ, Beutler E, Erslev AJ, et al., eds. *Hematology.* New York: McGraw-Hill, 1990:1285–1290.
68. Nemerson Y, Williams WJ. Biochemistry of plasma coagulation factors. In: Williams WJ, Beutler E, Erslev AJ, et al., eds. *Hematology.* New York: McGraw-Hill, 1990:1267–1284.
69. Esmon NL, Owen WG, Esmon CT. Isolation of a membrane-bound cofactor for thrombin-catalyzed activation of protein C. *J Biol Chem* 1982;257:859–864.
70. Francis CW, Marder VJ. Physiologic regulation and pathologic disorders of fibrinolysis. In: Colman RW, Hirsh J, Marder VJ, et al., eds. *Hemostasis and thrombosis: basic principles and clinical practice.* Philadelphia: JB Lippincott, 1987:358–379.
71. Collen D, Lijnen HR. Molecular and cellular basis of fibrinolysis. In: Hoffman R, Benz EJ Jr, Shattil SJ, et al., eds. *Hematology: basic principles and practice.* New York: Churchill Livingstone, 1991:1232–1242.
72. Badimon L, Badimon JJ, Galvez A, et al. Influence of arterial damage and wall shear rate on platelet deposition. *Ex vivo* study in swine model. *Arteriosclerosis* 1986;6:312–320.
73. Badimon L, Badimon JJ. Mechanism of arterial thrombosis in non-parallel streamlines: platelet grow at the apex of stenotic severely injured vessel wall. Experimental study in the pig model. *J Clin Invest* 1989;84:1134–1144.
74. Lassila R, Badimon JJ, Vallbhajosula S, et al. Dynamic monitoring of platelet deposition on severely damaged vessel wall in flowing blood. Effects of different stenosis on thrombus growth. *Arteriosclerosis* 1990;10:306–315.
75. Drake TA, Morrissey JH, Edgington TS. Selective cellular expression

of tissue factor in human tissues: implication of hemostasis and thrombosis. *Am J Pathol* 1989;134:1087–1097.

76. Wilcox JN, Smith SM, Schwartz SM, et al. Localization of tissue factor in the normal vessel wall and atherosclerotic plaque. *Proc Natl Acad Sci USA* 1989;86:2839–2843.

77. Fuster V, Chesebro JH. Mechanisms of unstable angina. *N Engl J Med* 1986;315:1023–1025.

78. Fernández-Ortiz A, Badimon JJ, Falk E, et al. Characterization of the relative thrombogenicity of atherosclerotic plaque components: implications for consequences of plaque rupture. *J Am Coll Cardiol* 1994;23:1562–1569.

79. Toschi V, Gallo R, Lettino M, et al. Tissue factor modulates the thrombogenicity of human atherosclerotic plaques. *Circulation* 1997;95:594–599.

80. Badimon JJ, Lettino M, Toschi V, et al. Local inhibition of tissue factor reduces the thrombogenicity of disrupted human atherosclerotic plaques. Effects of TFPI on plaque thrombogenicity under flow conditions. *Circulation* 1999;99:1780–1787.

81. Sánchez-Gómez S, Casani L, Vilahur G, et al. FFR-rFVIIa inhibits thrombosis triggered by ruptured and eroded vessel wall. *Thromb Haemost* 2001;OC999 (abst).

82. Badimon JJ, Fernández-Ortiz A, Meyer B, et al. Different response to balloon angioplasty of carotid and coronary arteries: effects on acute platelet deposition and intimal thickening. *Atherosclerosis* 1998;140:307–314.

83. Van de Werf F, Arnold AE, and the European Cooperative Study Group for Recombinant Tissue-Type Plasminogen Activator (rt-PA). Effect of intravenous tissue plasminogen activator on infarct size, left ventricular function and survival in patients with acute myocardial infarction. *Br Med J* 1988;297:374–379.

84. Van Lierde J, De Geest H, Verstraete M, et al. Angiographic assessment of the infarct-related residual coronary stenosis after spontaneous or therapeutic thrombolysis. *J Am Coll Cardiol* 1990;16:1545–1549.

85. Fuster V, Stein B, Badimon L, et al. Atherosclerotic plaque rupture and thrombosis: evolving concepts. *Circulation* 1990;82[Suppl II]:47–59.

86. Davies SW, Marchant B, Lyon JP, et al. Coronary lesion morphology in acute myocardial infarction: demonstration of early remodeling after streptokinase treatment. *J Am Coll Cardiol* 1990;16:1079–1086.

87. Badimon L, Badimon JJ, Lasilla R, et al. Thrombin inhibition by hirudin decreases platelet thrombus growth on areas of severe vessel wall injury. *J Am Coll Cardiol* 1989;13:145A.

88. Waller BF, Rothbaum DA, Pinkerton CA, et al. Status of the myocardium and infarct-related coronary artery in 19 necropsy patients with acute recanalization using pharmacologic (streptokinase, r-tissue plasminogen activator), mechanical (percutaneous transluminal coronary angioplasty) or combined types of reperfusion therapy. *J Am Coll Cardiol* 1987;9:785–801.

89. Meyer BJ, Badimon JJ, Mailhac A, et al. Inhibition of growth of thrombus on fresh mural thrombus: targeting optimal therapy. *Circulation* 1994;90:2432–2438.

90. Meyer B, Badimon JJ, Chesebro JH, et al. Dissolution of mural thrombus by specific thrombin inhibition with r-hirudin: comparison with Heparin and Aspirin. *Circulation* 1998;97:681–685.

91. Badimon L, Meyer BJ, Badimon JJ. Thrombin in arterial thrombosis. *Haemostasis* 1994;24:69–80.

92. Graham DJ, Alexander JJ. The effects of thrombin on bovine aortic endothelial and smooth muscle cells. *J Vasc Surg* 1990;11:307–313.

93. Nelken NA, Soifer SJ, O'Keefe J, et al. Thrombin receptor expression in normal and atherosclerotic human arteries. *J Clin Invest* 1992;90:1614–1621.

94. Hedin U, Frebelius S, Sanchez J, et al. Antithrombin III inhibits thrombin-induced proliferation in human arterial smooth muscle cells. *Arterioscler Thromb* 1994;14:254–260.

95. Varela O, Martínez-González J, Badimon L. Smooth muscle cells response to alpha-thrombin depends on its arterial origin: comparison among different species. *Eur J Clin Invest* 1998;28:313–323.

96. Sarembock IJ, Gertz SD, Gimple LW, et al. Effectiveness of recombinant desulphatohirudin in reducing restenosis after balloon angioplasty of atherosclerotic femoral arteries in rabbits. *Circulation* 1991;84:232–243.

97. Martinez-Gonzalez J, Rius J, Castello A, et al. Neuron-derived orphan receptor-1 (NOR-1) modulates vascular smooth muscle cell proliferation. *Circ Res* 2003;92:96–103.

CHAPTER 42

Coronary Spasm and Atherothrombosis

Thomas F. Lüscher, Georg Noll, Lukas Spieker, Roberto Corti, and Carl J. Pepine

Key Words: Atherothrombosis; coronary spasm; endothelium; vascular smooth muscle; vasomotion; vasospasm.

In 1959, Prinzmetal and colleagues (1,2) described a new syndrome consisting of chest pain that developed at rest and often occurred in the early morning hours. The pain was associated with ST-segment elevations in the electrocardiogram (ECG) and was relieved by nitroglycerin. They named the syndrome "variant angina" and suggested that it was caused by a spasm of a major epicardial coronary artery.

Subsequently, coronary spasm has been documented angiographically in most patients with variant angina (3–7). In addition, coronary constriction has been recognized as an important factor in the pathogenesis of many other ischemia-related coronary syndromes (8,9). Although the phenomenon has been well characterized clinically and angiographically, the cause of coronary spasm remains enigmatic. Moreover, it even appears uncertain whether all increases in coronary vascular tone occurring in acute ischemic syndromes can be explained by a single factor or rather represent a heterogeneous entity ranging from normal coronary vasomotion in a narrowed vascular segment to "true spasm" with total or near-total occlusion of an angiographically normal or mildly atherothrombotic coronary artery (8).

In patients with variant angina, vasospasm is often, but not always, a localized phenomenon that repeatedly affects the same coronary vascular segment either spontaneously or after provocation (Fig. 42–1). Thus, a local dysfunction of the blood vessel wall at the site of spasm must be involved. Accordingly, alterations of local neurogenic control, vascular smooth muscle function, the endothelium, or even blood cells have been implicated. Sometimes, however, spasm may affect multiple sites in the same or different arteries, diffuse sites, or even migrate from site to site. These cases are difficult to explain by a local dysfunction theory.

CORONARY VASOMOTION AND VASOSPASM

Coronary arteries are able to contract and relax through various mechanisms. Normally, even *in vitro* coronary arteries exhibit spontaneous tone—that is, the vascular smooth muscle is contracted to some degree, a phenomenon that can be demonstrated by application of vasodilators. Constriction therefore is a normal phenomenon in the coronary circulation and is not necessarily pathologic (Fig. 42–2). Under certain disease conditions, however, vasoconstriction becomes dominant and may contribute to symptoms such as angina pectoris. The degree of vasoconstriction occurring

    T. F. Lüscher: Division of Cardiology, Ramistrasse 100, 8091 Zurich, Switzerland.
    G. Noll: Cardiology, Ramistrasse 100, 8091 Zurich, Switzerland.
    L. Spieker: Cardiology, Ramistrasse 100, 8091 Zurich, Switzerland.
    R. Corti: Cardiology, Ramistrasse 100, 8091 Zurich, Switzerland.
    C. J. Pepine: Division of Cardiovascular Medicine, University of Florida, Box 100277, 1600 Archer Road, Gainesville, Florida 32610.

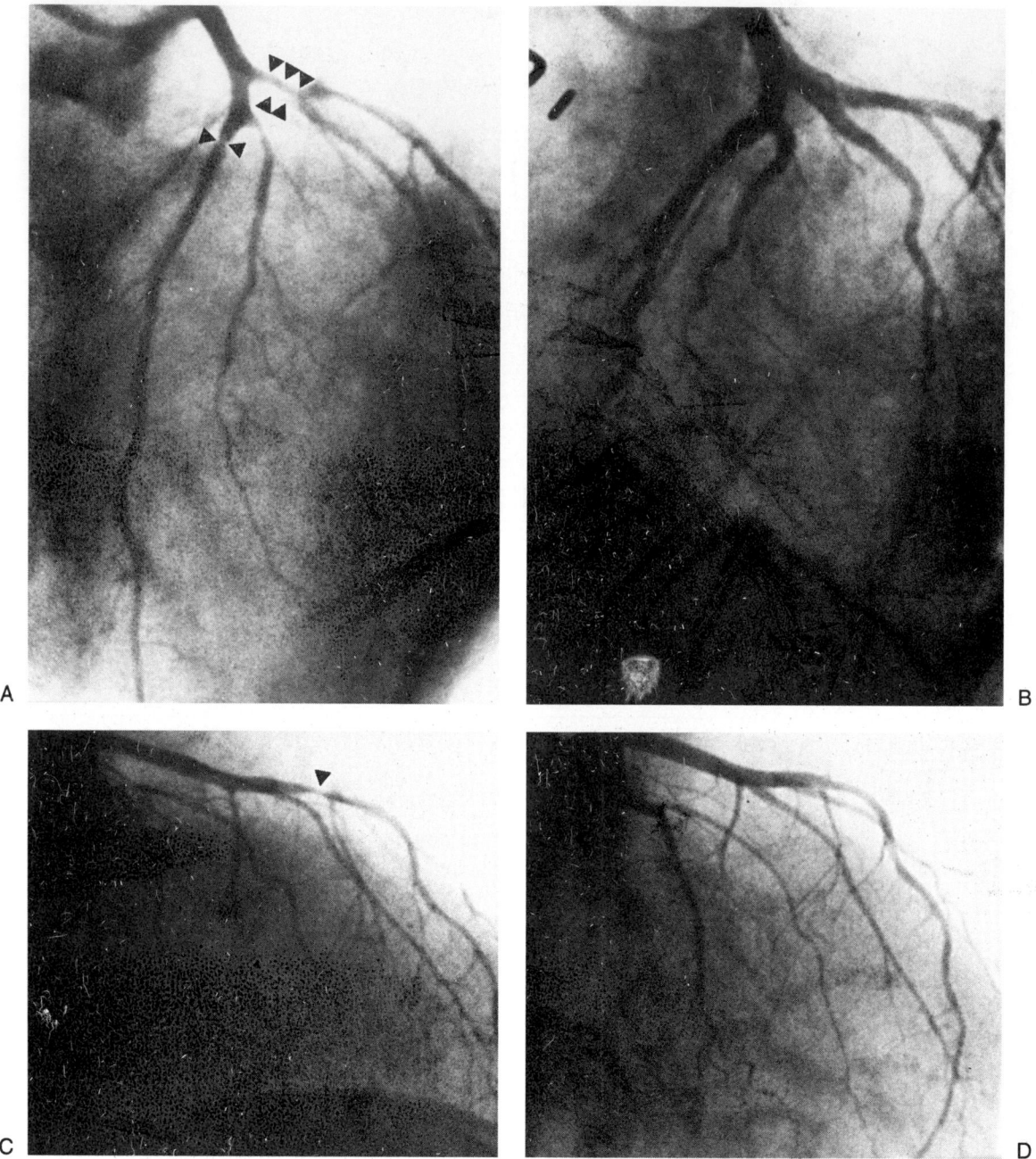

FIG. 42–1. Examples of coronary spasm. **Top row:** Multivessel spasm. **A:** Spontaneously occurring spasm involving the proximal left anterior descending (single pair of *arrowheads*), first diagonal branch *(double arrowheads),* and second diagonal branch (no arrows), as well as the proximal portion of the left circumflex artery *(triple arrowheads).* **B:** Resolution of spasm at these sites after intracoronary nitroglycerin. **Bottom row:** Single-vessel spasm. **C:** Ergonovine-induced spasm localized to a single site in the midleft anterior descending artery *(arrow).* **D:** Resolution after nitroglycerin.

under these conditions may differ considerably in different syndromes and in different patients. In certain patients, coronary constriction may be only slightly increased, and hence may not bother the patient under resting conditions, but it may alter the threshold for angina during exercise. As most coronary lesions are eccentric (10), diseased segments are able to relax and constrict to various stimuli. On the other end of this spectrum are patients in whom coronary constriction is so severe that angina occurs even under resting conditions. Under these conditions, a near-total or total occlusion of the coronary artery can be demonstrated angiographically (Fig. 42–1).

Some authors have restricted the expression "coronary spasm" to total occlusion of a coronary artery. However,

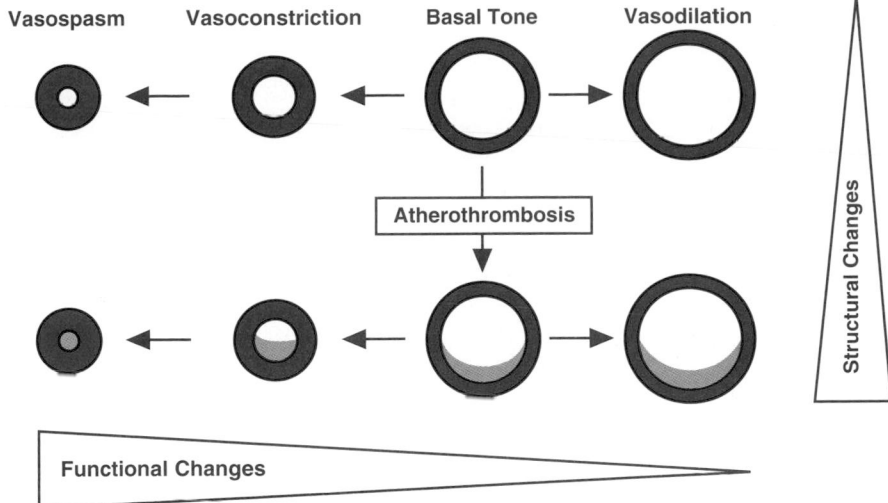

FIG. 42–2. Role of structural and functional changes of the coronary artery as determinant of coronary obstruction. Coronary diameter can change as a result of vasoconstriction and vasodilation of normal **(upper line)** and atherothrombotic vessel **(lower line).** "True" coronary spasm is the extreme of the responses.

more recent studies clearly suggest that increased constriction contributes to a large variety of coronary syndromes (although total occlusion occurs less commonly [11,12]) and that the difference between hyperconstriction and true coronary spasm is gradual. At this time, there is no definitive evidence for different pathogenetic mechanisms.

CONTROL OF CORONARY VASCULAR TONE

The coronary circulation is regulated by endothelial mediators, neurotransmitters, and the response of vascular smooth muscle cells to these agents (see Lüscher and Vanhoutte [13]). The contribution of each mechanism to coronary vascular tone differs in large epicardial and intramyocardial coronary arteries. Also, the contribution of certain mediators and the expression of receptors may differ in the coronary circulation as compared with other parts of the body.

Endothelial Mediators

Nitric Oxide

Endothelium-dependent relaxations occur *in vitro* and *in vivo;* neurotransmitters, hormones, and substances derived from platelets and the coagulation system can elicit these responses (Fig. 42–3) (13–19). Furthermore, mechanical factors such as shear stress induce endothelium-dependent vasodilation (20,21). The relaxations are mediated by a diffusible substance with a half-life of a few seconds (15,22), the so-called endothelium-derived relaxing factor (15), which has been identified as nitric oxide (NO) (23–25).

Endothelium-derived nitric oxide (EDNO) is formed from L-arginine by oxidation of its guanidine nitrogen termi-

nal by the enzyme NO synthase (26,27). Several isoforms of the enzyme have been described, occurring not only in endothelial cells but also in platelets (28), macrophages (29), vascular smooth muscle cells (30–32), and the brain (33). In addition, an inducible enzyme exists in vascular smooth muscle, endothelium, and macrophages. The enzyme is induced by cytokines such as endotoxin, interleukin (IL)-1β, and tumor necrosis factor, and hence may be activated in inflammatory processes and endotoxin shock.

Endothelium-dependent relaxations are inhibited by analogs of L-arginine such as L-N^G-monomethyl arginine (L-NMMA) and are restored by L- but not D-arginine (Fig. 42–4) (34). In quiescent arteries, L-NMMA causes endothelium-dependent contractions (35,36). In intact organs, inhibition of NO formation by L-arginine methyl ester (L-NAME) markedly decreases local blood flow (37). In humans, local infusion of L-NMMA into the brachial artery induces an increase in forearm vascular resistance. When infused intravenously, L-NMMA induces long-lasting increases in blood pressure that are reversed by L-arginine (38). The vasculature thus is in a constant state of dilation as a result of continuous basal endothelial release of NO.

Of particular interest is the endogenous inhibitor of the L-arginine NO pathway, asymmetric dimethylarginine (39). An increased production or elimination, or both, of this both locally and systemically acting endogenous inhibitor could profoundly affect the function of the cardiovascular system, for instance, in patients with renal failure (39).

EDNO leads to an increase in cyclic 3′,5′-guanosine monophosphate (cGMP) in vascular smooth muscle cells and platelets through activation of soluble guanylate cyclase (40). Methylene blue, an inhibitor of this enzyme, prevents production of cGMP and inhibits endothelium-dependent relaxations (13).

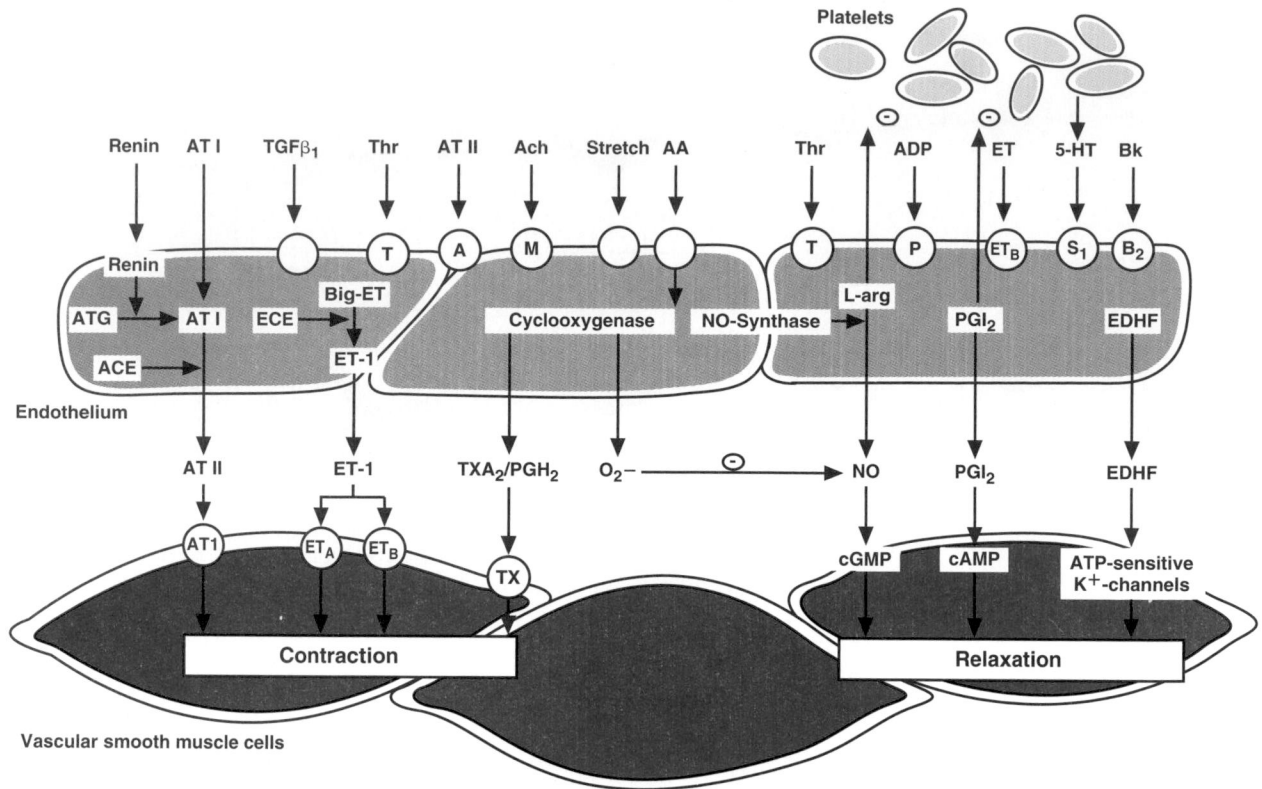

FIG. 42–3. Endothelium-derived vasoactive substances. The endothelium is a source of relaxing **(right)** and contracting factors **(left)**. AA, arachidonic acid; ACE, angiotensin converting enzyme; Ach, acetylcholine; ADP, adenosine diphosphate; AT, angiotensin; ATG, angiotensinogen; ATP, adenosine triphosphate; Bk, bradykinin; cAMP/cGMP, cyclic adenosine/guanosine monophosphate; ECE, endothelin-converting enzyme; EDHF, endothelium-derived hyperpolarizing factor; 5-HT, 5-hydroxytryptamine (serotonin); ET, endothelin; L-arg, L-arginine; NO, nitric oxide; O_2^-, superoxide radical; PGH$_2$, prostacyclin H$_2$; PGI$_2$, prostacyclin; TGFβ$_1$, transforming growth factor-β$_1$; Thr, thrombin; TXA$_2$, thromboxane A$_2$. *Circles* represent receptors. (Modified from Lüscher TF, Boulanger CM, Dohi Y, et al. Endothelium-derived contracting factors. *Hypertension* 1992;19:117–130, by permission of the American Heart Association.)

In platelets, an increase of intracellular cGMP is associated with reduced adhesion and aggregation. Therefore, EDNO causes both vasodilatation and platelet deactivation, thereby representing an important antithrombotic feature of the endothelium. Most interestingly, platelets release substances such as adenosine diphosphate and triphosphate and serotonin, which activate the release of NO and prostacyclin from the endothelium (Fig. 42–5) (16,18,41). Furthermore, thrombin, the major enzyme of the coagulation cascade, stimulates the formation of NO and prostacyclin by the endothelium of human arteries (17,42). Hence, at sites where platelets and the coagulation cascade are activated, intact endothelial cells, in turn, cause vasodilation and platelet inhibition, thereby preventing vasoconstriction and thrombus formation.

Vasodilator Prostaglandins

Prostacyclin is the major product of vascular cyclooxygenase (43). It is formed primarily in the intima but also in the media and adventitia in response to shear stress, hypoxia,

and several mediators that also lead to the formation of EDNO. In most blood vessels, the contribution of prostacyclin to endothelium-dependent relaxations is negligible (18,34). Prostacyclin increases cyclic 3′,5′-adenosine monophosphate (cAMP) in smooth muscle and platelets (44), where it inhibits platelet aggregation (Fig. 42–3). In human platelets, EDNO and prostacyclin synergistically inhibit aggregation (45).

Endothelium-derived Hyperpolarizing Factor

EDNO cannot explain all endothelium-dependent responses (13,46). In the porcine coronary artery, endothelium-dependent relaxations to serotonin are inhibited by L-NMMA, hemoglobin, or methylene blue, but the response to bradykinin is only partially affected by the inhibitors of the L-arginine pathways (Fig. 42–6) (34,35). Relaxations resistant to inhibitors of the NO pathway are even more prominent in intramyocardial vessels (35). In the canine coronary and mesenteric artery, acetylcholine causes endothelium-depen-

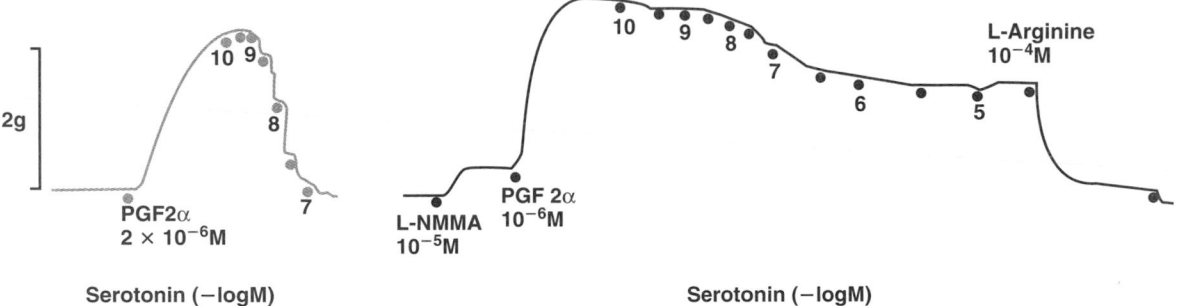

FIG. 42–4. Responses of isolated porcine coronary artery to serotonin (5-hydroxytryptamine [5-HT]) under control conditions **(left)** and after inhibition of nitric oxide formation by L-N^G-monomethyl arginine (L-NMMA; **right**). (Data from Richard V, Tanner FC, Tschudi M, et al. Different activation of L-arginine pathway by bradykinin, serotonin, and clonidine in coronary arteries. *Am J Physiol* 1990;259:H1433–H1439, with permission).

dent hyperpolarization, an effect not shared by NO (47–49); although under certain conditions NO may also hyperpolarize cells (50–52). Hence, an endothelium-dependent hyperpolarizing factor of unknown chemical structure has been proposed (Fig. 42–3) (13,46,53).

Endothelins

Among the peptides endothelin-1, 2, and 3, endothelial cells appear to produce exclusively the 21–amino acid peptide endothelin-1 (54–56). Preproendothelin is converted to big en-

dothelin (54); its conversion to endothelin-1 by the endothelin-converting enzyme is necessary for development of full vascular activity (54–56). The expression of messenger RNA and release of the peptide is stimulated by thrombin, transforming growth factor β_1, IL-1, epinephrine, angiotensin II, arginine vasopressin, calcium ionophore, and phorbol ester (Fig. 42–7) (55–59).

Endothelin-1 is a potent vasoconstrictor (54,60–63). Endothelin causes dilation at smaller and marked contractions at greater concentrations (Fig. 42–8) (37,62,64,65). Small vessels, where local blood flow is regulated, are particularly

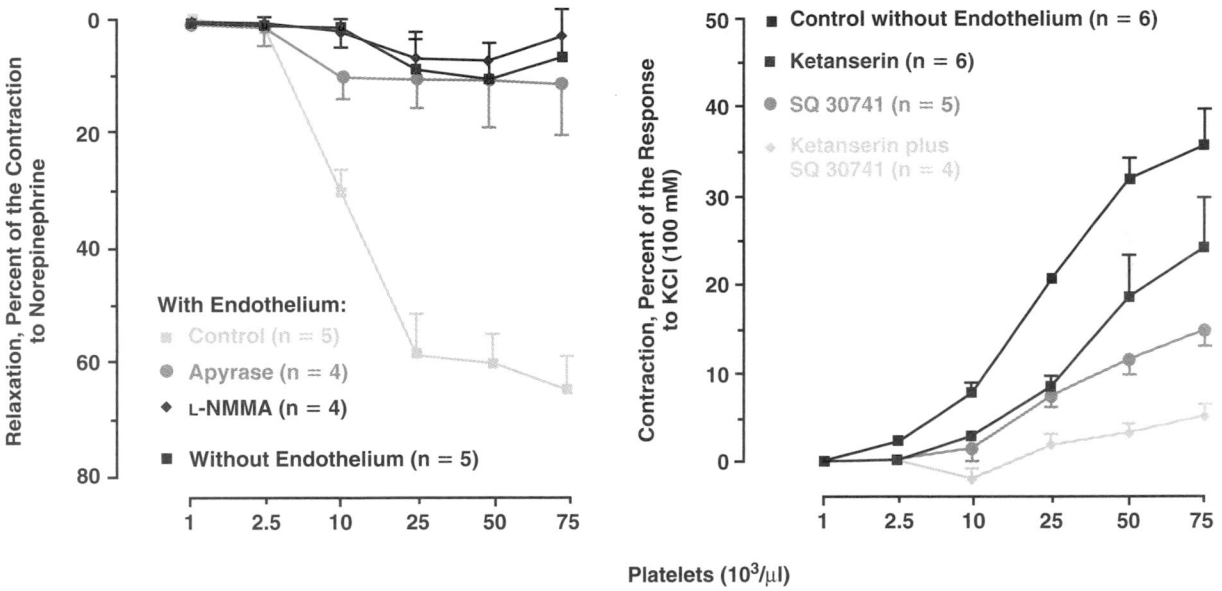

FIG. 42–5. Effects of aggregating platelets in human internal mammary artery. In vessels contracted with norepinephrine **(left)**, aggregating platelets cause endothelium-dependent relaxations that are prevented by L-N^G-monomethyl arginine (L-NMMA; an inhibitor of nitric formation) or apyrase (an enzyme that breaks down adenosine triphosphate/diphosphate). In quiescent preparations without endothelium **(right)**, platelets cause only contractions that are reduced by ketanserin (an antagonist of 5-hydroxytryptamine [serotonin] type 2 [5-HT$_2$] receptor) or SQ30741 (a thromboxane receptor antagonist). (Modified from Yang ZH, Stulz P, von Segesser L, et al. Different interactions of platelets with arterial and venous coronary bypass vessels. *Lancet* 1991;337:939–943, with permission.)

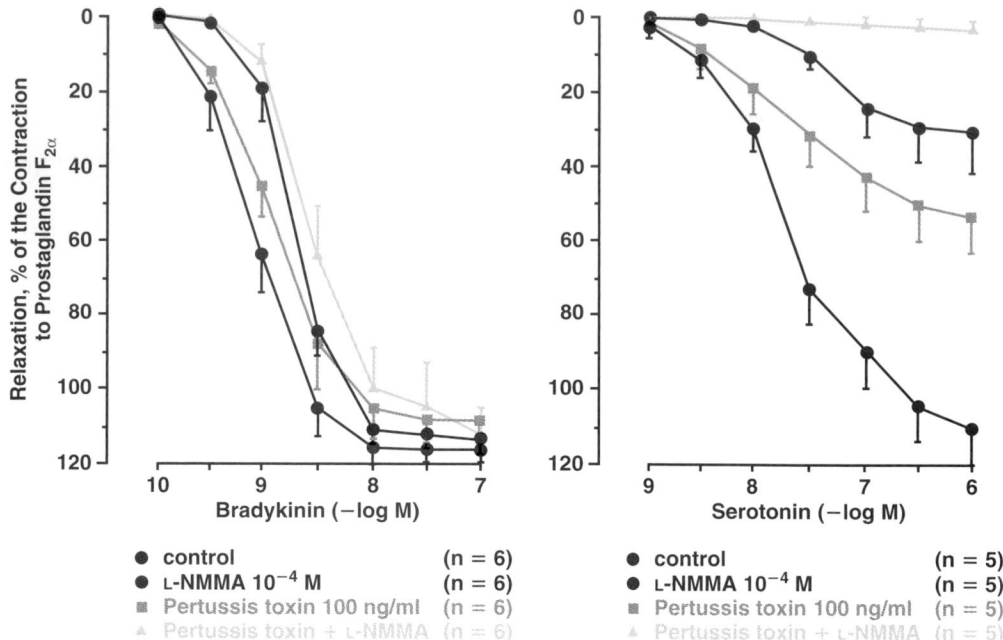

FIG. 42–6. Endothelium-dependent relaxations to bradykinin in porcine coronary arteries. Bradykinin causes relaxations that are only minimally inhibited by the inhibitor of nitric oxide formation L-N^G-monomethyl arginine (L-NMMA; **right**) and by inactivation of G$_i$ proteins by pertussis toxin. In contrast, serotonin (5-hydroxytryptamine [5-HT]) is sensitive to both interventions. (From Richard V, Tanner FC, Tschudi M, et al. Different activation of L-arginine pathway by bradykinin, serotonin, and clonidine in coronary arteries. *Am J Physiol* 1990;259:H1433–H1439, with permission.)

sensitive to the vasoconstrictor effects of endothelin-1 (35,63,66).

Circulating levels of endothelin-1 are very low, suggesting that little of the peptide is formed under physiologic conditions (56,67,68). Indeed, three inhibitory mechanisms regulating endothelin production have been delineated: (a) cGMP-dependent inhibition mediated by EDNO, nitroglycerin, linsidomine, and atrial natriuretic peptide (13,57,58,69,70); (b) cAMP-dependent inhibition (70), and (c) an inhibitory factor produced by vascular smooth muscle cells (67). Endothelin can also release NO and prostacyclin from endothelial cells, which may represent a negative feedback mechanism (60,68). Indeed, the contractions to the peptide are enhanced after endothelial removal, indicating that basal production of EDNO reduces its response (13). Stimulation of the formation of EDNO by acetylcholine reverses endothelin-induced contractions in most blood vessels (13,71).

Two distinct endothelin receptors have been cloned: the ET$_A$ and ET$_B$ receptor (Fig. 42–9) (72,73). Endothelial cells express ET$_B$ receptors linked to the formation of NO (68) and prostacyclin (60) explaining the transient vasodilator effects of endothelin. In vascular smooth muscle, ET$_A$ and in part ET$_B$ receptors are mediating contraction and proliferation (74). Both specific ET$_A$ receptor antagonists, as well as combined ET$_A$ and ET$_B$ receptor antagonists, have been developed (37,74–78). These antagonists induce vasodilation indicating that endothelin contributes to blood pressure regulation (75,77–79).

Vasoconstrictor Prostaglandins

Exogenous arachidonic acid evokes endothelium-dependent contractions prevented by indomethacin (an inhibitor of cyclooxygenase) (Fig. 42–3) (19,36,80). The products of cyclooxygenase mediating the contractions are thromboxane A$_2$ in the case of acetylcholine and endoperoxides (prostaglandin H$_2$) in that of histamine (36). Thromboxane A$_2$ and endoperoxide activate both vascular smooth muscle and platelets, and hence counteract effects of NO and prostacyclin.

Furthermore, the cyclooxygenase pathway is a source of superoxide anions breaking down NO. Superoxide anions also provoke direct vasoconstriction (81,82). Thus, the cyclooxygenase pathway produces a variety of endothelium-derived contracting factors (Fig. 42–3) (13).

Vascular Smooth Muscle

Vascular smooth muscle cells regulate vascular tone reacting to circulating hormones, endothelial mediators, and neurotransmitters released from nerve endings, as well as substances released from circulating blood cells such as platelets, leukocytes, and monocytes. The response to such mediators usually involves binding to surface receptors, activation of signal transduction mechanisms, and increases in second messengers, which regulate the intracellular concentration of calcium. Calcium is a crucial ion regulating contractility of vascular smooth muscle cells (83).

0 1 2 3 4 hours

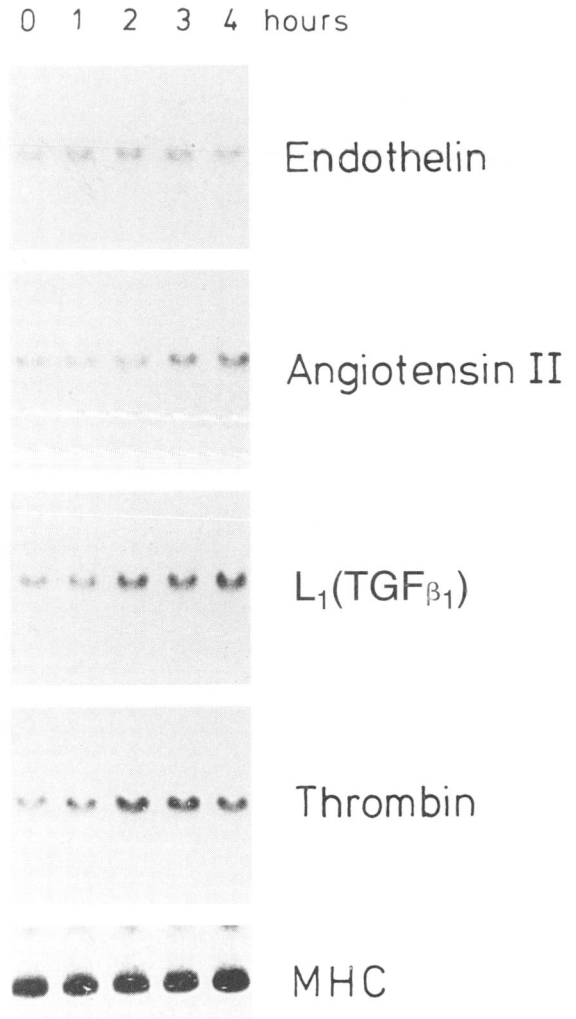

Endothelin

Angiotensin II

$L_1(TGF\beta_1)$

Thrombin

MHC

FIG. 42–7. Expression of endothelin messenger RNA in porcine aortic endothelial cells in culture after exposure to either endothelin, angiotensin II, transforming growth factor L_1 (TGFβ_1), or thrombin. MHC, major histocompatibility complex. (From Lüscher TF, Oemar BS, Boulanger CM, et al. Molecular and cellular biology of endothelin and its receptors—Part I. *J Hypertens* 1993;11:7–11, with permission.)

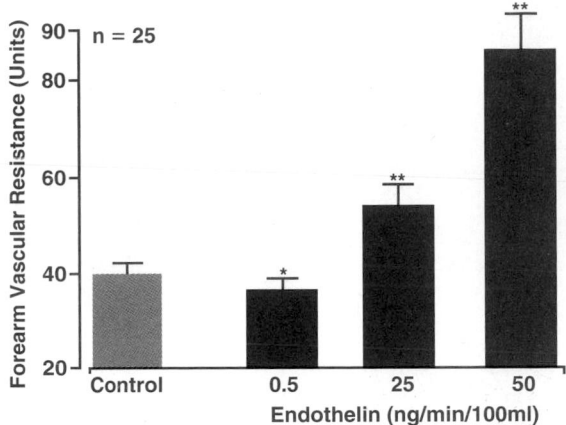

FIG. 42–8. Effects of intraarterial infusion of endothelin-1 on the forearm circulation of healthy human subjects. Endothelin causes a small decrease, followed by marked increases, in forearm vascular resistance. (Modified from Kiowski W, Lüscher TF, Linder L, et al. Endothelin-1-induced vasoconstriction in humans. Reversal by calcium channel blockade but not by nitrovasodilators or endothelium-derived relaxing factor. *Circulation* 1991;83:469–475, by permission of the American Heart Association.)

Sympathetic Activation

Sympathetic outflow to the resistance vessels is of utmost importance for determination of the level of vascular resistance and, in turn, local blood flow (14,84–88). Sympathetic outflow to blood vessel originates in neurons located in the lateral parts of the reticular formation of the brainstem—that is, the vasomotor center (14). Activity of the center is governed by baroreceptors (14,89) through the solitary nucleus tract. Neurons of the vasomotor center descend to the preganglionic neurons of the spinal cord. Outflow to the periphery is determined by interplay between pressor and depressor neurons (90). In the sympathetic ganglia, cholinergic preganglionic neurons interconnect with adrenergic post-

ganglionic neurons innervating the heart and the peripheral blood vessels (Fig. 42–10) (87,88). All mature blood vessels are innervated by postganglionic sympathetic nerves. The density of adrenergic innervation of blood vessels decreases progressively with age, whereas sympathetic activity of neurons increases with age (84,85,87,88,91).

Receptors

Most agonists derived from nerve endings, the circulating blood, platelets, or the endothelium (except NO; discussed earlier) exert their action in vascular smooth muscle by activating specific receptors (Fig. 42–10) (83). Important contractile receptors include α_1- and α_2-adrenergic receptors, 5-hydroxytryptamine-1 (5-HT$_1$)– and 5-HT$_2$–serotonergic receptors (92,93), thromboxane receptors (both activated after release of the mediators from aggregating platelets), ET$_A$ and ET$_B$ receptors, angiotensin type 1 (AT-1) receptors (94), and V$_1$ vasopressin receptors (95).

The most important neurotransmitter mediating effects of sympathetic neurons in the blood vessel wall is norepinephrine, but adenosine triphosphate and neuropeptide Y also can contribute under certain conditions (Fig. 42–10) (14,96). The release of adrenergic neurotransmitters is facilitated by epinephrine and angiotensin II, but it is inhibited by norepinephrine itself (through prejunctional α_2-adrenergic receptors), acetylcholine, 5-HT, histamine, purines, and prostanoids (14). Released norepinephrine interacts with postjunctional α_1- and α_2-adrenergic receptors.

Certain receptors on vascular smooth muscle, however, mediate vascular relaxation (e.g., 5-HT$_1$–serotonergic or prostacyclin receptors) (34,35,97,98). Epinephrine can acti-

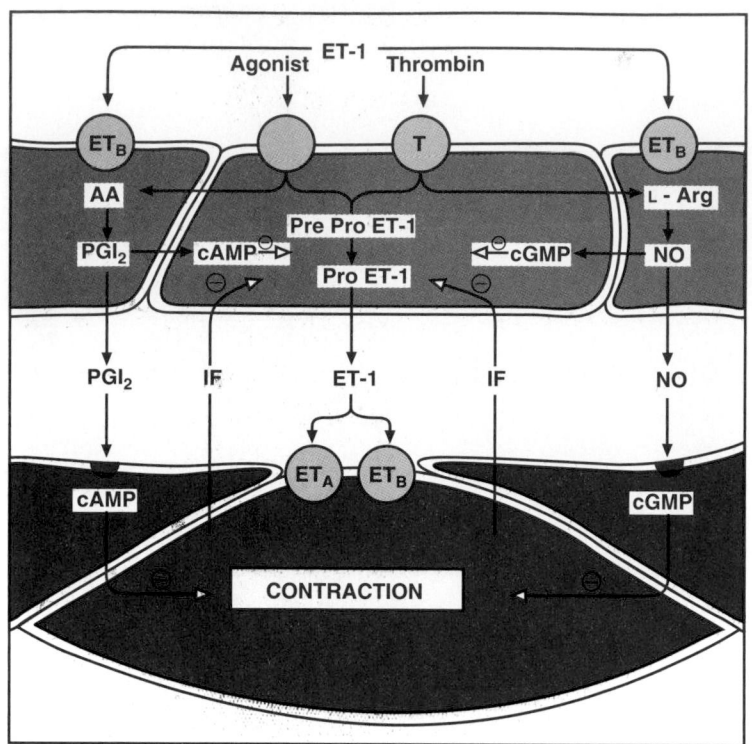

FIG. 42–9. Regulation of vascular endothelin (ET) production. Endothelin is formed from prepro-ET and big-ET through the endothelin-converting enzymes (ECEs) and activates specific receptors *(circles)*. The ET production is stimulated by thrombin (Thr) and many other receptor *(circles)* agonists. Its production is inhibited by nitric oxide (NO) formed from L-arginine (L-Arg), possibly by prostacyclin (PGI₂) and a putative inhibitory factor (IF) produced by vascular smooth muscle cells. AA, arachidonic acid; cAMP, cyclic adenosine monophosphate; cGMP, cyclic guanosine monophosphate. (Modified from Lüscher TF, Boulanger CM, Dohi Y, et al. Endothelium-derived contracting factors. *Hypertension* 1992;19:117–130, by permission of the American Heart Association.)

vate α_2-adrenergic receptors mediating relaxation of epicardial coronary arteries. As judged from the canine coronary circulation, α_2-adrenergic receptors are particularly important in proximal epicardial arteries, whereas the expression of α_1- and α_2-adrenergic receptors is sparse, except in distal segments of the coronary vascular tree (99). Normally, α-adrenergic stimulation (e.g., by psychological stress) provides flow-dependent release of vasodilating NO (100,101). Coronary spasm is usually localized to the proximal epicardial arteries.

We demonstrated that mental stress induces prolonged endothelial dysfunction, which is prevented by selective ET_A receptor antagonism (102), providing a novel and potential important link between mental stress and atherothrombotic vascular disease.

Signal Transduction Mechanisms

Activation of these receptors activates phospholipase C and, in turn, leads to formation of inositol triphosphate (IP_3) and diacylglycerol (DAG) (83,103). Whereas IP_3 releases intracellular calcium from sarcoplasmatic reticulum, DAG activates protein kinase C. Both events allow development of

contraction. Activation of sympathetic nerves leads to release not only of norepinephrine but also of adenosine triphosphate and neuropeptide Y (Fig. 42–10) (14,96). The latter potentiates the effects of norepinephrine (96). Similarly, endothelin-1 is able to potentiate contractions to serotonin in human coronary arteries (104).

Voltage-operated Calcium Channels

Voltage-operated calcium channels also importantly regulate vascular tone (83). These channels are activated with changes in membrane potential and allow extracellular calcium to enter the vascular smooth muscle cell. The channels are blocked by calcium antagonists of the dihydropyridine (e.g., nifedipine, amlodipine), phenylalkalanine (e.g., verapamil, mibefradil), or benzothiodiazepine type (e.g., diltiazem) (105). Certain receptors—for instance, endothelin receptors on vascular smooth muscle—are linked through a G_i protein to the channel, and thereby can increase influx of extracellular calcium into the cell (106). Thus, endothelin-induced contractions are reduced by calcium antagonists (107), particularly in smaller arteries (66,108).

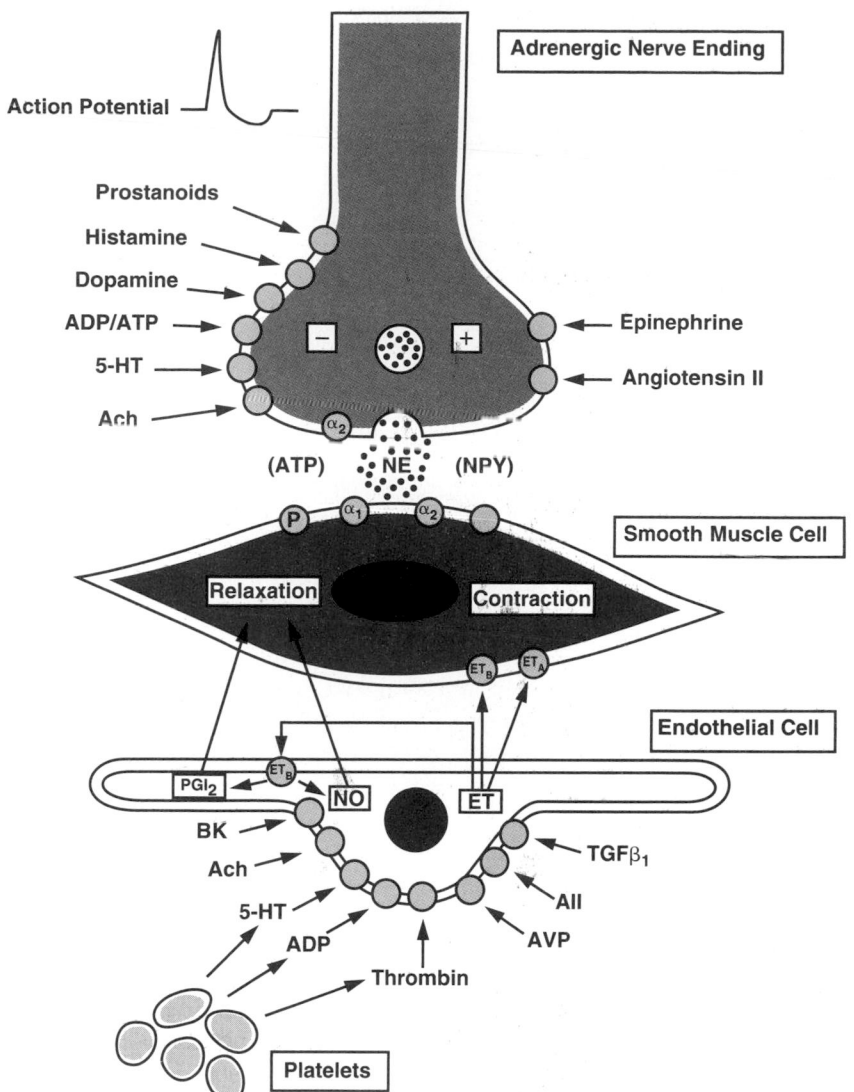

FIG. 42–10. Regulation of tone of vascular smooth muscle cells by adrenergic nerves and circulating and local factors. AII, angiotensin II; Ach, acetylcholine; ADP/ATP, adenosine diphosphate/triphosphate; AVP, arginine vasopressin; Bk, bradykinin; 5-HT, 5-hydroxytryptamine (serotonin); ET, endothelin; NO, nitric oxide; NPY, neuropeptide Y; P, purinergic receptor; PGI$_2$, prostacyclin; TGFβ$_1$, transforming growth factor-β$_1$; Thr, thrombin. *Circles* represent receptors.

CLINICAL ASPECTS

Symptoms and Clinical Presentation

The clinical hallmark of coronary constriction, as well as structural atherothrombotic changes of the blood vessel wall, is angina pectoris, caused by myocardial ischemia. Anginal pain typically is perceived in the precordial part of the chest, although atypical locations such as the upper part of the abdomen and parts of the back also occur. Radiation of pain into the left shoulder and arm and less frequently into the right arm and jaws is typical for chest pain of cardiac origin. However, most cardiac ischemia occurring during life occurs in the absence of angina pectoris (i.e., silent ischemia) (109,110). Ischemia occurs when the coronary artery is not able to maintain an adequate blood supply to

functioning myocardium. Coronary obstruction is determined by coronary vascular tone and thrombus formation within the lumen (Fig. 42–2).

In variant angina, coronary constriction is the overwhelming mechanism (1–3). With severe coronary constriction, myocardial infarction (MI) may ensue even in regions supplied by arterial segments with no or minimal atherothrombotic changes (6). The ECG shows ST-segment elevations as a reflection of transmural ischemia. Imaging techniques such as echocardiography or angiography reveal wall motion abnormalities of the involved myocardial segment.

In patients with obstructing coronary atherothrombosis, the structural obstruction per se sets a level of maximal blood flow that limits exercise performance of these patients. However, coronary constriction also contributes importantly (111). The latter explains why the ischemia threshold (i.e., level of exercise above which angina or ischemia occurs) varies in the same patient on different occasions. Indeed, activation of the sympathetic nervous system by cold temperature or psychological stress can cause paradoxic coronary constriction in patients with diseased coronary arteries (112), resulting in symptoms with minimal or no exertion. Typically, in patients with obstructive coronary disease, angina occurs on exertion, and the ECG typically reveals ST-segment depression with relief of symptoms at rest. Reversible motion abnormalities in the involved myocardial segment are used diagnostically in stress echocardiography (113,114).

Trigger Mechanisms

Several substances have been used in the catheterization laboratory to trigger coronary constriction. Most commonly, acetylcholine, histamine, or ergonovine is infused into the coronary circulation, and changes in diameter of epicardial coronary arteries are measured at angiography (115).

In patients with variant angina, coronary spasm can be provoked during angiography by methacholine and acetylcholine (116). Many patients with coronary artery disease exhibit more or less pronounced coronary constriction after infusion of acetylcholine, whereas mild vasodilation is observed in healthy individuals (Fig. 42–11) (11). Some patients, however, exhibit constriction at one site and dilation at other sites (117). In contrast to most other blood vessels, the human coronary artery exhibits marked contractions to

acetylcholine after removal of the endothelium because of the presence of excitatory muscarinic receptors on vascular smooth muscle (15,17,118,119).

Alternatively, serotonin is used to evoke coronary constriction, as this substance is released from aggregating platelets, activating serotonergic and α-adrenergic receptors. It is able to elicit coronary spasm in a considerable number of patients with variant angina not responsive to other tests.

Intracoronary histamine administration leads to dilation in normal humans through endothelial H_1-histaminergic receptors linked to release of NO (118,120,121). On vascular smooth muscle, however, contractile H_2-histaminergic receptors exist. In one report, in about half of the patients with variant angina studied, spasm was provoked by histamine (115).

Natural Course and Prognosis

The natural progressing course of atherothrombotic coronary artery disease is determined by lesion progression (which involves lipid accumulation, macrophage invasion and migration, and proliferation of vascular smooth muscle cells) (122–124) and, in particular, plaque rupture, constriction, and thrombus formation leading to prolonged obstruction of a major epicardial coronary artery. Plaque rupture appears particularly common in lipid-rich lesions (125,126). Immunologic stimuli and physical forces (e.g., with strenuous exercise) may also destabilize existing plaques. Plaque rupture and coronary occlusion eventually leads to MI with loss of functioning myocardium. Pump failure and arrhythmia are common causes of death under these conditions. Clinically, major determinants of prognosis in patients with coronary artery disease are the extent of coronary artery disease and the degree of functional impairment of the left ventricle.

In patients with variant angina, prognosis may be somewhat more favorable than in those with atherothrombotic coronary artery disease. However, the natural history of coronary spasm is unknown. The clinical course of patients with objective evidence for transient myocardial ischemia (e.g., ST segment elevation) and angiographically documented coronary spasm is best described as highly variable. Periods of exacerbation of transient ischemia (with and without symptoms) and ischemia-related events alternate with remission of ischemia and related events, often without identifiable reason. Long-term data reveal that outcome in the patient with coronary spasm is highly dependent on the presence and severity of associated coronary atherothrombosis (127,128). Over 3 to 5 years, those with coronary spasm and relatively minimal coronary atherothrombosis are at low risk (approximately 5%) for development of death or nonfatal MI. Patients with coronary spasm who have only one artery showing a 70% or greater "fixed" atherothrombotic obstruction are at low to moderate risk. Those with severe multivessel obstructions are at relatively high (approximately 30%) risk for these events. MI occurs most

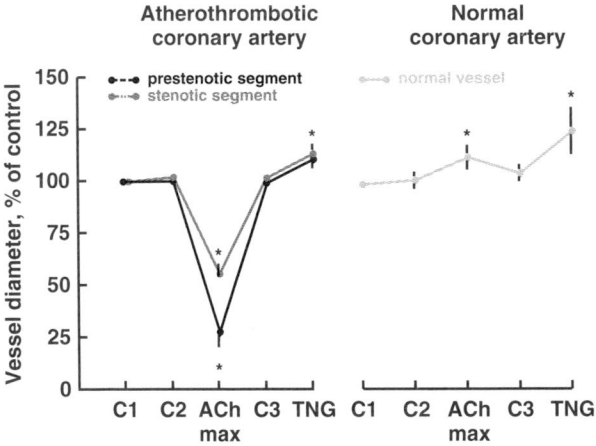

FIG. 42–11. Effects of intracoronary infusion of acetylcholine (ACh) on the arterial diameter of the left anterior descending coronary artery in healthy subjects and in patients with coronary artery disease. The response is expressed as percentage of the control arterial diameter. C1, C2, C3, control periods; *closed circles,* prestenotic or normal segments; *open circles,* stenotic segments; TNG, nitroglycerin. (Modified from Ludmer PL, Selwyn AP, Shook TL, et al. Paradoxical vasoconstriction induced by acetylcholine in atherosclerotic coronary arteries. *N Engl J Med* 1986;315:1046–1051, with permission.)

frequently shortly after the patient's initial presentation for rest angina and many times even before the diagnosis of coronary spasm has been given strong consideration. Patients with ventricular dysrhythmia during rest angina have approximately twice the risk for death as those without (129). Retrospective and prospective cohort studies suggest that calcium antagonists seem to have a beneficial effect on risk for adverse outcome events (127,128,130). Ischemia-related events may continue to occur, however, even when calcium antagonist therapy appears to control rest angina, and events tend to cluster in those with severe multivessel coronary disease (130,131).

MECHANISMS OF VASOSPASM

Although the cause of coronary spasm remains elusive, tremendous progress has been made in understanding local vascular mechanisms capable of causing coronary constriction. Most of these mechanisms involve dysfunction of mediators that are important in regulation of normal coronary vascular tone (discussed earlier).

Endothelium

The endothelium may be damaged by a wide variety of factors (e.g., hypertension, smoking, lipids) and even by intense smooth muscle contraction. As indicated earlier, alterations in the release or responsiveness, or both, of vascular smooth muscle to substances released by endothelial cells can profoundly affect contractile responses of coronary arteries (Fig. 42–3) (63). By definition, such endothelial dysfunction could involve local impairment in the release of relaxing factors or increased production of contracting factors by the endothelium. Furthermore, vascular smooth muscle cells may be hyperresponsive.

L-Arginine Pathway

In porcine coronary arteries, *in vivo* denudation of the endothelium with a balloon catheter is followed by a rapid regeneration of the endothelial layer within days (97). Also, endothelium-dependent relaxations to bradykinin, serotonin, and aggregating platelets recover at this point. However, 4 weeks after denudation (and lasting up to 5 months at least), the number of endothelial cells per given area is increased (Fig. 42–12) (97), and endothelium-dependent relaxations to serotonin, α_2-adrenergic agonists, and aggregating platelets are reduced (Fig. 42–13) (97). In contrast, endothelium-dependent relaxations to other agonists such as bradykinin, adenosine diphosphate, thrombin, platelet-activating factor, and the calcium ionophore A23187 are maintained. This indicates a very selective defect of certain receptor-operated mechanisms for release of NO in regenerated endothelial cells. Interestingly, this defect involves endothelial receptors that are sensitive to pertussis toxin (132), suggesting that in regenerated coronary endothelial cells,

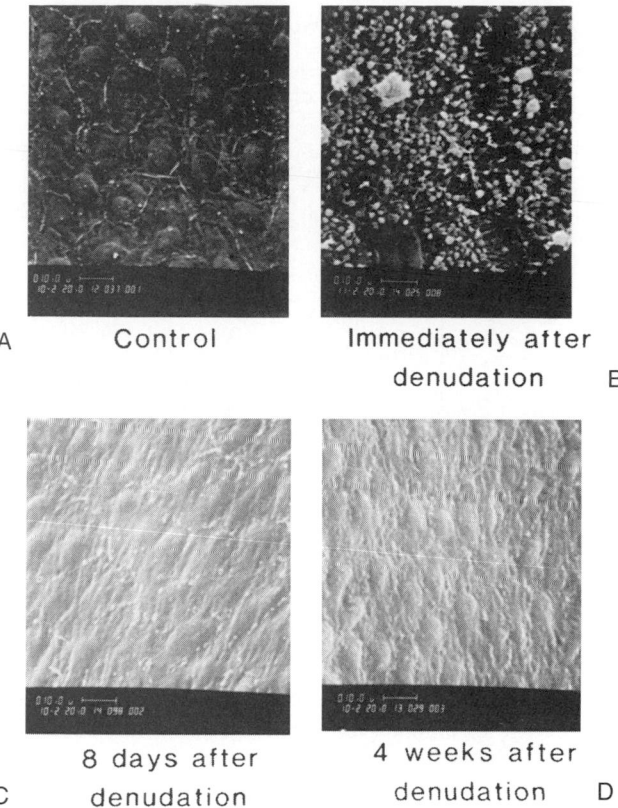

A   Control   Immediately after
                     denudation   B

8 days after   4 weeks after
C   denudation   denudation   D

FIG. 42–12. Scanning electron microscopy of porcine coronary arteries immediately **(B)**, 8 days **(C)**, and 4 weeks **(D)** after the endothelium had been removed *in vivo* with a balloon catheter. Note the adhesion of circulating blood cells in **B** and the increased number of endothelial cells in **D** as compared with **C**. (From Shimokawa H, Aarhus LL, Vanhoutte PM. Porcine coronary arteries with regenerated endothelium have a reduced endothelium-dependent responsiveness to aggregating platelets and serotonin. *Circ Res* 1987;61:256–270, by permission of the American Heart Association.)

expression or function of G_i proteins linked to 5-HT$_1$–serotonergic and α_2-adrenergic receptors is defective (133). More recent studies in the porcine coronary circulation demonstrated that ergonovine elicits similar responses as serotonin, and that regenerated endothelial cells also exhibit abnormal responses to this agonist (97,133,134). This is of particular interest because ergonovine is the most reliable substance to provoke vasospasm in patients with variant angina (115). Indeed, a loss of NO release from endothelium, with overwhelming effects on vascular smooth muscle contractile receptors, could explain the constrictor response to ergonovine in coronary segments prone to spasm, as well as rapid reversal by low doses of intracoronary nitrate. Structural changes at sites of mechanical endothelial denudation may also contribute. Indeed, myointimal thickening invariably occurs at sites of endothelial denudation (134). The increased muscle mass further increases vasoconstrictor responses.

In the pig, coronary spasm can be provoked with histamine several weeks after *in vivo* endothelial denudation in

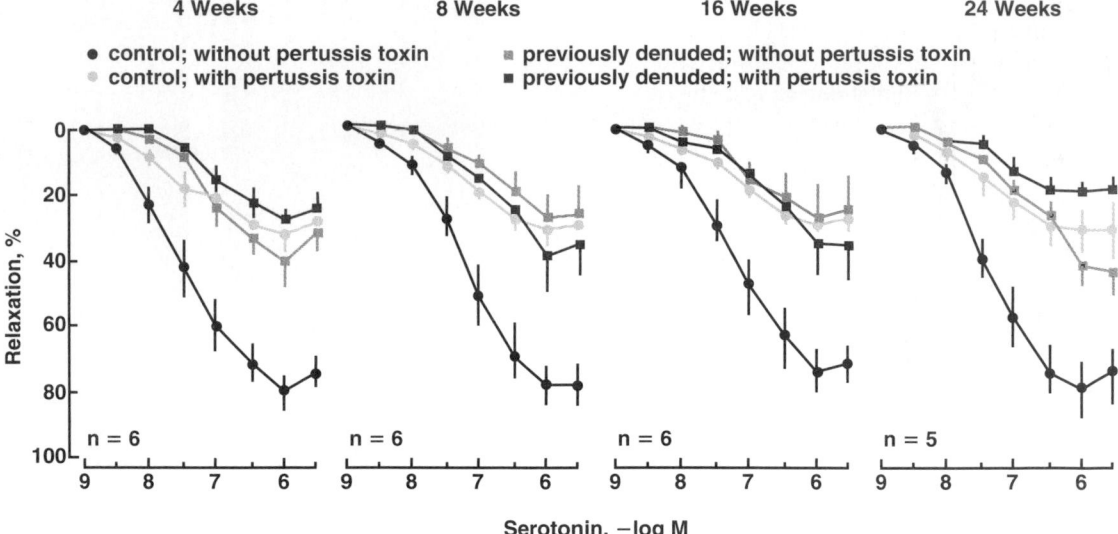

FIG. 42–13. Endothelium-dependent relaxations of porcine coronary arteries to serotonin in control preparations *(circles)* and arteries in which the endothelium had been previously denuded with a balloon catheter. The effect of pertussis toxin, an inhibitor of G_i proteins, also is shown. (From Shimokawa H, Flavahan NA, Vanhoutte PM. Natural course of the impairment of endothelium-dependent relaxations after balloon endothelium removal in porcine coronary arteries. Possible dysfunction of a pertussis toxin-sensitive G protein. *Circ Res* 1989;65:740–753, by permission of the American Heart Association.)

conjunction with an atherogenic diet (97). An increased number of adventitial mast cells, a major source of histamine, have been documented in a patient with coronary spasm (135). Also, coronary arteries from patients with coronary artery disease contain greater amounts of histamine, and they respond with vasoconstriction to the amine (136). As histamine also has a bimodal action in normal coronary arteries (i.e., release of EDNO through H_1-histaminergic receptors and direct vasoconstriction through H_2-histaminergic receptors (118,120), endothelial dysfunction leaving dominant activation of smooth muscle cells could explain some of these findings.

Abnormal coronary vasomotion in response to endothelial vasodilators also has been demonstrated with atherothrombotic coronary artery disease and no signs of variant angina. Indeed, acetylcholine causes vasoconstriction in most patients with coronary artery disease (Fig. 42–11) (11,137). Also, intracoronary infusion of serotonin elicits vasodilation in patients with normal coronary arteries but profound contraction in patients with coronary artery disease (Fig. 42–14) (12) or variant angina (138). In patients with coronary artery disease, the vasoconstriction to serotonin can be inhibited with the 5-HT_2-serotonergic antagonist ketanserin (12). In contrast, ketanserin does not prevent ergonovine-induced coronary spasm in patients with variant angina (139). Hence, either 5-HT_2–serotonergic receptors are not involved in variant angina or ergonovine predominantly activates other serotonergic or adrenergic receptors. *In vitro* studies have demonstrated that contractile 5-HT_1–serotonergic receptors on

vascular smooth muscle may importantly contribute to the response to serotonin in human coronary arteries (93).

Prostacyclin

Prostacyclin is a vasodilator in the coronary circulation. However, at least in the pig, prostacyclin contributes little to endothelium-dependent relaxations of coronary arteries (34). In most patients with variant angina, intravenous prostacyclin does not influence the number, severity, or duration of spontaneous or provoked coronary vasospasm (140).

Vasoconstrictor Prostaglandins

In isolated quiescent porcine coronary arteries studied as ring preparations in organ chambers, serotonin causes contractions with or without endothelium (34,35,97). In arteries with regenerated endothelium, contractions to serotonin are enhanced as compared with preparations with either normal endothelium or those without endothelium (97). These findings suggest that endothelium produces a contracting factor under these conditions, most likely one derived from the cyclooxygenase pathway.

Endothelin

Endothelin causes profound constriction of coronary arteries (discussed earlier). However, the time course of its response is slow but sustained and does not resemble the rapid vaso-

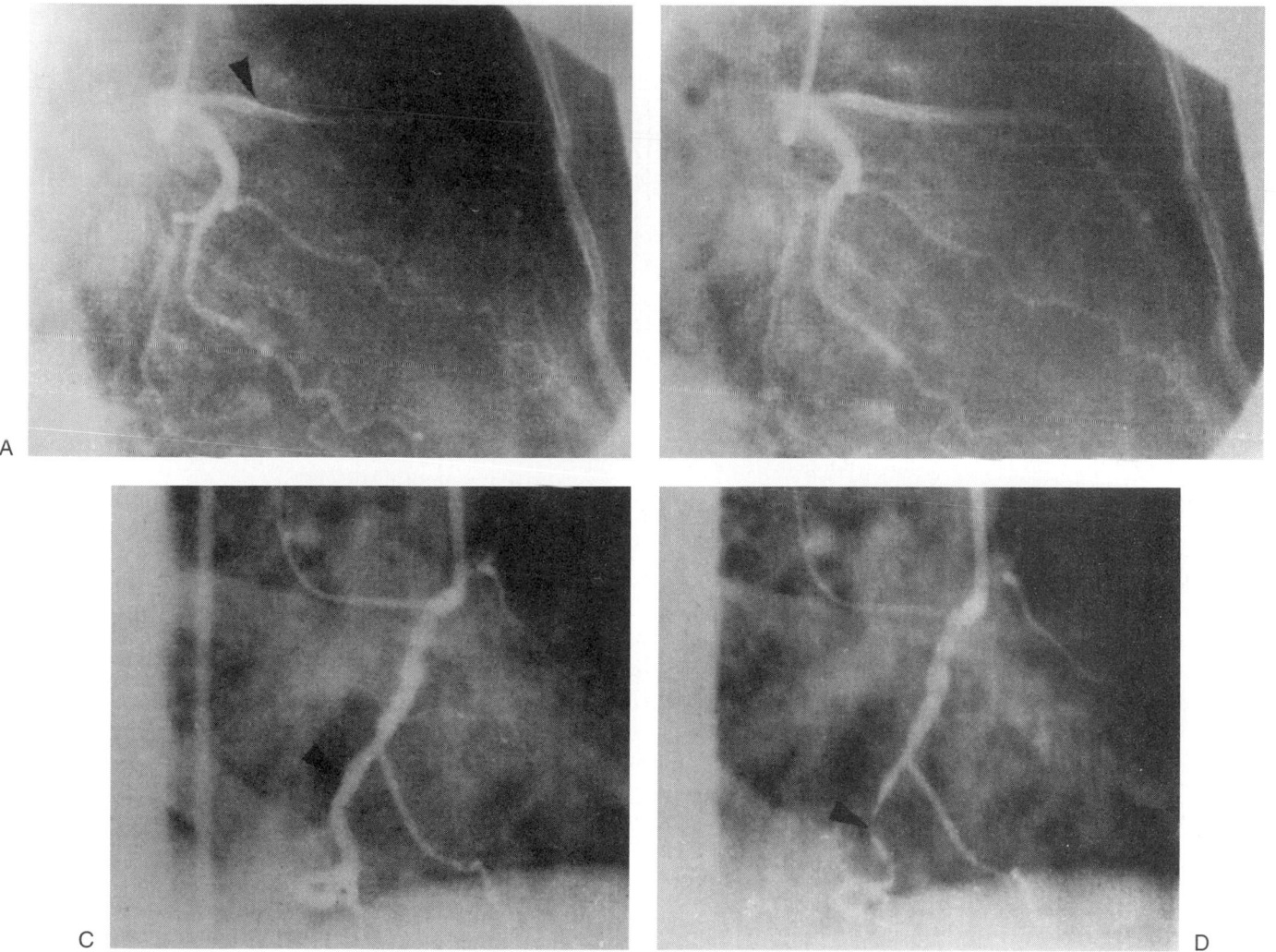

FIG. 42–14. Effects of intracoronary infusion of serotonin on the arterial diameter of the left anterior descending coronary artery in a patient with normal coronary arteries before **(A)** and after **(B)** application of the drug. Note the small vasodilation in response to serotonin. In contrast, in a patient with coronary artery disease **(C)**, serotonin causes contraction **(D)**. (Modified from Golino P, Piscione F, Willerson JT, et al. Divergent effects of serotonin on coronary-artery dimensions and blood flow in patients with coronary atherosclerosis and control patients. *N Engl J Med* 1991;324:641–648, by permission.)

constriction elicited in patients with variant angina after mechanical stimulation or activation with acetylcholine, histamine, or ergonovine (54). However, endothelin, particularly low and threshold concentrations, at which its own contractile effects are absent, is able to potentiate contractions to serotonin of human coronary arteries (Fig. 42–15) (104). Endothelin appears to increase the sensitivity of vascular smooth muscle to calcium. This could explain the generalized hypercontractility that occurs in certain patients with coronary artery disease and in selected patients with variant angina.

In patients with variant angina and provocable coronary vasospasm, there are increased venous and coronary sinus levels of endothelin-1 (Fig. 42–16) (141). Interestingly, endothelin plasma levels in the coronary sinus decreased rather than increased during the attack, possibly as a result of reduced flow in the affected coronary segment. In contrast, in patients with clinical findings consistent with variant angina but not provocable vasospasm, systemic venous plasma levels of the peptide were within the normal range. Interestingly, not only in coronary sinus but also in venous samples endothelin levels were twice as high in provocable than in nonprovocable patients (141). Furthermore, patients with coronary spasm do have a greater incidence of Raynaud's phenomenon, migraine (141), and ocular vasospasm than those without the disease, suggesting some generalized tendency of the vascular system to react with organ-specific focal contraction in response to certain stimuli. Endothelin

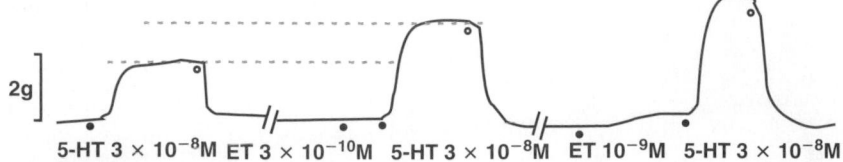

FIG. 42–15. Potentiating effects of threshold concentrations of endothelin-1 on contractions induced by serotonin (5-hydroxytryptamine [5-HT]) in human coronary artery. (From Yang ZH, Richard V, von SL, et al. Threshold concentrations of endothelin-1 potentiate contractions to norepinephrine and serotonin in human arteries. A new mechanism of vasospasm? *Circulation* 1990;82:188–195, by permission of the American Heart Association.)

may contribute to a generalized vasoconstrictor tendency, and the local trigger mechanism may not necessarily be directly related to the action of the peptide.

Endothelin contributes to the pathogenesis of atherothrombotic vascular disease. In atherothrombotic human blood vessels, endothelin production is increased (Fig. 42–17) (see also color insert) (142–144), but expression of endothelin receptors is down-regulated (143). A most likely stimulus is oxidized low-density lipoprotein, which increases endothelin gene expression and release of the peptide (Fig. 42–18) (145). In addition to endothelial cells, vascular smooth muscle cells, particularly those that migrated into the intima during the atherothrombotic process, also produce endothelin (146). Both plasma endothelin levels and vascular endothelin production are increased in patients with hyperlipidemia and in patients with clinically relevant atherothrombosis correlating with the extent of the atherothrombotic process (144). Furthermore, lesions removed from the coronary circulation (by atherectomy) of patients with coronary artery disease do exhibit marked staining for endothelin-1 (142), particularly in patients with unstable angina, suggesting that endothelin contributes to the abnormal vasomotion in these patients (142). Triggers of endothe-

lin production in patients with acute coronary syndromes might include ischemia (147) and thrombin (54–58).

Vascular Smooth Muscle

Hypercontractility of vascular smooth muscle may arise at sites where the continuous vasodilator tone of EDNO is lacking or in segments in which the responsiveness of vascular smooth muscle cells to contractile stimuli is increased. An increased smooth muscle cell mass with augmented contractions to a receptor-independent vasoconstrictor such as potassium chloride has been observed after endothelial injury (134). In the rabbit, cholesterol-induced atherothrombosis is associated with increased vasoconstrictor responses to serotonin. Oxidized low-density lipoprotein may cause contraction not only through inactivation of the NO pathway but also through direct stimulation of vascular smooth muscle (148).

Neuronal Mechanisms

Overactivity of the sympathetic nervous system as a cause of variant angina has been suspected by several investiga-

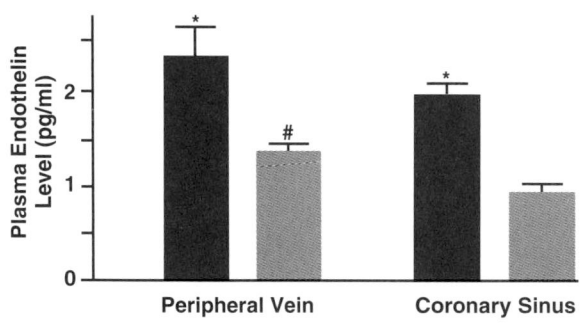

FIG. 42–16. Endothelin levels in the coronary sinus and peripheral vein in patients with *(dark bars)* or without *(light bars)* provocable coronary spasm at angiography. *Significant difference versus patients without spasms. #Significant difference versus coronary sinus data. (Data from Toyo-oka T, Aizawa T, Suzuki N, et al. Increased plasma level of endothelin-1 and coronary spasm induction in patients with vasospastic angina pectoris. *Circulation* 1991;83:476–483, by permission of the American Heart Association.)

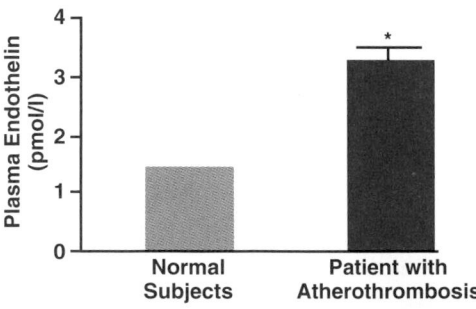

FIG. 42–17. Endothelin in patients with atherothrombosis Plasma levels of endothelin-1 are significantly greater in patients with atherothrombosis. Endothelin-1 can be detected immunohistochemically in endothelial cells and in the intima and media of arteries of patients with atherothrombosis. (Modified from Lerman A, Edwards BS, Hallett JW, et al. Circulating and tissue endothelin immunoreactivity in advanced atherosclerosis. *N Engl J Med* 1991;325:997–1001, by permission.) (See color insert for Fig. 42–17B.)

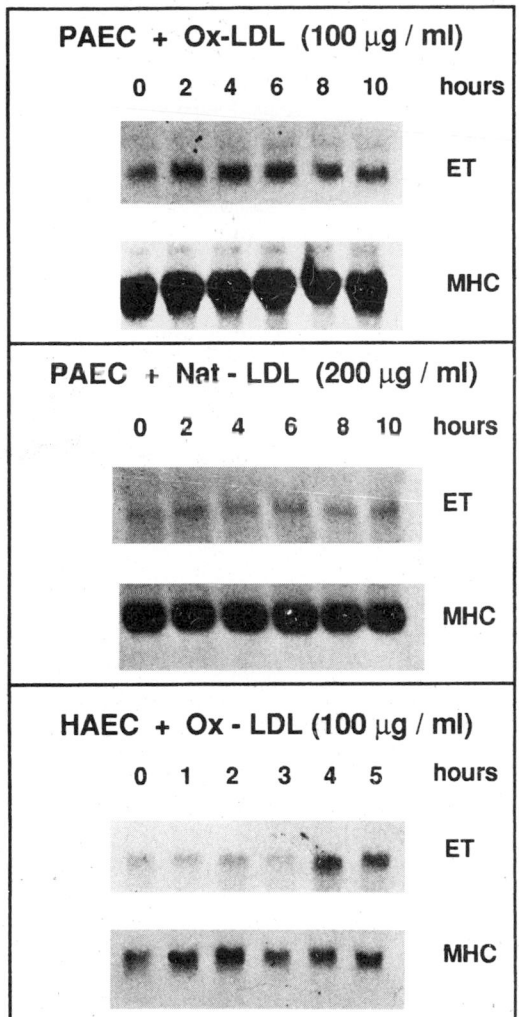

FIG. 42–18. Stimulation of endothelin (ET) gene expression by oxidized low-density lipoproteins (Ox-LDL), but not native LDL (Nat-LDL). Shown is a Northern blot with a cDNA probe for ET in endothelial cells in culture from the porcine aorta (PAEC) and human aorta (HAEC). Major histocompatibility complex (MHC) served as control. (Modified from Boulanger CM, Tanner FC, Bea ML, et al. Oxidized low density lipoproteins induce mRNA expression and release of endothelin from human and porcine endothelium. *Circ Res* 1992;70: 1191–1197, by permission of the American Heart Association.)

tors. However, in patients with coronary spasm, the response to the α_1-adrenergic agonist phenylephrine is normal, and α-adrenergic antagonists are ineffective in experimental models and in patients (140,149). Furthermore, sympathetic activation, such as during exercise, is not a typical trigger mechanism in patients with coronary spasm.

The sympathetic nervous system, however, does contribute to the ischemia threshold in patients with coronary atherothrombosis. For example, the cold pressor test (a strong activator of the sympathetic nervous system) causes no change or a small increase in coronary vascular diameter in cases without atherothrombosis, but marked constriction

is observed in patients with coronary atherothrombosis (112). During bicycle exercise, flow-dependent vasodilation of normal coronary segments occurs, but diseased segments exhibit paradoxic vasoconstriction (111). In the human forearm circulation, flow-dependent vasodilation is abolished after inhibition of NO synthesis by intraarterial administration of L-NMMA (101). Hence, it appears that lack of NO production in diseased coronary segments unmasks a vasoconstrictor mechanism. Because the paradoxic vasoconstriction during exercise can be blocked by phentolamine or a calcium antagonist, this vasoconstrictor mechanism is likely to be mediated by activation of the sympathetic nervous system. Abnormal coronary vasomotion during exercise may importantly contribute to exercise-induced angina in patients with atherothrombotic coronary disease.

THERAPEUTIC ASPECTS

General Considerations

Certain general considerations should be taken into account when treating patients with coronary artery spasm in any setting. Contributing factors that have been associated with precipitation of exacerbation of coronary artery spasm include exposure to cold, smoking, and emotional stress. These factors should be removed whenever possible. Known vasoconstrictors should be avoided, and patients should be cautioned against use of over-the-counter sympathomimetics. Recent withdrawal of nitrates, calcium or calcium antagonists, or α-adrenergic blocking agents should be sought as a possible exacerbating factor. Cocaine and other illicit drugs have become an increasingly important cause of vasomotor-related myocardial ischemia (150).

In patients with variant angina, therapy primarily aims at preventing or reversing coronary constriction. Currently available drugs that relax coronary vascular smooth muscle effectively are nitrates and calcium antagonists (105). Other vasodilators such as potassium channel openers and hydralazine have been for use in susceptible patients, but these have largely been abandoned because they cause a reflex tachycardia, which may aggravate myocardial ischemia. Newer drugs such as endothelin receptor antagonists (151) or AT-1 antagonists (94) have not been evaluated yet in patients with known or suspected spasm.

In patients with atherothrombotic coronary artery disease and increased vasomotion, nitrates and calcium antagonists are also useful in reversing coronary constriction and relieving angina pectoris and signs of ischemia (152,153). Rarely, the angina threshold of patients with coronary spasm may also be lowered by drugs with little vascular action that decrease heart rate and myocardial oxygen consumption (i.e., β-blockers), but when a fixed obstruction coexists with spasm, these patients often benefit. Furthermore, the antianginal effects of nitrates are not only related to coronary dilation but also to reduction in preload of the ventricle. Inhibition of platelet function or coagulation is an important part of therapy of patients with atherothrombotic coronary artery disease, because these drugs have been shown to reduce the risk for MI and death (154–158). Ideally, drugs should be able to interfere with the atherothrombotic process itself. This, however, is much more difficult to achieve, although calcium antagonists (159–161) and angiotensin-converting enzyme inhibitors do exert some inhibitory effects on plaque formation (162).

Specific Drugs

Calcium Channel Blockers

Calcium channel blockers inhibit inflow of extracellular calcium into the smooth muscle cell, thereby causing profound vasodilation (discussed earlier). Three different classes of calcium channel blockers exist: (a) phenylalkalanines, (b) dihydropyridines, and (c) benzothiodiazepines (106). The prototype of phenylalkalanines is verapamil, whereas mibefradil interferes not only with L-type, but also with T-type calcium channels (163). Furthermore, although verapamil exhibits negative inotropic and electrophysiologic effects, mibefradil lacks these properties. Nifedipine is the classical dihydropyridine; newer compounds such as amlodipine, felodipine, isradipine, and nicardipine exhibit marked vascular selectivity (i.e., they are more potent vasodilators and lack negative inotropic effects at clinically used dosages) (105). Finally, diltiazem is the representative of the benzothiodiazepines and exhibits both vasodilation and negative inotropism. That the three classes of calcium channel blockers bind to different and distinct parts of the L-type calcium channel may explain why, under certain conditions (e.g., in patients with severe coronary spasm), combination therapy may be useful. The drugs have been used successfully to relieve symptoms in patients with both variant angina (alone or in combination) and exercise-induced angina.

Short-term controlled trials have demonstrated that calcium antagonists used alone or in combination are effective for management of recurrent ischemic episodes in the early phase of illness (164,165) (Fig. 42–19). Comparison studies (166,167) showed similar responses to prevent ischemic episodes among the three first-generation calcium antagonists (diltiazem, nifedipine, and verapamil) when the same patients are exposed to the different agents in adequate doses; however, adverse experiences were less frequent with diltiazem (167) (Fig. 42–20). When the patient is nonresponsive, addition of another calcium antagonist may be helpful, but the risk for negative side effects may also increase (167,168).

Whether prognosis of patients after MI is favorably affected is uncertain. Indeed, a large trial with diltiazem showed no benefit (169), and another with verapamil found a favorable response only in patients without heart failure (170).

Nitrates

Ever since Thomas Lauder Brunton (171) successfully used nitrate of amyl in patients with angina pectoris, nitrates have been a standard therapy in patients with atherothrombotic coronary artery disease and also in those with variant angina. The drugs act by releasing NO from their molecule (172), which, in turn, activates guanylate cyclase and leads to the formation of cGMP (Fig. 42–3; discussed earlier). Hence, nitrates act similarly to EDNO and are a substitute for the endogenous nitrovasodilator in disease states with reduced formation of NO in the blood vessel wall.

In vessels without endothelium, or after inhibition of the endogenous NO formation, nitrovasodilators are particularly effective vasodilators (173,174). With progressing atherothrombotic coronary artery disease, the response of vascular smooth muscle to nitrates usually is reduced (41).

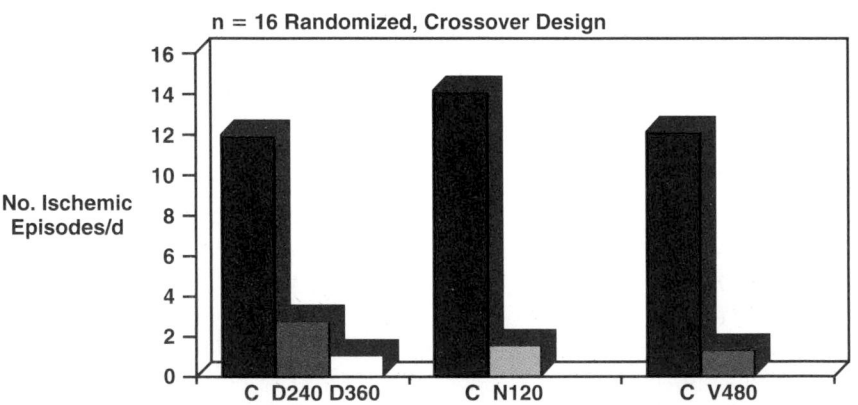

FIG. 42–19. Comparison of diltiazem (240 and 360 mg/day [D240 and D360]), nifedipine (120 mg/day [N120]), and verapamil (480 mg/day [V480]) given to the same patients with variant angina. Note that each of the first-generation calcium antagonists decreased the number of ischemic episodes per day in a similar fashion in this randomized crossover design. C, control. (From Turitto G, Pezzella A, Prati PL. [Diltiazem in spontaneous angina: comparison with nifedipine and verapamil]. *G Ital Cardiol* 1985;15: 1079–1084, with permission.)

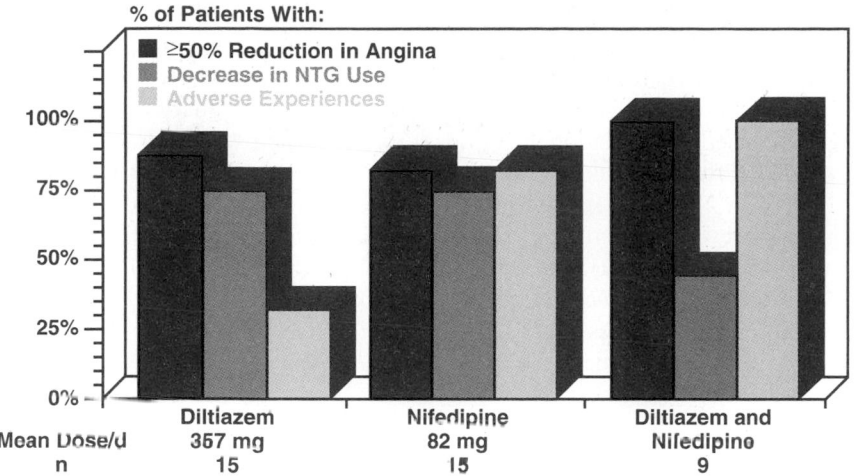

FIG. 42–20. Comparison of diltiazem and nifedipine monotherapy and combination therapy in the same patients with coronary spasm. Diltiazem (mean dose 357 mg/day) and nifedipine (mean dose 82 mg/day) monotherapy were both associated with significant reductions in the proportion of patients showing a 50% or greater reduction in angina *(left hand column of each group)* in 15 patients. Likewise, the decrease in nitroglycerin use (NTG; *bars in the middle of each group)* paralleled this antianginal effect. Frequency of adverse experiences, however, was greater with nifedipine monotherapy than with diltiazem monotherapy. When diltiazem and nifedipine were combined in nine patients *(bars to the right in each group),* there was an increase in the proportion of patients with reduction in angina, but adverse experiences occurred in every patient exposed to the combination. (From Prida XE, Gelman JS, Feldman RL, et al. Comparison of diltiazem and nifedipine alone and in combination in patients with coronary artery spasm. *J Am Coll Cardiol* 1987;9:412–419, with permission.)

The potency of nitrates is reduced by nitrate tolerance (i.e., the loss of vasodilator effects with prolonged application of the drugs) (175). Nitrate tolerance can occur as a result of counter-regulatory mechanisms stimulated by the drugs (i.e., activation of the sympathetic nervous system and the renin-angiotensin system), decreased biotransformation of organic nitrates (because of reduced availability of sulfhydryl groups and other mechanisms), and possibly a reduced activity of guanylate cyclase (175). Nitrovasodilators that do not require enzymatic biotransformation and spontaneously release NO from their molecule (i.e., molsidomine) appear to be less prone to tolerance (176). Clinically, intermittent therapy with a nitrate-free window of at least 8 hours has been recommended.

In patients with variant angina occurring in the catheterization laboratory, intracoronary nitroglycerin rapidly reverses spasm. Intravenous nitrates are useful for patients with frequently recurring spasms. Sublingual and oral preparations are useful for relieving an acute episode and preventing episodes that cluster into one portion of the day (usually the early morning). But, in general, when used in a dosing schedule that is designed to limit tolerance, nitrates should be combined with calcium antagonists for maximal benefit to control spasm.

New Compounds

Newly developed compounds that may be promising in patients with abnormal coronary vasoconstriction are endothe- lin receptor antagonists and angiotensin receptor antagonists.

Specific endothelin antagonists interfering with ET_A, ET_A/ET_B, or ET_B receptors have been synthesized (17). Some of these compounds are active orally (e.g., darusentan and bosentan) (75,78,151,177). Data in patients with variant angina are lacking. That plasma levels of endothelin are increased in patients with variant angina (Fig. 42–16) (134) and also in patients with atherothrombosis (Fig. 42–17) (142–147) suggests that the drugs might be useful tools to interfere with increased coronary vasoconstriction.

Angiotensin II is a potent vasoconstrictor that binds to specific receptors on vascular smooth muscle cells to exert its effects. Up to four angiotensin receptors exist (94), but it appears that in vascular smooth muscle cells, vasoconstriction, as well as migration and proliferation, is exclusively mediated by angiotensin receptor subtype 1. Data in patients with atherothrombotic coronary artery disease or variant angina are lacking (178,179).

Current Recommendations

Acute Setting

As noted earlier, coronary spasm can play an important role in the pathogenesis of unstable or periinfarction angina syndromes. Thus, spasm should be considered in the treatment strategies used for management of all coronary care unit patients presenting with myocardial ischemia at rest in whom spasm has not been excluded. Accordingly, in the acute setting, the initial agent of choice is intravenous nitroglycerin. We initiate therapy with an intravenous bolus of 400 μg followed by an infusion. The infusion rate is started at 5 to 10 μg per minute and titrated to achieve resolution of signs and symptoms of ischemia. The infusion should not be targeted to any arbitrary reduction in blood pressure because, potentially, such a strategy may provoke ischemia by reducing coronary perfusion pressure while causing a reflex increase in heart rate in patients with fixed obstructive lesions. Acute ischemia caused by coronary spasm is rapidly relieved by intravenous nitroglycerin, and coronary spasm is sensitive to nitrates; thus, continuous high blood levels are neither needed nor desirable if tolerance is to be minimized (128). We anticoagulate with intravenous heparin, based on the association of thrombus formation with acute ischemic syndromes and the proven beneficial effect of heparin in such patient groups (158). We also add low-dose aspirin (100 mg/day).

Shortly after parenteral nitrates are started, oral calcium antagonists are instituted. The choice of calcium antagonist is usually not critical. Verapamil and diltiazem are more potent negative inotropes than the dihydropyridines and should be avoided in patients with either bradyarrhythmia or severe impairment of left ventricular function. Dihydropyridine compounds are more potent peripheral vasodilators than either verapamil or diltiazem and should not be used in patients who are hypotensive.

In the rare instance that acute ischemia caused by coronary spasm appears refractory to intravenous nitroglycerin and a calcium antagonist, a second calcium antagonist may be added. Logic would dictate combining a dihydropyridine with a heart rate–slowing compound (diltiazem or verapamil). Intravenous administration of either diltiazem or verapamil can be used (180,181), although care must be taken to avoid systemic hypotension in this setting. However, if hypotension occurs, restoration of blood pressure may be achieved by fluid administration and down-titration of the dose of nitroglycerin. We have, on rare occasion, given calcium antagonists directly into a coronary artery when spasm has been refractory to all other measures.

When acute ischemia is controlled in the critical care setting, parenteral nitrates should be changed to oral or topical preparations, administered on an eccentric dosing schedule with a 10- to 12-hour nitrate-free window. Because attacks tend to cluster between 12 AM and 8 AM (182,183), the nitrate-free window should be positioned during the afternoon and early evening hours. Interestingly, there is diurnal fluctuation in endothelial function, which is associated with variation in the frequency of ischemic episodes (184).

Some patients with coronary spasm, initially well controlled, may have recurrent ischemia while receiving the measures cited earlier. When recurrent episodes are either frequent or prolonged, and sufficient time has elapsed since the first angiogram for possible changes in anatomy, repeat coronary angiography may be considered to define the coronary anatomy and guide other therapy if indicated. If the episodes are frequent or prolonged, placement of an intraaortic balloon pump may be useful while the patient is prepared for coronary angiography. When refractory spasm is associated with intracoronary thrombus, thrombolytic therapy may be helpful. When refractory spasm is associated with severe atherothrombotic stenosis, adjunct revascularization may be considered.

Adjunctive Revascularization

Coronary artery bypass surgery can be an effective adjunct to calcium antagonist therapy in selected patients with recurrent spasm limited to the site of an important atherothrombotic narrowing (185,186). However, if spasm involves multiple vessels, is diffuse in the same vessel, is migrating to different vessels, or is not associated with important atherothrombotic obstruction, coronary bypass surgery is not indicated. In any patient with suspected coronary spasm undergoing operation, it is essential to provide effective pharmacologic prophylaxis against coronary spasm before, during, and after surgery (185). The frequency of graft occlusion and perioperative MI is greater in patients with spasm than in those without spasm. Coronary bypass surgery has been combined with denervation (plexectomy), but there is no objective evidence from controlled trials that this improves results.

Infrequently, percutaneous coronary intervention may be an adjunct to pharmacologic therapy in managing selected patients with coronary spasm limited to the site of an important atherothrombotic narrowing (187). Angioplasty is not indicated if spasm involves multiple sites or different vessels. Care should be exercised in patients with dynamic stenosis because of a risk for restenosis (188).

Ambulatory Setting

Treatment principles for coronary spasm in ambulatory patients are similar to those outlined in the acute setting and differ only in the routes by which medications are administered. Oral nitrates and calcium antagonists remain the mainstays of chronic ambulatory treatment, with sublingual nitroglycerin used to relieve acute episodes. At our institution, we have found that after several months of combination treatment some patients do well with only calcium antagonist monotherapy. However, because the clinical course of patients with coronary spasm is highly variable and typically displays periods of exacerbation and remission even with seemingly optimal therapy, regular evaluation of treatment regimens is necessary. During flares of activity, our approach is to increase doses of calcium antagonists and nitrates; several different calcium antagonists may be used in combination to take advantage of each agent's different properties and to minimize side effects seen when very large doses of a single agent are used. Sublingual nitroglycerin is used to relieve acute episodes. After several symptom-free months, one calcium antagonist is discontinued, and, with continued remission, the second is discontinued.

Monitoring Therapy

After institution of an effective ambulatory treatment regimen, several options are available to follow patients with coronary spasm. Monitoring symptoms may be sufficient for many patients, but there is evidence that as many as 90% of all ischemia-related episodes in patients with coronary spasm may be asymptomatic. In addition, the natural history of Prinzmetal's angina may be difficult to predict. Thus, it is helpful to attempt a more objective assessment of therapeutic efficacy, especially in patients with severe ischemia or ischemia-related sequelae such as tachydysrhythmia, pump dysfunction, or conduction disturbances related to coronary spasm. Repeat catheterization with ergonovine provocation during therapy to assess efficacy could be considered, but this strategy has not been compared with a less invasive strategy documenting therapeutic success and has obvious disadvantages with regard to costs, risks, and discomfort. Repeated ambulatory ECG monitoring of the ST segment is probably the best current objective method to follow therapy in patients with coronary spasm. If spasm-related dysrhythmias are present in a given patient, these too can be used to follow the adequacy of therapy and the possibility for spontaneous remission. Clearly, ischemia-associated dysrhythmias should be managed by prevention of ischemia rather than by attempting to suppress the rhythm disturbance with antiarrhythmic agents. Recent data demonstrate that preconditioning by transient ischemia induces a significant protection against ischemia-induced complex ventricular arrhythmias in patients with variant angina (189). This beneficial effect is not related to a reduction in either severity or duration of ischemia, suggesting that arrhythmic protection is a direct consequence of preconditioning rather than an epiphenomenon of ischemic protection.

FUTURE DIRECTIONS

Coronary vasomotion is an important regulatory mechanism that allows the coronary circulation to adapt blood flow to the oxygen requirements of the myocardium under different physiologic conditions. In disease states such as variant angina and exercise-induced angina, the regulation of coronary vascular tone becomes abnormal. Abnormal coronary vasomotion importantly contributes to symptoms and prognosis of these patients. The understanding of the cellular and molecular mechanisms regulating coronary tone has improved dramatically in the last decade. This allowed for the development of new and more dynamic concepts of atherothrombotic coronary artery disease and variant angina. This should lead to more effective drugs, some of which are already in clinical development, to treat these patients. At this point, nitrates and calcium channel blockers alone or in combination are most effective to relieve vasospasm in pa-

tients with variant angina or to increase vasoconstriction in patients with atherothrombotic coronary artery disease.

REFERENCES

1. Prinzmetal M, Ekmekci A, Kennamer R, et al. Variant form of angina pectoris. *JAMA* 1960;174:1794–1800.
2. Prinzmetal M, Kennamer R, Merliss R, et al. A variant form of angina pectoris. *Am J Med* 1959;27:375–388.
3. Wiener L, Kasparian H, Duca PR, et al. Spectrum of coronary arterial spasm. Clinical, angiographic and myocardial metabolic experience in 29 cases. *Am J Cardiol* 1976;38:945–955.
4. Dhurandhar RW, Watt DL, Silver MD, et al. Prinzmetal's variant form of angina with arteriographic evidence of coronary arterial spasm. *Am J Cardiol* 1972;30:902–905.
5. Oliva PB, Potts DE, Pluss RG. Coronary arterial spasm in Prinzmetal angina. Documentation by coronary arteriography. *N Engl J Med* 1973;288:745–751.
6. Maseri A, L'Abbate A, Baroldi G, et al. Coronary vasospasm as a possible cause of myocardial infarction. A conclusion derived from the study of "preinfarction" angina. *N Engl J Med* 1978;299:1271–1277.
7. Vincent GM, Anderson JL, Marshall HW. Coronary spasm producing coronary thrombosis and myocardial infarction. *N Engl J Med* 1983;309:220–223.
8. Hillis LD, Braunwald E. Coronary-artery spasm. *N Engl J Med* 1978;299:695–702.
9. Maseri A, Severi S, Nes MD, et al. "Variant" angina: one aspect of a continuous spectrum of vasospastic myocardial ischemia. Pathogenetic mechanisms, estimated incidence and clinical and coronary arteriographic findings in 138 patients. *Am J Cardiol* 1978;42:1019–1035.
10. Rafflenbeul W, Nellessen U, Galvao P, et al. [Progression and regression of coronary sclerosis in the angiographic image]. *Z Kardiol* 1984;73[Suppl 2]:33–40.
11. Ludmer PL, Selwyn AP, Shook TL, et al. Paradoxical vasoconstriction induced by acetylcholine in atherosclerotic coronary arteries. *N Engl J Med* 1986;315:1046–1051.
12. Golino P, Piscione F, Willerson JT, et al. Divergent effects of serotonin on coronary-artery dimensions and blood flow in patients with coronary atherosclerosis and control patients. *N Engl J Med* 1991;324:641–648.
13. Lüscher TF, Vanhoutte PM. *The endothelium: modulator of cardiovascular function*. Boca Raton, FL: CRC Press, 1990.
14. Vanhoutte PM, Lüscher TF. Peripheral mechanisms in cardiovascular regulation: transmitters, receptors and the endothelium. In: Zanchetti RC, Tarazzi, eds. *Handbook of hypertension, Vol 8*. Amsterdam: Elsevier, 1986:96–123.
15. Furchgott RF, Zawadzki JV. The obligatory role of endothelial cells in the relaxation of arterial smooth muscle by acetylcholine. *Nature* 1980;299:373–376.
16. Cohen RA, Shepherd JT, Vanhoutte PM. Inhibitory role of the endothelium in the response of isolated coronary arteries to platelets. *Science* 1983;221:273–274.
17. Lüscher TF, Diederich D, Siebenmann R, et al. Difference between endothelium-dependent relaxation in arterial and in venous coronary bypass grafts. *N Engl J Med* 1988;319:462–467.
18. Yang ZH, Stulz P, von Segesser L, et al. Different interactions of platelets with arterial and venous coronary bypass vessels. *Lancet* 1991;337:939–943.
19. De Mey JG, Claeys M, Vanhoutte PM. Endothelium-dependent inhibitory effects of acetylcholine, adenosine diphosphate, thrombin and arachidonic acid in the canine femoral artery. *J Pharm Exp Ther* 1982;222:166–173.
20. Rubanyi GM, Romero JC, Vanhoutte PM. Flow-induced release of endothelium-derived relaxing factor. *Am J Physiol* 1986;250:H1145–H1149.
21. Pohl U, Holtz J, Busse R, et al. Crucial role of endothelium in the vasodilator response to increased flow in vivo. *Hypertension* 1986;8:37–44.
22. Rubanyi GM, Vanhoutte PM. Superoxide anions and hyperoxia inactivate endothelium-derived relaxing factor. *Am J Physiol* 1986;250:H822–H827.

23. Furchgott RF. Studies on relaxation of rabbit aorta by sodium nitrite: the basis for the proposal that acid-activable inhibitory factor from bovine retractor penis is inorganic nitrite and the endothelium-derived relaxing factor is nitric oxide. In: Vanhoutte PM, ed. *Vasodilation: vascular smooth muscle, peptides, autonomic nerves and endothelium.* New York: Raven Press, 1988:401–414.

24. Palmer RM, Ferrige AG, Moncada S. Nitric oxide release accounts for the biological activity of endothelium-derived relaxing factor. *Nature* 1987;327:524–526.

25. Ignarro LJ, Byrns RE, Buga GM, et al. Pharmacological evidence that endothelium-derived relaxing factor is nitric oxide: use of pyrogallol and superoxide dismutase to study endothelium-dependent and nitric oxide-elicited vascular smooth muscle relaxation. *J Pharmacol Exp Ther* 1988;244:181–189.

26. Palmer RM, Ashton DS, Moncada S. Vascular endothelial cells synthesize nitric oxide from L-arginine. *Nature* 1988;333:664–666.

27. Bredt DS, Hwang PM, Glatt CE, et al. Cloned and expressed nitric oxide synthase structurally resembles cytochrome P-450 reductase. *Nature* 1991;351:714–718.

28. Radomski MW, Palmer RM, Moncada S. An L-arginine/nitric oxide pathway present in human platelets regulates aggregation. *Proc Natl Acad Sci USA* 1990;87:5193–5197.

29. Hibbs J Jr, Taintor RR, Vavrin Z, et al. Nitric oxide: a cytotoxic activated macrophage effector molecule. *Biochem Biophys Res Commun* 1988;157:87–94.

30. Bernhardt J, Tschudi MR, Dohi Y, et al. Release of nitric oxide from human vascular smooth muscle cells. *Biochem Biophys Res Commun* 1991;180:907–912.

31. Julou-Schaeffer G, Gray GA, Fleming I, et al. Loss of vascular responsiveness induced by endotoxin involves L-arginine pathway. *Am J Physiol* 1990;259:1038–1043.

32. Wright CE, Rees DD, Moncada S. Protective and pathological roles of nitric oxide in endotoxin shock. *Cardiovasc Res* 1992;26:48–57.

33. Knowles RG, Palacios M, Palmer RM, et al. Formation of nitric oxide from L-arginine in the central nervous system: a transduction mechanism for stimulation of the soluble guanylate cyclase. *Proc Natl Acad Sci USA* 1989;86:5159–5162.

34. Richard V, Tanner FC, Tschudi M, et al. Different activation of L-arginine pathway by bradykinin, serotonin, and clonidine in coronary arteries. *Am J Physiol* 1990;259:H1433–H1439.

35. Tschudi M, Richard V, Bühler FR, et al. Importance of endothelium-derived nitric oxide in porcine coronary resistance arteries. *Am J Physiol* 1991;260:H13–H20.

36. Yang ZH, von Segesser L, Bauer E, et al. Different activation of the endothelial L-arginine and cyclooxygenase pathway in the human internal mammary artery and saphenous vein. *Circ Res* 1991;68:52–60.

37. Meyer P, Flammer J, Lüscher TF. Endothelium-dependent regulation of the ophthalmic microcirculation in the perfused porcine eye: role of nitric oxide and endothelins. *Invest Ophthalmol Vis Sci* 1993;34:3614–3621.

38. Rees DD, Palmer RMJ, Moncada S. Role of endothelium-derived nitric oxide in the regulation of blood pressure. *Proc Natl Acad Sci USA* 1989;86:3375–3378.

39. Vallance P, Leone A, Calver A, et al. Accumulation of an endogenous inhibitor of nitric oxide synthesis in chronic renal failure. *Lancet* 1992;339:572–575.

40. Rapoport RM, Draznin MB, Murad F. Endothelium-dependent relaxation in rat aorta may be mediated through cyclic GMP-dependent protein phosphorylation. *Nature* 1983;306:174–176.

41. Förstermann U, Mügge A, Bode SM, et al. Response of human coronary arteries to aggregating platelets: importance of endothelium-derived relaxing factor and prostanoids. *Circ Res* 1988;63:306–312.

42. Yang Z, Arnet U, Bauer E, et al. Thrombin-induced endothelium-dependent inhibition and direct activation of platelet-vessel wall interaction. Role of prostacyclin, nitric oxide, and thromboxane A2. *Circulation* 1994;89:2266–2272.

43. Moncada S, Vane VR. Pharmacology and endogenous roles of prostaglandin endoperoxides, thromboxane A2 and prostacyclin. *Pharmacol Rev* 1979;30:293–331.

44. Nakahata N, Suzuki T. Effects of prostaglandin E1, I2 and isoproterenol on the tissue cyclic AMP content in longitudinal muscle of rabbit intestine. *Prostaglandins* 1981;22:159–165.

45. Radomski MW, Palmer RM, Moncada S. Comparative pharmacology of endothelium-derived relaxing factor, nitric oxide and prostacyclin in platelets. *Br J Pharmacol* 1987;92:181–187.

46. Vanhoutte PM. Vascular physiology: the end of the quest? *Nature* 1987;327:459–460.

47. Nagao T, Vanhoutte PM. Hyperpolarization contributes to endothelium-dependent relaxations to acetylcholine in femoral veins of rats. *Am J Physiol* 1991;261:H1034–H1037.

48. Nagao T, Vanhoutte PM. Hyperpolarization as a mechanism for endothelium-dependent relaxations in the porcine coronary artery. *J Physiol (Lond)* 1992;445:355–367.

49. Feletou M, Vanhoutte PM. Endothelium-dependent hyperpolarization of canine coronary smooth muscle. *Br J Pharmacol* 1988;93:515–524.

50. Archer SL, Huang JM, Hampl V, et al. Nitric oxide and cGMP cause vasorelaxation by activation of a charybdotoxin-sensitive K channel by cGMP-dependent protein kinase. *Proc Natl Acad Sci USA* 1994;91:7583–7587.

51. Bolotina VM, Najibi S, Palacino JJ, et al. Nitric oxide directly activates calcium-dependent potassium channels in vascular smooth muscle. *Nature* 1994;368:850–853.

52. Tare M, Parkington HC, Coleman HA, et al. Hyperpolarization and relaxation of arterial smooth muscle caused by nitric oxide derived from the endothelium. *Nature* 1990;346:69–71.

53. Nakao K, Ogawa Y, Suga S, et al. Molecular biology and biochemistry of the natriuretic peptide system. II: Natriuretic peptide receptors. *J Hypertens* 1992;10:1111–1114.

54. Yanagisawa M, Kurihara H, Kimura S, et al. A novel potent vasoconstrictor peptide produced by vascular endothelial cells. *Nature* 1988;332:411–415.

55. Yanagisawa M, Masaki T. Molecular biology and biochemistry of the endothelins. *Trends Pharmacol Sci* 1989;10:374–378.

56. Lüscher TF, Boulanger CM, Dohi Y, et al. Endothelium-derived contracting factors. *Hypertension* 1992;19:117–130.

57. Boulanger C, Lüscher TF. Release of endothelin from the porcine aorta. Inhibition by endothelium-derived nitric oxide. *J Clin Invest* 1990;85:587–590.

58. Boulanger CM, Lüscher TF. Hirudin and nitrates inhibit the thrombin-induced release of endothelin from the intact porcine aorta. *Circ Res* 1991;68:1768–1772.

59. Dohi Y, Hahn AW, Boulanger CM, et al. Endothelin stimulated by angiotensin II augments contractility of spontaneously hypertensive rat resistance arteries. *Hypertension* 1992;19:131–137.

60. Dohi Y, Lüscher TF. Endothelin in hypertensive resistance arteries. Intraluminal and extraluminal dysfunction. *Hypertension* 1991;18:543–549.

61. Clarke JG, Larkin SW, Benjamin N, et al. Endothelin-1 is a potent long-lasting vasoconstrictor in dog peripheral vasculature in vivo. *J Cardiovasc Pharmacol* 1989;13:S211–S212.

62. Kiowski W, Lüscher TF, Linder L, et al. Endothelin-1-induced vasoconstriction in humans. Reversal by calcium channel blockade but not by nitrovasodilators or endothelium-derived relaxing factor. *Circulation* 1991;83:469–475.

63. Lüscher TF, Yang Z, Tschudi M, et al. Interaction between endothelin-1 and endothelium-derived relaxing factor in human arteries and veins. *Circ Res* 1990;66:1088–1094.

64. Neubauer S, Ertl G, Haas U, et al. Effects of endothelin-1 in isolated perfused rat heart. *J Cardiovasc Pharmacol* 1990;16:1–8.

65. Zaugg CE, Zhu P, Simper D, et al. Differential effects of endothelin-1 on normal and postischemic reperfused myocardium. *J Cardiovasc Pharmacol* 1993;22[Suppl 8]:S367–S370.

66. Kung CF, Tschudi MR, Noll G, et al. Differential effects of the calcium antagonist mibefradil in epicardial and intramyocardial coronary arteries. *J Cardiovasc Pharmacol* 1995;26:312–318.

67. Stewart DJ, Langleben D, Cernacek P, et al. Endothelin release is inhibited by coculture of endothelial cells with cells of vascular media. *Am J Physiol* 1990;259:H1928–H1932.

68. Wagner OF, Christ G, Wojta J, et al. Polar secretion of endothelin-1 by cultured endothelial cells. *J Biol Chem* 1992;267:16066–16068.

69. Saijonmaa O, Ristimaki A, Fyhrquist F. Atrial natriuretic peptide, nitroglycerine, and nitroprusside reduce basal and stimulated endothelin production from cultured endothelial cells. *Biochem Biophys Res Commun* 1990;173:514–520.

70. Yokokawa K, Kohno M, Yasunari K, et al. Endothelin-3 regulates endothelin-1 production in cultured human endothelial cells. *Hypertension* 1991;18:304–315.

71. Miller VM, Komori K, Burnett JJ, et al. Differential sensitivity to endothelin in canine arteries and veins. *Am J Physiol* 1989;257: H1127–H1131.
72. Arai H, Hori S, Aramori I, et al. Cloning and expression of a cDNA encoding an endothelin receptor. *Nature* 1990;348:730–732.
73. Sakurai T, Yanagisawa M, Takuwa Y, et al. Cloning of a cDNA encoding a non-isopeptide-selective subtype of the endothelin receptor. *Nature* 1990;348:732–735.
74. Seo B, Oemar BS, Siebenmann R, et al. Both ETA and ETB receptors mediate contraction to endothelin-1 in human blood vessels. *Circulation* 1994;89:1203–1208.
75. Clozel M, Breu V, Burri K, et al. Pathophysiologic role of endothelin revealed by the first orally active endothelin receptor antagonist. *Nature* 1993;365:759–761.
76. Bazil MK, Lappe RW, Webb RL. Pharmacologic characterization of an endothelinA (ETA) receptor antagonist in conscious rats. *J Cardiovasc Pharmacol* 1992;20:940–948.
77. Nishikibe M, Tsuchida S, Okada M, et al. Antihypertensive effect of a newly synthesized endothelin antagonist, BQ-123, in a genetic hypertensive model. *Life Sci* 1993;52:717–724.
78. Wenzel RR, Noll G, Lüscher TF. Endothelin receptor antagonists inhibit endothelin in human skin microcirculation. *Hypertension* 1994; 23:581–586.
79. Lüscher TF, Seo BG, Buhler FR. Potential role of endothelin in hypertension. Controversy on endothelin in hypertension. *Hypertension* 1993;21:752–757.
80. Miller VM, Vanhoutte PM. Endothelium-dependent contractions to arachidonic acid are mediated by products of cyclooxygenase. *Am J Physiol* 1985;248:H432–H437.
81. Katusic ZS, Vanhoutte PM. Superoxide anion is an endothelium-derived contracting factor. *Am J Physiol* 1989;257:H33–H37.
82. Vanhoutte PM, Katusic ZS. Endothelium-derived contracting factor: endothelin and/or superoxide anion? *Trends Pharmacol Sci* 1988;9: 229–230.
83. Somlyo AP, Somlyo AV. Signal transduction and regulation in smooth muscle. *Nature* 1994;372:231–236.
84. Berkowitz BA, Kohler C. Vascular catecholamines and aging. In: Bevan JA, Maxwell RA, Godfraind T, et al., eds. *Vascular neuroeffector mechanisms.* New York: Raven Press, 1980:335.
85. Wallin BG, Sundlöf G, Eriksson BM, et al. Plasma noradrenaline correlates to sympathetic muscle nerve activity in normotensive man. *Acta Physiol Scand* 1981;111:69–73.
86. Goldstein DS, Horwitz D, Keiser HR, et al. Plasma l-[3H]norepinephrine, d-[14C]norepinephrine, and d,l-[3H]isoproterenol kinetics in essential hypertension. *J Clin Invest* 1983;72:1748–1758.
87. Frewin DB, Hume WR, Waterson JG, et al. The histochemical localisation of sympathetic nerve endings in human gingival blood vessels. *Aust J Exp Biol Med Sci* 1971;49:573–580.
88. Gerke DC, Frewin DB, Soltys JS. Adrenergic innervation of human mesenteric blood vessels. *Aust J Exp Biol Med Sci* 1975;53: 241–243.
89. Spieker LE, Corti R, Binggeli C, et al. Baroreceptor dysfunction induced by nitric oxide synthase inhibition in humans. *J Am Coll Cardiol* 2000;36:213–218.
90. Corti R, Binggeli C, Sudano I, et al. The beauty and the beast: aspects of the autonomic nervous system. *News Physiol Sci* 2000;15: 125–129.
91. Waterson JG, Frewin DB, Soltys JS. Age-related differences in catecholamine fluorescence of human vascular tissue. *Blood Vessels* 1974;11:79–85.
92. Cohen RA. Role of autonomic nerves and endothelium in coronary vasospasm. *Prog Clin Biol Res* 1986;219:353–362.
93. Kaumann AJ, Frenken M, Posival H, et al. Variable participation of 5-HT1-like receptors and 5-HT2 receptors in serotonin-induced contraction of human isolated coronary arteries. 5-HT1-like receptors resemble cloned 5-HT1D beta receptors. *Circulation* 1994;90:1141–1153.
94. Timmermans PB, Chiu AT, Herblin WF, et al. Angiotensin II receptor subtypes. *Am J Hypertens* 1992;5:406–410.
95. Katusic ZS, Shepherd JT, Vanhoutte PM. Oxytocin causes endothelium-dependent relaxations of canine basilar arteries by activating V1-vasopressinergic receptors. *J Pharmacol Exp Ther* 1986;236: 166–170.
96. Ekblad E, Edvinsson L, Wahlestedt C, et al. Neuropeptide Y co-exists and co-operates with noradrenaline in perivascular nerve fibers. *Regul Pept* 1984;8:225–235.
97. Shimokawa H, Aarhus LL, Vanhoutte PM. Porcine coronary arteries with regenerated endothelium have a reduced endothelium-dependent responsiveness to aggregating platelets and serotonin. *Circ Res* 1987;61:256–270.
98. Cohen RA, Shepherd JT, Vanhoutte PM. 5-Hydroxytryptamine can mediate endothelium-dependent relaxation of coronary arteries. *Am J Physiol* 1983;245:H1077–H1080.
99. Cohen RA, Shepherd JT, Vanhoutte PM. Neurogenic cholinergic prejunctional inhibition of sympathetic beta adrenergic relaxation in the canine coronary artery. *J Pharmacol Exp Ther* 1984;229:417–421.
100. Cox DA, Vita JA, Treasure CB, et al. Atherosclerosis impairs flow-mediated dilation of coronary arteries in humans. *Circulation* 1989;80:458–465.
101. Joannides R, Haefeli WE, Linder L, et al. Nitric oxide is responsible for flow-dependent dilatation of human peripheral conduit arteries in vivo. *Circulation* 1995;91:1314–1319.
102. Spieker LE, Hurlimann D, Ruschitzka F, et al. Mental stress induces prolonged endothelial dysfunction via endothelin-A receptors. *Circulation* 2002;105:2817–2820.
103. Resink TJ, Scott-Burden T, Buhler FR. Endothelin stimulates phospholipase C in cultured vascular smooth muscle cells. *Biochem Biophys Res Commun* 1988;157:1360–1368.
104. Yang ZH, Richard V, von SL, et al. Threshold concentrations of endothelin-1 potentiate contractions to norepinephrine and serotonin in human arteries. A new mechanism of vasospasm? *Circulation* 1990;82:188–195.
105. Opie LH, Buhler FR, Fleckenstein A, et al. International Society and Federation of Cardiology: Working Group on Classification of Calcium Antagonists for Cardiovascular Disease. *Am J Cardiol* 1987;60:630–632.
106. Goto K, Kasuya Y, Matsuki N, et al. Endothelin activates the dihydropyridine-sensitive, voltage-dependent Ca(2+) channel in vascular smooth muscle. *Proc Natl Acad Sci USA* 1989;86:3915–3918.
107. Godfraind T, Mennig D, Bravo G, et al. Inhibition by amlodipine of activity evoked in isolated human coronary arteries by endothelin, prostaglandin F2 alpha and depolarization. *Am J Cardiol* 1989;64: 58I–64I.
108. Cauvin C, Tejerina M, Hwang O, et al. The effects of Ca2+ antagonists on isolated rat and rabbit mesenteric resistance vessels. What determines the sensitivity of agonist-activated vessels to Ca2+ antagonists? *Ann NY Acad Sci* 1988;522:338–350.
109. Schang SJ Jr, Pepine CJ. Transient asymptomatic S-T segment depression during daily activity. *Am J Cardiol* 1977;39:396–402.
110. Stern S, Tzivoni D. Early detection of silent ischaemic heart disease by 24-hour electrocardiographic monitoring of active subjects. *Br Heart J* 1974;36:481–486.
111. Gage JE, Hess OM, Murakami T, et al. Vasoconstriction of stenotic coronary arteries during dynamic exercise in patients with classic angina pectoris: reversibility by nitroglycerin. *Circulation* 1986;73: 865–876.
112. Zeiher AM, Drexler H, Wollschlaeger H, et al. Coronary vasomotion in response to sympathetic stimulation in humans: importance of the functional integrity of the endothelium. *J Am Coll Cardiol* 1989; 14:1181–1190.
113. Picano E. Stress echocardiography. From pathophysiological toy to diagnostic tool. *Circulation* 1992;85:1604–1612.
114. Picano E, Lattanzi F. Dipyridamole echocardiography. A new diagnostic window on coronary artery disease. *Circulation* 1991;83:III19–III26.
115. Kaski JC, Crea F, Meran D, et al. Local coronary supersensitivity to diverse vasoconstrictive stimuli in patients with variant angina. *Circulation* 1986;74:1255–1265.
116. Yasue H, Horio Y, Nakamura N, et al. Induction of coronary artery spasm by acetylcholine in patients with variant angina: possible role of the parasympathetic nervous system in the pathogenesis of coronary artery spasm. *Circulation* 1986;74:955–963.
117. el-Tamimi H, Mansour M, Wargovich TJ, et al. Constrictor and dilator responses to intracoronary acetylcholine in adjacent segments of the same coronary artery in patients with coronary artery disease. Endothelial function revisited. *Circulation* 1994;89:45–51.
118. Bossaller C, Habib GB, Yamamoto H, et al. Impaired muscarinic endothelium-dependent relaxation and cyclic guanosine 5'-mono-

phosphate formation in atherosclerotic human coronary artery and rabbit aorta. *J Clin Invest* 1987;79:170–174.

119. Kalsner S. Coronary artery reactivity in human vessels: some questions and some answers. *Fed Proc* 1985;44:321–325.

120. Yang Z, Diederich D, Schneider K, et al. Endothelium-derived relaxing factor and protection against contractions induced by histamine and serotonin in the human internal mammary artery and in the saphenous vein. *Circulation* 1989;80:1041–1048.

121. Vigorito C, Poto S, Picotti GB, et al. Effect of activation of the H1 receptor on coronary hemodynamics in man. *Circulation* 1986;73:1175–1182.

122. Blankenhorn DH, Nessim SA, Johnson RL, et al. Beneficial effects of combined colestipol-niacin therapy on coronary atherosclerosis and coronary venous bypass grafts [published erratum appears in JAMA 1988 May 13;259(18):2698]. *JAMA* 1987;257:3233–3240.

123. Brown G, Albers JJ, Fisher LD, et al. Regression of coronary artery disease as a result of intensive lipid-lowering therapy in men with high levels of apolipoprotein B. *N Engl J Med* 1990;323:1289–1298.

124. Ross R. The pathogenesis of atherosclerosis: a perspective for the 1990s. *Nature* 1993;362:801–809.

125. Fuster V, Corti R. Evolving concepts of atherothrombosis. In: Fuster V, ed. *Assessing and modifying the vulnerable atherosclerotic plaque.* Armonk, NY: Futura Publishing Company, 2002:1–27.

126. Fuster V, Fayad ZA, Badimon JJ. Acute coronary syndromes: biology. *Lancet* 1999;353[Suppl 2]:SII5–SII9.

127. Nakamura M, Takeshita A, Nose Y. Clinical characteristics associated with myocardial infarction, arrhythmias, and sudden death in patients with vasospastic angina. *Circulation* 1987;75:1110–1116.

128. Walling A, Waters DD, Miller DD, et al. Long-term prognosis of patients with variant angina. *Circulation* 1987;76:990–997.

129. Myerburg RJ, Kessler KM, Mallon SM, et al. Life-threatening ventricular arrhythmias in patients with silent myocardial ischemia due to coronary-artery spasm. *N Engl J Med* 1992;326:1451–1455.

130. Schroeder JS, Lamb IH, Bristow MR, et al. Prevention of cardiovascular events in variant angina by long-term diltiazem therapy. *J Am Coll Cardiol* 1983;1:1507–1511.

131. Pepine CJ, Feldman RL, Hill JA, et al. Clinical outcome after treatment of rest angina with calcium blockers: comparative experience during the initial year of therapy with diltiazem, nifedipine, and verapamil. *Am Heart J* 1983;106:1341–1347.

132. Flavahan NA, Shimokawa H, Vanhoutte PM. Pertussis toxin inhibits endothelium-dependent relaxations to certain agonists in porcine coronary arteries. *J Physiol (Lond)* 1989;408:549–560.

133. Shimokawa H, Flavahan NA, Vanhoutte PM. Natural course of the impairment of endothelium-dependent relaxations after balloon endothelium removal in porcine coronary arteries. Possible dysfunction of a pertussis toxin-sensitive G protein. *Circ Res* 1989;65:740–753.

134. Kawachi Y, Tomoike H, Maruoka Y, et al. Selective hypercontraction caused by ergonovine in the canine coronary artery under conditions of induced atherosclerosis. *Circulation* 1984;69:441–450.

135. Forman MB, Oates JA, Robertson D, et al. Increased adventitial mast cells in a patient with coronary spasm. *N Engl J Med* 1985;313:1138–1141.

136. Kalsner S, Richards R. Coronary arteries of cardiac patients are hyperreactive and contain stores of amines: a mechanism for coronary spasm. *Science* 1984;223:1435–1437.

137. Zeiher AM, Drexler H, Saurbier B, et al. Endothelium-mediated coronary blood flow modulation in humans. Effects of age, atherosclerosis, hypercholesterolemia, and hypertension. *J Clin Invest* 1993;92:652–662.

138. McFadden EP, Clarke JG, Davies GJ, et al. Effect of intracoronary serotonin on coronary vessels in patients with stable angina and patients with variant angina. *N Engl J Med* 1991;324:648–654.

139. Freedman SB, Chierchia S, Rodriguez-Plaza L, et al. Ergonovine-induced myocardial ischemia: no role for serotonergic receptors? *Circulation* 1984;70:178–183.

140. Chierchia S, Davies G, Berkenboom G, et al. Alpha-adrenergic receptors and coronary spasm: an elusive link. *Circulation* 1984;69:8–14.

141. Toyo-oka T, Aizawa T, Suzuki N, et al. Increased plasma level of endothelin-1 and coronary spasm induction in patients with vasospastic angina pectoris. *Circulation* 1991;83:476–483.

142. Zeiher AM, Ihling C, Pistorius K, et al. Increased tissue endothelin immunoreactivity in atherosclerotic lesions associated with acute coronary syndromes. *Lancet* 1994;344:1405–1406.

143. Winkles JA, Alberts GF, Brogi E, et al. Endothelin-1 and endothelin receptor mRNA expression in normal and atherosclerotic human arteries. *Biochem Biophys Res Commun* 1993;191:1081–1088.

144. Lerman A, Edwards BS, Hallett JW, et al. Circulating and tissue endothelin immunoreactivity in advanced atherosclerosis. *N Engl J Med* 1991;325:997–1001.

145. Boulanger CM, Tanner FC, Bea ML, et al. Oxidized low density lipoproteins induce mRNA expression and release of endothelin from human and porcine endothelium. *Circ Res* 1992;70:1191–1197.

146. Hahn AW, Resink TJ, Scott-Burden T, et al. Stimulation of endothelin mRNA and secretion in rat vascular smooth muscle cells: a novel autocrine function. *Cell Regul* 1990;1:649–659.

147. Rakugi H, Tabuchi Y, Nakamaru M, et al. Evidence for endothelin-1 release from resistance vessels of rats in response to hypoxia. *Biochem Biophys Res Commun* 1990;169:973–977.

148. Galle J, Bassenge E, Busse R. Oxidized low density lipoproteins potentiate vasoconstrictions to various agonists by direct interaction with vascular smooth muscle. *Circ Res* 1990;66:1287–1293.

149. Winniford MD, Filipchuk N, Hillis LD. Alpha-adrenergic blockade for variant angina: a long-term, double-blind, randomized trial. *Circulation* 1983;67:1185–1188.

150. Lange RA, Cigarroa RG, Yancy CW Jr, et al. Cocaine-induced coronary-artery vasoconstriction. *N Engl J Med* 1989;321:1557–1562.

151. Lüscher TF. Do we need endothelin antagonists? *Cardiovasc Res* 1993;27:2089–2093.

152. Taylor SH. Therapeutic targets in ischaemic heart disease. *Drugs* 1992;43:1–8.

153. Yusuf S, Held P, Furberg C. Update of effects of calcium antagonists in myocardial infarction or angina in light of the second Danish Verapamil Infarction Trial (DAVIT-II) and other recent studies. *Am J Cardiol* 1991;67:1295–1297.

154. Resnekov L, Chediak J, Hirsh J, et al. Antithrombotic agents in coronary artery disease. *Chest* 1989;95:52S–72S.

155. Lewis HD Jr, Davis JW, Archibald DG, et al. Protective effects of aspirin against acute myocardial infarction and death in men with unstable angina. Results of a Veterans Administration Cooperative Study. *N Engl J Med* 1983;309:396–403.

156. Cairns JA, Gent M, Singer J, et al. Aspirin, sulfinpyrazone, or both in unstable angina. Results of a Canadian multicenter trial. *N Engl J Med* 1985;313:1369–1375.

157. The RISC Group. Risk of myocardial infarction and death during treatment with low dose aspirin and intravenous heparin in men with unstable coronary artery disease. *Lancet* 1990;336:827–830.

158. Theroux P, Ouimet H, McCans J, et al. Aspirin, heparin, or both to treat acute unstable angina. *N Engl J Med* 1988;319:1105–1111.

159. Lichtlen PR, Hugenholtz PG, Rafflenbeul W, et al. Retardation of angiographic progression of coronary artery disease by nifedipine. Results of the International Nifedipine Trial on Antiatherosclerotic Therapy (INTACT). INTACT Group Investigators. *Lancet* 1990;335:1109–1113.

160. Loaldi A, Polese A, Montorsi P, et al. Comparison of nifedipine, propranolol and isosorbide dinitrate on angiographic progression and regression of coronary arterial narrowings in angina pectoris. *Am J Cardiol* 1989;64:433–439.

161. Henry PD, Bentley KI. Suppression of atherogenesis in cholesterol-fed rabbit treated with nifedipine. *J Clin Invest* 1981;68:1366–1369.

162. Chobanian AV, Haudenschild CC, Nickerson C, et al. Trandolapril inhibits atherosclerosis in the Watanabe heritable hyperlipidemic rabbit. *Hypertension* 1992;20:473–477.

163. Mishra SK, Hermsmeyer K. Selective inhibition of T-type Ca2+ channels by Ro 40-5967. *Circ Res* 1994;75:144–148.

164. Rosenthal SJ, Lamb IH, Schroeder JS, et al. Long-term efficacy of diltiazem for control of symptoms of coronary artery spasm. *Circ Res* 1983;52:I153–I157.

165. Johnson SM, Mauritson DR, Willerson JT, et al. A controlled trial of verapamil for Prinzmetal's variant angina. *N Engl J Med* 1981;304:862–866.

166. Turitto G, Pezzella A, Prati PL. [Diltiazem in spontaneous angina: comparison with nifedipine and verapamil]. *G Ital Cardiol* 1985;15:1079–1084.

167. Prida XE, Gelman JS, Feldman RL, et al. Comparison of diltiazem and nifedipine alone and in combination in patients with coronary artery spasm. *J Am Coll Cardiol* 1987;9:412–419.

168. Pepine CJ, Feldman RL, Whittle J, et al. Effect of diltiazem in pa-

tients with variant angina: a randomized double-blind trial. *Am Heart J* 1981;101:719–725.

169. The effect of diltiazem on mortality and reinfarction after myocardial infarction. The Multicenter Diltiazem Postinfarction Trial Research Group. *N Engl J Med* 1988;319:385–392.

170. The Danish Verapamil Infarction Trial II—DAVIT II: effect of verapamil on mortality and major events after acute myocardial infarction. *Am J Cardiol* 1990;66:779–785.

171. Brunton TL. On the use of nitrite of amyl in angina pectoris. *Lancet* 1867;II:97–98.

172. Feelisch M, Noack EA. Correlation between nitric oxide formation during degradation of organic nitrates and activation of guanylate cyclase. *Eur J Pharmacol* 1987;139:19–30.

173. Lüscher TF, Richard V, Yang Z. Interaction between endothelium-derived nitric oxide and SIN-1 in human and porcine blood vessels. *J Cardiovasc Pharmacol* 1989;14[Suppl 11]:S76–S80.

174. Dunne R, Pohl U, Mulsch A, et al. Modulation of the vasodilator action of SIN-1 by the endothelium. *J Cardiovasc Pharmacol* 1989;14[Suppl 11]:S81–S85.

175. Abrams J. Clinical aspects of nitrate tolerance. *Eur Heart J* 1991;12[Suppl E]:42–52.

176. Rudolf W, Dirschinger J. Clinical comparison of nitrates and sydnonimines. *Eur Heart J* 1991;12[Suppl E]:33–41.

177. Haynes WG, Webb DJ. Contribution of endogenous generation of endothelin-1 to basal vascular tone. *Lancet* 1994;344:852–854.

178. Brown MJ. Angiotensin receptor blockers in essential hypertension. *Lancet* 1993;342:1374–1375.

179. Brunner HR, Nussberger J, Burnier M, et al. Angiotensin II antagonists. *Clin Exp Hypertens* 1993;15:1221–1238.

180. Schamroth L. The clinical use of intravenous verapamil. *Am Heart J* 1980;100:1070–1075.

181. Joyal M, Feldman RL, Cremer K, et al. Systemic and coronary hemodynamic effects of combined intravenous diltiazem and nitroglycerin administration. *Am Heart J* 1987;113:1376–1382.

182. Masuda T, Ogawa H, Miyao Y, et al. Circadian variation in fibrinolytic activity in patients with variant angina. *Br Heart J* 1994;71:156–161.

183. Waters DD, Miller DD, Bouchard A, et al. Circadian variation in variant angina. *Am J Cardiol* 1984;54:61–64.

184. Kawano H, Motoyama T, Yasue H, et al. Endothelial function fluctuates with diurnal variation in the frequency of ischemic episodes in patients with variant angina. *J Am Coll Cardiol* 2002;40:266–270.

185. Katsumoto K, Niibori T. Prevention of coronary spasms during aortocoronary (A-C) bypass surgery for variant angina and effort angina with ST-elevation. *J Cardiovasc Surg (Torino)* 1988;29:343–348.

186. Kitamura S, Morita R, Kawachi K, et al. Different responses of coronary artery and internal mammary artery bypass grafts to ergonovine and nitroglycerin in variant angina. *Ann Thorac Surg* 1989;47:756–760.

187. Corcos T, David PR, Bourassa MG, et al. Percutaneous transluminal coronary angioplasty for the treatment of variant angina. *J Am Coll Cardiol* 1985;5:1046–1054.

188. Bertrand ME, LaBlanche JM, Thieuleux FA, et al. Comparative results of percutaneous transluminal coronary angioplasty in patients with dynamic versus fixed coronary stenosis. *J Am Coll Cardiol* 1986;8:504–508.

189. Pasceri V, Lanza GA, Patti G, et al. Preconditioning by transient myocardial ischemia confers protection against ischemia-induced ventricular arrhythmias in variant angina. *Circulation* 1996;94:1850–1856.

CHAPTER 43

Transplant Arteriosclerosis

David Gordon

Key Words: Adventitia; arteriosclerosis; artery; chronic rejection; endothelialitis; heart; lumen; lymphocyte; macrophage; smooth muscle cell; transplantation; transplant arteriosclerosis.

INTRODUCTION

Transplant arteriosclerosis is a diffuse and progressive thickening of the arterial intima that develops in the major and minor arteries of transplanted solid organs. Other commonly used synonyms for this disease include "graft arteriosclerosis," "accelerated atherosclerosis," "allograft arteriopathy," "transplant vasculopathy," and "chronic rejection." I prefer the term "transplant arteriosclerosis" because this refers to the specific arterial intimal lesions that develop in *transplanted* organs. In contrast, "graft arteriosclerosis" could also refer to the intimal thickening that occurs in bypass grafts (tissue and prosthetic grafts). Some authors have used "accelerated arteriosclerosis" to refer to bypass graft lesions and to the restenosis lesions that follow angioplasty. The term "chronic rejection" also encompasses other nonarterial lesions (e.g., loss of bile ducts and interstitial fibrosis in the liver, tubular atrophy, and interstitial fibrosis in the kidney).

Transplant arteriosclerotic lesions are progressive and frequently lead to severe arterial stenoses and occlusions. The result is sudden or progressive ischemic damage, or both, to

D. Gordon: Department of Pathology, University of Michigan, Ann Arbor, Michigan 48109.

the transplanted organ, with its eventual functional failure. This disease has become a major clinical problem with organ transplants, and at least for hearts, it is the major cause of graft failure (and too often patient death) 1 year after transplantation (1,2). This progressive disease occurs to variable degrees in all types of human solid organs that have been transplanted, including the heart, kidneys, liver, pancreas, and bowel. The pathology of this lesion is essentially the same in all of these organs, although quantitative differences may exist (e.g., lipid-laden foam cells appear to be more commonly seen in the arteries of transplanted livers) (3). This chapter refers to the arteriosclerosis that occurs in humans unrelated to transplantation, which is generally well modeled by animal models of hypercholesterolemia-induced arterial lesions, as "ordinary arteriosclerosis." Because several topographic and cellular similarities exist between transplant arteriosclerosis and ordinary arteriosclerosis, many of the theories and ideas concerning ordinary arteriosclerosis are now being applied to transplant arteriosclerosis (4,5). Finally, this clinical disease has been most heavily studied in reference to human heart transplants, probably because of causing sudden or eventual death of the affected patients, and given the lack of available transplant donors for retransplantation and the lack of suitable life-sustaining alternatives for the affected patients (unlike hemodialysis for unsuccessful renal transplants). Thus, this chapter focuses primarily on heart transplant arteriosclerosis, but also on the cell biology and pathology issues of this disease rather than on the detailed immunologic aspects. Several literature reviews of transplant arteriosclerosis are available (see References 4–14).

HUMAN PATHOLOGY

General Description and Cell Composition

Historically, transplant arteriosclerosis was first noticed in renal transplant patients, because kidney transplants were the first solid organ transplants generally performed (9,15). However, as transplants of other organs became more prevalent, this disease became a recognized clinical problem in all organ transplant areas. However, cell suspension transplants such as those of bone marrow do not appear to be associated with transplant arteriosclerosis, even in the face of recognized graft-versus-host disease (16–18).

Transplant arteriosclerosis has basically the same pathology in all affected transplant organs. In the heart, this manifests grossly as diffuse arterial narrowing that extends far down the arterial tree, involving second- and higher-order arterial branches, not just the epicardial coronary arteries, as is usually the case with ordinary arteriosclerosis. Thus, in addition to the surface epicardial coronary arteries, transplant arteriosclerosis also involves the penetrating intramyocardial branches. Histologic sections generally reveal a circumferentially uniform ("concentric") thickening of the intima that diffusely involves the affected arteries (Fig. 43–1) (see color insert). Although more prominent in size, its appearance is much like the diffuse intimal thickening that occurs normally in human epicardial coronary arteries (18–21) and may indeed be difficult to distinguish from the normal aging process in the earliest stages. Failure to appreciate diffuse intimal thickening as a normal aging process in the epicardial coronary arteries may lead to an overestimation of how soon after transplantation actual transplant arteriosclerosis starts. In humans, true early transplant arteriosclerosis is probably better appreciated in the penetrating intramyocardial arteries, which normally do not display such a prominent intima.

Despite the diffuse nature of transplant arteriosclerosis seen on angiography and in pathologic specimens, there is quite a variable degree of involvement within any one heart (and frequently on the same microscopic section), with some arteries of comparable size appearing normal and others only minimally diseased. This variability in arterial involvement has not been adequately explained, and I am not aware of any detailed topographic studies relating such lesions to the sites of features such as arterial branch points (as is the case for ordinary arteriosclerosis) (22). Animal models of heart transplants also frequently reveal a similar variable involvement of coronary arteries despite presumably all arterial branches being exposed to the same plasma and blood-borne cellular factors that might be responsible for this disease (Fig. 43–2) (see color insert).

Comparisons with Ordinary Arteriosclerosis

Similarities

A number of pathologic features exist in common between human transplant arteriosclerosis and human ordinary arteriosclerosis (4,6,9,23–31). These similarities and differences are summarized in Table 43–1. In regard to general topography, both processes primarily involve the arterial intima, causing its expansion. Although there may be variable fragmentation of the internal elastic lamina, this lamina is generally preserved in both lesion types, with relative sparing of the underlying media. Duplication and fragmentation of the internal elastica may be more common with ordinary arteriosclerosis. Both diseases also have variable numbers of inflammatory cells (lymphocytes, monocyte/macrophages) in the surrounding adventitia (3,32). Finally, with the possible exception of transplanted kidneys, there is generally a more prominent involvement of the proximal, large-, and medium-sized arteries, with decreasing involvement of third- and fourth-order branches down to the arteriole level (3). This is particularly the case with the heart, in which the epicardial coronary arteries and their first-order branches are the ones most likely to be affected, whereas the arterioles seen on endomyocardial biopsy are only rarely affected (23,32). Despite occasional reports (33), most investigators feel that the presence of signifi-

TABLE 43–1. *Comparison of pathologic features of ordinary arteriosclerosis with transplant arteriosclerosis in human organs*

Features	Ordinary arteriosclerosis	Transplant arteriosclerosis
Predilection for arterial branches	+++	−
Involves second- and third-order branches	+/−	+++
Concentric lesion morphology	+	+++
Eccentric lesion morphology	+++	+
Subendothelial inflammatory cell concentration	−	++
Fragmentation of the internal elastic lamina	++	+/−
Presence of necrotic core with cholesterol crystals	+++	+
Medial necrosis	+	+
Smooth muscle cells	+++	+++
Monocyte/macrophages	+++	+++
Foam cells	+++	+
T lymphocytes	+++	+++
B lymphocytes	+/−	+/−
Chronic inflammatory infiltrate in adventitia	+	++

cant cardiac transplant arteriosclerosis cannot be reliably detected on the basis of endomyocardial biopsy (2), and thus most heart transplant centers perform periodic coronary angiograms, with or without intravascular ultrasound studies, on their patients to detect this disease (14,34). Some endomyocardial biopsy findings such as focal vasculitis or arterial intimal thickening are believed by some to be predictive of later developing clinically significant transplant arteriosclerosis (33). Häyry and coworkers (13) reported that several biopsy findings can at least be statistically correlated with the prevalence of this disease, although the predictive value in the individual patient is not clear.

The similarities between ordinary arteriosclerosis and transplant arteriosclerosis at the cellular level are also striking (1,6,8,9,32,35–42). At the well developed, clinically significant stage, both types of human lesions are composed of numerous smooth muscle cells with their associated extracellular matrix elements (collagen, proteoglycans, and others). In addition, a significant population of monocyte/macrophages is present in both, and foam cells (macrophages with much lipid engorgement) also can be seen in both, especially if the transplant patient is hypercholesterolemic. Prominent foam cell intimal infiltrates also have been described with liver transplants (3). Significant populations of T lymphocytes are present in both, with a relative paucity of B lymphocytes (43). Finally, both lesions are also generally believed to be covered by luminal endothelial cells, although this is sometimes difficult to ascertain in human samples because of tissue acquisition artifacts. Certainly, focal breaks in the endothelial integrity, or in the fibrous cap, are thought to predispose to coronary thrombosis with ordinary coronary atherothrombosis, and thrombotic occlusions of transplant arteriosclerotic arteries certainly occur, often leading to silent myocardial infarcts in these patients with denervated hearts. Thus, from a cellular composition viewpoint, there are probably no significant *qualitative* differences between ordinary arteriosclerosis and transplant arteriosclerosis. This also has been borne out in animal models of these two diseases (hypercholesterolemia-induced atherothrombosis vs. transplanted heart or aortic arteriosclerosis; see later). Indeed, except for some mostly statistical and distributional differences described in the following section, the pathologist often is unable to distinguish transplant arteriosclerosis from ordinary arteriosclerosis on the basis of inspection of single artery sections alone.

Differences

Significant differences do exist in the morphology of ordinary arteriosclerosis versus transplant arteriosclerosis; however, these tend to be more quantitative than qualitative. Thus, as far as arterial topography is concerned, ordinary arteriosclerosis tends to involve the artery wall very focally and has a predilection for arterial branch points, particularly the low–shear stress regions just beyond and on the lateral aspects

of arterial branch bifurcations (22). Second- and third-order arterial branches and penetrating intramyocardial branches tend not to be involved. In contrast, for transplant arteriosclerosis most observers report no such branch point predilection. Instead, in humans and in animal models, the intimal involvement with transplant arteriosclerosis is described as being diffuse, often involving long segments of affected arteries, and extending into second- and third-order branches (3,6,23,44). The occasional finding of focal lesions in rat models of this disease (Fig. 43–2) suggests that focal transplant intimal lesions can be produced by a transplant environment (6,45,46).

On arterial cross sections, ordinary arteriosclerosis usually involves one part of the arterial wall circumference more heavily than other parts, producing prominent, "eccentric" lesions. In contrast, transplant arteriosclerosis is usually described as a diffuse, "concentric" intimal thickening involving the artery wall circumferentially (6,23,32). Although this generally is the case, there are certainly also numerous examples of "concentric" ordinary arteriosclerosis (47,48), and it is not uncommon to find prominent eccentric lesions in transplanted hearts. In the latter situation, there may be argument as to whether the "eccentric" transplant lesion represents transplant arteriosclerosis superimposed on a previously existing ordinary arteriosclerotic lesion. However, because usually it is not known what the pretransplant morphology was at such sites in humans, this hypothesis cannot be substantiated or disproved.

Finally, the features usually associated with complications of ordinary arteriosclerotic plaques—calcification, a large necrotic core with an overlying fibrous cap, neovascularization, and intraplaque hemorrhage—are generally absent from transplant arteriosclerotic lesions. Again, one can occasionally see such lesions in transplanted hearts, but the issue of the preexisting lesions at such sites remains. One potentially distinguishing feature is the occurrence in some (but not all) early transplant arteriosclerotic lesions of a marked concentration of lymphocytes and monocyte/macrophages in the immediate subendothelial space (Figs. 43–3 through 43–6) (see color insert). This prominent collection of mononuclear inflammatory cells has been termed "endothelialitis" by some investigators (43), although whether there is actual destruction or damage to the overlying endothelial cells suggesting that the inflammatory infiltrate is indeed directed toward the endothelium has not been clarified in human material (37). We have not seen this particular morphology in samples of ordinary atherothrombosis, and again it is not present in all cases of transplant arteriosclerosis.

CLINICAL RAMIFICATIONS OF TRANSPLANT ARTERIOSCLEROSIS

Incidence of the Human Disease

As a direct result of the orthotopic heart transplantation procedure in which the native heart is removed and a donor heart is sutured into its place, the new heart is necessarily denervated, because all of the nerve connections have been cut. Although some partial reinnervation is occasionally mentioned (14), most of these transplanted hearts remain functionally denervated for the lifetime of the graft (and patient). As a result, patients with significant transplant arteriosclerotic disease do not generally experience the common clinical warning symptom of angina that patients with ordinary coronary atherothrombosis experience (44). They are more likely to experience congestive heart failure (shortness of breath, fatigue, poor exercise tolerance) (14). However, such heart failure symptoms may also be produced by acute rejection of the myocardium or by fluid overload, particularly in patients with some degree of renal failure (e.g., from hypertension and cyclosporine effects). When these other disease processes are ruled out, the clinician may suspect significant transplant arteriosclerosis by exclusion. Unfortunately, sudden death may be the first distinct clinical manifestation of this disease.

Primarily for this reason, most transplant centers perform periodic coronary angiograms on heart transplant patients to assess this disease (44), making coronary transplant arteriosclerosis development far better studied clinically than that occurring in other solid organ transplants. From such serial angiographic studies, it has been estimated that the general incidence in transplant hearts increases approximately 10% per year after transplantation (11,13,49–51). At 5 years after transplantation, approximately half of the transplant hearts have some evidence of this disease (44,50,52). The angiographic description is usually one of very diffuse involvement along the courses of the major epicardial coronary arteries and their first-order branches. Pruning, obliteration, or both of smaller branches also is seen.

Unfortunately, angiography, which has been the mainstay of clinical assessments of coronary arterial narrowing for many years, is not by any means perfect and essentially provides an image of only the lumen and not the arterial wall components. Indeed, angiographic estimates of the onset and prevalence of transplant arteriosclerosis probably represent underestimates of the actual pathologically determined disease, primarily for three reasons. First, the earliest lesions are not angiographically detectable. Second, angiographic degrees of stenosis are usually based on comparisons with so-called normal coronary artery segments, and such segments often are difficult to find because of the diffuse nature of the disease, and undoubtedly many segments designated as normal are in fact narrowed (44). Indeed, this is a recognized problem even with ordinary arteriosclerosis (53). Quantitative angiographic measurements of lumen diameters, especially when there is a baseline angiogram for comparison, are an improvement in this regard. Third, as has been shown at least for ordinary coronary atherothrombosis, the artery wall is able to undergo a considerable amount of remodeling by expanding the contour of the media to maintain lumen dimensions in the face of an increasing volume of atherothrombotic intima (54,55). Thus, even quantitative angiography would be expected to underestimate the amount of intimal

disease seen by a pathologist on histologic examination. The extent to which such arterial remodeling occurs during the evolution of human transplant arteriosclerosis needs study. Finally, intravascular ultrasound can provide some information on lumen diameters and arterial layer dimensions and is an alternative technique for after the clinical development of this disease (34,44). It appears to be more sensitive than angiography in detecting early transplant arteriosclerosis, but it has other shortcomings such as being currently able to study only the more proximal, larger coronary artery branches (14). Studies using intravascular ultrasound generally corroborate the above angiographic impressions, indicating that significant disease starts developing during the first year of transplantation in many patients (14,34). As discussed earlier, however, even with ultrasound there may also be problems in identifying the onset of this disease; because in humans, variable degrees of progressive diffuse intimal thickening of at least the epicardial coronary arteries is a universal finding, even among nontransplanted and nonatherothrombotic hearts.

Finally, some investigators have demonstrated "endothelial dysfunction," defined as abnormal vasoreactivity in response to acetylcholine, in transplanted human hearts. This is thought to be caused by defective nitric oxide physiology in the arterial wall, similar to what is seen with ordinary arteriosclerotic arteries, and may be an early indication of this disease before clinically significant stenoses develop (56). However, this does not appear to be a routinely used method of the detection of this disease.

Risk Factors for Cardiac Transplant Arteriosclerosis

Several risk factors have been sought in relation to transplant arteriosclerosis (10,11,13). Indeed, many studies have shown no significant risk factor associations other than the survival time of the graft, as discussed earlier (11,43,57). With heart transplants, most are done either for end-stage ordinary coronary atherothrombotic disease or for idiopathic dilated cardiomyopathies (in which the coronary arteries are usually normal or only minimally affected by atherothrombosis). However, transplant arteriosclerosis appears in both groups of patients with similar incidence; thus, the original disease does not predict risk (6). Similarly, sex and age of the patient have not been well correlated with this disease (57); however, some have reported that the age of the *donor* heart may be related to disease development once this heart is transplanted (6,13,58). The degree of tissue mismatch also has been studied, and although some studies have suggested a relation between human leukocyte antigen (HLA) or ABO mismatch degree (58,59), others have found no such associations (6,35,57).

Because some of the transplanted patients have hypercholesterolemia, either endogenously or as a complication of immunosuppressive treatment, lipid profile factors that are risk factors for ordinary arteriosclerosis have been studied. This too is controversial, with some studies reporting that low-density lipoprotein (LDL) cholesterol correlates with the development of transplant arteriosclerosis (34), but with others finding no such strong association (6,57,60). Although foam cell macrophage infiltrates are occasionally described in human transplant arteriosclerotic lesions, on the basis of animal model studies, this may be more a case of coexisting hyperlipidemia giving a foam cell character to lesions that would likely develop anyway in the absence of hyperlipidemia (61–63). In rabbit models of transplant arteriosclerosis, hypercholesterolemia may exacerbate the disease in terms of the number and size of arterial lesions (64), but hypercholesterolemia is not a requirement for the development of this disease (61–63), as also evidenced by rat models of transplant arteriosclerosis that do not involve hypercholesterolemia (11–13). Transplant arteriosclerosis also develops in mouse models without hypercholesterolemia (65,66).

Some reports have suggested that the number of biopsy-demonstrated, acute cellular rejection episodes in the myocardium experienced by heart transplant patients correlated positively with the incidence of transplant arteriosclerosis (10,13,49,58,67). This is important because it may reflect suboptimal immunosuppressive control of acute cellular rejection, with a similar immunologic injury affecting the arteries. However, other studies have reported no such positive correlation between transplant arteriosclerosis and frequency of acute rejection episodes (10,23,56,68). Thus, this area remains controversial.

An interesting area of investigation has been the role of cytomegalovirus (CMV) infection. Several groups have reported striking positive correlations between the incidence of acute CMV viral infections (detected by increasing anti-CMV viral titers or by use of endomyocardial biopsies with immunocytochemical or polymerase chain reaction techniques) and transplant arteriosclerosis (13,44,57,69,70). This is of particular interest in view of previous work of Hajjar, the Fabricants, and others suggesting that herpes viruses also can be causative of ordinary arteriosclerosis (71–78). The potential roles played by CMV in the development of transplant arteriosclerosis have, however, not been elucidated, and few studies have found the CMV organism directly in involved arteries (70). Of interest, Häyry and colleagues (79,80) reported that a rat form of CMV induces platelet-derived growth factor (PDGF) gene expression associated with increased smooth muscle cell proliferation in their rat model of transplant arteriosclerosis. It should be noted that most of the general population has had previous exposure to CMV, and that many cases of active infection after transplantation probably reflect a resurgence of endogenous virus during immunosuppression, as opposed to truly new infections. It is also of interest that CMV infections have been correlated with the number of acute cellular rejection episodes, and it is unclear whether the positive association between rejection episodes and transplant arteriosclerosis reported by some investigators could have CMV infections as a basis. Thus, the causal role of CMV in transplant arteriosclerosis remains unclear.

Finally, some investigators have suggested that the loss of artery wall antithrombogenic features is a key event in the development of transplant arteriosclerosis, at least in transplanted human hearts. This is largely based on the positive association of the loss of microvascular plasminogen activator inhibitor-1, loss of vascular antithrombin, and the microvascular deposition of fibrin as seen in transplant monitoring endomyocardial biopsies, and the subsequent development of transplant arteriosclerosis in these same patients (68,81). Whether future treatments based on these ideas will prevent human transplant arteriosclerosis is unknown.

CELLULAR PATHOBIOLOGY AND EXPERIMENTAL STUDIES

Human Observational Studies

The sequence of cellular events in the development of the transplant arteriosclerotic lesion is less precisely described in humans than in animal models where the disease can be studied sequentially as it develops. However, here again, the general impression is that of an early inflammatory infiltration of the arterial intima by T lymphocytes and monocytes (Fig. 43–3), with later expansion of the intima by these cells. Subsequent increases in the smooth muscle and extracellular matrix components occur with time. Notably, early inflammatory infiltrates also are often seen in the arterial adventitia, which suggests that the adventitia may be an additional portal of entry of inflammatory cells into the artery wall (32). One confusing issue here is that the human coronary arteries normally start with some diffuse intimal thickening on which either ordinary arteriosclerosis or transplant arteriosclerosis occurs (18–21). This is unlike most animal models of this disease, which generally start with arteries with no significant numbers of preexisting intimal smooth muscle cells.

Animal Models Used

A number of animal models have been used to study transplant arteriosclerosis. Most of these have involved either the rat (11–13,82–86) or the rabbit (61,61,62,87–96). However, more recently, mouse models of this disease have been described (5,65,66,97,98). All of these model systems appear to reproduce the basic pathology of this lesion as seen in humans. Rats have probably been the most studied with respect to immune system mechanisms and have the advantage over rabbits of having several well defined and truly syngeneic strains. The rat, however, is not well suited for studies of the effects of hypercholesterolemia, at least compared with the rabbit or mouse. Rabbits appear to generate arterial lesions faster than rats but suffer somewhat from the decreased availability of reagents for study (e.g., cell type- and subtype-specific antibodies, cloned genes). They are, however, good for hypercholesterolemia studies as they are

with ordinary arteriosclerosis. The increased availability of transgenic mice and specific gene knockouts in the mouse have allowed many studies of transplant arteriosclerosis to be studied in detail in the mouse, particularly in elucidating molecular mechanisms and the importance of specific gene expressions in the evolution of this disease (5,65). Certainly the mouse has been the most heavily studied from a basic immunology viewpoint, and the availability of reagents for study is probably best with this species. The surgery for arterial or heart transplantation, however, is considerably more challenging in these small animals compared with rats and rabbits.

In all animal systems, two primary models of transplantation have been used. In *heterotopic heart transplantation* the recipient's heart is left *in situ,* and a donor heart is transplanted into the abdomen (or the neck). The groups led by Minick (61,96) and separately by Laden (99,100) were among the first to pursue transplant arteriosclerosis studies using these whole-heart transplantation systems. In this procedure, the donor heart's aorta is anastomosed to the abdominal aorta (or common carotid artery in the neck), the right atrial vena cava inflows are tied off, and for the transplanted heart's venous outflow, the pulmonary artery is anastomosed to the inferior vena cava (or jugular vein in the neck). Such hearts are thus perfused through their coronary arteries but, given their heterotopic nature, are not truly working hearts, because the recipient animal's own heart still supports the cardiac output for the whole animal. Whether this lack of "working heart" physiology has any bearing on the rate of development or character, or both, of transplant arteriosclerosis is unclear. However, such hearts certainly do develop transplant-associated arterial lesions. The left ventricular cavity, being a blind pouch with respect to blood flow, usually thromboses. Finally, most heart transplants in which significant histocompatibility differences exist between donor and recipient, require *some* sort of immunosuppression therapy to allow the heart to survive acute cellular rejection destruction long enough to develop significant arterial lesions (usually a few to several weeks of transplantation). Otherwise, uncontrolled acute rejection usually supervenes and destroys the heart within a few days.

With *straight arterial segment transplants* (86,97,101), a segment of artery (e.g., aorta) is anastomosed end-to-end to the arterial circulation, usually in the abdominal aortic position but sometimes in the common carotid position. The advantages of straight artery segment transplants over heart transplants include: (a) there is no whole organ to protect, and thus the sequence of cellular events can be studied in the absence of immunosuppressive therapy; (b) the straight segment allows for easier en face assessment of early leukocyte adhesion to the endothelial surface using techniques such as scanning electron microscopy, which is technically much more difficult in the curved and tortuous coronary arteries; (c) the straight segment allows for easier morphometric quantification of the area or volume of intimal thickening that develops, compared with the tortuous coronary arteries, which are frequently cut tangentially on tissue sections. As a result, much of the whole-heart transplant arteriosclerosis data are in the form of semiquantitative assessments of arterial involvement over different-sized arteries (e.g., "present/absent," percentage of vessels involved, or qualitative scores of degree of involvement); and (d) straight artery segments are more amenable to bulk biochemical studies of transplanted arterial tissue uncontaminated by surrounding organ tissue (e.g., RNA extraction for Northern blotting).

There are several disadvantages to using straight arterial segments. First, the commonly used straight segments are usually elastic arteries such as the aorta and not the more muscular arteries of the heart. Second, coronary flow patterns differ from straight artery segments and could conceivably have an effect on the development of transplant arteriosclerosis. Third, whole-heart preparations allow a comparison of the inflammatory events occurring at the artery wall with those occurring in the microvasculature and parenchymal cells of the transplanted organ. Although these models frequently use some immunosuppression, this is more analogous to the actual human situation in which all patients are on multidrug immunosuppression regimens. Finally, a potentially important difference that occurs in the straight artery segment models, but not to a significant degree in the whole-heart transplants, is a progressive loss of smooth muscle cells from the media of the transplanted segment, frequently with replacement by monocyte/macrophages (86,88,97,102). This finding has raised concern about the representative nature of such straight artery segments to the actual human disease. However, this loss of medial smooth muscle cells is generally reported when no immunosuppression is used and appears not to occur when immunosuppression with agents such as cyclosporine are used (103–105). In addition, some focal medial necrosis can be seen even in human cases on immunosuppression, although this may be called "vasculitis" as opposed to transplant arteriosclerosis (1,2,6,8,23,32). Because a prominent inflammatory infiltrate of the artery wall is clearly involved in the evolution of transplant arteriosclerosis, where "vasculitis" ends and "true transplant arteriosclerosis" begins is quite unclear. It is conceivable, however, that the development of transplant-associated intimal thickening may represent a balance between immune-mediated cell injury/death of arterial wall cells and arterial smooth muscle proliferation and extracellular matrix production. Intense vasculitic responses tend to promote arterial destruction without much proliferation, whereas more moderate rejection responses may allow the intimal proliferative and extracellular matrix aspects to predominate.

Cellular Sequence of Events

Despite the several different animal models and species used to study transplant arteriosclerosis, there is a general consensus on the cellular sequence of events. Most of the early sequence of events, as well as measures of cell proliferation, have necessarily come from animal experimental work, with some corroborative observations in human material. Although the general sequence of events here is the same

TRANSPLANT ARTERIOSCLEROSIS / 629

across various models, the times of occurrence vary depending on the model used (e.g., degree of immunologic mismatch) and on the type of immunosuppressive treatment (if any) used.

Endothelial Injury/Alteration

The earliest change after transplantation appears to be increased adhesion of mononuclear inflammatory cells to the luminal surface of the arterial endothelium. This has been shown most graphically by the scanning electron microscopy studies of Reidy and Bowyer (89,106) in which straight artery segments of rabbit aorta were transplanted. This early leukocyte adhesion becomes noticeable within 24 hours of transplantation, and a progressively increasing density of these cells is seen from that time onward. Morphologically, many of the cells appear to be monocytes and probably lymphocytes. As for the role of cell adhesion molecules, although this has been extensively studied in the myocardial and renal microvasculature during acute cellular rejection, there has been much less work done in the arteries. However, most relevant studies suggest an early increase in vascular cell adhesion molecule-1 and increased intercellular adhesion molecule-1 expression in such model systems (10,12,63,93,107). Both of these cell adhesion molecules are clearly relevant to the adhesion of lymphocytes and monocytes and probably play significant roles in this early leukocyte adhesion and entry, as they are believed to do with the initiation of ordinary arteriosclerosis (which has been suggested for the hypercholesterolemic rabbit model of ordinary arteriosclerosis) (108). In addition, some cell adhesion–blocking experiments in an attempt to inhibit transplant arteriosclerosis have shown a prolongation of heart graft survival from acute cellular rejection and some reduction in arterial involvement (92,109–111). When sought, upregulation of major histocompatibility complex (MHC) Class I antigens and early expression of MHC Class II antigens by the endothelium also are seen, as is Class II expression in transplanted artery smooth muscle (8,37,92,112).

These attached mononuclear inflammatory cells appear to migrate rapidly between the endothelial cells to gain access to the subendothelial space. This secondarily gives the endothelial surface an irregular contour, as seen on scanning electron microscopy (89), again not unlike that described for hypercholesterolemia models of ordinary arteriosclerosis (113,114). However, the fate of the allografted endothelium is much less clear. Although some human studies have mentioned that the arterial endothelium is (115) or is not damaged (37), this cannot be easily studied in human material, because good endothelial preservation for detailed study requires en face techniques and perfusion fixation, which is usually not possible with human samples. *Functional* endothelial damage may be an early change in humans based on endothelial dysfunction studies, and the degree of dysfunction may predict which patients are more likely to experience development of transplant arteriosclerosis (116). Some animal studies have indicated that focal or diffuse en-

dothelial damage does occur (83,91,117,118), but the majority of animal studies do not report significant, morphologic endothelial cell removal in transplanted arteries (46,63,93, 94,97,104,117,119). The presence of circulating antibodies to vimentin, an intracellular intermediate filament protein found in endothelial cells, has been suggested by some as evidence of endothelial injury in human heart transplants, and such circulating antibodies are correlated with the development of transplant arteriosclerosis (67). However, vimentin is not specific to endothelial cells and also is present in smooth muscle cells (120) and other cell types (121). More studies specifically looking at endothelial cell death and proliferation indices, as have been done for nontransplant animal studies (122 126), are needed.

Finally, studies that try to determine clearly whose endothelium (recipient or host) populates the luminal surface are few. A couple of human studies using either sex chromatin identification (in cases in which donor and recipient were of a different sex [35]) or specific anti-HLA antibodies (127) have suggested that whereas the inflammatory component in transplanted arteries is of recipient origin, most mesenchymal cells appear to be of allograft origin. However, these have not been of an appropriate resolution to address the origin of individual endothelial cells (could some be from the recipient, especially extending from the vascular anastomoses into the allograft vasculature?). It is perhaps hard to conceive of all of the allografted heart endothelium (arterial and microvascular) being destroyed and/or replaced and the heart remaining viable. Thus, although it is conceivable that, similar to hypercholesterolemia models of ordinary arteriosclerosis, the endothelium remains largely intact until either significant subendothelial deposits of cells or lesion complications such as thrombosis occur, or both, this area clearly needs much further investigation. As late events, severely stenosed arteries can become thrombosed, indicating either true endothelial loss or loss of the natural anticoagulant milieu of the artery wall in such diseased segments, similar to that described for transplanted microvasculature (68).

Intimal Expansion

The intima, which is usually just the potential space between the endothelium and the internal elastic lamina, soon becomes expanded by rapidly accumulating numbers of monocyte/macrophages and predominantly T lymphocytes. These progressively expand the intima by both a process of continued cellular influx and *in situ* proliferation as determined by thymidine labeling or other proliferation markers such as the proliferating cell nuclear antigen (Figs. 43–7 and 43–8) (see color insert) (13,86,97,100,128). This inflammatory cell proliferation is later followed by some proliferative activity among smooth muscle cells within the media, associated with subsequent migration of smooth muscle cells from the media into the intima. Once in the intima, these smooth muscle cells also continue to divide and begin elaborating extracellular matrix (including fibronectin and collagen), particularly in those intimal regions closest to the media. Thus, with time, the cellular character of the intima changes from a closely packed, inflammatory-rich cell mass to a later one enriched with smooth muscle cells, extracellular matrix, and a progressively decreasing cell density.

The time course of cell proliferation after transplantation has been best studied in the straight artery segment transplant models without immunosuppression (13,86,97,128) and appears to be self-limited, with peak proliferative indices occurring at approximately 15 to 30 days after transplantation, depending on the model. Notably, in our own studies (86) many of the proliferating cells did not mark with any of our available cell type markers and could therefore represent "dedifferentiated" smooth muscle cells or undefined cell types that are important to the development of this lesion. Thus, the overall pattern of smooth muscle proliferative activity has similarities to that described after mechanical injury to the artery wall in which there is a brief early burst of proliferative activity, followed by migration of cells into the intima and continued cell proliferation, followed by a prominent extracellular matrix synthesis and an expansion phase (129–131).

As mentioned earlier, despite transplant arteriosclerosis being viewed as a chronically progressive lesion ("chronic rejection"), the cell proliferation may be characterized by an initial self-limited burst of proliferative activity, followed by mostly extracellular matrix expansion in its later stages. Compared with the balloon injury rat carotid artery model, this transplant arteriosclerosis lesion develops over a longer period and has a much smaller peak in proliferative activity (6–7% of cells showing proliferative activity vs. 30–50% in the rat balloon injury model). But the sequence of early proliferation and later extracellular matrix expansion appears to be similar. This may have treatment implications if it can be shown that an abrogation of this early proliferative wave can inhibit this intimal thickening, just as has been shown for models of mechanical arterial injury.

Several types of extracellular matrix molecules are synthesized in transplant arteriosclerotic lesions, as is the case for ordinary arteriosclerosis development. This includes type I collagen, elastin, fibronectin, and probably several proteoglycans as being among the newly formed intimal matrix constituents. Clausell and coworkers (112) have drawn attention to the importance of endogenously synthesized fibronectin in pig and rabbit models of transplant arteriosclerosis. This molecule appears to have chemotactic activity for monocyte/macrophages and smooth muscle cells, and thus may serve to attract and trap both cell types within the developing neointima (112).

Finally, the growth factors that presumably drive this proliferative activity of inflammatory cells and smooth muscle cells are not fully known. However, several growth factors have been described as having a potential role. In human transplant arteriosclerosis lesions, we have seen intimal immunoreactivity for basic fibroblast growth factor (132) and the B form of PDGF. Other authors also have found evidence for other growth factors in transplant arteriosclerotic lesions, including PDGF, interleukin-1, and tumor necrosis factor (12,13,63,112). As with ordinary atherothrombosis development, there is proliferative activity among both smooth muscle elements and at least monocyte/macrophage elements (Figs. 43–7 and 43–8) (101), suggesting that both smooth muscle and inflammatory cell growth factors are involved.

Adventitial Alterations

The adventitia also develops a chronic inflammatory infiltrate after transplantation. This is seen in hearts (63) and is particularly prominent in straight artery segment transplants (86). The minimal-to-absent chronic inflammatory infiltrate in the adventitia associated with isografts further indicates that such lymphocyte and monocyte/macrophage infiltration of the adventitia is indeed transplant mediated and not simply a reaction to the trauma of surgery. With time, as the intima is being infiltrated by similar inflammatory cells, penetration of the media from the adventitia also is seen. Thus, at least for arteries, the transplant-associated cellular immune response appears to have two portals of entry into the artery wall: (a) through the surface endothelium and (b) through the adventitia. Although the adventitia is a relatively neglected area in both ordinary atherothrombosis and transplant arteriosclerosis studies, we have certainly seen prominent proliferative activity and type I collagen gene expression in this region (unpublished observations). Progressive scarring of the adventitia could conceivably affect arterial wall compliance and possibly interfere with the kind of compensatory dilatation described for ordinary arteriosclerosis to minimize encroachment on the lumen (5).

Medial Changes

In most heart models of transplant arteriosclerosis, the media is described as relatively undisturbed save for focal breaks in the internal elastica. However, as mentioned earlier, some human hearts do show focal destruction of the media or replacement by inflammatory cells and fibrosis, or both. In the straight artery segment models of transplant arteriosclerosis, if no immunosuppression is given, progressive necrosis of the media with loss of smooth muscle elements and often replacement by inflammatory cells is seen. This may lead to some degree of arterial dilatation (86). As discussed earlier, this is frequently prevented by immunosuppression (e.g., cyclosporine), which is usually used for the heart transplants.

Immunologic Aspects

A historical debate that remains is whether transplant arteriosclerosis is the result of primarily a humoral or a cell-mediated immunologic attack on the arterial wall. The similarity between these lesions and those induced experimentally in the arteries of serum sickness models (e.g., studies by Minick and coworkers [133–135] in which bovine serum albumin was injected into rabbits, with or without coincident hypercholesterolemia) would argue for a humorally-mediated arm. Support for this view also comes from the observations that immunosuppressive treatments such as cyclosporine, which are successful in treating cellular rejection, generally do not prevent transplant arteriosclerosis (46,49,103,105), although some inhibition of transplant arteriosclerosis with cyclosporine has been reported in rabbits (90). Some agents such as Imuran, which are better at inhibiting the humoral immune response, can reportedly inhibit transplant arteriosclerosis (99). Finally, as mentioned previously, in humans, there does not appear to be a good correlation between HLA mismatch and the development of cardiac transplant arteriosclerosis.

Arguments in favor of a primary role of the cell-mediated response include the identification of numerous activated T cells and up-regulation of MHC Class II expression within the transplanted arterial wall (3,8,12,36,37,37,43,63,86,92, 97,103,107,112,136,137). In addition, studies in rats in which the degree of MHC mismatch has been varied have been done at least for whole-heart transplants. However, here the complication appears to be survival of the myocardium from cellular rejection for a long enough period that one can see the later arterial changes (11,82). Thus, many such heart transplant models use minimal MHC differences and do not truly answer the question. Also, treatments that can inhibit cellular rejection do not necessarily also prevent transplant arteriosclerosis (e.g., transforming growth factor-β gene expression in a mouse heart transplant model [65], or tolerance induction because of CD40 ligand deficiency [66]). Further elucidation of the immunologic mechanisms of transplant arteriosclerosis is forthcoming from genetically engineered mouse studies (5,66), just as they have been used to discern the cellular immune components necessary for myocardial rejection (138–140).

Finally, rather than the above cellular versus humoral immunity paradigm debate, studies have suggested that different cellular immune responses may be at play. The parenchymal rejection that leads to myocyte cell loss appears to be mediated by cytolytic killer T cells working through Class I histocompatibility antigens. By contrast, the transplant arteriosclerosis development is more typified by a helper T cell–mediated and cytokine/growth factor–mediated mechanism, working through Class II histocompatibility antigens (4).

TREATMENT

Currently, short of retransplantation, there are no specific clinical treatments for transplant arteriosclerosis causing transplant organ failure. As discussed earlier, although modern immunosuppressive therapy is quite effective in controlling cellular rejection of the organ parenchyma, this has not significantly decreased the incidence of transplant arteriosclerosis. Because of the marked disparity between the demand for transplanted organs and their supply, this remains a critical problem. For heart transplant patients, this often means death of the patient while waiting for a second donor, and discussions continue on the ethics of providing a failing transplant patient with a second donor heart, often at the expense of providing that same donor heart to a needy individual who has not yet had the chance for survival through transplantation. Thus, effective treatments are being actively sought.

Except in selected cases, angioplasty (with or without stenting) or bypass surgery is generally not efficacious in treating the resultant coronary artery insufficiency, because given the usually diffuse distribution of the disease involvement of the coronary arterial tree, there is usually no good distal coronary artery with which to link (14). Interestingly, treatment with 3-hydroxy-3-methylglutaryl coenzyme A reductase inhibitors (or "statin" drugs) such as pravastatin (141) and simvastatin (142,143) have shown some promise in lessening the development and progression of this disease. There is evidence that hypercholesterolemia can act synergistically with the arterial immune reactions to promote transplant arteriosclerosis (64,101). However, the extent to which the efficacy of "statin" drugs is because of the reduction of plasma cholesterol levels including LDL cholesterol is not clear (141–143), because there is evidence of an antiinflammatory/immunosuppressive effect of these drugs as well (141,144), in addition to other properties that may inhibit arterial intimal thickening.

Some additional potential treatments also have been reported in animal model studies. Foegh and colleagues (91, 117) reported that the administration of estrogens to a rabbit straight artery segment model could reduce the amount of transplant intimal thickening seen. This is interesting in light of the lack of a sex predilection for this disease. These same investigators also reported that a somatostatin analog, Angiopeptin, can inhibit transplant intimal thickening (145, 146). Other authors have reported that whereas cyclosporine A alone does not have much inhibitory effect on a rat model of transplant arteriosclerosis, when used in combination with low–molecular weight heparin, it can inhibit transplant intimal thickening (46,105). Whether any of these treatments will gain clinical applicability currently is unclear.

Many of the proposed treatments have been aimed at inhibiting smooth muscle proliferation. The early burst in cell proliferation and subsequent phase of extracellular matrix synthesis may have important treatment ramifications in that inhibition of these rather early processes could conceivably inhibit the progressive intimal thickening seen in "chronic rejection." Perhaps self-limited treatments that abrogate early arterial wall proliferation, such as thymidine kinase gene expression with ganciclovir administration, may soon prove effective in this regard, similar to their demonstrated effectiveness in reducing intimal thickening after arterial injury (101,147). Similarly, increased focus should be directed at separately inhibiting the extracellular matrix synthesis phase of this disease.

FUTURE DIRECTIONS

As highlighted earlier, although a great deal has been learned about human and animal models of transplant arteriosclerosis, several unresolved issues remain with respect to how this disease develops. In humans and in rat hearts, the lesions are frequently spotty, as seen on histologic sections. Are there specific anatomic predilections? Could a superimposed injury such as ischemia/reperfusion at the time of transplantation act synergistically with allograft immune rejection to account for some of this focal nature and to exacerbate transplant arteriosclerosis? Most investigators have found no correlation between human donor heart ischemic time and who experiences development of the disease (11,148). However, all such hearts are necessarily ischemic to some degree, and at least one investigator has presented rat data in favor of such a synergism (149). Several growth factors have been identified in transplanted arterial tissue, but their direct correlation with ongoing cell proliferation needs to be determined. In addition, specific blocking experiments are needed to test their significance, as has been done for mechanical injury models of intimal thickening. Similar studies need to be done to elucidate the controls of extracellular matrix synthesis and to clarify the roles of specific cytokines in this disease.

The nature of solid organ transplantation, specifically placing the organ in a holding solution before transplantation, would seem to be particularly amenable to gene transfer methods aimed at immunosuppression or inhibition of the proliferative events leading to arterial occlusion. It is hoped that further elucidation of the growth factors and cytokines involved will help in this endeavor and open the way for more localized treatment of transplant patients without many of the systemic effects of current immunosuppressive therapy.

REFERENCES

1. Uys CJ, Rose AG. Pathologic findings in long-term cardiac transplants. *Arch Pathol Lab Med* 1984;108:112–116.
2. Chomette G, Auriol M, Cabrol C. Chronic rejection in human heart transplantation. *J Heart Transplant* 1988;7:292–297.
3. Demetris AJ, Zerbe T, Banner B. Morphology of solid organ allograft arteriopathy: identification of proliferating intimal cell populations. *Transplant Proc* 1989;21:3667–3669.
4. Libby P, Zhao DX. Allograft arteriosclerosis and immune-driven angiogenesis. *Circulation* 2003;107:1237–1239.
5. Libby P, Pober JS. Chronic rejection. *Immunity* 2001;14:387–397.
6. Billingham ME. Cardiac transplant atherosclerosis. *Transplant Proc* 1987;19:19–25.
7. Libby P, Salomon RN, Payne DD, et al. Functions of vascular wall cells related to development of transplantation-associated coronary arteriosclerosis. *Transplant Proc* 1989;21:3677–3684.
8. Schoen FJ, Libby P. Cardiac transplant graft arteriosclerosis. *Trends Cardiovasc Med* 1991;1:216–223.
9. Vollmer E, Roessner A. Renal transplant arteriopathy: similarities to atherosclerosis. In: Robenek H, Severs NJ, eds. *Cell interactions in atherosclerosis*. Boca Raton, FL: CRC Press, 1992:71–100.
10. Tilney NL, Whitley WD, Diamond JR, et al. Chronic rejection: an undefined conundrum. *Transplant* 1991;52:389–398.
11. Cramer DV. *Graft arteriosclerosis in heart transplantation*. Austin, TX: R.G. Landes Company, 1993:1–95.
12. Adams DH, Russell ME, Hancock WW, et al. Chronic rejection in experimental cardiac transplantation: studies in the Lewis-F344 model. *Immunological Rev* 1993;134:5–19.
13. Häyry P, Isoneimi H, Yilmaz S, et al. Chronic allograft rejection. *Immunological Rev* 1993;134:33–81.
14. Aranda JM, Hill J. Cardiac transplant vasculopathy. *Chest* 2000;118;1792–1800.
15. Hume DM, Merrill JP, Miller BF, et al. Experiences with renal homotransplantation in the human: report of nine cases. *J Clin Invest* 1955;34:327–382.
16. Sale GE. Bone marrow and thymic transplantation. In: Sale GE, ed. *The Pathology of organ transplantation*. Boston: Butterworths, 1990:229–259.
17. Armitage JO. Bone marrow transplantation. *N Engl J Med* 1994;330:827–838.
18. Stary HC. Macrophages, macrophage foam cells, and eccentric intimal thickening in coronary arteries of young children. *Atherosclerosis* 1987;64:91–108.
19. Velican C, Velican D. Intimal thickening in developing coronary arteries and its relevance to atherosclerotic involvement. *Atherosclerosis* 1976:23:345–355.
20. Hartman JD. Structural changes within the media of coronary arteries related to intimal thickening. *Am J Pathol* 1977;89:13–34.
21. Sims FH. A comparison of coronary and internal mammary arteries and implications of the results in the etiology of arteriosclerosis. *Am Heart J* 1983;105:560–566.
22. Glagov S, Zarins C, Giddens DP, et al. Hemodynamics and atherosclerosis. Insights and perspectives gained from studies of human arteries. *Arch Pathol Lab Med* 1988;112:1018–1031.
23. Rose AG, Viviers L, Odell JA. Pathology of chronic cardiac rejection: an analysis of the epicardial and intramyocardial coronary arteries and myocardial alterations in 43 human allografts. *Cardiovasc Pathol* 1993;2:7–19.
24. McGill HC. Persistent problems in the pathogenesis of atherosclerosis. *Arteriosclerosis* 1984;4:443–451.
25. Wissler RW. The evolution of the atherosclerotic plaque and its complications. In: Connor WE, Bristow JD, eds. *Coronary heart disease*. Philadelphia: JB Lippincott, 1985:193–214.
26. Ross R. The pathogenesis of atherosclerosis—an update. *N Engl J Med* 1986;314:488–500.
27. Velican C, Velican D. Natural history of coronary atherosclerosis as related to age. In: Velican C, Velican D, eds. *Natural history of coronary atherosclerosis*. Boca Raton, FL: CRC Press, 1989:279–352.
28. Stary HC. The sequence of cell and matrix changes in atherosclerotic lesions of coronary arteries in the first forty years of life. *Eur Heart J* 1990:11[Suppl E]:3–19.
29. Libby P, Hansson GK. Involvement of the immune system in human atherogenesis: current knowledge and unanswered questions. *Lab Invest* 1991;64:5–15.
30. Ross R. The pathogenesis of atherosclerosis: a perspective for the 1990s. *Nature* 1993;362:801–809.
31. Davies MJ, Woolf N. Atherosclerosis: what is it and why does it occur? *Br Heart J* 1993;69[Suppl]:S3–S11.
32. Gravanis MB. Allograft heart accelerated atherosclerosis: evidence for cell-mediated immunity in pathogenesis. *Mod Pathol* 1989;2:495–505.
33. Palmer DC, Tsai CC, Roodman ST, et al. Heart graft arteriosclerosis: an ominous finding on endomyocardial biopsy. *Transplant* 1985;39:385–388.
34. Progression of cardiac allograft vascular disease as assessed by serial intravascular ultrasound: correlation to immunological and nonimmunological risk factors. *Heart* 2000;84:494–498.
35. Beiber CP, Stinson EB. Cardiac transplantation in man. VII. Cardiac allograft pathology. *Circulation* 1970;41:753–772.
36. Oguma S, Banner B, Zerbe T, et al. Participation of dendritic cells in vascular lesions of chronic rejection of human allografts. *Lancet* 1988;2(8617):933–936.
37. Salomon RN, Hughes CC, Schoen FJ, et al. Human coronary transplantation-associated arteriosclerosis: evidence for a chronic immune reaction to activated graft endothelial cells. *Am J Pathol* 1991;138:791–798.
38. Jahn L, Kreuzer J, von Hodenberg E, et al. Cytokeratins 8 and 18 in smooth muscle cells: detection in human coronary artery, peripheral

vascular, and vein graft disease and in transplantation-associated arteriosclerosis. *Arterioscler Thromb* 1993;13:1631–1639.
39. Hansson GK, Jonasson L, Holm J, et al. Class II MHC antigen expression in the atherosclerotic plaque: smooth muscle cells express HLA-DR, HLA-DQ and the invariant gamma chain. *Clin Exp Immunol* 1986;64:261–268.
40. Gown AM, Tsukada T, Ross R. Human atherosclerosis. II. Immunocytochemical analysis of the cellular composition of human atherosclerotic lesions. *Am J Pathol* 1986;125:191–207.
41. Hansson GK, Holm J, Jonasson L. Detection of activated T lymphocytes in the human atherosclerotic plaque. *Am J Pathol* 1989;135:169–175.
42. Katsuda S, Coltrera MD, Ross R, et al. Human atherosclerosis: IV. Immunocytochemical analysis of cell activation and proliferation in lesions of young adults. *Am J Pathol* 1993;142:1787–1793.
43. Hruban RH, Beschorner WE, Baumgartner WA, et al. Accelerated arteriosclerosis in heart transplant recipients is associated with a T-lymphocyte-mediated endothelialitis. *Am J Pathol* 1990;137:871–882.
44. Schroeder JS, Gao S, Hunt SA, et al. Accelerated graft coronary artery disease: diagnosis and prevention. *J Heart Lung Transplant* 1992;11:S258–S266.
45. Sarris GE, Mitchell RS, Billingham ME, et al. Inhibition of accelerated cardiac allograft arteriosclerosis by fish oil. *J Thorac Cardiovasc Surg* 1989;97:841–855.
46. Aziz S, Tada Y, Gordon D, et al. A reduction in accelerated graft coronary disease and an improvement in cardiac allograft survival using low molecular weight heparin in combination with cyclosporine. *J Heart Lung Transplant* 1993;12:634–643.
47. Freudenberg H, Lichtlen PR. The normal wall segment in coronary stenosis—a postmortem study. *Z Kardiol* 1981;70:863–869.
48. Wissler RW, Vesselinovitch D. Atherosclerosis: relationship to coronary blood flow. *Am J Cardiol* 1983;52:2a–7a.
49. Uretsky BF, Murali S, Reddy PS, et al. Development of coronary artery disease in cardiac transplant patients receiving immunosuppressive therapy with cyclosporine and prednisone. *Circulation* 1987;76:827–834.
50. Paul LC. Chronic rejection of organ allografts: magnitude of the problem. *Transplant Proc* 1993;25:2024–2025.
51. Gao SZ, Schroeder JS, Alderman EL, et al. Clinical and laboratory correlates of accelerated coronary artery disease in the cardiac transplant patient. *Circulation* 1987;76:V56–V61.
52. Pascoe EA, Barnhart GR, Carter WH, et al. The prevalence of cardiac allograft arteriosclerosis. *Transplant* 1987;44:838–839.
53. Roberts WC. Coronary heart disease: a review of abnormalities observed in the coronary arteries. *Cardiovasc Med* 1977;2:29–48.
54. Glagov S, Weisenberg E, Zarins CK, et al. Compensatory enlargement of human atherosclerotic coronary arteries. *N Engl J Med* 1987;316:1371–1375.
55. Clarkson TB, Prichard RW, Morgan TM, et al. Remodeling of coronary arteries in human and nonhuman primates. *JAMA* 1994;271:289–294.
56. Fish RD, Nabel EG, Selwyn AP, et al. Responses of coronary arteries of cardiac transplant patients to acetylcholine. *J Clin Invest* 1987;81:21–31.
57. McDonald K, Rector TS, Braunlin EA, et al. Association of coronary artery disease in cardiac transplant recipients with cytomegalovirus infection. *Am J Cardiol* 1989;64:359–362.
58. Almond PS, Matas AJ, Gillingham K, et al. Predictors of chronic rejection in renal transplant recipients. *Transplant Proc* 1993;25:936.
59. Nakatani T, Aida H, Frazier OH, et al. Effect of ABO blood type on survival of heart transplant patients treated with cyclosporine. *J Heart Transplant* 1989;8:27–33.
60. Hess MJ, Hatillo A, Mohanakumar T, et al. Accelerated atherosclerosis in cardiac transplantation: role of cytotoxic B-cell antibodies and hyperlipidemia. *Circulation* 1983;68[Suppl II]:II-94–II-101.
61. Alonso DR, Starek PK, Minick CR. Studies on the pathogenesis of atheroarteriosclerosis induced in rabbit cardiac allografts by the synergy of graft rejection and hypercholesterolemia. *Am J Pathol* 1977;87:415–442.
62. Laden AM. Experimental atherosclerosis in rat and rabbit cardiac allografts. *Arch Pathol* 1972;93:240–245.
63. Tanaka H, Sukhova GK, Libby P. Interaction of the allogeneic state and hypercholesterolemia in arterial lesion formation in experimental cardiac allografts. *Arterioscler Thromb* 1994;14:734–745.
64. Interaction of the allogeneic state and hypercholesterolemia in arterial lesion formation in experimental cardiac allografts. *Arterioscler Thromb Vasc Biol* 1994;14:734–745.
65. Chan SY, Goodman RE, Szmuszkovicz JR, et al. DNA-liposome versus adenoviral mediated gene transfer of transforming growth factor β1 in vascularized cardiac allografts: differential sensitivity of CD4+ and CD8+ cells to transforming growth factor β1. *Transplantation* 2000;70:1292–1301.
66. Shimizu K, Schöenbeck U, Mach F, et al. Host CD40 ligand deficiency induces long-term allograft survival and donor-specific tolerance in mouse cardiac transplantation but does not prevent graft arteriosclerosis. *J Immunol* 2000;165:3506–3518.
67. Jurcevic S, Ainsworth ME, Pomerance A, et al. Antivimentin antibodies are an independent predictor of transplant-associated coronary artery disease after cardiac transplantation. *Transplantation* 2001;71:886–892.
68. Labarrere CA, Nelson DR, Park J. Pathologic markers of allograft arteriopathy: insight into the pathophysiology of cardiac allograft chronic rejection. *Curr Opin Cardiol* 2001;16:110–117.
69. Grattan MT, Moreno Cabral CE, Starnes VA, et al. Cytomegalovirus infection is associated with cardiac allograft rejection and atherosclerosis. *JAMA* 1989;261:3561–3566.
70. Wu T, Hruban RH, Ambinder RF, et al. Demonstration of cytomegalovirus nucleic acids in the coronary arteries of transplanted hearts. *Am J Pathol* 1992;140:739–747.
71. Hajjar DP. Viral pathogenesis of atherosclerosis: impact of molecular mimicry and viral genes. *Am J Pathol* 1991;139:1195–1211.
72. Hajjar DP, Pomerantz KB, Falcone DJ, et al. Herpes simplex virus infection in human arterial cells: implications in arteriosclerosis. *J Clin Invest* 1987;80:1317–1321.
73. Melnick JL, Dreesman GR, McCollum CH, et al. Cytomegalovirus antigen within human arterial smooth muscle cells. *Lancet* 1983;2:644–647.
74. Yamashiroya HM, Ghosh L, Yang R, et al. Herpesviridae in the coronary arteries and aorta of young trauma victims. *Am J Pathol* 1988;130:71–79.
75. Melnick JL, Adam E, DeBakey ME. Possible role of cytomegalovirus in atherogenesis. *JAMA* 1990;263:2204–2207.
76. Hendrix MG, Salimans MM, van Boven CP, et al. High prevalence of latently present cytomegalovirus in arterial walls of patients suffering from grade III atherosclerosis. *Am J Pathol* 1990;136:23–28.
77. Benditt EP, Barrett T, McDougall JK. Viruses in the etiology of atherosclerosis. *Proc Natl Acad Sci USA* 1983;80:6386–6389.
78. Hendrix MG, Dormans PH, Kitslaar P, et al. The presence of cytomegalovirus nucleic acids in arterial walls of atherosclerotic and nonatherosclerotic patients. *Am J Pathol* 1989;134:1151–1157.
79. Lemström KB, Bruning JH, Bruggeman CA, et al. Cytomegalovirus infection enhances smooth muscle cell proliferation and intimal thickening of rat aortic allografts. *J Clin Invest* 1993;92:549–558.
80. Lemström KB, Aho PT, Bruggeman CA, et al. Cytomegalovirus infection enhances mRNA expression of platelet-derived growth factor-BB and transforming growth factor-beta 1 in rat aortic allografts: possible mechanism for cytomegalovirus-enhanced graft arteriosclerosis. *Arterioscler Thromb* 1994;14:2043–2052.
81. Labarrere CA, Torry RJ, Nelson DR, et al. Vascular antithrombin and clinical outcome in heart transplant patients. *Am J Cardiol* 2001;87:425–431.
82. Cramer DV, Qian S, Harnaha J, et al. Cardiac transplantation in the rat. I. The effect of histocompatibility differences on graft arteriosclerosis. *Transplant* 1989;47:414–419.
83. Laden AM, Sinclair RA. Thickening of arterial intima in rat cardiac allografts. *Am J Pathol* 1971;63:69–84.
84. Lurie KG, Billingham ME, Jamieson SW, et al. Pathogenesis and prevention of graft arteriosclerosis in an experimental heart transplant model. *Transplant* 1981;31:41–47.
85. Halttunen J, Partanen T, Leszczynski D, et al. Rat aortic allografts: a model for chronic vascular rejection. *Transplant Proc* 1990;22:125.
86. Isik FF, McDonald TO, Ferguson M, et al. Transplant arteriosclerosis in a rat aortic model. *Am J Pathol* 1992;141:1139–1149.
87. Sasaguri S, Tsukada T, Hosoda Y. Immunocytochemical investigations of vessel allograft arteriosclerosis using smooth muscle cell- and macrophage-specific monoclonal antibodies. *Transplant* 1990;50:898–901.

88. Reddy GS, Cliff WJ. Morphologic changes in arterial grafts in rabbit ears. *Lab Invest* 1979;40:109–121.
89. Bowyer DE, Reidy MA. Scanning electron microscope studies of the endothelium of aortic allografts in the rabbit: morphological observations. *J Pathol* 1977;123:237–245.
90. Andersen HO, Madsen G, Nordestgaard BG, et al. Cyclosporin suppresses transplant arteriosclerosis in the aorta-allografted, cholesterol-clamped rabbit: suppression preceded by decrease in arterial lipoprotein permeability. *Arterioscler Thromb* 1994;14:944–950.
91. Cheng LP, Kuwahara M, Jacobson J, et al. Inhibition of myointimal hyperplasia and macrophage infiltration by estradiol in aorta allografts. *Transplant* 1991;52:967–972.
92. Sadahiro M, McDonald TO, Allen MD. Reduction in cellular and vascular rejection by blocking leukocyte adhesion molecule receptors. *Am J Pathol* 1993;142:675–683.
93. Tanaka H, Sukhova GK, Swanson SJ, et al. Endothelial and smooth muscle cells express leukocyte adhesion molecules heterogeneously during acute rejection of rabbit cardiac allografts. *Am J Pathol* 1994;144:938–951.
94. Eich DM, Nestler JE, Johnson DE, et al. Inhibition of accelerated coronary atherosclerosis with dehydroepiandrosterone in the heterotopic rabbit model of cardiac transplantation. *Circulation* 1993;87:261–269.
95. Hjelms E, Stender S. Accelerated cholesterol accumulation in homologous arterial transplants in cholesterol-fed rabbits: a surgical model to study transplantation atherosclerosis. *Arteriosol Thromb* 1992;12:771–779.
96. Minick CR, Murphy GE. Immunologic injury and atherosclerosis. *Adv Exp Med Biol* 1974;43:355–376.
97. Shi C, Russell ME, Bianchi C, et al. Murine model of accelerated transplant arteriosclerosis. *Circ Res* 1994;75:199–207.
98. Russell PS, Chase CM, Winn HJ, et al. Coronary atherosclerosis in transplanted mouse hearts: III. Effects of recipient treatment with a monoclonal antibody to interferon-γ. *Transplant* 1994;57:1367–1371.
99. Laden AM. The effects of treatment on the arterial lesions of rat and rabbit cardiac allografts. *Transplant* 1972;13:281–290.
100. Laden AM. Autoradiographic evidence for the origin of cells constituting arterial intimal thickening in experimental cardiac allografts. *J Reticuloendothelial Soc* 1972;11:524–533.
101. Graft permeabilization facilitates gene therapy of transplant arteriosclerosis in a rabbit model. *Circulation* 1998;98:1335–1341.
102. Häyry P, Mennander A, Tiisala S, et al. Rat aortic allografts: an experimental model for chronic transplant arteriosclerosis. *Transplant Proc* 1991;23:611–612.
103. Schmitz-Rixen T, Megerman J, Colvin RB, et al. Immunosuppressive treatment of aortic allografts. *J Vasc Surg* 1988;7:82–92.
104. Mennander A, Paavonen T, Häyry P. Intimal thickening and medial necrosis in allograft arteriosclerosis (chronic rejection) are independently regulated. *Arterioscler Thromb* 1993;13:1019–1025.
105. Plissonnier D, Amichot G, Lecagneux J, et al. Additive and synergistic effects of a low-molecular-weight, heparin-like molecule and low doses of cyclosporin in preventing arterial graft rejection in rats. *Arterioscler Thromb* 1993;13:112–119.
106. Reidy MA, Bowyer DE. Scanning electron-microscope studies of the endothelium of aortic allografts in the rabbit: effect of azathioprine, prednisolone, and promethazine on early cellular invasion. *J Pathol* 1978;124:1–5.
107. Tilney NL, Whitley WD, Tullius SG, et al. Serial analysis of cytokines, adhesion molecule expression, and humoral responses during development of chronic kidney allograft rejection in a new rat model. *Transplant Proc* 1993;25:861–862.
108. Li H, Cybulsky MI, Gimbrone MA, et al. An atherogenic diet rapidly induces VCAM-1, a cytokine-regulatable mononuclear leukocyte adhesion molecule, in rabbit aortic endothelium. *Arterioscler Thromb* 1993;13:197–204.
109. Cosimi AB, Conti D, Delmonico FL, et al. In vivo effects of monoclonal antibody to ICAM-1 (CD54) in nonhuman primates with renal allografts. *J Immunol* 1990;144:4604–4612.
110. Isobe M, Yagita H, Okumura K, et al. Specific acceptance of cardiac allograft after treatment with antibodies to ICAM-1 and LFA-1. *Science* 1992;255:1125–1127.
111. Orosz CG, Ohye RG, Pelletier RP, et al. Treatment with anti-vascular cell adhesion molecule 1 monoclonal antibody induces long-term murine cardiac allograft acceptance. *Transplant* 1993;56:453–460.
112. Clausell N, Molossi S, Rabinovitch M. Increased interleukin-1 beta and fibronectin expression are early features of the development of the postcardiac transplant coronary arteriopathy in piglets. *Am J Pathol* 1993;142:1772–1786.
113. Faggiotto A, Ross R, Harker L. Studies of hypercholesterolemia in the nonhuman primate. I. Changes that lead to fatty streak formation. *Arteriosclerosis* 1984;4:323–340.
114. Faggiotto A, Ross R. Studies of hypercholesterolemia in the nonhuman primate. II. Fatty streak conversion to fibrous plaque. *Arteriosclerosis* 1984;4:341–356.
115. Yowell RL, Hammond EH, Bristow MR, et al. Acute vascular rejection involving the major coronary arteries of a cardiac allograft. *J Heart Transplant* 1988;7:191–197.
116. Hollenberg SM, Klein LW, Parrillo JE, et al. Coronary endothelial dysfunction after heart transplantation predicts allograft vasculopathy and cardiac death. *Circulation* 2001;104:3091–3096.
117. Jacobsson J, Cheng L, Lyke K, et al. Effect of estradiol on accelerated atherosclerosis in rabbit heterotopic aortic allografts. *J Heart Lung Transplant* 1992;11:1188–1193.
118. Kosek JC, Beiber C, Lower RR. Heart graft arteriosclerosis. *Transplant Proc* 1971;3:512–514.
119. Kuwahara M, Jacobsson J, Kagan E, et al. Coronary artery ultrastructural changes in cardiac transplant atherosclerosis in the rabbit. *Transplant* 1991;52:759–765.
120. Gabbiani G, Schmid E, Winter S, et al. Vascular smooth muscle cells differ from other smooth muscle cells: predominance of vimentin filaments and a specific α-type actin. *Proc Natl Acad Sci USA* 1981;78:298–302.
121. Kuhn C, McDonald JA. The roles of the myofibroblast in idiopathic pulmonary fibrosis: ultrastructural and immunohistochemical features of sites of active extracellular matrix synthesis. *Am J Pathol* 1991;138:1257–1265.
122. Hansson GK, Chao S, Schwartz SM, et al. Aortic endothelial cell death and replication in normal and lipopolysaccharide-treated rats. *Am J Pathol* 1985;121:123–127.
123. Schwartz SM, Lombardi DM. Effect of chronic hypertension and antihypertensive therapy on endothelial cell replication in the spontaneously hypertensive rat. *Lab Invest* 1982;47:510–515.
124. Walker LN, Reidy MA, Bowyer DE. Morphology and cell kinetics of fatty streak lesion formation in the hypercholesterolemic rabbit. *Am J Pathol* 1986;125:450–459.
125. Reidy MA, Yoshida K, Harker LA, et al. Vascular injury: quantification of experimental focal endothelial denudation in rats using indium-111-labeled platelets. *Arteriosclerosis* 1986;6:305–311.
126. Hansson GK, Schwartz SM. Evidence for cell death in the vascular endothelium in vivo and in vitro. *Am J Pathol* 1983;112:278–286.
127. Kennedy LJ, Weissman IL. Dual origin of intimal cells in cardiac-allograft arteriosclerosis. *N Engl J Med* 1971;285:884–887.
128. Mennander A, Tiisala S, Halttunen J, et al. Chronic rejection in rat aortic allografts: an experimental model for transplant arteriosclerosis. *Arterioscler Thromb* 1991;11:671–680.
129. Clowes AW, Reidy MA, Clowes MM. Mechanisms of stenosis after arterial injury. *Lab Invest* 1983;49:208–215.
130. Clowes AW, Reidy MA, Clowes MM. Kinetics of cellular proliferation after arterial injury. I. Smooth muscle growth in the absence of endothelium. *Lab Invest* 1983;49:327–333.
131. Snow AD, Bolender RP, Wight TN, et al. Heparin modulates the composition of the extracellular matrix domain surrounding arterial smooth muscle cells. *Am J Pathol* 1990;137:313–330.
132. Isik FF, Valentine HA, McDonald TO, et al. Localization of bFGF in human transplant coronary atherosclerosis. *Ann NY Acad Sci* 1991;638:487–488.
133. Minick CR, Murphy GE, Campbell WG. Experimental induction of athero-arteriosclerosis by the synergy of allergic injury to arteries and lipid-rich diet. I. Effect of repeated injections of horse serum in rabbits fed a dietary cholesterol supplement. *J Exp Med* 1966;124:635–652.
134. Minick CR, Murphy GE. Experimental induction of atheroarteriosclerosis by the synergy of allergic injury to arteries and lipid-rich diet. II. Effect of repeatedly injected foreign protein in rabbits fed a lipid-rich, cholesterol-poor diet. *Am J Pathol* 1973;73:265–300.
135. Hardin NJ, Minick CR, Murphy GE. Experimental induction of atheroarteriosclerosis by the synergy of allergic injury to arteries and lipid-rich diet. III. The role of earlier acquired fibromuscular intimal thickening in the pathogenesis of later developing atherosclerosis. *Am J Pathol* 1973;73:301–327.

136. Gravanis MB, Ansari AA, Neckelman N, et al. Evidence of cell-mediated immunity in the pathogenesis of allograft heart arteriosclerosis. *J Am Coll Cardiol* 1990;15:127a.

137. Hancock WW, Whitley WD, Baldwin WM, et al. Cells, cytokines, adhesion molecules, and humoral responses in a rat model of chronic renal allograft rejection. *Transplant Proc* 1992;24:2315–2316.

138. Hall BM, Dorsch S, Roser B. The cellular basis of allograft rejection in vivo. 1. The cellular requirements for first-set rejection of heart grafts. *J Exp Med* 1978;148:878–889.

139. Hall BM, Dorsch S, Roser B. The cellular basis of allograft rejection in vivo. II. The nature of memory cells mediating second set heart graft rejection. *J Exp Med* 1978;148:890–902.

140. Hall BM, Saxe I, Dorsch S. The cellular basis of allograft rejection in vivo. III. Restoration of first-set rejection of heart grafts by T helper cells in irradiated rats. *Transplant* 1983;36:700–705.

141. Kobashigawa JA, Katznelson S, Laks H, et al. Effect of pravastatin on outcomes after cardiac transplantation. *N Engl J Med* 1995;333:621–627.

142. Wenke K, Meiser B, Thiery J, et al. Simvastatin reduces graft vessel disease and mortality after heart transplantation: a four-year randomized trial. *Circulation* 1997;96:1398–1402.

143. Wenke K, Meiser B, Thiery J, et al. Simvastatin initiated early after heart transplantation: 8-year prospective experience. *Circulation* 2003;107:93–97.

144. Sparrow CP, Burton CA, Hernandez M, et al. Simvastatin has anti-inflammatory and antiatherosclerotic activities independent of plasma cholesterol lowering. *Arterioscler Thromb Vasc Biol* 2001;21:115–121.

145. Foegh ML, Khirabadi BS, Chambers E, et al. Peptide inhibition of accelerated transplant atherosclerosis. *Transplant Proc* 1989;21:3674–3676.

146. Foegh ML. Accelerated cardiac transplant atherosclerosis/chronic rejection in rabbits: inhibition by Angiopeptin. *Transplant Proc* 1993;25:2095–2097.

147. Ohno T, Gordon D, San H, et al. Gene therapy for vascular smooth muscle cell proliferation after arterial injury. *Science* 1994;265:781–784.

148. Masetti P, DiSesa VJ, Schoen FJ, et al. Ischemic injury before heart transplantation does not cause coronary arteriopathy in experimental isografts. *J Heart Lung Transplant* 1991;10:597–599.

149. Wanders A, Akyürek ML, Waltenberger J, et al. Ischemia-induced transplant arteriosclerosis in the rat. *Arterioscler Thromb* 1995;15:145–155.

CHAPTER 44

Vascular Grafts and Their Sequelae

Larry W. Kraiss and Alexander W. Clowes

Key Words: Graft atherothrombosis; graft patency; total arterial revascularization; vasoactivity.

When the first edition of this textbook was published, the previous version of this chapter highlighted the superior performance of the internal thoracic artery (ITA) as a coronary bypass graft compared with the commonly used saphenous vein graft (SVG) (1). This principle remains unchallenged. In the last decade, as the deficiencies of the SVG became more apparent when compared with the ITA, coronary surgeons have increasingly substituted other arterial conduits for SVGs in coronary artery bypass graft (CABG) operations in the belief that these arteries would also outperform the vein graft (2). This practice is referred to as a philosophy of total arterial revascularization (3).

This chapter focuses on the biologic characteristics of the commonly used arterial conduits and contrasts them with those of the saphenous vein. The clinical performance of these grafts also is reviewed. Because SVGs are still a commonly used conduit (4), information concerning

optimization of their long-term performance also is presented.

TYPES OF CORONARY CONDUITS AND THEIR BIOLOGIC CHARACTERISTICS

The significant histologic and biologic features of the commonly used coronary bypass conduits are highlighted in Table 44–1.

Saphenous Vein Grafts

The most distinguishing histologic features of the saphenous vein are those that define it as vein: a relatively thin wall with a poorly developed medial layer and the presence of valves. The valves require reversal of the graft (most common) or lysis (less common) to permit antegrade arterial flow. Even with reversal, some authors have postulated that the valves are capable of producing "pressure traps" at certain points during the cardiac cycle that may accentuate wall stress in segments of the grafts just distal to the valves producing injury and promoting wall thickening in these areas (5).

Overall, SVGs appear to have more vasoconstrictive tone than do ITA conduits, exhibit more intense contractions in response to leukotrienes (5,6), exhibit more angiotensin-converting enzyme activity (7), and show evidence of endothelin-1 synthesis and responsiveness (8–10). Further-

L. W. Kraiss: Division of Vascular Surgery, Department of Surgery, University of Utah, 30 North 1900 East, Salt Lake City, Utah 84132.

A. W. Clowes: Division of Vascular Surgery, Department of Surgery (BB442-HSB), University of Washington, 1959 NE Pacific, Seattle, Washington 98195.

TABLE 44–1. *Biologic comparison of coronary artery bypass conduits*

Parameter	SVG	ITA	RA
Endothelial cells	Larger, thinner, less firmly anchored to subendothelium	Smaller, thicker, more firmly anchored	Similar to ITA
Tunica intima	More permeable	Less permeable	Less permeable
Internal elastic lamina	Poorly defined	Well defined	Intermediate between SVG and ITA
Elastic lamellae	Absent	Present	Present
Medial smooth muscle cells	Few, circular and longitudinal in arrangement, widely separated by collagen	Circular arrangement, orderly array with collagen, elastic fibers, and matrix	Similar to ITA, although media much thicker
Vasa vasorum	More anastomoses	Less anastomoses	Less anastomoses
Valves	Present	Absent	Absent
Express and respond to vasoconstrictors	High	Low	Medium
Express and respond to vasodilators, e.g., NO	Low	High	High
Flow-dependent remodeling after grafting in humans	No	Yes	Yes

ITA, internal thoracic artery; NO, nitric oxide; RA, radial artery; SVG, saphenous vein graft.

more, their ability to produce vasodilators such as nitric oxide (NO) when stimulated is inferior to the ITA (11). Because vasoconstrictive tone often is associated with a proliferative influence on smooth muscle cells, whereas vasodilators often double as growth inhibitors (12), the SVG may be particularly prone to develop intimal hyperplasia and subsequent atherothrombosis.

Another important histologic feature is a highly fenestrated, porous internal elastic lamina (IEL) (13,14). The porous nature of this layer, coupled with arterial pressure to which the vein is not accustomed, may help explain the increased rates of lipid transudation into the SVG wall compared with arterial conduits.

SVGs that have functioned as coronary grafts for several years develop lesions that contain lipid cores covered with thin fibrous caps that are indistinguishable from atherothrombotic lesions found in arteries (15–18). Whereas native coronary arteries involved with atherothrombosis tend to dilate to preserve luminal diameter as the plaque encroaches on the flow channel (19), SVGs do not (20). Such lesions are commonly observed in SVGs within 3 to 5 years of grafting (17,21,22). Thus, SVG atherothrombosis develops at a greatly accelerated pace compared with atherothrombotic lesions in native arteries. Atheromatous lesions in vein grafts are more commonly implicated than residual native coronary lesions as the cause of adverse cardiac events experienced by patients who have undergone prior CABG with SVGs (17,21,22).

The concept of the unstable atherothrombotic plaque, used to explain how moderately stenosing arterial plaques produce acute coronary syndromes, has also been applied to SVG atherothrombosis (17). This paradigm reinforces the theoretic benefits of measures to reduce the risk for native coronary plaque rupture, because the same measures might be expected to positively impact SVG function.

Internal Thoracic Artery

By virtue of its anatomic location and good size match with the native coronary arteries, the ITA was one of the first arterial conduits used as a coronary bypass graft (23). As its superior clinical performance became apparent, the biologic reasons for this superiority began to be investigated.

All arteries share certain histologic features that distinguish them from veins, primarily a thicker medial layer of smooth muscle cells subdivided by varying amounts of laminated elastin into lamellar units. Among the commonly used arterial conduits, the ITA contains significantly more elastin and a more obvious lamellar medial architecture (14). Some authors have hypothesized that its relatively high content of metabolically quiescent elastin renders the ITA more resistant to ischemia (24). The IEL of the ITA is well defined compared with that of the saphenous vein. When harvested from its anatomic location as a pedicled graft, its vasa vasorum remains relatively intact, perhaps helping to preserve this conduit from ischemia/reperfusion insults experienced by free grafts such as the SVG. When remnants are studied after harvest for use as coronary grafts, few ITAs show signs of preexisting atherothrombosis (25).

Functionally, the endothelial lining of the ITA appears to differ from that of the SVG and demonstrates a greater capacity for vasodilator production (NO and prostacyclin) compared with SVG endothelium (11). After being grafted into the coronary circulation, the ITA has been shown to remodel in adaptation to specific flow demands posed by the configuration of the revascularization (26). For instance, ITAs supplying multiple coronary beds through sequentially constructed anastomoses or composite T-graft configurations often enlarge and develop increased coronary flow reserve compared with what existed immediately after graft placement (27,28). In contrast, ITAs grafted to coronary vessels with moderate instead of critical degrees of stenosis tend to have smaller lumens or even fail, presumably as a result of competitive flow (29). All coronary bypass conduits experience increased risk for failure when grafted into coronary arteries with lesser degrees of stenosis. ITA grafts tolerate this situation better than any other available conduit, further attesting to the more functional nature of its endothelial lining (26).

Radial Artery

The radial artery (RA) is distinguished histologically from the ITA primarily by its markedly thicker, more muscular media (14) and paucity of elastic laminae. The IEL of the RA contains more fenestrae than the ITA. Several authors have postulated that the RA will thus be more prone to the development of atherothrombosis (7,14,24), although perioperative biopsies of RA remnants have not shown preexisting atheroma to be a significant problem (25).

Of all the commonly used arterial conduits, the RA has the thickest medial layer (14). Not unexpectedly, clinical and experimental studies have shown the RA to be the arterial conduit most prone to vasoconstriction regardless of the agonist (7,30,31). The luminal diameters of all the arterial conduits are smaller than SVGs, making perioperative vasospasm potentially a more clinically relevant problem when it occurs in arterial bypasses. The use of specific intraoperative and perioperative countermeasures against vasospasm has been credited as being responsible for the recent clinical success using the RA as a coronary bypass graft (25,31), although the need for these adjuncts has been questioned (32).

Although the RA is more vasoconstrictive than the ITA, its active vasodilating capacity appears to be equal to the ITA with equal relaxation responses when stimulated with endothelial-dependent and independent agonists (7). RAs from patients with diabetes respond equally well as RAs from those without diabetes (33). RA conduits contain more NO synthase and generate more NO with specific stimulation than do SVGs (25).

Consistent with experimental observations indicating that the RA and ITA behave similarly in tests of vasodilation, clinical studies have shown that the RA also is capable of flow-dependent remodeling after grafting (34). Also, like the ITA, the degree of postoperative luminal enlargement correlates negatively with competitive flow from native coronary arteries (26).

Other Conduits

The right gastroepiploic artery was the arterial conduit of second choice after the ITA until the recent popularization of the RA (4). Its anatomic location makes it suitable for use as a pedicled graft to the inferior wall of the heart. Histologically and physiologically, it occupies an intermediate position between the ITA and RA with few elastic lamellae but also a significantly thinner media than the RA (14). It is not as prone to vasospasm as the RA and also has been observed

to remodel in flow-dependent fashion on postoperative angiograms (26).

Other potential arterial conduits are the inferior epigastric artery and the subscapular arteries (4). The increased use of the RA has significantly reduced use of these vessels, and their biology is less completely characterized.

CLINICAL PERFORMANCE OF THE DIFFERENT TYPES OF CONDUITS

Saphenous Vein Grafts

In a large study in which patency was verified angiographically, 81% of SVGs were patent at 1 year, 75% at 5 years, and only ~50% at 15 years (35). Among the grafts open at 5 years, nearly half were visibly involved with disease. The proportion of diseased grafts increased to ~80% at the 15-year mark. These results are not significantly improved from those of another large postoperative angiographic study published by Loop and coworkers (36) 10 years earlier (Fig. 44–1). The relatively stable patency rates for SVGs over the last two decades, despite presumed improvements in the performance of CABG, suggest that the durability of the SVG is now more dependent on biologic factors rather than technical factors.

Internal Thoracic Artery

The patency and durability of the ITA as a coronary conduit surpasses that of SVGs (36) (Fig. 44–1). Long-term patency rates (5–15 years) well in excess of 90% are consistently reported (36–38). Late failure of an ITA graft is considered a rare event; early failures may reflect surgical errors in either technique (damage during harvest or construction of the anastomosis) or judgment (grafting to a vessel with significant competitive flow).

There is now widespread consensus that the left ITA (LITA) is the graft of choice and that this graft should be placed to the most important threatened coronary artery distribution (4,39). There is weaker consensus as to whether a second arterial graft should be the right ITA or another arterial conduit such as the RA (discussed later).

Radial Artery

After a disappointing early experience, the RA has regained popularity as a coronary graft in the last decade (39,40). There is strong rationale for its use: superior performance of arteries over SVGs, avoidance of potential sternotomy problems if the RA is used instead of the right ITA for a second graft, ease of procurement, adequate usable length (≤22 cm), avoidance of lower extremity incisions in patients with coexistent peripheral arterial disease, and good size match with native coronary arteries (39).

The largest reported series from Australia involved 8,420 RA conduits placed in a cohort of 6,646 consecutive patients

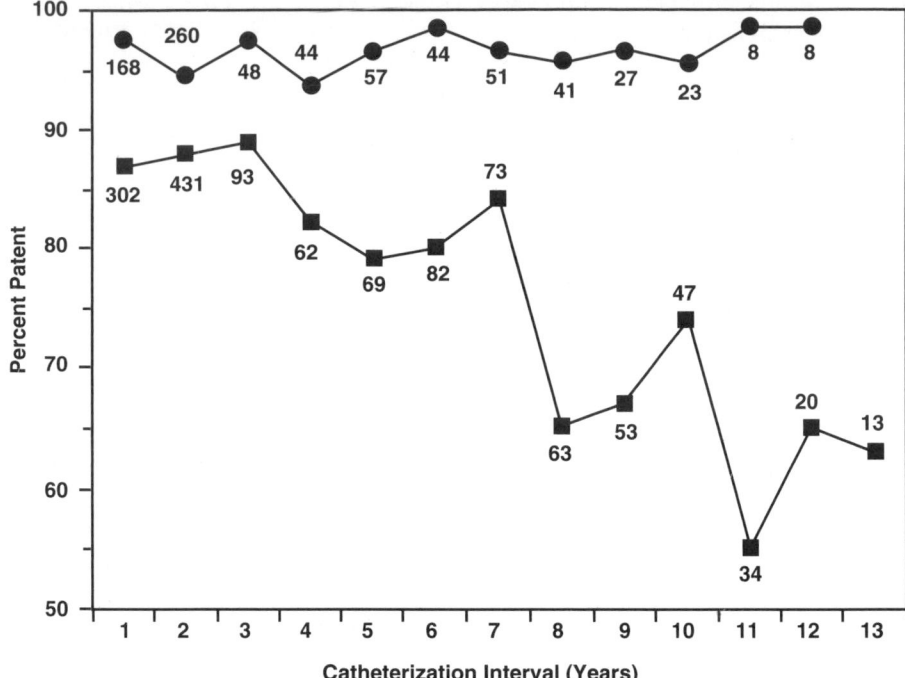

FIG. 44–1. Patency of internal thoracic (mammary) artery (*circles;* n = 855) and saphenous vein (*squares;* n = 1,445) grafts at 1-year intervals. The number of patients restudied at each interval is noted. (From Loop FD, Lytle BW, Cosgrove DM, et al. Influence of the internal-mammary-artery graft on 10-year survival and other cardiac events. *N Engl J Med* 1986;314:1–6, with permission.)

in whom 87% of all coronary anastomoses were artery–artery, reflecting the authors' commitment to total arterial revascularization (32). During follow-up of 14 ± 10 months, angiograms were obtained for various reasons on 271 patients in whom 280 RA conduits had been placed, representing 369 RA to coronary anastomoses. The overall anastomotic patency rate was 90% (333/369 anastomoses).

Longer follow-up of RA patency also is available from smaller cohorts. Acar and coworkers (41) reported on the first 102 consecutive patients to have received an RA coronary graft after the revival of this conduit's use. Most of these grafts were placed to the diagonal or circumflex distributions, whereas the left anterior descending (LAD) artery was revascularized with an ITA graft. Actuarial survival at 7 years for this group was ~90%. These authors requested that the first 102 patients treated with an RA graft undergo routine angiography 4 to 7 years after surgery to assess RA graft patency; 50 patients consented, including all who had recurrent symptoms. RA patency was found to be 83%, whereas ITA patency in the same patients was 91%.

In an Italian study, Iaco and coworkers (42) obtained angiographic follow-up of 72 patients (out of a total of 164) 48 ± 27 months (range, 6–96 months) after RA bypass. Eight-year actuarial survival was 83%. RA patency was 96% with

no difference noted if the RA was used as a composite graft attached to LITA (94%) or if the RA was attached proximally to the ascending aorta (100%). The RA was used to preferentially revascularize the lateral wall of the left ventricle. In this analysis, RA patency was essentially equivalent to ITA patency (100%) in the patients studied with angiography.

One-year patencies of ITA, RA, and SVGs were analyzed by Moran and coworkers (43). They performed follow-up angiography on 50 patients (out of 115) and found ITA patency to be 100%, RA patency 80%, and SVG patency 68%. *Post hoc* analysis showed that native coronary stenosis affected the patency of RA grafts. Average degree of stenosis in the coronary arteries (at the time of surgery) with patent RA grafts was 73%, whereas occluded RA grafts had been placed to coronary arteries with an average stenosis of only 40%. RA patency when grafted to coronary arteries with greater than 70% stenosis was 92%.

The role of target vessel and degree of native coronary stenosis also was addressed by Maniar and coworkers (44). In studying 231 RA anastomoses an average of 27 months after surgery (range, 2–70 months), they found that RA patency was best if directed to the LAD (83%) versus the circumflex (CIRC) (75%) or right coronary artery (73%). Furthermore, if the target artery stenosis was 90% to

100%, RA patency was 83% compared with 69% for artery stenosis of 71% to 89% or 57% for arteries 70% or less narrowed. On multivariate analysis, both target artery (LAD) and critical stenosis ($\geq$90%) were independent predictors of RA patency. Similar observations have been made by others (39).

In an attempt to directly compare the overall clinical effectiveness of using the RA versus SVG as the second graft (both combined with an ITA as primary graft), Cohen and coworkers (45) performed a case–control study. A total of 478 patients who received LITA+RA grafts were case-matched 1:2 with 956 patients receiving LITA+SVG. Both groups received SVGs as the third or fourth grafts, if necessary. Cases were matched for age, sex, Canadian Cardiovascular Society class, left ventricular function, number of diseased vessels, and timing of operation. The RA group was burdened with a greater prevalence of diabetes, hypertension, and peripheral vascular disease compared with the control group. Whereas overall survival at 36 months for the two groups was similar (RA 96% vs. SVG 92%), the RA group had significantly fewer perioperative myocardial infarctions and fewer late nonfatal cardiac events. On the basis of these results, the Radial Artery Patency Study (RAPS) is randomly assigning RA or SVG as the second conduit after the ITA to determine overall clinical efficacy (46).

Although of obvious theoretic concern, the risk for upper extremity or hand ischemia with the RA graft is low. When Allen's test is used to assess ulnar collateral adequacy, only 2% to 5% of RA are disqualified from potential use (39,47), and a significant postoperative problem attributed to the use of the RA is rare (~0.1%) (32,48).

Overall, the RA appears to be the preferred choice as the second arterial graft after the ITA is used to revascularize the LAD. There are a variety of theoretic reasons to choose this graft rather than the SVG, with numerous historical series demonstrating improved patency of the RA compared with SVGs. However, many of these series did not systematically study patency in the majority of patients who received an RA graft; therefore, these impressions are still based on angiographic study of only a fraction of patients receiving RA grafts. Most series also have not directly compared performance of RA with SVG; therefore, the results of the RAPS trial (46) should be eagerly anticipated.

Other Conduits

Other arterial conduits also have been investigated for use as a coronary graft. These include the right gastroepiploic and inferior epigastric arteries, although arteries as varied as the splenic, subscapular, lateral costal, left gastric, and lateral femoral circumflex also have been used, presumably in desperate situations (4,49).

Both the gastroepiploic and inferior epigastric arteries had their advocates in the late 1980s and early 1990s, although use of these grafts appear to have been supplanted by the RA, perhaps because of overall ease of use.

When necessary and when placed by a surgeon experienced in their use, clinical outcomes with the gastroepiploic artery have been acceptable, although a significant drawback is the need to combine a laparotomy with the cardiac procedure. Problems with intense vasospasm also have been encountered (50), although similar problems early in the use of RA grafts were overcome. Furthermore, these grafts are potentially vulnerable to injury during subsequent abdominal surgery (4).

The inferior epigastric artery also has been used as a free graft with 60% to 85% early patency (4). Usable length often is an issue because segments longer than 13 cm are rare (3,4).

Total Arterial Revascularization

The clearly demonstrated improved performance of the ITA graft led surgeons to surmise that total arterial revascularization would lead to improved postoperative outcomes compared with procedures that used SVGs as the second and succeeding grafts. Initial strategies to accomplish total arterial revascularization in patients with triple vessel disease used both ITAs. Because the RITA is generally too short to reach the circumflex distribution while still attached to the right subclavian artery, it was detached and anastomosed as a free graft based from the aorta or in a T configuration from the LITA (51). In particular, the T configuration permits revascularization of all three main coronary distributions with only two grafts using the detached RITA to sequentially bypass the circumflex and right coronary arteries (51).

A similar strategy of total arterial revascularization using the RA in place of the right ITA has produced overall results that equal or surpass that of other strategies (3). Use of the RA shortens the procedure because it can be harvested simultaneously with the LITA. Furthermore, it preserves the saphenous vein in patients with peripheral vascular disease and avoids the increased risk for sternal complications in some patients who have both ITAs harvested.

There are several compelling single institution reports that suggest use of two arterial grafts provides better clinical outcomes than procedures using only one (52–54). Although these are retrospective, nonrandomized studies, the consistency in their results is notable. In particular, the Cleveland Clinic experience (53) with bilateral ITA grafts showed superior survival of the double arterial graft cohort at 5-, 10-, and 15-year postoperative intervals and an even more significant advantage in freedom from reoperation (Fig. 44–2). Subgroup analysis showed that patients with diabetes and left ventricular dysfunction also enjoyed improved survival if they received bilateral ITA grafts (53).

The Toronto study showed that RA conduits performed just as well as the right ITA as the second graft and were associated with fewer sternal wound complications (52).

Although there is no prospective, randomized trial that supports the concept of total arterial revascularization, the approach clearly has theoretic advantages, and significant clinical data suggesting its superiority exist. The use of mul-

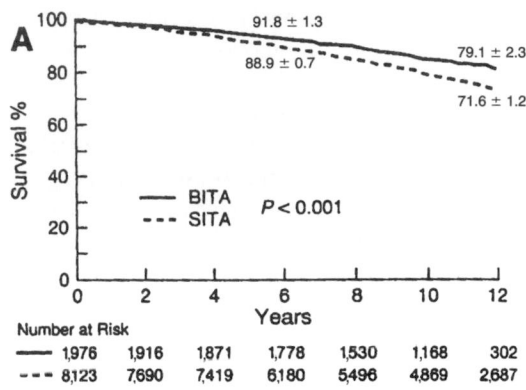

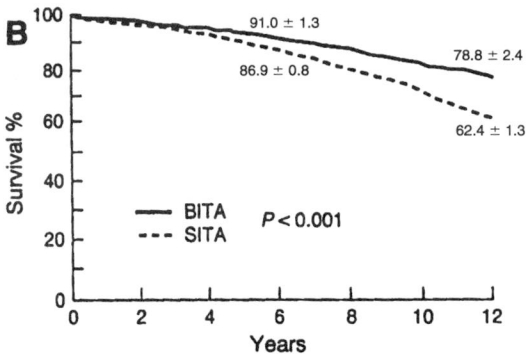

FIG. 44–2. Comparison of the bilateral internal thoracic artery (BITA) and single ITA (SITA) groups in terms of survival **(A)** and reoperation-free survival **(B).** Numbers of patients surviving at selected follow-up intervals are listed beneath **A.** (From Lytle BW, Blackstone EH, Loop FD, et al. Two internal thoracic artery grafts are better than one. *J Thorac Cardiovasc Surg* 1999;117:855–872, with permission).

tiple arterial conduits whenever possible in lieu of the SVG is a growing trend in cardiac surgery, and level 1 evidence will likely be available sometime in the next decade.

IMPROVING GRAFT PATENCY AND FUNCTION

SVG failure is an important clinical problem that affects up to 50% of vein grafts within 10 years after surgery (18). In addition, patients with SVG in place are more likely to experience subsequent ischemic episodes and need treatment for graft-related problems than for progression of disease within the native coronary system (21).

The Biology of Coronary Graft Failure

SVGs have an ~15% failure rate in the first year after grafting (Fig. 44–1) (17,18,36), probably because of thrombosis of the graft secondary to endothelial dysfunction produced by technical factors, harvest trauma, problems in the distal vascular bed or suboptimal quality (preexisting disease) of the conduit (17,21). Between Years 1 and 7 after surgery, relatively few SVGs fail, but graft loss accelerates after the fifth to seventh year (17,18,21). Pathologic changes between Years 1 and 7

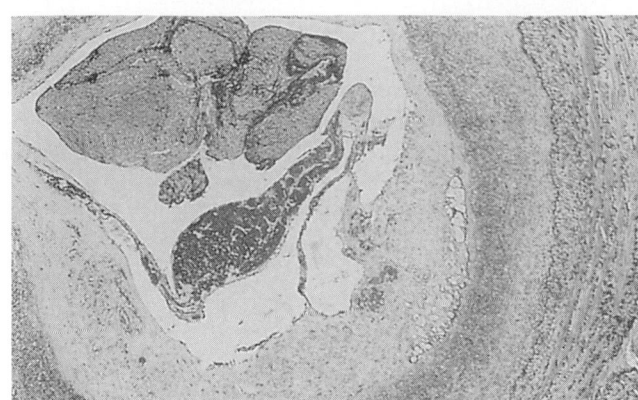

FIG. 44–3. Photomicrograph of a thrombosed saphenous vein graft to a coronary artery. The section is taken through a vein valve. The lumen contains thrombus. There are several distinct layers of thickening in the graft wall between the lumen and the internal elastic lamina. The luminal layer is composed of material consistent with atherothrombotic plaque and contains areas of foam cell accumulation. Movat stain, original magnification ×12.8. (Courtesy Russell Ross, University of Washington, Seattle, WA.)

are primarily those of intimal hyperplasia caused by migration of smooth muscle cells from the media and subsequent proliferation in the intimal compartment accompanied by extracellular matrix deposition. These changes then provide the background for vein graft atherothrombosis, a process that looks histologically almost exactly like arterial atherothrombosis with foam cell deposition, lipid accumulation, and plaque rupture (17,18) (Figs. 44–3 and 44–4). Up to 50% of SVGs have failed by the tenth postoperative year (18).

Atherothrombosis of SVGs is especially problematic because it occurs in accelerated fashion, the plaques are generally more fragile than in native arteries, and vein grafts do not have the compensatory mechanisms such as positive remodeling to mitigate the occlusive effects of the growing

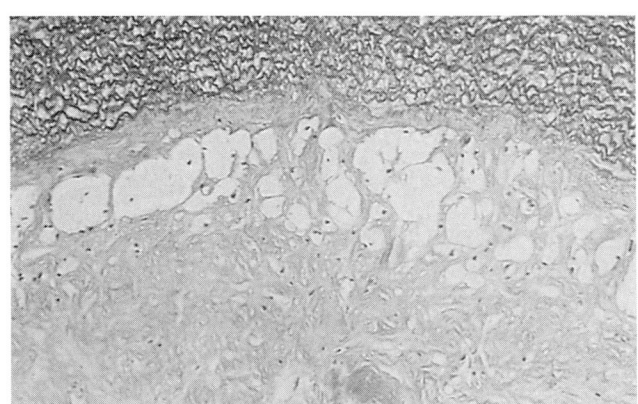

FIG. 44–4. Higher power view of the foam cell deposit described in Figure 44–3. Verhoeff-van Gieson stain, original magnification ×51.2. (Courtesy Russell Ross, University of Washington, Seattle, WA.)

plaque (17,26). The concept of the vulnerable plaque has been extended from native arterial atherothrombotic lesions to vein graft lesions (17). Although "triggers" for plaque rupture in vein grafts have not been specifically distinguished from those that rupture arterial plaques, it is thought that vein graft plaques are likely to rupture with significantly less force than native arterial plaques (17).

In contrast, ITA grafts appear to be relatively immune to atherothrombotic-type lesions, as evidenced by the relatively flat patency curves out to 10 to 15 years (36,53) (Fig. 44–1). After the 2% to 3% graft loss that occurs early, most likely from technical problems, ITA grafts are durable.

Whether non-ITA grafts such as the RA will prove to be as durable is difficult to predict. Early and midterm data suggesting that patency of the RA is only incrementally poorer than the ITA might indicate that these grafts are also relatively immune from atherothrombosis. Conversely, there are histologic differences that suggest the RA may be more susceptible to atherothrombosis. Large-scale follow-up of these grafts beyond 7 years (when SVG atherothrombosis is especially apparent) is necessary to answer this question.

Adjuncts to Improve Graft Patency and Function

Graft problems are more likely to determine clinical outcome in patients who have undergone coronary revascularization than is progression of native disease (17,21). Thus, it is natural that attempts to optimize graft function after initial placement would be important.

The early postoperative period up to 1 year claims 10% to 15% of all SVGs (17,18,21) that are placed and appears to be the time when ITA grafts are most vulnerable to failure. Technical factors related to graft placement and thrombosis appear to be the most likely opportunities for improving graft function in this period. Although there are no controlled trials evaluating particular techniques designed to minimize graft trauma during harvest and preparation, it is axiomatic among cardiovascular surgeons that minimal manipulation and gentle handling will result in a graft with the most functional endothelium possible.

SVG thrombosis in the first postoperative year can be minimized by institution of aspirin-based antiplatelet treatment within hours of surgery (21,55). Several randomized controlled trials of aspirin versus placebo demonstrated a 5% to 10% increased patency of SVGs in the treated group (55) over the first year but no benefit thereafter. Aspirin has never been shown to specifically improve ITA graft patency (55). However, the overall benefits of antiplatelet treatment on all-cause cardiovascular morbidity and mortality merit the indefinite use of aspirin in patients with clinically significant atherothrombosis (56). For patients with documented hypersensitivity or those who are otherwise intolerant of aspirin, clopidogrel is recommended (55).

There are no randomized controlled trials demonstrating the superiority of oral Coumadin derivatives over standard antiplatelet regimens (55).

The established risk factors for graft loss after the first year are smoking and hypercholesterolemia (57,58). Both are also well defined overall atherothrombotic risk factors. Although there are no randomized controlled trials demonstrating the benefits of smoking cessation in improving graft patency, it is hard to imagine that this would not be of benefit.

The Post Coronary Artery Bypass Graft Trial, based on a comparison of coronary angiograms an average of 4.3 years apart, found that aggressive reduction of cholesterol to a target low-density lipoprotein (LDL) of less than 100 mg/dl resulted in less atherothrombotic degeneration of SVGs including outright occlusions (59). The cholesterol-lowering regimen used lovastatin with cholestyramine if needed to achieve target LDL levels. The beneficial effect of cholesterol reduction was observed in all patient subgroups including young and old, smokers and nonsmokers, men and women, and those with hypertension, diabetes, and/or hypertriglyceridemia (60).

The Post Coronary Artery Bypass Graft Trial was also designed to detect a beneficial effect of low-dose anticoagulation (target international normalized ratio ≤ 2.0) on atherothrombotic SVG degeneration, and none was found (59). However, clinical follow-up of the same patient cohort at 7.5 years found that the patients assigned to low-dose Coumadin had fewer myocardial infarctions and a lower mortality rate (61). Because these later results were not angiographically controlled, it is not possible to state with certainty that the benefits of anticoagulation were because of improved graft function.

Because the historical performance of ITA grafts has been so good, it has been difficult to show effectiveness for postoperative strategies designed to specifically improve their function. However, soon after RA grafting became popular, many surgeons noted problems with spasm of this graft leading many to implement specific spasmolytic measures, often with calcium channel blockade, to prevent this problem in the early postoperative period (25,31,62). However, as experience with this graft accumulated, centers with large volumes have seen little problem with RA spasm in the perioperative period and do not routinely use systemic vasodilators (32).

NEW DIRECTIONS

Experience over the last two to three decades has clearly highlighted the limitations of the SVG. Some of these problems have been partially mitigated by the increasing use of arterial conduits. However, there remain limits to the availability of these potentially more desirable grafts. Thus, research continues into alternatives to SVG and autogenous artery.

Prosthetic Grafts

No prosthetic graft has ever functioned satisfactorily as a coronary graft (or in any other vascular bed that requires a small [≤4 mm] diameter conduit) with widespread use. These conduits are still sought because of their potential convenience and universal applicability. Two recent options under clinical investigation include a new polyurethane graft fabricated from the same biomaterial used in ventricular assist devices (63). Another option is the Perma-Flow conduit in which polytetrafluoroethylene (PTFE) is used to construct an aortocaval fistula with intervening side–side coronary anastomoses to the PTFE conduit (64,65). A restrictor placed distal to the coronary anastomoses but proximal to the caval outflow prevents high output failure and maintains arterial perfusion pressure to the grafted coronary arteries. Clinical experience with both grafts is preliminary, and their place in coronary revascularization remains unknown.

Tissue Engineering

Another approach in preclinical investigation uses tissue engineering techniques to "grow" functional arteries *in vitro* that can then be implanted into the arterial system to function as a bypass graft (66). Presumably, this strategy would use autologous cells to avoid problems with rejection seen with other vascular homografts. A potential drawback to this approach involves the amount of time that would be required between the decision to perform a revascularization and the ultimate availability of the customized autologous graft.

Rapamycin

No pharmacologic adjunct has been shown to significantly inhibit the intimal hyperplastic process that precedes and presumably leads to graft atherothrombosis (67–69). This also has been a problem with percutaneous interventions. Rapamycin-eluting stents have shown great promise in preventing poststenting restenosis (70,71). Use of rapamycin in bypass grafts may produce similar benefits, but no clinical studies currently have been published.

E2F Decoy

Another attempt to block cell proliferation that underlies intimal hyperplasia involves the use of antisense oligonucleotides to block E2F, a transcription factor that regulates expression of several cell cycle genes. The antisense treatment is applied to the vein graft *ex vivo* after harvesting but before implantation and exposure to arterial hemodynamic forces that are thought to partially underlie the intimal hyperplastic response in vein grafts (1,67). A preliminary safety analysis in patients undergoing infrainguinal bypass grafting has shown promising results (72) in terms of blockade of cell cycle activation and cell proliferation with an early, preliminary trend toward fewer graft occlusions. Larger, phase III trials are currently underway in both coronary and peripheral bypass grafting.

SUMMARY

SVGs, long the mainstay of coronary artery bypass grafting, remain the most commonly used conduit largely because of their availability and the frequent need to revascularize more vessels than there are arterial conduits. However, the SVG is clearly a biologically inferior conduit when compared with the ITA and is also perhaps inferior to the RA. Whenever possible, the graft of choice to the most critical coronary vascular bed should be the LITA. Its performance is currently unsurpassed. Over the last decade, many coronary surgeons have minimized their use of the SVG as the second graft in favor of a policy of total arterial revascularization (usually with the right ITA or the RA) whenever possible. Although there are many retrospective, single institution studies indicating the clinical superiority of this approach, there is as yet no compelling level 1 evidence from randomized controlled trials to confirm these widespread impressions. Until such data are available, the SVG is likely to remain a commonly used coronary conduit (4). The best proven strategy to prolong the life of SVGs involves antiplatelet therapy for at least the first postoperative year with aggressive attention to controlling classic atherothrombotic risk factors such as cigarette smoking and hypercholesterolemia.

REFERENCES

1. Kraiss LW, Clowes AW. Vascular grafts and their sequelae. In: Fuster V, Ross R, Topol EJ, eds. *Atherosclerosis and coronary artery disease.* Philadelphia: Lippincott-Raven, 1996:727–737.
2. Barner HB. New arterial conduits for coronary bypass surgery. *Semin Thorac Cardiovasc Surg* 1994;6:76–80.
3. Barner HB, Sundt TM 3rd, Bailey M, et al. Midterm results of complete arterial revascularization in more than 1,000 patients using an internal thoracic artery/radial artery T graft. *Ann Surg* 2001;234:447–452.
4. Mills NL. Arterial grafts for coronary artery bypass. *Adv Card Surg* 1997;9:195–216.
5. Mills NL, Everson CT. Vein graft failure. *Curr Opin Cardiol* 1995;10:562–568.
6. Allen SP, Chester AH, Dashwood MR, et al. Preferential vasoconstriction to cysteinyl leukotrienes in the human saphenous vein compared with the internal mammary artery. Implications for graft performance. *Circulation* 1994;90:515–524.
7. Chester AH, Amrani M, Borland JA. Vascular biology of the radial artery. *Curr Opin Cardiol* 1998;13:447–452.
8. Davenport AP, Maguire JJ. The endothelin system in human saphenous vein graft disease. *Curr Opin Pharmacol* 2001;1:176–182.
9. Dumont AS, Lovren F, McNeill JH, et al. Augmentation of endothelial function by endothelin antagonism in human saphenous vein conduits. *J Neurosurg* 2001;94:281–286.
10. Cracowski JL, Stanke-Labesque F, Sessa C, et al. Functional comparison of the human isolated femoral artery, internal mammary artery, gastroepiploic artery, and saphenous vein. *Can J Physiol Pharmacol* 1999;77:770–776.
11. Yang Z, Luscher TF. Basic cellular mechanisms of coronary bypass graft disease. *Eur Heart J* 1993;14:193–197.
12. Berk BC, Alexander RW. Vasoactive effects of growth factors. *Biochem Pharmacol* 1989;38:219–225.
13. Cox JL, Chiasson DA, Gotlieb AI. Stranger in a strange land: the pathogenesis of saphenous vein graft stenosis with emphasis on structural and functional differences between veins and arteries. *Prog Cardiovasc Dis* 1991;34:45–68.
14. van Son JA, Smedts F, Vincent JG, et al. Comparative anatomic studies

of various arterial conduits for myocardial revascularization. *J Thorac Cardiovasc Surg* 1990;99:703–707.

15. Lie JT, Lawrie GM, Morris GC Jr. Aortocoronary bypass saphenous vein graft atherosclerosis. Anatomic study of 99 vein grafts from normal and hyperlipoproteinemic patients up to 75 months postoperatively. *Am J Cardiol* 1977;40:906–914.

16. Neitzel GF, Barboriak JJ, Pintar K, et al. Atherosclerosis in aortocoronary bypass grafts. Morphologic study and risk factor analysis 6 to 12 years after surgery. *Arteriosclerosis* 1986;6:594–600.

17. Safian RD. Accelerated atherosclerosis in saphenous vein bypass grafts: a spectrum of diffuse plaque instability. *Prog Cardiovasc Dis* 2002;44:437–448.

18. Solymoss BC, Leung TK, Pelletier LC, et al. Pathologic changes in coronary artery saphenous vein grafts and related etiologic factors. *Cardiovasc Clin* 1991;21:45–65.

19. Glagov S, Weisenberg E, Zarins CK, et al. Compensatory enlargement of human atherosclerotic coronary arteries. *N Engl J Med* 1987;316:1371–1375.

20. Nishioka T, Luo H, Berglund H, et al. Absence of focal compensatory enlargement or constriction in diseased human coronary saphenous vein bypass grafts. An intravascular ultrasound study. *Circulation* 1996;93:683–690.

21. Schussheim AE, Fuster V. Antithrombotic therapy and venous graft disease. *Curr Opin Cardiol* 1998;13:459–464.

22. Motwani JG, Topol EJ. Aortocoronary saphenous vein graft disease: pathogenesis, predisposition, and prevention. *Circulation* 1998;97:916–931.

23. Barner HB, Sundt TM 3rd. Multiple arterial grafts and survival. *Curr Opin Cardiol* 1999;14:501–505.

24. Dzimiri N, Chester AH, Allen SP, et al. Vascular reactivity of arterial coronary artery bypass grafts—implications for their performance. *Clin Cardiol* 1996;19:165–171.

25. Buxton B, Fuller J, Gaer J, et al. The radial artery as a bypass graft. *Curr Opin Cardiol* 1996;11:591–598.

26. Barner HB. Remodeling of arterial conduits in coronary grafting. *Ann Thorac Surg* 2002;73:1341–1345.

27. Wendler O, Hennen B, Markwirth T, et al. T grafts with the right internal thoracic artery to left internal thoracic artery versus the left internal thoracic artery and radial artery: flow dynamics in the internal thoracic artery main stem. *J Thorac Cardiovasc Surg* 1999;118:841–848.

28. Akasaka T, Yoshikawa J, Yoshida K, et al. Flow capacity of internal mammary artery grafts: early restriction and later improvement assessed by Doppler guide wire. Comparison with saphenous vein grafts. *J Am Coll Cardiol* 1995;25:640–647.

29. Akasaka T, Yoshida K, Hozumi T, et al. Flow dynamics of angiographically no-flow patent internal mammary artery grafts. *J Am Coll Cardiol* 1998;31:1049–1056.

30. Chamiot-Clerc P, Copie X, Renaud JF, et al. Comparative reactivity and mechanical properties of human isolated internal mammary and radial arteries. *Cardiovasc Res* 1998;37:811–819.

31. Rosenfeldt FL, He GW, Buxton BF. Pharmacology of coronary artery bypass grafts. *Ann Thorac Surg* 1999;67:878–888.

32. Tatoulis J, Royse AG, Buxton BF, et al. The radial artery in coronary surgery: a 5-year experience—clinical and angiographic results. *Ann Thorac Surg* 2002;73:143–148.

33. Wendler O, Landwehr P, Bandner-Risch D, et al. Vasoreactivity of arterial grafts in the patient with diabetes mellitus: investigations on internal thoracic artery and radial artery conduits. *Eur J Cardiothorac Surg* 2001;20:305–311.

34. Gaudino M, Glieca F, Trani C, et al. Midterm endothelial function and remodeling of radial artery grafts anastomosed to the aorta. *J Thorac Cardiovasc Surg* 2000;120:298–301.

35. Fitzgibbon GM, Kafka HP, Leach AJ, et al. Coronary bypass graft fate and patient outcome: angiographic follow-up of 5,065 grafts related to survival and reoperation in 1,388 patients during 25 years. *J Am Coll Cardiol* 1996;28:616–626.

36. Loop FD, Lytle BW, Cosgrove DM, et al. Influence of the internal-mammary-artery graft on 10-year survival and other cardiac events. *N Engl J Med* 1986;314:1–6.

37. Lytle BW, Loop FD, Cosgrove DM, et al. Long-term (5 to 12 years) serial studies of internal mammary artery and saphenous vein coronary bypass grafts. *J Thorac Cardiovasc Surg* 1985;89:248–258.

38. Dion R, Glineur D, Derouck D, et al. Long-term clinical and angiographic follow-up of sequential internal thoracic artery grafting. *Eur J Cardiothorac Surg* 2000;17:407–414.

39. Tatoulis J, Buxton BF, Fuller JA, et al. The radial artery as a graft for coronary revascularization: techniques and follow-up. *Adv Card Surg* 1999;11:99–128.

40. Acar C, Jebara VA, Portoghese M, et al. Revival of the radial artery for coronary artery bypass grafting. *Ann Thorac Surg* 1992;54:652–659.

41. Acar C, Ramsheyi A, Pagny JY, et al. The radial artery for coronary artery bypass grafting: clinical and angiographic results at five years. *J Thorac Cardiovasc Surg* 1998;116:981–989.

42. Iaco AL, Teodori G, Di Giammarco G, et al. Radial artery for myocardial revascularization: long-term clinical and angiographic results. *Ann Thorac Surg* 2001;72:464–469.

43. Moran SV, Baeza R, Guarda E, et al. Predictors of radial artery patency for coronary bypass operations. *Ann Thorac Surg* 2001;72:1552–1556.

44. Maniar HS, Sundt TM, Barner HB, et al. Effect of target stenosis and location on radial artery graft patency. *J Thorac Cardiovasc Surg* 2002;123:45–52.

45. Cohen G, Tamariz MG, Sever JY, et al. The radial artery versus the saphenous vein graft in contemporary CABG: a case-matched study. *Ann Thorac Surg* 2001;71:180–185.

46. Fremes SE. Multicenter Radial Artery Patency Study (RAPS). Study design. *Control Clin Trials* 2000;21:397–413.

47. Buxton B, Windsor M, Komeda M, et al. How good is the radial artery as a bypass graft? *Coron Artery Dis* 1997;8:225–233.

48. Royse AG, Royse CF, Shah P, et al. Radial artery harvest technique, use and functional outcome. *Eur J Cardiothorac Surg* 1999;15:186–193.

49. Morgenstern DA, Mills NL. New conduits for coronary artery bypass. *Coron Artery Dis* 1993;4:677–681.

50. Mills NL, Hockmuth DR, Everson CT, et al. Right gastroepiploic artery used for coronary artery bypass grafting. Evaluation of flow characteristics and size. *J Thorac Cardiovasc Surg* 1993;106:579–585.

51. Tector AJ, Amundsen S, Schmahl TM, et al. Total revascularization with T grafts. *Ann Thorac Surg* 1994;57:33–38.

52. Borger MA, Cohen G, Buth KJ, et al. Multiple arterial grafts. Radial versus right internal thoracic arteries. *Circulation* 1998;98:II7–II13.

53. Lytle BW, Blackstone EH, Loop FD, et al. Two internal thoracic artery grafts are better than one. *J Thorac Cardiovasc Surg* 1999;117:855–872.

54. Endo M, Nishida H, Tomizawa Y, et al. Benefit of bilateral over single internal mammary artery grafts for multiple coronary artery bypass grafting. *Circulation* 2001;104:2164–2170.

55. Stein PD, Dalen JE, Goldman S, et al. Antithrombotic therapy in patients with saphenous vein and internal mammary artery bypass grafts. *Chest* 2001;119:278S–282S.

56. Collaborative overview of randomised trials of antiplatelet therapy—II: maintenance of vascular graft or arterial patency by antiplatelet therapy. Antiplatelet-Trialists'-Collaboration. *BMJ* 1994;308:159–168.

57. Solymoss BC, Nadeau P, Millette D, et al. Late thrombosis of saphenous vein coronary bypass grafts related to risk factors. *Circulation* 1988;78:I140–I143.

58. FitzGibbon GM, Leach AJ, Kafka HP. Atherosclerosis of coronary artery bypass grafts and smoking. *CMAJ* 1987;136:45–47.

59. The effect of aggressive lowering of low-density lipoprotein cholesterol levels and low-dose anticoagulation on obstructive changes in saphenous-vein coronary-artery bypass grafts. The Post Coronary Artery Bypass Graft Trial Investigators. *N Engl J Med* 1997;336:153–162.

60. Campeau L, Hunninghake DB, Knatterud GL, et al. Aggressive cholesterol lowering delays saphenous vein graft atherosclerosis in women, the elderly, and patients with associated risk factors. NHLBI post coronary artery bypass graft clinical trial. Post CABG Trial Investigators. *Circulation* 1999;99:3241–3247.

61. Knatterud GL, Rosenberg Y, Campeau L, et al. Long-term effects on clinical outcomes of aggressive lowering of low-density lipoprotein cholesterol levels and low-dose anticoagulation in the post coronary artery bypass graft trial. Post CABG Investigators. *Circulation* 2000;102:157–165.

62. Chardigny C, Jebara VA, Acar C, et al. Vasoreactivity of the radial artery. Comparison with the internal mammary and gastroepiploic arteries with implications for coronary artery surgery. *Circulation* 1993;88:II115–II127.

63. Farrar DJ. Development of a prosthetic coronary artery bypass graft. *Heart Surg Forum* 2000;3:36–40.

64. Emery RW, Mills NL, Teijeira FJ, et al. North American experience

with the Perma-Flow prosthetic coronary graft. *Ann Thorac Surg* 1996;62:691–695.

65. Weyand M, Kerber S, Schmid C, et al. Coronary artery bypass grafting with an expanded polytetrafluoroethylene graft. *Ann Thorac Surg* 1999;67:1240–1244.

66. Niklason LE, Gao J, Abbott WM, et al. Functional arteries grown in vitro. *Science* 1999;284:489–493.

67. Kraiss LW, Clowes AW. *Response of the arterial wall to injury and intimal hyperplasia.* In: Sidawy AN, Sumpio BE, DePalma RG, eds. *The basic science of vascular disease.* Armonk, NY: Futura Publishing, 1997:289–317.

68. Allaire E, Clowes AW. Endothelial cell injury in cardiovascular surgery: the intimal hyperplastic response. *Ann Thorac Surg* 1997;63:582–591.

69. Zubilewicz T, Wronski J, Bourriez A, et al. Injury in vascular surgery—the intimal hyperplastic response. *Med Sci Monit* 2001;7:316–324.

70. Sousa JE, Costa MA, Sousa AG, et al. Two-year angiographic and intravascular ultrasound follow-up after implantation of sirolimus-eluting stents in human coronary arteries. *Circulation* 2003;107:381–383.

71. Sousa JE, Costa MA, Abizaid AC, et al. Sustained suppression of neointimal proliferation by sirolimus-eluting stents: one-year angiographic and intravascular ultrasound follow-up. *Circulation* 2001;104:2007–2011.

72. Mann MJ, Whittemore AD, Donaldson MC, et al. Ex-vivo gene therapy of human vascular bypass grafts with E2F decoy: the PREVENT single-centre, randomised, controlled trial. *Lancet* 1999;354:1493–1498.

CHAPTER 45

Genomics and Gene Transfer

Santhi K. Ganesh and Elizabeth G. Nabel

Key Words: Gene therapy; gene transfer; genomics; genotyping; human genome; proteomics.

INTRODUCTION

The discovery of the structure and function of DNA in 1953 laid the foundation for molecular medicine. Molecular medicine currently uses molecular biology approaches and genetic information to formulate clinical diagnoses and treatments. This chapter reviews the application of molecular genetics to the diagnosis and treatment of atherothrombotic cardiovascular disease. The focus of this chapter begins with monogenic and polygenic causes of atherothrombosis. The applications of genotyping, genomics, and proteomics to atherothrombotic diseases are presented. Therapeutic applications of molecular genetics—that is, gene transfer and gene therapy—are then discussed. Vectors, animal models, and human trials are reviewed, and challenges to the field are discussed. A perspective on future directions in the genomics of atherothrombosis follows.

GENOMICS OF ATHEROTHROMBOSIS

Historically, the field of genetics has focused on monogenic disorders—that is, diseases caused by a single gene deletion or mutation. The sequencing of the human genome has pro-

---

    S. K. Ganesh: Cardiovascular Branch, National Heart, Lung, and Blood Institute, National Institutes of Health, Bethesda, Maryland 20892.

    E. G. Nabel: Cardiovascular Branch, National Heart, Lung, and Blood Institute, National Institutes of Health, Bethesda, Maryland 20892.

vided many new approaches to understanding the genetic susceptibility to rare and common cardiovascular diseases. Newer approaches include gene expression profiling by examining patterns of mRNA expression, protein expression profiling or proteomics, and determination of gene sequences or genotyping. Functional analysis of genes, also known as genomics, will be of particular importance in determining gene-based diagnosis, prevention, and therapy of diseases. Analysis of genes and their products is performed in the context of single gene function, as well as function of interconnected pathways and networks. Genomics provides detailed annotation of gene function for those genes that function as part of a complex regulatory network. Complex diseases are multigenic and require the application of approaches designed to examine genes at the sequence and functional level. Understanding the genetic basis for complex diseases, like atherothrombosis, requires an understanding of gene sequences, the proteins the genes encode, and the functions of these proteins.

Monogenetic Disorders

Medical genetics to date has focused on single gene or monogenic diseases, for which the cause of disease is traced to a missing or defective gene. Many disease-causing mutations in single genes are known (see the Online Mendelian Inheritance in Man database for a catalogue of human genes and genetic disorders available at: http://www.ncbi.nlm.nih.gov/omim; a glossary of terms is provided in Table 45–1). A mutation in a single gene inherited in an autosomal pattern is referred to as a "Mendelian" inheritance. Monogenic diseases are rare, although heterozygotes for some re-

TABLE 45–1. *Glossary*

Allele	An alternate form of a gene or genetic locus.
Allelic	A condition in which two phenotypically different traits are the result of different mutations in the same gene.
Alternative splicing	A regulatory mechanism by which variations in the incorporation of a gene's exons, or coding regions, into messenger RNA lead to the production of more than one related protein or isoform.
Codon	A three-base sequence of DNA or RNA that specifies a single amino acid.
Compound heterozygote	An individual with one mutation in one allele of a given gene and another mutation in the other allele of the same genre.
Epigenetic	Nonmutational phenomena, such as methylation or histone modification, that modify gene expression.
Exon	A region of a gene that does not code for a protein.
Genomics	The study of the functions and interactions of the genes in a genome.
Genotype	An individual's genetic makeup defined by his/her DNA sequence.
Haplotype	A group of nearby alleles that are inherited together.
Heterozygote	An individual with a genetic variation (mutation or other) in one copy of any given gene and absence of the variation in the other copy.
Homozygote	An individual with a genetic variation (mutation of other) in both copies of any given gene.
Intron	A region of a gene that does not code for a protein.
Linkage disequilibrium	The nonrandom association in a population of alleles at nearby loci. LD, aka allelic association, exists when alleles at two distinct locations in the genome are more highly associated than expected.

Mendelian distribution	The distribution of inheritance of two alleles in offspring. Example: Suppose one genetic locus has two alleles: A and a. Because each parent passes on one allele, inheritance can be predicted.
	    Mother: A-a (heterozygote)
	    Father: a-A (heterozygote)
	    Children: 25% A-A, 50% A-a, 25%, a-a
	    Mother: a-a (homozygote)
	    Father: a-A (heterozygote)
	    Children: 0% A-A, 50% A-a, 50% a-a

Monogenic	Caused by a mutation in a single gene.
Motif	A DNA sequence pattern within a gene that suggests possible function of the gene or corresponding protein(s), on the basis of similarity to sequences within known gene.
Mutation	A deletion or substitution in base pair sequence in a gene.
Phenotype	The clinical presentation or expression of a specific gene or set of genes, environmental factors, or both.
Polymorphism	A gene variant present in at least 1% of individuals. A single nucleotide polymorphism is variation at a single DNA base and has differing effects depending on the location. Single nucleotide polymorphisms are the most common polymorphism, numbering at an estimated 1.4 million in the human genome.
Positional cloning	Positional cloning determines the physical location of a disease-causing gene through genetics, or physical mapping techniques, or both. It has been most successfully applied in the study of Mendelian disorders. Using positional cloning, a causal gene can be identified without prior knowledge of its function.
Proteomics	The systematic study of the proteome, the proteins expressed by a genome.

cessive conditions are surprisingly common within defined populations. Although these diseases affect few individuals, insights gained from these diseases are applied to common disorders found in the general population.

Factor V Leiden (FVL) is one example in the field of atherothrombosis in which a single gene mutation has led to an understanding of the pathophysiology of arterial and venous thrombosis in common settings. A single base change in the factor V gene, from guanine to adenine at nucleotide position 1691, results in the synthesis of a protein with substitution of arginine with glutamine at position 506, termed FVL. FVL protein is more resistant to cleavage by activated protein C, preventing degradation and promoting clot formation. FVL is the most common genetic mutation predisposing to

venous thromboembolic disease, with a prevalence of 2% to 7% in European populations (1). Approximately 20% to 50% of patients with venous thromboembolic disease have a FVL mutation (2). FVL is inherited as an autosomal dominant trait with incomplete penetrance and variable expression. Approximately 80% of FVL homozygotes and 10% of FVL heterozygotes experience development of thrombosis in their lifetime (3). FVL mutation increases the risk for myocardial infarction (MI), stroke, and venous thrombosis in men (4). In a subset of patients, thrombosis is associated with coinheritance of gene mutations that modify the presentation of FVL (5–7). Identification of these gene modifiers is an active area of research that is essential to distinguish the 10% of heterozygous patients in whom serious thrombosis develops from the ~90% who are asymptomatic. FVL is one example of a monogenetic disorder with a reasonably high prevalence among patients with venous thrombosis and supports the concept that genetic mutations may underlie other athero-thrombotic diseases yet to be discovered.

Complex Trait Analysis

Single Nucleotide Polymorphisms

Human genetics is the study of human variation. On average, any two individuals share ~99.9% of their genomes. Individual variation arises from changes in gene structures, such as polymorphisms, mutations, and microsatellites. Single nucleotide polymorphisms (SNPs) are changes in single bases in a gene sequence. A mutation is a change in base pair (bp) sequence that causes disease or dysfunction. A microsatellite is a 1- to 6-bp sequence repeat. SNPs are the most common form of genetic variation, and there are an estimated 1.4 million SNPs in the human genome (8). SNPs may or may not lead to alterations in gene function. The difference between a SNP and a mutation depends on its prevalence in the population. A single base change is called a polymorphism if it is present in at least 1% of the population studied; a mutation is present in less than 1% of the population (9). Putative and confirmed SNPs are accessible through several public databases, such as dbSNP, a database maintained by the National Center for Biotechnology Information (http://www.ncbi.nlm.nih.gov/SNP/).

SNPs are associated with a disease due to either a direct effect of the SNP on the disease or linkage with a nearby susceptibility locus. An SNP may be a marker of disease susceptibility without causing any functional change in the gene product. SNPs tend to be grouped by genetic regions that are inherited *en bloc*. A set of SNPs that occur together in a given population is known as a haplotype. Haplotypes have important confounding effects on SNP association studies. If a SNP is associated with a disease, it is likely that the SNP is inherited as part of a haplotype in which other SNPs are also statistically associated with the disease. This nonrandom association of alleles is called linkage disequilibrium. Linkage disequilibrium exists when alleles at two distinct locations in the genome are inherited together more frequently than expected. Because a SNP may simply be a marker of disease predisposition rather than a causal agent, demonstration of altered gene function must be shown to prove causality (Fig. 45–1). The International Haplotype Mapping Project or "HapMap" was initiated in October 2002 to construct a genome-wide map of SNP clusters on the basis of DNA samples from different human populations (10). The HapMap will greatly assist genetic association studies. When all haplotypes are defined and a SNP is associated with a disease, the SNP haplotype partners can also be evaluated for contribution to the disease. In summary, SNPs provide insight into the genetic basis for disease for several reasons: They are direct causal agents of altered gene function; markers of disease, regardless of causality; and genome-wide markers for genetic studies because of their presence at high density throughout the genome.

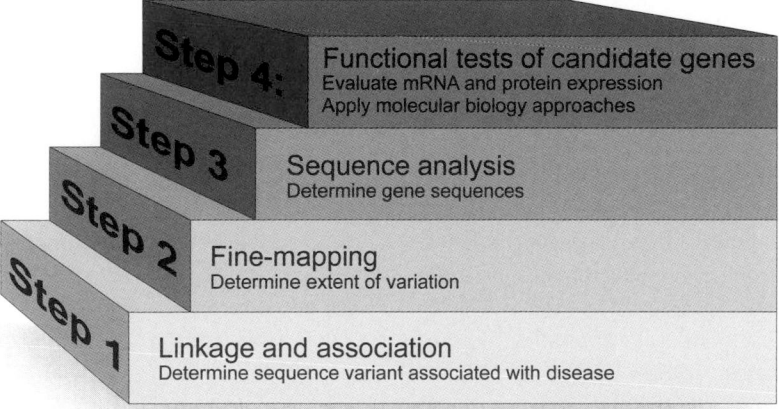

Burden of Proof for Genetic Association Studies

Step 4: Functional tests of candidate genes
Evaluate mRNA and protein expression
Apply molecular biology approaches

Step 3 Sequence analysis
Determine gene sequences

Step 2 Fine-mapping
Determine extent of variation

Step 1 Linkage and association
Determine sequence variant associated with disease

FIG. 45–1. Determining the functional consequences of associated single nucleotide polymorphisms by levels of experimental data. Four steps are essential for gene discovery in the analysis of complex traits. Step 1 is linkage and association of a portion of the genome with the disease. In step 2, various techniques, including linkage disequilibrium testing, may be applied to reduce the size of the genomic interval identified. Step 3 typically involves direct sequencing to identify DNA variations. Finally, step 4 establishes the functional importance of the identified variant. mRNA, messenger RNA. (Adapted from Glazier AM, Nadeau JH, Aitman TJ. Finding genes that underlie complex traits. *Science* 2002;298:941–942, with permission.) (See color insert for Fig. 45–2.)

Linkage Analysis and Association Studies

Two types of genetic studies examine inheritance: linkage analysis and association studies. Linkage studies are performed in families to examine for coinheritance of two traits passed down from parent to child. SNP analyses often reveal coinheritance of two alleles, which occur because genes encoding the two traits reside in close proximity to each other. The traits, or alleles, are linked. Linkage is determined by a LOD score—that is, the logarithm of the odds that markers are linked at a particular distance, divided by the odds that they are linked at 50% coinheritance (not linked at all). This approach is commonly applied to Mendelian traits. Allele-sharing methods also are used to compare similarity of alleles in closely affected individuals, such as affected sibling pairs.

For common disorders without clear Mendelian inheritance, which is typical of most common cardiovascular conditions, population-based association studies are used. Case–control studies provide adequate sample sizes for these investigations. Careful consideration of the most appropriate control population is necessary to draw conclusions and infer gene function from these studies. Known SNPs in candidate genes are investigated, using the alleles of a given SNP as variables, which are then associated with the presence or absence of disease or a particular outcome. If SNPs in a candidate gene are not known, then the gene is directly sequenced in a subset of the study and in control populations to determine which SNPs are differentially represented in the two populations. Confirmation of SNPs is then performed in the remainder of the population using polymerase chain reaction (PCR)–based techniques. This is called a *candidate gene approach*. One limitation of this approach is the bias inherent in selection of candidate genes. Only those genes known or of interest are often chosen for investigation. In contrast, identification of genes by a technique called positional cloning has frequently led to unanticipated discoveries.

The biologic effect of any one SNP is variable. Some SNPs cause biochemical changes in a metabolic pathway, whereas other SNPs lead to structural changes within cells. Other SNPs contribute subtly to an individual's phenotype and require the presence of one or more other genetic variants or an environmental stimulus to become apparent. Once genetic susceptibility to common human diseases is better understood, the role of environmental determinants are more readily determined.

Atherothrombosis and thrombosis are examples of complex diseases resulting from the interaction of inheritance and environment. Current research on complex cardiovascular traits focuses on identification of genetic variants that enhance genetic susceptibility to atherothrombosis. Several investigations have used genome-wide linkage analyses to derive specific DNA variations and susceptibility loci for coronary artery disease and known risk factors for atherothrombosis, including hypercholesterolemia, diabetes, and hypertension (11–24). One example of a genome-wide association study to determine specific genetic variants in

MI was performed by Yamada and colleagues (25). These investigators examined the prevalence of 112 polymorphisms in 71 candidate genes in 2,819 patients with MI and 2,242 control patients at 15 hospitals in Japan. A screening phase involving 909 participants was followed by a large-scale association study involving the other 4,152 participants. The analysis yielded one SNP association in men (C1019T in the *connexin 37* gene) and two in women (4G-668/5G in *plasminogen activator inhibitor type 1* gene and 5A-1171-6A in the *stromelysin-1* gene) that were statistically significant, suggesting that these SNPs may confer susceptibility to MI in this population (25). Another group performed a large-scale analysis of several thousand SNPs in a cohort of approximately 1,100 patients with MI compared with control subjects. Analyses pointed to a single 50 kilobase (kb) haplotype composed of 5 SNPs in genes encoding lymphotoxin-α (LTA), nuclear factor of light polypeptide gene enhancer in B cells, inhibitor-like 1, and human leukocyte antigen B–associated transcript 1. Homozygosity with respect to two SNPs in LTA was significantly associated with increased risk for MI. The investigators demonstrated *in vitro* functional consequence of the SNPs within the *LTA* gene to alter transcriptional level of *LTA* and increase induction of several adhesion molecules, including vascular cell adhesion molecule-1, providing a rationale based on altered gene function for why the associated SNPs may increase the risk for MI (26).

The GeneQuest study examined 62 candidate genes in individuals and family members with premature MI (men <55 years old and women <45 years old). A case–control approach was used to compare genomic sequences in 72 SNPs between persons with premature coronary artery disease and a control population. Interestingly, three variants in thrombospondin genes were identified—thrombospondin-4, 2, and 1—that were associated with premature MI. The mechanisms by which thrombospondin genes, which encode for platelet products, may be causal in MI is under investigation (27).

Genome-wide scans of SNPs are newer techniques performed on high-throughput platforms and assay for several thousand SNPs simultaneously. By taking advantage of the physical distribution of SNPs through the genome, chromosomal regions between SNPs are associated with a disease. With this technique, SNPs can be identified as biomarkers of disease. This approach will be an active area of research in the atherothrombosis field in the coming years.

Genomics

Genomics is the study of the function and interactions of genes within the genome. This is accomplished by investigation of gene sequences, as in the case of genome-wide SNP association studies. However, obtaining sequence information is only the first step in understanding how a genome functions. Gene function is examined at the level of gene products, mRNA and protein, with two approaches. The first approach is to investigate a hypothesis using mRNA or protein analysis. The second approach is gene discovery where the goal is to discover new genes and their function.

Gene Expression Profiling: Microarrays

Microarrays are techniques that permit detection of gene expression through analysis of RNA (Fig. 45–2) (see color insert). Three methods are used to profile gene expression: complementary DNA (cDNA) arrays, oligonucleotide arrays, and serial analysis of gene expression (SAGE). Microarrays are used for three purposes: discovery of genes and pathways involved in disease (hypothesis-generating); testing of specific hypotheses (hypothesis-confirming); and molecular fingerprinting of individual patients (28,29).

cDNA microarrays are created from probe cDNA libraries (500–5,000 bases) that are then hybridized to a target RNA. A cDNA microarray is constructed by spotting a cDNA corresponding to an individual gene, termed a probe, at a precise location on the microscope slide. To perform cDNA microarray analysis, RNAs are first isolated from target tissues and labeled with a fluorescent dye. Labeled RNA pools are hybridized to the cDNA microarray surface, along with a control sample. The two RNA samples compete for binding to each probe; RNA that matches the cDNA sequence binds or hybridizes to the individual cDNA spot on the microscope surface. The two samples on the microarray are compared, usually using a dual fluorescent dye system, such as Cy 3 and Cy 5, where each sample is labeled with one of the two dyes. The fluorescent images are compared using the signal intensities from the fluorescent dyes from each probe. The comparison reflects the ratios of RNA abundance for each expressed gene. Results between separate microarrays can be compared after application of normalization strategies that allow for standardization of interarray comparisons.

Oligonucleotide arrays are created by attachment of synthetic nucleotide probes (12- to 80-mer oligonucleotides) representative of unique portions of genes to an array surface. This type of array also requires synthesis of cDNA from the experimental mRNA sample but then additionally follows with an *in vitro* transcription step to create biotin-labeled cRNA that is hybridized to the microarray target. The microarray is treated with a fluorescent dye tagged to avidin and subjected to laser image analysis. As opposed to cDNA arrays, single samples are applied to each oligonucleotide microarray. Signal intensities are measured as a reflection of expression level for each expressed gene.

SAGE is a technique for global characterization of gene expression on the basis of direct sequencing of transcripts rather than an array platform. The strength of SAGE is the ability to analyze transcripts when the sequence is unknown. It requires approximately tenfold larger mRNA requirements for analysis and is relatively inefficient, even with automated sequencers, because the simplest two-sample comparison requires sequencing of 1.5×10^6 bases. These factors make it generally less suitable for cardiovascular ap-

plications compared with microarrays, despite its greater sensitivity for changes in expression level (30,31).

After acquisition of data by image processing, data are analyzed in three steps: normalization, filtering, and computation. Normalization accounts for technical factors, such as array manufacturing, differences in dye incorporation, and irregularities in probe distribution during hybridization, and it is performed to allow meaningful comparisons between individual arrays. Filtering of data refers to the selection of those data likely to represent significant findings. Typical criteria for filtering include assessment of signal quality and fold change in gene expression level. Differential gene expression in microarray analysis often is defined by a 1.5- to 2-fold difference in relative gene expression level. Once data has been normalized and filtered, various analytic approaches can be applied. Data analysis often is performed with a two-stage approach. The first stage simplifies the data by organizing gene expression by meaningful compartments using techniques such as clustering and principal components analysis. The second step is statistical analysis. Before any microarray data are taken at face value, significant findings should be validated with independent testing of RNA expression levels using quantitative reverse transcription PCR.

Clinical Uses of Microarrays

Microarrays have been used successfully in research applications designed to understand the pathophysiology of cardiac hypertrophy, heart failure, arrhythmias, and restenosis. Zohlnhofer and colleagues (32,33) identified clusters of differentially expressed genes from coronary artery neointima and peripheral blood leukocytes (PBLs) in patients with coronary restenosis, as compared with samples of normal coronary arteries. These investigators identified clusters of genes that were differentially up-regulated in the restenosis tissue, compared with the normal coronary artery samples. Cell proliferation, extracellular matrix, cell adhesion, and inflammatory genes were up-regulated in the restenosis samples. Many genes were expressed to a similar extent in neointimal tissue and PBLs, suggesting that PBLs might be a source of tissue for analysis in atherothrombosis when vascular tissue is not accessible.

Proteomics

The proteome is defined as the complement of proteins expressed by the genome. Investigation at the protein level is directly reflective of cellular function and alterations in disease states. Therefore, proteomic studies are functional genomic investigations. Tools used in proteomics are based on the human genome sequence and well established analytic methods that have been adapted for use in proteomics (Fig. 45–3). These tools allow profiling of proteins and determination of protein modifications for the purposes of defining disease mechanisms and biomarker discovery. Examples of proteomic applications in cardiovascular research include

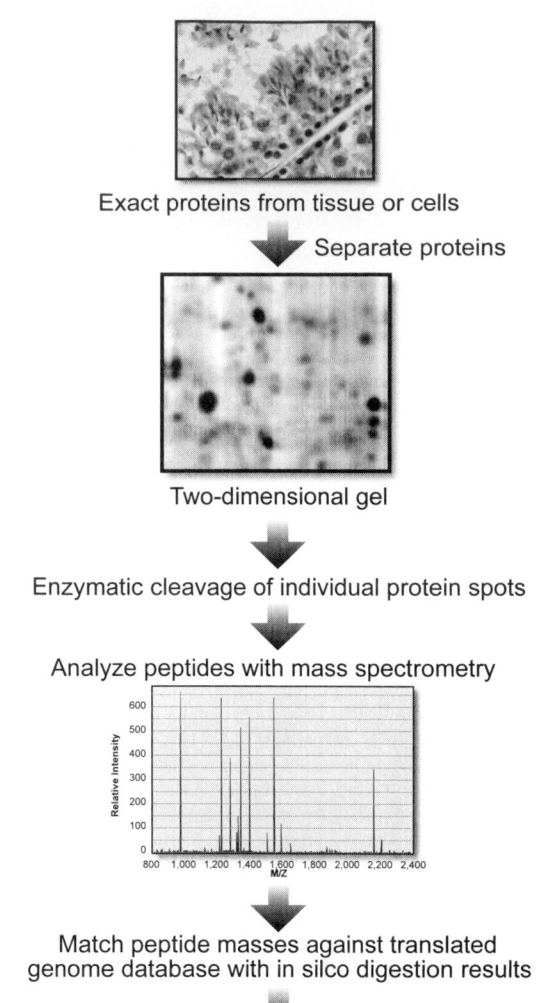

Exact proteins from tissue or cells

→ Separate proteins

Two-dimensional gel

Enzymatic cleavage of individual protein spots

Analyze peptides with mass spectrometry

Match peptide masses against translated genome database with in silco digestion results

Identify proteins

FIG. 45–3. Typical proteomic workflow for peptide mass fingerprinting. Proteins are isolated from the cells or tissue of interest and separated. In this example, two-dimensional gel electrophoresis is the separation method. Individual protein spots are then cut out of the gel and enzymatically digested into peptides of which mass is determined using mass spectrometry.

the determination of downstream effectors of protein kinase C signaling during myocardial preconditioning (34) and phosphatase-binding proteins in vascular smooth muscle cells (35). As proteomic technologies develop and applications in cardiovascular research broaden, significant understanding of disease mechanisms, prediction of responses to pharmacologic therapies, and biomarker discovery will be possible (36).

Summary

Cardiovascular research is in the midst of a significant transition that is being driven by the availability of DNA sequence information and genome-based technologies with which to

investigate diseases. Application of these technologies will establish functional relations between genes and diseases. The resulting understanding of molecular genetic mechanisms for atherothrombotic diseases holds promise for accurate disease detection, improved risk stratification of patients, and determination of novel therapeutic targets. Current research initiatives focus on the natural history of monogenic disorders in large numbers of patients with specific mutations, to identify persons at high risk for cardiovascular events, asymptomatic carriers in whom pharmacologic interventions will retard or prevent disease, and nonaffected family members whose concern about their health can be addressed. With regard to complex traits in more common cardiovascular diseases, genomics research is identifying functionally significant variations in DNA sequences that can establish a molecular diagnosis and influence patient outcome. Because therapeutic gene transfer requires thorough understanding of the functions of genes in disease pathogenesis, the determination of disease-causing gene targets in genomic investigations of atherothrombosis will enable these strategies in the field of atherothrombosis.

VASCULAR GENE TRANSFER

Gene transfer is the introduction and expression of recombinant genes in mammalian cells. The goal of gene transfer is to introduce recombinant genes into target cells to study the mechanisms and consequences of gene expression. Genes are transfected into cells using vectors. The recombinant gene undergoes transcription into RNA and translation into protein by host enzymes, culminating in the expression of the recombinant protein. The recombinant protein remains intracellular or is secreted into the extracellular space or circulation. Gene expression is transient or stable, depending on whether integration into chromosomes occurs. The efficiency of DNA uptake and gene expression, often referred to as transfection efficiency, is dependent on many factors, including delivery of DNA to the cell, uptake of DNA into the cytoplasm, degradation of DNA in endosomes, release of DNA from endosomes into the cytoplasm, transport to the nucleus, and persistence in the nucleus.

In vivo gene transfer is performed by cell-mediated or direct gene transfer methods. Cell-mediated or *ex vivo* gene transfer involves removing autologous cells from the host and transfecting the cells with the vector *in vitro* (37). Genetically modified cells are reintroduced into the host by infusion or injection. *Ex vivo* gene transfer permits the introduction of recombinant genetic material into a specific cell—for example, endothelial or smooth muscle cells—and analysis of recombinant gene expression within that cell type.

In vivo gene transfer uses the direct introduction of recombinant genes into target cells and tissues (38). Targeted gene transfer in the vasculature has been performed with cell-specific promoters to achieve gene expression within endothelial cells or smooth muscle cells (39). Both *ex vivo* and *in vivo* gene transfer approaches have been used in the development of animal models of vascular disease and in clinical trials of gene transfer to the cardiovascular system.

Vector Systems

Transfection of appropriate target cells represents the critical first step in gene transfer. As a result, development of gene transfer methods has represented a significant area of research in the field. Both viral and nonviral vectors have been used in vascular gene transfer studies. A common feature of these methods is the efficient delivery of genes into cells. Vectors differ, however, in the processing of foreign DNA and the frequency of integration into chromosomal DNA. In the case of retroviral and lentiviral vectors, the transferred sequences are stably integrated into the chromosomal DNA of the target cell. These vectors have been considered most often for *ex vivo* gene therapy. Other methods of gene transfer result primarily in the introduction of foreign DNA into target cell nuclei in an unintegrated form. These methods result in high, but transient, gene expression. These vectors, including adenovirus, adeno-associated virus (AAV), and cationic liposomes, have been used predominantly for *in vivo* gene transfer studies.

Retroviruses

Retroviruses were the first vectors used in gene transfer studies in the 1980s. Interest in retroviruses as vectors stemmed from the observation that these vectors can stably transduce up to 100% of target cells in culture (40). Retroviral vectors were used initially in vascular gene transfer studies, primarily in *ex vivo* studies (37). However, their use in the vasculature was limited because of low transfection efficiencies. More recently, retroviral vectors were used in gene therapy studies for treatment of severe combined immune deficiency. Unfortunately, in one trial, two children experienced the complication of retroviral insertion into an oncogenic site of chromosome X, leading to leukemia (41).

Adenovirus

Adenovirus types 2 and type 5 have been developed for use as viral vectors in gene therapy (42). The adenovirus genome is composed of linear, double-stranded DNA approximately 36 kb in length, which is divided into 100 map units, each of which is 360 bp in length. The DNA contains short inverted terminal repeats (ITRs) at the end of the genome that are required for viral DNA replication. The gene products are organized into early (E1-E4) and late (L1-L5) regions, on the basis of expression before or after initiation of DNA replication. Adenoviruses have a lytic life cycle that is characterized by attachment to an adenoviral glycoprotein receptor on mammalian target cells and entry into cells by receptor-mediated endocytosis. Adenoviruses escape lysosomal degradation by adenoviral capsid proteins,

and viral DNA translocates to the nucleus. Expression of viral genes depends on cellular transcription factors and expression of the adenoviral E1 region (early region), which encodes a transactivator of viral gene expression. During lytic infection, the viral genome replicates to several thousand copies per cell. The viral genome associates with core proteins and is packaged into capsids by self-assembling of major capsid proteins.

Replication-deficient adenoviral vectors developed for gene transfer contain deletions of the E1A and E1B regions. The E1 region regulates adenoviral transcription and is required for viral replication. Foreign cDNA inserted into the adenoviral genome as a replacement for the E1 region result in a replication-defective adenovirus. Adenoviral vectors are produced by homologous recombination in 293 cells or any cell line that contains an integrated copy of the adenoviral E1 region. A foreign cDNA with appropriate eukaryotic regulatory sequences is introduced into a bacterial plasmid that contains a small region of the left adenoviral genome (type 2 or type 5) that has been deleted of the native *E1* gene. The bacterial plasmid is cotransfected into 293 cells with an incomplete adenoviral genome. Homologous recombination between the two DNA generates a recombinant genome in which the E1 region is replaced by the foreign gene. Viral stock is propagated in 293 cells to high titer, generally 10^9 to 10^{10} plaque-forming units per milliliter.

Adenovirus types 2 and 5 produce a respiratory disease in humans. These subclasses of adenovirus are not associated with human malignancies. Live adenovirus vaccines have been used safely in human populations. Adenoviral vectors have several additional advantages, including efficient infection of mammalian cells and expression in nondividing cells *in vitro* and *in vivo*. These vectors are relatively stable and can be grown and concentrated to a high titer. Extrachromosomal replication of the vector greatly reduces the chance of mutation by random integration and dysregulation of host cellular genes.

Despite these advantages, there are several limitations to the use of adenoviral vectors for gene transfer experiments. Gene expression in vascular and myocardial cells after adenoviral infection usually persists for only several weeks (43–45). Although transient gene expression may be desirable for some vascular therapies, other vascular diseases may require long-term gene expression. Loss of foreign gene sequences has been observed in the liver (46), muscle (47), and other tissues after adenoviral infection. Transient expression may result from loss of viral genomic DNA, promoter extinction, or host immune responses.

The development of host immune response to adenoviral proteins has been a major limitation to use of these vectors *in vivo*. Most adults have neutralizing antibodies to one or more adenoviral serotypes. Viral infection of experimental animals results in neutralizing antibody titers directed against adenoviral capsid proteins (48). Although low levels of neutralizing antibodies do not appear to have adverse clinical effects, it remains to be determined whether host immune responses to the adenovirus will preclude repeated administrations of the same serotype of adenovirus. First-generation recombinant adenoviral vectors (deletion of *E1A* and *E1B* genes and partial deletion of *E3* genes) were used for *in vivo* gene therapy treatments for cystic fibrosis (49); however, in animal models, gene expression was transient and often associated with tissue inflammation, particularly in the liver and lung (50). Inactivation of the *E2A* gene has been associated with longer gene expression and less inflammation in lung and liver. In arterial gene transfer studies using adenoviral vectors, mononuclear inflammatory cell infiltrates have been observed in the adventitia of peripheral (51) and pulmonary (45) arteries, but no necrosis or vasculitis was observed. Infection of pulmonary arteries with adenovirus was associated with mild degrees of perivascular inflammation; however, pulmonary arteries instilled with saline or liposomes also exhibited mild accumulation of perivascular mononuclear cells (45).

Recombinant adenoviral vectors have been used to introduce genes into multiple cell lines *in vitro* and into tissue *in vivo*. Despite the current problems with generation of immune response to adenoviral capsid proteins, the adenoviral vectors are attractive vehicles for *in vivo* gene transfer because of their efficient infection of many mammalian cells, including nondividing quiescent cells. Whether adenoviral vectors will be used clinically is currently unknown.

Adeno-associated Virus

AAV is a defective human parvovirus with attractive properties for gene transfer. This virus can be prepared at high titers, is not normally pathogenic in humans, and can infect many cell types *in vitro* (52). The AAV genome is a single-stranded, linear, 5-kb DNA molecule. The wild-type AAV integrates in a site-specific fashion into a single 7-kb region on human chromosome 19. The AAV genome is flanked by 145-bp ITRs containing the sequences required for packaging, DNA replication, and integration. The coding region contains two open reading frames, which can be deleted and replaced with one or more transgenes plus transcriptional regulatory units (53). AAV vectors can accept transgene cassettes of only 4 to 5 kb; this limits the types of transgenes that can be used. Propagation of AAV vectors requires complex packaging, including AAV Rep and Cap proteins and five adenoviral proteins (i.e., E1A, E1B, E2A, E4, and VA). These complex packaging requirements have precluded construction of a helper cell line for AAV. Currently, vectors are constructed by cotransfection of cells with the AAV vector and a nonpackageable plasmid containing the AAV Rep and Cap proteins. This is followed by infection of the transfected cells with wild-type or mutant helper adenovirus. AAV is separated from contaminating adenovirus by heat treatment and equilibrium density gradation centrifugation. Protocols for constructing AAV vectors are described elsewhere (52).

AAV vectors infect a variety of cells *in vitro*, but their use *in vivo* has not been established. Their ability to transduce vascular endothelial cells and smooth muscle cells also remains unknown (54), and several problems are associated with their use. Lack of a packaging cell line and need for coinfection with adenovirus make it difficult to prepare large quantities of pure AAV vectors. Deletion of viral genes during vector construction limits the ability of these vectors to integrate in a site-specific manner, and it raises the possibility of insertional mutagenesis. AAV vectors are theoretically attractive, but considerable work is required before they can be implemented broadly (53).

Cationic Liposomes

Cationic lipids are preparations of positively charged lipids that spontaneously complex with negatively charged DNA to form DNA–lipid conjugates. The lipid component facilitates delivery of DNA to cells by fusion with plasmid membrane or with endosomal membranes after endocytosis. After release from endosomes, plasmid DNA is maintained in an extrachromosomal form.

Cationic liposomes have been used in arterial gene transfer studies *in vivo* in several animal models, including rats (55), rabbits (56), dogs (57), and pigs (38,58). There are several advantages of cationic liposomes, including a favorable safety profile. Liposome vectors contain no viral coding sequences. There are fewer cDNA size constraints in vector construction. Cationic liposomes have been administered intravenously and intraarterially with minimal biochemical, hemodynamic, or cardiac toxicity in animals or humans (59). Cationic liposome vectors are straightforward to prepare for experimental and clinical use.

In vitro, approximately 5% to 15% of endothelial cells and smooth muscle cells are transfected with liposome vectors (45). In porcine arteries *in vivo*, the efficiency of gene transfer is 0.1% to 1% of cells (38). After liposomal transfection, gene expression persists for approximately 1 month (45). Cell division is not required for liposome transfection, although the efficiency appears to be increased in proliferating vascular cells (56).

Hemagglutinating Virus of Japan Liposome Complexes

Another liposome vector involves the encapsulation of plasmid DNA and nuclear protein in liposomes fused with a heat-inactivated hemagglutinating virus of Japan (HVJ). HVJ is used to fuse DNA-loaded liposome vesicles with cell membranes. A nuclear protein, high mobility group I, often is included to facilitate migration of plasmid DNA to the nucleus. HVJ liposome gene transfer has been used in rat arterial models to investigate the function of angiotensin-converting enzyme and renin genes (55). In the rat carotid artery, this vector yields an efficiency greater than or equal to 30% of vascular cells without local toxicity.

In addition, HVJ liposomes have been used to deliver antisense oligonucleotides to rat carotid arteries, to inhibit vascular cell proliferation (60). It is likely that further modifications to vectors used for vascular gene transfer will include components of viral and nonviral vectors that optimize delivery, improve gene expression, and minimize toxic side effects.

Polymers

Nucleic acids and drugs have been applied to polymer gels coated onto stents or balloons and directly applied to arteries. Hydrogel catheters were developed to transmit plasmid DNA to rabbit arteries *in vivo* and to humans in clinical gene therapy trials (61). Over time, other polymers were developed associated with stenting of arteries, but many early polymers were associated with intense inflammatory reactions. Newer formulations have been successfully used in the development of drug-eluting stents (62,63).

Animal Models

Gene transfer has been successfully used to develop animal models of cardiovascular disease in many species, including mice, rats, rabbits, dogs, and pigs. The goals of these studies have been to define gene function and to develop potential new therapeutic strategies for vascular proliferative disorders. Two approaches have been used: *ex vivo* and *in vivo* gene transfer.

Ex Vivo *Gene Transfer*

Ex vivo gene transfer in the vasculature is the seeding of transduced cells onto denuded arteries or vascular prostheses. The feasibility of *ex vivo* gene transfer has been demonstrated using transfected autologous endothelial (37) and vascular smooth muscle (64) cells. One application of *ex vivo* gene transfer technology is the seeding of vascular prostheses, such as synthetic grafts and stents, with endothelial cells transduced to optimize fibrinolysis, thrombolysis, or both. Prosthetic devices have been seeded with endothelial cells encoding fibrinolytic genes such as tissue-type plasminogen activator and urokinase-type plasminogen activator (65). Further studies are required to define the usefulness of this approach.

Direct In Vivo *Gene Transfer*

Direct gene transfer into arteries has been performed in normal, injured, and atherothrombotic vessels of rats, rabbits, dogs, and pigs. Initial studies used retroviral and cationic liposome vectors. Studies in normal arteries of pigs (38), dogs (57), and rabbits (66) suggested an efficiency of gene transfer of approximately 0.1% to 1% of cells. Gene transfer into

balloon-injured arteries is higher, suggesting that ongoing cell proliferation at the time of transfection may improve the frequency of gene expression. After transfer of reporter genes, multiple layers in arteries are transfected, including the intima, media, and adventitia. However, regions of greatest gene expression are endothelial and smooth muscle cells in the intima, smooth muscle cells in the luminal region of the media, and connective tissues and capillary endothelial cells in the adventitia. Simple infusion of vector into normal arteries results in transfection of primarily intimal cells; the application of pressure to the vector infusate results in delivery of DNA vector transmurally with gene expression in the media. Several delivery catheters have been used in gene transfer studies, and the patterns of gene expression within an artery may differ depending on the design of the catheter (66). These catheters include the double-balloon catheter, porous balloon catheter, hydrogel catheter, and simple ligation techniques.

To improve gene transfer frequencies and expression in the vasculature, adenoviral vectors have been used. These first-generation adenoviral vectors, characterized by deletion of *E1A* and *E1B* genes and partial deletion of *E3* genes, result in a greater efficiency of gene transfer and expression in arteries *in vivo*. Adenoviral vectors encoding reporter genes have been infused in direct gene transfer experiments in the peripheral, coronary, and pulmonary vasculature in several species. Adenoviral infection of injured rat and porcine arteries results in reporter gene expression in endothelial cells and smooth muscle cells in the intima and media. The efficiency of gene transfer in intimal smooth muscle cells of injured rat arteries is reported to be 10% to 75% (67). A common finding in these studies is the transient nature of gene expression after adenoviral injection. Gene expression, measured by mRNA and protein expression, generally peaks at 1 to 2 weeks and is lost by 1 month.

Studies of Gene Expression and Function

Direct gene transfer has been used as a somatic transgenic model to define gene function in the vessel wall. In this system, recombinant genes are expressed in local arterial segments, and their biologic function is investigated. This approach has proved useful for the investigation of growth regulatory and cytokine genes, whose direct *in vivo* effects have been difficult to analyze (68).

Our laboratory has been interested in investigating the pathogenesis of smooth muscle cell proliferation *in vivo*. We examined the expression of growth factor genes in porcine arteries. These recombinant growth factor genes include platelet-derived growth factor B (PDGF-B), the secreted form of fibroblast growth factor-1 (FGF-1), and a secreted form of active transforming growth factor-β_1 (TGF-β_1). Arteries transfected with a *PDGF-B* gene demonstrated severe intimal thickening, characterized by increased intima-to-media area ratios, compared with control vessels transfected with a reporter gene (58). In contrast, expression of secreted FGF-1 was associated with expansion of the intima and intimal angiogenesis (69). The source of the intimal capillaries was luminal endothelial cells, because immunohistochemical studies identifying endothelial cells using von Willebrand factor (vWF) antibody revealed vWF staining in adventitial capillaries but not in luminal endothelial cells or in intimal capillary endothelial cells. Arteries transfected with a human TGF-β_1 gene demonstrated increased procollagen synthesis in the intima and media as early as 4 days after gene transfer (70). These findings suggested differential patterns of gene expression for these three growth factors. Although PDGF-B, FGF-1, and TGF-β_1 each stimulated vascular cell proliferation *in vivo,* they exerted different effects on smooth muscle cell proliferation, angiogenesis, and procollagen synthesis. These findings also suggested that intimal thickening is a common response to the expression of many growth factors and cytokines.

One approach to investigating the pathogenesis of vascular cell proliferation *in vivo* is to examine gene products that inhibit cell proliferation. One approach to the selective elimination of dividing cells was to express a herpes virus thymidine kinase (HSV-*tk*) gene in smooth muscle cells after balloon injury. Thymidine kinase, when expressed in transduced cells, converts ganciclovir, a nucleoside analog, into an active toxic form. The efficacy of an adenoviral vector encoding a herpes virus *tk* gene (ADV-*tk*) in altering the development of intimal hyperplasia after balloon injury was tested in a pig model of balloon injury (51). ADV-*tk* vectors were transfected into balloon-injured porcine arteries, and ganciclovir or saline treatment was administered 36 hours later. A significant reduction in BrdC labeling in intimal cells and in intima-to-media (I/M) area ratio was observed in vessels subjected to mild or severe injury in animals transduced with ADV-*tk* and treated with ganciclovir, compared with control groups. This reduction in I/M area ratio persisted 6 weeks after balloon injury, suggesting a prolonged effect. Similar reductions in cell proliferation were observed in rat models as well (71,72).

Additional approaches to limit smooth muscle cell proliferation after vascular injury could potentially include targeting of cell cycle inhibitors including the retinoblastoma gene product (Rb) (73), p21^{Cip1} (74,75), or p27^{Kip1} (76). The cell cycle inhibitors are potent regulators of smooth muscle cell and monocyte/macrophage proliferation and are important targets for restenosis (77,78). The role of constitutive or endothelium-derived nitric oxide synthase (NOS) in the regulation of smooth muscle cell proliferation also has been studied *in vivo.* Transfection of HVJ liposome vectors encoding endothelial cell–derived NOS (ecNOS) in injured rat carotid arteries was associated with local NO generation and a reduction in intimal thickening in ecNOS-transfected vessels compared with control vessels transfected with a reporter gene (79).

Angiogenesis

Therapeutic vascular growth involves the stimulation of angiogenesis, arteriogenesis, and lymphangiogenesis. Angiogenesis is the sprouting of new blood vessels from preexisting vessels. Arteriogenesis is the enlargement of muscular collateral blood vessels from preexisting arteriolar anastomoses, and often is referred to as *collateralization.* Lymphangiogenesis is the generation of new lymphatic vessels from preexisting ones. Multiple growth factors have been used to stimulate therapeutic vascular growth. Vascular endothelial growth factor A (VEGF-A) has been widely used in preclinical and clinical studies. Two splice variants, VEGF$_{165}$ and VEGF$_{121}$, have been consistently angiogenic in animal models (80) and have been evaluated in clinical trials (81). VEGF-B (82), VEGF-C (83), VEGF-D (84), VEGF-E (85), and placental growth factor (PlGF) (86) also have angiogenic activity in preclinical animal models. PlGF binds to VEGFR1 and has been implicated in angiogenesis under pathologic conditions (87). An important property of VEGF-A, VEGF-B, and PlGF is their chemotactic effect on monocytes and macrophages through activation of VEGFR1 in these cells. Interestingly, PlGF also promotes angiogenesis and arteriogenesis through mobilization of hematopoietic stem cells and endothelial progenitor cells (EPCs) from the bone marrow (87). The clinical relevance of VEGF-B, PlGF, and EPCs in the clinical treatment of ischemia remains undetermined.

VEGF-induced capillaries regress soon after cessation of treatment (88). Factors needed to stabilize newly formed vessels are not known, although clinical experience would suggest that blood flow is required to promote persistence of vessels. In addition, arterialization of new conduits and recruitment of pericytes are required to generate functional, persistent blood vessels. In addition, optimization of dose and duration of VEGF expression are key elements in moving from preclinical to successful clinical vascular growth therapy.

Other growth factors have been evaluated for their angiogenic properties. Angiopoietin-1 and VEGF gene transfer reportedly increase the size of collateral vessels, although angiopoietin-1 alone does not stimulate endothelial cell proliferation (89). The role of angiopoietin-1 and 2 in vascular gene therapy is unknown. The FGF family has 23 known members; of these, FGF-1, FGF-2, FGF-4, and FGF-5 have been used for angiogenesis studies (90). The FGFs stimulate the proliferation of mesodermal and neuroectodermal cells, including endothelial cells, smooth muscle cells, and myoblasts. FGFs and VEGFs have synergistic effects—that is, FGF-4–induced angiogenesis may be mediated in part by VEGF-A (91). Hepatocyte growth factor (HGF) induces angiogenesis in several animal models (92), and an HGF plasmid is in phase I clinical trials for peripheral vascular disease. Another strategy for the induction of angiogenesis *in vivo* is the expression of cellular genes or transcription factors that induce angiogenic factors. For example, endothelial and inducible NOS are important mediators of angiogenesis and arteriogenesis, but not lymphangiogenesis (88). Hypoxia-inducible factor-1α activates several angiogenic growth factors, including VEGF-A, VEGFR2, insulin-like growth factor-2, and erythropoietin (93). A leucine zipper transcription factor that activated VEGF transcription also has been described (94).

The concept of therapeutic vascular growth has been tested in several animal models of peripheral and myocardial ischemia, including *ex vivo* transduction of stem cells and EPCs (reviewed in References 80, 95, and 96). Several lessons have been learned from the preclinical animal studies when applied to human clinical trials. The efficiency of adenoviral-mediated VEGF and FGF delivery and vascular growth has been demonstrated in the myocardium and skeletal muscle. Proliferation and enlargement of capillaries has been observed, although cessation of therapy (or extinction of the transgene) leads to regression of most of the vessels. Importantly, expression of VEGF for more than 4 weeks led to sufficient vascular remodeling that new vessel growth persisted for several months after withdrawing VEGF treatment (97). In many animal models, hemodynamic factors and persistence of blood flow are important for stabilization of the newly formed vessels. In addition, it is important to remember that the predictive value of a preclinical animal model is inversely related to the animal size. Many applications and vectors work well in smaller animals, like mice and rats, but scale up to larger animals like pigs, dogs, and sheep has proven difficult. Finally, demonstration of efficacy in young, healthy animals may not predict responses in older patients with chronic diseases. Indeed, vascular growth is impaired in elderly and diabetic animals (98). Hence, many of the beneficial biologic effects reported in animals may not be achievable in humans, given current gene vector technologies.

CLINICAL TRIALS

Cardiovascular gene therapy trials have proceeded in two areas: vascular proliferative disease and angiogenesis. Vascular studies have used cell cycle inhibitors or NOS to inhibit vascular smooth muscle cell proliferation that leads to intimal hyperplasia and recurrent arterial and graft narrowing. A phase I/II trial, PREVENT, to prevent bypass graft failure after peripheral surgery was conducted using oligonucleotides mixed with a liposome vector targeted as decoys against the transcription factor E2F (99). The transcription factor E2F acts at the G_1/S phase cell cycle checkpoint, and blockage of E2F activation leads to G_1 arrest, inhibiting vascular smooth muscle cell proliferation. Patients were randomized to one of three groups—placebo, E2F decoys, and scrambled oligonucleotides—and the oligonucleotides were introduced into venous grafts at the time of peripheral bypass surgery. A statistically significant decrease in time to primary graft failure was observed in the E2F decoy group, although phase III studies will be required to validate these results. Other studies have evaluated the potential role of VEGF as an inhibitor of restenosis after angioplasty (100).

Stimulation of angiogenesis and arteriogenesis is required to improve perfusion of myocardial or skeletal muscle. Therapeutic angiogenesis trials conducted to date can be grouped into three phases. The initial group of phase I clinical trials used plasmid DNA (101–103) and adenoviruses (104,105) (Table 45–2) to induce angiogenesis for peripheral or myocardial ischemia. These phase I trials evaluated the vector and delivery approach (catheter or direct injection) in small numbers of patients. In general, the findings of these trials were consistent: No serious adverse events were encountered attributable to the gene vector or delivery device. With this demonstration of safety in place, the second phase of trials was conducted. These phase I/II trials evaluated larger numbers of patients and began to examine efficacy (106–114). Again, no major adverse events were reported, and, indeed, positive efficacy findings were reported, although it should be noted that many of these trials were not controlled. Collectively, these trials revealed several important clinical insights. Placebo effects are significant in treated patients, possibly because of altered hemodynamics, earlier mobilization, and perhaps better care. Meaningful clinical end points need to be predefined. Although these clinical results are promising, the findings are difficult to interpret in the absence of controlled, randomized trials. More recently, the third phase of clinical trials have gone forward—that is, randomized, placebo-controlled studies including larger number of patients and predefined clinical end points (115–123).

Currently, we do not know whether a gene therapy product will be approved by the U.S. Food and Drug Administration and clinically used to treat myocardial or peripheral ischemia, or both. Data from these phase III studies, as well as long-term follow-up, will be critical. A greater understanding of the pharmacokinetics will be required (124). To date, however, safety concerns present in other organ systems have not occurred, fortunately, in the cardiovascular system. We must, therefore, proceed with carefully conducted and evaluated trials.

FUTURE DIRECTIONS

Our understanding of the mechanisms by which single genes cause disease have been helpful to an understanding of the pathophysiology of complex common cardiovascular diseases. The challenge ahead is to understand in greater detail the genetic susceptibility to the common cardiovascular diseases. The tools of genomics, genotyping, and proteomics will provide approaches, but this exploration will require thoughtful, observant clinicians who detect unusual patterns of disease in their patients. Furthermore, we currently do not know whether genetic treatments will find a place in the everyday, pharmacologic armamentarium of

TABLE 45–2. *Clinical angiogenesis trials: phase II/III*

Trial	Therapeutic agent	Disease	n	End point	Results[a]	Reference
VIVA trial	Recombinant VEGF protein	CAD	178	ETT at 60 d	Negative	115
FIRST trial	Recombinant FGF-2 protein	CAD	337	ETT at 90 d	Negative	116
TRAFFIC trial	Recombinant FGF-2 protein	PVD	190	ETT at 90 d	Positive	117
GM-CSF trial	Recombinant GM-CSF protein	CAD	21	Invasive collateral flow Index at 2 weeks	Positive	118
AGENT trial	Adenovirus-FGF-4	CAD	79	ETT at 4 weeks	Positive[b]	119
VEGF PVD trial	Adenorivus-VEGF$_{165}$ Plasmid/liposome VEGF$_{165}$	PVD	54	Increased vascularity in angiography at 3 months	Positive	120
KAT trial	Adenovirus-VEGF$_{165}$ Plasmid/liposome VEGF$_{165}$	CAD	103	Improved myocardial perfusion at 6 months	Positive (adenovirus group only)	121
RAVE trial (Biobypass-PAD)	Adenovirus VEGF$_{121}$	PVD	105	Peak walking time at 12 weeks	Negative	122
Euroinject One Trial	Plasmid VEGF$_{165}$	CAD	74	Improved myocardial perfusion at 3 months	Negative[c]	123

AGENT, Angiogenic Gene Therapy; CAD, coronary artery disease; ETT, exercise tolerance test; FIRST, FGF Initiating Revascularization Trial; FGF, fibroblast growth factor; GM-CSF, granulocyte-monocyte colony-stimulating factor; KAT, Kuopio Angiogenesis Trial; PVD, peripheral vascular disease; RAVE, Regional Angiogenesis with Vascular Endothelial Growth Factor; TRAFFIC, therapeutic angiogenesis with recombinant fibroblast growth factor-2 for intermittent claudication; VEGF, vascular endothelial growth factor; VIVA, vascular endothelial growth factor for ischemia for vascular angiogenesis.

[a]Efficacy determined by protocol primary or secondary end point.
[b]Only one dose-group showed positive results.
[c]Positive results were obtained only after excluding results from two of the six study centers.
Adapted from Yla-Herttuala S, Alitalo K. Gene transfer as a tool to induce therapeutic vascular growth. *Nat Med* 2003;9:694–701, with permission.

cardiologists. Yet, the efforts of many physician-scientists to test gene therapies is now proceeding in a scientific manner using the principles of sound clinical trials design.

REFERENCES

1. Svensson PJ, Dahlback B. Resistance to activated protein C as a basis for venous thrombosis. *N Engl J Med* 1994;330:566–567.
2. Griffin JH, Evatt B, Wideman C, et al. Anticoagulant protein C pathway defective in majority of thrombophilic patients. *Blood* 1994;83: 2008–2009.
3. Rosendaal FR, Koster T, Vandenbroucke JP, et al. High risk of thrombosis in patients homozygous for factor V Leiden (activated protein C resistance). *Blood* 1995;85:1504–1508.
4. Ridker PM, Hennekens CH, Lindpaintner K, et al. Mutation in the gene coding for coagulation factor V and the risk of myocardial infarction, stroke, and venous thrombosis in apparently healthy men. *N Engl J Med* 1995;332:912–917.
5. Koeleman BP, Reitsma PH, Allaart CF, et al. Activated protein C resistance as an additional risk factor for thrombosis in protein C-deficient families. *Blood* 1994;84:1031–1035.
6. Zoller B, Berntsdotter A, Garcia de Frutos P, et al. Resistance to activated protein C as an additional genetic risk factor in hereditary deficiency of protein S. *Blood* 1995;85:3518–3523.
7. van Boven HH, Reitsma PH, Rosendaal FR, et al. Factor V Leiden (FV R506Q) in families with inherited antithrombin deficiency. *Thromb Haemost* 1996;75:417–421.
8. Sachidanandam R, Weissman D, Schmidt SC, et al., International SNP Map Working Group. A map of human genome sequence variation containing 1.42 million single nucleotide polymorphisms. *Nature* 2002;409:928–933.
9. Wang DG, Fan JB, Siao CJ, et al. Large-scale identification, mapping, and genotyping of single-nucleotide polymorphisms in the human genome. *Science* 1998;280:1077–1082.
10. Couzin J. Human genome. HapMap launched with pledges of $100 million. *Science* 2002;298:941–942.
11. Broeckel U, Hengstenberg C, Mayer B, et al. A comprehensive linkage analysis for myocardial infarction and its related risk factors. *Nat Genet* 2002;30:210–214.
12. Pajukanta P, Cargill M, Viitanen L, et al. Two loci on chromosomes 2 and X for premature coronary heart disease identified in early- and late-settlement populations of Finland. *Am J Hum Genet* 2000;67: 1481–1493.
13. Dahlen GH, Srinivasan SR, Stenlund H, et al. The importance of serum lipoprotein (a) as an independent risk factor for premature coronary artery disease in middle-aged black and white women from the United States. *J Intern Med* 1998;244:417–424.
14. Boerwinkle E, Leffert CC, Lin J, et al. Apolipoprotein (a) gene accounts for greater than 90% of the variation in plasma lipoprotein(a) concentrations. *J Clin Invest* 1992;90:52–60.
15. Pajukanta P, Nuotio I, Terwilliger JD, et al. Linkage of familial combined hyperlipidaemia to chromosome 1q21-q23. *Nat Genet* 1998;18: 369–373.
16. Vionnet N, Hani El-H, Dupont S, et al. Genomewide search for type 2 diabetes-susceptibility genes in French whites: evidence for a novel susceptibility locus for early-onset diabetes on chromosome 3q27-qter and independent replication of a type 2-diabetes locus on chromosome 1q21-q24. *Am J Hum Genet* 2000;67:1470–1480.
17. Ghosh S, Watanabe RM, Valle TT, et al. The Finland-United States investigation of non-insulin-dependent diabetes mellitus genetics (FUSION) study. I. An autosomal genome scan for genes that predispose to type 2 diabetes. *Am J Hum Genet* 2000;67:1174–1185.
18. Stoll M, Kwitek-Black AE, Cowley AW Jr, et al. New target regions for human hypertension via comparative genomics. *Genome Res* 2000;10:473–482.
19. Koschinsky ML, Boffa MB, Nesheim ME, et al. Association of a single nucleotide polymorphism in CPB2 encoding the thrombin-activatable fibrinolysis inhibitor (TAF1) with blood pressure. *Clin Genet* 2001;60;345–349.
20. Krushkal J, Xiong M, Ferrell R, et al. Linkage and association of adrenergic and dopamine receptor genes in the distal portion of the long arm of chromosome 5 with systolic blood pressure variation. *Hum Mol Genet* 1998;7:1379–1383.
21. Krushkal J, Ferrell R, Mockrin SC, et al. Genome-wide linkage analyses of systolic blood pressure using highly discordant siblings. *Circulation* 1999;23:1407–1410.
22. Mansfield TA, Simon DB, Farfel Z, et al. Mutilocus linkage of familial hyperkalaemia and hypertension, pseudohypoaldosteronism type II, to chromosomes 1q31-42 and 17p11-q21. *Nat Genet* 1997;16: 202–205.
23. Rieder MJ, Taylor SL, Clark AG, et al. Sequence variation in the human angiotensin converting enzyme. *Nat Genet* 1999;22:59–62.
24. Halushka MK, Fan JB, Bentley K, et al. Patterns of single-nucleotide polymorphisms in candidate genes for blood-pressure homeostasis. *Nat Genet* 1999;22:239–247.
25. Yamada Y, Izawa H, Ichihara S, et al. Prediction of the risk of myocardial infarction from polymorphisms in candidate genes. *N Engl J Med* 2002;347:1916–1923.
26. Ozaki K, Ohnishi Y, Iida A, et al. Functional SNPs in the lymphotoxin-alpha gene that are associated with susceptibility to myocardial infarction. *Nat Genet* 2002;32:650–654.
27. Topol EJ, McCarthy J, Gabriel S, et al. Single nucleotide polymorphisms in multiple novel thrombospondin genes may be associated with familial premature myocardial infarction. *Circulation* 2001;104: 2641–2644.
28. Lockhart DJ, Winzeler EA. Genomics, gene expression and DNA arrays. *Nature* 2000;405:827–836.
29. Ye SQ, Usher DC, Zhang LQ. Gene expression profiling of human diseases by serial analysis of gene expression. *J Biomed Sci* 2002;9: 384–394.
30. Velculescu VE, Vogelstein B, Kinzler KW. Analysing uncharted transcriptomes with SAGE. *Trends Genet* 2000;16:423–425.
31. Patino WD, Mian OY, Hwang PM. Serial analysis of gene expression: technical considerations and applications to cardiovascular biology. *Cir Res* 2002;91:565–569.
32. Zohlnhofer D, Richter T, Neumann F, et al. Transcriptome analysis reveals a role of interferon-gamma in human neointima formation. *Mol Cell* 2001;7:1059–1069.
33. Zohlnhofer D, Klein CA, Richter T, et al. Gene expression profiling of human stent-induced neointima by cDNA array analysis of microscopic specimens retrieved by helix cutter atherectomy: detection of FK506-binding protein 12 upregulation. *Circulation* 2001;103:1396–1402.
34. Ping P, Zhang J, Pierce WM Jr, et al. Functional proteomic analysis of protein kinase C epsilon signaling complexes in the normal heart and during cardioprotection. *Circ Res* 2001;88:59–62.
35. Damer CK, Partridge J, Pearson WR, et al. Rapid identification of protein phosphatase 1-binding proteins by mixed peptide sequencing and data base searching. Characterization of a novel holoenzymic form of protein phosphatase 1. *J Biol Chem* 1998;273:24396–24405.
36. Arrell DK, Neverova I, Van Eyk JE. Cardiovascular proteomics: evolution and potential. *Circ Res* 2001;88:763–773.
37. Nabel EG, Plautz G, Boyce FM, et al. Recombinant gene expression in vivo within endothelial cells of the arterial wall. *Science* 1989;244: 1342–1344.
38. Nabel EG, Plautz G, Nabel GJ. Site-specific gene expression in vivo by direct gene transfer into the arterial wall. *Science* 1990;249: 1285–1288.
39. Akyürek LM, Yang ZY, Aoki K, et al. SM22α promoter targets gene expression to vascular smooth muscle cells in vitro and in vivo. *Mol Med* 2000;11:983–991.
40. Miller AD. Retroviral vectors. *Curr Top Microbiol* 1992;158:1–24.
41. Marshall E. Second child in French trial is found to have leukemia. *Science* 2003;299:320.
42. Graham FL, Prevec L. Adenovirus-based expression vectors and recombinant vaccines. In: Ellis RW, ed. *Vaccines: new approaches to immunological problems*. Boston: Butterworth-Heinemann, 1992:363–390.
43. Lemarchand P, Jones M, Yamada I, et al. In vivo gene transfer and expression in normal uninjured blood vessels using replication-deficient recombinant adenovirus vectors. *Circ Res* 1993;72:1132–1138.
44. Guzman RJ, Lemarchand P, Crystal RG, et al. Efficient gene transfer into myocardium by direct injection of adenovirus vectors. *Circ Res* 1993;73:1202–1207.
45. Muller DW, Gordon D, San H, et al. Catheter-mediated pulmonary vascular gene transfer and expression. *Circ Res* 1994;75:1039–1049.

46. Jaffe HA, Danel C, Longenecker G, et al. Adenovirus-mediated in vivo gene transfer and expression in normal rat liver. *Nat Genet* 1992;1:372–378.

47. Stratford-Perricaudet LD, Makeh I, Perricaudet M, et al. Widespread long-term gene transfer to mouse skeletal muscles and heart. *J Clin Invest* 1992;90:626–630.

48. Natuk RJ, Chanda PK, Lubeck MD, et al. Adenovirus-human immunodeficiency virus (HIV) envelope recombinant vaccines elicit high-titered HIV-neutralizing antibodies in the dog model. *Proc Natl Acad Sci USA* 1992;89:7777–7781.

49. Zabner J, Couture LA, Gregory RJ, et al. Adenovirus-mediated gene transfer transiently corrects the chloride transport defect in nasal epithelia of patients with cystic fibrosis. *Cell* 1993;75:207–216.

50. Yang Y, Nunes FA, Berencsi K, et al. Cellular immunity to viral antigens limits E1-deleted adenoviruses for gene therapy. *Proc Natl Acad Sci USA* 1994;91:4407–4411.

51. Ohno T, Gordon D, San H, et al. Gene therapy for vascular smooth muscle cell proliferation after arterial injury. *Science* 1994;265:781–784.

52. Tal J. Adeno-associated virus-based vectors in gene therapy. *J Biomed Sci* 2000;7:279–291.

53. Rolling F, Samulski RJ. AAV as a viral vector for human gene therapy. Generation of recombinant virus. *Mol Biotechnol* 1995;3:9–15.

54. Lynch CM, Hara PS, Leonard JC, et al. Adeno-associated virus vectors for vascular gene delivery. *Circ Res* 1997;80:497–505.

55. Morishita R, Gibbons GH, Kaneda Y, et al. Novel and effective gene transfer technique for study of vascular renin angiotensin system. *J Clin Invest* 1993;91:2580–2585.

56. Takeshita S, Gai D, Leclerc G, et al. Increased gene expression after liposome-mediated arterial gene transfer associated with intimal smooth muscle gene proliferation. *J Clin Invest* 1994;93:652–661.

57. Lim CS, Chapman GD, Gammon RS, et al. Direct in vivo gene transfer into the coronary and peripheral vasculatures of the intact dog. *Circulation* 1991;83:2007–2011.

58. Nabel EG, Yang Z, Liptay S, et al. Recombinant platelet-derived growth factor B gene expression in porcine arteries induces intimal hyperplasia in vivo. *J Clin Invest* 1993;91:1822–1829.

59. San H, Yang ZY, Pompili VJ, et al. Safety and short-term toxicity of a novel cationic lipid formulation for human gene therapy. *Hum Gene Ther* 1993;4:781–788.

60. Morishita R, Gibbons GJ, Ellison KE, et al. Intimal hyperplasia after vascular injury is inhibited by antisense cdk 2 kinase oligonucleotides. *J Clin Invest* 1994;93:1458–1464.

61. Riessen R, Rahimizadeh H, Blessing E, et al. Arterial gene transfer using pure DNA applied directly to a hydrogel-coated angioplasty balloon. *Hum Gene Ther* 1993;4:749–758.

62. Sousa JE, Serruys PW, Costa MA. New frontiers in cardiology: drug-eluting stents: part I. *Circulation* 2003;107:2274–2279.

63. Sousa JE, Serruys PW, Costa MA. New frontiers in cardiology: drug-eluting stents: part II. *Circulation* 2003;107:2383–2389.

64. Plautz G, Nabel EG, Nabel GJ. Introduction of vascular smooth muscle cells expressing recombinant genes in vivo. *Circulation* 1991;83:578–583.

65. Podrazik RM, Whitehill TA, Ekhterae D, et al. High-level expression of recombinant human tPA in cultivated canine endothelial cells under varying conditions of retroviral gene transfer. *Ann Surg* 1992;216:233–240.

66. Willard JE, Landau C, Glamann B, et al. Genetic modification of the vessel wall. Comparison of surgical and catheter-based techniques for delivery of recombinant adenovirus. *Circulation* 1994;89:2190–2197.

67. Guzman RJ, Lemarchand P, Cystsal RG, et al. Efficient and selective adenovirus-mediated gene transfer into vascular neointima. *Circulation* 1993;88:2838–2848.

68. Nabel EG, Plautz G, Nabel GJ. Transduction of a foreign histocompatibility gene into the arterial wall induces vasculitis. *Proc Natl Acad Sci USA* 1992;89:5157–5161.

69. Nabel EG, Yang Z, Plautz G, et al. Recombinant fibroblast growth factor-1 promotes intimal hyperplasia and angiogenesis in arteries in vivo. *Nature* 1993;362:844–846.

70. Nabel EG, Shum L, Pompili VJ, et al. Direct gene transfer of transforming growth factor β1 into arteries stimulates fibrocellular hyperplasia. *Proc Natl Acad Sci USA* 1993;90:10759–10763.

71. Chang MW, Ohno T, Gordon D, et al. Adenovirus-mediated transfer of the herpes simplex virus thymidine kinase gene inhibits vascular smooth muscle cell proliferation and neointima formation following balloon angioplasty of the rat carotid artery. *Mol Med* 1995;1:172–181.

72. Guzman RJ, Hirschowitz EA, Brody SL, et al. In vivo suppression of injury-induced vascular smooth muscle cell accumulation using adenovirus-mediated transfer of herpes simplex thymidine kinase gene. *Proc Natl Acad Sci USA* 1994;91:10732–10736.

73. Chang MW, Barr E, Seltzer J, et al. Cytostatic gene therapy for vascular proliferative disorders using a constitutively active form of Rb. *Science* 1995;267:518–522.

74. Chang MW, Barr E, Lu MM, et al. Adenovirus-mediated overexpression of the cyclin/cyclin-dependent kinase inhibitor, p21 inhibits vascular smooth muscle cell proliferation and neointima formation in the rat carotid artery model of balloon angioplasty. *J Clin Invest* 1995;96:2260–2268.

75. Yang ZY, Perkins ND, Simari RD, et al. Role of the p21 cyclin-dependent kinase inhibitor in limiting intimal cell proliferation in response to arterial injury. *Proc Natl Acad Sci USA* 1996;93:7905–7910.

76. Tanner F, Akyurek L, San H, et al. Differential effects of cyclin-dependent kinase inhibitors on vascular smooth muscle cell proliferation. *Circulation* 2000;101:2022–2025.

77. Nabel EG. CDKs and CKIs: molecular targets for tissue remodelling. *Nat Rev Drug Discov* 2002;1:587–598.

78. Poon M, Badimon JJ, Fuster V. Overcoming restenosis with sirolimus: from alphabet soup to clinical reality. *Lancet* 2002;359:619–622.

79. von der Leyen H, Gibbons GH, Morishita R, et al. In vivo gene transfer to prevent hyperplasia after vascular injury: effect of overexpression of constitutive nitric oxide synthase. *Proc Natl Acad Sci USA* 1995;92:1137–1141.

80. Isner JM. Myocardial gene therapy. *Nature* 2002;415:234–239.

81. Yla-Herttuala S, Martin JF. Cardiovascular gene therapy. *Lancet* 2000;355:213–222.

82. Olofsson B, Pajusola K, Kaipainen A, et al. Vascular endothelial growth factor B, a novel growth factor for endothelial cells. *Proc Natl Acad Sci USA* 1996;93:2576–2581.

83. Joukov V, Pajusola K, Kaipainen A, et al. A novel vascular endothelial growth factor, VEGF-C, is a ligand for the Flt4 (VEGFR-3) and KDR (VEGFR-2) receptor tyrosine kinases. *EMBO J* 1996;15:290–298.

84. Achen MG, Jeltsch M, Kukk E, et al. Vascular endothelial growth factor D (VEGF-D) is a ligand for the tyrosine kinases VEGF receptor 2 (Flk1) and VEGF receptor 3 (Flt4). *Proc Natl Acad Sci USA* 1998;95:548–553.

85. Ogawa S, Oku A, Sawano A, et al. A novel type of vascular endothelial growth factor, VEGF-E (NZ-7 VEGF), preferentially utilized KDR/Flk-1 receptor and carries a potent mitotic activity without heparin-binding domain. *J Biol Chem* 1998;273:31273–31282.

86. Park JE, Chen HH, Winer J, et al. Placenta growth factor. Potentiation of vascular endothelial growth factor bioactivity, in vitro and in vivo, and high affinity binding to Flt-1 but not to Flk-1/KDR. *J Biol Chem* 1994;269:25646–25654.

87. Lutun A, Tjwa M, Moons L, et al. Revascularization of ischemic tissues by P1GF treatment, and inhibition of tumor angiogenesis, arthritis and atherosclerosis by anti-Flt1. *Nat Med* 2002;8:831–840.

88. Rissanen TT, Markkanen JE, Gruchala M, et al. VEGF-D is the strongest angiogenic and lymphangiogenic effector among VEGFs delivered into skeletal muscle via adenoviruses. *Circ Res* 2003;92:1098–1106.

89. Chae JK, Kim I, Lim ST, et al. Coadministration of angiopoietin-1 and vascular endothelial growth factor enhances collateral vascularization. *Arterioscler Thromb Vasc Biol* 2000;20:2573–2578.

90. Javerzat S, Auguste P, Bikfalvi A. The role of fibroblast growth factors in vascular development. *Trends Mol Med* 2002;8:483–489.

91. Rissanen TT, Markkanen JE, Arve K, et al. Fibroblast growth factor 4 induces vascular permeability, angiogenesis and arteriogenesis in a rabbit hindlimb ischemia model. *FASEB J* 2003;17:100–102.

92. Morishita R, Nakamura S, Hayashi S, et al. Therapeutic angiogenesis induced by human recombinant hepatocyte growth factoring rabbit hind limb ischemia model as cytokine supplement therapy. *Hypertension* 1999;33:1379–1384.

93. Vincent KA, Shyu KG, Luo Y, et al. Angiogenesis is induced in a rabbit model of hindlimb ischemia by naked DNA encoding an HIF-1alpha/VP16 hybrid transcription factor. *Circulation* 2000;102:2255–2261.

94. Rebar EJ, Huang Y, Hickey R, et al. Induction of angiogenesis is a mouse model using engineered transcription factors. *Nat Med* 2002;8:1427–1432.

95. Nabel EG. Stem cells combined with gene transfer for therapeutic vasculogenesis. *Circulation* 2002;105:672–674.

96. Yla-Herttuala S, Alitalo K. Gene transfer as a tool to induce therapeutic vascular growth. *Nat Med* 2003;9:694–701.

97. Dor Y, Djonov V, Abramovitch R, et al. Conditional switching of VEGF provides new insights into adult neovascularization and pro-angiogenic therapy. *EMBO J* 2002;21:1939–1947.

98. Schratzberger P, Walter DH, Rittig K, et al. Reversal of experimental diabetic neuropathy by VEGF gene transfer. *J Clin Invest* 2001;107:1083–1090.

99. Mann MJ, Whittemore AD, Donaldson MC, et al. Ex-vivo gene therapy of human vascular bypass grafts with E2F decoys: the PREVENT single-centre, randomized, controlled trial. *Lancet* 1999;354:1493–1498.

100. Laitinen M, Hartikainen J, Hiltunen MO, et al. Catheter-mediated vascular endothelial growth factor gene transfer to human coronary arteries after angioplasty. *Hum Gene Ther* 2000;11:263–270.

101. Isner JM, Pieczek A, Schainfeld R, et al. Clinical evidence of angiogenesis after arterial gene transfer of phVEGF165 in patient with ischaemic limb. *Lancet* 1996,348;370 374.

102. Baumgartner I, Pieczek A, Manor O, et al. Constitutive expression of phVEGF165 after intramuscular gene transfer promotes collateral vessel development in patients with critical limb ischemia. *Circulation* 1998;97:1114–1123.

103. Isner JM, Baumgartner I, Rauh G, et al. Treatment of thromboangiitis obliterans (Buerger's disease) by intramuscular gene transfer of vascular endothelial growth factor: preliminary clinical results. *J Vasc Surg* 1998;28:964–973.

104. Laitinen M, Makinen K, Manninen H, et al. Adenovirus-mediated gene transfer to lower limb artery of patients with chronic critical leg ischemia. *Hum Gene Ther* 1998;9:1481–1486.

105. Losordo DW, Vale PR, Symes JF, et al. Gene therapy for myocardial angiogenesis: initial clinical results with direct myocardial injection of phVEGF165 as sole therapy for myocardial ischemia. *Circulation* 1998;98:2800–2804.

106. Symes JF, Losordo DW, Vale PR, et al. Gene therapy with vascular endothelial growth factor for inoperable coronary artery disease. *Ann Thorac Surg* 1999;68:830–836.

107. Vale PR, Losordo DW, Milliken CE, et al. Left ventricular electromechanical mapping to assess efficacy of phVEGF(165) gene transfer for therapeutic angiogenesis in chronic myocardial ischemia. *Circulation* 2000;102:965–974.

108. Laitinen M, Hartikainen J, Kiltunen MO, et al. Catheter-mediated vascular endothelial growth factor gene transfer to human coronary arteries after angioplasty. *Hum Gene Ther* 2000;11:263–270.

109. Vale PR, Losordo DW, Milliken CE, et al. Randomized, single-blind, placebo-controlled pilot study of catheter-based myocardial gene transfer for therapeutic angiogenesis using left ventricular electromechanical mapping in patients with chronic myocardial ischemia. *Circulation* 2001;103:2138–2143.

110. Rajagopalan S, Shah M, Luciano A, et al. Adenovirus-mediated gene transfer of VEGF(121) improves lower-extremity endothelial function and flow reserve. *Circulation* 2001;104:753–755.

111. Sarkar N, Ruck A, Kallner G, et al. Effects of intramyocardial injection of phVEGF-A165 as sole therapy in patients with refractory coronary artery disease—12-month follow-up: angiogenic gene therapy. *J Intern Med* 2001;250:373–381.

112. Comerota AJ, Throm RC, Miller KA, et al. Naked plasmid DNA encoding fibroblast growth factor type 1 for the treatment of end-stage unreconstructible lower extremity ischemia: preliminary results of a phase I trial. *J Vasc Surg* 2002;35:930–936.

113. Losordo DW, Vale PR, Hendel RC, et al. Phase 1/2 placebo-controlled, double-blind, dose-escalating trial of myocardial vascular endothelial growth factor 2 gene transfer by catheter delivery in patients with chronic myocardial ischemia. *Circulation* 2002;105:2012–2018.

114. Shyu KG, Chang H, Wang BW, et al. Intramuscular vascular endothelial growth factor gene therapy in patients with chronic critical leg ischemia. *Am J Med* 2003;114:85–92.

115. Henry TD, Annex BH, McKendall GR, et al. The VIVA trial: vascular endothelial growth factor in ischemia for vascular angiogenesis. *Circulation* 2003;107:1359–1365.

116. Simons M, Annex BH, Laham RJ, et al. Pharmacological treatment of coronary artery fibroblast growth factor-2: double-blind, randomized, controlled clinical trial. *Circulation* 2002;105:788–793.

117. Lederman RJ, Mendelsohn FO, Anderson RD, et al. Therapeutic angiogenesis with recombinant fibroblast growth factor-2 for intermittent claudication (the TRAFFIC study): a randomized trial. *Lancet* 2002;359:2053–2058.

118. Seiler C, Pohl T, Wustmann K, et al. Promotion of collateral growth by granulocyte-macrophage colony-stimulating factor in patients with coronary artery disease: a randomized, double-blind, placebo-controlled study. *Circulation* 2001;104:2012–2017.

119. Grines CL, Watkins MW, Helmer G, et al. Angiogenic Gene Therapy (AGENT) trial in patients with stable angina pectoris. *Circulation* 2002;105:1291–1297.

120. Makinen K, Manninen H, Hedman M, et al. Increased vascularity detected by digital subtraction angiography after VEGF gene transfer to human lower limb artery: a randomized, placebo-controlled, double-blinded phase II study. *Mol Ther* 2002;6:127–133.

121. Hedman M, Hartikainen J, Syvanne M, et al. Safety and feasibility of catheter-based local intracoronary vascular endothelial growth factor gene transfer in the prevention of postangioplasty and in-stent restenosis and in the treatment of chronic myocardial ischemia: phase II results of the Kuopio Angiogenesis Trial (KAT). *Circulation* 2003;107:2677–2683.

122. Rajagopalan S, Mohler E 3rd, Lederman RJ, et al. Regional Angiogenesis with Vascular Endothelial Growth Factor (VEGF) in peripheral arterial disease: design of the RAVE trial. *Am Heart J* 2003;145:1114–1118.

123. Kastrup J. Euroinject One trial. Late breaking clinical trials sessions, American College of Cardiology 2003, Chicago. *J Am Coll Cardiol* 2003;41:1603.

124. Pislaru S, Janssens SP, Gersh BJ, et al. Defining gene transfer before expecting gene therapy: putting the horse before the cart. *Circulation* 2002;106:631–636.

CHAPTER 46

Nonatherothrombotic Coronary Artery Disease

Donald C. Harrison

Key Words: Congenital anomalies; coronary arteritis; coronary artery aneurysm; muscle bridges; myocardial oxygen demand/supply imbalance.

INTRODUCTION

Coronary artery disease caused by nonatherothrombotic processes has been recognized with increasing frequency as a result of the widespread use of new modalities for invasive and noninvasive imaging of the cardiovascular system. Congenital anomalies of the origin of coronary arteries, coronary artery aneurysms, coronary embolization, genetic metabolic

D. C. Harrison: Office of the Senior Vice President and Provost for Health Affairs Emeritus, University of Cincinnati Medical Center, P.O. Box 670669, Cincinnati, Ohio 45267-0669.

disorders, and coronary arteritis are all important causes of nonatherothrombotic disease. With the increasing use of catheter-based interventional techniques and the widespread use of coronary stents and brachytherapy for treating coronary artery disease, coronary dissection, coronary embolization, and coronary aneurysm are occurring with increasing frequency. The nonatherothrombotic diseases of coronary arteries are particularly important in younger individuals, even though they occur much more rarely than atherothrombotic disease, and it is important for practicing cardiologists to make the correct diagnosis to achieve successful therapeutic outcomes.

Ischemic heart disease (angina pectoris, myocardial infarction [MI], and sudden cardiac death) is almost always caused by narrowing of major coronary arteries by atherothrombosis, but in rare instances it may result from one of a

TABLE 46–1. *Nonatherothrombotic coronary artery disease*

1. Congenital anomalies of the coronary circulation
   a. Anomalous origin from the aorta
      i. Origin from the contralateral sinus of Valsalva
      ii. Single coronary artery
      iii. Atresia of the coronary ostium
   b. Anomalous origin from the pulmonary artery
   c. Coronary artery fistula
   d. Coronary artery aneurysm
2. Mechanical insults to the coronary circulation
   a. Coronary artery embolus
      i. Thrombus
      ii. Calcium plaques
      iii. Cardiac surgery
      iv. Coronary catheterization
      v. Coronary angioplasty
      vi. Prosthetic valves
      vii. Paradoxical (venous)
   b. Coronary artery dissection
   c. Coronary artery trauma
      i. Nonpenetrating trauma
      ii. Penetrating trauma
      iii. Trauma during cardiac catheterization or surgery
   d. Coronary thrombosis (polycythemia and other hypercoagulable states)
3. Progressive nonatherothrombotic coronary occlusive disease
   a. Coronary artery vasculitis
      i. Polyarteritis nodosa
      ii. Systemic lupus erythematosus
      iii. Wegener's granulomatosis
      iv. Takayasu's disease
      v. Kawasaki disease
      vi. Infection
   b. Intimal proliferation or fibrosis
      i. Ionizing radiation
      ii. Cardiac transplantation
      iii. Coronary angioplasty
      iv. Cocaine
      v. Treatment with methysergide
   c. Accumulation of metabolic substances
      i. Inborn errors of metabolism (Hurler's disease, Hunter's disease)
      ii. Amyloid accumulation
      iii. Homocystinuria
   d. Extrinsic coronary compression
      i. Muscle bridges
      ii. Primary or metastatic tumors
      iii. Aortic aneurysm
4. Miscellaneous
   a. Myocardial oxygen demand-supply imbalance
      i. Aortic stenosis
      ii. Carbon monoxide poisoning
      iii. Severe hypotension (prolonged)
   b. Substance abuse
      i. Cocaine
      ii. Amphetamines
   c. Coronary artery brachytherapy

Adapted from Harrison DC, Baim DS. Nonatherosclerotic coronary heart disease. In: Hurst JW, ed. *The heart,* 6th ed. New York: McGraw-Hill, 1990:1130–1139; Waller BF. Nonatherosclerotic coronary heart disease. In: Hurst JW, ed. *The heart,* 9th ed. New York: McGraw-Hill, 1998:1197–1240; and Alpert JS, Braunwald E. Acute myocardial infarction: pathological, pathophysiological and clinical manifestations. In: Braunwald E, ed. *Heart disease. A textbook of cardiovascular medicine.* Philadelphia: WB Saunders, 1984:1262–1300.

variety of nonatherothrombotic coronary artery pathologies (Table 46–1) (1–4). In societies outside the United States, there appears to be a greater prevalence of the nonatherothrombotic coronary syndromes. To use thrombolytic therapy and advanced interventional techniques such as stents and brachytherapy appropriately, recognition of these rarer forms of coronary artery disease is essential. However, these relatively uncommon disease processes pose several important problems for the clinician: (a) they often occur in patients in whom ischemic heart disease is uncommon, unsuspected, or masked by an underlying systemic disease; (b) they may occur in association with underlying atherothrombotic coronary artery disease; (c) they may require specialized noninvasive and invasive techniques for diagnosis; and (d) their natural histories, pathophysiologies, and optimal management are frequently incompletely understood. Because specific drug and device therapies have been shown to be effective in these syndromes, the physician should have an overall familiarity with the diagnosis and therapy of these nonatherothrombotic coronary artery diseases.

CLINICAL RECOGNITION OF NONATHEROTHROMBOTIC CORONARY DISEASE

The clinical recognition of nonatherothrombotic coronary disease is difficult because the clinical symptoms are quite similar to those occurring with atherothrombotic coronary disease. When the symptoms are chest pain, they are frequently overlooked in teenage and young patients, who may present on multiple occasions, and the diagnosis and definition of a cause occur only after acute myocardial infarction (AMI)for which no atherothrombotic process can be identified, or after coronary angiography in which no luminal atherothrombotic process can be visualized. The most helpful way for the physician to make the diagnosis is to recognize situations in which atherothrombosis is uncommon and suspect one of the diagnoses listed in Table 46–1. Clues that can be helpful are symptoms of coronary artery disease in young patients, especially those patients younger than 30 years, the absence of routine coronary risk factors, and the recognition and diagnosis of any of the associated diseases or conditions listed in Table 46–1.

Approximately 5% of all patients with AMI do not have documented atherothrombotic disease at the time of angiography or autopsy (5,6). A number of studies suggest that approximately 95% of all patients with fatal MI have at least one major coronary artery with more than 80% narrowing or total occlusion, with many patients having associated thrombosis. Approximately 5% of all patients at autopsy have normal coronary arteries. In those patients younger than 30 years, there is a threefold or fourfold increase in this number to as great as 20%. Of those patients who have AMI with normal or near normal coronary arteries, many probably have the syndrome of clinical coronary artery spasm.

CORONARY ARTERY SPASM

The frequency of coronary artery spasm in coronary arteries that are not involved with the atherothrombotic process is unknown. Studies have documented that MI may occur in this syndrome, and it appears to be greater in Oriental populations. Pathophysiologic studies have defined alterations in endothelial function as a signaling mechanism for the constriction of coronary arteries, and pharmacologic provocation during catheterization may be used to establish the diagnosis. Necropsy studies are rare, and in the largest reported series more patients had narrowing caused by plaque, even though it had not been detected during clinical study (7). Although the extent of lesions varied, serial sections of the area of spasm have demonstrated alterations in the arrangement of smooth muscle cells, which might make them susceptible to spasm (4). The clinical syndrome and pathophysiology are presented extensively by Lüscher and Pepine (see Chapter 42).

CONGENITAL ANOMALIES OF THE CORONARY CIRCULATION

Coronary artery anomalies/variations in the origin, course, and distribution of the coronary arteries are present in 1% to 2% of the population and are noted more frequently during life rather than necropsy (5–10). Ostial lesions, passage of a major artery between the walls of the pulmonary trunk and the aorta, the origin of a major artery from the pulmonary trunk, and myocardial bridges appear to produce more symptoms of ischemia and subsequent MI (11). These anomalies may make angiographic visualization of the coronary circulation more difficult and probably increase the risk for coronary artery trauma during cardiac surgery. Only a fraction of the patients in whom these congenital anomalies are present experience myocardial ischemia. The absence or presence of symptoms of ischemia depend on the origin of the coronary artery, the direction of blood flow at rest, and the alterations in flow that result during physical exertion, which in some cases may produce a true "coronary steal" syndrome. The anatomy and physiology of anomalies of the coronary arteries that produce the coronary steal syndrome have been defined. For a coronary steal, it is required to have a common coronary vessel to have a resistance to flow that supplies two myocardial regions in parallel and vasodilatation that is greater in one of the two parallel regions (12). The conditions are met when there is a single coronary artery. Drug therapy that results in differential vasodilatation in the two parallel vascular beds appears to be the mechanism for producing this phenomenon (13). If one vascular bed is already maximally dilated because of myocardial ischemia, and a coronary vasodilator drug is administered, there is an increase in coronary blood flow, but the increase to the normal vascular bed is greater, and the "steal" occurs because blood is differentially shunted from the ischemic area.

There are many variations in the anomalous origin of coronary arteries (4,5), and evaluation of each patient with a coronary anomaly must therefore include an anatomic classification, recognition of the particular anomaly as one capable of producing myocardial ischemia, and documentation that true ischemia is present by symptomatic or biochemical studies. In many symptomatic patients with coronary anomalies in whom ischemia can be documented by exercise testing, isotopic myocardial perfusion scanning, or transmyocardial metabolic testing, effective corrective cardiac surgery can usually be performed.

Anomalous Origin from the Aorta

In normal coronary circulation, the right coronary artery originates from a single ostium within the right sinus of Valsalva, and the left coronary artery originates from a single ostium within the left sinus of Valsalva (Fig. 46–1A) (5,14). Abnormally high or low locations of the coronary ostia and the presence within the appropriate sinus of Valsalva of separate ostia from the left anterior descending and circumflex coronary artery branches, or for the right coronary artery and its conus branch, are common minor variations that do not result in myocardial ischemia. Other anomalous patterns of coronary artery origin from the aorta are potential causes of myocardial ischemia even in the absence of atherothrombosis.

Origin from the Contralateral Sinus of Valsalva

When one of the coronary arteries originates from the contralateral sinus of Valsalva, this anomalous vessel must traverse the base of the heart to reach its territory of distribution, passing anterior to, posterior to, or between the aorta and pulmonary artery (Fig. 46–1B) (6–14). Acute angulation at the origin of the artery from the aorta may result in anatomic or functional constriction of the proximal portion of the anomalous coronary artery. Anomalous vessels passing between the aorta and pulmonary artery seem to carry an additional risk for ischemia, possibly as a result of being compressed between the great vessels, although this is unlikely at normal pulmonary artery pressure. Abnormal mechanical stresses or flow patterns that produce internal injury may enhance the development of coronary atherothrombosis in the anomalous segment.

Origin of the left coronary artery from the right sinus of Valsalva with passage of the proximal left coronary artery between the aorta and pulmonary artery is associated with an increased incidence of exercise-related sudden cardiac death in young patients. In an autopsy study of 33 patients with this anomaly, sudden death occurred in 9 (27%), generally without prior warning symptoms (14). Autopsy studies in sudden death victims without known atherothrombosis occurring during exercise show a high incidence of this syndrome. Some authors even recommend prophylactic coronary artery bypass surgery when this anomaly is detected in young patients (11,14).

In patients without coronary atherothrombosis, passage of the anomalous left coronary artery either anterior or poste-

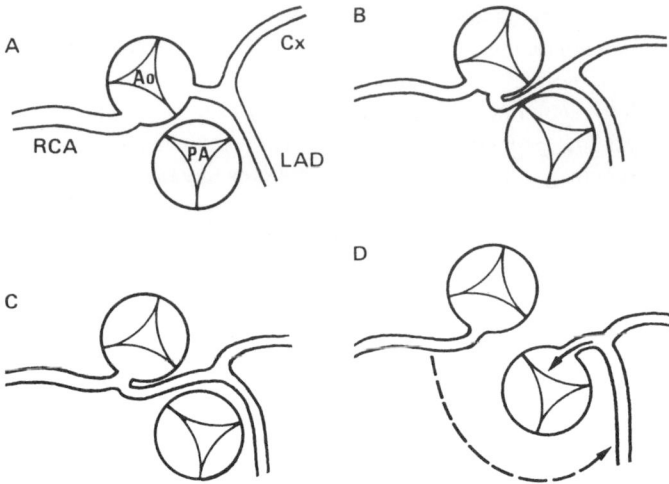

FIG. 46–1. Representative patterns of anomalous coronary artery origin. **A:** Normal coronary circulation with origin of the right coronary artery (RCA) from the right sinus of Valsalva and origin of the left coronary artery from the left sinus of Valsalva. The aorta (Ao), pulmonary artery (PA), and left anterior descending (LAD) and circumflex (Cx) branches of the left coronary artery are shown. **B:** Anomalous origin of the left coronary artery from the right sinus of Valsalva, with passage of the left main coronary artery between the aorta and pulmonary artery. **C:** Single coronary artery originating from the right sinus of Valsalva, with passage of the left main coronary artery between the aorta and pulmonary artery. **D:** Origin of the left coronary artery from the pulmonary artery, showing the development of collateral flow *(dotted arrow)* from the right coronary artery and the associated left-to-right shunt into the pulmonary artery *(solid arrow).*

rior to both great vessels has been associated with pacing-induced myocardial lactate production and angina pectoris but does not seem to carry a significant risk for sudden death. Angina pectoris also has been reported in patients in whom the right coronary artery originates from the left sinus of Valsalva, but confirmation of myocardial ischemia has been less complete in these patients than in patients with anomalous origin of the left coronary artery. The most common pattern of anomalous aortic origin—origin of the circumflex coronary artery from the right sinus of Valsalva or proximal right coronary artery—does not seem to impose independent ischemic risk.

Single Coronary Artery

Derivation of the entire coronary circulation from a single ostium is a rare coronary anomaly (Fig. 46–1C). In a study of 50,000 consecutive coronary angiograms, only 33 cases of a single coronary artery were described, yielding an incidence of 0.066% (15). Approximately 40% of patients with this anomaly have an associated congenital cardiac defect—that is, tetralogy of Fallot, transposition of the great vessels, or improper division of the truncus arteriosus (16). There is no clear sex predominance for this condition, and the frequency of occurrence of single left and single right coronary arteries is approximately equal (17). As in the case of anomalous origin from the contralateral sinus of Valsalva, one or more components of the coronary circulation system must cross the base of the heart to reach its territory of distribution, passing anterior to, posterior to, or between the great vessels. These transposed vessels may thereby be exposed to the risks of angulation, compression, accelerated atherothrombosis, and acute thrombosis. Because the entire myocardium is supplied by way of the single coronary artery, proximal coronary atherothrombosis poses the risk for global myocardial ischemia and death. Coronary atherothrombosis frequently develops in the single coronary artery syndrome but probably does not differ in incidence from the normal population.

Clinical manifestations of the single coronary artery anomaly depend in part on associated cardiac defects and atherothrombosis, but up to 15% of patients with only this anomaly develop severe cardiac complications by age 40 years (16). Angina pectoris and myocardial lactate production have been demonstrated in patients with a single coronary artery in the absence of coronary atherothrombosis or vessel passage between the aorta and pulmonary artery (17).

Atresia of the Coronary Ostium

Atresia or severe stenosis of one of the coronary ostia, often associated with hypoplasia of the proximal coronary artery, is a rare congenital coronary anomaly, with only seven reported cases (8,18). The absence of a second coronary ostium may lead to the incorrect diagnosis of a single coronary artery. Myocardial perfusion studies will differentiate inadequate flow to segments of the myocardium and establish the diagnosis. Because the involved vessel is dependent on collateral flow from the contralateral coronary artery, myocardial ischemia or MI may develop during infancy. In this sense, patients with ostial atresia bear an angiographic and clinical resemblance to patients with anomalous origin of a coronary artery from the pulmonary artery (discussed later). Successful coronary artery bypass grafting has been reported in a patient as young as 10 years old with ostial atresia (18).

Anomalous Origin from the Pulmonary Artery

Origin of a coronary artery from the pulmonary artery rather than from the aorta is a relatively uncommon but severe coronary anomaly. It should be recognized by pediatric cardiologists because it is generally treatable with surgery. In more than 90% of cases, it is the left coronary artery that originates from the pulmonary artery, generally from the left posterior pulmonary sinus (8). Generally, it is the left main coronary artery that has an anomalous origin and the right coronary arises correctly from the aorta (8) (Fig. 46–1D).

Origin of the right coronary artery, an accessory coronary artery, and both coronary arteries from the pulmonary artery have been described, the last of which is invariably fatal in the neonatal period (8,9,19).

As the pulmonary artery pressure decreases during the first weeks of life, perfusion of the anomalous coronary artery from the pulmonary artery decreases. Unless adequate collateral flow develops from the contralateral coronary artery, the territory of the anomalous vessel becomes ischemic. Angina pectoris or congestive heart failure with mitral regurgitation may then develop, often accompanied by electrocardiographic manifestations of myocardial ischemia or MI. This clinical picture, the infantile syndrome, develops in approximately 80% of affected patients, usually within the first 4 months of life (8,20,21). In the absence of surgical correction, this syndrome has an 80% first-year mortality rate, although the mortality rate is somewhat less with anomalous origin of the right coronary artery (19). Those patients who do not experience development of the infantile syndrome may present during childhood or adult life with congestive heart failure, asymptomatic murmur, mitral regurgitation, angina pectoris, or sudden death (8,20).

Patients surviving infancy tend to have extensive intercoronary collateral flow, with dilatation of both the normal and the anomalous vessels. This collateral flow reverses the direction of blood flow in the anomalous coronary artery, constituting a left-to-right shunt into the pulmonary artery. Despite extensive collateralization, electrocardiographic evidence of ischemia and pathologic evidence of subendocardial fibrosis usually persist.

Surgical correction of anomalous coronary artery origin from the pulmonary artery seeks to eliminate the left-to-right shunt and to establish an independent arterial blood supply to the anomalous vessel. Ligation of the anomalous vessel at its origin in combination with saphenous vein aortocoronary bypass grafting has been performed, but it is technically difficult in children younger than 2 years and is associated with a high rate of graft failure (21). The alternative method of correction, reimplantation of the anomalous vessel with the subclavian artery, seems more successful in infants. This anomaly is associated with high morbidity and mortality rates, and because suitable techniques are available, early surgical correction appears to be the treatment of choice.

Coronary Artery Fistula

The most common hemodynamically significant coronary artery anomaly is a direct anastomosis between a major coronary artery and one of the cardiac chambers or major great vessels, such as the superior vena cava, coronary sinus, or pulmonary artery. Fistulas from the right coronary artery are slightly more common than those from the left coronary artery, and bilateral fistulas are present in 4% to 5% of cases (Fig. 46–2) (22,23). Fistulas are recognized with increasing frequency because of the greater use of coronary angiography, three-dimensional echocardiographic studies, and magnetic resonance imaging (MRI) technologies. More than 90% of the fistulas drain into the venous circulation (the right ventricle in 41%; the right atrium in 26%; pulmonary artery in 17%; coronary sinus in 7%; superior vena cava in 1%) (24). The remaining fistulas drain into the arterial circulation (left atrium in 5%; left ventricle in 3%) (24). Multiple anastomoses between the involved coronary artery and the structure within the heart or great vessels into which it drains are possible. The involved coronary artery proximal to the fistula is markedly dilated, and flow through the fistula

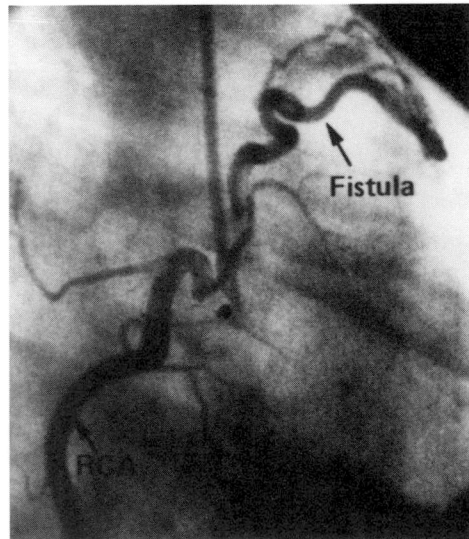 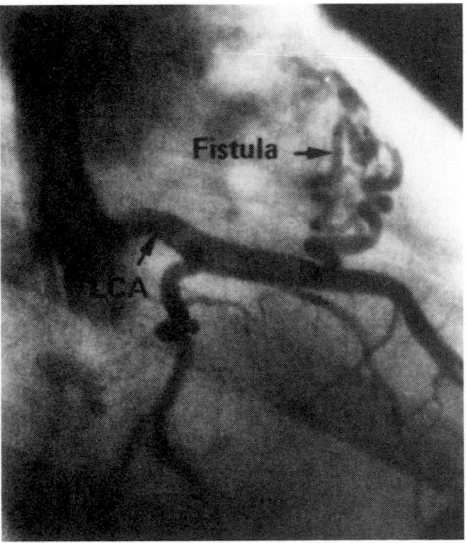

FIG. 46–2. Bilateral coronary artery to pulmonary artery fistula, originating from the proximal right coronary artery (RCA) and the left anterior descending branch of the left coronary artery (LCA), in an asymptomatic 29-year-old woman with a continuous heart murmur. No left-to-right shunt was detected by oximetry.

may be several times that delivering oxygen to the myocardium. When the fistula drains into the venous circulation, a significant left-to-right shunt may be present.

Runoff through a fistula may decrease intracoronary diastolic pressure and produce myocardial ischemia in some patients by a "coronary steal" phenomenon (8,9). Physical examination often reveals a continuous heart murmur, which brings approximately one-half of patients with coronary artery fistulas to seek medical attention. In a series of 58 patients, 21 had associated cardiac defects that brought them to diagnostic study (25).

In a large study of 171 neonates with pulmonary atresia, coronary artery–right ventricular fistulas were found in 45% of the patients, and right ventricular dependency was severe in 9% of the neonates. This again demonstrates the frequency of fistula associated with other congenital abnormalities of the heart.

Results of a chest radiograph are usually normal but may show evidence of pulmonary overcirculation when a large left-to-right shunt is present, mimicking a patent ductus arteriosus. Electrocardiographic abnormalities are uncommon. Diagnosis is best made by selective coronary angiography, particularly when catheterization to evaluate a continuous murmur has failed to disclose the expected anatomic abnormality. Fistulas may also result from cardiac trauma, cardiac interventions, cardiac surgery, endomyocardial biopsy, and pacemaker lead placement.

This is the most clinically recognized nonatherothrombotic coronary syndrome and merits understanding by all cardiologists. Most patients with coronary fistulas are asymptomatic and may be detected only by the presence of a murmur or an abnormal electrocardiogram (ECG); therefore, the decision regarding surgical correction of a fistula is complex. Ischemia has been documented in some patients with coronary fistulas and no atherothrombosis (8,9), and there is evidence that the majority of patients do become symptomatic with advancing age (23). In addition to angina and MI, congestive heart failure, bacterial endocarditis, and fistula rupture have been described. Because spontaneous fistula closure is rare, and the risk for surgical closure of the fistula is significantly less in patients younger than 20 years, some authorities have suggested elective fistula ligation in young patients, including those who are asymptomatic (23). A report of 58 patients showed surgery to be safe and effective with good long-term results (25). No deaths occurred in patients with isolated fistulas and no other congenital heart lesions. Antibiotic prophylaxis against bacterial endocarditis is recommended for all patients (22).

Muscle Bridge: Tunneling of Coronary Arteries into the Myocardium

In some patients, the major epicardial coronary arteries penetrate into the myocardium to be covered over with muscle bands. The intramyocardial segments of the large coronary arteries, particularly the left anterior descending artery, may be subject to systolic compression with cardiac contraction, or "milking" (Fig. 46–3). This pathologic finding has been known for several centuries, but only recently has it been shown to be of clinical relevance. Intramyocardial segments of the coronary arteries are present in approximately 20% of autopsied hearts (4,26), but angiographic evidence of systolic compression is reported in only 0.5% of patients undergoing coronary angiography for chest pain (27). In most cases, angiographic compression is a benign finding, but when a long vessel segment demonstrates systolic compression to less

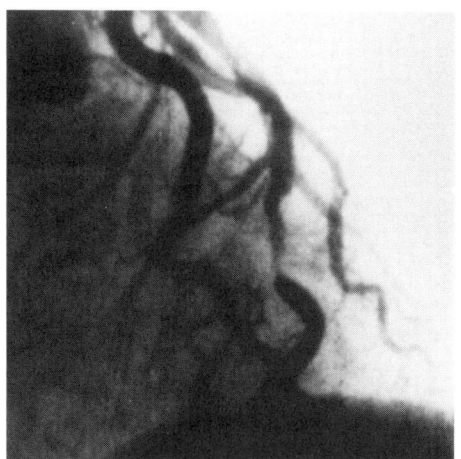
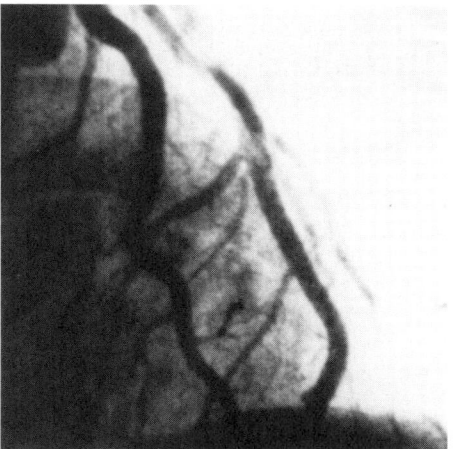

Systole   Diastole

FIG. 46–3. Systolic compression of the midleft anterior descending coronary artery by a muscle bridge with restoration of the normal coronary artery diameter during diastole in a young man with exercise-induced ventricular tachycardia. Treated with oral propranolol, the patient was free of both arrhythmia and electrocardiographic evidence of myocardial ischemia during maximal treadmill exercise testing. (Courtesy of Dr. John A. Michal, Santa Barbara, CA.)

than 25% of its diastolic diameter, ischemia may be revealed by exercise, by thallium-201 myocardial perfusion scanning, or by coronary sinus pacing metabolic evaluation, even in the absence of coronary atherothrombosis (27).

Because most coronary flow takes place during diastole, it is not clear how systolic compression alone results in myocardial ischemia. One possibility is that the compression results in abnormal vascular tone in the segment and coronary spasm. In some symptomatic patients, coronary compression may extend into early diastole, and excessive myocardial oxygen demand may be present as the result of associated left ventricular hypertrophy (27). Although muscle bridges are a congenital anomaly, symptoms of ischemia may not develop until middle age, which is likely because of associated changes in vascular tone.

Angina pectoris resulting from systolic coronary artery compression may respond to therapy with β-adrenergic blocking drugs, calcium channel-blocking agents, or both. When symptoms are refractory to medical therapy and when inducible ischemia has been unequivocally demonstrated, coronary bypass grafting or simple unroofing of the bridged coronary segment has resulted in relief of symptoms and normalization of myocardial perfusion and metabolism (27,28).

In one study, nine patients with obstruction to coronary artery flow caused by myocardial bridging underwent surgery after failure of medical therapy. Postoperative scintigraphic and angiographic studies demonstrated restoration of normal coronary flow and myocardial perfusion in all nine of these patients. The impaired flow occurred in the distribution of the left coronary descending artery in seven patients and in a diagonal branch in two patients. All patients are alive and asymptomatic (29).

CORONARY ARTERY ANEURYSM

Coronary artery aneurysms, localized areas of coronary dilatation relative to adjacent normal arterial segments, occur in approximately 1.5% of patients studied by autopsy or coronary angiography (30). The frequency of diagnosis depends on the definition as a true aneurysm or just ectatic segments in extensive coronary atherothrombosis. Acquired causes (Table 46–2) frequently result from intrinsic pathology of the arterial wall media or damage to it during a procedure. The aneurysms are frequently multiple, may attain a diameter of several centimeters, involve the right coronary artery more frequently than the left (31), and may be either congenital or acquired. Atherothrombosis, either by stenosis with poststenotic dilatation or by primary destruction of the coronary intima and media, accounts for a large percentage of coronary aneurysms in Western populations. Atherothrombotic damage may also produce diffuse coronary ectasia rather than focal coronary aneurysm (2). Other pathologic processes that damage the arterial wall, including dissection, trauma, coronary angioplasty, vasculitis, mycotic emboli, syphilis, and mucocutaneous lymph node syndrome, may

TABLE 46–2. *Causes of coronary aneurysms*

Atherothrombosis with vessel ectasia
Atherectomy
Dissection of coronary arteries
Angioplasty
Mycotic emboli
Kawasaki disease
Arteritis
Trauma
Congenital

Adapted from Waller BF. Nonatherosclerotic coronary heart disease. In: Hurst JW, ed. *The heart,* 9th ed. New York: McGraw-Hill, 1998:1197–1240.

also lead to aneurysm formation (30,31). More recently, coronary aneurysm has been reported with stent implantation (32,33) and after coronary brachytherapy. Coronary aneurysms may also be congenital in origin. The largest cause of coronary aneurysms in Oriental populations is Kawasaki disease (discussed later), but many cases are reported in U.S. pediatric populations as well. The course may be followed with intravascular ultrasound or electron beam tomography (34). Early therapy with aspirin in Kawasaki disease was reported to prevent the occurrence of coronary aneurysms (35), but this has been largely replaced with treatment with other antiinflammatory agents. Aneurysms are frequently detected with echocardiographic techniques, and treatment of the inflammatory disease frequently results in resolution of the aneurysms (36). Similar resolution has been noted in 188 cases followed with serial angiograms (37).

There are no reliable clinical features of coronary artery aneurysm, although a diastolic or continuous heart murmur may occasionally be present (30). Results of a chest radiograph may show a pericardiac mass or calcification, and MR and electron beam tomography are helpful, but coronary angiography is required for accurate diagnosis. The most frequent way in which these conditions are diagnosed is repeat coronary angiography after angioplasty or atherectomy.

The clinical course of patients with coronary artery aneurysms usually depends on the severity of the associated atherothrombotic stenoses. Even in the absence of stenosis, abnormal flow patterns within the aneurysm may lead to thrombus formation with subsequent vessel occlusion, distal thromboembolization, or MI (30). Cases have been reported in which a large intramyocardial aneurysm resulted in angina by a coronary steal mechanism. Rupture of a coronary aneurysm is a rare but serious complication.

Surgical therapy of combined stenotic and aneurysmal atherothrombosis consists of ligation of the involved vessel immediately beyond the aneurysm (to eliminate subsequent emboli) and aortocoronary bypass grafting to the distal vessel. Stents have been used to seal the ostia of aneurysms. Similar surgery has been suggested in patients without stenotic lesions and even in asymptomatic patients with coronary aneurysms (30). Anticoagulant or antiplatelet therapy may also be of value in this condition (2). Because aneurysmal changes are frequently present in other vessels, particularly the abdominal aorta, comprehensive arteriographic evaluation is recommended in patients with coronary artery aneurysms (30,31).

In inflammatory causes such as Kawasaki disease, surgery is generally not indicated because response to antiinflammatory drugs is usually good. Surgical correction with aortocoronary bypass and ligation of large aneurysms is indicated only with persistent myocardial ischemia.

MECHANICAL INSULTS TO THE CORONARY ARTERY CIRCULATION

Mechanical injury to coronary arteries has been recognized for centuries, but with the more widespread application of catheter-based interventions including stent placement and brachytherapy in coronary artery disease, the prevalence of these types of injuries has markedly increased. Early recognition of mechanical injury to coronary arteries may permit early thrombolytic therapy or surgical intervention to salvage viable myocardium.

Coronary Artery Embolus

The coronary arteries may be partially protected from embolic events by the acute angulation of the coronary ostia relative to the aortic stream and by their position behind the aortic valve leaflets during systole. When coronary artery emboli do occur (Table 46–3), the outcome is dictated by the size of the embolus and its position of impaction in the coronary circulation, which determines the magnitude of the ensuing infarctions. Small emboli tend to produce occlusion of a distal branch of one of the coronary arteries (most commonly the left anterior descending artery), resulting in a small area of myocardial necrosis that may not be clinically evident (38,39). Emboli may also be generated downstream when angioplasty or rotoblade opening of total occlusions

TABLE 46–3. *Causes of coronary arterial emboli*

Infective endocarditis (native or artificial valves)
Cardiac cavitary thrombus
   Left ventricle (myocardial infarction, cardiomyopathies, ventricular aneurysms)
   Left atrium (mitral stenosis, atrial fibrillation)
Cardiac tumors (myxomas)
Metastatic cancer
Calcific aortic or mitral valves
Coronary plaques or aneurysms
Coronary artery trauma
   Cardiac surgery
   Angioplasty and stent placement
   Atherectomy
During cardiac catheterization and angioplasty
Paradoxical
   Atrial septal defect with pulmonary hypertension
   Patent foramen ovale from thrombophlebitis
   Congenital heart disease

are being attempted. These small emboli appear to be relatively frequent. In one autopsy series, they were found in 13% of patients with histologically evident myocardial necrosis (39). Quite possibly these small emboli may trigger sudden death by producing small areas of ischemia that are arrhythmogenic. Larger coronary artery emboli are relatively less frequent but generally result in clinically apparent MI.

Coronary artery emboli should be considered in the differential diagnosis of acute myocardial ischemia in patients whose clinical condition predisposes them to arterial emboli, including patients with valvular heart disease (endocarditis, noninfected abnormal valve, prosthetic valve), mural thrombus (congestive cardiomyopathy, previous MI, atrial fibrillation), left-sided catheterization, or the anatomic potential for paradoxic embolization (38,39). Coronary emboli of a variety of materials, including tumor, myocardial or skeletal muscle, and materials used in cardiac surgery, also have been reported. Extracardiac emboli may also be present. In patients sustaining coronary emboli, prompt coronary angiography may show occlusion of the involved vessel, but restudy as soon as 1 month after the acute event may show renewed vessel patency as the result of lysis or recanalization of the embolus (38).

In the last 20 years, coronary embolism occurring with attempted transluminal angioplasty, stent placement, or the introduction of thrombolytic agents (streptokinase, tissue plasminogen activator, and others) into coronary arteries has been noted with increasing frequency. During the past several years with newer invasive techniques to treat coronary atherothrombosis such as atherectomy, rotobladers, stents, and lasers, emboli to the coronary arteries are more frequently reported. One report demonstrates the benefit of distal protection devices for acute and long-term follow-up (40). Because these patients have fresh thrombus in their coronary arteries and are undergoing acute infarction, it is difficult to separate the effects of progressive disease from the effects of embolizing the thrombus more distally. In such instances, where distal embolic material is noted with persistent symptoms, the administration of additional thrombolytic therapy is suggested. If flow is not restored promptly and loss of significant myocardium seems likely, bypass surgery is indicated.

The role of cardiac surgery in the treatment of acute coronary emboli has become commonplace when they occur during interventional cardiac procedures and threaten large segments of myocardium. When emboli occur during cardiac surgery, embolectomy appears to correct the myocardial ischemia. Embolectomy performed for emboli associated with endocarditis (41) or cardiac catheterization seems to have less influence on the evolution of MI. If the embolus is a result of thrombotic material dislodged from more proximal sites, thrombolytic therapy is indicated.

Coronary Artery Dissection

Hemorrhage into the coronary artery wall, with or without an associated intimal tear, forces the intima into the coronary lumen and may produce distal myocardial ischemia or frank infarction. Coronary artery dissections may occur by extension of aortic root dissection (secondary dissection) or may be limited to the coronary artery (primary dissection). Primary coronary artery dissections may occur as the result of diagnostic coronary angiography, coronary angioplasty, stent placement, cardiac surgery, or chest trauma (discussed later), or they may occur spontaneously. Earlier evident localized coronary dissection occurs in at least 30% of patients undergoing coronary angioplasty and may progress to abrupt vessel reclosure in the first hour after the procedure in 2% to 3% of patients (42). These percentages have decreased with better prediction of patients who require stents or atherectomy.

During the last two decades, the technologies available for treating coronary artery obstructions have improved significantly (43–46). There have been major modifications of the catheters and the balloon profiles, and the development of multiple stents (47,48) and the use of lasers, high-frequency rotobladers, and several techniques for atherectomy have been introduced (43). The selection of technologies available to the interventional cardiologist to remove obstructions in coronary arteries has expanded considerably during the last decade. Matching the correct lesion with the best technology available has resulted in vastly improved outcomes produced by interventional cardiologists.

As the number of coronary angioplasty procedures increased to a projected level of 125,000 in 1987, the frequency of coronary artery dissections reported also increased (49,50). By 2000, coronary interventional procedures increased to approximately 950,000 annually. The frequency of dissections of the coronary arteries has decreased progressively with the introduction of new technologies such as the low-profile balloon, smaller catheters, coronary stents (47,48), and techniques for better visualization of the placement of angioplasty catheters (43). In the National Heart, Lung and Blood Institute angiographic registry experience, 6.6% of patients required emergency surgery, among which 46% were operated on for coronary dissection (49). These figures have also decreased markedly as new interventional technologies and other approaches in interventional cardiology have become commonplace. Bypass surgery has a three to four times greater mortality rate in those patients requiring emergency surgery than in those having elective surgery (43,51), and although coronary dissection is a major cause of early occlusion of a successfully dilated coronary artery by percutaneous transluminal coronary angioplasty, the placement of stents has markedly reduced this complication. Some cardiologists believe that dissection is necessary to achieve a satisfactory long-term result (52,53).

Most spontaneous dissections occur in women, particularly in the peripartum period (46,54). Hypertension and coronary atherothrombotic involvement are infrequent, but changes resembling cystic medial necrosis may be present (54–56). The involved vessel is enlarged and ecchymotic and may rupture. The left anterior descending artery is in-

volved in three-fourths of cases, usually within 2 cm of its origin (56).

The diagnosis of coronary artery dissection during life relies on coronary angiography showing extravasation or delayed clearance of contrast, an intimal flap, or the presence of true and false lumina, but dissection may present simply as occlusion of the involved vessel (54,56).

CORONARY ARTERY TRAUMA

Nonpenetrating Blunt Trauma

Chest wall impact, frequently the result of vehicular trauma (of being thrown against the steering device), may lead to myocardial necrosis by direct myocardial contusion or by occlusive injury to the coronary arteries. This occlusive injury may be the result of coronary artery dissection, thrombosis, or rupture (57,58). Coronary artery fistulas or aneurysms may develop as late sequelae (59–61). The left anterior descending and right coronary arteries are most frequently involved. The ECG usually shows a pattern of AMI, but this finding does not distinguish between coronary occlusion and myocardial contusion. This distinction can be made by prompt coronary angiography, which should be performed promptly and followed by immediate revascularization (bypass surgery, thrombolytic therapy, or angioplasty performed on an emergency basis). Recovery is the rule, although left ventricular aneurysm formation is common.

Penetrating Trauma

Laceration of a coronary artery, as in a stab wound or small-caliber gunshot wound, may cause acute myocardial ischemia, although the immediate presentation is generally that of acute pericardial tamponade. The left anterior descending and right coronary arteries are most frequently involved. Laceration of small coronary artery branches may be treated with simple ligation without producing significant myocardial ischemia, but ligation of larger vessels often results in a large area of myocardial ischemia (manifested as immediate myocardial discoloration and hypokinesis), necessitating coronary artery bypass grafting (62). Development of a loud continuous murmur days to months after the original injury may signal the development of a coronary artery fistula. Surgical repair of these fistulas often is only transiently successful, with return of the murmur in the postoperative period; thus, surgery should be reserved for patients with evidence of hemodynamic compromise (60,61).

Trauma During Cardiac Catheterization or Surgery

Catheterization of the left side of the heart, particularly selective cannulation of the coronary arteries, is associated with a 0.1% to 0.2% incidence of MI as the result of coronary artery embolization (thrombus, dislodged plaque, air) or coronary artery dissection (63,64). Coronary artery dissection (particularly that which occurs during percutaneous transluminal angioplasty) and embolization have been reported without ischemic sequelae; but when they result in AMI with hypotension or refractory arrhythmia, urgent coronary artery bypass surgery may be life-saving (see "Coronary Artery Dissection"). Careful flushing technique and systemic heparinization during coronary angiography have minimized these complications. Laceration of a coronary artery is a potential but rare complication during pericardiocentesis.

CORONARY THROMBOSIS

Coronary thrombosis clearly plays an important role in the evolution of MI. When MI develops in the setting of coronary atherothrombosis, superimposed coronary thrombosis is nearly always present. In certain disorders involving thrombocytosis or platelet activation, including polycythemia vera, idiopathic thrombocytosis, thrombotic thrombocytopenia purpura, and multiple myeloma (65,66), AMI has occurred in the absence of significant underlying atherothrombosis. Although this circumstantial evidence points toward primary coronary thrombosis as the cause of infarction, the differentiation between *in situ* thrombosis and thromboembolus may be difficult. Although acute infarction as a complication of these diseases is rare, it should be considered by expert clinicians when the clinical symptoms appear.

PROGRESSIVE NONATHEROTHROMBOTIC CORONARY OCCLUSIVE DISEASE

There are a number of conditions that develop as progressive nonatherothrombotic coronary occlusion and that may result from coronary artery vasculitis (67), intimal proliferation or fibrosis, abnormal accumulation of metabolic substances (2), or extrinsic coronary artery compression. If large proximal coronary arteries are involved, angina pectoris or AMI may result, but clinical, angiographic, and even histologic differentiation of progressive nonatherothrombotic coronary occlusion from occlusive atherothrombosis may be difficult. When the small coronary vessels (0.1–1.0 mm in diameter) are involved, as they may be in diabetes mellitus, collagen vascular disease, cardiac transplantation, neuromuscular diseases (Friedreich's ataxia and progressive muscular dystrophy), rheumatoid arthritis, hypertrophic cardiomyopathy, thrombotic thrombocytopenic purpura, or homocystinuria, the patient may experience development of arrhythmias, conduction defects, chest pain, or sudden death despite angiographic normality of the large coronary arteries (68). A special syndrome of small-vessel coronary disease has been postulated, and patients with unexplained "ischemia" pain have been so categorized on the basis of endomyocardial biopsy studies. These unexplained ischemic syndromes have been called "syndrome X." Mosseri and colleagues (69) have studied ten autopsied patients with typical pictures of AMI who died within 25 days of the onset of symptoms.

The coronary arterial system showed little luminal narrowing, and no thrombotic material was observed in the coronary arteries, despite that the AMI was only 2 days old in five of the patients. A number of hypotheses have been proposed to explain the occurrence of infarction, which has been reported with increasing frequency, in these patients. These hypotheses include coronary artery disease in vessels too small to be visualized angiographically or a severe form of coronary artery spasm. These studies have shown intimal and medial changes in vessels 20 to 50 (m in diameter, but because there are changes from aging in the same vessels, the relation of pathology to a specific disease entity has been difficult to establish (69). The overall prevalence of small-vessel disease and the frequency with which it leads to clinical sequelae are not known, but cases of this "syndrome X" are being reported with increasing frequency.

Coronary Artery Vasculitis

Major coronary artery vasculitis is a rare event but may be suspected in conjunction with general medical conditions (Table 46–4). Myocardial ischemia and MI with or without associated coronary artery thrombosis may be the presenting manifestations. A useful classification of arteritis conditions on the basis of the type of coronary artery pathology has been proposed by Baroldi (70). Arteritis of the coronary arteries may result from direct extension from adjacent organs or tissue infections involving the heart, such as myocardial abscess from aortic valve endocarditis or pericardial tuberculosis. The coronary artery adventitial layer is involved directly in these cases. On the other hand, coronary arteritis may develop from hematogenous spread through the coronary lumen or through the vasa vasorum or may be caused by the immunologic reactions throughout the body. In these cases, the intimal layer of the coronary artery is involved in

TABLE 46–4. *Conditions producing coronary vasculitis*

Rheumatic fever
Giant cell arteritis
Polyarteritis nodosa
Tuberculosis
Leprosy
Mucocutaneous lymph node syndrome
Takayasu's disease
Malaria and schistosoma infection
Typhus
Infective endocarditis
Rheumatoid arthritis
Syphilis
Wegener's granulomatosis
Salmonella infections
Rickettsial infections
Systemic lupus erythematosus
Ankylosing spondylitis

From Waller BF. Nonatherosclerotic coronary heart disease. In: Hurst JW, ed. *The heart,* 9th ed. New York: McGraw-Hill, 1998:1197–1240, reproduced with permission.

the process. Baroldi (70) proposed the following morphologic and histologic findings as signs of coronary arteritis: (a) focal artery necrosis with or without calcification; (b) coronary artery thrombosis or recanalization of thrombus associated with underlying arteriosclerotic plaques; (c) rupture of vessel walls that are not associated with trauma or interventional procedures; (d) coronary artery wall thickening with secondary luminal narrowing; and (e) wall thickening with aneurysm formation.

A more extensive characterization of the vasculitides has been developed by Lie (71) in which the involvement of the coronary circulation is based on the size of arteries involved. Specific causes for some of the vasculitides are discussed later.

Tuberculosis

Tuberculous arteritis is most often noted in patients with pericardial or myocardial lesions, but it is rarely seen in developed countries (70,72). Tuberculous granulomas may also involve the adventitia, the intima, or the entire wall of the coronary artery. With the emergence of resistant forms of tuberculosis in patients with depressed immune systems, physicians should consider the possibility of this form of arteritis when patients with tuberculosis have chest pain.

Polyarteritis Nodosa

Polyarteritis nodosa is probably the most common cause of coronary vasculitis. It is a systemic necrotizing vasculitis that affects the media and small arteries and is most prevalent in men aged 30 to 60 years. Of 66 cases of polyarteritis nodosa reported by Holsinger and coworkers (73), 41 (62%) had involvement of epicardial coronary arteries, and 41 also had MIs of various sizes. The coronary lesions resemble necrotizing vascular lesions found elsewhere in the body with the demonstration of acute cellular-phase destruction of media and internal elastic membranes together with subsequent intimal proliferation and scars in the muscle of the heart. Coronary aneurysm formation or occlusion may lead to MI in these patients (58,73). Prompt medical therapy for the generalized disease is indicated.

Systemic Lupus Erythematosus

Systemic lupus erythematosus is a chronic multisystem disease that most commonly affects women between the ages of 20 and 40 years. Pericarditis and myocarditis are common and may lead to chest pain and electrocardiographic abnormalities. In addition, AMI has developed in several young patients with lupus erythematosus despite the absence of conventional coronary atherothrombosis risk factors (66, 74). Pathologic examination in these cases showed intimal fibrosis of the coronary arteries, but to what degree this was the result of coronary arteritis rather than atherothrombosis accelerated by the underlying disease or corticosteroid ther-

apy is unclear. In one reported case, however, progressive coronary occlusion was observed on sequential coronary angiograms performed several days apart and was attributed to coronary vasculitis (73). Coronary vasculitis also has been reported in pathologic studies of patients with rheumatoid arthritis and acute rheumatic fever (66). Occasionally, the process may be limited only to coronary arteries (75).

Buerger's Disease (*Thromboangiitis* Obliterans)

In Buerger's disease the epicardial coronary arteries have been shown to be involved with focal polymorphonuclear infiltrates, histiocytes, and giant cells with or without coronary thrombosis (76) or with only coronary thrombosis. In 30 cases studied by Sophir (76), only 1 patient had coronary involvement, whereas in 19 cases studied by others (77), 6 patients had coronary thrombosis.

Wegener's Granulomatosis

Wegener's granulomatosis is a necrotizing vasculitis that most commonly affects the respiratory tract and kidney. Cardiac involvement is rare, but fibrinoid necrosis of the small- and medium-sized coronary arteries has been described (67). One case of large-vessel coronary occlusion with MI has been reported (78).

Takayasu's Disease (Pulseless Disease)

Takayasu's disease is predominantly a disease of young Oriental women. Granulomatous panarteritis and fibrosis of the aorta and its large branches lead to stenosis of these vessels, associated with decreased pulse amplitude and vascular bruits. Involvement of the coronary ostia and proximal coronary arteries, which has been described in 16 patients, may lead to angina pectoris or MI (67). This disease is seen with greater frequency in areas such as the west coast of the United States, which has a large Oriental population. Successful coronary artery bypass grafting has been performed for this condition.

Kawasaki Disease (Mucocutaneous Lymph Node Syndrome)

Kawasaki disease, a clinical syndrome first described by Kawasaki in 1967, appears to be much more prevalent than first suspected (35–37). It is a febrile illness of infants and young children that produces sterile conjunctivitis, oral pharyngeal erythema, desquamative reaction of the extremities, and nonpurulent cervical adenopathy. In more than 20% of patients, intense vasculitis of the coronary vasa vasorum leads to inflammation of coronary arteries, coronary artery aneurysm, thrombosis, and severe stenotic scarring. In a large study of 1,100 patients with the disease, 262 (24%) had coronary artery involvement with most having a complete occlusion (79). The cause of the disease has been considered immunologic because of the nature of the vasculitis and the infiltration of mononuclear cells in the area of pan vasculitis. Several studies have identified abnormalities in T lymphocytes and in various ratios of OKT3$^+$, OKT4$^+$, and OKT8$^+$ cells in those patients with and without vasculitis (80). These abnormalities may identify those patients likely to develop coronary involvement and to need intense immunosuppression. Other studies have suggested that a retrovirus may be the pathogenic agent for Kawasaki disease (81,82).

Death from Kawasaki disease may result from myocardial ischemia or arrhythmias, frequently during the recovery phase. Coronary aneurysm or diffuse stenosis may present as myocardial ischemia in the later course of the disease. Early recognition and intense therapy with aspirin and immunosuppression has been postulated to reduce the sequelae of the active process. Coronary bypass grafting has been performed successfully on these patients, although continued scarring and aneurysm formation may occur (66,83,84). This disease appears to be becoming more prevalent worldwide and is noted in all racial groups.

Infection

Syphilis is the most common infectious disease affecting the coronary arteries. Up to one-fourth of patients with tertiary cardiovascular syphilis may have ostial stenosis of one or both coronary arteries in addition to involvement of the ascending aorta or aortic valve. The right coronary artery is most frequently affected. Angina and MI have resulted from syphilitic coronary disease (85).

Other infections that cause coronary arteritis only rarely include *Salmonella,* tuberculosis, and leprosy (1). Viral and rickettsial infections and parasitic infestation (malaria and schistomes) have caused abnormalities of the coronary intima and have been proposed as a cause of MI in some patients (71,86-90).

Intimal Proliferation or Fibrosis

Coronary arteries may be narrowed severely by a fibrous hyperplasia that produces myocardial ischemia and MI. This condition may be associated with fibromuscular hyperplasia of the renal arteries, the use of methysergide, ostial cannulation during cardiac surgery or angioplasty, and following aortic valve replacement (92,93). As many as 50% of patients undergoing cardiac transplantation experience development of significant epicardial coronary artery narrowing or total occlusion by intimal fibrous proliferation within 3 to 5 years after transplantation. MI and sudden death have resulted from this type of chronic rejection. This process is thought to be related to the cardiac rejection process, which serves as the basis for the fibrous hyperplasia. A similar process has been noted after balloon angioplasty (92,93). Waller and coworkers (94) reported a case of left main coronary fibrous proliferation occurring after balloon angio-

plasty of a lesion in the left anterior descending coronary artery. They postulated that this process resulted from the angioplasty procedure.

Ionizing Radiation

Therapeutic doses of ionizing radiation delivered to the heart may cause pericarditis or myocardial fibrosis. The level necessary to cause arteritis exceeds 6,000 rad. Animal experimentation suggests that cardiac radiation may also injure capillary walls and enhance the development of lesions resembling atherothrombotic plaque in animals fed lipid-rich diets. In a small number of young patients with no conventional risk factors for coronary atherothrombosis, acute AMI has been reported at varying intervals after therapeutic cardiac radiation (95). The relation between radiation and coronary atherothrombosis in these patients has not been established (96).

Coronary Artery Radiation with Beta and Gamma Sources

In the last 5 years or so, bradytherapy of coronary lesions with either beta or gamma sources has been used to inhibit restenosis after angioplasty or stent placement (97-100). Although the therapy has clearly reduced the incidence of restenosis, the procedure has shed light on the ability of radiation to damage coronary arteries and induce atherothrombosis. The so-called candy wrapper effect, which describes the area adjacent to each end of the radiation source field, shows extensive damage and narrowing caused by atherothrombosis (101). Radiation clearly can damage the intima and leads to accelerated atherothrombosis (102).

CARDIAC TRANSPLANTATION

A number of patients experience development of significant coronary fibrosis or atherothrombosis within 3 years of cardiac transplantation. The disease is almost always diffusely distributed in large and small coronary arteries. It is not usually treatable with angioplasty or bypass surgery, and it is not symptomatic with angina because of cardiac denervation, therefore it must be followed by periodic angiography. The lesions differ from native-vessel atherothrombosis. It may be immunologically mediated and probably related to chronic rejection occurring in the intima (103). Myocardial rejection is frequently associated with the graft atherothrombosis, as demonstrated by endomyocardial biopsy (104). Better means of immunosuppression with cyclosporine and its analogs have reduced the incidence of atherothrombosis after successful cardiac transplantation. Angina pectoris is absent because of cardiac denervation, but MI or sudden death may result. This process usually involves the epicardial coronary arteries and is therefore evident on coronary arteriography. Selective fibrosis of the smaller coronary vessels also has been reported. Intimal damage resulting from immunologic rejection is believed to be the initiating injury causing coronary artery disease after cardiac transplantation (105). In patients who do not experience clinical or biopsy evidence for rejection, there appears to be a smaller prevalence of coronary atherothrombosis. Studies using diet, lipid-lowering drugs, and exercise programs appear to show a longer survival for patients undergoing cardiac transplantation.

ACCUMULATION OF METABOLIC SUBSTANCES

Specific metabolic substances may accumulate in various body tissues as the result of an inborn error of metabolism. Deposition of these substances in the walls of large and small coronary arteries may narrow the vessel lumen and lead to myocardial ischemia. These diseases include the mucopolysaccharidoses (Hunter's and Hurler's diseases [(106]), gangliosidoses (Sandhoff's disease and G_{M1}), primary oxalosis, alkaptonuria, and Fabry's disease. Accentuated intimal proliferation of the coronary arteries has been reported in patients with homocystinuria and Friedreich's ataxia (1–5).

In patients with systemic amyloidosis, amyloid may be deposited in the walls of both large and small coronary arteries and may lead to focal myocardial necrosis. The clinical importance of such small areas of necrosis is unclear, but they may contribute to the myocardial dysfunction that results from extensive deposits of myeloid in the myocardium (107).

EXTRINSIC CORONARY ARTERY COMPRESSION

External compression of the coronary artery may cause progressive narrowing of the vessel lumen. This has been reported in patients with aneurysms of the sinus of Valsalva and in patients with epicardial tumor metastases (95). Systolic coronary compression by muscle bridges has been discussed previously.

SUBSTANCE ABUSE: COCAINE

Reports have documented that cocaine abuse may result in myocardial ischemia and MI in the absence of coronary artery disease. Both coronary artery thrombosis and coronary artery spasm have been reported in patients with cocaine abuse (108-113). A number of physiologic studies using coronary artery segments *in vivo* also have demonstrated the coronary constrictive capacity of cocaine. In some instances, there is underlying atherothrombotic plaque disease, but in many others the coronary arteries are totally normal. The syndrome has been associated with cocaine-induced coronary artery spasm or possibly primary thrombogenicity produced by cocaine and its metabolites.

Cocaine may also have progressive and long-term effects on coronary arteries. Simpson and Edwards (114) have reported severely narrowed coronary arteries by fibrointimal proliferation that was caused by focal vessel endothelial injury and platelet adherence and aggregation. Platelets liberate platelet-derived growth factors, which can produce intimal proliferative lesions similar to those seen in restenosis after angioplasty. Thus, it appears that cocaine-induced coronary spasm may produce endothelial disruption and promote platelet aggregation and further vasoconstriction, which can lead to MI.

MYOCARDIAL OXYGEN DEMAND/SUPPLY IMBALANCE

An abnormality of myocardial oxygen demand/supply balance is the basis for much of the reported chest pain in all types of atherothrombosis. But, in some instances, an imbalance may result without obstructive coronary artery disease. The classic example of a failure to deliver adequate oxygen supplies to the myocardium has been noted in carbon monoxide poisoning (115). This condition has been associated with extensive focal infarction in the presence of normal coronary arteries. Prolonged hypotensive shock may also produce extensive nontransmural necrosis, especially of papillary muscles, which may lead to rupture and severe mitral regurgitation.

The classic example of a situation in which there is increased myocardial wall tension requiring increased coronary oxygen supply, producing an imbalance, is aortic stenosis or hypertrophic obstructive cardiomyopathy. These increased myocardial oxygen demands, frequently associated with increased muscle mass of the heart, result in a limited blood supply and poor perfusion of the myocardium. This may result in decreased myocardial function and a syndrome known as the "stone heart syndrome" when it is of prolonged duration. Thyrotoxicosis also has been shown to result occasionally in fibrosis in the myocardium, which is likely the result of an imbalance in myocardial oxygen demands as compared with the supply available (116).

FUTURE DIRECTIONS

Even though congenital anomalies of the origin and course of coronary arteries are diagnosed with increasing frequency, because of more widely used interventional technologies, clinicians must be wise and vigilant as they see patients with unusual symptoms. Interventional cardiologists will probably account for increasing the incidence of coronary aneurysms, coronary dissections, and coronary embolizations. Distal protection devices will become more widely used as cardiologists open lesions in vein grafts and attempt opening of total occlusions.

The development of intimal injury by radiation (caused by brachytherapy) and by immune reactions as occurs in cardiac transplantation as the stimulus for accelerated atherothrombosis will add to our understanding. The restenosis syndrome that is so prominent will no doubt lead to successful new therapies such as drug eluting stents, gene and gene product transfers, and better drugs to suppress immune injury.

The recent questions of homocystine, viruses and chlamydia as etiologic agents in the development of atherogenesis need further epidemiologic study. Clinicians need to be aware that many systemic diseases may affect coronary arteries and lead to unusual symptoms. This is particularly true for multiple vasculitides and metabolic diseases that are rare but may be fatal if coronary artery involvement is not recognized and treated.

REFERENCES

1. Cheitlin MD, McAllister HA, DeCastro CM. Myocardial infarction without atherosclerosis. *JAMA* 1975;231:951–959.
2. Rozavi M. Unusual forms of coronary artery disease. *Cardiovasc Clin* 1975;7:25.
3. Neufeld HN, Blieden LC. Coronary artery disease in children. *Postgrad Med J* 1978;54:163–170.
4. Waller BF. Nonatherosclerotic coronary heart disease. In: Hurst JW, ed. *The heart*, 9th ed. New York: McGraw-Hill, 1998:1197–1240.
5. Waller BF. Atherosclerotic and nonatherosclerotic coronary artery factors in acute myocardial infarction. In: Pepine CF, ed. *Acute myocardial infarction*. Philadelphia: FA Davis, 1989:29–104.
6. Engel HJ, Torres C, Page HL Jr. Major variations in anatomical origin of the coronary arteries: angiographic observations in 4,250 patients without associated congenital heart disease. *Cathet Cardiovasc Diagn* 1975;1:157–161.
7. Isner JM, Donaldson RF. Coronary angiographic and morphologic correlation. In: Waller BF, ed. *Cardiac morphology. Cardiology clinics*. Philadelphia: WB Saunders, 1984:571–592.
8. Levin DC, Fellows KE, Abrams HL. Hemodynamically significant primary anomalies of the coronary arteries: angiographic aspects. *Circulation* 1978;58:25–34.
9. Roberts WC. Major anomalies of coronary arterial origin seen in adulthood. *Am Heart J* 1986;111:941–963.
10. Kimbiris D, Iskandrian AS, Segal B, et al. Anomalous aortic origin of coronary arteries. *Circulation* 1978;58:606–615.
11. Liberthson RR, Dinsmore RE, Fallon JT. Aberrant coronary artery origin from the aorta. Report of 18 patients, review of literature and delineation of natural history and management. *Circulation* 1979;59:748–754.
12. Becker LC. Conditions for vasodilatory-induced coronary steal in experimental myocardial ischemia. *Circulation* 1978;57:1103.
13. Muller JE, Gunther SJ. Nifedipine therapy for Prinzmetal angina. *Circulation* 1978;57:137.
14. Chaitman BR, Lesperance J, Saltiel J. Clinical, angiographic, and hemodynamic findings in patients with anomalous origin of the coronary arteries. *Circulation* 1976;53:122–131.
15. Desmet W, Vanhaecke J, Vrolix M, et al. Isolated single coronary artery: a review of 50,000 consecutive coronary angiographies. *Eur Heart J* 1992;13:1637–1640.
16. Sharbaugh AH, White RS. Single coronary artery. Analysis of the anatomic variation, clinical importance, and report of five cases. *JAMA* 1974;230:243–246.
17. Joswig BC, Warren SE, Vieweg WV, et al. Transmural myocardial infarction in the absence of coronary arterial luminal narrowing in a young man with single coronary arterial anomaly. *Cathet Cardiovasc Diagn* 1978;4:297–301.
18. Byrum CJ, Blackman MS, Schneider B, et al. Congenital atresia of the left coronary ostium and hypoplasia of the left main coronary artery. *Am Heart J* 1980;99:354–358.
19. Lerberg DB, Ogden JA, Zuberbuhler JR, et al. Anomalous origin of the right coronary artery from the pulmonary artery. *Ann Thorac Surg* 1979;27:87–94.
20. Wesselhoeft H, Fawcett JS, Johnson AL. Anomalous origin of the left coronary artery from the pulmonary trunk. *Circulation* 1968;38:403–425.
21. Richardson JV, Doty DB. Correction of anomalous origin of the left coronary artery. *J Thorac Cardiovasc Surg* 1979;77:699–703.
22. Baim DS, Kline H, Silverman JF. Bilateral coronary-pulmonary artery fistulae: report of five cases and review of the literature. *Circulation* 1982;65:810–815.
23. Liberthson RR, Sagar K, Berkoben JP, et al. Congenital coronary arteriovenous fistula: report of 13 patients. Review of the literature and delineation of the management. *Circulation* 1979;59:849–854.
24. Harrison DC, Baim DS. Nonatherosclerotic coronary heart disease. In: Hurst JW, ed. *The heart*, 6th ed. New York: McGraw-Hill, 1990:1130–1139.
25. Urrutia-S CO, Falaschi G, Ott DA, et al. Surgical management of 56 patients with congenital coronary artery fistulas. *Ann Thorac Surg* 1983;35:300–307.
26. Geiringer E. The mural coronary artery. *Am Heart J* 1951;41:359–368.
27. Noble J, Bourassa MG, Petitclerc R, et al. Myocardial bridging and milking effect of the left anterior descending coronary artery: normal variant or obstruction. *Am J Cardiol* 1976;37:993–999.
28. Grondin P, Bourassa MG, Noble J, et al. Successful course after supra-arterial myotomy for myocardial bridging and milking effect of the left anterior descending artery. *Ann Thorac Surg* 1977;24:422–429.
29. Iversen S, Hake U, Mayer E, et al. Surgical treatment of myocardial bridging causing coronary artery obstruction. *Scand J Thorac Cardiovasc Surg* 1992;26:107–111.
30. Glickel SZ, Maggs PR, Ellis FH Jr. Coronary artery aneurysm. *Ann Thorac Surg* 1978;25:372–376.
31. Befeler B, Aranda JM, Embi A, et al. Coronary artery aneurysms: study of the etiology, clinical course and effect on left ventricular function and prognosis. *Am J Med* 1977;62:597–607.
32. Yotsumoto G, Shimokawa S, Moriyama Y, et al. Coronary artery aneurysm after stent implantation. *Jpn J Thorac Cardiovasc Surg* 1999;47:339–341.
33. Berkalp B, Kervancioglu C, Oral D. Coronary artery aneurysm formation after balloon angioplasty and stent implantation. *Int J Cardiol* 1999;69:65–70.
34. Tomita H. Intravascular ultrasound and electron beam tomography of late developing coronary artery aneurysms after Kawasaki disease. *Catheter Cardiovasc Interv* 1999;47:114–115.
35. Daniels SR, Specker B, Capannari TE, et al. Correlates of coronary artery aneurysm formation in patients with Kawasaki disease. *Am J Dis Child* 1987;141:205–207.
36. Takahashi M, Mason W, Lewis AB. Regression of coronary aneurysms in patients with Kawasaki syndrome. *Circulation* 1987;75:387–394.
37. Kato H, Ichinose E, Kawasaki T. Myocardial infarction in Kawasaki disease: clinical analyses in 195 cases. *J Pediatr* 1986;108:923–927.
38. Roberts WC. Coronary embolism: a review of causes, consequences, and diagnostic considerations. *Cardiovasc Med* 1978;3:699–703.
39. Baim DS, Wahr D, George B, et al., Saphenous vein graft Angioplasty Free of Emboli Randomized (SAFER) Trial Investigators. Randomized trial of a distal embolic protection device during percutaneous intervention of saphenous vein aorto-coronary bypass grafts. *Circulation* 2002;105:1285–1290.
40. Prizel KR, Hutchins GM, Bulkley BH. Coronary artery embolism and myocardial infarction. *Ann Intern Med* 1978;88:155–161.
41. Pfeifer JF, Lipton MJ, Oury JH. Acute coronary embolism complicating bacterial endocarditis: operative treatment. *Am J Cardiol* 1976;37:920–922.
42. Baim DS. Percutaneous transluminal coronary angioplasty: analysis of unsuccessful procedures as a guide toward improved results. *Cardiovasc Intervent Radiol* 1982;5:186–193.
43. Bell MR, Garratt KN, Bresnahan JF, et al. Relation of deep arterial resection and coronary artery aneurysms after directional coronary atherectomy. *J Am Coll Cardiol* 1992;20:1474–1481.
44. Topol EJ, Leya F, Piinkerton CA, et al. A comparison of directional atherectomy with coronary angioplasty in patients with coronary artery disease. *N Engl J Med* 1993;329:221–227.
45. Adelman AG, Cohen EA, Kimball BP, et al. A comparison of directional atherectomy with balloon angioplasty for lesions of the left anterior descending coronary artery. *N Engl J Med* 1993;329:228–233.
46. Warth DC, Martin BL, O'Neil W, et al. Rotational atherectomy multicenter registry: acute results, complications and 6-month angiographic follow-up in 709 patients. *J Am Coll Cardiol* 1994;24:641–648.
47. Mehran R, Dangas G, Abizaid AS. Angiographic patterns of in-stent restenosis: classification and implications for long-term outcome. *Circulation* 1999;100:1872–1878.

48. Liistro F, Stankovic G, Di Mario C, et al. First clinical experience with a paclitaxel derivate-eluting polymer stent system implantation for in-stent restenosis: immediate and long-term clinical and angiographic outcome. *Circulation* 2002;105:1883–1886.

49. Cowley MJ, Dorris G, Kelsey SF, et al. Emergency coronary bypass surgery after coronary angioplasty: the National Heart, Lung and Blood Institute's percutaneous transluminal coronary angioplasty registry experience. *Am J Cardiol* 1984;53:22C–26C.

50. Ischinger T, Gruentzig AR, Meier B, et al. Coronary dissection and total coronary occlusion associated with percutaneous transluminal coronary angioplasty: significance of initial angiographic morphology of coronary stenoses. *Circulation* 1986;74:1371–1378.

51. Brahos GJ, Baker NH, Ewy HG, et al. Aortocoronary bypass following unsuccessful PTCA: experience in 100 consecutive patients. *Ann Thorac Surg* 1985;40:7–10.

52. Hoshino T, Yoshida H, Takayama S, et al. Significance of intimal tears in the mechanism of luminal enlargement in percutaneous transluminal coronary angioplasty: correlation of histologic and angiographic findings in postmortem human hearts. *Am Heart J* 1987;114:503–510.

53. Spring DA. Coronary artery dissection during PTCA: a necessary evil? *Cathet Cardiovasc Diagn* 1985;11:1–3.

54. Shaver PJ, Carrig TF, Baker WP. Postpartum coronary artery dissection. *Br Heart J* 1978;40:83–86.

55. Claudon DG, Claudon DB, Edwards JE. Primary dissecting aneurysm of coronary artery. *Circulation* 1972;45:259–266.

56. Smith JC. Dissecting aneurysms of coronary arteries. *Arch Pathol* 1975;99:117–121.

57. Ciraulo DA, Chesne RB. Coronary arterial dissection: an unrecognized cause of myocardial infarction, with subsequent coronary arterial patency. *Chest* 1978;73:677–679.

58. Allen RP, Liedtke AJ. The role of coronary artery injury and perfusion in the development of cardiac contusion secondary to nonpenetrating chest trauma. *J Trauma* 1979;19:153–156.

59. Cheitlin MD. Key references: cardiovascular trauma. Part I. *Circulation* 1982;65:1529–1532.

60. Cheitlin MD. Cardiovascular trauma. Part II. *Circulation* 1982;66:244–247.

61. Austin SM, Applefeld MM, Turney SZ, et al. Traumatic left anterior descending coronary artery to right ventricle fistula: report of two cases. *South Med J* 1977;70:581–584.

62. Espada R, Whisenand HH, Mattox KL, et al. Surgical management of penetrating injuries to the coronary arteries. *Surgery* 1975;78:755–760.

63. Sethi GK, Scott SM, Takaro T. Iatrogenic coronary artery stenosis following aortic valve replacement. *J Thorac Cardiovasc Surg* 1979;77:760–767.

64. Kennedy JW. Complications associated with cardiac catheterization and angiography. *Cathet Cardiovasc Diagn* 1982;8:5–11.

65. Virmani R, Popovsky MA, Roberts WC. Thrombocytosis, coronary thrombosis and acute myocardial infarction. *Am J Med* 1979;67:498–506.

66. Ridolfi RL, Hutchins GM, Bell WR. The heart and cardiac conduction system in thrombotic thrombocytopenia purpura. A clinicopathologic study of 17 autopsied patients. *Ann Intern Med* 1979;91:357–363.

67. Parillo JE, Fauci AS. Necrotizing vasculitis, coronary angiitis and the cardiologist. *Am Heart J* 1980;99:547–554.

68. James TN. Small arteries of the heart. *Circulation* 1977;56:2–14.

69. Mosseri M, Yarom R, Gotsman MS, et al. Histologic evidence for small-vessel coronary artery disease in patients with angina pectoris and patent large coronary arteries. *Circulation* 1986;74:964–972.

70. Baroldi G. Diseases of the coronary arteries. In: Silver MD, ed. *Cardiovascular pathology.* New York: Churchill Livingstone, 1983:341.

71. Lie JT. Coronary vasculitis: a review in the current scheme of classification of vasculitis. *Arch Pathol Lab Med* 1987;111:224–233.

72. Gouley BA, Bellet S, McMillan TM. Tuberculosis of the myocardium: report of six cases, with observations on involvement of coronary arteries. *Arch Intern Med* 1933;51:244–263.

73. Holsinger DR, Osmundson PJ, Edwards JE. The heart in periarteritis nodosa. *Circulation* 1962;25:610–618.

74. Meller J, Conde CA, Deppisch LM. Myocardial infarction due to coronary atherosclerosis in three young adults with systemic lupus erythematosus. *Am J Cardiol* 1975;35:309–314.

75. Douglas WA, Gardner MA, Carey LM, et al. Systemic lupus erythem-

atosus with vasculitis confined to the coronary arteries. *Aust NZ J Med* 2000;30:283–285.

76. Sophir O. Thromboangiitis obliterans of the coronary arteries and its relation to atherosclerosis. *Am Heart J* 1936;12:521–535.

77. Averbuck SH, Silbert S. Thromboangiitis obliterans: cause of death. *Arch Intern Med* 1934;54:436–465.

78. Gatenby PA, Lytton DG, Bulteau VG, et al. Myocardial infarction in Wegener's granulomatosis. *Aust NZ J Med* 1976;6:336–340.

79. Suzuki A, Kamlya T, Kuwahara N, et al. Coronary arterial lesions of Kawasaki disease: cardiac catheterization findings of 1100 cases. *Pediatr Cardiol* 1986;7:3–9.

80. Terai M, Kohno Y, Niwa K, et al. Imbalance among T-cell subsets in patients with coronary arterial aneurysms in Kawasaki disease. *Am J Cardiol* 1987;60:555–559.

81. Shulman ST, Rowley AH. Does Kawasaki disease have a retroviral aetiology? *Lancet* 1986;2:545–546.

82. Burns JC, Geha RS, Schneeberger EE, et al. Polymerase activity in lymphocyte culture supernatants from patients with Kawasaki disease. *Nature* 1986;323:814–816.

83. Onouchi Z, Shinichiro S, Kiyosawa N, et al. Aneurysms in the coronary arteries in Kawasaki disease: an angiographic study of 30 cases. *Circulation* 1982;66:6–13.

84. Fukushige J, Nihill MR, McNamara DG. Spectrum of cardiovascular lesions in mucocutaneous lymph node syndrome. *Am J Cardiol* 1980;45:98–107.

85. Holt S. Syphilitic ostial occlusion. *Br Heart J* 1977;39:469–470.

86. Merkel WC. Plasmodium falciparum malaria: the coronary and myocardial lesions observed in autopsy in two cases of acute fulminating *P. falciparum* infection. *Arch Pathol* 1946;41:290–298.

87. Gazayerli M. Unusual site of a schistosome worm in the circumflex branch of the left coronary artery. *J Egypt Med Assoc* 1939;22:34–39.

88. Allen AC, Spitz S. A comparative study of the pathology of scrub typhus (Tsutsugamuschi's disease) and other rickettsial diseases. *Am J Pathol* 1945;21:603–681.

89. Moe JB, Mosher DF, Kenyon RH, et al. Functional and morphological changes during experimental Rocky Mountain spotted fever in guinea pigs. *Lab Invest* 1976;35:235–245.

90. Sergent JS. Vasculitides associated with viral infections. *Clin Rheum Dis* 1980;6:339–350.

91. Burch GE, Shewey LL. Viral coronary arteritis and myocardial infarction. *Am Heart J* 1976;92:11–14.

92. Brill IC, Brodeur MT, Oyama AA. Myocardial infarction in two sisters less than 20 years old. *JAMA* 1971;217:1345–1348.

93. Trimble AS, Bigelow WG, Wigle ED. Coronary ostial stenosis: a late complication of coronary perfusion in open-heart surgery. *J Thorac Cardiovasc Surg* 1969;57:792–795.

94. Waller BF, Pinkerton CA, Foster LN. Morphologic evidence of accelerated left main coronary artery stenosis: a late complication of percutaneous transluminal angioplasty of the proximal left anterior descending coronary artery. *J Am Coll Cardiol* 1987;9:1019–1023.

95. Kopelson G, Herwig KJ. The etiologies of coronary artery disease in cancer patients. *Int J Radiat Oncol Biol Phys* 1978;4:895–906.

96. Fajardo LF. Radiation-induced coronary artery disease [editorial]. *Chest* 1977;71:563–564.

97. Grise MA, Massullo V, Jani S, et al. Five-year clinical follow-up after intracoronary radiation: results of a randomized clinical trial. *Circulation* 2002;105:2737–2740.

98. Moussavian M, Castereall P, Teirstein PS. Restenosis after angioplasty. *Curr Treatment Options Cardiovasc Med* 2001;3:103–112.

99. Raizner AE, Osterle SN, Waksman R. Inhibition of restenosis with β-emitting radiotherapy report of the proliferation reduction with vascular energy trial (PREVENT). *Circulation* 2000;102:951–958.

100. Verin V, Popowski Y, de Bruyne B. Endoluminal β-radiation therapy for the prevention of coronary restenosis after balloon angioplasty. *N Engl J Med* 2001;344:243–249.

101. Serruys PW, Kay IP. I like the candy, I hate the wrapper: the 32P radioactive stent. *Circulation* 2000;101:3–7.

102. Costa MA, Sabate M, van der Giessen WJ. Late coronary occlusion after intracoronary brachytherapy. *Circulation* 1999;100:789–792.

103. Frist WH, Oyer PE, Baldwin JC, et al. HLA antigen compatibility and cardiac transplant recipient survival. *Ann Thorac Surg* 1987;44:242–246.

104. Narrod J, Kormos R, Armitage J, et al. Acute rejection and plantation. *J Heart Transplant* 1988;7:71(abst).
105. Mason JW, Strefling A. Small vessel disease of the heart resulting in myocardial necrosis and death despite angiographically normal coronary arteries. *Am J Cardiol* 1979;44:171–176.
106. Brosius FC, Roberts WC. Coronary artery disease in the Hurler syndrome. *Am J Cardiol* 1981;47:649–653.
107. Smith RR, Hutchins GM. Ischemic heart disease secondary to amyloidosis of intramyocardial arteries. *Am J Cardiol* 1979;44:413–417.
108. Isner JM, Estes NA III, Thompson PD, et al. Acute cardiac events temporally related to cocaine abuse. *N Engl J Med* 1986;315:1438–1443.
109. Simpson RW, Edwards WD. Pathogenesis of cocaine-induced ischemic heart disease. *Arch Pathol Lab Med* 1986;110:479–484.
110. Zimmerman FH, Gustafson GM, Kemp HG. Recurrent myocardial infarction associated with cocaine abuse in a young man with normal coronary arteries: evidence for coronary artery spasm culminating in thrombosis. *J Am Coll Cardiol* 1987;9:964–978.
111. Smith HW, Liberman HA, Brody SL, et al. Acute myocardial infarction temporarily related to cocaine use. Clinical, angiographic and pathophysiologic observations. *Ann Intern Med* 1987;107:13–18.
112. Patel R, Haider B, Ahmed S, et al. Cocaine-related myocardial infarction: high prevalence of occlusive coronary thrombi without significant obstructive atherosclerosis. *Circulation* 1988;78[Suppl II]:II-436(abst).
113. Lange RA, Cigarroa RG, Yancy CW, et al. Cocaine-induced coronary artery vasoconstriction. *N Engl J Med* 1989;321:1557–1562.
114. Simpson RW, Edwards WD. Pathogenesis of cocaine-induced ischemic heart disease. Autopsy finding in a 21-year-old man. *Arch Pathol Lab Med* 1986;110:479–484.
115. Cheitlin MD, McAllister HA, deCastro CM. Myocardial infarction without atherosclerosis. *JAMA* 1975;231:951–959.
116. Gross II, Stenberg WH. Myocardial infarction without significant lesions of coronary arteries. *Arch Intern Med* 1939;64:249–267.

CHAPTER 47

The Microcirculation in Atherothrombotic Coronary Artery Disease

Richard O. Cannon III

Key Words: Coronary blood flow; coronary microcirculation; endothelium; hypercholesterolemia; myocardial ischemia; nitric oxide.

INTRODUCTION

Although the focus of clinical attention in coronary heart disease has been on atherothrombosis in epicardial coronary arteries, there is increasing evidence that dysfunction of the coronary microcirculation may contribute to myocardial ischemia. In this regard, epicardial coronary atherothrombosis is commonly associated with endothelial dysfunction that may extend to the coronary microcirculation, preventing appropriate regulation of coronary blood flow. An understanding of disease or dysfunction of the coronary microcirculation has led to consideration of therapies that may complement targeted treatment of epicardial atherothrombotic disease.

In this chapter, coronary microcirculation is defined as vessels too small to be imaged angiographically: intermediate-sized intramural arteries 100 to 300 μm in diameter, arterioles and collateral arteries 20 to 50 μm in diameter, and capillaries and venules less than 20 μm in diameter. This chapter initially discusses the role of the coronary microcir-

culation in the regulation of blood flow, with a focus on the importance of endothelium-derived relaxant factors, especially nitric oxide (NO). This is followed by studies of the coronary microcirculation in animal models of atherothrombosis. Human studies of coronary microvascular flow dynamics are discussed, with an emphasis on potential mechanisms for myocardial ischemia independent of significant obstructive disease of the epicardial arteries by atherothrombosis. Pharmacologic approaches for improving microvascular function are presented. Finally, there continues to be need for research further defining the role of microcirculation in myocardial ischemic syndromes, especially in the absence of obstructive coronary artery disease, and optimum treatment options to relieve ischemia and manage symptoms.

CORONARY MICROCIRCULATION IN ANIMALS

Contribution of Small Arteries to Vascular Resistance

Until recently, only the smallest component of the coronary arterial microcirculation—arterioles approximately 20 to 30 μm diameter—were believed to ordinarily impose any significant resistance to coronary flow. In response to surrounding myocardial metabolic conditions, arterioles dilate or constrict to match flow appropriate to myocardial oxygen demands. However, Chilian and coworkers (1,2), using an epicardial imaging system and micropuncture measurements of pressure

R. O. Cannon: Cardiovascular Branch, NHLBI, National Institutes of Health, Building 10, Room 7B-15, 10 Center Drive MSC 1650, Bethesda, Maryland 20892-1650.

in small subepicardial arteries of the beating cat heart, showed that 40% to 50% of the total coronary resistance is imposed by small arteries between 100 and 300 μm in diameter. In contrast, the arterioles accounted for only about 10% of the total basal coronary vascular resistance. This group also showed that coronary microvessels within the subepicardium may not respond uniformly to stimuli or agonists that affect coronary flow. For example, in response to reduction of coronary perfusion pressure, only arteries less than 100 μm in diameter dilated (larger vessels actually constricted) (3), whereas in response to the myocardial oxygen demands of pacing, all levels of microvessels dilated (4). The heterogeneity of microvascular responses may result from variability in the distribution of receptors, myogenic tone, and innervation, as well as other considerations (5). For technical reasons, these studies have been limited to the subepicardial microcirculation; the microvasculature at deeper levels within the myocardium may differ both in the relative contribution of small intramural arteries to resistance to coronary flow and in the vasomotor responses to neurohumoral stimuli.

Nitric Oxide and Regulation of Microvascular Tone

The discovery of endothelium-derived relaxing factors (6), NO in particular (7), has led to numerous studies of the role of NO in the coronary microcirculation. Inhibition of NO synthesis with N^G-monomethyl-L-arginine (L-NMMA) increases basal coronary vascular resistance and blunts the vasodilator response to the endothelium-dependent agonists acetylcholine and bradykinin in isolated perfused hearts (8,9). These responses to NO inhibition are reversible by addition of L-arginine, the substrate for NO synthesis within the endothelium by the enzyme nitric oxide synthase (NOS). L-NMMA administered systemically to the awake dog at doses that increase systemic blood pressure by blocking NO production in the systemic circulation also increases basal coronary vascular resistance (10). L-NMMA inhibits dilation of subepicardial arteries greater than 120 μm in diameter by the endothelium-dependent vasodilator acetylcholine, with partial inhibition of this response by L-NMMA in arteries less than 120 μm in diameter (11). In the anesthetized dog, NO inhibition with N-nitro-L-arginine attenuates acetylcholine-induced increases in coronary flow (12,13). Thus, animal studies indicate that coronary vascular resistance is decreased or increased by agonists that augment or inhibit NO production, respectively. Because the majority of coronary resistance is mediated by intramyocardial small arteries and arterioles, it seems likely that microvascular endothelial release of relaxant factors such as NO is important in regulating basal and agonist-stimulated coronary flood flow.

Atherothrombosis and the Coronary Microcirculation

Vascular strips or rings from large arteries of animals fed high-cholesterol diets exhibit impaired responses to endothelium-dependent vasodilators such as acetylcholine, with en-

dothelium-independent vasodilator responses to drugs such as nitroglycerin unaffected by atherothrombosis (14–16). Animal models of atherothrombosis also have revealed endothelial dysfunction of the small arteries of the heart. Small subepicardial arteries approximately 300 μm in diameter from cholesterol-fed rabbits contracted in vitro in response to doses of acetylcholine that produced relaxation in similar-sized small arteries from control animals, despite equal degrees of relaxation to a NO donor in the two groups of animals (17). Microscopic examination of the vascular segments used in the study showed the endothelium of the small arteries from hypercholesterolemic rabbits to be structurally intact and free of atherothrombosis, although small lipid deposits were seen within endothelial cells. The media of the arteries appeared unaltered by hypercholesterolemia. Small epicardial coronary arteries (122–222 μm in diameter) dissected from the hearts of cynomolgus monkeys fed an atherogenic diet were found to contract in response to acetylcholine, with impaired dilator responses to other endothelium-dependent vasodilator agonists such as bradykinin and calcium ionophore (which stimulates NO production within the endothelium without activation of cell surface receptors), compared with similar-sized small arteries from control animals, which dilated to all endothelium-dependent agonists (18). These responses were not affected by indomethacin, which blocks the synthesis of vasodilating prostaglandins. The responses of the small arteries to the endothelium-independent vasodilators adenosine and nitroprusside were no different between cholesterol-fed and control monkeys in this study. Histologic examination of the vascular segments showed no atherothrombosis involving the small arteries of the cholesterol-fed animals despite extensive atherothrombosis of the large arteries, although intracellular vacuoles were noted in the endothelium of small arteries from cholesterol-fed animals. Even smaller arteries (30–70 μm in diameter) have been isolated from hearts of cholesterol-fed pigs and studied in vitro (19). Compared with similar-sized microvessels from control animals, these vascular segments exhibited impaired responses to the endothelium-dependent vasodilators histamine, serotonin, and adenosine diphosphate and to increases in flow (shear stress), also an endothelium-dependent vasodilator stimulus. These abnormal responses were normalized by exposure of the vascular segments to L-arginine, the precursor for NO synthesis. Consistent with other studies, the microvascular endothelium from the cholesterol-fed animals often contained large lipid-laden vacuoles.

Mechanisms of Microvascular Endothelial Dysfunction

Investigations indicate that endothelial dysfunction in hypercholesterolemia and atherothrombosis may be selective for certain signal transduction pathways that link receptor activation on the endothelial cell surface to activation of NOS (20,21). For example, despite impaired vasodilator responses of vascular rings from hypercholesterolemic pigs to acetylcholine, an endothelium-dependent vasodilator that activates NO production through a pertussis toxin–sensitive, G_i protein–dependent signal transduction pathway, responses to other endothelium-dependent vasodilators such as bradykinin, which uses a different signal transduction pathway that is unaffected by pertussin toxin, are unimpaired, at least in animals with early atherothrombosis. Oxidatively modified, low-density lipoproteins, especially lysolecithin in the oxidized particle, may be responsible for inhibition of NO production by inhibiting signaling pathways or enzymatic activity of NOS (22,23).

Experimental studies suggest that NO synthesis may be limited under some situations by limited L-arginine availability. In normal endothelial cell metabolism, L-arginine is not rate-limiting in the enzymatic synthesis of NO, with cytosolic concentrations of this amino acid far exceeding the maximum rate of substrate use by NOS. However, accumulation of methylated arginines such as asymmetric dimethylarginine (ADMA), generated enzymatically from proteins that regulate RNA processing, may compete with L-arginine for the substrate binding site on NOS (24). Intracellular ADMA may increase as a result of reduced degradation by the enzyme dimethylarginine dimethylaminohydrolase (25). Because ADMA cannot serve as an active substrate to NOS, NO synthesis might be reduced if sufficient L-arginine were displaced. Additional mechanisms by which L-arginine bioavailability might be reduced include excess conversion to ornithine through enhanced activity of arginase (26) and inhibition of L-arginine into cells (27).

NO may also be degraded to biologically inactive nitrogen oxide compounds by the action of superoxide anions, which may be increased in hypercholesterolemia (28). The source of this free radical species, which may oxidize NO to toxic molecules such as peroxynitrite, may include oxidase enzyme systems. In experimental settings, NOS may become a generator of superoxide anions as well, as may occur in the absence of the cofactor tetrahydrobiopterin (29). Levels of this cofactor may be reduced in atherothrombosis, contributing to endothelial dysfunction, possibly by increased oxidation to dihydrobiopterin. Folate regenerates tetrahydrobiopterin, and may restore NO synthesis in this setting.

Thus, NO bioavailability may be reduced in experimental settings by a combination of reduced synthesis (which may be selective for specific signal transduction pathways) and accelerated degradation of NO, resulting in impaired endothelium-dependent vascular relaxation and dilation.

CORONARY VASCULAR STUDIES IN HUMANS

Methodologic Considerations

Unlike many of the animal studies described earlier, in which small arteries were directly visualized in beating hearts or studied *in vitro*, the coronary microcirculation in humans can be assessed only indirectly. Changes in coronary flow in response to an agonist in the absence of obstructive epicardial coronary artery disease or significant changes in epicardial coronary artery luminal diameter are generally interpreted to reflect vasomotor changes of the coronary microcirculation. These assumptions immediately raise several concerns. For example, what quantity of atherothrombotic disease or changes in luminal diameter in the epicardial coronary arteries can be considered "insignificant," and thus not limit coronary flow during stress? Gould (30) showed that focal stenoses of greater than 50% luminal diameter narrowing are required to affect pharmacologically stimulated coronary flow adversely. In humans, however, atherothrombosis may be diffuse, and lesions may be multiple and in series, thus making the detection of "significance" by a simple percentage stenosis at a given lesion site problematic. Indeed, a "50% stenosis" in humans may or may not adversely affect coronary flow responses to coronary microvascular vasodilators such as papaverine, suggesting that visual assessment of lesions "intermediate" in severity often is inaccurate (31), as confirmed by use of intravascular ultrasound. With regard to changes in luminal diameter of epicardial arteries, the resistance to coronary flow is inversely related to the diameter of the epicardial artery to the fourth power and directly related to the length of the arterial segment analyzed. For a normal epicardial artery, small changes in the diameter will have little impact on coronary resistance (ignoring compensatory changes in microvascular tone). However, diffuse narrowing of an epicardial vessel in response to an agonist may result in some resistance to coronary flow, especially if superimposed on "insignificant" coronary artery disease. Accordingly, the contribution of the epicardial coronary arteries to coronary resistance can be confidently excluded only in the absence of coronary artery disease or constriction of epicardial arteries in response to an agonist.

Measurement of coronary flow, which is necessary for assessment of microvascular function, has been accomplished in the catheterization laboratory with intracoronary Doppler measurements of flow velocity, a technique thoroughly validated in animals and experimental flow models (32,33). Instantaneous changes in flow velocity can be recorded after intracoronary administration of agonists such as acetylcholine and adenosine. Flow velocity measurements require simultaneous quantitative angiography to derive volume flow. Quantitative angiography, even if it uses computerized edge detection techniques, necessitates geometric assumptions about the artery, which may not be valid in patients with coronary artery disease.

Positron emission tomography (PET) provides noninvasive measurement of regional myocardial perfusion using flow tracers such as ^{15}O-labeled water and has been used to assess coronary flow reserve in response to vasodilators such as dipyridamole (34,35). However, in addition to limited availability, PET cannot be used to assess endothelium-dependent agonists such as acetylcholine that require administration into a coronary artery. Furthermore, interpretation of a limited flow response to a vasodilator agonist as being caused by microvascular dysfunction requires knowledge of the absence of coronary artery disease in the patient undergoing testing. Cardiac magnetic resonance imaging can provide estimates of relative changes in blood flow, before and during administration of a microvascular dilator such as adenosine, with resolution sufficient to compare subendocardial versus subepicardial responses (36,37).

Atherothrombosis and the Coronary Circulation in Humans

As discussed previously in this chapter, atherothrombosis can impair endothelium-dependent vasodilator responses in large arteries (including coronary arteries) of animals fed high-cholesterol diets. Ludmer and coworkers (38) reported that epicardial coronary arteries in humans with significant coronary artery disease constricted both at sites of significant disease and at sites of plaquing in response to acetylcholine, as opposed to vasodilation in coronary arteries of patients without any evidence of coronary artery disease. In contrast to the different responses of these two patient groups to acetylcholine, responses to nitroglycerin were similar, indicating unimpaired smooth muscle responsiveness to NO in atherothrombotic arteries. Patients with atheromatous plaquing or "nonsignificant" coronary artery disease also exhibit constrictor responses of epicardial arteries to intracoronary acetylcholine (38–41). Studies also have shown that angiographically normal coronary arteries of patients with significant atherothrombotic disease involving other arteries also constrict in response to intracoronary acetylcholine in doses that cause dilation of epicardial arteries in patients with entirely normal coronary angiograms (42). Even risk factors for atherothrombosis such as hypercholesterolemia, male sex, age, and family history of coronary artery disease have been associated with constrictor responses of the epicardial coronary arteries to acetylcholine in patients with normal-appearing coronary angiograms (40,43,44). These observations are compatible with the concept that endothelial dysfunction of epicardial coronary arteries may precede development of atherothrombotic disease that is either angiographically apparent or of sufficient obstructive severity to cause myocardial ischemia and angina pectoris.

Several studies of epicardial coronary responses to endothelium-dependent and independent vasodilators in patients with early atherothrombosis also reported the effects of these agonists on coronary blood flow. Zeiher and coworkers (40) found a smaller decrease in coronary resistance (coronary flow derived from intracoronary Doppler flow velocity measurement) in response to intracoronary acetylcholine (range, 0.72–7.2 μg/min) in nine patients with hypercholesterolemia (average cholesterol, 281 mg/dL) but smooth epicardial coronary arteries, compared with 29 normocholesterolemic patients either without angiographic evidence for coronary artery disease or with "early" athero-

thrombosis only. Coronary resistance responses to the endothelium-independent vasodilator papaverine were unaffected by hypercholesterolemia. In the patients with hypercholesterolemia, acetylcholine resulted in a 35% decrease in epicardial coronary artery area. Egashira and coworkers (41) reported that coronary flow (intracoronary Doppler flow velocity measurement) responses to intracoronary acetylcholine (range, 1–30 μg/min) in 12 patients with "mild" (<40% stenosis) epicardial coronary atherothrombosis were impaired compared with 16 patients with normal coronary angiograms, with similar responses to the endothelium-independent vasodilator papaverine. The greatest dose of acetylcholine used in this study was associated with a 26% reduction in arterial cross-sectional area in the patients with atherothrombosis. By univariate analysis, hypertension, hypercholesterolemia, age greater than 50 years, and total number of coronary risk factors were associated with the impaired increase in coronary flow in response to acetylcholine.

The constrictor effects of acetylcholine on epicardial arteries and limited dilator effects of this agonist within the microcirculation of patients with early atherothrombosis or its risk factors are consistent with reduced NO bioactivity within the entire extent of the coronary arterial circulation. To prove this possibility, Quyyumi and coworkers (44) infused L-NMMA into coronary arteries of patients with normal coronary angiograms, although most had one or more risk factors for atherothrombosis (Fig. 47–1). Inhibition of NO synthesis caused a 10% to 15% constriction of epicardial arteries and a 15% to 20% reduction in coronary blood flow in patients who had normal-appearing coronary angiograms and no risk factors for atherothrombosis. In contrast, patients with risk factors had less of a constrictor effect on the coronary circulation, consistent with reduced NO bioactivity. Furthermore, coinfusion of L-NMMA with acetylcholine caused greater attenuation of the dilator effects of this agonist in patients without risk factors than those with risk factors, indicating that the effect of acetylcholine on normal arteries, regardless of size, is largely mediated through enhanced NO release (Fig. 47–2).

The authors of these studies concluded that risk factors for atherothrombosis cause microvascular endothelial dysfunction. Although the reduction in epicardial cross-sectional area in response to acetylcholine might have contributed to the limited flow increase in response to acetylcholine in these studies, the results are consistent with the animal studies described earlier in this chapter regarding the impact of hypercholesterolemia on the coronary microcirculation. Furthermore, the results are also consistent with responses to the same agonists in the forearms of patients with hypertension and hypercholesterolemia, a vascular bed generally spared from large-artery atherothrombosis (45–47).

Activities commonly encountered by patients with coronary artery disease may adversely affect the coronary microcirculation. To assess the coronary microvascular response to increased cardiac work and to determine whether NO

artery "without significant obstruction," the 16 patients who experienced a cardiovascular event (cardiovascular death, unstable angina, myocardial infarction, ischemic stroke, coronary or peripheral artery revascularization over a median follow-up period of 7.7 years) had greater constrictor responses to acetylcholine and cold pressor testing and more blunted flow-mediated dilation than the remaining cohort. The epicardial dilator response to nitroglycerin also was more blunted in these 16 patients compared with the remainder, suggesting a more generalized lack of responsiveness to NO. Suwaidi and coworkers (56) found that coronary microvascular endothelial dysfunction in patients with mildly diseased coronary arteries (all lesions <40% luminal narrowing by intravascular ultrasound) has adverse prognostic implications as well. They reported that of the 42 patients whose coronary blood flow actually decreased during intracoronary acetylcholine infusion, 6 (14%) experienced cardiac events (cardiac death, myocardial infarction, congestive heart failure, coronary revascularization), as compared with no events in the remaining 115 patients over a mean follow-up of 28 months. The coronary flow response to adenosine was more limited in the group with reduced blood flow in response to acetylcholine compared with the others. Because vasodilator effect of adenosine on the microcirculation is largely endothelium-independent, dysfunction of microvascular smooth muscle may also be present. More recently, Halcox and coworkers (57) reported the prognostic implications of coronary endothelial testing in 132 patients with coronary artery disease (with testing performed in a "nondiseased" artery) and in 176 patients with "normal" coronary arteries. Over a mean follow-up of 46 months, the 35 patients with acute cardiovascular events (cardiovascular death, acute coronary syndrome, ischemic stroke) had more abnormal coronary microvascular responsiveness to acetylcholine than the remaining study participants (Fig. 47–4). Patients with cardiovascular events tended to have less vasodilation in response to sodium nitroprusside and to adenosine, suggesting coexisting microvascular smooth muscle dysfunction, as noted in other studies. Report of an association between increased levels of C-reactive protein in serum and forearm microvascular dysfunction in patients (all male) with coronary artery disease suggests that endothelial dysfunction may result from chronic inflammation within the arterial circulation (58).

Reversibility of Coronary Microvascular Dysfunction

Several groups have reported that coronary microvascular dysfunction may be reversible with pharmacologic intervention, including statins (59), L-arginine (60–63), estrogen (64,65), α-adrenoceptor blockade (66), angiotensin-converting enzyme (ACE) inhibitor therapy (67), and vitamin C (68). Thus, Egashira and coworkers (59) administered the pravastatin, 10 to 20 mg daily, to patients with hypercholesterolemia with coronary artery disease after percutaneous coronary angioplasty. At the follow-up study approximately 6 months later,

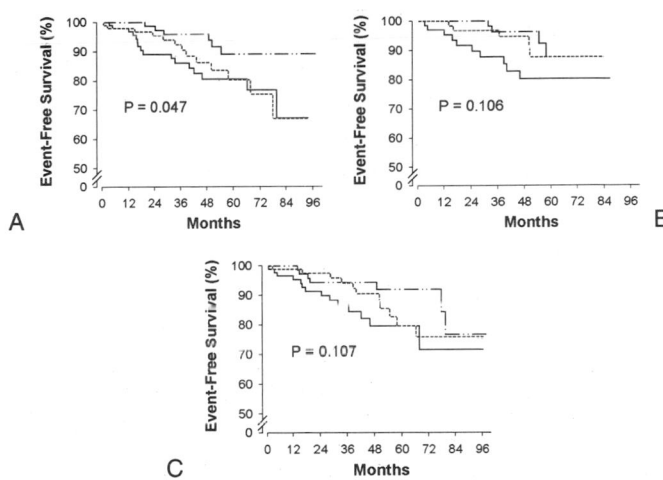

FIG. 47–4. Relation between microvascular coronary vasomotor function and acute cardiovascular events. Kaplan-Meier analyses demonstrate proportion of patients surviving free from events during the follow-up period. Study cohort is divided into tertiles according to the change in coronary vascular resistance with acetylcholine (A), sodium nitroprusside (B), and adenosine (C). Dashed and dotted lines represent tertile with the greatest decrease in coronary vascular resistance (greatest increase in coronary blood flow); dashed lines represent tertile with intermediate response; and solid lines represent tertile with least vasodilation in response to these agonists. (From Halcox JPJ, Schenke WH, Zalos G, et al. Prognostic value of coronary vascular endothelial dysfunction. Circulation 2002;106:653–658, with permission.)

epicardial and microvascular endothelium-dependent vasomotor responses to acetylcholine were improved compared with the pretreatment study. The coronary flow response to the endothelium-independent vasodilator papaverine was unaltered by treatment. Improved coronary microvascular endothelial function with statins may account in part for reduced ambulatory ischemia (69,70) and prolonged survival (71,72) in patients with coronary atherothrombosis. However, whether similar links among improved coronary microvascular endothelial function, reduced ambulatory ischemia, and prolonged survival exist with other therapies is less certain. For example, ACE inhibitors may prolong life in patients at risk for atherothrombosis (73), but do not prevent ambulatory or treadmill exercise ischemia (74). Benefit of estrogen therapy to exercise ischemia has not been reproducible in postmenopausal women (75,76), and hormone replacement therapy did not reduce cardiovascular events in women with coronary artery disease (77), probably because of biologic effects independent of endothelial vasodilator function (e.g., coagulation activation, inflammation) that may increase the risk for coronary thrombosis. Although one group reported that L-arginine improved symptoms in patients with chest pain and coronary microvascular endothelial dysfunction, no objective measures of inducible ischemia were reported (63). Whether L-arginine or vitamin C reduces cardiovascular events is unknown.

Thus, not all therapies that benefit microvascular endothelial function also improve myocardial blood flow sufficient to prevent ischemia. Furthermore, biologic effects other than improved endothelial function may determine whether a therapy reduces cardiovascular events, including mortality.

SUMMARY AND FUTURE RESEARCH DIRECTIONS

The coronary microcirculation, which cannot be assessed angiographically, contributes importantly to coronary flow regulation, largely through synthesis and release of NO. Atherothrombosis of the epicardial coronary arteries may coexist with evidence of microvascular endothelial dysfunction in humans. Common activities such as mental stress, smoking, and exercise may have adverse effects on the coronary microcirculation in patients with coronary artery disease and contribute to myocardial ischemia. Future research directions include proving causality between coronary microvascular dysfunction and inducible myocardial ischemia, especially in patients who have normal-appearing coronary arteries by angiography. Therapies that might improve microvascular endothelial vasomotor responsiveness, such as statins, L-arginine, and vitamin C, should be tested in patients with evidence of microvascular dysfunction, especially those with evidence of ischemia during stress.

REFERENCES

1. Chilian WM, Eastham CL, Marcus ML. Microvascular distribution of coronary vascular resistance in beating left ventricle. Am J Physiol 1986;251:H779–H788.
2. Chilian WM, Layne SM, Klausner EC, et al. Redistribution of coronary microvascular resistance produced by dipyridamole. Am J Physiol 1989;256:H383–H390.
3. Kanatsuka H, Lamping KG, Eastham CL, et al. Heterogeneous changes in epimyocardial microvascular size during graded coronary stenosis. Evidence of the microvascular site for anticoagulation. Circ Res 1990;66:389–396.
4. Kanatsuka H, Lamping KG, Eastham CL, et al. Comparison of the effects of increased myocardial oxygen consumption and adenosine on the coronary microvascular resistance. Circ Res 1989;65:1296–1305.
5. Marcus ML, Chilian WM, Kanatsuka H, et al. Understanding the coronary circulation through studies at the microvascular level. Circulation 1990;82:1–7.
6. Furchgott RF, Zawadzki JV. The obligatory role of endothelial cells in the relaxation of arterial smooth muscle by acetylcholine. Nature 1980;288:373–376.
7. Palmer RM, Ferrige AG, Moncada S. Nitric oxide release accounts for the biological activity of endothelium-derived relaxant factor. Nature 1987;327:524–526.
8. Amezcua JL, Palmer RM, de Souza BM, et al. Nitric oxide synthesized from L-arginine regulates vascular tone in the coronary circulation of the rabbit. Br J Pharmacol 1989;97:1119–1124.
9. Levi R, Gross SS, Lamparter B, et al. Evidence that L-arginine is the biosynthetic precursor of vascular and cardiac nitric oxide. In: Moncada S, Higgs EA, eds. Nitric oxide from L-arginine: a bioregulatory system. Amsterdam: Exerpta Medica, 1990:35–45.
10. Chu A, Chambers DE, Lin CC, et al. Effects of inhibition of nitric oxide formation on basal vasomotion and endothelium-dependent responses of the coronary arteries in awake dogs. J Clin Invest 1991;87:1964–1968.
11. Komaru T, Lamping KG, Eastham CL, et al. Effect of an arginine analogue on acetylcholine-induced coronary microvascular dilatation in dogs. Am J Physiol 1991;261:H2001–H2007.
12. Woodman OL, Dusting GJ. N-Nitro-L-arginine causes coronary vaso-
constriction and inhibits endothelium-dependent vasodilatation in anesthetized greyhounds. Br J Pharmacol 1991;103:1407–1410.
13. Broten TP, Miyashiro JK, Moncada S, et al. Role of endothelium-derived relaxing factor in parasympathetic coronary vasodilation. Am J Physiol 1992;262:H1579–H1584.
14. Habib JR, Bossaler C, Wells G, et al. Preservation of endothelium-dependent vascular relaxation in cholesterol-fed rabbit by treatment with the calcium channel blocker PN 200110. Circ Res 1986;58:305–309.
15. Verbeuren TJ, Jordaens FH, Zonnekeyn LL, et al. Effect of hypercholesterolemia on vascular reactivity in the rabbit: I. Endothelium-dependent and endothelium-independent contractions and relaxations in isolated arteries of control and hypercholesterolemic rabbits. Circ Res 1986;58:552–564.
16. Freiman PC, Mitchell GC, Heistad DD, et al. Atherosclerosis impairs endothelium-dependent vascular relaxation to acetylcholine and thrombin in primates. Circ Res 1986;58:783–789.
17. Osborne JA, Siegman MJ, Sedar AW, et al. Lack of endothelium-dependent relaxation in coronary resistance arteries of cholesterol-fed rabbits. Am J Physiol 1989;256:C591–C597.
18. Selke FW, Armstrong ML, Harrison DG. Endothelium-dependent vascular relaxation is abnormal in the coronary microcirculation of atherosclerotic primates. Circulation 1990;81:1586–1593.
19. Kuo L, Davis MJ, Cannon MS, et al. Pathophysiological consequences of atherosclerosis extend into the coronary microcirculation. Restoration of endothelium-dependent responses by L-arginine. Circ Res 1992;70:465–476.
20. Cohen RA, Zitnay KM, Haudenschild CC, et al. Loss of selective endothelial cell vasoactive functions caused by hypercholesterolemia in pig coronary arteries. Circ Res 1988;63:903–910.
21. Shimokawa H, Flavahan NA, Vanhoutte PM. Loss of endothelial pertussis toxin-sensitive G protein function in atherosclerotic porcine coronary arteries. Circulation 1991;83:652–660.
22. Kugiyama K, Kerns SA, Morrisett JD, et al. Impairment of endothelium-dependent arterial relaxation by lysolecithin in modified low-density lipoproteins. Nature 1990;344:160–162.
23. Flavahan NA. Atherosclerosis or lipoprotein-induced endothelial dysfunction: potential mechanisms underlying reduction in EDRF/nitric oxide activity. Circulation 1992;85:1927–1938.
24. Vallance P, Leone A, Calver A, et al. Accumulation of an endogenous inhibitor of nitric oxide synthase in chronic renal failure. Lancet 1992;339:572–575.
25. Ito A, Tsao PS, Adimoolam S, et al. Novel mechanism for endothelial dysfunction: dysregulation of dimethylarginine dimethylaminohydrolase. Circulation 1999;99:3092–3095.
26. Buga GM, Singh R, Pervin S, et al. Arginase activity in endothelial cells: inhibition by N^G-hydroxy-L-arginine during high-output NO production. Am J Physiol 1996;271:H1988–H1998.
27. Kikuta K, Sawamura T, Miwa T, et al. High-affinity arginine transport of bovine aortic endothelial cells is impaired by lysophosphatidylcholine. Circ Res 1998;83:1088–1096.
28. Minor RL, Myers PR, Guerra R, et al. Diet-induced atherosclerosis increases the release of nitrogen oxides from rabbit aorta. J Clin Invest 1990;86:2109–2116.
29. Vasquez-Vivar J, Kalyanaraman B, Martásek P, et al. Superoxide generation by endothelial nitric oxide synthase: the influence of cofactors. Proc Natl Acad Sci USA 1998;95:9220–9225.
30. Gould KL, Lipscomb K. Effects of coronary stenosis on coronary flow reserve and resistance. Am J Cardiol 1974;34:48–55.
31. White CW, Wright CB, Doty DB, et al. Does visual interpretation of the coronary arteriogram predict the physiologic importance of a coronary stenosis? N Engl J Med 1984;310:819–824.
32. Wilson RF, Laughlin DE, Ackell PH, et al. Transluminal, subselective measurement of coronary artery blood flow velocity and vasodilator reserve in man. Circulation 1985;72:82–92.
33. Doucette JW, Corl PD, Payne HM, et al. Validation of a Doppler guide wire for intravascular measurement of coronary artery flow velocity. Circulation 1992;85:1899–1911.
34. Demer LL, Gould KL, Goldstein RA, et al. Assessment of coronary artery disease severity by positron emission tomography. Comparison with quantitative arteriography in 193 patients. Circulation 1989;79:825–835.
35. Uren NG, Melin JA, De Bruyne B, et al. Relation between myocardial blood flow and the severity of coronary artery stenoses. N Engl J Med 1994;330:1782–1788.
36. Schwitter J, Nanz D, Kneifel S, et al. Assessment of myocardial perfu-

sion in coronary artery disease by magnetic resonance: a comparison with positron emission tomography and coronary angiography. *Circulation* 2001;103:2230–2235.

37. Panting JR, Gatehouse PD, Guang-Zhong Y, et al. Abnormal subendocardial perfusion in cardiac syndrome X detected by cardiovascular magnetic resonance imaging. *N Engl J Med* 2002;346:1948–1953.

38. Ludmer PL, Selwyn AP, Shook TL, et al. Paradoxical vasoconstriction induced by acetylcholine in atherosclerotic coronary arteries. *N Engl J Med* 1986;315:1046–1051.

39. Hodgson JM, Marshall JJ. Direct vasoconstriction and endothelium-dependent vasodilation. Mechanisms of acetylcholine effects on coronary flow and arterial diameter in patients with nonstenotic coronary arteries. *Circulation* 1989;79:1043–1051.

40. Zeiher AM, Drexler H, Wollschlager H, et al. Modulation of coronary vasomotor tone in humans. Progressive endothelial dysfunction with different early stages of coronary atherosclerosis. *Circulation* 1991;83:391–401.

41. Egashira K, Inou T, Hirooka Y, et al. Impaired coronary blood flow response to acetylcholine in patients with coronary risk factors and proximal atherosclerotic lesions. *J Clin Invest* 1993;91:29–37.

42. Werns SW, Walton JA, Hsia HH, et al. Evidence of endothelial dysfunction in angiographically normal coronary arteries of patients with coronary artery disease. *Circulation* 1989;79:287–291.

43. Vita JA, Treasure CB, Nabel EG, et al. Coronary vasomotor response to acetylcholine relates to risk factors for coronary artery disease. *Circulation* 1990;81:491–497.

44. Quyyumi AA, Dakak N, Andrews NP, et al. Nitric oxide in the human coronary circulation. Impact of risk factors for coronary atherosclerosis. *J Clin Invest* 1995;95:1747–1755.

45. Creager MA, Cooke JP, Mendelsohn ME, et al. Impaired vasodilation of forearm resistance vessels in hypercholesterolemic humans. *J Clin Invest* 1990;86:228–234.

46. Casino PR, Kilcoyne CM, Quyyumi AA, et al. The role of nitric oxide in the endothelium-dependent vasodilation of hypercholesterolemic patients. *Circulation* 1993;88:2541–2547.

47. Panza JA, Quyyumi AA, Brush JE Jr, et al. Abnormal endothelium-dependent vascular relaxation in patients with essential hypertension. *N Engl J Med* 1990;323:22–27.

48. Quyyumi AA, Dakak N, Andrews NP, et al. Contribution of nitric oxide to metabolic coronary vasodilation in the human heart. *Circulation* 1995;92:320–326.

49. Yeung AC, Vekshtein VI, Krantz DS, et al. The effect of atherosclerosis on the vasomotor response of coronary arteries to mental stress. *N Engl J Med* 1991;325:1551–1556.

50. Quillen JE, Rossen JD, Oskarsson HJ, et al. Acute effect of cigarette smoking on the coronary circulation: constriction of epicardial and resistance vessels. *J Am Coll Cardiol* 1993;22:642–647.

51. Egashira K, Inou T, Hirooka Y, et al. Evidence of impaired endothelium-dependent coronary vasodilation in patients with angina pectoris and normal coronary angiograms. *N Engl J Med* 1993;328:1659–1664.

52. Zeiher AM, Krause T, Schachinger V, et al. Impaired endothelium-dependent vasodilation of coronary resistance vessels is associated with exercise-induced myocardial ischemia. *Circulation* 1995;91:2345–2352.

53. Hasdai D, Gibbons RJ, Holmes DR Jr, et al. Coronary endothelial dysfunction in humans is associated with myocardial perfusion defects. *Circulation* 1997;96:3390–3395.

54. Buchthal SD, den Hollander JA, Merz CN, et al. Abnormal myocardial phosphorous-31 nuclear magnetic resonance spectroscopy in women with chest pain but normal coronary angiograms. *N Engl J Med* 2000;342:829–835.

55. Schachinger V, Britten MB, Zeiher AM. Prognostic impact of coronary vasodilator dysfunction on adverse long-term outcome of coronary heart disease. *Circulation* 2000;101:1899–1906.

56. Suwaidi JA, Hamasaki S, Higano ST, et al. Long-term follow-up of patients with mild coronary artery disease and endothelial dysfunction. *Circulation* 2000;101:948–954.

57. Halcox JP, Schenke WH, Zalos G, et al. Prognostic value of coronary vascular endothelial dysfunction. *Circulation* 2002;106:653–658.

58. Fichhtlscherer S, Rosenberger G, Walter DH, et al. Elevated C-reactive protein and impaired endothelial vasoreactivity in patients with coronary artery disease. *Circulation* 2000;102:1000–1006.

59. Egashira K, Hirooka Y, Kai H, et al. Reduction in serum cholesterol with pravastatin improves endothelium-dependent vasomotion in patients with hypercholesterolemia. *Circulation* 1994;89:2519–2524.

60. Drexler H, Zeiher AM, Meinzer K, et al. Correction of endothelial dysfunction in coronary microcirculation of hypercholesterolemic patients by L-arginine. *Lancet* 1991;338:1546–1550.

61. Dubois-Rande JL, Zelinsky R, Roudot F, et al. Effects of infusion of L-arginine into the left anterior descending coronary artery on acetylcholine-induced vasoconstriction of human atheromatous coronary arteries. *Am J Cardiol* 1992;70:1269–1275.

62. Quyyumi AA, Dakak N, Gilligan DM, et al. Effect of L-arginine on human coronary endothelium-dependent and physiologic vasodilation. *J Am Coll Cardiol* 1997;30:1220–1227.

63. Lerman A, Burnett JC Jr, Higano ST, et al. Long-term L-arginine supplementation improves small-vessel coronary endothelial function in humans. *Circulation* 1999;97:2123–2128.

64. Reis SE, Gloth ST, Blumenthal RS, et al. Ethinyl estradiol acutely attenuates abnormal coronary vasomotor responses to acetylcholine in postmenopausal women. *Circulation* 1994;89:52–60.

65. Gilligan DM, Quyyumi AA, Cannon RO. Effects of physiological levels of estrogen on coronary vasomotor function in postmenopausal women. *Circulation* 1994;89:2545–2551.

66. Dakak N, Quyyumi AA, Eisenhofer G, et al. Sympathetically-mediated effects of mental stress on the cardiac microcirculation of patients with coronary artery disease. *Am J Cardiol* 1995;76:125–130.

67. Schlaifer JD, Wargovich TJ, O'Neill B, et al. Effects of quinapril on coronary blood flow in coronary artery disease patients with endothelial dysfunction. TREND Investigators. Trial on Reversing Endothelial Dysfunction. *Am J Cardiol* 1997;80:1594–1597.

68. Kaufmann PA, Gnecchi-Ruscone T, di Terlizzi M, et al. Coronary heart disease in smokers: vitamin C restores coronary microcirculatory function. *Circulation* 2000;102:1233–1238.

69. van Boven AJ, Jukema JW, Zwinderman AH, et al. Reduction of transient myocardial ischemia with pravastatin in addition to the conventional treatment in patients with angina pectoris. REGRESS Study Group. *Circulation* 1996;94:1503–1505.

70. Andrews TC, Raby K, Barry J, et al. Effect of cholesterol reduction on myocardial ischemia in patients with coronary disease. *Circulation* 1997;95:324–328.

71. Randomized trial of cholesterol-lowering in 4444 patients with coronary heart disease: the Scandinavian Simvastatin Survival Study (4S). *Lancet* 1994;344:1383–1389.

72. Sacks FM, Pfeffer MA, Moye LA, et al. The effect of pravastatin on coronary events after myocardial infarction in patients with average cholesterol levels. *N Engl J Med* 1996;335:1001–1009.

73. Yusuf S, Sleight P, Pogue J, et al. Effects of an angiotensin-converting-enzyme inhibitor, ramipril, on cardiovascular events in high-risk patients. The Heart Outcomes Prevention Evaluation Study Investigators. *N Engl J Med* 2000;342:145–153.

74. van den Heuvel AF, van Gilst WH, van Veldhuisen DJ, et al. Long-term anti-ischemic effects of angiotensin-converting enzyme inhibition in patients with myocardial infarction. Captopril And Thrombolysis Study (CATS) Investigators. *J Am Coll Cardiol* 1997;30:400–405.

75. Rosano GM, Sarrel PM, Poole-Wilson PA, et al. Beneficial effect of oestrogen on exercise-induced myocardial ischemia in women with coronary artery disease. *Lancet* 1993;342:133–136.

76. Al-Khalili F, Landgren BM, Eksborg S, et al. Does sublingual 17β-estradiol have any effects on exercise capacity and myocardial ischemia in postmenopausal women with stable coronary artery disease? *Eur Heart J* 1998;19:1019–1026.

77. Hulley S, Grady D, Bush T, et al. Randomized trial of estrogen plus progestin for secondary prevention of coronary heart disease in postmenopausal women. Heart and Estrogen/progestin Replacement Study (HERS) Research Group. *JAMA* 1998;280:605–613.

Markers and Evolving Imaging of Atherothrombotic Disease

CHAPTER 48

Inflammatory Markers

Gavin J. Blake, Peter Libby, and Paul M. Ridker

Key Words: C-reactive protein; cell adhesion; cytokines; proatherogenic enzymes; risk prediction.

INTRODUCTION

The past decade has seen a dramatic shift in the understanding of atherogenesis. Previously thought of as a disease of bland lipid accumulation, advances in basic science have illuminated the pivotal role of inflammatory processes in the pathogenesis of atherothrombosis and its complications (1,2). The biology of the atherothrombotic plaque, rather than the degree of luminal stenosis, is now recognized as a pivotal feature in determining plaque stability. Inflammatory processes play a central role in mediating all phases of atherothrombosis, from initial recruitment of circulating leukocytes to the vascular endothelium, to eventual rupture of the unstable plaque. Attempts to translate the evolving understanding of atherothrombosis into clinical practice have

focused attention on whether plasma levels of markers of inflammation can predict those individuals who are at high risk for plaque rupture.

CENTRAL ROLE OF INFLAMMATION IN ATHEROGENESIS

Compelling laboratory evidence has emerged that inflammatory processes mediate the initiation and evolution of the atherothrombotic lesion, as well as contributing decisively to the ultimate development of acute ischemic syndromes (3). The normal vascular endothelium does not in general support the binding of leukocytes. However, shortly after the initiation of an atherogenic diet, the endothelium begins to express adhesion molecules that selectively bind to circulating leukocytes. These cell adhesion molecules (CAMs) include the selectins and members of the immunoglobulin superfamily, intercellular adhesion molecule-1 (ICAM-1) and vascular cell adhesion molecule-1 (VCAM-1). P- and E-selectin mediate a transient rolling interaction with the endothelium, whereas ICAM-1 and VCAM-1 mediate stronger attachment (4). Proinflammatory cytokines such as monocyte chemoattractant protein-1 (MCP-1) expressed within atheroma provide a chemotactic stimulus to adherent monocytes, directing their migration into the intima (5,6). Here the leukocytes contribute to the local inflammatory response, with macrophages expressing receptors for modified lipoproteins, and macrophage colony-stimulating factor combining with MCP-1, among other factors, to augment the differentiation of monocytes into macrophage foam cells (7,8).

G. J. Blake: Department of Cardiology, Mater Misericordiae University Hospital, Eccles Street, Dublin 7, Ireland.

P. Libby: Cardiovascular Division, Brigham and Women's Hospital, Donald W. Reynolds Clinical Research Center, Department of Medicine, Brigham and Woman's Hospital and Harvard Medical School, 77 Avenue Louis Pasteur, NRB 741, Boston, Massachusetts 02115.

P. M Ridker: Center for Cardiovascular Disease Prevention, Brigham and Women's Hospital, Donald W. Reynolds Clinical Research Center, Department of Medicine, Brigham and Woman's Hospital and Harvard Medical School, 900 Commonwealth Avenue East, Boston, Massachusetts 02155.

T-cell activation further amplifies the inflammatory response by expression of interferon-γ and lymphotoxin. Macrophages, T cells, and smooth muscle cells produce the pluripotent cytokine tumor necrosis factor-α (TNF-α), which like interferon-γ and interleukin-1 (IL-1) stimulates IL-6 expression. As this inflammatory process evolves, the activated leukocytes and arterial cells can release a variety of peptide growth factors that can promote replication of the smooth muscle cells and contribute to production by these cells of a dense extracellular matrix characteristic of the advanced atherothrombotic lesion (2).

As the atherothrombotic lesion matures, accumulation of foam cells typically leads to the formation of a lipid pool rich in prothrombotic tissue factor (4). Smooth muscle cells produce collagen that contributes to the tensile strength of the fibrous cap, shielding the circulating blood from the prothrombotic lipid pool. Platelet-derived growth factor and transforming growth factor-β increase the rate of collagen production. Conversely, interferon-γ arrests collagen synthesis by smooth muscle cells, whereas activated macrophages abundant in atheroma can produce proteolytic enzymes capable of degrading the collagen in the fibrous cap, rendering the cap thin and prone to rupture (1). Thus, a dynamic balance prevails between collagen synthesis and breakdown.

Given the pivotal role of inflammatory processes in mediating the initiation, development, and eventual complications of atherothrombosis, attention has focused on whether plasma levels of markers of inflammation can predict cardiovascular risk. The remainder of this chapter focuses on this issue.

POTENTIAL USE OF INFLAMMATORY MARKERS FOR CARDIOVASCULAR RISK PREDICTION

Cholesterol screening is the single blood test routinely performed for cardiovascular risk assessment. However, less than half of all individuals with myocardial infarction (MI) have overt hyperlipidemia. Thus, improved methods of risk prediction, which could add to the predictive value of established cholesterol screening, are urgently required. In light of the central role of inflammatory processes in atherogenesis, attention has focused on whether a variety of plasma markers of inflammation can help to predict individuals who are at high risk for plaque rupture (9). Candidate markers include CAMs, primary cytokines such as TNF-α, messenger cytokines such as IL-6 and IL-18, proatherogenic enzymes such as lipoprotein-associated phospholipase A_2 (LpPLA$_2$), and downstream markers of the inflammatory response such as the acute-phase reactant C-reactive protein (CRP).

Cell Adhesion Molecules

In view of their role in the initial recruitment of leukocytes to the diseased endothelium, CAMs are promising candidate markers of underlying vascular inflammation. After cellular activation by cytokines, endothelial cells and leukocytes shed CAMs into plasma permitting measurement of levels of circulating CAMs. In this regard, plasma levels of soluble P-selectin have been shown to be an independent predictor of future cardiovascular risk in a large-scale prospective study of apparently healthy women enrolled in the Women's Health Study (10). The risk for future cardiovascular events among women in the highest quartile of P-selectin was 2.2 times greater than those in the lowest quartile, an effect that was independent of traditional risk factors.

The Physicians' Health Study reported similar data regarding the predictive value of ICAM-1 for future MI among apparently healthy men, with a relative risk of 1.8 for those in the highest quartile of ICAM-1 compared with those in the lowest quartile (11). The Atherosclerosis Risk In Communities (ARIC) study also found that baseline levels of ICAM-1 independently predicted future risk in a generally healthy population (12). However, in neither the Physicians' Health Study nor the ARIC study did plasma levels of VCAM-1 predict future risk among healthy individuals (12,13). Similarly, ICAM-1 but not VCAM-1 predicts incident peripheral vascular disease (14). In contrast, in a population with previously documented coronary disease, baseline plasma levels of both VCAM-1 and ICAM-1 were increased among those who died because of cardiovascular causes (15). Indeed, in this cohort with established atherothrombosis, VCAM-1 was the stronger predictor of risk, suggesting that there may be important differences between the biologic roles of different CAMs at various stages of atherogenesis. ICAM-1 is expressed by many types of cells, and thus may be a less specific marker than VCAM-1, which is mainly expressed in atherothrombotic plaques by activated endothelial cells and smooth muscle cells. Thus, the predictive value of VCAM-1 may be most marked among those patients with established atherothrombosis at the time of measurement.

Data regarding the prognostic value of CAMs have been reported from the British Regional Heart Study (16). Although levels of ICAM-1, VCAM-1, and P-selectin were increased among those individuals who subsequently developed coronary disease, the predictive value of these parameters was attenuated and was not significant in adjusted analyses. Little is known about the mechanism of CAM release from the vascular endothelium, and thus measurement of CAM levels on a single peripheral blood sample may not accurately reflect their biologic importance at the vascular endothelium (17).

Inflammatory Cytokines

IL-1, IL-6, and TNF-α play an important role in the genesis and amplification of the inflammatory cascade. Evidence in support of the role of inflammatory processes in acute coronary syndromes comes from data showing that increased levels of IL-1 receptor antagonist and IL-6 at 48 hours after presentation with acute coronary syndromes are associated with an adverse in-hospital prognosis, even among patients without an increase in troponin (18). Further work from the Physicians' Health Study has found that increasing levels of IL-6 also predict future cardiovascular events, with those patients in the top quartile of IL-6 having a 2.3-fold increased risk compared with those in the lowest quartile (19). Furthermore, increases of TNF-α in the stable phase after MI were associated with an increased risk for recurrent coronary events (20). The plasma half-life of TNF-α, however, is short, a factor that may limit its potential clinical use.

Other, more recently recognized inflammatory cytokines may also predict cardiovascular risk. First identified as an interferon γ inducing factor in 1995, IL-18 plays a pivotal role in the processes of innate and acquired immunity because of its ability to induce interferon-γ production in T lymphocytes and natural killer cells (21). Cells in human atheroma express IL-18, and this cytokine exerts proinflammatory effects on vascular cells and leukocytes. Clinical data show that IL-18 levels were a strong independent predictor of death from cardiovascular causes among 1,229 patients with documented coronary artery disease (CAD) (22).

Macrophage inhibitory cytokine-1 (MIC-1) is part of the transforming growth factor-β superfamily and was first cloned in 1997 (23). Although not expressed in resting macrophages, stimulation of macrophages by several inflammatory mediators such as TNF-α, IL-1, and macrophage colony-stimulating factor induce its expression. Recent data suggest that MIC-1 concentrations were greater at baseline among apparently healthy women who subsequently experienced development of cardiovascular events than among those who did not (24). The predictive value of MIC-1 did not depend on traditional cardiovascular risk factors and was at least additive to CRP. These data suggest that MIC-1 and CRP may represent different aspects of the inflammatory response, and that perhaps each is active at different times in plaque evolution. Further data are required to more clearly delineate the potential predictive value of these more recently recognized inflammatory cytokines.

Proatherogenic Enzymes

LpPLA$_2$ circulates in association with low-density lipoprotein (LDL) cholesterol and may contribute to atherogenesis by hydrolyzing oxidized phospholipids into proatherogenic fragments and by generating lysolecithin, which has proinflammatory activity. The West of Scotland study group reported that baseline levels of LpPLA$_2$ were an independent predictor of risk for incident cardiovascular events among a cohort of hyperlipidemic men (25). In another study among women at lower risk, baseline levels of LpPLA$_2$ also were increased among women who subsequently experienced development of cardiovascular events compared with those who did not (26). However, in this cohort, LpPLA$_2$ levels correlated highly with LDL cholesterol levels; thus, in adjusted analyses, the predictive value of LpPLA$_2$ was markedly attenuated and not significant. In contrast, CRP remained a significant predictor in adjusted analyses in this cohort.

Myeloperoxidase (MPO) levels may also be increased among individuals with CAD. MPO is an enzyme secreted by a variety of inflammatory cells including neutrophils, a subpopulation of blood monocytes, and tissue macrophages such as those found in atherothrombotic plaque. The enzyme is not released until leukocyte activation and degranulation. MPO may contribute to endothelial dysfunction by acting as a nitric oxide (NO) sink and may convert LDL into a high-uptake form leading to foam cell formation. Case–control data suggest that increasing levels of leukocyte-MPO and blood-MPO significantly predict risk for CAD such that after adjustment for Framingham score and white cell count (WCC), those in the top quartile of blood-MPO had a 20-fold greater risk for CAD than those in the lowest quartile (27). Prospective data are needed to directly test the hypothesis that levels of MPO may portend cardiovascular risk.

Pregnancy-associated plasma protein A (PAPP-A) is a zinc-binding metalloproteinase that is a specific activator of insulin-like growth factor, a mediator of atherothrombosis. Among eight patients who died suddenly of cardiac causes, PAPP-A was abundantly expressed in ruptured and eroded unstable plaques, but was absent or minimally expressed in stable plaques (28). In plaques with large lipid cores and cap rupture, staining for PAPP-A revealed that PAPP-A occurred mostly in the inflamed shoulder region. In a small case–control study, circulating levels of PAPP-A also were greater among patients with unstable angina or acute MI than among those with stable angina (28). As with MPO, these data require assessment in larger, prospective cohorts.

C-REACTIVE PROTEIN: MARKER OR MEDIATOR?

With regard to cardiovascular risk prediction, CRP has been the most extensively studied of all markers of inflammation. Produced mainly by the liver in response to IL-6, CRP has been thought of as a downstream marker of the inflammatory cascade. Emerging data, however, suggest that CRP may play a more direct role in atherogenesis. CRP localizes with the complement membrane attack complex in early atherothrombotic tissue (29), and levels of mRNA encoding both CRP and certain complement factors increase in atherothrombotic plaque (30). Smooth muscle cells and macrophages appear to be the main producers, illustrating that CRP can be produced by extrahepatic mechanisms.

CRP opsonization of LDL mediates LDL uptake by macrophages (31), and CRP stimulates monocyte release of other proinflammatory cytokines such as IL-1, IL-6, and TNF-α (32). Furthermore, high concentrations of CRP cause ICAM-1 and VCAM-1 expression by endothelial cells and also mediate MCP-1 induction, an effect that is inhibited by fenofibrate (33,34). In addition, CRP has the ability to sensitize endothelial cells to destruction by cytotoxic CD4$^+$ T cells (35).

Recent data provide further evidence that CRP may play a part in directly mediating atherogenesis. Verma and colleagues (36) have illustrated that increased secretion of endothelin-1 (ET-1) and IL-6 may mediate the proatherothrombotic effects of CRP (36). Incubation of human saphenous vein endothelial cells with recombinant CRP resulted in a marked increase in ICAM-1 and VCAM-1 expression and MCP-1 production. These effects were mediated in part through increased secretion of IL-6 and ET-1 and were attenuated by both IL-6 antagonism and the endothelin antagonist bosentan. ET-1 is one of the most potent endogenous vasoconstrictors and mediates a host of proatherogenic responses including endothelial dysfunction, vasomotor contraction, leukocyte and platelet activation, and cellular proliferation (37). In addition, it augments the action of other vasoactive agents such as angiotensin II, norepinephrine, and serotonin. As discussed earlier, IL-6 is a pivotal messenger cytokine in the inflammatory cascade and is the main stimulus for the hepatic production of CRP. Thus, a positive feedback system may exist whereby CRP stimulates its own local synthesis through IL-6–dependent mechanisms.

Further work from this group has shown that CRP, at concentrations known to predict increased cardiovascular risk, directly quenches the production of NO by endothelial cells, at least in part through the posttranscriptional effect of endothelial NO synthase on mRNA stability (38). This effect also has been demonstrated by Venugopal and colleagues (39). Diminished NO bioactivity, in turn, can inhibit angiogenesis under some conditions, an important compensatory mechanism in chronic ischemia. NO derived from endothelial NO synthase is the key endothelium-derived relaxing factor that maintains vascular tone and reactivity. NO opposes the actions of potent vasoconstrictors such as angiotensin II and ET-1, and thus promotes arterial vasodilatation. In addi-

tion, NO inhibits smooth muscle cell proliferation, LDL oxidation, platelet adhesion and aggregation, and monocyte adhesion (40,41). Thus, through decrease of NO synthesis and augmentation of the vasoconstrictor ET-1 and the proatherogenic cytokine IL-6, CRP appears to mediate several processes crucial to the development and progression of vascular dysfunction and atherothrombosis.

C-REACTIVE PROTEIN AND CARDIOVASCULAR RISK PREDICTION

There is now robust evidence from numerous large-scale prospective studies among men and women that CRP predicts a variety of cardiovascular outcomes in numerous clinical settings. In the primary prevention setting, CRP has emerged as a strong independent determinant of future MI, stroke, cardiovascular death, need for coronary revascularization, development of peripheral vascular disease, and sudden cardiac death (Fig. 48–1) (42–53). In these studies, those subjects with CRP levels in the top quartile have had a twofold to fourfold increased risk compared with the lowest quartile. Furthermore, CRP predicts risk among patients with stable and unstable angina (54–61), in the chronic phase after MI (62), and among patients undergoing revascularization procedures (63–67). Importantly, among those patients presenting with acute coronary syndromes, the predictive value of CRP is independent of, and additive to, that of established markers of myocyte necrosis, such as troponin.

An analysis from the Women's Health Study sought to compare the predictive value of CRP with other markers of inflammation and traditional lipid predictors among appar-

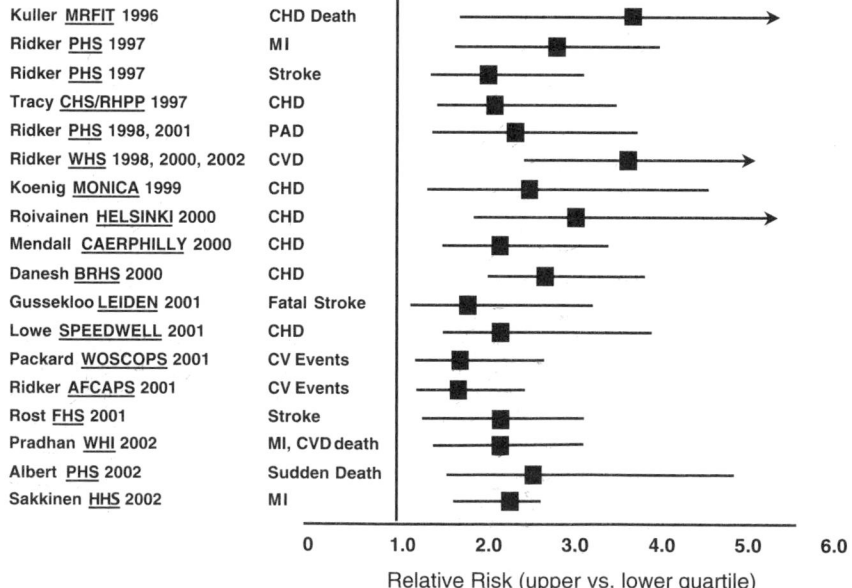

FIG. 48–1. Prospective studies of C-reactive protein and future cardiovascular events among healthy individuals. Risk estimates and 95% confidence intervals are calculated by comparison of the top versus the bottom quartile within each study group. CHD, coronary heart disease; CV, cardiovascular; CVD, cardiovascular disease; MI, myocardial infarction; PAD, peripheral arterial disease, (Reprinted from Ridker PM. Clinical application of C-reactive protein for cardiovascular disease detection and prevention. *Circulation* 2003;107:363–369, with permission.)

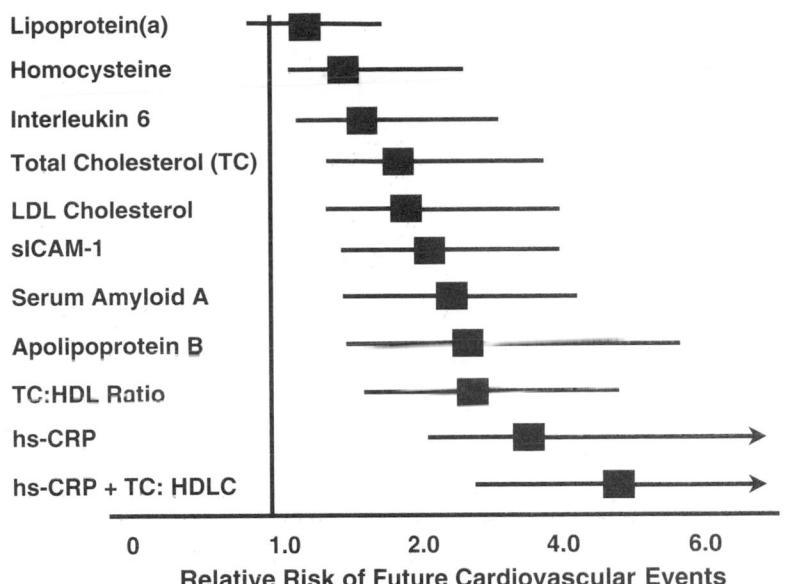

FIG. 48–2. Adjusted relative risks of future cardiovascular events for the highest compared with the lowest quartile of each risk marker among apparently healthy women. CRP, C-reactive protein; HDL, high-density lipoprotein; HDLC, high-density lipoprotein cholesterol; ICAM, intercellular adhesion molecule; LDL, low-density lipoprotein. (Adapted from Ridker PM, Hennekens CH, Buring JE, et al. C-reactive protein and other markers of inflammation in the prediction of cardiovascular disease in women. *N Engl J Med* 2000;342:836–843, with permission.)

ently healthy women (Fig. 48–2) (47). Baseline levels of CRP, serum amyloid A (SAA), IL-6, and ICAM-1 were each significantly increased at baseline among women who subsequently experienced development of cardiovascular events compared with those who did not. In multivariable analyses, matched for age and smoking and adjusted for other traditional risk factors, only CRP and the total cholesterol:HDL cholesterol ratio were independent predictors of risk. Interestingly, the combination of any inflammatory marker with lipid testing significantly improved on risk prediction on the basis of lipid testing alone. This type of observation suggests that inflammatory stimuli beyond the classically measured lipid levels can contribute to cardiovascular risk. Furthermore, even among those with LDL cholesterol less than 130 mg/dL, who are not targeted for preventive measures in the current guidelines, women with increased levels of a marker of inflammation had increased risk for future events, an effect that was most marked for CRP.

Although the results of this and other studies have been remarkably consistent, limitations inherent to the nested case–control design have made it difficult to directly assess the relative merit of CRP. In particular, population-based cutoff points and prospective cohort data directly comparing the predictive value of CRP to LDL cholesterol have been lacking, and nested case–control studies cannot provide data regarding population attributable risk. To address these deficiencies, CRP and LDL cholesterol were measured in all 27,939 participants of the Women's Health Study who provided baseline blood samples and had been followed for incident cardiovascular events over a mean period of 8 years (68). The distribution of CRP levels was found to be very

similar to those reported in previous U.S. and European studies with a median value of 1.52 mg/dL. After adjustment for age, smoking, diabetes, blood pressure, and use of hormone replacement therapy, the multivariable relative risks of incident cardiovascular events for increasing quintiles of CRP were 1.0, 1.4, 1.6, 2.0, and 2.3 ($p < 0.001$), whereas the comparable risk associated with increasing quintiles of LDL cholesterol were 1.0, 0.9, 1.1, 1.3, and 1.5 ($p < 0.001$). In crude models evaluating the total cohort, the calculated area under the receiver operating curve (ROC) was 0.64 for CRP and 0.60 for LDL cholesterol. In models including other risk factors, the ability of the CRP model to discriminate events from nonevents was virtually identical to that of the LDL cholesterol model (area under ROC for both = 0.81). However, CRP and LDL cholesterol were minimally correlated ($r = 0.08$), suggesting again that each marker was detecting different high-risk groups.

Notably, 77% of all events occurred among those patients with LDL cholesterol less than 160 mg/dL, and 46% occurred among those with LDL cholesterol less than 130 mg/dL. After the total cohort was divided into four groups on the basis of median CRP and median LDL cholesterol levels, the adjusted relative risks for the low CRP/low LDL, low CRP/high LDL, high CRP/low LDL, and high CRP/high LDL groups were 1.0, 1.5, 1.5, and 2.1 with corresponding age-adjusted event rates of 1.3, 2.0, 2.6, and 3.0 per 1,000 person-years of follow-up, respectively (Fig. 48–3). Furthermore, at all levels of estimated Framingham 10-year risk and at all levels of LDL cholesterol, CRP remained predictive of future cardiovascular risk (Fig. 48–4) (68).

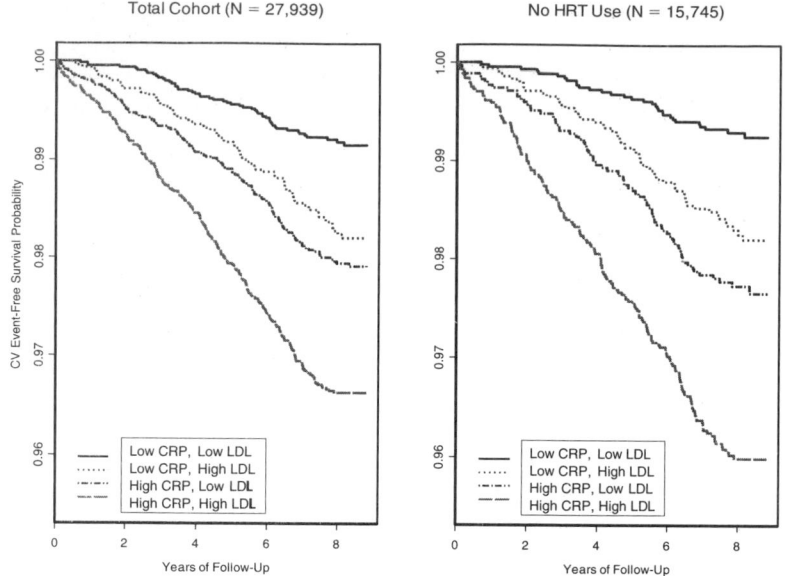

FIG. 48–3. Cardiovascular (CV) event–free survival curves with C-reactive protein (CRP) levels greater than or less than 1.52 mg/L and low-density lipoprotein (LDL) cholesterol levels greater than or less than 123.8 mg/dL, the respective study medians for each biomarker among nonhormone replacement therapy using women who participated in the Women's Health Study. HRT, hormone replacement therapy. (Reprinted from Ridker PM, Rifai N, Rose L, et al. Comparison of C-reactive protein and LDL cholesterol levels in the prediction of first cardiovascular events. *N Engl J Med* 2002;347:1557–1565, with permission.)

These data have important implications for the detection and prevention of cardiovascular disease. Women in the high CRP/low LDL subgroup were at greater absolute risk than those in the high LDL/low CRP subgroup, yet only the latter group is likely to receive aggressive prevention under current guidelines. These observations suggest that a continued reliance solely on LDL cholesterol does not optimally target preventive strategies, and that combining a test for CRP with established lipid screening should improve identification of those individuals at increased risk for cardiovascular disease.

RELATION OF C-REACTIVE PROTEIN TO OTHER CARDIOVASCULAR RISK FACTORS

Obesity is associated with increased CRP levels (69). This observation is in keeping with adipose tissue being an abundant source of cytokines such as TNF-α and of IL-6, which,

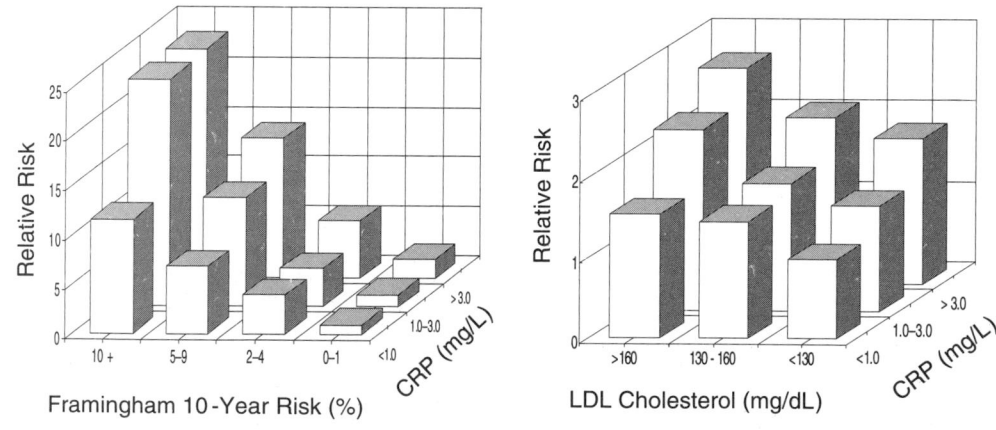

FIG. 48–4. Adjusted relative risks of cardiovascular disease according to levels of C-reactive protein (CRP) and the estimated 10-year risk based on the Framingham risk score as currently defined by the National Cholesterol Education Program and according to levels of C-reactive protein and categories of low-density lipoprotein (LDL) cholesterol. (Adapted from Ridker PM, Rifai N, Rose L, et al. Comparison of C-reactive protein and LDL cholesterol levels in the prediction of first cardiovascular events. *N Engl J Med* 2002;347:1557–1565, with permission.)

in turn, is a proximate stimulus for hepatic production of CRP (70). In a study of obese women, CRP independently predicted urinary 8-iso prostaglandin $F_2\alpha$ (a marker of *in vivo* lipid peroxidation) and 11-dehydrothromboxane B_2 (a marker of *in vivo* platelet activation) excretion (71). Furthermore, among women with android obesity (waist-to-hip ratio $\geq$ 0.86), successful weight loss was associated with a significant reduction in CRP, urinary 8-iso prostaglandin $F_2\alpha$, and 11-dehydrothromboxane B_2.

Data also suggest that CRP levels associate inversely with the degree of physical activity (72). Diabetics, smokers, and those with hypertension also have increased CRP levels (73,74). Thus, intensification of standard preventive measures such as weight loss, exercise, smoking cessation, dietary modification, and blood pressure control would seem particularly prudent among those individuals with increased CRP levels.

Recent data also indicate that baseline levels of CRP and IL-6 may also predict the future onset on type II diabetes among apparently healthy women (75). After adjustment for body mass index and other risk factors, women with CRP levels in the highest quartile had a greater than fourfold increased risk for development of type II diabetes. This observation, together with basic research showing an important role for inflammation in the pathogenesis of diabetes, suggests that the causes of type II diabetes and cardiovascular disease may share a common inflammatory basis (76).

Given the evolving epidemic of the metabolic syndrome in western societies, the proportion of cardiovascular events attributable to this condition is likely to increase dramatically. In this regard, each of the attributes of the metabolic syndrome is associated with increased levels of CRP. For example, among 14,719 apparently healthy women not taking hormone replacement therapy, baseline levels of CRP increased in a stepwise fashion for those with 0, 1, 2, 3, 4, or 5 characteristics of the metabolic syndrome (77). Over 8 years of follow-up, cardiovascular event–free survival was similar based on those subjects with CRP greater than or less than 3 mg/L or based on those subjects with three or more characteristics of the metabolic syndrome (Fig. 48–5). However, in analyses restricted to those 3,597 women defined by Adult Treatment Panel III (ATP III) as having the metabolic syndrome, baseline CRP levels differentiated between individuals at low and high risk, with age-adjusted incident rates of cardiovascular disease of 3.4 among those with baseline CRP less than 3.0 mg/L and 5.9 per 1,000 person-years among those with baseline CRP greater than 3.0 mg/L. These data suggest that CRP adds clinically important information to the ATP III definition of the metabolic syndrome.

Targeted Therapies for Patients with High C-Reactive Protein

Although there is currently robust evidence that CRP predicts future cardiovascular risk, emerging data also suggest the use of CRP to target established preventive measures to those individuals at greatest risk. For instance, the benefits

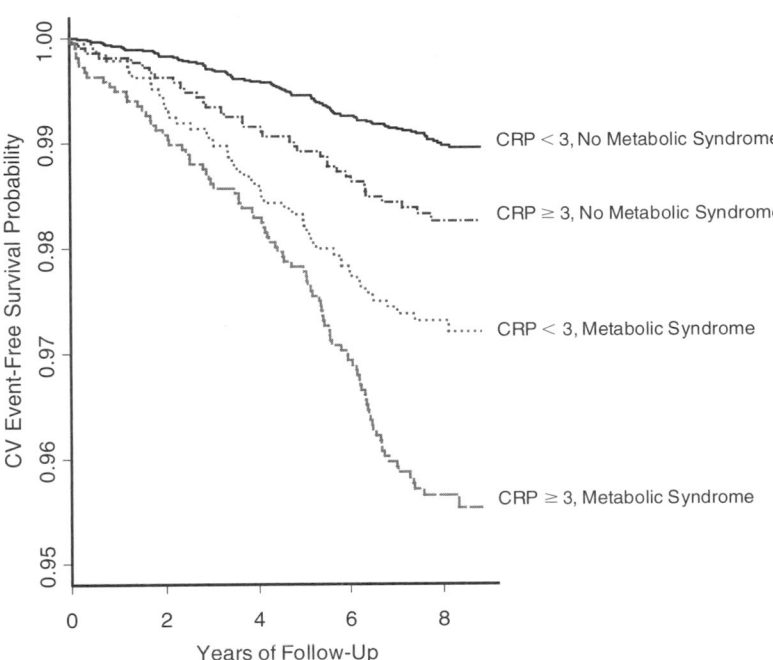

FIG. 48–5. Cardiovascular (CV) event–free survival according to the presence or absence of the metabolic syndrome and according to C-reactive proteins (CRP) levels greater or less than 3 mg/L. (Reprinted from Ridker PM, Buring JE, Cook NR, et al. C-reactive protein, the metabolic syndrome, and risk of incident cardiovascular events: an 8-year follow-up of 14,719 initially healthy American women. *Circulation* 2003;107:391–397, with permission.)

of aspirin may be greatest among those with the greatest CRP levels. In a large randomized trial of aspirin for the primary prevention of cardiovascular disease among men, the magnitude of benefit of aspirin for the prevention of MI was directly related to baseline CRP levels, specifically the risk reduction for aspirin of 56% among those in the highest quartile of CRP, whereas the risk reduction was small (14%; $p = 0.8$) and nonsignificant among those with the lowest quartile of CRP (44). These data suggest that aspirin prevents ischemic events through antiinflammatory and antiplatelet effects. Similarly, in a study of patients presenting with acute coronary syndromes, CRP strongly predicted future risk among those patients who did not receive pretreatment with aspirin, but not among those who did receive pretreatment with aspirin (78). The direct effect of aspirin on CRP levels remains controversial (79,80).

In observational data, the benefits of clopidogrel among patients undergoing percutaneous coronary intervention (PCI) also may be greatest among those with increased CRP levels (81), although no randomized trials are available to test this hypothesis. Intriguingly, clopidogrel decreases expression of P-selectin (82) and in one study also decreased the adenosine diphosphate–induced expression of CD40 ligand, a pivotal proinflammatory mediator of activated platelets. The antiplatelet and antiinflammatory actions of clopidogrel are thus likely to be closely linked, with platelet inhibition disrupting inflammatory pathways, and antiinflammatory effects reducing platelet activation (83). Interestingly, increased plasma levels of CD40 ligand also appear to confer increased cardiovascular risk, and recent data suggest that patients with evidence of lipid pool in carotid atheroma on magnetic resonance imaging also have increased CD40 ligand levels (84,85).

With regard to the preceding discussion of CRP and the metabolic syndrome, recent data also suggest that rosiglitazone directly reduces CRP levels (86). This is an intriguing observation given that this peroxisome proliferator-activated receptor-γ inhibitor is already established as standard care for those with type II diabetes.

Evidence from laboratory studies indicates that statins have potent antiinflammatory effects (87–89). In this regard, several studies have shown that statin therapy decreases CRP levels (90–94). This action appears to be a class effect and to be independent of any lipid-decreasing effect of statins. The first clinical trial evidence that the antiinflammatory actions of statins may be of practical importance came from the Cholesterol and Recurrent Events (CARE) study, a randomized trial of pravastatin versus placebo for the secondary prevention of cardiovascular events. Post-MI patients with a persistent inflammatory response as evidenced by an increased level of CRP or SAA were at increased risk for recurrent events (62). Furthermore, the proportion of recurrent events prevented by pravastatin was 54% among those with evidence of persistent inflammation and 25% among those without. More recent reports of the nonrandomized use of statins among patients undergoing stent implantation also have shown a similar pattern with the greatest benefit of statin therapy seen among those with the greatest CRP levels (95).

An analysis from the Air Force/Texas Coronary Atherosclerosis Prevention Study (AFCAPS/TexCAPS) study, a randomized trial of lovastatin versus placebo for the primary prevention of cardiovascular events, sought to test the hypothesis that the benefits of statin therapy are greatest among those with increased CRP levels in the primary prevention setting (94). Individuals were divided into four groups according to median CRP (1.6 mg/L) and median LDL-cholesterol levels (149 mg/dL). Individuals with LDL cholesterol greater than 149 mg/dL were at high risk and benefited substantially from randomization to lovastatin, irrespective of CRP levels. Those individuals with low LDL cholesterol and low CRP levels were at low risk and showed no benefit with lovastatin therapy compared with placebo. In contrast, those with low LDL cholesterol but high CRP had markedly increased risk, and the benefits of lovastatin therapy were similar to that seen among those with increased LDL cholesterol levels. These data, although hypothesis-generating, suggest that CRP testing could serve as a method to target statin therapy among individuals without overtly increased LDL cholesterol levels, who nonetheless have increased risk for future cardiovascular events. Exploratory analyses suggest that the potential gains from such a strategy could be substantial and could apply to many millions of adults in the United States who do not currently meet National Cholesterol Education Program guidelines for statin therapy (96).

REMAINING QUESTIONS AND FUTURE DIRECTIONS

On the basis of the combined data outlined earlier, the Centers for Disease Control is drawing up recommendations regarding the use of CRP for primary cardiovascular risk assessment (97). The cutoff points for CRP of less than 1, 1 to 3, and greater than 3 mg/L will be used to denote low, intermediate, and high risk, respectively. With regard to targeted preventive therapies, there is currently an urgent need for randomized trials designed to test directly the hypothesis that the benefits of statins are increased among those individuals with high CRP levels (98).

Further research also is needed to clarify other issues. The precise trigger to increased CRP levels among patients presenting with acute coronary syndromes remains unknown. Data suggest that focal plaque rupture may not be the cause, but rather that increased CRP levels may be a marker of hyperresponsiveness of the inflammatory system to even minor stimuli. For example, CRP levels do not change after balloon angioplasty in patients with stable or unstable coronary disease who have normal preprocedural levels, but they do increase after angioplasty in unstable patients with increased CRP preprocedural levels (99). Moreover, even diagnostic angiography without intervention caused an increase in CRP levels among patients with increased levels at baseline.

The optimal cutoff points for defining increased risk among those patients presenting with acute coronary syndromes also remain unclear. Moreover, no data are currently available to indicate if monitoring serial CRP levels is useful to detect a reduction in cardiovascular risk. Further trials are required to resolve these questions.

In conclusion, advances in basic research have illuminated the role of inflammation in atherothrombosis (3). The translation of these advances into clinical studies has identified several plasma markers of inflammation as predictors of future cardiovascular events. There is now compelling evidence that CRP strongly predicts cardiovascular risk, independently of, but additively with, lipid values. However, no evidence to date establishes that decreasing CRP levels reduces cardiovascular risk. Harnessing the basic and clinical biology of inflammation in atherothrombosis discussed here should refine our predictive ability, aid rational and cost-effective deployment of preventive strategies, and also promote the development and evaluation of novel therapies to reduce the overall impact of atherothrombosis and its complications.

REFERENCES

1. Libby P. Current concepts of the pathogenesis of the acute coronary syndromes. *Circulation* 2001;104:365–372.
2. Ross R. Atherosclerosis—an inflammatory disease. *N Engl J Med* 1999;340:115–126.
3. Libby P. Inflammation in atherosclerosis. *Nature* 2002;420:868–874.
4. Libby P, Ridker PM, Maseri A. Inflammation and atherosclerosis. *Circulation* 2002;105:1135–1143.
5. Boring L, Gosling J, Cleary M, et al. Decreased lesion formation in CCR2-/- mice reveals a role for chemokines in the initiation of atherosclerosis. *Nature* 1998;394:894–897.
6. Gu L, Okada Y, Clinton SK, et al. Absence of monocyte chemoattractant protein-1 reduces atherosclerosis in low density lipoprotein receptor-deficient mice. *Mol Cell* 1998;2:275–281.
7. Smith JD, Trogan E, Ginsberg M, et al. Decreased atherosclerosis in mice deficient in both macrophage colony-stimulating factor (op) and apolipoprotein E. *Proc Natl Acad Sci USA* 1995;92:8264–8268.
8. Qiao JH, Tripathi J, Mishra NK, et al. Role of macrophage colony-stimulating factor in atherosclerosis: studies of osteopetrotic mice. *Am J Pathol* 1997;150:1687–1699.
9. Blake GJ, Ridker PM. Novel clinical markers of vascular wall inflammation. *Circ Res* 2001;89:763–771.
10. Ridker PM, Buring JE, Rifai N. Soluble P-selectin and the risk of future cardiovascular events. *Circulation* 2001;103:491–495.
11. Ridker PM, Hennekens CH, Roitman-Johnson B, et al. Plasma concentration of soluble intercellular adhesion molecule 1 and risks of future myocardial infarction in apparently healthy men. *Lancet* 1998;351:88–92.
12. Hwang SJ, Ballantyne CM, Sharrett AR, et al. Circulating adhesion molecules VCAM-1, ICAM-1, and E-selectin in carotid atherosclerosis and incident coronary heart disease cases: the Atherosclerosis Risk In Communities (ARIC) study. *Circulation* 1997;96:4219–4225.
13. de Lemos JA, Hennekens CH, Ridker PM. Plasma concentration of soluble vascular cell adhesion molecule-1 and subsequent cardiovascular risk. *J Am Coll Cardiol* 2000;36:423–426.
14. Pradhan AD, Rifai N, Ridker PM. Soluble intercellular adhesion molecule-1 and soluble vascular adhesion molecule-1 and the development of symptomatic peripheral vascular disease in men. *Circulation* 2002;106:820–825.
15. Blankenberg S, Rupprecht HJ, Bickel C, et al. Circulating cell adhesion molecules and death in patients with coronary artery disease. *Circulation* 2001;104:1336–1342.
16. Malik I, Danesh J, Whincup P, et al. Soluble adhesion molecules and prediction of coronary heart disease: a prospective study and meta-analysis. *Lancet* 2001;358:971–976.
17. Ridker PM. Role of inflammatory biomarkers in prediction of coronary heart disease. *Lancet* 2001;358:946–948.
18. Biasucci LM, Liuzzo G, Fantuzzi G, et al. Increasing levels of interleukin (IL)-1Ra and IL-6 during the first 2 days of hospitalization in unstable angina are associated with increased risk of in-hospital coronary events. *Circulation* 1999;99:2079–2084.
19. Ridker PM, Rifai N, Stampfer MJ, et al. Plasma concentration of interleukin-6 and the risk of future myocardial infarction among apparently healthy Men. *Circulation* 2000;101:1767–1772.
20. Ridker PM, Rifai N, Pfeffer M, et al. Elevation of tumor necrosis factor-alpha and increased risk of recurrent coronary events after myocardial infarction. *Circulation* 2000;101:2149–2153.
21. Okamura H, Tsutsi H, Komatsu T, et al. Cloning of a new cytokine that induces IFN-gamma production by T cells. *Nature* 1995;378:88–91.
22. Blankenberg S, Tiret L, Bickel C, et al. Interleukin-18 is a strong predictor of cardiovascular death in stable and unstable angina. *Circulation* 2002;106:24–30.
23. Bootcov MR, Bauskin AR, Valenzuela SM, et al. MIC-1, a novel macrophage inhibitory cytokine, is a divergent member of the TGF-beta superfamily. *Proc Natl Acad Sci USA* 1997;94:11514–11519.
24. Brown DA, Breit SN, Buring J, et al. Concentration in plasma of macrophage inhibitory cytokine-1 and risk of cardiovascular events in women: a nested case-control study. *Lancet* 2002;359:2159–2163.
25. Packard CJ, O'Reilly DS, Caslake MJ, et al. Lipoprotein-associated phospholipase A2 as an independent predictor of coronary heart disease. West of Scotland Coronary Prevention Study Group. *N Engl J Med* 2000;343:1148–1155.
26. Blake GJ, Dada N, Fox JC, et al. A prospective evaluation of lipoprotein-associated phospholipase A(2) levels and the risk of future cardiovascular events in women. *J Am Coll Cardiol* 2001;38:1302–1306.
27. Zhang R, Brennan ML, Fu X, et al. Association between myeloperoxidase levels and risk of coronary artery disease. *JAMA* 2001;286:2136–2142.
28. Bayes-Genis A, Conover CA, Overgaard MT, et al. Pregnancy-associated plasma protein A as a marker of acute coronary syndromes. *N Engl J Med* 2001;345:1022–1029.
29. Torzewski J, Torzewski M, Bowyer DE, et al. C-reactive protein frequently colocalizes with the terminal complement complex in the intima of early atherosclerotic lesions of human coronary arteries. *Arterioscler Thromb Vasc Biol* 1998;18:1386–1392.
30. Yasojima K, Schwab C, McGeer EG, et al. Generation of C-reactive protein and complement components in atherosclerotic plaques. *Am J Pathol* 2001;158:1039–1051.
31. Zwaka TP, Hombach V, Torzewski J. C-reactive protein-mediated low density lipoprotein uptake by macrophages: implications for atherosclerosis. *Circulation* 2001;103:1194–1197.
32. Ballou SP, Lozanski G. Induction of inflammatory cytokine release from cultured human monocytes by C-reactive protein. *Cytokine* 1992;4:361–368.
33. Pasceri V, Willerson JT, Yeh ET. Direct proinflammatory effect of C-reactive protein on human endothelial cells. *Circulation* 2000;102:2165–2168.
34. Pasceri V, Chang J, Willerson JT, et al. Modulation of c-reactive protein-mediated monocyte chemoattractant protein-1 induction in human endothelial cells by anti-atherosclerosis drugs. *Circulation* 2001;103:2531–2534.
35. Nakajima T, Schulte S, Warrington KJ, et al. T-cell-mediated lysis of endothelial cells in acute coronary syndromes. *Circulation* 2002;105:570–575.
36. Verma S, Li SH, Badiwala MV, et al. Endothelin antagonism and interleukin-6 inhibition attenuate the proatherogenic effects of C-reactive protein. *Circulation* 2002;105:1890–1896.
37. Miyauchi T, Masaki T. Pathophysiology of endothelin in the cardiovascular system. *Annu Rev Physiol* 1999;61:391–415.
38. Verma S, Wang CH, Li SH, et al. A self-fulfilling prophecy: C-reactive protein attenuates nitric oxide production and inhibits angiogenesis. *Circulation* 2002;106:913–919.
39. Venugopal SK, Devaraj S, Yuhanna I, et al. Demonstration that C-reactive protein decreases eNOS expression and bioactivity in human aortic endothelial cells. *Circulation* 2002;106:1439–1441.
40. Wever RM, Luscher TF, Cosentino F, et al. Atherosclerosis and the two faces of endothelial nitric oxide synthase. *Circulation* 1998;97:108–112.

41. Loscalzo J. Nitric oxide and vascular disease. *N Engl J Med* 1995; 333:251–253.
42. Koenig W, Sund M, Frohlich M, et al. C-Reactive protein, a sensitive marker of inflammation, predicts future risk of coronary heart disease in initially healthy middle-aged men: results from the MONICA (Monitoring Trends and Determinants in Cardiovascular Disease) Augsburg Cohort Study, 1984 to 1992. *Circulation* 1999;99:237–242.
43. Kuller LH, Tracy RP, Shaten J, et al. Relation of C-reactive protein and coronary heart disease in the MRFIT nested case-control study. Multiple Risk Factor Intervention Trial. *Am J Epidemiol* 1996;144:537–547.
44. Ridker PM, Cushman M, Stampfer MJ, et al. Inflammation, aspirin, and the risk of cardiovascular disease in apparently healthy men [published erratum appears in N Engl J Med 1997 Jul 31;337(5):356]. *N Engl J Med* 1997;336:973–979.
45. Ridker PM, Cushman M, Stampfer MJ, et al. Plasma concentration of C-reactive protein and risk of developing peripheral vascular disease. *Circulation* 1998;97:425–428.
46. Ridker PM, Buring JE, Shih J, et al. Prospective study of C-reactive protein and the risk of future cardiovascular events among apparently healthy women. *Circulation* 1998;98:731–733.
47. Ridker PM, Hennekens CH, Buring JE, et al. C-reactive protein and other markers of inflammation in the prediction of cardiovascular disease in women. *N Engl J Med* 2000;342:836–843.
48. Ridker PM, Stampfer MJ, Rifai N. Novel risk factors for systemic atherosclerosis: a comparison of C-reactive protein, fibrinogen, homocysteine, lipoprotein(a), and standard cholesterol screening as predictors of peripheral arterial disease. *JAMA* 2001;285:2481–2485.
49. Tracy RP, Lemaitre RN, Psaty BM, et al. Relationship of C-reactive protein to risk of cardiovascular disease in the elderly. Results from the Cardiovascular Health Study and the Rural Health Promotion Project. *Arterioscler Thromb Vasc Biol* 1997;17:1121–1127.
50. Danesh J, Whincup P, Walker M, et al. Low grade inflammation and coronary heart disease: prospective study and updated meta-analyses. *BMJ* 2000;321:199–204.
51. Harris TB, Ferrucci L, Tracy RP, et al. Associations of elevated interleukin-6 and C-reactive protein levels with mortality in the elderly. *Am J Med* 1999;106:506–512.
52. Lowe GD, Yarnell JW, Rumley A, et al. C-reactive protein, fibrin D-dimer, and incident ischemic heart disease in the Speedwell study: are inflammation and fibrin turnover linked in pathogenesis? *Arterioscler Thromb Vasc Biol* 2001;21:603–610.
53. Albert C, Ma J, Rifai N, et al. Prospective study of C-reactive protein, homocysteine, and plasma lipid levels as predictors of sudden cardiac death. *Circulation* 2002;105:2595–2599.
54. Zebrack JS, Muhlestein JB, Horne BD, et al. C-reactive protein and angiographic coronary artery disease: independent and additive predictors of risk in subjects with angina. *J Am Coll Cardiol* 2002;39:632–637.
55. Morrow DA, Rifai N, Antman EM, et al. C-reactive protein is a potent predictor of mortality independently of and in combination with troponin T in acute coronary syndromes: a TIMI 11A substudy. Thrombolysis in Myocardial Infarction. *J Am Coll Cardiol* 1998;31:1460–1465.
56. Liuzzo G, Biasucci LM, Gallimore JR, et al. The prognostic value of C-reactive protein and serum amyloid a protein in severe unstable angina. *N Engl J Med* 1994;331:417–424.
57. Biasucci LM, Liuzzo G, Grillo RL, et al. Elevated levels of C-reactive protein at discharge in patients with unstable angina predict recurrent instability. *Circulation* 1999;99:855–860.
58. Toss H, Lindahl B, Siegbahn A, et al. Prognostic influence of increased fibrinogen and C-reactive protein levels in unstable coronary artery disease. FRISC Study Group. Fragmin during Instability in Coronary Artery Disease. *Circulation* 1997;96:4204–4210.
59. Lindahl B, Toss H, Siegbahn A, et al. Markers of myocardial damage and inflammation in relation to long-term mortality in unstable coronary artery disease. FRISC Study Group. Fragmin during Instability in Coronary Artery Disease. *N Engl J Med* 2000;343:1139–1147.
60. Haverkate F, Thompson SG, Pyke SD, et al. Production of C-reactive protein and risk of coronary events in stable and unstable angina. European Concerted Action on Thrombosis and Disabilities Angina Pectoris Study Group. *Lancet* 1997;349:462–466.
61. Heeschen C, Hamm CW, Bruemmer J, et al. Predictive value of C-reactive protein and troponin T in patients with unstable angina: a comparative analysis. CAPTURE Investigators. Chimeric c7E3 AntiPlatelet Therapy in Unstable angina REfractory to standard treatment trial. *J Am Coll Cardiol* 2000;35:1535–1542.
62. Ridker PM, Rifai N, Pfeffer MA, et al. Inflammation, pravastatin, and the risk of coronary events after myocardial infarction in patients with average cholesterol levels. Cholesterol and Recurrent Events (CARE) Investigators. *Circulation* 1998;98:839–844.
63. Mueller C, Buettner HJ, Hodgson JM, et al. Inflammation and long-term mortality after non-ST elevation acute coronary syndrome treated with a very early invasive strategy in 1042 consecutive patients. *Circulation* 2002;105:1412–1415.
64. Chew DP, Bhatt DL, Robbins MA, et al. Incremental prognostic value of elevated baseline C-reactive protein among established markers of risk in percutaneous coronary intervention. *Circulation* 2001;104:992–997.
65. Buffon A, Liuzzo G, Biasucci LM, et al. Preprocedural serum levels of C-reactive protein predict early complications and late restenosis after coronary angioplasty. *J Am Coll Cardiol* 1999;34:1512–1521.
66. Ellis SG, Chew D, Chan A, et al. Death following creatine kinase-MB elevation after coronary intervention: identification of an early risk period: importance of creatine kinase-MB level, completeness of revascularization, ventricular function, and probable benefit of statin therapy. *Circulation* 2002;106:1205–1210.
67. Milazzo D, Biasucci LM, Luciani N, et al. Elevated levels of C-reactive protein before coronary artery bypass grafting predict recurrence of ischemic events. *Am J Cardiol* 1999;84:459–461,A9.
68. Ridker PM, Rifai N, Rose L, et al. Comparison of C-reactive protein and LDL cholesterol levels in the prediction of first cardiovascular events. *N Engl J Med* 2002;347:1557–1565.
69. Visser M, Bouter LM, McQuillan GM, et al. Elevated C-reactive protein levels in overweight and obese adults. *JAMA* 1999;282:2131–2135.
70. Yudkin JS, Stehouwer CD, Emeis JJ, et al. C-reactive protein in healthy subjects: associations with obesity, insulin resistance, and endothelial dysfunction: a potential role for cytokines originating from adipose tissue? *Arterioscler Thromb Vasc Biol* 1999;19:972–978.
71. Davi G, Guagnano MT, Ciabattoni G, et al. Platelet activation in obese women: role of inflammation and oxidant stress. *JAMA* 2002;288:2008–2014.
72. Ford ES. Does exercise reduce inflammation? Physical activity and C-reactive protein among U.S. adults. *Epidemiology* 2002;13:561–568.
73. Bermudez EA, Rifai N, Buring JE, et al. Relation between markers of systemic vascular inflammation and smoking in women. *Am J Cardiol* 2002;89:1117–1119.
74. Bermudez EA, Rifai N, Buring J, et al. Interrelationships among circulating interleukin-6, C-reactive protein, and traditional cardiovascular risk factors in women. *Arterioscler Thromb Vasc Biol* 2002;22:1668–1673.
75. Pradhan AD, Manson JE, Rifai N, et al. C-reactive protein, interleukin 6, and risk of developing type 2 diabetes mellitus. *JAMA* 2001;286:327–334.
76. Pradhan AD, Ridker PM. Do atherosclerosis and type 2 diabetes share a common inflammatory basis? *Eur Heart J* 2002;23:831–834.
77. Ridker PM, Buring JE, Cook NR, et al. C-reactive protein, the metabolic syndrome, and risk of incident cardiovascular events: an 8-year follow-up of 14,719 initially healthy American women. *Circulation* 2003;107:391–397.
78. Kennon S, Price CP, Mills PG, et al. The effect of aspirin on C-reactive protein as a marker of risk in unstable angina. *J Am Coll Cardiol* 2001;37:1266–1270.
79. Feldman M, Jialal I, Devaraj S, et al. Effects of low-dose aspirin on serum C-reactive protein and thromboxane B2 concentrations: a placebo-controlled study using a highly sensitive C-reactive protein assay. *J Am Coll Cardiol* 2001;37:2036–2041.
80. Ikonomidis I, Andreotti F, Economou E, et al. Increased proinflammatory cytokines in patients with chronic stable angina and their reduction by aspirin. *Circulation* 1999;100:793–798.
81. Chew DP, Bhatt DL, Robbins MA, et al. Effect of clopidogrel added to aspirin before percutaneous coronary intervention on the risk associated with C-reactive protein. *Am J Cardiol* 2001;88:672–674.
82. Moshfegh K, Redondo M, Julmy F, et al. Antiplatelet effects of clopidogrel compared with aspirin after myocardial infarction: enhanced inhibitory effects of combination therapy. *J Am Coll Cardiol* 2000;36:699–705.
83. Libby P, Simon DI. Inflammation and thrombosis: the clot thickens. *Circulation* 2001;103:1718–1720.
84. Schonbeck U, Varo N, Libby P, et al. Soluble CD40L and cardiovascular risk in women. *Circulation* 2001;104:2266–2268.
85. Blake GJ, Ostfeld RJ, Yucel EK, et al. Soluble CD40 ligand levels indi-

cate lipid accumulation in carotid atheroma: an in vivo study with high-resolution MRI. *Arterioscler Thromb Vasc Biol* 2003;23:e11–e14.

86. Haffner SM, Greenberg AS, Weston WM, et al. Effect of rosiglitazone treatment on nontraditional markers of cardiovascular disease in patients with type 2 diabetes mellitus. *Circulation* 2002;106:679–684.

87. Sukhova GK, Williams JK, Libby P. Statins reduce inflammation in atheroma of nonhuman primates independent of effects on serum cholesterol. *Arterioscler Thromb Vasc Biol* 2002;22:1452–1458.

88. Fukumoto Y, Libby P, Rabkin E, et al. Statins alter smooth muscle cell accumulation and collagen content in established atheroma of Watanabe heritable hyperlipidemic rabbits. *Circulation* 2001;103:993–999.

89. Crisby M, Nordin-Fredriksson G, Shah PK, et al. Pravastatin treatment increases collagen content and decreases lipid content, inflammation, metalloproteinases, and cell death in human carotid plaques: implications for plaque stabilization. *Circulation* 2001;103:926–933.

90. Albert M, Danielson E, Rifai N, et al. Effect of statin therapy on C-reactive protein levels. The Pravastatin Inflammation/CRP Evaluation (PRINCE): a Randomized Trial and Cohort Study. *JAMA* 2001;286:64–70.

91. Jialal I, Stein D, Balis D, et al. Effect of hydroxymethyl glutaryl coenzyme a reductase inhibitor therapy on high sensitive C-reactive protein levels. *Circulation* 2001;103:1933–1935.

92. Ridker PM, Rifai N, Pfeffer MA, et al. Long-term effects of pravastatin on plasma concentration of C-reactive protein. The Cholesterol and Recurrent Events (CARE) Investigators. *Circulation* 1999;100:230–235.

93. Ridker PM, Rifai N, Lowenthal SP. Rapid reduction in C-reactive protein with cerivastatin among 785 patients with primary hypercholesterolemia. *Circulation* 2001;103:1191–1193.

94. Ridker PM, Rifai N, Clearfield M, et al. Measurement of C-reactive protein for the targeting of statin therapy in the primary prevention of acute coronary events. *N Engl J Med* 2001;344:1959–1965.

95. Walter DH, Fichtlscherer S, Britten MB, et al. Statin therapy, inflammation and recurrent coronary events in patients following coronary stent implantation. *J Am Coll Cardiol* 2001;38:2006–2012.

96. Blake GJ, Ridker PM, Kuntz KM. Projected life-expectancy gains with statin therapy for individuals with elevated C-reactive protein levels. *J Am Coll Cardiol* 2002;40:49–55.

97. Centers for Disease Control/American Heart Association workshop on inflammatory markers and cardiovascular disease: application to clinical and public health practice, Atlanta, March 14-15, 2002. Atlanta, GA: Atlanta Centers for Disease Control and Prevention, 2002.

98. Ridker PM. Should statin therapy be considered for patients with elevated C-reactive protein? The need for a definitive clinical trial. *Eur Heart J* 2001;22:2135–2137.

99. Liuzzo G, Buffon A, Biasucci LM, et al. Enhanced inflammatory response to coronary angioplasty in patients with severe unstable angina. *Circulation* 1998;98:2370–2376.

CHAPTER 49

Evolving Invasive and Noninvasive Imaging Techniques in Atherothrombotic Disease

Robin P. Choudhury, Valentin Fuster, and Zahi A. Fayad

Key Words: Imaging techniques; intravascular ultrasound; magnetic resonance imaging; molecular imaging.

The recognition of atherothrombosis in the pathogenesis of acute coronary syndromes has generated a desire to identify and characterize atherothrombotic plaque and to develop new imaging modalities that will help to identify plaques that are prone to provoke acute atherothrombotic events through erosion or rupture. Plaque characterization may facilitate the targeted administration of treatments to prevent the complications of atherothrombosis. Atherothrombosis imaging techniques are

R. P. Choudhury: Department of Cardiovascular Medicine, Level 5, John Radcliffe Hospital, Oxford, OX3 9DU, United Kingdom.

V. Fuster: The Zena and Michael A. Wiener Cardiovascular Institute, The Marie-Josée and Henry R. Kravis Cardiovascular Health Center, Mount Sinai School of Medicine, Box 1030, New York, New York.

Z. A. Fayad: Department of Radiology and Medicine (Cardiology), The Zena and Michael A. Wiener Cardiovascular Institute, The Marie-Josée and Henry R. Kravis Cardiovascular Health Center, Mount Sinai School of Medicine, One Gustave L. Levy Place, Imaging Science Laboratories, Box 1234, New York, New York 10029.

evolving rapidly. Here, we address the rationale for plaque imaging and describe the characteristics of plaque using evolving and experimental imaging techniques. Current and future applications including real-time vascular intervention, new contrast agents, and molecular imaging are also discussed. Other chapters in this book deal with computed tomography (CT) and magnetic resonance imaging (MRI) in greater detail.

X-ray arteriography images arterial lumen and some features of arterial wall (such as dissection, ulceration, and adherent thrombus) with excellent spatial and temporal resolution, and it is well suited to the diagnosis and percutaneous treatment of symptomatic coronary and carotid stenoses. However, arteriography gives little information about plaque composition or character and does not provide information that is useful in predicting pathologic behavior of plaques or their response to disease-modifying treatment. Pathologic studies have determined the plaque types at greatest risk for acute rupture or erosion (1,2). In particular, the presence of a large extracellular lipid core, thin fibrous cap, and inflammatory cell infiltrate characterize such plaques (3–5).

Evolving invasive and noninvasive techniques have the potential to image atherothrombotic plaque, to determine its composition and microanatomy, and to predict pathophysiologic behavior.

TABLE 49–1. *Comparison of novel imaging modalities used for the characterization of atherothrombotic plaque*

Modality	Setting	Vessel	French gauge, F	Spatial resolution, μm	Depth, μm	Imaging time	Lipid core Sensitivity, %	Specificity, %	Author (reference)
IB-IVUS	PM	Coronary	3.2	~40 × ~40 × 100	2,000	—	100	—	Kawasaki et al., 2002 (9)
40 MHz IVUS	PM	Coronary	3.0	—	—	—	65	95	Prati et al., 2001 (8)
Elastography	In vivo	Coronary	4.3	~200 radial	—	10 frames s⁻¹	—	—	Carlier et al., 2002 (11)
OCT	PM	Aorta, carotid/coronary	3.2	10 × 20	~2,500	4–8 frames s⁻¹	~90	~90	Yabushita et al., 2002 (17)
NIR spectroscopy	PM	Aorta	N/A	7,800 × 7,800	2,000	120 s	90	93	Moreno et al., 2002 (21)
Raman spectroscopy	Explant	Coronary	N/A	~100 × ~100	1500	10–100 s	—	—	Romer et al., 1998 (142)
Thermography	In vivo	Human coronary	4	500 × 500	—	—	—	—	Stefanadis et al., 1999 (38)
Intravascular MRI	In vivo	Rabbit aorta	4.3	156 × 156 × 3,000	N/A	10–15 min	N/A	N/A	Worthley et al., 2003 (96)
Non invasive MRI	In vivo	Human coronary	N/A	500 × 500 × 3,000	N/A	~20 s/slice	—	—	Fayad et al., 2000 (77)
Non invasive MRI	In vivo	Human carotid	N/A	250 × 250 × 2,000	N/A	—	98	100	Yuan et al., 2001 (73)

Some sensitivity and specificity calculations are based on small numbers and should be interpreted with caution.

IB-IVUS, integrated backscatter intravascular ultrasound; IVUS, intravascular ultrasound; MRI, magnetic resonance imaging; N/A, data not applicable; NIR, near infrared; OCT, optical coherence tomography; PM, postmortem; —, data not available.

INTRAVASCULAR ULTRASOUND

Intravascular ultrasound (IVUS) is an invasive technique that requires a transluminal catheter, typically 2.6 to 3.0 F (diameter, 0.89–1.0 mm), containing a miniaturized ultrasound transducer. At 30 MHz, the wavelength is ~50 μm, giving a practical axial spatial resolution of approximately 150 to 200 μm. A fundamental difference in approach between IVUS and arteriography is that the former images vessel wall and plaque directly, not in relief superimposed on radiographic contrast in the vessel lumen. Such direct imaging is a common feature of the evolving modalities under discussion. A further important advantage over arteriography is the systematic acquisition of tomographic data that are not limited to two-dimensional projections.

Abrupt changes in acoustic impedance that occur at the interface between tissue types produce strong ultrasound reflection and generate an apparent border between anatomic compartments of the vessel wall. This occurs most markedly between the lumen and endothelium and between media and external elastic lamina. Within the coronary arterial wall, atherothrombotic lesions can be detected, quantified (including volumetric analysis), and partially characterized. Lesions of low echogenicity correspond to areas of fibromuscular plaque or to diffuse lipid infiltration. Brightly echogenic areas correspond to densely fibrous plaque (although fibrous caps are generally too thin to be resolved with IVUS), and intensely bright echogenicity represents calcified areas (6,7). Thus, plaque appearances by IVUS are not absolutely specific in determining composition, and it is not possible to identify reliably fibrous cap or lipid core (8; see Table 49–1). Sensitivity of IVUS in determining plaque composition in real time may be improved by technical advancement, such as use of integrated backscatter (9) or by enhanced data analysis, including the application of mathematic algorithms to create tissue maps from radiofrequency data (10).

IVUS provides, at best, an *in vivo* approximation to histologic analysis of vessel wall and has not yet been shown capable of predicting plaque behavior in prospective studies. It is, however, one of the few imaging modalities discussed in this chapter that is in widespread routine clinical use in the context of atherosclerosis and thrombosis imaging.

INTRAVASCULAR ULTRASOUND ELASTOGRAPHY

In IVUS elastography, data are derived from mechanophysical properties of arterial wall and plaque. Using an IVUS catheter, radiofrequency data are obtained at two levels of intraarterial pressure. An estimation of deformation can be obtained from comparison of the signals acquired with and without the application of a stress. Strain is then computed as the displacement derivative and can be mapped as a two-dimensional image, the elastogram (11). Thus, elastography does not provide direct evidence about plaque composition, but rather about its mechanical properties. Preliminary studies in human coronary and femoral arteries *ex vivo* suggested that plaque composition may be inferred from IVUS elastography (12). More recently, *in vivo*, IVUS elastography examination (20 MHz) of the iliac and femoral arteries in Yucatan pigs has been used to determine the mechanoelastic properties of arterial wall. A temporal resolution of 30 frames per second with radial spatial resolution of ~200 μm was obtained. This initial study has suggested high sensitivity (≤100%) and specificity (≤80%) of elastography for the detection of fatty lesions, which display greater average strain values than fibrous lesions (13) (Fig. 49–1) (see color insert). Such results compare favorably with sensitivity of conventional IVUS in detecting lipid-rich lesions (14), even at a relatively high frequency (8). Early results for IVUS elastography are promising in peripheral arteries, but the technique is potentially limited by problems of catheter motion during cardiac contraction. This can be minimized by obtaining data from two points in diastole, where movement is minimal, but intraarterial pressure differences (approximately 5 mm Hg) are sufficient to provide strain data (11). Potential strain distortion caused by vessel branching and intracoronary stents in the index or adjacent arterial segment remains to be evaluated. Application of this invasive technique also is limited by lengthy data acquisition and processing.

OPTICAL COHERENCE TOMOGRAPHY

Intravascular optical coherence tomography (OCT) is a recently developed invasive optical imaging technique that uses back-reflected infrared light. Samples that have greater heterogeneity of optical index of refraction exhibit stronger optical scattering and, therefore, stronger OCT signal. Importantly, signal from lipid and fibrous tissue give significantly different refractive indices (15). Initial feasibility studies showed marked heterogeneity in human coronary arteries (16). A subsequent study has investigated the ability of OCT to discern plaque components (17). A training series of images identified fibrous plaques as homogeneous signal-rich area, whereas fibrocalcific plaque was signal-poor, with well defined borders. Lipid-rich plaque also appeared signal-poor but was distinguished from fibrocalcific plaque by the presence of ill-defined borders. Using these appearances to classify in categoric fashion cross sections of aorta, carotid arteries, and coronary arteries, good agreement was achieved for OCT and histopathologic examination. Although OCT provides excellent axial (10 μm) and lateral (20 μm) spatial resolution, it has relatively limited tissue penetration (1 to 2 mm), and a significant false-negative rate for the detection of lipid-rich plaque has been attributed to this (17). The technique has been shown to be feasible and safe for human coronary artery imaging *in vivo* (18). Using a modified 3.2 F IVUS catheter, images with clearly superior resolution to IVUS at 30 MHz could be obtained in 5 to 10 minutes additional procedure time (Fig. 49–2). Because

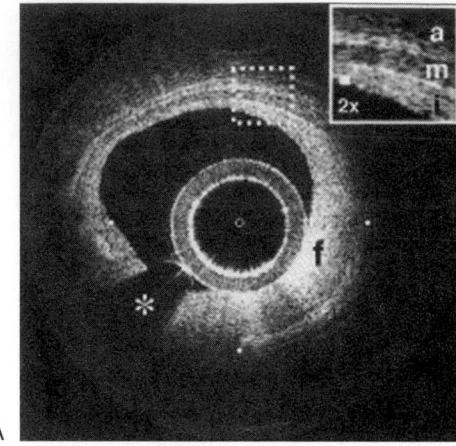

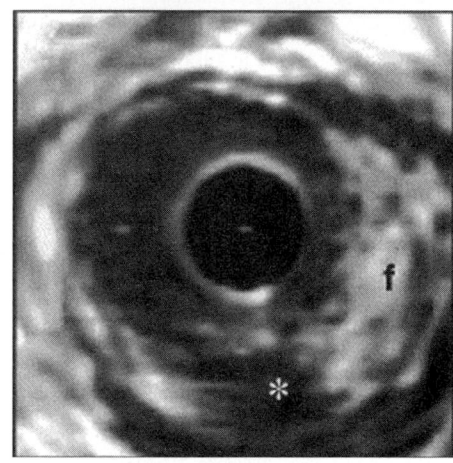

FIG. 49–2. Fibrous coronary plaque imaged *in vivo* by optical coherence tomography (OCT) **(A)** and intravascular ultrasound (IVUS) **(B)**. **A:** From 9 to 2 o'clock, this OCT image demonstrates visualization of the intima (with intimal hyperplasia [*i*]), media *(m)*, and adventitia *(a)*. The internal and external elastic laminae are visible as signal-rich lines bordering the media *(inset)*. A plaque extending from 2 to 9 o'clock contains a homogeneous, signal-rich region consistent with a fibrous plaque *(f)* that is partially obscured by a guidewire shadow artifact *(asterisk)*. **B:** In the corresponding IVUS image, the fibrous plaque *(f)* also is visualized. Tick marks are 1 mm. (Reproduced from Jang IK, Bouma BE, Kang DH, et al. Visualization of coronary atherosclerotic plaques in patients using optical coherence tomography: comparison with intravascular ultrasound. *J Am Coll Cardiol* 2002;39:604–609, with permission.)

blood distorts appearances under OCT, imaging was obtained during saline flushes through the coronary guide catheter. Systematic imaging throughout a prolonged coronary segment would not be practical using this technique and may require occlusion balloon techniques of the sort used in coronary angioscopy (19). OCT also is limited by relatively low temporal resolution (4 frames/second), which renders it susceptible to corruption by motion artifact *in vivo* in coronary arteries. As stated previously, the presence of macrophages in coronary atherothrombotic plaques is associated with plaque vulnerability. Because OCT signal in-

creases with the number of refractive index mismatches in tissue, caps containing mismatches would be expected to show multiple high-signal areas. This has been explored in a preliminary study that demonstrated high OCT signal in selected areas of plaques immunostaining positively for the macrophage marker CD68 (20). The high degree of spatial resolution of this technique provides compelling images, and further developments are awaited with interest.

NEAR INFRARED SPECTROSCOPY

Near infrared spectroscopy (NIR) is an invasive technique based on the absorbance of light by organic molecules. Reflectance spectra between 400 and 2,400 nm allow detailed analysis of chemical composition. NIR can provide simultaneous multicomponent chemical analysis of biologic tissue within 1 second (21). Organic chemicals possess characteristic absorbance at different wavelengths and mathematic analysis with computer-aided pattern recognition has allowed different plaque components to be identified (21–23). In the study of Moreno and coworkers (21), qualitative tissue data were obtained from formalin-fixed, postmortem samples of human aorta. NIR was reported to detect lipid core (sensitivity 90%, specificity 93%), thin fibrous cap (sensitivity 77%, specificity 93%), and inflammatory cells (sensitivity 84%, specificity 89%) (Table 49–1). As the authors pointed out, the histologic validation, on the basis of adjacent 5-μ histologic sections, may not precisely reflect the NIR signal obtained from a gross tissue segment. Data were obtained from a region of vessel with a surface area of 78 mm^2; thus, the effective spatial resolution of NIR is substantially less than other techniques and currently is not sufficient to provide useful images of coronary arteries, although NIR does have the advantage of relatively deep tissue penetration ($\approx$2 mm). NIR spectra have been measured through fiber optic–based systems 1 to 4 mm in diameter to explore the feasibility of a coronary catheter-mounted system. This technique can quantify plaque cholesterol (22,23) and, less precisely, plaque collagen content (23). Although image acquisition is relatively rapid (1 second), even this is too long to avoid potential motion artifact *in vivo* in coronary arteries; furthermore, the effects of blood on laser light attenuation and the ability of NIR to characterize plaque *in vivo* is not clearly established, although initial reports are favorable (24). Finally, the read out from NIR is spectroscopic, not primarily topographic, and this important feature may limit its application clinically unless combined with another imaging modality. Although there are encouraging features, this technique remains experimental.

RAMAN SPECTROSCOPY

When a photon encounters a molecule, the vibrational energy of the molecule is changed and scattered light is emitted at an altered frequency. This gives rise to Raman spectra with a range of well defined peaks corresponding specifically to different molecules within a tissue (25). This principle has been applied to the characterization of biologic tissue, using near infrared laser excitation (750–1,064 nm wavelength range), and specifically to quantify components of atherothrombotic plaque (26). Combing the emission characteristics of plaque elements, Brennan and coworkers (27) devised a model to measure relative quantities of cholesterol, cholesteryl esters, triglycerides and phospholipids, and calcium salts in small volumes (1 mm^3) of human coronary artery homogenates on the basis of a linear superposition of spectra of individual plaque components. Application of this model has enabled quantification of these same components in fresh intact human explant heart coronary arteries and correlation with plaque type (nonatherothrombotic, noncalcified plaque and calcified plaque) assessed by histopathology (28). With contemporary near infrared laser excitation and spectrophotograph/charge–coupled cameras, Raman spectroscopic data can be acquired in approximately 10 to 100 seconds (28,29), a timeframe that poses problems for *in vivo* imaging in moving structures. In addition, the three plaque types (discussed earlier) that Raman spectroscopy has been shown to identify may not be the strongest predictors of plaque behavior (29). Furthermore, quantification of plaque components alone, without detailed morphologic data, is of limited use because it is not only composition but microanatomy of the plaque that determines susceptibility to rupture or erosion. Development of fiber optic catheter–mounted systems (30) for use *in vivo,* particularly in combination with IVUS (31) or other imaging modalities, may prove fruitful. Indeed, the first application *in vivo* in the presence of luminal blood has been described (25,32).

THERMOGRAPHY

Inflammation is important in the pathogenesis of atherothrombosis (33), and infiltration with inflammatory cells, particularly macrophages, has been associated with plaque rupture in human coronary arteries (4,34). Because heat generation is a cardinal feature of inflammation, techniques have been developed to measure temperature (and thermal heterogeneity) on the surface of atherothrombotic plaques. Casscells and coworkers (35) used a 24-gauge needle thermistor applied to the surface of fresh human carotid plaque obtained at endarterectomy. Some areas of plaque showed temperature increase by up to 2.2°C. Furthermore, there was a positive correlation between plaque surface temperature and inflammatory cell density (35). Although macrophage infiltration and plaque temperature correlate, it remains uncertain whether macrophages are the source of the heat or whether the correlation reflects concurrent processes such as neovascularization of plaque, which might also increase temperature and is also associated with plaque vulnerability (36,37). Development of catheter-based systems has allowed translation to the *in vivo* human setting. Stefanadis and coworkers (38) reported a 0.457-mm thermistor probe

mounted on a 3-F monorail device passed into coronary arteries over a standard guidewire. Apposition to the vessel wall was attained by hydrofoil on the opposite side of the catheter to the thermistor. Plaque surface temperature was greater in atheromatous versus normal vessels but did not vary with degree of angiographic stenosis. Significantly, however, plaque temperature was greater than background temperature in patients who had presented with unstable angina and acute myocardial infarction (AMI) (38). In this

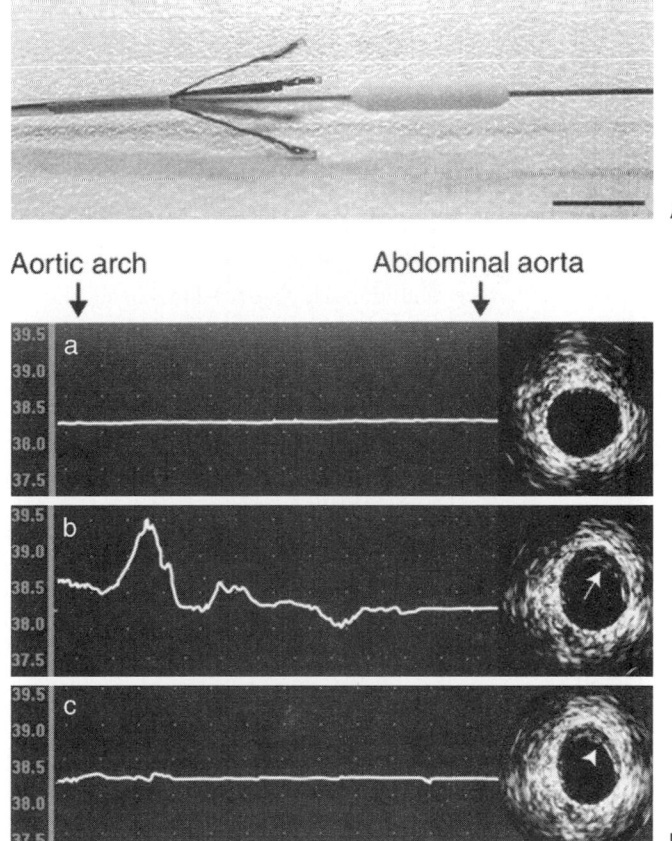

FIG. 49–3. **A:** Close-up photograph of the thermography catheter illustrating the engaged distal end of the catheter, with the four thermistors widely expanded (each at 90°C). Scale bar = 1 cm. **B:** Examples of *in vivo* temperature measurements of the endoaortic surface in rabbits. **a:** In control rabbits at 6 months, temperature differences are absent along the aortic wall. Intravascular ultrasound (IVUS) image illustrates the absence of plaque formation. **b:** In atherothrombotic rabbits at 6 months, marked temperature variations up to greater than 1°C are apparent along the endoluminal surface of the aortic wall. IVUS demonstrates plaque formation at the level of the proximal descending aorta just distal from the arch *(arrow).* **c:** In atherothrombotic rabbits after 3 months of dietary cholesterol reduction, temperature heterogeneity is absent, although IVUS (taken at the same level as in **b**) demonstrates the presence of a similar plaque *(arrowhead).* (Reproduced from Verheye S, De Meyer GR, Van Langenhove G, et al. In vivo temperature heterogeneity of atherosclerotic plaques is determined by plaque composition. *Circulation* 2002;105:1596–1601, with permission.)

study, there was no way to verify consistent contact of thermistor and vessel wall. Thermal heterogeneity may therefore have originated in variable plaque contact, although as noted by the authors, this effect would have been expected to apply to all patient groups and would not account for the relative increases in patients with stable angina versus normal coronary arteries or acute coronary syndromes. Initial results, in a small number of studies, appear encouraging. Technical advances, including catheters designed to ensure consistent and controllable wall apposition (Fig. 49–3) (39), perhaps with guidance of a collateral imaging modality (40), may remove doubts about measurement reliability. Further data are required to address sensitivity and specificity of the technique and, importantly, to investigate the relation between plaque temperature and prospective events.

SURFACE AND TRANSESOPHAGEAL ULTRASOUND

Measurements of carotid and aortic wall thickness, as well as qualitative and quantitative analysis of plaque, can be determined by surface and transesophageal ultrasound. Echogenicity of the plaque reflects its characteristics. Hypoechoic heterogeneous plaque is associated with both intraplaque hemorrhage and lipids, whereas hyperechoic homogeneous plaque is mostly fibrous (6).

The North American Symptomatic Carotid Endarterectomy Trial and the Asymptomatic Carotid Artery Stenosis Study have shown that the degree of stenosis and its hemodynamic consequences play a significant role in producing stroke (41,42). High-resolution (<0.4 mm axial), real-time B-mode ultrasonography with Doppler flow imaging has emerged as the modality of choice for examining the carotid arteries (43).

Using 8-MHz or larger transducers, B-mode ultrasonography can be used for measuring intima-media thickness (IMT) of large- and medium-sized peripheral arteries like the carotid, femoral, or radial arteries. Because of the physical principles of a diagnostic ultrasonography, the measurement is reliable only at the far arterial wall and does not indicate whether the thickening is caused by intima or media infiltration and/or hypertrophy (44). Like other ultrasonography methods, this technique is operator dependent and has low reproducibility.

Several studies have found that carotid and aortic atherothrombosis are markers for coronary atherothrombosis (45–47). Patients with symptomatic coronary artery disease (CAD) have increased IMT compared with asymptomatic control subjects (48). Carotid wall thickening also was found in patients with silent ischemia (49). The relation between IMT and CAD severity is constant but rather weak (50). Nevertheless, large prospective studies have demonstrated that IMT may be a useful marker of CAD progression. For example, the Cardiovascular Health Study found associations between carotid IMT and the incidence of new MI or stroke in patients 65 years or older (46). Prevention

trials of lipid-lowering treatments using IMT as a surrogate end point have shown that retardation in the progress of IMT correlates with a reduction of clinical end points (51,52).

Examination of the aorta by B-mode ultrasonography (53) and transesophageal echocardiography (TEE) have been used as predictors of CAD and cardiovascular risk (54). Using TEE, the French Study of Aortic Plaques in Stroke (FAPS) group (54,55) found a significantly increased risk for all vascular events for patients who had noncalcified aortic plaques greater than 4 mm in thickness. TEE-detected aortic plaque has been correlated with a greater prevalence of CAD and the presence of significant angiographic coronary artery stenosis (45). In addition, the lack of aortic plaque on TEE has been shown to be predictive of the absence of CAD (56).

Ultrasonic contrast agents have been introduced to improve image resolution and specificity (57–59). For example, acoustic liposomes conjugated with monoclonal antibodies can be used for plaque component-targeted imaging. The liposome formulation also has been modified to allow site-specific drug (60) or gene delivery (61).

MAGNETIC RESONANCE IMAGING

Noninvasive Magnetic Resonance Imaging

In MRI, after administration of a radiofrequency pulse, emitted radiofrequency signal differs between the nuclei of different atoms and further varies according to the molecular environment of the nuclei. Through this means it is possible to obtain quantitative information about specific molecules of interest within a given tissue (62–65).

Using a combination of inherent MRI contrast generated in so-called T1-weighted, T2-weighted, and proton density-weighted images, it has been possible to determine both plaque anatomy and composition in experimental animals (66,67), in *ex vivo* specimens (68–70), and in human aorta (71) and carotid arteries (70,72).

Fayad and coworkers (71) found good correlation of multicontrast MRI with aortic plaque quantification and characterization using TEE. In a study of 22 patients undergoing carotid endarterectomy (with a best voxel size of $254 \times 254 \times 1,000 \ \mu m^3$), thick fibrous caps were seen as a dark band between the lumen (white) and the vessel wall (gray) (72). The presence of a thin cap was inferred from the absence of any discernible dark band. Plaque rupture was identified *in vivo* by MRI in eight of the nine cases in which it was subsequently identified on the atherectomy specimens. Also, in human carotid arteries that were imaged *in vivo*, Yuan and coworkers (73) have identified lipid core with 85% sensitivity and 92% specificity using time of flight–based bright blood and spin-echo–based black blood multicontrast techniques (Table 49–1). Although lipid-rich necrotic cores were typically hypointense with T2-weighted images, this was variable, and, as reported previously (68), the comparison of vessel wall appearances under different contrast weightings provided greatest diagnostic yield.

The same authors have demonstrated clinical significance of carotid plaque characterization (74). In a case–control study of patients undergoing carotid endarterectomy, a recent (within 90 days) history of transient ischemic attack or stroke was strongly associated with the presence of thin or ruptured plaque identified before surgery by MRI. Compared with a thick fibrous cap, the risk for recent ischemic neurologic symptoms was increased by an impressive 23-fold in cases where ruptured plaque was identified. These encouraging observations will pave the way for studies that prospectively examine plaque behavior.

Coronary Artery Imaging with Magnetic Resonance Imaging

Coronary arteries have been imaged *in vivo* by MRI (75–78). Coronary imaging poses considerable technical difficulties. The coronary arteries are relatively small and have a tortuous and unpredictable course. In addition, to obtain MR images, cardiac and respiratory motion must be overcome. Use of MR navigator echoes that assess cardiac or diaphragmatic position accounts for movement and eliminates the time constraint imposed by imaging in a single breath hold, as shown in a multicenter study of coronary MR angiography (79). This provides longer effective image acquisition to enable submillimeter spatial resolution (75). Botnar and coworkers (78) have further refined their three-dimensional coronary wall imaging technique by the application of a local inversion technique, improving contrast between lumen and vessel wall in a series of normal subjects and attaining a resolution of $0.66 \times 0.66 \times 2$ mm^3 (78). Current coronary MRI techniques have limited spatial resolution mainly because of available signal-to-noise ratio (SNR). One way directly to increase the SNR is to improve the receiver coils. This was shown by Fayad and coworkers (80) using a four-element anterior phased-array coil that enabled in a series of patients *in vivo* coronary wall imaging at a resolution of $0.39 \times 0.39 \times 2$ mm^3.

Plaque Imaging with Gadolinium Contrast-enhanced Magnetic Resonance

New microvessels form in atherothrombotic plaque, and these may be associated with features of inflammation, such as up-regulation of adhesion molecules and leukocyte infiltration (37). The presence of new vessels also has been associated with carotid plaque instability (81). These vessels may also be abnormally permeable, allowing the extravasation of plasma proteins, such as albumin and fibrinogen (82,83). In published reports, contrast MRI has used these features to aid plaque characterization (Fig. 49–4) (84). On T1-weighted images of carotid arteries, a gadolinium-based contrast agent has been reported to enhance differentially areas rich in plaque microvascularization and may offer a further means of distinguishing necrotic core and fibrous cap and of highlighting at-risk plaque (85). Dynamic contrast-

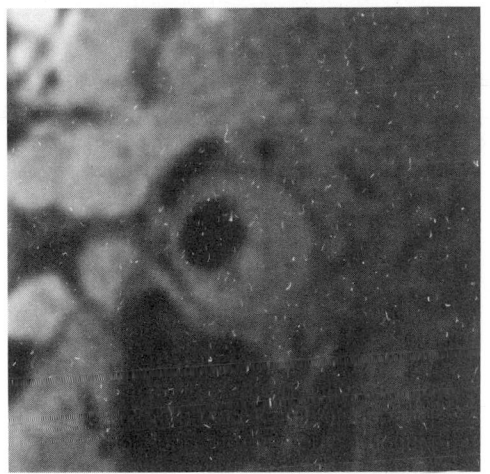

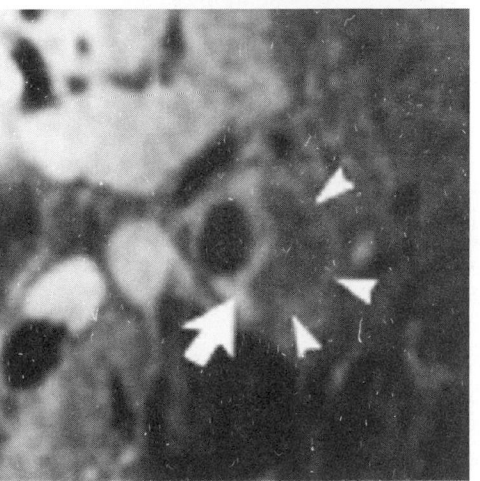

FIG. 49–4. *In vivo* human common carotid artery magnetic resonance images of plaque before **(A)** and after contrast (Gd-DTPA; 0.1 m*M*/kg) **(B)** images. A double-inversion recovery, T1-weighted fast spin-echo images with fat saturation was used. The postcontrast image in **B** demonstrates heterogeneous enhancement (*arrows* represent enhancement along the margin of the lumen, *arrowheads* represent enhancement along the outer wall of the atheroma). Scale bars = 1 cm. (Reproduced from Wasserman BA, Smith WI, Trout HH 3rd, et al. Carotid artery atherosclerosis: in vivo morphologic characterization with gadolinium-enhanced double-oblique MR imaging initial results. *Radiology* 2002;223:566–573, with permission.)

enhanced MRI may also allow quantification of neovasculature (86). It has been speculated that plaque enhancement reflects not only increased plaque vascularity (87), but also a leakiness of these microvessels, which suggests active inflammation (88).

In Vivo Monitoring of Therapy with Magnetic Resonance Imaging

In vivo MRI can be used to measure the effect of lipid-decreasing therapy (statins) in asymptomatic, hypercholesterolemic patients with carotid and aortic atherothrombosis (89). Atherosclerotic plaques were visualized and measured with MRI at different time points after initiation of lipid-decreasing therapy. Significant regression of atherosclerotic lesions was observed. There was a decrease in the vessel wall area but no change in the lumen area at 12 months. A longer follow-up showed a continued reduction on arterial wall area and even a small, but significant, increase in the arterial lumen at 24 months (90). Along similar lines, a case–control study demonstrated substantially reduced carotid plaque lipid content in patients treated for 10 years with an aggressive lipid-reducing regimen compared with untreated control subjects (91).

Intravascular Magnetic Resonance Imaging

An alternative way to improve SNR, and thus spatial resolution, is through the use of intravascular MR coils, which provide direct contact between the imaging coil and the vessel wall (Fig. 49–5). This allows the plaque to be within the

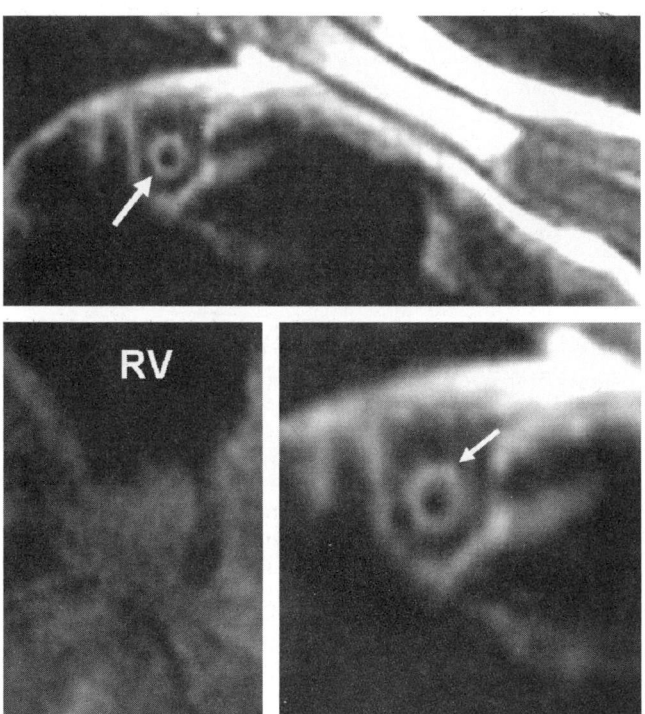

FIG. 49–5. Very high-resolution *in vivo* coronary wall magnetic resonance images of a patient with a plaque *(arrows)* in the right coronary artery. The images were obtained using the custom built four-element anterior phased-array chest coil. The images are obtained using the electrocardiogram-gated fast spin-echo sequence black-blood imaging with the double inversion recovery preparation pulses. Imaging parameters: repetition time, 1 RR interval; echo time, 42 ms; slice thickness, 4 mm; acquisition matrix, 512 × 512; field of view, 20 cm; number of signals averaged, 2; echo train length, 32; receiver bandwidth, ±64 kHz. A chemical shift suppression pulse was used to suppress the signal from perivascular fat. The inplane spatial resolution was ~390 × 390 × μm^2. The *insert* represents a magnified view of the right coronary artery plaque. RV, right ventricle.

area of maximal coil sensitivity. Problems related to intravascular MR include artifacts caused by blood flow and arterial wall pulsation, radial signal fall off, and poor flexibility (92). Zimmerman-Paul and colleagues (93,94) used a wire loop enclosed in an inflatable balloon to immobilize the coil against the vessel wall. An important limitation of such balloon techniques is the requirement for arterial occlusion for several minutes during imaging. This is not feasible for clinical imaging in human coronary or carotid arteries. Possible solutions include shorter imaging times or a new catheter design to allow distal perfusion during image acquisition (95,96). A nonocclusive MRI coil mounted on a 4.3-F over-the-wire catheter has been shown capable of obtaining images in rabbits *in vivo* and without image degradation because of motion artifact (96). Improved SNR provided 156 × 156 μm^2 inplane resolution (Fig. 49–6). Future work may extend this technique to study human coronary arteries.

Thrombus Imaging with Magnetic Resonance Imaging

Plaque rupture or erosion exposes the prothrombotic core to circulating blood (1,5), which can lead to acute vessel occlusion and MI, unstable angina, or death. Evidence suggests that layering and organization of thrombus may be responsible for plaque progression (2). Johnstone and coworkers (97) have identified the location and size of plaque-associated mural thrombus *in vivo* in an atherothrombotic rabbit model. Rapid, noninvasive identification and age characterization of thrombus may be clinically useful, for example, if treatment risk versus benefit was related to the timing and location of a thrombotic event. Time-related changes in the water diffusion properties of thrombus have been identified using pulse field gradient methods (98). MR signal intensities of hemorrhage and "altered blood" depend on the structure of hemoglobin and its oxidation state (99). For example, the generation of methemoglobin within evolving thrombus is known to cause T1 shortening. This phenomenon has been exploited for the detection of fresh thrombus in the setting of deep vein thrombosis (100,101), pulmonary embolus (102), and acute carotid thrombus (87). In these studies, direct imaging of thrombus against a suppressed background using a three-dimensional magnetization-prepared rapid gradient-echo (103) has been found to be effective in the imaging of thrombus.

The potential of MRI to detect arterial thrombotic obstruction and to define thrombus age has been recently evaluated using black-blood T1- and T2-weighted images (104). Carotid thrombi were induced in swine by arterial injury. Serial high-resolution *in vivo* MR images were obtained at 6 hours, 1 day, and 1, 2, 3, 6, and 9 weeks. Thrombus appearance and relative signal intensity revealed characteristic temporal changes in the MR images, reflecting histologic changes in the composition. Age definition using visual appearance was highly accurate (Pearson's χ^2 with 4 *df* ranging 96–132 and Cohen's κ 0.81–0.94).

Contrast agents that characterize thrombus are under development: Fibrin can be identified by lipid-encapsulated

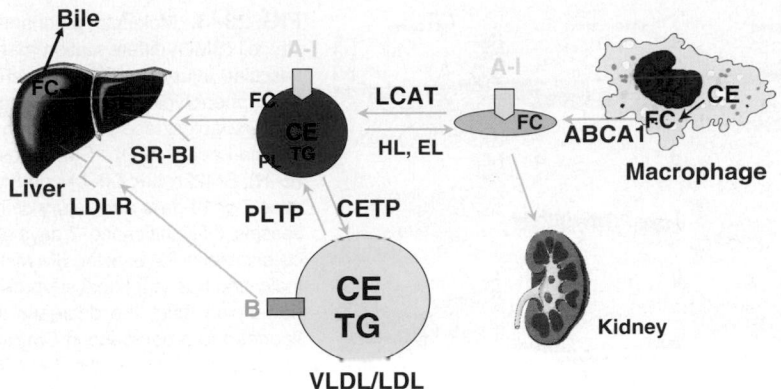

FIG. 7–1. High-density lipoprotein (HDL) metabolism and reverse cholesterol transport. Macrophages (and other peripheral cells) hydrolyze stored cholesteryl ester (CE) to free cholesterol (FC). Lipid-poor apoA-I promotes the cellular efflux of FC and phospholipid (PL) through a transport process facilitated by the cellular protein ATP-binding cassette protein A1 (ABCA1). FC is esterified to CE within the HDL particle by the enzyme lecithin cholesterol acyltransferase (LCAT). HDL CE and FC can be taken up selectively by the liver through the action of the scavenger receptor class BI (SR-BI). The liver secretes free cholesterol directly into the bile or converts it to bile acids, which are then secreted into the bile. Ultimately, biliary sterols are excreted in the feces, completing the reverse cholesterol transport pathway. HDL CE can also be selectively transferred to apoB-containing lipoproteins in exchange for triglyceride through the action of cholesteryl ester transfer protein (CETP) and then taken up by the liver via the LDL receptor. The phospholipid transfer protein (PLTP) mediates the transfer of phospholipids among lipoproteins, particularly from apoB-containing lipoproteins to HDL. Hepatic lipase (HL) and endothelial lipase (EL) hydrolyze HDL lipids, generating smaller HDL particles and promoting the catabolism of apoA-I by the kidneys. LDLR, low density lipoprotein receptor.

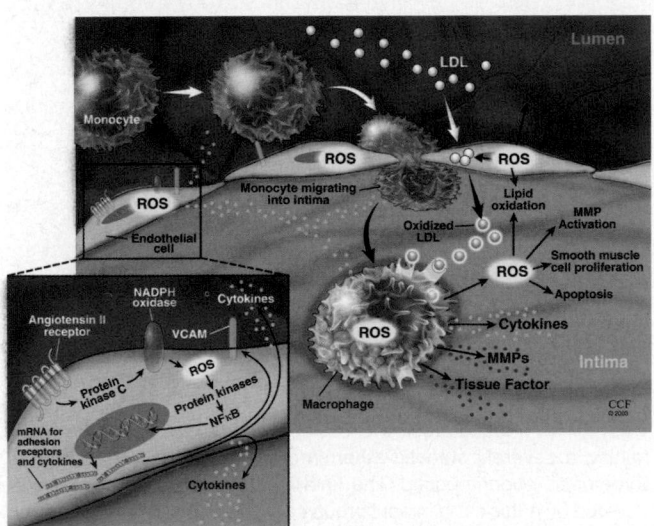

FIG. 21–1. Schematic representation of reactive oxygen species (ROS) involvement in the developing atherothrombotic lesion. LDL, low-density lipoprotein; MMP, matrix metalloproteinase; NADPH, nicotinamide adenine dinucleotide phosphate; NF-κB, nuclear factor-kappaB; VCAM, vascular cell adhesion molecule.

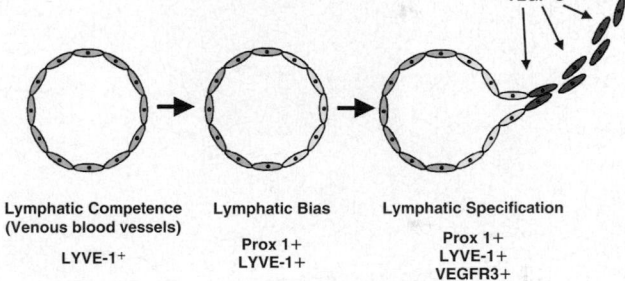

FIG. 24–3. A proposed model for lymphatic emergence from venous endothelium. Lymphatic endothelium emerges from *competent* venous endothelium expressing LYVE-1. Polarized expression of *Prox-1* on a subset of venous endothelial cells *biases* these cells toward producing lymphatic endothelium and induces or allows continued maintenance of the expression of a number of different lymphatic endothelial cell (*LEC*) genes including *VEGFR3*, the receptor for the lymphangiogenic factor VEGF-C. VEGF, Vascular endothelial growth factor. (See Oliver et al. [3] for a more comprehensive discussion of this model.) (Modified from Oliver G, Detmar M. The rediscovery of the lymphatic system: old and new insights into the development and biological function of the lymphatic vasculature. *Genes Dev* 2002;16:773–783.)

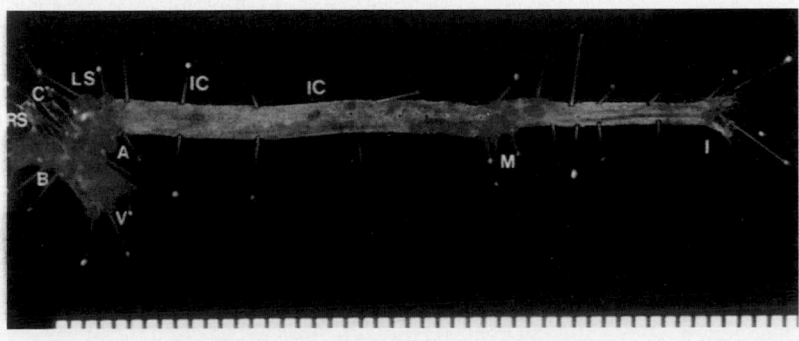

FIG. 25–3. Atherosclerosis in the apolipoprotein E (apoE)–deficient mouse. An aorta from an apoE-deficient mouse stained for lipid with oil red O. A, small curvature of the aortic arch; B, brachiocephalic trunk; C, common carotid; I, iliac bifurcation; IC, intercoastal arteries; LS, left subclavian; M, mesenteric and renal arteries; RS, right subclavian; V, aortic valve. (Reproduced from Palinski W, Ord VA, Plump AS, et al. Apolipoprotein E-deficient mice are a model of lipoprotein oxidation in atherogenesis: demonstration of oxidation-specific epitopes in lesions and high titers of autoantibodies to malondialdehyde-lysine in serum. *Arterioscler Thromb* 1994;14:606–616, with permission.)

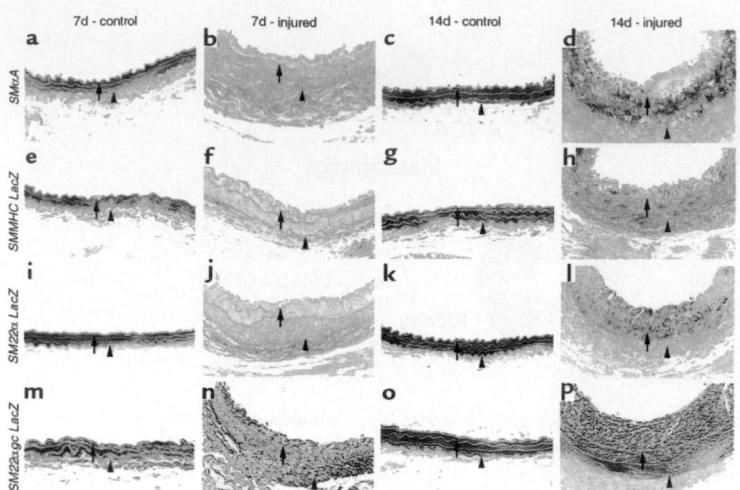

FIG. 28–3. Molecular mechanisms of decreased smooth muscle cell (SMC) differentiation marker expression associated with vascular injury—a novel experimental approach to studying SMC phenotypic modulation. Light micrographic images showing β-galactosidase staining of mouse carotid arteries from SM α-actin-LacZ **(A–D)**, SM myosin heavy chain (MHC)-LacZ **(E–H)**, SM22α-LacZ **(I–L)** and SM22αgc-LacZ **(M–P)** transgenic mice 7 or 14 days after injury or in uninjured contralateral carotid vessels. Of significance, 7 days after injury, LacZ activity was undetectable in SM α-actin, SM MHC, and SM22α transgenic mice indicating transcriptional suppression of the transgene. Although not shown here, the decrease in transgene expression corresponded to a decrease in SM α-actin and SM MHC protein expression and SM α-actin, SM MHC, and SM22α mRNA. By 14 days after injury, transgene activity was observed to increase within isolated subpopulations of SMCs with staining for the SM α-actin transgene greater than that for either the SM MHC or SM22α transgenes. These data show the dynamic nature of phenotypic switching of SMC genes during injury induced phenotypic switching. Mutation of the G/C-rich cis regulatory element positioned between two CArGs in the SM22α promoter (SM22αgc-LacZ) completely abrogated suppression of SM22α transgene at both 7 and 14 days after injury (compare LacZ staining in **J** vs. **N** and **L** vs. **P**), thus providing direct evidence for a role for the G/C repressor and some unknown transcription factor(s), possibly Sp1 or Sp1-like transcription factor(s), in injury-induced suppression of SM22α and the concomitant phenotypic modulation of the SMC. (Reprinted from Regan CP, Adam PJ, Madsen CS, et al. Molecular mechanisms of decreased smooth muscle cell differentiation marker expression after vascular injury. *J Clin Invest* 2000;106:1139–1147, with permission.)

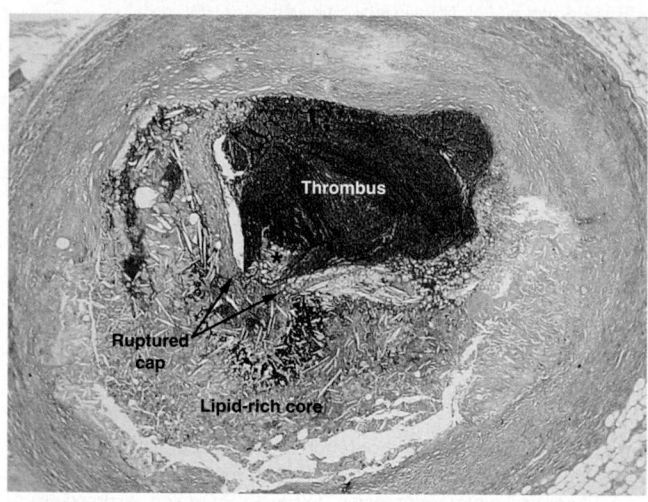

FIG. 31–1. Plaque rupture. Cross-sectioned coronary artery containing a lipid-rich atherothrombotic plaque with occlusive thrombosis superimposed. The fibrous cap covering the lipid-rich core is ruptured (between *arrows*) exposing the core (known to contain tissue factor) for the blood in the lumen. Atheromatous plaque content is displaced through the gap in the cap into the lumen (cholesterol crystals at *asterisk*), clearly indicating the sequence of events: Plaque rupture preceded thrombus formation. Trichrome stain, rendering thrombus (lumen) and hemorrhage (plaque) *red* and collagen *blue*.

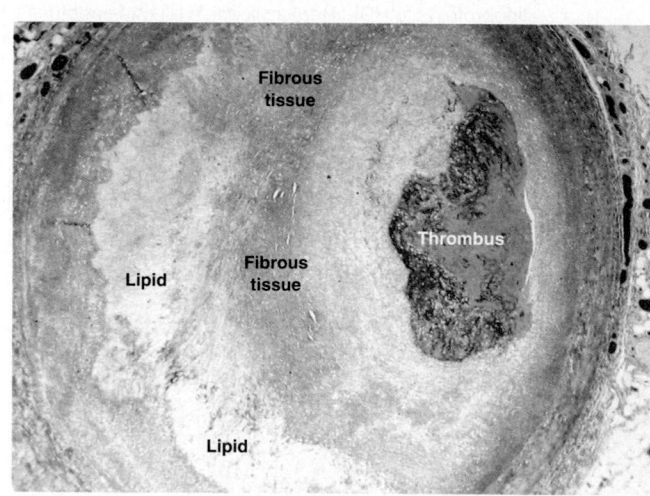

FIG. 31–2. Plaque erosion. Cross section of a coronary artery containing a severely stenotic atherothrombotic plaque with occlusive thrombosis superimposed. The lipid located deep in the plaque is covered by a thick and intact fibrous cap. The endothelium is missing at the plaque–thrombus interface, but the plaque surface is otherwise intact. Thus, there is no obvious local cause (plaque rupture) of thrombosis. Trichrome stain, rendering thrombus *red,* collagen *blue,* and lipid *colorless.*

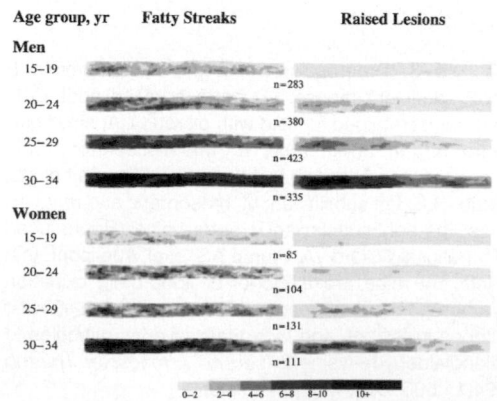

FIG. 32–2. Topographic prevalence map of fatty streaks and raised lesions in the right coronary artery of men and women by 5-year age groups. Color scale indicates prevalence. (Adapted from McGill HC Jr, Herderick EE, McMahan CA, et al. Atherosclerosis in youth. *Minerva Pediatr* 2002;54:437–447, with permission.)

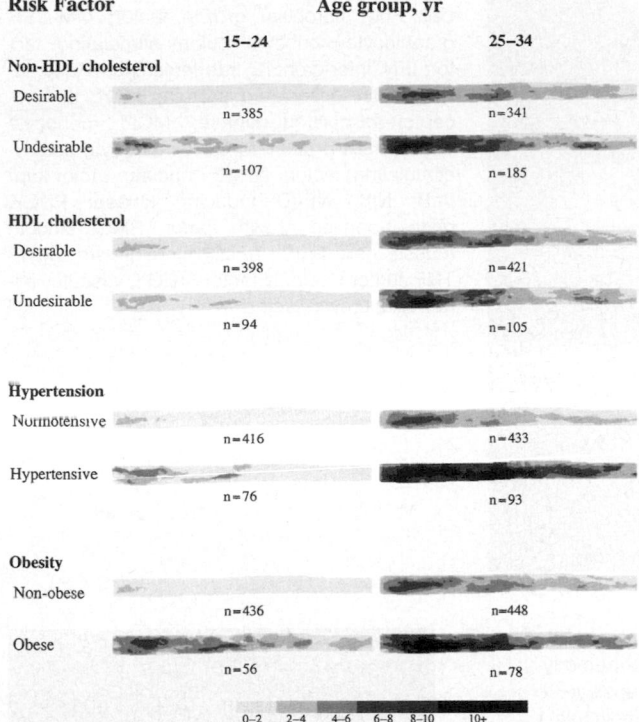

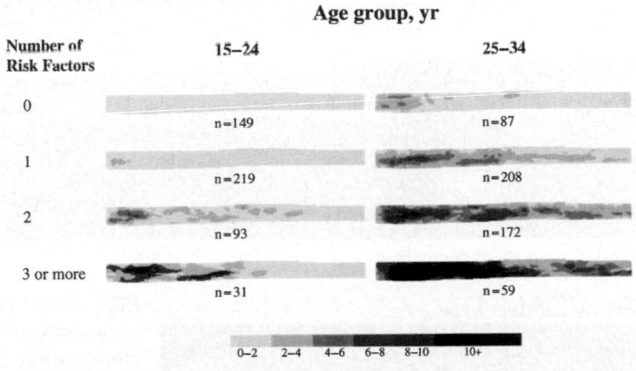

FIG. 32–4. Topographic prevalence map of raised lesions in the right coronary artery of men by 10-year age groups, high and low non–high-density lipoprotein (HDL) cholesterol, high and low HDL cholesterol, hypertension, and obesity. Color scale indicates prevalence. (Adapted from McGill HC Jr, Herderick EE, McMahan CA, et al. Atherosclerosis in youth. *Minerva Pediatr* 2002;54:437–447, with permission.)

FIG. 32–6. Prevalence map of raised lesions in the right coronary arteries of men by number of risk factors present and 10-year age groups. Color scale indicates prevalence. (Adapted from McGill HC Jr, Herderick EE, McMahan CA, et al. Atherosclerosis in youth. *Minerva Pediatr* 2002;54:437–447, with permission.)

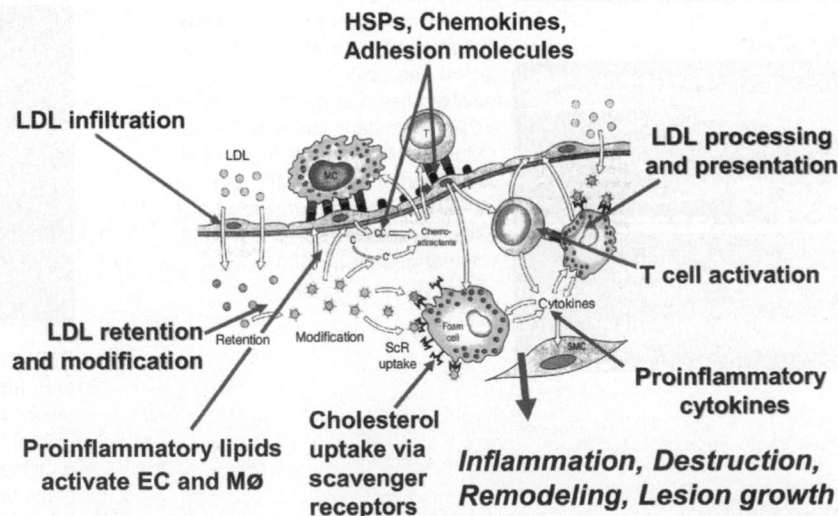

FIG. 36–1. Postulated recruitment and activation of immunocompetent cells in the early atherothrombotic lesion. Endothelial cells are stimulated to express vascular cell adhesion molecule-1, possibly by lysophosphatidylcholine or other components of LDL oxidized in the intima. Monocytes (*MC*) and T lymphocytes (*T*) adhere to endothelial VCAM-1 and other leukocyte adhesion molecules. They are stimulated chemotactically to enter the intima by chemokines such as macrophage chemoattractant protein-1, a potent chemotactic agent that is produced locally in the atherothrombotic plaque. The chemotactic complement fragment, C5a, is produced during complement activation (*C*), which may be secondary to low-density lipoprotein (*LDL*) oxidation (oxidized cholesterol) and may participate in recruitment of bloodborne cells. Antigen-specific T cells are activated by monocyte-derived macrophages (*Mø*) in the lesion. Both cell types produce cytokines that act on endothelial cells (*EC*), smooth muscle cells (*SMC*), macrophages, and foam cells to regulate adhesion molecule expression, chemotaxis, procoagulant activity, proliferation, contractility, and cholesterol uptake. In addition, EC and SMC release cytokines that act on both inflammatory and vascular cells. Vascular-derived cytokines are not indicated in the figure. HSPs, heat shock proteins; ScR; scavenger receptor.

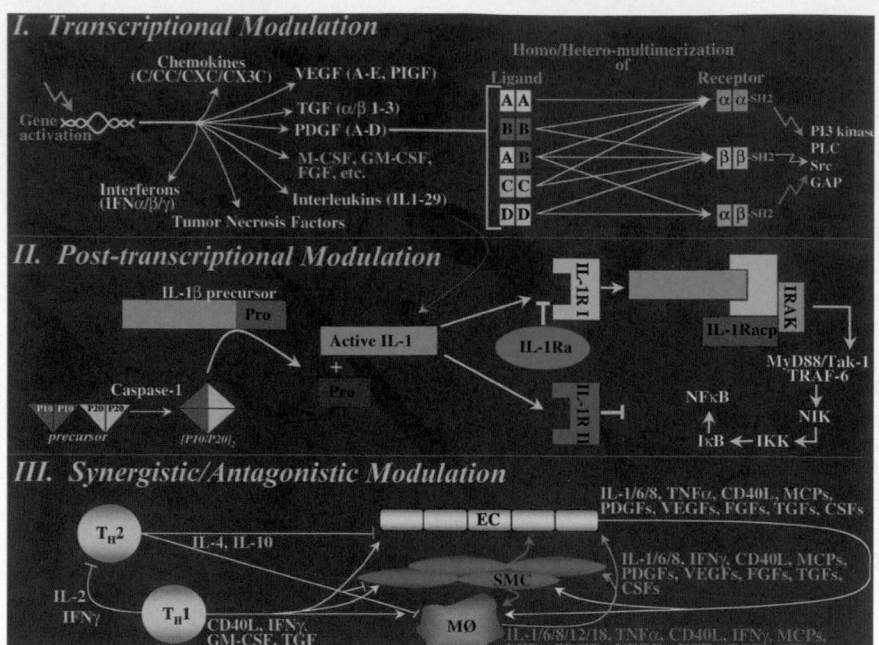

FIG. 38–1. Control mechanisms of the biologic activity of growth factors and cytokines. CSF, colony-stimulating factor; EC, endothelial cell; FGF, fibroblast growth factor; GM-CSF, granulocyte-monocyte colony-stimulating factor; IFN, interferon; IL, interleukin; IL-1Racp, IL-1 receptor–associated protein; IRAK, IL-1 receptor–associated kinase; MCP, monocyte chemotactic protein; M-CSF, monocyte colony-stimulating factor; NF-(B, nuclear factor-kappaB; NIK, NF-(B inducing kinase; PDGF, platelet-derived growth factor; SMC, smooth muscle cell; TGF, transforming growth factor; TNF, tumor necrosis factor; VEGF, vascular endothelial growth factor.

A. VCAM-1+/+

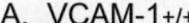

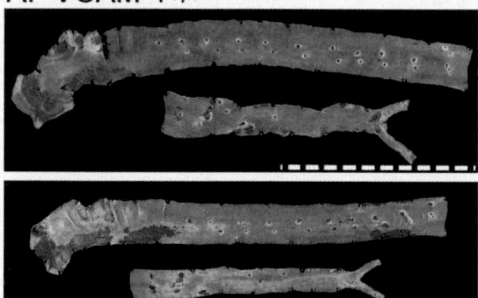

B. VCAM-1D4D/D4D

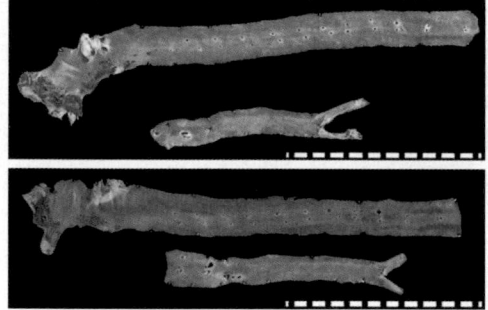

FIG. 39–2. Atherothrombosis in mice localizes to sites of hemodynamic stress and is sensitive to vascular cell adhesion molecule-1 (VCAM-1) expression and function. Highly localized lesion production (red, oil red O staining of lipid) in the aortae of low-density lipoprotein receptor knockout mice, without **(A)** and with **(B)** a mutation of the *VCAM-1* gene that reduced both expression and affinity of the adhesion molecule for counter-receptor. The inner curvature of the aorta is highly affected, as well as other reproducible sites, but much less so in VCAM-1 mutant animals. (From Cybulsky MI, Iiyama K, Li H, et al. A major role for VCAM-1, but not ICAM-1, in early atherosclerosis. *J Clin Invest* 2001;107:1255–1262, with permission.)

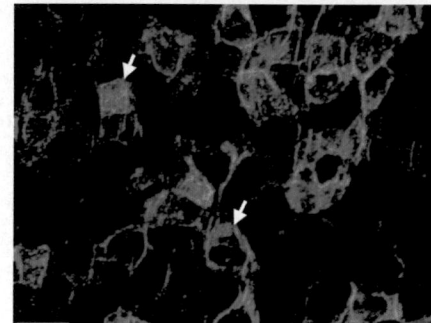

FIG. 39–4. Cross section of a human coronary artery 11 months after heart transplantation. The prominent diffuse and concentric intimal thickening has narrowed the lumen to a central slit (*arrow*). Hematoxylin and eosin stain, original magnification ×60.

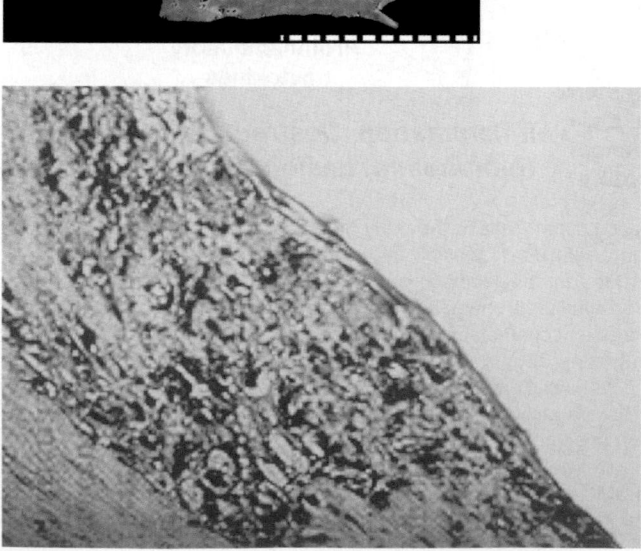

FIG. 42–17. Endothelin in patients with atherothrombosis. Plasma levels of endothelin-1 are significantly greater in patients with atherothrombosis. Endothelin-1 can be detected immunohistochemically in endothelial cells and in the intima and media of arteries of patients with atherothrombosis. (Modified from Lerman A, Edwards BS, Hallett JW, et al. Circulating and tissue endothelin immunoreactivity in advanced atherosclerosis. *N Engl J Med* 1991;325:997–1001, by permission.)

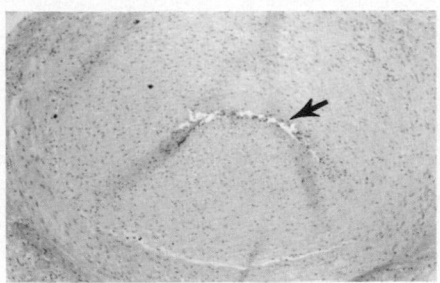

FIG. 43–1. Cross section of a human coronary artery 11 months after heart transplantation. The prominent diffuse and concentric intimal thickening has narrowed the lumen to a central slit (*arrow*). Hematoxylin and eosin stain, original magnification ×60.

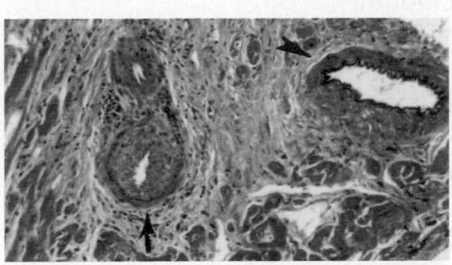

FIG. 43–2. Rat heart allograft obtained approximately 70 days after transplantation, showing one artery affected by transplant arteriosclerosis (*arrow*) and a nearby artery profile, which is normal in appearance (*arrowhead*). Hematoxylin and eosin stain, original magnification ×115.

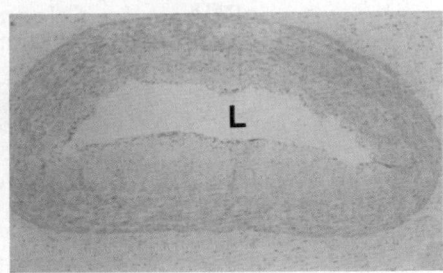

FIG. 43–3. Serial sections of an affected human coronary artery taken a few months after transplantation. Hematoxylin andeosin–stained section showing some diffuse intimal thickening, but a noncompromised lumen (*L*). A fibrotic adventitia (*A*) with some inflammation is present. Methyl green nuclear counterstain, original magnification ×24.

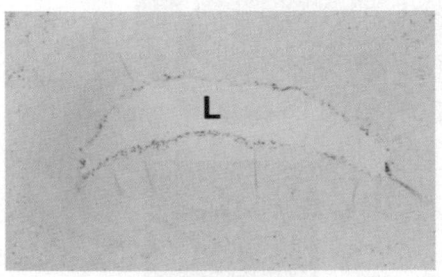

FIG. 43–4. Serial sections of an affected human coronary artery taken a few months after transplantation. CD45 antibody reaction for lymphocytes and monocytes showing a thin periluminal accumulation of inflammatory cells, just underneath the endothelium. Scattered lymphocytes in adventitia (*A*) also are seen. This pattern has been termed "endothelialitis" by some investigators. Methyl green nuclear counterstain, original magnification ×24. L, lumen.

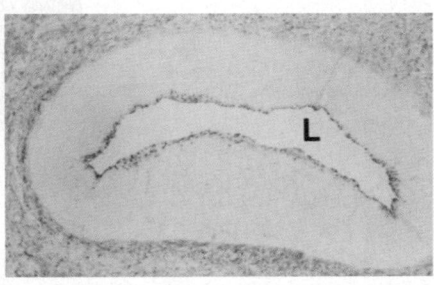

FIG. 43–5. Serial sections of an affected human coronary artery taken a few months after transplantation. HAM56 antibody reaction for macrophages showing a similar periluminal collection. Scattered macrophages in the adventitia (*A*) are also seen. Methyl green nuclear counterstain, original magnification ×24. L, lumen.

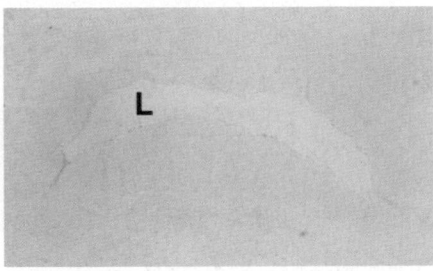

FIG. 43–6. Serial sections of an affected human coronary artery taken a few months after transplantation. CD20 antibody for B cells showing no appreciable number of B lymphocytes in this tissue. Methyl green nuclear counterstain, original magnification ×24. L, lumen.

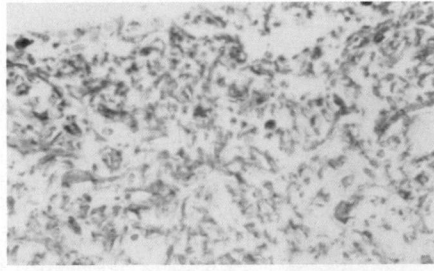

FIG. 43–7. Human transplant arteriosclerosis lesion from heart 3 years after transplantation. Here a double stain for smooth muscle cells (anti–smooth muscle (-actin as blue reaction product) and the proliferating cell nuclear antigen (PCNA; brown reaction product, e.g., *arrow*). The artery lumen (*L*) is at the top. Neutral red nuclear counterstain, original magnification ×370.

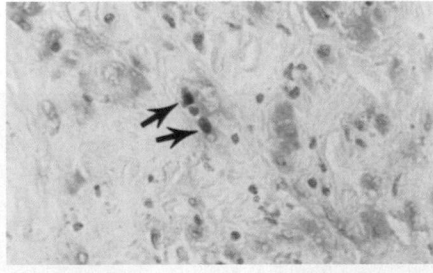

FIG. 43–8. Human transplant arteriosclerosis lesion from a heart 2 years after transplantation. Here a double immunolabeling for CD68 positive macrophages (blue reaction product) and the proliferating cell nuclear antigen (PCNA; brown reaction product, see *arrow*) has been performed indicating several intimal macrophages in this area, two of which show proliferative activity (*arrows*). Neutral red nuclear counterstain, original magnification ×370.

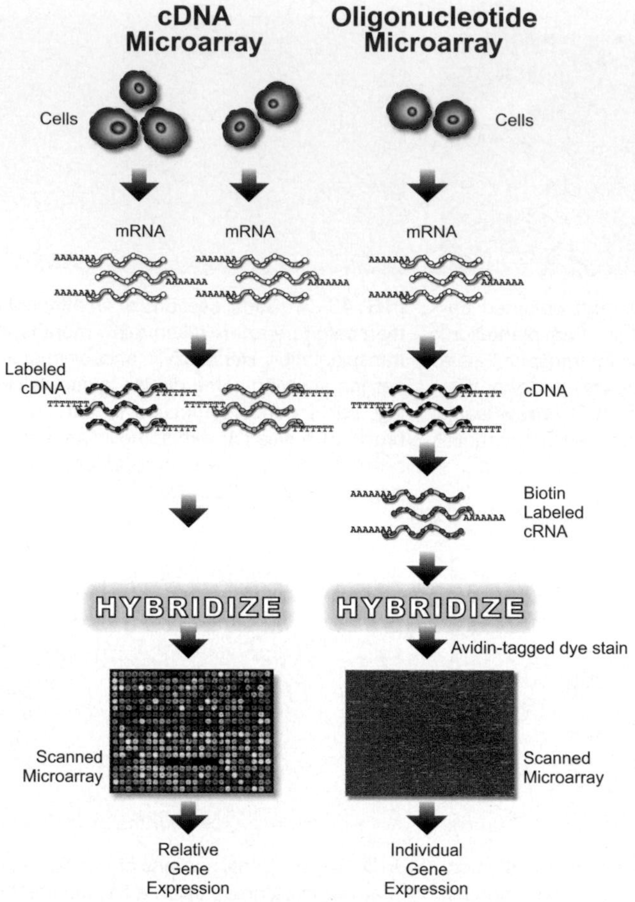

cDNA Microarray **Oligonucleotide Microarray**

Cells

mRNA   mRNA   mRNA

Labeled
cDNA

cDNA

Biotin
Labeled
cRNA

HYBRIDIZE   HYBRIDIZE

Avidin-tagged dye stain

Scanned
Microarray

Scanned
Microarray

Relative
Gene
Expression

Individual
Gene
Expression

FIG. 45–2. Differential expression of messenger RNA (mRNA) by cells and gene expression profiling using DNA microarrays. After mRNA is isolated from cells or tissues, it can be analyzed using complementary DNA (cDNA) microarrays, in which two-sample comparisons are made, or oligonucleotide microarrays, in which the gene expression profile of an individual sample is assessed.

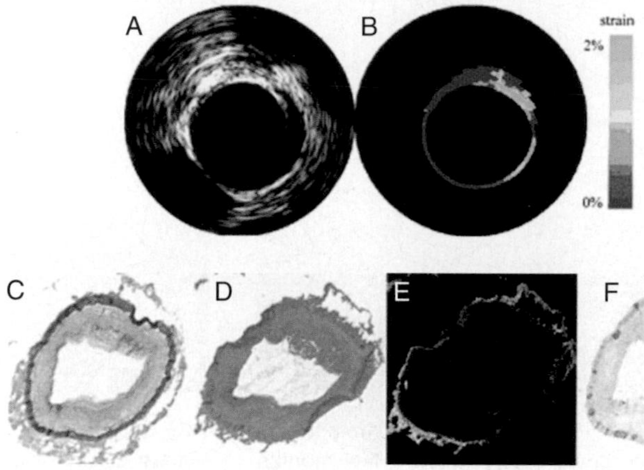

A   B   strain
2%

0%

C   D   E   F

FIG. 49–1. Intravascular ultrasound (IVUS) echogram **(A)** and elastogram **(B)** of an early fatty plaque. The strain in this plaque is high, which indicates soft material. Histology (elastin-van Gieson **[C]**, picro-Sirius red **[D]**, picro-Sirius red imaged with polarized light microscopy **[E]**, and acid phosphatase **[F]**) reveals a lack of collagen in this plaque and a heavy staining of macrophages. The geometry of the cross section is distorted because of shrinkage caused by freezing. (Reproduced from de Korte CL, Sierevogel MJ, Mastik F, et al. Identification of atherosclerotic plaque components with intravascular ultrasound elastography in vivo: a Yucatan Pig Study. *Circulation* 2002;105:1627–1630, with permission.)

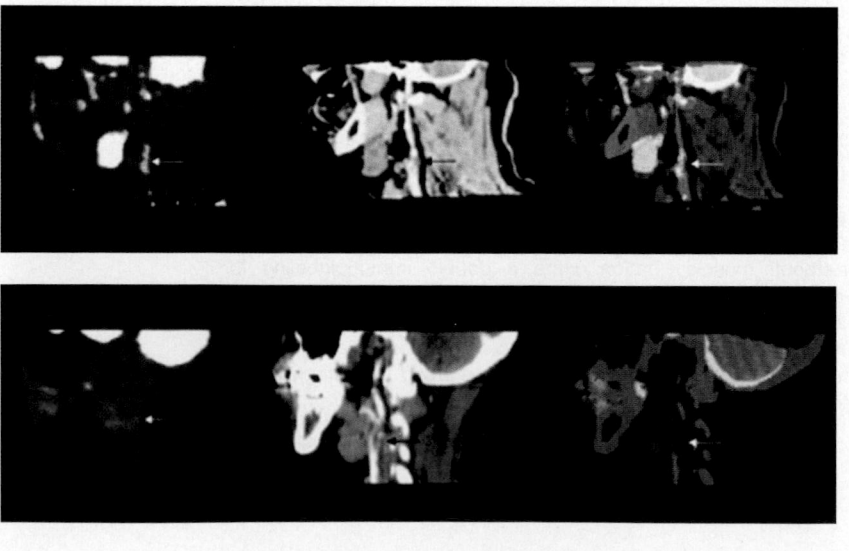

FIG. 49–7. The **upper row** (*left to right*) shows positron emission tomography (PET), contrast computed tomography (CT), and coregistered PET/CT images in the sagittal plane from a 63-year-old man who had experienced two episodes of left-sided hemiparesis. Angiography demonstrated stenosis of the proximal right internal carotid artery; this was confirmed on the CT image (*black arrow*). The *white arrows* show [^{18}F]-fluorodeoxyglucose (^{18}FDG) uptake at the level of the plaque in the carotid artery. As expected, there was high ^{18}FDG uptake in the brain, jaw muscles, and facial soft tissues. The **bottom row** (*left to right*) demonstrates a low level of ^{18}FDG uptake in an asymptomatic carotid stenosis. The *black arrow* highlights the stenosis on the CT angiogram, and the *white arrows* demonstrate minimal ^{18}FDG accumulation at this site on the ^{18}FDG-PET and coregistered PET/CT images. (Reproduced from Tsimikas S, Palinski W, Halpern SE, et al. Radiolabeled MDA2, an oxidation-specific, monoclonal antibody, identifies native atherosclerotic lesions in vivo. *J Nucl Cardiol* 1999;6:41–53, with permission.)

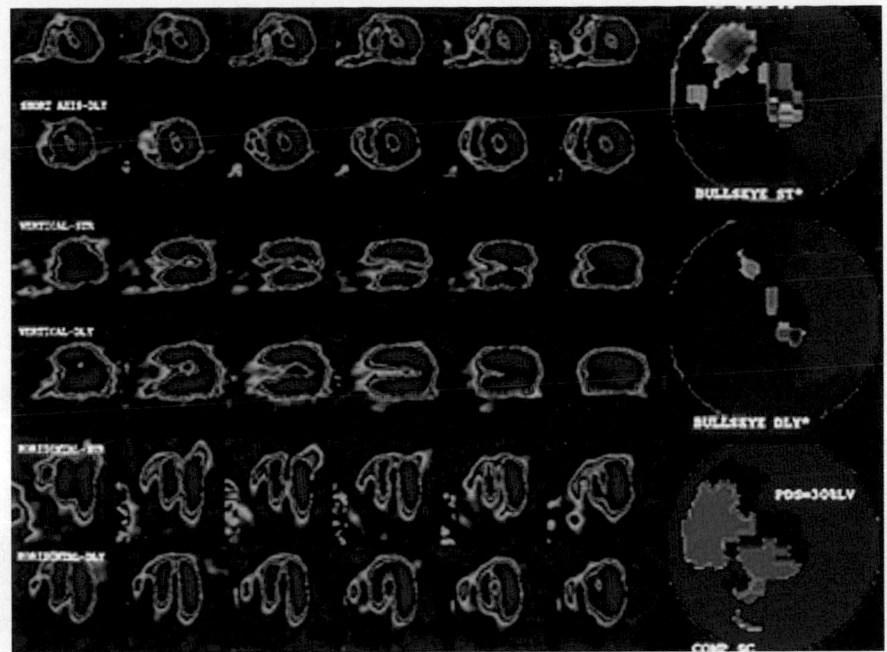

FIG. 51–6. Electron beam computed tomography and single photon emission computed tomography (SPECT) images of a 52-year-old, asymptomatic, hypertensive, hyperlipidemic man who had a high-risk CACS of 780. Calcium is shown as intensely *white areas* within all of the three coronary arteries. The treadmill test was terminated at 11 minutes because of patient fatigue, and the 12-lead electrocardiogram showed no evidence of ischemia at peak exercise. SPECT demonstrated a large, predominantly reversible 30% perfusion defect within the left anterior descending (LAD) coronary artery vascular territory. Coronary angiography showed subtotal stenosis of the proximal LAD coronary artery and 50% stenosis of the mid-right coronary artery. The patient underwent successful angioplasty and stenting of the LAD coronary artery. Results of repeat-exercise SPECT 6 months later was entirely normal. DLY, delay; PDS, perfusion defect size; STR, stress.

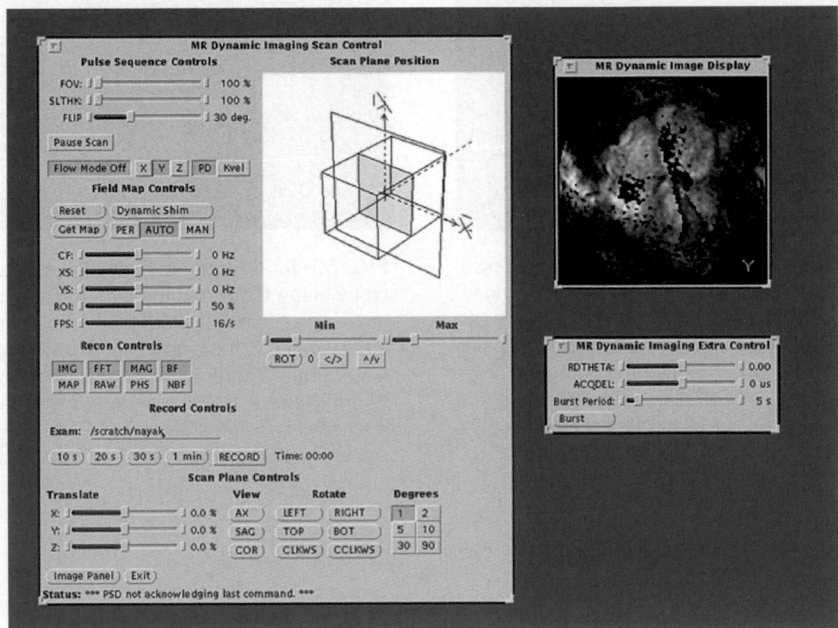

FIG. 52–2. A graphic user interface window of the real-time system including scan control, image display, imaging extra control, and imaging display. (From Nayak KS, Pauly JM, Kerr AB, et al. Real-time color flow MRI. *Magn Reson Med* 2000;43;251–258, with permission.)

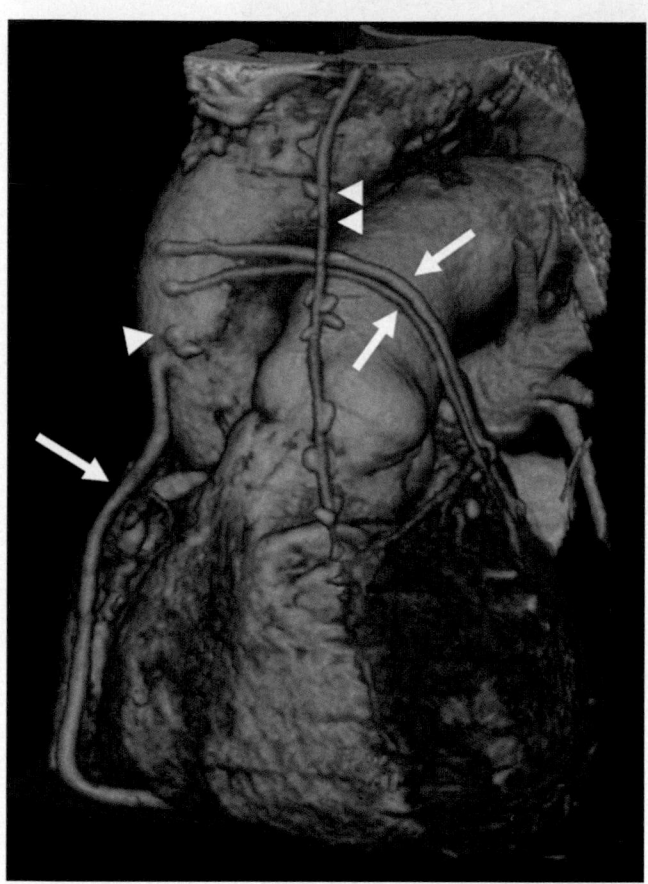

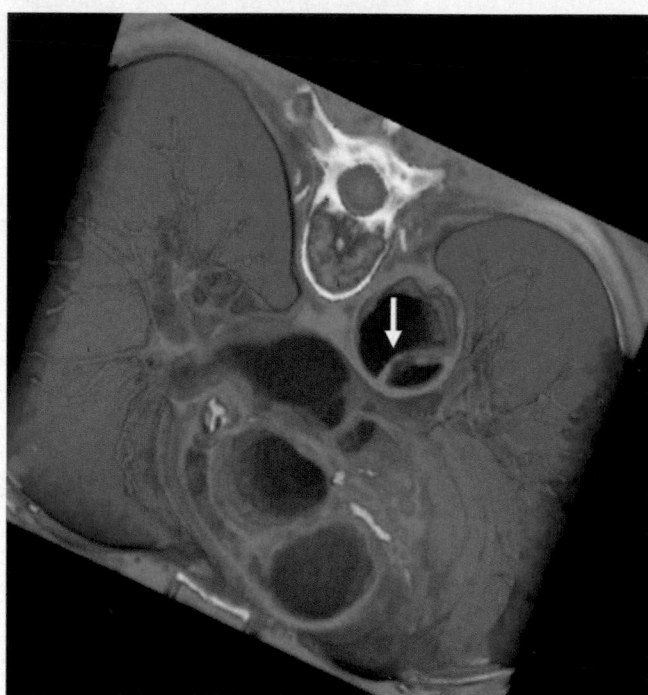

FIG. 53–3. Contrast-enhanced, 16-detector-row computed tomography bypass angiography. The three-dimensional volume-rendering reconstruction technique depicts three patent venous bypass grafts (*arrows*), one proximally occluded venous bypass graft (*arrowhead*), and a patent arterial bypass graft (*double arrowheads*). (From Wintersperger BJ, Nikolaou K, Jakobs TF, et al. Cardiac multidetector-row computed tomography: initial experience using 16 detector-row systems. *Crit Rev Comput Tomogr* 2003;44:27–45, with permission.)

FIG. 53–6. Contrast-enhanced multidetector-row computed tomography of the thoracic aorta. Single-slice images show a dissection of the aorta, originating from the aortic arch and extending distally into the descending thoracic aorta. A color-coded volume-rendering technique gives a three-dimensional overview of the thoracic anatomy. (From Huber A, Matzko M, Wintersperger BJ, et al. [Reconstruction methods in postprocessing of CT- and MR-angiography of the aorta]. *Radiologe* 2001;41:689–694, with permission.)

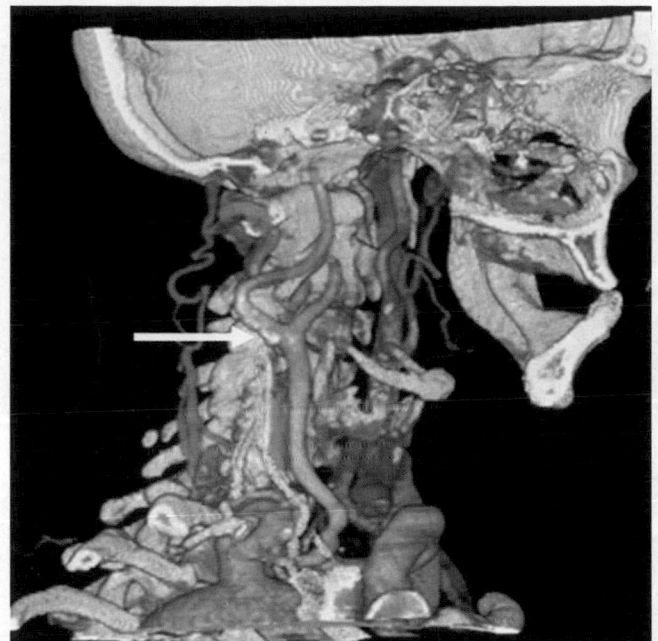

FIG. 53–9. Contrast-enhanced multidetector-row tomography of the supraaortal vessels. Maximum intensity projection and volume-rendering technique of the right carotid artery both reveal a calcified lesion at the height of the bifurcation, but no significant stenosis (*arrows*). (Courtesy of C. R. Becker, Ludwig-Maximilians-University, Munich, Germany.)

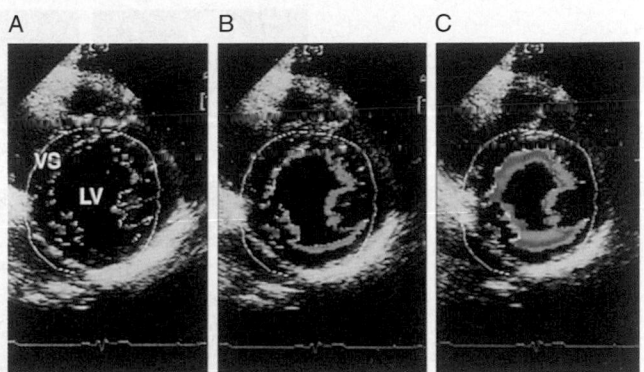

FIG. 60–5. A–C: Sequential frames during systole, illustrating a progressive color-encoded display of the inward movement of the endocardium by color kinesis. LV, left ventricle; VS, ventricular septum. (Courtesy of the American Society of Echocardiography.)

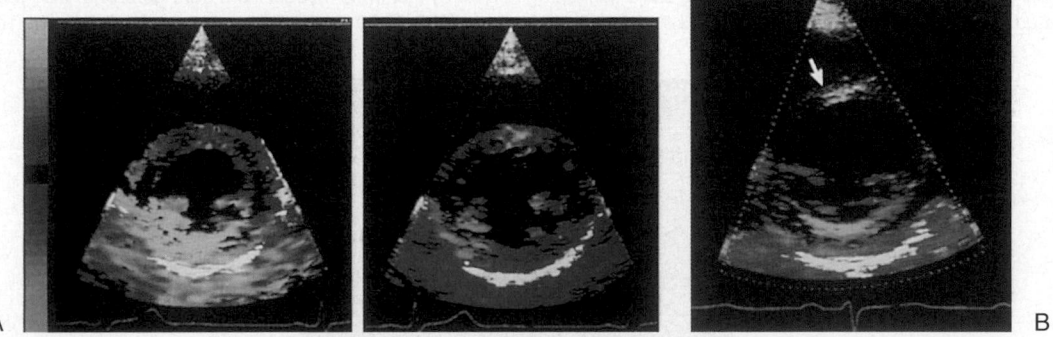

FIG. 60–4. A: Tissue Doppler images, parasternal short-axis view, of the left ventricle (LV) in a healthy subject. **Left:** During mid-systole, the anteroseptal wall appears *bright blue* and the posterior wall *bright red,* indicating good contraction toward the center of the ventricle. **Right:** In early diastole, the anteroseptal wall appears to be *bright red* and the posterior wall *bright blue,* indicating movement away from the center of the ventricle. **B:** Tissue Doppler image, parasternal short-axis view, of the LV in a patient with anteroseptal myocardial infarction. During mid-systole, the anteroseptal wall shows no color (*arrow*), indicating akinetic wall motion. (Courtesy of the American College of Cardiology.)

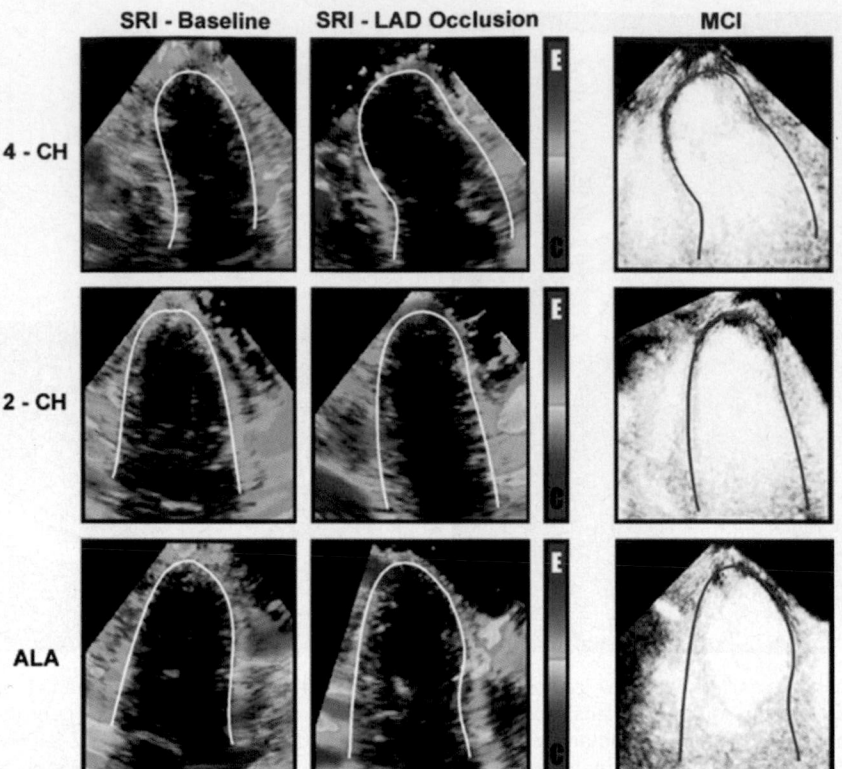

FIG. 60–7. A–C: Apical strain rate imaging (*SRI*) views at baseline and during acute left anterior descending coronary artery (*LAD*) occlusion at the end of the isovolumic relaxation period. The color bars (yellow-red and cyan-blue) indicate compression (*C*) and expansion (*E*) strain rates, respectively. Compared with baseline, SRI views after LAD occlusion demonstrate persisting, high-intensity compression patterns (i.e., red or orange hues) in the apical region. Myocardial contrast images (MCI) on the *right* were acquired in the same views (apical 4-chamber [*4-CH*], 2-chamber [*2-CH*], and long axis [*ALA*]), and delineated in the same way as the SRI occlusion views. The MCI data demonstrate the distribution of the perfusion pattern. The perfusion defect appears dark and is spatially consistent with the distribution of the persisting compression patterns. The SRI and MCI data within the myocardial midline were interactively delineated (*white* and *red outlines,* respectively). (From Jamal F, Kukulski T, D'hooge J, et al. Abnormal postsystolic thickening in acutely ischemic myocardium during coronary angioplasty: a velocity, strain, strain rate Doppler myocardial imaging study. J Am Soc Echocardiogr 1999;12:994–996, by permission from Elsevier.)

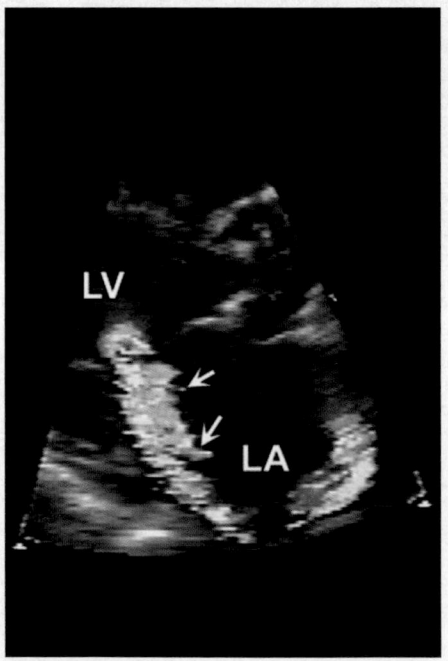

FIG. 60–21. Transthoracic parasternal long-axis view in a patient with severe ischemic mitral regurgitation after inferior myocardial infarction. Color Doppler showing severe posteriorly directed jet of mitral regurgitation (*white arrows*). LA, left atrium; LV, left ventricle. (Courtesy of Dr. William K. Freeman, Mayo Clinic, Rochester, MN.)

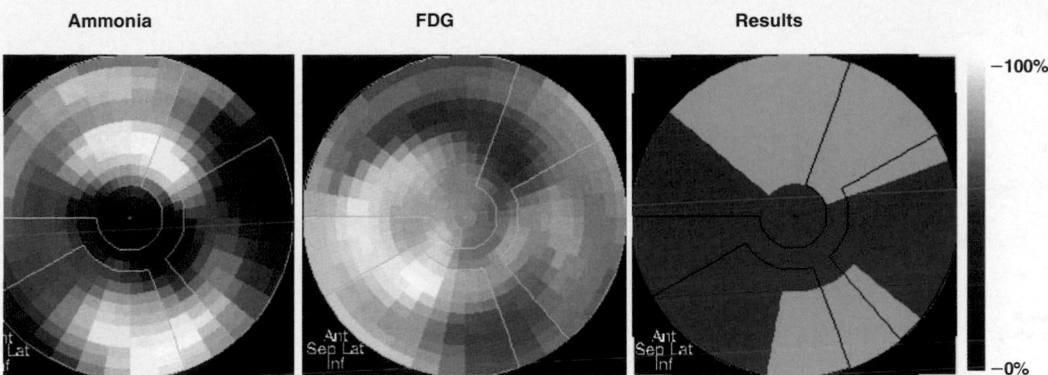

FIG. 64–7. Polar map display of the myocardial distribution of blood flow (nitrogen-13 ammonia) and of glucose utilization (fluorine-18 deoxyglucose [FDG]) in a patient with a prior myocardial infarction. The difference polar map (**right, results**) displays the types of blood flow metabolism patterns together with their location and geographic extent (*green* represent normal; *blue* represents mismatch, *red* represents match). In this patient, the ammonia polar images demonstrate diminished perfusion of the interventricular septum that, however, as seen on the FDG polar map, is associated with increased glucose utilization, resulting in an extensive blood flow–metabolism mismatch. The polar maps were constructed using the Munich Heart Software.

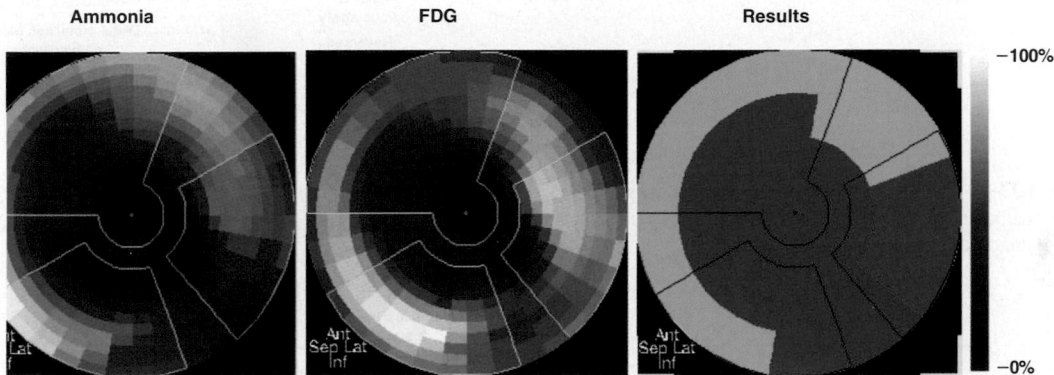

FIG. 64–8. Polar map displays of the distribution of myocardial blood flow and glucose utilization in a patient with a prior anterior myocardial infarction. Both myocardial blood flow and glucose utilization are severely reduced in the anterior wall and the apex of the left ventricular myocardium, resulting in an extensive blood flow–metabolism match (*red*). A relatively small region of a mismatch is noted in the lateral wall (*blue*). FDG, fluorine-18 deoxyglucose.

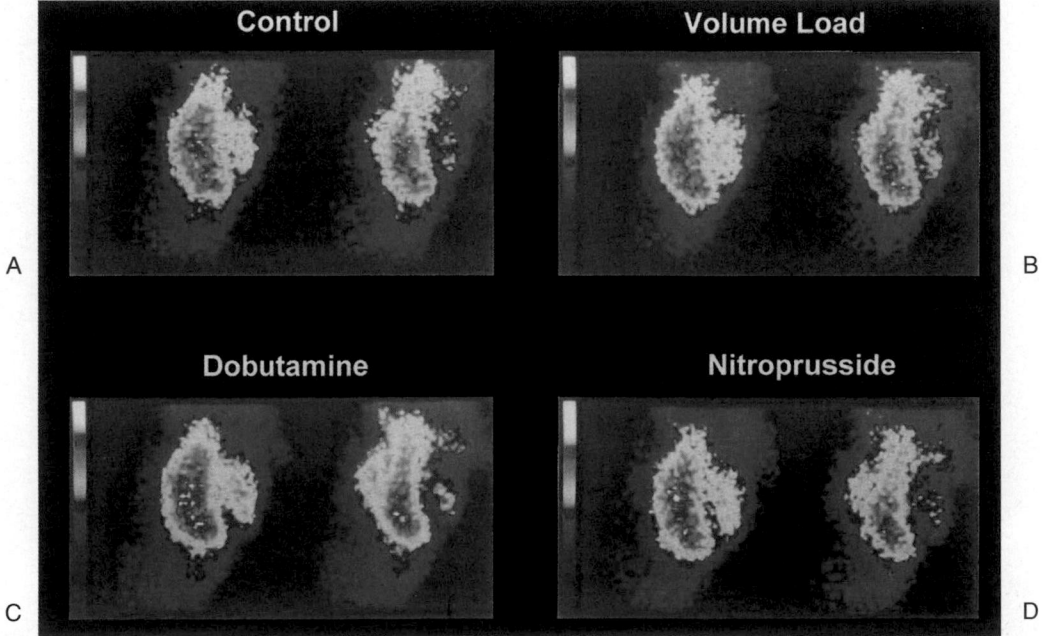

FIG. 75–9. Radionuclide angiogram demonstrating end-diastolic and end-systolic images of the right and left ventricles at baseline **(A)** and after volume load **(B)**, dobutamine **(C)**, and nitroprusside **(D)** infusions. The right ventricular apex and lateral wall are akinetic, whereas high outflow tract demonstrates normal contractility, all of which are unchanged by volume and nitroprusside but markedly improved by dobutamine resulting in a significant increase in right ventricular ejection fraction (Fig. 75–10). (From Dell'Italia LJ, Starling MR, Blumhardt R, et al. Comparative effects of volume loading, dobutamine and nitroprusside in patients with predominant right ventricular infarction. *Circulation* 1985;72:1327–1335, with permission.)

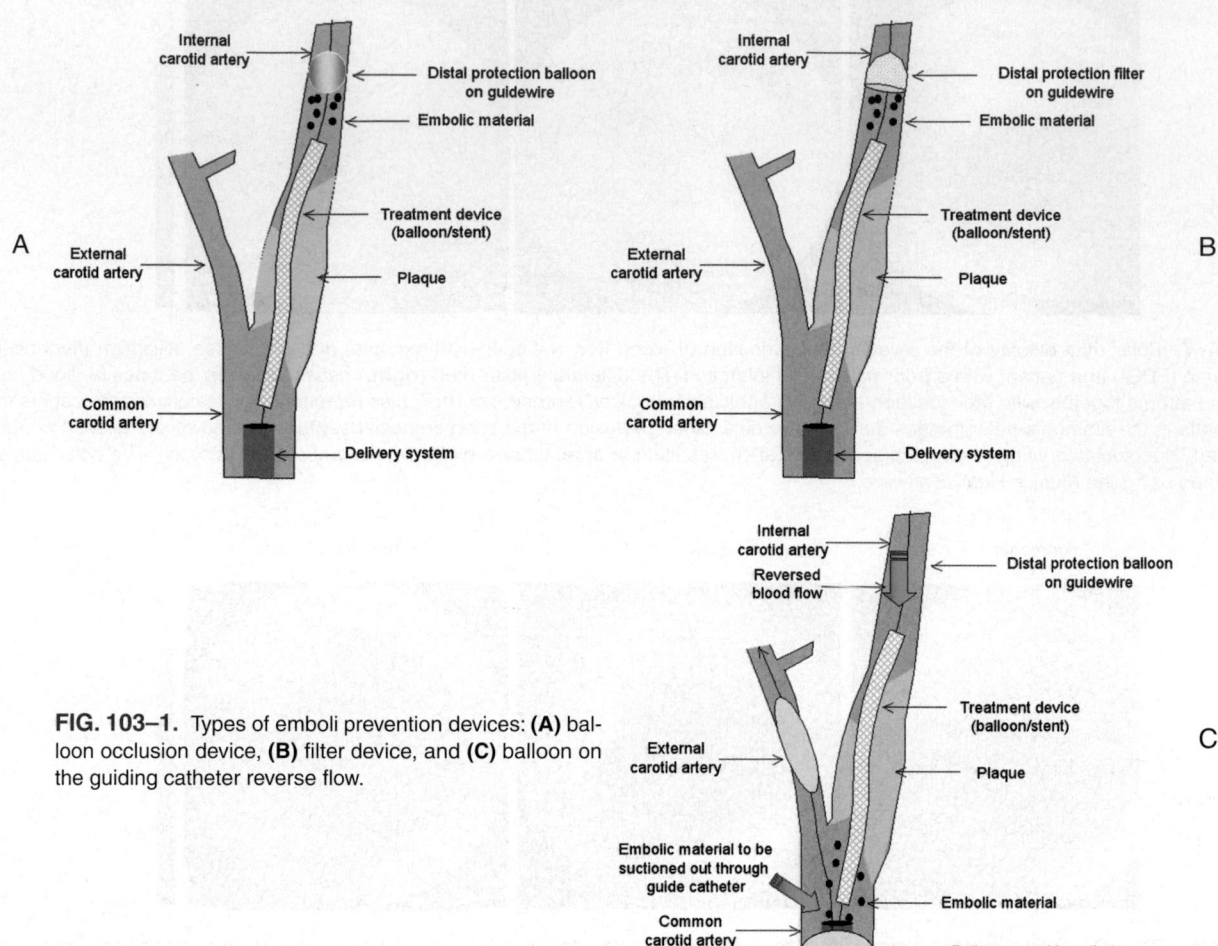

FIG. 103–1. Types of emboli prevention devices: **(A)** balloon occlusion device, **(B)** filter device, and **(C)** balloon on the guiding catheter reverse flow.

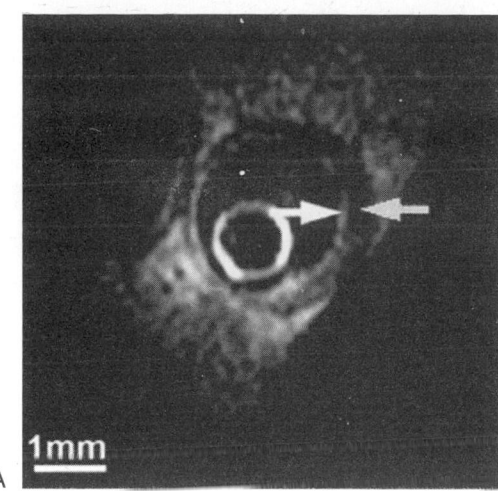

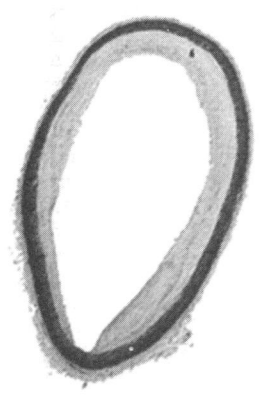

FIG. 49–6. Comparison of intravenous magnetic resonance (MR) coil image (T2W) with the corresponding histopathology section demonstrating the excellent agreement between the two for plaque morphology. Furthermore, one can appreciate the bright luminal fibrous cap *(arrow pointing to the right)* from the darker lipidic region *(arrow pointing to the left)* with the resolution obtained with the intravenous MR coil. (Reproduced from Ocali O, Atalar E. Intravascular magnetic resonance imaging using a loopless catheter antenna. *Magn Reson Med* 1997;37:112–118, with permission.) (See color insert for Fig. 49–7.)

perfluorocarbon paramagnetic nanoparticles *in vitro* (105, 106) and *in vivo* (106), or by a paramagnetic dendrimeric contrast agent (107), whereas activated platelets have been targeted through the interaction of a ultrasmall superparamagnetic particles of iron oxide (USPIO)-arginine-glycine-aspartic acid (RGD) peptide construct with the $\alpha_{IIb}\beta_3$ receptor (108).

Magnetic Resonance–guided Vascular Intervention

High-resolution images of vessel wall, excellent delineation of perivascular soft tissue structures, inherent versatility of multiple plane viewing, virtual real-time images and the ability to acquire angiographic and hemodynamic data make MRI an exceptionally promising platform for intravascular intervention (109). Preliminary studies have indicated the feasibility of MR-guided percutaneous angioplasty in rabbit aorta (110), and stent deployment in pig femoral (111), rabbit aorta (92), and pig coronary arteries (112), and for monitoring of catheter-based gene therapy in pig femoral artery (113). In humans, intraoperative MR has been shown to be safe and effective for intracranial neurosurgery (114), though *trans*-vascular applications are, thus far, limited (115). MR-guided coronary intervention is a relatively distant objective.

MOLECULAR IMAGING OF PLAQUE

Determination of plaque composition in the modalities discussed earlier is based on evaluation of a wide range of inherent physical properties of the tissues of the arterial wall. An alternative approach is to image plaque through the introduction of contrast agents that are targeted to specific sites or processes and provide output data that, ideally, can be precisely localized and quantified. An increasing appreciation of cellular and molecular events within atherothrombotic plaque has been accompanied by imaginative application of imaging tools to spawn a new field of "molecular imaging" (116–119).

Nuclear Scintigraphic Techniques

The potential diagnostic utility of radiotracers for imaging atherothrombotic lesions has been examined in animal models and in humans (120). For example, technetium-99m–labeled oxidized low-density lipoprotein (oxLDL) particles (121) have been shown to localize to human carotid atherothrombotic plaque using noninvasive tomographic scintigraphy, and autoradiography of endarterectomized carotid artery showed radiolabeled oxLDL localized to macrophages (122). Alternative approaches have used radiolabeled peptide fragments (123) and monoclonal antibodies (124) directed at plaque components. Nuclear techniques can be limited *in vivo* where labeled particles are cleared slowly from circulating blood and contribute a low target to background scintigraphic ratio. A further disadvantage of *in vivo* scintigraphy is relatively poor spatial resolution and paucity of anatomic information about the plaque. Anatomic information can be enhanced by coregistration of scintigraphic images with CT or MRI (125).

Positron emission tomography (PET) and single photon emission computed tomography benefit from imaging agents that can be detected in extremely low concentration (picomolar range) and provide excellent sensitivity for application to molecular imaging, but with less spatial resolution than other technologies (126). After intravenous injection, of [^{18}F]-fluorodeoxyglucose (^{18}FDG), a glucose analog that marks active glycolysis, Rudd and coworkers (125) demonstrated its accumulation in the plaques of patients with symptomatic carotid atherothrombosis and confirmed their noninvasive [18]FDG-positron emission tomography ([18]FDG-PET) findings by autoradiography after carotid endarterectomy (Fig. 49–7) (see color insert). Others have shown correlation between plaque macrophage content and signal from [18]FDG-PET (127).

Targeted Contrast-enhanced Magnetic Resonance Imaging

In contrast to PET, MRI provides excellent spatial resolution but is inherently limited by SNR. Much interest is focussed on the development of contrast-enhancing molecular probes for use in high-resolution MRI (117,128).

Contrast agents that specifically identify components of vulnerable plaque are of considerable interest. Macrophage-rich areas are a pathologic correlate of unstable plaque (4). Small SPIO and USPIO have T1-shortening properties and are taken up avidly by macrophages. In some small studies, injection of USPIO into hyperlipidemic rabbits was associated with accumulation in macrophages and, after 2 hours (129) to 5 days (130), the appearance of signal voids studded on the luminal surface of the aorta. Similar appearances have been observed incidentally in the aorta and intrapelvic arteries of humans that have received USPIO for oncologic imaging (131). This type of specific cellular targeting approach warrants further investigation.

Magnetic Resonance Imaging and Molecular Imaging

Louie and coworkers (132) developed a MR contrast agent capable of reporting activity of a β-galactosidase. The paramagnetic agent (abbreviated EgadMe) requires interaction with a water molecule to generate increased MR signal in T1-weighted images. In the resting state, however, its interaction with water is prevented by the attachment of galactopyranose, a "blocking group" that is susceptible to enzymatic cleavage by β-galactosidase. The subsequent association of water with EgadMe results in an increase of T1 signal by ~60%. Using this approach it was possible to localize the lineage of a cell injected with β-galactosidase mRNA in early embryonic development. The ability to image areas in which β-galactosidase is active may be of considerable use in the study of transgenic animals and in mapping sites of expression in vivo in gene therapy. Moreover, this technique may represent a paradigm of intelligent contrast agents that are activated in response to specific biologic events. EgadMe and its successors may be conjugated with blocking units that are substrates for other enzymes. In the context of atherothrombosis, matrix metalloproteinases (MMPs) digest collagen, elastin, and other matrix components. MMPs have the additional advantage of extracellular activity, thus circumventing the problem of intracellular access by contrast agents.

The endothelial cell surface protein vascular cell adhesion molecule-1 (VCAM-1) or intercellular adhesion molecule-1 (ICAM-1) is up-regulated in atherothrombotic plaque (133, 134) and in areas of artery prone to lesion formation (135). Exposure to circulating blood renders such molecules potential targets for monoclonal antibody–conjugated intravascular MR contrast agents. Antibodies conjugated to paramagnetic liposomes have been used to image, *ex vivo*, ICAM expression in a murine model of multiple sclerosis (136) and $\alpha_v\beta_3$ integrin expression as a marker of angiogenesis (137, 138). Where cells are accessible to blood, perhaps as a consequence of abnormal vascular permeability in plaques, imaging specific receptor expression using contrast–ligand constructs also should be feasible (139).

Enzyme Activity

Chen and coworkers (140) have developed fluorescent imaging probes that can be injected intravenously in an inactive or "quenched" form. After site-specific cleavage by proteolytic enzymes, the probe become brightly fluorescent and could be imaged by near infrared spectroscopy. This technique imaged cathepsin B activity in the atherothrombotic plaques of apolipoprotein E–deficient mice, but it is amenable to modification for broader application. Indeed, the same principle has been applied to image the activity of thrombin, a serine protease that plays a key role in thrombosis (141).

CONCLUSIONS

Imaging is key to the diagnosis and treatment of atherothrombotic disease and in determining both response to treatment and prognosis. New invasive and noninvasive imaging techniques described here begin the important task of atherothrombosis characterization. Most of the modalities described may be viewed as in the developmental stage, and the particular advantages and limitations of each have been discussed. It is not yet possible to predict in which of the many experimental techniques refinement and further development will lead to clinical application. The ideal modality will provide safe, rapid, high-resolution images that describe the anatomy and microanatomy of the arterial wall, plaque, and associated structures, most notably thrombus. It will inform on plaque composition and will provide insight into cellular and molecular processes, including inflammation and enzymic activity. Finally, it must be affordable, accessible, and compatible with imaging modalities and commonly used devices, including metallic intravascular stents.

REFERENCES

1. Farb A, Burke AP, Tang AL, et al. Coronary plaque erosion without rupture into a lipid core. A frequent cause of coronary thrombosis in sudden coronary death. *Circulation* 1996;93:1354–1363.
2. Virmani R, Kolodgie FD, Burke AP, et al. Lessons from sudden coronary death: a comprehensive morphological classification scheme for atherosclerotic lesions. *Arterioscler Thromb Vasc Biol* 2000;20:1262–1275.

3. Richardson PD, Davies MJ, Born GV. Influence of plaque configuration and stress distribution on fissuring of coronary atherosclerotic plaques. *Lancet* 1989;2:941–944.

4. Moreno PR, Falk E, Palacios IF, et al. Macrophage infiltration in acute coronary syndromes. Implications for plaque rupture. *Circulation* 1994;90:775–778.

5. Falk E, Shah PK, Fuster V. Coronary plaque disruption. *Circulation* 1995;92:657–671.

6. Nissen SE, Yock P. Intravascular ultrasound: novel pathophysiological insights and current clinical applications. *Circulation* 2001;103:604–616.

7. Nissen SE. Application of intravascular ultrasound to characterize coronary artery disease and assess the progression or regression of atherosclerosis. *Am J Cardiol* 2002;89:24B–31B.

8. Prati F, Arbustini E, Labellarte A, et al. Correlation between high frequency intravascular ultrasound and histomorphology in human coronary arteries. *Heart* 2001;85:567–570.

9. Kawasaki M, Takatsu H, Noda T, et al. In vivo quantitative tissue characterization of human coronary arterial plaques by use of integrated backscatter intravascular ultrasound and comparison with angioscopic findings. *Circulation* 2002;105:2487–2492.

10. Nair A, Kuban BD, Tuzcu EM, et al. Coronary plaque classification with intravascular ultrasound radiofrequency data analysis. *Circulation* 2002;106:2200–2206.

11. Carlier SG, de Korte CL, Brusseau E, et al. Imaging of atherosclerosis. Elastography. *J Cardiovasc Risk* 2002;9:237–245.

12. de Korte CL, Pasterkamp G, van der Steen AF, et al. Characterization of plaque components with intravascular ultrasound elastography in human femoral and coronary arteries in vitro. *Circulation* 2000;102:617–623.

13. de Korte CL, Sierevogel MJ, Mastik F, et al. Identification of atherosclerotic plaque components with intravascular ultrasound elastography in vivo: a Yucatan Pig Study. *Circulation* 2002;105:1627–1630.

14. Komiyama N, Berry GJ, Kolz ML, et al. Tissue characterization of atherosclerotic plaques by intravascular ultrasound radiofrequency signal analysis: an in vitro study of human coronary arteries. *Am Heart J* 2000;140:565–574.

15. Tearney GJ, Brezinski ME, Southern JF, et al. Determination of the refractive index of highly scattering human tissue by optical coherence tomography. *Opt Lett* 1995;20:2258–2260.

16. Brezinski ME, Tearney GJ, Bouma BE, et al. Optical coherence tomography for optical biopsy: properties and demonstration of vascular pathology. *Circulation* 1996;93:1206–1213.

17. Yabushita H, Bouma BE, Houser SL, et al. Characterization of human atherosclerosis by optical coherence tomography. *Circulation* 2002;106:1640–1645.

18. Jang IK, Bouma BE, Kang DH, et al. Visualization of coronary atherosclerotic plaques in patients using optical coherence tomography: comparison with intravascular ultrasound. *J Am Coll Cardiol* 2002;39:604–609.

19. Franzen D, Sechtem U, Hopp HW. Comparison of angioscopic, intravascular ultrasonic, and angiographic detection of thrombus in coronary stenosis. *Am J Cardiol* 1998;82:1273–1275,A9.

20. Tearney GJ, Yabushita H, Houser SL, et al. Quantification of macrophage content in atherosclerotic plaques by optical coherence tomography. *Circulation* 2003;107:113–119.

21. Moreno PR, Lodder RA, Purushothaman KR, et al. Detection of lipid pool, thin fibrous cap, and inflammatory cells in human aortic atherosclerotic plaques by near-infrared spectroscopy. *Circulation* 2002;105:923–927.

22. Jaross W, Neumeister V, Lattke P, et al. Determination of cholesterol in atherosclerotic plaques using near infrared diffuse reflection spectroscopy. *Atherosclerosis* 1999;147:327–337.

23. Neumeister V, Scheibe M, Lattke P, et al. Determination of the cholesterol-collagen ratio of arterial atherosclerotic plaques using near infrared spectroscopy as a possible measure of plaque stability. *Atherosclerosis* 2002;165:251–257.

24. Cassis LA, Lodder RA. Near-IR imaging of atheromas in living arterial tissue. *Anal Chem* 1993;65:1247–1256.

25. van de Poll SW, Romer TJ, Puppels GJ, et al. Imaging of atherosclerosis. Raman spectroscopy of atherosclerosis. *J Cardiovasc Risk* 2002;9:255–261.

26. Manoharan R, Baraga JJ, Feld MS, et al. Quantitative histochemical analysis of human artery using Raman spectroscopy. *J Photochem Photobiol B* 1992;16:211–233.

27. Brennan JF 3rd, Romer TJ, Lees RS, et al. Determination of human coronary artery composition by Raman spectroscopy. *Circulation* 1997;96:99–105.

28. Romer TJ, Brennan JF 3rd, Fitzmaurice M, et al. Histopathology of human coronary atherosclerosis by quantifying its chemical composition with Raman spectroscopy. *Circulation* 1998;97:878–885.

29. Buschman HP, Motz JT, Deinum G, et al. Diagnosis of human coronary atherosclerosis by morphology-based Raman spectroscopy. *Cardiovasc Pathol* 2001;10:59–68.

30. Brennan JF, Wang Y, Dasari RR, et al. Near infrared Raman spectrometer systems for human tissue studies. *Appl Spectrosc* 1997;51:201–208.

31. Romer TJ, Brennan JF 3rd, Puppels GJ, et al. Intravascular ultrasound combined with Raman spectroscopy to localize and quantify cholesterol and calcium salts in atherosclerotic coronary arteries. *Arterioscler Thromb Vasc Biol* 2000;20:478–483.

32. Buschman HP, Marple ET, Wach ML, et al. In vivo determination of the molecular composition of artery wall by intravascular Raman spectroscopy. *Anal Chem* 2000;72:3771–3775.

33. Ross R. Atherosclerosis—an inflammatory disease. *N Engl J Med* 1999;340:115–126.

34. van der Wal A, Becker A, van der Loos C, et al. Site of intimal rupture or erosion of thrombosed coronary atherosclerotic plaques is characterized by an inflammatory process irrespective of the dominant plaque morphology. *Circulation* 1994;89:36–44.

35. Casscells W, Hathorn B, David M, et al. Thermal detection of cellular infiltrates in living atherosclerotic plaques: possible implications for plaque rupture and thrombosis. *Lancet* 1996;347:1447–1451.

36. Verheye S, Diamantopoulos L, Serruys PW, et al. Imaging of atherosclerosis. Intravascular imaging of the vulnerable atherosclerotic plaque: spotlight on temperature measurement. *J Cardiovasc Risk* 2002;9:247–254.

37. de Boer OJ, van der Wal AC, Teeling P, et al. Leucocyte recruitment in rupture prone regions of lipid-rich plaques: a prominent role for neovascularization? *Cardiovasc Res* 1999;41:443–449.

38. Stefanadis C, Diamantopoulos L, Vlachopoulos C, et al. Thermal heterogeneity within human atherosclerotic coronary arteries detected in vivo: a new method of detection by application of a special thermography catheter. *Circulation* 1999;99:1965–1971.

39. Verheye S, De Meyer GR, Van Langenhove G, et al. In vivo temperature heterogeneity of atherosclerotic plaques is determined by plaque composition. *Circulation* 2002;105:1596–1601.

40. Naghavi M, Melling M, Gul K, et al. First prototype of a 4 French 180 degree side-viewing infra-red fibre optic catheter for thermal imaging of atherosclerotic plaque. *J Am Coll Cardiol* 2001;37:3A.

41. Barnett HJ, Taylor DW, Eliasziw M, et al. Benefit of carotid endarterectomy in patients with symptomatic moderate or severe stenosis. North American Symptomatic Carotid Endarterectomy Trial Collaborators. *N Engl J Med* 1998;339:1415–1425.

42. Endarterectomy for asymptomatic carotid stenosis. Executive Committee for the Asymptomatic Carotid Atherosclerosis Study. *JAMA* 1995;273:1421–1428.

43. Weinberger J, Ramos L, Ambrose JA, et al. Morphologic and dynamic changes of atherosclerotic plaque at the carotid artery bifurcation: sequential imaging by real time B-mode ultrasonography. *J Am Coll Cardiol* 1988;12:1515–1521.

44. Pignoli P, Tremoli E, Poli A, et al. Intimal plus medial thickness of the arterial wall: a direct measurement with ultrasound imaging. *Circulation* 1986;74:1399–1406.

45. Fazio GP, Redberg RF, Winslow T, et al. Transesophageal echocardiographically detected atherosclerotic aortic plaque is a marker for coronary artery disease. *J Am Coll Cardiol* 1993;21:144–150.

46. O'Leary DH, Polak JF, Kronmal RA, et al. Carotid-artery intima and media thickness as a risk factor for myocardial infarction and stroke in older adults. Cardiovascular Health Study Collaborative Research Group. *N Engl J Med* 1999;340:14–22.

47. Khoury Z, Schwartz R, Gottlieb S, et al. Relation of coronary artery disease to atherosclerotic disease in the aorta, carotid, and femoral arteries evaluated by ultrasound. *Am J Cardiol* 1997;80:1429–1433.

48. Burke GL, Evans GW, Riley WA, et al. Arterial wall thickness is associated with prevalent cardiovascular disease in middle-aged adults. The Atherosclerosis Risk in Communities (ARIC) Study. *Stroke* 1995;26:386–391.

49. Nagai Y, Metter EJ, Earley CJ, et al. Increased carotid artery intimal-

medial thickness in asymptomatic older subjects with exercise-induced myocardial ischemia. *Circulation* 1998;98:1504–1509.

50. Crouse JR 3rd, Craven TE, Hagaman AP, et al. Association of coronary disease with segment-specific intimal-medial thickening of the extracranial carotid artery. *Circulation* 1995;92:1141–1147.

51. Salonen R, Nyyssonen K, Porkkala E, et al. Kuopio Atherosclerosis Prevention Study (KAPS). A population-based primary preventive trial of the effect of LDL lowering on atherosclerotic progression in carotid and femoral arteries. *Circulation* 1995;92:1758–1764.

52. de Groot E, Jukema JW, Montauban van Swijndregt AD, et al. B-mode ultrasound assessment of pravastatin treatment effect on carotid and femoral artery walls and its correlations with coronary arteriographic findings: a report of the Regression Growth Evaluation Statin Study (REGRESS). *J Am Coll Cardiol* 1998;31:1561–1567.

53. Weinberger J, Azhar S, Danisi F, et al. A new noninvasive technique for imaging atherosclerotic plaque in the aortic arch of stroke patients by transcutaneous real-time B-mode ultrasonography: an initial report. *Stroke* 1998;29:673–676.

54. Atherosclerotic disease of the aortic arch as a risk factor for recurrent ischemic stroke. The French Study of Aortic Plaques in Stroke Group. *N Engl J Med* 1996;334:1216–1221.

55. Cohen A, Tzourio C, Bertrand B, et al. Aortic plaque morphology and vascular events: a follow-up study in patients with ischemic stroke. FAPS Investigators. French Study of Aortic Plaques in Stroke. *Circulation* 1997;96:3838–3841.

56. Parthenakis F, Skalidis E, Simantirakis E, et al. Absence of atherosclerotic lesions in the thoracic aorta indicates absence of significant coronary artery disease. *Am J Cardiol* 1996;77:1118–1121.

57. Lanza GM, Wallace KD, Scott MJ, et al. A novel site-targeted ultrasonic contrast agent with broad biomedical application. *Circulation* 1996;94:3334–3340.

58. Lindner JR, Song J, Xu F, et al. Noninvasive ultrasound imaging of inflammation using microbubbles targeted to activated leukocytes. *Circulation* 2000;102:2745–2750.

59. Demos SM, Alkan-Onyuksel H, Kane BJ, et al. In vivo targeting of acoustically reflective liposomes for intravascular and transvascular ultrasonic enhancement. *J Am Coll Cardiol* 1999;33:867–875.

60. Tiukinhoy SD, Huang S, Khan AA, et al. Novel acoustic drug-encapsulated liposomes for site-specific delivery. *J Am Coll Cardiol* 2001;37:256A.

61. Tiukinhoy SD, Mahowald ME, Shively VP, et al. Development of echogenic, plasmid-incorporated, tissue-targeted cationic liposomes that can be used for directed gene delivery. *Invest Radiol* 2000;35:732–738.

62. Mitchell DG. *MRI principles*. Philadelphia: WB Saunders, 1999.

63. Wood ML, Wehrli FW. Principles of magnetic resonance imaging. In: Stark DD, Bradley WG Jr, eds. *Magnetic resonance imaging*. St. Louis: Mosby, 1999.

64. Fayad ZA, Fuster V. Clinical imaging of the high-risk or vulnerable atherosclerotic plaque. *Circ Res* 2001;89:305–316.

65. Choudhury RP, Fuster V, Badimon JJ, et al. MRI and characterization of atherosclerotic plaque: emerging applications and molecular imaging. *Arterioscler Thromb Vasc Biol* 2002;22:1065–1074.

66. Skinner MP, Yuan C, Mitsumori L, et al. Serial magnetic resonance imaging of experimental atherosclerosis detects lesion fine structure, progression and complications in vivo. *Nat Med* 1995;1:69–73.

67. Helft G, Worthley SG, Fuster V, et al. Atherosclerotic aortic component quantification by noninvasive magnetic resonance imaging: an in vivo study in rabbits. *J Am Coll Cardiol* 2001;37:1149–1154.

68. Shinnar M, Fallon JT, Wehrli S, et al. The diagnostic accuracy of ex vivo MRI for human atherosclerotic plaque characterization. *Arterioscler Thromb Vasc Biol* 1999;19:2756–2761.

69. Toussaint JF, Southern JF, Fuster V, et al. T2-weighted contrast for NMR characterization of human atherosclerosis. *Arterioscler Thromb Vasc Biol* 1995;15:1533–1542.

70. Toussaint JF, LaMuraglia GM, Southern JF, et al. Magnetic resonance images lipid, fibrous, calcified, hemorrhagic, and thrombotic components of human atherosclerosis in vivo. *Circulation* 1996;94:932–938.

71. Fayad ZA, Nahar T, Fallon JT, et al. In vivo magnetic resonance evaluation of atherosclerotic plaques in the human thoracic aorta: a comparison with transesophageal echocardiography. *Circulation* 2000;101:2503–2509.

72. Hatsukami TS, Ross R, Polissar NL, et al. Visualization of fibrous cap thickness and rupture in human atherosclerotic carotid plaque in vivo with high-resolution magnetic resonance imaging. *Circulation* 2000;102:959–964.

73. Yuan C, Mitsumori LM, Ferguson MS, et al. In vivo accuracy of multispectral magnetic resonance imaging for identifying lipid-rich necrotic cores and intraplaque hemorrhage in advanced human carotid plaques. *Circulation* 2001;104:2051–2056.

74. Yuan C, Zhang SX, Polissar NL, et al. Identification of fibrous cap rupture with magnetic resonance imaging is highly associated with recent transient ischemic attack or stroke. *Circulation* 2002;105:181–185.

75. Botnar RM, Stuber M, Danias PG, et al. Improved coronary artery definition with T2-weighted, free-breathing, three-dimensional coronary MRA. *Circulation* 1999;99:3139–3148.

76. Botnar RM, Stuber M, Kissinger KV, et al. Noninvasive coronary vessel wall and plaque imaging with magnetic resonance imaging. *Circulation* 2000;102:2582–2587.

77. Fayad ZA, Fuster V, Fallon JT, et al. Noninvasive in vivo human coronary artery lumen and wall imaging using black-blood magnetic resonance imaging. *Circulation* 2000;102:506–510.

78. Botnar RM, Kim WY, Bornert P, et al. 3D coronary vessel wall imaging utilizing a local inversion technique with spiral image acquisition. *Magn Reson Med* 2001;46:848–854.

79. Kim WY, Danias PG, Stuber M, et al. Coronary magnetic resonance angiography for the detection of coronary stenoses. *N Engl J Med* 2001;345:1863–1869.

80. Fayad ZA, Hardy CJ, Giaquinto R, et al. Improved high resolution MRI of human coronary artery lumen and plaque with a new cardiac coil. *Circulation* 2000;102:II-399.

81. McCarthy MJ, Loftus IM, Thompson MM, et al. Angiogenesis and the atherosclerotic carotid plaque: an association between symptomatology and plaque morphology. *J Vasc Surg* 1999;30:261–268.

82. Zhang Y, Cliff WJ, Schoefl GI, et al. Immunohistochemical study of intimal microvessels in coronary atherosclerosis. *Am J Pathol* 1993;143:164–172.

83. Ware JA. Too many vessels? Not enough? The wrong kind? The VEGF debate continues. *Nat Med* 2001;7:403–404.

84. Wasserman BA, Smith WI, Trout HH 3rd, et al. Carotid artery atherosclerosis: in vivo morphologic characterization with gadolinium-enhanced double-oblique MR imaging initial results. *Radiology* 2002;223:566–573.

85. Yuan C, Kerwin WS, Ferguson MS, et al. Contrast-enhanced high resolution MRI for atherosclerotic carotid artery tissue characterization. *J Magn Reson Imaging* 2002;15:62–67.

86. Kerwin W, Hooker A, Spilker M, et al. Quantitative magnetic resonance imaging analysis of neovasculature volume in carotid atherosclerotic plaque. *Circulation* 2003;107:851–856.

87. Lin W, Abendschein DR, Haacke EM. Contrast-enhanced magnetic resonance angiography of carotid arterial wall in pigs. *J Magn Reson Imaging* 1997;7:183–190.

88. Maki JH, Wilson GJ, Lauffer RB, et al. Apparent vessel wall inflammation detected using MS-325, a blood pool contrast agent. *Proc Intl Soc Mag Reson Med* 2001;9:639.

89. Corti R, Fayad ZA, Fuster V, et al. Effects of lipid-lowering by simvastatin on human atherosclerotic lesions: a longitudinal study by high-resolution, noninvasive magnetic resonance imaging. *Circulation* 2001;104:249–252.

90. Corti R, Fuster V, Fayad ZA, et al. Lipid lowering by simvastatin induces regression of human atherosclerotic lesions: two years' follow-up by high-resolution noninvasive magnetic resonance imaging. *Circulation* 2002;106:2884–2887.

91. Zhao XQ, Yuan C, Hatsukami TS, et al. Effects of prolonged intensive lipid-lowering therapy on the characteristics of carotid atherosclerotic plaques in vivo by MRI: a case-control study. *Arterioscler Thromb Vasc Biol* 2001;21:1623–1629.

92. Lardo AC, Yang X, Fayad ZA, et al. High resolution intravascular imaging following magnetic resonance guided aortic stent placement. *Circulation* 2001;104:II-764.

93. Zimmermann GG, Erhart P, Schneider J, et al. Intravascular MR imaging of atherosclerotic plaque: ex vivo analysis of human femoral arteries with histologic correlation. *Radiology* 1997;204:769–774.

94. Zimmermann-Paul GG, Quick HH, Vogt P, et al. High-resolution intravascular magnetic resonance imaging: monitoring of plaque formation in heritable hyperlipidemic rabbits. *Circulation* 1999;99:1054–1061.

95. Ocali O, Atalar E. Intravascular magnetic resonance imaging using a loopless catheter antenna. *Magn Reson Med* 1997;37:112–118.

96. Worthley SG, Helft G, Fuster V, et al. A novel nonobstructive intravascular MRI coil: in vivo imaging of experimental atherosclerosis. *Arterioscler Thromb Vasc Biol* 2003;23:346–350.

97. Johnstone MT, Botnar RM, Perez AS, et al. In vivo magnetic resonance imaging of experimental thrombosis in a rabbit model. *Arterioscler Thromb Vasc Biol* 2001;21:1556–1560.

98. Toussaint JF, Southern JF, Fuster V, et al. Water diffusion properties of human atherosclerosis and thrombosis measured by pulse field gradient nuclear magnetic resonance. *Arterioscler Thromb Vasc Biol* 1997; 17:542–546.

99. Bradley WG Jr. MR appearance of hemorrhage in the brain. *Radiology* 1993;189.15–26.

100. Moody AR. Direct imaging of deep-vein thrombosis with magnetic resonance imaging. *Lancet* 1997;350:1073.

101. Fraser DG, Moody AR, Morgan PS, et al. Diagnosis of lower-limb deep venous thrombosis: a prospective blinded study of magnetic resonance direct thrombus imaging. *Ann Intern Med* 2002;136:89–98.

102. Moody AR, Liddicoat A, Krarup K Magnetic resonance pulmonary angiography and direct imaging of embolus for the detection of pulmonary emboli. *Invest Radiol* 1997;32:431–440.

103. Mugler JP 3rd, Brookeman JR. Three-dimensional magnetization-prepared rapid gradient-echo imaging (3D MP RAGE). *Magn Reson Med* 1990;15:152–157.

104. Corti R, Osende JI, Fayad ZA, et al. In vivo noninvasive detection and age definition of arterial thrombus by MRI. *J Am Coll Cardiol* 2002; 39:1366–1373.

105. Yu X, Song SK, Chen J, et al. High-resolution MRI characterization of human thrombus using a novel fibrin-targeted paramagnetic nanoparticle contrast agent. *Magn Reson Med* 2000;44:867–872.

106. Flacke S, Fischer S, Scott MJ, et al. Novel MRI contrast agent for molecular imaging of fibrin: implications for detecting vulnerable plaques. *Circulation* 2001;104:1280–1285.

107. Lauffer RB, Graham PB, Lahti KM, et al. Direct clot detection with MRI using a novel fibrin-targeted gadolinium agent. *Circulation* 2000;102:II-375.

108. Johansson LO, Bjornerud A, Ahlstrom HK, et al. A targeted contrast agent for magnetic resonance imaging of thrombus: implications of spatial resolution. *J Magn Reson Imaging* 2001;13:615–618.

109. Ladd ME, Quick HH, Debatin JF. Interventional MRA and intravascular imaging. *J Magn Reson Imaging* 2000;12:534–546.

110. Yang X, Atalar E. Intravascular MR imaging-guided balloon angioplasty with an MR imaging guide wire: feasibility study in rabbits. *Radiology* 2000;217:501–506.

111. Dion YM, Ben El Kadi H, Boudoux C, et al. Endovascular procedures under near-real-time magnetic resonance imaging guidance: an experimental feasibility study. *J Vasc Surg* 2000;32:1006–1014.

112. Spuentrup E, Ruebben A, Schaeffter T, et al. Magnetic resonance-guided coronary artery stent placement in a swine model. *Circulation* 2002;105:874–879.

113. Yang X, Atalar E, Li D, et al. Magnetic resonance imaging permits in vivo monitoring of catheter-based vascular gene therapy. *Circulation* 2001;104:1588–1590.

114. Schwartz RB, Hsu L, Wong TZ, et al. Intraoperative MR imaging guidance for intracranial neurosurgery: experience with the first 200 cases. *Radiology* 1999;211:477–488.

115. Smits HF, Bos C, van der Weide R, et al. Endovascular interventional MR: balloon angioplasty in a hemodialysis access flow phantom. *J Vasc Interv Radiol* 1998;9:840–845.

116. Rudin M, Weissleder R. Molecular imaging in drug discovery and development. *Nat Rev Drug Discov* 2003;2:123–131.

117. Weissleder R, Mahmood U. Molecular imaging. *Radiology* 2001;219: 316–333.

118. Wickline SA, Lanza GM. Molecular imaging, targeted therapeutics, and nanoscience. *J Cell Biochem Suppl* 2002;39:90–97.

119. Wickline SA, Lanza GM. Nanotechnology for molecular imaging and targeted therapy. *Circulation* 2003;107:1092–1095.

120. Vallabhajosula S, Fuster V. Atherosclerosis: imaging techniques and the evolving role of nuclear medicine. *J Nucl Med* 1997;38:1788–1796.

121. Iuliano L, Signore A, Vallabhajosula S, et al. Preparation and biodistribution of 99m technetium labelled oxidized LDL in man. *Atherosclerosis* 1996;126:131–141.

122. Iuliano L, Mauriello A, Sbarigia E, et al. Radiolabeled native low-density lipoprotein injected into patients with carotid stenosis accumulates in macrophages of atherosclerotic plaque: effect of vitamin E supplementation. *Circulation* 2000;101:1249–1254.

123. Hardoff R, Braegelmann F, Zanzonico P, et al. External imaging of atherosclerosis in rabbits using an 123I-labeled synthetic peptide fragment. *J Clin Pharmacol* 1993;33:1039–1047.

124. Tsimikas S, Palinski W, Halpern SE, et al. Radiolabeled MDA2, an oxidation-specific, monoclonal antibody, identifies native atherosclerotic lesions in vivo. *J Nucl Cardiol* 1999;6:41–53.

125. Rudd JH, Warburton EA, Fryer TD, et al. Imaging atherosclerotic plaque inflammation with [18F]-fluorodeoxyglucose positron emission tomography. *Circulation* 2002;105:2708–2711.

126. Sharma V, Luker GD, Piwnica-Worms D. Molecular imaging of gene expression and protein function in vivo with PET and SPECT. *J Magn Reson Imaging* 2002;16:336–351.

127. Helft G, Worthley SG, Zhang ZY, et al. Non-invasive in vivo imaging of atherosclerotic lesions using Fluorine-18 deoxyglucose (18-FDG) PET correlates with macrophage content in a rabbit model. *Circulation* 1999;100:I-311.

128. Aime S, Cabella C, Colombatto S, et al. Insights into the use of paramagnetic Gd(III) complexes in MR-molecular imaging investigations. *J Magn Reson Imaging* 2002;16:394–406.

129. Schmitz SA, Coupland SE, Gust R, et al. Superparamagnetic iron oxide-enhanced MRI of atherosclerotic plaques in Watanabe hereditable hyperlipidemic rabbits. *Invest Radiol* 2000;35:460–471.

130. Ruehm SG, Corot C, Vogt P, et al. Magnetic resonance imaging of atherosclerotic plaque with ultrasmall superparamagnetic particles of iron oxide in hyperlipidemic rabbits. *Circulation* 2001;103:415–422.

131. Schmitz SA, Taupitz M, Wagner S, et al. USPIO-enhanced magnetic resonance imaging of atherosclerotic plaques. *Eur Radiol* 2001;11:195.

132. Louie AY, Huber MM, Ahrens ET, et al. In vivo visualization of gene expression using magnetic resonance imaging. *Nat Biotechnol* 2000; 18:321–325.

133. Davies MJ, Gordon JL, Gearing AJ, et al. The expression of the adhesion molecules ICAM-1, VCAM-1, PECAM, and E-selectin in human atherosclerosis. *J Pathol* 1993;171:223–229.

134. Wood KM, Cadogan MD, Ramshaw AL, et al. The distribution of adhesion molecules in human atherosclerosis. *Histopathology* 1993;22: 437–444.

135. Nakashima Y, Raines EW, Plump AS, et al. Upregulation of VCAM-1 and ICAM-1 at atherosclerosis-prone sites on the endothelium in the ApoE-deficient mouse. *Arterioscler Thromb Vasc Biol* 1998;18:842–851.

136. Sipkins DA, Gijbels K, Tropper FD, et al. ICAM-1 expression in autoimmune encephalitis visualized using magnetic resonance imaging. *J Neuroimmunol* 2000;104:1–9.

137. Sipkins DA, Cheresh DA, Kazemi MR, et al. Detection of tumor angiogenesis in vivo by alphaVbeta3-targeted magnetic resonance imaging. *Nat Med* 1998;4:623–626.

138. Anderson SA, Rader RK, Westlin WF, et al. Magnetic resonance contrast enhancement of neovasculature with alpha(v)beta(3)-targeted nanoparticles. *Magn Reson Med* 2000;44:433–439.

139. Nunn AD, Linder KE, Tweedle MF. Can receptors be imaged with MRI agents? *Q J Nucl Med* 1997;41:155–162.

140. Chen J, Tung CH, Mahmood U, et al. In vivo imaging of proteolytic activity in atherosclerosis. *Circulation* 2002;105:2766–2771.

141. Jaffer FA, Tung CH, Gerszten RE, et al. In vivo imaging of thrombin activity in experimental thrombi with thrombin-sensitive near-infrared molecular probe. 2002;22:1929–1935.

142. Romer TJ, Brennan JF 3rd, Schut TC, et al. Raman spectroscopy for quantifying cholesterol in intact coronary artery wall. *Atherosclerosis* 1998;141:117–124.

CHAPTER 50

Endovascular Assessment of the High-Risk Plaque

Anthony C. De Franco, E. Murat Tuzcu, Paul Shoenhagen, and Steven E. Nissen

Key Words: Acute coronary syndrome; atheroma characterization; intravascular ultrasound; plaque rupture.

INTRODUCTION

Previous paradigms of coronary artery disease characterized atherothrombosis as a *focal* process on the basis of the angiographic appearance of focal lesions. However, insights from new imaging modalities demonstrate that coronary artery disease is most often diffuse and involves most or all of the coronary system. The contemporary paradigm also proposes that atheroma *composition* and its *inflammatory state* are critical determinants of outcome. Thus, a vital challenge is the early detection of unstable plaques, because identifica-

A. C. De Franco: McLaren Heart and Vascular Center, Division of Cardiology, McLaren Regional Medical Center; Department of Medicine, Michigan State University, Flint, Michigan.
E. M. Tuzcu: Intravascular Ultrasound Laboratory; Department of Medicine, The Cleveland Clinic Foundation, Cleveland, Ohio.
P. Shoenhagen: Department of Radiology and Cardiovascular Medicine, The Cleveland Clinic Foundation, Cleveland, Ohio.
S. E. Nissen: Division of Cardiology, Cleveland Clinic Foundation; Department of Medicine, The Cleveland Clinic Foundation, Cleveland, Ohio.

tion of vulnerable arteries before an event would allow interventions targeted at stabilization. This challenge is complex, because "vulnerable" lesions are presumably at a temporary stage of evolution, and their spatial and temporal distribution is dynamic.

Necropsy studies suggest that *plaque rupture* or *erosion* appear to be the initiating event in the majority of acute coronary syndromes (ACSs) (1–4). Libby and coworkers (4a) described these lesions as containing "a lipid-rich core in the central portion of an eccentric plaque" with a "thin, friable fibrous cap." Virmani and coworkers (5,6) extended this concept by proposing that most precursor lesions associated with rupture are "thin-cap fibroatheromas" with a cap thickness of less than 65 microns infiltrated by macrophages. These investigators described several plaque morphologies associated with ACS, including some with a small plaque burden, large eccentric or concentric lipid cores, and previously healed ruptures (7). *Plaque erosion* refers to the desquamation of endothelial cells and also can cause ACS by exposing the subendothelial layers to platelets and the coagulation system (8,9). The least common lesion associated with ACS is the calcified nodule (discussed later).

Any imaging modality used to identify lesions at risk for rupture must be able to identify some or all of these features

TABLE 50–1. *Endoluminal imaging of the coronary artery*

	Luminal percent stenosis	Total plaque volume	Surface features: cap thickness, rupture, and others	Lipid content	Fibrous tissue content	Calcium	Thrombus	Detection of inflammation
Angiography	+++	−	+	−	−	+	+	−
IVUS	+++	++++	+++	++	++	+++	+	−
Elastography	−	−	++	?	?	?	−	−
Angioscopy	−	−	++++	++	+	−	++++	+
Thermography	−	−	−	−	−	−	−	+++
OCT	−	−	+++	+++	+++	+++	?	++
Raman and NIR spectroscopy	−	−	−	++	++	?	?	?

IVUS, intravascular ultrasound; NIR, near-infrared spectroscopy; OCT, optical coherence tomography.

(Table 50–1). This chapter reviews several *in vivo* technologies for identifying the artery and the patient at risk, emphasizing the concepts that these modalities bring to the current paradigm of atherothrombosis.

RATIONALE FOR NEW IMAGING MODALITIES

Limitations of Conventional Angiographic Assessment

Angiography has many limitations in the assessment of coronary atherothrombosis (see detailed discussion in Chapter 91). Four limitations are relevant to the assessment of the vulnerable artery: underestimation of disease extent, inaccuracy in assessing irregular lumen shapes, inability to determine plaque composition and inflammatory state, and the inability to assess remodeling. In these areas, new technologies may add incremental information to the concepts of plaque rupture and the risk for ACS.

Extent of Disease

Patients with coronary disease have a much larger volume of atheroma than is apparent angiographically because coronary atherothrombosis often is diffuse, eliminating truly normal reference segments (Fig. 50–1). Thus, when angiography identifies a "focal" lesion, the "normal reference" is usually diseased (10). By the time a patient presents with

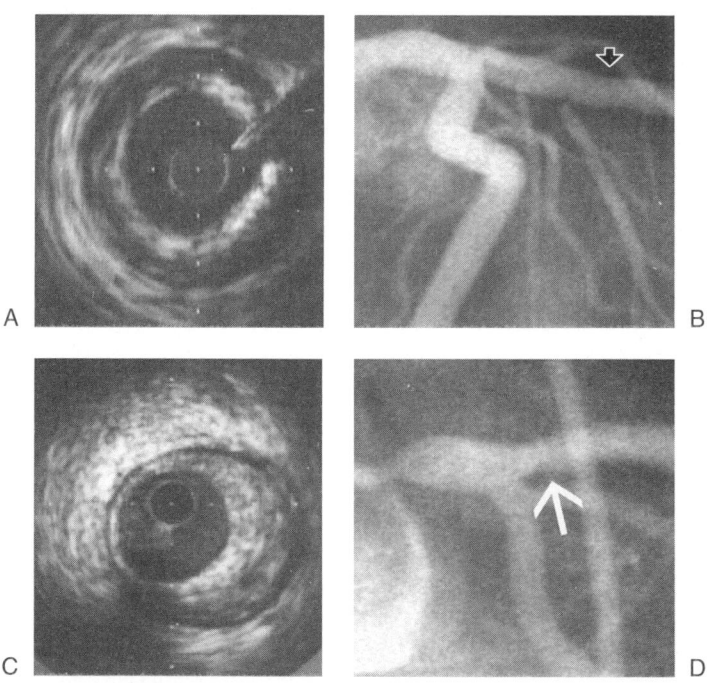

FIG. 50–1. Angiography often underestimates the amount of atheroma present. **A:** Ultrasound demonstrates a significant amount of atheroma, with approximately 40% cross-sectional narrowing of the external elastic membrane cross-sectional area (EEM CSA). At the corresponding site on the angiogram **(B),** only a mild luminal narrowing is present. **C:** Ultrasound demonstrates large, eccentric atheroma occupying nearly 50% of the EEM CSA. The corresponding site on the angiogram **(D)** shows only a mild narrowing.

clinical disease, ultrasound usually reveals so much atheroma that it is more accurate to refer to *segments* of the diseased artery rather than to an *individual* plaque. Another striking feature is the complete sparing of some coronary segments, even in patients with advanced disease.

Lumen Shape

Atheroma rupture often involves disruption of the luminal surface, creating fractures and cavities within the wall and irregular, sometimes bizarre, lumen shapes. Because angiography merely represents a lumen silhouette, it does not reveal the complexity of these irregular segments (11) (Fig. 50–2). In the early 1980s, Ambrose and coworkers (12,13) described angiographic characteristics of unstable plaques, such as irregular borders and intraluminal filling defects. For the next decade, these features remained the only clues to identify lesions responsible for ACS. However, clinicians recognized that many patients with ACS do not have any lesion with these features; conversely, some patients undergoing elective angiography had lesions with these features even though their angina was "stable." Plaque erosion also is associated with ACS, but erosion also is below the resolution limits of both angiography and intravascular ultrasound (IVUS).

Atheroma Composition and Inflammatory State

Most atherothrombotic segments consist predominantly of collagen and intercellular matrix with little or no signs of in-

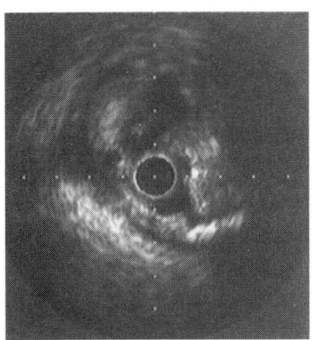
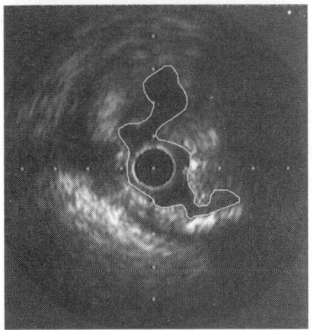

FIG. 50–2. Lumen shape affects the accuracy of angiography. Depending on the viewing angle, this eccentric lumen would project a markedly different degree of narrowing.

flammation. Although such regions may (or may not) contain angiographic narrowing, the current notion is that they have a low probability of rupture. A smaller proportion of atherothrombotic segments contain large amounts of cholesterol, lipid cells, and inflammatory cells and are presumably passing through a different phase of the process. These areas have several possible outcomes. Some may "heal" without rupture or erosion. Others may rupture but cause no ischemic consequences; they may "heal" and become part of the diffuse process. Others may rupture and result in transient or sustained occlusion. Presumably, in any of these situations some lesions heal with a residual luminal narrowing and others do not.

This concept of the dynamic evolution of coronary atheroma poses two challenges to imaging modalities that attempt to identify the unstable plaque. First, plaque evolution is thought to be continuous, with segments of the coronary atheroma in different stages of evolution. If plaque rupture is an *uncommon* event that frequently leads to occlusion, the imaging modality must have a high specificity in diagnosing rupture-prone areas. Conversely, if plaque rupture is a *common* event that infrequently results in clinical events, many plaque ruptures may be clinically silent. The technology used would need to have a high sensitivity to diagnose lesions at risk, because no clinical event would confirm the significance of the underlying lesion. Second, systemic factors (such as conventional and emerging risk factors, inflammatory mediators, and so on) may modulate the incidence of unstable plaques ruptures. If interventions are designed to decrease the frequency with which unstable plaques appear in the coronary system, then the "ideal" endoluminal technology would need to measure the "background" incidence of unstable plaques (i.e., before rupture or risk factor intervention), as well as any change in the number, morphology, or inflammatory state after risk factor intervention. Although this "ideal" technology does not currently exist, the devices discussed in this chapter can provide insight into these processes. Individual differences in platelet aggregation and thrombosis may also influence the risk for an acute event (5).

The underlying composition of a diseased segment of a coronary atheroma is thought to determine its potential for rupture. Atherothrombosis is a disease of the arterial *wall*. Thus, even though the number of stenosed coronary arteries has prognostic value, the determination of "stenosis severity" is merely a surrogate for disease burden. Angiography cannot reveal information about plaque composition, although in a minority of cases it can identify some features of plaque rupture.

If the concept of atheroma evolution through different stages is accurate, it has two implications for the imaging modalities discussed in this chapter: It presumes (a) that some features distinguish high-risk from low-risk segments and (b) that the same technique can identify these features. Any technology to assess "vulnerability" must address this issue.

INTRAVASCULAR ULTRASOUND

IVUS equipment and technique is discussed in detail in Chapter 91. IVUS is useful for evaluating potentially unstable plaque because of its tomographic orientation, its ability to measure lumen shape accurately, and its ability to examine the vessel wall itself, where the disease is located.

Normal Anatomy

The strength and signal quality of the ultrasound beam returning to the transducer determines what structural features the scanner depicts. Tissue acoustic impedance determines signal amplitude and image intensity. In normal arteries, collagen and elastin are highly reflective; thus, the internal elastic lamina and the external elastic membrane (EEM) appear bright white, as does adventitia, with its high collagen content. The relative reflectance of the adventitia serves as a reference to which other structures can be compared. In contrast, the media of coronary arteries consists predominantly of smooth muscle cells and reflects little of the signal. Thus, the typical appearance of a normal coronary artery consists of three layers (Fig. 50–3).

Early Disease and Remodeling

Atherothrombosis disrupts the IVUS appearance of the vessel; intimal thickness greater than 200 microns represents disease. Small to moderate atheromas often have a homogenous appearance, with intermediate signal intensity. Most

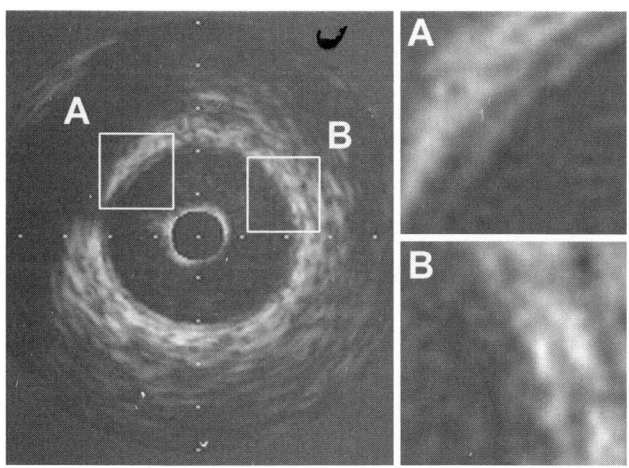

FIG. 50–3. A normal coronary artery assessed with intravascular ultrasound. A normal artery can be either trilaminar **(A)** or monolayered **(B)** depending on the angle of the ultrasound beam, the reflectance of the internal elastic lamina, or the thickness (histologically) of the intimal area. The bright, innermost layer caused by the reflections of the internal elastic lamina, a sonolucent *(black)* inner band caused by the low level of backscatter from the media, and a bright outer layer of adventitia. In other segments the internal elastic membrane is not dense enough to reflect the signal (particularly if the signal is off-axis) and the vessel appears monolaminar **(B)**.

early atheromas are eccentrically located. Necropsy and ultrasound studies indicate that atherothrombosis often begins on the side of the vessel opposite to bifurcations, in regions of low shear stress (14). As atheroma accumulates, the thickness of this zone increases, typically to 1 to 2 mm or more. At this stage, the homogenous ultrasound image often is replaced by regions of variable signal intensity. This may correspond to the network of collagen that buttresses the plaque seen in pathology specimens or to regions containing greater lipid content. As atherothrombosis advances, the media thins and, in some cases, is obliterated.

Ultrasound has reinforced the concept, first established by necropsy studies in the 1950s, that atherothrombosis begins in youth and is associated with risk factors from this age. By studying cardiac transplant recipients, Tuzcu and coworkers (14) documented atherothrombosis (defined as intimal thickness ≥0.5 mm) in the majority of donors by the third decade of life. In these young subjects, atherothrombosis was usually focal (85%) and located predominantly near bifurcations (14).

Remodeling refers to changes within the EEM area in normal or near-normal reference segments versus more severe lesions. In an autopsy study of human arteries, Glagov and coworkers (15) described *positive remodeling,* in which the cross-sectional area (CSA) within the EEM *increases* as plaque accumulates. These authors suggested that this might be "compensatory" because lumen size and shape was preserved until atheroma volume exceeded 30% to 40% of the EEM CSA (15). Ultrasound demonstrates that this process can be substantial (Fig. 50–4). Remodeling may be highly variable from one patient to another and even from one site versus another in the same artery. Positively remodeled atheroma may *not* encroach on the lumen and can escape angiographic detection.

Negative remodeling refers to a decrease in EEM CSA compared with the reference site. Approximately 20% severe stenoses are caused by "shrinkage" of the EEM area in addition to atheroma accumulation (10).

Multiple reports have demonstrated a consistent relation among positive remodeling, plaque rupture, and ACSs, whereas negative remodeling is more frequently associated with stable angina (Fig. 50–4) (16,17). Although some have speculated that the biochemical mechanisms responsible for positive remodeling may be related to the propensity for weakening of the fibrous cap and rupture (18,19), this association requires additional study.

"Stable" versus "Unstable" Coronary Atheroma: Ultrasound Morphology

In both early disease (such as in young transplant donors) and in patients with overt coronary disease, most atherothrombotic segments examined by ultrasound are thought to be relatively "stable." Ultrasonographers characterize lesions into three classes (Fig. 50–5). "Hard" plaques are more echodense than adventitia; these lesions are con-

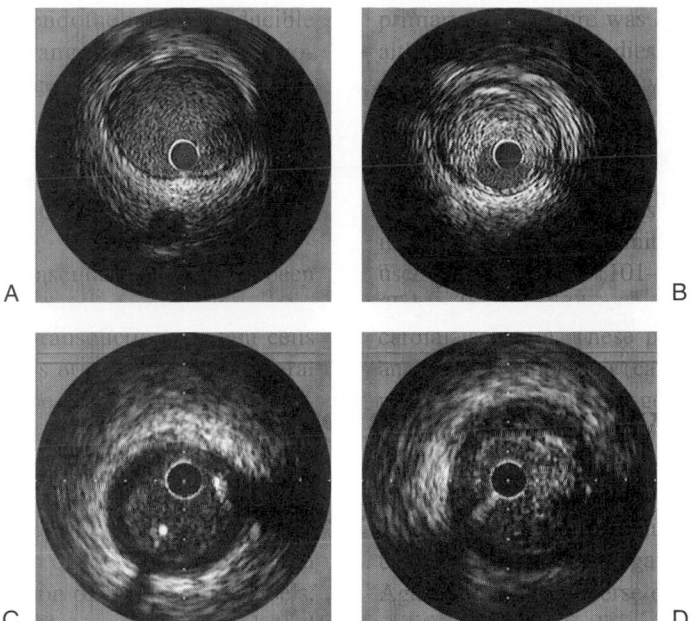

FIG. 50–4. Remodeling and plaque rupture. **A, B:** The reference external elastic membrane cross-sectional area (EEM CSA) **(A)** is larger than the site of the adjacent stenosis **(B),** illustrating negative remodeling at the lesion site. **C, D:** The reference EEM CSA **(C)** is smaller than the site of the adjacent stenosis **(D),** illustrating marked positive remodeling at the lesion site. Positive remodeling is associated with plaque rupture and lesions of acute coronary syndromes.

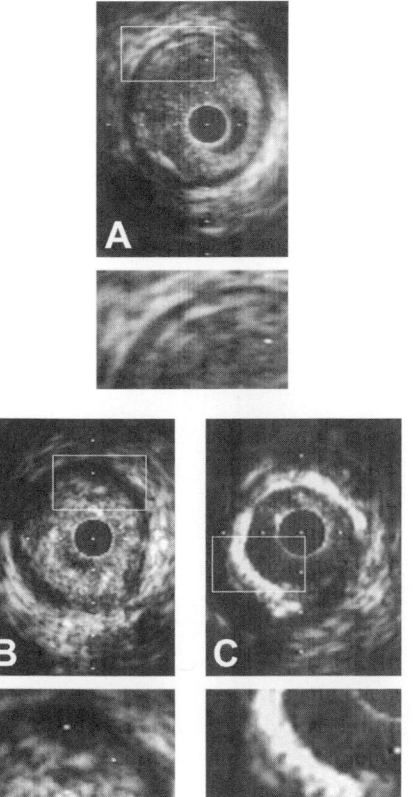

FIG. 50–5. Types of atheroma by intravascular ultrasound. Intravascular ultrasonographers classify plaque as soft **(A),** fibrous **(B),** or hard **(C).** These classes often are considered to be lipid-rich, fibrous, and calcific/fibrocalcific, respectively.

sidered to contain mostly collagen. Calcification is inferred when there is overt shadowing of the acoustic signal, but focal calcification may be present even in the absence of overt shadowing. "Fibrous" plaques have an acoustic density similar to the surrounding adventitia; these regions also are presumed to consist predominantly of collagen.

In contrast, lesions associated with ACS often have "soft" or echolucent sections (20,21), defined as areas less dense than adventitia. These segments are thought to contain more lipid and cholesterol on the basis of histopathology correlation studies. In some specimens, ultrasound demonstrates echolucent "pools" within the plaque. These areas often reflect little of the signal and appear as black or light-gray voids within the atheroma (Fig. 50–6). Such lesions have been associated with an increased risk for "no-reflow" and acute occlusion during intervention for acute myocardial infarction (MI), presumably because of an increased risk for embolization and dissection (22–24). Although small series have suggested minor differences in the ultrasonographic characteristics of atheroma from patients with different risk factors profiles, these data are inconclusive.

Necropsy studies define many plaque rupture areas as "thin-cap fibroatheromas" that have a necrotic core with an overlying thin fibrous cap (<65 mm) consisting of type I collagen, infiltrated by macrophages (7). Ultrasound can identify some "thin-cap" lesions. In some specimens, the "cap" appears thin and echolucent; these areas may be more vulnerable to rupture but do not have evidence of disruption at the time of examination.

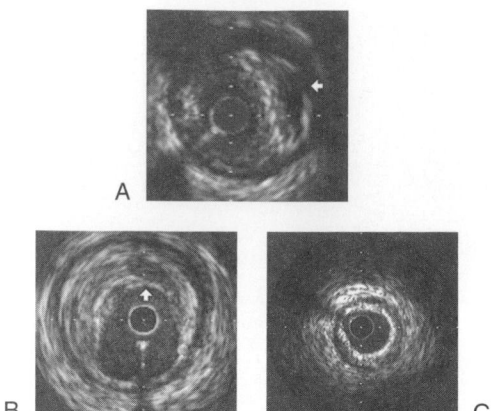

FIG. 50–6. Examples of thin-cap fibroatheromas with necrotic cores. In some plaques, as in **A,** the fibrous cap overlying the necrotic core *(arrow)* is relatively thick and presumably more resistant to rupture. In **B,** there is obvious thinning of the fibrous cap *(arrow);* this is considered to represent a vulnerable atheroma. In **C,** there appears to be a thick fibrous cap overlying a circumferential echolucent area; however, such an appearance can sometimes be caused by dropout of the ultrasound signal or other technical factors, rather than a circumferential "necrotic core."

Although the classification of plaques into "hard," "fibrous," and "soft" is useful for anticipating interventional devices response, and although ultrasonographic studies suggest good correlation with histology, the IVUS image does not represent *actual* histology. For example, the sensitivity and specificity of features suggestive of a "necrotic core" are unknown. System settings may affect the ability to detect such areas or they may depict a "necrotic core" when one is not actually present (25). Alteration in the dynamic range (grayscale) and gain of the system, the position of the transducer in relation to the area in question, and other factors may alter the sensitivity and specificity of the finding (26). Attenuation (dropout) of the ultrasound signal beyond a particularly dense or partially calcified fibrous cap or other imaging artifacts can create the illusion of a "necrotic core" or lipid-laden plaque when in fact the lipid content is low. Conversely, histopathologically documented lipid pools may escape IVUS detection (27). Greater frequency transducers or more sophisticated analysis of the ultrasound signal (discussed later) may improve the certainty with which unstable plaques are diagnosed.

Plaque Rupture: Ultrasound Appearance

The most reliable identification of an unstable plaque by ultrasound is when one or more features of plaque rupture are evident (Fig. 50–7). In patients with ACS, areas of spontaneous dissection or disruption of the plaque surface, or both, often are visible (28). Large echolucent areas may be contiguous with the lumen and may have pedunculated tissue. Such features are considered to be pathognomonic of plaque rupture. Many such sites contain echolucent areas, thought to represent lipid-laden or necrotic tissue or thrombus. In other specimens, the echolucent cavity appears empty; in these cases, the atheromatous material is presumed to have embolized (29).

Angioscopic and necropsy studies confirm that thrombus is present in more than 80% of plaque ruptures. Unfortunately,

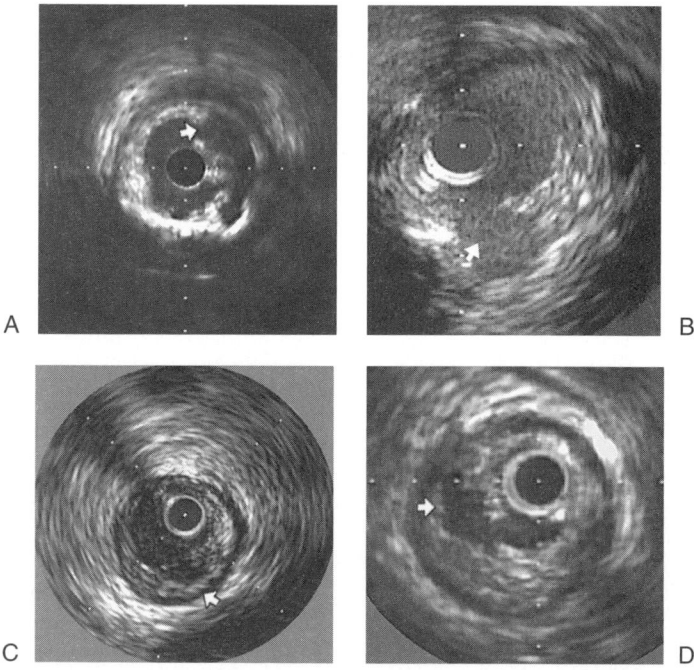

FIG. 50–7. A–D: Examples of plaque ruptures. *Arrows* in each specimen indicate the site of atheroma rupture.

current ultrasound systems are unable to diagnosis thrombus accurately because thrombus usually has an echodensity similar to "soft" plaque. In contrast, when a patient presents with an ACS and features of plaque rupture are evident (disruption overlying an echolucent zone), ultrasound can suggest the presence of fresh thrombus because it often has a characteristic scintillating appearance. Older, organized, laminated thrombus usually lacks any of these features and can be impossible to differentiate from plaque. Although enhancements to ultrasonic systems are in development, angioscopy is the only method to reliably identify thrombus *in vivo*.

Acute Coronary Syndromes: Insights from Ultrasound

Findings in Acute Coronary Syndromes

In general, ultrasound studies have supported the concepts of plaque rupture in the pathology literature. Ultrasound during ACSs suggests that culprit lesions are usually echolucent, eccentric, and positively remodeled. Hodgson and coworkers (20) reported that patients with unstable angina had more echolucent regions than those with stable angina. Bocksch and coworkers (30) compared 25 patients with acute MI to 15 control subjects with stable angina. The culprit lesion in patients with MI was smaller in CSA and the majority (>85%) were eccentric, compared with only one-third in those with stable angina. Fuchs and coworkers (31) demonstrated that patients with troponin level increases have a greater plaque burden, larger lesion and reference EEM areas (more remodeling), and a greater incidence of thrombus than in those without troponin level increases, suggesting more complex lesions and more diffuse disease.

The current paradigm of plaque rupture proposes that most ACS lesions are only mildly narrowed before rupture (32). Both necropsy studies and mathematical models suggest that the "shoulder" region of crescent-shaped, eccentric plaques (at the junction of plaque with more normal vessel wall) is the weakest segment structurally and the most prone to rupture. Flow disturbances near critical stenoses or side branches may predispose these areas to rupture, even if they are less severely narrowed. In a series of 257 patients, Maehara and coworkers (33) reported that the majority of incidentally diagnosed plaque ruptures were either near critical stenoses (<5 mm away) or side branches (<2 mm), and most of the tears were found in the "shoulders." Occasionally, rupture extends longitudinally, resulting in a long spontaneous dissection (28) (Fig. 50–8).

Davies has suggested that most plaque ruptures are clinically silent—that is, plaque rupture is a *common* event that *uncommonly* undergoes complete occlusion—and anecdotal IVUS observations support this concept. During routine imaging of a chronic, fibrocalcific, lesion in one coronary segment, it is common to observe incidentally sites with features of plaque rupture. These often are occult angiographically. Maehara and coworkers studied 254 patients presenting for elective intervention with preprocedural

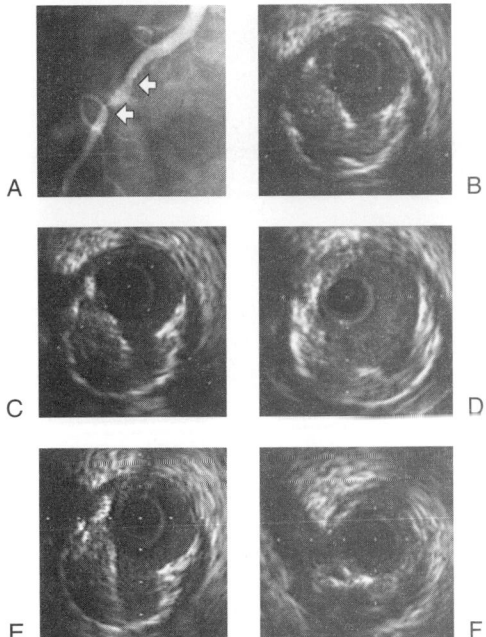

FIG. 50–8. Plaque rupture proximal to the site of a severe stenosis. This patient presented with new-onset angina; the angiogram demonstrated a severe stenosis and a "hazy" intermediate lesion proximal to the stenosis (**A**, *top arrow*). Ultrasound revealed an extensive spontaneous plaque rupture extending longitudinally through the vessel. **B–F:** Sequential ultrasound images obtained from the points indicated by the *arrows* on the angiogram. In **B** and **F** (at the "ends" of the tear), small defects in the fibrous cap are visible. In the images from the center of the plaque (**C–E**), a deep fissure is evident.

IVUS imaging. Slightly less than half had unstable angina and one-third had recent MI; the remainder had stable angina or no symptoms. Ultrasound signs of plaque rupture occurred not only in patients with ACS; 22% of the detected ruptures occurred in patients with stable angina or no symptoms. Ruptures often had preserved lumen areas; thus, they were usually *not* the most severe stenosis.

Recent ultrasound studies have called into question several angiographic "hallmarks" of ACSs. First, the angiographic "site" of plaque rupture often is incorrect. In patients with ST-segment elevation MI, the meniscus of the thrombus often does not coincide with the actual plaque rupture site. In the Controlled Abciximab and Device Investigation to Lower Late Angioplasty Complications (CADILLAC) trial of infarct angioplasty, an ultrasound substudy revealed that a plaque rupture was evident *proximal* to the stented segment (the site presumed to be responsible for the MI angiographically) in 20% of cases (34). In a provocative study, Rioufol and coworkers (35) performed IVUS in all 3 vessels in 25 patients with ACS. On the basis of the angiographic appearance, stents were deployed on the site of plaque rupture in only 40% of cases. In addition, more than 2.0 plaque ruptures on average were evident per patient. Other studies also have suggested that multiple plaque ruptures are common (33,36) (Fig. 50–9).

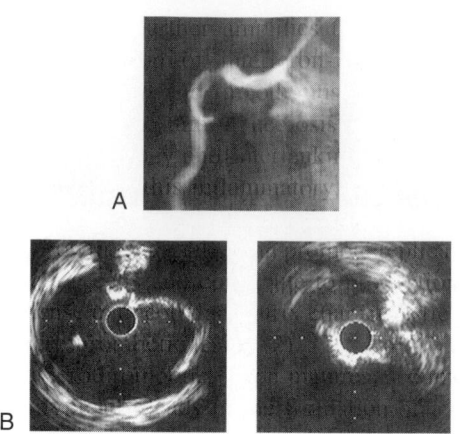

FIG. 50–9. Calcified intraluminal nodule presenting as an acute coronary syndrome. Some lesions with a "classic" angiographic appearance of unstable plaque have unsuspected features by ultrasound. This patient presented with a subendocardial infarction; the only angiographic finding **(A)** was a large intraluminal filling defect in the proximal right coronary artery consistent with thrombus. Ultrasound **(B:** Distal reference site; **C:** at the site of the angiographic filling defect) revealed an extensive, heavily calcified mass protruding into the lumen over the length of the lesion, indicating that the "thrombus" was actually a calcified intraluminal nodule.

Finally, calcium has been considered a hallmark of "old" atherothrombotic lesions; however, necropsy and IVUS studies suggest that calcium often is present in minimally diseased segments in young subjects (37) and in ACS lesions (28). Many ruptured plaques contain calcium, although it may be in a "fragmented" or "speckled" pattern (7). In 43 patients with unstable angina, 54% had either mild or heavily calcific deposits by IVUS at the suspected culprit lesion site (38). It is possible that in some lesions focal calcification predisposes to dissection by initiating cleavage planes (39).

Ultrasound and the Prediction of Acute Coronary Syndromes

A common limitation of ultrasound studies is that they are restricted to sites that have already ruptured. There has been only one systematic study that compared ultrasonic morphologic findings with *subsequent* coronary syndromes. Yamagishi and coworkers (40) studied 106 patients with intracoronary ultrasound; during 18 months of follow-up, ACS developed 12 patients. Ten of the 12 contained hypoechogenic areas at baseline and all were eccentric. Although the percent plaque area (the percentage of the vessel at the lesion site occupied by atheroma) was greater than that of adjacent sites, lumen dimensions were similar to other segments of the vessel. The authors concluded that larger, more eccentric plaques with areas of low echogenicity could become vulnerable during follow-up despite preserved lumen area. This observation supports the concept that mildly stenotic lesions may be more prone to rupture.

Limitations of Ultrasound: What Can *Not* Be Seen

Although ultrasound provides unique insights into ACSs, current technology has limitations. Imaging patients with ACS is more difficult than in stable patients; the need to reestablish coronary flow often precludes imaging before intervention. Virmani (40a) reports that some precursor lesions have cap thickness less than 65 microns; this is near the resolution of current systems. Plaque erosion is below the resolution of current systems. Catheters are still approximately 1 mm in size, precluding imaging of very distal and small vessels. The limitations in diagnosing thrombus have been discussed. There also is a potential for publication bias toward those articles that support current notions of "vulnerable" plaque and plaque rupture, findings that do not support this paradigm may be less likely to be reported. Finally, most of our knowledge of vulnerable plaques comes from specimens that have already ruptured; thus, the applicability of these findings to "vulnerable" plaques that have not yet ruptured remains uncertain.

Future Developments in Intravascular Ultrasound

Atherothrombosis Regression Studies

Anecdotal evidence suggests that coronary atherothrombosis may, in some cases, progress rapidly (Fig. 50–10); in other cases, regression may be possible. Several small regression studies have been completed. Takagi and coworkers (41) randomized 36 patients with ACS to conventional risk factor modification with or without pravastatin at a fixed dose of 10 mg. At 3 years, there were no significant changes in either group angiographically, but by IVUS, the statin group had a 9% *decrease* in atheroma area, whereas the conventionally treated group had a 41% *increase* in atheroma area. Small, hypothesis-generating studies such as this justify larger, more definitive studies of atherothrombosis stabilization and regression. Schartl and coworkers (42) randomized 139 patients to atorvastatin or "usual care" (which could include statin therapy). After 12 months, mean LDL cholesterol was reduced from 155 to 86 mg/dL in the atorvastatin group and from 166 to 140 mg/dL in the usual care group. Atheroma echogenicity (considered to be a marker of lower lipid content and stability) increased to a larger extent in the atorvastatin group than in the usual care group. There was a trend toward reduced plaque volume in the atorvastatin group compared with the usual care group.

Risk factor modification has been associated with favorable coronary remodeling and improved endothelial function. LDL-apheresis plus lipid-lowering therapy in Japanese patients with familial hypercholesterolemia was associated with improvements in minimal luminal diameter and smaller plaque areas at follow-up compared with patients

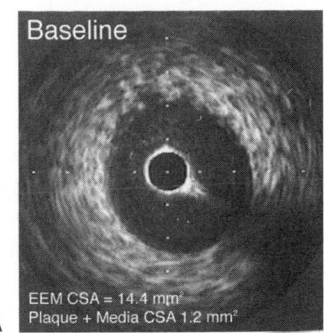

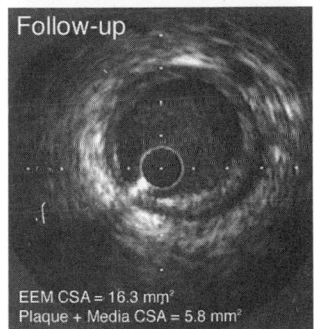

FIG. 50–10. Example of rapid progression of disease. Baseline **(A)** and follow-up at 18 months **(B)** in the same site in the same patient demonstrates that atherothrombosis can develop rapidly at a previously normal site. CSA, cross-sectional area; EEM CSA, external elastic membrane cross-sectional area.

treated with medication alone (43). Hamasaki and coworkers (44) studied 101 patients with normal or only mildly diseased (<30% angiographic narrowing) left anterior descending segments with IVUS and assessed endothelial function with intracoronary acetylcholine. Patients who had reduced their total cholesterol level to less than 240 mg/dL with medical therapy and those whose initial values were below this level (not on treatment at the time of study) had larger mean EEM CSAs and a greater increase in acetylcholine-induced vasodilation than did patients with a total cholesterol level greater than 240 mg/dL. Mean atheroma areas were similar in patients regardless of enhanced remodeling or changes in endothelial function. Thus, coronary regression may involve favorable remodeling of the EEM CSA together with improved endothelial function, even without measurable differences in plaque volume.

Whether more versus less aggressive lipid-lowering will lead to long-term stabilization or regression of atherothrombosis is currently being tested in the Reversal of Atherosclerosis with Aggressive Lipid Lowering (REVERSAL) trial, a prospective, randomized, double-blind multicenter study (45). This study has randomized patients to either 80 mg atorvastatin (with an expected target LDL of 70–80 mg/dL) versus 40 mg pravastatin (with an expected target LDL of 90–100 mg/dL). All patients had IVUS at baseline and at 18 months to assess the primary end point, the percent change in atheroma volume. Other secondary end points include new lesion development

and the development of "vulnerable" plaques. The study has completed enrollment and final data are anticipated in 2003.

Tissue Characterization

In commercially available ultrasound systems, the ultrasound signal is processed to create the image. However, this signal contains much more information than what is displayed. Complex mathematical algorithms called *backscatter* or *tissue analysis* can extract this information. These intrinsic characteristics of the backscattered ultrasound signals include the amplitude distribution, frequency response, and power spectrum density of the signal, and they convey information about tissue types that would otherwise appear similar on conventional ultrasound images.

Accordingly, spectral analysis of the unprocessed radiofrequency signal may improve on the current, limited ability of ultrasound systems to delineate the contents of individual plaques. Early *in vitro* studies suggest that backscatter analysis can improve the diagnosis of thrombus (46) and may be able to discriminate carotid plaques from symptomatic versus asymptomatic patients (47). A more sophisticated mathematical analysis of backscattered ultrasound signals *in vitro* reported exquisite discrimination of intraplaque histopathology including lipid-rich areas, moderate and dense fibrotic tissue, and calcified deposits (48).

Although the ability of computer-based analysis of the unprocessed radiofrequency backscatter to differentiate the histologic components of the normal and diseased vessel is investigational, investigators are optimistic that it will eventually offer the ability to discern detailed characterization of both stable and unstable atheroma *in vivo*.

Elastography

IVUS elastography is a technique that can differentiate the mechanical properties of different plaques. ECG-gated ultrasound images are acquired simultaneously with intracoronary pressure. Strain characteristics are used to infer tissue components. Preliminary studies *in vitro* suggest that elastography can differentiate fibrous and lipid-rich plaques, and the technique appears feasible in humans (49). Investigators must still overcome technical challenges, such as catheter motion during systole.

CORONARY ANGIOSCOPY

Coronary angioscopy uses small fiber-optic filaments for direct inspection of the surface characteristics and intraluminal morphology of human coronaries. The images are presented on a television monitor in color, enabling detailed examination of the vessel surface. Angioscopy can differentiate between platelet-rich and fibrin-rich thrombus, stable plaque versus those with evidence of rupture, and can identify intraplaque hemorrhage and coronary dissection. Much of this information is unobtainable by other techniques. For example, initial angioscopy studies of the early 1980s correlated unstable angina and the presence of the intraluminal thrombus (50).

Equipment and Technique

The development of a coronary angioscope small and flexible enough to steer safely over a guidewire through tortuous coronary segments is technically challenging. The device has four separate lumens. One lumen inflates a balloon to temporarily occlude flow, because angioscopy requires a blood-free field; thus, the operator must complete the examination quickly to minimize ischemia. An irrigation lumen clears the coronary of residual blood. A third lumen has an optical fibers light source. Finally, a fourth lumen contains fibers that transmit the image. This device is advanced over a conventional, 0.014-inch angioplasty guidewire and can be moved over 5 cm of the vessel; this is necessary because the depth of field is 0.5 mm. Although angioscopy currently is rarely used clinically, it is important for the research of coronary pathophysiology.

Angioscopy Insights into Acute Coronary Syndromes

Thrombus

In an early intraoperative coronary angioscopy study, Sherman and coworkers (50) demonstrated differences in the intraluminal appearance of stable versus unstable coronary atheromas. In all ten patients with unstable angina, there were distinctive intimal abnormalities. Four patients had "complex plaque," and seven had intraluminal thrombus. Angiography detected only one of four complex plaques and only one of seven thrombi. Neither complex plaques nor thrombi were observed in any patient with stable coronary disease. This study established the association of unstable coronary syndromes with plaque ulcerations and thrombosis. These findings were subsequently replicated with percutaneous angioscopy.

Angioscopy also can differentiate platelet-rich from fibrin-rich thrombi. The typical thrombus in patients with unstable angina is grayish white, suggesting the predominance of platelets; whereas in patients with acute MI, red thrombi predominate, suggesting an erythrocyte- and fibrin-rich clot (51). These observations support the hypothesis that platelet aggregation is an important step in the initiation of the unstable syndromes. However, technical limitations of the angioscopy hardware may not always render color accurately; quantitative colorimetric analysis has been proposed to overcome this potential variability.

Surface Color and Atheroma Composition

Surface color and characteristics are a predictor of underlying morphology. Stable plaques typically have a smooth appearance, an increased contour, and are grayish white. Yellow is more frequently seen in disrupted plaque sections and in association with ACSs. Thieme and coworkers (52) examined 44 patients with stable or unstable angina and the angiographic and angioscopic findings were compared with atherectomy specimens from the same sites. In patients with unstable angina, 89% had yellow, lipid-rich plaques, and 39% had thrombus. Patients with stable angina had both yellow plaque (57%) and grayish white lesions (43%), the latter demonstrating either degeneration (64%) or fibrous plaque (14%) histologically. Only 11% of those patients with stable angina had thrombus (52).

Angioscopic studies also support the concept that multiple sections of coronary tree may contain "vulnerable" plaques simultaneously. Yellow plaques often are diffusely distributed throughout the examined artery. One study demonstrated that patients with predominantly yellow plaques were found to have greater LDL cholesterol and apolipoprotein B lipoprotein levels (53). In a study of patients with MI, all three coronary arteries were diffusely diseased angioscopically and had multiple yellow, though nondisrupted, plaques. Yellow plaques were equally prevalent in infarct and noninfarct arteries, whereas thrombus was present in more than 80% of infarct arteries and in only 2% of noninfarct arteries (54). Van Belle and coworkers (55) imaged 56 patients with angioscopy between 24 hours and 4 weeks after MI. Their findings suggest that healing of the infarct-related lesion requires longer than 1 month, and "unstable" yellow plaques and thrombus are common during the first month *after* infarction. Ueda and coworkers (56) imaged 85 patients with an acute MI and at 1, 6, and 18 months. The mean color grade of the culprit lesion decreased progressively from yellow to white; most of the change occurred during the first 6 months and appeared delayed in patients with diabetes and in patients with hyperlipidemia. The incidence of thrombus also decreased progressively from 93% at the time of ACS to 12% at 18 months (56).

Evidence of stabilization also can be studied angioscopically, although the technique is not amenable to large series. One small study suggested that bezafibrate alters the predominant atheroma color during 6 months of treatment. Ohsawa and coworkers (57) compared 21 plaques in 14 patients treated with bezafibrate to 14 plaques in 10 control patients. After 6 months, a "vulnerability score" (including color and surface characteristics) improved in the treated patients, coincident with an increase in HDL.

Surface Irregularities

Angioscopy can detail surface irregularities that can predict adverse outcomes after angioplasty. Feld and coworkers (58) reported that angioscopic evidence of plaque disruption or thrombus was independently associated with adverse outcomes after coronary intervention. Because stents were used in only a small minority, the relevance of these findings to contemporary intervention is less certain. Intimal disruption may also play a role in patients with coronary spasm; one angioscopy study of ten patients with vasospastic angina demonstrated that 40% had intimal injuries such as hemorrhage, flap, thrombus, or an ulcer at the site of spasm (59). An example of a plaque rupture visualized by both IVUS and angioscopy is illustrated in Figure 50–11. Plaque regions with irregular or disrupted surface areas and that are associated with ACSs are positively remodeled, confirming IVUS studies (60). Takano and coworkers (61) combined ultrasound, angioscopy, and elastography to compare 27 patients with yellow plaques and 11 control subjects with white plaques. Yellow plaques were not only positively remodeled, but their distensibility index was significantly greater. These data suggest that lipid rich, positively remodeled sections of atheroma may be structurally weak, predisposing to rupture (61).

Surface irregularities are even more dramatic in degenerated saphenous vein grafts. Necropsy studies have shown that such conduits often contain friable and sometimes frankly necrotic atheromatous material, intraluminal thrombus, or both. These findings often escape angiographic detection but can be quite vivid with angioscopy (62), and probably account for the greater incidence of "no-reflow" in the absence of distal protection devices.

Limitations of Coronary Angioscopy

Angioscopy is limited to the proximal and mid-segments of relatively straight coronary arteries; it is difficult to advance these catheters through tortuous segments and into small distal branches. The most proximal segments of the coronaries—a common site for plaque rupture—are also not amenable to examination, because target segments must be 20 mm or more distal to the occlusion balloon. Angioscopy

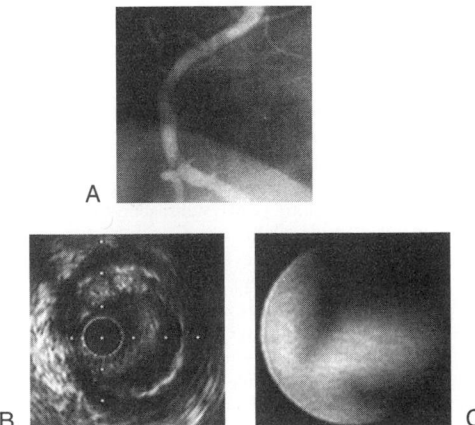

FIG. 50–11. Adjunctive imaging during an acute coronary syndrome. Angiography (A) reveals an intraluminal filling defect. Ultrasound (B) suggests a plaque rupture, with a pedunculated mass separated from the rest of the atheroma. Angioscopy (C) confirms that this mass is the site of plaque rupture.

reveals only the surface characteristics and the color of plaques at or immediately below the vessel surface. Although surface characteristics appear to be related to ACS, the incremental value of this information compared with other technologies (such as ultrasound backscatter analysis, optical coherence tomography [OCT], and other techniques) is unknown. Ischemia during balloon occlusion limits examination time, and transient occlusion may produce artifacts. The flaps and fronds of protruding tissue may not occur until the occlusion balloon depressurizes the vessel; thus, these findings may not reflect actual morphology. Finally, although the identification of red thrombus and dissection has acceptable interobserver agreement, other angioscopic diagnoses have greater interobserver variability.

INVESTIGATIONAL ENDOLUMINAL TECHNOLOGIES

Some lesions associated with an ACSs and thrombosis are "fibrous," with thick caps and without any demonstrable lipid core (23,31,63). Thus, ultrasound or angioscopy may not identify all "vulnerable" plaques. New technologies attempt to address this limitation by characterizing other features of vulnerable lesions.

Thermography

Inflammation is an important characteristic of lesions at risk for ACSs, and the heat released from these inflamed plaques may predict the risk for rupture (64). Casscells and coworkers (65) used a needle thermistor to demonstrate that 37% of excised plaques had regions that were substantially warmer (0.4–2.2°C) than other areas. The temperature increase correlated positively with inflammatory cell density. Catheter-based systems for use *in vivo* have a spatial resolution of 500 μm and an accuracy of 0.05°C. When patients with stable disease versus unstable angina versus acute MI are studied, progressively greater temperatures and greater thermal heterogeneity have been reported (66). Whether thermography will have clinical application depends on whether the device can be made easier to use and atraumatic.

Optical Coherence Tomography

OCT uses an *interferometer* to measure the intensity of reflected infrared light. Although the depth of penetration is less than ultrasound (only 1–2 mm), resolution is greater (5–20 microns), and may allow better detection of thin-cap atheromas. *In vitro* studies suggest a strong correlation with actual histology and superior definition of structural detail compared with IVUS, with a greater than 90% sensitivity and specificity for predicting the presence of lipid-rich plaques (67). In autopsy specimens, OCT also was able to quantify macrophage infiltration within fibrous caps (68). Initial *in vivo* studies suggest that OCT may have a greater sensitivity than conventional ultrasound in identifying potential lipid pools (69). Image acquisition times will need to be less for this to become a practical research or clinical tool.

Raman and Infrared Spectroscopy

In Raman spectroscopy, a laser illuminates the target tissue and the spectra of the reflected light is used to characterize its chemical composition. The relative quantities of calcification, cholesterol, and fibrous tissue can be inferred (70,71). Because Raman spectroscopy is a one-dimensional technique—that is, it can not provide information about depth—research is directed at combining this information with other modalities, such as ultrasound (70). Thus, the technical challenges that must be overcome before this becomes a more widely used research tool are substantial, including blood absorption of the laser light, strong background fluorescence, and relatively long acquisition times.

Near-infrared spectroscopy (NIR) analyzes the reflected signal from an infrared light source. Unlike Raman spectroscopy, tissue penetration is deeper, but the technique is one-dimensional. In human aortic specimens obtained at necropsy, NIR spectroscopy had a high sensitivity and specificity for identifying lipid pools, thin caps, and the presence of inflammatory cells (72). As with Raman spectroscopy, NIR may need to be combined with other modalities to provide depth information.

CONCLUSIONS

The conventional paradigm of coronary artery disease as a focal process was the direct result of the limitations of angiographic assessment; instead, necropsy and new imaging modalities confirm that coronary disease is most often diffuse. However, focal segments within a diffusely diseased vessel may exhibit unique morphologic characteristics or may be more intensely involved in the inflammatory aspects of the disease. IVUS is a practical technique to assess many of these morphologic changes, and newer endoluminal modalities may detect the signs of inflammation. In addition, an individual may have segments of the same artery at different stages of the disease at any one time, with some segments relatively inert; others involved in rupture, erosion, or healing from these events; and others in an earlier, "rupture-prone" stage. Muller and coworkers (73) first coined the term "vulnerable plaque" in the early 1990s in an attempt to characterize which lesions are likely to rupture. However, insights from new imaging modalities suggest that the dynamic and diffuse process of coronary atheroma evolution may make it more appropriate to refer to the vulnerable *artery*, or, perhaps even more accurately, to the vulnerable *patient*. Finally, given the diverse morphologies of plaques associated with ACSs, multiple approaches, rather than a single, "ideal" endoluminal technology, may be required for optimal identification of the plaque, the artery, and the patients at greatest risk. Whatever the ultimate ap-

proach, endoluminal assessment and risk stratification of the coronary system will hopefully allow pharmacologic and other interventions to be targeted to reduce subsequent events.

REFERENCES

1. Davies MJ, Thomas AC. Plaque fissuring—the cause of acute myocardial infarction, sudden ischaemic death, and crescendo angina. *Br Heart J* 1985;53:363–373.
2. Davies MJ. Anatomic features in victims of sudden coronary death. Coronary artery pathology. *Circulation* 1992;85[1 Suppl]:I19–I24.
3. Falk E, Shah PK, Fuster V. Coronary plaque disruption. *Circulation* 1995;92:657–671.
4. Davies MJ. The composition of coronary-artery plaques. *N Engl J Med* 1997;336:1312–1314.
4a. Libby P. What have we learned about the biology of atherosclerosis? The role of inflammation. *Am J Cardiol* 2001;88:3J–6J.
5. Topol EJ, McCarthy J, Gabriel S, et al. Single nucleotide polymorphisms in multiple novel thrombospondin genes may be associated with familial premature myocardial infarction. *Circulation* 2001;104:2641–2644.
6. Virmani R, Kolodgie FD, Burke AP, et al. Lessons from sudden coronary death: a comprehensive morphological classification scheme for atherosclerotic lesions. *Arterioscler Thromb Vasc Biol* 2000;20:1262–1275.
7. Kolodgie FD, Burke AP, Farb A, et al. The thin-cap fibroatheroma: a type of vulnerable plaque: the major precursor lesion to acute coronary syndromes. *Curr Opin Cardiol* 2001;16:285–292.
8. Farb A, Burke AP, Tang AL, et al. Coronary plaque erosion without rupture into a lipid core. A frequent cause of coronary thrombosis in sudden coronary death. *Circulation* 1996;93:1354–1363.
9. Virmani R, Burke AP, Farb A. Sudden cardiac death. *Cardiovasc Pathol* 2001;10:211–218.
10. Mintz GS, Painter JA, Pichard AD, et al. Atherosclerosis in angiographically "normal" coronary artery reference segments: an intravascular ultrasound study with clinical correlations. *J Am Coll Cardiol* 1995;25:1479–1485.
11. Berkalp B, Badak O, Schoenhagen P, et al. Influence of various percutaneous coronary interventional devices on postinterventional luminal shape and plaque surface characteristics as determined by intravascular ultrasound. *Am J Cardiol* 2003;19:1269–1272.
12. Ambrose JA, Winters SL, Stern A, et al. Angiographic morphology and the pathogenesis of unstable angina pectoris. *J Am Coll Cardiol* 1985;5:609–616.
13. Gorlin R, Fuster V, Ambrose J. Anatomic-physiologic links between acute coronary syndromes. *Circulation* 1986;74:6–9.
14. Tuzcu EM, Hobbs RE, Rincon G, et al. Occult and frequent transmission of atherosclerotic coronary disease with cardiac transplantation. Insights from intravascular ultrasound. *Circulation* 1995;91:1706–1713.
15. Glagov S, Weisenberg E, Zarins C, et al. Compensatory enlargement of human coronary arteries. *N Engl J Med* 1987;316:1371–1375.
16. Schoenhagen P, Ziada KM, Kapadia SR, et al. Extent and direction of arterial remodeling in stable versus unstable coronary syndromes: an intravascular ultrasound study. *Circulation* 2000;101:598–603.
17. von Birgelen C, Klinkhart W, Mintz GS, et al. Plaque distribution and vascular remodeling of ruptured and nonruptured coronary plaques in the same vessel: an intravascular ultrasound study in vivo. *J Am Coll Cardiol* 2001;37:1864–1870.
18. Varnava AM, Mills PG, Davies MJ. Relationship between coronary artery remodeling and plaque vulnerability. *Circulation* 2002;105:939–943.
19. Schoenhagen P, Vince DG, Ziada KM, et al. Relation of matrix-metalloproteinase 3 found in coronary lesion samples retrieved by directional coronary atherectomy to intravascular ultrasound observations on coronary remodeling. *Am J Cardiol* 2002;89:1354–1359.
20. Hodgson JM, Reddy KG, Suneja R, et al. Intracoronary ultrasound imaging: correlation of plaque morphology with angiography, clinical syndrome and procedural results in patients undergoing coronary angioplasty. *J Am Coll Cardiol* 1993;21:35–44.
21. Kearney P, Erbel R, Rupprecht H, et al. Differences in the morphology of unstable and stable coronary lesions and their impact on the mechanisms of angioplasty. An in vivo study with intravascular ultrasound. *Eur Heart J* 1995;17:721–730.
22. Tanaka A, Kawarabayashi T, Nishibori Y, et al. No-reflow phenomenon

and lesion morphology in patients with acute myocardial infarction. *Circulation* 2002;105:2148–2152.

23. Tanaka A, Kawarabayashi T, Taguchi H, et al. Use of preintervention intravascular ultrasound in patients with acute myocardial infarction. *Am J Cardiol* 2002;89:257–261.

24. Fukuda D, Tanaka A, Shimada K, et al. Predicting angiographic distal embolization following percutaneous coronary intervention in patients with acute myocardial infarction. *Am J Cardiol* 2003;91:403–407.

25. Di Mario C, Gorge G, Peters R, et al. Clinical application and image interpretation in intracoronary ultrasound. Study Group on Intracoronary Imaging of the Working Group of Coronary Circulation and of the Subgroup on Intravascular Ultrasound of the Working Group of Echocardiography of the European Society of Cardiology. *Eur Heart J* 1998; 19:207–229.

26. Hiro T, Leung C, de Guzman S, et al. Are "soft echoes" really soft? Intravascular ultrasound assessment of mechanical properties in human atherosclerotic tissue. *Am Heart J* 1997;133:1–7.

27. Prati F, Arbustini E, Labellarte A, et al. Correlation between high frequency intravascular ultrasound and histomorphology in human coronary arteries. *Heart* 2001;85:567–570.

28. Maehara A, Mintz GS, Castagna MT, et al. Intravascular ultrasound assessment of spontaneous coronary artery dissection. *Am J Cardiol* 2002;89:466–468.

29. von Birgelen C, Klinkhart W, Mintz GS, et al. Size of emptied plaque cavity following spontaneous rupture is related to coronary dimensions, not to the degree of lumen narrowing. A study with intravascular ultrasound in vivo. *Heart* 2000;84:483–488.

30. Bocksch W, Schartl M, Beckmann S, et al. Intravascular ultrasound imaging in patients with acute myocardial infarction. *Eur Heart J* 1995;19[Suppl J]:46–52.

31. Fuchs S, Stabile E, Mintz GS, et al. Intravascular ultrasound findings in patients with acute coronary syndromes with and without elevated troponin I level. *Am J Cardiol* 2002;89:1111–1113.

32. Ambrose JA, Tannenbaum MA, Alexopoulos D, et al. Angiographic progression of coronary artery disease and the development of myocardial infarction. *J Am Coll Cardiol* 1988;12:56–62.

33. Maehara A, Mintz GS, Bui AB, et al. Morphologic and angiographic features of coronary plaque rupture detected by intravascular ultrasound. *J Am Coll Cardiol* 2002;40:904–910.

34. Schoenhagen P, Stone GW, Nissen SE, et al. Coronary plaque morphology and frequency of ulceration distant from culprit lesions in patients with unstable and stable presentation. *Arterioscler Thromb Vasc Biol* 2003;23:1895–1900.

35. Rioufol G, Finet G, Ginon I, et al. Multiple atherosclerotic plaque rupture in acute coronary syndrome: a three-vessel intravascular ultrasound study. *Circulation* 2002;106:804–808.

36. Goldstein JA, Demetriou D, Grines CL, et al. Multiple complex coronary plaques in patients with acute myocardial infarction. *N Engl J Med* 2000;343:915–922.

37. Gutfinger DE, Leung CY, Hiro T, et al. In vitro atherosclerotic plaque and calcium quantitation by intravascular ultrasound and electron-beam computed tomography. *Am Heart J* 1996;131:899–906.

38. De Servi S, Arbustini E, Marsico F, et al. Correlation between clinical and morphologic findings in unstable angina. *Am J Cardiol* 1996; 77:128–132.

39. Huang H, Virmani R, Younis H, et al. The impact of calcification on the biomechanical stability of atherosclerotic plaques. *Circulation* 2001; 103:1051–1056.

40. Yamagishi M, Terashima M, Awano K, et al. Morphology of vulnerable coronary plaque: insights from follow-up of patients examined by intravascular ultrasound before an acute coronary syndrome. *J Am Coll Cardiol* 2000;35:106–111.

40a. Virmani R, Burke AP, Farb A. Plaque rupture and plaque erosion. *Thromb Haemost* 1999;82[Suppl 1]:1–3.

41. Takagi T, Yoshida K, Akasaka T, et al. Intravascular ultrasound analysis of reduction in progression of coronary narrowing by treatment with pravastatin. *Am J Cardiol* 1997;79:1673–1676.

42. Schartl M, Bocksch W, Koschyk DH, et al. Use of intravascular ultrasound to compare effects of different strategies of lipid-lowering therapy on plaque volume and composition in patients with coronary artery disease. *Circulation* 2001;104:387–392.

43. Matsuzaki M, Hiramori K, Imaizumi T, et al. Intravascular ultrasound evaluation of coronary plaque regression by low density lipoprotein-apheresis in familial hypercholesterolemia: the Low Density Lipoprotein-Apheresis Coronary Morphology and Reserve Trial (LACMART). *J Am Coll Cardiol* 2002;40:220–227.

44. Hamasaki S, Higano ST, Suwaidi JA, et al. Cholesterol-lowering treatment is associated with improvement in coronary vascular remodeling and endothelial function in patients with normal or mildly diseased coronary arteries. *Arterioscler Thromb Vasc Biol* 2000;20:737–743.

45. Nissen SE. Rationale for a postintervention continuum of care: insights from intravascular ultrasound. *Am J Cardiol* 2000;86(4B):12H–17H.

46. Komiyama N, Chronos NA, Uren NG, et al. The progression of thrombus in an ex-vivo shunt model evaluated by intravascular ultrasound radiofrequency analysis. *Ultrasound Med Biol* 1999;25:561–566.

47. Lee DJ, Sigel B, Swami VK, et al. Determination of carotid plaque risk by ultrasonic tissue characterization. *Ultrasound Med Biol* 1998;24:1291–1299.

48. Nair A, Kuban BD, Tuzcu EM, et al. Coronary plaque classification with intravascular ultrasound radiofrequency data analysis. *Circulation* 2002;106:2200–2206.

49. de Korte CL, Carlier SG, Mastik F, et al. Morphological and mechanical information of coronary arteries obtained with intravascular elastography: feasibility study in vivo. *Eur Heart J* 2002;23:405–413.

50. Sherman CT, Litvack F, Grundfest W, et al. Coronary angioscopy in patients with unstable angina pectoris. *N Engl J Med* 1986;315:913–919.

51. Mizuno K, Satomura K, Miyamoto A, et al. Angioscopic evaluation of coronary-artery thrombi in acute coronary syndromes. *N Engl J Med* 1992;326:287–291.

52. Thieme T, Wernecke KD, Meyer R, et al. Angioscopic evaluation of atherosclerotic plaques: validation by histomorphologic analysis and association with stable and unstable coronary syndromes. *J Am Coll Cardiol* 1996;28:1–6.

53. Kitamura K, Mizuno K, Miyamoto A, et al. Serum lipid profiles and the presence of yellow plaque in coronary lesions in vivo. *Am J Cardiol* 1997;79:676–679.

54. Asakura M, Ueda Y, Yamaguchi O, et al. Extensive development of vulnerable plaques as a pan-coronary process in patients with myocardial infarction: an angioscopic study. *J Am Coll Cardiol* 2001; 37:1284–1288.

55. Van Belle E, Lablanche JM, Bauters C, et al. Coronary angioscopic findings in the infarct-related vessel within 1 month of acute myocardial infarction: natural history and the effect of thrombolysis. *Circulation* 1998;97:26–33.

56. Ueda Y, Asakura M, Yamaguchi O, et al. The healing process of infarct-related plaques. Insights from 18 months of serial angioscopic follow-up. *J Am Coll Cardiol* 2001;38:1916–1922.

57. Ohsawa D, Uchida Y, Fujimori Y, et al. Angioscopic evaluation of stabilizing effects of an antilipemic agent, bezafibrate, on coronary plaques in patients with coronary artery disease: a multicenter prospective study. *Jpn Heart J* 2002;43:319–331.

58. Feld S, Ganim M, Carell ES, et al. Comparison of angioscopy, intravascular ultrasound imaging and quantitative coronary angiography in predicting clinical outcome after coronary intervention in high risk patients. *J Am Coll Cardiol* 1996;28:97–105.

59. Etsuda H, Mizuno K, Arakawa K, et al. Angioscopy in variant angina: coronary artery spasm and intimal injury. *Lancet* 1993;342:1322–1324.

60. Smits PC, Pasterkamp G, de Jaegere PP, et al. Angioscopic complex lesions are predominantly compensatory enlarged: an angioscopy and intracoronary ultrasound study. *Cardiovasc Res* 1999;41:458–464.

61. Takano M, Mizuno K, Okamatsu K, et al. Mechanical and structural characteristics of vulnerable plaques: analysis by coronary angioscopy and intravascular ultrasound. *J Am Coll Cardiol* 2001;38:99–104.

62. White CJ, Ramee SR, Collins TJ, et al. Percutaneous angioscopy of saphenous vein coronary bypass grafts. *J Am Coll Cardiol* 1993;21: 1181–1185.

63. Virmani R, Burke AP, Kolodgie FD, et al. Vulnerable plaque: the pathology of unstable coronary lesions. *J Interv Cardiol* 2002;15:439–446.

64. van der Wal AC, Becker AE, van der Loos CM, et al. Site of intimal rupture or erosion of thrombosed coronary atherosclerotic plaques is characterized by an inflammatory process irrespective of the dominant plaque morphology. *Circulation* 1994;89:36–44.

65. Casscells W, Hathorn B, David M, et al. Thermal detection of cellular infiltrates in living atherosclerotic plaques: possible implications for plaque rupture and thrombosis. *Lancet* 1996;347:1447–1451.

66. Stefanadis C, Diamantopoulos L, Vlachopoulos C, et al. Thermal heterogeneity within human atherosclerotic coronary arteries detected in vivo: a new method of detection by application of a special thermography catheter. *Circulation* 1999;99:1965–1971.

67. Yabushita H, Bouma BE, Houser SL, et al. Characterization of human atherosclerosis by optical coherence tomography. *Circulation* 2002; 106:1640–1645.

68. Tearney GJ, Yabushita H, Houser SL, et al. Quantification of macrophage content in atherosclerotic plaques by optical coherence tomography. *Circulation* 2003;107:113–119.

69. Jang IK, Bouma BE, Kang DH, et al. Visualization of coronary atherosclerotic plaques in patients using optical coherence tomography: comparison with intravascular ultrasound. *J Am Coll Cardiol* 2002;39: 604–609.

70. Romer TJ, Brennan JF 3rd, Puppels GJ, et al. Intravascular ultrasound combined with Raman spectroscopy to localize and quantify cholesterol and calcium salts in atherosclerotic coronary arteries. *Arterioscler Thromb Vasc Biol* 2000;20:478–483.

71. Buschman HP, Deinum G, Motz JT, et al. Raman microspectroscopy of human coronary atherosclerosis: biochemical assessment of cellular and extracellular morphologic structures in situ. *Cardiovasc Pathol* 2001;10:69–82.

72. Moreno PR, Lodder RA, Purushothaman KR, et al. Detection of lipid pool, thin fibrous cap, and inflammatory cells in human aortic atherosclerotic plaques by near-infrared spectroscopy. *Circulation* 2002;105: 923–927.

73. Muller JE, Abela GS, Nesto RW, et al. Triggers, acute risk factors and vulnerable plaques: the lexicon of a new frontier. *J Am Coll Cardiol* 1994;23:809–813.

74. Virmani R, Burke AP, Farb A, et al. Pathology of the unstable plaque. *Prog Cardiovasc Dis* 2002;44:349–356.

75. Duissaillant G, Mintz G, Pichard A, et al. Intravascular ultrasound identification of calcified intraluminal lesions misdiagnosed as thrombi by coronary angiography. *Am Heart J* 1996;132:687–689.

CHAPTER 51

Computed Tomography of the Heart

John J. Mahmarian

Key Words: Atherosclerosis; cardiac computed tomography; coronary calcification; myocardial ischemia; risk stratification.

INTRODUCTION

Computed tomography (CT) is a noninvasive technique that can detect the presence of early atherothrombosis based on the presence and extent of coronary artery calcification. Recent advancements also allow for contrast angiography of the coronary arteries (1–8). Enhanced imaging speed combined with electrocardiographic (ECG) gating can produce literally "freeze-frame" images of the heart, obviating most of the blur caused by motion artifact during systole and diastole. This is of paramount importance when obtaining both contrast-enhanced images of the coronary arteries or quantifying coronary artery calcium. Mechanical CT and electron beam CT (EBCT) scanners are currently available for performing cardiac evaluations.

TECHNICAL CONSIDERATIONS

Mechanical Computed Tomography

Advancements in CT technology have improved image acquisition speed and patient throughput. Traditional mechanical CT scanners produce images by rotating an x-ray table around

J. J. Mahmarian: Department of Medicine, Section of Cardiology, Baylor College of Medicine; Methodist DeBakey Heart Center, Nuclear Cardiology Laboratory, The Methodist Hospital, 6550 Fannin Street, SM-1256, Houston, Texas 77030-2717.

a circular gantry through which the patient advances on a moving couch. In the step-and-shoot CT mode, an obligatory 15-second delay occurs between each slice acquisition. To complete a standard 40-slice cardiac study, 2 scan acquisitions of 20 slices each must be obtained from 2 separate breath holds. This may lead to spatial misalignment of CT data from motion artifacts and differences in the depth of inspiration. With spiral CT scanners, the x-ray tube continuously rotates around the patient as the couch moves through the gantry, thus eliminating incremental stops and allowing completion of a cardiac scan within one breath hold. The introduction of multi-row spiral CT detector systems currently allows acquisition of four simultaneous images of 2.5 mm in thickness.

Improvements in gantry rotation speeds and development of partial reconstruction algorithms have reduced effective single-image acquisition time to ≈300 ms. However, image acquisition within 50 ms is required to completely avoid cardiac motion artifacts (9,10). The coronary arteries also move independently throughout the cardiac cycle and even at slow heart rates (i.e., <70 beats/min) exhibit significant translational motion (up to 60 mm/s for the right coronary artery) (10,11).

To potentially compensate for image blur, retrospective and prospective gating can be performed with either spiral or nonspiral CT using single row or multirow detector arrays. Retrospective gating with spiral CT uses acquisition of multiple images throughout each cardiac cycle. With multidetector spiral systems, temporal resolution may be further improved by selecting specific partial image sector data from different heartbeats and detector rings so as to reconstruct a complete 240-degree image data set. Retrospective gating allows one to "pick and choose" images with the least amount of motion-related distortion before final image reconstruction. However, this oversampling leads to significant and unnecessary excess radiation exposure to the patient. The typical radiation exposure from an EBCT study is less than 1.0 rad (12), whereas multidetector CT scanners using retrospective gating can increase exposure $\approx$13-fold (13). Prospective gating during either spiral or nonspiral acquisitions uses image triggering only at a specific temporal location of the cardiac cycle, thereby significantly reducing radiation exposure. Gating works relatively well at slow heart rates (i.e., <60 beats/min) where the R-R interval is greater than 1,000 ms and when the fastest imaging protocols are used. However, at faster heart rates, a 300- to 500-ms acquisition effectively covers most of the cardiac cycle, thus obviating any potential benefit from gating the image acquisition.

Electron Beam Computed Tomography

EBCT uses an electron beam (current: 630 MA, voltage: 130 kV) that is magnetically swept along a series of tungsten targets located beneath the patient at a 210-degree arc. The resultant x-rays generated beneath the patient are then attenuated as they pass through the thorax and recorded by a series of two twin-fixed detector arrays arranged in a semicircle above the patient. Because EBCT has no moving parts, as found in mechanical CT scanners, imaging time is complete within 50 ms, which is the time required for the electron beam to sweep along the tungsten targets. Incorporating rapid acquisition time and prospective gating allows for a nearly "freeze-frame" image of the myocardium and coronary arteries. With current EBCT scanners, image acquisition is complete within one single breath hold.

DETECTION OF CORONARY ARTERY CALCIFICATION

Mechanical CT imaging protocols vary widely among different camera systems and manufacturers. Generally, 40 consecutive 2.5- to 3-mm-thick images are acquired. Calcified lesions are defined as two or three adjacent pixels with a tomographic density of either $\geq$90 or $\geq$130 Hounsfield units (HU). Effective pixel size for a reconstruction matrix of 512 $\times$ 512 pixels with a common field of view of 26 cm is 0.26 mm^2. The traditional Agatston scoring system multiplies each calcified lesion by a density factor as follows: 1 for lesions 130 to 199 HU; 2 for lesions 200 to 299 HU; 3 for lesions 300 to 399 HU; and 4 for lesions 400 HU or greater. The modified system begins scoring at the 90-HU threshold. The total coronary artery calcium score (CACS) is calculated as the sum of each calcified plaque over all the tomographic slices.

The standard EBCT imaging protocol is to acquire approximately 40 consecutive 3-mm-thick images at a rate of 100 ms per image from the base of the heart to just below the carina. Images are obtained at end-inspiration with ECG triggering typically at 80% of the R-R interval. Image pixel size using a 512 $\times$ 512 reconstruction matrix is 0.26 or 0.34 mm^2 based on a 26 or 30 cm field of view, respectively. All calcified lesions covering two or three adjacent pixels with a density of 130 HU or greater are summed to calculate the CACS (Fig. 51–1). The Agatston-derived CACS correlates extremely well with the calcified areas found in individual coronary arteries as determined by histomorphometric measurements ($r = 0.96$, $p < 0.0001$) (14). No comparable data are available with mechanical CT. Furthermore, considerable variance exists between EBCT and mechanical CT–derived CACSs (Table 51–1) (15–20).

CORONARY ARTERY CALCIFICATION AND ATHEROTHROMBOTIC PLAQUE BURDEN

Coronary artery calcification signifies the presence of coronary atherothrombosis (21,22), and the CACS severity is directly related to the total atherothrombotic plaque burden present in the epicardial coronary arteries (21,22). Calcification is an active, organized, and regulated process occurring during atherothrombotic plaque development where calcium phosphate, in the form of hydroxyapatite, precipitates in atherothrombotic coronary arteries in a similar fashion as observed in bone mineralization (23–25). Coronary calcification begins early in life but progresses variably with age. Even among elderly men and women, some 30% will have a CACS less than 100 and $\approx$10% a normal study (26,27). Although lack of calcification does not categorically exclude the presence of atherothrombotic plaque, calcification occurs exclusively

TABLE 51–1. *Electron beam computed tomography versus mechanical computed tomography*

Author (reference)	Year	Patients, n	Age, yr	Average Ca^{2+} score	Mechanical CT technique	Gating	Detectors, n	Difference
Becker et al. (15)	1999	50	61	983	Nonspiral	No	Single	42%
Budoff et al. (16)	2001	33	54	52	Nonspiral	No	Single	84%
Becker et al. (17)	2000	50	62	—	Nonspiral	Prospective	Single	25%
Carr et al. (18)	2000	36	68	432	Spiral	Retrospective	Single	17%
Goldin et al. (19)	2001	70	48	70	Spiral	Retrospective	Single	28%
Becker et al. (20)	2001	88	63	793	Spiral	Prospective	4	32%

Ca^{2+}, calcium; CT, computed tomography.

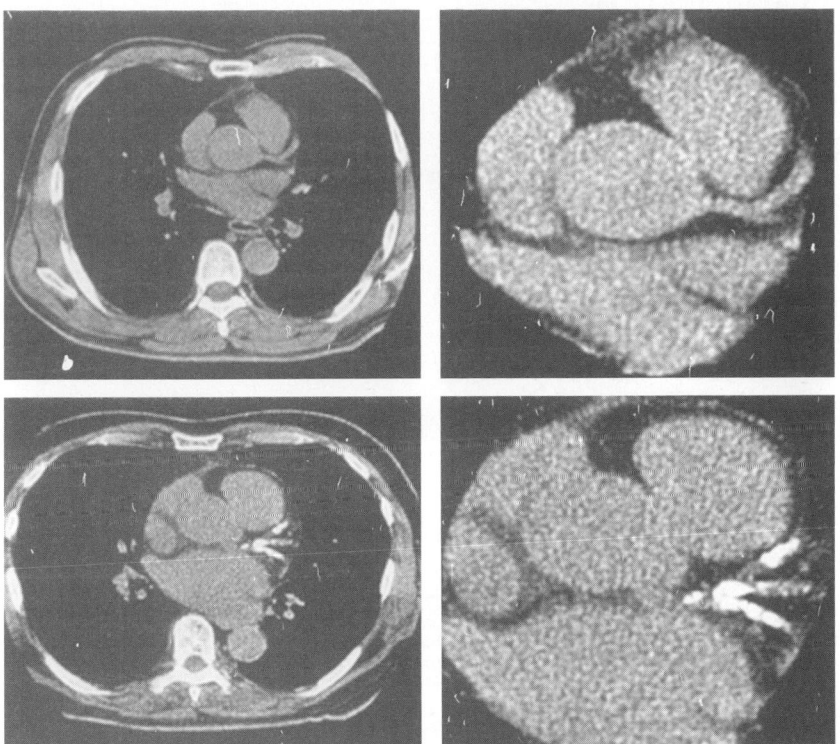

FIG. 51–1. Single-slice noncontrast electron beam computed tomography scan of a healthy subject **(top)** and an individual with severe coronary artery calcification **(bottom).** Calcium is shown as intensely *white areas* within the coronary arteries. (Reprinted from Mahmarian JJ. Computed tomography of the heart. In: Fuster V, et al., eds. *Hurst's the heart,* 10th ed. New York: McGraw-Hill, 2000:567–587.)

in atherothrombotic arteries and is not found in normal coronary arteries.

The presence and extent of histologically determined atherothrombotic plaque area has been compared with the total calcium area as assessed by EBCT from autopsied hearts (21). A strong linear correlation exists between total coronary artery atherothrombotic plaque burden and the extent of coronary artery calcification (Fig. 51–2). However, total plaque area is approximately fivefold greater than total calcified area (21).

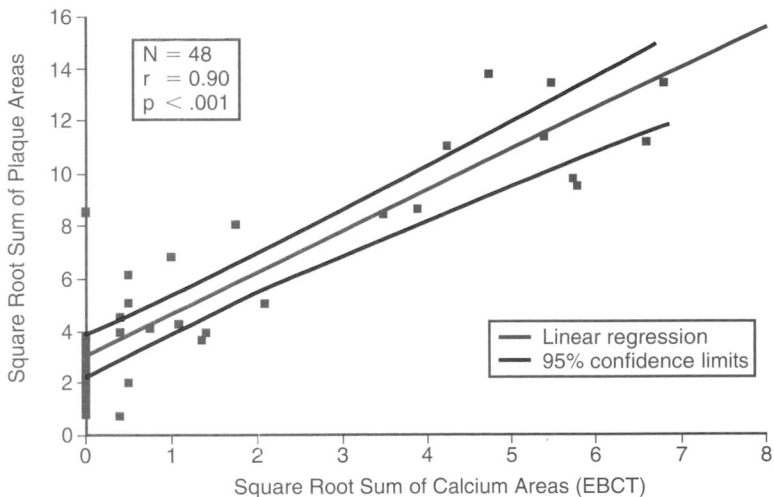

FIG. 51–2. Comparison of the square root sum of total coronary calcium area (mm) by electron beam computed tomography (EBCT) to actual atherothrombotic plaque area (mm) for 38 individual coronary arteries. The linear regression line and 95% confidence intervals are shown. (Redrawn from Rumberger JA, Simons DB, Fitzpatrick LA, et al. Coronary artery calcium area by electron-beam computed tomography and coronary atherosclerotic plaque area: a histopathologic correlative study. *Circulation* 1995;92:2157–2162, with permission.)

CORONARY ARTERY CALCIFICATION AND STENOSIS SEVERITY

Significant (>50%) coronary artery stenosis by angiography is almost universally associated with the presence of coronary artery calcium as assessed by EBCT. However, the extent of coronary artery calcification cannot be used to accurately estimate the severity of angiographic stenosis (22). Coronary artery remodeling occurs with increasing plaque burden, so as to increase luminal diameter and maintain patency (28,29). Nonetheless, noncalcified plaques at autopsy are almost universally associated with insignificant coronary artery stenosis (22).

Clinical trials confirm the relation between CACS severity and the presence of significant (≥50%) coronary artery disease (CAD) (30–45). In the 15 largest studies evaluating EBCT and coronary angiography, the overall sensitivity and specificity for detecting obstructive (>50%) CAD were 97% and 39%, respectively (30–44) (Table 51–2). The likelihood of multivessel and left main CAD increases with the CACS in both men and women (36,46). Haberl and coworkers (44) performed EBCT within 30 days of coronary angiography in 1,764 patients who had suspected CAD. Only 5 of 940 patients (0.5%) with significant (≥50%) coronary artery stenosis had a normal EBCT. Although differences in CACS were noted among men and women, EBCT did predict CAD equally well in both sexes, on the basis of age-specific CACS thresholds (44) (Fig. 51–3).

The poor specificity of EBCT can be reconciled by the fact that the presence of coronary calcification confirms the presence of atherothrombotic plaque, which may not necessarily be obstructive in nature. The CACS severity may be a better barometer of obstructive CAD than the mere presence of cal-

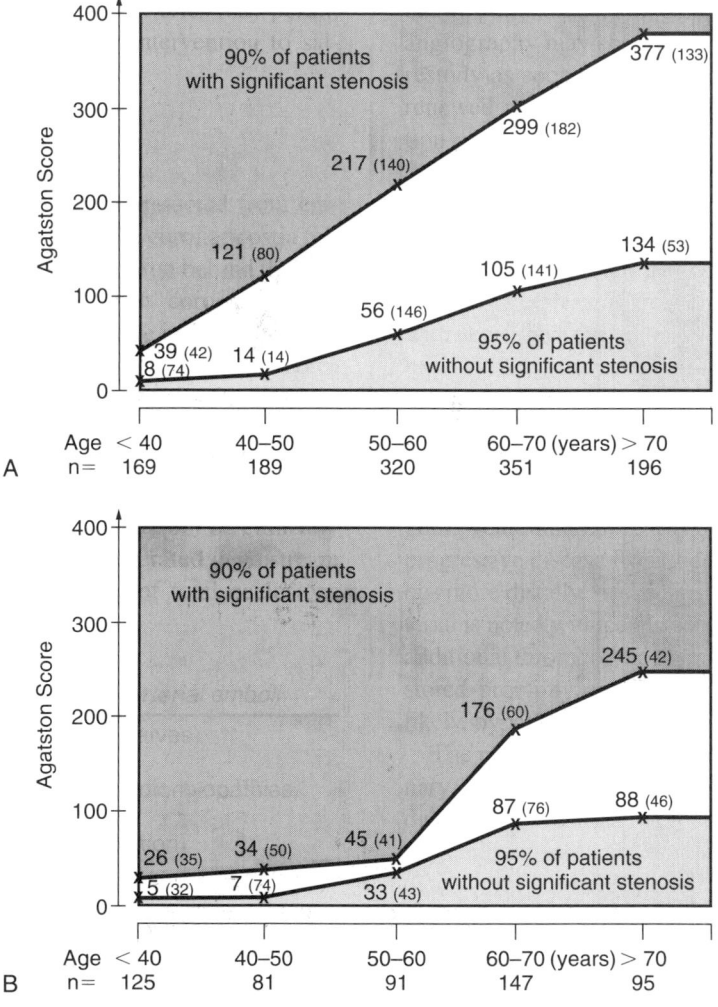

FIG. 51–3. Diagnostic yield of calcium screening in symptomatic men **(A)** and women **(B).** The lower scores define the calcium score thresholds for the 95% of patients without significant stenoses. The higher scores give the calcium score thresholds for the 90% of patients with significant stenoses. Within the central area, the diagnosis is uncertain. The numbers in parentheses give the number of patients within the area. For example, a man at the age of 50 years is probably free of coronary stenosis if his score is less than 56. At score values greater than 217, he bears a high risk for stenosis. (Reprinted from Haberl R, Becker A, Leber A, et al. Correlation of coronary calcification and angiographically documented stenoses in patients with suspected coronary artery disease: results of 1,764 patients. *J Am Coll Cardiol* 2001;37:451–457, with permission.)

TABLE 51–2. *Accuracy of electron beam computed tomography coronary artery calcification in detecting significant (>50%) coronary artery stenosis as defined by angiography*

Investigator (reference)	Year	Subjects, n	Sensitivity, %	Specificity, %	Positive predictive accuracy	Negative predictive accuracy
Agatston et al. (30)	1990	584	96	51	31	98
Breen et al. (31)	1992	100	100	47	63	100
Bielak et al. (32)	1994	160	96	45	57	93
Kaufman et al. (33)	1995	160	93	67	81	86
Rumberger et al. (34)	1995	139	98	39	59	97
Braun et al. (35)	1996	102	93	73	93	73
Budoff et al. (36)	1996	710	95	44	72	84
Detrano et al. (37)	1996	491	95	31	51	89
Fallavollita et al. (38)	1994	106	85	45	66	70
Baumgart et al. (39)	1997	57	97	21	50	86
Schmermund et al. (40)	1997	118	95	88	99	58
Kennedy et al. (41)	1998	368	96	31	51	90
Bielak et al. (42)	2000	213	99	39	64	98
Shavelle et al. (43)	2000	97	96	47	80	82
Haberl et al. (44)	2001	1,764	99	30	62	98
Total		5,169	97	39	61	92

cium in that specificity improves at greater calcium score thresholds. Several reports in patients referred for coronary angiography found that a CACS greater than 100 best predicted obstructive CAD with an equally high sensitivity and specificity of ≈80% (42,44,45,47,48). There appears to be a threshold CACS above which most patients will have significant coronary artery stenosis. The accuracy for identifying significant CAD on the basis of CACS may be further improved by incorporating age, sex (42,44,45), and traditional risk factor information (46,48). However, despite these refine-ments, the CACS is still too imprecise to be used as a definitive criterion for proceeding directly to coronary angiography.

CORONARY ARTERY CALCIFICATION AND MYOCARDIAL ISCHEMIA

Although patients with a normal EBCT are highly unlikely to have significant CAD and generally require no further cardiac testing, there is ongoing controversy how best to proceed in patients with an abnormal EBCT who will have

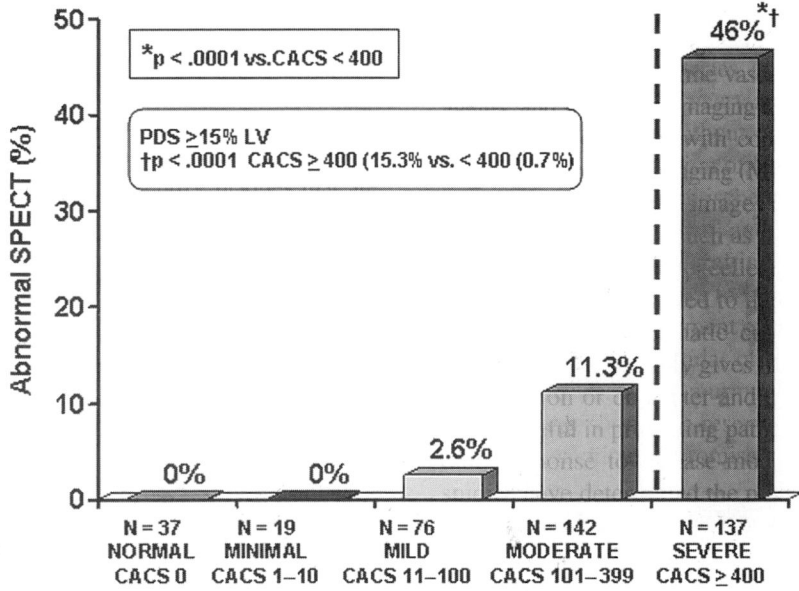

FIG. 51–4. Single photon emission computed tomography (SPECT) results based on total coronary artery calcium score (CACS). Few subjects with CACS less than 400 had abnormal SPECT (6.6%), and most (99.3%) had only a small (<15%) stress-induced perfusion defect size (PDS). LV, left ventricle. (Redrawn from He ZX, Hedrick TD, Pratt CM, et al. Severity of coronary artery calcification by electron beam computed tomography predicts silent myocardial ischemia. *Circulation* 2000;101:244–251, with permission.)

varying CACS severities. To proceed with invasive testing in this latter population is not warranted based on the significant overlap between CACS and the presence of obstructive CAD. An alternative approach might be to perform noninvasive testing in selected patients at high risk for having myocardial ischemia on the basis of specific CACS thresholds. Stress myocardial perfusion imaging is one such well established noninvasive technique for detecting the presence and determining the prognostic significance of CAD on the basis of the extent of inducible myocardial ischemia (49,50). Although not recommended as a screening test in asymptomatic patients because of the low prevalence of a positive test result (<5%) (51,52), perfusion imaging might be used as a secondary test to identify myocardial ischemia once a certain threshold of atherothrombotic plaque burden has been identified by EBCT.

A trial explored the complementary role of EBCT and stress myocardial perfusion single photon emission computed tomography (SPECT) for identifying both preclinical CAD and silent myocardial ischemia in a generally asymptomatic population who had risk factors for CAD development (53). Among the 3,895 subjects who had EBCT, 411 also underwent stress SPECT within a close temporal period (median 17 days). Although only 22% of 374 subjects with an abnormal EBCT were abnormal by SPECT, the likelihood of an abnormal SPECT increased dramatically with the total CACS (Fig. 51–4). Whereas less than 1% of subjects with a total CACS less than 100 had an abnormal SPECT, this was observed in 46% of those with scores of 400 or greater. The total CACS was the best single predictor of an abnormal stress SPECT study. Large ischemic left ventricular perfusion defects (i.e., ≥15%) were virtually confined to subjects who had a CACS score of 400 or greater. Miranda and coworkers (54) confirmed these findings in 233 consecutive asymptomatic patients who had EBCT and SPECT. No patients with a CACS less than 100 had an abnormal SPECT; whereas 4.1% with a moderate (101–400) CACS and 15% with a CACS of 400 or greater had an abnormal SPECT. The best CACS cutoff point for predicting an abnormal SPECT in this study was also 400 (54).

CORONARY ARTERY CALCIFICATION: PROGNOSTIC IMPLICATIONS

The likelihood of plaque rupture and the development of acute cardiovascular events is related to the total atherothrombotic plaque burden (55,56). Because there is a strong relation between CACS severity, the extent of atherothrombotic plaque, and the presence of silent myocardial ischemia, it would seem intuitive that the CACS should predict risk for subsequent cardiovascular events among otherwise heterogeneous patient populations with cardiac risk factors, thereby potentially guiding therapeutics.

The prognostic value of the EBCT-derived CACS has been studied in both symptomatic (57,58) and asymptomatic patients (59–66). Detrano and coworkers followed 422

symptomatic patients for 30 ± 12 months after EBCT and coronary angiography (57). Cardiac events were tenfold greater in patients with a CACS greater than 75th percentile for age (9.5%) versus those less than the 25th percentile (0.9%). Patients with a CACS greater than 100 had a significantly lower infarct-free survival rate than those with lower scores ($p = 0.009$). Keelan and coworkers (58) studied 288 symptomatic patients referred for coronary angiography. Patients with a CACS greater than 100 had a 3.2-fold greater relative risk for death or myocardial infarction (MI) as compared with those with a lower CACS (95% confidence limit, 1.17–8.71). Patient age and the CACS were the only independent predictors of these hard cardiac events.

Arad and coworkers (60) followed 1,173 asymptomatic subjects for 19 months after an initial screening with EBCT of whom 18 patients (1.53%) had 26 cardiac events, including 1 death, 7 nonfatal MIs, and 17 coronary revascularization procedures. No events occurred in subjects with a normal study, and the event rate was negligible (0.2%) among those with a CACS less than 100. However, the cardiac event rate progressively increased as the CACS increased from greater than 100 (5.5%) to greater than 160 (7.1%) and greater than 680 (14%). These results have now been extended to 3.6 years with a 5%, 7%, and 13% hard cardiac

TABLE 51–3. *Multivariate analyses of the association of coronary artery calcium scores and self-reported traditional coronary disease risk factors with all events*

Variable	Odds ratio (95% CI)
Independent of EBCT	
Increased cholesterol	3.9 (1.3–11.7)
Hypertension	2.8 (1.2–6.5)
Diabetes	5.4 (2.0–14.9)
With EBCT CACS ≥ 80	
CACS > 80	14.3 (4.9–42.3)
Age > 55 years	3.3 (1.3–8.4)
Increased cholesterol	4.0 (1.3–12.2)
Hypertension	2.6 (1.1–6.1)
Diabetes	4.8 (1.6–13.9)
With EBCT CACS ≥ 160	
CACS > 160	19.7 (6.9–56.4)
Age > 55 years	4.5 (1.6–12.2)
Increased cholesterol	3.7 (1.2–11.5)
Hypertension	3.0 (1.2–7.4)
Diabetes	5.8 (2.1–19.7)
With EBCT CACS ≥ 600	
CACS > 600	20.2 (7.3–55.8)
Age > 55 years	2.9 (1.1–7.9)
Increased cholesterol	3.5 (1.1–10.8)
Hypertension	2.9 (1.2–7.3)
Diabetes	4.4 (1.4–13.7)

Analyses were performed with and without the coronary artery calcium scores (CACS).

CI, confidence interval; EBCT, electron beam computed tomography; OR, odds ratio.

Reprinted from Arad Y, Spadaro LA, Goodman K, et al. Prediction of coronary events with electron beam computed tomography. *J Am Coll Cardiol* 2000;36:1253–1260, with permission.

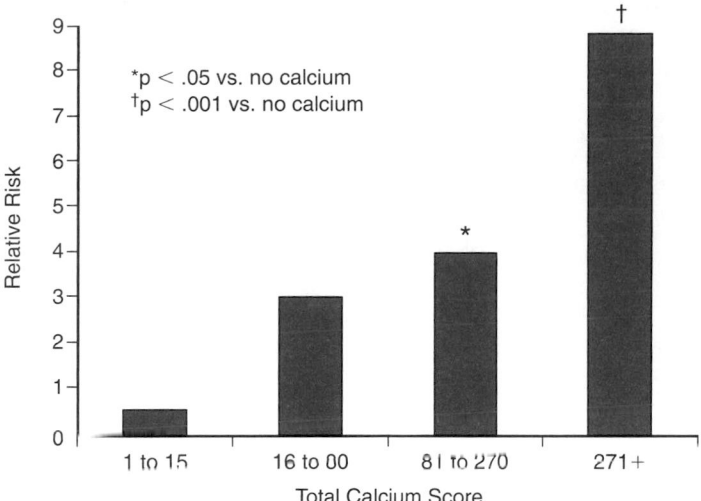

FIG. 51–5. Relative risks for total cardiovascular events in patients at various total calcium score quartiles versus those without calcium adjusting for age, sex, hypertension, hyperlipidemia, smoking history, and diabetes. (Redrawn from Wong ND, Hsu JC, Detrano RC, et al. Coronary artery calcium evaluation by electron beam computed tomography and its relation to new cardiovascular events. *Am J Cardiol* 2000;86:495–498, with permission.)

event rate in individuals with a CACS of 80 or greater, 160 or greater, and 600 or greater, respectively (61). Subjects with a CACS of 80 or greater had a 22-fold greater risk for death or MI as compared with those with lower scores (95% confidence interval [CI], 5.1–77.4). The total event rate was 10.9% among individuals in the greater (>75th) percentile of CACS (i.e., >97) versus 0.8% for those below this threshold. Multivariate analysis identified patient age, hypertension, diabetes, and hyperlipidemia as significant clinical risk predictors. The CACS remained the best single predictor of risk after adjustment for these variables (Table 51–3). Wong and coworkers (62) also showed that the CACS severity predicted subsequent events independent of age, sex, and patient risk factor profile (Fig. 51–5).

Raggi and coworkers (63) reported on 172 patients who had EBCT within 60 days of an unheralded MI and in 632 asymptomatic patients who were referred for a screening with EBCT and then followed for 32 ± 7 months (63). About 96% of all patients with infarction had abnormal EBCT results, and the CACS was 100 or greater in 62% and 400 or greater in 47% of patients. In the cohort of 632 asymptomatic patients, both the absolute CACS and the age-/sex-adjusted relative CACS percentiles predicted subsequent death and nonfatal MI. Hard cardiac events occurred in only 0.3% of subjects with a normal EBCT, but this increased to 10.8% in those with a CACS of 100 or greater and to 13% in those with a CACS greater than 400. Likewise, individuals in the lower 50th percentile for CACS severity had a total cardiac event rate of only 1.1% as compared with 8.2% in those with a CACS greater than the 50th percentile (Table 51–4). A very high CACS of 1,000 or greater may portend a particularly high risk for death or MI (i.e., 25%/year) (64).

The very low cardiac event rate in subjects with a CACS less than 100 is consistent with angiographic studies indicating a comparably low likelihood of significant CAD and an extremely low incidence of stress-induced myocardial ischemia (<1%) in such individuals (53,54). The increasing number of cardiac events with an ever-increasing CACS also is consistent with the dramatic increase in the incidence of stress-induced myocardial ischemia when scores exceed 400 (53,54). The CACS may provide complementary prognostic information to that obtained by the Framingham risk model (65). Combining EBCT results with biochemical markers, such as C-reactive protein, may more precisely define risk than either test alone (65). Currently, there are no published data using mechanical CT-derived CACS for assessing prognosis.

TABLE 51–4. *Cardiac event rates in asymptomatic subjects based on absolute and relative coronary artery calcium scores*

	Event rate (death/NFMI)
Absolute calcium score	
0	0.3% (1/292)
1–99	5.5% (12/219)
100–400	10.8% (8/74)
>400	12.8% (6/47)
Calcium score percentile	
<50th	1.1% (4/351)
>50th	8.2% (23/281)
>75th	10.5% (19/181)
>90th	11.8% (11/93)

NFMI, nonfatal myocardial infarction.
Adapted from Raggi P, Callister TQ, Cooil B, et al. Identification of patients at increased risk of first unheralded acute myocardial infarction by electron-beam computed tomography. *Circulation* 2000;101:850–855, with permission.

SCREENING FOR CORONARY ARTERY DISEASE USING ELECTRON BEAM COMPUTED TOMOGRAPHY

Traditional risk factor analysis indirectly infers risk based on the likelihood of significant atherothrombosis (67,68), whereas EBCT can directly measure the presence and severity of atherothrombotic burden based on the CACS. A modest relation exists between the number of cardiac risk factors and the presence of coronary artery calcification by EBCT. However, in one series, 40% of men and 30% of women without traditional risk factors had coronary artery calcification, whereas 26% of men and 36% of women with greater than three risk factors did not (69). Hecht and coworkers (70) demonstrated that 76% of asymptomatic subjects with an abnormal EBCT had a low-density lipoprotein (LDL) cholesterol level less than 160 mg/dL and, therefore, would not meet National Cholesterol Education Program (NCEP) II guidelines for lipid-lowering therapy. Conversely, 52% of patients with an LDL cholesterol level less than 130 mg/dL

and 46% with an LDL level less than 100 mg/dL had an abnormal EBCT. In the Healthy Women Study, risk factor analysis was imprecise at predicting coronary calcification in postmenopausal women (71). Although the constellation of high LDL, low high-density lipoprotein (HDL), and cigarette smoking predicted coronary artery calcification, this risk factor profile was observed in only 6% of all women studied. Conversely, 20% of women in the lowest risk profile (i.e., nonsmokers, LDL cholesterol level <130 mg/dL, and HDL cholesterol level >60 mg/dL) had calcium by EBCT. Hecht and coworkers (72) likewise showed that 42% of women 55 years or younger and 48% older than 55 years who were at low risk on the basis of NCEP II guidelines (i.e., LDL cholesterol level <130 and HDL level ≥35 mg/dL) had an abnormal EBCT (72).

The results of these aforementioned studies and the growing wealth of prognostic information further support the role of EBCT as an initial screening test beyond risk factor analysis alone for identifying subjects with varying degrees of coronary atherothrombosis. Some studies also emphasize the potential effectiveness of selectively combining stress myocardial perfusion imaging with EBCT in the anticipated small 10% of asymptomatic subjects who will have a high (≥400) CACS, so as to specifically identify those with silent myocardial ischemia (53,54). This testing strategy may prove to be optimal on the basis of the known prognostic value of perfusion imaging and the superior sensitivity of EBCT over the former for detecting preclinical CAD (Fig. 51–6) (see also color insert). Although the cost effectiveness of using EBCT as a screening test demands further clinical investigation, it has been proposed that the CACS might be used to guide therapeutics and recommends the need for additional diagnostic testing (73) (Fig. 51–7).

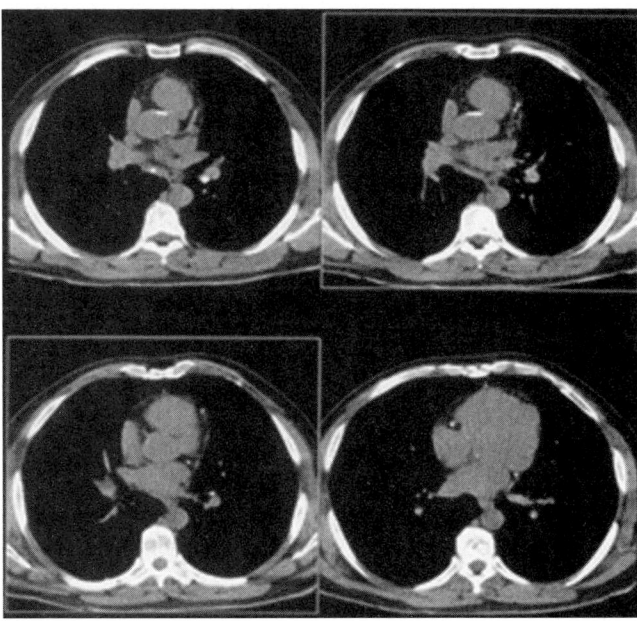

FIG. 51–6. Electron beam computed tomography **(A)** and single photon emission computed tomography (SPECT) **(B)** images of a 52-year-old, asymptomatic, hypertensive, hyperlipidemic man who had a high-risk CACS of 780. Calcium is shown as intensely *white areas* within all of the three coronary arteries. The treadmill test was terminated at 11 minutes because of patient fatigue, and the 12-lead electrocardiogram showed no evidence of ischemia at peak exercise. SPECT demonstrated a large, predominantly reversible 30% perfusion defect within the left anterior descending (LAD) coronary artery vascular territory. Coronary angiography showed subtotal stenosis of the proximal LAD coronary artery and 50% stenosis of the mid-right coronary artery. The patient underwent successful angioplasty and stenting of the LAD coronary artery. Results of repeat-exercise SPECT 6 months later was entirely normal. DLY, delay; PDS, perfusion defect size; STR, stress. (See color insert for Fig. 51–6B.)

TRACKING CHANGES IN ELECTRON BEAM COMPUTED TOMOGRAPHY–DERIVED CALCIUM SCORES

Sequential testing with EBCT may be useful in detecting the rate of progression of coronary atherothrombosis (74,75) or in tracking treatment effects based on lack of progression in the EBCT-derived CACS (75–77). For sequential testing to have clinical relevance, the biologic changes being studied must be greater than the inherent variability of the test result. Furthermore, the variability of the technique when performing sequential imaging in individual patients must be well defined.

Electron Beam Computed Tomography Reproducibility

The interobserver and intraobserver reproducibility of EBCT is excellent when recalculating the CACS on a single study (78,79). However, the variability in CACS associated with sequential imaging has ranged from 19% to 49% in different patient series (16,18,80–85). EBCT reproducibility is dependent on multiple technical factors, such as variability in ECG

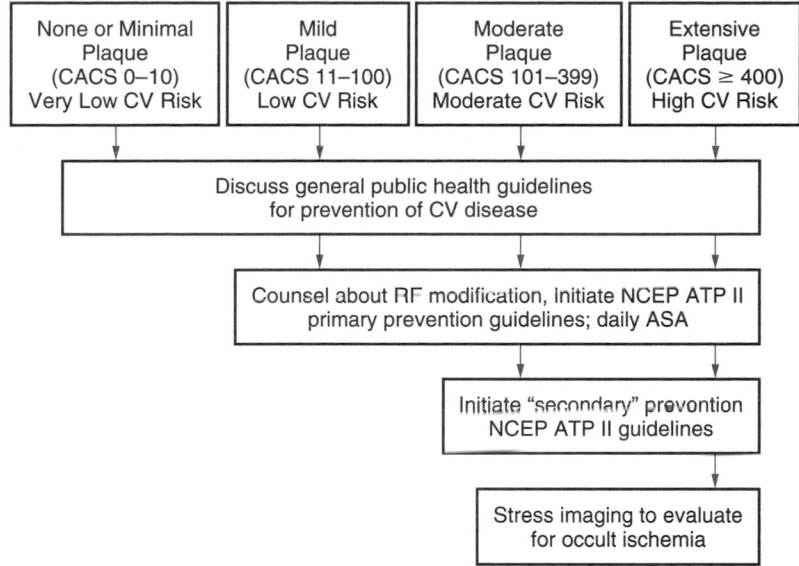

FIG. 51–7. Recommended electron beam computed tomography coronary artery calcium score (CACS) guidelines. ASA, acetylsalicylic acid; CV, cardiovascular; NCEP ATP II, National Cholesterol Education Program (Adult Treatment Panel II); RF, radiofrequency. (Adapted from Rumberger JA, Brundage BH, Rader DJ, et al. Electron beam computed tomographic coronary calcium scanning: a review and guidelines for use in asymptomatic persons. *Mayo Clin Proc* 1999;74:243–252, with permission.)

triggering, patient motion, respiratory variation, and cardiac motion, which may lead to partial volume effects and image noise. Over the years, technical advances and improvements in calcium scoring methodologies have reduced interscan variability. Achenbach and coworkers (84), using state-of-the-art EBCT imaging, reported an interscan variability of only 19.9% ± 36% with a median Agatston score variability of 7.8%. As in previous studies, there was a strong inverse relation between the initial CACS value and interscan reproducibility with the largest percent variation occurring in patients with the lowest CACS (Table 51–5). The variability for a CACS of 100 or greater was minimal at 10.5% ± 10.4% with a median variability of only 7.1%.

The traditional Agatston scoring system has been challenged by more recently proposed area (84–86) and volu-

metric scoring methods (87). The volumetric method uses isotropic interpolation to calculate the volume of calcified plaque area with a density of 130 HU or greater (87); rather than generating a CACS based on an arbitrary maximal plaque attenuation coefficient (i.e., Agatston method) (78). The calcified area method directly measures and sums the area (in mm²) of all coronary artery lesions. The volumetric and calcified area methods are more reproducible than the Agatston method (84,86,87) probably because of a reduction in partial volume effects and image noise on scan results.

In the largest series to date, Bielak and coworkers (85) defined the reproducibility of sequential EBCT imaging in 1,376 patients where scanning was performed minutes apart. The total calcified area method was used to define scan re-

TABLE 51–5. *Comparison of interscan variability for the Agatston score and volumetric score depending on amount of calcification in 120 patients*

Agatston score	Patients, n	Agatston score variability (%)	Volumetric score variability (%)
≥0	120	19.9 ± 36.0 (7.8)	16.2 ± 29.6 (5.7)
≥0.1	102	23.5 ± 39.5 (10.3)	19.9 ± 31.2 (8.3)
≥10	87	16.5 ± 22.7 (8.8)	18.0 ± 24.6 (9.1)
≥50	70	11.5 ± 11.1 (7.5)	11.6 ± 11.2 (6.6)
≥100	62	10.5 ± 10.4 (7.1)	11.4 ± 11.0 (6.6)
≥400	31	9.5 ± 9.1* (7.3)	7.3 ± 8.8.0* (4.9)
≥1000	11	8.3 ± 6.9 (6.2)	6.1 ± 4.9 (5.9)

Values are expressed as mean ± SD (median).
*Volumetric score variability significantly lower than Agatston score variability.
Reprinted from Achenbach S, Ropers D, Mohlenkamp S, et al. Variability of repeated coronary artery calcium measurements by electron beam tomography. *Am J Cardiol* 2001;87:210–213, with permission.

producibility. The mean calcified area was 60.6 ± 154.1 mm^2 on Scan 1 versus 59.8 ± 149.1 mm^2 on Scan 2 with a correlation coefficient between scans of 0.98 ($p < 0.001$). The absolute difference in calcified area between scans was greatest at higher scores, whereas the relative percent difference was most pronounced at low scores. This large data set is the first to allow calculation of 95% CIs for individual changes in sequential scores for calcified areas ranging as low as 5 mm^2 to more than 1000 mm^2.

Despite improvements in image acquisition and processing, cardiac motion still remains an important source of scan variability. Optimizing ECG triggering when cardiac motion is at a nadir (i.e., 30–50% of the R-R interval) may further improve reproducibility (86). Using a variable ECG trigger based on resting heart rate may significantly reduce inter-scan variability as compared with when image acquisition is triggered at the standard 80% R-R interval, and particularly in patients with small (2–10 mm^2) calcium burdens (15.3% vs. 23.2%, respectively; $p < 0.01$). To date, there are no studies evaluating the reproducibility of sequential imaging with mechanical CT scanning.

Tracking Calcium Progression

Reproducibility data suggest that the area or volumetric methods may be able to track temporal changes in coronary atherothrombosis and assess the effects of pharmacologic therapy on plaque progression using serial EBCT imaging. In asymptomatic subjects with an abnormal EBCT, CACS progression is approximately 30% per year, which is significantly greater than the inherent variability in EBCT calcium score measurements (75,88). However, patients without detectable calcium have a low likelihood of further progression. In the series by Budoff and coworkers (75), only 11 of 81 patients (14%) with a normal EBCT study developed calcification over 1 to 6 years of follow-up, and 82% had a subsequent score less than 10 (75). Repeat scanning in patients with a normal EBCT study is probably not warranted for at least 3 to 5 years after the baseline study.

Retrospective studies indicate that progression of coronary artery calcification can be significantly reduced with lipid-lowering therapy. Budoff and coworkers (75) performed repeat imaging in 299 patients 2.2 ± 11 years after baseline EBCT. The rate of progression in the Agatston-derived CACS was significantly less in treated (15% $\pm$ 8%/year) versus untreated (39% $\pm$ 12%/year) subjects with hyperlipidemia ($p < 0.001$). Callister and coworkers (76) studied 149 asymptomatic patients with hyperlipidemia who had a screening EBCT study and repeat imaging at 13.7 $\pm$ 0.6 months. The calcium score was calculated using the volumetric method. In the 44 untreated patients (mean LDL level 147 ± 22 mg/dL) and the 40 treated patients with an LDL cholesterol level greater than 120 (mean 139 ± 18 mg/dL), the calcium scores increased by 53% $\pm$ 36% and 25% $\pm$ 22%, respectively. However, in the 65 treated patients with a resultant LDL level less than 120 (mean 100 ± 17 mg/dL), the calcium score decreased by 7% $\pm$ 23%.

These results were confirmed in a prospective study where 66 untreated subjects with hyperlipidemia (LDL cholesterol level >130 mg/dL) had a baseline EBCT repeated at 14 $\pm$ 2.4 months (77). A third EBCT scan was then performed after 12 months of cerivastatin (0.3 mg/day). The calcium score was calculated on all three studies using both the volumetric and Agatston methods. Cerivastatin significantly decreased total (244 $\pm$ 32 vs. 188 $\pm$ 78 mg/dL) and LDL (164 $\pm$ 30 vs. 107 $\pm$ 21 mg/dL) cholesterol levels, with a subsequent reduction in calcium progression (Fig. 51–8). This was most dramatic in patients who maintained an LDL cholesterol

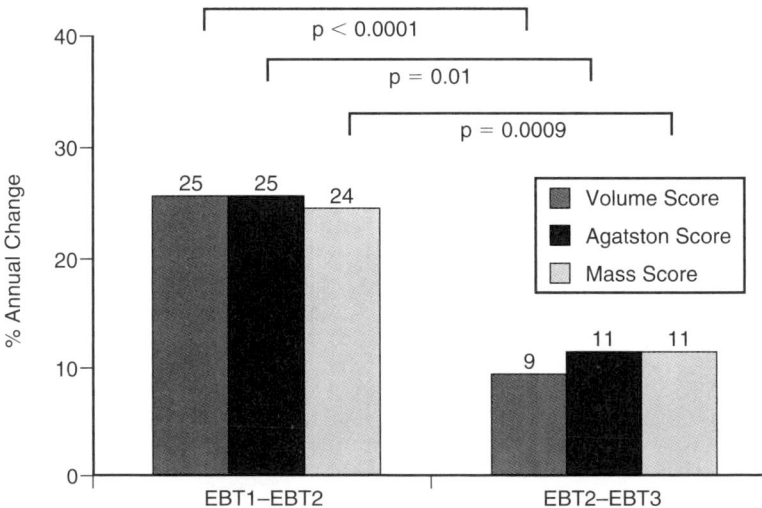

FIG. 51–8. Median annualized relative increase in volume, Agatston, and mass scores during the untreated (electron beam T1 [EBT1] to EBT2) and the treatment period (EBT2 to EBT3). (Redrawn from Achenbach S, Ropers D, Pohle K, et al. Influence of lipid-lowering therapy on the progression of coronary artery calcification: a prospective evaluation. *Circulation* 2002;106:1077–1082, with permission.)

level less than 100 mg/dL where the rate of calcium progression was effectively halted (median change −3.4%, volume score; 0%, Agatston score).

These studies indicate that the effects of lipid reduction therapy on calcium progression can be assessed using serial EBCT imaging. It is conceivable that sequential EBCT imaging may be able to track subsequent individual patient risk for cardiac events on the basis of either the annual rate of calcium progression or on reaching a certain "threshold" of CACS. Ongoing large prospective trials, such as the Multi Ethnic Study of Atherosclerosis, will better define the role of sequential EBCT imaging in assessing therapeutics and subsequent outcome (89).

REFERENCES

1. Rensing BJ, Bongaerts A, van Geuns RJ, et al. Intravenous coronary angiography by electron beam computed tomography: a clinical evaluation. *Circulation* 1998;98:2509–2512.
2. Achenbach S, Moshage W, Ropers D, et al. Value of electron-beam computed tomography for the noninvasive detection of high-grade coronary-artery stenoses and occlusions. *N Engl J Med* 1998;339:1964–1971.
3. Budoff MJ, Oudiz RJ, Zalace CP, et al. Intravenous three-dimensional coronary angiography using contrast enhanced electron beam computed tomography. *Am J Cardiol* 1999;83:840–845.
4. Schmermund A, Rensing BJ, Sheedy PF, et al. Intravenous electron-beam computed tomographic coronary angiography for segmental analysis of coronary artery stenosis. *J Am Coll Cardiol* 1998;31:1547–1554.
5. Reddy G, Chernoff DM, Adams JR, et al. Coronary artery stenoses: assessment with contrast-enhanced electron beam CT and axial reconstructions. *Radiology* 1998;208:167–172.
6. Achenbach S, Ulzheimer S, Baum U, et al. Noninvasive coronary angiography by retrospectively ECG-gated multislice spiral CT. *Circulation* 2000;102:2823–2828.
7. Nieman K, Rensing BJ, vanGeuns RJ, et al. Usefulness of multislice computed tomography for detecting obstructive coronary artery disease. *Am J Cardiol* 2002;89:913–918.
8. Achenbach S, Giesler T, Ropers D, et al. Detection of coronary artery stenoses by contrast-enhanced, retrospectively electrocardiographically-gated, multislice spiral computed tomography. *Circulation* 2001;103:2535–2538.
9. Boyd DP, Lipton MJ. Cardiac computed tomography. *Proc IEEE Nucl Sci* 1983;71:298–307.
10. Lu B, Mao SS, Zhuang N, et al. Coronary artery motion during the cardiac cycle and optimal ECG triggering for coronary artery imaging. *Invest Radiol* 2001;36:250–256.
11. Achenbach S, Ropers D, Holle J, et al. In-plane coronary arterial motion velocity. Measurement with electron-beam CT. *Radiology* 2000;216:457–463.
12. McCollough CH, Zink FE, Morin RL. Radiation dosimetry for electron beam CT. *Radiology* 1994;192:637–642.
13. Horiguchi J, Nakanishi T, Ito K. Quantification of coronary artery calcium using multidetector CT and a retrospective ECG-gating reconstruction algorithm. *Am J Roentgenol* 2001;177:1429–1435.
14. Mautner GC, Mautner SL, Froehlich J, et al. Coronary artery calcification: assessment with electron beam CT and histomorphometric correlation. *Radiology* 1994;192:619–623.
15. Becker CR, Knez A, Jakobs TF, et al. Detection and quantification of coronary artery calcification with electron-beam and conventional CT. *Eur Radiol* 1999;9:620–624.
16. Budoff MJ, Mao S, Zalace CP, et al. Comparison of spiral and electron beam tomography in the evaluation of coronary calcification in asymptomatic persons. *Int J Cardiol* 2001;77:181–188.
17. Becker CR, Jakobs TF, Aydemir S, et al. Helical and single-slice conventional CT versus electron beam CT for the quantification of coronary artery calcification. *AJR Am J Roentgenol* 2000;174:543–547.
18. Carr JJ, Crouse JR 3rd, Goff DC Jr, et al. Evaluation of subsecond gated helical CT for quantification of coronary artery calcium and comparison with electron beam CT. *AJR Am J Roentgenol* 2000;174:915–921.
19. Goldin JG, Yoon HC, Greaser LE 3rd, et al. Spiral versus electron-beam CT for coronary artery calcium scoring. *Radiology* 2001;221:213–221.
20. Becker CR, Kleffel T, Crispin A, et al. Coronary artery calcium measurement: agreement of multirow detector and electron beam CT. *AJR Am J Roentgenol* 2001;176:1295–1298.
21. Rumberger JA, Simons DB, Fitzpatrick LA, et al. Coronary artery calcium area by electron-beam computed tomography and coronary atherosclerotic plaque area: a histopathologic correlative study. *Circulation* 1995;92:2157–2162.
22. Sangiorgi G, Rumberger JA, Severson A, et al. Arterial calcification and not lumen stenosis is highly correlated with atherosclerotic plaque burden in humans: a histologic study of 723 coronary artery segments using nondecalcifying methodology. *J Am Coll Cardiol* 1998;31:126–133.
23. Ikeda T, Shirasawa T, Esaki Y, et al. Osteopontin mRNA is expressed by smooth muscle-derived foam cells in human atherosclerotic lesions of the aorta. *J Clin Invest* 1993;92:2814–2820.
24. Fitzpatrick LA, Severson A, Edwards WD, et al. Diffuse calcification in human coronary arteries: association of osteopontin with atherosclerosis. *J Clin Invest* 1994;94:1597–1604.
25. Hirota S, Imakita M, Kohri K, et al. Expression of osteopontin messenger RNA by macrophages in atherosclerotic plaques: a possible association with calcification. *Am J Pathol* 1993;143:1003–1008.
26. Janowitz WR, Agatston AS, Kaplan G, et al. Differences in prevalence and extent of coronary artery calcium detected by ultrafast computed tomography in asymptomatic men and women: relation to age and risk factors. *Am J Cardiol* 1993;72:247–254.
27. Newman AB, Naydeck BL, Sutton-Tyrrell K, et al. Coronary artery calcification in older adults to age 99. Prevalence and risk factors. *Circulation* 2001;104:2679–2684.
28. Glagov S, Weisenberg BA, Zarins CK, et al. Compensatory enlargement of human atherosclerotic coronary arteries. *N Engl J Med* 1987;316:1371–1375.
29. Clarkson TB, Prichard RW, Morgan TM, et al. Remodeling of coronary arteries in human and non human primates. *JAMA* 1994;271:289–294.
30. Agatston AS, Janowitz WR, Hildner FJ, et al. Quantification of coronary artery calcium using ultrafast computed tomography. *J Am Coll Cardiol* 1990;15:827–832.
31. Breen JF, Sheedy PF, Schwartz RS, et al. Coronary artery calcification detected with ultrafast CT as an indication of coronary artery disease. *Radiology* 1992;185:435–439.
32. Bielak LW, Kaufmann RB, Moll PP, et al. Small lesions in the heart identified at electron beam CT: calcification or noise? *Radiology* 1994;192:631–636.
33. Kaufmann RB, Sheedy PF, Maher JE, et al. Quantity of coronary artery calcium detected by electron beam computed tomography in asymptomatic subjects and angiographically studied patients. *Mayo Clin Proc* 1995;70:223–232.
34. Rumberger JA, Sheedy PF, Breen JF, et al. Coronary calcium, as determined by electron beam computed tomography, and coronary disease on arteriogram. Effect of patient's sex on diagnosis. *Circulation* 1995;91:1363–1367.
35. Braun J, Oldendorf M, Moshage W, et al. Electron beam computed tomography in the evaluation of cardiac calcification in chronic dialysis patients. *Am J Kidney Dis* 1996;27:394–401.
36. Budoff MJ, Georgiou D, Brody A, et al. Ultrafast computed tomography as a diagnostic modality in the detection of coronary artery disease. A multicenter study. *Circulation* 1996;93:898–904.
37. Detrano R, Hsiai T, Wang S, et al. Prognostic value of coronary calcification and angiographic stenoses in patients undergoing coronary angiography. *J Am Coll Cardiol* 1996;27:285–290.
38. Fallavollita JA, Brody AS, Bunnell IL, et al. Fast computed tomography detection of coronary calcification in the diagnosis of coronary artery disease. Comparison with angiography in patients <50 years old. *Circulation* 1994;89:285–290.
39. Baumgart D, Schmermund A, George G, et al. Comparison of electron beam computed tomography with intracoronary ultrasound and coronary angiography for detection of coronary atherosclerosis. *J Am Coll Cardiol* 1997;30:57–64.
40. Schmermund A, Baumgart D, Gorge D, et al. Coronary artery calcium in acute coronary syndromes: a comparative study of electron-beam computed tomography, coronary angiography, and intracoronary ultra-

sound in survivors of acute myocardial infarction and unstable angina. *Circulation* 1997;96:1461–1469.

41. Kennedy J, Shavelle R, Wang S, et al. Coronary calcium and standard risk factors in symptomatic patients referred for coronary angiography. *Am Heart J* 1998;135:696–702.

42. Bielak LF, Rumberger JA, Sheedy PF, et al. Probabilistic model for prediction of angiographically defined obstructive coronary artery disease using electron beam computed tomography calcium score strata. *Circulation* 2000;102:380–385.

43. Shavelle DM, Budoff MJ, LaMont DH, et al. Exercise testing and electron beam computed tomography in the evaluation of coronary artery disease. *J Am Coll Cardiol* 2000;36:32–38.

44. Haberl R, Becker A, Leber A, et al. Correlation of coronary calcification and angiographically documented stenoses in patients with suspected coronary artery disease: results of 1,764 patients. *J Am Coll Cardiol* 2001;37:451–457.

45. Budoff MJ, Diamond GA, Raggi P, et al. Continuous probabilistic prediction of angiographically significant coronary artery disease using electron beam tomography. *Circulation* 2002;105:1791–1796.

46. Schmermund A, Bailey KR, Rumberger JA, et al. An algorithm for noninvasive identification of angiographic three-vessel and/or left main coronary artery disease in symptomatic patients on the basis of cardiac risk and electron-beam computed tomographic calcium scores. *J Am Coll Cardiol* 1999;33:444–452.

47. Rumberger JA, Sheedy PF, Breen JF, et al. Electron beam computed tomographic coronary calcium score cutpoints and severity of associated angiographic lumen stenosis. *J Am Coll Cardiol* 1997;29:1542–1548.

48. Guerci AD, Spadaro LA, Goodman KJ, et al. Comparison of electron beam computed tomography scanning and conventional risk factor assessment for the prediction of angiographic coronary artery disease. *J Am Coll Cardiol* 1998;32:673–679.

49. Iskandrian AS, Chae SC, Heo J, et al. Independent and incremental prognostic value of exercise single-photon emission computed tomographic (SPECT) thallium imaging in coronary artery disease. *J Am Coll Cardiol* 1993;22:665–670.

50. Hachamovitch R, Berman DS, Kiat H, et al. Exercise myocardial perfusion SPECT in patients without known coronary artery disease. Incremental prognostic value and use in risk stratification. *Circulation* 1996;93:905–914.

51. Blumenthal RS, Becker DM, Moy TF, et al. Exercise thallium tomography predicts future clinically manifest coronary heart disease in a high-risk asymptomatic population. *Circulation* 1996;93:915–923.

52. Fleg JL, Gerstenblith G, Zonderman AB, et al. Prevalence and prognostic significance of exercise-induced silent myocardial ischemia detected by thallium scintigraphy and electrocardiography in asymptomatic volunteers. *Circulation* 1990;81:428–436.

53. He ZX, Hedrick TD, Pratt CM, et al. Severity of coronary artery calcification by electron beam computed tomography predicts silent myocardial ischemia. *Circulation* 2000;101:244–251.

54. Miranda RS, Schisterman EF, Gallagher AM, et al. The extent of coronary calcium by electron beam computed tomography discriminates the likelihood of abnormal myocardial perfusion SPECT. *Circulation* 2000;102[Suppl II]:II-543(abst).

55. Ringqvist I, Fisher LD, Mock M, et al. Prognostic value of angiographic indices of coronary artery disease from the Coronary Artery Surgery Study (CASS). *J Clin Invest* 1983;71:1854–1866.

56. Emond M, Mock MB, Davis KB, et al. Long-term survival of medically treated patients in the Coronary Artery Surgery Study (CASS) Registry. *Circulation* 1994;90:2645–2657.

57. Detrano R, Hsiai T, Wang S, et al. Prognostic value of coronary calcification and angiographic stenoses in patients undergoing coronary angiography. *J Am Coll Cardiol* 1996;27:285–290.

58. Keelan PC, Bielak LF, Ashai K, et al. Long-term prognostic value of coronary calcification detected by electron-beam computed tomography in patients undergoing coronary angiography. *Circulation* 2001;104:412–417.

59. Secci A, Wong N, Tang W, et al. Electron beam computed tomographic coronary calcium as a predictor of coronary events: comparison of two protocols. *Circulation* 1997;96:1122–1129.

60. Arad Y, Spadaro LA, Goodman K, et al. Predictive value of electron beam computed tomography of the coronary arteries. 19-month follow-up of 1173 asymptomatic subjects. *Circulation* 1996;93:1951–1953.

61. Arad Y, Spadaro LA, Goodman K, et al. Prediction of coronary events with electron beam computed tomography. *J Am Coll Cardiol* 2000;36:1253–1260.

62. Wong ND, Hsu JC, Detrano RC, et al. Coronary artery calcium evaluation by electron beam computed tomography and its relation to new cardiovascular events. *Am J Cardiol* 2000;86:495–498.

63. Raggi P, Callister TQ, Cooil B, et al. Identification of patients at increased risk of first unheralded acute myocardial infarction by electron-beam computed tomography. *Circulation* 2000;101:850–855.

64. Wayhs R, Zelinger A, Raggi P. High coronary artery calcium scores pose an extremely elevated risk for hard events. *J Am Coll Cardiol* 2002;39:225–230.

65. Taylor AJ, Burke AP, O'Malley PG, et al. A comparison of the Framingham risk index, coronary artery calcification, and culprit plaque morphology in sudden cardiac death. *Circulation* 2000;101:1243–1248.

66. Park R, Detrano R, Xiang M, et al. Combined use of computed tomography coronary calcium scores and C-reactive protein levels in predicting cardiovascular events in nondiabetic individuals. *Circulation* 2002;106:2073–2077.

67. Califf RM, Armstrong PW, Carver JR, et al. 27th Bethesda Conference: matching the intensity of risk factor management with the hazard for coronary disease events. Task Force 5. Stratification of patients into high, medium and low risk subgroups for purposes of risk factor management. *J Am Coll Cardiol* 1996;27:1007–1019.

68. Wilson PW, D'Agostino RB, Levy D, et al. Prediction of coronary heart disease using risk factor categories. *Circulation* 1998;97:1837–1847.

69. Wong ND, Kouwabunpat D, Vo AN, et al. Coronary calcium and atherosclerosis by ultrafast computed tomography in asymptomatic men and women: relation to age and risk factors. *Am Heart J* 1994;127:422–430.

70. Hecht HS, Superko HR, Smith LK, et al. Relation of coronary artery calcium identified by electron beam tomography to serum lipoprotein levels and implications for treatment. *Am J Cardiol* 2001;87:406–412.

71. Kuller LH, Matthews KA, Sutton-Tyrrell K, et al. Coronary and aortic calcification among women 8 years after menopause and their premenopausal risk factors: the healthy women study. *Arterioscler Thromb Vasc Biol* 1999;19:2189–2198.

72. Hecht HS, Superko HR. Electron beam tomography and national cholesterol education program guidelines in asymptomatic women. *J Am Coll Cardiol* 2001;37:1506–1511.

73. Rumberger JA, Brundage BH, Rader DJ, et al. Electron beam computed tomographic coronary calcium scanning: a review and guidelines for use in asymptomatic persons. *Mayo Clin Proc* 1999;74:243–252.

74. Janowitz WR, Agatston AS, Viamonte M Jr. Comparison of serial quantitative evaluation of calcified coronary artery plaque by ultrafast computed tomography in persons with and without obstructive coronary artery disease. *Am J Cardiol* 1991;68:1–6.

75. Budoff MJ, Lane KL, Bakhsheshi H, et al. Rates of progression of coronary calcium by electron beam tomography. *Am J Cardiol* 2000;86:8–11.

76. Callister TQ, Raggi P, Cooil B, et al. Effect of HMG-CoA reductase inhibitors on coronary artery disease as assessed by electron-beam computed tomography. *N Engl J Med* 1998;339:1972–1978.

77. Achenbach S, Ropers D, Pohle K, et al. Influence of lipid-lowering therapy on the progression of coronary artery calcification: a prospective evaluation. *Circulation* 2002;106:1077–1082.

78. Agatston AS, Janowitz WR, Hildner FJ, et al. Quantification of coronary artery calcium using ultrafast computed tomography. *J Am Coll Cardiol* 1990;15:827–832.

79. Kajinami K, Seki H, Takekoshi N, et al. Quantification of coronary artery calcification using ultrafast computed tomography: reproducibility of measurements. *Coron Artery Dis* 1993;4:1103–1108.

80. Bielak LF, Kaufmann RB, Moll PP, et al. Small lesions in the heart identified at electron beam CT: calcification or noise? *Radiology* 1994;192:631–636.

81. Devries S, Wolfkiel C, Shah V, et al. Reproducibility of the measurement of coronary calcium with ultrafast computed tomography. *Am J Cardiol* 1995;75:973–975.

82. Yoon HC, Goldin JG, Greaser LE 3rd, et al. Interscan variation in coronary artery calcium quantification in a large asymptomatic patient population. *AJR Am J Roentgenol* 2000;174:803–809.

83. Wang S, Detrano RC, Secci A, et al. Detection of coronary calcification with electron-beam computed tomography: evaluation of interexamination reproducibility and comparison of three image-acquisition protocols. *Am Heart J* 1996;132:550–558.

84. Achenbach S, Ropers D, Mohlenkamp S, et al. Variability of repeated coronary artery calcium measurements by electron beam tomography. *Am J Cardiol* 2001;87:210–213.

85. Bielak LF, Sheedy PF, Peyser PA. Coronary artery calcification mea-

sured at electron-beam CT: agreement in dual scan runs and change over time. *Radiology* 2001;218:224–229.

86. Mao S, Budoff MJ, Bakhsheshi H, et al. Improved reproducibility of coronary artery calcium scoring by electron beam tomography with a new electrocardiographic trigger method. *Invest Radiol* 2001;36:363–367.

87. Callister TQ, Cooil B, Raya SP, et al. Coronary artery disease: im-proved reproducibility of calcium scoring with an electron-beam CT volumetric method. *Radiology* 1998;208:807–814.

88. Maher JE, Bielak LF, Raz JA, et al. Progression of coronary artery cal-cification: a pilot study. *Mayo Clin Proc* 1999;74:347–355.

89. Bild DE, Bluemke DA, Burke GL, et al. Multi-ethnic study of athero-sclerosis: objectives and design. *Am J Epidemiol* 2002;156:871–881.

CHAPTER 52

Magnetic Resonance Imaging of the Heart in Coronary Artery Disease

Phillip C. Yang, Michael Poon, James A. Vitarius, and Gerald M. Pohost

Key Words: Comprehensive examination; coronary artery; myocardial perfusion; myocardial viability; wall motion.

INTRODUCTION

The diagnosis of coronary artery disease (CAD) by noninvasive imaging has been one of the most important clinical goals in cardiovascular medicine. Numerous approaches have been developed and evaluated. Stress echocardiography detects myocardial ischemia by examining induced wall motion abnormalities with stress. Radionuclide studies provide indirect assessment of CAD by demonstrating stress-induced abnormalities in myocardial perfusion. Coronary angiography is an imaging technique that allows direct visualization of the coronary artery using x-ray with cardiac

P. C. Yang: Department of Medicine, Division of Cardiovascular Medicine, Stanford University School of Medicine, 300 Pasteur Drive, H2157, Stanford, California 94305-5233.

M. Poon: Division of Cardiovascular Medicine, Department of Medicine, Mount Sinai Medical Center, New York, New York.

J. A. Vitarius: Division of Cardiovascular Medicine, Department of Medicine, Mount Sinai Medical Center, New York, New York.

G. M. Pohost: Division of Cardiovascular Medicine, Department of Medicine, Keck School of Medicine, University of Southern California, Los Angeles, California.

catheterization. However, technologic advances are approaching relative maturity in each diagnostic modality.

Coronary angiography is considered the current gold standard for the assessment of ischemic heart disease by directly imaging the coronary arteries. Clinical decision regarding surgical, percutaneous, or medical therapy is based frequently on angiographic results. More than one million procedures are performed annually in the United States, with up to 20% of studies showing no evidence of significant disease (1). The major limitation of this technique is the associated morbidity and mortality rates ranging from 0.02% to 0.1% of cases (2). In addition, the technique requires ionizing x-ray irradiation and provides only projective images of the coronary artery lumen. No substantial information is available to characterize atherothrombotic plaque within the coronary arterial wall or vascular function. Echocardiography is the most commonly used diagnostic imaging method. It is portable, interactive, and provides real-time image display. It generates diagnostic and prognostic information by observing the effect of stress on wall motion. If blood supply is limited because of significant coronary stenosis, wall motion deteriorates with stress. However, it is well known that at least 15% of echocardiographic studies are considered suboptimal because of inadequate acoustic window (3). A similar limitation is interpreting stress echocardiography. Interinstitutional agreement in interpreting stress echocardiography has been reported to be highly dependent on image quality (4). As image quality deteriorated, the percent agreement among the readers declined from 100% to 43%. More importantly, more than 20% of the studies were classified in the lowest image quality group with an interobserver agreement of no more than 57%. In a metaanalysis of published data of stress echocardiography from 1990 to 1997, sensitivity and specificity to detect CAD approached 85% and 77%, respectively (5).

An increase by more than 2.5-fold in normal coronary artery flow during stress or vasodilator infusion has been the cornerstone of modern myocardial perfusion imaging (6). The flow restriction caused by interference with normal increase in myocardial blood flow is the basis to myocardial perfusion imaging. By spatially mapping the distribution of the radioactivity within the myocardium, segmental differences in myocardial perfusion can be determined. The two principal radionuclides used in myocardial perfusion imaging are thallium-201 (^{201}Th) and technetium-99m. The low-energy ^{201}Th has lower photon energy in the 68 to 82 KeV range producing more scatter and lower spatial resolution compared with technetium-based agents. Attenuation artifacts due to liver and breast or those related to lung and liver uptake lead to reduced specificity in conditions such as left main or three vessel diseases. Metaanalysis of the published clinical studies from 1990 to 1997 of exercise radionuclide test reported sensitivity of 87% and specificity of 64% for detection of CAD (5).

The limitations of stress echocardiography and radionuclide testing result in more than 300,000 unnecessary coronary angiograms annually (1). A rapid, robust, safe, and cost-effective alternative is necessary. An integrated diagnostic platform that enables comprehensive evaluation of coronary anatomy, cardiac function, myocardial perfusion, and viability in a single, noninvasive, and complication-free setting should improve the current state for diagnosing and prognosticating in ischemic heart disease.

COMPREHENSIVE EXAMINATION OF ISCHEMIA USING MAGNETIC RESONANCE IMAGING

Magnetic resonance imaging (MRI) holds promise to allow an integrated and comprehensive evaluation of ischemic heart disease. Submillimeter resolution, exquisite soft tissue contrast, and arbitrary viewing of any tomographic plane are now possible noninvasively without ionizing radiation in routine clinical setting (7). MRI provides flexible imaging capability because of its ability to combine the chemical sensitivity of nuclear magnetic resonance with high spatial and temporal resolution. The potential of MRI lies in its ability to detect a wide range of physical and chemical processes including flow, motion, morphology, and tissue composition. The realization of this imaging technology in the routine practice of cardiology will enable integrated assessment of myocardial perfusion, global and regional ventricular function, direct visualization of the coronary arter-

ies, and detection of nonviable myocardium and scar. MR also can generate spectra that show the relative distribution of the high-energy phosphates adenosine triphosphate and phosphocreatine and their response to stress-induced ischemia insult.

The concept of comprehensive cardiovascular examination or "one-stop shop" has existed for nearly a decade (8). Although realization of such potential has been reported in the literature and claimed by manufacturers of MR scanners, routine clinical implementation has not been widespread. Challenges still remain including time requirements, reliability, and robustness of such examination. This chapter addresses these critical issues facing cardiovascular MRI (CMR) by examining recent technical advances, resultant clinical implementation, and potential future developments.

TECHNICAL CONSIDERATIONS

Hardware

Advances in hardware have been critical in rapid imaging necessary in cardiovascular applications. All applications discussed in this chapter have been performed in a CMR scanner with field strength of 1.5 Tesla (T) unless stated otherwise. The cryogenic superconducting magnet generates 1.5-T main magnetic field (B_0). Within the conventional cylindrical magnet, there are several layers of coils including superconducting "shim coils" to maintain homogeneity of the main magnetic field known as B_0, active shield coils to restrict the magnetic field to the scan room, and gradient coils to generate small differences in magnetic field from "point-to-point," which allows spatial encoding. The magnitude of B_0 (e.g., 1.5 T) is an important determinant of signal-to-noise ratio (SNR). An advantage of the trend toward B_0 of 3.0 T is improvement in SNR. The peak gradient strength and the slew rate (time required to switch the gradient from zero to maximum strength) of the gradient coils frequently determine the temporal and spatial resolution achievable in cardiovascular applications (9). Rapid, high-resolution imaging of dynamic cardiovascular function and anatomy is highly dependent on gradient characteristics. For example, coronary artery image resolution using spiral acquisition has been implemented in different gradient amplitude. Earlier maximum gradient amplitudes of 10 mT per meter using a slew rate of 16 mT per meter per millisecond yielded a spatial resolution of 1.1 to 1.3 mm. The newest high-performance gradient system with gradient amplitude to 40 mT per meter, using a slew rate of 150 mT per meter per millisecond, yielded a resolution in the range of 0.5 to 0.6 mm.

Software

Image acquisition software that specifies the gradient amplitudes, timing of radiofrequency (RF) pulses, and direction of gradient magnetization is known as a pulse sequence. The two most commonly used pulse sequences for cardiovascular applications are spin echo (SE) and gradient recalled echo (GRE) sequences. The SE sequence generates images in which blood pool appears dark relative to surrounding soft tissue such as myocardium. The sequence uses 2 RF pulses to generate signal. The first pulse excites the sensitive hydrogen protons nucleus followed by the second T2-weighted refocusing pulse to produce coherent signal. Typical timing between the two pulses known as the echo time (TE) is 20 to 30 ms for the first pulse and 50 to 90 ms for the second pulse. The SE sequence is used to assess morphology in valvular, congenital, pericardial, and other cardiovascular diseases. The GRE sequence leads to increased signal intensity of blood pool (bright blood). The sequence is commonly used to image ventricular function. It uses a single low flip-angle RF pulse refocused by the gradient coil to produce a coherent MR signal (10). Typical timing for a GRE sequence is a TE of 2 to 8 ms allowing acquisition every 20 to 40 ms using cardiac gating to image multiple phases of the cardiac cycle for cine display. Soft tissue contrast obtained with this technique is less when compared with an SE sequence.

Recent developments in pulse sequence design using high-performance gradient coils have provided a means to use an older pulse sequence known as steady-state free precession (SSFP). The SSFP sequence enhances the contrast between blood and myocardium through preservation of both longitudinal and transverse magnetizations by refocusing the gradients in all three axes (11). The steady state achieved by the magnetization provides high-quality images using both T_1 and T_2 relaxation times. Other advances including echoplanar imaging (EPI), also first developed more than two decades ago, improve imaging efficiency (12). Instead of acquiring multiple segmented k-space (data space) lines per cardiac cycle, EPI acquires the complete data sets usually after a SE or GRE sequence. All data required to form a complete image can be acquired rapidly within 30 to 40 ms. However, sensitivity of this technique to field inhomogeneities and flow limits usefulness of EPI in cardiovascular applications (13). Variations of the original EPI approach provide great potential in cardiovascular applications. Interleaved or multishot EPI uses several echoes to cover the data space to significantly reduce image artifact (14). Another strategy for rapid imaging is the spiral acquisition technique (15). This non-Cartesian acquisition technique generates images by sampling the data space from the center and spiraling outward. This method provides several advantages (13). High temporal resolution is achieved through efficient data collection resulting in shorter acquisition time. Shorter acquisition time reduces blurring. Improved spatial resolution is obtained through full, rather than partial, coverage of k-space. Image artifacts are reduced through lower sensitivity to flow by using short TE. Also, the requirement of fewer excitations per heartbeat leads to a greater SNR. Finally, contrast is enhanced by more robust fat suppression through spectral–spatial excitation (16). Data space coverage of EPI and spiral acquisition techniques with comparative images of

the right coronary artery using identical GRE pulse sequence are depicted in Figure 52–1.

Real-time interactive imaging (RT) represents one of the most significant advances in software development for cardiovascular application. A rapid acquisition method using EPI paved the way to RT (17). Currently, this method allows acquisition of a complete image within a period as short as 40 ms yielding a rate of 25 images per second. However, this method requires more complex hardware, produces a lower SNR, and leads to a lower resolution and artifacts from flow motion (13). Real-time image reconstruction also is essential. The sliding window reconstruction experimented with the possibility of real-time CMR image display on conventional scanners using fast low-angle shot (FLASH) or gradient recalled acquisition in steady state (GRASS) sequences (18). A clinically robust and reliable system enabled by ultrafast image acquisition eliminated the need for cardiac or respiratory gating, allowed interactive selection of scan plane, and provided real-time image reconstruction and display for instantaneous image-based feedback (19). The approach required only a modest hardware upgrade to a conventional 1.5-T MRI scanner. The rapid access of raw data and direct control of reconstruction and display generated interactive images with lag time of less than 500 ms. An example of such interactive protocol enabling manipulations of scan parameters and images is shown in Figure 52–2 (see color insert).

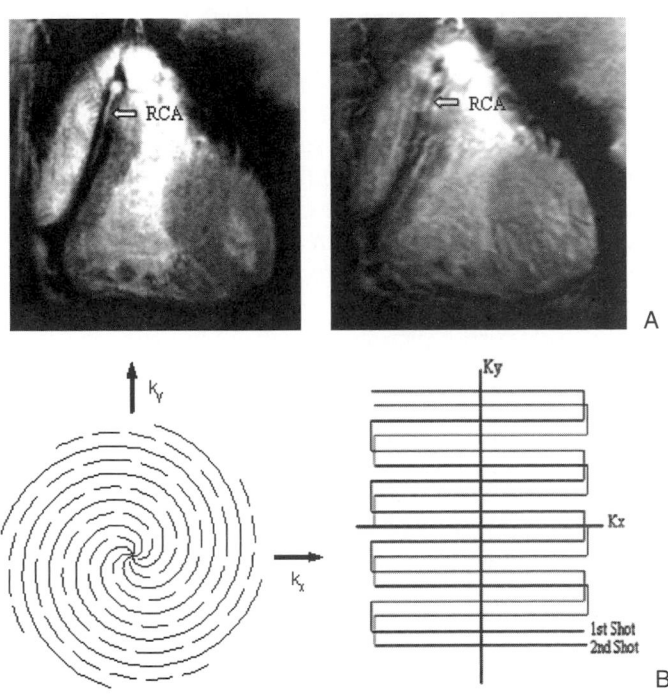

FIG. 52–1. Comparative data space coverage and corresponding images of the right coronary artery (RCA) using identical gradient recalled echo pulse sequence **(A)** echoplanar imaging and **(B)** spiral imaging. (Courtesy of C. Meyer, Stanford University, Stanford, CA.) (See color insert for Fig. 52–2.)

IMAGING OF WALL MOTION AND VENTRICULAR FUNCTION

Technical Considerations

The normal heart wall thickness varies from 0.6 to 1.2 cm. Wall motion is approximately 2.5 cm per second during systole and 10 cm per second during early diastole (20). It is necessary to have a temporal resolution of 20 to 30 frames per second to adequately evaluate wall motion caused by ventricular wall and respiratory motion (21). Cine images of the heart have been available since the early development of GRE MRI (22). Because of the inefficient acquisition of *k*-space, these temporally averaged images are acquired over a 2- to 4-minute interval. Although these early methods sometimes produced spectacular moving images of the heart, the poor temporal resolution resulting in cardiac and respiratory motion artifacts have made the method impractical for routine clinical applications. Subsequent fast imaging techniques allow cine acquisitions during a 15- to 20-second breath hold with a temporal resolution around 80 to 100 ms (23). Routine clinical implementation of regional wall motion using MR has become increasingly common in the more technically advanced medical centers.

Clinical Development

CMR imaging at rest provides the optimal means to assess ventricular volumes to quantitate left ventricular (LV) ejection fraction, LV end-systolic and end-diastolic volumes, and right ventricular (RV) volumes. Imaging at stress and rest provides a means to detect significant CAD or assess viability in asynergic segments. One of the first studies using dobutamine stress CMR to detect significant CAD consisted of 25 patients starting at 5 μg per kilogram per minute to a maximum of 20 μg per kilogram per minute (24). The detection of new wall motion abnormalities induced during dobutamine infusion corresponded with the location of reversible ischemia on thallium myocardial perfusion imaging in 95% of the patients. A similar study was performed in 39 patients with CAD and in 10 normal control patients generating sensitivity and specificity of 91% and 80%, respectively (25). Similar comparison between dobutamine CMR and technetium-sestamibi single photon emission computed tomography (SPECT) studies showed similar sensitivity and specificity (26). Although only intermediate doses of dobutamine infusion and limited imaging time were achieved at peak stress, comparable sensitivity and specificity to other noninvasive stress imaging protocols were achieved. Recently, a prospective, blinded study in 208 consecutive patients with suspected CAD using peak dobutamine dose and rapid imaging technique with breath holding was conducted (27). Dobutamine stress echocardiography (DSE) with harmonic imaging and dobutamine stress MRI (DMR) were performed before cardiac catheterization. DMR at peak dobutamine infusion increased the sensitivity from 74.3% to 86.2% and specificity from 69.8% to 85.7% (both *p* < 0.05) when compared with DSE. Similarly, a study consisting of 153 consecutively enrolled patients with suboptimal DSE image quality was conducted with peak dobutamine dose DMR with a breath hold acquisition (28). In comparison to coronary angiography, sensitivity and specificity of 83% and 83%, respectively, were achieved in patients with suboptimal DSE. Although these results show tremendous promise, the need for breath hold and cardiac-gating limits routine clinical implementation.

Future Directions

Current imaging protocols are suboptimal at peak stress when patients may become symptomatic or even unstable. A method allowing rapid intuitive adjustment to provide the optimal imaging plane with real-time dynamic display of the selected images would be a substantive improvement. Under stress conditions, ventricular and atrial arrhythmias may occur, breath holding is not always well tolerated, and continuous monitoring to detect wall motion abnormalities can be useful (29). RT imaging eliminates the need for cardiac-gating and breath holding and allows continuous monitoring of wall motion. The clinical utility of RT assessment of regional and global wall motion abnormality has already been demonstrated (30). The images of global and regional LV

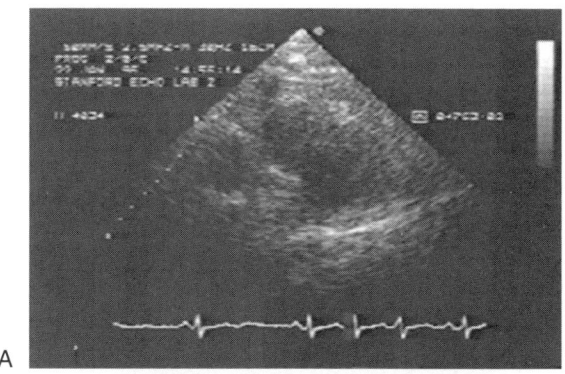

A

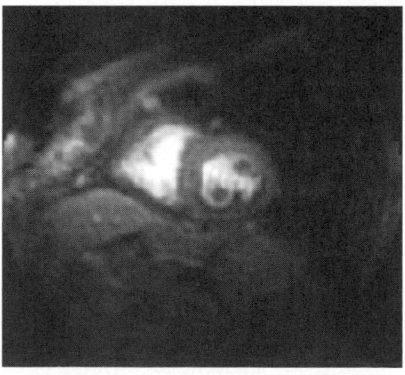

B

FIG. 52–3. Suboptimal image quality of the heart obtained by **(A)** echocardiography and **(B)** corresponding real-time image of the same patient. (From Yang P, Kerr A, Liu A, et al. New real-time interactive cardiac magnetic resonance imaging system complements echocardiography. *J Am Coll Cardiol* 1998;32:2049–2056, with permission.)

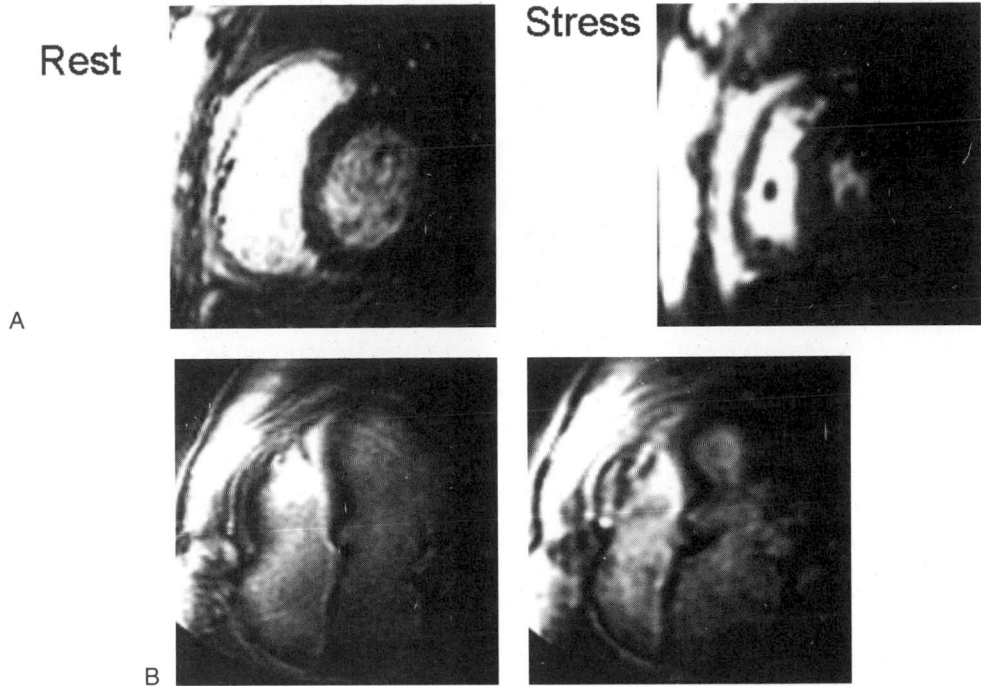

FIG. 52–4. Sample images of real-time interactive imaging equipped with steady-state free precession obtained at rest and stress conditions in **(A)** short-axis and **(B)** four-chamber views. (From Nguyen PK, Nayak, KS, Narayan, G, et al. *J Cardiovascular Magn Reson* 2003;5:68–69, with permission.)

function obtained in 85 patients using RT were compared with echocardiography. This clinical trial demonstrated that the RT detected wall motion abnormality as accurately as echocardiography. It also demonstrated that RT significantly improved the visualization of wall segments in patients with suboptimal echocardiography image quality. Using echocardiography, 38% of all wall segments were visualized adequately in suboptimal studies, whereas when using RT, 97% were adequately imaged ($p < 0.001$). Similar improvement was seen in patients with congenital heart or pulmonary disease who frequently have suboptimal echocardiography. Sample images are shown in Figure 52–3. On the basis of these findings, RT equipped with SSFP (RT-SSFP) with a temporal resolution of 10 to 20 frames per second and a spatial resolution of 2 to 3 mm have been developed to perform the entire DMR study in real time. Preliminary results in ten consecutive patients using the RT-SSFP have demonstrated high correlation with DSE evaluation of stress-induced wall motion abnormalities (31). Sample RT-SSFP images of systole and diastole at rest and stress wall motion are shown in Figure 52–4.

MYOCARDIAL PERFUSION IMAGING

Technical Considerations

Qualitative evaluation of perfusion was described more than a decade ago using first-pass gadolinium-diethylenetriamine penta-acetic acid (DTPA) (Gd-DTPA) contrast agent (32).

CMR perfusion imaging methods have steadily improved over the past several years. However, subsequent studies suggest that qualitative evaluation may not be superior to SPECT radionuclide imaging (33). Excellent quantitative multicompartment models of perfusion have long been known from physiologic investigations. CMR evaluation of perfusion using multicompartmental models have been described (34). These investigators were among the first to describe quantitative approaches in MR first-pass imaging in humans. They used a straightforward model assuming a linear relation between time course for appearance of contrast agent and amount of contrast agent injected without any change in the distribution of contrast agent during the signal measurement (35). By analyzing the relation between the myocardial intensity curve and the curve representing the supply of contrast agent to the myocardium, blood flow was approximated quantitatively. More recently, a semiquantitative measurement of perfusion using a linear fit to determine the up slope of the signal intensity–time curve has been developed. The signal intensity–time curve of each myocardial segment is corrected for the input function by dividing the signal intensity–time curve of each segment with the curve from LV cavity (36).

The quantitative assessment of perfusion requires dynamic imaging of the heart with adequate spatial coverage of the entire ventricle. At least 3 to 4 levels of the heart must be acquired. Because the capillary transit time through myocardium is about 3 to 4 seconds, temporal resolution of at least 2 to 4 short-axis images per second is required for adequate analysis (37). Newer techniques have been developed to improve the spatial coverage of the heart. A multishot EPI technique capable of covering the entire heart in contiguous 10-mm slices every 2 cardiac cycles with an in-plane resolution of 1.5 × 1.5 mm was developed (38). More recently, a new imaging technique using interleaved gradient echo/echoplanar imaging sequence was modified for and applied to dynamic contrast-enhanced imaging of the heart. Using interleaved gradient echo/echoplanar imaging, images with a nominal in-plane resolution of approximately 3 × 4 mm can be acquired in 100 ms, enabling 8 slices per heartbeat at a heart rate of 60 beats per minute. Acquisition characteristics to perform quantitative first-pass perfusion imaging with adequate LV coverage is possible (39). Furthermore, MR first-pass requires a T1-weighted sequence to enhance the perfusion image using Gd-based contrast agents in the myocardium. Various approaches have been used including volumetric imaging and planar tomographic sequences to optimize contrast between myocardium and blood pool (40–42).

Clinical Development

Although theoretically superior to radionuclide perfusion studies, clinical implementation of perfusion imaging with CMR has been limited. The initial observations in human studies suggested a difference in the kinetics of contrast agent uptake between normal and ischemic myocardium during resting conditions (43). Subsequently, successful detection of a 20% difference in blood flow was reported (44). MR perfusion studies in human subjects using the vasodilator dipyridamole demonstrated a close correlation with sestamibi-SPECT studies in single vessel disease (45). A prospective study assessed MR perfusion reserve in 34 patients using a model to determine the up slope of the signal intensity–time curve with the first pass of Gd-DTPA (36). Sensitivity, specificity, and diagnostic accuracy of 90%,

83%, and 87%, respectively, were determined using 75% or greater as the threshold for significant stenosis. Furthermore, a comparative study of CMR and positron emission tomography (PET) to coronary angiography in 48 patients and 18 healthy subjects was performed using a hybrid EPI multislice, saturation recovery sequence (46). Up slope of myocardial contrast agent was measured generating sensitivity and specificity of 91% and 94%, respectively, when compared with PET and 87% and 85%, respectively, when compared with coronary angiography.

Future Directions

The technical challenge associated with detection of myocardial ischemia in MR first-pass is to image the entire heart quickly under conditions of stress. In patients in whom symptoms of ischemia develop, the length of the induced state of stress must be minimized. Improvements are necessary in the areas of temporal and spatial resolution, volumetric coverage, and simultaneous imaging of wall motion and myocardial perfusion. Improvements in temporal and spatial resolution may be achieved with innovative reconstruction strategies involving the use of assumptions to reconstruct the image using partial data sets. Using homodyne detection of image reconstruction, partial k-space acquisitions may be used to reduce scan time and to improve spatial resolution (47). Acquisition techniques such as circular echoplanar imaging and variable-density spiral imaging have been developed (48,49). An alternative strategy uses a partial field of view (FOV) undersampling the data space to generate an image with a reduced FOV (50).

Current qualitative myocardial perfusion sequences using vasodilator infusion acquire three or more slice locations per cardiac cycle to ensure broad coverage. However, because of the need for higher temporal resolution, quantitative meth-

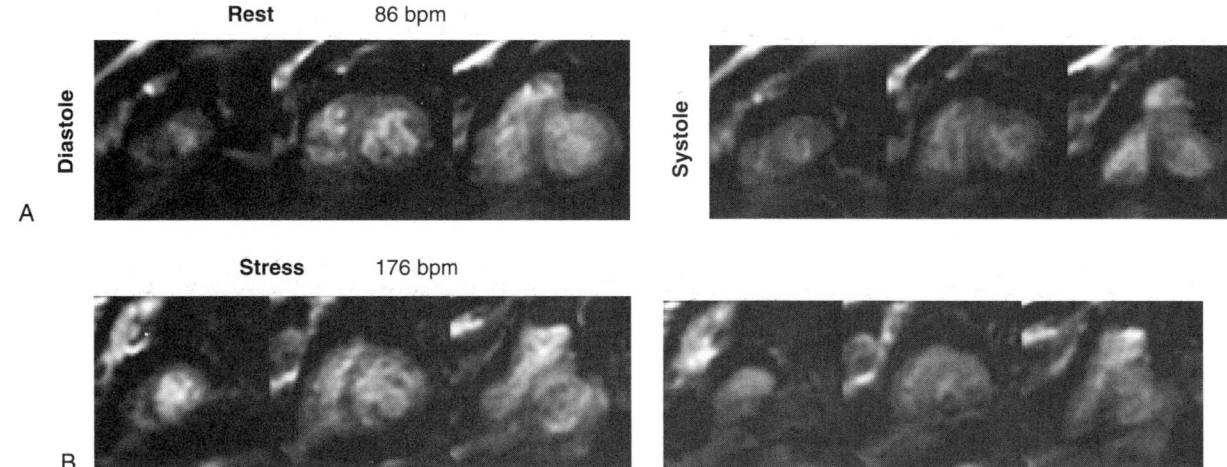

FIG. 52–5. Multi-slice images at diastole and systole obtained in **(A)** rest and **(B)** stress. (From Nayak K, Pauly J, Nishimura D, et al. Rapid ventricular assessment using real-time interactive multislice MRI. *Magn Reson Med* 2001;45:371–375, with permission.)

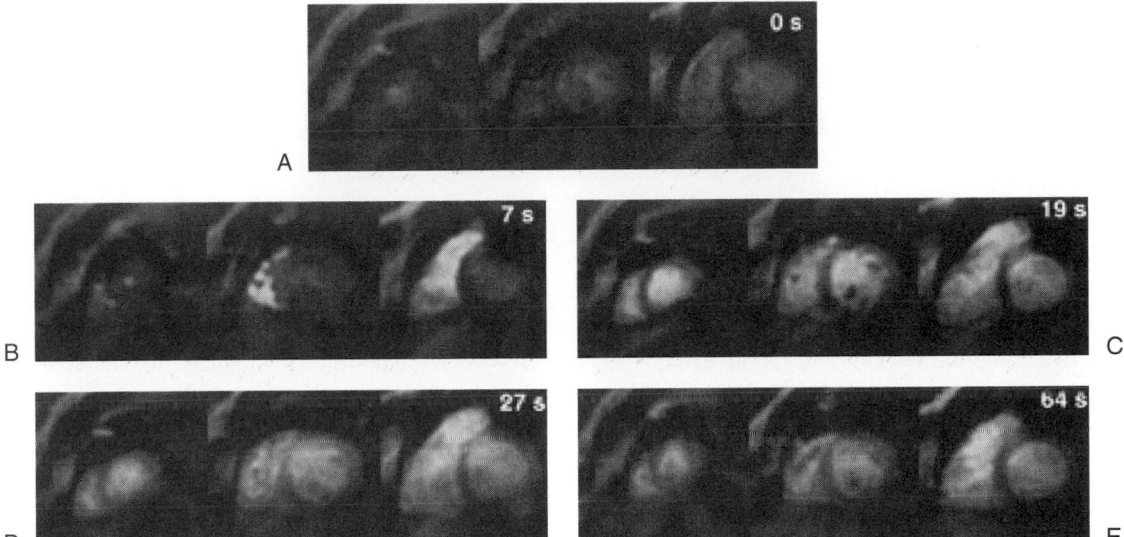

FIG. 52–6. Multislice images obtained simultaneously at the apex, midventricle, and base demonstrating first-pass perfusion **(A)** before injection, **(B)** right ventricular enhancement, **(C)** left ventricular enhancement, **(D)** myocardial enhancement, and **(E)** contrast washout. (From Nayak K, Pauly J, Nishimura D, et al. Rapid ventricular assessment using real-time interactive multislice MRI. *Magn Reson Med* 2001;45:371–375, with permission.)

ods suffer from limited coverage (35). Furthermore, these sequences are unable to provide adequate coverage of the heart during pharmacologic stress when cardiac cycles decrease to 350 to 400 ms. To provide adequate volumetric coverage and temporal resolution, an innovative RT multislice imaging sequence has been developed using a partial *k*-space circular EPI approach (51). This sequence allows imaging of three slices (apex, mid, and base) at frame rates of 16 frames per second with spatial resolution of 3 mm. It is possible to image both wall motion and myocardial perfusion simultaneously in all three myocardial slices. Preliminary studies on healthy volunteers have demonstrated reliable imaging of stress wall motion in tachycardia range with increased signal intensity in the myocardium from contrast perfusion (52). Sample RT multislice images of contrast enhancement and wall motion of the myocardial walls acquired simultaneously at rest and stress are shown in Figures 52–5 and 52–6.

CORONARY ARTERY IMAGING

Technical Considerations

Optimal spatial and temporal resolution, accurate motion compensation, wide anatomic coverage, and high signal and contrast-to-noise ratios are the inherent challenges in MR coronary angiography (MRCA). Fundamental problems with coronary angiography are their small size (<4 mm), tortuosity, competing MR signals from adjacent epicardial fat and myocardium, and the constant dyssynchrony between cardiac and respiratory motions (53). Attempts to improve one imaging parameter usually occur at the expense of another.

Significant technical developments have occurred in recent years to address these problems. Both two- (2D) and three-dimensional (3D) image acquisitions have become possible (15,54–57). Although the 2D techniques are easy to implement, image blurring, slice misregistration, and inadequate coverage of the coronary arterial tree occur (53). The 3D techniques designed to address these limitations, however, usually result in prolonged acquisition time, reduced contrast, and requirement for sophisticated respiratory motion compensation techniques (58). Acquisition strategies have evolved from rectilinear segmented *k*-space to more complex echoplanar and spiral imaging (13,15,54). Each approach, however, has its own limitation: Segmented *k*-space uses MR signal inefficiently, EPI is susceptible to flow artifact, and spiral imaging is sensitive to off-peak spectral resonance (59–61). Motion compensation has evolved from simple breath hold to more complex navigator-echo techniques (62–64). These advanced methods designed to improve patient comfort and compliance have not preserved the image quality consistently (65,66). Multiple strategies including T2 prep, SSFP, magnetization transfer, and intravascular contrast have been designed to improve contrast (67–70). Finally, innovations including sensitivity encoding (SENSE) and simultaneous acquisition of spatial harmonics (SMASH) have been attempted to improve temporal resolution (71,72).

Although high-quality images of the coronary arteries have been obtained with various techniques, clinical application of these techniques has not achieved consistent coronary coverage, image quality, motion sensitivity, and lesion detection. Clinical trials have produced variable results (53,73,74). Currently, MRCA is not yet in a form that can be widely used as a routine clinical test for the detection of CAD. Nevertheless, improvements are being made. Newer magnets using higher magnetic fields such as 3 T also should help to improve MRCA.

Clinical Development

Initial attempts at MRCA used SE with electrocardiogram-gating (75,76). In 1991, a fast breath hold technique was adopted for coronary angiography (62). This technique, combined with the contrast mechanism of selective inversion recovery, overcame the respiratory motion artifacts associated with previous attempts at coronary artery imaging. Subsequently, using fat saturation, Edelman (54) used a similar breath hold protocol using a segmented k-space fast gradient echo approach enabling partial imaging of the coronary artery. Subsequently, an alternative strategy of fast spiral readout coupled with spectral–spatial excitation was developed (15).

More recent developments have focused on multislice 2D and volumetric 3D coverage through ultrafast imaging techniques to improve on earlier clinical experience. The progress enabled contiguous slices and higher signal in one acquisition. Although the total imaging time was shorter than with 2D methods, a longer acquisition time made breath hold protocols problematic; respiratory motion compensation techniques were required. As early as 1993, a free-breathing method using averages of multiple acquisitions enabled a 64-mm-thick volume with fat saturation and magnetization transfer (77). A navigator-echo approach for coronary artery imaging led to improved 3D imaging with the development of a diminished variance algorithm (DVA) (78). This method analyzes the histogram of the respiratory positions from a complete set of data, then it reacquires the data from the most corrupt locations. Other methods to compensate for respiratory motion include retrospective or prospective sorting of the images to accept images acquired within a certain gating window (± 3–5 mm).

Clinical implementation of innovative 2D and 3D imaging sequences followed. A multislice 2D imaging using a spiral acquisition and real-time localization imaged 5 to 15 slices with 3 to 5 cm in thickness while maintaining acquisition time of 37 ms per slice during a single breath hold (79,80). Another technique combined 3D segmented k-space and EPI acquisition technique with prospective navigator gating (81). In addition, a spherical stack of 3D spiral imaging combined with DVA was implemented (82). Furthermore, a breath hold sequence involving volumetric coronary angiography with targeted volume scanning (VCATS) using combined 3D segmented EPI and turbo FLASH localized and imaged targeted volumes (74). More recently, a technique combining 3D VCATS and true fast imaging with steady-state free precession for improved contrast between blood and myocardium was proposed (56). Although each approach provided unique advantages, no specific technique allowed a truly robust method to accurately and routinely

detect significant CAD. Representative coronary artery images acquired using multislice 2D spiral and 3D turbo field echo–EPI techniques are shown in Figure 52–7.

Future Directions

The most pressing question regarding MRCA currently is how this imaging technique can become clinically reliable and routinely useful. Clearly, impressive progress has been made. However, this imaging application has yet to meet the high standards required for routine clinical implementation. To achieve this objective, developments focused on further improving contrast and signal, temporal and spatial resolution, and scan protocol are underway.

One of the most pressing issues is to achieve maximum contrast to distinguish the blood vessels from the adjacent myocardium, fat, and blood, while also delineating the thrombus and plaque in the vessels to detect coronary lesions. Fat suppression consists primarily of fat presaturation (16,61). Muscle suppression consists of magnetization transfer and T2 preparation to improve intrinsic contrast (67,69). Intravascular contrast agents may improve some of the problems related to reduced contrast and signal. The T1 shortening effects of the agents enhance contrast without significant loss to signal. Several agents have undergone clinical trials. These agents include MS-325 (Angiomark; EPIX medical, Cambridge, MA), NC100150 (Clariscan; Nycomed-Amersham, Buckingshire, UK), and B-22956/1 (Bracco Imaging Spa, Milano, Italy). Although only phase I and II trial results are available, significant improvement in contrast-to-noise ratio has been observed (81,83,84). Finally, novel imaging sequences including SSFP and fast spin echo (FSE; black blood) offer improved contrast. Although still preliminary, investigators using a 3D breath hold SSFP sequence and a 3D dual-inversion FSE (black-blood) sequence have lead to substantial improvement in contrast (56,85).

Another challenge in MRCA relates to optimization of signal. 3D imaging prolongs acquisition time and enhances signal (63). Improvement in receiver coil design also will lead to improved signal. For example, a load-optimized phased array coil with an ability to select the region of sensitivity for the targeted anatomy will minimize noise volume and eliminate the need for coil repositioning (86). In addition, a higher field magnet such as a 3-T magnet promises potential increase in SNR (87–89). Preliminary imaging of the coronaries at 3 T has been performed with remarkable results as shown in Figure 52–8. However, 3-T imaging is not without technical challenges. The readout duration is limited by the larger susceptibility effects leading to off-resonance blurring. Shortened RF pulses and TE may improve both flow characteristics and T2 signal loss.

An equally critical issue in MRCA is improvement in temporal and spatial resolution. Over the last decade, segmented k-space imaging has dominated MRCA (53,54,90). Most notably, a multicenter trial has demonstrated encour-

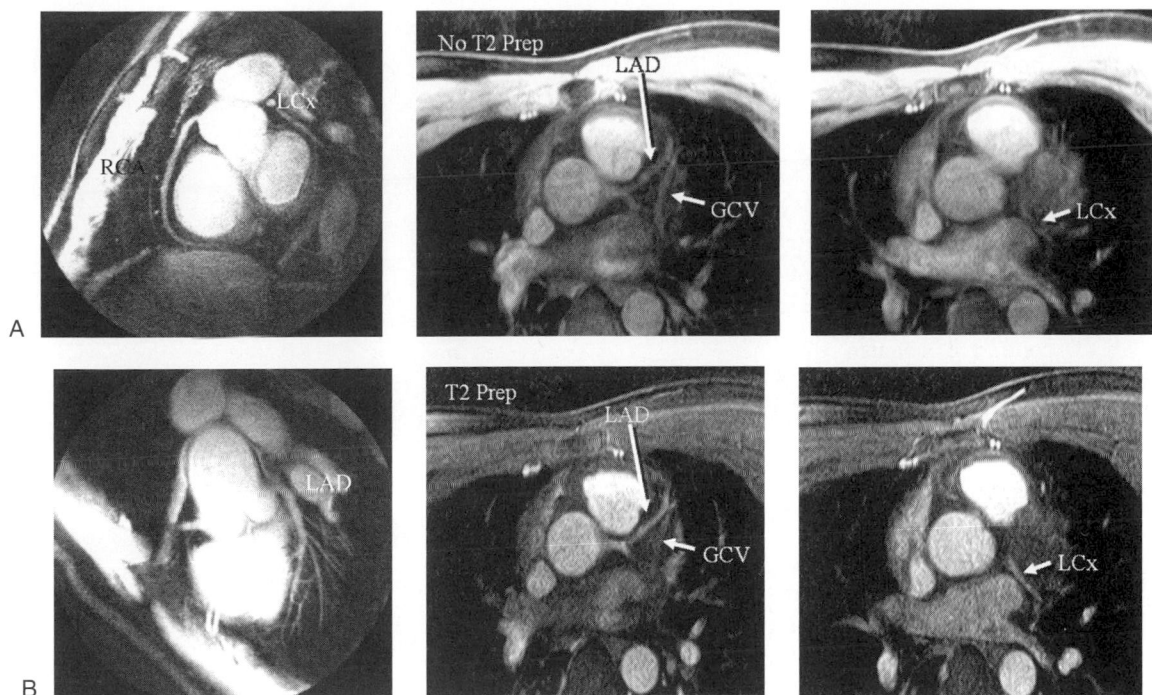

FIG. 52–7. Representative images of the coronary arteries using **(A)** two-dimensional spiral and **(B)** three-dimensional turbo field echo–echoplanar imaging techniques. GCV, greater cardial vein; LAD, left anterior descending; LCx, left circumflex artery. (A: From Yang P, Meyer C, Kerr A, et al. Spiral magnetic resonance coronary angiography with real-time localization. *J Am Coll Cardiol* 2003;41: 1134–1141, with permission; B: From Botnar R, Stuber M, Danias P, et al. Improved coronary artery definition with T2-weighted, free-breathing, three-dimensional coronary MRA. *Circulation* 1999;99: 3139–3148, with permission.)

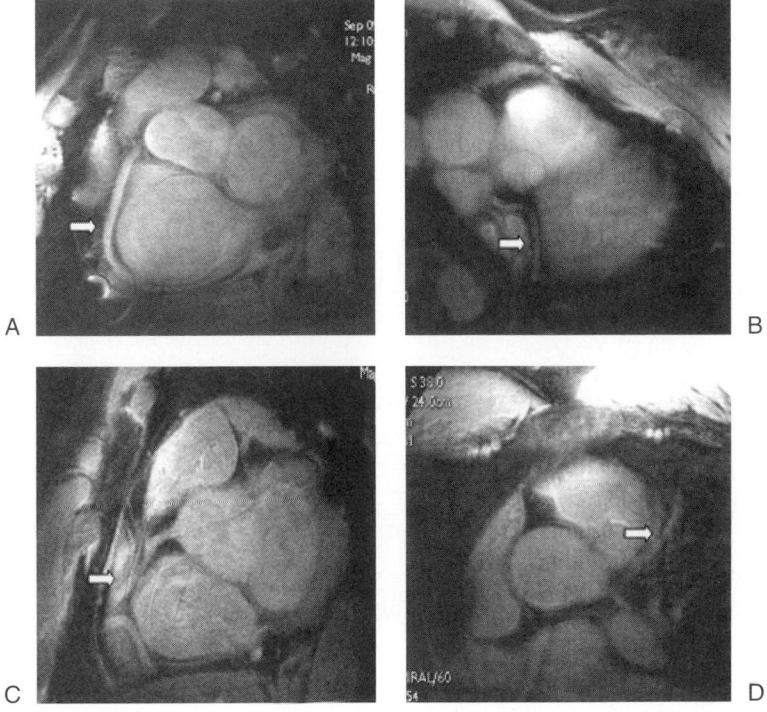

FIG. 52–8. Representative 3-T images of the coronary arteries: **(A)** right coronary, **(B)** left circumflex, **(C)** right coronary, and **(D)** left anterior descending arteries with mild stenosis. (From Yang P, Nguyen P, Shimakana A, et al. *J Cardiovascular Magn Reson* 2003;5:19–20, with permission.)

aging results, but it was hampered by low specificity (91). Application of more complex *k*-space acquisitions has demonstrated improvements in recent years (92). Several preliminary studies have reported improved temporal and spatial resolution in MRCA using the spiral *k*-space acquisitions (59–61,92). The first clinical trial of MRCA using a spiral *k*-space acquisition demonstrated good coverage, consistent image quality, and clinically acceptable sensitivity and specificity (93). Another approach to enhance temporal resolution involves parallel imaging. The technique accelerates image acquisition using spatial encoding from multiple detector coils by supplementing the encoding supplied by the gradient system. The two most common parallel imaging methods are SMASH and spatial SENSE (71,72).

Finally, for MRCA to become a clinical reality, a more time-efficient, operator-friendly, and patient-compliant scan protocol is essential. The RT system will substantially improve the way MRCA is performed. The RT images of the coronary arteries without cardiac-gating or respiratory motion compensation with a spatial resolution of 1.25 mm^2 and a temporal resolution of 190 ms have been achieved (94). Another innovative approach is the implementation of MRCA using a novel real-time architecture (95). This integrated system dynamically reconfigures pulse sequences on a per-acquisition basis and switch between phased array coils in real-time. The conventional MR scanners consist of sequencers that proceed through each acquisition on the basis of downloaded waveforms and timing commands. Using a modern PC (personal computer), a sequencer that is capable of running selected parameters of different pulse sequences simultaneously has been designed. A clinical study of 38 patients using this system switched dynamically between spiral real-time localization and high-resolution imaging in 1 repetition time (96). Preliminary results suggest improved sensitivity and specificity of detecting CAD of 83% and 90%, respectively. Furthermore, using two-element coronary coils, the image quality of the distal right coronary, left anterior descending, and left circumflex arteries were improved substantially. Sample RT coronary images are shown in Figure 52–9.

Myocardial Viability

Several features characterize viable myocardium including: (a) the preservation of contractile function; (b) maintenance of normal high-energy phosphates; (c) demonstration of myocardial cell membrane integrity; (d) maintenance of anaerobic glycolysis. Viable myocardium may appear dysfunctional as a result of either acute reversible ischemic insult (myocardial stunning) or chronic gradual decrease in blood supply (hibernating myocardium). After acute myocardial injury, the entire process of scarring usually takes up to 4 months to develop from the time of acute injury (97). The presence of hibernating myocardium has a substantial impact on the 4.7 million patients in the United States with ischemic heart failure. Optimal management of these patients may reduce mortality (40,000 deaths per

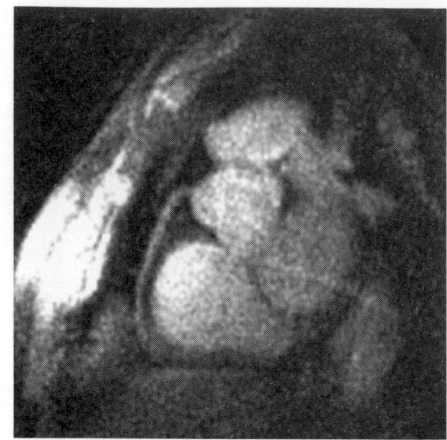

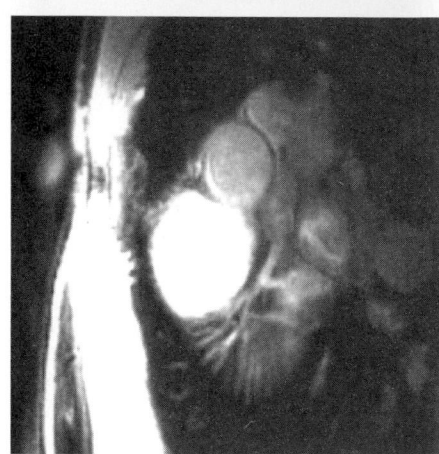

FIG. 52–9. Images of the coronary arteries using **(A)** real-time and **(B)** adaptive real-time imaging systems. (A: From Nayak K, Yang P, Pauly J, et al. Real-time interactive MRA. *Magn Reson Med* 2001;46:430–435; B: From Engvall J, Narayan G, Nguyen P, et al. *J Cardiovasc Magn Reson* 2003;5:290–291, with permission.)

year in the United States), and cost-effective strategies may significantly reduce the $20 billion annual expense associated with the condition (98). The concept that myocardial dysfunction can be reversed with catheter or surgical intervention has revolutionized the treatment of ischemic heart disease over the last two decades. Areas of heart muscle that are hypokinetic, akinetic, or dyskinetic at rest, once thought to be evidence of irreversible damage, may be viable. Diamond and Rahimtoola (99,100) originally coined the term "hibernation" in the late 1970s and early 1980s. The restoration of function, predicted with the aid of radionuclide methods using single photon thallium-201 and C-deoxyglucose dobutamine-stimulated echocardiography and dobutamine-stimulated MRI, had widespread application in the fields of ischemia-related LV dysfunction. The importance of reversing hibernation and other sequelae of CAD is considerable (101).

The term *hibernating myocardium* is generally accepted to mean areas of heart muscle, usually LV, whose function is impaired at rest but can be improved with medical or surgical intervention (including percutaneous coronary intervention or coronary artery bypass surgery). *Hibernation* implies wall motion abnormality caused by reduction of blood flow through a coronary artery with a "tight stenosis" (102). Dysfunctional hibernating myocardium is reversible, at least in part with revascularization and separation of this entity with reperfusion after coronary occlusion. The myocardium frequently remains asynergic for hours to days. This phenomenon is known as myocardial stunning and again the muscle is viable. It can be expected that one-third of revascularized myocardium will exhibit improvement in function. Furthermore, the prevalence of hibernating myocardium in ischemic cardiomyopathy with severely reduced ejection fraction is estimated to be 50% (103), although wall motion might not improve with revascularization if the problem has been long term.

The usefulness of MR techniques in the study of viable myocardium described by a metaanalysis by Bax and coworkers (104) is substantial. Certain parameters derived from resting MRI like end-diastolic wall thickness, systolic wall thickening, and contrast enhancement on delayed images obtained approximately 10 minutes after Gd-chelate appear to be markers of viability. In addition to cine stress MRI after inotropic stimulation and to viability, MR is evolving as a perfusion imaging methodology (Gd-chelate contrast agent is given by power injector and by serial rapid imaging is used to tract the distribution of the contrast agent into and out of the myocardium during the administration of dobutamine compared with perfusion in the nondobutamine stimulated states) (104).

Myocardial Delayed Contrast Enhancement

All the current conventional ultrasound and radionuclide-based imaging modalities for the assessment of cardiac viability have one major limitation: They cannot accurately depict scanned or acutely damaged myocardium. Gd-chelate contrast agent is accumulated and is retained in nonviable or scarred myocardium (Fig. 53–3). In an experimental model, the presence of either early hypoenhancement or delayed enhancement transmurally correlates with the loss of contractile reserve in response to low-dose dobutamine infusion (105). Kim and coworkers (106) correlated the percent of transmural extent of delayed contrast enhancement with the recovery of systolic wall thickening after surgical or percutaneous revascularization—the smaller the area of late enhancement, the greater the probability for mechanical improvement. Saeed and coworkers (107) used a necrosis-specific agent to show that the area of delayed contrast enhancement overestimated the true infarct zone, indicating that Gd-containing contrast agent not only demonstrated irreversible damage but also detected a periinfarct zone that is potentially viable (107).

Another consideration in predicting the extent of myocardial recovery after acute myocardial infarction is the *no-reflow phenomenon*. This term is used to describe a situation in which recanalization of a coronary artery may or may not occur, but, because of severe damage to distal vasculature, there is no reperfusion, and therefore functional activity is not restored. Delayed contrast enhancement can be used to identify the microvascular obstruction that characterizes the no-reflow phenomenon. Wu and coworkers (108) showed that a microvascular obstruction delayed contrast enhancement demonstrating as a hypoenhancement of contrast agent. This pattern predicted a significantly worse prognosis over a 2-year follow-up period. It is clear that some blood flow is essential to show delayed contrast enhancement, and, in the presence of no perfusion, the Gd agent cannot enter

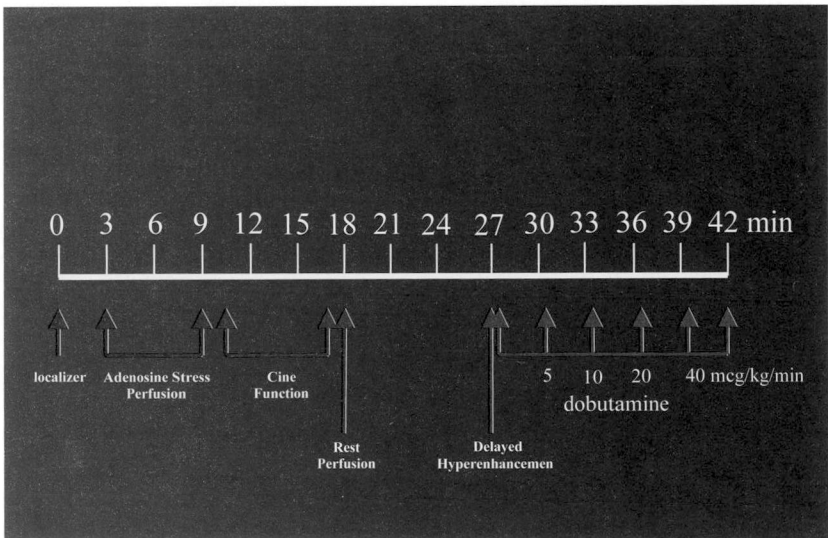

FIG. 52–10. Schematic depicts the time sequences for the combined perfusion, viability, and function stress magnetic resonance imaging protocol. (From Poon M, Fuster V, Fayad Z. Cardiac magnetic resonance imaging: a "one-stop-shop" evaluation of myocardial dysfunction. *Curr Opin Cardiol* 2002;17: 663–670, with permission.)

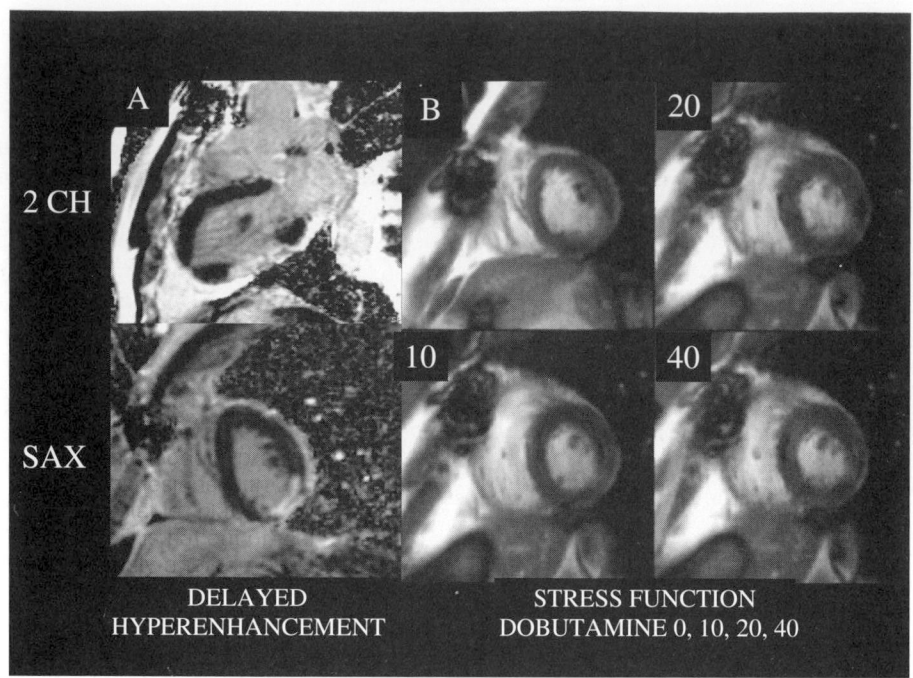

FIG. 52–11. A: Delayed hyperenhancement of the inferobasal region of the left ventricle consistent with nonviable myocardium. **B:** Stress dobutamine study was performed immediately after the acquisition of the delayed hyperenhancement images shown in **A.** Lack of normal thickening of the inferobasal region (with residual contrast hyperenhancement in the inferobasal region) in response to escalating doses of dobutamine (from 10–40 μg/kg/min). (Courtesy of M. Poon, Mount Sinai School of Medicine, New York, NY.)

the territory leading to the appearance of annular low signal intensity.

Accordingly, MRI as a single imaging modality is capable of assessing with high resolution cardiac function, perfusion, and viability—a task that usually requires radionuclide and echocardiography. In a study comparing MRI with fluorodeoxyglucose-PET in the assessment of cardiac viability, Lauerma and coworkers (109) reported that the combination of dobutamine stress, first-pass perfusion, and contrast enhancement was the best approach for detecting cardiac viability in patients with multivessel CAD. Poon and coworkers (110) developed and tested a protocol that evaluates myocardial perfusion, function, and viability in the same setting over a period of about 45 minutes (Fig. 52–10). This imaging protocol takes advantage of the short half-life of adenosine (a vasodilator and thus a perfusion agent), delayed contrast enhancement, and stress dobutamine (a positive inotropic agent) and allows for the infusion of both vasodilator and stress agent in a relatively short time interval to complete the resting and stress function and perfusion analyses of a given patient (Fig. 52–11).

Currently, the application of CMR for the evaluation of hibernating myocardium is still limited to specialized imaging centers with advanced equipment and trained personnel. As the hardware and software continue to advance, a "one-stop shop" approach for the assessment of the patient with ischemic heart disease (function, perfusion, and viability) will be feasible.

CONCLUSIONS

Clinical implementation of the comprehensive CMR examination in patients with possible ischemic heart disease has been challenging but provides the most cost-effective use for CMR. Currently, CMR is the most reliable method for the evaluation of LV (and RV) function with the potential to evaluate wall stress. With intravenous contrast agent administration, perfusion can be assessed followed by evaluation of nonviable myocardium and scar. Finally, coronary angiography and evaluation of the high-energy phosphates will be feasible. Comprehensive evaluation of cardiac ischemia using CMR will provide accurate imaging of cardiac function and anatomy data. This development may lead to a wide array of diagnostic information including detection of preclinical ischemic disease and accurate therapeutic guidance after myocardial infarction.

REFERENCES

1. Johnson L, Lozner E, Johnson S, et al. Coronary arteriography 1984-1987: a report of the Registry of the Society for Cardiac Angiography and Interventions. I. Results and complications. *Cathet Cardiovasc Diagn* 1989;17:5–10.
2. Lozner E, Johnson L, Johnson S, et al. Coronary arteriography 1984-1987: a report of the Registry of the Society for Cardiac Angiography and Interventions. II. An analysis of 218 deaths related to coronary arteriography. *Cathet Cardiovasc Diagn* 1989;17: 11–14.
3. Crouse L, Cheirif J, Hanly D, et al. Opacification and border delineation improvement in patients with suboptimal endocardial border

definition in routine echocardiography: results of the Phase III Albunex Multicenter Trial. *J Am Coll Cardiol* 1993;22:1494–1500.

4. Hoffman R, Lethen H, Marwick T, et al. Analysis of interinstitutional observer agreement in interpretation of dobutamine stress echocardiograms. *J Am Coll Cardiol* 1996;27:330–336.

5. Fleischmann K, Hunink M, Kuntz K, et al. Exercise echocardiography or exercise SPECT imaging? A meta-analysis of diagnostic test performance. *JAMA* 1998;280:913–920.

6. Gould K, Lipscomb K. Effects of coronary stenoses on coronary flow reserve and resistance. *Am J Cardiol* 1974;34:48–55.

7. Cranney G, Lotan C, Pohost G. *Cardiovascular applications of magnetic resonance imaging.* Boston: Little, Brown and Company, 1991.

8. Blackwell G, Pohost G. The evolving role of MRI in the assessment of coronary artery disease. *Am J Cardiol* 1995;75:74D–78D.

9. Schmitt F, Arz W. An ultra-high performance gradient system for cardio and neuro MR imaging. *Proceedings of the International Society for Magnetic Resonance in Medicine,* 7th Annual Meeting, Philadelphia, PA, April 1999:470.

10. Atkinson D, Edelman R. Cineangiography of the heart in a single breath hold with a segmented turbo-FLASH sequence. *Radiology* 1991;178:357–360.

11. Sekihara K. Steady-state magnetization in rapid NMR imaging using small flip angles and short repetition intervals. *IEEE Trans Med Imaging* 1987;6:157–164.

12. Mansfield P. Multi-planar image formation using NMR spin echos. *J Physics C: Solid State Physics* 1977:L55–L58.

13. Nishimura D, Irarrazabal P, Meyer C. A velocity k-space analysis of flow effects in echo-planar and spiral imaging. *Magn Reson Med* 1995;33:549–556.

14. McKinnon G. Ultrafast interleaved gradient-echoplanar imaging on a standard scanner. *Magn Reson Med* 1993;30:609–616.

15. Meyer C, Hu B, Nishimura D, et al. Fast spiral coronary artery imaging. *Magn Reson Med* 1992;28:202–213.

16. Meyer C, Pauly J, Macovski A, et al. Simultaneous spatial and spectral selective excitation. *Magn Reson Med* 1990;35:521–531.

17. Mansfield P. Real-time echo-planar imaging by NMR. *Br Med Bull* 1984:187–189.

18. Riederer S, Tasciyan T, Farzaneh F, et al. MR fluoroscopy: technical feasibility. *Magn Reson Med* 1988;8:1–15.

19. Kerr A, Pauly J, Hu B, et al. Real-time interactive MRI on a conventional scanner. *Magn Reson Med* 1997;38:355–367.

20. Matsuda T, Yamada H, Kida M, et al. Is 300 msec too long for cardiac MR imaging? Feasibility study demonstrating changes in left ventricular cross-sectional area with use of single-shot turboFLASH imaging. *Radiology* 1994;190:353–362.

21. Bove A, Ziskin M, Freeman E, et al. Selection of optimum cineradiographic frame rate: relation to accuracy of cardiac measurements. *Invest Radiol* 1970;5:329–335.

22. Pflugfelder P, Sechtem U, White R. Quantification of regional myocardial function by rapid cine MR imaging. *AJR Am J Roentgenol* 1988;150:523–539.

23. Martin E, Anthon R, Pohost G. Imaging cardiac structure and pump function. *Cardiol Clin* 1998:135–159.

24. Pennell D, Underwood S, Manzara C, et al. Magnetic resonance imaging during dobutamine stress in coronary artery disease. *Am J Cardiol* 1992;70:34–40.

25. Van Rugge F, Holman E, van der Wall E, et al. Quantitation of global and regional left ventricular function by cine magnetic resonance imaging during dobutamine stress in normal human subjects. *Eur Heart J* 1993;14:456–463.

26. Baer F, Smolarz K, Theissen P, et al. Identification of hemodynamically significant coronary artery stenoses by dipyridamole-magnetic resonance imaging and 99mTc-methoxyisobutyl-isonitrile-SPECT. *Int J Card Imaging* 1993;9:133–145.

27. Nagel E, Lehmkuhl H, Bocksch W, et al. Noninvasive diagnosis of ischemia-induced wall motion abnormalities with the use of high-dose dobutamine stress MRI: comparison with dobutamine stress echocardiography. *Circulation* 1999;16:763–770.

28. Hundely W, Hamilton C, Thomas M, et al. Utility of fast cine magnetic resonance imaging and display for the detection of myocardial ischemia in patients not well suited for second harmonic stress echocardiography. *Circulation* 1999;100:1697–1702.

29. Mertes H, Sawada S, Ryan T, et al. Symptoms, adverse effects, and complications associated with dobutamine stress echocardiography: experience in 1118 patients. *Circulation* 1993;88:15–19.

30. Yang P, Kerr A, Liu A, et al. New real-time interactive cardiac magnetic resonance imaging system complements echocardiography. *J Am Coll Cardiol* 1998;32:2049–2056.

31. Nguyen P, Nayak K, Narayan G, et al. Dobutamine stress MR with spiral real time SSFP reliably detects wall motion abnormalities. *J Cardiovasc Magn Reson* 2003;5:68–69.

32. Schaefer S, van Tyen R, Saloner D. Evaluation of myocardial perfusion in humans. *Radiology* 1992;185:795–801.

33. Eichenberger A, Schuiki E, Kochli V, et al. Ischemic heart disease: assessment with gadolinium-enhanced ultrafast MR imaging and dipyridamole stress. *J Magn Reson Imaging* 1994;4:425–431.

34. Wilke N, Simm C, Zhang J. Contrast-enhanced first pass myocardial perfusion imaging: correlation between myocardial blood flow in dogs at rest and during hyperemia. *Magn Reson Med* 1993;29:485–497.

35. Wilke N, Jerosch-Herold M, Wang Y. Myocardial perfusion reserve: assessment with multi-section, quantitative first-pass MR imaging. *Radiology* 1997;204:373–384.

36. Al-Saadi N, Nagel E, Gross M, et al. Noninvasive detection of myocardial ischemia from perfusion reserve based on cardiovascular magnetic resonance. *Circulation* 2000;101:1379–1383.

37. Kroll K, Wilke N, Jerosch-Herold M, et al. Accuracy of modeling of regional myocardial flows from residue functions of an intravascular indicator. *Am J Physiol* 1996;40:H1643–H1655.

38. Debatin J, McKinnon G, von Schulthess G. Technical note—approach to myocardial perfusion with echo planar imaging. *MAGMA* 1996;4:7–11.

39. Reeder S, Atalar E, Faranesh A, et al. Multi-echo segmented k-space imaging: an optimized hybrid sequence for ultrafast cardiac imaging. *Magn Reson Med* 1999;41:375–385.

40. Arai A. Magnetic resonance first-pass myocardial perfusion imaging. *Top Magn Reson Imaging* 2000;11:383–398.

41. Slavin G, Wolff S, Gupta S. First pass myocardial perfusion imaging using interleaved notched saturation. *Proceedings of the International Society for Magnetic Resonance in Medicine,* 8th Annual Meeting, Denver, CO, April 2000:36.

42. Reeder S, Atalay M, McVeigh E, et al. Quantitative cardiac perfusion: a noninvasive spin-labeling method that exploits coronary vessel geometry. *Radiology* 1996;200:177–184.

43. Manning W, Atkinson D, Grossman W, et al. First-pass nuclear magnetic resonance imaging studies using gadolinium-DTPA in patients with coronary artery disease. *J Am Coll Cardiol* 1991;18:959–965.

44. Kivelitz D, Bis K, Wilke N. Quantitative MR first pass perfusion imaging demonstrates coronary artery patency post interventions. *Radiology* 1997;205[Suppl]:253.

45. Matheijssen N, Louwerenburg H, van Rugge F, et al. Comparison of ultrafast dipyridamole magnetic resonance imaging with dipyridamole sestamibi SPECT for detection of perfusion abnormalities in patients with one-vessel coronary artery disease: assessment by quantitative model fitting. *Magn Reson Med* 1996;35:221–228.

46. Schwitter J, Nanz D, Kneifel S, et al. Assessment of myocardial perfusion in coronary artery disease by magnetic resonance: a comparison with positron emission tomography and coronary angiography. *Circulation* 2001;103:2230–2235.

47. Noll D, Nishimura D, Macovski A. Homodyne detection in magnetic resonance imaging. *IEEE Trans Med Imaging* 1991;10:629–637.

48. Pauly J, Butts R, Luk Pat G, et al. A circular echo planar pulse sequence. *Proceedings of the International Society for Magnetic Resonance in Medicine,* 3rd Annual Meeting, Nice, France, August 1995:106.

49. Lee J, Hargreaves B, Nishimura D. Fast 3D imaging using variable density spiral trajectories. *Proceedings of the International Society for Magnetic Resonance in Medicine,* 9th Annual Meeting, Glasgow, Scotland, April 2001:1777.

50. Sedarat H, Kerr A, Pauly J, et al. Improved temporal resolution in FOV-limited dynamic spiral imaging. *Proceedings of the International Society for Magnetic Resonance in Medicine,* 6th Annual Meeting, Sydney, Australia, April 1998:1973.

51. Nayak K, Pauly J, Nishimura D, et al. Rapid ventricular assessment using real-time interactive multislice MRI. *Magn Reson Med* 2001; 45:371–375.

52. Yang P, Nayak K, Kaji S, et al. Simultaneous evaluation of exercise-stress wall motion and myocardial perfusion using real-time interac-

tive multislice MRI—clinical validation. *J Cardiovasc Magn Reson* 2002;4:49.

53. Manning W, Li W, Edelman R. A preliminary report comparing magnetic resonance coronary angiography with conventional angiography. *N Engl J Med* 1993;328:828–832.

54. Edelman R, Manning W, Burstein D, et al. Coronary arteries: breath-hold MR angiography. *Radiology* 1991;181:641–643.

55. Botnar R, Stuber M, Danias P, et al. Improved coronary artery definition with T2-weighted, free-breathing, three-dimensional coronary MRA. *Circulation* 1999;99:3139–3148.

56. Deshapande V, Shea S, Laub G, et al. 3D Magnetization-prepared true-FISP: a new technique for imaging coronary arteries. *Magn Reson Med* 2001;46:494–502.

57. Li D, Carr J, Shea S, et al. Coronary arteries: magnetization-prepared contrast-enhanced three-dimensional volume-targeted breath-hold MR angiography. *Radiology* 2001;219:270–277.

58. Botnar R, Stuber M, Danias P, et al. A fast 3D approach for coronary MRA. *J Magn Reson Imaging* 1999;10:821–825.

59. Taylor A, Keegan J, Jhooti P, et al. A comparison between segmented k-space FLASH and interleaved spiral MR coronary angiography sequences. *J Magn Reson Imaging* 2000;11:394–400.

60. Keegan J, Gatehouse P, Taylor A, et al. Coronary artery imaging in 0.5-tesla scanner: implementation of real-time, navigator echo-controlled segmented k-space FLASH and interleaved spiral sequences. *Magn Reson Med* 1999;41:392–399.

61. Bornert P, Stuber M, Botnar R, et al. Direct comparison of 3D spiral vs. cartesian gradient-echo coronary magnetic resonance angiography. *Magn Reson Med* 2001;46:789–794.

62. Wang S, Hu B, Macovski A, et al. Coronary angiography using fast selective inversion recovery. *Magn Reson Med* 1991;18:417–423.

63. Sachs T, Meyer C, Irarrazabal P, et al. The diminishing variance algorithm for real-time reduction of motion artifact in MRI. *Magn Reson Med* 1995;34:412–422.

64. Wang Y, Watts R, Mitchell I, et al. Coronary MR angiography: selection of acquisition window of minimal cardiac motion with electrocardiography-triggered navigator cardiac motion prescanning—initial results. *Radiology* 2001;218:580–585.

65. McConnell M, Khasgiwala V, Savord B, et al. Comparison of respiratory suppression methods and navigator locations for MR coronary angiography. *AJR Am J Roentgenol* 1997;168:1369–1375.

66. Taylor A, Keegan J, Jhooti P, et al. Differences between normal subjects and patients with coronary artery disease for three different MR coronary angiography respiratory suppression techniques. *J Magn Reson Imaging* 1999;9:786–793.

67. Brittain J, Hu B, Wright G, et al. Coronary angiography with magnetization prepared T2 contrast. *Magn Reson Med* 1995;33:689–696.

68. Vasanawala S, Pauly J, Nishimura D. Fluctuating equilibrium MRI. *Magn Reson Med* 1999;42:876–883.

69. Hu B, Conolly S, Wright G, et al. Pulsed saturation transfer contrast. *Magn Reson Med* 1992;33:689–696.

70. Lorenz C, Johansson L. Contrast-enhanced coronary MRA. *J Magn Reson Imaging* 1999;10:703–708.

71. Pruessmann KP, Weiger M, Scheidegger MB, et al. SENSE: sensitivity encoding for fast MRI. *Magn Reson Med* 1999;42:952–962.

72. Sodickson D, Griswold M, Jakob P. SMASH imaging. *Magn Reson Imaging Clin N Am* 1999;7:237–254.

73. Paschal C, Haacke E, Adler L. Three-dimensional MR imaging of the coronary arteries: preliminary clinical experience. *J Magn Reson Imaging* 1993;3:491–500.

74. van Geuns R, Wielopolski P, de Bruin H, et al. MR coronary angiography with breath-hold targeted volumes: preliminary clinical results. *Radiology* 2000;217:270–277.

75. Lieberman L, Botti R, Nelson A. Magnetic resonance of the heart. *Radiol Clin North Am* 1984;22:847–858.

76. Paulin S, von Schulthess G, Fossel E. Magnetic resonance of the heart. *AJR Am J Roentenol* 1987;148:665–670.

77. Li D, Pascal C, Haacke E, et al. Coronary arteries: three dimensional MR imaging with fat saturation and magnetization transfer contrast. *Radiology* 1993;187:401–406.

78. Sachs T, Meyer C, Pauly J, et al. Real-time interactive 3D-DVA for robust coronary MRA. *IEEE Trans Med Imaging* 2000;19:73–79.

79. Meyer C, Hu B, Kerr A, et al. High-resolution multislice spiral coronary angiography with real-time interactive localization. *Proceedings*

80. Hu B, Meyer C, Macovski A, et al. Multi-slice spiral magnetic resonance coronary angiography. *Proceedings of the International Society for Magnetic Resonance in Medicine,* 4th Annual Meeting, New York, NY, April 1996:176.

81. Stuber M, Botnar RM, Danias PG, et al. Contrast agent-enhanced, free-breathing, three-dimensional coronary magnetic resonance angiography. *J Magn Reson Imaging* 1999;10:790–799.

82. Thedens D, Irarrazabal P, Sachs T, et al. Fast magnetic resonance coronary angiography with a three-dimensional stack of spiral trajectory. *Magn Reson Med* 1999;41:1170–1179.

83. Taylor AM, Panting JR, Keegan J, et al. Safety and preliminary findings with the intravascular contrast agent NC100150 injection for MR coronary angiography. *J Magn Reson Imaging* 1999;9:220–227.

84. Cavagna F, La Noce A, Maggioni F, et al. MR coronary angiography with the new intravascular contrast agent B-22956/1: first human experience. *Proceedings of the International Society for Magnetic Resonance in Medicine,* 10th Annual Meeting, Honolulu, HI, May 2002:114.

85. Stuber M, Botnar RM, Spuentrup E, et al. Three-dimensional high-resolution fast spin-echo coronary magnetic resonance angiography. *Magn Reson Med* 2001;45:206–211.

86. Fayad Z, Connick T, Axel L. An improved quadrature or phased-array coil for MR cardiac imaging. *Magn Reson Med* 1995;34:186–193.

87. Yang P, Nguyen P, Shimakawa A, et al. Spiral MR coronary angiography with real-time localization at 3T. *J Am Coll Cardiol* 2003;41: 432A.

88. Stuber M, Botnar R, Larmerichs R, et al. A preliminary report on in-vivo coronary MRA at 3T in humans. *Proceedings of the International Society for Magnetic Resonance in Medicine,* 10th Annual Meeting, Honolulu, HI, May 2002:116.

89. Huber M, Kozerke S, Pruessmann K, et al. Sensitivity encoding in free-breathing navigator-gated 3D coronary MRA at 3T. *Proceedings of the International Society for Magnetic Resonance in Medicine,* 10th Annual Meeting, Honolulu, HI, May 2002:115.

90. Pennell D, Bogren H, Keegan J, et al. Assessment of coronary artery stenosis by magnetic resonance imaging. *Heart* 1996;75:127–133.

91. Kim W, Danias P, Stuber M, et al. Coronary magnetic resonance angiography for the detection of coronary stenoses. *N Engl J Med* 2001;345:1863–1869.

92. Maintz D, Botnar R, Heindel W, et al. Coronary magnetic resonance angiography: an objective quantitative comparison between four different MR techniques. *Proceedings of the International Society for Magnetic Resonance in Medicine,* 10th Annual Meeting, Honolulu, HI, May 2002:108.

93. Yang P, Meyer C, Kerr A, et al. Spiral magnetic resonance coronary angiography with real-time localization. *J Am Coll Cardiol* 2003;41: 1134–1141.

94. Nayak K, Yang P, Pauly J, et al. Real-time interactive MRA. *Magn Reson Med* 2001;46:430–435.

95. Santos J, Wright G, Yang P, et al. Adaptive architecture of real-time imaging systems. *Proceedings of the International Society for Magnetic Resonance in Medicine,* 10th Annual Meeting, Honolulu, HI, May 2002:468.

96. Nguyen P, Santos J, Scott G, et al. Adaptive real-time MR coronary angiography: first prospective clinical trial. *J Cardiovasc Magn Reson* 2003;5:228–229.

97. Baer FM, Voth E, LaRosee K, et al. Comparison of dobutamine trans-esophageal echocardiography and dobutamine magnetic resonance imaging for detection of residual myocardial viability. *Am J Cardiol* 1996;78:415–419.

98. Iskander S, Iskandrian AE. Prognostic utility of myocardial viability assessment. *Am J Cardiol* 1999;83:696–702,A7.

99. Wijns W, Vatner SF, Camici PG. Hibernating myocardium. *N Engl J Med* 1998;339:173–181.

100. Rahimtoola SH. The hibernating myocardium. *Am Heart J* 1989;117: 211–221.

101. Ho KK, Pinsky JL, Kannel WB, et al. The epidemiology of heart failure: the Framingham Study. *J Am Coll Cardiol* 1993;22[4 Suppl A]: 6A–13A.

102. Udelson JE, Criss D. Assessment of regional viability in the infarct zone following myocardial infarction. *J Thromb Thrombolysis* 1997;4: 207–216.

103. al-Mohammad A, Mahy IR, Norton MY, et al. Prevalence of hibernat-

ing myocardium in patients with severely impaired ischaemic left ventricles. *Heart* 1998;80:559–564.

104. Bax JJ, de Roos A, van Der Wall EE. Assessment of myocardial viability by MRI. *J Magn Reson Imaging* 1999;10:418–422.

105. Cornel JH, Bax JJ, Elhendy A, et al. Agreement and disagreement between "metabolic viability" and "contractile reserve" in akinetic myocardium. *J Nucl Cardiol* 1999;6:383–388.

106. Kim RJ, Hillenbrand HB, Judd RM. Evaluation of myocardial viability by MRI. *Herz* 2000;25:417–430.

107. Saeed M, Lund G, Wendland MF, et al. Magnetic resonance characterization of the peri-infarction zone of reperfused myocardial infarc-tion with necrosis-specific and extracellular nonspecific contrast media. *Circulation* 2001;103:871–876.

108. Wu KC, Zerhouni EA, Judd RM, et al. Prognostic significance of microvascular obstruction by magnetic resonance imaging in patients with acute myocardial infarction. *Circulation* 1998;97:765–772.

109. Lauerma K, Niemi P, Hanninen H, et al. Multimodality MR imaging assessment of myocardial viability: combination of first-pass and late contrast enhancement to wall motion dynamics and comparison with FDG PET-initial experience. *Radiology* 2000;217:729–736.

110. Poon M FV, Fayad Z. Diagnosis of hibernating myocardium with cardiac MRI. *Curr Opin Cardiol* 2002;17:663–670.

CHAPTER 53

Noninvasive Imaging of the Vascular System

The Role of Magnetic Resonance Imaging and Computed Tomography

Konstantin Nikolaou, Michael Poon, Valentin Fuster, and Zahi A. Fayad

K. Nikolaou: Department of Clinical Radiology, University of Munich, Grosshadern, Germany; and Departments of Radiology and Medicine (Cardiology), Imaging Science Laboratories, The Zena and Michael A. Wiener Cardiovascular Institute, The Marie-Josée and Henry R. Kravis Cardiovascular Health Center, Mount Sinai School of Medicine, New York, New York.

M. Poon: The Zena and Michael A. Wiener Cardiovascular Institute, The Marie-Josée and Henry R. Kravis Cardiovascular Health Center, Mount Sinai School of Medicine, Cabrini Medical Center, New York, New York.

V. Fuster: The Zena and Michael A. Wiener Cardiovascular Institute, The Marie-Josée and Henry R. Kravis Cardiovascular Health Center, Mount Sinai School of Medicine, New York, New York.

Z. A. Fayad: Departments of Radiology and Medicine (Cardiology), Imaging Science Laboratories, The Zena and Michael A. Wiener Cardiovascular Institute, The Marie-Josée and Henry R. Kravis Cardiovascular Health Center, Mount Sinai School of Medicine, One Gustave L. Levy Place, Box 1234, New York, New York 10029.

Key Words: Computed tomography; magnetic resonance imaging; vascular.

INTRODUCTION

Magnetic Resonance Angiography

Magnetic resonance angiography (MRA) has evolved rapidly since its introduction more than 15 years ago. Initially, noncontrast-enhanced MRA techniques found their way into clinical routine for imaging vascular morphology (1). These initial noncontrast-enhanced approaches, in principle, can be divided into two subgroups: "black-blood" and "bright-blood" sequences (2). Although black-blood techniques based on signal voids within vessels containing flowing spins can confirm vessel patency, they remain of limited use in the assessment of vascular morphology. They are currently gaining acceptance, however, regarding the evaluation of vascular walls (3). Bright-blood MRA techniques are generally divided into those influenced by the effect of blood flow onto the signal amplitude (time of flight [TOF]) (4) and those based on the flow effect onto phase (phase contrast) (5). The flow dependence and associated artifacts inherent to these techniques have restricted the clinical use of these MRA techniques to the extracranial and intracranial arterial system and the portal venous system mainly. With the advent of high-performance gradient systems, a new promising MRA strategy has been developed: contrast-enhanced MRA (CE-MRA) using gadolinium chelates. It is based on the combination of rapid three-dimensional (3D) imaging and the T1-shortening effect of intravenously infused paramagnetic contrast (6). These techniques have been proven to give an extensive and diagnostically accurate evaluation of extracranial, thoracic, abdominal, and peripheral vessels (7). The possibilities for obtaining data in the thorax and abdomen within one breath hold, the resulting high contrast between vessel lumen and surrounding soft tissue, and the inherent 3D nature of the images allow for diagnostically relevant image quality. In many centers, contrast-enhanced 3D MRA has widely replaced the conventional x-ray angiography for the clarification of pathologies in arterial vessels (8).

Parallel acquisition technique (PAT), or partially parallel acquisition, is a new magnetic resonance technique based on the parallel use of more than one receiver coil to acquire image data with less phase-encoding steps than in conventional imaging. Advantages of parallel acquisitions techniques are acceleration of imaging, reduction of motion artifacts, and decrease of susceptibility sensitivity (9,10), making them ideally suited for high signal-to-noise applications like CE-MRA. First clinical applications of PATs recently have been tested, as described later.

Computed Tomography Angiography

Since spiral (i.e., helical) computed tomography (SCT) had been established in clinical routine in the early 1990s, computed tomography (CT) has matured to a volume scanning modality. 3D postprocessing methods like volume rendering techniques were clinically successful because of the availability of continuous volume data from spiral scanning (11). However, in practice, the spiral data sets suffered from a considerable mismatch between the transverse (in-plane) and the longitudinal (out-of-plane) spatial resolution. That is, the isotropic 3D volume element (voxel) could not be realized (12). Similarly, in routine practice a number of limitations still remained which prevented the scanning protocol to be fully adapted to the diagnostic needs (13). The advent of multidetector-row CT systems (MDCT) is the first real quantum leap in CT since the introduction of SCT (14). In general terms, the capabilities of SCT can be expanded in various ways: to scan anatomic volumes with standard techniques at significantly reduced scan times, to scan larger

volumes previously not accessible in practical scan times, or to scan anatomic volumes with high axial resolution (narrow collimation) to closely approach the isotropic voxel of high-quality data sets for excellent 3D postprocessing and diagnosis.

In addition, the faster gantry rotation time of the new MDCT systems of 500 ms or less revolutionized the CT application for diagnosis of moving organs. Particularly attractive is the cardiac CT application to freeze heart motion by combining rapid "partial-scan" techniques with electrocardiographic (ECG)-triggering (15). ECG gating of multislice spiral scans of the heart provides continuous 3D data sets during diastole. In combination with dedicated spiral reconstruction algorithms, which are optimized for a temporal resolution of 210 to 250 ms, significant advances have been reported for the diagnosis of coronary anatomy (16–19). Besides cardiac CT, the advantages of MDCT for assessing the vasculature in general are substantial. MDCT allows reduction of iodinated contrast utilization, improves spatial resolution, and shows less pulsation artifacts and greater coverage than SCT. MDCT technology has substantially improved computed tomography angiography (CTA) of extracranial, thoracic, abdominal, pulmonary, and peripheral vasculature (20–22).

Another promising technique specialized on cardiac imaging is electron beam computed tomography (EBCT). EBCT has mainly been used for accurate quantitation of coronary artery calcium, scanning the entire heart in a single breath hold from rapid (100 ms) tomographic scans done in synchrony with the heart cycle (23). Further indications can be noninvasive coronary artery imaging and assessment of coronary artery bypass grafts. In other vascular territories, EBCT has not been implemented extensively.

CORONARY ARTERIES

Noninvasive Coronary Angiography

Background

The small size and fast motion of the coronary arteries tests the effectiveness of any noninvasive diagnostic imaging modality. Currently, no cross-sectional imaging modality has proven itself capable of depicting the coronary arteries with a sufficient high temporal and spatial resolution for a consistent and adequate image quality, as well as that of x-ray angiography. Alternative modalities like EBCT, magnetic resonance imaging (MRI), and 4-detector-row CT (4DCT) systems have all been tested for their ability to reliably detect significant coronary artery stenoses, with varying results and conclusions (24,25). In some studies, good diagnostic results have been reported. However, in most reports, the number of vessel segments or patients excluded, because of being unable to assess as a direct result of the limitations in image quality, were considerably high (ranging between 5% and 30%) (26,27). In addition, the assessment was usually limited to the proximal and middle segments of the vessels. Active research development to overcome the technical barriers of EBCT and MRI are ongoing. Currently, both MR and EBCT appear to be outperformed by 16-detector-row CT (16DCT). For the first time, 16DCT has arrived as a robust and reliable noninvasive imaging modality that is capable of producing consistent and high-quality images of the coronary arteries in most patients.

Magnetic Resonance Angiography of the Coronary Arteries

Although several noninvasive imaging modalities have been tested clinically for the detection of coronary artery lesions, MRI deserves special attention. MRI can deliver high-resolution images with superb contrast characteristics in any desired orientation, especially suited to study the coronary anatomy. In addition, functional parameters like myocardial function or perfusion under rest and pharmacologic stress can be used to complement the evaluation of suspected coronary artery lesion. Coronary arteries are surrounded by epicardial fat; thus, using bright-blood techniques, fat-suppression is essential for adequate visualization of the vessel. Further improvements to enhance the coronary artery to myocardium contrast include additional preparatory pulses such as magnetization transfer (28) and T2 preparation (29) are likely to improve the overall image quality.

Since the publication of first clinical results in 1993 (30), noninvasive coronary MRA has undergone numerous technical improvements and innovations. Three major groups or "generations" of coronary MRA techniques have been proposed by several authors (31,32). Of all the imaging techniques available, two-dimensional (2D) breath hold magnetic resonance coronary angiography (MRCA) scans (33–35), 3D respiratory-gated MRCA (36–38) (Fig. 53–1), and breath hold 3D MRCA (39,40) have been evaluated most extensively. A multicenter study using a 3D prospective respiratory navigator approach has been presented, reporting an acceptable overall sensitivity of 82% for significant stenoses (≥50%) in proximal and middle vessel segments and a diagnostic accuracy of 75% for diagnosing coronary artery disease (CAD) (41). Still, after 10 years of preclinical trials using these different coronary MRA techniques, no technique has yet emerged as superior and can provide a sensitivity and specificity for coronary lesion detection that compares with traditional x-ray coronary angiography (Table 53–1).

To date, MRI methods continue to improve. Advanced second-generation coronary MRA techniques using navigator pulse feedback, 3D *k*-space reordering (42), or adaptive prospective correction of slice position with signal averaging (43) improve the reliability and image quality, thus increasing the sensitivity of the technique. The third-generation noncontrast-enhanced (40) and contrast-enhanced (44,45) 3D breath hold techniques appear fast and easy to use. These and other various new MRCA techniques await further clinical trials to determine their effectiveness. Recent studies on 2D fast spin echo (FSE) black blood techniques report maximized signal for coronary MRA at no loss in image spatial

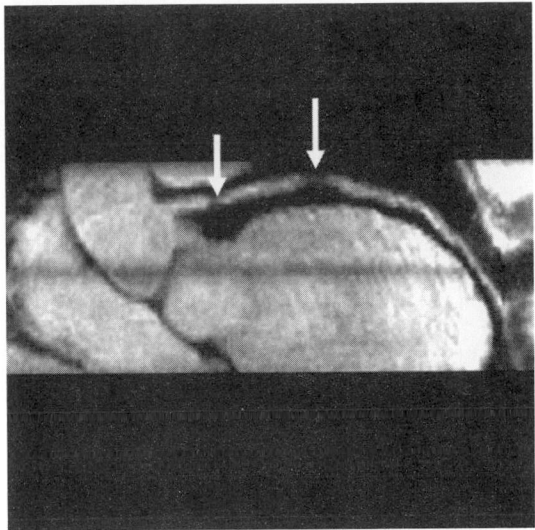

A

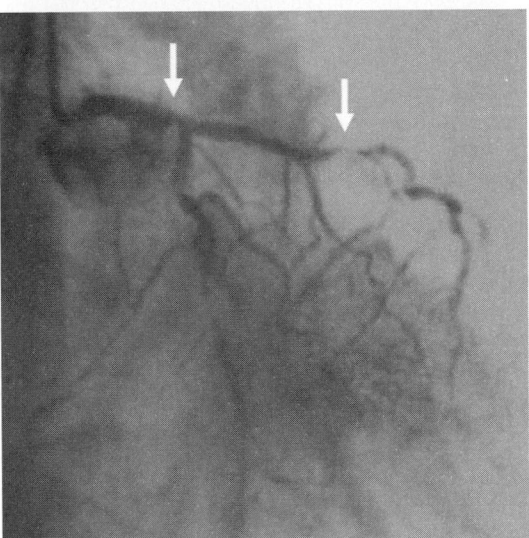

B

FIG. 53–1. Multiplanar reconstruction of a noncontrast-enhanced time-of-flight magnetic resonance data set **(A)** in a 62-year-old male patient depicts significant stenoses in the distal part of the left main coronary artery and an extended stenosis in the proximal part of the left anterior descending coronary artery **(A,** *arrows*). The conventional coronary angiography **(B)** confirms these lesions *(arrows)*. (From Nikolaou K, Huber A, Knez A, et al. Navigator echo-based respiratory gating for 3D-MR coronary angiography: reduction of scan time using a slice-interpolation technique. *J Comput Assist Tomogr* 2001;25:378–387, with permission.)

resolution. This suggests that the extension of black-blood coronary MRA with a 3D imaging technique would allow for a further signal increase (46). Segmented 3D steady-state free precession sequences also were described as a promising technique with substantially increased signal-to-noise ratio (SNR) and contrast-to-noise ratio for coronary artery imaging compared with conventional 3D gradient echo techniques with the same imaging time (47). New intravascular contrast agents may provide the long-awaited boost for reliable MRCA. Initial studies on animals (48) and in healthy volunteers (49) have shown promising results. In addition, the ma-

TABLE 53–1. *Sensitivity and specificity of magnetic resonance angiography and computed tomography angiography for the detection of significant coronary artery stenoses (>75%): results of a selection of clinical trials as compared with conventional angiography*

Author (reference)	Technique	Patients, n	Sensitivity, %	Specificity, %
Regenfus et al. 2003 (185)	MRA	61	85	90
Plein et al. 2003 (186)	MRA	40	74	88
Watanabe et al. 2002 (187)	MRA	22	80	85
Kim et al. 2001 (188)	MRA	109	93	42
Nikolaou et al. 2001 (37)	MRA	40	72	60
Ropers et al. 2003 (188a)	MDCTA (16)	77	92	93
Nieman et al. 2002 (18)	MDCTA (16)	59	95	86
Knez et al. 2001 (189)	MDCTA (4)	44	78	98
Nieman et al. 2001 (53)	MCDTA (4)	35	81	97
Achenbach et al. 2001 (26)	MCDTA (4)	64	85	76
Nikolaou et al. 2002 (27)	EBCTA	20	85	77
Achenbach et al. 2000 (190)	EBCTA	36	92	94
Budoff et al. 1999 (191)	EBCTA	52	78	91
Schmermund et al. 1998 (192)	EBCTA	28	82	88
Nakanishi et al. 1997 (193)	EBCTA	37	74	94

4, 4-detector-rows; 16, 16-detector-rows; EBCTA, electron-beam computed tomography angiography; MDCTA, multidetector-row computed tomography angiography.

jority of MRI manufacturers now offer dedicated cardiac scanners with strong imaging gradients (>30 mT/m) and fast rise times (>150 mT/m/ms) optimized for a smaller effective imaging field of view to provide greater speed and a better SNR. Introduction of parallel MRI acquisition techniques, such as simultaneous acquisition of spatial harmonics (SMASH) (50) and sensitivity encoding (SENSE) (51) may provide additional speed enhancement required to shorten imaging time.

Currently, established clinical applications include the evaluation of the patency of coronary artery bypass grafts (see "Noninvasive Imaging of Coronary Bypass Grafts") and the imaging of anomalous coronary arteries (52). The capability to reliably detect significant coronary artery stenoses in proximal and middle vessel segments with an acceptable sensitivity using any of the techniques currently available is still being discussed with significant differences in opinion. As the MR techniques continue to improve, the long-term value of MRCA cannot be underestimated despite the advent of MDCT coronary angiography.

Computed Tomography Angiography of the Coronary Arteries

The introduction of 4DCT scanner systems in 1998 had a major impact on noninvasive imaging of the coronary arteries (53). The introduction of its immediate successor, 16DCT systems, in 2002 has continued the dominant role of CT in current noninvasive coronary imaging. There are several advantages of the 16DCT scanner for angiographic examinations in general and especially for the coronary arteries (54). First, the gantry rotation time in 16DCT for cardiac investigations is 420 ms, allowing for 210-ms exposure time up to a heart rate of 65 beats per minute. This is a 20% gain in temporal resolution over that of a 4-channel detector sys-

tem. With greater heart rates and multisegment reconstruction algorithms, the exposure time varies between 105 and 210 ms, depending on the heart rate. Second, the spatial resolution along the z-axis improves by 25%, being now 0.75 mm as opposed to the 1.0 mm acquired previously on a 4DCT. Inplane resolution has remained the same, but still, using 16DCT, almost isotropic voxels can now be acquired with a voxel size of about $0.6 \times 0.6 \times 0.75$ mm. Thereby, beam-hardening artifacts of stents or of calcium deposits in the vessel wall might be decreased because of reduced partial volume effects. Thus, depiction and delineation of calcified and noncalcified plaques is improved. Third, and probably most important, the complete heart can now be depicted in a significantly shorter breath hold time of less than 20 s, compared with 35 to 40 seconds breath hold time on a 4DCT. This results in a considerable reduction of motion artifacts. Additional advantages of this shorter scan time are less venous contrast enhancement and a smaller contrast dose. The well tolerated examination can be performed within 15 minutes and requires no hospital admission. Concerning radiation exposure, the increase in dosage comparing 4DCT with 16DCT coronary angiography is not significant, being around 4 mSv (milliSievert) for 4DCT and 5 mSv for 16DCT, if prospective tube current modulation is used. Using this technique, the tube current is decreased during systole. Thereby, radiation exposure can be reduced by half at low heart rates (55). β-Blocker preparation in patients with heart rates greater than 65 beats per minute is mandatory to ensure motion-free image quality. Using 16DCT with short acquisition times, contrast timing should be more accurate, resulting in less contrast agent needed. For contrast enhancement of the coronaries, the amount of contrast can be reduced significantly using 16DCT, being now 80 mL of contrast in comparison to 120 mL for 4DCT, according to a previously published protocol (19). The continuous data acquisition of a coronary MDCT data set allows slice reconstruction at different time positions within the cardiac cycle. Images are typically reviewed on the basis of the cross-sectional images in combination with 3D reconstructions (Fig. 53–2) (56).

Clinical studies using 4DCT scanners have reported sensitivities and specificities for significant coronary artery stenoses (>75%) of 78% to 85% and 76% to 98%, respectively (Table 53–1). These reports showed promising results but were not robust enough to consistently produce reliable coronary imaging. Up to 30% of the proximal and middle coronary segments could not be interpreted because of insufficient image quality. Initial clinical studies on 16DCT coronary angiography report high sensitivities and specificities of 92% to 95% and 86% to 93%, respectively (Table 53–1). Most remarkably, the number of poorly assessable segments was very low, indicating the robustness of this technique.

Despite the promising initial experiences with 16DCT coronary angiography, there are still certain limitations to the technique. Currently, MDCT coronary angiography is not reliable in patients with arrhythmias, with moderate to high heart rates not amenable to β-blockade, or with severely calcified vessels. Severe calcifications are still causing partial volume and beam-hardening artifacts, despite the improvement in spatial resolution, resulting in false-negative results compared with cardiac x-ray angiography. In segments with extensive calcifications, significant coronary artery stenoses can neither be concluded nor ruled out. Although 16DCT has outstandingly high spatial resolution among noninvasive imaging modalities, small-caliber vessel can still lead to false-positive findings compared with x-ray coronary angiography. Coronary stents can now be well visualized using 16DCT. Insight into the patency of the stent lumen is not only plausible but, in most patients with adequately slow heart rates, it can be confirmed or excluded. However, the degree of in-stent stenoses does not seem to be assessable at this juncture.

The main advantage of 16DCT compared with 4DCT angiography of the coronary arteries seems to be the increased number of investigations with sufficiently good image quality. This robustness of its clinical application also can be ascertained by the shorter breath holding time, 20% improved temporal resolution, and the decreasing need of β-blocker for heart rate control. However, MDCT has yet to achieve the quantitative accuracy of x-ray–based imaging techniques. Nevertheless, it does allow noninvasive detection and exclusion of significant coronary obstructions. From the currently published studies on coronary MDCT, the negative predictive value compared with coronary x-ray angiography was in the range of 96% to 98%. This high negative predictive value indicates that MDCT may be an ideal tool to rule out CAD in low-prevalence populations such as in symptomatic patients with atypical chest pain. However, MDCT currently appears not to be suited to determine disease severity or progression in patients with CAD with typical angina or positive evidence of significant myocardial ischemia on exercise testing or after coronary intervention. Diagnosis of these patients would still be determined most accurately by conventional x-ray angiography that would also allow percutaneous coronary interventions in the same session.

Another promising CT technique for cardiac imaging and coronary angiography is EBCT. EBCT has been mainly used for accurate quantification of coronary artery calcium, scanning the entire heart in a single breath hold from rapid (100 ms) tomographic scans done in synchrony with the heart cycle (23). In various clinical studies, the sensitivity and specificity reported for the detection of significant coro-

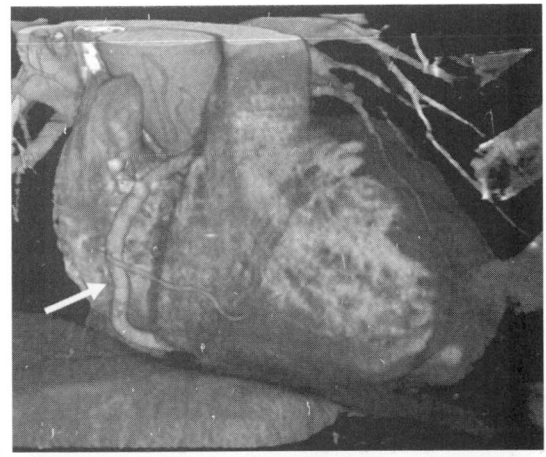

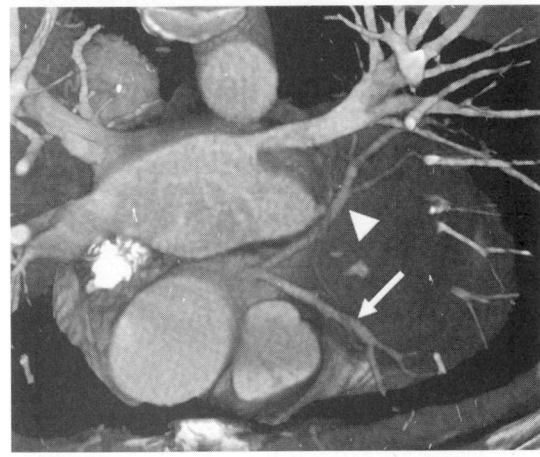

FIG. 53–2. Three-dimensional volume-rendering technique of a contrast-enhanced multidetector-row computed tomography coronary angiography data set. The spatial resolution achievable with this technique is sufficient for a reliable depiction of the proximal and middle segments of the coronary arteries including side branches, as seen on the right-anterior oblique view **(A),** depicting the right coronary artery *(arrow),* or on the view from the top **(B),** delineating the course of the left anterior descending *(arrow)* and circumflex *(arrowhead)* coronary artery. No significant stenoses could be found in this patient with atypical chest pain. (From Becker CR. Assessment of coronary arteries with CT. *Radiol Clin North Am* 2002;40:773–782,vi, with permission.) (See color insert for Fig. 53–3.)

nary artery stenoses was 74% to 92% and 77% to 94%, respectively (Table 53–1). Next-generation ECBT scanners will combine a greater temporal resolution of up to 50 ms with reduced slice thicknesses (i.e., greater spatial resolution), but, currently, no reports on the potential clinical advantages of these new scanners are available.

Noninvasive Imaging of Coronary Bypass Grafts

Background

Coronary artery bypass graft surgery is a frequently performed revascularization procedure in patients with multivessel CAD. The clinical outcome after bypass surgery depends on the status of the grafts after surgery. Initially, most patients are free of angina, but patients may experience chest pain as a result of acute occlusion early after surgery or gradual progression of atherothrombosis in the long term. Coronary angiography is the gold standard to evaluate the status of graft patency, but this is an invasive procedure that includes x-ray exposure, brief hospitalization after procedure to monitor any vascular complications, and a small risk for potentially serious complications. These disadvantages make the use of coronary angiography less attractive as a diagnostic screening tool for patients with bypass grafts who present with postoperative angina. The need for alternative noninvasive diagnostic methods is apparent (57).

Magnetic Resonance Imaging of Bypass Grafts

MRI is a noninvasive alternative method that allows direct visualization of coronary bypass grafts. Previously, 2D spin echo and gradient echo MR techniques and 3D breath hold CE-MRA techniques have enabled the evaluation of graft patency, but these techniques as a whole could only differentiate between graft patency and occlusion (Table 53–2). The visualization of different graft segments and the detection of graft stenosis remains difficult (58). Future ap-

proaches, such as navigator-gated fast MR techniques resulting in high-resolution angiography in combination with breath hold MR flow mapping with high temporal resolution, might allow a comprehensive evaluation of bypass graft stenosis and function (59). The assessment of bypass graft morphology and function allows a complete evaluation of the graft status. Navigator-gated 3D MRA may be the best approach to achieve high-resolution volume images of grafts, because image time is not limited by the duration of a breath hold. For an optimal assessment of graft function during pharmacologic stress, an MR sequence with short acquisition duration may be preferable. This would allow subsequent flow reserve measurements in different grafts and in different graft segments with minimal patient discomfort (60).

Computed Tomography Imaging of Bypass Grafts

Two alternative CT techniques—MDCT and EBCT—are considered useful in the noninvasive evaluation of coronary artery bypass grafts. With the faster speed of 16DCT systems, CTA of bypasses can now be performed with thin collimations. Depicting a range from the aortic arch to the base of the heart with a 0.75-mm collimation currently takes 25 to 30 seconds. Using ECG triggering, a high-quality angiography, even of small-caliber arterial bypasses, with motion-free depiction of the insertion of the bypass vessel to the grafted coronary artery is now feasible (Fig. 53–3) (see color insert). Thus far only a few clinical studies on the assessment of bypass grafts using MDCT have been published. A study reporting a sensitivity and specificity of 97% and 98%, respectively, for the evaluation of graft patency was published (61). More extensive experience has been gathered using EBCT for this indication (62–64). CT allows the functional analysis of the bypass graft in addition to flow measurements in the grafted vessels (65). Table 53–2 gives a comprehensive overview of the recent clinical CT studies on the assessment of coronary bypass grafts using different CT techniques.

TABLE 53–2. *Sensitivity and specificity of magnetic resonance angiography and computed tomography angiography for the detection of coronary bypass occlusion: results of a selection of clinical trials as compared with conventional angiography*

Author (reference)	Technique	Patients, n	Sensitivity, %	Specificity, %
Vetter et al. 2001 (194)	MRA	30	96	67
Engelmann et al. 2000 (195)	MRA	40	76–100	NA
Molinari et al. 2000 (196)	MRA	51	91	97
Brenner et al. 1999 (197)	MRA	85	90	94
Wintersperger et al. 1998 (198)	MRA	27	96	67
Enzweiler et al. 2003 (63)	EBCTA	37	92	96
Tello et al. 2002 (65)	SCTA	26	96	100
Ropers et al. 2001 (61)	MDCTA	65	97	98
Achenbach et al. 1997 (62)	EBCTA	25	100	97
Knez et al. 1996 (64)	EBCTA	30	95	89

EBCTA, electron beam computed tomography angiography; MDCTA, multidetector-row computed tomography angiography; SCTA, spiral (single-slice) computed tomography angiography.

TABLE 53–3. *Sensitivity and specificity of magnetic resonance angiography and computed tomography angiography for the detection of thromboembolic events in the pulmonary vasculature: results of a selection of clinical trials as compared with conventional angiography*

Author (reference)	Technique	Patients, n	Sensitivity, %	Specificity, %
Oudkerk et al. 2002 (199)	MRA	118	77	98
Goyen et al. 2001 (200)	MRA	8	100	75
Kruger et al. 2001 (201)	MRA	50	100	n./a.
Kreitner et al. 2000 (202)	MRA	20	87	100
Gupta et al. 1999 (203)	MRA	36	85	96
Perrier et al. 2001 (204)	CTA	299	70	91
Blachere et al. 2000 (205)	CTA	179	94	95
Qanadli et al. 2000 (206)	CTA	158	90	94
Remy-Jardin et al. 2000 (207)	CTA	370	96	100
Kim et al. 1999 (208)	CTA	110	92	96

CTA, computed tomography angiography, MRA, magnetic resonance angiography.

PULMONARY ARTERIES

Background

The diagnosis of pulmonary embolism (PE) remains difficult in clinical practice because clinical findings are nonspecific and all available objective tests have practical or clinical limitations (66). Pulmonary x-ray angiography remains the gold standard diagnostic test, but it is invasive, sometimes difficult to interpret because it can give false-negative results, and is not readily available in many centers (67). Various combinations of noninvasive aids to diagnosis, including assessment of clinical probability of PE, plasma D-dimer concentrations, ventilation-perfusion lung scanning, and venous compression ultrasonography of the legs, have

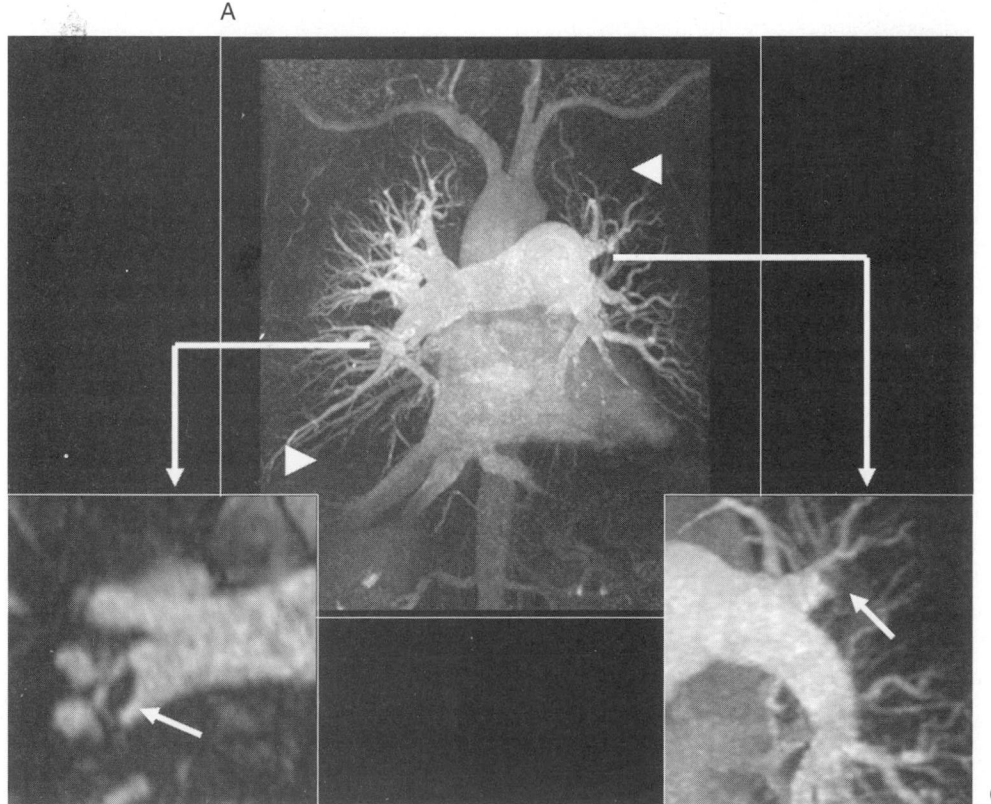

FIG. 53–4. Three-dimensional, contrast-enhanced, high-resolution magnetic resonance angiography of the pulmonary vasculature in a 47-year-old patient with secondary pulmonary hypertension caused by recurrent pulmonary embolism. The maximum intensity projection **(A)** shows reduction of peripheral pulmonary vessels in the region of the upper left and lower right lobe **(A,** *arrowheads*). Enlarged coronal views of the single angiographic images reveal thromboembolic clots in the lower right **(B)** and upper left **(C)** pulmonary artery. (From Nikolaou K, Schoenberg SO, Nittka M, et al. Magnetic resonance imaging in the diagnosis of pulmonary arterial hypertension: high resolution angiography and fast perfusion imaging using Intelligent Parallel Acquisition Techniques (IPAT). *Radiology* 2002;225:473, with permission.)

been developed and validated to reduce the need for pulmonary angiography. Nevertheless, this procedure is still necessary in a significant percentage of patients for whom there is high clinical suspicion of PE even after a combination of all the available noninvasive diagnostic tests have been used (67). In addition to being an invasive test, conventional x-ray angiography carries a risk for major complications of 1% and a mortality risk of 0.5% (68). In the last decade, SCT and MRA have become a viable alternative to conventional angiography in the diagnosis of acute and chronic PE (69).

Magnetic Resonance Angiography of the Pulmonary Arteries

CE-MRI uses even safer contrast agents (i.e., gadolinium chelates) than CT and does not involve radiation exposure. In addition, MRI allows for the depiction of functional aspects like perfusion and ventilation, which may further aid in the (differential) diagnosis of PE and thus appropriate patient care and treatment (70,71). This diagnostic technique is improving constantly, and by contrast-enhanced breath hold techniques, pulmonary vessel can be visualized effectively in most cases (72). A number of clinical studies have reported high sensitivities and specificities for the detection of pulmonary emboli as compared with conventional pulmonary angiography (Table 53–3) (Fig. 53–4). However, MRA is still time consuming, and patients with acute PE might not be stable enough to undergo this procedure. Although faster scanning techniques have permitted MRA to be performed in shorter times than before, MRA does not yield optimal image quality in individuals who are unable to hold their breath. Motion-compensated, or real-time, techniques with radial k-space scanning may offer potential in these patients and has been tested with satisfying diagnostic accuracy (69). In conclusion, MRI is a promising diagnostic tool, but to date it has not had a widespread clinical utility in emergency medicine and in critically ill patients, mainly because of its long examination time, difficulties in patient monitoring, higher costs, and limited availability of MR in most community-based medical centers. It has a role in the assessment of the stable patient with chronic lung disease in the diagnostic workup of pulmonary hypertension and in ruling out right to left cardiac shunt.

Computed Tomography Angiography of the Pulmonary Arteries

Conventional x-ray angiography in many institutions has been replaced by SCT, which is more readily available and yields lower procedure-associated risks. Sensitivity of SCT is about 90% for central, lobar, or segmental pulmonary emboli (Table 53–3). CTA has been proven to be an accurate, safe, noninvasive, easily and rapidly performed, widely accepted, and cost-effective technique for direct detection and demonstration of intraluminal PE (73). Depending on the

patient's clinical status and the CT technology available, a 4- to 40-second breath hold is required to scan the entire pulmonary vasculature. The ability to accurately rule out the presence of PE is an undisputed advantage of CT. Examination of the leg veins may be indicated in negative CT. The widespread use of MDCT is expected to increase acquisition speed, image quality, and overall accuracy of the test (Fig. 53–5). Follow-up studies of patients without anticoagulation are mandatory. SCT pulmonary angiography should be considered the initial imaging modality of choice, particularly in subgroups of patients who are known to be associated with a high rate of nondiagnostic ventilation-perfusion scans, such as hospitalized patients, patients with a history of cardiopulmonary disease, or patients with abnormal chest radiograph results.

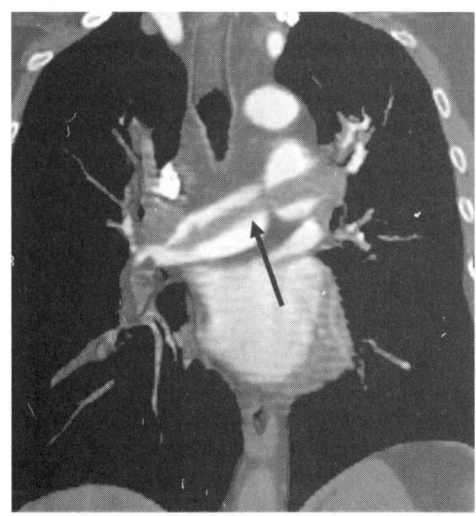

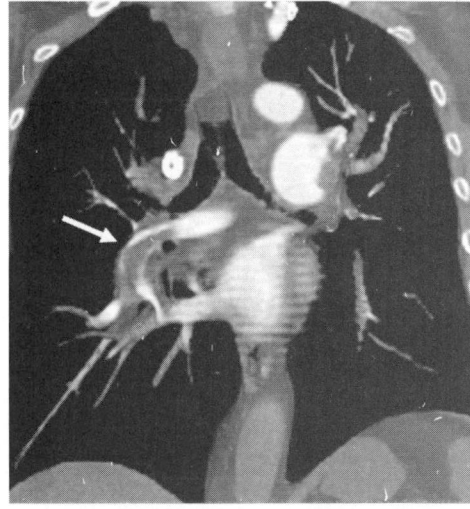

FIG. 53–5. Contrast-enhanced multidetector-row computed tomography pulmonary angiography depicting a large thromboembolic clot in the central pulmonary artery (**A,** *arrow*), extending into the lower right lobe pulmonary artery (**B,** *arrow*). (From Schoepf UJ, Kessler MA, Rieger CT, et al. Multislice CT imaging of pulmonary embolism. *Eur Radiol* 2001;11: 2278–2286, with permission.)

AORTA

Aortic Dissection

Acute aortic dissection is a challenging clinical emergency that may have catastrophic consequences if not diagnosed and treated promptly. There are 10 to 20 cases per million per year and, left untreated, 36% to 72% of patients die within 48 hours and 62% to 91% die within 1 week of diagnosis (74). However, technical advances in noninvasive imaging have heralded significant improvements in early diagnosis and treatment planning. Gadolinium-enhanced MRA has been established as a safe and reliable technique for evaluation of stenoses in the thoracic and abdominal aorta and major aortic branch arteries (75). However, aortic dissection is potentially life threatening and has routinely been evaluated with x-ray angiography and more recently with SCT. Both modalities have typically been chosen because of their availability and rapid examination times. Previously, emergency MR evaluation for aortic injury or disease was impractical and unsafe because of prolonged examination times (76). The choice of imaging technique still remains controversial. Each imaging modality has certain advantages and disadvantages with respect to accuracy, speed, convenience, risk, and cost, but no single modality is superior to all others in all situations. Single-slice or even multi-slice SCT is currently available in most hospitals, usually on an emergency basis. It is both sensitive and specific in the diagnosis of aortic dissection, and its accuracy has been improved by the recent availability of ultrafast scanning and 3D reconstruction (77) (Fig. 53–6) (see also color insert). However, it is unable to provide hemodynamic information and relies on the use of nephrotoxic contrast agents. In contrast, MRI offers improved anatomic delineation of the aorta and can provide high-quality images in several planes (Fig. 53–7). It does not require the use of nephrotoxic contrast agents, but it is relatively expensive and is not as readily available as conventional CT. Furthermore, MRI is contraindicated in patients with pacemakers and certain metallic prosthetic heart valves, and it may be inappropriate in hemodynamically unstable patients, who may be intubated and receiving intravenous medication with continuous arterial pressure monitoring. Total examination time for a complete diagnostic MR evaluation of the aorta has been reported to be between 10 and 45 minutes and is therefore suitable only for medically stable patients. With the combination of steady-state gradient echo techniques and advanced gradient hardware, the stage has been set for the introduction of a family of high-speed pulse sequences with favorable vascular imaging properties. Imaging of the aorta can be achieved in significant shorter time with adequate diagnostic quality, and the imaging time can be reduced to 10 minutes or less (78). In cases where endoluminal repair or fenestration is considered, x-ray angiography is still a preferred imaging modality that allows assessment of the access arteries (usually the iliacs), measurement of the aorta to permit selection of the correct device length and diameter, confirmation of

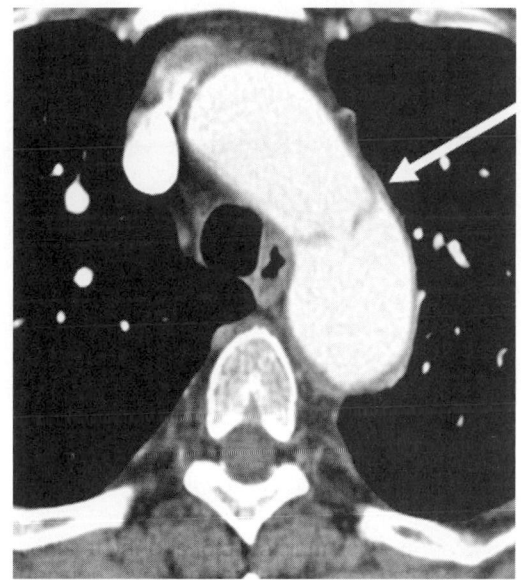

A

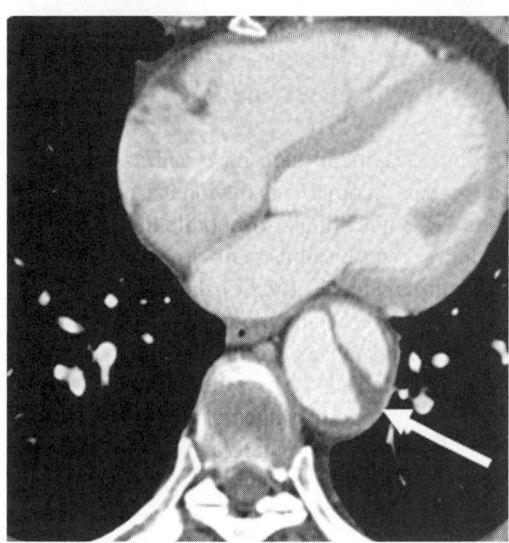

B

FIG. 53–6. Contrast-enhanced multidetector-row computed tomography of the thoracic aorta. Single-slice images (**A** and **B**) show a dissection of the aorta, originating from the aortic arch (**A,** *arrow*) and extending distally into the descending thoracic aorta (**B,** *arrow*). A color-coded volume-rendering technique **(C)** gives a three-dimensional overview of the thoracic anatomy. (From Huber A, Matzko M, Wintersperger BJ, et al. [Reconstruction methods in postprocessing of CT- and MR-angiography of the aorta]. *Radiologe* 2001;41:689–694, with permission.) (See color insert for Fig. 53–6C.)

branch vessel involvement, and assessment of bilateral luminal manometry before fenestration (79).

Aortic Aneurysm

Thoracic Aortic Aneurysm

Although thoracic aortic aneurysms expand at a slower rate than abdominal aortic aneurysms (AAAs), surgical repair is contemplated when thoracic aneurysms reach a diameter of

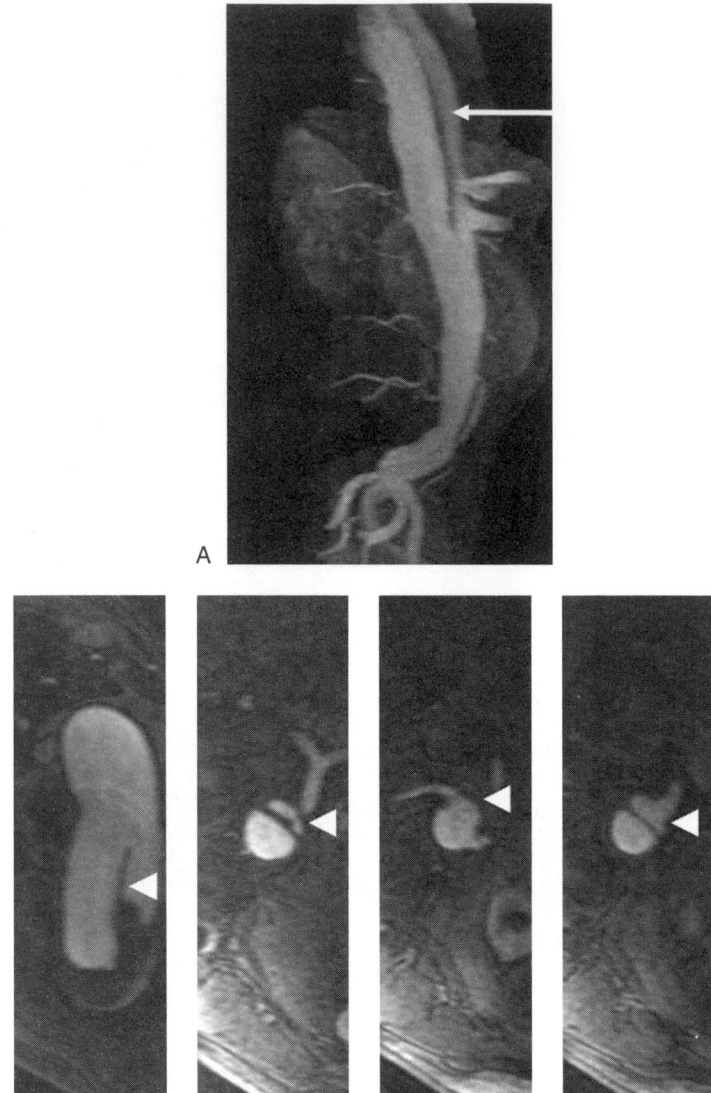

A

B

FIG. 53–7. Contrast-enhanced magnetic resonance angiography of the thoracica and abdominal aorta in a 57-year-old patient. The maximum intensity projection **(A)** shows a dissecting membrane in the abdominal aorta *(arrow).* The axial images **(B)** demonstrate the extent of the dissection *(arrowheads)* and allow a clear allocation of the true and the false vessel lumen to the origins of the abdominal vessels. (From Huber A, Matzko M, Wintersperger BJ, et al. [Reconstruction methods in postprocessing of CT- and MR-angiography of the aorta]. *Radiologe* 2001;41:689–694, with permission.)

5 to 6 cm, depending on their shape and their cause (80). Aneurysms of the thoracic aorta may be classified according to their localization (sinus of Valsalva, ascending aorta, aortic arch, descending aorta), their etiology (congenital, atherothrombotic, luetic, mycotic, traumatic, inflammatory), or their shape (saccular, fusiform, dissecting). For the thoracic aorta, a diameter exceeding 4 cm is generally considered aneurysmal. When a fusiform aneurysm exceeds 6 cm in diameter, the risk for rupture is increased, and surgical repair is recommended for patients who can tolerate major surgery. For those who cannot tolerate surgery, endoluminal stenting may be considered. Saccular aneurysms, mycotic aneurysms, and aneurysms that are rapidly increasing in size at a rate exceeding 1 cm per year also are thought to have an increased risk for rupture (81).

Magnetic Resonance Angiography of Thoracic Aneurysms

3D CE-MRA provides a comprehensive overview of the thoracic vascular anatomy, particularly the relation of aortic aneurysms to branch vessel origins (76). Both true and false aneurysms are equally well depicted. A study correlating 3D CE-MRA with conventional angiography and surgical exploration demonstrated a diagnostic accuracy of 100% for assessing size and extent of the aneurysm and its relation to aortic branches (82). By evaluating the entire aorta, 3D MRA clearly delineates the number of aneurysms present. Arterial phase MRA, however, contains little information about the morphology of the aortic wall. It displays the lumen but may fail to show the full extent of an aneurysm such as the area that is partially thrombosed. 3D MRA should therefore be complemented by postcontrast acquisitions.

The remaining contrast within the blood permits easy differentiation between flowing blood and thrombus. The aortic wall also can be assessed. Enhancement of the aortic wall and surrounding soft tissues is indicative of an inflammatory process as found in mycotic aneurysms or aortitis (83). Involvement of the aortic valve should always be considered in the presence of an aneurysm affecting the ascending aorta. Here, the acquisition of cine True-FISP (Fast Imaging with Steady-State Precession) sequences in a plane along the axis of the aortic outflow tract can determine if aortic stenosis, regurgitation, or both are present.

Computed Tomography Angiography of Thoracic Aneurysms

CTA also is a useful tool for diagnosing thoracic aortic aneurysms, determining their extent, and predicting appropriate management. Although the diagnosis of aortic aneurysms is readily made from transverse sections, an assessment of the extent of the lesion, particularly when the brachiocephalic branches are involved, is facilitated by an assessment of reconstruction techniques like maximum-intensity projections, multiplanar reconstructions, or volume-rendering techniques. SCT can facilitate surgical planning by delineating the extent of the aneurysm and the involvement of aortic branches (84). Because of the tortuosity and curvature of the thoracic aorta, aneurysm sizing is performed most accurately when double-oblique images are generated perpendicular to the aortic flow lumen. The major challenge of this approach is that data concerning the risk for aneurysm rupture and expansion rate are based on measurements made from transverse sections, where true diameters can be overestimated. MDCT provides the same information regarding aneurysm size and extent of mural thrombus available with conventional, single-slice SCT; however, the volumetric acquisition of thinner slices allows multiplanar and 3D renderings to be generated perpendicular to the long axis of the aneurysm, resulting in greater accuracy of the aneurysm size measurements (85).

Abdominal Aortic Aneurysm

AAAs are characteristically fusiform in configuration, although occasionally a saccular aneurysm may be seen (86). Evaluation of patients with AAA should include a systematic description of the following morphologic details: (a) the relation of the aneurysm to the main and accessory renal, iliac, superior, and inferior mesenteric arteries; (b) the extension of the aneurysm into the common, external, or internal iliac arteries to determine the type and length of prosthetic graft used; and (c) the evaluation of coexistent iliac or renal occlusive disease (87). Conventional x-ray aortography traditionally has been the imaging modality of choice before resection of AAAs. However, advantages of cross-sectional imaging provided by MR or CT compared with x-ray angiography are well established. CTA has been the preferred modality for cross-sectional imaging of the abdominal aorta. 3D CE-MRA, however, has overcome limitations inherent to conventional MR techniques including long imaging times and reduced vessel-to-background contrast in regions of slow flow.

Magnetic Resonance Angiography of Abdominal Aortic Aneurysms

Previously, the use of MRI in the assessment of patients with AAA has been limited (88). Noncontrast-enhanced bright blood and black blood, gradient echo and spin echo MRA techniques depend on flow effects to create contrast between vessels and background tissue. The complex and frequently slow flow patterns typically seen within AAA result in signal loss and may lead to difficulties in distinguishing between slow flow and thrombus. To prevent saturation effects, images must be acquired in a plane perpendicular to the vessels, resulting in long imaging times with consequent image degradation caused by respiratory artifacts and patient motion. CE-MRA techniques are essentially flow independent (89). Imaging can be performed in any plane allowing rapid acquisitions covering a large field of view during a single breath hold. Analysis of an aneurysmal aorta should always be based on the arterial phase 3D CE-MRA displaying the aortic lumen in combination with delayed, postcontrast scans depicting the thrombosed portion of the lumen (90). These delayed scans also evaluate enhancement of the aortic wall and surrounding tissues in inflammatory or mycotic aneurysms. With CE-MRA, all details of the aneurysmal morphology are well depicted. The large coronal field of view reveals extension of the aneurysm into the iliac arteries. Multiplanar reformations help to unfold even highly tortuous vascular morphology. On the basis of subvolume maximal intensity projection (MIPs) and multiplanar reformations, exact dimension of the aneurysm can be determined before any surgical or percutaneous intervention. MRA also is effective in demonstrating the status of renal arterial origins and their relation to the aortic aneurysm. High diagnostic accuracy of 3D CE-MRA regarding morphologic analysis of AAAs has been confirmed by several clinical studies (91–93).

Computed Tomography Angiography of Abdominal Aortic Aneurysms

CT has been advocated in the preoperative evaluation of AAA (94). It is noninvasive, more accurate than conventional angiography for predicting AAA size, and superior to angiography in its ability to demonstrate mural thrombus within an aneurysm, inflammatory aneurysms, perianeurysmal blood caused by contained rupture, and coexistent nonvascular abdominal disease (95). Single-slice SCT has been shown to enable an accurate depiction of the aneurysm neck relative to aortic branch vessels and an evaluation of the aortic branch vessels themselves (96). Juxtarenal and suprarenal extension of AAA can be missed on x-ray angiography because of the presence of mural thrombus and atheroma at the proximal neck. The ability of CTA to identify renal artery stenoses in the presence of AAAs has been reported with a 94% sensitivity and 96% specificity for significant stenoses greater than 50% (96). The introduction of MDCT with adapted contrast injection protocols has further increased image quality and diagnostic accuracy (97). MDCT provides the same information regarding aneurysm size and extent of mural thrombus available with single-slice helical CT; however, the volumetric acquisition of thinner slices allows multiplanar and 3D renderings to be generated perpendicular to the long axis of the aneurysm, resulting in greater accuracy of the aneurysm size measurements (85).

Mesenteric Arteries

Magnetic Resonance Angiography of the Abdominal Vasculature

The resolution of 3D contrast MRA is sufficient to accurately evaluate the origins of splanchnic arteries, including the celiac axis and superior mesenteric artery (SMA) (92). With fast scanners capable of high-resolution imaging during a breath hold, the inferior mesenteric artery (IMA) may also be evaluated. In patients with complicated anatomy or when the celiac axis and SMA do not arise directly anteriorly from the aorta, the 3D nature of MRA (or CTA) makes it easier to evaluate mesenteric artery origins compared with conventional angiography. Combining 3D CE-MRA with flow-measuring techniques allows comprehensive assessment of mesenteric arterial anatomy and function. MRA is already capable of displaying the main visceral vessels with excellent diagnostic accuracy (98). Still, the spatial resolution achievable with selective catheter angiography remains considerably better for smaller branch vessels. Accordingly, current clinical applications of 3D CE MRA in the splanchnic circulation focus on clinical situations that require assessment of the proximal celiac axis and SMA, including mesenteric ischemia, visceral artery aneurysms, tumor encasement, anatomic variations, and preliver/postliver transplantation. Diseases primarily involving the smaller splanchnic branch vessels, including polyarteritis nodosa, lupus, thromboangiitis obliterans, and other forms of vasculitis, as well as GI bleeding, are better evaluated by conventional x-ray angiography (99).

Computed Tomography Angiography of the Abdominal Vasculature

SCT and MDCT offer distinct advantages in the imaging of the mesenteric vasculature, including the SMA, superior mesenteric vein, IMA, and inferior mesenteric vein and their major branches. The faster scanning and narrower collimation allow data acquisition during optimal opacification of the mesenteric vessels and their branches on both axial and 3D reformatted images (100). These technologic advances,

coupled with rapid intravenous injection of contrast material, improve the quality of the data set available for 3D image reconstruction and manipulation. 3D angiographic parameters can be optimized to routinely display, in considerable detail, the mesenteric vasculature.

Currently, x-ray angiography can be almost completely avoided as a diagnostic tool for most abdominal indications. MDCT typically allows better visualization of arterial and venous branching as compared with MRA, thereby improving detection of involvement of the more distal portions of the mesenteric vessels (101). Visualization of the vasculature is greatly improved with 3D volume rendering, which can display a given vessel in the optimal plane; evaluation of the arteries and veins may be limited if only axial images are obtained. Still, in certain situations in which very small vessels need to be visualized, x-ray angiography does remain the diagnostic modality of choice, which is mainly the case for acute gastrointestinal bleeding, polyarteritis, or the search for the origin of the great radicular artery of the spine.

Vascular tumor involvement can be defined as either occlusion or narrowing of a vessel, usually with an associated soft-tissue mass surrounding the area of involvement (102). Collateral vessels may be present and are a useful secondary sign of vascular involvement. CTA is based on a contrast-enhanced SCT scan covering the whole abdomen. No tissue suppression is used. Thus, a CTA scan itself displays all surrounding structures and makes diagnostic evaluation of soft tissues possible without the requirement for additional data acquisition (no further examination time is needed, as would be the case for MRA). In contrast to MRA, CTA is able to distinguish directly between calcified and noncalcified plaques. Thus, it provides valuable information for the planning of angioplasty procedures (103). Although x-ray angiography has historically been the procedure of choice for the diagnosis of mesenteric ischemia, MDCT can now play a significant role. Thrombosis of the main vessels can easily be seen at axial imaging, often with associated collateral vessels, depending on its chronicity. For evaluation of more distal branches of the mesenteric vessels and of narrowing or plaque at the origin of the arteries, 3D imaging offers a distinct advantage. 3D images lead to improved complex vascular maps, which are useful in cancer staging, surgical planning, and evaluating patients with suspected mesenteric ischemia (101).

CAROTID ARTERIES

Background

Atherothrombosis of the carotid arteries results in significant morbidity and mortality. The North American Symptomatic Carotid Endarterectomy Trial (NASCET) multicenter trials have shown the benefit of carotid endarterectomy for patients with significant (104) and nonsignificant carotid artery stenoses (105). Other studies also have provided convincing

TABLE 53–4. *Sensitivity and specificity of magnetic resonance angiography and computed tomography angiography for the detection of significant carotid artery stenoses (>75%): results of a selection of clinical trials as compared with conventional angiography*

Reference	Technique	Carotids, n	Sensitivity, %	Specificity, %
Johnson et al. 2000 (209)	MRA	76	94	95
Serfaty et al. 2000 (210)	MRA	63	94	85
Sardanelli et al. 1999 (211)	MRA	56	100	100
Scarabino et al. 1998 (110)	MRA	46	100	100
Leclerc et al. 1998 (212)	MRA	54	100	98
Anderson et al. 2000 (213)	CTA	80	77	92
Leclerc et al. 1999 (214)	CTA	44	100	97
Marcus et al. 1999 (215)	CTA	46	93	97
Verhoek et al. 1999 (216)	CTA	38	100	100
Magarelli et al. 1998 (217)	CTA	40	92	98

CTA, computed tomography angiography; MRA, magnetic resonance angiography.

evidence that a decision regarding therapy should be made on the basis of the degree of stenosis (106). Accurate measurement of stenosis severity is a clinically important parameter in determining the need for surgery in these patients. X-ray angiography has been the gold standard for diagnosis of carotid bulb disease. However, this modality provides projection images of the carotid bulb, which leads to variation in the measurement of the percent stenosis depending on the observer or the projection. Also, the associated direct and indirect costs and increased procedural risk has prompted the development of other less invasive imaging techniques. Noninvasive imaging tools of extracranial carotid disease include Doppler ultrasound, MRA, and CTA. In many centers, these modalities have become standard in the preoperative evaluation of carotid artery stenosis. MRA and CTA allow the rapid acquisition of data that can be reconstructed into 2D and 3D images. High-resolution axial images can provide a cross-sectional view of the carotid vessel and atherothrombotic plaques. MIP allows data to be reconstructed into images that closely resemble conventional x-ray angiograms and can be rotated 360 degrees to be viewed from any angle. With both modalities, by using both axial and MIP images, extensive information regarding the carotid bifurcation and plaque characteristics can be obtained.

Magnetic Resonance Angiography of the Carotid Arteries

MRA of the carotid arteries was initially implemented using 2D and 3D TOF techniques, and good results for the detection of extracerebral arterial disease were reported (107–109). However, TOF imaging involves long acquisition times and can result in overestimation of stenosis (110,111). More recently, CE-MRA has become the state-of-the-art technique for imaging the carotid circulation. Several studies have shown CE-MRA to have high sensitivities and specificities in revealing carotid artery stenosis (Table 53–4). Previous MR techniques have not clearly visualized the entire carotid circulation, including the circle of Willis and aortic branch vessels, on a single study, which is now feasible (Fig. 53–8). In addition, breath holding has been

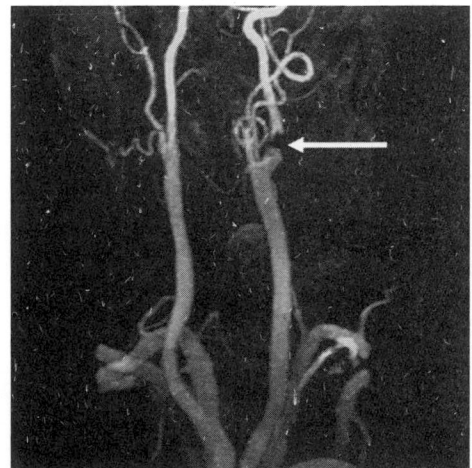

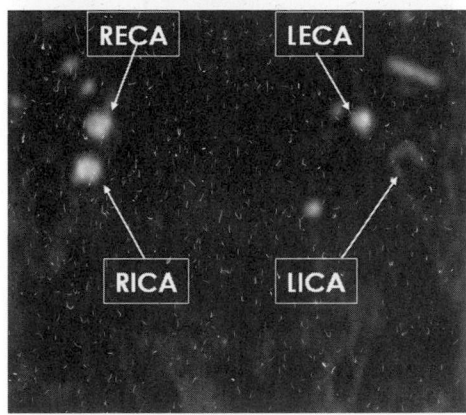

FIG. 53–8. Three-dimensional, contrast-enhanced magnetic resonance angiography of the supraaortic vessels. A complex stenosis of the proximal left internal carotid artery is revealed by the maximum intensity projection image (**A,** *arrow*), with no obvious patent lumen, but contrast enhancement of the vessel distal to the stenosis. Using the three-dimensional nature of the image data acquired with MRI, cross-sectional reconstructions at this location can be performed (**B**), demonstrating a high-grade stenosis with a small rim of contrast flow around the complex plaque. RECA/LECA, Right/left external carotid artery; RICA/LICA, right/left internal carotid artery. (Courtesy of J. Scheidler, Ludwig-Maximilians-University, Munich, Germany.)

used variably in MRA of the carotid arteries and arch vessels, the implication being that these vessels are unaffected by respiratory motion (112).

It has been reported that differentiation of high-grade stenoses and total vessel occlusions can be difficult on MR angiograms of the carotid arteries, because the flow characteristics of high-grade stenoses might lead to a signal void in the area of stenoses and might mimic total vessel occlusion (113). Also, early venous enhancement in the carotid circulation can interfere with visualization of the arterial system unless the contrast bolus is accurately timed to the arterial phase, because the timing window for a true arterial phase is only 6 to 8 seconds in duration (114). Introduction of new MR acquisition strategies that can significantly shorten the total acquisition time of a high-resolution angiography has been done to overcome this problem, namely parallel imaging techniques (10). Another approach is the use of time-resolved techniques. This way, multiple short acquisition of the carotid vasculature is performed, providing true arterial phased images and the additional information of flow dynamics (115,116), but at the cost of a decrease in spatial resolution. Other new acquisition techniques alter the way of selecting the information from k-space to enhance spatial resolution and suppress venous overlap at the same time. Elliptical centric acquisition, a recently developed technique,

acquires the high-contrast elements within k-space before venous enhancement, which results in a relative suppression of venous signal intensity (114). Using modern imaging approaches described earlier in this chapter, isotropic submillimeter voxel sizes can be achieved, covering the complete carotid vasculature in a short acquisition time for true arterial contrast.

Computed Tomography Angiography of the Carotid Arteries

In addition to MRA, CTA has been introduced as a noninvasive imaging procedure for detection of significant carotid artery stenoses. Intravenous application of iodine contrast is required, and imaging is not dependent on flow characteristics. Thus, severely stenotic but patent vessels can be accurately visualized. Axial images can be magnified to examine plaque morphology and to avoid artifacts created by dense calcifications. Using single-slice helical CT systems, CTA has been previously reported to have a diagnostic accuracy approaching 90% (117). Nevertheless, single-slice scanners had limitations in temporal and spatial resolution. The advantages of 4-channel MDCT were significant (118) (Fig. 53–9) (see also color insert). Studies on the newest generation of 16-slice multidetector-row systems have reported

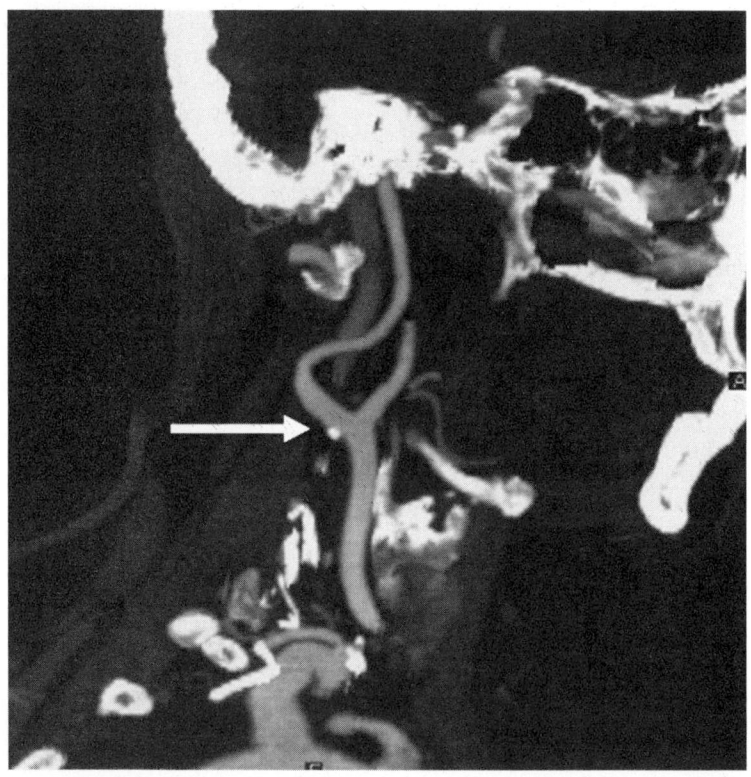

FIG. 53–9. Contrast-enhanced multidetector-row computed tomography of the supraaortal vessels. Maximum intensity projection **(A)** and volume-rendering technique **(B)** of the right carotid artery both reveal a calcified lesion at the height of the bifurcation, but no significant stenosis *(arrows)*. (Courtesy of C. R. Becker, Ludwig-Maximilians-University, Munich, Germany.) (See color insert for Fig. 53–9B.)

further improvements. A scan range of 30 cm currently can be covered in an acquisition time of just 9 seconds, allowing for imaging the whole lengths of the carotid artery from the aortic arch to the circle of Willis in a true arterial phase. The voxel size can be reduced to 0.3 mm^3 (0.6 × 0.6 × 0.75 mm). Preliminary results have demonstrated the potential of this technique to replace conventional x-ray angiography of the carotid arteries (119). Using adapted contrast injection protocols, a comprehensive evaluation of the extracranial and intracranial arterial system and of the intracerebral veins is feasible in a single CT scan (120). Calcifications of the carotids, especially in the region of the carotid bulb, may be a limitation of CTA because of overestimation of calcifications inherent to the CT technique. Some authors suggest manual segmentation or multiplanar reformatting for the assessment of the true arterial lumen in the area of heavy calcifications (121). The improvements in spatial resolution using 16DCT systems will further improve delineation of calcified plaques. Table 53–4 gives an overview of recent clinical studies on the value of CTA for the detection of significant stenoses of the carotid arteries.

Conclusions

In conclusion, contrast-enhanced CTA and MRA are reliable and fast techniques to evaluate the degree of carotid artery stenosis. Both modalities have some substantial benefits, including their 3D nature and lack of invasiveness, compared with conventional x-ray angiography. CTA is an inexpensive and easily accessible technique. Limiting factors are the use of iodine contrast agents and ionizing radiation. By using CE-MRA and fast imaging techniques, the carotid arteries can be rapidly imaged from the aortic arch to the skull base without significant interference from flow artifacts. A close correlation between gadolinium-enhanced MRA, CTA, and x-ray angiography in the evaluation of the degree of carotid stenosis was reported in several studies (Table 53–4). Technologic developments are rapid for both MR and CT imaging modalities, which will lead to even further improvement of their performance.

PERIPHERAL VESSELS

Magnetic Resonance Angiography of the Peripheral Vessels

Successful surgical and endovascular arterial revascularization is dependent on accurate and detailed imaging of the location and degree of the occlusive arterial lesions. X-ray angiography has been considered as the imaging standard in evaluating peripheral arteries and planning treatment of lower limb ischaemia. However, x-ray angiography has been questioned as the gold standard because it may fail to reveal patent infrapopliteal vessels in patients with multisegmental occlusive lesions and low inflow pressure (122). Further-

more, a noninvasive alternative to x-ray angiography is attractive because of a small but significant (2–3%) risk for serious complications using the transfemoral technique (123).

Several studies concerning MRA before surgical and endovascular treatment have been reported using noncontrast-enhanced time-of-flight magnetic resonance angiography (TOF-MRA) (124,125). However, TOF-MRA faces several drawbacks. Imaging of the iliac arteries is complicated by their curved course relative to the acquisition plane, causing inplane saturation effects that can lead to false-positive diagnosis of stenoses and occlusions. Misreadings caused by pulsation artifacts have been reported. TOF-MRA requires an acquisition time of approximately 60 to 120 minutes for a full lower limb examination. Therefore, the TOF-MRA technique has never become a common alternative to x-ray angiography, except in a few highly experienced centers. The introduction of CE-MRA has overcome many of these limitations (126). In CE-MRA, the inflow pressure is not as essential as in TOF-MRA or conventional contrast arteriography. Because of short echo times, CE-MRA reduces the examination time and minimizes clip artifacts and artifacts caused by movements. The total examination time is now less than 30 minutes for a full lower limb examination. A standard 1.5 Tesla MR system is satisfactory, and special coils are not obligatory; however, a dedicated lower extremity coil is beneficial in imaging small distal vessels (127). CE-MRA can be performed as a multistation examination, using a single infusion of contrast, followed by series of MRA images at three stations using special moving table techniques (128,129) (Fig. 53–10). Alternatively, MRA can be performed as one to three series of separate contrast injections and image acquisitions, using image subtraction to eliminate the effect of the preceding contrast injection (130). Using only one station, selective images with a minimum of venous or tissue signal can be preformed—that is, visualizing distal runoff (127). Currently, no single method has emerged as the preferred option, each having different strengths and weaknesses (131). In various clinical studies CE-MRA was found to be superior to duplex ultrasound and highly accurate compared with conventional arteriography, with pooled values of sensitivity of 81% to 100% and specificities of 83% to 99% (Table 53–5).

In conclusion, when reviewing the literature, the agreement between x-ray angiography and CE-MRA in patients facing vascular reconstruction is good, and CE-MRA is proven to be a promising noninvasive alternative to x-ray angiography in presurgical evaluation. CE-MRA is currently the "state-of-the-art" MRA technique, overcoming the troublesome aortoiliac region, reducing the examination time, and increasing the accuracy compared with the TOF-MRA technique. In selected patients, both CE-MRA and TOF-MRA can demonstrate patent runoff vessels not seen on x-ray angiography, possibly increasing the limb salvage rate. It is expected in the foreseeable future that the clinical demand of CE-MRA will gradually increase. New MRI tech-

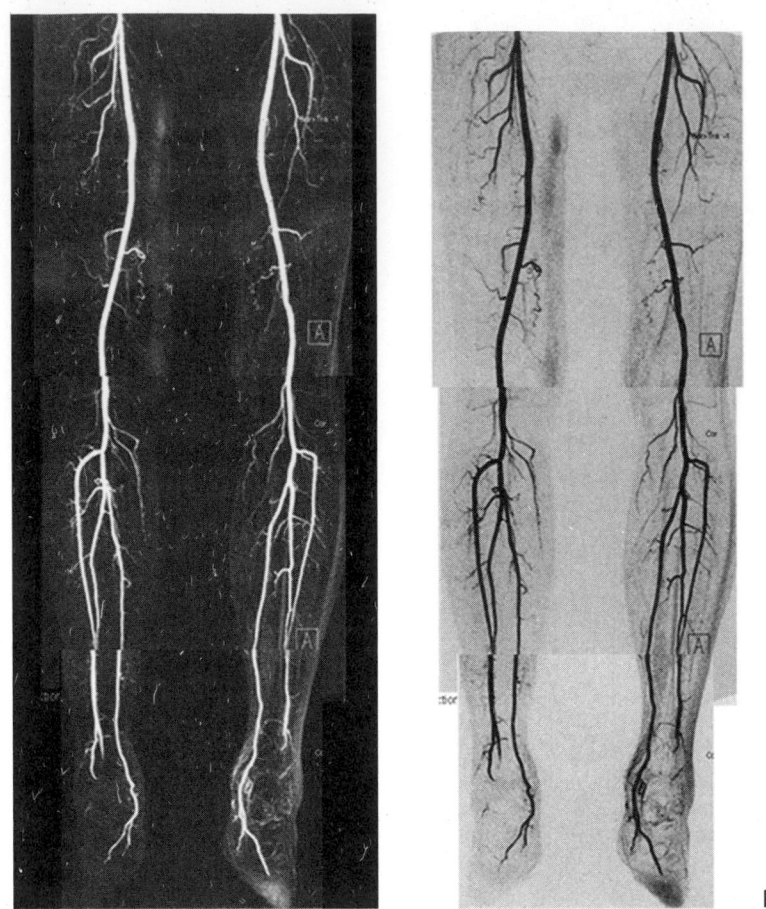

FIG. 53–10. Contrast-enhanced magnetic resonance angiography (MRA) of the peripheral runoff vessels using a three-step, moving-table technique, without detection of any significant stenosis. Maximum-intensity projection reconstructions of subtracted MRA data sets can be composed to a full angiogram of the peripheral vessels from the distal aorta to the ankle joint **(A).** Inverting the image, an angiographic image can be obtained similar to a conventional x-ray angiography **(B).** (From Huber A, Scheidler J, Wintersperger B, et al. Moving-table MR angiography of the peripheral runoff vessels: comparison of body coil and dedicated phased array coil systems. *AJR Am J Roentgenol* 2003;180:1365–1373, with permission.)

TABLE 53–5. *Sensitivity and specificity of magnetic resonance angiography and computed tomography angiography for the detection of significant stenoses of peripheral arteries (>75%): results of a selection of clinical trials as compared with conventional angiography*

Author (reference)	Technique	Patients, n	Sensitivity, %	Specificity, %
Ruehm et al. 2000 (218)	MRA	61	92	98
Huber et al. 2000 (219)	MRA	24	100	98
Meaney et al. 1999 (220)	MRA	20	81	91
Sueyoshi et al. 1999 (221)	MRA	23	97	99
Yamashita et al. 1998 (222)	MRA	20	96	83
Martin et al. 2003 (135)	MDCTA (4)	41	98	97
Ofer et al. 2003 (223)	MDCTA (4)	18	91	92
Rieker et al. 1997 (224)	SCTA	30	93	99
Raptopoulos et al. 1996 (225)	SCTA	39	93	96
Lawrence et al. 1995 (226)	SCTA	6	93	96

4, 4-detector-rows; MDCTA, multidetector computed tomography angiography; SCTA, spiral computed tomography angiography.

niques such as parallel imaging acquisitions are likely to further refine peripheral MRA techniques (132).

Computed Tomography Angiography of the Peripheral Vessels

Until the recent introduction of MDCT, CTA was limited to not more than 40 cm of craniocaudal coverage during a single intravenous contrast injection. Although this distance was sufficient for imaging the majority of systemic arteries, it was insufficient for studying the arterial inflow and runoff of the lower extremities. MDCT with four channels of simultaneous acquisition has eliminated this limitation (133). MDCTA is now able to assess lower extremity arterial inflow and runoff, offering shorter acquisition times, lower doses of contrast medium, and improved spatial resolution for assessing smaller arterial branches (21). The newest 16DCT systems are able to cover a range of up to 150 cm in less than 40 seconds with a 0.75-mm slice thickness, acquiring a total of about 1,500 axial images (134) (Fig. 53–11). A number of clinical studies on the implementation of SCT and MDCT for the assessment of peripheral arterial disease have been published, reporting sensitivities of 91% to 98% and speci-

ficities of 92% to 99% for significant stenoses greater than 75% (Table 53–5). Severe diffuse calcifications may lead to misinterpretations by CT, leading to both false-positive and false-negative results (85). The inability of conventional angiography to show calf vessels in patients with proximal occlusions is well documented, and it has been indicated that MDCTA may allow better visualization of calf vessels in these patients, because a systemic contrast bolus is used and because image quality is largely unaffected by patient motion (135). The high level of interobserver agreement in the currently published clinical trials indicates that the results as determined by MDCTA are highly reproducible. With the 16-detector scanners, lower extremity MDCTA can now be performed with thinner collimation. Imaging protocols on 4-detector scanners have to use high table speed to cover the full range of the peripheral runoff, which, in some cases, can lead to insufficient opacification of distal calf vessels. Slowing table speed by using a narrower slice thickness on the 16DCT systems reduces this problem of 4-detector scanners. An important consideration in the implementation of CT is that of radiation dose. In the first clinical study on peripheral MDCTA, calculated radiation dose of MDCTA was 3.9 times less than that with x-ray angiography (21). Clearly, radiation

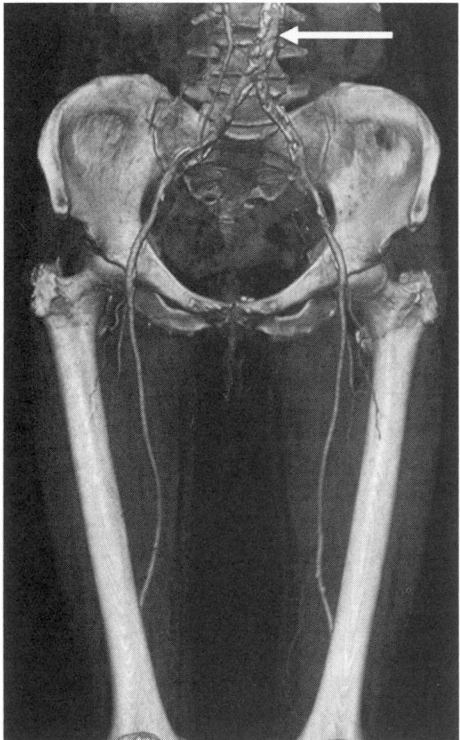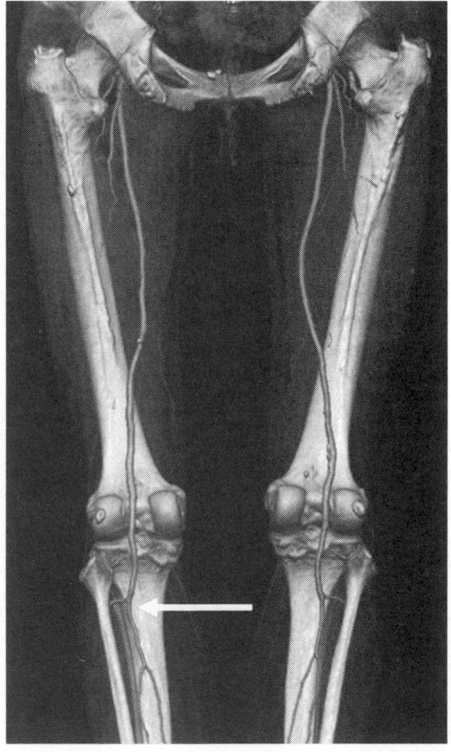

FIG. 53–11. 16-Detector-row computed tomography angiography of the peripheral vasculature in a 55-year-old male patient acquiring 1,500 images in an acquisition time shorter than 40 seconds with 0.75-mm slice thickness. Significant calcifications are demonstrated in the abdominal aorta *(arrow)*, but patent arteries are depicted on both sides along the course of the upper and lower legs **(A** and **B)**. Using volume-rendering techniques **(A** and **B)**, three-dimensional reconstruction is fast and easy, but bony structures are still visible, so various rotational views need to be obtained for full delineation of the peripheral vessels. (From Wintersperger BJ, Herzog P, Jakobs TF, et al. Initial experience with the clinical use of a 16 detector row CT system. *Crit Rev Comput Tomogr* 2002;43:283–316, with permission.)

doses will vary greatly depending on the technique used and the patient body habitus. As MDCTA continues to improve, techniques must be further refined to minimize radiation exposure without compromising image quality. Nevertheless, MDCTA, at its relatively early stage of development, has already offered a clear advantage to x-ray angiography with regard to radiation dose. MDCT may be more sensitive than x-ray angiography in identifying patent vessels distal to severe occlusions, but this difference in sensitivity will have to be evaluated by comparing these two techniques with a more sensitive reference standard such as MRA or intraoperative angiography. Validation of MDCTA requires further investigation regarding its effect on clinical decision making, patient outcomes, and cost-effectiveness. However, MDCTA of the lower extremities appears to be a promising new diagnostic test that will likely have an important role in the investigation of peripheral vascular disease.

PLAQUE IMAGING

Plaque Imaging of the Coronary Arteries

Background

Currently available imaging techniques for the diagnosis of CAD are subject to several limitations. Conventional coronary angiography, widely accepted as the gold standard for the detection of CAD, demonstrates the degree of luminal narrowing, but fails to visualize the coronary artery wall. It has been shown that plaque composition rather than the severity of an actual stenosis predicts the risk for plaque rupture and acute clinical complications of CAD (136–138). Thus, new imaging techniques that can image the arterial wall and characterize different lesion types may allow for identification and follow-up of patients at risk and for selecting appropriate therapeutic strategies (139).

Currently, a number of imaging modalities are used to study atherothrombosis and to assess luminal diameter, wall thickness, and plaque volume (140). Two noninvasive imaging modalities, CT and MRI, have been introduced to the study of atherothrombosis. Both have been shown to be capable of imaging vessel wall structures and differentiate various stages of atherothrombotic wall changes. The latest generation of MDCT scanners allow for quantitative measurement of atherothrombotic burden including calcified and noncalcified plaques (141) and characterization of the plaque components (142). MRI has been applied in various *in vivo* human studies to image atherothrombotic plaques in carotid (143,144) and aortic (145) atherothrombotic disease. Initial *in vivo* studies in human coronary arteries have used noninvasive, black blood, spin echo techniques with breath holding (146) or a real-time navigator for respiratory gating (147).

By possibly combining the advantages of both techniques, detecting significant coronary artery stenoses and describing the plaque composition at the same time, information could be provided that may predict cardiovascular risk, facilitate further study of atherothrombosis progression

and its response to therapy, and provide an important parameter for the assessment of subclinical disease.

Magnetic Resonance Plaque Imaging of the Coronary Arteries

High-resolution MR has emerged as the potential leading noninvasive *in vivo* imaging modality for atherothrombotic plaque characterization. MR differentiates plaque components on the basis of biophysical and biochemical parameters such as chemical composition and concentration, water content, physical state, molecular motion, and diffusion (148). With a combination of multicontrast MRI sequences, differentiation of fibrocellular, lipid-rich, and calcified regions of the atherothrombotic coronary plaque is feasible, as shown in an *ex vivo* study on human coronary arteries in correlation to histopathology (149). *In vivo* studies of coronary artery plaques are obviously more challenging. Preliminary studies in a pig model showed that the difficulties of coronary wall imaging are the result of a combination of cardiac and respiratory motion artifacts, nonlinear course, small size, and location (150). A human *in vivo* coronary MR plaque imaging study conducted by Fayad and coworkers (151) was performed during breath holding to minimize respiratory motion with a resolution of $0.46 \times 0.46 \times 2.0$ mm^3. Figure 53–12 shows *in vivo* MR coronary plaque images. To alleviate the need for the patient to hold his or her breath, Botnar and coworkers (152) combined the black blood FSE method and a real-time navigator for respiratory gating and real-time slice position correction. A near isotropic spatial resolution ($0.7 \times 0.7 \times 0.8$ mm^3) was achieved with the use of a 2D local inversion and black blood preparatory pulses (152). This method provided a quick way to image a long segment of the coronary artery wall and may be useful for rapid coronary plaque burden measurements. Future studies are needed to further address these advanced imaging techniques.

As shown in animal experimental studies (153,154), MR also is a powerful tool to serially and noninvasively investigate the progression and regression of atherothrombotic lesions *in vivo*. In asymptomatic, untreated patients with hypercholesterolemia with carotid and aortic atherothrombosis, Corti and coworkers (155) have shown that MR can be used to measure the efficacy of lipid-lowering therapy using a statin. Atherothrombotic plaques were assessed with MR at different times after lipid-lowering therapy. Significant regression of atherothrombotic lesions was observed. However, there are no longitudinal human *in vivo* studies on the alteration of coronary atherothrombotic plaques in response to lipid reduction therapy over time.

Computed Tomography Plaque Imaging of the Coronary Arteries

Primary requisites for the assessment of atherothrombotic calcified and noncalcified coronary plaques are similar to the requirements for a high-quality CTA of the coronaries—

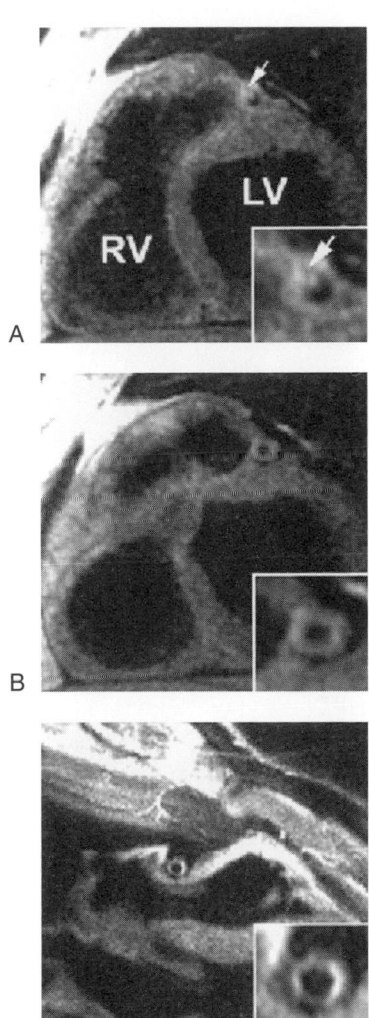

FIG. 53–12. *In vivo,* magnetic resonance, black blood, cross-sectional images of human coronary arteries demonstrating a plaque presumably with deposition of fat (**A,** *arrow*), a concentric fibrotic lesion (**B**) in the left anterior descending artery, and an ectatic, but atherothrombotic, right coronary artery (**C**). LV, left ventricle; RV, right ventricle. (From Fayad ZA, Fuster V, Nikolaou K, et al. Computed tomography and magnetic resonance imaging for noninvasive coronary angiography and plaque imaging: current and potential future concepts. *Circulation* 2002;106:2026–2034, with permission.)

that is, achieving both high spatial and high temporal resolution at the same time. Compared with low-pressure arterial systems such as the pulmonary arteries where calcifications are absent and the injection rate can be increased to visualize the smallest arterial branches, in coronary arteries, the opacification must not exceed ~300 HU for a reliable depiction and judgment of calcifications. Optimization of vessel contrast-to-noise also is mandatory for sufficient visualization of noncalcified plaques. Methods to enhance the contrast-to-noise in the vessel wall include either the use of a test bolus setting (20 mL + 50 mL NaCl) or a bolus tracking. Because nonenhanced blood on CT has similar attenuation (50–70 HU) to noncalcified plaques, this type of lesion

can only be detected after administration of contrast media. Therefore, a vessel enhancement significantly greater than the CT values of noncalcified lesions (150 HU) must be achieved to allow for reliable detection of noncalcified plaques. A target attenuation of 200 HU seems best suited to fulfill this requirement. With this vessel enhancement, calcified coronary lesions remain detectable because their attenuation is significantly greater (156).

CT has become an established method for noninvasive and highly sensitive detection of coronary artery calcifications (157). It was shown that CT has the potential to identify noncalcified plaques *in vivo* in the coronary arteries (Fig. 53–13) (19,158,159). Various imaging features of noncalcified and calcified plaques depicted with CT correlate with histopathologic stages of atherothrombosis defined by the American Heart Association (160), as demonstrated in an *ex vivo* study on human hearts (149). Intravascular ultrasound (IVUS) is the reference standard for detecting and evaluating atherothrombotic plaques *in vivo*. For plaques with and without signs of calcification detected on IVUS, EBCT without contrast enhancement yielded a sensitivity of 97% and 47% and a specificity of 80% and 75%, respectively (161). In an *in vivo* study on contrast-enhanced MDCT versus IVUS for the accuracy in determining coronary lesion configuration, Schroeder and coworkers (156) reported a good correlation of these two modalities. MDCT was able to differentiate between soft, intermediate, and calcified plaques, as compared with IVUS, with significant differences in CT attenuation values. In studies on MDCT of *ex vivo* coronary arteries versus histopathology as the gold standard, a good correlation again was found. Lipid-rich, fibrous, and calcified plaques were differentiated reliably (162). Acute intravascular thrombi also can be detected *in vivo,* with a typical appearance of the irregular thrombus with typically low attenuation numbers in the range of 20 to 30 HU. In addition, new software applications enable the quantification of noncalcified atherothrombotic lesions *in vivo* (141).

Future Potentials of Magnetic Resonance and Computed Tomography for Plaque Imaging

Thinner slices, such as those obtained with 3D MR acquisition techniques, could further improve artery wall imaging (152). Additional MR techniques, such as water diffusion weighting (163), magnetization transfer weighting (164), steady-state free precession sequences (165), contrast enhancement (166), and molecular imaging (167,168) may provide complementary structural information and allow more detailed plaque characterization. New and improved blood suppression methods (152) are necessary for accurate plaque imaging, especially in the carotid artery bifurcation.

CE-MRA with the use of gadolinium-based contrast agents may provide additional information for plaque characterization by identifying neovascularization in the atherothrombotic plaque and potentially may improve the

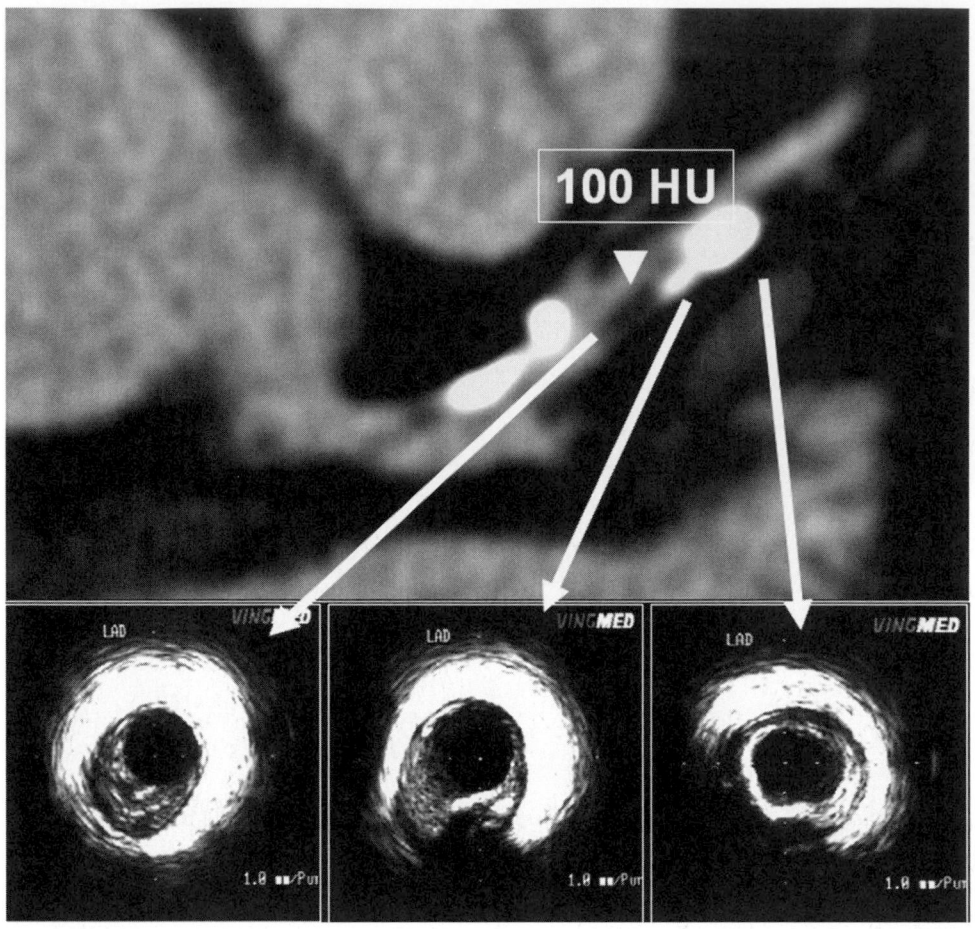

FIG. 53–13. Correlation of computed tomography angiography of the coronary arteries with intravascular ultrasound illustrates the ability of multidetector-row computed tomography (MDCT) to demonstrate calcified and noncalcified coronary plaques. The contrast-enhanced MDCT image **(top)** shows extensive calcified plaques along the course of the proximal left anterior descending coronary artery (LAD), as well as a noncalcified plaque in this area, with a density of about 100 Hounsfield Units (HU). Corresponding intravascular ultrasound images **(bottom)** confirm the presence of a noncalcified, fibrotic plaque. (From Becker CR, Ohnesorge BM, Schoepf UJ, et al. Current development of cardiac imaging with multidetector-row CT. *Eur J Radiol* 2000;36:97–103, with permission.)

differentiation between necrotic core and fibrous tissue (166). Furthermore, other nonspecific and specific contrast agents may facilitate accurate plaque constituent characterization and the identification of specific molecular and biologic activity (167,168). One example for promising specific contrast agents are fibrin-specific contrast agents, allowing for reliable detection of thrombotic material and for longitudinal study of thrombus progression or regression (169).

The next generation of MDCT scanners will most probably allow for even faster gantry rotation and simultaneous acquisition of more than 16 slices. The breath hold time may decrease to less than 10 s, thus reducing the necessary volume of contrast media (e.g., 60 mL) needed for sufficient enhancement of the coronary arteries. The temporal and spatial resolution may most likely further decrease to ideally 100 ms and 0.6-mm slice thickness for true isotropic voxel sizes. These enhancements may help in the detection, differentiation, and reliable quantification of calcified and noncal-

cified coronary artery plaques. Reduction of spatial resolution and new image reconstruction algorithms should further reduce beam hardening artifacts and partial volume effects caused by calcifications and improve the assessment of complex mixed plaques. Further optimization of multisegmental reconstruction algorithms (170,171) may allow the investigation of patients with higher heart rates without any loss in image quality.

Conclusion

Both high-resolution MRI and MDCT have specific advantages in the detection and differentiation of atherothrombotic vessel wall changes. Using dedicated MRI techniques, a greater inplane resolution can be achieved, and in combination with multi-echo sequences, a more detailed analysis of different plaque types and plaque components is feasible. MRI does not have beam-hardening artifacts and partial volume effects caused by calcifications, which allows for superior differentiation of mixed plaques with calcified and non-calcified components. The major disadvantages of MRI are its inherent limitations in *in vivo* imaging, because the image quality suffers greatly because of patient movement and breathing artifacts and the significantly longer image acquisition times. This is the main reason why, in an *in vivo* setting, a detailed analysis of coronary artery plaques is not currently feasible, and only limited regions of the coronary artery tree can be depicted (146).

Currently, MDCT is easier and faster to perform in an *in vivo* setting and is less sensitive to artifacts caused by patient movement or breathing, despite a relatively long acquisition window of 210 to 250 ms per heartbeat. Modern MDCT

scanners with 16-detector-rows allow for *in vivo* investigation of the entire coronary artery tree with 0.75-mm slice thickness within 1 short breath hold, achieving a nearly isotropic submillimeter voxel size, with typically better out-of-plane resolution compared with MRI.

A promising approach to the noninvasive assessment of coronary artery plaques may be the implementation of combined MRI and CT in a complementary algorithm. The advantage of MDCT is the potentially complete assessment of the entire coronary artery tree within a short scan time, and MRI offers excellent soft tissue contrast. However, because of the limited scan range and long examination time for MRI, MDCT may be used first to localize suspicious CAD lesions in the coronary arteries. With the knowledge of the

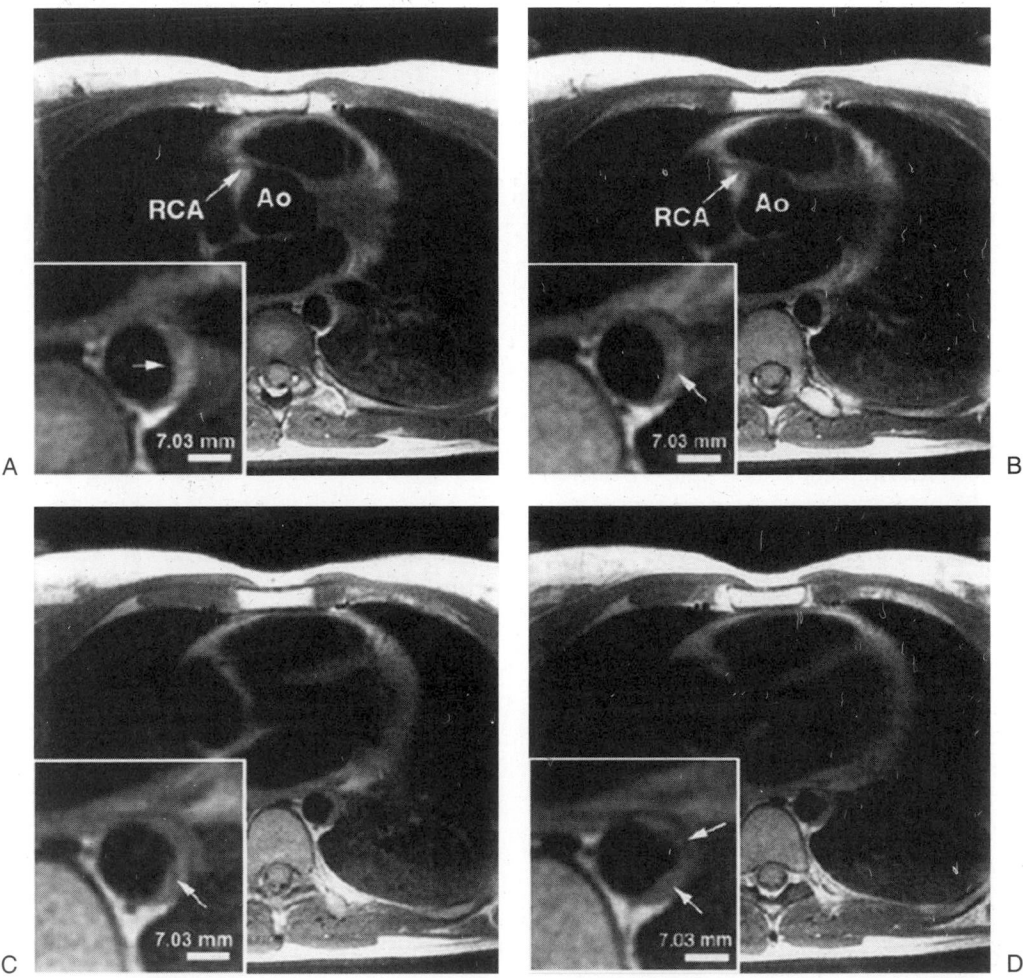

FIG. 53–14. Magnetic resonance (MR) plaque imaging of the thoracic aorta. T2-weighted MR images from a patient with severe diffuse disease in the descending thoracic aorta. Plaques are different in appearance and characteristics from one location to another. *Insets* in each panel represent magnified view of descending thoracic aorta. **A:** Type Vc (fibrotic) plaque. **B:** Type Vb (calcified) plaque. **C,D:** Lipid-rich plaques (type IV/Va). MR images are 5 mm in thickness and acquired with no interslice gap and are displayed cephalad **(A)** to caudal **(D)**. Origin of right coronary artery (RCA) is clearly seen taking off from aortic root (Ao). *Arrows* in insets indicate plaque and its components. (From Fayad ZA, Nahar T, Fallon JT, et al. In vivo magnetic resonance evaluation of atherosclerotic plaques in the human thoracic aorta: a comparison with transesophageal echocardiography. *Circulation* 2000;101:2503–2509, with permission.)

problematic site in the coronary arteries obtained from MDCT, the lesion characteristic can then be assessed in greater detail using MRI. A comprehensive study of atherothrombosis could involve a calcium screening measurement, contrast-enhanced CT for noncalcified plaque burden and stenosis assessment, and multicontrast MR plaque characterization for a detailed analysis and follow-up of the composition of coronary atherothrombotic lesions. The clinical utility of such a noninvasive combined CT and MR approach needs to be validated prospectively in large clinical trials.

Plaque Imaging of the Carotid Arteries

Other factors in addition to the degree of stenosis alone also are important in determining whether a carotid lesion will remain clinically silent. Plaques that are more prone to disruption, fracture, or fissuring may be associated with a greater risk for embolization, occlusion, and consequent ischemic neurologic events (172). In contrast to coronary artery vulnerable plaques that are often characterized by high lipid content and a thin fibrous cap, high-risk plaques in carotid arteries typically are severely stenotic. Currently, the term *high risk* is used rather than the classic term *vulnerable,* which only implies the presence of a lipid-rich core. High-risk carotid plaques are heterogeneous, very fibrous, and not necessarily lipid-rich (173). This is why increasing emphasis is put on the tissue characterization of the carotid artery wall, using MRI (173,174) (Fig. 53–8) and contrast-enhanced MDCT (Fig. 53–9) (175–177). These study findings emphasize the importance of accurate delineation of the morphology of the carotid bifurcation, as well as the degree of stenosis. The inability of conventional x-ray angiography to depict plaque ulceration is well documented (178), because it is an imaging technique for depicting the vessel lumen only and it also has only a limited number of views that are typically obtained. MRI has been shown to reliably identify plaque composition in the carotid artery vessel wall, using multicontrast, high-resolution, spin echo–based MR sequences (140,179,180). For black blood sequences, the signal from the blood flow is rendered black by the use of preparatory pulses to better visualize the adjacent vessel wall. Hatsukami and coworkers (181) introduced the use of bright blood TOF imaging for the visualization of the fibrous cap thickness and morphologic integrity. This sequence provides enhancement of the signal from flowing blood and a mixture of T1 and proton density contrast weighting that highlights the fibrous cap. MRA and high-resolution black blood imaging of the vessel wall can be combined. MRA demonstrates the severity of stenotic lesions and their spatial distribution, whereas the high-resolution wall characterization techniques may show the composition of the plaques and may facilitate the risk stratification and selection of the treatment modality. Improvements in spatial resolution have been possible with the design of new phased-array coils tailored for carotid imaging

(182) and new imaging sequences such as long echo train FSE imaging with "velocity-selective" flow suppression (183). CT, however, also has been shown to differentiate different tissue types in the carotid artery wall (175,176) and to reliably assess vessel wall thickness (177). Contrast-enhanced MDCT was able to differentiate between calcified, fibrous, and lipid plaque components with moderate to high sensitivity and specificity (176). Yet, it does not reach the

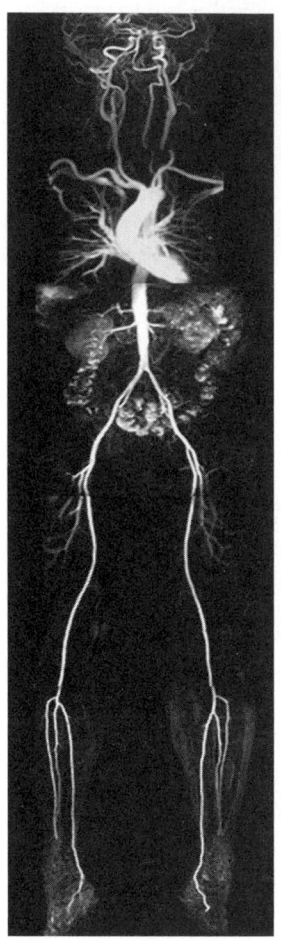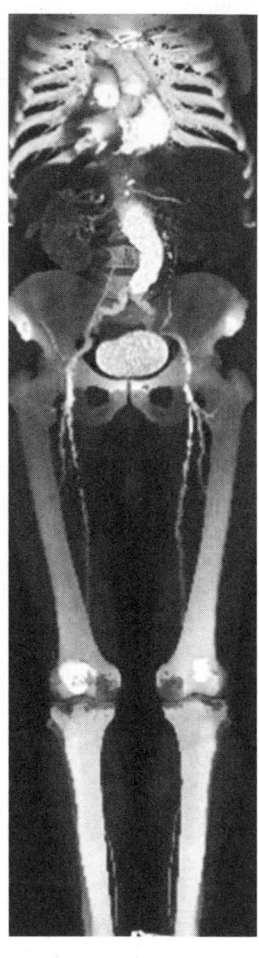

A   B

FIG. 53–15. Both magnetic resonance angiography (MRA) **(A)** and multidetector-row computed tomography (MDCT) **(B)** are able to provide whole-body angiographic images. For whole-body MRA, multicontrast injections are necessary for depiction of the thoracic, supraaortal, and distal runoff vessels. This way, high-resolution images with a high diagnostic accuracy can be obtained, and the image data sets can be composed to a whole-body angiographic image (**A**, maximum-intensity-projections [MIP]). Modern 16-detector-row CT systems can cover a range of 150 cm in a scan time shorter than 20 seconds with a 1.5-mm collimation, enabling the acquisition of a whole-body angiography from the thoracic aorta to the ankle joint with a single injection of contrast agent and in a true arterial phase (**B**, volume rendering technique). (A: Courtesy of K. Nikolaou, Ludwig-Maximilians-University, Munich, Germany; B: From Wintersperger BJ, Herzog P, Jakobs TF, et al. Initial experience with the clinical use of a 16 detector row CT system. *Crit Rev Comput Tomogr* 2002;43:283–316, with permission.)

potential of tissue characterization that is inherent to MRI, and inplane spatial resolution still will have to be improved for a more reliable assessment of plaque components and for identification of plaques at risk.

Plaque Imaging of the Aorta

Autopsy studies have shown that the amount of atherothrombotic plaque in the thoracic aorta directly correlates with the degree of atherothrombotic disease in the coronary arteries. Furthermore, thoracic aortic atherothrombosis is a stronger predictor of CAD than conventional risk factors and is also a marker of increased mortality, stroke, and visceral thromboembolic events. Examination of the descending thoracic aorta by transesophageal echocardiography (TEE) and by fast CT is used to predict CAD and cardiovascular risk. It could be shown that MR findings compare well with those obtained from TEE imaging (184). Therefore, MR may be a powerful noninvasive imaging tool for direct noninvasive assessment of aortic atherothrombotic plaque thickness, extent, and composition (Fig. 53–14). MR may allow the serial evaluation of progression and therapy-induced regression of atherothrombotic plaques.

CONCLUSIONS

In conclusion, for most vascular territories, diagnostic angiography can be performed in the near future using noninvasive methods such as MRA or CTA. The comprehensive assessment of the complete vascular system is an appealing new application for both techniques (Fig. 53–15). Both modalities offer significant advantages for certain vascular territories but with significant drawbacks inherent to both noninvasive imaging modalities. In the peripheral circulation, MRA might be the imaging modality of choice. CTA plays an important role in pulmonary and coronary imaging. MRA is more suited for elective diagnosis rather than clinical emergencies. Both noninvasive imaging technologies are rapidly improving. Thus, it is difficult to predict which modality will dominate the future clinical applications and indications because both modalities are undergoing rapid evolution in hardware, principal acquisition techniques, postprocessing tools, and specific contrast agents. It is rather safe to conclude that the future of catheter-based, x-ray angiography will mostly be downgraded to an adjunctive role in the diagnosis of various vascular diseases or primarily as a conduit to the increasing number of catheter-based cardiovascular interventions.

REFERENCES

1. Moran PR, Moran RA, Karstaedt N. Verification and evaluation of internal flow and motion. True magnetic resonance imaging by the phase gradient modulation method. *Radiology* 1985;154:433–441.
2. Dumoulin CL, Hart HR Jr. Magnetic resonance angiography. *Radiology* 1986;161:717–720.
3. Quick HH, Debatin JF, Ladd ME. MR imaging of the vessel wall. *Eur Radiol* 2002;12:889–900.
4. Kucharczyk W, Kelly WM, Davis DO, et al. Intracranial lesions: flow-related enhancement on MR images using time-of-flight effects. *Radiology* 1986;161:767–772.
5. O'Donnell M. NMR blood flow imaging using multiecho, phase contrast sequences. *Med Phys* 1985;12:59–64.
6. Prince MR. Gadolinium-enhanced MR aortography. *Radiology* 1994; 191:155–164.
7. Debatin JF, Hany TF. MR-based assessment of vascular morphology and function. *Eur Radiol* 1998;8:528–539.
8. Carroll TJ, Grist TM. Technical developments in MR angiography. *Radiol Clin North Am* 2002;40:921–951.
9. Griswold MA, Jakob PM, Heidemann RM, et al. Generalized autocalibrating partially parallel acquisitions (GRAPPA). *Magn Reson Med* 2002;47:1202–1210.
10. Sodickson DK, McKenzie CA, Li W, et al. Contrast-enhanced 3D MR angiography with simultaneous acquisition of spatial harmonics: a pilot study. *Radiology* 2000;217:284–289.
11. Kalender WA, Seissler W, Klotz E, et al. Spiral volumetric CT with single-breath-hold technique, continuous transport, and continuous scanner rotation. *Radiology* 1990;176:181–183.
12. Mahesh M. Search for isotropic resolution in CT from conventional through multiple-row detector. *Radiographics* 2002;22:949–962.
13. Brink JA. Technical aspects of helical (spiral) CT. *Radiol Clin North Am* 1995;33:825–841.
14. Klingenbeck-Regn K, Schaller S, Flohr T, et al. Subsecond multi-slice computed tomography: basics and applications. *Eur J Radiol* 1999; 31:110–124.
15. Kachelriess M, Ulzheimer S, Kalender WA. ECG-correlated imaging of the heart with subsecond multislice spiral CT. *IEEE Trans Med Imaging* 2000;19:888–901.
16. Knez A, Becker C, Ohnesorge B, et al. Noninvasive detection of coronary artery stenosis by multislice helical computed tomography. *Circulation* 2000;101:221–222.
17. Nieman K, Oudkerk M, Rensing BJ, et al. Coronary angiography with multi-slice computed tomography. *Lancet* 2001;357:599–603.
18. Nieman K, Cademartiri F, Lemos P, et al. Reliable noninvasive coronary angiography with fast submillimeter multislice spiral computed tomography. *Circulation* 2002;106:2051–2054.
19. Becker CR, Ohnesorge BM, Schoepf UJ, et al. Current development of cardiac imaging with multidetector-row CT. *Eur J Radiol* 2000;36: 97–103.
20. Rubin GD, Armerding MD, Dake MD, et al. Cost identification of abdominal aortic aneurysm imaging by using time and motion analyses. *Radiology* 2000;215:63–70.
21. Rubin GD, Schmidt AJ, Logan LJ, et al. Multi-detector row CT angiography of lower extremity arterial inflow and runoff: initial experience. *Radiology* 2001;221:146–158.
22. Hirai T, Korogi Y, Ono K, et al. Maximum stenosis of extracranial internal carotid artery: effect of luminal morphology on stenosis measurement by using CT angiography and conventional DSA. *Radiology* 2001;221:802–809.
23. Rumberger JA. Tomographic (plaque) imaging: state of the art. *Am J Cardiol* 2001;88(2A):66E–69E.
24. Bunce NH, Lorenz CH, Pennell DJ. MR coronary angiography: 2001 update. *Rays* 2001;26:61–69.
25. Gaylord GM. Computed tomographic and magnetic resonance coronary angiography: are you ready? *Radiol Manage* 2002;24:16–20.
26. Achenbach S, Giesler T, Ropers D, et al. Detection of coronary artery stenoses by contrast-enhanced, retrospectively electrocardiographically-gated, multislice spiral computed tomography. *Circulation* 2001;103: 2535–2538.
27. Nikolaou K, Huber A, Knez A, et al. Intraindividual comparison of contrast-enhanced electron-beam computed tomography and navigator-echo-based magnetic resonance imaging for noninvasive coronary artery angiography. *Eur Radiol* 2002;12:1663–1671.
28. Li D, Paschal CB, Haacke EM, et al. Coronary arteries: three-dimensional MR imaging with fat saturation and magnetization transfer contrast. *Radiology* 1993;187:401–406.
29. Botnar RM, Stuber M, Danias PG, et al. Improved coronary artery definition with T2-weighted, free-breathing, three-dimensional coronary MRA. *Circulation* 1999;99:3139–3148.
30. Manning WJ, Li W, Edelman RR. A preliminary report comparing

magnetic resonance coronary angiography with conventional angiography. *N Engl J Med* 1993;328:828–832.

31. Duerinckx AJ. Imaging of coronary artery disease—MR. *J Thorac Imaging* 2001;16:25–34.

32. Wielopolski PA, van Geuns RJ, de Feyter PJ, et al. Coronary arteries. *Eur Radiol* 2000;10:12–35.

33. Duerinckx A, Urman MK. Two-dimensional coronary MR angiography: analysis of initial clinical results. *Radiology* 1996;193:731–738.

34. Pennell DJ, Bogren HG, Keegan J, et al. Assessment of coronary artery stenosis by magnetic resonance imaging. *Heart* 1996;75:127–133.

35. Post JC, van Rossum AC, Hofman MB, et al. Clinical utility of two-dimensional magnetic resonance angiography in detecting coronary artery disease. *Eur Heart J* 1997;18:426–433.

36. Huber A, Nikolaou K, Gonschior P, et al. Navigator echo-based respiratory gating for three-dimensional MR coronary angiography: results from healthy volunteers and patients with proximal coronary artery stenoses. *AJR Am J Roentgenol* 1999;173:95–101.

37. Nikolaou K, Huber A, Knez A, et al. Navigator echo-based respiratory gating for 3D-MR coronary angiography: reduction of scan time using a slice-interpolation technique. *J Comput Assist Tomogr* 2001;25:378–387.

38. Sommer T, Hofer U, Hackenbroch M, et al. [Submillimeter 3D coronary MR angiography with real-time navigator correction in 107 patients with suspected coronary artery disease]. *Rofo Fortschr Geb Rontgenstr Neuen Bildgeb Verfahr* 2002;174:459–466. German.

39. Regenfus M, Ropers D, Achenbach S, et al. Noninvasive detection of coronary artery stenosis using contrast-enhanced three-dimensional breath-hold magnetic resonance coronary angiography. *J Am Coll Cardiol* 2000;36:44–50.

40. van Geuns RJ, Wielopolski PA, de Bruin HG, et al. MR coronary angiography with breath-hold targeted volumes: preliminary clinical results. *Radiology* 2000;217:270–277.

41. Manning WJ, Kim YK, Danias PG, et al. Comparison of 3D coronary MRA with X-ray angiography for detection of coronary stenoses: a prospective international multicenter study. *Circulation* 2001;104:II-374.

42. Huber ME, Hengesbach D, Botnar RM, et al. Motion artifact reduction and vessel enhancement for free-breathing navigator-gated coronary MRA using 3D k-space reordering. *Magn Reson Med* 2001;45:645–652.

43. Hardy CJ, Saranathan M, Zhu Y, et al. Coronary angiography by real-time MRI with adaptive averaging. *Magn Reson Med* 2000;44:940–946.

44. Kessler W, Laub G, Achenbach S, et al. Coronary arteries: MR angiography with fast contrast-enhanced three-dimensional breath-hold imaging—initial experience. *Radiology* 1999;210:566–572.

45. Li D, Carr JC, Shea SM, et al. Coronary arteries: magnetization-prepared contrast-enhanced three-dimensional volume-targeted breath-hold MR angiography. *Radiology* 2001;219:270–277.

46. Stuber M, Botnar RM, Kissinger KV, et al. Free-breathing black-blood coronary MR angiography: initial results. *Radiology* 2001;219:278–283.

47. Deshpande VS, Shea SM, Laub G, et al. 3D magnetization-prepared true-FISP: a new technique for imaging coronary arteries. *Magn Reson Med* 2001;46:494–502.

48. Li D, Zheng J, Weinmann HJ. Contrast-enhanced MR imaging of coronary arteries: comparison of intra- and extravascular contrast agents in swine. *Radiology* 2001;218:670–678.

49. Sandstede JJ, Pabst T, Wacker C, et al. Breath-hold 3D MR coronary angiography with a new intravascular contrast agent (feruglose)—first clinical experiences. *Magn Reson Imaging* 2001;19:201–205.

50. Sodickson DK, McKenzie CA, Li W, et al. Contrast-enhanced 3D MR angiography with simultaneous acquisition of spatial harmonics: a pilot study. *Radiology* 2000;217:284–289.

51. Pruessmann KP, Weiger M, Scheidegger MB, et al. SENSE: sensitivity encoding for fast MRI. *Magn Reson Med* 1999;42:952–962.

52. Taylor AM, Thorne SA, Rubens MB, et al. Coronary artery imaging in grown up congenital heart disease: complementary role of magnetic resonance and x-ray coronary angiography. *Circulation* 2000;101:1670–1678.

53. Nieman K, Oudkerk M, Rensing BJ, et al. Coronary angiography with multi-slice computed tomography. *Lancet* 2001;357:599–603.

54. Wintersperger BJ, Nikolaou K, Jakobs TF, et al. Cardiac multidetector-row computed tomography: initial experience using 16 detector-row systems. *Crit Rev Comput Tomogr* 2003;44:27–45.

55. Jakobs TF, Becker CR, Ohnesorge B, et al. Multislice helical CT of the heart with retrospective ECG gating: reduction of radiation exposure by ECG-controlled tube current modulation. *Eur Radiol* 2002;12:1081–1086.

56. Vogl TJ, Abolmaali ND, Diebold T, et al. Techniques for the detection of coronary atherosclerosis: multi-detector row CT coronary angiography. *Radiology* 2002;223:212–220.

57. Sarjeant JM, Rabinovitch M. Understanding and treating vein graft atherosclerosis. *Cardiovasc Pathol* 2002;11:263–271.

58. Langerak SE, Kunz P, De Roos A, et al. Evaluation of coronary artery bypass grafts by magnetic resonance imaging. *J Magn Reson Imaging* 1999;10:434–441.

59. Langerak SE, Vliegen HW, De Roos A, et al. Detection of vein graft disease using high-resolution magnetic resonance angiography. *Circulation* 2002;105:328–333.

60. Wittlinger T, Voigtlander T, Kreitner KF, et al. Non-invasive magnetic resonance imaging of coronary bypass grafts. Comparison of the haste- and navigator techniques with conventional coronary angiography. *Int J Cardiovasc Imaging* 2002;18:469–477.

61. Ropers D, Ulzheimer S, Wenkel E, et al. Investigation of aortocoronary artery bypass grafts by multislice spiral computed tomography with electrocardiographic-gated image reconstruction. *Am J Cardiol* 2001;88:792–795.

62. Achenbach S, Moshage W, Ropers D, et al. Noninvasive, three-dimensional visualization of coronary artery bypass grafts by electron beam tomography. *Am J Cardiol* 1997;79:856–861.

63. Enzweiler CN, Wiese TH, Petersein J, et al. Diameter changes of occluded venous coronary artery bypass grafts in electron beam tomography: preliminary findings. *Eur J Cardiothorac Surg* 2003;23:347–353.

64. Knez A, von Smekal A, Haberl R, et al. [The value of ultrafast computerized tomography in detection of the patency of coronary bypasses]. *Z Kardiol* 1996;85:629–634. German.

65. Tello R, Hartnell GG, Costello P, et al. Coronary artery bypass graft flow: qualitative evaluation with cine single-detector row CT and comparison with findings at angiography. *Radiology* 2002;224:913–918.

66. Hyers TM. Venous thromboembolism. *Am J Respir Crit Care Med* 1999;159:1–14.

67. Perrier A, Desmarais S, Miron MJ, et al. Non-invasive diagnosis of venous thromboembolism in outpatients. *Lancet* 1999;353:190–195.

68. Stein PD, Athanasoulis C, Alavi A, et al. Complications and validity of pulmonary angiography in acute pulmonary embolism. *Circulation* 1992;85:462–468.

69. Haage P, Piroth W, Krombach G, et al. Pulmonary embolism: comparison of angiography with spiral computed tomography, magnetic resonance angiography, and real-time magnetic resonance imaging. *Am J Respir Crit Care Med* 2003;167:729–734.

70. Mai VM, Bankier AA, Prasad PV, et al. MR ventilation-perfusion imaging of human lung using oxygen-enhanced and arterial spin labeling techniques. *J Magn Reson Imaging* 2001;14:574–579.

71. Kauczor HU, Hanke A, van Beek EJ. Assessment of lung ventilation by MR imaging: current status and future perspectives. *Eur Radiol* 2002;12:1962–1970.

72. Meaney JF, Johansson LO, Ahlstrom H, et al. Pulmonary magnetic resonance angiography. *J Magn Reson Imaging* 1999;10:326–338.

73. Ghaye B, Remy J, Remy-Jardin M. Non-traumatic thoracic emergencies: CT diagnosis of acute pulmonary embolism: the first 10 years. *Eur Radiol* 2002;12:1886–1905.

74. Prendergast BD, Boon NA, Buckenham T. Aortic dissection: advances in imaging and endoluminal repair. *Cardiovasc Interv Radiol* 2002;25:85–97.

75. Ho VB, Prince MR. Thoracic MR aortography: imaging techniques and strategies. *Radiographics* 1998;18:287–309.

76. Krinsky GA, Rofsky NM, DeCorato DR, et al. Thoracic aorta: comparison of gadolinium-enhanced three-dimensional MR angiography with conventional MR imaging. *Radiology* 1997;202:183–193.

77. LePage MA, Quint LE, Sonnad SS, et al. Aortic dissection: CT features that distinguish true lumen from false lumen. *AJR Am J Roentgenol* 2001;177:207–211.

78. Pereles FS, McCarthy RM, Baskaran V, et al. Thoracic aortic dissection and aneurysm: evaluation with nonenhanced true FISP MR angiography in less than 4 minutes. *Radiology* 2002;223:270–274.

79. Moore AG, Eagle KA, Bruckman D, et al. Choice of computed tomography, transesophageal echocardiography, magnetic resonance imaging, and aortography in acute aortic dissection: International Registry of Acute Aortic Dissection (IRAD). *Am J Cardiol* 2002;89:1235–1238.

80. Dapunt OE, Galla JD, Sadeghi AM, et al. The natural history of thoracic aortic aneurysms. *J Thorac Cardiovasc Surg* 1994;107:1323–1332.

81. Elefteriades JA. Natural history of thoracic aortic aneurysms: indications for surgery, and surgical versus nonsurgical risks. *Ann Thorac Surg* 2002;74:S1877–S1880.

82. Prince MR, Narasimham DL, Jacoby WT, et al. Three-dimensional gadolinium-enhanced MR angiography of the thoracic aorta. *AJR Am J Roentgenol* 1996;166:1387–1397.

83. Anbarasu A, Harris PL, McWilliams RG. The role of gadolinium-enhanced MR imaging in the preoperative evaluation of inflammatory abdominal aortic aneurysm. *Eur Radiol* 2002;12[Suppl 4]:S192–S195.

84. Quint LE, Francis IR, Williams DM, et al. Evaluation of thoracic aortic disease with the use of helical CT and multiplanar reconstructions: comparison with surgical findings. *Radiology* 1996;201:37–41.

85. Rubin GD. MDCT imaging of the aorta and peripheral vessels. *Eur J Radiol* 2003;45[Suppl 1]:S42–S49.

86. Coselli JS, Conklin LD, LeMaire SA. Thoracoabdominal aortic aneurysm repair: review and update of current strategies. *Ann Thorac Surg* 2002;74:S1881–S1884.

87. LaRoy LL, Cormier PJ, Matalon TA, et al. Imaging of abdominal aortic aneurysms. *AJR Am J Roentgenol* 1989;152:785–792.

88. Yucel EK. MR angiography for evaluation of abdominal aortic aneurysm: has the time come? *Radiology* 1994;192:321–323.

89. Prince MR, Yucel EK, Kaufman JA, et al. Dynamic gadolinium-enhanced three-dimensional abdominal MR arteriography. *J Magn Reson Imaging* 1993;3:877–881.

90. Ludman CN, Yusuf SW, Whitaker SC, et al. Feasibility of using dynamic contrast-enhanced magnetic resonance angiography as the sole imaging modality prior to endovascular repair of abdominal aortic aneurysms. *Eur J Vasc Endovasc Surg* 2000;19:524–530.

91. Petersen MJ, Cambria RP, Kaufman JA, et al. Magnetic resonance angiography in the preoperative evaluation of abdominal aortic aneurysms. *J Vasc Surg* 1995;21:891–898.

92. Prince MR, Narasimham DL, Stanley JC, et al. Breath-hold gadolinium-enhanced MR angiography of the abdominal aorta and its major branches. *Radiology* 1995;197:785–792.

93. Hany TF, Debatin JF, Leung DA, et al. Evaluation of the aortoiliac and renal arteries: comparison of breath-hold, contrast-enhanced, three-dimensional MR angiography with conventional catheter angiography. *Radiology* 1997;204:357–362.

94. Papanicolaou N, Wittenberg J, Ferrucci JT Jr, et al. Preoperative evaluation of abdominal aortic aneurysms by computed tomography. *AJR Am J Roentgenol* 1986;146:711–715.

95. Bandyk DF. Preoperative imaging of aortic aneurysms. Conventional and digital subtraction angiography, computed tomography scanning, and magnetic resonance imaging. *Surg Clin North Am* 1989;69:721–735.

96. Van Hoe L, Baert AL, Gryspeerdt S, et al. Supra- and juxtarenal aneurysms of the abdominal aorta: preoperative assessment with thin-section spiral CT. *Radiology* 1996;198:443–448.

97. Fleischmann D, Rubin GD, Bankier AA, et al. Improved uniformity of aortic enhancement with customized contrast medium injection protocols at CT angiography. *Radiology* 2000;214:363–371.

98. Meaney JF, Prince MR, Nostrant TT, et al. Gadolinium-enhanced MR angiography of visceral arteries in patients with suspected chronic mesenteric ischemia. *J Magn Reson Imaging* 1997;7:171–176.

99. Carlos RC, Stanley JC, Stafford-Johnson D, et al. Interobserver variability in the evaluation of chronic mesenteric ischemia with gadolinium-enhanced MR angiography. *Acad Radiol* 2001;8:879–887.

100. Horton KM, Fishman EK. 3D CT angiography of the celiac and superior mesenteric arteries with multidetector CT data sets: preliminary observations. *Abdom Imaging* 2000;25:523–525.

101. Horton KM, Fishman EK. Volume-rendered 3D CT of the mesenteric vasculature: normal anatomy, anatomic variants, and pathologic conditions. *Radiographics* 2002;22:161–172.

102. Fishman EK, Horton KM, Urban BA. Multidetector CT angiography in the evaluation of pancreatic carcinoma: preliminary observations. *J Comput Assist Tomogr* 2000;24:849–853.

103. Horton KM, Fishman EK. CT angiography of the GI tract. *Gastrointest Endosc* 2002;55[7 Suppl]:S37–S41.

104. Clinical alert: benefit of carotid endarterectomy for patients with high-grade stenosis of the internal carotid artery. National Institute of Neurological Disorders and Stroke and Trauma Division. North American Symptomatic Carotid Endarterectomy Trial (NASCET) investigators. *Stroke* 1991;22:816–817.

105. Hallett JW Jr, Pietropaoli JA Jr, Ilstrup DM, et al. Comparison of North American Symptomatic Carotid Endarterectomy Trial and population-based outcomes for carotid endarterectomy. *J Vasc Surg* 1998;27:845–850.

106. Rothwell PM, Gutnikov SA, Warlow CP. Reanalysis of the final results of the European Carotid Surgery Trial. *Stroke* 2003;34:514–523.

107. Polak JF, Bajakian RL, O'Leary DH, et al. Detection of internal carotid artery stenosis: comparison of MR angiography, color Doppler sonography, and arteriography. *Radiology* 1992;182:35–40.

108. Heiserman JE, Drayer BP, Fram EK, et al. Carotid artery stenosis: clinical efficacy of two-dimensional time-of-flight MR angiography. *Radiology* 1992;182:761–768.

109. Carriero A, Scarabino T, Magarelli N, et al. High-resolution magnetic resonance angiography of the internal carotid artery: 2D vs 3D TOF in stenotic disease. *Eur Radiol* 1998;8:1370–1372.

110. Scarabino T, Carriero A, Magarelli N, et al. MR angiography in carotid stenosis: a comparison of three techniques. *Eur J Radiol* 1998;28:117–125.

111. Huston J, Lewis BD, Wiebers DO, et al. Carotid artery: prospective blinded comparison of two-dimensional time-of-flight MR angiography with conventional angiography and duplex US. *Radiology* 1993;186:339–344.

112. Carr JC, Ma J, Desphande V, et al. High-resolution breath-hold contrast-enhanced MR angiography of the entire carotid circulation. *AJR Am J Roentgenol* 2002;178:543–549.

113. Remonda L, Senn P, Barth A, et al. Contrast-enhanced 3D MR angiography of the carotid artery: comparison with conventional digital subtraction angiography. *AJNR Am J Neuroradiol* 2002;23:213–219.

114. Huston J, Fain SB, Wald JT, et al. Carotid artery: elliptic centric contrast-enhanced MR angiography compared with conventional angiography. *Radiology* 2001;218:138–143.

115. Golay X, Brown SJ, Itoh R, et al. Time-resolved contrast-enhanced carotid MR angiography using sensitivity encoding (SENSE). *AJNR Am J Neuroradiol* 2001;22:1615–1619.

116. Lenhart M, Framme N, Volk M, et al. Time-resolved contrast-enhanced magnetic resonance angiography of the carotid arteries: diagnostic accuracy and inter-observer variability compared with selective catheter angiography. *Invest Radiol* 2002;37:535–541.

117. Schwartz RB, Jones KM, Chernoff DM, et al. Common carotid artery bifurcation: evaluation with spiral CT. Work in progress. *Radiology* 1992;185:513–519.

118. Jones TR, Kaplan RT, Lane B, et al. Single- versus multi-detector row CT of the brain: quality assessment. *Radiology* 2001;219:750–755.

119. Lell M, Wildberger JE, Heuschmid M, et al. [CT-angiography of the carotid artery: first results with a novel 16-slice-spiral-CT scanner]. *Rofo Fortschr Geb Rontgenstr Neuen Bildgeb Verfahr* 2002;174:1165–1169. German.

120. Ertl-Wagner B, Hoffmann RT, Bruning R, et al. [CT-angiographic evaluation of intracranial aneurysms—a review of the literature and first experiences with 4- and 16-slice multi detector CT scanners]. *Radiologe* 2002;42:892–897. German.

121. Magarelli N, Scarabino T, Simeone AL, et al. Carotid stenosis: a comparison between MR and spiral CT angiography. *Neuroradiology* 1998;40:367–373.

122. Koelemay MJ, Lijmer JG, Stoker J, et al. Magnetic resonance angiography for the evaluation of lower extremity arterial disease: a meta-analysis. *JAMA* 2001;285:1338–1345.

123. Egglin TK, O'Moore PV, Feinstein AR, et al. Complications of peripheral arteriography: a new system to identify patients at increased risk. *J Vasc Surg* 1995;22:787–794.

124. Ho KY, de Haan MW, Oei TK, et al. MR angiography of the iliac and upper femoral arteries using four different inflow techniques. *AJR Am J Roentgenol* 1997;169:45–53.

125. Huber TS, Back MR, Ballinger RJ, et al. Utility of magnetic resonance arteriography for distal lower extremity revascularization. *J Vasc Surg* 1997;26:415–423.

126. Eiberg JP, Lundorf E, Thomsen C, et al. Peripheral vascular surgery and magnetic resonance arteriography—a review. *Eur J Vasc Endovasc Surg* 2001;22:396–402.

127. Sharafuddin MJ, Stolpen AH, Sun S, et al. High-resolution multiphase contrast-enhanced three-dimensional MR angiography compared with two-dimensional time-of-flight MR angiography for the

identification of pedal vessels. *J Vasc Interv Radiol* 2002;13: 695–702.

128. Ruehm SG, Goyen M, Barkhausen J, et al. Rapid magnetic resonance angiography for detection of atherosclerosis. *Lancet* 2001;357:1086–1091.

129. Shetty AN, Bis KG, Duerinckx AJ, et al. Lower extremity MR angiography: universal retrofitting of high-field-strength systems with stepping kinematic imaging platforms initial experience. *Radiology* 2002;222:284–291.

130. Hany TF, Carroll TJ, Omary RA, et al. Aorta and runoff vessels: single-injection MR angiography with automated table movement compared with multiinjection time-resolved MR angiography—initial results. *Radiology* 2001;221:266–272.

131. Prince MR, Grist TM, Debatin JF. *3D contrast MR angiography,* 3rd ed. New York: Springer-Verlag, 2003.

132. Maki JH, Wilson GJ, Eubank WB, et al. Utilizing SENSE to achieve lower station sub-millimeter isotropic resolution and minimal venous enhancement in peripheral MR angiography. *J Magn Reson Imaging* 2002;15:484–491.

133. Rubin GD, Shiau MC, Schmidt AJ, et al. Computed tomographic angiography: historical perspective and new state-of-the-art using multi detector-row helical computed tomography. *J Comput Assist Tomogr* 1999;23[Suppl 1]:83–90.

134. Wintersperger BJ, Herzog P, Jakobs TF, et al. Initial experience with the clinical use of a 16 detector row CT system. *Crit Rev Comput Tomogr* 2002;43:283–316.

135. Martin ML, Tay KH, Flak B, et al. Multidetector CT angiography of the aortoiliac system and lower extremities: a prospective comparison with digital subtraction angiography. *AJR Am J Roentgenol* 2003;180:1085–1091.

136. Virmani R, Kolodgie FD, Burke AP, et al. Lessons from sudden coronary death: a comprehensive morphological classification scheme for atherosclerotic lesions. *Arterioscler Thromb Vasc Biol* 2000;20:1262–1275.

137. Fuster V, Badimon L, Badimon JJ, et al. The pathogenesis of coronary artery disease and the acute coronary syndromes (2). *N Engl J Med* 1992;326:310–318.

138. Fuster V, Badimon L, Badimon JJ, et al. The pathogenesis of coronary artery disease and the acute coronary syndromes (1). *N Engl J Med* 1992;326:242–250.

139. Pasterkamp G, Falk E, Woutman H, et al. Techniques characterizing the coronary atherosclerotic plaque: influence on clinical decision making? *J Am Coll Cardiol* 2000;36:13–21.

140. Fayad ZA, Fuster V. Clinical imaging of the high-risk or vulnerable atherosclerotic plaque. *Circ Res* 2001;89:305–316.

141. Nikolaou K, Becker CR, Wintersperger BJ, et al. Assessment of non-calcified vessel-wall changes in the coronary arteries using contrast-enhanced multirow-detector computed tomography. *Radiology* 2002;225:632.

142. Fayad ZA, Fuster V, Nikolaou K, et al. Computed tomography and magnetic resonance imaging for noninvasive coronary angiography and plaque imaging: current and potential future concepts. *Circulation* 2002;106:2026–2034.

143. Toussaint JF, LaMuraglia GM, Southern JF, et al. Magnetic resonance images lipid, fibrous, calcified, hemorrhagic, and thrombotic components of human atherosclerosis in vivo. *Circulation* 1996;94:932–938.

144. Yuan C, Beach KW, Smith LH Jr, et al. Measurement of atherosclerotic carotid plaque size in vivo using high resolution magnetic resonance imaging. *Circulation* 1998;98:2666–2671.

145. Fayad ZA, Nahar T, Fallon JT, et al. In vivo magnetic resonance evaluation of atherosclerotic plaques in the human thoracic aorta: a comparison with transesophageal echocardiography. *Circulation* 2000;101:2503–2509.

146. Fayad ZA, Fuster V, Fallon JT, et al. Noninvasive in vivo human coronary artery lumen and wall imaging using black-blood magnetic resonance imaging. *Circulation* 2000;102:506–510.

147. Botnar R, Stuber M, Kissinger K, et al. Noninvasive coronary vessel wall and plaque imaging with magnetic resonance imaging. *Circulation* 2000;102:2582–2587.

148. Toussaint JF, LaMuraglia GM, Southern JF, et al. Magnetic resonance images lipid, fibrous, calcified, hemorrhagic, and thrombotic components of human atherosclerosis in vivo. *Circulation* 1996;94:932–938.

149. Nikolaou K, Becker CR, Muders M. High-resolution magnetic resonance and multi-slice CT imaging of coronary artery plaques in human ex vivo coronary arteries. *Radiology* 2001;221:503.

150. Worthley SG, Helft G, Fuster V, et al. Noninvasive in vivo magnetic resonance imaging of experimental coronary artery lesions in a porcine model. *Circulation* 2000;101:2956–2961.

151. Fayad ZA, Fuster V, Fallon JT, et al. Noninvasive in vivo human coronary artery lumen and wall imaging using black-blood magnetic resonance imaging. *Circulation* 2000;102:506–510.

152. Botnar RM, Kim WY, Bornert P, et al. 3D coronary vessel wall imaging utilizing a local inversion technique with spiral image acquisition. *Magn Reson Med* 2001;46:848–854.

153. McConnell MV, Aikawa M, Maier SE, et al. MRI of rabbit atherosclerosis in response to dietary cholesterol lowering. *Arterioscler Thromb Vasc Biol* 1999;19:1956–1959.

154. Helft G, Worthley SG, Fuster V, et al. Progression and regression of atherosclerotic lesions: monitoring with serial noninvasive magnetic resonance imaging. *Circulation* 2002;105:993–998.

155. Corti R, Fayad ZA, Fuster V, et al. Effects of lipid-lowering by simvastatin on human atherosclerotic lesions: a longitudinal study by high-resolution, noninvasive magnetic resonance imaging. *Circulation* 2001;104:249–252.

156. Schroeder S, Kopp AF, Baumbach A, et al. Noninvasive detection and evaluation of atherosclerotic coronary plaques with multislice computed tomography. *J Am Coll Cardiol* 2001;37:1430–1435.

157. Becker CR, Knez A, Jakobs TF, et al. Detection and quantification of coronary artery calcification with electron-beam and conventional CT. *Eur Radiol* 1999;9:620–624.

158. Becker CR, Knez A, Leber A, et al. [Angiography with multi-slice spiral CT. Detecting plaque, before it causes symptoms]. *MMW Fortschr Med* 2001;143:30–32. German.

159. Becker CR, Knez A, Ohnesorge B, et al. Imaging of noncalcified coronary plaques using helical CT with retrospective ECG gating. *AJR Am J Roentgenol* 2000;175:423–424.

160. Stary HC. Natural history and histological classification of atherosclerotic lesions: an update. *Arterioscler Thromb Vasc Biol* 2000;20:1177–1178.

161. Baumgart D, Schmermund A, Goerge G, et al. Comparison of electron beam computed tomography with intracoronary ultrasound and coronary angiography for detection of coronary atherosclerosis. *J Am Coll Cardiol* 1997;30:57–64.

162. Becker CR, Nikolaou K, Muders M, et al. Ex vivo coronary atherosclerotic plaque characterization with multi-detector-row CT. *Eur Radiol* 2003;13:2094–2098.

163. Toussaint JF, Southern JF, Fuster V, et al. Water diffusion properties of human atherosclerosis and thrombosis measured by pulse field gradient nuclear magnetic resonance. *Arterioscler Thromb Vasc Biol* 1997;17:542–546.

164. Yuan C, Mitsumori LM, Beach KW, et al. Carotid atherosclerotic plaque: noninvasive MR characterization and identification of vulnerable lesions. *Radiology* 2001;221:285–299.

165. Coombs BD, Rapp JH, Ursell PC, et al. Structure of plaque at carotid bifurcation: high-resolution MRI with histological correlation. *Stroke* 2001;32:2516–2521.

166. Yuan C, Kerwin WS, Ferguson MS, et al. Contrast-enhanced high resolution MRI for atherosclerotic carotid artery tissue characterization. *J Magn Reson Imaging* 2002;15:62–67.

167. Ruehm SG, Corot C, Vogt P, et al. Magnetic resonance imaging of atherosclerotic plaque with ultrasmall superparamagnetic particles of iron oxide in hyperlipidemic rabbits. *Circulation* 2001;103:415–422.

168. Flacke S, Fischer S, Scott MJ, et al. Novel MRI contrast agent for molecular imaging of fibrin: implications for detecting vulnerable plaques. *Circulation* 2001;104:1280–1285.

169. Yu X, Song SK, Chen J, et al. High-resolution MRI characterization of human thrombus using a novel fibrin-targeted paramagnetic nanoparticle contrast agent. *Magn Reson Med* 2000;44:867–872.

170. Halliburton SS, Stillman AE, Flohr T, et al. Do segmented reconstruction algorithms for cardiac multi-slice computed tomography improve image quality? *Herz* 2003;28:20–31.

171. Flohr T, Kuttner A, Bruder H, et al. Performance evaluation of a multi-slice CT system with 16-slice detector and increased gantry rotation speed for isotropic submillimeter imaging of the heart. *Herz* 2003;28:7–19.

172. Hatsukami TS, Ferguson MS, Beach KW, et al. Carotid plaque morphology and clinical events. *Stroke* 1997;28:95–100.

173. Fayad ZA, Fuster V. Clinical imaging of the high-risk or vulnerable atherosclerotic plaque. *Circ Res* 2001;89:305–316.

174. Yuan C, Mitsumori LM, Beach KW, et al. Carotid atherosclerotic plaque: noninvasive MR characterization and identification of vulnerable lesions. *Radiology* 2001;221:285–299.

175. Estes JM, Quist WC, Lo Gerfo FW, et al. Noninvasive characterization of plaque morphology using helical computed tomography. *J Cardiovasc Surg (Torino)* 1998;39:527–534.

176. Oliver TB, Lammie GA, Wright AR, et al. Atherosclerotic plaque at the carotid bifurcation: CT angiographic appearance with histopathologic correlation. *AJNR Am J Neuroradiol* 1999;20:897–901.

177. Porsche C, Walker L, Mendelow AD, et al. Assessment of vessel wall thickness in carotid atherosclerosis using spiral CT angiography. *Eur J Vasc Endovasc Surg* 2002;23:437–440.

178. Comerota AJ, Katz ML, White JV, et al. The preoperative diagnosis of the ulcerated carotid atheroma. *J Vasc Surg* 1990;11:505–510.

179. Toussaint JF, LaMuraglia GM, Southern JF, et al. Magnetic resonance images lipid, fibrous, calcified, hemorrhagic, and thrombotic components of human atherosclerosis in vivo. *Circulation* 1996;94:932–938.

180. Yuan C, Beach KW, Smith LH Jr, et al. Measurement of atherosclerotic carotid plaque size in vivo using high resolution magnetic resonance imaging. *Circulation* 1998;98:2666–2671.

181. Hatsukami TS, Ross R, Polissar NL, et al. Visualization of fibrous cap thickness and rupture in human atherosclerotic carotid plaque in vivo with high-resolution magnetic resonance imaging. *Circulation* 2000;102:959–964.

182. Hayes CE, Mathis CM, Yuan C. Surface coil phased arrays for high-resolution imaging of the carotid arteries. *J Magn Reson Imaging* 1996;6:109–112.

183. Fayad ZA, Nahar T, Fallon JT, et al. In vivo magnetic resonance evaluation of atherosclerotic plaques in the human thoracic aorta: a comparison with transesophageal echocardiography. *Circulation* 2000;101:2503–2509.

184. Fayad ZA, Nahar T, Fallon JT, et al. In vivo MR evaluation of atherosclerotic plaques in the human thoracic aorta: a comparison with TEE. *Circulation* 2000;101:2503–2509.

185. Regenfus M, Ropers D, Achenbach S, et al. Diagnostic value of maximum intensity projections versus source images for assessment of contrast-enhanced three-dimensional breath-hold magnetic resonance coronary angiography. *Invest Radiol* 2003;38:200–206.

186. Plein S, Jones TR, Ridgway JP, et al. Three-dimensional coronary MR angiography performed with subject-specific cardiac acquisition windows and motion-adapted respiratory gating. *AJR Am J Roentgenol* 2003;180:505–512.

187. Watanabe Y, Nagayama M, Amoh Y, et al. High-resolution selective three-dimensional magnetic resonance coronary angiography with navigator-echo technique: segment-by-segment evaluation of coronary artery stenosis. *J Magn Reson Imaging* 2002;16:238–245.

188. Kim WY, Danias PG, Stuber M, et al. Coronary magnetic resonance angiography for the detection of coronary stenoses. *N Engl J Med* 2001;345:1863–1869.

188a. Ropers D, Baum U, Pohle K, et al. Detection of coronary artery stenoses with thin-slice multi-detector row spiral computed tomography and multiplanar reconstruction. *Circulation* 2003;107:664–666.

189. Knez A, Becker CR, Leber A, et al. Usefulness of multislice spiral computed tomography angiography for determination of coronary artery stenoses. *Am J Cardiol* 2001;88:1191–1194.

190. Achenbach S, Ropers D, Regenfus M, et al. Contrast enhanced electron beam computed tomography to analyse the coronary arteries in patients after acute myocardial infarction. *Heart* 2000;84:489–493.

191. Budoff MJ, Oudiz RJ, Zalace CP, et al. Intravenous three-dimensional coronary angiography using contrast enhanced electron beam computed tomography. *Am J Cardiol* 1999;83:840–845.

192. Schmermund A, Rensing BJ, Sheedy PF, et al. Intravenous electron-beam computed tomographic coronary angiography for segmental analysis of coronary artery stenoses. *J Am Coll Cardiol* 1998;31:1547–1554.

193. Nakanishi T, Ito K, Imazu M, et al. Evaluation of coronary artery stenoses using electron-beam CT and multiplanar reformation. *J Comput Assist Tomogr* 1997;21:121–127.

194. Vetter HO, Driever R, Mertens H, et al. Contrast-enhanced magnetic resonance angiography of mammary artery grafts after minimally invasive coronary bypass surgery. *Ann Thorac Surg* 2001;71:1229–1232.

195. Engelmann MG, Knez A, von Smekal A, et al. Non-invasive coronary bypass graft imaging after multivessel revascularisation. *Int J Cardiol* 2000;76:65–74.

196. Molinari G, Sardanelli F, Zandrino F, et al. Value of navigator echo magnetic resonance angiography in detecting occlusion/patency of arterial and venous, single and sequential coronary bypass grafts. *Int J Card Imaging* 2000;16:149–160.

197. Brenner P, Wintersperger B, von Smekal A, et al. Detection of coronary artery bypass graft patency by contrast enhanced magnetic resonance angiography. *Eur J Cardiothorac Surg* 1999;15:389–393.

198. Wintersperger BJ, Engelmann MG, von Smekal A, et al. Patency of coronary bypass grafts: assessment with breath-hold contrast-enhanced MR angiography—value of a non-electrocardiographically triggered technique. *Radiology* 1998;208:345–351.

199. Oudkerk M, van Beek EJ, Wielopolski P, et al. Comparison of contrast-enhanced magnetic resonance angiography and conventional pulmonary angiography for the diagnosis of pulmonary embolism: a prospective study. *Lancet* 2002;359:1643–1647.

200. Goyen M, Ruehm SG, Jagenburg A, et al. Pulmonary arteriovenous malformation: characterization with time-resolved ultrafast 3D MR angiography. *J Magn Reson Imaging* 2001;13:458–460.

201. Kruger S, Haage P, Hoffmann R, et al. Diagnosis of pulmonary arterial hypertension and pulmonary embolism with magnetic resonance angiography. *Chest* 2001;120:1556–1561.

202. Kreitner KF, Ley S, Kauczor HU, et al. [Contrast media enhanced three dimensional MR angiography of the pulmonary arteries in patients with chronic recurrent pulmonary embolism—comparison with selective intra-arterial DSA]. *Rofo Fortschr Geb Rontgenstr Neuen Bildgeb Verfahr* 2000;172:122–128. German.

203. Gupta A, Frazer CK, Ferguson JM, et al. Acute pulmonary embolism: diagnosis with MR angiography. *Radiology* 1999;210:353–359.

204. Perrier A, Howarth N, Didier D, et al. Performance of helical computed tomography in unselected outpatients with suspected pulmonary embolism. *Ann Intern Med* 2001;135:88–97.

205. Blachere H, Latrabe V, Montaudon M, et al. Pulmonary embolism revealed on helical CT angiography: comparison with ventilation-perfusion radionuclide lung scanning. *AJR Am J Roentgenol* 2000;174:1041–1047.

206. Qanadli SD, Hajjam ME, Mesurolle B, et al. Pulmonary embolism detection: prospective evaluation of dual-section helical CT versus selective pulmonary arteriography in 157 patients. *Radiology* 2000;217:447–455.

207. Remy-Jardin M, Remy J, Baghaie F, et al. Clinical value of thin collimation in the diagnostic workup of pulmonary embolism. *AJR Am J Roentgenol* 2000;175:407–411.

208. Kim KI, Muller NL, Mayo JR. Clinically suspected pulmonary embolism: utility of spiral CT. *Radiology* 1999;210:693–697.

209. Johnson MB, Wilkinson ID, Wattam J, et al. Comparison of Doppler ultrasound, magnetic resonance angiographic techniques and catheter angiography in evaluation of carotid stenosis. *Clin Radiol* 2000;55:912–920.

210. Serfaty JM, Chirossel P, Chevallier JM, et al. Accuracy of three-dimensional gadolinium-enhanced MR angiography in the assessment of extracranial carotid artery disease. *AJR Am J Roentgenol* 2000;175:455–463.

211. Sardanelli F, Zandrino F, Parodi RC, et al. MR angiography of internal carotid arteries: breath-hold Gd-enhanced 3D fast imaging with steady-state precession versus unenhanced 2D and 3D time-of-flight techniques. *J Comput Assist Tomogr* 1999;23:208–215.

212. Leclerc X, Martinat P, Godefroy O, et al. Contrast-enhanced three-dimensional fast imaging with steady-state precession (FISP) MR angiography of supraaortic vessels: preliminary results. *AJNR Am J Neuroradiol* 1998;19:1405–1413.

213. Anderson GB, Ashforth R, Steinke DE, et al. CT angiography for the detection and characterization of carotid artery bifurcation disease. *Stroke* 2000;31:2168–2174.

214. Leclerc X, Godefroy O, Lucas C, et al. Internal carotid arterial stenosis: CT angiography with volume rendering. *Radiology* 1999;210:673–682.

215. Marcus CD, Ladam-Marcus VJ, Bigot JL, et al. Carotid arterial stenosis: evaluation at CT angiography with the volume-rendering technique. *Radiology* 1999;211:775–780.

216. Verhoek G, Costello P, Khoo EW, et al. Carotid bifurcation CT angiography: assessment of interactive volume rendering. *J Comput Assist Tomogr* 1999;23:590–596.

217. Magarelli N, Scarabino T, Simeone AL, et al. Carotid stenosis: a com-

parison between MR and spiral CT angiography. *Neuroradiology* 1998;40:367–373.

218. Ruehm SG, Hany TF, Pfammatter T, et al. Pelvic and lower extremity arterial imaging: diagnostic performance of three-dimensional contrast-enhanced MR angiography. *AJR Am J Roentgenol* 2000;174: 1127–1135.

219. Huber A, Heuck A, Baur A, et al. Dynamic contrast-enhanced MR angiography from the distal aorta to the ankle joint with a step-by-step technique. *AJR Am J Roentgenol* 2000;175:1291–1298.

220. Meaney JF, Ridgway JP, Chakraverty S, et al. Stepping-table gadolinium-enhanced digital subtraction MR angiography of the aorta and lower extremity arteries: preliminary experience. *Radiology* 1999;211: 59–67.

221. Sueyoshi E, Sakamoto I, Matsuoka Y, et al. Aortoiliac and lower extremity arteries: comparison of three-dimensional dynamic contrast-enhanced subtraction MR angiography and conventional angiography. *Radiology* 1999;210:683–688.

222. Yamashita Y, Mitsuzaki K, Ogata I, et al. Three-dimensional high-resolution dynamic contrast-enhanced MR angiography of the pelvis and lower extremities with use of a phased array coil and subtraction: diagnostic accuracy. *J Magn Reson Imaging* 1998;8:1066–1072.

223. Ofer A, Nitecki SS, Linn S, et al. Multidetector CT angiography of peripheral vascular disease: a prospective comparison with intraarterial digital subtraction angiography. *AJR Am J Roentgenol* 2003;180: 719–724.

224. Rieker O, Duber C, Neufang A, et al. CT angiography versus intraarterial digital subtraction angiography for assessment of aortoiliac occlusive disease. *AJR Am J Roentgenol* 1997;169:1133–1138.

225. Raptopoulos V, Rosen MP, Kent KC, et al. Sequential helical CT angiography of aortoiliac disease. *AJR Am J Roentgenol* 1996;166: 1347–1354.

226. Lawrence JA, Kim D, Kent KC, et al. Lower extremity spiral CT angiography versus catheter angiography. *Radiology* 1995;194:903–908.

Acute Coronary Syndromes

Pathophysiology and Pathogenesis

CHAPTER 54

Definitions of Acute Coronary Syndromes

Hitinder S. Gurm and Eric J. Topol

Key Words: Acute coronary syndrome; coronary thrombosis; non-ST elevation myocardial infarction; platelet; ST elevation myocardial infarction; unstable angina.

INTRODUCTION

Coronary artery disease (CAD) is the leading cause of death in the western world. It is estimated that 30% of all deaths worldwide can be ascribed to cardiovascular causes, and this percentage is expected to increase further as the incidence of cardiovascular disease (CVD) in the developing world increases secondary to lifestyle changes. Every fifth death in the United States can be directly ascribed to CAD (1). More than 1.1 million people will have a myocardial infarction (MI) in a given year, and nearly 500,000 will suffer sudden cardiac death. According to Centers for Disease Control computations, elimination of all forms of CVD would increase the average life expectancy by almost 7 years (2,3).

H. S. Gurm: F 25, Department of Cardiovascular Medicine, Cleveland Clinic Foundation, Cleveland, Ohio.

E. J. Topol: Department of Cardiovascular Medicine, Cleveland Clinic Foundation, Cleveland, Ohio.

CAD is almost synonymous with atherothrombosis, although a small number of patients will have other underlying etiologic factors. Coronary atherothrombosis can clinically manifest in myriad fashions, ranging from totally asymptomatic to rapidly fatal. Clinically manifest CAD may present as stable angina, acute coronary syndrome (ACS), or sudden cardiac death. This review focuses on the definition of ACS and its various components.

ACUTE CORONARY SYNDROME

ACS is an umbrella term that encompasses patients who have evidence of myonecrosis or are believed to be at high risk for myonecrosis in the immediate future. This term thus covers patients with unstable angina (UA), non-ST elevation myocardial infarction (non-STEMI), and ST elevation myocardial infarction (STEMI) (Fig. 54–1). These patients share a common pathophysiology with key distinctive features that translate into vital differences in therapeutic approach and impart differing prognosis. The concept of ACS provides a simplified diagnosis to approach a patient with chest pain and helps to rationalize therapeutic intervention on the basis of clinical evidence (Fig. 54–2).

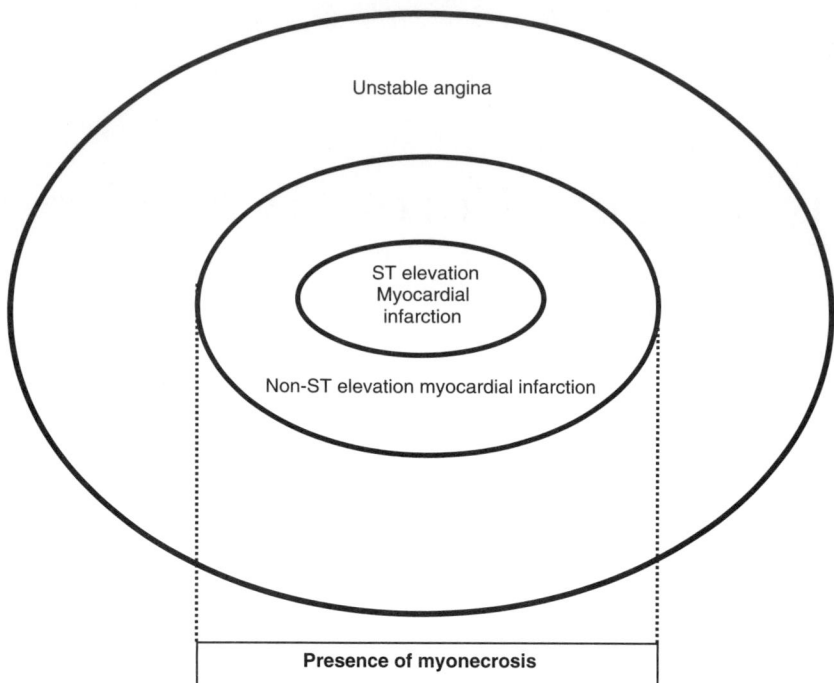

FIG. 54–1. The continuum of acute coronary syndrome.

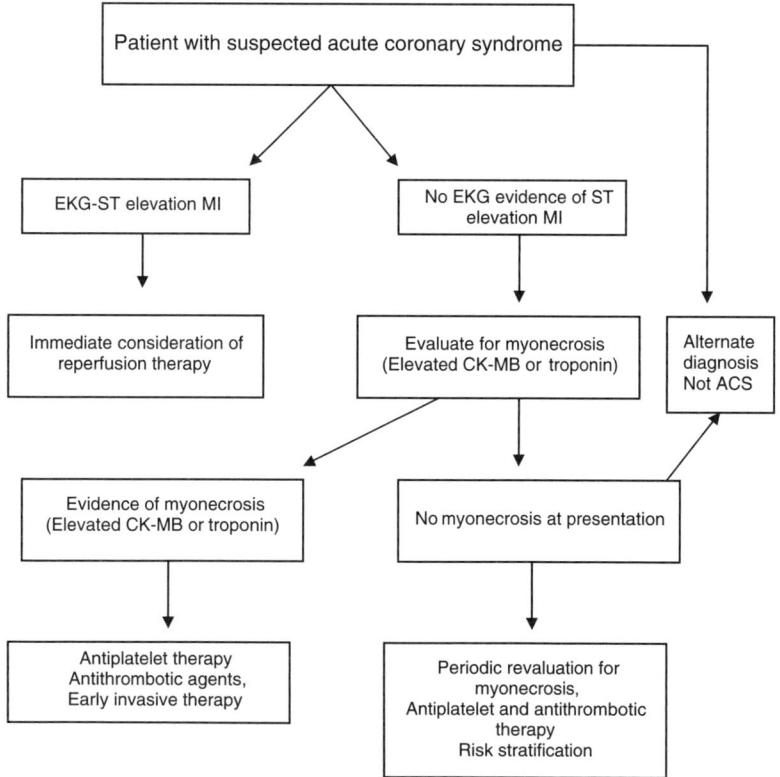

FIG. 54–2. Approach to suspected acute coronary syndrome (ACS). CK-MB, creatinine kinase–MB; EKG, electrocardiogram; MI, myocardial infarction.

DEFINITIONS OF COMPONENTS OF ACUTE CORONARY SYNDROME

Unstable Angina

UA is a syndrome complex that has been variously described as preinfarction angina, intermediate coronary syndrome, and accelerated angina during the early 20th century (4–8). Currently, UA is the more commonly used term and has been defined by the clinical presentation of chest pain that is believed to be of ischemic origin and has one of the three characteristics: (a) rest angina (pain that comes on at rest and is usually prolonged); (b) new-onset severe angina (severe angina is usually used to denote pain of Canadian Cardiovascular Society [CCS] Class III severity); and (c) previously diagnosed angina that is distinctly increasing in frequency or occurring at a lower degree of exertion (increase in angina severity of more than one CCS class to at least CCS III) (9,10). Because of the heterogeneous population of patients that make up UA, these patients often are subclassified based on clinical features that suggest a greater risk for early complications. The commonly used Braunwald classification was initially introduced in 1989 (11) (Table 54–1) and has been subsequently validated in prospective studies as a useful prognosticating tool (12,13).

Non-ST Elevation Myocardial Infarction

Non-STEMI occupies the middle ground between UA and STEMI. It is defined by presence of myonecrosis—either in the shape of increased troponin levels (defined as a value greater than 99th percentile of a reference control group) or creatinine kinase–MB isoenzyme increase (defined as a value exceeding the 99th percentile of a reference control group) and absence of electrocardiographic (ECG) changes suggestive of STEMI (9,10,14).

ST Elevation Myocardial Infarction

STEMI is defined by the occurrence of new or presumed new ST elevation in two or more contiguous leads that is 0.2 mV or greater in leads V_1, V_2, and V_3 and greater than 0.1 mV in other leads or the occurrence of a new-onset left bundle branch block (14). These patients usually have ongoing occlusion of an epicardial coronary artery and need consideration of immediate reperfusion therapy. Presence of pathologic Q waves is a marker of established MI and usually follows STEMI when reperfusion does not occur in a timely fashion. Some patients with non-STEMI also will develop Q waves and other patients will present with Q waves without a clear history of ACS. A pathologic Q wave is defined as any Q wave in V_1–V_3 or any Q wave in any other two contiguous leads 30 ms or longer and 1 mm or more in depth (14).

Pathophysiology

ACS is the clinical reflection of MI. The pathogenesis of MI and its triggers is discussed in detail in Chapters 54 through 57, but this chapter briefly summarizes pathologic factors that underlie ACS and are determinants of its specific presentations. Patients with ACS have one or more of the following underlying etiologic factors: (a) a nonocclusive or an occlusive thrombus on a preexisting plaque, (b) vasoconstriction or dynamic obstruction, (c) progressive mechanical obstruction, (d) inflammation, and (e) secondary UA (10, 15,16).

Supply/Demand Mismatch

The supply/demand mismatch of blood supply and balance may be caused by limitation of supply, an increase in demand, or commonly both. The patients with predominantly

TABLE 54–1. *Braunwald classification of unstable angina*

Severity	Classification circumstances		
	A. Develops in presence of extracardiac condition that intensifies myocardial ischemia (secondary UA)	B. Develops in absence of extracardiac condition (primary UA)	C. Develops within 2 weeks after AMI (postinfarction UA)
I. New onset of severe angina or accelerated angina; no rest pain	IA	IB	IC
II. Angina at rest within past month but not within preceding 48 h (angina at rest, subacute)	IIA	IIB	IIC
III. Angina at rest within 48 h (angina at rest, acute)	IIIA	IIIB	IIIC

Patients with unstable angina (UA) may also be divided into three groups depending on whether UA occurs (a) in the absence of treatment for chronic stable angina, (b) during treatment for chronic stable angina, or (c) despite maximal antiischemic drug therapy. These three groups may be designed by subscripts 1, 2, or 3, respectively. Patients with UA may be further divided into those with and without transient ST–T-wave changes during pain.
AMI, acute myocardial infarction.
From Braunwald E. Unstable angina. A classification. *Circulation* 1989;80:410–414.

an increase in oxygen demand typically in the background of a fixed coronary stenosis usually have Braunwald Class I UA. There is frequently a secondary cause that may precipitate such an event, and some of these causes are listed in Table 54–2. MI is rarely caused by such a supply/demand mismatch and is more likely to be secondary to atherothrombosis. However, in rare cases, some of the above listed causes or other pathologies may lead to a MI (Table 54–3).

Atherothrombosis

Most cases of ACS have atherothrombotic coronary occlusion as the underlying mechanism of myocardial ischaemia. The inciting event in this cascade is plaque disruption, which with its attendant superimposed thrombosis and associated vasoconstriction impairs coronary perfusion and may be complicated by distal embolization. The association of intimal disruption and thrombosis with MI was recognized approximately 70 years ago (17).The association was strongly contested in the following years and even the veritable Osler's textbook of medicine in its bicentennial edition cast doubt on the validity of this association (18).

> It is often called coronary occlusion, but as in occasional patient no obstruction of a coronary artery can be found, and in another there is occlusion but no infarct and no symptoms, and since symptoms are caused more directly by the myocardial than coronary lesion, it is preferable to use the term, cardiac infarction.

Subsequently, better autopsy techniques and meticulously carried out studies demonstrated coronary thrombi in most patients with fatal MI (19). Intimal rupture with plaque hemorrhage and superimposed intraluminal thrombosis was confirmed to underlie most cases of MI.

A postmortem study of 77 coronary lesions demonstrated that lesion with histologic evidence of rupture, hemorrhage, and thrombosis demonstrated irregular borders and intraluminal lucency, thus providing an angiographic surrogate of an

TABLE 54–2. *Secondary precipitants of myocardial ischemia*

Increased myocardial oxygen demand
- Fever
- Thyrotoxicosis
- Tachycardia
- Malignant hypertension
- Pheochromocytoma
- Aortic stenosis
- High-output state
- Pregnancy
- Drugs: cocaine, amphetamine

Decreased oxygen supply
- Anemia
- Hypoxemia
- Carbon monoxide poisoning
- Polycythemia vera
- Hyperviscosity syndromes

TABLE 54–3. *Causes of myocardial infarction in patients without atherothrombosis*

Nonatherothrombotic coronary occlusion
- Spasm-Prinzmetal's angina
- Aortic dissection with coronary ostial involvement
- Coronary artery dissection
- Anomalous coronary artery origin

Embolization
- Endocarditis
- Cardiac myxoma
- Cardiac thromboembolism (prosthetic valve, atrial fibrillation, left ventricle or atrial thrombus)
- Iatrogenic during coronary artery catheterization (air, thrombus, atheroma)

Inadequate myocardial oxygenation
- Carbon monoxide poisoning
- Sustained hypotension

Others
- Arteritis
- Trauma
- Cocaine

unstable plaque (20). This association was subsequently confirmed by Ambrose and colleagues (21), and angiographic evidence of lesion complexity provided a surrogate of plaque instability.

Whereas earlier studies of UA suggested a fixed thrombotic occlusion secondary to plaque disruption, studies done in the 1970s suggested a pivotal role for vasospasm induced by platelet aggregation (22,23). Demonstration of amelioration of these changes with aspirin (22) in dogs suggested a potential role for prostaglandin metabolism, and a role for aspirin as a therapeutic agent was hypothesized. Hirsh and colleagues (24) demonstrated increased production of thromboxane in the coronary beds of patients with UA, whereas other authors demonstrated an increase in tissue serotonin, suggesting a role for platelet-mediated vasospasm in UA (25).

In an autopsy study of 25 cases of MI, Falk demonstrated a layered structure of the thrombus, suggesting episodes of thrombosis with progressive luminal encroachment and a final occlusive thrombus in a majority of patients. Furthermore, most patients had evidence of platelet microembolization distal to the thrombus, suggesting a period of thrombus instability and spontaneous fragmentation (26).

It was speculated that all patients with ACS have luminal obstruction, and patients with UA and non-STEMI differed from STEMI in early spontaneous restoration of flow (27). Based on animal models, a flow occlusion of less than 20 minutes was considered to cause UA, 20 minutes to 2 hours caused non–Q-wave MI, and greater than 2 hour caused Q-wave MI (28–30). On the basis of these lines of evidence, it can be argued that ACS spectrum can be pathologically explained by plaque instability that does not cause necrosis on one end of the spectrum but does cause total occlusion and ST elevation on the other end. Patients who have delayed spontaneous restoration of flow and those who have small amount of myocardial necrosis caused by microembolization lie between these two extremes. Patients with UA may have nonocclusive thrombi with limited or no embolization in the presence of a disrupted plaque that leads to a reduction in myocardial perfusion and produce chest pain (31). Transient vasoocclusion by either thrombosis or secondary to platelet-mediated vasoconstrictors may explain the waxing and waning nature of chest pain. In patients with non–Q-wave MI, the occlusion is more prolonged and by definition is associated with irreversible cell death. The degree of myonecrosis is limited, however, by spontaneous recanalization or presence of collaterals (31,32). Some patients with patent epicardial vessels and evidence of myonecrosis have areas of microinfarcts probably secondary to microembolization. STEMI is almost always secondary to a totally occluded vessel that provides total or near-total cessation of flow to the distal myocardial bed. The atherothrombotic plaque associated with ACS is angiographically usually a minor to moderate plaque, suggesting that it is the acute process associated with plaque disruption and superimposed thrombosis that is responsible for the morbidity and mortality associated with coronary atherothrombosis (33,34).

It, however, remains unclear as to why the severity of plaque rupture or the thrombotic response shows such variability in different patients. The thrombotic response does not follow any correlation to the degree of plaque rupture (28,35). Patients with large ulcerative plaque lesions often demonstrate flat nonocclusive thrombi, whereas minimal fissures can be associated with a large thrombotic burden. Furthermore, most occlusive thrombi appear to develop in a layered fashion (26,28), although the nature of the final occlusive layer and factors that precipitate it remain ill defined. In a German autopsy study, it was demonstrated that 85% of the occlusive thrombi were rich in fibrin and red blood cells, whereas 15% were pure platelet thrombi (36). Extrusion of plaque components was usually associated with a fibrin-rich or a mixed thrombus (35–37).

Angioscopic studies also have corroborated and extended such findings. In a study by Sherman and colleagues (38) of 10 patients with stable angina and 10 patients with UA, patients with accelerated angina had complex plaque and those with rest pain had evidence of thrombosis. Such findings were not seen in patients with stable angina. In another angioscopic study from Japan, Mizuo and colleagues (39,40) demonstrated that the thrombus in UA was more likely to be a pale or a grey thrombus (suggesting predominantly platelet origin), whereas in those with acute MI it was more likely to a red thrombus. A larger study from the same group demonstrated occlusive thrombi in those with MI and nonocclusive thrombi in those with UA. Further plaque associated with ACS was more likely to be xanthomatous and ulcerative (41).

This would suggest that the coagulation pathway is more likely to be activated in patients with STEMI. This may be related to the nature of the plaque component exposed to the lumen at time of plaque disruption. Lipid-rich core is more likely to express tissue factor (42), and inhibition of tissue factor reduced platelet and thrombin deposition at site of plaque rupture (43). Patients with MI (44) or UA (45) are more likely to express tissue factor activity in their plaques as compared with patients with stable angina. Furthermore, plasma levels of tissue factor have been demonstrated to be greater in patients with UA or MI (46) as compared with patients with stable angina or healthy control subjects (47). Although this provides a putative link to coagulation activation, tissue factor by virtue of its platelet-activating effects cannot be solely used to explain the red clot. The factors that determine why one specific plaque rupture leads to red clot whereas another does not remain to be fully elucidated (35).

These findings would suggest that UA is more likely to respond to antiplatelet therapy, whereas STEMI responds to fibrinolytic agents. This has been borne out in numerous clinical studies. Use of fibrinolytic therapy fails to provide angiographic improvement in UA (48,49), although it provided life-saving thrombolysis in those patients with ST elevation MI (50–54). Similarly, patients with non-STEMI, given their underlying platelet-based thrombi and microemboli, would be expected to benefit from potent platelet inhibition, as has been borne out in studies of glycoprotein IIb/IIIa inhibition (55) and clopidogrel (56).

Serologic Evidence of Thrombosis in Acute Coronary Syndrome

Although it is customary to measure markers of myonecrosis to provide risk stratification of patients with ACS, other researchers have investigated differences in markers of thrombosis and inflammation in patients with ACS. The association between increase in tissue factor and clinical presentation in ACS has been discussed earlier. In a small study, Soejima and colleagues (57) demonstrated an association between higher tissue factor and need for revascularization in patients with chest pain. A provocative study from France found that monocyte-associated tissue factor activity was increased in patients with UA compared with those with MI or stable angina pectoris. This may suggest that different inflammatory components have differing roles across the spectrum of ACS (58). Other investigators have focused on fibrinopeptide A—a polypeptide cleaved from fibrinogen as it is cleaved to fibrin by thrombin—and prothrombin fragments 1+2 (F1+2) as markers of thrombosis. In separate studies, the levels of both fibrinopeptide A and F1+2 were greater in patients with ACS when compared with control subjects (59–63).

CLINICAL SPECTRUM

Demographics

The demographic spectrum of ACS is difficult to define because the definition of various components has undergone changes with time. Studies that enroll across the spectrum of ACS are more useful but do not provide a complete picture secondary to predefined exclusion criteria and selection bias associated with clinical trials. Since routine determination of troponin is a more recent phenomenon, patients with UA in earlier studies have a worse outcome secondary to inclusion of those who are likely to have troponin level increase and a correspondingly increased mortality hazard. Comparing patients enrolled in Global Use of Strategies to Open Occluded Coronary Arteries (GUSTO) IIb trial of ACS, those with ST elevation were younger and more likely to be men, less likely to have prior MI or coronary revascularization, and had a greater incidence of previously diagnosed diabetes, hypertension, and hyperlipidemia (64). However, there was no difference in clinical severity as determined by the Killip class.

Studies that have focused on non-ST segment ACS provide a glimpse of the other end of the spectrum. In a secondary analysis of the Thrombolysis in Myocardial Ischemia (TIMI) IIIB trial, Antman and colleagues (65) demonstrated a worse prognosis in non-ST elevation ACS in those with troponin level increase compared with those with no evidence of myonecrosis. No difference in age, race, or sex was noted, but patients with troponin level increase were less likely to have previously diagnosed angina, hypertension, or MI. They were, however, more likely to have more extensive ECG changes (65).

Coronary Anatomy

Angiographic assessment of coronary arteries in patients with ACS has confirmed the role played by plaque disruption and thrombosis (21,33,34). Patients with UA often have more extensive disease, with some studies reporting up to 50% of patients having three-vessel disease and another 35% having two-vessel disease (66). A study from the Veterans Affairs Non-Q-Wave Infarction Strategies in-Hospital (VANQWISH) core laboratory found that a single-culprit lesion could be identified in only 49% of patients, whereas 37% of patients had no identifiable culprit (37%) and 14% had multiple apparent culprit lesions. Furthermore, an isolated incomplete occlusion of the infarct-related artery was found in 36% of patients, and a single acute occlusion of the infarct-related artery was found in 13%. Patients without an identifiable culprit lesion had severe diffuse CAD but lacked complex lesion morphology (67). An earlier study by DeWood and coworkers (68) suggested that the incidence of coronary occlusion was greater in patients studied later after non–Q-wave MI and approached 40% in those studies after 72 hours of symptom onset. A study by Keen and colleagues (69) compared patients with Q-wave and non–Q-wave MI who were studied within 6 hours of symptom onset. Patients with Q-wave MI were more likely to have thrombus (84% vs. 43%) and complete occlusion (91% vs. 39%), but they were less likely to have collaterals feeding the infarct-related vessel as compared with those patients with a non–Q-wave MI. Investigators at Rush Heart Institute compared a cohort of patients who had angiography performed before and after MI and found that subsequent non–Q-wave

MI occurred at sites of either minimal luminal narrowing or nonulcerated severe stenosis. Q-wave MIs, in contrast, occurred at the site of a moderate eccentric and ulcerated stenosis (70).

Studies using intravascular ultrasound (IVUS) have demonstrated that patients with unstable clinical presentation have larger plaque and are more likely to have positive remodeling (71). A small study from Japan demonstrated that the degree of positive remodeling showed a gradient being maximum in patients with acute MI, intermediate in those with UA, and least in patients with stable CAD (72). Another study demonstrated greater volume of soft plaque in patients with MI as compared with those with UA (73).

Treatment and Outcome

The treatment of UA and MI is discussed in greater length in Chapters 65 through 70. This review focuses on key similarities and differences in approach based on the pathophysiology of ACS.

Pathophysiology-based Medical Therapy

The key pathologic chains in ACS involve plaque disruption, thrombosis, vasoconstriction, and embolization. The success of preventing plaque disruption as evident by treatment of hyperlipidemia impacts on the entire spectrum of ACS. Randomization to simvastatin in the Heart Protection Study (HPS) was associated with a significant reduction in death, fatal or nonfatal MI, need for coronary or peripheral revascularization, and hospitalization for UA (74). Similar benefits of modification of coronary risk factors can be expected to impact across the entire spectrum of ACS.

Antiplatelet and Antithrombotic Therapy

Platelets and the coagulation cascade are central to the thrombotic response associated with ACS. Given the preeminence of platelets in ACS, platelet suppression plays a key role in treatment across the entire spectrum of ACS (75).

Aspirin

Aspirin is the oldest known inhibitor of platelet action. Its usefulness has been demonstrated across the entire spectrum of ACS. A Veteran's Administration study found that aspirin use decreases the risk for death or MI in patients with UA by almost 50% (76). In a Canadian study of 555 men with UA, aspirin was associated with a similar significant reduction in both death and MI (77). Another Canadian study compared heparin with aspirin and found similar benefits from either as compared with placebo in a cohort of men with UA (78). Similar marked benefits of aspirin were demonstrated in acute MI by the Second International Study of Infarct Survival (ISIS-2) investigators (79).

Thienopyridines

In a large trial of UA/non-STEMI, 12,562 patients were randomized to clopidogrel or placebo in addition to aspirin (56). There was a 20% relative reduction in the composite of death, MI, or stroke, although there was a slight excess of bleeding complication in patients receiving clopidogrel. The role of clopidogrel in STEMI remains to be defined. It is commonly administered to patients undergoing primary percutaneous coronary intervention (PCI) who are anticipated to undergo intracoronary stenting. There are no data supporting or refuting its use in combination with fibrinolytic therapy.

Glycoprotein IIb/IIIa Inhibitors

The use of glycoprotein IIb/IIIa inhibitors in the setting of UA/non-STEMI was studied in seven large trials (c7E3 Fab Antiplatelet Therapy in Unstable Refractory Angina [CAPTURE] [80], Platelet Receptor Inhibition in Ischemic Syndrome Management [PRISM] [81], Platelet Receptor Inhibition in Ischemic Syndrome Management in Patients Limited by Unstable Signs and Symptoms [PRISM-PLUS] [82], Platelet Glycoprotein IIb/IIIa in Unstable Angina: Receptor Suppression Using Integrilin Therapy [PURSUIT] [83], Platelet IIb/IIIa Antagonism for the Reduction of Acute coronary syndrome events in a Global Organization Network [PARAGON-A] [84], PARAGON B [85] and GUSTO IV [86]). Use of abciximab in GUSTO IV was associated with an increase in adverse outcome, whereas use of small molecules in other trials was associated with a modest reduction in death and recurrent MI. Further analysis demonstrated that the benefits of glycoprotein IIb/IIIa inhibitors were more evident in patients with increased troponin levels (87,88), patients undergoing PCI (55,89), or patients with diabetes (90). Use of these agents in combination with fibrinolytics was initially tested in two pilot studies in patients with STEMI (91,92). Although improved angiographic outcome was evident, in larger studies this did not translate into a mortality benefit (50,53), although consistent reduction in key secondary ischemic end points was noted. Thus, these agents are specifically of value in patients with non-STEMI where platelet aggregation and microembolization play such a vital role and are of limited value in patients with UA. This may be related to that degree of inhibition associated with use of aspirin and heparin may be sufficient to calm the relatively lesser degree of platelet activation, and the added benefit of further platelet inhibition would not translate into reduction in adverse clinical events. The patients with STEMI, however, have clear evidence of reduction in important clinical end points when these agents are used in combination with fibrinolytics or in the setting of primary PCI (93).

Antithrombins

Antithrombin agents are routinely used in the treatment of ACS. Heparin, the first agent to be used, was demonstrated in patients with UA to be superior to placebo in preventing recurrent MI or death (78). A metaanalysis of number of smaller studies suggested a trend toward improved clinical course in patients randomized to heparin and aspirin compared with those randomized to aspirin alone (94). Heparin is commonly used in addition to glycoprotein IIb/IIIa inhibitors, and its role was supported by the increased mortality noted in the tirofiban alone arm of PRISM-PLUS. Heparin is also routinely used in addition to fibrinolytic therapy and appears to be most efficacious when the PTT is maintained between 50 and 70 seconds (95). The role of heparin in patients receiving streptokinase is less well established given the increased bleeding complications associated with its use in Gruppo Italiano per lo Studio della Sopravvivenza nell'Infarto Miocardico (GISSI) II and ISIS-III studies (96,97).

Low–Molecular Weight Heparin

Studies of low–molecular weight heparin (LMWH) in UA/non-STEMI have produced mixed results. Although the benefit of these agents over placebo was established in the Fragmin during Instability in Coronary Artery Disease (FRISC) trial (98), trials comparing LMWH with unfractionated heparin have produced more mixed results. Two trials of enoxaparin suggest beneficial reduction in clinical end points (99,100) whereas a metaanalysis of five trials did not find a benefit of LWMH over unfractionated heparin (101). Increased troponin levels identified patients who appeared to benefit from dalteparin in FRISC study (102). There is limited data on use of LMWH in patients with STEMI. Assessment of the Safety and Efficacy of a New Thrombolytic Regimen (ASSENT)-III randomized patients to enoxaparin, heparin, or abciximab in addition to tenecteplase and demonstrated improved clinical outcome in patients randomized to enoxaparin (50) compared with those randomized to unfractionated heparin.

Fibrinolytic Therapy

The response of patients with ACS to fibrinolytic therapy is markedly influenced by the specific presentation of ACS. Although such therapy has been clearly demonstrated to be life saving in patients with STEMI (50–52,79,96,97), most studies indicate a trend toward worse outcome in patients with UA/non-STEMI (103). This can be explained based on the lack of fibrin preponderance in the thrombosis associated with UA/non-STEMI and paradoxic platelet stimulation associated with fibrinolytics that translate into lack of efficacy and increased propensity to local thrombosis with its attendant increased risk for MI and death. As previously discussed, STEMI is associated with red clot that is fibrin rich and thus forms an ideal substrate for a fibrinolytic agent.

OUTCOME

The outcome of ACS is dependent both on the hemodynamic impact of the presenting event and the premorbid state. Although it is difficult to compare outcomes across trials, some useful assumptions can be made from major studies. Studies of glycoprotein IIb/IIIa inhibition in UA/non-STEMI provide a comparison of patients with and without myonecrosis. The incidence of death or MI varies between trials secondary to difference in the inclusion criteria and is usually less than in patients in the community (Fig. 54–3). In a metaanalysis of six trials of glycoprotein IIb/IIIa inhibitors in ACS, Boersma and colleagues (55) described a 1.2% mortality rate at 5 days and a 3.6% mortality rate at 30 days among a cohort of 31,402 patients from 41 countries. The mortality associated with STEMI also varies on the basis of enrollment criteria of different trials. The GUSTO V trial with a 30-day mortality rate of 5.9% in the reteplase group and 5.6% in the arm randomized to a combination of abciximab and half-dose reteplase had one of the lowest mortality rates ever reported in a clinical trial. The 1-year mortality rate in the earlier GUSTO I (104) and III (105) trials has ranged from 9% to 11%. The mortality rate at 1 year in GUSTO V (STEMI) was 8.38% (106), whereas in GUSTO IV (non-STEMI ACS) it was 8.3% (107), suggesting that although the two ends of ACS have differing early hazards of mortality, the long-term hazard of mortality is relatively similar. The decrease in mortality seen in GUSTO V compared with the earlier GUSTO trials may be secondary to either difference in patient population or improved outcome associated with better secondary prevention.

Data from the community is more representative of a wider patient population but is confounded by absence of rigid quality control and adjudication of end points common to clinical trials. The Global Registry of Acute Coronary Events (GRACE) has collected data from 11,543 patients enrolled in 14 countries (108). The inhouse mortality rate among patients with STEMI was 7%, whereas it was 6% in patients with non-STEMI, and 3% in patients with UA. These data, however, reflect wide differences in practice and do not represent current state of the art (109). Similarly, data from the National Registry of Myocardial Infarction 1, 2, and 3 suggest that the prevalence of non–Q-wave MI has increased from 45% to 63% of all patients with MI between 1994 and 1999. The inhospital mortality in this group is much greater being of the order of 11.2% in the early 1990s and declining to 9.4% in 1999 (110). These high mortality rates highlight the grave burden imposed by ACS and suggest the need for ongoing efforts to develop better therapeutic interventions and better deployment of the current therapeutic armamentarium.

SUMMARY

The term ACS has served the purpose of unifying a group of patients with similar pathophysiology and therapy, but it also has introduced an element of confusion. The continuum of ACS shares a common pathogenesis and a similar risk factor profile. The short-term risk associated with ACS increases as the severity of ischemic injury reflected by myonecrosis increases. There are three distinct components of ACS: UA, non-STEMI, and STEMI. The difference in the preeminence of platelet in non-STEMI ACS versus fibrin-rich clot in STEMI translates into differing response to fibrinolytic therapy. The increased age of patients with non-STEMI associated with a greater preponderance of comorbidities and more extensive CAD translates into equalization of long-term mortality associated with ACS. Increasing use of proven preventive agents such as aspirin and statins and better risk factor modification may be shifting the pendulum of ACS from

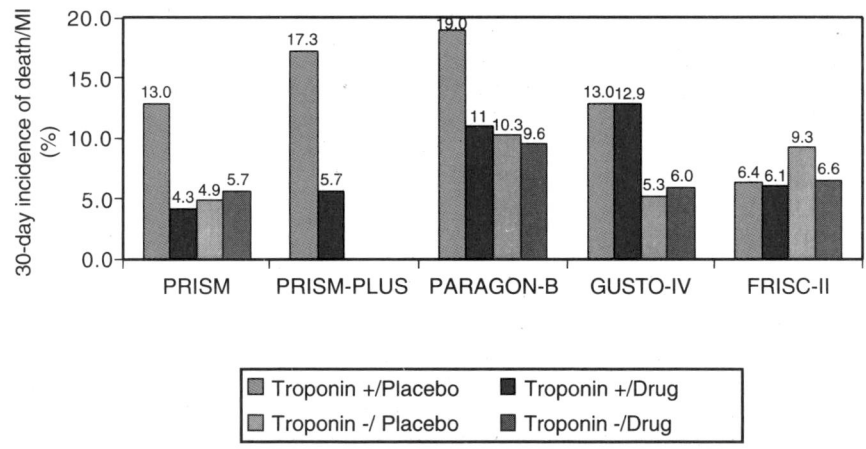

FIG. 54–3. Thirty-day incidence of death/myocardial infarction (MI) in five recent trials in patients with non-ST elevation acute coronary syndrome. FRISC, Fragmin during Instability in Coronary Artery Disease; GUSTO, Global Use of Strategies to Open Occluded Coronary Arteries; PARAGON, Platelet IIb/IIIa Antagonism for the Reduction of Acute coronary syndrome events in a Global Organization Network; PRISM, Platelet Receptor Inhibition in Ischemic Syndrome Management; PRISM-PLUS, Platelet Receptor Inhibition in Ischemic Syndrome Management in Patients Limited by Unstable Signs and Symptoms.

STEMI to a preponderance of non-STEMI ACS. Given the economic and social burden associated with ACS, efforts must be continued to better delineate patients with varying pathogenesis and prognosis within the subgroups of ACS to better target therapeutic interventions. Better definition of similarities and differences across this spectrum will facilitate research and help provide better clinical care that translates into better clinical outcomes.

REFERENCES

1. American Heart Association. *Heart disease and stroke statistics—2004 update* [accessed January 6, 2003]. Dallas, TX: American Heart Association; 2003. Available at: http://www.americanheart.org/presenter.jhtml?identifier=1928.
2. Anderson RN. US decennial life tables for 1989-91, vol 1 no 4, United States life tables eliminating certain causes of death [accessed March 10, 2003]. National Center for Health Statistics. Hyattsville, MD; 1999. Available at: http://www.cdc.gov/nchs/data/lifetables/life89_1_4.pdf.
3. Anderson RN. US decennial life tables for 1989-91, vol 1 no 4, United States life tables eliminating certain causes of death. National Center for Health Statistics. Hyattsville, MD; 1999.
4. Sampson JJ, Eliaser M. The diagnosis of impending acute coronary artery occlusion. *Am Heart J* 1937;13:675.
5. Levy H. The natural history of changing patterns of angina pectoris. *Ann Intern Med* 1956;44:1123.
6. Beamish RE, Storrie VM. Impending myocardial infarction: recognition and management. *Circulation* 1960;21:1107.
7. Vakil RJ. Intermediate coronary syndrome. *Circulation* 1961;24:557.
8. Wood P. Acute and subacute coronary insufficiency. *Br Med J* 1961;1:1779.
9. Braunwald E, Antman EM, Beasley JW, et al. ACC/AHA guidelines for the management of patients with unstable angina and non-ST-segment elevation myocardial infarction. A report of the American College of Cardiology/American Heart Association Task Force on Practice Guidelines (Committee on the Management of Patients With Unstable Angina). *J Am Coll Cardiol* 2000;36:970–1062.
10. Braunwald E, Antman EM, Beasley JW, et al. ACC/AHA guidelines for the management of patients with unstable angina and non-ST-segment elevation myocardial infarction: executive summary and recommendations. A report of the American College of Cardiology/American Heart Association task force on practice guidelines (Committee on the Management of Patients With Unstable Angina). *Circulation* 2000;102:1193–1209.
11. Braunwald E. Unstable angina. A classification. *Circulation* 1989;80:410–414.
12. Calvin JE, Klein LW, VandenBerg BJ, et al. Risk stratification in unstable angina. Prospective validation of the Braunwald classification. *JAMA* 1995;273:136–141.
13. Ahmed WH, Bittl JA, Braunwald E. Relation between clinical presentation and angiographic findings in unstable angina pectoris, and comparison with that in stable angina. *Am J Cardiol* 1993;72:544–550.
14. Alpert JS, Thygesen K, Antman E, et al. Myocardial infarction redefined—a consensus document of The Joint European Society of Cardiology/American College of Cardiology Committee for the redefinition of myocardial infarction. *J Am Coll Cardiol* 2000;36:959–969.
15. Braunwald E, Califf RM, Cannon CP, et al. Redefining medical treatment in the management of unstable angina. *Am J Med* 2000;108:41–53.
16. Hamm CW, Braunwald E. A classification of unstable angina revisited. *Circulation* 2000;102:118–122.
17. Saphir O, Priest WS, Hamburger WW, et al. Coronary arteriosclerosis, coronary thrombosis, and the resulting myocardial changes: an evaluation of their respective clinical pictures including the electrocardiographic records, based on the anatomical findings. *Am Heart J* 1935;10:567–595.
18. Christian HA. Cardiac (myocardial) infarction. In: *The principles and practice of medicine,* 14th ed. New York: D. Appleton-Century Company, 1942:1091.
19. Chandler AB, Chapman I, Erhardt LR, et al. Coronary thrombosis in myocardial infarction. Report of a workshop on the role of coronary thrombosis in the pathogenesis of acute myocardial infarction. *Am J Cardiol* 1974;34:823–833.
20. Levin DC, Fallon JT. Significance of the angiographic morphology of localized coronary stenoses: histopathologic correlations. *Circulation* 1982;66:316–320.
21. Ambrose JA, Winters SL, Stern A, et al. Angiographic morphology and the pathogenesis of unstable angina pectoris. *J Am Coll Cardiol* 1985;5:609–616.
22. Folts JD, Crowell EB Jr, Rowe GG. Platelet aggregation in partially obstructed vessels and its elimination with aspirin. *Circulation* 1976;54:365–370.
23. Maseri A, L'Abbate A, Baroldi G, et al. Coronary vasospasm as a possible cause of myocardial infarction. A conclusion derived from the study of "preinfarction" angina. *N Engl J Med* 1978;299:1271–1277.
24. Hirsh PD, Hillis LD, Campbell WB, et al. Release of prostaglandins and thromboxane into the coronary circulation in patients with ischemic heart disease. *N Engl J Med* 1981;304:685–691.
25. Ashton JH, Benedict CR, Fitzgerald C, et al. Serotonin as a mediator of cyclic flow variations in stenosed canine coronary arteries. *Circulation* 1986;73:572–578.
26. Falk E. Unstable angina with fatal outcome: dynamic coronary thrombosis leading to infarction and/or sudden death. Autopsy evidence of recurrent mural thrombosis with peripheral embolization culminating in total vascular occlusion. *Circulation* 1985;71:699–708.
27. Gorlin R, Fuster V, Ambrose JA. Anatomic-physiologic links between acute coronary syndromes. *Circulation* 1986;74:6–9.
28. Davies MJ, Thomas AC. Plaque fissuring—the cause of acute myocardial infarction, sudden ischaemic death, and crescendo angina. *Br Heart J* 1985;53:363–373.
29. Willerson JT, Hillis LD, Winniford M, et al. Speculation regarding mechanisms responsible for acute ischemic heart disease syndromes. *J Am Coll Cardiol* 1986;8:245–250.
30. Reimer KA, Lowe JE, Rasmussen MM, et al. The wavefront phenomenon of ischemic cell death. 1. Myocardial infarct size vs duration of coronary occlusion in dogs. *Circulation* 1977;56:786–794.
31. Fuster V, Badimon L, Badimon JJ, et al. The pathogenesis of coronary artery disease and the acute coronary syndromes (2). *N Engl J Med* 1992;326:310–318.
32. Fuster V, Badimon L, Badimon JJ, et al. The pathogenesis of coronary artery disease and the acute coronary syndromes (1). *N Engl J Med* 1992;326:242–250.
33. Ambrose JA, Tannenbaum MA, Alexopoulos D, et al. Angiographic progression of coronary artery disease and the development of myocardial infarction. *J Am Coll Cardiol* 1988;12:56–62.
34. Ambrose JA, Winters SL, Arora RR, et al. Angiographic evolution of coronary artery morphology in unstable angina. *J Am Coll Cardiol* 1986;7:472–478.
35. Rentrop KP. Thrombi in acute coronary syndromes: revisited and revised. *Circulation* 2000;101:1619–1626.
36. Sinapius D. [Morphology of occlusive coronary thrombi. Localization, length, composition, growth]. *Dtsch Med Wochenschr* 1972;97:544–546. German.
37. Sinapius D. [Relationship between coronary-artery thrombosis and myocardial infarction]. *Dtsch Med Wochenschr* 1972;97:443–448. German.
38. Sherman CT, Litvack F, Grundfest W, et al. Coronary angioscopy in patients with unstable angina pectoris. *N Engl J Med* 1986;315:913–919.
39. Mizuno K, Hikita H, Miyamoto A, et al. The pathogenesis of an impending infarction and its treatment—an angioscopic analysis. *Jpn Circ J* 1992;56:1160–1165.
40. Mizuno K, Satomura K, Miyamoto A, et al. Angioscopic evaluation of coronary-artery thrombi in acute coronary syndromes. *N Engl J Med* 1992;326:287–291.
41. Mizuno K, Miyamoto A, Satomura K, et al. Angioscopic coronary macromorphology in patients with acute coronary disorders. *Lancet* 1991;337:809–812.
42. Toschi V, Gallo R, Lettino M, et al. Tissue factor modulates the thrombogenicity of human atherosclerotic plaques. *Circulation* 1997;95:594–599.
43. Badimon JJ, Lettino M, Toschi V, et al. Local inhibition of tissue factor reduces the thrombogenicity of disrupted human atherosclerotic plaques: effects of tissue factor pathway inhibitor on plaque thrombogenicity under flow conditions. *Circulation* 1999;99:1780–1787.

44. Ardissino D, Merlini PA, Ariens R, et al. Tissue-factor antigen and activity in human coronary atherosclerotic plaques. *Lancet* 1997;349: 769–771.

45. Annex BH, Denning SM, Channon KM, et al. Differential expression of tissue factor protein in directional atherectomy specimens from patients with stable and unstable coronary syndromes. *Circulation* 1995; 91:619–622.

46. Suefuji H, Ogawa H, Yasue H, et al. Increased plasma tissue factor levels in acute myocardial infarction. *Am Heart J* 1997;134:253–259.

47. Misumi K, Ogawa H, Yasue H, et al. Comparison of plasma tissue factor levels in unstable and stable angina pectoris. *Am J Cardiol* 1998;81:22–26.

48. Early effects of tissue-type plasminogen activator added to conventional therapy on the culprit coronary lesion in patients presenting with ischemic cardiac pain at rest. Results of the Thrombolysis in Myocardial Ischemia (TIMI IIIA) Trial. *Circulation* 1993;87:38–52.

49. Rentrop P, Blanke H, Karsch KR, et al. Selective intracoronary thrombolysis in acute myocardial infarction and unstable angina pectoris. *Circulation* 1981;63:307–317.

50. Assessment of the Safety and Efficacy of a New Thrombolytic Regimen (ASSENT)-3 Investigators. Efficacy and safety of tenecteplase in combination with enoxaparin, abciximab, or unfractionated heparin: the ASSENT-3 randomised trial in acute myocardial infarction. *Lancet* 2001;358:605–613.

51. An international randomized trial comparing four thrombolytic strategies for acute myocardial infarction. The GUSTO Investigators. *N Engl J Med* 1993;329:673–682.

52. A comparison of reteplase with alteplase for acute myocardial infarction. The Global Use of Strategies to Open Occluded Coronary Arteries (GUSTO III) Investigators. *N Engl J Med* 1997;337:1118–1123.

53. Topol EJ. Reperfusion therapy for acute myocardial infarction with fibrinolytic therapy or combination reduced fibrinolytic therapy and platelet glycoprotein IIb/IIIa inhibition: the GUSTO V randomised trial. *Lancet* 2001;357:1905–1914.

54. Stampfer MJ, Goldhaber SZ, Yusuf S, et al. Effect of intravenous streptokinase on acute myocardial infarction: pooled results from randomized trials. *N Engl J Med* 1982;307:1180–1182.

55. Boersma E, Harrington RA, Moliterno DJ, et al. Platelet glycoprotein IIb/IIIa inhibitors in acute coronary syndromes: a meta-analysis of all major randomised clinical trials. *Lancet* 2002;359:189–198.

56. Yusuf S, Zhao F, Mehta SR, et al. Effects of clopidogrel in addition to aspirin in patients with acute coronary syndromes without ST-segment elevation. *N Engl J Med* 2001;345:494–502.

57. Soejima H, Ogawa H, Yasue H, et al. Heightened tissue factor associated with tissue factor pathway inhibitor and prognosis in patients with unstable angina. *Circulation* 1999;99:2908–2913.

58. Jude B, Agraou B, McFadden EP, et al. Evidence for time-dependent activation of monocytes in the systemic circulation in unstable angina but not in acute myocardial infarction or in stable angina. *Circulation* 1994;90:1662–1668.

59. Wilensky RL, Bourdillon PD, Vix VA, et al. Intracoronary artery thrombus formation in unstable angina: a clinical, biochemical and angiographic correlation. *J Am Coll Cardiol* 1993;21:692–699.

60. Merlini PA, Bauer KA, Oltrona L, et al. Persistent activation of coagulation mechanism in unstable angina and myocardial infarction. *Circulation* 1994;90:61–68.

61. Merlini PA, Ardissino D, Oltrona L, et al. Heightened thrombin formation but normal plasma levels of activated factor VII in patients with acute coronary syndromes. *Arterioscler Thromb Vasc Biol* 1995;15:1675–1679.

62. Gallino A, Haeberli A, Baur HR, et al. Fibrin formation and platelet aggregation in patients with severe coronary artery disease: relationship with the degree of myocardial ischemia. *Circulation* 1985;72:27–30.

63. Theroux P, Latour JG, Leger-Gauthier C, et al. Fibrinopeptide A and platelet factor levels in unstable angina pectoris. *Circulation* 1987;75: 156–162.

64. A comparison of recombinant hirudin with heparin for the treatment of acute coronary syndromes. The Global Use of Strategies to Open Occluded Coronary Arteries (GUSTO) IIb investigators. *N Engl J Med* 1996;335:775–782.

65. Antman EM, Tanasijevic MJ, Thompson B, et al. Cardiac-specific troponin I levels to predict the risk of mortality in patients with acute coronary syndromes. *N Engl J Med* 1996;335:1342–1349.

66. Alison HW, Russell RO Jr, Mantle JA, et al. Coronary anatomy and arteriography in patients with unstable angina pectoris. *Am J Cardiol* 1978;41:204–209.

67. Kerensky RA, Wade M, Deedwania P, et al. Revisiting the culprit lesion in non-Q-wave myocardial infarction. Results from the VANQWISH trial angiographic core laboratory. *J Am Coll Cardiol* 2002;39:1456–1463.

68. DeWood MA, Stifter WF, Simpson CS, et al. Coronary arteriographic findings soon after non-Q-wave myocardial infarction. *N Engl J Med* 1986;315:417–423.

69. Keen WD, Savage MP, Fischman DL, et al. Comparison of coronary angiographic findings during the first six hours of non-Q-wave and Q-wave myocardial infarction. *Am J Cardiol* 1994;74:324–328.

70. Dacanay S, Kennedy HL, Uretz E, et al. Morphological and quantitative angiographic analyses of progression of coronary stenoses. A comparison of Q-wave and non-Q-wave myocardial infarction. *Circulation* 1994;90:1739–1746.

71. Schoenhagen P, Ziada KM, Kapadia SR, et al. Extent and direction of arterial remodeling in stable versus unstable coronary syndromes: an intravascular ultrasound study. *Circulation* 2000;101:598–603.

72. Nakamura M, Nishikawa H, Mukai S, et al. Impact of coronary artery remodeling on clinical presentation of coronary artery disease: an intravascular ultrasound study. *J Am Coll Cardiol* 2001;37:63–69.

73. Namiki N, Uchiyama T, Nagai Y, et al. Graphical comparison of coronary arterial culprit lesions in acute myocardial infarction and unstable angina pectoris. *Intern Med* 1999;38:849–855.

74. Heart Protection Study Collaborative Group. MRC/BHF Heart Protection Study of cholesterol lowering with simvastatin in 20,536 high-risk individuals: a randomised placebo-controlled trial. *Lancet* 2002; 360:7–22.

75. Topol EJ. Toward a new frontier in myocardial reperfusion therapy: emerging platelet preeminence. *Circulation* 1998;97:211–218.

76. Lewis HD Jr, Davis JW, Archibald DG, et al. Protective effects of aspirin against acute myocardial infarction and death in men with unstable angina. Results of a Veterans Administration Cooperative Study. *N Engl J Med* 1983;309:396–403.

77. Cairns JA, Gent M, Singer J, et al. Aspirin, sulfinpyrazone, or both in unstable angina. Results of a Canadian multicenter trial. *N Engl J Med* 1985;313:1369–1375.

78. Theroux P, Ouimet H, McCans J, et al. Aspirin, heparin, or both to treat acute unstable angina. *N Engl J Med* 1988;319:1105–1111.

79. Randomised trial of intravenous streptokinase, oral aspirin, both, or neither among 17,187 cases of suspected acute myocardial infarction: ISIS-2. ISIS-2 (Second International Study of Infarct Survival) Collaborative Group. *Lancet* 1988;2:349–360.

80. Randomised placebo-controlled trial of abciximab before and during coronary intervention in refractory unstable angina: the CAPTURE Study. CAPTURE Investigators. *Lancet* 1997;349:1429–1435.

81. A comparison of aspirin plus tirofiban with aspirin plus heparin for unstable angina. Platelet Receptor Inhibition in Ischemic Syndrome Management (PRISM) Study Investigators. *N Engl J Med* 1998;338: 1498–1505.

82. Inhibition of the platelet glycoprotein IIb/IIIa receptor with tirofiban in unstable angina and non-Q-wave myocardial infarction. Platelet Receptor Inhibition in Ischemic Syndrome Management in Patients Limited by Unstable Signs and Symptoms (PRISM-PLUS) Study Investigators. *N Engl J Med* 1998;338:1488–1497.

83. Inhibition of platelet glycoprotein IIb/IIIa with eptifibatide in patients with acute coronary syndromes. The PURSUIT Trial Investigators. Platelet Glycoprotein IIb/IIIa in Unstable Angina: Receptor Suppression Using Integrilin Therapy. *N Engl J Med* 1998;339:436–443.

84. International, randomized, controlled trial of lamifiban (a platelet glycoprotein IIb/IIIa inhibitor), heparin, or both in unstable angina. The PARAGON Investigators. Platelet IIb/IIIa Antagonism for the Reduction of Acute coronary syndrome events in a Global Organization Network. *Circulation* 1998;97:2386–2395.

85. Randomized, placebo-controlled trial of titrated intravenous lamifiban for acute coronary syndromes. *Circulation* 2002;105:316–321.

86. Simoons ML. Effect of glycoprotein IIb/IIIa receptor blocker abciximab on outcome in patients with acute coronary syndromes without early coronary revascularisation: the GUSTO IV-ACS randomised trial. *Lancet* 2001;357:1915–1924.

87. Hamm CW, Heeschen C, Goldmann B, et al. Benefit of abciximab in patients with refractory unstable angina in relation to serum troponin T levels. c7E3 Fab Antiplatelet Therapy in Unstable Refractory

Angina (CAPTURE) Study Investigators. *N Engl J Med* 1999;340: 1623–1629.

88. Heeschen C, Hamm CW, Goldmann B, et al. Troponin concentrations for stratification of patients with acute coronary syndromes in relation to therapeutic efficacy of tirofiban. PRISM Study Investigators. Platelet Receptor Inhibition in Ischemic Syndrome Management. *Lancet* 1999;354:1757–1762.

89. Roffi M, Chew DP, Mukherjee D, et al. Platelet glycoprotein IIb/IIIa inhibition in acute coronary syndromes. Gradient of benefit related to the revascularization strategy. *Eur Heart J* 2002;23:1441–1448.

90. Roffi M, Chew DP, Mukherjee D, et al. Platelet glycoprotein IIb/IIIa inhibitors reduce mortality in diabetic patients with non-ST-segment-elevation acute coronary syndromes. *Circulation* 2001;104:2767–2771.

91. Trial of abciximab with and without low-dose reteplase for acute myocardial infarction. Strategies for Patency Enhancement in the Emergency Department (SPEED) Group. *Circulation* 2000;101:2788–2794.

92. Antman EM, Giugliano RP, Gibson CM, et al. Abciximab facilitates the rate and extent of thrombolysis: results of the Thrombolysis In Myocardial Infarction (TIMI) 14 trial. The TIMI 14 Investigators. *Circulation* 1999;99:2720–2732.

93. Montalescot G, Barragan P, Wittenberg O, et al. Platelet glycoprotein IIb/IIIa inhibition with coronary stenting for acute myocardial infarction. *N Engl J Med* 2001;344:1895–1903.

94. Oler A, Whooley MA, Oler J, et al. Adding heparin to aspirin reduces the incidence of myocardial infarction and death in patients with unstable angina. A meta-analysis. *JAMA* 1996;276:811–815.

95. Granger CB, Hirsch J, Califf RM, et al. Activated partial thromboplastin time and outcome after thrombolytic therapy for acute myocardial infarction: results from the GUSTO-I trial. *Circulation* 1996;93:870–878.

96. In-hospital mortality and clinical course of 20,891 patients with suspected acute myocardial infarction randomised between alteplase and streptokinase with or without heparin. The International Study Group (ISIS-3 Investigators). *Lancet* 1990;336:71–75.

97. GISSI-2: a factorial randomised trial of alteplase versus streptokinase and heparin versus no heparin among 12,490 patients with acute myocardial infarction. Gruppo Italiano per lo Studio della Sopravvivenza nell'Infarto Miocardico (GISSI-2 Investigators). *Lancet* 1990;336: 65–71.

98. Low-molecular-weight heparin during instability in coronary artery disease, Fragmin during Instability in Coronary Artery Disease (FRISC) study group. FRISC Investigators. *Lancet* 1996;347:561–568.

99. Cohen M, Demers C, Gurfinkel EP, et al. A comparison of low-molecular-weight heparin with unfractionated heparin for unstable coronary artery disease. Efficacy and Safety of Subcutaneous Enoxaparin in Non-Q-Wave Coronary Events Study Group. *N Engl J Med* 1997;337:447–452.

100. Antman EM, McCabe CH, Gurfinkel EP, et al. Enoxaparin prevents death and cardiac ischemic events in unstable angina/non-Q-wave myocardial infarction. Results of the thrombolysis in myocardial infarction (TIMI) 11B trial. *Circulation* 1999;100:1593–1601.

101. Eikelboom JW, Anand SS, Malmberg K, et al. Unfractionated heparin and low-molecular-weight heparin in acute coronary syndrome without ST elevation: a meta-analysis. *Lancet* 2000;355:1936–1942.

102. Lindahl B, Venge P, Wallentin L. Troponin T identifies patients with unstable coronary artery disease who benefit from long-term antithrombotic protection. Fragmin in Unstable Coronary Artery Disease (FRISC) Study Group. *J Am Coll Cardiol* 1997;29:43–48.

103. Indications for fibrinolytic therapy in suspected acute myocardial infarction: collaborative overview of early mortality and major morbidity results from all randomised trials of more than 1000 patients. Fibrinolytic Therapy Trialists' (FTT) Collaborative Group. *Lancet* 1994;343: 311–322.

104. Califf RM, White HD, Van de Werf F, et al. One-year results from the Global Utilization of Streptokinase and TPA for Occluded Coronary Arteries (GUSTO-I) trial. GUSTO-I Investigators. *Circulation* 1996;94: 1233–1238.

105. Topol EJ, Ohman EM, Armstrong PW, et al. Survival outcomes 1 year after reperfusion therapy with either alteplase or reteplase for acute myocardial infarction: results from the Global Utilization of Streptokinase and t-PA for Occluded Coronary Arteries (GUSTO) III Trial. *Circulation* 2000;102:1761–1765.

106. Lincoff AM, Califf RM, Van de Werf F, et al. Mortality at 1 year with combination platelet glycoprotein IIb/IIIa inhibition and reduced-dose fibrinolytic therapy vs conventional fibrinolytic therapy for acute myocardial infarction: GUSTO V randomized trial. *JAMA* 2002;288: 2130–2135.

107. Ottervanger JP, Armstrong P, Barnathan ES, et al. Long-term results after the glycoprotein IIb/IIIa inhibitor abciximab in unstable angina: one-year survival in the GUSTO IV-ACS (Global Use of Strategies To Open Occluded Coronary Arteries IV—Acute Coronary Syndrome) Trial. *Circulation* 2003;107:437–442.

108. Steg PG, Goldberg RJ, Gore JM, et al. Baseline characteristics, management practices, and in-hospital outcomes of patients hospitalized with acute coronary syndromes in the Global Registry of Acute Coronary Events (GRACE). *Am J Cardiol* 2002;90:358–363.

109. Fox KA, Goodman SG, Klein W, et al. Management of acute coronary syndromes. Variations in practice and outcome; findings from the Global Registry of Acute Coronary Events (GRACE). *Eur Heart J* 2002;23:1177–1189.

110. Rogers WJ, Canto JG, Lambrew CT, et al. Temporal trends in the treatment of over 1.5 million patients with myocardial infarction in the US from 1990 through 1999: the National Registry of Myocardial Infarction 1, 2 and 3. *J Am Coll Cardiol* 2000;36:2056–2063.

CHAPTER 55

Pathology of Myocardial Ischemia, Infarction, Reperfusion, and Sudden Death

Renu Virmani and Allen P. Burke

Key Words: Ischemic preconditioning; myocardial infarction; no-reflow; pathology; reperfusion; sudden death.

EPIDEMIOLOGY AND ETIOLOGIC FACTORS

Despite recent declines in the incidence of acute myocardial infarction (AMI), more than 1.5 million Americans still experience an acute infarct annually (1). Women are older at presentation, have more concomitant disease, and present later in the course of their AMI (2). Black individuals have a greater risk for complications and mortality after AMI and have experienced as a group a smaller decrease in mortality in the latter half of the twentieth century as compared with white individuals (3). The major cause of AMI in both sexes and all races is coronary atherothrombosis with superimposed luminal thrombus, which accounts for greater than 80% of all infarcts. MIs resulting from nonatherothrombotic diseases of the coronary arteries are rare.

Factors Affecting Mortality

Mortality after AMI is greatest in patients older than 65 years (4); patients aged 65 to 74 years have a greater mortality than patients younger than 65 years, independent of infarct size (5,6). Although men have a fivefold greater risk of MI than women between the ages of 45 to 54 years, this differential decreases to a twofold difference in the eighth decade of life, and women have a greater mortality than men after an MI at all age ranges.

The opinions or assertions contained herein are the private views of the authors and are not to be construed as official or reflecting the views of the Department of the Army, the Department of the Air Force, or the Department of Defense.

R. Virmani: Department of Cardiovascular Pathology, Armed Forces Institute of Pathology, 6825 16th Street, NW, Washington, DC 20306-6000.
A. P. Burke: Department of Cardiovascular Pathology, Armed Forces Institute of Pathology, 6825 16th Street, NW, Washington, DC 20306-6000.

Recent Declines in Death Rates from Acute Myocardial Infarction

Deaths from MI caused by coronary heart disease among 35- to 74-year-old residents of four communities in the United States have decreased. There has been a significant decrease in the death rate and case fatality rate for AMI in persons 45 to 64 years of age in the United States from 1970 through 1995 (7,8). In-hospital mortality rates have decreased 5.1% per year, whereas out-of-hospital mortality rates have declined by 3.6% per year, with the greatest decline seen in white men followed by white women, black women, and black men (9). The in-hospital and late survival rates of patients with AMI have improved remarkably from the 1970s to early 1980s from 16% to 8% to 10% in the early 1990s. The reasons for this decrease are multifactorial and include myocardial salvage from reperfusion, small infarction, and remodeling (10). However, the incidence of cardiogenic shock in community studies has not declined (11). The complications of myocardial infarction (MI) may manifest immediately or may appear late, and they are dependent of the location and extent of infarction. The acute complications consist of arrhythmias and sudden death, cardiogenic shock, infarct extension, fibrinous pericarditis, cardiac rupture including papillary muscle rupture, and mural thrombus and embolization.

CLINICAL DIAGNOSIS OF ACUTE MYOCARDIAL INFARCTION

Clinical criteria for the diagnosis of AMI include at least two of the following three changes: (a) a history of chest pain or discomfort; (b) an increase and subsequent decrease in serum cardiac enzymes; and (c) the development of electrocardiographic (ECG) abnormalities (new Q waves or ST segment or T-wave changes) on serially obtained ECGs (12). Because the ECG lacks sufficient sensitivity and specificity to detect myocardial necrosis, the presence of myocardial injury often is dependent on the release of cardiac-specific serum markers such as troponin T, troponin I, and CK-MB (13–16). It has been shown that infarct size generally correlates with the peak increase in serum creatine kinase-MB (CK-MB) level (17). Recently, it has been appreciated that the clinical presentation of AMI differs significantly in women (18).

Normal Cardiac Metabolism

The normal function of the heart muscle is supported by high rates of combustion of carbon fuel and oxygen consumption. Under normal aerobic conditions, 60% to 80% of cardiac adenosine triphosphate (ATP) is derived from fatty acids, the remainder coming from the oxidation of glucose and lactate (19). Almost all of the ATP formed comes from oxidative phosphorylation in the mitochondria; only a small amount of ATP (<2%) is synthesized by glycolysis. Approximately two-thirds of the ATP used by the heart goes to contractile shortening, and the remaining one-third is used by sarcoplasmic reticulum Ca^{2+} ATPase and other ion pumps.

Myocardial Ischemia

Myocardial ischemia, defined as insufficient oxygen for the synthesis of ATP at the normal rate, dramatically changes fuel metabolism. About 30% to 60% of normal coronary flow results in an increase in uptake of glucose, which is not readily oxidized in the mitochondria but is converted to lactate. As a consequence of lactate accumulation, ATP content decreases, intracellular pH decreases, and contractile work decreases. Paradoxically, the ischemic tissue continues to derive 50% to 70% of its energy from the oxidation of fatty acids (19). Although biochemical and functional abnormalities begin almost immediately at onset of ischemia, severe loss of myocardial contractility occurs within 60 seconds, whereas other changes take a more protracted course; for example, the loss of viability (irreversible injury) takes at least 20 to 40 minutes after total occlusion of blood flow.

Duration of Occlusion and Infarct Development

In the dog model of coronary occlusion, myocardial necrosis progresses as a "wave front phenomenon," resulting in increasing extent of myocardial necrosis after durations of occlusion of 40 minutes, 3 hours, and permanently for 4 days (Fig. 55–1A) (20). After only 15 minutes of occlusion, no infarct occurs. At 40 minutes, the infarct is subendocardial, involving only the papillary muscle, resulting in 28% of the myocardium at risk. At 3 hours after coronary artery occlusion and reperfusion the infarct is significantly smaller compared with nonreperfused permanently occluded infarct (62% of area at risk). The infarct size is the greatest in permanent occlusion, becoming transmural involving 75% of the area at risk (21) (Fig. 55–1B). In the dog model, it is impossible to achieve 100% infarcted area at risk because of species-related native collaterals. In humans, it has been shown that approximately 40% of patients with AMI have well developed collateral circulation (22).

THE NO-REFLOW PHENOMENON

The no-reflow phenomenon was originally described by Kloner and coworkers (23) in an experimental canine model of MI. They demonstrated homogenous distribution of thioflavin S dye after 40 minutes of ischemia and reperfusion. However, after 90 minutes of ischemia, areas of no-reflow were identified primarily in the subendocardial regions as zones that do not stain with thioflavin S. By electron microscopy, swollen endothelial protrusions and membrane-bound intraluminal bodies obstruct the capillary lumen and plug the capillaries by red cells, neutrophils, and platelet and fibrin thrombi. The term *reperfusion injury* was used to describe increasing degrees or extent of the ischemic injury as assessed by contractile performance, the arrhythmogenic threshold, conversion of reversible to irreversible myocyte injury, and microvessel dysfunction. Studies have shown that angiographic no-reflow is a strong predictor of

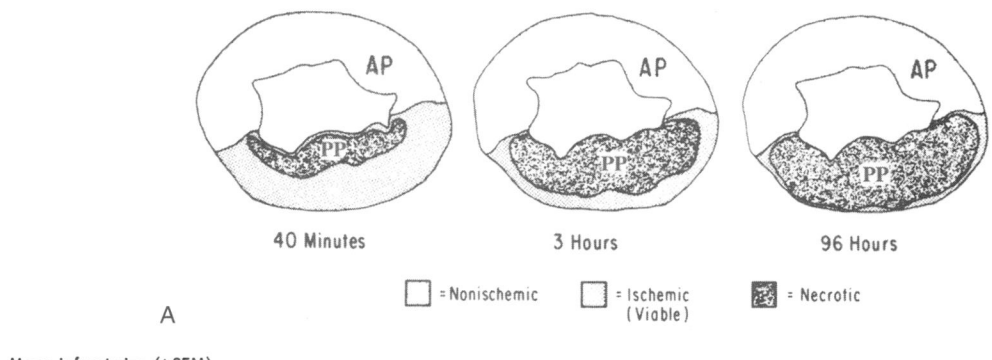

A

B

FIG. 55–1. **A:** Progression of cell death versus time after experimental occlusion of the left circumflex coronary artery in the dog. Necrosis occurs first in the subendocardial region of the myocardium. With extension of the occlusion time, a wave front of cell death moves from the subendocardial zone across the wall to involve progressively more of the transmural thickness of the ischemic zone. **B:** Infarct size variation with increasing duration of coronary occlusion. Infarct size dramatically increases from 40 minutes to 3 hours; however, there is little increase between 3 and 6 hours and between 6 and 96 hours of coronary artery occlusion. AP, anterior; LCC, left circumflex coronary bed; PP, posterior. (From Reimer KA, Jennings RB. The "wavefront phenomenon" of myocardial ischemic cell death. II. Transmural progression of necrosis with the framework of ischemic bed size (myocardium at risk) and collateral flow. *Lab Invest* 1979;40:633–644, with permission.)

major cardiac events, such as congestive heart failure, malignant arrhythmias, and cardiac death after AMI.

Collaterals and the Extent of Myocardial Damage

The extent of coronary collateral flow is one of the principal determinants of infarct size. Absence of myocardial ischemia (revealed by ECG changes or angina during transient coronary balloon occlusion) is associated with presence of well developed collateral vessels, suggesting that the patients with well developed collateral vessels have a small risk for development of AMI on abrupt closure of the culprit coronary artery (24). It is not uncommon to see chronic total coronary occlusion at autopsy and an absence of MI in the distribution of that artery, presumably because of well developed collaterals. Collaterals have been shown to be better developed in patients with angina and in younger individuals as compared with older patients with acute infarcts (22).

The presence of collaterals may also affect the course of infarct healing. If there is good collateral blood flow locally, healing will be relatively rapid, especially at the lateral borders where viable myocardium interdigitates with necrotic myocardium. There may be various levels of healing within an infarct, because of differences in blood flow in adjoining vascular beds caused by variable extent of coronary narrowing. The border areas may show hemorrhage and contraction band necrosis, depending on regional variations in blood flow. Systemic factors that influence repair of myocardium are the systemic blood pressure and cardiac output, which are severely decreased in heart of patients with multisystem failure.

Ischemic Preconditioning and Size of Myocardial Infarct

Ischemic preconditioning was first described in 1986 when it was discovered that canine myocardial infarct size was markedly reduced if it follows four brief episodes of 5 minutes of occlusion followed by 5 minutes of reperfusion (25). The original description of preconditioning was applied only to infarct size reduction; this definition is now extended to cardiac function and arrhythmias (26). Preconditioning also has been observed with only one episode of brief occlusion followed by reperfusion. If the duration between ischemic preconditioning and the long duration of occlusion is extended to 24 to 96 hours, the protective effect is not significantly marked (27). Infarct size in the absence of preconditioning is almost entirely related to collateral blood flow, given equal duration of occlusion.

The mechanisms of preconditioning in reducing the energy demand of the myocardium are unclear. Intermittent aortic cross-clamping during coronary artery bypass surgery results in preservation of ATP levels within the left ventricle (28). Repeated balloon inflations of 60 to 90 seconds in patients undergoing percutaneous transluminal coronary angioplasty have been associated with decreasing chest pain, reduced ST segment elevation, and decreased lactate production with subsequent inflations in patients with or without collaterals (29). This preconditioning effect was noted only in patients with angina beginning within 24 hours of infarction and was manifest as smaller infarct size (30).

The mediators of preconditioning are believed to involve the K_{ATP} channel and specific isoforms of protein kinase

C (PKC). The protective effect of temporary ischemia can be blocked by pretreatment of the myocardium with inhibitors of K_{ATP} channel, such as glibenclamide and 5-hydrocydeconate (31,32). Similarly, inhibitors of PKC and tyrosine kinase, but not PKC alone, will prevent ischemic preconditioning. Agonists of adenosine (A_1 receptor) will pharmacologically precondition the heart against ischemia (33). The benefits of preconditioning cannot be applied to patients with AMI, because the therapy needs to be instituted before coronary occlusion. However, it may be useful if administered before cardioplegia or to heart before removal for transplantation (32).

Size of Infarct and Development of Heart Failure

Loss of perfusion results in two zones of myocardial damage: a central zone with no flow or very low flow and a zone of collateral vessels in a surrounding marginal zone. The survival of the marginal zone is dependent on the level of ischemia and the duration of ischemia. Because infarct size is an important determinant of survival and development of congestive heart failure, efforts have been directed to limit infarct size by early reperfusion, reduction of myocardial oxygen demand, and prevention of reperfusion injury. In 1971, Page and coworkers (34) showed that infarcts of 40% or greater of left ventricle are predictors of cardiogenic shock and death.

Electron Microscopic Changes in Myocardial Ischemia

Electron microscopic criteria for reversible versus irreversible MI injury are well established in animal models. There is, however, species-specific variation in the time course of these uniform changes (35,36). Reversible injury is defined as injury that can be reversed to normal functioning state without any structural damage, if the offending agent is removed (37).

Reversibly injured myocytes are swollen from the osmotic leakage through damaged cell membranes, and there is a decrease in glycogen content (21,38). The cell membrane is morphologically intact as no breaks can be identified. The mitochondria are swollen, with loss of normal dense mitochondrial granules and incomplete clearing of the mitochondrial matrix, but without amorphous or granular flocculent densities (Fig. 55–2A). The myocyte fibrils are thinned, and I-bands are prominent secondary to noncontracting ischemic myofibrils (21). The nuclei show mild condensation of chromatin at the nucleoplasm.

Irreversibly injured myocytes contain shrunken nuclei with marked chromatin margination (Fig. 55–2B). The two hallmarks of irreversible injury are cell membrane breaks and mitochondrial presence of small osmiophilic amorphous densities (21,35). The densities are composed of lipid, denatured proteins, and calcium (35,39,40). The cell membrane breaks are small and are associated with subsarcolemmal blebs of edema fluid (21).

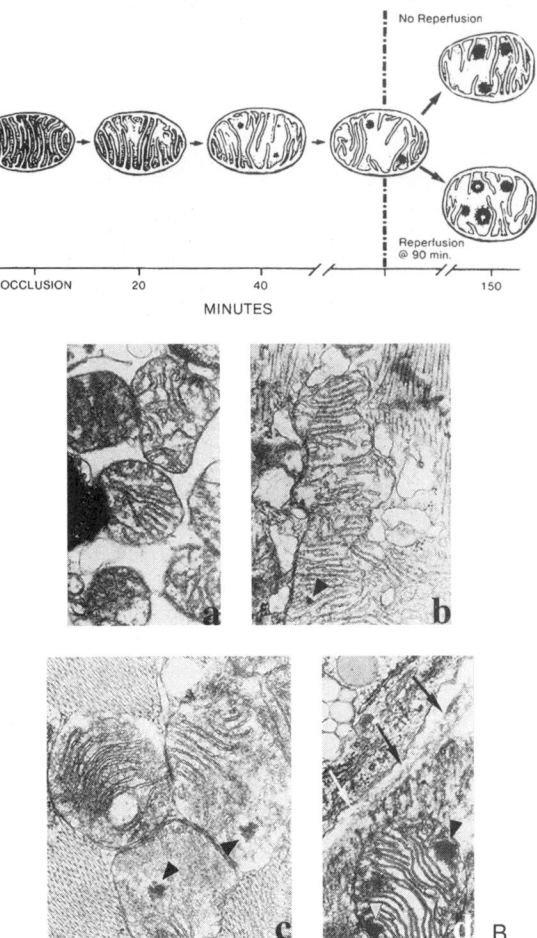

FIG. 55–2. A: Sequential changes within mitochondria with varying time intervals of myocardial ischemia. At 20 minutes of ischemia, there is mild mitochondrial swelling. Matrix spaces between cristae show disorganization. At 40 minutes of ischemia, there is greater mitochondrial swelling, and prominent amorphous matrix densities are present, which indicate irreversible injury. With longer duration of coronary occlusion, mitochondria show larger amorphous matrix densities, and they also become more numerous. On reperfusion, both amorphous and granular densities are seen. Granular densities, however, seem larger and more fully developed. B: Electron micrographs showing progressive changes in mitochondria as a result of ischemia in the canine model. a: Mitochondria showing reversible changes of ischemia after 10 minutes of coronary occlusion and reperfusion: mitochondria are swollen, there is clearing of mitochondrial matrix, and some cristae show disorganization. b: Similar changes as in A, with only one of the mitochondria showing amorphous matrix densities (arrowhead) after 90 minutes of ischemia. c: Note the presence of large amorphous matrix densities (arrowheads) in two of the three mitochondria in a dog with 120 minutes of coronary occlusion. d: Ischemic myocyte with mitochondria containing multiple large amorphous matrix densities (arrowheads) after 3 days of permanent coronary occlusion. Note the break in the plasmalemma (arrow). (A: Adapted from Jennings RB, Ganote CE. Structural changes in myocardium during acute ischemia. *Circ Res* 1974;35[Suppl 3]:156–172, by permission from the American Heart Association; B: Reproduced from Virmani R, Forman MB, Kolodgie FD. Myocardial reperfusion injury. Histopathological effects of perfluorochemical. *Circulation* 1990;81:IV57–IV68, by permission from the American Heart Association.)

GROSS PATHOLOGY OF ACUTE MYOCARDIAL INFARCTION

Without special studies, the earliest changes of AMI are not detected until 12 hours after the onset of irreversible ischemia. The first change is pallor of the myocardium. Earlier irreversible changes can be detected grossly by the use of tetrazolium salt solutions (nitro-blue tetrazolium [NBT] and 2,3,5-triphenyltetrazolium chloride [TTC]), which form a colored precipitate on gross section of normal fresh myocardium (Fig. 55–3). The basis for the color reaction (red for TTC, and blue in NBT) is the presence of dehydrogenase-mediated oxidation, which is depleted in ischemic tissue. In the dog, acute myocardial infarct can be detected by NBT as early as 2 to 3 hours; in the pig, the time interval is shorter because of poor collaterals (11). In humans, the necrotic myocardium can be detected within 2 to 3 hours after infarct by immersion of the fresh heart slices in solution of TTC or NBT. An autopsy study demonstrated that TTC staining had a sensitivity of 77% and a specificity of 93% compared with routine histologic diagnosis. The predictive values of positive and negative test using TTC were 81% and 91%, respectively (42).

In the human, there is little change in the gross evolution of AMI between 12 and 24 hours, except for enhancement of the pallor (Fig. 55–4A). If there has been no reperfusion, the area of the infarct is better defined at 2 to 3 days with a central area of yellow discoloration that is surrounded by a thin rim of highly vascularized hyperemia (Fig. 55–4B through D). At 5 to 7 days, the regions are much more distinct, with a central soft area and a depressed hyperemic border (43–45). At 1 to 2 weeks, the infarct begins to heal with infiltration by macrophages and early fibroblasts at the margins. At the same time the infarct begins to be more depressed, especially at the margins where organization takes place, and there is white hue borders (Table 55–1) (Fig. 55–4E). Healing may be complete as early as 4 to 6 weeks in small infarcts, or it may take as long as 2 to 3 months when the area of infarction is large. Healed infarcts are white from the scarring, and the ventricular wall may or may not be thinned (aneurysmal). In general, infarcts that are trans-

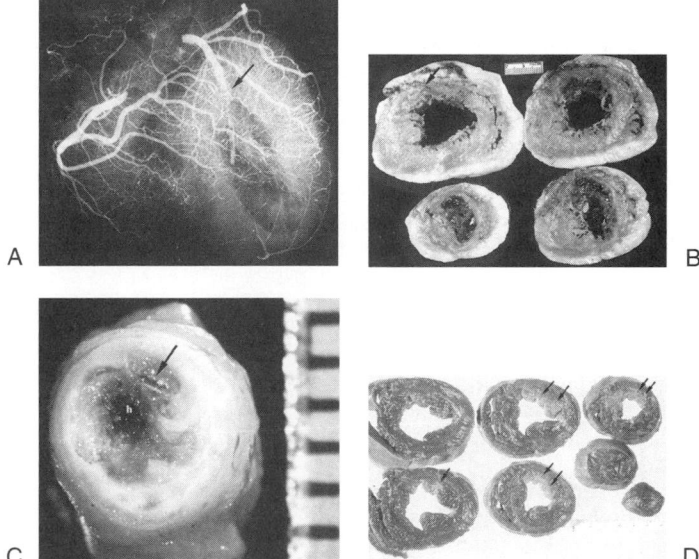

FIG. 55–3. Regional distribution of vascular supply to the ventricles with right coronary artery dominance. **A:** Postmortem angiogram of the heart in a patient with acute myocardial infarction with total occlusion *(arrow)* of the proximal left anterior descending coronary artery in a 65-year-old woman who presented with persistent chest pain of 6 hours in duration. **B:** At autopsy, she had a hemopericardium with rupture site *(arrow)* identified on the anterior wall of the left ventricle. Note extensive hemorrhagic transmural infarction involving the anterior wall of the left ventricle near the base of the heart *(top slices)* and extending into the septum in the mid and apical slices *(bottom slices)*. **C:** A gross photograph of the left anterior descending coronary artery showing hemorrhage into the necrotic core and a greater than 90% luminal narrowing; barium is seen within the lumen *(arrow)*. **D:** Dog heart slices after 15-minute incubation in 2% triphenyltetrazolium chloride (TTC) at 37°C. The animal had undergone 60 minutes of left anterior descending (LAD) coronary artery occlusion distal to the first diagonal branch followed by reperfusion and was killed at 24 hours. Injecting monastery dye after reocclusion of the LAD just before death identified the myocardium at risk for infarction. The heart was sliced and then immersed in TTC. The viable myocardium at risk stains red and the area not at risk is blue-red, whereas the infarcted region is creamy white *(arrows)*. (Virmani R, Burke AP, Farb A, Atkinson J, eds. Pathology of myocardial infarction. *In: Cardiovascular pathology,* 2nd ed. Major problems in pathology series, vol 40. Philadelphia: WB Saunders Company, 2001, with permission.)

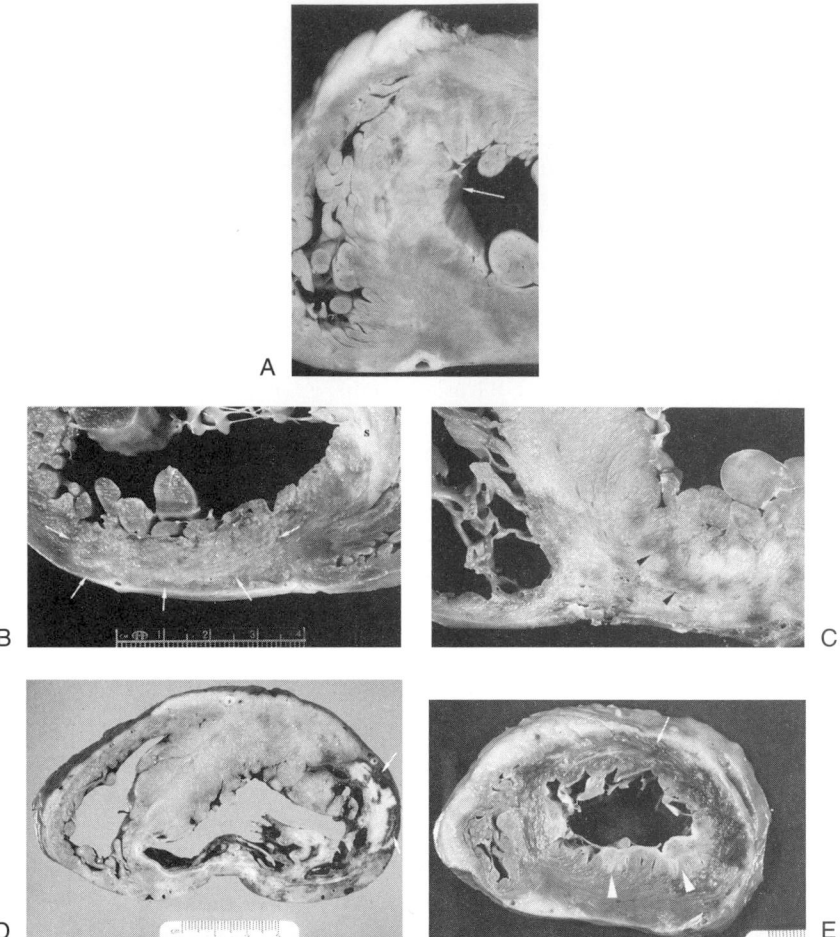

FIG. 55–4. Gross photographs of the hearts with varying ages of acute myocardial infarction. **A:** A 50-year-old man with hyperlipidemia and hypertension who presented with unstable angina, underwent emergency percutaneous transluminal coronary angioplasty (PTCA) of the left anterior descending artery (LAD), and died 20 hours after onset of chest pain. At autopsy, the patient had a pale ill-defined, slightly raised region in the anterior ventricular septum suggestive of an acute transmural infarct *(arrow)*, which was confirmed by the presence of hypereosinophilic myocytes localized to the septum with sparing of the subendocardial myocytes. The LAD at the PTCA site was totally occluded by a luminal thrombus and an underlying 60% atherothrombotic lesion. **B:** Another high power of a different acute transmural myocardial infarct involving the posterior wall of the heart, well defined pale, creamy tan, slightly raised infarct. Note absence of hyperemia in the border region; the infarct is 24 to 36 hours old. An older infarct can be seen in the septum (s). **C:** An older infarct dated 36 to 72 hours showing hyperemic areas *(arrowheads)* surrounding the subendocardial infarct (age 3 days), with paler area in the outer half of the posterior wall of the left ventricle (infarct extension). The more recent infarct involves the posterior portion of the ventricular septum and the posterior wall of the right ventricle (36–48 hours). **D:** Gross photograph of a heart slice close to the base of the heart shows 1-week-old acute transmural myocardial infarct involving the posterolateral wall of the heart. Note the marked pale region in the inner two-thirds of the infarct with surrounding prominent hyperemic zone *(arrows)*. Also present is a healed transmural myocardial infarct involving the posterior wall and posteroseptal region of the heart. The patient died in severe congestive heart failure. **E:** Gross photograph of a transmural healing myocardial infarct involving the septum, anterior, and lateral wall of the left ventricle in an apical slice of the heart. Note the depressed, gelatinous appearance *(arrow)* of the infarct, which is 3 weeks old. Focal areas of scarring can be seen *(arrowheads)*. (From Virmani R, Burke AP, Farb A, Atkinson J, eds. Pathology of myocardial infarction. *In: Cardiovascular pathology,* 2nd ed. Major problems in pathology series, vol 40. Philadelphia: WB Saunders Company, 2001, with permission.)

TABLE 55–1. *Gross and microscopic evolution of reperfused and nonreperfused acute myocardial infarct*

Time of occlusion	Permanent occlusion/no reperfusion		Reperfusion after occlusion	
	Gross	Histologic	Gross	Histologic
12 h	No change pallor	Wavy fibers	Mottled, prominent hemorrhage	CBN
24–48 hours	Pallor: yellow, soft	Hypereosinophilic fibers, PMNs at borders	Prominent hemorrhage	Hypereosinophilic fibers + CBN + PMNs + hemorrhage throughout
3–5 d	Yellow center, hyperemic borders	Large number of PMNs at border, coagulation necrosis, loss of nuclei	Prominent hemorrhage	Aggressive phagocytosis profuse fibroblast infiltration + collagen
6–10 d	Yellow, depressed central infarct, tan-red margins	Mummified fibers in center, macrophage phagocytosis + granulation tissue at borders	Depressed red-brown infarct with gray-white intermingled	Aggressive healing with greater collagen
10–14 d	Gray-red borders, infiltrating central tan-yellow infarct if large	Marked granulation tissue, collagen deposition, subendocardial myocyte sparing	Gray-white intermingled with brown	Aggressive healing with greater collagen
2–8 wk	Gelatinous to gray white scar, greater healing at border zone	Collagen deposition with prominent large capillaries	White intermingled with groups of myocytes with red myocardium	Collagen intermingled with groups of myocytes

CBN, contraction band necrosis; PMN, polymorphonuclear leukocyte.
From Virmani R, Burke AP, Farb A, Atkinson J, eds. Pathology of myocardial infarction. *In: Cardiovascular pathology*, 2nd ed. Major problems in pathology series, vol 40. Philadelphia: WB Saunders Company, 2001, with permission.

mural and confluent are likely to result in thinning, whereas subendocardial and nonconfluent infarcts are not.

In the current era of thrombolytic therapy, the natural evolution of AMI has been significantly altered. The reperfused infarcted region will appear red from trapping of the red cells and hemorrhage from the rupture of the necrotic capillaries (Fig. 55–5). The time course of gross changes is compressed in reperfused infarcts, with the hemorrhagic appearance occurring as early as 24 hours, and organization occurring within 1 week. In contrast to nonreperfused infarcts, a yellow necrotic area with a hyperemic border does not form.

Histology of Early Nonreperfused Infarction

The earliest morphologic characteristic of nonreperfused infarction that can be discerned, between 12 to 24 hours after onset of irreversible myocyte damage, is the hypereosinophilic myocyte (Fig. 55–6A through C). The myocyte striations appear normal, and some chromatin condensation may be seen in the nucleus. In experimentally-induced infarction, the appearance of "wavy fibers" may be the result of stretching of the ischemic noncontractile fibers by the adjoining viable contracting myocytes (46). Although wavy fibers may occur experimentally earlier than hypereosinophilia, they are often a nonspecific artifact in the human, and therefore must be interpreted with caution. The early myocyte changes of hypereosinophilia and wavy fiber change are best appreciated by hematoxylin and eosin staining. In animal models, another early histologic change is interstitial edema; however, this change is difficult to appreciate in human autopsy hearts.

Other stains that have been used to detect MI within 6 to 8 hours include hematoxylin-basic fuchsin-picric acid. However, this technique has not proven to be reliably sensitive or specific in humans. Immunohistochemical techniques using antibodies against creatine kinase, ceruloplasmin, myoglobin, C-reactive protein, complement complex (C5b-9), fibronectin, and others have been used with variable success (41).

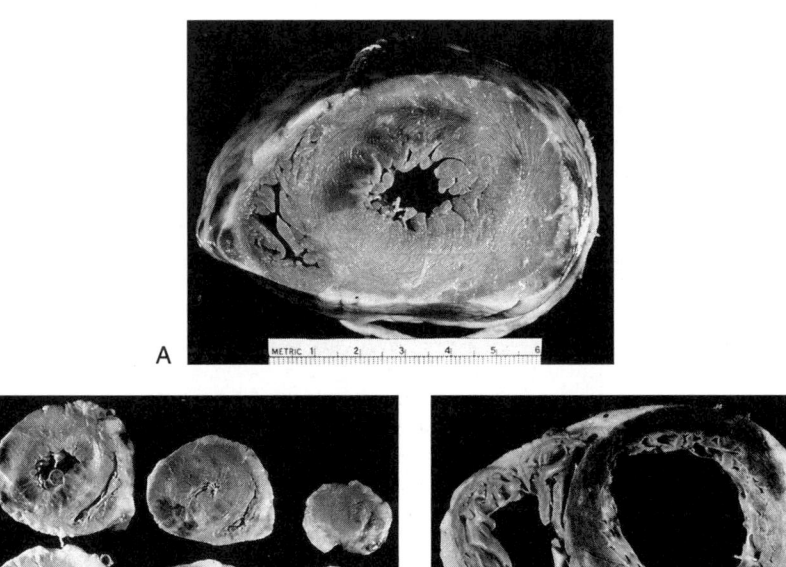

FIG. 55–5. A 47-year-old black man presented with unstable angina that evolved into a Q-wave infarct. **A:** On catheterization, the patient had a total occlusion of the left anterior descending coronary artery and severe stenosis of the right and left circumflex coronary arteries, and underwent emergency bypass graft to all three vessels. He died secondary to refractory arrhythmias on his third day in the hospital. Note the subendocardial hyperemic region in the anteroseptal wall of the left ventricle. **B:** The patient presented with acute myocardial infarction of 6 hours in duration, received streptokinase in the emergency room, and died 2 days after successful reperfusion of a cerebral bleed. Note a hemorrhagic transmural infarct involves the posteroseptal wall of the left ventricle, extending from the base to the apex of the heart with approximately 20% to 25% of the myocardium infarcted. **C:** A 60-year-old man admitted with onset of chest pain while mowing the lawn did not seek medical treatment until 8 hours after onset of chest pain. He received streptokinase, experienced development of arrhythmias, was treated with lidocaine, went into cardiogenic shock, and died 3 days after infarction. Note transmural confluent hemorrhagic infarct of the anteroseptal wall of the left ventricle involving at least 40% of the left ventricle. (From Virmani R, Burke AP, Farb A, Atkinson J, eds. Pathology of myocardial infarction. *In: Cardiovascular pathology,* 2nd ed. Major problems in pathology series, vol 40. Philadelphia: WB Saunders Company, 2001, with permission.)

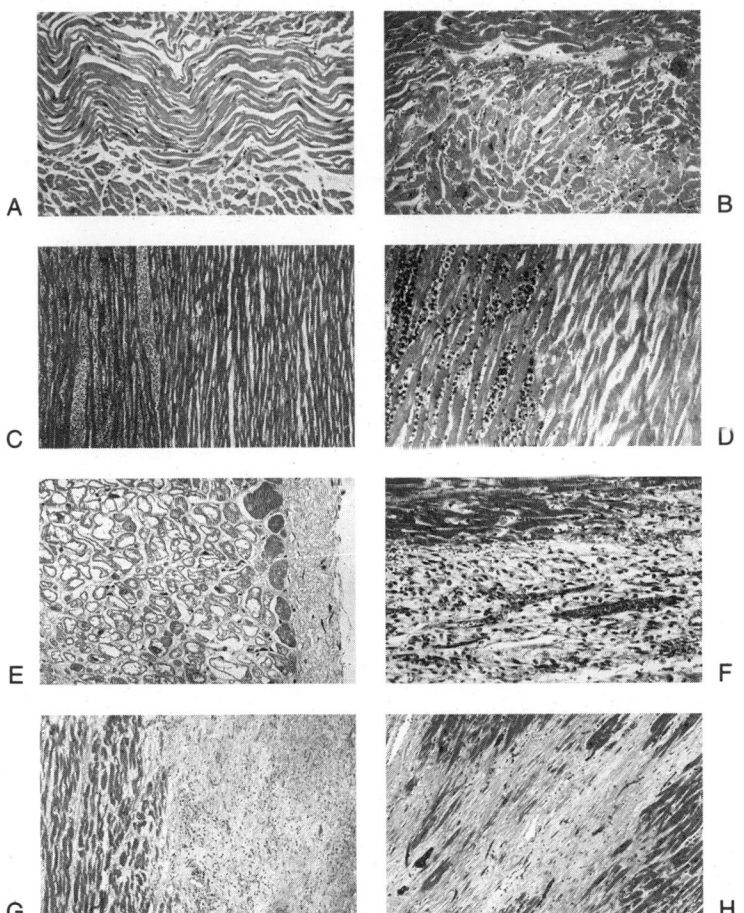

FIG. 55–6. Histologic characteristics of myocardial infarction after total occlusion of a coronary artery. **A:** The earliest change seen is within 12 hours after the onset of chest pain and has been described as wavy fibers with elongation of myocytes and narrowing of the myocyte diameter. **B:** Hypereosinophilic myocyte fibers representing early features of coagulation necrosis can be seen between 12 and 24 hours after onset of chest pain, the nucleus is intact, and the cross-striation are well seen. **C:** By 48 to 72 hours, the neutrophils are now concentrated at the border of the infarcted and viable myocardium; the extent of neutrophil infiltration depends on the collateral flow and the extent of coronary perfusion of the adjacent bed. The central zone of infarction now shows all the features of coagulation necrosis with karyolysis and loss of cross-striations. **D:** Photomicrograph showing high-power view of the border zone of a 5-day-old infarct with marked neutrophil infiltration that has undergone karyopyknosis and karyorrhexis, and the adjoining infarcted myocardium shows coagulation necrosis with loss of nuclei and cross-striations. **E:** A high-power view of the subendocardial region, which is usually ischemic but viable showing myocyte vacuolization and loss of myofibrils. **F:** Almost complete removal of the necrotic myocardium, note presence of neovascular channels and surrounding macrophages and few lymphocytes (granulation tissue) at 7 to 10 days after acute myocardial infarction. **G:** The infarct is heavily infiltrated with fibroblasts with early collagen deposition and interspersed neocapillaries and few lymphocytes; infarct age is 3 to 4 weeks. **H:** A fully healed infarct with dense collagen and few interspersed myocytes at the border region of the healed infarct. Infarct age may be 6 weeks and greater. (From Virmani R, Burke AP, Farb A, Atkinson J, eds. Pathology of myocardial infarction. *In: Cardiovascular pathology,* 2nd ed. Major problems in pathology series, vol 40. Philadelphia: WB Saunders Company, 2001, with permission.)

Histology of Developing Nonreperfused Infarction

An inflammatory response marks the second stage of acute ischemia, after the initial hallmarks of myocyte damage. Neutrophil infiltration is present by 24 hours at the border areas of acute infarcts and becomes prominent by 48 hours (Fig. 55–6D through F). As the infarct progresses between 24 and 48 hours, coagulation necrosis is established with nuclear pyknosis of myocytes, early karyorrhexis (nuclear

dust), and karyolysis. Karyorrhexis is especially prominent in smaller infarcts. The myocyte striations are initially preserved, whereas the sarcomeres elongate, but disappear by 3 to 5 days, beginning in the central zones. Loss of myocyte striations is best appreciated by Mallory's trichrome stain.

After the initial stages of myocyte necrosis and acute inflammation, macrophages, endothelial cell ingrowth, and fibroblasts begin to appear in the border area at approximately

5 days, 1 week, and 2 weeks, respectively. By 1 week, neutrophils decline and granulation tissue is established with angiogenesis and infiltration by lymphocytes and plasma cells. Although lymphocytes may be seen as early as 2 to 3 days, they are not prominent in any stage of infarct evolution. Eosinophils may be seen within the inflammatory infiltrate but are only present in 24% of infarcts (47). There is phagocytic removal of the necrotic myocytes by macrophages, and pigment is seen within macrophages.

There is continued removal of the necrotic myocytes as angiogenesis and macrophage infiltration continue, and fibroblasts replace the necrotic areas with collagen. Fibroblasts are established by the second week, but their appearance may be seen as early as Day 4 at the periphery of the infarct. The healing continues, and depending on the extent of necrosis, may be complete as early as 4 weeks. In general, complete healing is accomplished by 8 weeks (Fig. 55–6G and H). If ingrowth of capillaries within the central portion of the infarct is incomplete, the central area of infarction remains unhealed and contains metabolically inactive, mummified myocytes. Areas of myocyte mummification may persist for months or even years after healing is complete in the border regions. For this reason, it is important to evaluate the age of the infarct by examining the border with noninfarcted muscle.

LIGHT MICROSCOPIC APPEARANCE OF REPERFUSED ACUTE MYOCARDIAL INFARCTION

If thrombolytic treatment is successfully accomplished within 4 to 6 hours after onset of chest pain or ECG changes, the extent of infarct is significantly lessened and may be confined to the subendocardium. Histologically, there is a confluent area of hemorrhage within the subendocardium, the size of which depends of the extent of reperfusion and duration of the ischemic time, both of which affect the degree of capillary necrosis and leakage. Myocytes demonstrate extensive contraction band necrosis. Within a few hours of reperfusion, neutrophils are evident within the area of necrosis, but they are usually sparse (Fig. 55–7A). In contrast to nonreperfused infarcts, neutrophils do not show concentration at the margins. However, reperfused infarcts often demonstrate areas of necrosis at the periphery with interdigitation with noninfarcted myocardium.

Similar to humans, the amount of myocardium that can be salvaged in the dog model depends on the duration of total occlusion of the artery supplying the area of infarction. The maximal salvage is possible, as is the case with humans, if the artery is opened within 6 hours. The myocardium in the dog after 90 minutes of occlusion followed by reperfusion and death at 24 hours shows a hemorrhagic infarct limited to the area of occlusion, which is subendocardial in extent. Hemorrhage occurs when the myocardial blood flow during the occlusion period is less than one-fifth of normal. As in human infarcts, the myocytes are thin, hypereosinophilic, devoid of nuclei, or showing karyorrhexis,

with ill-defined borders and interspersed areas of interstitial hemorrhage (Fig. 55–7B). There is a diffuse but mild neutrophil infiltration (Fig. 55–7C) with occasional calcified myocytes (Fig. 55–7D). Within 2 to 3 days, macrophage infiltration is obvious (Fig. 55–7E and F) with phagocytosis of necrotic myocytes and early stages of granulation tissue. The infarct healing in the dog is more rapid than that in humans, most likely because of collaterals and a lack of underlying myocardial disease secondary to diffuse epicardial atherothrombosis.

Similar to the dog, macrophages begin to appear in human myocardial infarcts by the second or third day, and stromal cells show enlarged nuclei and nucleoli by Days 3 and 4. Neutrophil debris, which may be concentrated at the border areas in cases of incomplete reperfusion, is seen by 3 to 5 days. Angiogenesis with a lymphoplasmacytic response is prominent at this stage, and myocytolysis, or loss of cross striations, occurs (Fig. 55–7G and H). Fibroblasts appear almost as early as angiogenesis, with an accelerated rate of healing as compared with nonreperfused infarcts. By 1 week there is collagen deposition with disappearance of neutrophils and prominence of macrophages containing pigment derived from ingested myocytes and red blood cells (Fig. 55–7H). Subendocardial infarcts may be fully healed as early as 2 to 3 weeks.

Larger infarcts, and those reperfused after 6 hours, take longer to heal. Infarcts reperfused after 6 hours show larger areas of hemorrhage as compared with occlusions with more immediate reperfusion. However, myocytes maintain their striations, become stretched and elongated, and, as they do not respond to calcium influx, do not show significant contraction band necrosis. Despite that reperfusion should occur within 6 hours of occlusion for maximal myocyte salvage, there appears to be some benefit in opening an artery regardless of the duration of coronary occlusion.

Hibernating Myocardium

The concept of hibernation myocardium arose from the observation, initially reported by Rahimtoola and coworkers (48), that coronary artery bypass graft surgery resulted in significant improvement in left ventricular function in a subset of patients with depressed ventricular performance. The definition of hibernating myocardium, which is distinct from the stunned myocardium, is "resting left ventricular function due to reduced coronary blood flow that can be partially or completely reversed by myocardial revascularization and/or by reducing myocardial oxygen demand" (49,50). The clinical determination of hibernating myocardium (as well as stunned myocardium, another form of reversible ischemic injury) is important, because revascularization of irreversibly damaged myocardium is of little benefit. The relative merits of different imaging techniques, including nuclear medicine imaging and magnetic resonance, have been reviewed (51). Coronary revascularization by percutaneous angioplasty has shown improvement of left

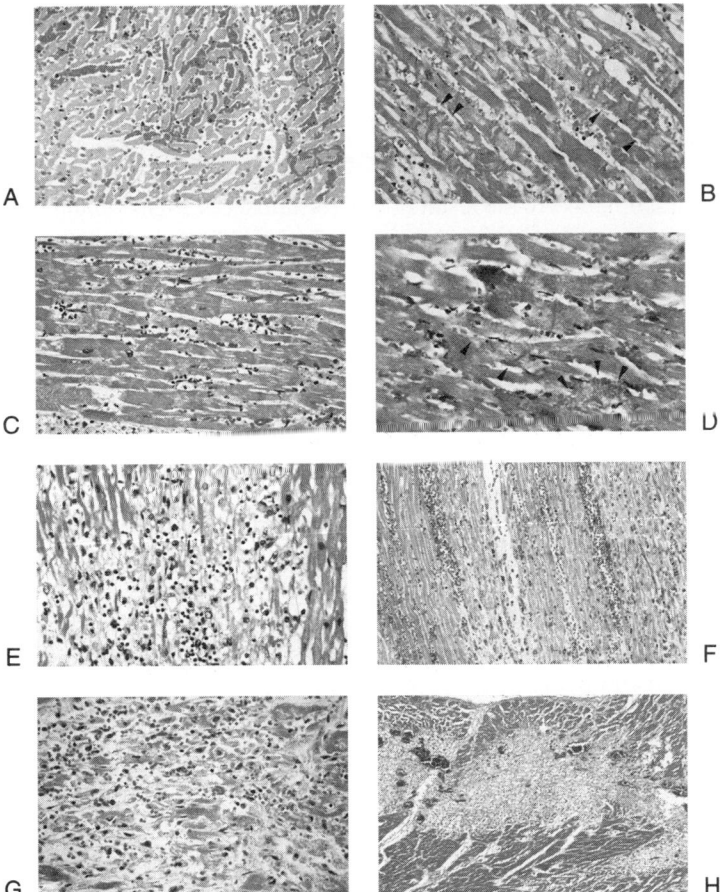

FIG. 55–7. Histologic characteristics of a reperfused infarct after occlusion and reperfusion either with thrombolysis (tissue plasminogen activator, streptokinase, or IIb/IIIa) or balloon angioplasty with or without stenting or surgical revascularization. **A:** A cross section of myocytes shows necrosis with interstitial hemorrhage. Note pale myocyte nuclei and early neutrophil infiltration. **B:** Myocytes cut longitudinally in a patient who was admitted with chest pain of 2 hours in duration followed by infusion of streptokinase. The patient died within 6 hours. Note the extensive contraction band necrosis (dark bands alternating with lighter bands, *arrowheads*), a hallmark of reperfusion injury. There are interstitial red cells and a few neutrophils, which were scattered throughout the infarct. **C:** Note the number of neutrophils is greater than in the previous example. There is mild red cell extravasation and contraction band necrosis. The duration of chest pain was 3 hours before reperfusion, and the patient died 24 hours later. **D:** It is not uncommon to see single or a few necrotic myocytes with calcification *(arrowheads)* in patients with reperfused infarcts. **E:** Note the presence of macrophages and lymphocytes with early dissolution of the necrotic myocytes. These areas of necrosis are interdigitating with viable noninfarcted myocardium (4- to 5-day-old reperfused infarct). **F:** Note interstitial hemorrhage and infiltrating macrophages seen in the lower one-fifth and the right one-third of the photomicrograph. **G:** High-power view of another infarct showing dissolution of the infarct and replacement with macrophages and early angiogenesis. Hemorrhage is still present, but no neutrophils are seen (5- to 7-day infarct). **H:** Low-power view of a healing infarct at 7 to 10 days. Note angiogenesis and early replacement fibrosis. (From Virmani R, Burke AP, Farb A, Atkinson J, eds. Pathology of myocardial infarction. *In: Cardiovascular pathology,* 2nd ed. Major problems in pathology series, vol 40. Philadelphia: WB Saunders Company, 2001, with permission.)

ventricular wall motion in patients with hibernation myocardium, which disappears with restenosis (52).

In the course of acute subendocardial infarcts or at the border regions of transmural infarcts, a viable subendocardial layer is spared, generally consisting of five to ten layers of subendocardial myocytes. Myofibrillar loss, which is a result of ischemia not severe enough to cause cell death, is prominent in this subendocardial zone. Morphologically, hibernating myocytes show loss of contractile elements, espe-

cially in the perinuclear region, and occasionally throughout the cytoplasm. The space left by the dissolution of the myofibrils is occupied by glycogen, as evidenced by the strong positivity for the periodic acid-Schiff reagent. Ultrastructurally, there is depletion of sarcomeres, most pronounced in the perinuclear region, with increased glycogen. The nuclei are enlarged, with a tortuous nuclear membrane and evenly distributed heterochromatin. The mitochondria are elongated, shrunken, and osmiophilic (53). There are no morphologic hallmarks of postischemic stunned myocardium, which is defined entirely by clinical criteria (32,54).

Relation of Myocardial Ischemia and Epicardial Coronary Artery Disease

More than 90% of acute myocardial infarcts are the result of thrombosis occurring at the site of atherothrombotic plaque. Arbustini and coworkers (55) found coronary thrombi in 98% of patients dying with clinically documented AMI, a rate that is similar to previous autopsy series (56–58). Angiographic studies have shown that "culprit" lesions are not necessarily sites of maximal luminal narrowing, underscoring the need for imaging of plaques that are prone to thrombosis (59).

The nature of thrombosis overlying coronary artery plaques is morphologically diverse. Autopsy studies of patients dying of severe coronary disease, emphasizing patients dying suddenly and unexpectedly, have shown that coronary thrombosis is most frequently the result of plaque rupture (65%) and less frequently of plaque erosion (30–35%), and uncommonly from calcified nodule (2–5%) (60, 61). Arbustini and coworkers (55) confirmed a high rate of plaque erosion in hospitalized patients dying of complications of AMI. There are sex differences in the causation of coronary thrombi leading to acute myocardial infarcts, as Arbustini and coworkers (55) showed that 37% of thrombi in women were erosive compared with only 18% in men. Although an individual severe stenosis is more likely to become occluded by a thrombus than a lesion with less severe stenosis, the less severely narrowed plaques give rise to more occlusions, as there are many more sites that are mild to moderately narrowed (62). We have observed that 82% of fatal plaque erosions occur in coronary segments with relatively little stenosis (<79% cross-sectional area narrowing) compared with only 57% of plaque ruptures. The most frequent (approximately 50%) culprit coronary artery of infarction at autopsy is the left anterior descending artery, followed by the right coronary artery (30–45%) and then the left circumflex (15–20%) (61).

Arrhythmias and Effect of Ischemia on the Specialized Conduction System

Arrhythmias occurring after AMI may be the result of instability in the working myocardium or ischemia of the areas of the specialized conduction system. Tachyarrhythmias that occur during AMI often result from reperfusion, altered automatic tone, or hemodynamic instability. Bradyarrhythmias during the first few hours of AMI are triggered from inferior MI and are usually benign. Ventricular tachyarrhythmias most likely arise from the adjoining ischemic but noninfarcted myocardium. In this acidotic arrhythmogenic zone, there is the release of metabolites such as potassium, calcium, and catecholamines, with low levels of ATP and hypoxemia (63,64). Later in the course of MI, arrhythmias

may occur as a result of scar tissue surrounding viable myocytes (65).

The conduction system is relatively protected against ischemic injury because conduction fibers are relatively inactive metabolically, as their function is not to provide contractility but rather the propagation of the impulse (66,67). Conduction disturbances (right bundle branch block and left anterior fascicular block) resulting from anterior MI are associated with high mortality caused by necrosis of the conduction system. The site of conduction system disturbance caused by ischemia is related to vascular supply. The atrioventricular node is supplied from the right coronary artery in 90% of cases and left circumflex in 10% (68). The bundle of His is supplied from the atrioventricular branch of the right coronary artery, and a small contribution comes from the septal perforator of the left anterior descending artery. The His bundle divides into the right and left bundle branches, and the right bundle branch receives most of its blood from the septal perforators of the left anterior descending artery, but there may be collaterals from the right and left circumflex arteries. The left anterior branch receives its blood supply from the septal perforators from the left anterior descending artery and is particularly susceptible to ischemia or infarction. The proximal portion of the left posterior fascicle receives its blood supply from the atrioventricular nodal artery and from the septal perforators of the left anterior descending artery. The distal portion of posterior fascicle is supplied from two sources and includes the anterior and posterior septal perforating arteries.

Cardiogenic Shock

Cardiogenic shock is the most common cause of death in patients hospitalized with AMI, with a mortality rate of approximately 10%. Cardiogenic shock is caused by decreased systemic cardiac output in the presence of adequate intravascular volume. Cardiogenic shock after MI usually occurs if there is loss of at least 40% of the left ventricular mass, either acutely or in combination with scarred myocardium from previously healed infarcts (34,69,70). In about 10% of patients who experience development of cardiogenic shock, shock occurs before hospitalization immediately on presentation. Much more commonly, shock develops while the patient is in the hospital, presumably from infarct extension (71,72). Cardiogenic shock accounts for 44% of short-term deaths after MI. The remainder of deaths results from cardiac rupture (26%) and arrhythmias (16%) (65). Patients with extension of infarction (reinfarction) into subendocardial zones remote from the larger infarct may experience development of cardiogenic shock. In turn, cardiogenic shock renders the remaining viable myocardium prone to ischemic necrosis because of poor perfusion (73).

Infarction of the Right Ventricle

Right ventricular infarction is a common complication of inferior transmural MI, occurring in 14% to 60% of patients.

Right ventricular infarcts commonly involve the inferior/posterior wall, posterior septum, and posterior right ventricular wall contiguously, with rare extension to the anterolateral right ventricle (74,75). More than three-fourths of right ventricular infarctions occur in patients with inferior left ventricular infarcts and right ventricular hypertrophy (76). Isolated right ventricular infarction may infrequently occur in the absence of coronary disease in patients with chronic lung disease and right ventricular hypertrophy (77). Atrial infarction occurs in 10% of all left ventricular inferior wall infarcts and typically involves the right atrium (78).

Cardiac Rupture After Acute Myocardial Infarction

The overall incidence of postinfarct ventricular free wall rupture is approximately 2% to 3% (79–81). Risk factors for cardiac rupture after MI include multivessel atherothrombotic disease, female sex and age older than 60 years, hypertension, absence of hypertrophy and previous infarction, poor collateral flow, the presence of a transmural infarct involving at least 20% of the wall, and location of the infarct in the midanterior or lateral wall of the left ventricle (82–87). There is some evidence that rupture is less frequent in cigarette smokers (79).

Cardiac rupture usually occurs in the first few days (1–4 days) after the infarct when coagulation necrosis and neutrophilic infiltration are at their peak and have weakened the left ventricular wall (88,89). Ruptures usually are not seen beyond 10 days after healing occurs. However, ruptures in infarcts with healing generally occur in the center of the infarct, unlike earlier ruptures (88,89).

Left ventricular wall rupture is seven times more common than right ventricle rupture (88,89) (Fig. 55–8A and B). Infarcts with rupture contain more extensive inflammation and are more likely to demonstrate eosinophils (30% eosinophilic infiltration compared with 12% eosinophilic infiltration in nonruptured infarcts (90). However, at least 13% to 28% rupture occurs within 24 hours of onset of infarction when inflammation and necrosis are not prominent (91). Rupture most frequently occurs at the border of the infarcted region with the viable myocardium.

Reperfusion therapy has reduced the incidence of cardiac rupture. However, late thrombolytic therapy may increase the risk for cardiac rupture (Fig. 55–8C). There is some evidence that primary coronary angioplasty reduces the incidence of free wall rupture, as compared with patients treated with thrombolysis alone (92–94).

Almost half of the deaths from cardiac rupture occur as out-of-hospital sudden deaths and therefore are never seen by the clinician (91). In a series of patients who survived free wall rupture after AMI, there was an equal incidence of free wall and septal ruptures, with papillary muscle rupture occurring 25% as frequently as either free wall or septal rupture (95). In this series, delayed hospitalization and undue in-hospital activity appeared to increase the risk for rupture (95).

Rupture of the free wall usually leads to hemopericardium and death when it occurs resulting from cardiac tamponade. Infrequently, pseudoaneurysm may form, preventing lethal hemopericardium. Ruptures of the ventricular septum have been classified into simple or complex (Fig. 55–8D through F). Simple ruptures have a discrete defect and a direct through-and-through communication across the septum, are usually associated with anterior MI, and are located in the apex. Complex ruptures are characterized by extensive hemorrhage with irregular serpiginous borders of the necrotic muscle, usually occur in inferior infarcts, and involve the basal inferoposterior septum (96). The mortality rate of septal rupture in the prethrombolytic era was extremely high, with a 50% mortality rate in surgically treated patients and a 90% rate in those treated medically. The mortality rates have not declined significantly since the introduction of thrombolysis. Patients with septal rupture from inferior rather than anterior MI have the shortest survival time.

Rupture of papillary muscle is less common than septal or free wall rupture and may occur as a complication of small subendocardial or larger transmural MIs (97,98). More than 80% of infarcts underlying papillary muscle rupture involve the posteromedial muscle, which has a single blood supply from the right coronary artery (Figure 55–8G). Because the anterolateral papillary muscle has a dual blood supply from the left anterior descending and the left circumflex coronary artery, it rarely undergoes isolated ischemic rupture (88,98,99). The patient with papillary muscle rupture presents with sudden mitral regurgitation with variable severity. Complete transection of a left ventricular papillary muscle is incompatible with survival because of massive sudden mitral regurgitation (89).

Infarct Extension and Expansion

Two related but distinct complications of MI are infarct extension and infarct expansion. Infarct extension results from an incremental increase in absolute necrotic myocardium and may be the result of infarction remote from the original infarct in either the right or left ventricle (Fig. 55–9). It has been suggested that the more general term *recurrent infarction* be used for infarct extension (100). Infarct extension usually occurs between 2 and 10 days after infarction, at a time when ECG changes are evolving and the troponin I or T is still high. However, the rapidly decreasing serum CK-MB after the first 24 hours may be useful for the detection of infarct extension along with new Q wave on ECG. The risk factors associated with infarct expansion are cardiogenic shock, subendocardial infarct, female sex, and previous infarcts (101,102).

Infarct expansion is the thinning of the area of the infarcted region and is not an increase in myocardial necrosis. In contrast, infarct expansion is caused by stretching of myocyte bundles reducing the density of myocytes in the area of the infarcted wall, resulting in loss of tissue within the

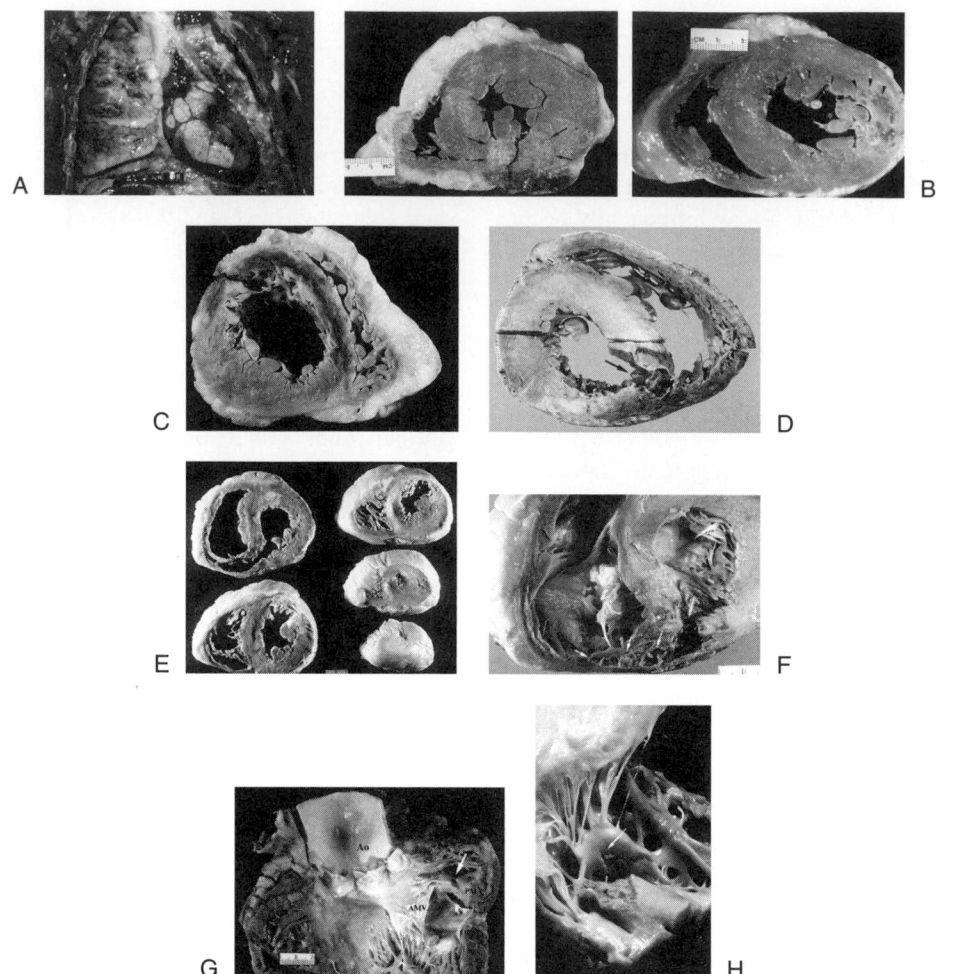

FIG. 55–8. Ruptured acute myocardial infarction. **A:** Hemopericardium in a 70-year-old man with a history of chest pain and diagnosis of acute transmural infarction who died suddenly while walking to the bathroom 24 hours after hospital admission. The pericardium contained 300 mL blood, and a rupture site was identified on the posterior wall of the left ventricle **(B1).** Note an early transmural infarct (pale area on the posterior wall, *arrows*) with rupture site close to the viable myocardium but within the infarct zone. **B2:** A lateral wall rupture. Note the rupture site is close to the viable and the infarcted myocardium *(arrowheads).* **C:** A 50-year-old man presented with chest pain of 7 hours in duration. He received streptokinase and underwent balloon angioplasty of the proximal left anterior descending coronary artery. At autopsy, the patient had hemopericardium and a transmural hemorrhagic reperfused infarct involving the anteroseptal wall of left ventricle. The rupture occurred close to the viable myocardium on the anterior wall. **D:** Rupture of the posterior ventricular septum *(arrow)* 2 weeks after an acute myocardial infarction. The patient died of severe congestive heart failure, and the diagnosis of ventricular septal rupture was clinically missed. (A four-chamber cut had been made before bread loaf). **E:** Ventricular septal rupture involving the inferobasal portion of the heart, which extends through the posterior septum and into the right ventricular, causing a dissection of the posterior wall of the right ventricle. **F:** High-power view of the inferobasal portion of the heart showing the rupture through the septum extending into the right ventricle and piercing the right ventricular wall *(arrow* along the rupture tract). **G:** A patient with transmural myocardial infarction of the posterior wall of the left ventricle with rupture of one of the two heads of posteromedial *(PM)* papillary muscle *(arrow).* The base of the heart has been opened along the left ventricular outflow tract. **H:** High-power view showing total severance of one of the papillary heads *(arrow)* of the posteromedial papillary muscle. AMV, anterior mitral leaflet; Ao, aorta. (From Virmani R, Burke AP, Farb A, Atkinson J, eds. Pathology of myocardial infarction. *In: Cardiovascular pathology,* 2nd ed. Major problems in pathology series, vol 40. Philadelphia: WB Saunders Company, 2001, with permission.)

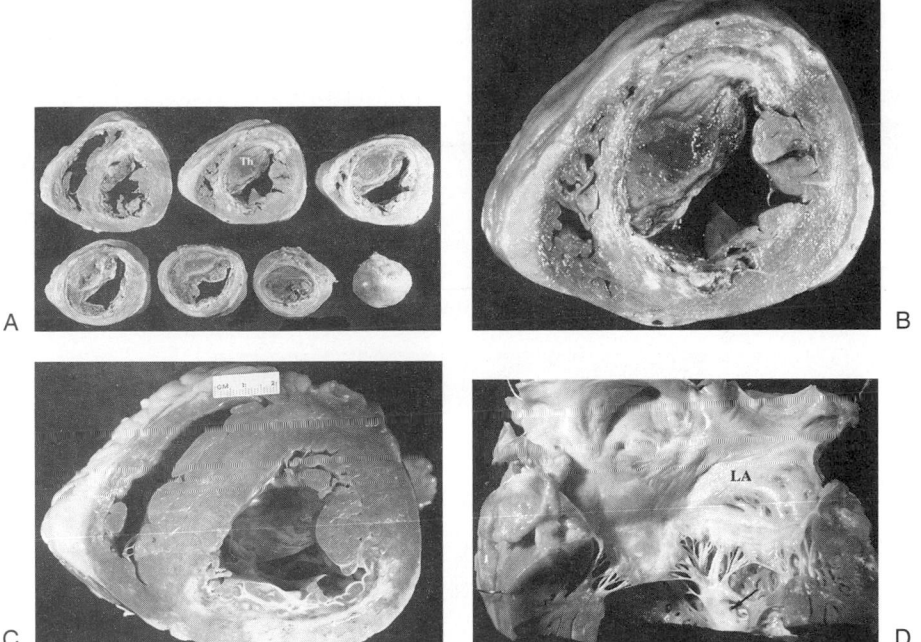

FIG. 55–9. Thrombus left ventricle with healed myocardial infarct. **A:** Ventricular slices of a heart with healed myocardial infarction involving the anteroseptal wall of the left ventricle with extension from the base to the apex. Note dilatation of the left ventricular cavity and presence of an organizing thrombus *(Th).* **B:** Close-up view of the basal ventricular slice (middle slice from top row in **A**), not large transmural healed infarct with overlying organizing infarct. At autopsy, patient had multiple infarcts in the kidneys and one in the spleen. **C:** A 60-year-old man with congestive heart failure and mitral regurgitation had a healed myocardial infarction of the posterolateral wall of the left ventricle at autopsy. **D:** Note scarred and thinned posteromedial papillary muscle *(arrow)* whereas the anterolateral papillary muscle is hypertrophied. Note dilated left atrium *(LA).* (From Virmani R, Burke AP, Farb A, Atkinson J, eds. Pathology of myocardial infarction. *In: Cardiovascular pathology,* 2nd ed. Major problems in pathology series, vol 40. Philadelphia: WB Saunders Company, 2001, with permission.)

necrotic myocardium (103). Infarct expansion typically results in dilatation and thinning of the infarct and is associated with heart failure, ventricular aneurysm, and high mortality. Risk factors for infarct expansion are anterior transmural infarcts and life-threatening arrhythmias (104). Another term often applied to infarct expansion is ventricular remodeling, and it involves remodeling of both the infarcted and the noninfarcted myocardium. As so defined, infarct expansion is a combination of changes of left ventricular dilation and hypertrophy of noninfarcted myocardium (105,106).

Development of Aneurysms After Myocardial Infarction

One outcome of free wall rupture after AMI is the development of a pseudoaneurysm. False aneurysms have a small neck, derived from a prior rupture of the ventricle contained by the adherent pericardium. The wall of the false aneurysm is formed by fibrous pericardium, not from the left ventricular MI and healing. The aneurysm is usually filled by a thrombus, which is organizing (Fig. 55–10A). False aneurysms often require urgent surgical repair because of propensity to rupture, and they also predispose to congestive heart failure. The presence of hypertension and the use of steroids

and nonsteroidal antiinflammatory drugs may promote aneurysm formation (107).

True aneurysms result when large acute transmural myocardial infarcts undergo expansion (108,109). The pulsatile force from the blood in the cavity stretches and thins the necrotic muscle, which heals forming the wall of a true aneurysm (110). An aneurysm is defined clinically as a discrete thinned segment of the left ventricle that protrudes during both systole and diastole and has a broad neck (Fig. 55–10B through D). Morphologically, the wall of a true aneurysm develops after MI and consists of fibrous tissue with or without interspersed myocytes.

The incidence of true aneurysm after an MI is 5% to 10% and is more frequent in transmural infarction than subendocardial infarction (89). Aneurysms are usually associated with two-vessel or multivessel coronary disease with poorly developed collaterals (111). Four of five aneurysms involve the anteroapical wall of the left ventricle (88) and are four times more frequent in this wall than in the inferior or posterior wall (89). The pericardium is usually adherent to the aneurysm and may calcify. In contrast to pseudoaneurysms (Fig. 55–10E and F), true aneurysms rarely rupture (Fig. 55–10G) (112). The cavity of the aneurysm usually contains

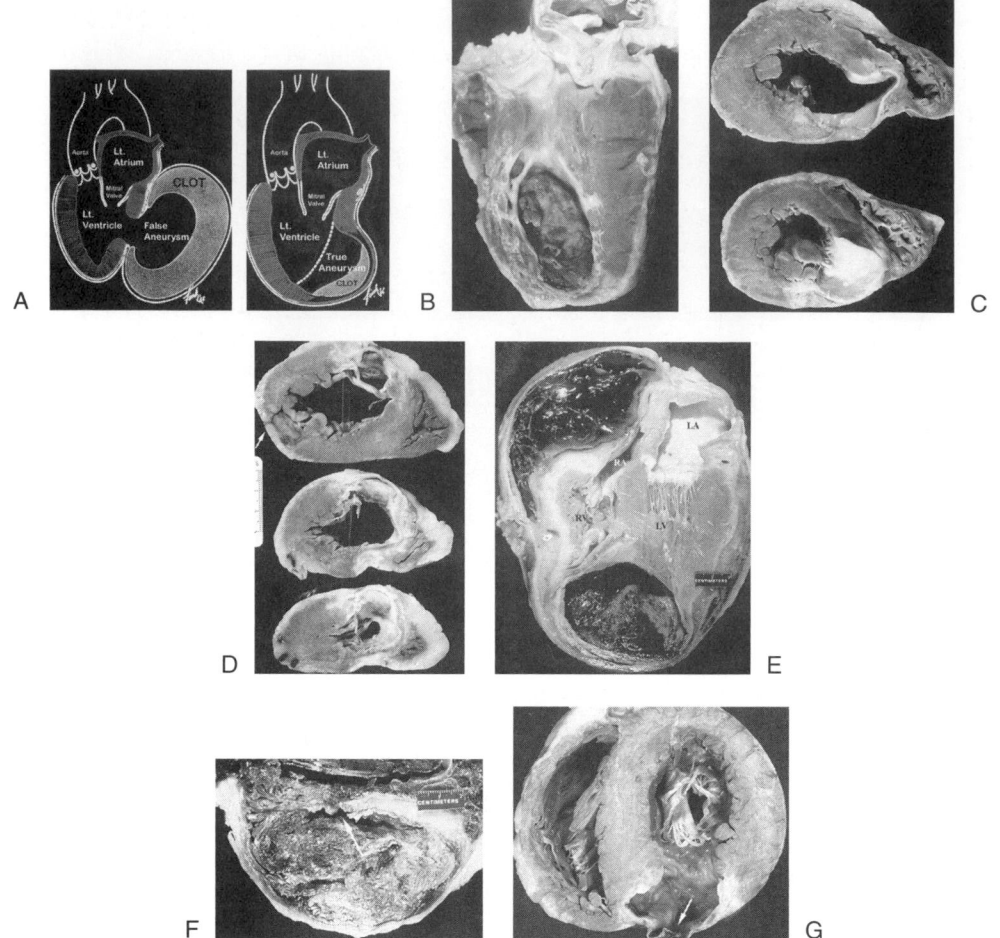

FIG. 55–10. A: Diagram of a false *(left)* and a true *(right)* aneurysm. Note a rupture of the left ventricular wall with the blood contained by the pericardial wall. The left ventricle does not form the wall of the aneurysm, and the neck of the aneurysm is narrow. The wall of the true aneurysm is formed by the wall of the infarcted myocardium, and the neck of the aneurysm is wide. **B:** A true aneurysm is seen at the apex of the heart involving the anteroseptal apical two-thirds of the left ventricle. The aneurysm is filled with a thrombus, and there is endocardial thickening around the edges of the infarct. **C:** Healed transmural infarction of the posteroseptal wall of the left ventricle, note the thinned and bulging aneurysm of the posterior and septal wall with marked endocardial thickening. No thrombus was identified within the cavity of the aneurysm. **D:** A 54-year-old man died suddenly without any significant medical history. At autopsy, there was cardiac tamponade with ventricular rupture of the posterolateral wall *(arrow)* secondary to a transmural acute infarction. Ventricular slices of the heart showing presence of a localized small anterior aneurysm from a healed myocardial infarction involving the anterior and septal wall of the left ventricle. Note organizing thrombus in the aneurysmal cavity. **E:** False aneurysm. A 47-year-old man presented with sudden-onset shortness of breath and died in the emergency room. At autopsy, there was a loculated hemopericardium and a left ventricular anteroapical aneurysm secondary to a healed myocardial infarction with overlying thrombus. Four-chamber cut of the heart showed extensive adhesions between the visceral and the parietal pericardium, and loculated fresh blood was present in the pericardial space above the right atrium *(RA)* and right ventricle *(RV)*, as well as organizing hemorrhage around the heart. **F:** A deeper posterior cut revealed the rupture site in the aneurysmal wall *(arrow)*. Note the narrow, communicating neck of the true aneurysm with the false aneurysm. A diagnosis of rupture of a true aneurysm with a secondary false aneurysm was made. **G:** Rupture of a healed inferior wall aneurysm *(arrow)* in a 56-year-old man who experienced development of chest pain and died while undergoing a stress test. At autopsy, there was hemopericardium (500 mL). LA, left atrium; LV, left ventricle. (A: Courtesy Dr. William C. Roberts, Baylor Heart and Vascular Institute, Baylor University Medical Center, Dallas, TX; B–G: From Virmani R, Burke AP, Farb A, Atkinson J, eds. Pathology of myocardial infarction. *In: Cardiovascular pathology,* 2nd ed. Major problems in pathology series, vol 40. Philadelphia: WB Saunders Company, 2001, with permission.)

an organizing thrombus, and the patient may present with embolic complications. The mortality rate is six times greater in patients with than without aneurysm (113).

More than half of pseudoaneurysms are located in the posterior or inferior walls, whereas true aneurysms generally involve the anterior wall. Reasons for these differences have been speculated to be because large inferoposterior infarcts that could lead to aneurysms are more often fatal, and posterior rupture is more often contained by the pericardium allowing pseudoaneurysm to develop (114).

Mills and coworkers (115) suggested that aneurysmectomy should be performed in patients having true aneurysms because of poor prognosis. They reported a 27% 3-year survival in an autopsy series and a 70% survival in the Coronary Artery Surgery Study. The survival rate of patients with pseudoaneurysm is also greater after surgery.

Postinfarct Pericarditis

Pericardial effusion is reported in 25% of patients with acute myocardial infarcts and is more common in patients with anterior MI, large infarcts, and congestive heart failure (116,117). Pericardial effusion secondary to AMI may occur as a transudative effusion, or as an exudate, in association with acute pericarditis. Pericardial effusion after MI usually takes several months to reabsorb.

After infarction, pericarditis occurs less often than pericardial effusion and is seen only in transmural AMI. Pericarditis, in contrast to postinfarction effusions, may be localized to the area of necrosis and is accompanied by chest pain. Pericarditis consists of fibrin deposition in addition to inflammation and may be present from the first day after infarction to as late as 6 weeks. Risk factors for the development of postinfarction pericarditis include heparinization and thrombolytic therapy (118). Pericardial involvement is related to infarct size and is associated with poor prognosis. Postinfarction syndrome (Dressler's syndrome) consists of pleuropericardial chest pain, friction rub, fever, leukocytosis, and pulmonary infiltrates, occurs weeks to months after MI, and often is recurrent. It is reported to occur in 3% to 4% of all patients with MI (89). At autopsy, there is localized fibrinous pericarditis together with neutrophil infiltration. The cause of Dressler's syndrome is unknown, but antibodies to cardiac tissue have been reported, suggesting an immunologic process (119). The incidence of postinfarction syndrome since the institution of thrombolytic therapy has markedly reduced; however, the reasons for this reduction are unclear.

Congestive Heart Failure After Acute Myocardial Infarction

The survival rate has improved from 28% to 56% after hospitalization for MI. Enhances in medical care have primarily benefited younger patients compared with patients with diabetes and older patients (120). Patients with large AMI and persistent ischemia are the most likely to experience devel-

opment of heart failure. Severity of congestive heart failure is a predictor of mortality (121). Congestive heart failure usually occurs in the presence of two- or three-vessel disease and may develop even in the presence of well developed collaterals (122). Grossly, the atria and the ventricles are dilated and the ventricle shows either a large healed infarct or multiple smaller infarcts with or without a transmural scar (123). Scarring of the inferior wall of the left ventricle often involves the posteromedial papillary muscle, which gives rise to mitral regurgitation contributing to congestive heart failure (123). Microscopically, the subendocardial regions of ischemia will show myocytes with myofibrillar loss that are rich in glycogen, suggesting a state of "hibernation" (discussed earlier) (124). Sometimes it is difficult to differentiate ischemic cardiomyopathy from idiopathic dilated cardiomyopathy when infarcts are few and small and only one-vessel disease is present; in such situations, we tend to use the term idiopathic dilated cardiomyopathy with incidental coronary artery disease (125).

MURAL THROMBUS AND EMBOLIZATION

Mural thrombus forming on the endocardial surface over the area of the acute infarction occurs in 20% of all patients. However, the incidence is 40% for anterior infarcts and 60% for apical infarcts (126–130). Patients with left ventricular thrombi have poorer global left ventricular function and poorer prognosis compared with those without thrombi (126). The poor prognosis is secondary to complications of a large infarct and not from emboli (127). It has been reported that those patients who form thrombi have endocardial inflammation during the phase of acute infarction. The thrombi tend to organize, but the superficial portions may embolize in about 10% of cases (126). The usual sites of symptomatic embolization are the brain, eyes, kidney, spleen, bowel, legs, and coronary arteries. Symptomatic emboli are usually caused by larger fragments, whereas small particles of thrombus that embolize generally do not cause symptoms (128). The risk for embolization is greatest in the first few weeks of AMI (129). Anticoagulation has been show to reduce the incidence of left ventricular thrombus formation (89).

REFERENCES

1. Tavazzi L. Clinical epidemiology of acute myocardial infarction. *Am Heart J* 1999;138:48–54.
2. Mendelson MA, Hendel RC. Myocardial infarction in women. *Cardiology* 1995;86:272–285.
3. Williams JE, Massing M, Rosamond WD, et al. Racial disparities in CHD mortality from 1968-1992 in the state economic areas surrounding the ARIC study communities. Atherosclerosis Risk in Communities. *Ann Epidemiol* 1999;9:472–480.
4. Pashos CL, Newhouse JP, McNeil BJ. Temporal changes in the care and outcomes of elderly patients with acute myocardial infarction, 1987 through 1990. *JAMA* 1993;270:1832–1836.
5. Miller TD, Christian TF, Hodge DO, et al. Comparison of acute myocardial infarct size to two-year mortality in patients <65 to those > or =65 years of age. *Am J Cardiol* 1999;84:1170–1175.

6. Rosamond WD, Chambless LE, Folsom AR. Survival trends, coronary event rates, and the MONICA project. Monitoring trends and determinants in cardiovascular disease. *Lancet* 1999;354:864–865.

7. Levy D, Thom TJ. Death rates from coronary disease—progress and a puzzling paradox. *N Engl J Med* 1998;339:915–917.

8. Beller GA. Coronary heart disease in the first 30 years of the 21st century: challenges and opportunities: the 33rd Annual James B. Herrick Lecture of the Council on Clinical Cardiology of the American Heart Association. *Circulation* 2001;103:2428–2435.

9. Rosamond WD, Chambless LE, Folsom AR, et al. Trends in the incidence of myocardial infarction and in mortality due to coronary heart disease, 1987 to 1994. *N Engl J Med* 1998;339:861–867.

10. Hohnloser SH, Gersh BJ. Changing late prognosis of acute myocardial infarction: impact on management of ventricular arrhythmias in the era of reperfusion and the implantable cardioverter-defibrillator. *Circulation* 2003;107:941–946.

11. Menon V, Hochman JS. Management of cardiogenic shock complicating acute myocardial infarction. *Heart* 2002;88:531–537.

12. Tunstall-Pedoe H, Kuulasmaa K, Amouyel P, et al. Myocardial infarction and coronary deaths in the World Health Organization MONICA Project. Registration procedures, event rates, and case-fatality rates in 38 populations from 21 countries in four continents. *Circulation* 1994;90:583–612.

13. Hedges JR, Young GP, Henkel GF, et al. Serial ECGs are less accurate than serial CK-MB results for emergency department diagnosis of myocardial infarction. *Ann Emerg Med* 1992;21:1445–1450.

14. Young GP, Gibler WB, Hedges JR, et al. Serial creatine kinase-MB results are a sensitive indicator of acute myocardial infarction in chest pain patients with nondiagnostic electrocardiograms: the second Emergency Medicine Cardiac Research Group Study. *Acad Emerg Med* 1997;4:869–877.

15. Morrow DA, Rifai N, Tanasijevic MJ, et al. Clinical efficacy of three assays for cardiac troponin I for risk stratification in acute coronary syndromes: a Thrombolysis In Myocardial Infarction (TIMI) 11B Substudy. *Clin Chem* 2000;46:453–460.

16. Antman EM, Grudzien C, Sacks DB. Evaluation of a rapid bedside assay for detection of serum cardiac troponin T. *JAMA* 1995;273:1279–1282.

17. Hackel DB, Reimer KA, Ideker RE, et al. Comparison of enzymatic and anatomic estimates of myocardial infarct size in man. *Circulation* 1984;70:824–835.

18. Zucker DR, Griffith JL, Beshansky JR, et al. Presentations of acute myocardial infarction in men and women. *J Gen Intern Med* 1997;12:79–87.

19. Stanley WC. Cardiac energetics during ischaemia and the rationale for metabolic interventions. *Coron Artery Dis* 2001;12:S3–S7.

20. Reimer KA, Jennings RB. The "wavefront phenomenon" of myocardial ischemic cell death. II. Transmural progression of necrosis within the framework of ischemic bed size (myocardium at risk) and collateral flow. *Lab Invest* 1979;40:633–644.

21. Jennings RB, Steenbergen C Jr, Reimer KA. Myocardial ischemia and reperfusion. *Monogr Pathol* 1995;37:47–80.

22. Fujita M, Nakae I, Kihara Y, et al. Determinants of collateral development in patients with acute myocardial infarction. *Clin Cardiol* 1999;22:595–599.

23. Kloner RA, Ganote CE, Jennings RB. The "no-reflow" phenomenon after temporary coronary occlusion in the dog. *J Clin Invest* 1974;54:1496–1508.

24. Miwa K, Fujita M, Kameyama T, et al. Absence of myocardial ischemia during sudden controlled occlusion of coronary arteries in patients with well-developed collateral vessels. *Coron Artery Dis* 1999;10:459–463.

25. Murry CE, Jennings RB, Reimer KA. Preconditioning with ischemia: a delay of lethal cell injury in ischemic myocardium. *Circulation* 1986;74:1124–1136.

26. Hagar JM, Hale SL, Kloner RA. Effect of preconditioning ischemia on reperfusion arrhythmias after coronary artery occlusion and reperfusion in the rat. *Circ Res* 1991;68:61–68.

27. Kuzuya T, Hoshida S, Yamashita N, et al. Delayed effects of sublethal ischemia on the acquisition of tolerance to ischemia. *Circ Res* 1993;72:1293–1299.

28. Yellon DM, Alkhulaifi AM, Pugsley WB. Preconditioning the human myocardium. *Lancet* 1993;342:276–277.

29. Kloner RA, Yellon D. Does ischemic preconditioning occur in patients? *J Am Coll Cardiol* 1994;24:1133–1142.

30. Kloner RA, Shook T, Antman EM, et al. Prospective temporal analysis of the onset of preinfarction angina versus outcome: an ancillary study in TIMI-9B. *Circulation* 1998;97:1042–1045.

31. Critz SD, Liu GS, Chujo M, et al. Pinacidil but not nicorandil opens ATP-sensitive K+ channels and protects against simulated ischemia in rabbit myocytes. *J Mol Cell Cardiol* 1997;29:1123–1130.

32. Kloner RA, Jennings RB. Consequences of brief ischemia: stunning, preconditioning, and their clinical implications: part 2. *Circulation* 2001;104:3158–3167.

33. Takano H, Bolli R, Black RG Jr, et al. A(1) or A(3) adenosine receptors induce late preconditioning against infarction in conscious rabbits by different mechanisms. *Circ Res* 2001;88:520–528.

34. Page DL, Caulfield JB, Kastor JA, et al. Myocardial changes associated with cardiogenic shock. *N Engl J Med* 1971;285:133–137.

35. Jennings RB, Ganote CE. Structural changes in myocardium during acute ischemia. *Circ Res* 1974;35[Suppl 3]:156–172.

36. Jennings RB, Ganote CE, Reimer KA. Ischemic tissue injury. *Am J Pathol* 1975;81:179–198.

37. Virmani R, Forman MB, Kolodgie FD. Myocardial reperfusion injury. Histopathological effects of perfluorochemical. *Circulation* 1990;81:IV57–IV68.

38. Jennings RB. Acute myocardial ischemic injury. Ultrastructural and biochemical studies of the early phase of lethal injury. *Arch Inst Cardiol Mex* 1980;50:365–371.

39. Buja LM, Fattor RA, Miller JC, et al. Effects of calcium loading and impaired energy production on metabolic and ultrastructural features of cell injury in cultured neonatal rat cardiac myocytes. *Lab Invest* 1990;63:320–331.

40. Buja LM, Burton KP, Chien KR, et al. Altered calcium homeostasis and membrane integrity in myocardial cell injury. *Adv Exp Med Biol* 1988;232:115–124.

41. Vargas SO, Sampson BA, Schoen FJ. Pathologic detection of early myocardial infarction: a critical review of the evolution and usefulness of modern techniques. *Mod Pathol* 1999;12:635–645.

42. Adegboyega PA, Adesokan A, Haque AK, et al. Sensitivity and specificity of triphenyl tetrazolium chloride in the gross diagnosis of acute myocardial infarcts. *Arch Pathol Lab Med* 1997;121:1063–1068.

43. Schoen FJ. *The heart*, 6th ed. Philadelphia: WB Saunders Company, 1999.

44. Mallory GK, White PD, Salcedo-Salgar J. The speed of healing of myocardial infarction: a study of the pathologic anatomy in seventy-two cases. *Am Heart J* 1939;18:647–671.

45. Lodge-Patch I. The aging of cardiac infarcts, and its influence on cardiac rupture. *Br Heart J* 1951;13:37–42.

46. Bouchardy B, Majno G. Histopathology of early myocardial infarcts. A new approach. *Am J Pathol* 1974;74:301–330.

47. Cowan MJ, Reichenbach D, Turner P, et al. Cellular response of the evolving myocardial infarction after therapeutic coronary artery reperfusion. *Hum Pathol* 1991;22:154–163.

48. Rahimtoola SH, Grunkemeier GL, Teply JF, et al. Changes in coronary bypass surgery leading to improved survival. *JAMA* 1981;246:1912–1916.

49. Rahimtoola SH. The hibernating myocardium. *Am Heart J* 1989;117:211–221.

50. Rahimtoola SH. Concept and evaluation of hibernating myocardium. *Annu Rev Med* 1999;50:75–86.

51. Thornhill RE, Prato FS, Wisenberg G. The assessment of myocardial viability: a review of current diagnostic imaging approaches. *J Cardiovasc Magn Reson* 2002;4:381–410.

52. Fath-Ordoubadi F, Beatt KJ, Spyrou N, et al. Efficacy of coronary angioplasty for the treatment of hibernating myocardium. *Heart* 1999;82:210–216.

53. Vanoverschelde JL, Wijns W, Depre C, et al. Mechanisms of chronic regional postischemic dysfunction in humans. New insights from the study of noninfarcted collateral-dependent myocardium. *Circulation* 1993;87:1513–1523.

54. Kloner RA, Jennings RB. Consequences of brief ischemia: stunning, preconditioning, and their clinical implications: part 1. *Circulation* 2001;104:2981–2989.

55. Arbustini E, Dal Bello B, Morbini P, et al. Plaque erosion is a major substrate for coronary thrombosis in acute myocardial infarction. *Heart* 1999;82:269–272.

56. Davies MJ. Acute coronary thrombosis—the role of plaque disruption and its initiation and prevention. *Eur Heart J* 1995;16:3–7.
57. Falk E. Morphologic features of unstable atherothrombotic plaques underlying acute coronary syndromes. *Am J Cardiol* 1989;63:114E–120E.
58. Kragel AH, Gertz SD, Roberts WC. Morphologic comparison of frequency and types of acute lesions in the major epicardial coronary arteries in unstable angina pectoris, sudden coronary death and acute myocardial infarction. *J Am Coll Cardiol* 1991;18:801–808.
59. Little WC. Angiographic assessment of the culprit coronary artery lesion before acute myocardial infarction. *Am J Cardiol* 1990;66:44G–47G.
60. Farb A, Burke AP, Tang AL, et al. Coronary plaque erosion without rupture into a lipid core. A frequent cause of coronary thrombosis in sudden coronary death. *Circulation* 1996;93:1354–1363.
61. Virmani R, Kolodgie FD, Burke AP, et al. Lessons from sudden coronary death: a comprehensive morphological classification scheme for atherosclerotic lesions. *Arterioscler Thromb Vasc Biol* 2000;20:1262–1275.
62. Falk E, Shah PK, Fuster V. Coronary plaque disruption. *Circulation* 1995;92:657–671.
63. Corr PB, Gillis RA. Autonomic neural influences on the dysrhythmias resulting from myocardial infarction. *Circ Res* 1978;43:1–9.
64. Corr PB, Sobel BE. Mechanisms contributing to dysrhythmias induced by ischemia and their therapeutic implications. *Adv Cardiol* 1978;(22):110–129.
65. Stevenson WG, Linssen GC, Havenith MG, et al. The spectrum of death after myocardial infarction: a necropsy study. *Am Heart J* 1989;118:1182–1188.
66. Bloor CM, White FC. Coronary artery reperfusion: effects of occlusion duration on reactive hyperemia responses. *Basic Res Cardiol* 1975;70:148–158.
67. Bloor CM, Ehsani A, White FC, et al. Ventricular fibrillation threshold in acute myocardial infarction and its relation to myocardial infarct size. *Cardiovasc Res* 1975;9:468–472.
68. Zimetbaum PJ, Josephson ME. Use of the electrocardiogram in acute myocardial infarction. *N Engl J Med* 2003;348:933–940.
69. Mark DB, Naylor CD, Hlatky MA, et al. Use of medical resources and quality of life after acute myocardial infarction in Canada and the United States. *N Engl J Med* 1994;331:1130–1135.
70. Califf RM, Bengtson JR. Cardiogenic shock. *N Engl J Med* 1994;330:1724–1730.
71. Holmes DR Jr, Califf RM, Topol EJ. Lessons we have learned from the GUSTO trial. Global Utilization of Streptokinase and Tissue Plasminogen Activator for Occluded Arteries. *J Am Coll Cardiol* 1995;25:10S–17S.
72. Holmes DR Jr, Bates ER, Kleiman NS, et al. Contemporary reperfusion therapy for cardiogenic shock: the GUSTO-I trial experience. The GUSTO-I Investigators. Global Utilization of Streptokinase and Tissue Plasminogen Activator for Occluded Coronary Arteries. *J Am Coll Cardiol* 1995;26:668–674.
73. Gutovitz AL, Sobel BE, Roberts R. Progressive nature of myocardial injury in selected patients with cardiogenic shock. *Am J Cardiol* 1978;41:469–475.
74. Isner JM, Roberts WC. Right ventricular infarction complicating left ventricular infarction secondary to coronary heart disease. Frequency, location, associated findings and significance from analysis of 236 necropsy patients with acute or healed myocardial infarction. *Am J Cardiol* 1978;42:885–894.
75. Goldstein JA. Pathophysiology and management of right heart ischemia. *J Am Coll Cardiol* 2002;40:841–853.
76. Forman MB, Wilson BH, Sheller JR, et al. Right ventricular hypertrophy is an important determinant of right ventricular infarction complicating acute inferior left ventricular infarction. *J Am Coll Cardiol* 1987;10:1180–1187.
77. Kopelman HA, Forman MB, Wilson BH, et al. Right ventricular myocardial infarction in patients with chronic lung disease: possible role of right ventricular hypertrophy. *J Am Coll Cardiol* 1985;5:1302–1307.
78. Lazar EJ, Goldberger J, Peled H, et al. Atrial infarction: diagnosis and management. *Am Heart J* 1988;116:1058–1063.
79. Moreno R, Lopez de Sa E, Lopez-Sendon JL, et al. Frequency of left ventricular free-wall rupture in patients with acute myocardial infarction treated with primary angioplasty. *Am J Cardiol* 2000;85:757–760,A8.
80. Davis N, Sistino JJ. Review of ventricular rupture: key concepts and diagnostic tools for success. *Perfusion* 2002;17:63–67.
81. Polic S, Perkovic D, Stula I, et al. Early cardiac rupture following streptokinase in patients with acute myocardial infarction: retrospective cohort study. *Croat Med J* 2000;41:303–305.
82. Mann JM, Roberts WC. Rupture of the left ventricular free wall during acute myocardial infarction: analysis of 138 necropsy patients and comparison with 50 necropsy patients with acute myocardial infarction without rupture. *Am J Cardiol* 1988;62:847–859.
83. Reeder GS. Acute myocardial infarction: enhancing the results of reperfusion therapy. *Mayo Clin Proc* 1995;70:1185–1190.
84. Pohjola-Sintonen S, Muller JE, Stone PH, et al. Ventricular septal and free wall rupture complicating acute myocardial infarction: experience in the Multicenter Investigation of Limitation of Infarct Size. *Am Heart J* 1989;117:809–818.
85. Reddy SG, Roberts WC. Frequency of rupture of the left ventricular free wall or ventricular septum among necropsy cases of fatal acute myocardial infarction since introduction of coronary care units. *Am J Cardiol* 1989;63:906–911.
86. Shapira I, Isakov A, Burke M, et al. Cardiac rupture in patients with acute myocardial infarction. *Chest* 1987;92:219–223.
87. Oliva PB, Hammill SC, Edwards WD. Cardiac rupture, a clinically predictable complication of acute myocardial infarction: report of 70 cases with clinicopathologic correlations. *J Am Coll Cardiol* 1993;22:720–726.
88. Edwards WD. *Pathology of myocardial infarction and reperfusion*, 1st ed. New York: Elsevier, 1991.
89. Antman EM, Braunwald E. *Acute myocardial infarction*, 5th ed. Philadelphia: WB Saunders Company, 1997.
90. Atkinson JB, Robinowitz M, McAllister HA, et al. Association of eosinophils with cardiac rupture. *Hum Pathol* 1985;16:562–568.
91. Batts KP, Ackermann DM, Edwards WD. Postinfarction rupture of the left ventricular free wall: clinicopathologic correlates in 100 consecutive autopsy cases. *Hum Pathol* 1990;21:530–535.
92. Moreno R, Lopez-Sendon J, Garcia E, et al. Primary angioplasty reduces the risk of left ventricular free wall rupture compared with thrombolysis in patients with acute myocardial infarction. *J Am Coll Cardiol* 2002;39:598–603.
93. Solodky A, Behar S, Herz I, et al. Comparison of incidence of cardiac rupture among patients with acute myocardial infarction treated by thrombolysis versus percutaneous transluminal coronary angioplasty. *Am J Cardiol* 2001;87:1105–1108,A9.
94. Bartoletti A, Fantini A, Meucci F, et al. Primary coronary angioplasty in acute myocardial infarction: is it possible to prevent postinfarction cardiac rupture? *Ital Heart J* 2000;1:400–406.
95. Figueras J, Cortadellas J, Calvo F, et al. Relevance of delayed hospital admission on development of cardiac rupture during acute myocardial infarction: study in 225 patients with free wall, septal or papillary muscle rupture. *J Am Coll Cardiol* 1998;32:135–139.
96. Birnbaum Y, Fishbein MC, Blanche C, et al. Ventricular septal rupture after acute myocardial infarction. *N Engl J Med* 2002;347:1426–1432.
97. Reeder GS. Identification and treatment of complications of myocardial infarction. *Mayo Clin Proc* 1995;70:880–884.
98. Barbour DJ, Roberts WC. Rupture of a left ventricular papillary muscle during acute myocardial infarction: analysis of 22 necropsy patients. *J Am Coll Cardiol* 1986;8:558–565.
99. Wei JY, Hutchins GM. The pathogenesis of papillary muscle rupture complicating myocardial infarction: hemorrhage accompanying contraction band necrosis. *Lab Invest* 1978;39:204–209.
100. Califf RM. Myocardial reperfusion: is it ever too late? *J Am Coll Cardiol* 1989;13:1130–1132.
101. Comparison of invasive and conservative strategies after treatment with intravenous tissue plasminogen activator in acute myocardial infarction. Results of the thrombolysis in myocardial infarction (TIMI) phase II trial. The TIMI Study Group. *N Engl J Med* 1989;320:618–627.
102. Ellis SG, Topol EJ, George BS, et al. Recurrent ischemia without warning. Analysis of risk factors for in-hospital ischemic events following successful thrombolysis with intravenous tissue plasminogen activator. *Circulation* 1989;80:1159–1165.
103. Weisman HF, Bush DE, Mannisi JA, et al. Cellular mechanisms of myocardial infarct expansion. *Circulation* 1988;78:186–201.
104. Weisman HF, Healy B. Myocardial infarct expansion, infarct extension, and reinfarction: pathophysiologic concepts. *Prog Cardiovasc Dis* 1987;30:73–110.
105. Gaudron P, Eilles C, Ertl G, et al. Adaptation to cardiac dysfunction after myocardial infarction. *Circulation* 1993;87:IV83–IV89.

106. Gaudron P, Eilles C, Kugler I, et al. Progressive left ventricular dysfunction and remodeling after myocardial infarction. Potential mechanisms and early predictors. *Circulation* 1993;87:755–763.
107. Friedman BM, Dunn MI. Postinfarction ventricular aneurysms. *Clin Cardiol* 1995;18:505–511.
108. Erlebacher JA, Weiss JL, Weisfeldt ML, et al. Early dilation of the infarcted segment in acute transmural myocardial infarction: role of infarct expansion in acute left ventricular enlargement. *J Am Coll Cardiol* 1984;4:201–208.
109. Erlebacher JA, Richter RC, Alonso DR, et al. Early infarct expansion: structural or functional? *J Am Coll Cardiol* 1985;6:839–844.
110. Hamer DH, Lindsay J Jr. Redefining true ventricular aneurysm. *Am J Cardiol* 1989;64:1192–1194.
111. Forman MB, Collins HW, Kopelman HA, et al. Determinants of left ventricular aneurysm formation after anterior myocardial infarction: a clinical and angiographic study. *J Am Coll Cardiol* 1986;8:1256–1262.
112. Vlodaver Z, Coe JI, Edwards JE. True and false left ventricular aneurysms. Propensity for the altter to rupture. *Circulation* 1975;51:567–572.
113. Meizlish JL, Berger HJ, Plankey M, et al. Functional left ventricular aneurysm formation after acute anterior transmural myocardial infarction. Incidence, natural history, and prognostic implications. *N Engl J Med* 1984;311:1001–1006.
114. Brown SL, Gropler RJ, Harris KM. Distinguishing left ventricular aneurysm from pseudoaneurysm. A review of the literature. *Chest* 1997;111:1403–1409.
115. Mills NL, Everson CT, Hockmuth DR. Technical advances in the treatment of left ventricular aneurysm. *Ann Thorac Surg* 1993;55:792–800.
116. Galve E, Garcia-Del-Castillo H, Evangelista A, et al. Pericardial effusion in the course of myocardial infarction: incidence, natural history, and clinical relevance. *Circulation* 1986;73:294–299.
117. Sugiura T, Iwasaka T, Takayama Y, et al. Factors associated with pericardial effusion in acute Q wave myocardial infarction. *Circulation* 1990;81:477–481.
118. Erhardt LR. Clinical and pathological observations in different types of acute myocardial infarction. *Acta Med Scand Suppl* 1974;560:1–78.
119. Uuskiula MM, Lamp KM, Martin SI. Relation between the clinical course of acute myocardial infarction and specific sensitization of lymphocytes and lymphotoxin production. *Kardiologiia* 1987;27:57–60.
120. Ali AS, Rybicki BA, Alam M, et al. Clinical predictors of heart failure in patients with first acute myocardial infarction. *Am Heart J* 1999;138:1133–1139.
121. Pantely GA, Bristow JD. Ischemic cardiomyopathy. *Prog Cardiovasc Dis* 1984;27:95–114.
122. Schuster EH, Bulkley BH. Ischemic cardiomyopathy: a clinicopathologic study of fourteen patients. *Am Heart J* 1980;100:506–512.
123. Virmani R, Roberts WC. Quantification of coronary arterial narrowing and of left ventricular myocardial scarring in healed myocardial infarction with chronic, eventually fatal, congestive cardiac failure. *Am J Med* 1980;68:831–838.
124. Kloner RA, Bolli R, Marban E, et al. Medical and cellular implications of stunning, hibernation, and preconditioning: an NHLBI workshop. *Circulation* 1998;97:1848–1867.
125. Atkinson JB, Virmani R. Congestive heart failure due to coronary artery disease without myocardial infarction: clinicopathologic description of an unusual cardiomyopathy. *Hum Pathol* 1989;20:1155–1162.
126. Keeley EC, Hillis LD. Left ventricular mural thrombus after acute myocardial infarction. *Clin Cardiol* 1996;19:83–86.
127. Fuster V, Halperin JL. Left ventricular thrombi and cerebral embolism. *N Engl J Med* 1989;320:392–394.
128. Meltzer RS, Visser CA, Fuster V. Intracardiac thrombi and systemic embolization. *Ann Intern Med* 1986;104:689–698.
129. Kupper AJ, Verheugt FW, Peels CH, et al. Left ventricular thrombus incidence and behavior studied by serial two-dimensional echocardiography in acute anterior myocardial infarction: left ventricular wall motion, systemic embolism and oral anticoagulation. *J Am Coll Cardiol* 1989;13:1514–1520.
130. Visser CA, Kan G, Meltzer RS, et al. Incidence, timing and prognostic value of left ventricular aneurysm formation after myocardial infarction: a prospective, serial echocardiographic study of 158 patients. *Am J Cardiol* 1986,57:729–732.

CHAPTER 56

The Pathophysiology and Biochemistry of Myocardial Ischemia, Necrosis, and Reperfusion

Yoshifumi Naka, David M. Stern, and David J. Pinsky

Key Words: Apoptosis, ischemia; myocardial stunning; myocyte; necrosis; neutrophils; no-reflow phenomenon; reperfusion; reperfusion arrhythmias; vascular homeostasis; vascular reperfusion injury.

INTRODUCTION

The human heart, an organ only the size of a clenched fist, must pump nearly 4,000 L blood daily to sustain life. It can do so only if there is a continual supply of fresh blood to provide oxygen and nutrients, as well as to remove metabolic waste. Interruption of this blood supply, even for brief periods, sets a panoply of homeostatic mechanisms into motion, which immediately break the work performed by the heart to limit the

Y. Naka: Division of Surgery, Department of Surgery, College of Physicians and Surgeons of Columbia University, Milstein Hospital Building 7-435, 177 Fort Washington Avenue, New York, New York 10032.

D. M. Stern: School of Medicine AA152, Medical College of Georgia, 1120 15th Street, Augusta, Georgia 30912-4750.

D. J. Pinsky: Department of Cardiovascular Medicine, Cardiovascular Center, University of Michigan Health Systems, 3119N Taubman Center, 1500 E. Medical Center Drive, Ann Arbor, Michigan 48109-0366.

resulting damage. Even so, because of the heart's rich vascularity, specific vascular homeostatic mechanisms are perturbed, which can lead to irreversible myocardial damage. Even on reestablishment of blood flow in the large conduit epicardial arteries, further damage may result as a consequence of reperfusion injury. Reperfusion injury, which shares many features characteristic of the inflammatory response, comes about because of interactions of a number of different cell types and components of the coagulation and complement systems, which combine to form a toxic milieu in which myocytes may not survive. It is currently recognized that the cardiac myocyte that is unable to survive the period of oxygen/nutrient deprivation or the onslaught of toxic cells and substances dies by one of two primary modes of death: necrosis or apoptosis. Understanding the mechanisms that lead to myocyte death and the mechanisms by which cardiac myocytes die has led to the development of novel therapeutic interventions designed to mitigate the pathophysiologic processes that accompany myocardial ischemia and reperfusion.

PATHOLOGIC SUBSTRATE

Myocardial ischemia is defined simply as an arterial oxygen supply that is insufficient to meet the metabolic demands of the tissue (1). Shortly after cessation of blood flow to a region of the heart, tissue myoglobin oxygen stores are consumed, the partial pressure of oxygen in the region declines (2), and that region of cardiac muscle that is ischemic loses its ability to maintain its normal (negative) resting membrane potential (3). Adenosine triphosphate (ATP) stores are depleted (4), mechanical contraction ceases (3), and cardiac myocytes arrest in the relaxed state, perhaps as the result of passive stretch imposed by adjacent nonischemic (contracting) muscle (5). These changes are accompanied by increases in tissue lactate (4,6), H^+ ions (7), phosphate (6), and potassium (8,9). During ischemia, cytosolic calcium levels are only slightly increased, although mitochondrial calcium is increased (10). Arterioles become maximally dilated (11), but if blood flow is insufficient for as little as 20 minutes, early stages of myocardial necrosis may be observed (12). If early reperfusion ensues, however, mechanical function can return (13). In the current era of pharmacologic or percutaneous coronary intervention, rapid restoration of blood flow can result in a rapid reversal of many of these changes and a resumption of contractility, albeit sometimes transiently depressed. This is called *myocardial stunning,* wherein there is a postischemic flow–function mismatch, such that perfusion appears normal when examined by scintigraphy or Doppler, yet myocardial contractility remains temporarily impaired.

The earliest structural changes seen in the heart during ischemia are a decrease in the size and number of glycogen granules present within the myocytes, consumed by the relatively inefficient processes of anaerobic metabolism (14–16). Microscopic examination reveals that myofibrils are relaxed, presumably stretched by the tugging of adjacent nonischemic cells (17). Intracellular edema develops, with concomitant swelling of the t-tubules, sarcoplasmic reticulum, and mitochondria (14–16). This edema is manifest as an increase in myocardial water content, small during the first 15 minutes after coronary artery occlusion, but increasing by nearly 50% by 75 minutes in an *in situ* model of coronary occlusion in the pig (18,19). Part of this increased myocardial water content during ischemia is the result of interstitial edema (20), which has been interpreted as resulting from increased microvascular permeability (21) as a consequence of the retraction of the lateral margins of vascular endothelial cells, thereby enlarging intercellular spaces (22).

IRREVERSIBLE MYOCYTE DEATH

Irreversible myocyte death is part of pathologic processes that occur incrementally over the early minutes to hours of ischemia; it is difficult to define exactly when myocytes cross the threshold of irreversibility—that is, the degree of ischemia that makes it inevitable that they will die. A working definition of *irreversibility* has been proposed as an ischemic insult of such severity that cells will continue to degenerate/necrose even after restoration of blood flow (23). The degree of ischemia and the duration of ischemia are both important factors in determining the point of irreversibility,

with severe reductions of arterial flow causing irreversibility as early as 20 minutes after onset (23). Histologically, irreversible cell death is characterized by ultrastructural changes that include the development of contraction bands (24–26) and amorphous densities within the mitochondria (24). Numerous plasma markers of myocyte death have been used with varying degrees of success to quantify the degree of myocardial necrosis in patients. In addition to traditional markers such as lactate dehydrogenase, creatinine phosphokinase, and serum glutamic oxaloacetic transaminase, myoglobin, troponin T, troponin I, and cardiac-specific myosin light chains have been used as markers of cardiomyocyte death (27). In the last decade, there has been an evolution of the use of these markers, on the basis of sensitivity and specificity of the assay systems as well as the temporal characteristics of their release. Creatine phosphokinase (MB fraction), long the mainstay of clinical practice for the detection of myocardial infarction (MI), has been largely supplanted by measurement of cardiac troponin. Although the kinetics of release and detection vary among the different markers, they share in common the feature that their increases in plasma reflect a loss of myocyte membrane integrity. Reperfusion of an ischemic area may also contribute to a rapid washout of these markers into peripheral blood, resulting in earlier peaks, complicating an analysis of extent of infarction (28).

REPERFUSION

Definitions

Restoration of blood flow to a previously ischemic zone causes profound physiologic changes in both myocytes and the local vasculature in the reperfused zone. Collectively, these changes may promote further tissue damage in a process called *reperfusion injury.* Although there are numerous experimental models of reperfusion injury, it has been impossible to define exactly those cells that were otherwise destined to live after ischemia alone, but were killed by the process of reperfusion (29). Reperfusion of ischemic myocardium halts the advancing wave front of ischemic myocyte death, with an exponential decay in the number of myocytes that may be salvaged as ischemic time lengthens (30), so that clinical reperfusion should be attempted even in the face of potential reperfusion injury. Clinical trials of patients receiving thrombolytic therapy or percutaneous coronary intervention to restore epicardial coronary artery patency in the setting of acute myocardial infarction (AMI) have demonstrated that timely reperfusion is beneficial (14). Despite these consistent data showing the beneficial effects of early reperfusion, there is a significant body of experimental literature suggesting that improving the reperfusion milieu might have an additive benefit. It is quite possible that future therapy for AMI will consist of timely mechanical- or thrombolytic-driven reperfusion and an optimal reperfusion cocktail.

The term reperfusion injury encompasses a spectrum of changes, which can be categorized into four separate components (29). *Lethal reperfusion injury* refers to the death of myocytes that is attributed to reperfusion per se, rather than to the preceding period of ischemia. *Vascular reperfusion injury* includes a progressive deterioration of blood flow secondary to vascular damage, thrombosis, and neutrophil plugging during reperfusion, which is accompanied by a deterioration of the normal ability of the coronary vasculature to dilate in times of need, referred to as coronary flow reserve. This latter aspect may be largely secondary to the production of reactive oxygen intermediates, which rapidly quench available nitric oxide (NO), leading to a failure of endothelium-dependent vasodilation (31,32). *Myocardial stunning* comprises a third category of reperfusion injury, representing a delayed failure of return of normal myocardial contractility, even when blood flow has been adequately restored. Ventricular tachycardia or fibrillation may herald the onset of reperfusion, and represents a final form of reperfusion injury termed *reperfusion arrhythmias* (33,34).

Mechanisms

Reoxygenation of endothelial cells is associated with a burst of oxygen free radical production both from endothelial cells (32) and the heart itself (35–37). This oxygen free radical production appears to peak within minutes of reperfusion and continues for hours at lower levels (38–40), producing such toxic species as superoxide, hydroxyl anion, and hydrogen peroxide. These highly reactive molecules may result in lipid peroxidation, membrane dysfunction, and further increases in membrane permeability beyond those observed during ischemia alone (41). The biochemical source of these free radicals remains controversial, however. Although xanthine oxidase has been repeatedly implicated in their production (42), this enzyme is virtually undetectable in human myocardial tissue (43–45). Other likely sources include mitochondria (46), recruited neutrophils (47), or transition metal–catalyzed formation of hydroxyl radical by the Haber–Weiss pathway (48).

Evidence for the formation of reactive oxygen intermediates in the human heart also abounds. Malondialdehyde, a detectable byproduct of lipid peroxidation (49), has been shown to increase in coronary sinus blood after percutaneous coronary angioplasty (50). When peripheral venous blood was sampled in the setting of MI 2 hours after streptokinase administration, levels of thiobarbituric acid–reactive substances (a measure of malondialdehyde levels) increased only in those patients in whom coronary artery patency was reestablished (51). Although there is little controversy regarding the generation of oxygen free radicals during reperfusion, there remains some skepticism regarding the clinical benefits of scavenging these free radicals as adjunctive therapy in managing clinical reperfusion. Although canine studies have demonstrated benefit by the use of superoxide dismutase linked to polyethylene glycol to prolong its half-life in the circulation (52), the effectiveness of this strategy may be improved by adding catalase (53) to

eliminate the hydrogen peroxide generated by the dismutation of superoxide.

At a cellular level, reperfusion of an ischemic zone results in an explosive increase in intracellular sodium and calcium, with a concomitant abrupt cellular swelling (54–56). A *calcium paradox* has been described, wherein there is little increase in free intracellular calcium during ischemia, but a tenfold increase within 10 minutes of reperfusion (57). These processes appear to accelerate myocyte necrosis, although this may occur only in cells otherwise destined to die (56). The end result is that calcium precipitates in mitochondria (56), intracellular vesicles and subsarcolemmal blebs form (54,56), and contraction bands appear (56). Reperfusion injury is not limited to cardiac myocytes, however, as there is significant vascular involvement as well. Thrombosis and hemorrhage are seen in areas of reperfused myocardium (58), as well as neutrophil adhesion to the reperfused endothelium (32,59,60). Edema of microvascular endothelial cells is observed, with endothelial blebs and gaps that may expose blood to the tissue factor–rich procoagulant subendothelium, accelerating thrombosis (58).

These processes contribute to the *no-reflow phenomenon*, wherein blood flow does not return to preischemic levels even after release of the coronary artery occlusion (29,58). In instances particularly where the ischemic phase has been severe or prolonged, no-reflow worsens as time elapses after reperfusion (61). This implicates an important role for recruited effector mechanisms, such as progressive microcirculatory thrombosis, vasomotor dysfunction, and neutrophil recruitment (29). The no-reflow phenomenon is more than simply a laboratory observation. Thallium-201– and Tc-99m–labeled microsphere studies in humans show that perfusion defects persist even for several weeks after successful thrombolysis of coronary artery occlusions in humans (62).

After successful reperfusion, myocytes often do not immediately regain normal contractile function. This postischemic dysfunction of viable myocytes is called *myocardial stunning* (63). Even if flow is adequately restored, myocardial stunning reflects the presence of a flow/function mismatch (64,65).

MECHANISMS OF ISCHEMIA/REPERFUSION–INDUCED MYOCYTE DEATH

Numerous mechanisms have been proposed to explain the final common pathway by which myocytes die during ischemia and reperfusion. Because of the unavailability of molecular oxygen during the period of ischemia, maintaining the myocyte energy charge of ATP is relegated to relatively inefficient glycolytic processes. As ATP demands overtake ATP supply, cellular energy charge is depleted, resulting in an inability of metabolic pumps to maintain normal ion gradients (4). Cytosolic calcium overload is thought to be an important mediator of ischemic contracture (66) and myocyte death (67). Depletion of ATP also can result in depletion of the reduced form of glutathione (GSH), which serves as a physiologic defense against cellular oxidant stress (67). Depletion of GSH, with the concomitant accumulation of the oxidized form of glutathione, impairs the detoxifying functions of glutathione peroxidase (68), which normally removes hydrogen peroxide (10,67,68). Protons are generated (6,69), which also may contribute to the toxic intracellular milieu. Activation of phospholipase A_2 by ischemia can turn membrane phospholipids such as lecithin into highly detergent-like lysophospholipid micelles (70). Oxygen-derived free radicals may not only directly oxidize membrane lipids and cause membrane dysfunction, but may further inhibit glycolysis and contribute to calcium overload (71).

Recent evidence suggests that reperfused myocytes may undergo programmed cell death *(apoptosis),* a process wherein endogenous nucleases are activated by specific genes within the cardiac myocytes, cleaving DNA into characteristic 200–base pair fragments (72). Apoptosis is an active process that involves a cascade of events triggered by diverse stimuli. Among these, reactive oxygen intermediates (generated during reperfusion) are an especially important trigger for cardiac myocyte apoptosis. Other apoptotic death signals in cardiac myocytes include tumor necrosis factor (TNF) receptor and FAS-FAS ligand signaling, as well as NO/p53-mediated pathways that may have as their basis self-regulatory mechanisms triggered by the presence of damaged DNA. The apoptosis program is actuated by one or several cysteine proteases (caspases). Mitochondria, with which cardiac myocytes are richly endowed, play an important role in the apoptosis program, because when triggered they undergo a characteristic permeability transition that eventuates in the release of cytochrome C and execution of the death cascade. Apoptotic cardiac myocytes can be found in the infarcted zone of human myocardial infarcts (particularly at the periphery, the region wherein the fate of myocytes may hang in the life/death balance depending on signals detected from both the internal and the external environment). Apoptotic cardiac myocytes also have been detected in the setting of dilated cardiomyopathy, which leads to the obvious (yet unresolved) question as to whether it may contribute to its pathogenesis. It becomes that there are an extraordinary number of paths down which a myocyte might progress in a march toward death, and some checkpoints, when passed, are irreversible. Interfering with paths leading to necrosis or death receptor signaling is a provocative strategy for treating and preventing irreversible cardiac myocyte death.

ROLE OF THE ENDOTHELIUM

Myocardial cells do not live in isolation, but rather in the context of the other cells and stromal elements, which *in toto* comprise the heart. Considerations of the biochemistry of myocardial ischemia and reperfusion would be incomplete without specific attention to the important role of the vasculature in these processes. Endothelial cells play a cardinal role in orchestrating the complex vascular processes

that maintain *vascular homeostasis,* wherein nutrient supply and waste elimination are in balance, and leukocyte traffic is maintained in a steady state. Endothelial cells line both the cardiac macrovasculature and microvasculature, providing the nonwetting surface over which blood must continually flow. They do not simply serve as passive conduits for blood, but actively maintain normal barrier properties of the blood vessel wall, regulating blood fluidity by preventing coagulation, controlling blood vessel luminal diameter by modulating vasomotor tone of the underlying vascular smooth muscle, and orchestrating neutrophil adhesion and egress into the underlying tissue. Dysfunction of any of these important endothelial functions may be observed in the setting of cardiac ischemia and reperfusion, where it may lead to the characteristic highly permeable, prothrombotic, and proinflammatory phenotype of the ischemic and reperfused vascular wall. Because the period of hypoxia is an important component of the ischemic period, understanding the responses of endothelial cells to hypoxia and reoxygenation has helped to elucidate mechanisms of endothelial cell dysfunction that are relevant to the period of cardiac ischemia and reperfusion.

Barrier Function

Under physiologic conditions, endothelial cells are normally tightly adherent to one another, forming the characteristic cobblestone appearance of unperturbed endothelium. This endothelial surface forms a barrier to the passage of solutes and the cellular components of the blood. Endothelial barrier function can be measured as electrical conductivity of endothelial cell monolayers, as well as by the passage of radiolabeled solutes of various sizes across endothelial cell monolayers. When endothelial cells are exposed to a period of hypoxia of the same severity as accompanies cardiac ischemia, they undergo changes in their actin-based cytoskeleton, leading to retraction of their lateral margins (73). This forms large gaps (1–3 μM) between apposing endothelial cells (73,74) through which large solutes may readily pass. Permeability to small molecules such as sorbitol increases, and even large molecules such as albumin have greater permeability across the hypoxic endothelial cell monolayer (73). This may be manifest as leakage of large intravascular proteins into the interstitial space, similar to the transvascular protein leakage observed in the lungs of rats exposed to hypoxia (75). The loss of endothelial barrier function is dependent both on the duration of exposure of the monolayer to hypoxia and the absolute level of hypoxia (73,74).

When the relation between levels of hypoxia and endothelial cell hyperpermeability was explored further, it was determined that the increased permeability only occurred at lower oxygen tensions. In parallel with the increased endothelial cell permeability (as oxygen tension declined), a decrease in cyclic adenosine monophosphate (cAMP) levels within the endothelial cells was noted, caused by a reduction of both basal and stimulated adenylate cyclase activity (76). Restoration of levels of the second messenger cyclic nucleotide cAMP using a membrane-permeable cAMP analog, dibutyryl-cAMP, restored endothelial barrier function in a dose-dependent manner (76). Similarly, other disparate means of increasing the activity of the cAMP second messenger pathway, such as protein kinase A activation or pertussis toxin treatment, likewise normalized endothelial cell permeability under conditions of hypoxia (76,77). Studies in multiple laboratories support these observations (78–81), with phosphodiesterase inhibition being particularly effective at reducing capillary hyperpermeability in an isolated perfused rabbit lung model (82).

Vasomotor Tone

Not only does the hypoxia-induced decrease in endothelial cell cAMP levels have implications with respect to endothelial cell barrier function, but cAMP is as an important component of the intrinsic vasodilator response of vascular smooth muscle (83). When vascular smooth muscle was studied under hypoxic conditions, a similar decrease in cAMP levels was noted, although in these cells, it appears that this was caused by increased activity of types III and IV phosphodiesterase (60). These observations may have important implications for the no-reflow phenomenon, especially considering that reactive oxygen intermediates increase the activity of *phosphodiesterases in vitro* (84), which may compound the vasoconstrictive effects of low vascular cAMP levels during reperfusion. In a global cardiac model of ischemia and reperfusion in the rat, restoration of the cAMP second messenger pathway using cAMP analogs, phosphodiesterase inhibitors, or activators of the cAMP-dependent protein kinase enhanced cardiac preservation in parallel with improving blood flow after reperfusion (60), suggesting the potential relevance of these observations to the ischemic heart.

In addition to cAMP, endothelium-derived relaxation factor (EDRF, identified as NO [85]) subserves a critical vasodilatory role that is under endothelial control. Although during hypoxic exposure, NO synthesis precedes unabated, reoxygenation results in a rapid decline in available NO levels, largely because of the rapid quenching effects of superoxide anion generated during reoxygenation (32). These observations are entirely consistent with the rapid decline of coronary vascular EDRF bioactivity (31) or NO levels by direct measurement (32) observed within minutes of reperfusion. Similarly, endocardial NO levels also plummet during reperfusion (32) (Fig. 56–1). This rapid decline in available NO levels has far-ranging implications beyond simple vasoconstriction, because NO also serves to attenuate neutrophil adhesion to the endothelium (86), to prevent platelet aggregation (87), and to maintain endothelial barrier function (88).

To demonstrate the potential relevance of these observations to human cardiac preservation, a preservation solution was designed that incorporated dibutyryl-cAMP and nitro-

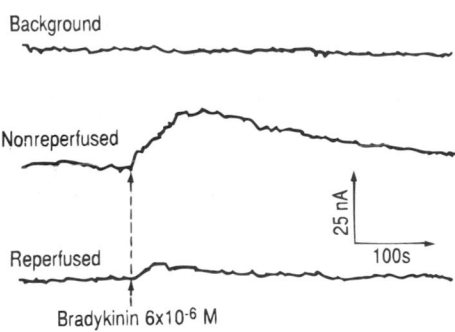

FIG. 56–1. Endocardial nitric oxide levels measured *in situ* after ischemia and reperfusion. A porphyrin microsensor that is highly sensitive and specific for nitric oxide (26) was embedded in the septal endocardium, and bradykinin was applied. Nitric oxide levels are significantly less after a period of ischemia and reperfusion than in nonreperfused endocardium (peak levels at the endocardial surface were 0.65 μM after bradykinin challenge in the nonreperfused endocardium). Application of superoxide dismutase increased endocardial nitric oxide levels, suggesting that superoxide quenches available nitric oxide during reperfusion. (Adapted from Pinsky DJ, Oz MC, Koga S, et al. Cardiac preservation is enhanced in a heterotopic rat transplant model by supplementing the nitric oxide pathway. *J Clin Invest* 1994;93:2291–2297, with permission.)

glycerin to augment both the cAMP and NO/cyclic guanosine monophosphate second messenger pathways. These experiments enabled unprecedented 24-hour preservation of primate hearts with simple *ex vivo* hypothermic storage (89), suggesting the potential clinical relevance of these second messenger pathways to the preservation of ischemic human hearts. Although the mechanisms of benefit continue to be evaluated, it appears as if augmentation of blood flow (32, 60), reduction of neutrophil infiltration (32,60), reduction of oxidant stress, and reduction of platelet aggregation during reperfusion are of paramount importance.

Balance between Forces Promoting and Suppressing Coagulation and Fibrinolysis

Quiescent endothelium maintains an anticoagulant phenotype by a number of different mechanisms, which serve to maintain blood fluidity. The nonwetting endothelial surface prevents contact of the coagulation system with highly procoagulant subendothelial matrix, rich in collagen and tissue factor (90). Under physiologic conditions, quiescent endothelial cells constitutively express the membrane-spanning protein thrombomodulin, which binds to thrombin to accelerate local production of the anticoagulant protein C (91). In addition, local production of NO potently inhibits platelet aggregation (87,92).

Hypoxic exposure activates endothelium to shift the balance to the procoagulant phenotype. Gaps that form between apposing endothelial cells are sufficiently large to permit contact of the bloodborne coagulation elements with procoagulant subendothelial collagen and tissue factor. Hypoxia selectively modulates endothelial cell expression of certain proteins such as thrombomodulin, which is significantly reduced (both message and activity) after endothelial cell exposure to hypoxia (73). Decreased thrombomodulin elicited by a period of oxygen deprivation would be expected to prime the vessel wall for procoagulant events, as an antithrombotic mechanism is compromised. *De novo* synthesis of interleukin-1 (IL-1) by hypoxic macrophages (93) or endothelial cells (94) within the heart also can promote endothelial cell expression of tissue factor (95), a powerful endogenous procoagulant that combines with factor VIIa to activate the extrinsic pathway of coagulation. In addition, there is increased secretion of the procoagulant polypeptide von Willebrand factor by endothelial cells exposed to hypoxia or ischemia/reperfusion, as occurs in the vasculature of human hearts during myocardial preservation (96). The marked depression of NO levels during reperfusion (31,32), brought about because of rapid quenching by superoxide anion, also would be expected to contribute to the prothrombotic state by fostering platelet aggregation.

The growth of a nascent thrombus is critically dependent on competing forces that exist within the confines of the vascular lumen. Accretion occurs because of deposition of platelets and fibrin, together with other cellular and proteinaceous elements of blood that are trapped within the growing fibrin mesh. In the setting of ischemia, competing pathways that promote dissolution of the growing thrombus are suppressed, thereby greatly amplifying the speed and amount of thrombus accretion. The most important of the antifibrinolytic pathways involves the activation of endogenous plasminogen by the tissue-type plasminogen activator (t-PA), thereby forming plasmin, which cleaves fibrin. Under normal conditions, the fibrinolytic cascade is under constant check by an inhibitory system. t-PA complexes with plasminogen activator inhibitor-1 (PAI-1), a 52-kD serine protease inhibitor that is the main inhibitor of t-PA in human plasma. These molecules and cascades are important to understand in the context of myocardial ischemia and reperfusion, because ischemia induces changes in the production of these molecules. Hypoxia causes an increase in the transcription of PAI-1 message and a reduction in degradation of PAI-1 message, resulting in an increase in PAI-1 protein and activity. This results in a net suppression of fibrinolysis that eventuates in a net suppression of fibrinolysis that promotes the accretion of thrombus. Another reason that it is important to understand these net competing forces is that PAI-1 secretion, produced by platelets or other cells of the vascular wall, is a major reason for thrombolysis resistance in the setting of AMI.

Recent data demonstrate that of the many potential triggers for hypoxic/ischemic induction of tissue factor and PAI-1, one particular transcription factor stands out as potentially a central effector mechanism. Hypoxia causes induction of this transcription factor, early growth response gene-1 *(Egr-1)*, which sets in motion many downstream events that are characteristic of the coagulant or inflammatory response. Many of the genes that are triggered by *Egr-1* have been identified as having a pathologic role in the setting of ischemia and reperfusion; these include PAI-1 and tissue factor, as well as cytokines, chemokines, and adhesion receptors (including intercellular adhesion molecule-1 [ICAM-1]). Ischemia-driven induction of *Egr-1* may represent a master switch that coordinates diverse pathologic responses to myocardial ischemia and reperfusion.

CYTOKINE PRODUCTION/ADHESION MOLECULE EXPRESSION

Leukocytes have been ascribed a central role in the tissue damage that occurs in ischemic syndromes (97–101). Multiple cytokines act synergistically to draw leukocytes into loci of hypoxic vascular injury. These proinflammatory cytokines include IL-1 (102,103), TNF (104), and IL-8 (104, 105). Endothelial cells subjected to hypoxia demonstrate *de novo* synthesis of IL-1, with steadily increasing levels peaking within 16 hours of hypoxic exposure in *in vitro* experiments, with increased plasma levels in mice exposed to hypoxia reaching a peak within 6–8 hours of hypoxic exposure (94). In similar experiments, IL-8 transcripts and antigen and activity were increased in endothelial cell culture supernatants and in blood vessels exposed to a hypoxic environment (106) (Fig. 56–2). In addition, reoxygenated human mononuclear phagocytes, present in abundance in the reperfused heart, likewise synthesize and release IL-1 (93).

Both IL-1 and TNF have the potential to set in motion events leading to increased expression of leukocyte adherence molecules on the endothelial cell surface (95), as well as the further production of neutrophil chemoattractant substances (104). IL-1 synthesis induces endothelial expression of ICAM-1 and E-selectin, both of which can be blocked by preventing IL-1 synthesis (using antisense oligomers for IL-1α) or by blocking it at the ligand-receptor level (using blocking antibodies or IL-1 receptor antagonist) (94). These results have been corroborated by several investigative groups, who have shown that anoxia/reoxygenation induces neutrophil adherence to cultured endothelial cells (107) and that platelet activating factor may also play a role in this neutrophil adherence (108,109).

A very potent ischemia/reperfusion-driven mechanism that promotes neutrophil adhesion in the earliest moments after reperfusion is that mediated by endothelial surface expression of P-selectin. Together with von Willebrand factor, P-selectin is stored in subplasmalemmal granules within endothelial cells, called Weibel–Palade bodies (110–112). Increases in calcium within endothelial cells, such as occur with thrombin or histamine receptor stimulation (113), promote rapid surface expression of P-selectin (114). Exposure of endothelial cells to reactive oxygen intermediates, which are formed in abundance during coronary reperfusion (35,36), promotes expression of P-selectin at the endothelial cell surface (115), which may rapidly cause neutrophil adhesion (116) during reperfusion. The importance of P-selectin

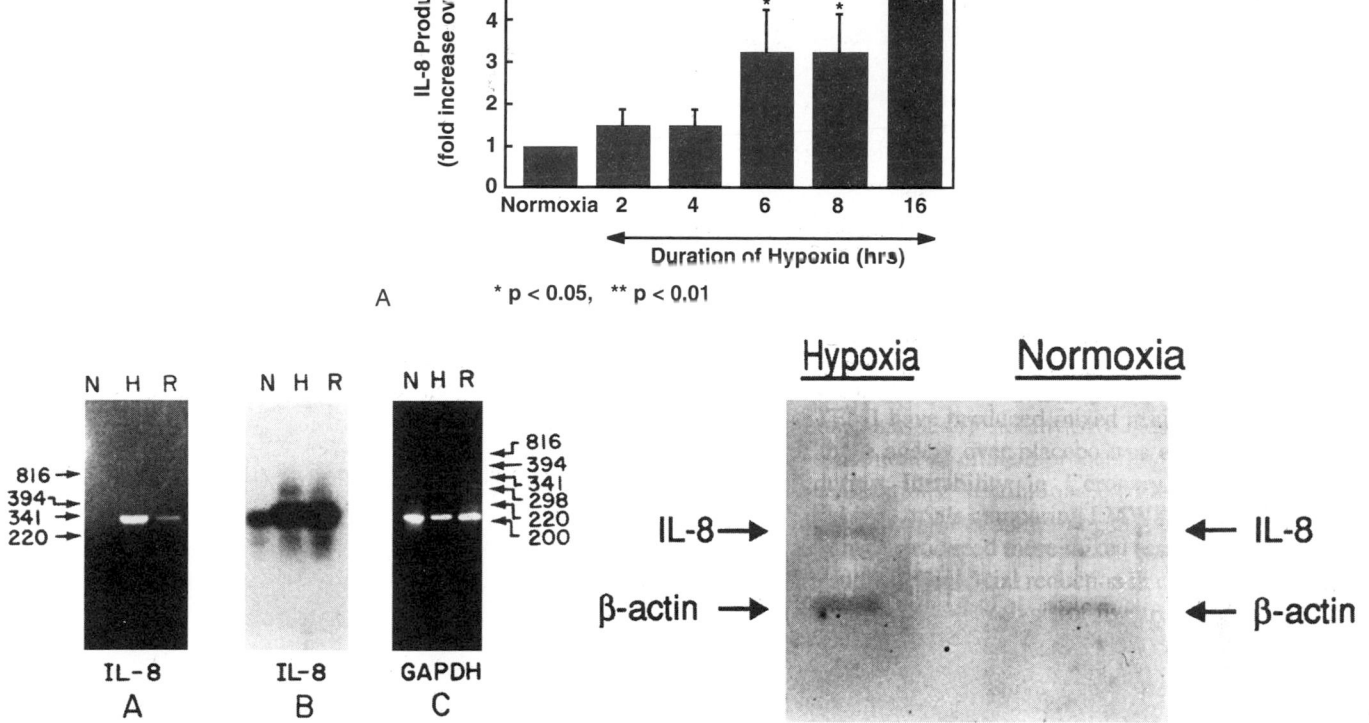

FIG. 56–2. Hypoxia-induced production of endothelial interleukin-8 (IL-8). **A:** Enzyme-linked immunosorbent assay demonstrates an increase in IL-8 antigen after hypoxic exposure of human umbilical vein endothelial cells. **B:** IL-8 message is likewise increased in hypoxia, as demonstrated by polymerase chain reaction **(left),** and Southern blotting of amplicons to confirm their identity **(middle),** compared with control glyceraldehyde phosphate dehydrogenase (GAPDH) message **(right). C:** Nuclear run-on assay further confirming an up-regulation of IL-8 transcripts in hypoxia **(left)** compared with control β-actin transcripts **(right).** H, hypoxia; N, normoxia; R, reoxygenation. (Adapted from Karakurum M, Shreeniwas R, Chen J, et al. Hypoxic induction of interleukin-8 gene expression in human endothelial cells. *J Clin Invest* 1994;93:1564–1570, with permission.)

in cardiac ischemia and reperfusion has been verified in a number of animal models, including mouse, rats, and cats (117) (Fig. 56–3).

ROLE OF NEUTROPHILS AND PROINFLAMMATORY CYTOKINES

Neutrophils (polymorphonuclear leukocytes [PMNs]) play a cardinal role in reperfusion-induced tissue damage in the heart (101,118–123). It is not surprising that neutrophils may be toxic to tissues in which they accumulate, because they serve an important role in the initial clearing of debris after an ischemic event. On recruitment to ischemic/reperfused tissue, they release numerous cytotoxic lysosomal enzymes with which to carry out these functions, including elastase, the metalloproteinase collagenase and gelatinase, neutral proteases, and heparinase (124). In addition, recruited neutrophils may be activated by cytokines and che-

motactic factors to undergo a respiratory burst, which elicits a sudden release of toxic reactive oxygen metabolites such as superoxide anion, chloramine, hypochlorous acid, hydroxyl radical, and hydrogen peroxide (124). Multiple studies have demonstrated that either depleting neutrophils before ischemia/reperfusion (118) or interfering with neutrophil adhesion to the endothelium can limit infarct size in experimental animals (125,126). Even in models of global cardiac ischemia/reperfusion, such as occurs during heart transplantation, therapies that interfere with neutrophil adhesion and reduce the extent of graft myeloperoxidase activity (which serves as a semiquantitative index of graft neutrophil accumulation) are associated with improved graft survival (32, 60) (Fig. 56–4).

The process of PMN recruitment into the ischemic and reperfused vasculature occurs in several phases, controlled principally by endothelial cell/PMN interactions. Neutrophils are first attracted into an ischemic or reperfused milieu

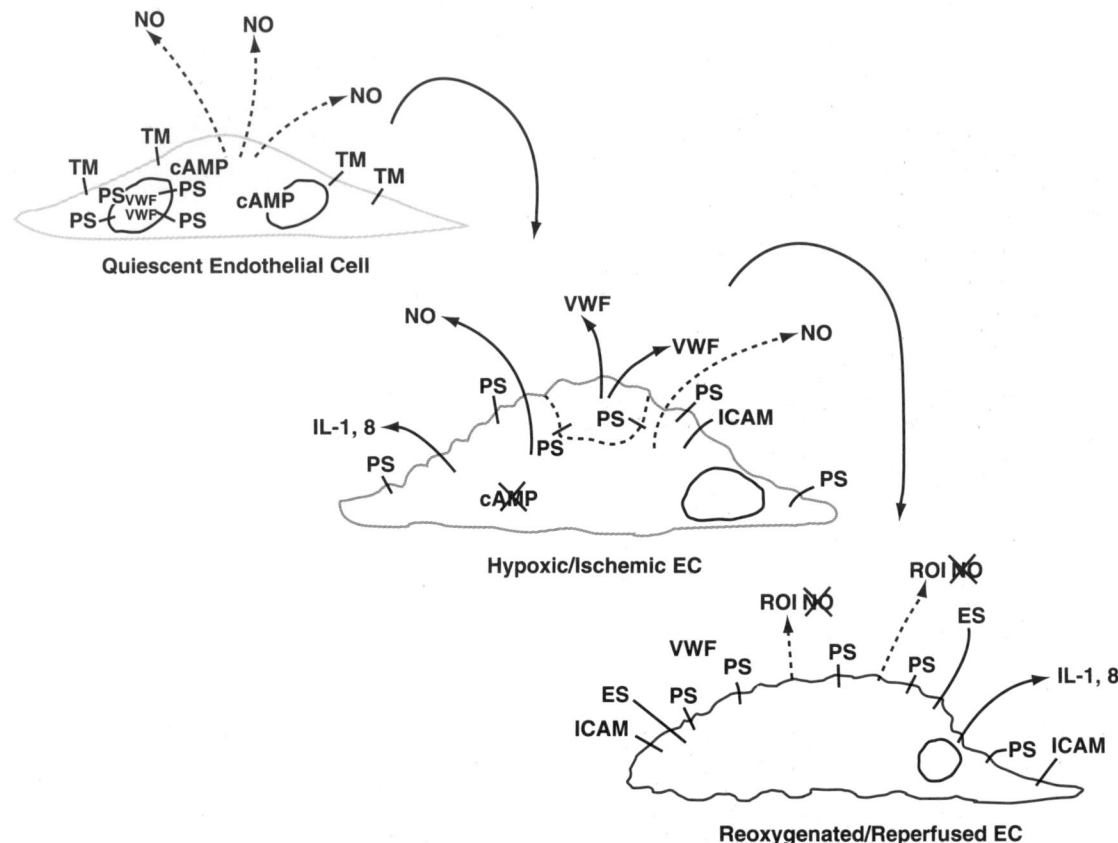

FIG. 56–3. Schematic representation of endothelial perturbations during hypoxia and reoxygenation. During hypoxia and reoxygenation, endothelial cyclic adenosine monophosphate (cAMP) levels decrease, and endothelial cells secrete proinflammatory cytokines such as interleukin-1 (IL-1) and IL-8 and procoagulant von Willebrand factor (vWF) and express neutrophil adhesion molecules on their surface (E-selectin [ES]; P-selectin [PS]; intercellular adhesion molecule-1 [ICAM]). In addition, surface expression of the anticoagulant cofactor thrombomodulin (TM) is reduced. Reoxygenation is associated with the production of reactive oxygen intermediates (ROIs), which can rapidly quench nitric oxide (NO), making it unavailable to perform its vasodilatory, antiplatelet, antipermeability, and antineutrophil functions. EC, endothelial cell.

by specific chemoattractants, such as the activated complement components C3a and C5a (124), as well as the specific neutrophil chemoattractant IL-8 (127), which not only recruits neutrophils, but also activates them (128,129) and promotes their emigration from the vasculature (127). Circulating neutrophils that localize to an ischemic and reperfused area first adhere to the activated endothelial surface in a decelerating, rolling type of adhesive process mediated by a group of glycoprotein adhesion receptors known as the selectins. L-selectin is expressed (and shed) by the neutrophil. Endothelial P-selectin engages its cognate glycoprotein ligand on the neutrophil, which is composed of P-selectin glycoprotein ligand-1 (PSGL-1) and the attached carbohydrate moiety (sialyl-Lewis^x) (130). The interaction between neutrophil PSGL-1/sLe^x and endothelial P-selectin brings the neutrophils into close approximation with the endothelial surface. Once so tethered, other adhesive interactions become dominant, especially that mediated by ICAM-1 on the endothelial cell engaging β_2 integrins (CD11/CD18) on the

neutrophil (124). Further elements of the hypoxic/ischemic vascular milieu that also contribute to the generalized proinflammatory state include such cytokines as IL-1, which upregulates endothelial cell expression of ICAM-1 (131), platelet-activating factor (a lipid mediator of inflammation induced by hypoxia), and E-selectin (94), which further supports PMN adhesion.

Many strategies designed to block neutrophil adhesion have been successful in experimental models of ischemia and reperfusion, although, to date, human studies have failed to demonstrate utility. Conceptually, one might envision the optimal use of an antiadhesive strategy as that which is given as adjunctive therapy with thrombolysis. Antibody to IL-8 administered to rabbits limits pulmonary reperfusion injury (132). Anti–P-selectin treatment not only attenuates reperfusion injury in the rabbit ear (133), but limits myocardial infarct size in a feline model (117). In other models of cardiac ischemia and reperfusion, anti-β_2 integrin (98,126) or anti–ICAM-1 (125) therapy has been shown to

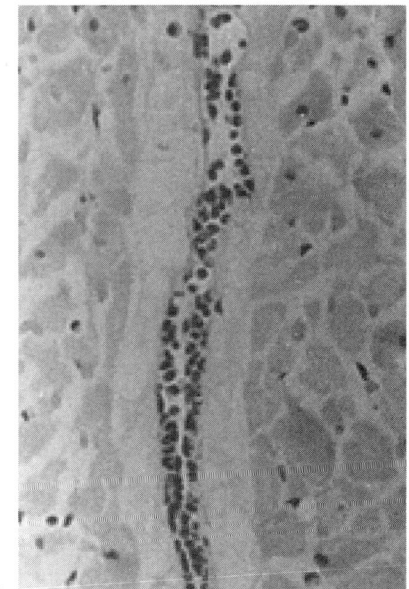

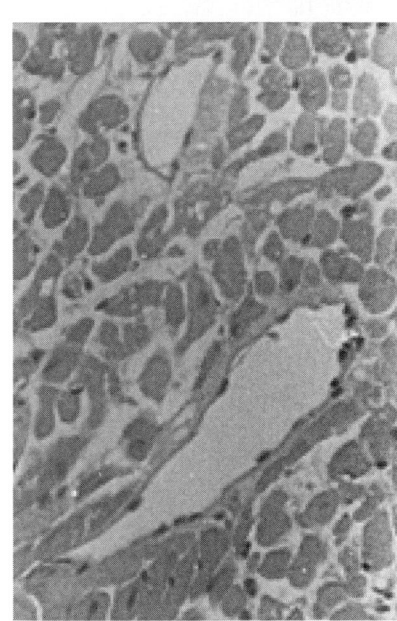

FIG. 56–4. Neutrophil infiltration into the heart after reperfusion. Using a model of global cardiac ischemia and reperfusion, one can see neutrophils adhere to the endothelial lining of blood vessels as early as 10 minutes after reperfusion **(left).** This neutrophil recruitment can be blocked by using nitroglycerin during the ischemic period, which acts as a nitric oxide donor to reduce neutrophil adherence to the reperfused vasculature **(right).** These results were corroborated by tissue myeloperoxidase activity, measured by a chromogenic assay that quantifies the presence of the neutrophil-specific enzyme myeloperoxidase. (Adapted from Pinsky DJ, Oz MC, Koga S, et al. Cardiac preservation is enhanced in a heterotopic rat transplant model by supplementing the nitric oxide pathway. *J Clin Invest* 1994;93:2291–2297, with permission.)

be similarly effective. In addition to antibody therapy, novel antiadhesion strategies also are being considered for the treatment of ischemia and reperfusion, including administration of the oligosaccharide counterligand for P-selectin (sialyl-Lewis^x) (134), recombinant soluble PSGL-1, antisense ICAM-1 (used in the setting of renal ischemia/reperfusion), and others.

ROLE OF THE COMPLEMENT CASCADE

The complement system represents an essential component of the innate immune system, a primitive and highly conserved pattern recognition system that consists of three principal arms: the classical, the alternative, and the lectin (sometimes called the mannose-binding protein) pathways. These cascades are activated either because of a cognate interaction (such as occurs with a specific domain on the Fc tail of complement-fixing antibodies), a pattern recognition interaction, or by a proteolytic event. Once activated, components self-assemble and trigger a proteolytic cascade not dissimilar to that which is responsible for activation of coagulation. Pathways converge at the complement component C3, the cleavage of which leads to the formation of anaphylatoxins (C3a and C5a) and the amphiphilic membrane attack complex (MAC), consisting of complement components C5b-C9. Anaphylatoxins are potent leukocyte chemoattractants, which serve to amplify the inflammatory milieu. The MAC adheres to membrane phospholipids and essentially punches gaping holes in cells, resulting in rapid target-cell lysis.

Activation of complement has been implicated in the pathogenesis of ischemia/reperfusion injury in a number of different organs. In the heart, a potential role for complement activation was suggested more than a quarter of a century ago in studies of MI in rats (135). Decomplementation of experimental animals (by administration of cobra venom factor) before experimental infarction significantly reduced myocardial necrosis after ischemia and reperfusion (122, 136). Ischemia and reperfusion itself is sufficient to trigger complement activation, which may be deleterious to myocytes by amplification of the inflammatory milieu by way of further neutrophil recruitment and activation, or by local generation and insertion of the MAC into bystander myocytes. Deposition of MAC has been noted in areas of MI, with relatively little deposition in adjacent nonischemic areas (137). Even sublytic amounts of C5b-C9 may trigger endothelial cell Weibel–Palade body exocytosis, with concomitant translocation of P-selectin to the endothelial surface, which may further contribute to neutrophil adhesion (138). Local activation of complement is deleterious to the heart, as has been shown in a number of studies (122, 139,140). It has been more difficult, however, from a clinical standpoint to prove that complement inhibition is in fact protective. Several strategies for complement blockade have emerged, ranging from use of C1 esterase inhibitor to use of soluble complement receptor type 1, which lacks cytosolic and transmembrane domains, to protect against postischemic myocardial inflammation and necrosis (141). Although a number of experimental studies have demonstrated clear (and sometimes striking) preclinical utility, there has not yet been a successful anticomplement therapy that has passed into the clinical therapeutic realm.

CONCLUSION

The pathophysiology and biochemistry of cardiac ischemia, necrosis, and reperfusion can be seen as a complex interplay between intrinsic and programmed responses of myocytes and their surrounding cellular and humoral milieu. Various proinflammatory and procoagulant vascular effector mechanisms, as well as intrinsic cardiac myocyte death cascades, contribute to the ultimate outcome after MI. Cellular effector mechanisms (including neutrophils) and humoral mechanisms (including the complement and coagulation cascades) are activated during the processes of ischemia and reperfusion. The cardiac vasculature plays a critical modulatory role in these events, with the period of hypoxia/ischemia emerging as an important priming event for the subsequent endothelial cell dysfunction and proinflammatory milieu that follows a period of myocardial ischemia and reperfusion. Novel strategies designed to abrogate endothelial dysfunction and to limit the consequences of neutrophil adhesion and complement activation are likely to play important adjunctive roles together with thrombolytic therapy in the future treatment of AMI.

ACKNOWLEDGMENTS

This work was supported in part by the National Institutes of Health grants R01HL60900 and R01HL69448. The editorial assistance provided by Debbie Ventura during manuscript preparation is gratefully acknowledged.

REFERENCES

1. Jennings RB. Myocardial ischemia observations, definitions, and speculations. *J Mol Cell Cardiol* 1970;1:345–349.
2. Sayen JJ, Sheldon WF, Pierce G, et al. Polarigraphic oxygen, the epicardial electrocardiogram and muscle contraction in experimental acute regional ischemia of the left ventricle. *Circ Res* 1958;6:779–798.
3. Jennings RB. Early phase of myocardial ischemic injury and infarction. *Am J Cardiol* 1969;24:753–765.
4. Braasch W, Gudbjarnason S, Puri PS, et al. Early changes in energy metabolism in the myocardium following acute coronary artery occlusion in anesthetized dogs. *Circ Res* 1968;23:429–438.
5. Kloner RA, Ellis SG, Lange R, et al. Studies of experimental coronary artery reperfusion. effects on infarct size, myocardial function, biochemistry, ultrastructure and microvascular damage. *Circulation* 1983;68:8–15.
6. Hersdon PB, Kaltenbach JP, Jennings RB. Fine structural and biochemical changes in dog myocardium during autolysis. *Am J Pathol* 1969;57:539–557.
7. Krug A. Der Fruhnachweis des Herzinfarktes durch Bestimmung der Wasserstoffionenkonzentration im Herzmuskel mit Idicatorpapier. *Virchows Arch* 1965;338:339–341.
8. Harris AS, Bisteni A, Russell RA, et al. Excitatory factors in ventricular tachycardia resulting from myocardial ischemia: potassium is a major excitant. *Science* 1954;119:200–203.
9. Case RB, Nasser MG, Crampton RS. Biochemical aspects of early myocardial ischemia. *Am J Cardiol* 1969;24:766–775.
10. Ferrari R, Ceconi C, Curello S, et al. Myocardial damage during ischaemia and reperfusion. *Eur Heart J* 1993;14[Suppl G]:G25–G30.
11. Berne RM, Rubio R. Acute coronary occlusion: early changes that induce coronary dilatation and the development of collateral circulation. *Am J Cardiol* 1969;24:776–781.
12. Jennings RB, Sommers HM, Smyth GA, et al. Myocardial necrosis induced by temporary occlusion of a coronary artery in the dog. *Arch Pathol* 1960;70:68–78.
13. Tennant R, Wiggers CJ. The effect of coronary occlusion on myocardial contraction. *Am J Physiol* 1935;112:351–361.
14. Sobel RE. Acute myocardial infarction. In: Pasternak RC, Braunwald E, eds. *Heart disease: a textbook of cardiovascular medicine.* Philadelphia: WB Saunders Company, 1992:1200–1272.
15. Kloner RA, Rude RE, Carlson N, et al. Ultrastructural evidence of microvascular damage and myocardial cell injury after coronary artery occlusion: which comes first? *Circulation* 1980;62:945–952.
16. Kloner RA, DeBoer LW, Carlson N, et al. The effect of verapamil on myocardial ultrastructure during and following release of coronary artery occlusion. *Exp Mol Pathol* 1982;36:277–286.
17. Jennings RB, Reimer KA. Salvage of ischemic myocardium. *Mod Concepts Cardiovasc Dis* 1974;43:125–130.
18. Garcia-Dorado D, Oliveras J. Myocardial oedema: a preventable cause of reperfusion injury? *Cardiovasc Res* 1993;27:1555–1563.
19. Garcia-Dorado D, Theroux P, Munoz R, et al. Favorable effects of hyperosmotic reperfusion on myocardial edema and infarct size. *Am J Physiol* 1992;262:H17–H22.
20. Steenbergen C, Hill ML, Jennings RB. Volume regulation and plasma membrane injury in aerobic, anaerobic, and ischemic myocardium in vitro. Effects of osmotic cell swelling on plasma membrane integrity. *Circ Res* 1985;57:864–875.
21. Dauber IM, Vanbenthuysen KM, McMurtry IF, et al. Functional coronary microvascular injury evident as increased permeability due to brief ischemia and reperfusion. *Circ Res* 1990;66:986–998.
22. Pilati CF. Macromolecular transport in canine coronary microvasculature. *Am J Physiol* 1990;258:H748–H753.
23. Jennings RB, Ganote CE, Reimer KA. Ischemic tissue injury. *Am J Pathol* 1975;81:179–198.
24. Jennings RB, Schaper J, Hill ML, et al. Effect of reperfusion late in the phase of reversible ischemic injury. Changes in cell volume, electrolytes, metabolites, and ultrastructure. *Circ Res* 1985;56:262–278.
25. Baroldi G. Different types of myocardial necrosis in coronary heart disease: a pathophysiologic review of their functional significance. *Am Heart J* 1975;89:742–752.
26. Hutchins GM, Bulkley BH. Correlation of myocardial contraction band necrosis and vascular patency. A study of coronary artery bypass graft anastomoses at branch points. *Lab Invest* 1977;36:642–648.
27. Adams JE, Abendschein DR, Jaffe AS. Biochemical markers of myocardial injury. Is MB creatine kinase the choice for the 1990s? *Circulation* 1993;88:750–763.
28. Devries SR, Jaffe AS, Geltman EM, et al. Enzymatic estimation of the extent of irreversible myocardial injury early after reperfusion. *Am Heart J* 1989;117:31–36.
29. Kloner RA. Does reperfusion injury exist in humans? *J Am Coll Cardiol* 1993;21:537–545.
30. Reimer KA, Vander Heide RS, Richard VJ. Reperfusion in acute myocardial infarction: effect of timing and modulating factors in experimental models. *Am J Cardiol* 1993;72:13G–21G.
31. Lefer AM, Tsao PS, Lefer DJ, et al. Role of endothelial dysfunction in the pathogenesis of reperfusion injury after myocardial ischemia. *FASEB J* 1991;5:2029–2034.
32. Pinsky DJ, Oz MC, Koga S, et al. Cardiac preservation is enhanced in a heterotopic rat transplant model by supplementing the nitric oxide pathway. *J Clin Invest* 1994;93:2291–2297.
33. Manning AS, Hearse DJ. Reperfusion-induced arrhythmias: mechanisms and prevention. *J Mol Cell Cardiol* 1984;16:497–518.
34. Hale SL, Lange R, Alker KJ, et al. Correlates of reperfusion ventricular fibrillation in dogs. *Am J Cardiol* 1984;53:1397–1400.
35. Zweier JL, Kuppusamy P, Lutty GA. Measurement of endothelial cell free radical generation: evidence for a central mechanism of free radical injury in postischemic tissues. *Proc Natl Acad Sci USA* 1988;85:4046–4050.
36. Babbs CF, Cregor MD, Turek JJ, et al. Endothelial superoxide pro-

duction in the isolated rat heart during early reperfusion after ischemia. A histochemical study. *Am J Pathol* 1991;139:1069–1080.

37. Kramer JH, Arroyo CM, Dickens BF, et al. Spin-trapping evidence that graded myocardial ischemia alters post-ischemic superoxide production. *Free Radic Biol Med* 1987;3:153–159.

38. McCord JM. Free radicals and myocardial ischemia: overview and outlook. *Free Radic Biol Med* 1988;4:9–14.

39. Zweier JL, Rayburn BK, Flaherty JT, et al. Recombinant superoxide dismutase reduces oxygen free radical concentrations in reperfused myocardium. *J Clin Invest* 1987;80:1728–1734.

40. Bolli R, Patel BS, Jeroudi MO, et al. Demonstration of free radical generation in "stunned" myocardium of intact dogs with the use of the spin trap alpha-phenyl N-tert-butyl nitrone. *J Clin Invest* 1988;82:476–485.

41. McCord JM. Oxygen-derived free radicals in postischemic tissue injury. *N Engl J Med* 1985;312:159–163.

42. McCord JM, Roy RS, Schaffer SW. Free radicals and myocardial ischemia. The role of xanthine oxidase. *Adv Myocardiol* 1985;5:183–189.

43. Eddy J, Stewart R, Jones H, et al. Xantine oxidase is detected in ischemic rat heart but not in human hearts. *Physiologist* 1986;29:166–170.

44. Eddy LJ, Stewart JR, Jones HP, et al. Free radical-producing enzyme, xanthine oxidase, is undetectable in human hearts. *Am J Physiol* 1987;253:H709–H711.

45. Muxfeldt M, Schaper W. The activity of xanthine oxidase in heart of pigs, guinea pigs, rabbits, rats, and humans. *Basic Res Cardiol* 1987;82:486–492.

46. Boveris A, Chance B. The mitochondrial generation of hydrogen peroxide. General properties and effect of hyperbaric oxygen. *Biochem J* 1973;134:707–716.

47. Lucchesi BR, Werns SW, Fantone JC. The role of the neutrophil and free radicals in ischemic myocardial injury. *J Mol Cell Cardiol* 1989;21:1241–1251.

48. Halliwell B. Oxidants and human disease: some new concepts. *FASEB J* 1987;1:358–364.

49. Gutteridge JM. Aspects to consider when detecting and measuring lipid peroxidation. *Free Radic Res Commun* 1986;1:173–184.

50. Roberts MJ, Young IS, Trouton TG, et al. Transient release of lipid peroxides after coronary artery balloon angioplasty. *Lancet* 1990;336:143–145.

51. Davies SW, Ranjadayalan K, Wickens DG, et al. Lipid peroxidation associated with successful thrombolysis. *Lancet* 1990;335:741–743.

52. Tamura Y, Chi LG, Driscoll EM Jr, et al. Superoxide dismutase conjugated to polyethylene glycol provides sustained protection against myocardial ischemia/reperfusion injury in canine heart. *Circ Res* 1988;63:944–959.

53. Jolly SR, Kane WJ, Bailie MB, et al. Canine myocardial reperfusion injury. Its reduction by the combined administration of superoxide dismutase and catalase. *Circ Res* 1984;54:277–285.

54. Whalen DA Jr, Hamilton DG, Ganote CE, et al. Effect of a transient period of ischemia on myocardial cells. I. Effects on cell volume regulation. *Am J Pathol* 1974;74:381–397.

55. Shen AC, Jennings RB. Kinetics of calcium accumulation in acute myocardial ischemic injury. *Am J Pathol* 1972;67:441–452.

56. Kloner RA, Ganote CE, Whalen DA Jr, et al. Effect of a transient period of ischemia on myocardial cells. II. Fine structure during the first few minutes of reflow. *Am J Pathol* 1974;74:399–422.

57. Shen AC, Jennings RB. Myocardial calcium and magnesium in acute ischemic injury. *Am J Pathol* 1972;67:417–420.

58. Kloner R, Ganote C, Jennings R. The "no-reflow" phenomenon after temporary coronary occlusion in the dog. *J Clin Invest* 1974;54:1496–1508.

59. Engler RL, Schmid-Schoenbein GW, Pavelec RS. Leukocyte capillary plugging in myocardial ischemia and reperfusion in the dog. *Am J Pathol* 1983;111:98–111.

60. Pinsky D, Oz M, Liao H, et al. Restoration of the cAMP second messenger pathway enhances cardiac preservation for transplantation in a heterotopic rat model. *J Clin Invest* 1993;92:2994–3002.

61. Komamura K, Kitakaze M, Nishida K, et al. Progressive decreases in coronary vein flow during reperfusion in acute myocardial infarction: clinical documentation of the no reflow phenomenon after successful thrombolysis. *J Am Coll Cardiol* 1994;24:370–377.

62. Schofer J, Montz R, Mathey DG. Scintigraphic evidence of the "no reflow" phenomenon in human beings after coronary thrombolysis. *J Am Coll Cardiol* 1985;5:593–598.

63. Braunwald E, Kloner RA. The stunned myocardium: prolonged, postischemic ventricular dysfunction. *Circulation* 1982;66:1146–1149.

64. Takeishi Y, Tono-oka I, Kubota I, et al. Functional recovery of hibernating myocardium after coronary bypass surgery: does it coincide with improvement in perfusion? *Am Heart J* 1991;122:665–670.

65. Stack RS, Phillips HR, Grierson DS, et al. Functional improvement of jeopardized myocardium following intracoronary streptokinase infusion in acute myocardial infarction. *J Clin Invest* 1983;72:84–95.

66. Owen P, Dennis S, Opie LH. Glucose flux rate regulates onset of ischemic contracture in globally underperfused rat hearts. *Circ Res* 1990;66:344–354.

67. Opie LH. The mechanism of myocyte death in ischaemia. *Eur Heart J* 1993;14[Suppl G]:G31–G33.

68. Ferrari R, Alfieri O, Curello S, et al. Occurrence of oxidative stress during reperfusion of the human heart. *Circulation* 1990;81:201–211.

69. Dennis SC, Gevers W, Opie LH. Protons in ischemia: where do they come from; where do they go to? *J Mol Cell Cardiol* 1991;23:1077–1086.

70. Corr PB, Gross RW, Sobel BE. Arrhythmogenic amphiphilic lipids and the myocardial cell membrane. *J Mol Cell Cardiol* 1982;14:619–626.

71. Corretti MC, Koretsune Y, Kusuoka H, et al. Glycolytic inhibition and calcium overload as consequences of exogenously generated free radicals in rabbit hearts. *J Clin Invest* 1991;88:1014–1025.

72. Gottlieb RA, Burleson KO, Kloner RA, et al. Reperfusion injury induces apoptosis in rabbit cardiomyocytes. *J Clin Invest* 1994;94:1621–1628.

73. Ogawa S, Gerlach H, Esposito C, et al. Hypoxia modulates the barrier and coagulant function of cultured bovine endothelium. Increased monolayer permeability and induction of procoagulant properties. *J Clin Invest* 1990;85:1090–1098.

74. Ogawa S, Shreeniwas R, Brett J, et al. The effect of hypoxia on capillary endothelial cell function: modulation of barrier and coagulant function. *Br J Haematol* 1990;75:517–524.

75. Stelzner TJ, O'Brien RF, Sato K, et al. Hypoxia-induced increases in pulmonary transvascular protein escape in rats. Modulation by glucocorticoids. *J Clin Invest* 1988;82:1840–1847.

76. Ogawa S, Koga S, Kuwabara K, et al. Hypoxia-induced increased permeability of endothelial monolayers occurs through lowering of cellular cAMP levels. *Am J Physiol* 1992;262:C546–C554.

77. Beebe S, Corbin J. Cyclic nucleotide-dependent protein kinases. In: *The enzymes.* New York: Academic Press, 1986:43–111.

78. Minnear FL, Johnson A, Malik AB. Beta-adrenergic modulation of pulmonary transvascular fluid and protein exchange. *J Appl Physiol* 1986;60:266–274.

79. Minnear FL, DeMichele MA, Moon DG, et al. Isoproterenol reduces thrombin-induced pulmonary endothelial permeability in vitro. *Am J Physiol* 1989;257:H1613–H1623.

80. Farrukh IS, Gurtner GH, Michael JR. Pharmacological modification of pulmonary vascular injury: possible role of cAMP. *J Appl Physiol* 1987;62:47–54.

81. Stelzner TJ, Weil JV, O'Brien RF. Role of cyclic adenosine monophosphate in the induction of endothelial barrier properties. *J Cell Physiol* 1989;139:157–166.

82. Adkins WK, Barnard JW, May S, et al. Compounds that increase cAMP prevent ischemia-reperfusion pulmonary capillary injury. *J Appl Physiol* 1992;72:492–497.

83. Haynes J Jr, Robinson J, Saunders L, et al. Role of cAMP-dependent protein kinase in cAMP-mediated vasodilation. *Am J Physiol* 1992;262:H511–H516.

84. Suttorp N, Weber U, Weisch T, et al. Role of phosphodiesterase in the regulation of endothelial permeability in vitro. *J Clin Invest* 1993;91:1421–1428.

85. Feelisch M, te Poel M, Zamora R, et al. Understanding the controversy over the identity of EDRF. *Nature* 1994;368:62–65.

86. Kubes P, Suzuki M, Granger DN. Nitric oxide: an endogenous modulator of leukocyte adhesion. *Proc Natl Acad Sci USA* 1991;88:4651–4655.

87. Radomski MW, Palmer RM, Moncada S. Endogenous nitric oxide inhibits human platelet adhesion to vascular endothelium. *Lancet* 1987;2:1057–1058.

88. Kubes P, Granger DN. Nitric oxide modulates microvascular permeability. *Am J Physiol* 1992;262:H611–H615.

89. Oz MC, Pinsky DJ, Koga S, et al. Novel preservation solution permits 24-hour preservation in rat and baboon cardiac transplant models. *Circulation* 1993;88[pt 2]:291–297.

90. Gerlach H, Clauss M, Ogawa S, et al. Perturbation of endothelial bar-

rier and coagulant properties by environmental factors. In: *Endothelial cell dysfunction*. New York: Plenum Press, 1991:525–545.

91. Esmon C. The regulation of natural anticoagulant pathways. *Science* 1987;235:1348–1352.

92. Broekman MJ, Eiroa A, Marcus A. Inhibition of human platelet reactivity by endothelium-derived relaxing factor from human umbilical vein endothelial cells in suspension: blockade of aggregation and secretion by an aspirin-insensitive mechanism. *Blood* 1991;78:1033–1040.

93. Koga S, Ogawa S, Kuwabara K, et al. Synthesis and release of interleukin 1 by reoxygenated human mononuclear phagocytes. *J Clin Invest* 1992;90:1007–1015.

94. Shreeniwas R, Koga S, Karakurum M, et al. Hypoxia-mediated induction of endothelial cell interleukin-1a. An autocrine mechanism promoting expression of leukocyte adhesion molecules on the vessel surface. *J Clin Invest* 1992;90:2333–2339.

95. Pober J. Cytokine-mediated activation of vascular endothelium. *Am J Pathol* 1988;133:416–422.

96. Oz M, Rose E, Michler R, et al. Coronary vascular endothelium may release contents of Weibel-Palade bodies but does not shed membrane proteins during cardiac surgery. *Circulation* 1993;88[Suppl]:I-247–I-250.

97. Horgan MJ, Wright SD, Malik AB. Antibody against leukocyte integrin (CD18) prevents reperfusion-induced lung vascular injury. *Am J Physiol* 1990;259:L315–L319.

98. Simpson PJ, Todd RF, Fantone JC, et al. Reduction of experimental canine myocardial reperfusion injury by a monoclonal antibody (anti-Mo1, anti-CD11b) that inhibits leukocyte adhesion. *J Clin Invest* 1988;81:624–629.

99. Repine JE, Cheronis JC, Rodell TC, et al. Pulmonary oxygen toxicity and ischemia-reperfusion injury. A mechanism in common involving xanthine oxidase and neutrophils. *Am Rev Respir Dis* 1987;136:483–485.

100. Colletti LM, Remick DG, Burtch GD, et al. Role of tumor necrosis factor-alpha in the pathophysiologic alterations after hepatic ischemia/reperfusion injury in the rat. *J Clin Invest* 1990;85:1936–1943.

101. Dreyer WJ, Michael LH, West M, et al. Neutrophil accumulation in ischemic canine myocardium. Insights into time course, distribution, and mechanism of localization during early reperfusion. *Circulation* 1991;84:400–411.

102. Dinarello CA. Interleukin-1 and its biologically related cytokines. *Adv Immunol* 1989;44:153–205.

103. Sherry B, Cerami A. Cachectin/tumor necrosis factor exerts endocrine, paracrine, and autocrine control of inflammatory responses. *J Cell Biol* 1988;107:1269–1277.

104. Strieter RM, Kunkel SL, Showell HJ, et al. Endothelial cell gene expression of a neutrophil chemotactic factor by TNF-alpha, LPS, and IL-1 beta. *Science* 1989;243:1467–1469.

105. Baggiolini M, Walz A, Kunkel SL. Neutrophil-activating peptide-1/interleukin 8, a novel cytokine that activates neutrophils. *J Clin Invest* 1989;84:1045–1049.

106. Karakurum M, Shreeniwas R, Chen J, et al. Hypoxic induction of interleukin-8 gene expression in human endothelial cells. *J Clin Invest* 1994;93:1564–1570.

107. Yoshida N, Granger DN, Anderson DC, et al. Anoxia/reoxygenation-induced neutrophil adherence to cultured endothelial cells. *Am J Physiol* 1992;262:H1891–H1898.

108. Arnould T, Michiels C, Remacle J. Increased PMN adherence on endothelial cells after hypoxia: involvement of PAF, CD18/CD11b, and ICAM-1. *Am J Physiol* 1993;264:C1102–C1110.

109. Kubes P, Ibbotson G, Russell J, et al. Role of platelet-activating factor in ischemia/reperfusion-induced leukocyte adherence. *Am J Physiol* 1990;259:G300–G305.

110. Hattori R, Hamilton K, Fugate R, et al. Stimulated secretion of endothelial vWF is accompanied by rapid redistribution to cell surface of the intercellular granule membrane protein GMP-140. *J Biol Chem* 1989;264:7768–7771.

111. McEver RP, Beckstead JH, Moore KL, et al. GMP-140, a platelet a-Granule membrane protein, is also synthesized by vascular endothelial cell and is localized in Weibel-Palade bodies. *J Clin Invest* 1989;84:92–99.

112. Ewenstein BM, Warhol MJ, Handin RI, et al. Composition of the von Willebrand factor storage organelle (Weibel-Palade body) isolated from cultured human umbilical vein endothelial cells. *J Cell Biol* 1987;104:1423–1433.

113. Birch KA, Pober JS, Zavoico GB, et al. Calcium/calmodulin trans-

duces thrombin-stimulated secretion: studies in intact and minimally permeabilized human umbilical vein endothelial cells. *J Cell Biol* 1992;118:1501–1510.

114. Lorant DE, Patel KD, McIntyre TM, et al. Coexpression of GMP-140 and PAF by endothelium stimulated by histamine or thrombin: a juxtacrine system for adhesion and activation of neutrophils. *J Cell Biol* 1991;115:223–234.

115. Patel KD, Zimmerman GA, Prescott SM, et al. Oxygen radicals induce human endothelial cells to express GMP-140 and bind neutrophils. *J Cell Biol* 1991;112:749–759.

116. Geng JG, Bevilacqua MP, Moore KL, et al. Rapid neutrophil adhesion to activated endothelium mediated by GMP-140. *Nature* 1990;343:757–760.

117. Weyrich AS, Ma XY, Lefer DJ, et al. In vivo neutralization of P-selectin protects feline heart and endothelium in myocardial ischemia and reperfusion injury. *J Clin Invest* 1993;91:2620–2629.

118. Romson J, Hook B, Kunkel S, et al. Reduction of the extent of ischemic myocardial injury by neutrophil depletion in the dog. *Circulation* 1983;67:1016–1023.

119. Mullane KM, Read N, Salmon JS, et al. Role of leukocytes in acute myocardial infarction in anesthetized dogs: relationship to myocardial salvage by anti-inflammatory drugs. *J Pharmacol Exp Ther* 1984;228:510–521.

120. Lucchesi B, Mullane K. Leukocytes and ischemia-induced myocardial injury. *Ann Rev Pharmacol Toxicol* 1986;26:201–224.

121. Entman M, Michael L, Rossen R, et al. Inflammation in the course of early myocardial ischemia. *FASEB J* 1991;5:2529–2537.

122. Crawford MH, Grover FL, Kolb WP, et al. Complement and neutrophil activation in the pathogenesis of ischemic myocardial injury. *Circulation* 1988;78:1449–1458.

123. Granger DN. Role of xanthine oxidase and granulocytes in ischemia-reperfusion injury. *Am J Physiol* 1988;255:H1269–H1275.

124. Kilgore KS, Lucchesi BR. Reperfusion injury after myocardial infarction: the role of free radicals and the inflammatory response. *Clin Biochem* 1993;359:370.

125. Ma XL, Lefer DJ, Lefer A, et al. Cardiac protective effects of a monoclonal antibody to intercellular adhesion molecule-1 in myocardial ischemia and reperfusion. *Circulation* 1992;86:937–946.

126. Ma XL, Tsao PS, Lefer AM. Antibody to CD-18 exerts endothelial and cardiac protective effects in myocardial ischemia and reperfusion. *J Clin Invest* 1991;88:1237–1243.

127. Rot A. Endothelial cell binding of NAP-1/IL-8: role in neutrophil emigration. *Immunol Today* 1992;13:291–294.

128. Peveri P, Walz A, Dewald B, et al. A novel neutrophil-activating factor produced by human mononuclear phagocytes. *J Exp Med* 1988;167:1547–1549.

129. Detmers PA, Lo SK, Olsen-Egbert E, et al. Neutrophil-activating protein 1/interleukin 8 stimulates the binding activity of the leukocyte adhesion receptor CD11b/CD18 on human neutrophils. *J Exp Med* 1990;171:1155–1562.

130. Mayadas TN, Johnson RC, Rayburn H, et al. Leukoctye rolling and extravasation are severely compromised in P selectin-deficient mice. *Cell* 1993;74:541–554.

131. Vadas MA, Gamble JR. Regulation of the adhesion of neutrophils to endothelium. *Biochem Pharmacol* 1990;40:1683–1687.

132. Sekido N, Mukaida N, Harada A, et al. Prevention of lung reperfusion injury in rabbits by a monoclonal antibody against interleukin-8. *Nature* 1993;365:654–657.

133. Winn RK, Liggitt D, Vedder NB, et al. Anti-P-selectin monoclonal antibody attenuates reperfusion injury to the rabbit ear. *J Clin Invest* 1993;92:2042–2047.

134. Mulligan MS, Paulson JC, de Frees S, et al. Protective effects of oligosaccharides in P-selectin-dependent lung injury. *Nature* 1993;364:149–151.

135. Hill JH, Ward P. The physiologic role of C3 leukotactic fragments in myocardial infarcts of rats. *J Exp Med* 1971;133:885–900.

136. Maroko PR, Carpenter CB, Chiariello M, et al. Reduction by cobra venom factor of myocardial necrosis after coronary artery occlusion. *J Clin Invest* 1978;61:661–670.

137. Schafer H, Mathey D, Hugo F, et al. Deposition of the terminal C5b-9 complement complex in infarcted area of human myocardium. *J Immunol* 1986;137:1945–1949.

138. Hattori R, Hamilton KK, McEver RP, et al. Complement proteins C5b-9 induce secretion of high molecular weight multimers of en-

dothelial von Willebrand factor and translocation of granule membrane protein GMP-140 to the cell surface. *J Biol Chem* 1989;264: 9053–9060.

139. Homeister JW, Satoh P, Lucchesi BR. Effects of complement activation in the isolated heart. Role of the terminal complement components. *Circ Res* 1992;71:303–319.

140. Homeister JW, Satoh PS, Kilgore KS, et al. Soluble complement receptor type 1 prevents human complement-mediated damage of the rabbit isolated heart. *J Immunol* 1993;150:1055–1064.

141. Weisman HF, Bartow T, Leppo MK, et al. Soluble human complement receptor type 1: in vivo inhibitor of complement suppression post-ischemic myocardial inflammation and necrosis. *Science* 1990;249:146–151.

CHAPTER 57

Triggering of Onset of Myocardial Infarction and Sudden Cardiac Death

Geoffrey H. Tofler, Simon P. Eggleton, Murray A. Mittleman, and James E. Muller

Key Words: Arrhythmia; circadian rhythm; endothelium; myocardial infarction; plaques; sudden cardiac death; thrombosis; triggering.

INTRODUCTION

Over the last two decades, substantial information has been obtained indicating that the onset of myocardial infarction (MI), as well as of sudden cardiac death (SCD), often is triggered by activities of the patient (1–3). This information helps to illuminate the mechanisms linking a previously quiescent atherothrombotic plaque to the acute coronary syndromes (4). The increased prospects for success in this field of study result from the multiple advances in understanding of acute coronary artery disease achieved during the 1980s and continued through the 1990s. The work of DeWood and coworkers (5) clearly established that acute thrombosis leads to MI. Davies and Thomas (6), Falk (7), and others, building on the pioneering studies of Constantinides in the 1960s (8), identified

the pathoanatomic role of plaque disruption and thrombosis in SCD, unstable angina, and in MI. Fuster and colleagues characterized the types of arterial injury likely to produce thrombosis (9), and Willerson and coworkers (10) identified interventions capable of modifying conversion of chronic to acute disease in experimental animals. Randomized clinical trials have demonstrated that aspirin (11), β-blocking agents (12), lipid-lowering regimens (13), and angiotensin-converting enzyme inhibitors (14) can prevent MI, but the mechanism of the beneficial effect is not fully explained. It also is recognized that the entire sequence of plaque disruption and occlusive thrombosis often begins in lesions previously causing less than 50% reduction of the diameter of the arterial lumen (15,16).

Although these gains in understanding are impressive, the field of triggering remains relatively unexplored, and only a small fraction of its potential benefit has been realized (17,18). Exploration of this aspect of coronary artery disease is of great importance, not because all triggering activities could or necessarily should be avoided, but because a better understanding of mechanism of onset would create new opportunities for prevention. Preventative methods include avoidance of some high-risk activities, developing pharmacologic and other strategies to interrupt the linkage between a trigger and its pathologic consequences, or the provision of defibrillators at cost-effective locations.

G. H. Tofler: Royal North Shore Hospital, Sydney, Australia.

S. P. Eggleton: Royal North Shore Hospital, Sydney, Australia.

M. A. Mittleman: Beth Israel Deaconess Medical Center, Boston, Massachusetts.

J. E. Muller: Massachusetts General Hospital, Boston, Massachusetts.

HISTORY OF THE TRIGGERING CONCEPT

In their original clinical description of acute MI in 1910, Obraztsov and Strazhesko (19) noted "direct events often precipitated the disease: the infarct began in one case on climbing a high staircase, in another during an unpleasant conversation, and in a third during emotional distress associated with a heated card game." In the 1930s and later, larger studies revealed that MI often occurred without an obvious precipitating event, thus challenging their view (14,20). However, studies conducted with modern epidemiologic methods and with the insight provided by new understanding of the pathogenesis of MI indicate that the original concept of Obraztsov and Strazhesko may be correct.

CIRCADIAN VARIATION OF MYOCARDIAL INFARCTION AND SUDDEN CARDIAC DEATH

The evidence that MI does not occur randomly throughout the day but shows a prominent increased morning frequency supports the concept that daily activities are important triggers. Data indicating that the onset of MI is more likely to occur in the morning come from numerous studies from different geographic areas (1,21–23). In the Multicenter Investigation of Limitation of Infarct Size (MILIS) (1) (Fig. 57–1), a threefold difference was seen between the maximum of 45 infarcts between 9 and 10 AM and a minimum of 15 between 11 PM and 12 AM. In the Intravenous Streptoki-

nase in Acute Myocardial Infarction (ISAM) Study (21), MI was four times more likely to occur between 8 and 9 AM than between 12 and 1 AM. The finding of these two studies is further supported by Goldberg and coworkers (23), who reported that the increased incidence of MI occurs within the first 4 hours after awakening and onset of activity.

The first direct evidence of circadian variation of SCD was reported in 1987 from an analysis of mortality records of the Massachusetts population (2). The time of day of death in this population showed a distinct circadian variation with a primary peak in the late morning from 9 to 11 AM and a minor secondary peak in the late afternoon. This was confirmed in subjects enrolled in the Framingham Heart Study (24). In a study of SCD conducted in Germany, (25) patients demonstrating an initial rhythm of ventricular tachycardia or ventricular fibrillation showed a marked circadian variation in occurrence, whereas the time of death of patients whose initial finding was electromechanical dissociation or asystole was relatively evenly distributed throughout the day. A morning peak of ventricular tachycardia has been documented by Twidale and coworkers (26) and has been confirmed in studies of implantable cardioverter-defibrillators (27,28).

Stroke also shows a primary morning increase (29,30). Transient myocardial ischemia also demonstrates a peak incidence between 6 AM and 12 PM (31). Parker and coworkers (32) have shown that delay of morning activity delays the onset of the transient ischemia peak. A smaller, evening

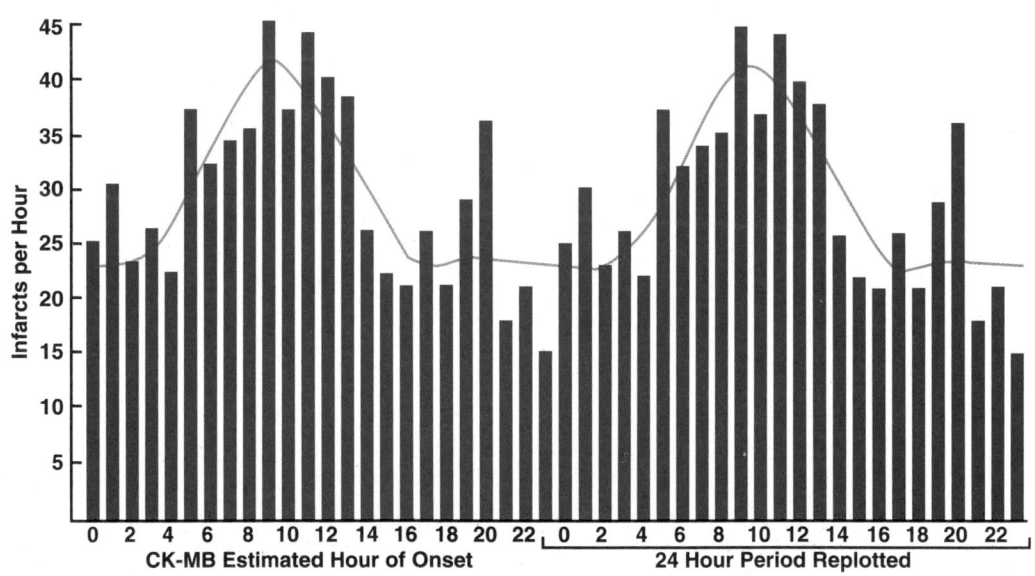

FIG. 57–1. Hourly frequency of onset of myocardial infarction (MI) as determined by the creatine kinase-MB method. **Left:** The number of infarctions beginning during each of the 24 hours of the day. **Right:** The identical data as the **left** are plotted again to permit appreciation of the relation between the end and beginning of the day. A two-harmonic regression equation for the frequency of onset of MI has been fitted to the data *(curved line)*. A primary peak incidence of infarction occurs at 9 AM, and a secondary peak occurs at 8 PM. (From Muller Muller JE, Stone PH, Turi ZG, et al. Circadian variation in the frequency of onset of acute myocardial infarction. *N Engl J Med* 1985;313:1315–1322, with permission.)

peak of both MI and SCD appears in some studies. Its cause is unknown and requires further investigation. A weekly variation also has been described with a peak frequency occurring on Mondays (33).

EPIDEMIOLOGIC EVIDENCE THAT ACTIVITIES TRIGGER DISEASE ONSET

Increasingly convincing evidence has been obtained indicating that certain activities trigger disease onset. Data on possible triggering activities collected from 849 patients enrolled in the MILIS Study (34) suggested frequent triggering. Possible triggers were reported by 48.5% of patients, 13.6% of whom reported two or more triggers. The triggers included emotional upset (18.8%), moderate physical activity (14.4%), heavy physical activity (8.7%), lack of sleep (8.0%), overeating (6.9%), sexual activity (1.2%), surgery (0.4%), and miscellaneous triggers (6.6%). These data are similar to those reported by Sumiyoshi and coworkers (35).

Although these and other observational studies (36) suggest that triggers of MI are present, the above mentioned studies suffer from a lack of control data. To assess the relative risk of an MI occurring after a common stressor such as physical exercise, it is essential to estimate the expected level of activity in the hours before the MI. Adjustment for usual exposure also is needed for comparisons of possible triggering between groups because differences clearly exist in the likelihood of patients with specific characteristics, such as older age and performing activities such as heavy physical exertion. These and other methodologic limitations of earlier studies led to the development of the case–crossover study design by Maclure (37) and Mittleman and coworkers (38). This enables estimation of the relative risk of an MI after a potential trigger. This risk is calculated as the observed frequency of the activity during a designated hazard period (the hour before the MI) compared with its expected frequency on the basis of the individual's usual frequency of exertion (Fig. 57–2).

Physical Activity as a Trigger of Myocardial Infarction

The level of physical activity at onset of MI was determined in 3,339 patients entered into the Thrombolysis in Myocardial Infarction (TIMI) II Study (36). Moderate or marked physical activity occurred at onset of MI in 18.7% of patients, more than could be expected from the proportionally much smaller fraction of the 24 hours that the subjects engage in moderate or marked activity. The importance of physical activity as a trigger was confirmed by the Determinants of Onset of Myocardial Infarction Study (ONSET), using the case–crossover methodology. By the use of this

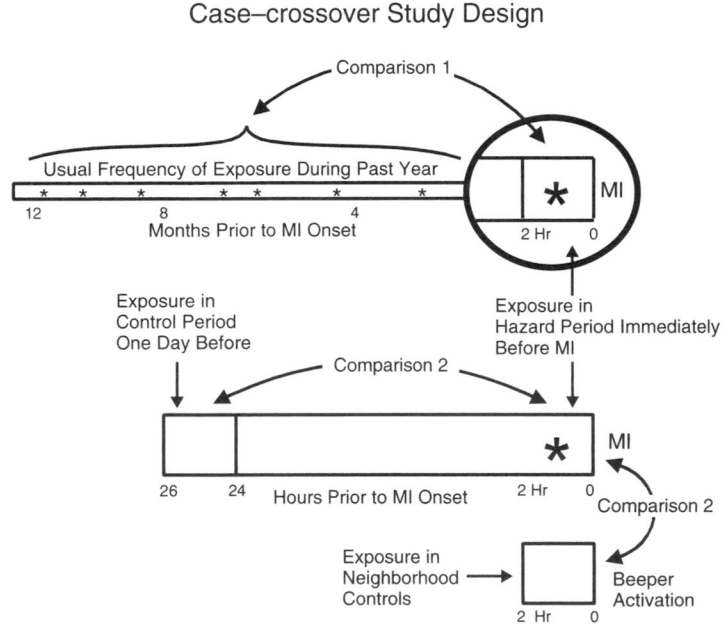

FIG. 57–2. Schematic representation of the case–crossover study design. The 2-hour period before MI onset is defined as the "hazard period." *Comparison 1* contrasts exposure to potential triggering activities (such as episodes of anger) in the hazard period with the frequency of exposure expected based on the reported usual frequency over the year before MI. In *Comparison 2*, exposure in the hazard period is compared with exposure in the "control period" at the same time on the preceding day. Together, the two methods of control information permit assessment of recall and other biases inherent in the study of triggering.

method, heavy exertion (exertion estimated to be > 6 metabolic equivalents [METS]) produced a 5.9-fold increase in risk (95% confidence interval [CI], 4.6–7.7) for MI in the subsequent hour (38). The risk for MI onset during heavy exertion was significantly greater in those who were sedentary (107-fold) compared with those who regularly exercised (2-fold) (Fig. 57–3). Willich and coworkers (39) found similar results.

Psychological Stress as a Trigger of Myocardial Infarction

Anger

Although abundant anecdotal evidence links acute psychological stress with onset of MI, there has been little controlled study of this acute phenomenon. Prior studies have focused on chronic risk and have yielded sometimes contradictory results (40–42). In the ONSET study, data on outbursts of anger were collected in 1,623 patients. Anger corresponding to levels greater than 4 in a 7-level self-report scale was reported by 14% of patients within 26 hours before MI onset. Using the same study design described for the study of physical exertion, the risk for MI onset was increased in the 2 hours after an outburst of anger, with a rela-

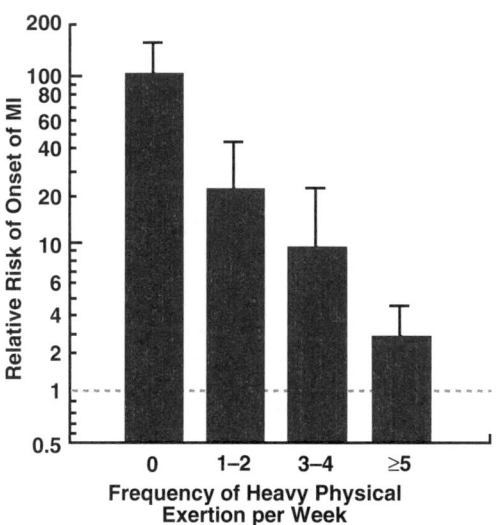

FIG. 57–3. Modification of the relative risk for myocardial infarction (MI) by usual frequency of heavy exertion (defined as ≥6 metabolic equivalents). The relative risks for heavy physical exertion are shown for subgroups of patients whose habitual frequency of heavy physical exertion is less than 1, 1 to 2, 3 to 4, and 5 or more episodes per week. Sedentary individuals experienced an extreme relative risk (107), whereas those who exerted themselves 5 or more times per week had an increase in risk only 2.4 times over baseline (p < 0.001). *Error bars* indicate 95% confidence intervals. (From Mittleman MA, Maclure M, Tofler GH, et al. Triggering of acute myocardial infarction by heavy physical exertion. Protection against triggering by regular exertion. Determinants of Myocardial Infarction Onset Study Investigators. *N Engl J Med* 1993;329:1677–1683, with permission.)

tive risk of 2.3 (95% CI, 1.7–3.2) (43). The Stockholm Heart Epidemiology Program (SHEEP) found an even greater increased risk for MI (relative risk, 9.0) after an episode of anger (44).

Bereavement

Several studies link life events such as bereavement with an increased risk for MI (45,46). In the ONSET study, a 14-fold increased relative risk of nonfatal MI was observed in the 24 hours after the death of a close family member (47). An increase in risk persisted beyond 1 month compared with baseline.

Acute Population Stress

An increased relative risk for acute MI (2.4) and cardiac death was observed after the 1994 Los Angeles earthquake, which occurred in the early morning, compared with the weeks before the disaster or the same day the previous year (48) (Fig. 57–4). During the initial 8 days after six blizzards in Massachusetts from 1974 to 1978, a 22% increase in ischemic deaths per day was reported in comparison with preceding and subsequent control weeks (49). During the 1991 Gulf War, the cardiovascular effects of the psychological stress induced by Scud missile attacks could be evaluated. During the first week of missile attacks on Israel, MI developed in 20 civilians in the area of one hospital compared with only eight during a control period (50). One study indicated an increase in cardiovascular events at the time of a football final (51).

Sexual Activity as a Trigger of Myocardial Infarction

In the ONSET study, the relative risk of an MI occurring in the 2 hours after sexual activity was 2.5 (95% CI, 1.7–3.7) compared with baseline risk (52). The relative risk was not greater among patients with a history of angina or infarction than that observed in those without prior cardiac disease. A similar doubling of relative risk with sexual activity was found in the SHEEP study (53). Effect modification by frequency of regular exertion also was noted, such that sedentary individuals had a fourfold increase in relative risk.

Consideration of sexual activity as a trigger allows discussion of the difference between relative risk and absolute risk. Relative risk provides a clue to mechanism, whereas absolute risk has practical implications for the individual subject. Because the baseline absolute risk of an MI in any given hour is extremely low (approximately 1 chance in 1,000,000 per hour for a healthy asymptomatic 50-year-old individual, or 10 chances in 1,000,000 per hour for a patient with a prior MI), doubling of baseline risk would produce only a small increase in absolute risk and should not be a factor in the decision of an asymptomatic cardiac patient to engage in sexual activity. Nonetheless, there is additional benefit in embarking on an exercise program, be-

Northridge Earthquake, 1994
Deaths from CVD

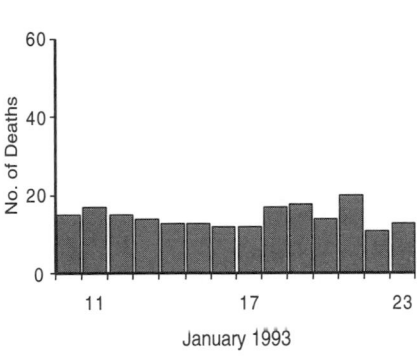
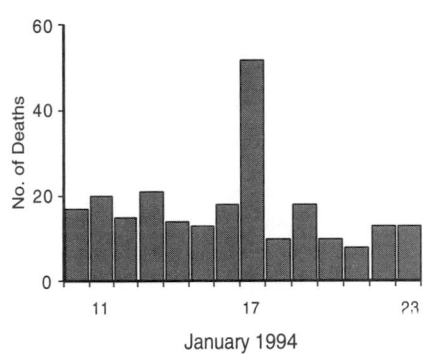

FIG. 57–4. Significant increase In the number of cases of sudden cardiac death on January 17, the day of the Northridge earthquake. CVD, cardiovascular disease. (From Leor J, Poole WK, Kloner RA. Sudden cardiac death triggered by an earthquake. *N Engl J Med* 1996;334:413–419, with permission)

cause the relative risk of sexual activity is further reduced in active individuals.

Recreational Drugs

MI and SCD after cocaine use have been reported, partly because of prothrombotic effects (54). In the ONSET study, cocaine use within 1 hour of symptoms of MI was associated with a 24-fold increase in relative risk (55). The ONSET study also showed that marijuana use led to a fourfold increase in relative risk for MI (56). Marijuana is associated with reduced vagal tone and an increased heart rate.

Heavy Meals

The secondary evening peak seen in some circadian studies of MI raises the possibility that a lipid-laden evening meal might be a contributing factor. Data are limited, but analysis from ONSET suggested an increase in relative risk for MI after a heavy fat meal (57). A prothrombotic changed induced by the triglycerides may be a contributing factor (58).

Respiratory Infection

The seasonal variation in MI and cardiac death, with a peak in winter months, could be due in part to respiratory infections (59). Although data are limited, Spokick and colleagues (60) found a doubling in relative risk for MI during respiratory infection in a case–control study. Days of high pollution also are associated with increased cardiovascular event rates.

Triggering of Sudden Cardiac Death

Although controlled studies of triggering activities are limited for SCD, several observational studies suggest that physical or mental stress may trigger SCD. In a controlled study, Thompson and coworkers (61) identified an age-adjusted risk for SCD during jogging of 7 (95% CI, 4–26) compared with the estimated rate during sedentary activities (61). Siscovick and coworkers (62) found that among men with low levels of habitual activity, the relative risk for SCD during vigorous activity was 56 (95% CI, 23–31); among men with high levels of habitual activity, it was 5 (95% CI, 2–14) (62). Mental stress also has been implicated as a trigger of SCD. Myers and Dewar (45) reported that in 40 of 100 cases, sudden death occurred within 24 hours after acute psychological stress. In patients after MI, depression was a significant predictor of subsequent sudden death (27). The ability of implantable defibrillators to identify circadian changes led Tofler and colleagues (63) to initiate the case–crossover Triggers of Ventricular Arrhythmia (TOVA) pilot study to provide further insight into triggers of SCD. Data from the TOVA study indicate the utility of such a study design.

PHYSIOLOGIC PROCESSES THAT MIGHT TRIGGER DISEASE ONSET

A variety of mechanisms, alone or in combination, could account for the morning increase in MI onset (3). A morning arterial pressure surge could initiate plaque disruption (64). An increase in coronary arterial tone could worsen the flow reduction produced by a fixed stenosis. The combination of increases in arterial pressure and coronary tone increase could result in increased shear stress (force directed against the endothelium resulting from increased coronary blood flow velocity), thus predisposing a vulnerable plaque to disrupt. Other prothrombotic processes, including increased platelet adhesion, increased blood viscosity, and increased platelet aggregability (65), have been described. Such a thrombotic tendency added to a reduced fibrinolytic activity in the morning (66) could increase the likelihood that an otherwise harmless mural thrombus overlying a small plaque fissure would propagate and occlude the coronary lumen. It remains unclear if the 24-hour periodicity of disease onset results from a true endogenous circadian rhythm or from the daily rest–activity cycle. Cortisol secretion is an endogenous circadian process not dependent on daily activity (67), whereas the morning platelet aggregability increase is abolished if the subjects remain at bed rest (68). Although the peak incidence of disease onset occurs in the morning, it is likely that similar physiologic processes trigger disease onset at other times of the day. The peak morning incidence of infarct onset probably results from the synchronization of potential triggers in the morning, whereas a smaller secondary evening peak may result from synchronization for an additional trigger, such as the evening meal.

Evidence suggests a prominent role for the autonomic nervous system in triggering SCD. Laboratory studies have demonstrated a reduced threshold for ventricular fibrillation in dogs subjected to acute psychological stress (69). The relation between platelet activity and sympathetic activation has been investigated in an animal model developed by Folts and coworkers (70). Thrombotic tendency can be increased by epinephrine infusion and decreased by sympatholytic interventions. This model exemplifies the importance of sympathetic activity in the pathogenesis of SCD and suggests a possible physiologic link between stressors causing sympathetic activation and the occurrence of fatal arrhythmias.

EFFECT OF DRUG THERAPY ON CIRCADIAN VARIATION AND TRIGGERING OF DISEASE ONSET

For nonfatal MI and SCD, β-adrenergic blockade selectively decreases the morning peak of events (1). In Beta Blocker Heart Attack Trial (BHAT), in which patients were randomly assigned to β-blockade or placebo, β-blockade demonstrated a selective beneficial effect against the occurrence of SCD in the morning (71). Observations of the timing of infarction in patients taking aspirin therapy, but not by random assignment, before their infarction have yielded mixed results. However, a randomized study in which the effect has been studied has demonstrated a selective morning decrease in nonfatal MI in patients receiving aspirin therapy (72). Data have been obtained indicating that aspirin may diminish the ability of anger to trigger infarction (43). Studies of silent myocardial ischemia have demonstrated that β-blockade, but not a short-acting calcium channel blocker, attenuates the morning increase (73).

MODEL OF TRIGGERING OF ACUTE CARDIOVASCULAR EVENTS

The information on triggering has provided the basis for a general theory of onset of coronary thrombosis (74). The hypothesis presented in Figure 57–5 adds the concept of triggering activities to the general scheme of the role of thrombosis in the acute coronary syndromes (6,7,9,10,75).

It is proposed that the initial step leading to disease onset is the development of a vulnerable atherothrombotic plaque. Plaque vulnerability is defined functionally as the susceptibility of a plaque to disruption. Development of such vulnerability is presumably a dynamic, potentially reversible disorder caused by several factors including changes in plaque constituents or its blood supply through vasa vasorum or changes in the functional integrity of the overlying endothelium, or both, in part from increased macrophage activity and thinning of the plaque collagen cap. Onset of MI might begin when a physical or mental stress produces a hemodynamic change that is sufficient to disrupt a vulnerable plaque. Vasoconstrictive, thrombogenic, and shear forces might then lead to coronary occlusion. A synergistic combination of triggering activities may account for thrombosis when each activity alone may not exceed the threshold for causation of infarction. For example, physical exertion (producing a minor plaque disruption) followed by cigarette smoking (producing an increase in coronary artery vasoconstriction and a relatively hypercoagulable state) (76) may be needed to cause occlusive thrombosis and disease onset. Also, the response of a healthy individual to a potential trigger may differ from that observed in an individual with a condition predisposing to MI. For example, patients with hypertension demonstrate a greater increase in vascular resistance after infusion of norepinephrine than healthy individuals (77). Patients with atherosclerosis may demonstrate a paradoxic vasoconstrictor response in response to acetylcholine infusion (78) and an impaired increase in fibrinolytic potential with exercise (79).

The findings of circadian variation and triggering also have led to the concept of an acute risk factor that supplements the traditional concept of a chronic risk factor. The acute risk factor is defined as the pathophysiologic change (vasoconstrictive, hemodynamic, or prothrombotic) potentially leading to occlusive coronary thrombosis. It results from a combination of an external stress (physical or mental) and the individual's reactivity to that stress. Although the extent of atherothrombosis changes slowly with time (chronic risk factor), hemodynamic, vasoconstrictive, and prothrombotic forces (acute risk factors) may be rapidly generated by external stresses.

The model presented earlier also serves as a mechanism through which thrombosis produces SCD. In addition, it is likely that triggers cause SCD through several other mechanisms. First, the trigger and increased sympathetic activation may decrease the threshold of the myocardium for a fatal arrhythmia. Second, the trigger may act on the conducting system of the heart, thereby predisposing to a fatal arrhythmia. Third, in conditions with hypertrophic cardiomyopathy or significant valvular disease, a triggering activity may lead to death through hemodynamic mechanisms. In addition, the adequacy of the collateral circulation and the condition of the microcirculation may play critical roles in determining whether a total coronary occlusion leads to a lethal cardiac arrhythmia (80).

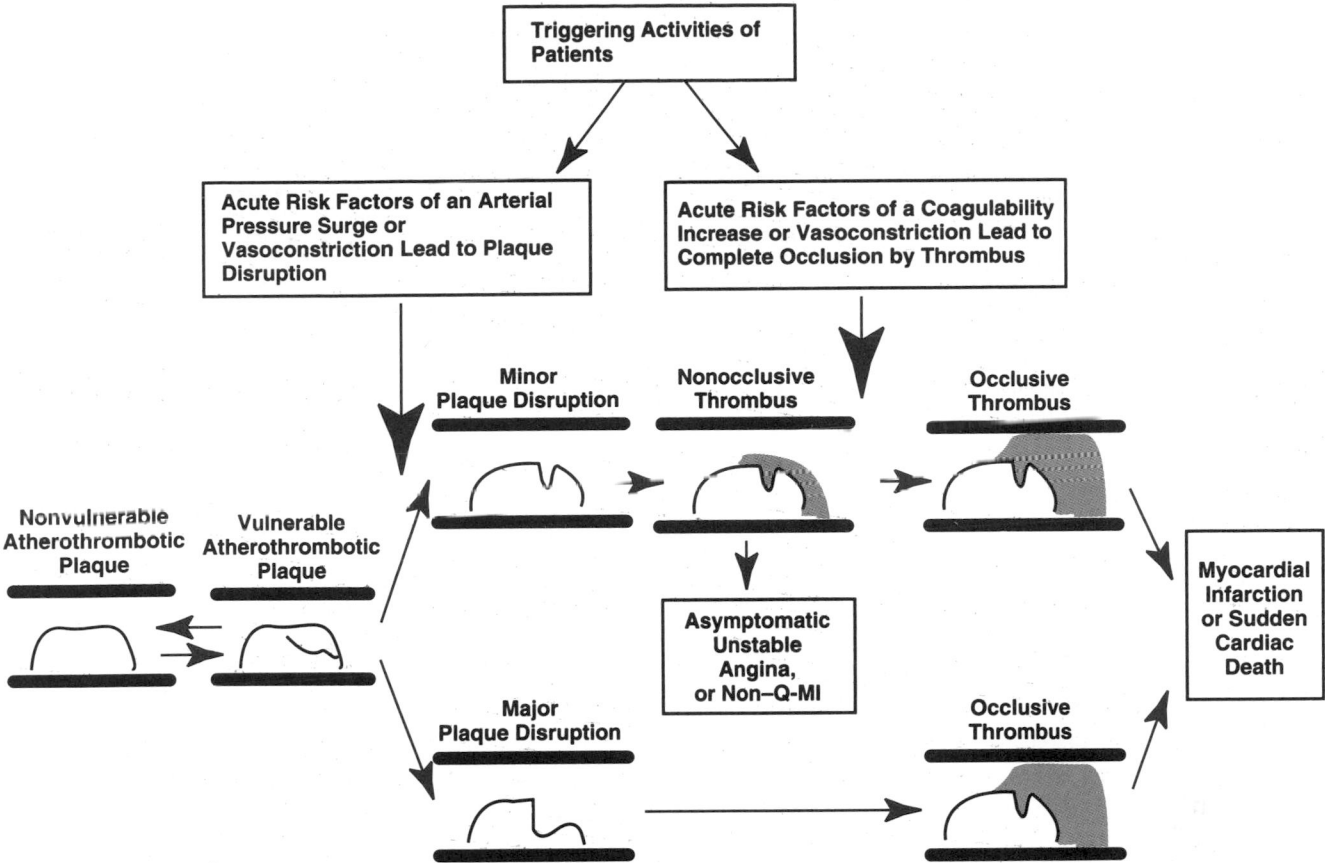

FIG. 57–5. Illustration of a hypothetic method by which daily activities may trigger coronary thrombosis. Three triggering mechanisms are presented: (a) physical or mental stress producing hemodynamic changes leading to plaque rupture; (b) activities causing a coagulability increase; and (c) stimuli leading to vasoconstriction. MI, myocardial infarction. (From Muller JE, Abela GS, Nesto RW, et al. Triggers, acute risk factors and vulnerable plaques: the lexicon of a new frontier. *J Am Coll Cardiol* 1994;23: 809–813, with permission.)

CLINICAL IMPLICATIONS OF CIRCADIAN VARIATION AND TRIGGERING

Although the circadian variation of cardiovascular disease onset has now been well described, there is no clear evidence that stressors occurring in the morning have a greater risk than stressors occurring at other times of day (81). Rather, the morning period may be a time of increased confluence of triggering activities. The following clinical implications can be gained from this field of study:

1. Avoidance of High-Risk Activity: Avoidance of drugs such as cocaine and marijuana should eliminate the increased transient cardiovascular risk associated with their use. Limiting exposure to the outside atmosphere during days of high pollution also is appropriate, particularly among individuals with coronary artery disease. Sedentary individuals should be aware of the increased relative risk for MI during heavy exertion. The reduced relative risk for MI being induced by heavy exertion among regular exercisers supports other evidence that regular exertion is protective. Avoidance of situations

provoking severe emotional distress or anger may be useful, as would be psychological assistance to modify acute anger responses. Flu and pneumococcal vaccines to reduce the risk for a respiratory infection would be recommended, particularly to individuals with known cardiovascular disease.

2. Strategies to Interrupt the Link between a Trigger and Its Pathologic Consequences: The current state of knowledge of the morning increase and triggering of disease onset raises the question as to whether pharmacologic therapy should be altered to prevent triggering. For β-blockade, the data appear sufficient to justify selection of an agent that will provide adequate 24-hour protection, particularly in the morning hours. This recommendation is based on substantial evidence, but it is important to note that there has not been, and there is unlikely to be, a randomized trial comparing the ability of a long-acting β-blocker versus a shorter-acting agent to prevent cardiovascular events. For aspirin, the issue of morning protection is moot because aspirin provides suppression of morning

platelet activity for approximately 3 days. For other agents, it seems reasonable that pharmacologic protection should be provided during the morning hours for patients already receiving antiischemic and antihypertensive therapy. Furthermore, although not well studied, it would be logical that increased cardioprotective medication during times of heightened transient risk would be beneficial.

3. Discussion of Absolute Risk versus Relative Risk in Triggering Activities: It is important to consider and discuss with patients the difference between relative risk and the absolute risk of experiencing an event during exertion or any other potential trigger. Although there may exist a sixfold increase in the relative risk of an infarction during exercise, this generally translates to only a small increase in absolute risk because baseline risk is low and the period of increased risk is short. The absolute risk that an individual would experience an MI in the hour after exertion might increase from approximately 5 in 1,000,000 to 30 in 1,000,000 after heavy exertion. The well recognized benefits of regular exertion support a recommendation that patients exercise regardless of the time of day.

4. Defibrillators in Cost-effective Places: The demonstration that the risk for SCD increases with physical and mental stress supports the role for defibrillators in public places. They are now being increasingly placed in airline terminals (82) and provided at sporting arenas.

CONCLUSION

The primary significance of the recognition of triggering and circadian variation of disease onset are the clues provided for understanding of disease onset and the new opportunities for prevention that such knowledge would provide. Further epidemiologic studies must be conducted to better characterize the role and frequency of identifiable triggers and their modifiers. The certainty with which an activity can be identified as a trigger also will vary in individual cases. In a patient whose plaque is only slightly vulnerable, the activity required to produce disease onset may be extreme, and the activity can be recognized as a trigger by its intensity. However, in a patient with an extremely vulnerable plaque, even nonstrenuous, routine, daily activities such as eating a heavy meal may be sufficient to trigger the cascade leading to infarction. On the clinical level, increased study of the relation between daily activities and potentially triggering physiologic responses could clarify the manner in which these processes cause disease onset. Techniques to identify vulnerable plaques might be used to characterize the plaques responsible for disease onset. Such studies might lead to the possibility that vulnerable plaques could be recognized before their disruption. On the basic science level, there is a need for complete characterization of the control mechanisms of potentially adverse and beneficial physiologic processes pertinent to triggering.

Greater understanding of triggering mechanisms should facilitate progress in the prevention of clinical coronary artery disease. The means of prevention would not be to eliminate all potential triggering activities—an undesirable and unattainable goal—but to design regimens that can be evaluated in randomized studies for their ability to sever the link between potential triggering activity and development of MI and SCD.

REFERENCES

1. Muller JE, Stone PH, Turi ZG, et al. Circadian variation in the frequency of onset of acute myocardial infarction. N Engl J Med 1985; 313:1315–1322.
2. Muller JE, Ludmer PL, Willich SN, et al. Circadian variation in the frequency of sudden cardiac death. Circulation 1987;75:131–138.
3. Muller JE, Tofler GH, Stone PH. Circadian variation and triggers of onset of acute cardiovascular disease. Circulation 1989;79:733–743.
4. MacIsaac AI, Thomas JD, Topol EJ. Toward the quiescent coronary plaque. J Am Coll Cardiol 1993;22:1228–1241.
5. DeWood MA, Spores J, Notske R, et al. Prevalence of total coronary occlusion during the early hours of transmural myocardial infarction. N Engl J Med 1980;303:897–902.
6. Davies MJ, Thomas A. Thrombosis and acute coronary-artery lesions in sudden cardiac ischemic death. N Engl J Med 1984;310:1137–1140.
7. Falk E. Plaque rupture with severe pre-existing stenosis precipitating coronary thrombosis. Characteristics of coronary atherosclerotic plaques underlying fatal occlusive thrombi. Br Heart J 1983;50:127–134.
8. Constantinides P. Plaque fissure in human coronary thrombosis. J Atheroscler Res 1966;1:1–17.
9. Ip JH, Fuster V, Badimon L, et al. Syndromes of accelerated atherosclerosis: role of vascular injury and smooth muscle cell proliferation. J Am Coll Cardiol 1990;15:1667–1687.
10. Willerson JT, Campbell WB, Winniford MD, et al. Conversion from chronic to acute coronary artery disease: speculation regarding mechanisms. Am J Cardiol 1984;54:1349–1354.
11. Final report of aspirin component of ongoing Physicians' Health Study. Steering Committee of the Physicians' Health Study Research Group. N Engl J Med 1989;321:129–135.
12. Willich SN, Pohjola-Sintonen S, Bhatia SJ, et al. Suppression of silent ischemia by metoprolol without alteration of morning increase of platelet aggregability in patients with stable coronary artery disease. Circulation 1989;79:557–565.
13. Downs JR, Clearfield M, Weis S, et al. Primary prevention of acute coronary events with lovastatin in men and women with average cholesterol levels: results of the AFCAPS/TexCAPS. JAMA 1998;279:1383–1389.
14. Effects of an angiotensin-converting-enzyme inhibitor, Ramipril, on cardiovascular events in high-risk patients. N Engl J Med 2000;342:145–153.
15. Little WC, Constantinescu M, Applegate RJ, et al. Can coronary angiography predict the site of a subsequent myocardial infarction in patients with mild-to-moderate coronary artery disease? Circulation 1988;78[5 Pt 1]:1157–1166.
16. Brown BG, Gallery CA, Badger RS, et al. Incomplete lysis of thrombus in the moderate underlying atherosclerotic lesion during intracoronary infusion of streptokinase for acute myocardial infarction: quantitative angiographic observations. Circulation 1986;73:653–661.
17. American Heart Association. 1992 Heart and stroke facts. Dallas, TX: American Heart Association, 2002.
18. Muller JE, Tofler GH. Circadian variation and cardiovascular disease. N Engl J Med 1991;325:1038–1039.
19. Obraztsov VP, Strazhesko ND. The symptomatology and diagnosis of coronary thrombosis. In: Vorobeva VA, Konchalovski MP, eds. Works of the First Congress of Russian Therapists. Comradeship Typography of A.E. Mamontov. 1910:26–43.
20. Master AM. The role of effort and occupation (including physicians) in coronary occlusion. JAMA 1960;174:942–948.
21. Willich SN, Linderer T, Wegscheider K, et al. Increased morning incidence of myocardial infarction in the ISAM Study: absence with prior beta-adrenergic blockade. Circulation 1989;80:853–858.

22. Thompson DR, Blandford RL, Sutton TW, et al. Time of onset of chest pain in acute myocardial infarction. *Int J Cardiol* 1985;7:139–148.

23. Goldberg RJ, Brady P, Muller JE, et al. Time of onset of symptoms of acute myocardial infarction. *Am J Cardiol* 1990;66:140–144.

24. Willich SN, Levy D, Rocco MB, et al. Circadian variation in the incidence of sudden cardiac death in the Framingham Heart Study population. *Am J Cardiol* 1987;60:801–806.

25. Arntz HR, Willich SN, Oeff M, et al. Circadian variation of sudden cardiac death reflects age-related variability in ventricular fibrillation. *Circulation* 1993;88:2284–2289.

26. Twidale N, Taylor S, Hekkle WF, et al. Morning increase in the time of onset of sustained ventricular tachycardia. *Am J Cardiol* 1989;64:1204–1206.

27. Lampert R, Rosenfeld L, Batsford W, et al. Circadian variation of sustained ventricular tachycardia in patients with coronary artery disease and implantable cardioverter-defibrillators. *Circulation* 1994;90:241–247.

28. Tofler GH, Gebara OC, Mittleman MA, et al. Morning peak in ventricular tachyarrhythmias detected by time of implantable cardioverter/defibrillator therapy. The CPI Investigators. *Circulation* 1995;92:1203–1208.

29. Tsementzis SA, Gill JS, Hitchcock ER, et al. Diurnal variation of and activity during the onset of stroke. *Neurosurgery* 1985;17:901–904.

30. Marler JR, Price TR, Clark GL, et al. Morning increase in onset of ischemic stroke. *Stroke* 1989;20:473–476.

31. Rocco MB, Barry J, Campbell S, et al. Circadian variation of transient myocardial ischemia in patients with coronary artery disease. *Circulation* 1987;75:395–400.

32. Parker JD, Testa MA, Jimenez AH, et al. Morning increase in ambulatory ischemia in patients with stable coronary artery disease. Importance of physical activity and increased cardiac demand. *Circulation* 1994;89:604–614.

33. Gnecchi-Ruscone T. Morning and Monday: critical periods for the onset of acute myocardial infarction: the GISSI 2 study experience. *Eur Heart J* 1994;15:882–887.

34. Tofler GH, Stone PH, Maclure M, et al. Analysis of possible triggers of acute myocardial infarction (The MILIS Study). *Am J Cardiol* 1990;66:22–27.

35. Sumiyoshi T. Evaluation of clinical factors involved in onset of myocardial infarction. *Jpn Circulation* 1986;50:164–173.

36. Tofler GH, Muller JE, Stone PH, et al. Modifiers of timing and possible triggers in the Thrombolysis in Myocardial Infarction Phase II (TIMI II) study group. *J Am Coll Cardiol* 1992;20:1049–1055.

37. Maclure M. The case-crossover design: a method for studying transient effects on the risk of acute events. *Am J Epidemiol* 1991;133:144–153.

38. Mittleman MA, Maclure M, Tofler GH, et al. Triggering of acute myocardial infarction by heavy physical exertion. Protection against triggering by regular exertion. Determinants of Myocardial Infarction Onset Study Investigators. *N Engl J Med* 1993;329:1677–1683.

39. Willich SN, Lewis M, Lowel H, et al. Physical exertion as a trigger of acute myocardial infarction. Triggers and Mechanisms of Myocardial Infarction Study Group. *N Engl J Med* 1993;329:1684–1690.

40. Eaker ED. Use of questionnaires, interviews, and psychological tests in epidemiological studies of coronary heart disease. *Eur Heart J* 1988;9:698–704.

41. Chang PP, Ford DE, Meoni IC, et al. Anger in young men and subsequent cardiovascular disease: the Precursors Study. *Arch Intern Med* 2002;162:901.

42. Williams JE, Paton CC, Siegler IC, et al. Anger proneness predicts coronary heart disease risk: prospective analysis from the Atherosclerosis in Communities (ARIC) Study. *Circulation* 2000;101:2034.

43. Mittleman MA, Maclure M, Sherwood JB, et al. Triggering of acute myocardial infarction onset by episodes of anger. *Circulation* 1995;92:1720–1725.

44. Moller J, Hallqvist J, Diderichsen F, et al. Do episodes of anger trigger myocardial infarction? A case-crossover analysis in the Stockholm Heart Epidemiology Program (SHEEP). *Psychosomatic Medicine* 1999;61:842–849.

45. Myers A, Dewar HA. Circumstances attending 100 sudden deaths from coronary artery disease with coroner's necropsies. *Br Heart J* 1975;37:1133–1143.

46. Parkes CM, Benjamin B, Fitzgerald R. Broken heart: statistical study of increased mortality among widowers. *Br Med J* 1969;1:740–743.

47. Mittleman MA, Maclure M, Sherwood JB, et al. Death of a significant person increased the risk of acute myocardial infarction onset. *Circulation* 1996;93:621A.

48. Leor J, Poole WK, Kloner RA. Sudden cardiac death triggered by an earthquake. *N Engl J Med* 1996;334:413–419.

49. Glass RI, Zack MM Jr. Increase in deaths from ischemic heart diseases after blizzards. *Lancet* 1979;1:485.

50. Meisel SR, Kutz I, Dayan KI, et al. Effect of Iraqi missile war on incidence of acute myocardial infarction and sudden death in Israeli civilians. *Lancet* 1991;338:660–661.

51. Witte DR, Bois MI, Hoes AW, et al. Cardiovascular mortality in Dutch men during 1996 European football championship: longitudinal population study. *Br Med J* 2000;321:1552–1554.

52. Muller JE, Mittleman MA, Maclure M, et al. Triggering myocardial infarction by sexual activity: low absolute risk and prevention by regular physical exertion. *JAMA* 1996;275:1405–1409.

53. Moller J, Ahlborn A, Hulting J, et al. Sexual activity as a trigger of myocardial infarction: a case-crossover analysis in the Stockholm heart Epidemiology Program (SHEEP). *Heart* 2001;86:387–390.

54. Siegel AJ, Sholar MB, Mendelson JH, et al. Cocaine-induced erythrocytosis and increase in von Willebrand factor. *Arch Intern Med* 1999;159:1925–1930.

55. Mittleman MA, Mintzer D, Maclure M, et al. Triggering of myocardial infarction by cocaine. *Circulation* 1999;99:2737–2741.

56. Mittleman MA, Lewis RA, Maclure M, et al. Triggering myocardial infarction by Marijuana. *Circulation* 2001;103:2805–2809.

57. Lopez-Jimenez F, Mittleman MA, Maclure M, et al. Triggering of acute myocardial infarction by heavy meals. *Circulation* 2000;102:II-612.

58. Miller GJ, Martin JC, Mitropolous KA. Plasma factor VII is activated by post-prandial triglyceridemia irrespective of dietary fat composition. *Atherosclerosis* 1991;86:163–166.

59. Woodhouse PR, Khaw KT, Plummer M, et al. Seasonal variation of plasma fibrinogen and factor VII activity in the elderly: winter infections and death from cardiovascular disease. *Lancet* 1994;343:435–439.

60. Spodick DH, Flessas AP, Johnson MM. Association of acute respiratory symptoms with onset of acute myocardial infarction: prospective investigation of 150 consecutive patients and matched control patients. *Am J Cardiol* 1984;53:481–482.

61. Thompson PD, Funk EJ, Carleton RA, et al. Incidence of death during jogging in Rhode Island from 1975 through 1980. *JAMA* 1982;247:2535–2538.

62. Siscovick DS, Weiss NS, Fletcher RH, et al. The incidence of primary cardiac arrest during vigorous exercise. *N Engl J Med* 1984;311:874–877.

63. Mittleman MA, Rich DQ, Wang PJ, et al. Moderate exertion as a trigger of ICD discharge for UT/UF. *Circulation* 2003;108:617A.

64. Millar-Craig MW, Bishop CN, Raftery EB. Circadian variation of blood pressure. *Lancet* 1978;I:795–797.

65. Tofler GH, Brezinski D, Schafer AI, et al. Concurrent morning increase in platelet aggregability and the risk of myocardial infarction and sudden cardiac death. *N Engl J Med* 1987;316:1514–1518.

66. Andreotti F, Davies GJ, Hackett DR. Major circadian fluctuations in fibrinolytic factors and possible relevance to time of onset of myocardial infarction, sudden cardiac death and stroke. *Am J Cardiol* 1988;62:635–637.

67. Weitzman ED, Fukushima D, Nogeire C, et al. Twenty-four hour pattern of the episodic secretion of cortisol in normal subjects. *J Clin Endo Metab* 1971;33:14–22.

68. Winther K, Hillegass W, Tofler GH, et al. Effects on platelet aggregation and fibrinolytic activity during upright posture and exercise in healthy men. *Am J Cardiol* 1992;70:1051–1055.

69. Corbalan R, Verrier R, Lown B. Psychological stress and ventricular arrhythmias during myocardial infarction in the conscious dog. *Am J Cardiol* 1974;34:692–696.

70. Folts JD, Stamler J, Loscalzo J. Intravenous nitroglycerin infusion inhibits cyclic blood flow responses caused by periodic platelet thrombus formation in stenosed canine coronary arteries. *Circulation* 1991;83:2122–2127.

71. Peters RW, Muller JE, Goldstein S, et al. Propranolol and the morning increase in the frequency of sudden cardiac death (BHAT Study). *Am J Cardiol* 1989;63:1518–1520.

72. Ridker PM, Manson JE, Buring JE, et al. Circadian variation of acute myocardial infarction and the effect of low-dose aspirin in a randomized trial of physicians. *Circulation* 1990;82:897–902.

73. Mulcahy D, Keegan J, Cunningham D, et al. Circadian variation of total ischaemic burden and its alteration with anti-anginal agents. *Lancet* 1988;2:755–759.

74. Muller JE, Abela GS, Nesto RW, et al. Triggers, acute risk factors and vulnerable plaques: the lexicon of a new frontier. *J Am Coll Cardiol* 1994;23:809–813.

75. Fuster V, Badimon L, Badimon JJ, et al. The pathogenesis of coronary artery disease and the acute coronary syndromes. *N Engl J Med* 1992;326:310–318.

76. Belch JJ, McArdle BM, Burns P, et al. The effects of acute smoking on platelet behaviour, fibrinolysis and haemorheology in habitual smokers. *Thromb Haemost* 1984;51:6–8.

77. Egan B, Schork N, Panis R, et al. Vascular structure enhances regional resistance responses in mild essential hypertension. *J Hypertension* 1988;6:41–48.

78. Ludmer PL, Selwyn AP, Shook TL, et al. Paradoxical vasoconstriction induced by acetylcholine in atherosclerotic coronary arteries. *N Engl J Med* 1986;315:1046–1051.

79. Khann PK, Seth HN, Balasubramanian V, et al. Effect of submaximal exercise on fibrinolytic activity in ischemic heart disease. *Br Med J* 1975;2:910–912.

80. Fuster V, Frye RL, Kennedy MA, et al. The role of collateral circulation in the various coronary syndromes. *Circulation* 1979;59:1137–1144.

81. Murray PM, Herrington DM, Pettus CW, et al. Should patients with heart disease exercise in the morning or afternoon? *Arch Intern Med* 1993;153:833–836.

82. O'Rourke MF, Donaldson E, Geddes JS. An Airline Cardiac Arrest Program. *Circulation* 1997;96:2849–2853.

Clinical Presentation

CHAPTER 58

Clinical Presentation and Diagnostic Evaluation of Unstable Angina and Non–ST-Segment Elevation Myocardial Infarction

Robert M. Califf and Daniel B. Mark

Key Words: Angina; diagnosis; electrocardiography; myocardial infarction; prognosis.

INTRODUCTION

The pathophysiology of acute ischemic heart disease has been extensively reviewed in Chapters 55 and 56. The goal of this chapter is to review the elements of the history, physical examination, electrocardiogram (ECG) results, and laboratory evaluation that are important for appropriate diagnostic and therapeutic decision-making for these patients.

The 1994 Clinical Practice Guideline for Unstable Angina defined unstable angina as a clinical syndrome that lies between stable angina and acute myocardial infarction (AMI) and has three principal clinical presentations: prolonged rest angina, usually longer than 20 minutes; new-onset severe angina, Canadian Cardiovascular Society Class (CCSC) III or greater within the previous 2 months; or increasing angina that is more frequent, longer in duration, or lower in threshold and is CCSC III or greater (1). This definition was intended for use at the time of initial patient evaluation, before definitive laboratory tests became available. It therefore deliberately included patients who would later be diagnosed with AMI and those who would later be determined to have noncardiac chest pain.

The 2000 American College of Cardiology (ACC)/American Heart Association (AHA) Guidelines further emphasized the continuum of acute coronary disease by using the term unstable angina/non–ST-elevation myocardial infarction (NSTEMI) to designate a syndrome usually (but not always) caused by atherothrombotic coronary disease and associated with an increased risk for MI and death (2). Another term now in common usage is acute coronary syndromes (ACS), which includes both AMI (both ST-elevation and non–ST-elevation forms) and unstable angina. As discussed later in this chapter, the distinction of greatest initial therapeutic importance is between ST-elevation AMI

R. M. Califf: Department of Medicine, Division of Cardiology, Duke University Medical Center, Duke Clinical Research Institute, 2400 Pratt Street, Room 0311, Durham, North Carolina 27715.

D. B. Mark: Department of Medicine, Division of Cardiology, Duke University Medical Center, Duke Clinical Research Institute, 2400 Pratt Street, Room 0311, Durham, North Carolina 27715.

and other forms of ACS. Subsequent distinctions among NSTEMI and unstable angina are made during the first 8 to 12 hours after presentation, using cardiac marker data. Identification of patients initially considered to have unstable angina who actually have a noncoronary cause for their symptoms is usually accomplished within 72 hours of initial evaluation.

ASSESSMENT OF DIAGNOSIS: GENERAL CONSIDERATIONS

Often in the early evaluation of the patient with ACS, the diagnosis of coronary artery disease has not yet been made. Serum cardiac markers are not yet available or often are still negative. As a result, the clinician must answer two important and related questions to decide on a therapeutic strategy. First, what is the likelihood that the patient's symptoms reflect active atherothrombotic coronary artery disease (the diagnostic question)? Second, what is the likelihood that the patient's symptoms represent a high-risk condition that may lead to early death or MI (the prognostic question)? We consider the general aspects of the diagnostic question in this section and address the prognostic question in the next section.

Clinical History

Whether the initial contact with the patient is by telephone, at the office, or in the emergency department (ED), the physician must ask a series of directed questions to ascertain whether reported symptoms could represent cardiac ischemia. Multiple studies have examined the importance of key historical factors in predicting the angiographic diagnosis of coronary artery disease (3–5). The five major factors from the initial history and physical examination useful for the diagnosis of coronary artery disease in patients without known disease, in order of importance, are the assessment of the anginal symptoms by the physician; prior MI by history, ECG, or both; sex; age; and number of cardiac risk factors present (diabetes, smoking, hypercholesterolemia, hypertension).

Typical or definite angina is characteristically described by patients as deep, poorly localized chest or arm discomfort. It is reproducibly associated with physical exertion or emotional stress and relieved promptly (i.e., within 5 minutes) by rest or sublingual nitroglycerin. Discomfort at rest with all the features of typical angina except for an exertional component should be considered definite angina for purposes of estimating coronary disease likelihood. Although the principal symptom of coronary disease is commonly referred to as "chest pain," some patients may not consider their ischemic symptoms painful. Instead, these patients report a difficult-to-describe sense of discomfort in their thorax. Severe dyspnea accompanying chest discomfort may indicate a high-risk situation (discussed later), but other associated symptoms such as nausea, sweating, or palpitations are not particularly useful for diagnosis.

Some patients may have no discomfort in the chest but instead have jaw, neck, ear, or arm discomfort. With a clear relation to exertion or stress or prompt relief by nitroglycerin, these symptoms should be considered equivalent to angina. Without such a history, a high degree of suspicion is helpful in reaching the correct diagnosis in these difficult situations. Other difficult presentations of the patient with possible unstable angina include those without any chest or equivalent discomfort. Most common among these latter presentations is isolated, unexplained, new-onset, or worsening exertional dyspnea; other atypical presentations include nausea and vomiting and diaphoresis. Atypical presentations have particularly been noted to be more frequent among elderly patients and also are more common in women and individuals with diabetes. The physician's assessment of the patient's symptoms should conclude with a summary assessment that assigns the patient to one of the following four categories: definite angina, probable angina, probably not angina, and not angina (6).

The major features suggesting a diagnosis of "not angina" include the following:

- Pleuritic chest pain, a sharp or knifelike pain brought on by respiratory movements
- Primary or sole location of the discomfort in the middle or lower abdominal region
- Pain localized with one finger
- Pain fully reproduced by movement or palpation of the chest wall or arms
- Constant pain lasting for days
- Brief episodes of pain lasting for a few seconds or less
- Pain radiating into the lower extremities.

Notably, however, even with such uncharacteristic symptoms, acute ischemic heart disease cannot be completely eliminated as a possibility. In the Multicenter Chest Pain Study, acute ischemia was the diagnosis in 22% of ED patients with sharp or stabbing chest pain and in 13% of patients with some pleuritic qualities to their pain. In addition, 7% of patients whose pain was fully reproduced by palpation were ultimately diagnosed with acute ischemic heart disease (7).

Evidence of a prior MI, from either the history or pathologic Q waves on the resting ECG, or a history of resuscitation from sudden cardiac death indicates a high likelihood of significant coronary artery disease. For any given clinical presentation, older patients have a greater likelihood of coronary artery disease than younger patients, and, at any age, men have a greater likelihood of coronary artery disease than do women.

In stable, symptomatic patients and asymptomatic subjects, cardiovascular risk factors are modestly predictive of the likelihood of coronary disease (3,5). Diabetes mellitus is the risk factor most closely correlated with coronary disease, but cigarette smoking, hypercholesterolemia, and hypertension also are important. A history of premature coronary artery disease (age < 55 years) in a parent or sibling has been inconsistently identified as a major risk factor. Family history may either signify a genetic predisposition to coronary artery disease or reflect the end result of a shared environment or lifestyle, or both.

In the patient with acute ischemic heart disease presenting in the ED, risk factors have been found to be only weakly predictive of the likelihood of acute ischemia. In men, diabetes and family history were the strongest factors in one study, followed by smoking history; in women, no risk factor was a significant predictor of acute ischemia, possibly because of insufficient statistical power (8). A common mistake in this setting is for the clinician to base a decision about treatment and admission for patients on the presence or absence of risk factors. The key concept is that traditional risk factors are far less important in patients with suspected unstable angina than are the patient's symptoms and ECG findings. Risk factor data become important later in the course as the basis for instituting aggressive medical therapy, modifying the usual therapy (particularly if there is a history of significant hypertension), or prescribing lifestyle modification.

Variant angina (Prinzmetal's angina) is an uncommon clinical syndrome of pain at rest and reversible ST-segment elevation without evidence of resulting MI. The prevalence of this disorder is quite low in the United States, and it may be difficult to diagnose on initial presentation. About one quarter of these patients have "insignificant" coronary disease, and their symptoms reflect episodic coronary vasospasm. In such patients, the diagnosis of variant angina indicates the need for specific management strategies, particularly the use of calcium-channel blockers and nitrates and avoidance of β-blockers. In the United States, however, three-quarters or more of patients with variant angina have significant subtotal stenosis of the culprit coronary vessel with a ruptured plaque; their management is identical to other patients with unstable angina (9,10). With the increased use of diagnostic catheterization over the last decade, the diagnostic designation of variant angina in the United States appears to have decreased. In addition, the effect of troponin testing on the requirement that MI be ruled out to confirm the diagnosis of variant angina has not been studied.

Cocaine use is an increasingly important cause of chest pain and ACS (11). There were 175,000 cocaine-related visits to EDs in 2000, 40% of which involved chest pain (11). Cocaine can induce myocardial ischemia by at least three possible mechanisms: by increasing myocardial oxygen demand; by reducing myocardial oxygen supply, secondary to coronary vasospasm or coronary thrombosis, or both; and through direct myocardial toxicity. In patients who are known to use cocaine, however, the clinician should not rule out underlying significant coronary artery disease, even if they are otherwise considered "too young" to have significant coronary disease.

If the physician believes that the patient's acute discomfort could represent myocardial ischemia, the initial physical examination should be brief and directed so that appropriate decisions about therapy can be made quickly. It is desirable to complete the directed history, physical examination, and ECG within 20 minutes of ED arrival. If the patient is having ongoing chest discomfort, an ECG should be obtained within 10 minutes.

Physical Examination

As in any physical examination of an ill patient, the level of consciousness should be noted first. Then the heart rate and rhythm should be assessed, followed by blood pressure measurement (in both arms) and temperature.

The cardiac physical examination has substantially less to contribute to the diagnosis of coronary artery disease than does the clinical history. Hypotension may indicate cardiogenic shock or some other high-risk problem and deserves the most aggressive diagnostic and therapeutic efforts possible until resolved. Although cardiogenic shock is typically regarded as a complication of STEMI, it may occur in up to 5% of patients with NSTEMI and carries the same adverse prognostic significance (12). Major findings on physical examination that are of diagnostic use include a transient S_3 or S_4, a mitral regurgitation murmur, or precordial lift during an episode of discomfort. Such factors are uncommon, but, if found, signify high likelihood of obstructive coronary disease. Presence of bruits or pulse deficits over the carotid or peripheral arteries suggesting extracardiac vascular disease also identifies a patient with a greater likelihood of significant coronary disease.

A brief abdominal examination is indicated to develop clues about gastrointestinal diagnoses, such as perforated ulcer or ruptured gallbladder, which can masquerade as discomfort in the chest. A brief neurologic examination provides an essential baseline against which new neurologic abnormalities can be identified in the setting of fibrinolytic and anticoagulant therapies. Focal neurologic deficits should prompt immediate detailed evaluation, given that ~2% of patients with MI will have a stroke during the same admission (13,14).

Having concluded the history and physical examination and having examined the ECG, the clinician should briefly consider the common life-threatening diagnoses that can masquerade as acute ischemia. Pulmonary embolism may be differentiated by the pleuritic nature of the chest pain, the nonspecific nature of the ECG, and hypoxemia. Aortic dissection often is described as a "tearing" or "ripping" sensation down the back and is sometimes accompanied by a difference in blood pressure in the arms, reduced or absent pulses, a murmur of aortic regurgitation, or a widened mediastinum on chest radiograph. Classic features often are absent for both pulmonary embolism and dissection, and a high index of suspicion should be maintained until an alternative diagnosis is firmly established (15). Pericardial tamponade leads to the classic finding of tachycardia, hypotension with a pulsus paradoxus, and distended neck veins without pulmonary rales. Acute pericarditis can be sometimes difficult to distinguish from acute ischemia, but the discomfort of pericarditis is characteristically pleuritic in nature, and the diagnosis is supported by finding a friction rub and diffuse ST-segment elevation on the ECG. Mistaking pericarditis for AMI and giving fibrinolytic therapy may lead to pericardial tamponade, although this is not inevitable (16). Acute pneumothorax is less common but requires emergency treatment. Asymmetrically diminished breath sounds, pleuritic pain, and a primary symptom of acute dyspnea should speed performance and examination of the chest radiograph.

Electrocardiographic Findings Useful for Diagnosis

A careful examination of the ECG by a trained interpreter is one of the critical steps in the diagnosis of unstable angina (17). A recording made during the patient's presenting symptoms is particularly useful. Transient ST- or T-wave changes that develop during a symptomatic episode at rest and resolve when the patient becomes asymptomatic are strong evidence for an ischemic cause and a high likelihood of underlying severe coronary disease. Diagnostic accuracy is improved if a patient's prior ECG is available for comparison (18). ST-segment and, to a lesser extent, T-wave changes are the primary elements on which an ECG diagnosis of acute ischemic heart disease is based. ST-segment elevation of 1 mm or greater in two or more contiguous leads indicates a diagnosis of AMI until proven otherwise and the need for prompt reperfusion therapy. The common ECG imitators of STEMI include acute pericarditis, early repolarization, left ventricular aneurysm, and left ventricular hypertrophy.

ST-segment depression of 0.5 to 1 mm or more typically indicates ischemia or non–Q-wave infarction. In a cohort of 2,457 patients with non–ST-segment elevation ACS enrolled in the Fast Revascularisation during InStability in Coronary artery disease (FRISC)-II study, 45% of the patients with ST-segment depression of 0.5 mm or more had three-vessel or left main coronary disease compared with 22% of the patients without ST-segment depression ($p < 0.001$) (19). Less than 10% of patients with ST-segment depression had no significant coronary disease, whereas almost 20% without admission ST changes had such findings at angiography. Isolated T-wave inversions had a diagnostic significance in this study similar to that of no ST-segment or T-wave changes.

In earlier studies, significant T-wave inversions (i.e., ≥ 2 mm) in precordial leads with dominant R waves indicated significant stenosis of the left anterior descending coronary artery in most of the unstable angina cases studied (20). Unfortunately, T-wave changes have received substantially less attention in the contemporary literature than ST-segment changes.

Established Q waves of 0.04 seconds or longer are less useful for the diagnosis of ACS, although they do indicate a high likelihood of significant coronary disease with prior MI. Importantly, isolated, 0.04-second Q waves in lead III may be a normal finding. Of patients who satisfy the criteria for NSTEMI, up to 25% will evolve Q waves in follow-up ECGs.

Nonspecific ST- and T-wave changes, usually defined as ST depression or T-wave inversion of less than 1 mm, are less useful than the foregoing in the diagnosis of ACS. In the Multicenter Chest Pain Study, these nonspecific changes

TABLE 58–1. *Likelihood of significant coronary artery disease in patients with symptoms suggesting unstable angina*

High likelihood (e.g., 0.85–0.99)	Intermediate likelihood (e.g., 0.15–0.84)	Low likelihood (e.g., 0.01–0.14)
Any of the following features:	*No high-likelihood features and any of the following:*	*No high- or intermediate-likelihood features but may have the following:*
History of prior MI or sudden death or other known history of CAD	Definite angina: men <60 or women <70 years of age	Chest pain classified as probably not angina
Definite angina: men ≥60 or women ≥70 years old	Probable angina: men ≥60 or women ≥70 years old	One risk factor other than diabetes
Transient hemodynamic or ECG changes during pain	Chest pain probably not angina in patients with diabetes	T-wave flattening or inversion <2 mm in leads with dominant R waves
Variant angina (pain with reversible ST-segment elevation)	Chest pain probably not angina and two or three risk factors other than diabetes[a]	Normal ECG
ST-segment elevation or depression ≥1 mm	Extracardiac vascular disease	
Marked symmetrical T-wave inversion in multiple precordial leads	ST depression 0.05–1 mm	
	T-wave inversion ≥2 mm in leads with dominant R waves	

Likelihood of significant coronary artery disease (CAD) is a complex, multivariable problem that cannot be fully specified within the confines of this table. Therefore, the table is meant to illustrate major relations rather than offer rigid algorithms.

ECG, electrocardiogram; MI, myocardial infarction.

[a]Coronary artery disease risk factors include diabetes, smoking, hypertension, and elevated cholesterol.

Adapted from Braunwald E, Mark DB, Jones RH, et al. *Unstable angina: diagnosis and management.* Rockville, MD: U.S. Department of Health and Human Services, 1994, with permission.

were associated with a *lesser* likelihood of MI or unstable angina, although not sufficiently to exclude either diagnosis reliably (7). The Multicenter Acute Ischemia Predictive Instrument Trial showed similar findings (21). In this later study, together with elevation or depression of the ST segment of 1 mm or greater, ST-segment "straightening" (horizontal or downsloping ST segments with slight depression suggesting acute ischemia) was significantly predictive of the presence of acute ischemia.

Even completely normal ECG results in the ED does not exclude the possibility of acute ischemia, given that 1% to 6% of patients with such a finding in the presence of suggestive symptoms will eventually be found to have had an AMI, and 4% or more will be found to have unstable angina (17,22).

Summary

The clinical and ECG findings that are important in deciding about the likelihood of significant coronary artery disease in patients with suspected non-ST-segment elevation ACS can be integrated into a summary statement about the likelihood of disease in the individual patient. For illustrative purposes, Table 58–1 summarizes the major clinical factors important in this determination (1). This table can be used to supplement the general clinical impression about the patient in determining whether the patient's symptoms reflect a low, intermediate, or high likelihood of coronary disease.

ASSESSMENT OF PROGNOSIS: GENERAL CONSIDERATIONS

Clinical Findings Related to Short-Term Prognosis

Although patients with unstable angina as a group are at increased risk for cardiac death or nonfatal MI, they are heterogeneous with regard to prognosis. The clinician's initial assessment of prognosis is crucial in setting the pace of the evaluation and early treatment decisions of patients with symptoms compatible with acute ischemia (Table 58–2) (1). Clearly one of the important prognostic factors is the likelihood of coronary artery disease, which has been discussed in the previous section. Patients with a high likelihood of coronary disease are at greater risk for a major cardiac event than patients with a lower likelihood. Thus, determining the likelihood of coronary disease is the initial step in assessing prognosis in this population. The other two major elements of the prognostic assessment relate to the recent tempo of the patient's clinical course and the patient's likelihood of survival if an acute ischemic event occurs.

The tempo of the patient's disease is judged from the cardiac history, the 12-lead ECG, and, whenever possible, from examination of the patient during a symptomatic episode.

The key elements of the history are the current frequency of episodes, the change in frequency over the last 2 months (and particularly the last week), the pattern of change in severity or duration of symptoms, the occurrence of any episode lasting longer than 20 minutes, a pattern of progression from effort- or stress-related symptoms to symptoms occurring at rest, new onset of nocturnal symptoms, or a significant decrease in the amount of stress or effort needed to provoke symptoms (23,24). New-onset angina identifies patients with an increased risk for cardiac events, but this risk is completely defined by the other variables from the history described earlier (23,25).

An examination of the patient during an episode of presumed myocardial ischemia can be quite useful. The key prognostic elements from the physical examination at this time would include any evidence of acute congestive heart failure (i.e., new or worsening rales, an S_3), a new or worsening mitral regurgitation murmur, and systemic hypotension.

Clinical Factors Affecting Both Short-Term and Long-Term Prognosis

The four major factors related to the likelihood of survival if an acute ischemic event occurs are left ventricular function, extent of obstructive coronary artery disease, age, and comorbid conditions, particularly renal insufficiency. The extent of left ventricular dysfunction is the single strongest predictor of cardiac death in patients with coronary disease. This relation reflects the decreased cardiac reserve available in patients with preexisting left ventricular dysfunction, which makes them substantially less tolerant of further ischemia or infarction. The extent of coronary disease defines both the likelihood of an acute coronary event (i.e., the general likelihood of a plaque event) and the likely availability of collateral supply to the affected zone and adequate blood supply to the nonaffected zone if such an event occurs. Thus, ischemic coronary events are both more frequent and more likely to be fatal in patients with advanced coronary disease of all three arteries than in patients with single-vessel disease (26,27). Advanced age represents an independent risk factor that may relate to the decreased reserve of cardiac function during stress observed in the elderly and to diminished function of other important organ systems (28). Major comorbid conditions that substantially influence the survival of patients with ACS include renal dysfunction, chronic obstructive lung disease, cerebral vascular disease, malignancy, and other chronic systemic illnesses.

Renal dysfunction deserves special consideration because of its increasing prevalence, its recent recognition as a major risk factor, and the critical importance of adjusting drug doses when it is present. In one study of 19,304 patients with non–ST-segment elevation ACS pooled from four clinical trials, 42% of patients had abnormal renal function (creati-

TABLE 58–2. *Short-term risk for death or nonfatal myocardial infarction in patients with symptoms suggesting unstable angina*

High risk	Intermediate risk	Low risk
At least one of the following features must be present:	*No high-risk feature, but must have any of the following:*	*No high- or intermediate-risk feature, but may have any of the following features:*
Prolonged ongoing (>20 min) rest pain	Prolonged (>20 min) rest angina, now resolved, with moderate or high likelihood of CAD	Increased anginal frequency, severity, or duration
Pulmonary edema, most likely related to ischemia	Nocturnal angina	Angina provoked at a lower threshold
Angina at rest with dynamic ST-segment changes ≥0.5 mm	Angina with dynamic T-wave changes (>0.2 mV)	New-onset angina with onset 2 weeks to 2 months before presentation
Angina with new or worsening mitral regurgitation murmur, S_3, new/worsening rales, or hypotension	New-onset CCSC III or IV angina in the last 2 weeks with moderate or high likelihood of CAD	Normal or unchanged ECG
Age >75 years	Pathologic Q waves, or resting ST-segment depression ≥0.5 mV	
Troponin T or I level >0.1 ng/mL	Age >65 years	

Estimation of the short-term risks for death and nonfatal myocardial infarction in unstable angina is a complex multivariable problem that cannot be fully specified within the confines of this table. Therefore, the table is meant to offer general guidance and illustration rather than rigid algorithms.

CAD, coronary artery disease; CCSC, Canadian Cardiovascular Society classification; ECG, electrocardiogram.

Adapted from Braunwald E, Mark DB, Jones RH, et al. *Unstable angina: diagnosis and management*. Rockville, MD: U.S. Department of Health and Human Services, 1994, with permission.

nine clearance < 70 mL/min) (29). Abnormal renal function was an independent predictor of death and MI at all time points within 6 months.

Electrocardiographic Findings Related to Prognosis

The 12-lead ECG is the most important universally available diagnostic test for evaluating patients with unstable symptoms compatible with ischemia. The presence and extent of ST-segment changes, in particular, convey important diagnostic and prognostic information in patients with acute ischemic syndromes. A 12-lead ECG recorded during symptoms is of particular value. The major prognostic ECG changes are reviewed in this section.

Transient ST-Segment Elevation

ST-segment elevation represents a dynamic underlying pathophysiology involving both thrombosis and endogenous thrombolysis. In a small proportion of patients, the ST-segment elevation resolves before reperfusion therapy can be started; this sequence of events occurred in 2% to 3% of patients in the Global Utilization of Streptokinase and TPA for Occluded coronary arteries (GUSTO-I) trial (30). In the Research group on InStability in Coronary artery disease (RISC) study, men with transient ST-segment elevation had a 16% rate of death or myocardial infarction at 1 year, compared with 8% in patients with a normal ECG and the same qualifying symptoms (31). This syndrome, often previously classified as Prinzmetal's angina (32), has been associated with a high rate of critical coronary stenosis and a high risk for early progression to MI or death (9,10). Such patients should be considered as having

a high-risk form of unstable angina and treated as such with antiplatelet and antithrombin therapy.

Bundle Branch Block

Patients with ongoing prolonged acute ischemic symptoms and left bundle branch block on the ECG not known to be old should be treated like similar patients with ST-segment elevation (see Chapter 66). The evidence from the Fibrinolytic Therapy Trialists' overview is that fibrinolytic therapy in these patients is associated with a substantial reduction in mortality that is at least equal to and possibly even greater than that seen in patients with ST-segment elevation (33). In patients with left bundle branch block and AMI, a validated scoring system has been developed to distinguish patients with AMI from those without MI (34). In this score, patients with ST-segment elevation of 1 mm or greater concordant with QRS polarity receive 5 points; patients with ST-segment depression of 1 mm or greater in lead V_1, V_2, or V_3 receive 3 points; and patients with ST-segment elevation of 5 mm or greater discordant with QRS polarity receive 2 points. A score of more than 2 points is associated with a greater than 50% likelihood of AMI.

ST-segment elevation in the presence of right bundle branch block is more easily interpreted, particularly changes in the inferior leads. The diffuse ST-segment abnormalities and particularly precordial ST-segment depression that are typical of right bundle branch block, however, can make the determination of other acute ischemic changes quite difficult. Importantly, patients with right bundle branch block in the GUSTO-I trial had a mortality rate of 16% at 30 days, which was much greater than the overall mortality rate for the trial of 7% (35).

ST-Segment Depression

The presence and severity of ST-segment depression provides crucial prognostic information in patients with ACS. In the RISC study cited earlier in this chapter, the 24% of patients who had ST-segment depression also had a 12% risk for death or MI at 30 days compared with 3.4% in patients with no ST- or T-wave changes (31). This group also had the greatest rate of recurrence of Class III or IV angina, with a 33.8% recurrence rate compared with 19.2% in those with ST-segment elevation, 24.4% in patients with T-wave inversion, and 16.5% in those without ECG changes.

In the Global Use of Strategies To Open occluded arteries in acute coronary syndromes (GUSTO-IIb) study of 12,142 patients with ischemic symptoms at rest accompanied by ECG signs of ischemia, ST-segment depression was associated with a 10.5% rate of death or nonfatal MI at 30 days compared with a 5.5% rate in patients with T-wave inversion alone (36). Similarly, in the FRISC-II ECG substudy, ST-segment depression was associated with a significantly greater rate of death or MI at 12 months (19). In the Thrombolysis In Myocardial Ischemia (TIMI)-IIIB ECG Registry study, ST-segment deviation of 0.5 mm had a greater adverse prognostic effect than 2 mm or more of ST-segment deviation (10.7% rate of death or MI at 42 days vs. 2.8%, respectively; $p = 0.0001$), which may partly reflect the role of chance in this sample (37). In a cohort of 367 patients with non–ST-segment elevation ACS followed for an average of 4.3 years, the magnitude of ST-segment depression stratified prognosis well: Survival rates were 53%, 77%, and 82% for patients with 2-mm or more, 1-mm, and 0.5-mm ST-segment depression, respectively (38). On the basis of these findings, the 2000 ACC/AHA guidelines placed ACS patients with 0.5 mm or greater ST-segment deviation in the high-risk subgroup (2).

A common and difficult issue arises when patients arrive with ST-segment abnormalities that are of uncertain duration. Most evidence indicates that active ST-segment shifts with symptoms identify the population at greatest risk. Patients with chronically abnormal ST segments also have a high risk for negative outcomes, if the new symptoms truly indicate acute myocardial ischemia.

An interesting and important observation by several investigators is that when diffuse ST-segment depression in present in up to eight leads with ST-segment elevation in lead aVR, critical left main stenosis should be suspected (39,40). In this setting, particularly with evidence of pump dysfunction, emergency angiography and intraaortic balloon pumping should be considered.

T-Wave Inversion

For purposes of establishing prognosis, T-wave inversion has been less well studied than ST depression. In the RISC study, isolated T-wave inversion was found in 31% of patients; these patients had a smaller risk for death or MI compared with patients with ST-segment depression or elevation, but a much greater risk compared with patients with no ST-segment or T-wave abnormalities. In the GUSTO-IIb study, isolated T-wave inversions conferred the lowest risk among the cohort of ACS patients (all of whom had either ST-segment or T-wave changes) (36). In the TIMI-IIIB Registry study, T-wave inversion did not add to the clinical history in predicting outcomes (37).

Normal or Nonspecific Electrocardiograms

Several early reports have indicated that in the absence of ST-segment shift, T-wave inversion, or conduction disturbances, the prognosis is good, even when patients have positive cardiac markers (41–43). In the RISC study of 237 such patients (representing 21% of the population), only 3.4% died or had an MI within 30 days, despite having symptoms convincing enough to enter them into a clinical trial of therapy for unstable angina or non–Q-wave MI. Angina reoccurred in 16% of these patients compared with 24% of patients with T-wave inversion and 34% of patients with ST-segment depression. In the TIMI-IIIB ECG Registry study, about half of patients enrolled had no ST-segment or T-wave changes (37). This high prevalence rate may reflect partly the oversampling in this registry of women and minorities. The rate of in-hospital death or MI for patients without ECG changes was 1.6%, equivalent to that for patients with isolated T-wave changes.

Serum Markers of Cardiac Necrosis

The lethal manifestations of ischemic heart disease generally are sequelae of myocardial necrosis, so that the early diagnosis of patients with ongoing necrosis enables the clinician to make a rapid triage decision to institute more aggressive care. Most patients with acute myocardial necrosis do not have ST-segment elevation, and most patients with chest pain but no ST-segment elevation do not have acute myocardial necrosis. The proper use of serum cardiac markers of necrosis is therefore essential to high-quality management of these patients. Table 58–3 contains a list of available markers for myocardial necrosis and their characteristics (44).

TABLE 58–3. *Plasma markers of myocardial necrosis*

Marker	Cardiac specificity	Initial increase, h	Peak, h	Return to normal
Myoglobin	0	2	4–6	24–48 h
CK-MB mass	1+	4	24	48–72 h
Troponin T	2+	3	12–24	10–14 d
Troponin I	2+	3	24	7–10 d

CK, creatine kinase.

Troponins

Troponins have now replaced creatine kinase (CK)-MB as the gold standard for diagnosis of myocardial necrosis (2). Troponin T and troponin I fragments of the myocardial contractile apparatus appear in the serum within 3 to 12 hours after irreversible myocyte injury and have a long half-life (Fig. 58–1) (45). Because the troponins in skeletal muscle are immunologically distinct from those in cardiac muscle, cardiac troponins are extremely specific for myocardial necrosis. Thus, cardiac troponin is undetectable in the serum of healthy subjects; even minor degrees of troponin level increase are significant given the use of an assay with sufficient precision (46). Troponin markers are usually positive when the CK-MB is positive. Even more important, when the CK-MB is negative or borderline, a positive troponin value has been associated with a substantial increase in the risk for death and other complications (47).

Interpretation of serum troponin testing must be performed in conjunction with the clinical history. Thus, a negative troponin in a patient within 2 hours of symptom onset cannot be used to exclude the diagnosis of ACS. If the initial troponin level is negative in a patient suspected to have ACS, it should be repeated at 8 to 12 hours after the onset of the symptoms that brought the patient to the ED. Conversely, a patient who had severe symptoms 4 days ago but is now symptom-free and has a positive troponin and negative CK-MB is probably more than 72 hours beyond the occurrence of acute myocardial necrosis.

If the troponin level is unequivocally positive, there currently is little clinical value in continuing to repeat the test (as was routinely done with CK-MB), because the level may

TABLE 58–4. *Potential causes of increased troponin level in the absence of overt coronary artery disease*

Congestive heart failure (severe)
Hypertension (severe)
Hypotension/shock
Renal failure
Cardiac trauma
Inflammatory cardiac disease
Infiltrative cardiac disease
Pulmonary embolism
Cardiotoxicity from chemotherapeutic agents

stay unchanged for several days and take more than 1 week to return to normal. In addition, although the absolute level of troponin elevation has prognostic information beyond the simple assessment of the test as "positive," as is discussed later, most clinical risk stratification algorithms consider the test simply as positive or not positive (48).

The use of routine troponin testing instead of or in addition to CK-MB has resulted in a significant increase in the diagnosis of NSTEMI and a decrease in the diagnosis of unstable angina. In some patients with small increases of troponin, a nonatherothrombotic process may be responsible (Table 58–4) (49,50). For example, patients with left ventricular hypertrophy who present with marked increase in blood pressure may have a minimally positive troponin test, presumably because of severe left ventricular strain with a small amount of myocardial necrosis. This also can be seen in patients with end-stage renal disease and in those with heart failure who experience development of volume overload (51).

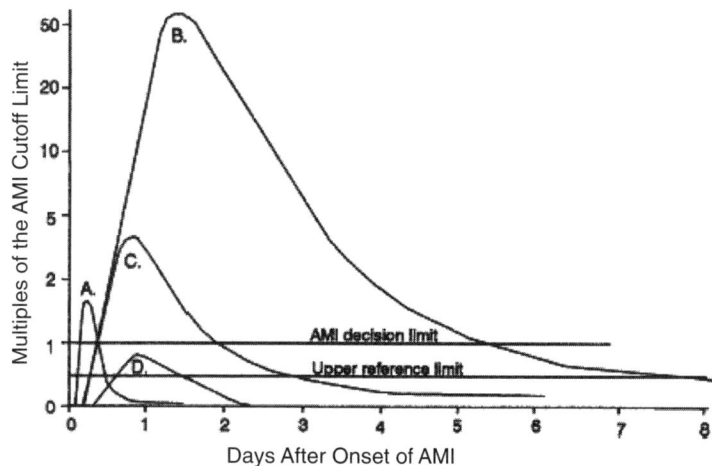

FIG. 58–1. Appearance of cardiac biomarkers in the serum by time from symptom onset. Peak A, early release of myoglobin or creatine kinase (CK)-MB isoforms after myocardial infarction (MI); peak B, cardiac troponin after MI; peak C, CK-MB after MI; peak D, cardiac troponin after unstable angina. Data are plotted on a relative scale, where 1.0 is set at the MI cutoff concentration. AMI, acute myocardial infarction. (From Wu AHB, Apple FS, Gibler WB, et al. National Academy of Clinical Biochemistry Standards of Laboratory Practice: recommendations for the use of cardiac markers in coronary artery diseases. *Clin Chem* 1999;45:1104–1121, with permission.)

Creatine Kinase MB Fraction

CK-MB is generally released into the serum within 3 to 12 hours after onset of coronary occlusion, peaks within 24 hours, and returns to normal within 48 to 72 hours. Several factors can affect the time to appearance (reperfusion, right ventricular infarction), peak levels (infarct size, right ventricular infarction, reperfusion), and half-life (renal failure). As with troponins, an initially negative CK-MB determination cannot be used to exclude the presence of acute myocardial necrosis. In addition, unlike troponins, CK-MB can be detected in the blood of healthy individuals and also is present in small quantities in noncardiac muscles (including those of the small intestine, tongue, diaphragm, prostate, and uterus). The primary clinical utility of CK-MB levels currently is in detection of reinfarction in a patient who already has an increased troponin level.

Myoglobin

Because of its appearance in the serum early after the onset of myocardial necrosis (within 1–4 hours) and its high sensitivity, myoglobin is an attractive molecule for early diagnosis of myocardial necrosis (52). However, the clinical utility of confirming the diagnosis of NSTEMI 1 or 2 hours earlier has not been shown. Serum myoglobin was an independent predictor of 6-month mortality, but not (re)infarction, in the TIMI databases (53).

Novel Markers

A recent substudy of GUSTO-IV showed that levels of N-terminal pro-brain natriuretic peptide (NT-proBNP) measured early after presentation can predict 1-year mortality independent of standard clinical risk factors (54). In the Treat Angina with Aggrastat and determine Cost of Therapy with an Invasive or Conservative Strategy (TACTICS-TIMI 18) study, elevated BNP levels predicted later death and heart failure, independent of troponin I and clinical risk factors (55).

Several new tests show promise for detecting ischemia before infarction or necrosis develops. The Albumin Cobalt Binding (ACB) test was approved by the U.S. Food and Drug Administration (FDA) for use in the ED. This test is based on the observation that ischemia reduces the ability of the N-terminal region of human albumin to bind cobalt. Clinically, it is hypothesized that this test has abnormal results in patients with ACS hours before any markers of myocardial necrosis are detectable. In one preliminary study of 256 patients with ACS, the ACB test at presentation had a negative predictive value of 96% for predicting subsequent troponin negative status, whereas the positive predictive value was 33% (56). Because the ACB test may be positive in the absence of irreversible cellular damage, a positive troponin test is not the ideal gold standard to assess its perfor-

mance. Another interesting marker undergoing clinical evaluation is nourin-1, a cardiac-specific chemotactic factor generated in response to the earliest phase of ischemia.

Multimarker Strategies

Several groups have investigated the clinical utility of a bedside multimarker testing strategy in ACS. In the CHest pain Evaluation by Creatine Kinase-MB, Myoglobin, And Troponin I (CHECKMATE) study, Newby and colleagues evaluated such a bedside multimarker strategy versus local laboratory testing (52). Myoglobin, CK-MB, and troponin I were measured in 1,005 patients at 0, 3, 6, 9 12, and 16 to 24 hours after admission to a chest pain unit (CPU). At 24 hours, significantly more patients were positive by the bedside multimarker strategy than by local laboratory testing (24% vs. 9%, $p = 0.001$). Time to positivity was reduced by about 1 hour. In addition, the multimarker strategy showed a substantially stronger relation with 30-day death or MI. Other studies have shown the value of combining troponin testing with ST-/T-wave analysis for risk stratification (57). Both factors are included in the TIMI risk score (discussed in the next section).

In 450 patients enrolled in Orbofiban in Patients with Unstable coronary Syndromes (OPUS-TIMI 16), increased levels of troponin I, C-reactive protein, and BNP each contributed prognostic information about the risk for death, MI, or heart failure at 30 days and at time points up to 10 months (58). The prognostic value of the number of increased biomarkers at presentation was validated in 1,635 patients enrolled in TACTICS-TIMI 18.

Other markers that have been investigated as prognostic factors in ACS include serum amyloid A, plasma and urinary fibrinopeptide A, and serum myosin light chains (59,60).

Risk Stratification Models

Because of the limited accuracy of clinical risk stratification as performed by the physician, investigators have attempted to develop mathematically based decision aids and newer diagnostic techniques to optimize the initial triage of patients with unstable ACS. Two generations of risk stratification models can be distinguished. The first, represented by the Multicenter Chest Pain Study and the Multicenter Predictive Instrument Trial, included only clinical and ECG factors and were focused on decision-making in the ED. More recent models, represented by the TIMI and Platelet glycoprotein IIb/IIIa in Unstable angina: Receptor Suppression Using Integrilin Therapy (PURSUIT) risk scores, include cardiac marker results and are focused on longer-term management decisions in patients admitted to the hospital because of ACS.

The Multicenter Chest Pain Study developed a model using data from the history, physical examination, and ECG of 12,140 patients with chest pain to predict the probability of

AMI and to assist decisions about triage to the intensive care unit (ICU) (61). In this model, the features associated with a greater probability of AMI included duration of symptoms less than 48 hours before ED evaluation, history of angina or prior MI, pain duration of 1 hour or longer, pain worse than prior angina or equivalent to prior MI, age 40 years or older, ST-segment or T-wave changes of ischemia or a strain not known to be old, and radiation of pain to the neck, left shoulder, or left arm. Features associated with a lower probability of AMI included radiation of pain to the back, abdomen, or legs; "stabbing" quality of pain; and reproduction of pain by palpation. Combinations of these various characteristics yielded 14 subgroups with probabilities of AMI ranging from 1% to 77%. In a prospective validation study, the Multicenter Chest Pain Study model stratified 36% of patients arriving at the ED with acute ischemic symptoms into a low-risk subgroup (Fig. 58–2) (62). After a 12-hour observation period, 81% of these subjects at low risk remained free of recurrent symptoms and had at least one normal and no abnormal cardiac enzyme levels; these uncomplicated, low-risk patients were judged suitable for further evaluation in an unmonitored hospital bed. In this cohort, evidence of AMI was eventually obtained in 0.5% of patients, whereas 0.6% died of cardiac causes during the hospitalization, all after Day 3. Using the prospective data from 10,682 patients within the Multicenter Chest Pain Study (1984–1986), Goldman and colleagues (63) developed a model to predict the risk for major cardiac events within 72 hours requiring hospitalization in an ICU. This model, which was prospectively validated in 4,676 patients (1990–1994), does not include biomarker test results. Although it would be reasonable to regard a positive biomarker (particularly troponin) as placing patients in the intermediate- or high-risk group, it would be useful to have data validating the predictive power of this model in marker-negative patients.

Pozen and colleagues (21) developed and validated a quantitative predictive instrument to improve the diagnosis of acute cardiac ischemia (unstable angina or AMI) for triage decisions in the ED. An updated version of this model identified seven major predictive factors useful in making this determination: age; sex; the presence or absence of chest pain or pressure or left arm pain, whether chest pain or pressure was the patient's most important presenting symptom; the presence of Q waves; the presence and degree of ST-segment elevation and depression; and the presence and degree of T-wave peaking or inversion (64). This model was found to have a sensitivity of 95% and a specificity of 78%

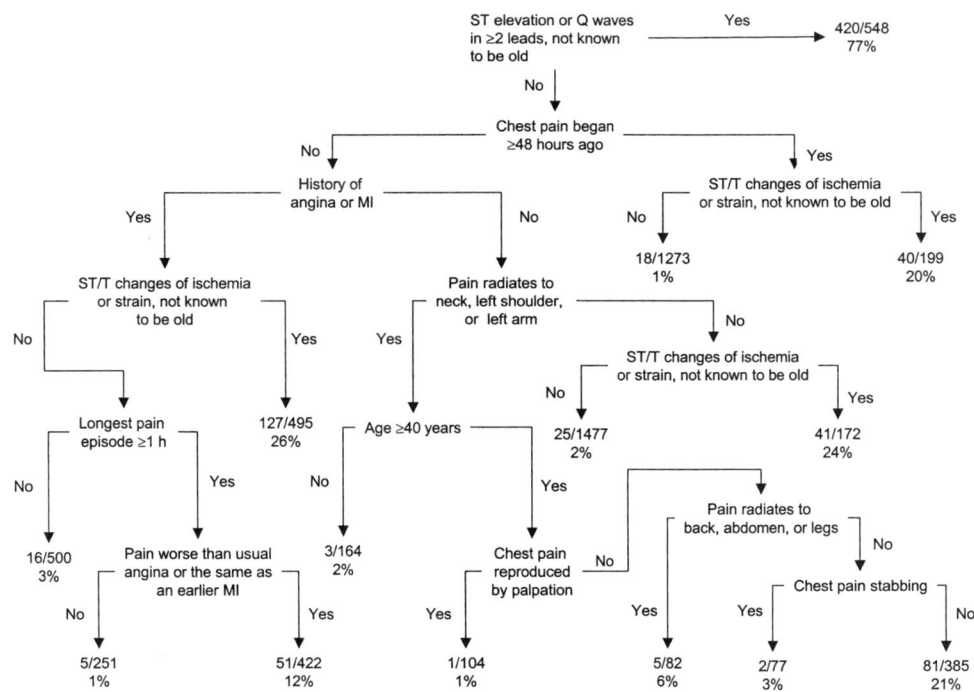

FIG. 58–2. Prospectively validated multivariate algorithm to predict a patient's risk for acute myocardial infarction (MI) on the basis of emergency room data. Patients can be assigned to 1 of 14 subgroups, each of which has been classified as having a low (≤7%) or a high (>7%) risk for acute MI. The values shown for each subgroup are the numbers of patients with acute MI, divided by the total number of patients in a subgroup of 6,149 patients enrolled in the Multicenter Chest Pain Study, with the corresponding percentages. "Pain worse than usual angina" denotes worse in frequency, severity, duration, or failure to respond to usual measures. (From Lee TH, Juarez G, Cook EF, et al. Ruling out acute myocardial infarction. A prospective multicenter validation of a 12-hour strategy for patients at low risk. *N Engl J Med* 1991;324:1239–1246, with permission.)

for the diagnosis of acute cardiac ischemia. In a multicenter, controlled trial, the use of this Acute Cardiac Ischemia Time-Insensitive Predictive Instrument (ACI-TIPI) was associated with reduced hospitalization among ED patients without ACS (65). Admission rates for patients with ACS were not altered.

In contrast with the Goldman/Lee models and the Pozen/Selker models, which were designed to assist with ED triage, the TIMI and PURSUIT risk scores focus on patients admitted with an initial diagnosis of ACS. In some cases, these and similar risk scores have been used to identify *post hoc* subgroups whose members appear to derive particular benefit from more aggressive therapies for ACS. The TIMI risk score uses seven factors (including elevated serum markers) to predict the risk for complications (death, MI, severe recurrent ischemia) at 14 days in patients with non–ST-segment elevation ACS (66). These factors, which are each given equal weight (1 if present, 0 if absent) are: age 65 years or older; three or more risk factors for coronary disease; known significant coronary disease; ST-segment deviation on the presentation ECG; severe anginal symptoms (e.g., two or more anginal events in last 24 hours); use of aspirin in last 7 days; and increased serum markers (CK-MB or troponin). The score has been validated in multiple independent cohorts (67).

In the TIMI-IIIB cohort of 1,473 patients with non–ST-segment elevation ACS, a separate risk score based on age, increased CK-MB, history of accelerated angina, and ST-segment depression of 0.1 mV or more identified a subset of high-risk patients who appeared to derive particular benefit from an early invasive management strategy (68). In the TACTICS-TIMI 18 study, patients with troponin I levels of 0.1 mg/mL or more showed a significant reduction in composite event rate (death, MI, readmission for ACS) with early invasive in contrast to early conservative therapy (66).

The PURSUIT risk score was developed to predict 30-day death and (re)infarction in 9,461 patients with ACS (69). Major predictors of mortality included age, heart rate, systolic blood pressure, ST-segment depression, signs of heart failure, and ruling-in for an MI. The predictive accuracy of the model was better for 30-day death than for 30-day reinfarction.

Because complex scores are unlikely to be used by busy clinicians, some investigators have presented simplified risk scores on the basis of two or three variables. One example of this is the work of Kaul and colleagues using the Platelet IIb/IIIa Antagonism for the Reduction of Acute coronary syndrome events in a Global Organization Network (PARAGON)-B database (70). In 959 patients with ACS, the amount of ST-segment depression on the presenting ECG (classified as none, 1 mm, ≥2 mm) and an increased troponin T level (≥0.1 mg/mL) stratified 6-month rates of death or MI. A troponin test that was positive within 6 hours of symptom onset was associated with a worse prognosis than one that turned positive later. In contrast, a follow-up ECG showing 2 mm or greater ST-segment depression was associated with a worse prognosis than if this finding was present on the initial ECG. In the FRISC-II ECG substudy, the presence of ST-segment depression at arrival identified a subgroup that derived significant benefit from the early invasive management strategy (19).

OTHER DIAGNOSTIC AND PROGNOSTIC TESTS

ST-Segment Monitoring

The available information on ambulatory or continuous ICU monitoring for ischemia in patients with unstable angina does not provide a clear indication of its clinical value. Gottlieb and colleagues (71) initially reported that 37 of 60 patients with unstable angina had recurrent silent myocardial ischemia while in the hospital for treatment of unstable angina, and this finding was associated with a fivefold increase in the risk for MI (16% vs. 3%). Similar findings were reported in the setting of unstable angina by Langer and colleagues (72), who also showed a relation between the duration of ischemia and prognosis. An in-depth follow-up study from Sydney, however, found little independent importance of silent ischemia (73). These investigators reported that although silent ischemia was common, symptomatic ischemia was a much better predictor of adverse outcomes.

In an analysis of data on 119 patients at intermediate risk with chest pain at the Mayo Clinic (Rochester, MN), the use of continuous ECG monitoring was of limited clinical value (74). Ischemic ST-segment changes, seen in 16 patients, had minimal effect on diagnostic or prognostic stratification. In a substudy of FRISC-II, 629 patients with ACS underwent continuous 12-lead ECG or vectorcardiography for the first 24 hours after hospital admission (75). In the 34% of patients with ischemic ST-segment changes, dalteparin therapy was associated with a 34% lower rate of death, MI, or revascularization. In contrast, in patients without ischemic changes, no therapeutic benefit was seen for dalteparin.

Echocardiography

Without risk to the patient, the echocardiogram assesses the presence and extent of left ventricular dysfunction and, if present, the extent of any valvular dysfunction (particularly mitral regurgitation, which often has an ischemic cause). Focal wall–motion abnormalities, like diagnostic Q waves on the ECG, are associated with a high likelihood of significant coronary disease. As noted earlier, significant left ventricular dysfunction is a major adverse prognostic finding.

In a prospective study of decision-making for 100 patients in the ED, senior physicians were asked to provide their level of confidence in patient diagnosis, treatment, and disposition decisions before and after an echocardiogram was performed (76). The test results changed diagnostic impressions in 37% of cases, treatment plans in 25%, and disposition plans in 11%. In addition, physician confidence in their assessment and plans was improved in 50%. A different perspective is provided by a study from a large ED in Singapore. This study examined the prognostic utility of echocardiography in the evaluation of 1,112 patients with chest pain who had normal serial CK-MB levels and no ECG changes (77). Only 18 patients had wall–motion abnormalities. All the adverse events during follow-up occurred in patients with a negative rest echocardiogram. These data suggest that patients who are at low risk on the basis of standard criteria (reviewed earlier in this chapter) do not derive significant benefit from resting echocardiography.

Chest Radiograph

The chest radiograph usually provides little useful information to aid in acute decision-making unless heart failure, aortic dissection, or pneumothorax is suspected. In most patients with a normal physical examination, results of the chest radiograph will be normal or nonspecific. Nevertheless, the patient with a great enough suspicion of unstable angina or a related diagnosis to warrant hospital admission should have a chest radiograph to assess for evidence of cardiomegaly or pulmonary edema, which would merit a greater level of monitoring and therapeutic intervention.

Cardiac Catheterization

Two main strategies have evolved to address the inhospital risk stratification of patients admitted with ACS. The *early conservative* approach uses selective use of invasive procedures and substitutes noninvasive testing such as stress testing for the remainder. In this strategy, early referral to cardiac catheterization is recommended for high-risk groups believed more likely to benefit from early revascularization (Table 58–5) (2). The *early invasive* approach is a plan of routine angiography unless the patient has a contraindication. Four clinical trials have now compared varying versions of these strategies in non–ST-segment elevation ACS.

TABLE 58–5. *High-risk groups whose members should be considered for early referral to cardiac catheterization in the early conservative strategy*

Recurrent angina/ischemia at rest or with low-level activities, despite antiischemic therapy
Recurrent angina/ischemia with signs or symptoms of heart failure or new/worsening mitral regurgitation
High-risk findings on stress testing
Ejection fraction depressed (e.g., <40%)
Hemodynamic instability
Sustained ventricular tachycardia
Prior coronary artery bypass surgery
Percutaneous coronary intervention within the last 6 months

Adapted from Braunwald E, Antman EM, Beasley JW, et al. ACC/AHA guidelines for the management of patients with unstable angina and non-ST-segment elevation myocardial infarction: executive summary and recommendations. *J Am Coll Cardiol* 2000;36:970–1062, with permission.

In the TIMI-IIIB trial, 1,473 patients with symptoms of acute ischemia who did not have ST-segment elevation but had either an abnormal ECG or known previous coronary disease were randomized to either the early conservative or the early invasive strategy (78). At 42 days, the rates of death, nonfatal MI, or their combination did not differ significantly between the two strategies. The FRISC-II trial used a conservative version of the early conservative strategy, with only 10% of patients referred for angiography (79). In contrast, 57% of the patients in the TIMI-IIIB early conservative arm were referred for angiography during the index admission.

The most recent trial in this area is the TACTICS-TIMI 18 trial, which enrolled 2,220 patients with non–ST-segment elevation ACS (80). During the index admission, 51% of patients in the early conservative arm and 97% of patients in the early invasive arm underwent diagnostic angiography. All patients received tirofiban therapy, and coronary stenting was routinely used in percutaneous revascularization procedures. At 6 months, the early invasive arm had 2 fewer deaths per 1,000 patients treated and 20 fewer nonfatal MIs per 1,000 patients treated. As reviewed earlier, patients with high-risk features, such as a positive troponin level, ST-segment deviation, or a TIMI risk score of 3 or greater derived a larger therapeutic benefit from the early invasive strategy. In contrast, patients without these features showed no benefit. These findings constitute the basis for the revision of the ACC/AHA guidelines regarding referral of patients at high risk to early angiography when using the early conservative strategy (81).

Stress Testing

When the early conservative approach is selected and the patient has none of the high-risk indications for coronary angiography in Table 58–5, noninvasive stress testing is usually performed to identify additional patients who need invasive study and possible revascularization. Testing also can provide a guide to the need for additional medical therapy and a basis for prescribing a rational exercise program. Finally, the patient often will benefit from the reassurance provided by "passing" an exercise test, a concept that has been referred to as self-efficacy (82).

Various tests are available using combinations of exercise versus pharmacologic stress, ECG monitoring, and perfusion or ventricular function imaging. Unfortunately, little solid information is available to guide the clinician in selecting one form of testing over another. The 2000 ACC/AHA guidelines recommend testing within 72 hours of admission in patients treated with the early conservative approach who do not develop recurrent ischemia and who have been free of symptoms of angina or heart failure for 48 hours (2). The guidelines also recommend the treadmill exercise test as the standard test for patients without confounding ECG abnormalities (resting ST-segment abnormalities or conduction disturbances). Patients who appear unlikely to be able to exercise adequately should be stressed with a pharmacologic agent, whereas those with abnormal ECG results at rest should undergo either perfusion imaging or ventricular function testing as part of their exercise test. As shown in Table 58–6, a large number of patients have now undergone noninvasive studies after unstable angina, and the gamut of possible tests has been evaluated (1,83–90). All of these studies can segregate patients into high-risk and low-risk populations, but differences in operating characteristics of the tests are not adequate to justify a choice on scientific considerations. Rather, the local expertise and cost should be considered, because the degree of expertise varies considerably depending on the training and orientation of the noninvasive testing laboratory (91).

CHEST PAIN UNITS AND EMERGENCY DEPARTMENT TRIAGE

Given the large numbers of patients with symptoms compatible with acute ischemia seen in EDs, a systematic approach to their evaluation and treatment seems attractive from the perspectives of both cost-efficient management and patient outcomes. In particular, the uncertainty about whether myocardial necrosis is occurring, with its attendant risk for sudden complications, has led to the common policy of admitting patients with a low probability of AMI to the ICU. In a registry of 10,689 patients with chest pain seen in the EDs of 10 U.S. centers during 1993, 2.1% of patients with AMI and 2.3% of those with unstable angina were mistakenly sent home (92). These patients had substantially greater mortality than their hospitalized counterparts. Thus, the patients who were misdiagnosed were clearly not a lower risk subset. Factors most strongly correlated with a missed ED diagnosis included female sex, age younger than 55 years, nonwhite race, dyspnea as a presenting complaint, and a normal or nondiagnostic ECG. The extent to which the routine use of troponin testing has reduced the rate of missed ACS cases in the ED remains uncertain.

To improve the quality of care for patients with chest pain in the ED, many institutions have developed protocols for the systematic collection of history, physical examination, ECG, and serum biomarker data. Investigators at the Mayo Clinic tested admission to a CPU versus standard hospital admission in 424 patients at intermediate risk with unstable angina (93). The CPU arm used an explicit protocol that included aspirin, heparin, continuous ST-segment monitoring, serial CK-MB levels, and an exercise ECG or imaging stress test. Patients with positive test results were hospitalized. There was no difference in adverse events at 30 days in the two arms, but resource use was less at 6 months with the CPU strategy. At Cook County Hospital (Chicago, IL), the use of a validated clinical decision rule significantly improved the triage decisions of ED physicians, especially for patients at very low risk (94).

Contemporary CPU protocols consist of two main stages: (a) initial risk stratification (8–12 hours) with clinical, ECG, and serum marker data; and (b) exercise or stress testing for subjects who are judged to have low risk from the initial data (95). Numerous studies have examined alternative exercise/stress testing strategies in this context. The available data suggest that exercise testing in the ED is safe in patients properly identified as being at low risk (95). In addition, for patients who have an interpretable ECG response, there is no evidence that an imaging exercise test is required.

Some CPU protocols have explored the addition of imaging at rest to the standard clinical ECG marker evaluation. In a randomized trial of 2,475 patients with chest pain and normal or nondiagnostic ECGs, Udelson and colleagues (96) observed that results of acute resting perfusion imaging were associated with fewer unnecessary hospitalizations (admission rates of 52% vs. 42%). Other investigators have evaluated the use of resting cardiac echocardiography and resting cardiac magnetic resonance imaging in the ED (97).

SUMMARY

Patients with a constellation of signs, symptoms, or both compatible with acute ischemia are labeled as having ACS until a more definitive evaluation can be accomplished. On

TABLE 58-6. *Noninvasive studies in patients with unstable angina reporting ten or more cardiac events (cardiac death or myocardial infarction) during follow-up*

Study	Inclusion criteria	Low risk, n	High risk, n
Moss et al. (83)	30% unstable angina, 26% non–Q-wave MI	893	23
Swahn et al. (84)	100% unstable angina	247	145
Severi et al. (85)	100% unstable angina	199	175
Madsen et al. (86)	100% unstable angina	118	98
Nyman et al. (87)	100% unstable angina	366	374
Krone et al. (88)	100% non–Q-wave MI	85	7
Moss et al. (83)	30% unstable angina, 26% non–Q-wave MI	876	20
Madsen et al. (86)	100% unstable angina	129	29
Gibson et al. (89)	36% non–Q-wave MI, 64% MI	133	108
Younis et al. (90)	58% unstable angina, 42% MI	14	54

MI, myocardial infarction.
From Braunwald E, Mark DB, Jones RH, et al. *Unstable angina: diagnosis and management.* Rockville, MD: U.S. Department of Health and Human Services, 1994, with permission.

the basis of immediate history, physical examination, ECG, and chest radiograph, a rapid decision about reperfusion therapy can be arrived at, and obvious alternative diagnoses can be made. Cardiac marker, angiographic, and functional testing data can be used to place the patient into various risk strata, from which appropriate logistical and therapeutic decisions can be made. Subsequent chapters address the therapeutics of ACS in greater detail.

REFERENCES

1. Braunwald E, Mark DB, Jones RH, et al. *Unstable angina: diagnosis and management.* Rockville, MD: U.S. Department of Health and Human Services, 1994.
2. Braunwald E, Antman EM, Beasley JW, et al. ACC/AHA guidelines for the management of patients with unstable angina and non-ST-segment elevation myocardial infarction: executive summary and recommendations. *J Am Coll Cardiol* 2000;36:970–1062.
3. Chaitman BR, Bourassa MG, Davis K, et al. Angiographic prevalence of high risk coronary artery disease in patient subsets (CASS). *Circulation* 1981;64:360–367.
4. Pryor DB, Harrell FE Jr, Lee KL, et al. Estimating the likelihood of significant coronary artery disease. *Am J Med* 1983;75:771–780.
5. Pryor DB, Shaw L, McCants CB, et al. Value of the history and physical in identifying patients at increased risk for coronary artery disease. *Ann Intern Med* 1993;118:81–90.
6. Principle Investigators of CASS. Coronary artery surgery study (CASS), National Heart, Lung, and Blood Institute. *Circulation* 1981;63:1–81.
7. Lee TH, Cook EF, Weisberg M, et al. Acute chest pain in the emergency room. Identification and examination of low risk patients. *Arch Intern Med* 1985;145:65–69.
8. Jayes RL, Beshansky JR, D'Agostino RB, et al. Do patients' coronary risk factor reports predict acute cardiac ischemia in the emergency department? *J Clin Epidemiol* 1992;45:621–626.
9. Mark DB, Califf RM, Morris KG, et al. Clinical characteristics and long term survival of patients with variant angina. *Circulation* 1984;69:880–888.
10. Waters DD, Miller DD, Szlachcic J, et al. Factors influencing the long term prognosis of treated patients with variant angina. *Circulation* 1983;68:258–265.
11. Weber JE, Shofer FS, Larkin GL, et al. Validation of a brief observation period for patients with cocaine-associated chest pain. *N Engl J Med* 2003;348:510–517.
12. Holmes DR Jr, Berger PB, Hochman JS, et al. Cardiogenic shock in patients with acute ischemic syndromes with and without ST-segment elevation. *Circulation* 1999;100:2067–2073.
13. Weaver WD, Eisenberg MS, Martin JS, et al. Myocardial infarction triage and intervention project—phase I: patient characteristics and feasibility of prehospital initiation of thrombolytic therapy. *J Am Coll Cardiol* 1990;15:925–931.
14. Komrad MS, Coffey CE, Coffey KS, et al. Myocardial infarction and stroke. *Neurology* 1984;34:1403–1409.
15. Hagan PG, Nienaber CA, Isselbacher EM, et al. The International Registry of Acute Aortic Dissection (IRAD): new insights into an old disease. *JAMA* 2000;283:897–903.
16. Millaire A, de Groote P, Decoulx E, et al. Outcome after thrombolytic therapy of nine cases of myopericarditis misdiagnosed as myocardial infarction. *Eur Heart J* 1995;16:333–338.
17. Rouan GW, Lee TH, Cook EF, et al. Clinical characteristics and outcome of acute myocardial infarction in patients with initially normal or nonspecific electrocardiograms (a report from the Multicenter Chest Pain Study). *Am J Cardiol* 1989;64:1087–1092.
18. Lee TH, Cook EF, Weisberg MC, et al. Impact of the availability of a prior electrocardiogram on the triage of the patient with acute chest pain. *J Gen Intern Med* 1990;5:381–388.
19. Diderholm E, Andren B, Frostfeldt G, et al. ST depression in ECG at entry indicates severe coronary lesions and large benefits of an early invasive treatment strategy in unstable coronary artery disease: the FRISC II ECG substudy. *Eur Heart J* 2002;23:41–49.
20. Haines DE, Raabe DS, Gundel WD, et al. Anatomic and prognostic significance of new T-wave inversion in unstable angina. *Am J Cardiol* 1983;52:14–18.
21. Pozen MW, D'Agostino RB, Selker HP, et al. A predictive instrument to improve coronary care unit admission practices in acute ischemic heart disease. A prospective multicenter clinical trial. *N Engl J Med* 1984;310:1273–1278.
22. McCarthy BD, Beshansky JR, D'Agostino RB, et al. Missed diagnoses of acute myocardial infarction in the emergency department: results from a multicenter study. *Ann Emerg Med* 1993;22:579–582.
23. Califf RM, Mark DB, Harrell FE Jr, et al. Importance of clinical measures of ischemia in the prognosis of patients with documented coronary artery disease. *J Am Coll Cardiol* 1988;11:20–26.
24. De Servi S, Arbustini E, Marsico F, et al. Correlation between clinical and morphologic findings in unstable angina. *Am J Cardiol* 1996;77:128–132.
25. White LD, Lee TH, Cook EF, et al. Comparison of the natural history of new onset and exacerbated chronic ischemic heart disease. *J Am Coll Cardiol* 1990;16:304–310.
26. Wilcox I, Ben Freedman S, Li JN, et al. Comparison of exercise stress testing with ambulatory electrocardiographic monitoring in the detection of myocardial ischemia after unstable angina pectoris. *Am J Cardiol* 1991;67:89–91.
27. Grines CL, Topol EJ, Califf RM, et al. Prognostic implications and predictors of enhanced regional wall motion of the noninfarct zone after thrombolysis and angioplasty therapy of acute myocardial infarction. The TAMI Study Groups. *Circulation* 1989;80:245–253.
28. Lee KL, Woodlief LH, Topol EJ, et al. Predictors of 30 day mortality in the era of reperfusion for acute myocardial infarction: results from an international trial of 41,021 patients. The GUSTO I Investigators. *Circulation* 1995;91:1659–1668.
29. Al Suwaidi J, Reddan DN, Williams K, et al. Prognostic implications of abnormalities in renal function in patients with acute coronary syndromes. *Circulation* 2002;106:974–980.
30. Langer A, Krucoff MW, Klootwijk P, et al. Noninvasive assessment of speed and stability of infarct-related artery reperfusion: results of the GUSTO ST segment monitoring study. *J Am Coll Cardiol* 1995;25:1552–1557.
31. Nyman I, Areskog M, Areskog NH, et al. Very early risk stratification by electrocardiogram at rest in men with suspected unstable coronary heart disease. *J Intern Med* 1993;234:293–301.
32. Prinzmetal M, Kennamer R, Merliss R, et al. Angina pectoris and variant angina pectoris. *Am J Med* 1959;1:375–388.
33. Fibrinolytic Therapy Trialists' Collaborative Group. Indications for fibrinolytic therapy in suspected acute myocardial infarction. *Lancet* 1994;343:311–322.
34. Sgarbossa EB, Pinski SL, Barbagelata A, et al. Electrocardiographic diagnosis of evolving acute myocardial infarction in the presence of left bundle-branch block (Erratum in N Engl J Med 1996;334:931). *N Engl J Med* 1996;334:481–487.
35. Hathaway WR, Peterson ED, Wagner GS, et al. Prognostic significance of the initial electrocardiogram in patients with acute myocardial infarction. *JAMA* 1998;279:387–391.
36. Savonitto S, Ardissino D, Granger CB, et al. Prognostic value of the admission electrocardiogram in acute coronary syndromes. *JAMA* 1999;281:707–713.
37. Cannon CP, McCabe CH, Stone PH, et al. The electrocardiogram predicts one-year outcome of patients with unstable angina and non-Q wave myocardial infarction: results of the TIMI III Registry ECG Ancillary Study. *J Am Coll Cardiol* 1997;30:133–140.
38. Hyde TA, French JK, Wong CK, et al. Four-year survival of patients with acute coronary syndromes without ST-segment elevation and prognostic significance of 0.5-mm ST-segment depression. *Am J Cardiol* 1999;84:379–385.
39. Braat SH, Gorgels AP, Bar FW, et al. Value of the ST T segment in lead V4R in inferior wall acute myocardial infarction to predict the site of coronary arterial occlusion. *Am J Cardiol* 1988;62:140–142.
40. Frierson JH, Dimas AP, Metzdorff MT, et al. Critical left main stenosis presenting as diffuse ST segment depression. *Am Heart J* 1993;125:1773–1777.
41. Brush JE Jr, Brand DA, Acampora D, et al. Use of the initial electrocardiogram to predict in hospital complications of acute myocardial infarction. *N Engl J Med* 1985;312:1137–1141.
42. Slater DK, Hlatky MA, Mark DB, et al. Outcome in suspected acute

myocardial infarction with normal or minimally abnormal admission electrocardiographic findings. *Am J Cardiol* 1987;60:766–770.

43. Stark ME, Vacek JL. The initial electrocardiogram during admission for myocardial infarction. Use as a predictor of clinical course and facility utilization. *Arch Intern Med* 1987;147:843–846.

44. Ohman EM, Christenson RH. Noninvasive assessment of myocardial reperfusion and reocclusion. In: Topol EJ, Serruys PW, eds. *Current review of interventional cardiology,* 2nd ed. Philadelphia: Current Medicine, 1994:151–169.

45. Wu AH, Apple FS, Gibler WB, et al. National Academy of Clinical Biochemistry Standards of Laboratory Practice: recommendations for the use of cardiac markers in coronary artery diseases. *Clin Chem* 1999;45:1104–1121.

46. Alpert JS, Thygesen K, Antman E, et al. Myocardial infarction redefined—a consensus document of The Joint European Society of Cardiology/American College of Cardiology Committee for the redefinition of myocardial infarction (Erratum in J Am Coll Cardiol 2001;37:973). *J Am Coll Cardiol* 2000;36:959–969.

47. Antman EM. Decision making with cardiac troponin tests *N Engl J Med* 2002;346:2079–2082.

48. Ohman EM, Armstrong PW, Christenson RH, et al. Cardiac troponin T levels for risk stratification in acute myocardial ischemia. *N Engl J Med* 1996;335:1333–1341.

49. Newby LK, Alpert JS, Ohman EM, et al. Changing the diagnosis of acute myocardial infarction: implications for practice and clinical investigations. *Am Heart J* 2002;144:957–980.

50. Califf RM, Ohman EM. The diagnosis of acute myocardial infarction. *Chest* 1992;101:106S–115S.

51. Del Carlo CH, O'Connor CM. Cardiac troponins in congestive heart failure. *Am Heart J* 1999;138:646–653.

52. Newby LK, Storrow AB, Gibler WB, et al. Bedside multimarker testing for risk stratification in chest pain units: the CHest pain Evaluation by Creatine Kinase-MB, Myoglobin, And Troponin I (CHECKMATE) study. *Circulation* 2001;103:1832–1837.

53. de Lemos JA, Morrow DA, Gibson CM. The prognostic value of serum myoglobin in patients with non-ST-segment elevation acute coronary syndromes. Results from the TIMI 11B and TACTICS-TIMI 18 studies. *J Am Coll Cardiol* 2002;40:238–244.

54. James SK, Lindahl B, Siegbahn A, et al. N-Terminal pro-brain natriuretic peptide and other risk markers for the separate prediction of mortality and subsequent myocardial infarction in patients with unstable coronary artery disease. *Circulation* 2003;108:275–281.

55. Morrow DA, de Lemos JA, Sabatine MS, et al. Evaluation of B-type natriuretic peptide for risk assessment in unstable angina/non-ST-elevation myocardial infarction: B-type natriuretic peptide and prognosis in TACTICS-TIMI 18 (Erratum in J Am Coll Cardiol 2003;41:1852). *J Am Coll Cardiol* 2003;41:1264–1272.

56. Christenson RH, Duh SH, Sanhai WR, et al. Characteristics of an Albumin Cobalt Binding Test for assessment of acute coronary syndrome patients: a multicenter study. *Clin Chem* 2001;47:464–470.

57. Jernberg T, Lindahl B. A combination of troponin T and 12-lead electrocardiography: a valuable tool for early prediction of long-term mortality in patients with chest pain without ST-segment elevation. *Am Heart J* 2002;144:804–810.

58. Sabatine MS, Morrow DA, de Lemos JA, et al. Multimarker approach to risk stratification in non-ST elevation acute coronary syndromes: simultaneous assessment of troponin I, C-reactive protein, and B-type natriuretic peptide. *Circulation* 2002;105:1760–1763.

59. Ardissino D, Merlini PA, Gamba G, et al. Thrombin activity and early outcome in unstable angina pectoris. *Circulation* 1996;93:1634–1639.

60. Sonel A, Sasseen BM, Fineberg N, et al. Prospective study correlating fibrinopeptide A, troponin I, myoglobin, and myosin light chain levels with early and late ischemic events in consecutive patients presenting to the emergency department with chest pain. *Circulation* 2000;102:1107–1113.

61. Goldman L, Cook EF, Brand DA, et al. A computer protocol to predict myocardial infarction in emergency department patients with chest pain. *N Engl J Med* 1988;318:797–803.

62. Lee TH, Juarez G, Cook EF, et al. Ruling out acute myocardial infarction. A prospective multicenter validation of a 12-hour strategy for patients at low risk. *N Engl J Med* 1991;324:1239–1246.

63. Goldman L, Cook EF, Johnson PA, et al. Prediction of the need for intensive care in patients who come to the emergency departments with acute chest pain. *N Engl J Med* 1996;334:1498–1504.

64. Selker HP, Griffith JL, D'Agostino RB. A tool for judging coronary care unit admission appropriateness, valid for both real time and retrospective use. A time sensitive predictive instrument (TIPI) for acute cardiac ischemia: a multicenter study. *Med Care* 1991;29:610–627.

65. Selker HP, Beshansky JR, Griffith JL, et al. Use of the acute cardiac ischemia time-insensitive predictive instrument (ACI-TIPI) to assist with triage of patients with chest pain or other symptoms suggestive of acute cardiac ischemia. A multicenter, controlled clinical trial. *Ann Intern Med* 1998;129:845–855.

66. Antman EM, Cohen M, Bernink PJ, et al. The TIMI risk score for unstable angina/non-ST elevation MI: a method for prognostication and therapeutic decision making. *JAMA* 2000;284:835–842.

67. Solomon DH, Stone PH, Glynn RJ, et al. Use of risk stratification to identify patients with unstable angina likeliest to benefit from an invasive versus conservative management strategy. *J Am Coll Cardiol* 2001;38:969–976.

68. Morrow DA, Cannon CP, Rifai N, et al. Ability of minor elevations of troponins I and T to predict benefit from an early invasive strategy in patients with unstable angina and non-ST elevation myocardial infarction: results from a randomized trial. *JAMA* 2001;286:2405–2412.

69. Boersma E, Pieper KS, Steyerberg EW, et al. Predictors of outcome in patients with acute coronary syndromes without persistent ST-segment elevation. Results from an international trial of 9461 patients. *Circulation* 2000;101:2557–2567.

70. Kaul P, Newby LK, Fu Y, et al. Troponin T and quantitative ST-segment depression offer complementary prognostic information in the risk stratification of acute coronary syndrome patients. *J Am Coll Cardiol* 2003;41:371–380.

71. Gottlieb SO, Weisfeldt ML, Ouyang P, et al. Silent ischemia as a marker for early unfavorable outcomes in patients with unstable angina. *N Engl J Med* 1986;314:1214–1219.

72. Langer A, Minkowitz J, Dorian P, et al. Pathophysiology and prognostic significance of Holter detected ST segment depression after myocardial infarction. Tissue Plasminogen Activator: Toronto (TPAT) Study Group. *J Am Coll Cardiol* 1992;20:1313–1317.

73. Wilcox I, Ben Freedman S, Kelly DT, et al. Clinical significance of silent ischemia in unstable angina pectoris. *Am J Cardiol* 1990;65:1313–1316.

74. Decker WW, Prina LD, Smars PA, et al. Continuous 12-lead electrocardiographic monitoring in an emergency department chest pain unit: an assessment of potential clinical effect. *Ann Emerg Med* 2003;41:342–351.

75. Jernberg T, Abrahamsson P, Lindahl B, et al. Continuous multilead ST-monitoring identifies patients with unstable coronary artery disease who benefit from extended antithrombotic treatment. *Eur Heart J* 2002;23:1093–1101.

76. Levitt MA, Jan BA. The effect of real time 2-D-echocardiography on medical decision-making in the emergency department. *J Emerg Med* 2002;22:229–233.

77. Lim SH, Sayre MR, Gibler WB. 2-D echocardiography prediction of adverse events in ED patients with chest pain. *Am J Emerg Med* 2003;21:106–110.

78. Effects of tissue plasminogen activator and a comparison of early invasive and conservative strategies in unstable angina and non-Q-wave myocardial infarction. Results of the TIMI IIIB Trial. Thrombolysis in Myocardial Ischemia. *Circulation* 1994;89:1545–1556.

79. Invasive compared with non-invasive treatment in unstable coronary-artery disease: FRISC II prospective randomised multicentre study. FRagmin and Fast Revascularisation during InStability in Coronary artery disease Investigators. *Lancet* 1999;354:708–715.

80. Cannon CP, Weintraub WS, Demopoulos LA, et al. Comparison of early invasive and conservative strategies in patients with unstable coronary syndromes treated with the glycoprotein IIb/IIIa inhibitor tirofiban. *N Engl J Med* 2001;344:1879–1887.

81. Braunwald E, Antman EM, Beasley JW, et al. ACC/AHA 2002 guideline update for the management of patients with unstable angina and non-ST-segment elevation myocardial infarction. *J Am Coll Cardiol* 2002;40:366–374.

82. Ewart CK, Taylor CB, Reese LB, et al. Effects of early postmyocardial infarction exercise testing on self-perception and subsequent physical activity. *Am J Cardiol* 1983;51:1076–1080.

83. Moss AJ, Goldstein RE, Hall WJ, et al. Detection and significance of myocardial ischemia in stable patients after recovery from an acute coronary event. Multicenter Myocardial Ischemia Research Group. *JAMA* 1993;269:2379–2385.

84. Swahn E, Areskog M. Berglund U, et al. Predictive importance of clin-

ical findings and a predischarge exercise test in patients with suspected unstable coronary artery disease. *Am J Cardiol* 1987;59:208–214.

85. Severi S, Orsini E. Marraccini P, et al. The basal electrocardiogram and the exercise stress test in assessing prognosis in patients with unstable angina. *Eur Heart J* 1988;9:441–446.

86. Madsen JK, Thomsen BL, Mellemgaard K, et al. Independent prognostic risk factors for patients referred because of suspected acute myocardial infarction without confirmed diagnosis. Prognosis after discharge in relation to medical history and non invasive investigations. *Eur Heart J* 1988;9:611–618.

87. Nyman I, Larsson H, Areskog M, et al. The predictive value of silent ischemia at an exercise test before discharge after an episode of unstable coronary artery disease. RISC Study Group. *Am Heart J* 1992;123:324–331.

88. Krone RJ, Dwyer EM, Greenberg H, et al. Risk stratification in patients with first non Q wave infarction: limited value of the early low level exercise test after uncomplicated infarcts. *J Am Coll Cardiol* 1989;14:31–37.

89. Gibson RS, Beller GA, Gheorghiade M, et al. The prevalence and clinical significance of residual myocardial ischemia 2 weeks after uncomplicated non Q wave infarction: a prospective natural history study. *Circulation* 1986;73:1186–1198.

90. Younis LT, Byers S, Shaw L, et al. Prognostic value of intravenous dipyridamole thallium scintigraphy after an acute myocardial ischemic event. *Am J Cardiol* 1989;64:161–166.

91. Zabalgoitia M, Ismaeil M. Diagnostic and prognostic use of stress echo in acute coronary syndromes including emergency department imaging. *Echocardiography* 2000;17:479–493.

92. Pope JH, Aufderheide TP, Ruthazer R, et al. Missed diagnoses of acute cardiac ischemia in the emergency department. *N Engl J Med* 2000;342:1163–1170.

93. Farkouh ME, Smars PA, Reeder GS, et al. A clinical trial of a chest-pain observation unit for patients with unstable angina. *N Engl J Med* 1998;339:1882–1888.

94. Reilly BM, Evans AT, Schaider JJ, et al. Impact of a clinical decision rule on hospital triage of patients with suspected acute cardiac ischemia in the emergency department. *JAMA* 2002;288:342–350.

95. Stein RA, Chaitman BR, Balady GJ, et al. Safety and utility of exercise testing in emergency room chest pain centers: an advisory from the Committee on Exercise, Rehabilitation, and Prevention, Council on Clinical Cardiology, American Heart Association. *Circulation* 2000;102:1463–1467.

96. Udelson JE, Beshansky JR, Ballin DS, et al. Myocardial perfusion imaging for evaluation and triage of patients with suspected acute cardiac ischemia: a randomized controlled trial (Erratum in JAMA 2003;289:178). *JAMA* 2002;288:2693–2700.

97. Kwong RY, Schussheim AE, Rekhraj S, et al. Detecting acute coronary syndrome in the emergency department with cardiac magnetic resonance imaging. *Circulation* 2003;107:531–537.

CHAPTER 59

Clinical Presentation and Diagnostic Evaluation of ST-Segment Elevation Myocardial Infarction

Gordon S. Huggins and Patrick T. O'Gara

Key Words: Arrhythmias and heart block; diabetes mellitus; elderly; electrocardiography; mechanical complications; myocardial infarction; myocardial reperfusion; risk stratification; serum biomarkers.

INTRODUCTION

Coronary heart disease (CHD) is the leading cause of death in the United States. An estimated 1.5 million individuals have a myocardial infarction (MI) each year, one-third of which are fatal. The majority of deaths occur before hospital treatment; in-hospital mortality rates average 10% and are greater among the elderly and patients with diabetes. An additional 10% of hospital survivors will die within the first year after infarction. Reinfarction rates approach 10% to 15% within the first year, the greatest number of which occur within the first 6 to 12 weeks after the index event.

    G. S. Huggins: Molecular Cardiology Research Institute, Cardiology Division, Tufts-New England Medical Center, Boston, Massachusetts 02111.
    P. T. O'Gara: Cardiovascular Division, Department of Medicine, Brigham and Women's Hospital/Harvard Medical School, Boston, Massachusetts 02115.

There has been a steady and significant decline in age-adjusted mortality rates for patients with cardiovascular disease over the last three decades. Much of this improvement can be related to risk factor modification, including programs directed at smoking cessation and blood pressure (BP) control, but advances in coronary care, such as acute reperfusion and arrhythmia intervention, also have contributed. Since 1984, mortality rates after MI have decreased to 5.0% and 17.6%, for patients younger and older than 65 years of age, respectively (1). Further improvements in survival will depend on more aggressive implementation of preventive measures, better public education and awareness, and more rapid diagnosis and treatment. The latter depends primarily on an appropriate clinical index of suspicion and streamlined system approaches to acute care.

CLINICAL FEATURES

History

History remains the most important element of the initial evaluation. Patients with MI usually report constant chest discomfort, albeit of waxing and waning intensity. It most commonly has a pressing or squeezing character and is felt in a retrosternal location. Often, it can radiate to the ulnar aspect of the left arm or to the jaw. Most patients will provide an antecedent history of a similar chest discomfort occurring transiently hours to days before the pain became more intense. Differentiating the time of chest pain onset from the time that it became more intense or prolonged may help to establish temporally the initiation of infarction. Patients with a history of angina will usually describe their discomfort as similar in quality, yet more severe, uncharacteristically prolonged, and less responsive to nitroglycerin. Many patients will emphasize that their discomfort does not manifest as "pain," but rather as "pressure" or "tightness."

MI often is associated with diaphoresis; many patients describe the onset of a "cold sweat." Patients may develop a drenching sweat when pulmonary edema intervenes. Inferior MI is frequently accompanied by gastrointestinal symptoms of abdominal bloating, the urge to defecate, nausea, and emesis. Syncope and near-syncope in the setting of MI should be characterized by their postural nature, rapidity of onset, and the awareness of premonitory palpitations. A higher clinical index of suspicion is warranted in the elderly and in patients with diabetes, who may not report chest discomfort, but rather present with dyspnea, confusion, or syncope.

Prolonged myocardial ischemia leading to infarction stems from a critical imbalance between oxygen supply and demand. Although emphasis usually is placed on vulnerable plaque rupture and thrombotic vessel occlusion, the initial evaluation should take into account those factors that may precipitate sustained increases in oxygen demand that cannot be met in the setting of fixed atherothrombotic coronary artery disease (CAD). These include fever, sepsis, anemia, thyrotoxicosis, and arrhythmia, such as rapid atrial fibrillation (AF). Cocaine exposure may not only cause tachycardia and hypertension, but may also precipitate coronary vasospasm, dissection, and platelet activation. Specific inquiry regarding cocaine use, and urine toxicology screening, should be pursued for all patients at risk, especially those without obvious attributes for atherothrombotic disease. Other nonatherothrombotic causes of MI include embolism of thrombotic or vegetative material in the setting of valvular heart disease, infective endocarditis, AF spontaneous coronary dissection, and arteritis.

Chest pain, when considered in isolation, is not strongly predictive of MI. The Myocardial Infarction Triage and Intervention (MITI) Project enrolled 522 patients with chest pain in a trial of prehospital administration of thrombolytic therapy. Acute MI (AMI) was diagnosed in only one fifth of patients with chest pain of presumed cardiac origin (2). The Multicenter Chest Pain Study investigators reviewed the characteristics of chest pain predictive of MI in 596 patients. They found that chest pain described as a "pressure" or "burning" was most commonly associated with MI, whereas chest pain that was positional, pleuritic, or reproduced by palpation was rarely reported (3). Finally, it is worth noting

that as many as 25% of MIs are detected retrospectively by electrocardiographic (ECG) analysis during an unrelated evaluation. Patients with silent MI may be prone to silent ischemia, and detailed questioning may identify a noteworthy historical event in only half of such patients.

The resolution of chest pain is an imprecise gauge of vessel patency after thrombolysis. Patients with angiographically patent infarct related arteries (IRAs) often continue to have chest pain and persistent ST-segment elevation, perhaps secondary to distal embolization and impaired microvascular tissue perfusion. Angiographic, echocardiographic, and ECG indices of tissue perfusion are predictive of outcome.

Triggers of Myocardial Infarction

There is a circadian distribution of MI, sudden death, stroke, and transient myocardial ischemia, with the greatest peak in the first few morning hours after awakening. Plasma catecholamine and cortisol levels also have a diurnal variation that parallels the daily pattern of the ischemic threshold in patients with angina. In addition, there is a marked increase in epinephrine- and adenosine diphosphate–induced platelet aggregability in the early morning, which can be reduced by the prior use of aspirin (4). MIs with onset in the early morning hours tend to be larger than those that occur at other times. There are also seasonal (e.g., winter) and weekly (e.g., Monday) peaks in the distribution of MI (5).

Heavy physical exertion immediately preceding the onset of chest pain has been identified as a trigger for MI. Patients with MI are more likely to have engaged in strenuous physical exercise within 1 hour of the event; routine heavy exertion three to four times per week can decrease the risk for effort-related MI by tenfold (6). Emotionally upsetting events may also serve as triggers for MI (7).

Coronary Risk Factors and Myocardial Infarction

Patients with chest pain should be evaluated considering the likelihood that CAD is present. Detailed reviews of coronary risk factors are offered in other chapters in this textbook, as well as many published scientific statements and conference reports (8,9). Briefly, advancing age is characterized by an increasing burden of atherothrombosis. Women are relatively protected from CAD until menopause, after which their risk approximates that for men. Women lose their protective advantage if menopause occurs prematurely or if they have diabetes. A family history of premature CAD, such as MI in male kindred members younger than 55 years of age, is an independent risk factor for cardiovascular death, especially for men. The prevalence of CHD is tenfold greater among patients with diabetes versus nondiabetic patients. Prognosis after MI is adversely affected by diabetes. Both systolic and diastolic hypertension are independent risk factors, with a log-linear relation between the diastolic BP and the incidence of cardiovascular disease. The risk for development of CHD is directly related to the levels of total and low-density lipoprotein cholesterol and is inversely related to the level of high-density lipoprotein cholesterol. The importance of triglycerides has been recognized in the most recent National Cholesterol Education Program/Adult Treatment Panel III (NCEP/ATPIII) recommendations (9). Smoking is a potent risk factor for both sudden death and MI. There is no safe degree of cigarette consumption; a habit of four or fewer cigarettes per day is positively associated with a risk for MI.

Physical Examination

The physical examination is frequently overlooked, but it may provide important corroborative or prognostic information. Attention should be focused on the vital signs, general appearance, venous pressure, arterial pulses, lung sounds, heart sounds, and extremities. Commonly, the examination is relatively unchanged or unremarkable because any abnormal physical findings may have antedated the acute event, or the associated pathophysiologic impairments are not severe enough to have caused any noticeable derangements.

The heart rate is usually normal or slightly fast, but may be slow in patients with inferior MI. An irregular rhythm may be a clue to the presence of premature beats, advanced atrioventricular (AV) block, or AF. Careful measurement of the BP, in both arms, is critical to the institution of appropriate medical therapy. Hypotension may imply cardiogenic shock. It is frequently seen in patients with inferior MI and is usually responsive to volume resuscitation. A higher BP allows for the acute administration of nitrates and intravenous β-blockers, whereas severe hypertension (BP > 180/110 mm Hg) is a contraindication to thrombolytic therapy. The heart rate and BP at time of presentation of acute ST-segment elevation MI (STEMI) are important determinants of prognosis. The Thrombolysis in Myocardial Infarction (TIMI) risk score $(HR*(Age/10)^2/$ systolic BP) integrates hemodynamic and age variables at the time of presentation and provides an estimate of prognosis for patients with ST-segment myocardial infarction (STEMI) (10).

The jugular venous pressure is usually low or normal, but it may be increased when right ventricular (RV) involvement complicates the course of an inferior MI or when left ventricular (LV) dysfunction is advanced. A paradoxic increase in the jugular venous pressure with inspiration (Kussmaul's sign), indicative of reduced RV diastolic compliance, is a sensitive and specific indicator of RV MI. A prominent Y descent and a right-sided S3 may also be present. These findings are highly preload dependent and may not be evident without volume challenge in patients with hypovolemia.

Careful examination of the arterial pulses and the abdominal aorta is an essential component of the initial evaluation. It will inform appropriate planning for mechanical interventions such as percutaneous coronary intervention (PCI) and intraaortic balloon counterpulsation. Examination of the carotid pulse may provide clues regarding the presence of associated cardiac lesions, such as aortic stenosis, as well as an appreciation of overall pump performance. Elderly patients have less compliant carotid arteries, which may retain a normal contour even in the presence of reduced output. Reduced or absent pulses or the presence of vascular bruits, or both, may reflect more widespread atherothrombotic disease. Compromise of the left internal mammary artery from high-grade proximal left subclavian artery disease, a potential cause of angina in patients after coronary artery bypass graft (CABG) surgery, often can be inferred from the physical examination findings. Notation also should be made of the presence and quality of the lower extremity veins.

The breath sounds, together with the systolic BP and a general sense of the adequacy of peripheral perfusion, can be used in the prognostic index originally developed by Killip and Kimball (11) to predict hospital outcome (Table 59–1). This simple classification scheme has maintained its usefulness for more than four decades. Signs of pulmonary congestion are potentially ominous.

Cardiac murmurs may be fixed or transient; the latter category would include the murmur of mitral regurgitation caused by ischemic papillary muscle dysfunction. It is usually heard best between the lower left sternal border and apex, more often with a decrescendo or diamond-shaped than holosystolic configuration. S4 and S3 gallops sounds reflect diastolic and systolic impairment, respectively. A pericardial friction rub, if heard at presentation, would imply that the acute event occurred days, rather than hours, before admission. Pericardial friction rubs are more common after ST-segment elevation than non-STEMI.

TABLE 59–1. *Killip classification of heart failure*

Class	Physical finding	Chest radiography
1	No clinical finding of congestive heart failure	Clear lung fields
2	Inspiratory rales, increased jugular venous pressure, S3 gallop without pulmonary edema	Cephalization of pulmonary vasculature, Kerley B lines
3	Frank pulmonary edema without hypotension	Alveolar pulmonary edema
4	Cardiogenic shock: systemic hypotension accompanied by diminished organ perfusion and/or pulmonary edema	Pulmonary edema, cardiomegaly may be present

Adapted from Killip T 3rd, Kimball JT. Treatment of myocardial infarction in a coronary care unit. A two year experience with 250 patients. *Am J Cardiol* 1967;20:457–464, with permission.

Electrocardiogram

The diagnosis of MI relies on the demonstration of characteristic ECG and serum biomarker changes. Karlson and coworkers (12) assessed the additive benefit of the ECG in 7,157 consecutive patients with chest pain. The presence of a normal ECG was associated with MI in only 6% of patients, whereas ischemic ECG changes in the setting of chest pain were associated with MI in 88% of patients. The incidence rate of AMI in the setting of a normal or nonspecific ECG can range from less than 1% to 17%, and it depends on the specific characteristics of the presenting symptoms (13). Goldman and coworkers (14) integrated historical features (pretest probability) with ECG findings in a computer algorithm to predict MI and used this tool prospectively to analyze 4,770 patients with chest pain in the emergency department. The sensitivity and specificity of this combined analysis for the detection of MI were 88% and 74%, respectively.

Acute ST-segment elevation has a relatively high positive predictive value for MI (Fig. 59–1), whereas the combination of ST-segment depression, T-wave abnormalities, or both consistent with ischemia has a lower predictive value (15). Misdiagnosis of AMI is frequent among patients with nonspecific ECG changes and those with changes caused by pericarditis, LV aneurysm, left ventricular hypertrophy (LVH) with strain, intraventricular conduction delay, drugs known to effect the ECG, electrolyte disturbances, or normal early repolarization. Patients with MI who have normal or nonspecific ECG findings have fewer complications.

AMI associated with ST-segment elevation is usually associated with the evolution of new, pathologic Q waves in the same anatomic distribution (Fig. 59–2). Variants include loss of R wave and splintering of the QRS complex. At presentation, these ST-segment elevations, in concert with typical chest pain, constitute the major criteria for the use of acute reperfusion therapy. New or presumed new left bundle branch block, a less common presenting finding, also is considered an indication for such treatment. Non-STEMI is not usually accompanied by Q-wave development (Fig. 59–3). The absence of acute ST-segment elevation (or new left bundle branch block) is a contraindication to the use of thrombolytic therapy, except in the instance of true posterior MI. STE (Q-wave) MIs were previously termed *transmural,* whereas non-STE (non–Q-wave) MIs were referred to as *nontransmural* or *subendocardial.* Such pathologic distinctions are imprecise. Confinement of the MI to the subendocardial zone is observed in only about half of patients studied at autopsy after non-STEMI. STEMIs are anatomically larger and result in lower ejection fractions and greater hospital mortality rates. Non-STEMIs are best thought of as incomplete events with greater subsequent rates of recurrent ischemia, reinfarction, and late death, particularly in the absence of therapeutic PCI. Indeed, by 1 year, mortality rates for STEMIs and non-STEMIs are comparable. Some non-

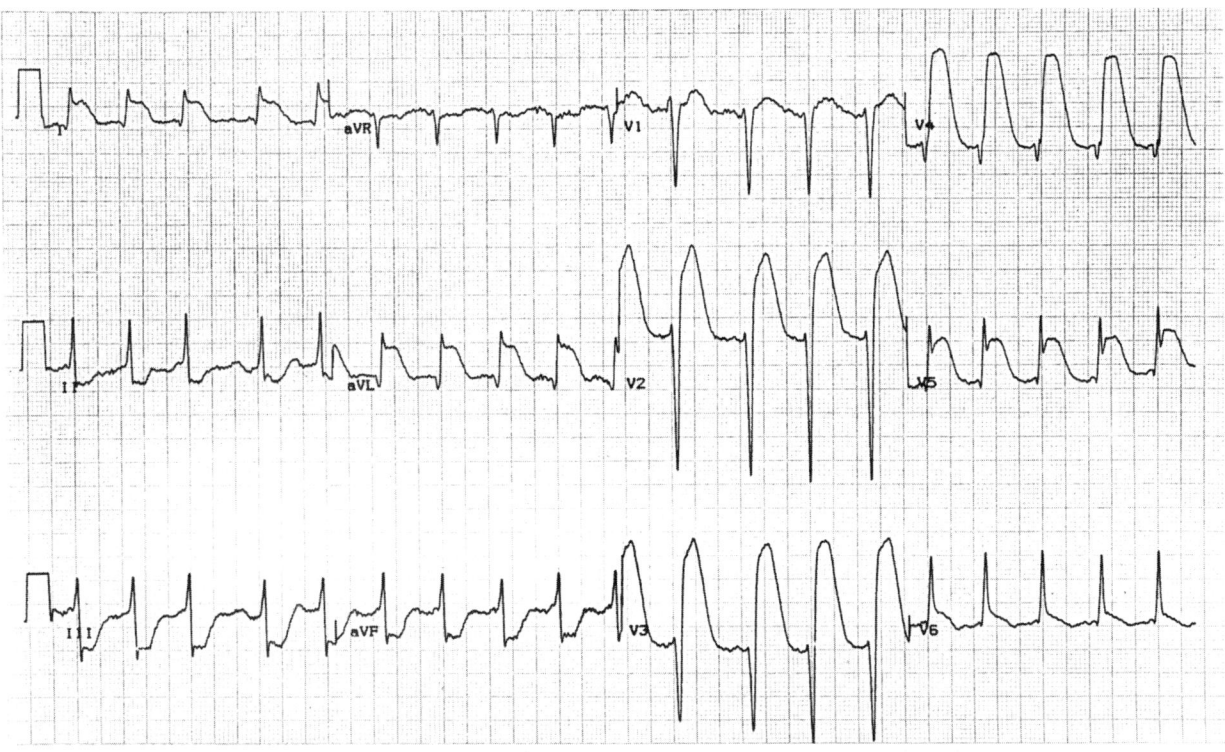

FIG. 59–1. Anterior myocardial infarction (MI). Electrocardiogram after initial resuscitation from ventricular fibrillation with acute anterolateral ST-segment elevation, loss of R wave through V_4, and reciprocal ST-segment depression in the inferior leads (2, 3, aVF).

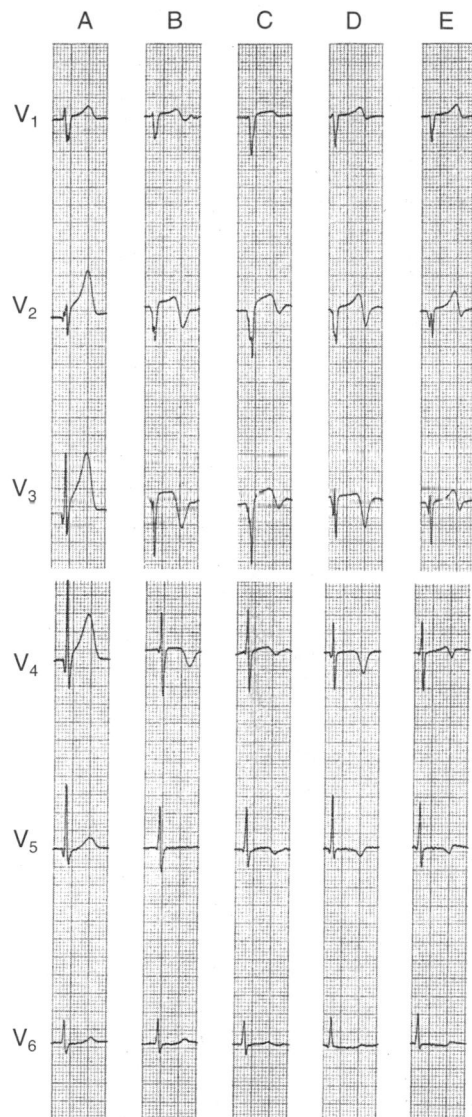

FIG. 59–2. ST-segment elevation (STE) anteroseptal myocardial infarction (MI) evolution. Serial electrocardiograms on presentation **(A)**, 1 day **(B)**, 1 week **(C)**, 1 month **(D)**, and 1 year **(E)** after an STE anteroseptal MI treated successfully with recombinant tissue-type plasminogen activator within 4 hours of symptom onset. There are hyperacute T-wave changes in leads V_2 to V_4 on presentation; STE persists in V_2 to V_3 for at least 1 week. Precordial leads V_2 to V_3 evolve Q waves with terminal T-wave inversions. Repolarization abnormalities extend to lead V_5.

STEMIs may initially be limited in size by spontaneous thrombolysis with early reflow or by the presence of coronary collaterals subserving the infarct zone. Notably, many of these natural history observations regarding the differences between STEMI and non-STEMI antedate the current era of aggressive reperfusion and PCI.

Acute ST-segment elevations often are accompanied by reciprocal ST-segment depressions in the ECG leads corresponding to the contralateral LV wall. For example, an acute injury pattern in the inferior leads (2, 3, and aVF) can be ac-companied by precordial (V_1–V_4) ST-segment depressions, the significance of which is frequently debated. Such con-comitant ST-segment depressions could represent true posterior wall involvement, reciprocal changes, or anterior ischemia (Fig. 59–4). This last entity, also referred to as "ischemia at a distance," portends a more ominous progno-sis. True posterior wall involvement is the most common cause of these precordial changes, but neither the ECG nor vectorcardiography can distinguish among the various etio-logic factors. Echocardiography can provide corroborative and perhaps discriminatory information regarding regional wall motion. Regardless of the precise cause, inferior MIs accompanied by precordial ST-segment depressions are anatomically larger than inferior MIs without these ST-segment shifts, and they result in lower LV ejection fractions and a more complicated hospital course (16).

Presentation with bundle branch block can obscure the di-agnosis of MI particularly if a prior ECG is not available for comparison. ST-segment deviation concordant to the QRS deflection (ST-segment elevation with positive QRS or ST-segment depression with negative QRS) is highly predictive of MI in the setting of bundle branch block (17). Although ST-segment deviation opposite to that of the QRS deflection (negative QRS complex with ST-segment elevation) can be normal, ST-segment elevation in excess of 5 mm with a neg-ative QRS has moderate to high probability for MI (18). In the Global Utilization of Streptokinase and t-PA [tissue-type plasminogen activator] for Occluded Coronary Arteries (GUSTO-I) trial, 1.6% of patients had bundle branch block. These patients were more likely to die in the hospital or to experience development of cardiogenic shock (17). Finally, resolution of the bundle branch block portended a better prognosis than persistent bundle branch block.

The addition of leads V_4R, V_8, and V_9 to the screening ECG may improve the diagnostic yield by enhancing detec-tion of RV and posterior MI, respectively (19). RV MI oc-curs in approximately 30% to 40% of patients with inferior STEMI. Correlation of autopsy findings with premortem ECGs in patients with RV MI and LV MI found that ST-segment elevation of 0.5 mm in V_4R was highly sensitive for the diagnosis of RV MI. Zehender and coworkers (20) re-ported a sensitivity of 88% and a specificity of 78% for 1.0-mm ST-segment elevation in V_4R (83% accuracy). These authors found that ST-segment elevation in V_4R strongly predicts the development of several major in-hospital complications, including shock, high-grade AV block, ventricular fibrillation (VF), and death (20). Early di-agnosis of RV involvement may greatly affect management. All patients with inferior STEMI should have an ECG with right-sided leads.

Prognosis after MI is critically dependent on the extent of myocardial necrosis, which, in turn, is the principal determi-nant of LV function. The primary goal in the management of patients with STEMI is the reestablishment and mainte-nance of normal epicardial and microvascular flow, to re-duce infarct size, preserve LV function, and improve sur-

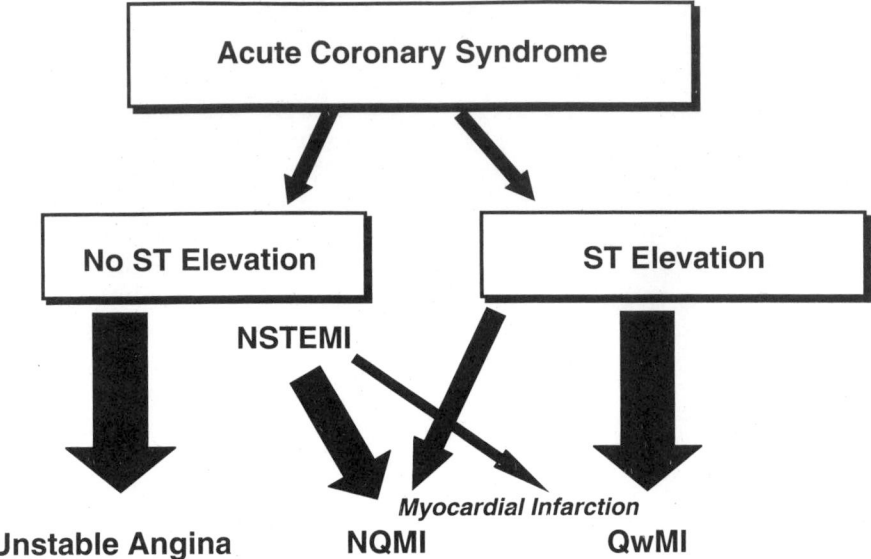

FIG. 59–3. Electrocardiographic progression of acute coronary syndromes. The majority *(large arrows)* of patients presenting without ST-segment elevation *(STE)* are subsequently classified as having unstable angina or non-STE (non–Q-wave) myocardial infarction *(NSTEMI)*, whereas few patients *(narrow arrow)* experience development of Q-wave MI *(QwMI)*. By comparison the majority of patients with STE evolve a QwMI, unless there is successful infarct-related artery reflow. NQMI, non–Q-wave myocardial infarction. (Adapted from Antman EM, Braunwald E. Acute myocardial infarction. In: Braunwald EB, ed. *Heart disease: a textbook of cardiovascular medicine.* Philadelphia: WB Saunders Company, 1996, with permission.)

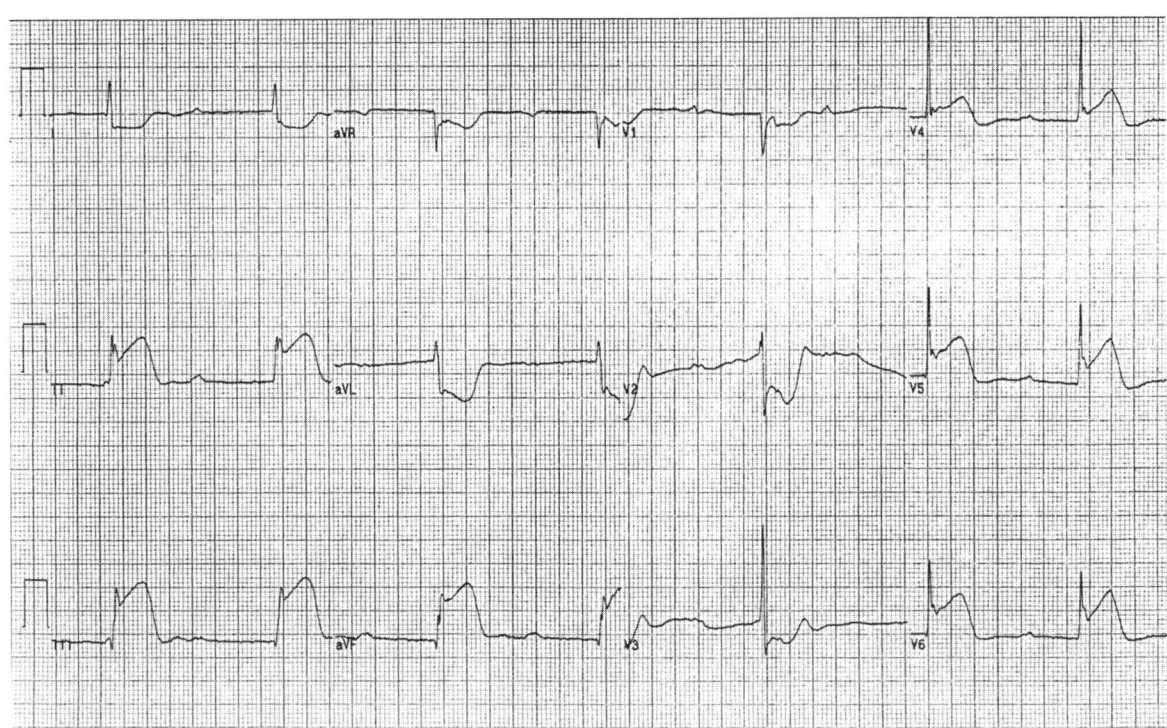

FIG. 59–4. Acute inferior–posterior–apical myocardial infarction complicated by complete heart block. Cardiac catheterization demonstrated subtotal occlusion of a large and dominant right coronary artery just after the acute right ventricular marginal branch. The right coronary artery supplied the inferior septum and most of the posterior wall. There was no significant disease involving the left coronary artery.

vival. IRA patency may also have a beneficial effect on LV remodeling (21,22), heart failure, and the risk for sudden death (23). Crude noninvasive indices of IRA patency include the resolution of chest pain, improvement in or resolution of ST-segment elevation, and early serologic marker release. Improvement in ECG abnormalities is the most useful indicator. Barbash and coworkers (24) studied the change in ST-segment elevation in 286 patients receiving recombinant tissue-type plasminogen activator (rt-PA) within 4 hours of chest pain onset. When the ST-segment elevation resolved within 1 hour of therapy, there was greater preservation of LV function, with a reduction in the incidence of heart failure and improved survival at 3 months. The Gruppo Italiano per lo Studio della Sopravvivenza nell'Infarto Miocardico II (GISSI-2) investigators found that a greater than 50% reduction in the amplitude of ST-segment elevation 4 hours after the initiation of thrombolytic therapy was associated with improved survival at 30 days (25). The greatest survival benefit was noted in patients who had complete resolution of ST-segment elevation within 4 hours of the initiation of thrombolytic therapy. The Israeli Study of Early Intervention in Myocardial Infarction investigators also found that patients with a greater than 70% reduction in the amplitude of ST-segment elevation had significantly reduced morbidity and mortality rates (26). Clemmensen and coworkers (27) compared the ST-segment elevation on the initial ECG performed within 6 hours of the onset of chest pain with a preangiographic ECG to correlate patency with injury current more precisely. They found that a 20% or greater decrease in ST-segment elevation predicted arterial patency with a sensitivity of 88% and a specificity of 80%. Although greater reductions in ST-segment elevation had a greater specificity, sensitivity decreased. The analysis of ST-segment change is inexact. Persistent ST elevation, despite IRA patency, has been well described. Angiographic and contrast echocardiographic studies have correlated this finding to reduced tissue or microvascular flow. Excellent flow in the epicardial IRA and normal microvascular flow correlates with a 70% or greater decrease from peak ST elevation, and identifies a subset of patients with an excellent prognosis (28,29). Even among patients with normal (TIMI Grade 3) epicardial flow, those with reduced tissue perfusion scores incur greater mortality risk (30).

Serologic Markers

Previously, the World Health Organization (WHO) defined MI on the basis of two of three characteristics: typical symptoms, diagnostic ECG changes, and increased serum creatine kinase (CK) levels. This definition proved less specific than intended. After the development of highly specific and sensitive serologic markers of myocardial necrosis (cardiac troponins), a joint European Society of Cardiology/American College of Cardiology consensus panel revised the definition of MI in 2000 (31). One major change was the absolute requirement for the finding of a typical increase and

decrease in biochemical markers of myocardial necrosis, in combination with either ischemic symptoms, ECG changes, or the need for coronary intervention.

The myocardial-specific isoforms of troponin T and I are the preferred serologic markers for the detection of MI. Cardiac troponin T and I isoforms are critical regulatory components of the contractile apparatus and are distinct from skeletal muscle isoforms. The cardiac isoforms are expressed in the myocardium of both normal and myopathic hearts (32). Unlike CK-MB, cardiac troponin T and I are not expressed in skeletal muscle, and may therefore identify cardiac muscle damage in the setting of rhabdomyolysis and after extraordinarily strenuous exercise (33). Both troponin T and I have a unique two-compartment kinetic model of release. Troponin T can appear in the serum as early as 3 hours after the onset of symptoms, reflecting its acute release from free cytosolic stores. Serum levels remain increased for as long as 130 hours because of the continued release of troponin bound to the contractile apparatus (34).

Because basal serum troponin levels are low, even small amounts of myocardial necrosis can be detected. Presentation with an increased cardiac troponin T level identifies a population at risk for death within 30 days (35), even among patients with renal dysfunction (36). Increases of troponin T or I in the serum of patients with acute coronary syndromes (ACSs) are directly proportional to adverse outcomes (37,38). Although the troponins have a unique role in the diagnosis of recent or latent infarction, because serum levels remain increased for up to 14 days, they are less sensitive to the detection of early reinfarction.

Serum CK and the predominantly myocardial-specific isoenzyme CK-MB were the previous gold standards for diagnosis. Skeletal muscle CK exists almost entirely as the MM isoenzyme, whereas CK-BB predominates in brain. CK-MB comprises 15% to 30% of the total myocardial CK activity and accounts for as much as 2% of the total CK activity in skeletal muscle. The use of CK and CK-MB assays is limited by the potential for false-positive increases caused by skeletal muscle disease, such as acute rhabdomyolysis, polymyositis, or Duchenne's muscular dystrophy, which may increase the absolute level of the CK-MB above the reference range in the absence of MI. Other conditions that interfere with CK-MB release, clearance, or both, such as hypothyroidism and renal failure, may also falsely increase the serum CK-MB level (39). CK and CK-MB are released quickly after myonecrosis, and increased levels may be detected within 6 hours of infarction (40). CK-MB is useful for the detection of early reinfarction. Analysis of CK-MB and CK-MM "subisoforms" may allow for detection of myocardial necrosis within 6 hours of symptom onset. Assays for CK-MM are not routinely available for clinical use.

More recently, investigators analyzed the prognostic information provided by multiple serologic markers, especially in the setting of non–ST-segment elevation ACS. ACSs often are the end result of chronic vessel wall inflammation, which can be monitored by high-sensitivity

C-reactive protein (hs-CRP) levels. Increased levels of hs-CRP adversely affect short- and intermediate-term outcome (41), as does a greater admission white blood cell count (42). Subclinical and overt LV dysfunction increases serum levels of the B-type natriuretic protein. Increasing numbers of increased markers (troponin I, hs-CRP, and B-type natriuretic protein) predict an adverse outcome (43). Increases of troponin T and B-type natriuretic protein also can identify patients at high risk for cardiac death (44,45).

Reperfusion is associated with the more rapid release of markers of myocardial necrosis, and the times to peak level of both CK and CK-MB are shortened in the setting of successful reperfusion. Myoglobin is a nonselective muscle protein released rapidly after infarct artery reflow. Early washout of myoglobin in conjunction with resolution of chest pain and ECG injury current identifies a low-risk population (46,47). Although myoglobin is limited as a marker for MI, a fourfold or greater increase in myoglobin 60 minutes after the initiation of thrombolytic therapy identifies more than 90% of patients with patent IRAs (48). A time to peak CK level of less than 4 hours also is highly predictive of patency after thrombolysis. Levels that peak beyond 16 hours are usually indicative of persistent vessel occlusion. Similarly, a rapid increase to peak troponin levels may also predict reflow (49).

Clinical Risk Score

As individual markers of prognosis have been validated, investigators have sought to create a composite algorithm to better refine the prediction of outcome. The TIMI investigators derived a risk score that weighs equally the presence of at least three coronary risk factors: age older than 65 years and a history of CAD, with clinical and laboratory findings, including ST-segment deviation, recurrent symptoms of angina, and aspirin use and increased cardiac biomarkers. This simple integer score provides a bedside risk assessment for patients with both STEMI and non-STEMI (10,50). For patients with STEMI, mortality risk correlates strongly with the TIMI score over a rather wide range of composite scores (Fig. 59–5) (50).

Imaging Studies in Acute Myocardial Infarction

Several imaging studies can be used to determine the likelihood of MI when the ECG is not diagnostic. Echocardiography is clearly the most readily available, portable, and efficient imaging modality for use in the diagnostic and prognostic evaluation of patients with suspected MI. It need not be applied routinely in the emergency department setting, but it may have its greatest diagnostic utility in the assessment of patients with ambiguous clinical and ECG features, before the results of serologic assays become available. Abnormal systolic wall thickening and motion can indicate severely ischemic or recently infarcted myocardium. Numerous studies have shown that nearly all patients with AMI have a new wall motion abnormality noted on echocardiography. Importantly, a completely normal echocardiogram in the setting of chest pain has

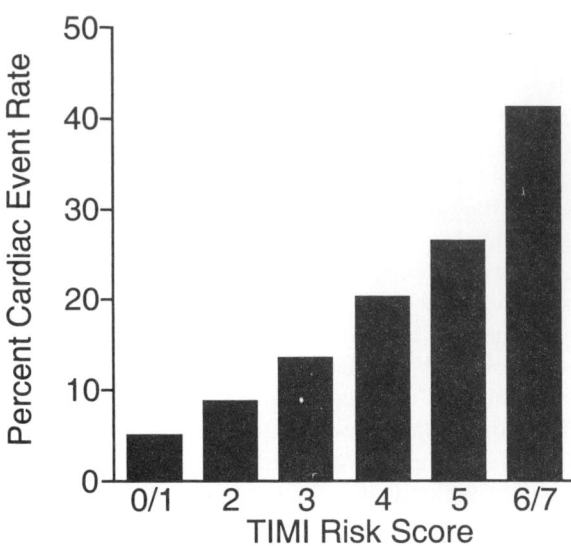

FIG. 59–5. Thrombolysis in Myocardial Infarction (TIMI) risk score predicts cardiac event rates. Increasing TIMI risk score correlated significantly with cardiac event rates, including mortality, myocardial infarction, and severe recurrent ischemia prompting urgent revascularization. (Adapted from Antman EM, Cohen M, Bernink PJ, et al. The TIMI risk score for unstable angina/non-ST elevation MI: a method for prognostication and therapeutic decision making. *JAMA* 2000;284:835–842.)

high negative predictive value. Preexistent regional wall motion abnormalities limit the specificity and positive predictive value of echocardiography.

Radionuclide imaging also has been applied to the study of patients with chest pain and suspected MI (51). Technetium-99m sestamibi (^{99m}Tc MIBI) is retained by the myocardium in proportion to its blood flow with minimal, if any, redistribution, thereby providing a "snapshot in time" of coronary blood flow. Normal myocardial scintigraphy has high negative predictive value, and a normal emergency department ^{99m}Tc MIBI scan correlates well with the absence of CAD (52). The presence of preexistent scar or significant soft tissue attenuation may produce falsely positive or equivocal images and limit the specificity of this technique. Infarct avid imaging with ^{99m}Tc pyrophosphate and radiolabeled antimyosin antibodies relies on the demonstration of necrotic rather than viable myocardium; the former technique is generally of historical interest, whereas the latter is restricted to research applications.

Invasive and noninvasive cardiac imaging studies have an invaluable role in the evaluation and management of patients during the course of MI. Predischarge noninvasive testing is discussed in Chapters 78–80. Urgent echocardiography is indicated for the assessment of suspected LV pump failure, mitral regurgitation, myocardial rupture, and tamponade. Coronary angiography as a prelude to revascularization is undertaken before PCI in high to intermediate risk non–ST-segment elevation ACSs and in patients with recurrent ischemia, heart failure, or late ventricular tachycardia (VT). Correlation of angiographic findings with noninvasive markers of viability (echo, nuclear, positron emission tomography, magnetic resonance) is indicated to inform decisions regarding revascularization in patients with severely reduced LV systolic function. Coronary angiography also is performed before urgent surgery in selected patients with cardiogenic shock caused by LV pump failure, as well as in those with ventricular rupture (53–55).

EARLY COMPLICATIONS

Heart Failure

Symptoms and signs of left heart failure may be present on admission or may develop several days to weeks after an MI. The development of heart failure is a risk factor for early death. Heart failure may be indicative of a large infarction with systolic dysfunction, a small infarction superimposed on several previous scars, acute mitral regurgitation, or diastolic dysfunction.

In their initial description of 250 patients with MI, Killip and Kimball (11) reported hospital mortality rates of 17% and 38% for patients with heart failure (Class 2) and pulmonary edema (Class 3), respectively, compared with only 6% for patients without heart failure. The Multicenter Postinfarction Research Group prospectively analyzed 866 patients for clinical risk factors affecting mortality after MI. The finding of inspiratory crackles involving more than the basal lung fields and the presence of pulmonary congestion on chest radiograph at presentation were significant risk factors for death within 6 months. In this registry, anterior MI was more commonly associated with heart failure than inferior MI (56).

Acute pulmonary edema is usually associated with depressed LV systolic function; isolated diastolic dysfunction is less common. Acute mitral regurgitation may cause pulmonary edema, in which case global systolic function need not be depressed (57). Other patients with advanced CAD (e.g., left main or severe proximal three-vessel disease) may experience development of transient, global dysfunction with pulmonary edema, yet their resting ejection fraction may be in the normal range when measured under nonischemic conditions. Similar observations pertain to patients with abrupt and severe increases of systemic BP with relatively small increases in cardiac biomarkers.

The initial ECG can provide a rough estimate of infarct size and the potential for the development of systolic heart failure. The arithmetic sum of the amplitude of individual lead ST-segment elevations can identify patients with lower ejection fractions who are at increased risk for in-hospital death, especially in the absence of reperfusion therapy (16). The absolute magnitude of ST-segment elevation is less helpful in inferior than in anterior MI. As previously noted, precordial ST-segment depressions that occur with inferior STEMI may reflect reciprocal changes, posterior involvement, or anterior ischemia. Precordial ST-segment depressions accompanying an ST-segment elevation inferior MI

are markers of a greater extent of inferior, apical, and posterolateral myocardial damage (58).

Anterior STEMIs are more frequently associated with pulmonary congestion and LV ejection fraction less than 0.40 than are nonanterior STEMIs. Nevertheless, there is a similar 1-year mortality rate for patients with anterior and inferior/posterior STEMIs (59). Patients with more extensive Q-wave development are at greater risk for heart failure and early death. The extent of Q-wave development after successful thrombolysis is a poor predictor of the resultant degree of LV dysfunction (60,61).

Mitral Regurgitation

Normal papillary muscle function is dependent on an adequate blood supply and the integrity of the supporting myocardium. The posteromedial papillary muscle is involved far more frequently than the anterolateral papillary muscle because of its singular blood supply. Chamber enlargement, annular dilatation, and displacement of the papillary muscles contribute to mitral regurgitation in the majority of cases. Mitral regurgitation can complicate both anterior and inferior MI, and it has a major impact on 1-year survival.

The TIMI Study Group reviewed the long-term effects of mitral regurgitation in 206 patients in the early reperfusion era (62). Mitral regurgitation was present in 27 (13%) patients; 20 patients had anterior MI. The presence of mitral regurgitation was not related to the peak CK level, chamber size, or filling pressures. Only 2 of the 27 patients had an audible murmur. The unadjusted relative risk for cardiovascular death at 1 year was 12.2 for patients with any mitral regurgitation (62). Tcheng and coworkers (63) reported similar observations among 1,480 consecutive patients admitted to Duke University Medical Center (Durham, North Carolina) between 1986 and 1990. Fifty patients had moderately severe or severe mitral regurgitation, the presence of which was associated with a 30-day mortality rate of 24% and a 1-year mortality rate of 52%. Half of these patients could not be identified by physical examination as having mitral regurgitation (63). Mitral regurgitation can wax and wane in intensity during the first 10 days after MI, often independently of the presence or absence of improved coronary flow after reperfusion. Leor and coworkers (64) reported conflicting results in a smaller cohort of patients with first inferior MI. These investigators found a reduced incidence of mitral regurgitation after thrombolytic therapy. The impact of PCI on the development of mitral regurgitation has been less well studied.

Heart Block

Advanced AV block may contribute significantly to in-hospital morbidity and mortality. The AV node is supplied by the dominant coronary artery, most often the right. The precise cause(s) of AV nodal dysfunction in the setting of MI is/are unknown. It does not appear to be explained solely by the vagal influences of the Bezold–Jarisch reflex (65).

The incidence of advanced heart block in the first 24 hours of acute inferior MI can approach 20%. In the TIMI II Trial, the overall incidence was 12%; half of these patients had AV block at presentation, whereas the other half developed significant heart block within 24 hours. Heart block was a marker for larger infarct size, lower ejection fraction, and greater risk for death (66). The Worcester Heart Attack Study Group reported a relative risk of in-hospital death of 2.10 for patients with heart block compared with those without heart block. After hospital discharge, however, there was no independent effect of AV block on mortality (67).

The Multicenter Investigation of the Limitation of Infarct Size (MILIS) study group developed a complete heart block (CHB) risk score, on the basis of their observations among 698 patients with AMI (68). The CHB risk score assigned one point to each of the following: first-degree AV block, Mobitz I block, Mobitz II block, right bundle branch block, left bundle branch block, left anterior hemiblock, and left posterior hemiblock, assuming each had equal predictive value for the subsequent risk for CHB. The risk score was simply the summation of individual points. In the absence of ECG abnormalities, these investigators found the incidence of CHB to be 1.2%. The incidence of CHB with one, two, or three or more risk factors was 7.8%, 25.0%, and 36.4%, respectively. Despite the previous perception that CHB develops after gradually increasing AV block, several patients were identified with first-degree AV block or Mobitz I block as the only antecedent sign.

Patients who experience development of acute bundle branch block are at greater risk for heart failure and death. Whereas the AV node is supplied by the dominant coronary artery, septal perforator branches from the left anterior descending coronary artery supply the left and right bundle branches. In the setting of an anteroseptal MI, the development of bundle branch block usually reflects proximal occlusion of the left anterior descending coronary artery. Of particular concern is the development of alternating bundle branch block or the combination of right bundle branch block with left posterior hemiblock. These conduction disturbances are associated with an increased incidence of more extensive CAD, larger infarctions, and greater mortality. The cardiac rhythm should be monitored closely for the development of bradyarrhythmias during AMI to allow for the timely application of temporary pacing as indicated (58). Mobitz type II second-degree AV block, new bifascicular block with first-degree heart block, alternating bundle branch block, symptomatic bradycardia not responsive to atropine, and asystole are American College of Cardiology/ American Heart Association (ACC/AHA) Class I indications for pacing (53). Patients with heart block frequently require temporary pacing, but permanent devices are only rarely necessary.

Sudden Death and Acute Myocardial Infarction

Sudden cardiac death claims the lives of 300,000 to 400,000 people each year in the United States and all too often (up to 25% of cases) is the first manifestation of CHD. Sudden death usually results from ischemic VF. In the setting of MI, two relatively broad categories of VF have been defined. VF or VT is defined as "primary" when it occurs within the first 48 hours after infarction in patients without heart failure or shock, whereas "secondary" VT/VF is usually associated with prior MI, scar formation, and/or severe LV pump dysfunction. Among patients with MI complicated by significant ventricular arrhythmia, one-third of arrhythmic events occur within the first 24 hours and one-half of events occur within the first 48 hours. The two most powerful predictors of poor outcome are heart failure and cardiogenic shock (69). Sustained monomorphic primary VT is less common than VF (70).

The GISSI study investigators reported a 2.8% incidence rate of primary VF among 11,712 patients with AMI, and 3.1% in patients receiving thrombolytic therapy (71). There was a relatively lower incidence of VF among older patients, perhaps because of more chronic or better collateralized CAD. Although the in-hospital mortality rate was more than twice as high for patients with versus without primary VF, no difference in mortality was observed at 6 months (72). Presentation with hypokalemia and hypotension are independent risk factors for primary VF (71). Although the incidence of primary VF has remained constant, hospital survival has improved (73).

Mechanical Complications

Cardiogenic shock caused by primary LV pump failure complicates the course of approximately 7% to 10% of patients with AMI. It may be present on admission or may develop over the course of the first week (74). It represents the leading cause of death from MI in the modern era. Rupture involving the ventricular free wall, interventricular septum, or papillary muscle most often occurs 2 to 7 days after the acute event. RV infarction may complicate the course of as many as 30% of patients with inferior STEMI and is evident at the time of presentation. The special features of these complications, their presentation, and their diagnosis are more fully discussed elsewhere in Chapters 74 and 75.

SPECIAL CIRCUMSTANCES

Acute Myocardial Infarction in Women

CHD constitutes the leading cause of death for women in the United States. It has long been appreciated that women, as compared with men, are prone to worse outcomes after MI, as well as after invasive coronary therapies such as PCI and bypass surgery (75). The reasons for these sex-related differences are multifactorial. At time of presentation with MI, women are, on average, 5 to 8 years older than men and more often have hypertension and diabetes (76). They also are more likely to experience development of congestive heart failure and non-STEMI (77). Although smoking has traditionally been more common among men, its use has increased significantly among women. Finally, women may experience comparatively longer delays in seeking medical attention possibly related to socioeconomic factors, such as family or elder care needs (78). As a result, they may derive less benefit from acute reperfusion therapies.

Debate continues as to whether female sex is an independent risk factor for post-MI death or whether the observed sex differences can be explained by other factors. In the MILIS study, female sex was an independent risk factor for mortality, especially among black women (79). After adjustment for age, prior MI, heart failure, and infarct location, the Secondary Prevention Reinfarction Israeli Nifedipine Trial (SPRINT) study investigators found the relative risks of in-hospital and 1 year mortality for women to be 1.72 (95% confidence interval [CI] 1.45–2.04) and 1.32 (CI 1.05–1.66), respectively (80). This sex difference also was observed in thrombolytic trials. In their combined metaanalysis of large-scale, placebo-controlled thrombolytic trials, the Fibrinolytic Therapy Trialists' Collaborative Group reported 35-day mortality rates of 10.1% and 16.0%, respectively, for men and women control patients versus 8.2% and 14.1% for those allocated fibrinolysis (81). The GUSTO IIb study found that women had more complications during hospitalization and were more likely to die within 30 days. However, after adjustment for the type of coronary syndrome and other baseline variables, this association was no longer significant. In fact, women were more likely to survive an episode of unstable angina (82). The SHould we emergently revascularize Occluded Coronaries for cardiogenic shocK (SHOCK) Registry found that women with cardiogenic shock were more likely than men to have mechanical complications such as acute mitral regurgitation or ventricular septal rupture than men (83). After adjustment for treatment and demographic features, women were no more likely to die of cardiogenic shock than men. Analysis of the TIMI IIIB trial of unstable angina and non-STEMI confirmed that women have greater comorbidity than men, and that adverse outcomes in women are more related to the severity of illness than sex (84).

Several studies have documented that women undergo fewer invasive procedures after MI than men (85). This difference raises the question as to whether the frequency of the use of such procedures is inappropriately low in women or inappropriately high in men. Once angiography is performed, comparable proportions of men and women are sponsored for PCI, bypass surgery, or both (86). Women with MI appear to have equivalent degrees of CAD when compared with their male counterparts (78). When adjusted for demographic, clinical, and hospital characteristics, women have the same rates of catheterization as men (87). Older studies have suggested that perhaps because of their more advanced age, greater prevalence of comorbid illnesses, and smaller body sizes, women fared less well after such procedures and experienced greater rates of death or major complications, or both (75,88). Newer studies have found that although procedural complications and recurrent angina are more common in women, there is no excess risk for death or MI in women treated invasively for ACSs (89,90).

Myocardial Infarction in the Elderly

The elderly comprise the fastest-growing segment of the U.S. population. Currently, more than half of all patients with AMI, and approximately 80% of those with fatal MI, are older than 65 years of age. The majority of fatalities occur in patients older than 75 years of age (1). Increasing age is associated with an exponential increase in both in-hospital and postdischarge mortality rates (91). Although 30-day and 1-year mortality rates have decreased significantly for the Medicare population, elderly patients still face a 20% to 30% risk for death after MI (92).

Women comprise a disproportionate majority of the elderly population. In addition, there is a greater prevalence among this population of previous MI, heart failure, and recurrent angina (93,94). As previously noted, older patients may have more atypical features, such as dyspnea, weakness, confusion, and syncope. Similar to patients with diabetes, their perception of pain often is altered. As a result, they present relatively later and may be ineligible for acute reperfusion therapy. Factors that contribute to the significantly less frequent use of thrombolysis in the elderly population include the lack of qualifying ECG changes and the presence of comorbid illnesses that are contraindications to its use, particularly active gastrointestinal bleeding or a history of recent stroke. With or without thrombolysis, the elderly face a substantially greater risk for stroke from a variety of causes: LV mural thrombus, AF, concomitant carotid artery atherothrombosis, and intracerebral small-vessel angiopathy. When thrombolytic therapy is provided, the risk for intracranial hemorrhage is exacerbated by the presence of systemic hypertension, a wide pulse pressure, small body size, female sex, and preferential use of rt-PA (95).

Although thrombolytic therapy causes a greater relative reduction in mortality among younger patients, the absolute reduction of mortality with the use of thrombolytic therapy is more pronounced in older patients up to age 75 years. There is likely benefit from thrombolytic therapy in patients older than 75 years, but this has been less well studied (53). Efforts are needed to ensure that such treatment, when indicated, is provided promptly and efficiently unless primary PCI is an option. Age alone is not a contraindication to either strategy. In this regard, it is important to note that the use of thrombolytic drugs in the National Registry of Myocardial Infarction (1990–1993) decreased progressively with age older than 60 years to 11% of patients in the eighth decade and 4% in the ninth decade of life (96). These data are similar to the MITI experience, in which only 5% of patients older than 75 years received thrombolytic therapy (97). The use of thrombolytic therapy for STEMI patients older than 75 years is a Class IIA recommendation of the ACC/AHA (53).

The impact of interventional procedures on outcomes in the elderly population has been difficult to assess. Although some studies have suggested that the recent decline in death rates for this age group is most strongly related to a population decline in the incidence of AMI, other studies have implied that the acute care available at referral centers has contributed significantly. Rates of angiography, PCI, and bypass surgery among the elderly have all increased significantly (92), in parallel with a decline in national mortality rates, suggesting improved outcomes after treatment (98). The elderly incur a greater risk for procedural complications, but the reported rates of death and MI after PCI are generally acceptable (99). The reduction in the risk for intracranial hemorrhage with PCI, as compared with thrombolysis, is a major advantage. Subsequent quality of life is an important determinant of outcome. Longer term rates of recurrent angina, MI, and death are important considerations.

Diabetes Mellitus and Myocardial Infarction

Obesity has contributed to the worsening epidemic of adult-onset (type 2) diabetes mellitus in the United States. More than 10 million individuals in the United States are diagnosed with diabetes and about 5 million more individuals likely have undiagnosed diabetes (8). Although juvenile-onset (Type I) diabetes mellitus also is a potent risk factor for vascular disease, the prevalence of type 2 diabetes is considerably greater. The long-term survival of patients with diabetes, but without clinically overt CAD, is similar to that of patients without diabetes who have demonstrated CAD (100,101). The presence of diabetes alone is considered a CHD risk equivalent. Diabetes damages endothelium, accelerates atherothrombosis, and contributes adversely to vulnerable plaque rupture and platelet activation (102). Patients with diabetes have a heavier burden of atherothrombotic disease, advanced endothelial dysfunction, and relative resistance to several of the standard antithrombotic treatments used in the management of ACS (54).

Patients with diabetes are notorious for their inability to perceive chest pain and are more likely to present with atypical features. Critical time may be lost in seeking or directing medical attention, because thoughts may be initially mistakenly focused on the possibility of hypoglycemic/hyperglycemic reactions. Patients with diabetes constitute a high-risk group with an excess incidence of heart failure, shock, reinfarction, arrhythmias, and death, both early and late after MI (103,104). These patients commonly have hypertension and LVH that predispose to heart failure during ACS (54). Interestingly, reanalysis of the Survival and Ventricular Enlargement (SAVE) study found that despite having a greater incidence of heart failure, patients with diabetes had relatively less LV remodeling (105). This discrepancy may be explained further by the influence of the cardiomyopathic changes caused by diabetes, in addition to that caused by CAD, LVH, or both. Diabetes is known to increase myocardial fibrosis and LVH, as well as adversely affect myocyte metabolism, which can affect LV systolic and diastolic function after MI.

In the acute phase of MI, the goals of rapidly reestablishing IRA patency and tissue perfusion are the same for patients with and without diabetes (54). Considering the prothrombotic effects of diabetes, aggressive antiplatelet and antithrombotic treatments in the acute setting may be particularly effective (102). Surgical revascularization of the patient with diabetes and multivessel disease, especially with LAD involvement, may be more effective than PCI (54). This observation is to be reexamined with the more widespread use of intracoronary stents.

Perioperative Myocardial Infarction

Noncardiac surgery poses a considerable threat to the cardiovascular system and may predispose to myocardial ischemia and infarction, usually within the first 48 to 72 hours after surgery. Pathophysiologically, myocardial ischemia/infarction can result from excess oxygen demand or a prothrombotic tendency induced by the surgical procedure, or both. In the setting of residual anesthesia, narcotic analgesia, and sedatives, chest pain may be absent and a high clinical index of suspicion is necessary. Worsening heart failure, hypotension, atrial arrhythmias, or confusion may be the major manifestations of such perioperative events (106).

The risk for perioperative cardiac complications can be inferred from a preoperative assessment on the basis of clinical features, exercise or pharmacologic stress testing, and radionuclide or echocardiographic imaging. Independent predictors of increased cardiac risk are age older than 70 years, MI within 6 months, a history of heart failure, diabetes, critical aortic stenosis, emergency surgery, and poor medical condition. Symptoms of exertional angina may be underappreciated, especially in the setting of diabetes or claudication. The presence of an increased jugular venous pressure and a third heart sound also identify patients at high risk (107). Patients considered at low or intermediate clinical risk can be further studied by means of adjunctive stress testing with or without diagnostic imaging as indicated. The demonstration of stress-induced ischemia, particularly if multisegmental or accompanied by evidence of LV dysfunction, confers greater risk (108,109).

The postoperative development of ST-segment depressions, T-wave inversions, or both is a frequent indicator of ischemia; frank ST-segment elevations are uncommon. These ECG changes may precede the onset of chest pain or pulmonary edema by several hours. Such ischemia is the most powerful predictor of an adverse cardiac event (death, MI, unstable angina, heart failure, or VT) (110). The cardiac troponins are the preferred biomarkers for the assessment of perioperative ischemia and infarction (111).

Cocaine-induced Myocardial Infarction

Cocaine abuse has reached widespread proportions. The inhalation of the highly addictive alkaloidal "crack" cocaine results in a large delivered dose, thus increasing the risk for cardiovascular complications. Cocaine increases the release and inhibits the presynaptic reuptake of catecholamines in both the peripheral and central nervous systems. Serum catecholamine levels are increased and postsynaptic stimulation is markedly enhanced. Cocaine also inhibits sodium channels and produces a local anesthetic effect.

Coronary artery vasoconstriction may develop in response to the increased α-adrenergic receptor stimulation that occurs after the use of cocaine with a resultant decrease in luminal diameter and impairment of coronary blood flow (112). Although none of the traditional cardiovascular risk factors has been strongly associated with cocaine-induced MI, tobacco use greatly increases its vasoconstrictive effect (113). The vasoconstrictive influences of cocaine may also be potentiated by β-adrenergic receptor blockade, which results in unopposed α-adrenergic receptor stimulation (114). Nitrates and calcium channel blockers may reverse the vasoconstriction. Intense cocaine-induced vasoconstriction may produce neointimal hyperplasia and premature atherothrombosis in epicardial coronary arteries. This may predispose to regional infarction secondary to either prolonged vasoconstriction, similar to that seen with vasospastic angina, or conventional plaque rupture and large-vessel thrombus formation (115). Cocaine exposure also enhances platelet aggregation. Alternatively, intensive microvascular vasospasm may produce diffuse ischemia and global LV dysfunction (116). Some asymptomatic men with a long-term history of "crack" cocaine abuse have increased LV mass and LVH, albeit with preserved systolic function (117).

Chest pain is a frequent complaint among cocaine users who present for hospital evaluation. Myocardial ischemia can occur on a substrate of increased oxygen demand (tachycardia, hypertension) in the setting of reduced supply through one or more of the mechanisms described earlier. Atherothrombotic CAD is present in only a minority of patients, and an inflammatory myocarditis, similar to that seen with pheochromocytoma, has been described rarely. The presence of traditional cardiac risk factors is more commonly found in patients with cocaine-induced MI who have underlying CAD (118). Ventricular arrhythmias, sudden death, or both may occur. Interestingly, the length of time between cocaine use and the onset of pain indicative of MI may be prolonged, suggesting that its secondary effects on endothelium and platelets may be causative (119). Evaluation of nontraumatic chest pain in a recent cocaine user is hampered by frequent abnormalities on the resting ECG and increased CK-MB caused by rhabdomyolysis. Nevertheless, patients with cocaine-related chest pain who do not have acute ECG changes or increased troponin levels and who are free of cardiovascular complications after 9 to 12 hours of observation are at low risk for MI and can be safely discharged (112,120).

FUTURE DIRECTIONS

The appropriate treatment of MI begins with its prompt recognition. The elements of the history, physical examination, and ECG should enable the experienced clinician to render an accurate diagnosis in the majority of circumstances. Yet, there are several patient subgroups in which the signs and symptoms of MI are masked by the presence of comorbid conditions, such as diabetes mellitus or advanced age. A high index of suspicion and the knowledge of prior probabilities are necessary tools for accurate diagnosis. Serologic markers are helpful in a retrospective sense. Acute imaging studies can provide both diagnostic and prognostic insight. Initial risk assessment can begin with the appreciation and recognition of several demographic and clinical attributes that are ascertainable at presentation—for example, age, sex, diabetes mellitus, prior MI, prior PCI/CABG, aspirin use, heart rate, BP, the presence of heart failure, mitral regurgitation, peripheral vascular disease, the extent and severity of ECG changes, and arrhythmias. Concern has been raised that we have reached an irreducible mortality rate for AMI. There remains great interest in the early, prehospital administration of pharmacologic agents to speed reperfusion or enhance the early benefit of primary PCI, or both. We continue to explore the appropriate mix and duration of post-MI antithrombotic therapies. Most importantly, local efforts to close the gap between the advances discovered in the large trials of AMI and their application in practice must continue. Programs of primary and secondary prevention, including aggressive efforts to control obesity and type 2 diabetes, will be paramount.

REFERENCES

1. Gillum RF. Trends in acute myocardial infarction and coronary heart disease death in the United States. *J Am Coll Cardiol* 1994;23: 1273–1277.
2. Weaver WD, Eisenberg MS, Martin JS, et al. Myocardial Infarction Triage and Intervention Project—phase I: patient characteristics and feasibility of prehospital initiation of thrombolytic therapy. *J Am Coll Cardiol* 1990;15:925–931.
3. Lee TH, Cook EF, Weisberg M, et al. Acute chest pain in the emergency room. Identification and examination of low-risk patients. *Arch Intern Med* 1985;145:65–69.
4. Ridker PM, Manson JE, Buring JE, et al. Circadian variation of acute myocardial infarction and the effect of low-dose aspirin in a randomized trial of physicians. *Circulation* 1990;82:897–902.
5. Willich SN, Lowel H, Lewis M, et al. Weekly variation of acute myocardial infarction. Increased Monday risk in the working population. *Circulation* 1994;90:87–93.
6. Mittleman MA, Maclure M, Tofler GH, et al. Triggering of acute myocardial infarction by heavy physical exertion. Protection against triggering by regular exertion. Determinants of Myocardial Infarction Onset Study Investigators. *N Engl J Med* 1993;329:1677–1683.
7. Willich SN, Lewis M, Lowel H, et al. Physical exertion as a trigger of acute myocardial infarction. Triggers and Mechanisms of Myocardial Infarction Study Group. *N Engl J Med* 1993;329:1684–1690.
8. Grundy SM, Pasternak R, Greenland P, et al. Assessment of cardiovascular risk by use of multiple-risk-factor assessment equations: a statement for healthcare professionals from the American Heart Association and the American College of Cardiology. *Circulation* 1999; 100:1481–1492.
9. Smith SC Jr, Blair SN, Bonow RO, et al. AHA/ACC Scientific Statement: AHA/ACC guidelines for preventing heart attack and death in patients with atherosclerotic cardiovascular disease: 2001 update: a statement for healthcare professionals from the American Heart Association and the American College of Cardiology. *Circulation* 2001; 104:1577–1579.
10. Morrow DA, Antman EM, Giugliano RP, et al. A simple risk index for

rapid initial triage of patients with ST-elevation myocardial infarction: an InTIME II substudy. *Lancet* 2001;358:1571–1575.

11. Killip T 3rd, Kimball JT. Treatment of myocardial infarction in a coronary care unit. A two year experience with 250 patients. *Am J Cardiol* 1967;20:457–464.

12. Karlson BW, Herlitz J, Wiklund O, et al. Early prediction of acute myocardial infarction from clinical history, examination and electrocardiogram in the emergency room. *Am J Cardiol* 1991;68:171–175.

13. Rouan GW, Lee TH, Cook EF, et al. Clinical characteristics and outcome of acute myocardial infarction in patients with initially normal or nonspecific electrocardiograms (a report from the Multicenter Chest Pain Study). *Am J Cardiol* 1989;64:1087–1092.

14. Goldman L, Cook EF, Brand DA, et al. A computer protocol to predict myocardial infarction in emergency department patients with chest pain. *N Engl J Med* 1988;318:797–803.

15. Lee TH, Weisberg MC, Brand DA, et al. Candidates for thrombolysis among emergency room patients with acute chest pain. Potential true- and false-positive rates. *Ann Intern Med* 1989;110:957–962.

16. Willems JL, Willems RJ, Willems GM, et al. Significance of initial ST segment elevation and depression for the management of thrombolytic therapy in acute myocardial infarction. European Cooperative Study Group for Recombinant Tissue-Type Plasminogen Activator. *Circulation* 1990;82:1147–1158.

17. Sgarbossa EB, Pinski SL, Topol EJ, et al. Acute myocardial infarction and complete bundle branch block at hospital admission: clinical characteristics and outcome in the thrombolytic era. GUSTO-I Investigators. Global Utilization of Streptokinase and t-PA [tissue-type plasminogen activator] for Occluded Coronary Arteries. *J Am Coll Cardiol* 1998;31:105–110.

18. Sgarbossa EB, Pinski SL, Barbagelata A, et al. Electrocardiographic diagnosis of evolving acute myocardial infarction in the presence of left bundle-branch block. GUSTO-1 (Global Utilization of Streptokinase and Tissue Plasminogen Activator for Occluded Coronary Arteries) Investigators. *N Engl J Med* 1996;334:481–487.

19. Zalenski RJ, Cooke D, Rydman R, et al. Assessing the diagnostic value of an ECG containing leads V4R, V8, and V9: the 15-lead ECG. *Ann Emerg Med* 1993;22:786–793.

20. Zehender M, Kasper W, Kauder E, et al. Right ventricular infarction as an independent predictor of prognosis after acute inferior myocardial infarction. *N Engl J Med* 1993;328:981–988.

21. McKay RG, Pfeffer MA, Pasternak RC, et al. Left ventricular remodeling after myocardial infarction: a corollary to infarct expansion. *Circulation* 1986;74:693–702.

22. Pfeffer MA, Lamas GA, Vaughan DE, et al. Effect of captopril on progressive ventricular dilatation after anterior myocardial infarction. *N Engl J Med* 1988;319:80–86.

23. Cigarroa RG, Lange RA, Hillis LD. Prognosis after acute myocardial infarction in patients with and without residual anterograde coronary blood flow. *Am J Cardiol* 1989;64:155–160.

24. Barbash GI, Roth A, Hod H, et al. Rapid resolution of ST elevation and prediction of clinical outcome in patients undergoing thrombolysis with alteplase (recombinant tissue-type plasminogen activator): results of the Israeli Study of Early Intervention in Myocardial Infarction. *Br Heart J* 1990;64:241–247.

25. Mauri F, Maggioni AP, Franzosi MG, et al. A simple electrocardiographic predictor of the outcome of patients with acute myocardial infarction treated with a thrombolytic agent. A Gruppo Italiano per lo Studio della Sopravvivenza nell'Infarto Miocardico (GISSI-2)-Derived Analysis. *J Am Coll Cardiol* 1994;24:600–607.

26. Schroder R, Dissmann R, Bruggemann T, et al. Extent of early ST segment elevation resolution: a simple but strong predictor of outcome in patients with acute myocardial infarction. *J Am Coll Cardiol* 1994;24:384–391.

27. Clemmensen P, Ohman EM, Sevilla DC, et al. Changes in standard electrocardiographic ST-segment elevation predictive of successful reperfusion in acute myocardial infarction. *Am J Cardiol* 1990;66:1407–1411.

28. Gibson CM, Cannon CP, Murphy SA, et al. Relationship of TIMI myocardial perfusion grade to mortality after administration of thrombolytic drugs. *Circulation* 2000;101:125–130.

29. de Lemos JA, Antman EM, Gibson CM, et al. Abciximab improves both epicardial flow and myocardial reperfusion in ST-elevation myocardial infarction. Observations from the TIMI 14 trial. *Circulation* 2000;101:239–243.

30. de Lemos JA. ST-Segment resolution as a marker of epicardial and

31. Alpert JS, Thygesen K, Antman E, et al. Myocardial infarction redefined—a consensus document of The Joint European Society of Cardiology/American College of Cardiology Committee for the redefinition of myocardial infarction. *J Am Coll Cardiol* 2000;36:959–969.

32. Sasse S, Brand NJ, Kyprianou P, et al. Troponin I gene expression during human cardiac development and in end-stage heart failure. *Circ Res* 1993;72:932–938.

33. Mair J, Wohlfarter T, Koller A, et al. Serum cardiac troponin T after extraordinary endurance exercise. *Lancet* 1992;340:1048.

34. Katus HA, Remppis A, Neumann FJ, et al. Diagnostic efficiency of troponin T measurements in acute myocardial infarction. *Circulation* 1991;83:902–912.

35. Ohman EM, Armstrong PW, Christenson RH, et al. Cardiac troponin T levels for risk stratification in acute myocardial ischemia. GUSTO IIA Investigators. *N Engl J Med* 1996;335:1333–1341.

36. Aviles RJ, Askari AT, Lindahl B, et al. Troponin T levels in patients with acute coronary syndromes, with or without renal dysfunction. *N Engl J Med* 2002;346:2047–2052.

37. Hamm CW, Ravkilde J, Gerhardt W, et al. The prognostic value of serum troponin T in unstable angina. *N Engl J Med* 1992;327:146–150.

38. Antman EM, Tanasijevic MJ, Thompson B, et al. Cardiac-specific troponin I levels to predict the risk of mortality in patients with acute coronary syndromes. *N Engl J Med* 1996;335:1342–1349.

39. Adams JE 3rd, Bodor GS, Davila-Roman VG, et al. Cardiac troponin I. A marker with high specificity for cardiac injury. *Circulation* 1993; 88:101–106.

40. Zimmerman J, Fromm R, Meyer D, et al. Diagnostic marker cooperative study for the diagnosis of myocardial infarction. *Circulation* 1999;99:1671–1677.

41. Morrow DA, Rifai N, Antman EM, et al. C-reactive protein is a potent predictor of mortality independently of and in combination with troponin T in acute coronary syndromes: a TIMI 11A substudy. Thrombolysis in Myocardial Infarction. *J Am Coll Cardiol* 1998;31: 1460–1465.

42. Sabatine MS, Morrow DA, Cannon CP, et al. Relationship between baseline white blood cell count and degree of coronary artery disease and mortality in patients with acute coronary syndromes: a TACTICS-TIMI 18 (Treat Angina with Aggrastat and determine Cost of Therapy with an Invasive or Conservative Strategy—Thrombolysis in Myocardial Infarction 18 trial) substudy. *J Am Coll Cardiol* 2002;40:1761–1768.

43. Sabatine MS, Morrow DA, de Lemos JA, et al. Multimarker approach to risk stratification in non-ST elevation acute coronary syndromes: simultaneous assessment of troponin I, C-reactive protein, and B-type natriuretic peptide. *Circulation* 2002;105:1760–1763.

44. de Lemos JA, Morrow DA, Bentley JH, et al. The prognostic value of B-type natriuretic peptide in patients with acute coronary syndromes. *N Engl J Med* 2001;345:1014–1021.

45. Ishii J, Nomura M, Nakamura Y, et al. Risk stratification using a combination of cardiac troponin T and brain natriuretic peptide in patients hospitalized for worsening chronic heart failure. *Am J Cardiol* 2002; 89:691–695.

46. De Lemos JA, Antman EM, Giugliano RP, et al. Very early risk stratification after thrombolytic therapy with a bedside myoglobin assay and the 12-lead electrocardiogram. *Am Heart J* 2000;140:373–378.

47. de Lemos JA, Morrow DA, Gibson CM, et al. Early noninvasive detection of failed epicardial reperfusion after fibrinolytic therapy. *Am J Cardiol* 2001;88:353–358.

48. Tanasijevic MJ, Cannon CP, Antman EM, et al. Myoglobin, creatine-kinase-MB and cardiac troponin-I 60-minute ratios predict infarct-related artery patency after thrombolysis for acute myocardial infarction: results from the Thrombolysis in Myocardial Infarction study (TIMI) 10B. *J Am Coll Cardiol* 1999;34:739–747.

49. Abe S, Arima S, Yamashita T, et al. Early assessment of reperfusion therapy using cardiac troponin T. *J Am Coll Cardiol* 1994;23:1382–1389.

50. Antman EM, Cohen M, Bernink PJ, et al. The TIMI risk score for unstable angina/non-ST elevation MI: a method for prognostication and therapeutic decision making. *JAMA* 2000;284:835–842.

51. Udelson JE, Beshansky JR, Selker HP. Sestamibi imaging to triage patients with acute chest pain. *JAMA* 2003;289:1381–1382.

52. Varetto T, Cantalupi D, Altieri A, et al. Emergency room technetium-99m sestamibi imaging to rule out acute myocardial ischemic events

in patients with nondiagnostic electrocardiograms. *J Am Coll Cardiol* 1993;22:1804–1808.

53. Ryan TJ, Antman EM, Brooks NH, et al. 1999 update: ACC/AHA guidelines for the management of patients with acute myocardial infarction. A report of the American College of Cardiology/American Heart Association Task Force on Practice Guidelines (Committee on Management of Acute Myocardial Infarction). *J Am Coll Cardiol* 1999;34:890–911.

54. Braunwald E, Antman E, Beasley J, et al. ACC/AHA 2002 guideline update for the management of patients with unstable angina and non-ST-segment elevation myocardial infarction—summary article. A report of the American College of Cardiology/American Heart Association task force on practice guidelines (Committee on the Management of Patients With Unstable Angina). *J Am Coll Cardiol* 2002;40:1366.

55. Ryan TJ, Anderson JL, Antman EM, et al. ACC/AHA guidelines for the management of patients with acute myocardial infarction: executive summary. A report of the American College of Cardiology/American Heart Association Task Force on Practice Guidelines (Committee on Management of Acute Myocardial Infarction) *Circulation* 1996;94:2341–2350.

56. Dwyer EM Jr, Greenberg H, Case RD. Association between transient pulmonary congestion during acute myocardial infarction and high incidence of death in six months. *Am J Cardiol* 1986;58:900–905.

57. Stone GW, Griffin B, Shah PK, et al. Prevalence of unsuspected mitral regurgitation and left ventricular diastolic dysfunction in patients with coronary artery disease and acute pulmonary edema associated with normal or depressed left ventricular systolic function. *Am J Cardiol* 1991;67:37–41.

58. Zimetbaum PJ, Josephson ME. Use of the electrocardiogram in acute myocardial infarction. *N Engl J Med* 2003;348:933–940.

59. Benhorin J, Moss AJ, Oakes D, et al. The prognostic significance of first myocardial infarction type (Q wave versus non-Q wave) and Q wave location. The Multicenter Diltiazem Post-Infarction Research Group. *J Am Coll Cardiol* 1990;15:1201–1207.

60. Mikell FL, Petrovich J, Snyder MC, et al. Reliability of Q-wave formation and QRS score in predicting regional and global left ventricular performance in acute myocardial infarction with successful reperfusion. *Am J Cardiol* 1986;57:923–926.

61. Roubin GS, Shen WF, Kelly DT, et al. The QRS scoring system for estimating myocardial infarct size: clinical, angiographic and prognostic correlations. *J Am Coll Cardiol* 1983;2:38–44.

62. Lehmann KG, Francis CK, Dodge HT. Mitral regurgitation in early myocardial infarction. Incidence, clinical detection, and prognostic implications. TIMI Study Group. *Ann Intern Med* 1992;117:10–17.

63. Tcheng JE, Jackman JD Jr, Nelson CL, et al. Outcome of patients sustaining acute ischemic mitral regurgitation during myocardial infarction. *Ann Intern Med* 1992;117:18–24.

64. Leor J, Feinberg MS, Vered Z, et al. Effect of thrombolytic therapy on the evolution of significant mitral regurgitation in patients with a first inferior myocardial infarction. *J Am Coll Cardiol* 1993;21:1661–1666.

65. Koren G, Weiss AT, Ben-David Y, et al. Bradycardia and hypotension following reperfusion with streptokinase (Bezold-Jarisch reflex): a sign of coronary thrombolysis and myocardial salvage. *Am Heart J* 1986;112:468–471.

66. Berger PB, Ruocco NA Jr, Ryan TJ, et al. Incidence and prognostic implications of heart block complicating inferior myocardial infarction treated with thrombolytic therapy: results from TIMI II. *J Am Coll Cardiol* 1992;20:533–540.

67. Goldberg RJ, Zevallos JC, Yarzebski J, et al. Prognosis of acute myocardial infarction complicated by complete heart block (the Worcester Heart Attack Study). *Am J Cardiol* 1992;69:1135–1141.

68. Lamas GA, Muller JE, Turi ZG, et al. A simplified method to predict occurrence of complete heart block during acute myocardial infarction. *Am J Cardiol* 1986;57:1213–1219.

69. Goldberg RJ, Gore JM, Haffajee CI, et al. Outcome after cardiac arrest during acute myocardial infarction. *Am J Cardiol* 1987;59:251–255.

70. Mont L, Cinca J, Blanch P, et al. Predisposing factors and prognostic value of sustained monomorphic ventricular tachycardia in the early phase of acute myocardial infarction. *J Am Coll Cardiol* 1996;28:1670–1676.

71. Volpi A, Cavalli A, Santoro L, et al. Incidence and prognosis of early primary ventricular fibrillation in acute myocardial infarction—results of the Gruppo Italiano per lo Studio della Sopravvivenza nell'Infarto Miocardico (GISSI-2) database. *Am J Cardiol* 1998;82:265–271.

72. Volpi A, Cavalli A, Franzosi MG, et al. One-year prognosis of primary ventricular fibrillation complicating acute myocardial infarction. The GISSI (Gruppo Italiano per lo Studio della Streptochinasi nell'Infarto miocardico) Investigators. *Am J Cardiol* 1989;63:1174–1178.

73. Thompson CA, Yarzebski J, Goldberg RJ, et al. Changes over time in the incidence and case-fatality rates of primary ventricular fibrillation complicating acute myocardial infarction: perspectives from the Worcester Heart Attack Study. *Am Heart J* 2000;139:1014–1021.

74. Goldberg RJ, Gore JM, Alpert JS, et al. Cardiogenic shock after acute myocardial infarction. Incidence and mortality from a community-wide perspective, 1975 to 1988. *N Engl J Med* 1991;325:1117–1122.

75. Eysmann SB, Douglas PS. Reperfusion and revascularization strategies for coronary artery disease in women. *JAMA* 1992;268:1903–1907.

76. Tsuyuki RT, Teo KK, Ikuta RM, et al. Mortality risk and patterns of practice in 2,070 patients with acute myocardial infarction, 1987-92. Relative importance of age, sex, and medical therapy. *Chest* 1994;105:1687–1692.

77. Dittrich H, Gilpin E, Nicod P, et al. Acute myocardial infarction in women: influence of gender on mortality and prognostic variables. *Am J Cardiol* 1988;62:1–7.

78. Jenkins JS, Flaker GC, Nolte B, et al. Causes of higher in-hospital mortality in women than in men after acute myocardial infarction. *Am J Cardiol* 1994;73:319–322.

79. Tofler GH, Stone PH, Muller JE, et al. Effects of gender and race on prognosis after myocardial infarction: adverse prognosis for women, particularly black women. *J Am Coll Cardiol* 1987;9:473–482.

80. Greenland P, Reicher-Reiss H, Goldbourt U, et al. In-hospital and 1-year mortality in 1,524 women after myocardial infarction. Comparison with 4,315 men. *Circulation* 1991;83:484–491.

81. Indications for fibrinolytic therapy in suspected acute myocardial infarction: collaborative overview of early mortality and major morbidity results from all randomised trials of more than 1000 patients. Fibrinolytic Therapy Trialists' (FTT) Collaborative Group. *Lancet* 1994;343:311–322.

82. Hochman JS, Tamis JE, Thompson TD, et al. Sex, clinical presentation, and outcome in patients with acute coronary syndromes. Global Use of Strategies to Open Occluded Coronary Arteries in Acute Coronary Syndromes IIb Investigators. *N Engl J Med* 1999;341:226–232.

83. Wong SC, Sleeper LA, Monrad ES, et al. Absence of gender differences in clinical outcomes in patients with cardiogenic shock complicating acute myocardial infarction. A report from the SHOCK Trial Registry. *J Am Coll Cardiol* 2001;38:1395–1401.

84. Hochman JS, McCabe CH, Stone PH, et al. Outcome and profile of women and men presenting with acute coronary syndromes: a report from TIMI IIIB. TIMI Investigators. Thrombolysis in Myocardial Infarction. *J Am Coll Cardiol* 1997;30:141–148.

85. Shaw LJ, Miller DD, Romeis JC, et al. Gender differences in the noninvasive evaluation and management of patients with suspected coronary artery disease. *Ann Intern Med* 1994;120:559–566.

86. Maynard C, Litwin PE, Martin JS, et al. Gender differences in the treatment and outcome of acute myocardial infarction. Results from the Myocardial Infarction Triage and Intervention Registry. *Arch Intern Med* 1992;152:972–976.

87. Rathore SS, Wang Y, Radford MJ, et al. Sex differences in cardiac catheterization after acute myocardial infarction: the role of procedure appropriateness. *Ann Intern Med* 2002;137:487–493.

88. Weintraub WS, Wenger NK, Kosinski AS, et al. Percutaneous transluminal coronary angioplasty in women compared with men. *J Am Coll Cardiol* 1994;24:81–90.

89. Robertson T, Kennard ED, Mehta S, et al. Influence of gender on in-hospital clinical and angiographic outcomes and on one-year follow-up in the New Approaches to Coronary Intervention (NACI) registry. *Am J Cardiol* 1997;80:26K–39K.

90. Keelan ET, Nunez BD, Grill DE, et al. Comparison of immediate and long-term outcome of coronary angioplasty performed for unstable angina and rest pain in men and women. *Mayo Clin Proc* 1997;72:5–12.

91. Maggioni AP, Maseri A, Fresco C, et al. Age-related increase in mortality among patients with first myocardial infarctions treated with thrombolysis. The Investigators of the Gruppo Italiano per lo Studio della Sopravvivenza nell'Infarto Miocardico (GISSI-2). *N Engl J Med* 1993;329:1442–1448.

92. Pashos CL, Newhouse JP, McNeil BJ. Temporal changes in the care and outcomes of elderly patients with acute myocardial infarction, 1987 through 1990. *JAMA* 1993;270:1832–1836.

93. Rich MW, Bosner MS, Chung MK, et al. Is age an independent predictor of early and late mortality in patients with acute myocardial infarction? *Am J Med* 1992;92:7–13.

94. Smith SC Jr, Gilpin E, Ahnve S, et al. Outlook after acute myocardial infarction in the very elderly compared with that in patients aged 65 to 75 years. *J Am Coll Cardiol* 1990;16:784–792.

95. Maggioni AP, Franzosi MG, Santoro E, et al. The risk of stroke in patients with acute myocardial infarction after thrombolytic and antithrombotic treatment. Gruppo Italiano per lo Studio della Sopravvivenza nell'Infarto Miocardico II (GISSI-2), and The International Study Group. *N Engl J Med* 1992;327:1–6.

96. Rogers WJ, Bowlby LJ, Chandra NC, et al. Treatment of myocardial infarction in the United States (1990 to 1993). Observations from the National Registry of Myocardial Infarction. *Circulation* 1994;90:2103–2114.

97. Weaver WD, Litwin PE, Martin JS, et al. Effect of age on use of thrombolytic therapy and mortality in acute myocardial infarction. The MITI Project Group. *J Am Coll Cardiol* 1991;18:657–662.

98. Peterson ED, Jollis JG, Bebchuk JD, et al. Changes in mortality after myocardial revascularization in the elderly. The national Medicare experience. *Ann Intern Med* 1994;121:919–927.

99. Nasser TK, Fry ET, Annan K, et al. Comparison of six-month outcome of coronary artery stenting in patients <65, 65-75, and >75 years of age. *Am J Cardiol* 1997;80:998–1001.

100. Haffner SM, Lehto S, Ronnemaa T, et al. Mortality from coronary heart disease in subjects with type 2 diabetes and in nondiabetic subjects with and without prior myocardial infarction. *N Engl J Med* 1998;339:229–234.

101. Cho E, Rimm EB, Stampfer MJ, et al. The impact of diabetes mellitus and prior myocardial infarction on mortality from all causes and from coronary heart disease in men. *J Am Coll Cardiol* 2002;40:954–960.

102. Beckman JA, Creager MA, Libby P. Diabetes and atherosclerosis: epidemiology, pathophysiology, and management. *JAMA* 2002;287:2570–2581.

103. Barbash GI, White HD, Modan M, et al. Significance of diabetes mellitus in patients with acute myocardial infarction receiving thrombolytic therapy. Investigators of the International Tissue Plasminogen Activator/Streptokinase Mortality Trial. *J Am Coll Cardiol* 1993;22:707–713.

104. Zuanetti G, Latini R, Maggioni AP, et al. Influence of diabetes on mortality in acute myocardial infarction: data from the GISSI-2 study. *J Am Coll Cardiol* 1993;22:1788–1794.

105. Solomon SD, St John Sutton M, Lamas GA, et al. Ventricular remodeling does not accompany the development of heart failure in diabetic patients after myocardial infarction. *Circulation* 2002;106:1251–1255.

106. Abraham SA, Coles NA, Coley CM, et al. Coronary risk of noncardiac surgery. *Prog Cardiovasc Dis* 1991;34:205–234.

107. Goldman L, Caldera DL, Nussbaum SR, et al. Multifactorial index of cardiac risk in noncardiac surgical procedures. *N Engl J Med* 1977;297:845–850.

108. Eagle KA, Coley CM, Newell JB, et al. Combining clinical and thallium data optimizes preoperative assessment of cardiac risk before major vascular surgery. *Ann Intern Med* 1989;110:859–866.

109. Wong T, Detsky AS. Preoperative cardiac risk assessment for patients having peripheral vascular surgery. *Ann Intern Med* 1992;116:743–753.

110. Mangano DT, Browner WS, Hollenberg M, et al. Association of perioperative myocardial ischemia with cardiac morbidity and mortality in men undergoing noncardiac surgery. The Study of Perioperative Ischemia Research Group. *N Engl J Med* 1990;323:1781–1788.

111. Adams JE 3rd, Sicard GA, Allen BT, et al. Diagnosis of perioperative myocardial infarction with measurement of cardiac troponin I. *N Engl J Med* 1994;330:670–674.

112. Lange RA, Hillis LD. Cardiovascular complications of cocaine use. *N Engl J Med* 2001;345:351–358.

113. Moliterno DJ, Lange RA, Gerard RD, et al. Influence of intranasal cocaine on plasma constituents associated with endogenous thrombosis and thrombolysis. *Am J Med* 1994;96:492–496.

114. Brogan WC 3rd, Lange RA, Kim AS, et al. Alleviation of cocaine-induced coronary vasoconstriction by nitroglycerin. *J Am Coll Cardiol* 1991;18:581–586.

115. Om A, Warner M, Sabri N, et al. Frequency of coronary artery disease and left ventricle dysfunction in cocaine users. *Am J Cardiol* 1992;69:1549–1552.

116. Minor RL Jr, Scott BD, Brown DD, et al. Cocaine-induced myocardial infarction in patients with normal coronary arteries. *Ann Intern Med* 1991;115:797–806.

117. Chakko S, Fernandez A, Mellman TA, et al. Cardiac manifestations of cocaine abuse: a cross-sectional study of asymptomatic men with a history of long-term abuse of "crack" cocaine. *J Am Coll Cardiol* 1992;20:1168–1174.

118. Hollander JE, Shih RD, Hoffman RS, et al. Predictors of coronary artery disease in patients with cocaine-associated myocardial infarction. Cocaine-Associated Myocardial Infarction (CAMI) Study Group. *Am J Med* 1997;102:158–163.

119. Amin M, Gabelman G, Karpel J, et al. Acute myocardial infarction and chest pain syndromes after cocaine use. *Am J Cardiol* 1990;66:1434–1437.

120. Weber JE, Shofer FS, Larkin GL, et al. Validation of a brief observation period for patients with cocaine-associated chest pain. *N Engl J Med* 2003;348:510–517.

CHAPTER 60

The Role of Echocardiography

Joseph F. Malouf

Key Words: Coronary artery disease; echocardiography; myocardial infarction.

INTRODUCTION

Two-dimensional Doppler echocardiography is widely used in the evaluation of patients with coronary artery disease (1). Rapid identification of the effects of myocardial ischemia or infarction on both regional and global left ventricular function can be performed by imaging the entire myocardium in real time from multiple tomographic planes (1), thus facilitating therapeutic decision-making, as well as providing prognostic information. In patients with unstable hemodynamics, two-dimensional and Doppler echocardiography can rapidly identify the underlying cause so that appropriate interventions can be undertaken (1). Analysis of intracardiac flow velocities by Doppler echocardiography allows measurement of hemodynamic variables, such as cardiac output and left ventricular filling pressures, thus usually obviating the need for invasive hemodynamic monitoring (1). Technologic innovations, including tissue Doppler and myocardial contrast echocardiography, have opened "new windows" for the assessment of left ventricular function and myocardial viability (1). The purpose of this chapter is to review the cur-

rent and future role of echocardiography in the evaluation and management of patients with coronary artery disease in general and myocardial infarction (MI) in particular.

ECHOCARDIOGRAPHIC ASSESSMENT OF REGIONAL AND GLOBAL LEFT VENTRICULAR FUNCTION

Resting left ventricular size and systolic function are the most important outcome predictors in patients with coronary artery disease (2,3). In the past, the reference standard for determination of left ventricular size and function was quantitative left ventriculography. However, this method has the inherent limitations of any invasive technique, including discomfort and risk to the patient. Radionuclide angiography is a noninvasive method for examining left ventricular size and function, but it is limited to evaluation of endocardial motion. Two-dimensional echocardiography has become the imaging modality of choice for assessment of left ventricular size and both regional and global left ventricular systolic function, because of its ability to noninvasively visualize endocardial motion and myocardial thickening (1).

Regional Wall Motion Analysis

The heart is not fixed in the chest cavity, and thus moves relative to the echo transducer. Both translation and rotation of

J. F. Malouf: Division of Cardiovascular Diseases, Gonda 6-411, Mayo Clinic, 200 First St. SW, Rochester, Minnesota 55905.

the heart occur throughout the cardiac cycle, and there is temporal and spatial heterogeneity of contraction in the normal heart (4,5). These inherent characteristics of cardiac motion and contractility create difficulties in applying a quantitative computer model for the detection of abnormalities of endocardial motion or wall thickening.

Subjective visual interpretation of regional wall motion abnormalities on two-dimensional echocardiography by an experienced echocardiographer overcomes many of the problems inherent in computer analysis. Endocardial borders that are not readily apparent on still-frame images can be seen better on real-time images. Visual interpretation incorporates the degree of myocardial thickening and endocardial motion and compares favorably with cineangiography (6,7) and radionuclide angiography (8). The thinned and calcified appearance of an old transmural infarction is thus readily apparent. A major limitation of two-dimensional echocardiography is the inability to visualize all segments of the myocardium in patients with poor acoustic windows (e.g., obesity, lung disease, chest deformities, and breast implants). Advances in ultrasound image acquisition, including second harmonic imaging (Fig. 60–1) and contrast echocardiography (Fig. 60–2), have markedly enhanced endocardial definition (1).

A wall motion score index is used to obtain a semiquantitative estimate of the extent of wall motion abnormality and, hence, severity of global systolic dysfunction. (1). This method consists of dividing the myocardium into segments and then assigning each segment a score depending on the absence, presence, and severity of regional abnormality. The wall motion score index is thus the mean of sum of all the individual segment scores. The American Society of Echocardiography has published a standardized nomenclature for determining a wall motion score index (1). In this well accepted model the left ventricle is divided into 16 segments (6

at the basal level, 6 at the midpapillary muscle level, and 4 at the apical level). Each segment is assigned a score from 1 to 5 as follows: 1, normal; 2, hypokinesis; 3, severe hypokinesis or akinesis; 4, dyskinesis; and 5, aneurysm. The wall motion score index is the arithmetic mean of the segment scores (Fig. 60–3). Thus, a normally contracting left ventricle would have a wall motion score index of 1, and a wall motion score index greater than 2 is indicative of a large area of contractile dysfunction (1). Transmural infarction of the myocardium can be recognized on two-dimensional echocardiography by akinesis of the involved region. However, akinesis may also be observed during ischemia or after nontransmural (non–Q-wave) MI, because myocardial contractility ceases when greater than 20% of myocardial thickness is affected (9). The wall motion score index is a more accurate descriptor of left ventricular function in patients with coronary artery disease than is the global ejection fraction, because of the segmental changes that exist in this disease (7). In experienced laboratories, the wall motion score index is a reproducible measurement with acceptable intraobserver and interobserver variability.

A major technologic advance in the echocardiographic assessment of wall motion abnormalities has been the development of digital imaging (1). Most commonly, 8 frames per systolic cycle are captured at 50-millisecond intervals. These can then be stored and displayed in a side-by-side or quad-screen format allowing visualization of multiple views and comparison of rest and stress images. Moreover, side-by-side comparison of digital images allows for serial follow-up including assessment of adequacy of medical or catheter-based intervention. Digital imaging will soon become the standard technique for storing and displaying two-dimensional echocardiographic images. Evolving techniques for assessment of regional myocardial function include tissue Doppler imaging

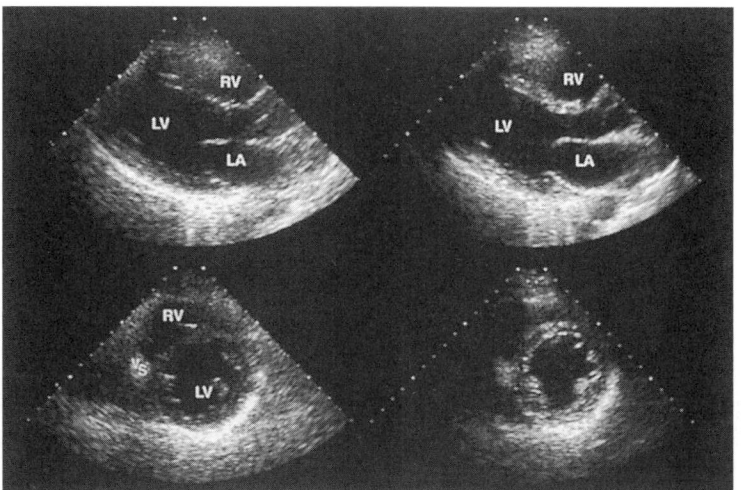

FIG. 60–1. Demonstration of better visualization of the left ventricular *(LV)* endocardial border by native harmonic imaging. Parasternal long-axis views **(top panels)** and short-axis views **(bottom panels)** were scanned by fundamental imaging (2.5 MHz; **left panels)** and by native harmonic imaging **(right panels)** for comparison. LA, left atrium; RV, right ventricle; VS, ventricular septum. (Courtesy of Mayo Foundation, Rochester, MN.)

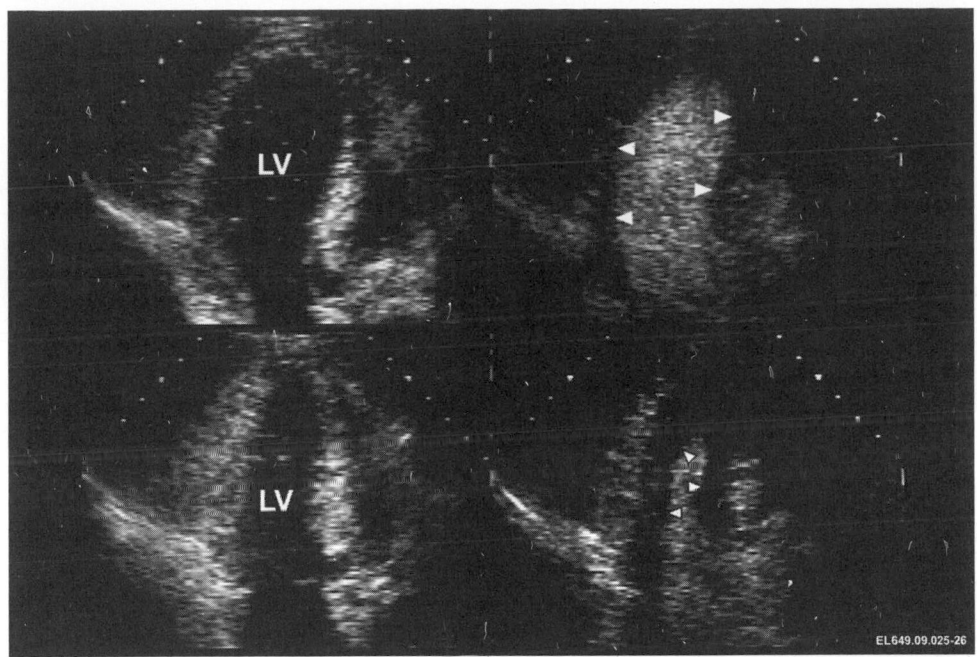

FIG. 60–2. Apical long-axis views of the left ventricle *(LV)* in diastole **(top)** and systole **(bottom)** showing markedly enhanced endocardial definition *(arrowheads)* after administration of a contrast agent (Definity Health, St. Louis Park, MN).

(1,10–13), color kinesis (1,14), automated border detection (1,15), and strain rate imaging (13). With tissue Doppler imaging (Fig. 60–4) (see color insert), recording of the low *myocardial* velocities is possible. Color coding allows appreciation of the contractility and direction of motion of the various myocardial segments. Thus, whereas a bright color is assigned to normally contracting segments, the absence of color is indicative of akinesis. Color kinesis (Fig. 60–5) (see color insert) and automated border detection (Fig. 60–6) provide real-time display of LV *endocardial* motion. Major limitations include poor endocardial definition and translational motion of the heart. Strain rate imaging (Fig. 60–7) (see color insert) depicts regional deformation and is less susceptible to cardiac translation and tethering (13). The acoustic properties of ischemic or infarcted myocardium are altered either as a result of collagen deposition or decreased perfusion (16). Tissue characterization techniques can detect these altered acoustic properties. Although still largely an investigational tool, tissue characterization has been used to identify abnormal myocardium in humans after MI (16).

Stress Echocardiography

Stress (exercise or pharmacologic) echocardiography has become a well accepted diagnostic method for evaluating patients with coronary artery disease (1). The basic premise of stress echocardiography is simple: Stress-induced ischemia results in regional wall motion abnormalities that precede the onset of symptoms and electrocardiographic changes (17). Stress-induced increase in left ventricular end-systolic volume, decrease in global systolic function, or both, in the ab-

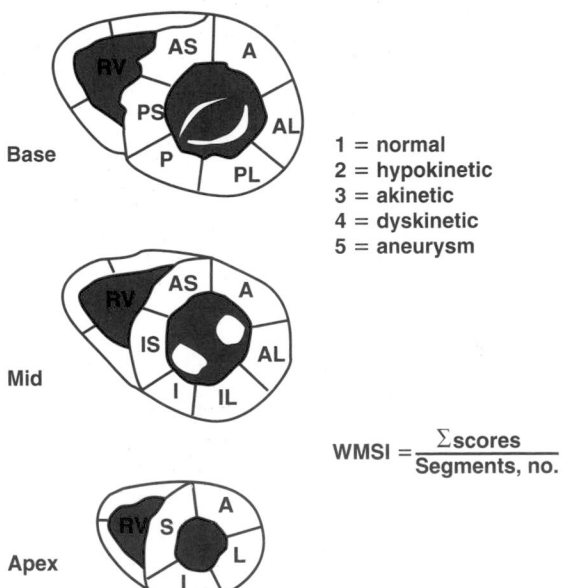

1 = normal
2 = hypokinetic
3 = akinetic
4 = dyskinetic
5 = aneurysm

$$WMSI = \frac{\Sigma\, scores}{Segments,\ no.}$$

FIG. 60–3. Determination of the wall motion score index (WMSI). The left ventricle is divided into 16 segments, as suggested by the American Society of Echocardiography. There are six segments at the basal level, six segments at the midlevel, and four segments at the apex. Each segment is assigned a score of 1 to 5. The WMSI is the arithmetic mean of the individual scores. A, anterior; AL, anterolateral; AS, anteroseptal; P, posterior; PL, posterolateral; PS, posteroseptal; RV, right ventricle; WMSI, wall motion score index. (Modified from the American Society of Echocardiography Committee on Standards, Subcommittee on Quantitation of Two-Dimensional Echocardiograms, by permission of the American Society of Echocardiography.) (See color insert for Figs. 60–4 and 60–5.)

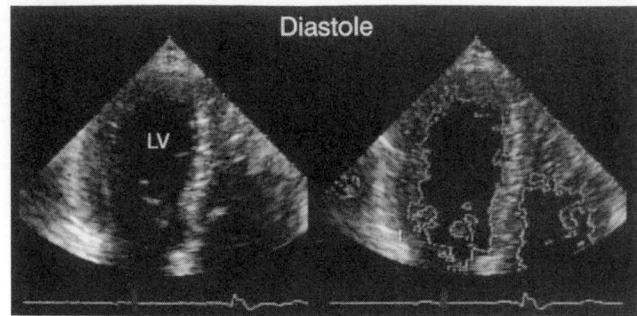
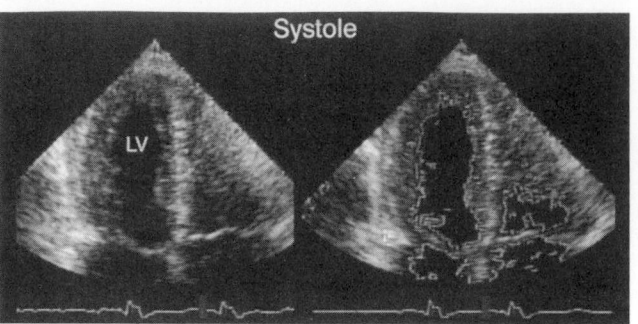

FIG. 60–6. A,B: Ultrasound backscatter differs markedly between the myocardium and intracavitary blood pool. Therefore, the endocardial border is defined where a greater than preestablished threshold difference in backscatter is identified. The borders are identified and *dotted*. Connection of the endocardial dots creates an endocardial border in real time throughout the cardiac cycle. LV, left ventricle. (Courtesy of Mayo Foundation, Rochester, MN.) (See color insert for Fig. 60–7.)

sence of a marked hypertensive response, are indicative of severe ischemia and multivessel disease (1,18). The sensitivity and specificity of stress echocardiography compare favorably with those of thallium or sestamibi stress testing for the diagnosis of coronary artery disease (1,19). The basal inferior wall and basal inferior interventricular septum are the two most difficult regions to evaluate for wall motion abnormalities because of their unique geometry. Tissue Doppler imaging of these two segments may be helpful in differentiating normal from ischemic or infarcted myocardium (11).

Global Left Ventricular Function Analysis

Multiple methods for measuring left ventricular volume and ejection fraction have been proposed. These have consisted of extrapolations from M-mode measurements, visual estimates, and, most recently, quantitative two-dimensional echocardiography. The M-mode measurements provide an "ice pick" view of the heart at the midcavitary level only. Although these M-mode measurements may be of benefit in evaluating patients with normally contracting myocardium and in those with diffuse global hypokinesis, they are of little value in patients with multiple regional wall motion abnormalities. Visual assessment of left ventricular function (normal or hyperdynamic vs. mild to severely depressed) and visual estimates of the left ventricular ejection fraction can be provided by experienced echocardiographers and compare favorably with cineangiography. However, visual estimate of the ejection fraction is not sensitive enough to detect subtle changes that may occur in global left ventricular systolic function after an event or intervention.

Quantitative two-dimensional echocardiography has been made possible by such technologic advances as digital imaging, online cineloop capabilities, and online computer software. By storing echocardiographic views in either a digital format or on a cineloop, echocardiographers are able to trace accurately the endocardial borders in systole and end-diastole. By applying mathematical formulas to the traced endocardial circumferences, the end-systolic volume, end-diastolic vol-

ume, and ejection fraction can be calculated. The American Society of Echocardiography (1) recommends the modified Simpson method to estimate ventricular volume from two orthogonal apical views (Fig. 60–8). With this formula, the true left ventricular volume is slightly underestimated, probably related to foreshortening of the apex. Real-time automatic border detection of the left ventricular endocardium (Fig. 60–6) is another quantitative method that takes advantage of the marked differences in ultrasound backscatter properties of myocardium and blood (1). A major limitation for all volumetric techniques remains adequate endocardial border definition.

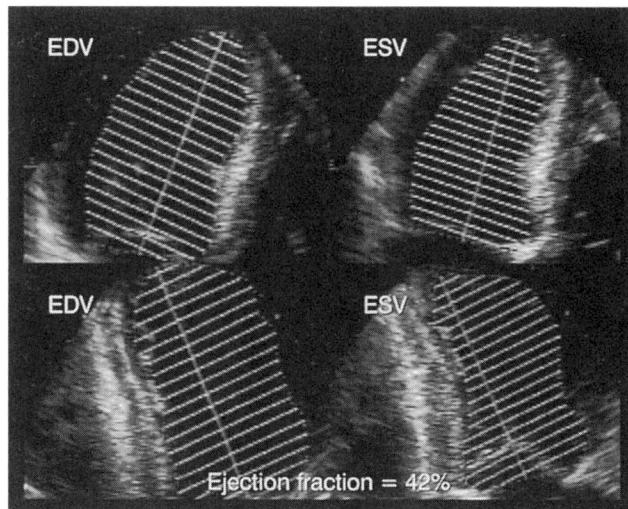

FIG. 60–8. Still frames of two orthogonal views (apical four-chamber **[top]** and apical two-chamber **[bottom]** views) to calculate the left ventricular *(LV)* volume and ejection fraction using a modified Simpson method. End-diastolic *(EDV)* and end-systolic *(ESV)* frames illustrate 20 cylinders (disks) of equal height. When the endocardial border and the long-axis (vertical line to the short-axis lines) are identified, a fixed number of cylinders are created, and the volumes of the cylinders are summed to estimate ventricular volume. (Courtesy of Mayo Foundation, Rochester, MN.)

Hemodynamic Assessment

Knowledge of the hemodynamic state of the left ventricle is essential for treatment of unstable patients with acute myocardial infarction (AMI). The development several decades ago of the balloon-tipped flotation catheter provided the ability to measure both left ventricular filling pressures and cardiac output from catheterization of the right side of the heart at the bedside. Hemodynamic subsets emerged from these measurements and formed the basis for institution of proper treatment options (20). However, catheterization of the right side of the heart has its own inherent risks (21) and causes discomfort to the patient.

Echo–Doppler assessment of intracardiac hemodynamics is now readily feasible. The accuracy of Doppler-derived measurements of the cardiac output and pulmonary artery systolic pressure has been validated (1). Doppler-derived mitral flow velocity curves are invaluable for diastolic function assessment because they reflect changes in loading conditions, relaxation, and compliance of the left ventricle. Thus, the early rapid filling phase (E in Fig. 60–9) and late postatrial (A in Fig. 60–9) contraction mitral flow velocities reflect the corresponding transmitral pressure gradients (1). The interval from the peak of the E velocity to its nadir corresponds to the time required for equilibration of left atrial and left ventricular pressures during early diastole and is referred to as the deceleration time (Fig. 60–9). Doppler-derived pulmonary vein velocities and early diastolic mitral annular velocity provide incremental information regarding left ventricular filling (1). The hemodynamic information obtained by echo–Doppler techniques is invaluable for the treatment of critically ill patients and frequently obviates the need for right heart catheterization.

Echocardiography as a Prognostic Tool

The information provided by stress echocardiography in patients with known or suspected coronary artery disease may have significant prognostic implications (7,22–27). The location (for example, left anterior descending distribution) (27) and extent and severity of stress-induced left ventricular dysfunction (25) have been reported to have an independent and incremental predictive value for subsequent hard cardiac events (death or nonfatal MI). Moreover, in patients with multivessel disease, functional assessment of disease severity by stress echocardiography may be a better predictor of adverse events than anatomic assessment using angiography (22).

Numerous studies have shown that the wall motion score index has prognostic value in patients with AMI (28) and in the posthospital phase after MI (8,29–31). After MI, however, the extent of wall motion abnormality visualized on two-dimensional echocardiography may overestimate the true area of infarction (32). This may be because of a "tethering" effect in which the infarcted muscle fibers act as parallel mechanical resistors to impede contraction of the adjacent normal segments (33) or residual ischemia involving the border segments of the infarcted zone. Early detection of regional wall motion abnormalities by two-dimensional echocardiography is predictive of future cardiac events or the need for revascularization in patients with acute chest pain and a nondiagnostic electrocardiogram and may be superior to cardiac enzyme markers (34).

Resting left ventricular ejection fraction is a key determinant of prognosis after MI (2). In patients with an ejection fraction less than 40%, the left ventricular size and specifically end-systolic volume provide additive prognostic value. The finding of left ventricular systolic dysfunction on two-dimensional echocardiography in patients presenting to the emergency department for cardiac-related symptoms was shown to be predictive of a sixfold increased incidence of early events and a fourfold increased incidence of late events (35). Compared with the clinical history and electrocardiogram, echocardiographic data provided incremental prognostic information (35). With the availability of digital technology, two-dimensional echocardiography has become an ideal method for serial quantitative measurement of left ventricular volumes and ejection fraction (1). Two-dimensional echocardiographic measurement of left ventricular volumes and ejection fraction between 3 and 5 days after infarction is highly predictive of early and late mortality, especially when combined with clinical variables (36,37). The measurement of left ventricular volume within several days after infarction correlates with the follow-up volume measured at 1 year (38). Doppler-derived myocardial performance indices have been shown to be predictive of cardiac events after MI (39,40).

Two-dimensional echocardiography and Doppler assessment of left ventricular diastolic function in patients with

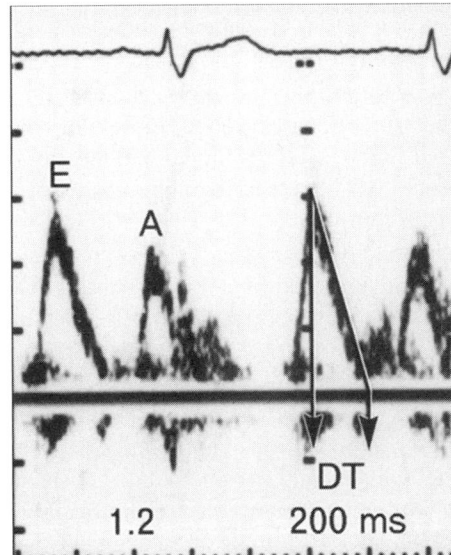

FIG. 60–9. Normal mitral inflow Doppler signal. A, late filling wave due to atrial contraction; DT, deceleration time; E, early rapid filling wave. (Courtesy of Mayo Foundation, Rochester, MN.)

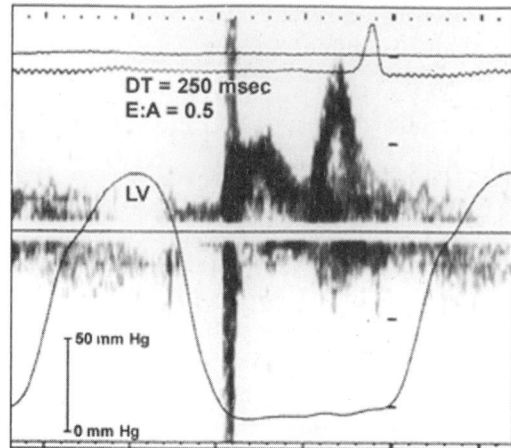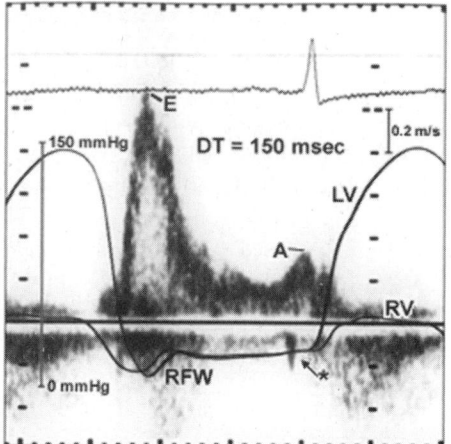

FIG. 60–10. Actual intracardiac pressure tracings and corresponding diastolic Doppler recordings of mitral inflow velocities. **Left:** Typical abnormal left ventricular relaxation pattern characterized by prolonged deceleration time (DT), decreased E velocity, increased A velocity and E/A ratio less than 1. **Right:** Typical restrictive left ventricular diastolic filling pattern characterized by shortened DT, increased E velocity, decreased A velocity, and E/A ratio greater than 2. LV, left ventricle; RFW, rapid filling wave; RV, right ventricle. (Courtesy of Dr. Rick A. Nishimura, Mayo Clinic, Rochester, MN.)

coronary artery disease also can have important prognostic implications. Three abnormal diastolic filling patterns have been identified: abnormal relaxation, pseudonormal, and restrictive (1) (Fig. 60–10). They are associated with progressive increase in the mean left ventricular diastolic pressure and pulmonary artery systolic pressure (1). In patients with severe left ventricular systolic dysfunction undergoing coronary artery bypass graft surgery, restrictive left ventricular diastolic dysfunction is a strong predictor of perioperative morbidity and mortality and lack of significant improvement in left ventricular systolic function (41). Restrictive left ventricular filling may also be the single best predictor of in-hospital heart failure or cardiac death after MI and adds significantly to clinical and echocardiographic markers of systolic dysfunction (42–44). After AMI, pseudonormal and restrictive filling patterns are associated with greater infarct size and lower left ventricular ejection fraction. Exercise capacity is reduced regardless of severity of left ventricular diastolic dysfunction, even when systolic function is preserved (45).

Infarct expansion and remodeling occur after transmural MI and have clinically important prognostic implications. Infarct expansion occurs within minutes after the onset of MI (46). The length of an infarct segment can expand as much as 65%. Accordingly, regional dilatation followed by progressive global left ventricular dilatation and systolic dysfunction may occur; such progression portends a poor prognosis (47,48). Visual assessment of the myocardium with two-dimensional echocardiography is unable to identify subtle early changes of infarct expansion but can readily assess the later changes of regional wall thinning and dilatation that occur days to weeks after MI (49). Two-dimensional echocardiography may also be useful in assessing the impact of early drug intervention on postinfarc-

tion left ventricular remodeling (50). Small non–Q-wave (nontransmural) MIs may not be detected as visible wall motion abnormalities (51). Imaging advances including tissue Doppler imaging (1,10–13), strain rate imaging (13), automated border detection (1,15), and color kinesis (1,14) may prove to be clinically useful for assessing subtle regional wall motion abnormalities.

ROLE OF ECHOCARDIOGRAPHY IN ACUTE MYOCARDIAL INFARCTION IN THE REPERFUSION ERA

Mega trials have convincingly shown that timely restoration of coronary blood flow in patients with AMI significantly decreases mortality (52,53). The method of reperfusion and the optimal agent are discussed elsewhere in this textbook and are therefore not considered further in this chapter. However, with the need to institute rapid therapy in patients with suspected MI, echocardiography has assumed a new and prominent role.

The decision to proceed with reperfusion therapy (thrombolytics or catheter-based intervention) during AMI is contingent on establishing a correct diagnosis of MI and the anticipated benefits are a direct function of the amount of myocardium at risk. In patients with chest pain and nonspecific ST-/T-wave changes or uninterpretable electrocardiograms caused by conduction abnormalities or paced rhythm, echocardiography can aid in the rapid diagnosis of MI (54). In patients with unambiguous electrocardiographic changes of AMI, the site and magnitude of ST-segment changes may be a poor indicator of the amount of myocardium at risk (55). The degree of wall motion abnormality on a two-dimensional echocardiographic study, in contrast, provides a direct assessment of the amount of myocardium at risk.

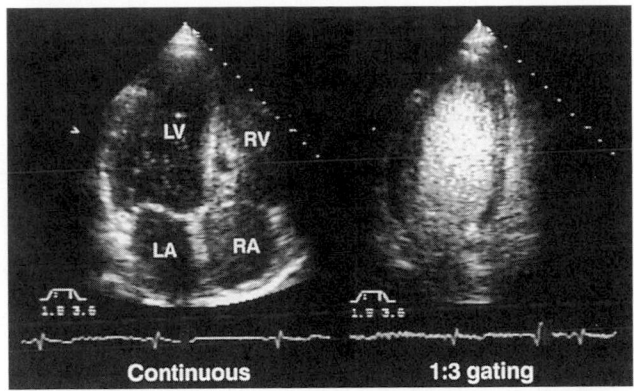

FIG. 60–11. Apical four-chamber view of second harmonic imaging during infusion of perfluorocarbon-exposed sonicated dextrose albumin (PESDA). **Left:** Continuous imaging shows contrast in the right heart chambers but not much in the left ventricular (LV) cavity and myocardium. **Right:** 1:3 Gating transient-response imaging shows contrast in the ventricular septum and lateral myocardium, as well as in the LV cavity. LA, left atrium; RA, right atrium; RV, right ventricle. (Courtesy of Mayo Foundation, Rochester, MN.)

Prompt intervention must be considered if there is a large amount of myocardium at risk. Alternatively, if there is a small region of wall motion abnormality or no wall motion abnormality, the patient may not benefit from acute reperfusion therapy or the risks of any intervention will likely outweigh the potential benefits, or both. Other causes of chest pain (e.g., aortic dissection, pericarditis, and pulmonary embolism) that mimic MI may be rapidly diagnosed with two-dimensional echocardiography (1).

Myocardial contrast echocardiography may soon prove to be a clinically useful bedside technique for the assessment of the myocardium at risk during AMI (1,56–59). With this technique, highly echo-reflective microbubbles can be injected into a peripheral vein. These microbubbles then enter the right side of the heart, pulmonary circulation, and left side of the heart and eventually flow through the coronary arteries. As they traverse the intramyocardial microvascular beds, they produce enhancement of the myocardium on two-dimensional echocardiography (Fig. 60–11). Myocardial contrast echocardiography can be used to predict the ultimate infarct size at the time of coronary occlusion (60–62). The area of contrast enhancement seen on echocardiography after direct injection into a coronary vessel defines its true perfusion zone (60). In the presence of a completely occluded coronary artery, the total area at risk can be measured directly from the area not enhanced by the contrast agent. The microbubbles used are small enough to act like red blood cells and not get trapped in arterioles, therefore there is no adverse hemodynamic change from capillary blockage (63,64).

MYOCARDIAL VIABILITY

The detection of viable myocardium has important therapeutic and prognostic implications (64). Viable myocardium can be either hibernating or stunned (1). The former refers to dysfunctional myocardium caused by down-regulation of function in response to chronic ischemia. Recovery of contractile function is expected after revascularization (catheter-based or surgical). The latter refers to persistence of regional abnormalities despite adequate reperfusion of the occluded artery. Recovery of function occurs with time.

There are simple echocardiographic clues to the presence of viable myocardium. Preserved wall thickness of the dysfunctional segment indicates viability (1). In contrast, a segment that is thin and echo-dense is considered scarred (1), and an end-diastolic wall thickness less than 6 mm excludes the potential for recovery of function in hibernating segments (65). Other viability indicators include left ventricular dysfunction that is disproportionate to infarct size as assessed by cardiac enzymes or perfusion defect size and absence of restrictive left ventricular diastolic filling in patients with ischemic cardiomyopathy (66).

Viable myocardium, whether stunned or hibernating, demonstrates increased contractility in response to low or inotropic doses of dobutamine (1) (Fig. 60–12). However, in response to high or chronotropic doses of dobutamine, viable myocardium can have one of two responses (1) (Fig. 60–12). In the first response, there is sustained and improved contractility of the dysfunctional myocardial segment if the coronary artery that supplies that segment is patent, as occurs after thrombolysis. In the second response, a biphasic response is observed. This is characterized by initial improvement in contractility with low doses of dobutamine followed by deterioration in function with high doses of dobutamine in the case of hibernating myocardium or if there is a flow-limiting residual stenosis in the infarct-related artery after thrombolysis (1). Dobutamine stress echocardiography is reliable in predicting recovery of viable myocardium even after delayed revascularization (67). Compared with positron emission tomography, the currently accepted "gold standard" for the detection of viable myocardium and thallium perfusion imag-

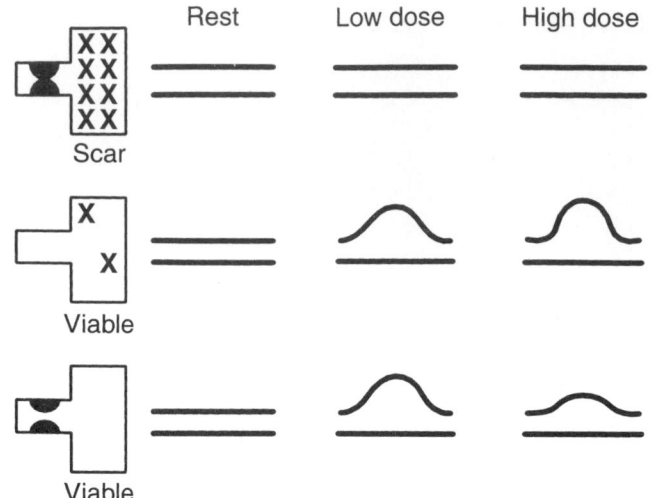

Rest   Low dose   High dose

Scar

Viable

Viable

FIG. 60–12. Myocardial response to a low dose and a high dose of dobutamine in three different clinical scenarios, with resting akinetic segment. **Top:** When myocardium is scarred, with no myocardial viability, there is no myocardial thickening at rest with either a low dose or a high dose of dobutamine. **Middle:** If myocardium is viable with no stenosis of the coronary artery subtending the akinetic myocardium, myocardial contractility increases continuously with low and high doses of dobutamine. **Bottom:** If the myocardium is viable but the coronary artery that supplies the myocardium is severely stenotic, myocardial contractility improves initially with low-dose dobutamine but worsens with high doses. This is a typical biphasic response. (Courtesy of Mayo Foundation, Rochester, MN.)

ing, dobutamine stress echocardiography appears to be less sensitive but more specific (68,69). For patients able to exercise, low-level exercise echocardiography is comparable to low-dose dobutamine stress echocardiography for detecting contractile reserve and predicting reversible dysfunction after AMI (70,71). The presence of myocardial viability early after AMI is predictive of recurrent in-hospital ischemic events and unstable angina after discharge (72). Tissue characterization and tissue Doppler imaging may allow rapid estimation of the transmural extent of viable myocardium after reperfusion for AMI (73,74).

An intact microvascular circulation is at the very foundation of myocardial viability. Through sequential enhancement of the endocardium and myocardium, myocardial contrast echocardiography allows for the simultaneous assessment of the extent of microvascular integrity and corresponding regional myocardial contractility in real time (1,75). After reperfusion for AMI, homogenous myocardial contrast opacification predicts the presence of contractile reserve in akinetic segments (Figs. 60–13 and 60–14). In contrast, the lack of myocardial contrast enhancement is indicative of extensive myocardial necrosis and microcirculatory damage ("no-reflow phenomenon") and portends a poor outcome for the affected segment (76,77) (Fig. 60–15). Assessment of both the size of the area at risk during AMI and microvascular integrity soon after thrombolytics or catheter-based intervention allows better determination of the efficacy of reperfusion therapy (78,79). However, myocardial

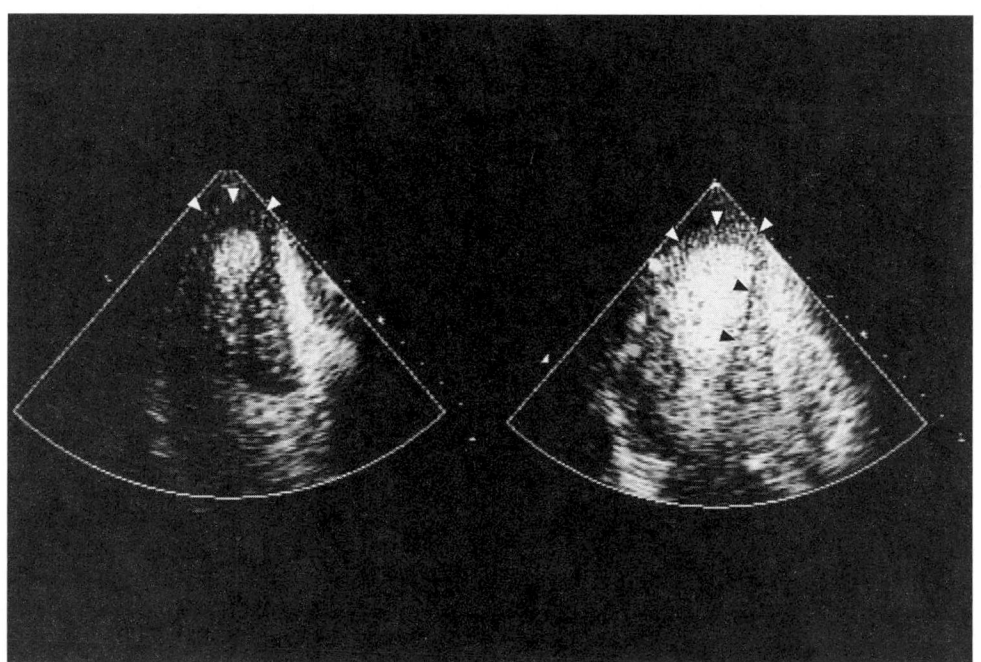

FIG. 60–13. Apical four-chamber view in a patient with acute apical myocardial infarction treated with thrombolytic therapy. **Left:** Contrast (Optison; Amersham, Princeton, NJ) is initially seen in the right and left ventricular cavities but not left ventricular apical myocardium *(white arrowheads)*. **Right:** With power Doppler, homogenous uptake of contrast is seen throughout the left ventricular apex *(white arrowheads)* and interventricular septum *(black arrowheads)*. (Courtesy of Drs. Graham Hillis and Jae K. Oh, Mayo Clinic, Rochester, MN.)

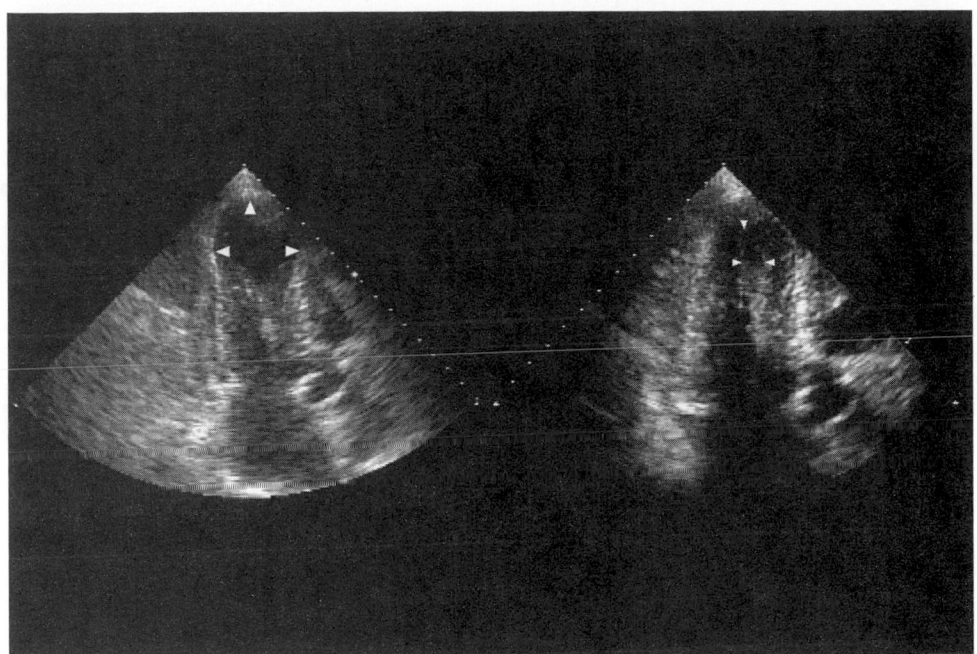

FIG. 60–14. Two-chamber, long-axis view in same patient as in Figure 60–13. Immediately after thrombolytic therapy, the left ventricular apex *(white arrowheads)* is dilated and akinetic **(left).** A few months later, there is complete recovery of apical anatomy and function **(right).** (Courtesy of Drs. Graham Hillis and Jae Oh, Mayo Clinic, Rochester, MN.)

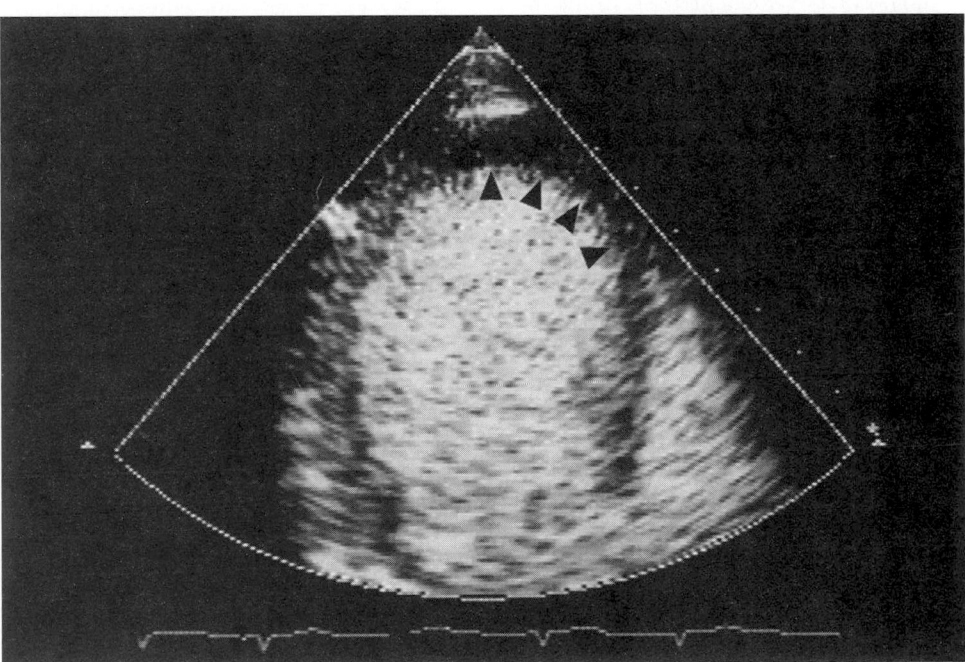

FIG. 60–15. Apical four-chamber view in a patient with acute anteroseptal myocardial infarction treated with reperfusion therapy. After opacification of the right and left ventricular cavities, there is contrast (Optison; Amersham, Princeton, NJ) enhancement of the mid to basal segments of the inferior interventricular septum and anterolateral wall. However, a large apical perfusion defect is clearly visible *(black arrowheads).* (Courtesy of Drs. Graham Hillis and Jae Oh, Mayo Clinic, Rochester, MN.)

contrast enhancement, even when complete, may underestimate the severity of microvascular damage because of reactive hyperemia (80,81). Moreover, the optimal timing for assessing microvascular integrity after AMI remains unclear (82). Nonetheless, studies have shown that myocardial contrast echocardiography compares favorably with low-dose dobutamine stress echocardiography for detecting hibernating myocardium and in predicting recovery of regional left ventricular dysfunction after AMI (83,84). Importantly, intravenous contrast administration appears to be as reliable as intracoronary injections for the detection of viable myocardium (85). Technical innovations, including pulse inversion imaging and power Doppler, have brought myocardial contrast echocardiography one step closer to becoming a practical reality (75,86,87). It remains to be determined how different combinations of low-dose dobutamine, myocardial contrast echocardiography, and tissue characterization will impact the sensitivity and specificity for the detection of viable myocardium.

USE OF ECHOCARDIOGRAPHY IN THE PREDISMISSAL PHASE

The most important outcome predictors after AMI are patency of the infarct-related artery and recovery of myocardial perfusion and both the extent of coronary artery disease and severity of left ventricular systolic dysfunction. All of these prognostic indicators can be reliably assessed by a combination of rest and stress two-dimensional echocardiography. Pharmacologic (dobutamine, dipyridamole) stress echocardiography is being increasingly used before hospital dismissal to identify high-grade residual stenosis in the infarct-related artery after thrombolysis and to detect significant multivessel disease (88) with comparable results to quantitative technetium-99m sestamibi single-photon emission computed tomography (89). Compared with predischarge submaximal treadmill exercise test alone or in the form of submaximal exercise echocardiography, standard pharmacologic stress echocardiography appears to be better at risk stratification after AMI and provides incremental prognostic information (90–92). Prehospital discharge dobutamine stress echocardiography is an accurate tool for prediction of late recovery of myocardial perfusion after AMI treated with thrombolysis (93). In the elderly, inducible ischemia during dobutamine stress echocardiography within 10 days after uncomplicated AMI portends a poor prognosis (94). Importantly, a negative dobutamine stress echocardiogram after uncomplicated AMI has been associated with good short- and long-term outcomes (95).

COMPLICATIONS OF ACUTE MYOCARDIAL INFARCTION

Echocardiography is currently the procedure of choice for the detection of AMI–related complications (1). Transthoracic echocardiography performed at the bedside should be

the first procedure used in hemodynamically unstable patients. If there are suboptimal images from the transthoracic approach, transesophageal echocardiography provides high-resolution images in nearly all critically ill patients (1,96, 97). The combination of transthoracic and transesophageal echocardiography obviates the need for cardiac catheterization in almost all cases.

Cardiogenic Shock

Cardiogenic shock carries a poor prognosis unless the cause is reversible. Visualization of hyperdynamic systolic left ventricular function on two-dimensional echocardiography in critically ill patients indicates the presence of a mechanical mechanism (papillary muscle rupture, ventricular septal defect, and free wall rupture) for the hemodynamic deterioration (98). It is essential to identify these mechanical complications of infarction quickly because urgent operation may be lifesaving (98–100). A reversible *functional* cause for cardiogenic shock after AMI is dynamic left ventricular outflow obstruction with or without associated severe mitral regurgitation (Fig. 60–16) (101,102). The proposed mechanism is compensatory hyperkinesis of the unaffected basal segments in patients with a large apical infarct (101,102).

Papillary Muscle Rupture

Papillary muscle rupture, either partial or complete, is a mechanical complication of MI that causes severe mitral regurgitation (1). It most commonly is associated with an inferior MI, because of the single blood supply of the posteromedial papillary muscle. Both partial and complete rupture of the papillary muscle can be seen on two-dimensional echocardiography (Fig. 60–17). The former gives the appearance of

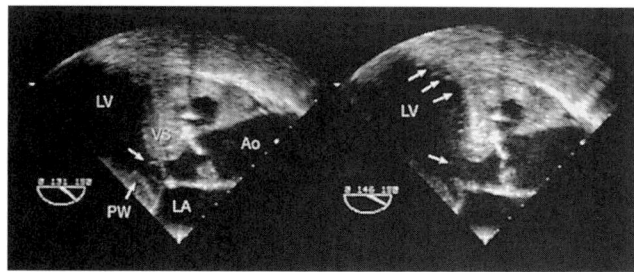

FIG. 60–16. Transesophageal systolic frame of long-axis view in a 72-year-old woman with chest pain, hypotension, and systolic murmur. **Left:** Note large apical aneurysm, hyperdynamic inferobasal area *(upward arrow)* resulting in systolic anterior motion of the mitral valve *(downward arrow)*, and dynamic left ventricular (LV) outflow tract obstruction. **Right:** With infusion of phenylephrine (α-agonist), LV outflow tract obstruction *(single arrow)* is less and hemodynamics are improved. Apical aneurysm *(three arrows)* is not improved. Ao, aorta; PW, posterior wall; VS, ventricular septum. (Courtesy of Mayo Foundation, Rochester, MN.)

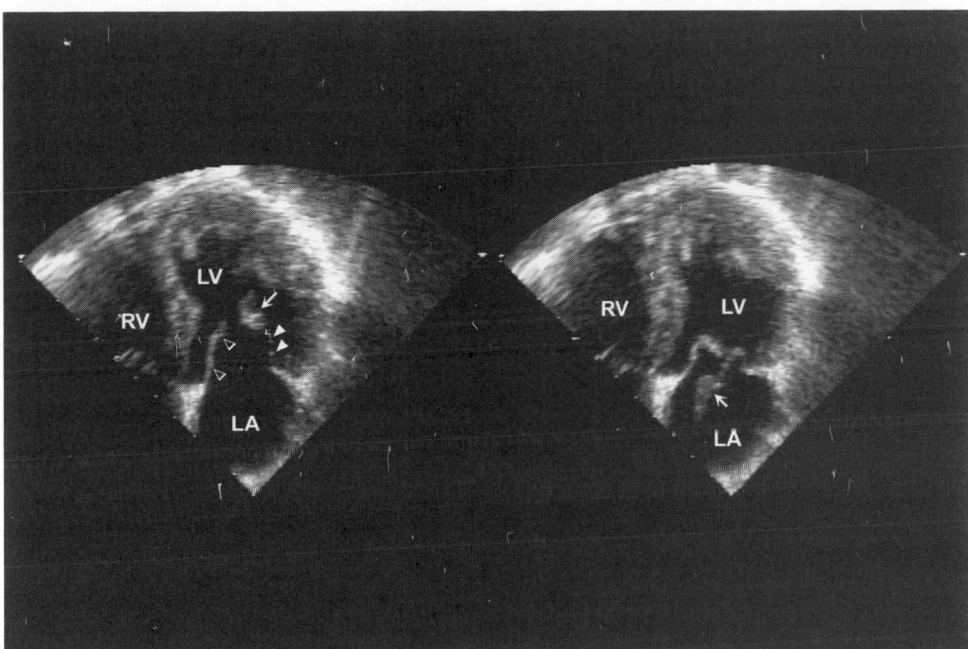

FIG. 60–17. Horizontal four-chamber transesophageal view in a patient with severe mitral regurgitation secondary to complete papillary muscle rupture. The severed papillary muscle head is seen as a large echo-density *(white arrow)* within the left ventricular cavity attached to the posterior mitral leaflet *(white arrowheads)* in diastole **(left)** and swinging into the left atrium in systole **(right).** *Black arrowheads with white border* point to the anterior mitral leaflet. LA, left atrium; LV, left ventricle; RV, right ventricle. (Courtesy of Dr. Sharonne N. Hayes, Mayo Clinic, Rochester, MN.)

a tear in the muscle head, whereas the latter typically presents as a flail mitral valve leaflet with secondary severe mitral regurgitation on color flow imaging. The severed head of the papillary muscle may also be seen attached to the mitral leaflets as an echo density swinging in and out of the left atrium (Fig. 60–17).

Free Wall Rupture

Free wall rupture is the most common type of myocardial rupture after MI and is usually associated with a small infarct. It is most commonly seen in older women with hypertension and usually presents with acute electromechanical dissociation and death. However, a subepicardial aneurysm may develop if rupture is contained by the epicardium (Fig. 60–18) (1). Rarely, rupture occurs into the pericardium with subsequent tamponade and a transient period of hypotension before death. Prompt diagnosis of pericardial tamponade can be made with two-dimensional echocardiography. Echocardiographically directed pericardiocentesis (103) followed by emergency operation may be lifesaving (104).

Pseudoaneurysm

A pseudoaneurysm is a contained free wall rupture with the pericardium forming the outer wall of the aneurysm (Fig. 60–19) (105). A pseudoaneurysm is usually characterized by a small neck communication between the left ventricle and aneurysmal cavities, but the communication may be wide (105). A typical to-and-fro pattern of blood flow at site of rupture can be detected by Doppler (105). When there is associated pericardial effusion, color flow Doppler or contrast echocardiography can help to determine whether the effusion is simply a reaction to the pseudoaneurysm or the first sign of impending rupture.

Postinfarction Ventricular Septal Defect

Ventricular septal defect is a mechanical complication of MI that also causes rapid hemodynamic deterioration. The location of the MI determines the type of rupture (99,100, 106,107). The septal defect associated with an anterior MI is usually a simple type of rupture near the apex of the left ventricle. In contrast, a complex serpiginous rupture of the septum occurs with an inferior MI at the base of the heart (Fig. 60–20) and is frequently associated with right ventricular involvement (106,107). Direct visualization of the septal defect by precordial echocardiography is possible in more than two-thirds of patients (96). However, two-dimensional echocardiography alone may not always be able to detect small serpiginous septal ruptures. With color flow imaging, a high-velocity turbulent flow through the defect can be detected in nearly all patients with postinfarct septal defects (96, 108–110).

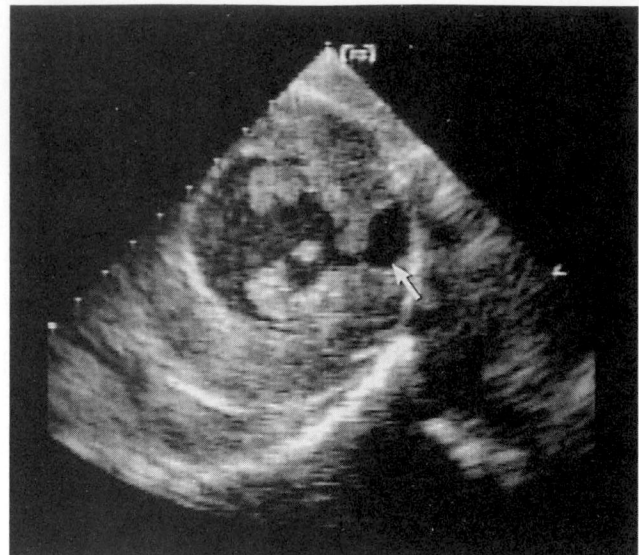

FIG. 60–18. Transesophageal transgastric view of the left ventricle in a patient with incomplete rupture of the myocardium, resulting in a subepicardial aneurysm *(arrow).* The cavity was contained by the epicardial layer. (Courtesy of Mayo Foundation, Rochester, MN.)

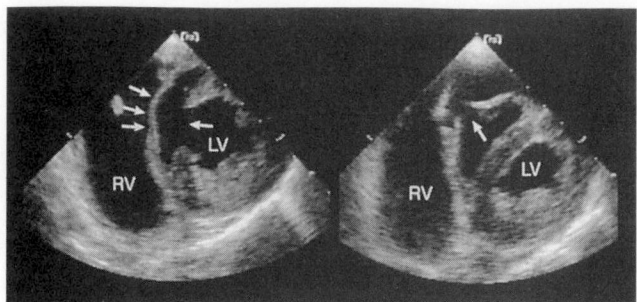

FIG. 60–20. Postinfarction ventricular septal rupture. Transesophageal transgastric view of the left ventricle *(LV)* demonstrating a serpiginous tear of the ventricular septum. **Left:** The tear in the left side of the ventricular septum *(single arrow* in LV), with dissection into the myocardium; the right side of the septum was intact *(three arrows).* **Right:** A tear in the right side of the ventricular septum, more toward the apical level *(arrow).* RV, right ventricle. (Courtesy of Mayo Foundation, Rochester, MN.)

men ovale, the markedly increased right atrial pressure can result in significant right-to-left shunting with secondary hypoxemia (1).

Right Ventricular Infarction

Right ventricular infarction is a common complication of inferior MI (111). The diagnosis of right ventricular infarction can be made on two-dimensional echocardiography by demonstrating enlargement and akinesis of the right ventricle (112,113). Two-dimensional echocardiography has a greater sensitivity and specificity than clinical and electrocardiography alone for making the diagnosis (113). In severe cases, there is right ventricular dilatation and even severe tricuspid regurgitation because of annular dilatation. Abnormal diastolic filling of the right side of the heart in patients with right ventricular infarction can be assessed from the tricuspid flow velocity curves (1). In the presence of a patent fora-

Left Ventricular Thrombus

Left ventricular thrombus was a common complication of anterior MI in the prereperfusion era (114,115), but its prevalence has significantly decreased after the routine use of thrombolytics (1). Care must be taken to differentiate a thrombus from other echo-densities, such as aberrant chordae or other artifacts, seen on two-dimensional echocardiography in the left ventricular apex. Noninvasive left ventriculography using contrast agents can be helpful in this regard. Ultrasonic characteristics of the thrombus, including its mobility and degree of protrusion into the left ventricular cavity, may identify patients at even greater risk for emboli (116). Intramyocardial dissecting hematoma is a rare complication of AMI that may be confused with intracavitary thrombus and pseudoaneurysm (117).

Ischemic Mitral Regurgitation

Functional mitral regurgitation, a frequent complication of left ventricular systolic dysfunction, is associated with a structurally normal mitral valve apparatus (118). Functional mitral regurgitation often is silent but can be detected by echocardiography. When the underlying etiologic factor is coronary artery disease, functional mitral regurgitation is referred to as ischemic mitral regurgitation. Severe ischemic mitral regurgitation portends a poor prognosis, underscoring the importance of having a clear understanding of its underlying anatomic determinants (118). Data suggest that the presence and severity of ischemic mitral regurgitation are unrelated to the severity of global left ventricular systolic dysfunction and are more a function of local left ventricular

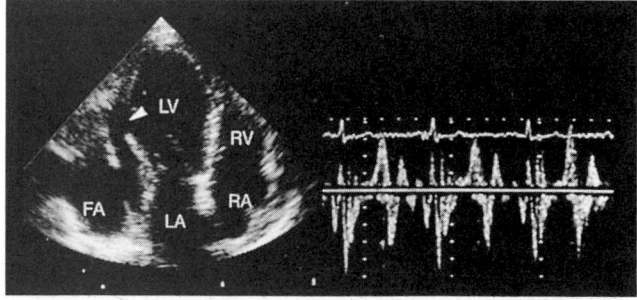

FIG. 60–19. Left: Apical four-chamber imaging of a free wall rupture (arrowhead) resulting in a false aneurysm (FA). **Right:** Pulsed-wave Doppler at site of rupture shows to-and-fro blood flow velocities. LA, left atrium; LV, left ventricle; RA, right atrium; RV, right ventricle. (Courtesy of Mayo Foundation, Rochester, MN.)

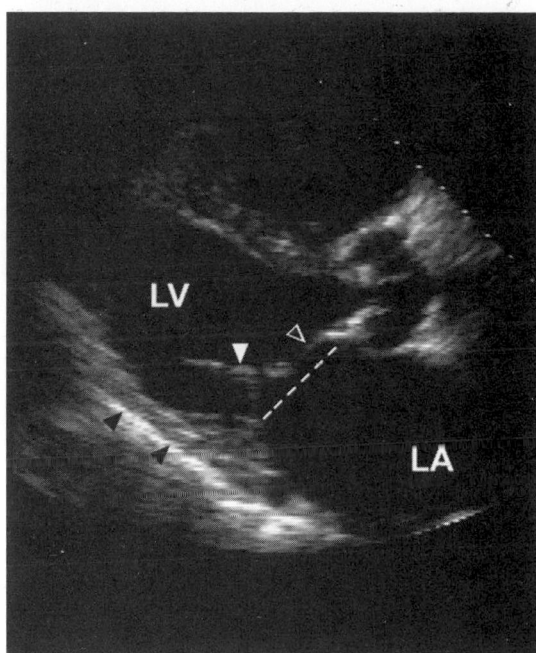

FIG. 60–21. Transthoracic parasternal long-axis view in a patient with severe ischemic mitral regurgitation after inferior myocardial infarction. **Left:** Tethering of the posterior mitral leaflet *(white arrowhead)* has caused mitral valve tenting and prolapse of the anterior leaflet *(black arrowhead with white border)*. *Black arrowheads* point to the infarcted mid and basal segments of the inferolateral wall. The *dashed white line* shows the plane of the mitral anulus. **Right:** Color Doppler showing severe posteriorly directed jet of mitral regurgitation *(white arrows)*. LA, left atrium; LV, left ventricle. (Courtesy of Dr. William K. Freeman, Mayo Clinic, Rochester, MN.) (See color insert for right side of Fig. 60–21.)

remodeling (118). After a MI, apical and posterior displacement of papillary muscles may cause tethering of the mitral valve leaflets and secondary valve tenting (Fig. 60–21) (see also color insert). The magnitude of mitral tenting correlates with mitral regurgitation severity and can be readily measured by two-dimensional echocardiography (118). Using Doppler methods, severity of ischemic mitral regurgitation can be quantified (119). Surgical correction of apical and posterior displacements of papillary muscles to minimize mitral valve tenting combined with mitral annuloplasty may provide rational approaches to correcting ischemic mitral regurgitation (118,119).

SUMMARY

Two-dimensional and Doppler echocardiography are increasingly important in the evaluation and management of patients with AMI. The impetus to rapidly institute reperfusion therapy has made echocardiography an essential part of the coronary intensive care unit in helping to decide whether to initiate thrombolytic therapy and to rule out conditions that mimic MI. Evaluation of residual ischemia in survivors of MI can be helped by the ability to image the myocardium

during stress, whether induced by exercise or pharmacologically. The evaluation of hemodynamically unstable patients can now be performed rapidly and accurately at the bedside with two-dimensional and Doppler echocardiography. New and emerging technologies including tissue Doppler imaging, tissue characterization, and myocardial contrast echocardiography have great potential for aiding in the clinical management of patients with MI. Ultrasonographic imaging advances may ultimately allow accurate assessment of coronary artery flow and the detection of subclinical atherothrombosis using transthoracic echocardiography (120,121). Because two-dimensional echocardiography relies on multiple tomographic slices through the myocardium, the images obtained with this technique readily lend themselves to computerized three-dimensional reconstruction (117). Rapid advances in computer technology and image resolution are helping make this technique a reality (122–124).

REFERENCES

1. Oh JK, Seward JB, Tajik AJ. *The echo manual,* 4th ed. Philadelphia: Lippincott-Raven, 1999.
2. Hammermeister KE, DeRouen TA, Dodge HT. Variables predictive of survival in patients with coronary disease. Selection by univariate and multivariate analyses from the clinical, electrocardiographic, exercise, arteriographic, and quantitative angiographic evaluations. *Circulation* 1979;59:421–430.
3. White HD, Norris RM, Brown MA, et al. Left ventricular end-systolic volume as the major determinant of survival after recovery from myocardial infarction. *Circulation* 1987;76:44–51.
4. Haendchen RV, Wyatt HL, Maurer G, et al. Quantitation of regional cardiac function by two-dimensional echocardiography. I. Patterns of contraction in the normal left ventricle. *Circulation* 1983;67:1234–1245.
5. Weyman AE, Franklin TD Jr, Hogan RD, et al. Importance of temporal heterogeneity in assessing the contraction abnormalities associated with acute myocardial ischemia. *Circulation* 1984;70:102–112.
6. Kisslo JA, Robertson D, Gilbert BW, et al. A comparison of real-time, two dimensional echocardiography and cineangiography in detecting left ventricular asynergy. *Circulation* 1977;55:134–141.
7. Shiina A, Tajik AJ, Smith HC, et al. Prognostic significance of regional wall motion abnormality in patients with prior myocardial infarction: a prospective correlative study of two-dimensional echocardiography and angiography. *Mayo Clin Proc* 1986;61:254–262.
8. Van Reet RE, Quinones MA, Poliner LR, et al. Comparison of two-dimensional echocardiography with gated radionuclide ventriculography in the evaluation of global and regional left ventricular function in acute myocardial infarction. *J Am Coll Cardiol* 1984;3:243–252.
9. Lieberman AN, Weiss JL, Jugdutt BI, et al. Two-dimensional echocardiography and infarct size: relationship of regional wall motion and thickening to the extent of myocardial infarction in the dog. *Circulation* 1981;63:739–746.
10. Fukuda K, Oki T, Tabata T, et al. Regional left ventricular wall motion abnormalities in myocardial infarction and mitral annular descent velocities studied with pulsed tissue Doppler imaging. *J Am Soc Echocardiogr* 1998;11:841–848.
11. Naqvi TZ, Neyman G, Broyde A, et al. Myocardial Doppler tissue imaging: findings in inferior myocardial infarction and left ventricular hypertrophy–wall motion assessment. *J Am Soc Echocardiogr* 2001; 14:867–873.
12. Derumeaux G, Loufoua J, Pontier G, et al. Tissue Doppler imaging differentiates transmural from nontransmural acute myocardial infarction after reperfusion therapy. *Circulation* 2001;103:589–596.
13. Abraham TP, Nishimura RA, Holmes DR, et al. Strain rate imaging for assessment of regional myocardial function: results from a clinical model of septal ablation. *Circulation* 2002;105:1403–1406.
14. Vermes E, Guyon P, Weingrod M, et al. Assessment of left ventricular

regional wall motion by color kinesis technique: comparison with angiographic findings. *Echocardiography* 2000;17:521–527.

15. Fujino T, Ono S, Murata K, et al. New method of on-line quantification of regional wall motion with automated segmental motion analysis. *J Am Soc Echocardiogr* 2001;14:892–901.

16. Neskovic AN, Mojsilovic A, Jovanovic T, et al. Myocardial tissue characterization after acute myocardial infarction with wavelet image decomposition: a novel approach for the detection of myocardial viability in the early postinfarction period. *Circulation* 1998;98:634–641.

17. Armstrong WF. Stress echocardiography: introduction, history, and methods. *Prog Cardiovasc Dis* 1997;39:499–522.

18. Ha JW, Juracan EM, Mahoney DW, et al. Hypertensive response to exercise: a potential cause for new wall motion abnormality in the absence of coronary artery disease. *J Am Coll Cardiol* 2002;39:323–327.

19. Quinones MA, Verani MS, Haichin RM, et al. Exercise echocardiography versus 201Tl single-photon emission computed tomography in evaluation of coronary artery disease. Analysis of 292 patients. *Circulation* 1992;85:1026–1031.

20. Forrester JS, Diamond G, Chatterjee K, et al. Medical therapy of acute myocardial infarction by application of hemodynamic subsets (second of two parts). *N Engl J Med* 1976;295:1404–1413.

21. Foote GA, Schabel SI, Hodges M. Pulmonary complications of the flow-directed balloon-tipped catheter. *N Engl J Med* 1974;290:927–931.

22. Carlos ME, Smart SC, Wynsen JC, et al. Dobutamine stress echocardiography for risk stratification after myocardial infarction. *Circulation* 1997;95:1402–1410.

23. Cortigiani L, Picano E, Landi P, et al. Value of pharmacologic stress echocardiography in risk stratification of patients with single-vessel disease: a report from the Echo-Persantine and Echo-Dobutamine International Cooperative Studies. *J Am Coll Cardiol* 1998;32:69–74.

24. Krivokapich J, Child JS, Walter DO, et al. Prognostic value of dobutamine stress echocardiography in predicting cardiac events in patients with known or suspected coronary artery disease. *J Am Coll Cardiol* 1999;33:708–716.

25. McCully RB, Roger VL, Mahoney DW, et al. Outcome after abnormal exercise echocardiography for patients with good exercise capacity: prognostic importance of the extent and severity of exercise-related left ventricular dysfunction. *J Am Coll Cardiol* 2002;39:1345–1352.

26. Arruda-Olson AM, Juracan EM, Mahoney DW, et al. Prognostic value of exercise echocardiography in 5,798 patients: is there a gender difference? *J Am Coll Cardiol* 2002;39:625–631.

27. Elhendy A, Mahoney DW, Khandheria BK, et al. Prognostic significance of the location of wall motion abnormalities during exercise echocardiography. *J Am Coll Cardiol* 2002;40:1623–1629.

28. Nishimura RA, Tajik AJ, Shub C, et al. Role of two-dimensional echocardiography in the prediction of in-hospital complications after acute myocardial infarction. *J Am Coll Cardiol* 1984;4:1080–1087.

29. Bhatnagar SK, Moussa MA, Al-Yusuf AR. The role of prehospital discharge two-dimensional echocardiography in determining the prognosis of survivors of first myocardial infarction. *Am Heart J* 1985;109:472–477.

30. Nishimura RA, Reeder GS, Miller FA, et al. Prognostic value of predischarge 2-dimensional echocardiogram after acute myocardial infarction. *Am J Cardiol* 1984;53:429–432.

31. Carluccio E, Tommasi S, Bentivoglio M, et al. Usefulness of the severity and extent of wall motion abnormalities as prognostic markers of an adverse outcome after a first myocardial infarction treated with thrombolytic therapy. *Am J Cardiol* 2000;85:411–415.

32. Shen WK, Khandheria BK, Edwards WD, et al. Value and limitations of two-dimensional echocardiography in predicting myocardial infarct size. *Am J Cardiol* 1991;68:1143–1149.

33. Wyatt HL, Forrester JS, da Luz PL, et al. Functional abnormalities in nonoccluded regions of myocardium after experimental coronary occlusion. *Am J Cardiol* 1976;37:366–372.

34. Muscholl MW, Oswald M, Mayer C, et al. Prognostic value of 2D echocardiography in patients presenting with acute chest pain and non-diagnostic ECG for ST-elevation myocardial infarction. *Int J Cardiol* 2002;84:217–225.

35. Sabia P, Abbott RD, Afrookteh A, et al. Importance of two-dimensional echocardiographic assessment of left ventricular systolic function in patients presenting to the emergency room with cardiac-related symptoms. *Circulation* 1991;84:1615–1624.

36. Launbjerg J, Berning J, Fruergaard P, et al. Sensitivity and specificity of echocardiographic identification of patients eligible for safe early

discharge after acute myocardial infarction. *Am Heart J* 1992;124:846–853.

37. Berning J, Launbjerg J, Appleyard M. Echocardiographic algorithms for admission and predischarge prediction of mortality in acute myocardial infarction. *Am J Cardiol* 1992;69:1538–1544.

38. Abernethy M, Sharpe N, Smith H, et al. Echocardiographic prediction of left ventricular volume after myocardial infarction. *J Am Coll Cardiol* 1991;17:1527–1532.

39. Moller JE, Sondergaard E, Poulsen SH, et al. The Doppler echocardiographic myocardial performance index predicts left-ventricular dilation and cardiac death after myocardial infarction. *Cardiology* 2001;95:105–111.

40. Moller JE, Sondergaard E, Poulsen SH, et al. Serial Doppler echocardiographic assessment of left and right ventricular performance after a first myocardial infarction. *J Am Soc Echocardiogr* 2001;14:249–255.

41. Vaskelyte J, Stoskute N, Kinduris S, et al. Coronary artery bypass grafting in patients with severe left ventricular dysfunction: predictive significance of left ventricular diastolic filling pattern. *Eur J Echocardiogr* 2001;2:62–7.

42. Oh JK, Ding ZP, Gersh BJ, et al. Restrictive left ventricular diastolic filling identifies patients with heart failure after acute myocardial infarction. *J Am Soc Echocardiogr* 1992;5:497–503.

43. Nijland F, Kamp O, Karreman AJ, et al. Prognostic implications of restrictive left ventricular filling in acute myocardial infarction: a serial Doppler echocardiographic study. *J Am Coll Cardiol* 1997;30:1618–1624.

44. Moller JE, Sondergaard E, Seward JB, et al. Ratio of left ventricular peak E-wave velocity to flow propagation velocity assessed by color M-mode Doppler echocardiography in first myocardial infarction: prognostic and clinical implications. *J Am Coll Cardiol* 2000;35:363–370.

45. De Sutter J, De Mey S, De Backer J, et al. Diastolic dysfunction, infarct size, and exercise capacity in remote myocardial infarction: a combined approach of mitral E-wave deceleration time and color M-mode flow propagation velocity. *Am J Cardiol* 2002;89:593–595.

46. Schuster EH, Bulkley BH. Expansion of transmural myocardial infarction: a pathophysiologic factor in cardiac rupture. *Circulation* 1979;60:1532–1538.

47. Erlebacher JA, Weiss JL, Weisfeldt ML, et al. Early dilation of the infarcted segment in acute transmural myocardial infarction: role of infarct expansion in acute left ventricular enlargement. *J Am Coll Cardiol* 1984;4:201–208.

48. McKay RG, Pfeffer MA, Pasternak RC, et al. Left ventricular remodeling after myocardial infarction: a corollary to infarct expansion. *Circulation* 1986;74:693–702.

49. Sakai Y, Tsunoda K, Ishibashi I, et al. Time course of left ventricular remodeling after myocardial infarction: a two-dimensional echocardiographic study. *Jpn Circ J* 2000;64:421–429.

50. Ricci R, Coletta C, Ceci V, et al. Effect of early treatment with captopril and metoprolol singly and together on postinfarction left ventricular remodeling. *Am Heart J* 2001;142:E5.

51. Loh IK, Charuzi Y, Beeder C, et al. Early diagnosis of nontransmural myocardial infarction by two-dimensional echocardiography. *Am Heart J* 1982;104:963–968.

52. Effectiveness of intravenous thrombolytic treatment in acute myocardial infarction. Gruppo Italiano per lo Studio della Streptochinasi nell'Infarto Miocardico (GISSI). *Lancet* 1986;1:397–402.

53. Randomised trial of intravenous streptokinase, oral aspirin, both, or neither among 17,187 cases of suspected acute myocardial infarction: ISIS-2. ISIS-2 (Second International Study of Infarct Survival) Collaborative Group. *Lancet* 1988;2:349–360.

54. Oh JK, Miller FA, Shub C, et al. Evaluation of acute chest pain syndromes by two-dimensional echocardiography: its potential application in the selection of patients for acute reperfusion therapy. *Mayo Clin Proc* 1987;62:59–66.

55. Christian TF, Gibbons RJ, Gersh BJ. Effect of infarct location on myocardial salvage assessed by technetium-99m isonitrile. *J Am Coll Cardiol* 1991;17:1303–1308.

56. Kaul S, Glasheen W, Ruddy TD, et al. The importance of defining left ventricular area at risk in vivo during acute myocardial infarction: an experimental evaluation with myocardial contrast two-dimensional echocardiography. *Circulation* 1987;75:1249–1260.

57. Kaul S, Pandian NG, Gillam LD, et al. Contrast echocardiography in acute myocardial ischemia. III. An in vivo comparison of the extent of

abnormal wall motion with the area at risk for necrosis. *J Am Coll Cardiol* 1986;7:383–392.

58. Porter TR, Li S, Jiang L, et al. Real-time visualization of myocardial perfusion and wall thickening in human beings with intravenous ultrasonographic contrast and accelerated intermittent harmonic imaging. *J Am Soc Echocardiogr* 1999;12:266–271.

59. Kaul S. Myocardial contrast echocardiography: basic principles. *Prog Cardiovasc Dis* 2001;44:1–11.

60. Kaul S, Gillam LD, Weyman AE. Contrast echocardiography in acute myocardial ischemia. II. The effect of site of injection of contrast agent on the estimation of area at risk for necrosis after coronary occlusion. *J Am Coll Cardiol* 1985;6:825–830.

61. Coggins MP, Sklenar J, Le DE, et al. Noninvasive prediction of ultimate infarct size at the time of acute coronary occlusion based on the extent and magnitude of collateral-derived myocardial blood flow. *Circulation* 2001;104:2471–2477.

62. Villanueva FS, Myocardial contrast echocardiography in acute myocardial infarction. *Am J Cardiol* 2002;90[Suppl 10A]:38J–47J.

63. Keller MW, Glasheen W, Teja K, et al. Myocardial contrast echocardiography without significant hemodynamic effects or reactive hyperemia: a major advantage in the imaging of regional myocardial perfusion. *J Am Coll Cardiol* 1988;12:1039–1047.

64. Moore CA, Smucker ML, Kaul S. Myocardial contrast echocardiography in humans: I. Safety—a comparison with routine coronary arteriography. *J Am Coll Cardiol* 1986;8:1066–1072.

65. Cwajg JM, Cwajg E, Nagueh SF, et al. End-diastolic wall thickness as a predictor of recovery of function in myocardial hibernation: relation to rest-redistribution T1-201 tomography and dobutamine stress echocardiography. *J Am Coll Cardiol* 2000;35:1152–1161.

66. Yong Y, Nagueh SF, Shimoni S, et al. Deceleration time in ischemic cardiomyopathy: relation to echocardiographic and scintigraphic indices of myocardial viability and functional recovery after revascularization. *Circulation* 2001;103:1232–1237.

67. Monin JL, Garot J, Scherrer-Crosbie M, et al. Prediction of functional recovery of viable myocardium after delayed revascularization in postinfarction patients: accuracy of dobutamine stress echocardiography and influence of long-term vessel patency. *J Am Coll Cardiol* 1999;34:1012–1019.

68. Tani T, Teragaki M, Watanabe H, et al. Prediction of functional recovery in patients with myocardial infarction after revascularization—comparison of low-dose dobutamine stress echocardiography with fluorine-18 fluorodeoxyglucose positron emission tomography. *Jpn Circ J* 2001;65:177–181.

69. Dangas G, Machac J, Goldman ME, et al. Evaluation of myocardial viability in asymptomatic patients early after infarction with perfusion/metabolism single-photon-emission computed tomographic imaging and dobutamine echocardiography. *Coron Artery Dis* 2000;11:409–414.

70. Hoffer EP, Dewe W, Celentano C, et al. Low-level exercise echocardiography detects contractile reserve and predicts reversible dysfunction after acute myocardial infarction: comparison with low-dose dobutamine echocardiography. *J Am Coll Cardiol* 1999;34:989–997.

71. Haghani K, Shapiro S, Ginzton LE. Low-level exercise echocardiography identifies contractile reserve in patients with a recent myocardial infarction: comparison with dobutamine stress echocardiography. *J Am Soc Echocardiogr* 2002;15:671–677.

72. Nijland F, Kamp O, Verhorst PM, et al. In-hospital and long-term prognostic value of viable myocardium detected by dobutamine echocardiography early after acute myocardial infarction and its relation to indicators of left ventricular systolic dysfunction. *Am J Cardiol* 2001;88:949–955.

73. Takiuchi S, Ito H, Iwakura K, et al. Ultrasonic tissue characterization predicts myocardial viability in early stage of reperfused acute myocardial infarction. *Circulation* 1998;97:356–362.

74. Pislaru C, Bruce CJ, Belohlavek M, et al. Intracardiac measurement of pre-ejection myocardial velocities estimates the transmural extent of viable myocardium early after reperfusion in acute myocardial infarction. *J Am Coll Cardiol* 2001;38:1748–1756.

75. Zoghbi WA. Evaluation of myocardial viability with contrast echocardiography. *Am J Cardiol* 2002;90[Suppl 10A]:65J–71J.

76. Kloner RA, Ganote CE, Jennings RB. The "no-reflow" phenomenon after temporary coronary occlusion in the dog. *J Clin Invest* 1974;54:1496–1508.

77. Kloner RA, Rude RE, Carlson N, et al. Ultrastructural evidence of mi-

crovascular damage and myocardial cell injury after coronary artery occlusion: which comes first? *Circulation* 1980;62:945–952.

78. Sakuma T, Hayashi Y, Sumii K, et al. Prediction of short- and intermediate-term prognoses of patients with acute myocardial infarction using myocardial contrast echocardiography one day after recanalization. *J Am Coll Cardiol* 1998;32:890–897.

79. Kamp O, Lepper W, Vanoverschelde JL, et al. Serial evaluation of perfusion defects in patients with a first acute myocardial infarction referred for primary PTCA using intravenous myocardial contrast echocardiography. *Eur Heart J* 2001;22:1485–1495.

80. Asanuma T, Tanabe K, Ochiai K, et al. Relationship between progressive microvascular damage and intramyocardial hemorrhage in patients with reperfused anterior myocardial infarction: myocardial contrast echocardiographic study. *Circulation* 1997;96:448–453.

81. Kaul S. Assessing the myocardium after attempted reperfusion: should we bother? *Circulation* 1998;98:625–627.

82. Sakuma T, Otsuka M, Okimoto T, et al. Optimal time for predicting myocardial viability after successful primary angioplasty in acute myocardial infarction: a study using myocardial contrast echocardiography. *Am J Cardiol* 2001;87:687–692.

83. Iwakura K, Ito H, Nishikawa N, et al. Use of echocardiography for predicting myocardial viability in patients with reperfused anterior wall myocardial infarction. *Am J Cardiol* 2000;85:744–748.

84. Main ML, Magalski A, Morris BA, et al. Combined assessment of microvascular integrity and contractile reserve improves differentiation of stunning and necrosis after acute anterior wall myocardial infarction. *J Am Coll Cardiol* 2002;40:1079–1084.

85. Agati L, Funaro S, Bilotta F. Assessment of no-reflow phenomenon after acute myocardial infarction with harmonic angiography and intravenous pump infusion with Levovist: comparison with intracoronary contrast injection. *J Am Soc Echocardiogr* 2001;14:773–781.

86. Main ML, Magalski A, Chee NK, et al. Full-motion pulse inversion power Doppler contrast echocardiography differentiates stunning from necrosis and predicts recovery of left ventricular function after acute myocardial infarction. *J Am Coll Cardiol* 2001;38:1390–1394.

87. Swinburn JM, Senior R. Real time contrast echocardiography—a new bedside technique to predict contractile reserve early after acute myocardial infarction. *Eur J Echocardiogr* 2002;3:95–99.

88. Previtali M, Fetiveau R, Lanzarini L, et al. Prognostic value of myocardial viability and ischemia detected by dobutamine stress echocardiography early after acute myocardial infarction treated with thrombolysis. *J Am Coll Cardiol* 1998;32:380–386.

89. Lancellotti P, Benoit T, Rigo P, et al. Dobutamine stress echocardiography versus quantitative technetium-99m sestamibi SPECT for detecting residual stenosis and multivessel disease after myocardial infarction. *Heart* 2001;86:510–515.

90. Sicari R, Landi P, Picano E, et al. Exercise-electrocardiography and/or pharmacological stress echocardiography for non-invasive risk stratification early after uncomplicated myocardial infarction. A prospective international large scale multicentre study. *Eur Heart J* 2002;23:1030–1037.

91. Schroder K, Voller H, Dingerkus H, et al. Comparison of the diagnostic potential of four echocardiographic stress tests shortly after acute myocardial infarction: submaximal exercise, transesophageal atrial pacing, dipyridamole, and dobutamine-atropine. *Am J Cardiol* 1996;77:909–914.

92. Salustri A, Ciavatti M, Seccareccia F, et al. Prediction of cardiac events after uncomplicated acute myocardial infarction by clinical variables and dobutamine stress test. *J Am Coll Cardiol* 1999;34:435–440.

93. Samad BA, Hojer J, Bouvier F, et al. Spontaneous delayed recovery of perfusion after thrombolyzed acute myocardial infarction: is it predictable before discharge? *J Am Soc Echocardiogr* 2001;14:902–909.

94. de la Torre MM, San Roman JA, Bermejo J, et al. Prognostic power of dobutamine echocardiography after uncomplicated acute myocardial infarction in the elderly. *Chest* 2001;120:1200–1205.

95. Bigi R, Cortigiani L, Mariani PR, et al. Sustained favorable long-term prognosis of negative stress echocardiography following uncomplicated myocardial infarction. *Am J Cardiol* 2002;90:149–152.

96. Kishon Y, Iqbal A, Oh JK, et al. Evolution of echocardiographic modalities in detection of postmyocardial infarction ventricular septal defect and papillary muscle rupture: study of 62 patients. *Am Heart J* 1993;126:667–675.

97. Koenig K, Kasper W, Hofmann T, et al. Transesophageal echocardiography for diagnosis of rupture of the ventricular septum or left ven-

tricular papillary muscle during acute myocardial infarction. *Am J Cardiol* 1987;59:362.

98. Nishimura RA, Schaff HV, Gersh BJ, et al. Early repair of mechanical complications after acute myocardial infarction. *JAMA* 1986;256:47–50.

99. Radford MJ, Johnson RA, Daggett WM Jr, et al. Ventricular septal rupture: a review of clinical and physiologic features and an analysis of survival. *Circulation* 1981;64:545–553.

100. Montoya A, McKeever L, Scanlon P, et al. Early repair of ventricular septal rupture after infarction. *Am J Cardiol* 1980;45:345–348.

101. Di Chiara A, Plewka M, Fioretti PM. Systolic anterior movement of mitral valve during acute apical myocardial infarction: an unusual mechanism of acute mitral regurgitation. *J Am Soc Echocardiogr* 1999;12:1117–1121.

102. Haley JH, Sinak LJ, Tajik AJ, et al. Dynamic left ventricular outflow tract obstruction in acute coronary syndromes: an important cause of new systolic murmur and cardiogenic shock. *Mayo Clin Proc* 1999; 74:901–906.

103. Tsang TS, Enriquez-Sarano M, Freeman WK, et al. Consecutive 1127 therapeutic echocardiographically guided pericardiocenteses: clinical profile, practice patterns, and outcomes spanning 21 years. *Mayo Clin Proc* 2002;77:429–436.

104. Oliva PB, Hammill SC, Edwards WD. Cardiac rupture, a clinically predictable complication of acute myocardial infarction: report of 70 cases with clinicopathologic correlations. *J Am Coll Cardiol* 1993;22:720–726.

105. Yeo TC, Malouf JF, Reeder GS, et al. Clinical characteristics and outcome in postinfarction pseudoaneurysm. *Am J Cardiol* 1999;84:592–595,A8.

106. Moore CA, Nygaard TW, Kaiser DL, et al. Postinfarction ventricular septal rupture: the importance of location of infarction and right ventricular function in determining survival. *Circulation* 1986;74:45–55.

107. Edwards BS, Edwards WD, Edwards JE. Ventricular septal rupture complicating acute myocardial infarction: identification of simple and complex types in 53 autopsied hearts. *Am J Cardiol* 1984;54:1201–1205.

108. Miyatake K, Okamoto M, Kinoshita N, et al. Doppler echocardiographic features of ventricular septal rupture in myocardial infarction. *J Am Coll Cardiol* 1985;5:182–187.

109. Helmcke F, Mahan EF 3rd, Nanda NC, et al. Two-dimensional echocardiography and Doppler color flow mapping in the diagnosis and prognosis of ventricular septal rupture. *Circulation* 1990;81:1775–1783.

110. Fortin DF, Sheikh KH, Kisslo J. The utility of echocardiography in the diagnostic strategy of postinfarction ventricular septal rupture: a comparison of two-dimensional echocardiography versus Doppler color flow imaging. *Am Heart J* 1991;121:25–32.

111. Zehender M, Kasper W, Kauder E, et al. Right ventricular infarction as an independent predictor of prognosis after acute inferior myocardial infarction. *N Engl J Med* 1993;328:981–988.

112. Panidis IP, Ren JF, Kotler MN, et al. Two-dimensional echocardiographic estimation of right ventricular ejection fraction in patients with coronary artery disease. *J Am Coll Cardiol* 1983;2:911–918.

113. Bellamy GR, Rasmussen HH, Nasser FN, et al. Value of two-dimensional echocardiography, electrocardiography, and clinical signs in detecting right ventricular infarction. *Am Heart J* 1986;112:304–309.

114. Spirito P, Bellotti P, Chiarella F, et al. Prognostic significance and natural history of left ventricular thrombi in patients with acute anterior myocardial infarction: a two-dimensional echocardiographic study. *Circulation* 1985;72:774–780.

115. Nihoyannopoulos P, Smith GC, Maseri A, et al. The natural history of left ventricular thrombus in myocardial infarction: a rationale in support of masterly inactivity. *J Am Coll Cardiol* 1989;14:903–911.

116. Jugdutt BI, Sivaram CA. Prospective two-dimensional echocardiographic evaluation of left ventricular thrombus and embolism after acute myocardial infarction. *J Am Coll Cardiol* 1989;13:554–564.

117. Vargas-Barron J, Roldan FJ, Romero-Cardenas A, et al. Two- and three-dimensional transesophageal echocardiographic diagnosis of intramyocardial dissecting hematoma after myocardial infarction. *J Am Soc Echocardiogr* 2001;14:637–640.

118. Yiu SF, Enriquez-Sarano M, Tribouilloy C, et al. Determinants of the degree of functional mitral regurgitation in patients with systolic left ventricular dysfunction: a quantitative clinical study. *Circulation* 2000;102:1400–1406.

119. Grigioni F, Enriquez-Sarano M, Zehr KJ, et al. Ischemic mitral regurgitation: long-term outcome and prognostic implications with quantitative Doppler assessment. *Circulation* 2001;103:1759–1764.

120. Gradus-Pizlo I, Sawada SG, Wright D, et al. Detection of subclinical coronary atherosclerosis using two-dimensional, high-resolution transthoracic echocardiography. *J Am Coll Cardiol* 2001;37:1422–1429.

121. Gradus-Pizlo I, Feigenbaum H. Imaging of the left anterior descending coronary artery by high-frequency transthoracic and epicardial echocardiography. *Am J Cardiol* 2002;90:28L–31L.

122. Collins M, Hsieh A, Ohazama CJ, et al. Assessment of regional wall motion abnormalities with real-time 3-dimensional echocardiography. *J Am Soc Echocardiogr* 1999;12:7–14.

123. Bock AP, Genov A, Zotz RJ. Free-hand four-dimensional echocardiography: a diagnostic tool in coronary artery disease. *Echocardiography* 2002;19:135–137.

124. Yao J, Cao QL, Masani N, et al. Three-dimensional echocardiographic estimation of infarct mass based on quantification of dysfunctional left ventricular mass. *Circulation* 1997;96:1660–1666.

CHAPTER 61

The Role of Radionuclide Imaging

George A. Beller

Key Words: Hypoperfusion; myocardial infarction; myocardial perfusion; necrosis; radionuclide angiography; reperfusion; scintigraphy; single-photon emission computed tomography; ventriculography.

INTRODUCTION

Nuclear cardiology techniques used in the resting state or in conjunction with exercise or pharmacologic stress have been proven useful for detection of acute myocardial injury, distinguishing of myocardial necrosis from ischemia, determination of infarct size, assessment of myocardial salvage and infarct zone viability after reperfusion therapy, and risk stratification before discharge in patients presenting with suspected or proven acute myocardial infarction (AMI). The emergence of gated single-photon emission computed tomographic (SPECT) imaging and the approval of new technetium-99m (^{99m}Tc)-labeled perfusion agents have permitted enhanced localization and sizing of zones of myocardial infarction (MI) and assessment of regional and global function, which have substantial prognostic value. Positron emission tomography (PET) using [^{18}F]-fluorodeoxyglucose (FDG) has allowed determination of myocardial viability in zones of MI that demonstrate abnormal systolic function.

G. A. Beller: Department of Medicine, Cardiovascular Division, University of Virginia Health System, P.O. Box 800158, Charlottesville, Virginia 22908-0158.

Both conventional radionuclide and PET techniques can identify viability in stunned myocardium in patients experiencing an acute infarction who have undergone reperfusion therapy.

MYOCARDIAL PERFUSION IMAGING: TECHNIQUES AND RADIOPHARMACEUTICALS

Instrumentation

Single-Photon Emission Computed Tomography Imaging

SPECT imaging yields tomographic images of slices of the heart without interference of activity from noncardiac overlapping myocardial regions. Data are collected about the heart from multiple views, using camera rotation around the body, which then are used to construct tomograms through the heart. The tomographic approach is an improvement over the planar approach in contrast resolution and assists in the enhanced detection of small regions of hypoperfusion (e.g., subendocardial infarction). The overlap of normal and abnormal segments on planar images makes detection and localization of small zones of infarction difficult. Because SPECT images are free of background, lesion contrast is higher, and the size of defects is made greater by tomographic reconstructed views compared with the planar anterior, 45-degree left anterior oblique (LAO), and 70-degree LAO projections. It must be mentioned, however, that the cost of improvement in contrast resolution is a loss of spatial resolution.

Tomographic SPECT imaging is best accomplished with a large field-of-view gamma camera equipped with a low-energy, general purpose collimator. Detector orbits can be elliptical or circular and can be either 180 or 360 degrees. The 180-degree orbit is characterized by high spatial and contrast resolution, whereas the 360-degree orbit is associated with enhanced field uniformity. Typically in an 180-degree orbit, the camera makes 32 or 64 stops for 40 seconds each image acquisition. Each of the projections is corrected for field nonuniformity and for misalignment of the mechanical center of rotation with respect to the reconstruction matrix.

After the orbit is complete, the series of planar images taken at different angles around the patient are "backprojected" into the transverse axial images, which are slices that are oriented perpendicular to the axis of rotation. Backprojection is undertaken to reconstruct transverse tomograms encompassing the heart from apex to base. These transaxial images correspond to the long axis of the patient. The transaxial images are then reoriented to produce horizontal long-axis and vertical long-axis images. The final images are displayed in a slice-by-slice format for visual analysis. Figure 61–1 shows normal short-axis, vertical long-axis, and horizontal long-axis SPECT tomograms.

Quantitation of Single-Photon Emission Computed Tomography Images

Computer-assisted quantitative scan analysis can enhance the detection of myocardial perfusion defects on SPECT reconstructed images (1). One of the most common techniques for quantitating myocardial perfusion is the use of two-dimensional polar maps. These polar maps are constructed by mapping sequential maximal-count circumferential profiles, ranging from apex to the base of the heart, into successive rings on a polar map display. The apex is placed in the center of the map, and the base of the heart is displayed at its periphery. This polar map also is referred to as a "bull's-eye plot." This plot consists of a series of 15 concentric circles made from the 15 profiles interpolated from 12 slices from apex to base. Bull's-eyes are constructed for both stress and rest images and can be used for determination of defect size. Normalization of bull's-eye plots can be accomplished by comparison with a normal database obtained from subjects with a low probability of coronary artery disease (CAD).

Electrocardiographic Single-Photon Emission Computed Tomography Imaging

Electrocardiographic (ECG) gating of SPECT ^{99m}Tc-sestamibi or ^{99m}Tc-tetrofosmin images permits accurate assessment of regional wall motion or thickening and measurement of the left ventricular ejection fraction (LVEF). An excellent correlation between the SPECT LVEF and LVEF calculated by contrast ventriculography ($r = 0.93$) has been reported (2,3). Interpretation of gated SPECT images im-

proves the specificity of the radionuclide technique because defects produced by attenuation artifacts show preservation of systolic thickening, whereas nonreversible defects secondary to myocardial scar tend to show abnormal wall thickening in the defect region (4). The SPECT-determined LVEF and the end-diastolic volume provided incremental prognostic value over perfusion imaging variables alone in predicting cardiac death (5). The cardiac death rate per year was 0.96% in patients with a mild to moderate stress perfusion defect and a SPECT LVEF of 45% or more compared with 9.2% per year in such patients whose LVEF was less than 45%. In another study by this group (6), the LVEF measured on the poststress SPECT images was the best predictor of subsequent cardiac death, whereas the amount of ischemia was the best predictor of nonfatal MI. Significant postexercise LV regional dysfunction, consistent with stunning, occurs in regions of severe stress-induced ischemia (7). Presence of regional dysfunction in areas that show no significant perfusion defects identifies patients with high-risk coronary lesions on angiography (8).

Radionuclide Angiography

Radionuclide angiography or ventriculography is a technique that allows the noninvasive assessment of left ventricular (LV) and right ventricular (RV) function, and for the most part is undertaken using a single-crystal gamma scintillation camera (9). The two methods used for radionuclide angiography are the "first-pass" and the "equilibrium." Both techniques use gating in the acquisition, permitting the display of a series of images depicting changes in radioactivity occurring within the LV and RV blood pools during the cardiac cycle. The radionuclide angiogram can be displayed in a cineformat and can be digitized in the form of a relative volume curve. This volume curve is based on the principle that a change in radioactivity is proportional to the change in blood volume, and when background corrections have been performed, the time–activity curve within the LV blood pool represents the average change in blood volume during the cardiac cycle. Chamber size and segmental wall motion can be subjectively evaluated from the radionuclide angiogram, and computer-derived global and regional ejection fractions (EFs) can be measured. For adequately assessing regional wall motion using the equilibrium technique, anterior, 45-degree LAO, and 70-degree LAO projections are obtained. The area-counts technique for calculation of LVEF correlates well with the LVEF assessed from contrast ventriculography in the same patients. Similarly, there is excellent reproducibility and intraobserver variability by measuring the LVEF from radionuclide angiograms (10).

The RVEF is better assessed using the first-pass method in which a single bolus is injected rapidly through the intravenous route, and analysis is limited to the initial transient of the radioactive bolus through the central circulation. For first-pass studies, a multicrystal scintillation camera is preferable to the single-crystal Anger camera, because high

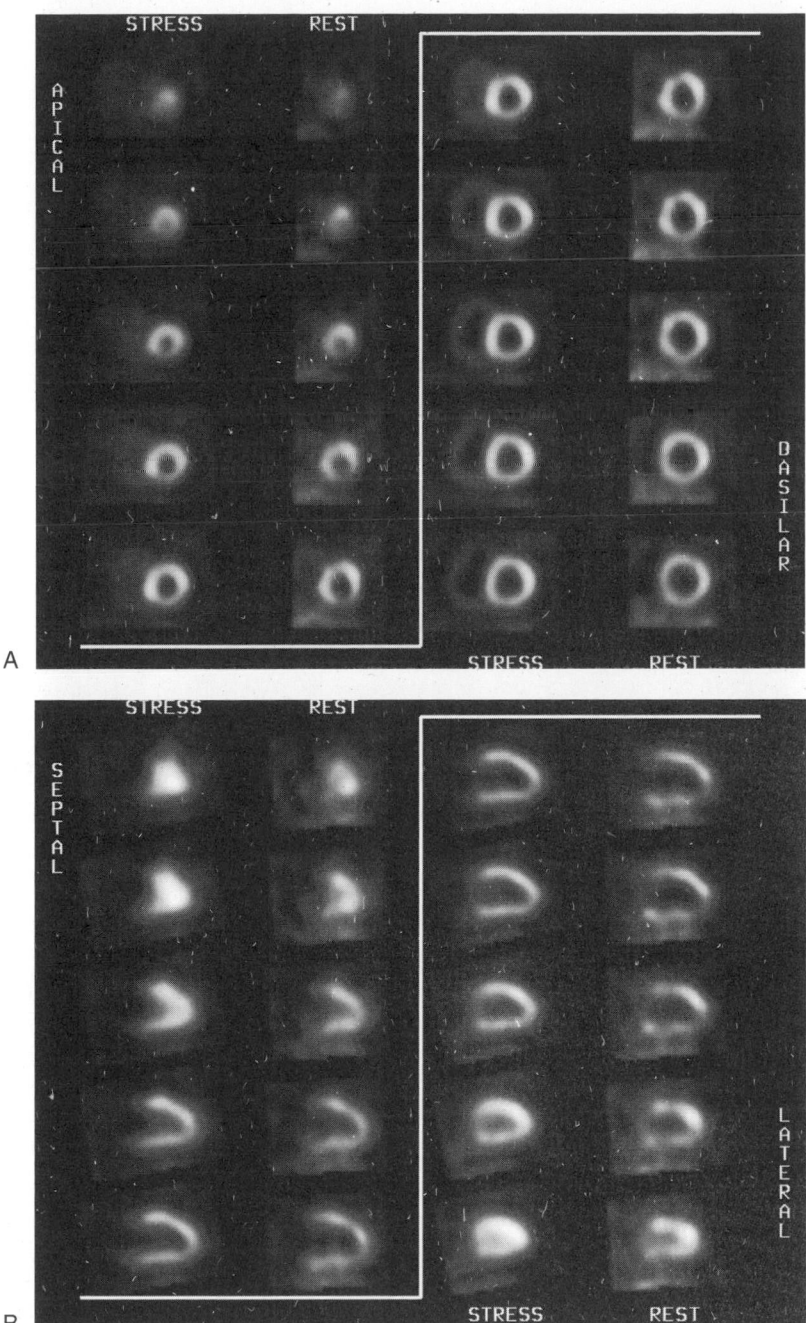

FIG. 61–1. A: Normal stress **(left column)** and rest **(right column)** short-axis single-photon emission computed tomography tomograms from apex **(top left)** to the base. Note uniform technetium-99m (^{99m}Tc)-sestamibi uptake in all myocardial segments. **B:** Vertical long-axis stress and rest tomograms from the same patient from the septal **(top left)** to the lateral **(bottom right)** region of the left ventricle. Note uniform uptake of ^{99m}Tc-sestamibi in all segments. **C:** Stress and rest horizontal long-axis tomograms from the same patient with the inferior slices **(top left)** to the superior slices **(bottom right).** As with the previous views, shown in **A** and **B,** note the uniform ^{99m}Tc-sestamibi uptake in all segments.

count rates are obtainable with the multicrystal instrument. EFs of the RV and LV are measured with the first-pass approach by delineating the regions of the blood pool of the LV and RV chambers on the computer display and deriving the time–activity curve as the bolus of radioactivity traverses the heart. The LVEF is determined by averaging several in-

dividual beats or from a summed cardiac cycle by adding several beats. RVEF measurements using the first-pass technique are perhaps most useful in the setting of MI for quantitating RV dysfunction in patients experiencing acute inferior/posterior infarction with suspected RV involvement. Estimates of valvular regurgitation and detection of left-to-

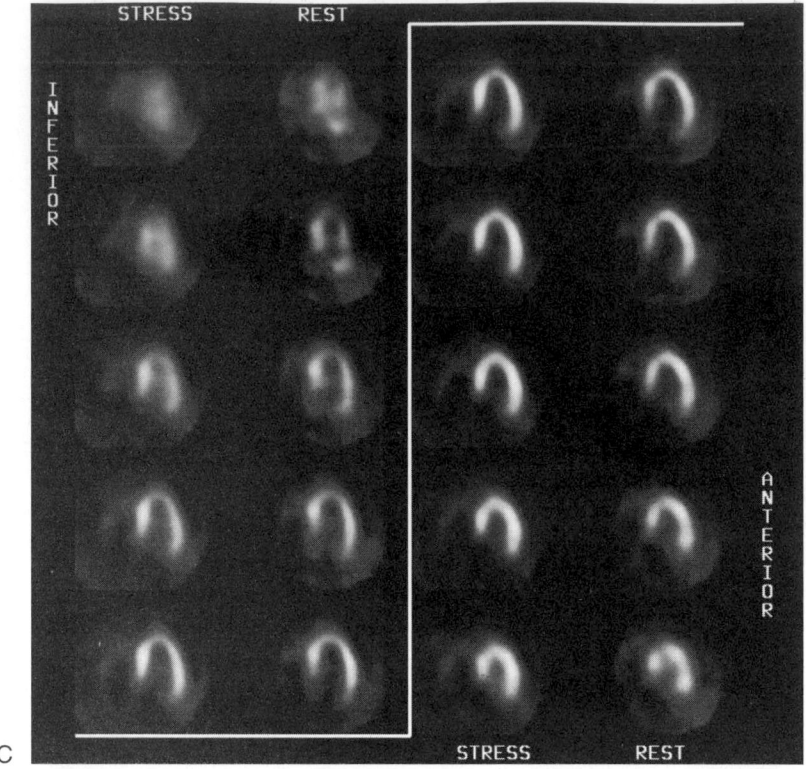

FIG. 61-1. *Continued.*

right shunts also can be accomplished by radionuclide angiography techniques.

The LVEF measured by radionuclide angiography is a powerful predictor of prognosis after AMI (11). The 6-month mortality rate after MI in the study by Burns and coworkers (12) was greatest (11%) in the subgroup with an LVEF less than 30%. The mortality rate was only 0.7% in the 603 patients with an LVEF of 50% or greater (12).

Ventricular diastolic function also can be evaluated by radionuclide angiography techniques by measuring rate of ventricular filling, peak filling rate, and time-to-peak filling derived from the high–temporal resolution volume curve of the LV.

Radionuclide Agents

In recent years, new ^{99m}Tc-labeled perfusion agents have been introduced into clinical practice, which enhance the specificity of SPECT perfusion imaging and provide additional diagnostic and prognostic information regarding regional and global LV function. The image quality obtained with these new Tc-labeled radionuclides, such as ^{99m}Tc-sestamibi and ^{99m}Tc-tetrofosmin, was superior to that of images obtained with thallium-201 (^{201}Tl) because of the more favorable physical characteristics of Tc imaging with a gamma camera. With ^{99m}Tc, doses of 10 to 20 times greater than those that are feasible with ^{201}Tl can be administered, providing images with greater count density. [99m]Tc demon-

strates less scatter and attenuation than ^{201}Tl, which is associated with fewer image artifacts in patients with no underlying CAD.

Experimental studies have shown that the uptake of ^{99m}Tc-sestamibi and ^{99m}Tc-tetrofosmin is proportional to regional myocardial blood flow but plateaus earlier at hyperemic flows than [201]Tl. This is because of a lower myocardial first-pass extraction fraction for these ^{99m}Tc-labeled perfusion agents compared with [201]Tl. In addition, the first-pass myocardial extraction fraction of ^{99m}Tc-tetrofosmin is less than ^{99m}Tc-sestamibi by approximately 10% to 15%. This may be a factor contributing to its lower sensitivity for detecting mild to moderate stenoses with a vasodilator stress. A new ^{99m}Tc-labeled perfusion agent, ^{99m}Tc-NOET, currently in clinical trials, shows a greater first-pass extraction than ^{99m}Tc-sestamibi or ^{99m}Tc-tetrofosmin and redistributes after a single intravenous injection similar to ^{201}Tl but faster.

When ^{201}Tl is injected during peak stress, there is delayed redistribution that is characterized by filling in of perfusion defects in ischemic regions of 3 to 4 hours. No significant redistribution after a single tracer injection is observed after administration of ^{99m}Tc-sestamibi or ^{99m}Tc-tetrofosmin. Therefore, separate injections at rest and with exercise are undertaken to identify zones of reversible ischemia. This is accomplished by using either a 2-day protocol (particularly in obese individuals), in which the stress and resting studies are performed on separate days. For these studies, high doses (30 mCi) are given for the stress and for the rest injections, yielding high-quality studies with adequate count density. For the majority of patients, a same-day study was performed, in which a low dose (7–10 mCi) of the ^{99m}Tc-labeled imaging agent is given at rest and 25 to 30 mCi of the agent are administered during stress several hours later. With respect to the same-day study, regional and global function is quantitated on the images obtained after stress (which are required in the resting state usually 30 minutes to 1 hour after tracer injection at peak treadmill or bicycle exercise, or at peak pharmacologic stress). Figure 61–2 shows stress and rest ^{99m}Tc-sestamibi SPECT images showing reversible apical and anteroseptal defects consistent with inducible ischemia in the supply zone of the left anterior descending coronary artery. The percent change in defect magnitude in the affected segments is shown below the images.

As mentioned previously, the accuracy of SPECT imaging is significantly influenced by the presence of tissue attenuation that produces artifacts that can mimic true defects, reducing the specificity of the test for CAD detection. Attenuation artifacts most often appear as fixed defects on SPECT images, which might be difficult to distinguish from defects attributed to MI. As mentioned previously, gating the images to evaluate thickening from end-diastole to end-systole is one way to differentiate attenuation artifacts from scar. Another way in which artifacts can be diminished is using a technique that corrects for soft tissue attenuation. Major artifacts encountered include breast attenuation artifacts pro-

ducing diminished tracer uptake in the anterior wall and upper septum. False-positive reversible defects can be produced if there is "shifting" breast attenuation from stress to rest images. For the most part, however, breast attenuation artifacts produce fixed (nonreversible) defects. In addition, conventional SPECT imaging is influenced by artifacts caused by inferior wall or posterior wall attenuation. Increased count densities in the inferior wall can occur secondary to high concentration of ^{99m}Tc in the subdiaphragmatic abdominal viscera, including liver, spleen, stomach, and loops of bowel. Such visceral activity adjacent to the heart may scatter into the LV wall, resulting in falsely increased count densities.

A number of solutions for attenuation correction are currently being evaluated in the clinical setting. The attenuation-corrected images that are produced by the software programs have been shown to improve the normalcy rate for stress SPECT imaging, as well as specificity. Attenuation-corrected images improve the quality of ^{201}Tl scintigraphy and SPECT imaging using the ^{99m}Tc tracers. Shotwell and coworkers (13) applied attenuation correction on SPECT ^{201}Tl imaging using a triple-headed camera with fan-beam collimation and reported a significant increase in normalcy rate (88% vs. 74%, $p = 0.009$) compared with nonattenuation-corrected images. Attenuation correction also improved the detection rate of patients with significant coronary artery stenoses (90% vs. 71%, $p = 0.016$). Interestingly, the addition of scatter correction yielded no incremental improve-

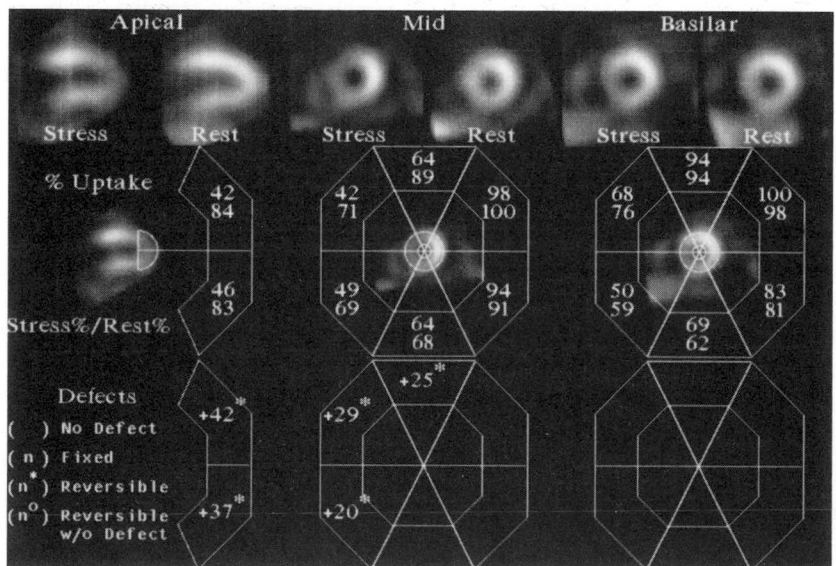

FIG. 61–2. Stress and rest quantitative technetium-99m (^{99m}Tc)-sestamibi images in a patient with reversible defects in the apex and in the anteroseptal region. The *numbers on the top* of each pair represent the percent ^{99m}Tc-sestamibi uptake in that segment during stress. The *bottom number* of each pair represents the percent ^{99m}Tc-sestamibi uptake after the resting injection of the tracer. Note that in the anteroapical region, ^{99m}Tc-sestamibi uptake improved from 42% of the area showing the greatest uptake (normalized at 100%) to 84% at rest, yielding a 42% reversible defect. The percent defect magnitudes are shown in the segments at the bottom of the figure. The abnormal segments are in the distribution of the left anterior descending coronary artery. The *asterisks* represent that the abnormalities represent more than two standard deviations from the normal database.

ment in the detection rate of stenotic vessels or the normalcy rate.

Links and colleagues (14) reported that the combination of ECG gating and attenuation correction provided the greatest diagnostic accuracy for detection of abnormal vascular territories. Identification of left main coronary disease was reported to be enhanced using attenuation-corrected SPECT, compared with uncorrected SPECT (15). It should be pointed out that attenuation-corrected SPECT imaging requires greater complexity and more imaging time than conventional SPECT imaging. This is because a transmission map is acquired separately from the patient emission data.

Not all studies have shown substantial value for simultaneously acquired transmission and emission radionuclide data for attenuation correction and incorporating scatter correction. Although the normalcy rate was significantly improved on the attenuation-corrected images (96% vs. 86%) in one multicenter study (16), the ability to detect multivessel disease was reduced with attenuation/scatter correction. Reduced sensitivity but improved specificity for right coronary lesions was observed using attenuation/scatter-correction methodology. Thus, more work and clinical research need to be undertaken to determine if such advances in technology can truly add value in improving the overall accuracy for SPECT imaging of ischemia and infarction.

[^{18}F]-Fluorodeoxyglucose Single-Photon Emission Computed Tomography for Evaluating Myocardial Viability

In recent years, high-energy SPECT imaging with 511-keV collimators has been introduced to evaluate both perfusion and FDG uptake with one system at one session using a dual-isotope imaging approach. Coincidence imaging using a gamma camera was subsequently introduced to improve this dual-imaging technique because the 511-keV, high-energy collimator resulted in low resolution and counting statistics with respect to the perfusion tracer, often being ^{99m}Tc-sestamibi.

Several studies in the literature compared FDG SPECT with FDG PET in patients with chronic CAD. These studies consistently showed good agreement between PET and SPECT in the assessment of viable myocardium (17).

Diagnosis of Myocardial Infarction in the Emergency Department Using Single-Photon Emission Computed Tomography Imaging

Each year, more than 6 million patients come to emergency departments in the United States with chest pain or symptoms suggestive of an acute coronary syndrome. Until recently, the majority of these patients (>50%) were admitted to the hospital because the initial clinical examination, resting ECG results, and initial cardiac enzyme levels were insufficient to eliminate the possibility of AMI or unstable angina. The cost of admitting patients to the hospital to rule out an acute coronary syndrome for patients without this entity is approximately $12 billion per year. Conversely, of patients who are discharged from the emergency department who present with chest pain, approximately 5% to 10% have an unrecognized MI with an annual mortality rate of 6% to 8%, and others have unstable angina or CAD resulting in a subsequent hospital admission. These latter patients represent a group with a high litigation risk.

To improve the efficacy and efficiency of treating patients in the emergency department, specialized chest pain centers have emerged, and new clinical pathways with new cardiac markers and noninvasive diagnostic technologies have been introduced to distinguish patients without CAD from those with CAD.

New biochemical serum markers have emerged that have played a major role in the diagnosis and risk stratification of patients presenting to the emergency department with a suspected acute coronary syndrome with a nondiagnostic resting ECG showing neither ST-segment elevation nor ischemic ST-segment depression (18). The cardiac troponins have received the greatest attention recently as serum markers that are clinically useful in excluding myocardial damage in patients with a suspected acute coronary syndrome. Serial troponin I measurements over 8 to 10 hours, for example, have yielded an excellent negative predictive value for ruling out MI when creatine kinase (CK-MB) is used as the gold standard. Circulating troponins I and T are not ordinarily detected in serum, even in patients with extensive skeletal muscle necrosis. The circulating levels of troponins remain increased for days after infarction. One important caveat with respect to the measurement of serum troponins to rule out myocardial damage is that only approximately 30% of patients presenting to an emergency department with chest pain and a suspected acute coronary syndrome have positive values when the first blood sample is drawn on admission. Therefore, such patients must be observed for at least 8 to 10 hours with serial troponin measurements to definitively diagnose or exclude myocardial damage (i.e., infarction) as a cause of the chest pain.

Acute myocardial perfusion imaging in the emergency department with either ^{99m}Tc-sestamibi or ^{99m}Tc-tetrofosmin in patients with chest pain have shown a high sensitivity and negative predictive value for detection of acute myocardial ischemia. With this approach, one of the ^{99m}Tc-labeled perfusion agents is injected during chest pain or soon after the resolution of pain, with images acquired 30 to 60 minutes later. A negative gated SPECT image when the radiopharmaceutical is administered in the emergency department in such patients has an approximate 98% negative predictive value for ruling out "acute infarction."

In one multicenter randomized trial, 357 patients presenting to 6 centers with symptoms suggestive of myocardial ischemia and a nondiagnostic ECG underwent ^{99m}Tc-tetrofosmin SPECT during or within 6 hours of symptoms (19). Follow-up evaluation was undertaken during hospitalization and 30 days after discharge. In these patients, 57% of the images were normal and 43% abnormal. Of the 20 patients (6%) with an AMI during the hospital period, 18 had abnormal images (sensitivity 90%), whereas only 2 had normal images (negative predictive value 99%). Using a normal SPECT image as a criterion not to admit patients from the emergency department would have resulted in a 57% reduction in hospital admissions, with a mean cost savings per patient of $4,258.

The only randomized study regarding the utility of myocardial perfusion imaging for evaluation and triage of patients with suspected acute cardiac ischemia using acute SPECT imaging was reported by Udelson and coworkers (20). Among 2,475 adult emergency department patients with chest pain or other symptoms suggestive of acute cardiac ischemia and with a normal or nondiagnostic initial ECG, 1,260 were randomly assigned for usual care and 1,215 were assigned to an acute resting ^{99m}Tc SPECT imaging strategy. The study showed that the acute imaging strategy improved triage decision-making in that unnecessary hospitalization of patients without acute cardiac ischemia was reduced (42% vs. 52%) without affecting the appropriate hospitalization of patients with acute cardiac ischemia.

Several studies have compared the results of acute rest myocardial perfusion imaging with serial CK-MB and troponin analysis (21,22). The sensitivity for detecting AMI was similar between the two strategies, but acute resting myocardial perfusion imaging was positive earlier after

presentation. This is because cardiac markers require 6 to 12 hours to become maximally positive, whereas rest myocardial perfusion imaging reflects the status of myocardial blood flow at the time the radiopharmaceutical is injected. Another study by Swinburn and coworkers (23) showed that the combination of troponin T and SPECT is the best model for early prediction of cardiac events in patients with acute chest pain. Figure 61–3 shows event-free survival curves demonstrating the increased risk associated with an abnormal gated SPECT scan in addition to an increased troponin T level.

Many patients will have negative troponin assays and normal resting gated SPECT perfusion scans but will still have underlying CAD that may or may not have been the cause of the emergency presentation. Therefore, most groups perform stress testing, with or without myocardial imaging, after an AMI or an unstable coronary syndrome is excluded. Such patients referred for early stress testing, often directly from the emergency department, have normal or nondiagnostic serial ECGs, no troponin level increase, and a low-to-intermediate likelihood of an acute coronary syndrome. Some who have had resting perfusion imaging are at an even smaller risk for an acute coronary syndrome because the perfusion scan was interpreted as normal. A percentage of these patients will demonstrate stress exercise or pharmacologic stress-induced ischemia on testing, which necessitates further management decisions, with either referral for car-

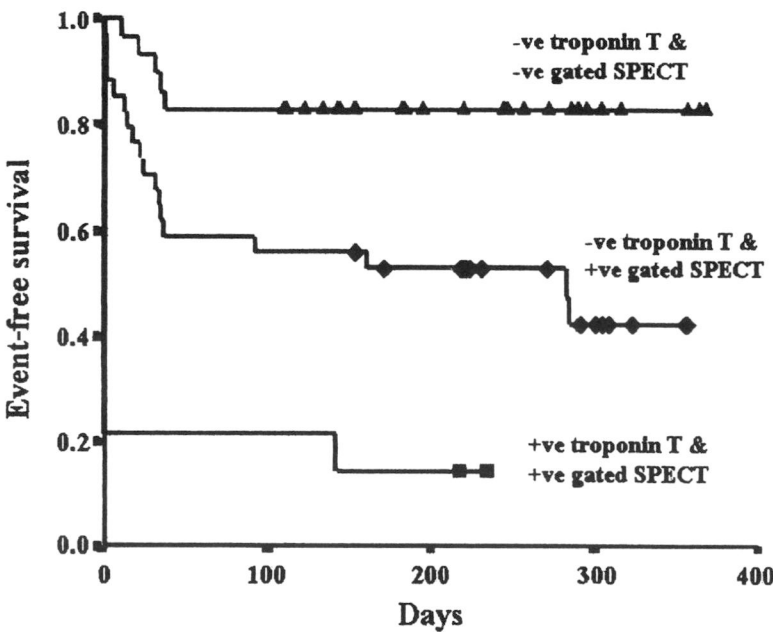

FIG. 61–3. Event-free survival curves demonstrating the increased risk associated with an abnormal gated technetium-99m-sestamibi single-photon emission computed tomography (SPECT) performed in patients during or soon after an episode of chest pain. Note the increase in risk associated with a positive gated SPECT and the additional increase in risk with troponin T positivity. All troponin-positive patients had abnormal gated SPECT scans. −ve, negative; +ve, positive. (From Swinburn JM, Stubbs P, Soman P, et al. Rapid assessment of patients with non-ST-segment elevation acute chest pain: troponins, inflammatory markers, or perfusion imaging? *J Nucl Cardiol* 2002;9:491–499, with permission.)

diac catheterization or medical therapy. Amsterdam and coworkers (24) reported that immediate exercise testing of patients presenting to the emergency department for chest pain and evidence of low clinical risk is safe and provides important information for determining those patients who require admission and those who can be discharged with the condition of further outpatient evaluation. They performed sign- or symptom-limited exercise in 1,000 patients presenting to the emergency department with chest pain compatible with a cardiac cause but clinical evidence of low risk on initial assessment. Of these patients, the test results were positive for ischemia in 13%, negative in 64%, and nondiagnostic in 23%. Most importantly, there were no adverse effects of exercise testing.

Quantification of Infarct Size

^{99m}Tc-sestamibi or ^{99m}Tc-tetrofosmin imaging may be successfully used for sizing of AMI and precisely localizing the zone of myocardial injury. In experimental studies, ^{99m}Tc-sestamibi scintigraphic defect size in dogs undergoing coronary occlusion and reperfusion correlates well with pathologic infarct size as determined by histochemistry (25,26). Resting SPECT ^{99m}Tc-sestamibi has been successfully used for determination of infarct size in clinical studies (27). ^{99m}Tc-sestamibi infarct size on SPECT correlates well with other variables traditionally used to clinically estimate infarct size including LVEF, end-systolic volume, regional wall motion, CK-MB release, and infarct size measured by ^{201}Tl. Figure 61–4 shows the relation between ^{99m}Tc-sestamibi infarct size measured at discharge and the end-systolic volume of the LV measured 1 year later by CT scanning (28). The correlation was highly statistically significant

($r = 0.80$; $p = 0.0005$). Medrano and coworkers (29) reported a close correlation between the extent of fibrosis in human hearts explanted for cardiac transplantation from patients with ischemic cardiomyopathy and the perfusion defect size measured by *ex vivo* SPECT imaging after intravenous administration of ^{99m}Tc-sestamibi antiharvesting of the heart. Finally, ^{99m}Tc-sestamibi infarct size was associated with subsequent cardiac mortality in a study by Miller and coworkers (30). Patients with infarct size of 12% or greater had a substantially greater mortality rate compared with patients with an infarct size of less than 12% (Fig. 61–5). Figure 61–6 shows images in a patient with a large posterior infarction with a nonreversible defect seen on stress and rest images. This patient has a high probability of experiencing remodeling of the LV over time. No significant ischemia is provoked, which is reflected by the absence of a reversible defect.

Resting ^{99m}Tc-sestamibi imaging has been used as a measurement of myocardial salvage and infarct size in several randomized clinical trials (31). The Acute Myocardial Infarction Study of Adenosine (AMISTAD) trial was designed to test the hypothesis that adenosine as an adjunct to thrombolysis would reduce myocardial infarct size in patients with ST-segment elevation MI. The primary end point of SPECT infarct size was determined by ^{99m}Tc-sestamibi imaging 6 ± 1 days after enrollment. In this study, there was a 33% relative reduction in infarct size with adenosine. A 67% relative reduction in infarct size was seen in patients with anterior infarction, but no reduction was seen in patients with infarcts localized elsewhere. Thus, this study showed that adjunct administration of adenosine with thrombolytic therapy resulted in a significant reduction in infarct size.

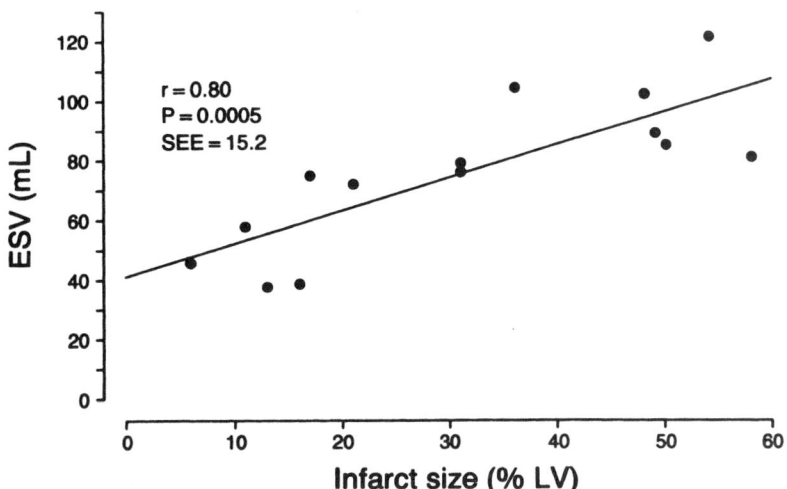

FIG. 61–4. Correlation between infarct size (percentage of left ventricle) determined by technetium-99m (^{99m}Tc)-sestamibi rest imaging and the end-systolic volume (ESV) of the left ventricle 1 year later. The correlation between ^{99m}Tc-sestamibi infarct size and ESV was 0.80. SEE, standard error of the mean. (From Chareonthaitawee P, Christian TF, Hirose K, et al. Relation of initial infarct size to extent of left ventricular remodeling in the year after acute myocardial infarction. *J Am Coll Cardiol* 1995;25:567–573, with permission.)

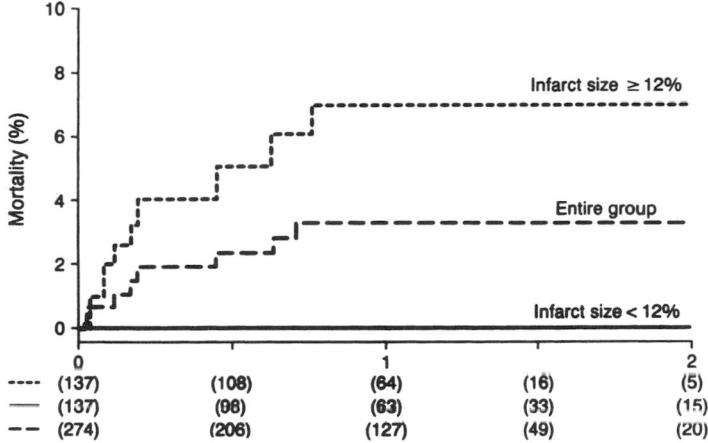

FIG. 61–5. Two-year survival in 274 patients with varying infarct sizes as measured by technetium-99m-sestamibi rest imaging. Patients with an infarct size of 12% or greater had a 7% mortality rate over 2 years, whereas patients with an infarct size of less than 12% had a 0% mortality rate over 2 years. (From Miller TD, Christian TF, Hopfenspirger MR, et al. Infarct size after acute myocardial infarction measured by quantitative tomographic ^{99m}Tc sestamibi imaging predicts subsequent mortality. *Circulation* 1995; 92:334–341, with permission.)

Resting ^{99m}Tc SPECT imaging was used to quantitate infarct size in patients receiving an inhibitor of the CD11/CD18 integrin receptor on neutrophils during reperfusion therapy with primary angioplasty (32). Experimental studies have previously shown that inhibition of the CD11/CD18 leukocyte integrin receptor results in a significant reduction in infarct size (33,34). Despite promise from these experimental studies, no difference in infarct size was observed in patients receiving placebo versus patients receiving a low dose and a high dose of the CD11/CD18 antibody directed against the integrin receptor. Infarct size was 16% in the placebo group and 16.6% in the high-dose, antibody-treated group.

Determination of Myocardial Viability Using Radionuclide Imaging

The noninvasive assessment of myocardial viability has been proven to be clinically useful for distinguishing viable but stunned or hibernating myocardium from myocardial necrosis and scar in patients with chronic ischemic heart disease or a recent MI (35–37). The accurate noninvasive determination of viability is critically important for clinical decision-making because it allows for selection of patients with CAD and resting LV dysfunction who benefit most from revascularization strategies.

After MI, regional dysfunction in the infarct zone can be attributed to either irreversible myocardial injury, stunned myocardium that will recover function most often observed after coronary reperfusion, and hibernating myocardium caused by chronic low-flow ischemia in the distribution of a residual high-grade infarct vessel stenosis.

A number of techniques have emerged for the clinical assessment of myocardial viability using radionuclide techniques. Myocardial perfusion and integrity of cell membranes can be assessed with quantitative SPECT using either ^{201}Tl or one of the ^{99m}Tc-labeled agents. Demonstration of the uptake of either more than 50% or more than 60% of these tracers by dysfunctional myocardium is reflective of viability. Perfusion and metabolism can be assessed simultaneously with PET with nitrogen-13 ammonia as the flow tracer and FDG as the metabolic tracer. A "mismatch" pattern showing diminished perfusion with corresponding enhanced uptake of FDG is indicative of viability. As reviewed earlier in this chapter, SPECT also can be used to assess perfusion and metabolism using high-energy (511 keV) collimators. The greater the uptake is of ^{201}Tl or ^{99m}Tc-tetrofosmin in dysfunctional myocardium, the greater the chance for recovery of function, either spontaneously in the presence of stunned myocardium or after revascularization in the instance of a flow-limiting stenosis that is either bypassed or opened with percutaneous coronary angioplasty. Figure 61–7 shows survival free of cardiac transplantation in patients with CAD with predominantly viable myocardium versus patients with predominantly nonviable myocardium who underwent coronary artery bypass surgery (38). Segmental viability was determined before surgery by quantitative ^{201}Tl scintigraphy. In another study (39), the clinical outcome of patients with prior MI and LV dysfunction was assessed after they underwent ^{99m}Tc-sestamibi SPECT and FDG SPECT for viability testing. As shown in Figure 61–8, the event-free survival was significantly better in patients with viable myocardium who underwent revascularization than patients with viability who were treated medically. In contrast, survival was comparable in revascularized versus medically-treated patients who had nonviable myocardium.

The evaluation of myocardial perfusion with gated SPECT using ^{201}Tl in combination with the evaluation of

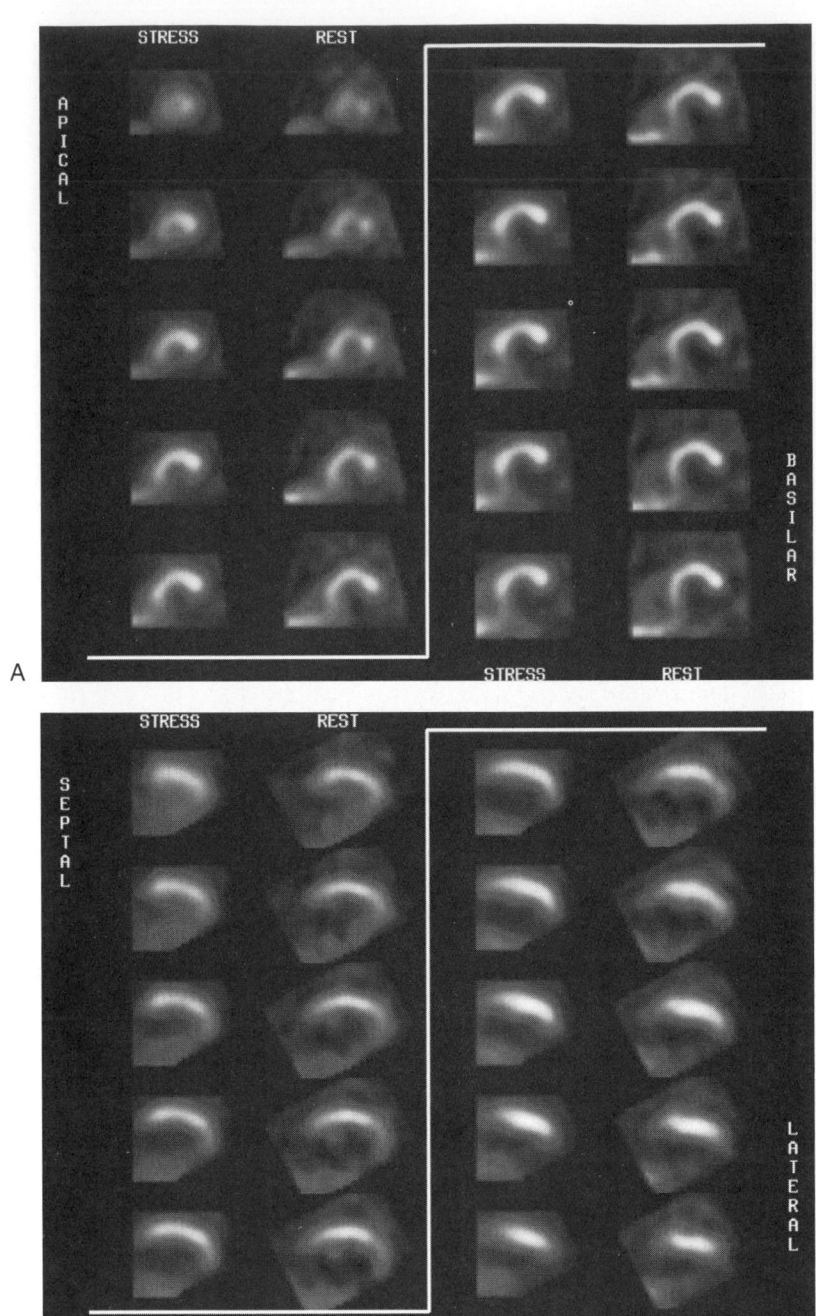

FIG. 61–6. A: Stress and rest short-axis tomograms in a patient with a posterior myocardial infarction. Note the nonreversible inferior and inferolateral defects. There are no areas of stress-induced ischemia characterized by defect reversibility. **B:** Stress and rest technetium-99m (^{99m}Tc)-sestamibi vertical long-axis tomograms showing a severe reduction in ^{99m}Tc-sestamibi activity in the posterior wall. Again, no evidence of inducible ischemia is observed. **C:** Stress and rest horizontal long-axis tomograms showing that the defect involves the inferior and inferolateral regions.

contractile reserve by means of low-dose dobutamine echocardiography is reported to show incremental value for viability detection and prediction of improved function in dyssynergic regions over perfusion assessment alone (40).

Stunned myocardium can be prospectively identified using ^{99m}Tc-sestamibi–based measurements of infarct size (41). A group of patients can be identified for whom the EF at hospital discharge is significantly less than would be expected

from the ^{99m}Tc-sestamibi defect size—a surrogate measure of infarct size. Patients with this "mismatch stunned" pattern, who had discharge EFs less than those predicted by infarct size demonstrated a significant improvement in EF at 6 weeks from 41% to 47%. In patients with a totally occluded infarct vessel after infarction, ^{201}Tl viability imaging can predict recoverable myocardium with a reasonable degree of accuracy, which can help select those patients benefiting most

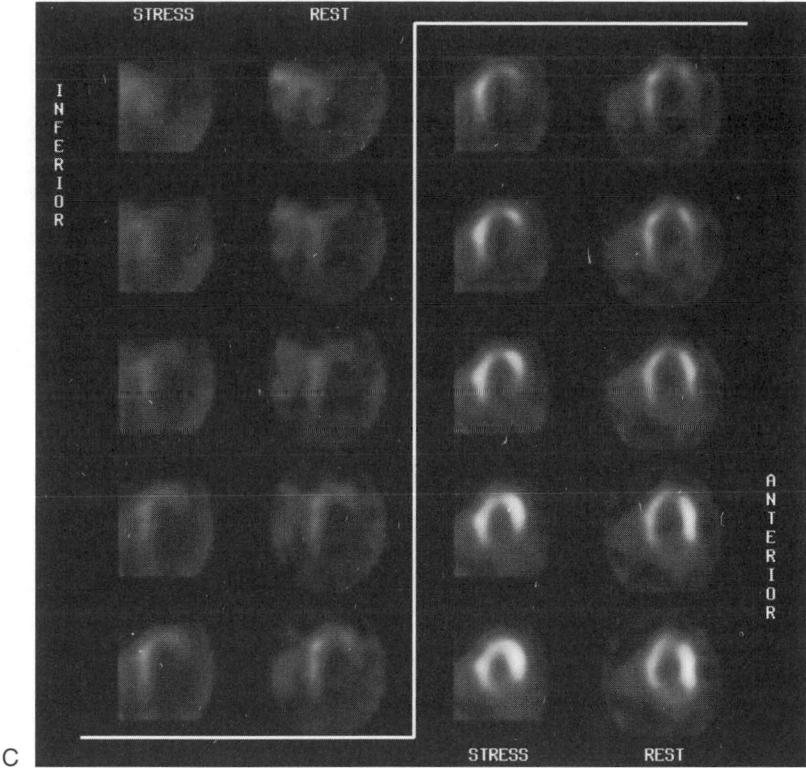

FIG. 61–6. *Continued.*

from revascularization (42). In this study, among 41 abnormal wall motion segments in the infarct territories, the sensitivity of ^{201}Tl imaging for prediction of recovery of regional function was 89%. All patients with occluded arteries underwent percutaneous coronary angioplasty. After reperfused

MI, the degree of LV dilation and LV remodeling is inversely related to the extent of residual myocardial viability in the infarct zone (43).

Thus, resting SPECT perfusion imaging can provide useful information regarding localization and sizing of MI. In

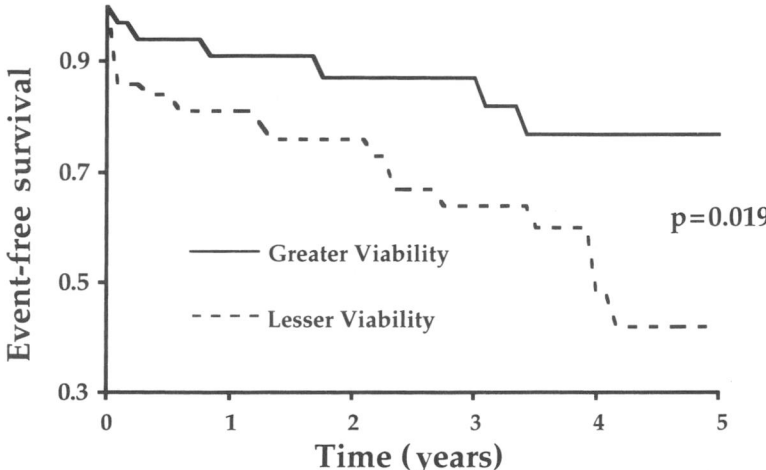

FIG. 61–7. Event-free survival of cardiac transplantation in patients with predominantly viable myocardium versus patients with predominantly nonviable myocardium, all who underwent coronary artery bypass graft surgery for severe multivessel coronary artery disease. Viability was assessed quantitatively using the percent uptake of thallium-201 on rest and delayed redistribution imaging. (From Pagley PR, Beller GA, Watson DD, et al. Improved outcome after coronary bypass surgery in patients with ischemic cardiomyopathy and residual myocardial viability. *Circulation* 1997;96:793–800, with permission.)

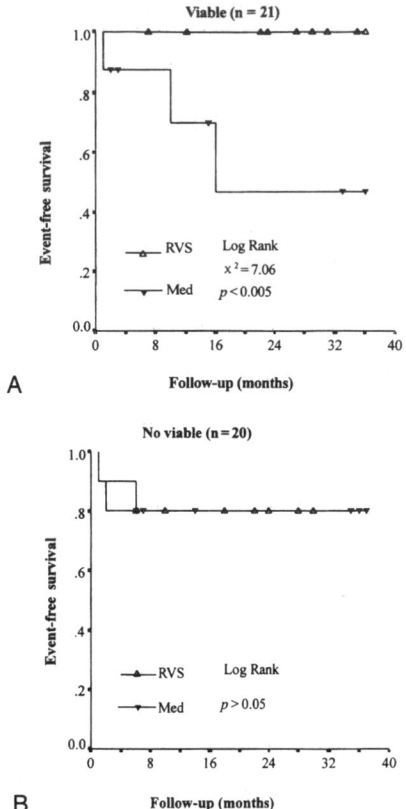

FIG. 61–8. Event-free survival in patients with predominantly viable myocardium **(A)** treated with revascularization *(RVS)* versus those with viable myocardium treated medically *(Med)*. **B:** Event-free survival in patients with nonviable myocardium treated either with revascularization or medically. Note that patients with predominantly viable myocardium who underwent revascularization had the best event-free survival during 40 months of follow-up. Those with the worst event-free survival were patients with predominantly viable myocardium treated medically. (From Zhang X, Liu XJ, Wu Q, et al. Clinical outcome of patients with previous myocardial infarction and left ventricular dysfunction assessed with myocardial ⁹⁹ᵐTc-MIBI SPECT and ¹⁸F-FDG PET. *J Nucl Med* 2001;42:1166–1173, with permission.)

addition, myocardial viability within the zone of infarction can be determined by the magnitude of tracer uptake using SPECT imaging or the presence of preserved myocardial FDG uptake on PET or FDG SPECT. As cited in the literature, the infarct size does have significant prognostic importance in that the larger the infarct size is, the greater the subsequent mortality rate is. The larger the area is of nonviability on resting radionuclide imaging, the greater the probability is of infarct expansion and LV remodeling characterized by cardiac dilatation and further diminution in LVEF. For patients with residual infarct vessel stenoses, the extent of viability can predict subsequent improvement, or lack thereof, in regional function after revascularization. (The role of stress perfusion imaging using radionuclide agents is discussed in Chapter 78.)

Resting Myocardial Perfusion Imaging for Assessment of Coronary Reperfusion

Myocardial perfusion imaging may provide useful information in the early and late assessment of MI patients who have received thrombolytic agents (44,45). Because ²⁰¹Tl uptake requires preserved nutrient flow and a viable cell membrane, the demonstration of substantial ²⁰¹Tl uptake on postreperfusion scintigraphy in the distribution of the previously occluded and reperfused vessel would reflect myocardial salvage and preserved viability.

Serial resting ²⁰¹Tl scintigraphy has been used to evaluate the efficacy of thrombolytic therapy in patients with AMI (46–51). Several investigators administered ²⁰¹Tl intravenously at acute presentation and obtained prethrombolysis images during the phase of coronary occlusion (46,47). Subsequently, delayed "redistribution" images were obtained after the administration of the thrombolytic agent. Each of these studies found that patients demonstrating successful reperfusion had greater delayed ²⁰¹Tl uptake and smaller final ²⁰¹Tl defects compared with scintigraphic findings in patients who did not respond to reperfusion. Many limitations exist with respect to the use of prethrombolysis and postthrombolysis resting ²⁰¹Tlscintigraphy to determine the size of the initial risk area and the amount of salvage after reflow. It may take as long as 30 to 40 minutes to obtain pretreatment SPECT ²⁰¹Tl images, which would unduly delay the administration of the thrombolytic agent. In addition, the nuclear cardiology laboratory may be located at a substantial distance from the emergency department, necessitating transport of an acute infarct patient out of the critical care treatment area. Currently, rest ²⁰¹Tl scintigraphy is more likely to be used 24 hours or later after admission for acute infarction to assess the extent of residual viable myocardium. In patients with a depression of LVEF, substantial delayed ²⁰¹Tl uptake in infarct zones of asynergy suggests viable but still underperfused myocardium. Such patients may benefit from coronary angioplasty of a high-grade, infarct-related stenosis with subsequent improvement in myocardial perfusion and function.

An attractive alternative to rest ²⁰¹Tl scintigraphy for assessment of myocardial salvage after thrombolytic therapy is the use of ⁹⁹ᵐTc sestamibi imaging (52–58). Because this agent does not substantially redistribute over time, it can be administered just before thrombolytic therapy, and imaging can be postponed several hours until thrombolytic drug administration has been completed. The images obtained several hours after tracer injection reflect the perfusion pattern at the time of administration when the infarct vessel was still occluded. This "snapshot" of the perfusion pattern reflects the "area at risk" in the supply region of the infarct-related artery. Imaging can be delayed for as long as 6 hours after injection, and the images acquired will still delineate the risk area corresponding to perfusion when the infarct artery was occluded. A second injection of ⁹⁹ᵐTc-sestamibi is administered some time after thrombolytic therapy, which reflects infarct size, and the change in defect extent from the pretreatment to the posttreatment images reflects the amount of myocardial salvage.

This serial imaging approach to assessing myocardial salvage after reperfusion has been tested in the clinical research setting, where serial ^{99m}Tc-sestamibi imaging was used to assess efficacy of thrombolytic therapy in patients with AMI in the Thrombolysis in Myocardial Infarction (TIMI) II study. Wackers and coworkers (53) performed serial ^{99m}Tc-sestamibi imaging in patients with an acute myocardial injury characterized by ST-segment elevation on the initial admission ECG. The ^{99m}Tc-sestamibi was administered before thrombolysis, and imaging was performed several hours later. The postreperfusion images were obtained 18 to 48 hours after thrombolytic therapy. Patients demonstrating myocardial salvage had a reduction in ^{99m}Tc-sestamibi defect size.

Gibbons and coworkers (54) undertook a similar study, but they used SPECT ^{99m}Tc-sestamibi imaging rather than the planar technique used by Wackers and coworkers (53); however, similar findings were obtained. A subsequent study from the same group demonstrated that the change in defect area varied significantly with both infarct location and infarct vessel patency (55). Defect extent and severity were significantly greater for anterior than for lateral or inferior infarctions (57).

The ^{99m}Tc-sestamibi defect size will continue to diminish from images obtained at 18 to 48 hours after reperfusion to images obtained 1 week later (56). This diminution in defect size might be explained by enhanced antegrade flow or presence of collateral flow, by improvement in regional systolic function, thereby diminishing the partial volume effect, or by enhanced intracellular transport of ^{99m}Tc-sestamibi with resolution of ischemia.

[99m]Tc-sestamibi imaging also has been used to evaluate the reduction in the area of myocardium at risk with immediate angioplasty (58–60). Behrenbeck and coworkers (58) found that the acute defect size before angioplasty was 48% ± 17% of the LV and diminished significantly to 29% ± 19% on repeat images obtained 6 to 10 days after acute balloon dilatation of the infarct-related vessel. Gibbons and coworkers (59) reported that myocardial salvage, reflected by the percent of the LV showing a reduction in defect size on serial ^{99m}Tc-sestamibi images, was similar in patients randomized to immediate angioplasty and patients who underwent only thrombolytic therapy. The greater the collateral flow is at the time of initial catheterization, the greater the amount is of myocardial salvage after angioplasty, as assessed by serial ^{99m}Tc-sestamibi imaging. ^{99m}Tc-sestamibi uptake in the zone of infarction after stenting of the infarct vessel correlated well with coronary flow reserve (CFR) using a Doppler guide wire at the time of catheterization (61). ^{99m}Tc-sestamibi uptake was significantly greater in patients with a CFR of 2.0 or greater compared with patients with a CFR less than 2.0 (Fig. 61–9). All ten patients with CFR greater than 2.0 had ^{99m}Tc-sestamibi uptake of more than 50% in the infarct region perfused by the stented infarct vessel. Finally, ^{99m}Tc-sestamibi imaging after reperfusion therapy provides information that is predictive of the LVEF at 1-year of follow-up (62). The EF at the time of discharge may not accurately reflect perfusion defect size because the effects of stunning have not yet resolved.

SUMMARY

Radionuclide imaging techniques have been proven to be useful in the diagnosis of acute or remote MI, identifying the

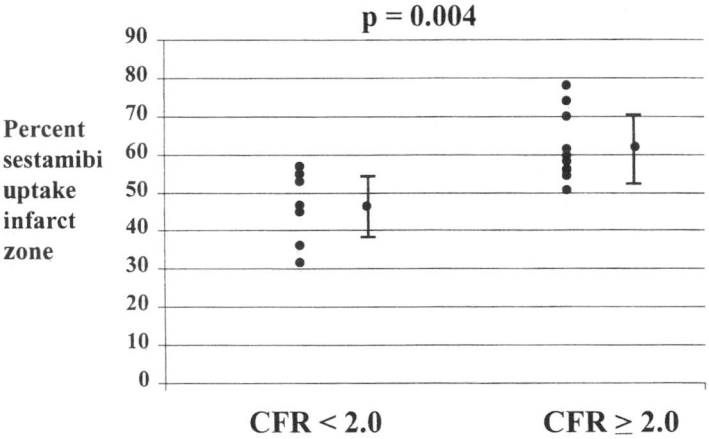

FIG. 61–9. Percent technetium-99m (^{99m}Tc)-sestamibi uptake in the infarct zone after stenting of the infarct-related vessel versus coronary flow reserve (CFR) measured at the time of cardiac catheterization using a Doppler-tipped guide wire. In this study, all patients with a CFR greater than 2.0 had preserved viability in the infarct zone defined as an average ^{99m}Tc-sestamibi uptake greater than 50%. (From Ragosta M, Powers ER, Samady H, et al. Relationship between extent of residual myocardial viability and coronary flow reserve in patients with recent myocardial infarction. *Am Heart J* 2001;141:456–462, with permission.)

precise location of infarction, sizing an acute infarction, evaluating residual viability in infarct zones, and determining the extent of global and regional myocardial dysfunction. Perhaps the most used of the nuclear cardiology techniques is myocardial perfusion imaging with ^{201}Tl or one of the new ^{99m}Tc-labeled agents. In this era of health care system reform, these techniques must be used in a cost-effective manner and contribute to the decision-making process. Myocardial perfusion or function imaging in the early hours after the onset of symptoms of AMI is rarely necessary because the diagnosis of infarction can be well established by conventional quantitation of CK-MB enzyme release and inspection of serial ECGs. Rest perfusion imaging may be more contributory to patient management later in the course of hospitalization when issues such as extent of myocardial viability and determination of residual ischemia are raised (the latter is discussed elsewhere in this textbook). The application of resting myocardial perfusion imaging for assessment of myocardial salvage after coronary reperfusion should still be considered investigational. Nevertheless, a single resting perfusion scan can be used to distinguish stunned from irreversible myocardial injury after thrombolytic therapy or immediate angioplasty. Finally, the role of acute imaging in the emergency department for distinguishing ischemic from nonischemic origins of undiagnosed chest pain also is under investigation and may prove to be useful in certain patient subgroups. The routine imaging of such patients is certainly not warranted.

REFERENCES

1. Garcia EV. Quantitative myocardial perfusion single-photon emission computed tomographic imaging: *Quo vadis* (where do we go from here)? *J Nucl Cardiol* 1994;1:83–93.
2. Van Kriekinge SD, Berman DS, Germano G. Automatic quantification of left ventricular ejection fraction from gated blood pool SPECT. *J Nucl Cardiol* 1999;6:498–506.
3. Smith WH, Kastner RJ, Calnon DA, et al. Quantitative gated single photon emission computed tomography imaging: a counts-based method for display and measurement of regional and global ventricular systolic function. *J Nucl Cardiol* 1997;4:451–463.
4. Smanio PE, Watson DD, Segalla DL, et al. Value of gating of technetium-99m sestamibi single-photon emission computed tomographic imaging. *J Am Coll Cardiol* 1997;30:1687–1692.
5. Sharir T, Germano G, Kavanagh PB, et al. Incremental prognostic value of post-stress left ventricular ejection fraction and volume by gated myocardial perfusion single photon emission computed tomography. *Circulation* 1999;100:1035–1042.
6. Sharir T, Germano G, Kang X, et al. Prediction of myocardial infarction versus cardiac death by gated myocardial perfusion SPECT: risk stratification by the amount of stress-induced ischemia and the post-stress ejection fraction. *J Nucl Med* 2001;42:831–837.
7. Paul AK, Hasegawa S, Yoshioka J, et al. Characteristics of regional myocardial stunning after exercise in gated myocardial SPECT. *J Nucl Cardiol* 2002;9:388–394.
8. Sharir T, Bacher-Stier C, Dhar S, et al. Identification of severe and extensive coronary artery disease by postexercise regional wall motion abnormalities in Tc-99m sestamibi gated single-photon emission computed tomography. *Am J Cardiol* 2000;86:1171–1175.
9. Zaret B, Berger H. Radionuclide studies of ventricular performance in coronary artery disease. In: Yu PN, Goodwin JF, eds. *Progress in cardiology, vol 12.* Philadelphia: Lea and Febiger, 1983;33–58.
10. Burow RD, Strauss HW, Singleton R, et al. Analysis of left ventricular function from multiple gated acquisition cardiac blood pool imaging: comparison to contrast angiography. *Circulation* 1977;56:1024–1028.
11. Multicenter Postinfarction Research Group. Risk stratification and survival after myocardial infarction. *N Engl J Med* 1983;309:331–336.
12. Burns RJ, Gibbons RJ, Yi Q, et al. The relationships of left ventricular ejection fraction, end-systolic volume index and infarct size to six-month mortality after hospital discharge following myocardial infarction treated by thrombolysis. *J Am Coll Cardiol* 2002;39:30–36.
13. Shotwell M, Singh BM, Fortman C, et al. Improved coronary disease detection with quantitative attenuation-corrected Tl-201 images. *J Nucl Cardiol* 2002;9:52–62.
14. Links JM, DePuey EG, Taillefer R, et al. Attenuation correction and gating synergistically improve the diagnostic accuracy of myocardial perfusion SPECT. *J Nucl Cardiol* 2002;9:183–187.
15. Duvernoy CS, Ficaro EP, Karabajakian MZ, et al. Improved detection of left main coronary artery disease with attenuation-corrected SPECT. *J Nucl Cardiol* 2000;7:639–648.
16. Hendel RC, Berman DS, Cullom SJ, et al. Multicenter clinical trial to evaluate the efficacy of correction for photon attenuation and scatter in SPECT myocardial perfusion imaging. *Circulation* 1999;99:2742–2749.
17. Bax JJ, Wijns W. Fluorodeoxyglucose imaging to assess myocardial viability: PET, SPECT or gamma camera coincidence imaging? *J Nucl Med* 1999;40:1893–1895.
18. Hamm CW. Cardiac biomarkers for rapid evaluation of chest pain. *Circulation* 2001;104:1454–1456.
19. Heller CV, Stowers SA, Hendel RC, et al. Clinical value of acute rest technetium-99m tetrofosmin tomographic myocardial perfusion imaging in patients with acute chest pain and nondiagnostic electrocardiograms. *J Am Coll Cardiol* 1998;31:1011–1017.
20. Udelson JE, Beshansky JR, Ballin DS, et al. Myocardial perfusion imaging for evaluation and triage of patients with suspected acute cardiac ischemia: a randomized controlled trial. *JAMA* 2002;288:2693–2700.
21. Kontos MC, Jesse RL, Anderson FP, et al. Comparison of myocardial perfusion imaging and cardiac troponin I in patients admitted to the emergency department with chest pain. *Circulation* 1999;99:2073–2078.
22. Duca MD, Giri S, Wu AH, et al. Comparison of acute rest myocardial perfusion imaging and serum markers of myocardial injury in patients with chest pain syndromes. *J Nucl Cardiol* 1999;6:570–576.
23. Swinburn JM, Stubbs P, Soman P, et al. Rapid assessment of patients with non-ST-segment elevation acute chest pain: troponins, inflammatory markers, or perfusion imaging? *J Nucl Cardiol* 2002;9:491–499.
24. Amsterdam EA, Kirk JD, Diercks DB, et al. Immediate exercise testing to evaluate low-risk patients presenting to the emergency department with chest pain. *J Am Coll Cardiol* 2002;40:251–256.
25. Verani MS, Jeroudi MO, Mahmarian JJ, et al. Quantification of myocardial infarction during coronary occlusion and myocardial salvage after reperfusion using cardiac imaging with technetium-99m hexakis 2-methoxyisobutyl isonitrile. *J Am Coll Cardiol* 1988;12:1573–1581.
26. Sinusas AJ, Trautman KA, Bergin JD, et al. Quantification of area at risk during coronary occlusion and degree of myocardial salvage after reperfusion with technetium-99m methoxyisobutyl isonitrile. *Circulation* 1990;82:1424–1437.
27. Gibbons RJ, Miller TD, Christian TF. Infarct size measured by single photon emission computed tomographic imaging with (99m)Tc-sestamibi: a measure of the efficacy of therapy in acute myocardial infarction. *Circulation* 2000;10:101–108.
28. Chareonthaitawee P, Christian TF, Hirose K, et al. Relation of initial infarct size to extent of left ventricular remodeling in the year after acute myocardial infarction. *J Am Coll Cardiol* 1995;25:567–573.
29. Medrano R, Lowry RW, Young JB, et al. Assessment of myocardial viability with 99mTc sestamibi in patients undergoing cardiac transplantation. A scintigraphic/pathological study. *Circulation* 1996;94:1010–1017.
30. Miller TD, Christian TF, Hopfenspirger MR, et al. Infarct size after acute myocardial infarction measured by quantitative tomographic (99m)Tc sestamibi imaging predicts subsequent mortality. *Circulation* 1995;92:334–341.
31. Mahaffey KW, Puma JA, Barbagelata NA, et al. Adenosine as an adjunct to thrombolytic therapy for acute myocardial infarction: results of a multicenter, randomized, placebo-controlled trial: the Acute Myocardial Infarction STudy of ADenosine (AMISTAD) trial. *J Am Coll Cardiol* 1999;34:1711–1720.
32. Faxon DP, Gibbons RJ, Chronos NA, et al. The effect of blockade of the CD11/CD18 integrin receptor on infarct size in patients with acute

myocardial infarction treated with direct angioplasty: the results of the HALT-MI study. *J Am Coll Cardiol* 2002;40:1199–1204.

33. Lefer DJ, Shandelya SM, Serrano CV Jr, et al. Cardioprotective actions of a monoclonal antibody against CD-18 in myocardial ischemia-reperfusion injury. *Circulation* 1993;88:1779–1787.

34. Palazzo AJ, Jones SP, Girod WG, et al. Myocardial ischemia-reperfusion injury in CD18- and ICAM-1–deficient mice. *Am J Physiol* 1998;275[6 Pt 2]:H2300–H2307.

35. Hendel RC, Chaudhry FA, Bonow RO. Myocardial viability. *Curr Probl Cardiol* 1996;21:145–221.

36. Beller GA. Noninvasive assessment of myocardial viability. *N Engl J Med* 2000;343:1488–1490.

37. Di Carli MF. Assessment of myocardial viability after myocardial infarction. *J Nucl Cardiol* 2002;9:229–235.

38. Pagley PR, Beller GA, Watson DD, et al. Improved outcome after coronary bypass surgery in patients with ischemic cardiomyopathy and residual myocardial viability. *Circulation* 1997;96:793–800.

39. Zhang X, Liu XJ, Wu Q, et al. Clinical outcome of patients with previous myocardial infarction and left ventricular dysfunction assessed with myocardial (99m)Tc-MIBI SPECT and (18)F-FDG PET. *J Nucl Med* 2001;42:1166–1173.

40. Simoes MV, de Almeida-Filho OC, Pintya AO, et al. Prediction of left ventricular wall motion recovery after acute myocardial infarction by Tl-201 gated SPECT: incremental value of integrated contractile reserve assessment. *J Nucl Cardiol* 2002;9:294–303.

41. Christian TF, Gitter MJ, Miller TD, et al. Prospective identification of myocardial stunning using technetium-99m sestamibi-based measurements of infarct size. *J Am Coll Cardiol* 1997;30:1633–1640.

42. Beanlands RS, Labinaz M, Ruddy TD, et al. Establishing an approach for patients with recent coronary occlusion: identification of viable myocardium. *J Nucl Cardiol* 1999;6:298–305.

43. Bolognese L, Cerisano G, Buonamici P, et al. Influence of infarct-zone viability on left ventricular remodeling after acute myocardial infarction. *Circulation* 1997;96:3353–3359.

44. Beller GA. Role of myocardial perfusion imaging in evaluating thrombolytic therapy for acute myocardial infarction. *J Am Coll Cardiol* 1987;9:661–668.

45. Beller GA. Myocardial reperfusion imaging: basic principles and clinical applications. *Am J Cardiac Imaging* 1993;7:11–23.

46. Reduto LA, Freund GC, Garcia JM, et al. Coronary artery reperfusion in acute myocardial infarction: beneficial effects of intracoronary streptokinase on left ventricular salvage and performance. *Am Heart J* 1981;102:1168–1177.

47. De Coster PM, Melin JA, Detry JM, et al. Coronary artery reperfusion in acute myocardial infarction: assessment by pre- and postintervention thallium-201 myocardial perfusion imaging. *Am J Cardiol* 1985;55:889–895.

48. Schwarz F, Hofmann M, Schuler G, et al. Thrombolysis in acute myocardial infarction: effect of intravenous followed by intracoronary streptokinase application on estimates of infarct size. *Am J Cardiol* 1984;53:1505–1510.

49. Schuler G, Schwarz F, Hoffmann M, et al. Thrombolysis in acute myocardial infarction using intracoronary streptokinase: assessment by thallium-201 scintigraphy. *Circulation* 1982;66:658–664.

50. Ritchie JL, Davis KB, Williams DL, et al. Global and regional left ventricular function and tomographic radionuclide perfusion: the Western Washington Intracoronary Streptokinase in Myocardial Infarction Trial. *Circulation* 1984;70:867–875.

51. Krause T, Kasper W, Meinertz T, et al. Comparison in acute myocardial infarction of anisoylated plasminogen streptokinase activator complex versus heparin evaluated by simultaneous thallium-201/technetium-99m pyrophosphate tomography. *Am J Cardiol* 1993;71:8–13.

52. Christian TF, Clements IP, Gibbons RJ. Noninvasive identification of myocardium at risk in patients with acute myocardial infarction and nondiagnostic electrocardiograms with technetium-99m sestamibi. *Circulation* 1991;83:1615–1620.

53. Wackers FJ, Gibbons RJ, Verani MS, et al. Serial quantitative planar technetium-99m isonitrile imaging in acute myocardial infarction: efficacy for noninvasive assessment of thrombolytic therapy. *J Am Coll Cardiol* 1989;14:861–873.

54. Gibbons RJ, Verani JS, Behrenbeck T, et al. Feasibility of tomographic (99m)Tc-hexakis-2-methoxy-2-methylpropyl-isonitrile imaging for the assessment of myocardial area at risk and the effect of treatment in acute myocardial infarction. *Circulation* 1989;80:1277–1286.

55. Gibson WS, Christian TF, Pellikka PA, et al. Serial tomographic imaging with technetium-99m sestamibi for the assessment of infarct-related arterial patency following reperfusion therapy. *J Nucl Med* 1992;33:2080–2085.

56. Pellikka PA, Behrenbeck T, Verani MS, et al. Serial changes in myocardial perfusion using tomographic technetium-99m-hexakis-2-methoxy-2-methylpropyl-isonitrile imaging following reperfusion therapy of myocardial infarction. *J Nucl Med* 1990;31:1269–1275.

57. Christian TF, Gibbons RJ, Gersh BJ. Effect of infarct location on myocardial salvage assessed by technetium-99m isonitrile. *J Am Coll Cardiol* 1991;17:1303–1308.

58. Behrenbeck T, Pellikka PA, Huber KC, et al. Primary angioplasty in myocardial infarction: assessment of improved myocardial perfusion with technetium-99m sestamibi. *J Am Coll Cardiol* 1991;17:365–372.

59. Gibbons RJ, Holmes DR, Reeder GS, et al., for the Mayo Coronary Care Unit and Catheterization Laboratory Groups. Immediate angioplasty compared with the administration of a thrombolytic agent followed by conservative treatment for myocardial infarction. *N Engl J Med* 1993;328:685–691.

60. Clements IP, Christian TF, Higano ST, et al. Residual flow to the infarct zone as a determinant of infarct size after direct angioplasty. *Circulation* 1993;88:1527–1533.

61. Ragosta M, Powers ER, Samady H, et al. Relationship between extent of residual myocardial viability and coronary flow reserve in patients with recent myocardial infarction. *Am Heart J* 2001;141:456–462.

62. Christian TF, Behrenbeck T, Gersh BJ, et al. Relation of left ventricular volume and function over one year after acute myocardial infarction to infarct size determined by technetium-99m sestamibi. *Am J Cardiol* 1991;68:21–26.

CHAPTER 62

The Role of Hemodynamic Assessment

William Ganz, Prediman K. Shah, and James S. Forrester

Key Words: Acute myocardial infarction; cardiac output; central venous pressure; hemodynamics; hypoperfusion; pulmonary capillary pressure; right atrial pressure; right ventricular failure; Starling function curve; tricuspid regurgitation.

INTRODUCTION

Acute myocardial infarction (AMI) causes derangement in cardiovascular hemodynamics. For the clinical cardiologist, the four most important hemodynamic changes are increased

W. Ganz: Division of Cardiology, Department of Medicine, UCLA David Geffen School of Medicine, Cedars-Sinai Medical Center, Los Angeles, California 90048-0750.

P. K. Shah: Division of Cardiology, Department of Medicine, UCLA David Geffen School of Medicine, Cedars-Sinai Medical Center, Los Angeles, California 90048-0750.

J. S. Forrester: Division of Cardiology, Department of Medicine, UCLA David Geffen School of Medicine, Cedars-Sinai Medical Center, Los Angeles, California 90048-0750.

right atrial pressure, increased pulmonary capillary pressure, decreased cardiac output, and decreased systemic arterial pressure. Because each of these hemodynamic changes have specific clinical manifestations, careful bedside assessment is an excellent method for determination of the magnitude of cardiac dysfunction. This assessment is critical in patients with acute infarction, because in-hospital prognosis is directly related to the magnitude of cardiac dysfunction (1), and because the type and magnitude of cardiac dysfunction right heart failure, pulmonary congestion, and peripheral hypoperfusion determine the choice of therapy (2,3). There are, however, clinical conditions in which bedside evaluation may not be sufficiently reliable for diagnosis or management. In general, these conditions fall into one of three categories: clinical instability, the use of drugs that cause rapid hemodynamic changes, and the need for a specific anatomic diagnosis. This chapter discusses how normal cardiac function is deranged by acute infarction, how disordered cardiac hemodynamics determine both the clinical state and choice of therapy, the diagnosis of clinical syndromes by hemodynamics, and the technical details of hemodynamic monitoring.

REGULATION OF CARDIAC FUNCTION

Regulatory Factors for Normal Cardiac Function

The factors controlling function of the intact heart have been defined by the study of isolated mammalian heart muscle. When cardiac muscle is stimulated to contract, how much it shortens is determined by three factors: preload, afterload, and contractility. As the resting length (preload) of a cardiac muscle is increased, the force it develops during contraction increases. The relation is not linear. As the unstretched muscle initially lengthens, it shortens proportionately more; but with further increase in length, a plateau is reached beyond which no further increase in force of contraction occurs. Once contraction begins, shortening is determined by the resistance against which the muscle must contract (afterload) and by the intrinsic contractility of the muscle.

Preload, afterload, and contractility have direct analogies in the intact heart. Preload is represented by the end-diastolic volume of the left ventricle and is most commonly estimated clinically by the left ventricular end-diastolic pressure. Afterload, the force the left ventricle develops during contraction, is represented by arterial or left ventricular systolic pressure. Although contractility is not generally measured in the intact hearts, the rate of increase of left ventricular pressure is a rough estimate of contractility. These interrelations are expressed in the family of Starling function curves. Therapeutic manipulation of the Starling function curve is the basis for treatment of disordered hemodynamics in AMI.

Transition from Normal to Abnormal Cardiac Function

The transition from normal cardiac function to heart failure is a subtle continuum. Heart failure occurs when the infarct-induced decrease in cardiac performance exceeds the ability of these mechanisms to compensate. The acute compensatory responses are those that also control normal cardiac function, whereas the chronic compensatory responses are involved only in nonphysiologic conditions. Therefore, in the progression from normal function to heart failure, there is a usual sequence of clinical events. In general, the autonomic nervous system is the first to be used in response to acute heart failure. Autonomic nervous system activation increases peripheral vascular resistance, heart rate, and myocardial contractility. The infarct-induced reduction in function combined with the compensatory increase in vascular resistance cause an increase in end-diastolic volume and activation of the Starling mechanism. When these acute compensatory mechanisms fail, chronic renal retention of sodium and water is activated. When heart failure persists beyond several days, these acute and subacute compensatory responses tend to diminish in intensity and effectiveness and are replaced by cardiac dilation and hypertrophy.

HEMODYNAMIC–CLINICAL CORRELATION

Relation of Altered Cardiac Function to the Clinical State

Regardless of either the cause of acute heart failure or the magnitude of compensatory responses, the three fundamental alterations in cardiac hemodynamics—increased right atrial pressure, increased pulmonary capillary pressure, and decreased cardiac output—determine the type of presentation, prognosis, and therapy. Each of these parameters may change independently, and each is responsible for a different set of symptoms.

Understanding the relation between hemodynamics and clinical presentation has practical bedside relevance. Physical signs change less rapidly than hemodynamics and are difficult to quantify. Thus, during management of critically ill patients, direct hemodynamic measurements can be used to predict the subsequent clinical response. A typical example is clearance of rales and x-ray evidence of pulmonary congestion a day after pulmonary capillary pressure reduction by intravenous vasodilator therapy.

Increased Right Atrial Pressure: The Cause of Venous Congestion

Right atrial pressure is equivalent to both right ventricular diastolic pressure (when the triscupid valve is open, and the right atrium and right ventricle are common chambers) and the central venous pressure. Reduced right atrial pressure is generally secondary to hypovolemia or venodilation. Increased pressure has three principal causes: right ventricular failure, tricuspid regurgitation, and pericardial tamponade. The increased right atrial pressure presents clinically as jugular venous distention, hepatic enlargement, and peripheral edema. In AMI, increased right atrial pressure may reflect right heart failure, most frequently caused by right ventricular infarction and less commonly by pulmonary venous hypertension, resulting from severe left heart failure or acute valvular regurgitation. Right atrial pressure also is increased in the presence of cardiac tamponade and after pulmonary embolism.

Increased Pulmonary Capillary Pressure: The Cause of Pulmonary Congestion

As left ventricular diastolic volume increases with acute left heart failure, so does left ventricular diastolic pressure. Retrograde transmission results in increased pulmonary capillary pressure, which is manifest clinically as the symptoms and signs of pulmonary congestion. In the acute setup, the severity of acute pulmonary congestion is related to the magnitude of increase in pulmonary capillary pressure. A rough guideline for acute congestion is as follows (4):

18 to 20 mm Hg: onset of pulmonary congestion
21 to 25 mm Hg: moderate congestion

26 to 30 mm Hg: severe congestion
Greater than 30 mm Hg: onset of acute pulmonary edema

Although this progression remains unchanged in chronic pulmonary congestion, the magnitude of pulmonary capillary pressure increase required to produce such signs may be significantly greater, because of lymphatic enlargement (5) and decrease in capillary permeability.

Decreased Cardiac Output: The Cause of Peripheral Hypoperfusion

Reduction in cardiac output presents as decreased perfusion of organs, most dramatically the skin, kidney, and brain, resulting in cold, clammy skin, oliguria, and anxiety, lethargy, or coma. The severity of peripheral hypoperfusion relates to the depression in cardiac output. To normalize for differences of body size, cardiac output is divided by body surface area to obtain cardiac index. A rough guideline for the relation of cardiac index to acute peripheral hypoperfusion is as follows (2,3):

2.5 to 3.5 L/min/m^2: "normal" range
2.0 to 2.2 L/min/m^2: onset of peripheral hypoperfusion
1.8 to 2.0 L/min/m^2: onset of cardiogenic shock

As with pulmonary congestion, the ability of the body to withstand chronic depression of cardiac output can be remarkable. Patients with moderately severe chronic heart failure can present with a level of cardiac index that would be lethal in acute heart failure.

CLASSIFICATION OF HEMODYNAMIC DYSFUNCTION

The classification of patients by the magnitude of clinical dysfunction has prognostic value. The most widely used method of classifying cardiac dysfunction is the Killip classification (6), based on physical findings on admission: Class I—no signs of left heart failure; Class II—S3 gallop, signs of pulmonary congestion limited to the basal lung segments, or both; Class III—acute pulmonary edema; and Class IV—cardiogenic shock. This classification scheme has the advantage of simplicity.

There is an important relation between clinical evaluation and cardiac hemodynamics. Cardiac index, a measure of contractile force, represents the y-axis of the Starling function curve. Pulmonary capillary pressure, a measure of left ventricular volume, represents the x-axis of the curve. On the basis of this correlation, four hemodynamic subsets are established, each with a different prognosis (Table 62–1). Because hemodynamics have clinical correlates, patients with AMI can be classified into either clinical or hemodynamic subsets on the basis of the type of information available at the bedside. The four clinical subsets of patients with AMI are as follows: subset I—no evidence of either peripheral hypoperfusion or pulmonary congestion; subset II—

TABLE 62–1. *Prognostic hemodynamic subsets in acute myocardial infarction*

Hemodynamic profile	In-hospital mortality, %
PCW ≤ 18 mm Hg CI > 2.2 L/min/m^2	3
PCW > 18 mm Hg CI ≥ 2.2 L/min/m^2	9
PCW > 18 mm Hg CI < 2.2 L/min/m^2	23
PCW > 18 mm Hg CI < 2.2 L/min/m^2	51

CI, cardiac index; PCW, pulmonary capillary wedge pressure.

pulmonary congestion, but no systemic hypoperfusion; subset III—systemic hypoperfusion with no signs of pulmonary congestion (in this subset are found patients in whom hypovolemia dominates and also patients with right ventricular infarction and minimal involvement of the left ventricle); subset IV—both pulmonary congestion and systemic hypoperfusion. Because depressed cardiac output causes hypoperfusion and increased pulmonary capillary pressure causes pulmonary congestion, patients also were independently classified into four parallel hemodynamic subsets.

The usefulness of these classifications lies in that there are clearly significant differences among subsets in terms of mortality. Decreased cardiac index increases the mortality of AMI 5- to 15-fold, depending on whether the pulmonary capillary pressure is increased, and there is a corresponding increase in mortality with clinical evidence of systemic hypoperfusion. Similarly, increased pulmonary capillary pressure increases mortality 2- to 15-fold, depending on the concomitant presence of decreased cardiac output. Correspondingly, there is an increase in mortality with clinical evidence of pulmonary congestion and peripheral hypoperfusion.

APPROACH TO HEMODYNAMIC THERAPY IN ACUTE MYOCARDIAL INFARCTION

In addition to thrombolytic and antiarrhythmic therapy (as discussed in other chapters), hemodynamic therapy often is necessary. The selection of therapy requires assessment of the magnitude of pulmonary congestion and peripheral hypoperfusion, because agents can be selected to alter pulmonary capillary pressure, cardiac output, or arterial pressure in various combinations. Signs of increased pulmonary capillary pressure typically precede signs of decreased cardiac output and reduction in blood pressure.

In patients with uncomplicated AMI, serial clinical evaluation is usually sufficient. Hemodynamic monitoring is used (a) to determine the role of left ventricular failure, hypovolemia, right ventricular failure, valvular insufficiency, cardiac tamponade, pulmonary embolism, septal or free wall rupture, in severe hypotension, or pulmonary edema; (b) to select the appropriate therapy; and (c) to assess the response to therapy.

It is possible to predict reasonably the response to a given therapy in an individual with infarction-induced failure. To accomplish this, one must know the two major determinants of this response: (a) the resting level of cardiac function and (b) the mechanism of action of the drug, which varies with the level of cardiac function and the state of compensatory response mechanisms. For selection of therapy, it is useful to consider therapeutic agents in three classes: diuretics, vasodilators, and inotropic agents. This classification is particularly suitable in clinical practice, because although there are substantial variations in the magnitude of effects, the direction of the hemodynamic response to various drugs within each clinical category is similar.

Diuretic Agents

Diuretic agents reduce pulmonary capillary pressure with little change in cardiac output or heart rate in patients with heart failure. Diuresis decreases intravascular volume with a consequent decrease in left ventricular volume and pressure. This leads to a reduction in pulmonary capillary pressure and relief of pulmonary congestion. When pulmonary capillary pressure is reduced from greater levels to 15 to 18 mm Hg, little change in cardiac output occurs. As pulmonary capillary pressure is reduced from this range to lower levels, however, a substantial decrease in cardiac output may occur, as the left ventricle descends on its Starling function curve (7,8). Diuretics, therefore, are preferred in patients who have pulmonary congestion without peripheral hypoperfusion.

Peripheral Vasodilators

Peripheral vasodilators are dramatically effective in improving cardiac hemodynamics in patients with heart failure (9,10). Cardiac output increases substantially, pulmonary capillary pressure decreases, and there is little change in heart rate. Reduction in resistance to ejection results in an increase in ejection fraction, which is translated into an increase in stroke volume, and cardiac output. The increase in systolic emptying leads to a decreased left ventricular diastolic volume and pressure and decreased pulmonary capillary pressure.

As is the case for diuretic agents, the effect of peripheral vasodilators differs among patients in the heart failure subsets and those classified as healthy. Peripheral vasodilators increase stroke volume in patients with increased pulmonary capillary pressure, but decrease stroke volume and increase heart rate in patients with normal or low pulmonary capillary pressure. These differences are a direct outcome of the resting level of cardiac function. Arterial dilation leads to reduction in resistance to ejection (afterload), and venodilation causes venous pooling; both cause reduction in left ventricular volume (preload). In the healthy heart, these two effects lead to reduced stroke volume by the Starling effect. In contrast, in patients with heart failure, ejection fraction increases with decreased afterload, and venous pooling causes a decrease in left ventricular volume. Initially, the reduced left ventricular volume does not reduce stroke volume, because the heart is operating on the flat portion of the Starling function curve.

The hemodynamic response to vasodilators follows a three-step progression determined by infusion rate. At low doses, cardiac output increases and pulmonary capillary pressure decreases. There is little change in arterial pressure because the increase in stroke volume and cardiac output balances the decrease in resistance. As infusion rate is increased to the medium range, cardiac output further increases and pulmonary capillary pressure decreases with a concomitant decline in arterial pressure. With high infusion rates, profound vasodilation occurs, leading to reduction in pulmonary capillary pressure, cardiac output, and arterial pressure. It is at this latter level that peripheral vasodilators change from being dramatically effective to potentially lethal by seriously compromising coronary perfusion. For this reason there are two clinical rules to follow during vasodilator infusion: Arterial pressure should be maintained, and heart rate should not be increased by more than 10%.

Inotropic Agents

Drugs in the inotropic agent class exert their effect predominantly by increasing myocardial contractility. Some also are peripheral vasodilators and can increase cardiac output by this mechanism, whereas other drugs cause peripheral constriction. Some agents also selectively dilate the renal vascular bed, thereby augmenting renal function.

Inotropic agents generally become progressively less effective as the magnitude of the left ventricular failure increases. Administration of inotropic agents to patients in cardiogenic shock frequently results in little change in either cardiac output or pulmonary capillary pressure because with an extensive ischemia and necrosis, there is little myocardium to respond to inotropic stimulation. Furthermore, the remaining nonischemic and noninfarcted muscle may be functioning at near-maximum potential as a result of endogenous catecholamine release secondary to diminished cardiac output. When the capability of the heart to respond to inotropic stimulation is substantially reduced, inotropic agents that increase peripheral vascular resistance may actually cause a decrease in cardiac output and an increase in pulmonary capillary pressure, and they may even precipitate acute pulmonary edema. Ironically, therefore, the patients who most require therapy show the least response, whereas those who do not require therapy tend to exhibit the desired effect. Because the hemodynamic response to inotropic therapy frequently diminishes with time and long-term results have been poor, this therapy has increasingly become a short-term method of circulatory support before treatment with more definitive procedures such as emergency angioplasty or cardiac surgery.

SPECIFIC DIAGNOSES MADE BY HEMODYNAMIC MEASUREMENTS

Right Ventricular Infarction

Right ventricular infarction is caused by occlusion of the right coronary artery proximal to the origin of the right ventricular branches. Frequently it is clinically silent, that is, overshadowed by the more extensive left ventricular involvement (11,12). In 30% to 40% of patients, however, right ventricular infarction may cause profound hypotension, mimicking cardiogenic shock (13). The key to recognition of this syndrome is the absence of pulmonary congestion in the presence of inferior myocardial infarction, especially when accompanied by increased jugular venous pressure.

Characteristic hemodynamic changes include a narrowed pulse pressure in the pulmonary artery and increase of right atrial pressure. There may be a steep right atrial y descent with a paradoxic increase in right atrial pressure during inspiration, a dip, and a plateau during diastole in the right ventricular pressure tracing (Fig. 62–1). The level of pulmonary capillary pressure depends on the extent of coexisting left ventricular infarction. Cardiac output is depressed. Rarely there is a right-to-left shunt across a patent foramen ovale (14,15). Echocardiography and radionuclide ventriculography demonstrate disproportionate right ventricular di-

lation, regional right ventricular wall motion abnormalities, and a depressed right ventricular ejection fraction.

Cardiac Tamponade

Tamponade complicating AMI is less common in the thrombolytic era, because timely reperfusion prevents the wave front of myocardial necrosis from reaching the epicardium. However, when transmural necrosis develops, hemorrhagic pericardial exudate may accumulate rapidly, resulting in tamponade. Clinically, the patient is hypotensive, tachycardic, and dyspneic. Right atrial, right ventricular diastolic, pulmonary artery diastolic, and mean pulmonary capillary wedge pressures are increased and characteristically equal. Right atrial pressure tracings may demonstrate a prominent x descent, caused by the diminished cardiac volume and a blunted, absent, or even reversed y descent. Stroke volume and cardiac output are decreased. Arterial blood pressure is reduced and may exhibit pulsus paradoxus (Fig. 62–2).

Massive Pulmonary Embolism

In the era of early patient mobilization and routine antithrombotic and thrombolytic therapy, pulmonary embolism is a rare complication of AMI. When pulmonary embolism occurs and is massive, it presents as acute worsening

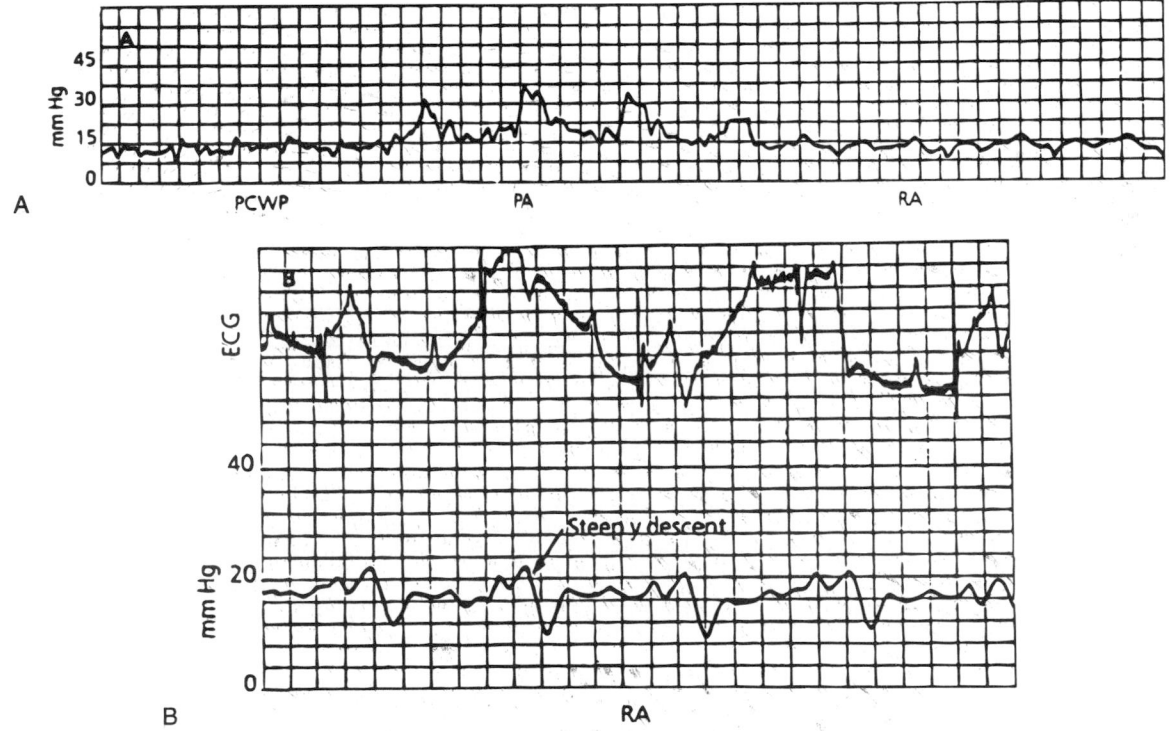

FIG. 62–1. **A:** Right atrial (RA) pressure is increased to the level of pulmonary capillary wedge pressure (PCWP). The pulmonary artery (PA) and the pulmonary capillary wedge pressures are normal in this patient with predominant right ventricular infarction. **B:** Also characteristic of right atrial pressure tracing: a steep y descent followed by a diastolic plateau. ECG, electrocardiogram. (From Swan HJC, Shah PK. The Swan–Ganz catheter; indications for insertion. *J Crit Illn* 1986;1:54–61, with permission.)

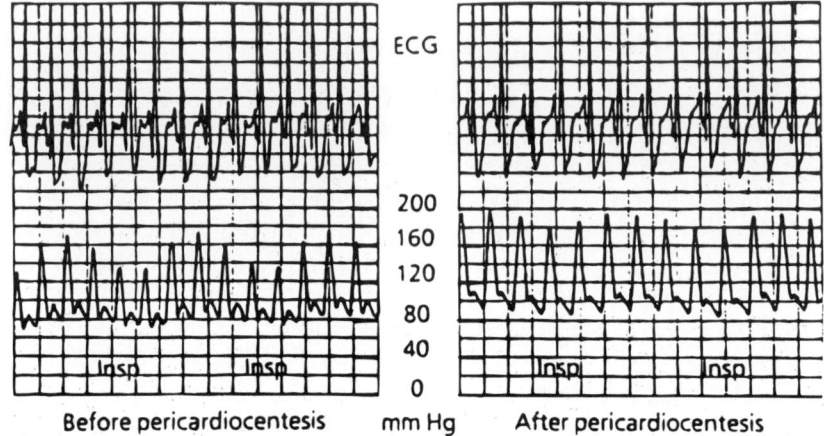

FIG. 62–2. A prominent pulsus paradoxus that is markedly diminished after pericardiocentesis in a patient with pericardial tamponade. Note also the increase in systolic blood pressure and the pressure amplitude after pericardiocentesis. ECG, electrocardiogram; Insp, inspiration. (From Swan HJC, Shah PK. The Swan–Ganz catheter; indications for insertion. *J Crit Illn* 1986;1:54–61, with permission.)

of dyspnea, associated with cyanosis and increase of jugular venous pressure. Hemodynamic assessment reveals increased pulmonary systolic and diastolic pressure, the latter caused by increased pulmonary vascular resistance, and increased right ventricular end-diastolic and right atrial pressures. In the absence of prior pulmonary disease, the nonhypertrophic right ventricle rarely generates pulmonary artery (systolic) pressure in excess of 35 to 40 mm Hg (16). The level of pulmonary capillary wedge pressure depends on the degree of left ventricular dysfunction caused by the myocardial infarction (17). Pulmonary embolization does not directly affect the level of pulmonary capillary wedge pres-

sure, which may actually decrease because of a decrease in cardiac output. When systemic hypotension is severe, pulmonary embolism may mimic cardiogenic shock (18). A shocklike state with increased pulmonary artery pressure and pulmonary diastolic pressure significantly exceeding the level of pulmonary capillary wedge pressure suggests the correct diagnosis (Fig. 62–3).

Acute Mitral Regurgitation

Acute mitral regurgitation may result from ischemia or necrosis of the left ventricular papillary muscles and the ad-

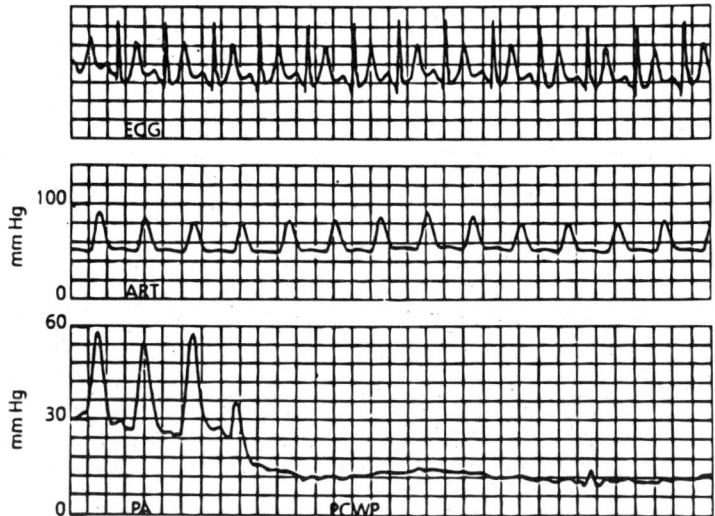

FIG. 62–3. A patient in shock after massive pulmonary embolism. Radial artery pressure *(ART)* was low, and the pulmonary artery *(PA)* pressure was acutely increased, but the pulmonary artery wedge pressure *(PCWP)* was normal, ruling out cardiogenic shock from left ventricular involvement. ECG, electrocardiogram. (From Swan HJC, Shah PK. The Swan–Ganz catheter; indications for insertion. *J Crit Illn* 1986;1:54–61, with permission.)

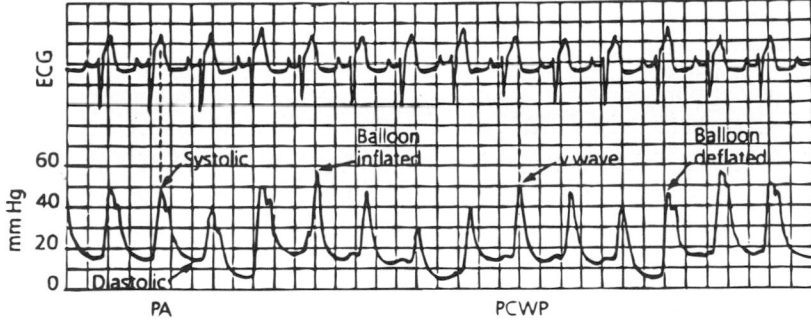

FIG. 62–4. The double peak of the pulmonary artery *(PA)* systolic pressure consists of the PA systolic wave and the tall v wave transmitted from the left atrium. When the balloon is inflated to record pulmonary capillary wedge pressure *(PCWP),* the PA systolic wave disappears and the tall v wave remains. ECG, electrocardiogram. (From Swan HJC, Shah PK. The Swan–Ganz catheter; Indications for insertion. *J Crit Illn* 1986;1:54–61, with permission.)

jacent left ventricular myocardium or from rupture of the papillary muscle (19–21). Papillary muscle necrosis causes severe mitral regurgitation and rapidly deteriorating hemodynamics. Papillary muscle dysfunction is rarely sufficient to cause severe mitral regurgitation unless the contractile function of the left ventricular myocardium contiguous to the base of the papillary muscles also is impaired.

A large v wave transmitted to both the pulmonary capillary and the pulmonary artery is typical of acute mitral regurgitation (22–24) (Fig. 62–4). Large v waves may also occur in the absence of mitral regurgitation caused by acute volume overload (25–27)—for example, in a patient with ruptured interventricular septum and a left-to-right shunt. In the latter instances the onset and the peak of the v wave usually appear later compared with the early systolic appearance of the regurgitant v wave of mitral insufficiency. In acute mitral regurgitation the mean pulmonary capillary

wedge pressure may be greater than the pulmonary artery diastolic pressure. As the atrium dilates in chronic mitral insufficiency, the large v wave tends to diminish in size.

Ventricular Septal Rupture

Ventricular septal rupture presents with recurrent chest pain, dyspnea, and severe left ventricular failure, accompanied by a new harsh, loud holosystolic murmur and a palpable thrill. The left-to-right interventricular shunt causes right ventricular volume overload and an increase in pulmonary artery blood flow, but with reduced forward cardiac output. Under these circumstances, the thermodilution technique that measures pulmonary artery blood flow yields erroneously high cardiac output values. A large v wave may be seen on the pulmonary capillary wedge pressure waveform, suggesting mitral insufficiency (27). The v wave is a consequence of

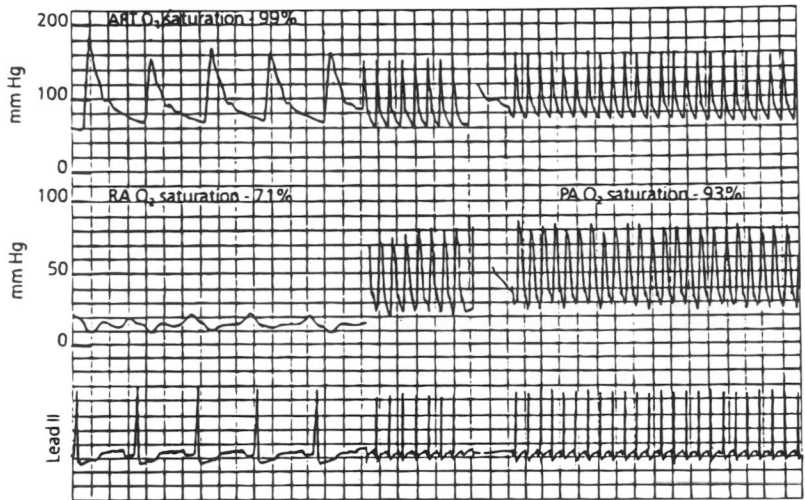

FIG. 62–5. In this patient with acute ventricular septal rupture, the step-up of oxygen saturation from 71% of the right atrial *(RA)* blood to 93% of the pulmonary arterial *(PA)* blood permits differentiation from acute mitral regurgitation. ART, arterial blood. (Swan HJC, Shah PK. The Swan–Ganz catheter; indications for insertion. *J Crit Illn* 1986;1:54–61, with permission.)

markedly increased blood flow into the left atrium, which reaches the limit of its distensibility and transmits pressure retrograde to the pulmonary venous system. Differentiation of acute ventricular septal rupture from acute mitral regurgitation is readily made by demonstration of a step-up in blood oxygen saturation between the right atrial and pulmonary arterial blood (Fig. 62–5).

TECHNIQUES OF HEMODYNAMIC ASSESSMENT

Systemic Arterial Pressure Monitoring

There are several indications for intraarterial monitoring in AMI. Noninvasive methods for blood pressure determination, although adequate in most patients, may be inaccurate in profoundly hypotensive patients and in patients with severe peripheral vasoconstriction. These methods are inadequate for rapid assessment of response to potent vasoactive drugs, particularly when the arterial pressure is unstable.

Three sites are used for entry into the arterial system. The *radial artery* is most frequently used for establishing an arterial line. Before catheter insertion, Allen's test should be applied to confirm the presence of adequate collateral blood flow if the radial artery becomes occluded. In most patients, an 18- to 20-gauge, 4-cm-long, plastic catheter is adequate. The *brachial* and *femoral arteries* are less preferred for long-term cannulation, although the femoral artery may be easiest to locate and cannulate in profoundly hypotensive patients. The femoral artery may also more accurately reflect central perfusion pressure in severely vasoconstricted patients. Femoral artery cannulation is best performed using the Seldinger technique and a 10- to 15-cm-long cannula.

Maintenance of sterility during and after catheter insertion, frequent inspection of the area of insertion, frequent change of dressing, aspiration before catheter flushing, and continuous display of an adequate arterial pressure waveform are essential steps in minimizing complications such as hemorrhage, thrombosis, infection, embolization, and aneurysm formation.

Flow-directed Right-Heart Catheterization

Pulmonary artery catheters (28) used in coronary care units are usually 110 cm in length, 7 or 7.5 F in diameter, with a balloon at the tip and a thermistor proximal to the balloon (29,30). Newer versions of catheters have additional options. Some catheters have a lumen reserved for insertion of probes for pacing the right atrium or the right ventricle, or both. The most recent modification allows measurement of cardiac output at 30-second intervals with a continuously updated display (31). The catheter has a thermal filament located in the right ventricle, which inputs small amounts of heat. The resulting increase in blood temperature is detected by a thermistor in the pulmonary artery, to produce a "thermal washout" curve. No injection of fluid is necessary. An-

other modification of the pulmonary artery catheter has an opening 10 cm from the tip. When this lumen transmits right ventricular pressure waveform, the catheter tip is less than 10 cm inside the pulmonary artery, and the position is safe for balloon inflation. Conversely, transmission of a pulmonary artery pressure waveform indicates distal migration of the catheter to a position that may be unsafe for balloon inflation. This so-called position-monitoring catheter (32, 33) may help to avoid damaging the pulmonary artery, a serious complication of flow-directed catheterization.

Flow-directed catheters can be inserted at the bedside; however, fluoroscopic guidance is preferable in patients with dilated right heart chambers, severe pulmonary hypertension, or severe tricuspid regurgitation. Before insertion, the catheter shaft should be inspected and the balloon inflated under water to test for integrity and symmetry of inflation. The right internal jugular vein is most frequently used for insertion of flow-directed catheters; the subclavian, the external jugular, the femoral, and the basilic veins are less preferred. The catheter is advanced into the right or left main pulmonary artery. The catheter is in a proper position when its tip is not evident beyond the silhouette of the mediastinal structures.

SOURCES OF ERROR AND COMPLICATIONS IN HEMODYNAMIC MONITORING

Correct interpretation of measurements requires careful attention to their technical quality and physiologic validity. *Technical* causes of pressure waveform distortion include (a) inadequate system frequency response, (b) underdamping, (c) overdamping, (d) catheter whip, and (e) catheter tip occlusion. *Physiologic* sources of error include (a) inappropriate phlebostatic level, (b) ventilatory effects, (c) positive end-expiratory pressure (PEEP), and (d) misplacement of the catheter tip. These physiologic sources of error are further discussed later.

Inappropriate Phlebostatic Level

Failure to rezero at the phlebostatic axis (midaxillary line in the fourth intercostal space) after a change in the patient's position may result in inaccuracy of measurements.

Ventilatory Effects

During normal quiet breathing there is a change in intrathoracic pressure that is superimposed on the pressure recording. Therefore, pressures should be assessed at end-expiration, when air flow is minimal and the intrathoracic pressure practically equals atmospheric pressure. In patients with breathing difficulty, the baseline variations between inspiration and expiration may be dramatic and breath holding may be impossible. In these patients, pressures are best evaluated from pressure tracings recorded over several respiratory cycles at end-expiration.

Positive End-Expiratory Pressure

Mechanical ventilation using high alveolar pressures interferes with hemodynamic measurements in two ways: (a) by transmission of extravascular pressure to the intravascular structures and to the catheter tip, and (b) by hemodynamic alterations caused by intermittent or continuous obstruction of pulmonary capillaries (34–36). There is no ideal way to correct for these distortions. Brief discontinuation or reduction of PEEP is associated with risks to the patients' health, and it is not a solution because it alters the hemodynamic status (37,38). One can measure intrathoracic pressure using an esophageal balloon (39) or a fluid-filled pleural catheter (40) and subtract the measured value from the pulmonary capillary wedge pressure. This is impractical and may even be inaccurate because the intrathoracic pressure at the tips of the pleural and the intravascular catheters may not be identical because of differences in regional lung compliance.

Catheter Tip in Nonzone 3 Position

Gravity affects the distribution of blood flow in the lungs. In the uppermost portions of zone 1 (apex in an upright person, the anterior chest in the supine position), the alveolar pressure may exceed pulmonary capillary pressure. Therefore, pressure must be obtained from the dependent zone 3 portion of the lung (41). Nonzone 3 conditions may prevail over a greater portion of the lung and render hemodynamic measurements inaccurate when the capillary pressure is low (e.g., in hypovolemia) or when the alveolar pressure is increased (e.g., during mechanical ventilation). Two criteria can be used to assess the appropriateness of catheter tip position. First, a damped wedge pressure tracing suggests nonzone 3 conditions if technical causes of damping can be ruled out. Second, on a lateral chest roentgenogram, visualization of the catheter tip below the level of the left atrium indicates a zone 3 position.

Complications of Flow-directed Pulmonary Artery Catheterization

During insertion, accidental puncture of the carotid or subclavian artery may cause bleeding. Pneumothorax occurs most frequently in association with the subclavian vein approach and is less common with the internal jugular vein approach. Atrial and ventricular arrhythmias, induced by physical contact of the catheter tip with a chamber wall, are usually short-lasting. Right bundle branch block or complete heart block in patients with preexisting left bundle branch block can occur. In the latter situation, prophylactic insertion of either a pacing catheter or a pulmonary artery catheter with a special lumen for insertion of a right ventricular pacing probe is recommended. A standby external pacemaker may obviate the need for prophylactic pacemaker insertion. Knotting of the pulmonary artery catheter around the cardiac structures by itself or another intravascular

catheter may occur when an excessive length of the catheter is inserted.

The most serious complication is perforation or rupture of the pulmonary artery (42). It occurs (a) in patients with long-standing pulmonary hypertension and (b) in patients of advanced age. The complication is particularly dangerous in patients receiving anticoagulants. Inflation of the balloon after the catheter tip has migrated into a small distal pulmonary artery branch is one mechanism of rupture. Perforation of the arterial wall by the catheter tip when the balloon inflates asymmetrically and forces the tip to impinge on the wall is another mechanism. During cardiopulmonary bypass, the catheter may be displaced by the surgeon into a small distal branch, and a hypothermia-stiffened catheter may perforate the vessel wall. Keeping the catheter in a proximal position in the right or left main pulmonary artery helps to avoid this serious complication.

SUMMARY

Two hemodynamic abnormalities that accompany AMI—reduction of cardiac output and increase of pulmonary capillary pressure—are primarily responsible for mortality and morbidity and for clinical signs and symptoms of power failure.

Increase of pulmonary capillary pressure is manifested clinically as pulmonary congestion. The failing left ventricle is able to eject a progressively smaller fraction of its volume, resulting in an increased diastolic volume. This leads to an increase in left ventricular diastolic pressure, which is transmitted retrograde into the pulmonary capillaries. The increase in pulmonary capillary pressure leads to an accelerated transudation of fluid from the lumen of the capillary into the interstitium and ultimately into the alveoli, producing acute pulmonary edema, which can be detected by auscultation at the bedside or by radiologic examination.

When pump function is further compromised by infarction, the heart can no longer maintain an adequate cardiac output. This is manifest clinically as peripheral hypoperfusion, and it is frequently, but not always, accompanied by systemic hypotension and a compensatory tachycardia. Hypoperfusion of the brain leads to an altered mental status, whereas hypoperfusion of the kidneys produces oliguria and occasionally renal failure. In response to decreased arterial pressure, peripheral vasoconstriction occurs, resulting in cold and cyanotic skin. Profound hypotension can cause cardiac hypoperfusion and can lead to extension of the infarction. Severe hypotension and peripheral hypoperfusion also can be produced by extensive infarction of the right ventricle. Hemodynamics can be assessed with reasonable accuracy by simple noninvasive clinical evaluation. Bedside evaluation of hemodynamics is the basis for both prognosis and choice of therapy. In unstable patients, particularly those in whom potent intravenous pharmacologic therapy is used, direct hemodynamic monitoring is a valuable guide to therapy.

FUTURE DIRECTIONS

The management of AMI has been changed dramatically with the introduction of early thrombolysis and angioplasty, which limit the extent of infarction and the magnitude of hemodynamic dysfunction. With decrease in both mortality and catastrophic complications such as cardiogenic shock has come a concomitant decrease in the need for invasive hemodynamic monitoring. Careful bedside evaluation of cardiac hemodynamics, as represented by clinical signs and symptoms, remains crucial to excellent patient management. The type and magnitude of cardiac dysfunction, right heart failure, pulmonary congestion, and peripheral hypoperfusion will continue to determine the choice of pharmacologic therapies.

REFERENCES

1. Forrester J, Diamond G, Swan HJ. Correlative classification of clinical and hemodynamic function after acute myocardial infarction. *Am J Cardiol* 1977;39:137–145.
2. Forrester JS, Diamond G, Chatterjee K, et al. Medical therapy of acute myocardial infarction by the application of hemodynamic subsets (first of two parts). *N Engl J Med* 1976;295:1356–1362.
3. Forrester JS, Diamond G, Chatterjee K, et al. Medical therapy of acute myocardial infarction by application of hemodynamic subsets (second of two parts). *N Engl J Med* 1976;295:1404–1413.
4. McHugh TJ, Adler L, Zion D, et al. Simultaneous hemodynamic, radiologic and physiologic evaluation of left ventricle failure in acute myocardial infarction. *Chest* 1970;58:285–289.
5. Sampson JJ, Leeds SE, Uhley HN, et al. Studies of lymph flow and changes in pulmonary structures as indexes of circulatory changes in experimental pulmonary edema. *Israel J Med Sci* 1969;5:826–830.
6. Killip T, Kimbal JT. Treatment of myocardial infarction in a coronary care unit: a two year experience with 250 patients. *Am J Cardiol* 1967;20:457–464.
7. Crexells C, Chatterjee K, Forrester JS, et al. Optimal level of left heart filling pressures in acute myocardial infarction. *N Engl J Med* 1973; 289:1263–1266.
8. Forrester J, Diamond G, McHugh T, et al. Filling pressures in the right and left sides of the heart in myocardial infarction. *N Engl J Med* 1971;285:190–193.
9. Franciosa JB, Buiha NM, Limas CJ, et al. Improved left ventricle function during nitroprusside infusion in acute myocardial infarction. *Lancet* 1972;1:650–654.
10. Chatterjee K, Swan HJ, Kaushik US, et al. Effects of vasodilator therapy for severe pump failure in acute myocardial infarction on short-term and late prognosis. *Circulation* 1976;53:797–802.
11. Cohn JN, Guiha NH, Broder MI, et al. Right ventricular infarction. Clinical and hemodynamic features. *Am J Cardiol* 1974;33:209–214.
12. Rackley CE, Russel RO. Right ventricular function in acute myocardial infarction. *Am J Cardiol* 1974;33:927–929.
13. Lloyd EA, Gersh BJ, Kennelly BM. Hemodynamic spectrum of dominant right ventricular infarction in 19 patients. *Am J Cardiol* 1982;48: 1016–1022.
14. Morris AL, Donen N. Hypoxia and intracardiac right to left shunt complicating inferior myocardial infarction with right ventricular extension. *Arch Intern Med* 1978;138:1405–1406.
15. Manno BV, Bemis CE, Carver J, et al. Right ventricular infarction complicated by right to left shunt. *J Am Coll Cardiol* 1983;1:554–557.
16. McIntyre KM, Sasahara AA. The hemodynamic response to pulmonary embolism in patients with prior cardiopulmonary disease. *Am J Cardiol* 1971;28:288–294.
17. Jenkins BS, Bradley RD, Branthwaite MA. Evaluation of pulmonary end-diastolic pressure as an indirect estimate of left atrial mean pressure. *Circulation* 1970;42:75–78.
18. The urokinase-pulmonary embolism trial. A national cooperative study. *Circulation* 1973;47[Suppl I]:I-51–I-59.
19. Shelburne JC, Rubinstein D, Gorlin R. A reappraisal of papillary muscle dysfunction: correlative clinical and angiographic study. *Am J Med* 1969;46:862–871.
20. Nishimura RA, Schaff HV, Shuh C, et al. Papillary muscle rupture complicating acute myocardial infarction: analysis of 17 patients. *Am J Cardiol* 1983;51:373–377.
21. Clements SD, Story WE, Hurst JW, et al. Ruptured papillary muscle, a complication of acute myocardial infarction: clinical presentation, diagnosis and treatment. *Clin Cardiol* 1985;8:93–103.
22. Levinson DC, Wilburne M, Meehan JP, et al. Evidence for retrograde trans-pulmonary propagation of the v (or regurgitant) wave in mitral insufficiency. *Am J Cardiol* 1958;2:159–169.
23. Tatooles CJ, Gault JH, Mason DT, et al. Reflux of oxygenated blood into the pulmonary artery in severe mitral regurgitation. *Am Heart J* 1968;75:102–106.
24. Grose R, Strain J, Cohen MV. Pulmonary arterial v waves in mitral regurgitation: clinical and experimental observations. *Circulation* 1984; 69:214–222.
25. Pichard AD, Kay R, Smith H, et al. Large v waves in pulmonary wedge pressure tracing in the absence of mitral regurgitation. *Am J Cardiol* 1982;50:1044–1050.
26. Fuchs RM, Heuser RR, Yin FC, et al. Limitations of pulmonary wedge v waves in diagnosing mitral regurgitation *Am J Cardiol* 1982;49:849–854.
27. Downes TR, Hackshaw BT, Kahl FR. Frequency of large v waves in the pulmonary artery wedge pressure in ventricular septal defect of acquired (during acute myocardial infarction) or congenital origin. *Am J Cardiol* 1987;60:415–417.
28. Swan HJ, Ganz W, Forrester JS, et al. Catheterization of the heart in man with use of a flow-directed balloon-tipped catheter. *N Engl J Med* 1970;283:477–481.
29. Ganz W, Donoso R, Marcus HS, et al. A new technique for measurement of cardiac output by thermodilution in man. *Am J Cardiol* 1971;27:392–396.
30. Forrester JS, Ganz W, Diamond G, et al. Thermodilution cardiac output determination with a single flow-directed catheter. *Am Heart J* 1972; 83:306–311.
31. Yelderman ML, Ramsay MA, Quinn MD, et al. Continuous thermodilution cardiac output measurement in intensive care unit patients. *J Cardiothorac Vasc Anesth* 1992;6:270–724.
32. Santora T, Ganz W, Gold J, et al. New method for monitoring pulmonary artery catheter location. *Crit Care Med* 1991;19:422–426.
33. Robertie PG, Johnston WE, Williamson MK, et al. Clinical utility of a position monitoring catheter in the pulmonary artery. *Anesthesiology* 1991;74:440–445.
34. Downs JB, Douglas ME. Assessment of cardiac filling pressure during continuous positive-pressure ventilation. *Crit Care Med* 1980;8:285–292.
35. Tooker J, Huseby J, Butler J. The effects of Swan–Ganz catheter height on the wedge pressure–left atrial pressure relationship in edema during positive pressure ventilation. *Am Rev Respir Dis* 1978;117:721–726.
36. Shasby DM, Dauber IM, Pfister S, et al. Swan–Ganz catheter location and left atrial pressure determine the accuracy of the wedge pressure when positive end-expiratory pressure is used. *Chest* 1981;80:666–670.
37. De Campo T, Civetta JM. The effect of short-term discontinuation of high-level PEEP in patients with acute respiratory failure. *Crit Care Med* 1979;7:47–49.
38. Luterman A, Horovitz JH, Carrico CJ, et al. Withdrawal from positive end-expiratory pressure. *Surgery* 1978;83:328–332.
39. Craven KD, Wood LD. Extrapericardial and esophageal pressures with positive end-expiratory pressure in dogs. *J Appl Physiol* 1981;51:798–805.
40. Marini J, O'Quinn R, Culver BH, et al. Estimation of transmural cardiac pressures during ventilation with PEEP. *J Appl Physiol* 1982;53:384–391.
41. West JB, Dollery CT, Naimark A. Distribution of blood flow in isolated lung: relation to vascular and alveolar pressures. *J Appl Physiol* 1964; 19:713–724.
42. Barash PG, Nardi D, Hammond G. Catheter-induced pulmonary artery perforation—mechanisms, management, and modification. *J Thorac Card Surg* 1981;82:5–12.

CHAPTER 63

The Role of Cardiac Magnetic Resonance in the Clinical Presentation of Acute Coronary Syndromes

Michael Poon, Javier Sanz, and Philip T. Zhao

Key Words: Cardiac; ischemia; magnetic resonance imaging.

INTRODUCTION

Cardiovascular disease remains the leading cause of death in most developed countries for both men and women, particularly coronary artery disease (CAD), which accounts for about one-fifth of total mortality. Despite great progress made in medical therapy, the incidence of CAD has progressively increased over the past decades and is predicted to grow because of the increasing size of the aging population (1). The evaluation of the patient with symptoms or risk factors for ischemic heart disease (IHD) is aimed to establishing the diagnosis, prognosis, and appropriate therapeutic measures. Cardiac magnetic resonance (CMR) has emerged as a multipurpose imaging modality for the assessment of IHD, a major complication of CAD.

M. Poon: The Zena and Michael A. Wiener Cardiovascular Institute, The Marie-Josée and Henry R. Kravis Cardiovascular Health Center, Mount Sinai School of Medicine, Cardiovascular Medicine and Integrated Imaging Program, Cabrini Medical Center, 227 East 19th Street, Room 549B, New York, New York 10003.

J. Sanz: The Zena and Michael A. Wiener Cardiovascular Institute, The Marie-Josée and Henry R. Kravis Cardiovascular Health Center, Mount Sinai School of Medicine, New York, New York.

P. T. Zhao: The Zena and Michael A. Wiener Cardiovascular Institute, The Marie-Josée and Henry R. Kravis Cardiovascular Health Center, Mount Sinai School of Medicine, New York, New York.

In 1945, Felix Bloch (2) and Edward Mills Purcell (3) separately developed the technique of nuclear magnetic resonance (NMR) spectroscopy to analyze the composition of different chemical compounds. This Nobel Prize–winning concept gained a new dimension in the medical and pharmaceutical communities during the 1960s and 1970s through the contributions of Drs. Lauterbur (4) and Damadian (5) and other researchers. The transition from the single dimension of NMR spectroscopy to the second dimension of spatial orientation formed the foundation of current magnetic resonance imaging (MRI). The medical applications of MRI have already become conventional in assessing the workings of the inner body. Specifically, using MRI to assess the cardiovascular system has tremendously improved the diagnostic capability and capacity of cardiology. Further improvements in CMR imaging afford great potential for more effective and efficient methods of diagnosing cardiac diseases.

BASIC MAGNETIC RESONANCE PHYSICS

The physics of generating MRI depends on the random distribution of water and fat protons (^{1}H) within the body and the spin of those protons. In essence, MRI uses the property of magnetic field gradients across the body to make the frequency of ^{1}H spins a function of position that can be mapped into graphic interpretation (6). The magnet coil within the MRI produces a stable strong magnetic field, B_s, that forces the ^{1}H protons to rotate randomly around a specific axis in a cone-shaped fashion. A separate weak magnetic field, B_w, oscillating at a specific Larmor frequency, is then applied perpendicularly to the strong magnetic field to displace the ^{1}H spins to a transverse plane where they rotate in a coherent fashion (in phase). Because this second magnetic field is much lower in energy and is applied only transiently, a transverse magnetization wave is created. Once the B_w field is turned off and ^{1}H protons start to realign with B_s, the transverse magnetization signals can be detected. The frequency of these signals is then determined using a Fourier transform, and the amplitude in relation with time is calculated. The reversion of the ^{1}H proton system to randomization produces dampened oscillations; these decays are known as magnetic relaxation or free induction decay. This process proceeds through two pathways. One pathway is the realignment of the spins with B_s with loss of energy to the surrounding environment, which is known as spin–lattice relaxation and is called longitudinal relaxation rate (T1). The second pathway is the randomization of the phase of the spins, also known as spin–spin relaxation (T2). There is also a T2*, which is defined as the combined impact of the molecular spin–spin interactions (T2) and other dephasing processes that include field inhomogeneity and cardiac/respiratory motions. These three basic relaxation processes—T1, T2, and T2*—are essential in the generation of optimal image contrast and sequences to optimize the evaluation of cardiac anatomy, function, and physiology (7).

One of the most attractive capabilities of MRI is the possibility to resolve between tissues. The interpreted data from the resonance of the ^{1}H protons depend not only on the concentration of spins but also on molecular differences between water and fat protons in specific tissues that result in different magnetic relaxation times. These differences account for the variation of contrast between normal and infarct tissues, for example; thus, MRI makes the distinction of various tissues of health or disease possible.

BASIC CARDIAC MAGNETIC RESONANCE IMAGING SEQUENCES

For clinically acceptable CMR images, there must be relatively high spatial (<2 mm) and temporal (<50 ms) resolutions (8). The cornerstone of the CMR procedure is the pulse sequence, which determines the timing of image acquisition, signal-to-noise ratio, contrast-to-noise ratio, and image artifacts within the targeted frame. The two basic pulse sequences are the spin echo and gradient echo.

Spin-Echo (Dark-Blood) Sequence

A unique feature of spin-echo sequence is a "black-blood" image in which rapidly flowing blood appears dark, whereas stagnant tissues appear brighter. This happens as a result of a 90-/180-degree slice-selective/refocusing pulse pair, which affects only the spins that have not moved from the slice between both radiofrequency (RF) excitations. Systolic blood flow is usually darker than diastolic flow because the arterial blood pulsates with each heartbeat. The spin-echo sequence is relatively insensitive to magnetic field inhomogeneities produced by small metallic implants like vascular stents and clips. Compared with gradient-echo, a spin-echo sequence offers greater tissue contrast but a slower imaging speed. Its main use is the anatomic delineation of the pericardium, vascular structures, and mediastinum (Fig. 63–1) (8).

Gradient-Echo (Bright-Blood) Sequence

Gradient-echo sequence is the more widely used pulse because of its greater versatility. Acquisition of the entire *k*-

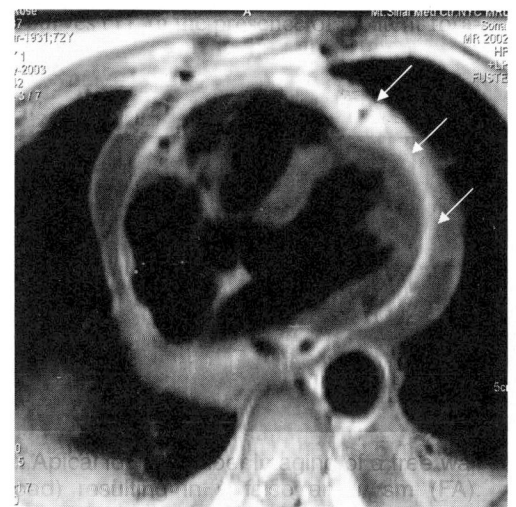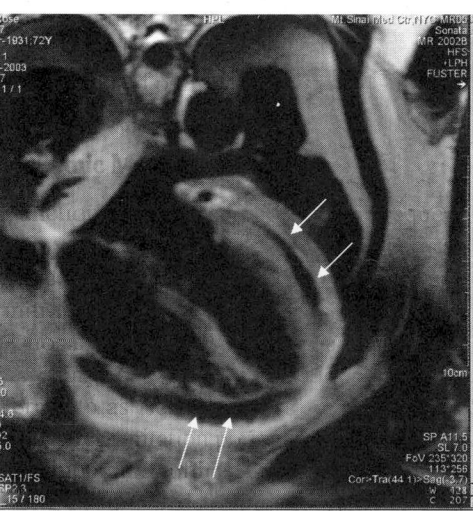

FIG. 63–1. Dark-blood imaging. T2-weighted images of the heart without **(A)** and with **(B)** fat saturation showing the pericardial fat *(arrows)* separating the myocardium from the thickened isodense pericardial fluid.

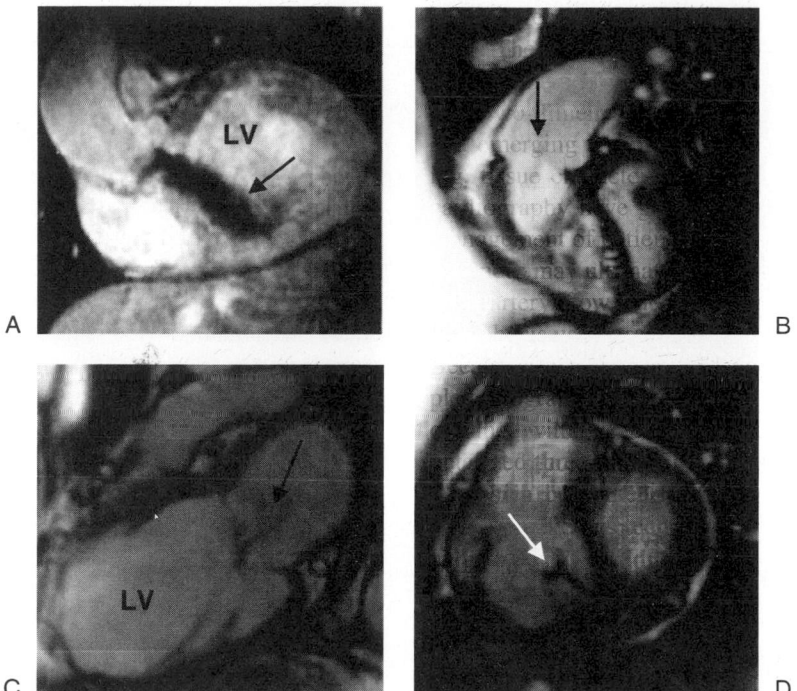

FIG. 63–2. Bright-blood imaging. **A:** Gradient-echo sequence showing signal void caused by high-velocity turbulent regurgitant flow *(red arrow)* into the left ventricle *(LV)* as a result of severe aortic insufficiency. **B:** True-fast imaging with steady-state precession (True-FISP) bright-blood sequence showing significant pulmonary insufficiency *(red arrow)* into the right ventricle in the right ventricular outflow tract view. **C:** True FISP bright-blood sequence showing significant mitral insufficiency *(red arrow)* into the left atrium in the LV two-chamber view. **D:** True FISP bright-blood sequence showing significant tricuspid insufficiency *(red arrow))* into the right atrium in the short-axis view.

space occurs by a series of signal echoes generated by slice-selective RF pulses, each of which is followed by a phase-encoding gradient and a readout gradient. This readout gradient is modified so that it causes the spins to rephase (substituting the role of the 180-degree RF pulse in the spin-echo sequence). The gradient echo is faster than spin echo because less time is required between spin excitation and signal detection (the 180-degree pulse is absent). The rapid repetition of excitations can cause signal saturation (loss) of spins in the slice. Blood flowing during the interpulse is exposed to less RF pulses, and therefore generates a greater signal than multiple excited stagnant tissues. Thus, a window of saturation is established that results in the "bright-blood" images characteristic of gradient-echo sequence (8). However, shorter acquisition times and saturation effects reduce the tissue contrast compared with spin-echo sequence. Another disadvantage of gradient-echo sequence is its extreme sensitivity to magnetic field inhomogeneities, which interferes with the qualitative perspective of the image. Common applications of gradient-echo sequence include ventricular function assessment, myocardial perfusion assessment, valvular motion and valvular regurgitation, and coronary artery imaging (Fig. 63–2). In general, gradient-echo sequence usage in cardiology is much more effective and efficient at providing solid and clear images of real-time heart function.

ASSESSMENT OF ISCHEMIC HEART DISEASE

IHD is the leading cause of mortality in the United States with more than 500,000 deaths per year, almost 200,000 of which are secondary to myocardial infarction (MI) (9). In the evaluation of the patient with symptoms or risk factors for IHD, it is necessary to establish the diagnosis, prognosis, and appropriate therapeutic measures. Several parameters need to be evaluated: biventricular function; presence and extent of ischemia; presence or absence of infarcted versus viable myocytes; and number, location, and severity of coronary stenoses. Ideally, the diagnostic test should provide reliable information for all of these parameters and should be safe and nondestructive or minimally invasive. Currently, the diagnostic approach to IHD can be time-consuming and laborious, and the results often are imprecise at best. Many unnecessary invasive procedures are performed as a direct consequence of the lack of a more accurate noninvasive diagnostic imaging modality for the assessment of this common cardiac problem.

Assessment of Cardiac Function

Assessment of cardiac function is a critical part of the management of many cardiac disorders including CAD, valvular heart disease, and cardiomyopathy. Currently, there is substantial evidence to indicate the use of CMR as a highly accurate and effective imaging modality in the assessments of global and regional cardiac function. Therefore, CMR is being increasingly recognized as the gold standard for the noninvasive evaluation of cardiac function (10,11), including left ventricular (LV) mass, end-diastolic volume (EDV), end-systolic volume (ESV), and ejection fraction. This is because of the high spatial, temporal, and contrast resolution of the technique, together with excellent reproducibility (12). In addition, it is possible to obtain static or moving images in any plane without exposure to ionizing radiation or contrast agents.

The two current methods for the measurement of end-diastolic and end-systolic LV volumes are an adaptation of the area–length measurements used in echocardiography and the stacking of contiguous tomographic slices. The former method assumes the left ventricle as an ellipsoid where the area (A) of the LV endocardial border can be traced and the length (L) from the apex to the mitral annulus can be measured. The equation $0.85A^2/L$ is then used to calculate the volume. However, this method fails in the same respect with echocardiography in its need for geometric assumptions and its inability to account for regional wall motion abnormalities (13). The second method applies Simpson's rule to a collection of short-axis contiguous covering the left ventricle from base to apex (Fig. 63–3). The volume is calculated to be the sum of the endocardial areas multiplied by the distance between the centers of individual slices. As no geometric assumptions are made, this method is more effective and accurate (13,14). By subtracting the ESV from the EDV, the stroke volume can be calculated. Multiplying the stroke volume by the heart rate then yields the cardiac output. The resultant cardiac output from CMR studies correlates well with that determined from catheterization laboratory (15). LV mass can be estimated from the volume of the myocardium multiplied by the specific gravity of the myocardium (1.05).

Global and regional wall motion abnormalities are important factors in the pathophysiology of numerous cardiovascular diseases, particularly CAD. CMR has proven an excellent noninvasive modality for the evaluation of segmental contractility, both qualitatively and quantitatively (16). If the volumes mentioned previously are measured over the entire cardiac cycle, time–volume curves can be derived, and estimates of diastolic performance (such as ventricular filling rate) are obtained (17). Phase–velocity mapping, a technique used for flow quantification, has been used to analyze transmitral and pulmonary vein flow patterns in the assessment of LV diastolic function (18).

Myocardial Perfusion

The initial work by Manning and others (19,20) demonstrated the feasibility of analyzing the first pass of an intravascular gadolinium-based contrast agent through the myocardium. Areas with hampered perfusion show decreased or late enhancement (Fig. 63–4) (21). Signal intensity versus time curves can be obtained, and different parameters, such as peak intensity, time to peak, and up-slope, provide semiquantitative estimations of blood flow. In combination with pharmacologic stressors like adenosine and dipyridamole, coronary flow reserve can be similarly measured. Using these approaches, several groups have reported promising results in the detection of IHD (22–25). Because current contrast agents diffuse into the interstitial space, signal changes reflect a mixture of myocardial perfusion and diffusion properties. The advent of newer purely intravascular agents may further improve the diagnostic capabilities of CMR perfusion analysis (26). Another application of contrast first-pass evaluation is the assessment of microvascular integrity in the setting of MI. Microvascular occlusion can be visualized as a hypoperfused area within the necrotic region and is an indicator of poor prognosis in survivors of a MI (27). Other authors have used CMR perfusion to detect

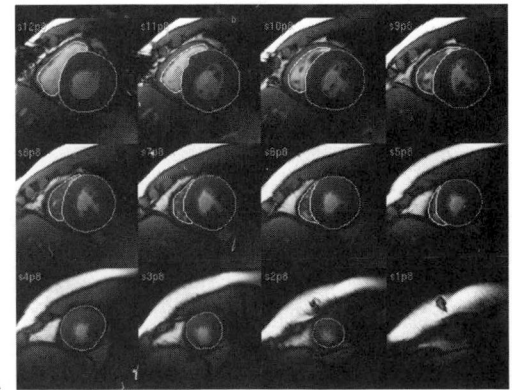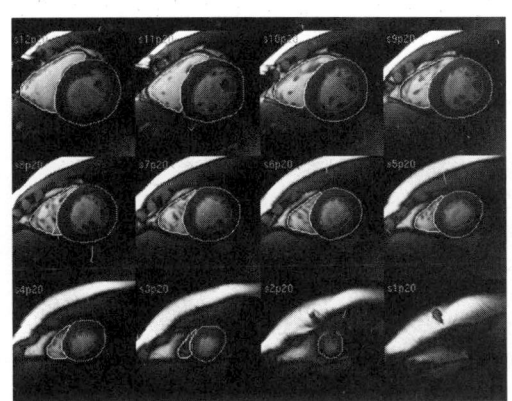

FIG. 63–3. Quantitative analysis of cardiac function by cardiac magnetic resonance. Twelve separate cine gradient-echo acquisitions in the short-axis of the end-systole **(A)** and end-diastole **(B)** were taken for the calculation of the ejection fraction based on modified Simpson's method.

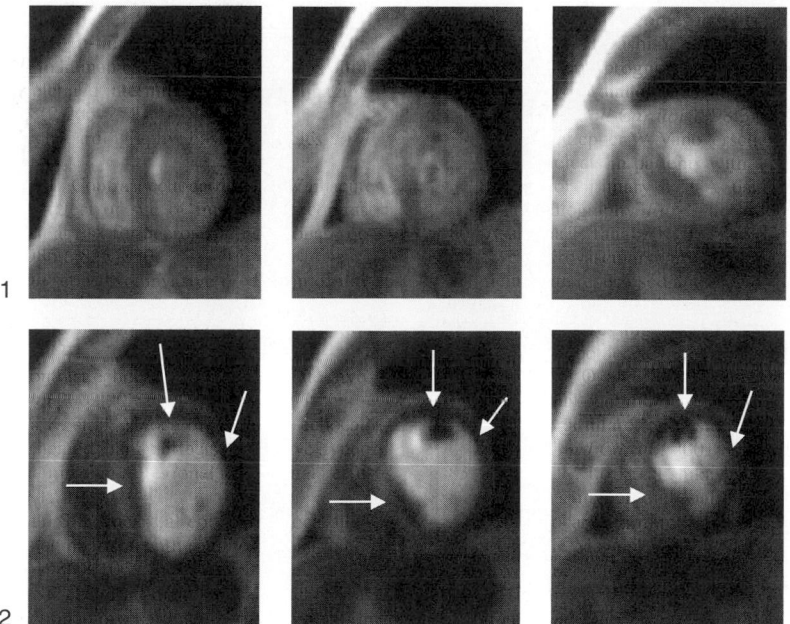

FIG. 63–4. Adenosine stress cardiac magnetic resonance. **1:** Resting perfusion study at three levels of the heart (*A,* upper segment; *B,* mid-ventricle; *C,* lower segment). **2:** Adenosine stress perfusion study showing hypoperfusion *(arrows)* to anterior, septal, and lateral wall in all three levels of the heart.

myocardial viability and to predict functional recovery after revascularization (28).

Dobutamine Stress Cardiac Magnetic Resonance

In a similar fashion as with echocardiography, the contractile response of myocardial segments to increasing doses of intravenous dobutamine is used in conjunction with CMR to evaluate ventricular ischemia and viability. Overall sensitivities and specificities of 80% to 90% and 80% to 100%, respectively, have been reported in the detection of coronary stenosis (29–31). In this regard, CMR has been proven superior to dobutamine echocardiography probably because of increased image quality (Fig. 63–5) (31). Therefore, it has been proposed as a particular useful alternative in subjects with a poor acoustic window (32). The quantification of wall thickening and myocardial strain with tagging is more accurate than visual assessment alone (33). From a prognostic viewpoint, inducible ischemia predicts a greater cardiac risk in patients with LV dysfunction (34) or those undergoing noncardiac surgery (35).

Contractile reserve in dysfunctional segments is a specific marker of viability that can be revealed by an infusion of low doses of dobutamine. There is evidence supporting its use in predicting spontaneous functional recovery after MI (36) or after revascularization in hibernating areas (37).

Contrast-enhanced Cardiac Magnetic Resonance

On the basis of the high contrast and high spatial resolution of nonenhanced CMR, it is possible to visualize infarcted areas because of their different magnetic properties as compared with normal, viable myocardium. In the setting of acute MI, there is tissue edema that leads to increased T1 and T2 times, so the infarction can be seen as a brighter area on T2-weighted images (38). However, the contrast between tissues is relatively small and tends to disappear as the infarction becomes chronic (39). At the same time, because severely ischemic but nonnecrotic tissue also can be edematous, regions with reversible injury may show signal enhancement (40).

The observation that gadolinium-DTPA (Gd-DTPA) has differential effects on the relaxation times of normal and infarcted myocardium (41) led to its application for the visualization of MI. Contrast-enhanced MRI increases tissue contrast significantly and is useful in the acute or chronic setting (39). The acquisition of images 5 to 30 minutes after the administration of an intravenous bolus of Gd-DTPA results in the delineation of the necrotic area as a region with increased signal intensity in T1-weighted images, a phenomenon known as *delayed hyperenhancement* (Fig. 63–6). The mechanism that leads to the signal enhancement is not completely elucidated, although several factors are known to play a role. Several investigators have reported an increment in gadolinium concentration in the infarcted tissue (42,43). Different mechanisms can potentially explain the accumulation of contrast in the necrotic area. An increase in the volume of distribution of Gd-DTPA as a result of an almost doubled extracellular volume in the area of MI has been reported (44). This is secondary not only to the presence of interstitial edema but also to the disruption of cellular membranes allowing the access of the contrast to the intracellular space (45,46). Therefore, the underlying mechanism for the detection of necrosis is, as in the case of nuclear techniques, the loss of membrane in-

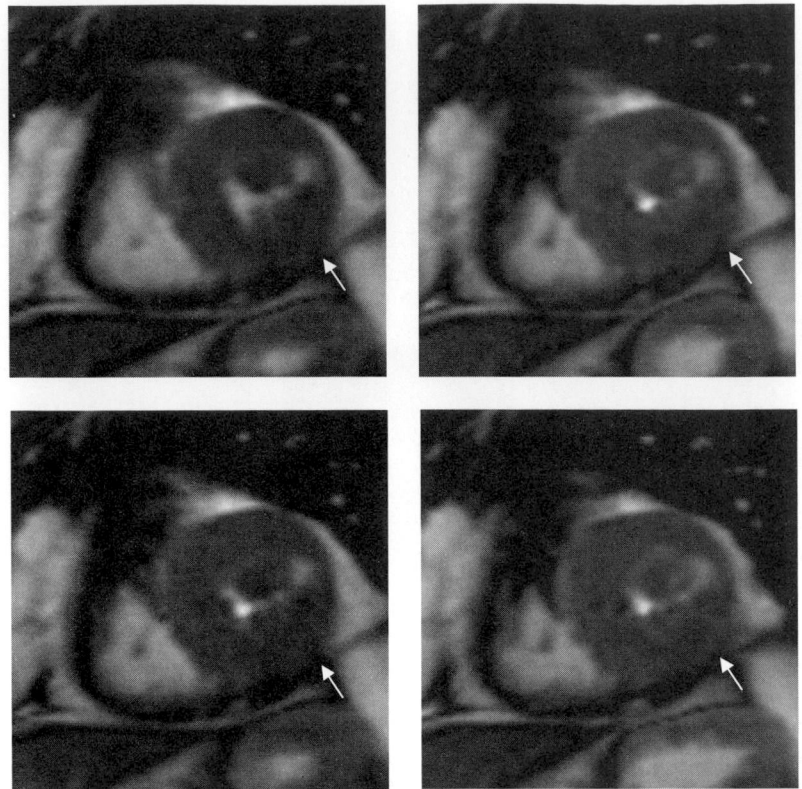

FIG. 63–5. Dobutamine stress cardiac magnetic resonance imaging together with the infusion of region *(white arrow)* of hyperenhanced myocardium in the lateral wall which failed to contract in response to low and high doses of dobutamine.

tegrity, a reliable marker of cellular death. It has been shown that the T1- and T2-shortening effect of gadolinium is more prominent in healthy as compared with infarcted canine myocardium shortly after the injection, but the relation is reversed after 5 minutes (41). This suggests that the delivery of the drug to the necrotic region is delayed. Judd and coworkers (47) demonstrated that whereas there is normally a constant relation between signal intensity in the myocardium and the blood pool, this ratio increases in infarcted areas, suggesting an impaired washout of the contrast agent. In summary, the decrease in capillary density together with a significant increase in "extracellular" space (edema and

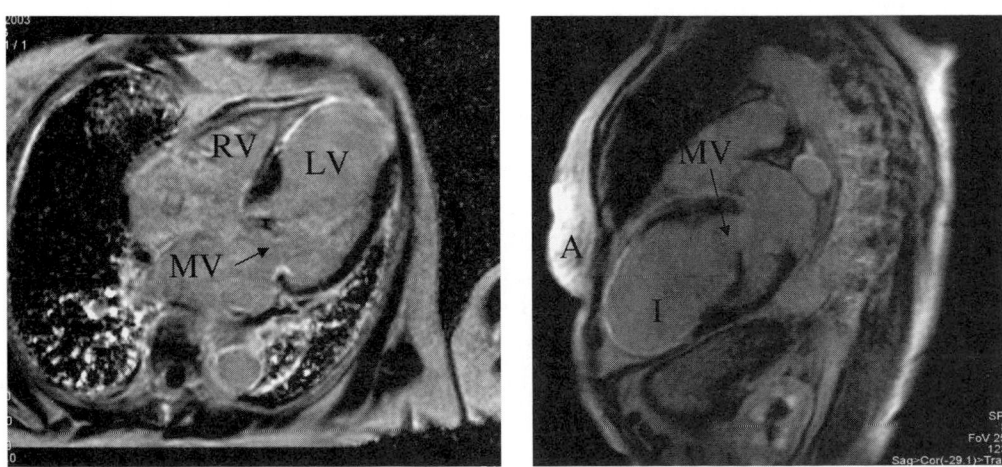

FIG. 63–6. Delayed hyperenhancement. Extensive scarring, bright hyperenhanced area, shown in four- **(A)** and two-chamber **(B)** view. A, anterior wall; I, inferior wall; LV, left ventricle; MV, mitral valve; RV, right ventricle.

membrane rupture) explain the slow diffusion and the delay in wash-in and wash-out of the contrast agent (45).

Studies comparing the spatial distribution of the hyperenhanced area with the pathologic specimens have proven an almost identical distribution (48). With the high spatial resolution of CMR it is possible to detect infarctions as small as 1 g myocardial tissue, even in areas with preserved contractility that would probably be missed by other imaging methods (49,50). The technique compares favorably with other well established techniques such as single-photon emission computed tomography (SPECT) or positron emission tomography in the detection of scar (51,52). The absence of hyperenhancement is a marker of cellular membrane integrity, and therefore a marker of viability that correlates well with thallium SPECT imaging or dobutamine echocardiography (53). The degree of viability can be estimated by quantifying the transmural extent of hyperenhancement, which is inversely related to the probability of functional recovery after MI (54) or revascularization (55).

Coronary Magnetic Resonance Angiography

Magnetic resonance angiography (MRA) of the coronary tree has emerged as an enormously attractive noninvasive diagnostic modality for the visualization of coronary stenoses. Nevertheless, it still remains a major challenge because of the constant cardiac and respiratory motion and small-caliber and tortuous course of the coronary arteries. Most laboratories currently use two- or three-dimensional gradient-echo sequences with *k*-space segmentation implemented with navigator echoes to compensate for respiratory motion. Using this approach, a recent multicenter trial demonstrated good accuracy, although limited to the proximal and mid segments, for the detection of severe CAD as compared with conventional coronary angiography (56). Results will probably be improved with the use of several technical implementations such as newer MR pulse sequences (57), spiral data acquisition (58), higher magnetic fields (59), and contrast-enhanced MRA with conventional extracellular agents (60) or newer intravascular molecules (61,62).

Another significant strength of CMR is its ability to image not only the vascular lumen but also vessel wall structures usually inaccessible by other noninvasive modalities. High-resolution black-blood studies enable the visualization of coronary artery plaques and vessel remodeling before the development of significant stenoses (63,64).

CONCLUSIONS

Thorough assessment of patients with CAD requires good clinical judgment and the practice of evidence-based medicine. Advances in noninvasive imaging have contributed greatly to the diagnostic accuracy of various stages of IHD. However, a typical diagnostic evaluation of symptomatic CAD includes the use of multiple imaging modalities that are expensive and time-consuming. MRI has become an im-

portant conventional medical imaging modality with exceptionally high spatial and temporal resolution. With current advanced cardiac gating, magnetic gradient, and coil design, CMR has taken on an important clinical role as a reliable quantitative noninvasive tool for the assessment of cardiac morphology, function, viability in health and disease. Its current limitations include high hardware/software costs and limited training centers for technologists and clinicians. However, with the pace of current advancements in MRI coil design and magnet technology, as well as better software programs to process and evaluate data, CMR may soon become as readily available as the cardiac catheterization laboratory.

ACKNOWLEDGMENTS

This work is supported in part by the Mount Sinai School of Medicine Consortium for Cardiovascular Imaging Technology (New York, NY). Dr. Sanz is supported by a research grant from the Spanish Society of Cardiology.

REFERENCES

1. American Heart Association. *Heart disease and stroke statistics—2003 update.* Dallas, TX: American Heart Association, 2002.
2. Bloch R, Hensen WW, Packard ME. Nuclear induction. *Phys Rev* 1946;69:127.
3. Purcell EM, Torrey HC, Pound RV. Resonance absorption by nuclear magnetic moments in a solid. *Phys Rev* 1946;69:37–38.
4. Lauterbur PC. Image formation by induced local interactions: examples employing nuclear magnetic resonance. *Nature* 1973;242:190–191.
5. Damadian R. Field focusing n.m.r. (FONAR) and the formation of chemical images in man. *Philos Trans R Soc Lond B Biol Sci* 1980;289:489–500.
6. Basic principles of MRI. In: Bradley WG, ed. *MRI the basics.* Philadelphia: Lippincott Williams & Wilkins, 1997:17–31.
7. Balaban RS. The physics of image generation by magnetic resonance. In: Manning WJ, Pennell DJ, eds. *Cardiovascular magnetic resonance.* Philadelphia: Churchill Livingstone, 2002:3–17.
8. Sodickson DK. Clinical cardiovascular magnetic resonance imaging techniques. In: Manning WJ, Pennell DJ, eds. *Cardiovascular magnetic resonance.* Philadelphia: Churchill Livingstone, 2002:18–30.
9. Arias E, Smith BL. Deaths: preliminary data for 2001. *Natl Vital Stat Rep* 2003;51:1–44.
10. Peshock RM, Willet D, Sayad D, et al. Quantitation of cardiac function by MRI. In: Boxt LM, ed. *MRI clinics of North America.* 1996.
11. Pennell D. Cardiovascular magnetic resonance. *Heart* 2001;85:581–589.
12. Pattynama PM, Lamb HJ, van der Velde EA, et al. Left ventricular measurements with cine and spin-echo MR imaging: a study of reproducibility with variance component analysis. *Radiology* 1993;187:261–268.
13. Chuang ML, Hibberd MG, Salton CJ, et al. Importance of imaging method over imaging modality in noninvasive determination of left ventricular volumes and ejection fraction: assessment by two- and three-dimensional echocardiography and magnetic resonance imaging. *J Am Coll Cardiol* 2000;35:477–484.
14. Shapiro EP, Rogers WJ, Beyar R, et al. Determination of left ventricular mass by magnetic resonance imaging in hearts deformed by acute infarction. *Circulation* 1989;79:706–711.
15. Hundley WG, Meshack BM, Willett DL, et al. Comparison of quantitation of left ventricular volume, ejection fraction, and cardiac output in patients with atrial fibrillation by cine magnetic resonance imaging versus invasive measurements. *Am J Cardiol* 1996;78:1119–1123.
16. Kwong RY, Schussheim AE, Rekhraj S, et al. Detecting acute coronary syndrome in the emergency department with cardiac magnetic resonance imaging. *Circulation* 2003;107:531–537.
17. Hoffmann U, Globits S, Stefenelli T, et al. The effects of ACE inhibitor

therapy on left ventricular myocardial mass and diastolic filling in previously untreated hypertensive patients: a cine MRI study. *J Magn Reson Imaging* 2001;14:16–22.

18. Hartiala JJ, Mostbeck GH, Foster E, et al. Velocity-encoded cine MRI in the evaluation of left ventricular diastolic function: measurement of mitral valve and pulmonary vein flow velocities and flow volume across the mitral valve. *Am Heart J* 1993;125:1054–1066.

19. Atkinson DJ, Burstein D, Edelman RR. First-pass cardiac perfusion: evaluation with ultrafast MR imaging. *Radiology* 1990;174:757–762.

20. Manning WJ, Atkinson DJ, Grossman W, et al. First-pass nuclear magnetic resonance imaging studies using gadolinium-DTPA in patients with coronary artery disease. *J Am Coll Cardiol* 1991;18:959–965.

21. Sensky PR, Samani NJ, Reek C, et al. Magnetic resonance perfusion imaging in patients with coronary artery disease: a qualitative approach. *Int J Cardiovasc Imaging* 2002;18:373–386.

22. Schwitter J, Nanz D, Kneifel S, et al. Assessment of myocardial perfusion in coronary artery disease by magnetic resonance: a comparison with positron emission tomography and coronary angiography. *Circulation* 2001;103:2230–2235.

23. Nagel E, Klein C, Paetsch I, et al. Magnetic resonance perfusion measurements for the noninvasive detection of coronary artery disease. *Circulation* 2003;108:432–437.

24. Ibrahim T, Nekolla SG, Schreiber K, et al. Assessment of coronary flow reserve: comparison between contrast-enhanced magnetic resonance imaging and positron emission tomography. *J Am Coll Cardiol* 2002;39:864–870.

25. Al-Saadi N, Nagel E, Gross M, et al. Noninvasive detection of myocardial ischemia from perfusion reserve based on cardiovascular magnetic resonance. *Circulation* 2000;101:1379–1383.

26. Kraitchman DL, Chin BB, Heldman AW, et al. MRI detection of myocardial perfusion defects due to coronary artery stenosis with MS-325. *J Magn Reson Imaging* 2002;15:149–158.

27. Wu KC, Zerhouni EA, Judd RM, et al. Prognostic significance of microvascular obstruction by magnetic resonance imaging in patients with acute myocardial infarction. *Circulation* 1998;97:765–772.

28. Lauerma K, Niemi P, Hanninen H, et al. Multimodality MR imaging assessment of myocardial viability: combination of first-pass and late contrast enhancement to wall motion dynamics and comparison with FDG PET-initial experience. *Radiology* 2000;217:729–736.

29. van Rugge FP, van der Wall EE, de Roos A, et al. Dobutamine stress magnetic resonance imaging for detection of coronary artery disease. *J Am Coll Cardiol* 1993;22:431–439.

30. van Rugge FP, van der Wall EE, Spanjersberg SJ, et al. Magnetic resonance imaging during dobutamine stress for detection and localization of coronary artery disease. Quantitative wall motion analysis using a modification of the centerline method. *Circulation* 1994;90:127–138.

31. Nagel E, Lehmkuhl HB, Bocksch W, et al. Noninvasive diagnosis of ischemia-induced wall motion abnormalities with the use of high-dose dobutamine stress MRI: comparison with dobutamine stress echocardiography. *Circulation* 1999;99:763–770.

32. Hundley WG, Hamilton CA, Thomas MS, et al. Utility of fast cine magnetic resonance imaging and display for the detection of myocardial ischemia in patients not well suited for second harmonic stress echocardiography. *Circulation* 1999;100:1697–1702.

33. Kuijpers D, Ho KY, van Dijkman PR, et al. Dobutamine cardiovascular magnetic resonance for the detection of myocardial ischemia with the use of myocardial tagging. *Circulation* 2003;107:1592–1597.

34. Hundley WG, Morgan TM, Neagle CM, et al. Magnetic resonance imaging determination of cardiac prognosis. *Circulation* 2002;106:2328–2333.

35. Rerkpattanapipat P, Morgan TM, Neagle CM, et al. Assessment of preoperative cardiac risk with magnetic resonance imaging. *Am J Cardiol* 2002;90:416–419.

36. Baer FM, Theissen P, Crnac J, et al. Head to head comparison of dobutamine-transoesophageal echocardiography and dobutamine-magnetic resonance imaging for the prediction of left ventricular functional recovery in patients with chronic coronary artery disease. *Eur Heart J* 2000;21:981–991.

37. Baer FM, Theissen P, Schneider CA, et al. Dobutamine magnetic resonance imaging predicts contractile recovery of chronically dysfunctional myocardium after successful revascularization. *J Am Coll Cardiol* 1998;31:1040–1048.

38. Fisher MR, McNamara MT, Higgins CB. Acute myocardial infarction: MR evaluation in 29 patients. *AJR Am J Roentgenol* 1987;148:247–251.

39. Schulz-Menger J, Gross M, Messroghli D, et al. Cardiovascular magnetic resonance of acute myocardial infarction at a very early stage. *J Am Coll Cardiol* 2003;42:513–518.

40. Bouchard A, Reeves RC, Cranney G, et al. Assessment of myocardial infarct size by means of T2-weighted 1H nuclear magnetic resonance imaging. *Am Heart J* 1989;117:281–289.

41. Wesbey GE, Higgins CB, McNamara MT, et al. Effect of gadolinium-DTPA on the magnetic relaxation times of normal and infarcted myocardium. *Radiology* 1984;153:165–169.

42. Inoue S, Murakami Y, Ochiai K, et al. The contributory role of interstitial water in Gd-DTPA-enhanced MRI in myocardial infarction. *J Magn Reson Imaging* 1999;9:215–219.

43. Rehwald WG, Fieno DS, Chen EL, et al. Myocardial magnetic resonance imaging contrast agent concentrations after reversible and irreversible ischemic injury. *Circulation* 2002;105:224–229.

44. Lima JA, Judd RM, Bazille A, et al. Regional heterogeneity of human myocardial infarcts demonstrated by contrast-enhanced MRI. Potential mechanisms. *Circulation* 1995;92:1117–1125.

45. Kim RJ, Chen EL, Lima JA, et al. Myocardial Gd-DTPA kinetics determine MRI contrast enhancement and reflect the extent and severity of myocardial injury after acute reperfused infarction. *Circulation* 1996;94:3318–3326.

46. Arheden H, Saeed M, Higgins CB, et al. Measurement of the distribution volume of gadopentetate dimeglumine at echo-planar MR imaging to quantify myocardial infarction: comparison with 99mTc-DTPA autoradiography in rats. *Radiology* 1999;211:698–708.

47. Judd RM, Lugo-Olivieri CH, Arai M, et al. Physiological basis of myocardial contrast enhancement in fast magnetic resonance images of 2-day-old reperfused canine infarcts. *Circulation* 1995;92:1902–1910.

48. Fieno DS, Kim RJ, Chen EL, et al. Contrast-enhanced magnetic resonance imaging of myocardium at risk: distinction between reversible and irreversible injury throughout infarct healing. *J Am Coll Cardiol* 2000;36:1985–1991.

49. Ricciardi MJ, Wu E, Davidson CJ, et al. Visualization of discrete microinfarction after percutaneous coronary intervention associated with mild creatine kinase-MB elevation. *Circulation* 2001;103:2780–2783.

50. Wu E, Judd RM, Vargas JD, et al. Visualisation of presence, location, and transmural extent of healed Q-wave and non-Q-wave myocardial infarction. *Lancet* 2001;357:21–28.

51. Klein C, Nekolla SG, Bengel FM, et al. Assessment of myocardial viability with contrast-enhanced magnetic resonance imaging: comparison with positron emission tomography. *Circulation* 2002;105:162–167.

52. Wagner A, Mahrholdt H, Holly TA, et al. Contrast-enhanced MRI and routine single photon emission computed tomography (SPECT) perfusion imaging for detection of subendocardial myocardial infarcts: an imaging study. *Lancet* 2003;361:374–379.

53. Ramani K, Judd RM, Holly TA, et al. Contrast magnetic resonance imaging in the assessment of myocardial viability in patients with stable coronary artery disease and left ventricular dysfunction. *Circulation* 1998;98:2687–2694.

54. Choi KM, Kim RJ, Gubernikoff G, et al. Transmural extent of acute myocardial infarction predicts long-term improvement in contractile function. *Circulation* 2001;104:1101–1107.

55. Kim RJ, Wu E, Rafael A, et al. The use of contrast-enhanced magnetic resonance imaging to identify reversible myocardial dysfunction. *N Engl J Med* 2000;343:1445–1453.

56. Kim WY, Danias PG, Stuber M, et al. Coronary magnetic resonance angiography for the detection of coronary stenoses. *N Engl J Med* 2001;345:1863–1869.

57. Bunce NH, Lorenz CH, John AS, et al. Coronary artery bypass graft patency: assessment with true fast imaging with steady-state precession versus gadolinium-enhanced MR angiography. *Radiology* 2003;227:440–446.

58. Yang PC, Meyer CH, Terashima M, et al. Spiral magnetic resonance coronary angiography with rapid real-time localization. *J Am Coll Cardiol* 2003;41:1134–1141.

59. Stuber M, Botnar RM, Fischer SE, et al. Preliminary report on in vivo coronary MRA at 3 Tesla in humans. *Magn Reson Med* 2002;48:425–429.

60. Regenfus M, Ropers D, Achenbach S, et al. Comparison of contrast-enhanced breath-hold and free-breathing respiratory-gated imaging in three-dimensional magnetic resonance coronary angiography. *Am J Cardiol* 2002;90:725–730.

61. Bunce NH, Keegan J, Gatehouse PD, et al. Initial experience with the

intravascular contrast agent NC100150-injection (Clariscan) for breath-hold and navigator-gated magnetic resonance coronary artery imaging. *J Magn Reson Imaging* 2002;16:217–223.

62. Taupitz M, Schnorr J, Wagner S, et al. Coronary MR angiography: experimental results with a monomer-stabilized blood pool contrast medium. *Radiology* 2002;222:120–126.

63. Kim WY, Stuber M, Bornert P, et al. Three-dimensional black-blood cardiac magnetic resonance coronary vessel wall imaging detects positive arterial remodeling in patients with nonsignificant coronary artery disease. *Circulation* 2002;106:296–299.

64. Fayad ZA, Fuster V, Fallon JT, et al. Noninvasive in vivo human coronary artery lumen and wall imaging using black-blood magnetic resonance imaging. *Circulation* 2000;102:506–510.

CHAPTER 64

The Role of Positron Emission Tomography

Heinrich R. Schelbert and Thomas H. Schindler

Key Words: Coronary artery disease; hibernation; ischemic cardiomyopathy; positron emission tomography; stunning; viability.

INTRODUCTION

Positron emission tomography (PET) expands the scope of available noninvasive studies of the human heart with standard nuclear medicine techniques. Combining the virtually photon attenuation–free high-spatial resolution images and the high temporal sampling capability of PET with positron-emitting radiotracers and tracer kinetic principles, regional functional processes can be measured noninvasively in absolute units. These noninvasive probes of PET extend beyond measurements of myocardial blood flow (MBF) and include assays of the myocardium's substrate metabolism, oxygen consumption, and neuronal activity. Applied to the

Supported in part by research grants HL 29845 and HL 33177, National Institutes of Health, and an Investigative Group Award by the Greater Los Angeles Affiliate of the American Heart Association.

H. R. Schelbert: Department of Molecular and Medical Pharmacology, David Geffen School of Medicine at UCLA, 650 Charles E. Young Drive South, University of California at Los Angeles, Los Angeles, California 90095-6948.
T. H. Schindler: Department of Molecular and Medical Pharmacology, David Geffen School of Medicine at UCLA, 650 Charles E. Young Drive South, University of California at Los Angeles, Los Angeles, California 90095-6948.

human heart, investigations with PET have explored effects of coronary atherosclerosis on myocardial blood flow or uncovered regional alterations of blood flow and substrate metabolism that are unique to acute and "chronic" ischemia. Moreover, PET has been proven useful in the diagnosis and management of patients with cardiovascular disease. This chapter begins with a description of methodologic aspects of PET, continues with a review of observations made with PET in patients with acute myocardial infarction (AMI), and concludes with an examination of the clinical utility of this imaging modality in patients after infarction and ischemic cardiomyopathy.

TOOLS OF POSITRON EMISSION TOMOGRAPHY

Many of the short-lived positron emitters represent radioactive isotopes of elements that constitute living matter (Table 64–1). They are incorporated into physiologically active substances without modifying their biologic properties. Synthesized at high specific activities, minute quantities of mass of tracer produce images of high diagnostic quality without interfering with the very process to be studied. Table 64–2 lists the four major groups of positron-emitting tracers that have been applied to the study of the human myocardium.

Tracers of Myocardial Blood Flow

The majority of human studies have relied on oxygen-15 (^{15}O) water, nitrogen-13 (^{13}N) ammonia, rubidium-82

TABLE 64–1. *Positron emitting isotopes used in cardiac positron emission tomography studies*

Isotope	Production	Half-life, min
^{15}O (Oxygen-15)	Cyclotron	2.07
^{13}N (Nitrogen-13)	Cyclotron	9.96
^{11}C (Carbon-11)	Cyclotron	20.40
^{18}F (Fluorine-18)	Cyclotron	109.70
^{82}Rb (Rubidium-82)	Generator (^{82}Sr[a])	1.25
^{38}K (Potassium-38)	Cyclotron	7.70
^{62}Cu (Copper-62)	Generator (^{62}In[a])	9.73

[a]Parent isotope.

(^{82}Rb), and, to a lesser extent, potassium-38 (^{38}K) (Table 64–2).

Oxygen-15 Water

The radiotracer ^{15}O water meets most closely the criteria of an ideal tracer of blood flow (1). It is metabolically inert. The capillary and sarcolemmal membranes do not exert a significant barrier effect so that the tracer exchanges freely between blood and tissue; the myocardial uptake of ^{15}O water, therefore, correlates linearly with blood flow (1). Because water equilibrates rapidly among blood, myocardium, and adjacent tissues, delineation of the myocardium requires subtraction of the tracer activity in the blood pool and the vascular space of the myocardium. This is accomplished through near simultaneous imaging of the water space with ^{15}O water and the blood pool with ^{15}O- or ^{11}C-labeled carbon monoxide bound to hemoglobin. Myocardial and blood pool time–activity curves are derived from rapid serially acquired images. Fitted with a single-compartment tracer kinetic model, regional MBF can be quantified in milliliters per minute per gram (2,3).

Another potentially exciting use of ^{15}O water includes the water perfusable tissue index (PTI) (4). The index assumes that only normal or viable myocardium, not necrotic myocardium or scar tissue, exchanges water rapidly. It thus delineates the fraction of nonviable or scar tissue in a given myocardial region or segment. The PTI is derived from a transmission image, depicting the tissue volume and density, a labeled carbon monoxide blood pool image, used to subtract the vascular spaces, and an ^{15}O water image for determining the fraction of the extravascular tissue volume that is capable of exchanging water rapidly. As expected, scar tissue in regions of prior myocardial infarction (MI) results in a decrease of the PTI (5), and, in animals (6), the PTI was found to correlate inversely with the fraction of tissue fibrosis.

TABLE 64–2. *Positron-emitting tracers used for the study of human myocardial infarction*

PET tracer	Tracer kinetics of metabolism	Functional aspect evaluated
Myocardial blood flow		
^{15}O water	Metabolically inert; no significant barrier effect	Uptake correlates linearly with MBF (mL/min · g^{-1})
^{13}N ammonia	Trapping by glutamine synthetase reaction	Uptake correlates nonlinearly with MBF (mL/min · g^{-1})
^{82}Rb, ^{38}K	Active transport by Na$^+$-K$^+$ ATPase	Nonlinear correlation with MBF (mL/min · g^{-1})
Substrate metabolism		
^{11}C glucose	Glucose uptake and turnover	Glucose metabolism
^{18}F 2-deoxyglucose	Trapped after hexokinase-mediated phosphorylation to glucose-6-phosphate	Glucose utilization (μmol/min · g^{-1})
^{11}C palmitate	Flow-dependent uptake followed by biexponential clearance	Qualitative fatty acid metabolism; size and slope of the rapid phase correspond to fatty acid oxidation and of the slow phase correspond to fatty acid entering endogenous lipid pools
^{18}F flouro-6-thia-heptadeconic acid	Flow-dependent uptake followed by metabolic trapping	Thought to trace FFA fraction committed to oxidation
^{15}O oxygen	Myocardial oxygen extraction	Myocardial oxygen consumption
^{11}C acetate	Flow-dependent uptake followed by biexponential clearance; flux rate through tricarboxylic acid cycle	Rate of oxidative metabolism as approximation of myocardial oxygen consumption
Special aspects		
^{18}F misonidazole	Becomes trapped in hypoxic tissue	Tissue hypoxia/ischemia
Neuronal control		
^{11}C meta-hydroxyephedrine	Norepinephrine analog; enters adrenergic neuron through uptake II mechanism	Adrenergic neuron density or function

ATPase, adenosine triphosphatase; ^{11}C, carbon-11; ^{18}F, fluorine-18; FFA, free fatty acid; ^{38}K, potassium-38; MBF, myocardial blood flow; ^{13}N, nitrogen-13; ^{15}O, oxygen-15; PET, positron emission tomography; ^{82}Rb, rubidium-82.

Nitrogen-13 Ammonia

[13]N ammonia diffuses freely across the capillary membranes (7,8) and becomes trapped in the myocardium mostly through the glutamate to glutamine reaction (9–11). The rate of metabolic trapping competes with back-diffusion of ammonia from the myocardium into blood. The rate of metabolic trapping appears to be relatively constant, but back-diffusion of ammonia depends on blood flow. Hence, retention of tracer label in the myocardium declines nonlinearly with increasing flow so that its myocardial net uptake correlates with MBF in a curvilinear fashion (9). Trapping of ^{13}N ammonia in the human myocardium is usually complete within 2 minutes of intravenous administration. For measurements of MBF, the initial image data are acquired in rapid sequence. Blood pool and myocardial time–activity curves derived from these images are fitted with a two-compartment tracer kinetic model that corrects for the nonlinearity of the tracer net uptake and yields MBF (mL/min $\cdot$ g^{-1}) (12–15). Because of the longer physical half-life of [13]N (10 minutes), static, high-diagnostic quality images of the relative distribution of MBF are obtained.

Rubidium-82

[82]Rb is a radioactive cation (Rb^{+}) that is generator produced. As a potassium analog, it is transported actively into myocytes. Because of a barrier effect of the capillary and sarcolemmal membranes, the tracer first-pass extraction fraction (the fraction of tracer crossing the capillary membranes during a single tracer transit through the coronary circulation) declines curvilinearly with greater flows. Hence, the myocardial tracer net uptake is correlated nonlinearly with MBF (16–18). Through use of tracer kinetic models, estimates of MBF (mL/min $\cdot$ g^{-1}) can be obtained, although such estimates appear to underestimate flows in the hyperemic range (19). As a distinct advantage, [82]Rb can be delivered intravenously through a pushbutton-operated infusion system at preselected dosages and infusion rates.

In addition to [38]K (19–21), use of flow tracers like copper-62–labeled pyruvaldehyde N^{4}-methylthiosernicarbazone (20, 22,23) or technetium-94m teboroxime (24) appear promising but remain in an exploratory state.

Tracers of Myocardial Substrate Metabolism

The most widely used and applied tracers to the study of human myocardial ischemia have been ^{11}C acetate, ^{11}C palmitate, and fluorine-18 (^{18}F) deoxyglucose (Table 64–2).

Carbon-11 Acetate

Because of its relatively straightforward metabolism, ^{11}C acetate affords an assessment of flux rates of substrate through the tricarboxylic acid (TCA) cycle as the final oxidative pathway shared by several fuel substrates. Administered in-travenously, the tracer is initially retained in the myocardium in proportion to blood flow (25). The ^{11}C label leaves the myocardium in the form of carbon dioxide liberated during the second turn of acetate metabolites through the TCA cycle (26). The rate of release from the myocardium is correlated linearly with myocardial oxygen consumption (MVO$_2$), as demonstrated in animals (27–30), or to the rate–pressure product as an index of cardiac work, as demonstrated in humans (31–33). Accordingly, estimates of regional MVO$_2$ are derived by monoexponential or biexponential least-square fitting of the regional myocardial time–activity curves obtained from regions of interest assigned to the serially acquired PET images. The slow-clearance phase reflects incorporation of the ^{11}C label into a slow-turnover pool of glutamine. Estimates of oxidative metabolism in human myocardium can be obtained readily by monoexponential fitting of the early portion of the clearance curve; the slope is usually referred to as k_{mono}. The approach yields only rates of flux rather than of the true mass flux of substrate through the TCA cycle. Furthermore, the clearance rate of tracer from the myocardium depends on the pool sizes of TCA cycle metabolites. Studies in isolated rabbit hearts have identified the glutamate pool as the largest one (26); the size of this pool together with the rate of substrate flux through it determines k_{mono} or the initial rate of tracer clearance from the myocardium. The sum of all pool sizes remains relatively constant during ischemia, hypoxia, or both so that k_{mono} reflects rather reliably the TCA cycle activity (27,29).

O-15 Molecular Oxygen

Measurements of the mass flux of oxygen—that is, of MVO$_2$ (μmol/min $\cdot$ g^{-1})—are indeed possible with [15]O oxygen. Although technically demanding, [15]O is administered by inhalation; the extraction of the radioactive oxygen by myocardium is determined from serially acquired serial PET images. Combined with measurements of MBF with the [15]O water method, the MVO$_2$ is estimated from the product of the oxygen extraction and MBF. Estimates of the oxygen consumption by this noninvasive approach in human myocardium were found to be comparable to those obtained invasively with the coronary sinus catheter technique and the Fick principle (34,35).

Carbon-11 Palmitate

[11]C palmitate was one of the first tracers developed specifically for cardiac PET studies (36,37). Its initial uptake in myocardium depends on blood flow. The unidirectional esterification palmitate to palmityl-coenzyme A effectively sequesters the tracer into the myocardium. A fraction of tracer then enters endogenous lipid pools (diglycerides and triglycerides, phospholipids, and others); the remaining fraction proceeds through the carnitine shuttle to the inner mitochondrial membrane for β-oxidation to C-2 fragments and fur-

ther to final oxidation in the TCA cycle (38–40) with release of tracer label from the myocardium in the form of carbon dioxide. The fractional distribution of tracer label between the large, slow-turnover pool of endogenous lipids and a small, rapid-turnover pool of oxidation accounts for the characteristic biexponential clearance curve morphology. The size and slope of the rapid-clearance phase correspond to the fraction of labeled palmitate that enters immediate oxidation and its rate of oxidation, whereas the slow-clearance curve component (defined again by its relative size and slope) reflects the fraction of tracer that has been incorporated into the large endogenous lipid pools (38).

The fractional distribution of tracer between these two major pools depends on the substrate preference of the myocardium. If, as is the case during fasting, myocardium preferentially oxidizes free fatty acid (FFA), then the relative size of the rapid-clearance phase is large and its slope is steep. Conversely, if myocardium oxidizes disproportionately more glucose than FFA, then both the size and slope of the rapid-clearance phase decline. Furthermore, when energy demand increases as, for example, with greater cardiac work, oxidation of FFA may increase as reflected by an increase in the size and slope of the rapid-clearance phase (41). Back-diffusion of nonmetabolized ^{11}C palmitate may limit the accuracy of estimates of FFA oxidation (39,42). Also, because the Carbon-16 palmitate is only one of many long-chain fatty acids consumed by myocardium. Nevertheless, measurements of myocardial FFA consumption appear possible. Through use of tracer compartment models and serial image acquisition and from arterial FFA concentrations, estimates of the myocardial uptake of FFA and its oxidation (in units of $\mu mol/min \cdot g^{-1}$) are available (43).

Fluorine-18 Fluoro-6-Thia-Heptadecanoic Acid

^{18}F fluoro-6-thia-heptadecanoic acid has been developed as a tracer of myocardial fatty acid metabolism (44). It is thought to track the fraction of FFA that immediately becomes oxidized. Again, the initial uptake of the radiotracer in myocardium largely depends on blood flow. However, different from ^{11}C palmitate, the activated radiotracer is a poor substrate for β-oxidation so that the tracer becomes essentially trapped in the myocardium. From the rate of radiotracer accumulation in the myocardium (as a function of the arterial radiotracer concentration or the arterial tracer input function), MBF and the arterial plasma FFA concentration, estimates of the myocardial FFA uptake can be determined (45,46).

Fluorine-18 2-Fluoro-2-Deoxyglucose

Developed for measurements of regional cerebral glucose metabolism initially with autoradiography labeled with ^{14}C (47) and subsequently with PET (48), the glucose analog permits measurements of the myocardial exogenous glucose utilization (49,50). ^{18}F 2-fluoro-2-deoxyglucose traces the initial transmembranous exchange of glucose and the hexo-

kinase-mediated phosphorylation to glucose-6-phosphate (47). Unlike glucose, its tracee, the phosphorylated tracer is a poor substrate for glycogen synthesis, glycolysis, and the fructose pentose shunt. Furthermore, because dephosphorylation in the myocardium is slow and the compound is rather impermeable to the cell membrane, the ^{18}F label becomes virtually trapped in the myocardium. Images recorded about 30 to 40 minutes after tracer injection, when most of the tracer is in its phosphorylated form in the myocardium (51), reflect the relative distribution of exogenous glucose utilization rates in the myocardium. Regional glucose utilization rates ($\mu mol/min \cdot g^{-1}$) in myocardium can be estimated by fitting regional myocardial time–activity curves derived from serially acquired images using a unidirectional transport compartment model (47,50,52). The operational equation requires knowledge of the arterial glucose concentration and includes a "lumped constant" that adjusts for differences in the transmembranous exchange and phosphorylation rates between glucose and ^{18}F deoxyglucose (50). Although there is some debate on the constancy of this lumped constant, it nevertheless appears to be relatively independent of the heart's preferential substrate selection and of insulin concentrations (53–55).

Carbon-11 Glucose

Different from ^{18}F deoxyglucose, which traces only the initial transmembranous exchange of glucose and its hexokinase-mediated phosphorylation to glucose-6-phosphate, and thus offers little if any information on its subsequent metabolism, such information is available with ^{11}C glucose. Time-dependent ^{11}C activity concentrations in myocardium and arterial blood after intravenous radiotracer administrations are derived from serially acquired PET images and provide estimates of the radiotracer net uptake and clearance rates in the myocardium and, when adjusted to the arterial glucose concentration, offer estimates of the myocardial glucose utilization and metabolism (56–58).

Ischemia-specific Tracers

Misonidazole, labeled with ^{18}F, targets ischemic/hypoxic myocardium (59). Animal studies demonstrated selective uptake in acutely ischemic but not in reperfused or necrotic myocardium (59). Although encouraging, subsequent studies in patients with ischemic heart disease similarly showed increased uptake of ^{18}F-labeled misonidazole in hypoperfused myocardium. However, the selectively increased uptake in hypoperfused myocardium barely exceeded blood pool activity (60) so that the agent has thus far failed to gain clinical acceptance.

Tracers of Adrenergic Neuron Function and Density

^{11}C-labeled meta-hydroxyephedrine has been extensively evaluated in animals and in humans (61). The agent traces the uptake 1 mechanism of norepinephrine and accumulates in the storage granules of adrenergic neuron terminals (62). However, images of the myocardial ^{11}C hydroxyephedrine uptake do not distinguish between absence and dysfunction of adrenergic neurons. Yet, such distinction may become possible if the tracer is combined with the more recently synthesized ^{11}C-labeled norepinephrine (63,64). Importantly, radiotracer concentrations in the myocardium correlate with those of norepinephrine and tracer kinetics with uptake and release of norepinephrine in myocardium (61,63, 65,66).

POSITRON EMISSION TOMOGRAPHY IMAGING AND IMAGE DISPLAY

Technical Considerations

PET images are virtually free of photon attenuation artifacts; this together with a high spatial and temporal resolution renders PET superior to single-photon emission computed tomography (SPECT). Before image acquisition, attenuation of photons is measured directly by recording transmission images that during the reconstruction of the emission images serve to correct for measured (rather than assumed) photon attenuation. Modern tomographs acquire as many as 47 transaxial slices simultaneously, with a slice thickness of about 3 to 4 mm. The intrinsic in-plane resolution approaches the theoretic limits and is about 3 to 4 mm. The axial field of view of newer tomographs is usually about 15 to 16 cm. The transaxially acquired image sets are reoriented into short- and long-axis cuts of the left ventricular myocardium (12,67–69). Three-dimensional displays of the left ventricular myocardium are available (70), although most PET facilities now display the relative distribution of tracer concentrations in the left ventricular myocardium in the form of two-dimensional polar maps.

The distribution of functional processes can be displayed in the form of "parametric images" where color codes reflect regional rates of, for example, blood flow or glucose utilization in milliliters blood or micromole glucose per minute per gram myocardium (52,70,71). The high temporal resolution permits rapid (dynamic) acquisition of serial images at sampling rates of 1 to 12 seconds. It is thus possible to measure noninvasively rapid changes in tracer concentrations in the myocardium and the arterial blood. Regional tissue time–activity curves derived through regions of interest assigned to the serially acquired images are fitted with appropriate tracer kinetic models and afford noninvasive measurements of regional functional processes.

Yet, there are limitations. First, the images depict only the concentrations of the radiolabel, but not those of the chemical species that contain the radiolabel. The metabolic fate of the tracer label must therefore be carefully delineated and must be predictable. Second, the effective spatial resolution of current tomographs, after image filtering, precludes the evaluation of transmural myocardial gradients of tracer con-

centrations. Furthermore, the "partial volume effect" (72) leads to an underrepresentation of the "true myocardial tracer concentrations." Yet, they can be obtained if the myocardial wall thickness (e.g., by magnetic resonance imaging, computed tomography [CT], or echocardiography) and the performance characteristics of the tomograph are known (73,74). Because the myocardial wall thickness varies regionally, myocardial tracer concentrations may appear heterogeneous. Such artifactual heterogeneity is especially apparent on transaxial images because the image planes traverse the myocardial wall at different angles. Image reorientation into short-axis cuts diminishes this effect. In dysfunctional segments, impaired or absent systolic thickening reduces the "average wall thickness," thus causing artifactual reductions in regional tracer uptake (75). Thus, a regional wall motion abnormality alone, even if true tracer uptake were normal, may cause the appearance of a tracer uptake defect. Obviously, the same mechanism accentuates the severity of, for example, an existing blood flow defect. The severity of such "defects" depends inversely on the resolution capability of the imaging system and is less prominent with the modem high-resolution scanners. This shortcoming is not unique to PET, but also applies to SPECT or, for that matter, to all imaging modalities.

Image Acquisition

PET studies typically begin with acquisition of transaxial transmission images using a rotating rod containing a positron-emitting isotope. Acquisition times typically range from 15 to 20 minutes. The new hybrid PET/CT imaging system substantially shortens the time required for attenuation correction. The transaxial CT images of the chest serve to map the distribution of photon attenuation and are used for correction of the emission images for photon attenuation. The positron-emitting tracer is then administered, usually intravenously. If functional processes are to be quantified, acquisition of serial sets of transaxial images begins at the time of tracer injection and continues, depending on the specific tracer, for 20 to 60 minutes. Typically, acquisition of a dynamic ^{13}N ammonia study and a ^{18}F deoxyglucose study requires 20 minutes and about 60 to 90 minutes, respectively. If only the relative tracer uptake is to be imaged, time for clearance of tracer from the blood and for uptake into the myocardium is allowed. Usually, this time interval amounts to about 5 minutes for ^{13}N ammonia and about 30 to 40 minutes for ^{18}F deoxyglucose. Static images are then recorded for about 15 to 20 minutes.

Studies with intravenous ^{11}C acetate and ^{11}C palmitate are typically acquired in the dynamic mode because metabolic information is derived from the initial tracer uptake and the subsequent clearance pattern from the myocardium. Time–activity curves are derived from regions of interest assigned on the serial images to the left ventricular blood pool and the myocardium.

Finally, gated image acquisition also is available with PET and has been shown to allow measurements of left ventricular volumes and ejection fractions and assessments of regional wall motion and thickening (72,76–78).

POSITRON EMISSION TOMOGRAPHY INVESTIGATIONS IN MYOCARDIAL ISCHEMIA

Observations in Animal Experiments

Early animal experimental studies explored whether known alterations of substrate metabolism during acute myocardial ischemia could indeed be demonstrated noninvasively with PET. These studies used ^{11}C palmitate, ^{18}F deoxyglucose, and ^{13}N ammonia. Acute, moderate ischemia had long been known to suppress oxidation of FFA and to accelerate glycolysis and, possibly, exogenous glucose utilization (79). Canine studies had demonstrated in moderate ischemia enhanced glucose extraction and glycolytic activity as evidenced by lactate release (80). Studies with PET indicated that the known suppression of FFA oxidation could indeed be demonstrated with ^{11}C palmitate. The relative size and slope of the rapid-clearance phase markedly declined in acutely ischemic segments (39,41). Pacing-induced tachycardia in the presence of severe, experimentally induced coronary stenosis resulted in segmental flow defects that selectively accumulated ^{18}F deoxyglucose, consistent with increased glucose utilization and, presumably, glycolytic activity (81). Although ^{18}F deoxyglucose uptake in normal myocardium could be altered by manipulating circulating substrate levels, corresponding changes in acutely ischemic myocardium were markedly attenuated. The latter implied that local mechanisms modulated effects of systemic regulatory mechanisms of substrate interaction and selection. Other studies in acute, experimentally induced ischemia demonstrated preserved ^{18}F deoxyglucose uptake in acutely ischemic myocardium with moderately reduced flows (82). Even for flow reductions of 60% to 80% less than that in normal myocardium, ^{18}F deoxyglucose uptake remained substantially greater than blood flow (82). The preserved glucose utilization in hypoperfused myocardium reflects an increase in glucose utilization that corresponds to the operational term of "blood flow–glucose metabolism mismatch," as observed subsequently in human myocardium (83). The observation implied further that glucose metabolism, or at least utilization, can be maintained despite marked reductions in blood flow. Clearance rates of ^{11}C acetate from the acutely ischemic or from postischemic canine myocardium were found to be diminished (84), consistent with a decrease in oxidative metabolism. These observations provided a framework for exploring regional alterations in blood flow and substrate metabolism in acutely infarcted myocardium in humans.

Increases in glucose utilization relative to blood flow, thought initially to be characteristic of acute myocardial ischemia, were found to persist even after reperfusion, and thus after the acute ischemia had resolved. For example, despite full restoration of MBF at 24 hours after a transient 3-hour coronary occlusion, glucose extraction in postischemic myocardium remained significantly increased (85,86). Although glucose oxidation in reperfused myocardium no longer differed from that in remote myocardium, rates of anaerobic glycolysis remained increased in postischemic myocardium and most likely accounted for the regional increase in ^{18}F deoxyglucose uptake.

Findings in Acute Myocardial Infarction in Humans

Ischemia and infarction injure myocardium heterogeneously. The subendocardial layer sustains the most severe insult, whereas islands of necrotic tissue coexist with islands of normal and islands of ischemic but reversibly injured tissue in the remainder of the myocardial wall. As demonstrated with the PTI in 11 patients admitted within 4 hours of onset of acute symptoms, submitted to successful thrombolysis and patent infarct vessels at 24 hours, the fraction of myocardium rendered necrotic ranged from 0% to 63% (87). The fraction of irreversibly injured tissue was significantly less in myocardial segments with than without subsequent recovery of contractile function. Notably, all 11 patients developed Q waves on electrocardiography despite the large variability of irreversible tissue injury.

Fifteen consecutive patients with AMI studied with PET before the era of thrombolysis or angioplasty invariably exhibited regional flow defects at the site of abnormal wall motion or of ECG changes characteristic of AMI (88). Infarct regions revealed reduced ^{11}C palmitate uptake; relative to remote myocardium, clearance of ^{11}C palmitate from infarcted myocardial regions was markedly delayed (Fig. 64–1). The fraction of tracer entering the slow-turnover pool was markedly increased at the expense of the fraction entering the rapid-turnover pool, implying reduced fatty acid oxidation and increased fatty acid storage. Importantly, half of the infarct segments exhibited regionally increased ^{18}F deoxyglucose uptake either relative to that in remote myocardium or relative to blood flow. The other half of infarct segments revealed concordant reductions in ^{13}N ammonia and in ^{18}F deoxyglucose uptake. These concordant reductions were referred to by their operational terms as perfusion–metabolism matches, whereas flow reductions associated with increased ^{18}F deoxyglucose uptake were defined as "mismatches."

"Mismatches" in patients with chronic coronary artery disease signify a potentially reversible impairment of contractile function, whereas "matches" characteristically are associated with irreversibly impaired contractile function (89). Differences between AMI and chronic coronary artery disease should lead to caution in extrapolating the significance of findings in patients with chronic coronary artery disease to those with AMI. Observations in patients early after infarction (90,91) appear to support the validity of the concept of blood flow–metabolism patterns as indices of reversible and irreversible dysfunction in AMI.

Other studies have explored the quantitative relations between regional MBF, oxidative metabolism and oxidative

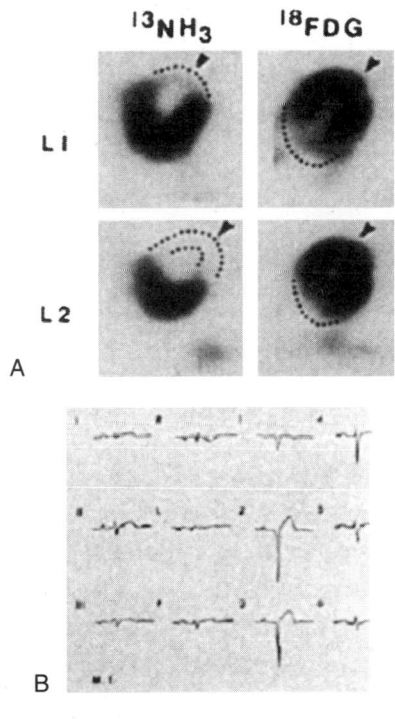

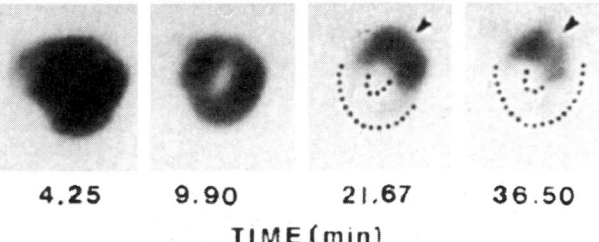

$^{13}NH_3$ $\quad$ ^{18}FDG

L I

L 2

A

B

^{11}C PALMITIC ACID

4.25 $\quad$ 9.90 $\quad$ 21.67 $\quad$ 36.50

C $\quad\quad\quad$ TIME (min)

FIG. 64–1. Regional myocardial blood flow, glucose utilization, and fatty acid metabolism in a patient with recent acute anteroseptal myocardial infarction. **A:** Transaxial images through the mid and inferior portions of the left ventricle (L2 and L2). The N-13 ammonia images ($^{13}NH_3$) reveal an extensive and severe flow defect in the anterior wall, whereas, as seen on the corresponding fluorine-18 deoxyglucose (^{18}FDG) images, glucose utilization is preserved or even enhanced (blood flow–metabolism mismatch). **B:** The patient's 12-lead electrocardiogram with Q waves in V_1 and V_2 and a loss of the R wave in the remaining precordial leads. **C:** Serially acquired transaxial images of carbon-11 (^{11}C) palmitate. Note the modestly reduced uptake of a tracer in the anterior wall at the 9.9-minute image; however, as the subsequently acquired images demonstrate, clearance of ^{11}C palmitate from the infarct territory is markedly delayed as a sign of impaired fatty acid oxidation when compared with the clearance of C-11 acetate in remote myocardium. (From Brunken RC, Schwaiger M, Schelbert HR. PET detection of residual, viable tissue in acute MI. *Appl Radiol* 1985;14:82.)

metabolism, and glucose utilization in patients early after infarction at an average of 3.6 ± 1.6 days after onset of acute symptoms (92). Perfusion defects were identified by quantitative polar map approaches. The majority of patients revealed flow defects that corresponded in location to ECG and wall motion abnormalities. The absence of flow defects in some patients was attributed to prior angioplasty. The quantitative polar map approach identified 51 anatomic regions with hypoperfusion. Of these, 29 exhibited blood flow–metabolism mismatches (57%) and 22 blood flow–metabolism matches (43%) (examples are shown in Figures 64–2 through 64–8) (see also color insert).

In remote myocardium, blood flow averaged 0.83 ± 0.20 mL/min · g^{-1} and k_{mono}, an index of oxidative metabolism, averaged 0.63 ± 0.12 min^{-1}. Both values are similar to those in healthy volunteers (93,94). Furthermore, MBF correlated with oxidative metabolism, and both were related to the rate–pressure product used as index of cardiac work. No such correlation between cardiac work and blood flow or oxidative metabolism was found for "infarcted myocardium." Of greater interest are observed correlations among regional measurements of blood flow, oxidative metabolism, and glucose utilization rate. As depicted in Figure 64–9, regional glucose utilization rates were unrelated to regional MBF. Several reasons account for this. Rates of exogenous glucose utilization in remote myocardium varied considerably among patients. Although all patients received oral glucose to stimulate insulin secretion, thus enhancing myocardial ^{18}F deoxyglucose uptake, other factors—for example, increased serum catecholamine and FFA levels frequently present early after an AMI (95)—may have suppressed glucose utilization by remote myocardium. The variability implies that control of glucose uptake and of substrate selection in "hypoperfused, infarcted" myocardium differs from that in remote myocardium. Mechanisms possibly accounting for the regional differences include regional alterations in expression of glucose transporters and in key regulatory enzymes of the glucose metabolic pathway. Similar attenuated responses have been noted by other investigators studying patients with ^{18}F deoxyglucose in the fasted and in the glucose-loaded state (96). When rates of glucose utilization in hypoperfused myocardium were normalized to those in remote myocardium, normal glucose metabolic rates declined with lower MBF (Fig. 64–9B). Yet, there was considerable scatter of the data about the regression line in segments with intermediate flow reductions. The "variability" of glucose uptake relative to flow implies regional variations in glucose extraction and, especially, increases in glucose extraction that are consistent with the qualitatively observed blood flow–metabolism mismatch. Conversely, proportionate decreases in flow and glucose utilization suggest that glucose extraction remained constant and corresponded to the qualitatively observed blood flow–metabolism match.

As depicted in Figure 64–10, oxidative metabolism correlated significantly with blood flow. However, the correlation was not linear but "biphasic." Oxidative metabolism as

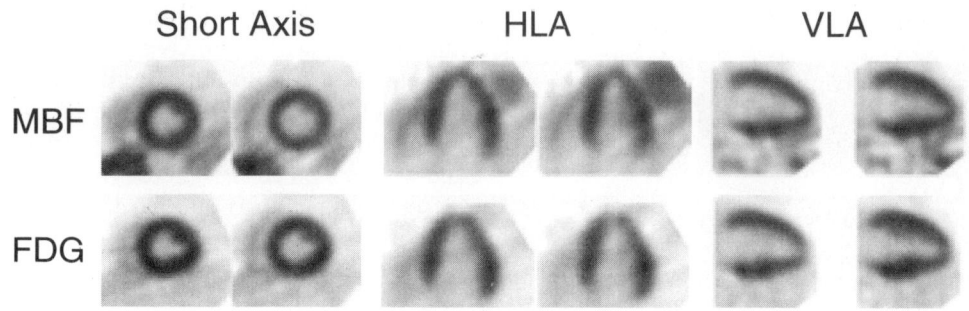

FIG. 64–2. Myocardial blood flow (MBF) and fluorine-18 deoxyglucose (FDG) images in a healthy volunteer. Short-axis together with horizontal (HLA) and vertical long-axis (VLA) images are shown. Note the homogeneous distribution of both tracers in the left ventricular myocardium.

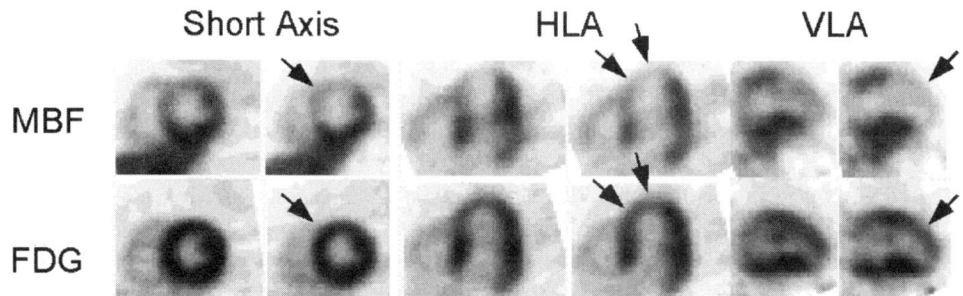

FIG. 64–3. Images of myocardial perfusion with ¹³N ammonia and myocardial glucose utilization with fluorine-18 deoxyglucose (FDG) in a patient with ischemic cardiomyopathy, demonstrating a "mismatch." Again, short-axis and vertical (VLA) and horizontal long-axis (HLA) images of the left ventricular myocardium are shown. Note the decreased perfusion in the anteroseptal anterior and anterolateral wall but the preserved FDG uptake in these regions. MBF, myocardial blood flow.

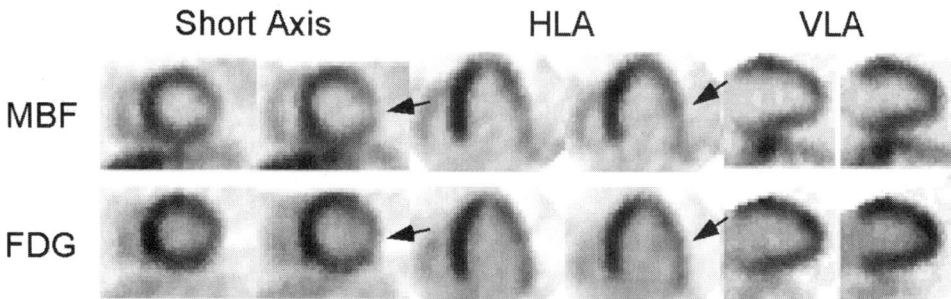

FIG. 64–4. Images of myocardial blood flow (MBF) and glucose metabolism in a patient with ischemic cardiomyopathy showing a "match." Short-axis and horizontal (HLA) and vertical long-axis (VLA) images are shown. Note the severely decreased perfusion in the anterior, anterolateral, and lateral walls that is associated with a proportionate reduction in fluorine-18 deoxyglucose (FDG) uptake.

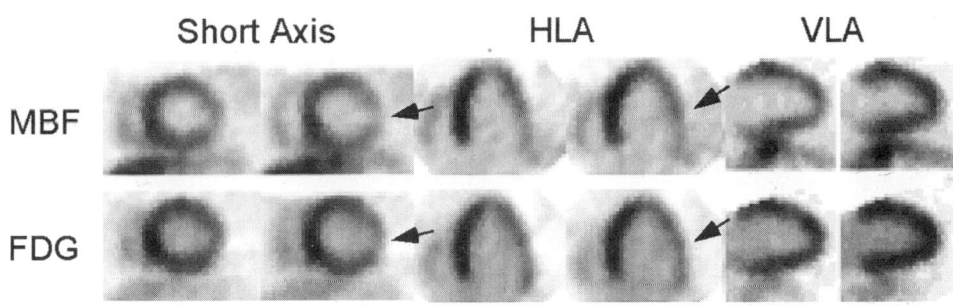

FIG. 64–5. Three contiguous cross-sectional images of myocardial blood flow (MBF) at rest **(upper panel),** during dipyridamole stress **(middle panel),** and of fluorine-18 (^{18}F) deoxyglucose uptake. On the resting images, myocardial perfusion is relatively homogenous. During hyperemia, there is a stress-induced flow defect in the lateral wall *(arrows)* that is on the ^{18}F deoxyglucose image associated with regionally enhanced glucose utilization. This pattern is most likely consistent with myocardial stunning.

defined by k_{mono} of the ^{11}C acetate clearance rate declined disproportionately less than blood flow to values of 0.56 mL/min · g^{-1}. Further flow reductions below this threshold were associated with a precipitous decline in oxidative metabolism. The biphasic relation between blood flow and oxidative metabolism (oxygen consumption) was unexpected in view of the widely held notion of a direct linear relation between them (97). It is, however, consistent with findings in a more recent study that, based on animal experimental studies, modeled the relation among coronary blood flow and pressure, O_2 extraction and consumption, and autoregulation (98). On the basis of this analysis, the biphasic relation can be attributed to a progressive increase in O_2 extraction as blood flow decreases until a maximum is reached.

It is possible to estimate the O_2 extraction from these data, at least indirectly. Use of the correlation between ^{11}C acetate clearance rates and MVO_2 in canine myocardium (29) appears to underestimate MVO_2 as reported for human myocardium (99). If, however, the clearance rates are adjusted to humans by using the rate–pressure product as the common denominator (29,99) and, furthermore, if an average O_2 extraction fraction of 62% is used for baseline flows (99), then, as depicted in Figure 64–11, the O_2 extraction increases to a maximum of 93% at a flow of 0.56 mL/min · g^{-1}.

Blood flow and oxidative metabolism were significantly reduced in "infarct regions" in patients early after infarction (92). Yet, the severity of these reductions differed between regions with and without blood flow–metabolism mismatches. In "mismatch" regions, blood flow was reduced by 35% ± 20%, and oxidative metabolism (as determined from k_{mono} of the acetate clearance curve) was reduced by only 16% ± 5%. These reductions were significantly greater in infarct regions with "matches," with an average flow reduction of 58% ± 18% and an average reduction in oxidative metabolism of 48% ± 19%. Other investigations reported similar reductions. For example, in 11 patients of whom 5 underwent prompt thrombolysis, who were studied from 4 to 9 days (mean 6 days) after the acute infarction, "viable" infarct regions revealed about a 23% reduction in blood flow and about a 26% decrease in oxidative metabolism (100). In "nonviable myocardium," flow was reduced by about 36%, and oxidative metabolism was reduced by about 55%. Viable and nonviable myocardium in that study were defined by the outcome in regional systolic wall motion After angioplasty. In another study (101), the initial uptake of ^{11}C acetate and its subsequent clearance was determined in 18 pa-

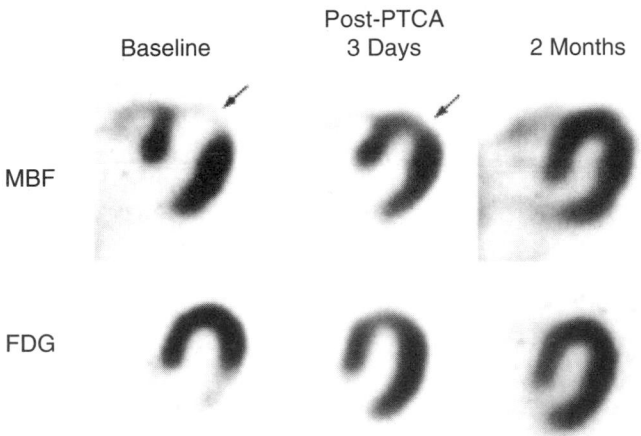

FIG. 64–6. Blood flow metabolism mismatch in a patient with subtotal occlusion of the proximal left anterior descending coronary artery. **Left:** Markedly decreased perfusion in the anterior wall **(top,** *arrows*), but enhanced fluorine-18 (^{18}F) deoxyglucose uptake **(bottom). Middle and right:** Follow-up studies in the same patient after coronary angioplasty. Note the marked improvement in perfusion to the anterior wall and the normalization of ^{18}F deoxyglucose uptake. At baseline, there was akinesis of the anterior wall. After restoration of resting myocardial blood flow after angioplasty, wall motion normalized, whereas myocardial blood flow and glucose utilization became normal. (See color insert for Figs. 64–7 and 64–8.)

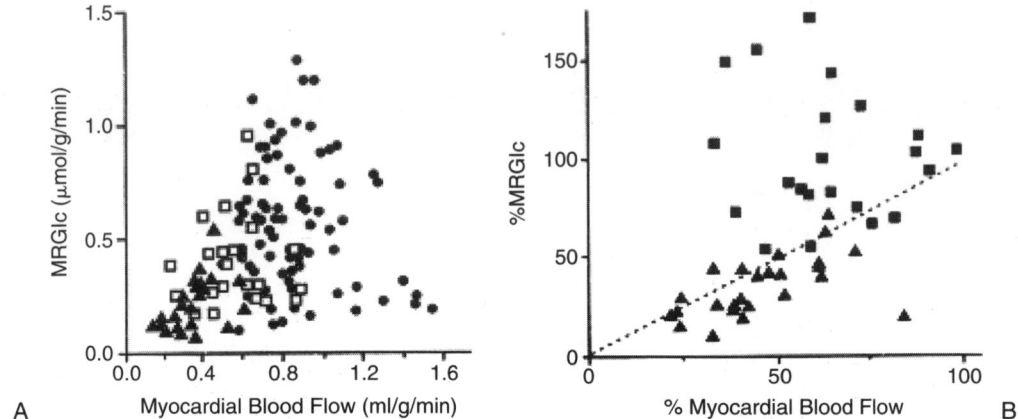

FIG. 64–9. Relation between myocardial blood flow and exogenous glucose utilization (MRGlc). **A:** There is no significant correlation between the two parameters. **B:** After normalizing blood flow and glucose utilization rates in infarct territories to those in normal remote myocardium, relative glucose utilization rates are correlated linearly with blood flow in infarct territories with blood flow–metabolism matches *(closed triangles)*. However, the relative glucose utilization rates markedly exceed blood flow in regions with blood flow–metabolism mismatches *(open rectangles)*. (From Czernin J, Prenta G, Brunken R. Regional blood flow, oxidative metabolism, and glucose utilization in patients with recent myocardial infarction. *Circulation* 1993;88:884–895.)

tients at an average of 4 ± 2 days after hospital admission. All patients had been submitted to thrombolysis within less than 24 hours of onset of acute symptoms. The initial uptake of ^{11}C acetate served as a measure of relative regional blood flow. The authors note again a regional reduction in oxidative metabolism in infarct regions, yet point to discrepancies between relative flow and ^{11}C acetate clearance rates. In some regions, flow and oxidative metabolism were reduced concordantly, whereas in others, flow was reduced more severely than oxidative metabolism. In other regions again,

oxidative metabolism appeared to be suppressed more severely than blood flow.

Myocardial Adrenergic Innervation

Studies with ^{11}C metahydroxyephedrine and PET further demonstrated the effects of an AMI on regional adrenergic neuron density, function, or both (102). In 16 patients studied with PET at an average of 7 ± 3 days after an AMI, the geographic extent of reduced ^{11}C hydroxyephedrine uptake

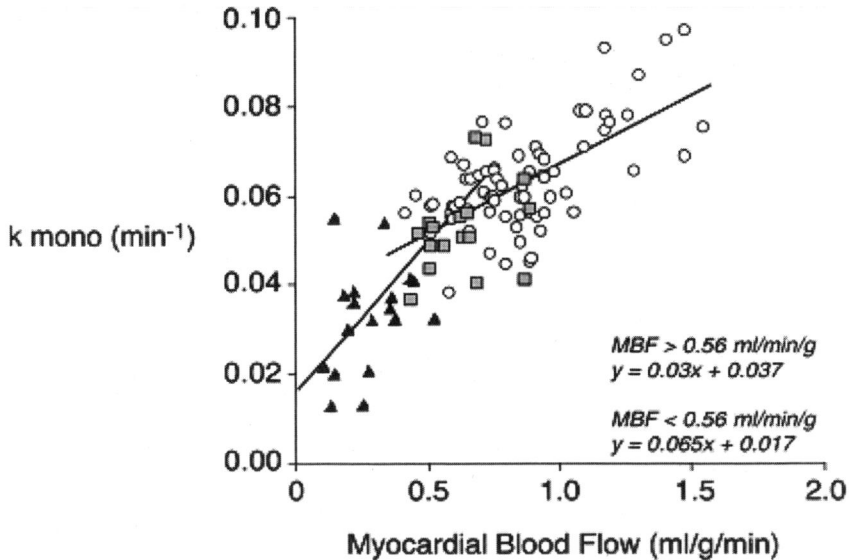

FIG. 64–10. Relation between oxidative metabolism (carbon-11 acetate clearance rate defined as k_{mono}) and myocardial blood flow (MBF) in patients early after infarction. *Solid circles* represent normal myocardium; *open rectangles* represent infarct territories with blood flow–metabolism mismatches; and *solid triangles* represent infarct territories with blood flow–metabolism matches. Note the biphasic correlation between flow and oxidative metabolism.

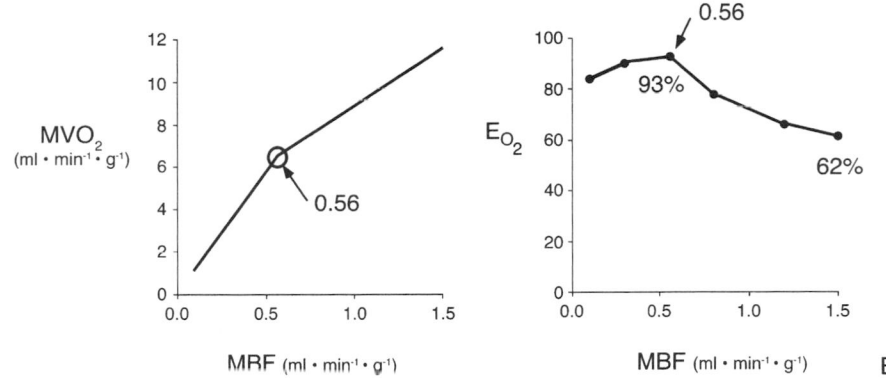

FIG. 64-11. Myocardial oxygen consumption, oxygen extraction, and myocardial blood flow **A:** The correlation between myocardial oxygen consumption (derived after converting k_{mono} to MVO_2) and myocardial blood flow. Again, note the biphasic correlation. **B:** Assuming an extraction fraction of oxygen (E_{O2}) of 62% in normal myocardium, the oxygen extraction fraction progressively increases to 93% for flow reductions down to 0.56 mL/min · g^{-1}.

consistently exceeded the extent of the infarct-related flow defect. For example, the blood flow defect involved an average of 17% ± 17% of the left ventricular myocardium, whereas the ^{11}C hydroxyephedrine uptake defect averaged 31% ± 15% ($p < 0.05$). The uptake defect was similar for Q-wave and non–Q-wave infarctions, despite significantly smaller blood flow defects in non–Q-wave than in Q-wave infarctions (3.5% ± 2.5% vs. 31% ± 11%).

Summary and Conclusions

The water PTI demonstrated that despite prompt thrombolytic therapy the fraction of myocardium surviving the ischemic insult varies greatly. A consistent finding on PET is the regional reduction in blood flow. Immediate revascularization appears to decrease the prevalence of flow defects; however, even if blood flow has been restored fully, an apparent defect may be present because of a partial volume–related underestimation of true tracer tissue concentration caused by a persistent wall motion abnormality. Blood flow and oxidative metabolism remain correlated in infarct regions, but in a biphasic relation; a progressive increase in the extraction of oxygen as a compensatory mechanism seems to account for the biphasic correlation. Regional ^{18}F deoxyglucose uptake and thus use of exogenous glucose are enhanced in about half of the infarct regions; greater extraction and thus reliance on the more oxygen-efficient glucose may represent, in addition to the increase in O_2 extraction, another compensatory mechanism that contributes to tissue survival when blood flow and oxygen supply are limited. The disparities between blood flow and oxidative metabolism and glucose utilization in early postinfarction myocardium raise questions on whether they identify different types of tissue injury. Follow-up studies have provided answers, at least to some extent, as to whether these discrepancies represent ongoing ischemia, stunning, or even hibernation.

Transition from Acute to Chronic Alterations

Investigations with PET have confirmed the dynamic nature of an AMI. PET studies also have demonstrated how therapeutic interventions modify the "natural history" or course of an evolving MI. In some patients, concordant reductions in blood flow and glucose utilization early after the acute event subsequently convert to a blood flow–metabolism mismatch without significant improvements in regional contractile function (91). In other instances, blood flow–metabolism mismatches resolve and contractile function improves when reexamined after several months. In other patients again, flow to "infarct regions" was found to be normal at the time of the initial PET study during the early postinfarction period (21,87,92,101), presumably because coronary blood flow had been successfully restored through angioplasty or thrombolysis. These observations suggest that regional alterations in blood flow, oxidative metabolism, and glucose utilization and their interrelations as described with PET early after an AMI may depend on the severity and duration of the ischemic injury. Although such explanation awaits confirmation, preliminary findings in canine experiments appear to support this notion (103). These studies noted a close correlation between the severity of the flow reduction during an acute coronary occlusion and altered blood flow and oxidative metabolism after reperfusion.

Of interest are long-term changes in patients studied initially within 72 hours after an AMI (88). Follow-up studies with two-dimensional echocardiography in 12 patients at an average of 6 ± 5 weeks after the acute event indicated that contractile function had failed to recover in all eight segments with regional flow–metabolism matches but had improved or even normalized in four of eight segments with early postinfarction mismatches. Repeat studies with PET in some patients without improvement in regional contractile function revealed a conversion of the initially present mismatch to a match at the time of the follow-up examination.

Conversely, blood flow–metabolism mismatches may persist for prolonged periods. In 15 patients examined with PET within 3 months after an AMI (average 2.9 weeks), only 2 of the 17 infarct territories were normal, whereas 9 territories (53%) exhibited blood flow–metabolism matches. Importantly, six infarct territories revealed "mismatches" or "matches" coexisting with "mismatches" (35%) (83). Similarly, in a group of 15 patients with a first anterior MI, all submitted to early thrombolysis, and only 8 of the infarct territories exhibited blood flow–metabolism matches when studied at an average of 6.0 ± 3.6 weeks after the acute event (104). In contrast, seven of the infarct territories exhibited a central "match" associated with an adjacent "mismatch" (two territories) or a central blood flow–metabolism mismatch (seven territories). Blood flow was similar in both types of infarct territories (104). Other studies again report regionally enhanced ^{18}F deoxyglucose uptake in the infarct territory even years after an AMI, although the incidence of such enhanced uptake declines with time (105,106). Conversely, in patients with chronic coronary artery disease evaluated for myocardial viability, regionally enhanced ^{18}F deoxyglucose uptake is frequently found to be located in areas of prior MI (83).

It thus appears that patterns of MBF and metabolism and their changes over time vary greatly among patients. In some patients, an initial pattern of a match may subsequently convert to a mismatch, possibly because of a severe, though transient, ischemic injury and indicate the reversibility of impairments of contractile function. Furthermore, patterns of flow metabolism mismatches may persist for long periods after an AMI, although clinical implications and underlying mechanisms of persistent metabolic alterations remain poorly understood. Possible explanations include the following: (a) regional alterations in autonomic neuronal control; (b) continued compromise of resting or stress MBF, or both, resulting in myocardial stunning or hibernation; and (c) functional and especially structural alterations related to the severity of the ischemic injury and requiring time for repair.

Sympathetic Denervation

Findings with ^{11}C hydroxyephedrine and PET in patients early after infarction suggest that adrenergic neurons are highly sensitive to ischemia. Regional reductions in myocardial ^{11}C hydroxyephedrine uptake were located in the infarct regions, but they exceeded in size the extent of the "risk myocardium," suggesting that transient and mild flow reductions may lead to neuronal injury (107). Sympathetic denervation may modify regional myocardial substrate selection as findings in human orthotopic cardiac transplants indicate. For example, glucose utilization rates measured with ^{18}F deoxyglucose were about 10% greater in denervated than in reinnervated myocardial regions of cardiac transplants (108).

Severity of the Ischemic Injury

The relation between the severity of an acute ischemic/reperfusion injury and the rate of recovery of metabolic alter-

ations remains to be explored. However, observations in patients with ischemic cardiomyopathy suggest such dependency. Contractile function after coronary revascularization improved more slowly in myocardial regions with more severely reduced perfusion at baseline (109,110). Furthermore, delays in recovery of contractile function appear to be correlated with the degree of structural alterations including myocardial fibrosis and perinuclear loss of contractile proteins with replacement by glycogen granules in myocytes (also referred to as "hibernating myocytes") (111). If, in fact, more severe flow reductions are associated with greater structural alterations, then the observed persistence of an increased ^{18}F deoxyglucose uptake in revascularized myocardial regions with more severely reduced blood flow at rest might implicate structural alterations as a possible explanation (112).

Myocardial Stunning and Hibernation

If the "at risk" myocardium continues to be subtended by coronary vessels with flow-limiting stenoses, stunning and hibernation may ensue (113,114). Residual coronary lesions preclude adequate flow increases in response to increases in demand. Transient, though repetitive, episodes of ischemia may lead to chronic impairment of contractile function (115). Regional ^{18}F deoxyglucose may remain normal or may be increased while resting flow is normal, whereas the myocardial flow reserve is diminished. The severity of contractile dysfunction has been found to depend on the degree of attenuation of the flow reserve and, in turn, on the severity of the upstream coronary stenosis, as PET measurements of MBF in patients with coronary artery disease have demonstrated (116,117). By contrast, myocardial hibernation as a down-regulation of contractile function and an adaptation of substrate metabolism in response to diminished blood flow at rest characteristically exhibits a regional reduction in MBF at rest that is associated with an increase in glucose extraction, and thus an increase in ^{18}F deoxyglucose uptake. Although the subject of considerable controversy, the concept of hibernation has received support by findings in chronically instrumented animals. In these studies, mild reductions in MBF at rest at 3 to 5 months after instrumentation were associated with impaired contractile function and enhanced glucose extraction without, however, producing fibrosis or scar tissue (118–122). Hypoperfused and dysfunctional myocardium continued to extract lactate, and thus did not reveal metabolic evidence of ischemia. Oxygen consumption was found to be diminished, although in proportion to blood flow, and appeared to indicate a resetting of the myocardium's substrate metabolism that also protected it against ischemia (123). The animal experimental findings also prompted formulation of a unifying concept in which progression of stunning to hibernation was mostly driven by changes in myocardial flow reserve (118,123). A progressive decline and, ultimately, complete loss of flow reserve together with a decrease in resting flow are thought to be responsible for the progression of stunning to hibernation (Fig. 64–12).

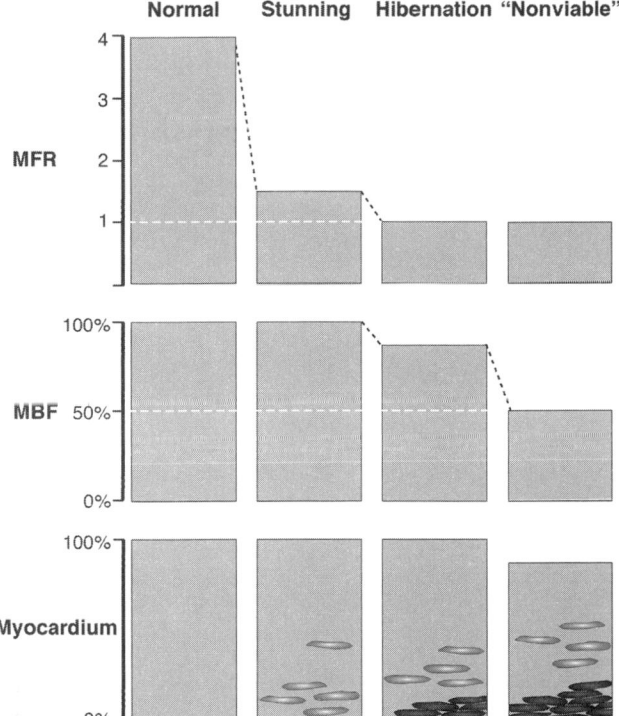

FIG. 64–12. Schematic, highly simplified depiction of the progression of myocardial stunning to myocardial hibernation and further to "nonviability" or loss of reversibility of contractile function. **Top:** The myocardial flow reserve (MFR). **Middle:** The myocardial blood at rest (MBF; normal = 100%). **Bottom:** The thickness and some histopathologic features of the myocardium (*light cells* represent "hibernating myocytes"; *dark structures* represent scar tissue and fibrosis). With increasing severity of the coronary stenosis, the flow reserve in the dependent downstream myocardium progressively declines and leads to ischemic stunning and chronic impairment of contractile function while "hibernating" or "dedifferentiated" myocytes appear. As the stenosis severity further increases, the flow reserve becomes more severely compromised and finally may be absent (MFR = 1), whereas MBF might decline at rest, representing myocardial hibernation. "Hibernating" myocytes are present and tissue fibrosis develops. Continued loss of myocytes caused by necrosis and apoptosis may be associated with continued progression of tissue fibrosis so that the thickness of the myocardium declines. Once fibrosis occupies more than 35% of the myocardial wall, the impairment of contractile function becomes irreversible.

Whether a true state of hibernation, as found in animal experiments, can indeed be maintained indefinitely and whether it exists in the more complex situation of human coronary artery disease remains uncertain. Several clinical observations suggest that this is not the case. For example, for the same perfusion metabolism pattern (i.e., similar reduction in flow and similar increase in ^{18}F deoxyglucose uptake), the degree of structural alterations can vary considerably (124). Second, the fractions of abnormal myocytes and, in particular, of fibrosis appear to increase with the duration of "hibernation." One study, for example, reports a significant correlation between the fractional tissue amount of fibrosis and the duration

of congestive heart failure symptoms used as surrogate for the presence of hibernating myocardium (125). Third, contractile function is less likely to recover if revascularization of viable myocardium with mismatched perfusion and metabolism is delayed (126,127). Finally, tissue assays of "mismatched" dysfunctional myocardium present evidence for increased expression of intercellular matrix proteins and of decreased expression of contractile and cytoskeletal proteins (128). These findings imply continuous and progressive loss of myocytes that is paralleled by progress fibrosis and scar formation and accounts for the transition from a reversible to an irreversible impairment of contractile function.

In postinfarction myocardium, different mechanisms may account for the augmented glucose utilization observed early after the infarction as compared with that during later follow-up (see also Fig. 64–13). For example, early postinfarction mismatches in territories supplied by patent infarct vessels may reflect "stunning." Even an early postinfarction "match" may be consistent with possibly metabolic stunning, as demonstrated in chronic dog experiments (85). When studied immediately after reperfusion after a 3-hour coronary occlusion, both blood flow and ^{18}F deoxyglucose uptake were depressed, but reverted to "mismatches" when restudied 24 hours later, followed by a gradual improvement in contractile function (86). However, the persistence of a blood flow–metabolism mismatch over prolonged periods, as observed in other studies (129), most likely represents "hibernation" (114). Conversely, flow may remain inadequately low so that ischemia still present early after the acute event progresses slowly to necrosis and scar tissue formation.

If, in fact, myocardium survives the initial ischemic insult and enters a chronically altered state of hibernation, it remains unclear whether the mechanisms accounting for the enhanced glucose uptake can indeed be extrapolated from those operating during acute myocardial ischemia. What is known is that this chronically altered state is associated on biopsy studies with morphologically abnormal (or hibernating) myocytes (129, 130). Uncertain is whether such "hibernating" or, as referred to by others, "dedifferentiated" myocytes (131) represent the morphologic correlate of the enhanced glucose uptake or whether the increased ^{18}F deoxyglucose uptake reflects an increase in the rate of glycolysis that is uncoupled from oxidation of glucose (132). Increases in glycolytic flux rates might be driven by translocation or enhanced expression of membrane glucose transporters and up-regulation of key regulatory enzymes along the glycolytic pathway (133–136). More teleologic explanations argue that glycolytic production of high-energy adenosine triphosphate located strategically in the proximity of the cellular and sarcolemmal membranes may be critical for maintaining transmembranous ion concentration gradients (i.e., for sodium and potassium) and calcium fluxes to prevent ischemic contracture and to assure cell survival (137).

Summary and Conclusions

The ischemic insult of an AMI often results in cell death and subsequent replacement by scar tissue. However, because of

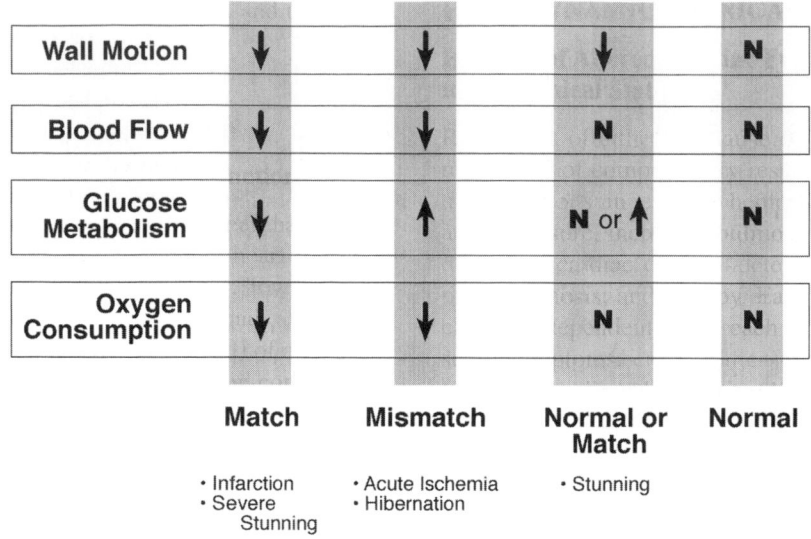

FIG. 64–13. Myocardial blood flow and metabolism patterns observed with positron emission tomography in patients early after infarction. A blood flow–metabolism match is associated with concordant moderate to severe reductions (↓) in myocardial blood flow, oxygen consumption, and glucose utilization. Furthermore, systolic wall motion is impaired. In a blood flow–metabolism match, there can be a similar impairment in regional systolic wall motion associated with reductions in myocardial blood flow, and oxygen consumption. However, glucose utilization is normal (N) or even increased (↑) when compared with remote and presumably normal myocardium. Infarct territories may also appear normal on positron emission tomography or may exhibit modest decreases in blood flow and oxygen consumption if systolic wall motion is impaired. In this situation, the metabolic rate of the glucose might be either decreased or increased. This pattern might represent stunned myocardium, and the wall motion abnormality might lead to an artifactual reduction in regional tracer uptake. Oxidative metabolism may be reduced in parallel with the impairment in regional function.

the heterogeneity of the insult, islands of normal or of compromised yet viable cells can survive the initial ischemic attack. PET images then reveal severe to moderate reductions in blood flow and metabolism. Conversely, incomplete occlusion, recanalization of the infarct vessel, or, possibly, preexisting collaterals may protect cells against death. Depending on the magnitude of residual blood flow, myocardial stunning may ensue and function may recover spontaneously. Yet, if flow remains low, myocardium may downregulate its contractile function, adjust its substrate metabolism, and enter a state of "hibernation." Alternatively, blood flow remains inadequate, and initially surviving yet ischemic myocardium subsequently dies and is replaced by scar tissue. Regardless of the ultimate outcome, the presence of "viable" or surviving myocardium early after an AMI can be identified by PET as a blood flow–metabolism mismatch pattern and by relatively well preserved oxidative metabolism. Thus, there is a time window during which interventional restoration of blood flow can salvage compromised myocardium and improve or even normalize regional contractile function.

Diagnostic and Clinical Implications

The time window for salvaging of injured yet surviving myocardium may vary considerably and may range from days to weeks or even months. Blood flow–metabolism mismatches may persist for long periods after an AMI (83,104) or, conversely, rapidly convert to "matches," suggesting progression of ischemia to necrosis and scar tissue formation (88). Therapeutically, these observations imply that blood flow to the infarct territory should be improved or restored as soon as possible.

Most investigations agree that the magnitude of flow reductions alone does not distinguish between irreversibly injured and potentially salvageable and irreversibly injured myocardium (87,88,100). The severity of an impairment in regional systolic wall motion appears to be an equally unreliable criterion, because wall motion is equally reduced in "mismatches" and "matches" (83,88). In addition, electrocardiographic criteria such as Q waves fail to discriminate adequately between an irreversible transmural injury and potential reversibility of contractile function (83,88,92). One investigation in patients studied 42 days after the AMI further failed to observe a correlation between blood flow–metabolism patterns and thallium-201 (^{201}Tl) redistribution findings in myocardial infarct regions (104). Another, though preliminary, study also suggested that a rest redistributing defect on planar ^{201}Tl scintigraphy is highly specific for viable myocardium, but fixed defects markedly underestimate the presence of viable myocardium (138). In aggregate, these findings imply that conventional diagnostic approaches failed to identify reliably ischemically injured, though potentially salvageable, myocardium.

One approach to predict the recovery of regional contractile function is the PTI. For example, Yamamoto and coworkers (87) demonstrated if the PTI in postinfarction myocardium exceeds 0.7 (i.e., <30% of the myocardium has been injured irreversibly) and if the infarct vessel is patent, then systolic wall motion will improve after revascularization. Conversely, if the fraction of irreversibly injured myocardium exceeded 30%, systolic wall motion will remain impaired. Because the patients in this study had undergone thrombolytic therapy early after the onset of symptoms, the perfusable tissue fraction in these patients most likely represented stunned myocardium. It also remains unclear whether the PTI per se will distinguish among normal, stunned, and hibernating myocardium.

Characteristically, either stunned or hibernating myocardium exhibits preserved or enhanced exogenous glucose utilization on PET imaging with ^{18}F deoxyglucose. Ideally, stunning can be distinguished from hibernation by evaluating regional MBF (Fig. 64–13). By definition, stunned myocardium exhibits normal blood flow, and ischemic or hibernating myocardium exhibits reduced blood flow. However, even if blood flow is normal, it may appear to be reduced on

the images because of the partial volume–related underestimation of regional tracer concentrations (discussed earlier). It also is possible that stunning and hibernation may coexist. A persistent, severe coronary stenosis of the infarct vessel may result in "repetitive stunning," as proposed in chronic coronary artery disease (130). The flow reserve is limited so severely that repeated increases in demand may result in transient ischemic episodes, followed by stunning and slow recovery of contractile function, interrupted by renewed ischemic episodes, so that a more chronic impairment of contractile function ensues, whereas resting blood flow is relatively well preserved.

Identification of such "altered states" by PET can guide therapy in patients early after infarction (Fig. 64–14). Normal blood flow at rest and a relatively well preserved MBF reserve as tested with pharmacologic interventions such as dipyridamole or adenosine can identify myocardium as only stunned; alternatively, the absence of a hemodynamically significant stenosis of the infarct vessel on angiography similarly would demonstrate that stunning accounts for the regional increase in ^{18}F deoxyglucose uptake and that contractile function will recover spontaneously (88,139).

However, reduced blood flow at rest, loss or marked attenuation of myocardial flow reserve, together with preserved

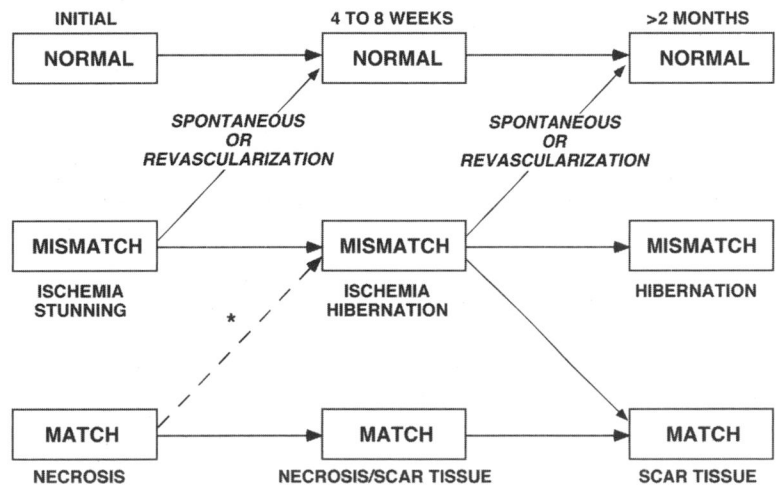

FIG. 64–14. Clinical relevance and therapeutic implications of various blood flow–metabolism patterns in infarct territories. Infarct regions with normal blood flow and metabolism might have recovered fully at the time of the initial positron emission tomography studies because of either spontaneous or therapeutic revascularization. When restudied, these parameters usually remain normal and no additional interventions are needed. A blood flow–metabolism mismatch pattern might represent ongoing ischemia or stunned myocardium. Depending on either spontaneous or interventional revascularization, this pattern might revert to normal when studied after 4 to 6 weeks following the infarction. Conversely, a mismatch might initially persist as evidence of persistent myocardial ischemia or hibernation. To prevent progression of ischemia to necrosis, revascularization is required. This is likely to result in an improvement in regional contractile function and an improvement in blood flow and metabolism. A mismatch observed after 4 to 6 weeks may also be related to repetitive stunning, where again relief of the culprit lesion might result in an improvement in contractile function, as well as in regional blood flow and metabolism. A blood flow–metabolism match pattern usually indicates the presence of necrosis, which on follow-up study persists and indicates the development of scar tissue. In some instances, presumably because of a severe ischemic injury, an initial match might subsequently revert to a blood flow–metabolism mismatch especially when residual is available. A further improvement or normalization might be achievable if revascularization is instituted.

glucose utilization more likely indicate the presence of hibernating myocardium or ischemia progressing to necrosis. In these instances, PET during the early postinfarction period can identify potentially salvageable myocardium. Interventional revascularization then is likely to result in a long-term improvement in contractile function (91).

Several studies support the predictive power of blood flow–glucose metabolism patterns in patients after infarction. For example, contractile function remained depressed or even deteriorated in "match" regions, but it improved in half of the regions with early postinfarction "mismatches" (88). Notably, none of the 13 patients in that study underwent interventional revascularization. Yet, in a more recent study of 11 patients, all of whom underwent coronary angioplasty after the initial PET study, a "mismatch" was 84% accurate in predicting an improvement in contractile function. Conversely, "matches" predicted with 70% accuracy that function would not recover (100). Lastly, in 10 patients studied with PET at 3.7 and again at 97 days after the acute infarction, blood flow, oxidative metabolism, and regional wall motion improved in all 11 "mismatch" regions. Conversely, contractile function, as well as blood flow and oxidative metabolism, remained unchanged in the 10 "match" regions (91).

Another approach for identifying reversible contractile dysfunction entails the assessment of regional oxidative metabolism with ^{11}C acetate (100). As demonstrated in 11 patients early after infarction after prompt coronary thrombolysis, oxidative metabolism as determined with PET within 4 to 9 days after the acute event predicted the long-term functional outcome after coronary angioplasty (90). MBF was similar in segments with and without long-term recovery of contractile function. However, oxidative metabolism in recovery segments, although reduced relative to that in remote myocardium, was significantly greater than in segments that did not recover function. In contrast, another study (100) suggested that the level of oxidative metabolism alone may be of limited predictive accuracy. Because of this, oxidative rates should be evaluated together with reductions in MBF to predict more accurately the potential revascularization outcome in regional contractile function.

SUMMARY AND FUTURE DEVELOPMENTS

Initial investigations with PET on regional MBF and substrate metabolism in acutely infarcted myocardium demonstrated various patterns of flow and metabolism that most likely correlated with the duration and severity of the ischemic insult and with restoration of blood flow. These findings attest to the dynamic nature of an AMI and, at the same time, offer diagnostic possibilities for identifying potentially salvageable myocardium. They also pose new questions. For example, what mechanisms account for the enhanced glucose utilization? Why does the enhanced glucose utilization persist in some instances despite adequate restoration of MBF having been restored adequately

(86,104,140)? Furthermore, does the persistence of a blood flow–metabolism mismatch render the patient more vulnerable to lethal arrhythmias? These questions warrant further investigations, which in fact might be answered, at least to some extent, with already established or emerging PET approaches. Techniques for the exploration of neuronal function with labeled catecholamine analogs or the quantification of regional β-receptor densities and affinities are on the horizon. Also, markers of the myocardium's state of tissue oxygenation have been developed. Although still unsatisfactory, the proposed electrochemical modifications of these agents are likely to render these tracers clinically useful. However, analytic probes available with PET might also become useful for examining the effects of treatment, not only related to mechanical revascularization, but also to vasodilatory drugs, unloading agents, substances that directly affect the ischemic process, as well as receptor agonists and blockers.

ACKNOWLEDGMENTS

The author thanks Diane Martin, Akiyaa Nickelson, and Jim Strommer for preparing the illustrations and Ashley Denault for her skillful assistance in preparing the manuscript.

REFERENCES

1. Bergmann SR, Fox KA, Rand AL, et al. Quantification of regional myocardial blood flow in vivo with H215O. Circulation 1984;70:724–733.
2. Bergmann SR, Herrero P, Markham J, et al. Noninvasive quantitation of myocardial blood flow in human subjects with oxygen-15-labeled water and positron emission tomography. J Am Coll Cardiol 1989;14:639–652.
3. Araujo LI, Lammertsma AA, Rhodes CG, et al. Noninvasive quantification of regional myocardial blood flow in coronary artery disease with oxygen-15-labeled carbon dioxide inhalation and positron emission tomography. Circulation 1991;83:875–885.
4. Iida H, Rhodes C, de Silva R, et al. Myocardial tissue fraction—correction for partial volume effects and measure of tissue viability. J Nucl Med 1991;32:2169–2175.
5. Gerber BL, Melin JA, Bol A, et al. Nitrogen-13-ammonia and oxygen-15-water estimates of absolute myocardial perfusion in left ventricular ischemic dysfunction. J Nucl Med 1998;39:1655–1662.
6. Iida H, Tamura Y, Kitamura K, et al. Histochemical correlates of (15)O-water-perfusable tissue fraction in experimental canine studies of old myocardial infarction. J Nucl Med 2000;41:1737–1745.
7. Schelbert HR, Phelps ME, Hoffman EJ, et al. Regional myocardial perfusion assessed with N-13 labeled ammonia and positron emission computerized axial tomography. Am J Cardiol 1979;43:209–218.
8. Schelbert H. Principles of positron emission tomography. In: Marcus ML, Skorton DJ, Wolf GL, eds. Cardiac imaging. Philadelphia: WB Saunders, 1991:1140–1168.
9. Schelbert HR, Phelps ME, Huang SC, et al. N-13 ammonia as an indicator of myocardial blood flow. Circulation 1981;63:1259–1272.
10. Krivokapich J, Barrio JR, Phelps ME, et al. Kinetic characterization of 13NH3 and [13N]glutamine metabolism in rabbit heart. Am J Physiol 1984;246:H267–H273.
11. Krivokapich J, Huang SC, Phelps ME, et al. Dependence of 13NH3 myocardial extraction and clearance on flow and metabolism. Am J Physiol 1982;242:H536–H542.
12. Kuhle WG, Porenta G, Huang SC, et al. Quantification of regional myocardial blood flow using 13N-ammonia and reoriented dynamic positron emission tomographic imaging. Circulation 1992;86:1004–1017.
13. Muzik O, Beanlands RS, Hutchins GD, et al. Validation of nitrogen-

13-ammonia tracer kinetic model for quantification of myocardial blood flow using PET. *J Nucl Med* 1993;34:83–91.

14. Bol A, Melin JA, Vanoverschelde JL, et al. Direct comparison of [13N]ammonia and [15O]water estimates of perfusion with quantification of regional myocardial blood flow by microspheres. *Circulation* 1993;87:512–525.

15. Bellina CR, Parodi O, Camici P, et al. Simultaneous in vitro and in vivo validation of nitrogen-13-ammonia for the assessment of regional myocardial blood flow. *J Nucl Med* 1990;31:1335–1343.

16. Budinger TF, Derenzo SE, Huesman RH, et al. Quantitative myocardial flow extraction data using gated ECT. *J Nucl Med* 1981;21:16.

17. Goldstein RA, Mullani NA, Marani SK, et al. Myocardial perfusion with rubidium-82. II. Effects of metabolic and pharmacologic interventions. *J Nucl Med* 1983;24:907–915.

18. Mullani NA, Goldstein RA, Gould KL, et al. Myocardial perfusion with rubidium-82. I. Measurement of extraction fraction and flow with external detectors. *J Nucl Med* 1983;24:898–906.

19. Herrero P, Markham J, Shelton ME, et al. Noninvasive quantification of regional myocardial perfusion with rubidium-82 and positron emission tomography. Exploration of a mathematical model. *Circulation* 1990;82:1377–1386.

20. Melon PG, Brihaye C, Degueldre C, et al. Myocardial kinetics of potassium-38 in humans and comparison with copper-62-PTSM. *J Nucl Med* 1994;35:1116–1122.

21. Pierard LA, De Landsheere CM, Berthe C, et al. Identification of viable myocardium by echocardiography during dobutamine infusion in patients with myocardial infarction after thrombolytic therapy: comparison with positron emission tomography. *J Am Coll Cardiol* 1990;15:1021–1031.

22. Beanlands RS, Muzik O, Mintun M, et al. The kinetics of copper-62-PTSM in the normal human heart. *J Nucl Med* 1992;33:684–690.

23. Herrero P, Markham J, Weinheimer CJ, et al. Quantification of regional myocardial perfusion with generator-produced 62Cu-PTSM and positron emission tomography. *Circulation* 1993;87:173–183.

24. Nickles RJ, Nunn AD, Stone CK, et al. Technetium-94m-teboroxime: synthesis, dosimetry and initial PET imaging studies. *J Nucl Med* 1993;34:1058–1066.

25. Chan SY, Brunken RC, Phelps ME, et al. Use of the metabolic tracer carbon-11-acetate for evaluation of regional myocardial perfusion. *J Nucl Med* 1991;32:665–672.

26. Ng CK, Huang SC, Schelbert HR, et al. Validation of a model for [1-11C]acetate as a tracer of cardiac oxidative metabolism. *Am J Physiol* 1994;266:H1304–H1315.

27. Buxton DB, Schwaiger M, Nguyen A, et al. Radiolabeled acetate as a tracer of myocardial tricarboxylic acid cycle flux. *Circ Res* 1988;63:628–634.

28. Brown M, Marshall DR, Sobel BE, et al. Delineation of myocardial oxygen utilization with carbon-11-labeled acetate. *Circulation* 1987;76:687–696.

29. Buxton DB, Nienaber CA, Luxen A, et al. Noninvasive quantitation of regional myocardial oxygen consumption in vivo with [1-11C]acetate and dynamic positron emission tomography. *Circulation* 1989;79:134–142.

30. Brown MA, Myears DW, Bergmann SR. Noninvasive assessment of canine myocardial oxidative metabolism with carbon-11 acetate and positron emission tomography. *J Am Coll Cardiol* 1988;12:1054–1063.

31. Armbrecht JJ, Buxton DB, Brunken RC, et al. Regional myocardial oxygen consumption determined noninvasively in humans with [1-11C]acetate and dynamic positron tomography. *Circulation* 1989;80:863–872.

32. Henes CG, Bergmann SR, Walsh MN, et al. Assessment of myocardial oxidative metabolic reserve with positron emission tomography and carbon-11 acetate. *J Nucl Med* 1989;30:1489–1499.

33. Tamaki N, Magata Y, Takahashi N, et al. Oxidative metabolism in the myocardium in normal subjects during dobutamine infusion. *Eur J Nucl Med* 1993;20:231–237.

34. Yamamoto Y, de Silva R, Rhodes CG, et al. Noninvasive quantification of regional myocardial metabolic rate of oxygen by 15O2 inhalation and positron emission tomography. Experimental validation. *Circulation* 1996;94:808–816.

35. Iida H, Rhodes CG, Araujo LI, et al. Noninvasive quantification of regional myocardial metabolic rate for oxygen by use of 15O2 inhalation and positron emission tomography. Theory, error analysis, and application in humans. *Circulation* 1996;94:792–807.

36. Hoffman EJ, Phelps ME, Weiss ES, et al. Transaxial tomographic imaging of canine myocardium with 11C-palmitic acid. *J Nucl Med* 1977;18:57–61.

37. Klein MS, Goldstein RA, Welch MJ, et al. External assessment of myocardial metabolism with [11C]palmitate in rabbit hearts. *Am J Physiol* 1979;237:H51–H58.

38. Rosamond TL, Abendschein DR, Sobel BE, et al. Metabolic fate of radiolabeled palmitate in ischemic canine myocardium: implications for positron emission tomography. *J Nucl Med* 1987;28:1322–1329.

39. Schon HR, Schelbert HR, Najafi A, et al. C-11 labeled palmitic acid for the noninvasive evaluation of regional myocardial fatty acid metabolism with positron-computed tomography. II. Kinetics of C-11 palmitic acid in acutely ischemic myocardium. *Am Heart J* 1982;103:548–561.

40. Schon HR, Schelbert HR, Robinson G, et al. C-11 labeled palmitic acid for the noninvasive evaluation of regional myocardial fatty acid metabolism with positron-computed tomography. I. Kinetics of C-11 palmitic acid in normal myocardium. *Am Heart J* 1982;103:532–547.

41. Schelbert HR, Henze E, Schon HR, et al. C-11 palmitate for the noninvasive evaluation of regional myocardial fatty acid metabolism with positron computed tomography. III. In vivo demonstration of the effects of substrate availability on myocardial metabolism. *Am Heart J* 1983;105:492–504.

42. Fox KA, Abendschein DR, Ambos HD, et al. Efflux of metabolized and nonmetabolized fatty acid from canine myocardium. Implications for quantifying myocardial metabolism tomographically. *Circ Res* 1985;57:232–243.

43. Bergmann SR, Weinheimer CJ, Markham J, et al. Quantitation of myocardial fatty acid metabolism using PET. *J Nucl Med* 1996;37:1723–1730.

44. DeGrado TR, Wang S, Holden JE, et al. Synthesis and preliminary evaluation of (18)F-labeled 4-thia palmitate as a PET tracer of myocardial fatty acid oxidation. *Nucl Med Biol* 2000;27:221–231.

45. Mäki MT, Haaparanta M, Nuutila P, et al. Free fatty acid uptake in the myocardium and skeletal muscle using fluorine-18-fluoro-6-thia-heptadecanoic acid. *J Nucl Med* 1998;39:1320–1327.

46. Taylor M, Wallhaus TR, Degrado TR, et al. An evaluation of myocardial fatty acid and glucose uptake using PET with [18F]fluoro-6-thia-heptadecanoic acid and. *J Nucl Med* 2001;42:55–62.

47. Sokoloff L, Reivich M, Kennedy C, et al. The [14C]deoxyglucose method for the measurement of local cerebral glucose utilization: theory, procedure, and normal values in the conscious and anesthetized albino rat. *J Neurochem* 1977;28:897–916.

48. Phelps ME, Huang SC, Hoffman EJ, et al. Tomographic measurement of local cerebral glucose metabolic rate in humans with (F-18)2-fluoro-2-deoxy-D-glucose: validation of method. *Ann Neurol* 1979;6:371–388.

49. Phelps ME, Hoffman EJ, Selin C, et al. Investigation of [18F]2-fluoro-2-deoxyglucose for the measure of myocardial glucose metabolism. *J Nucl Med* 1978;19:1311–1319.

50. Ratib O, Phelps ME, Huang SC, et al. Positron tomography with deoxyglucose for estimating local myocardial glucose metabolism. *J Nucl Med* 1982;23:577–586.

51. Krivokapich J, Huang SC, Selin CE, et al. Fluorodeoxyglucose rate constants, lumped constant, and glucose metabolic rate in rabbit heart. *Am J Physiol* 1987;252:H777–H787.

52. Choi Y, Hawkins RA, Huang SC, et al. Parametric images of myocardial metabolic rate of glucose generated from dynamic cardiac PET and 2-[18F]fluoro-2-deoxy-d-glucose studies. *J Nucl Med* 1991;32:733–738.

53. Ng CK, Holden JE, DeGrado TR, et al. Sensitivity of myocardial fluorodeoxyglucose lumped constant to glucose and insulin. *Am J Physiol* 1991;260:H593–H603.

54. Russell RR 3rd, Mrus JM, Mommessin JI, et al. Compartmentation of hexokinase in rat heart. A critical factor for tracer kinetic analysis of myocardial glucose metabolism. *J Clin Invest* 1992;90:1972–1977.

55. Krivokapich J, Huang SC, Phelps ME, et al. Estimation of rabbit myocardial metabolic rate for glucose using fluorodeoxyglucose. *Am J Physiol* 1982;243:H884–H895.

56. Herrero P, Weinheimer CJ, Dence C, et al. Quantification of myocardial glucose utilization by PET and 1-carbon-11-glucose. *J Nucl Cardiol* 2002;9:5–14.

57. Herrero P, Sharp TL, Dence C, et al. Comparison of 1-(11)C-glucose

and (18)F-FDG for quantifying myocardial glucose use with PET. *J Nucl Med* 2002;43:1530–1541.

58. Davila-Roman VG, Vedala G, Herrero P, et al. Altered myocardial fatty acid and glucose metabolism in idiopathic dilated cardiomyopathy. *J Am Coll Cardiol* 2002;40:271–277.

59. Shelton ME, Dence CS, Hwang DR, et al. In vivo delineation of myocardial hypoxia during coronary occlusion using fluorine-18 fluoromisonidazole and positron emission tomography: a potential approach for identification of jeopardized myocardium. *J Am Coll Cardiol* 1990;16:477–485.

60. Martin GV, Caldwell JH, Graham MM, et al. Noninvasive detection of hypoxic myocardium using fluorine-18-fluoromisonidazole and positron emission tomography. *J Nucl Med* 1992;33:2202–2208.

61. Schwaiger M, Kalff V, Rosenspire K, et al. Noninvasive evaluation of sympathetic nervous system in human heart by positron emission tomography. *Circulation* 1990;82:457–464.

62. Schwaiger M, Hutchins GD, Kalff V, et al. Evidence for regional catecholamine uptake and storage sites in the transplanted human heart by positron emission tomography. *J Clin Invest* 1991;87:1681–1690.

63. Schwaiger M, Wieland D, Muzik O, et al. Comparison of C-11 epinephrine and C-11 HED for evaluation of sympathetic neurons of the heart. *J Nucl Med* 1993;34.

64. Corbett JR, Chiao P-C, del Rosario R, et al. Mapping neuronal enzyme function of the human heart with C-11 phenylephrine. *J Nucl Med* 1994;35:109 (abst).

65. DeGrado TR, Hutchins GD, Toorongian SA, et al. Myocardial kinetics of carbon-11-meta-hydroxyephedrine: retention mechanisms and effects of norepinephrine. *J Nucl Med* 1993;34:1287–1293.

66. Ungerer M, Hartmann F, Karoglan M, et al. Regional in vivo and in vitro characterization of autonomic innervation in cardiomyopathic human heart. *Circulation* 1998;97:174–180.

67. Hicks K, Ganti G, Mullani N, et al. Automated quantitation of three-dimensional cardiac positron emission tomography for routine clinical use. *J Nucl Med* 1989;30:1787–1797.

68. Kuhle WG, Porenta G, Huang SC, et al. Issues in the quantitation of reoriented cardiac PET images. *J Nucl Med* 1992;33:1235–1242.

69. Porenta G, Kuhle W, Czernin J, et al. Semiquantitative assessment of myocardial blood flow and viability using polar map displays of cardiac PET images. *J Nucl Med* 1992;33:1628–1636.

70. Laubenbacher C, Rothley J, Sitomer J, et al. An automated analysis program for the evaluation of cardiac PET studies: initial results in the detection and localization of coronary artery disease using nitrogen-13-ammonia. *J Nucl Med* 1993;34:968–978.

71. Choi Y, Huang SC, Hawkins RA, et al. A simplified method for quantification of myocardial blood flow using nitrogen-13-ammonia and dynamic PET. *J Nucl Med* 1993;34:488–497.

72. Hoffman EJ, Phelps ME, Wisenberg G, et al. Electrocardiographic gating in positron emission computed tomography. *J Comput Assist Tomogr* 1979;3:733–739.

73. Henze E, Huang SC, Ratib O, et al. Measurements of regional tissue and blood-pool radiotracer concentrations from serial tomographic images of the heart. *J Nucl Med* 1983;24:987–996.

74. Gambhir SS. Quantitation of the physical factors affecting the tracer kinetic modeling of cardiac position emission tomography data. Los Angeles: University of California, Los Angeles, 1990.

75. Parodi O, Schelbert HR, Schwaiger M, et al. Cardiac emission computed tomography: underestimation of regional tracer concentrations due to wall motion abnormalities. *J Comput Assist Tomogr* 1984;8:1083–1092.

76. Boyd HL, Gunn RN, Marinho NV, et al. Non-invasive measurement of left ventricular volumes and function by gated positron emission tomography. *Eur J Nucl Med* 1996;23:1594–1602.

77. Yamashita K, Tamaki N, Yonekura Y, et al. Quantitative analysis of regional wall motion by gated myocardial positron emission tomography: validation and comparison with left ventriculography. *J Nucl Med* 1989;30:1775–1786.

78. Hattori N, Bengel FM, Mehilli J, et al. Global and regional functional measurements with gated FDG PET in comparison with left ventriculography. *Eur J Nucl Med* 2001;28:221–229.

79. Liedtke AJ. Alterations of carbohydrate and lipid metabolism in the acutely ischemic heart. *Prog Cardiovasc Dis* 1981;23:321–336.

80. Opie LH, Owen P, Riemersma RA. Relative rates of oxidation of glucose and free fatty acids by ischaemic and non-ischaemic myocardium after coronary artery ligation in the dog. *Eur J Clin Invest* 1973;3:419–435.

81. Schelbert H, Phelps M, Selin C, et al. Regional myocardial ischemia assessed by 18Fluoro-2-deoxyglucose and positron emission computed tomography. In: Kreuzer H, Parmley WW, Rentrop P, Heiss HW, eds. *Quantification of myocardial ischemia.* New York: Gerhard Witzstrock Publishing House, 1980:437–447.

82. Kalff V, Schwaiger M, Nguyen N, et al. The relationship between myocardial blood flow and glucose uptake in ischemic canine myocardium determined with fluorine-18-deoxyglucose. *J Nucl Med* 1992;33:1346–1353.

83. Marshall RC, Tillisch JH, Phelps ME, et al. Identification and differentiation of resting myocardial ischemia and infarction in man with positron computed tomography, 18F-labeled fluorodeoxyglucose and N-13 ammonia. *Circulation* 1983;67:766–778.

84. Armbrecht JJ, Buxton DB, Schelbert HR. Validation of [1-11C]acetate as a tracer for noninvasive assessment of oxidative metabolism with positron emission tomography in normal, ischemic, postischemic, and hyperemic canine myocardium. *Circulation* 1990;81:1594–1605.

85. Schwaiger M, Schelbert HR, Ellison D, et al. Sustained regional abnormalities in cardiac metabolism after transient ischemia in the chronic dog model. *J Am Coll Cardiol* 1985;6:336–347.

86. Schwaiger M, Neese RA, Araujo L, et al. Sustained nonoxidative glucose utilization and depletion of glycogen in reperfused canine myocardium. *J Am Coll Cardiol* 1989;13:745–754.

87. Yamamoto Y, De Silva R, Rhodes C, et al. A new strategy for the assessment of viable myocardium and regional myocardial blood flow using ^{15}O-water and dynamic positron emission tomography. *Circulation* 1992;86:167–178.

88. Schwaiger M, Brunken R, Grover-McKay M, et al. Regional myocardial metabolism in patients with acute myocardial infarction assessed by positron emission tomography. *J Am Coll Cardiol* 1986;8:800–808.

89. Tillisch J, Brunken R, Marshall R, et al. Reversibility of cardiac wall-motion abnormalities predicted by positron tomography. *N Engl J Med* 1986;314:884–888.

90. Gropler RJ, Geltman EM, Sampathkumaran K, et al. Comparison of carbon-11-acetate with fluorine-18-fluorodeoxyglucose for delineating viable myocardium by positron emission tomography. *J Am Coll Cardiol* 1993;22:1587–1597.

91. Czernin J, Porenta G, Brunken R, et al. Metabolic and functional fate of viable myocardium by PET early after acute infarction. *J Am Coll Cardiol* 1991;17 (abst).

92. Czernin J, Porenta G, Brunken R, et al. Regional blood flow, oxidative metabolism, and glucose utilization in patients with recent myocardial infarction. *Circulation* 1993;88:884–895.

93. Czernin J, Muller P, Chan S, et al. Influence of age and hemodynamics on myocardial blood flow and flow reserve. *Circulation* 1993;88:62–69.

94. Krivokapich J, Smith GT, Huang SC, et al. 13N ammonia myocardial imaging at rest and with exercise in normal volunteers. Quantification of absolute myocardial perfusion with dynamic positron emission tomography. *Circulation* 1989;80:1328–1337.

95. Mueller HS, Ayres SM. Metabolic response of the heart in acute myocardial infarction in man. *Am J Cardiol* 1978;42:363–371.

96. Henrich M, Vester E, Julicher F, et al. Myocardial glucose metabolism in patients with a coronary artery occlusion: a FDG-PET study in the fasted state and after glucose load. *J Nucl Med* 1991;32:909.

97. Berne R, Rubio R. Coronary circulation. In: Berne R, ed. *Handbook of physiology, section 2: the cardiovascular system, vol I. The heart.* Bethesda, MD: American Physiological Society, 1979:873–952.

98. Feigl EO, Neat GW, Huang AH. Interrelations between coronary artery pressure, myocardial metabolism and coronary blood flow. *J Mol Cell Cardiol* 1990;22:375–390.

99. Holmberg S, Serzysko W, Varnauskas E. Coronary circulation during heavy exercise in control subjects and patients with coronary heart disease. *Acta Med Scand* 1971;190:465–480.

100. Gropler RJ, Siegel BA, Sampathkumaran K, et al. Dependence of recovery of contractile function on maintenance of oxidative metabolism after myocardial infarction. *J Am Coll Cardiol* 1992;19:989–997.

101. Hicks RJ, Melon P, Kalff V, et al. Metabolic imaging by positron emission tomography early after myocardial infarction as a predictor of recovery of myocardial function after reperfusion. *J Nucl Cardiol* 1994;1:124–137.

102. Allman KC, Wieland DM, Muzik O, et al. Carbon-11 hydroxyephedrine with positron emission tomography for serial assessment of

cardiac adrenergic neuronal function after acute myocardial infarction in humans. *J Am Coll Cardiol* 1993;22:368–375.

103. Hashimoto T, Buxton DB, Krivokapich J, et al. Responses of blood flow, oxygen consumption, and contractile function to inotropic stimulation in stunned canine myocardium. *Am Heart J* 1994;127:1250–1262.

104. Vanoverschelde JL, Melin JA, Bol A, et al. Regional oxidative metabolism in patients after recovery from reperfused anterior myocardial infarction. Relation to regional blood flow and glucose uptake. *Circulation* 1992;85:9–21.

105. Fragasso G, Chierchia SL, Lucignani G, et al. Time dependence of residual tissue viability after myocardial infarction assessed by [18F]fluorodeoxyglucose and positron emission tomography. *Am J Cardiol* 1993;72:131G–139G.

106. Fragasso G, Chierchia SL, Landoni C, et al. Regional glucose utilization in infarcted and remote myocardium: its relation to coronary anatomy and perfusion. *Nucl Med Commun* 1998;19:625–632.

107. Matsunari I, Schricke U, Bengel FM, et al. Extent of cardiac sympathetic neuronal damage is determined by the area of ischemia in patients with acute coronary syndromes. *Circulation* 2000;101:2579–2585.

108. Bengel FM, Permanetter B, Ungerer M, et al. Alterations of the sympathetic nervous system and metabolic performance of the cardiomyopathic heart. *Eur J Nucl Med Mol Imaging* 2002;29:198–202.

109. Haas F, Augustin N, Holper K, et al. Time course and extent of improvement of dysfunctioning myocardium in patients with coronary artery disease and severely depressed left ventricular function after revascularization: correlation with positron emission tomographic findings. *J Am Coll Cardiol* 2000;36:1927–1934.

110. Bax JJ, Visser FC, Poldermans D, et al. Time course of functional recovery of stunned and hibernating segments after surgical revascularization. *Circulation* 2001;104:I314–I318.

111. Haas F, Jennen L, Heinzmann U, et al. Ischemically compromised myocardium displays different time-courses of functional recovery: correlation with morphological alterations? *Eur J Cardiothorac Surg* 2001;20:290–298.

112. Marwick TH, MacIntyre WJ, Lafont A, et al. Metabolic responses of hibernating and infarcted myocardium to revascularization. A follow-up study of regional perfusion, function, and metabolism. *Circulation* 1992;85:1347–1353.

113. Braunwald E, Kloner RA. The stunned myocardium: prolonged, postischemic ventricular dysfunction. *Circulation* 1982;66:1146–1149.

114. Rahimtoola SH. A perspective on the three large multicenter randomized clinical trials of coronary bypass surgery for chronic stable angina. *Circulation* 1985;72:V123–V135.

115. Bolli R. Myocardial 'stunning' in man. *Circulation* 1992;86:1671–1691.

116. Barnes E, Dutka DP, Khan M, et al. Effect of repeated episodes of reversible myocardial ischemia on myocardial blood flow and function in humans. *Am J Physiol Heart Circ Physiol* 2002;282:H1603–H1608.

117. Barnes E, Hall RJ, Dutka DP, et al. Absolute blood flow and oxygen consumption in stunned myocardium in patients with coronary artery disease. *J Am Coll Cardiol* 2002;39:420–427.

118. Canty JM Jr, Fallavollita JA. Chronic hibernation and chronic stunning: a continuum. *J Nucl Cardiol* 2000;7:509–527.

119. Canty JM Jr, Fallavollita JA. Resting myocardial flow in hibernating myocardium: validating animal models of human pathophysiology. *Am J Physiol* 1999;277:H417–H422.

120. Fallavollita JA, Canty JM Jr. Differential 18F-2-deoxyglucose uptake in viable dysfunctional myocardium with normal resting perfusion: evidence for chronic stunning in pigs. *Circulation* 1999;99:2798–2805.

121. Fallavollita JA, Canty JM Jr. Ischemic cardiomyopathy in pigs with two-vessel occlusion and viable, chronically dysfunctional myocardium. *Am J Physiol Heart Circ Physiol* 2002;282:H1370–H1379.

122. Fallavollita JA, Perry BJ, Canty JM Jr. 18F-2-deoxyglucose deposition and regional flow in pigs with chronically dysfunctional myocardium. Evidence for transmural variations in chronic hibernating myocardium. *Circulation* 1997;95:1900–1909.

123. Fallavollita JA, Malm BJ, Canty JM Jr. Hibernating myocardium retains metabolic and contractile reserve despite regional reductions in flow, function, and oxygen consumption at rest. *Circ Res* 2003;92:48–55.

124. Schwarz ER, Schaper J, vom Dahl J, et al. Myocyte degeneration and cell death in hibernating human myocardium. *J Am Coll Cardiol* 1996;27:1577–1585.

125. Schwarz ER, Schoendube FA, Kostin S, et al. Prolonged myocardial hibernation exacerbates cardiomyocyte degeneration and impairs recovery of function after revascularization. *J Am Coll Cardiol* 1998;31:1018–1026.

126. Beanlands RS, Hendry PJ, Masters RG, et al. Delay in revascularization is associated with increased mortality rate in patients with severe left ventricular dysfunction and viable myocardium on fluorine 18-fluorodeoxyglucose positron emission tomography imaging. *Circulation* 1998;98:II51–II56.

127. Bax JJ, Schinkel AF, Elhendy A, et al. Delayed revascularization has an adverse effect on outcome in patients with viable myocardium. *J Am Coll Cardiol* 2003;41:504.

128. Elsasser A, Schlepper M, Klovekorn WP, et al. Hibernating myocardium: an incomplete adaptation to ischemia. *Circulation* 1997;96:2920–2931.

129. Flameng W, Suy R, Schwarz F, et al. Ultrastructural correlates of left ventricular contraction abnormalities in patients with chronic ischemic heart disease: determinants of reversible segmental asynergy postrevascularization surgery. *Am Heart J* 1981;102:846–857.

130. Vanoverschelde JL, Wijns W, Depre C, et al. Mechanisms of chronic regional postischemic dysfunction in humans. New insights from the study of noninfarcted collateral-dependent myocardium. *Circulation* 1993;87:1513–1523.

131. Ausma J, Thone F, Dispersyn GD, et al. Dedifferentiated cardiomyocytes from chronic hibernating myocardium are ischemia-tolerant. *Mol Cell Biochem* 1998;186:159–168.

132. Lopaschuk GD, Rebeyka IM, Allard MF. Metabolic modulation: a means to mend a broken heart. *Circulation* 2002;105:140–142.

133. Brosius FC 3rd, Liu Y, Nguyen N, et al. Persistent myocardial ischemia increases GLUT1 glucose transporter expression in both ischemic and non-ischemic heart regions. *J Mol Cell Cardiol* 1997;29:1675–1685.

134. Brosius FC 3rd, Nguyen N, Egert S, et al. Increased sarcolemmal glucose transporter abundance in myocardial ischemia. *Am J Cardiol* 1997;80:77A–84A.

135. Vogt AM, Elsasser A, Nef H, et al. Increased glycolysis as protective adaptation of energy depleted, degenerating human hibernating myocardium. *Mol Cell Biochem* 2003;242:101–107.

136. Vogt AM, Nef H, Schaper J, et al. Metabolic control analysis of anaerobic glycolysis in human hibernating myocardium replaces traditional concepts of flux control. *FEBS Lett* 2002;517:245–250.

137. Opie LH. Myocardial ischemia—metabolic pathways and implications of increased glycolysis. *Cardiovasc Drugs Ther* 1990;4[Suppl 4]:777–790.

138. Kotler T, Neienaber C, Lew A, et al. Early post-thrombolysis assessment of necrosis and viability with rest-redistribution thallium scintigraphy: correlation with positron emission tomography (PET). *J Am Coll Cardiol* 1989;13 (abst).

139. Schwaiger M, Brunken RC, Krivokapich J, et al. Beneficial effect of residual anterograde flow on tissue viability as assessed by positron emission tomography in patients with myocardial infarction. *Eur Heart J* 1987;8:981–988.

140. Hashimoto T, Kambara H, Fudo T, et al. Increased fluorine-18 deoxyglucose uptake after percutaneous transluminal coronary angioplasty in recently infarcted myocardium. *Am J Cardiol* 1989;63:743–744.

Management

CHAPTER 65

Medical Management of Unstable Angina and Non–ST-Segment Elevation Myocardial Infarction

Eugene Braunwald and Daniel B. Mark

Risk Stratification	**Antiischemic Therapy**
Antiplatelet Therapy	Nitrates
Aspirin	β-Blockers
Clopidogrel	Calcium Channel Blockers
Glycoprotein IIb/IIIa Antagonists	Angiotensin-converting Enzyme Inhibitors
Anticoagulants	**Management of Lower Risk Patients**
Unfractionated Heparin	**Prehospital Discharge and Postdischarge Care**
Low–Molecular Weight Heparin	**References**

Key Words: Antiischemic therapy; antiplatelet therapy; clopidogrel; glycoprotein IIb/IIIa antagonists; low molecular-weight heparin.

Unstable angina and non–ST-segment elevation myocardial infarction (UA/non-STEMI, also referred to as non-STEMI–acute coronary syndrome [ACS]) is a heterogeneous disorder of varied cause and severity. Because a large fraction of adverse events in these patients occur during the first hours or days after the initial event, immediate assessment of patients known to have or suspected of having UA/non-STEMI is essential. Both the careful clinical assessment and 12-lead electrocardiogram (ECG) are central to diagnosis and risk stratification. Therefore, patients with symptoms that suggest ACS should not be evaluated solely over the telephone, but instead they should be referred immediately to a facility that allows assessment by a physician, the recording of a 12-lead ECG, and, if necessary, the administration of emergency care (1). The clinical presentation

and diagnostic evaluation of patients with UA/non-STEMI are discussed in Chapter 58.

RISK STRATIFICATION

Once the diagnosis of UA/non-STEMI is established or strongly suspected, management should be directed by the estimated risk (Fig. 65–1). Therefore, risk stratification is of critical importance. The following three approaches may be used when the patient is initially seen, usually in the emergency department:

1. Table 65–1 lists features of high-, intermediate-, and low-risk UA/non-STEMI derived from Agency for Health Care Policy and Research and American College of Cardiology/American Heart Association guidelines (1,2,2a).
2. The Thrombolysis In Myocardial Infarction (TIMI) risk score for UA/non-STEMI (Fig. 65–2) is a simple, convenient, and useful instrument for risk stratification that was derived from one large trial and validated in four additional trials (3–5). It consists of the simple integer sum of seven risk factors derived from a multivariate analysis of baseline variables, each of which contributes approximately equally to adverse outcome—that is, death, reinfarction, or recurrent se-

E. Braunwald: TIMI Study Group, 350 Longwood Avenue, Boston, Massachusetts 02115.

D. B. Mark: Duke Clinical Research Institute, 2400 Pratt Avenue, Rm 0311, Durham, North Carolina 27705.

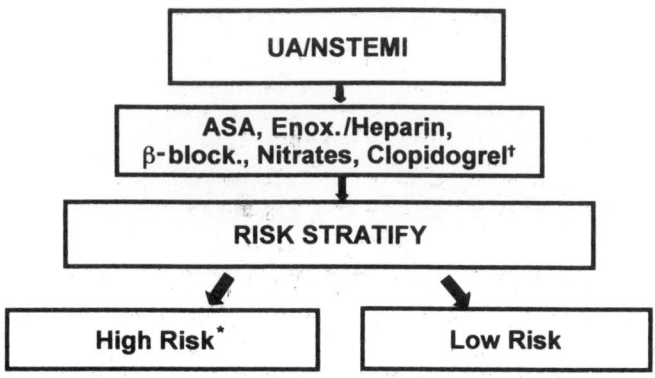

FIG. 65–1. Algorithm for the management of patient with unstable angina (UA)/non–ST-segment elevation myocardial infarction (NSTEMI). Patients in whom this diagnosis is confirmed or suspected are treated with aspirin (ASA), heparin (enoxaparin [enox.] preferred to unfractionated heparin), β-blockade, nitrates, and clopidogrel. They are then risk stratified, and their subsequent management is dictated by their risk category. CABG, coronary artery bypass grafting; dysf, dysfunction; LV, left ventricular; Trop, troponin; VT, ventricular tachycardia.

vere ischemia requiring urgent revascularization. The risk for such an adverse outcome ranged from 5% in patients with a score of 0 or 1 to 41% with a score of 6 or 7.

3. The third approach is a recently proposed multimarker laboratory approach that depends on ascertainment of three biomarkers: troponin, C-reactive protein, and brain natriuretic peptide (6). Increase of each of these three biomarkers independently increases the risk for adverse outcomes by 1.5- to 2-fold (Fig. 65–3). How-

ever, they must be considered together with the clinical findings.

Irrespective of which of these approaches is applied, patients who present within 6 hours of the onset of chest pain with a negative troponin should have the test repeated 6 to 8 hours later, before it is deemed to be negative.

It is recommended that patients considered to be at high risk (Table 65–1; i.e., patients with a TIMI risk score ≥5 or with two or more abnormally increased biomarkers) be admit-

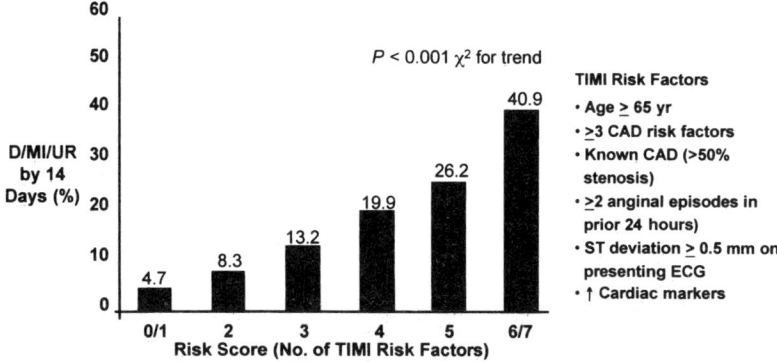

FIG. 65–2. Thrombolysis In Myocardial Infarction (TIMI) risk score for unstable angina/non–ST-segment elevation myocardial infarction. The risk factors are shown on the right and the risk for death *(D)*, myocardial infarction *(MI)*, or urgent revascularization *(UR)* is shown along the vertical axis. CAD, coronary artery disease; ECG, electrocardiogram. (Adapted from Antman EM, Cohen M, Bernink PJ, et al. The TIMI risk score for unstable angina/non-ST elevation MI: a method for prognostication and therapeutic decision making. *JAMA* 2000;284:835–842, with permission.)

TABLE 65–1. *Short-term risk of death or nonfatal MI in patients with unstable angina*

Feature	High risk (at least 3 of the following features must be present)	Intermediate risk (no high-risk feature but must have 1 of the following features)	Lower risk (no high- or intermediate-risk feature but may have any of the following features)
History	Accelerating tempo of ischemic symptoms in preceding 48 hours	Prior MI, peripheral or cerebrovascular disease, or CABG; prior aspirin use	
Character of pain	Prolonged ongoing (>20 min) rest pain	Prolonged (>20 min) rest angina, now resolved, with moderate or high likelihood of CAD Rest angina (<20 min or relieved with rest or sublingual nitroglycerin)	New-onset or progressive CCS Class III or IV angina in the past 2 weeks with moderate or high likelihood of CAD.
Clinical findings	Pulmonary edema, most likely related to ischemia New or worsening MR murmur S$_3$ or new/worsening rales Hypotension, bradycardia, tachycardia Age >75 yrs	Age >70 yrs	
ECG findings	Angina at rest with transient ST-segment changes >0.05 mV Bundle-branch block, new or presumed new Sustained ventricular tachycardia	T-wave inversions >0.2 mV Pathologic Q-waves	Normal or unchanged ECG during an episode of chest discomfort
Cardiac markers	Elevated (e.g., TnT or TnI >0.1 ng/mL)	Slightly elevated (e.g., TnT >0.01 but <0.1 ng/mL)	Normal

CABG, coronary artery bypass graft; CAD, coronary artery disease; CCS, Canadian Cardiovascular Society; ECG, electrocardiogram; MI, myocardial infarction; MR, mitral regurgitation; TnT, troponin T; and TnI, troponin I.

Adapted from Braunwald E, Antman EM, Beasley JW, et al. ACC/AHA guidelines for the management of patients with unstable angina-non-ST segment elevation myocardial infarction: A report of the American College of Cardiology/American Heart Association Task Force on Practice Guidelines (Committee on the Management of Patients with Unstable Angina). *J Am Coll Cardiol* 2000;36:970–1062, with permission.

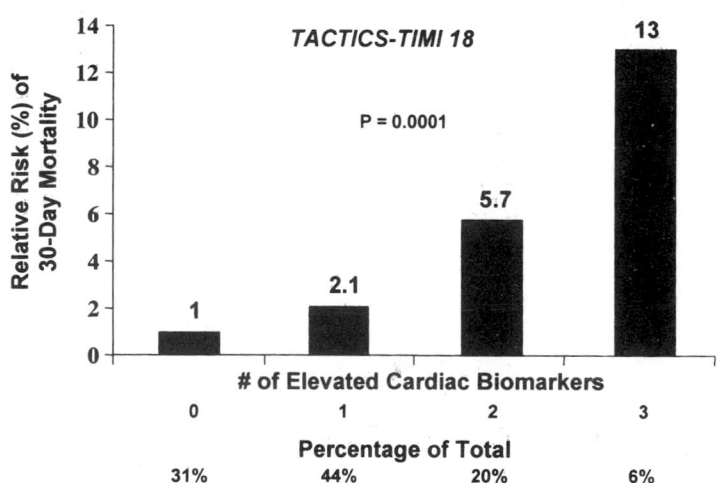

FIG. 65–3. Relative risks of 30-day mortality with zero, one, two, or three abnormally elevated biomarkers. BNP, brain natriuretic protein; CRP, C-reactive protein; cTnI, cardiac specific troponin I; TIMI, Thrombolysis In Myocardial Infarction. (Modified from Sabatine MS, Morrow DA, deLemos J, et al. Multimarker approach to risk stratification in non-ST elevation acute coronary syndromes: simultaneous assessment of troponin I, C-reactive protein, and B-type natriuretic peptide. *Circulation* 2002;105:1760–1763, with permission.)

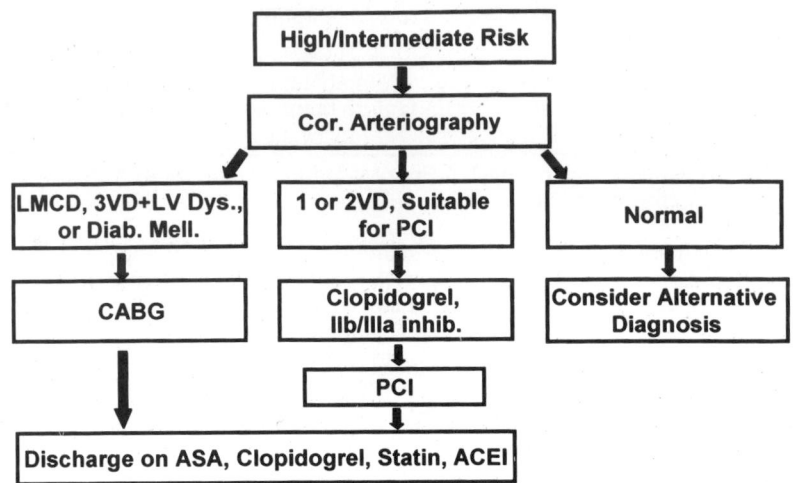

FIG. 65–4. Algorithm for the management of patients at high and intermediate risk with unstable angina/non–ST-segment elevation myocardial infarction. ACEI, angiotensin-converting enzyme inhibitor; ASA, aspirin; CABG, coronary artery bypass grafting; Diab. Mell., diabetes mellitus; LMCD, left main coronary artery disease; LV Dys., left ventricular dysfunction; PCI, percutaneous coronary intervention; 3VD, three-vessel disease.

ted immediately to a cardiac intensive care unit, whereas patients at intermediate risk (as described in Table 65–1; i.e., patients with a TIMI risk score of 3 or 4 or with one abnormal biomarker) also should be admitted to the hospital where they can usually be managed in a monitored bed without intensive care facilities. Patients with ACS deemed to be at lower risk (Table 65–1; i.e., patients who have a TIMI risk score ≤ 2 without an increased biomarker) may be managed as outpatients (discussed later), but they should be seen and reevaluated within 72 hours of presentation to determine their response to initial therapy and need for additional workup. Patients in whom the diagnosis, risk level, or both are not clear and in whom further observation and testing are required may be admitted to "chest pain units" or "short-stay emergency department coronary care units," where critical pathways are used to guide evaluation and subsequent triage. Such units provide the additional diagnostic evidence that allows many patients at low risk to avoid hospital admission (1).

The hospital management of patients with UA/non-STEMI at high or intermediate risk is summarized in Figure 65–4 and may be divided into four components: (a) antiplatelet therapy; (b) antithrombin therapy; (c) antiischemic therapy; and (d) coronary revascularization. The first three components are described in this chapter; coronary revascularization is discussed in Chapter 68.

ANTIPLATELET THERAPY

Given the central role of coronary thrombosis in the pathogenesis of UA/non-STEMI, and the important role played by platelets and thrombin in the generation and propagation of these thrombi (see Chapters 55 and 56), a combination of antiplatelet and antithrombin therapies play a central role in management. Three classes of antiplatelet agents and two

antithrombin agents are available for the management of UA/non-STEMI.

Aspirin

Aspirin is an irreversible inhibitor of platelet cyclooxygenase-1 that prevents the formation of thromboxane A_2, a potent activator of platelets. A pooled analysis of four separate placebo-controlled trials on 3,114 patients with UA/non-STEMI revealed that assignment to aspirin was associated with a reduction of death or myocardial infarction (MI) by 56% from 11.7% to 5.2% (Fig. 65–5). (7) Therefore, all patients with established or suspected UA/non-STEMI without contraindications should be taking aspirin. In patients not already receiving aspirin, an initial dose of 162 to 325 mg of a nonenteric formulation should be followed by 75 to 162 mg per day of an enteric or nonenteric formulation; the latter also should be continued in patients who experience development of UA/non-STEMI while already taking aspirin. Contraindications include allergy, active bleeding, high bleeding risk, or uncontrolled hypertension. For patients with severe gastrointestinal intolerance, clopidogrel may be selected as an alternative.

Clopidogrel

Clopidogrel is a thienopyridine derivative that inhibits the binding of adenosine diphosphate (ADP) to the platelet P2Y12 receptor, blocking ADP-induced inhibition of adenylate cyclase and cyclic ADP formation, thereby interfering with platelet activation. Clopidogrel has replaced ticlopidine, an earlier thienopyridine, because of a better safety profile and a more rapid onset of action. The effects of

Treatment	Number of trials	Number of patients
Aspirin	4	3,114
Heparin	4	1,547
Beta - Blockers	5	4,700
Thrombolytic Therapy	12	2,376
Calcium Blockade	5	956
ACE Inhibitors	1	2,395

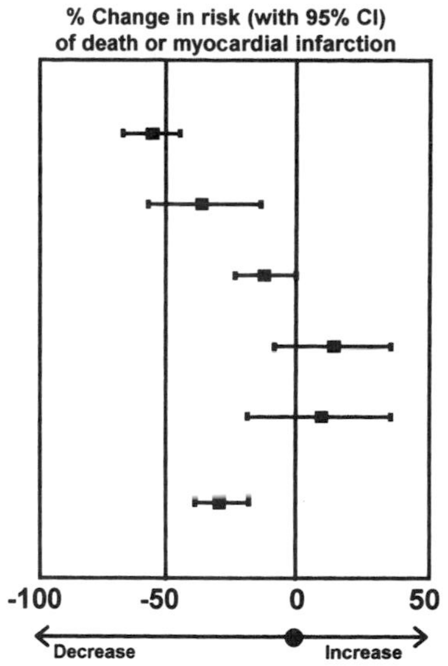

FIG. 65–5. Percent change in risk for death or myocardial infarction (with 95% confidence intervals [CI]) of common therapies for unstable angina, determined by pooling data from randomized clinical trials. ACE, angiotensin-converting enzyme. (Adapted from Granger CB, Califf RM. Stabilizing the unstable artery. In: Califf RM, Wagner GS, eds. *Acute coronary care,* 2nd ed. St. Louis: Mosby–Year Book, 1995: 525–541, with permission.)

adding clopidogrel to aspirin were studied in the Clopidogrel in Unstable angina to prevent Recurrent Events (CURE) trial, a double-blind, randomized trial in which 12,562 patients were treated for an average of 9 months (8). The composite of cardiovascular death, MI, or stroke occurred in 11.5% of patients randomized to placebo and was reduced significantly by 20% to 9.3% in those assigned to clopidogrel (Fig. 65–6A). Evidence for efficacy was observed by 6 hours (Fig. 65–6B) (9). However, major bleeding occurred significantly more frequently in the patients assigned to clopidogrel (3.7%) than placebo (2.7%), and this excess was greater in patients receiving greater doses of aspirin (>162 mg/d) and in patients who underwent coronary artery bypass grafting within the first 5 days after clopidogrel was discontinued (8).

A substudy of CURE (Percutaneous Coronary Intervention–Clopidogrel in Unstable angina to prevent Recurrent Events [PCI-CURE] [10]) was conducted on 2,658 patients who underwent PCI; all patients received open-label thienopyridine for 4 weeks after the procedure. Those patients who received (blinded) clopidogrel before and recommencing 4 weeks after PCI exhibited a significant 31% reduction in death or MI compared with those who received a placebo during these periods. In the Clopidogrel for the Reduction of Events During Observation (CREDO) trial (11), a second trial of clopidogrel in 2,116 patients (55% of whom had UA/non-STEMI) who were to undergo PCI, clopidogrel pretreatment (3–24 hours before PCI) and continued treatment for up to 1 year after PCI was associated with a significant (27%) reduction in death, MI, or stroke. Patients who received pretreatment 6 to 24 hours before PCI showed a 39% reduction compared with placebo.

It is recommended that clopidogrel be administered, in addition to aspirin, to all patients with UA/non-STEMI without contraindication (a high risk for bleeding) in whom an early (<24–36 hours) interventional approach is not planned (4). A loading dose of 300 mg followed by 75 mg daily is suggested (Table 65–2). In patients who will undergo early catheterization, clopidogrel should be held until the need for urgent coronary artery bypass surgery can be excluded to avoid the excess bleeding risks associated with this drug. Clopidogrel may then be administered on the catheterization table or given immediately after the procedure. On the basis of the CURE and CREDO trials, clopidogrel should be continued for at least 9 to 12 months. Although the question has not yet been addressed in a clinical trial, and costs need to be considered, it is reasonable to consider continuing this drug beyond 1 year in patients at high risk for recurrent events. When elective coronary artery bypass surgery or other elective surgery is required, clopidogrel, which is an irreversible inhibitor of platelet activation, should be held for at least 5 days and preferably for 7 days before surgery (4). Clopidogrel without aspirin is indicated in patients who are intolerant of the latter.

Glycoprotein IIb/IIIa Antagonists

After activation of platelets, their glycoprotein (GP) IIb/IIIa surface receptors undergo a change in configuration that enhances their affinity for binding to fibrinogen, leading to platelet aggregation and enhancing thrombus formation. GPIIb/IIIa antagonists occupy these receptors, thereby inhibiting the aggregation of platelets, regardless of their mech-

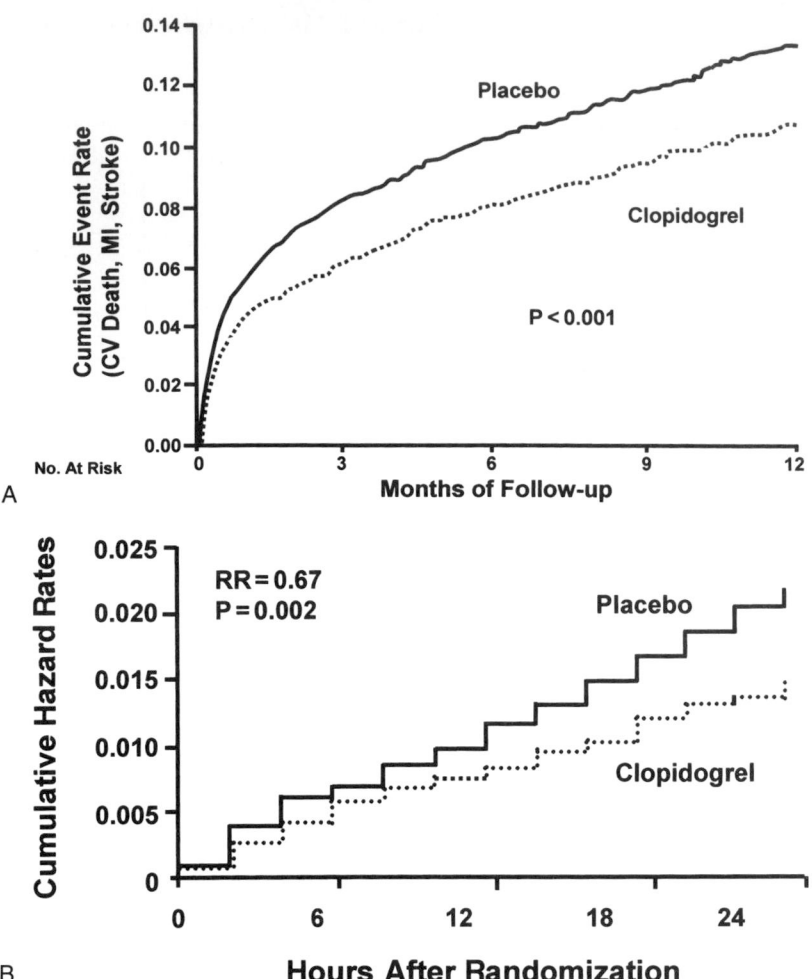

FIG. 65–6. Cumulative event rates for the first primary outcome of cardiovascular (CV) death, nonfatal myocardial infarction (MI), or stroke during the 12 months **(A)** and 24 hours **(B)** of the Clopidogrel in Unstable angina to prevent Recurrent Events (CURE) trial (8). (A: From Yusuf S, Zhao F, Mehta SR, et al. Effects of clopidogrel in addition to aspirin in patients with acute coronary syndromes without ST-segment elevation. *N Engl J Med* 2001;345:494–502, with permission; B: From Berger PB, Steinhubl S. Clinical Implications of Percutaneous Coronary Intervention-Clopidogrel in Unstable angina to prevent Recurrent Events (PCI-CURE) study: a US perspective. *Circulation* 2002;106:2284–2287, with permission.).

TABLE 65–2. *Clinical use of antithrombotic therapy*

Oral antiplatelet therapy	
Aspirin	Initial dose of 162–325 mg nonenteric formulation followed by 75–160 mg/d of an enteric or a nonenteric formulation
Clopidogrel (Plavix)	75 mg/d; a loading dose of 4–8 tablets (300–600 mg) can be used when rapid onset of action is required
Heparins	
Dalteparin (Fragmin)	120 IU/kg subcutaneously every 12 hours (maximum 10,000 IU twice daily)
Enoxaparin (Lovenox)	1 mg/kg subcutaneously every 12 hours; the first dose may be preceded by a 30-mg IV bolus
Heparin (UFH)	Bolus 60–70 U/kg (maximum 5,000 U) IV followed by infusion of $12–15 \text{ U} \cdot \text{kg}^{-1} \cdot \text{hours}^{-1}$ (maximum 1,000 U/hours) titrated to aPTT 1.5–2.5 times control
Intravenous antiplatelet therapy	
Abciximab (ReoPro)	0.25 mg/kg bolus followed by infusion of $0.125 \text{ mcg} \cdot \text{kg}^{-1} \cdot \text{min}^{-1}$ (maximum 10 mcg/min) for 12 to 24 hours
Eptifibatide (Integrilin)	180 mcg/kg bolus followed by infusion of $2.0 \text{ mcg} \cdot \text{kg}^{-1} \cdot \text{min}^{-1}$ for 72 to 96 hours[a]
Tirofiban (Aggrastat)	$0.4 \text{ mcg} \cdot \text{kg}^{-1} \cdot \text{min}^{-1}$ for 30 minutes followed by infusion of $0.1 \text{ mcg} \cdot \text{kg}^{-1} \cdot \text{min}^{-1}$ for 48 to 96 hours[a]

[a]Different dose regimens were tested in recent clinical trials before percutaneous interventions.

Adapted from Braunwald E, Antman EM, Beasley JW, et al. ACC/AHA guidelines for the management of patients with unstable angina-non-ST segment elevation myocardial infarction: A report of the American College of Cardiology/American Heart Association Task Force on Practice Guidelines (Committee on the Management of Patients with Unstable Angina). *J Am Coll Cardiol* 2000;36:970–1062, with permission.

anism(s) of activation. Three GPIIb/IIIa antagonists, each of which exhibits strong affinity for the receptors, are available:

1. Abciximab: a Fab fragment of a humanized murine antibody
2. Eptifibatide: a cyclic heptapeptide
3. Tirofiban: a nonpeptide mimetic of the fibrinogen binding site to the receptor.

Abciximab is administered as a bolus and followed by a 12- to 24-hour infusion. Eptifibatide and tirofiban are synthetic, small molecular antagonists with short half-lives and require continuous intravenous infusion for 48 to 96 hours (Table 65–2).

The efficacy of these agents in patients with UA/non-STEMI undergoing PCI has been shown clearly in several trials (2) and is discussed in Chapter 68. More problematic is the role of GPIIb/IIIa antagonists without scheduled PCI. In a metaanalysis of 31,302 such patients enrolled into placebo-controlled trials (12), only a small, although significant, overall benefit with these agents was observed (odds ratio for death or MI, 0.91). This modest benefit was limited largely to those patients (38% of the total) who, although not scheduled for such, actually underwent PCI. Conversely, in the 62% of the patients who did not undergo PCI, there was no significant reduction in adverse outcomes in patients assigned to a GPIIb/IIIa inhibitor compared with placebo. Not unexpectedly, however, there was a significantly greater bleeding rate in patients who received the platelet antagonists (2.4%) compared with those who received placebo (1.4%).

On the basis of these observations and on the totality of evidence currently available, GPIIb/IIIa receptor antagonists are advised in patients at high risk with UA/non-STEMI without excessive bleeding risks in whom catheterization with the intention of carrying out PCI is planned. The antagonists may be administered before or during the procedure. These drugs are not indicated in patients with UA/non-STEMI who are not at high risk and in whom early PCI is not planned. The administration of eptifibatide or tirofiban in patients at high risk in whom PCI is not planned is optional, but abciximab should not be administered to these patients (4).

GPIIb/IIIa receptor antagonists, aspirin, and clopidogrel act through different mechanisms and appear to have additive efficacies. Although more information on this point is required, observations of subgroups of patients in the CURE (8) and CREDO (11) trials suggest that the bleeding risk of GPIIb/IIIa antagonists does not appear to be increased in patients who are receiving clopidogrel (in addition to aspirin and heparin), and when patients at high risk for bleeding are excluded, triple antiplatelet therapy (aspirin + clopidogrel + a GPIIb/IIIa antagonist) may be used in patients with UA/non-STEMI undergoing PCI.

ANTICOAGULANTS

Unfractionated Heparin

Unfractionated heparin (UFH) is a mixture of glycosaminoglycans with saccharide chains of varying lengths that accel-

erates the actions of antithrombin, a circulatory protein that acts primarily to inactivate thrombin (factor IIa) (see Chapter 69). The addition of UFH to aspirin has been studied in seven randomized trials. In four of these trials suitable for metaanalysis, the incidence of death or MI at 1 week was reduced significantly by 62% from 5.5% in those receiving aspirin alone to 2.6% in those in whom UFH was added (2). On the basis of these findings and that the additional benefits of clopidogrel and GPIIb/IIIa antagonists described earlier were all observed together with aspirin and UFH, the addition of UFH has been standard therapy for patients with UA/non-STEMI for more than 15 years.

However, there are serious limitations to the use of UFH (13). Although it blocks circulating thrombin, it does not inhibit clot-bound thrombin or thrombin generation. UFH binds nonspecifically to and is inactivated by platelets, vascular endothelium, fibrin, platelet factor 4, and a variety of circulating proteins, and it has a short plasma half-life. Therefore, the anticoagulant effect is variable, and the administration of UFH requires the monitoring of the activated partial thromboplastin time (aPTT) and continuous intravenous infusion. After administration of a bolus of 60 to 70 U per kilogram (maximum 5,000 U) and after 6 hours of infusion of 12 to 15 U per kilogram per minute, the aPTT should be measured and, if necessary, the dose adjusted to an aPTT that ranges from 1.5 to 2.5 times control. Once the target aPTT has been achieved, an aPTT should be remeasured every 24 hours, as well as 6 hours after each dose adjustment. Treatment should be continued for 2 to 5 days. The major complication of administration of UFH is hemorrhage. Heparin-induced thrombocytopenia (HIT) is a well documented, although infrequent, adverse effect and is thought to be caused by heparin or antibody-induced platelet aggregation that can cause thrombosis or excessive bleeding, or both.

Low–Molecular Weight Heparin

Given the aforementioned disadvantages of UFH, there has been increasing interest in heparin preparations without these problems. Low–molecular weight heparins (LMWHs) are fragments of depolymerized UFH, which bind to and inactivate not only factor IIa (thrombin) but also factor Xa, which generates thrombin (13). Because LMWHs are not inactivated by platelet factor 4 and are less inactivated by endothelial cells and plasma proteins than is UFH, they have a predictable and prolonged anticoagulant effect, do not require monitoring, generate a much lower incidence of HIT, and can be administered by the subcutaneous route once or twice daily.

UFH and LMWH have been compared in UA/non-STEMI in four randomized clinical trials. No differences were found for dalteparin or nadroparin (2). However, a prespecified metaanalysis of two trials comprising 7,081 patients using enoxaparin revealed a significant reduction in death or MI (odds ratio, 0.77 at 1 week) (14). It also has been shown that enoxaparin is well tolerated in combination with GPIIb/IIIa inhibitors (13). In the INTegrilin and Enoxaparin Randomized assessment of Acute Coronary syndromes Treatment (INTERACT) trial, enoxaparin was compared with UFH in 746 patients with UA/non-STEMI receiving aspirin and eptifibatide (15). Noncoronary bypass–related major bleeding was significantly less in the enoxaparin group than in the UFH group (1.8% vs. 4.6%). Also, the rates of death or nonfatal MI at 30 days and of ischemia on a continuous Holter were each reduced almost by half in the enoxaparin arm.

In a meta-analysis of 22,000 patients with non-ST segment elevation acute coronary syndrome, Enoxaparin was more effective than unfractionated heparin in preventing death or myocardial infarction and did not increase major bleeding (16). Although no large "head-to-head" comparisons between different LMWHs have been carried out, on the basis of the large amount of evidence with enoxaparin, the substitution of this LMWH for UFH is recommended (4).

ANTIISCHEMIC THERAPY

Nitrates

The beneficial effect of nitroglycerin in acute ischemic heart disease is attributed to its reduction of myocardial oxygen demand by decreasing both preload and afterload and relieving coronary vasoconstriction. Organic nitrates promote the formation of nitric oxide, the so-called endogenous endothelium-derived relaxing factor. Atherothrombosis depletes endogenous nitric oxide from the arterial endothelium, and nitrate therapy may rectify this deficiency. Nitroglycerin also appears to exert a platelet-inhibiting effect, although the clinical significance, if any, of this action in patients receiving concomitant antiplatelet therapy is undefined.

Nitroglycerin is one of the mainstays of therapy for symptomatic ischemia in patients with UA/non-STEMI. Sublingual nitroglycerin tablets are used in the emergency department or, if available, en route, to relieve any ongoing symptoms. Patients whose symptoms are not relieved fully with three sublingual nitroglycerin tablets (0.4 mg) taken 5 minutes apart and the administration of an intravenous β-blocker (discussed later), as well as all patients without hypotension with UA/non-STEMI, may benefit from intravenous nitroglycerin. This should be started at a dose of 5 to 10 μg per minute by continuous infusion and titrated up by 10 μg per minute every 5 to 10 minutes until symptoms are relieved, limiting side effects are encountered (headache or hypotension with systolic blood pressure <100 mm Hg or more than 25% below starting mean arterial pressure), or a ceiling of 200 μg per minute is reached.

Topical, oral, or buccal nitrates are acceptable alternatives for patients without ongoing or refractory symptoms. Also, patients on intravenous nitroglycerin should be switched to oral or topical nitrate therapy once they have been free of symptoms for 24 hours. Tolerance to nitrates is dose and duration dependent and typically becomes significant after 24 hours of continuous therapy. Responsiveness can be restored by increasing the dose of intravenous nitroglycerin or switching the patient to a nonparenteral form of therapy and using a nitrate-free period. As long as the patient continues to have symptoms, the former option should be selected. Nonparenteral nitrates should be given with a 6- to 8-hour nitrate-free interval.

Despite the central role of nitrate therapy in UA/non-STEMI, there have been no large, randomized, placebo-controlled trials that address the efficacy of these drugs in the reduction of cardiac events. Thus, the rationale for their use in UA/non-STEMI is extrapolated from pathophysiologic principles, relatively small studies of efficacy, and clinical experience, which has shown a rapid relief of ischemic discomfort, especially with intravenous nitroglycerin in a large majority of patients (1,2).

β-Blockers

The effectiveness of β-adrenoceptor blockers in relieving symptoms of myocardial ischemia is related to their blockade of the myocardial β_1 receptors with resulting reductions in heart rate, contractility, blood pressure, and, consequently, myocardial oxygen demand. These agents also have been reported to blunt the circadian morning increase in serious ischemic events (17). Contraindications include a history of bronchoconstriction, the presence of advanced first-degree (PR interval >0.24 seconds) or higher atrioventricular block, hypotension (systolic blood pressure <100 mm Hg), and sinus bradycardia (heart rate <50 bpm).

Initial studies of β-blockers in acute ischemic heart disease were small and uncontrolled. Episodes of ischemia were reduced. Metaanalysis of the available trials indicated a 13% reduction in the risk for progression to acute MI (18), but no clear mortality benefit in UA was demonstrated. However, randomized trials in acute or recent MI and in stable angina with silent ischemia have all shown a mortality benefit for β-blockers (19), and their utility in prevention and control of recurrent ischemic symptoms has been shown. Thus, the overall rationale for the use of β-blockers in UA/non-STEMI is sufficiently compelling to make them a part of the routine care of such patients who have no contraindications to their use (1,2,7). They are particularly useful in patients with evidence of high adrenergic tone with attendant sinus tachycardia, hypertension, or both.

The choice of agent is based primarily on pharmacokinetics and side effects. There is no evidence that any particular β-blocker is more effective than any other in acute ischemic syndromes, although β-blockers with partial agonist activity should be avoided. One popular regimen is to administer intravenous metoprolol (5 mg over 1 minute) and, if it is tolerated, repeat every 5 minutes for a total of 15 mg followed by 100 mg orally twice daily. The duration of benefits with long-term oral therapy remains undefined, but in patients with acute MI, it appears to last for at least 5 years. It is reasonable to extrapolate these findings to UA as long as the drug is well tolerated.

Calcium Channel Blockers

Calcium channel blockers act by blocking the inward flux of calcium through cell membranes, thereby reducing myocardial contractility, decreasing atrioventricular conduction, relaxing vascular smooth muscle, and in the case of several of these agents, reducing heart rate. Their benefits in relieving ischemic symptoms are believed to result from variable combinations of reduced myocardial oxygen demand produced by decreased afterload and contractility and improved myocardial blood supply through coronary vasodilatation. Adverse effects include bradycardia, atrioventricular block, hypotension, and heart failure.

In randomized trials in patients with UA, the efficacy of calcium channel blockers in relieving ischemic symptoms appears to be equivalent to that of β-blockers (20). Three metaanalyses of the effects of calcium channel blockers on death or nonfatal MI in UA showed no benefit (7,19,21). However, the data for verapamil alone suggest a beneficial effect (22). The Diltiazem Reinfarction Study (DRS) in patients with non–Q-wave MI (23) and the Multicenter Diltiazem Postinfarction Trial (MDPIT) (24) also pointed to benefit in these patients. Current evidence for the benefit of calcium channel blockers in UA/non-STEMI is limited to control of ongoing or recurrent ischemia in patients who do not respond adequately to nitrates and β-blockers or who have contraindications to the latter (1,2). However, because they are effective antihypertensive agents, calcium blockers are especially useful in patients with UA/non-STEMI with hypertension. These agents should be avoided in patients with pulmonary edema or significant left ventricular dysfunction. In addition, studies using short-acting nifedipine as monotherapy have reported an unfavorable trend in cardiac events (25). Thus, this agent is not recommended in the absence of concurrent β-blockade.

Angiotensin-converting Enzyme Inhibitors

Angiotensin-converting enzyme inhibition has been shown to reduce mortality in a wide spectrum of patients with coronary artery disease, including MI, and previous UA/non-STEMI. These drugs are indicated in most patients with UA/non-STEMI, especially those with hypertension, left ventricular dysfunction, diabetes mellitus, or other high-risk features (26).

MANAGEMENT OF LOWER RISK PATIENTS

Patients with ACS considered to be at lower risk as defined in Table 65–1, a TIMI risk score of 2 or less (2) or without one elevated biomarker (4), should undergo exercise or pharmacologic stress testing before discharge from the emergency department or chest pain center, or they should undergo such testing within 72 hours of discharge (Fig. 65–7). A low-level exercise test can be carried out in patients who have been free of rest pain for more than 12 hours. In patients with a negative stress test an alternative diagnosis (including variant angina) should be considered. Patients with a "high-risk" stress test (27) should promptly undergo coronary angiography, and the findings should dictate the recommendation for revascularization. Coronary angiography is optional for patients with a positive but not high-risk stress test. Details of noninvasive test selection and interpretation are presented in Chapter 88.

PREHOSPITAL DISCHARGE AND POSTDISCHARGE CARE

Although the medical measures described earlier, when coupled with coronary revascularization (see Chapter 68), have improved the early outcome in of patients with UA/non-STEMI, these patients often have advanced multivessel coronary artery disease. Thus, secondary prevention is of critical

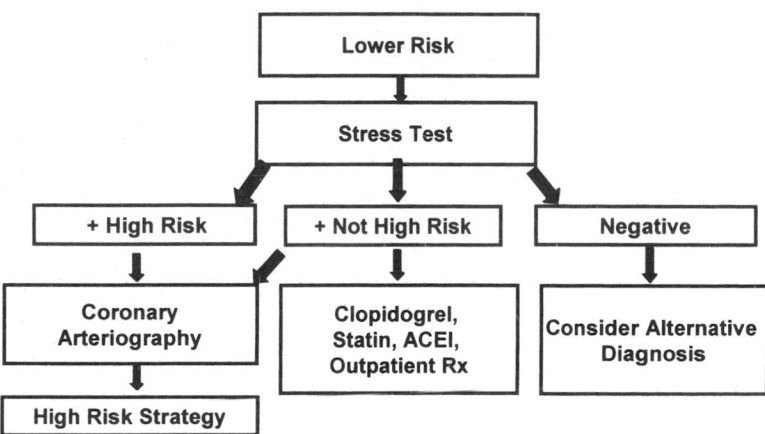

FIG. 65–7. Algorithm for the management of lower risk patients with unstable angina/non–ST-segment elevation myocardial infarction. ACEI, angiotensin-converting enzyme inhibitor; Rx, prescription.

importance and should be started before hospital discharge. Contemporary secondary prevention has a number of components:

1. *Lipid management* (see Chapters 11 and 84): All patients should be placed on an American Heart Association Step 1 diet and, irrespective of their total or low-density lipoprotein cholesterol concentrations, they also should be placed on intensive statin therapy (27a) (or continued on one if they were already receiving such a drug on admission) (2). Although the precise timing of commencing statin therapy and the dosage are still under investigation, it is clear that long-term compliance is improved if the drug is begun before hospital discharge (28), and it is advisable to do so, irrespective of whether coronary revascularization has been carried out (29). A fibrate or niacin should be added if high-density lipoprotein is less than 40 mg/dL. (4)

2. *Control of other risk factors* (see Chapter 84): The diagnosis of UA/non-STEMI should serve as a "wake up call" to intensify control of other coronary risk factors as well, including achievement of optimal weight, smoking cessation, and intensive treatment of hypertension and diabetes mellitus. Fasting blood sugar and hemoglobin A1C measurements should be obtained to detect previously unrecognized diabetes.

3. *Antiplatelet therapy:* Aspirin (75–162 mg/d) and clopidogrel (75 mg/d) should be continued, the former permanently and the latter for at least 9 months.

4. *Antiischemic therapy:* Patients with UA/non-STEMI who do not undergo coronary revascularization are frequently left with chronic stable angina and require antiischemic therapy with nitrates and β-blockers. Calcium blockers are advisable in patients who cannot tolerate β-blockers or in patients with angina despite nitrates and β-blockers. Angiotensin-converting enzyme inhibitors, if started during hospitalization, should be continued. Patients with persistent angina will require reevaluation for revascularization.

REFERENCES

1. Braunwald E, Mark DB, Jones RH, et al. *Unstable angina: diagnosis and management.* Rockville, MD: Agency for Health Care Policy and Research and the National Heart, Lung, and Blood Institute, US Public Health Service, US Department of Health and Human Services; 1994:1. DHHS Publication no. 94-0602.
2. Braunwald E, Antman EM, Beasley JW, et al. ACC/AHA guidelines update for the management of patients with unstable angina and non-ST-segment elevation myocardial infarction: a report of the American College of Cardiology/American Heart Association Task Force on Practice Guidelines (Committee on the Management of Patients with Unstable Angina). 2002. Available at: http://www.acc.org/clinical/guidelines/unstable/unstable.pdf. Accessed on August 10, 2004.
2a. Braunwald E. Application of current guidelines to the management of unstable angina and non-ST segment elevation myocardial infarction. *Circulation* 2003;108[Suppl III]:III–28–III–37.
3. Antman EM, Cohen M, Bernink PJ, et al. The TIMI risk score for unstable angina/non-ST elevation MI: a method for prognostication and therapeutic decision making. *JAMA* 2000;284:835–842.
4. Braunwald E, Antman EM, Beasley JW, et al. ACC/AHA guideline update for the management of patients with unstable angina and non-ST-segment elevation myocardial infarction—2002: summary article. *J Am Coll Cardiol* 2002;40:1366–1374.
5. Budaj A, Yusuf S, Mehta SR, et al. Benefit of clopidogrel in patients with acute coronary syndromes without ST-segment elevation in various risk groups. *Circulation* 2002;106:1622–1626.
6. Sabatine MS, Morrow DA, deLemos J, et al. Multimarker approach to risk stratification in non-ST elevation acute coronary syndromes: simultaneous assessment of troponin I, C-reactive protein, and B-type natriuretic peptide. *Circulation* 2002;105:1760–1763.
7. Granger CB, Califf RM. Stabilizing the unstable artery. In: Califf RM, Wagner GS, eds. *Acute coronary care,* 2nd ed. St. Louis: Mosby–Year Book, 1995:525–541.
8. Yusuf S, Zhao F, Mehta SR, et al. Effects of clopidogrel in addition to aspirin in patients with acute coronary syndromes without ST-segment elevation. *N Engl J Med* 2001;345:494–502.
9. Yusuf S, Mehta SR, Zhau F, et al. Early and late effects of clopidogrel in patients with acute coronary syndromes. *Circulation* 2003;107:966–972.
10. Mehta SR, Yusuf S, Peters RJ, et al. Effects of pretreatment with clopidogrel and aspirin followed by long-term therapy in patients undergoing percutaneous coronary intervention: the PCI-CURE study. *Lancet* 2001;358:527–533.
11. Steinhubl SR, Berger PD, Mann JT III, et al.. Early and sustained dual oral antiplatelet therapy following percutaneous coronary intervention: a randomized controlled trial. The CREDO Investigators. Clopidogrel for the Reduction of Events During Observation. *JAMA* 2002;288:2411–2420.
12. Boersma E, Harrington RA, Moliterno DJ, et al. Platelet glycoprotein IIb/IIIa inhibitors in acute coronary syndromes: a meta-analysis of all major randomised clinical trials. *Lancet* 2002;359:189–198.
13. Wong GC, Giugliano RP, Antman EM. Use of low-molecular-weight heparins in the management of acute coronary artery syndromes and percutaneous coronary intervention. *JAMA* 2003;289:331–342.
14. Antman EM, Cohen M, Radley D, et al. Assessment of the treatment effect of Enoxaparin for unstable angina/non-Q wave myocardial infarction: TIMI 11B ESSENCE meta-analysis. *Circulation* 1999;100:1602–1608.
15. Goodman DG, Fitchett D, Armstrong PW, et al. Randomized evaluation of the safety and efficacy of enoxaparin vs. unfractionated heparin in high risk patients with non-ST segment elevation acute coronary syndromes receiving the glycoprotein IIb/IIIa inhibitor eptifibatide. *Circulation* 2003;107:238–244.
16. Petersen JL, Mahaffey KW, Hasselblad V, et al. A systematic overview of efficacy and bleeding complications among patients randomized to enoxaparin or unfractionated heparin for antithrombin therapy in non-ST-segment elevation acute coronary syndromes. *JAMA* 2004;292:89–100.
17. Muller JE, Tofler GH, Stone PH. Circadian variation and triggers of onset of acute cardiovascular disease. *Circulation* 1989;79:733–743.
18. Yusuf S, Wittes J, Friedman L. Overview of results of randomized clinical trials in heart disease. I. Treatments following myocardial infarction. *JAMA* 1988;260:2088–2093.
19. Yusuf S, Wittes J, Friedman L. Overview of results of randomized clinical trials in heart disease. II. Unstable angina, heart failure, primary prevention with aspirin, and risk factor modification. *JAMA* 1988;260:2259–2263.
20. Theroux P, Taeymans Y, Morissette D, et al. A randomized study comparing propranolol and diltiazem in the treatment of unstable angina. *J Am Coll Cardiol* 1985;5:717–722.
21. Held PH, Yusuf S, Furberg CD. Calcium channel blockers in acute myocardial infarction and unstable angina: an overview. *BMJ* 1989;299:1187–1192.
22. Pepine CJ, Faich G, Makuch R. Verapamil use in patients with cardiovascular disease: an overview of randomized trials. *Clin Cardiol* 1998;28:633–641.
23. Gibson RS, Boden WE, Theroux P, et al. Diltiazem and reinfarction in patients with non-Q-wave myocardial infarction: results of a double-blind, randomized, multicenter trial. *N Engl J Med* 1986;315:423–429.
24. Boden WE, Krone RJ, Kleiger RE, et al. Electrocardiographic subset analysis of diltiazem administration on long-term outcome after acute myocardial infarction. The Multicenter Diltiazem Post-Infarction Trial Research Group. *Am J Cardiol* 1991;67:335–342.
25. Furberg CD, Psaty BM, Meyer JV. Nidefipine: dose-related increase in

mortality in patients with coronary heart disease. *Circulation* 1995;92: 1326–1331.

26. Yusuf S, Sleight P, Pogue J, et al. Effects of an angiotensin-converting-enzyme inhibitor, ramipril, on cardiovascular events in high-risk patients. The Heart Outcomes Prevention Evaluation Study Investigators. *N Engl J Med* 2000;342:145–153.

27. Gibbons RJ, Abrams J, Chatterjee K, et al. ACC/AHA 2002 guideline update for the management of patients with chronic stable angina. 2002. Available at: http://www.acc.org/clinical/guidelines/stable/stable.pdf. Accessed on August 10, 2004.

27a. Cannon CP, Braunwald E, McCabe CH, et al. Intensive versus moderate lipid lowering with statins after acute coronary syndromes. *N Engl J Med* 2004;350:1495–1504.

28. Faronow GC, Ballantyne CM. In-hospital initiation of lipid-lowering therapy for patients with coronary heart disease: the time is now. *Circulation* 2001;103:2768–2770.

29. Serruys PW, de Feyter P, Macaya C, et al. Fluvastatin for prevention of cardiac events following successful first percutaneous coronary intervention: a randomized controlled trial. *JAMA* 2002;287:3215–3222.

CHAPTER 66

Medical Management of ST-Segment Elevation Acute Myocardial Infarction

Álvaro Avezum, Alexandre Biasi Cavalcanti, and Leopoldo Soares Piegas

<table>
<tr><td>

Clinical Course of Acute Myocardial Infarction
General Measures
Specific Pharmacologic Agents
  β-Blockers
  Angiotensin-converting Enzyme Inhibitors
  Aldosterone Blockers
  Angiotensin II Receptor Blockers

</td><td>

Nitrates
Statins
Magnesium
Calcium Antagonists
Prophylactic Antiarrhythmic Therapy
Summary
References

</td></tr>
</table>

Key Words: Adjunctive therapy; clinical practice; evidence-based medicine; myocardial infarction; treatment.

The management of ST-segment elevation acute myocardial infarction (AMI) has changed significantly in recent years. Milestones in advancement were the introduction of coronary care units in the 1960s, fibrinolytics and aspirin in the 1980s, and the increasing use of percutaneous coronary interventions since the 1990s. All these improvements have contributed to reduce mortality rates. However, long-term prevention of new major clinical events has evolved enormously with the verification of the beneficial role of aspirin, β-blockers, angiotensin-converting enzyme (ACE) inhibitors, and statins. Reducing the use of potentially harmful therapies such as Class I antiarrhythmic agents and calcium channel blockers also would help to avoid deaths. More than any other area in medicine, cardiology has had plenty of randomized controlled trials (RCTs) that have helped to estab-

lish robust and relevant evidence to guide treatment. Certainly, the management of patients with AMI will continue to improve with results from new clinical trials; nonetheless, the major challenge for the clinician treating patients with AMI is to apply current evidence in the clinical practice. This review focuses on the management of AMI in patients with ST-segment elevation. First, key aspects of the clinical course of AMI and the different approaches to treatment are discussed. Sequentially, basic mechanisms of action, rationale for use, and clinical evidence for most of available pharmacologic agents that have shown to improve the prognosis when used for the routine treatment of AMI (β-blockers, ACE inhibitors, and statins), those that can alleviate symptoms (nitrates, opioids), and those without clear evidence of benefit or with evidence of harm when routinely used, including magnesium, calcium antagonists, and Class I antiarrhythmics, are summarized. Reperfusion and antithrombotic therapies are discussed in other chapters in this textbook.

The management of ST elevation AMI has changed dramatically over the past decades and is continuously evolving. The introduction of coronary care units in the 1960s, fibrinolytics and aspirin in the 1980s, and the increasing use of percutaneous coronary interventions since the 1990s have contributed to a striking decrease in mortality rates (1–3). In addition, treatment with aspirin, β-blockers, ACE inhibitors, and statins has improved the long-term care of patients surviving an AMI (4–7).

The optimal care of patients with AMI should be based on robust and reliable evidence derived from RCTs (8) and sys-

Á. Avezum: Dante Pazzanese Institute of Cardiology, Research Division Director, Av. Dante Pazzanese, 500, São Paulo, SP, Brazil, 04012-909; and Clinical Research Center-Albert Einstein Education and Research Institute, Albert Einstein Hospital, Av. Albert Einstein, 627/701–São Paulo, SP, Brazil, 05651-901.

A. B. Cavalcanti: Clinical Research Center–Albert Einstein Education and Research Institute, Albert Einstein Hospital, Av. Albert Einstein, 627/701–São Paulo, SP, Brazil 05651-901.

L. S. Piegas: Dante Pazzanese Institute of Cardiology, Director, Av. Dante Pazzanese, 500, São Paulo, SP, Brazil, 04012-909.

tematic overviews (9,10) of RCTs of sufficient size to detect moderate but medically worthwhile risk reductions (e.g., 10%, 15%, or 20%) in the incidence of major adverse outcomes. Despite a large amount of accumulated evidence coming from RCTs and systematic overviews on the benefits of therapeutic interventions on major outcomes such as death and recurrent MI, these scientific evidences have not been adequately implemented in clinical practice, thus failing to prevent adverse events in patients who experience an AMI (11,12). Therefore, we are facing a substantial gap between what we already know (best available scientific evidence) and what we should implement during the daily clinical practice.

This review focuses on the management of AMI in patients with ST-segment elevation. First, this chapter outlines key aspects of the clinical course of AMI and provides an overall framework for the different approaches to treatment. Next it summarizes the basic mechanisms of action, theoretic rationale, and clinical evidence for a number of pharmacologic agents that have been shown to improve the prognosis when used for the routine treatment of AMI (β-blockers, ACE inhibitors, and statins), those that can help to alleviate symptoms (nitrates, opioids), and those for which there is no evidence of benefit or sometimes harm when used routinely, including magnesium, calcium antagonists, and antiarrhythmic therapy. Reperfusion and antithrombotic therapies are discussed in other chapters in this textbook.

CLINICAL COURSE OF ACUTE MYOCARDIAL INFARCTION

It is estimated that between 20% and 30% of patients die within the first hour or so of the onset of symptoms of AMI, and this fatality rate probably has not changed over the last 30 years (13–16). During the initial few days after the AMI, the risk for death decreases, although it still remains substantially increased. The very early deaths are thought to be chiefly from ventricular fibrillation, although it is possible that a significant proportion may result from asystole, bradyarrhythmias, or cardiac rupture (17). These very early deaths may be avoided by preventing the occurrence of AMI and by prompt supportive treatment. In the absence of evidence of coronary disease, efforts at preventing AMI have focused on modifying conventional risk factors such as cigarette smoking, hyperlipidemia, hypertension, obesity, diabetes, and promoting healthy lifestyle behaviors such as aerobic exercise, reducing fat and calorie intake, and eating more fruit and vegetables. This approach is equally, if not more, important for people with documented coronary artery disease.

Early recognition leading to rapid hospitalization and appropriate treatment of patients with suspected AMI and unstable angina is an important part of reducing the burden of death and disability from acute coronary syndromes. The combined approaches of prevention and early treatment

have had a substantial impact on deaths from AMI in several Western countries. For example, deaths from ischemic heart disease have declined by 30% to 35% in both the United States and Canada over the last three decades (18–20). Part of this improvement reflects lower in-hospital case fatality rates after AMI and can be attributed to greater rates of fibrinolytic therapy, aspirin, and β-blocker use and to improvements in supportive therapy and interventions (21). Although the in-hospital case fatality rate has declined substantially in recent decades, it still remains high at about 10% to 15% when data are obtained from a broad range of hospitals (22). These data indicate a continuing need for efforts to develop new approaches to reducing mortality and morbidity.

Survivors of a myocardial infarction (MI) still face a substantial excess risk for further cardiovascular events including an increase in mortality. The long-term outcomes for ST-segment elevation and non–ST-segment elevation MIs are similar (23). Mortality rates after unrecognized and recognized infarctions also are similar (24).

The morbidity burden of AMI also is high. In 6 years the recurrence of an AMI is about 21% and 33% for men and women, respectively (23,25). Heart failure develops in 21% of men and 30% of women (25).

In summary, measures to improve survival for people with AMI include early hospitalization and rapid initiation of proven therapies such as reperfusion with percutaneous coronary intervention or fibrinolytics, within an appropriate time delay, aspirin, β-blockers, and ACE inhibitors. Reducing the use of potentially harmful therapies such as Class I antiarrhythmic agents and calcium channel blockers also would help to avoid some of the early deaths.

GENERAL MEASURES

The approach to the patient with suspected acute coronary syndrome involves early and rapid diagnosis, early risk stratification, relief of pain, assessment of hemodynamic status and appropriate treatment if needed, and prevention or treatment of cardiac arrest, death reinfarction, and heart failure. The prompt recognition of an ST-segment elevation MI is crucial in this early phase, because the benefits of mechanical or pharmacologic reperfusion interventions, the cornerstone of the treatment, are highly time dependent.

The routine measures that must be promptly initiated for every patient with chest pain, suggesting an acute coronary syndrome, is to monitor the electrocardiogram, to obtain an intravenous access, and to supplement oxygen if the patient is experiencing breathlessness, with blood oxygen saturation 90% or less or with signs of heart failure or shock. It also is recommended to monitor the pulse oximetry. An ECG and a short history should be obtained as early as possible (Table 66–1).

Among the initial goals in the treatment of patients with AMI are the relief of chest pain, breathlessness, and anxiety. Treatment of pain can be done with opioids and nitroglyc-

TABLE 66–1. *Routine measures for the management of all the patients with chest pain suggestive of an acute coronary syndrome*

- Supplemental oxygen, especially if the patient experiences breathlessness or has blood oxygen saturation ≤90%
- Intravenous access
- Pain relief (opioids and nitroglycerin)
- Electrocardiography monitoring
- Electrocardiogram obtained and interpreted within 10 minutes of arrival in the emergency department

erin. There is no evidence from randomized clinical trials comparing the two approaches. However, trials that compared nitrates with placebo in the acute phase did not show a survival benefit for the group that received nitrates (26,27). Morphine is the opioid most commonly used for this purpose, with an initial intravenous dose of 4 to 8 mg, and repeated doses of 2 mg at 5-minute intervals, as needed (28). Besides alleviating the pain, they reduce anxiety and, if present, pulmonary congestion. Common side effects are nausea, vomiting, hypotension, bradycardia, and respiratory depression. In the event of important side effects, especially respiratory depression, naloxone can be used. Nitrates can be used alternatively or if inadequate response to opioids occurs (29).

Patients with a ST-segment elevation MI should be admitted to an intensive care unit (if possible, a coronary care unit), although the initial management, including reperfusion therapy, should be initiated either at the emergency department, or at the catheterization laboratory, if percutaneous coronary intervention is the strategy of choice. In uncomplicated cases, bed rest may only be necessary for 24 to 48 hours, and the duration of hospital stay may be as short as 4 to 5 days, depending on facilities for risk stratification and early rehabilitation (30).

SPECIFIC PHARMACOLOGIC AGENTS

β-Blockers

β-Adrenoceptor blocking drugs, or β-blockers, have been available for clinical use for about four decades. In 1948, Ahlquist (31) described the α and β receptors responsible for adrenergic responses. α Receptors are mainly stimulated by epinephrine, and peripheral artery vasoconstriction is the most important vascular response. β receptors can be divided into β_1 receptors, which are predominantly found in the heart, and β_2 receptors, which are found in bronchial, uterine, and vascular smooth muscle (32). β_2 Receptors also have been described in the heart, but their functional significance is unclear. Vascular effects mediated through the β receptors pathways include vasodilatation and myocardial stimulation, but β receptor stimulation also inhibits uterine and bronchial smooth muscle contraction. β Receptors also are involved in a number of metabolic and hor-

monal processes including glucose metabolism and renin secretion (33).

Rationale for Use of β-Blockers

β-Blockers reduce oxygen demand by decreasing heart rate and blood pressure. They may also oppose the potential direct adverse effects of sympathetic activation in AMI and have useful antiarrhythmic properties. Experimental studies of β-blocker use in AMI have shown decreased epicardial ST-segment elevation, Q-wave development, and cardiac enzyme release, as well as a reduction in infarct size (34). Clinical studies of β-blockers in AMI have generally confirmed these findings and have provided evidence of a decrease in the frequency and recurrence of chest pain and cardiac rupture (35–38). In addition, a decrease in early ventricular fibrillation also has been demonstrated (39). β-Blockers also inhibit the left ventricular remodeling and improve its hemodynamic function, especially the diastolic function with a less restrictive pattern (40,41).

Evidence for Use of β-Blockers

The largest trial of the use of early intravenous β-blockers was ISIS-1 (International Studies of Infarct Survival), which included 16,027 patients and evaluated the effects of intravenous atenolol started within 12 hours of the onset of chest pain followed by 7 days of oral atenolol, compared with standard therapy in the treatment of AMI (42). Vascular mortality during the treatment period (Days 0–7) was significantly less in the treated group compared with the control group (3.89% vs. 4.75%, respectively; 15% mortality rate reduction [95% confidence interval (CI), 1–27%; $p < 0.04$) (Table 66–2). The reduction in mortality was most marked during the first 2 days after the initiation of therapy (25%; $p < 0.003$) and was chiefly a result of reduction in cardiac rupture and ventricular fibrillation (43). Similar mortality results were obtained in another large trial involving 5,778 patients, the Metoprolol In Acute Myocardial Infarction (MIAMI) trial (44). Although the overall results were not significant (13% mortality reduction, 95% CI 8% to 33%; $p = 0.29$), they were very consistent with the ISIS-1 results. A systematic review performed by Yusuf and colleagues (7) pooling the results of all 27 available randomized trials indicates that such treatment reduces mortality by 13% ($p < 0.02$; 95% CI, −2% to −25%), nonfatal reinfarction by 19% ($p < 0.01$; 95% CI, −5% to 33%), and nonfatal cardiac arrest by 19% ($p < 0.02$; 95% CI, −2% to −30%) in the first week (42). These data indicate a 16% reduction in the risk for experiencing one of these major events ($p < 0.0002$).

The Thrombolysis In Myocardial Infarction (TIMI) II-B study compared the effect of immediate intravenous versus delayed (started 6 days later) oral metoprolol in 1,434 patients undergoing thrombolytic therapy with tissue plasminogen activator (t-PA) (45). There was a lower incidence of reinfarction (2.7% vs. 5.1 %; $p = 0.02$) and recurrent

TABLE 66–2. *Recommended β-blockers after myocardial infarction*

Drug	Intravenous dosage	Initial oral dosage	Target oral dosage
Propranolol	—	40 mg t.i.d.	180–240 mg/d in 3–4 divided doses
Metoprolol	5 mg 3 times at 2-min interval	50 mg b.i.d.	100 mg b.i.d.
Atenolol	5 mg over 5 min; repeat 5 min later	50 mg daily	100 mg daily
Timolol	—	5 mg b.i.d.	10 mg b.i.d.
Carvedilol	—	6.25 mg b.i.d.	25 mg b.i.d.

Achievement of the target dose often is limited by hypotension and bradycardia; therefore, the clinical response dictates the adjustment of the drug dose.

chest pain (18.8% vs. 24.1%; $p < 0.02$) at 6 days in the group receiving immediate intravenous metoprolol. Intracranial hemorrhage also occurred less frequently in the early metoprolol group than in the delayed group (0.3% vs. 1.4%, respectively; $p < 0.03$).

A more recent systematic review of β-blockers trials in AMI, including two trials done in the postthrombolytic era, confirmed a survival benefit for those who were allocated to receive long-term β-blockers (23% reduction in mortality rates; 95% CI, 15–31%) (5).

Benefits of β-blockade in reducing mortality and morbidity also are seen in patients with "relative contraindications" to such therapy, as patients with mild to moderate chronic obstructive lung disease (COPD) or asthma are not on β-agonist therapy (46,47).

Earlier studies of β-blockers in AMI generally did not include patients with asymptomatic left ventricular dysfunction or heart failure (42,44). The Carvedilol Post-Infarct Survival Control in LV Dysfunction (CAPRICORN) trial was the first trial to study the effects of a β-blocker, carvedilol (it also blocks α-adrenergic receptors), in patients with AMI and a left ventricular ejection fraction of 40% or less (48). Carvedilol was started at 6.25 mg twice daily and up-titrated to 25 mg twice daily. Compared with the placebo group, those patients who received carvedilol did not have a different incidence in the primary end points of all-cause mortality or hospitalization for cardiovascular causes (35% vs. 37%; hazard ratio, 0.92; 95% CI, 0.80–1.07), although there were statistically significant reductions in the other primary end points of all-cause mortality alone (12% vs. 15%; hazard ratio, 0.77; 95% CI, 0.60–0.98; $p = 0.03$), and also in the secondary end point of nonfatal MI (3% vs. 6%; hazard ratio, 0.59%; 95% CI, 0.39–0.90; $p = 0.014$).

Short-Term versus Long-Term Trials

Although the long-term benefit of oral therapy with β-blockers is clearly established, the short-term benefit and the intravenous administration are still under debate. Prethrombolysis era trials and systematic reviews reported a reduction in short-term mortality (7,42,44). The studies with intravenous administration of β-blockers in patients submitted to fibrinolytics did not detect a survival benefit (45,49); however, they were not conclusive because of the small number of events observed, and, consequently, lack of ade-

quate statistical power. A systematic review that pooled the prethrombolytic and postthrombolytic era studies found no survival benefit in the short term (5); however, early use of intravenous β-blockers decreased the incidence of recurrent MI, chest pain, and intracerebral hemorrhage observed even in the most recent trials (42,44,45).

Different β-Blockers in Acute Myocardial Infarction

Propranolol, metoprolol, timolol, carvedilol, and atenolol are among the drugs best tested in RCTs (5,42,44,45,48). For early intravenous use, metoprolol and atenolol can be administered. For oral long-term administration, any drug, without intrinsic sympathomimetic activity, may be used. Drugs with proven benefits in mortality are propranolol and timolol (5), although another study found no difference among propranolol, metoprolol, and atenolol (50). For patients after MI with left ventricular dysfunction, long-term use of carvedilol offers benefit on survival improvement (48).

One major issue for the treatment of patients with AMI is the underuse of β-blockers, because a large amount of patients with AMI do not receive them, despite the overwhelming evidence of the beneficial effect of β-blocker therapy. Between 80% and 90% of patients with acute AMI are eligible for β-blocker treatment (46); but in a large international registry, only 72% were discharged from the hospital using β-blockers (51). Several factors contribute to the underuse of β-blockers after AMI. Exaggerated concern of adverse effects may play a pivotal role, as demonstrated by the smaller chance of patients with COPD, the very elderly, those with heart failure or left ventricular dysfunction, and insulin-dependent diabetics receiving β-blockers. These patients at high risk for adverse outcomes after AMI can benefit from β-blockade (46).

Recommendations

All patients without absolute contraindications should be treated with a β-blocker. Intravenous β-blockers in the early treatment should be offered to all patients with AMI. More important, however, is to reassure long-term oral β-blocker treatment, because it has been established that it can positively affect survival and risk for other major cardiovascular events in the treated patients.

Angiotensin-converting Enzyme Inhibitors

The renin-angiotensin-aldosterone system is substantially activated within 72 hours from the onset of AMI (52–54). Angiotensin II can adversely affect the balance of myocardial oxygen demand and supply by causing coronary vasoconstriction (thereby decreasing myocardial blood flow), increasing the heart inotropic state, and increasing ventricular wall stress. After AMI, prognosis is substantially influenced by the occurrence and extent of left ventricular dilatation, which is associated with an increased risk for congestive heart failure, myocardial aneurysm formation, cardiac rupture, and death (55–58). A major precipitating cause of ventricular dilatation is early infarct expansion, which can start in the first few days after AMI (57,59,60). Later progressive ventricular dilatation, which is usually associated with larger infarcts, starts during the first few months after AMI and may be the result of increased wall stress, produced by remodeling of the infarcted and noninfarcted areas (61). ACE is abnormally increased in the edges of the infarct zone, generating high amounts of angiotensin II, which plays a pivotal role in the remodeling process. Experimental studies have shown that ACE inhibitors may reduce infarct size, ventricular wall stress, and subsequent ventricular dilatation in AMI (61–64).

The clinical benefits associated with ACE inhibitors after AMI are mostly attributed to inhibition of the left ventricular remodeling process though inhibitions in the conversion of angiotensin I to angiotensin II. However, it is likely that ACE inhibitors play additional direct mechanisms on the heart and vasculature that are important, including the following: improvement in endothelial function (65); preservation of ischemic preconditioning (66); antagonizing the direct effects of angiotensin II on vasoconstriction and proliferation of vascular smooth muscle cells (67); reduction in the risk for plaque rupture (68); reduction of left ventricular hypertrophy (67); improvement in the oxygen supply/demand ratio (69); favorable effects in fibrinolysis by means of reductions in the plasminogen activator inhibitor 1 and increases in t-PA (70,71); and reduction in the procoagulant activity and in the inflammatory response (72). All these properties favor the reduction of ischemia and recurrence of infarctions.

Evidence for Use of Angiotensin-converting Enzyme Inhibitors

The effect of ACE inhibitors in mortality reduction of patients who experienced an AMI is definitively proven by a substantial body of evidence from well conducted and adequately powered RCTs (26,27,73–77) and systematic overviews (78,79). Several clinical trials showed an improvement in left ventricular ejection fraction after an AMI in those patients randomized to receive an ACE inhibitor compared with placebo (26,27,73–79).

More important, however, is the finding of reduced mortality in most of the studies that evaluated both the early and the long-term use of ACE inhibitors. In a systematic overview (78) of the early treatment of AMI with ACE inhibitors, almost 100,000 patients from four trials (26,27,76,80) were pooled. In these studies, the ACE inhibitor or the placebo was started within the acute phase (0–36 hours) and maintained for up to 4 to 6 weeks. The 30-day mortality rate was reduced from 7.6% in the control group to 7.1% in the treated group, corresponding to a 7% relative risk reduction (95% CI, 2–11%; $p < 0.004$). The number of patients needed to treat (NNT) to avoid 1 death was 200. The relative reduction in mortality risk was generally consistent across different subgroups. Therefore, the greatest benefit was derived for the high absolute risk group, such as those with anterior infarction (NNT = 94), with heart failure (NNT = 71), or with heart rate of 100 spm or greater (NNT = 44). This systematic review also showed that most of the benefit occurred in the first days, when mortality is greater. A total of 40% of the 30-day survival advantage was achieved on Day 1, and 80% of the deaths were avoided in the first week of treatment. Therefore, it is important to start ACE inhibitors in the first day to give the maximum benefit to the patients, although it is possible to wait 2 to 12 hours until the patient has received other therapies such as reperfusion, β-blockers, and opioids and have optimum hemodynamic status.

The effects of the long-term use of an ACE inhibitor in patients who survived an AMI were evaluated in three RCTs with more than 1,000 patients each (73,74,77). Data for the 5,966 patients included in these trials were pooled in a systematic overview (79). The patients had evidence of left ventricular dysfunction or heart failure and started receiving an ACE inhibitor between 3 and 16 days after AMI. The treatment lasted for a minimum of 12 months. After a median follow-up of 31 months, there were 23.4% of deaths in the ACE inhibitor versus 29.1% in the control group (odds ratio [OR] = 0.74; 95% CI, 0.66–0.83; $p < 0.0001$). To avoid 1 death, about 15 patients would need to be treated for 31 months (NNT = 15). Consistent with the overview of short-term trials, the benefits were apparent soon after randomization: In 6 weeks, the relative risk reduction for death was 32.8%. The risk for readmission for heart failure (OR, 0.73; 95% CI, 0.63–0.85; NNT = 28) and recurrent AMI (OR, 0.8; 95% CI, 0.64–0.94; NNT = 71) also was reduced by ACE inhibitors. Other features such as age, sex, initial blood pressure or heart rate, and treatment (receiving or not receiving aspirin, β-blockers, diuretics) did not modify the beneficial response to ACE inhibitors in patients after AMI.

The observation of reduced risk for recurrent AMI in patients receiving ACE inhibitors in the post-AMI study, Survival And Ventricular Enlargement (SAVE), and the Studies of Left Ventricular Dysfunction (SOLVD) studies irrespective of the left ventricular function had been used as the rationale for the conduction of the Heart Outcomes Prevention Evaluation (HOPE) study (81). In this trial, an ACE inhibitor, ramipril, was compared with placebo in patients who were at high risk for cardiovascular events but who did not have heart failure or left ventricular dysfunction. Inclusion criteria were evidence of atherothrombotic disease (coronary artery disease, stroke, peripheral vascular disease) or patients with diabetes with another cardiovascular risk factor. A total of 9,297 patients were randomly assigned to receive ramipril (10 mg once daily) or placebo for a mean of 5 years. The primary outcome, a composite of MI, stroke, or death from cardiovascular causes, occurred in 14.0% of patients in the ramipril group and 17.8% of patients in the placebo group (relative risk, 0.78%; 95% CI, 0.70–0.86; $p < 0.001$). The NNT was 26. When analyzed separately, all the end points were significantly reduced in the group that received ramipril compared with the placebo group: Death from cardiovascular causes was 6.1% versus 8.1% (relative risk, 0.74; 95% CI, 0.64–0.84; $p < 0.001$); AMI was 9.9 versus 12.3 (relative risk, 0.80; 95% CI, 0.70–0.90; $p < 0.001$); and stroke was 3.4% versus 4.9% (relative risk, 0.68; 95% CI, 0.56–0.84; $p < 0.001$). The risk for death from any cause also was reduced by ramipril: 10.4% versus 12.2% (relative risk, 0.84; 95% CI, 0.75–0.95; $p = 0.005$). Subgroup analysis demonstrated a beneficial effect of ramipril on the composite outcome in all the predefined subgroups: diabetics and nondiabetics, women and men, patients with or without evidence of cardiovascular disease, patients younger or older than 65 years old, those with or without hypertension, and those with or without microalbuminuria. There also were benefits irrespective of aspirin use. Therefore, in a large randomized trial, it was demonstrated that in patients with evidence of atherothrombotic disease or at high risk for development of cardiovascular events, but without heart failure or left ventricular systolic dysfunction, the use of an ACE inhibitor is beneficial to reduce major complications.

The best studied ACE inhibitors in the short-term after an AMI are lisinopril (26), captopril (27,73,76), zofenopril (75), and enalapril (80); in the long-term, they are captopril (73), ramipril (74), and trandolapril (77); and, in the long-term for patients without heart failure or left ventricular dysfunction, ramipril is the best studied inhibitor (81). Thus, to expect reproduction of the benefits seen in the clinical trials, it is necessary to use the tested drugs and, most important, to prescribe the drug according to the protocols used in the trials reported (Table 66–3).

TABLE 66–3. *Recommended angiotensin-converting enzyme inhibitors after myocardial infarction*

Angiotensin-converting enzyme (reference)	Initial dose	Target dosage
Lisinopril (26)	5 mg	10 mg once per day
Captopril (27,73,76)	6.25 mg	50 mg b.i.d.
Enalapril (80)	2.5 mg	10 mg b.i.d.
Ramipril (74,81)	2.5 mg	10 mg once per day
Trandolapril (77)	1 mg	2–4 mg once per day
Zofenopril (75)	7.5 mg	30 mg b.i.d.

Recommendations

On the basis of current evidence, it is recommended that all patients who experienced an AMI receive an ACE inhibitor within the first 24 hours and be continued long-term on this therapy. The benefits of ACE inhibitors were demonstrated in patients already receiving other proven therapies, such as aspirin and β-blockers. Therefore, they must be considered additive and not substitute therapies. Clinically significant hypotension in the setting of adequate preload, pregnancy, and hypersensitivity are the main contraindications to use of an ACE inhibitor. The most common adverse reactions are hypotension, cough, and worsening of renal function. To avoid hypotension, it is recommended to start with low doses and increase steadily to achieve a full dose. Unnecessary use of nitrates for patients without chest pain is a common cause of hypotension, limiting the use of ACE inhibitors. Nitrates do not improve the prognosis of patients with AMI, but ACE inhibitors do, and, therefore, nitrates should not be used routinely but should be reserved for patients with AMI with ongoing chest pain (26,27). Currently, there is unequivocal evidence on the benefits of ACE inhibitor therapy for patients who experienced an AMI. However, the actual worldwide prescription is much less than would be expected. In a report from the Global Registry of Acute Coronary Events (GRACE) evaluating the treatment of 11,543 patients with acute coronary syndrome in 14 countries, from 1999 to 2001, only 66% of patients with ST-segment elevation AMI received ACE inhibitors during admission, and this proportion was even less (60%) at discharge (51).

Aldosterone Blockers

Serum levels of aldosterone are generally increased in patients with heart failure, and local production of aldosterone also occurs in the heart, proportionally to the severity of heart failure (82). The actions of aldosterone can be deleterious for patients with ventricular dysfunction because in addition to causing retention of sodium and loss of potassium and magnesium, it increases sympathetic activation; inhibits parasympathetic axis, stimulates cardiac and vascular hypertrophy, fibrosis, and remodeling; and increases cardiac arrhythmias (83–85). Spironolactone, an aldosterone receptor blocker, reduces mortality and morbidity in patients with severe heart failure (86). The role of blocking aldosterone in patients with heart failure after AMI was tested in the Eplerenone Post-acute myocardial infarction Heart failure Efficacy and SUrvival Study (EPHESUS) trial (87). Eplerenone, a selective aldosterone blocker, was compared with placebo in 6,642 patients with left ventricular ejection fraction of 40% or less and signs of heart failure (clinical or radiologic). The study drug was started 3 to 14 days after AMI. After a mean follow-up of 16 months, the primary end point, death, occurred in 478 (14.4%) patients in the eplerenone group and 554 (16.7%) patients in the placebo group (relative risk, 0.85; 95% CI, 0.75–0.96; $p = 0.008$; NNT = 44). Cardiovascular death plus hospitalization because of cardiovascular events was another evaluated end point, and it was also reduced in the eplerenone group (relative risk, 0.87; 95% CI, 0.72–0.94; $p = 0.005$; NNT = 30). On the basis of the results of the EPHESUS trial and considering the evidence from experimental studies and clinical studies in patients with heart failure, eplerenone may be considered for patients with AMI who have left ventricular ejection fraction less than 40% and heart failure, after reassuring that β-blockers and ACE inhibitors have been already prescribed. The initial dosage is 25 mg once daily and should be increased to 50 mg after 4 weeks if there are no adverse reactions.

Angiotensin II Receptor Blockers

Blockade of angiotensin II is incomplete during ACE inhibition (88); therefore, a more complete blockade of angiotensin II action, by direct inhibition of its receptor, would seem potentially beneficial. This hypothesis was tested in the Optimal Trial In Myocardial infarction with Angiotensin II Antagonist Losartan (OPTIMAAL) trial, which was a RCT that evaluated 5,477 patients, 60 years of age or older, with signs of heart failure within 10 days of an AMI (89). Patients were assigned to receive captopril (target dosage of 50 mg three times daily) or losartan (50 mg once daily). All-cause mortality was the primary end point, and it occurred in 499 patients (18%) in the losartan group versus 447 patients (16%) in the captopril group (relative risk, 1.13; 95% CI, 0.99–1.28; $p = 0.07$). There were no significant differences in other efficacy end points. Because there was a trend to increase the risk for death in the losartan group, the ACE inhibitors remain the first choice treatment for patients after having AMI.

The role of the combination of an angiotensin II receptor blocker with ACE inhibitors in patients with AMI is currently unknown, but it is being evaluated in the Valsartan in Acute Myocardial Infarction Trial (VALIANT) study (90).

Nitrates

Organic nitrates are vasodilators that have effects on both the venous and arterial systems. The biologically active substance is nitric oxide (NO), produced by nitrates through a series of enzymatic steps. NO exerts its actions through direct effects on vascular smooth muscle. Prolonged exposure of vascular smooth muscle to organic nitrates attenuates its hemodynamic response, a condition known as "tolerance" (91,92). The syndrome and etiology of nitrate tolerance is still being investigated, but depletion of certain key substrates involved in the production of NO at a cellular level (e.g., sulfhydryl groups) may decrease NO production and may be one cause of loss of effect of nitrates. In the acute phase of MI, nitrates might improve oxygenation of the ischemic zone by improving the balance of epicardial to endocardial blood flow. They also reduce preload and afterload, thereby decreasing myocardial work and oxygen demand (93–95). Experimental studies of nitrates in AMI have shown a reduction in infarct size and improved regional myocardial function (96–98). Nitrates also have been shown to be useful for pain relief in AMI in conjunction with narcotic analgesics.

Clinical Studies

Several clinical studies have shown favorable effects of nitrates on infarct size, left ventricular function, and clinical events (mortality and major morbidity) before the routine use of thrombolytic therapy and aspirin (99–102). Most of the RCTs were individually too small to assess adequately the effects of nitrates on important clinical outcomes, and this information is summarized in a systematic overview of ten RCTs (seven using intravenous nitroglycerin and three using intravenous nitroprusside [103–110] involving 2,042 patients published in 1988 [111]). When taken together, these trials suggest that nitrates may reduce the mortality rate after AMI by up to 35% (95% CI, 28–49%; $p < 0.001$), and similar data were available from less patients for oral nitrates, although the estimate of treatment effect was somewhat lower at about 20% and was not statistically significant (111,112). The greatest reduction in mortality occurred during the first week or so of follow-up, with a nonsignificant further reduction after this early period. More recent evidence has come from two megatrials that have investigated nitrate therapy in the context of routine use of thrombolytic therapy and aspirin (under a background of liberal use of nontrial nitrates, whenever thought to be clinically indicated, leading to contamination). The Gruppo Italiano per lo Studio della Sopravvivenza nell'Infarto Miocardico (GISSI)-3 trial randomized 19,394 patients to a 24-hour infusion of nitroglycerin (starting within 24 hours of pain onset) followed by topical nitroglycerin, 10 mg daily for 6 weeks (with the patch removed at bedtime allowing a 10-hour nitrate-free interval to avoid tolerance), or to control (26). About 50% of patients in the control group received nontrial intravenous nitrates in the first day or so. There was a slight, nonsignificant reduction in mortality at 6 weeks in the group randomized to nitrate therapy compared with control (6.52% vs. 6.92%, respectively; OR, 0.94; 95% CI, 0.84–1.05), with a similar result in the prespecified combined end point of death plus left ventricular dysfunction or clinical heart failure (15.9% vs. 16.7%; OR, 0.94; 95% CI, 0.87–1.02). In GISSI-3, the effects of the ACE inhibitor lisinopril also were compared with control in a 2 × 2 factorial design (for results, see the section on ACE inhibitors later in this chapter).

The other megatrial, ISIS-4, compared 28-day treatment of controlled-release oral isosorbide mononitrate with placebo control (as well as intravenous magnesium sulphate versus control and the ACE inhibitor captopril versus placebo control in a $2 \times 2 \times 2$ factorial design) in 58,000 patients with suspected AMI (27). The controlled-release nitrate in ISIS-4 has a dose-release profile in which most of the active drug is released within 12 hours of administration, with a relatively "nitrate-poor" period at night, which is designed to avoid the development of tolerance. Mononitrates are active after oral administration by largely avoiding the "first-pass" metabolism through the liver and reach peak plasma concentrations after about 1 hour (113). The results of ISIS-4 were remarkably consistent with GISSI-3, with a small, nonsignificant reduction in 35-day mortality in the mononitrate group compared with placebo (7.26% vs. 7.47%, respectively). However, as in GISSI-3, about 50% of patients in the control group received nontrial intravenous nitrates during the first 24 to 48 hours after randomization. The combined data from all the RCTs of nitrate versus control show that there is a clinically small (5.8% to 2.6%) relative reduction in mortality that is just statistically significant ($p = 0.02$). In both GISSI-3 and ISIS-4, the power to detect any real beneficial effects of routine nitrate therapy was probably reduced by extensive early use ($>$50%) of nontrial nitrate during the first day or so in the control groups. This may explain the much smaller effect size seen in these trial results compared with the metaanalysis of older trials.

Both recent large trials confirmed that nitrate therapy, whether given intravenously or orally, is safe and well tolerated when started in the acute phase of MI. The results of these studies do not support the routine use of nitrates, but this approach is not substantially refuted by the way in which the trials were designed (i.e., allowing extensive use of early, nontrial intravenous nitrates, named contamination). In any case, nitrates are clinically useful agents for selected patients with AMI, especially those with continuing ischemic symptoms or heart failure.

Statins

Several trials have demonstrated the beneficial effects of statin therapy on morbidity and mortality for patients with previous AMI (114–116). Evidence from observational studies indicates that the lower the low-density lipoprotein (LDL) cholesterol level, the lower the risk is for coronary heart disease, without a threshold below which additional reductions are not accompanied by reduced risk (117). The large clinical trial Heart Protection Study could confirm this observation (118). The Heart Protection Study included 20,536 adults (40–80 years old) with high risk for occlusive cardiovascular events and randomized them to treatment with simvastatin (40 mg daily) or placebo. There was no lower LDL-cholesterol threshold in the inclusion criteria. After 5 years, all-cause mortality was reduced in the simvastatin group (12.9% vs. 14.7%; relative risk, 0.87; 95% CI, 0.81–0.84; $p = 0.0003$; NNT = 55) largely because of a reduction in coronary deaths and in other vascular deaths. Reduction of about 25% was observed for AMI, stroke, and coronary or noncoronary revascularization. The propor-

tional reduction in events was similar and significant in all the subgroups evaluated, even in those who had initial LDL cholesterol less than 116 mg/dL.

A question that remains unanswered is whether beginning statins in the acute post-MI phase is safe and effective. Secondary prevention trials have evaluated statins started 3 months after an AMI. However, several mechanisms are proposed for the beneficial effects of statins that do not involve lipid reduction and that, altogether, could possibly have a favorable effect on plaque stability and reduction of thrombosis (119). This rationale prompted the accomplishment of the Myocardial Ischaemia Reduction with Aggressive Cholesterol Lowering (MIRACL) study to evaluate the role of statins in acute coronary syndromes (120). In this trial, 3,086 adults with non–ST-segment elevation acute coronary syndromes were randomized to receive 80 mg atorvastatin or placebo between 1 and 4 days after hospital admission. The primary end point, a combination of death, nonfatal AMI, cardiac arrest with resuscitation, and recurrent symptomatic ischemia with objective evidence and requiring hospitalization, was reduced in the group receiving atorvastatin (14.8% vs. 17.4%; relative risk, 0.84; 95% CI, 0.70–1.00; $p = 0.048$). This benefit was caused by a reduction in symptomatic ischemia, but no reduction was observed on death, nonfatal AMI, or cardiac arrest rates. Another study was presented that involved early statin treatment for unstable angina and AMI; however, it was prematurely stopped by commercial reasons, and after including 3,408 patients, there was no difference in clinical events after a month (121).

Therefore, current evidence is actually not conclusive, and the results of other ongoing trials are necessary to clarify this question. Nevertheless, many authors advocate early statin therapy for ACS based on the possible nonlipid effects of statins plus evidence of greater adherence if the treatment is started in the hospital (122). Conversely, withdrawal of statin in patients already using the drug when admitted is not recommended on the basis of results from observational studies that have demonstrated it is associated with significantly increased risk for death and recurrent AMI (hazard ratio, 2.93; 95% CI, 1.64–6.27; $p = 0.005$) (123).

Magnesium

Several actions of magnesium could contribute toward a cardioprotective effect when given in AMI. These actions include a coronary vasodilator action, reduced myocardial oxygen demand by decreasing peripheral vascular resistance and sinus node slowing, platelet inhibition, preservation of high-energy phosphate supplies, prevention of calcium overload in ischemic myocardium, limitation of oxygen-derived free radicals injury, and suppression of arrhythmias during ischemia and reperfusion (124–129). There is evidence from experimental studies that magnesium supplements might also reduce infarct size by limiting reperfusion injury (124,129–131). The original rationale for using magnesium in AMI was to reduce the incidence of serious arrhythmias. Seven small RCTs have been combined in a metaanalysis (all conducted in patients not routinely treated with thrombolytic and antiplatelet therapy) with a total of 1,300 patients and only 78 deaths (132–138). This metaanalysis suggested a substantial benefit with magnesium (risk reduction of 55%; 95% CI, 29–72%; $p < 0.001$) (139). The second Leicester Intravenous Magnesium Intervention Trial (LIMIT-2) investigated the effects of intravenous magnesium versus placebo control in 2,316 patients and demonstrated a borderline statistically significant benefit with magnesium on mortality (7.8% in the magnesium group vs. 10.3% in the control group; risk reduction, 24%; 95% CI, 1–43%; $p < 0.04$) (140) that persisted on longer term follow-up (mean 2.7 years) with a risk reduction in cardiovascular mortality of 21% (95% CI, 5–35%; $p = 0.01$) (141). The data on magnesium therefore appeared to be promising on the basis of experimental data, the initial safety and efficacy data, and that the regimens tested were simple and inexpensive.

The ISIS-4 study has reported on the effects of intravenous magnesium sulfate versus control in 58,000 patients with suspected AMI (27). The results demonstrated a nonsignificant adverse effect of magnesium on mortality, which sharply contradicted the previous evidence from the metaanalysis (139) and LIMIT-2 (140). At 35 days of follow-up, there were 2,216 deaths out of 29,009 patients in the group receiving magnesium compared with 2,103 deaths out of 29,034 patients who received standard treatment (7.64% vs. 7.24%; OR, 1.06; 95% CI, 1.00–1.13; $p = 0.07$). This lack of benefit was consistent across all major subgroups, including patients treated early or those treated later and those receiving or not receiving concomitant thrombolytic therapy. There has been much debate in attempting to reconcile these apparently discrepant pieces of information about the efficacy of magnesium in AMI. A potential explanation to this conflicting data among the results of the systematic review of the smaller trials plus experimental evidence and the results of ISIS-4 is that the alleged benefit of magnesium in MI lies on limiting reperfusion injury, and this could only happen if magnesium is administered before, simultaneously, or early after reperfusion, be it fibrinolysis or primary angioplasty. In the ISIS-4 trial, magnesium sulfate was administered after fibrinolytics, and the randomization occurred at a median of 8 hours from onset of chest pain. Therefore, the magnesium blood level increases occurred out of the therapeutic window (142). However, the lack of benefit in ISIS-4 was consistent across all major subgroups, including patients treated very early or those treated later and those treated or not treated with thrombolytic therapy. Further analysis of ISIS-4 indicates that there was no evidence of benefit of magnesium even among the 10,252 patients randomized within 3 hours of symptom onset. In these patients, it is likely that recanalization of the infarct-related coronary artery and the infusion of magnesium should have been almost simultaneous. The most recent Magnesium in Coronary Arteries (MAGIC) trial tested if the magnesium treatment would be able to prevent short-term mortality when administered early to patients with ST-segment elevation AMI (143). The early administra-

tion of magnesium was compared with placebo in 6,213 patients. No differences in outcomes were detected between the two groups, or even in the various subgroups analyzed.

After exploring the possible role of magnesium in more than 68,000 patients, in several trials and different settings, it can be concluded that this drug offers no benefit as routine treatment for AMI. Also, there is no particular subgroup in which this drug should be indicated, except when there is documented magnesium deficit or for the treatment of polymorphic ventricular arrhythmias with a prolonged baseline QT interval (Torsades de pointes) (144). In conclusion, currently, intravenous magnesium cannot be recommended as a routine therapy for the treatment of AMI.

Calcium Antagonists

The concentration of intracellular calcium ions is now recognized to be a key regulator and messenger for a number of important cellular functions. The movement of calcium, across the cellular membrane, is carefully controlled by the calcium current, the sodium–calcium exchange mechanism, and other active and passive processes (145,146). Influx of calcium into cells through the calcium current plays an important role in cardiac contraction, generation of impulses in the sinus and atrioventricular nodes, and regulation of the tone of vascular smooth muscle, including coronary arteries and peripheral resistance arterioles (147). The influx of excess calcium into cells during ischemia has been found to be associated with increased cellular damage. Therefore, preventing these adverse events during ischemia theoretically might be expected to reduce infarct size and perhaps improve ventricular function. Calcium channel antagonists specifically regulate the voltage-dependent entry of calcium ions in the myocardium, nodal tissue, and vascular smooth muscle by blocking the slow calcium channels through a direct action (148).

Calcium antagonists have been classified by taking into account their structural and pharmacologic differences. On the basis of chemical grouping, there are the phenylalkylamines (e.g., verapamil), the benzothiazepines (e.g., diltiazem), and the dihydropyridines (e.g., nifedipine). These groups have different molecular structures and bind to different sites on the sarcolemma. These differences may account for the spectrum of clinical effects of the three agents.

Potential beneficial mechanisms of action include (a) reduction of oxygen demand by decreasing blood pressure and myocardial contractility; (b) dilation of coronary vessels and prevention of calcium overload of ischemic cells; (c) reduction in experimental infarct size; (d) reduction in incidence of arrhythmias; (e) increase in endocardial perfusion; and (f) reduction in "stunning" of ischemic myocardium (149).

Clinical Studies

There is no clear clinical evidence supporting the routine use of calcium antagonists in AMI. None of the trials has indicated a reduction in mortality, although there is some evidence for preventing reinfarction with the nondihydropyridine compounds. Data are available from a metaanalysis of 23 randomized trials in a total of 19,600 patients (150–152). Seven studies included more than 1,000 patients, whereas most evaluated less than 200 patients. Although six different agents have been tested, most data come from trials of nifedipine, diltiazem, and verapamil. The Trial of Nifedipine in Acute Myocardial Infarction (TRENT) study compared the effect on mortality of nifedipine for 1 month versus placebo in 4,491 patients with suspected MI (70% of patients were entered into the study within 8 hours of the onset of chest pain) (153). Mortality was 6.3% in the placebo group and 6.7% in the nifedipine-treated group (NS*), and the reinfarction rates were 1.5% and 2.2% (NS), respectively. The Secondary Prevention Reinfarction Israeli Nifedipine Trial (SPRINT) assessed the efficacy of nifedipine in 2,276 patients between 7 and 21 days after AMI (154). The mortality rate during an average of 10 months of follow-up was 5.7% in the placebo group and 5.8% in the nifedipine-treated group (NS), and nonfatal recurrent MI was 4.8% and 4.4% (NS), respectively. Patients at greater risk were recruited in the SPRINT-II trial, which was stopped when 1,358 patients were randomized because of a trend toward increased early mortality in the nifedipine-treated group (15.8% vs. 12.6%) (155).

Three small trials of early administration of diltiazem evaluated the effects of treatment on infarct size. Two of these trials reported nonsignificantly lower enzyme levels in the diltiazem group, and one trial found a significant increase in infarct size in the diltiazem group. Another moderate-sized trial, Incomplete Infarction Trial of European Research Collaborators Evaluating Prognosis post-Thrombolysis (INTERCEPT), was a study with 874 patients after AMI submitted to thrombolysis (156). These patients were randomized to diltiazem or placebo. The primary end point, a combination of cardiac death, nonfatal reinfarction, or refractory ischemia, was less common in the diltiazem group, but the difference was not statistically significant and was largely because of a reduction in refractory ischemia. There were no differences in the incidences of either cardiac death or reinfarction.

The Multicenter Diltiazem Postinfarction Trial Research Group was the only large trial studying the effects of diltiazem on mortality and reinfarction. A total of 2,446 patients were randomly assigned to receive either diltiazem or placebo starting 3 to 15 days after the onset of MI, and these patients were followed for 12 to 52 months (mean 25 months). Total mortality rates were nearly identical between the two treatment groups (13.5% in both groups), and the reinfarction rate was 8% in the diltiazem group versus 9.4% in the placebo group (NS) (157).

The Danish Verapamil Infarction Trial I (DAVIT I) included 1,436 patients who received verapamil or placebo intravenously and continued orally over the following 6 months. After 6 months, mortality was 12.8% in the verapamil group

versus 13.8% in the placebo group (NS), and the reinfarction rate was 7% versus 8.3% (NS), respectively (158). The DAVIT II trial examined whether treatment with verapamil from the second week after an AMI and continued for 12 to 18 months (mean 16 months) might reduce total mortality and reinfarction. Mortality was 11.1% in the verapamil group and 13.8% in the placebo group (NS), and the reinfarction rates were 9.6% and 11.9% (NS), respectively (159,160).

In summary, none of 23 individual RCTs was able to detect a statistically significant difference in mortality or reinfarction with calcium channel blockers. The overall pooled data showed no indication of benefit with respect to mortality with any single drug. If diltiazem and verapamil data are combined, there is a 5% reduction in the odds of death (95% CI, −18% to 9%; NS), and reinfarction rates are reduced by 21% (95% CI, −33% to −6%; $p < 0.01$) (150). The combined data on the dihydropyridine calcium antagonists indicate a slight but definite increase in mortality and reinfarction (150,151).

The use of calcium antagonists in patients with AMI has been declining. Data from the National Registry of Myocardial Infarction reported that calcium antagonist use in the United States declined from 44% in 1990 to 31% in 1993 (161). Although used less often than previously, rates of calcium antagonists use are still greater than one would expect based on the lack of evidence supporting their utilization.

Recommendations

Both diltiazem and verapamil may reduce the risk for reinfarction, but there is no indication that any of the calcium antagonists reduce mortality after AMI, and there is evidence that the dihydropyridine calcium antagonists may increase both mortality and reinfarction. Therefore, the prophylactic use of calcium channel blockers during the early phase of AMI cannot be recommended. If, however, a calcium antagonist has to be used for a specific indication (e.g., relief of angina despite β-blockers and nitrates), then it would be preferable to use verapamil or diltiazem.

Prophylactic Antiarrhythmic Therapy

The presence of frequent and repetitive ventricular arrhythmias in the recovery phase of AMI is a marker of increased risk for mortality and cardiac arrest independent of reduced ventricular function and silent or manifest myocardial ischemia (162,163). These observations provide a rationale for the prophylactic use of antiarrhythmic therapy for patients with MI.

Class I Agents

There have been several trials evaluating the effects of Class I antiarrhythmic agents on mortality rates after AMI (164). The largest of these trials, the CAST (Cardiac Arrhythmia Suppression Trial), evaluated the effects of antiarrhythmic therapy with encainide and flecainide (Class IC agents, eval-

---

*Throughout this chapter "NS" means "not statistically significant."

uated in CAST I) and moricizine (Class IA agent, evaluated in CAST II) in patients with asymptomatic or mildly symptomatic ventricular arrhythmias after AMI (165,166). The results of the main trials of Class I agents are summarized below.

Class IA

The CAST II study showed a greater mortality among patients who received moricizine compared with those who received placebo (166,167). This study was divided into two phases: an early phase involving 1,325 patients within 14 days after MI, and a long-term phase follow-up period involving 1,155 patients. During the first 14-day period of treatment, there was a significant excess of mortality excess in the moricizine group compared with the placebo group (2.6% vs. 0.45%, respectively; $p = 0.02$), and at the completion of the long-term phase there was a slight, nonsignificant excess of mortality in the moricizine group (8.4% vs. 7.3%; $p = 0.40$). Overall, the data from 18 RCTs, including 6,582 patients, showed a trend toward an excess in mortality among patients assigned to Class IA agents (quinidine, procainamide, disopyramide, imipramine, and moricizine) compared with those among control subjects (OR, 1.19; 95% CI, 0.99(1.44; $p = 0.07$) (164).

Class IB

In a metaanalysis by MacMahon and coworkers (168), 14 randomized trials of lidocaine versus control were included, with a total of 9,155 patients. Nine trials evaluated intravenous lidocaine (2,194 patients), and five trials evaluated intramuscular lidocaine (6,961 patients) (168). The data from all trials indicated a 35% reduction in the odds of development of ventricular fibrillation (in the lidocaine group, 95% CI: 0.56–0.03; $p < 0.04$), but early mortality was 38% greater among lidocaine-treated patients compared with control patients (82/4,616 [1.8%] vs. 55/4,539 [1.2%], respectively; 95% CI, 0.02–0.95; $p < 0.10$). This increase in mortality may be in part caused by an increased risk for asystole. Another metaanalysis evaluating Class 1B agents showed an excess of mortality of 15% with lidocaine (17 trials; 95% CI, 0.9–1.47; $p = 0.27$) and a mortality increase of 2% with tocainide, phenytoin, and mexiletine (15 trials; 95% CI, 0.77–1.25; $p = 0.88$). The overall mortality rate increase for 32 trials of Class IB agents involving 14,013 patients was about 6% (95% CI, 0.89–1.26; $p = 0.50$) (164).

Class IC

In CAST I, which involved 1,498 patients, there was a significant excess of mortality in patients allocated to receive encainide or flecainide compared with placebo (165). After a mean follow-up of 10 months, the mortality rates were 8.3% in the active treatment group and 3.5% in the placebo group ($p = 0.0004$). When the data from eight trials of Class IC

agents were combined (aprindine, encainide, and flecainide), which involved 2,538 patients, there was a trend toward an excess of mortality in the treated group compared with the control group (OR, 1.31; 95% CI, 0.95–1.79; $p = 0.10$) (164).

A summary metaanalysis of Class I agents, involving 59 randomized trials with a total of 23,229 patients, showed mortality rates of 5.6% in the treated group versus 5.0% in the control group (OR, 1.14; 95% CI, 1.01–1.28; $p = 0.03$) (164). These data indicate that all Class I antiarrhythmic agents have the potential to increase mortality. Therefore, they should not be routinely used. Intravenous lidocaine and procainamide have a role in the treatment of sustained stable ventricular tachycardia and ventricular fibrillation, but they should not be used to treat ventricular premature beats or nonsustained ventricular tachycardia (169).

Class II Agents

β-blockers, when used during an AMI or long term after an infarction, have been shown to reduce total mortality and sudden death. However, the antiarrhythmic properties of β-blockers may be only partly responsible for the observed benefit with these drugs. It is possible that their ability to reduce ischemia, decrease heart rate, reduce myocardial wall or coronary plaque rupture, and prevent reinfarction may be important mechanisms. A metaanalysis of data from 53 trials (short- and long-term) involving 53,268 patients showed a significant overall reduction in mortality (OR, 0.81; 95% CI, 0.75–0.87; $p = 0.00001$) (164). Because β-blockers have been clearly shown to reduce mortality after MI, these agents should currently be the drug of choice in the secondary prevention of sudden death after infarction (5,7,170).

Class III Agents

Dofetilide, sotalol, azimilide, and amiodarone are the Class III agents that have been studied in patients after MI.

The Survival With Oral d-Sotalol (SWORD) trial evaluated d-sotalol, an isomer of d,l-sotalol that has no β-blocking activity, in 3,121 patients. The trial was prematurely stopped because of an excess of mortality in the sotalol group (5.0% vs. 3.1%; relative risk, 1.65; 95% CI, 1.15–2.36; $p = 0.006$) (171).

Dofetilide was tested in the Danish Investigations of Arrhythmia and Mortality on Dofetilide (DIAMOND) trial (172) in 1,510 patients with left ventricular dysfunction after recent AMI. Compared with placebo, dofetilide was not superior in avoiding all-cause death or arrhythmic death. Another Class III agent, azimilide, also had no effect on all-cause mortality as evidenced in a trial that included 3,381 patients after MI with left ventricular dysfunction (173).

Amiodarone, a Class III agent with multiple actions including β-blockade, has been tested in several trials in patients after AMI. The larger trials were the Canadian Amiodarone Myocardial Infarction Arrhythmia Trial (CAMIAT) and the European Myocardial Infarct Amiodarone Trial (EMIAT) (174,175). CAMIAT compared amiodarone with placebo in 1,202 survivors of AMI who had frequent (≥10 per hour) or repetitive ventricular premature beats. The primary end point, resuscitated ventricular fibrillation or arrhythmic death, occurred less often in patients assigned to amiodarone than placebo (4.5% vs. 6.9%; risk relative reduction [RRR], 38.2%; 95% CI, 2.1–62.6; $p = 0.03$; NNT = 42). No difference in all-cause mortality was observed (174). In the EMIAT, patients with recent AMI and left ventricular systolic dysfunction (left ventricular ejection fraction ≤40%) were randomized to treatment with amiodarone or placebo (175). The primary end point was all-cause mortality, and it was similar in both groups. In addition, amiodarone reduced arrhythmic death. In both studies, the treatment was started at least 5 days from admission to the coronary care unit. Early permanent discontinuation of study drug because of adverse effects was common in EMIAT and CAMIAT. Hypothyroidism, sleep disturbances, and gastrointestinal, pulmonary, skin, hepatic, visual, and neurologic abnormalities were more common in the amiodarone group (174,175).

A metaanalysis of 13 RCTs of prophylactic amiodarone in patients with recent MI or congestive heart failure (most of the patients also had previous AMI) found an all-cause mortality reduction with amiodarone of 13% (OR, 0.87; 95% CI, 0.78–0.99; $p = 0.03$) (176). Although when considering only the post-MI trials, the difference in total mortality is no longer significant (OR, 0.92; 95% CI, 0.78–1.08; $p = 0.43$).

Class IV Agents

As has been previously discussed, the metaanalysis of calcium channel blockers, which involved 20,342 patients, showed a nonsignificant trend toward a greater mortality rate in the treated group compared with the control group (OR, 1.04; 95% CI, 0.95–1.14; $p = 0.41$). A metaanalysis of trials of agents that on average increase heart rate (dihydropyridine calcium channel blockers, e.g., nifedipine), which involved 10,272 patients, showed a trend toward increased mortality in the treated group compared with the control group (OR, 1.16; 95% CI, 0.99–1.35; $p = 0.06$). Trials of agents that tend to decrease heart rate (e.g., verapamil and diltiazem), which involved 8,444 patients, showed a modest, nonsignificant decrease in mortality (OR, 0.95; 95% CI, 0.82–1.09; $p = 0.46$) (150).

These data indicate that until there is clear proof of a reduction in mortality with a specific agent, it may be reasonable to view all Class I antiarrhythmic agents as being potentially harmful. β-Blockers (Class II antiarrhythmic agents) are clearly beneficial in the acute and chronic phase of MI. Class III antiarrhythmic should not be routinely used in patients after MI. For the purpose of symptom control in patients with frequent ventricular arrhythmias that are already on β-blockers or do not tolerate them, amiodarone may be indicated. There is no clear evidence to support the prophylactic use of the Class IV antiarrhythmic agents (calcium channel blockers) after AMI.

Metabolic Modulation

Therapies aimed at reducing the amount of necrosis after coronary occlusion may address two different aims: to obtain reperfusion, and to protect ischemic myocytes. In recent years, most of the efforts have focused on the first approach, and few were able to attain the second goal (e.g., β-blockers). Glucose-insulin-potassium (GIK) infusion possibly will be a therapeutic option for this clinical scenario. In fact, this treatment was proposed more than 40 years ago by Sodi-Pallares and coworkers (177), who observed that the systemic administration of GIK shortened the electrocardiographic evolution of an AMI and improved early survival.

The initial rationale for GIK therapy was based on that insulin enhances glucose uptake for glycolytic energy production and stimulates potassium reuptake through stimulation of the sodium-potassium adenosine triphosphatase pump. However, the physiologic relevance of this effect is probably small, and, currently, many additional mechanisms have been listed as a potential explanation to a beneficial effect of the GIK solution (178–180).

The preliminary clinical evidence on the role of GIK in the treatment of AMI comes from relatively small studies. A metaanalysis involving 1,932 patients from 9 clinical trials found GIK to be associated with reduced in-hospital mortality (16% for GIK vs. 21% for placebo; OR, 0.72; 95% CI, 0.57–0.90; $p = 0.004$; NNT = 20) (181).

The efficacy of the GIK solution was explored in a study that included 407 patients within 24 hours from the onset of AMI to determine the efficacy and safety of GIK in AMI (182). There was no statistically significant difference in the occurrence of major and minor in-hospital events, although a reduction in mortality was observed (relative risk, 0.34; 95% CI, 0.15–0.78; $p = 0.008$) in the subgroup of 252 patients (61.9%) treated with reperfusion strategies. The other two studies did not show clinical benefits of GIK in the management of AMI (183,184). The positive results on the initial metaanalysis and in certain subgroups of the subsequent trials (181–183), the inexpensive cost of treatment, and the lack of power of these initial studies justify larger trials to definitely answer this question (GIK-2 and Clinical trial of Reviparin and mEtabolic modulation in Acute myocardial infarction Treatment Evaluation Study [CREATE] studies). However, currently, there is no robust evidence to support the routine use of GIK in the treatment of AMI.

In patients with diabetes admitted to the hospital because of AMI, the use of a solution of insulin–glucose followed by a 6-month intensive insulin scheme to control blood glucose was compared with conventional treatment in patients in the Diabetes Mellitus, Insulin Glucose Infusion in Acute Myocardial Infarction (DIGAMI) study (185). After a mean follow-up of 3.4 years, 33% of the patients assigned to the insulin protocol died compared with 44% in the control group (relative risk, 0.72; 95% CI, 0.55–0.92; $p = 0.011$; NNT = 9).

Development of hyperglycemia is a common response to stress, and it does not seem to be just an epiphenomenon, but an independent marker of increased mortality and morbidity

(186,187). It is possible that strict blood glucose control with insulin infusion may be helpful to protect not only patients with diabetes who have an AMI, but also patients without diabetes.

SUMMARY

On the basis of current available evidence, the general approach to the management of patients with AMI comprises early hospitalization with rapid institution of reperfusion therapy and intravenous β-blockers to appropriate patients. Aspirin should be given to all patients unless there are definite contraindications. All these treatments should be administered as early as possible to all eligible patients, ideally within 15 to 30 minutes after presentation to hospital and definitely within 1 hour. After stabilization of the patient, ACE inhibitors should be considered (starting at low doses and titrating up to greater doses over a few days) for all patients without contraindications (e.g., hypotension), and especially for patients with evidence of heart failure or left ventricular dysfunction or those at high risk for development of left ventricular dysfunction (e.g., patients with large MIs or history of prior MI). Aspirin and β-blockers should be continued long term, and ACE inhibitors also should be continued long term for patients with left ventricular dysfunction or heart failure after MI, as well as for all patients older than 55 years. Some physicians may consider use of intravenous nitrates (e.g., for patients with ongoing ischemia) or heparin (e.g., after fibrin-specific agents, such as recombinant t-PA, reteplase, and tenecteplase, postinfarction angina, and large MIs).

Coronary angiography and revascularization should be considered in appropriately selected patients at high risk, and these strategies are discussed elsewhere in this textbook. These efforts should be complemented by a strategy of aggressive efforts at risk factor modification (smoking cessation, blood pressure and weight control, increased exercise, and lipid-lowering therapy). Mortality and morbidity also are likely to be improved by avoiding or minimizing the use of potentially harmful therapies such as Class I antiarrhythmic agents and some of calcium antagonist agents. The combined effects of all these approaches are likely to have a substantial beneficial impact on the short- and long-term prognosis of patients after AMI.

Future directions in the overall approach for patients with AMI will be refined by ongoing and subsequent large-scale clinical trials. However, the current challenge for clinicians for treating patients with AMI is not lack of available evidence of beneficial treatments, but rather the application of this knowledge to daily clinical practice.

REFERENCES

1. Lee TH, Goldman L. The coronary care unit turns 25: historical trends and future directions. *Ann Intern Med* 1988;108.887–894.
2. Indications for fibrinolytic therapy in suspected acute myocardial infarction: collaborative overview of early mortality and major morbidity results from all randomised trials of more than 1000 patients. Fibrinolytic Therapy Trialists' (FTT) Collaborative Group. *Lancet* 1994; 343:311–322.
3. Keeley EC, Boura JA, Grines CL. Primary angioplasty versus intravenous thrombolytic therapy for acute myocardial infarction: a quantitative review of 23 randomised trials. *Lancet* 2003;361:13–20.
4. Antithrombotic Trialists' Collaboration. Collaborative meta-analysis of randomised trials of antiplatelet therapy for prevention of death, myocardial infarction, and stroke in high risk patients. *BMJ* 2002; 324:71–86.
5. Freemantle N, Cleland J, Young P, et al. Beta blockade after myocardial infarction: systematic review and meta regression analysis. *BMJ* 1999;318:1730–1737.
6. Latini R, Tognoni G, Maggioni AP, et al. Clinical effects of early angiotensin-converting enzyme inhibitor treatment for acute myocardial infarction are similar in the presence and absence of aspirin: systematic overview of individual data from 96712 randomized patients. Angiotensin-converting Enzyme Inhibitor Myocardial Infarction Collaborative Group. *J Am Coll Cardiol* 2000;35:1801–1807.
7. Yusuf S, Peto R, Lewis J, et al. Beta blockade during and after myocardial infarction: an overview of the randomized trials. *Prog Cardiovasc Dis* 1985;27:335–371.
8. Yusuf S, Collins R, Peto R. Why do we need some large, simple randomized trials? *Stat Med* 1984;3:409–420.
9. Collins R, Gray R, Godwin J, et al. Avoidance of large biases and large random errors in the assessment of moderate treatment effects: the need for systematic overviews. *Stat Med* 1987;6:245–250.
10. Yusuf S. Obtaining medically meaningful answers from an overview of randomized clinical trials. *Stat Med* 1987;6:281–286.
11. European Action on Secondary Prevention by Intervention to Reduce Events (EUROASPIRE) I and II Group. Clinical reality of coronary prevention guidelines: a comparison of EUROASPIRE I and II in nine countries. *Lancet* 2001;357:995–1001.
12. Eagle KA, Goodman SG, Avezum A, et al. Practice variation and missed opportunities for reperfusion in ST-segment-elevation myocardial infarction: findings from the Global Registry of Acute Coronary Events (GRACE). *Lancet* 2002;359:373–377.
13. McNeilly RH, Pemberton J. Duration of last attack in 998 fatal cases of coronary artery disease and its relation to possible cardiac resuscitation. *Br Med J* 1968;3:139.
14. Huikuri HV, Castellanos A, Myerburg RJ. Sudden death due to cardiac arrhythmias. *N Engl J Med* 2001;345:1473–1482.
15. Norris RM. Fatality outside hospital from acute coronary events in three British districts, 1994–5. United Kingdom Heart Attack Study Collaborative Group. *BMJ* 1998;316:1065–1067.
16. Law MR, Watt HC, Wald NJ. The underlying risk of death after myocardial infarction in the absence of treatment. *Arch Intern Med* 2002;162:2405–2410.
17. Pantridge JF, Webb SW, Adgey AA, et al. The first hour after the onset of acute myocardial infarction. In: Yu PN, Goodwin JF, eds. *Progress in cardiology.* Philadelphia: Lea & Febiger, 1974:174.
18. National Heart Lung and Blood Institute. *Vital statistics of the United States.* Rockville, MD: National Center for Health Statistics, 1986.
19. Stamler J. The marked decline in coronary heart disease mortality rates in the United States, 1968-1981: summary of findings and possible explanations. *Cardiology* 1985;72:11–22.
20. Heart and Stroke Foundation of Canada. *Cardiovascular disease in Canada.* Toronto: Heart and Stroke Foundation of Canada, 1991.
21. Tunstall-Pedoe H, Kuulasmaa K, Mahonen M, et al. Contribution of trends in survival and coronary-event rates to changes in coronary heart disease mortality: 10-year results from 37 WHO MONICA project populations. Monitoring trends and determinants in cardiovascular disease. *Lancet* 1999;353:1547–1557.
22. Rogers WJ, Canto JG, Lambrew CT, et al. Temporal trends in the treatment of over 1.5 million patients with myocardial infarction in the US from 1990 through 1999: the National Registry of Myocardial Infarction 1, 2 and 3. *J Am Coll Cardiol* 2000;36:2056–2063.
23. Berger CJ, Murabito JM, Evans JC, et al. Prognosis after first myocardial infarction. Comparison of Q-wave and non-Q-wave myocardial infarction in the Framingham Heart Study. *JAMA* 1992;268:1545–1551.
24. Sheifer SE, Manolio TA, Gersh, BJ. Unrecognized myocardial infarction. *Ann Intern Med* 2001;135:801–811.
25. Thom TJ, Kannel WB, Silbershatz S, et al. Incidence, prevalence, and mortality of cardiovascular diseases in the United States. In: Alexan-

der RW, Schlant RC, Fuster V, Roberts R, eds. *Hurst's the heart,* 9th ed. New York: McGraw Hill, 1998:3.

26. Gruppo Italiano per lo Studio della Sopravvivenza nell'Infarto Miocardico. GISSI-3: effects of lisinopril and transdermal glyceryl trinitrate singly and together on 6-week mortality and ventricular function after acute myocardial infarction. *Lancet* 1994;343:1115–1122.

27. ISIS-4 Collaborative Group. ISIS-4: a randomised factorial trial assessing early oral captopril, oral mononitrate, and intravenous magnesium sulphate in 58,050 patients with suspected acute myocardial infarction. ISIS-4 (Fourth International Study of Infarct Survival) Collaborative Group. *Lancet* 1995;345:669–685.

28. Herlitz J, Hjalmarson A, Waagstein F. Treatment of pain in acute myocardial infarction. *Br Heart J* 1989;61:9.

29. Van de Werf F, Ardissino D, Betriu A, et al. Management of acute myocardial infarction in patients presenting with ST-segment elevation. *Eur Heart J* 2003;24:28–66.

30. Newby LK, Califf RM. Redefining uncomplicated myocardial infarction in the thrombolytic era. GUSTO Investigators. *Circulation* 1994; 90:1–110.

31. Ahlquist RP. A study of the adrenotropic receptors. *Am J Physiol* 1948;153:586–600.

32. Andersson KE. Drugs blocking adrenoceptors. *Acta Med Scand* 1982;665[Suppl]:9–17.

33. Eichhorn EJ, McGhie AL, Bedotto JB, et al. Effects of bucindolol on neurohormonal activation in congestive heart failure. *Am J Cardiol* 1991;67:67–73.

34. Maroko PR, Kjekshus J, Sobel BE, et al. Factors influencing infarct size following experimental coronary artery occlusions. *Circulation* 1971;43:67–82.

35. Rossi PR, Yusuf S, Ramsdale D, et al. Reduction of ventricular arrhythmias by early intravenous atenolol in suspected acute myocardial infarction. *Br Med J* 1983;286:506–510.

36. Ramsdale D, Faragher EB, Bennett D, et al. Ischemic pain relief in patients with acute myocardial infarction by intravenous atenolol. *Am Heart J* 1982;103:459–467.

37. Yusuf S, Lopez R, Sleight P. Effect of atenolol on recovery of electrocardiographic signs of myocardial infarction. *Lancet* 1979;2:868–869.

38. Yusuf S, Sleight P, Rossi PR, et al. Reduction in infarct size, arrhythmias, chest pain, and morbidity by early intravenous beta-blockade in suspected acute myocardial infarction. *Circulation* 1983;67[Pt 2]:32–41.

39. Norris RM, Barnaby PF, Brown MA, et al. Prevention of ventricular fibrillation during acute myocardial infarction by intravenous propranolol. *Lancet* 1984;2:883–886.

40. Galcera-Tomas J, Castillo-Soria FJ, Villegas-Garcia M, et al. Effects of early use of atenolol or captopril on infarct size and ventricular volume: a double-blind comparison in patients with acute anterior myocardial infarction. *Circulation* 2001;103:813–819.

41. Poulsen SH, Jensen SE, Egstrup K. Effects of long-term adrenergic beta-blockade on left ventricular diastolic filling in patients with acute myocardial infarction. *Am Heart J* 1999;138:710–720.

42. Randomised trial of intravenous atenolol among 16027 cases of suspected acute myocardial infarction: ISIS-1. First International Study of Infarct Survival Collaborative Group. *Lancet* 1986;2:57–66.

43. Mechanisms for the early mortality reduction produced by beta-blockade started early in acute myocardial infarction: ISIS-1. ISIS-1 (First International Study of Infarct Survival) Collaborative Group. *Lancet* 1988;1:921–923.

44. Metoprolol in acute myocardial infarction (MIAMI). A randomiozed placebo controlled international trial. The MIAMI Trial Research Group. *Eur Heart J* 1985;6:199–226.

45. Roberts R, Rogers WJ, Mueller HS, et al. Immediate versus deferred beta-blockade following thrombolytic therapy in patients with acute myocardial infarction. Results of the Thrombolysis in Myocardial Infarction (TIMI) II-B Study. *Circulation* 1991;83:422–437.

46. Gottlieb SS, McCarter RJ, Vogel RA. Effect of beta-blockade on mortality among high-risk and low-risk patients after myocardial infarction. *N Engl J Med* 1998; 339:489–497.

47. Chen J, Radford MJ, Wang Y, et al. Effectiveness of beta-blocker therapy after acute myocardial infarction in elderly patients with chronic obstructive pulmonary disease or asthma. *J Am Coll Cardiol* 2001;37:1950–1956.

48. Dargie HJ. Effect of carvedilol on outcome after myocardial infarction in patients with left-ventricular dysfunction: the CAPRICORN randomised trial. *Lancet* 2001;357:1385–1390.

49. Van de Werf F, Janssens L, Brzostek T, et al. Short-term effects of early intravenous treatment with a beta-adrenergic blocking agent or a specific bradycardiac agent in patients with acute myocardial infarction receiving thrombolytic therapy. *J Am Coll Cardiol* 1993;22:407–416.

50. Gottlieb SS, McCarter RJ. Comparative effects of three beta blockers (atenolol, metoprolol, and propranolol) on survival after acute myocardial infarction. *Am J Cardiol* 2001;87:823–826.

51. Steg PG, Goldberg R, Gore J, et al. Baseline characteristics, management practices, and in-hospital outcomes of patients hospitalized with acute coronary syndromes in the Global Registry of Acute Coronary Events (GRACE). *Am J Cardiol* 2002;90:358.

52. McAlpine HM, Morton JJ, Leckie B, et al. Neuroendocrine activation after acute myocardial infarction. *Br Heart J* 1988;60:117–124.

53. Ceremuzynski L. Hormonal and metabolic reactions evoked by acute myocardial infarction. *Circ Res* 1981;48:767–776.

54. Michorowski BL, Ceremuzynski L. The renin-angiotensin-aldosterone system and the clinical course of acute myocardial infarction. *Eur Heart J* 1983;4:259–264.

55. White HD, Norris RM, Brown MA, et al. Left ventricular end-systolic volume as the major determinant of survival after recovery from myocardial infarction. *Circulation* 1987;76:44–51.

56. Pfeffer MA, Braunwald E. Ventricular remodeling after myocardial infarction. Experimental observations and clinical implications. *Circulation* 1990;81:1161–1172.

57. Schuster EH, Bulkley BH. Expansion of transmural myocardial infarction: a pathophysiologic factor in cardiac rupture. *Circulation* 1979;60:1532–1538.

58. Jugdutt BI, Michorowski BL. Role of infarct expansion in rupture of the ventricular septum after acute myocardial infarction: a two dimensional echocardiographic study. *Clin Cardiol* 1987;10:641–652.

59. Nolan SE, Mannisi JA, Bush DE, et al. Increased afterload aggravates infarct expansion after acute myocardial infarction. *J Am Coll Cardiol* 1988;12:1318–1325.

60. Sutton MG, Sharpe N. Left ventricular remodeling after myocardial infarction: pathophysiology and therapy. *Circulation* 2000;101:2981–2988.

61. McKay RG, Pfeffer MA, Pasternak RC, et al. Left ventricular remodeling after myocardial infarction: a corollary to infarct expansion. *Circulation* 1986;74:693–702.

62. Ertl G, Kloner RA, Alexander RA, et al. Limitation of experimental infarct size by an angiotensin-converting enzyme inhibitor. *Circulation* 1982;65:40–48.

63. Gay RG. Early and late effects of captopril treatment after large myocardial infarction in rats. *J Am Coll Cardiol* 1990;16:967–977.

64. Pfeffer JM, Pfeffer MA, Braunwald E. Influence of chronic captopril therapy on the infarcted left ventricle of the rat. *Circ Rev* 1985;57: 84–95.

65. Mancini GB, Henry GC, Macaya C, et al. Angiotensin-converting enzyme inhibition with quinapril improves endothelial vasomotor dysfunction in patients with coronary artery disease. The TREND (Trial on Reversing Endothelial Dysfunction) Study. *Circulation* 1996;94:258–265.

66. Miki T, Miura T, Tsuchida A, et al. Cardioprotective mechanism of ischemic preconditioning is impaired by postinfarct ventricular remodeling through angiotensin II type 1 receptor activation. *Circulation* 2000;102:458–463.

67. Lonn EM, Yusuf S, Jha P, et al. The emerging role of angiotensin-converting enzyme inhibitors in cardiac and vascular protection. *Circulation* 1994;90:2056–2069.

68. Schieffer B, Schieffer E, Hilfiker-Kleiner D, et al. Expression of angiotensin II and interleukin 6 in human coronary atherosclerotic plaques: potential implications for inflammation and plaque instability. *Circulation* 2000;101:1372–1378.

69. Schneider CA, Voth E, Moka D, et al. Improvement of myocardial blood flow to ischemic regions by angiotensin-converting enzyme inhibition with quinaprilat IV: a study using [15O] water dobutamine stress positron emission tomography. *J Am Coll Cardiol* 1999;34:1005–1011.

70. Boman KO, Jansson JH, Nyhlen KA, et al. Improved fibrinolysis after one year of treatment with enalapril in men and women with uncomplicated myocardial infarction. *Thromb Haemost* 2002;87:311–316.

71. Minai K, Matsumoto T, Horie H, et al. Bradykinin stimulates the release of tissue plasminogen activator in human coronary circulation: effects of angiotensin-converting enzyme inhibitors. *J Am Coll Cardiol* 2001;37:1565–1570.

72. Soejima H, Ogawa H, Yasue H, et al. Angiotensin-converting enzyme

inhibition reduces monocyte chemoattractant protein-1 and tissue factor levels in patients with myocardial infarction. *J Am Coll Cardiol* 1999;34:983–988.

73. Pfeffer MA, Braunwald E, Moye LA, et al. Effect of captopril on mortality and morbidity in patients with left ventricular dysfunction after myocardial infarction. Results of the survival and ventricular enlargement trial. The SAVE Investigators. *N Engl J Med* 1992;327:669–677.

74. Effect of ramipril on mortality and morbidity of survivors of acute myocardial infarction with clinical evidence of heart failure. The Acute Infarction Ramipril Efficacy (AIRE) Study Investigators. *Lancet* 1993;342:821–828.

75. Ambrosioni E, Borghi C, Magnani B. The effect of the angiotensin-converting-enzyme inhibitor zofenopril on mortality and morbidity after anterior myocardial infarction. Survival of Myocardial Infarction Long-Term Evaluation (SMILE) Study Investigators. *N Engl J Med* 1995;332:80–85.

76. Oral captopril versus placebo among 13,634 patients with suspected acute myocardial infarction: interim report from the Chinese Cardiac Study (CCS-1). *Lancet* 1995;345:686–687.

77. Kober L, Torp-Pedersen C, Carlsen JE, et al. A clinical trial of the angiotensin-converting-enzyme inhibitor trandolapril in patients with left ventricular dysfunction after myocardial infarction. *N Engl J Med* 1995;333:1670–1676.

78. Indications for ACE inhibitors in the early treatment of acute myocardial infarction: systematic overview of individual data from 100,000 patients in randomized trials. ACE Inhibitor Myocardial Infarction Collaborative Group. *Circulation* 1998;97:2202–2212.

79. Flather MD, Yusuf S, Kober L, et al. Long-term ACE-inhibitor therapy in patients with heart failure or left-ventricular dysfunction: a systematic overview of data from individual patients. *Lancet* 2000;355:1575–1581.

80. Swedberg K, Held P, Kjekshus J, et al. Effects of the early administration of enalapril on mortality in patients with acute myocardial infarction: results of the Cooperative New Scandinavian Enalapril Survival Study II (CONSENSUS II). *N Engl J Med* 1992;327:678–684.

81. Yusuf S, Sleight P, Pogue J, et al. Effects of an angiotensin-converting-enzyme inhibitor, ramipril, on cardiovascular events in high-risk patients. The Heart Outcomes Prevention Evaluation Study Investigators. *N Engl J Med* 2000;342:145–153.

82. Mizuno Y, Yoshimura M, Yasue H, et al. Aldosterone production is activated in failing ventricle in humans. *Circulation* 2001;103:72–77.

83. Lijnen P, Petrov V. Induction of cardiac fibrosis by aldosterone. *J Mol Cell Cardiol* 2000;32:865–879.

84. Fullerton MJ, Funder JW. Aldosterone and cardiac fibrosis: in vitro studies. *Cardiovasc Res* 1994;28:1863–1867.

85. Pitt D. ACE inhibitor co-therapy in patients with heart failure: rationale for the Randomized Aldactone Evaluation Study (RALES). *Eur Heart J* 1995;16[Suppl N]:107–110.

86. Pitt B, Zannad F, Remme WJ, et al. The effect of spironolactone on morbidity and mortality in patients with severe heart failure. Randomized Aldactone Evaluation Study Investigators. *N Engl J Med* 1999;341:709–717.

87. Pitt B, Remme W, Zannad F, et al., for the Eplerenone Post-Acute Myocardial Infarction Heart Failure Efficacy and Survival Study Investigators. Eplerenone, a selective aldosterone blocker, in patients with left ventricular dysfunction after myocardial infarction. *N Engl J Med* 2003;348:1309–1321.

88. Wolny A, Clozel J, Rein J, et al. Functional and biochemical analysis of angiotensin II forming pathways in the human heart. *Circ Res* 1997;80:219–227.

89. Dickstein K, Kjekshus J, the OPTIMAAL Steering Committee, for the OPTIMAAL Study Group. Effects of losartan and captopril on mortality and morbidity in high-risk patients after acute myocardial infarction: the OPTIMAAL randomised trial. Optimal Trial in Myocardial Infarction with Angiotensin II Antagonist Losartan. *Lancet* 2002;360:752–760.

90. Pfeffer MA, McMurray J, Leizorovicz A, et al. Valsartan in acute myocardial infarction trial (VALIANT): rationale and design. *Am Heart J* 2000;140:727–750.

91. Thadani U, Manyari D, Parker JO, et al. Tolerance to circulatory effects of oral isosorbide dinitrate. Rate of development and cross tolerance to glyceryl trinitrate. *Circulation* 1980;61:526–535.

92. Armstrong PW, Moffat JA. Tolerance to organic nitrate: clinical and experimental perspective. *Am J Med* 1983;74[Suppl]:73.

93. Rezakovic DZ, Rutishauser W, Pavicic L, et al. Different hemody-

namic actions of trinitroglycerin and isosorbide dinitrate in patients with acute myocardial infarction. *Eur Heart J* 1983;4:718–723.

94. Abrams J. Hemodynamic effects of nitroglycerin and long acting nitrates. *Am Heart J* 1985;110:216.

95. Garadah T, Ghaisas NK, Mehana N, et al. Impact of intravenous nitroglycerin on pulsed Doppler indexes of left ventricular filling in acute anterior myocardial infarction. *Am Heart J* 1998;136:812–817.

96. Jugdutt BI, Becker LC, Hutchins OM, et al. Effect of intravenous nitroglycerin on collateral blood flow and infarct size in the conscious dog. *Circulation* 1981;63:17–28.

97. Flaherty JT. Intravenous nitroglycerin in acute myocardial infarction. *Cardiovasc Rev Rep* 1990;11:46.

98. Kjekshus J. Nitrates in acute myocardial infarction. *Drugs* 1987;33:140–146.

99. Jugdutt BI, Warnica JW. Intravenous nitroglycerin therapy to limit myocardial infarct size, expansion and complications. Effect of timing, dosage, and infarct location. *Circulation* 1988;78:906–909.

100. Hills LD, Davis C, Khuri SF. The effect of nitroglycerin and nitroprusside on ischemic injury during acute myocardial infarction. *Circulation* 1976;54:766–773.

101. Shell WE, Sobel BE. Protection of jeopardized ischemic myocardium by reduction of ventricular after load. *N Engl J Med* 1974;291:481–486.

102. Conti CR. Nitrate therapy for ischaemic heart disease. *Eur Heart J* 1986;6[Suppl A]:3–11.

103. Hockings BE, Cope GD, Clarke GM, et al. Randomised controlled trial of vasodilator therapy after myocardial infarction. *Am J Cardiol* 1981;48:354–351.

104. Durrer JD, Lie KI, van Capelle FJ, et al. Effect of sodium nitroprusside on mortality in acute myocardial infarction. *N Engl J Med* 1982;306:1121–1128.

105. Cohn JN, Franciosa JA, Francis GS, et al. Effect of short-term infusion of sodium nitroprusside on mortality rate in acute myocardial infarction complicated by left ventricular failure. Results of a VA Cooperative Study. *N Engl J Med* 1982;306:1129–1136.

106. Chiche P, Baligadoo SJ, Derrida JP. A randomised trial of prolonged nitroglycerin infusion in acute myocardial infarction. *Circulation* 1979;59,60[Suppl II]:165.

107. Bussman WD, Passek D, Seidel W, et al. Reduction of CK and CK-MB indexes of infarct size by intravenous nitroglycerin. *Circulation* 1981;63:615–622.

108. Flaherty JT, Becker LC, Bulkley BH, et al. A randomized prospective trial of IV nitroglycerin in patients with acute myocardial infarction. *Circulation* 1983;68:576–588.

109. Jaffe AS, Geltman EM, Tiefenbrunn AJ, et al. Reduction of infarct size in patients with inferior infarction with IV glyceryl trinitrate. A randomized study. *Br Heart J* 1983;49:452–460.

110. Lis Y, Bennet D, Lambert G, et al. A preliminary double-blind study of IV nitroglycerin in acute myocardial infarction. *Intens Care Med* 1984;10:179–184.

111. Yusuf S, Collins R, MacMahon S, et al. Effect of intravenous nitrates on mortality in acute myocardial infarction: an overview of the randomized trials. *Lancet* 1988;1:1088–1092.

112. Fitzgerald LJ, Bennett ED. The effects of oral isosorbide mononitrate on mortality following acute myocardial infarction. A multicentre study. *Eur Heart J* 1990;11:120–126.

113. Kendall MJ. Long-term therapeutic efficacy with once-daily isosorbide-5-mononitrate (Imdur). *J Clin Pharm Ther* 1990;15:169–185.

114. Sacks FM, Pfeffer MA, Moye LA, et al. The effect of pravastatin on coronary events after myocardial infarction in patients with average cholesterol levels. Cholesterol and Recurrent Events Trial investigators. *N Engl J Med* 1996;335:1001–1009.

115. Prevention of cardiovascular events and death with pravastatin in patients with coronary heart disease and a broad range of initial cholesterol levels. The Long-Term Intervention with Pravastatin in Ischaemic Disease (LIPID) Study Group. *N Engl J Med* 1998;339:1349–1357.

116. Randomised trial of cholesterol lowering in 4444 patients with coronary heart disease: the Scandinavian Simvastatin Survival Study (4S). *Lancet* 1994;344:1383–1389.

117. Stamler J, Wentworth D, Neaton JD. Is relationship between serum cholesterol and risk of premature death from coronary heart disease continuous and graded? Findings in 356,222 primary screenees of the Multiple Risk Factor Intervention Trial (MRFIT). *JAMA* 1986;256:2823–2828.

118. Heart Protection Study Collaborative Group. MRC/BHF Heart Protection Study of cholesterol lowering with simvastatin in 20,536 high-

risk individuals: a randomised placebo-controlled trial. *Lancet* 2002; 360:7–22.

119. Rosenson RS, Tangeny CC. Antiatherothrombotic properties of statins: implications for cardiovascular event reduction. *JAMA* 1998;279: 1643–1650.

120. Schwartz GG, Olsson AG, Ezekowitz MD, et al. Effects of atorvastatin on early recurrent ischemic events in acute coronary syndromes. The MIRACL Study: a randomized controlled trial. *JAMA* 2001;285: 1711–1718.

121. Thompson PL, Meredith I, Amerena J, et al. Effect of pravastatin compared with placebo initiated within 24 hours of onset of acute myocardial infarction or unstable angina: the Pravastatin in Acute Coronary Treatment (PACT) trial. *Am Heart J* 2004;148:e2.

122. Muhlestein JB, Horne BD, Bair TL, et al. Usefulness of in-hospital prescription of statin agents after angiographic diagnosis of coronary artery disease in improving continued compliance and reduced mortality. *Am J Cardiol* 2001;87:257–261.

123. Heeschen C, Hamm CW, Laufs U, et al. Withdrawal of statins increases event rates in patients with acute coronary syndromes. *Circulation* 2002;105:1446–1452.

124. Woods KL. Possible pharmacological actions of magnesium in acute myocardial infarction. *Br J Clin Pharmacol* 1991;32:3–10.

125. Ferrari R, Albenini A, Curello S, et al. Myocardial recovery during post-ischaemic reperfusion: effects of nifedipine, calcium and magnesium. *J Mol Cell Cardiol* 1986;18:487–498.

126. Altura BT, Altura BM. Endothelium-dependent relaxation in coronary arteries requires magnesium ions. *Br J Pharmacol* 1987;91: 449–451.

127. Haverkamp W, Hindricks G, Keteller T, et al. Prophylactic antiarrhythmic and antifibrillatory effects of intravenous magnesium sulphate during acute myocardial ischaemia. *Eur Heart J* 1988;9:228.

128. Ferrara N, Longobardi G, Leosco PA, et al. Electrical and mechanical actions of magnesium sulfate during ischemia and reperfusion on isolated perfused rat heart. *Arch Int Pharmacodyn* 1988;293:84–96.

129. du Toit EF, Opie LH. Modulation of severity of reperfusion stunning in the isolated rat heart by agents altering calcium flux at reperfusion. *Circ Res* 1992;70:960–967.

130. Christensen CW, Rieder MA, Silverstein EL, et al. Magnesium sulfate reduces myocardial infarct size when administered prior to but not after coronary reperfusion in a canine model. *Circulation* 1995;92:2617–2621.

131. Herzog WR, Scholssberg ML, MacMurdy KS, et al. Timing of magnesium therapy affects experimental infarct size. *Circulation* 1995;92: 2622–2626.

132. Morton BC, Nair RC, Smith FM, et al. Magnesium therapy in acute myocardial infarction—a double blind study. *Magnesium* 1984;3: 346–352.

133. Rasmussen HS, Norregard P, Lindeneg O, et al. Intravenous magnesium after acute myocardial infarction. *Lancet* 1986;1:234–235.

134. Smith LF, Heagerty AM, Bing RF, et al. Intravenous infusion of magnesium sulphate after acute myocardial infarction: effects on arrhythmias and mortality. *Int J Cardiol* 1986;12:175–180.

135. Abraham AS, Rosenmann D, Kramer M, et al. Magnesium in the prevention of lethal arrhythmias in acute myocardial infarction. *Arch Intern Med* 1987;147:753–755.

136. Feldstedt M, Boesgard S, Bouchelouche P, et al. Magnesium substitution in acute ischaemic heart syndromes. *Eur Heart J* 1991;12: 1215–1218.

137. Shechter M, Hod H, Marks N, et al. Magnesium therapy and mortality in acute myocardial infarction. *Am J Cardiol* 1990;66:271–274.

138. Ceremuzynski L, Jurgiel R, Kulakowski P, et al. Threatening arrhythmias in acute myocardial infarction are prevented by intravenous magnesium sulfate. *Am Heart J* 1989;118:1333–1334.

139. Teo KT, Yusuf S, Collins R, et al. Effects of intravenous magnesium in suspected acute myocardial infarction: overview of randomised trials. *Br Med J* 1991;303:1499–1503.

140. Woods KL, Fletcher S, Roffe C, et al. Intravenous magnesium sulphate in suspected acute myocardial infarction: results of the second Leicester Intravenous Magnesium Intervention Trial (LIMIT-2). *Lancet* 1992;339:1553–1558.

141. Woods KL, Fletcher S. Long-term outcome after intravenous magnesium sulphate in suspected acute myocardial infarction: the second Leicester Intravenous Magnesium Intervention Trial (LIMIT-2). *Lancet* 1994;343:816–819.

142. Antman EM. Magnesium in acute MI: timing is critical. *Circulation* 1995;92:2367–2372.

143. The Magnesium in Coronary Arteries (MAGIC) Trial Investigators. Early administration of intravenous magnesium to high-risk patients with acute myocardial infarction in the Magnesium in Coronary Arteries (MAGIC) Trial: a randomized controlled trial. *Lancet* 2002; 360:1189–1196.

144. Ryan TJ, Antman EM, Brooks NH, et al. 1999 update: ACC/AHA guidelines for the management of patients with acute myocardial infarction. A report of the American College of Cardiology/American Heart Association Task Force on Practice Guidelines (Committee on Management of Acute Myocardial Infarction). *J Am Coll Cardiol* 1999;34:890–911.

145. Deck KA, Kem R, Trautwein W. Voltage clamp technique in mammalian cardiac fiber. *Pflugers Arch* 1964;280:50–62.

146. Reuter H. The dependence of slow inward current in Purkinje fibers on the extracellular calcium concentration. *J Physiol* 1967;192:479–492.

147. Fabiato A. Calcium-induced release of calcium from the cardiac sarcoplasmic reticulum. *Am J Physiol* 1983;245:C1–C14.

148. Godfraind T, Miller R, Wibo M. Calcium antagonism and calcium entry blockade. *Pharmacol Rev* 1986;38:321–416.

149. Opie LH. Myocardial stunning: a role for calcium antagonists during reperfusion. *Cardiovasc Res* 1992;26:20–24.

150. Held P, Yusuf S. Effects of β-blockers and calcium channel blockers in acute myocardial infarction. *Eur Heart J* 1993;14[Suppl F]:18–25.

151. Yusuf S, Furberg CD. Effects of calcium-channel blockers on survival after myocardial infarction. *Cardiovasc Drugs Ther* 1987;1:343–344.

152. Yusuf S, Held P, Furberg C. Update of effects of calcium antagonists in myocardial infarction or angina in light of the second Danish verapamil infarction trial (DAVIT-11) and other recent studies. *Am J Cardiol* 1991;67:1295–1297.

153. Wilcox RG, Hampton JR, Banks DC, et al. Trial of early nifedipine in acute myocardial infarction: the TRENT Study. *Br Med J* 1986;293: 1204–1208.

154. Secondary prevention reinfarction Israeli nifedipine trial (SPRINT). A randomised intervention trial of nifedipine in patients with acute myocardial infarction. The Israeli Sprint Study Group. *Eur Heart J* 1988;9:354–364.

155. The SPRINT Study Group. The secondary prevention reinfarction Israeli nifedipine trial (SPRINT) II: design, methods, results. *Eur Heart J* 1988;9[Suppl I]:350.

156. Boden WE, van Gilst WH, Scheldewaert RG, et al. Diltiazem in acute myocardial infarction treated with thrombolytic agents: a randomised placebo-controlled trial. Incomplete Infarction Trial of European Research Collaborators Evaluating Prognosis post-Thrombolysis (INTERCEPT). *Lancet* 2000;355:1751–1756.

157. The effect of diltiazem on mortality and reinfarction after myocardial infarction. The Multicenter Diltiazem Postinfarction Trial Research Group. *N Engl J Med* 1988;319:385–392.

158. Verapamil in acute myocardial infarction. The Danish Group on Verapamil in Myocardial Infarction. *Eur Heart J* 1984;5:516–528.

159. Effect of verapamil on mortality and major events after acute myocardial infarction (the Danish Verapamil Infarction Trial—DAVIT II). *Am J Cardiol* 1990;66:779–785.

160. The Danish Group on Verapamil in Myocardial Infarction. Secondary prevention with verapamil after myocardial infarction. *Am J Cardiol* 1990;66:331–401.

161. Rogers WJ, Bowlby LJ, Chandra NC, et al., for the Participants in the National Registry of Myocardial Infarction. Treatment of myocardial infarction in the United States (1990 to 1993). Observations from the National Registry of Myocardial Infarction. *Circulation* 1994;90:2103–2114.

162. Jensen G, Torp-Pedersen C. Prognosis of ventricular fibrillation in hospital. *Eur Heart J* 1992;13:1185–1188.

163. Maggioni AP, Zuanetti A, Franzosi MA, et al. Prevalence and prognostic significance of ventricular arrhythmias after acute myocardial infarction in the fibrinolytic era: GISSI-2 results. *Circulation* 1993; 87:312–322.

164. Teo KK, Yusuf S, Furberg CD. Effects of prophylactic antiarrhythmic drug therapy in acute myoardial infarction. *JAMA* 1993;270:1589–1595.

165. Echt DS, Liebson PR, Mitchell LB, et al. Mortality and morbidity in patients receiving encainaide, flecainide or placebo. The Cardiac Arrhythmia Suppression Trial. *N Engl J Med* 1991;324:781–788.

166. Effect of the antiarrhythmic agent moricizine on the survival after myocardial infarction. The Cardiac Arrhythmia Suppression Trial II Investigators. *N Engl J Med* 1992;327:227–233.
167. Greene HL, Roden DM, Katz RJ, et al. The Cardiac Arrhythmia Suppression Trial: first CAST . . . then CAST-II. *J Am Coll Cardiol* 1992;19:894–898.
168. MacMahon S, Collins R, Peto R, et al. Effects of prophylactic lidocaine in suspected acute myocardial infarction. *JAMA* 1988;260:1910–1916.
169. Guidelines 2000 for Cardiopulmonary Resuscitation and Emergency Cardiovascular Care. Part 6: advanced cardiovascular life support: 7D: the tachycardia algorithms. The American Heart Association in collaboration with the International Liaison Committee on Resuscitation. *Circulation* 2000;102[8 Suppl]:I158–I165.
170. Sleight P. Use of beta adrenoceptor blockade during and after acute myocardial infarction. *Annu Rev Med* 1986;37:415–425.
171. Waldo AL, Camm AJ, deRuyter H, et al. Effect of d-sotalol on mortality in patients with left ventricular dysfunction after recent and remote myocardial infarction. The SWORD Investigators. Survival With Oral d-Sotalol. *Lancet* 1996;348:7–12.
172. Kober L, Bloch Thomsen PE, Moller M, et al. Effect of dofetilide in patients with recent myocardial infarction and left-ventricular dysfunction: a randomised trial. *Lancet* 2000;356:2052.
173. Pratt CM, Singh SN, Al-Khalidi HR, et al. The efficacy of azimilide in the treatment of atrial fibrillation in the presence of left ventricular systolic dysfunction: results from the Azimilide Postinfarct Survival Evaluation (ALIVE) trial. *J Am Coll Cardiol* 2004;43:1211–1216.
174. Cairns JA, Connolly SJ, Roberts R, et al. Randomised trial of outcome after myocardial infarction in patients with frequent or repetitive ventricular premature depolarisations: CAMIAT. Canadian Amiodarone Myocardial Infarction Arrhythmia Trial Investigators. *Lancet* 1997;349:675–682.
175. Julian DG, Camm AJ, Frangin G, et al. Randomised trial of effect of amiodarone on mortality in patients with left-ventricular dysfunction after recent myocardial infarction: EMIAT. European Myocardial Infarct Amiodarone Trial Investigators. *Lancet* 1997;349:667–674.
176. Effect of prophylactic amiodarone on mortality after acute myocardial infarction and in congestive heart failure: meta-analysis of individual data from 6500 patients in randomised trials. Amiodarone Trials Meta-Analysis Investigators. *Lancet* 1997;350:1417–1424.
177. Sodi-Pallares D, Testelli M, Fishleder F. Effects of an intravenous infusion of a potassium-insulin-glucose solution on the electrocardiographic signs of myocardial infarction. *Am J Cardiol* 1962;9:166.
178. Eberli FR, Weinberg EO, Grice WN, et al. Protective effect of increased glycolytic substrate against systolic and diastolic dysfunction and increased coronary resistance from prolonged global underperfusion and reperfusion in isolated rabbit hearts perfused with erythrocyte suspensions. *Circ Res* 1991;68:466–481.
179. Xu KY, Zweier JL, Becker LC. Functional coupling between glycolysis and sarcoplasmic reticulum Ca2+ transport. *Circ Res* 1995;77:88–97.
180. Oliver MF, Opie LH. Effects of glucose and fatty acids on myocardial ischaemia and arrhythmias. *Lancet* 1994;343:155–158.
181. Fath-Ordoubadi F, Beatt KJ. Glucose-insulin-potassium therapy for treatment of acute myocardial infarction: an overview of randomized placebo-controlled trials. *Circulation* 1997;96:1152.
182. Diaz R, Paolasso EA, Piegas LS, et al. Metabolic modulation of acute myocardial infarction. The ECLA (Estudios Cardiologicos Latinamerica) Collaborative Group. *Circulation* 1998;98:2227–2234.
183. Ceremuzynski L, Budaj A, Czepiel A, et al. Low-dose glucose-insulin-potassium is ineffective in acute myocardial infarction: results of a randomized multicenter Pol-GIK trial. *Cardiovasc Drugs Ther* 1999;13:191–200.
184. Van der Horst JC, Zijlstra F, van't Hof AW, et al. Glucose-insulin-potassium infusion in patients treated with primary angioplasty for acute myocardial infarction: the glucose-insulin-potassium study: a randomized trial. *J Am Coll Cardiol* 2003;42:784–791.
185. Malmberg K. Prospective randomised study of intensive insulin treatment on long term survival after acute myocardial infarction in patients with diabetes mellitus. DIGAMI (Diabetes Mellitus, Insulin Glucose Infusion in Acute Myocardial Infarction) Study Group. *BMJ* 1997;314:1512–1515.
186. Wahab NN, Cowden EA, Pearce NJ, et al. Is blood glucose an independent predictor of mortality in acute myocardial infarction in the thrombolytic era? *J Am Coll Cardiol* 2002;40:1748–1754.
187. Capes S, Hunt D, Malmberg K, et al. Stress hyperglycaemia and increased risk of death after myocardial infarction in patients with and without diabetes: a systematic overview. *Lancet* 2000;355:773–778.

CHAPTER 67

Thrombolytic Therapy

Frank J. Zidar and A. Michael Lincoff

Key Words: Diabetes mellitus; fibrin; hypertension; intermittent coronary patency; myocardial infarction; plasmin; recanalization; reocclusion; reperfusion.

INTRODUCTION

Approximately 1.5 million patients experience acute myocardial infarction (AMI) in the United States each year. Although myocardial infarction (MI) had been suspected for nearly a century to originate with coronary thrombosis (1), the pathogenesis of this process remained controversial (2) until DeWood and associates (3) demonstrated that coronary occlusion and thrombus might be detected in most patients with infarction and ST-segment elevation. Plaque rupture in an inflammatory milieu, with exposure of thrombogenic lipids and components of the subendothelium, appears to be the initiating event. This results in platelet adhesion, activation, aggregation, thrombin generation, and fibrin deposition, with formation of occlusive thrombus.

Classic experiments in dogs demonstrated the "wave front" phenomenon of myocardial necrosis during acute coronary occlusion (4,5), wherein cell death begins to occur almost immediately, but a period of 4 hours or more is required before all tissue within the distribution of the occluded vessel is destroyed. Therefore, the rationale for reperfusion therapy in the setting of acute infarction is that rapid clot lysis and restoration of blood flow may interrupt the process of myocardial necrosis, thus limiting infarct size, preserving ventricular function, and ultimately decreasing mortality. The fibrinolytic properties of an extract of β-hemolytic Streptococcus have been recognized since 1933 (6), and initial attempts to recanalize occluded coronary vessels during AMI with this agent were published as early as 1958 (7). The several small-scale studies that followed testing intravenous streptokinase (SK) for acute infarction in the 1960s and early 1970s in retrospect had many methodologic flaws, including inadequate sample sizes, enrollment of late-presenting patients, or overly conservative drug dosing; pooled results, however, suggested significant mortality benefit despite increased risk for hemorrhagic complications (8).

The current era of thrombolytic therapy was ushered in by the seminal angiographic demonstrations of successful myocardial reperfusion by intracoronary fibrinolysis in 1976 (9) and 1979 (10), prompting a number of studies using the intracoronary route of administration to minimize the bleeding risk associated with these agents. Recognition of the logistic difficulties that would be imposed by emergency catheteri-

F. J. Zidar: Division of Cardiology, Duke University Medical Center, Box 3157, Durham, North Carolina 27710.

A. M. Lincoff: Department of Cardiovascular Medicine, F25, The Cleveland Clinic Foundation, 9500 Euclid Avenue, Cleveland, Ohio 44195.

zation to affect intracoronary fibrinolytic administration in all patients with acute infarction led to the investigation of intravenous fibrinolytic therapy, with a series of large-scale, placebo-controlled, randomized trials demonstrating unequivocal efficacy among more than 50,000 patients (11). Pharmacologic reperfusion strategies have evolved to include adjuvant therapies, which concurrently and potently block platelet activation and aggregation or enhance thrombin inhibition. With advanced molecular and recombinant technology, fibrinolytic agents have evolved to become more easily administered, more fibrin-specific, and even resistant to inhibition.

THROMBOLYTIC AGENTS

The fibrinolytic agents act as direct or indirect plasminogen activators, resulting in conversion of this proenzyme to its active form (plasmin), which, in turn, catalyzes the degradation of fibrin or fibrinogen and clot dissolution. These agents may be conceptually dichotomized as "fibrin-specific" and "nonfibrin-specific" activators. Nonspecific activators such as SK, urokinase, or anistreplase convert both circulating and clot-bound plasminogen to plasmin, resulting not only in lysis of fibrin within the clot, but also in substantial systemic fibrinogenolysis, fibrinogenemia, and increase in circulating fibrin degradation products (12). By virtue of their relative selectivity for the plasminogen–fibrin binary complex, the fibrin-selective agents, in contrast, preferentially result in lysis of fibrin at the clot surface with sparing of circulating fibrinogen (12). As a result of selective genetic deletions and mutations in wild type tissue plasminogen activator (t-PA), several third generation thrombolytic agents currently exist. These genetic modifications specifically decrease plasma clearance, increase or decrease fibrin specificity, and confer resistance to inhibition by plasminogen activator inhibitor-1 (PAI-1), whereas still maintaining effective plasminogen activation (Table 67–1).

SK, although not an enzyme, does form a stoichiometric complex with plasminogen, which, in turn, converts uncomplexed plasminogen to plasmin (13). SK is nonfibrin-specific, and administration of the full 1.5-MU dose over 30 to 60 minutes results in a "systemic lytic state" with a decrease in circulating fibrinogen levels to less than 20% of baseline (12). Most humans have some level of preformed antistreptococcal antibodies, which result in mild allergic reactions (fever, urticaria, rash) in about 4% of patients (14); neutralizing antibodies to SK develop after administration and persist for up to 4 years or longer (15), although the clinical significance of this laboratory parameter in terms of diminished thrombolytic efficacy or safety on second exposure has yet to be demonstrated. Hypotension occurs frequently during SK administration, resulting in a mean systolic blood pressure decrease of 35 mm Hg and requiring vasopressor support in 7% to 10% of patients, although this phenomenon is likely caused by bradykinin release rather than allergic response (16).

Anistreplase (anisoylated plasminogen streptokinase activator complex [APSAC]) is an anisoylated derivative of the SK-plasminogen complex, and therefore is a direct plasminogen activator. The anisoylated form of this SK-plasminogen complex is inactive and protected from circulating inhibitors until it is activated by deacylation within the circulation, thus prolonging its half-life to nearly 100 minutes and allowing bolus administration (30 U). This agent is nonfibrin-specific and retains the antigenic and hypotensive properties of its SK moiety.

Urokinase is a naturally occurring, nonfibrin-specific, direct plasminogen activator first isolated from human urine. This agent is synthesized from human kidney tissue culture, and therefore does not share the antigenic properties of SK. Urokinase has not been systematically tested in mortality trials and is not formally approved by the U.S. Food and Drug Administration for intravenous administration in the treatment of AMI.

Staphylokinase (SAK) is a protein produced by *Staphylococcus aureus,* which efficiently activates plasminogen. Small phase II angiographic studies have shown safety and efficacy of a single bolus administration compared with alteplase (17). The high fibrin specificity of SAK makes it an appealing thrombolytic agent; however, despite genetic modifications, issues of antigenicity persist (17,18). Its use has been limited to clinical trials.

t-PA is a naturally occurring protease (containing 537 amino acids) produced by human vascular endothelial cells, and it is considered a key endogenous mediator of intravascular plasminogen activation (19). The activity of this direct plasminogen activator is counter-regulated by circulating inhibitors, particularly PAI-1 and α_2 antiplasmin. Unlike SK, t-PA is not antigenic and is not associated with allergic reactions. The distinguishing feature of t-PA is the relative fibrin specificity, because of its affinity for the fibrin–plasminogen binary complex; at conventional doses, serum fibrinogen levels decrease by only about 50%, with minimal increase in circulating fibrin degradation products (12). The relative fibrin specificity of t-PA appears to enhance the speed with which this agent achieves coronary recanalization relative to the nonspecific agents, as well as improve the ability of t-PA to lyse relatively aged clots (20). In contrast, coronary reocclusion and hemorrhagic complications (including intracranial hemorrhage [ICH]) appear to occur more frequently after administration of t-PA compared with the nonspecific agents; these important issues are discussed later in this chapter. Two commercial forms of recombinant tissue plasminogen activator have been produced, predominantly single-chain (alteplase) and double-chain (duteplase) versions, which appear to be functionally equivalent. The alteplase form has been approved for use in the United States. Alteplase is administered as a "front-loaded" 90-minute infusion because of its short half-life of 4 minutes. In the Global Utilization of Streptokinase and t-PA for Occluded Arteries (GUSTO) trial, a 15 mg intravenous bolus was given followed by a weight-adjusted maintenance regimen of 0.75

TABLE 67–1. *Characteristics of fibrinolytic agents*

Agents	Source	Metabolism	Half-life, min	Fibrin specificity	Dosing	Antigenic	Approximate hospital cost	Comments
Streptokinase	Group C β-hemolytic *Streptococcus*	Hepatic	$t_{1/2\alpha} = 23$	+	60-min infusion	Yes	$200	
Anistreplase	Anisoylated derivative of plasminogen–streptokinase complex	Hepatic	$t_{1/2\alpha} = 95$	+	10-min infusion	Yes	$1,500	
Staphylokinase	*Staphylococcus aureus*, recombinant	Plasma	$t_{1/2\alpha} = 6$	++++	30-min infusion	Yes	NA	
Alteplase	Recombinant	Hepatic	$t_{1/2\alpha} = 4$	+++	90-min infusion	No	$2,200	
Reteplase	Recombinant/mutation	Renal	$t_{1/2\alpha} = 16$	++	Double bolus	No	$2,200	
Lanoteplase	Recombinant/mutation	Hepatic	$t_{1/2\alpha} = 30$	++	Single bolus	No	NA	Increased ICH
Tenecteplase	Recombinant/mutation	Hepatic	$t_{1/2\alpha} = 18$	++++	Single bolus	No	$2,200	Resistant to PAI-I

ICH, Intracranial hemorrhage; NA, not available; PAI-1, plasminogen activator inhibitor-1.

mg per kilogram over 30 minutes (not to exceed 50 mg) and then 0.50 mg per kilogram over 60 minutes (not to exceed 35 mg) (21). This dosing regimen, often referred to as accelerated alteplase, became the standard of therapy against which third generation fibrinolytic agents were assessed for equivalence.

Reteplase (r-PA) is genetic variant of wild type t-PA with a deletion of the sequence altering plasma clearance and fibrin specificity. With a half-life of 16 minutes, it can be administered as a double bolus of 10 mg given 30 minutes apart (22). With the deletion of amino acids 4 through 175, the plasmin cleavage site is maintained, but the tertiary structure that imparts the high fibrin affinity of wild type t-PA is affected and fibrin affinity is decreased (23). Thus, r-PA has a lower affinity for fibrin than wild type t-PA.

Lanoteplase (n-PA) is a genetic variant of wild type t-PA with a deletion of the sequence conferring fibrin specificity, resulting in a decreased fibrin selectivity compared with t-PA. It has the longest half-life of the t-PA derivatives, 30 minutes, allowing for single bolus administration. The phase II Intravenous n-PA for Treatment of Infarcting Myocardium Early (InTIME) trial found 120 kU per kilogram to be the optimal dose achieving maximum infarct-related artery patency and Thrombolysis in Myocardial Infarction (TIMI) III flow (24). An increased incidence of hemorrhagic stroke was seen in the phase III InTIME-II trial (25). The potential causes for this increased ICH incidence are discussed later in this chapter. n-PA is not currently available for clinical use.

Tenecteplase (TNK–t-PA) is a mutant version of t-PA specifically modified using three distinct amino acid substitutions to alter fibrin binding and plasma clearance. Two mutations in the tertiary structure which imparts the high fibrin affinity of wild type t-PA, result in a 14-fold increase in fibrin affinity, markedly minimizing systemic plasminogen activation (26,27). The decreased clearance of TNK–t-PA allows for single bolus administration. A unique feature of this engineered agent is its resistance to PAI-1, a major regulator of the fibrinolytic system. TNK–t-PA may also induce less of a prothrombotic state after lysis, as measured by thrombin-antithrombin complex; whereas SK and alteplase administration resulted in a fourfold and twofold increase in thrombin-antithrombin complex, respectively; no change was seen with TNK–t-PA (28).

Bolus Fibrinolysis

An advantage of longer acting third generation thrombolytic agents is the relative ease of administration as a simple single or double bolus injection, whereas prior agents required a sustained infusion with or without a loading dose. Easier administration may make prehospital therapy feasible, leading to more rapid treatment of ST-segment elevation MI, and improved survival (29,30); this advance in thrombolytic therapy is currently being evaluated. Bolus therapy also seems to result in fewer medication errors. Of the 41,021 patients treated in the GUSTO-I trial with alteplase or SK, 12% had a medication error (31). The Assessment of the Safety of a New Thrombolytic (ASSENT)-2 study revealed a greater frequency of dosing errors with alteplase versus single bolus TNK–t-PA (32). In the InTIME-II trial, there were more dosing errors in the alteplase group than in the single bolus n-PA group (7.3% vs. 5.7%; $p \leq 0.001$) (25). These errors may be associated with an increase in 30-day mortality and increased ICH (31,33). Simplification of fibrinolytic therapy as a bolus dose has become increasingly important as new combination regimens with glycoprotein (GP) IIb/IIIa inhibitors and antithrombin agents evolve.

CLINICAL EFFICACY OF THROMBOLYTIC AGENTS

Various end points have been used to evaluate and compare the clinical usefulness of different thrombolytic regimens in the setting of AMI. Although the most important goal of thrombolytic therapy for infarction is that of mortality reduction, "megatrials" enrolling tens of thousands of patients are required to detect significant improvements in the risk for this relatively infrequent event. On the basis of the intuitive paradigm, whereby thrombolytic therapy would be expected to produce mortality reduction through restoration of infarct vessel patency and myocardial salvage, these latter two end points also have been used in the assessment of thrombolytic efficacy. Although the relations among patency, left ventricular function, and mortality remain to be precisely defined, these parameters may either individually or in combination serve as clinically relevant measures of therapeutic benefit. The failures with thrombolytic therapy have led to an increased focus on the successful reperfusion of the microvasculature, not just the infarct-related epicardial vessel. The techniques available to measure complete myocardial reperfusion, including corrected TIMI frame count (CTFC), TIMI myocardial perfusion grade (TMPG), ST-segment monitoring, and myocardial contrast echocardiography (MCE), are reviewed in this chapter.

Patency: Epicardial and Microvascular Reperfusion

Epicardial Patency

The primary angiographic end point addressed by many of the clinical thrombolytic trials has been that of infarct vessel patency, despite the limitations inherent in this "snapshot" angiographic view that often fails to reflect adequately the dynamic nature of coronary recanalization or the potential for dissociation between epicardial coronary reflow and tissue-level myocardial reperfusion. Early animal experiments demonstrated that administration of t-PA resulted in more rapid clot lysis than did that of SK, although patency with both agents reached a similar plateau at later periods (34). Numerous angiographic studies, summarized in a comprehensive review by Granger and colleagues (35), have reported rates of infarct vessel patency produced in patients by the first and second generation thrombolytic agents. During the first 24 hours after AMI, angiography reveals an open infarct-related artery in only 9% to 29% of patients who have not received reperfusion therapy (20,36,37). At the historical 90-minute window of observation after initiation of thrombolytic therapy, infarct vessel patency (TIMI 2 or 3 flow) is achieved least frequently after treatment with intravenous SK (43–64%) (20,38) and in nearly equal proportions of patients receiving t-PA in "standard" dosages (63–79%) (36,39–42) or anistreplase (55–73%) (38,43).

Superior infarct vessel patency was obtained using an accelerated dosing regimen of alteplase initially proposed by Neuhaus and colleagues (44), in which the majority of the dose (~60–70%) was administered over 30 minutes with the balance over the subsequent hour (compared with administration over 3 hours). Using this alteplase "front-loading" technique, it was found that 90-minute patency rates ranged from 82% to 91% (mean 85%) (44–48). In numerous phase II angiographic studies performed using third generation fibrinolytic agents, 90-minute patency rates (TIMI 2 or 3 flow) have been quite similar despite the agent used—r-PA (83–85%) (22,49), n-PA (83%) (24), or TNK–t-PA (75–88%) (27,50) (Table 67–2).

It has become apparent that "patency" is not simply a dichotomous event, but the quality of coronary recanalization may be more properly viewed as a continuum ranging from an absence of distal coronary blood flow to complete normalization of myocardial perfusion. As initially proposed by the TIMI study group, angiographic outcome after thrombolysis may be classified according to the extent of contrast penetration beyond the coronary lesion: TIMI 0—with no flow; TIMI 1—with minimal penetration of contrast; TIMI 2—with delayed flow of contrast that nevertheless fills the infarct vessel; and TIMI 3—brisk and complete flow (20). By this scheme, arteries with TIMI Grade 0 or 1 flow were regarded as occluded, whereas those exhibiting Grade 2 or 3 flow were initially considered patent.

Several studies have demonstrated that TIMI 2 and TIMI 3 flow are not functionally equivalent (51–54). Among more than 1,200 patients enrolled in different phases of the Thrombolysis and Angioplasty in Myocardial Infarction (TAMI) trials (54), the presence of TIMI 2 rather than TIMI 3 flow at 90-minute angiography was associated with significantly less myocardial salvage, an increased incidence of congestive heart failure and recurrent myocardial ischemia, and a trend toward greater risk for death (6.1% for TIMI 2 vs. 4.3% for TIMI 3). The significant relation between TIMI flow grade and mortality was documented among patients in the GUSTO Angiographic Substudy (Fig. 67–1) (51). The relative frequency of Grade 2 and 3 flow in coronary arteries considered to be patent after infarction has been remarkably consistent across various reports (Table 67–2).

Consistently less angiograms demonstrated TIMI 3 flow at 60-minute versus 90-minute end points. In view of the critical importance of early initiation of thrombolytic therapy, it may be inferred that a greater rapidity of infarct artery recanalization also would confer a substantial benefit in terms of survival and preservation of ventricular function. Thus, rather than at 90 minutes, optimal reperfusion should be more ap-

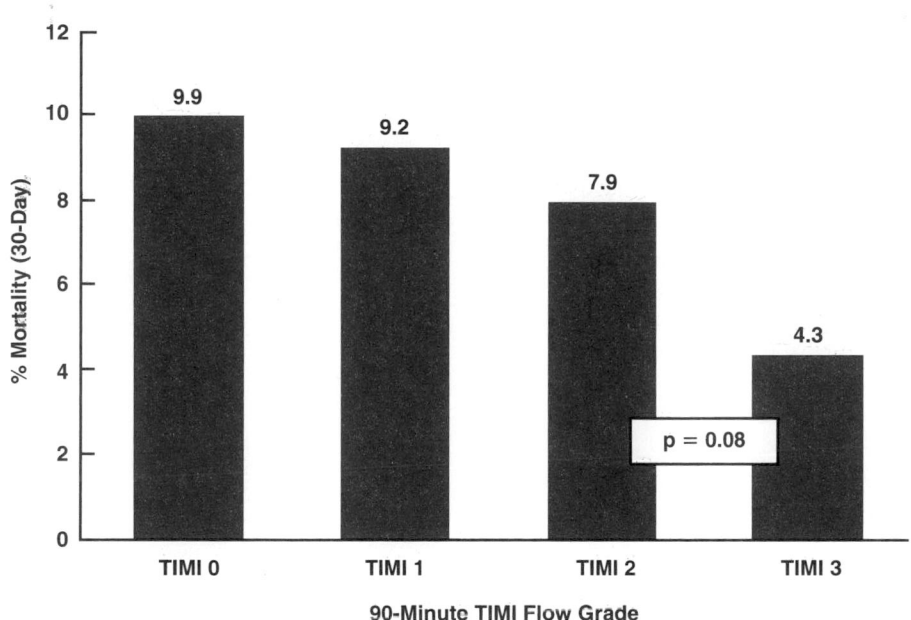

FIG. 67–1. Relation between 30-day mortality and 90-minute infarct vessel patency (defined by Thrombolysis in Myocardial Infarction [TIMI] flow) in the Global Utilization of Streptokinase and t-PA for Occluded Arteries (GUSTO) Angiographic Substudy (51). There is a substantial gradient in mortality with improved patency grade.

TABLE 67–2. Patency and thrombolysis in myocardial infarction 3 flow of fibrin-specific agents

Trial (year)	Thrombolytic regimen	Time to treatment	Time to angiography, min	Patients undergoing catheterization, n	Patency, % patients with TIMI 2 or 3	TIMI 3, %	TIMI 2, %
TAPS (1992)	Accelerated rt-PA (100 mg/90 min)	162 min	60	199	73	54%	19
			90	199	84	72	12
Neuhaus et al. (1989)	Accelerated rt-PA (100 mg/90 min)	<6 h	60	73	74	59%	15
			90	74	91	78	12
RAAMI (1991)	"Standard" rt-PA (100 mg/3 h)	168 min	60	86	63	40%	23
			90	122	77	54	23
	Accelerated rt-PA (100 mg/90 min)	162 min	60	87	76	62%	14
			90	128	81	62	20
TAMI (1992)	"Standard" rt-PA	?	—	—	—	—	—
	Accelerated rt-PA, rt-PA + urokinase, Urokinase		90	1,229	72	55	17
TIMI 4 (1993)	Accelerated rt-PA	?	—	—	—	—	—
	Anistreplase		—	—	—	—	—
	Anistreplase + rt-PA		90	210	76	47	29
STAR (1995)	r-staphylokinase (10 or 20 mg/30 min)	161 min	90	48	75	60	15
	Accelerated rt-PA (100 mg/90 min)	158 min	90	52	77	54	23
RAPID (1995)	"Standard" rt-PA (100 mg/3 h)	186 min	60	101	66	33%	33
			90	145	77	49	28
	Reteplase (10 mg double bolus)	180 min	60	98	78	51%	27
			90	142	85	63	22
RAPID II (1996)	Accelerated rt-PA (100 mg/90 min)	150 min	60	121	66	37%	29
			90	157	73	45	28
	Reteplase (10 mg/double bolus)	144 min	60	115	82	51%	31
			90	146	83	60	24
Vanderschueren et al. (1997)	r-staphylokinase (15-mg double bolus)	163 min	—	—	—	—	—
			90	50	84	68	16
	Accelerated rt-PA (100 mg/90 min)	186 min	—	—	—	—	—
			90	52	79	54	25
InTIME (1998)	Accelerated rt-PA (100 mg/90 min)	192 min	60	107	66	37%	29
			90		71	25	46
	Lanoteplase (120 kU/kg bolus)	186 min	60	102	72	47%	25
			90		83	26	57
TIMI 10B (1998)	Accelerated rt-PA (100 mg/90 min)	94 min	60	170	79	48%	31
			90	311	82	63	19
	TNK–t-PA (40-mg bolus)	94 min	60	88	75	55%	21
			90	148	79	63	16

InTIME, Intravenous n-PA for Treatment of Infarcting Myocardium Early; RAAMI, Randomized Angiographic trial of recombinant tissue-type plasminogen activator (Alteplase) in Myocardial Infarction; rt-PA, recombinant tissue-type plasminogen activator (alteplase); TAPS, rt-PA–APSAC Patency Study; TAMI, Thrombolysis and Angioplasty in Myocardial Infarction; TIMI, Thrombolysis in Myocardial Infarction; TNK–t-PA, tenecteplase.

propriately judged as the restoration of angiographic patency as quickly as possible after administration of fibrinolytic agents. Sixty-minute TIMI 3 flow rates became an accepted angiographic end point and have been reported in several angiographic studies (Table 67–2) (17,18,22,24,27,44–46,49, 50,54,55). Among patients enrolled in thrombolytic trials undergoing angiography 60 minutes after therapy with accelerated dosages of alteplase, 54% (range 37–62%) were found to have TIMI 3 flow (24,27,44–46,49,50,54,55). Among more than 3,000 patients enrolled in randomized, controlled, angiographic studies performed using third generation thrombolytic agents, 60-minute TIMI 3 flow rates were quite similar despite the agent used—r-PA (51%) (22,49), n-PA (47%) (24), or TNK-t-PA (55%) (27,50). Thus, by the criteria of rapid and complete restoration of coronary patency, only half of patients appear to achieve optimal reperfusion, despite more fibrin-specific fibrinolytic agents.

More quantifiable methods of assessing epicardial vessel flow have confirmed the relation with clinical outcomes. CTFC quantifies the number of cine frames required for dye to reach standardized distal coronary landmarks, with a correction for the greater length of the left anterior descending artery (56). In a study of 1,248 patients from the TIMI 4, 10, and 10B trials, a multivariate model revealed a 0.7% increase in absolute mortality at 30 days for every 10-frame increase in CTFC (57). Patients with TIMI 3 flow (or CTFC < 40) after lysis also were stratified based on CTFC, showing CTFC less than 20 was associated with a 7.9% incidence of in-hospital adverse events, whereas the event rate was 15.5% with CTFC of 20 to 40 (57). CTFC remains a predictor of mortality even at 2-year follow-up. In a multivariate model, which corrected for previously identified correlates of death (age, sex, pulse, anterior infarction, and any percutaneous coronary intervention [PCI] during initial hospitalization), CTFC (hazard ratio 0.90 per 10-frame decrease, $p = 0.01$) was associated with a reduced 2-year mortality rate (58).

Reocclusion

Although timely restoration of coronary patency may result in substantial preservation of myocardium during acute infarction, this benefit may be attenuated by subsequent occurrence of reocclusion. The clinical consequences of reocclusion depend on the extent of initial salvage of jeopardized myocardium and the adequacy of collateral coronary flow. In a series of 91 patients with reocclusion documented angiographically 0.5 to 38 days after successful thrombolysis (with or without adjunctive angioplasty) in the TAMI trials (59), reocclusion was associated with a greater in-hospital mortality rate (11.0% vs. 4.5%; $p = 0.001$), less recovery of global or infarct zone left ventricular function, and greater rates of pulmonary edema, hypotension, respiratory failure, and atrioventricular block than was sustained infarct artery patency. It is likely that thrombotic reocclusion is mediated primarily by the interaction of a number of hematologic factors (60–63).

The reported incidences of reocclusion with the different fibrinolytic agents vary considerably, in part related to the use of aspirin and heparin and the methods by which reocclusion was detected. There exist clear data that reocclusion after treatment with the fibrin-specific agent alteplase occurs more frequently than after therapy with nonfibrin-specific agents such as SK, APSAC, or urokinase (Fig. 67–2). In a pooled analysis of more than 1,100 patients, all of whom received aspirin and intravenous heparin, the reocclusion rate with alteplase at 13% was nearly twice that with the other agents (35). This increased risk for reocclusion may be, in part, because of the shorter half-life and the diminished systemic fibrinogen breakdown with alteplase than with nonspecific agents. The role of heparin and antiplatelet therapy in the prevention of reocclusion and recurrent ischemia during thrombolysis is addressed later in this chapter together with the discussion of other adjunctive agents.

Although reocclusion has been variably reported to negate the preservation of ventricular function and reduction in mortality achieved by successful thrombolysis (59,64), these data are confounded by the use of varying adjunctive pharmacotherapy, the frequency of mechanical reperfusion, and the methods (timing) by which reocclusion was detected (at 24 hours, discharge, or 3–6 months). It also is important to consider that a therapeutic intervention that provides increased early patency will result in more vessels available for reocclusion. Nonetheless, although in-hospital reocclusion rates may be in excess of 10% among patients treated with the fibrin-specific agent alteplase (35), it is sobering to note that late reocclusion of 25% to 30% of previously patent infarct-related arteries was documented by coronary angiography performed 3 to 6 months after hospital discharge in the TAMI-6 and the Anti-thrombotics in the Prevention of Reocclusion in Coronary Thrombolysis (APRICOT) trials (65,66).

A phenomenon observed in experimental models that may also play a role in the degradation of thrombolytic efficacy in humans is that of intermittent coronary patency. Oscillatory reflow and occlusion after successful coronary thrombolysis may be demonstrated by serial angiography (67–69) or inferred from continuous electrocardiographic monitoring (69–72) in 16% to 58% of patients (Fig. 67–3). This process appears to be primarily caused by thrombin activity (73) and obstructive platelet aggregation at the site of plaque rupture, followed by dislodgement and embolization (61,74). Although the clinical significance of cyclic coronary flow after thrombolytic reperfusion remains to be clearly defined, this finding has been associated with reduced myocardial salvage and poor long-term coronary patency (70,71), as well as a trend toward greater 1-year mortality rates (70). Continuous ST-segment monitoring may provide a better understanding of the complex and dynamic nature of reperfusion (75).

Microvascular Flow

Patency of the epicardial infarct-related artery is a less than ideal tool to assess the success of thrombolysis because it

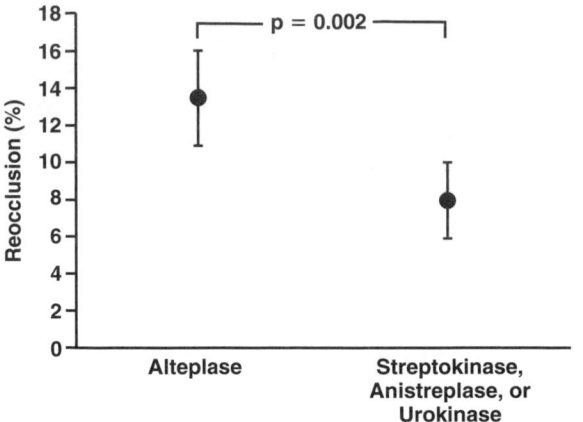

FIG. 67–2. Pooled analysis of angiographic reocclusion rates from 1,173 patients enrolled in randomized trials comparing alteplase with nonfibrin-specific agents; reocclusion rates were greater after alteplase (*p* = 0.002). (From Granger CB, Califf RM, Topol EJ. Thrombolytic therapy for acute myocardial infarction, a review. *Drugs* 1992;44:293–325, with permission.)

does not account for flow in the microvasculature and reperfusion of the myocardium on a cellular or tissue level. The move from epicardial TIMI flow to assessing microvascular reperfusion began with the development of MCE, a technique wherein microbubbles are injected into the circulation and perfusion of the subserved myocardium is assessed by surface echocardiography. Work with MCE has provided evidence that epicardial artery recanalization as determined by angiography may be dissociated from tissue-level reperfusion. Ito and associates (76) used this imaging technique to demonstrate the absence of myocardial reflow, despite a patent infarct artery, in 23% of 39 patients with acute anterior MI treated with direct coronary angioplasty or thrombolysis. Patients without microcirculatory reflow had significantly less recovery of global or regional left ventricular function than those in whom myocardial perfusion had been restored. In a larger series of 86 patients with an anterior MI and with TIMI 3 flow at initial angiogram, a significant improvement in left ventricular function at 1 month was seen only in those patients who had normal microcirculatory reflow (77). Newer contrast agents that can be injected intravenously have been developed (78,79), and small clinical studies are underway (80). MCE dramatically demonstrated the importance of com-

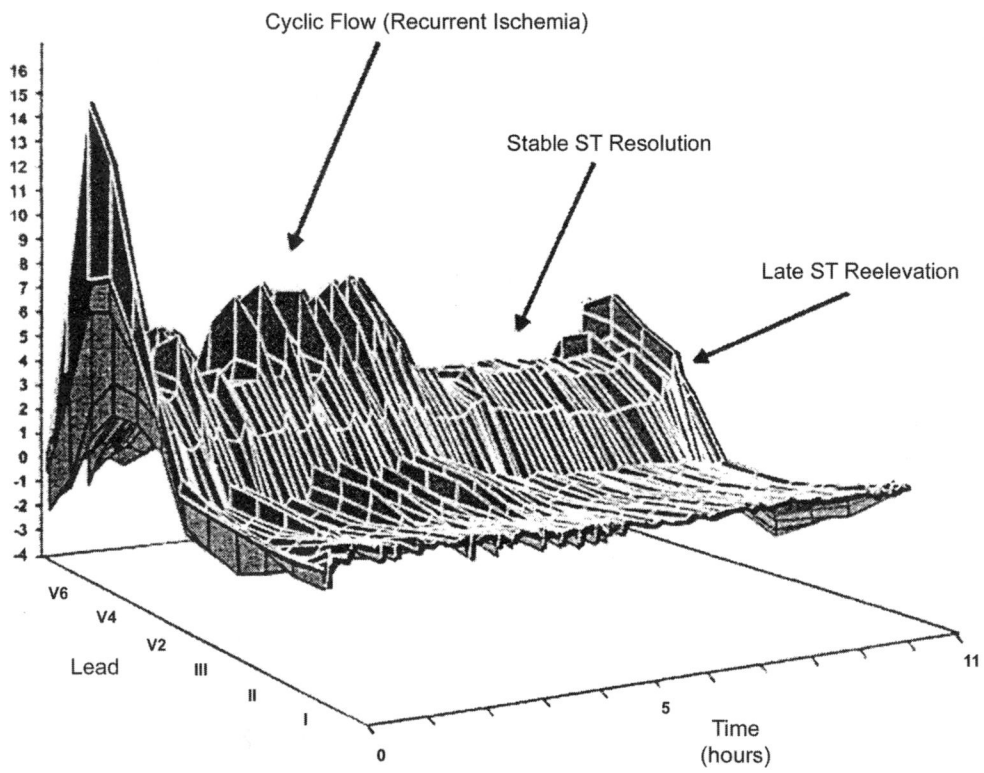

FIG. 67–3. Transient recurrent ST-segment elevations, likely representing cyclic infarct artery flow, detected by continuous 12-lead electrocardiographic monitoring in a patient after thrombolytic therapy in the Global Utilization of Streptokinase and t-PA for Occluded Arteries (GUSTO) trial. (From Lincoff AM, Topol EJ. Illusion of reperfusion. Does anyone achieve optimal reperfusion during acute myocardial infarction? [Erratum appears in *Circulation* 1993;88:1361–1374.] *Circulation* 1993;87:1792–1805, with permission.)

plete reperfusion of the microvasculature by the correlation to improved clinical outcomes. Other markers of microvascular reperfusion include TMPG and ST-segment resolution.

The TMPG is an angiographic method for assessing the status of the microcirculation after reperfusion therapy. TMPG quantifies the microvascular blush: TMPG 0—no blush; TPMG 1—dye stains the myocardium and persists on the next injection; TPMG 2—stains the myocardium but washes out slowly so that dye is strongly persistent at the end of the injection; TPMG 3—normal entrance/exit of dye so that it is mildly persistent at the end of the injection (81). The TMPG was obtained for the 762 patients in the TIMI 10B trial, and a 30-day mortality gradient was seen across the perfusion grades—TMPG 3 (2.0%), TMPG 2 (4.4%), TMPG 0/1 (6.0%, three-way $p = 0.05$). TMPG also predicted 30-day mortality independent of TIMI flow. TMPG is a powerful predictor of mortality even at 2-year follow-up. In a multivariate model that corrected for previously identified correlates of death (age, sex, pulse, anterior infarction, and any PCI during initial hospitalization), TMPG 2 or 3 (hazard ratio, 0.46; $p = 0.02$) was associated with a reduced 2-year mortality rate (58).

Resolution of ST-segment elevation has been considered a marker of epicardial *and* microvascular reperfusion. ST-segment resolution is an accurate predictor of both short- and long-term mortality and congestive heart failure in patients after thrombolytic therapy (82,83). Data from three randomized trials including more than 3,500 patients receiving thrombol-

ysis reveal a consistent relation between the degree of ST-segment resolution and subsequent 35-day mortality (Fig. 67–4) (72). In addition to the degree of ST-segment resolution, the time to ST-segment resolution also predicts 1-year mortality. Comparing ST-segment resolution at 60 versus 90 minutes in the 1,797 patients enrolled in the InTIME-II trial, investigators showed a 2.7% versus 4.7% 1-year mortality (84). In studies using TMP grading, patients with normal epicardial flow and persistent ST-segment elevation had lower TMPGs indicative of impaired microvascular perfusion (85,86). Given availability of the electrocardiogram and accessibility and technical limitations of angiography, ST-segment resolution would appear to be an attractive option to determine the success of microvascular reperfusion and to identify patients in need of mechanical reperfusion. Unfortunately, even among patients with "complete" (≥70%) ST-segment elevation, only 70% to 80% will have TIMI 3 flow (87). Thus, ST-segment elevation accurately predicts patency but not always complete (epicardial and microvascular) reperfusion. Moreover, because of the dynamic nature of reperfusion, the ideal time to measure ST-segment resolution after thrombolysis remains controversial.

Left Ventricular Function

Despite identification of left ventricular ejection fraction as an important predictor of long-term mortality after AMI (88), the use of this parameter as an end point for evaluation

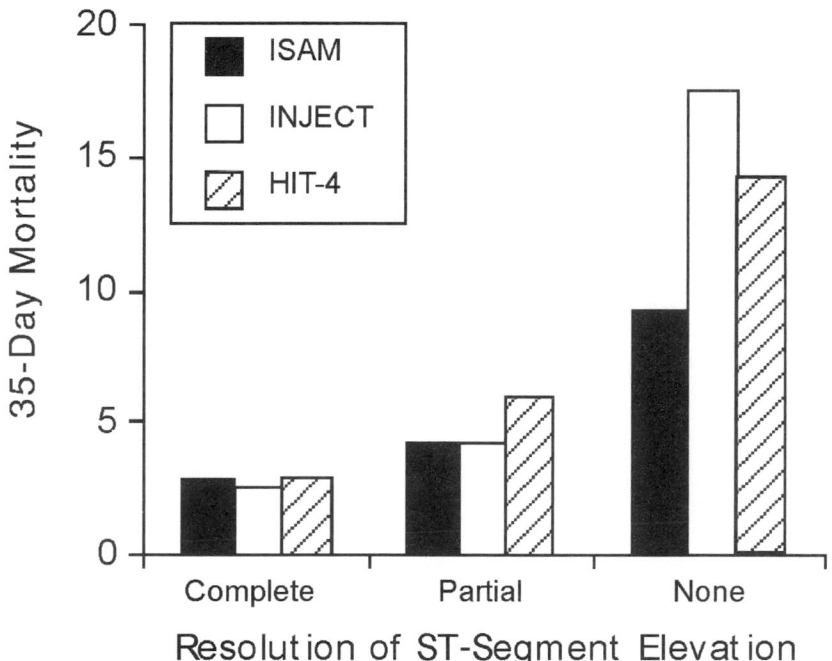

FIG. 67–4. In three studies of acute myocardial infarction, the degree of ST-segment resolution at 180 minutes after thrombolytic therapy was associated with 35-day mortality. Data from the Hirudin for Improvement of Thrombolysis (HIT)–4 (158), International Joint Efficacy Comparison of Thrombolytics (INJECT) study (112), and Intravenous Streptokinase in Acute Myocardial Infarction (ISAM) trial (94).

of thrombolytic therapy has proven to be problematic. Differences in left ventricular function among treatment groups may be obscured by many factors, including the relatively high proportion of missing values from the patients with the worst prognosis who die, those referred for coronary bypass surgery, those who did not undergo catheterization, or those part of technically inadequate studies. Moreover, the average ejection fraction in a cohort of patients treated with thrombolysis may actually be reduced relative to control therapy, because of inclusion of values obtained from the sickest patients who might otherwise have died had thrombolytic therapy not been administered (89). In addition, compensatory hyperkinesis of noninfarcted segments of the left ventricle early in the course of infarction tends to limit the extent to which global ejection fraction reflects infarct size.

Interpretation of left ventricular function data derived from the various thrombolytic trials is therefore complex and has been discussed in detail elsewhere (35). However, the important points may be summarized as follows. First, trials comparing thrombolytic with control therapy have in general demonstrated improvements in ejection fraction with thrombolysis, although the magnitude of benefit has been modest and variable. Second, the differences in ejection fraction between lytic and control groups do not improve (and, if anything, appear to narrow) over time (Fig. 67–5). Third, the magnitudes of improvement in left ventricular function and infarct vessel patency appear to be related, with ventricular function most highly correlated with early patency rather than with thrombolytic treatment per se (90–92). Fourth, there is, however, essentially no correlation between the improvement in ejection fraction and the reduc-

tion in mortality produced by thrombolytic therapy (93). Fifth, most trials attempting to compare fibrinolytic agents have failed to demonstrate a difference with regard to left ventricular ejection fraction.

Mortality: Thrombolytic versus "Conventional" Therapy

The benefit of thrombolytic therapy in the setting of AMI was demonstrated in the most unequivocal and relevant manner by five major placebo-controlled, randomized trials that used the reduction in short-term (3–5 weeks) mortality as their primary end point (14,29,94–96). Despite different entry criteria, fibrinolytic agents, adjunctive therapies, and follow-up periods, the highly concordant results of these trials, at least during the first 6 hours of MI, demonstrated a pooled mortality reduction of 27% among more than 28,000 patients (Fig. 67–6). The landmark Gruppo Italiano per lo Studio della Streptochinasi nell'Infarto Miocardico (GISSI-1) trial of 11,806 patients treated with SK or conventional therapy (not placebo) within 12 hours of symptom onset (29) was the first study to show definitively a reduction in mortality with thrombolytic therapy during AMI (Fig. 67–7A), representing approximately 23 lives saved per 1,000 patients treated. This mortality benefit of thrombolysis was preserved by 1-year follow-up (17.2% in the SK group vs. 19.0% among control subjects; $p = 0.008$) (97). The Second International Study of Infarct Survival (ISIS-2) (14) extended these findings by demonstrating the critical importance of aspirin therapy among 17,187 patients randomized in a 2 × 2 factorial design to receive placebo, aspirin (160 mg on the first day, continued indefinitely), SK, or aspirin

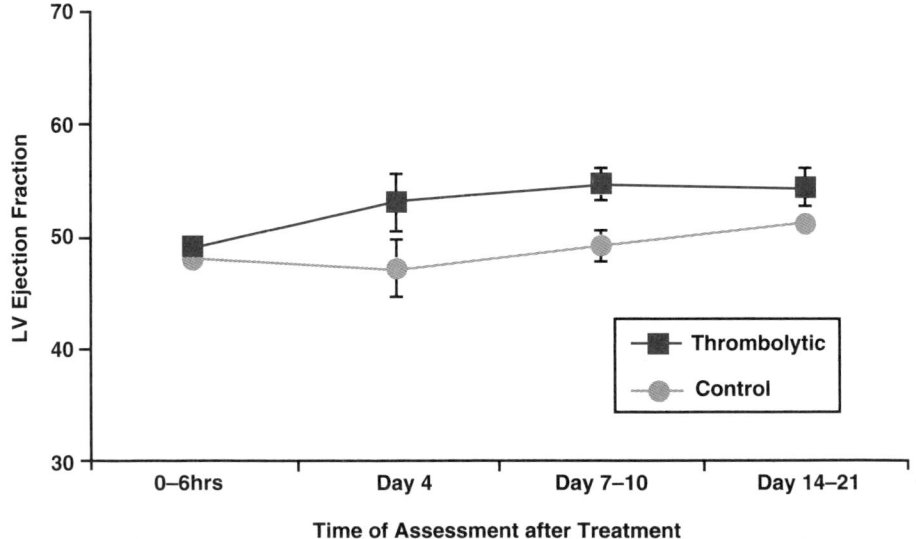

FIG. 67–5. Pooled analysis of left ventricular (LV) ejection fraction from 3,066 ventriculographic observations during randomized trials of thrombolytic therapy versus control. Thrombolysis results in significantly greater ejection fractions at each time point. (From Granger CB, Califf RM, Topol EJ. Thrombolytic therapy for acute myocardial infarction, a review. *Drugs* 1992;44:293–325, with permission.)

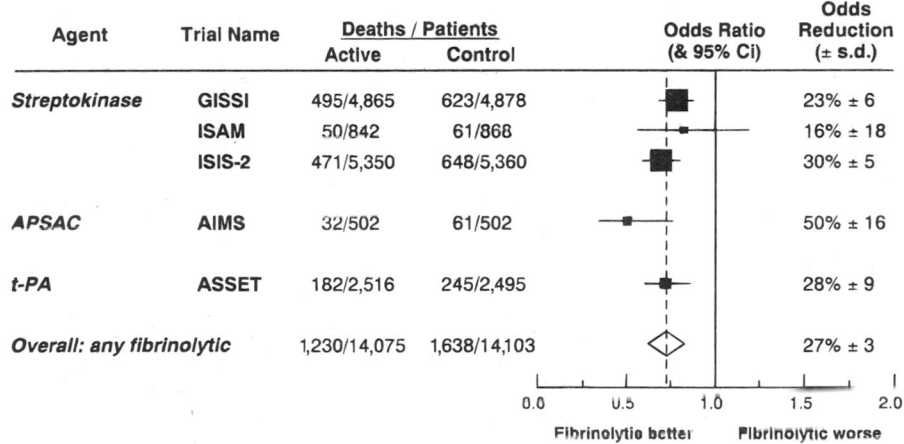

Agent	Trial Name	Deaths / Patients		Odds Ratio (& 95% Ci)	Odds Reduction (± s.d.)
		Active	Control		
Streptokinase	GISSI	495/4,865	623/4,878		23% ± 6
	ISAM	50/842	61/868		16% ± 18
	ISIS-2	471/5,350	648/5,360		30% ± 5
APSAC	AIMS	32/502	61/502		50% ± 16
t-PA	ASSET	182/2,516	245/2,495		28% ± 9
Overall: any fibrinolytic		1,230/14,075	1,638/14,103		27% ± 3

0.0   0.5   1.0   1.5   2.0

Fibrinolytic better   Fibrinolytic worse

FIG. 67–6. Reduction in mortality (3–5 weeks) among patients treated within 6 hours of symptom onset in the five major placebo-controlled trials of thrombolytic therapy. AIMS, Anistreplase Intervention Mortality Study; APSAC, anistreplase (anisoylated plasminogen streptokinase activator complex); ASSET, Anglo-Scandinavian Study of Early Thrombolysis; CI, confidence interval; GISSI, Gruppo Italiano per lo Studio della Streptochinasi nell'Infarto Miocardico; ISAM, Intravenous Streptokinase in Acute Myocardial Infarction; ISIS-2, Second International Study of Infarct Survival; t-PA, tissue plasminogen activator. (From Granger CB, Califf RM, Topol EJ. Thrombolytic therapy for acute myocardial infarction, a review. *Drugs* 1992;44:293–325, with permission.)

plus SK. Aspirin produced a relative reduction (23%) in mortality that was equal to that of SK (24%) and was additive when the two drugs were administered together (42%) (Fig. 67–7B).

The Anglo-Scandinavian Study of Early Thrombolysis (ASSET) examined the efficacy of alteplase plus heparin compared with placebo plus heparin among 5,011 patients, with a 26% mortality rate reduction due to thrombolytic therapy despite administration of alteplase over a relatively long infusion time (100 mg over 5 hours) and no use of aspirin in this early study (96). A subsequent randomized, placebo-controlled trial of alteplase infused over 3 hours

with both heparin and aspirin demonstrated a 51% mortality rate reduction (98).

The Fibrinolytic Therapy Trialists' (FTT) Collaborative Group reported the pooled data from all nine controlled trials of fibrinolytic therapy, which each randomized more than 1,000 patients (11). Among these 58,600 patients, fibrinolytic therapy produced a highly significant 18% mortality rate reduction during the first 35 days, with a highly concordant mortality benefit among nearly every patient subgroup examined.

Mortality data derived from collaborative analyses of the major placebo-controlled thrombolytic trials (11,99) have

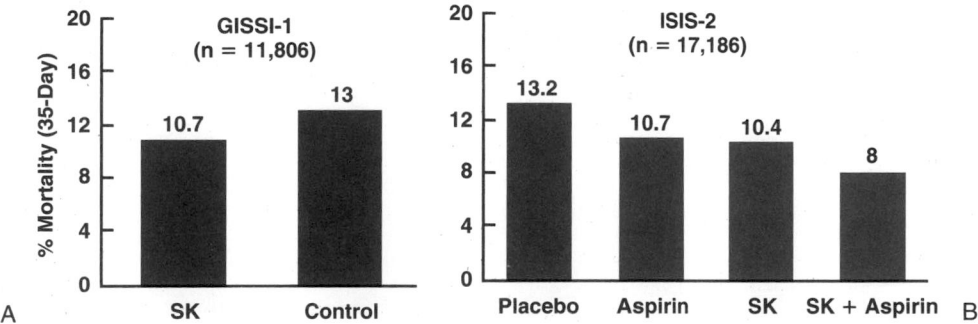

FIG. 67–7. A: Mortality (21 days) reduction with streptokinase versus conventional therapy in Gruppo Italiano per lo Studio della Streptochinasi nell'Infarto Miocardico (GISSI)-1. **B:** Data from Second International Study of Infarct Survival (ISIS-2) demonstrating reduction in 5-week vascular mortality compared with placebo by aspirin, streptokinase (SK), or the combination of aspirin and SK. (A: From Gruppo Italiano per lo Studio della Streptochinasi nell'Infarto Miocardico (GISSI). Effectiveness of intravenous thrombolytic treatment in acute myocardial infarction. *Lancet* 1986;1:397–401, with permission; B: from ISIS-2 (Second International Study of Infarct Survival) Collaborative Group. Randomized trial of intravenous streptokinase, oral aspirin, both, or neither among 17,187 cases of suspected acute myocardial infarction: ISIS-2. *Lancet* 1988;2:349–360, with permission.)

demonstrated the phenomenon of the "early hazard." During the first day of hospitalization for acute infarction, patients who receive thrombolytic therapy are actually paradoxically at greater risk for mortality than those receiving conventional therapy (Fig. 67–8). Mortality rates on subsequent days are greater in the patients not receiving thrombolytics, thus leading to the net observed mortality benefit of thrombolytic therapy. The cause of the early hazard is unknown, although investigators have suggested that reperfusion injury and early cardiac rupture may play a role.

Mortality: Comparative Thrombolytic Studies Using Alteplase

With the first phase of large-scale, randomized, mortality trials demonstrating the efficacy of thrombolysis compared with conventional therapy, subsequent research has been directed at defining and refining the optimal thrombolytic and adjunctive agents to achieve coronary reperfusion and to reduce mortality during acute infarction. The superior early patency rates obtained with alteplase as compared with other thrombolytic agents and the paradigm of the "open-vessel hypothesis" led to an expectation of improved clinical benefit with this agent as well. Two large trials, GISSI-2/International and ISIS-3, set out to test this hypothesis. In the GISSI-2/International study, 20,891 patients were randomized within 6 hours of onset of MI with ST-segment elevation to receive alteplase (conventional dosing of 100 mg over 3 hours) or SK, with a subrandomization to subcutaneous heparin (12,500 U twice daily) initiated 12 hours after thrombolysis or no heparin (100,101). All patients received aspirin. This trial found no difference in mortality rates at 30

to 35 days between patients treated with alteplase or SK (Fig. 67–9A). The ISIS-3 trial enrolled 41,299 patients within 24 hours of symptoms consistent with acute infarction, although without electrocardiographic criteria, to therapy with SK, conventional dosing of the duteplase form of t-PA (0.6 MU/kg over 3 hours), or anistreplase (102); all patients received aspirin, and a subrandomization to subcutaneous heparin or no heparin, initiated 4 hours after initiation of thrombolysis, also was carried out in this trial. As with the GISSI-2/International study, ISIS-3 30-day mortality rates among patients receiving SK, alteplase, or anistreplase were the same (Fig. 67–9B).

In neither the GISSI-2/International nor the ISIS-3 study did the addition of subcutaneous heparin to aspirin confer mortality benefit with any of the three thrombolytic agents. In GISSI-2, heparin was associated with an increased risk for "major" bleeds (1.0% vs. 0.5%), whereas in ISIS-3, "definite" or "probable" ICH was significantly greater in patients receiving subcutaneous heparin (0.56% vs. 0.40%). Moreover, both of these studies demonstrated that alteplase rather than SK therapy was associated with an increased risk for total stroke (1.3% vs. 1.0% in GISSI-2) or ICH (0.7% vs. 0.3% in ISIS-3).

The findings of the GISSI-2/International and ISIS-3 studies among more than 60,000 patients led to an apparent thrombolytic paradox, where despite that alteplase was known to open arteries faster than SK, it was not found to save more lives. This conclusion had been defended by reference to the "catch-up phenomenon" of coronary patency (Fig. 67–10), with the suggestion that the speed of restoration of patency is not as important as that most vessels will ultimately become open with any thrombolytic agent

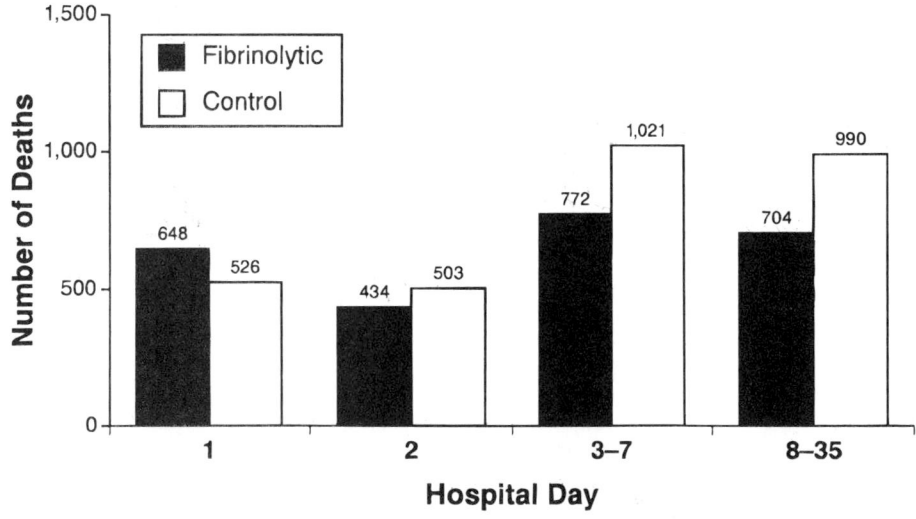

FIG. 67–8. Data from an overview of seven major randomized, controlled, thrombolytic trials (11), demonstrating the paradoxically increased mortality risk during the first day of hospitalization among patients treated with streptokinase or alteplase, compared with placebo therapy ("early hazard"). (From Lincoff AM, Topol EJ. Illusion of reperfusion. Does anyone achieve optimal reperfusion during acute myocardial infarction? [Erratum appears in *Circulation* 1993;88:1361–1374.] *Circulation* 1993;87:1792–1805, with permission.)

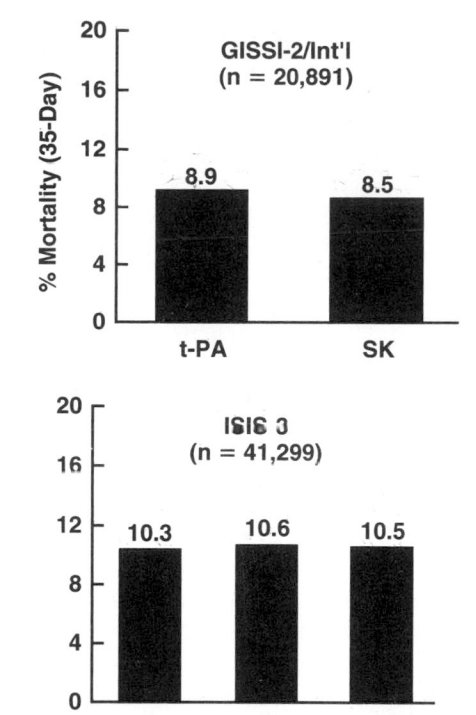

FIG. 67–9. A: Mortality (30- to 35-day) data from Gruppo Italiano per lo Studio della Streptochinasi nell'Infarto Miocardico (GISSI)-2/International Study (100,101) demonstrating no difference in mortality among patients treated with conventional dosing of alteplase or streptokinase (SK). **B:** Mortality (35-day) data from the Third International Study of Infarct Survival (ISIS-3) trial (102), again showing no differences among patients treated with alteplase, SK, or anistreplase (APSAC).

(103,104). There are other potential explanations for the observed lack of correlation between mortality reduction and choice of thrombolytic agent in the GISSI-2 and ISIS-3 studies, which are concordant with the paradigm of early infarct vessel recanalization. First, although the velocity of recanalization is greater with alteplase than with SK or anistreplase, sustained patency with the fibrin-specific alteplase appears to be critically dependent on adequate and consistent thrombin inhibition by heparin (105–107). Both the GISSI-2/International and ISIS-3 trials used heparin by subcutaneous injection, initiated in a delayed fashion after administration of thrombolytic therapy. The inadequacies of the subcutaneous route of heparin therapy have been documented, both in terms of delayed (108) and widely variable (109) degrees of anticoagulation. Second, the accelerated "front-loading" technique of administration of alteplase produces substantially greater and more rapid infarct vessel recanalization than the conventional alteplase regimen used in the GISSI-2 and ISIS-3 studies (46,47), suggesting that these megatrials did not test the optimal means of achieving infarct artery reperfusion.

The GUSTO-I trial was therefore undertaken to test directly the hypothesis that rapid, complete, and sustained coronary reperfusion would result in mortality reduction relative to conventional thrombolytic therapy (21). More than 41,000 patients were randomized within 6 hours of onset of symptoms of AMI to one of four treatment strategies. The reference arm of SK (1.5 MU over 60 minutes) with subcutaneous heparin (12,500 U twice daily) was that used in ISIS-3, whereas a second treatment arm used SK with intravenous heparin to assess the incremental benefit derived from intravenous heparin with SK. The third strategy used the regimen known to achieve infarct vessel patency most

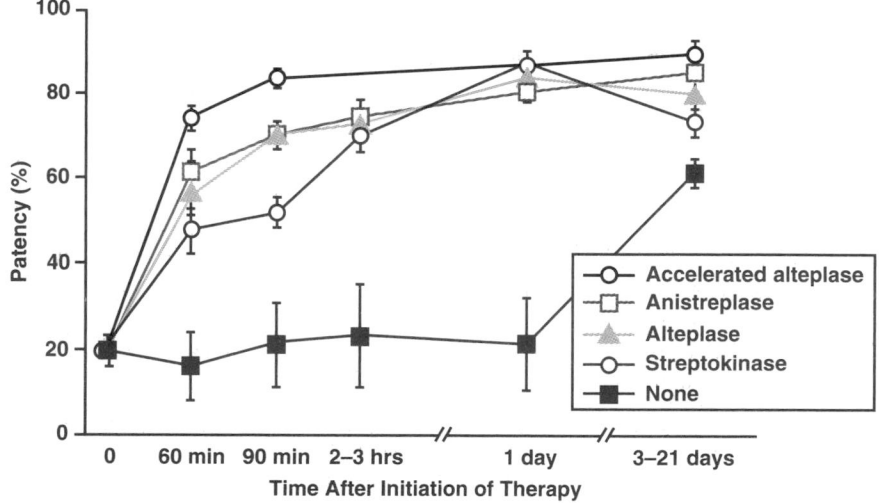

FIG. 67–10. Pooled analysis of patency rates over time after various thrombolytic agents among more than 13,728 angiographic observations. Patency rates are greatest after accelerated alteplase, roughly equal after conventional alteplase or anistreplase, and lowest after streptokinase, although the "catch-up" phenomenon is apparent after 2 to 3 hours. (From Granger CB, Califf RM, Topol EJ. Thrombolytic therapy for acute myocardial infarction, a review. *Drugs* 1992;44:293–325, with permission.)

rapidly, that of accelerated, weight-adjusted dosing of alteplase (15-mg bolus, 0.75 mg/kg over 30 minutes, then 0.50 mg/kg over 60 minutes) with intravenous heparin. Finally, a combined alteplase (1 mg/kg over 60 minutes) and SK (1 MU over 60 minutes) arm with intravenous heparin was included, on the basis of pilot data indicating that such a combination might effectively reduce the risk for reocclusion.

Compared with the treatment arms of SK with either subcutaneous or intravenous heparin or the combination of alteplase and SK, accelerated alteplase resulted in a highly significant 14% relative reduction in the primary end point of 30-day mortality, representing 9 to 11 lives saved per 1,000 patients treated (Fig. 67–11). This benefit of accelerated alteplase relative to the other treatment arms was consistent across nearly every patient subgroup examined both prospectively and retrospectively, with the possible exceptions of patients presenting more than 6 hours after symptom onset and patients with Killip Class IV cardiogenic shock (although the number of patients in these subgroups was small). When considered from the standpoint that thrombolysis resulted in approximately 28 lives saved per 1,000 patients treated in the original landmark placebo-controlled trials, the incremental 9 to 11 lives saved with the use of accelerated alteplase and intravenous heparin in GUSTO-I represented a substantial (~36%) clinically relevant improvement in the efficacy of this form of therapy.

Framed within the GUSTO-I main trial was an angiographic substudy of 2,431 patients randomized to undergo angiography to assess vessel patency at various time points ranging from 90 minutes to 7 days (51). By the traditional 90-minute time point, a substantially and significantly greater proportion of arteries was patent in the accelerated alteplase group (Fig. 67–12). Reocclusion rates were low

and not different in the four groups, ranging from 7.7% with SK plus subcutaneous heparin to 5.3% with alteplase plus SK. This angiographic substudy demonstrating the best patency in the alteplase group provided the mechanistic data to explain differences in mortality noted in the main clinical trial. When mortality rates were assessed as a function of the status of the infarct vessel at 90 minutes, regardless of the treatment used to achieve that status, there was a highly significant association between infarct vessel patency and survival (Fig. 67–1). GUSTO-I, therefore, confirmed the "open-vessel hypothesis" that mortality benefit from thrombolysis is a result of achievement of rapid, complete, and sustained infarct vessel patency.

Mortality reduction with more aggressive thrombolytic regimens in GUSTO-I was obtained at the price of a "stroke gradient," where the rates of total stroke, ICH, fatal stroke, and disabling stroke were all heightened by increasing aggressiveness of thrombolytic therapy. Disabling strokes were least frequent in the SK group with subcutaneous heparin (0.25%) and were greatest in the accelerated alteplase group (0.41%). To reconcile the opposing outcomes of mortality benefit versus increased risk for stroke, the concept "net clinical benefit" is used. Compared with either the SK arm or the pooled SK data, accelerated alteplase resulted in a mortality benefit of 9 to 11 lives saved per 1,000 patients treated. Subtracted from this mortality benefit was the number of patients who experienced nonfatal disabling stroke, an additional 1 patient per 1,000 treated with alteplase rather than SK. Thus, even with the slight excess of disabling stroke in the alteplase group, there was nevertheless a net clinical benefit of 9 lives saved without disabling stroke per 1,000 patients treated with accelerated alteplase rather than SK.

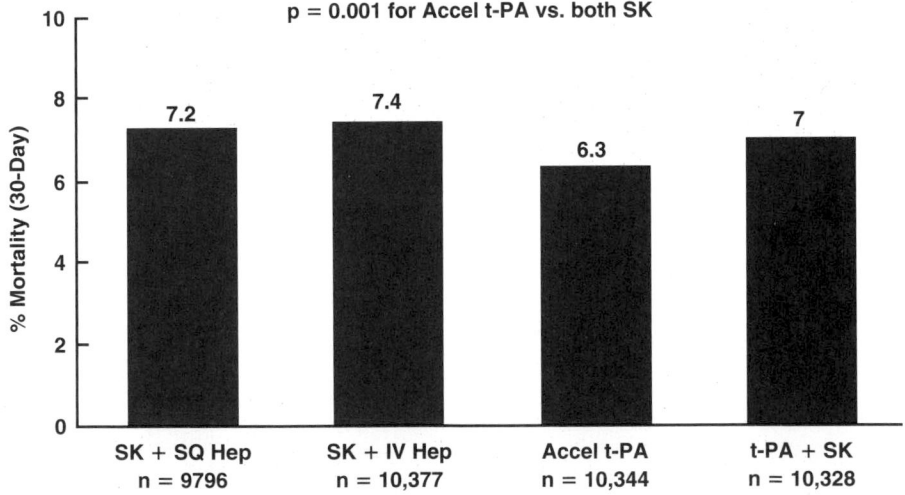

FIG. 67–11. The 30-day mortality rates for the four treatment arms in the Global Utilization of Streptokinase and t-PA for Occluded Arteries (GUSTO)-I trial. The accelerated (Accel) alteplase with intravenous (IV) heparin strategy resulted in a highly significant reduction in mortality compared with the other three groups (21). Hep, heparin; IV, intravenous; SK, streptokinase; SQ, subcutaneous; t-PA, tissue plasminogen activator.

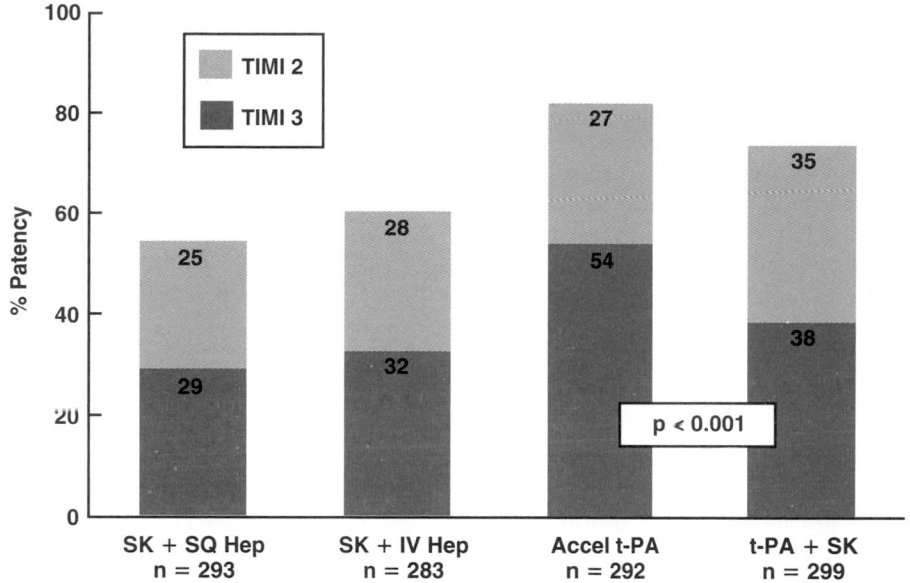

FIG. 67–12. Patency rates for the four treatment groups in the Global Utilization of Streptokinase and t-PA for Occluded Arteries (GUSTO)-I Angiographic Substudy. By 90 minutes, patency (defined as Thrombolysis in Myocardial Infarction [TIMI] 3 flow or as TIMI 2 + 3 flow) was significantly better among patients treated with accelerated (Accel) alteplase (51). Hep, heparin; IV, intravenous; SK, streptokinase; SQ, subcutaneous; t-PA, tissue plasminogen activator.

The large sample size in the GUSTO-I trial lent itself to outcome modeling to determine the predictors of mortality after thrombolytic therapy. Several patient characteristics, such as age, Killip class, infarct location, systolic blood pressure, and heart rate were shown to be strong predictors of 30-day mortality and are listed in Table 67–3 (110).

TABLE 67–3. *Predictors of 30-day mortality in the Global Utilization of Streptokinase and t-PA for Occluded Arteries (GUSTO) trial*

Patient characteristics	Adjusted χ^2	p
Age	717	<0.00001
Systolic blood pressure	550	<0.00001
Killip class	350 (3 df)	<0.00001
Heart rate, bpm	272 (2 df)	<0.00001
Location of infarction	143 (2 df)	<0.00001
Prior infarction	64	<0.00001
Age by Killip class interaction	29	<0.00001
Height, cm	31 (4 df)	<0.00001
Time to treatment	23	<0.00001
Diabetes	21	<0.00001
Weight, kg	16	<0.0001
Smoking	22 (2 df)	<0.0001
Choice of fibrinolytic therapy	15 (3 df)	<0.0001
Prior bypass surgery	16	<0.0001
Hypertension	14	<0.01
Prior cerebrovascular disease	10	<0.01

df, degrees of freedom.
Adapted from Lee KL, Woodlief LH, Topol EJ, et al. Predictors of 30-day mortality in the era of reperfusion for acute myocardial infarction. Results from an international trial of 41,021 patients. GUSTO-I Investigators. *Circulation* 1995;91: 1659–1668, with permission.

Mortality: Comparative Thrombolytic Studies Using Third Generation Thrombolytic Agents

GUSTO-I tested and proved the superiority of accelerated alteplase, at that time a novel agent and approach, versus established treatment. Once unequivocal benefit of lysis was established, it became unethical to randomize new therapies in a placebo-controlled design. Thus, a different trial method and statistical approach, known as equivalence testing, was used with many of the third generation fibrinolytic agents. This method assumes that the differences between outcomes with two treatments should be less than a certain prespecified value to be considered equivalent. Because the absolute mortality benefit observed with fibrinolytic therapy over placebo in controlled trials was 2% (11), studies have adopted an absolute mortality difference of half that for placebo (i.e., a 1% reduction) to be equivalent. Therefore, a new therapy is considered to have equivalent efficacy if it has an absolute mortality rate and 95% confidence intervals within 1% of the established therapy, assuming a similar safety profile is observed (111).

The efficacy of r-PA was assessed in two large-scale, phase III trials: the International Joint Efficacy Comparison of Thrombolytics (INJECT) study and the GUSTO-III trial. The INJECT study, an equivalence trial comparing SK with r-PA (two 10-MU bolus doses 30 minutes apart) in 6,010 patients, showed a 35-day mortality rate of 9.02% with r-PA versus 9.53% with SK. The absolute mortality reduction (0.5%; 95% confidence intervals, −1.98 to 0.96) satisfied the criterion for equivalency, suggesting that r-PA is at least as effective as SK and superior to placebo (112). This led to the GUSTO-III trial, which enrolled more than 15,000 patients in 20 countries and randomized them in a 2:1 ratio to receive r-PA (two 10-MU bolus doses) or accelerated alteplase (up to 100 mg over 90 minutes). The trial's hypothesis—that 30-day mortality would be less with r-PA versus alteplase—was based on the phase II RAPID trial, which showed improved patency with r-PA (49). Compared with alteplase, r-PA did not provide additional survival benefit at 30 days (7.47% for r-PA vs. 7.24% for alteplase; $p = 0.54$; odds ratio, 1.03) and had no significant impact on the combined end point of death or nonfatal, disabling stroke (7.89% for r-PA vs. 7.91% for alteplase; $p = 0.97$; odds ratio, 1.0) (113). The absolute mortality difference of 0.23% in favor of alteplase and the broad 95% confidence intervals around that difference did not meet the strict predetermined definition of equivalence. Thus, r-PA cannot be considered equivalent to alteplase on the basis of GUSTO-III results. One-year follow-up revealed no significant difference in mortality (11.1% for r-PA vs. 11.2% for alteplase; $p = 0.77$) (114).

n-PA was tested in a large, phase III, randomized equivalence trial (25). A total of 15,078 patients were treated with n-PA using the 120-kU per kilogram dose, determined from the phase II angiographic study (24) to achieve best patency, versus accelerated alteplase. Overall 30 day mortality was similar between the two agents (6.7% for n-PA vs. 6.6% for alteplase; $p < 0.05$ for equivalence). ICH rates, however, were significantly greater with n-PA compared with alteplase (1.13% vs. 0.62%; $p < 0.003$) (25). n-PA, therefore, has not been approved for clinical use.

The ASSENT and TIMI 10 trials investigated TNK–t-PA dosing, safety, and efficacy. TIMI 10B, with 886 patients, was a phase II angiographic and dose finding study; ASSENT, with 3,325 enrolled patients, was a parallel safety study of TNK–t-PA. The TIMI 10B Investigators found that a 40-mg bolus of TNK–t-PA provided similar TIMI 3 flow rates and frame counts compared with alteplase, and that weight adjustment of TNK–t-PA achieved optimal reperfusion (27,115). After the heparin dosing regimen was modified (with earlier titration at 6 hours), rates of serious bleeding and ICH with weight-adjusted TNK–t-PA were similar to rates with accelerated alteplase regimen (27,116). The large phase III equivalence trial, ASSENT-2, enrolled 16,949 patients. A weight-based, single bolus of TNK–t-PA was found to be equivalent to accelerated alteplase on the basis of 30-day mortality rates (6.18% for TNK–t-PA vs. 6.15% for alteplase) and absolute mortality reduction (primary analysis: 0.028%; p value for equivalence = 0.006). Rates of ICH were similar (~0.9%), although fewer non-cerebral bleeding complications (26.4% vs. 29.0%; p = 0.0003) and fewer blood transfusions (4.3% vs. 5.9%; p = 0.0002) were observed with TNK–t-PA. The 30-day mortality rate among patients treated more than 4 hours after the onset of symptoms was significantly less in the patients who received TNK–t-PA (7% vs. 9%) (32). It was proposed by the trial investigators that this apparent benefit among late treated patients may be related to the increased fibrin specificity of TNK–t-PA compared with alteplase. A similar trend of survival favoring a more fibrin-specific agent, alteplase, was noted among late treated patients in GUSTO-III.

CONTROVERSIES AND COMPLICATIONS

The global effectiveness of reperfusion therapy remains limited in that most patients hospitalized with acute infarction are considered ineligible for thrombolytic administration. The National Registry of Myocardial Infarction (NRMI)-2 Investigators identified 272,651 patients presenting to the emergency departments (EDs) of 1,470 participating hospitals with a MI. Among these patients, 84,663 were eligible for thrombolytic therapy as defined by the following: presentation less than 6 hours after symptom onset, ST-segment elevation or left bundle branch block on the initial electrocardiogram, and no contraindications to thrombolytic therapy. Using these strict criteria, only 31% of these were considered to be eligible for reperfusion therapy after exclusions (117). Importantly, criteria for exclusion of patients from thrombolytic therapy are based in large part on overly restrictive protocols of the early randomized trials or untested assumptions regarding inadequate potential for benefit or excessive bleeding risk in certain subgroups of patients. In fact, mortality among patients with infarction who are deemed ineligible for thrombolysis is substantially greater than in those who are received treatment; in one analysis of 1,206 patients screened for inclusion in the TIMI 2B trial (118), the in-hospital mortality rate among the 163 patients who received alteplase was only 2.5%, whereas among the patients excluded for various reasons, mortality rates ranged from 10% to 25%. Thus, thrombolytic treatment has generally been applied to patients at relatively low risk, with exclusion of those patient subsets at high risk who may derive the most substantial survival benefit from reperfusion therapy (117).

There is little controversy regarding the benefit of thrombolytic therapy among patients younger than 76 years with ischemic chest pain of less than 6 hours in duration and electrocardiographic ST-segment elevations (119). Similarly, there is nearly universal agreement that a number of medical comorbidities, such as intracranial neoplasm, arteriovenous fistula or aneurysm, recent craniospinal trauma or surgery, severe bleeding diatheses, coagulopathy or thrombocytopenia, aortic dissection, or history of hemorrhagic cerebrovascular accident, likely are life threatening and pose prohibitively high risks for ICH with thrombolytic administration. A substantial proportion of patients with acute infarction, however, fall into one or more categories for whom the treatment with thrombolytic therapy has been more controversial. Although data suggest that for many of these patients, the benefit of thrombolysis has been under appreciated.

Advanced Age

In early trials of thrombolytic therapy, patients older than 75 years of age were frequently excluded because of a perception of increased risk for major bleeding complications (120,121) and speculation that thrombolysis may be less effective in elderly than in younger patients. Thus, nearly 15% of patients with acute infarction were considered ineligible for thrombolytic therapy on the basis of age (122), despite clear evidence of a marked increase in baseline risk for mortality with increasing age (ranging from <2% among patients <40 years to >18% among those ≥75 years) (123, 124). The two major placebo-controlled mortality trials of SK, GISSI (29) and ISIS-2 (14), had no upper age limit, however, and active lytic treatment resulted in substantial mortality reductions in all age groups in these two trials (Table 67–4). Importantly, although older patients experienced more modest relative mortality reductions than their younger counterparts (which did not quite reach statistical significance in GISSI), the absolute mortality benefits were actually greatest in the most elderly patients as a consequence of their greatest baseline risk (125). Similarly, whereas the relative mortality reduction caused by alteplase rather than SK therapy among elderly (75 years old) patients in GUSTO was less than that in younger patients, the absolute mortality benefit was greater in the elderly group (21).

Notably, the incidence of hemorrhagic stroke associated with thrombolysis also appears to grow with increasing patient age (126–128). An analysis by Krumholz and associates (129), however, demonstrated that even for a wide range of possible rates of lethal or incapacitating complications, the net clinical benefit of thrombolytic therapy among elderly patients remains quite favorable. Thus, although many older patients may be unsuitable for treatment with fibrinolytic agents because of other medical comorbidities, advanced senescence, late presentation, or nondiagnostic electrocardiographic findings, the data suggest that age per se is an inappropriate exclusionary criterion for thrombolytic therapy, and that, as with younger patients, an individualized approach to evaluation and treatment is required. Fortunately, the percentage of patients older than 75 years in thrombolytic trials has been increasing (113), and no longer are upper age limits used as an exclusion criterion.

Late Presentation

On the basis of experimental and clinical studies demonstrating minimal myocardial salvage when thrombolysis is administered more than 4 hours after coronary occlusion (4), approximately 41% of patients with acute infarction have been excluded from thrombolytic treatment because of presentation greater than 6 hours after the onset of ischemic symptoms (117). In the ISIS-2 trial, however, a significant reduction in mortality was observed among patients treated with SK between 5 and 24 hours after onset of pain (14), whereas a nonsignificant trend toward decreased mortality also was evident among a smaller cohort of patients treated between 6 and 9 hours in the GISSI study (29).

Therefore, three randomized, placebo-controlled trials have directly addressed the role of thrombolytic therapy among patients presenting after the traditional 6-hour time window. The TAMI-6 study group found that among 197 patients with 6 to 24 hours of anginal symptoms and ST-segment elevation randomized to alteplase or placebo, there was no difference in left ventricular systolic function at 6 months (65). The Late Assessment of Thrombolytic Efficacy (LATE) study compared alteplase with placebo in 5,709 patients presenting 6 to 24 hours after acute infarction (130). Mortality at 35 days was reduced with alteplase therapy from 11.9% to 8.7% among patients treated between 6 and 12 hours of symptom onset (p = 0.033), a 27% relative mortality reduction. Only a small, nonsignificant reduction in death rates was observed in those patients presenting after 12 hours. These mortality reductions were associated with only a modest excess of nonfatal strokes (1.3% vs. 0.7%) in the thrombolytic group. A similar, although nonsignificant, 12% benefit among patients randomized within 6 to 12 hours of infarction was observed with SK therapy in the Estudios Multicentrico Estreptoquinasa Republica Americas Sud (EMERAS) trial (131), whereas again there was no trend toward mortality reduction in those patients treated later. In aggregate, these trials thus provide strong evidence of benefit with thrombolysis for patients treated up to 12 hours from symptom onset.

TABLE 67–4. *Mortality as a function of age in the Gruppo Italiano per lo Studio della Streptochinasi nell'Infarto Miocardico and Second International Study of Infarct Survival trials*

| Trial | Patient age, yr | Mortality rate | | Mortality reduction with SK | |
		Streptokinase	Control	Relative, %	Absolute (lives saved/1,000)
GISSI (SK alone)	<60	5.7	7.7	26	20
	60–69	16.6	18.1	8	15
	>70	28.9	33.1	13	42
ISIS-2 (SK + aspirin)	<65	3.7	6.2	40	25
	65–75	9.1	16.1	43	70
	>75	15.8	23.8	34	80

GISSI, Gruppo Italiano per lo Studio della Streptochinasi nell'Infarto Miocardico; ISIS, Second International Study of Infarct Survival; SK, streptokinase.
Adapted from Sherry S, Marder VJ. Mistaken guidelines for thrombolytic therapy of acute myocardial infarction in the elderly. *J Am Coll Cardiol* 1991;17:1237–1238, with permission.

1004 / Chapter 67

In the ASSENT-2 and GUSTO-III trials, patients who were treated more than 4 hours after their symptom onset had lower 30-day mortality rates when treated with more fibrin-specific agents (32,113). Similar angiographic patency findings have been observed among patients presenting after 4 hours of symptoms (20,40). With the hypothesis that increased fibrin specificity achieves better fibrinolysis in more mature coronary thrombosis, agents such as TNK–t-PA, or potentially SAK, may have a future role in application of thrombolysis for patients with prolonged symptoms or late presentation.

Infarct Location and Size

Because of the lower baseline mortality rate among patients with inferior rather than anterior infarctions, many individual mortality trials have been underpowered to detect an unequivocal benefit in these patients. The metaanalysis by FTT, however, demonstrated a reduction in mortality of 8 lives per 1,000 patients with inferior infarction treated (11), a somewhat modest improvement compared with the 37 lives saved per 1,000 patients with anterior infarction. It has become apparent that the magnitude of benefit derived from fibrinolytic therapy is more dependent on the size of the infarction rather than the anatomic location. An analysis derived from GISSI experience (132) demonstrated a distinct gradient in absolute mortality benefit according to the extent of infarction as measured by the number of ECG leads with ST-segment elevation. Thus, thrombolysis is likely to be beneficial in patients with inferior MI, particularly in those with extensive myocardium in jeopardy.

Hypertension

A history of stable systemic hypertension has never been demonstrated to be a risk factor for ICH in patients treated with thrombolytic therapy (126,128) and should not constitute a criterion for exclusion. There are data to suggest, however, that hemorrhagic stroke risk may be associated with hypertension at presentation. A large-scale analysis by the GISSI group implicated increase of diastolic blood pressure to greater 110 mm Hg at the time of admission with a significant fivefold increase in the incidence of hemorrhagic stroke (128); systolic hypertension in this study, however, was associated with only a nonsignificant trend toward increased stroke risk after multivariate adjustment. Similarly, in the FTT report, a systolic blood pressure greater than 175 mm Hg was associated with a trend toward increased stroke risk, although, importantly, there remained a substantial mortality benefit among these patients as well (11). Most phase III studies assessing clinical benefit and harm of thrombolytic therapy currently exclude patients with systolic blood pressure greater that 180 mm Hg or diastolic blood pressure greater than 110 mm Hg on repeated measurements at presentation. Thus, although the exact role of thrombolytic therapy among patients with systemic hyper-

tension on admission remains to be defined, refractory or diastolic increases in blood pressure should be considered to represent contraindications to thrombolytic therapy.

Intracranial Hemorrhage

The major risk of thrombolytic therapy is ICH. This tragic complication usually occurs in the first 24 hours and is associated with high morbidity and mortality (133,134). Age is the greatest predictor among the several patient characteristics that are associated with greater risk for ICH after thrombolysis. Using data from 71,073 patients from NRMI-2, multivariable modeling that demonstrated advanced age, female sex, African-American ethnicity, systolic blood pressure of 140 mm Hg or greater, diastolic blood pressure of 100 mm Hg or greater, history of stroke, and low body weight were significantly associated with ICH (Fig. 67–13) (134). The multivariable analysis of predictors of ICH performed by the GUSTO-I investigators demonstrated the continuous nature of these predictors of ICH, specifically age, blood pressure, and weight (Fig. 67–14) (133). Although ICH was a rare occurrence in GUSTO-I, there was an increased incidence in the patients who received alteplase (0.5% for SK vs. 0.7% for alteplase) (21). As more fibrin-selective agents, such as TNK–t-PA, are used, a trend toward a decrease in ICH has been observed. In ASSENT-2, patients older than 75 years had an incidence rate of ICH of 1.7% in the TNK–t-PA group and 2.6% in the alteplase group (32). Similarly, GUSTO-III Investigators observed a trend toward a greater rate of ICH in patients older than 75 years treated with the relatively less fibrin-specific r-PA versus those treated with who received alteplase (2.5% vs. 1.7%; odds ratio, 1.55; $p = 0.21$) (113). Among thin (<67 kg), elderly women, a group identified in several studies as at increased risk for ICH (134–136), the rate of ICH in ASSENT-2 was 1.1% with TNK–t-PA and 3.0% with alteplase (multivariate-adjusted odds ratio, 0.30; 95% confidence intervals, 0.09–0.98; $p < 0.05$) (135). The level of anticoagulation with intravenous heparin, as measured by activated partial thromboplastin time, also influences the rate of ICH (32,137). Increased rates of ICH among patients treated with hirudin and heparin in conjunction with thrombolysis in the GUSTO-IIa (138), TIMI-9a (137), and Hirudin for improvement of thrombolysis (HIT)-III (139) trials emphasize the risks of more potent anticoagulation in combination with thrombolysis. The 1999 American College of Cardiology/American Heart Association (ACC/AHA) guidelines on the management of patients with AMI recommend the "judicious use" of unfractionated heparin for at least 48 hours when alteplase is the chosen thrombolytic agent and to target the activated partial thromboplastin time (aPTT) to a range of 50 to 70 seconds. Excessive risk of ICH has been associated with bolus thrombolysis in one metaanalysis (140), although a pooled review of more than 30,000 patients concluded that no evidence exists of excess ICH with TNK–t-PA or r-PA versus accelerated al-

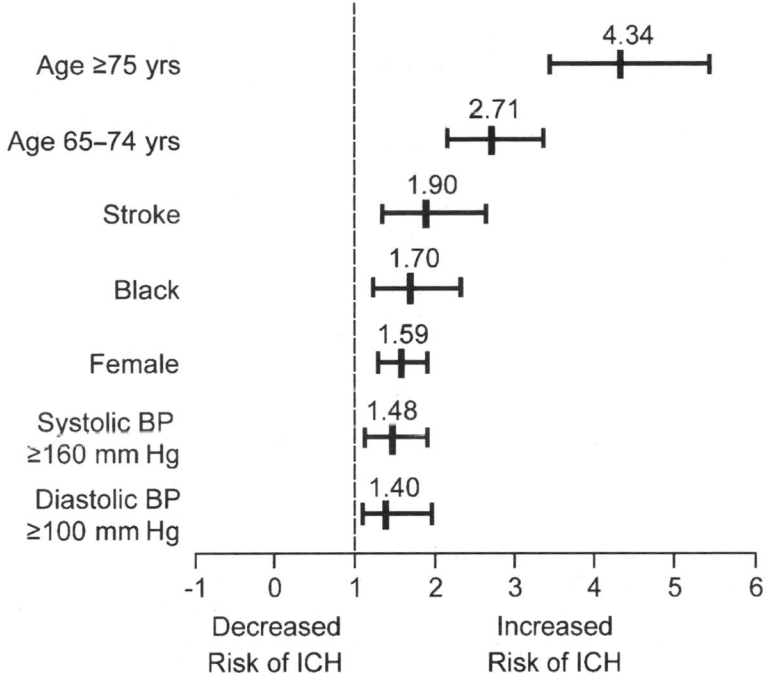

FIG. 67–13. Predictors of intracerebral hemorrhage from the National Registry of Myocardial Infarction-2 multivariate model. BP, blood pressure; ICH, intracranial hemorrhage. (Adapted from Gurwitz JH, Gore JM, Goldberg RJ, et al. Risk for intracranial hemorrhage after tissue plasminogen activator treatment for acute myocardial infarction. Participants in the National Registry of Myocardial Infarction 2. *Ann Intern Med* 1998;129:597–604, with permission.)

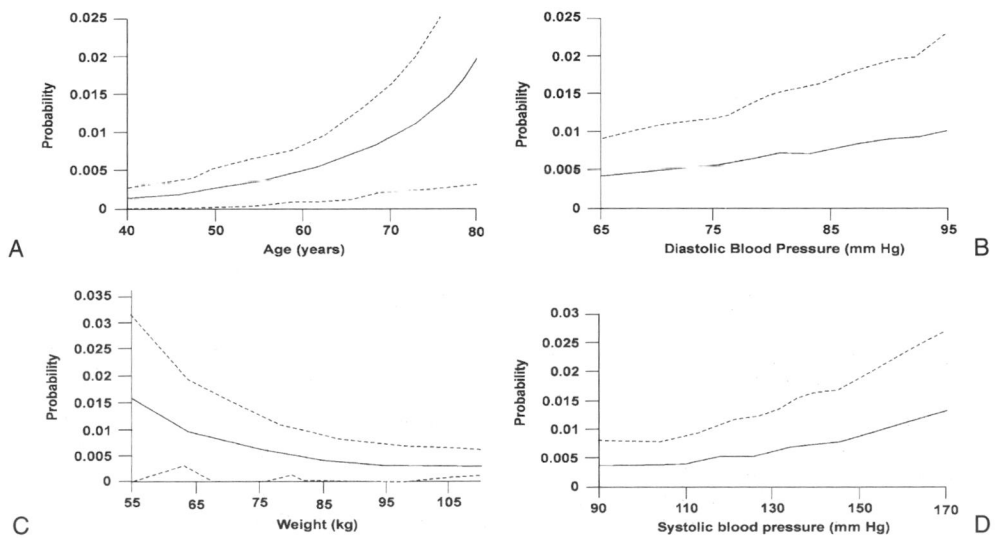

FIG. 67–14. Graphs demonstrate the continuous relation between intracerebral hemorrhage and age **(A)**, diastolic blood pressure **(B)**, weight **(C)**, and systolic blood pressure **(D)** as derived from Global Utilization of Streptokinase and t-PA for Occluded Arteries (GUSTO)-I multivariate modeling. (From Gore JM, Granger CB, Simoons ML, et al. Stroke after thrombolysis. Mortality and functional outcome in the GUSTO-I trial. *Circulation* 1995;92:2811–2818, with permission.)

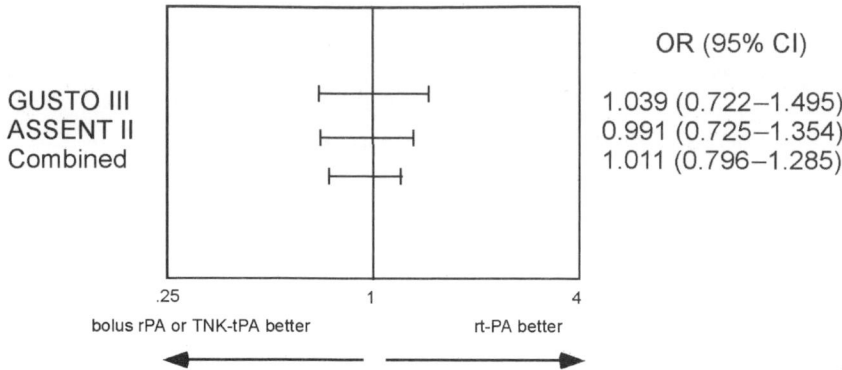

	OR (95% CI)
GUSTO III	1.039 (0.722–1.495)
ASSENT II	0.991 (0.725–1.354)
Combined	1.011 (0.796–1.285)

.25   1   4

bolus rPA or TNK-tPA better   rt-PA better

FIG. 67–15. Odds ratios (OR) and 95% confidence intervals (CI) comparing intracranial hemorrhage rates among patients treated with reteplase (r-PA; Global Utilization of Streptokinase and t-PA for Occluded Arteries [GUSTO-III] [113]) and tenecteplase (TNK-tPA; Assessment of the Safety of a New Thrombolytic [ASSENT]-II] [32]) with accelerated alteplase (rt-PA) demonstrating no difference in intracranial hemorrhage incidence. (From Armstrong PW, Granger C, Van de Werf F. Bolus fibrinolysis: risk, benefit, and opportunities. *Circulation* 2001;103:1171–1173, with permission.)

teplase (Fig. 67–15) (141). As clinical trial exclusion criteria become less restrictive—that is, enrolling more elderly and hypertensive patients—the incidence of ICH has slowly increased (142), requiring careful and vigilant analysis with studies powered to assess this important outcome.

ADJUVANT THERAPY

The thrombotic milieu that occurs within the coronary artery in the setting of AMI has been described by DeWood (3) and observed angioscopically. There exists a clear procoagulant effect of plasminogen activators associated with the exposure of clot bound thrombin (Fig. 67–16). This stimulus leads to an increase in platelet activation and aggregation. The goal of this adjunctive pharmacotherapy is to facilitate rapid, complete reperfusion of myocardium at a tissue-level and to prevent reocclusion and reinfarction.

Antithrombin Agents

Antithrombin agents are an important component of pharmacologic reperfusion therapy as plasminogen activators lyse fibrin from the fibrin–thrombin clot and expose free thrombin, a potent platelet activator. Since the early thrombolytic trials with fibrin-specific agents, aspirin and unfractionated intravenous heparin have been widely used. There are few data to support the need for heparin therapy in conjunction with nonfibrin-specific agents such as SK (21, 101,102). In contrast, five relatively small-scale randomized angiographic trials have examined the influence of heparin on infarct vessel patency after reperfusion therapy with alteplase (42,105–107,143). Although immediate administration of heparin does not appear to accelerate or enhance early (90-minute) infarct vessel patency (42), intravenous administration of heparin has been associated with improvements in patency at later time points (18–80 hours), likely because of inhibition of reocclusion (105–107). Notably,

however, is that the two trials demonstrating the greatest magnitude of difference between groups treated with and without heparin used only low-dose or no adjunctive aspirin therapy (106,107). Administration of heparin for longer than 24 hours after alteplase therapy did not provide incremental benefit over a 1-day heparin infusion followed by aspirin plus dipyridamole in the National Heart Foundation Study (143), suggesting that the period of greatest risk for reocclusion is the first 24 hours after thrombolysis, during which time heparin anticoagulation provides the greatest salutary effect on patency.

A systematic overview was performed of six randomized controlled trials comparing intravenous heparin to placebo as an adjunct to thrombolytic therapy to assess clinical outcomes. Among 1,735 patients, there was a nonsignificant 9% relative reduction in odds of death at discharge (5.1% for intravenous heparin vs. 5.6% for control; odds ratio, 0.91; 95% confidence intervals, 0.59–1.39) (144). The wide confidence intervals and limited power of the overview preclude supportive statements regarding the effect of intravenous heparin on mortality. There was no significant difference in events among patients receiving alteplase, SK, APSAC, or aspirin. Similar rates for recurrent ischemia, infarction, and ICH were observed among randomized patients. In the absence of large randomized controlled trials, the clinical effect of intravenous heparin as an adjunct to thrombolytic therapy remains unproven, despite observed improvements in infarct-related artery patency.

The improvement in patency produced by heparin therapy after thrombolysis with alteplase appears to be critically tied to the adequacy of anticoagulation. In the Heparin Aspirin Reperfusion Trial (HART) (145) and European Cooperative Study Group (ECSG-6) trial (146), clear dose–response relations were demonstrated between aPTT values and infarct vessel patency (Fig. 67–17). This observed dependence of patency on both the level and consistency of anticoagulation with heparin is particularly germane in that several studies

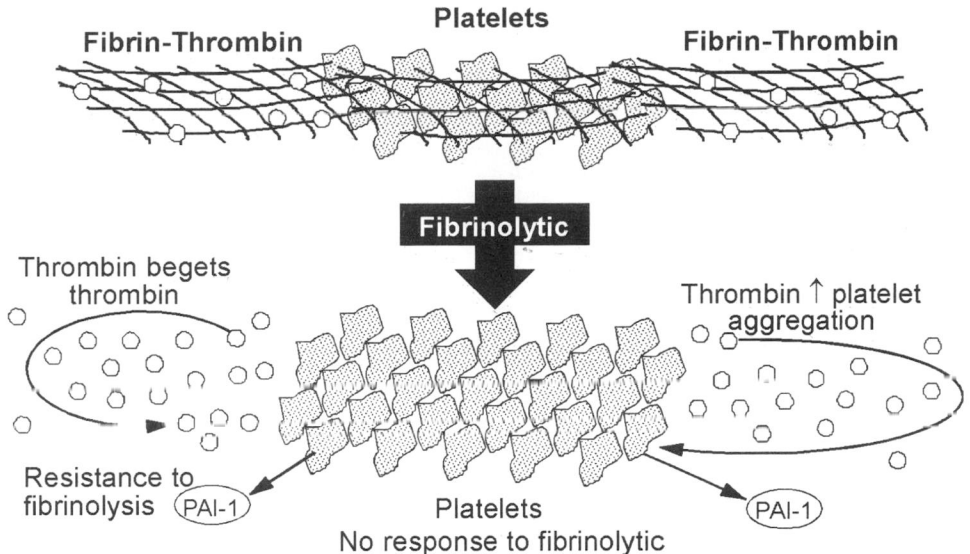

FIG. 67–16. Prothrombotic effects of fibrinolytic therapy. Coronary thrombus is composed of a platelet core with fibrin–thrombin admixture (*white* and *red* clot). After fibrinolytic therapy, there is exposure of free thrombin, which autocatalytically begets more thrombin and strongly promotes platelet aggregation (note more platelet mass). Platelets themselves are resistant to fibrinolytic therapy and furthermore secrete large amounts of platelet activator inhibitor (PAI)-1, which is a potent antagonist to fibrinolysis. (From Topol EJ. Toward a new frontier in myocardial reperfusion therapy: emerging platelet preeminence. *Circulation* 1998;97:211–218, with permission.)

have shown that many or even a majority of patients receiving heparin are not adequately anticoagulated, even on "standard" intravenous (145,146), and particularly on subcutaneous (147), heparin doses.

With observations from trials comparing third generation fibrinolytics, the InTIME-II and ASSENT-2 Investigators demonstrated a clear relation between lower aPTT peak levels in the setting of thrombolysis and a lower incidence of ICH (25,32). As a result, the ACC/AHA guidelines were updated in 1999, providing a Class IIa recommendation for unfractionated heparin in the setting of thrombolytic therapy, using a 60-U per kilogram intravenous bolus (maximum

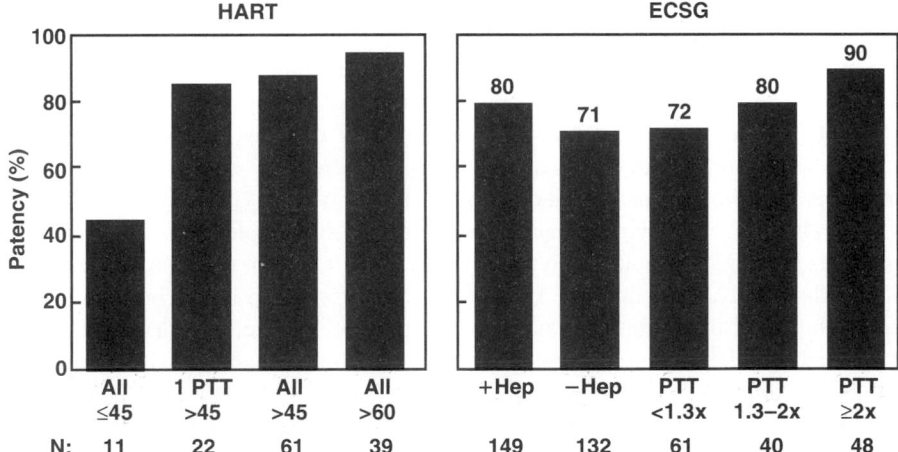

FIG. 67–17. Relation between partial thromboplastin time (PTT) and infarct vessel patency in the Heparin Aspirin Reperfusion Trial (HART) and European Cooperative Study Group (ECSG) trial of intravenous heparin (Hep) therapy with alteplase. (From Hsia J, Kleiman N, Aguirre F, et al. Heparin-induced prolongation of partial thromboplastin time after thrombolysis: relation to coronary artery patency. *J Am Coll Cardiol* 1992;20:31–35, with permission; and Arnout J, Simoons M, de Bono D, et al. Correlation between level of heparinization and patency of the infarct-related coronary artery after treatment of acute myocardial infarction with alteplase (rt-PA). *J Am Coll Cardiol* 1992;20:513–519, with permission.)

4,000 U), a maintenance infusion of 12 U per kilogram per hour (maximum 1,000 U/h), and a target aPTT of 50 to 70 seconds over 48 hours with titration beginning at 3 hours (148). Some investigators also advise no upward titration of the heparin dose during the first 6 hours.

Low–molecular weight heparins (LMWHs) have been studied as a substitute for unfractionated heparin with thrombolytic therapy. As a class, LMWHs have several potential benefits over unfractionated heparin. They have more predictable pharmacokinetics, have greater inhibition of more proximal reactions in the coagulation cascade, are less protein bound, have less potential for platelet activation, and may require no monitoring (149). LMWH have been tested during thrombolytic trials with full- or half-dose TNK–t-PA, with full- or half-dose r-PA, and with concurrent platelet GPIIb/IIIa blockade. The Enoxaparin as Adjunctive Antithrombin Therapy for ST-Elevation Myocardial Infarction (ENTIRE-TIMI 23) trial used 60-minute angiograms in 415 patients to study enoxaparin with full-dose TNK–t-PA and half-dose TNK–t-PA plus abciximab. A decreased enoxaparin dose was used with the TNK–t-PA/abciximab arm. Enoxaparin produced similar angiographic outcomes (TIMI 3 flow rates and frame counts) compared with UFH, but it was associated with a lower composite end point of death or nonfatal MI at 30 days (10.7% with UFH vs. 5.0% with enoxaparin; $p = 0.012$). This benefit was achieved with similar risk for major hemorrhage (150). As an antithrombin adjunct to full-dose thrombolysis, an enoxaparin regimen of 30-mg intravenous bolus and 1 mg per kilogram every 12 hours was evaluated among 400 patients in the Low Molecular Weight Heparin and Unfractionated Heparin Adjunctive to t-PA Thrombolysis and Aspirin (HART) II and among 6,095 patients in the ASSENT-3 trials (151,152). In ASSENT-3, enoxaparin-treated patients had a lower 30-day composite efficacy and safety end point (mortality, in-hospital reinfarction or ischemia, ICH, major bleeding) compared with patients receiving UFH (14% vs. 17%; $p = 0.003$). More major bleeding complications and transfusions were seen in the patients treated with enoxaparin compared with patients treated with UFH, although these differences were not significant (151). The optimal dose of enoxaparin to be used with thrombolysis and whether this benefit can be extrapolated to other LMWHs requires further study.

Direct thrombin inhibitors are attractive potential replacements for heparin during thrombolysis because of a more specific and sustained inhibition of thrombin generation of fibrin and thrombin-induced platelet activation, and their ability to inhibit clot-bound thrombin (153–155). Hirudin is a protein derived from the leech, *Hirudo medicinalis*, which binds thrombin in a nearly irreversible fashion (154). Three large trials comparing hirudin with heparin during thrombolysis showed no significant difference in 30-day mortality among the more than 15,000 patients, although there were trends toward lower rates of reinfarction in patients treated with hirudin (156–158). The GUSTO-IIa and TIMI-9a trials were stopped because of increased incidence of ICH and restarted with lower hirudin dosing as GUSTO-IIb and TIMI-9b (156,157). Bivalirudin (previously Hirulog), a synthetic molecule derived from hirudin, was studied in the largest study of direct thrombin inhibition during thrombolysis, the Hirulog and Early Reperfusion or Occlusion (HERO)-2 trial; of 17,073 patients receiving SK randomized to bivalirudin or UFH, no difference in 30-day mortality was observed, although the adjudicated 96-hour reinfarction rate was decreased by 30% (159). Among the more than 30,000 patients tested in all trials of direct thrombin inhibitors, no significant differences in major bleeding occurred, although there was a consistently significant increase in minor and moderate bleeding events among patients treated with hirudin or bivalirudin (156–159). Thus, the theoretic advantages of direct thrombin inhibitors have yet to translate into clinical benefit in this setting.

Antiplatelet Agents

The benefit of aspirin during AMI was clearly established in the ISIS–2 trial, where aspirin alone resulted in a mortality reduction similar to that of SK, with additive benefit when the two agents were used in combination (14). In a meta-analysis of 32 studies in which patients were treated with either SK or alteplase for acute infarction, aspirin therapy was associated with 56% and 39% reductions in the risks for recurrent ischemia or angiographic reocclusion, respectively (101). The magnitude of this beneficial effect was independent of the choice of either alteplase or SK. The mortality benefit of aspirin therapy is incontrovertible, but often under appreciated. Measurements of hospital performance indicators have shown that as many as 15% to 20% of patients with AMI still fail to receive aspirin therapy (160). Aspirin therapy likely plays a salutary role in many stages of the process of coronary occlusion and reperfusion, from modest effect on platelet aggregation and enhanced epicardial patency to minimizing reperfusion injury and stabilizing endothelial function. It is this profound effect of a simple intervention that focused the attention of researchers on the pivotal role that the platelet plays in not only MI but all acute coronary syndromes, leading to the clinical application of platelet GPIIb/IIIa inhibitors and other aggressive antiplatelet therapies.

Strategies for more profound inhibition of platelet activity have focused on the integrin GPIIb/IIIa receptor on the platelet surface, which binds von Willebrand factor and cross-links adjacent platelets as the final common pathway to platelet aggregation (161). Pharmacologic compounds directed against GPIIb/IIIa block this receptor, prevent binding of circulating adhesion molecules, and potently inhibit platelet aggregation (162). These agents have been extensively studied in placebo-controlled, randomized trials in the setting of unstable ischemic syndromes and percutaneous coronary revascularization. Given the unequivocal benefit of antiplatelet therapy with aspirin, the apparent "ceiling" of infarct-related artery patency with plasminogen activators, and the clinical benefits observed with GPIIb/IIIa inhibitors in other acute coronary syndromes, trials with these agents in the setting of ST-segment elevation MI were performed. Gold (163) and others (164–173) have shown that the dose of fibrinolytic therapy can be substantially reduced when combined with GPIIb/IIa inhibitors. Moreover, substudy analyses of TIMI 14 patients have shown improved outcomes, specifically greater ST-segment resolution with PCI, reduced dose alteplase and abciximab versus PCI and full-dose alteplase (54% vs. 8%,; $p = 0.002$) (174). After two angiographic trials—TIMI-14 trial (175) and Strategies for Patency Enhancement in the Emergency Department (SPEED) trial (176)—demonstrated improved patency rates in patients treated with the GPIIb/IIIa inhibitor, abciximab, and reduced-dose thrombolytic therapy, the critical issue of mortality benefit with combination therapy was explored in the GUSTO-V trial. The ASSENT-3 trial also assessed adjunctive therapy with abciximab in a smaller format (151). Importantly, in both trials there was no significant difference in 30-day mortality rates among the more than 22,000 patients randomized (GUSTO-V: 5.6%, half-dose r-PA and abciximab; 5.9%, r-PA alone; $p = 0.43$; ASSENT-3: 6.6%, half-dose TNK–t-PA and abciximab; 6.0%, TNK–t-PA alone; $p = 0.25$). A reduction in the incidence of reinfarction, recurrent ischemia, and urgent revascularization was observed, but this did not translate into a reduction in 30-day or 1-year mortality. Combination therapy was associated with an increase in rates of nonintracranial bleeding (GUSTO-V: 4.6% vs. 2.3%, $p < 0.001$; ASSENT-3: 4.4% vs. 2.2%, $p = 0.0005$) (151,177). Rates of ICH were not increased by combination therapy in the overall cohort of both trials, although elderly patients (>75 years old) did have a high risk for ICH with abciximab and thrombolytic therapy. The large phase III trials have thus far been limited to abciximab, a chimeric Fab monoclonal antibody fragment, and efficacy of other GPIIb/IIIa inhibitors such as eptifibatide, a cyclic heptapeptide, or tirofiban, a nonpeptide mimetic, remain to be defined in this setting.

TIME TO TREATMENT

Notwithstanding the enhancements in the "state-of-the-art" thrombolytic treatment that have resulted from improved fibrinolysis and adjuvant therapy, there remain several important limitations to the effectiveness of current myocardial reperfusion therapy. Regardless of the thrombolytic regimen used, several lines of evidence demonstrate that the most profound benefit from reperfusion therapy may be derived if that therapy is administered as early as possible after the onset of ischemic symptoms. The value of early infarct vessel recanalization was apparent even in the GISSI (29) and ISIS-2 (178) placebo-controlled trials of SK (Fig. 67–18). Patients enrolled within 1 hour of symptom onset enjoyed a nearly 50% reduction in mortality with lytic therapy, whereas among patients treated later, mortality reduction was only 23%. Studies with prehospital thrombolysis have

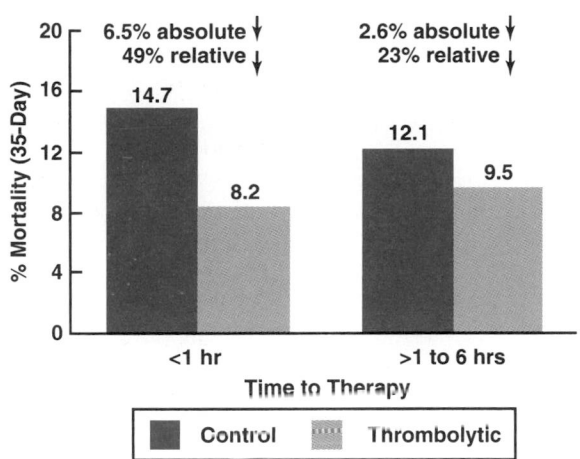

FIG. 67–18. Pooled results of Gruppo Italiano per lo Studio della Streptochinasi nell'Infarto Miocardico (GISSI) and International Study of Infarct Survival (ISIS)-2 trials of streptokinase versus conventional therapy, demonstrating enhanced mortality reduction among patients treated with streptokinase within 1 hour of symptom onset (49% relative reduction) as compared with patients treated after 1 hour (23% mortality reduction).

supported the hypothesis that very early reperfusion therapy may produce marked improvements in mortality. The largest trial of prehospital thrombolysis by the European Myocardial Infarction Project (EMIP) Group randomized nearly 5,500 patients to prehospital or emergency room administration of anistreplase in a placebo-controlled fashion (179). With prehospital thrombolysis leading to a median 55-minute decrease in the time to therapy, this study demonstrated a significant 16% reduction in the risk for cardiac death (8.3% vs. 9.8%; $p = 0.049$). Similarly, short-term (3-month) mortality was reduced by an impressive 49% (8.0% vs. 15.5%; $p = 0.04$) by domiciliary rather than in-hospital thrombolytic therapy among 311 patients in the Grampian Region Early Anistreplase Trial (GREAT), in which substantial treatment delays within the hospital resulted in a median time savings of 139 minutes by domiciliary thrombolytic administration (180). A metaanalysis of 6 randomized controlled trials of prehospital thrombolysis pooled data from 6,434 patients and demonstrated a significant reduction in all-cause mortality at discharge with prehospital thrombolytic therapy (odds ratio, 0.83; 95% confidence intervals, 0.70–0.98; Fig. 67–19) (181). Interestingly, the results were similar regardless of the field provider experience (emergency medical personnel vs. physician), suggesting that an early reperfusion strategy might be suitable in the U.S. healthcare system, where physicians do not routinely travel with emergency medical teams.

These and other data point to the existence of a so-called golden first hour—that is, a time window during which thrombolytic therapy is likely to result in the most significant mortality benefits because of extensive myocardial salvage (Fig. 67–20). In the period thereafter, to at least 12

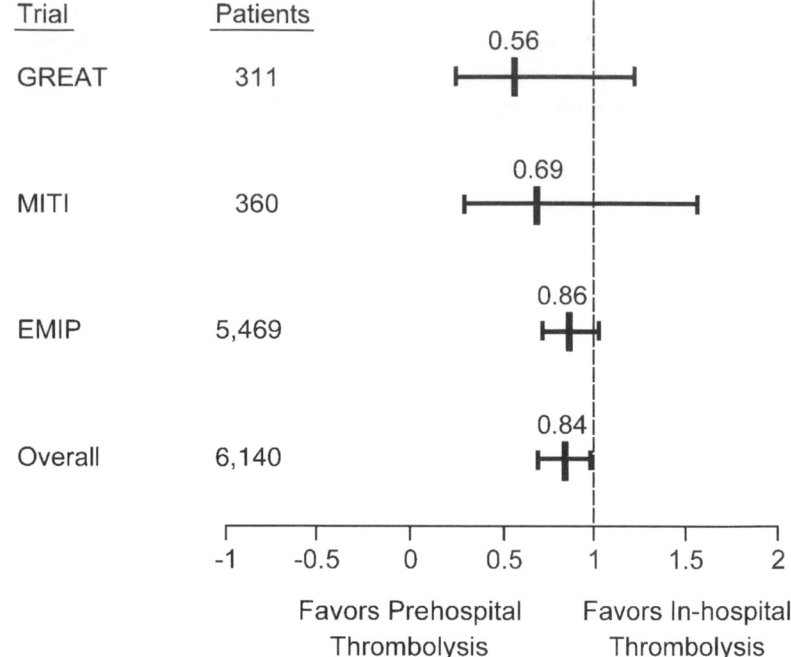

FIG. 67–19. Pooled data from a metaanalysis of randomized controlled trials of prehospital thrombolysis demonstrated a significant reduction in all-cause mortality at discharge with prehospital thrombolytic therapy. EMIP, European Myocardial Infarction Project; GREAT, Grampian Region Early Anistreplase Trial; MITI, Myocardial Infarction and Triage Intervention Project. (Adapted from Morrison LJ, Verbeek PR, McDonald AC, et al. Mortality and prehospital thrombolysis for acute myocardial infarction: a metaanalysis. *JAMA* 2000;283:2686–2692, with permission.)

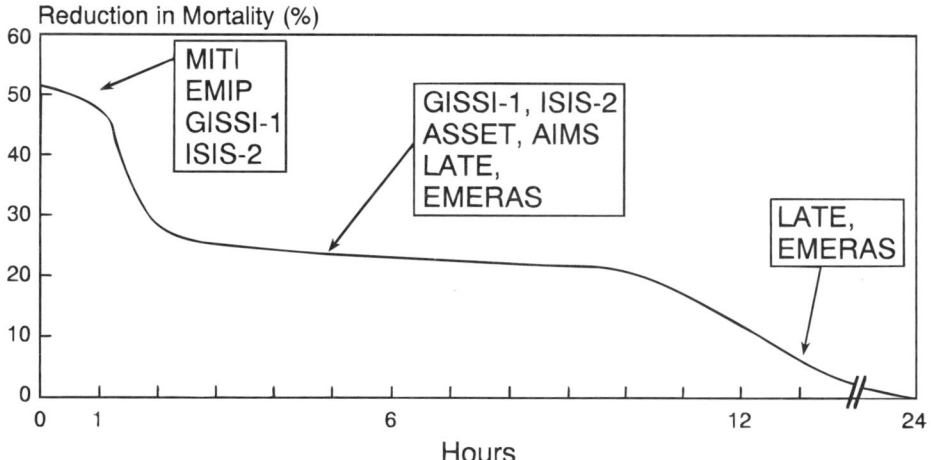

FIG. 67–20. Plot of relative mortality reduction (%) derived from thrombolytic therapy as a function of the elapsed time between onset of symptoms and initiation of thrombolytic agent. Clinical trials from which these data are extrapolated are noted. A greater than 50% reduction in mortality is noted during the "golden first hour," after which mortality benefit declines to a plateau of approximately 25% reduction until 12 hours after symptom onset. Beyond 12 hours, significant survival benefit has not been demonstrated with thrombolytic administration. AIMS, Anistreplase Intervention Mortality Study (95); ASSET, Anglo-Scandinavian Study of Early Thrombolysis (96); EMERAS, Estudios Multicentrico Estreptoquinasa Republica Americas Sud (131); EMIP, European Myocardial Infarction Project (108); GISSI-1, Gruppo Italiano per lo Studio della Streptochinasi nell-Infarto Miocardico (29); ISIS-2, Second International Study of Infarct Survival (14); LATE, Late Assessment of Thrombolytic Efficacy (130); MITI, Myocardial Infarction and Triage Intervention Project (197). (From Lincoff AM, Topol EJ. Illusion of reperfusion. Does anyone achieve optimal reperfusion during acute myocardial infarction? [Erratum appears in *Circulation* 1993;88:1361–1374.] *Circulation* 1993;87:1792–1805, with permission.)

hours, there is a lesser extent of benefit from infarct vessel recanalization, because of both time-dependent and time-independent mechanisms. It appears, in fact, that very early initiation of therapy results in a more profound improvement in clinical outcome than all other modification of thrombolytic regimens or adjunctive interventions combined. Yet it is noteworthy that despite recognition of the exceptional value of reperfusion therapy administered within that first hour, only a small minority of patients with acute infarction actually receive very early therapy. Improvements in ED triage systems can improve the time from patient arrival to reperfusion ("door-to-needle" time) (182,183); however, the majority of the time before reperfusion lies in the substantial delay before the patient's ED presentation. A review of the NRMI-2 by Goldberg and coworkers (184) found that among the more than 69,000 patients with MI in 1997, only 20% of patients were seen in an ED within the first "golden" hour since onset of symptoms. The median time to ED presentation, 2.1 hours, remained unchanged during the NRMI-2 observational period from 1994 to 1997. Impressively, prehospital thrombolytic therapy trials have demonstrated that the time from activation of emergency medical services to thrombolytic therapy can be as short as 27 to 31 minutes (185,186).

Although efficiently delivered and rapidly acting thrombolytic regimens may have a modest effect on reducing the total time to myocardial reperfusion, the most profound benefit with reperfusion therapy may be derived from improvements in the currently dismal performance in initiating therapy through enhanced efforts toward public education.

THE FUTURE

The validation of the open-vessel hypothesis and improvements in techniques to critically assess the true quality and stability of myocardial reperfusion have led to an appreciation of the weaknesses of the current state of thrombolytic therapy for AMI. The concurrent study of primary angioplasty in the setting of AMI led to a perplexing landscape for the physician triaging patients with acute ST-segment elevation MI. Unfortunately, a dichotomy evolved where the two reperfusion strategies were not seen as complementary. This was fostered by experience with increasing bleeding complications when percutaneous interventions were performed as a "rescue" procedure after failure of full-dose thrombolysis. Studies such as the SPEED trial (176), the Plasminogen Activator Compatibility Trial (PACT) (187), and the GUSTO-V trial (177) have provided reassurance that percutaneous intervention after early administration of a thrombolytic with or without a platelet GPIIb/IIIa inhibitor is a tenable reperfusion strategy. The term *facilitated* PCI has been used to describe a number of different management strategies that aim to use pharmacologic agents to improve the outcome of early PCI in AMIs, but it has most commonly been used to denote treatment with reduced dose fibrinolytic therapy and GPIIb/IIIa inhibitor before a planned, immediate PCI (188). This approach unites two different reperfusion strategies and may provide the clinical benefits not seen in large trials of reduced-dose fibrinolysis and GPIIb/IIIa inhibitors alone. Facilitated PCI may also provide a means of overcoming delays in bringing patients to PCI and offer a reperfusion strategy for those institutions without catheterization laboratories to initiate before transfer. A facilitated PCI strategy is currently under evaluation in two clinical trials: Facilitated Intervention with Enhanced Speed to Stop Events (FINESSE) and Tenecteplase and Integrilin for Event Reduction (TIGER).

The pharmacology of thrombolytic agents has matured in the last decade as recombinant DNA technology created third generation mutants of wild type t-PA that have longer half-lives, increased fibrin specificity, and resistance to PAI-1. These agents are likely nearing a plateau in their ability to achieve epicardial patency. Adjuvant therapy has evolved to include effective inhibitors of thrombin and platelet activation. As epicardial vessel patency is optimized, there is an increased focus on the microvasculature and "complete" myocardial reperfusion. Just as adjunctive GPIIb/IIIa inhibitors may relieve microvascular obstruction caused by platelet-thrombin microemboli, other adjunctive agents may improve myocardial reperfusion. With the exception of work with adenosine and its analogs (189–191), several studies attempting to pharmacologically minimize reperfusion injury have been proven unsuccessful (192–196). Further study is warranted to evaluate other potential agents that may improve endothelial function, minimize the inflammatory response to myocyte necrosis, and prepare the injured or ischemic myocardium for prompt reperfusion perhaps through a facilitated PCI strategy.

REFERENCES

1. Herrick JB. Certain clinical features of sudden obstruction of the coronary arteries. *JAMA* 1912;59:2015–2020.
2. Friedberg C, Horn H. Acute myocardial infarction not due to coronary artery occlusion. *JAMA* 1939;112:1675–1679.
3. DeWood MA, Spores J, Notske R, et al. Prevalence of total coronary occlusion during the early hours of transmural myocardial infarction. *N Engl J Med* 1980;303:897–902.
4. Reimer KA, Lowe JE, Rasmussen MM, et al. The wavefront phenomenon of ischemic cell death. Myocardial infarct size vs. duration of coronary occlusion in dogs. *Circulation* 1977;56:786–794.
5. Reimer KA, Jennings RB. The "wavefront phenomenon" of myocardial ischemic cell death. II. Transmural progression of necrosis within the framework of ischemic bed size (myocardium at risk) and collateral flow. *Lab Invest* 1979;40:633–644.
6. Tillett WS, Garner RI. The fibrinolytic activity of hemolytic streptococci. *J Exp Med* 1933;58:485–502.
7. Fletcher AP, Alkjaersig N, Smyrniotis FE, et al. Treatment of patients suffering from early myocardial infarction with massive and prolonged streptokinase therapy. *Trans Assoc Am Physicians* 1958;71:287–296.
8. Yusuf S, Collins R, Peto R, et al. Intravenous and intracoronary fibrinolytic therapy in acute myocardial infarction: overview of results on mortality, reinfarction, and side effects from 33 randomized controlled trials. *Eur Heart J* 1985;6:556–585.
9. Chazov EI, Mateeva LS, Mazaev AV, et al. Intracoronary administration of fibrinolysis in acute myocardial infarction. *Ter Arkh* 1976;48:8–19.
10. Rentrop KT, Blanke H, Karsch KR, et al. Initial experience with

transluminal recanalization of the recently occluded infarct-related artery in acute myocardial infarction: comparison with conventionally treated patients. *Clin Cardiol* 1979;2:92–105.

11. Indications for fibrinolytic therapy in suspected acute myocardial infarction: collaborative overview of early mortality and major morbidity results from all randomised trials of more than 1000 patients. Fibrinolytic Therapy Trialists' (FTT) Collaborative Group. *Lancet* 1994; 343:311–322.

12. Collen D, Bounameaux H, De Cock F, et al. Analysis of coagulation and fibrinolysis during intravenous infusion of recombinant human tissue-type plasminogen activator in patients with acute myocardial infarction. *Circulation* 1986;73:511–517.

13. Davies MC, Englert ME, De Renzo EC. Interaction of streptokinase and human plasminogen. I. Combining of streptokinase and plasminogen observe in the ultracentrifuge under a variety of experimental conditions. *J Biol Chem* 1964;239:2651–2656.

14. Randomized trial of intravenous streptokinase, oral aspirin, both, or neither among 17,187 cases of suspected acute myocardial infarction: ISIS-2. ISIS-2 (Second International Study of Infarct Survival) Collaborative Group. *Lancet* 1988;2:349–360.

15. Fears R, Ferres H, Glasgow E, et al. Monitoring of streptokinase resistance titre in acute myocardial infarction patients up to 30 months after giving streptokinase or anistreplase and related studies to measure specific antistreptokinase IgG. *Br Heart J* 1992;68:167–170.

16. Lew AS, Laramee P, Cercek P, et al. The hypotensive effect of intravenous streptokinase in patients with acute myocardial infarction. *Circulation* 1985;72:1321–1326.

17. Vanderschueren S, Barrios L, Kerdschinai P, et al. A randomized trial of recombinant staphylokinase versus alteplase for coronary artery patency in acute myocardial infarction. The STAR Trial Group. *Circulation* 1995;92:2044–2049.

18. Vanderschueren S, Dens J, Kerdsinchai P, et al. Randomized coronary patency trial of double-bolus recombinant staphylokinase versus front-loaded alteplase in acute myocardial infarction. *Am Heart J* 1997;134:213–219.

19. Loscalzo J, Braunwald E. Tissue plasminogen activator. *N Engl J Med* 1988;319:925–931.

20. Chesebro JH, Knatterud G, Roberts R, et al. Thrombolysis in Myocardial Infarction (TIMI) Trial, phase I: a comparison between intravenous tissue plasminogen activator and intravenous streptokinase. *Circulation* 1987;76:142–154.

21. An international randomized trial comparing four thrombolytic strategies for acute myocardial infarction. GUSTO Investigators. *N Engl J Med* 1993;329:673–682.

22. Smalling RW, Bode C, Kalbfleisch J, et al. More rapid, complete, and stable coronary thrombolysis with bolus administration of reteplase compared with alteplase infusion in acute myocardial infarction. *Circulation* 1995;91:2725–2732.

23. Wu Z, Van de Werf F, Stassen T, et al. Pharmacokinetics and coronary thrombolytic properties of two human tissue-type plasminogen activator variants lacking the finger-like, growth factor-like, and first kringle domains (amino acids 6-173) in a canine model. *J Cardiovasc Pharmacol* 1990;16:197–203.

24. den Heijer P, Vermeer F, Ambrosioni E, et al. Evaluation of a weight-adjusted single-bolus plasminogen activator in patients with myocardial infarction: a double-blind, randomized angiographic trial of lanoteplase versus alteplase. *Circulation* 1998;98:2117–2125.

25. Intravenous NPA for the treatment of infarcting myocardium early; InTIME-II, a double-blind comparison of single-bolus lanoteplase vs accelerated alteplase for the treatment of patients with acute myocardial infarction. InTime Investigators. *Eur Heart J* 2000;21:2005–2013.

26. Keyt BA, Paoni NF, Refino CJ, et al. A faster-acting and more potent form of tissue plasminogen activator. *Proc Natl Acad Sci USA* 1994; 91:3670–3674.

27. Cannon CP, Gibson CM, McCabe CH, et al. TNK-tissue plasminogen activator compared with front-loaded alteplase in acute myocardial infarction. Results of the TIMI 10B trial. *Circulation* 1998;98:2805–2814.

28. DeMarco E, Rebuzzi AG, Quaranta G, et al. Lack of procoagulant effect after TNK-plasminogen activator in patients with acute myocardial infarction. *Eur Heart J* 1998;19:5.

29. Gruppo Italiano per lo Studio della Streptochinasi nell'Infarto Miocardico (GISSI). Effectiveness of intravenous thrombolytic treatment in acute myocardial infarction. *Lancet* 1986;1:397–401.

30. Effects of tissue plasminogen activator and a comparison of early in-

31. Vorchheimer DA, Baruch L, Thompson TD. North American versus Non-North American streptokinase use in GUSTO-I: impact of protocol deviation on mortality benefit of t-PA. *Circulation* 1997;96[Suppl]: I–535(abst).

32. Single-bolus tenecteplase compared with front-loaded alteplase in acute myocardial infarction: the ASSENT-2 double-blind randomised trial. ASSENT-2 (Assessment of the Safety and Efficacy of a New Thrombolytic) Investigators. *Lancet* 1999;354:716–722.

33. Granger CB, Van de Werf F, Armstrong PW. Caution is needed in interpreting the impact of dosing errors: a case study from ASSENT 2. *Circulation* 2000;102[Suppl]:II–590(abst).

34. Topol EJ, Ciuffo AA, Pearson TA, et al. Thrombolysis with recombinant tissue plasminogen activator in atherosclerotic thrombotic occlusion. *J Am Coll Cardiol* 1985;5:85–91.

35. Granger CB, Califf RM, Topol EJ. Thrombolytic therapy for acute myocardial infarction, a review. *Drugs* 1992;44:293–325.

36. Topol EJ, Morris DC, Smalling RW, et al. A multicenter, randomized, placebo-controlled trial of a new form of intravenous recombinant tissue-type plasminogen activator (Activase) in acute myocardial infarction. *J Am Coll Cardiol* 1987;9:1205–1213.

37. Anderson JL, Marshall HW, Askins JC, et al. A randomized trial of intravenous and intracoronary streptokinase in patients with acute myocardial infarction. *Circulation* 1984;70:606–618.

38. Hogg KJ, Gemmill JD, Burns JM, et al. Angiographic patency study of anistreplase versus streptokinase in acute myocardial infarction. *Lancet* 1990;335:254–258.

39. Neuhaus KL, Tebbe U, Gottwik M, et al. Intravenous recombinant tissue plasminogen activator (rt-PA) and urokinase in acute myocardial infarction: results of the German Activator Urokinase Study (GAUS). *J Am Coll Cardiol* 1988;12:581–587.

40. The Thrombolysis in Myocardial Infarction (TIMI) trial. Phase I findings. TIMI Study Group. *N Engl J Med* 1985;312:932–936.

41. Immediate vs. delayed catheterization and angioplasty following thrombolytic therapy for acute myocardial infarction. TIMI IIA results. TIMI Research Group. *JAMA* 1988;260:2849–2858.

42. Topol EJ, George BS, Kereiakes DJ, et al. A randomized controlled trial of intravenous tissue plasminogen activator and early intravenous heparin in acute myocardial infarction. *Circulation* 1989;79:281–286.

43. Neuhaus K-L, von Essen R, Tebbe U, et al. Improved thrombolysis in acute myocardial infarction with front-loaded administration of alteplase: results of the rt-PA-APSAC Patency Study (TAPS). *J Am Coll Cardiol* 1992;19:885–891.

44. Neuhaus KL, Feuerer W, Jeep-Tebbe S, et al. Improved thrombolysis with a modified dose regimen of recombinant tissue-type plasminogen activator. *J Am Coll Cardiol* 1989;14:1566–1569.

45. Neuhaus KL, Von Essen R, Tebbe U, et al. Improved thrombolysis in acute myocardial infarction with front-loaded administration of alteplase: results of the rt-PA-APSAC Patency Study (TAPS). *J Am Coll Cardiol* 1992;19:885–891.

46. Carney RJ, Murphy GA, Brandt TR, et al. Randomized angiographic trial of recombinant tissue-type plasminogen activator (alteplase) in myocardial infarction. *J Am Coll Cardiol* 1992;20:17–23.

47. Smalling RW, Schumacher R, Morris D, et al. Improved infarct-related arterial patency after high dose, weight-adjusted, rapid infusion of tissue-type plasminogen activator in myocardial infarction: results of a multicenter randomized trial of two dosage regimens. *J Am Coll Cardiol* 1990;15:915–921.

48. Wall TC, Califf RM, George BS, et al. Accelerated plasminogen activator dose regimens for coronary thrombolysis. *J Am Coll Cardiol* 1992;19:482–489.

49. Bode C, Smalling RW, Berg G, et al. Randomized comparison of coronary thrombolysis achieved with double-bolus reteplase (recombinant plasminogen activator) and front-loaded, accelerated alteplase (recombinant tissue plasminogen activator) in patients with acute myocardial infarction. The RAPID II Investigators. *Circulation* 1996;94: 891–898.

50. Cannon CP, McCabe CH, Gibson CM, et al. TNK-tissue plasminogen activator in acute myocardial infarction. Results of the thrombolysis in myocardial infarction (TIMI) 10A dose-ranging trial. *Circulation* 1997;95:351–356.

51. The effects of tissue plasminogen activator, streptokinase, or both on

coronary-artery patency, ventricular function, and survival after acute myocardial infarction. GUSTO Angiographic Investigators. *N Engl J Med* 1993;329:1615–1622.

52. Anderson JL, Karagounis LA, Becker LC, et al. TIMI perfusion grade 3 but not grade 2 results in improved outcome after thrombolysis for myocardial infarction. Ventriculographic, enzymatic, and electrocardiographic evidence from the TEAM-3 study. TEAM-3 Investigators. *Circulation* 1993;87:1829–1839.

53. Karagounis L, Sorensen SG, Menlove RL, et al. Does thrombolysis in myocardial infarction (TIMI) perfusion grade 2 represent a mostly patent artery or a mostly occluded artery? Enzymatic and electrocardiographic evidence from the TEAM-2 study. *J Am Coll Cardiol* 1992;19:1–10.

54. Lincoff AM, Topol EJ, Califf RM, et al. Significance of a coronary artery with thrombolysis in myocardial infarction grade 2 flow "patency" (outcome in the thrombolysis and angioplasty in myocardial infarction trials). Thrombolysis and Angioplasty in Myocardial Infarction Study Group. *Am J Cardiol* 1995;75:871–876.

55. Gibson CM, Cannon CP, Piana RN, et al. Angiographic predictors of reocclusion after thrombolysis: results from the Thrombolysis in Myocardial Infarction (TIMI) 4 trial. *J Am Coll Cardiol* 1995;25:582–589.

56. Gibson CM, Cannon CP, Daley WL, et al. TIMI frame count. A quantitative method of assessing coronary artery flow. *Circulation* 1996;93:879–888.

57. Gibson C, Murphy S, Rizzo M, et al. Relationship between TIMI frame count and clinical outcomes after thrombolytic administration. *Circulation* 1999;99:1945–1950.

58. Gibson CM, Cannon CP, Murphy SA, et al. Relationship of the TIMI myocardial perfusion grades, flow grades, frame count, and percutaneous coronary intervention to long-term outcomes after thrombolytic administration in acute myocardial infarction. *Circulation* 2002;105:1909–1913.

59. Ohman EM, Califf RM, Topol EJ, et al. Consequences of reocclusion after successful reperfusion therapy in acute myocardial infarction. *Circulation* 1990;82:781–791.

60. Gash AK, Spann JF, Sherry S, et al. Factors influencing reocclusion after coronary thrombolysis for acute myocardial infarction. *Am J Cardiol* 1986;57:175–177.

61. Golino P, Ashton JH, Glas-Greenwalt P, et al. Mediation of reocclusion by thromboxane A_2 and serotonin after thrombolysis with tissue-type plasminogen activator in a canine preparation of coronary thrombosis. *Circulation* 1988;77:678–684.

62. Weitz JI, Hudoba M, Massel D, et al. Clot-bound thrombin is protected from inhibition by heparin-antithrombin III but is susceptible to inactivation by antithrombin III independent inhibitors. *J Clin Invest* 1990;86:385–391.

63. Fitzgerald DJ, Catella F, Roy L, et al. Marked platelet activation in vivo after intravenous streptokinase in patients with acute myocardial infarction. *Circulation* 1988;77:142–150.

64. Lim MJ, Gallagher MA, Ziadeh M, et al. Effect of coronary reocclusion after initial reperfusion on ventricular function and infarct size. *J Am Coll Cardiol* 1991;18:879–885.

65. Topol EJ, Califf RM, Vandormael M, et al. A randomized trial of late reperfusion therapy for acute myocardial infarction. *Circulation* 1992;85:2090–2099.

66. Meijer A, Verheugt FW, Werter CJ, et al. Aspirin versus coumadin in the prevention of reocclusion and recurrent ischemia after successful thrombolysis: a prospective placebo-controlled angiographic study. Results of the APRICOT study. *Circulation* 1993;87:1524–1530.

67. Grines CL, Topol EJ, Bates ER, et al. Infarct vessel status after intravenous tissue plasminogen activator and acute coronary angioplasty: prediction of clinical outcome. *Am Heart J* 1988;115:1–7.

68. Davies GJ, Chierchia S, Maseri A. Prevention of myocardial infarction by very early treatment with intracoronary streptokinase: some clinical observations. *N Engl J Med* 1984;311:1488–1492.

69. Hackett D, Davies G, Chierchia S, et al. Intermittent coronary occlusion in acute myocardial infarction. Value of combined thrombolytic and vasodilator therapy. *N Engl J Med* 1987;317:1055–1059.

70. Dellborg M, Topol EJ, Swedberg K. Dynamic QRS complex and ST segment vectorcardiographic monitoring can identify vessel patency in patients with acute myocardial infarction treated with reperfusion therapy. *Am Heart J* 1991;122.943–948.

71. Kwon KI, Freedman B, Wilxos I, et al. The unstable ST segment early after thrombolysis for acute infarction and its usefulness as a marker of recurrent coronary occlusion. *Am J Cardiol* 1991;67:109–115.

72. Roe MT, Ohman EM, Maas AC, et al. Shifting the open-artery hypothesis downstream: the quest for optimal reperfusion. *J Am Coll Cardiol* 2001;37:9–18.

73. Eidt JF, Allison P, Noble S, et al. Thrombin is an important mediator of platelet aggregation in stenosed canine coronary arteries with endothelial injury. *J Clin Invest* 1992;84:18–27.

74. Schumacher WA, Buda AJ, Lucchesi BR. Streptokinase thrombolysis in experimental coronary artery thrombosis: pattern of reflow and effect of a stenosis. *Int J Cardiol* 1984;6:615–627.

75. Klootwijk P, Langer A, Meij S, et al. Non-invasive prediction of reperfusion and coronary artery patency by continuous ST segment monitoring in the GUSTO-I trial. *Eur Heart J* 1996;17:689–698.

76. Ito H, Tomooka T, Sakai N, et al. Lack of myocardial perfusion immediately after successful thrombolysis. A predictor of poor recovery of left ventricular function in anterior myocardial infarction. *Circulation* 1992;85:1699–1705.

77. Ito H, Okamura A, Iwakura K, et al. Myocardial perfusion patterns related to thrombolysis in myocardial infarction perfusion grades after coronary angioplasty in patients with acute anterior wall myocardial infarction. *Circulation* 1996;93:1993–1999.

78. Porter TR, Li S, Oster R, et al. The clinical implications of no reflow demonstrated with intravenous perfluorocarbon containing microbubbles following restoration of Thrombolysis In Myocardial Infarction (TIMI) 3 flow in patients with acute myocardial infarction. *Am J Cardiol* 1998;82:1173–1177.

79. Meza M, Greener Y, Hunt R, et al. Myocardial contrast echocardiography: reliable, safe, and efficacious myocardial perfusion assessment after intravenous injections of a new echocardiographic contrast agent. *Am Heart J* 1996;132:871–881.

80. Lepper W, Kamp O, Vanoverschelde JL, et al. Intravenous myocardial contrast echocardiography predicts left ventricular remodeling in patients with acute myocardial infarction. *J Am Soc Echocardiogr* 2002;15:849–856.

81. Gibson CM, Cannon CP, Murphy SA, et al. Relationship of TIMI myocardial perfusion grade to mortality after administration of thrombolytic drugs. *Circulation* 2000;101:125–130.

82. Schroder R, Dissmann R, Bruggemann T, et al. Extent of early ST segment elevation resolution: a simple but strong predictor of outcome in patients with acute myocardial infarction. *J Am Coll Cardiol* 1994;24:384–391.

83. Schroder R, Wegscheider K, Schroder K, et al. Extent of early ST segment elevation resolution: a strong predictor of outcome in patients with acute myocardial infarction and a sensitive measure to compare thrombolytic regimens. A substudy of the International Joint Efficacy Comparison of Thrombolytics (INJECT) Trial Group. *J Am Coll Cardiol* 1995;26:1657–1664.

84. de Lemos JA, Antman EM, Giugliano RP, et al. Comparison of a 60-versus 90-minute determination of ST-segment resolution after thrombolytic therapy for acute myocardial infarction. In TIME-II Investigators. Intravenous nPA for Treatment of Infarcting Myocardium Early-II. *Am J Cardiol* 2000;86:1235–1237,A5.

85. de Lemos JA, Gibson CM, Antman EM. Correlation between the TIMI myocardial perfusion grade and ST segment resolution after fibrinolytic therapy. *Circulation* 2000;102[Suppl]:II–775(abst).

86. van 't Hof AW, Liem A, Suryapranata H, et al. Angiographic assessment of myocardial reperfusion in patients treated with primary angioplasty for acute myocardial infarction: myocardial blush grade. Zwolle Myocardial Infarction Study Group. *Circulation* 1998;97:2302–2306.

87. de Lemos JA, Antman EM, Giugliano RP, et al. ST-segment resolution and infarct-related artery patency and flow after thrombolytic therapy. Thrombolysis in Myocardial Infarction (TIMI) 14 investigators. *Am J Cardiol* 2000;85:299–304.

88. Risk stratification and survival after myocardial infarction. Multicenter Postinfarction Research Group. *N Engl J Med* 1983;309:331–336.

89. Van de Werf F. Discrepancies between the effects of coronary reperfusion on survival and left ventricular function. *Lancet* 1989;1:1367–1369.

90. Sheehan FH, Braunwald E, Canner P, et al. The effect of intravenous thrombolytic therapy on left ventricular function: a report on tissue-type plasminogen activator and streptokinase from the Thrombolysis in Myocardial Infarction (TIMI Phase I) trial. *Circulation* 1987;75:817–829.

91. Shroder R, Neuhaus KL, Linderer T, et al. Impact of late coronary artery reperfusion on left ventricular function one month after acute myocardial infarction (results of the ISAM study). *Am J Cardiol* 1989;64:878–884.

92. Morgan CD, Roberts RS, Haq A, et al. Coronary patency, infarct size and left ventricular function after thrombolytic therapy for acute myocardial infarction: results from the Tissue Plasminogen Activator: Toronto (TPAT) placebo-controlled trial. *J Am Coll Cardiol* 1991;17: 1451–1457.

93. Califf RM, Harrelson-Woodlief L, Topol EJ. Left ventricular ejection fraction may not be useful as an end point of thrombolytic therapy comparative trials. *Circulation* 1990;82:1847–1853.

94. A prospective trial of intravenous streptokinase in acute myocardial infarction (ISAM). ISAM Study Group. *N Engl J Med* 1986;314: 1465–1471.

95. Effect of intravenous APSAC on mortality after acute myocardial infarction: preliminary report of a placebo-controlled clinical trial. AIMS Trial Study Group. *Lancet* 1988;1:545–549.

96. Wilcox RG, Olsson CG, Skene AM, et al. Trial of tissue plasminogen activator for mortality reduction in acute myocardial infarction. Anglo-Scandinavian Study of Early Thrombolysis (ASSET). *Lancet* 1988;2:525–530.

97. Gruppo Italiano per lo Studio della Streptochinasi nell'Infarto Miocardico (GISSI). Long-term effects of intravenous thrombolysis in acute myocardial infarction: final report of the GISSI study. *Lancet* 1987;8564:871–874.

98. Van de Werf F, Arnold AE. Intravenous tissue plasminogen activator and size of infarct, left ventricular function, and survival in acute myocardial infarction. European Cooperative Study Group. *Br Med J* 1988;297:1374–1379.

99. Mauri F, DeBiase AM, Franzosi MG, et al. In-hospital causes of death in the patients admitted to the GISSI study. *G Ital Cardiol* 1987;17: 37–44.

100. In-hospital mortality and clinical course of 20,891 patients with suspected acute myocardial infarction randomised between alteplase and streptokinase with or without heparin. International Study Group. *Lancet* 1990;336:71–75.

101. Gruppo Italiano per lo Studio dell Sopravvivenza nell'Infarto Miocardico. GISSI-2: a factorial randomized trial of alteplase versus streptokinase and heparin versus no heparin among 12,490 patients with acute myocardial infarction. *Lancet* 1990;336:65–71.

102. ISIS-3 (Third International Study of Infarct Survival) Collaborative Group. ISIS-3: a randomised comparison of streptokinase vs tissue plasminogen activator vs anistreplase and of aspirin plus heparin vs aspirin alone among 41,229 cases of suspected acute myocardial infarction. *Lancet* 1992;339:753–770.

103. Braunwald E. Myocardial reperfusion, limitation of infarct size, reduction of left ventricular dysfunction, and improved survival: should the paradigm be expanded? *Circulation* 1989;79:441–444.

104. Fortin DG, Califf RM. Long-term survival from acute myocardial infarction: salutary effect of an open vessel. *Am J Med* 1990;88: 1-9N–1-15N.

105. de Bono DP, Simoons ML, Tijssen J, et al. Effect of early intravenous heparin on coronary patency, infarct size, and bleeding complications after alteplase thrombolysis: results of a randomised double blind European Cooperative Study Group (ECSG-6). *Br Heart J* 1992;67: 122–128.

106. Hsia J, Hamilton WP, Kleiman N, et al. A comparison between heparin and low-dose aspirin as adjunctive therapy with tissue plasminogen activator for acute myocardial infarction. *N Engl J Med* 1990;323: 1433–1437.

107. Bleich SD, Nichols TC, Schumacher RR, et al. Effect of heparin on coronary arterial patency after thrombolysis with tissue plasminogen activator in acute myocardial infarction. *Am J Cardiol* 1990;66: 1412–1417.

108. Hull RD, Raskob GE, Hirsch J, et al. Continuous intravenous heparin compared with intermittent subcutaneous heparin in the initial treatment of proximal vein thrombosis. *N Engl J Med* 1986;315: 1109–1114.

109. Kroon C, ten Hove WR, de Boer A, et al. Highly variable anticoagulant response after subcutaneous administration of high-dose (12,500 IU) heparin in patients with myocardial infarction and healthy volunteers. *Circulation* 1992;86:1370–1375.

110. Lee KL, Woodlief LH, Topol EJ, et al. Predictors of 30-day mortality in the era of reperfusion for acute myocardial infarction. Results from an international trial of 41,021 patients. GUSTO-I Investigators. *Circulation* 1995;91:1659–1668.

111. Ohman EM, Harrington RA, Cannon CP, et al. Intravenous thrombolysis in acute myocardial infarction. *Chest* 2001;119:253S–277S.

112. Randomised, double-blind comparison of reteplase double-bolus administration with streptokinase in acute myocardial infarction (INJECT): trial to investigate equivalence. International Joint Efficacy Comparison of Thrombolytics. *Lancet* 1995;346:329–336.

113. A comparison of reteplase with alteplase for acute myocardial infarction. The Global Use of Strategies to Open Occluded Coronary Arteries (GUSTO III) Investigators. *N Engl J Med* 1997;337:1118–1123.

114. Topol EJ, Ohman EM, Armstrong PW, et al. Survival outcomes 1 year after reperfusion therapy with either alteplase or reteplase for acute myocardial infarction: results from the Global Utilization of Streptokinase and t-PA for Occluded Coronary Arteries (GUSTO) III Trial. *Circulation* 2000;102:1761–1765.

115. Gibson CM, Cannon CP, Murphy SA, et al. Weight-adjusted dosing of TNK-tissue plasminogen activator and its relation to angiographic outcomes in the thrombolysis in myocardial infarction 10B trial. TIMI 10B Investigators. *Am J Cardiol* 1999;84:976–980.

116. Van de Werf F, Cannon CP, Luyten A, et al. Safety assessment of single-bolus administration of TNK tissue-plasminogen activator in acute myocardial infarction: the ASSENT-1 trial. The ASSENT-1 Investigators. *Am Heart J* 1999;137:786–791.

117. Barron HV, Bowlby LJ, Breen T, et al. Use of reperfusion therapy for acute myocardial infarction in the United States: data from the National Registry of Myocardial Infarction 2. *Circulation* 1998;97: 1150–1156.

118. Cragg DR, Friedman HZ, Bonema JD, et al. Outcome of patients with acute myocardial infarction who are ineligible for thrombolytic therapy. *Ann Intern Med* 1991;115:173–177.

119. Gunnar RM, Bourdillon PD, Dixon DW, et al. Guidelines for the early management of patients with acute myocardial infarction. A report of the American College of Cardiology/American Heart Association Task Force on Assessment of Diagnostic and Therapeutic Cardiovascular Procedures. *J Am Coll Cardiol* 1990;16:249–292.

120. Chaitman BR, Thompson B, Wittry MD, et al. The use of tissue-type plasminogen activator for acute myocardial infarction in the elderly: results from Thrombolysis in Myocardial Infarction Phase I, open label studies and Thrombolysis in Myocardial Infarction Phase II Pilot Study. *J Am Coll Cardiol* 1989;14:1159–1165.

121. Lew AS, Hod H, Cercek B, et al. Mortality and morbidity rates of patients older and younger than 75 years with acute myocardial infarction treated with intravenous streptokinase. *Am J Cardiol* 1987;59:1–5.

122. Muller DW, Topol EJ. Selection of patients with acute myocardial infarction for thrombolytic therapy. *Ann Intern Med* 1990;113:949–960.

123. Weaver WD, Litwin PE, Martin JS, et al. Effect of age on use of thrombolytic therapy and mortality in acute myocardial infarction. *J Am Coll Cardiol* 1991;18:657–662.

124. Maggioni AP, Maseri A, Fresco C, et al. Age-related increase in mortality among patients with first myocardial infarctions treated with thrombolysis. *N Engl J Med* 1993;329:1442–1448.

125. Sherry S, Marder VJ. Mistaken guidelines for thrombolytic therapy of acute myocardial infarction in the elderly. *J Am Coll Cardiol* 1991;17:1237–1238.

126. De Jaegere P, Arnold AA, Balk AH, et al. Intracranial hemorrhage in association with thrombolytic therapy: incidence and clinical predictive factors. *J Am Coll Cardiol* 1992;19:289–294.

127. Gore JM, Sloan M, Price TR, et al. Intracerebral hemorrhage, cerebral infarction, and subdural hematoma after acute myocardial infarction and thrombolytic therapy in the thrombolysis in myocardial infarction study. *Circulation* 1991;83:448–459.

128. Maggioni AP, Franzosi MG, Santoro E, et al. The risk of stroke in patients with acute myocardial infarction after thrombolytic and antithrombotic treatment. *N Engl J Med* 1992;327:1–6.

129. Krumholz HM, Pasternak RC, Weinstein MC, et al. Cost effectiveness of thrombolytic therapy with streptokinase in elderly patients with suspected acute myocardial infarction. *N Engl J Med* 1992;327:7–13.

130. Late assessment of thrombolytic efficacy (LATE) study with alteplase 6-24 hours after onset of acute myocardial infarction. LATE Study Group. *Lancet* 1993;342:759–766.

131. Randomised trial of late thrombolysis in patients with suspected acute myocardial infarction. EMERAS (Estudio Multicentrico Estreptoquinasa Republicas de America del Sur) Collaborative Group. *Lancet* 1993;342:767–772.

132. Mauri R, Gasparini M, Barbonaglia L, et al. Prognostic significance of the extent of myocardial injury in acute myocardial infarction treated by streptokinase (the GISSI trial). *Am J Cardiol* 1989;63: 1291–1295.

133. Gore JM, Granger CB, Simoons ML, et al. Stroke after thrombolysis. Mortality and functional outcome in the GUSTO-I trial. *Circulation* 1995;92:2811–2818.

134. Gurwitz JH, Gore JM, Goldberg RJ, et al. Risk for intracranial hemorrhage after tissue plasminogen activator treatment for acute myocardial infarction. Participants in the National Registry of Myocardial Infarction 2. *Ann Intern Med* 1998;129:597–604.

135. Barron HV, Fox NL, Berioli S. Comparison of intracranial hemorrhage rates in patients treated with rt-PA and TNK t-PA: impact of gender, age, and low body weight. *Circulation* 1999;100:I-1.

136. Simoons ML, Maggioni AP, Knatterud G, et al. Individual risk assessment for intracranial haemorrhage during thrombolytic therapy. *Lancet* 1993;342:1523–1528.

137. Antman EM. Hirudin in acute myocardial infarction. Safety report from the thrombolysis and thrombin inhibition in myocardial infarction (TIMI) 9A trial. TIMI 9A Investigators. *Circulation* 1994;90:1624–1630.

138. Randomized trial of intravenous heparin versus recombinant hirudin for acute coronary syndromes. The Global Use of Strategies To Open occluded coronary arteries (GUSTO) IIa investigators. GUSTO II Investigators. *Circulation* 1994;90:1631–1637.

139. Neuhaus KL, Essen RV, Tebbe U, et al. Safety observations from the pilot phase of the randomized r-Hirudin for improvement of thrombolysis (HIT-III) study. A study of the Arbeitsgemeinschaft Leitender Kardiologischer Krankenhausarzte (ALKK). *Circulation* 1994;90:1638–1642.

140. Mehta SR, Eikelboom JW, Yusuf S. Risk of intracranial haemorrhage with bolus versus infusion thrombolytic therapy: a meta-analysis. *Lancet* 2000;356:449–454.

141. Armstrong PW, Granger C, Van de Werf F. Bolus fibrinolysis: risk, benefit, and opportunities. *Circulation* 2001;103:1171–1173.

142. Rogers WJ, Bowlby LJ, Chandra NC, et al. Treatment of myocardial infarction in the United States (1990 to 1993). Observations from the National Registry of Myocardial Infarction. *Circulation* 1994;90:2103–2114.

143. Thompson PL, Aylward PE, Federman J, et al. A randomized comparison of intravenous heparin with oral aspirin and dipyridamole 24 hours after recombinant tissue-type plasminogen activator for acute myocardial infarction. *Circulation* 1991;83:1534–1542.

144. Mahaffey KW, Granger CB, Collins R, et al. Overview of randomized trials of intravenous heparin in patients with acute myocardial infarction treated with thrombolytic therapy. *Am J Cardiol* 1996;77:551–556.

145. Hsia J, Kleiman N, Aguirre F, et al. Heparin-induced prolongation of partial thromboplastin time after thrombolysis: relation to coronary artery patency. *J Am Coll Cardiol* 1992;20:31–35.

146. Arnout J, Simoons M, de Bono D, et al. Correlation between level of heparinization and patency of the infarct-related coronary artery after treatment of acute myocardial infarction with alteplase (rt-PA). *J Am Coll Cardiol* 1992;20:513–519.

147. Turpie AG, Robinson JG, Doyle DJ, et al. Comparison of high-dose with low-dose subcutaneous heparin to prevent left ventricular mural thrombosis in patients with acute transmural anterior myocardial infarction. *N Engl J Med* 1989;320:352–357.

148. Ryan TJ, Antman EM, Brooks NH, et al. 1999 update: ACC/AHA Guidelines for the Management of Patients With Acute Myocardial Infarction: Executive Summary and Recommendations: A report of the American College of Cardiology/American Heart Association Task Force on Practice Guidelines (Committee on Management of Acute Myocardial Infarction). *Circulation* 1999;100:1016–1030.

149. Direct thrombin inhibitors in acute coronary syndromes: principal results of a meta-analysis based on individual patients' data. Direct Thrombin Inhibitors Trialists' Collaborative Group. *Lancet* 2002;359: 294–302.

150. Antman EM, Berline JA. Declining incidence of ventricular fibrillation in myocardial infarction. Implications for the prophylactic use of lidocaine. *Circulation* 1992;86:764–773.

151. Efficacy and safety of tenecteplase in combination with enoxaparin, abciximab, or unfractionated heparin: the ASSENT-3 randomised trial in acute myocardial infarction. ASSENT-3 (Assessment of the Safety and Efficacy of a New Thrombolytic) Investigators. *Lancet* 2001;358: 605–613.

152. Ross AM, Molhoek P, Lundergan C, et al. Randomized comparison of enoxaparin, a low-molecular-weight heparin, with unfractionated heparin adjunctive to recombinant tissue plasminogen activator thrombolysis and aspirin: second trial of Heparin and Aspirin Reperfusion Therapy (HART II). *Circulation* 2001;104:648–652.

153. Rydel TJ, Ravichandran KG, Tulinsky A, et al. The structure of a complex of recombinant hirudin and human alpha-thrombin. *Science* 1990;249:277–280.

154. Markwardt F. Hirudin and derivatives as anticoagulant agents. *Thromb Haemost* 1991;66:141–152.

155. Weitz JI, Hudoba M, Massel D, et al. Clot-bound thrombin is protected from inhibition by heparin-antithrombin III but is susceptible to inactivation by antithrombin III-independent inhibitors. *J Clin Invest* 1990;86:385–391.

156. Antman EM. Hirudin in acute myocardial infarction. Thrombolysis and Thrombin Inhibition in Myocardial Infarction (TIMI) 9B Trial. TIMI 9B Investigators. *Circulation* 1996;94:911–921.

157. Metz BK, White HD, Granger CB, et al. Randomized comparison of direct thrombin inhibition versus heparin in conjunction with fibrinolytic therapy for acute myocardial infarction: results from the GUSTO-IIb Trial. Global Use of Strategies to Open Occluded Coronary Arteries in Acute Coronary Syndromes (GUSTO-IIb) Investigators. *J Am Coll Cardiol* 1998;31:1493–1498.

158. Neuhaus KL, Molhoek GP, Zeymer U, et al. Recombinant hirudin (lepirudin) for the improvement of thrombolysis with streptokinase in patients with acute myocardial infarction: results of the HIT-4 trial. *J Am Coll Cardiol* 1999;34:966–973.

159. Thrombin-specific anticoagulation with bivalirudin versus heparin in patients receiving fibrinolytic therapy for acute myocardial infarction: the HERO-2 randomised trial. HERO (Hirulog and Early Reperfusion or Occlusion)-2 Trial Investigators. *Lancet* 2001;358:1855–1863.

160. Mehta RH, Montoye CK, Gallogly M, et al. Improving quality of care for acute myocardial infarction: The Guidelines Applied in Practice (GAP) Initiative. *JAMA* 2002;287:1269–1276.

161. Phillips DR, Charo IF, Parise LV, et al. The platelet membrane glycoprotein IIb/IIIa complex. *Blood* 1988;71:831–843.

162. Lefkovits J, Ivanhoe R, Anderson K, et al. Platelet IIb/IIIa receptor inhibition during PTCA for acute myocardial infarction: insights from the EPIC trial. *Circulation* 1994;90[Suppl]:I–564(abst).

163. Gold HK, Coller BS, Yasuda T, et al. Rapid and sustained coronary artery recanalization with combined bolus injection of recombinant tissue-type plasminogen activator and monoclonal antiplatelet GPIIb/IIIa antibody in a canine preparation. *Circulation* 1988;77:670–677.

164. Shebuski RJ, Stabilito IJ, Sitko GR, et al. Acceleration of recombinant tissue-type plasminogen activator-induced thrombolysis and prevention of reocclusion by the combination of heparin and the arg-gly-asp-containing peptide bitistatin in a canine model of coronary thrombosis. *Circulation* 1990;82:169–177.

165. Yasuda T, Gold HK, Leinbach RC, et al. Lysis of plasminogen activator-resistant platelet-rich coronary artery thrombus with combined bolus injection of recombinant tissue-type plasminogen activator and antiplatelet GPIIb/IIIa antibody. *J Am Coll Cardiol* 1990;16:1728–1735.

166. Yasuda T, Gold HK, Leinbach RC, et al. Kistrin, a polypeptide platelet GPIIb/IIIa receptor antagonist, enhances and sustains coronary arterial thrombolysis with recombinant tissue-type plasminogen activator in a canine preparation. *Circulation* 1991;83:1038–1047.

167. Mickelson JK, Simpson PJ, Cronin M, et al. Antiplatelet antibody [7E3 F(ab')$_2$] prevents rethrombosis after recombinant tissue-type plasminogen activator-induced coronary artery thrombolysis in a canine model. *Circulation* 1990;81:617–627.

168. Holahan MA, Mellott MJ, Garsky VM, et al. Prevention of reocclusion following tissue type plasminogen activator-induced thrombolysis by the RGD-containing peptide, echistatin, in a canine model of coronary thrombosis. *Pharmacology* 1991;42:340–348.

169. Modi NB, Reynolds T, Baughman SA, et al. Pharmacokinetics and pharmacodynamics of TP-9201, a gpIIbIIIa antagonist, administered in combination with recombinant tissue-type plasminogen activator, heparin, and aspirin in beagles. *J Cardiovasc Pharmacol* 1996;27:105–112.

170. Nicolini FA, Lee P, Rios G, et al. Combination of platelet fibrinogen receptor antagonist and direct thrombin inhibitor at low doses markedly improves thrombolysis. *Circulation* 1994;89:1802–1809.

171. Roux SP, Tschopp TB, Kuhn H, et al. Effects of heparin, aspirin and a synthetic platelet glycoprotein IIb-IIIa receptor antagonist (Ro 43-5054) on coronary artery reperfusion and reocclusion after thrombolysis with tissue-type plasminogen activator in the dog. *J Pharmacol Exp Ther* 1992;264:501–508.

172. Lu HR, Gold HK, Wu Z, et al. G4120, an Arg-Gly-Asp containing pentapeptide, enhances arterial eversion graft recanalization with recombinant tissue-type plasminogen activator in dogs. *Thromb Haemost* 1992;67:686–691.

173. Yasuda T, Gold HK, Kohmura C, et al. Intravenous and endobronchial administration of G4120, a cyclic Arg-Gly-Asp-containing platelet GPIIb/IIIa receptor-blocking pentapeptide, enhances and sustains coronary arterial thrombolysis with rt-PA in a canine preparation. *Arterioscler Thromb* 1993;13:738–747.

174. de Lemos JA, Gibson CM, Antman EM, et al. Abciximab and early adjunctive percutaneous coronary intervention are associated with improved ST-segment resolution after thrombolysis: observations from the TIMI 14 Trial. *Am Heart J* 2001;141:592–598.

175. Antman E, Guigliano R, Gibson C, et al. Abciximab facilitates the rate and extent of thrombolysis results of the thrombolysis in myocardial infarction (TIMI) 14 trial. *Circulation* 1999;99:2720–2732.

176. SPEED (Strategies for Patency Enhancement in the Emergency Department) Group. Trial of abciximab with and without low-dose reteplase for acute myocardial infarction. *Circulation* 2000;101:2788–2794.

177. Reperfusion therapy for acute myocardial infarction with fibrinolytic therapy or combination reduced fibrinolytic therapy and platelet glycoprotein IIb/IIIa inhibition: the GUSTO V randomised trial. GUSTO V Investigators. *Lancet* 2001;357:1905–1914.

178. Randomized trial of intravenous streptokinase, oral aspirin, both, or neither among 17,187 cases of suspected acute myocardial infarction: ISIS-2. ISIS-2 (Second International Study of Infarct Survival) Collaborative Group. *J Am Coll Cardiol* 1988;12[6 Suppl A]:3A–13A.

179. Prehospital thrombolytic therapy in patients with suspected acute myocardial infarction. European Myocardial Infarction Project Group. *N Engl J Med* 1993;329:383–389.

180. Feasibility, safety, and efficacy of domiciliary thrombolysis by general practitioners: Grampian region early anistreplase trial. GREAT Group. *BMJ* 1992;305:548–553.

181. Morrison LJ, Verbeek PR, McDonald AC, et al. Mortality and prehospital thrombolysis for acute myocardial infarction: a meta-analysis. *JAMA* 2000;283:2686–2692.

182. Rogers WJ, Canto JG, Lambrew CT, et al. Temporal trends in the treatment of over 1.5 million patients with myocardial infarction in the US from 1990 through 1999: the National Registry of Myocardial Infarction 1, 2 and 3. *J Am Coll Cardiol* 2000;36:2056–2063.

183. Gersh BJ, Anderson JL. Thrombolysis and myocardial salvage. *Circulation* 1993;88:296–306.

184. Goldberg RJ, Gurwitz JH, Gore JM. Duration of, and temporal trends (1994-1997) in, prehospital delay in patients with acute myocardial infarction: the second National Registry of Myocardial Infarction. *Arch Intern Med* 1999;159:2141–2147.

185. Bonnefoy E, Lapostolle F, Leizorovicz A, et al. Primary angioplasty versus prehospital fibrinolysis in acute myocardial infarction: a randomised study. *Lancet* 2002;360:825–829.

186. Morrow DA, Antman EM, Sayah A, et al. Evaluation of the time saved by prehospital initiation of reteplase for ST-elevation myocardial infarction: results of The Early Retavase-Thrombolysis in Myocardial Infarction (ER-TIMI) 19 trial. *J Am Coll Cardiol* 2002;40:71–77.

187. Ross AM, Coyne KS, Reiner JS, et al. A randomized trial comparing primary angioplasty with a strategy of short-acting thrombolysis and immediate planned rescue angioplasty in acute myocardial infarction: the PACT trial. PACT investigators. Plasminogen-activator Angioplasty Compatibility Trial. *J Am Coll Cardiol* 1999;34:1954–1962.

188. Li RH, Herrmann HC. Facilitated percutaneous coronary intervention: a novel concept in expediting and improving acute myocardial infarction care. *Am Heart J* 2000;140:S125–S135.

189. Mahaffey KW, Puma JA, Barbagelata A, et al. Adenosine as an adjunct to thrombolytic therapy for acute myocardial infarction. *J Am Coll Cardiol* 1999;34:1711–1720.

190. Budde JM, Velez DA, Zhao Z, et al. Comparative study of AMP579 and adenosine in inhibition of neutrophil-mediated vascular and myocardial injury during 24 h of reperfusion. *Cardiovasc Res* 2000;47:294–305.

191. Kopecky SL, Aviles RJ, Bell MR, et al. A randomized, double-blinded, placebo-controlled, dose-ranging study measuring the effect of an adenosine agonist on infarct size reduction in patients undergoing primary percutaneous transluminal coronary angioplasty: the ADMIRE (AmP579 Delivery for Myocardial Infarction REduction) study. *Am Heart J* 2003;146:146–152.

192. Topol EJ, Ellis SG, Califf RM, et al. Combined tissue-type plasminogen activator and prostacyclin therapy for acute myocardial infarction. *J Am Coll Cardiol* 1989;14:877–884.

193. Wall TC, Califf RM, Blankenship J, et al. Intravenous fluosol in the treatment of acute myocardial infarction. Results of the thrombolysis and angioplasty in myocardial infarction 9 trial. *Circulation* 1994;90:114–120.

194. ISIS-4 (Fourth International Study of Infarct Survival) Collaborative Group. ISIS-4: a randomised factorial trial assessing early oral captopril, oral mononitrate, and intravenous magnesium sulphate in 58,050 patients with suspected acute myocardial infarction. ISIS-4 (Fourth International Study of Infarct Survival) Collaborative Group. *Lancet* 1995;345:669–685.

195. Effects of RheothRx on mortality, morbidity, left ventricular function, and infarct size in patients with acute myocardial infarction. Collaborative Organization for RheothRx Evaluation (CORE). *Circulation* 1997;96:192–201.

196. Faxon DP, Gibbons RJ, Chronos NA, et al. The effect of blockade of the CD11/CD18 integrin receptor on infarct size in patients with acute myocardial infarction treated with direct angioplasty: the results of the HALT-MI study. *J Am Coll Cardiol* 2002;40:1199–1204.

197. Weaver WD, Cerqueira M, Hallstrom AP, et al. Prehospital-initiated vs hospital-initiated thrombolytic therapy. *JAMA* 1993;270:1211–1216.

CHAPTER 68

The Role of Percutaneous
Coronary Intervention

Pim J. de Feyter and Patrick W. Serruys

Key Words: Acute coronary syndrome; coronary athero-thrombosis; percutaneous coronary intervention; stent-implantation.

Since the introduction of percutaneous coronary intervention (PCI) in 1977, the scope of the technique has broadened to include patients with stable angina and patients with acute coronary syndromes (1–3).

Initially using balloon angioplasty only, the procedure was associated with a rather high procedural complication rate; but with the introduction of stent implantation and adjunctive treatment with platelet glycoprotein (GP) 2b/3a inhibitors and thienopyridienes, the procedure has become safe, with a predictable result. Acute coronary syndromes are common causes of emergency hospital admissions and a

major cause of mortality worldwide (4–8). Over recent years significant advances have been made in therapeutic interventions and new drugs for acute coronary syndromes, but many patients are refractory to medical treatment and require revascularization, whereas primary PCI may be more efficacious than thrombolytic treatment in acute ST-segment elevation myocardial infarction (STEMI) (9).

This chapter reviews the in-hospital and late outcomes of current PCI techniques for the treatment of unstable coronary artery disease (CAD), emphasizes the role of an early risk-stratification strategy and PCI, discusses the merits of an early invasive treatment strategy versus an early conservative treatment strategy, and provides the early and late outcomes of primary PCI for acute myocardial infarction (AMI).

DEFINITION OF UNSTABLE CORONARY
ARTERY DISEASE

Acute coronary syndromes encompass STEMI, non ST-segment elevation myocardial infarction (non-STEMI), and unstable angina. An acute coronary syndrome is a clinical manifestation occurring in pathologically far-

P. J. de Feyter: Thoraxcenter, room Bd 410, Erasmus Medical Centre, Dr. Molewaterplein 40, 3015 GD Rotterdam, The Netherlands.
P. W. Serruys: Thoraxcenter, room Bd 404, Erasmus Medical Centre, Dr. Molewaterplein 40, 3015 GD Rotterdam, The Netherlands.

advanced coronary lesions that, however, are often nonobstructive. Inflammation plays a central role in the progression of atherothrombosis and the processes leading to intracoronary thrombosis (10–16). It is now apparent that acute coronary syndromes share a common pathophysiologic substrate with atherothrombotic plaque rupture or erosion and superimposed thrombosis and distal embolization.

This chapter discusses separately STEMI and unstable CAD, which constitutes two components: non-STEMI and unstable angina. Non-STEMI is distinguished from UA by the presence of increases of cardiac enzymes: on the basis of increased levels of troponin I or T. About 30% of the patients previously considered to have unstable angina on the basis of normal CK-MB levels are currently considered to have a myocardial infarction (MI) on the basis of increased troponin levels.

Non-STEMI and UA have a wide range of clinical, electrocardiographic, biochemical, and angiographic manifestations, and therefore exhibit a variable prognosis (6). This makes it difficult to propose simple guidelines that are generally applicable to this wide range of patients, and it does reflect the differences in European and American guidelines for the management of the acute coronary syndromes *without* persistent ST-segment elevation (17,18).

PERCUTANEOUS TREATMENT OF UNSTABLE CORONARY ARTERY DISEASE

Rationale of Percutaneous Coronary Intervention

PCI in patients with unstable CAD is performed to prevent or interrupt the rapid ongoing process of an unstable lesion progressing to total occlusion resulting in ongoing ischemia, myocardial necrosis, or coronary death (19–25).

Balloon angioplasty enlarges the lumen by mechanical disruption of the plaque, increase of the total vessel circumference, and mechanical dissolution of the superimposed intracoronary thrombus (26). Currently, stent implantation, which is technically easy to use, resulting in a safe and predictable procedural outcome, and which has reduced late restenosis, is considered the optimal treatment strategy (27–30).

Intracoronary stenting improves suboptimal angioplasty outcome and may prevent distal embolization of friable thrombotic material because of its scaffolding properties. Balloon angioplasty and stenting creates an optimal coronary lumen and coronary flow dynamics. This reduces the high-shear rate forces occurring within a narrow coronary lumen, which are known to stimulate platelet activation and aggregation, and thus may be helpful in further stabilizing the unstable plaque.

PCI of an unstable plaque may prevent progression of the coronary narrowing. Plaque disruption often results in an increase of plaque burden, which may be accompanied by negative remodeling, both of which contribute to a significant decrease in coronary lumen (31–33).

Percutaneous treatment of an unstable lesion may be associated with an increased risk for early adverse events because of mechanical manipulation of the highly thrombogenetic unstable lesion and distal embolization of thrombotic or necrotic material (34). Adjunctive treatment with platelet GPIIb/IIIa inhibitors has been shown to significantly reduce PCI-related major complications (35,36).

Risk Stratification

Patients with unstable CAD are heterogeneous in their clinical presentation, resulting in a variable prognosis. This variation may be explained by the use of differences in definition, inherent wide variation of clinical manifestation, and management and treatment of these patients. From large, published, randomized studies, information can be gathered about the prognosis of patients with unstable CAD, who were treated with aspirin, heparin, and varying antiischemic medications. The overall mortality rate at 48 hours, 7 days, 30 days, and 6 months was on average 0.3%, 1.7%, 3.7%, and 6.4%, respectively. The combined death and nonfatal MI rate was 2.4%, 8.7%, 11.3%, and 16.3%, respectively (37–46). However, these prognostic data represent an average number of a heterogeneous population that consists of a range of subgroups with different risks. Prognosis is mainly determined by clinical manifestation, baseline electrocardiogram, and release of cardiac-specific enzymes.

The revised Braunwald risk stratification, which is based on the severity of angina and clinical circumstances during which angina occurs and the release of cardiac-specific protein troponin T, often is used (47–52). The incorporation of troponin T is important, and according to this revised stratification, the 30-day risk for death and MI may be up to 20% in Class IIIb troponin-positive and less than 2% in Class IIIb troponin-negative patients (Table 68–1).

TABLE 68–1. *Braunwald revisited classification—adapted for percutaneous coronary intervention*

Severity UA	Class B primary UA	Class C post-MI UA within 2 wk after MI
I New onset of angina or accelerated angina; no rest pain	IB	IC
II Angina at rest within past month but not within past 48 h	IIB	IIC
III Angina at rest within 48 h	IIIB: T-negative IIIB: T-positive	IIIC

MI, myocardial infarction; T, troponin; UA, unstable angina.

TABLE 68–2. *Baseline electrocardiogram*

Incidence of death/myocardial infarction at 30 d	
T-wave inversion	5.5%
ST-segment elevation	9.4%
ST-segment depression	10.5%
ST-segment depression/elevation	12.4%

The prognosis of patients with unstable angina is better than those with non-STEMI. The 1-year mortality rate for unstable angina was 7% and was 11% for non-STEMI, whereas the 6-month (re)infarction rate was 6.2% versus 9.8% (53).

The ST-segment and T-wave changes of the baseline electrocardiogram are an important prognostic indicator (Table 68–2) (54). In addition, mortality is related to the number of leads with ST-segment changes and the magnitude of ST-segment deflection (55).

The cardiac-specific proteins troponin T and I are sensitive markers of myocardial cell injury, and they are highly predictive of short- and long-term adverse events (56–61). There appears to be a quantitative relation between troponin T release and the risk for death within 42 days (Fig. 68–1) (58). The acute-phase protein, C-reactive protein (CRP), a marker of inflammation, also is an indicator of short- and long-term adverse cardiac events (62–65). And the B-type natriuretic peptide also is associated with a greater rate of death and recurrent ischemic events in acute coronary syndromes (66). Combination of troponin, C-reactive protein and, B-type natriuretic peptide provides a powerful broad risk stratification (67).

A risk score based on easily obtainable baseline variables was developed that is highly useful in identifying patients at high risk who may benefit most from an early revascularization strategy (Fig. 68–2) (68).

Risk for Major Adverse Coronary Event during Percutaneous Coronary Intervention for Unstable Coronary Artery Disease

Balloon angioplasty, without adjunctive treatment with platelet GPIIb/IIIa inhibitors or stent implantation, was associated with a greater major adverse coronary event (MACE) rate in unstable patients than in stable patients (3,69–72).

The introduction of adjunctive treatment with platelet GPIIb/IIIa inhibitors and stent implantation has significantly improved the safety of the procedure and has more or less equalized the MACE rate in patients with stable and unstable angina (73–76). However, the MACE rate continues to be greater in subsets of patients with unstable angina, such as those refractory to medical treatment or early post-MI unstable angina (77,78). The risk for MACE appears to be greater in angiographic complex, ulcerated, or thrombotic lesions; bifurcation lesions or severe calcified lesions; and in patients with increased levels of troponin (79–82). Obviously, additional severe comorbidity, notably diabetes mellitus (83), severe renal dysfunction, or old age will increase the risk.

It is estimated that the risk for MACE during PCI for unstable CAD may be 2% to 5% for those at low risk, between 5% and 10% for those at intermediate risk, and 10% to 15% for those at high risk. Severe comorbidity may further increase this risk.

Outcome of Percutaneous Coronary Intervention for Unstable Coronary Artery Disease

Modern PCI is based on two major effective techniques: balloon angioplasty and stent implantation. Adjunctive treatment with platelet GPIIb/IIIa inhibition has significantly reduced the major complication rate during the procedure and the 30-day outcome after balloon angioplasty, as was clearly

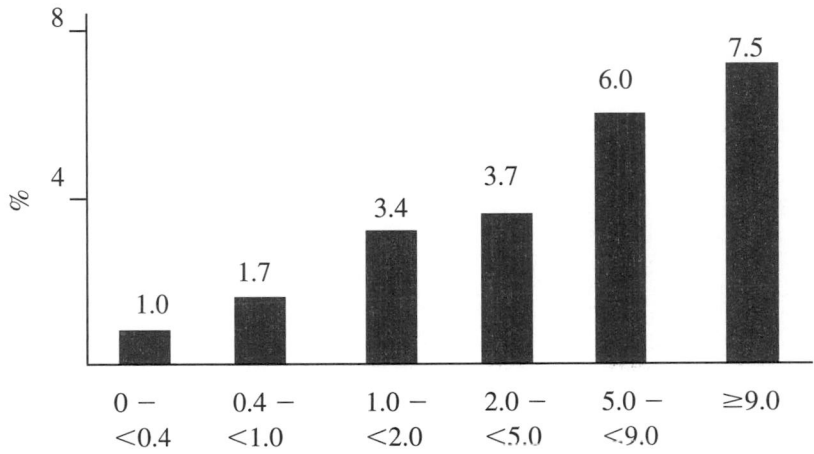

FIG. 68–1. Mortality at 42 days in relation to troponin release at baseline. (Adapted from Antman EM, Tanasijevic MJ, Thompson B, et al. Cardiac-specific troponin I levels to predict the risk of mortality in patients with acute coronary syndromes. *N Engl J Med* 1996;335:1342–1349, with permission.)

- Age 65 yrs
- Anginal events
- ST-segment deviation
- Elevated serum cardiac markers
- 3 Risk factors CAD
- Aspirin use (prior 7 days)
- Prior coronary stenosis (>50%)

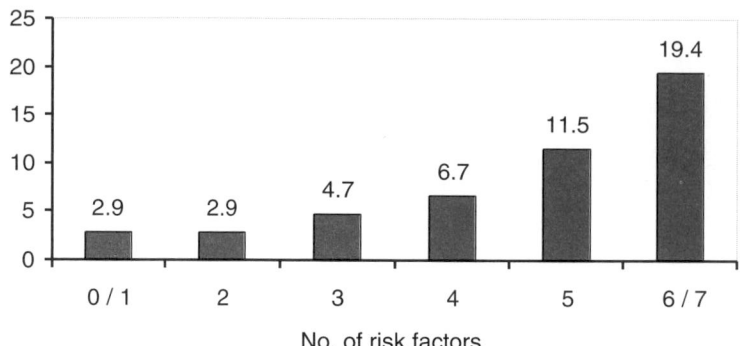

FIG. 68–2. Thrombolysis in Myocardial Ischemia (TIMI) predictive risk score. CAD, coronary artery disease. (From Antman EM, Cohen M, Bernick PJ, et al. The TIMI risk score for unstable angina/non-ST-elevation MI: a method for prognostification and therapeutic decision making. *JAMA* 2000;284:835–842, with permission.)

demonstrated in major randomized trials (Table 68–3) (41,42,44,75,77). However, this beneficial effect was less striking at 6 months.

Stent implantation was relatively safe in patients with unstable CAD, even in patients who required multiple stent implantation (Table 68–4) (84–89). The initially rather high frequency of subacute thrombotic stent occlusion has been significantly reduced by the combined treatment of aspirin and ticlopidin or clopidogrel, and it has been reduced to less than 1% (90–94). Currently, the treatment with clopidogrel is preferred because the classic study demonstrated superior safety and tolerability of clopidogrel compared with tidopidine (95).

In subgroup analyses of the BElgium NEtherland STENT (BENESTENT) trial, the EPI-STENT trial, and the Enhanced Suppression of Platelet Receptor GP IIb/IIIa using Integrelin Trial (ESPRIT) trial, it was shown that the combination of stent implantation with GPIIb/IIIa inhibitor was superior than stent alone or a combination of balloon and a GPIIb/IIIa inhibitor (Tables 68–5 through 68–7) in various subsets of patients with unstable CAD (96–98).

Stent implantation has significantly reduced the 6-month restenosis rate in patients with unstable CAD. The restenosis rate varies from 11% to 27% (96,97,99). The 1-year outcome after stent implantation is comparable for stable and unstable angina, with the exception of the occurrence of non–Q-wave MI, which is slightly greater in unstable patients (Table 68–8).

Troponin Release to Guide Therapy

It has been shown that patients with troponin increase are more likely than those without to have distal emboli in the microvasculature and to have left ventricular dysfunction (100).

TABLE 68–3. *Balloon angioplasty and glycoprotein IIb/IIIa inhibitors for unstable coronary artery disease: 30-day death/myocardial infarction outcome*

Trial	Treatment	Placebo (n)	GPIIB/IIIa (n)
Epilog[a]	Abciximab	11.7% (663)	6.1% (634) and 4.7% (610)[b]
CAPTURE[a]	Abciximab	15.9% (635)	11.3% (630)
PRISM	Tirofiban	9.1% (352)	7.2% (348)
PRISM PLUS	Tirofiban	10.2% (236)	5.9% (239)
PURSUIT	Eptifibatide	16.7% (606)	11.6% (622)

CAPTURE, c7E3 Fab Antiplatelet Therapy in Unstable Refractory Angina; Epilog, Evaluation in Ptca to Improve Long-term Outcome with abciximab Gp IIb/IIIa blockade; PRISM, Platelet Receptor Inhibition in Ischemic Syndrome Management; PURSUIT, Platelet Glycoprotein IIb/IIIa in Unstable angina: Receptor Suppression Using Integrin Therapy.
[a]Combined end point: death/myocardial infarction/urgent revascularization.
[b]Plus/minus standard dose of heparin.

TABLE 68–4. *Stent implantation in unstable coronary artery disease*

Author (reference)	Patients, n	Death, %	Myocardial infarction, %	Abrupt occlusion, %	Emergency surgery, %
Robinson et al. (84)	83	0	2.7	3.6	7.2
Marzocchi et al. (85)	132	0	4.5	6.8	4.5
Chauhan et al. (86)	110	0	4.5	3.6	0.9
Alfonso et al. (87)	86	6	6.0	1.0	0
Madan et al. (88)	156	0.6	1.9	1.9	1.9
Kornowski et al. (89)	334	1.0	0.6	0.6	3.0

Trials have shown that patients with increased troponin levels specifically benefitted from treatment with low–molecular weight heparin (82,101), GPIIb/IIIa blockers (41–43,79,80) (Fig. 68–3), or an early invasive strategy (15,102).

However, the relation between the magnitude of troponin increase and treatment benefit is not simple. It appears that low troponin levels gain little benefit, intermediate levels gain greatest benefit, and greatest levels gain almost no benefit because these levels represent a large amount of irreversible myocardial necrosis (103).

Early Invasive Strategy versus Ischemia-guided Conservative Strategy

Several earlier trials, the Thrombolysis in Myocardial Ischemia (TIMI)-IIIb (104), the Veterans Affairs Non-Q-Wave Infarction Strategies in Hospital (VANQWISH) trial (105), and the Medicine versus Angiography in Thrombolytic Exclusion (MATE) trial (106), have shown that an ischemia-driven conservative strategy was safe and effective in patients with unstable CAD and that an aggressive invasive treatment strategy was not superior. These studies were criticized, because the revascularization frequency was relatively high in the conservative arms, or patients who deserved revascularization did not receive this treatment, whereas those who underwent surgery had a high operative mortality rate (11.9%).

Three recently conducted trials, using state-of-the-art interventional techniques and modern anti platelet therapy, demonstrated unequivocally that early invasive strategy was superior to an early conservative strategy (45,107–109). The patients in the Fragmin during Instability in Coronary Artery Disease (FRISC)-II trial were high-risk patients with ST-segment depression or T-wave charges and evidence of CK-

MB release or troponin T release. Early revascularization was achieved in more than 70% of the patients (Table 68–9). The 6-month and 1-year combined death and MI rate was statistically significantly less in favor of the early invasive strategy (Table 68–9 and Fig. 68–4). This favorable effect was predominantly achieved in male patients only, whereas almost no effect was noted in female patients. The rate with use of stents was 65% and with platelet GPIIb/IIIa inhibitors was 10%.

The Treat angina with Aggrastat and determine Cost of Therapy with an Invasive of Conserative Strategy (TACTICS-TIMI) 18 trial enrolled 2,220 unstable patients who had ST-segment depression greater than 1 mm, troponin T release, or both. All patients were treated with aspirin, heparin, a β-blocker, and tirofiban (Aggrastat), a GPIIb/IIIA inhibitor. Coronary angiography and revascularization were performed within 4 to 48 hours of chest pain in the invasive arm (Table 68–10). The major adverse event rate at 180 days was significantly less in the invasive strategy arm than in the conservative strategy (15.9% vs. 19.4%). The Value of first day angiography/angioplasty In evolving Non-st segment elevation myocardial infarction: an Open multicenter randomized trial (VINO) trial investigated whether an early invasive strategy—that is, coronary angiography and PCI of the culprit lesion on the same day of admission—in patients with a non-STEMI was superior to an initial conservative strategy. A total of 131 patients were randomized, and revascularization was performed in 47% of the 64 patients who were assigned to the early invasive strategy. Mortality, myocardial reinfarction, or the combined death and reinfarction rates were significantly less at 30 days and at 6 months in the invasive strategy arm (Table 68–11) (109).

A risk stratification, on the basis of the release of troponins, demonstrated that patients likeliest to benefit from an early invasive treatment strategy had increased levels of

TABLE 68–5. *BENESTENT trial: subanalysis of unstable angina*

Follow up at 400 days	Balloon (79)	Stent (96)
Composite end point (death/MI/CABG/rePTCA)	21.5%	6.3%
Restenosis (>5%)	35%	18%

BENESTENT, BElgium NEtherland STENT; CABG, coronary artery bypass grafting; MI, myocardial infarction; PTCA, porcutaneous transluminal coronary angioplasty.

TABLE 68–6. *EPI-STENT trial: 30-day end point for death, myocardial infarction, urgent revascularization*

	Stent + placebo, %	Balloon + abciximab, %	Stent + abciximab, %
Stable angina	11.5	7.9	4.4
UA < 6 mo	11.3	6.5	4.7
UA < 7 d	11.1	9.4	5.2
UA < 48 h	14.8	7.3	4.5

EPI-STENT, Evaluation of Platelet IIb/IIIa Inhibitor for STENTing; UA, unstable angina.

TABLE 68–7. *ESPRIT trial: death, myocardial infarction, and urgent revascularization at 48 hours*

	Stable angina, (n)	ACS > 2 d (n)	ACS ≤ 2 d (n)	STEMI ≤ 7 d (n)
Stent + placebo	7.2% (387)	11.1% (333)	15.0% (140)	20.4% (49)
Stent + Eptifibatide	5.4% (407)	5.7% (331)	7.9% (139)	11.4% (44)

ACS, acute coronary syndrome; ESPRIT, Enhanced Suppression of Platelet Receptor GP IIb/IIIa using Integrelin Trial; STEMI, ST-segment elevation myocardial infarction.

TABLE 68–8. *One-year outcome after coronary stenting in unstable angina*

	Unstable angina (1,475)	Stable angina (2,369)	Odds ratio (95% CI)
Death	4.5%	4.1%	1.13 (0.82–1.55)
Nonfatal MI	4.7%	2.8%	1.74 (1.23–2.45)
Q-wave MI	1.3%	1.2%	1.05 (0.59–1.88)
Non–Q-wave MI	3.2%	1.7%	1.87 (1.22–2.86)
Target vessel revascularization	20.7%	18.8%	1.13 (0.96–1.33)
Angiographic restenosis	33.2%	33.8%	0.97 (0.83–1.14)
Any adverse clinical event	27.5%	23.9%	1.21 (1.04–1.40)

Performed in 80% of the patients.
CI, confidence interval; MI, myocardial infarction.
From Mehilli J, Kastrati A, Dirschinger J, et al. Clinical and angiographic results of 1 year follow-up after coronary artery stenting in unstable angina. *J Am Coll Cardiol* 2001[Suppl]:53A(abst).

TABLE 68–9. *Fragmin during Instability in Coronary Artery Disease (FRISC) II trial: revascularization strategies in high-risk unstable angina*

Outcome	Invasive strategy (n = 1215)	Conservative strategy (n = 1229)	p
Revascularization			
<10 d	71%	9%	
<6 mo	78%	38%	
Death at 6 mo			
All patients	1.9%	3.0%	0.10
Males	1.5%	3.2%	0.03
Females	2.9%	2.6%	0.75
Death/Myocardial infarction at 6 months			
All patients	9.5%	12%	0.04
Males	9.1%	13.9%	0.002

TABLE 68–10. *TACTICS-TIMI 18: revascularization strategies for acute coronary syndromes*

	Invasive strategy (4–48 h) (n = 1114)	Conservative strategy (n = 1106)	p
Revascularization	64%	36%	
End point at 180 d			
Death	3.3%	3.5%	NS
MI	4.8%	6.9%	0.03
Death/MI	7.3%	9.5%	0.05
Readmission to hospital for ACS	11%	13.7%	0.054
Composite end point	15.9%	19.4%	0.025

ACS, acute coronary syndrome; MI, myocardial infarction; NS, not significant; TACTICS-TIMI, Treat angina with Aggrastat and determine Cost of Therapy with an Invasive of Conservative Strategy.

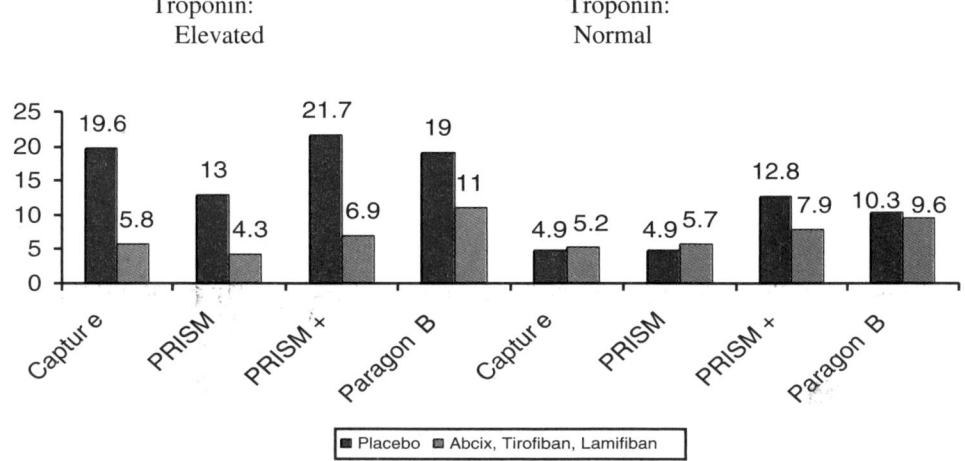

FIG. 68–3. Troponin release and outcome (death/myocardial infarction at 1 month) in patients with unstable coronary artery disease. Capture, c7E3 Fab Antiplatelet Therapy in Unstable Refractory Angina; Paragon, Paragon stent versus Palmaz-Schatz stent for treatment of coronary stenoses; PRISM, Platelet Receptor Inhibition in Ischemic Syndrome Management.

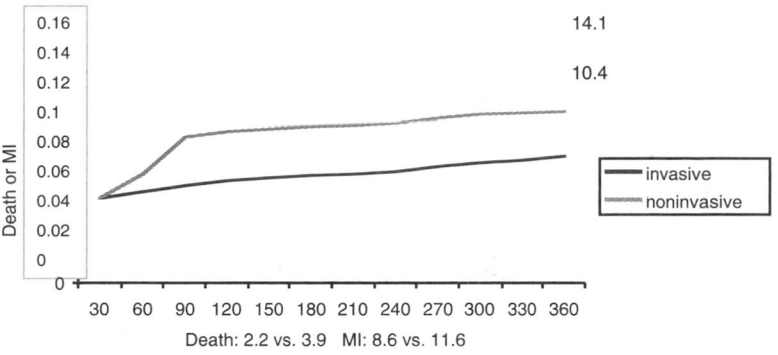

Death: 2.2 vs. 3.9   MI: 8.6 vs. 11.6

FIG. 68–4. One-year follow up of Fragmin during Instability in Coronary Artery Disease (FRISC)-II patients. (Adapted from FRISC-Trial: FRagmin and Fast Revascularization during InStability in Coronary artery disease Investigators. *Lancet* 1999;354:708–715.)

troponin, whereas patients with normal or low troponin levels had almost no benefit of an early invasive strategy (108) (Fig. 68–5). Also, patients with ST-segment depression or a high TIMI risk score (Fig. 68–2) benefitted more from an early invasive treatment strategy, as was shown in a subanalysis of the TIMI-IIIb, the FRISC-II, and TACTICS-TIMI-18 trials (104,107,110,111).

Surgery versus Percutaneous Coronary Intervention in Multivessel Disease and Unstable Coronary Artery Disease

Recently, revascularization of patients with unstable CAD, be it bypass surgery or PCI, has been associated with a greater frequency of periprocedural complications compared with patients with stable angina. This has changed with current approaches, as was demonstrated in the randomized Arterial Revascularization Therapies Study (ARTS) trial. The ARTS trial investigated whether the outcome of an intervention with stenting in patients with multivessel disease and stable and unstable angina was different from the outcome of modern bypass surgery using arterial grafting if possible (112). In terms of 1-year death, cardiovascular accident, and MI rates, there was no difference between stenting or surgery both in stable

and unstable patients (Table 68–12). However, there was a need for more repeat procedures in the stented group.

Notably, severe refractory unstable patients or patients with left main disease were not included into this trial; therefore, the outcome may not be applicable to all subsets of unstable angina. Also important is that the outcome of the ARTS trial demonstrated that "instability" in the majority of unstable patients no longer acts as a risk factor for revascularization.

Long-Term Outcome after Percutaneous Coronary Intervention—Sex Differences?

The long-term outcome after balloon angioplasty, in terms of death, reinfarction, and repeat revascularization, for unstable angina is relatively good (113–115). Data are conflicting about the influence of sex on the long-term outcome. In the FRISC-II trial, it was shown that in women with unstable CAD, undergoing an early aggressive invasive treatment did not reduce the risk compared with early conservative strategy (116). However, this was not confirmed in the TACTICS trial, in which the adverse event rate after an invasive strat-

TABLE 68–11. *VINO study: early invasive versus conservative strategy in non–ST-segment elevation myocardial infarction*

	Invasive strategy (64)	Conservative strategy (67)	p
30 d			
Death	1.6%	7.5%	0.2
RE-MI	1.6%	7.5%	0.2
Death/re-MI	3.1%	10.4%	0.16
6 mo			
Death	3.1%	13.4%	0.03
Re-MI	3.1%	14.9%	0.02
Death/re-MI	6.3%	22.4%	0.001

MI, myocardial infarction; VINO, Value of first day angiography/angioplasty In evloving Non-st segment elevation myocardial infarction: an Open multicenter randomized trial.

TABLE 68–12. *Frequency of Major Cardiac Events at 1 year*

	Stented angioplasty, %		CABG, %	
	Stable (n = 374)	Unstable (n = 226)	Stable (n = 381)	Unstable (n = 224)
Death	2.4	2.7	3.2	2.2
CVA	2.1	0.4	1.3	3.1
MI	5.1	5.8	2.9	5.8
Q-wave	4.3	5.3	2.9	4.9
Non–Q-wave	0.8	0.4	0	0.9
CABG[a]	3.7	6.2	0.3	0.9
Repeat PCI[a]	13.1	10.6	3.2	2.7
No MACE[b]	73.5	74.3	89.2	85.3

CABG, coronary artery bypass grafting; CVA, cardiovascular accident; MACE, major adverse coronary event; MI, myocardial infarction; PCI, percutaneous coronary intervention.

All bypass patients versus stented patients: [a]p < 0.01; [b]p < 0.001.

Troponin: Positive   Troponin: Negative

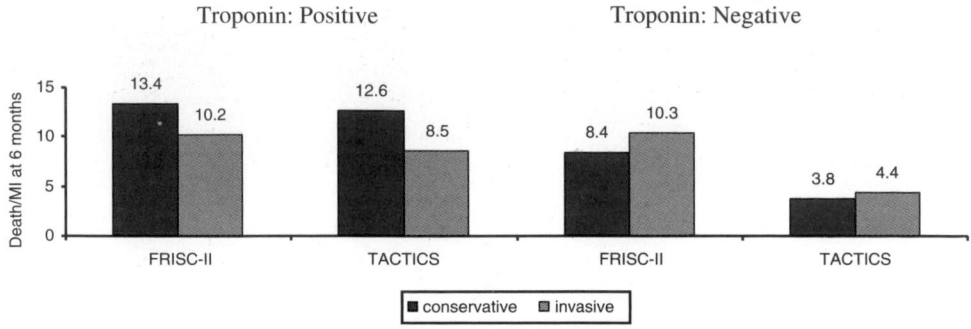

FIG. 68–5. Benefit of an early invasive strategy according to troponin levels. FRISC, Fragmin during Instability in Coronary Artery Disease; MI, myocardial infarction; TACTICS, Treat angina with Aggrastat and determine Cost of Therapy with an Invasive of Conservative Strategy.

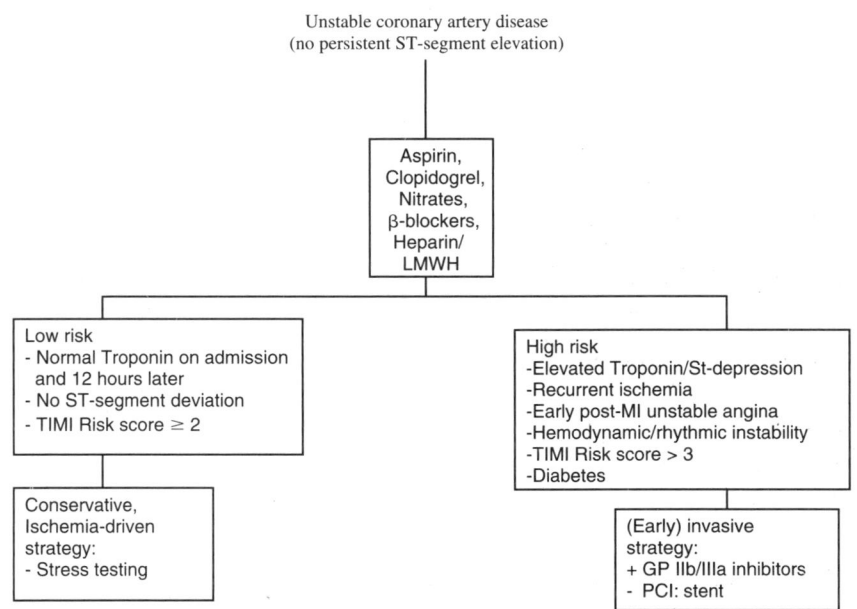

FIG. 68–6. Management of unstable coronary artery disease. GP, glycoprotein; LMWH, low–molecular weight heparin; MI, myocardial infarction; PCI, percutaneous coronary intervention; TIMI, Thrombolytics in Myocardial Infarction.

TABLE 68–13. *Direct stenting versus direct balloon angioplasty for acute myocardial infarction*

Author (reference)	n	Angiographic success, %		6-Mo mortality/REMI		Event-free survival at 1 year, %		Target vessel revascularization	
		Stent	Balloon	Stent	Balloon	Stent	Balloon	Stent	Balloon
Zwolle (122)	452	98	96	3.0/1	9/7	95	80	4	17
Grami (123)	104	98	94	3.8/NA	15/NA	83	65	14	21
Fresco (124)	150	75	75	1.0/1.5	4/3	91	72	17	43
Stent-PAMI (125)	900	NA	NA	4.2/2.4	2.7/2.2	87	80	7.7	17
Stentim-2 (126)	211	86	83	2/4	1/5.5	81	72	17	27

GRAMI, Gianturco-Roubin in Acute Myocardial Infarction; NA, not applicable; PAMI, Primary Angioplasty in Myocardial Infarction.

TABLE 68–14. *Odds of adverse event at 6 to 12 months: stenting versus balloon for myocardial infarction*

| | Stent versus Balloon | | |
	Odds ratio	95% Confidence interval	p
Death	1.04	0.75–1.44	0.9
Reinfarction	0.71	0.47–1.08	0.13
Target vessel revascularization	0.43	0.36–0.52	< 0.001

From Zhu MM, Feit A, Chadow H, et al. Primary stent implantation compared with primary balloon angioplasty for acute myocardial infarction: a meta-analysis of randomized clinical trials. *Am J Cardiol* 2001;88;297–301

egy was reduced in both men and women to an almost equal rate (15.3% vs. 17.0%; *p* = not significant) (108). A prospective study of 1,450 consecutive unstable patients, who were followed for a mean of 20 months with respect to the occurrence of death or nonfatal MI, demonstrated that the long-term outcome after very early aggressive revascularization was better for women than for men (7.0% vs. 10.5%; *p* = 0.045) (117).

Thus, although the data about differences in long-term outcome between men and women are unclear, this should not dissuade one from performing PCI when clinically indicated in both men and women.

Place of Percutaneous Coronary Intervention in the Management of Unstable Coronary Artery Disease

Patients admitted to the hospital with unstable CAD (no persistent ST-segment elevation) should receive pharmacologic treatment to relief ischemia and to stabilize the unstable plaque (Fig. 68–6). The measurement of cardiac troponins plays an important role to distinguish unstable angina from a MI, to establish the prognosis (low vs. high risk according to European guidelines), and to guide treatment (institution of GPIIb/IIIa or early invasive strategy) (17,18).

In patients with low risk, a conservative, ischemia-driven strategy is recommended. These patients should undergo stress testing, preferably before discharge (118). Those patients with provocable ischemia should undergo coronary angioplasty with subsequent revascularization.

Patients at high risk are referred for early angioplasty and revascularization. If planned for PCI, they should receive GPIIb/IIIa before and during the procedure (119). PCI is indicated in one- or two-vessel disease and often includes stent implantation. Bypass surgery is indicated in left main and three-vessel disease. An attempt should be made to use arterial grafts.

In very elderly patients or in patients with concomitant severe comorbidity, catheter-based treatment of the ischemia-related lesion only may be preferred.

After stent implantation, a combined treatment of aspirin and thienopyridienes (ticlopidine or clopidogrel) is recommended to prevent the occurrence of subacute thrombotic occlusion.

Long-term treatment should include measures to prevent cardiac events. These must include lifestyle changes, in particular, cessation of smoking, aspirin, and cholesterol reduction (120).

Percutaneous Treatment of ST-Segment Elevation Myocardial Infarction

The rationale for primary coronary intervention is the immediate reopening of the included infarct vessel to preserve left ventricular myocardium, reduce infarct size, and thus reduce mortality and morbidity. It has been shown that primary balloon angioplasty is superior to thrombolytic treatment. In a metaanalysis, there was an absolute reduction of 2.1% in short-term mortality and an absolute reduction of 4.7% in short-term mortality and reinfarction (121). The occurrence of stroke was less in the primary percutaneous transluminal coronary angioplasty group than the thrombolytic group (0.8% vs. 2.0%). Primary stenting has further increased the efficacy of percutaneous catheter-based treatment by reducing the early and late reocclusion restenosis rate (122–126) (Table 68–13). A recent metaanalysis concerning 2,050 patients randomized to stenting and 2,070 randomized to balloon angioplasty revealed that mortality was similar for both techniques, but reinfarction and target vessel revascularization were less in stented patients (127) (Table 68–14). The role of adjunctive treatment with a platelet GPIIb/IIIa blockers is unclear. Three randomized trials addressed this issue, but the outcomes were conflicting (Table 68–15) (128–130).

The ReoPro and Primary PTCA Organization and Randomized Trial (RAPPORT) and Controlled Abciximab and

TABLE 68–15. *Abciximab and percutaneous coronary intervention for acute myocardial infarction: 6 months*

Trial (reference)	Re-MI abciximab	Placebo	TVR abciximab	Placebo	Composite abciximab	End point placebo
Rapport (129)	—	—	—	—	28%	28%
Admiral (128)	2.0%	4.0%	18%	24%	23%	34%
Cadillac (130)	0%	0%	7.5%	7.5%	11%	11%

Stenting versus stenting + abciximab.
ADMIRAL, Abciximab before Direct angioplasty and stenting in Myocardial Infarction Regarding Acute and Long-term follow-up; CADILLAC, Controlled Abciximab and Device Investigation to Lower Late Angioplasty Complications; RAPPORT, ReoPro and Primary PTCA Organization and Randomized Trial; TVR, target vessel revascularization.

TABLE 68–16. *Outcome of patients with early, immediate, and late presentation treated by primary coronary angioplasty or thrombolytic treatment*

Presentation	Primary angioplasty[a] (n = 1,302)	Thrombolytic therapy[a] (n = 1,333)
Early: <2 h	5.8%	12.5%
Intermediate: 2–4 h	8.6%	14.2%
Late: >4 h	7.7%	19.4%

[a]Primary end point: combined death, reinfarction, and stroke at 30 days.

Device Investigation to Lower Late Angioplasty Complications (CADILLAC) trials did not show any benefit, whereas the smaller Abciximab before Direct angioplasty and stenting in Myocardial Infarction Regarding Acute and Long-term follow-up (ADMIRAL) trial showed benefit of the adjunctive use of abciximab. There is clear evidence that early treatment, particularly within the first "golden" hour, results in a considerable mortality benefit. However, this seems particularly true for thrombolytic treatment but does not seem to be true for primary coronary angioplasty. Pooled data from 10 randomized trials of primary angioplasty (1,302 subjects) versus thrombolytic treatment (1,333 subjects) were analyzed (Table 68–16) (131). Primary angioplasty was associated with a consistently lower major adverse cardiac event rate, irrespective of time of presentation in patients with an AMI. Cardiogenic shock in the course of an AMI continues to be associated with an extremely high mortality and morbidity rate, even though primary intervention has decreased these rates compared with medical treatment. The 6- and 12-month mortality rate was less in the primary intervention group than in the medical group (50.3% vs. 63.1% and 55% vs. 70%, respectively) (132). The debate about treatment with thrombolysis or percutaneous catheter-based therapy is still continuing. It is generally accepted that primary intervention is superior, but the availability of such treatment is limited, the logistics to transport these acute patients to intervention facilities is complicated, and the financial costs involved are staggering.

Currently, it seems a reasonable approach to perform primary intervention in patients with access to a coronary intervention facility or in patients with a contraindication to thrombolytic treatment and to offer thrombolytic treatment to the remaining patients with an AMI.

REFERENCES

1. Gruntzig AR, Senning A, Siegenthaler WE. Nonoperative dilatation of coronary-artery stenosis: percutaneous transluminal coronary angioplasty. *N Engl J Med* 1979;301:61–68.
2. Bittl J. Medical progress: advances in coronary angioplasty. *N Engl J Med* 1996;335:1290–1302.
3. de Feyter PJ, Serruys PW, van den Brand M, et al. Emergency coronary angioplasty in refractory unstable angina. *N Engl J Med* 1985;313:342–346.
4. Fox KA, Cokkinos DV, Deckers J, et al. The ENACT study: a pan-European survey of acute coronary syndromes. European Network for Acute Coronary Treatment. *Eur Heart J* 2000;21:1440–1449.
5. Tunstall-Pedoe H, Kuulasmaa K, Mahonen M, et al. Contribution of trends in survival and coronary-event rates to changes in coronary heart disease mortality: 10-year results from 37 WHO MONICA Project populations. *Lancet* 1999;353:1547–1557.
6. Collinson J, Flather MD, Fox KA, et al. Clinical outcomes, risk stratification and practice patterns of unstable angina and myocardial infarction without ST elevation: Prospective Registry of Acute Ischaemic Syndromes in the UK (PRAIS-UK). *Eur Heart J* 2000;21:1450–1457.
7. Hasdai D, Behar S, Wallentin L, et al. A prospective survey of the characteristics, treatments and outcomes of patients with acute coronary syndromes in Europe and the Mediterranean basin. The Euro Heart Survey of Acute Coronary Syndromes (Euro Heart Survey ACS). *Eur Heart J* 2002;23:1190–1201.
8. Fox KA, Goodman SG, Klein W, et al. Management of acute coronary syndromes. Variations in practice and outcome. Findings from the Global Registry of Acute Coronary Events (GRACE). *Eur Heart J* 2002;23:1177–1189.
9. Maynard SJ, Scott GO, Riddell JW, et al. Management of acute coronary syndromes. *BMJ* 2000;321:220–223.
10. Davies MJ. Stability and instability: two faces of coronary atherosclerosis. The Paul Dudley White Lecture 1995. *Circulation* 1996;94:2013–2020.
11. Falk E, Shah PK, Fuster V. Coronary plaque disruption. *Circulation* 1995;92:657–671.
12. Fuster V, Lewis A. Conner Memorial Lecture. Mechanisms leading to myocardial infarction: insights from studies of vascular biology. *Circulation* 1994;90:2126–2146.
13. Ross R. Atherosclerosis—an inflammatory disease. *N Engl J Med* 1999;340:115–126.
14. Virmani R, Kolodgie FD, Burke AP, et al. Lessons from sudden coronary death: a comprehensive morphological classification scheme for atherosclerotic lesions. *Arterioscler Thromb Vasc Biol* 2000;20:1262–1275.
15. Libby P. Current concepts of the pathogenesis of the acute coronary syndromes. *Circulation* 2001;104:365–372.
16. van der Wal AC, Becker AE, van der Loos CM, et al. Site of intimal rupture or erosion of thrombosed coronary atherosclerotic plaques is characterized by an inflammatory process irrespective of the dominant plaque morphology. *Circulation* 1994;89:36–44.
17. Bertrand ME, Simoons ML, Fox KA, et al. Management of acute coronary syndromes: acute coronary syndromes without persistent ST segment elevation; recommendations of the Task Force of the European Society of Cardiology. *Eur Heart J* 2000;21:1406–1432.
18. Braunwald E, Antman EM, Beasley JW, et al. ACC/AHA guideline update for the management of patients with unstable angina and non-ST-segment elevation myocardial infarction—2002: summary article: a report of the American College of Cardiology/American Heart Association Task Force on Practice Guidelines (Committee on the Management of Patients With Unstable Angina). *Circulation* 2002;106:1893–1900.
19. Neill WA, Wharton TP Jr, Fluri-Lundeen J, et al. Acute coronary insufficiency—coronary occlusion after intermittent ischemic attacks. *N Engl J Med* 1980;302:1157–1162.
20. DeWood M, Spores J, Notske R, et al. Prevalence of total coronary occlusion during the early hours of transmural myocardial infarction. *N Engl J Med* 1980;303:897–902.
21. Rafflenbeul W, Smith LR, Rogers WJ, et al. Quantitative coronary arteriography. Coronary anatomy of patients with unstable angina pectoris reexamined 1 year after optimal medical therapy. *Am J Cardiol* 1979;43:699–707.
22. Moise A, Theroux P, Taeymans Y, et al. Unstable angina and progression of coronary atherosclerosis. *N Engl J Med* 1983;309:685–689.
23. Kaski JC, Chester MR, Chen L, et al. Rapid angiographic progression of coronary artery disease in patients with angina pectoris. The role of complex stenosis morphology. *Circulation* 1995;92:2058–2065.
24. Yokoya K, Takatsu H, Suzuki T, et al. Process of progression of coronary artery lesions from mild or moderate stenosis to moderate or severe stenosis: a study based on four serial coronary arteriograms per year. *Circulation* 1999;100:903–909.
25. Ojio S, Takatsu H, Tanaka T, et al. Considerable time from the onset of plaque rupture and/or thrombi until the onset of acute myo-

cardial infarction in humans: coronary angiographic findings within 1 week before the onset of infarction. *Circulation* 2000;102: 2063–2069.

26. Block PC, Myler RK, Stertzer S, et al. Morphology after transluminal angioplasty in human beings. *N Engl J Med* 1981;305:382–385.

27. Sigwart U, Puel J, Mirkovitch V, et al. Intravascular stents to prevent occlusion and restenosis after transluminal angioplasty. *N Engl J Med* 1987;316:701–706.

28. Kimmel SE, Localio AR, Krone RJ, et al. The effects of contemporary use of coronary stents on in-hospital mortality. Registry Committee of the Society for Cardiac Angiography and Interventions. *J Am Coll Cardiol* 2001;37:499–504.

29. Williams DO, Holubkov R, Yeh W, et al. Percutaneous coronary intervention in the current era compared with 1985-1986: the National Heart, Lung, and Blood Institute Registries. *Circulation* 2000;102: 2945–2951.

30. Windecker S, Meier B. Intervention in coronary artery disease. *Heart* 2000;83:481–190.

31. Mann JM, Davies MJ. Vulnerable plaque. Relation of characteristics to degree of stenosis in human coronary arteries. *Circulation* 1996;94:928–931.

32. Mann J, Davies MJ. Mechanisms of progression in native coronary artery disease: role of healed plaque disruption. *Heart* 1999;82:265–268.

33. Burke AP, Kolodgie FD, Farb A, et al. Healed plaque ruptures and sudden coronary death: evidence that subclinical rupture has a role in plaque progression. *Circulation* 2001;103:934–940.

34. Topol EJ, Yadav JS. Recognition of the importance of embolization in atherosclerotic vascular disease. *Circulation* 2000;101:570–580.

35. Lincoff AM, Califf RM, Topol EJ. Platelet glycoprotein IIb/IIIa receptor blockade in coronary artery disease. *J Am Coll Cardiol* 2000;35:1103–1115.

36. Bhatt DL, Topol EJ. Current role of platelet glycoprotein IIb/IIIa inhibitors in acute coronary syndromes. *JAMA* 2000;284:1549–1558.

37. A comparison of recombinant hirudin with heparin for the treatment of acute coronary syndromes. The Global Use of Strategies to Open Occluded Coronary Arteries (GUSTO) IIb investigators. *N Engl J Med* 1996;335:775–782.

38. Low-molecular-weight heparin during instability in coronary artery disease. Fragmin during Instability in Coronary Artery Disease (FRISC) study group. *Lancet* 1996;347:561–568.

39. Klein W, Buchwald A, Hillis SE, et al. Comparison of low-molecular-weight heparin with unfractionated heparin acutely and with placebo for 6 weeks in the management of unstable coronary artery disease. Fragmin in unstable coronary artery disease study (FRIC). *Circulation* 1997;96:61–68.

40. Cohen M, Demers C, Gurfinkel EP, et al. A comparison of low-molecular-weight heparin with unfractionated heparin for unstable coronary artery disease. Efficacy and Safety of Subcutaneous Enoxaparin in Non-Q-Wave Coronary Events Study Group. *N Engl J Med* 1997;337:447–452.

41. Inhibition of the platelet glycoprotein IIb/IIIa receptor with tirofiban in unstable angina and non-Q-wave myocardial infarction. Platelet Receptor Inhibition in Ischemic Syndrome Management in Patients Limited by Unstable Signs and Symptoms (PRISM-PLUS) Study Investigators. *N Engl J Med* 1998;338:1488–1497.

42. A comparison of aspirin plus tirofiban with aspirin plus heparin for unstable angina. Platelet Receptor Inhibition in Ischemic Syndrome Management Study Investigators. *N Engl J Med* 1998;338:1498–1505.

43. International, randomized, controlled trial of lamifiban (a platelet glycoprotein iib/iiia inhibitor), heparin, or both in unstable angina. The PARAGON Investigators. Platelet IIb/IIIa Antagonism for the Reduction of Acute coronary syndrome events in a Global Organization Network. *Circulation* 1998;97:2386–2395.

44. Inhibition of platelet glycoprotein IIb/IIIa with eptifibatide in patients with acute coronary syndromes. The PURSUIT Trial Investigators. Platelet Glycoprotein IIb/IIIa in Unstable Angina: Receptor Suppression Using Integrin Therapy. *N Engl J Med* 1998;339:436–443.

45. Invasive compared with non-invasive treatment in unstable coronary-artery disease: FRISC II prospective randomised multicentre study. FRagmin and Fast Revascularisation during InStability in Coronary artery disease Investigators. *Lancet* 1999;354:708–715.

46. Effects of recombinant hirudin (lepirudin) compared with heparin on death, myocardial infarction, refractory angina, and revascularisation procedures in patients with acute myocardial ischaemia without ST elevation: a randomised trial. Organisation to Assess Strategies for Ischemia Syndromes (OASIS-2) Investigators. *Lancet* 1999;353:429–438.

47. Braunwald E. Unstable angina. A classification. *Circulation* 1989; 80:410–414.

48. Ahmed WH, Bittl JA, Braunwald E. Relation between clinical presentation and angiographic findings in unstable angina pectoris, and comparison with that in stable angina. *Am J Cardiol* 1993;72:544–550.

49. Depre C, Wijns W, Robert AM, et al. Pathology of unstable plaque: correlation with the clinical severity of acute coronary syndromes. *J Am Coll Cardiol* 1997;30:694–702.

50. van Miltenburg-van Zijl AJ, Simoons ML, Veerhoek RJ, et al. Incidence and follow-up of Braunwald subgroups in unstable angina pectoris. *J Am Coll Cardiol* 1995;25:1286–1292.

51. Calvin JE, Klein LW, VandenBerg BJ, et al. Risk stratification in unstable angina. Prospective validation of the Braunwald classification. *JAMA* 1995;273:136–141.

52. Hamm CW, Braunwald E. A classification of unstable angina revisited. *Circulation* 2000;102:118–122.

53. Armstrong PW, Fu Y, Chang WC, et al. Acute coronary syndromes in the GUSTO-IIb trial: prognostic insights and impact of recurrent ischemia. The GUSTO-IIb Investigators. *Circulation* 1998;98:1860–1868.

54. Savonitto S, Ardissino D, Granger CB, et al. Prognostic value of the admission electrocardiogram in acute coronary syndromes. *JAMA* 1999;281:707–713.

55. Topol E. Patient stratification and its predictive value for cardiac events. *Eur Heart J* 1998;19[Suppl K]:K5–K7.

56. Lindahl B, Venge P, Wallentin L. Relation between troponin T and the risk of subsequent cardiac events in unstable coronary artery disease. The FRISC study group. *Circulation* 1996;93:1651–1657.

57. Ohman EM, Armstrong PW, Christenson RH, et al. Cardiac troponin T levels for risk stratification in acute myocardial ischemia. GUSTO IIA Investigators. *N Engl J Med* 1996;335:1333–1341.

58. Antman EM, Tanasijevic MJ, Thompson B, et al. Cardiac-specific troponin I levels to predict the risk of mortality in patients with acute coronary syndromes. *N Engl J Med* 1996;335:1342–1349.

59. Hamm CW, Goldmann BU, Heeschen C, et al. Emergency room triage of patients with acute chest pain by means of rapid testing for cardiac troponin T or troponin I. *N Engl J Med* 1997;337:1648–1653.

60. Holmvang L, Luscher MS, Clemmensen P, et al. Very early risk stratification using combined ECG and biochemical assessment in patients with unstable coronary artery disease (a thrombin inhibition in myocardial ischemia [TRIM] substudy). The TRIM Study Group. *Circulation* 1998;98:2004–2009.

61. Newby LK, Christenson RH, Ohman EM, et al. Value of serial troponin T measures for early and late risk stratification in patients with acute coronary syndromes. The GUSTO-IIa Investigators. *Circulation* 1998;98:1853–1859.

62. Lindahl B, Toss H, Siegbahn A, et al. Markers of myocardial damage and inflammation in relation to long-term mortality in unstable coronary artery disease. FRISC Study Group. Fragmin during Instability in Coronary Artery Disease. *N Engl J Med* 2000;343:1139–1147.

63. de Winter RJ, Bholasingh R, Lijmer JG, et al. Independent prognostic value of C-reactive protein and troponin I in patients with unstable angina or non-Q-wave myocardial infarction. *Cardiovasc Res* 1999;42: 240–245.

64. Lagrand WK, Visser CA, Hermens WT, et al. C-reactive protein as a cardiovascular risk factor: more than an epiphenomenon? *Circulation* 1999;100:96–102.

65. Toss H, Lindahl B, Siegbahn A, et al. Prognostic influence of increased fibrinogen and C-reactive protein levels in unstable coronary artery disease. FRISC Study Group. Fragmin during Instability in Coronary Artery Disease. *Circulation* 1997;96:4204–4210.

66. de Lemos JA, Morrow DA, Bentley JH, et al. The prognostic value of B-type natriuretic peptide in patients with acute coronary syndromes. *N Engl J Med* 2001;345:1014–1021.

67. Sabatine MS, Morrow DA, de Lemos JA, et al. Multimarker approach to risk stratification in non-ST elevation acute coronary syndromes: simultaneous assessment of troponin I, C-reactive protein, and B-type natriuretic peptide. *Circulation* 2002;105:1760–1763.

68. Antman EM, Cohen M, Bernink PJ, et al. The TIMI risk score for unstable angina/non-ST elevation MI: a method for prognostication and therapeutic decision making. *JAMA* 2000;284:835–842.

69. de Feyter PJ, Suryapranata H, Serruys PW, et al. Coronary angioplasty for unstable angina: immediate and late results in 200 consecutive patients with identification of risk factors for unfavorable early and late outcome. *J Am Coll Cardiol* 1988;12:324–333.

70. de Feyter PJ, Serruys PW, Soward A, et al. Coronary angioplasty for early postinfarction unstable angina. *Circulation* 1986;74:1365–1370.

71. Holmes DR Jr, Holubkov R, Vlietstra RE, et al. Comparison of complications during percutaneous transluminal coronary angioplasty from 1977 to 1981 and from 1985 to 1986: the National Heart, Lung, and Blood Institute Percutaneous Transluminal Coronary Angioplasty Registry. *J Am Coll Cardiol* 1988;12:1149–1155.

72. Bentivoglio LG, Detre K, Yeh W, et al. Outcome of percutaneous transluminal coronary angioplasty in subsets of unstable angina pectoris. A report of the 1985-1986 National Heart, Lung, and Blood Institute Percutaneous Transluminal Coronary Angioplasty Registry. *J Am Coll Cardiol* 1994;24:1195–1206.

73. Singh M, Rihal CS, Berger PB, et al. Improving outcome over time of percutaneous coronary interventions in unstable angina. *J Am Coll Cardiol* 2000;36:674–678.

74. Use of a Monoclonal antibody directed against the platelet glycoprotein IIb/IIIa receptor in high-risk coronary angioplasty. The EPIC Invesigation. *N Engl J Med* 1994;330:956–961.

75. Platelet glycoprotein IIb/IIIa receptor blockade and low-dose heparin during percutaneous coronary revascularization. The EPILOG Investigators. *N Engl J Med* 1997;336:1689–1697.

76. Effects of platelet glycoprotein IIB/IIIa blockade with tirofiban on adverse cardiac events in patients with unstable angina or acute myocardial infarction undergoing coronary angioplasty. The RESTORE Investigators. Randomized Efficacy Study of Tirofiban for Outcomes and REstenosis. *Circulation* 1997;96:1445–1453.

77. Randomised placebo-controlled trial of abciximab before and during coronary intervention in refractory unstable angina: the CAPTURE Study. *Lancet* 1997;349:1429–1435.

78. Lincoff AM, Califf RM, Anderson KM, et al. Evidence for prevention of death and myocardial infarction with platelet membrane glycoprotein IIb/IIIa receptor blockade by abciximab (c7E3 Fab) among patients with unstable angina undergoing percutaneous coronary revascularization. EPIC Investigators. Evaluation of 7E3 in Preventing Ischemic Complications. *J Am Coll Cardiol* 1997;30:149–156.

79. Hamm CW, Heeschen C, Goldmann B, et al. Benefit of abciximab in patients with refractory unstable angina in relation to serum troponin T levels. c7E3 Fab Antiplatelet Therapy in Unstable Refractory Angina (CAPTURE) Study Investigators. *N Engl J Med* 1999;340:1623–1629.

80. Heeschen C, Hamm CW, Goldmann B, et al. Troponin concentrations for stratification of patients with acute coronary syndromes in relation to therapeutic efficacy of tirofiban. PRISM Study Investigators. Platelet Receptor Inhibition in Ischemic Syndrome Management. *Lancet* 1999;354:1757–1762.

81. Newby LK, Ohman EM, Christenson RH, et al. Benefit of glycoprotein IIb/IIIa inhibition in patients with acute coronary syndromes and troponin t-positive status: the paragon-B troponin T substudy. *Circulation* 2001;103:2891–2896.

82. Morrow DA, Antman EM, Tanasijevic M, et al. Cardiac troponin I for stratification of early outcomes and the efficacy of enoxaparin in unstable angina: a TIMI-11B substudy. *J Am Coll Cardiol* 2000;36:1812–1817.

83. Kip KE, Faxon DP, Detre KM, et al. Coronary angioplasty in diabetic patients. The National Heart, Lung, and Blood Institute Percutaneous Transluminal Coronary Angioplasty Registry. *Circulation* 1996;94:1818–1825.

84. Robinson NM, Thomas MR, Wainwright RJ, et al. Is unstable angina a contraindication to intracoronary stent insertion? *J Invasive Cardiol* 1996;8:351–356.

85. Marzocchi A, Piovaccari G, Marrozzini C, et al. Results of coronary stenting for unstable versus stable angina pectoris. *Am J Cardiol* 1997;79:1314–1318.

86. Chauhan A, Vu E, Ricci DR, et al. Multiple coronary stenting in unstable angina: early and late clinical outcomes. *Cathet Cardiovasc Diagn* 1998;43:11–16.

87. Alfonso F, Rodriguez P, Phillips P, et al. Clinical and angiographic implications of coronary stenting in thrombus-containing lesions. *J Am Coll Cardiol* 1997;29:725–733.

88. Madan M, Marquis JF, de May MR, et al. Coronary stenting in unstable angina: early and late clinical outcomes. *Can J Cardiol* 1998;14:1109–1114.

89. Kornowski R, Hong MK, Saucedo J, et al. Procedural results and long-term clinical outcomes following coronary stenting in perimyocardial infarction syndromes. *Am J Cardiol* 1998;82:1163–1167.

90. Schömig A, Neumann FJ, Kastrati A, et al. A randomized comparison of antiplatelet and anticoagulant therapy after the placement of coronary-artery stents. *N Engl J Med* 1996;334:1084–1089.

91. Leon MB, Baim DS, Popma JJ, et al. A clinical trial comparing three antithrombotic-drug regimens after coronary-artery stenting. Stent Anticoagulation Restenosis Study Investigators. *N Engl J Med* 1998;339:1665–1671.

92. Bertrand ME, Legrand V, Boland J, et al. Randomized multicenter comparison of conventional anticoagulation versus antiplatelet therapy in unplanned and elective coronary stenting. The full anticoagulation versus aspirin and ticlopidine (fantastic) study. *Circulation* 1998;98:1597–1603.

93. Urban P, Macaya C, Rupprecht HJ, et al. Randomized evaluation of anticoagulation versus antiplatelet therapy after coronary stent implantation in high-risk patients: the multicenter aspirin and ticlopidine trial after intracoronary stenting (MATTIS). *Circulation* 1998;98:2126–2132.

94. Cutlip DE, Baim DS, Ho KK, et al. Stent thrombosis in the modern era: a pooled analysis of multicenter coronary stent clinical trials. *Circulation* 2001;103:1967–1971.

95. Bertrand ME, Rupprecht HJ, Urban P, et al. Double-blind study of the safety of clopidogrel with and without a loading dose in combination with aspirin compared with ticlopidine in combination with aspirin after coronary stenting: the clopidogrel aspirin stent international cooperative study (CLASSICS). *Circulation* 2000;102:624–629.

96. Serruys PW, van Hout B, Bonnier H, et al. Randomised comparison of implantation of heparin-coated stents with balloon angioplasty in selected patients with coronary artery disease (Benestent II). *Lancet* 1998;352:673–681.

97. Randomised placebo-controlled and balloon-angioplasty-controlled trial to assess safety of coronary stenting with use of platelet glycoprotein-IIb/IIIa blockade. The EPISTENT Investigators. Evaluation of Platelet IIb/IIIa Inhibitor for Stenting. *Lancet* 1998;352:87–92.

98. ESPRIT Investigators. Enhanced Suppression of the Platelet IIb/IIIa Receptor with Integrilin Therapy. Novel dosing regimen of eptifibatide in planned coronary stent implantation (ESPRIT): a randomised, placebo-controlled trial. *Lancet* 2000;356:2037–2044.

99. Lincoff AM, Califf RM, Moliterno DJ, et al. Complementary clinical benefits of coronary-artery stenting and blockade of platelet glycoprotein IIb/IIIa receptors. Evaluation of Platelet IIb/IIIa Inhibition in Stenting Investigators. *N Engl J Med* 1999;341:319–327.

100. Lindahl B, Diderholm E, Lagerqvist B, et al. Mechanisms behind the prognostic value of troponin T in unstable coronary artery disease: a FRISC II substudy. *J Am Coll Cardiol* 2001;38:979–986.

101. Lindahl B, Venge P, Wallentin L. Troponin T identifies patients with unstable coronary artery disease who benefit from long-term antithrombotic protection. Fragmin in Unstable Coronary Artery Disease (FRISC) Study Group. *J Am Coll Cardiol* 1997;29:43–48.

102. Morrow DA, Cannon CP, Rifai N, et al. Ability of minor elevations of troponins I and T to predict benefit from an early invasive strategy in patients with unstable angina and non-ST elevation myocardial infarction: results from a randomized trial. *JAMA* 2001;286:2405–2412.

103. Antman EM. Troponin measurements in ischemic heart disease: more than just a black and white picture. *J Am Coll Cardiol* 2001;38:987–990.

104. Effects of tissue plasminogen activator and a comparison of early invasive and conservative strategies in unstable angina and non-Q-wave myocardial infarction. Results of the TIMI IIIB Trial. Thrombolysis in Myocardial Ischemia. *Circulation* 1994;89:1545–1556.

105. Boden WE, O'Rourke RA, Crawford MH, et al. Outcomes in patients with acute non-Q-wave myocardial infarction randomly assigned to an invasive as compared with a conservative management strategy. Veterans Affairs Non-Q-Wave Infarction Strategies in Hospital (VANQWISH) Trial Investigators. *N Engl J Med* 1998;338:1785–1792.

106. McCullough P, O'Neill WW, Graham M, et al. A prospective randomized trial of triage angiography in acute coronary syndromes ineligible for thrombolytic therapy. Results of the medicine versus angiography in thrombolytic exclusion (MATE) trial. *J Am Coll Cardiol* 1998;32:596–605.

107. Wallentin L, Lagerqvist B, Husted S, et al. Outcome at 1 year after an invasive compared with a non-invasive strategy in unstable coronary-

artery disease: the FRISC II invasive randomised trial. FRISC II Investigators. Fast Revascularisation during Instability in Coronary artery disease. *Lancet* 2000;356:9–16.

108. Cannon CP, Weintraub WS, Demopoulos LA, et al. Comparison of early invasive and conservative strategies in patients with unstable coronary syndromes treated with the glycoprotein IIb/IIIa inhibitor tirofiban. *N Engl J Med* 2001;344:1879–1887.

109. Spacek R, Widimsky P, Straka Z, et al. Value of first day angiography/angioplasty in evolving non-ST segment elevation myocardial infarction: an open multicenter randomized trial. The VINO Study. *Eur Heart J* 2002;23:230–238.

110. Solomon DH, Stone PH, Glynn RJ, et al. Use of risk stratification to identify patients with unstable angina likeliest to benefit from an invasive versus conservative management strategy. *J Am Coll Cardiol* 2001;38:969–976.

111. Diderholm E, Andren B, Frostfeldt G, et al. ST depression in ECG at entry indicates severe coronary lesions and large benefits of an early invasive treatment strategy in unstable coronary artery disease, the FRISC II ECG substudy. The Fast Revascularisation during InStability in Coronary artery disease. *Eur Heart J* 2002;23:41–49.

112. de Feyter PJ, Serruys PW, Unger F, et al. Bypass surgery versus stenting for the treatment of multivessel disease in patients with unstable angina compared with stable angina. *Circulation* 2002;105:2367–2372.

113. Rupprecht HJ, Brennecke R, Kottmeyer M, et al. Short- and long-term outcome after PTCA in patients with stable and unstable angina. *Eur Heart J* 1990;11:964–973.

114. Ruygrok PN, de Jaegere PT, van Domburg RT, et al. Clinical outcome 10 years after attempted percutaneous transluminal coronary angioplasty in 856 patients. *J Am Coll Cardiol* 1996;27:1669–1677.

115. Keelan ET, Nunez BD, Grill DE, et al. Comparison of immediate and long-term outcome of coronary angioplasty performed for unstable angina and rest pain in men and women. *Mayo Clin Proc* 1997;72:5–12.

116. Lagerqvist B, Safstrom K, Stahle E, et al. Is early invasive treatment of unstable coronary artery disease equally effective for both women and men? FRISC II Study Group Investigators. *J Am Coll Cardiol* 2001;38:41–48.

117. Mueller C, Neumann FJ, Roskamm H, et al. Women do have an improved long-term outcome after non-ST-elevation acute coronary syndromes treated very early and predominantly with percutaneous coronary intervention: a prospective study in 1,450 consecutive patients. *J Am Coll Cardiol* 2002;40:245–250.

118. Coplan NL, Wallach ID. The role of exercise testing for evaluating patients with unstable angina. *Am Heart J* 1992;124:252–256.

119. Boersma E, Akkerhuis KM, Theroux P, et al. Platelet glycoprotein IIb/IIIa receptor inhibition in non-ST-elevation acute coronary syndromes: early benefit during medical treatment only, with additional protection during percutaneous coronary intervention. *Circulation* 1999;100:2045–2048.

120. Serruys PW, de Feyter P, Macaya C, et al. Fluvastatin for prevention of cardiac events following successful first percutaneous coronary intervention: a randomized controlled trial. *JAMA* 2002;287:3215–3222.

121. Weaver WD, Simes RJ, Betriu A, et al. Comparison of primary coronary angioplasty and intravenous thrombolytic therapy for acute myocardial infarction: a quantitative review. *JAMA* 1997;278:2093–2098.

122. Suryapranata H, van't Hof AW, Hoorntje JC, et al. Randomized comparison of coronary stenting with balloon angioplasty in selected patients with acute myocardial infarction. *Circulation* 1998;97:2502–2505.

123. Rodriguez A, Bernardi V, Fernandez M, et al. In-hospital and late results of coronary stents versus conventional balloon angioplasty in acute myocardial infarction (GRAMI trial). Gianturco-Roubin in Acute Myocardial Infarction. *Am J Cardiol* 1998;81:1286–1291.

124. Antoniucci D, Santoro GM, Bolognese L, et al. A clinical trial comparing primary stenting of the infarct-related artery with optimal primary angioplasty for acute myocardial infarction: results from the Florence Randomized Elective Stenting in Acute Coronary Occlusions (FRESCO) trial. *J Am Coll Cardiol* 1998;31:1234–1239.

125. Grines CL, Cox DA, Stone GW, et al. Coronary angioplasty with or without stent implantation for acute myocardial infarction. Stent Primary Angioplasty in Myocardial Infarction Study Group. *N Engl J Med* 1999;341:1949–1956.

126. Maillard L, Hamon M, Khalife K, et al. A comparison of systematic stenting and conventional balloon angioplasty during primary percutaneous transluminal coronary angioplasty for acute myocardial infarction. STENTIM-2 Investigators. *J Am Coll Cardiol* 2000;35:1729–1736.

127. Zhu MM, Feit A, Chadow H, et al. Primary stent implantation compared with primary balloon angioplasty for acute myocardial infarction: a meta-analysis of randomized clinical trials. *Am J Cardiol* 2001;88:297–301.

128. Brener SJ, Barr LA, Burchenal JE, et al. Randomized, placebo-controlled trial of platelet glycoprotein IIb/IIIa blockade with primary angioplasty for acute myocardial infarction. ReoPro and Primary PTCA Organization and Randomized Trial (RAPPORT) Investigators. *Circulation* 1998;98:734–741.

129. Montalescot G, Barragan P, Wittenberg O, et al. Platelet glycoprotein IIb/IIIa inhibition with coronary stenting for acute myocardial infarction. *N Engl J Med* 2001;344:1895–1903.

130. Stone GW, Grines CL, Cox DA, et al. Comparison of angioplasty with stenting, with or without abciximab, in acute myocardial infarction. *N Engl J Med* 2002;346:957–966.

131. Zijlstra F, Patel A, Jones M, et al. Clinical characteristics and outcome of patients with early (<2 h), intermediate (2–4 h) and late (>4 h) presentation treated by primary coronary angioplasty or thrombolytic therapy for acute myocardial infarction. *Eur Heart J* 2002;23:550–557.

132. Hochman JS, Sleeper LA, White HD, et al. One-year survival following early revascularization for cardiogenic shock. *JAMA* 2001;285:190–192.

CHAPTER 69

Antithrombotics During the Acute Phase

W. Lane Duvall and David A. Vorchheimer

Key Words: Antiplatelet therapy; antithrombotic therapy; fibrinolytic therapy; myocardial infarction; percutaneous coronary intervention.

INTRODUCTION

Numerous alternatives for reperfusion therapy and concurrent antithrombotic therapy currently exist. Decisions regarding reperfusion therapy are based on the clinical presentation of the acute coronary syndrome (ACS), ST-segment elevation myocardial infarction (STEMI) versus non–STEMIs, availability of resources such as catheterization laboratories, and patient characteristics. The concurrent antithrombotic regimen is then guided by the reperfusion strategy used.

ST-SEGMENT ELEVATION MYOCARDIAL INFARCTION

Aspirin

Multiple clinical trials over the last fifteen years have established aspirin as one of the most cost-effective therapies for acute myocardial infarction (AMI). Aspirin exerts its an-

tiplatelet effect by irreversibly acetylating the enzyme cyclooxygenase, thereby inhibiting the production of thromboxane A_2, a potent promoter of platelet aggregation. Aspirin as antiplatelet therapy has been shown to reduce both reinfarction and mortality during MI.

The Second International Study of Infarct Survival (ISIS-2) trial was the definitive study responsible for establishing the efficacy of aspirin in reducing cardiovascular events during and immediately after AMI (1). More than 17,000 patients were randomized to receive either aspirin (160 mg/d for 1 month) or placebo, and at 5 weeks, vascular mortality was reduced by 23% ($p < 0.0001$), stroke by 36%, and reinfarction by 44% in the patients treated with aspirin. The study found no differences in the rates of major bleeding or cerebral hemorrhage between the two groups. Aspirin was effective at all time points studied in the trial: when given in the first 4 hours after MI (mortality reduction 25%), after the 12 hours (mortality reduction 21%), or after 12 to 24 hours (mortality reduction 21%).

The Antithrombotic Trialists' Collaboration reviewed 15 trials of 19,288 patients with suspected AMI, nearly all of whom were in the ISIS-2 trial (2). Treatment with antiplatelet therapy, mostly 160 mg aspirin daily, for mean of duration of 1 month resulted in 38 less serious vascular events, 13 less reinfarctions ($p < 0.0001$), 23 less vascular deaths ($p < 0.0001$), and 2 fewer strokes ($p = 0.02$) per 1,000 patients treated. These benefits were far in excess of the risk for major extracranial bleeds, which was estimated to be about 1 to 2 additional bleeds per 1,000 patients treated with aspirin.

W. L. Duvall: Mount Sinai Medical Center, The Zena and Michael A. Wiener Cardiovascular Institute, One Gustave L. Levy Place, Box 1030, New York, New York 10029.

D. A. Vorchheimer: Mount Sinai Medical Center, The Zena and Michael A. Wiener Cardiovascular Institute, One Gustave L. Levy Place, Box 1030, New York, New York 10029.

Antithrombotic Therapy in Conjunction with Fibrinolytic Therapy

Antiplatelet Agents

Aspirin

The ISIS-2 trial also examined the combination of aspirin and fibrinolytics (streptokinase) in more than 17,000 patients (1). The 5-week vascular mortality rate was reduced by 23% by aspirin alone, by 25% in those treated with streptokinase alone, and by 42% in those treated with aspirin and streptokinase.

Combination of Glycoprotein IIb/IIIa and Fibrinolytic

Treatment directed at both the thrombus with a fibrinolytic agent and the platelet aggregate with a glycoprotein (GP) IIb/IIIa inhibitor might achieve more rapid, more complete, and more sustained coronary reperfusion.

Several dose-ranging patency pilot studies established the prospect of improved outcomes with abciximab combination therapy. The Strategies for Patency Enhancement in the Emergency Department (SPEED) (3) enrolled 530 patients and the Thrombolysis in Myocardial Infarction (TIMI) 14 trial (4) evaluated 888 patients with STEMI. In the two trials, regimens of abciximab alone, abciximab plus various doses of reteplase, standard-dose reteplase, accelerated-dose alteplase, or abciximab plus reduced doses of alteplase or streptokinase were all studied. In SPEED, TIMI 3 flow at 90 minutes was significantly improved with the best combination of abciximab, reteplase, and heparin over controls (61% combination vs. 47% reteplase vs. 27% abciximab). In TIMI 14, the most promising regimen involved reduced-dose alteplase plus abciximab, which resulted in TIMI 3 flow at 90 minutes in 77% of subjects. There was no significant increase in hemorrhagic complications in the combined therapy group. These pilot studies were not powered to detect differences in clinical outcomes, but on the basis of data from Global Use of Strategies To Open Occluded Coronary Arteries (GUSTO) I, a 23% improvement in TIMI 3 flow at 90 minutes would be associated with a 1% decrease in mortality (5,6).

The GUSTO V trial enrolled 16,588 patients with STEMI of less than 6 hours in duration and randomly assigned them to either standard-dose reteplase or half-dose reteplase plus full-dose abciximab (7). At 30 days, the reteplase plus abciximab arm had a nonsignificant 0.3% absolute (5.9% vs. 5.6%) and 5% relative reduction in the primary end point of mortality and nonsignificant reductions in most secondary end points. The secondary end point that did reach statistical significance was a 34% reduction (2.3% vs. 3.5%; $p < 0.0001$) in reinfarction at 7 days. This benefit was achieved at a cost of statistically significant increases in mild and severe bleeding (overall 13.7% vs. 24.6%) and blood transfusions in the combination group (Fig. 69–1). Although there was no difference in mortality between the two treatment

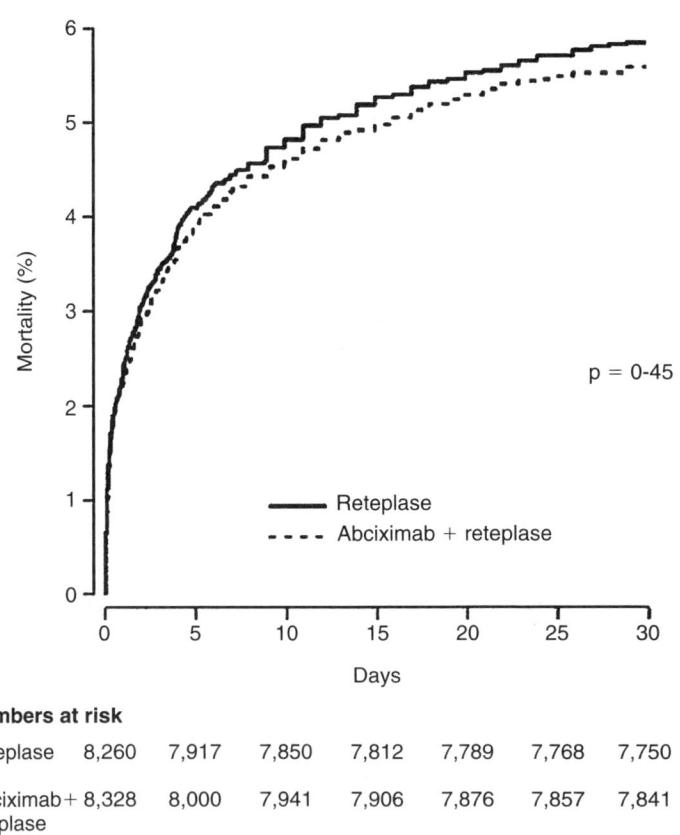

Numbers at risk

Reteplase	8,260	7,917	7,850	7,812	7,789	7,768	7,750
Abiciximab+ reteplase	8,328	8,000	7,941	7,906	7,876	7,857	7,841

FIG. 69–1. Kaplan-Meier mortality curves at 30 days for reteplase versus abciximab plus half-dose reteplase in the Global Use of Strategies To Open Occluded Coronary Arteries (GUSTO) V trial (7).

groups at 1 year of follow up, patients who experienced re-infarction had a significant increase in 1-year mortality (22.6% vs. 8.0%; $p < 0.001$) (8).

The Assessment of the Safety and Efficacy of a New Thrombolytic Regimen (ASSENT)-3 trial examined abciximab in combination with another fibrinolytic agent, tenecteplase (9). The study randomized 4,065 patients with STEMI of less than 6 hours duration to either standard-dose tenecteplase or half-dose tenecteplase plus abciximab. The half-dose tenecteplase plus abciximab group was found to have a 28% reduction in the primary end point (a composite of death, in-hospital reinfarction, or in-hospital refractory ischemia at 30 days) compared with the standard-dose group (11.1% vs. 15.4%; $p = 0.0001$). The majority of the benefit was derived from a reduction in reinfarction and refractory ischemia because there was no statistically significant difference in mortality. Although there were no differences in the rate of intracranial hemorrhages, there was a significant increase in the rate of major bleeding in the abciximab arm (4.4% vs. 2.2%; $p = 0.0005$) (Fig. 69–2).

The small molecule GPIIb/IIIa inhibitor eptifibatide has been studied in conjunction with fibrinolytics in somewhat less detail than abciximab. The Integrilin to Minimize Platelet Aggregation and Prevent Coronary Thrombosis in Acute Myocardial Infarction (IMPACT-AMI) trial (10) and the Integrilin and Low-Dose Thrombolysis in Acute Myocardial Infarction (INTRO-AMI) trial (11) studied 180 patients and 649 patients, respectively, with STEMI of less than 6 hours in duration. The most promising dose combinations in both studies demonstrated significantly increased rates of TIMI 3 flow at 60 or 90 minutes with the tissue plasminogen activator (t-PA) plus eptifibatide compared with

t-PA alone (66% vs. 39%, $p = 0.006$ for IMPACT-AMI; and 56% vs. 40%, $p = 0.04$ for INTRO-AMI). There was no statistically significant increase in major bleeding with combination therapy in either study. In contrast, another dose-ranging study with streptokinase of 181 patients by Ronner and coworkers (12) showed no statistically significant improvement in TIMI 3 flow at 90 minutes, and there was a significant increase in major and minor bleeding and transfusion requirements with eptifibatide.

The currently unpublished Integrilin and Tenecteplase in Acute Myocardial Infarction (INTEGRITI) trial studied the effects of reduced-dose tenecteplase for the treatment of acute STEMI in 350 patients. INTEGRITI is the first trial of eptifibatide combined with fibrinolytics with clinical end points. This study showed that combination therapy improved ST-segment recovery, TIMI flow, and TIMI frame count compared with fibrinolytic alone (13–16).

Lamifiban, another small-molecule GPIIb/IIIa inhibitor, has only been studied in conjunction with fibrinolytics in a single small dose–ranging study. Lamifiban was evaluated in 353 subjects with STEMIs treated with streptokinase or t-PA in the Platelet Aggregation Receptor Antagonist Dose Investigation and Reperfusion Gain in Myocardial Infarction (PARADIGM) trial (17). Although the study was not powered to detect clinical differences between the groups, it did demonstrate improvement in the speed and stability of ST-segment resolution as measured by continuous electrocardiographic (ECG) monitoring, but at the cost of an increase in major bleeding episodes.

Recommendations. Currently, the role of GPIIb/IIIa inhibitors in conjunction with reduced-dose fibrinolytics is being studied, but recent trials demonstrate certain reproducible

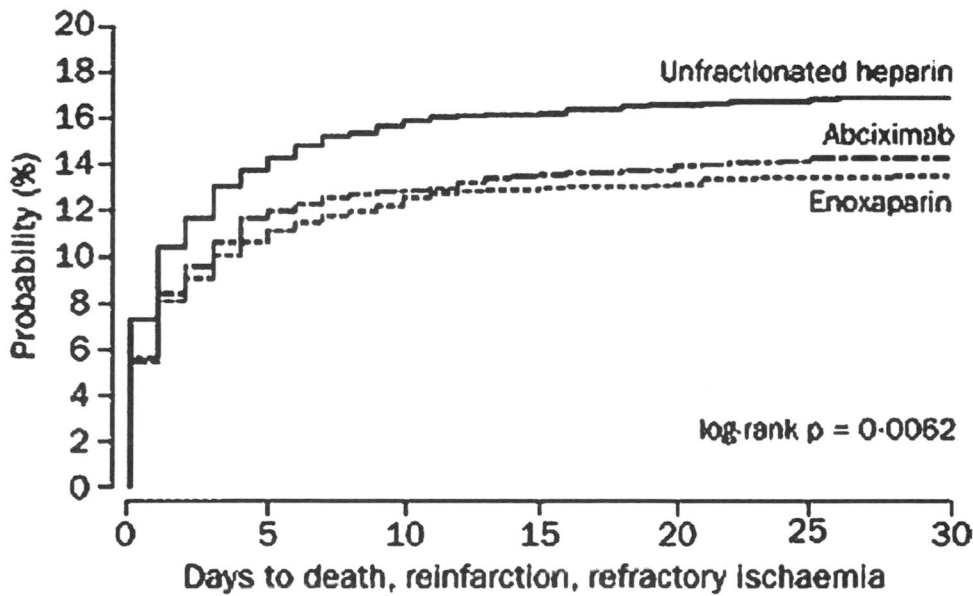

FIG. 69–2. Kaplan-Meier efficacy plus safety curves at 30 days for tenecteplase plus unfractionated heparin, enoxaparin, or abciximab in the Assessment of the Safety and Efficacy of a New Thrombolytic Regimen (ASSENT)-3 trial (9).

findings. Combination therapy consistently results in less re-infarction without corresponding reductions in mortality, but at the expense of increased bleeding. Future studies will need to address the issues of why decreased rates of reinfarction do not translate into decreased mortality, why there appears to be a difference in efficacy with the fibrinolytic agent used, and how to use this combination in an aging population who is at increased risk for bleeding complications. Whether this reperfusion strategy will play a role in the future without being incorporated into a facilitated percutaneous intervention framework remains to be seen.

Antithrombin Therapy

Unfractionated Heparin

Unfractionated heparin consists of a heterogeneous mixture of glycosaminoglycans with molecular weights ranging from approximately 3,000 to 30,000 and only about one-third of these molecules are active anticoagulants (18). Heparin functions as an anticoagulant by interacting with antithrombin III, thereby increasing its ability to bind to and neutralize thrombin and other activated clotting factors. However, thrombin that is already fibrin bound is relatively protected from inactivation by heparin.

Although the ISIS-2 trial was designed to study the benefits of aspirin and fibrinolytic in the setting of STEMI, the protocol did not mandate or specify the use of heparin. As such, approximately two-thirds of patients received some form of heparin in a nonrandomized manor in addition to aspirin and streptokinase, which resulted in a 5-week mortality rate of 9.8% in those who received no heparin, 7.6% in those treated who received subcutaneous heparin, and 6.4% in those who received intravenous heparin (1).

The large-scale Gruppo Italiano per lo Studio della Sopravvivenza nell'Infarto Miocardico (GISSI)-2/International t-PA versus Streptokinase Mortality Trial (19,20) with 20,891 patients and the ISIS-3 trial (21) with 41,299 subjects were designed to specifically address the issue of the coadministration of heparin with fibrinolytics. Both trials used fibrinolytic and subcutaneous heparin at a dose of 12,500 U every 12 hours, and a pooled analysis of these two studies showed a mortality rate at 35 days of 10.6% without heparin and 10.2% with heparin (21). There was, however, a slight but significant decrease in mortality in GISSI-2 and in reinfarction in ISIS-3 to fuel further study. The overall failure to find significant benefit from heparin was thought to be because of subtherapeutic anticoagulation caused by suboptimal heparin regimens. The dose administered in the trials was relatively conservative; the subcutaneous route resulted in delayed onset of therapeutic effect and was initiated relatively late (4 hours in ISIS-3 and 12 hours in GISSI-2/International t-PA versus Streptokinase Mortality Trial).

The GUSTO I trial was partially designed to answer the question regarding subcutaneous heparin, intravenous heparin, or neither in conjunction with fibrinolytics (5). Of the

41,021 patients enrolled in GUSTO I, 20,251 were randomized to streptokinase plus aspirin with either subcutaneous heparin (12,500 U twice daily starting 4 hours after the start of fibrinolytics) or intravenous heparin (5,000 U followed by 1,000 U/h started immediately). The 30-day mortality rate and rate of disabling stroke were 7.2% and 0.5% with subcutaneous heparin and 7.4% and 0.5%, respectively, with intravenous heparin (p = not significant [NS]). All 10,396 patients receiving t-PA and aspirin were treated with intravenous heparin and had a 30-day mortality rate and rate of disabling stroke of 6.3% and 0.6%, respectively. This study found that there was no benefit of intravenous heparin over subcutaneous heparin when streptokinase and aspirin were used and that there was even a trend toward increased bleeding with intravenous heparin.

Two overviews attempted to pool data from multiple studies to clarify the role of heparin in AMI treated with fibrinolytics. Mahaffey and coworkers (22) analyzed 6 randomized trials of 1,735 patients receiving intravenous heparin versus placebo and found an in-hospital mortality of 5.1% with heparin versus 5.6% with placebo. No significant difference was found with streptokinase versus t-PA, or with or without aspirin therapy. Although there was no significant reduction in reinfarction or recurrent ischemia, there was a trend toward increased risk for intracranial bleeding and a clear increased risk in overall bleeding. Because of these adverse consequences and the absolute benefit of only 5 deaths per 1,000 patients treated, the authors concluded that there was not enough data to support or refute the routine use of intravenous heparin. The overview by Collins and coworkers (23) pooled data from 26 studies of heparin versus placebo, the majority of patients coming from GISSI-2 and ISIS-3. They found that in the absence of aspirin, heparin reduced mortality by 25%, whereas in the presence of aspirin, mortality was only reduced by 6%. No difference was found between subcutaneous and intravenous heparin, and there was again a nonsignificant increase in stroke and a clear increase in major bleeding. These authors concluded that the current evidence from trials does not justify the routine addition of heparin to aspirin with fibrinolytic therapy.

Analysis of almost 30,000 patients from the GUSTO I study revealed a relation between the activated partial thromboplastin time (aPTT) and clinical outcomes in patients treated with fibrinolytic (t-PA and streptokinase) and intravenous heparin (24). At 12 hours, the aPTT associated with the lowest 30-day mortality, stroke, and bleeding rates was 50 to 70 seconds, and aPTTs greater than 70 seconds were found to be associated with greater likelihood of mortality, stroke, bleeding, and reinfarction (Fig. 69–3).

Recommendations. The current recommendations from the American College of Cardiology/American Heart Association (ACC/AHA) on the use of heparin in patients with AMI undergoing reperfusion therapy with fibrinolytics (Class IIa and IIb) vary depending on the type of fibrinolytic—selective or nonselective (25). In patients treated with a selective agent such as alteplase, intravenous heparin

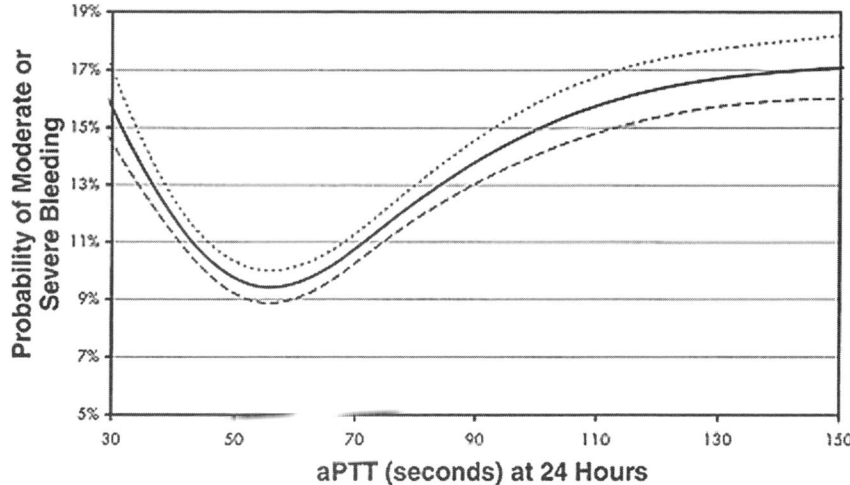

FIG. 69–3. Activated partial thromboplastin time (aPTT) versus probability of bleeding at 24 hours with 95% confidence intervals marked from the Global Use of Strategies To Open Occluded Coronary Arteries (GUSTO) I trial (24).

as an initial bolus of 60 U per kilogram and subsequent maintenance infusion of 12 U per kilogram per hour (with a maximum of 4,000-U bolus and 1,000 U/hr infusion in patients weighing >70 kg) adjusted to maintain the aPTT at 50 to 70 seconds is recommended for 48 hours with consideration of longer therapy in patients at high risk for thromboembolism. For nonselective agents such as streptokinase, intravenous heparin adjusted to maintain the aPTT at 50 to 70 seconds is recommended in patients at high risk for systemic emboli. Heparin should be withheld for 6 hours after fibrinolytic and not started until the aPTT decreases to less than 70. In patients not at high risk, subcutaneous heparin at doses of 7,500 to 12,500 U twice daily is recommended until the patient is ambulatory.

Low–Molecular Weight Heparin

Low–molecular weight heparin (LMWH) has several advantages over standard, unfractionated heparin: It has a more predictable anticoagulant effect, provides a simpler route of administration, requires no monitoring of anticoagulation, is resistant to inhibition by activated platelets, and has a lower incidence of heparin-induced thrombocytopenia.

LMWH has only recently been studied in combination with fibrinolytics and aspirin. Data from the GUSTO I trial found that although intravenous heparin partly suppresses the increased thrombin activity associated with thrombolysis, it does not inhibit thrombin, suggesting that perhaps other more specific antithrombin agents might be more effective than unfractionated heparin (26). With its greater inhibition of thrombin generation, simpler route of administration, more predictable anticoagulant effect, and lack of monitoring requirements, LMWH might be superior to unfractionated heparin after fibrinolytics (27). Enoxaparin is currently the only LMWH with consistently positive large-scale trial data supporting its use in this context, but dal-

teparin also is starting to accumulate results from smaller clinical trials.

Patency Studies. The Second Trial of Heparin and Aspirin Reperfusion Therapy (HART II) was the initial patency trial enrolling 400 patients undergoing fibrinolytic therapy (t-PA) to either enoxaparin or unfractionated heparin (28). Enoxaparin was found not to be inferior to unfractionated heparin overall with a trend toward benefit in 90-minute patency rates (80.1% vs. 75.1%) and in reocclusion rates at 5 to 7 days (5.9% vs. 9.8%). The Acute Myocardial Infarction-Streptokinase (AMI-SK) study examined enoxaparin in combination with streptokinase in 496 patients with STEMI (29). Treatment with enoxaparin resulted in improved TIMI 3 flow rates at 8 days (70% vs. 58%; $p = 0.01$), improved ST-segment resolution at 180 minutes, and improved composite clinical end point of death, reinfarction, and recurrent angina at 30 days (13% vs. 21%; $p = 0.03$). The Enoxaparin and TNK–t-PA With or Without GP-IIb/IIIa Inhibitor as Reperfusion Strategy in ST Elevation MI (ENTIRE)-TIMI 23 evaluated enoxaparin versus unfractionated heparin in the setting of either full-dose tenecteplase or half-dose tenecteplase plus abciximab (30). In the 483 patients enrolled, there was similar TIMI 3 flow rates at 60 minutes (51% vs. 50%) with enoxaparin and unfractionated heparin, but at 30 days of follow-up there was a significant reduction in death and MI in the enoxaparin group (10.7% vs. 5.0%; $p = 0.012$). There was a nonsignificant increase in major hemorrhage with enoxaparin (5.2% vs. 3.8%). In a small clinical outcomes trial of 300 patients receiving alteplase for acute STEMI, subjects were randomized to enoxaparin or unfractionated heparin for 4 days (31). At 90 days, there was a 10% absolute reduction in the composite end point of death, reinfarction, or unstable angina (36% vs. 26%; $p = 0.04$) with no significant differences in major bleeding.

Dalteparin has been evaluated in three small pilot studies with rather equivocal results. The first and largest study was the Fragmin in Acute Myocardial Infarction (FRAMI) trial, which randomized 776 subjects to dalteparin versus placebo during hospitalization in patients treated with streptokinase for STEMI (32). Although the trial end point was rates of thromboembolism and not coronary events, safety analysis revealed an increased risk for major (2.9% vs. 0.3%; $p = 0.006$) and minor bleeding (14.8% vs. 1.8%; $p < 0.001$). The Biochemical Markers in Acute Coronary Syndromes (BIOMACS II) study randomized 101 patients treated with streptokinase to placebo or two doses of dalteparin and found a nonsignificant trend toward improved TIMI 3 flow at 24 hours and ST-segment monitoring (33). Finally, the ASSENT-PLUS trial examined 434 patients treated with reteplase and given either dalteparin or unfractionated heparin as adjuvant therapy (34). TIMI 3 flow at 4 to 7 days demonstrated a trend toward improvement with dalteparin as compared with unfractionated heparin without a significant increase in bleeding.

Clinical Studies. The ASSENT-3 trial included the first large-scale trial of enoxaparin compared with unfractionated heparin in patients with AMI presenting within 6 hours of symptom onset treated with tenecteplase and aspirin (9). More than 2,000 patients were randomized to each group and followed for the composite primary end point of 30-day mortality, in-hospital reinfarction, and in-hospital refractory ischemia in addition to safety end points. The study found a significant 26% relative risk reduction (RRR; 95% confidence interval [CI], 13–37%; $p = 0.0002$) with enoxaparin, which was driven by significant reductions in reinfarction and refractory ischemia. Although there was also a significant reduction (19%) in the combined efficacy and safety end points, the enoxaparin group had a greater incidence of major bleeding than the unfractionated heparin group (3.0% vs. 2.2%; $p = 0.0005$). Interestingly, the RRR in efficacy plus safety end points achieved with enoxaparin was greater than that achieved with half-dose tenecteplase plus abciximab (19% vs. 16%).

Recommendations. Although still under investigation without recommendations from any major society, the combination of LMWH with fibrinolytics seems extremely promising. In addition to simplifying therapy by obviating the need to monitor anticoagulation, LMWH reduces reinfarction and recurrent ischemia with only a small increase in bleeding. Currently, the only agent to show reproducible and significant benefit in this area has been enoxaparin. There is no evidence to suggest that the benefits seen with enoxaparin are generalizable to the remainder of the LMWH class. Given the concern regarding potential hemorrhagic complications whenever any antithrombotic is combined with a fibrinolytic, the clinical data would suggest that enoxaparin would be the LMWH used in combination with lytics.

Direct Thrombin Inhibitors

The direct thrombin inhibitors represent another group of antithrombotic agents that have potential mechanistic ad-

vantages over standard unfractionated heparin when used as therapy for ACSs. Unlike unfractionated heparin, direct thrombin inhibitors do not require cofactors, can neutralize clot-bound thrombin, and are not inactivated by plasma proteins or platelet factor 4 (18). Hirudin and Hirulog/bivalirudin form a bivalent complex with thrombin blocking both the active site and the substrate recognition ecosite. Several other synthetic univalent direct thrombin inhibitors have been developed that block only the active site of thrombin. Early dose-ranging pilot studies such as TIMI 5 (hirudin with t-PA) (35) and TIMI 6 (hirudin with streptokinase) (36) returned promising results with improved angiographic findings and low rates of adverse events.

After the preliminary observations of the TIMI 9a (37) and GUSTO IIa (38), trials were designed to examine the role of hirudin in STEMI treated with fibrinolytics. Both studies used a high dose of hirudin based on TIMI 5 data and an aggressive weight-based heparin dosing scheme, and, as a result, experienced an excess of intracranial bleeding in both groups causing the studies to be terminated prematurely by their data and safety monitoring committees. These studies were reconfigured and resumed with lower doses of hirudin and heparin as TIMI 9b and GUSTO IIb. TIMI 9b (39) studied 3,002 patients, whereas the 4,131 patients among the more than 12,000 subjects enrolled in GUSTO IIb (40) who received either t-PA or streptokinase within 12 hours of symptom onset were randomized to either hirudin or unfractionated heparin. At 30 days, the primary end point (death, recurrent MI, congestive heart failure, or cardiogenic shock) in TIMI 9b was reached in 11.9% of the patients treated with heparin and in 12.9% of the patients treated with hirudin ($p = $ NS), whereas in GUSTO IIb, the primary end point (death and MI) occurred in 11.3% of the heparin group and 9.9% of the hirudin group ($p = 0.13$). The occurrence of major bleeding episodes was not significantly different between the two agents.

Hirudin also was studied concurrently on a smaller scale in the Hirudin for the Improvement of Thrombolysis (HIT) trials. HIT-I (41) and HIT-II (42) were dose-ranging patency studies that established the efficacy and safety of hirudin in about 200 patients. HIT-III (43) was similar to TIMI 9a and GUSTO IIa in that it was terminated early because of an increased incidence of intracranial bleeding after only 302 patients of a planned 7,000 were enrolled. Finally, HIT-4 studied 1,208 patients treated with streptokinase within 6 hours of symptom onset and found no significant differences in the 30-day occurrence of death, stroke, MI, or their composite (44).

The Hirulog Early Reperfusion/Occlusion (HERO) trial was a dose-ranging pilot study of Hirulog in patients with STEMI treated with streptokinase (45). Four hundred twelve patients were randomly assigned to receive either unfractionated heparin or two doses of Hirulog. Superior patency rates were achieved with Hirulog as TIMI 3 flow was 35% (95% CI, 28–44%) with heparin, 46% (95% CI, 38–55%) with low-dose Hirulog, and 48% (95% CI, 40–57%) with high-dose Hirulog (heparin vs. Hirulog, $p = 0.023$; heparin vs. high-dose Hirulog, $p = 0.03$). These results led to the larger HERO-2 study, which randomized 17,073 patients with acute STEMI presenting within 6 hours of symptoms and treated with streptokinase to either unfractionated heparin or bivalirudin (previously Hirulog) (46). The primary end point of 30-day mortality was reached in 10.8% of the bivalirudin group and 10.9% of the heparin group ($p = $ NS). There were fewer reinfarctions at 96 hours with bivalirudin (1.6% vs. 2.3%; $p = 0.001$), which was a prespecified secondary end point of the study. Again the rates of major bleeding were similar between groups, but the rate of minor bleeding was increased with bivalirudin.

A pooled analysis by the Organization to Assess Strategies for Ischemic Syndromes (OASIS) investigators of hirudin versus unfractionated heparin with fibrinolytic therapy found a nonsignificant RRR of 11% to 12% at 72 hours, 7 days, and 35 days ($p = $ NS) (47) (Fig. 69–4). A meta-analysis of direct thrombin inhibitors in the management of ACSs compared with unfractionated heparin including 11 randomized trials and almost 36,000 patients was published in 2002 (48). Although direct thrombin inhibitors were found to have a significantly lower risk for death or MI at the end of treatment and at 30 days, the study did not analyze ST-segment elevation and non–ST-segment elevation ACSs separately.

Other synthetic direct thrombin inhibitors have been developed and have been the subject of ongoing clinical trials. These univalent inhibitors represent a potential trend toward future therapy and drug development, but they are not currently approved for therapy.

Argatroban, a synthetic nonpeptide arginine derivative, has been studied in several dose-ranging, pilot patency studies. In the Argatroban in Acute Myocardial Infarction (ARGAMI) study, a total of 162 patients being treated for STEMI with alteplase were treated with either argatroban or unfractionated heparin and found to have similar safety and efficacy profiles (49). In the Myocardial Infarction with Novastan and t-PA (MINT) study, 125 patients treated with t-PA were randomized to argatroban or unfractionated heparin and found improved TIMI grade 3 flow rates in the high-dose argatroban group versus heparin (57.1% vs. 20.0%; $p = 0.03$), whereas major bleeding and combined clinical end points also were nonsignificantly reduced (50,51). Efegatran, another synthetic arginine derivative, also has been evaluated in two small trials. The Efegatran and Streptokinase to Canalize Arteries like Accelerated tPa (ESCALAT) trial analyzed 245 subjects in a dose-ranging, patency trial comparing efegatran and streptokinase with unfractionated heparin and t-PA and found no improvement in TIMI flow, clinical outcomes, or safety with efegatran (52). The Promotion of Reperfusion in Myocardial Infarction Evolution (PRIME) trial also evaluated at 336 patients with STEMIs treated with alteplase and found no clear advantage of efegatran over unfractionated heparin (53). Finally, the synthetic pentasaccharide (ORG31540/SR9017A) was evaluated in 333 patients with STEMI treated with alteplase and demonstrated similar TIMI flow rates at 90 min-

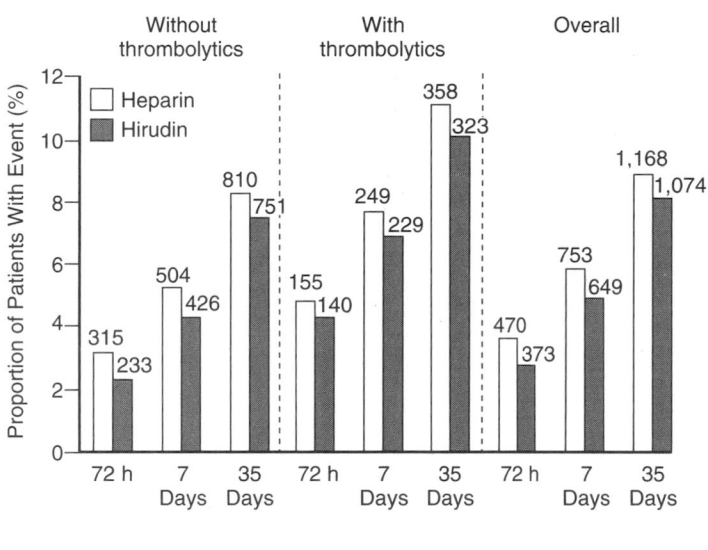

FIG. 69–4. Pooled analysis of all large trials of hirudin verus heparin in acute ST-segment elevation myocardial infarction (Thrombolysis in Myocardial Infarction [TIMI] 9b and Global Use of Strategies To Open Occluded Coronary Arteries [GUSTO] IIb) and in acute non–ST-segment elevation myocardial infarction (Organization to Assess Strategies for Ischemic Syndromes [OASIS] pilot, OASIS-2, and GUSTO IIb) (47).

utes and a trend toward improved patency at 5 to 7 days. There were less revascularizations during 30 days of follow-up with the Xa inhibitor than with heparin (39% vs. 51%; $p = 0.054$) and no difference in intracranial hemorrhage or blood transfusions (54).

Recommendations. Despite their superior thrombin inhibition, hirudin and Hirulog/bivalirudin have not shown marked improvements over unfractionated heparin in clinical trials. A current view is that direct thrombin inhibitors are more potent than unfractionated heparin as inhibitors of thrombin activity; heparin is the more effective inhibitor of thrombin generation (55). During thrombolysis, thrombin is elaborated, and this thrombin is inhibited by hirudin. However, small amounts of fibrin-bound thrombin may be transiently protected from the action of hirudin and could lead to further fibrin production, platelet activation, and thrombus formation. This corresponds with the observation that the only benefit seen with hirudin in the overall GUSTO IIb cohort occurred during hirudin administration in the first 24 to 48 hours, and once the medication was stopped this benefit eroded. The majority of these direct thrombin inhibitors have been used in conjunction with streptokinase, which is not used as extensively in the United States as it is in Canada and Europe, and there is less compelling data regarding its use with t-PA. As a result, hirudin and bivalirudin are not recommended or approved for use as antithrombotic therapy with fibrinolytics.

Antithrombotic Therapy with Percutaneous Coronary Intervention as the Primary Strategy

Antiplatelet Therapy

Aspirin

The current ACC/AHA guidelines recommend the routine use of aspirin at the time of primary percutaneous intervention for AMI because aspirin reduces the frequency of ischemic complications after coronary angioplasty (56). Although the minimum effective aspirin dosage in the setting of coronary angioplasty has not been established, a dose of 80 to 325 mg, given at least 2 hours before percutaneous coronary intervention (PCI) is recommended (56). Only the thienopyridine derivatives, ticlopidine and clopidogrel, have been routinely used as alternative antiplatelet agents in aspirin-sensitive patients during coronary angioplasty.

Glycoprotein IIb/IIIa Inhibitors

Abciximab is the GPIIb/IIIa inhibitor that has been most thoroughly evaluated for use in conjunction with percutaneous intervention in the setting of AMI, whereas eptifibatide is beginning to accumulate data in this setting.

The ReoPro in Acute Myocardial Infarction and Primary PTCA Organization and Randomized Trial (RAPPORT) study was the first to look at the use of GPIIb/IIIa inhibitors in this setting (57). The trial randomized 483 patients who presented for primary angioplasty with acute STEMI of less than 12 hours in duration to abciximab bolus plus 12-hour infusion or placebo. By intention-to-treat analysis there was no significant difference between the two groups in the composite end point of death, reinfarction, or target vessel revascularization at 6 months, 30 days, and 7 days. However, there was a trend toward benefit with abciximab treatment that became even more apparent in the treated patient analysis. Abciximab provided most of its benefit by significantly reducing the need for urgent target vessel revascularization by 78% at 7 days, by 74% at 30 days, and by 62% at 6 months, and also by reducing the need for "unplanned bailout" stenting by 42%. Unfortunately, there was a near doubling of major bleeding (16.6% vs. 9.5%) and transfusion requirements (13.7% vs. 7.9%) in the abciximab group, which may have been related to the heparin dose and late sheath removal.

The Abciximab before Direct Angioplasty and Stenting in Myocardial Infarction Regarding Acute and Long-Term Follow-up (ADMIRAL) trial randomized 300 patients with STEMI scheduled to undergo primary intracoronary stenting to either abciximab or placebo (58). The primary composite end point of death, reinfarction, or urgent target vessel revascularization was reduced by 59% in the abciximab group (6.0% vs. 14.6%; $p = 0.01$) at 30 days, and the benefit persisted to the 6-month follow-up. The clinical outcome was linked to the incidence of angiographic TIMI 3 flow, which was significantly greater in the abciximab group before the procedure, immediately afterward, and at 6 months. Subjects with Diabetes who received abciximab had a statistically significant reduction in mortality (0% vs. 16.7%; $p = 0.02$) and in the composite of death, reinfarction, and any revascularization (20.7% vs. 50.0%; $p = 0.02$) at 6 months (Fig. 69–5).

The Controlled Abciximab and Device Investigation to Lower Late Angioplasty Complications (CADILLAC) study enrolled 2,082 patients with STEMI and followed them for 6 months for the occurrence of the primary end point of death, reinfarction, urgent target vessel revascularization, and stroke (59). Patients were randomized using a 2×2 factorial design: stent plus abciximab, percutaneous transluminal coronary angioplasty (PTCA) plus abciximab, stent plus placebo, and PTCA plus placebo. At 6 months the major finding was that the composite end point was roughly halved with stent placement compared with PTCA (20.0% with PTCA, 16.5% with PTCA plus abciximab, 11.5% with stenting, and 10.2% with stenting plus abciximab), as was angiographically determined restenosis (40.8% vs. 22.2%). The reduction in primary end point was entirely because of differences in rates of target vessel revascularization, not reductions in death, reinfarction, or even TIMI 3 flow. Only stenting compared with PTCA demonstrated any statistical benefit in this study, as the comparison of abciximab versus placebo only showed trends toward benefit. This decreased efficacy of abciximab compared with the ADMIRAL study has been partially attributed to the low-risk population enrolled, as reflected by the much lower mortality rate when compared with other primary PCI trials.

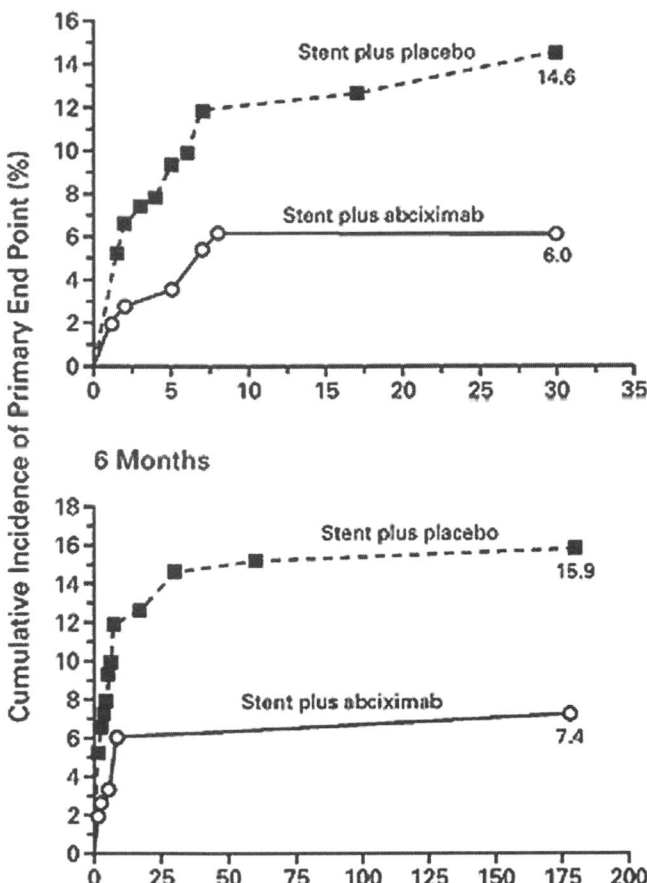

FIG. 69–5. Kaplan-Meier curves of the primary end point of death, reinfarction, or urgent target vessel revascularization at 30 days and 6 months in the Abciximab before Direct Angioplasty and Stenting in Myocardial Infarction Regarding Acute and Long-Term Follow-up (ADMIRAL) trial (58).

Limited data involving eptifibatide consists mostly of substudies and pilot studies. The Emergency Room Administration of Eptifibatide before Primary Angioplasty (RAPIER) trial was a pilot study of 60 patients with STEMI to be treated with primary angioplasty randomized to either eptifibatide pretreatment or routine care (60). Pretreatment resulted in TIMI 2 or 3 flow in 57% of patients compared with 13% in the control group ($p = 0.001$) and a reduced time from angiography to balloon inflation (10 vs. 22 minutes). A substudy of 333 patients in the INTRO-AMI trial involved immediate percutaneous intervention in patients with STEMI treated with eptifibatide plus reduced-dose t-PA (61). The corrected TIMI frame count was significantly less in patients after percutaneous intervention facilitated by eptifibatide plus t-PA and compared with t-PA alone (17.8% vs. 23.5%; $p = 0.0001$). The corrected frame count also was less after percutaneous intervention in the group pretreated with eptifibatide plus t-PA (17.8% vs. 20.0%; $p = 0.02$), and procedural success was greater if the artery was open at the time of intervention (86% vs. 68%; $p = 0.002$). The INTEGRITI trial included 153 patients who underwent facilitated percu-

taneous intervention for STEMI after eptifibatide and reduced-dose tenecteplase (14). Facilitated intervention was associated with a high rate of vessel patency (TIMI 3 flow of 91% and TIMI 2 flow of 9%) and myocardial tissue reperfusion (82% complete ST resolution 90 minutes later).

Recommendations. Currently, the role of GPIIb/IIIa inhibitors in the setting of STEMI treated primarily by percutaneous intervention is still the subject of ongoing studies. Numerous studies have proven the superiority of primary percutaneous intervention over fibrinolytics even in the setting of delaying therapy while awaiting transfer to a facility that can perform percutaneous interventions (62). This practice of direct intervention as the primary reperfusion strategy replacing fibrinolytics is likely to progress as the population ages (increased bleeding risks with fibrinolytics will pose contraindication to lysis for greater proportions of patients with MI) and as more data emerges for performing percutaneous intervention in centers without surgical backup (63). Currently, GPIIb/IIIa inhibition is integral to the practice of percutaneous intervention, especially in cohorts of patients at high risk. Unresolved issues include whether to start the GPIIb/IIIa inhibitor early at presentation or instead wait until the intervention is to be performed. Currently, abciximab would seem to be the preferred agent because it has the strongest body of evidence in its favor, whereas eptifibatide is currently being studied in further depth.

Antithrombin Therapy

Unfractionated Heparin

Heparin is an important therapeutic component of PCI because therapeutic levels of anticoagulation with heparin are roughly correlated with therapeutic efficacy in the reduction of complications during coronary angioplasty. The 2001 ACC/AHA guidelines for percutaneous intervention recommend that in those patients who do not receive GPIIb/IIIa inhibitors, sufficient unfractionated heparin should be given during coronary angioplasty to achieve an ACT of 250 to 300 seconds with the HemoTec (Medtronic Hemotec, Minneapolis, MN) device and 300 to 350 seconds with the Hemochron (International Technidyne, Edison, NJ) device. The unfractionated heparin bolus should be reduced to 50 to 70 U per kilogram when GPIIb/IIIa inhibitors are given to achieve a target ACT of 200 seconds using either the HemoTec or Hemochron device (56).

NON–ST-SEGMENT ELEVATION MYOCARDIAL INFARCTION

Antiplatelet Therapy

Aspirin

Based on the previously mentioned data demonstrating the benefit of aspirin therapy to reduce both reinfarction and mortality during MI, the ACC/AHA guidelines for unstable angina and non–STEMI establish aspirin therapy as level of evidence

A (64). They state that "aspirin should be administered as soon as possible after presentation and continued indefinitely."

Clopidogrel

The Clopidogrel in Unstable Angina to Prevent Recurrent Events (CURE) trial studied the combination of clopidogrel plus aspirin as the primary antiplatelet therapy of non–STEMIs (65). The study randomized 12,562 patients who presented within 24 hours of the onset of chest pain with either ECG changes or increased cardiac enzymes to either clopidogrel (300 mg load then 75 mg daily) or placebo in addition to aspirin (75–325 mg daily). Patients were treated for a mean duration of 9 months and followed for a primary outcome of a composite of cardiovascular death, MI, or stroke. During hospitalization, there were significant reductions in severe ischemia, recurrent angina, and congestive heart failure with clopidogrel, and at 30 days, there was a 21% RRR (95% CI, 8–33%), which persisted at 1 year 20% (95% CI, 0.10–0.28; $p < 0.001$). There were significantly more patients with major (3.7% vs. 2.7%) and minor (5.1% vs. 2.4%) bleeding in the clopidogrel group than the placebo group, and a retrospective analysis showed that the risk for major or life-threatening bleeding was dependent on the aspirin dose (66). The major limit to the universal applicability of this approach was the trial's setting in a mostly European environment of noninvasive management in which only 5.9% to 7.2% of patients received glycoprotein IIb/IIIa inhibitors and only about 20% underwent a revascularization procedure during their hospitalization. This conservative management environment differs from the strategy of early catheterization and revascularization that is prevalent in North America.

A nonrandomized, observational substudy of the CURE study, PCI-CURE, involved 2,658 patients presenting with non–ST-segment elevation ACS who underwent PCI during the CURE study (67). Patients were pretreated with a median of 10 days of study therapy, received 2 to 4 weeks of open-label thienopyridine after PCI, and continued with the study drug for a mean of 8 months. At 30 days, there was a significant 30% (95% CI, 3–50%; $p = 0.03$) RRR in the primary composite end point of cardiovascular death, MI, or urgent target vessel revascularization with clopidogrel plus aspirin pretreatment versus aspirin alone. There continued to be a reduction in cardiovascular deaths or MIs from PCI to the end of follow-up (RRR, 25%; 95% CI, 0–44%; $p = 0.047$) and over the entire length of the study (RRR, 31%; 95% CI, 13–46%; $p = 0.002$). There was no difference in major bleeding between the groups at 30 days or 8 months even in patients that received GPIIb/IIIa inhibitors.

The Clopidogrel for the Reduction of Events During Observation (CREDO) trial was not specifically a trial of ACSs, but it did enroll a patient population that included 53% with unstable angina and 13% with recent MIs (68). The study investigated pretreatment with clopidogrel and long-term clopidogrel combined with aspirin to prevent cardiovascular

events in 2,116 subjects undergoing elective percutaneous intervention. Patients were randomized to 300 mg clopidogrel 3 to 24 hours before intervention versus placebo, and at 28 days did not have a significant reduction in the composite primary end point of death, MI, or urgent target vessel revascularization (18.5% RR; $p = 0.23$). However, in the prespecified subgroup of patients that received the loading dose at least 6 hours before intervention, there was a 38.6% ($p = 0.051$) reduction in events. The second aspect of the study compared patients who continued clopidogrel (75 mg daily) from Day 29 to 12 months with patients taking placebo with all subjects receiving daily aspirin (81–325 mg). At 1 year, there was a 26.9% RRR (95% CI, 3.9–44.4%; $p = 0.02$) in the composite end point of death, MI, and stroke (Fig. 69–6). The benefit occurred beyond the standard 28-day period of treatment as there was a 37.4% (95% CI, 1.8–60.1%; $p = 0.04$) RRR from 4 weeks to 1 year. There was a trend toward an increase in major bleeding in the clopidogrel group (8.8% vs. 6.7%; $p = 0.7$) with approximately two-thirds of all major bleeding events occurring in patients undergoing coronary artery bypass graft (CABG).

Glycoprotein IIb/IIIa Inhibitors

The Platelet Glycoprotein IIb/IIIa in Unstable Angina: Receptor Suppression Using Integrilin Therapy (PURSUIT) trial was the largest of the non–ST-segment elevation ACS studies (69). The study enrolled 10,948 patients who presented with chest pain at rest within 24 hours and either ECG changes or positive cardiac enzymes and randomized them to either placebo or eptifibatide for 72 to 96 hours. The study protocol recommended that all patients receive aspirin and heparin, but cardiac catheterization and revascularization were performed at the discretion of the treating physician. Treatment resulted in a statistically significant 10% reduction in the composite end point of death or MI at 30 days (15.7% vs. 14.2%; $p = 0.04$). This absolute benefit of 1.2% to 1.5% was apparent by 96 hours and persisted up to 6 months (70). Among the four predefined geographic regions involved in the trial, the greatest treatment benefit (and greatest use of percutaneous intervention) was observed among the 4,358 North American patients (11.7% vs. 15.0%). There was a 1.5% increase in the rate of major bleeding ($p = 0.02$) in the eptifibatide group, but there was no difference in the rate of thrombocytopenia.

The Platelet Receptor Inhibition for Ischemic Syndrome Management (PRISM) trial was the first of two studies evaluating tirofiban in ACS (71). This study enrolled 3,232 patients who were at somewhat lower risk than in other trials and who had chest pain at rest or with minimal exertion within 24 hours with either ECG changes, positive cardiac enzymes, or a history of coronary artery disease. Patients were randomized to either tirofiban or heparin for 48 hours, and a conservative strategy was encouraged as catheterization and revascularization during study drug infusion were discouraged. Treatment with tirofiban reduced the compos-

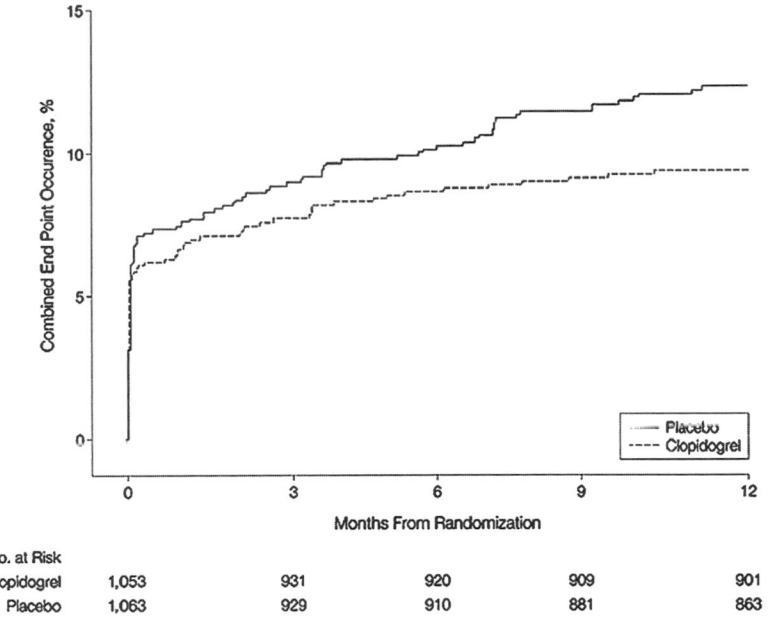

FIG. 69–6. Kaplan-Meier curves of the combined end point of death, myocardial infarction, or stroke at 1 year for aspirin plus clopidogrel versus aspirin in the Clopidogrel for the Reduction of Events During Observation (CREDO) trial (68).

ite end point of death, MI, and refractory ischemia at 48 hours by 32% (5.6% vs. 3.8%; $p = 0.01$). However, at 30 days, this benefit was no longer present. In a retrospective analysis of the data looking at troponin-positive patients, treatment with tirofiban demonstrated significant reduction in death and MI over heparin at 48 hours (3.4% vs. 0.3%) and at 30 days (13.0% vs. 4.3%; $p < 0.001$) (72). The second trial, Platelet Receptor Inhibition for Ischemic Syndrome Management in Patients Limited by Unstable Signs and Symptoms (PRISM-PLUS), randomized 1,915 patients who were at greater risk than in PRISM and who had chest pain at rest or with minimal exertion within 12 hours with either ECG changes or positive cardiac enzymes to heparin, tirofiban, or both (73). An early invasive strategy was encouraged consisting of a 48-hour study drug pretreatment period followed by catheterization and revascularization, if possible. Compared with heparin alone, treatment with tirofiban plus heparin resulted in a 32% risk reduction in the composite of death, MI, and refractory ischemia at 7 days (17.9% vs. 12.9%; $p = 0.004$), which was maintained at 30 days and 6 months. The tirofiban monotherapy arm was terminated prematurely after interim analysis because of excessive mortality at 7 days compared with heparin (4.6% vs. 1.1%; $p = 0.012$), a treatment effect not seen in PRISM.

The Platelet IIb/IIIa Antagonism for the Reduction of Acute Coronary Syndromes in a Global Organization Network (PARAGON) A trial was a dose-ranging precursor to the larger B trial, which represents the major research work on the small molecule lamifiban in non–ST-segment elevation ACS. PARAGON A enrolled 2,282 patients who had chest pain at rest within 12 hours with ECG changes and ran-

domly assigned them to 72 hours of 1 of 5 strategies: high-dose lamifiban with heparin, high-dose lamifiban without heparin, low-dose lamifiban with heparin, low-dose lamifiban without heparin, or heparin alone (74). Catheterization and revascularization were discouraged within the first 48 hours. The study found no significant differences in the primary end point at 30 days of death or MI in any of the groups, and when compared with heparin, high-dose lamifiban significantly increased hemorrhagic events. PARAGON B enrolled 5,225 patients who were randomized to lamifiban with a dose tailored to their creatinine clearance or placebo with the thought that the renally-excreted lamifiban needed to be more accurately dosed to be effective (75,76). There was only a nonsignificant trend toward benefit in the lamifiban group compared with heparin at 30 days. The one positive finding was that in the subgroup of troponin-positive patients, there was a 43% reduction in death, MI, and severe recurrent ischemia at 30 days (19.4% vs. 11.0%; $p = 0.01$) in those who received lamifiban (77).

The GUSTO IV ACS trial enrolled 7,800 patients who presented with anginal symptoms within 24 hours with either a positive troponin or ST-segment depression and were randomized to either abciximab bolus plus 48-hour infusion, abciximab bolus plus 24-hour infusion, or placebo (78). The study protocol espoused a conservative strategy by discouraging early catheterization and revascularization unless severe refractory ischemia occurred. At 30 days, the composite end point of death or MI was not statistically different across the three groups, and even among the subgroup with positive troponin there was no clinical benefit with abciximab. The results of this study demonstrate that abciximab is not appropriate therapy for patients with ACS who are not undergoing PCI.

Recommendations. Current 2002 ACC/AHA guidelines for antithrombotic therapy during non–STEMI reflect the concept that antithrombotic therapy depends on the reperfusion strategy used (64). The one generalization that can be made is that aspirin at a dose of at least 325 mg should be given to all patients who do not have a hypersensitivity reaction. For patients in whom early percutaneous intervention is planned, GPIIb/IIIa inhibition with either a small molecule started upstream in the emergency department or abciximab started in the catheterization laboratory is recommended. Aspirin and clopidogrel should be used for at least 1 year after percutaneous intervention. Given the increased risk for bleeding during CABG with combination aspirin and clopidogrel seen in PCI-CURE and CREDO and the lack of substantial benefit with a clopidogrel loading dose in CREDO, clopidogrel should be delayed until after the diagnostic catheterization is completed and CABG is excluded as a revascularization alternative. In patients for whom a conservative, noninterventional approach is planned, aspirin plus clopidogrel initially and continued for at least 9 months would be the treatment of choice. The benefit of GPIIb/IIIa blockade is proportional to the patient's risk and eventual use of percutaneous intervention (79), and as such the choice of using GPIIb/IIIa inhibitor should be individualized depending on patient risk.

Antithrombin Therapy

Unfractionated Heparin

Unfractionated heparin together with aspirin are current mainstays of therapy in unstable angina and non–STEMI. Several early studies established the superiority of heparin over placebo in these conditions (80–83), but they are no longer clinically relevant as combination therapy with aspirin is the current clinical standard. Interestingly, several of these trials compared continuous intravenous heparin to

aspirin therapy and suggested that heparin was superior to aspirin alone. The Canadian aspirin-heparin trial of 479 patients with unstable angina found a nonsignificant reduction in MI at a mean follow-up of 6 days in the patients who received heparin (0.8% vs. 3.3%) (81). Another trial by Theroux and coworkers (84) with 484 patients found a similar reduction of 2.9% (0.8% vs. 3.7%) in the rate of MI at 5 days in the heparin group. Data from individual trials was inconclusive regarding any benefit of combination heparin and aspirin over aspirin alone, so in 1996 a meta-analysis reviewed six studies to attempt to overcome the limitations of the smaller studies (85). A 33% reduction in MI or death during drug treatment period was found in the pooled analysis but with confidence intervals that crossed unity (95% CI, (2% to 56%), which left the question somewhat unanswered.

Low–Molecular Weight Heparin

Two large-scale clinical trials have established the superiority of enoxaparin over unfractionated heparin in unstable angina and non–Q-wave MI, whereas the results of trials involving dalteparin and nadroparin have been less definitive (86) (Fig. 69–7).

The Efficacy and Safety of Subcutaneous Enoxaparin in Non-Q-Wave Coronary Events Study (ESSENCE) randomized 3,171 patients with ischemic chest pain at rest within 24 hours and either ST-segment depression or previously documented history of coronary artery disease to either enoxaparin (1 mg/kg twice daily) or standard unfractionated heparin for 2 to 8 days (87). At 48 hours, there was no difference in the composite end point of death, MI, or recurrent angina. However, by 14 days, the enoxaparin group demonstrated a 16.2% risk reduction in the composite end point with a 16.6% event rate compared with 19.8% in the unfractionated heparin group ($p = 0.019$), and there continued to be a significant reduction at 30 days (15%; $p = 0.016$) and even at 1-year follow-up (10%; $p = 0.022$) (88). The reduction in the

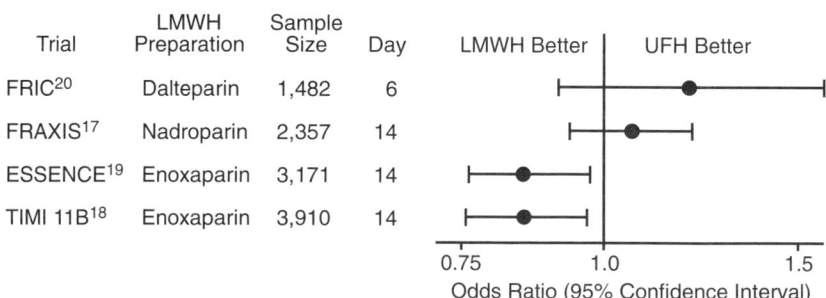

FIG. 69–7. Effects of low–molecular weight heparins (LMWH) in the major unstable angina/non–ST-segment elevation myocardial infarction trials on the composite end point of death, myocardial infarction, and recurrent ischemia (86). ESSENCE, Efficacy and Safety of Subcutaneous Enoxaparin in Non-Q-Wave Coronary Events Study; FRAXIS, FRAXiparine in Ischaemic Syndrome; FRIC, Fragmin in Unstable Coronary Artery Disease; TIMI, Thrombolysis in Myocardial Infarction; UFH, unfractionated heparin.

composite end point was powered by statistically significant reductions in MI and recurrent angina at the different time points. There was a nonsignificant trend toward a reduction in major bleeding in the enoxaparin group (6.5% vs. 7.0%), but there was an increase in minor bleeding caused mainly by ecchymosis at the injection site. An economic assessment of the patients randomized in the United States showed a cost savings for enoxaparin therapy over unfractionated heparin in addition to the clinical outcomes (89). The TIMI 11B trial again randomized 3,910 patients with ischemic pain at rest within 24 hours and either a history of coronary artery disease, ST-segment depression, or increased cardiac enzymes to enoxaparin or unfractionated heparin for 3 to 8 days while hospitalized and then to either continued enoxaparin (40 or 60 mg twice daily) or placebo as an outpatient through Day 43 (90). At 8 days, the enoxaparin group demonstrated a 14.6% risk reduction ($p = 0.048$) in the composite end point of death, MI, or urgent revascularization, and at 43 days, there was a 12.3% reduction ($p = 0.048$). Again, there were no differences in the rate of major hemorrhage during initial hospitalization between the two groups, but during the outpatient phase, enoxaparin did show an increase compared with placebo (2.9% vs. 1.5%; $p = 0.021$). Two metaanalyses of the ESSENCE and TIMI 11B data (91,92) found that there were statistically significant reductions in the composite end points of death and MI and death, MI, and urgent revascularization at Days 8, 14, and 43. At 1 year, however, the only benefit that persisted was a reduction in death, MI, and urgent revascularization (Fig. 69–8).

The Fragmin in Unstable Coronary Artery Disease (FRIC) study (93) and the Low-Molecular-Weight Heparin (Fragmin) During Instability in Coronary Artery Disease (FRISC) trial (94) both compared dalteparin (120 U/kg twice daily) with unfractionated heparin for the acute treatment of unstable angina and non–Q-wave MI. FRIC randomized 1,482 patients, whereas FRISC enrolled 1,506 subjects with chest pain within 72 hours and ECG evidence of ischemia to compare the two agents during the first 5 to 7 days after hospitalization and then dalteparin (7,500 U subcutaneously daily) to aspirin alone during the following 35 to 45 days. The FRIC investigators did not find any significant advantage to dalteparin during either time period, whereas the FRISC group found that dalteparin was superior at both 6 days and 40 days. After 6 days, there was a significant 64% RRR ($p = 0.001$) in the primary end point of death or MI with dalteparin therapy that lost statistical significance at 40 days (25% RRR; $p = 0.07$) and 5 months. Again, there was no difference in major bleeding, even during the outpatient period, and an increase in minor bleeding caused by ecchymosis.

The FRAXiparine in Ischaemic Syndrome (FRAXIS) study evaluated the LMWH nadroparin in 3,468 patients with unstable angina or non–Q-wave MIs defined as chest pain within 48 hours and characteristic ECG changes (95). Subjects were randomized to either unfractionated heparin, nadroparin (86 IU/kg twice daily) for 6 days, or nadroparin for 14 days. At Day 14, there were no statistically significant differences between the groups in the primary end point of cardiac death, MI, or refractory/recurrent angina. Although there was no difference in major bleeding rates between the patients treated with LMWH versus unfractionated heparin for a 6-day course, increased bleeding was seen among patients treated for 14 days.

Direct Thrombin Inhibitors

Direct thrombin inhibitors also have been studied in the setting of unstable angina and non–STEMIs. In the OASIS pilot

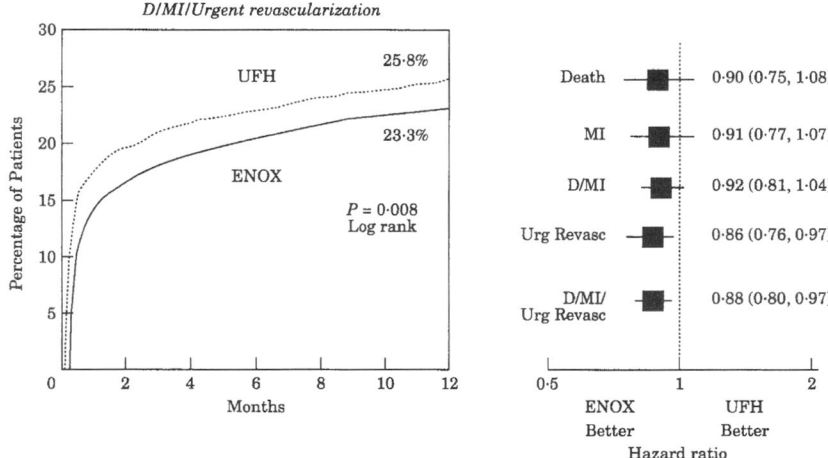

FIG. 69–8. Metaanalysis of the treatment effect of enoxaparin (ENOX) versus unfractionated heparin (UFH) up to 1 year in the Efficacy and Safety of Subcutaneous Enoxaparin in Non-Q-Wave Coronary Events Study (ESSENCE) and Thrombolysis in Myocardial Infarction (TIMI) 11b trials. Kaplan-Meier curves of the composite end point and point estimates of the hazard ratio for each of the individual elements of the composite end point (90). D, death; MI, myocardial infarction.

study, 909 patients with unstable angina or non–ST-segment MI were randomized to unfractionated heparin or two doses of hirudin and were followed for the occurrence of cardiovascular death, MI, or refractory angina at 7 days (96). At 7 days, 6.5% of patients in the heparin group, 4.4% in the low-dose hirudin, and 3.0% in the medium-dose hirudin group experienced the composite end point (low dose: $p = 0.267$; medium dose: $p = 0.047$). OASIS-2 then randomized more than 10,000 patients to the medium-dose hirudin and observed them for the primary outcome of cardiovascular death or MI at 7 days (47). Although there was only a nonsignificant trend toward benefit with hirudin for the primary end point (3.6% vs. 4.2%; $p = 0.077$), once refractory angina was added, the composite end point became significant (6.7% vs. 5.6%; $p = 0.0125$). There was, however, an increase in major bleeding with hirudin (1.2% vs. 0.7%; $p = 0.01$).

GUSTO IIb examined 8,011 patients with non–STEMI out of a total of 12,142 enrolled (40). At 30 days, there was no difference between the groups in the occurrence of death or MI with hirudin versus unfractionated heparin (8.3% vs. 9.1%; $p = 0.22$). There were significant increases in major and moderate bleeding with hirudin in these patients with non–ST-segment MI. A combined analysis by the OASIS investigators of hirudin versus unfractionated heparin used without fibrinolytics (OASIS, OASIS-2, and GUSTO IIb) found a 28% RRR of cardiac events at 72 hours ($p = 0.0002$), 17% at 7 days ($p = 0.004$), and 10% at 35 days ($p = 0.057$) with hirudin (47) (Fig. 69–4).

A metaanalysis of direct thrombin inhibitors in the management of ACSs compared with unfractionated heparin including 11 randomized trials and almost 36,000 patients was published in 2002 (48). Although direct thrombin inhibitors were found to have a significantly lower risk for death or MI at the end of treatment and at 30 days, the study did not analyze ST-segment elevation and non–ST-segment elevation ACSs separately.

Although not strictly studies of unstable angina or non–ST-segment MI, direct thrombin inhibitors, particularly bivalirudin, have been studied in the setting of PCI (97–102). The largest and most recent of these trials, the Randomized Evaluation in PCI Linking Angiomax to Reduced Clinical Events (REPLACE)-2, randomized 6,010 patients undergoing urgent or elective PCI to either bivalirudin with provisional GPIIb/IIIa inhibition or unfractionated heparin plus planned GPIIb/IIIa blockade (102). Of the subjects enrolled, 35% had unstable angina and 8% had AMI. At 30 days, the primary composite end point of death, MI, urgent repeat revascularization, or major bleeding occurred in 9.2% of the bivalirudin group and 10.0% of the heparin group (odds ratio, 0.92; 95% CI, 0.77–1.09; $p = 0.32$), which met prespecified statistical criteria for noninferiority to heparin. Bivalirudin, however, demonstrated a significant reduction in major bleeding rates compared with unfractionated heparin (2.4% vs. 4.1%; $p < 0.001$).

Only two of the univalent direct thrombin inhibitors have been studied in the setting of unstable angina and non–ST-

segment MI. Five doses of efegatran were studied in 432 patients with unstable angina, and no benefit was seen with regard to continuous ECG ischemia monitoring or clinical outcomes such as death, MI, recurrent angina, or coronary revascularization when compared with unfractionated heparin (103). The largest dose-ranging study involved inogatran, a low–molecular weight selective thrombin inhibitor, in 1,209 patients with unstable angina or non–Q-wave MIs in the Thrombin inhibition in Myocardial Ischaemia (TRIM) study (104). Patients were randomized to receive one of three doses of inogatran or unfractionated heparin for 3 days. The study showed no benefit of inogatran over unfractionated heparin at 30 days, and, in fact, unfractionated heparin was superior to inogatran at 3 and 7 days.

Recommendations. Current 2002 ACC/AHA guidelines for the treatment of unstable angina and non–STEMI recommend that subcutaneous LMWH or intravenous unfractionated heparin be added to antiplatelet therapy as a Class I recommendation (64). Because of the compelling results of the ESSENCE and TIMI 11B trials, the ACC/AHA guidelines state in a Class IIa recommendation that enoxaparin is preferable to unfractionated heparin in the absence of renal failure and unless CABG is planned within 24 hours. Emerging data now support the safety and efficacy of LMWH with GPIIb/IIIa inhibitors (105–108) and with PCI (109–112), which had previously hindered the use of LMWH in this situation. Given its ease of use and its clinical superiority, LMWH should replace unfractionated heparin in non–STEMI and unstable angina.

Currently, although there appears to be greater clinical efficacy for the direct thrombin inhibitors, albeit at the cost of increased bleeding, they have not been approved for use in this setting. The only compelling clinical data for direct thrombin inhibitors is limited to the catheterization laboratory (102). It is unknown whether the direct thrombin inhibitors will prove to have any advantage over the already proven LMWH exclusive of the catheterization laboratory.

REFERENCES

1. Randomised trial of intravenous streptokinase, oral aspirin, both, or neither among 17,187 cases of suspected acute myocardial infarction: ISIS-2. ISIS-2 (Second International Study of Infarct Survival) Collaborative Group. *Lancet* 1988;2:349–360.
2. Collaborative meta-analysis of randomised trials of antiplatelet therapy for prevention of death, myocardial infarction, and stroke in high risk patients. *BMJ* 2002;324:71–86.
3. Trial of abciximab with and without low-dose reteplase for acute myocardial infarction. Strategies for Patency Enhancement in the Emergency Department (SPEED) Group. *Circulation* 2000;101:2788–2794.
4. Antman EM, Giugliano RP, Gibson CM, et al. Abciximab facilitates the rate and extent of thrombolysis: results of the thrombolysis in myocardial infarction (TIMI) 14 trial. The TIMI 14 Investigators. *Circulation* 1999;99:2720–2732.
5. An international randomized trial comparing four thrombolytic strategies for acute myocardial infarction. The GUSTO investigators. *N Engl J Med* 1993;329:673–682.
6. The effects of tissue plasminogen activator, streptokinase, or both on coronary-artery patency, ventricular function, and survival after acute myocardial infarction. The GUSTO Angiographic Investigators. *N Engl J Med* 1993;329:1615–1622.

7. Topol EJ. Reperfusion therapy for acute myocardial infarction with fibrinolytic therapy or combination reduced fibrinolytic therapy and platelet glycoprotein IIb/IIIa inhibition: the GUSTO V randomised trial. *Lancet* 2001;357:1905–1914.

8. Lincoff AM, Califf RM, Van de Werf F, et al. Mortality at 1 year with combination platelet glycoprotein IIb/IIIa inhibition and reduced-dose fibrinolytic therapy vs conventional fibrinolytic therapy for acute myocardial infarction: GUSTO V randomized trial. *JAMA* 2002;288:2130–2135.

9. Efficacy and safety of tenecteplase in combination with enoxaparin, abciximab, or unfractionated heparin: the ASSENT-3 randomised trial in acute myocardial infarction. *Lancet* 2001;358:605–613.

10. Ohman EM, Kleiman NS, Gacioch G, et al. Combined accelerated tissue-plasminogen activator and platelet glycoprotein IIb/IIIa integrin receptor blockade with Integrilin in acute myocardial infarction. Results of a randomized, placebo-controlled, dose-ranging trial. IMPACT-AMI Investigators. *Circulation* 1997;95:846–854.

11. Brener SJ, Zeymer U, Adgey AA, et al. Eptifibatide and low-dose tissue plasminogen activator in acute myocardial infarction: the integrelin and low-dose thrombolysis in acute myocardial infarction (INTRO AMI) trial. *J Am Coll Cardiol* 2002;39:377–386.

12. Ronner E, van Kesteren HA, Zijnen P, et al. Safety and efficacy of eptifibatide vs placebo in patients receiving thrombolytic therapy with streptokinase for acute myocardial infarction; a phase II dose escalation, randomized, double-blind study. *Eur Heart J* 2000;21:1530–1536.

13. Roe MT, Green C, Crater S, et al. Improved speed and stability of reperfusion with reduced-dose tenecteplase and eptifibatide for acute myocardial infarction. *Circulation* 2002;106[Suppl]:II-629.

14. Zeymer U, Roe MT, Giugliano RP, et al. Effects of facilitated percutaneous coronary intervention on myocardial perfusion and clinical outcome in patients treated with reduced dose tenecteplase and eptifibatide for acute myocardial infarction. *Circulation* 2002;106[Suppl]:II-445.

15. Gibson CM, Murphy SA, Marble SJ, et al. Combination therapy with eptifibatide and TNK is associated with an improved rate of dye entry into the myocardium (TIMI myocardial frame count) in ST elevation myocardial infarction (STEMI): an INTEGRITI substudy. *Circulation* 2002;106[Suppl]:II-363.

16. Giugliano RP, Roe MT, Zeymer U, et al. Restoration of epicardial and myocardial perfusion in acute ST-elevation myocardial infarction with combination eptifibatide + reduced-dose tenecteplase: dose-finding results from the INTEGRITI trial. *Circulation* 2001;104[Suppl]:II-538.

17. Combining thrombolysis with the platelet glycoprotein IIb/IIIa inhibitor lamifiban: results of the Platelet Aggregation Receptor Antagonist Dose Investigation and Reperfusion Gain in Myocardial Infarction (PARADIGM) trial. *J Am Coll Cardiol* 1998;32:2003–2010.

18. Levine GN, Ali MN, Schafer AI. Antithrombotic therapy in patients with acute coronary syndromes. *Arch Intern Med* 2001;161:937–948.

19. In-hospital mortality and clinical course of 20,891 patients with suspected acute myocardial infarction randomised between alteplase and streptokinase with or without heparin. The International Study Group. *Lancet* 1990;336:71–75.

20. GISSI-2: a factorial randomised trial of alteplase versus streptokinase and heparin versus no heparin among 12,490 patients with acute myocardial infarction. Gruppo Italiano per lo Studio della Sopravvivenza nell'Infarto Miocardico. *Lancet* 1990;336:65–71.

21. ISIS-3: a randomised comparison of streptokinase vs tissue plasminogen activator vs anistreplase and of aspirin plus heparin vs aspirin alone among 41,299 cases of suspected acute myocardial infarction. ISIS-3 (Third International Study of Infarct Survival) Collaborative Group. *Lancet* 1992;339:753–770.

22. Mahaffey KW, Granger CB, Collins R, et al. Overview of randomized trials of intravenous heparin in patients with acute myocardial infarction treated with thrombolytic therapy. *Am J Cardiol* 1996;77:551–556.

23. Collins R, MacMahon S, Flather M, et al. Clinical effects of anticoagulant therapy in suspected acute myocardial infarction: systematic overview of randomised trials. *BMJ* 1996;313:652–659.

24. Granger CB, Hirsch J, Califf RM, et al. Activated partial thromboplastin time and outcome after thrombolytic therapy for acute myocardial infarction: results from the GUSTO-I trial. *Circulation* 1996;93:870–878.

25. Ryan TJ, Antman EM, Brooks NH, et al. 1999 update. ACC/AHA Guidelines for the Management of Patients With Acute Myocardial Infarction: Executive Summary and Recommendations: a report of the American College of Cardiology/American Heart Association Task Force on Practice Guidelines (Committee on Management of Acute Myocardial Infarction). *Circulation* 1999;100:1016–1030.

26. Granger CB, Becker R, Tracy RP, et al. Thrombin generation, inhibition and clinical outcomes in patients with acute myocardial infarction treated with thrombolytic therapy and heparin: results from the GUSTO-I Trial. GUSTO-I Hemostasis Substudy Group. Global Utilization of Streptokinase and TPA for Occluded Coronary Arteries. *J Am Coll Cardiol* 1998;31:497–505.

27. Becker RC, Bovill EG, Seghatchian MJ, et al. Pathobiology of thrombin in acute coronary syndromes. *Am Heart J* 1998;136:S19–S31.

28. Ross AM, Molhoek P, Lundergan C, et al. Randomized comparison of enoxaparin, a low-molecular-weight heparin, with unfractionated heparin adjunctive to recombinant tissue plasminogen activator thrombolysis and aspirin: second trial of Heparin and Aspirin Reperfusion Therapy (HART II). *Circulation* 2001;104:648–652.

29. Simoons M, Krzeminska-Pakula M, Alonso A, et al. Improved reperfusion and clinical outcome with enoxaparin as an adjunct to strep tokinase thrombolysis in acute myocardial infarction. The AMI-SK study. *Eur Heart J* 2002;23:1282.

30. Antman EM, Louwerenburg HW, Baars HF, et al. Enoxaparin as adjunctive antithrombin therapy for ST-elevation myocardial infarction: results of the ENTIRE-Thrombolysis in Myocardial Infarction (TIMI) 23 Trial. *Circulation* 2002;105:1642–1649.

31. Baird SH, Menown IB, McBride SJ, et al. Randomized comparison of enoxaparin with unfractionated heparin following fibrinolytic therapy for acute myocardial infarction. *Eur Heart J* 2002;23:627–632.

32. Kontny F, Dale J, Abildgaard U, et al. Randomized trial of low molecular weight heparin (dalteparin) in prevention of left ventricular thrombus formation and arterial embolism after acute anterior myocardial infarction: the Fragmin in Acute Myocardial Infarction (FRAMI) Study. *J Am Coll Cardiol* 1997;30:962–969.

33. Frostfeldt G, Ahlberg G, Gustafsson G, et al. Low molecular weight heparin (dalteparin) as adjuvant treatment of thrombolysis in acute myocardial infarction—a pilot study: biochemical markers in acute coronary syndromes (BIOMACS II). *J Am Coll Cardiol* 1999;33:627–633.

34. Wallentin L, Dellborg DM, Lindahl B, et al. The low-molecular-weight heparin dalteparin as adjuvant therapy in acute myocardial infarction: the ASSENT PLUS study. *Clin Cardiol* 2001;24:I12–I14.

35. Cannon CP, McCabe CH, Henry TD, et al. A pilot trial of recombinant desulfatohirudin compared with heparin in conjunction with tissue-type plasminogen activator and aspirin for acute myocardial infarction: results of the Thrombolysis in Myocardial Infarction (TIMI) 5 trial. *J Am Coll Cardiol* 1994;23:993–1003.

36. Lee LV. Initial experience with hirudin and streptokinase in acute myocardial infarction: results of the Thrombolysis in Myocardial Infarction (TIMI) 6 trial. *Am J Cardiol* 1995;75:7–13.

37. Antman EM. Hirudin in acute myocardial infarction. Safety report from the Thrombolysis and Thrombin Inhibition in Myocardial Infarction (TIMI) 9A Trial. *Circulation* 1994;90:1624–1630.

38. Randomized trial of intravenous heparin versus recombinant hirudin for acute coronary syndromes. The Global Use of Strategies to Open Occluded Coronary Arteries (GUSTO) IIa Investigators. *Circulation* 1994;90:1631–1637.

39. Antman EM. Hirudin in acute myocardial infarction. Thrombolysis and Thrombin Inhibition in Myocardial Infarction (TIMI) 9B trial. *Circulation* 1996;94:911–921.

40. A comparison of recombinant hirudin with heparin for the treatment of acute coronary syndromes. The Global Use of Strategies to Open Occluded Coronary Arteries (GUSTO) IIb Investigators. *N Engl J Med* 1996;335:775–782.

41. Zeymer U, von Essen R, Tebbe U, et al. Recombinant hirudin and front-loaded alteplase in acute myocardial infarction: final results of a pilot study. HIT-I (hirudin for the improvement of thrombolysis). *Eur Heart J* 1995;16[Suppl D]:22–27.

42. von Essen R, Zeymer U, Tebbe U, et al. HBW 023 (recombinant hirudin) for the acceleration of thrombolysis and prevention of coronary reocclusion in acute myocardial infarction: results of a dose-finding study (HIT-II) by the Arbeitsgemeinschaft Leitender Kardiologischer Krankenhausarzte. *Coron Artery Dis* 1998;9:265–272.

43. Neuhaus KL, von Essen R, Tebbe U, et al. Safety observations from the pilot phase of the randomized r-Hirudin for Improvement of Thrombolysis (HIT-III) study. A study of the Arbeitsgemeinschaft

Leitender Kardiologischer Krankenhausarzte (ALKK). *Circulation* 1994;90:1638–1642.

44. Neuhaus KL, Molhoek GP, Zeymer U, et al. Recombinant hirudin (lepirudin) for the improvement of thrombolysis with streptokinase in patients with acute myocardial infarction: results of the HIT-4 trial. *J Am Coll Cardiol* 1999;34:966–973.

45. White HD, Aylward PE, Frey MJ, et al. Randomized, double-blind comparison of hirulog versus heparin in patients receiving streptokinase and aspirin for acute myocardial infarction (HERO). Hirulog Early Reperfusion/Occlusion (HERO) Trial Investigators. *Circulation* 1997;96:2155–2161.

46. White H. Thrombin-specific anticoagulation with bivalirudin versus heparin in patients receiving fibrinolytic therapy for acute myocardial infarction: the HERO-2 randomised trial. *Lancet* 2001;358:1855–1863.

47. Effects of recombinant hirudin (lepirudin) compared with heparin on death, myocardial infarction, refractory angina, and revascularisation procedures in patients with acute myocardial ischaemia without ST elevation: a randomised trial. Organisation to Assess Strategies for Ischemic Syndromes (OASIS-2) Investigators. *Lancet* 1999;353:429–438.

48. Direct thrombin inhibitors in acute coronary syndromes: principal results of a meta-analysis based on individual patients' data. *Lancet* 2002;359:294–302.

49. Vermeer F, Vahanian A, Fels PW, et al. Argatroban and alteplase in patients with acute myocardial infarction: the ARGAMI Study. *J Thromb Thrombolysis* 2000;10:233–240.

50. Serebruany VL, Jang IK, Giugliano RP, et al. A Randomized, Blinded Study of Two Doses of Novastan® (Brand of Argatroban) Versus Heparin as Adjunctive Therapy to Recombinant Tissue Plasminogen Activator (Accelerated Administration) in Acute Myocardial Infarction: Rationale and Design of the Myocardial Infarction using Novastan® and T-PA (MINT) Study. *J Thromb Thrombolysis* 1998;5:49–52.

51. Jang IK, Brown DF, Giugliano RP, et al. A multicenter, randomized study of argatroban versus heparin as adjunct to tissue plasminogen activator (TPA) in acute myocardial infarction: myocardial infarction with novastan and TPA (MINT) study. *J Am Coll Cardiol* 1999;33:1879–1885.

52. Fung AY, Lorch G, Cambier PA, et al. Efegatran sulfate as an adjunct to streptokinase versus heparin as an adjunct to tissue plasminogen activator in patients with acute myocardial infarction. ESCALAT Investigators. *Am Heart J* 1999;138:696–704.

53. Multicenter, dose-ranging study of efegatran sulfate versus heparin with thrombolysis for acute myocardial infarction: the Promotion of Reperfusion in Myocardial Infarction Evolution (PRIME) trial. *Am Heart J* 2002;143:95–105.

54. Coussement PK, Bassand JP, Convens C, et al. A synthetic factor-Xa inhibitor (ORG31540/SR9017A) as an adjunct to fibrinolysis in acute myocardial infarction. The PENTALYSE study. *Eur Heart J* 2001;22:1716–1724.

55. Loscalzo J. Thrombin inhibitors in fibrinolysis. A Hobson's choice of alternatives. *Circulation* 1996;94:863–865.

56. Smith SC Jr, Dove JT, Jacobs AK, et al. ACC/AHA guidelines for percutaneous coronary intervention (revision of the 1993 PTCA guidelines)—executive summary: a report of the American College of Cardiology/American Heart Association task force on practice guidelines (Committee to revise the 1993 guidelines for percutaneous transluminal coronary angioplasty) endorsed by the Society for Cardiac Angiography and Interventions. *Circulation* 2001;103:3019–3041.

57. Brener SJ, Barr LA, Burchenal JE, et al. Randomized, placebo-controlled trial of platelet glycoprotein IIb/IIIa blockade with primary angioplasty for acute myocardial infarction. ReoPro and Primary PTCA Organization and Randomized Trial (RAPPORT) Investigators. *Circulation* 1998;98:734–741.

58. Montalescot G, Barragan P, Wittenberg O, et al. Platelet glycoprotein IIb/IIIa inhibition with coronary stenting for acute myocardial infarction. *N Engl J Med* 2001;344:1895–1903.

59. Stone GW, Grines CL, Cox DA, et al. Comparison of angioplasty with stenting, with or without abciximab, in acute myocardial infarction. *N Engl J Med* 2002;346:957–966.

60. Cutlip DE, Cove CJ, Irons D, et al. Emergency room administration of eptifibatide before primary angioplasty for ST elevation acute myocardial infarction and its effect on baseline coronary flow and procedure outcomes. *Am J Cardiol* 2001;88:62–64.

61. L'Allier PL, Brener SJ. Evidence of more complete arterial patency with immediate percutaneous intervention and eptifibatide plus re-

duced-dose t-PA in acute myocardial infarction. Final results from the INTRO-AMI trial. *Circulation* 2001;104[Suppl]:II-465.

62. Keeley EC, Boura JA, Grines CL. Primary angioplasty versus intravenous thrombolytic therapy for acute myocardial infarction: a quantitative review of 23 randomised trials. *Lancet* 2003;361:13–20.

63. Aversano T, Aversano LT, Passamani E, et al. Thrombolytic therapy vs primary percutaneous coronary intervention for myocardial infarction in patients presenting to hospitals without on-site cardiac surgery: a randomized controlled trial. *JAMA* 2002;287:1943–1951.

64. Braunwald E, Antman EM, Beasley JW, et al. ACC/AHA guideline update for the management of patients with unstable angina and non-ST-segment elevation myocardial infarction—2002: summary article: a report of the American College of Cardiology/American Heart Association Task Force on Practice Guidelines (Committee on the Management of Patients With Unstable Angina). *Circulation* 2002;106:1893–1900.

65. Yusuf S, Zhao F, Mehta SR, et al. Effects of clopidogrel in addition to aspirin in patients with acute coronary syndromes without ST-segment elevation. *N Engl J Med* 2001;345:494–502.

66. Peters RJ, Zao F, Lewis BS, et al. Aspirin dose and bleeding events in the CURE study. *Eur Heart J* 2002;23:510.

67. Mehta SR, Yusuf S, Peters RJ, et al. Effects of pretreatment with clopidogrel and aspirin followed by long-term therapy in patients undergoing percutaneous coronary intervention: the PCI-CURE study. *Lancet* 2001;358:527–533.

68. Steinhubl SR, Berger PB, Mann JR 3rd, et al. Early and sustained dual oral antiplatelet therapy following percutaneous coronary intervention: a randomized controlled trial. *JAMA* 2002;288:2411–2420.

69. Inhibition of platelet glycoprotein IIb/IIIa with eptifibatide in patients with acute coronary syndromes. The PURSUIT Trial Investigators. Platelet Glycoprotein IIb/IIIa in Unstable Angina: Receptor Suppression Using Integrilin Therapy. *N Engl J Med* 1998;339:436–443.

70. Harrington RA, Lincoff MA, Berdan LG, et al. Maintenance of clinical benefit at six-months in patients treated with the platelet glycoprotein IIb/IIIa inhibitor eptifibatide versus placebo during an acute ischemic coronary event. *Circulation* 1998;98:I-359.

71. A comparison of aspirin plus tirofiban with aspirin plus heparin for unstable angina. Platelet Receptor Inhibition in Ischemic Syndrome Management (PRISM) Study Investigators. *N Engl J Med* 1998;338:1498–1505.

72. Heeschen C, Hamm CW, Goldmann B, et al. Troponin concentrations for stratification of patients with acute coronary syndromes in relation to therapeutic efficacy of tirofiban. PRISM Study Investigators. Platelet Receptor Inhibition in Ischemic Syndrome Management. *Lancet* 1999;354:1757–1762.

73. Inhibition of the platelet glycoprotein IIb/IIIa receptor with tirofiban in unstable angina and non-Q-wave myocardial infarction. Platelet Receptor Inhibition in Ischemic Syndrome Management in Patients Limited by Unstable Signs and Symptoms (PRISM-PLUS) Study Investigators. *N Engl J Med* 1998;338:1488–1497.

74. International, randomized, controlled trial of lamifiban (a platelet glycoprotein IIb/IIIa inhibitor), heparin, or both in unstable angina. The PARAGON Investigators. Platelet IIb/IIIa Antagonism for the Reduction of Acute coronary syndrome events in a Global Organization Network. *Circulation* 1998;97:2386–2395.

75. Moliterno DJ. Patient-specific dosing of IIb/IIIa antagonists during acute coronary syndromes: rationale and design of the PARAGON B study. The PARAGON B International Steering Committee. *Am Heart J* 2000;139:563–566.

76. Harrington RA. PARAGON B. 49th Annual Scientific Session of the American College of Cardiology; Anaheim, CA; March 2000.

77. Newby LK, Ohman EM, Christenson RH, et al. Benefit of glycoprotein IIb/IIIa inhibition in patients with acute coronary syndromes and troponin t-positive status: the paragon-B troponin T substudy. *Circulation* 2001;103:2891–2896.

78. Simoons ML. Effect of glycoprotein IIb/IIIa receptor blocker abciximab on outcome in patients with acute coronary syndromes without early coronary revascularisation: the GUSTO IV-ACS randomised trial. *Lancet* 2001;357:1915–1924.

79. Roffi M, Chew DP, Mukherjee D, et al. Platelet glycoprotein IIb/IIIa inhibition in acute coronary syndromes. Gradient of benefit related to the revascularization strategy. *Eur Heart J* 2002;23:1441–1448.

80. Telford AM, Wilson C. Trial of heparin versus atenolol in prevention

of myocardial infarction in intermediate coronary syndrome. *Lancet* 1981;1:1225–1228.

81. Theroux P, Ouimet H, McCans J, et al. Aspirin, heparin, or both to treat acute unstable angina. *N Engl J Med* 1988;319:1105–1111.

82. Risk of myocardial infarction and death during treatment with low dose aspirin and intravenous heparin in men with unstable coronary artery disease. The RISC Group. *Lancet* 1990;336:827–830.

83. Neri Serneri GG, Gensini GF, Poggesi L, et al. Effect of heparin, aspirin, or alteplase in reduction of myocardial ischaemia in refractory unstable angina. *Lancet* 1990;335:615–618.

84. Theroux P, Waters D, Qiu S, et al. Aspirin versus heparin to prevent myocardial infarction during the acute phase of unstable angina. *Circulation* 1993;88:2045–2048.

85. Oler A, Whooley MA, Oler J, et al. Adding heparin to aspirin reduces the incidence of myocardial infarction and death in patients with unstable angina. A meta-analysis. *JAMA* 1996;276:811–815.

86. Wong GC, Giugliano RP, Antman EM. Use of low-molecular-weight heparins in the management of acute coronary syndromes and percutaneous coronary intervention. *JAMA* 2003;289:331–342.

87. Cohen M, Demers C, Gurfinkel EP, et al. A comparison of low-molecular-weight heparin with unfractionated heparin for unstable coronary artery disease. Efficacy and Safety of Subcutaneous Enoxaparin in Non-Q-Wave Coronary Events Study Group. *N Engl J Med* 1997;337:447–452.

88. Goodman SG, Cohen M, Bigonzi F, et al. Randomized trial of low molecular weight heparin (enoxaparin) versus unfractionated heparin for unstable coronary artery disease: one-year results of the ESSENCE Study. Efficacy and Safety of Subcutaneous Enoxaparin in Non-Q Wave Coronary Events. *J Am Coll Cardiol* 2000;36:693–698.

89. Mark DB, Cowper PA, Berkowitz SD, et al. Economic assessment of low-molecular-weight heparin (enoxaparin) versus unfractionated heparin in acute coronary syndrome patients: results from the ESSENCE randomized trial. Efficacy and Safety of Subcutaneous Enoxaparin in Non-Q wave Coronary Events [unstable angina or non-Q-wave myocardial infarction]. *Circulation* 1998;97:1702–1707.

90. Antman EM, McCabe CH, Gurfinkel EP, et al. Enoxaparin prevents death and cardiac ischemic events in unstable angina/non-Q-wave myocardial infarction. Results of the thrombolysis in myocardial infarction (TIMI) 11B trial. *Circulation* 1999;100:1593–1601.

91. Antman EM, Cohen M, McCabe C, et al. Enoxaparin is superior to unfractionated heparin for preventing clinical events at 1-year follow-up of TIMI 11B and ESSENCE. *Eur Heart J* 2002;23:308–314.

92. Antman EM, Cohen M, Radley D, et al. Assessment of the treatment effect of enoxaparin for unstable angina/non-Q-wave myocardial infarction. TIMI 11B-ESSENCE meta-analysis. *Circulation* 1999;100: 1602–1608.

93. Klein W, Buchwald A, Hillis WS, et al. Fragmin in unstable angina pectoris or in non-Q-wave acute myocardial infarction (the FRIC study). Fragmin in Unstable Coronary Artery Disease. *Am J Cardiol* 1997;80:30E–34E.

94. Swahn E, Wallentin L. Low-molecular-weight heparin (Fragmin) during instability in coronary artery disease (FRISC). FRISC Study Group. *Am J Cardiol* 1997;80:25E–29E.

95. Comparison of two treatment durations (6 days and 14 days) of a low molecular weight heparin with a 6-day treatment of unfractionated heparin in the initial management of unstable angina or non-Q wave myocardial infarction: FRAX.I.S. (FRAxiparine in Ischaemic Syndrome). *Eur Heart J* 1999;20:1553–1562.

96. Comparison of the effects of two doses of recombinant hirudin compared with heparin in patients with acute myocardial ischemia without ST elevation: a pilot study. Organization to Assess Strategies for Ischemic Syndromes (OASIS) Investigators. *Circulation* 1997;96: 769–777.

97. Serruys PW, Herrman JP, Simon R, et al. A comparison of hirudin with heparin in the prevention of restenosis after coronary angioplasty. Helvetica Investigators. *N Engl J Med* 1995;333:757–763.

98. Bittl JA, Strony J, Brinker JA, et al. Treatment with bivalirudin (Hirulog) as compared with heparin during coronary angioplasty for unstable or postinfarction angina. Hirulog Angioplasty Study Investigators. *N Engl J Med* 1995;333:764–769.

99. Bittl JA, Feit F. A randomized comparison of bivalirudin and heparin in patients undergoing coronary angioplasty for postinfarction angina. Hirulog Angioplasty Study Investigators. *Am J Cardiol* 1998;82:43P–49P.

100. Bittl JA, Chaitman BR, Feit F, et al. Bivalirudin versus heparin during coronary angioplasty for unstable or postinfarction angina: final report reanalysis of the Bivalirudin Angioplasty Study. *Am Heart J* 2001;142:952–959.

101. Lincoff AM, Kleiman NS, Kottke-Marchant K, et al. Bivalirudin with planned or provisional abciximab versus low-dose heparin and abciximab during percutaneous coronary revascularization: results of the Comparison of Abciximab Complications with Hirulog for Ischemic Events Trial (CACHET). *Am Heart J* 2002;143:847–853.

102. Lincoff AM, Bittl JA, Harrington RA, et al. Bivalirudin and provisional glycoprotein IIb/IIIa blockade compared with heparin and planned glycoprotein IIb/IIIa blockade during percutaneous coronary intervention: REPLACE-2 randomized trial. *JAMA* 2003;289:853–863.

103. Klootwijk P, Lenderink T, Meij S, et al. Anticoagulant properties, clinical efficacy and safety of efegatran, a direct thrombin inhibitor, in patients with unstable angina. *Eur Heart J* 1999;20:1101–1111.

104. A low molecular weight, selective thrombin inhibitor, inogatran, vs heparin, in unstable coronary artery disease in 1209 patients. A double-blind, randomized, dose-finding study. Thrombin inhibition in Myocardial Ischaemia (TRIM) study group. *Eur Heart J* 1997;18: 1416–1425.

105. Cohen M, Theroux P, Borzak S, et al. Randomized double-blind safety study of enoxaparin versus unfractionated heparin in patients with non-ST-segment elevation acute coronary syndromes treated with tirofiban and aspirin: the ACUTE II study. The Antithrombotic Combination Using Tirofiban and Enoxaparin. *Am Heart J* 2002; 144:470–477.

106. Ferguson JJ. The use of enoxaparin and IIb/IIIa antagonists in acute coronary syndromes; including PCI: final results of the NICE 3 study. *J Am Coll Cardiol* 2001;37[Suppl A]:365A.

107. James S, Armstrong P, Califf R, et al. Safety and efficacy of abciximab combined with dalteparin in treatment of acute coronary syndromes. *Eur Heart J* 2002;23:1538–1545.

108. Mukherjee D, Mahaffey KW, Moliterno DJ, et al. Promise of combined low-molecular-weight heparin and platelet glycoprotein IIb/IIIa inhibition: results from Platelet IIb/IIIa Antagonist for the Reduction of Acute coronary syndrome events in a Global Organization Network B (PARAGON B). *Am Heart J* 2002;144:995–1002.

109. Collet JP, Montalescot G, Lison L, et al. Percutaneous coronary intervention after subcutaneous enoxaparin pretreatment in patients with unstable angina pectoris. *Circulation* 2001;103:658–663.

110. Fox KA, Antman EM, Cohen M, et al. Comparison of enoxaparin versus unfractionated heparin in patients with unstable angina pectoris/non-ST-segment elevation acute myocardial infarction having subsequent percutaneous coronary intervention. *Am J Cardiol* 2002;90:477–482.

111. Invasive compared with non-invasive treatment in unstable coronary-artery disease: FRISC II prospective randomised multicentre study. FRagmin and Fast Revascularisation during InStability in Coronary artery disease Investigators. *Lancet* 1999;354:708–715.

112. Goodman SG, Fitchett D, Armstrong PW, et al. Randomized evaluation of the safety and efficacy of enoxaparin versus unfractionated heparin in high-risk patients with non-ST-segment elevation acute coronary syndromes receiving the glycoprotein IIb/IIIa inhibitor eptifibatide. *Circulation* 2003;107:238–244.

CHAPTER 70

Ischemic Ventricular Arrhythmias

Mina K. Chung and David O. Martin

Key Words: Idioventricular rhythm; ischemia; monomorphic ventricular tachycardia; nonsustained ventricular tachycardia; polymorphic ventricular tachycardia; ventricular arrhythmia.

INTRODUCTION

Ventricular arrhythmias associated with ischemic heart disease can be categorized into those that occur during the acute, reperfusion, subacute, or chronic phases of myocardial ischemia or infarction. During the first hours of acute ischemia or infarction, frequent premature ventricular complexes (PVCs), ventricular tachycardia (VT), or ventricular fibrillation (VF) may be observed. After the first 6 to 24 hours, the incidence of unstable, rapid ventricular arrhythmia decreases. Coronary reperfusion, particularly after the use of thrombolytic therapy or percutaneous intervention, has been associated with accelerated idioventricular rhythms (AIVRs) and ventricular tachyarrhythmias. In the subacute, chronic, or healing phase of myocardial infarction (MI), PVCs, nonsustained VT, sustained monomorphic VT, or late VF may develop.

M. K. Chung: Department of Cardiovascular Medicine, The Cleveland Clinic Foundation, Cleveland, Ohio.

D. O. Martin: Department of Cardiovascular Medicine, The Cleveland Clinic Foundation, Cleveland, Ohio.

INCIDENCE AND PROGNOSIS OF SPECIFIC ARRHYTHMIAS

Premature Ventricular Complexes

Isolated PVCs are the most frequently detected ventricular arrhythmia in the general population, even in the absence of MI. They have a reported incidence rate after acute MI ranging from 5% to 100% (1–7). The greatest incidence is reported in the first 24 to 72 hours after infarction; it declines thereafter, but a secondary increase may be noted after 1 to 3 weeks. Frequent or complex ventricular ectopy detected after the acute phase of MI has been associated with increased mortality, particularly in the presence of left ventricular dysfunction (3,8–10). Bigger and coworkers (11) related the outcome of 766 patients after infarction to left ventricular function and the frequency of ventricular arrhythmias detected by Holter monitoring. Over a mean follow-up period of 22 months, the 2-year mortality rate increased from 6% to 16% as PVC frequency increased from 1 to 10 per hour. In the thrombolytic era, the Gruppo Italiano per lo Studio della Streptochinasi nell'Infarto miocardico (GISSI)-2 study obtained 24-hour Holter recordings before hospital discharge in 8,676 patients after MI. After 6-month follow-up, adjusted analysis showed that more than 10 PVCs per hour was a significant predictor of total (relative risk, 1.62) and sudden (relative risk, 2.24) mortality.

Accelerated Idioventricular Rhythm

AIVR is a form of ectopic or automatic ventricular arrhythmia. This condition is characterized by a ventricular rate that is slower than traditionally defined VT. Generally, the heart rate is less than 100 beats per minute, but some authors have used heart rate less than 120 beats per minute. This arrhythmia has been associated with myocardial reperfusion after coronary occlusion. In trials of thrombolytic therapy that used continuous ambulatory electrocardiographic (ECG) monitoring during the acute phase of MI, AIVR has been reported to occur with an incidence of 77% to 90% (12). In trials documenting coronary perfusion status by acute coronary angiography after thrombolytic therapy, the incidence rate of AIVR has generally been greater in reperfused (43–90%) than in nonreperfused patients (0–57%) (5). Although AIVR has been reported to be a marker for coronary reperfusion, it also is observed in patients without documented reperfusion. Its role in the prediction of coronary reperfusion after thrombolysis is discussed later. Although AIVR can cause loss of atrioventricular synchrony, it is usually brief, spontaneously terminating, and not hemodynamically compromising. Thus, treatment is not generally required.

Ventricular Tachycardia

The pathophysiologic mechanisms and prognostic significance of ventricular tachyarrhythmias after MI vary according to the timing, duration, rate, morphology, and hemodynamic tolerance of the arrhythmia. VT is classified by its duration, rate, morphology, and frequency. VT is generally defined as three or more consecutive ventricular beats with a rate of 100 or more beats per minute. Nonsustained VT consists of three or more beats that spontaneously terminate within 30 seconds without hemodynamic deterioration. Sustained VT is defined as tachycardia lasting more than 30 seconds or tachycardia requiring intervention because of hemodynamic compromise. VT may be described as polymorphic: consisting of varying QRS morphologies, width, and polarity; monomorphic: consisting of QRS complexes of similar appearance and axis; or pleomorphic: displaying more than one type of monomorphic tachycardia. Tachycardia frequency may be described as paroxysmal, repetitive, or incessant. Ventricular arrhythmias may also be classified as primary or secondary, with the latter occurring in association with cardiac failure, hypotension, or shock.

Nonsustained Ventricular Tachycardia

In the first 24 to 48 hours of MI, nonsustained VT may be monomorphic or polymorphic and of rapid rate (>200 beats/min). Nonsustained VT may result from electrical instability of the infarction, recurrent ischemia, or coronary reperfusion. In trials that used continuous ambulatory ECG monitoring, the incidence rate of nonsustained VT in the acute phase of MI treated with thrombolytic agents ranged from 60% to 90% (5,12–15). A metaanalysis of ventricular arrhythmias in trials of thrombolytic therapy for acute MI reported an incidence rate of VT (nonsustained or sustained) occurring any time during hospitalization of 10.8% in patients treated with thrombolysis and 7.5% in patients treated with placebo (16).

The prognosis of VT occurring within the acute phase of MI was examined by de Soyza and coworkers (17), who reported that VT occurring within the first 24 hours of acute MI was not predictive of long-term mortality. Eldar and coworkers (18) reported that the mortality of Killip Class I patients with primary nonsustained VT, detected during the first 48 hours of acute MI, was not significantly different at 1 year when compared with similar patients without VT. In-hospital mortality was less in the nonsustained VT group (3.7% vs. 5.4%). They also noted that polymorphic VT occurred in 6% of patients with primary nonsustained VT but in 50% of patients with primary sustained VT. In-hospital mortality was greater in patients with sustained tachycardia (21% vs. 3.7%).

In contrast, nonsustained VT detected in the subacute or chronic phase of MI has been associated with increased overall and sudden death mortality in most studies (8,19,20).The GISSI-2 study (3) was analyzed for the prognostic significance of ventricular arrhythmias in the fibrinolytic era and found that despite the mortality reduction achieved by thrombolysis, frequent or complex ventricular arrhythmias again remained an independent risk factor for long-term mortality. Frequent or complex ventricular arrhythmias were associated with a twofold to threefold increase in total and sudden mortality. However, although nonsustained VT was associated with greater mortality risk in the univariate analysis, it did not retain prognostic significance after multivariate analysis. Similarly, in the Survival Trial of Antiarrhythmic Therapy in Congestive Heart Failure (CHF-STAT) (21) Veterans Administration study, which included patients with ischemic and nonischemic cardiomyopathy, nonsustained VT was a univariate predictor of mortality, but the only independent predictor was left ventricular ejection fraction (LVEF). Thus, frequent or complex ventricular arrhythmias detected after the acute phase of MI are associated with a twofold to threefold increase in overall and sudden death mortality. Although the incidence of these arrhythmias increases with worsening left ventricular function, they appear to be independent risk factors for mortality in some studies. However, in patients after thrombolysis or with severe heart failure, nonsustained VT may not provide prognostic information independent of left ventricular dysfunction.

Polymorphic Ventricular Tachycardia

Polymorphic VT is characterized by a rapid rate (>200 beats/min) and varying QRS morphology. VT that occurs in association with acute ischemia tends to be polymorphic and usually nonsustained but may degenerate into VF. In the setting of acute MI, polymorphic VT is not usually related to electrolyte imbalance, drug toxicity, QT-interval prolongation, or long-short initiation sequences as is typically seen with Torsade de pointes (22). It is infrequently observed with a reported incidence of 0.5% to 2% (5,18,22,23). Wolfe and coworkers (22) reported 11 patients with polymorphic VT occurring 1 to 13 days after MI. They found evidence of associated myocardial ischemia and described a poor prognosis. In contrast, Birnbaum and coworkers (23) suggested that polymorphic VT occurring within the first 4 hours of MI may represent a form of reperfusion arrhythmia. In their series of seven patients, six of whom had received thrombolytic therapy, a rapid decline in ST segment elevation was observed shortly after the polymorphic VT, and no further episodes of ventricular arrhythmias was detected during the remainder of the hospital stay. Polymorphic VT usually subsided 24 to 48 hours after MI. The late occurrence of this rhythm may suggest the need for evaluation and treatment of recurrent ischemia.

Sustained Monomorphic Ventricular Tachycardia

Sustained monomorphic VT occurs less commonly in the acute phase of MI. Few studies have analyzed the prognosis of primary sustained VT occurring within the first 48 hours of acute MI. In most analyses, this arrhythmia has been grouped with VF. In the prethrombolysis era, the Multicenter Investigation of the Limitation of Infarct Size (MILIS) trial (24) reported that primary VT/VF occurring within the first 72 hours of infarction did not predict greater mortality. However, Eldar and coworkers (18) reported that Killip Class I patients with primary sustained VT occurring within the first 48 hours of MI demonstrated increased in-hospital mortality (21%) compared with similar patients with nonsustained VT (4%) and a trend toward increased mortality compared with patients without primary VT (9.6%). Although a trend toward greater overall 1-year mortality was recorded (25% for sustained VT group vs. 15% for without VT group), mortality of hospital survivors did not change. The Thrombolysis in Myocardial Infarction (TIMI) phase II trial reported an increase in early mortality rates (20.4% vs. 1.6% at 21 days) in patients with primary VT/VF occurring within the first 24 hours after thrombolytic therapy, even in the absence of congestive heart failure or hypotension (25). Notably, these arrhythmias were associated with a greater rate of occlusion of the infarct-related artery. Among patients surviving 21 days, 1-year mortality was not different from that in those patients who had not experienced VT/VF. However, in the larger Global Use of Streptokinase t-PA for Occluded Coronary Arteries (GUSTO-I) study of 40,895 patients, 4,188 patients had sustained VT or VF, or both (26). In-hospital and 30-day mortality rates were greater in patients with sustained VT/VF, occurring either early (<2 days) or late (>2 days). These patients also had greater late mortality rates. Even hospital survivors with VT or VT/VF had greater mortality rates at 1 year. Thus, sustained VT oc-

curring in the acute phase of MI can be associated with increased short- and long-term mortality.

Because of earlier studies, VT/VF occurring in the setting of acute infarction had been considered an arrhythmia associated with a reversible or transient cause. However, data from the GUSTO-I study (26), as well as the Antiarrhythmics versus Implantable Defibrillators (AVID) trial registry (27), suggest that hemodynamically significant sustained ventricular arrhythmias occurring in the setting of such reversible or transient causes may still be associated with increased mortality. In AVID, this was the case despite a greater rate of revascularization performed in these patients compared with the primary VT/VF population randomized in AVID. In view of these results, patients with VT/VF occurring in such settings with significant left ventricular dysfunction may warrant consideration of electrophysiologic testing, implantation of an implantable cardioverter-defibrillator (ICD), or both.

In contrast, the risk for long-term mortality has been well established to be considerably increased by sustained VT occurring later in the course of acute MI. The occurrence of sustained VT after the first 48 hours is typically associated with significant left ventricular dysfunction and multivessel coronary artery disease (CAD) (28,29). ICD implantation or further electrophysiologic testing is generally indicated because of the high possibility of arrhythmia recurrence if specific treatment is not initiated. Complete evaluation may also include assessment of the need for revascularization. Urgent revascularization may be required for incessant or refractory VT in the setting of recurrent ischemia.

Ventricular Fibrillation

Because patients who experience out-of-hospital VF associated with MI often do not survive, the incidence of VF associated with the acute phase of MI is underestimated in the literature. VF may be classified as early versus late (occurring >48 hours after the onset of infarction) or primary versus secondary (resulting from shock, hypotension, or heart failure). The reported incidence of VF associated with acute MI ranges from 2% to 15% (12,16,24,25,30–36) with a peak incidence occurring in the first hours after MI. The reported incidence of primary VF ranges from 2% to 7% (24, 25,30–32,34,35), and that of secondary VF from 2% to 4% (24,33,37,38). The prognosis of patients in whom VF develops during the course of acute MI is decreased compared with that of patients without VF. Although primary VF, or early VF occurring within the first 48 hours of infarction, was reported to carry no significant impact on short- or long-term prognosis in the MILIS study (24), several other studies have demonstrated that patients with primary VF have at least a twofold (range 1.1–32.2) increase in risk for hospital mortality compared with patients without VF (25,31, 32,34,35). Late or secondary VF occurring during hospitalization for MI is usually associated with significant left ventricular dysfunction and at least a twofold to threefold greater in-hospital mortality rate (24,30,33,37,38). In most studies, survivors of in-hospital VF carry a similar long-term prognosis as hospital survivors who have not experienced this arrhythmia (24,25,31,32,37–39).

Thrombolysis and Ventricular Arrhythmias

Reperfusion Ventricular Arrhythmias

Although the overall mortality rate of acute MI has been decreased by thrombolytic therapy, an increased risk for death during the first hospital day was noted in several studies (40,41). These findings raised the concern that thrombolytic therapy may increase potentially life-threatening reperfusion-induced arrhythmias (42). Reperfusion arrhythmias can be defined as arrhythmias that develop within seconds after restoration of coronary artery blood to ischemic or infarcted myocardium (43). Animal models of ischemia and reperfusion have been associated with a high probability of reperfusion arrhythmias that often degenerate into VF. However, studies in humans have shown that although arrhythmias are common after thrombolysis, they are less severe than those observed in animal models and are not predictive of the time of reperfusion (42,43). Postulated explanations for these differences include the longer time of coronary occlusion in humans and possibly a slower rate of reperfusion (42). An analysis of intracoronary thrombolysis in humans suggested that the incidence of reperfusion-associated VT or VF is low (6%, range 0–17%) and more likely to occur when the interval from the onset of infarction to thrombolytic therapy is short (43).

Several authors have examined controlled trials of thrombolysis to determine if a greater frequency of arrhythmias occurs after thrombolytic therapy with successful reperfusion. Most studies have shown that the incidences of AIVR and VT are generally greater in patients with documented coronary reperfusion (43–90% and 85–100%) than in patients with persistent coronary occlusion (0–57% and 25–71%) (5,6,14,44–47). Goldberg and coworkers (44) studied 21 patients treated with intracoronary streptokinase and lidocaine. Transient arrhythmias were observed in 12 of 17 patients with documented restoration of coronary flow. The most frequent arrhythmia noted was AIVR. Sinus bradycardia and atrioventricular block with hypotension occurred during reperfusion of arteries supplying the inferoposterior left ventricle. In the Intravenous Streptokinase in Acute Myocardial Infarction (ISAM) trial (48), no lidocaine was routinely given. Bradycardia, frequent PVCs, ventricular couplets, ventricular salvos (three to five beats in a row), and AIVR occurred more frequently in the group treated with streptokinase.

The incidence of malignant arrhythmias also has been studied after thrombolysis. The incidence rate of VF in randomized controlled trials of thrombolytic therapy for acute MI ranges from 0% to 7.5% in control groups and 0% to 9.3% in thrombolytic-treated groups (15,16,48–52). In a metaanalysis of these trials by Solomon and coworkers (16),

VF in patients treated with thrombolysis versus placebo was not increased within the first 6 hours (3.15% vs. 3.23%) or the first day (2.99% vs. 2.99%) after MI. With thrombolytic therapy the overall incidence rate of VF occurring at any time during hospitalization for MI was decreased (5.04% vs. 6.01%; $p < 0.0001$), whereas that of in-hospital VT was increased (10.8% vs. 7.5%; $p < 0.0001$).

In summary, although the incidence rates of AIVR and VT have been found to be greater in reperfused than in non-reperfused patients in most studies, there is little support that malignant ventricular arrhythmias occur more commonly after thrombolysis. Analysis of the incidence of early VF suggests that thrombolytic therapy does not increase the risk for acute, life-threatening ventricular arrhythmias and that the overall incidence of VF occurring during hospitalization appears to be decreased. These findings suggest that concurrent prophylactic antiarrhythmic drugs immediately after thrombolysis are not necessary.

The use of AIVR and other ventricular arrhythmias to predict the occurrence of reperfusion remains controversial. Methodology has been problematic in some studies because of imprecise determination of reperfusion, late angiography, inconsistent use of lidocaine, and lack of quantitative monitoring of arrhythmias. AIVR has been found to be predictive of reperfusion in some (44,46,53,54) but not all (55,56) studies. Coronary patency can be present without the occurrence of these arrhythmias (54). In addition, AIVR may occur in patients with occluded infarct-related arteries. This may be partly related to reperfusion followed by reocclusion by the time of follow-up angiography (57). Greater specificity for reperfusion has been reported for early, longer, frequent, or repetitive runs of AIVR (12,13,57). However, reperfusion arrhythmias have not been found to be independent predictors of reperfusion when other clinical indicators, such as resolution of ST-segment elevation, reduction of chest pain, or early peaking of cardiac enzymes, are considered (53,58,59). In summary, ventricular arrhythmias are common in patients with evolving MI and thrombolysis. However, they are an insensitive and nonspecific marker of successful reperfusion.

Late Ventricular Arrhythmias

The prognostic significance of late ventricular arrhythmias after MI in the thrombolytic era has been addressed by Maggioni and coworkers (GISSI-2) (3). They analyzed 24-hour Holter monitors obtained before hospital discharge in 8,676 patients treated with thrombolytic therapy. Ventricular arrhythmias were detected in 64% of patients, with 44.4% of patients demonstrating 1 to 10 PVCs per hour, 19.7% with more than 10 PVCs per hour, 6.8% with nonsustained VT, 33.3% with complex ventricular arrhythmias (>10 PVCs/h, ventricular couplets, or nonsustained VT), and 0.1% with sustained VT. At 6 months, total and sudden death mortality rate was 3% and 0.98%, respectively. Mortality in patients with under one PVC per hour was 2%, 1 to 10 PVCs per hour was 2.7%, more than 10 PVCs per hour was 5.5%, complex ventricular arrhythmias was 4.8%, nonsustained VT was 4.9%, and sustained VT was 16.7%. Nonsustained VT, although a univariate predictor of mortality, was not found to be an independent predictor of prognosis in the adjusted analysis of this study. However, as reported in prethrombolytic era literature, frequent ventricular arrhythmias were confirmed as significant independent predictors of total and sudden death mortality.

Thrombolytic therapy has been associated with a decreased incidence of noninvasive and invasive predictors of arrhythmogenic substrate. Most, but not all, studies have demonstrated a decreased incidence of late potentials in patients treated with thrombolytic agents (60–66), particularly in patients with evidence of coronary repertusion (62,64,65, 67–70). In addition, nonrandomized studies have shown a lower rate of sustained ventricular arrhythmias inducible by programmed ventricular stimulation (71–74).

MANAGEMENT OF VENTRICULAR ARRHYTHMIAS AFTER MYOCARDIAL INFARCTION

Acute management of ventricular arrhythmias after MI depends on the hemodynamic status of the patient, the presence of ongoing or recurrent ischemia or other precipitating factors, and the timing of the arrhythmias in relation to ischemia or infarction. Chronic management requires an assessment of the prognostic significance of these arrhythmias. Assessment and treatment for the risk for potentially life-threatening ventricular arrhythmias are key components of management of ventricular arrhythmias after ischemia or infarction.

Acute Management

Premature Ventricular Complexes

Single ventricular ectopic beats typically do not require therapy. Frequent, complex, and early coupled ventricular premature depolarizations or nonsustained VT have been interpreted as "warning arrhythmias" for the development of more severe sustained ventricular arrhythmias. However, several studies have demonstrated that ventricular ectopy is not an accurate predictor of VF in the acute phase of MI (7,75), and suppression of these arrhythmias does not assure prevention of sustained ventricular arrhythmias.

Ventricular Tachycardia

The appropriate management of VT depends on the clinical presentation. Nonsustained VT that is brief, asymptomatic, and infrequent does not require acute intervention. If arrhythmic episodes are rapid, symptomatic, prolonged, or hemodynamically unstable, antiarrhythmic drug treatment may be required, and evaluation for ischemia should be considered.

In hemodynamically stable patients with sustained monomorphic VT, intravenous antiarrhythmic drug loading may be attempted. In patients with preserved left ventricular function, procainamide is substantially more effective than lidocaine (76–78). In patients with reduced left ventricular function, amiodarone and lidocaine are both acceptable first-line therapies (77,78). Synchronized direct current cardioversion of monomorphic VT can be successful at energies less than 100 J, but acceleration to rapid VT or VF can occur. Sedation should be administered in conscious patients before electrical cardioversion.

Sustained VT that is hemodynamically unstable or symptomatic (e.g., associated with acute ischemia, hypotension, or pulmonary edema) should be electrically cardioverted. Rapid or polymorphic VT and VF typically require higher energy shocks than monomorphic VT (79).

Patients with refractory, recurring, or incessant VT should be considered for emergent revascularization or catheter or surgical ablation. Correction of hypoxemia, acidosis, and electrolyte imbalances should be routine for patients with ventricular arrhythmias. Evaluation for and minimization of ischemia should be performed for refractory VT and may include use of β-adrenergic blockade, nitrates, minimization of inotropic agents, and revascularization. Magnesium supplementation also has been advocated in selected patients and is discussed later. Intravenous amiodarone may be helpful.

Ventricular Fibrillation

VF should be immediately defibrillated with a high-energy (200–360 J monophasic or 150–200 J biphasic) unsynchronized shock, which should be repeated if unsuccessful. Neurologic recovery and overall survival are inversely correlated with the time interval before successful defibrillation. Amiodarone, lidocaine, or procainamide may be administered intravenously for persistent or recurrent VF (80,81). Intravenous amiodarone has been shown to be superior to placebo for treatment of out-of-hospital cardiac arrest in the Amiodarone in Out-of-Hospital Resuscitation of Refractory Sustained Ventricular Tachycardia (ARREST) trial, in which 44% of patients treated with amiodarone survived to hospital admission, compared with 34% of patients who received placebo ($p = 0.03$) (82). Intravenous amiodarone also has been shown to be more effective than intravenous lidocaine for out-of-hospital shock-resistant VF in the Amiodarone versus Lidocaine in Prehospital Ventricular Fibrillation Evaluation (ALIVE) trial (83). In this study, 347 patients with VF resistant to three shocks, intravenous epinephrine and another shock, or recurrent VF after a successful defibrillation, were randomized to intravenous amiodarone or lidocaine plus matching placebos. The primary end point, survival to hospital admission, was 22.8% in the amiodarone and 12.0% in the lidocaine arm ($p = 0.009$).

Treatment for drug refractory polymorphic VT or VF should include attempts to reduce ischemia, including β-adrenergic blockade, minimization of inotropic agents, intraaortic balloon pumping, and emergency revascularization with percutaneous coronary intervention or coronary artery bypass surgery. Electrolyte and metabolic imbalances, including hypokalemia, hypoxia, and acidosis, should routinely be corrected. Magnesium sulfate in suspected hypomagnesemic states or severe refractory VF may be beneficial.

Vasopressors also have been studied. A dose of 40 U vasopressin intravenously also was shown to be superior to 1 mg epinephrine intravenously in a pilot study of 40 patients with shock-resistant VF (84). Survival to hospital admission was 70% in the vasopressin and 35% in the epinephrine arm. Survival to hospital discharge was 40% in the vasopressin and 15% in the epinephrine group. However, in a larger study of vasopressin versus epinephrine in 200 patients, there were no significant survival advantages observed (85).

Prophylactic Antiarrhythmic Therapy in the Acute Infarct Period

Role of Prophylactic Lidocaine

The use of lidocaine for the prophylaxis of VF in patients with suspected acute MI has been controversial. An early study by Lie and coworkers (86) reported no instances of VF in a lidocaine-treated group (0/107 patients) but an unusually high incidence of VF in a placebo-treated group (11/105 patients). Although a review of 14 trials by MacMahon and coworkers (87) showed a 35% reduction in the odds of VF development with lidocaine treatment ($p < 0.04$; 95% confidence interval [CI], 56% to 3%), there was no significant difference in mortality, and there was a trend toward an increase in early mortality (one-third greater) among patients treated with lidocaine. These findings were confirmed in a metaanalysis by Hine and coworkers (88) of six prehospital- and eight hospital-phase randomized controlled trials of lidocaine prophylaxis. Other studies also have suggested potential for an increase in mortality (89). An analysis of 43,706 patients who underwent thrombolysis in GUSTO-I or GISSI-IIB showed a decrease in VF in the United States but no adjusted improvement in mortality (90). In addition, Antman and Berlin (36) reviewed 18 randomized controlled trials of lidocaine prophylaxis in acute MI and found that the incidence of VF in control groups decreased from 4.51% in 1970 to 0.35% in 1990 and decreased from 4.32% to 0.11% in lidocaine-treated groups. This suggests that the current risk for development of VF is relatively low. In summary, most studies show a small decrease in the incidence of VF but no improvement in mortality. Prophylactic lidocaine may best be reserved for patients with a strong suspicion of acute MI and when defibrillation capabilities are not immediately or reliably available.

Prophylaxis for Reperfusion Arrhythmias

The practice of prophylactic treatment for reperfusion arrhythmias remains unproven. Lidocaine has shown no bene-

fit in the prevention of reperfusion arrhythmias (5,46). Early use of β-adrenergic blockade also has not shown significant benefit (12,91). In fact, a trend toward a greater incidence of AIVR has been reported, possibly from the bradycardia effect of these drugs (12).

β-Adrenergic Blockade and Acute Ventricular Arrhythmias

Activation of the sympathetic nervous system can potentiate the risk for ventricular arrhythmias and sudden death, particularly during ischemia (92). β-Adrenergic blockers are thus logical agents to reduce arrhythmias and sudden death in patients with MI. Indeed, chronic use of β-blockers in patients after MI has been shown to decrease mortality and the rate of reinfarction in multiple trials. The effect of intravenous β-blockers on early mortality and arrhythmias during the acute phases of MI has been addressed in several trials. The results have been less impressive than those seen with chronic use of β-blockers. The Goteborg Metoprolol Trial (93–95) showed a significant decrease in the incidence of VF in patients treated with metoprolol (6/698 metoprolol-treated patients vs. 17/697 control patients; $p < 0.05$). Significant decreases in the incidence of VF also have been reported in a trial of propranolol after MI (2/364 propranolol-treated patients vs. 14/371 control patients experienced development of VF; $p = 0.006$) (96). Nonsignificant trends toward a decrease in incidence of VF were noted in the First International Study of Infarct Survival (ISIS-1) trial (97) using atenolol and the Metoprolol In Acute Myocardial Infarction (MIAMI) trial (98) using metoprolol. In a pooled analysis of 27 studies with more than 26,000 patients, β-blockers resulted in a 13% reduction in early mortality and a 15% reduction in VF after MI (99). Other studies have shown a decrease in other ventricular arrhythmias, such as ventricular ectopy, in patients treated with β-blockers (100–103). β-Blockers with intrinsic sympathomimetic activity appear to be less effective (94,104).

The effect of β-blockers used in conjunction with thrombolytic agents on ventricular arrhythmias has been less significant. In the TIMI IIB trial of immediate versus deferred β-blocker therapy after thrombolysis, the addition of a β-blocker to thrombolytic therapy did not further decrease the incidence of fatal arrhythmias compared with thrombolytic therapy alone (105). Hohnloser and coworkers (91) studied the effects of β-blockade on arrhythmias during the acute phase of reperfusion therapy and found no significant difference in ventricular arrhythmias with early β-blockade. Van de Werf and coworkers (106) and Heidbuchel and coworkers (12) studied the early administration of atenolol or alinidine, a specific bradycardic agent, in patients receiving thrombolytic therapy and found no significant differences in the incidence of arrhythmias with either agent during the first 24 hours. In addition, a greater incidence of nonfatal pulmonary edema was noted in the atenolol group. Thus, the routine use of β-blockers for prevention of VF in acute MI is probably not justified in patients treated with thrombolysis. However, their use may be justified for the limitation of infarct size, secondary prevention of recurrent infarction, and improvement in long-term mortality.

Magnesium Repletion and Supplementation

Magnesium in pharmacologic concentrations can cause systemic, coronary, and pulmonary vasodilation, calcium antagonism, platelet inhibition, and antiarrhythmic effects (107,108). Myocardial protection from ischemic injury in experimental models of ischemia and reperfusion may occur from enhanced preservation of mitochondrial function through inhibition of mitochondrial calcium overload and preservation of intracellular adenosine triphosphate and creatine phosphate (109). There is evidence that patients with acute MI may be relatively deficient in magnesium (108, 110–112). In patients with acute MI, magnesium has been reported to decrease the incidence of arrhythmias (113–117) and to reduce mortality (107,116–119). However, some studies have failed to show a decrease in arrhythmias (107, 118,120,121), even with a decrease in mortality (107,118, 122), and an increase in AV conduction disturbances associated with magnesium administration has been reported (120). The large second Leicester Intravenous Magnesium Intervention Trial (LIMIT-2) study (107) randomized 2,316 patients with suspected acute MI to intravenous magnesium or saline and found a 24% reduction in the 28-day mortality of the treated group that was independent of the use of thrombolysis. Thogersen and coworkers (123) reported a decrease in cardiac mortality in patients with MI receiving a magnesium infusion. However, this mortality benefit was demonstrated only in patients not treated with thrombolysis. The largest study to date, ISIS-4 (124), a trial of 58,050 patients after acute MI, failed to demonstrate any beneficial effect of magnesium administration. These data do not support the routine prophylactic use of magnesium in acute MI.

In contrast, magnesium has been shown to be useful in the acute treatment of Torsade de pointes (125) and is potentially useful in the treatment of resistant VF or VT (126), although randomized trials of magnesium for refractory VF in cardiac arrest patients did not show a benefit (127,128). Caution should be exercised in patients with preexistent AV block or severe renal failure, because magnesium has been reported to exacerbate AV block in these conditions.

Long-Term Management

The risk for sudden and total cardiac death after an acute cardiac event is greatest during the first 6 to 24 months after the event (129). Thus, assessment and management of risk for sudden death are critical after MI. Factors that have been associated with a high risk for sudden death and that have been used for risk stratification and targeting of patients for these therapies have included: left ventricular dysfunction, frequent or complex ventricular ectopy or nonsus-

tained VT (discussed earlier), late potentials on signal averaged ECGs, abnormal heart rate variability, abnormal T-wave alternans, and inducible sustained monomorphic VT by programmed ventricular stimulation. Randomized clinical trials have tested the impact of empiric antiarrhythmic drug or ICD implantation on mortality in patients assessed to be at high risk after MI.

Major Trials on Empiric Antiarrhythmic Drug Use after Myocardial Infarction

β-Adrenergic Blockers and Survival after Myocardial Infarction

β-Adrenergic blockers have been well established to improve long-term survival in patients after MI (104,130–132). Gottlieb and coworkers (132) reviewed 201,752 patients with MI, abstracted by the Cooperative Cardiovascular Project, sponsored by the Health Care Financing Administration. After adjusted analysis, β-adrenergic blocker use was associated with a 40% reduction in mortality during the 2 years after MI. Reduction in mortality was seen across all subgroups studied. These data confirm earlier randomized trials of β-blockers after MI demonstrating improvement in survival (93,130,133).

Empiric Suppression of Premature Ventricular Complexes and Nonsustained Ventricular Tachycardia after Myocardial Infarction with Class I Antiarrhythmic Drugs

Although ventricular arrhythmias are markers of a poorer prognosis, empiric suppressive treatment with antiarrhythmic drugs has not been demonstrated to improve mortality. The Cardiac Arrhythmia Suppression Trial (CAST) was designed to test the hypothesis that suppression of asymptomatic or mildly symptomatic ventricular arrhythmias with antiarrhythmic drugs after MI reduces the rate of death from arrhythmia (134,135). The population studied included patients with prior MI (6 days to 2 years); 6 or more PVCs per hour, but no nonsustained VT of 15 beats or greater at 120 or more beats per minute; and LVEF of 55% or less if within 90 days of MI or LVEF of 40% or less if more than 90 days after MI (mean LVEF 40%). Despite adequate suppression of ventricular arrhythmias during ambulatory ECG monitoring, treatment with encainide and flecainide was associated with a 2.64-fold increase in the relative risk from arrhythmic death or cardiac arrest and a 2.38-fold increase in the relative risk of death or cardiac arrest from all causes. The trial was continued in CAST II (135), using moricizine, but was stopped prematurely because a short-term dose-titration trial demonstrated an increase in mortality associated with moricizine use, and it was statistically unlikely that the long-term trial would show a benefit from treatment. CAST was important in demonstrating that suppression of asymptomatic or mildly symptomatic PVCs with Class I antiarrhythmic drugs did not improve survival and may carry an excess risk for mortality in patients with LV dysfunction after MI. In addition, the potential risk for delayed proarrhythmia, despite initial efficacy and tolerance in PVC suppression, was suggested.

These disappointing results also have been encountered in several other trials of Class I antiarrhythmic agents and have been summarized in reviews (136,137). A metaanalysis of antiarrhythmic therapy on mortality after MI demonstrated that empiric therapy with Class I antiarrhythmic drugs failed to reduce mortality in patients after MI and in patients with frequent or complex ventricular arrhythmias. In this metaanalysis, the only antiarrhythmic agents that improved postinfarction survival were the β-adrenergic blocking agents; trials also suggest a potential benefit or at least no excessive mortality in some patient populations from amiodarone (136,138–142).

Empiric Amiodarone after Myocardial Infarction

Several studies have examined the role of empiric amiodarone in the reduction of mortality after MI. The earliest studies suggested mortality benefits in patients treated with amiodarone (139–144). A metaanalysis (145) using the results of four trials suggested that the prophylactic administration of low-dose amiodarone to patients after acute MI reduces the incidence of sudden cardiac death and total mortality, although the benefits might be limited to patients with preserved LV function.

The two largest randomized trials of amiodarone after MI also suggest that amiodarone may reduce arrhythmic death. The *Canadian Amiodarone Myocardial Infarction Arrhythmia Trial (CAMIAT)* (146) enrolled 1,202 patients who had an acute MI within 6 to 45 days and 10 or more PVCs per hour or any VT run (3 beats > 100 beats/min) by ambulatory monitoring. Patients were randomized to amiodarone or placebo. Amiodarone dosage was 10 mg per kilogram per day for 2 weeks, then 400 mg per day or 300 mg per day if older than 75 years or less than 55 kg in weight. Dosage was decreased if side effects occurred or PVCs were suppressed (absence of VT; 80–90% PVC suppression). The minimum dose was 200 mg 5 to 7 days per week. The primary end point was arrhythmic death or resuscitated VF with secondary end points including arrhythmic death, nonarrhythmic cardiac death, and all-cause mortality. The discontinuation rate was 42.3% in the amiodarone group and 28.5% in the placebo group. In these patients with recent acute MI and frequent or repetitive PVCs, after a mean follow-up period of 1.79 years, amiodarone significantly decreased arrhythmic death or resuscitated VF (corrected incidence of 4.5% for amiodarone and 6.9% for placebo; $p = 0.016$). There was a 48.5% relative risk reduction by efficacy analysis and a 38.2% reduction by intent-to-treat analysis. Favorable trends also were seen in relative risk reduction for arrhythmic death (32.6% efficacy analysis; 29.3% intent-to-treat analysis), cardiac mortality (27.4% by efficacy analysis and 22% by intent-to-treat analysis), and all-cause mortality (21.2% by efficacy analysis).

Similar findings were reported by the *European Myocardial Infarction Amiodarone Trial (EMIAT)* (147). This study enrolled 1,486 patients within 5 to 21 days of MI with poor LV function (LVEF ≤ 40%) but no arrhythmia criteria for study entry. Patients were randomized (743 patients each arm) to amiodarone (800 mg/d × 14 days, then 400 mg/d × 3 months, then 200 mg daily) or placebo. The primary end point was all-cause mortality by intent-to-treat analysis. Secondary end points included total cardiac mortality, arrhythmic death, and arrhythmic death plus resuscitated cardiac arrest. At a median of 21 months of follow-up, there was no significant difference in total or cardiac mortality between the groups. Amiodarone was associated with a 35% risk reduction in arrhythmic death ($p = 0.05$) and 32% risk reduction in arrhythmic death plus resuscitated cardiac arrest ($p = 0.05$). During the trial, 38.5% of the amiodarone group and 21.4% of the placebo group had discontinued the study medication. Analysis by treatment again showed no significant differences in total or cardiac mortality, but it did show significant decreases in arrhythmic death ($p = 0.02$; 45% risk reduction) and arrhythmic death plus resuscitated cardiac arrest ($p = 0.006$; 45% risk reduction). Thus, although there was no significant difference in the primary end point of total mortality, decreases in arrhythmic death and cardiac arrest were seen. There was a high rate of discontinuation of amiodarone, with a significant incidence of side effects. This was similar to the findings in CAMIAT.

The results of these two large trials are remarkably similar. Amiodarone did not significantly decrease total mortality, although favorable trends were noted. However, it does appear to decrease arrhythmic deaths and arrhythmic end points in patients after MI. Its use also was associated with a relatively high rate of discontinuation (40%), largely because of adverse side effects. At this time, these results do not support the routine use of amiodarone after MI. Use of amiodarone in this group should be individualized, may provide some benefits in reducing arrhythmia end points, and at least does not appear to be associated with increased mortality.

Empiric Use of Other Class III Antiarrhythmic Drugs after Myocardial Infarction

The potential benefits and efficacy of amiodarone have led to efforts to develop other Class III antiarrhythmic agents without the potential toxicities associated with amiodarone. An early double-blind, placebo-controlled trial of d,l-sotalol for 1 year after MI showed an 18% lower mortality rate in the sotalol group (7.3% in 64 patients on sotalol vs. 8.9% in 52 patients on placebo), although the difference was not statistically significant (148). The rate of definite MI was 41% less in the sotalol group ($p < 0.05$). This led to a trial using d-sotalol, which had antiarrhythmic Class III activity, but lacked the β-blocking properties of d,l-sotalol. The *Survival With Oral D-Sotalol (SWORD)* trial thus tested the hypothesis that a prophylactic antiarrhythmic Class III drug after MI could reduce mortality (149). The patient population studied included patients with LVEF of 40% or less and recent MI (6 days to 6 weeks) or remote MI with symptomatic heart failure. Patients were randomized to d-sotalol (100–200 mg twice daily) or placebo. This trial was stopped prematurely after recruitment of 3,121 patients. There was increased mortality in patients receiving d-sotalol (5.0% d-sotalol, 3.1% placebo, relative risk 1.65; $p = 0.006$). The increased mortality was accounted for by an increase in presumed arrhythmic deaths (relative risk 1.77; $p = 0.008$). The effect was greater in patients with LVEF of 30% or less (relative risk 4.0; $p = 0.007$). The trend toward improved survival and the reduction in MI seen in the d,l-sotalol study may have been attributable to the β-blocking effects of d,l-sotalol.

The implications of CAST and SWORD have been multiple. The practice of empiric suppression of asymptomatic PVCs has essentially been abolished, and Class IC drugs are now avoided in patients with significant structural heart disease. Encainide was withdrawn from the market, d-sotalol was never released to the market, and there has been slowing of Class III drug development programs. Design of future trials also has been impacted by the low mortality rates seen in the placebo groups of CAST and SWORD.

Two other Class III antiarrhythmic drugs, dofetilide and azimilide, have been studied in trials of survival after MI. Dofetilide, an I_{Kr} potassium channel blocker, was studied by the Danish Investigations of Arrhythmia and Mortality on Dofetilide (DIAMOND) study group. In DIAMOND-MI (150), 1,510 patients with wall motion index of 1.2 or less, corresponding to an LVEF 35% or less, and recent (within 7 days) MI were randomized to dofetilide or placebo. For the first 187 patients, dofetilide dosage was 0.5 mg twice daily for patients in sinus rhythm and 0.25 mg twice daily for those in atrial fibrillation. Subsequent dosage adjustments were made for patients with reduced creatinine clearance. All patients were monitored in hospital for the first 72 hours of treatment. Seven cases of Torsade de pointes occurred in the dofetilide group. However, no significant differences were found between groups in the primary end point, all-cause mortality, or total arrhythmic death. Dofetilide was more effective than placebo in converting patients with atrial fibrillation or flutter at study entry to sinus rhythm. Azimilide, an I_{Kr} and I_{Ks} potassium channel blocker, was studied in the ALIVE trial (151), which randomized 3,717 patients with recent (5–21 days) MI and LVEF of 15% to 35% to 75 mg or 100 mg azimilide daily or placebo. Results showed no significant difference in all-cause mortality or arrhythmic death at 1 year. Incidences of Torsade de pointes and neutropenia were slightly higher on azimilide, although fewer patients on azimilide developed atrial fibrillation. Low heart rate variability identified a higher risk group.

Summary

In summary, empiric antiarrhythmic therapy with either Class I or III antiarrhythmic drugs has failed to demonstrate benefits in improving overall mortality after MI. Class I drugs and d-sotalol were associated with increased mortality. Dofetilide and azimilide have been associated with no significant effect on overall or arrhythmic mortality. Amiodarone was not shown to improve overall mortality, but may improve arrhythmic mortality. Thus, current results do not support the routine empiric use of Class I or III antiarrhythmic drugs to improve mortality after MI. The only antiarrhythmic class shown to improve survival after MI has been the β-adrenergic blockers.

Implantable Cardioverter-Defibrillator versus Medical Therapy for Primary Prevention of Sudden Death

Several large randomized trials have been performed comparing conventional medical therapy with ICD therapy for the primary prevention of sudden death in patients with ischemic heart disease.

The Coronary Artery Bypass Graft (CABG)-Patch Trial (152) was an early primary prevention trial that randomized 900 patients undergoing coronary artery bypass surgery with LVEF of 35% or less and an abnormal preoperative signal averaged ECG to no therapy or ICD implantation. After a mean follow-up period of 32 months, no significant difference in mortality rates was found. Slow enrollment hampered this trial, and since its inception significant advances in ICD therapy have been made, including more common use of transvenous, nonthoracotomy lead systems and biphasic waveforms.

In contrast to this study and to the antiarrhythmic drug trials, more recent major randomized trials have supported the use of ICDs for the primary prevention of sudden death in patients with ischemic heart disease. The Multicenter Automatic Defibrillator Implantation Trial (MADIT) (153) and the Multicenter Unsustained Tachycardia Trial (MUSTT) (154) both demonstrated a benefit in mortality reduction with ICD implantation.

In the MADIT study (153), 196 patients with LVEF of 35% or less, prior MI (>3 weeks), nonsustained VT (3–30 beats >120 bpm), and inducible nonsuppressible ventricular tachyarrhythmia at electrophysiology study were randomized to ICD implantation or conventional medical therapy. Exclusion criteria included MI within 3 weeks, coronary artery bypass graft within the last 2 months, percutaneous transluminal coronary angioplasty within the last 3 months, active myocardial ischemia, New York Heart Association (NYHA) Class IV, or history of sustained VT/VF. Patients underwent standard electrophysiologic testing consisting of up to two or three extrastimuli at two right ventricular sites. The end point was inducible, reproducible sustained VT or VF. After induction, intravenous procainamide was administered, and patients were eligible for randomization if sustained VT or VF remained inducible. In the conventional therapy group, 80% of patients received amiodarone, 11% received a Class I antiarrhythmic drug, and 7% received sotalol. The study was terminated with a 54% reduction in mortality rate in the ICD group after a mean follow-up period of 27 months ($p = 0.009$). These results suggested that the MADIT screening criteria could identify a group of patients after MI at high risk for death—that is, patients with nonsustained VT, LVEF of 35% or less, and inducible but not suppressible VT. In these high-risk patients, ICD implantation significantly improved survival compared with medical therapy.

In *MUSTT* (154), patients with CAD, LVEF of 40% or less, and asymptomatic nonsustained VT underwent electrophysiologic testing. The qualifying nonsustained VT occurred at least 4 days after the most recent MI or revascularization procedure. Patients who had an inducible sustained ventricular tachyarrhythmia (sustained monomorphic VT induced by any protocol method; or sustained polymorphic VT, fibrillation, or flutter induced with single or double extrastimuli) were randomized to electrophysiologic-guided antiarrhythmic therapy, including drugs and ICDs, or no antiarrhythmic therapy. In the 704 patients randomized, there was a 27% reduction in risk for the primary end point of cardiac arrest or arrhythmic death (primary end point reached in 25% of the patients assigned to electrophysiologic-guided therapy and 32% of patients assigned to no antiarrhythmic therapy; relative risk 0.73; 95% CI, 0.53–0.99). The 5-year estimates of overall mortality were 42% and 48%, respectively (p = not significant). However, overall mortality was significantly less in patients who received treatment with ICDs (relative risk 0.24; 95% CI, 0.13–0.45).

In a third primary prevention trial, *MADIT II* (155), 1,232 patients with prior MI and LVEF of 30% or less were randomized in a 3:2 ratio to ICD implantation or conventional medical therapy. The presence of nonsustained VT or electrophysiology study was not required for entry into the study. Patients included were at least 1 month after MI and 3 months after revascularization. A 31% reduction in mortality was observed in the ICD arm after a mean follow-up time of 20 months (19.8% mortality rate for conventional therapy vs. 14.2% for the ICD group; hazard ratio, 0.69; 95% CI, 0.51–0.93).

Two primary prevention trials, *Sudden Cardiac Death in Heart Failure Trial (SCD-HeFT)* and *Defibrillator In Acute Myocardial Infarction Trial (DINAMIT),* have been preliminarily reported. SCD-HeFT was a three-arm trial that randomized patients with NYHA Class II and III heart failure and reduced left ventricular function (LVEF ≤ 35%) with no history of sustained VT or VF and with ischemic or nonischemic cardiomyopathy. Patients were randomized to receive a control placebo versus amiodarone (double-blinded) versus a single lead, pectoral ICD. The primary end point is all-cause mortality after a minimum of 2.5 years of follow-up. Preliminary results report superiority of ICD therapy over amiodarone and placebo. No significant survival benefit was derived from amiodarone compared to placebo use. DINAMIT enrolled patients with recent MI (6–40 days), LVEF ≤ 35%, decreased heart rate variability, and no intercurrent CABG or 3-vessel percutaneous transluminal coronary angioplasty to ICD or no ICD implantation. Preliminary results showed no significant difference in overall mortality. A significant reduction in arrhythmic death in the ICD group was offset by a higher risk in nonarrhythmic deaths.

In summary, studies have demonstrated that certain patients at high risk who have ischemic heart disease have reduced mortality with prophylactic ICD implantation. The implications are potentially widespread. Screening patients who would be considered ICD candidates and who have had an MI can be recommended. In general, patients who fulfill criteria for high potential risk and who do not have major comorbidities should be referred for ICD implantation, electrophysiologic testing, or both. In patients with CAD and LVEF of 30% or less, MADIT II results justify ICD implantation without need for an electrophysiologic study or nonsustained VT. Results of MUSTT and MADIT support electrophysiologic testing in patients with CAD, LVEF of 31% to 40%, and nonsustained VT with subsequent ICD implantation if sustained ventricular tachyarrhythmia is induced. Other medical therapies shown to improve mortality, including β-adrenergic blockers, angiotensin-converting enzyme inhibitors, aspirin, and cholesterol-lowering medications, such as statins, also should be used.

Implantable Cardioverter-Defibrillator versus Medical Therapy for Secondary Prevention of Sudden Death

Patients who have survived sudden cardiac arrest or sustained ventricular arrhythmias in the absence of reversible causes are known to be at high risk for recurrent sustained ventricular arrhythmias. Several secondary prevention trials have been reported and are reviewed in Chapter 72. Because of the known high risk that precludes use of an untreated control group, these studies generally compared types of therapies, such as ICD versus antiarrhythmic drug therapy. These studies have established ICD therapy as the treatment of choice for most patients who have survived a life-threatening ventricular arrhythmia.

The *AVID* trial (156) compared antiarrhythmic drug therapy with ICD implantation in 1,013 patients who were resuscitated from VF, had sustained VT with syncope, or sustained VT with LVEF of 40% or less and symptoms suggesting severe hemodynamic compromise caused by the arrhythmia. Patients who underwent revascularization were required to have LVEF of 40% or less. Patients were randomized to ICD implantation or Class III antiarrhythmic drug therapy, mostly using empiric amiodarone. Overall survival was greater in the ICD group compared with the antiarrhythmic drug group with 39%, 27%, and 31% reductions in mortality rate at 1, 2, and 3 years, respectively. A subgroup analysis showed no statistically significant advantage of ICD implantation in patients with LVEF greater than 35% (157). However, in an analysis of patients who were ineligible for randomization because of VT/VF believed to be caused by a transient or correctable cause (including new Q-wave or non–Q-wave MI or other ischemic event representing 65.8% of the 278 patients studied in this category), mortality remained high and no different or worse than in the primary VT/VF population followed in the randomized AVID trial (27). These findings occurred despite a greater mean LVEF, younger age, and greater revascularization rate in the transient and correctable cause group.

Similar findings have been reported by smaller trials, including the *Cardiac Arrest Study Hamburg (CASH)* (158) and the *Canadian Implantable Defibrillator Study (CIDS)* (159). CASH (158) compared metoprolol, amiodarone, and propafenone versus ICD implantation in survivors of cardiac arrest. Propafenone was removed after the first 58 patients because of excessive mortality, but the study continued randomization of 288 patients to its other arms. After a mean follow-up of 57 months, there was a strong trend toward better overall survival in the patients assigned to ICD therapy compared with drug therapy ($p = 0.081$; hazard ratio, 0.766). In CIDS, 659 patients were enrolled with resuscitated VF or VT, sustained VT causing syncope, sustained VT of 150 or more beats per minute causing near syncope or angina with LVEF of 35% or less, or unmonitored syncope with subsequent spontaneous VT of 10 seconds or longer or sustained monomorphic VT ($\geq$30 seconds) induced by programmed ventricular stimulation. Patients were randomized to ICD or amiodarone therapy. ICD implantation was associated with trends toward a reduction in overall risk for death (10.2% per year to 8.3% per year; 19.7% relative risk reduction; $p = 0.142$) and risk for arrhythmic death (4.5% per year to 3.0% per year; 32.8% relative risk reduction; $p = 0.094$).

These studies support the use of ICD implantation as primary therapy for patients surviving spontaneous life-threatening ventricular arrhythmias.

SUMMARY

Ventricular arrhythmias associated with acute MI range from asymptomatic ventricular ectopy to potentially life-threatening VF. The acute management of these arrhythmias is dependent on the hemodynamic status of the patient and the presence of ongoing or recurrent ischemia. Their long-term prognosis depends on their timing in relation to the acute infarction and the degree of ventricular dysfunction. Asymptomatic PVCs and nonsustained VT generally do not require acute therapy. AIVRs have been associated with coronary reperfusion but do not have sufficient specificity or sensitivity to serve as reliable markers of coronary reperfusion. They generally do not require intervention. Trials of thrombolysis in acute MI have not demonstrated an increase in life-threatening ventricular arrhythmias from reperfusion, and no long-term consequences of reperfusion arrhythmias have been documented. Early VT or VF is associated with increased in-hospital mortality and may also signify worsened long-term prognosis. Acute therapy may require direct current countershock, antiarrhythmic therapy, correction of electrolyte and metabolic imbalances, and/or assessment for and treatment of recurrent or ongoing ischemia. Although the use of prophylactic lidocaine may produce a small decrease in incidence of VF, it has not been shown to improve mortality, and significant adverse effects can occur. Other medical therapies that have been shown to improve mortality, including β-adrenergic blockers, angiotensin-converting enzyme inhibitors, aspirin, and cholesterol-lowering medications, should be used concomitantly in appropriate patients after MI.

Assessment and management of the risk for sudden cardiac death before hospital discharge are critical to the management of patients surviving acute MI. Significant left ventricular dysfunction is a key risk factor with or without frequent PVCs or nonsustained VT. Empiric antiarrhythmic therapy with Class I or III antiarrhythmic agents has not been shown to improve overall mortality, although amiodarone may reduce arrhythmic death. The only antiarrhythmic agents demonstrated to improve mortality after MI have been the β-adrenergic blockers. On the basis of studies of prophylactic ICD implantation for the primary prevention of death in patients at high risk after MI, screening of patients who would be considered ICD candidates and who have had MI is recommended to assess for significant LV dysfunction and the presence of other risk factors, including nonsustained VT. In general, patients who fulfill criteria for high potential risk should be referred for ICD implantation, electrophysiologic testing, or both. In patients with CAD and LVEF of 30% or less, ICD implantation may be justified without need for other studies. In patients with CAD, LVEF of 31% to 40%, and nonsustained VT, electrophysiologic testing is supported with subsequent ICD implantation if sustained ventricular tachyarrhythmia is induced. In patients who have survived a cardiac arrest or sustained ventricular tachyarrhythmias in the subacute or chronic phase after acute MI, ICD implantation is indicated in the absence of other contraindications or severe comorbidities. In patients who survive cardiac arrest or sustained ventricular tachyarrhythmias in the acute phase of MI (within 24–48 hours), ICD implantation, electrophysiologic testing, or both may also be warranted, as data suggest these patients may remain at risk despite presence of a reversible arrhythmia.

REFERENCES

1. Connolly SJ, Cairns JA. Prevalence and predictors of ventricular premature complexes in survivors of acute myocardial infarction. CAMIAT Pilot Study Group. Canadian Amiodarone Myocardial Infarction Arrhythmia Trial. *Am J Cardiol* 1992;69:408–411.
2. Kostis JB, Wilson AC, Sanders MR, et al. Prognostic significance of ventricular ectopic activity in survivors of acute myocardial infarction who receive propranolol. *Am J Cardiol* 1988;61:975–978.
3. Maggioni AP, Zuanetti G, Franzosi MG, et al. Prevalence and prognostic significance of ventricular arrhythmias after acute myocardial infarction in the fibrinolytic era. GISSI-2 results. *Circulation* 1993;87:312–322.
4. Moss AJ, Davis HT, DeCamilla J, et al. Ventricular ectopic beats and their relation to sudden and nonsudden cardiac death after myocardial infarction. *Circulation* 1979;60:998–1003.
5. Gressin V, Louvard Y, Pezzano M, et al. Holter recording of ventricular arrhythmias during intravenous thrombolysis for acute myocardial infarction. *Am J Cardiol* 1992;69:152–159.
6. Cercek B, Lew AS, Laramee P, et al. Time course and characteristics of ventricular arrhythmias after reperfusion in acute myocardial infarction. *Am J Cardiol* 1987;60:214–218.
7. Lie KI, Wellens HJ, Downar E, et al. Observations on patients with primary ventricular fibrillation complicating acute myocardial infarction. *Circulation* 1975;52:755–759.
8. Mukharji J, Rude RE, Poole WK, et al. Risk factors for sudden death after acute myocardial infarction: two-year follow-up. *Am J Cardiol* 1984;54:31–36.
9. Moss AJ, DeCamilla J, Mietlowski W, et al. Prognostic grading and

significance of ventricular premature beats after recovery from myocardial infarction. *Circulation* 1975;52:III204–III210.

10. Ruberman W, Weinblatt E, Goldberg JD, et al. Ventricular premature complexes and sudden death after myocardial infarction. *Circulation* 1981;64:297–305.

11. Bigger JT Jr, Fleiss JL, Kleiger R, et al. The relationships among ventricular arrhythmias, left ventricular dysfunction, and mortality in the 2 years after myocardial infarction. *Circulation* 1984;69:250–258.

12. Heidbuchel H, Tack J, Vanneste L, et al. Significance of arrhythmias during the first 24 hours of acute myocardial infarction treated with alteplase and effect of early administration of a beta-blocker or a bradycardiac agent on their incidence. *Circulation* 1994;89:1051–1059.

13. Zehender M, Utzolino S, Furtwangler A, et al. Time course and interrelation of reperfusion-induced ST changes and ventricular arrhythmias in acute myocardial infarction. *Am J Cardiol* 1991;68:1138–1142.

14. Miller FC, Krucoff MW, Satler LF, et al. Ventricular arrhythmias during reperfusion. *Am Heart J* 1986;112:928–932.

15. Alexopoulos D, Collins R, Adamopoulos S, et al. Holter monitoring of ventricular arrhythmias in a randomised, controlled study of intravenous streptokinase in acute myocardial infarction. *Br Heart J* 1991;65:9–13.

16. Solomon SD, Ridker PM, Antman EM. Ventricular arrhythmias in trials of thrombolytic therapy for acute myocardial infarction. A meta-analysis. *Circulation* 1993;88:2575–2581.

17. de Soyza N, Bennett FA, Murphy ML, et al. The relationship of paroxysmal ventricular tachycardia complicating the acute phase and ventricular arrhythmia during the late hospital phase of myocardial infarction to long-term survival. *Am J Med* 1978;64:377–381.

18. Eldar M, Sievner Z, Goldbourt U, et al. Primary ventricular tachycardia in acute myocardial infarction: clinical characteristics and mortality. The SPRINT Study Group. *Ann Intern Med* 1992;117:31–36.

19. Bigger JT Jr, Weld FM, Rolnitzky LM. Prevalence, characteristics and significance of ventricular tachycardia (three or more complexes) detected with ambulatory electrocardiographic recording in the late hospital phase of acute myocardial infarction. *Am J Cardiol* 1981;48:815–823.

20. Anderson KP, DeCamilla J, Moss AJ. Clinical significance of ventricular tachycardia (3 beats or longer) detected during ambulatory monitoring after myocardial infarction. *Circulation* 1978;57:890–897.

21. Singh SN, Fisher SG, Carson PE, et al. Prevalence and significance of nonsustained ventricular tachycardia in patients with premature ventricular contractions and heart failure treated with vasodilator therapy. Department of Veterans Affairs CHF STAT Investigators. *J Am Coll Cardiol* 1998;32:942–947.

22. Wolfe CL, Nibley C, Bhandari A, et al. Polymorphous ventricular tachycardia associated with acute myocardial infarction. *Circulation* 1991;84:1543–1551.

23. Birnbaum Y, Sclarovsky S, Ben-Ami R, et al. Polymorphous ventricular tachycardia early after acute myocardial infarction. *Am J Cardiol* 1993;71:745–749.

24. Tofler GH, Stone PH, Muller JE, et al. Prognosis after cardiac arrest due to ventricular tachycardia or ventricular fibrillation associated with acute myocardial infarction (the MILIS Study). Multicenter Investigation of the Limitation of Infarct Size. *Am J Cardiol* 1987;60:755–761.

25. Berger PB, Ruocco NA, Ryan TJ, et al. Incidence and significance of ventricular tachycardia and fibrillation in the absence of hypotension or heart failure in acute myocardial infarction treated with recombinant tissue-type plasminogen activator: results from the Thrombolysis in Myocardial Infarction (TIMI) Phase II trial. *J Am Coll Cardiol* 1993;22:1773–1779.

26. Newby KH, Thompson T, Stebbins A, et al. Sustained ventricular arrhythmias in patients receiving thrombolytic therapy: incidence and outcomes. The GUSTO Investigators. *Circulation* 1998;98:2567–2573.

27. Wyse DG, Friedman PL, Brodsky MA, et al. Life-threatening ventricular arrhythmias due to transient or correctable causes: high risk for death in follow-up. *J Am Coll Cardiol* 2001;38:1718–1724.

28. Kleiman RB, Miller JM, Buxton AE, et al. Prognosis following sustained ventricular tachycardia occurring early after myocardial infarction. *Am J Cardiol* 1988;62:528–533.

29. Willems AR, Tijssen JG, van Capelle FJ, et al. Determinants of prognosis in symptomatic ventricular tachycardia or ventricular fibrillation late after myocardial infarction. The Dutch Ventricular Tachycardia Study Group of the Interuniversity Cardiology Institute of The Netherlands. *J Am Coll Cardiol* 1990;16:521–530.

30. Lawrie DM, Higgins MR, Godman MJ, et al. Ventricular fibrillation complicating acute myocardial infarction. *Lancet* 1968;2:523–528.

31. Nicod P, Gilpin E, Dittrich H, et al. Late clinical outcome in patients with early ventricular fibrillation after myocardial infarction. *J Am Coll Cardiol* 1988;11:464–470.

32. Behar S, Goldbourt U, Reicher-Reiss H, et al. Prognosis of acute myocardial infarction complicated by primary ventricular fibrillation. Principal Investigators of the SPRINT Study. *Am J Cardiol* 1990;66:1208–1211.

33. Jensen GV, Torp-Pedersen C, Kober L, et al. Prognosis of late versus early ventricular fibrillation in acute myocardial infarction. *Am J Cardiol* 1990;66:10–15.

34. Volpi A, Maggioni A, Franzosi MG, et al. In-hospital prognosis of patients with acute myocardial infarction complicated by primary ventricular fibrillation. *N Engl J Med* 1987;317:257–261.

35. Chiriboga D, Yarzebski J, Goldberg RJ, et al. Temporal trends (1975 through 1990) in the incidence and case-fatality rates of primary ventricular fibrillation complicating acute myocardial infarction. A communitywide perspective. *Circulation* 1994;89:998–1003.

36. Antman EM, Berlin JA. Declining incidence of ventricular fibrillation in myocardial infarction. Implications for the prophylactic use of lidocaine. *Circulation* 1992;86:764–773.

37. Behar S, Reicher-Reiss H, Shechter M, et al. Frequency and prognostic significance of secondary ventricular fibrillation complicating acute myocardial infarction. SPRINT Study Group. *Am J Cardiol* 1993;71:152–156.

38. Volpi A, Cavalli A, Santoro E, et al. Incidence and prognosis of secondary ventricular fibrillation in acute myocardial infarction. Evidence for a protective effect of thrombolytic therapy. GISSI Investigators. *Circulation* 1990;82:1279–1288.

39. Volpi A, Cavalli A, Franzosi MG, et al. One-year prognosis of primary ventricular fibrillation complicating acute myocardial infarction. The GISSI (Gruppo Italiano per lo Studio della Streptochinasi nell'Infarto miocardico) investigators. *Am J Cardiol* 1989;63:1174–1178.

40. Kleiman NS, Terrin M, Mueller H, et al. Mechanisms of early death despite thrombolytic therapy: experience from the Thrombolysis in Myocardial Infarction Phase II (TIMI II) study. *J Am Coll Cardiol* 1992;19:1129–1135.

41. Yusuf S, Sleight P, Held P, et al. Routine medical management of acute myocardial infarction. Lessons from overviews of recent randomized controlled trials. *Circulation* 1990;82:II117–II134.

42. Krumholz HM, Goldberger AL. Reperfusion arrhythmias after thrombolysis. Electrophysiologic tempest, or much ado about nothing. *Chest* 1991;99:135S–140S.

43. Kloner RA. Does reperfusion injury exist in humans? *J Am Coll Cardiol* 1993;21:537–545.

44. Goldberg S, Greenspon AJ, Urban PL, et al. Reperfusion arrhythmia: a marker of restoration of antegrade flow during intracoronary thrombolysis for acute myocardial infarction. *Am Heart J* 1983;105:26–32.

45. Cercek B, Horvat M. Arrhythmias with brief, high-dose intravenous streptokinase infusion in acute myocardial infarction. *Eur Heart J* 1985;6:109–113.

46. Gorgels AP, Vos MA, Letsch IS, et al. Usefulness of the accelerated idioventricular rhythm as a marker for myocardial necrosis and reperfusion during thrombolytic therapy in acute myocardial infarction. *Am J Cardiol* 1988;61:231–235.

47. Ganz W, Geft I, Shah PK, et al. Intravenous streptokinase in evolving acute myocardial infarction. *Am J Cardiol* 1984;53:1209–1216.

48. A prospective trial of intravenous streptokinase in acute myocardial infarction (I.S.A.M.). Mortality, morbidity, and infarct size at 21 days. The ISAM Study Group. *N Engl J Med* 1986;314:1465–1471.

49. Wilcox RG, von der Lippe G, Olsson CG, et al. Trial of tissue plasminogen activator for mortality reduction in acute myocardial infarction. Anglo-Scandinavian Study of Early Thrombolysis (ASSET). *Lancet* 1988;2:525–530.

50. Wilcox RG, Eastgate J, Harrison E, et al. Ventricular arrhythmias during treatment with alteplase (recombinant tissue plasminogen activator) in suspected acute myocardial infarction. *Br Heart J* 1991;65:4–8.

51. Effectiveness of intravenous thrombolytic treatment in acute myocardial infarction. Gruppo Italiano per lo Studio della Streptochinasi nell'Infarto Miocardico (GISSI). *Lancet* 1986;1:397–402.

52. Randomised trial of intravenous streptokinase, oral aspirin, both, or neither among 17,187 cases of suspected acute myocardial infarction: ISIS-2. ISIS-2 (Second International Study of Infarct Survival) Collaborative Group. *Lancet* 1988;2:349–360.

53. Hohnloser SH, Zabel M, Kasper W, et al. Assessment of coronary artery patency after thrombolytic therapy: accurate prediction utilizing the combined analysis of three noninvasive markers. *J Am Coll Cardiol* 1991;18:44–49.

54. Six AJ, Louwerenburg JH, Kingma JH, et al. Predictive value of ventricular arrhythmias for patency of the infarct-related coronary artery after thrombolytic therapy. *Br Heart J* 1991;66:143–146.

55. Hackett D, McKenna W, Davies G, et al. Reperfusion arrhythmias are rare during acute myocardial infarction and thrombolysis in man. *Int J Cardiol* 1990;29:205–213.

56. Gore JM, Ball SP, Corrao JM, et al. Arrhythmias in the assessment of coronary artery reperfusion following thrombolytic therapy. *Chest* 1988;94:727–730.

57. Gressin V, Gorgels A, Louvard Y, et al. ST-segment normalization time and ventricular arrhythmias as electrocardiographic markers of reperfusion during intravenous thrombolysis for acute myocardial infarction. *Am J Cardiol* 1993;71:1436–1439.

58. Califf RM, O'Neil W, Stack RS, et al. Failure of simple clinical measurements to predict perfusion status after intravenous thrombolysis. *Ann Intern Med* 1988;108:658–662.

59. Kircher BJ, Topol EJ, O'Neill WW, et al. Prediction of infarct coronary artery recanalization after intravenous thrombolytic therapy. *Am J Cardiol* 1987;59:513–515.

60. Tobe TJ, de Langen CD, Crijns HJ, et al. Effects of streptokinase during acute myocardial infarction on the signal-averaged electrocardiogram and on the frequency of late arrhythmias. *Am J Cardiol* 1993;72:647–651.

61. Pedretti R, Laporta A, Etro MD, et al. Influence of thrombolysis on signal-averaged electrocardiogram and late arrhythmic events after acute myocardial infarction. *Am J Cardiol* 1992;69:866–872.

62. Chew EW, Morton P, Murtagh JG, et al. Intravenous streptokinase for acute myocardial infarction reduces the occurrence of ventricular late potentials. *Br Heart J* 1990;64:5–8.

63. Eldar M, Leor J, Hod H, et al. Effect of thrombolysis on the evolution of late potentials within 10 days of infarction. *Br Heart J* 1990;63:273–276.

64. Zimmermann M, Adamec R, Ciaroni S. Reduction in the frequency of ventricular late potentials after acute myocardial infarction by early thrombolytic therapy. *Am J Cardiol* 1991;67:697–703.

65. Gang ES, Lew AS, Hong M, et al. Decreased incidence of ventricular late potentials after successful thrombolytic therapy for acute myocardial infarction. *N Engl J Med* 1989;321:712–716.

66. Turitto G, Risa AL, Zanchi E, et al. The signal-averaged electrocardiogram and ventricular arrhythmias after thrombolysis for acute myocardial infarction. *J Am Coll Cardiol* 1990;15:1270–1276.

67. Vatterott PJ, Hammill SC, Bailey KR, et al. Late potentials on signal-averaged electrocardiograms and patency of the infarct-related artery in survivors of acute myocardial infarction. *J Am Coll Cardiol* 1991;17:330–337.

68. Lange RA, Cigarroa RG, Wells PJ, et al. Influence of anterograde flow in the infarct artery on the incidence of late potentials after acute myocardial infarction. *Am J Cardiol* 1990;65:554–558.

69. Tranchesi B Jr, Verstraete M, Van de Werf F, et al. Usefulness of high-frequency analysis of signal-averaged surface electrocardiograms in acute myocardial infarction before and after coronary thrombolysis for assessing coronary reperfusion. *Am J Cardiol* 1990;66:1196–1198.

70. Leor J, Hod H, Rotstein Z, et al. Effects of thrombolysis on the 12-lead signal-averaged ECG in the early postinfarction period. *Am Heart J* 1990;120:495–502.

71. Pedretti RF, Colombo E, Sarzi Braga S, et al. Effect of thrombolysis on heart rate variability and life-threatening ventricular arrhythmias in survivors of acute myocardial infarction. *J Am Coll Cardiol* 1994;23:19–26.

72. Sager PT, Perlmutter RA, Rosenfeld LE, et al. Electrophysiologic effects of thrombolytic therapy in patients with a transmural anterior myocardial infarction complicated by left ventricular aneurysm formation. *J Am Coll Cardiol* 1988;12:19–24.

73. Kersschot IE, Brugada P, Ramentol M, et al. Effects of early reperfusion in acute myocardial infarction on arrhythmias induced by programmed stimulation: a prospective, randomized study. *J Am Coll Cardiol* 1986;7:1234–1242.

74. Bourke JP, Young AA, Richards DA, et al. Reduction in incidence of inducible ventricular tachycardia after myocardial infarction by treatment with streptokinase during infarct evolution. *J Am Coll Cardiol* 1990;16:1703–1710.

75. El-Sherif N, Myerburg RJ, Scherlag BJ, et al. Electrocardiographic antecedents of primary ventricular fibrillation. Value of the R-on-T phenomenon in myocardial infarction. *Br Heart J* 1976;38:415–422.

76. Gorgels AP, van den Dool A, Hofs A, et al. Comparison of procainamide and lidocaine in terminating sustained monomorphic ventricular tachycardia. *Am J Cardiol* 1996;78:43–46.

77. Kern KB, Halperin HR, Field J. New guidelines for cardiopulmonary resuscitation and emergency cardiac care: changes in the management of cardiac arrest. *JAMA* 2001;285:1267–1269.

78. Guidelines 2000 for Cardiopulmonary Resuscitation and Emergency Cardiovascular Care. Part 6: advanced cardiovascular life support: 7D: the tachycardia algorithms. The American Heart Association in collaboration with the International Liaison Committee on Resuscitation. *Circulation* 2000;102:I1-384.

79. Kerber RE, Kienzle MG, Olshansky B, et al. Ventricular tachycardia rate and morphology determine energy and current requirements for transthoracic cardioversion. *Circulation* 1992;85:158–163.

80. Kowey PR, Levine JH, Herre JM, et al. Randomized, double-blind comparison of intravenous amiodarone and bretylium in the treatment of patients with recurrent, hemodynamically destabilizing ventricular tachycardia or fibrillation. The Intravenous Amiodarone Multicenter Investigators Group. *Circulation* 1995;92:3255–3263.

81. Levine JH, Massumi A, Scheinman MM, et al. Intravenous amiodarone for recurrent sustained hypotensive ventricular tachyarrhythmias. Intravenous Amiodarone Multicenter Trial Group. *J Am Coll Cardiol* 1996;27:67–75.

82. Kudenchuk PJ, Cobb LA, Copass MK, et al. Amiodarone for resuscitation after out-of-hospital cardiac arrest due to ventricular fibrillation. *N Engl J Med* 1999;341:871–878.

83. Dorian P, Cass D, Schwartz B, et al. Amiodarone as compared with lidocaine for shock-resistant ventricular fibrillation. *N Engl J Med* 2002;346:884–890.

84. Lindner KH, Dirks B, Strohmenger HU, et al. Randomised comparison of epinephrine and vasopressin in patients with out-of-hospital ventricular fibrillation. *Lancet* 1997;349:535–537.

85. Stiell IG, Hebert PC, Wells GA, et al. Vasopressin versus epinephrine for inhospital cardiac arrest: a randomised controlled trial. *Lancet* 2001;358:105–109.

86. Lie KI, Wellens HJ, van Capelle FJ, et al. Lidocaine in the prevention of primary ventricular fibrillation. A double-blind, randomized study of 212 consecutive patients. *N Engl J Med* 1974;291:1324–1326.

87. MacMahon S, Collins R, Peto R, et al. Effects of prophylactic lidocaine in suspected acute myocardial infarction. An overview of results from the randomized, controlled trials. *JAMA* 1988;260:1910–1916.

88. Hine LK, Laird N, Hewitt P, et al. Meta-analytic evidence against prophylactic use of lidocaine in acute myocardial infarction. *Arch Intern Med* 1989;149:2694–2698.

89. Sadowski ZP, Alexander JH, Skrabucha B, et al. Multicenter randomized trial and a systematic overview of lidocaine in acute myocardial infarction. *Am Heart J* 1999;137:792–798.

90. Alexander JH, Granger CB, Sadowski Z, et al. Prophylactic lidocaine use in acute myocardial infarction: incidence and outcomes from two international trials. The GUSTO-I and GUSTO-IIb Investigators. *Am Heart J* 1999;137:799–805.

91. Hohnloser SH, Zabel M, Olschewski M, et al. Arrhythmias during the acute phase of reperfusion therapy for acute myocardial infarction: effects of beta-adrenergic blockade. *Am Heart J* 1992;123:1530–1535.

92. Podrid PJ, Fuchs T, Candinas R. Role of the sympathetic nervous system in the genesis of ventricular arrhythmia. *Circulation* 1990;82:I103–I113.

93. Hjalmarson A, Elmfeldt D, Herlitz J, et al. Effect on mortality of metoprolol in acute myocardial infarction. A double-blind randomised trial. *Lancet* 1981;2:823–827.

94. Hjalmarson A, Olsson G. Myocardial infarction. Effects of beta-blockade. *Circulation* 1991;84:VI101–VI107.

95. Ryden L, Arinicgo R, Arman K, et al. A double-blind trial of metoprolol in acute myocardial infarction. Effects on ventricular tachyarrhythmias. *N Engl J Med* 1983;308:614–618.

96. Norris RM, Barnaby PF, Brown MA, et al. Prevention of ventricular fibrillation during acute myocardial infarction by intravenous propranolol. *Lancet* 1984;2:883–886.
97. Randomised trial of intravenous atenolol among 16 027 cases of suspected acute myocardial infarction: ISIS-1. First International Study of Infarct Survival Collaborative Group. *Lancet* 1986;2:57–66.
98. Metoprolol in acute myocardial infarction (MIAMI). A randomised placebo-controlled international trial. The MIAMI Trial Research Group. *Eur Heart J* 1985;6:199–226.
99. Yusuf S, Wittes J, Friedman L. Overview of results of randomized clinical trials in heart disease. I. Treatments following myocardial infarction. *JAMA* 1988;260:2088–2093.
100. Yusuf S, Sleight P, Rossi P, et al. Reduction in infarct size, arrhythmias and chest pain by early intravenous beta blockade in suspected acute myocardial infarction. *Circulation* 1983;67:I32–I41.
101. Murray DP, Murray RG, Littler WA. The effects of metoprolol given early in acute myocardial infarction on ventricular arrhythmias. *Eur Heart J* 1986;7:217–222.
102. Olsson G, Held P. Early intravenous beta blockade and thrombolytics in acute myocardial infarction. *Am J Cardiol* 1993;72:156G–160G.
103. Lichstein E, Morganroth J, Harrist R, et al. Effect of propranolol on ventricular arrhythmia. The beta-blocker heart attack trial experience. *Circulation* 1983;67:I5–I10.
104. Yusuf S, Peto R, Lewis J, et al. Beta blockade during and after myocardial infarction: an overview of the randomized trials. *Prog Cardiovasc Dis* 1985;27:335–371.
105. Roberts R, Rogers WJ, Mueller HS, et al. Immediate versus deferred beta-blockade following thrombolytic therapy in patients with acute myocardial infarction. Results of the Thrombolysis in Myocardial Infarction (TIMI) II-B Study. *Circulation* 1991;83:422–437.
106. Van de Werf F, Janssens L, Brzostek T, et al. Short-term effects of early intravenous treatment with a beta-adrenergic blocking agent or a specific bradycardiac agent in patients with acute myocardial infarction receiving thrombolytic therapy. *J Am Coll Cardiol* 1993;22:407–416.
107. Woods KL, Fletcher S, Roffe C, et al. Intravenous magnesium sulphate in suspected acute myocardial infarction: results of the second Leicester Intravenous Magnesium Intervention Trial (LIMIT-2). *Lancet* 1992;339:1553–1558.
108. Shechter M, Kaplinsky E, Rabinowitz B. The rationale of magnesium supplementation in acute myocardial infarction. A review of the literature. *Arch Intern Med* 1992;152:2189–2196.
109. Woods KL. Possible pharmacological actions of magnesium in acute myocardial infarction. *Br J Clin Pharmacol* 1991;32:3–10.
110. Ryzen E, Elkayam U, Rude RK. Low blood mononuclear cell magnesium in intensive cardiac care unit patients. *Am Heart J* 1986;111:475–480.
111. Rasmussen HS, McNair P, Goransson L, et al. Magnesium deficiency in patients with ischemic heart disease with and without acute myocardial infarction uncovered by an intravenous loading test. *Arch Intern Med* 1988;148:329–332.
112. Abraham AS, Eylath U, Weinstein M, et al. Serum magnesium levels in patients with acute myocardial infarction. *N Engl J Med* 1977;296:862–863.
113. Smith LF, Heagerty AM, Bing RF, et al. Intravenous infusion of magnesium sulphate after acute myocardial infarction: effects on arrhythmias and mortality. *Int J Cardiol* 1986;12:175–183.
114. Abraham AS, Rosenmann D, Kramer M, et al. Magnesium in the prevention of lethal arrhythmias in acute myocardial infarction. *Arch Intern Med* 1987;147:753–755.
115. Ceremuzynski L, Jurgiel R, Kulakowski P, et al. Threatening arrhythmias in acute myocardial infarction are prevented by intravenous magnesium sulfate. *Am Heart J* 1989;118:1333–1334.
116. Rasmussen HS, McNair P, Norregard P, et al. Intravenous magnesium in acute myocardial infarction. *Lancet* 1986;1:234–236.
117. Thogersen AM, Johnson O, Wester PO. Effects of intravenous magnesium sulphate in suspected acute myocardial infarction on acute arrhythmias and long-term outcome. *Int J Cardiol* 1995;49:143–151.
118. Shechter M, Hod H, Marks N, et al. Beneficial effect of magnesium sulfate in acute myocardial infarction. *Am J Cardiol* 1990;66:271–274.
119. Teo KK, Yusuf S, Collins R, et al. Effects of intravenous magnesium in suspected acute myocardial infarction: overview of randomised trials. *BMJ* 1991;303:1499–1503.
120. Feldstedt M, Boesgaard S, Bouchelouche P, et al. Magnesium substi-
121. Santoro GM, Antoniucci D, Bolognese L, et al. A randomized study of intravenous magnesium in acute myocardial infarction treated with direct coronary angioplasty. *Am Heart J* 2000;140:891–897.
122. Ziegelstein RC, Hilbe JM, French WJ, et al. Magnesium use in the treatment of acute myocardial infarction in the United States (observations from the Second National Registry of Myocardial Infarction). *Am J Cardiol* 2001;87:7–10.
123. Thogersen AM, Johnson O, Wester PO. Effects of magnesium infusion on thrombolytic and non-thrombolytic treated patients with acute myocardial infarction. *Int J Cardiol* 1993;39:13–22.
124. ISIS-4: a randomised factorial trial assessing early oral captopril, oral mononitrate, and intravenous magnesium sulphate in 58,050 patients with suspected acute myocardial infarction. ISIS-4 (Fourth International Study of Infarct Survival) Collaborative Group. *Lancet* 1995;345:669–685.
125. Tzivoni D, Keren A, Cohen AM, et al. Magnesium therapy for torsades de pointes. *Am J Cardiol* 1984;53:528–530.
126. Iseri LT, Chung P, Tobis J. Magnesium therapy for intractable ventricular tachyarrhythmias in normomagnesemic patients. *West J Med* 1983;138:823–828.
127. Fatovich DM, Prentice DA, Dobb GJ. Magnesium in cardiac arrest (the magic trial). *Resuscitation* 1997;35:237–241.
128. Hassan TB, Jagger C, Barnett DB. A randomised trial to investigate the efficacy of magnesium sulphate for refractory ventricular fibrillation. *Emerg Med J* 2002;19:57–62.
129. Myerburg RJ, Kessler KM, Castellanos A. Sudden cardiac death: epidemiology, transient risk, and intervention assessment. *Ann Intern Med* 1993;119:1187–1197.
130. The beta-blocker heart attack trial. beta-Blocker Heart Attack Study Group. *JAMA* 1981;246:2073–2074.
131. Huikuri HV, Castellanos A, Myerburg RJ. Sudden death due to cardiac arrhythmias. *N Engl J Med* 2001;345:1473–1482.
132. Gottlieb SS, McCarter RJ, Vogel RA. Effect of beta-blockade on mortality among high-risk and low-risk patients after myocardial infarction. *N Engl J Med* 1998;339:489–497.
133. Timolol-induced reduction in mortality and reinfarction in patients surviving acute myocardial infarction. *N Engl J Med* 1981;304:801–807.
134. Echt DS, Liebson PR, Mitchell LB, et al. Mortality and morbidity in patients receiving encainide, flecainide, or placebo. The Cardiac Arrhythmia Suppression Trial. *N Engl J Med* 1991;324:781–788.
135. Effect of the antiarrhythmic agent moricizine on survival after myocardial infarction. The Cardiac Arrhythmia Suppression Trial II Investigators. *N Engl J Med* 1992;327:227–233.
136. Nademanee K, Singh BN, Stevenson WG, et al. Amiodarone and post-MI patients. *Circulation* 1993;88:764–774.
137. Hine LK, Laird NM, Hewitt P, et al. Meta-analysis of empirical long-term antiarrhythmic therapy after myocardial infarction. *JAMA* 1989;262:3037–3040.
138. Teo KK, Yusuf S, Furberg CD. Effects of prophylactic antiarrhythmic drug therapy in acute myocardial infarction. An overview of results from randomized controlled trials. *JAMA* 1993;270:1589–1595.
139. Ceremuzynski L, Kleczar E, Krzeminska-Pakula M, et al. Effect of amiodarone on mortality after myocardial infarction: a double-blind, placebo-controlled, pilot study. *J Am Coll Cardiol* 1992;20:1056–1062.
140. Burkart F, Pfisterer M, Kiowski W, et al. Effect of antiarrhythmic therapy on mortality in survivors of myocardial infarction with asymptomatic complex ventricular arrhythmias: Basel Antiarrhythmic Study of Infarct Survival (BASIS). *J Am Coll Cardiol* 1990;16:1711–1718.
141. Cairns JA, Connolly SJ, Gent M, et al. Post-myocardial infarction mortality in patients with ventricular premature depolarizations. Canadian Amiodarone Myocardial Infarction Arrhythmia Trial Pilot Study. *Circulation* 1991;84:550–557.
142. Pfisterer M, Kiowski W, Burckhardt D, et al. Beneficial effect of amiodarone on cardiac mortality in patients with asymptomatic complex ventricular arrhythmias after acute myocardial infarction and preserved but not impaired left ventricular function. *Am J Cardiol* 1992;69:1399–1402.
143. Pfisterer ME, Kiowski W, Brunner H, et al. Long-term benefit of 1-year amiodarone treatment for persistent complex ventricular arrhythmias after myocardial infarction. *Circulation* 1993;87:309–311.
144. Navarro-Lopez F, Cosin J, Marrugat J, et al. Comparison of the effects

of amiodarone versus metoprolol on the frequency of ventricular arrhythmias and on mortality after acute myocardial infarction. SSSD Investigators. Spanish Study on Sudden Death. *Am J Cardiol* 1993; 72:1243–1248.

145. Zarembski DG, Nolan PE Jr, Slack MK, et al. Empiric long-term amiodarone prophylaxis following myocardial infarction. A meta-analysis. *Arch Intern Med* 1993;153:2661–2667.

146. Cairns JA, Connolly SJ, Roberts R, et al. Randomised trial of outcome after myocardial infarction in patients with frequent or repetitive ventricular premature depolarisations: CAMIAT. Canadian Amiodarone Myocardial Infarction Arrhythmia Trial Investigators. *Lancet* 1997;349:675–682.

147. Julian DG, Camm AJ, Frangin G, et al. Randomised trial of effect of amiodarone on mortality in patients with left-ventricular dysfunction after recent myocardial infarction: EMIAT. European Myocardial Infarct Amiodarone Trial Investigators. *Lancet* 1997;349:667–674.

148. Julian DG, Prescott RJ, Jackson FS, et al. Controlled trial of sotalol for one year after myocardial infarction. *Lancet* 1982;1:1142–1147.

149. Waldo AL, Camm AJ, deRuyter H, et al. Effect of d-sotalol on mortality in patients with left ventricular dysfunction after recent and remote myocardial infarction. The SWORD Investigators. Survival With Oral d-Sotalol. *Lancet* 1996;348:7–12.

150. Kober L, Bloch Thomsen PE, Moller M, et al. Effect of dofetilide in patients with recent myocardial infarction and left-ventricular dysfunction: a randomised trial. *Lancet* 2000;356:2052–2058.

151. Camm AJ, Pratt CM, Schwartz PJ, et al. Mortality in patients after a recent myocardial infarction. A randomized placebo-controlled trial of azimilide using heart rate variability for risk stratification. *Circulation* 2004;109:990–996.

152. Bigger JT Jr. Prophylactic use of implanted cardiac defibrillators in patients at high risk for ventricular arrhythmias after coronary-artery bypass graft surgery. Coronary Artery Bypass Graft (CABG) Patch Trial Investigators. *N Engl J Med* 1997;337:1569–1575.

153. Moss AJ, Hall WJ, Cannom DS, et al. Improved survival with an implanted defibrillator in patients with coronary disease at high risk for ventricular arrhythmia. Multicenter Automatic Defibrillator Implantation Trial Investigators. *N Engl J Med* 1996;335:1933–1940.

154. Buxton AE, Lee KL, Fisher JD, et al. A randomized study of the prevention of sudden death in patients with coronary artery disease. Multicenter Unsustained Tachycardia Trial Investigators. *N Engl J Med* 1999;341:1882–1890.

155. Moss AJ, Zareba W, Hall WJ, et al. Prophylactic implantation of a defibrillator in patients with myocardial infarction and reduced ejection fraction. *N Engl J Med* 2002;346:877–883.

156. A comparison of antiarrhythmic-drug therapy with implantable defibrillators in patients resuscitated from near-fatal ventricular arrhythmias. The Antiarrhythmics versus Implantable Defibrillators (AVID) Investigators. Investigators TAvIDA, *N Engl J Med* 1997;337:1576–1583.

157. Domanski MJ, Sakseena S, Epstein AE, et al. Relative effectiveness of the implantable cardioverter-defibrillator and antiarrhythmic drugs in patients with varying degrees of left ventricular dysfunction who have survived malignant ventricular arrhythmias. AVID Investigators. Antiarrhythmics Versus Implantable Defibrillators. *J Am Coll Cardiol* 1999;34:1090–1095.

158. Kuck KH, Cappato R, Siebels J, et al. Randomized comparison of antiarrhythmic drug therapy with implantable defibrillators in patients resuscitated from cardiac arrest: the Cardiac Arrest Study Hamburg (CASH). *Circulation* 2000;102:748–754.

159. Connolly SJ, Gent M, Roberts RS, et al. Canadian implantable defibrillator study (CIDS): a randomized trial of the implantable cardioverter defibrillator against amiodarone. *Circulation* 2000;101:1297–1302.

CHAPTER 71

Atherothrombosis, The Conduction System, and Cardiac Pacing

S. Serge Barold and J. Warren Harthorne

Key Words: Acute myocardial infarction; arrhythmia; atrioventricular block; cardiac pacing; electrocardiography; thrombolysis.

INTRODUCTION

There is little doubt that disorders of cardiac conduction, in the form of either impulse generation or transmission, can occur in acute ischemic syndromes secondary to occlusive coronary disease (1,2), coronary spasm in variant angina (3,4), or transient occlusion caused by a myocardial bridge (5). Less clear is the correlation between chronic conduction system disease involving "sick sinus syndrome," the fascicular blocks, and variable degrees of chronic atrioventricular (AV) block and causative coronary arterial obstruction in an aging population of patients (6). Indeed, many of the disease states involving the cardiac conduction system that culminate in pacemaker prescription are the consequence of senescent changes that affect the sinoatrial node (7), the AV node (8), or the lower ramifications of the His-Purkinje system (9,10). Sick sinus syndrome is

almost never caused by acute myocardial infarction (MI). However, myocardial ischemia can rarely cause sinus node hibernation potentially reversible with angioplasty (11).

In acute MI, AV block is a marker for infarct size. AV block is more common in inferior MI than anterior MI (12–14). High-degree AV block (defined as second- or third-degree block in this chapter) is associated in both the prethrombolytic and thrombolytic era with larger infarcts, greater incidence of complications, and mortality (13–16). With anterior wall infarction, the implications of damage to the cardiac conduction system are ominous, and mortality is seldom altered by temporary cardiac pacing, although such intervention may stabilize the patient so that interventional angiographic procedures including surgical bypass may be considered. Patients who experience development of second- or third-degree AV block with a non–Q-wave MI have a poor hospital course, larger infarcts, and a high mortality that require an early aggressive approach soon after admission (17).

ACUTE INFERIOR MYOCARDIAL INFARCTION

Pathology of Atrioventricular Block

Bilbao and coworkers (18) described the pathologic findings in the hearts of 44 patients who died of acute posterior MI

S. S. Barold: Division of Cardiology, University of South Florida College of Medicine, and Tampa General Hospital, Tampa, Florida.

J. W. Harthorne: Massachusetts General Hospital, Boston, Massachusetts.

(third-degree AV block was found in 26 cases, and second-degree AV block in 4, i.e., 30 hearts with AV block). The authors found a close correlation between the occurrence of AV block and necrosis of the prenodal (supranodal) atrial myocardial fibers. Twenty-nine of 30 hearts with AV block (97%) showed ischemic lesions involving the atrial prenodal fibers. Only 11 of these 29 hearts revealed acute changes in the AV node, in the His bundle, or in both. Eleven of the 14 hearts in the group without AV block also showed no lesions in the prenodal atrial myocardium, whereas 3 showed acute prenodal myocardial necrosis. Nineteen cases with necrosis of the atrial prenodal myocardium were associated with an otherwise normal conduction system, and AV block was recorded in 18 of these 19 patients. Isolated necrosis of the specialized conduction system was not present without necrosis of the atrial prenodal fibers. The response of AV block to pharmacologic therapy or spontaneous reversion was correlated with the absence of acute lesions in the conduction system. Seventy-five percent of AV blocks that responded to treatment did not have necrosis of the specialized conduction system. There was no correlation between chronic lesions and AV block.

Hackel and coworkers (19) reported an autopsy study of 17 hearts with inferior MI with complete heart block (CHB) and 5 without CHB. There was predominant necrosis of the proximal part of the conduction system located anteriorly. In the CHB group, the atrial approaches to the AV node were involved with infarction in 9 of 17 cases, the AV node in 4 of 17 cases, the His bundle in 2 cases, and the posterior left

bundle in 3 cases. In those without AV block, only one of the hearts showed slight necrotic changes in the atrial approach to the AV node. The observation of Hackel and coworkers (19) confirmed those of Bilbao and coworkers (18) in that inferior wall MI tends to affect mainly the atrial approaches to the AV node, to a lesser degree the AV node itself, and more rarely the His bundle.

Ohkawa and Hackel (20) studied seven hearts from patients who died of right ventricular (RV) MI with AV block (six with posterior MI and one with anterior MI). They found necrosis of the AV node in three cases, His bundle in two cases, left bundle in three cases, and right bundle in one case. Although the number of patients was small, these observations correlate with the greater occurrence of second- and third-degree AV block in patients with RV MI.

Atrioventricular Block in the Prethrombolytic Era

High-degree AV block occurs in about 18% to 20% of patients with acute inferior wall MI (Table 71–1). Complete AV block constitutes approximately 60% of high-degree AV block in this situation. Table 71–2 shows how in the prethrombolytic era the mortality of inferior MI complicated by high-degree AV block averaged 21% (range 11–44%) compared with 9% (range 4–15%) in inferior MI without high-degree AV block. In the prethrombolytic era, the mortality of inferior MI complicated by complete AV block was 33% (range 0–45%) compared with 11% (range

TABLE 71–1. *Incidence of second- and third-degree heart block in acute inferior infarction: prethrombolytic era*

Study (reference)	Patients, n	Second-degree, %	Third-degree, %	Second- and third-degree, %
Rotman et al. (21)	181	7	18	25
Jewitt (22)	128	16	12	28
Julian et al. (23)	44	9	16	25
Stock and Macken (24)	130	5	8	13
Tans et al. (25)	843	6	11	17
Bassan et al. (26)	51	10	8	18
Gupta et al. (27)	80	?	15	?
Brown et al. (28)	160	?	8	?
Nicod et al. (29)	749	?	13	?
Kaul et al. (30)	82	?	?	34
Feigl et al. (31)	288	?	?	13
Braat et al. (32)	67	?	?	28
Dubois et al. (33)	477	10	10	20
Norris (34)	96	?	?	27
Courter et al. (35)	35	?	?	26
Katz et al. (36)	167	8	6	14
Gupta et al. (37)	410	6	9	15
McDonald et al. (38)	356	?	?	12
Mavric et al. (39)	243	?	16	?
Behar et al. (40)	2,273	6	11	17
Goldberg et al. (41)	2,241	?	8	?
Total				18

A few patients received thrombolytic therapy in the reports of Mavric et al. (39) and Goldberg et al. (41). The use of thrombolytic therapy was not stated in the report of McDonald et al. (38).

Adapted from Berger PB, Ryan TJ. Inferior wall myocardial infarction high-risk subgroups. *Circulation* 1990;81:401–410, with permission.

TABLE 71–2. *Hospital mortality in acute inferior myocardial infarction complicated by second- and third-degree heart block: prethrombolytic era*

Study	Year	AV block, n	Mortality rate, %	No AV block, n	Mortality rate, %
McDonald et al. (38)	1990	44	20	312	7
Dubois et al. (33)	1989	88	24	359	4
Kaul et al. (30)	1986	28	11	54	6
Sclarovsky et al. (42)	1984	76	13	?	?
Strasberg et al. (43)	1984	26	15	113	6
Tans et al. (25)	1980	144	22	699	9
Gupta et al. (27)	1976	60	28	?	?
Rotman et al. (21)	1973	45	24	136	15
Beregovich et al. (44)	1969	13	23	?	?
Norris (34)	1969	26	19	?	?
Chatterjeee et al. (45)	1969	65	23	?	?
Friedberg et al. (46)	1900	16	44	?	?
Total			21		9

AV, atrioventricular.
Adapted from Berger PB, Ryan TJ. Inferior wall myocardial infarction high-risk subgroups. *Circulation* 1990;81:401–410, with permission.

6% to 14%) in patients without high-degree AV block or without complete AV block (considered together according to data analysis in the various reports; Table 71–3). Berger and Ryan (54) have emphasized that few of the patients reported in the literature were believed to have died as a direct consequence of their heart block (although many died with persistent heart block) or from treatment of the heart block.

High-degree AV block in inferior MI is associated with a greater incidence of the following: (a) right and left ventricular dysfunction (15,30,43,55), left ventricular failure (25, 29,33,39–41,55,56), cardiogenic shock, and sustained hypotension (15,25,40,41,55); (b) atrial or ventricular arrhythmias (33,40,41,55); and (c) increased peak creatine phosphokinase (15,29,37–39,41,57) (except in the study of

Dubois and coworkers [33]) and serum glutamic oxaloacetic transaminase (SGOT) levels (25,40) and larger infarct size (57). All these complications reflect more extensive myocardial damage in patients with high-degree AV block compared with those without AV block—that is, AV block is a marker for a larger infarct size. Furthermore, in some studies, CHB appears to be an independent predictor of increased in-hospital mortality in acute MI (29,38,55,56).

Early versus Late Development of Atrioventricular Blocks

There are two patterns of occurrence of AV block in acute inferior MI. One study suggested that the time of appearance of AV block does not seem to affect the prognosis of in-hospital patients with acute inferior MI (58).

TABLE 71–3. *Hospital mortality in acute inferior myocardial infarction complicated by complete heart block: prethrombolytic era*

Study	Year	AV block, n	Mortality rate, %	No AV block, n	Mortality rate, %
Behar et al. (40)	1993	251	37	1890 (2/3)	11
Goldberg et al. (41)	1992	186	42	2241 (3)	14
Mavric et al. (39)	1990	39	26	204 (3)	11
Nicod et al. (29)	1988	95	24	654 (3)	6
Rodrigues et al. (47)	1987	111	32	?	?
Tans et al. (25)	1980	94	21	699 (2/3)	9
Gupta et al. (27)	1978	12	42	?	?
Leth et al. (48)	1974	36	22	?	?
Christiansen et al. (49)	1973	16	19	?	?
Kostuk and Beanlands (50)	1970	20	45	?	?
Brown et al. (28)	1969	16	25	?	?
Lassers and Julian (51)	1968	33	27	?	?
Gregory and Grace (52)	1968	16	31	?	?
Stock and Macken (24)	1968	11	0	?	?
Paulk and Hurst (53)	1966	32	41	?	?
Total			33		11

AV, atrioventricular.
Adapted from Berger PB, Ryan TJ. Inferior wall myocardial infarction high-risk subgroups. *Circulation* 1990;81:401–410, with permission.

Early-Onset Atrioventricular Block

Early-onset AV block develops in the first 6 hours from the onset of symptoms and often is present at the time of admission to the hospital. About 40% of the patients who experience development of high-degree AV block during hospitalization actually present with it on admission. The AV block often occurs abruptly, in contrast with the gradual onset of the late form of AV block, and usually presents with complete AV block and a slow ventricular rate. The duration of AV block is relatively short (<12 hours). Early AV block probably results from hypervagotonia and often responds favorably to atropine, although Sclarovsky and coworkers (42) found that only one-third of their patients responded to atropine. As a rule, this type of AV block rarely requires temporary pacing.

Late Atrioventricular Block

Late AV block occurs beyond 6 hours, generally in the first 3 days, and rarely develops as late as the fifth day. This form of AV block evolves gradually, progressing from first- and second-degree AV block (type I second-degree AV block and 2:1 AV block). It is not vagally mediated and does not generally respond to atropine. Rather, it reflects ischemia or metabolic abnormalities of the AV node. The AV block usually persists for a few days, sometimes as long as 16 days, but rarely longer. About 65% of all patients who experience development of early or late high-degree AV block do so within 24 hours of admission; but in about 35% of patients, AV block occurs after 24 hours (25,27,29,31–33,42,50). A few patients experience development of both early and late AV block with intervening 1:1 AV conduction. Patients with complete AV block within 6 hours of symptom onset and a reperfused inferior MI have a better prognosis and less myocardial damage if the atrial rate of 75 beats per minute or less than when the atrial rate is greater than 75 beats per minute (59).

Long-Term Prognosis of Atrioventricular Block

All studies involving more than 25 patients with AV block indicate that in the prethrombolytic era, patients who survived inferior MI complicated by second- or third-degree AV blocks demonstrated no increased long-term mortality when compared with patients who never developed second- or third-degree AV block (29,33,40,41,60).

Atrioventricular Block in the Thrombolytic Era

Berger and coworkers (56) studied 1,786 patients with acute inferior MI enrolled in the Thrombolysis in Myocardial Infarction (TIMI) II trial who received recombinant tissue plasminogen activator (t-PA) within 4 hours of the onset of symptoms. High-degree AV block (second- or third-degree) occurred in 214 patients (12%); 113 patients demonstrated high-degree AV block on admission (6.3%), and 101 (5.7%) experienced development of high-degree AV block in the first 24 hours after treatment with t-PA. The right coronary artery was more often the infarct-related artery among patients with compared with patients without high-degree AV block. Furthermore, occlusion of the infarct-related artery was more frequent in patients with high-degree AV block compared with those without high-degree AV block after treatment with t-PA. The 21-day mortality rate among the patients with high-degree AV block at the time of admission was 7.1% compared with 2.7% among patients without AV block. In contrast, the 21-day mortality rate increased to 9.9% in patients in whom high-degree AV block developed by 24 hours after hospital admission compared with 2.2% in patients without AV block by 24 hours. Follow-up data suggest that 1-year mortality after hospital discharge was increased in survivors who experienced development of high-degree AV block by 24 hours (not on admission) after thrombolytic therapy (14.9%) compared with survivors who did not (4.2%; $p = 0.001$). In contrast, 1-year mortality after hospital discharge was not increased in survivors in whom high-degree AV block developed on admission (before receiving thrombolytic therapy) compared with survivors in the control group without early (or entry) high-degree AV block.

The Thrombolysis and Angioplasty in Acute Myocardial Infarction (TAMI) investigators studied 373 patients with acute inferior MI on the basis of total occlusion of the right coronary artery demonstrated by angiography (55). Patients with acute occlusion of other arteries were excluded. Fifty patients (13.4%) experienced development of complete AV block—complete AV block occurred in 27 patients (7.2%) before and in 23 patients (6.2%) in the 24 hours after thrombolytic therapy. The incidence of *complete* AV block is greater in this study than others in the thrombolytic era probably because of a selected patient population with total occlusion of the right coronary artery (13,14,55,56). Complete AV block was of brief duration (<12 hours) in 75% of patients and lasted a median of only 2.5 hours. The mortality rate among patients with complete AV block was 20% compared with 4% among patients without complete AV block ($p < 0.001$). Acute patency rates of the right coronary artery after thrombolytic therapy were similar in patients with or without AV block. However, the reocclusion rate was greater in patients with complete AV block (29% vs. 16%; $p = 0.03$). After a median follow-up period of 22 months, the mortality of survivors was unaffected by the development of complete AV block during hospitalization compared with survivors without complete AV block.

Although the impact of the TAMI and TIMI studies on the incidence of AV block was unimpressive, the hospital mortality rates of TAMI patients with complete AV block (55) and that of TIMI patients in whom second- or third-degree AV block developed within the first 24 hours (56) were less than the 22% for patients with second- or third-degree AV block and the 33% for patients with complete AV block from pooled data reported in the prethrombolytic era (Tables 71–2 and 71–3).

Two major studies since the TIMI and TAMI studies have yielded important data about AV block in the thrombolytic era.

1. In the large study of Rathore and coworkers (13) involving 106,780 Medicare patients (≥65 years of age), AV block was more likely to be associated with a history of smoking, diabetes, and slightly older age.

2. The overall incidence of AV block (defined as either second- and third-degree, or only third-degree) has diminished in the thrombolytic era compared with historical control subjects and in patients actually not given thrombolytic therapy (13,14). The lower incidence of AV block in the thrombolytic era in patients not given thrombolytic therapy suggests that other factors such as changes in the management of MI are involved.

3. The frequency of AV block is greater in patients with inferior MI receiving thrombolytic therapy than in those without therapy (13,14). Harpaz and coworkers (14) (who classified AV block in terms of only complete AV block) found that thrombolytic therapy imparts a twofold risk for AV block when thrombolytic therapy is administered in patients with an acute inferior MI. It is unknown whether the duration of AV block was shorter with thrombolytic therapy in the recent reports. Furthermore, there are no data about the impact of thrombolytic therapy on the need for permanent pacing in this setting. The benefit of thrombolytic therapy in anterior MI complicated by AV block is unclear, but the data of Rathore and coworkers (13) (who classified AV block in terms of second-and third-degree block) suggest no significant reduction in the incidence of AV block (3.1% with thrombolytic therapy vs. 2.7% with no therapy in a group of more than 2,000 patients with acute anterior MI and AV block).

4. AV block in patients treated with thrombolytics still carries a poor prognosis for in-hospital mortality (13,14). Thrombolytic therapy in acute anterior MI complicated by AV block probably does not improve in-hospital mortality compared with no therapy. However, the results of the large study of Rathore and coworkers (13) strongly suggest that patients with acute inferior MI and AV block exhibit a significantly lower in-hospital mortality with thrombolytic therapy compared with those receiving no treatment (18.9% vs. 32.9%). This was confirmed in two other studies (15,16). However, Harpaz and coworkers (14) in a smaller study (122 cases of complete AV block, 13 with anterior MI) found no difference in the 7-day and 30-day adjusted mortality rates when the treated and untreated groups (all MI sites) were compared.

5. The large Medicare study of Rathore and coworkers (13) showed that thrombolytic therapy in patients with inferior MI and AV block produced the same 1-year mortality rate as patients with inferior MI and no AV block (7.0% vs. 6.7%). The 1-year mortality rate of patients who did not receive thrombolysis was the same regardless of whether the acute phase had been complicated by AV block (23.1% vs. 20.0%), a finding similar to previous data from the prethrombolytic era. There was no significant change in the 1-year mortality rate in the study of Harpaz and coworkers (14) (122 cases of AV block as above) when patients with AV block who received thrombolysis were compared with those who did not receive this therapy. These results are in keeping with the data from TAMI study and those of Rathore and coworkers (13) in the thrombolytic era and mimic the data from the prethrombolytic era (55,56).

Mechanism of Atrioventricular Block

Two different mechanisms have been proposed for the development of AV block in inferior wall MI: first, reversible or irreversible ischemic injury to the AV node and His bundle; and, second, abnormal autonomic reflexes (Bezold-Jarisch reflex) (61) precipitated by ischemia and leading to excessive vagal tone (54,62).

Total occlusion of the proximal portion of the right coronary artery occurs in about 70% of cases of inferior wall MI. Yet, right coronary occlusion does not cause necrosis of the AV node, which appears resistant to hypoxic damage. Furthermore, the observation that only 20% of inferior infarctions are associated with second- or third-degree AV block, or both, and that right coronary artery occlusion occurs proximal to the origin of the AV nodal artery (the right coronary artery gives rise to the AV nodal artery in 90% of cases) suggest that the mechanism of AV block is not simply related to infarction or ischemia of the AV node (54). Lack of necrosis of the AV node may be related to collateral circulation from the septal perforator branch of the left anterior descending artery (26).

The Bezold-Jarisch reflex reflects increased vagal tone as a result of stimulation of afferent nerves adjacent to the AV node during ischemia or necrosis. This mechanism does not explain the increased infarct size in patients with heart block and the occurrence of heart block frequently without sinus slowing.

Two other explanations have been proposed on the basis of chemical mediators that might account for the association of AV block with larger infarcts: (a) local hyperkalemia released by ischemic cells; and (b) adenosine released by ischemic cells and shown to produce AV block in animal models (63,64).

A number of reports have indicated that aminophylline, a competitive adenosine antagonist (which blocks specific extracellular adenosine receptors not affected by atropine), can reverse some cases of atropine-resistant late AV block (after 24 hours) in acute inferior MI, suggesting a metabolic cause in some cases (65–70). Aminophylline does not produce sympathetic potentiation (71,72).

Right Ventricular Infarction and Atrioventricular Block

The incidence of RV dysfunction in inferior MI may be as high as 40% to 50% (30,39,43,73). The diagnosis of RV MI using ST-segment elevation in lead V_4R identifies a subgroup of patients with acute inferior MI at a greater risk for development of AV block (second-degree, third-degree, or both) even without hemodynamic evidence of RV failure (30,32,39,43,73). Mehta and coworkers (73) studied 1,129 patients with acute inferior MI (638 without RV MI and 491 with RV MI). Ninety-six percent of the patients received thrombolytic therapy. The authors found a 9% incidence rate of high-degree AV block in patients without RV MI compared with 21% when there was RV involvement. The increased risk for AV block was related to the presence of RV MI itself rather than the extent of left ventricular damage. Mehta and coworkers (73) also conducted a metaanalysis of 1,198 patients (6 studies) with RVMI that included their 491 patients. Compared with patients who did not have RV myocardial involvement, those with RV MI were at a significantly greater risk for death, cardiogenic shock, ventricular tachyarrhythmia, and high-degree AV block.

Normally, the RV is a compliant chamber whose performance depends more on afterload than preload. An RVMI causes an acute increase in diastolic stiffness (compliance) so that the RV then becomes more dependent on preload. The infarcted RV acts more or less as a passive conduit for the atrial pump. The atrial systolic pressure may become greater than the pulmonary artery diastolic pressure so that passive flow through the RV occurs at end-diastole. Indeed, the A wave generated by atrial systole can be transmitted directly into the pulmonary artery. Furthermore, dilatation of the RV with its poor systolic function can impair left ventricular filling by increasing the intrapericardial pressure. Hypotension or shock in RVMI can be partly or entirely a result of AV block and loss of AV synchrony. Ventricular pacing may not improve hemodynamics because of the missing crucial synchronized atrial contribution to the RV preload. Sequential AV pacing with restoration of AV synchrony can cause a dramatic increase in blood pressure, cardiac output, and stroke volume (74–81). AV synchrony also decreases intrapericardial pressure by the appropriately timed decline in atrial volume during ventricular end-diastole, thereby providing space within the pericardium for additional filling of the atria. External transthoracic pacing can be successful and life-saving in patients with an inferior MI complicated by RV MI in whom transvenous endocardial pacing of the RV is unsuccessful because of the capability of transthoracic depolarization of the left ventricle rather than the infarcted and unresponsive RV (82).

Electrocardiographic Characteristics of Atrioventricular Block

Lamas and coworkers (83) analyzed data from 698 patients with proven acute MI and proposed a scoring system to pre-

dict the occurrence of CHB to simplify the decision process related to the use of prophylactic temporary pacing. There were 19 patients with alleged Mobitz type II second-degree AV block and they claimed that six patients with narrow QRS complexes demonstrated both type I and type II second-degree AV block—an exceedingly rare combination with a narrow QRS complex. The relatively high incidence of type II second-degree AV block without associated bundle branch block (BBB) in the study of Lamas and coworkers (83) is difficult to understand. Other workers have indicated, also incorrectly, that narrow QRS type II second-degree AV block can occur in acute inferior wall MI (84–92). Because Lamas and coworkers (83) did not define type II second-degree AV block in their study, it appears that they incorrectly called second-degree type II AV block what was really type I AV block (with atypical sequences of apparent type II AV block caused by hypervagotonia) or even advanced AV block (e.g., 2:1 AV block). The incidence rate of type II second-degree AV block is about 1% or less in all types of acute MI; yet, Lamas and coworkers (83) found an incidence rate of 3% (19 patients) in 698 patients (which included non–Q-wave MIs), suggesting that they may have overestimated the number of patients with true type II AV block (93–97).

AV block associated with inferior MI is almost always located in the AV node. A wide QRS complex with AV block in an inferior MI does not mean that the AV block is not in the AV node (98). Infranodal AV block in acute inferior MI is quite rare, but its occurrence should not be surprising in view of the pathologic changes observed in the His bundle at autopsy (18–20,99). Few cases of AV block within the His bundle have been reported (100–113), some preceded by second-degree type I AV block on the surface electrocardiogram (102–104). Patients with infranodal AV block may exhibit a variety of abnormalities demonstrable only with an electrophysiologic study, including: (a) infranodal third-degree AV block (100,101,104); (b) second-degree AV block below the site of recording of the His bundle potential (e.g., 2:1 AV block) (102,111–113; Guerot and coworkers [114] reported one case of second-degree type II intra-Hisian block in inferior MI, but previous electrocardiograms clearly demonstrated that the block antedated the MI); (c) first-degree intra-Hisian block with prolongation of the HV interval (105–108,110,112); and (d) split His bundle potentials reflecting delay in intra-Hisian conduction (101,103,111,112).

The documentation of intra- and infra-Hisian blocks in inferior MI suggests that true type II second-degree AV block is theoretically possible in this situation. Yet, we could not find any published electrocardiograms showing true Mobitz type II second-degree AV block in the literature concerning AV block during inferior wall MI, even in the patients exhibiting a variety of infranodal conduction disturbances (97). In 1984, Sclarovsky and coworkers (42) found no cases of type II second-degree AV block in 76 patients with advanced AV block (second and third degree) in the setting of acute inferior MI. Behar and coworkers (60) could not find a single case of type II second-degree AV block in 132 patients with second-degree AV block in inferior wall acute MI. In 1980, Scheinman and Gonzalez (115) wrote that "classic type II AV block has not been documented in patients with acute inferior myocardial infarction," and this statement is still currently true. Type II second-degree AV block in acute MI occurs invariably in patients with anterior MI complicated by BBB (116–118).

Alternating Wenckebach Atrioventricular Block

Alternating Wenckebach AV block occurs in the setting of 2:1 AV block when there is progressive increase in the PR interval of the conducted sinus impulses until two or more consecutive impulses are blocked and the pattern generally repeats itself (119–121). Alternating Wenckebach periods are caused by multilevel block in the AV node. Alternating Wenckebach AV block occurs in about 2% of patients with acute inferior MI. Atropine can expose latent advanced degrees of AV block in acute inferior MI and may induce alternating Wenckebach AV block (122,123). Atropine should not be administered in alternating Wenckebach AV block because an increase in the atrial rate without associated improvement in AV conduction may precipitate even greater degrees of AV block and hypotension. Isoproterenol also is ineffective. Most, if not all, patients with alternating Wenckebach block appear to need a temporary pacemaker, and atropine should not be given unless the pacemaker is already in place. Patients with alternating Wenckebach block have a high incidence of syncope, high-degree AV block, hemodynamic deterioration, and death (123).

ACUTE ANTERIOR MYOCARDIAL INFARCTION

Pathophysiology of Atrioventricular Block

Anterior wall MI complicated by AV block occurs with extensive necrosis of the septum, the His bundle, and bundle branches in the setting of severe left ventricular dysfunction. The high mortality rate reflects myocardial damage and accompanying pump failure rather than the conduction abnormality. The transition from 1:1 AV conduction to CHB often is abrupt, and the resulting idioventricular rhythm often is slow and unreliable at rates of 30 to 40 per minute. The mortality of anterior MI and AV block is high (80%) because of the extent of myocardial damage. Narrow QRS type II second-degree block has not been reported as a complication of acute anterior wall MI. Narrow QRS AV block can occur in acute anterior wall MI during vomiting or other strong vagal stimulation, when the block is AV nodal, transient, and does not require specific therapy. BBB occurs in about 8% to 13% of patients with acute anterior MI. Patients who experience development of BBB and transient second- or third-degree AV block during anterior MI have a high in-hospital mortality rate and are at a high risk for sudden death after hospital discharge. Sudden death usually results from malignant ventricular tachyarrhythmias and less commonly is re-

lated to complete AV block with ventricular asystole, although the latter can occasionally precipitate a ventricular tachyarrhythmia. The impact of thrombolytic therapy on the incidence of second- and third-degree AV block in acute anterior MI currently remains largely unknown.

INDICATIONS FOR TEMPORARY PACING IN ACUTE MYOCARDIAL INFARCTION

The role of temporary pacing in acute MI remains controversial because the risk-to-benefit ratio is unclear. Death is generally not related directly to the conduction disturbance, and the ultimate prognosis depends more on MI size than the degree of AV block. On the basis of survival statistics alone, it is not clear that temporary or permanent cardiac pacing offers a positive impact on the prognosis of patients with ischemically mediated cardiac conduction system disease. Despite the evidence that patients with inferior MI complicated by AV block do not need permanent cardiac pacing and that those with anterior MI complicated by AV block have a gloomy prognosis with or without permanent pacemakers, there does appear to be a role for pacing in a small subset of this population, and certain guidelines and principles are pertinent. Tables 71–4 and 71–5 outline the indications for temporary pacing according to the American College of Cardiology/American Heart Association (ACC/AHA) guidelines (124,125).

Acute Inferior Myocardial Infarction

AV block in acute inferior MI is relatively benign. Most hemodynamically stable patients with second-degree AV block can be treated without pacing but require monitoring. In third-degree AV block, the AV junctional rhythm exhibits a narrow QRS complex in more than 70% of cases with an adequate rate (50–60 per minute), often without associated hemodynamic compromise. The ventricular rate is slower

TABLE 71–4. *Classification of indications for pacing according to the American College of Cardiology/American Heart Association Guidelines*

Class I: Conditions for which there is general agreement that permanent pacemakers (or antitachycardia devices) should be implanted.
Class II: Conditions for which permanent pacemakers (or antitachycardia devices) are frequently used but there is a divergence of opinion with respect to the necessity of their insertion.
Class III: Conditions for which there is general agreement that pacemakers (or antitachycardia devices) are not necessary.

Data from Gregoratos G, Cheitlin MD, Conill A, et al. ACC/AHA guidelines for implantation of cardiac pacemakers and antiarrhythmia devices: a report of the American College of Cardiology/American Heart Association Task Force on Practice Guidelines (Committee on Pacemaker Implantation). *J Am Coll Cardiol* 1998;3:1175–1209.

TABLE 71–5. *Temporary pacing in acute myocardial infarction*

Pacing recommendations in these revised guidelines place more emphasis on transcutaneous pacing. The newly available transcutaneous pacemaker systems are suitable for providing standby pacing in acute MI, especially for those not requiring immediate pacing and at only moderate risk for progression to AV block, and do not entail the difficulty in application and risk for complications of intravenous systems. Transcutaneous technology also is well suited to patients receiving thrombolytic therapy, reducing the need for vascular interventions.

Recommendations for Placement of Transcutaneous Patches[a] and Active (Demand) Transcutaneous Pacing Patches[b]:

Class I

1. Sinus bradycardia (rate <50 beats/min) with symptoms of hypotension (systolic blood pressure <80 mm Hg) unresponsive to drug therapy[a]
2. Mobitz type II second-degree AV block[b]
3. Third-degree heart block[a]
4. Bilateral BBB (alternating BBB, or right BBB and alternating LAFB, LPFB; irrespective of time of onset)[a]
5. Newly acquired or age-indeterminate left BBB, left BBB and LAFB, right BBB and LPFB[a]
6. Right or left BBB and first-degree AV block[a]

Class IIa

1. Stable bradycardia (systolic blood pressure >90 mm Hg, no hemodynamic compromise, or compromise responsive to initial drug therapy)[a]
2. Newly acquired or age-indeterminate right BBB[a]

Class IIb

1. Newly acquired or age-indeterminate first-degree AV block[a]

Class III

1. Uncomplicated acute MI without evidence of conduction system disease.

Transcutaneous systems are available that use a single pair of adequately sized, multifunctional electrodes that allow electrocardiographic monitoring, transcutaneous pacing, and defibrillation as needed. These systems may be used in a standby mode in potentially unstable patients. Because transcutaneous pacing may be uncomfortable, especially when prolonged, it is intended to be prophylactic and temporary. A transvenous pacing electrode should be placed in patients who require ongoing pacing and in those with a high probability of requiring pacing (risk for AV block ≥30%). Thus, transcutaneous pacing systems have allowed both the broadening of the application of standby pacing and the narrowing of the application of transvenous pacing. Technical aspects of transcutaneous pacing are reviewed elsewhere. The revised recommendations reflect this change.

Reccmmendations for Temporary Transvenous Pacing[c]:

Class I
1. Asystole
2. Symptomatic bradycardia (includes sinus bradycardia with hypotension and type I second-degree AV block with hypotension not responsive to atropine)
3. Bilateral BBB (alternating BBB or right BBB with alternating LAFB/LPFB; any age)
4. New or indeterminate age bifascicular block (right BBB with LAFB or LPFB, or left BBB) with first-degree AV block
5. Mobitz type II second-degree AV block

Class IIa (note also "Recommendations for Transcutaneous Standby Pacing" above)
1. Right BBB and LAFB or LPFB (new or indeterminate)
2. Right BBB with first-degree AV block
3. Left BBB, new or indeterminate
4. Incessant VT, for atrial or ventricular overdrive pacing
5. Recurrent sinus pauses (>3 seconds) not responsive to atropine

Class IIb
1. Bifascicular block of indeterminate age
2. New or age-indeterminate isolated right BBB

Class III
1. First-degree heart block
2. Type I second-degree AV block with normal hemodynamics
3. Accelerated idioventricular rhythm
4. BBB or fascicular block known to exist before acute MI

AV, atrioventricular; BBB, bundle branch block; LAFB, left anterior fascicular block; LPFB, left posterior fascicular block; MI, myocardial infarction; VT, ventricular tachycardia

[a]Transcutaneous patches applied; system may be attached and activated within a brief time if needed. Transcutaneous pacing may be helpful as an urgent expedient. Because it is associated with significant pain, high-risk patients likely to require pacing should receive a temporary pacemaker.

[b]Apply patches and attach system; system is in either active or standby mode to allow immediate use on demand as required. In facilities in which transvenous pacing or expertise are not available to place an intravenous system, consideration should be given to transporting the patient to one equipped and competent in placing transvenous systems.

[c]It should be noted that in choosing an intravenous pacemaker system, patients with substantially depressed ventricular performance, including right ventricular infarction, may respond better to atrial/AV sequential pacing than ventricular pacing.

From Ryan TJ, Anderson JL, Antman EM, et al. ACC/AHA guidelines for the management of patients infarction; executive summary. A report of the American College of Cardiology/American Heart Association Task Force on Practice guidelines (Committee on Management of Acute Myocardial Infarction). *Circulation* 1996;94:2341–2350, with permission; and Ryan TJ, Antman EM, Brooks NH, et al. 1999 update: ACC/AHA guidelines for the management of patients with acute myocardial infarction. A report of the American College of Cardiology/American Heart Association Task Force on Practice guidelines (Committee on Management of Acute Myocardial Infarction). *J Am Coll Cardiol* 1999;34:890–911, with permission.

when the QRS complex is wide. The AV block is transient and often resolves within a week. Temporary pacing is rarely necessary in hemodynamically stable patients with complete AV block and a ventricular rate of about 40 to 45 per minute in the absence of ventricular arrhythmia. Temporary pacing is indicated in second- or third-degree AV block only in the presence of an excessively slow ventricular rate (<40), ventricular arrhythmia requiring antiarrhythmic agents (also for overdrive suppression of bradycardia-dependent ventricular arrhythmias), hypotension, signs of hypoperfusion, or congestive heart failure. Patients with AV block and RV MI often require dual-chamber pacing (74–81).

Acute Anterior Myocardial Infarction

Second- or third-degree AV block is almost invariably preceded by an intraventricular conduction disorder and often occurs 12 to 24 hours after the onset of MI, but also on the second or third day. AV block in anterior MI almost always involves the His-Purkinje system and occasionally occurs in the form of second-degree AV block (Mobitz type II, 2:1, or higher degree AV block) before the appearance of complete AV block. In acute MI, wide QRS type II block occurs only in anterior infarction. Narrow QRS type II second-degree AV block has not been reported as a complication of acute anterior MI. Type I second-degree AV block in the setting of an anterior MI is rare and may be caused by hypervagotonia such as during vomiting, in which case it requires no therapy. However, it may also occur from disease of the His-Purkinje system, in which case it will almost invariably progress to 2:1 and complete AV block, for which temporary pacing is required. All patients with second- or third-degree heart block and anterior MI should receive temporary pacing, although the mortality rate is quite high; improvement of eventual survival is controversial because the conduction disturbances generally occur in patients with large infarcts. Nevertheless, pacing protects against hypotension that may minimize infarct extension and malignant ventricular arrhythmias, particularly when dual-chamber pacing is used. Prophylactic pacing also is generally recommended in the presence of new right BBB with left anterior hemiblock, right BBB with left posterior hemiblock, left BBB with first-degree AV block, and alternating right and left BBB because these patients are at greater risk for progression to complete atrioventricular block. The transition from 1:1 AV conduction with an intraventricular conduction disorder to complete AV block often is sudden, and prolonged asystole is common. The resulting idioventricular rhythm (wide QRS) often is slow and unreliable (30–40 per minute). The role of pacing for right BBB with normal axis or left BBB with normal P-R interval is more controversial. Preexisting right or left BBB is usually not an indication for temporary pacing.

The advent of reliable external transcutaneous pacing has diminished the need in many patients for prophylactic temporary RV pacing in acute MI, an important consideration in patients treated with thrombolytic therapy and anticoagulants.

PERMANENT PACING AFTER ACUTE MYOCARDIAL INFARCTION

The requirement for temporary pacing in acute MI does not by itself constitute an indication for permanent pacing. Unlike many other indications, the need for permanent pacing after acute MI does not necessarily depend on the presence of symptoms. The 1999 ACC/AHA guidelines for the treatment of acute MI, and the 1998 ACC/AHA guidelines (updated but unchanged in 2002), introduced "persistent and symptomatic AV block" as a new Class I indication for pacing (124–127). This statement is vague and ignores the simple fact that any form of AV block in acute MI can be symptomatic before it resolves completely as in inferior MI.

Atrioventricular Block in Inferior Myocardial Infarction

The 1998 and 2002 ACC/AHA guidelines classify persistent AV nodal block as a Class II indication (Table 71–4) without defining what "persistent" means, a limitation that also appears in the ACC/AHA guidelines for the treatment of acute MI. It is therefore possible that pacemakers may be implanted unnecessarily considering the wide latitude of the ACC/AHA recommendation. It cannot be concluded at this juncture whether in the thrombolytic era less permanent pacemakers will be required in survivors of second- or third-degree AV block, or both, but the need should be less than 2%. The guidelines should state categorically that permanent pacing is almost never needed in patients with inferior MI and narrow QRS AV block. Even relatively uncommon intra-Hisian block in inferior MI is almost always reversible and rarely requires permanent pacing (25,29,55,56). The term *persistent* has been interpreted by some workers to mean 14 to 16 days, a cutoff point that seems satisfactory. More conservative workers have indicated that pacemaker implantation should not be considered unless second- or third-degree AV block is present 3 weeks after MI (128). On the basis of the 14- to 16-day criterion, the need for permanent pacing in survivors who experience development of second- or third-degree AV block, or both, should not exceed 1% to 2% of the entire AV block group, regardless of whether they are treated with thrombolytics (128). Lie and Durrer (129) stated more than two decades ago that "there is little controversy over the indications for permanent pacing in conduction disturbance following inferior infarctions, since these are always transient and do not have a tendency to recur. Permanent pacing is generally not necessary in this setting." This statement remains true today.

As a rule, permanent pacing should not be implanted when AV block is prolonged to facilitate mobilization and rehabilitation, because most patients with persistent CHB during inferior MI may not be truly pacemaker-dependent if the pacing rate is gradually decreased so as to allow the emergence of a spontaneous rhythm, often with an acceptable rate, and hemodynamic stability.

Transient second-degree AV block (nodal) with BBB in acute inferior wall MI does not require a permanent pacemaker. Rarely, a patient with preexistent right BBB and left anterior hemiblock presents with an acute inferior MI complicated by left posterior hemiblock and the development of CHB in the His-Purkinje system. A permanent pacemaker seems justified in this situation.

Atrioventricular Block in Anterior Myocardial Infarction

Table 71–6 presents the Class I indications (Table 71–4) for permanent pacing modified from the 1998 and the identical 2002 ACC/AHA guidelines (126,127). Transient or persis-

TABLE 71–6. *Guidelines for implantation of cardiac pacemakers after acute myocardial infarction*

Class I	
A	Persistent or transient second-degree or complete AV block in the His-Purkinje system
B	Alternating left bundle branch block and right bundle branch block with 1:1 AV conduction
Class II	
	Persistent advanced or complete AV block at the AV node (>16 days)
Class III	
A	Transient AV conduction disturbances without intraventricular conductions defects
B	Transient AV block in the presence of isolated left anterior hemiblock
C	Acquired left anterior hemiblock, bundle branch block, or bifascicular block with or without first-degree AV block, but in the absence of second-degree or complete AV block
D	Transient second-degree or complete AV block and associated bundle branch block in acute inferior myocardial infarction[a]

AV, atrioventricular.

[a]Transient AV block in inferior myocardial infarction is virtually always in the AV node or His bundle and almost never requires permanent pacing even if associated with permanent bundle branch block. Therefore, transient advanced AV block and associated bundle branch block should not be classified as a Class I indication, unless there is firm evidence of transient second- or third-degree AV block in the His-Purkinje system).

Adapted from Gregoratos G, Cheitlin MD, Conill A, et al. ACC/AHA guidelines for implantation of cardiac pacemakers and antiarrhythmia devices: a report of the American College of Cardiology/American Heart Association Task Force on Practice Guidelines (Committee on Pacemaker Implantation). *J Am Coll Cardiol* 1998;3:1175–1209, with permission; and Braunwald E, Antman EM, Beasley JW, et al. ACC/AHA 2002 guideline update for the management of patients with unstable angina and non-ST-segment elevation myocardial infarction—summary article: a report of the American College of Cardiology/American Heart Association task force on practice guidelines (Committee on the Management of Patients with Unstable Angina). *J Am Coll Cardiol* 2002;40:1366–1374, with permission.

tent second-degree AV block of any form and associated BBB in acute *anterior* wall MI are almost certainly infranodal, and a permanent pacemaker is indicated if vagal block is excluded. Such patients have a high in-hospital mortality rate and are at a high risk for sudden death after hospital discharge. Sudden death usually is caused by malignant ventricular tachyarrhythmias and is less commonly related to the development of complete AV block with prolonged ventricular asystole (although the latter can occasionally precipitate a ventricular tachyarrhythmia).

The use of permanent pacing in patients with transient trifascicular AV block during acute anterior MI remains controversial (116,130–141). In 1978, Roos and Dunning (136) put this problem into perspective by pointing out the following: (a) that about 10% of patients reaching the hospital with acute anterior MI experience development of BBB; (b) that approximately one-third of these patients progress to CHB; and (c) that 80% of patients with transient or permanent CHB die in the hospital. Thus, less than 1% of patients with an acute anterior MI who survive the first 4 weeks are possible candidates for permanent pacing. By analyzing the available literature, Roos and Dunning (136) concluded that late sudden death in patients in whom transient AV develops block could possibly be reduced by permanent pacing. In the same year, the study of Hindman and coworkers (137,138), involving a relatively large number of patients, also suggested a reduction in sudden death mortality by implantation of a permanent pacemaker in patients who experienced development of BBB and transient AV block during acute anterior MI. A 1983 review of the subject pooling patients from the available literature also suggested that permanent pacing might be helpful (116). The number of patients in all the trials has been far too small to make firm conclusions about the role of permanent pacing. Thus, permanent pacing, with the aim of preventing sudden death from asystole or the induction of ventricular tachyarrhythmias by the resultant bradycardia, although still controversial, should nevertheless be considered in patients who experience development of transient trifascicular block (with either complete or second-degree block) and eventual return of 1:1 AV conduction.

The 1998 and 2002 ACC/AHA guidelines (126,127) recommend that in transient second- or third-degree AV block with BBB an electrophysiologic study should be considered to assess the site and extent of heart block in uncertain cases. Missing from these new guidelines is how to interpret the data from such a study in the decision-making process of whether to implant a permanent pacemaker.

Permanent antibradycardia pacing is not indicated in patients with acute anterior MI and residual bundle branch or bifascicular block without documented transient second- or third-degree AV block because there is no appreciable risk for late development of complete AV block. Measurement of the HV interval does not predict which patients will experience development of progressive conduction system disease. However, prophylactic permanent pacing also should be considered in the absence of transient second- or third-degree AV block if alternating BBB occurs during acute MI.

INTRAVENTRICULAR CONDUCTION DELAY WITHOUT ATRIOVENTRICULAR BLOCK

New-onset BBB, especially right BBB, usually occurs in anterior infarction and is associated with a substantially increased in-hospital and 1-year mortality (142–145). Right BBB is an independent prognostic factor in acute MI (143). The prognosis of preexisting BBB carries a better prognosis (142). The advent of thrombolytic therapy seems to have reduced the incidence of persistent BBB or bifascicular but has led to an increase in reversible or transient BBB (142,146). Persistent BBB carries a much worse prognosis than transient BBB (142,146,147). New-onset persistent right BBB in acute inferior MI increases short- and long-term mortality (148).

Permanent pacing is not needed in most patients with acute anterior MI and residual intraventricular conduction disorders without documented AV block (with the possible exceptions of alternating BBB and right BBB and left posterior hemiblock) because there is no appreciable risk for late development of CHB. Patients were allocated at random to permanent pacing and a control group in the prospective study of Watson and coworkers (130) involving 50 patients surviving 2 weeks after anterior MI with right BBB with either left anterior or left posterior hemiblock but without AV block at any stage. This study included no patients with CHB or transient AV block and showed no benefit from prophylactic pacing during a follow-up period of 5 years. Measurements of the HV interval at the time of pacemaker placement failed to predict which patients in whom progressive conduction system disease would develop. In this study, ventricular tachycardia was an important cause of death. Pagnoni and coworkers (140) also demonstrated the stability of HV conduction by means of sequential HV determinations in patients with anterior MI and intraventricular conduction disorder without transient CHB. Thus, it appears that once established during acute MI, lesions in the bundle branch system tend to remain constant and generally do not progress with time.

Some questions remain unanswered. Although we advise prophylactic permanent pacing in the absence of transient second- or third-degree AV block in patients with alternating BBB or those with right BBB and left posterior hemiblock, this practice cannot be fully justified on the basis of existing data. Because of the high incidence of deaths in the first 6 weeks after MI from ventricular tachyarrhythmias rather than AV block, an automatic implantable cardioverter-defibrillator that offers "back-up" dual-chamber pacing (when or if available) would seem more appropriate especially in the presence of a low left ventricular ejection fraction (149).

Atrioventricular Block Related to Myocardial Ischemia

At Rest

Transient AV block may rarely be caused by myocardial ischemia. The development of AV block at rest in so-called Prinzmetal angina is well known (3,150–154). It may occasionally present as syncope without prior chest pain (150) and may then be detected with Holter monitoring in association with ST-segment elevation. A permanent pacemaker should be considered only when revascularization is not feasible or there is drug-refractory spasm in anatomically patent coronary arteries.

On Exertion

Permanent pacing is recommended as a Class I indication in symptomatic or asymptomatic patients with exercise-induced AV block (absent at rest) because most cases are caused by tachycardia-dependent block in the His-Purkinje system (155–157) and carry a poor prognosis in terms of the development of complete AV block. This form of AV block often is reproducible in the electrophysiologic laboratory by rapid atrial pacing (provided the atrial rate is increased gradually to avoid functional infra-Hisian block) because it is tachycardia-dependent and rarely caused by AV nodal disease. AV block secondary to myocardial ischemia occurring during exercise (or spontaneously) is rare and does not require pacing unless ischemia cannot be alleviated (158–161).

REFERENCES

1. Stephens MR, Fadayomi MO, Gavies GJ, et al. The clinical features and significance of bifascicular block complicating myocardial infarction. *Eur J Cardiol* 1975;3:289–296.
2. Parameswaran R, Ohe T, Goldberg H. Sinus node dysfunction in acute myocardial infarction. *Br Heart J* 1976;38:93–96.
3. Haywood LJ, Ventkataramen K. Prinzmetal angina, multifocal ischemia, recurrent AV block, and bradycardia with patent coronary arteries responsive to verapamil. *J Electrocardiol* 1991;24:177–183.
4. Bashour TT, Hakim O, Ennis AL, et al. Coronary artery spasm with sinus node dysfunction and syncope. *Arch Intern Med* 1982;142:1719–1721.
5. den Dulk K, Brugada P, Braat S, et al. Myocardial bridging as a cause of paroxysmal atrioventricular block. *J Am Coll Cardiol* 1983;1:965–969.
6. Hsueh CW, Lee WL, Chen YT, et al. The incidence of coronary disease in patients with symptomatic bradyarrhythmias. *Jpn Heart J* 2001;42:417–423.
7. Lev M. Aging changes in the human sinoatrial node. *J Gerontol* 1954;9:1–9.
8. Lev M, Unger PN. The pathology of the conduction system in acquired heart disease. *Arch Pathol* 1955;60:502.
9. Lev M. The pathology of complete atrioventricular block. *Prog Cardiovasc Dis* 1964;6:317–325.
10. Lev M, Bharati S. Atrioventricular and intraventricular conduction disease. *Arch Intern Med* 1975;135:405–410.
11. Bashour TT, Chen F, Feeney J. Ischemic sinus node hibernation: resolution following angioplasty. *Am Heart J* 1991;122:1156–1158.
12. Escosteguy CC, Carvalho Mde A, Medronho Rde A, et al. Bundle branch and atrioventricular block as complications of acute myocardial infarction in the thrombolytic era. *Arq Bras Cardiol* 2001;76:291–296.
13. Rathore SS, Gersh BJ, Berger PB, et al. Acute myocardial infarction

complicated by heart block in the elderly: prevalence and outcomes. *Am Heart J* 2002;141:47–54.

14. Harpaz D, Behar S, Gottlieb S, et al. Complete atrioventricular block complicating acute myocardial infarction in the thrombolytic era. SPRINT Study Group and the Israeli Thrombolytic Survey Group. Secondary Prevention Reinfarction Israeli Nifedipine Trial. *J Am Coll Cardiol* 1999;34:1721–1728.

15. Melgarejo Moreno A, Galcera Tomas J, Garcia Alberola A, et al. The prognostic significance of complete atrioventricular block in patients with acute inferior myocardial infarct. A study in the era of thrombolytics. *Rev Esp Cardiol* 1997;50:397–405.

16. Melgarejo Moreno A, Galcera Tomas J, Garcia Alberola A, et al. Prognostic significance of advanced atrioventricular block in patients with acute myocardial infarction. *Med Clin (Barc)* 2000;114:321–325.

17. Haim M, Hod H, Kaplinsky E, et al. Frequency and prognostic significance of high-degree atrioventricular block in patients with a first non-Q wave acute myocardial infarction. The SPRINT Study Group. Second Prevention reinfarction Israeli Nifedipine trial. *Am J Cardiol* 1997;79:674–676.

18. Bilbao FJ, Zabalza IE, Vilanova JR, et al. Atrioventricular block in posterior acute myocardial infarction: a clinicopathologic correlation. *Circulation* 1987;75:733–736.

19. Hackel DB, Sevilla MD, Mikat EM, et al. Comparison of patients with acute anterior or posterior myocardial infarcts with or without complete heart block. *Am J Cardiovasc Pathol* 1988;2:105–126.

20. Ohkawa S, Hackel DB. Anatomic studies of the conduction system in right ventricular infarction. *Jpn Heart J* 1982;23[Suppl]:184–186.

21. Rotman M, Wagner GS, Waugh RA. Significance of high degree atrioventricular block in acute posterior myocardial infarction. *Circulation* 1973;47:257–262.

22. Jewitt D. The genesis of cardiac arrhythmias in acute myocardial infarction. *Prog Cardiol* 1972;1:61–94.

23. Julian DJ, Valentine PA, Miller GG. Disturbances of rate, rhythm and conduction in acute myocardial infarction. *Am J Med* 1964;37:915–927.

24. Stock RJ, Macken RJ. Observations on heart block during continuous electrocardiographic monitoring in myocardial infarction. *Circulation* 1968;38:993–1005.

25. Tans AC, Lie KI, Durrer D. Clinical setting and prognostic significance of high degree atrioventricular block in acute inferior myocardial infarction: a study of 144 patients. *Am Heart J* 1980;99:4–8.

26. Bassan R, Maig IG, Bozza A, et al. Atrioventricular block in acute inferior wall myocardial infarction: harbinger of associated obstruction of the left anterior descending coronary artery. *J Am Coll Cardiol* 1986;8:773–778.

27. Gupta MC, Singh MM, Wahal PK, et al. Complete heart block complicating acute myocardial infarction. *Angiology* 1978;10:749–757.

28. Brown RW, Hunt D, Sloman JG. The natural history of atrioventricular conduction defects in acute myocardial infarction. *Am Heart J* 1969;78:460–466.

29. Nicod P, Gilpin E, Dittrich H, et al. Long-term outcome in patients with inferior myocardial infarction and complete atrioventricular block. *J Am Coll Cardiol* 1988;12:589–594.

30. Kaul V, Haron H, Malhotra A, et al. Significance of advanced atrioventricular block in acute myocardial infarction: a study based on ventricular function and Holter monitoring. *Int J Cardiol* 1986;11:187–193.

31. Feigl D, Ashkenasy J, Kishon Y. Early and late atrioventricular block in acute inferior myocardial infarction. *J Am Coll Cardiol* 1984;4:35–38.

32. Braat SH, De Zwaan C, Brugada P, et al. Right ventricular involvement with acute inferior wall myocardial infarction identifies high risk of developing atrioventricular nodal conduction disturbances. *Am Heart J* 1984;107:1183–1187.

33. Dubois C, Pierard LA, Smeets JP, et al. Long-term prognostic significance of atrioventricular block in inferior acute myocardial infarction. *Eur Heart J* 1989;10:816–820.

34. Norris RM. Heart block in posterior and anterior myocardial infarction. *Br Heart J* 1969;31:352–356.

35. Courter SR, Moffat J, Fowler NO. Advanced atrioventricular block in acute myocardial infarction. *Circulation* 1963;27:1034–1042.

36. Katz R, Conroy RM, Robinson K, et al. The aetiology and prognostic implications of reciprocal changes in acute myocardial infarction. *Br Heart J* 1986;55:423–427.

37. Gupta PK, Lichstein E, Chadda KD. Heart block complicating acute inferior wall myocardial infarction. *Chest* 1976;69:599–604.

38. McDonald K, O'Sullivan JJ, Conroy RM, et al. Heart block as a predictor of in-hospital death in both acute inferior and acute anterior myocardial infarction. *Q J Med* 1990;74:277–282.

39. Mavric Z, Zaputovic L, Matana A, et al. Prognostic significance of complete atrioventricular block in patients with acute inferior myocardial infarction with and without right ventricular involvement. *Am Heart J* 1990;119:823–828.

40. Behar S, Zissman E, Zion M, et al. Complete atrioventricular block complicating inferior acute wall myocardial infarction short- and long-term prognosis. *Am Heart J* 1993;125:1622–1626.

41. Goldberg RJ, Zevallos JC, Yarzebski J, et al. Prognosis of acute myocardial infarction complicated by complete heart block (the Worcester Heart Attack Study). *Am J Cardiol* 1992;69:1135–1141.

42. Sclarovsky S, Strasberg B, Hirshberg A, et al. Advanced early and late atrioventricular block in acute inferior wall myocardial infarction. *Am Heart J* 1984;108:19–24.

43. Strasberg B, Pinchas A, Arditti A, et al. Left and right ventricular function in inferior acute myocardial infarction and significance of advanced atrioventricular block. *Am J Cardiol* 1984;54:985–987.

44. Beregovich J, Fenig S, Lasser J, et al. Management of acute myocardial infarction complicated by advanced atrioventricular block. *Am J Cardiol* 1969;23:54–65.

45. Chatterjee K, Leatham A, Harris A. The risk of pacing after infarction and current recommendations. *Lancet* 1969;2:1061–1063.

46. Friedberg CK, Cohen H, Donoso E. Advanced heart block as a complication of acute myocardial infarction: role of pacemaker therapy. *Prog Cardiovasc Dis* 1968;10:466–481.

47. Rodrigues RD, Vidaillet HJ, Hlatky MA. Long-term prognosis of complete heart block during acute myocardial infarction. *Circulation* 1987;76[Suppl IV]:IV-283.

48. Leth A, Hansen JF, Meibom J. Acute myocardial infarction complicated by third degree atrioventricular block treated with temporary pacemaker: hospital and long-term survival in 57 patients. *Acta Med Scand* 1974;195:391–395.

49. Christiansen I, Haghelt T, Amtorp O. Complete heart block in acute myocardial infarction: drug therapy. *Am Heart J* 1973;85:162–166.

50. Kostuk WJ, Beanlands DS. Complete heart block associated with acute myocardial infarction. *Am J Cardiol* 1970;26:380–384.

51. Lassers BW, Julian DG. Artificial pacing in management of complete heart block complicating acute myocardial infarction. *Br Med J* 1968; 20:142–146.

52. Gregory JJ, Grace WJ. The management of sinus bradycardia, nodal rhythm and heart block for the prevention of cardiac arrest in acute myocardial infarction. *Prog Cardiovasc Dis* 1968;10: 505–517.

53. Paulk EA, Hurst JW. Complete heart block in acute myocardial infarction. *Am J Cardiol* 1966;17:695–706.

54. Berger PB, Ryan TJ. Inferior wall myocardial infarction high-risk subgroups. *Circulation* 1990;81:401–410.

55. Clemmenson P, Bates ER, Califf RM, et al. Complete atrioventricular block complicating inferior wall acute myocardial infarction treated with reperfusion therapy. TAMI Study Group. *Am J Cardiol* 1991; 67:225–230.

56. Berger PB, Ruocco NA Jr, Ryan TJ, et al. Incidence and prognostic implications of heart block complicating inferior wall myocardial infarction treated with thrombolytic therapy: results from TIMI II. TIMI Investigators. *J Am Coll Cardiol* 1992;20:533–540.

57. Opolski G, Kraska T, Ostrzycki A, et al. The effect of infarct size on atrioventricular and intraventricular conduction disturbances in acute myocardial infarction. *Int J Cardiol* 1986;10:141–147.

58. Altun A, Ozkan B, Gurcagan A, et al. Early and late advanced atrioventricular block in acute inferior myocardial infarction. *Coron Artery Dis* 1998;9:1–4.

59. Kosuge M, Kimura K, Ishikawa T, et al. Clinical features of patients with reperfused inferior wall acute myocardial infarction complicated by early complete atrioventricular block. *Am J Cardiol* 2001;88: 1187–1191.

60. Behar S, Zissman E, Zion M, et al. Prognostic significance of second-degree block in inferior wall acute myocardial infarction. SPRINT Study Group. *Am J Cardiol* 1993;72:831–834.

61. Mark AL. The Bezold-Jarisch reflex revisited: clinical implications of inhibitory reflexes originating in the heart. *J Am Coll Cardiol* 1983;1: 90–102.

62. Berger PB, Bell MR. Heart block in inferior myocardial infarction. *Cardiology* 1991;8:49–51.
63. Belardinelli L, Belloni FL, Rubio R, et al. Atrioventricular conduction disturbances during hypoxia. Possible role of adenosine in rabbit and guinea pig heart. *Circulation Res* 1980;47:684–691.
64. Belardinelli L, Mattos EC, Berne RM. Evidence for adenosine mediation of atrioventricular block in the ischemic canine myocardium. *J Clin Invest* 1981;68:195–205.
65. Wesley RC, Lerman B, DiMarco JP, et al. Mechanisms of atropine-resistant atrioventricular block during inferior myocardial infarction: possible role of adenosine. *J Am Coll Cardiol* 1986;8:1232–1234.
66. Shah PK, Nalos P, Peter T. Atropine-resistant post-infarction complete AV block: possible role of adenosine and improvement with aminophylline. *Am Heart J* 1987;131:194–195.
67. Gupta A, Jain A, Kala SC. Role of aminophylline in atropine-resistant atrioventricular block. *J Assoc Physicians India* 1991;39:214.
68. Strasberg B, Bassevich R, Mager A, et al. Effects of aminophylline on atrioventricular conduction in patients with late atrioventricular block during inferior wall acute myocardial infarction. *Am J Cardiol* 1991;67:527–528.
69. Altun A, Kirdar C, Ozbay G. Effect of aminiphylline in patients with atropine-resistant advanced atrioventricular block during acute inferior myocardial infarction. *Clin Cardiol* 1998;21:759–762.
70. Goodfellow J, Walker PR. Reversal of atropine-resistant atrioventricular block with intravenous aminophylline in the early phase of inferior wall acute myocardial infarction following treatment with streptokinase. *Eur Heart J* 1995;16:862–865.
71. Favale S, DiBiase M, Rizzo U, et al. Effect of adenosine and adenosine 5' triphosphate on atrioventricular conduction in patients. *J Am Coll Cardiol* 1985;5:1212–1219.
72. Belardinelli L, Fenton RA, West A, et al. Extracellular action of adenosine and antagonism by aminophylline on the atrioventricular conduction of isolated perfused guinea pig and rat hearts. *Circulation Res* 1982;51:569–579.
73. Mehta SR, Eikelboom JW, Natarajan MK, et al. Impact of right ventricular involvement on mortality and morbidity in patients with inferior myocardial infarction. *J Am Coll Cardiol* 2001;37:37–43.
74. Burks JM, Calder JR Jr, Roland DL. Sinus arrest in diaphragmatic myocardial infarction: treatment of power failure with atrial pacing. *Pacing Clin Electrophysiol* 1979;2:553–559.
75. Love JC, Haffajee CI, Gore JM, et al. Reversibility of hypotension and shock by atrial or atrioventricular sequential pacing in patients with right ventricular infarction. *Am Heart J* 1984;108:5–13.
76. Sheron N, Clarke M. Temporary sequential atrioventricular pacing in myocardial infarction. *Postgrad Med J* 1987;63:121–122.
77. Isner JM, Fisher GP, Del Negro AA, et al. Right ventricular infarction with hemodynamic decompensation due to transient loss of active atrial augmentation. Successful treatment with atrial pacing. *Am Heart J* 1981;102:792–794.
78. Topol EJ, Goldschlager N, Ports TA, et al. Hemodynamic benefit of atrial pacing in right ventricular myocardial infarction. *Ann Intern Med* 1982;96:594–597.
79. Matagni M. Temporary physiologic pacing in inferior wall acute myocardial infarction with right ventricular damage. *Am J Cardiol* 1987;59:1207–1208.
80. Abraham KA, Brown MA, Norris RM. Right ventricular infarction, bradyarrhythmias and cardiogenic shock: importance of atrial or atrioventricular sequential pacing. *Aust NZ J Med* 1985;15:52–54.
81. Love JC, Haffajee CI, Gore JM, et al. Reversibility of hypotension and shock by atrial or atrioventricular sequential pacing in right ventricular infarction. *Am Heart J* 1984;108:5–13.
82. Little T. External cardiac pacing in right ventricular infarction. *Ann Emerg Med* 1988;17:640–642.
83. Lamas GA, Muller JE, Turi ZG, et al., the MILIS Study Group. A simplified method to predict occurrence of complete heart block during acute myocardial infarction. *Am J Cardiol* 1986;57:1213–1219.
84. Haft JI. Clinical implications of atrioventricular and intraventricular conduction abnormalities II. Acute myocardial infarction. *Cardiovasc Clin* 1977;8:65–77.
85. Schamroth L. Acute inferior myocardial infarction. Mobitz Type II second degree AV block. In: Schamroth L. *The disorders of cardiac rhythms,* 2nd ed. St. Louis: Blackwell Scientific Publications, 1980:538–539.
86. Silber EN. Ischemic heart disease. In: Silber EN. *Heart disease,* 2nd ed. New York: Macmillan, 1987:1011–1116.
87. Hayes DL. Indications for permanent pacing. In: Furman S, Hayes DL, Holmes DR, eds. *A practice of cardiac pacing,* 3rd ed. Mount Kisco, NY: Futura Publishing, 1993:1–28.
88. Silver MD, Goldschlager N. Temporary transvenous cardiac pacing in the critical care setting. *Chest* 1988;93:607–613.
89. Willerson JT. Acute myocardial infarction. In: Wyngaarden JB, Smith LH, eds. *Cecil textbook of medicine.* Philadelphia: WB Saunders, 1988:329–337.
90. Andreoli TE, Carpenter CJ, Plum F, et al. Arrhythmias. In: Andreoli TE, Carpenter CJ, Plum F, et al., eds. *Cecil essentials of medicine,* 2nd ed. Philadelphia: WB Saunders, 1990:80–105.
91. Ellenbogen KA, Peters RW. Indications for permanent and temporary cardiac pacing. In: Ellenbogen KA, ed. *Cardiac pacing.* Boston: Blackwell Scientific Publications, 1992:1–3.
92. Alpert JS. Conduction disturbances: temporary and permanent pacing in patients with acute myocardial infarction. In Gersh BJ, Rahimtoola SH, eds. *Acute myocardial infarction.* New York: Elsevier, 1991:249–258.
93. Definition of terms related to cardiac rhythm. *Am Heart J* 1978;95:796–806.
94. Surawicz B, Uhley H, Borun R, et al. Optimal electrocardiography. Tenth Bethesda Conference co-sponsored by the American College of Cardiology and the Health Resources Administration of the Department of Health, Education, and Welfare Task Force I. Standardization of terminology and interpretation. *Am J Cardiol* 1978;41:130–144.
95. Puech P, Wainwright RJ. Clinical electrophysiology of atrioventricular block. *Cardiol Clin* 1983;1:209–224.
96. Barold SS. ACC/AHA guidelines for implantation of cardiac pacemakers: how accurate are the definitions of atrioventricular and intraventricular conduction blocks? *Pacing Clin Electrophysiol* 1993;16:1221–1226.
97. Barold SS. Narrow QRS mobility type II second-degree AV block in acute myocardial infarction. True or false? *Am J Cardiol* 1991;67:1291–1294.
98. Lie KI, Wellens HJ, Schuilenberg RM, et al. Mechanism and significance of widened QRS complexes during complete atrioventricular block in acute inferior myocardial infarction. *Am J Cardiol* 1974;33:833–839.
99. Hunt D, Lie JT, Vohra J, et al. Histopathology of heart block complicating acute myocardial infarction. Correlation with the His bundle electrogram. *Circulation* 1973;48:1252–1261.
100. Gupta PK, Lichstein E, Chadda KD. Heart block complicating acute inferior wall myocardial infarction. *Chest* 1976;69:599–604.
101. Rizzon P, DiBiase M. Intra-His bundle block in acute myocardial infarction. Report of two cases. *J Electrocardiol* 1977;10:197–200.
102. Rosen KM, Loeb HS, Chuquimia R, et al. Site of heart block in acute myocardial infarction. *Circulation* 1970;42:925–933.
103. Nasrallah AT, Beard EF. Intra-His bundle branch block complicating acute myocardial infarction. *Chest* 1976;69:420–422.
104. Bashour TT, Fahdul H, Cheng TO. Complete heart block with normal QRS duration occurring distal to the His bundle in acute inferior myocardial infarction. *J Electrocardiol* 1975;8:185–190.
105. Touboul P, Clement C, Porte J, et al. Etude electrophysiologique des troubles de conduction auriculo-ventriculaires dans l'infarctus myocardique recent. *Arch Mal Coeur* 1972;65:1287–1298.
106. Aizawa Y, Hayaski S, Hosokawa O, et al. His bundle electrogram in the convalescent stage of inferior myocardial infarction complicated with complete AV block. *J Electrocardiol* 1982;15:127–130.
107. Harper R, Hunt D, Vohra J, et al. His bundle electrogram in patients with acute myocardial infarction complicated by atrioventricular or intraventricular conduction disturbances. *Br Heart J* 1975;37:705–710.
108. Gould L, Reddy CV, Kim SG, et al. His bundle electrogram in patients with acute myocardial infarction. *Pacing Clin Electrophysiol* 1979;2:428–434.
109. Casella G, Buttaforro A, Pavia L, et al. Prognostic value of split His bundle potentials during acute myocardial infarction. In: Pérez Gómez F, ed. *Cardiac pacing, electrophysiology, tachyarrhythmias.* Mount Kisco, NY: Futura Publishing, 1985:311–315.
110. Puech P, Grolleau R. Particularités rhythmique au cours des blocs AV. In: Puech P, Grolleau R. *L'Activité du Faisceau de His Normale et Pathologique.* Paris: Sandoz, 1972:146–147.
111. Cadabes A, O'Callaghan AC, Jorda CF, et al. Bloqueo auriculo-ventricular intra-His en el infarto de miocardio aguda. *Rev Esp Cardiol* 1979;32:199–202.

112. Sanz RR, Somolino FM, Ceballos AA, et al. El bloqueo intrahisiano en el infarto de miocardio subagudo. *Rev Esp Cardiol* 1982;35:331–337.
113. Guerot CI, Valère PE, Castillo A, et al. Aspects inhabituels des blocs auriculo-ventriculaires au cours de l'infarctus du myocarde. *Coeur* 1973;4:441–454.
114. Guerot CI, Valère PE, Coste A, et al. Blocs auriculo–ventriculaire localise au tronc du faisceau de His: lebloc tronculaire. *Ann Cardiol Angeiol* 1972;21:143–152.
115. Scheinman MM, Gonzalez RP. Fascicular block and acute myocardial infarction. *JAMA* 1980;244:2646–2649.
116. Codini MA. Conduction disturbances in acute myocardial infarction. The use of pacemaker therapy. *Clin Prog Pacing Electrophysiol* 1983; 1:142–155.
117. El-Sherif N, Scherlag B, Lazzara R. Second-degree atrioventricular block in the His-Purkinje system following acute myocardial infarction, clinical observations on its evolution. *Chest* 1977;71: 615 623.
118. El-Sherif N, Amat-Y-Leon F, Schonfield C, et al. Normalization of bundle branch block patterns by distal His bundle pacing. Clinical and experimental evidence of longitudinal dissociation in the pathologic His bundle. *Circulation* 1978;57:473–483.
119. Kosowsky B, Latif P, Radoff AM. Multilevel atrioventricular block. *Circulation* 1976;54:914–921.
120. Littmann L, Svenson RH. Atrioventricular alternating Wenckebach periodicity: conduction patterns in multilevel block. *Am J Cardiol* 1982;49:855–862.
121. Castellanos A, Sung RJ, Aldrich JL, et al. Electrocardiographic manifestations and clinical significance of atrioventricular nodal alternating Wenckebach periods: a possible indication for prophylactic pacing. *Chest* 1978;73:69–74.
122. Castellanos A, Garcia H, Rozanski JJ, et al. Atropine-induced multilevel block in acute myocardial infarction. *Pacing Clin Electrophysiol* 1981;4:528–537.
123. Lewin RF, Kusneic J, Sclarovsky S, et al. Alternating Wenckebach periods in acute inferior wall myocardial infarction. Clinical, electrocardiographic and therapeutic characterization. *Pacing Clin Electrophysiol* 1986;9:468–475.
124. Ryan TJ, Anderson JL, Antman EM, et al. ACC/AHA guidelines for the management of patients infarction; executive summary. A report of the American College of Cardiology/American Heart Association Task Force on Practice guidelines (Committee on Management of Acute Myocardial Infarction). *Circulation* 1996;94: 2341–2350.
125. Ryan TJ, Antman EM, Brooks NH, et al. 1999 update: ACC/AHA guidelines for the management of patients with acute myocardial infarction. A report of the American College of Cardiology/American Heart Association Task Force on Practice guidelines (Committee on Management of Acute Myocardial Infarction). *J Am Coll Cardiol* 1999;34:890–911.
126. Gregoratos G, Cheitlin MD, Conill A, et al. ACC/AHA guidelines for implantation of cardiac pacemakers and antiarrhythmia devices: a report of the American College of Cardiology/American Heart Association Task Force on Practice Guidelines (Committee on Pacemaker Implantation). *J Am Coll Cardiol* 1998;3:1175–1209.
127. Gregoratos G, Abrams J, Epstein AE, et al. ACC/AHA/NASPE 2002 Guideline Update for Implantation of Cardiac Pacemakers and Antiarrhythmia Devices—summary article: a report of the American College of Cardiology/American Heart Association Task Force on Practice Guidelines (ACC/AHA/NASPE Committee to Update the 1998 Pacemaker Guidelines). *J Am Coll Cardiol* 2002;40:1703–1719.
128. Barold SS. American College of Cardiology/American Heart Association guidelines for pacemaker implantation after acute myocardial infarction. What is persistent block at the AV node? *Am J Cardiol* 1997;80:770–774.
129. Lie KI, Durrer D. Indications of temporary and permanent pacing in ischemic conduction disturbances. In: Samet P, El-Sherif N, eds. *Cardiac pacing*, 2nd ed. New York: Grune & Stratton, 1980:45.
130. Watson RD, Glover DR, Page AJ, et al. The Birmingham trial of permanent pacing in patients with intraventricular conduction disorders after myocardial infarction. *Am Heart J* 1984;108:496–501.
131. Grigg L, Pitt A, Kertes P, et al. The role of permanent pacing after anterior myocardial infarction complicated by transient atrioventricular block. *Aust NZ J Med* 1988;18:685–688.
132. Klein RC, Vera Z, Mason DT. Intraventricular conduction defects in acute myocardial infarction: Incidence, prognosis, and therapy. *Am Heart J* 1984;108:1007–1013.
133. Edhag O, Berfeldt L, Edvardsson N, et al. Pacemaker dependence in patients with bifascicular block during acute anterior myocardial infarction. *Br Heart J* 1984;52:408–412.
134. Murphy E, DeMots H, McAnulty J, et al. Prophylactic permanent pacemakers for transient heart block during myocardial infarction? Results of a prospective study. *Am J Cardiol* 1982;49:952.
135. Talwar KK, Kalra GS, Dogra B, et al. Prophylactic permanent pacemaker implantation in patients with anterior wall myocardial infarction complicated by bundle branch block and transient AV block. A prospective long-term study. *Indian Heart J* 1987;39:22–25.
136. Roos JC, Dunning AJ. Bundle branch block. *Eur J Cardiol* 1978;6: 403–424.
137. Hindman MC, Wagner GS, JaRo M, et al. The clinical significance of bundle branch block complicating acute myocardial infarction. 1, Clinical characteristics, hospital mortality, and one year followup. *Circulation* 1978;58:679 688.
138. Hindman MC, Wagner GS, Jaro M, et al. The clinical significance of bundle branch block. 2. Indications for temporary and permanent pacemaker insertion. *Circulation* 1978;58:689–699.
139. Hauer RNW, Lie KI, Liem KL, et al. Long-term prognosis in patients with bundle branch block complicating acute anteroseptal infarction. *Am J Cardiol* 1982;49:1581–1585.
140. Pagnoni F, Finzia A, Valentini R, et al. Long-term prognostic significance and electrophysiologic evolution of intraventricular conduction disturbances complicating acute myocardial infarction. *Pacing Clin Electrophysiol* 1986;9:91–100.
141. Peters RW. Modern coronary care. In: Francis GS, Alpert JS, eds. *Heart block in acute myocardial infarction*. Boston: Little, Brown and Company, 1990:177–193.
142. Melgarejo-Moreno A, Galcera-Tomas J, Garcia-Alberola A, et al. Incidence, clinical characteristics, and prognostic significance of right bundle branch block in acute myocardial infarction; a study in the thrombolytic era. *Circulation* 1997;96:1139–1144.
143. Simmons GR, Sgarbossa E, Wagner G, et al. Atrioventricular and intraventricular conduction disorders in acute myocardial infarction: a reappraisal in the thrombolytic era. *Pacing Clin Electrophysiol* 1998;21:2651–2663.
144. Melgarejo-Moreno A, Galcera-Tomas J, Garcia-Alberola A. Prognostic significance of bundle branch block in acute myocardial infarction: the importance of location and time of appearance. *Clin Cardiol* 2001;24:371–376.
145. Go AS, Barron HV, Rundle AC, et al. Bundle branch block and in-hospital mortality in acute myocardial infarction. National Registry of Myocardial Infarction 2 Investigators. *Ann Intern Med* 1998;129: 690–697.
146. Newby KH, Pisano E, Krucoff MW, et al. Incidence and clinical relevance of the occurrence of bundle-branch block in patients treated with thrombolytic therapy. *Circulation* 1996;94:2424–2428.
147. Sgarbossa EB, Pinski SL, Topol EJ, et al. Acute myocardial infarction and complete bundle branch block hospital admission: clinical characteristics and outcome in the thrombolytic era. GUSTO-I Investigators. Global Utilization of Streptokinase and t-PA [tissue-type plasminogen activator] for Occluded Coronary Arteries. *J Am Coll Cardiol* 1998;31:105–110.
148. Hod H, Goldbourt U, Behar S. Bundle branch block in acute Q wave inferior wall myocardial infarction. A high risk subgroup of inferior myocardial infarction patients. The SPRINT Study Group. Secondary Prevention Reinfarction Israeli Nifedipine Trial. *Eur Heart J* 1995; 16:471–477.
149. Moss AJ, Zareba W, Hall WJ, et al. Prophylactic implantation of a defibrillator in patients with myocardial infarction and reduc4ed ejection fraction. *N Engl J Med* 2002;346:877–883.
150. Underwood RD, Caracciolo E, Bjerregaard P, et al. Syncope as the initial symptom of silent coronary vasospasm. *Am Heart J* 1994;128:1241–1245.
151. Drakos SG, Anastasiou-Nana MI, Nanas JN. Exacerbation of variant angina by metoprolol resulting in syncope due to transient atrioventricular block. *Int J Cardiol* 2002;82:83–85.
152. Kovac JD, Murgatroyd FD, Skehan JD. Recurrent syncope due to complete atrioventricular block, a rare presenting symptom of otherwise silent coronary artery disease: successful treatment by PTCA. *Cathet Cardiovac Diagn* 1997;42:216–218.
153. Underdorben M, Haag M, Fuerste T, et al. Vasospasm in smooth coro-

nary arteries as a cause of asystole and syncope. *Cathet Cardiovasc Diagn* 1997;41:430–434.

154. Ujhelyi E, Bohm A, Toth C, et al. Prinmetal angina pectoris associated with 3rd degree atrioventricular block. *Orv Hetil* 2001;142:1809–1811.

155. Barold SS, Falkoff MD, Ong LS, et al. Atrioventricular block. In: Barold SS, Mugica J, eds. *New perspectives in cardiac pacing 2.* Mount Kisco, NY: Futura Publishing Company, 1991:23–52.

156. Sumiyoshi M, Nakata Y, Yasuda M, et al. Clinical and electrophysiologic features of exercise-induced atrioventricular block. *Am Heart J* 1996;132:1277–1281.

157. Luscure M, Dechandol AM, Lagorge P, et al. Blocs auriculo-ventriculaires d'effort. *Ann Cardiol Abgeiol* 1995;44:486–492.

158. Deaner A, Fluck D, Timmis AD. Exertional atrioventricular block presenting with recurrent syncope: successful treatment by coronary angioplasty. *Heart* 1996;75:640–641.

159. Madeiros A, Iturralde P, Millan F, et al. A complete atrioventricular block during exertion. *Arch Inst Cardiol Mex* 1999;69:250–257.

160. Rumoroso JR, Montes Orbe PM, Cembellin JC, et al. Exercise-induced atrioventricular block. Significance of the ischemic component. Report of 4 new cases. *Rev Esp Cardiol* 1997;50:278–282.

161. Finzi A, Bruno A, Perondi R. Exercise-induced paroxysmal atrioventricular block during nuclear perfusion stress testing: evidence for transient ischemia of the conduction system. *G Ital Cardiol* 1999;29:1313–1317.

CHAPTER 72

Sudden Cardiac Death

Rafael F. Sequeira, Jeffrey D. Simmons, and Robert J. Myerburg

Key Words: Antiarrhythmic therapy; automatic implantable cardioverter-defibrillator; electrophysiologic testing; sudden cardiac death; ventricular fibrillation; ventricular tachycardia.

INTRODUCTION

Sudden cardiac death (SCD) remains a complex major health problem in the industrialized world. This chapter deals with its definition and epidemiology, followed by a discussion of the various substrates associated with the syndrome. Other areas of discussion that follow include the pathophysiology of SCD and identification and management of patients at increased risk. The final section deals with different modes of therapy and future directions.

DEFINITION

SCD remains a complex major health problem in the industrialized world. It accounts for approximately 20% to 25% of all nontraumatic deaths and 50% of deaths from coronary artery disease (CAD) (1–4). In the United States, approximately 300,000 SCDs occur annually, with at least one-third of these in individuals younger than 65 years (2,3,5). Mechanisms of SCD are heterogeneous. It is usually a consequence of the interaction of a number of complex factors in various subsets of patients (6). Thus, not surprisingly, no generally accepted definition exists (1,5). Those proposed have involved differences in the time interval from onset of symptoms to death, use of information on location of death, inclusion or exclusion of unwitnessed deaths, consideration of the unexpected nature of the event, and disease history (5,6). This heterogeneity of definition of SCD makes difficult the interpretation and comparison of different studies of this disorder and the

R. F. Sequeira: Division of Cardiology, Department of Medicine, University of Miami/Jackson Memorial Hospital, Miami, Florida 33136.
J. D. Simmons: Mount Sinai Medical Center, Division of Electrophysiology, Florida 33140.
R. J. Myerburg: Division of Cardiology, Department of Medicine, University of Miami/Jackson Memorial Hospital, Miami, Florida 33136.

formulation of a hypothesis for its pathophysiologic mechanism (4,6,7).

Myerburg (1) has defined SCD as natural death from cardiac causes, heralded by abrupt loss of consciousness within 1 hour of the onset of symptoms in a person with or without preexisting heart disease, but in whom the time and mode of death are unexpected. This definition, which combines the key elements of "natural," "rapid," and "unexpected," incorporates all of the essential elements.

EPIDEMIOLOGY

Over the last 20 years, the incidence of SCD has ranged from 300,000 to 350,000 annually in the United States. However, more recent attempts to more accurately estimate the incidence of SCD have been undertaken by the National Center for Health Statistics (NCHS) and the National Heart, Lung and Blood Institute (NHLBI). The source of the information and its accuracy greatly influences the final estimate. For example, in the NCHS study (which used death certificate data and a broad inclusion of all causes of SCD), the annual incidence was estimated at 460,000 events with more than 50% of all cardiac deaths defined as sudden (8). In contrast, The American Heart Association statistical handbook (which used narrower ICD-9 based definitions of SCD) suggests an incidence of 220,000 SCDs annually on the basis of coronary heart disease diagnoses (2). Whatever the estimate of the "true" annual incidence, the population pool from which the coronary and noncoronary SCD events derive continues to grow. This raises the question as to whether the time has come to establish a better vital statistic recording system from which more accurate information regarding SCD would be available. This investment would greatly advance future healthcare expenditure planning and assist in further clinical research endeavors (5,6,9).

Age, Sex, and Race

The incidence of SCD increases with age and is two to three times greater in men than in women (10). The proportion of sudden death from CAD decreases with increasing age. In the Framingham Study, 62% of all CAD deaths were sudden in men aged 45 to 54 years, declining to 58% in those aged 55 to 65 years and to 42% in the 65- to 74-year age group (10). In Kuller's series, 72% of deaths from CAD in the 20- to 39-year age group were sudden (11).

Limited studies using death certificates and autopsy data indicate that more blacks than whites die out of the hospital or experience out-of-hospital cardiac arrest. This has not been confirmed in broader populations. Out-of-hospital deaths may be related to lack of access to emergency cardiac care or to delay in the prehospital phase of acute myocardial infarction (MI) care (12–14).

Circadian Variation

A circadian variation related to time of awakening, with a major peak in midmorning and a lesser one in the afternoon/late evening, has been found for SCD (15–19). Similar patterns have been described for MI, transient ischemia, and ventricular and supraventricular arrhythmias (18). The Beta-Blocker Heart Attack Trial (BHAT) demonstrated a peak between 8 and 11 AM in both the propranolol and the placebo groups (20). The peaks were less prominent in the β-blocker group, suggesting an effect of propranolol on the circadian variation.

Mechanisms proposed for the increased morning incidence of SCD and other ischemic events point to increases in sympathetic activity with its known consequences, associated with awakening and assumption of the erect posture (18–20).

Psychosocial Factors

A number of studies suggest that vigorous physical activity in rare instances may trigger SCD (21,22). The confidence limits around the estimated risk for SCD in this setting are wide, and the incidence data indicate an extremely low risk. Several studies have identified an increase in informant-reported life stress either immediately before SCD or during the weeks preceding the event (23,24). The effect of stress on a population as a result of imminent warfare showed a doubling in sudden out-of-hospital deaths when compared with a similar controlled calendar period 1 year before commencement of hostilities (24).

SUBSTRATE ASSOCIATED WITH SUDDEN CARDIAC DEATHS

Atherothrombotic Coronary Artery Disease

Atherothrombotic CAD exceeds all other causes for SCD, accounting for 80% of events (25–27). In the Framingham Study, more than 50% of coronary mortality was related to SCD, and CAD and cardiac failure were the two most important risk factors for subsequent SCD (28). In men without a history of previous CAD, risk factors for SCD were similar to those for all coronary events. In men with known CAD, the only independent risk factors for SCD were the electrocardiographic abnormalities of left ventricular hypertrophy and intraventricular conduction delay reflecting left ventricular dysfunction secondary to ischemic damage (1,6,28).

Autopsy and angiographic data are consistent with epidemiologic evidence affirming the importance of CAD (25–27). Narrowing of more than 75% by cross-sectional area of at least one vessel is found in more than 90% of patients, and involvement of all three vessels is found in 60% to 65% or patients (29,30). In angiographic studies of survivors of out-of-hospital cardiac arrest, 60% to 80% have

75% or more stenosis of two or more coronary arteries, and more than 50% have three-vessel disease (31).

With increased awareness that plaque rupture or fissuring with consequent thrombus formation plays a crucial role in the pathophysiology of the acute ischemic syndromes, attention has focused on the morphology of coronary lesions and presence or absence of thrombus in victims of SCD.

The most frequent postmortem coronary angiographic lesions in victims of SCD are type II stenoses, identical to those found in acute MI after thrombolysis and in unstable angina (32). Rupture of an atherothrombotic plaque was found in more than 90% of patients dying of SCD, defined as death within 6 hours of onset of symptoms (26,31). These are characterized as eccentric lesions with ragged edges. Survivors of cardiac arrest who are not inducible at electrophysiologic testing or who do not have a significant akinetic or dyskinetic ventricular segment also have been shown to have a significant prevalence of type II angiographic lesions (31).

Left Ventricular Function

Left ventricular dysfunction as an indicator of myocardium vulnerable to lethal ventricular arrhythmias is an important predictor of SCD in patients with CAD (26,32) (Fig. 72–1). In studies involving more than 3,000 patients after MI, there was a strong association among left ventricular ejection fraction (LVEF), ambient ventricular arrhythmias, and death. Both ejection fraction (EF) and ventricular arrhythmias that served as independent predictors of mortality, with no statistical interaction (32,33). The increased risk for LVEF was measured at 40%, but the greatest rate of change of risk was between 30% and 40%. Although an EF of 30% or less was the most

important predictor for SCD, it had a low specificity. In the Multicenter Post-Infarction Program (MPIP), depressed left ventricular function predicted deaths occurring within the first 6 months after MI, whereas ventricular arrhythmias were more powerful for predicting later mortality (33).

Ambient Ventricular Arrhythmias in Chronic Ischemic Heart Disease

Most forms of ambient ventricular activity are of no significance in the absence of structural heart disease (34). However, when present in people older than 30 years, they select a subgroup with a greater probability of CAD and SCD. Most studies have identified both form and frequency of ventricular ectopic activity as indicators of risk, but no uniform classification exists. Although a frequency cutoff of 10 premature ventricular complexes (PVCs) is most frequently cited as a threshold level for increased risk, some have used cutoffs in the range of 1 to 9 PVCs per hour, 10 PVCs per 1,000 sinus beats, and more than 20 PVCs per hour (35). Previously it was thought that forms suggestive of high risk included multiform PVCs, bigeminy, and the R-on-T phenomenon, but these are now believed to have no independent prognostic significance, and more recent large studies have focused on the quantitative assessment of PVCs and the presence or absence of nonsustained ventricular tachycardia (VT). Most investigators have emphasized that salvos of three or more PVCs are the most powerful predictor (34,36,37). Subgroup analysis of the placebo arm of the Cardiac Arrhythmia Suppression Trial (CAST) suggested increased mortality risk among those patients with nonsustained VT and EF equal to or less than 30% (38).

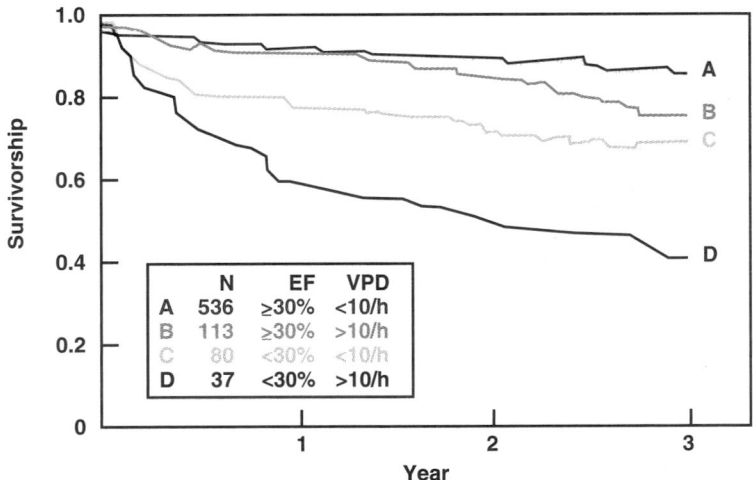

FIG. 72–1. Survival during 3 years of follow-up after acute myocardial infarction as a function of left ventricular dysfunction and ventricular arrhythmias. The survival curves were calculated as Kaplan-Meier estimates. With greater premature ventricular complex frequency and lower ejection fraction (EF), the mortality rate increases. VPD, ventricular premature depolarizations. (From Bigger JT, Fleis JL, Kleijer R, et al. The relationship among ventricular arrhythmia, left ventricular dysfunction, and mortality in the 2 years after myocardial infarction. *Circulation* 1984;69:250–258, with permission.)

The prevalence of hemodynamically tolerated sustained VT in the general population is unknown. Reasons for this lack of information include lack of a standardized approach to grading arrhythmia-related symptoms and nonreporting of symptoms or hemodynamic status during VT. Pooled data from the electrophysiologic literature indicate that roughly half of the cases of sustained VT referred for treatment are hemodynamically tolerated (39,40).

Sustained Tachyarrhythmia

Hemodynamically tolerated sustained VT occurs typically in men (85%) with a mean age of 63 years and with a history of previous MI in at least 80% of cases. Mean LVEF is typically about 34%, and as many as 50% to 70% of patients are taking oral antiarrhythmic medication at presentation. In various studies, VT rates from 170 to 190 beats per minute have been recorded, with rates in some cases as high as 240 to 270 beats per minute. The tachyarrhythmia may last from 30 minutes to 24 hours with an average of some 6 hours before medical evaluation. Electrophysiologic testing in this population group reveals inducible VT in more than 95% of patients, a rate comparable to that in patients presenting with poorly tolerated sustained VT. Whereas sustained VT is the most commonly induced arrhythmia, "nonclinical" uniform VT morphologies may be induced in more than 50% of cases. These latter VTs may at times be faster than the "clinical" arrhythmia (40,41).

Brugada and coworkers (42), reporting outcomes in 200 patients after MI, noted that hemodynamically tolerated sustained VT occurring in patients in NYHA Class I or II 2 months after MI had an excellent prognosis. There were no SCDs in 55 patients and only 1 nonsudden cardiac death.

Given the inconsistencies in data reporting and analysis, firm conclusions on the significance of hemodynamically tolerated sustained VT in the genesis of SCD are not possible at this time. Most information supports the notion that patients with CAD with spontaneous hemodynamically tolerated sustained VT have a relatively lower short- and long-term sudden death mortality rate than patients with poorly tolerated sustained VT or cardiac arrest.

Myocardial Hypertrophy

The Framingham Study suggested that left ventricular hypertrophy was a risk factor for SCD (7). Other studies have confirmed this observation and reinforced its role as a risk factor in both the presence and absence of CAD (43,44). Patients with primary hypertrophic cardiomyopathy and left or right ventricular hypertrophy secondary to a variety of causes are at increased risk for SCD (44–46). In patients with CAD who die suddenly, autopsy studies have revealed coexisting left ventricular hypertrophy in as many as 75% of the victims, with the severity of the hypertrophy bearing no relation to the severity of the CAD (43). Left ventricular hypertrophy predisposes to high-grade ventricular ectopy and

TABLE 72–1. *Other cardiovascular diseases associated with sudden cardiac death*

Coronary arteries
  Anomalous coronary arteries
  Coronary artery embolism
  Coronary arteritis
  Coronary dissection
  Coronary spasm
Cardiomyopathies
  Nonischemic dilated cardiomyopathy
  Hypertrophic cardiomyopathy
Inflammatory and infiltrative diseases of the heart
  Myocarditis
  Chronic granulomatous diseases
  Sarcoid
  Collagen vascular disease
Arrhythmogenic right ventricular dysplasia
Valvular heart disease
  Aortic stenosis
  Mitral valve prolapse
Congenital heart disease
  Eisenmenger's syndrome
  Postsurgical repair
Electrical abnormalities
  Prolonged QT interval syndromes
  Wolff-Parkinson-White syndrome
  Brugada syndrome
Miscellaneous
  Catecholamine-dependent
  "Voodoo death"
  Idiopathic ventricular fibrillation

electrophysiologic instability (47). Prolonged recovery of excitability and other abnormalities of the hypertrophied myocyte in response to ischemia and reperfusion have been demonstrated, and these may contribute to electrophysiologic heterogenicity (48,49).

Cardiac Disease Other Than Coronary Atherothrombotic Heart Disease

Although SCD is most commonly associated with coronary heart disease and its consequences, it may also occur in the setting of a wide variety of other disorders (Table 72–1).

PATHOPHYSIOLOGY OF SUDDEN CARDIAC DEATH

Ventricular fibrillation (VF) and VT are most likely to occur in hearts with preexisting or acutely evolving structural abnormalities, or both (27–29). CAD is responsible for more than 80% of the structural defects, with cardiomyopathies accounting for 10% to 15% and valvular heart disease accounting for most of the remainder (27). Structurally, the alterations have been categorized under healing and healed MI, myocardial fibrosis, ventricular hypertrophy, and structural electrophysiologic abnormalities such as bypass tracts.

From monitoring patients during acute MI, Lown and Wolfe (27a) observed a relation between the incidence and complexity of ventricular arrhythmias and the development of VF; they termed these "warning arrhythmias," and Lown proposed a grading system for these arrhythmias that was widely accepted. This became the basis for the PVC hypothesis. Simply stated, "Premature ventricular complexes are triggers for VF, and this risk is increased with more frequent and/or complex PVC forms." The advent of Holter monitoring revealed that in patients with prior MI, there was a positive correlation between the risk for sudden death and the frequency and complexity of PVCs (32,33,36,50) (Table 72–2).

Controlled studies, however, have revealed that suppression of ventricular ectopic activity does not equate with prevention of death, and, indeed, in some cases as in the CAST, active antiarrhythmic drugs were associated with an increased risk (38). Experience with programmed electrical stimulation also has shown that even in those patients with easily inducible sustained arrhythmias and frequent PVCs, special circumstances are required to initiate spontaneous clinical events. These observations and other experimental data suggest that there is no simple relation between PVCs and VT and/or VF (51,52).

Advances in the delineation of the mechanisms underlying SCD suggest an important role for triggering events at the onset of cardiac arrest. This hypothesis is strengthened by the observation of a circadian variation in its incidence (15,16). The morning increase in the occurrence of SCD and other related events suggest causation by identifiable triggers. Pathologic findings in the coronary arteries of patients with SCD, identification of morphologic and functional abnormalities of myocardial tissue that increase its arrhythmogenic potential, and recognition of the significance of increased platelet aggregability, decreased fibrinolytic activity, and other blood components involved in thrombogenesis have increased our understanding of the pathophysiology of SCD (53).

Myerburg and coworkers (51) have proposed the structure/function concept to explain the interaction between PVC, VT/VF, and the susceptible myocardium. It states that the initiation of sustained tachyarrhythmias requires both a preexisting structural abnormality that provides the condition for establishing pathways or foci responsible for sustained arrhythmias and a modification of the preexisting abnormality by functional changes at a specific point in time. The functional changes alter a stable electrophysiologic abnormality, converting it to an unstable state because of transient changes in electrophysiology. Programmed electrical stimulation supports this concept. As we stress the importance of a structural substrate in the genesis of lethal ventricular arrhythmias, it is of note that approximately one-third of SCD survivors are noninducible at electrophysiologic study (54). Modification of this electrophysiologic substrate by triggering events such as ischemia, hemodynamic variables, autonomic tone, electrolyte imbalance, and antiarrhythmic drugs facilitates the sustenance of ventricular arrhythmias (51).

Structural Abnormalities and Triggering Mechanisms

All forms of structural heart disease are associated with SCD (25–28). Functional factors that can modulate the structurally based pathophysiology include the consequences of transient ischemia and reperfusion, hemodynamic and metabolic abnormalities, autonomic fluctuations, and the effects of toxic substances in the heart (51,55) (Fig. 72–2).

Coronary Artery Disease and Sudden Cardiac Death Triggering Factors

The majority of episodes of SCD occur in patients with CAD and left ventricular dysfunction secondary to previous MI (27,56,57). The terminal arrhythmia may begin as a sustained monomorphic VT that degenerates into hemodynamically unstable VT. In others, a brief period of polymorphic VT degenerates directly into VF. In only 15% to 20% is there evidence of acute MI, although coronary vascular lesions suggesting active ischemia are considerably more common (26,27,31,58,59).

TABLE 72–2. *Association of frequent or complex premature ventricular complexes and sudden cardiac death after myocardial infarction*

Study (reference)	Patients, n	Follow-up, mo	SCD, % With frequent PVCs[a]	SCD, % Without frequent PVCs	SCD, % With complex PVCs[b]	SCD, % Without complex PVCs	Sensitivity/ Specificity	PPV, %
Ruberman (36)	1,739	42	15	5			54/76	15
	1,739	42			16	6	57/67	16
Bigger (32)	819	22	12	6			33/81	12
	819	22			13	5	48/73	13
Ridker (112)	533	18	13	4			34/87	13
Farrell (86)	416	20	54[c]	18[c]			54/82	16

PPV, positive predictive value; PVC, premature ventricular complex; SCD, sudden cardiac death.
[a]PVCs ≥ 10 per hour.
[b]Bigeminy, pairs, multiform, R on T.
[c]Including sudden cardiac death and sustained ventricular tachycardia.

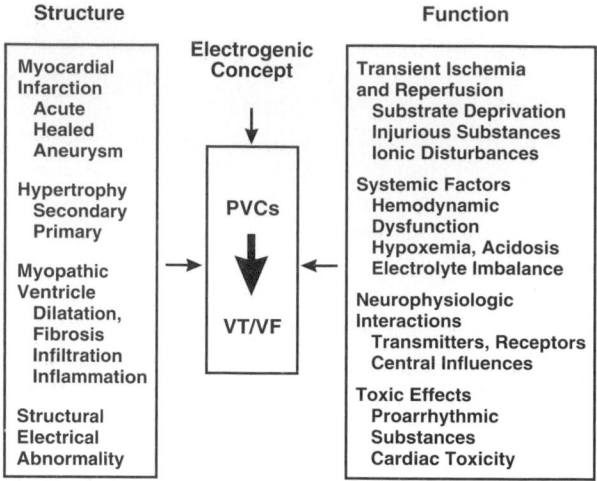

FIG. 72–2. Structure, function, and the pathogenesis of sudden cardiac death. Functional alterations of the structural cardiac abnormalities "substrate" by one or more inciting influences may convert premature ventricular complexes (PVCs), which are pathophysiologically innocuous, into triggering events for ventricular tachycardia or fibrillation (VT/VF). (From Myerburg RJ, Kessler KM, Bassett AL, et al. A biological approach to sudden cardiac death: structure, function and cause. *Am J Cardiol* 1989;63:1512–1516, with permission.)

Various lines of evidence suggest a different physiologic substrate between those presenting primarily with VT and those with VF (52). Greater extent of structural damage (previous MI or LV aneurysm), inducible arrhythmias, abnormalities of endocardial activation, and greater prevalence of late potentials have been demonstrated among patients with sustained monomorphic VT as compared with VF and polymorphic VT (52,54,60). It is in this latter group that triggering factors more likely play a major role. Additional support for a triggering mechanism, particularly in this latter group, is offered by the evaluation of CABG on noninducibility of previously inducible arrhythmias in cardiac arrest survivors and patients with life-threatening arrhythmias. In two published series, coronary revascularization suppressed inducibility in a greater percentage of patients in whom the inducible arrhythmia was VF but in only a small percentage of patients in whom the inducible arrhythmia was inducible monomorphic VT (61–63).

Ischemia and Reperfusion as Triggers

The extent of CAD, morphologic characteristics, and presence of intracoronary thrombi in victims and survivors of SCD has been described earlier (26,27,29,30). The electrophysiologic effect of acute ischemia and its relation to VF has been clearly demonstrated (58,64,65). Clinically, marked transient ischemia is associated with the risk for VT, ventricular flutter, or rapid polymorphic VT (37,64–66). Slow or stable monomorphic VT is usually associated with a substrate such as healed MI (66,67). Importantly, reperfusion, although

affecting reversal of the electrophysiologic consequences of ischemia, may in itself lead to specific patterns of membrane disturbance (64,68). Experimentally, periods of ischemia lasting 5 to 30 minutes are those most likely to result in potentially dangerous electrical disturbances. Furthermore, reperfusion arrhythmias can generate in a much smaller mass of tissue than is required for reentry (49,64–66).

Ambulatory ECG tracings recorded at the time of SCD have provided insight into the arrhythmic mechanism and role of ischemia (67,68). Estimates of the presence of ischemia before SCD, based on these tracings, have ranged from 10% to 50%. Given the limitations of ambulatory monitoring in the detection of myocardial ischemia, these studies may underestimate its true incidence.

Exercise-induced painless myocardial ischemia has been demonstrated in some survivors of VF (69). Silent ischemia on exercise testing predicted subsequent SCD among Coronary Artery Surgery Study (CASS) registry patients with three-vessel disease (70). In a study of 17 survivors of exercise-induced cardiac arrest, Campricotti and coworkers (66) pointed out that in all patients this event was associated with unstable angina, asymptomatic ST-segment depression, or acute coronary artery occlusion.

At least one-third of survivors of cardiac arrest are found to be noninducible at electrophysiologic study (54,71). Noninducible survivors with significant CAD or coronary artery spasm have an excellent prognosis when treated for the underlying CAD (72,73).

Prinzmetal "variant angina" serves as a useful model of paroxysmal transmural myocardial ischemia. Miller and coworkers (64), reviewing the clinical characteristics associated with sudden death in patients with variant angina, found serious rhythm disturbances in approximately 45% of subjects during ischemic episodes. On follow-up, SCD occurred in 42% of patients with arrhythmias during ischemic episodes but in only 6% of those without ischemia-induced arrhythmias. These data have been corroborated in another study that showed that most arrhythmias occurred during the resolution phase of ST-segment elevation, and thus presumably were caused by reperfusion (65).

Randomized controlled trials of β-blocker therapy, and in particular those without sympathetic activity, after acute MI have consistently demonstrated a decrease in total mortality, primarily linked to a reduction in SCD (74). Other antiischemic agents such as calcium blockers or pure antiarrhythmic agents have not been shown to have any effect on SCD after MI (75). β-Blockers have complex actions, and the mechanism of protection by them is likely to be multifactorial with a decisive role for its antiischemic effect (76,77).

Some investigators have argued against a role for ischemia in the pathophysiology of SCD, supporting instead the importance of the substrate (58,78,79). These investigators have identified the presence of late potentials and EF less than 40% as the most important predictors of VT or VF and have suggested that electrophysiologic triggers play a critical role in the spontaneous initiation of VT or VF leading to SCD.

Autonomic Triggers

Several lines of evidence suggest that disturbances of autonomic nervous system activity is accompanied by an increased risk for SCD, although the mechanism whereby ventricular arrhythmias are precipitated is not completely understood (80–83). During myocardial ischemia, the discharge frequency of vagal and sympathetic sensory endings in the LV is increased (80–83). Sympathetic hyperactivity facilitates the onset of malignant ventricular arrhythmias and favors a thrombotic tendency, whereas vagal activation exerts an antifibrillatory effect. Disturbances of autonomic function may occur at several levels (83). Experimental data and clinical studies suggest that cardiac abnormalities that predispose to the risk for SCD are accompanied by regional changes in autonomic function within the heart itself (80,81). Many physiologic variables possibly involved in triggering cardiac arrest are closely associated with function of the autonomic system (15,53). After MI, heart rate variability and baroreflex sensitivity, markers of tonic and reflex vagal activity, respectively, often are reduced (84–86). This reduction in protective vagal activity has been found to be associated with a greater mortality rate and, in particular, SCD after MI. It has been suggested that the reduction in SCD by β-blockers is a consequence of attenuation of the effects of denervation supersensitivity on dispersion of refractoriness, conduction changes, and other electrophysiologic properties of the myocardial cells, as well as through a central vagotonic effect (87–89).

Toxic Triggers: Proarrhythmia

That antiarrhythmic drugs can in themselves be proarrhythmic was first recognized with quinidine (90). Numerous examples also have been seen in the electrophysiologic laboratory, where nonsustained VT has been converted to sustained VT after antiarrhythmic therapy. The CAST emphasized the consequences of this known effect. Mechanisms proposed for drug-induced tachyarrhythmias include promotion of reentry and the induction of delayed and early afterdepolarizations (52).

Certain groups of patients are known to be at a greater risk. In patients with structural heart disease and significant LV dysfunction who have demonstrated preexisting VT or VF, agents that block the sodium channel are more likely to cause serious proarrhythmias (91,92). Evidence from animal models of ischemic heart disease and detailed analyses of the CAST study indicate that antiarrhythmic agents may facilitate malignant arrhythmias when ischemia develops (52, 92–94).

The reported association between cocaine and SCD suggests that cocaine may cause lethal arrhythmias (95–97). This agent has been shown *in vitro* and *in vivo* to cause repolarization abnormalities. Arrhythmias secondary to vasospasm-related ischemia, reperfusion, or both may be the mechanism in some abnormalities.

IDENTIFICATION OF POPULATIONS AT RISK

Risk Factor Assessment

In patients with CAD, ventricular ectopy, left ventricular dysfunction, and certain electrocardiographic changes are associated with an enhanced risk for SCD (1,10,35). Although these predictors have statistical significance in identifying groups of patients, they are far from satisfactory in both sensitivity and specificity when applied to the population at large (98–100) (Fig. 72–2).

Furthermore, the risk for SCD does not appear to be linear as a function of time after a change in cardiovascular status (101). In recent reports, a reduced EF was the only predictor for early-phase recurrence, and persistent inducibility was the strongest predictor for late-phase recurrence (102,103) (Fig. 72–3). In addition, many investigators have demonstrated a temporal variability of ventricular arrhythmias with resulting influence on risk stratification (104,105). Pepine and coworkers (68), in patients with stable cardiac disease, found that the spontaneous variation in PVC frequency was 48% from hour to hour, 23% from day to day, and 37% between repeated 3-day monitoring periods.

In addition to hourly and daily variability, biologic variability also has been documented for ventricular arrhythmias. This variation is of particular relevance in the patient after infarction (105,106). Application of preventive measures therefore requires identification of high-risk groups and an appreciation and study of the changing time dependence of various predictors for SCD.

Coronary Artery Disease

Eighty percent of SCDs in the United States and Europe occur in patients with CAD (25–27). In 20% to 25% of patients,

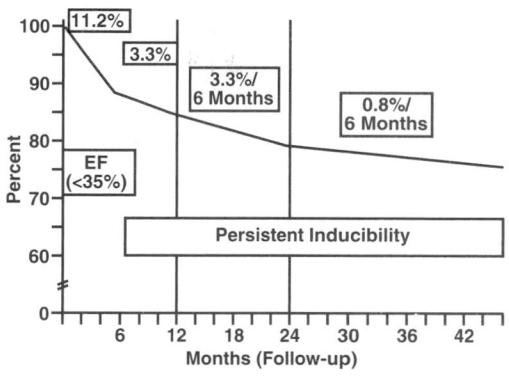

FIG. 72–3. Survival curve showing time dependence of risk for recurrence among survivors of cardiac arrest. Risk was greatest in the first 6 months. A low ejection fraction (EF) was the most powerful predictor of death during the first 6 months, but, subsequently, persistent inducibility during programmed stimulation, despite drug therapy or surgery, was the most powerful predictor. (From Myerburg RJ, Kessler KM, Castellanos. Sudden cardiac death: epidemiology, transient risk, and intervention assessment. *Ann Intern Med* 1993;119: 1187–1195, with permission.)

SCD may be the first and only manifestation of the underlying disease. Healed MIs are a common finding at autopsy, with the incidence ranging from 40% to more than 70%, even in those with no previous clinical history (1,2,4,27). Narrowing of more than 75% by cross-sectional area of at least one vessel is found in more than 90% of patients, and involvement of all three vessels is found in more than 60%. Left ventricular dysfunction also is a common finding. Systolic blood pressure, cholesterol, cigarette smoking, heart rate, electrocardiographic abnormalities, and left ventricular hemodynamics such as wedge pressure and stroke work index do not appear to be risk factors (102,103). Male sex and left ventricular dysfunction do appear to be independently associated with SCD (7,28,32).

Plaque destabilization with consequent erosion or rupture leads to the clinical expression of the acute coronary syndromes (56,58,107). In a number of studies, an association of SCD with the acute coronary syndromes has been demonstrated (31,58,107). Inflammatory markers have been shown to be a predictor of risk for plaque destabilization (108–112). Thus, the ability to identify the individual at risk for plaque rupture, in advance of its clinical expression, might provide a useful method for identifying individuals at potential risk for SCD.

Survivors of Cardiac Arrest

Up to 30% of cardiac arrest victims who have out-of-hospital resuscitation efforts may survive (102,103). These survivors are at greatest risk for recurrence. In early series, the rates ranged from 22% in a mean follow-up of 2 months to 45% at 2 years, but this has improved significantly during the last decade (104,113).

Absence of acute MI identifies a group at particularly high risk. The 1- and 2-year mortality rates in patients surviving cardiac arrest with associated MI are 0% and 14%, whereas in those without MI, they are 32% and 43% (114). Most of these deaths are sudden. VF is the first documented rhythm in 60% to 85% of patients resuscitated from SCD (104) and is found even more frequently if the underlying heart disease is CAD. This rhythm is associated with the best short-term survival to hospital admission and accounts for the greatest proportion of survivors of out-of-hospital cardiac arrest (114,115).

Data from Holter monitoring have shown that rapid VT is most commonly the initial arrhythmia, followed by degeneration to polymorphic VT and VF (67,116,117). Bradyarrhythmias, asystole, and electromechanical dissociation are more frequently found as causes of SCD in patients with severe congestive heart failure. These terminal rhythms indicate a poor short-term prognosis (118–120).

Left ventricular function is the strongest independent predictor for recurrence and long-term survival after out-of-hospital cardiac arrest (113). It is also predictive of successful suppression of inducible ventricular arrhythmias during serial drug testing (121). In a study of 154 cardiac arrest survivors, the 5-year mortality rate was 4% in those with LVEF greater than 50%, 48% in those with LVEF of 35% to 50%, and 70% in those with LVEF less than 35% (122).

Up to 50% to 60% of out-of-hospital survivors of SCD die early after hospitalization. Most die of sepsis and anoxic encephalopathy, with cardiogenic shock and heart failure second most frequent cause. Recurrent cardiac arrhythmias, sustained VT, and VF account for only 5% to 10% of early deaths. Ventricular premature beats or nonsustained VT is fairly common and is seen in up to 80% of the survivors (113). The role of ventricular ectopy as a predictor for subsequent SCD remains unclear. Although earlier studies (113,115,123) had shown nonsustained VT after cardiac arrest to be associated with a greater incidence of recurrent SCD, more recent studies suggest that complex ventricular ectopy after SCD is a marker of underlying cardiac disease, particularly LV dysfunction, and does not have a useful predictor value for subsequent death (50, 113,115,123).

In survivors of SCD with underlying CAD, sustained ventricular arrhythmias are induced in up to 70% at baseline electrophysiologic testing (60,124). This incidence depends on the degree of LV dysfunction, the presenting arrhythmias, and the aggressiveness of the stimulation protocol used (125). The role of premature extrasystole (PES) for risk stratification and therapy guidance in survivors of out-of-hospital cardiac arrest has been extensively studied (124,126). However, because of varying definitions of SCD used, the nonuniform substrate, and the different stimulation protocols, comparison of studies has been difficult, and therefore its value is difficult to assess. In this heterogeneous population, where CAD accounts for more than 70%, induction of arrhythmias at baseline PES is predictive of total cardiac mortality but does not predict recurrent cardiac arrest. Persistent inducibility of VT or VF on antiarrhythmic drugs, coupled with reduced LVEF, however, is strongly predictive of both total cardiac mortality and recurrent cardiac arrest (60,127,128). The predictive value of PES in cardiac arrest survivors with nonischemic heart disease remains controversial (47,129,130).

The inability to induce any ventricular arrhythmia at baseline PES is generally associated with better LV function, a lower incidence of CAD, and a better long-term outcome (47,60,129). Patients with no inducible arrhythmias and significant CAD with preserved LV function who undergo revascularization have an excellent prognosis.

MANAGEMENT OF PATIENTS AT INCREASED RISK FOR SUDDEN CARDIAC DEATH

Cardiac Arrest Survivors

The refinement of implantable cardioverter-defibrillator (ICD) technology has pushed the management of cardiac arrest survivors away from electrophysiologic testing and antiarrhythmic drug therapy and toward device-based therapy for secondary prevention of cardiac arrest. With the knowl-

TABLE 72–3. *Noninvasive methods for evaluation of patients at risk for sudden cardiac death*

Ambulatory Holter monitoring
Signal-averaged electrocardiogram
Heart rate variability
Exercise testing

edge that 30% of patients successfully resuscitated from cardiac arrest in the absence of a new ST-segment elevation MI will have a recurrent cardiac arrest within the first year of follow-up, several randomized trials worldwide were performed comparing the ICD with antiarrhythmic drugs in secondary prevention of SCD. In the United States, the National Institutes of Health (NIH)–sponsored AVID (Amiodarone Versus Implantable Defibrillators) trial randomized patients with cardiac arrest and symptomatic VT to receive amiodarone or ICD as initial therapy (131). A 38% reduction in total mortality was noted for the ICD group compared with the arrhythmic group. Similar studies from Canada and Europe have confirmed the superiority of the ICD as initial therapy for cardiac arrest survivors and transvenous implantation techniques have made the operative mortality rate less than 1%. Therefore, in patients who do not have an obvious explanation for cardiac arrhythmia precipitating cardiac arrest (e.g., ST-segment elevation MI within first 48 hours of cardiac arrest, offending drug leading to polymorphic VT), ICD therapy has been accepted as a first-line standard therapy. Patients with rarer causes of cardiac arrest (e.g., hypertrophic or dilated cardiomyopathy, right ventricular dysplasia, long QT syndrome, Brugada syndrome) also are considered ICD candidates, given the unpredictability of the underlying cardiac substrate for producing cardiac arrest.

Primary Prevention of Sudden Cardiac Death in Patients at "High Risk"

Several methods of noninvasive cardiac evaluation have been proposed to detect an additional increased risk for future ventricular tachydysrhythmia and SCD in patients at risk for increased total cardiac mortality stratified by decreased left ventricular function (Table 72–3). Coronary revascularization in the CASS proved that treatment of myocardial ischemia decreased risk for cardiac mortality threefold compared with medical therapy in "high-risk" groups (Fig. 72–4) (109). Ambient nonsustained VT and decreased heart rate variability detected by ambulatory monitoring and fractionated electrical activation of the left ventricle detected by signal-averaged electrocardiogram have been noted to identify an increased risk for symptomatic ventricular arrhythmia or inducibility of VT at electrophysiologic testing. The positive predictive power, however, has been poor, leading to uncertainty in clinical application.

More recently, clinical research has explored the use of the ICD as primary therapy for the patient subgroups at greatest risk for SCD. The Multicenter Automatic Defibrillator Implantation Trial (MADIT) trial randomized patients who had LVEF less than 35%, previous MI, nonsustained VT on ambulatory monitoring, and inducible VT at electrophysiologic testing to standard medical therapy or ICD implantation (132). A total mortality rate for ICD implantation was noted and has been confirmed by similar randomized studies in the range of 20% to 30% mortality reduction over 2 to 3 years. ICD therapy was tested further in the MADIT-II trial, which randomized patients with previous MI and LVEF less than 30% to ICD or standard medical therapy (133). Again, ICD therapy improved total mortality, sug-

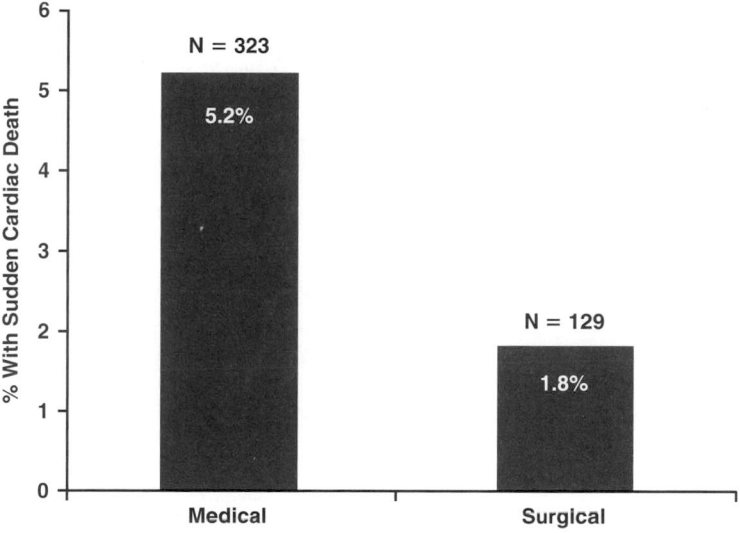

FIG. 72–4. Incidence of sudden cardiac death in 13,476 medically and surgically treated Coronary Artery Surgical Study (CASS) patients. (Modified from Holmes DR, Davis K, Gersh BJ, et al. Risk factor profiles of patients with sudden cardiac death and deaths from other causes. A report from the Coronary Artery Surgery Study (CASS). *J Am Cardiol* 1989;13:524–531, with permission.)

gesting an increased risk for arrhythmic death in this patient group.

Unfortunately, significant clinical uncertainty (secondary to lack of clinical research data) remains for primary prevention of cardiac arrest in patient subgroups other than those with ischemic heart disease. Generally speaking, indicators of increased risk for SCD for the nonischemic cardiomyopathies and inherited disorders include syncope, documented ventricular tachydysrhythmia, or family history of SCD. Significant clinical judgment on a case-by-case basis is still necessary, given the unpredictability of the arrhythmic cardiac substrate, but most patients at high enough risk are considered candidates for ICD implantation, given the lack of other alternative therapies.

FUTURE DIRECTIONS IN THE APPROACH TO SUDDEN CARDIAC DEATH

The ability to predict and prevent SCD is currently limited by the frequency with which SCD is either the first clinical manifestation of previously unrecognized disease (approximately 30% of all SCDs) or occurs in patients considered at low risk because of the absence of specific high-risk markers (approximately 33% of all SCDs). To make progress in the future, it will be necessary to find new markers of risk that are highly specific for SCD as an expression of CAD or other disorders. One avenue that offers promise in this regard is the evolution of the field of genetic electrophysiology, which offers the hope of translation to genetic epidemiology (134). With the discovery of a number of gene loci that encode arrhythmia risk in specific arrhythmic syndromes such as long QT interval syndrome, Brugada syndrome, "idiopathic" VF, and right ventricular dysplasia, candidate genes for studying the expression of risk among the more general population have emerged. With the recognition that many (if not most) proarrhythmic responses associated with a "acquired" long QT interval syndrome are actually genetically based abnormalities of ion channel function with low penetrance until an inciting factor is present, the notion that such genetic abnormalities may predispose to specific arrhythmic risk has emerged. One study highlighted the presence of a genetic variant among approximately 13% of the black population, who appear predisposed to arrhythmias generally and to drug-induced arrhythmias in particular. This variation in the gene encoding the cardiac sodium channel appears to be more prevalent among patients in arrhythmia clinics and is consistent with epidemiologic data that suggest that SCDs as a specific manifestation of an acute coronary syndrome is familial. The sodium channel abnormality in the black population is an example that is leading investigators to seek other polymorphisms or genetic variants among other segments of the population that may predispose to risk for arrhythmia. This leads to the emerging field of genetic epidemiology and will likely incorporate other genetic markers of risks for acute coronary syndromes such as variations in the thrombotic cascade or

inflammatory responses, as well as atherogenesis. Taken cumulatively, the construction of a risk profile based on complex system analysis of multigenic modifiers of disease expression leads to the hope of identifying patients susceptible to the risk for sudden death far in advance of disease expression (99).

REFERENCES

1. Myerburg RJ, Castellanos A. Cardiac arrest and sudden cardiac death. In: Braunwald E, ed. *Heart disease: a textbook of cardiovascular medicine,* 6th ed. Philadelphia: WB Saunders, 2001:890–931.
2. American Heart Association. *2001 heart and stroke statistical update.* Dallas, TX: American Heart Association, 2000.
3. Cobb LA, Fahrenbruch CE, Olsufka M, et al. Changing incidence of out-of-hospital ventricular fibrillation, 1980-2000. *JAMA* 2002;288:3008–3013.
4. Zheng ZJ, Croft JB, Giles WH, et al. Sudden cardiac death in the United States, 1989 to 1998. *Circulation* 2001;104:2158–2163.
5. Every NR, Parsons L, Hlatsky MA, et al. Use and accuracy of state death certificates for clarification of sudden deaths in high-risk populations. *Am Heart J* 1997;134:1129–1132.
6. Myerburg RJ. Sudden cardiac death: exploring the limits of our knowledge. *J Cardiovasc Electrophysiol* 2001;12:369–381.
7. Doyle JT, Kannel WB, McNamara PM, et al. Factors related to suddenness of coronary death: combined Albany-Framingham studies. *Am J Cardiol* 1976;37:1073–1078.
8. National Center for Health Statistics. *Vital statistics of the United States, 1984, vol 11. Mortality, part A.* Washington, DC: Public Health Service, U.S. Government Printing Office, 1987. Department of Health and Human Services [DHHS] Publication no. (PHS) 87-1122.
9. Priori SG, Borggrefe M, Camm AJ, et al. Unexplained cardiac arrest: the need for a prospective registry. *Eur Heart J* 1992;13:1445–1446.
10. Schatzkin A, Cupples LA, Heeren T, et al. Sudden death in the Framingham Heart Study: differences in incidence and risk factors by sex and coronary disease status. *Am J Epidemiol* 1984;120:888–889.
11. Kuller L, Lilienfeld A, Fischer R. Sudden and unexpected deaths in young adults: an epidemiologic study. *JAMA* 1966;198:158–165.
12. McCord C, Freeman HP. Excess mortality in Harlem. *N Engl J Med* 1990;322:173–177.
13. Clark LT, Bellam SV, Shah AH, et al. Analysis of prehospital delay among inner-city patients with symptoms of myocardial infarction: implications for therapeutic intervention. *J Natl Med Assoc* 1992;84:931–937.
14. Maynard C, Fisher LD, Passamani ER. Survival of black persons compared with white persons in the Coronary Artery Surgery Study (CASS). *Am J Cardiol* 1987;60:513–518.
15. Willich SN, Goldberg RJ, Maclure M. Increased onset of sudden cardiac death in the first 3 hours after awakening. *Am J Cardiol* 1992;70:58–65.
16. Muller JE, Ludmer PL, Willich SN, et al. Circadian variation in the frequency of sudden cardiac death. *Circulation* 1987;75:131–138.
17. Roberts W, Peters L, Brent M, et al. Circadian pattern of arrhythmic death in patients receiving encainide, flecainide, or moricizine in the Cardiac Arrhythmia Suppression Trial (CAST). *J Am Coll Cardiol* 1994;23:283–289.
18. Muller JE, Tofler SH, Stone PH. Circadian variation and triggers of onset of acute cardiovascular disease. *Circulation* 1989;79:733–743.
19. Andreotti F, Davies SJ, Hoekett DR, et al. Major circadian fluctuations in fibrinolytic factors and possible relevance to time of onset of myocardial infarction, sudden cardiac death and stroke. *Am J Cardiol* 1988;62:635–637.
20. Peters RW. Propranolol and the morning increase in sudden cardiac death: the Beta-Blocker Heart Attack Trial experience. *Am J Cardiol* 1990;65:579–599.
21. Maclure M, Sherwood J, Mittleman M, et al. Myocardial infarction onset study: triggering of onset of myocardial infarction by heavy exertion. *Circulation* 1991;84[Suppl II]:II-61.
22. Willich SN, Lowell H, Lewis M, et al. TRIMM Study Group: exertional and physical activity is associated with increased risk of myocardial infarction. *J Am Coll Cardiol* 1993;21[Suppl A]:437A.

23. Karmack T, Jennings JR. Biobehavioral factors in sudden cardiac death. *Psychol Bull* 1991;109:42–75.

24. Meisel SR, Kutz I, Dayan KI, et al. Effect of Iraqi missile war on incidence of acute myocardial infarction and sudden death in Israeli civilians. *Lancet* 1991;338:660–661.

25. Thomas A, Knapman P, Krikler D, et al. Community study of the causes of "natural" sudden death. *Br Med J* 1988;297:1453–1456.

26. Davies M. Pathological view of sudden cardiac death. *Br Heart J* 1981;45:88–96.

27. Virami R, Roberts WC. Sudden cardiac death. *Hum Pathol* 1987;18: 485–492.

27a. Lown B, Wolf M. Approaches to sudden death from coronary heart disease. *Circulation* 1971;44:130–142.

28. Kannel WB, Thomas HE. Sudden coronary death. The Framingham Study. *Ann NY Acad Sci* 1982;382:3–20.

29. Warners C, Robert S. Sudden coronary death: relation of amount and distribution of coronary narrowing at necropsy to previous symptoms of myocardial ischemia, left ventricular scarring, and heart weight. *Am J Cardiol* 1984;54:65–73.

30. Roberts W, Potkin B, Johns D, et al. Mode of death frequency of healed and acute myocardial infarction, number of major epicardial coronary arteries severely narrowed by atherosclerotic plaque, and heart weight in fatal atherosclerotic coronary artery disease. Analysis of 889 patients studied at necropsy. *J Am Cardiol* 1990;15:196–203.

31. Davies M, Thomas A. Thrombosis and acute coronary artery lesions in sudden cardiac ischaemic death. *N Engl J Med* 1984;30:1137–1140.

32. Bigger JT, Fleis JL, Kleijer R, et al. The relationship among ventricular arrhythmia, left ventricular dysfunction, and mortality in the 2 years after myocardial infarction. *Circulation* 1984;69:250–258.

33. Risk stratification and survival after myocardial infarction. *N Engl J Med* 1983;309:331–336.

34. Kennedy HL, Whitlock JA, Sprague MK, et al. Long-term follow-up of asymptomatic healthy subjects with frequent and complex ventricular ectopy. *N Engl J Med* 1985;312:193–196.

35. Myerburg RJ, Kessler KM, Luceri RM, et al. Classification of ventricular arrhythmias based on parallel hierarchies of frequency and form. *Am J Cardiol* 1984;54:1355–1358.

36. Ruberman W, Weinblatt E, Frank CW, et al. Repeated 1-hour electrocardiographic monitoring of survivors of myocardial infarction at 6-month intervals. Arrhythmia detection and relation to prognosis. *Am J Cardiol* 1981;47:1197–1203.

37. Follansbee WP, Michelson EL, Morganroth RJ. Non-sustained ventricular tachycardia in ambulatory patients. Characteristics and association with sudden cardiac death. *Ann Intern Med* 1980;92:741–747.

38. Greene HL, Roden DM, Katz RJ, et al. The Cardiac Arrhythmia Suppression Trial. First CAST . . . then CAST II. *J Am Coll Cardiol* 1992;19:894–898.

39. Kadish AH, Buxton AE, Waxman HL, et al. Usefulness of electrophysiologic study to determine the clinical tolerance of arrhythmic recurrences during amiodarone therapy. *J Am Coll Cardiol* 1987;10:90–96.

40. Buxton AE, Waxman HL, Marchlinski FE, et al. Role of triple extrastimuli during electrophysiologic study of patients with documented sustained ventricular tachyarrhythmias. *Circulation* 1984;69:532–540.

41. Steinman RT, Lehman MH, Zheutin T, et al. Long-term outcome of electrophysiologically-guided therapy for haemodynamically-tolerated sustained ventricular tachycardia in coronary artery disease. *J Am Coll Cardiol* 1990;15:123A.

42. Brugada P, Talaju M, Smeets J, et al. The value of the clinical history to assess prognosis of patients with ventricular tachycardia or ventricular fibrillation after myocardial infarction. *Eur Heart J* 1989;10:747–752.

43. Rissanen V, Romo M, Siltanen P. Prehospital sudden death from ischaemic heart disease: a postmortem study. *Br Heart J* 1978;40: 1025–1033.

44. Koren MJ, Devereux RB, Casale PN, et al. Relation of left ventricular mass and geometry to morbidity and mortality in uncomplicated essential hypertension. *Ann Intern Med* 11991;4:345–352.

45. Maron BJ, Roberts WC, Epstein SE. Sudden death in hypertrophic cardiomyopathy: a profile of 78 patients. *Circulation* 1982;65:1388–1394.

46. McKenna WJ, Camm AJ. Sudden death in hypertrophic cardiomyopathy. *Circulation* 1989;80:1489–1492.

47. Fogoron RN, Elson JJ, Bonnet CA, et al. Long-term outcome of survivors of cardiac arrest whose therapy is guided by electrophysiologic testing. *J Am Coll Cardiol* 1991;19:780–788.

48. Kowey PR, Friehling TD, Sewter J, et al. Electrophysiological effects

49. Kuo C, Munakata K, Reddy CP, et al. Characteristics and possible mechanism of ventricular arrhythmia dependent on the dispersion of action potential durations. *Circulation* 1983;67:1356 1367.

50. Bigger JT, Weld FM, Rolnitzky LM. Prevalence, characteristics and significance of ventricular tachycardia (three or more complexes detected with ambulatory electrocardiographic recording) in the late hospital phase of acute myocardial infarction. *Am J Cardiol* 1981;48:815–819.

51. Myerburg RJ, Kessler KM, Bassett AL, et al. A biological approach to sudden cardiac death: structure, function and cause. *Am J Cardiol* 1989;63:1512–1516.

52. Akhtar M, Breithardt GM, Coumel P, et al. CAST and beyond: implications of the Cardiac Arrhythmia Suppression Trial. *Circulation* 1990;81:1123–1127.

53. Andreotti HF, Davies GJ, Hackett DR, et al. Major circadian fluctuations in fibrinolytic factors and possible relevance to time of onset of myocardial infarction, sudden cardiac death and stroke. *Am J Cardiol* 1988;62:635–637.

54. Roy D, Waxman HL, Kienzle MG, et al. Clinical characteristics and long-term follow-up in 119 survivors of cardiac arrest. Relation to inducibility at electrophysiologic testing. *Am J Cardiol* 1983;52:969–974.

55. Myerburg RJ, Kessler KM, Castellanos A. Interactions between structure and function in sudden cardiac death. In: Akhlar M, Myerberg RJ, Ruskin JN, eds. *Sudden cardiac death: prevalence, mechanisms, and approaches to diagnosis and management.* Baltimore, MD: Williams & Wilkins, 1994;32–50.

56. Taylor AJ, Burke AP, O'Malley PG, et al. A comparison of the Framingham risk index, coronary artery calcification, and culprit plaque morphology in sudden cardiac death. *Circulation* 2000;101:1243–1248.

57. Liberthson RR, Nagel EL, Hirschman JC, et al. Pathophysiologic observations in prehospital ventricular fibrillation and sudden cardiac death. *Circulation* 1974;49:790–798.

58. Mehta D, Curwin J, Gomes A, et al. Sudden death in coronary artery disease: acute ischemia versus myocardial substrate. *Circulation* 1997;96:3215–3223.

59. Warnes CA, Roberts WC. Sudden coronary death: relation of amount and distribution of coronary narrowing at necropsy to previous symptoms of myocardial ischemia, left ventricular scarring, and heart weight. *Am J Cardiol* 1984;54:65–73.

60. Wilber DJ, Goran H, Finkelstein D. Out-of-hospital cardiac arrest: use of electrophysiologic testing in the prediction of long-term outcome. *N Engl J Med* 1988;318:19–24.

61. Kelly P, Ruskin JN, Vlahakes GJ, et al. Surgical coronary revascularization in survivors of pre-hospital cardiac arrest: its effect on ventricular arrhythmias and long-term survival. *J Am Coll Cardiol* 1990;15: 267–273.

62. Kron IL, Lerman BB, Haines DE, et al. Coronary bypass grafting in patients with ventricular fibrillation. *Ann Thorac Surg* 1989;48:85–89.

63. Ricks WB, Winkle RA, Shumway NE, et al. Surgical management of life-threatening ventricular arrhythmias in patients with coronary artery disease. *Circulation* 1977;56:38–42.

64. Miller DD, Waters DD, Szlachcic J, et al. Clinical characteristics associated with sudden death in patients with variant angina. *Circulation* 1982;66:588–589.

65. Previtali M, Klevsy C, Salerno SA, et al. Ventricular tachyarrhythmias in Prinzmetal's variant angina. Clinical significance and relation to the degree and time course of ST-segment elevation. *Am J Cardiol* 1983;52:19–22.

66. Campricotti R, Taverne R, El Gamel M. Clinical and angiographic observations on resuscitated victims of exercise-related sudden ischemic death. *Am J Cardiol* 1991;68:47–50.

67. Bayes' de Luna A, Coumel P, Leclercq JF. Ambulatory sudden death: mechanisms of production of fatal arrhythmia on the basis of data from 157 cases. *Am Heart J* 1989;117:151–159.

68. Pepine CJ, Morganroth J, McDonald JT, et al. Sudden death during ambulatory electrocardiographic monitoring. *Am J Cardiol* 1991;68: 785–788.

69. Sharma B, Asinger R, Francis GS, et al. Demonstration of exercise-induced painless myocardial ischemia in survivors of out-of-hospital ventricular fibrillation. *Am J Cardiol* 1987;59:740–745.

70. Weiner DA, Ryan TJ, McCabe CH, et al. Risk of developing an acute myocardial infarction or sudden coronary death in patients with exercise-induced silent myocardial ischemia. A report from the Coronary

Artery Surgery Study (CASS) Registry. *Am J Cardiol* 1988;63:1155–1158.

71. McLaren CJ, Gersh BJ, Sugrue DD, et al. Out-of-hospital cardiac arrest in patients without clinically significant coronary artery disease. Comparison of clinical, electrophysiological, and survival characteristics with those in similar patients who have clinically significant coronary artery disease. *Br Heart J* 1987;58:583–589.

72. Morady F, DiCarlo L, Winston S, et al. Clinical features and prognosis of patients with out-of-hospital cardiac arrest and a normal electrophysiologic study. *J Am Coll Cardiol* 1984;4:39.

73. Kehoe R, Tommaso C, Zehutlin T, et al. Factors determining programmed stimulation responses and long-term arrhythmic outcome in survivors of ventricular fibrillation with ischemic heart disease. *Am Heart J* 1988;116:355–363.

74. Yusuf S, Peto R, Lewis J, et al. Beta blockade during and after myocardial infarction: an overview of the randomized trials. *Prog Cardiovasc Diagn* 1985;27:335–371.

75. Held PH, Yusuf S, Furberg CD. Calcium channel blockers in acute myocardial infarction and unstable angina: an overview. *Br Med J* 1989;299:1187–1190.

76. Singh BN. Advantages of beta blockers versus antiarrhythmic agents and calcium antagonists in secondary prevention after myocardial infarction. *Am J Cardiol* 1990;66:9C.

77. Frishman WH, Lazar EJ. Reduction of mortality, sudden death and nonfatal reinfarction with beta-adrenergic blockers in survivors of acute myocardial infarction. A new hypothesis regarding the cardioprotective action of beta-adrenergic blockade. *Am J Cardiol* 1990;66:669–672.

78. Meissner MD, Akhtar M, Lehmann MH. Nonischemic sudden tachyarrhythmic death in atherosclerotic heart disease. *Circulation* 1991;84:905–912.

79. Gomes JA, Alexopoulos D, Winters SL, et al. The role of silent ischemia, the arrhythmic substrate and the short-long sequence in the genesis of sudden cardiac death. *J Am Coll Cardiol* 1989;14:1618–1625.

80. Schwartz PJ, Priori SG. Sympathetic nervous system and cardiac arrhythmias. In: Zipes D, Jalife J, eds. *Cardiac electrophysiology: from cell to bedside.* Philadelphia: WB Saunders, 1990:330–343.

81. Schwartz PJ, Stramba-Badiale M. Parasympathetic nervous system and cardiac arrhythmias. In: Kulbertus HE, Frank G, eds. *Neurocardiology.* Mount Kisco, NY: Futura, 1988:179–200.

82. Corr PB, Yamada KA, Witkowski FX. Mechanisms controlling autonomic function and their relation to arrhythmogenesis. In: Fozzard HA, Hales E, Jennings RB, et al., eds. *The heart and cardiovascular system, vol II.* New York: Raven Press, 1986:1343–1403.

83. Schwartz PT, La Rovere MT, Vanoli E. Autonomic nervous system and sudden cardiac death. Experimental basis and clinical observations for post-myocardial infarction risk stratification. *Circulation* 1992;85[Suppl 1]:77–91.

84. Schneider RA, Costiloe JP. Relationship of sinus arrhythmia to age and its prognostic significance in ischemic heart disease. *Clin Res* 1965;13:1213–1219.

85. Kleiger RE, Miller JP, Briggs JT Jr, et al. Decreased heart rate variability and its association with increased mortality after myocardial infarction. *Am J Cardiol* 1987;60:86–89.

86. Farrell TG, Bashier Y, Cripps T, et al. Risk stratification for arrhythmic events in post infarction patients based on heart rate variability, ambulatory electrocardiographic variables and signal averaged electrocardiogram. *J Am Coll Cardiol* 1991;18:683–687.

87. Zipes D. Changes in innervation patterns and autonomic responsiveness in myocardial infarction. In: Rosen MR, Janse MJ, Wit AL, eds. *Cardiac electrophysiology: a textbook.* Mount Kisco, NY: Futura Publishing, 1990:915–931.

88. Bittner SB, Smith SE. Beta-adrenoreceptor antagonists increase sinus arrhythmia, a vagotonic effect. *Br J Clin Pharmacol* 1986;22:691–695.

89. La Rovere MT, Bigger JT Jr, Marcus FI, et al. Baroreflex sensitivity and heart-rate variability in prediction of total cardiac mortality after myocardial infarction. ATRAMI (Autonomic Tone and Reflexes After Myocardial Infarction) Investigators. *Lancet* 1998;351:478–484.

90. Kerr WC, Bender WL. Paroxysmal ventricular fibrillation with cardiac recovery in a case of auricular fibrillation and complete heart block while under quinidine sulfate therapy. *Heart* 1921;9:269.

91. Lazzara R. Pharmacological triggers of sudden death. In: Akhlar M, Myerberg RJ, Ruskin JN, eds. *Sudden cardiac death: prevalence, mechanisms and approaches to diagnosis and management.* Philadelphia: Williams & Wilkins, 1994:394–406.

92. Splawski I, Timothy KW, Tateyama M, et al. Variant of SCN5A sodium channel implicated in risk of cardiac arrhythmia. *Science* 2002;297:1333–1336.

93. Sesti F, Abbott GW, Wei J, et al. A common polymorphism associated with antibiotic-induced cardiac arrhythmia. *Proc Natl Acad Sci USA* 2000;97:10613–10618.

94. Napolitano C, Schwartz PJ, Brown AM, et al. Evidence for a cardiac ion channel mutation underlying drug-induced QT prolongation and life-threatening arrhythmias. *J Cardiovasc Electrophysiol* 2000;11:691–696.

95. Inoue H, Zipes DP. Cocaine-induced supersensitivity and arrhythmogenesis. *J Am Coll Cardiol* 1988;11:867–874.

96. Kloner RA, Hale S, Alker K, et al. The effects of acute and chronic cocaine use on the heart. *Circulation* 1992;85:407–419.

97. Kimura S, Bassett AL, Xi H, et al. Early afterdepolarizations and triggered activity induced by cocaine. A possible mechanism of cocaine arrhythmogenesis. *Circulation* 1992;85:2227–2235.

98. Myerburg RJ, Kessler KM, Castellanos. Sudden cardiac death: epidemiology, transient risk, and intervention assessment. *Ann Intern Med* 1993;119:1187–1195.

99. Myerburg RJ. Scientific gaps in the prediction and prevention of sudden cardiac death. *J Cardiovasc Electrophysiol* 2002;13:709–723.

100. Jouven X, Desnos M, Guerot C, et al. Predicting sudden death in the population: the Paris Prospective Study I. *Circulation* 1999;99:1978–1983.

101. Myerburg RJ, Kessler KM, Castellanos A. Interactions between structure and function in sudden cardiac death. In: Akhlar M, Myerberg RJ, Ruskin JN, eds. *Sudden cardiac death: prevalence, mechanisms, and approaches to diagnosis and management.* Baltimore: Williams & Wilkins, 1994:32–50.

102. Cupples LA, Gagnon DR, Kannel WB. Long and short-term risk of sudden coronary death. *Circulation* 1992;85[Suppl 1]:111–118.

103. Hurwitz JL, Josephson ME. Sudden cardiac death in patients with chronic coronary heart disease. *Circulation* 1992;85[Suppl I]:I-43–I-49.

104. Eisenberg MS, Cummins RO, Larsen MP. Numerators, denominators and survival rates: reporting survival from out-of-hospital cardiac arrest. *Am J Emerg Med* 1991;9:544–546.

105. Pratt CM, Slymen DJ, Wierman AM, et al. Analysis of the spontaneous variability of ventricular arrhythmias: consecutive ambulatory electrocardiographic recordings of ventricular tachycardia. *Am J Cardiol* 1985;56:67–72.

106. Klieger RF, Miller JP, Thanavero S, et al. Relationship between clinical features of acute myocardial infarction and ventricular runs two weeks to one year following infarction. *Circulation* 1981;63:64–70.

107. Davies MJ: Anatomic features in victims of sudden coronary death. Coronary artery pathology. *Circulation* 1992;85[Suppl]:I-19–I-24.

108. Braunwald E. Cardiovascular medicine at the turn of the millennium: triumphs, concerns, and opportunities. *N Engl J Med* 1997;337:1360–1369.

109. Holmes DR, Davis K, Gersh BJ, et al. Risk factor profiles of patients with sudden cardiac death and deaths from other causes. A report from the Coronary Artery Surgery Study (CASS). *J Am Cardiol* 1989;13:524–531.

110. Koenig W, Sund M, Fröhlich M, et al. C-reactive protein, a sensitive marker of inflammation, predicts future risk of coronary heart disease in initially healthy middle-aged men: results from the MONICA (Monitoring Trends and Determinants in Cardiovascular Disease) Augsburg Cohort Study, 1984 to 1992. *Circulation* 1999;99:237–242.

111. Ridker PM, Rifai N, Clearfield M, et al., Air Force/Texas Coronary Atherosclerosis Prevention Study Investigators. Measurement of C-reactive protein for the targeting of statin therapy in the primary prevention of acute coronary events. *N Engl J Med* 2001;344:1959–1965.

112. Ridker PM, Cushman M, Stampfer MJ, et al. Inflammation, aspirin, and the risk of cardiovascular disease in apparently healthy men [Erratum in: *N Engl J Med* 1997;337:356]. *N Engl J Med* 1997;336:973–979.

113. Myerburg RJ, Kessler KM, Estes D, et al. Long term survival after prehospital cardiac arrest: analysis of outcome during an 8 year study. *Circulation* 1984;70:538–546.

114. Goldberg R, Szklo M, Tonascia JA, et al. Acute myocardial infarction: prognosis complicated by ventricular fibrillation or cardiac arrest. *JAMA* 1979;241:2024–2027.

115. Myerburg RJ, Conde CA, Sung RJ, et al. Clinical, electrophysiologic and hemodynamic profile of patients resuscitated from prehospital cardiac arrest. *Am J Med* 1980;68:568–576.

116. Pratt CM, Francis MJ, Luck GC, et al. Analysis of ambulatory electrocardiograms in 15 patients during spontaneous ventricular fibrillation with special reference to preceding arrhythmic events. *J Am Coll Cardiol* 1983;2:789–797.

117. Kempf FC, Josephson ME. Cardiac arrest recorded on ambulatory electrocardiograms. *Am J Cardiol* 1984;53:1577–1582.

118. Packer M. Sudden unexpected death in patients with congestive heart failure: a second frontier. *Circulation* 1985;72:681–685.

119. Luu M, Stevenson WG, Stevenson LW, et al. Diverse mechanisms of unexpected cardiac arrest in advanced heart failure. *Circulation* 1989;80:1675–1680.

120. Chakko CS, Gheorghiade M. Ventricular arrhythmias in severe heart failure: incidence, significance, and effectiveness of antiarrhythmic therapy. *Am Heart J* 1985;109:497–504.

121. Stevenson WG, Brugada P, Waldecker B, et al. Clinical, angiographic and electrophysiologic findings in patients with aborted sudden death as compared with patients with sustained ventricular tachycardia after myocardial infarction. *Circulation* 1985;71:1146–1152.

122. Ritchie JL, Hallstrom AP, Troughbaugh JC, et al. Out-of-hospital sudden coronary death: rest and exercise radionuclide left ventricular function in survivors. *Am J Cardiol* 1985;55:645–651.

123. Weaver WD, Cobb LA, Hallstrom AP. Ambulatory arrhythmias in resuscitated victims of cardiac arrest. *Circulation* 1982;66:212–218.

124. Akhtar M, Garan H, Lehmann MH, et al. Sudden cardiac death. Management of high-risk patients. *Ann Intern Med* 1991;114:499–512.

125. Freedman RA, Swerdlow CD, Soderholm DV, et al. Prognostic significance of arrhythmia inducibility or noninducibility at initial electrophysiologic study in survivors of cardiac arrest. *Am J Cardiol* 1988;61:578–582.

126. Adhar GC, Larson LW, Bardy GH, et al. Sustained ventricular arrhythmias: differences between survivors of cardiac arrest and patients with recurrent sustained ventricular tachycardia. *J Am Coll Cardiol* 1988;12:159–165.

127. Furukawa T, Rozanski J, Nogami A, et al. Time-dependent risk of and predictors for cardiac arrest recurrence in survivors of out-of-hospital cardiac arrest with chronic coronary artery disease. *Circulation* 1989;80:599–608.

128. Wilber DJ, Kelly E, Garan H, et al. Determinants of inducible ventricular arrhythmias in survivors of out-of-hospital cardiac arrest. *Circulation* 1986;75[Suppl II]:II-482.

129. Trouton TG, Powell AC, Krislnan S, et al. Inducibility of ventricular arrhythmias at baseline electrophysiologic study in cardiac arrest survivors. *J Am Coll Cardiol* 1993;2:327A.

130. Kron J, Hart M, Schnal BS, et al. Idiopathic dilated cardiomyopathy: role of programmed electrical stimulation and Holter monitoring in predicting those at risk for sudden cardiac death. *Chest* 1988;93:85–90.

131. A comparison of antiarrhythmic-drug therapy with implantable defibrillators in patients resuscitated from near-fatal ventricular arrhythmias. The Antiarrhythmics versus Implantable Defibrillators (AVID) Investigators. *N Engl J Med* 1997;337:1576–1583.

132. Moss AJ, Hall WJ, Cannom DS, et al. Improved survival with an implanted defibrillator in patient with coronary disease at high risk for ventricular arrhythmia. Multicenter Automatic Defibrillator Implantation Trial Investigators. *N Engl J Med* 1996;335:1933–1940.

133. Moss AJ, Zareba W, Hall WJ, et al. Prophylactic implantation of a defibrillator in patients with myocardial infarction and reduced ejection fraction. *N Engl J Med* 2002;346:877–883.

134. Bonow R, Clark EB, Curfman GD, et al. Task force on strategic research direction: clinical science subgroup. *Circulation* 2002;106:e162–e166.

CHAPTER 73

Cardiogenic Shock

John C. Wang and Patrick T. O'Gara

Key Words: Cardiogenic shock; pump failure; revascularization; shock trial.

Cardiogenic shock caused by left ventricular (LV) pump failure is the leading cause of death after myocardial infarction (MI) (1,2). Despite significant advances in coronary care over the last three decades, its incidence has remained essentially unchanged and the associated mortality distressingly high (3). The recognition of cardiogenic shock should initiate a rapid sequence of evaluation and treatment strategies designed to achieve prompt myocardial reperfusion, but only when the anticipated benefit of such an invasive approach justifies the enormous clinical and financial costs it engenders. Earlier identification of patients at particularly high risk for pump failure and more rapid access to expert percutaneous coronary intervention (PCI) are critical components of any care pathway.

DEFINITION

Cardiogenic shock is a low-output state characterized by increased intracardiac filling pressures and peripheral hypoperfusion. It most commonly results from a critical loss of functioning myocardium after one or more infarctions. Non-

atherothrombotic causes of myocardial necrosis and replacement, such as myocarditis, dilated cardiomyopathy, or contusion, can be readily distinguished. Severe LV systolic dysfunction after MI must be distinguished from several other mechanical complications that can result in cardiogenic shock (Table 73–1): papillary muscle rupture with severe mitral regurgitation, interventricular septal rupture with acute left to right shunting, LV free wall rupture with hemopericardium and tamponade, and the syndrome of right ventricular infarction. In the SHOCK (SHould we emergently revascularize Occluded Coronaries for shocK) trial registry of 1,190 patients with cardiogenic shock, 78.5% had predominant LV failure, 6.9% had severe mitral regurgitation, 3.9% had ventricular septal rupture, 2.8% had isolated right ventricular shock, 1.4% had tamponade from free wall rupture, and 6.7% had shock from other causes (4). The special features of these particular entities are reviewed in Chapters 74 and 75. Hemopericardium with tamponade after thrombolysis, without identifiable rupture, also has been reported (5). Shock may complicate the course of severe aortic stenosis with advanced LV dysfunction and may occur with massive pulmonary embolism. The following discussion focuses on post-MI shock caused by LV failure.

Cardiogenic shock is manifested clinically by systemic hypotension (systolic blood pressure <90 mm Hg) with signs of pulmonary congestion and tissue hypoperfusion (oliguria [urine output <30 mL/h]; cool, clammy skin with mottling or livedo reticularis; and/or depressed mentation). Although various hemodynamic criteria have been proposed, most authorities would agree that the triad of systemic hypotension (systolic blood pressure <90 mm Hg or

J. C. Wang: Interventional Cardiology, Midatlantic Cardiovascular Associates, P. A., Department of Medicine, St. Joseph Medical Center, O'Dea Medical Arts Bldg., 7505 Osler Drive, Suite 103, Towson, Maryland 21204.
P. T. O'Gara: Brigham and Women's Hospital, Harvard Medical School.

TABLE 73–1. *Complications causing postinfarction cardiogenic shock*

Predominant left ventricular failure
Papillary muscle rupture
Ventricular septal rupture
Left ventricular free wall rupture with tamponade
Right ventricular infarction
Hemopericardium and tamponade after thrombolysis or
   perforation

mean arterial pressure <60 mm Hg without response to fluid resuscitation), increased left-heart filling pressures (mean pulmonary capillary wedge pressure ≥18 mm Hg), and depressed cardiac output (cardiac index ≤2.0 L/min/m²) adequately defines the diagnosis. Many case series and patient registries suffer from the lack of an applied and uniform definition.

EPIDEMIOLOGY

The true incidence of cardiogenic shock is difficult to ascertain. Reported rates have ranged from 2% to 20% during the last three decades (3,6–12). In the Multicenter Investigation of the Limitation of Infarct Size (MILIS) Study, 4.5% of patients had cardiogenic shock at the time of hospital admission; another 7.1% (60/845) of patients experienced development of shock during hospitalization, with the greatest incidence on Day 0, although the condition of half of the patients deteriorated more than 24 hours after admission (8). Among the 9,076 patients admitted to 16 community hospitals in the Worcester Heart Attack Study between 1975 and 1997, the overall incidence rate of cardiogenic shock averaged 7.1% over the 23-year study period (Fig. 73–1) (3). Multivariate adjusted analysis revealed nonsignificant trends in the risk for development of shock over the study period, supporting the relatively constant incidence of cardiogenic

shock in patients with acute MI (3). Cardiogenic shock occurred in 2,972 (7.2%) of 41,021 patients enrolled in the Global Utilization of Streptokinase and Tissue Plasminogen Activator for Occluded Coronary Arteries (GUSTO-I) trial (12). Most patients (89%) experienced development of shock after admission, usually within 48 hours; only 11% had shock at presentation.

In a landmark 1967 description of their early coronary care experience, Killip and Kimball (6) reported a high mortality rate (81%) among 47 patients with post-MI shock (19% of the total patients studied). The SHOCK registry investigators reported an in-hospital mortality rate of 60% (4), whereas the Worcester Heart Attack Study in-hospital case fatality rates in patients with cardiogenic shock averaged 71.7% over 23 years (3). Interestingly, the in-hospital mortality rate remained relatively constant in the Worcester Heart Attack Study until the mid-1990s. Multivariable regression analysis demonstrated considerable improvement in in-hospital survival thereafter (50–55%) (Fig. 73–2). This improvement in survival coincided with the more aggressive treatment of acute coronary syndromes with both invasive (i.e., PCI, coronary artery bypass grafting [CABG], and intraaortic balloon counterpulsation [IABP]) and pharmacologic therapies (3). Holmes and coworkers (13) stratified patients with cardiogenic shock who were enrolled in GUSTO-I by country of treatment (1,891 patients treated in the United States, 1,081 patients treated in other countries). These investigators demonstrated more aggressive use of diagnostic and therapeutic procedures in the United States compared with other countries: cardiac catheterization (58% vs. 23%); PCI (26% vs. 8%); IABP (25% vs. 7%); right-heart catheterization (57% vs. 22%); and ventilatory support (54% vs. 38%) (13). This more aggressive treatment strategy in the United States was associated with improved adjusted 30-day (50% vs. 66%; *p* < 0.001) and 1-year (56% vs. 70%; hazard ratio, 0.69; 95% confidence interval [CI], 0.63–0.75; *p* < 0.001) mortality rates (13), lending further

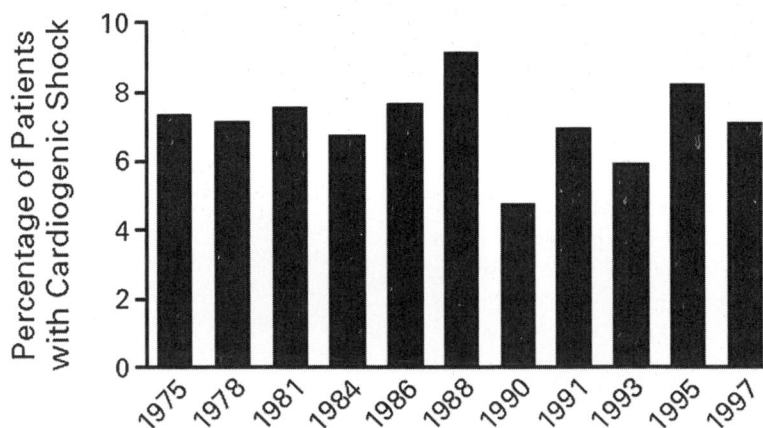

FIG. 73–1. Temporal trends in the incidence of cardiogenic shock in patients with acute myocardial infarction. (From Goldberg RJ, Samad NA, Yarzebski J, et al. Temporal trends in cardiogenic shock complicating acute myocardial infarction. *N Engl J Med* 1999;340:1162–1168, with permission.)

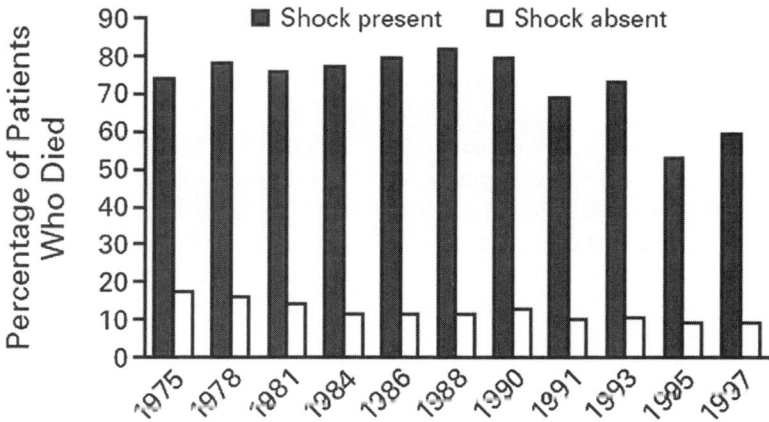

FIG. 73–2. Temporal trends in in-hospital mortality rates among patients with acute myocardial infarction according to the presence or absence of cardiogenic shock. (From Goldberg RJ, Samad NA, Yarzebski J, et al. Temporal trends in cardiogenic shock complicating acute myocardial infarction. *N Engl J Med* 1999;340:1162–1168, with permission.)

support and impetus to the early recognition and aggressive treatment of cardiogenic shock complicating acute MI.

PATHOPHYSIOLOGY

LV pump failure is generally associated with the pathologic demonstration of a loss of 40% or more of functioning myocardium (14,15). This extensive destruction can be the result of a single, large infarction or may represent the cumulative result of a relatively smaller infarction superimposed on numerous prior insults. What follows is a complex interplay among several processes involving neurohormonal regulatory systems, progressively declining pump function, and microcirculatory derangements (Fig. 73–3) (16–19). In the absence of intervention, a vicious cycle of repetitive injury is established that will eventuate in pump failure and, most commonly, death. Indeed, such patients are susceptible to "piecemeal" myocardial necrosis reflected clinically by a relatively greater and more prolonged myocardial-specific creatine kinase (CK-MB) release or a propensity to infarct extension after the initial event, or both (18,20).

The systemic hypotension that derives from the depression of cardiac output triggers a variety of compensatory responses. Activation of sympathetic outflow through baroreceptor mechanisms results in an increase in heart rate and peripheral vasoconstriction with redistribution of the circulating blood volume more centrally to the brain and heart. Renal blood flow is reduced with further redistribution away from the renal cortex, mediated largely by α_1-adrenergic mechanisms and sympathetic renal nerve activity. Renin release results ultimately in the generation of angiotensin II, a potent vasoconstrictor, and the concomitant release of aldosterone from the adrenal cortex with the retention of Na^+ and water by the kidney. Antidiuretic hormone (vasopressin) is released centrally in response to the perceived reduction in systemic pressure with further conservation of water and systemic vasoconstriction. Cerebral blood flow may be maintained

through autoregulation by which cerebral vascular resistance decreases in relation to the initial decrease in perfusion pressure. However, this mechanism is eventually overwhelmed once flow decreases to less than 50% of normal values (mean arterial pressure ≤50 mm Hg) (21).

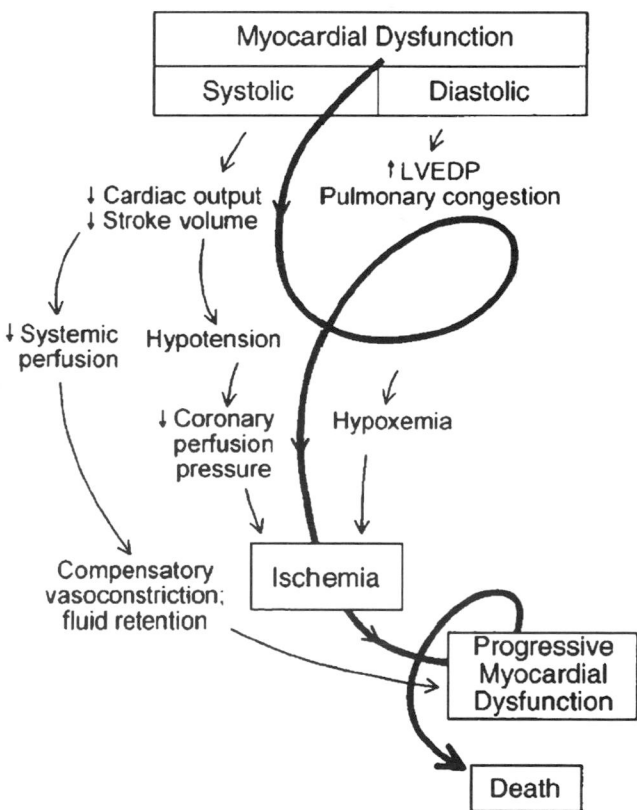

FIG. 73–3. The downward spiral in cardiogenic shock. LVEDP, left ventricular end-diastolic pressure. (From Hollenberg SM, Kavinsky CJ, Parrillo JE. Cardiogenic shock. *Ann Intern Med* 1999;131:47–59, with permission.)

Myocardial pump performance will depend on the relative contributions to output of the infarct zone, the vulnerable periinfarct border, and remote areas uninvolved by the acute process. Oxygen delivery throughout the myocardium is impaired for several reasons including: (a) diminished forward pressure secondary to the decrease in cardiac output; (b) a further reduction in the coronary perfusion gradient (diastolic pressure time index) because of the associated increase in LV end-diastolic volume and pressure (22); and (c) microcirculatory obstruction caused by intraluminal debris (fragmented plaque, platelet/fibrin thrombi), edema with luminal compression, and impairment/exhaustion of vasodilator reserve. The infarct zone itself, especially if transmural and anatomically large, undergoes a process of thinning and expansion because of tissue loss, myocardial slippage, and disruption of individual myocytes. In its extreme form, rupture may occur (18).

The periinfarct zone is susceptible to eventual ischemic attack and inclusion in the process of injury through an imbalance of myocardial oxygen supply/demand. Reduced coronary perfusion pressure and oxygen delivery, increased regional and global wall stress, and enhanced catecholamine stimulation provide the requisite ingredients for progressive injury.

The function of areas of myocardium remote from the infarct zone is a critical determinant of pump performance and survival (23,24). The normal response includes dilation, hypertrophy, and compensatory hyperkinesis. When this process is impaired, however, outcomes are significantly jeopardized. The noninfarct zone may be fibrotic and scarred from prior injury. Alternatively, perfusion to this zone may be compromised by interruption of collateral flow from the infarct vessel and by coexistent disease in the individual artery subtending the noninfarct zone itself. "Ischemia at a distance" portends a poor outcome (25).

Autopsy studies have shown that the majority of patients who die with cardiogenic shock have multivessel coronary artery disease (CAD) (26), most commonly with involvement of the left anterior descending coronary artery. In the prereperfusion era, persistent occlusion of the infarct vessel was the rule (14,15).

CLINICAL FEATURES

The typical patient with cardiogenic shock caused by LV failure has an anterior ST-segment elevation MI (STEMI) accompanied by hypotension, tachycardia, and pulmonary congestion, with one or more of the several signs of peripheral hypoperfusion discussed earlier in this chapter. The multivariate predictors for the development of cardiogenic shock identified in the MILIS study by Hands and coworkers (8) included age older than 65 years ($p = 0.007$), the presence of diabetes mellitus ($p = 0.011$), and a history of previous MI ($p = 0.012$). Female sex, although identified as a univariate predictor, did not prove to be a significant independent predictor of shock in multivariate logistic regression analysis. The remaining multivariate predictors of shock were admission LV ejection fraction less than 35% ($p = 0.007$) and peak CK-MB greater than 160 IU/L ($p = 0.008$) (8). The probability of development of cardiogenic shock was 1.7%, 3.9%, 8.6%, 17.9%, 33.7%, and 54.4%, respectively, for patients with 0 to 5 independent risk factors (8).

Most of the patients in the MILIS study in whom cardiogenic shock developed had predominant LV failure. Indeed, ventricular septal rupture and mitral regurgitation comprised only 5.1% and 10.3%, respectively, of the total patients with cardiogenic shock (8). The important pathophysiologic role of infarct extension was again emphasized by the finding that 23.3% of the 60 patients who experienced development of shock had enzymatic evidence of reinfarction, defined as a secondary reelevation of the CK-MB fraction 48 hours after initial onset (8). This definition likely underestimates the true incidence of infarct extension, because it excludes patients who may have had recurrent injury within the first 48 hours. According to the authors, infarct extension was documented to have occurred before or at the time of onset of cardiogenic shock in most patients (8). Reinfarction occurred in 11% of GUSTO-I patients in whom shock developed versus only 3% of patients who did not experience cardiogenic shock ($p < 0.0001$) (12).

Additional risk factors for the development of cardiogenic shock include blood lactate levels (27), anterior location of MI, history of angina, and prior treatment for congestive heart failure (11,26,28).

Cardiogenic shock developed a median of 6.2 hours after the onset of MI in the SHOCK registry and varied by culprit artery (left main, median 1.7 hours; right, 3.5 hours; circumflex, 3.9 hours; left anterior descending, 11 hours; saphenous vein graft, 10.9 hours) (29). Early shock (74.1%), defined as occurring less than 24 hours after MI onset, was associated with chest pain at shock onset, ST-segment elevation in two or more leads, multiple infarct locations, inferior MI, left main disease, and smoking. In-hospital mortality rate was greater for early versus late shock (62% vs. 53.6%; $p = 0.022$) (29).

Although cardiogenic shock complicates the course of STEMI more often, it has been reported to occur with unstable angina and non–STEMI (30–32). Holmes and coworkers (32) studied the 12,084 patients (4,092 with ST-segment elevation and 7,991 without ST-segment elevation) in GUSTO-IIb who did not present with cardiogenic shock. Cardiogenic shock developed in 4.2% of patients with STEMI, compared with only 2.5% of patients without ST-segment elevation (odds ratio [OR], 0.58; 95% CI, 0.47–0.72; $p < 0.001$) (32). Nevertheless, when compared with patients with STEMI and shock, patients without ST-segment elevation were older, more frequently had diabetes mellitus, prior MI, prior coronary bypass surgery, prior heart failure, recurrent ischemia, and three-vessel CAD, but had less TIMI Grade 0 flow at angiography (32). The 30-day mortality rate was greater for patients with non–ST-segment elevation and shock (73% non–ST-segment elevation vs. 63% ST-segment elevation; $p = 0.050$) (32).

Similar findings were reported from the SHOCK registry. Of the 881 patients with cardiogenic shock caused by predominant LV failure, 729 had STEMI and 152 had non–STEMI. Compared with patients with STEMI, patients with non–STEMI were significantly older and greater incidences of prior MIs, heart failure, azotemia, coronary bypass surgery, peripheral vascular disease, three-vessel CAD, and recurrent ischemia (31). In-hospital mortality rates were similarly high for both groups (62.5% non–STEMI vs. 60.4% ST-elevation MI) (31).

CLINICAL ASSESSMENT

The initial clinical assessment should include careful notation of vital signs, heart rhythm, venous pressure, breath sounds, heart sounds, peripheral and carotid pulses, extremities, skin, and neurologic function. The electrocardiogram may reveal obvious injury in an anatomic zone, most commonly anterior, but also can demonstrate global ST-segment depressions of only moderate severity or a nondiagnostic intraventricular conduction delay. Chest radiography provides information regarding heart size and pulmonary vascularity, the latter ranging from normal to bilateral alveolar edema. As a general rule, a large heart size implies a more chronic process with LV systolic dysfunction. Early risk assessment is critical and can begin with readily ascertainable medical history, examination, and laboratory data. It has been estimated that 90% of the risk for 30-day mortality after MI can be attributed to the composite of age, systolic blood pressure, Killip class, heart rate, and location of MI (33). Identification of patients at high risk should dictate prompt application of aggressive therapies when appropriate.

Once an aggressive strategy is deemed both justifiable (as a function of age and other comorbidities) and feasible, further diagnostic testing should commence immediately, while resuscitative measures are instituted (Fig. 73–4). Two-dimensional Doppler echocardiography can be a valuable first step, providing information regarding LV size and shape, regional and global function, valve structure and function, pericardial pathology (e.g., hemopericardium caused by free wall rupture), and confirmation of ventricular septal or papillary muscle rupture when clinically suspected. Doppler echocardiography provides important prognostic information in patients with cardiogenic shock. In a multivariate analysis of the SHOCK trial, Picard and coworkers (34) showed that both LV ejection fraction (<28%; 1-year OR for death, 4.04; $p = 0.005$) and mitral regurgitation severity (≥2 vs. <2; 1-year OR for death, 6.64; $p = 0.0003$) were both independent predictors of 30-day and 1-year mortality. The performance of Doppler echocardiography should not, however, delay the preparations necessary for right- and left-heart catheterization, coronary angiography, and, in selected patients, left ventriculography. Right-heart catheterization may be preferentially performed through the right internal jugular vein so that the Swan-Ganz catheter can be left in place to guide subsequent pharmacologic therapy. Alternatively, if time does not allow or if the patient may have re-

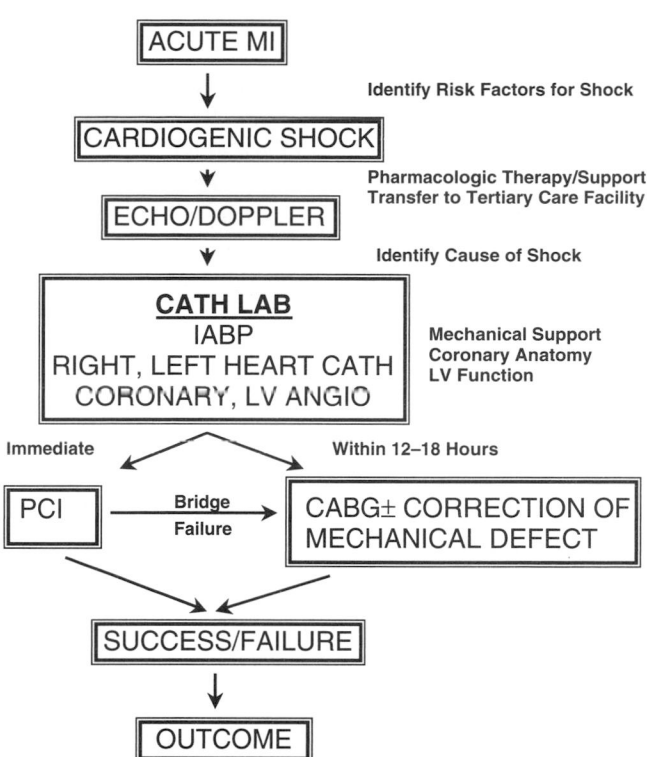

FIG. 73–4. General approach to the patient with postinfarction cardiogenic shock. Algorithm should be applied selectively to appropriate patients. ANGIO, angiography; CABG, coronary artery bypass graft surgery; CATH, catheterization; IABP, intraaortic balloon counterpulsation; LV, left ventricular; MI, myocardial infarction; PCI, percutaneous coronary intervention.

ceived a thrombolytic agent, right-heart catheterization should be performed through the right common femoral vein. Right heart pressures, oxygen saturations, and cardiac output should be quickly acquired by means of which the diagnosis of cardiogenic shock can be established and appropriate treatment initiated (35). Arterial access is typically achieved through the right common femoral artery. The operator also must decide whether the patient requires mechanical stabilization with IABP or even percutaneous bypass before to the performance of coronary angiography and left ventriculography. If so, arterial access also must be obtained through the left common femoral artery. The exact sequence of coronary arteriographic injections varies among operators, although most would choose to opacify the noninfarct vessel initially to screen for the presence of collateral channels. On completion of the diagnostic catheter study, a definitive treatment plan can be instituted.

MANAGEMENT

Pharmacologic

Initial medical measures are aimed at optimization of the volume status, manipulation of preload and afterload, and enhancement of myocardial contractility, all as guided by the measurements of pressures, resistances, and outputs derived through the Swan-Ganz catheter and an indwelling arterial catheter. By definition, the pulmonary capillary wedge pressure is increased in cardiogenic shock. Efforts to reduce it and to alleviate pulmonary congestion with diuretics are usually limited by a low systemic blood pressure. A similar limitation may apply to the use of vasodilators such as nitroglycerin and nitroprusside. If and when patients recover from their initial injury, these agents can help to optimize cardiac output and systemic blood flow. The dominant effect of nitroglycerin is to increase systemic venous capacitance with a resultant decrease in ventricular preload and wall tension, but it is also useful as a coronary vasodilator and has the additional benefit of increasing collateral blood flow. Nitroprusside, however, has more powerful preload- and afterload-reducing effects, but it may create a coronary "steal" phenomenon (36). Toxicity may develop in relation to the infusion dose and duration, as well as renal function.

Intravenous inotropic agents are the cornerstones of pharmacologic management. The choice of individual agents varies among physicians (and institutions), but a few general principles should apply. First, the effects of any single drug should be assessed by serial and repeated measurements of heart rate, blood pressure, rhythm, cardiac output, and systemic vascular resistance as a function of dose, to establish the optimum infusion rate. Second, if either an adverse or no effect is observed, a second agent should be chosen. Third, it is frequently necessary to combine inotropic agents in variable doses to achieve the optimum effect.

Dopamine in low doses (1–2 μg/kg/min) activates dopaminergic receptors in the mesentery and kidney with corresponding increases in splanchnic and renal blood flow (37). Yet, even at these low doses, cardiac stimulation can occur. Contrary to previously held beliefs, it appears unlikely that low-dose dopamine in this setting improves renal function independent of its salutary effects on cardiac output. Mid-range doses of dopamine (4–10 μg/kg/min) activate β_1-adrenergic cardiac receptors and peripheral β_2 receptors and cause an increase in contractility (as assessed by cardiac output) and a mild decrease in peripheral vascular resistance. Use of this drug in this dose range can be limited by tachycardia and arrhythmias. Higher doses of dopamine exert predominant α effects with peripheral vasoconstriction and may not offer any special advantages (37).

Dobutamine is a useful β-adrenergic agonist that can increase myocardial contractility and cardiac output, augment coronary and collateral blood flow, and decrease LV filling pressures, usually without the same arrhythmogenic cost seen with dopamine (38,39). On rare occasions, β_2-adrenergic stimulation results in unwanted peripheral vasodilation, necessitating a reduction in dose.

The intravenous phosphodiesterase inhibitors amrinone and milrinone are usually reserved for patients who have not fully responded to dopamine or dobutamine, or both (40). Drug tolerance and thrombocytopenia are relative concerns with their use. The use of oral forms of phosphodiesterase inhibitors has been associated with increased mortality among patients with chronic heart failure caused by ischemic cardiomyopathy (41,42).

When significant hypotension exists and the blood pressure requires immediate restoration, norepinephrine (levarterenol) is the drug of choice. Although its effects are predominantly mediated through α-adrenergic stimulation, concomitant augmentation of myocardial contractility does occur to a lesser extent. Neo-Synephrine, in contrast, is essentially a pure α agonist. These vasopressor medications should only be delivered centrally.

The choice of which particular inotropic or vasopressor drug to use clinically often is the subject of some debate. For example, will an infusion of dobutamine result in excessive myocardial stimulation with further increases in myocardial oxygen demand and hence worsening ischemia? Conversely, the associated decrease in LV cavity size may decrease wall tension and myocardial oxygen demand. Will the increase in ventricular afterload achieved with norepinephrine lead to further compromise of pump function, or will the associated increase in coronary perfusion pressure augment myocardial blood flow? Certainly, these are important concerns, but the clinician's first obligation is to restore the circulation (i.e., systemic blood pressure) as quickly as possible and reassess the clinical response on the basis of the data derived from hemodynamic measurements.

Simultaneous with these pharmacologic interventions, efforts may be needed to protect the airway in an obtunded patient, to perform intubation, to provide mechanical ventilation and oxygenation, and to correct arterial acidemia.

Intraaortic Balloon Pumping

IABP is instituted either during or immediately after the diagnostic catheterization. In the absence of a contraindication (severe peripheral vascular disease, ≥2+/4+ aortic regurgitation, or aortic dissection), IABP can be a highly effective means of temporary mechanical support, the net result of which is an improvement in cardiac output by as much as 20% and a decrease in left-sided filling pressures (43–47). Deflation of the balloon at the onset of systole results in a significant reduction in LV afterload. Inflation during diastole increases the coronary perfusion gradient (aortic diastolic pressure minus LV diastolic pressure), but whether this increase in driving pressure translates into augmented coronary blood flow beyond a critical stenosis remains unclear. Kern and coworkers (48) reported that IABP decreased systolic pressure (6% ± 10%; $p < 0.001$) and increased diastolic pressure (80% ± 30%; $p < 0.001$) from baseline in 19 selected patients, 9 of whom had acute MI with shock (Fig. 73–5). Coronary blood flow velocity was measured using a Doppler-tipped (20-MHz) angiographic catheter or a 3-F intracoronary Doppler catheter positioned in the normal proximal coronary artery segment. Peak phasic and mean coronary flow velocity, as well as the diastolic flow velocity

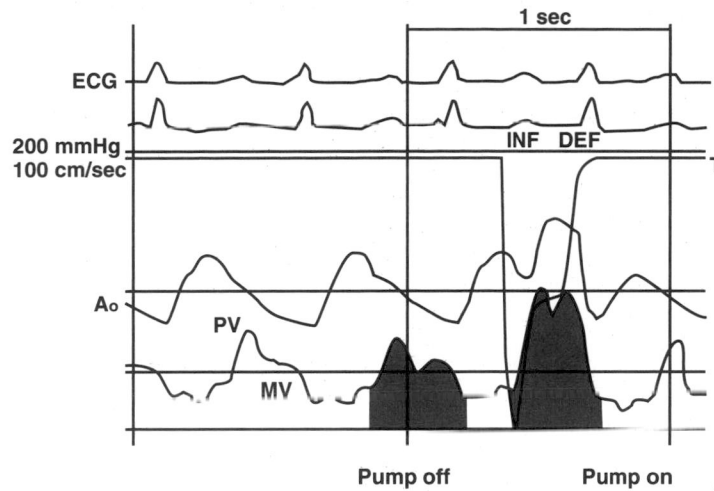

FIG. 73–5. Electrocardiogram (ECG), aortic pressure tracing (Ao), and phasic (PV) and mean (MV) flow velocity signals demonstrating the effects of intraaortic balloon pumping. Note the increase in aortic diastolic pressure and phasic and mean flow velocities with balloon inflation. *Shaded areas,* the diastolic flow velocity integrals. DEF, deflation of the balloon; INF, inflation of the balloon; T, timing signal. (Reproduced from Kern M, Aguirre FV, Tatineni S, et al. Enhanced coronary blood flow velocity during intraaortic balloon counterpulsation in critically ill patients. *J Am Coll Cardiol* 1993; 21:359–368, with the permission of the publisher.)

integral, were all significantly ($p < 0.001$) increased during IABP (48). The increase in the diastolic flow velocity integral was greatest in patients with baseline systolic pressure of 90 mm Hg or less. Larger increases in flow velocity corresponded to longer durations of balloon inflations. The authors were careful, however, to emphasize that their findings pertained to changes in flow velocity proximal to coronary stenosis and that they could not extrapolate these observations to events distal to an obstruction (48). Enhanced proximal flow may nevertheless be helpful, for example, in the use of IABP to reduce the incidence of abrupt vessel closure after complex direct or salvage percutaneous transluminal coronary angioplasty before the availability of stents (49).

Several observational studies have shown a beneficial effect of IABP in patients with cardiogenic shock (50–53). Sanborn and coworkers (50) reported from the SHOCK registry that patients who were selected for IABP had lower in-hospital mortality rates than those who did not receive IABP (50% vs. 72%; $p < 0.0001$). However, after adjusting for the increased revascularization rates in patients who received IABP, the difference in mortality was no longer significant ($p = 0.313$) (50). Similarly, Anderson and coworkers (51) reported on the use of IABP in the GUSTO-I study population. Of the 310 patients with shock, 68 (22%) had an intraaortic balloon pump placed within 24 hours. The trend toward lower 30-day mortality in this group also was no longer significant after adjusting for differences in baseline patient characteristics ($p = 0.11$) (51).

IABP was used in 7,268 (31%) patients with cardiogenic shock in the National Registry of Myocardial Infarction 2.

When used with thrombolysis in this cohort, IABP was associated with a decrease in the OR for death of 18% (OR, 0.82; 95% CI, 0.72–0.93) (52). Interestingly, a survival benefit was not observed when IABP was combined with primary PCI (45% vs. 47%) (52). In contrast to these findings, Brodie and coworkers (53) showed that cardiogenic shock was the strongest independent predictor of adverse events in the catheterization laboratory (OR, 2.18; 95% CI, 1.58–3.02). IABP before PCI was associated with a significant reduction in such events (14.5% vs. 35.1%; $p = 0.009$) (53). These observational studies illustrate the common problems of bias and confounding by indication, and until a randomized controlled trial is conducted, the additive benefit of IABP in patients with cardiogenic shock after MI will remain unknown.

Complications associated with the use of IABP have decreased with continued refinements in catheter design and flexibility. The most frequent problems encountered include limb ischemia, bleeding, and transient thrombocytopenia caused by consumption (54). Delirium may complicate the course of as many as one-third of patients who require prolonged IABP support (55).

Thrombolysis

Despite the beneficial effect of the timely administration of thrombolytic therapy in patients with STEMI, pharmacologic reperfusion has provided disappointing in patients with cardiogenic shock. Patients with shock were underrepresented in the major randomized trials (56) (Table 73–2)

TABLE 73–2. *Thrombolysis in cardiogenic shock*

Trial (reference)	Year	n[a]	Treatment	Reperfusion	Mortality
Dioguardi et al. (57)	1971	34	Intravenous SK	NR	NR
Society for Cardiac Angiography (59)	1985	44	Intracoronary SK	43%	42% successful vs. 84% failed thrombolysis; total 66%
GISSI-I (7)	1986	280	Intravenous SK	NR	69.9% SK vs. 70.1% placebo
International Study Group (9)	1990	322	Intravenous SK vs. rt-PA	NR	64.9% SK vs. 78.1% rt-PA
Bengtson et al. (60)	1992	69	Intravenous SK, rt-PA, UK, or combination	47%	58% did not respond to thrombolysis treated medically; 38% did not respond to thrombolysis treated with PCI or CABG

CABG, coronary artery bypass graft surgery; NR, not reported; PCI, percutaneous coronary intervention; rt-PA, recombinant tissue plasminogen activator; SK, streptokinase; UK, urokinase.
[a]Number of patients with cardiogenic shock.
Adapted from Col NF, Gurwitz JH, Alpert JS, et al. Frequency of inclusion of patients with cardiogenic shock in trials of thrombolytic therapy. *Am J Cardiol* 1994;73:149–157, with permission.

and subgroup analysis may not provide an accurate assessment of efficacy and safety.

In an early randomized trial of intravenous streptokinase (SK) reported by Dioguardi and coworkers (57), 34 of 321 (10.6%) patients had cardiogenic shock, but survival data were not provided. Mathey and coworkers (58) reported successful reperfusion and survival in three patients with cardiogenic shock who received intracoronary SK. The Society for Cardiac Angiography (SCAI) intracoronary SK registry included 44 patients with cardiogenic shock. The overall mortality rate was 66%, but 42% for those 19 patients (43%) with successful reperfusion versus 84% for patients with shock with failed reperfusion (59). Of 200 consecutive patients with pump failure after MI admitted to Duke University Medical Center between January 1987 and December 1988, 69 patients (35%) received intravenous thrombolytic therapy before cardiac catheterization performed after a median of 2.9 hours. Patency of the infarct-related artery was documented in 33 of the 69 patients (47%) (60). Low-patency rates after thrombolysis in patients with shock likely relate to the associated reduction in cardiac output and coronary perfusion pressure, although the extent of coronary thrombus burden may also play a role.

Data regarding outcomes in patients with cardiogenic shock from the major randomized trials of thrombolysis are limited. The Gruppo Italiano per lo Studio della Streptochinasi nell'Infarto Miocardico (GISSI-1) trial included 280 Killip Class IV patients at entry, comprising 2.4% of the total number of patients studied (n = 11,806) (7). The 30-day mortality rate was 69.9% for the 146 patients treated with SK versus 70.1% for the 134 patients randomized to placebo (7). A total of 323 (1.6%) of the 20,768 patients enrolled in the International Trial were designated Killip Class IV (9). Hospital mortality rates were 64.9% for patients randomized to SK plus aspirin versus 78.1% for patients treated with alteplase (recombinant tissue plasminogen activator [rt-PA]) plus aspirin (9). In GUSTO-I, the 30-day mortality rates were 57% and 55%, respectively, for patients with shock at

entry and for those who experienced shock during hospitalization (vs. 3% for patients who did not have cardiogenic shock). There was a trend toward improved mortality for patients who experienced development of shock and were treated with SK plus subcutaneous heparin (51%), compared with patients who received rt-PA (57%; $p = 0.061$) (12). The significance of this apparent superiority of SK over rt-PA is unclear, as these overall mortality rates did not differ substantially from those observed among historical and placebo control groups. Others observed, however, that the confidence limits for the treatment effects of thrombolysis in patients with cardiogenic shock (Killip Class IV) overlap the expected effect of such therapy in all treatment groups (19,61).

It was initially difficult to reconcile this apparent lack of efficacy of thrombolytic therapy in patients with cardiogenic shock with the generally accepted notion that such treatment should have had its greatest benefit among patients with anatomically large infarctions. Indeed, successful thrombolysis with intracoronary SK in the Western Washington trial was associated with the greatest relative survival benefit at 1 year for those patients with the most substantial reductions in LV ejection fraction at entry (62). Several trials showed a lower incidence of the in-hospital development of congestive heart failure for patients treated with thrombolysis versus those patients who received placebo (63–66). A significantly smaller number of patients treated with accelerated-dose rt-PA and heparin (5.5%) in GUSTO-I had cardiogenic shock, compared with patients treated with SK plus subcutaneous heparin (7.4%), SK plus intravenous heparin (6.9%), and combination SK plus rt-PA (6.3%) ($p < 0.001$ for accelerated rt-PA vs. both SK groups) (10,12). In addition, patients in the GUSTO-I trial who experienced shock had a longer time to therapy compared with patients without shock (3.20 ± 1.75 vs. 3.09 ± 1.62 hour; $p = 0.01$) (12). Finally, the Fibrinolytic Therapy Trialists' Collaborative Group, in their combined analysis of 9 controlled trials each of which randomized more than 1,000 patients, emphasized that fibrinolytic therapy did result in an absolute mortality reduction for those patients at high risk who presented with systolic blood pressure less than 100 mm Hg, heart rate greater than 100 beats per minute, or both, certainly some of whom would likely have satisfied the clinical definition of cardiogenic shock (61). The presence of shock, therefore, should not be considered a contraindication to fibrinolytic therapy, although primary PCI is now the preferred treatment strategy when readily available (67).

Coronary Angioplasty

Given the generally unfavorable results with thrombolytic therapy in patients with cardiogenic shock, interest turned to methods of mechanical revascularization, namely PCI and CABG surgery. PCI is more readily available and can be performed more expeditiously, whereas CABG surgery offers a more controlled method of reperfusion, and cardiac surgery affords an opportunity to repair other mechanical complications should they coexist. There have been more than 23 retrospective studies comprising 926 patients that examined the use of PCI (Table 73–3). The early, individual study sizes ranged from 7 to 175 patients, not all patients had primary pump failure as the cause of cardiogenic shock, many patients received either intravenous or intracoronary thrombolytic therapy in addition to PCI, and several patients required CABG surgery either immediately or a few days after its performance. Berger and coworkers (68) performed a subgroup analysis of 2,200 GUSTO-I patients with cardiogenic shock. The 30-day mortality rate was 38% in the 406 patients who underwent early angiography and were referred within 24 hours for PCI (n – 175), bypass surgery (n = 36), both (n = 22), or neither (n = 173), compared with 62% in the 1,794 patients who did were not referred for revascularization ($p = 0.001$) (68). Even after adjusting for differences in baseline characteristics, the use of an aggressive strategy remained independently associated with reduced 30-day (OR, 0.43; 95% CI, 0.34–0.54; $p = 0.001$) (68) and 1-year (OR, 0.60; 95% CI, 0.40–0.90; $p = 0.007$) mortality rates (69).

The SHOCK investigators performed the first randomized controlled trial comparing emergent revascularization (n = 152) with initial medical stabilization (n = 150) in patients with shock caused by LV failure complicating MI (70). Baseline characteristics were well balanced between the two groups (mean age 66 years, 32% women, 31% diabetes mellitus, and 55% transferred from another hospital). Among the patients randomized to revascularization, 64% underwent PCI (37.5% received coronary stents), whereas 36% underwent bypass surgery (70). For these patients randomized to the emergency revascularization arm, the median time from randomization to PCI was 0.9 hours and 2.7 hours to surgery. In contrast, 32 patients (21.3%) assigned to medical therapy group ultimately underwent delayed revascularization a median of 102.8 hours after randomization. The SHOCK trial had a 90% power to detect a 20% absolute dif-

TABLE 73–3. *Percutaneous coronary intervention in cardiogenic shock*

Study (reference)	Year	Patients, n	Overall survival, %	Reperfusion rate, %	Survival after successful PCI, %	Survival after unsuccessful PCI, %
O'Neill et al. (102)	1985	27	70	89	75	33
Shani et al. (103)	1986	9	67	67	83	0
Heuser et al. (104)	1986	10	70	60	83	25
Disler et al. (105)	1987	7	43	71	60	0
Landin et al. (106)	1988	34	59	79	70	14
Laramee et al. (107)	1988	39	59	86	NR	NR
Lee et al. (108)	1988	24	50	54	77	18
Verna et al. (109)	1989	7	86	100	86	—
Kaplan et al. (110)	1990	88	58	61	65	29
Meyer et al. (111)	1990	25	53	88	59	0
Brodie et al. (112)	1991	22	50	68	NR	NR
Lee et al. (113)	1991	69	55	71	69	20
Bengtson et al. (60)	1992	44	57	84	62	29
Gacioch et al. (92)	1992	48	55	73	61	7
Hibbard et al. (114)	1992	45	56	62	71	29
Moosvi et al. (115)	1992	38	NR	78	56	8
Yamamoto et al. (116)	1992	26	38	76	56	10
Seydoux et al. (117)	1992	21	57	85	67	0
Laney et al. (118)	1993	52	81	94	86	0
Morrison et al. (119)	1995	17	47	71	67	0
Eltchaninoff et al. (120)	1995	33	64	75	76	25
Berger et al. (68)	1997	175	75	75	65	19[a]
Antoniucci et al. (121)	1998	66	74	94	79	0

NR, not reported; PCI, percutaneous coronary intervention
[a]Includes patients who had PCI only; excludes patients who had PCI followed by coronary artery bypass grafting.
Adapted from Hollenberg SM, Kavinsky CJ, Parrillo JE. Cardiogenic shock. *Ann Intern Med* 1999;131:47–59, with permission.

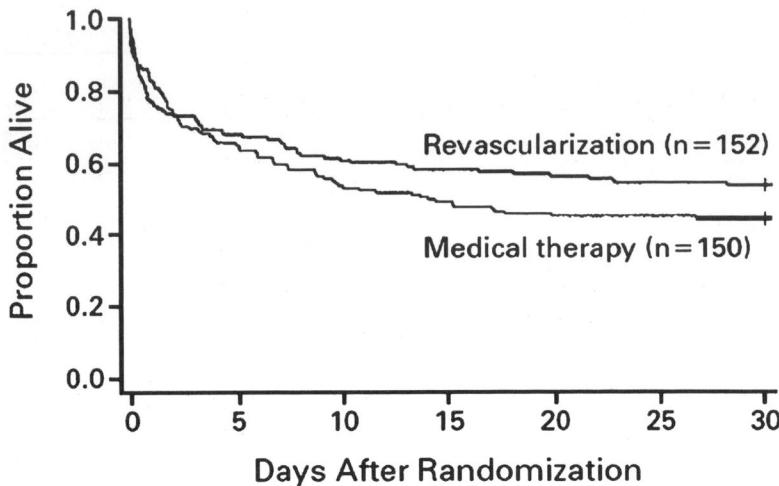

FIG. 73–6. Overall 30-day survival in the SHould we emergently revascularize Occluded Coronaries for shocK (SHOCK) study. The 30-day survival rate was 53.3% for patients assigned to revascularization and 44.0% those assigned to medical therapy. (From Hochman JS, Sleeper LA, Webb JG, et al. Early revascularization in acute myocardial infarction complicated by cardiogenic shock. SHOCK Investigators. Should We Emergently Revascularize Occluded Coronaries for Cardiogenic Shock. *N Engl J Med* 1999;341:625–634, with permission.)

ference between the two groups with an overall type I error of 0.05. The primary end point, overall mortality 30 days after randomization, was not significantly different between the two groups (46.7% revascularization vs. 56% medical stabilization; risk difference −9.3%; $p = 0.11$) (70). However, both 6-month (50.3% vs. 63.1%; $p = 0.027$) and 1-year (53.3% vs. 66.4%; $p < 0.03$) mortality rates were less in the revascularization arm when compared with the medical therapy arm (70,71) (Figs. 73–6 and 73–7). Interestingly, when examining 10 prespecified subgroups, age (<75 years vs. ≥75 years) interacted significantly ($p < 0.03$) with treatment strategy, and the survival benefit of the emergent revascularization strategy was only evident for patients younger than 75 years (71). This significant interaction must

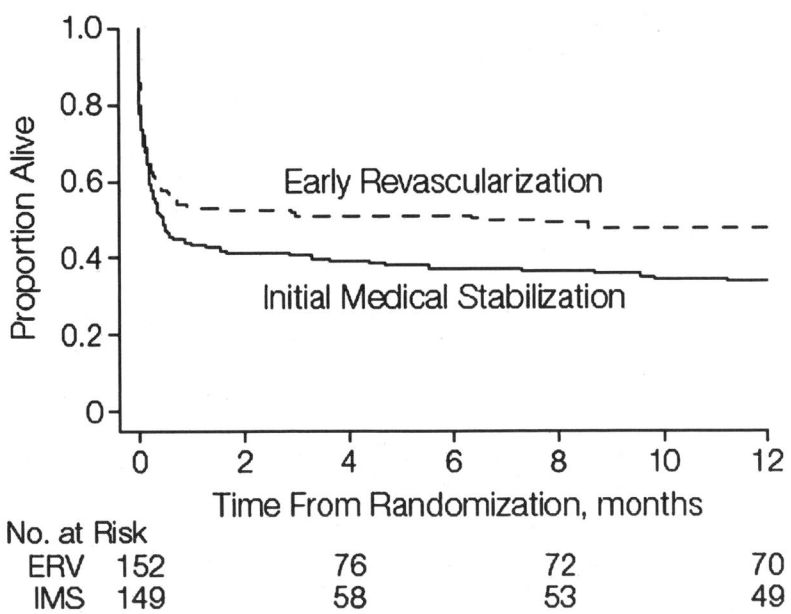

No. at Risk

ERV	152	76	72	70
IMS	149	58	53	49

FIG. 73–7. SHould we emergently revascularize Occluded Coronaries for shocK (SHOCK) trial. Kaplan-Meier survival curve 1-year after randomization (71). Survival estimates for early revascularization (ERV; n = 152) and initial medical stabilization (IMS; n = 149) groups. Log rank test: $p = 0.04$. (From Hochman JS, Sleeper LA, White HD, et al. One-year survival following early revascularization for cardiogenic shock. *JAMA* 2001;285:190–192, with permission.)

factor into the decision-making process when formulating an overall treatment strategy for an individual patient.

Given these findings, most authorities would currently recommend primary PCI with or without adjunctive IABP as the treatment of choice for patients with MI with cardiogenic shock, provided that cardiac catheterization facilities, technical expertise, and surgical backup are promptly available (within 60 minutes). Attention should be restricted initially to the infarct vessel. A successful PCI could then serve as a bridge to later PCI of critically stenosed noninfarct vessels or to CABG surgery, as deemed appropriate by the anatomic findings. In the majority of centers where emergency catheterization, angiography, PCI, and surgery are not readily available, intravenous thrombolytic or glycoprotein IIB/IIIA (depending on the anticipated time delay) therapy should be instituted, and the patient should be prepared for immediate transfer to an accepting facility where such procedures can be performed (72).

Coronary Artery Bypass Graft Surgery

Earlier surgical reports that described the experience with CABG suffered from small sample sizes, selection bias, inconsistent definitions of cardiogenic shock, and lack of a standardized operative approach (73–87) (Table 73–4). Early results were not particularly favorable. The field was energized by DeWood and coworkers' 1980 report (81) of a 25% hospital mortality rate for a small (n = 12) group of patients managed with IABP and surgical revascularization within 16 hours of symptom onset. Two larger series reported in 1986 included a total of 84 patients and documented a similarly low 27% short-term mortality rate (83,84). Most impressive was the 1989 report from UCLA summarizing the results for 80 consecutive patients who underwent emergency CABG

TABLE 73–4. *Coronary artery bypass graft surgery in cardiogenic shock*

Study (reference)	Year	n	Short-term mortality (%)
Mundth et al. (73)	1973	33	20/33 (61)
Miller et al. (74)	1974	12	7/12 (58)
Willerson et al. (75)	1975	3	2/3 (67)
Johnson et al. (76)	1977	5	3/5 (60)
Ehrich et al. (77)	1977	3	2/3 (67)
Bardet et al. (78)	1977	4	2/4 (50)
O'Rourke et al. (79)	1979	6	4/6 (67)
Subramanian et al. (80)	1980	20	9/20 (45)
DeWood et al. (81)	1980	19	8/19 (42)
Kirklin et al. (82)	1985	1	0/1 (0)
Phillips et al. (83)	1986	34	8/34 (24)
Laks et al. (84)	1986	50	15/50 (30)
Guyton et al. (85)	1987	9	2/9 (22)
Bolooki et al. (86)	1989	7	3/7 (43)
Allen et al. (87)	1989	80	14/80 (17)
Total		289	99/289 (34)

Adapted from Bates ER, Topol EJ. Limitations of thrombolytic therapy for acute myocardial infarction complicated by congestive heart failure and cardiogenic shock. *J Am Coll Cardiol* 1991;18:1077–1084, with permission.

surgery for post-MI shock (87). Operative strategies included the use of warm, substrate-enriched blood cardioplegia, multidose cold cardioplegia replenishment, a standardized order of bypass grafting, warm blood reperfusate, and a generous allotment of time on continued extracorporeal circulation after completion of the proximal anastomoses. The total perioperative (30-day) mortality rate was 17%, but only 7% (3/45) for patients who underwent surgery within 18 hours of the onset of shock versus 31% (11/35) for those patients for whom surgery was delayed beyond 18 hours (87) (Fig. 73–8). Preoperative organ failure complicated the course of 9

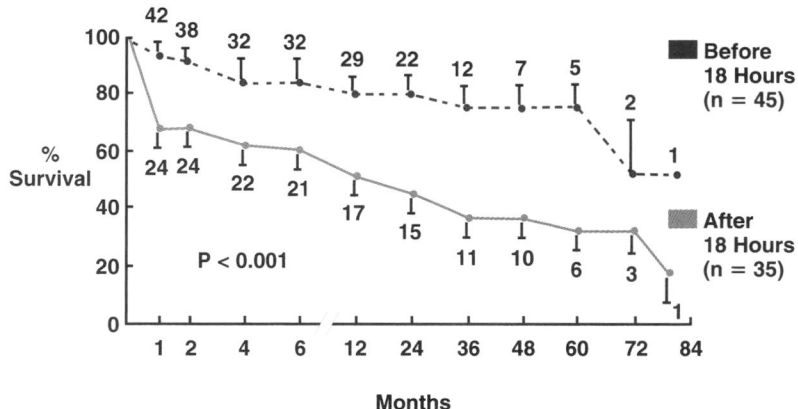

FIG. 73–8. Influence of the timing of operation (coronary artery bypass grafting) on survival of postinfarction cardiogenic shock patients at UCLA from 1982 to 1988. Thirty-day survival rates were 93% and 69%, respectively, for patients who underwent surgery before and after 18 hours of the onset of shock. (From Allen BS, Rosenkranz E, Buckberg GD, et al. Studies on prolonged acute regional ischemia. VI. Myocardial infarction with left ventricular power failure: a medical/surgical emergency requiring urgent revascularization with maximal protection of remote muscle. *J Thorac Cardiovasc Surg* 1989;98[5 Pt 1]:691–703, with permission.)

of the 35 patients (26%) in the delayed group, but did not occur in patients who underwent early surgery (87). Such results substantiate the observation made by Mundth and coworkers in 1973 (73) that appropriate candidates for emergency surgery have better outcomes when surgery is performed earlier in their course. These rather astounding results, derived from a retrospective analysis, have not been duplicated. Other groups have used more novel techniques of myocardial protection, such as retrograde coronary sinus perfusion, in an effort to limit the process of ischemic injury (88). Bolooki (89) has maintained that reperfusion injury is not a clinical problem.

The use of CABG surgery has been restricted by a variety of factors, including its limited availability, the delays inherent in its planning and performance, the need for high-level technical support, cost, and an appropriate reluctance among many surgeons to undertake a procedure with a predictably high perioperative mortality risk. Coronary bypass surgery is usually reserved for patients who are not candidates for PCI (e.g., patients with left main CAD), for those with associated mechanical lesions, and for patients with multivessel disease who have been stabilized by primary PCI of the infarct-related artery. Advances in the timely and effective performance of PCI, including stents and adjunctive antithrombotic therapies, have made this strategy the treatment of choice whenever feasible. Standards regarding operator and institutional performance metrics have been published.

OTHER SUPPORTIVE THERAPIES

The mechanical hemodynamic support provided by IABP may at times prove inadequate. Percutaneous cardiopulmonary support (PCS) has been used to maintain cardiac output while patients with cardiogenic shock undergo high-risk PCI (90). Shawl and coworkers (91) reported the use of PCS in eight patients (aged 42 to 80 years) with cardiogenic shock complicating MI. Successful PCI was performed on 15 of 16 lesions. One patient died, whereas the remaining seven patients were successfully weaned from PCS and were alive and asymptomatic at 2.2-month follow-up (91). Such success was not duplicated by several other groups (92–94). The use of PCS is time-limited to a matter of hours and, more specifically, to the time necessary to perform high-risk PCI. Consequently, other support devices have been used in selected patients to maintain the circulation.

The Hemopump is a catheter-mounted, motor-driven turbine (17,000–25,000 g) that is placed under fluoroscopic guidance across the aortic valve into the left ventricle. Insertion requires surgical construction of a femoral artery sleeve graft and the relative absence of aortoiliofemoral occlusive disease. The Hemopump (Johnson and Johnson, NJ) can pump blood from the left ventricle into the aorta in a nonpulsatile manner at a rate up to 3.5 L per minute for as long as 7 days. Associated complications include bleeding, hemolysis, limb ischemia, and ventricular ectopy. In the small series reported by Gacioch

and coworkers (92), only two of seven (29%) patients with the Hemopump insertion survived to discharge (95).

Extracorporeal membrane oxygenation has been used under a variety of clinical circumstances for temporary circulatory support (96,97). Percutaneous insertion techniques similar to those for PCS are available, and flow rates of 3 to 5 L per minute can be achieved. Bleeding is a common complication, as full-dose heparin anticoagulation is necessary. A left atrial–femoral artery system also has been deployed percutaneously (98). Transseptal puncture is required, but the need for an oxygenator is eliminated. This system may have the advantage of reducing stasis within the left heart chambers when ventricular ejection is severely reduced, thereby decreasing the risk for intracardiac thrombus formation.

External pulsatile ventricular assist devices have been used almost exclusively for temporary support as a bridge to transplantation (43,99). Right, left, or biventricular assist can be accomplished. Thoracotomy with cannulation of the right atrium and pulmonary artery for right ventricular support, the left atrium or LV apex and aorta for LV support, or their combination is required. Bleeding, thromboembolism, renal failure, and infection are the most common complications. Orthotopic cardiac transplantation is an attractive idea for carefully selected patients with post-MI cardiogenic shock. Park and coworkers (100) reported seven patients who had LV assist devices implanted for cardiogenic shock complicating acute MI. Six patients were transplanted successfully, and five of the original seven patients were alive and well at a mean follow-up of 898 days (100). Champagnac and coworkers (101) reported a 70% long-term survival rate for 15 patients (mean age 49 years) who underwent transplantation at an average of 15 days after MI, 6 of whom required interim mechanical circulatory assistance (101). The application of cardiac transplantation to the care of patients with shock remains severely restricted by the shortage of donors, which has plagued its more widespread use for patients with chronic heart failure.

PREVENTION

With the recognition that cardiogenic shock caused by LV pump failure is the most common cause of death after MI and that a substantial proportion of patients experience development of shock after presentation, efforts must be redoubled to identify early those patients at greatest risk (1,8,11). Aggressive reperfusion strategies, which require the combined input of cardiologists and cardiac surgeons, should be instituted promptly, in conjunction with appropriate pharmacologic and mechanical therapies necessary to support the circulation.

An equally important challenge for the clinician is to establish the appropriateness of such aggressive, highly invasive, and costly therapy for an individual patient (19). Experience would suggest that severe comorbidity, functional disability, or advanced age would mitigate against such an approach. Advance care directives seem the exception rather than the rule. Most often, the clinician is faced with an extremely difficult decision with insufficient or ambiguous information and a severe time constraint. Although there is no substitute for judgment, every effort should be made to engage the patient or surrogate, or both, in a careful discussion of the nature of the problem, the expected outcomes, and any individual (patient) preferences. It also is critical to readdress these issues daily, particularly when progress has not been achieved (19).

FUTURE DIRECTIONS

The events leading to the development of cardiogenic shock from predominant LV failure after MI are well understood. Early recognition of the patient at high risk and the timely application of reperfusion strategies in appropriately selected patients are critical elements of any management algorithm. Adjunctive medical therapy to limit infarct size and to attenuate the process of reperfusion injury is useful. Prevention strategies directed against the vulnerable plaque in at-risk patients should reduce the burden of MI and the associated risk for pump failure.

As changes in healthcare policy, delivery, and financing continue to evolve, it is possible that the invasive and costly care engendered by these strategies will become more restricted. It will remain necessary to identify that subgroup of patients who will derive the greatest benefit from such aggressive care.

REFERENCES

1. Kleiman NS, Terrin M, Mueller H, et al. Mechanisms of early death despite thrombolytic therapy: experience from the Thrombolysis in Myocardial Infarction Phase II (TIMI II) study. *J Am Coll Cardiol* 1992;19:1129–1135.
2. Norris R. The changing natural history and prognosis of acute myocardial infarction. In: Gersh BJ, Rahimtoola SH, eds. *Acute myocardial infarction.* New York: Elsevier, 1991:87–97.
3. Goldberg RJ, Samad NA, Yarzebski J, et al. Temporal trends in cardiogenic shock complicating acute myocardial infarction. *N Engl J Med* 1999;340:1162–1168.
4. Hochman JS, Buller CE, Sleeper LA, et al. Cardiogenic shock complicating acute myocardial infarction—etiologies, management and outcome: a report from the SHOCK Trial Registry. SHould we emergently revascularize Occluded Coronaries for cardiogenic shocK? *J Am Coll Cardiol* 2000;36[3 Suppl A]:1063–1070.
5. Renkin J, de Bruyne B, Benit E, et al. Cardiac tamponade early after thrombolysis for acute myocardial infarction: a rare but not reported hemorrhagic complication. *J Am Coll Cardiol* 1991;17:280–285.
6. Killip T 3rd, Kimball JT. Treatment of myocardial infarction in a coronary care unit. A two year experience with 250 patients. *Am J Cardiol* 1967;20:457–464.
7. Effectiveness of intravenous thrombolytic treatment in acute myocardial infarction. Gruppo Italiano per lo Studio della Streptochinasi nell'Infarto Miocardico (GISSI). *Lancet* 1986;1:397–402.
8. Hands ME, Rutherford JD, Muller JE, et al. The in-hospital development of cardiogenic shock after myocardial infarction: incidence, predictors of occurrence, outcome and prognostic factors. The MILIS Study Group. *J Am Coll Cardiol* 1989;14:40–48.
9. In-hospital mortality and clinical course of 20,891 patients with suspected acute myocardial infarction randomised between alteplase and streptokinase with or without heparin. The International Study Group. *Lancet* 1990;336:71–75.
10. An international randomized trial comparing four thrombolytic strategies for acute myocardial infarction. The GUSTO investigators. *N Engl J Med* 1993;329:673–682.
11. Leor J, Goldbourt U, Reicher-Reiss H, et al. Cardiogenic shock complicating acute myocardial infarction in patients without heart failure on admission: incidence, risk factors, and outcome. SPRINT Study Group. *Am J Med* 1993;94:265–273.
12. Holmes DR Jr, Bates ER, Kleiman NS, et al. Contemporary reperfusion therapy for cardiogenic shock: the GUSTO-I trial experience. The GUSTO-I Investigators. Global Utilization of Streptokinase and Tissue Plasminogen Activator for Occluded Coronary Arteries. *J Am Coll Cardiol* 1995;26:668–674.
13. Holmes DR Jr, Califf RM, Van de Werf F, et al. Difference in countries' use of resources and clinical outcome for patients with cardiogenic shock after myocardial infarction: results from the GUSTO trial. *Lancet* 1997;349:75–78.
14. Alonso DR, Scheidt S, Post M, et al. Pathophysiology of cardiogenic shock. Quantification of myocardial necrosis, clinical, pathologic and electrocardiographic correlations. *Circulation* 1973;48:588–596.
15. Page DL, Caulfield JB, Kastor JA, et al. Myocardial changes associated with cardiogenic shock. *N Engl J Med* 1971;285:133–137.
16. Hollenberg SM, Kavinsky CJ, Parrillo JE. Cardiogenic shock. *Ann Intern Med* 1999;131:47–59.
17. Pasternak RC, Braunwald E. Acute myocardial infarction. In: Wilson JD, ed. *Harrison's principles of internal medicine,* 12th ed. New York: McGraw-Hill, 1991:953–963.
18. Pasternak RC, Braunwald E, Sobel BE. Acute myocardial infarction. In: Braunwald E, ed. *Heart disease: a textbook of cardiovascular medicine,* 4th ed. Philadelphia: WB Saunders, 1992:1200–1291.
19. Califf RM, Bengtson JR. Cardiogenic shock. *N Engl J Med* 1994;330:1724–1730.
20. Gutovitz AL, Sobel BE, Roberts R. Progressive nature of myocardial injury in selected patients with cardiogenic shock. *Am J Cardiol* 1978;41:469–475.
21. Weil MH, Von Planta M, Rackow E. Acute circulatory failure. In: Braunwald E, ed. *Heart disease: a textbook of cardiovascular medicine,* 4th ed. Philadelphia: WB Saunders, 1992:569–587.
22. Berne RM, Rubio R. Coronary circulation. In: Berne RM, Sperelakis N, Geiger SR, eds. *Handbook of physiology; section 2, the cardiovascular system.* Bethesda, MD: American Physiological Society, 1979:873–952.
23. Grines CL, Topol EJ, Califf RM, et al. Prognostic implications and predictors of enhanced regional wall motion of the noninfarct zone after thrombolysis and angioplasty therapy of acute myocardial infarction. The TAMI Study Groups. *Circulation* 1989;80:245–253.
24. Frid DJ, et al. Undercompensation: the role of the non-infarct related zone in the pathogenesis of cardiogenic shock. *Circulation* 1990;82[Suppl III]:III-430(abst).
25. Schuster EH, Bulkley BH. Early post-infarction angina. Ischemia at a distance and ischemia in the infarct zone. *N Engl J Med* 1981;305:1101–1105.
26. Wackers FJ, Lie KI, Becker AE, et al. Coronary artery disease in patients dying from cardiogenic shock or congestive heart failure in the setting of acute myocardial infarction. *Br Heart J* 1976;38:906–910.
27. Mavric Z, Zaputovic L, Zagar D, et al. Usefulness of blood lactate as a predictor of shock development in acute myocardial infarction. *Am J Cardiol* 1991;67:565–568.
28. Scheidt S, Ascheim R, Killip T 3rd. Shock after acute myocardial infarction. A clinical and hemodynamic profile. *Am J Cardiol* 1970;26:556–564.
29. Webb JG, Sleeper LA, Buller CE, et al. Implications of the timing of onset of cardiogenic shock after acute myocardial infarction: a report from the SHOCK Trial Registry. SHould we emergently revascularize Occluded Coronaries for cardiogenic shocK? *J Am Coll Cardiol* 2000;36[3 Suppl A]:1084–1090.
30. Hasdai D, Topol EJ, Califf RM, et al. Cardiogenic shock complicating acute coronary syndromes. *Lancet* 2000;356:749–756.
31. Jacobs AK, French JK, Col J, et al. Cardiogenic shock with non-ST-segment elevation myocardial infarction: a report from the SHOCK Trial Registry. SHould we emergently revascularize Occluded coronaries for Cardiogenic shocK? *J Am Coll Cardiol* 2000;36[3 Suppl A]:1091–1096.
32. Holmes DR Jr, Berger PB, Hochman JS, et al. Cardiogenic shock in patients with acute ischemic syndromes with and without ST-segment elevation. *Circulation* 1999;100:2067–2073.
33. Ryan TJ, Anderson JL, Antman EM, et al. ACC/AHA guidelines for

the management of patients with acute myocardial infarction. A report of the American College of Cardiology/American Heart Association Task Force on Practice Guidelines (Committee on Management of Acute Myocardial Infarction). *J Am Coll Cardiol* 1996;28:1328–1428.

34. Picard MH, Davidoff R, Sleeper LA, et al. Echocardiographic predictors of survival and response to early revascularization in cardiogenic shock. *Circulation* 2003;107:279–284.

35. Forrester JS, Diamond G, Chatterjee K, et al. Medical therapy of acute myocardial infarction by application of hemodynamic subsets (second of two parts). *N Engl J Med* 1976;295:1404–1413.

36. Becker LC, Fortuin NJ, Pitt B. Effect of ischemia and antianginal drugs on the distribution of radioactive microspheres in the canine left ventricle. *Circ Res* 1971;28:263–269.

37. Hoffman BB, Lefkowitz RJ. Catecholamines and sympathomimetics drugs. In: Gilman AG, Rall TW, Nies AS, et al., eds. *Goodman and Gilman's the pharmacological basis of therapeutics,* 8th ed. New York: Permagon Press, 1990:187–220.

38. Gillespie TA, Ambos HD, Sobel BE, et al. Effects of dobutamine in patients with acute myocardial infarction. *Am J Cardiol* 1977;39:588–594.

39. Goldstein RA, Passamani ER, Roberts R. A comparison of digoxin and dobutamine in patients with acute infarction and cardiac failure. *N Engl J Med* 1980;303:846–850.

40. Monrad ES, Baim DS, Smith HS, et al. Milrinone, dobutamine, and nitroprusside: comparative effects on hemodynamics and myocardial energetics in patients with severe congestive heart failure. *Circulation* 1986;73[3 Pt 2]:III168–III174.

41. Packer M, Carver JR, Rodeheffer RJ, et al. Effect of oral milrinone on mortality in severe chronic heart failure. The PROMISE Study Research Group. *N Engl J Med* 1991;325:1468–1475.

42. Dec GW, Fifer MA, Herrmann HC, et al. Long-term outcome of enoximone therapy in patients with refractory heart failure. *Am Heart J* 1993;125[2 Pt 1]:423–429.

43. Pennington DG, Swartz MT. Assisted circulation and mechanical hearts. In: Braunwald E, ed. *Heart disease: a textbook of cardiovascular medicine,* 4th ed. Philadelphia: WB Saunders, 1992:535–550.

44. Sanders CA, Buckley MJ, Leinbach RC, et al. Mechanical circulatory assistance. Current status and experience with combining circulatory assistance, emergency coronary angiography, and acute myocardial revascularization. *Circulation* 1972;45:1292–1313.

45. Dunkman WB, Leinbach RC, Buckley MJ, et al. Clinical and hemodynamic results of intraaortic balloon pumping and surgery for cardiogenic shock. *Circulation* 1972;46:465–477.

46. Leinbach RC, Gold HK, Dinsmore RE, et al. The role of angiography in cardiogenic shock. *Circulation* 1973;48[1 Suppl]:III95–III98.

47. Bolooki H. Physiology in balloon pumping. In: Balooki H, ed. *Clinical application of intra-aortic balloon pump.* Mount Kisco, NY: Futura, 1984:57–126.

48. Kern MJ, Aguirre FV, Tatineni S, et al. Enhanced coronary blood flow velocity during intraaortic balloon counterpulsation in critically ill patients. *J Am Coll Cardiol* 1993;21:359–368.

49. Ohman EM, George BS, White CJ, et al. Use of aortic counterpulsation to improve sustained coronary artery patency during acute myocardial infarction. Results of a randomized trial. The Randomized IABP Study Group. *Circulation* 1994;90:792–799.

50. Sanborn TA, Sleeper LA, Bates ER, et al. Impact of thrombolysis, intra-aortic balloon pump counterpulsation, and their combination in cardiogenic shock complicating acute myocardial infarction: a report from the SHOCK Trial Registry. SHould we emergently revascularize Occluded Coronaries for cardiogenic shocK? *J Am Coll Cardiol* 2000;36[3 Suppl A]:1123–1129.

51. Anderson RD, Ohman EM, Holmes DR Jr, et al. Use of intraaortic balloon counterpulsation in patients presenting with cardiogenic shock: observations from the GUSTO-I Study. Global Utilization of Streptokinase and TPA for Occluded Coronary Arteries. *J Am Coll Cardiol* 1997;30:708–715.

52. Barron HV, Every NR, Parsons LS, et al. The use of intra-aortic balloon counterpulsation in patients with cardiogenic shock complicating acute myocardial infarction: data from the National Registry of Myocardial Infarction 2. *Am Heart J* 2001;141:933–939.

53. Brodie BR, Stuckey TD, Hansen C, et al. Intra-aortic balloon counterpulsation before primary percutaneous transluminal coronary angioplasty reduces catheterization laboratory events in high-risk patients with acute myocardial infarction. *Am J Cardiol* 1999;84:18–23.

54. Goldberger M, Tabak SW, Shah PK. Clinical experience with intra-aortic balloon counterpulsation in 112 consecutive patients. *Am Heart J* 1986;111:497–502.

55. Sanders KM, Stern TA, O'Gara PT, et al. Delirium during intra-aortic balloon pump therapy. Incidence and management. *Psychosomatics* 1992;33:35–44.

56. Col NF, Gurwitz JH, Alpert JS, et al. Frequency of inclusion of patients with cardiogenic shock in trials of thrombolytic therapy. *Am J Cardiol* 1994;73:149–157.

57. Dioguardi N, Lotto A, Nevi GF, et al. Controlled trial of streptokinase and heparin in acute myocardial infarction. *Lancet* 1971;2:891–895.

58. Mathey DG, Kuck KH, Tilsner V, et al. Non surgical coronary artery recanalization in acute transmural myocardial infarction. *Circulation* 1981;63:489–497.

59. Kennedy JW, Gensini GG, Timmis GC, et al. Acute myocardial infarction treated with intracoronary streptokinase: a report of the Society for Cardiac Angiography. *Am J Cardiol* 1985;55:871–877.

60. Bengtson JR, Kaplan AJ, Pieper KS, et al. Prognosis in cardiogenic shock after acute myocardial infarction in the interventional era. *J Am Coll Cardiol* 1992;20:1482–1489.

61. Indications for fibrinolytic therapy in suspected acute myocardial infarction: collaborative overview of early mortality and major morbidity results from all randomised trials of more than 1000 patients. Fibrinolytic Therapy Trialists' (FTT) Collaborative Group. *Lancet* 1994;343:311–322.

62. Stadius ML, Davis K, Maynard C, et al. Risk stratification for 1 year survival based on characteristics identified in the early hours of acute myocardial infarction. The Western Washington Intracoronary Streptokinase Trial. *Circulation* 1986;74:703–711.

63. Simoons ML, Serruys PW, van den Brand M, et al. Early thrombolysis in acute myocardial infarction: limitation of infarct size and improved survival. *J Am Coll Cardiol* 1986;7:717–728.

64. Guerci AD, Gerstenblith G, Brinker JA, et al. A randomized trial of intravenous tissue plasminogen activator for acute myocardial infarction with subsequent randomization to elective coronary angioplasty. *N Engl J Med* 1987;317:1613–1618.

65. Bassand JP, Machecourt J, Cassagnes J, et al. Multicenter trial of intravenous anisoylated plasminogen streptokinase activator complex (APSAC) in acute myocardial infarction: effects on infarct size and left ventricular function. *J Am Coll Cardiol* 1989;13:988–997.

66. Bates ER, Topol EJ. Limitations of thrombolytic therapy for acute myocardial infarction complicated by congestive heart failure and cardiogenic shock. *J Am Coll Cardiol* 1991;18:1077–1084.

67. Keeley EC, Boura JA, Grines CL. Primary angioplasty versus intravenous thrombolytic therapy for acute myocardial infarction: a quantitative review of 23 randomised trials. *Lancet* 2003;361:13–20.

68. Berger PB, Holmes DR Jr, Stebbins AL, et al. Impact of an aggressive invasive catheterization and revascularization strategy on mortality in patients with cardiogenic shock in the Global Utilization of Streptokinase and Tissue Plasminogen Activator for Occluded Coronary Arteries (GUSTO-I) trial. An observational study. *Circulation* 1997;96:122–127.

69. Berger PB, Tuttle RH, Holmes DR Jr, et al. One-year survival among patients with acute myocardial infarction complicated by cardiogenic shock, and its relation to early revascularization: results from the GUSTO-I trial. *Circulation* 1999;99:873–878.

70. Hochman JS, Sleeper LA, Webb JG, et al. Early revascularization in acute myocardial infarction complicated by cardiogenic shock. SHOCK Investigators. Should We Emergently Revascularize Occluded Coronaries for Cardiogenic Shock. *N Engl J Med* 1999;341:625–634.

71. Hochman JS, Sleeper LA, White HD, et al. One-year survival following early revascularization for cardiogenic shock. *JAMA* 2001;285:190–192.

72. Ryan TJ, Antman EM, Brooks NH, et al. 1999 update: ACC/AHA guidelines for the management of patients with acute myocardial infarction. A report of the American College of Cardiology/American Heart Association Task Force on Practice Guidelines (Committee on Management of Acute Myocardial Infarction). *J Am Coll Cardiol* 1999;34:890–911.

73. Mundth ED, Buckley MJ, Leinbach RC, et al. Surgical intervention for the complications of acute myocardial ischemia. *Ann Surg* 1973;178:379–390.

74. Miller MG, Hedley-White J, Weintraub RM, et al. Surgery for cardiogenic shock. *Lancet* 1974;2:1342–1345.

75. Willerson JT, Buja LM. Intraaortic balloon counterpulsation in pa-

tients in cardiogenic shock, medically refractory left ventricular failure and/or recurrent ventricular tachycardia. *Am J Med* 1975;58: 183–191.

76. Johnson SA, Scanlon PJ, Loeb HS, et al. Treatment of cardiogenic shock in myocardial infarction by intraaortic balloon counterpulsation surgery. *Am J Med* 1977;62:687–692.

77. Ehrich DA, Biddle TL, Kronenberg MW, et al. The hemodynamic response to intra-aortic balloon counterpulsation in patients with cardiogenic shock complicating acute myocardial infarction. *Am Heart J* 1977;93:274–279.

78. Bardet J, Masquet C, Kahn JC, et al. Clinical and hemodynamic results of intraortic balloon counterpulsation and surgery for cardiogenic shock. *Am Heart J* 1977;93:280–288.

79. O'Rourke MF, Sammel N, Chang VP. Arterial counterpulsation in severe refractory heart failure complicating acute myocardial infarction. *Br Heart J* 1979;41:308–316.

80. Subramanian VA, Roberts AJ, Zema MJ, et al. Cardiogenic shock following acute myocardial infarction; late functional results after emergency cardiac surgery. *NY State J Med* 1980;80:947–952.

81. DeWood MA, Notske RN, Hensley GR, et al. Intraaortic balloon counterpulsation with and without reperfusion for myocardial infarction shock. *Circulation* 1980;61:1105–1012.

82. Kirklin JK, Blackstone EH, Zorn GL. Intermediate-term results of coronary artery bypass grafting for acute myocardial infarction. *Circulation* 1985;72[Suppl II]:175–178.

83. Phillips SJ, Zeff RH, Skinner JR, et al. Reperfusion protocol and results in 738 patients with evolving myocardial infarction. *Ann Thorac Surg* 1986;41:119–125.

84. Laks H, Rosenkranz E, Buckberg GD. Surgical treatment of cardiogenic shock after myocardial infarction. *Circulation* 1986;74[Suppl III]:III11–III16.

85. Guyton RA, Arcidi JM, Langford DA. Emergency coronary bypass for cardiogenic shock. *Circulation* 1987;76[Suppl V]:V22–V27.

86. Bolooki H. Emergency cardiac procedures in patients in cardiogenic shock due to complications of coronary artery disease. *Circulation* 1989;79[Suppl I]:I137–I148.

87. Allen BS, Rosenkranz E, Buckberg GD, et al. Studies on prolonged acute regional ischemia. VI. Myocardial infarction with left ventricular power failure: a medical/surgical emergency requiring urgent revascularization with maximal protection of remote muscle. *J Thorac Cardiovasc Surg* 1989;98[5 Pt 1]:691–703.

88. Lust RM, Beggerly CE, Morrison RF. Improved protection of chronically inflow-limited myocardium with retrograde coronary sinus cardioplegia. *Circulation* 1988;78[Suppl III]:III217–III223.

89. Bolooki H. Surgical treatment of complications of acute myocardial infarction. *JAMA* 1990;263:1237–1240.

90. Shawl FA, Domanski MJ, Hernandez TJ, et al. Emergency percutaneous cardiopulmonary bypass support in cardiogenic shock from acute myocardial infarction. *Am J Cardiol* 1989;64:967–970.

91. Shawl FA. Percutaneous cardiopulmonary support in high-risk angioplasty. *Cardiol Clin* 1989;7:865–875.

92. Gacioch GM, Ellis SG, Lee L, et al. Cardiogenic shock complicating acute myocardial infarction: the use of coronary angioplasty and the integration of the new support devices into patient management. *J Am Coll Cardiol* 1992;19:647–653.

93. Rees MR, Browne T, Sivananthan UM, et al. Cardiac resuscitation with percutaneous cardiopulmonary support. *Lancet* 1992;340:513–514.

94. Matsuwaka R, Sakakibara T, Shintani H, et al. Emergency cardiopulmonary bypass support in patients with severe cardiogenic shock after acute myocardial infarction. *Heart Vessels* 1996;11:27–29.

95. Wampler RK, Moise JC, Frazier OH, et al. In vivo evaluation of a peripheral vascular access axial flow blood pump. *ASAIO Trans* 1988;34:450–454.

96. Pennington DG, Merjavy JP, Codd JE. Extracorporeal membrane oxygenation for patients with cardiogenic shock. *Circulation* 1984; 70[Suppl]:130–137.

97. Reichman RT, Joyo CI, Dembitsky WP, et al. Improved patient survival after cardiac arrest using a cardiopulmonary support system. *Ann Thorac Surg* 1990;49:101–105.

98. Laschinger JC, Cunningham JN Jr, Catinella FP, et al. 'Pulsatile' left atrial-femoral artery bypass. A new method of preventing extension of myocardial infarction. *Arch Surg* 1983;118:965–969.

99. Farrar DJ, Hill JD, Gray LA Jr, et al. Heterotopic prosthetic ventricles as a bridge to cardiac transplantation. A multicenter study in 29 patients. *N Engl J Med* 1988;318:333–340.

100. Park SJ, Nguyen DQ, Bank AJ, et al. Left ventricular assist device bridge therapy for acute myocardial infarction. *Ann Thorac Surg* 2000;69:1146–1151.

101. Champagnac D, Claudel JP, Chevalier JP, et al. Primary cardiogenic shock during acute myocardial infarction: results of emergency cardiac transplantation. *Eur Heart J* 1993;14:925–929.

102. O'Neill W, et al. Coronary angioplasty therapy of cardiogenic shock complicating acute myocardial infarction. *Circulation* 1985; 72[Suppl II]:309.

103. Shani J, et al. Percutaneous transluminal coronary angioplasty in cardiogenic shock. *J Am Coll Cardiol* 1986;7:149A.

104. Heuser RR, et al. Coronary angioplasty in the treatment of cardiogenic shock: the therapy of choice. *J Am Coll Cardiol* 1986;7:219A.

105. Disler L, Haitas B, Benjamin J, et al. Cardiogenic shock in evolving myocardial infarction: treatment by angioplasty and streptokinase. *Heart Lung* 1987;16[6 Pt 1]:649–652.

106. Landin RJ, et al. Hospital mortality of patients undergoing emergency angioplasty for acute myocardial infarction: relationship of mortality to cardiogenic shock and unsuccessful angioplasty. *Circulation* 1988; 78[Suppl II]:II-9.

107. Laramee LA, et al. Coronary angioplasty for cardiogenic shock following myocardial infarction. *Circulation* 1988;78[Suppl II]:II-634.

108. Lee L, Bates ER, Pitt B, et al. Percutaneous transluminal coronary angioplasty improves survival in acute myocardial infarction complicated by cardiogenic shock. *Circulation* 1988;78:1345–1351.

109. Verna E, Repetto S, Boscarini M, et al. Emergency coronary angioplasty in patients with severe left ventricular dysfunction or cardiogenic shock after acute myocardial infarction. *Eur Heart J* 1989;10: 958–966.

110. Kaplan AJ, et al. Reperfusion improves survival in patients with cardiogenic shock after acute myocardial infarction. *J Am Coll Cardiol* 1990;15:155A.

111. Meyer P, Blanc P, Baudouy M, et al. [Treatment of primary cardiogenic shock by coronary transluminal angioplasty during the acute phase of myocardial infarction]. *Arch Mal Coeur Vaiss* 1990;83:329–334.

112. Brodie BR, Weintraub RA, Stuckey TD, et al. Outcomes of direct coronary angioplasty for acute myocardial infarction in candidates and non-candidates for thrombolytic therapy. *Am J Cardiol* 1991;67:7–12.

113. Lee L, Erbel R, Brown TM, et al. Multicenter registry of angioplasty therapy of cardiogenic shock: initial and long-term survival. *J Am Coll Cardiol* 1991;17:599–603.

114. Hibbard MD, Holmes DR Jr, Bailey KR, et al. Percutaneous transluminal coronary angioplasty in patients with cardiogenic shock. *J Am Coll Cardiol* 1992;19:639–646.

115. Moosvi AR, Khaja F, Villanueva L, et al. Early revascularization improves survival in cardiogenic shock complicating acute myocardial infarction. *J Am Coll Cardiol* 1992;19:907–914.

116. Yamamoto H, Hayashi Y, Oka Y, et al. Efficacy of percutaneous transluminal coronary angioplasty in patients with acute myocardial infarction complicated by cardiogenic shock. *Jpn Circ J* 1992;56:815–821.

117. Seydoux C, Goy JJ, Beuret P, et al. Effectiveness of percutaneous transluminal coronary angioplasty in cardiogenic shock during acute myocardial infarction. *Am J Cardiol* 1992;69:968–969.

118. Laney PL, et al. Follow-up exercise function in patients presenting with cardiogenic shock and acute transmural myocardial infarction. *J Am Coll Cardiol* 1993;21:77A.

119. Morrison DC, Silverstein R, Luchi M, et al. Systolic blood pressure response to percutaneous transluminal coronary angioplasty for cardiogenic shock. *Am J Cardiol* 1995;76:313–314.

120. Eltchaninoff H, Simpfendorfer C, Franco I, et al. Early and 1-year survival rates in acute myocardial infarction complicated by cardiogenic shock: a retrospective study comparing coronary angioplasty with medical treatment. *Am Heart J* 1995;130[3 Pt 1]:459–464.

121. Antoniucci D, Valenti R, Santoro GM, et al. Systematic direct angioplasty and stent-supported direct angioplasty therapy for cardiogenic shock complicating acute myocardial infarction: in-hospital and long-term survival. *J Am Coll Cardiol* 1998;31:294–300.

CHAPTER 74

Mechanical Complication of Acute Myocardial Infarction

Randi Rose

Key Words: Cardiac rupture; left ventricular aneurysm; left ventricular thrombus; mitral regurgitation; myocardial infarction; papllary muscle dysfunction.

INTRODUCTION

In the reperfusion era, the 30-day mortality rate and overall complications of acute myocardial infarction (AMI) have been substantially reduced (1,2). Unfortunately, there has been no significant decrease in the incidence rate of cardiogenic shock, which has remained at 7% to 10% over the last 20 years (3). Cardiogenic shock still remains the leading cause of death in patients admitted to the hospital for AMI (4). In the majority of these patients, the problem is one of overwhelming left ventricular damage, and their prognosis is quite poor (5). There is, however, a small but significant subgroup of patients with cardiogenic shock for which the prognosis can be substantially improved if prompt recognition and management is achieved. This subgroup comprises the mechanical complications of AMI, including ventricular free wall rupture, ventricular septal rupture, papillary muscle rupture, and ventricular false aneurysm formation. As a group,

R. Rose: The Zena and Michael A. Wiener Cardiovascular Institute, Mount Sinai Hospital, One Gustave L. Levy Place, Box 1030, New York, New York 10029-6574.

they are probably responsible for about 15% of all deaths from AMI (5). Although conservative treatment of these complications carries a mortality rate of greater than 80%, with surgical correction, patients can extend their 5-year survival rates to 65% (6). Sudden or progressive hemodynamic deterioration with low cardiac output, or both, should lead to the prompt consideration of these defects and the rapid institution of diagnostic and therapeutic measures. The clinical and hemodynamic profiles of the common mechanical defects that occur are summarized in Table 74–1.

VENTRICULAR FREE WALL RUPTURE

Incidence and Timing

Left ventricular free wall rupture occurs in 1% to 3% of all patients with AMI and is involved in approximately 10% to 15% of all infarct deaths, accounting for up to one-third of in-hospital deaths (4). Free wall rupture is second only to cardiac failure and is ahead of arrhythmia as a cause of in-hospital mortality (7). The incidence of free wall rupture in cases of fatal AMI is about ten times that of septal or papillary muscle rupture (6). The peak incidence of rupture occurs 3 to 5 days after the MI (8). In an analysis of patients who received a thrombolytic agent, the time course to rupture was noted to be accelerated, as 62% of patients ruptured within 1 day (9).

TABLE 74–1. *Characteristics of ventricular septal rupture, rupture of the ventricular free wall, and papillary muscle rupture*

Characteristic	Ventricular septal rupture	Rupture of ventricular free wall	Papillary muscle rupture
Incidence rate	1–3% without reperfusion therapy, 0.2–0.34% with thrombolytic therapy, 3.9% among patients with cardiogenic shock	0.8–6.2%, thrombolytic therapy does not reduce risk; primary PTCA seems to reduce risk	About 1% (posteromedial more frequent than anterolateral papillary muscle)
Time course	3–7 days without reperfusion therapy; median, 24 hours with thrombolysis	1–7 days without reperfusion therapy; mean, 2.7 days with thrombolysis	Median, 1 day (range 1–14 days)
Clinical manifestations	Chest pain, shortness of breath, hypotension	Anginal, pleuritic, or pericardial chest pain, syncope, hypotension, arrhythmia, nausea, restlessness, hypotension, sudden death	Abrupt onset of shortness of breath and pulmonary edema; hypotension
Physical findings	Harsh holosystolic murmur, thrill (+), S3, accentuated second heart sound, pulmonary edema, RV and LV failure, cardiogenic shock	Jugular venous distension (29% of patients), pulsus paradoxus (47%), electromechanical dissociation, cardiogenic shock	A soft murmur in some cases, no thrill, variable signs of RV overload, severe pulmonary edema, cardiogenic shock
Echocardiographic findings	Ventricular septal rupture, left-to-right shunt on color flow Doppler echocardiography through the ventricular septum, pattern of RV overload	>5 mm pericardial effusion not visualized in all cases, layered high-acoustic echoes within pericardium (blood clot), direct visualization of tear, signs of tamponade	Hypercontractile LV, torn papillary muscle or chordae tendinea, flail leaflet, severe mitral regurgitation on color flow Doppler echocardiography
Right heart catheterization	Increase in oxygen saturation from RA to RV, large V waves	Ventriculography insensitive, classic signs of tamponade not always present (equalization of diastolic pressures among cardiac chambers)	No increase in oxygen saturation from the RA to RV, large V waves, very high pulmonary capillary wedge pressures

LV, left ventricle; PTCA, percutaneous transluminal coronary angioplasty; RA, right atrium; RV, right ventricle.
From Birnbaum Y, Fishbein MC, Blanche C, et al. Current concepts: ventricular septal rupture after acute myocardial infarction. *N Engl J Med* 2002;347:1426–1432, with permission.)

Risk Factors

Several risk factors for rupture have been identified. Advanced age, first transmural MI, hypertension, and female sex have all been shown to be independently associated with cardiac rupture (8–10). Although prior use of corticosteroids or nonsteroidal antiinflammatory agents have been implicated as a predisposing factor for rupture as a result of impaired infarct healing and fibrosis, observational studies have not been consistent in this regard (11).

The rupture rate is three times greater in patients having their first MI, perhaps because the presence of scarring may offer some degree of protection against rupture during a later infarction (12). Increased outflow resistance manifested as hypertension or significant aortic stenosis may increase rupture by increasing mechanical stress on the infarcted tissue (13). The explanation for the enhanced risk for the female sex is unclear, but may be as simple as that because MIs occur at more advanced ages in women, they may rupture proportionally more often in women then men.

Although prompt reperfusion therapy is thought to decrease the incidence of rupture, delayed reperfusion may be associated with an increased risk for rupture (14). Although contradictory data exist, timely thrombolytic therapy seems not to increase the risk for free wall rupture (10). Data do, however, suggest that in patients with AMI, primary angioplasty reduces the risk for free wall rupture in comparison with thrombolysis (15). The reduction in the rate of free wall rupture achieved by primary angioplasty is probably a result of the earlier and more effective coronary recanalization.

Other protective factors include the early use of medications such as β-blockers and angiotensin-converting enzyme (ACE) inhibitors. Such therapies may help to prevent early infarct expansion and thinning, which predisposes to cardiac rupture (16). In International Study of Infarct Survival (ISIS-I), patients treated with intravenous β-blocker had a significant reduction in early in-hospital mortality that was related almost entirely to a lower rate of rupture (17). **In Thrombolysis in Myocardial Infarction (TIMI) 9, by multivariate analysis,**

ACE inhibitor or β-blocker use was inversely associated with cardiac rupture (14).

Pathophysiology

Zones of extensive myocardial necrosis are characterized by a marked reduction in collagen fibers, a process that begins within hours of the infarction. Infarct expansion, in these areas of reduced collagen fibers, leading to acute dilatation and thinning of the ventricular wall, has been thought to be the underlying pathophysiologic factor responsible for cardiac rupture.

Clinical and pathologic studies have demonstrated that ventricular free wall ruptures may take an acute, subacute, or chronic course (12,18–22). In the first instance, an abrupt transmural tear produces cardiac tamponade and is rapidly fatal. In subacute ventricular free wall rupture, the cardiac tamponade is less severe as a gradual or incomplete rupture of the infarcted area leads to slow or repetitive bleeding into the pericardial sac. Chronic rupture occurs with the formation of a false aneurysm.

Most patients with free wall rupture identified at autopsy have complete occlusion or incomplete reperfusion of the infarct-related artery (23). Rupture is, therefore, most likely to occur in the setting of a transmural infarction (Fig. 74–1).

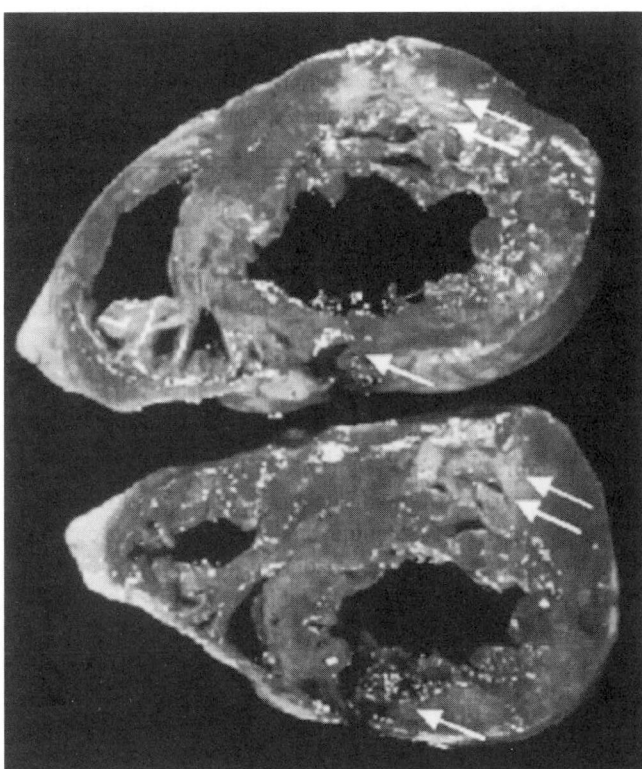

FIG. 74–1. Photograph of a left ventricular free wall rupture in a patient approximately 5 days after an acute anteroseptal myocardial infarction *(arrow)*. Note the old posterior myocardial infarction *(double arrow)*. (Courtesy of Dr. John T. Fallon, Department of Pathology, Mount Sinai Hospital, New York, NY.)

Approximately half of ruptures are serpiginous rather than simple tears (7). The most common site of rupture is the lateral aspect of the ventricle (7). The left anterior descending or left circumflex artery is the culprit vessel more often in those with free wall rupture or tamponade (10,24).

Clinical Features

Free wall rupture usually presents as a catastrophic event with rapid hemodynamic deterioration and shock from a combination of impaired ventricular systolic function and tamponade. Previously, the diagnosis was always made on the basis of the clinical picture: sudden loss of consciousness, jugular venous distension, cyanosis, rhythm changes, electromechanical dissociation, respiratory arrest, and death. Cardiac rupture, however, does not always present such a dramatic picture and is dependent on the type of rupture. Up to 40% of cases occur subacutely, over a matter of hours, not minutes, allowing the astute clinician the opportunity for recognition and management of this life-threatening event (25). More subtle symptoms occurring hours or days before the final event include unexplained hypotension, transient bradycardia, and some electrocardiographic features such as persistent ST-segment elevation and T waves failing to invert in the same leads (26–28).

Echocardiography remains the diagnostic modality of choice. The presence of pericardial fluid, diastolic compression of the ventricular chambers, dissecting hematoma of the ventricular wall, an echo-dense mass in the pericardial space, and direct visualization of the wall defect are highly suggestive features of myocardial rupture (22,29–31). Administration of a contrast agent can be useful in demonstrating active bleeding into the pericardium and may limit the number of false-positives with two-dimensional Doppler echocardiography alone (32).

Hemopericardium by pericardiocentesis is a reliable finding in cardiac rupture; however, the procedure is not without its own risks, and a negative tap should not deter clinicians with a high index of suspicion.

Treatment

Once the diagnosis is confirmed, an inotropic agent and infusion of fluids should be initiated immediately, while preparations for surgical intervention are made. The use of an intraaortic balloon pump is controversial, although it may be required as a bridge to surgery. Pericardiocentesis, as a therapeutic measure, appears to be of little benefit as hemopericardium tends to reaccumulate rapidly, and the clotting process quickly develops into the set for pericardial drainage. Coronary angiography is an unwarranted procedure in patients who are hemodynamically unstable (33–36).

Simple surgical procedures, especially when cardiopulmonary bypass can be avoided, seem preferable to complex repair as the operation is performed only a few days after an AMI and frequently after a period of cardiogenic shock.

Principles of repair of left ventricular free wall rupture are to stop the bleeding, to anchor the repair on healthy tissue, and to minimize distortion of heart geometry (7,33,34). Surgical options include infarct excision and closure of the created defect with interrupted suture or covering the rupture zone and surrounding infarct with Teflon or Dacron patches (7,36,37). Epicardial patching of the bleeding area is easy to perform, does not require unloading of the heart, and effectively controls bleeding (38). Furthermore, when performing the more traditional technique of infarctectomy and repair using cardiopulmonary bypass, it is often difficult to distinguish the border between viable myocardium and infarct. Only a general estimation of size is required with the application of a patch and glue (38).

Surgical repair of the rupture site is the definitive treatment for cardiac rupture. Operative mortality is high; however, those who survive the perioperative period generally have a good long-term prognosis (33). Long-term survival may become even more common as clinical predicting factors and early diagnosis are better established, allowing for earlier attempts at surgical repair (33).

VENTRICULAR SEPTAL RUPTURE

Incidence and Risk Factors

Ventricular septal rupture complicating AMI is uncommon, with a reported incidence in the prethrombolytic era of 1% to 3% (39–41). With the advent of thrombolytic therapy, this number has significantly decreased with only 84 of 41,021 (0.2%) patients in the Global Utilization of Streptokinase and TPA for Occluded Coronary Arteries (GUSTO-I) trial identified as having confirmed septal defects (42). Thrombolytic therapy appears to reduce the overall incidence of septal rupture by restoring vessel patency, salvaging myocardium, and preventing ongoing infarct expansion—a prerequisite for septal rupture.

Advanced age (>70 years), anterior infarct location, and female sex have all been shown to be important predictors of septal rupture (11,40,43,44). These clinical characteristics have been shown to be independent risk factors for septal rupture in both the prethrombolytic and thrombolytic era.

Time Course

Although ventricular septal rupture is occurring with less frequency in the thrombolytic era, the timing appears to be accelerated. Presentation of septal rupture in the prethrombolytic era typically occurred within the first week at a median time from 3 to 5 days (41,45–47). Thrombolytic therapy appears to accelerate the occurrence of rupture to within 24 to 48 hours of treatment. The median time from MI onset to septal rupture in patients receiving thrombolysis in both the GUSTO-I and SHould we emergently revascularize Occluded Coronaries for cardiogenic shocK? (SHOCK) trial was 1 day and 16 hours, respectively (42,48).

Becker and colleagues postulate that although thrombolysis may prevent the occurrence of transmural necrosis, it may cause myocardial hemorrhage so that if a septal rupture were to occur, its time course would be accelerated (4). However, in a study of more than 3,700 patients with AMI given thrombolytics, aspirin, and adjunctive anticoagulation therapy, there was no identifiable association between the mechanism or intensity of anticoagulation and cardiac rupture (14). Rather, the apparent acceleration of the occurrence of postinfarction septal rupture may be because of the positive impact of thrombolytic therapy in reducing the incidence of late post-MI septal ruptures.

Pathophysiology

Angiographic data show that patients who experience development of septal rupture after AMI are more likely to have total occlusion of the infarct artery (41,42,49). In the GUSTO-I study, total occlusion of the infarct-related artery was documented in 57% of patients with septal rupture, compared with 18% of those without septal rupture (42). In the SHOCK trial, all culprit vessels had more than 90% stenosis, and the overwhelming majority (22/26) exhibited TIMI grade 0 or 1 flow (48). Collaterals also appear to be less evident in patients with ventricular septal rupture (44,50). The absence of collateral flow to the infarcted area creates a milieu for extensive transmural myocardial necrosis, predisposing to rupture. These findings suggest that the pathophysiology of acute septal rupture involves sudden, severe ischemia, leading to extensive, transmural myocardial necrosis. Without reperfusion, disintegration of the necrotic myocardium is hastened by the attraction of neutrophils that release lytic enzymes.

Necroscopy evaluation of postinfarct ventricular rupture shows two distinct morphologic variations (47,51) (Fig. 74–2). Simple ruptures have a direct through-and-through tear in the septal myocardium. The perforation is at the same level on both sides of the septum. Septal ruptures in patients with anterior MI are generally apical and simple. Complex ruptures are characterized by serpiginous tracts through the septal myocardium and are usually associated with extensive hemorrhage (47,51). Ventricular septal defects associated with inferior infarctions are more likely to be complex and located toward the base of the heart. Complex ventricular septal defects are more likely to be associated with free wall rupture.

Clinical Features

Ventricular septal rupture is usually associated with sudden hemodynamic deterioration and cardiogenic shock. Patients often complain of recurrent or protracted chest pain preceding myocardial rupture (24). As opposed to left ventricular free wall rupture, ventricular septal rupture is more likely (20–30%) to be associated with complete heart block, right bundle branch block, and atrial fibrillation (24).

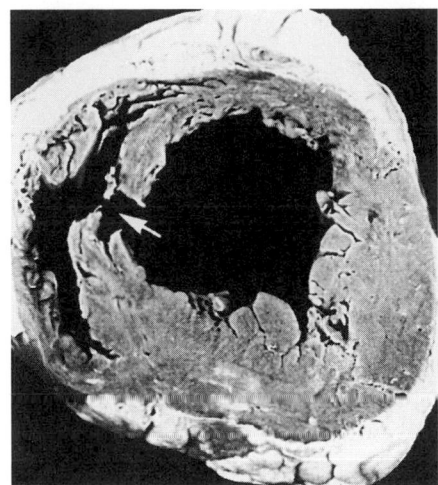 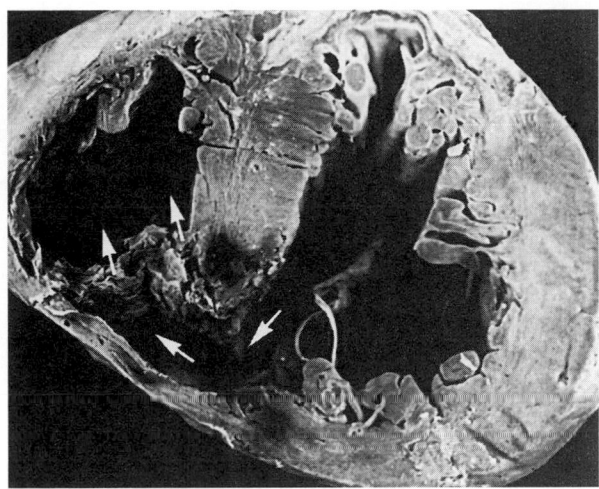

FIG. 74–2. Left: Cross section viewed from the apex of the ventricular portion of the heart. A simple rupture of the ventricular septum is apparent as are scars of an old inferior myocardial infarction. **Right:** Complex septal rupture with laceration and hemorrhage in the region of the inferobasal septum and involvement of the right ventricular free wall with additional rupture.

A ruptured interventricular septum is characterized by the appearance of a loud holosystolic murmur best heard at the lower left sternal border that may be accompanied by a thrill (52). As arterial pressure decreases, the thrill may be absent and the murmur more difficult to identify. It may be difficult on clinical grounds to distinguish between acute mitral regurgitation and rupture of the ventricular septum in patients with AMI who experience development of a loud holosystolic murmur. The location of the murmur and thrill may be able to aid in this differentiation. The murmur and thrill of a septal rupture are generally more prominent at the left sternal border, whereas the murmur and thrill of mitral regurgitation are usually more prominent at the apex. This differentiation can be made most readily by color flow Doppler echocardiography.

Right heart catheterization also can be used in the evaluation of patients with septal rupture (53). Patients with ventricular septal ruptures demonstrate a "step-up" in oxygen saturation of greater than 5% in blood samples from the right ventricle and pulmonary artery compared with those from the right atrium. Rarely, a "step-up" in oxygen saturation in the peripheral pulmonary artery may be present in some cases of severe mitral regurgitation (54). Echocardiography has greatly reduced the value of right heart catheterization as a diagnostic tool (Fig. 74–3).

Treatment

Medical stabilization with hemodynamic monitoring is important in the preparation of the patient for further diagnostic studies and surgical repair. Invasive monitoring with a right heart catheterization allows for the determination of initial treatment options. Unless the patient is hypotensive, vasodilator therapy with either nitroprusside or nitroglycerin should be initiated. If vasodilator therapy is not tolerated, in-

traaortic balloon counterpulsation should be rapidly instituted (53). Preoperative intraaortic balloon pump will increase cardiac output and decrease the left-to-right shunt, and also will improve coronary perfusion.

Attempts to stabilize the patient medically are only temporizing; surgical intervention is required. Mortality with this complication remains extremely high despite improvements in medical therapy. In the GUSTO-I study, 30-day and 1-year mortality rates were 94% and 97%, respectively, in patients treated medically (42). In the SHOCK trial, only 1 of the 24 patients managed medically survived (48). Mortality appears to be worse in patients with cardiogenic shock. In the GUSTO-I trial, all patients with ventricular septal rupture who had pulmonary congestion (Killip Class III or IV) at admission died within 30 days; the mortality rate was 27% among patients with septal rupture who were in Killip Class I or II (42). Another independent predictor of early mortality is the time period from infarction to rupture. Earlier rupture, usually associated with more extensive myocardial damage, portends a worse prognosis even in the absence of overt shock before surgery (44). Most reports identify septal ruptures associated with posterior infarcts as having a worse outcome than those with anterior infarcts (40,42,45,55). This is probably related to that posterior infarcts are more likely to be associated with complex septal ruptures located in the inferobasal portion of the septum; an area that is difficult to access surgically (47). Right ventricular infarction and dysfunction, more commonly associated with posterior infarcts, also have been shown to be a poor prognostic indicator (55). Nevertheless, this mortality difference based on infarct location is not a universal finding (44,56). Deja and coworkers (44), in their retrospective analysis of 117 patients who underwent postinfarction septal rupture repair, found similar mortality in the anterior and posterior groups (34% vs. 35%). David and Armstrong (56)

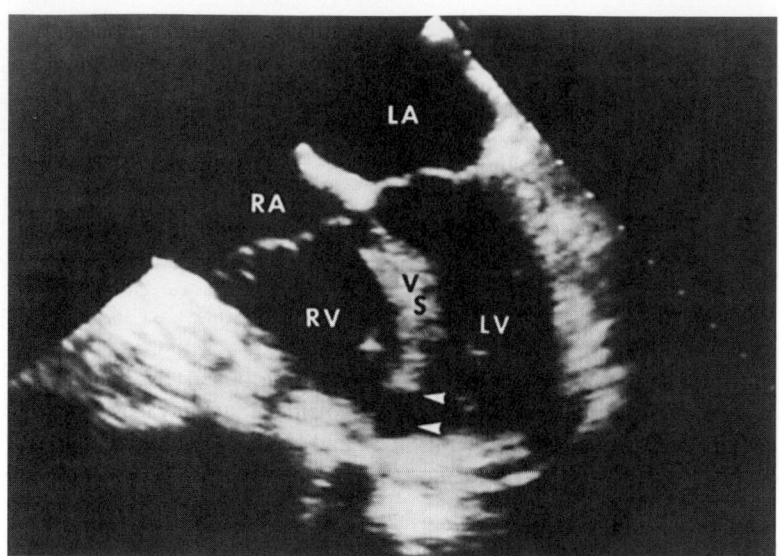

FIG. 74–3. Transesophageal echocardiogram showing an apical ventricular septal defect *(arrowheads).* LA, left atrium; LV, left ventricle; RA right atrium; RV, right ventricle; VS, ventricular septum.

found that repair of the septal rupture by infarct exclusion (securing a pericardial patch to the endocardium of the left ventricle all around the necrotic myocardium to exclude the septal defect and the infarct from the left ventricular cavity) resulted in similar survival/mortality in both septal rupture locations.

The timing of surgery for acute septal rupture has been a source of controversy for years. It had long been believed that delaying surgery for 3 to 6 weeks after an AMI allowed for tissue healing before surgical repair and was associated with a reduction in perioperative mortality (57). However, this apparent improvement in surgical mortality is more likely to be the result of selection bias as sicker patients would have died before surgery. In fact, it is now recognized that prompt surgical repair after a period of medical stabilization is necessary in all patients with septal rupture regardless of presenting hemodynamic status. The poor outcome of patients with ventricular septal rupture and cardiogenic shock in the SHOCK trial would tend to support the Class I indication for urgent early surgical intervention before shock onset (48,53). Surgical survival is predicted by early surgery, short duration of shock, and mild degrees of right ventricular impairment (44,58,59).

The need for concomitant coronary revascularization remains a controversial question. Several studies have failed to show a relation between coronary artery bypass grafting and perioperative mortality (44,60). Preoperative cardiac catheterization for assessment of coronary anatomy seems appropriate in patients in Killip Class I and II who are hemodynamically stable, and coronary artery bypass grafting should be considered in patients with two- or three-vessel coronary artery disease. There are some data to suggest that concomitant revascularization may improve late survival (59,61). However, patients in Killip Class III or IV should proceed directly

to surgery. In a small group of patients with cardiogenic shock in the SHOCK trial, there was no additional benefit of concomitant bypass surgery (48).

Most septal ruptures can be repaired with direct closure, although some large and complex defects may require patch placement. The septal rupture should be accessed through the infarcted myocardium, and all necrotic and friable material should be removed to avoid a residual septal defect, postoperative hemorrhage, or both (62). Favorable experience with a newer technique of excluding the infarction and rupture site from the left ventricular cavity, which has the benefit of avoiding direct incision of the ventricles, has been described by David and Armstrong (56). Exposure of the septum through the right atrium has similar appeal (63). Surgical repair may also involve correction of mitral regurgitation with a mitral valve repair or replacement if indicated (62). Percutaneous closure as an alternative to reoperation in residual or recurrent postinfarction ventricular septal defects has been described (64–66). More experience is needed to assess its value as a primary closure technique or a bridge to surgery in acute ventricular septal rupture.

PAPILLARY MUSCLE RUPTURE

Incidence, Timing, and Risk Factors

Acute papillary muscle rupture is a rare complication of MI occurring slightly less frequently than ventricular septal rupture. It can be seen in approximately 0.5% to 5% of MIs (6). Papillary muscle dysfunction without rupture is much more common, however, occurring in 20% to 50% of autopsied cases (67). Papillary muscle rupture, an often fatal complication of AMI, accounts for approximately 5% of infarct-related deaths (6).

Papillary muscle rupture usually occurs 3 to 5 days after infarction. Risk factors for the development of papillary muscle rupture include female sex, advanced age, and inferior MI (5,24,68–70). Patients often present with single-vessel coronary artery disease and usually do not have a positive history for previous MI (69).

Pathophysiology

The clinical presentation of papillary muscle rupture is closely tied to the anatomy and blood supply of the anterolateral and posteromedial papillary muscles. The anterolateral papillary muscle is usually fed by a dual blood supply from the left anterior descending artery and circumflex artery. The posteromedial papillary muscle, in contrast, usually has a single blood supply from the right coronary artery, leaving it more susceptible to infarction, necrosis, and rupture in the setting of an AMI (71–73). Thus, rupture of the posteromedial muscle is 6 to 12 times more common than that of the anteromedial papillary muscle.

Anatomically, the posteromedial papillary muscle consists of one or two large common trunks and multiple smaller heads that give off chordae to both the anterior and posterior mitral valve leaflet (71,72). Complete transection of the papillary muscle at the common trunk may occur resulting in overwhelming mitral regurgitation, which is incompatible with life (Fig. 74–4). Partial tear of the common trunk, or rupture of one of the multiple heads of the papillary muscle, which is much more frequent, results in less severe deterioration, although the potential for additional rupture is present and may lead to unpredictable rapid decompensation (72). These observations indicate that acute severe mitral regurgitation may be the consequence of infarction or dysfunction of limited but exquisitely important myocardium.

Indeed, in the SHOCK registry, less than half of the mitral regurgitation cohort displayed clinically recognized ST-segment elevation or new Q waves, and left ventricular function was well preserved in many of these patients (70).

Clinical Features

The clinical presentation of a patient with an acute papillary muscle rupture is characterized by rapid hemodynamic deterioration, pulmonary edema, and cardiogenic shock. Lesser degrees of regurgitation caused by incomplete rupture of a papillary muscle head or rupture of chordae tendinea can be difficult to recognize. A murmur of mitral regurgitation may be present, but may be inaudible because of the rapid equalization of pressure between the left ventricle and the left atrium. Furthermore, the location of the murmur may be atypical because of the eccentric nature of the regurgitant jet. Differentiation between the systolic murmur of acute mitral regurgitation and that of an acute ventricular septal defect also can be difficult, although papillary muscle rupture is less commonly associated with a palpable thrill. Given the lack of any reliable features on physical examination, a heightened index of suspicion is crucial for the prompt recognition of this syndrome. The presence of cardiogenic shock or pulmonary edema in the patient with an acute inferior MI, particularly a first infarction, should always raise the possibility of acute mitral regurgitation and papillary muscle rupture. If the left ventricular function is relatively preserved, the likelihood of a mechanical complication as a cause for the deterioration is magnified.

Echocardiography is the initial diagnostic modality in the evaluation of acute mitral regurgitation (Fig. 74–5). Features suggestive of papillary muscle rupture include a flail mitral valve leaflet with systolic prolapse into the left atrium, a mo-

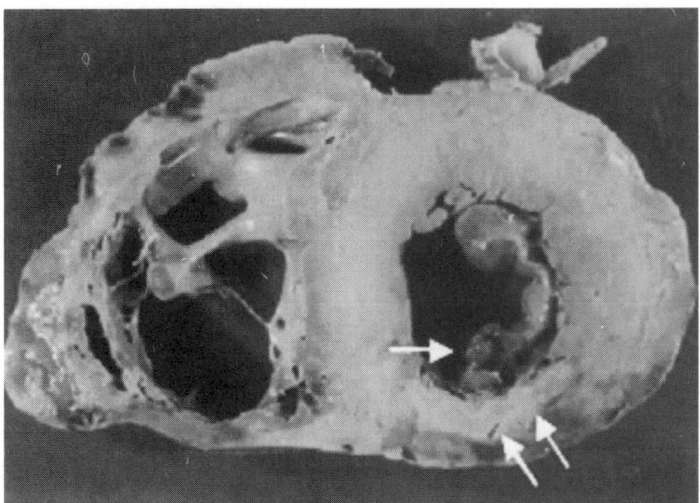

FIG. 74–4. Photograph of complete rupture of the posteromedial papillary muscle *(arrow)* in a patient approximately 3 days after a large inferoposterior myocardial infarction *(double arrow)*. (Courtesy of Dr. John T. Fallon, Department of Pathology, Mount Sinai Hospital, New York, NY.)

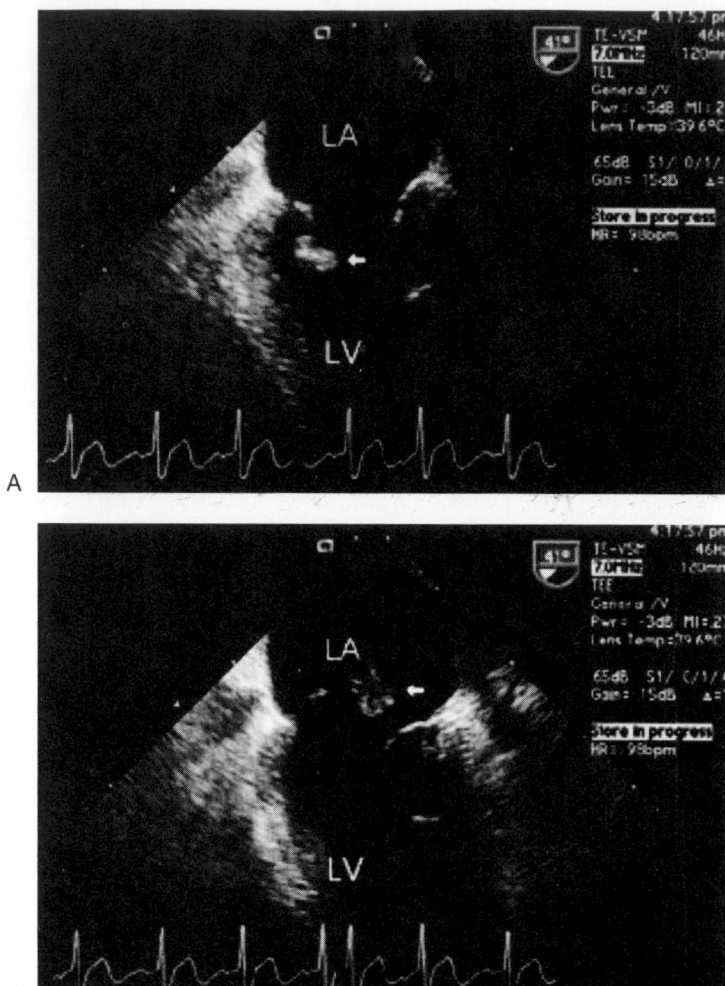

FIG. 74–5. Transesophageal echocardiogram demonstrating complete papillary muscle rupture. Entire head of papillary muscle *(arrowheads)* is shown during diastole **(A)** and systole **(B).** There is complete lack of coaptation of the mitral valve. LA, left atrium; LV, left ventricle. (Courtesy of Dr. Martin Goldman, Department of Cardiology, Mount Sinai Hospital, New York, NY.)

bile mass attached to the chordae tendinea and to the mitral valve, and an abnormal cutoff of one papillary muscle (74). Doppler and color flow examination can provide additional information in the form of the severity and mechanism of mitral regurgitation (75) (Fig. 74–6). The use of transesophageal echocardiogram in critically ill patients with equivocal or technically difficult transthoracic images remains an excellent option for more direct visualization of the mitral valve apparatus (76).

Right heart catheterization as a diagnostic tool has fallen out of favor. The presence of a large "V" wave on the pulmonary artery wedge pressure is not specific for acute mitral regurgitation because it may also be seen in patients with severe left ventricular dysfunction and decreased chamber compliance (77) (Fig. 74–7). A "step-up" in saturation from the right atrium to right ventricle and pulmonary artery, the "sin quo non" of ventricular septal rup-

ture, also has been seen in patients with papillary muscle rupture caused by the transmission of oxygenated blood retrograde across the pulmonary circulation (54). Likewise, cardiac catheterization and left ventriculography need not be performed merely to confirm the diagnosis unless other information such as coronary anatomy is required to guide surgical therapy in patients who are stable from a hemodynamic standpoint.

Treatment

The prognosis of papillary muscle rupture is poor. Approximately one-third of patients die within hours, 50% within 24 hours, and the mortality rate approaches 80% within 2 weeks (78,79). The management of patients with an acute papillary muscle rupture includes initial medical stabilization with inotropes, afterload reduction, and an

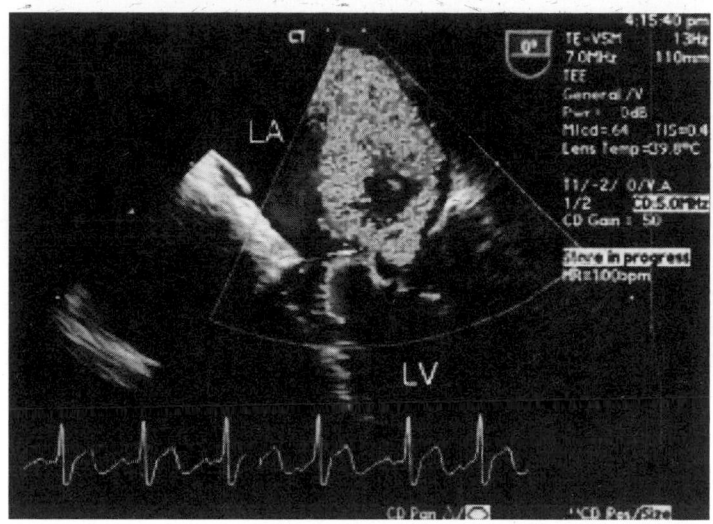

FIG. 74–6. Doppler echocardiography demonstrating severe mitral regurgitation as a result of complete papillary muscle rupture. (Courtesy of Dr. Martin Goldman, Department of Cardiology, Mount Sinai Hospital, New York, NY.)

intraaortic balloon pump. Surgical intervention with mitral valve repair or replacement should be instituted as early as possible after medical stabilization (80,81). The natural history of papillary muscle rupture is unpredictable, and apparent medical stabilization should not discourage clinicians from pursuing prompt surgical intervention. There are several reasons for sudden deterioration including progression from partial to complete rupture, recurrent ischemia, and cardiac decompensation. In a study from the Mayo Clinic, 50% of patients who were initially stabilized with medical therapy suddenly experienced deterioration in their condition and died (72). In the last decade, an early surgical approach has translated into a significant mortality rate reduction to less than 30% (80). When technically possible, the supporting structure of the mitral valve should be retained to more effectively preserve ventricular function.

LEFT VENTRICULAR FALSE ANEURYSM

Postinfarction pseudoaneurysm is a rare complication of AMI detected in less than 0.1% of cases (82). Incomplete rupture of the myocardium may occur when organizing thrombus and hematoma, together with pericardium, seal a rupture of the left ventricular free wall and prevent the development of a hemopericardium. Over time, this area of organized thrombus and pericardium can form a pseudoaneurysm that maintains communication with the cavity of the left ventricle. In contrast to true aneurysms, which always contain some myocardial elements in their walls, the walls of a pseudoaneurysm lack any elements of the original myocardial wall (Fig. 74–8). Inferior MIs account for approximately twice as many cases of pseudoaneurysms as anterior MIs (83). Thus, unlike true aneurysms, which have a propensity for the apex and anterior wall, false aneurysms are located more frequently on the posterolateral or di-

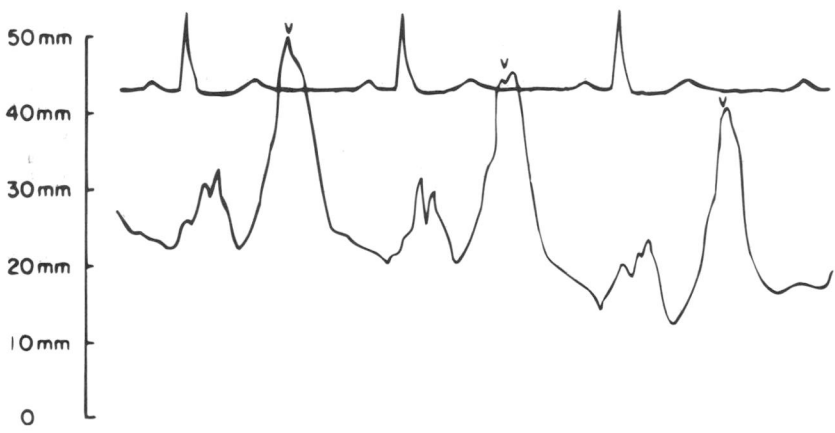

FIG. 74–7. Pulmonary capillary wedge tracing of a patient with large V waves.

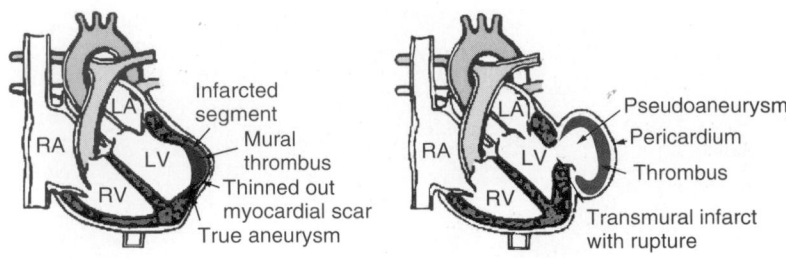

FIG. 74–8. Differences between a pseudoaneurysm and a true aneurysm. LA, left atrium; LV, left ventricle; RA, right atrium; RV, right ventricle. (From Shah PK. Complications of acute myocardial infarction. In: Parmley W, Chatterjee K, eds. *Cardiology.* Philadelphia: JB Lippincott, 1987, with permission.)

aphragmatic surface. Time of presentation can range from 3 to 80 days after an AMI.

The physical findings are nonspecific; therefore, clinical detection on the basis of physical examination can be difficult. A to-and-fro murmur may result from blood flow through the narrow neck. However, in up to 30% of patients with confirmed pseudoaneurysm, this finding is absent (83). A friction rub may also be present. Although most patients (>95%) have an abnormal electrocardiogram, ST-segment changes are nonspecific (83). The chest radiograph may demonstrate a bulge on the cardiac silhouette.

Two-dimensional echocardiography and angiography are the diagnostic modalities of choice (Fig. 74–9). The findings on the echocardiogram of an echo-free space that communicates with the left ventricular cavity by a narrow neck is highly suggestive of a pseudoaneurysm, especially if color Doppler records turbulent flow at the neck (84). Echocardiography can differentiate a pseudoaneurysm from a true aneurysm on the basis of a narrow opening between the ventricular chamber and the aneurysm with a ratio of the neck diameter to maximal aneurysm diameter of less than 0.5 (85). A ratio of 0.9 to 1.0 is usually more consistent with a true aneurysm (85). Angiographic findings that help to distinguish false aneurysms include a narrow orifice leading to a saccular aneurysm combined with the lack of surrounding coronary arteries (86). Frances and coworkers (83), in a literature review of 290 patients with left ventricular pseudoaneurysms, found that angiography revealed some abnormality 98% of the time and provided a definitive diagnosis in 87% of patients. Coronary angiography is necessary before surgery to evaluate the need for concomitant bypass grafting.

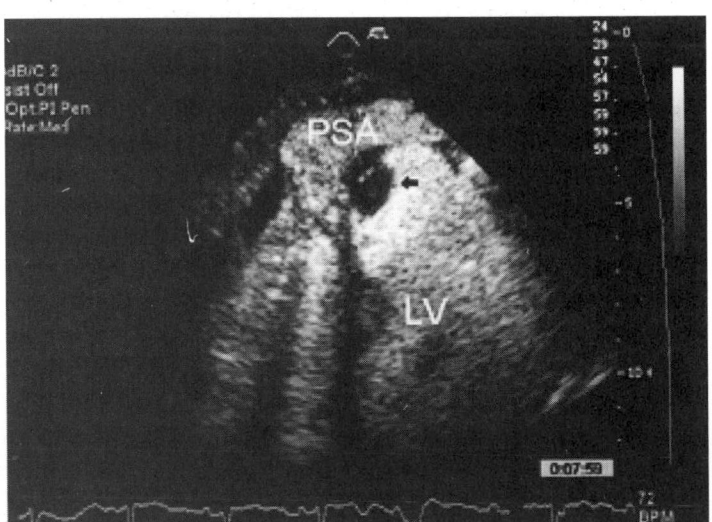

FIG. 74–9. Transthoracic echocardiogram with contrast showing an echo free space adjacent to the left ventricular apex. A small myocardial rupture was identified. Contrast imaging demonstrated shunting of blood between the left ventricle *(LV)* and the echo free space, enabling a diagnosis of left ventricular pseudoaneurysm (PSA) to be made. A left ventricular apical thrombus *(arrowhead)* also was present. (Courtesy of Dr. Martin Goldman, Department of Cardiology, Mount Sinai Hospital, New York, NY.)

The distinction between true and false aneurysms is important for therapeutic management. True aneurysms have a fibrotic wall that is highly resistant to rupture, and therefore does not mandate surgical intervention. Pseudoaneurysms, in contrast, initially consist of loose tissues that have a high propensity for secondary rupture. Prompt surgical correction is mandatory (50). In uncontrolled studies, mortality rates of medically treated patients with pseudoaneurysms were twice as high as those of their surgical counterparts (48% vs. 23%, respectively) (83). The principle of surgical repair is straightforward. Once the neck of the false aneurysm is dissected out, the perforation can be closed primarily or with patch repair (87). Manipulation and dissection around the false aneurysm should be avoided in an attempt to minimize the risk for bleeding and embolization (50). In acute cases, epicardial patching is an effective and reliable method (36).

As patients with false aneurysms often are more stable than those experiencing acute rupture, surgical repair can be combined with coronary artery bypass grafting with good outcomes. Concomitant mitral valve replacement, however, increases mortality significantly, likely related to that the presence of regurgitation requiring surgical intervention represents more extensive myocardial damage (88).

CONCLUSION

The relative infrequency of these mechanical complications of MI should not belie their importance as a potentially reversible cause of cardiogenic shock. Myocardial rupture tends to occur in patients with small areas of infarction and, as a result, well preserved left ventricular systolic function. The correction of the mechanical complication has the potential of leaving the patient with relatively preserved ventricular function and, as a result, a favorable long-term outcome. The entire diagnostic and therapeutic focus is to identify expeditiously patients who need surgical correction and for the surgery to be performed with minimal delay.

Ultimately, however, therapies directed specifically at prevention of rupture may be the best avenue for preventing deaths. Although prompt reperfusion therapy is thought to decrease the incidence of rupture, delayed reperfusion may be associated with an increased risk for rupture. Strategies aimed at decreasing the time from infarction to vessel patency are therefore at the cornerstone of any preventive measure. Furthermore, therapeutic agents targeted at reducing wall stress and therapies that decrease blood pressure and attenuate neurohormonal activation may prove promising avenues of ongoing research.

REFERENCES

1. Effectiveness of intravenous thrombolytic treatment in acute myocardial infarction. Gruppo Italiano per lo Studio della Streptochinasi nell'Infarto Miocardico (GISSI). *Lancet* 1986;1:397–402.
2. Randomised trial of intravenous streptokinase, oral aspirin, both, or neither among 17,187 cases of suspected acute myocardial infarction: ISIS-2. ISIS-2 (Second International Study of Infarct Survival) Collaborative Group. *Lancet* 1988;2:349–360.
3. Goldberg RJ, Samad NA, Yarzebski J, et al. Temporal trends in cardiogenic shock complicating acute myocardial infarction. *N Engl J Med* 1999;340:1162–1168.
4. Becker RC, Gore JM, Lambrew C, et al. A composite view of cardiac rupture in the United States National Registry of Myocardial Infarction. *J Am Coll Cardiol* 1996;27:1321–1326.
5. Hochman JS, Buller CE, Sleeper LA, et al. Cardiogenic shock complicating acute myocardial infarction—etiologies, management and outcome: a report from the SHOCK Trial Registry. SHould we emergently revascularize Occluded Coronaries for cardiogenic shocK? *J Am Coll Cardiol* 2000;36[3 Suppl A]:1063–1070.
6. Davis N, Sistino JJ. Review of ventricular rupture: key concepts and diagnostic tools for success. *Perfusion* 2002;17:63–67.
7. Park WM, Connery CP, Hochman JS, et al. Successful repair of myocardial free wall rupture after thrombolytic therapy for acute infarction. *Ann Thorac Surg* 2000;70:1345–1349.
8. Rasmussen S, Leth A, Kjoller E, et al. Cardiac rupture in acute myocardial infarction. A review of 72 consecutive cases. *Acta Med Scand* 1979;205(1–2):11–16.
9. Becker RC, Charlesworth A, Wilcox RG, et al. Cardiac rupture associated with thrombolytic therapy: impact of time to treatment in the Late Assessment of Thrombolytic Efficacy (LATE) study. *J Am Coll Cardiol* 1995;25:1063–1068.
10. Slater J, Brown RJ, Antonelli TA, et al. Cardiogenic shock due to cardiac free-wall rupture or tamponade after acute myocardial infarction: a report from the SHOCK Trial Registry. Should we emergently revascularize occluded coronaries for cardiogenic shock? *J Am Coll Cardiol* 2000;36[3 Suppl A]:1117–1122.
11. Shapira I, Isakov A, Burke M, et al. Cardiac rupture in patients with acute myocardial infarction. *Chest* 1987;92:219–223.
12. Reddy SG, Roberts WC. Frequency of rupture of the left ventricular free wall or ventricular septum among necropsy cases of fatal acute myocardial infarction since introduction of coronary care units. *Am J Cardiol* 1989;63:906–911.
13. Connery CP, Dumont HJ, Dervan JP, et al. Transmural myocardial infarction with coexisting critical aortic stenosis as an etiology for early myocardial rupture. *J Cardiovasc Surg (Torino)* 1994;35:53–56.
14. Becker RC, Hochman JS, Cannon CP, et al. Fatal cardiac rupture among patients treated with thrombolytic agents and adjunctive thrombin antagonists: observations from the Thrombolysis and Thrombin Inhibition in Myocardial Infarction 9 Study. *J Am Coll Cardiol* 1999;33:479–487.
15. Moreno R, Lopez-Sendon J, Garcia E, et al. Primary angioplasty reduces the risk of left ventricular free wall rupture compared with thrombolysis in patients with acute myocardial infarction. *J Am Coll Cardiol* 2002;39:598–603.
16. Ichihara S, Senbonmatsu T, Price E Jr, et al. Targeted deletion of angiotensin II type 2 receptor caused cardiac rupture after acute myocardial infarction. *Circulation* 2002;106:2244–2249.
17. Randomised trial of intravenous atenolol among 16 027 cases of suspected acute myocardial infarction: ISIS-1. First International Study of Infarct Survival Collaborative Group. *Lancet* 1986;2:57–66.
18. Balakumaran K, Verbaan CJ, Essed CE, et al. Ventricular free wall rupture: sudden, subacute, slow, sealed and stabilized varieties. *Eur Heart J* 1984;5:282–288.
19. Bates RJ, Beutler S, Resnekov L, et al. Cardiac rupture—challenge in diagnosis and management. *Am J Cardiol* 1977;40:429–437.
20. Lautsch EV, Lanks KW. Pathogenesis of cardiac rupture. *Arch Pathol* 1967;84:264–271.
21. Bashour T, Kabbini SS, Ellertson DG, et al. Surgical salvage of heart rupture: report of two cases and review of the literature. *Ann Thorac Surg* 1983;36:209–213.
22. Lopez-Sendon J, Gonzalez A, Lopez de Sa E, et al. Diagnosis of subacute ventricular wall rupture after acute myocardial infarction: sensitivity and specificity of clinical, hemodynamic and echocardiographic criteria. *J Am Coll Cardiol* 1992;19:1145–1153.
23. Cheriex EC, de Swart H, Dijkman LW, et al. Myocardial rupture after myocardial infarction is related to the perfusion status of the infarct-related coronary artery. *Am Heart J* 1995;129:644–650.
24. Figueras J, Cortadellas J, Soler-Soler J. Comparison of ventricular septal and left ventricular free wall rupture in acute myocardial infarction. *Am J Cardiol* 1998;81:495–497.

25. Raitt MH, Kraft CD, Gardner CJ, et al. Subacute ventricular free wall rupture complicating myocardial infarction. *Am Heart J* 1993;126:946–955.

26. Oliva PB, Hammill SC, Edwards WD. Cardiac rupture, a clinically predictable complication of acute myocardial infarction: report of 70 cases with clinicopathologic correlations. *J Am Coll Cardiol* 1993;22:720–726.

27. Varbella F, Bongioanni S, Sibona Masi A, et al. Subacute left ventricular free-wall rupture in early course of acute myocardial infarction. Clinical report of two cases and review of the literature. *G Ital Cardiol* 1999;29:163–170.

28. Purcaro A, Costantini C, Ciampani N, et al. Diagnostic criteria and management of subacute ventricular free wall rupture complicating acute myocardial infarction. *Am J Cardiol* 1997;80:397–405.

29. Desoutter P, Halphen C, Haiat R. Two-dimensional echographic visualization of free ventricular wall rupture in acute anterior myocardial infarction. *Am Heart J* 1984;108:1360–1361.

30. Hermoni Y, Engel PJ. Two-dimensional echocardiography in cardiac rupture. *Am J Cardiol* 1986;57:180–181.

31. Knopf WD, Talley JD, Murphy DA. An echo-dense mass in the pericardial space as a sign of left ventricular free wall rupture during acute myocardial infarction. *Am J Cardiol* 1987;59:1202.

32. Garcia-Fernandez MA, Macchioli RO, Moreno PM, et al. Use of contrast echocardiography in the diagnosis of subacute myocardial rupture after myocardial infarction. *J Am Soc Echocardiogr* 2001;14:945–947.

33. Reardon MJ, Carr CL, Diamond A, et al. Ischemic left ventricular free wall rupture: prediction, diagnosis, and treatment. *Ann Thorac Surg* 1997;64:1509–1513.

34. Sutherland FW, Guell FJ, Pathi VL, et al. Postinfarction ventricular free wall rupture: strategies for diagnosis and treatment. *Ann Thorac Surg* 1996;61:1281–1285.

35. McMullan MH, Maples MD, Kilgore TL Jr, et al. Surgical experience with left ventricular free wall rupture. *Ann Thorac Surg* 2001;71:1894–1899.

36. Pretre R, Benedikt P, Turina MI. Experience with postinfarction left ventricular free wall rupture. *Ann Thorac Surg* 2000;69:1342–1345.

37. Coletti G, Torracca L, Zogno M, et al. Surgical management of left ventricular free wall rupture after acute myocardial infarction. *Cardiovasc Surg* 1995;3:181–186.

38. Canovas SJ, Lim E, Hornero F, et al. Surgery for left ventricular free wall rupture: patch glue repair without extracorporeal circulation. *Eur J Cardiothorac Surg* 2003;23:639–641.

39. Pohjola-Sintonen S, Muller JE, Stone PH, et al. Ventricular septal and free wall rupture complicating acute myocardial infarction: experience in the Multicenter Investigation of Limitation of Infarct Size. *Am Heart J* 1989;117:809–818.

40. Radford MJ, Johnson RA, Daggett WM Jr, et al. Ventricular septal rupture: a review of clinical and physiologic features and an analysis of survival. *Circulation* 1981;64:545–553.

41. Topaz O, Taylor AL. Interventricular septal rupture complicating acute myocardial infarction: from pathophysiologic features to the role of invasive and noninvasive diagnostic modalities in current management. *Am J Med* 1992;93:683–688.

42. Crenshaw BS, Granger CB, Birnbaum Y, et al. Risk factors, angiographic patterns, and outcomes in patients with ventricular septal defect complicating acute myocardial infarction. GUSTO-I (Global Utilization of Streptokinase and TPA for Occluded Coronary Arteries) Trial Investigators. *Circulation* 2000;101:27–32.

43. Birnbaum Y, Fishbein MC, Blanche C, et al. Ventricular septal rupture after acute myocardial infarction. *N Engl J Med* 2002;347:1426–1432.

44. Deja MA, Szostek J, Widenka K, et al. Post infarction ventricular septal defect—can we do better? *Eur J Cardiothorac Surg* 2000;18:194–201.

45. Loisance DY, Lordez JM, Deleuze PH, et al. Acute postinfarction septal rupture: long-term results. *Ann Thorac Surg* 1991;52:474–478.

46. Lemery R, Smith HC, Giuliani ER, et al. Prognosis in rupture of the ventricular septum after acute myocardial infarction and role of early surgical intervention. *Am J Cardiol* 1992;70:147–151.

47. Edwards BS, Edwards WD, Edwards JE. Ventricular septal rupture complicating acute myocardial infarction: identification of simple and complex types in 53 autopsied hearts. *Am J Cardiol* 1984;54:1201–1205.

48. Menon V, Webb JG, Hillis LD, et al. Outcome and profile of ventricular septal rupture with cardiogenic shock after myocardial infarction: a report from the SHOCK Trial Registry. SHould we emergently revascularize Occluded Coronaries in cardiogenic shocK? *J Am Coll Cardiol* 2000;36[3 Suppl A]:1110–1116.

49. Skehan JD, Carey C, Norrell MS, et al. Patterns of coronary artery disease in post-infarction ventricular septal rupture. *Br Heart J* 1989;62:268–272.

50. Pretre R, Linka A, Jenni R, et al. Surgical treatment of acquired left ventricular pseudoaneurysms. *Ann Thorac Surg* 2000;70:553–557.

51. Mann JM, Roberts WC. Acquired ventricular septal defect during acute myocardial infarction: analysis of 38 unoperated necropsy patients and comparison with 50 unoperated necropsy patients without rupture. *Am J Cardiol* 1988;62:8–19.

52. Fox KA. Coronary disease. Acute coronary syndromes: presentation—clinical spectrum and management. *Heart* 2000;84:93–100.

53. Ryan TJ, Antman EM, Brooks NH, et al. 1999 update: ACC/AHA guidelines for the management of patients with acute myocardial infarction: executive summary and recommendations: a report of the American College of Cardiology/American Heart Association Task Force on Practice Guidelines (Committee on Management of Acute Myocardial Infarction). *Circulation* 1999;100:1016–1030.

54. Tatooles CJ, Gault JH, Mason DT, et al. Reflux of oxygenated blood into the pulmonary artery in severe mitral regurgitation. *Am Heart J* 1968;75:102–106.

55. Moore CA, Nygaard TW, Kaiser DL, et al. Postinfarction ventricular septal rupture: the importance of location of infarction and right ventricular function in determining survival. *Circulation* 1986;74:45–55.

56. David TE, Armstrong S. Surgical repair of postinfarction ventricular septal defect by infarct exclusion. *Semin Thorac Cardiovasc Surg* 1998;10:105–110.

57. Giuliani ER, Danielson GK, Pluth JR, et al. Postinfarction ventricular septal rupture: surgical considerations and results. *Circulation* 1974;49:455–459.

58. Held AC, Cole PL, Lipton B, et al. Rupture of the interventricular septum complicating acute myocardial infarction: a multicenter analysis of clinical findings and outcome. *Am Heart J* 1988;116[5 Pt 1]:1330–1336.

59. Cox FF, Plokker HW, Morshuis WJ, et al. Importance of coronary revascularization for late survival after postinfarction ventricular septal rupture. A reason to perform coronary angiography prior to surgery. *Eur Heart J* 1996;17:1841–1845.

60. Dalrymple-Hay MJ, Monro JL, Livesey SA, et al. Postinfarction ventricular septal rupture: the Wessex experience. *Semin Thorac Cardiovasc Surg* 1998;10:111–116.

61. Muehrcke DD, Daggett WM Jr, Buckley MJ, et al. Postinfarct ventricular septal defect repair: effect of coronary artery bypass grafting. *Ann Thorac Surg* 1992;54:876–883.

62. Madsen JC, Daggett WM Jr. Repair of postinfarction ventricular septal defects. *Semin Thorac Cardiovasc Surg* 1998;10:117–127.

63. Massetti M, Babatasi G, Le Page O, et al. Postinfarction ventricular septal rupture: early repair through the right atrial approach. *J Thorac Cardiovasc Surg* 2000;119[4 Pt 1]:784–789.

64. Landzberg MJ, Lock JE. Transcatheter management of ventricular septal rupture after myocardial infarction. *Semin Thorac Cardiovasc Surg* 1998;10:128–132.

65. Lee EM, Roberts DH, Walsh KP. Transcatheter closure of a residual postmyocardial infarction ventricular septal defect with the Amplatzer septal occluder. *Heart* 1998;80:522–524.

66. Lowe HC, Jang IK, Yoerger DM, et al. Compassionate use of the amplatzer ASD closure device for residual postinfarction ventricular septal rupture following surgical repair. *Catheter Cardiovasc Interv* 2003;59:230–233.

67. Coma-Canella I, Gamallo C, Onsurbe PM, et al. Anatomic findings in acute papillary muscle necrosis. *Am Heart J* 1989;118:1188–1192.

68. Hochman JS, Boland J, Sleeper LA, et al. Current spectrum of cardiogenic shock and effect of early revascularization on mortality. Results of an International Registry. SHOCK Registry Investigators. *Circulation* 1995;91:873–881.

69. Calvo FE, Figueras J, Cortadellas J, et al. Severe mitral regurgitation complicating acute myocardial infarction. Clinical and angiographic differences between patients with and without papillary muscle rupture. *Eur Heart J* 1997;18:1606–1610.

70. Thompson CR, Buller CE, Sleeper LA, et al. Cardiogenic shock due to acute severe mitral regurgitation complicating acute myocardial infarction: a report from the SHOCK Trial Registry. SHould we use emergently revascularize Occluded Coronaries in cardiogenic shocK? *J Am Coll Cardiol* 2000;36[3 Suppl A]:1104–1109.

71. Barbour DJ, Roberts WC. Rupture of a left ventricular papillary muscle

during acute myocardial infarction: analysis of 22 necropsy patients. *J Am Coll Cardiol* 1986;8:558–565.

72. Nishimura RA, Schaaf HV, Shub C, et al. Papillary muscle rupture complicating acute myocardial infarction: analysis of 17 patients. *Am J Cardiol* 1983;51:373–377.

73. Voci P, Bilotta F, Caretta Q, et al. Papillary muscle perfusion pattern. A hypothesis for ischemic papillary muscle dysfunction. *Circulation* 1995;91:1714–1718.

74. Erbel R, Schweizer P, Bardos P, et al. Two-dimensional echocardiographic diagnosis of papillary muscle rupture. *Chest* 1981;79:595–598.

75. Smyllie JH, Sutherland GR, Geuskens R, et al. Doppler color flow mapping in the diagnosis of ventricular septal rupture and acute mitral regurgitation after myocardial infarction. *J Am Coll Cardiol* 1990;15: 1449–1455.

76. Moursi MH, Bhatnagar SK, Vilacosta I, et al. Transesophageal echocardiographic assessment of papillary muscle rupture. *Circulation* 1996;94:1003–1009,

77. Fuchs RM, Heuser RR, Yin FC, et al. Limitations of pulmonary wedge V waves in diagnosing mitral regurgitation. *Am J Cardiol* 1982;49:849 854.

78. Wei JY, Hutchins GM, Bulkley BH. Papillary muscle rupture in fatal acute myocardial infarction: a potentially treatable form of cardiogenic shock. *Ann Intern Med* 1979;90:149–152.

79. Vlodaver Z, Edwards JE. Rupture of ventricular septum or papillary muscle complicating myocardial infarction. *Circulation* 1977;55:815–822.

80. Tavakoli R, Weber A, Vogt P, et al. Surgical management of acute mi-

tral valve regurgitation due to post-infarction papillary muscle rupture. *J Heart Valve Dis* 2002;11:20–26.

81. Chen Q, Darlymple-Hay MJ, Alexiou C, et al. Mitral valve surgery for acute papillary muscle rupture following myocardial infarction. *J Heart Valve Dis* 2002;11:27–31.

82. Csapo K, Voith L, Szuk T, et al. Postinfarction left ventricular pseudo-aneurysm. *Clin Cardiol* 1997;20:898–903.

83. Frances C, Romero A, Grady D. Left ventricular pseudoaneurysm. *J Am Coll Cardiol* 1998;32:557–561.

84. Brown SL, Gropler RJ, Harris KM. Distinguishing left ventricular aneurysm from pseudoaneurysm. A review of the literature. *Chest* 1997; 111:1403–1409.

85. Gatewood RP Jr, Nanda NC. Differentiation of left ventricular pseudoaneurysm from true aneurysm with two dimensional echocardiography. *Am J Cardiol* 1980;46:869–878.

86. al-Saadon K, Walley VM, Green M, et al. Angiographic diagnosis of true and false LV aneurysms after inferior wall myocardial infarction. *Cathet Cardiovasc Diagn* 1995;35:266 269.

87. Kollar A, Byrd BF 3rd, Lui HK, et al. Mitral valve replacement and endocavitary patch repair for a giant left ventricular pseudoaneurysm. *Ann Thorac Surg* 2001;71:2020–2022.

88. Komeda M, David TE. Surgical treatment of postinfarction false aneurysm of the left ventricle. *J Thorac Cardiovasc Surg* 1993;106: 1189–1191.

CHAPTER 75

Right Ventricular Myocardial Infarction

Robert A. O'Rourke and Louis J. Dell'Italia

Key Words: Inotropic therapy; jugular venous pressure; Kussmaul's sign; left ventricle; myocardial infarction; percutaneous coronary intervention; right ventricle; thrombolytic therapy; ventricular function; ventricular interaction.

INTRODUCTION

In 1930, Sanders (1) reported a patient with the previously undescribed clinical syndrome of hypotension, increased jugular venous pressure, and clear lung fields. A postmortem examination documented extensive right ventricular (RV) necrosis with minimal left ventricular (LV) involvement. For many subsequent decades, RV myocardial infarction (MI) was not recognized as an important manifestation of acute coronary artery disease, partially because of research in animals in which experimentally induced isolated RV damage caused no substantial changes in systemic venous pressure, pulmonary artery pressure, or cardiac output (2–5).

R. A. O'Rourke: Division of Cardiology, University of Texas Health Science Center at San Antonio, San Antonio, Texas 78284-7872.

L. J. Dell'Italia: Departments of Medicine and Physiology and Biophysics Division of Cardiology, and Birmingham Department of Veteran Affairs, University of Alabama at Birmingham, 901 19th Street South BMR2 432, Birmingham, Alabama 35294.

In 1974, Guiha and associates (6) demonstrated that extensive damage to the lateral wall of the canine right ventricle by cauterization produced RV dysfunction manifested as an increase of right-heart filling pressures that was evident only after a volume infusion. The same year, these investigators (7) published a classic report on RV infarction as a distinct clinical syndrome.

Subsequent milestones affecting the recognition and management of acute RV infarction include the descriptive postmortem studies of Isner and Roberts (8), data from Lopez-Sendon and associates (9) concerning the sensitivity and specificity of invasive hemodynamic criteria for the diagnosis of acute RV infarction, and the identification of the pathophysiologic mechanism for low cardiac output in acute RV MI (10,11). In the latter studies, acute right coronary artery occlusion in a dog model resulted in a disproportionate increase of right-heart filling pressures over left-heart filling pressures, causing an increase in RV size and a decrease in LV cavity dimensions. After the description of this pathophysiologic mechanism, different methods of treatment were investigated with the objective of unloading rather than maximally preloading the right ventricle using afterload reduction, intrapulmonary balloon counterpulsation, inotropic support and, most recently, RV assist devices (12,13).

RV MI is currently recognized as a common consequence of inferior LV infarction, its incidence in inferior infarction varying from as low as 10% to as high as 50%, depending on the noninvasive, hemodynamic, or postmortem criteria used (5,13–18).

RELEVANT ANATOMY AND PHYSIOLOGY

Although the cardiac output is the same for both ventricles, the muscle mass of the RV is about one-sixth that of the left ventricle, and it performs one-fourth of the stroke work because the pulmonary vascular resistance is one-tenth of the systemic vascular resistance (19). The RV is a crescent-shaped chamber comprising a sinus body and outflow tract, in contrast to the ellipsoidal concentric left ventricle. However, the interdependence of the two ventricles results from their shared interventricular septum and the surrounding pericardium (5,19).

In the absence of severe RV hypertrophy, the RV coronary blood flow occurs during both systole and diastole (5,19). The right coronary artery provides the predominant blood flow to the RV (Fig. 75–1). In most patients, the right coronary artery supplies blood flow to the RV outflow tract through the conus artery, to the RV lateral wall through the acute marginal branches, and to the posterior wall and interventricular septum through the posterior descending artery (5,19). In addition, the right coronary artery (depending on its dominance) provides a variable blood supply to the posterior wall of the LV. The left coronary artery usually supplies meager blood flow to the RV through small branches to

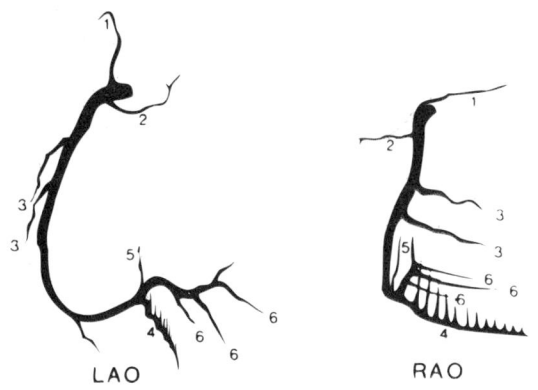

1. CONUS ARTERY
2. S-A NODE ARTERY
3. ACUTE MARGINAL ARTERY
4. POSTERIOR DESCENDING ARTERY WITH SEPTAL BRANCHES
5. A-V NODE ARTERY
6. POSTERIOR LEFT VENTRICULAR ARTERY

FIG. 75–1. A dominant right coronary artery and its branches as depicted in the left anterior oblique *(LAO)* and right anterior oblique *(RAO)* angiographic projections. *1,* Conus artery; *2,* sinoatrial node artery; *3,* acute marginal artery; *4,* posterior descending artery with septal branches; *5,* atrioventricular node artery; *6,* posterior left ventricular artery. (From Levin DC, Gardiner GA Jr. Complex and simple coronary artery stenoses: a new way to interpret coronary angiograms based on morphologic features of lesions. *Radiology* 1987;164:675–680.)

the RV anterior wall from the left anterior descending coronary artery.

PATHOGENESIS OF RIGHT VENTRICULAR INFARCTION

RV MI often results when there is an occlusion of the right coronary artery proximal to the acute marginal branches. The right coronary artery usually is the culprit vessel in RV MI, and more extensive RV myocardial necrosis is associated with proximal right coronary occlusions (14). RV MI may also occur because of a left circumflex coronary artery occlusion in patients who have a left-dominant coronary circulation. Occasionally, occlusion of the left anterior descending coronary artery may also result in an infarct of the anterior RV (14). RV ischemia or infarction often results from occlusion of a dominant right coronary artery with various degrees of RV ischemia, necrosis, or both, as described by Isner and Roberts (8) (Fig. 75–2):

Grade I: Necrosis of less than 50% of the RV posterior wall.
Grade II: Necrosis limited to but not involving more than 50% of the posterior wall.
Grade III: Necrosis of the posterior wall and less than 50% of the anterolateral wall.
Grade IV: Necrosis of the RV posterior wall and more than 50% of the anterolateral wall.

This pathologic classification explains how differing degrees of RV ischemic necrosis might have variable effects on the hemodynamic and noninvasive findings in RV MI. Also, these pathogenic studies indicate that necrosis of the RV is usually accompanied by only a small amount of LV posterior necrosis. Therefore, RV MI generally produces RV dysfunction with very little untoward effects on global LV systolic function. However, RV MI may occur in association with extensive anterior MI affecting the LV anterior wall and septum (14). In such instances, the RV necrosis, ischemia, or both involve only the anterior RV wall and are contiguous with the LV infarction (15,17).

Importantly, many right coronary artery occlusions do not result in significant RV necrosis and dysfunction. This is different from the left coronary circulation, where a much greater extent of LV necrosis occurs with left coronary artery occlusion. This dissimilarity likely is because of the different anatomy and physiology of the RV (Table 75–1). The reason for this difference may be due in part to the lesser RV myocardial oxygen demands during acute coronary artery occlusion to the lower pressure RV, the greater systolic/diastolic flow ratio in coronary vessels perfusing the RV, the increased ability of the RV to extract more oxygen during hemodynamic stress, possible direct perfusion of the RV by the thespian veins (18), and the presence of extensive anatomic collaterals that protect the RV from irreversible ischemic damage (20–26). More specifically, the RV with its thinner wall and lower operating pressures has a systolic–diastolic coronary blood flow ratio that is much greater than

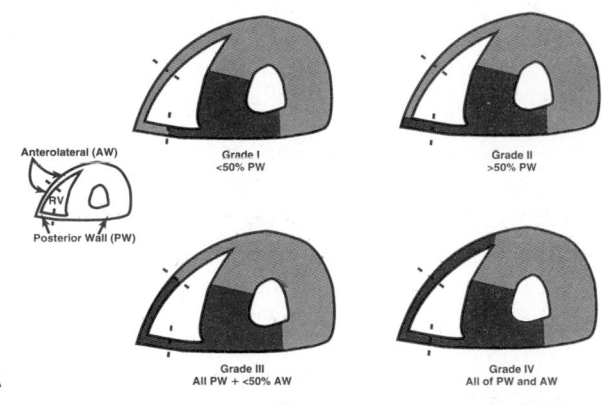

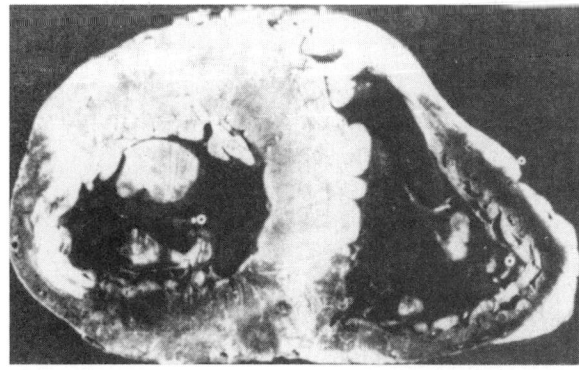

FIG. 75–2. Transverse slices of the right and left ventricles illustrating the scheme for grading the extent of right ventricular myocardial infarction. AW, anterolateral wall; PW, posterior wall. (From Isner J, Roberts WC. Right ventricular infarction complicating left ventricular infarction secondary to coronary heart disease. *Am J Cardiol* 1978;42:885–894, with permission.)

TABLE 75–1. *Reasons for less extensive right ventricular ischemia/necrosis*

Lower right ventricular myocardial oxygen demands
Greater systolic–diastolic right ventricular myocardial blood flow ratio
Increased ability of right ventricle to extract oxygen during stress
Presence of extensive anatomic collateral vessels

for the LV (20–23). In addition, animal studies have shown that the RV is capable of extracting increased amounts of oxygen during hemodynamic stress (24–27).

In several detailed postmortem studies (8,28), three quarters of all cardiac specimens with RV necrosis had a greater than 75% stenosis of the left anterior ascending artery, implying that the lack of sufficient left-to-right collateral coronary blood flow may be involved in the pathogenesis of RV MI. However, RV MI is a frequent occurrence in the absence of significant disease of the left coronary artery system. This may result from important variations in different hearts in the rate of collateral vessel development. In a study of 52 human hearts, Farrer-Brown (29) found a dominant right coronary circulation as expected in 49 of the 52 heart specimens. In general, the vascular density of the right ventricle was similar to that of the left ventricle and had a pattern like that of the LV anterolateral wall. Importantly, there were several potential sources of collateral blood supply to the right ventricle from the left coronary artery. Anatomic collaterals were demonstrated from the left anterior descending artery in the anterior margin of the RV free wall and apex, from the moderator band artery, and less often in the interventricular septum and posterior papillary muscle of the RV.

The studies of Haupt and associates (30) using postmortem hearts suggest that collateral blood flow to the right ventricle through the moderator band artery may protect against massive infarction in the presence of right coronary artery occlusion. The moderator band artery measured up to 1,000 microns in diameter and provided important blood supply to the anterior papillary muscle of the right ventricle. The protective benefit of collaterals has been previously suggested to explain the lower risk for development of RV MI in patients with acute inferior MI and antecedent angina (31).

Most patients with RV MI demonstrate proximal high-grade occlusion of the right coronary artery; whereas patients without RV MI had more distal right coronary artery lesions that spared the RV marginal branch vessels (32). Studies have demonstrated the importance of RV marginal branches that provide blood flow to the RV free wall (32,33). In these studies, the magnitude of RV dysfunction correlated with the extent of RV marginal branch flow impairment. In fact, failure to restore acute reperfusion of RV marginal branch flow by acute percutaneous intervention was associated with lack of recovery of RV function, as well as persistent hypotension and low cardiac output and high mortality (33). Whether selective recanalization of the RV marginal branches in patients with successful reperfusion of the main right coronary artery but persistently occluded RV marginal branches is beneficial requires further investigation.

Finally, RV MI has been reported to occur more commonly when there is antecedent RV hypertrophy both in human postmortem studies (34) and in pig models with gradual right coronary artery occlusion (35,36). This hypothesis is logical considering that the presence of hypertrophy increases RV myocardial oxygen demands and should result in more ischemic injury during acute right coronary occlusion. However, many autopsy studies have identified the frequent occurrence of RV MI in the complete absence of RV hypertrophy (37). In addition, Brooks and associates (38) showed histologic and hemodynamic evidence of RV MI without RV hypertrophy in a pig model using ligation rather than gradual occlusion of the right coronary artery. Thus, antecedent RV hypertrophy is not a prerequisite for RV MI. As indicated in Table 75–1, the intrinsic low myocardial oxygen demands, the ability to extract more oxygen at times of stress, the presence of coronary blood flow during both systole and diastole, and the existence of extensive anatomic collaterals may protect the RV myocardium from irreversible ischemic damage.

PATHOPHYSIOLOGY OF RIGHT VENTRICULAR INFARCTION

The hemodynamic consequences of RV MI include a combination of findings that indicate systolic and diastolic dysfunction of the RV (e.g., low cardiac output and a disproportionate increase of the RV filling pressures) compared with the left-sided filling pressures (9,13,39–46). Diminished RV systolic function often results in low cardiac output and hypotension. Decreased compliance of the RV causes an increased right atrial pressure (RAP), an increase in the RV filling pressure during inspiration (Kussmaul's sign), and a "severe noncompliant pattern" of the RAP waveform. The latter is characterized by "a" and "V" waves, which are equal in amplitude, and by a blunted x and y descent (Fig. 75–3). These abnormalities in right-sided filling pressure not only indicate the decreased compliance of the right atrial and ventricular myocardium throughout diastole, but also reflect the constraining effects of the pericardium resulting from acute RV distention. Thus, pericardial constraint and decreased RV compliance produce an increase in RAP during inspiration and a prominent "V" wave. The right atrial and RV waves subsequently increase to a plateau in the latter two-thirds of diastole (Fig. 75–3).

Cardiac Filling Pressures

The generally accepted hemodynamic criteria for significant RV MI originate from a combined autopsy/hemodynamic study performed by Lopez-Sendon and associates (9). Patients with RV MI may present with a spectrum of hemodynamic findings, which is not surprising considering the variable extent of RV necrosis resulting from right coronary artery occlusion. In the study by Lopez-Sendon and coworkers (9), 60 patients with acute infarction underwent hemodynamic monitoring before death, and all patients had subsequent postmortem examinations. RV necrosis was present in 22 of 60 heart specimens and correlated with a premortem RAP of 10 mm Hg or greater and a right atrial pressure/pulmonary artery wedge pressure (RAP:PAWP) ratio of 0.86 or greater. When these pressure measurements were accompanied by the "severe noncompliant pattern" of the RAP waveform, the sensitivity and specificity of detecting RV MI by invasive monitoring were 82% and 97%, respectively. However, these hemodynamic criteria were not present in 18% of the cases with well documented RV necrosis. A detailed analysis of the data indicates that 15 patients had a PAWP greater than 20 mm Hg, thus precluding further volume administration, and 10 of these 15 had acute necrosis or prior infarction of the LV anterior wall. In these patients with RV infarction, the usual close relation between the RAP and PAWP was not observed because there was concomitant im-

portant LV dysfunction, thus explaining the reduced sensitivity. However, when the function of both ventricles is reduced by myocardial necrosis, RAP often is persistently increased after appropriate diuresis or treatment with other agents that effectively reduce the filling pressure and unload the LV.

This and other studies (39–46) indicate that patients with RV MI may present with a spectrum of hemodynamic findings based on a determination of the RAP, the RAP:PAWP ratio, and a systolic arterial blood pressure of greater than or less than 100 mm Hg.

Two important clinical studies (39,40) documented that volume loading may increase the incidence of RV MI hemodynamics in patients with acute inferior MI. Subsequently, Dell'Italia and coworkers (46) studied 53 consecutive patients with acute inferior MI, 8 of whom had hemodynamic criteria consistent with RV MI at rest (RAP ≥ 10 mm Hg and RAP:PAWP ratio ≥ 0.8). An additional six patients experienced development of RV MI hemodynamics after volume loading with normal saline. Most patients with acute inferior infarction were hemodynamically stable and manifested no evidence of significant RV dysfunction. As previously mentioned, a few patients may present with increase of both RV and LV filling pressures because of coexisting LV MI.

While the severity of hemodynamic compromise in RV MI is related to the extent of RV contraction abnormalities, many patients have an adequate systemic arterial pressure in the presence of severe depression of RV systolic function. Accordingly, there must be other compensatory mechanisms for maintaining right heart blood flow in the presence of RV pump failure. Studies in an experimental animal model (47–49) and in patients (50) have determined that augmented right atrial contraction improves RV diastolic filling, RV systolic performance, and cardiac output. Conversely, the absence of enhanced right atrial transport because of ischemia or atrioventricular (AV) dyssynchrony diminishes RV filling, further impairs RV performance, and worsens the low cardiac output associated with RV dysfunction. The contribution of a forceful right atrial contraction to pulmonary blood flow has been demonstrated by the presence of premature opening of the pulmonic valve using M-mode echocardiography in patients with RV MI (51–53).

An increase and equalization of right and left heart pressures, together with an abnormal RAP waveform, can be caused by other cardiac disorders than RV infarction (19, 45). These can be subdivided into pathophysiologic conditions affecting predominantly RV diastolic or systolic function, or both. Those conditions that predominantly alter diastolic function include cardiac tamponade, constrictive pericarditis, and restrictive or infiltrative cardiomyopathy, all of which may be associated with normal or near-normal RV systolic function. In contrast, severe RV systolic dysfunction may result from pulmonary hypertension, secondary to acute or recurrent pulmonary thromboembolism, or

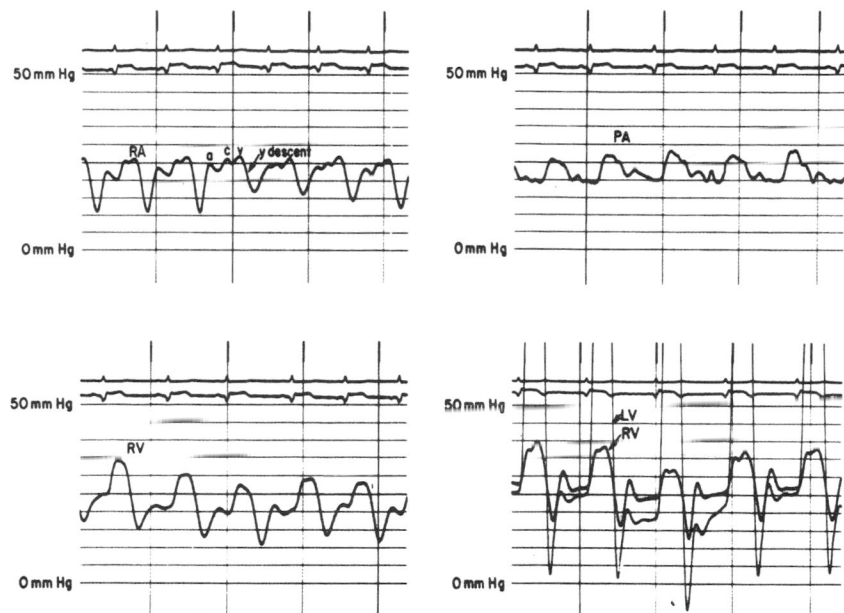

FIG. 75–3. Right atrial pressure waveform *(RA)* demonstrating the "severe noncompliant pattern" with diminished "a" wave. Pulmonary artery *(PA)* pressure demonstrating the small pulse pressure. Right ventricular *(RV)* pressure demonstrating a small pulse pressure and a "dip and plateau" pattern in diastole. Simultaneous RV and LV pressure demonstrating the increase and equalization of RV and LV diastolic filling pressures in a patient with RV myocardial infarction.

severe chronic obstructive lung disease. Also, severe chronic right and left heart failure may result in both increase and equalization of right and left heart filling pressures. Usually, an attentive history and detailed physical examination, together with an electrocardiogram or other noninvasive testing, will rule out potential cardiac disorders causing hemodynamic findings that may mimic RV MI.

Cardiac Output

In 1943, Starr and associates (2) first described the effects of RV damage on cardiac output and intracardiac pressures. In their animal model, the heart was suspended in a pericardial cradle, and there was no significant increase in venous pressure or decrease in cardiac output after cauterization of the RV lateral wall. Studies in other open-pericardial dog models showed the same results with no change in cardiac output resulting from RV injury as long as the pulmonary vascular resistance stayed normal (3,4,54). Thus, the incorrect perception arose that RV function was not essential to maintain circulatory stability and that the pressure pulse that developed in the RV after extensive destruction of its lateral wall might be generated by the LV.

After their classic description (7) of the clinical syndrome of RV MI in 1974, Guiha and colleagues (6) documented a small increase in RV filling pressures with a decrease in cardiac output after extensive cauterization of the RV lateral wall using an open-pericardial canine model. Although progressive volume infusion produced a greater increase in right-heart filling pressures than in left-heart filling pressures, it improved both systolic arterial pressure (SAP) and cardiac output. These results provided the rationale for volume administration in the treatment of RV MI with maximum benefit from the Frank Starling mechanism achieved by increasing RV preload. However, data from several clinical studies (12,55,56) indicate that volume loading does not uniformly produce an increase in cardiac output when given to patients with hemodynamic criteria for RV MI. In 36 patients with acute RV MI (RAP $\geq$ 10 mm Hg and not 5 mm Hg less than the PAWP), Lopez-Sendon and coworkers (55) infused volume until the PAWP increased more than 55 mm Hg. The individual response in cardiac output was highly variable, and the average cardiac output did not increase significantly in the 36 patients studied. No increase in cardiac output occurred either in those patients whose prevolume–infusion cardiac index was less than 2.2 L per minute per square meter or in those with a cardiac index greater than 2.2 L per minute per square meter. In a study of 13 patients with hemodynamic and radionuclide ventriculographic evidence of RV MI, Dell'Italia and coworkers (12) showed that progressive volume loading significantly increased RAP (11 $\pm$ 2 to 15 $\pm$ 2 mm Hg; $p < 0.001$) and PAWP (10 $\pm$ 4 to 15 $\pm$ 2 mm Hg; $p < 0.001$), but produced no significant change in cardiac output (1.9 $\pm$ 0.5 to 2.1 $\pm$ 0.4 L/min/m^2). Simultaneously obtained radionuclide ventriculographic studies documented an increase in RV end-diastolic volume, whereas LV end-diastolic volume remained unchanged. Thus, during volume loading, the PAWP did not accurately represent true LV preload or end-diastolic volume. Also, by increasing RV cavity size, volume loading may limit LV filling through the mechanism of ventricular interaction.

The importance of ventricular interaction in modifying the hemodynamics of RV infarction has been well documented in a closed-pericardial dog model. In the canine species, the right coronary artery supplies blood only to the RV free wall (10,11). After right coronary artery occlusion with the pericardium intact, the characteristic hemodynamic findings of RV MI resulted in the following: (a) increase and equalization of right- and left-sided filling pressures; (b) an increase in RV cavity size and a decrease in LV end-diastolic dimension; and (c) a decrease in cardiac output. With subsequent volume loading, the average LV end-diastolic pressure increased from 7 to 12 mm Hg with no significant change in LV cavity size; there was a small but significant increase in cardiac output. However, after the pericardium was removed, equalization of right and left heart diastolic pressures resolved, LV end-diastolic pressure decreased, and diastolic cavity size increased. Also, the cardiac output was significantly greater compared with the values measured after volume loading when the pericardium was intact. Thus, although the measured LV end-diastolic pressure increased significantly after volume loading, the actual LV transmural pressure (LV minus pericardial pressure) was reduced likely because of increased intrapericardial pressure. Furthermore, a study by Johnston and coworkers (57) demonstrated that volume expansion in dogs with an intact pericardium increased RV infarct size by twofold to threefold secondary to reduced periischemic collateral perfusion (57). The detrimental effect on infarct size was prevented by opening of the pericardium.

In a closed-chest canine model of RV MI, Sharkey and coworkers (58) embolized the right coronary artery selectively. After embolization, the transseptal pressure gradient reversed from 3 ± 1 to 1 ± 1 mm Hg ($p < 0.001$). In addition, the shape of the interventricular septum was flattened at end-diastole in the short-axis, two-dimensional, echocardiographic view as a result of the increased RV end-diastolic pressure (Fig. 75–4). Thus, despite a significant increase in LV end-diastolic pressure in both animal models, LV end-diastolic dimension decreased or did not change as LV filling pressures increased because of acute distention of the RV in the intact pericardial sac. Few studies, however, have actually evaluated the effect of right coronary artery occlusion on LV systolic function. In the dog, acute and chronic right coronary artery occlusion is a model of pure RV free wall ischemia (59,60), because the right coronary artery is a nondominant vessel and does not provide blood supply to the interventricular septum. Indeed, Goto and coworkers (61) demonstrated that indices of LV contractile performance (i.e., cardiac output, LV systolic pressure, peak plus LV dP/dt, and percent shortening) were similar at matched preloads in healthy dogs and those with RV MI. However, in a study of RV MI in pigs, where the right coronary artery is a dominant system as in humans, Brookes and coworkers

(62) demonstrated that acute right coronary artery occlusion caused a significant impairment in LV contractile function, manifested by a decrease in the slopes of the LV preload recruitable stroke work and the LV end-systolic pressure–volume relation (Fig. 75–4). Again, restoration of LV cavity geometry by either pericardiotomy or administration of dobutamine significantly improved LV performance.

LV geometry has important effects on systolic performance and may, in part, explain why volume loading in the context of RV dilatation may not improve overall cardiac function. Normalization of septal position could be promoted by reversing RV ischemia. Obviously, pericardiotomy cannot be offered in patients. It is of interest, however, that in pigs with acute right coronary artery occlusion, a modified Glenn shunt (superior vena cava to pulmonary artery) attenuated the LV dysfunction by limiting LV dilation and restoring LV cavity geometry (63). Nevertheless, in the setting of acute inferior MI, right coronary artery reperfusion resulted in a reversal to a normal septal position in patients having primary angioplasty in acute RV infarction (32). In addition, increasing LV systolic pressure generation could theoretically restore septal position and improve the septal contractile contribution to RV performance. Indeed, this mechanism has been suggested in a dog model of RV infarction (64) and in a pig model of acute RV MI after dobutamine infusion (62). Taken together, the interventricular septum has an important function in both RV and LV systolic and diastolic performance in the setting of acute right coronary artery occlusion through a combined mechanism of ischemia and ventricular interdependence (65) (Fig. 75–5).

PHYSICAL EXAMINATION

The early clinical detection of acute RV MI in patients with inferior wall MI often is essential to initiate appropriate therapy quickly in patients with hypotension or shock in whom intravenous fluids and drugs are needed before beginning invasive hemodynamic monitoring or noninvasive testing (66). Even for patients without hypotension or shock, it is important to recognize the likely presence of RV ischemia, infarction, or both to avoid diuretic or vasodilator therapy that will further decrease RV filling, and thus produce systemic arterial hypotension. Therefore, an accurate and deliberate physical examination often results in the correct early diagnosis of RV MI and the initiation of appropriate therapy for achieving and maintaining circulatory stability. All patients with an acute inferior wall MI should be suspected of having RV dysfunction, which occurs in 20% to 50% of such patients, depending on the gold standard criteria used. However, less than 10% of patients will have complications of hypotension or shock because the RV is remarkably resistant to extensive dysfunction, as discussed earlier.

As previously mentioned, the triad of hypotension, increased jugular venous pressure, and clear lung fields as physical examination indicators of RV MI in patients with

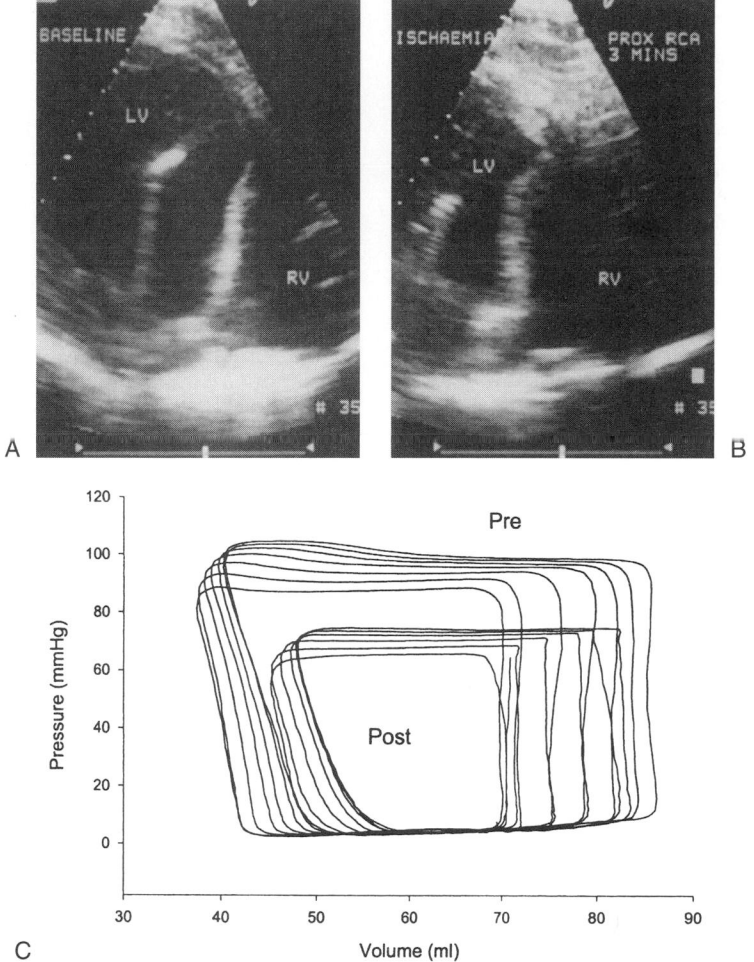

FIG. 75–4. **A and B:** Transesophageal echocardiogram in the pig showing change in septal position during right coronary artery occlusion with intact pericardium. **C:** Example of left ventricular (LV) pressure–volume cycles during inferior vena cava occlusion before *(Pre)* and after *(Post)* occlusion of the proximal right coronary artery *(RCA)*. RV, right ventricle. (From Brookes C, Ravn H, White P, et al. Acute right ventricular dilatation in response to ischemia significantly impairs left ventricular systolic performance. *Circulation* 1999;100:761–767, with permission.)

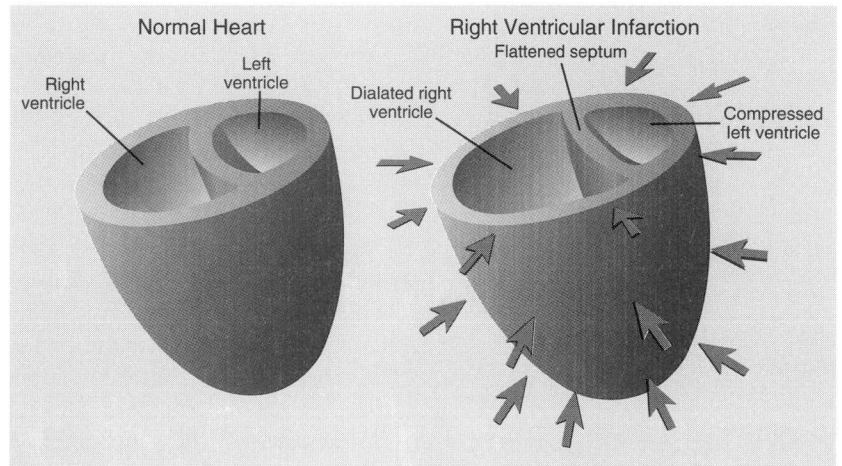

FIG. 75–5. Pathophysiologic mechanism underlying the low cardiac output state in right ventricular myocardial infarction. The low-output state is mediated by ventricular interaction (resulting in left shift of the septum and changes in left ventricular geometry) and the restraining effect of the pericardium *(arrows)* during acute right ventricular distension. (From Dell'Italia LJ. Reperfusion for right ventricular infarction. *N Engl J Med* 1998;338:978–980, with permission.)

acute inferior MI was first described in a group with RV infarction patients by Cohn and coworkers (7). Other reports have stressed the presence of Kussmaul's sign and various other clinical findings resulting from RV MI and systolic and diastolic dysfunction of the RV (39–42, 67–69) (Table 75–2).

Dell'Italia and coworkers (66) performed a detailed prospective clinical assessment in 53 consecutive patients with acute MI during the first 36 hours after the onset of symptoms. Eight patients were identified as having hemodynamics consistent with RV MI (RAP $\geq$ 10 mm Hg; RAP:PAWP ratio $\geq$ 0.8). On clinical assessment, the presence of both an increased jugular venous pressure ($\geq$8 cm H_2O) and Kussmaul's sign were the most sensitive (88%) and specific (100%) identifiers of hemodynamically important RV MI. The classic triad of hypotension, increased jugular venous pressure, and clear lung fields was only 25% sensitive but 96% specific, whereas an increased jugular venous pressure alone was more sensitive (88%) but less specific (69%) for RV MI. Accordingly, deliberate clinical assessment of the jugular venous pulse for pressure increase and for Kussmaul's sign provides a rapid diagnostic screen so that appropriate therapy may be initiated for the treatment of hypotension. Also, there is need for special caution in the administration of nitrates and morphine to avoid systemic arterial hypotension because of a deleterious decrease in right heart filling pressures with vasodilator therapy.

Several other findings on physical examination that often are present in patients with acute RV MI are listed in Table 75–2. Tricuspid regurgitation often results from RV chamber dilatation and tricuspid annulus enlargement. It may be identified by a systolic murmur of variable duration that is loudest at the lower left sternal border and often increases with inspiration. The murmur often is not holosystolic in patients without RV systolic hypertension. Other features of the physical examination indicating RV diastolic dysfunction include S_4 and S_3 heard best along the left sternal border and an abnormal waveform of the jugular venous pressure. In addition to indicating an increased RAP, the jugular veins may demonstrate an abnormal pattern manifested by an "a" and "V" wave, which are equal in magnitude, and a y descent that is greater than or equal to the x descent. These waveforms, reflecting a poorly compliant or nondistensible RV, may become more noticeable during inspiration or the abdominojugular reflex maneuver. A pulsus paradoxus may

TABLE 75–2. *Clinical findings associated with right ventricular infarction*

Hypotension, bradycardia
Increased jugular venous pressure
Kussmaul's sign
Abnormal jugular venous pressure pattern ($y \geq x$ descent)
Tricuspid regurgitation
Right ventricular S_3 and S_4
Pulsus paradoxus
High-grade atrioventricular block

be demonstrated by a careful recording of a greater than usual decrease in the systemic arterial pressure during inspiration by cuff sphygmomanometer. Bradyarrhythmias may result from sinus node ischemia and increased vagal tone; high-grade AV block often is caused by AV nodal ischemia. The subsequent loss of AV synchrony can potentiate hypotension and shock when RV dysfunction is present. The likelihood of high-grade AV block is greater in patients with acute inferior wall MI compared with those with anterior wall infarction (32,70), and this finding may be associated with a poorer prognosis (71). Whether RV myocardial ischemia or infarction is present, patients with inferior MI often experience development of bradycardia and hypotension presumably mediated by the cardioinhibitory reflexes (Bezold-Jarisch) arising from stimulation of vagal afferents in the ischemic LV inferoposterior wall (72). This effect is particularly evident during right coronary artery reperfusion through percutaneous coronary intervention (73) or thrombolysis (74).

The presence and severity of abnormal physical examination findings may be associated with RV MI and are dependent on the amount of RV dysfunction and dilatation. Increase of the jugular venous pressure and Kussmaul's sign provide the most accurate clinical markers of significant RV ischemia or necrosis. However, they occur with other causes of right heart failure as well. Although clinical findings of severe right heart failure such as hepatomegaly, pulsatile liver, ascites, and peripheral edema are rarely seen in the initial presentation of RV infarction, they may be present later resulting from tricuspid regurgitation caused by papillary muscle infarction or rupture (67–69).

TACHYARRHYTHMIAS IN RIGHT VENTRICULAR MYOCARDIAL INFARCTION

Studies have suggested that patients with acute RV MI have a greater incidence of ventricular arrhythmias (75–77). A study by Mehta and coworkers (78) in a large number of patients in the Collaborative Organization for RheothRx Evaluation (CORE) trial demonstrated that patients with inferior MI who also have RV myocardial involvement are at increased risk for death, shock, and arrhythmias. This increased risk is related to the presence of RV myocardial involvement itself rather than the extent of LV myocardial damage (78). Indeed, Bowers and coworkers (32) reported that ventricular arrhythmias were more common in patients with unsuccessful coronary reperfusion. It is of interest that RV MI in the dog causes sympathetic and vagal denervation at variable sites in the RV outflow tract: lateral and, to a lesser extent, septal sides of the viable periinfarct area (79). This pattern of denervation after RV MI differs from that of LV infarction and may be an important mechanism in the development of ventricular tachyarrhythmias in the acute stage of RV MI. Supraventricular tachyarrhythmias, including atrial fibrillation, are more common in those with RV dysfunction (80). Atrial infarction or ischemia, atrial distension, or an increased RAP may account for this trend.

INVASIVE HEMODYNAMIC MONITORING

Invasive hemodynamic monitoring usually confirms the clinical assessment by physical examination and identifies RV MI by a combination of findings that suggest systolic and diastolic dysfunction of the RV—for example, low cardiac output and a disproportionate increase of the RAP compared with the PAWP (9,39–46). Bedside measurements of right heart pressures including the PAWP and RAP, the recording of the direct systemic arterial pressure, and the measurement of cardiac output can be used to confirm the diagnosis of RV infarction and to guide various forms of therapy, including volume loading, vasodilator therapy, and the use of positive inotropic agents. In addition, the severe noncompliant pattern of the RAP waveform may be present at rest or only after a volume load or during inspiration. As mentioned earlier, the absence of an "a" wave on the right atrial waveform may be indicative of atrial infarction and portend a poor prognosis (50).

Studies evaluating hemodynamic function in the setting of acute inferior MI demonstrate that patients with RV MI may present with a spectrum of hemodynamic findings that are best summarized as follows:

1. RAP ≥ 10 mm Hg, RAP:PAWP ratio > 0.86, and SAP < 100 mm Hg
2. RAP ≥ 10 mm Hg, RAP : PAWP > 0.86, and SAP > 100 mm Hg
3. RAP ≥ 10 mm Hg and RAP : PAWP > 0.86 only after volume loading, with or without SAP > 100 mm Hg
4. RAP ≥ 10 mm Hg and RAP : PAWP > 0.86 caused by marked increase of the PAWP and greater amount of LV damage.

NONINVASIVE DIAGNOSIS

Electrocardiography, two-dimensional echocardiography, radionuclide ventriculography, and technetium pyrophosphate infarct-avid imaging have been the most commonly used noninvasive methods for identifying RV infarction in the setting of acute inferior wall MI. Using noninvasive techniques, workers have reported the incidence of RV MI in patients with inferior infarction to range between 25% and 50%. This variability is related to the inherent limitations of each technique and to the variability of criteria used in different studies for the diagnosis of RV infarction. Importantly, electrocardiography may provide a rapid diagnosis of RV MI, and radionuclide ventriculography and echocardiography may provide an assessment of pump function that complements invasive hemodynamic monitoring of patients in the coronary care unit.

The relative sensitivities and specificities of electrocardiography (81) and other noninvasive testing (46) for identifying patients with RV infarction are illustrated in Figure 75–6.

Electrocardiography

Most commonly, the V_{4R} lead placed in the fifth intercostal space in the right midclavicular line has been used for recording the electrocardiographic manifestations of acute RV injury (Fig. 75–7). A report by Erhardt and coworkers (82) indicates that ST-segment elevation of more than 1 mm in lead V_{4R} was a highly specific finding in 18 patients with RV infarction because of acute inferior infarction when compared with postmortem findings. In 16 surviving patients with ST-segment elevation in V_{4R}, there was a greater incidence of hypotension ($p < 0.05$) and right heart failure ($p > 0.01$) as compared with the remaining 58 survivors

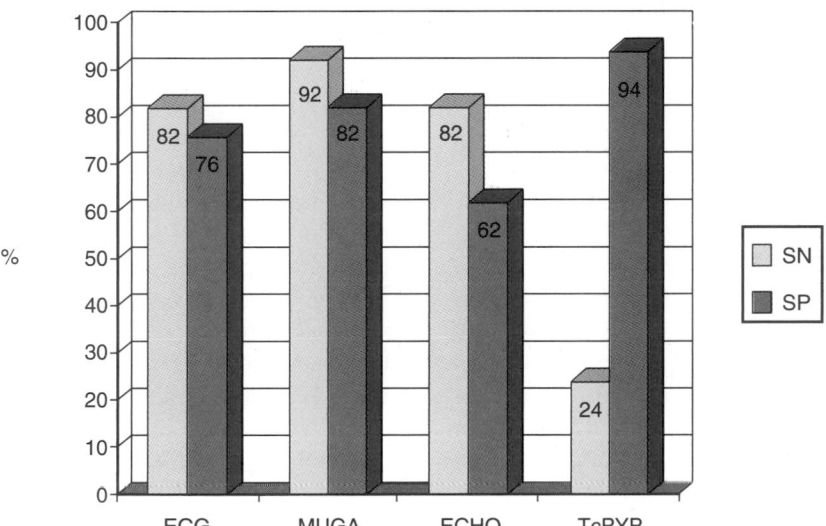

FIG. 75–6. Sensitivity *(SN)* and specificity *(SP)* of electrocardiography (81) and other noninvasive techniques (46) in diagnosing important right ventricular infarction. ECG, electrocardiograph; ECHO, echocardiography; MUGA, multigated acquisition; TcPYP, technetium pyrophosphate.

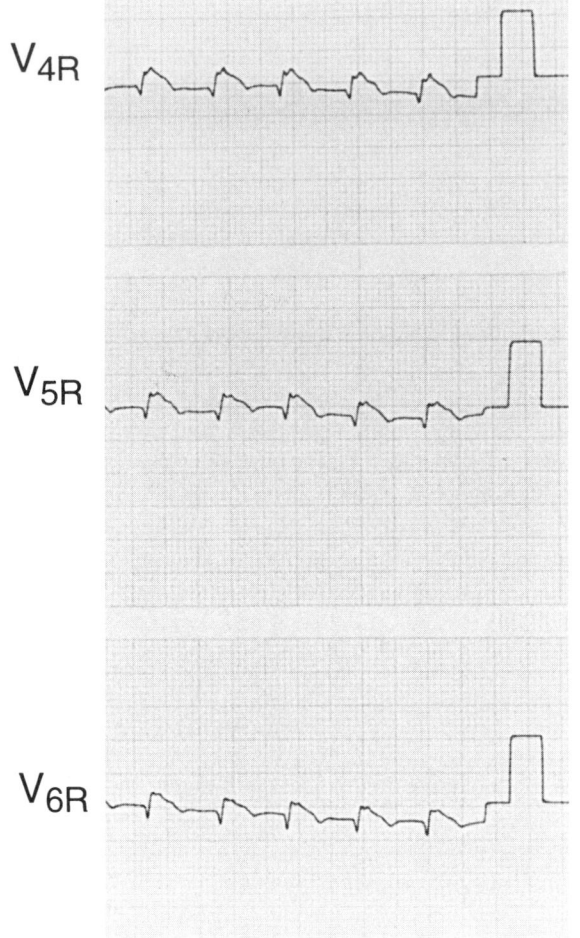

FIG. 75–7. Three right-sided precordial electrocardiographic leads showing Q waves and ST-segment elevation from a patient with right ventricular myocardial infarction.

with inferior infarction but no V_{4R} ST-segment elevation. In another study (83), transient ST-segment elevation in precordial lead V_1 occurred in 8 of 11 patients with acute inferior MI. RV infarction was documented by autopsy in five patients and by hemodynamic monitoring in the six others.

In a prospective study of 110 consecutive patients with acute inferior wall MI, Klein and coworkers (81) demonstrated greater than 0.5 mm ST-segment elevation in lead V_{4R} in 48 of 58 patients with hemodynamic or noninvasive evidence of RV MI (83% sensitivity) and in 12 of the remaining 52 patients with no evidence of RV MI (77% specificity) (Fig. 75–6). Multiple clinical reports during the last decade have shown a similar sensitivity and specificity. Data from these studies indicate that RV MI as defined by hemodynamic or noninvasive tests correlates best with ST-segment elevation greater than 1 mm in lead V_{4R} (84–88). However, all of these reports have indicated that this electrocardiographic finding often is transient, persisting for only 24 to 48 hours after the onset of chest pain; therefore, the sensitivity of ST-segment elevation in V_{4R} is time dependent. Also, cardiac diseases other than RV MI are associated with ST-

segment elevation in lead V_{4R}, including acute pulmonary embolism, LV hypertrophy, acute anteroseptal MI, pericarditis, and previous anterior MI with aneurysm formation.

An electrocardiographic pattern of ST-segment elevation in leads V_1BV_5 without Q waves but with minimal ST-segment elevation in the inferior leads was described in five patients with acute inferior wall MI by Geft and coworkers (89). Early catheterization within 4 hours of the onset of chest pain revealed proximal right coronary artery obstruction without significant left coronary artery disease in all five patients. Each patient also had technetium-99m pyrophosphate myocardial scintigraphy and radionuclide ventriculographic evidence of RV MI. Therefore, these electrocardiographic findings represent an early manifestation of predominant RV injury. The same investigators also produced RV infarction in a dog model and documented ST-segment elevations in $V_{4R}BV_{6R}$ leads in this model where the right coronary artery supplies the RV free wall and provides no blood supply to the LV posterior wall. However, when occlusion of the right coronary artery was followed by occlusion of the left circumflex coronary artery, ST-segment elevation in the right precordial leads that overlie the RV were suppressed. Thus, in this canine model, and probably in humans, LV necrosis appears to negate the ST-segment elevation associated with RV injury; it may also explain the uncommon occurrence of ST-segment elevation in early left precordial leads (V_1BV_3) (88,90) and its transient nature in the right precordial leads (V_{4R}), especially when RV necrosis is not extensive. Accordingly, although ST-segment elevation in the right precordial leads is a specific marker for RV necrosis, the sensitivity of this finding is limited by its transient appearance, which may be related to the relative proportion of RV compared with LV necrosis.

Despite the above limitations, studies have suggested that ST-segment elevation in right-sided precordial leads is a strong, independent predictor of major complications and in-hospital mortality (70,91–94). In a prospective study of 200 consecutive patients with acute inferior MI, Zehender and associates (70) demonstrated that the presence of ST-segment elevation of 1 mm or greater in lead V_{4R} identified subgroups of patients with increased hospital mortality ($p < 0.001$) and major complications ($p < 0.001$) including cardiogenic shock, ventricular fibrillation, third-degree block, and the need for temporary pacing. The in-hospital mortality rate after inferior MI was 19% for the group. However, two-thirds of the patients with inferior MI had contraindications to thrombolytic therapy, and these patients accounted for a substantial proportion of the high overall in-hospital mortality rate. Among the 36% who were suitable for thrombolytic therapy, the in-hospital mortality rate was 7%. Moreover, it is likely that some of the patients with electrocardiographic signs of RV dysfunction also had concomitant severe LV dysfunction (95). Because isolated inferior wall MI without complication is generally associated with a favorable prognosis, the early detection of RV infarction by recording lead V_{4R} has been recommended by some for quickly stratifying patients into low- and high-risk subgroups (94). As emphasized earlier, the diagnostic usefulness of right precordial ST-segment elevation is greatest during the first 10 hours after in acute inferior infarction. A complete electrocardiographic assessment should be obtained on all patients with inferior infarctions as soon after presentation as possible. In many hospitals, right-sided precordial leads are obtained routinely in all patients with inferior wall MIs.

Echocardiography

Early studies using M-mode echocardiography demonstrated an absolute increase in the RV end-diastolic dimension in many patients with RV infarction (40,42). The advent of two-dimensional echocardiography provided a method of assessing global RV size and performance, segmental wall motion, valvular structures, and LV size and performance (40,46,96–98). Lopez-Sendon and associates (98) assessed 63 consecutive patients with inferior MI by two-dimensional echocardiography and acute hemodynamic monitoring within 4 days of the onset of symptoms. Multiple views were used to examine the RV lateral wall and interventricular septum for evidence of akinesis or dyskinesis (Fig. 75–8). The number of asynergic RV wall segments correlated with the severity of RV hemodynamic dysfunction. A total of 32 patients met hemodynamic criteria for RV infarction, whereas the remaining 31 patients had no hemodynamic evidence during clinical observation. Importantly, 11 patients had abnormal two-dimensional echocardiographic evaluation but normal hemodynamic function.

In 53 consecutive patients with inferior MI studied by Dell'Italia and coworkers (46), two-dimensional echocardiography was a highly sensitive technique for documenting the presence of hemodynamically important RV MI by demonstrating segmental RV akinesis or dyskinesis. In this study, echocardiography also detected RV wall motion abnormalities in some patients who never developed hemodynamic criteria consistent with significant RV MI. The re-duced specificity of echocardiographic manifestations of RV motion abnormalities may reflect the superior sensitivity of a good quality two-dimensional echocardiography for detecting RV ischemia or infarction, or both, that does not result in hemodynamic impairment. Also, it is often difficult to assess regional wall motion abnormalities of the thin-walled RV accurately by this technique. Therefore, it is important to demonstrate both RV dilatation and the presence of akinesis or dyskinesis by echocardiography to define hemodynamically important RV MI with a high degree of accuracy.

Adequate visualization of the interventricular septum for recording its motion during diastole and systole is provided by both M-mode and two-dimensional echocardiography. Paradoxic septal motion has been recorded in many patients with severe RV MI (40,42,98) and in 14 of 16 patients with hemodynamically important RV MI (50). The interventricular septum is a major anatomic component of the RV chamber and contributes to RV systolic contraction (99,100). In a dog model of RV infarction, Goldstein and coworkers (47) demonstrated that the interventricular septum developed reversed curvature during diastole and that it bulged paradoxically into the RV during early systole, generating the initial peak of RV pressure and reducing its volume. Data from this animal study suggest that the reversed motion of the interventricular septum was associated with and related to the severity of RV lateral wall dysfunction. Paradoxic septal motion in RV MI is most likely caused by an early systolic transseptal pressure gradient, with the absence of RV contraction permitting an unopposed LV-septal pressure generation. In this situation, RV performance is dependent on LV-septal contraction transmitted through systolic interaction mediated by the interventricular septum. Furthermore, in this dog study, ischemic septal dysfunction decreased this mechanism of systolic interaction and further depressed both RV and LV function (47); whereas in patients, successful reperfusion of the right coronary artery in patients with RV MI restored normal septal motion (32).

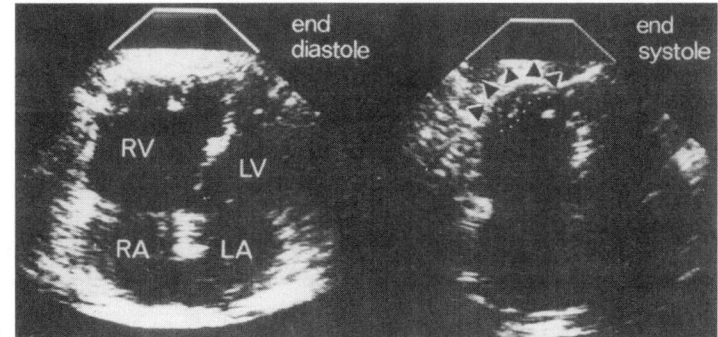

FIG. 75–8. End-diastolic (A) and end-systolic (B) two-dimensional echocardiographic four-chamber apical images of right ventricular (RV) myocardial infarction. There is dyskinesia of the lateral wall (arrows) and apex at end-systole and thrombus in the apex (arrows). LA, left atrium; LV, left ventricle; RA, right atrium. (From Lopez-Sendon J, Garcia-Fernandez MA, Coma-Canella I, et al. Segmental right ventricular function after acute myocardial infarction: two-dimensional echocardiographic study in 63 patients. Am J Cardiol 1983;51:390–396, with permission.) (See color insert for Fig. 75–9.)

The use of color Doppler flow recordings increases the diagnostic utility of two-dimensional echocardiography, because tricuspid and mitral valvular function and blood flow across a patent foramen ovale or ventricular septal defect may also be demonstrated at the bedside.

Radionuclide Ventriculography

The assessment of RV end-diastolic and end-systolic volumes and the RV ejection fraction is difficult to perform accurately using imaging techniques such as echocardiography that are geometry dependent. Radionuclide ventriculography offers an important advantage over other techniques because it is based on count density, and therefore can be used to evaluate RV performance relatively independent of geometry (Fig. 75–9) (see color insert). Use of either the first-past technique or multiple-gated equilibrium studies indicates that the incidence of RV dysfunction as determined by radionuclide ventriculography in patients with acute inferior MI is about 40% to 50% (101–106). RV dysfunction in these studies was defined as either RV enlargement or an ejection fraction value of less than 45%. However, most studies did not systematically examine RV wall motion, which is an important marker for identifying RV dysfunction caused by RV MI. The normal RV ejection fraction ranges between 35% and 75%, and many factors other than ischemia or infarction may reduce this measure of RV systolic performance. The most common causes are chronic obstructive lung disease, pulmonary emboli, valvular heart disease, or LV failure.

In a prospective evaluation, radionuclide ventriculography (Fig. 75–5) was 92% sensitive and 82% specific for identifying hemodynamically important RV MI when both a RV ejection fraction value of less than 40% and segmental wall motion abnormalities of akinesis or dyskinesis were used as radionuclide criteria for RV MI (46) (Fig. 75–8). Thus, by using the presence of depression in global RV performance and wall motion abnormalities of akinesis or dyskinesis as criteria, acute diagnosis of hemodynamically important RV MI can be made with a high degree of accuracy, the requirement of akinesis or dyskinesis improving the specificity for ischemia or infarction.

Depressed RV systolic performance may occur in association with acute anterior MI or in any cardiac disease when LV dysfunction results in pulmonary hypertension and an increase in RV afterload. Low RV ejection fraction values have been associated with symmetric depression of systolic contraction in the lateral, inferior, and apical LV wall segments in patients with anterior MI (106). In contrast, in patients with inferior infarction, the inferior and lateral LV wall segments are more severely depressed. Also, there is a linear correlation between RV ejection fraction and LV ejection fraction in patients with anterior MI (106). Therefore, an increased RV afterload caused by pulmonary venous congestion likely is responsible for acutely depressed RV performance when it occurs in patients with anterior MI. These findings emphasize the need for requiring RV segmental wall motion abnormalities and a reduction in systolic performance for the accurate diagnosis of RV MI by radionuclide ventriculography.

Technetium-99m Pyrophosphate Myocardial Scintigraphy

Technetium-99 myocardial infarct-avid imaging, when performed at an optimal time period after the onset of infarction, is a sensitive and specific marker for detecting LV MI. However, the application of this technique for the early diagnosis of RV infarction is limited because scans usually are not diagnostic until 72 hours after the onset of infarction. Documentation of RV MI has been reported to occur in approximately 40% of patients with acute inferior MI in one study (107). However, other studies have reported a much lower incidence in patients with inferior MI even when definite hemodynamic evidence of RV MI is documented (46). Potential problems with the use of this technique include the proper timing of the study after the onset of infarction and the interpretation of images, including uptake of radionuclide in noncardiac structures (chest wall, bone, and cartilage) that overlie the RV.

Other Noninvasive Testing

The efficacy of dual single-photon emission computed tomography (SPECT) with thallium-201 and technetium-99m pyrophosphate for the diagnosis of RV infarction has been reported. Using dual SPECT with simultaneous images taken 2 to 9 days after the onset of MI, Asano and associates (108) identified 30 RV infarctions among 198 patients with LV infarction. Technetium-99m pyrophosphate accumulation was mostly observed in the posterior wall of the right ventricle, and the prevalence of RV infarction was significantly lower in patients who achieved successfully early reperfusion with thrombolytic therapy than in those who did not (26.7% vs. 68.4%; $p < 0.01$).

Antunes and coworkers (109) studied 30 patients with acute inferior wall MI using simultaneous dual-isotope indium-111 antimyosin and thallium-201 (SPECT) within 2 days of admission. The indium antimyosin scan showed tracer update in the right ventricle in 14 patients (47%). A total of 13 patients had inferior wall thallium perfusion defects and antimyosin uptake. Simultaneous dual-isotope imaging aided in localizing necrosis to either the right coronary or left circumflex territory in diagnosing coexisting RV infarction and in detecting the rare entity of isolated RV infarction. Travin and coworkers (110) assessed the prevalence of RV perfusion defects after recent inferior wall MI in 33 patients who were studied 6 to 14 days after infarction with low-level exercise testing and technetium-99m sestamibi (SPECT) imaging. A quantitative method of defect detection was applied to the right ventricle. RV stress perfusion defects were identified in 10 (30%) of 33 patients with recent inferior MI, with 50% of the defects completely or partially normalizing on rest images, and thus consistent with ischemia rather than infarction. These data further emphasize the frequent occurrence of RV ischemia or infarction, or both, in patients with acute or recent inferior MI. Most recently, gadolinium-enhanced magnetic resonance imaging was equal to dual SPECT in sensitivity and specificity, but it provided better definition and spatial anatomy of heart (111).

TREATMENT

Volume Loading

As mentioned earlier in the discussion on pathophysiology of RV MI, most clinical studies have shown an insignificant increase in the mean cardiac index and blood pressure after a volume infusion (12,112,113). However, careful analysis of the data indicates a variable response among patients. This may reflect a differing initial volume status among patients with acute inferior MI. Some are relatively volume depleted and may benefit from a volume infusion. By contrast, other patients with a normal intravascular volume have no increment in cardiac index or blood pressure with a fluid load because RV preload is already maximal for maintaining RV stroke output. In patients with hemodynamically important RV infarction, an initial volume challenge of 300 to 600 mL normal saline over 10 to 15 minutes should be instituted through a central line or through a large-bore peripheral in-travenous site (12). In the absence of invasive hemodynamic monitoring, the initial volume infusion should be enough to improve SAP by increasing the RV preload. For patients unresponsive to an initial volume load, the further infusion of saline may be deleterious because increasing RV volume may prevent sufficient LV filling through the mechanism of ventricular interaction.

Inotropes

Because RV dilatation compromises LV size, it would seem prudent to unload the RV by a primary (inotropic therapy) mechanism. When this initial volume challenge fails to improve systemic arterial pressure, clinical studies have demonstrated that dobutamine therapy is usually effective in stabilizing hemodynamically compromised patients (12,114). To determine the relative efficacy of inotropic therapy or afterload reduction as adjunctive therapy to volume infusion, Dell'Italia and associates (12) studied the effects of dobutamine and nitroprusside in 13 patients with RV MI after volume loading with normal saline (Figs. 75–9 and 75–10). Dobutamine produced a statistically significant increase in cardiac index, stroke volume index, and RV ejection fraction when compared with nitroprusside. The data indicate that nitroprusside deleteriously decreased preload so that RV stroke volume was unchanged. In contrast, dobutamine maintained preload and augmented systolic performance, resulting in an increase in stroke output and RV ejection fraction with improvement in wall motion.

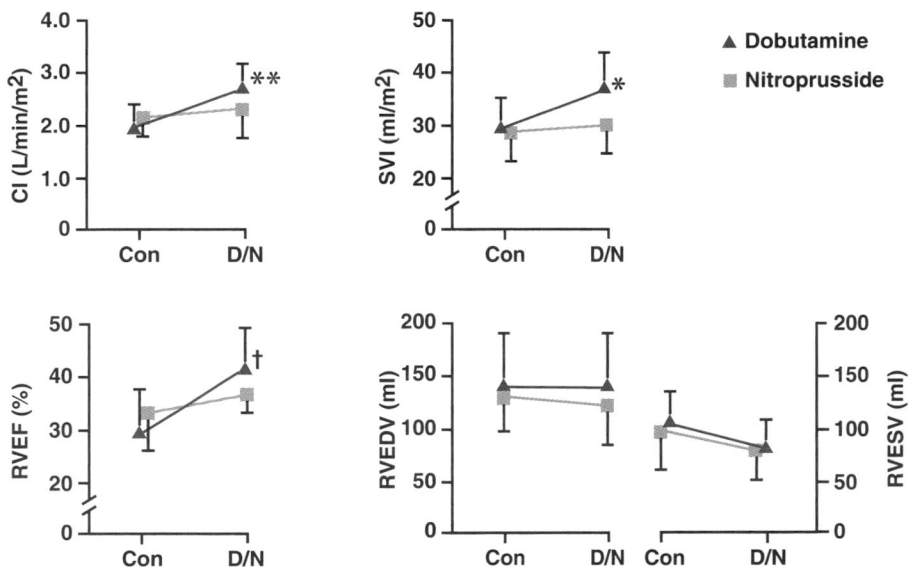

FIG. 75–10. Results of two-way analysis of variance comparing the effects of dobutamine *(D)* and nitroprusside *(N)* therapy on cardiac index *(CI)*, stroke volume index *(SVI)*, right ventricular ejection fraction *(RVEF)*, right ventricular end-diastolic volume *(RVEDV)*, and right ventricular end-systolic volume *(RVESV)* in the nine patients receiving both drugs as outlined in the protocol. Significant differences are noted as follows: $*p = 0.02$; $**p < 0.001$; $†p < 0.01$. (From Dell'Italia LJ, Starling MR, Blumhardt R, et al. Comparative effects of volume loading, dobutamine and nitroprusside in patients with predominant right ventricular infarction. *Circulation* 1985;72:1327–1335, with permission.)

The primary aim of inotropic therapy is the improvement of systemic arterial pressure. However, excessive doses of inotropes will only exacerbate the imbalance between myocardial oxygen demand and supply by increasing contractility and heart rate, thereby precipitating ischemia in the presence of left coronary artery disease. In patients who experience cardiogenic shock or are unresponsive to more than 20 μg per kilogram per minute of dobutamine, dopamine is the drug of choice because it has significantly greater α constrictive effects than dobutamine. However, dopamine has greater chronotropic effects than dobutamine and untoward increases in heart rate may further exacerbate angina. Currently, no animal or human study has compared the effects of the available parenteral positive inotropic agents in RV MI.

In the study by Dell'Italia and associates (12), radionuclide ventriculographic assessment of RV performance demonstrated that the augmentation in stroke output by dobutamine was because of better RV free wall contraction (Fig. 75–10). However, in the experimental dog model, Goldstein and coworkers (64,115) demonstrated augmented RV performance by increasing LV septal contraction. Importantly, these data indicate that if initial fluid loading increases right and left heart filling pressures without a significant improvement in cardiac output, additional volume is unlikely to improve cardiac output and dobutamine should be administered to improve RV systolic performance.

An improvement in cardiac index and mean arterial pressure has been reported after AV sequential pacing in patients with acute RV MI (116). These studies demonstrate the beneficial effect of atrial contraction on ventricular filling and stroke volume in the setting of acute MI. AV sequential pacing often is beneficial in patients who have persistent hypotension, high-grade AV block, or both, despite maximal therapy with inotropic agents and volume infusion.

Thrombolytic Therapy

Patients with inferior MI who also have RV myocardial involvement are at increased risk for death, shock, and arrhythmias (78). This increased risk is related to the presence of RV myocardial involvement itself rather than the extent of LV myocardial damage. Another study clearly demonstrated that the 8-year survival rate was significantly lower in patients with persistent RV dysfunction after acute inferior MI (117). Some studies demonstrated improved RV function with timely thrombolytic therapy (118–123), whereas others have demonstrated no benefit (124,125). However, Giannitsis and coworkers (123) demonstrated a high failure rate of thrombolytic therapy for acute inferior infarction with RV involvement. Thus, very proximal right coronary artery occlusions, which are most frequently associated with RV MI (31), may be problematic for delivery of adequate fibrinolytic agents. Taken together, the presence of hemodynamically important RV MI is associated with increased morbidity and mortality and may be best treated with primary angioplasty, which has been demonstrated to have remarkable immediate results (32,126).

COMPLICATIONS OF RIGHT VENTRICULAR MYOCARDIAL INFARCTION

The acute prognosis of RV MI often is worsened by its complications. Many case reports have described mild to severe arterial desaturation resulting from right-to-left shunting across an atrial septal defect or patent foramen ovale (127–130). With availability of current echo Doppler and color flow Doppler techniques, this important complication of RV MI can now be easily diagnosed at the bedside. In those patients who have hypoxemia, the differential diagnosis includes acute pulmonary embolism, because RV thrombus resulting from RV infarction may result in pulmonary emboli (131). Pulmonary perfusion scanning with macroaggregated albumin is a highly sensitive method for detecting intracardiac shunting as indicated by uptake of the radionuclide in the brain, thyroid, and kidneys. When interventricular septal rupture occurs secondary to acute inferior infarction, the acute and perioperative mortality is determined by the extent of RV ischemia (132–136).

BEDSIDE INDICATORS OF SHORT-TERM PROGNOSIS

Several studies have reported that the acute outcome of patients with RV MI is primarily determined by the amount of accompanying LV necrosis (137–139). In 27 patients with hemodynamic and radionuclide ventriculographic criteria for RV MI, extensive postmortem infarction of the right and left ventricles was found in all 3 patients who died within 72 hours of presentation (140). All three had 10 mm or more of summed ST-segment depression in leads V_1BV_4 that was disproportionate to the extent of ST-segment elevation in the inferior leads and, therefore, likely not caused by reciprocal changes. Such electrocardiographic changes most likely represent extensive LV posterior and lateral wall ischemia. This report and the data from other series (136–138) indicate that the early mortality of RV MI is not due principally to the severity of RV dysfunction, but rather to the presence of extensive LV or mechanical or electrical complications of MI, or both. However, it is has long been appreciated that patients die with hemodynamically important RV MI can also have a normal left coronary artery and normal LV systolic function.

Goldstein and coworkers (50) evaluated 16 patients with hemodynamically important RV MI confirmed by right-heart catheterization and two-dimensional echocardiography. The right atrial waveform had two characteristic patterns, depending on the amplitude of the "a" wave. These two distinct right atrial waveforms were associated with disparate clinical courses. Eight patients had prominent "a" waves and the remaining eight had depressed "a" waves.

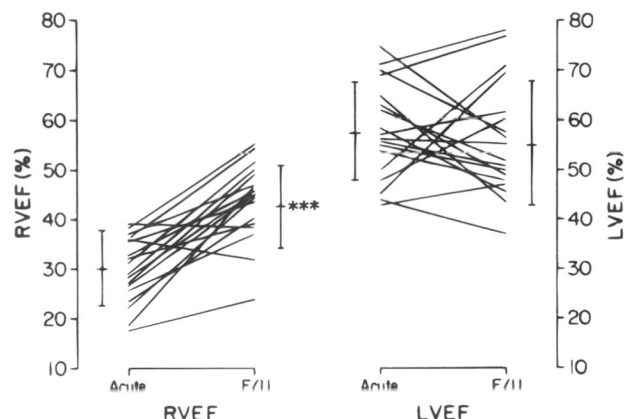

FIG. 75–11. Short-term and follow-up *(F/U)* resting, supine right ventricular ejection fraction *(RVEF)*, and left ventricular ejection fraction *(LVEF)* determinations in 18 survivors (group II). *p* < 0.001. (From Dell'Italia LJ, Lembo NJ, Starling MR, et al. Hemodynamically important right ventricular infarction: follow-up evaluation of right ventricular systolic function at rest and during exercise with radionuclide ventriculography and respiratory gas exchange. *Circulation* 1987;75: 996–1003, with permission.)

Those with augmented "a" waves had a greater average RV systolic pressure, a better mean cardiac output, and a more favorable response to volume and inotropic therapy, and less frequently required emergency revascularization for refractory shock. All differences were statistically significant. Coronary artery stenosis proximal to the major right atrial branches of the right or circumflex coronary artery was demonstrated in all six patients with diminished "a" waves and who had undergone coronary arteriography.

Interestingly, global LV function was near normal or normal in all but 2 of the 16 patients, and assessment of the interventricular septum echocardiographically revealed diastolic septal flattening in 10 patients and frank reversal of septal curvature during diastole in the remaining 6 patients. Definite systolic paradoxic septal motion was present in 14 of 16 patients and was difficult to assess in the remaining 2 patients because of technical limitations. Thus, all 16 patients had both hemodynamic and echocardiographic evidence of severe RV MI, and the loss of enhanced atrial transport contributed to a low cardiac output in 8 of the patients. The finding of a diminished "a" wave on the RAP waveform in patients with hemodynamically important RV MI may be an important acute prognostic indicator, even in the presence of well preserved LV systolic function.

LONG-TERM FOLLOW-UP OF RIGHT VENTRICULAR FUNCTION

It has been well documented that RV ejection fraction increases significantly in the recovery period in survivors after acute RV MI (46,140–142) (Fig. 75–11). Dell'Italia and as-

sociates (140) demonstrated that the response of the RV ejection fraction to exercise also is well preserved in patients 1 to 3 years after RV MI. This remarkable capacity of the right ventricle to regain systolic function after MI most likely explains the findings of Haines and associates (143), who reported that MI predominantly affecting the right ventricle was associated with excellent short- and long-term prognoses. They demonstrated that exercise tolerance as assessed by treadmill time, blood pressure–heart rate product, and peak work load in metabolic equivalent was comparable among 47 patients who had normal RV function, 12 patients with moderate dysfunction, and 50 patients with severe RV dysfunction as determined by radionuclide ventriculography before hospital discharge.

To elucidate further the factors affecting exercise capacity in patients with well documented RV infarction, Dell'Italia and coworkers (140) evaluated the response in the radionuclide right and left ventriculographic ejection fraction and the respiratory gas exchange analysis in patients 1 to 3 years after hemodynamically important RV MIs. The onset of anaerobic threshold during exercise correlated significantly with peak exercise RV ejection fraction ($r = 0.82$; $p < 0.02$; Fig. 75–12), but not with LV ejection fraction. Importantly, the baseline and exercise LV function were well preserved or normal in most of these patients. During upright exercise, as shown in Figure 75–13, the RV ejection fraction increased significantly from 41% ± 10% to 47% ± 12%, as did the LV ejection fraction (55% ± 15% to 60% ± 12%).

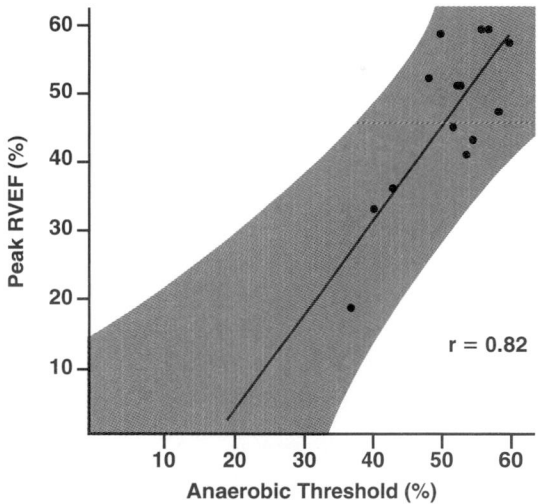

FIG. 75–12. Relation of peak exercise right ventricular ejection fraction *(RVEF)* to the anaerobic threshold in the 14 patients who underwent upright bicycle exercise with correlation coefficient *r* and 95% confidence intervals. (From Dell'Italia LJ, Lembo NJ, Starling MR, et al. Hemodynamically important right ventricular infarction: follow-up evaluation of right ventricular systolic function at rest and during exercise with radionuclide ventriculography and respiratory gas exchange. *Circulation* 1987;75:996–1003, with permission.)

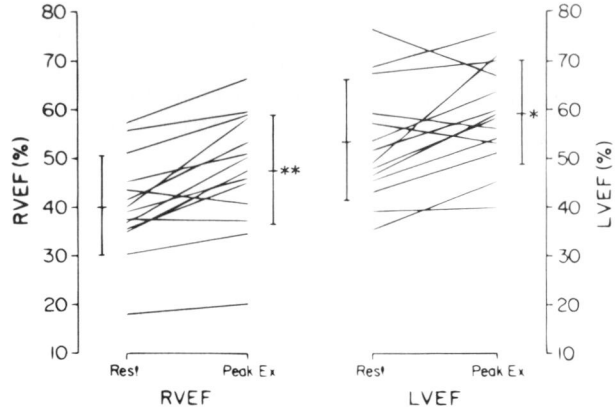

FIG. 75–13. Rest and peak exercise *(peak ex)* right ventricular ejection fraction *(RVEF)* and left ventricular ejection fraction *(LVEF)* in the 14 patients who underwent upright bicycle exercise. $*p < 0.05$; $**p < 0.01$. (From Dell'Italia LJ, Lembo NJ, Starling MR, et al. Hemodynamically important right ventricular infarction: follow-up evaluation of right ventricular systolic function at rest and during exercise with radionuclide ventriculography and respiratory gas exchange. *Circulation* 1987;75:996–1003, with permission.)

In this study, the direction and extent of change in RV ejection fraction correlated well with the change in LV ejection fraction ($r = 0.82$; $p < 0.02$). Deviations from this good correlation occurred only in patients who had a decreased 1-second forced expiratory volume and an abnormal ventilatory reserve during exercise as measured by respiratory gas exchange analysis. Thus, in the recovery phase after RV infarction, the RV ejection fraction often improves and the RV functional reserve usually is preserved during exercise in patients who are not limited by angina, pulmonary disease, or LV failure.

The importance of the right ventricle has even been emphasized in the prognosis of MI in general. In a published study from the Survival And Ventricular Enlargement (SAVE) trial, two-dimensional echocardiograms obtained in 416 patients with LV ejection fraction of 40% or less (mean 11.1 ± 3.2 days after MI) demonstrated that RV function was an independent predictor of death and the development of heart failure (144). Dobutamine stress is useful in assessing RV contractile reserve after acute MI (145,146). In fact, a reduced RV contractile reserve was related to proximal right coronary artery disease and is associated with stress-induced increased ST in VR leads (145). Taken together, the assessment of RV function not only at rest but also during stress may be an important prognostic indicator in patients with LV dysfunction after MI.

SUMMARY

These studies indicate that hemodynamic evidence of RV MI usually is associated with excellent short- and long-term prognoses. Although hemodynamic compromise and death can occur in the presence of RV MI alone, the prognosis in most cases is excellent as long as severe LV dysfunction is absent. This favorable prognosis is even more impressive considering that these prognostic studies were conducted before thrombolytic therapy and early direct coronary angioplasty were widely used. They affirm the remarkable resistance of the RV to necrosis in acute right coronary artery occlusion. However, the RV often may develop transient ischemic injury that sometimes produces reversible severe arterial hypotension. Accordingly, prompt recognition by physical examination or by the V_{4R} electrogram, appropriate treatment with judicious volume loading, and early inotropic therapy when needed are important in maintaining circulatory stability in preparation for immediate revascularization, preferably with acute coronary angioplasty. A careful clinical evaluation including risk stratification, noninvasive testing, and coronary arteriography, as appropriate, to rule out important left coronary artery disease, recurrent myocardial ischemia, and severe LV dysfunction before discharge results in excellent long-term survival.

REFERENCES

1. Sanders AO. Coronary thrombosis with complete heart-block and relative ventricular tachycardia: a case report. *Am Heart J* 1930;6:820–823.
2. Starr I, Jeffers WA, Meade RH. The absence of conspicuous increments of venous pressure after severe damage to the right ventricle of the dog, with a discussion of the relation between clinical congestive failure and heart disease. *Am Heart J* 1943;26:291–301.
3. Bakos AC. The question of the function of the right ventricular myocardium: an experimental study. *Circulation* 1950;1:724–731.
4. Kagan A. Dynamic responses of the right ventricle following extensive damage by cauterization. *Circulation* 1952;5:816–823.
5. Kinch JW, Ryan TJ. Right ventricular infarction. *N Engl J Med* 1994;330:1211–1217.
6. Guiha NH, Limas CJ, Cohn JN. Predominant right ventricular dysfunction after right ventricular destruction in the dog. *Am J Cardiol* 1974;33:243–257.
7. Cohn JN, Guiha NH, Broder MI, et al. Right ventricular infarction. *Am J Cardiol* 1974;33:209–214.
8. Isner J, Roberts WC. Right ventricular infarction complicating left ventricular infarction secondary to coronary heart disease. *Am J Cardiol* 1978;42:885–894.
9. Lopez-Sendon J, Coma-Cannella I, Gamallo C. Sensitivity and specificity of hemodynamic criteria in the diagnosis of acute right ventricular infarction. *Circulation* 1981;64:515–526.
10. Goldstein JA, Vlahakes GJ, Verrier ED, et al. The role of right ventricular systolic dysfunction and elevated intrapericardial pressure in the genesis of low output in experimental right ventricular infarction. *Circulation* 1982;65:513–522.
11. Goldstein JA, Vlahakes GJ, Verrier ED, et al. Volume loading improves low cardiac output in experimental right ventricular infarction. *J Am Coll Cardiol* 1983;2:270–278.
12. Dell'Italia LJ, Starling MR, Blumhardt R, et al. Comparative effects of volume loading, dobutamine and nitroprusside in patients with predominant right ventricular infarction. *Circulation* 1985;72:1327–1335.
13. O'Rourke RA, Dell'Italia LJ. Diagnosis and management of right ventricular myocardial infarction. *Curr Probl Cardiol* 2004;29:6–47.
14. Anderson FA, Falk E, Nielson D. Right ventricular infarction: frequency, size, and topography in coronary heart disease: a prospective study comprising 107 consecutive autopsies from a coronary care unit. *J Am Coll Cardiol* 1987;10:1223–1232.
15. Cabin HS, Clubb S, Wackers FJ, et al. Right ventricular myocardial infarction with anterior wall left ventricular infarction: an autopsy study. *Am Heart J* 1987;113:16–23.

16. Williams JF. Right ventricular infarction. *Clin Cardiol* 1990;13: 309–315.
17. Erhardt LR. Clinical and pathological observations in different types of acute myocardial infarction: a study of 84 patients deceased after treatment in a coronary care unit. *Acta Med Scand Suppl* 1974;26:7–78.
18. Setaro JF, Cabin HS. Right ventricular infarction. *Cardiol Clin* 1992;10:69–90.
19. Dell'Italia LJ. The right ventricle: anatomy, physiology and clinical importance. *Curr Prob Cardiol* 1991;16:659–720.
20. Bellamy RF, Lowensohn HS. Effect of systole on coronary pressure-flow relations in the right ventricle of the dog. *Am J Physiol* 1980; 238:H481–H486.
21. Cross CE. Right ventricular pressure and coronary flow. *Am J Physiol* 1962;202:12–16.
22. Hess DS, Bache RJ. Transmural right ventricular myocardial blood flow during systole in the awake dog. *Circ Res* 1979;45:88–94.
23. Lowensohn HS, Khoui EM, Gregg DE, et al. Phasic right coronary artery blood flow in conscious dogs with normal and elevated right ventricular pressures. *Circ Res* 1976;39:760–766.
24. Kusachi S, Nishiyama O, Yasuhara K, et al. Right and left ventricular oxygen metabolism in open-chest dogs. *Am J Physiol* 1982;24: H761–H766.
25. Takeda K, Haraoka S, Nagashima H. Myocardial oxygen metabolism of the right ventricle with volume loading and hypoperfusion. *Jpn Circ J* 1987;51:563–572.
26. Saito D, Yamada N, Kusachi S, et al. Coronary flow reserve and oxygen metabolism of the right ventricle. *Jpn Circ J* 1989;53:1310–1316.
27. Bian X, Fu M, Mallet RT, et al. Myocardial oxygen consumption modulates adenosine formation by canine right ventricle in absence of hypoxia. *J Mol Cell Cardiol* 2000;32:345–354.
28. Ratliff NB, Peter RH, Ramo BW, et al. A model for the production of right ventricular infarction. *Am J Pathol* 1970;58:471–479.
29. Farrer-Brown G. Vascular pattern of myocardium of right ventricle of human heart. *Br Heart J* 1968;30:679–686.
30. Haupt HM, Hutchins GM, Moore GW. Right ventricular infarction. Role of the moderator band artery in determining infarct size. *Circulation* 1983;67:1268–1272.
31. Shiraki H, Yoshikawa T, Anzai T, et al. Association between preinfarction angina and a lower risk of right ventricular infarction. *N Engl J Med* 1998;338:941–947.
32. Bowers TR, O'Neill WW, Grines C, et al. Effect of reperfusion on biventricular function and survival after right ventricular infarction. *N Engl J Med* 1998;338:933–940.
33. Bowers TR. O'Neill WW, Pica M, et al. Patterns of coronary compromise resulting in acute right ventricular ischemic dysfunction. *Circulation* 2002;106:1104–1109.
34. Wade WG. The pathogenesis of infarction of the right ventricle. *Br Heart J* 1959;21:545–554.
35. Ramo VW, Peter RH, Raliff N, et al. The natural history of right coronary arterial occlusion in the pig. *Am J Cardiol* 1970;26:156–161.
36. Ratliff NB, Hackel DB. Combined right and left ventricular infarction: pathogenesis and clinicopathologic correlations. *Am J Cardiol* 1980;45:217–221.
37. Horan LG, Flowers NC, Havelda CJ. Relation between right ventricular mass and cavity size: an analysis of 1500 human hearts. *Circulation* 1981;64:135–138.
38. Brooks H, Holland R, Al-Sadir J. Right ventricular performance during ischemia: an anatomic and hemodynamic analysis. *Am J Physiol* 1977;233:H505–H513.
39. Coma-Cannella I, Lopez-Sendon J. Ventricular compliance in ischemic right ventricular dysfunction. *Am J Cardiol* 1980;45:555–561.
40. Baigre RS, Hag A, Morgan CD, et al. The spectrum of right ventricular involvement in inferior wall myocardial infarction: a clinical, hemodynamic and noninvasive study. *J Am Coll Cardiol* 1983;1:1396–1404.
41. Cintron GB, Hernandez E, Linares E, et al. Bedside recognition, incidence and clinical course of right ventricular infarction. *Am J Cardiol* 1981;47:224–227.
42. Lorell B, Leinbach RC, Pohost GM, et al. Right ventricular infarction. Clinical diagnosis and differentiation from cardiac tamponade and pericardial constriction. *Am J Cardiol* 1979;43:465–471.
43. Coma-Canella I, Lopez-Sendon J, Gamallo C. Low output syndrome in right ventricular infarction. *Am Heart J* 1979;98:613–620.
44. Lloyd EA, Gersh BJ, Kennelly BM. Hemodynamic spectrum of "dominant" right ventricular infarction in 19 patients. *Am J Cardiol* 1981;48:1016–1021.

45. Jensen DP, Goolsby JP, Oliva PB. Hemodynamic pattern resembling pericardial construction after acute inferior myocardial infarction with right ventricular infarction. *Am J Cardiol* 1978;42: 858–861.
46. Dell'Italia LJ, Starling MR, Crawford MH, et al. Right ventricular infarction: identification by hemodynamic measurements before and after volume loading and correlation with noninvasive techniques. *J Am Coll Cardiol* 1984;4:931–939.
47. Goldstein JA, Harada A, Yagi Y, et al. Hemodynamic importance of systolic ventricular interaction, augmented right atrial contractility and atrioventricular synchrony in acute right ventricular dysfunction. *J Am Coll Cardiol* 1990;16:181–189.
48. Goldstein JA, Tweddell JS, Barzilai B, et al. Right atrial ischemia exacerbates hemodynamic compromise associated with experimental right ventricular dysfunction. *J Am Coll Cardiol* 1991;18:1564–1572.
49. Goldstein JA, Tweddell JS, Barzilai B, et al. Importance of left ventricular function and systolic ventricular interaction to right ventricular performance during acute right heart ischemia. *J Am Coll Cardiol* 1992;19:704–711.
50. Goldstein JA, Barzilai B, Rosamond TL, et al. Determinants of hemodynamic compromise with severe right ventricular infarction. *Circulation* 1990;82:359–368.
51. Coma-Canella I, Lopez-Sendon J, Oliver J. Premature pulmonic valve opening and inverted septal convexity in acute ischemic right ventricular dysfunction. *Am Heart J* 1981;101:684–685.
52. Lopez-Sendon J, Garcia AG, Marti JS, et al. Complete pulmonic valve opening during atrial contraction after right ventricular infarction. *Am J Cardiol* 1985;56:486–487.
53. Doyle T, Troup PJ, Wann LS. Mid-diastolic opening of the pulmonary valve after right ventricular infarction. *J Am Coll Cardiol* 1985;5: 366–368.
54. Donald DE, Essex HE. Pressure studies after inactivation of the major portion of the canine right ventricle. *Am J Physiol* 1954;176:155–161.
55. Lopez-Sendon J, Coma-Canella I, Adanez JV. Volume loading in patients with ischemic right ventricular dysfunction. *Eur Heart J* 1981;2:329–338.
56. Shah PK, Maddahi J, Berman DS, et al. Scintigraphically detected predominant right ventricular dysfunction in acute myocardial infarction: clinical and hemodynamic correlates and implications for therapy and prognosis. *J Am Coll Cardiol* 1985;6:1264–1272.
57. Johnston WE, Lin CY, Feerick AE, et al. Volume expansion increases right ventricular infarct size in dogs by reducing collateral perfusion. *Chest* 1996;109:494–503.
58. Sharkey SW, Shelley W, Carlyle PF, et al. M-mode and two-dimensional echocardiographic analysis of the septum in experimental right ventricular infarction: correlation with hemodynamic alterations. *Am Heart J* 1985;110:1210–1218.
59. Laster SB, Shelton TJ, Barzalai B, et al. Determinants of the recovery of right ventricular performance following experimental chronic right coronary artery occlusion. *Circulation* 1993;88:696–708.
60. Laster SB, Ohnishi Y, Saffitz JE, et al. Effects of reperfusion on ischemic right ventricular dysfunction. Disparate mechanisms of benefit related to duration of ischemia. *Circulation* 1994;90:1398–1409.
61. Goto Y, Yamamoto J, Saito M, et al. Effects of right ventricular ischemia on left ventricular geometry and the end-systolic pressure-volume relationship in the dog. *Circulation* 1985;72:1104–1114.
62. Brookes C, Ravn H, White P, et al. Acute right ventricular dilatation in response to ischemia significantly impairs left ventricular systolic performance. *Circulation* 1999;100:761–767.
63. Danton MH, Byrne JG, Flores KQ, et al. Modified Glenn connection for acutely ischemic right ventricular failure reverses secondary left ventricular dysfunction. *J Thorac Cardiovasc Surg* 2001;122: 80–91.
64. Goldstein JA, Tweddel JS, Barzlai B, et al. Importance of left ventricular function and systolic ventricular interaction in right ventricular performance during acute right heart ischemia. *J Am Coll Cardiol* 1992;19:704–711.
65. Dell'Italia LJ. Reperfusion for right ventricular infarction. *N Engl J Med* 1998;338:978–980.
66. Dell'Italia LJ, Starling MR, O'Rourke RA. Physical examination for exclusion of hemodynamically important right ventricular infarction. *Ann Intern Med* 1983;99:608–611.
67. Eisenberg S, Suyemoto J. Rupture of a papillary muscle of the tricuspid valve following acute myocardial infarction. *Circulation* 1964;30: 588–591.

68. McAllister RG, Friesinger GC, Sinclair-Smith BC. Tricuspid regurgitation following inferior myocardial infarction. *Arch Intern Med* 1976;136:95–99.

69. Zone DD, Botti RE. Right ventricular infarction with tricuspid insufficiency and chronic right heart failure. *Am J Cardiol* 1976;37:445–448.

70. Zehender M, Kasper W, Kauder E, et al. Right ventricular infarction as an independent predictor of prognosis after acute inferior myocardial infarction. *N Engl J Med* 1993;328:981–988.

71. Braat SH, de Zwann C, Brugada P, et al. Right ventricular involvement with acute inferior wall myocardial infarction identifies high risk of developing atrioventricular nodal conduction disturbances. *Am Heart J* 1984;107:1181–1187.

72. Mark A. The Bezold-Jarisch reflex revisited: clinical implications of inhibitory reflexes originating in the heart. *J Am Coll Cardiol* 1983; 1:90–102.

73. Gacioch GM, Topol EJ. Sudden paradoxic clinical deterioration during angioplasty of the occluded right coronary artery in acute myocardial infarction. *J Am Coll Cardiol* 1989;14:1202–1209.

74. Koren G, Weiss AT, Ben-David Y, et al. Bradycardia and hypotension following reperfusion with streptokinase (Bezold-Jarisch reflex): a sign of coronary thrombolysis and myocardial salvage. *Am Heart J* 1986;112:468–471.

75. Rechavia E, Strasberg B, Kusniec J, et al. The impact of right ventricular infarction on the prevalence of ventricular arrhythmias during acute inferior myocardial infarction. *Chest* 1990;98:1207–1209.

76. Pfisterer M, Emmenegger H, Soler M, et al. Prognostic significance of right ventricular ejection fraction for persistent complex ventricular arrhythmias and/or sudden death after first myocardial infarction: relation to infarct location, size and left ventricular function. *Eur Heart J* 1986;7:289–298.

77. Zehender M, Kasper W, Kauder E, et al. Eligibility for and benefit of thrombolytic therapy in inferior myocardial infarction: focus on the prognostic importance of right ventricular infarction. *J Am Coll Cardiol* 1994;24:362–369.

78. Meta M, Eikebloom J, Ntarajan M, et al. Impact of right ventricular involvement on mortality and morbidity in patients with inferior myocardial infarction. *J Am Coll Cardiol* 2001;37:37–43.

79. Elvan A, Zipes DP. Right ventricular infarction causes heterogeneous autonomic denervation of the viable peri-infarct area. *Circulation* 1998;97:484–492.

80. Rechavia E, Strasberg B, Mager A, et al. The incidence of atrial arrhythmias during inferior wall myocardial infarction with and without right ventricular involvement. *Am Heart J* 1992;124:387–391.

81. Klein HO, Tordjman T, Ninio R, et al. The early recognition of right ventricular infarction: diagnostic accuracy of the electrocardiographic V_{4R} lead. *Circulation* 1983;67:558–565.

82. Erhardt LR, Sjogern A, Wahlberg I. Single right-sided precordial lead in the diagnosis of right ventricular involvement in inferior myocardial infarction. *Am Heart J* 1976;91:571–576.

83. Chou T, Van Der Bel-Kahn J, Allen J, et al. Electrocardiographic diagnosis of right ventricular infarction. *Am J Med* 1981;70:1175–1180.

84. Croft CH, Nicod P, Corbett JR, et al. Detection of acute right ventricular infarction by right precordial electrocardiography. *Am J Cardiol* 1982;50:421–427.

85. Bratt SH, Brugada P, De Zwann C, et al. Value of electrocardiogram in diagnosing right ventricular involvement in patients with an acute inferior wall myocardial infarction. *Br Heart J* 1983;49:368–372.

86. Candell-Riera J, Figueras J, Valle V, et al. Right ventricular infarction: relationships between ST-segment elevation in V_4R and hemodynamic, scintigraphic and echocardiographic findings in patients with acute inferior myocardial infarction. *Am Heart J* 1981;101:281–287.

87. Morgera T, Alberti E, Silvestri F, et al. Right precordial ST and QRS changes in the diagnosis of right ventricular infarction. *Am Heart J* 1984;108:13–18.

88. Lopez-Sendon J, Coma-Canella I, Alcasena S, et al. Electrocardiographic findings in acute right ventricular infarction: sensitivity and specificity of electrocardiographic alterations in right precordial leads V_4R, V_3R, V_1, V_2 and V_3. *J Am Coll Cardiol* 1984;6:1273–1279.

89. Geft IL, Shah PK, Rodriguez L, et al. ST elevation in leads V_1 to V_5 may be caused by right coronary artery occlusion and acute right ventricular infarction. *Am J Cardiol* 1984;53:9911–9996.

90. Coma-Canella I, Lopez-Sendon J, Alcasena S, et al. Electrocardiographic alterations in leads V_1 to V_3 in the diagnosis of right and left ventricular infarction. *Am Heart J* 1986;112:940–946.

91. Wellens HJ. Right ventricular infarction. *N Engl J Med* 1993;328: 1036–1038.

92. Rodrigues EA, Dewhurst NG, Smart LM, et al. Diagnosis and prognosis of right ventricular infarction. *Br Heart J* 1986;56:19–26.

93. Anderson HR, Nielson D, Lund O, et al. Prognostic significance of right ventricular infarction diagnosed by ST elevation in right chest leads V_{3R} to V_{7R}. *Int J Cardiol* 1998;23:349–356.

94. Berger PB, Ryan TJ. Inferior myocardial infarction high-risk subgroups. *Circulation* 1990;81:401–411.

95. Shah PK. Right ventricular infarction. *N Engl J Med* 1993;329:1043.

96. D'Arcy B, Nanda NC. Two-dimensional echocardiographic features of right ventricular infarction. *Circulation* 1982;65:167–173.

97. Bellamy GR, Rasmussen HH, Nasser FN, et al. Value of two-dimensional echocardiography, electrocardiography and clinical signs in detecting right ventricular infarction. *Am Heart J* 1986;112:304–368.

98. Lopez-Sendon J, Garcia-Fernandez MA, Coma-Canella I, et al. Segmental right ventricular function after acute myocardial infarction: two-dimensional echocardiographic study in 63 patients. *Am J Cardiol* 1983;51:390–396.

99. Dell'Italia LJ, Santamore WP. Can indices of left ventricular function be applied to the right ventricle? *Prog Cardiovasc Dis* 1998;40:309–340.

100. Santamore WP, Dell'Italia LJ. Ventricular interdependence: significant left ventricular contributions to right ventricular systolic function. *Prog Cardiovasc Dis* 1998;40:289–308.

101. Rigo P, Murray M, Taylor DR. Right ventricular dysfunction detected by gated scintiphotography in patients with acute inferior myocardial infarction. *Circulation* 1975;52:268–274.

102. Sharpe DN, Botvinick EH, Shames DM, et al. The noninvasive diagnosis of right ventricular infarction. *Circulation* 1978;57:483–490.

103. Tobinick E, Schelbert HR, Henning H, et al. Right ventricular ejection fraction in patients with acute anterior and inferior myocardial infarction assessed by radionuclide angiography. *Circulation* 1978;57:1078–1084.

104. Reduto LA, Berger HJ, Cohen LS, et al. Sequential radionuclide assessment of left and right ventricular performance after acute transmural myocardial infarction. *Ann Intern Med* 1978;89:441–447.

105. Starling M, Dell'Italia LJ, O'Rourke RA, et al. First transit and equilibrium radionuclide angiography in inferior transmural myocardial infarction patients: criteria for the diagnosis of associated hemodynamically significant right ventricular infarction. *J Am Coll Cardiol* 1984;4:923–930.

106. Marmor A, Geltman EM, Biello DR, et al. Functional response of the right ventricle to myocardial infarction: dependence on the site of left ventricular infarction. *Circulation* 1981;64:1005–1011.

107. Wackers FJT, Lie KI, Sokole EB, et al. Prevalence of right ventricular involvement in inferior wall infarction assessed with myocardial imaging with thallium-201 and technetium-99m pyrophosphate. *Am J Cardiol* 1978;42:358–362.

108. Asano H, Sone T, Tsuboi H, et al. Diagnosis of right ventricular infarction by overlap images of simultaneous dual emission computed tomography using technetium-99m pyrophosphate and thallium-201. *Am J Cardiol* 1993;71:902–908.

109. Antunes ML, Johnson LL, Seldin DW, et al. Diagnosis of right ventricular acute myocardial infarction by dual isotope thallium-201 and indium-111 antimyosin SPECT imaging. *Am J Cardiol* 1992;70:426–431.

110. Travin MI, Malkin RD, Garber CE, et al. Prevalence of right ventricular perfusion defects after inferior myocardial infarction assessed by low-level exercise with technetium-99m sestamibi tomographic myocardial imaging. *Am Heart J* 1994;127:797–804.

111. Sato H, Murakami Y, Shimada T, et al. Detection of right ventricular infarction by gadolinium DTPA-enhanced magnetic resonance imaging. *Eur Hear J* 1995;16:1195–1199.

112. Siniorakis EE, Nikolaou NI, Sarantopoulos CD, et al. Volume loading in predominant right ventricular infarction: bedside haemodynamics using rapid response thermistors. *Eur Heart J* 1994;10:1340–1347.

113. Ferrario M, Poli A, Previtali M, et al. Hemodynamics of volume loading compared with dobutamine in severe right ventricular infarction. *Am J Cardiol* 1994;74:329–333.

114. Dhainaut JF, Ghannad E, Villemant D, et al. Role of tricuspid regurgitation and left ventricular damage in the treatment of right ventricular infarction-induced low cardiac output syndrome. *Am J Cardiol* 1990;66:289–295.

115. Goldstein JA, Harada A, Yagi Brazilai B, et al. Hemodynamic importance of systolic ventricular interaction, augmented right atrial contractility and atrioventricular synchrony in acute right ventricular dysfunction. *J Am Coll Cardiol* 1990;16:181–189.

116. Topol ES, Goldschlager N, Ports TA, et al. Hemodynamic benefit of atrial pacing in right ventricular myocardial infarction. *Ann Intern Med* 1982;96:594–597.

117. Sakata K, Yoshino H, Kurihara H, et al. Prognostic significance of persistent right ventricular dysfunction as assessed by radionuclide angiocardiography in patients with inferior wall acute myocardial infarction. *Am J Cardiol* 2000;85:939–944.

118. Schuler G, Hofmann M, Schwarz F, et al. Effect of successful thrombolytic therapy on right ventricular function in acute inferior wall myocardial infarction. *Am J Cardiol* 1984;54:951–957.

119. Verrani MS, Tortoledo FE, Batty JW, et al. Effect of coronary artery recanilization on right ventricular function patients with acute myocardial infarction. *J Am Coll Cardiol* 1985;5:1029–1035.

120. Kinn JW, Ajluni SC, Samyn JG, et al. Rapid hemodynamic improvement after reperfusion during right ventricular infarction. *J Am Coll Cardiol* 1995;26:1230–1234.

121. Zehender M, Kasper W, Kauder E, et al. Eligibility for and benefit of thrombolytic therapy in inferior myocardial infarction: focus on the prognostic importance of right ventricular infarction. *J Am Coll Cardiol* 1994;24:362–369.

122. Berger PB, Ruocco NA, Ryan RJ, et al. Frequency and significance of right ventricular myocardial infarction treated with thrombolytic therapy (results from the thrombolysis in myocardial infarction [TIMI II Trial]). *Am J Cardiol* 1993;71:1148–1152.

123. Giannitsis E, Potratz J, Wiegand U, et al. Impact of early accelerated dose tissue plasminogen activator on in-hospital patency of the infarcted vessel in patients with acute right ventricular infarction. *Heart* 1997;77:512–516.

124. Zeymer U, Neuhaus KL, Wegscheider K, et al. Effects of thrombolytic therapy in acute inferior myocardial infarction with or without right ventricular involvement. *J Am Coll Cardiol* 1998;32:876–881.

125. Roth A, Miller HI, Kaluski, et al. Early thrombolytic therapy does not enhance the recovery of the right ventricle in patients with acute inferior myocardial infarction and predominant right ventricular involvement. *Cardiology* 1990;77:40–49.

126. Goldstein JA. Pathophysiology and management of right heart ischemia. *J Am Coll Cardiol* 2002;40:841–853.

127. Stowers SA, Leiboff RH, Wasserman AG, et al. Right ventricular infarction complicated by right to left shunt. *Am J Cardiol* 1983;2:554–557.

128. Manno BV, Bhennis CE, Carver J, et al. Right ventricular infarction complicated by right to left shunt. *J Am Coll Cardiol* 1983;2:554–557.

129. Rietveld AP, Merrman L, Essed CE, et al. Right to left shunt, with severe hypoxemia at the atrial level in a patient with hemodynamically important right ventricular infarction. *J Am Coll Cardiol* 1983;2:776–779.

130. Laham RJ, Ho KK, Douglas PS, et al. Right ventricular infarction complicated by acute right-to-left shunting. *Am J Cardiol* 1994;74:824–826.

131. Stowers SA, Leiboff RH, Wasserman AG, et al. Right ventricular thrombus formation in association with acute myocardial infarction: diagnosis by two-dimensional echocardiography. *Am J Cardiol* 1983;52:912–913.

132. Radford MJ, Johnson RA, Daggett WM, et al. Ventricular septal rupture: a review of clinical and physiologic features and an analysis of survival. *Circulation* 1981;64:545–552.

133. Grose R, Spindola-Franco H. Right ventricular dysfunction in acute ventricular septal defect. *Am Heart J* 1981;101:67–74.

134. Fananapazir L, Bray CL, Dark JR, et al. Right ventricular dysfunction and surgical outcome in post-infarction ventricular septal defect. *Eur Heart J* 1983;4:157–167.

135. Moore CA, Nygaard TW, Kaiser DL, et al. Postinfarction ventricular septal rupture: the importance of location of infarction and right ventricular function in determining survival. *Circulation* 1986;74:45–55.

136. Cummings RG, Reimer KA, Califf R, et al. Quantitative analysis of right and left ventricular infarction in the presence of postinfarction ventricular septal defect. *Circulation* 1988;77:33–42.

137. Jugdutt BI, Sussex BA, Sivaram CA, et al. Right ventricular infarction: two-dimensional echocardiographic evaluation. *Am Heart J* 1984;107:505–518.

138. Legrand V, Rigo P, Demoulin JC, et al. Right ventricular myocardial infarction diagnosed by 99m pyrophosphate scintigraphy: clinical course and follow-up. *Eur Heart J* 1983;4:9–19.

139. Shah PK, Maddahi J, Staniloff HM, et al. Variable spectrum and prognostic implications of left and right ventricular ejection fractions in patients with and without heart failure after acute myocardial infarction. *Am J Cardiol* 1986;58:387–398.

140. Dell'Italia LJ, Lembo NJ, Starling MR, et al. Hemodynamically important right ventricular infarction: follow-up evaluation of right ventricular systolic function at rest and during exercise with radionuclide ventriculography and respiratory gas exchange. *Circulation* 1987;75:996–1003.

141. Yasuda T, Okada RD, Leinbach RC, et al. Serial evaluation of right ventricular dysfunction associated with acute inferior myocardial infarction. *Am Heart J* 1990;119:816–822.

142. Steele P, Kirch D, Ellis J, et al. Prompt return to normal of depressed right ventricular ejection fraction in acute inferior infarction. *Br Heart J* 1977;39:1319.

143. Haines DE, Beller GA, Watson DD, et al. A prospective clinical, scintigraphic, angiographic and functional evaluation of patients after inferior myocardial infarction with and without right ventricular dysfunction. *J Am Coll Cardiol* 1985;6:995–1003.

144. Zornoff LA, Skali H, Pfeffer MA, et al., SAVE Investigators. Right ventricular dysfunction and risk of heart failure and mortality after myocardial infarction. *J Am Coll Cardiol* 2002;39:1450–1455.

145. Coma-Canella I, del Val Gomez Martinez M, Terol I, et al. Radionuclide assessment of right ventricular contractile reserve after acute myocardial infarction. *Am J Cardiol* 1994;74:982–986.

146. San Roman JA, Vilacosta FI, Rollan MJ, et al. Right ventricular asynergy during dobutamine-atropine echocardiography. *J Am Coll Cardiol* 1997;30:430–435.

CHAPTER **76**

Acute Coronary Syndromes

The Role of Bypass Surgery in the Management of Unstable Angina and Acute Myocardial Infarction

Thoralf M. Sundt and Hartzell V. Schaff

Key Words: Acute myocardial infarction; coronary artery bypass; off-pump; unstable angina.

INTRODUCTION

The current standard of care in the management of most acute coronary syndromes is pharmacologic therapy with or without acute percutaneous coronary intervention (PCI). Indeed, many view PCI as the preferred first line of therapy in the management of an increasing segment of the spectrum of coronary artery disease. Coronary artery bypass (CAB) continues to play an important role, however, particularly for those patients with the most advanced ischemic disease. Even in the current era, CAB is performed during the index hospitalization for acute myocardial infarction (AMI) in 10% to 20% of patients in the United States (1) and Australia (2), although rates are less in Canada (3). An under-

T. M. Sundt: Mayo Clinic, 200 First Street SW, Rochester, Minnesota 55905.
H. V. Schaff: Mayo Clinic, 200 First Street SW, Rochester, Minnesota 55905.

standing of the risks and results of surgical intervention in the setting of acute coronary syndromes therefore remains relevant.

RATIONALE FOR SURGICAL REVASCULARIZATION IN ACUTE MYOCARDIAL INFARCTION

The pioneering work reported by DeWood and colleagues (4–11) and Phillips and associates (12,13) established the basis for the current practice of early revascularization for AMI. These investigators demonstrated that angiography was safe and that surgery was feasible, albeit at increased risk, over that for elective CAB. The early hospital mortality rate in their series of 701 patients undergoing CAB for AMI was 4.4%, with a somewhat greater risk for those with transmural infarction (5.2%) as compared with non–Q-wave infarction (3.1%) (4). The operative mortality rate in the setting of acute infarction reported in more contemporary series is remarkably similar; in 1997, Lee and associates (14) reported an overall 30-day mortality rate of 5.1% among 316 patients undergoing surgery within 21 days of infarction. Correlates with mortality included preoperative intraaortic balloon pump, depressed left ventricular function, and renal dysfunction. In 2000, Stone and colleagues (1) reported an operative mortality rate of 6.4% for emergent CAB after MI in the database from the Primary Angioplasty in Myocardial Infarction-2 Trial. Notably, the observed mortality rate in elective CAB in this study was only 2%, indicating that although acceptable, the operative mortality rate after AMI remains at least somewhat increased after AMI even in the current era.

These early studies also established a survival advantage among patients undergoing prompt revascularization as compared with medical therapy. DeWood and associates (10) examined the outcomes of 387 patients having medical or surgical treatment of AMI who were observed during follow-up at 10 to 13 years (mean 11.4). Medical and surgical patients were similar in regard to age, gender, previous MI, extent of infarction, number of vessels diseased, and clinical classification. For medical patients, hospital mortality was 11.5% (23 of 200) compared with 5.8% (11 of 187) for patients having emergency CAB ($p = 0.07$). Reperfusion within 6 hours of infarction was associated with an early mortality rate of 2% (2 of 100) compared with 10.3% (9 of 87) for patients who had surgical reperfusion more than 6 hours after the onset of chest pain.

The benefit of reperfusion in these studies extended into late follow-up. Among survivors of hospitalization, risk of subsequent sudden death for medical patients was 17.5% versus 7.4% for patients undergoing surgical revascularization ($p = 0.01$). After adjustment for risk factors by the Cox model, late survival of the surgically treated patients was 73% compared with 59% for the medical group ($p = 0.0007$). There was no difference in occurrence of late MI in the two groups, but mortality associated with reinfarction was considerably greater in patients who had no reperfusion (36.6% vs. 17.5%; $p = 0.04$). Furthermore, although regional function was improved among patients with anterior MI only if reflow was established early, late survival was improved by surgical reperfusion before or after the 6-hour mark from onset of chest pain (11). In contrast, among those with inferior wall Q-wave infarction, overall survival was enhanced only in patients who had early reperfusion.

TIMING OF CORONARY ARTERY BYPASS AFTER ACUTE MYOCARDIAL INFARCTION

Even if one accepts the advisability of early operation for unstable postinfarction angina, there remains an important, practical question of whether any delay (e.g., 1 or 2 weeks) will decrease operative mortality and morbidity if the patient demonstrates sufficient stability to permit elective operation. Unfortunately, all retrospective studies concerning the timing of CAB after MI are inherently flawed by bias in patient selection; highly unstable patients and those with large amounts of myocardium in jeopardy are more likely to have urgent revascularization compared with patients with less

severe coronary stenoses whose symptoms are reduced by medical treatment. It is self-evident that these too are the individuals at greatest perioperative risk. Despite these limitations, a number of studies have been reported and provide insight into this important question.

The argument in favor of delay is based in part on studies performed in the decade of the 1980s. Katz and coworkers (15) reviewed 145 patients having surgical revascularization within 4 weeks of MI; the overall operative mortality rate was 4.4%, and there was a 26% incidence rate of low cardiac output after surgery (defined as need for intraaortic balloon pumping or catecholamine support). Preoperative left ventricular failure, reduced left ventricular ejection fraction, and preoperative ischemia (need for intravenous nitroglycerin) were independent predictors of postoperative cardiac failure, but the time interval between MI and surgery was not an important predictor of postoperative cardiac failure. Hochberg and associates (16) studied the interaction of preoperative left ventricular dysfunction and interval to operation on operative risk. They reported no early deaths among 50 patients with preoperative ejection fraction greater than 50% who underwent coronary bypass within 4 weeks of MI. When preoperative ejection fraction was less than 50%, however, operative risk was 22% for patients who had revascularization within 7 weeks of infarction, and risk decreased from approximately 50% when surgery was undertaken within 2 weeks to 6% when surgery was 6 to 7 weeks after MI.

More recent evidence suggests that for nonemergent operations, there is little incremental risk for surgical revascularization early after MI. Sintek and associates (17) reported an operative mortality rate of 4.4% for 23 patients having surgery within 24 hours of AMI, 2.1% for 193 patients having revascularization between 3 and 7 days after infarction, and 1.4% for 284 patients undergoing revascularization between 1 week and 1 month after infarction. This is similar to the operative risk among 1,645 patients without recent infarction, for whom the mortality rate was 1.9%. The small difference in risk among the groups was neutralized when other risk factors (reoperation, sex, and age) were entered into a multivariate analysis. The authors concluded that nonemergency surgical revascularization can be undertaken safely at any time interval after AMI–certainly after 72 hours–with no increase in operative mortality and acceptable morbidity. These findings are similar to those reported by Phillips and coworkers (12,13) and Kirlin and associates (18) who found no relation between in-hospital mortality and the interval between infarct and operation.

Despite these reports, recent data from the New York State database support the notion that at least some additional risk is incurred for patients subjected to surgery during or early after MI. Using this database from 1991 to 1996, Lee and coworkers (19) found a steady decline in operative mortality as the interval between onset of infarction and surgical intervention increased. Patients undergoing revascularization with 6 hours had an observed mortality rate of

14.2%, whereas the rate for those undergoing surgery between 6 and 24 hours was 13.8%. The risk between 1 and 3 days was 7.9%, decreasing to 3.8% between 4 and 7 days, and 2.9% at 7 to 14 days. Multivariable analysis revealed revascularization within 3 days to be an independent risk factor for death.

As might be expected, perioperative risk appears to be related to the nature of the infarct. An early study by these same authors (20), again using the New York State database, indicated that although overall operative mortality did not differ between patients with acute transmural and nontransmural infarcts (mortality rate 3.1%), the risk of surgery was greater within the first 6 hours for nontransmural infarcts (11.5%) and within the first 24 hours for transmural infarcts (12.1% within 6 hours, 13.6% between 6 and 24 hours). The most powerful predictor of death in this study, however, was preoperative cardiogenic shock.

Should surgery be delayed, then, for elective revascularization after AMI? In clinical practice, timing of surgical intervention after MI often is dictated by the patient's response to antianginal therapy. Those patients who receive intensive medical therapy and continue to have angina at rest or with little activity should be referred for revascularization (21). If, in contrast, ischemic symptoms are promptly controlled with intravenous nitroglycerin and heparin, it may be reasonable to begin oral medications and gradually wean intravenous therapy. If patients remain free of ischemic symptoms, an interval of 7 to 10 days before revascularization may reduce the risk of surgery.

CORONARY ARTERY BYPASS FOR ACUTE INFARCTION IN THE SETTING OF SHOCK

It is quite clear that operative mortality is significant for patients in shock. The magnitude of this risk, as assessed in retrospective studies, is difficult to ascertain given the bias imposed by patient selection, as noted earlier. Athansuleas and coworkers (22) analyzed risk factors for early death among 83 patients having CAB during acute evolving MI. Time to reperfusion did not influence outcome, nor did the infarct-related artery. The overall mortality rate was 15.6%, however, and risk was increased in patients with cardiogenic shock, age older than 65 years, left ventricular ejection fraction less than or equal to 0.30, cardiac index less than 2.0 L per minute per square meter, and absent collateral flow. Allen and colleagues (23) reported an early mortality rate of 9% among 66 patients in preoperative shock treated surgically with controlled reperfusion using substrate-enhanced cardioplegia. Albes and colleagues (24) reported a 15.4% operative mortality rate among patients with acute infarction and postinfarction angina complicated by hemodynamic instability. Previous studies have also documented preoperative intraaortic balloon support, renal dysfunction, and depressed left ventricular function as risk factors (14).

More sobering data came from the Should We Emergently Revascularize Occluded Coronaries for Cardiogenic Shock (SHOCK) trial (25). In this multicenter trial, patients were prospectively randomized to emergent revascularization or initial medical stabilization. Overall, the 30-day mortality rate of patients undergoing revascularization was not significantly different from the medically treated group (46.7% vs. 56.0%). Of patients undergoing revascularization, 36% had surgical intervention with an observed mortality rate of 42.1% as compared with 45.3% among those undergoing PCI. The surgical group, as one would anticipate, had more extensive disease (left main or triple-vessel disease), and these patients were revascularized somewhat later than the PCI group (2.7 vs. 0.9 hours).

CORONARY ARTERY BYPASS EARLY AFTER THROMBOLYSIS

The emergence of thrombolytic therapy for MI has created a new subset of patients who are referred for coronary artery revascularization. Successful dissolution of intracoronary thrombus often reveals high-grade, fixed obstructions that are prone to reocclusion despite aggressive anticoagulation. Available data suggest that approximately 38% of patients treated with thrombolytic agents will undergo CAB during their initial hospitalization (26–32). Indications for surgery include residual high-grade stenoses after successful thrombolysis, unsuccessful reperfusion by thrombolytic therapy (or PCI), and/or discovery of severe, diffuse coronary artery disease (33). In the Thrombolysis and Angioplasty for Myocardial Infarction (TAMI) trial, emergency CAB was performed in 24 of 386 consecutive patients (6%); the surgery was prompted by left main or equivalent coronary artery disease (7 patients), coronary anatomy unsuitable for angioplasty (4 patients), or unsuccessful angioplasty (13 patients) (31). Other groups have chosen to proceed with CAB in preference to angioplasty as the primary therapy for patients with multivessel coronary disease who have received successful thrombolysis (30).

One specific concern with surgical revascularization early after thrombolysis is postoperative bleeding because of coagulopathy. The risk for postoperative bleeding appears to be related to the interval between thrombolytic therapy and surgery. In a literature survey, Lee and associates (34) found no increase in postoperative bleeding or mortality in 329 patients who had CAB from 3.3 to 16 days after streptokinase infusion. In their institutional experience, however, postoperative blood loss and use of blood and blood products were considerably greater in patients who had revascularization with 12 hours of thrombolysis compared with control subjects or those who had later surgery.

It has been hypothesized that the specificity of tissue plasminogen activator might preserve clotting factors and reduce bleeding complications. In the TAMI trial, however, excessive postoperative bleeding developed in 4 of 24 patients (16.6%; 70% confidence limits, 8.8–24.6%); coagulopathy, as a result of thrombolysis, was the probable cause of the bleeding in 2 patients (5.6%; 70% confidence limits,

2.5–14.1%) (31). The serine proteinase inhibitor aprotinin, a powerful antifibrinolytic that reduces postoperative bleeding in patients having primary coronary revascularization and in patients undergoing surgery for coronary bypass (35), may be particularly useful to reverse the lytic state in patients having coronary revascularization early after thrombolysis (36).

Thrombolytic therapy is typically followed by use of platelet inhibitors such as abciximab, tirofiban, or eptifibatide. Excessive bleeding after CAB has been reported within 12 hours after the use of abciximab, a monoclonal antibody that irreversibly binds to the glycoprotein IIb/IIIa receptor (37). When surgery is unavoidable in this circumstance, platelet transfusion should be anticipated and use of antifibrinolytics or off-pump surgery should be considered. Because tirofiban and eptifibatide are reversible antagonists, simple delay of surgery for 2 to 4 hours after discontinuing their use may be adequate to prevent excessive postoperative hemorrhage.

CORONARY ARTERY BYPASS FOR UNSTABLE ANGINA PECTORIS: RISKS

Early reports (38,39) of high operative mortality in unstable patients with AMI should be interpreted in the context of previous methods of preoperative care, anesthetic management, and myocardial protection which would be considered inadequate by contemporary standards. Furthermore, there is overlap of clinical syndromes between unstable angina and completed transmural (Q-wave) infarction, and it is likely that some patients in these previous reports had evolving MI rather than reversible ischemia.

Early after MI, occurrence of angina (or its physiologic equivalent) at rest or with little exercise identifies patients at high risk for recurrent infarction or cardiac death without revascularization. In the report by Schuster and Bulkley (40), the 6-month mortality rate was 44% for those patients with ischemia in the region of an AMI and 72% for patients in whom ischemia after AMI occurred in distant myocardium. In the short-term, prognosis for patients with subendocardial infarction may be better than that for patients with Q-wave infarction, but late events occur frequently. This is supported by the work of Hutter and colleagues (41), who found that risk for early death is less in patients with subendocardial MI compared with transmural infarction (9% vs. 12%), but risk for reinfarction after subendocardial infarction is 21% within 9 months. Marmor and associates (42) found that recurrent infarction developed in 42% of patients with subendocardial infarction, and the mortality rate (16%) was more than twice that observed in patients without recurrent ischemia.

Management of patients with unstable postinfarction angina has changed as techniques for revascularization have improved. Roberts and coworkers (43) advocated intensive medical stabilization of patients with postinfarction angina in hopes of decreasing operative mortality and perioperative myocardial damage. Although angina can be controlled in most instances, such patients will have restricted activities and will remain in continued jeopardy of further myocardial loss from critically narrowed vessels; unless the additional risk for balloon angioplasty or early surgical revascularization is substantial, both physicians and patients prefer definitive revascularization during the same hospital stay.

As data have accumulated it has become clear that operative risk is acceptably low for most subsets of patients with unstable postinfarction angina (44–50). Precise estimation of operative risk is difficult because some contemporary surgical reviews of CAB within 30 days of MI have included other clinical subgroups such as those with little or no angina but "compelling anatomy" (proximal high-grade narrowing of one or more of the three major vessels) who may have lower operative mortality, as well as patients with severe left ventricular failure who have high operative risk.

A reasonable estimate of perioperative risk in the current era for patients with unstable angina early after MI is 5% to 8%. This is certainly greater than the risk for patients with unstable angina without MI. In the experience of the University of Toronto from 1982 through 1987, the operative mortality rate for patients with unstable angina without recent MI was 4.0% (50) while that for patients with unstable angina and recent (<30 days) subendocardial MI was 8.3%. This risk increased to 17.5% for those patients with unstable angina and recent Q-wave MI.

For patients with unstable angina undergoing surgical revascularization early after MI, operative risk can be stratified further by the presence or absence of unstable hemodynamics and/or angina pectoris that is so severe that intraaortic balloon counterpulsation is necessary; such patients are at greatest risk for postoperative death. Naunheim and associates (51) reported operative risks of 6.1% for patients with unstable postinfarction angina without shock and 47.8% for revascularization in patients with severe postinfarction ischemia or infarct extension complicated by cardiogenic shock. Similarly, Connolly and coworkers (47) found that for patients undergoing CAB within 6 weeks of MI, the perioperative mortality rate was 28% in those with cardiogenic shock compared with 3.7% for those with unstable angina.

CORONARY ARTERY BYPASS FOR ACUTE CORONARY SYNDROMES: LONG-TERM BENEFITS

The long-term outlook after surgery for postinfarction angina is excellent. In a review of outcome of CAB for unstable angina, Rahimtoola and associates (52) reported that late postoperative survival was similar in patients with postinfarction angina compared with those having rest angina without recent infarction of progressive angina of recent onset; 5- and 10-year actuarial survival rates were 92% and 83%, respectively. In fact, survival of patients after CAB for unstable angina equals or exceeds that of patients undergoing surgery for stable angina. The 15-year survival rate after surgery for unstable angina was 59% compared with 55% for patients with stable angina before surgery.

Several studies have been directed toward defining the impact of revascularization for acute coronary syndromes on late outcomes. In the setting of a non–ST-segment elevation infarction, the recent randomized controlled trials (second Fragmin and Fast Revascularization During Instability in Coronary Artery Disease [FRISC II], Treat Angina with Aggrastat and Determine Cost of Therapy with an Invasive or Conservative Strategy [TACTICS], and VINO trials [53–55]) generally favor revascularization among high-risk (e.g., older patients, patients with diabetes, those with ST-segment depression on electrocardiogram, and those with increased creatine phospho kinase [CPK]-MB or serum troponins) patients. Two multicenter trials and one single-center randomized trial involving a total of 823 have specifically evaluated the relative merits of CAB surgery and medical therapy in unstable angina, although some subsets of patients (left main disease, ejection fraction <30%, and age >70 years) were not included. In the Veterans Administration (VA) cooperative study (56), although no difference in progression to Q-wave MI was observed, survival and freedom from recurrent angina were superior with surgery. Similarly, the National Cooperative Study Group Trial (57) showed no difference in progression to Q-wave MI, but less severe subsequent angina with surgery. Unlike the VA trial, however, there was no survival difference at 2 years (90% in both groups), although 32% of the medical group crossed over to surgery by 24 months. Finally, in the single-center study of 113 patients reported by Bertolasi and colleagues (58), there was less subsequent angina, fewer infarctions, and a survival benefit for surgery in short-term follow-up.

Subset analysis of the Thrombolysis in Myocardial Ischemia (TIMI) IIIB also has demonstrated a trend in favor of an aggressive approach to revascularization over medical therapy in patients at greater risk as characterized by an increased CPK-MB fraction (non–Q-wave myocardial infarction) (59).

In contrast, a greater early mortality rate—specifically a perioperative mortality rate of 7.7% among patients undergoing CAB—was observed in the Veterans Affairs Non–Q-Wave Infarcts and Strategies in Hospitals (VANQWISH) trial (60). The opposite result, however, was found in FRISC II (52). These investigators found a benefit with early revascularization, particularly among patients with increased troponin. The reasons for such different results among these studies are likely because of differences in patient populations studied. It is likely that the patients at greater risk benefit from an aggressive approach, whereas patients at lower risk have less to gain, but still risk adverse consequences. The results of the Randomized Intervention Trial (RITA) 3 also support an aggressive approach to revascularization because of lower rates of angina without increased risk for death or infarction (61). The results of the Danish trial in Acute Myocardial Infarction (DANAMI) study also support revascularization (62). In this study of patients with evidence of inducible ischemia after successful thrombolytic therapy for first-time MI, revascularization either by either surgical or percutaneous techniques resulted in less

risk for reinfarction or readmission with unstable angina or incidence of stable angina at 1-year follow-up compared with medical therapy.

CORONARY ARTERY BYPASS OR PERCUTANEOUS CORONARY INTERVENTION FOR ACUTE CORONARY SYNDROME?

Improvements in PCI techniques have, as noted earlier, placed interventional cardiology on the front line in the management of many patients with acute coronary syndrome. Several studies comparing PCI and CAB in the setting of ACS have been reported, all with similar results. When the results of PCI were compared with those of CAB in the DANAMI trial, despite more severe coronary artery disease in the therapeutic than the surgical group, there was no difference in survival at 2.4 years (63). Rates of recurrent angina (10.2% vs 25.6%; $p = 0.0002$) or repeat revascularization (0% vs. 15.4%) were less in the surgical patients. The Angina With Extremely Serious Operative Mortality Evaluation (AWESOME) trial (64) demonstrated no difference in 6-month or 3-year survival rates between PCI and CAB in the management of patients with postinfarction angina and at least one of five risk factors (prior heart surgery, infarct within 7 days, left ventricular ejection fraction <35%, age >70 years, preoperative intraaortic balloon) for adverse outcome with surgery. Similar results have been reported for the diabetic subgroup analysis (65) and for the subset with prior CAB (66).

The results reported by deFeyter and associates (67) from the University Hospital in Rotterdam confirmed those findings among 450 patients with unstable angina as compared with another 755 patients with stable angina. Patients in each group were randomized to CAB or PCI with stents. There was no difference at 1 year in death, MI, or stroke among patients in any of the four groups. As may be anticipated, however, the rate of reintervention was greater in the PCI groups than the CAB groups. Whether the advent of coated stents will impact this reintervention rate is a matter of speculation.

ROLE OF "OFF-PUMP" CORONARY ARTERY BYPASS IN ACUTE CORONARY SYNDROME

Advocates of "off-pump" or "beating heart" CAB argue that surgical mortality and morbidity rates can be reduced by avoiding the use of cardiopulmonary bypass. Although none of the randomized studies of off-pump versus on-pump CAB published thus far has demonstrated a reduction in perioperative death, stroke, or MI (68–73), enthusiasts argue that the advantage of this approach will become most apparent among patients at high risk. Those patients with recent MI or unstable angina should reasonably fall into this group.

Benetti (74), one of the true pioneers of this approach, reported no mortalities among 32 patients with acute transmural MIs operated off-pump over a 17-year period. These are excellent results, but no doubt this was a highly selective population. More recently, Mohr (75) reported an operative mortality rate of 1.7% among 57 patients with an AMI operated off-pump (75). Of these patients, 32 underwent surgery within 48 hours of infarction.

More recently, Meharwal and colleagues (76) reviewed more than 1,000 off-pump cases and compared the results with those obtained with cardiopulmonary bypass in more than 2,000 patients at their institution. Among the off-pump patients, 2% had an AMI and 37% had unstable angina pectoris. Although the patients with ACS were not examined as a subgroup, the observed mortality rate was no different between groups. This study can be taken as evidence that off-pump CAB may be done, but it does not demonstrate superiority. The same could be said of Bittner's (77) study of 57 patients judged "high risk" by virtue of a Parsonnet score greater than 15. In the study group, three-fourths of the patients had unstable angina and 10 had experienced MI within 24 hours. The mortality rate was an acceptable 3.5%, but there was no control group for comparison.

Finally, the study reported by Locker and associates (78) gives some reason for pause. In their nonrandomized study of 77 patients undergoing CAB within 48 hours of MI between 1992 and 1998, 37 patients had surgery on pump with an observed mortality rate of 24%. Among 40 patients having off-pump CAB, the mortality rate was 5%. Without doubt, the off-pump group had better early results, although the high mortality rate among on-pump patients, and accordingly the comparability of patients in both groups, must be questioned. Equally sobering are the statistics for late results, with lower rates of recurrent angina (0% vs. 15%), lower rates of reintervention (0% vs. 15%), and lower late mortality rates (0% vs. 22%) in the on-pump group as compared with off-pump.

In summary, as is the case in general for off-pump CAB, despite enthusiasm among its advocates, the place of off-pump CAB in the management of acute coronary system remains uncertain.

SUMMARY

Early studies of CAB in AMI established the effectiveness of early reperfusion in myocardial salvage. Indeed, basic concepts of pathogenesis of infarction and the critical role of intracoronary thrombus in acute coronary syndromes were defined in clinical studies of surgical revascularization. Although thrombolytic agents and PCI have superseded surgery for most patients with acute infarction, there remains an important role for CAB in patients with unsuccessful reperfusion, among who have postinfarction angina, and in subsets of patients with successful recanalization who have associated critical stenoses in other vessels or left main coronary artery narrowing, or both.

Patients with angina after MI should have prompt medical treatment and early angiography. Balloon angioplasty will

be possible in many patients with single-vessel involvement; however, American Heart Association Guidelines (79) continue to advocate CAB for patients with stenosis of the left main coronary artery ($\geq$50%) and/or significant narrowing in three major vessels or two vessels if the proximal left anterior descending is involved and there is evidence of ischemia or depressed left ventricular function (Class I indications). Surgery also should be considered (Class IIa indications) in patients with multiple stenoses of saphenous vein grafts, and in the presence of multivessel disease and diabetes mellitus. Either CAB or PCI is indicated in the presence of two-vessel disease when a large area of myocardium is at risk in the absence of proximal left anterior descending disease (Class I indications), and should be considered (Class IIa indications) in single-vessel disease with proximal left anterior descending stenosis or single- or double-vessel disease with a moderate area at risk.

From a practical standpoint, revascularization should be considered for all patients with persistent angina despite optimal medical management, which includes intravenous nitroglycerin and heparin; the only exceptions to this policy are those patients with advanced age and infirmity and/or serious associated medical illnesses. Intraaortic balloon support is used only for those patients who are hemodynamically unstable en route to surgery. For patients with multivessel coronary disease whose angina after MI is controlled medically, we generally advise early surgery if ventricular function is preserved; revascularization is delayed (>1 week) if left ventricular function is significantly impaired (ejection fraction <40%) in hopes of minimizing operative mortality. This policy seems prudent as long as patients whose surgery is postponed can be followed closely.

REFERENCES

1. Stone GW, Brodie BR, Griffin JJ, et al. Role of cardiac surgery in the hospital phase management of patients treated with primary angioplasty for acute myocardial infarction. *Am J Cardiol* 2000;85:1292–1296.
2. Koyama Y, Hansen PS, Hanratty CG, et al. Prevalence of coronary occlusion and outcome of an immediate invasive strategy in suspected acute myocardial infarction with and without ST-segment elevation. *Am J Cardiol* 2002;90:579–584.
3. Tu JV, Pashos CL, Naylor CD, et al. Use of cardiac procedures and outcomes in elderly patients with myocardial infarction in the United States and Canada 1997. *N Engl J Med* 1997;336:1500–1505.
4. DeWood MA, Spores J, Berg R Jr, et al. Acute myocardial infarction: a decade of experience with surgical reperfusion in 701 patients. *Circulation* 1983;68:II-8–II-16.
5. DeWood MA, Spores J, Notske RN, et al. Medical and surgical management of myocardial infarction. *Am J Cardiol* 1979;44:1356–1364.
6. DeWood MA, Heit J, Spores J, et al. Anterior transmural myocardial infarction: effects of surgical coronary reperfusion on global and regional left ventricular function. *J Am Coll Cardiol* 1983;1:1223–1234.
7. Berg R Jr, Selinger SL, Leonard JJ, et al. Acute evolving myocardial infarction. A surgical emergency. *J Thorac Cardiovasc Surg* 1984;88:902–906.
8. DeWood MA, Berg R Jr. The role of surgical reperfusion in myocardial infarction. *Cardiol Clin* 1984;2:113–122.
9. DeWood MA, Selinger SL, Coleman WS, et al. Surgical coronary reperfusion during acute myocardial infarction. *Cardiovasc Clin* 1987;17:91–103.
10. DeWood MA, Notske RN, Berg R Jr, et al. Medical and surgical man-

agement of early Q wave myocardial infarction. I. Effects of surgical reperfusion on survival, recurrent myocardial infarction, sudden death and functional class at 10 or more years of follow-up. *J Am Coll Cardiol* 1989;14:65–77.

11. DeWood MA, Leonard J, Grunwald RP, et al. Medical and surgical management of early Q wave myocardial infarction. II. Effects on mortality and global and regional left ventricular function at 10 or more years of follow-up. *J Am Coll Cardiol* 1989;14:78–90.

12. Phillips SJ, Kongtahworn C, Skinner JR, et al. Emergency coronary artery reperfusion: a choice therapy for evolving myocardial infarction. Results in 339 patients. *J Thorac Cardiovasc Surg* 1983;86:679–688.

13. Phillips SJ, Zeff RH, Kongtahworn C, et al. Surgery for evolving myocardial infarction. *JAMA* 1982;248:1325–1328.

14. Lee JH, Murrell HK, Strony J, et al. Risk analysis of coronary bypass surgery after acute myocardial infarction. *Surgery* 1997;122:675–680.

15. Katz NM, Kubanick TE, Ahmed SW, et al. Determinants of cardiac failure after coronary bypass surgery within 30 days of acute myocardial infarction. *Ann Thorac Surg* 1986;42:658–663.

16. Hochberg MS, Parsonnet V, Gielchinsky I, et al. Timing of coronary revascularization after acute myocardial infarction. Early and late results in patients revascularized within seven weeks. *J Thorac Cardiovasc Surg* 1984;88:914–921.

17. Sintek CF, Pfeffer TA, Khonsari S. Surgical revascularization after acute myocardial infarction. Does timing make a difference? *J Thorac Cardiovasc Surg* 1994;107:1317–1321.

18. Kirlin JK, Blackstone EH, Zorn GL Jr, et al. Intermediate-term results of coronary artery bypass grafting for acute myocardial infarction. *Circulation* 1985;72:II-175–II-178.

19. Lee DC, Oz MC, Weinberg AD, et al. Appropriate timing of surgical intervention after transmural acute myocardial infarction. *J Thorac Cardiovasc Surg* 2003;125:115–119.

20. Lee DC, Oz MC, Weinberg AD, et al. Optimal timing of revascularization: transmural versus nontransmural acute myocardial infarction. *Ann Thorac Surg* 2001;71:1197–1202.

21. Braunwald E, Jones RH, Mark DB, et al. Diagnosing and managing unstable angina. Agency for Health Care Policy and Research. *Circulation* 1994;90:613–622.

22. Athansuleas CL, Geer DA, Arciniegas JG, et al. A reappraisal of surgical intervention for acute myocardial infarction. *J Thorac Cardiovasc Surg* 1987;93:405–414.

23. Allen BS, Buckberg GD, Fontan FM, et al. Superiority of controlled reperfusion versus percutaneous transluminal coronary angioplasty in acute coronary occlusion. *J Thorac Cardiovasc Surg* 1993;105:864–884.

24. Albes JM, Gross M, Franke U, et al. Revascularization during acute myocardial infarction: risks and benefits revisited. *Ann Thorac Surg* 2002;74:102–108.

25. Hochman JS, Sleeper LA, Webb JG, et al. Early revascularization in acute myocardial infarction complicated by cardiogenic shock. SHOCK Investigators. Should We Emergently Revascularize Occluded Coronaries for Cardiogenic Shock. *N Engl J Med* 1999;341:625–634.

26. Wilson JM, Held JS, Wright CB, et al. Coronary artery bypass surgery following thrombolytic therapy for acute coronary thrombosis. *Ann Thorac Surg* 1984;37:212–217.

27. Rodewald G, Mathey D, Krebber HJ. Bypass surgery following thrombolytic therapy. *Z Kardiol* 1985;74:143–146.

28. Messmer BJ, von Essen R, Minale C, et al. Intracoronary thrombolysis and early bypass surgery for acute myocardial infarct: five years' experience. *Thorac Cardiovasc Surg* 1986;34:1–4.

29. Salem BI, Gowda S, Haikal M, et al. Early percutaneous transluminal coronary angioplasty or coronary bypass surgery following thrombolytic treatment of acute myocardial infarction. *Chest* 1987;91:648–653.

30. Taylor GJ, Moses HW, Katholi RE, et al. Six-year survival after coronary thrombolysis and early revascularization for acute myocardial infarction. *Am J Cardiol* 1992;70:26–30.

31. Kereiakes DJ, Topol EJ, George BS, et al. Favorable early and long-term prognosis following coronary bypass surgery therapy for myocardial infarction: results of a multicenter trial. TAMI Study Group. *Am Heart J* 1989;118:199–207.

32. Messmer BJ, Uebis R, Rieger C, et al. Late results after intracoronary thrombolysis and early bypass grafting for acute myocardial infarction. *J Thorac Cardiovasc Surg* 1989;97:10–18.

33. Barner HB, Lea JW 4th, Naunheim KS, et al. Emergency coronary bypass not associated with preoperative cardiogenic shock in failed an-

gioplasty, after thrombolysis, and for acute myocardial infarction. *Circulation* 1989;79:I-152–I-159.

34. Lee KF, Mandell J. Rankin JS, et al. Immediate versus delayed coronary grafting after streptokinase treatment. Postoperative blood loss and clinical results. *J Thorac Cardiovasc Surg* 1988;95:216–222.

35. Lemmer JH Jr, Stanford W, Bonney SL, et al. Aprotinin for coronary bypass operations: efficacy, safety, and influence on early saphenous graft patency: a multicenter, randomized, double-blind, placebo-controlled study. *J Thorac Cardiovasc Surg* 1994;107:543–553.

36. Efstratiadis T, Munsch C, Crossman D, et al. Aprotinin used in emergency coronary operation after streptokinase treatment. *Ann Thorac Surg* 1992;54:1022–1023.

37. Alvrez JM. Emergency coronary bypass grafting for failed percutaneous coronary artery stenting: increased costs and platelet transfusion requirements after the use of abciximab. *J Thorac Cardiovasc Surg* 1998;115:472–473.

38. Cheanvechai C, Effler DB, Loop FD, et al. Aortocoronary artery graft during early and late phases of acute myocardial infarction. *Ann Thorac Surg* 1973;16:249–260.

39. Dawson JT, Hall RJ, Hallman GL, et al. Mortality in patients undergoing coronary artery bypass surgery after myocardial infarction. *Am J Cardiol* 1974;33:483–486.

40. Schuster EH, Bulkley BH. Early post-infarction angina. Ischemia at a distance and ischemia in the infarct zone. *N Engl J Med* 1981;305:1101–1105.

41. Hutter AM Jr, DeSanctis RW, Flynn T, et al. Nontransmural myocardial infarction: a comparison of hospital and late clinical course of patients with that of matched patients with transmural anterior and transmural inferior myocardial infarction. *Am J Cardiol* 1981;48:595–602.

42. Marmor A, Sobel BE, Roberts R. Factors presaging early recurrent myocardial infarction ("extension"). *Am J Cardiol* 1981;48:603–610.

43. Roberts AJ, Sanders JH Jr, Moran JH, et al. The efficacy of medical stabilization prior to myocardial revascularization in early refractory postinfarction angina. *Ann Surg* 1983;197:91–98.

44. Breyer RH, Engelman RM, Rousou JA, et al. Postinfarction angina: an expanding subset of patients undergoing coronary artery bypass. *J Thorac Cardiovasc Surg* 1985;90:532–540.

45. Jones RN, Pifarre R, Sullivan HJ, et al. Early myocardial revascularization for postinfarction angina. *Ann Thorac Surg* 1987;44:159–163.

46. Naunheim KS, Kesler KA, Kanter KR, et al. Coronary artery bypass for recent infarction. Predictors of mortality. *Circulation* 1988;78:I122–I128.

47. Connolly MW, Gelbfish JS, Rose DM, et al. Early coronary artery bypass grafting for complicated acute myocardial infarction. *J Cardiovasc Surg (Torino)* 1988;29:375–382.

48. Kouchoukos NT, Murphy S, Philpott T, et al. Coronary artery bypass grafting for postinarction angina pectoris. *Circulation* 1989;79:I68–I72.

49. Gardner TJ, Stuart RS, Greene PS, et al. The risk of coronary bypass surgery for patients with postinfarction angina. *Circulation* 1989;79:I79–I80.

50. Fremes SE, Goldman BS, Weisel RD, et al. Recent preoperative myocardial infarction increases the risk of surgery for unstable angina. *J Cardiac Surg* 1991;6:2–12.

51. Naunheim KS, Kesler KA, Kanter KR, et al. Coronary artery bypass for recent infarction. Predictors of mortality. *Circulation* 1988;78:I122–I128.

52. Rahimtoola SH, Nunley D, Grunkemeier G, et al. Ten-year survival after coronary bypass surgery for unstable angina. *N Engl J Med* 1983;308:676–681.

53. Wallentin L, Lagerqvist B, Husted S, et al. Outcome at 1 year after an invasive compared with a non-invasive strategy in unstable coronary artery disease: the FRISC II invasive randomised trial, FRISC II Investigators. Fast revascularisation during instability in coronary artery disease. *Lancet* 2000;356:9–16.

54. Cannon CP, Wientraub WS, Demopoulos LA, et al. Comparison of early invasive and conservative strategies in patients with unstable coronary syndromes treated with the glycoprotein IIb/IIIa inhibitor tirofiban. *N Engl J Med* 2000;344:1879–1897.

55. Spacek R, Widimsky P, Straka Z, et al. Value of first day angiography/angioplasty in evolving non-ST segment elevation myocardial infarction: an open multicentre randomized trial. The VINO study. *Eur Heart J* 2002;23:230–238.

56. Luchi RJ, Scott SM, Deupree RH, et al. Comparison of medical and surgical treatment for unstable angina pectoris: results of a Veterans Administration cooperative study. *N Engl J Med* 1987;316:977.

57. Unstable angina pectoris: National Cooperative Study Group to Compare Surgical and Medical Therapy. *Am J Cardiol* 1978;42:839–848.

58. Bertolasi CA, Tronge JE, Riccitelli MA, et al. Natural history of unstable angina with medical or surgical therapy. *Chest* 1976;70:596–605.

59. Anderson HV, Cannon CP, Stone PH, et al. One-year results of the Thrombolysis in Myocardial Ischemia (TIMI) IIIB clinical trial. A randomized comparison of tissue-type plasminogen activator versus placebo and early invasive versus early conservative strategies in unstable angina and non-Q wave myocardial infarction. *J Am Coll Cardiol* 1995;26:1643–1650.

60. Boden WE, O'Rourke RA, Crawford MH, et al. Outcomes in patients with acute non-Q-wave myocardial infarction randomly assigned to an invasive as compared with a conservative management strategy. Veterans Affairs Non-Q-Wave Infarction Strategies in Hospital (VANQWISH) Trial Investigators. *N Engl J Med* 1998;338:1785–1792.

61. Fox KA, Poole-Wilson PA, Henderson RA, et al. Randomized Intervention Trial of Unstable Angina Investigators. Interventional versus conservative treatment for patients with unstable angina or non-ST-elevation myocardial infarction: the British Heart Foundation RITA 3 randomised trial. *Lancet* 2002;360:743–751.

62. Madsen JK, Grande P, Saunamaki K, et al. Danish multicenter randomized study of invasive versus conservative treatment in patients with inducible ischemia after thrombolysis in acute myocardial infarction (DANAMI). Danish trial in Acute Myocardial Infarction. *Circulation* 1997;96:748–755.

63. Hjelms E, Alstrup P, Paulsen PK, et al. CABG shortly after AMI treated with thrombolysis: an analysis of the surgical group and a comparison with PTCA in the DANAMI study. Danish multicenter randomized study of invasive versus conservative treatment in patients with inducible ischemia after thrombolysis in acute myocardial infarction. *Eur J Cardiothorac Surg* 1998;13:555–558.

64. Morrison DA, Sethi G, Sacks J, et al. Angina With Extremely Serious Operative Mortality Evaluation (AWESOME). Percutaneous coronary intervention versus coronary artery bypass graft surgery for patients with medically refractory myocardial ischemia and risk factors for adverse outcomes with bypass: a multicenter, randomized trial. Investigators of the Department of Veterans Affairs Cooperative Study #385, the Angina With Extremely Serious Operative Mortality Evaluation (AWESOME). *J Am Coll Cardiol* 2001;38:143–149.

65. Sedlis SP, Morrison DA, Loris JD, et al. Investigators of the Department of Veterans Affairs Cooperative Study #385, the Angina with Extremely Serious Operative Mortality Evaluation (AWESOME). Percutaneous coronary intervention versus coronary bypass graft surgery for diabetic patients with unstable angina and risk factors for adverse outcomes with bypass: outcome of diabetic patients in the AWESOME randomized trial and registry. *J Am Coll Cardiol* 2002;40:1555–1566.

66. Morrison DA, Sethi G, Sacks J, et al. Investigators of the Department of Veterans Affairs Cooperative Study #385, Angina with Extremely Serious Operative Mortality Evaluation. Percutaneous coronary intervention versus repeat bypass surgery for patients with medically refractor myocardial experience with post-CABG patients.

67. De Feyter PJ, Serruys PW, Under F, et al. Bypass surgery versus stenting for the treatment of multivessel disease in patients with unstable angina compared with stable angina. *Circulation* 2002;105:2367–2372.

68. Ascione R, Williams S, Lloyd CT, et al. Reduced postoperative blood loss and transfusion requirement after beating-heart coronary operations: a prospective randomized study. *J Thorac Cardiovasc Surg* 2001; 121:689–696.

69. Zamvar V, Williams D, Hall J, et al. Assessment of neurocognitive impairment after off-pump and on-pump techniques for coronary artery bypass graft surgery: prospective randomised controlled trial. *BMJ* 2002;325:1268.

70. Van Dijk D, Nierich AP, Jansen EW, et al., Octopus Study Group. Early outcome after off-pump versus on-pump coronary bypass surgery: results from a randomized study. *Circulation* 2001;104:1761–1766.

71. Angelini GD, Taylor FC, Reeves BC, et al. Early and midterm outcome after off-pump and on-pump surgery in Beating Heart Against Cardioplegic Arrest Studies (BHACAS 1 and 2): a pooled analysis of two randomised controlled trials. *Lancet* 2002;359:1194–1199.

72. Puskas JD, Williams WH, Duke PG, et al. Off-pump coronary artery bypass grafting provides complete revascularization while reducing myocardial injury, transfusion requirements and length of stay: prospective randomized comparison of 200 unselected patients having OPCAB versus conventional CABG. Presented at the 82nd Annual Meeting of the American Association for Thoracic Surgery; May 2002; Washington, DC.

73. Nathoe HM, van Dijk D, Jansen EW, et al., Octopus Study Group. A comparison of on-pump and off-pump coronary bypass surgery in low-risk patients. *N Engl J Med* 2003;348:394–402.

74. Benetti F, Mariani MA, Sani G, et al. Video-assisted minimally invasive coronary operations without cardiopulmonary bypass: a multicenter study. *J Thorac Cardiovasc Surg* 1996;112:1478–1484.

75. Mohr R, Moshkovitch Y, Shapira I, et al. Coronary artery bypass without cardiopulmonary bypass for patients with acute myocardial infarction. *J Thorac Cardiovasc Surg* 1999;118:50–56.

76. Meharwal ZS, Mishra YK, Kohli V, et al. Off-pump multivessel coronary artery surgery in high-risk patients. *Ann Thorac Surg* 2002;74: S1353–S1357.

77. Bittner HB, Savitt MA. Off pump coronary artery bypass grafting decreases morbidity and mortality in a selected group of high-risk patients. *Ann Thorac Surg* 2002;74:115–118.

78. Locker C, Shapira I, Paz Y, et al. Emergency myocardial revascularization for acute myocardial infarction: survival benefits of avoiding cardiopulmonary bypass. *Eur J Cardiothorac Surg* 2000;17:234–238.

79. American College of Cardiology/American Heart Association Task Force on Practice Guidelines (Committee on the Management of Patients with Unstable Angina). ACC/AHA guidelines for the management of patients with unstable angina and non-ST segment elevation myocardial infarction: executive summary and recommendations. *Catheter Cardiovasc Interv* 2000;51:505–521.

CHAPTER 77

Management of the Patient with Unstable Angina, Non–ST-Segment Elevation, and ST-Segment Elevation Myocardial Infarction after Initial Stabilization and after Discharge

Robert S. Gibson and James T. Willerson

Key Words: Angina; myocardial infarction; practice guidelines.

The term *acute coronary syndrome* (ACS) has evolved as a useful descriptor to refer to any constellation of clinical signs or symptoms compatible with acute myocardial ischemia. It encompasses acute myocardial infarction (AMI) with or without ST-segment elevation on the resting electrocardiogram (ECG), as well as unstable angina. In most cases, the pathophysiology involves a primary decrease in myocardial oxygen supply (1–15) caused by endothelial dysfunction and injury at the site of a vulnerable coronary artery plaque (6), with resultant intracoronary thrombus formation and associated vaso-

constriction (4–6,9–11). Patients with acute ST-segment elevation MI (STEMI) often have fissured or ulcerated atherothrombotic plaques and occlusive coronary artery thrombi (2,3) that persists for more than 2 hours. If pharmacologic lysis or catheter-based reperfusion is not promptly administered, many of these patients experience extensive, often transmural, myocardial damage. In contrast, patients with acute non–ST-segment elevation MI (non-STEMI) are much less likely to have permanently occlusive coronary artery thrombi (3); but like the patients with unstable angina, they have transient reductions in coronary blood flow followed by spontaneous reperfusion (15), this being more transient (minutes) in patients with unstable angina than in patients with non-STEMI. Therefore, it is not surprising that patients with non-STEMI usually have smaller infarcts, typically confined to the subendocardial surface, better left ventricular (LV) function, but more myocardium at risk within the perfusion zone of the infarct-related artery (IRA) than their nonreperfused STEMI counterparts (15–17).

R. S. Gibson: Department of Medicine, Division of Cardiology, University of Virginia, Charlottesville, Virginia.

J. T. Willerson: Texas Heart Institute, University of Texas Health Science Center, 7000 Fannin, Suite 1700, Houston, Texas 77030.

The American College of Cardiology (ACC), the American Heart Association (AHA), and the European Society of Cardiology (ESC) updated their practice guidelines for the management of patients with STEMI (18), non-STEMI, and unstable angina (19,20).The preceding chapters of this book discuss much of the evidence underlying these guidelines and have, by design, emphasized initial management strategies that are currently preferred, as well as the treatment of specific complications. This chapter summarizes the literature on risk-guided comprehensive care and secondary prevention strategies, giving priority to those areas where changes in ACC/AHA recommendations may be appropriate on the basis of new understanding and emerging evidence from recently reported clinical trials and the changing definitions of value in our constrained health care environment.

VALUE OF GUIDELINES APPLIED IN PRACTICE

The key action step and governmental mandate for clinical practice guidelines occurred in 1989 when the U.S. Congress created the Agency for Health Care Quality and Research. As a result, more than 900 guidelines have been produced during the last decade by various specialty organizations, including 18 by the ACC/AHA, which support optimal cardiovascular care. Clinical practice guidelines are intended to reflect the current trend in the practice of medicine, which is making a transition from practice patterns driven by pathophysiologic and nonquantitative reasoning to a broad belief in empiric evidence derived from large-scale randomized, controlled clinical trials (RCTs) (18–20). Guidelines should be viewed as tools for introducing scientific evidence into the clinical decision-making process, by describing a range of validated and generally acceptable approaches for the diagnosis, management, and prevention of specific diseases or conditions. Clinical practice guidelines are not intended to replace physician judgment and discretion, but rather to serve as an aid in helping the practicing physician in the following ways: (a) to identify those management strategies that provide the greatest protection against death, MI, stroke, recurrent ischemia, major arrhythmias, and heart failure; (b) to efficiently organize the relevant medical literature; (c) to reduce unjustified practice variability because of factors such as age, sex, ethnicity, geographic location, physician specialty, and type of hospital or health care organization (e.g., teaching status, and whether a hospital has an onsite cardiac catheterization laboratory); (d) to organize quality improvement efforts by focusing on actionable drivers of patient outcomes; and (e) to provide a framework for the creation of quality monitoring tools, including critical pathways, standardized order sets, patient information forms and discharge checklists (21–26).

The foundation of high-quality decision-making derives from a rigorous and expert analysis of available data that document the relative benefits and risks of specific management strategies that optimize patient outcomes, improve the efficiency of care, and favorably affect the overall cost of care through a focus of resources on the most effective strategies. Clinical practice guidelines provide physicians with much of this information, and several reports (26–31) have shown that guideline-concordant care is strongly linked to lower morbidity and better mortality outcomes for hospitalized patients with an ACS (Figs. 77–1 and 77–2). As valuable as guidelines are, they have several limitations, including the difficulty with timely updates that incorporate new evidence and its implication for clinical practice. In the field of cardiology, major trials are being performed at such a pace that important new findings relevant to clinical practice are common (32). For example, within months of the publication of the ACC/AHA guidelines on chronic heart failure (33), a randomized trial showed a survival advantage for LV assist devices (34), and initial data from several other randomized studies (35–37) appeared to show major benefits, and thus new indications for implantable defibrillators and biventricular pacing. Thus, continued familiarity with

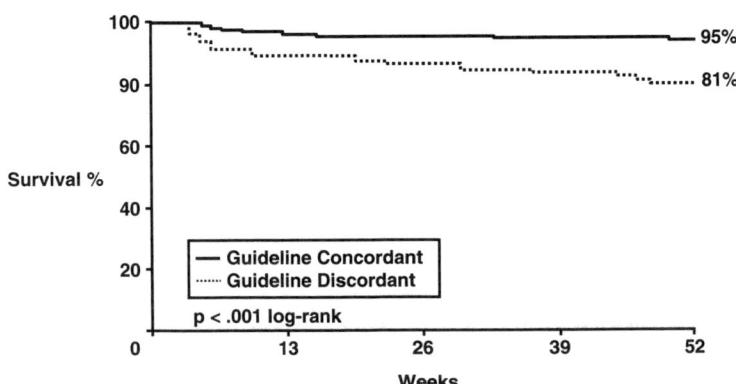

FIG. 77–1. Kaplan-Meier survival curves in patients with acute coronary syndrome showing improved survival among those who received guideline-concordant care (n = 189) versus those who did not (n = 86). (From Giugliano RP, Lloyd-Jones DM, Camargo CA Jr, et al. Association of unstable angina guideline care with improved survival. *Arch Intern Med* 2000;160:1775–1780, with permission.)

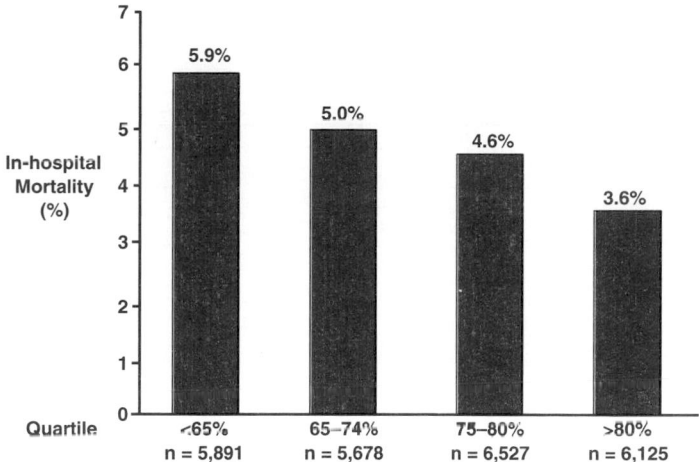

FIG. 77–2. Data from the Can Rapid risk stratification of Unstable angina patients Suppress ADverse outcomes with Early implementation of the ACC/AHA guidelines (CRUSADE) registry in 24,221 patients with acute coronary syndrome (ACS) provides a strong link between increased adherence to guidelines and improved clinical outcome. In-hospital mortality rates are depicted according to a composite adherence score that reflects compliance with the 2002 American College of Cardiology/American Heart Association guideline recommendations for acute management of patients with ACS without persistent ST-segment elevation. The composite adherence score equals the percent of time that care within the first 24 hours of hospital admission was delivered in accordance with the specific acute guideline-recommended therapies (i.e., aspirin, clopidogrel, an antithrombin [either unfractionated heparin or low–molecular weight heparin], β-blocker, and glycoprotein IIb/IIIa inhibitors). (From Harringston R, Smith S, Brindis R, et al. National Report from the Executive Committee of the CRUSADE National Quality Improvement Initiative. Newsletter. November 2002, pp. 1–4, with permission.)

the scientific literature remains necessary despite the existence of clinical practice guidelines.

ACUTE ANGIOGRAPHY AND INTERVENTIONAL THERAPY FOR ST-SEGMENT ELEVATION MYOCARDIAL INFARCTION

The *principles of practice* underlying a comprehensive management strategy of hospitalized patients with an ACS are summarized in Figure 77–3. As shown, the therapeutic goals during the first few hours after admission are somewhat different for the two patient populations. Among those with an acute STEMI, the most important goal is rapidly achieving Thrombolysis In Myocardial Infarction (TIMI) grade 3 flow in the IRA and effective perfusion at the myocapillary level, manifest as complete resolution of chest pain and the ST-segment elevation on the resting ECG. As discussed in Chapter 68, many studies have shown that IRA patency is best accomplished by a percutaneous coronary intervention (PCI). A major advance in the field of STEMI research in the last year or so (i.e., since the most recent clinical practice guideline update) has been the validation of acute angiography and PCI in three RCTs (38–40): (a) the Air Primary Angioplasty in Myocardial Infarction (Air PAMI) study; (b) the Primary Angioplasty in AMI Patients from General Community Hospitals Transported to PTCA Units versus Emergency Thrombolysis (PRAGUE-2) trial; and (c) the DANish multicenter randomized study of invasive versus conservative treatment in patients with inducible ischemia after thrombolysis in

Acute Myocardial Infarction (DANAMI)-2 study. Collectively, the results of these trials, as depicted in Figure 77–4, show a marked benefit with PCI compared with thrombolytic therapy, even after accounting for 1- to 2-hour treatment delays in transport. These findings argue strongly for increased use of mechanical reperfusion in patients with acute STEMI, especially when viewed in the context of previous studies and reports. The earlier reports include the following:

1. A metaanalysis by Weaver and coworkers (41) of 10 RCTs through 1997 demonstrated that a clear reduction in all cardiovascular end points, including death, MI, recurrent ischemia, stroke, and intracranial hemorrhage. The relative reduction in 30-day mortality alone was 34% (from 6.5% for thrombolysis to 4.4% for PCI; $p = 0.02$), indicating the potential of saving 2 lives for every 100 patients treated with PCI instead of thrombolysis. There was an even greater decrease in intracranial hemorrhage, which was reduced from 1.1% for patients treated with thrombolytic therapy to 0.1% for patients treated with PCI ($p < 0.001$).

2. There have now been several reports showing that these impressive results from highly selected "Centers of Excellence" can be duplicated under "real world" conditions. For example, in a study by Magid and coworkers (42) that included 62,299 patients enrolled in a national registry, a clear benefit with primary PCI was shown. When results were stratified based on the number of primary PCI procedures performed per year at each participating hospital, patients treated at the highest volume hospitals had the same mortality benefit (3.4% vs. 5.4%; $p < 0.001$) seen in the

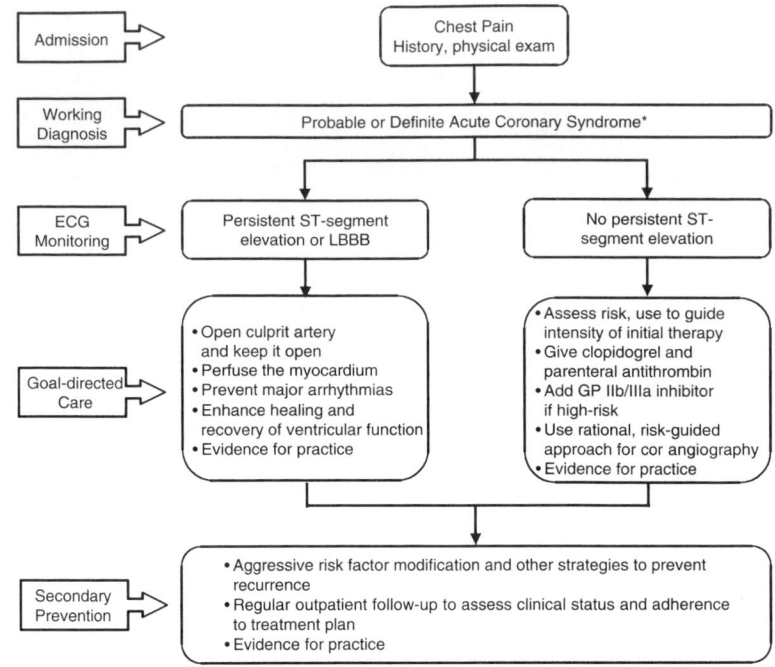

FIG. 77–3. Principles of practice underlying a comprehensive management strategy of hospitalized patients with acute coronary syndrome. ECG, electrocardiogram; GP, glycoprotein; LBBB, left bundle branch block.

randomized trials. Even at intermediate-volume hospitals—two middle quartiles of volume defined as 17 to 48 primary PCI procedures per year—there was a significant benefit of primary PCI (4.5% mortality vs. 5.9% for thrombolysis; $p <$ 0.001). Although the lowest volume centers (performing $\leq$ 16 primary PCI procedures per year) showed no mortality advantage, the total stroke rate was significantly lower with PCI (0.4% vs. 1.1% for thrombolysis; $p < 0.01$).

3. Preliminary data from the Atlantic Cardiovacular Patient Outcomes Research Team (C-PORT) study (43) suggest that this benefit may also extend to community hospitals that have initiated high-quality primary PCI programs despite not offering elective PCI or onsite surgical backup. Indeed, this RCT offers "proof of concept" that implementation of a comprehensive critical pathway with standardized order sets, checklists, and multidisciplinary training is effective in optimizing outcomes of patients with acute STEMI. The study re-

ported a significant reduction in both early and late cardiac events in patients treated with primary PCI as opposed to thrombolysis. At 6 weeks, the incidence of the composite end point of death, recurrent MI, and stroke was 10.7% in the PCI group and 17.7% in the thrombolytic therapy group. At 6 months, the rates were 12.4% versus 19.9% ($p = 0.03$). Mortality at 6 months was reduced by an absolute 2.3%, or 1 life saved for every 43 patients treated with PCI. Recurrent MI and stroke were each reduced by more than 50%, from 10.9% to 4.7%, and from 3.8% to 1.8%, respectively, at 6 months.

4. The work by Brodie and coworkers (44) and the Stent versus Thrombolysis for Occluded coronary arteries in Patients with Acute Myocardial Infarction (STOPAMI) investigators (45,46) showed no time-dependent worsening of myocardial salvage or mortality when PCI was delayed beyond 2 hours, thus supporting the emerging belief that the time delay in transferring patients with STEMI to tertiary

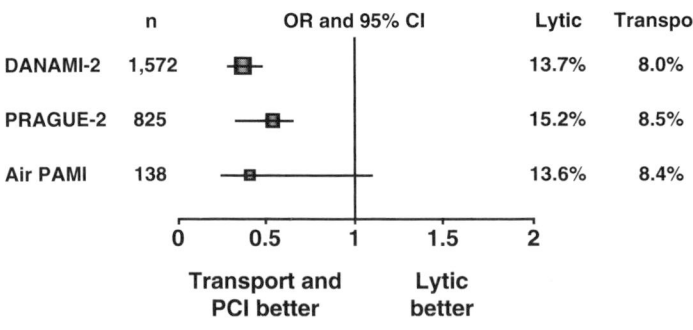

FIG. 77–4. Summary of three randomized, controlled trials comparing immediate thrombolysis versus a strategy of patient transport to nearest full-service hospital for percutaneous coronary intervention (PCI). Data show an approximate 40% reduction in death and myocardial with PCI. From Air Primary Angioplasty in Myocardial Infarction (Air-PAMI) (38), PRAGUE-2 (39) and DANAMI-2 (40) trials. CI, confidence interval; OR, odds ratio; PCI, percutaneous coronary intervention.

centers for primary PCI may be permissible if the procedure cannot be done within 2 to 3 hours of presentation.

5. During the past few years, important shifts have been taking place in PCI technique and adjunctive medical therapy, and these improvements are likely to widen the gap in therapeutic benefit. Indeed, one RCT of coronary stenting with platelet glycoprotein (GP) IIb/IIIa receptor blockade compared with front-loaded tissue plasminogen activator showed a 66% reduction in death, MI, or stroke with this more modern primary PCI strategy (47). Use of distal embolic protection devices during primary PCI may further improve outcomes (48).

As pointed out in two editorials by Cannon (49,50), the practical implications of these new findings are profound. First, if a community hospital makes a strong institutional commitment to establishing a comprehensive program, similar to what was done in the Atlantic C-PORT study (43), performance of primary PCI will be immensely beneficial to patients. Second, the collectively positive data on transfer of patients for primary PCI (Fig. 77–4), suggest it is time to change the approach of the emergency medical response system for acute STEMI. It has been the practice that patients with AMI are transported to the nearest acute care hospital so that they can be stabilized and treated appropriately. However, given the results of the five recently reported trials (38–40,43,46) and the 16 that preceded them (41, 51,52), this policy may need to be changed. In particular, it appears that there may be benefit in prompt transfer of patients from a community hospital that does not offer primary PCI to a nearby one that does. Conversely, an alternative model might be to regionalize AMI services (akin to what has been done for major trauma and high-risk perinatal services). In this model, patients found to have ST-segment elevation in the field on 12-lead ECGs would not necessarily be brought to the nearest hospital. Instead, such patients would be given appropriate pretreatment (e.g., aspirin, clopidogrel, and possibly a GPIIb/IIIa inhibitor) initiated in the ambulance and transferred directly to the nearest "MI center" with 24-hour, 7 days per week primary PCI capability,

thereby avoiding a second ambulance trip and minimizing time to reperfusion. This concept deserves public debate given the volume of MI cases relative to major trauma (Fig. 77–5). However, it is noteworthy that although there are numerous state-recognized trauma centers and many "regionalized" centers for high-risk pregnancy care, there are no identified MI centers in the United States.

Another major advantage of acute angiography, which is germane to the purpose of this chapter, is that it provides almost all of the information necessary for risk stratification and predischarge decision-making. Once the clinician has defined the extent of atherothrombotic coronary artery disease (CAD) and the degree of LV dysfunction, he or she is in a position to facilitate preparation for discharge from the hospital. For example, patients with treated single-vessel CAD and preserved left ventricular ejection fraction (LVEF) usually need no additional diagnostic testing, especially if their hospital course is uncomplicated, and can be discharged home on Day 2 or 3. As described later in this chapter, all patients after STEMI are candidates for either "comprehensive" or exercise-based cardiac rehabilitation, aggressive risk factor modification, and other interventions that have been shown to enhance freedom from future cardiac events.

EARLY INTERVENTIONAL THERAPY FOR NON–ST-SEGMENT ELEVATION MYOCARDIAL INFARCTION AND UNSTABLE ANGINA

Two distinct approaches have emerged over the last decade in the management of patients with non-STEMI and unstable angina (53,54). The *first* approach is an early invasive or "anatomy-driven" strategy consisting of prompt diagnostic coronary angiography within 6 to 48 hours in all patients followed by myocardial revascularization—generally with PCI and stenting, if coronary anatomy is amenable to this approach, or coronary artery bypass surgery if either left mainstem or proximal three-vessel disease with reduced LV function is found. The *second* approach is a watchful waiting or "ischemia-guided" strategy that consists of intensive

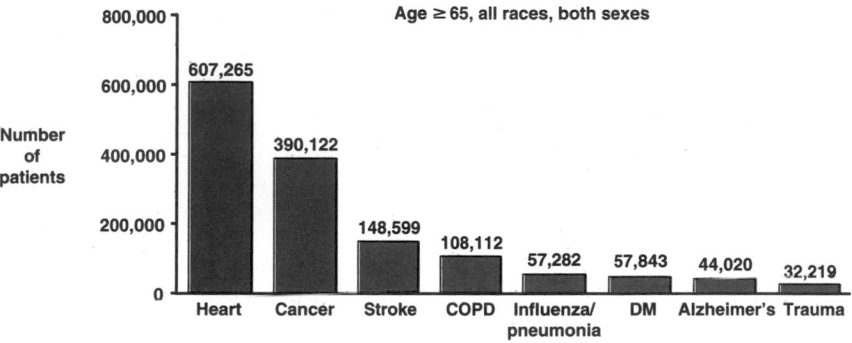

FIG. 77–5. 1999 Data showing the number of deaths in the elderly population in the United States from various causes. COPD, chronic obstructive pulmonary disease; DM, diabetes mellitus.

medical therapy with aggressive antiplatelet, antithrombin, and antiischemic drugs for a predefined treatment interval, usually for 24 to 48 hours, after which parenteral medications are discontinued and, if the patient remains symptom-free, exercise or pharmacologic stress testing is undertaken to delineate objective evidence of inducible ischemia. In this strategy, persistence or recurrence of ischemic symptoms, development of heart failure, hemodynamic instability or serious ventricular arrhythmias, or a positive predischarge stress test leads to cardiac catheterization and a more "selective" approach to revascularization.

Since 1994, there have been eight different randomized trials reported in the literature that have compared an early invasive strategy with an early conservative strategy in patients with non-STEMI or unstable angina (55–67). Three of these trials were relatively small (55–57), enrolling between 131 and 201 patients. Of the five major trials (58–62), each of which enrolled more than 900 patients, the frequency of recurrent angina was consistently reduced with early angiography followed by acute revascularization. Only two of the eight trials showed a significant effect on mortality outcome: One favored the conservative approach (59), and one favored the invasive approach (60). A composite analysis of all eight of these trials by Fox and coworkers (62) revealed substantial heterogeneity with respect to the risk ratios of death or MI at 1 year (Fig. 77–6). This analysis suggests an aggregate risk ratio of 0.88 (95% CI, 0.78–0.99), on the borderline of statistical significance. None of the trials provided strong evidence of superiority with anatomy-driven care for patients who were biomarker-negative (i.e., C-reactive protein [CRP]-negative, troponin–negative, or both) and for those without ST-segment depression. Thus, it is not possible to conclude that there is compelling evidence for universal benefit with invasive care regarding the mortality outcome or the combined end point of death and MI. As pointed out in a recent editorial by Yarlagadda and coworkers (54), this *may be* particularly true in women—a sizable and growing segment of the population with unstable coronary disease (63).

RISK STRATIFICATION AND SELECTION OF THERAPY

The assessment of patient prognosis is central to an efficient, cost-effective management strategy of patients with unstable angina or acute non-STEMI. As illustrated schematically in Figure 77–7, patients with symptomatic CAD can be characterized along a continuum of risk for cardiac events (68). Clearly, the ability to predict short-term prognosis in patients with a non-ST-segment elevation ACS offers the theoretic advantage of more appropriate, timely, and cost-effective decisions regarding the intensity of initial medical treatment and whether patients should be promptly triaged for early PCI. For example, when the risk for a major adverse cardiac event is low, cardiologists generally use conservative medical management. Conversely, when the risk for cardiac events is high, aggressive patient management, such as the performance of PCI or coronary artery bypass surgery, is strongly favored. Between these extremes of risk, however, reside a sizable number of patients who have an intermediate risk for cardiac events, which can be arbitrarily and roughly defined as a like-

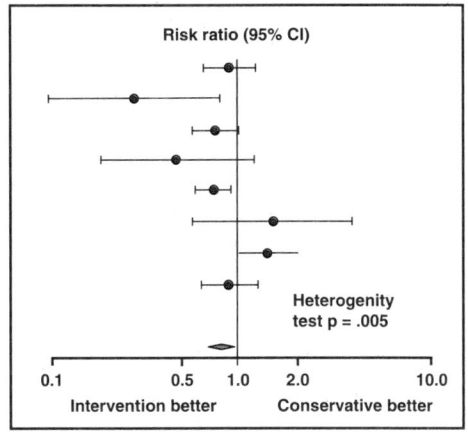

FIG. 77–6. Reported incidence of death, myocardial infarction (MI), or both in eight randomized trials of interventional versus conservative management for unstable angina or non–ST-segment elevation myocardial infarction. CI, confidence interval; FRISC, FRagmin and fast revascularization during InStability in Coronary artery disease; MATE, Medical versus Angiography in Thrombolytic Exclusion; RITA, Randomized Intervention Trial of unstable Angina; TACTICS-TIMI, Treat Angina with Aggrastat and Determine Cost of Therapy-Thrombolysis In Myocardial Infarction; TIMI, Thrombolysis In Myocardial Infarction; TRUCS, Treatment of refractory unstable angina in geographically isolated areas without cardiac surgery; VANQWISH, Veterans Affairs Non-Q-Wave Infarction Strategies In-Hospital; VINO, Value of First Day Angiography/Angioplasty in Evolving Non-ST Segment Elevation Myocardial Infarction. (From Fox KA, Poole-Wilson PA, Henderson RA, et al. Interventional versus conservative treatment for patients with unstable angina or non-ST-elevation myocardial infarction: the British Heart Foundation RITA 3 randomised trial. *Lancet* 2002;360:743–751, with permission.)

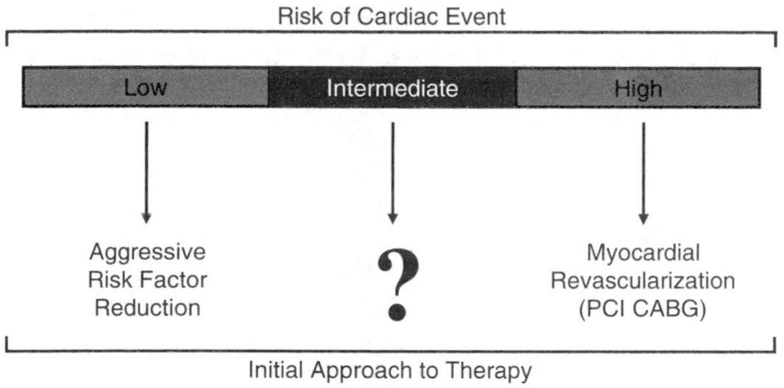

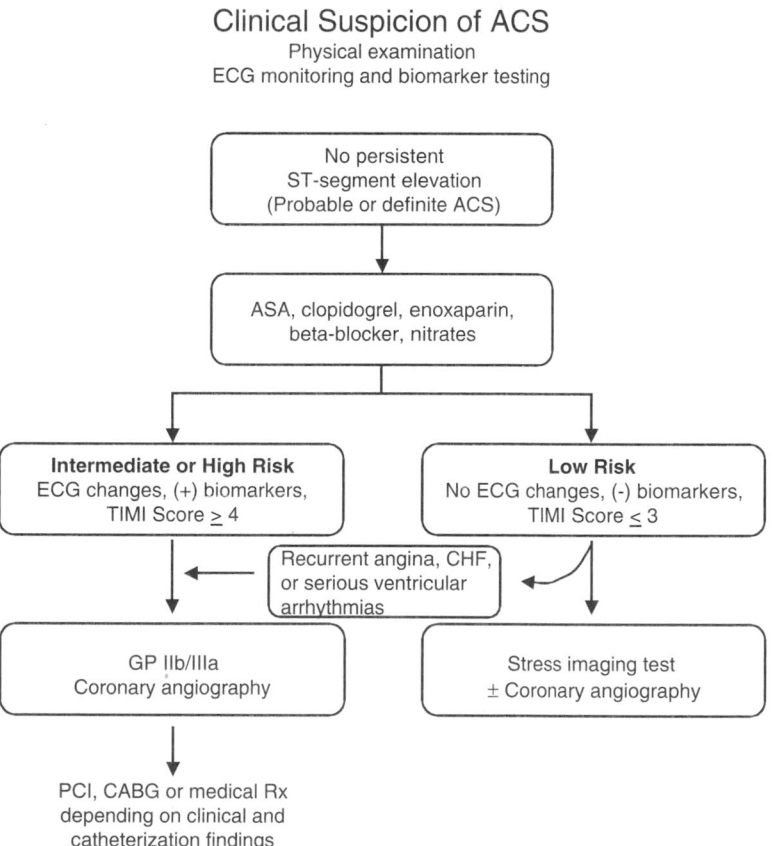

Risk of Cardiac Event

| Low | Intermediate | High |

Aggressive Risk Factor Reduction

?

Myocardial Revascularization (PCI CABG)

Initial Approach to Therapy

FIG. 77–7. Schematic diagram of relation between cardiac risk (for death or myocardial infarction) and selection of therapy for patients with established coronary artery disease, based on clinical data and results of noninvasive testing. CABG, coronary artery bypass graft; PCI, percutaneous coronary intervention. (Adapted from Yao S-S, Rozanski A. Myocardial perfusion scintigraphy in conjunction with exercise and pharmacologic stress: prognostic applications in the clinical management of patients with coronary artery disease. In: DePuey EG, Garcia EV, Berman DS, eds. *Cardiac SPECT imaging,* 2nd ed. Philadelphia: Lippincott Williams & Wilkins, 2001:264–296, with permission.)

lihood of from 2% to 10% of major cardiac events over the ensuing year. Decision-making with regard to such patients is challenging, because the indications for conservative versus aggressive treatment is most uncertain in this group.

The current ACC/AHA and ESC guidelines (19,20) reflect this philosophy of risk-guided decision-making for all patients with non-STEMI or unstable angina, beginning in the emergency department (ED) and continuing throughout the course of hospitalization. All three of these professional organizations acknowledge the highly heterogeneous nature of patients with non–ST-segment elevation ACS and, not surprisingly, guidelines introduced in 2002 endorsed both an

Clinical Suspicion of ACS
Physical examination
ECG monitoring and biomarker testing

No persistent ST-segment elevation (Probable or definite ACS)

ASA, clopidogrel, enoxaparin, beta-blocker, nitrates

Intermediate or High Risk
ECG changes, (+) biomarkers, TIMI Score $\geq$ 4

Low Risk
No ECG changes, (-) biomarkers, TIMI Score $\leq$ 3

Recurrent angina, CHF, or serious ventricular arrhythmias

GP IIb/IIIa
Coronary angiography

Stress imaging test ± Coronary angiography

PCI, CABG or medical Rx depending on clinical and catheterization findings

FIG. 77–8. Recommended management strategy in acute coronary syndromes without persistent ST-segment elevation. ACS, acute coronary syndrome; ASA, aspirin; CABG, coronary artery bypass graft; CHF, congestive heart failure; ECG, electrocardiogram; GP, glycoprotein; PCI, percutaneous coronary intervention; Rx, treatment; TIMI, Thrombolysis In Myocardial Infarction. (Adapted from Braunwald E, Antman EM, Beasley JW, et al. ACC/AHA 2002 guideline update for the management of patients with unstable angina and non-ST-segment elevation myocardial infarction. *J Am Coll Cardiol* 2002;40: 1366–1374; and Bertrand ME, Simoons ML, Fox KAA, et al. Management of acute coronary syndromes in patients presenting without persistent ST-segment elevation. The Task Force on the Management of Acute Coronary Syndromes of the European Society of Cardiology. *Eur Heart J* 2002;23:1809–1840, with permission.)

invasive approach (for high-risk patients) and the more conservative approach (for low-risk patients). As shown in Figure 77–8, it is now recommended that all patients with a diagnosis of "probable or definite" rest angina receive aspirin (325 mg, chewed), a loading dose of clopidogrel (300 mg), enoxaparin (1 mg/kg every 12 hours, unless serum creatinine is >2 mg/dL, in which case unfractionated heparin is used), as well as potent antiischemic therapy (usually a β-blocker combined with a nitrate) in the ED. The decision to use additional or adjunctive treatment is based on patient risk, which is determined in the ED from available clinical data, ECGs, and biomarker testing. Two categories, low- and intermediate- to high-risk patients, are identified. Patients at *low risk* include patients without dynamic ECG changes, who have negative troponin values and no recurrent angina. These patients receive baseline therapy, as described earlier, for a minimum of 24 to 36 hours and, in the absence of complications, undergo low-level stress testing to assess exercise capacity, LV function, and ischemic burden. As discussed in Chapter 78, this assessment is probably best accomplished with single-photon emission computed tomography (SPECT) technetium-99m–sestamibi myocardial perfusion scintigraphy, although stress echocardiography is an alternative. After this examination, coronary angiography and a revascularization procedure may be performed if significant inducible ischemia is found, an approach that is supported by the results of the DAMANI-1 trial (69). Patients at *intermediate-to high risk* include those patients with persistent or recurrent angina, ST-segment depression greater than 0.5 mm or deep T-wave inversions, increased troponin or CRP levels,

clinical heart failure or known LVEF less than 40%, or serious ventricular arrhythmias. Studies have shown that these patients benefit from infusion of a GPIIb/IIIa receptor inhibitor (30,31,70–79), in addition to baseline treatment, followed by prompt angiography. This examination is performed on an urgent basis in patients with ongoing ischemia and in those patients with hemodynamic instability or recurrent life-threatening arrhythmias. Otherwise, angiography can be safely deferred for 24 to 48 hours, during which time aggressive medical therapy is continued to facilitate "plaque passivation" as a prelude to PCI or surgical revascularization. The concept of plaque passivation has been advanced as a potential explanation for the improved clinical outcomes that may occur as a consequence of various pharmacologic interventions that improve endothelial function and vascular homeostasis and reduce both inflammation and microembolization (80–82).

The validity of the above approach derives from that many observational studies and RCTs have demonstrated the superiority of risk-guided decision-making in optimizing patient outcomes in an efficient and cost-effective manner (53,67,83–88). As shown in Figure 77–9, the Treat Angina with Aggrastat and Determine Cost of Therapy (TACTICS) trial (61) revealed the importance of admission ECG changes and biomarker status in predicting response to interventional therapy. This finding from this trial is noteworthy because all patients received "upstream" treatment with a GPIIb/IIIa receptor inhibitor, patients who were assigned to the early invasive strategy had angiography a mean of 22 hours after admission (vs. 5 to 7 days in the FRagmin and

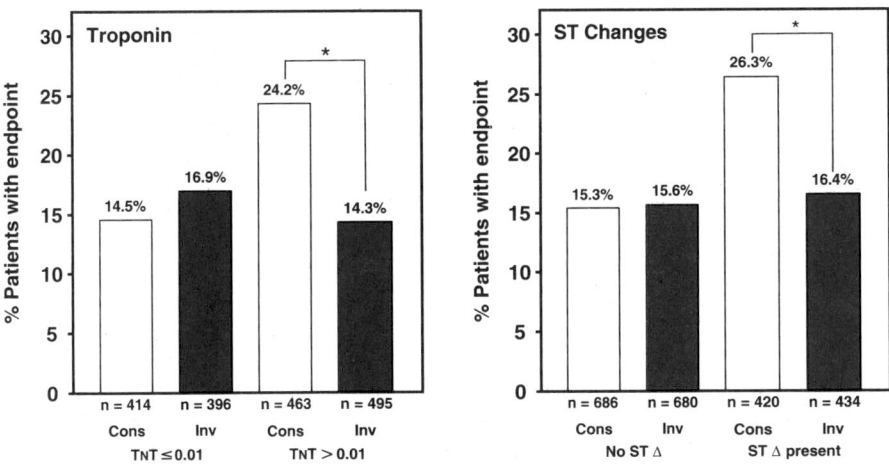

Endpoint = death, MI or rehospitalization for ACS at 6 months
p < .001 (interaction p < .001)

FIG. 77–9. Data from the Treat Angina with Aggrastat and Determine Cost of Therapy-Thrombolysis In Myocardial Infarction (TACTICS-TIMI) 18 trials. Rates of the primary end point of death, nonfatal myocardial infarction (MI), or rehospitalization for acute coronary syndrome (ACS) at 6 months are depicted according to treatment group assignment (invasive [*Inv*] or conservative [*Cons*] strategy), troponin level, and admission electrocardiographic findings. TnT, Troponin T. (From Cannon CP, Weintraub WS, Demopoulos LA, et al. Comparison of early invasive and conservative strategies in patients with unstable coronary syndromes treated with the glycoprotein IIb/IIIa inhibitor tirofiban. *N Engl J Med* 2001;344:1879–1887, with permission.)

fast revascularization during InStability in Coronary artery disease [FRISC]-II trial [60]), and all patients who were initially randomized to the conservative strategy arm were managed using a study protocol that was compliant with current ACC/AHA guidelines (e.g., patients were permitted to crossover to the invasive arm if their predischarge stress test provoked 1 mm or more of ischemic ST-segment depression or if the imaging study showed any high-risk finding) (66). As such, the results of the TACTICS trial are relevant to U.S. medical practice.

New Tools to Predict Cardiovascular Risk in Patients with Acute Coronary Syndrome

In recent years, several investigators have proposed use of new prediction models for assessing short- and long-term prognosis after STEMI (89–97), non-STEMI, and unstable angina (93–98). These models are based on a score that presumably provides enhanced discrimination of risk for future cardiac events, compared with what is currently recommended by the ACC/AHA and ESC (Table 77–1). These new scoring models have been derived from either clinical trials (e.g., the TIMI score (89,96), the Platelet Glycoprotein IIb/IIIa in Unstable angina: Receptor Suppression Using Integrilin Therapy trial [PURSUIT] score (97), the Global Utilization of Streptokinase and t-PA for Occluded coronary arteries [GUSTO] score (91), the FRISC score (98) and the Intravenous nPA Treatment of Infarcting Myocardium Early II [InTIME II] score [90]) or from registries and cohort studies (e.g., Predicting Risk of Death in Cardiac Disease Tool [PREDICT] (93,94) and the Cooperative Cardiovascular Project [CCP] scores [92]). They all differ with regard to their derivation population, the number and type of variables collected for score calculation, and meth-

TABLE 77–1. *Current guidelines for use of an invasive management strategy*

Patient characteristic	Endorsing organization[a]
New or presumably new ST-segment depression ≥ 0.5 mm, or transient ST-segment elevation	ACC/AHA and ESC
ECG pattern, which precludes assessment of ST-segment changes	ESC
Increased troponin T or I	ACC/AHA and ESC
Hemodynamic instability	ACC/AHA and ESC
Major arrhythmias—sustained ventricular tachycardia, repetitive nonsustained ventricular tachycardia or ventricular fibrillation	ACC/AHA and ESC
Recurrent angina/ischemia at rest or with low-level activities despite intensive medical therapy	ACC/AHA and ESC
Significant reduction in LV systolic function—LVEF < 0.40 on noninvasive study	ACC/AHA
High-risk findings on non-invasive stress testing	ACC/AHA and ESC
Diabetes mellitus	ESC
PCI within 6 months or prior CABG	ACC/AHA

For patients without persistent ST-segment elevation, and in the absence of contraindications for revascularization.

ACC, American College of Cardiology; AHA, American Heart Association; CABG, coronary artery bypass graft; ECG, electrocardiographic; ESC, European Society of Cardiology; LV, left ventricular; LVEF, left ventricular ejection fraction; PCI, percutaneous coronary intervention.

[a]Data from References 19 and 20.

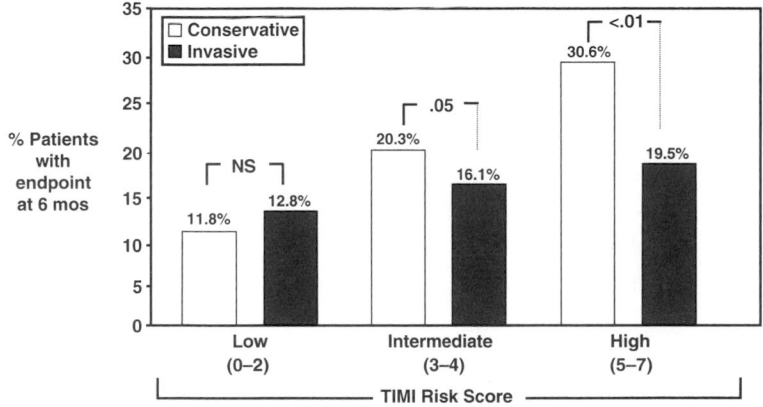

FIG. 77–10. Data from the Treat Angina with Aggrastat and Determine Cost of Therapy-Thrombolysis In Myocardial Infarction (TACTICS-TIMI) 18 trial showing the relative benefits of an invasive management strategy according to the TIMI risk score. NS, Not significant. (From Cannon CP, Weintraub WS, Demopoulos LA, et al. Comparison of early invasive and conservative strategies in patients with unstable coronary syndromes treated with the glycoprotein IIb/IIIa inhibitor tirofiban. *N Engl J Med* 2001;344:1879–1887; and Solomon DH, Stone PH, Glynn RJ, et al. Use of risk stratification to identify patients with unstable angina likeliest to benefit from an invasive versus conservative management strategy. *J Am Coll Cardiol* 2001;38:969–976, with permission.)

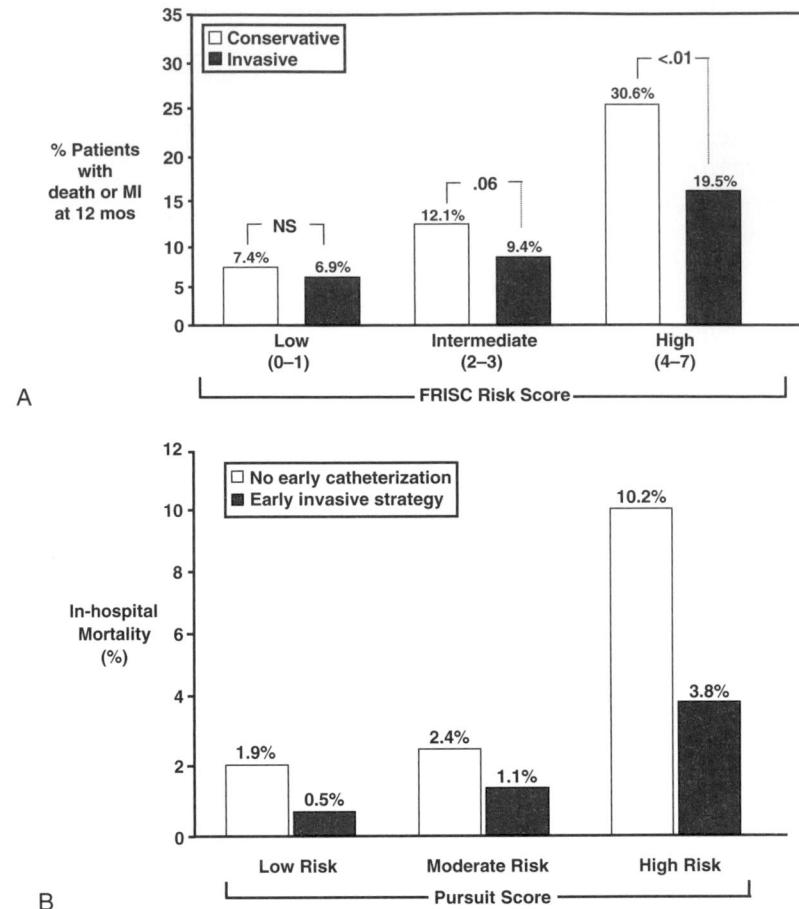

A

B

FIG. 77–11. Data from two studies illustrating the value of the FRagmin and fast revascularization during InStability in Coronary artery disease (FRISC) **(A)** and Platelet Glycoprotein IIb/IIIa in Unstable angina: Receptor Suppression Using Integrilin Therapy trial (PURSUIT) risk scores **(B)** in predicting benefit with an invasive management strategy. MI, myocardial infarction. (From Lagerqvist B, Diderholm E, Lindahl B, et al. High risk score predicts bad outcome in patients with unstable coronary artery disease: FRISCII sub-study. *Circulation* 2001;104[Suppl II]:II-648(abst); and Harringston R, Smith S, Brindis R, et al. National Report from the Executive Committee of the CRUSADE National Quality Improvement Initiative. Newsletter. November 2002, pp. 1–4, with permission.)

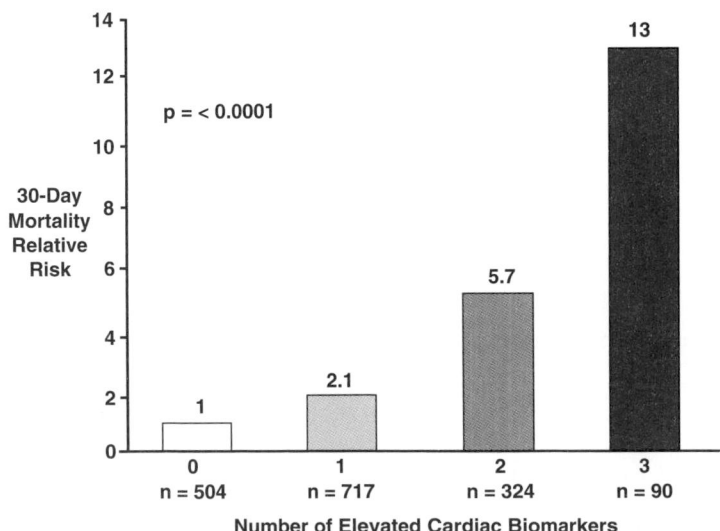

FIG. 77–12. Relative 30-day mortality risks in Treat Angina with Aggrastat and Determine Cost of Therapy-Thrombolysis In Myocardial Infarction (TACTICS-TIMI) 18 trial among patients stratified by the number of increased cardiac biomarkers. Biomarkers included troponin I, C-reactive protein, and B-type natriuretic peptide. (From Sabatine MS, Morrow DA, de Lemos JA, et al. Multimarker approach to risk stratification in non-ST elevation acute coronary syndromes. Simultaneous assessment of troponin I, C-reactive protein, and B-type natriuretic peptide. *Circulation* 2002;105:1760–1763, with permission.)

TABLE 77–2. *Risk evaluation schemes that predict prognosis in non–ST-segment elevation acute coronary syndrome*

TIMI risk score[a]		PURSUIT risk score[bc]		FRISC risk score[d]		GUSTO risk score[e]	
Age >65 y	1	Age, y:		Age ≥70 y	1	Age, y:	
≥3 CAD risk factors	1	50–59	0	CHF or LVEF ≤45%	1	50–60	2
≥50% angiographic stenosis	1	60–69	2(3)	Use of ≥2 antianginals before admission	1	61–70	4
ASA use ≤7 days	1	70–79	4(6)	Diabetes	1	71–80	6
≥2 anginal episodes in past 24 h	1	≥80	6(9)	↑ Troponin	1	>80	8
↑ Troponin or CK-MB	1	Male sex	1	↑ CRP	1	Prior CHF	2
ST-segment ↓ >0.5 mm	1	CCS Class III-IV	2	ST-segment ↓ ≥0.5 mm	1	Prior stroke/TIA	2
Maximum score	7	Pulse:		Maximum score	7	Prior MI, revascularization or angina	1
		100–119	1(2)			Pulse ≥ 90 beats/min	3
		≥120	2(5)			↑ CK-MB and troponin	3
		SBP:				↑ CRP (g/L):	
		81–100	1			10–20	1
		≤80	2			>20	2
		Rales	3			Creatinine > 1.4 mg/dL	2
		ST-segment ↓ ≥ 0.5 mm	3			↓ Hemoglobin	1
		Maximum score	25			Maximum score	25
C statistic = 0.65		**C statistic = 0.81**		**C statistic = NA**		**C statistic = 0.80**	
14-Day death, MI, or urgent revascularization		30-Day mortality		12-Month mortality		30-Day mortality	

ASA, aspirin; CAD, coronary artery disease; CHF, congestive heart failure; CK-MB, creatine kinase (MB fragment); CRP, C-reactive protein; FRISC, FRagmin and fast revascularization during InStability in Coronary artery disease; GUSTO, Global Utilization of Streptokinase and t-PA for Occluded coronary arteries; LVEF, left ventricular ejection fraction; SBP, systolic blood pressure; TIMI, Thrombolysis in Myocardial Infarction;
[a]Data from Reference 96.
[b]Data from Reference 97.
[c]With respect to age and heart rate in the Platelet Glycoprotein IIb/IIIa in Unstable angina: Receptor Suppression Using Integrilin Therapy (PURSUIT) model, there are separate points for enrollment diagnosis of unstable angina and non–ST-segment myocardial infarction (values in parentheses).
[d]Data from Reference 98.
[e]Data from Reference 91.

ods that have been used for clinical validation. Examples of four of these scoring models are shown in Table 77–2. It is perhaps noteworthy that none of these risk evaluation schemes included a "response to initial treatment" variable. Clearly, the management of patients with ACS is an interactive process that is guided by the individual physician's perception of patient risk, the anticipated reduction in risk by available therapies, and the response to such therapy. However, almost all prediction tools concentrate on risk assessment at the time of hospital admission; thus, response to initial therapy is not generally part of the model, neither are changes during hospitalization, such as recurrent ischemia.

Do these prediction tools provide incremental value in stratifying patients, and are they useful in making clinical decisions? Prediction tools may not only offer a simple method for estimating prognosis on admission, but they can help to identify the appropriate form of therapy if the optimal therapy has been shown to depend on the score. For example, in the TACTICS and TIMI IIIb trials (61,67), the benefit of an invasive strategy was not found at a low TIMI risk score, it was modest at the intermediate TIMI score, but it was marked at a high TIMI score (Fig. 77–10). Similarly, the application of both the FRISC (98) and the PURSUIT

risk evaluation schemes (30,97) have been validated as useful decision-making tools (Fig. 77–11, A and B).

Several new cardiac biomarkers have emerged as strong predictors of risk among patients with ACS and are currently routinely available to clinicians. Increased levels of troponin I and T, high-sensitivity CRP, and B-type natriuretic peptide each are associated with greater rates of death and recurrent ischemic events (99–103). In a report by Sabatine and coworkers (103), it was shown that a simple multimarker strategy that categorizes patients on the basis of the number of increased biomarkers at presentation allows risk stratification over a broad range of short- and long-term major cardiac events (Fig. 77–12).

SECONDARY PREVENTION STRATEGIES IN 2003

During the last 25 years, a large number of randomized, placebo-controlled clinical trials have been performed in patients with ACS. Almost all of these RCTs evaluated the effect of therapy on mortality, and many also assessed evidence of other benefits, such as reduction in new MI events, recurrent ischemia, stroke, or heart failure. Unfortunately, a sizable number of these trials evaluated therapeutic efficacy in large, undifferentiated ACS populations—that is, the RCT did not specify an *a priori* test of drug efficacy on the basis of biomarker status (positive vs. negative) or ECG type of infarction (STEMI vs. non-STEMI). In addition, many of the megatrials were conducted before widespread use of reperfusion therapy or at a time when aggressive "polypharmacy" was uncommon. Because of this, there is a relative paucity of data collected prospectively that adequately delineates the incremental therapeutic value, and cost-effectiveness, of specific secondary prevention strategies in specific subcategories of patients who have received contemporary management during their index hospitalization. Although the evidence supporting therapeutic lifestyle change and indefinite use of aspirin in the absence of allergy is indisputable, many other therapies continue to be surrounded by a degree of uncertainty. Table 77–3 summarizes the secondary prevention strategies that are currently recommended by the ACC/AHA (104,105).

Ticlopidine and Clopidogrel

For patients with significant allergy to aspirin, ticlopidine hydrochloride or clopidogrel bisulfate may be used. Both of these drugs are thienopyridines, and their mechanism of action differs from that of aspirin (106). Ticlopidine and clopidogrel both inhibit adenosine diphosphate (ADP)-mediated platelet activation, and because they act independently of aspirin, there will be a synergistic effect when either is used in combination with aspirin. Ticlopidine has been shown to reduce the rate of fatal and nonfatal MIs in patients with unstable angina (106,107).The onset of action of ticlopidine is delayed; its beneficial effect may not be evident until 1 to 2 weeks after the initial administration (106). Also, ticlopidine may induce neutropenia in 1% to 3% of patients or may cause severe dermatologic problems (106). Because clopidogrel has a more rapid onset of action (<2 hours), is more potent than ticlopidine in inhibiting ADP-mediated platelet activation, and almost never causes neutropenia, it is currently preferred. The Clopidogrel versus Aspirin in Patients at Risk of Ischemic Events (CAPRIE) trial showed that clopidogrel significantly decreased composite end points by 8.7% for as long as 3 years in comparison with aspirin (108). In the Clopidogrel in Unstable angina to prevent Recurrent Events (CURE) trial (109), 12,562 patients with a non–ST-segment elevation ACS were randomized to aspirin alone versus aspirin plus clopidogrel. Of these patients, only 2.3% were from U.S. centers, and most of the randomized patients received conservative or "ischemia-guided" management. As shown in Figure 77–13A, there was a 20% reduction in the combined primary end point of vascular death, MI, and stroke during an average follow-up of 9 months. This result, together with the findings of the PCI-CURE study (110), led the ACC/AHA and ESC in 2002 to recommend both aspirin and clopidogrel (75 mg/d) for a minimum of 30 days after non–ST-segment elevation ACS (19,20).

As pointed out by Berger and coworkers (111), there are several unresolved questions concerning the use of dual oral antiplatelet therapy, including the following: (a) whether treatment before PCI with clopidogrel remains beneficial if a GPIIb/IIIa receptor inhibitor is administered, or vice versa, and whether the benefit of aspirin, clopidogrel, and a GPIIb/IIIa antagonist is additive without an unacceptable bleeding risk; and (b) does prolonged clopidogrel therapy after PCI confer significant benefit? Other questions that have been raised concern the potential adverse interaction of clopidogrel with the synthetic statin, atorvastatin (112), and the cost to society of long-term dual antiplatelet therapy. Retrospective analysis of the Tirofiban [Aggrastat] and ReoPro Give similar Efficacy outcomes Trial (TARGET), a PCI study in which all patients with ACS received either abciximab or tirofiban, suggested that event rates were lower among patients pretreated with aspirin and clopidogrel (113). The Clopidogrel for the Reduction of Events During Observation (CREDO) trial (114) is the first large-scale prospective randomized trial to evaluate optimal initiation and duration of an ADP receptor antagonist with aspirin in patients undergoing an elective PCI. A total of 2,116 patients were recruited and randomized to either control therapy (325 mg/d aspirin plus 75 mg/d clopidogrel for 28 days after PCI, then 81–325 mg/d aspirin plus placebo for the remainder of the 1-year study) or to the active treatment arm (a 300-mg loading dose of clopidogrel and aspirin 3 to 24 hours before PCI, then the aspirin/clopidogrel combination for the full year after PCI). Of the two main findings of the CREDO trial, the first was that the clopidogrel loading dose given before PCI produced a reduction in events at 28 days that was nonsignificant except in the prespecified subgroup whose members received the 300-mg loading dose at least 6 hours before PCI. This subgroup enjoyed a borderline significant 38.6% relative reduction in the composite end point of death, MI, or urgent target vessel revascularization at 28 days ($p = 0.051$). The clopidogrel loading dose did not increase major or minor bleeding. The second main finding was that increasing the duration of clopidogrel from the standard 4 weeks to at least 1 year after PCI significantly reduces patients' risk for adverse ischemic events. Overall, there was a 26.8% relative reduction in the 1-year risk for death, MI, and stroke ($p = 0.01$), with similar reductions in risk for all three individual end points. Prolonged therapy was associated with a nonsignificant increase in major bleeding (8.8% vs. 6.7%; $p = 0.07$) with the majority of major bleeds in both study arms being related to the index PCI or coronary artery bypass surgery. Notably, approximately 45% of patients in CREDO received a GPIIb/IIIa antagonist at the time of PCI (either as bailout therapy or specified at the time of randomization). According to the CREDO investigators (114), data from this subset of patients "strongly suggest a complementary role of parenteral GPIIb/IIIa inhibition with dual oral anti-platelet therapy in the setting of PCI, without a concomitant increase in major bleeding." The authors add, however, that a definitive conclusion on this issue will have to await the results of the ongoing Intra-

TABLE 77–3. *American Heart Association/American College of Cardiology Secondary Prevention for Patients with Coronary and Other Vascular Disease 2001 Update*

Goals	Intervention recommendations
Smoking: complete cessation	Assess tobacco use. Strongly encourage patient and family to stop smoking and to avoid secondhand smoke. Provide counseling, pharmacologic therapy, including nicotine replacement and bupropion and formal smoking cessation programs as appropriate.
BP control: <140/90 mm Hg or <130/85 mm Hg if heart failure or renal insufficiency; <130/80 mm Hg if diabetes	Initiate lifestyle modification (weight control, physical activity, alcohol moderation, moderate sodium restriction, and emphasis on fruits, vegetables, and low-fat dairy products) in all patients with blood pressure ≥130 mm Hg systolic or 80 mm Hg diastolic. Add blood pressure medication, individualized to other patient requirements and characteristics (i.e., age, race, need for drugs with specific benefits) if blood pressure is not <140 mm Hg systolic or 90 mm Hg diastolic or if blood pressure is not <130 mm Hg systolic or 85 mm Hg diastolic for individuals with heart failure or renal insufficiency (<80 mm Hg diastolic for individuals with diabetes).
Lipid management Primary goal: LDL < 100 mg/dL	Start dietary therapy in all patients (<7% saturated fat and <200 mg/d cholesterol) and promote physical activity and weight management. Encourage increased consumption of ω3 fatty acids. Assess fasting lipid profile in all patients, and within 24 h of hospitalization for those with an acute event. If patients are hospitalized, consider adding drug therapy on discharge. Add drug therapy according to the following guide: LDL < 100 mg/dL (baseline or on-treatment): Further LDL-lowering therapy may not be required. Consider fibrate or niacin (if low HDL or high TG). LDL 100–129 mg/dL (baseline or on-treatment) therapeutic options: Intensity LDL-lowering therapy (statin or resin[a]). Fibrate or niacin (if low HDL or high TG). Consider combined drug therapy (statin + fibrate or niacin) (if low HDL or high TG). LDL ≥ 130 mg/dL (baseline or on-treatment): Intensity LDL-lowering therapy (statin or resin[a]). Add or increase drug therapy with lifestyle therapies.
Secondary goal: if TG (150 mg/dL, then non-HDL should be <130 mg/dL	If TG ≥150 mg/dL or HDL < 40 mg/dL: Emphasize weight management and physical activity. Advise smoking cessation. If TG = 200–499 mg/dL: Consider fibrate or niacin after LDL-lowering therapy.[a] If TG ≥ 500 mg/dL: Consider fibrate or niacin before LDL-lowering therapy.[a] Consider ω3 fatty acids as adjunct for high TG.
Physical activity—minimum: 30 minutes 3 to 4 d/wk	Assess risk, preferably with exercise tests, to guide perception. Encourage minimum of 30 to 60 min of activity preferably daily or at least 3 to 4 times/wk (walking, jogging, cycling, or other aerobic activity) supplemented by an increase in daily lifestyle activities (e.g., walking breaks at work, gardening, household work). Advise medically supervised programs for moderate- to high-risk patients.
Weight management: BMI 18.5–24.9 kg/m²	Calculate BMI and measure waist circumference as part of evaluation. Monitor response of BMI and waist circumference to therapy. Start weight management and physical activity as appropriate. Desirable BMI range is 18.5–24.9 kg/m². When BM ≥ 25 kg/m², goal for waist circumference is ≤40 inches in men and ≤35 inches in women.
Diabetes management: HbA1c < 7%	Appropriate hypoglycemic therapy to achieve near-normal fasting plasma glucose, as indicated by HbA1c. Treatment of other risks (e.g., physical activity, weight management, BP, and cholesterol management).
Antiplatelet agents/ anticoagulants	Start and continue indefinitely aspirin 75 to 325 mg/d if not contraindicated. Consider clopidogrel 75 mg/d or warfarin if aspirin contraindicated. Manage warfarin to international normalized ratio = 2.0 to 3.0 in post-MI patients when clinically indicated or for those not able to take aspirin or clopidogrel.
ACE inhibitors	Treat all patients indefinitely after MI; start early in stable high-risk patients (anterior MI, previous MI, Killip Class II [S₃ gallop, rales, radiographic CHF]). Consider chronic therapy for all other patients with coronary or other vascular disease unless contraindicated.
β-Blockers	Start in all post-MI and acute ischemic syndrome patients. Continue indefinitely. Observe usual contraindications. Use as needed to manage angina, rhythm, or blood pressure in all other patients.

ACE, angiotensin-converting enzyme; BMI, body mass index; BP, blood pressure; CHF, congestive heart failure; HbA1c, major fraction of hemoglobin A1c; HDL, high-density lipoprotein; LDL, low-density lipoprotein; MI, myocardial infarction; non-HDL cholesterol, total cholesterol minus high-density lipoprotein cholesterol; TG, triglycerides.
[a]The use of resin is relatively contraindicated when TG < 200 mg/dL.

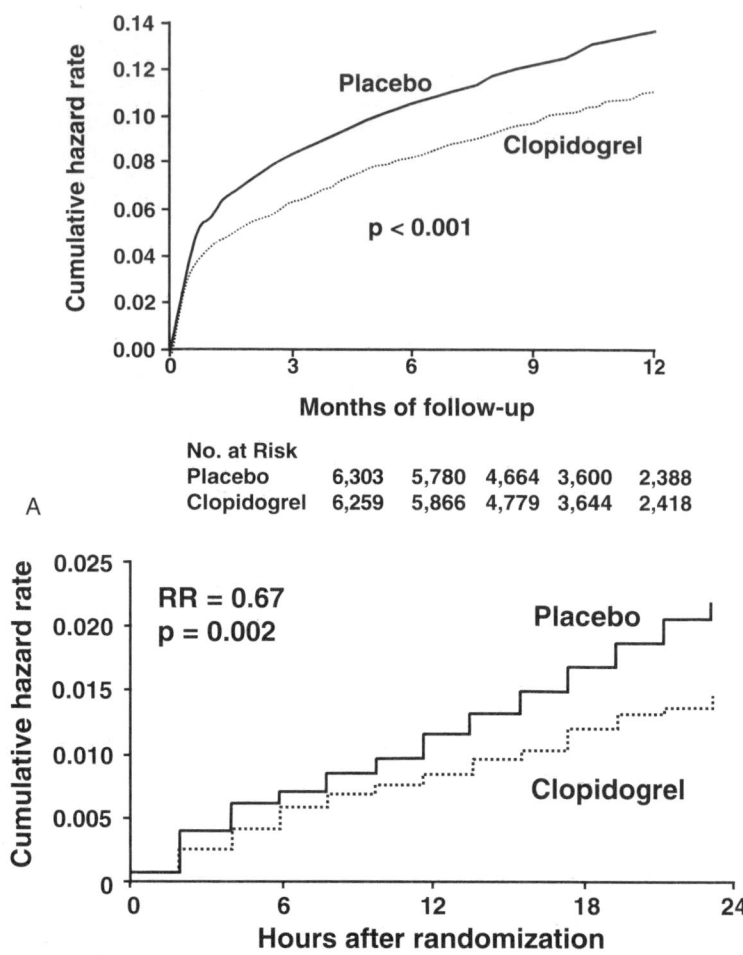

FIG. 77–13. Results of the Clopidogrel in Unstable angina to prevent Recurrent Events (CURE) trial show a highly significant effect with dual antiplatelet therapy with aspirin and clopidogrel on the composite primary end point of death, myocardial infarction (MI), and stroke **(A),** and on death/MI/stroke/severe ischemia in the first 24 hours after randomization **(B).** RR, relative risk. (From The Clopidogrel in Unstable Angina to Prevent Recurrent Events Trial Investigators. Effects of clopidogrel in addition to aspirin in patients with acute coronary syndromes without ST-segment elevation. *N Engl J Med* 2001;345:494–502; and Berger PB, Steinhubl S. Clinical implications of Percutaneous Coronary Intervention–Clopidogrel in Unstable Angina to Prevent Recurrent Events (PCI-CURE) Study. A US Perspective. *Circulation* 2002;106:2284–2287, with permission.)

coronary Stenting and Antithrombotic Regimen-Rapid Early Action for Coronary Treatment (ISAR-REACT) trial.

Based on available data, the following conclusions can be made: First, both clopidogrel and aspirin should routinely be started early and continued for the long term. As shown in Figure 77–13B, the benefits emerge rapidly; at the end of the first 24 hours in CURE, the clopidogrel group already had a 33% reduction in the combined end point of major vascular events plus refractory and severe angina. Second, clopidogrel prevents major MI events, not merely cardiac enzyme level increases. The incidence of Q-wave MI in CURE was reduced by 40% in the clopidogrel group. Third, the therapeutic benefits of clopidogrel are consistent regardless of whether patients are treated medically, by percutaneous intervention, or with coronary artery bypass surgery. Fourth, the benefits of clopidogrel accrue to all patients. A total of

60 subgroups have been examined, and none went in the wrong direction in terms of important outcomes. Fifth, the optimal aspirin dose for use with clopidogrel is 75 to 100 mg per day. The bleeding risk is less than with aspirin monotherapy at 325 mg per day; but when clopidogrel is used with aspirin at more than 100 mg per day, the bleeding risk increases significantly. Sixth, it is prudent to withhold clopidogrel for 4 to 5 days before bypass surgery. This reduces the need for transfusion. However, when surgery must be performed with aspirin and clopidogrel being administered, the excess bleeding risk is usually not prohibitive, amounting to 3 extra patients requiring transfusion per 100 treated. Seventh, further studies are needed to investigate potentially important drug–drug interactions, such as the one recently described with atorvastatin [112]; and eighth, the cost to society of dual antiplatelet therapy will probably be at least

neutral, because of fewer admissions and revascularization procedures.

Effects of β-Blockers, Nitrates, and Potassium Channel Activators

β-Blockers competitively inhibit the effects of circulating catecholamines on cell membrane β-adrenoreceptors (19, 20). They primarily decrease the oxygen demands of the heart by reducing the heart rate and myocardial contractility. This, in turn, increases the diastolic period with a corresponding increase in the time available for coronary perfusion. These drugs also reduce exercise-mediated increases in blood pressure and contractility, which, in turn, leads to decreased wall stress and lower oxygen demand. Therefore, this class of drugs is most effective during exercise or stress, or in the presence of increased sympathetic activity.

Evidence for a beneficial cardioprotective effect of β-blockers in unstable angina is based on limited and inconclusive randomized trial data, together with extrapolation from experience in stable angina and AMI. A metaanalysis of three small, placebo-controlled trials suggested that β-blocker treatment was associated with a 13% relative reduction in risk for progression to AMI (115). Although no significant effect on mortality in unstable angina was demonstrated in these relatively small trials, large RCTs of β-blockers in patients with acute or recent MI have shown a highly significant effect on mortality (116). In evaluating these post-MI trials, it is useful to divide β-blockers into those with intrinsic sympathomimetic activity (ISA), such as alprenolol, practolol, pindolol, and oxprenolol, and those without ISA, such as atenolol, carvedilol, metoprolol, propranolol, and timolol. Pooled data for β-blockers with ISA indicate a minimal (usually <5–10%) reduction in mortality. Studies of β-blockers without ISA have shown significantly greater benefit, typically a 25% to 30% reduction in all-cause mortality and an approximate 25% reduction in nonfatal reinfarction.

Although retrospective subgroup analysis should always be interpreted with caution (117), it is interesting that three of the largest β-blocker trials observed little or no benefit with treatment in patients with non-STEMI who did not evolve pathologic Q-waves on serial ECGs. The β-Blocker Heart Attack Trial (BHAT), for example, demonstrated reduced mortality and a lower reinfarction rate with propranolol in patients with Q-wave MI, but showed no effect on either end point in patients with non–Q-wave MI (118,119). Similarly, the Metoprolol In Acute Myocardial Infarction (MIAMI) trial found no reduction in mortality or reinfarction among the non–Q-wave group (120). By comparison, the Norwegian Timolol Trial showed prolonged survival in timolol-treated patients regardless of infarct type; however, the incidence of nonfatal reinfarction during long-term follow-up was reduced only in patients with Q-wave MI (121,122). In light of these findings, the routine use of prophylactic β-adrenergic blockade may not be justified for all normotensive patients recovering from a non–ST-segment elevation ACS, especially if LVEF is well preserved. Patients with STEMI without contraindications should probably receive prophylactic therapy with a β-blocker, and a strong case also can be made for patients with non-STEMI associated with low ejection fraction, increased heart rate or blood pressure, and persistent myocardial ischemia. The Carvedilol Post Infarction Survival Control in Left Ventricular Function (CAPRICORN) study evaluated the effect of carvedilol in 1,959 patients with AMI and LVEF less than 40%. Notably, the majority of patients in the STEMI cohort received reperfusion therapy, and 97% of these patients were discharged on an angiotensin-converting enzyme (ACE) inhibitor (123,124). Overall, carvedilol treatment reduced all-cause mortality by 23% (95% CI, 0.60–0.98; p < 0.03), nonfatal reinfarction by 41% (95% CI, 0.39–0.89; p < 0.01), and the composite death/MI end point by 29% (95% CI, 0.57–0.89; p = 0.002). All subcategories of patients benefited, including those with non-STEMI associated with low LVEF. Indeed, in this group, there was a 69% relative reduction in nonfatal reinfarction (124).

The ACC/AHA and ESC guidelines recommend β-blockers for all patients with ACS at the time of admission in the absence of contraindications. The intravenous route is preferred in patients with STEMI and in high-risk patients with non–ST-segment elevation, such as those with dynamic ST-segment depression or deep T-wave inversions. If there are concerns regarding patient tolerance, for example, in patients with pulmonary disease or significant LV dysfunction, a short-acting agent can be used for initial therapy. Initiation of parenteral β-blocker therapy requires frequent monitoring of vital signs and continuous ECG monitoring. Oral therapy should be subsequently instituted to achieve a resting heart rate between 50 and 60 beats per minute. In general, patients with significantly impaired atrioventricular conduction, a history of asthma, or severe acute LV dysfunction should not receive β-blockers.

The organic nitrates have been used in the management of ischemic heart disease since 1879, when nitroglycerin was first used for the relief of anginal pain (125). The primary action of nitrates is vasodilation that results from relaxation of vascular smooth muscle in veins, arteries, and arterioles, leading to a decrease in myocardial oxygen demand, greater epicardial coronary artery flow, and improvement in coronary collateral size and flow. Also, there is evidence suggesting that nitrates possess antiplatelet and antithrombotic properties (126–128), which may contribute to their anti-ischemic effects. There is good evidence that nitrate use in patients with unstable angina reduces or prevents symptoms (129), but there are no long-term trials to indicate whether nitrate therapy used alone alters prognosis.

Recently, the results of the Impact of Nicorandil in Angina (IONA) study (130) were published. This placebo-controlled trial addressed the question of whether treatment with an antianginal drug that has cytoprotective properties (nicorandil) improves clinical outcomes in 5,126 patients with chronic stable CAD and decreased LV function, diabetes, or hypertension. Nicorandil has two mechanisms of action; first, it has a nitrate-like vasodilator effect, and second, in cardiac mitochondria, nicorandil activates potassium–adenosine triphosphate channels that are cytoprotective during ischemia (131). Patients receiving sulphonylureas, which block the activation of mitochondrial potassium–adenosine triphosphate channels, were excluded from the study. During a mean follow-up of 1.6 years, nicorandil therapy (20 mg twice daily) significantly decreased the composite end point of cardiac death, nonfatal MI, and unstable angina by 17% (from 15.5% to 13.1%; odds ratio, 0.83; 95% CI, 0.72–0.97; $p = 0.014$). Because the benefit of nicorandil was observed when the drug was added to usual antianginal therapy (nitrates in most patients), IONA strongly suggests that clinical benefit is mediated, at least in part, through activation of mitochondrial potassium–adenosine triphosphate.

Effects of Calcium Channel Blockers

Calcium antagonists are a heterogeneous group of drugs that inhibit calcium ion movement through slow channels in cardiac and smooth muscle membranes by noncompetitive blockade of voltage-sensitive, L-type calcium channels. There are three major types of calcium antagonists: (a) the dihydropyridines (nifedipine, nicardipine, isradipine, felodipine and amlodipine); (b) the phenylalkylamines (verapamil); and (c) the modified benzothiazepines (diltiazem). All calcium antagonists are coronary vasodilators, prevent coronary spasm, and have some antiplatelet effect. In contrast to the dihydropyridines, both verapamil and diltiazem have prominent atrioventricular and sinus node effects and decrease heart rate. Calcium antagonists often are used to control ongoing or recurring ischemia-related symptoms or hypertension in patients who are already receiving adequate doses of nitrates and β-blockers, in patients who are unable to tolerate adequate doses of one or both of these agents, and in patients with variant angina. Rapid-release, short-acting dihydropyridines (e.g., nifedipine) must be avoided in the absence of adequate concurrent β-blockade in ACS because several RCTs suggest increased adverse outcomes (18–20).

During the last two decades, a number of studies have suggested a potential therapeutic benefit, both short and long term, with nondihydropyridine calcium channel blockers in patients with non-STEMI and preserved LV function (132). In 1984, the results of the Diltiazem Reinfarction Study (DRS) were reported; in 576 patients with acute non–Q-wave MI, treatment with diltiazem (360 mg/d) for up to 2 weeks was associated with a 50% reduction in reinfarction (primary end point), as well as refractory angina and recurrent angina associated with ECG changes (133,134). A prespecified subset analysis of the Multicenter Diltiazem Postinfarction Trial (MDPIT) showed lower mortality and reinfarction rates during an average follow-up of 24 months among patients with non–Q-wave MI and LVEF greater than 40% (135). More recently, a *post hoc* analysis of MDPIT and the second Danish Verapamil Infarction Trial (DAVIT-

II) (136) revealed a highly significant treatment-related effect on all-cause mortality and the composite end point of death or reinfarction in a similar cohort of patients who received a heart rate–decreasing calcium channel blocker (Fig. 77–14A and 77–14B).

Effect of Angiotensin-converting Enzyme Inhibitors

A universal role for ACE inhibitors in primary and secondary prevention has been suggested (137). The benefits of ACE inhibitors in the ACSs have been demonstrated in many large-scale trials, including Survival And Ventricular Enlargement (SAVE), International Study of Infarct Survival (ISIS)-4, Gruppo Italiano per lo Studio della Sopravvivenza nell'Infarto Miocardico (GISSI) 3, Acute Infarction Ramipril Efficacy (AIRE), and Trandolapril Cardiac Evaluation (TRACE) (138–142). Data from virtually all of these studies strongly suggest that the beneficial effects of ACE inhibition go beyond blood pressure control. This concept is supported by experimental data indicating that the advantage may also be related to plaque stabilization (137,143) and by the Heart Outcomes Prevention Evaluation (HOPE) trial (144), which showed a reduction of cardiovascular death from 8.1% to 6.1% (absolute risk reduction, 2%; relative risk reduction, 0.40; 95% CI, 0.64–0.87; $p < 0.001$) and MI (relative risk reduction, 0.80; 95% CI, 0.70–0.90; $p < 0.001$) over 4 to 6 years of follow-up. However, in HOPE, no benefit was observed in the subcategory of patients with unstable angina, but this may be merely chance (145). Other trials are ongoing to confirm these findings: European trial of Reduction Of cardiac events with Perindopril in stable coronary disease (EUROPA), and Prevention of Events with ACE inhibitors (PEACE), which may establish new strategies to prevent occurrence of ACSs. Currently, the main indications for use of ACE inhibitors in patients with ACS are as follows: (a) within the first 24 hours of onset of anterior STEMI, or if STEMI is associated with clinical congestive heart failure in the absence of significant contraindications (18); and (b) in all ACS patients, including those without ECG changes or positive biomarkers, if diabetes, hypertension, or an LVEF less than 40% exists (19,20). The results of the OPtimal Trial In Myocardial infarction with the Angiotensin II Antagonist Losartan (OPTIMAAL) study (146), taken in the context of Morality Data from the Losartan Heart Failure Survival (ELITE II) (147), reinforce the conclusion that ACE inhibitors, rather than an angiotensin receptor blocker, should remain the preferred treatment in these patient subcategories.

Lipid-lowering Therapy

The major lipid-lowering end point trials provide powerful evidence supporting the use of statin class drugs to improve patient outcomes across a wide range of patient types, including those recovering from ACS (148–156). In 1999, a metaanalysis of 2 primary and 3 secondary prevention trials

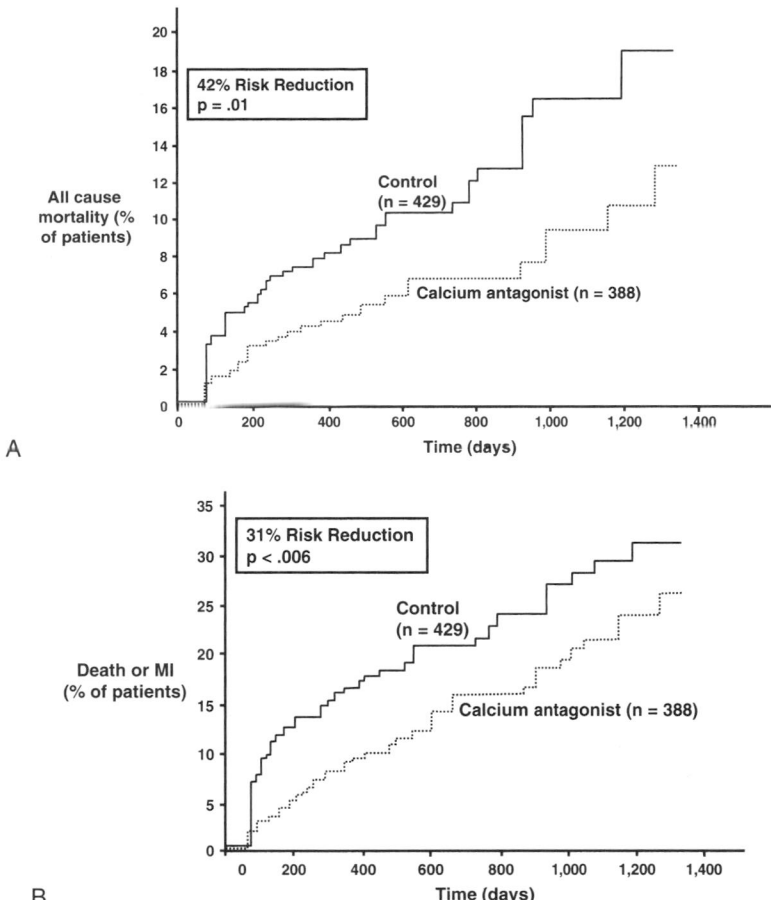

FIG. 77–14. Pooled analysis of the Multicenter Diltiazem Postinfarction Trial (MDPIT) and second Danish Verapamil Infarction Trial (DAVIT-2) trials. Cumulative all-cause mortality rate **(A)** and cardiac event rate **(B)** are depicted according to treatment group assignment for patients with non–Q-wave myocardial infarction (MI) and no pulmonary congestion. (From Gibson RS, Hansen JF, Messerli F, et al. Long-term effects of diltiazem and verapamil on mortality and cardiac events in non-Q-wave acute myocardial infarction without pulmonary congestion: post hoc subset analysis of the Multicenter Diltiazem Postinfarction Trial and the Second Danish Verapamil Infarction Trial Studies. *Am J Cardiol* 2000;86:275–279, with permission.)

showed the undeniable benefits of lipid reduction with statins in 30,817 patients with minimally to severely increased cholesterol levels (157). When the results of these five trials are pooled, statin treatment was associated with a 21% reduction in all-cause mortality (95% CI, 0.72–0.86; $p < 0.001$), a 27% reduction in vascular mortality (95% CI, 0.66–0.81; $p < 0.001$), a 29% reduction in fatal coronary events (95% CI, 0.64–0.80; $p < 0.001$), and a 31% reduction in major coronary events (95% CI, 0.64–0.74; $p < 0.001$). When the metaanalysis results were stratified by age and sex, reductions in vascular events were similar between men and women, and between patients ≥ 65 years and those younger than 65 years.

The landmark Heart Protection Study (HPS), because of its size (20,536 patients) and broad inclusion criteria, provided new information on the benefits of statin therapy in high-risk patient populations (154). It demonstrated substantial benefit not only in patients with established

CAD, but also in those without CAD who had cerebrovascular disease, peripheral arterial disease, treated hypertension, or diabetes, irrespective of blood lipid levels when treatment was initiated. During 5 years of follow-up, treatment-related significant reductions occurred in all-cause mortality (12%; $p = 0.0003$), coronary deaths (17%; $p = 0.0001$), cardiac death or nonfatal MI (27%; $p < 0.0001$), fatal and nonfatal stroke (25%; $p < 0.0001$), and revascularization procedures (24%; $p < 0.0001$). The HPS included large subgroups of women, elderly, patients with diabetes, and patients without diagnosed CAD but with previous transient ischemic attack/stroke or peripheral arterial disease; in all of these subgroups, the proportional decrease in vascular events was similar and statistically significant. The HPS also showed that decreasing low-density lipoprotein (LDL) cholesterol below the threshold levels in the guidelines of the ESC (158) and National Cholesterol Education Program-Adult Treatment Panel

(NCEP-ATP) III (159) may provide incremental benefit (Fig. 77–15). The impressive results seen among patients with baseline LDL levels less than 100 mg/dL are consistent with epidemiologic studies (160), previously reported RCTs (153,161–163), the Arterial Biology for the Investigation of the Treatment Effects of Reducing Cholesterol (ARBITER) trial (164), and the preliminary data from the Anglo-Scandinavian Cardiac Outcomes Trial (ASCOT) (165,166), all of which strongly support the emerging concept that more aggressive lipid therapy leads to greater benefit. Confirmation likely will come over the next few years, when several large RCTs testing the "lower is better" hypothesis reach completion. These include the Treating to New Targets (TNT) trial, the Study of the Effectiveness of Additional Reductions in Cholesterol and Homocysteine (SEARCH), and Incremental Decrease in Endpoints through Aggressive Lipid-Lowering (IDEAL) trial.

Although the vast majority of the statin megatrials did not study patients within 3 months of an acute coronary event, there seems to be adequate rationale and ample data to recommend statin therapy for all patients with ACS on hospital admission. Experimental models of ischemia and reperfusion have shown that statins reduce reperfusion injury and infarct size (167). It also has been demonstrated that statins: (a) decrease thrombus formation and facilitate fibrinolysis (168–170); (b) inhibit platelet reactivity and aggregation (168–171); (c) reduce thromboxane A_2 production (172); (d) improve endothelial function in patients with symptomatic CAD, including those with syndrome X, and significantly reduce objective evidence of inducible myocardial ischemia (173–177); (e) possibly stabilize plaques and make atheromas less susceptible to rupture by reducing cholesterol synthesis by macrophages (178), decreasing inflammatory cells (179), reducing matrix metalloproteinase activation (178), and promoting collagen accumulation in the fibrous cap (180); and (f) reduce serum levels of CRP and other inflammatory biomarkers (181–183) that predict adverse cardiovascular outcomes (184–187). Emerging data continue to substantiate CRP as an independent predictor of cardiac events in all patient populations, including those with ACS. For example, a baseline increase in CRP confers up to a threefold risk for MI in apparently healthy men (184) and a fourfold risk in healthy women (185). After an MI, greater

CRP levels correlate with significantly lower event-free survival rates and greater cardiac event rates (186). In patients undergoing percutaneous interventions, a baseline increase in CRP levels confers an almost fourfold risk for death or MI by 30 days (187). In a report by Walter and coworkers (188), it was shown that statin therapy abrogates the increased risk associated with increased CRP levels after coronary stent implantation.

As shown in Table 77–4, there is now a wealth of evidence from registries and observational studies that illustrate the potential "plaque stabilizing" effects of early statin therapy in patients with ACS (189–196). Moreover, in the last few years, there have been two RCTs testing the hypothesis that early statin therapy in patients with ACS is beneficial: the randomized Lipid-Coronary Artery Disease (L-CAD) trial and the Myocardial Ischemia Reduction with Aggressive Cholesterol Lowering (MIRACL) trial (197,198). Both trials showed benefit, and other studies have demonstrated that in-hospital prescription of statin drugs is rarely associated with adverse effects and greatly improves long-term compliance (26,199). Thus, a persuasive argument can be made for a recommendation that everyone without contraindication receive a statin on admission. Obviously, the choice of which statin to use should be based on strength of evidence, ideally obtained from well designed and properly executed RCTs, that demonstrates short- and long-term benefit on outcomes that matter to patients (e.g., death, MI, and stroke). As depicted in Table 77–5, there are substantial data showing benefit with "natural" statins (simvastatin, pravastatin, and lovastatin) and one "synthetic" statin (fluvastatin). To date, atorvastatin has not yet been shown to reduce mortality or MI, although several studies have demonstrated that this drug decreases the rate of recurrent or progressive angina (161,198), or both, and one would expect it to exert effects similar to other statins, especially because it is one of the most potent statins in its class.

Hormone Replacement Therapy in Postmenopausal Women

In numerous observational studies over the last 30 years comprising more than 600,000 women-years of follow-up, postmenopausal estrogen replacement, with or without a progestin, has been associated with reduced risk for coro-

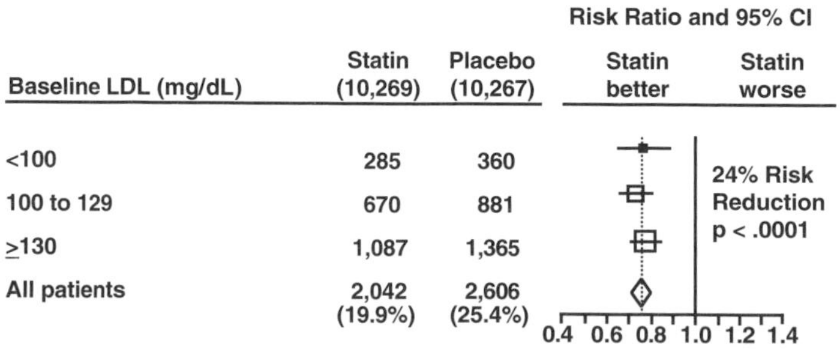

			Risk Ratio and 95% CI		
Baseline LDL (mg/dL)	Statin (10,269)	Placebo (10,267)	Statin better	Statin worse	
<100	285	360			24% Risk Reduction p < .0001
100 to 129	670	881			
≥130	1,087	1,365			
All patients	2,042 (19.9%)	2,606 (25.4%)			

0.4 0.6 0.8 1.0 1.2 1.4

FIG. 77–15. In the Heart Protection Study, when results were analyzed by baseline low-density lipoprotein (LDL) values, patients with LDL levels less than 100 mg/dL were found to benefit, as well as patients with LDL of 100 to 129 mg/dL and those with LDL of 130 mg/dL or greater. CI, confidence interval. (Adapted from Heart Protection Study Collaborative Group. MRC/BHF Heart Protection Study of cholesterol lowering with simvastatin in 20,536 high-risk individuals: a randomised placebo-controlled trial. *Lancet* 2002;360:7–22, with permission.)

TABLE 77–4. *Early statin therapy for plaque stabilization*

Observational study (reference)	Patients, n	End point	Risk reduction[a]	p
MITRA (189)	8,335	In-hospital mortality	13% ↓	<0.001
NRMI IV Registry (196)	174,635	In-hospital mortality	62% ↓	<0.001
PRISM (195)	1,616	30-day death/MI	55% ↓	<0.01
GUSTO/PURSUIT (191)	20,809	30-day mortality	50% ↓	<0.001
GERMAN PCI (190)	704	6-mo death/MI	87% ↓	<0.03
OPUS (193)	10,288	30-d mortality	69% ↓	<0.001
Swedish Registry (192)	19,599	12-mo mortality	25% ↓	<0.001
InTIME (194)	14,124	12-mo mortality	33% ↓	<0.001

GERMAN PCI, percutaneous coronary intervention; GUSTO, Global Utilization of Streptokinase and t-PA for Occluded coronary arteries; InTIME, Intravenous nPA Treatment of Infarcting Myocardium Early; MITRA, Maximal Individual Therapy in Acute Myocardial Infarction; NRMI, National Registry of Myocardial Infarction; OPUS, Orbofiban in Patients with Unstable Coronary Syndromes; PRISM, Platelet Receptor Inhibition In Ischemic Syndrome Management.
[a]Risk reduction of patients receiving early statin therapy compared with those who did not.

nary events, both in women with and without evidence of CAD (200–203). Estrogen exerts beneficial effects on LDL- and high-density lipoprotein (HDL) cholesterol, on vasomotor function, and on some aspects of the coagulation system (204). Yet, all six of the recently reported randomized trials of hormone replacement therapy (HRT) for secondary prevention failed to show any protective effect (205–211). Disturbingly, two of these trials showed a highly significant excess risk for death, MI, or stroke in the first 6 to 12 months after HRT initiation (205,206,208), and a third trial revealed a strong trend toward adverse outcome (211). This finding of early excess hazard also was seen in the Framingham study (212), and in five different registries, including the Coronary Drug Project (213,214), the Coumadin Aspirin Reinfarction Study (CARS) (215), the Nurse's Health Study (216), the Puget Sound Group Health Cooperative study (217), and the Kaiser Permanente Diabetes Registry (218). In addition, both of the primary prevention trials—the Women's Health Initiative (WHI) (219) and the Women's International Study of Long Duration Estrogen after Menopause (WISDOM)— reported excess early events and concluded that HRT should not be taken solely to prevent cardiovascular disease, osteoporosis, or other chronic diseases because the risks outweigh benefits. Notably, both primary prevention trials were termi-

nated prematurely because of excess risk in the group receiving HRT.

The causal relation between HRT and early ischemic events, including MI and fatal stroke, has not yet been fully explored, but it may relate to proinflammatory, prothrombotic, or proarrhythmic properties (220,221). The Estrogen Replacement and Atherosclerosis (ERA) trial found an associated increase in CRP levels and other prothrombotic molecules (207). Other studies have confirmed the adverse effect of oral conjugated equine estrogen on von Willebrand factor (221) and of various HRT regimens on serum CRP levels (Fig. 77–16) (222–224). Available data suggest the use of HRT should be discouraged in patients at risk for atherothrombotic events (225). This pessimism about HRT does not, however, imply pessimism about disease prevention in postmenopausal women. Many randomized trials that included women provide strong support for the use of therapeutic lifestyle change, regular exercise, antiplatelet agents, β-blockers, ACE inhibitors, and lipid-lowering drugs (226–230).

Can we predict who will benefit or will be harmed by HRT? In the future, it seems likely that clinicians will use genetic testing in determining the risk/benefit ratios of various drug therapies, including HRT (231). For example, it is

TABLE 77–5. *Effect of statin therapy on cardiac death and nonfatal myocardial infarction*

Randomized controlled trial (statin) (reference)	Patients, n	Relative risk reduction	Absolute risk reduction	NNT to prevent 1 event
4S (simvastatin) (148)	4,444	34%	8.5%	12
HPS (simvastatin) (154)	20,536	22%	5.5%	18
LIPID (pravastatin) (151)	9,014	23%	3.4%	30
CARE (pravastatin) (150)	4,159	24%	3.0%	34
WOSCOPS (pravastatin) (149)	6,595	29%	2.2%	46
LIPS (fluvastatin) (156)	1,677	31%	2.2%	46
PROSPER (pravastatin) (155)	5,804	19%	2.1%	48
AFCAPS/Tex CAPS (lovastatin) (152)	6,605	37%	2.0%	50

4S, Scandinavian Simvastatin Survival Study; AFCAPS/Tex CAPS, Air Force/Texas Coronary Atherosclerosis Prevention Study; CARE, Cholesterol And Recurrent Events; HPS, Heart Protection Study; LIPID, Long-term Intervention with Pravastatin in Ischaemic Disease; LIPS, Lescol Intervention Prevention Study; NNT, number needed to treat; PROSPER, Pravastatin in elderly individuals at risk of vascular disease; WOSCOPS, West Of Scotland COronary Prevention Study.

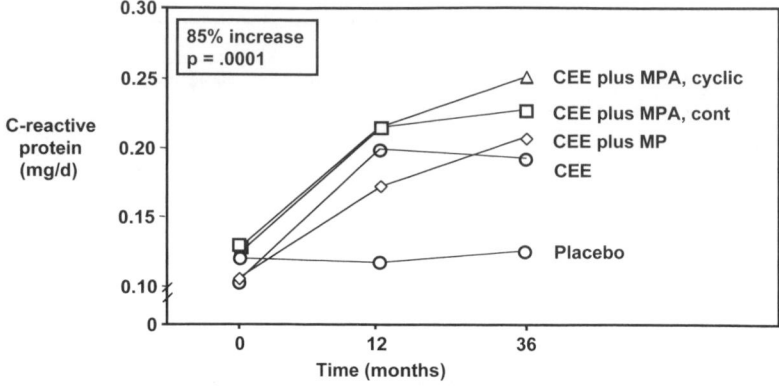

FIG. 77–16. Effect of placebo and four different hormone replacement therapy regimens on C-reactive protein levels in postmenopausal women. The regimens included: 0.625 mg/d conjugated equine estrogen (CEE); 0.625 mg/d CEE plus 10 mg/d medroxyprogesterone acetate (MPA), Days 1 through 12 each month, cyclic; 0.675 mg/d CEE plus 2.5 mg/d MPA, continuous; and 0.625 mg/d CEE plus 200 mg/d micronized progesterone (MP), Days 1 through 12 each month. (From Cushman M, Legault C, Barrett-Connor E, et al. Effect of postmenopausal hormones on inflammation-sensitive proteins: the Postmenopausal Estrogen/Progestin Interventions (PEPI) Study. *Circulation* 1999;100:717–722, with permission.)

known that the prothrombin G20210A mutation carried by approximately 5% of people increases the risk for venous and arterial thrombotic events. Psaty and coworkers (232) performed a case–control study to investigate the interaction between the prothrombin G20210A mutation and MI in HRT users with hypertension. These investigators estimated that women who carry the G20210A mutation and use HRT have a nearly 11-fold increased risk for MI if they are 80% compliant with their HRT regimen and a 20-fold increased risk if they are 100% compliant. A report by Glueck and coworkers (233) clarified the effect of exogenous estrogen on atherothrombotic vascular disease risk according to the presence or absence of the factor V Leiden mutation. Another report by Herrington and coworkers (234) illustrated the importance of estrogen receptor polymorphisms in predicting the effect of replacement estrogen on HDL cholesterol levels. Still other studies have shown the potential value of genetic testing in women for predicting risk for osteoporotic fractures, independent of bone mass (235), and for predicting response to cancer prevention therapies (236).

Raloxifene, a selective estrogen receptor modulator, is similar to estrogen in its effects on some CAD risk factors (decreasing total cholesterol, LDL cholesterol, and homocysteine) but dissimilar to others (not increasing triglyceride or CRP levels). Studies have shown that raloxifene reduces the risk for osteoporotic fractures by 50%, as well as the risk for invasive breast cancer by nearly 76% (237,238). An analysis of the Multiple Outcomes of Raloxifene Evaluation (MORE) study yielded an intriguing finding (239): As shown in Figure 77–17, healthy postmenopausal women with CAD risk factors had a significantly lower cardiac event rate if taking raloxifene compared with placebo. A large prospective trial, Raloxifene Use for The Heart (RUTH), is underway to confirm these findings (240).

Long-Term Oral Anticoagulation

Given its undeniable benefits and favorable safety profile, aspirin has become the initial antithrombotic agent of choice. Metaanalysis of a few small trials comparing moderate- to high-intensity anticoagulation with warfarin versus aspirin did not demonstrate a difference in efficacy, whereas bleeding was lower with aspirin (241). Interestingly, the Aspirin and Coumadin after Acute Coronary Syndromes (ASPECT-2; target International Normalized Ratio [INR]: 3–4) and WArfarin Re-Infarction Study (WARIS)-2 (target INR: 2.8–4.2) trials both reported that full-intensity anticoagulation as monotherapy was superior to aspirin alone in the secondary prevention of death, (re)infarction, and stroke (242,243). Thus, high-intensity oral anticoagulation appears to be an effective alternative for aspirin in the setting of well organized frequent INR monitoring. Among patients recovering from acute STEMI, if aspirin is contraindicated, oral anticoagulation with warfarin is the only effective long-term antithrombotic regimen evaluated to date.

Oral anticoagulation therapy at medium- to high- and low-intensity combined with aspirin has been tested in five clinical trials, comprising 20,656 patients (242–246). Results are mixed, with two trials showing incremental benefit compared with aspirin alone (242,243) and three trials showing no benefit (244–246). Unlike the situation mentioned earlier with patients with STEMI who are intolerant to aspirin, there is an effective alternative for patients recovering from non-STEMI or unstable angina. For these patients who can not take aspirin, 75 mg per day clopidogrel appears to be the currently preferred, practical, long-term alternative. With respect to the long-term benefits of clopidogrel (108–111,114), direct comparisons with oral anticoagulation, both as single agents and in addition to aspirin, currently have not been performed. We believe this is an important area for future research.

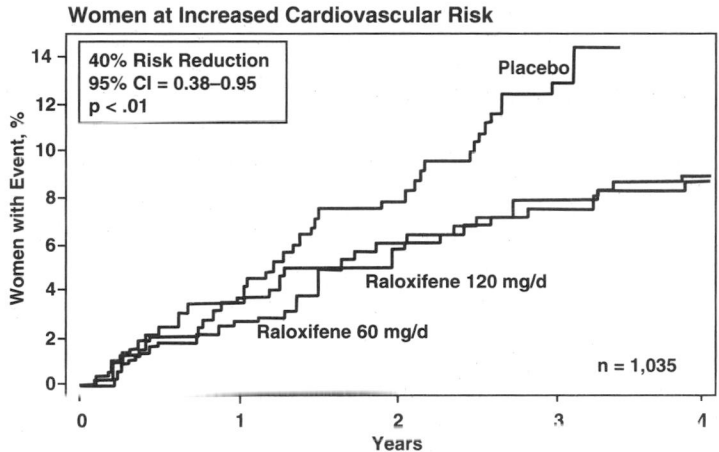

FIG. 77–17. Kaplan-Meier survival curves showing the cumulative incidence of cardiovascular events, according to treatment group assignment, in a subset of 1,035 high-risk postmenopausal women who were enrolled in the Multiple Outcomes of Raloxifene Evaluation (MORE) trial. The curves diverged beginning after the first year, which continued through 4 years. Compared with placebo, the Raloxifene groups had fewer events (12.9% vs 7.8%; odds ratio, 0.40; 95% confidence interval [CI], 0.38–0.95; p = 0.03). (From Barrett-Connor E, Grady D, Sashegyi A, et al. Raloxifene and cardiovascular events in osteoporotic postmenopausal women. Four-year results from the MORE (Multiple Outcomes of Raloxifene Evaluation) randomized trial. *JAMA* 2002;287:847–857, with permission.)

The reported results of the ASPECT and WARIS-2 trials not only established the need for a definitive trial of anticoagulant therapy in ACS, but they also raised the important possibility of a *threshold level* of anticoagulation for benefit. These two trials support a target level of anticoagulation approaching an INR of 3.0 (range 2.5–3.5) for anticoagulation monotherapy and 2.5 (range 2.0–3.0) for combination therapy with aspirin.

Other Therapeutic Considerations

Blood pressure control is an important goal, and patients with hypertension should be given explicit education on their target goal (<135/85 mm Hg in general, and <130/80 mm Hg if patient has diabetes, renal insufficiency or LVEF < 40%). Particular attention needs to be paid to smoking cessation. Daly and coworkers (247) quantified the long-term effects of smoking on patients with ACS. Men younger than 60 years who continued to smoke had a risk for death from all causes 5.4 times that of men who stopped smoking (p < 0.05). Referral to a smoking cessation program and the use of nicotine patches or gum is strongly recommended by the ACC/AHA and ESC, in part because studies have shown that these interventions substantially increase smoke-free time (248,249) and can significantly reduce ischemic burden by nuclear stress testing (250). Bupropion, an anxiolytic agent and a weak inhibitor of neuronal uptake of neurotransmitters, has been effective when added to brief regular counseling sessions in helping patients to quit smoking (248). Family members who live in the same household should be encouraged to stop smoking so as to reinforce the patient's effort and to decrease the risk for second-hand smoke.

The current ACC/AHA and ESC guidelines emphasize the importance of comprehensive cardiac rehabilitation and recommend that all survivors be referred to an appropriate outpatient program. Many studies have documented the effectiveness of these programs. In a metaanalysis of 10 RCTs, involving 10,971 patients, Taylor and coworkers (251) showed that "comprehensive" and "primarily exercise based" programs are associated with significant reductions in all-cause mortality, cardiac death, and systolic blood pressure, as well as improvements in lipid parameters and smoking cessation rates. Other studies have demonstrated that regular aerobic exercise prevents age-related declines in endothelial function (252), significantly retards carotid and coronary atherothrombosis as assessed by duplex ultrasound and electron beam computed tomography (253,254), improves myocardial blood flow reserve in patients recovering from AMI (255), and decreases blood pressure, fibrinogen, and CRP levels (256,257).

The randomized trial of insulin-glucose infusion followed by subcutaneous insulin treatment in diabetic patients with acute myocardial infarction (DIGAMI) demonstrated that tight glucose control in patients with diabetes during and after MI is associated with a lower acute and 1-year mortality rate in ACS (258). Tight glucose control, defined as HbA1c less than 7.0%, improves endothelial dysfunction, reduces microvascular complications, and has been shown to decrease major coronary events in newly detected type 2 diabetics without symptomatic macrovascular disease (259–262). In light of these data, it is not surprising that an HbA1c of less than 7% is strongly recommended by the ACC/AHA, ESC, and the American Diabetes Association (18–20,259).

Although there is an association between increased homocysteine blood levels and CAD, a reduction in homocysteine levels with folate has not yet been demonstrated to reduce the risk for major coronary events in patients with established CAD (263,264), except possibly in patients undergoing PCI (265). In 2002, the results of a large RCT were reported by Baker and coworkers (266). The aim of this trial was to determine whether high-dose folic acid (5 mg/d) prevents major adverse cardiac events in patients with either stable angina or recent ACS and angiographically documented CAD. A total of 1,882 patients were enrolled and followed for a median of 1.7 years. Treatment with folic acid significantly reduced plasma homocysteine from 11.2 + 6.9 to 9.7 + 5.3, but had no effect on the composite primary end point of cardiac death, nonfatal MI, and unplanned revascularization. Currently, there are inadequate data to support the routine use of folic acid supplementation in all patients with CAD and slightly increased homocysteine.

Oxidized LDL cholesterol is thought to play an important role in the pathogenesis of atherothrombosis, and several preclinical studies have found that α-tocopherol (vitamin E), a potent antioxidant, may delay onset and retard the progression of atherothrombosis (267–269). However, clinical outcome studies in humans have yielded conflicting results. To determine the effect of antioxidant therapy on long-term cardiovascular morbidity and mortality, the group from the Cleveland Clinic performed a metaanalysis of six RCTs that enrolled a total of 77,041 patients with CAD or who were at high risk for development of CAD (270). The pooled data showed no effect of vitamin E on all-cause mortality, cardiac death, or stroke. This lack of salutary effect was consistent across all major trials with a variety of vitamin doses and diverse patient populations. Furthermore, some indirect evidence suggests that antioxidant vitamin supplements might be harmful to patients with CAD. In one study of coronary patients with low HDL cholesterol, the combination of vitamins C and E plus β-carotene and selenium blunted the increase in HDL cholesterol and LDL particle size by simvastatin plus niacin treatment (163,271). A strong trend toward CAD regression was observed in the simvastatin plus niacin group, whereas minimal regression occurred when antioxidant vitamins were added (163). Vitamins C, E, and β-carotene also appeared to attenuate the reduced rate of restenosis after PCI produced by pretreatment with probucol (272). Given these results, the common use of vitamin E by consumers is actively discouraged by some physicians. An unanswered question, however, is whether vitamin E alone or combined vitamin E and C delays the development of atherothrombosis in patients who have not experienced an ACS.

During the last decade, many dietary trials in secondary prevention of coronary heart disease have reported impressive reductions in recurrence rates, ranging from 30% to 70% (273–275). The results of these trials were in contrast to previous dietary trials, which were aimed at reducing cholesterol by a low-cholesterol, low–saturated fat, high–polyunsaturated fat diet and failed to significantly improve the overall clinical prognosis of the dieters (276). The successful trials tested dietary patterns characterized by a low intake of total and saturated fat (273,274), and/or increased intake of fish (273) or plant ω3 fatty acids (274,275) and were not intended primarily to reduce blood cholesterol. Two of these trials (274,275) also included a high intake of fresh fruits and vegetables, legumes, and cereals containing large amounts of fiber and vegetable proteins. In 1999, the final report of the Lyon Diet Heart Study was published (277). This study was a randomized secondary prevention trial aimed at testing whether a Mediterranean-type diet, compared with a prudent Western-type diet, would be more effective in reducing recurrence after a first MI. The results were compelling in favor of the Mediterranean diet; during an average follow-up of 4 years, patients assigned to the Mediterranean diet had lower all-cause and cardiovascular mortality rates ($p = 0.01$), and a reduced rate of cardiac death combined with reinfarction ($p = 0.0001$). A second major trial confirmed the advantages of a Mediterranean diet versus a conventional Step 1 NCEP diet (278). In addition, the Lyon Diet study showed that major risk factors, such as high blood pressure and cholesterol, were independent and joint predictors of recurrent events, indicating that the Mediterranean dietary pattern did not alter, at least qualitatively, the usual relations between major risk factors and recurrence. It thus appears that a comprehensive strategy to decrease cardiovascular morbidity and mortality should include not only a cardioprotective diet but other interventions (e.g., pharmacologic) aimed at reducing modifiable risk factors.

An antiarrhythmic and antifibrillatory effect of ω3 fatty acids has been reported in many different animal studies and in laboratory experiments on isolated myocytes (279). Epidemiologic and clinical studies have suggested that ω3 fatty acids reduce the incidence of cardiovascular events, including sudden cardiac death (279–283). The most recent and largest of these trials was the GISSI-Prevenzione study (282). A total of 11,323 patients surviving a recent (<3 months) MI were randomly assigned to 850 mg per day ω3 fatty acid or placebo and optimal pharmacologic treatment and lifestyle advice and were followed for 12 months. Survival curves for (3 fatty acid treatment diverged early after randomization, and all-cause mortality was significantly decreased after only 3 months of treatment by 41% ($p = 0.037$). The early incidence of sudden death also was reduced by 53% ($p = 0.048$), and a similarly significant, although delayed, pattern after 6 to 8 months of treatment was observed for cardiovascular, cardiac, and coronary deaths. In light of this new information, the AHA issued an updated scientific statement (283) in November 2002. For the first time ever, the AHA recommends that a nutritional supplement (appropriately processed fish oil capsules containing ~1 g/d ω3 fatty acid) can be taken by patients with established CAD as an alternative to fish consumption. The guideline also states that people who need to reduce their triglyceride level—usually when it exceeds 200 mg/dL—can do so by taking 2 to 4 g ω3 fatty acids per day. Physicians should not misconstrue this recommendation as a blow

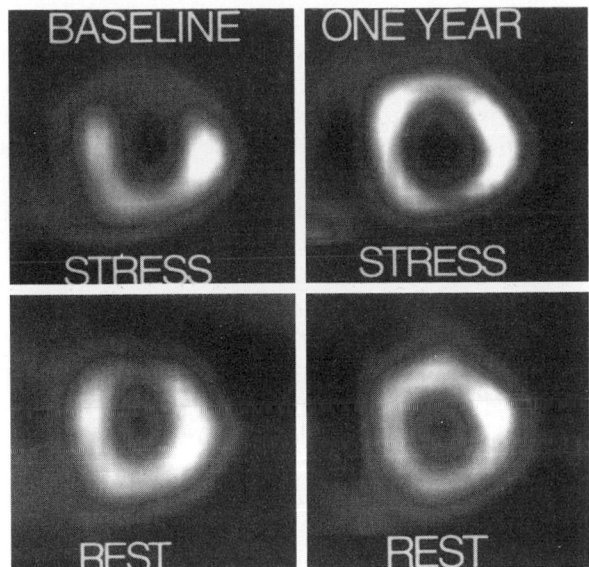

FIG. 77–18. Resolution of stress-induced myocardial ischemia during aggressive medical therapy as demonstrated by single-photon emission computed tomography technetium-99m–sestamibi imaging. (From O'Rourke RA, Chaudhuri T, Shaw L, et al. Resolution of stress-induced myocardial ischemia during aggressive medical therapy as demonstrated by single photon emission computed tomography imaging. *Circulation* 2001;103:2315, with permission.)

against drugs such as fibrates or niacin, which are the established agents for decreasing triglyceride levels.

Potential Impact of Aggressive Medical Treatment

Patients recovering from an ACS who have residual ischemia are at increased risk for subsequent cardiac events. As discussed in Chapter 78, the actual risk ratio depends on the quantified extent of ischemia and degree of LV dysfunction. Although antiplatelet drugs, lipid-lowering agents, β-blockers and possibly heart rate–reducing calcium channel blockers, and ACE inhibitors improve event-free survival after ACS, patients with residual ischemia generally undergo myocardial revascularization as the preferred approach. This therapeutic strategy is assumed to be optimal (69), when compared with "best" medical care, and is widely used in clinical practice. Whether this invasive approach is truly superior to intensive, contemporary medical management is unknown and is being evaluated in the multicenter Clinical Outcomes Utilizing Revascularization and Aggressive Drug Evaluation (COURAGE) trial.

During the last 5 years, there have been several intriguing reports showing the effects of various medical interventions on ischemia suppression, as assessed by ambulatory ECG monitoring, exercise electrocardiographic testing, stress myocardial perfusion SPECT imaging, dobutamine echocardiography, or positron emission tomography scanning techniques (175–177, 250,284–292). These studies have demonstrated a significant reduction in ischemic burden (Fig. 77–18) with intense lifestyle changes, statin class drugs, oral and transdermal nitroglycerin preparations, β-blockers, calcium channel blockers, and smoking cessation programs using a nicotine patch. The Asymptomatic Cardiac Ischemia Pilot (ACIP) study likewise showed that ischemia suppression can be achieved with combination medical therapy (293,294), although most patients in this study received less than two medications. In a small, but prospectively designed, randomized trial, Dakik and coworkers (295) demonstrated that intensive medical therapy and PCI were comparable at suppressing ischemia in stable patients after AMI (Fig. 77–19). Although the small sample size of this single-center pilot study precludes direct comparison of car-

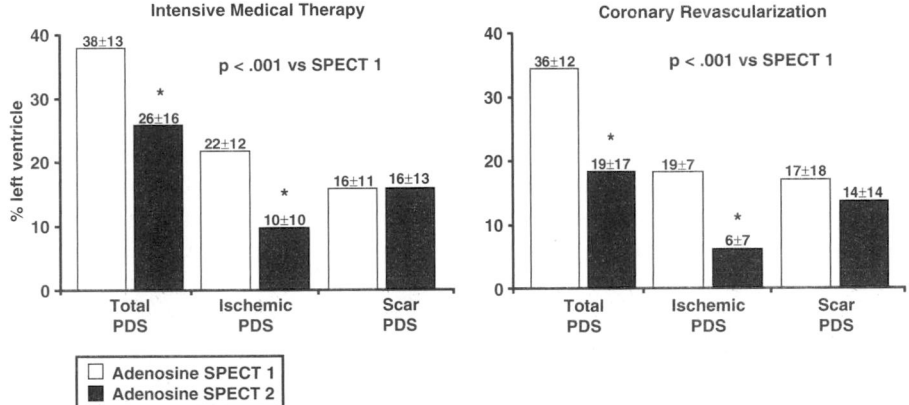

FIG. 77–19. Effect of intensive medical therapy versus coronary revascularization on perfusion defect scores (PDS), as assessed by sequential adenosine thallium-201 single-photon emission computed tomography (SPECT). The magnitude of the absolute reduction in total and ischemic PDS was similar in patients randomized to medical therapy (n = 22) and revascularization (n = 19). (From Dakik HA, Kleiman NS, Farmer JA, et al. Intensive medical therapy versus coronary angioplasty for suppression of myocardial ischemia in survivors of acute myocardial infarction. A prospective, randomized pilot study. *Circulation* 1998;98:2017–2023, with permission.)

diac event rates between the two treatment groups, it does illustrate the potential value of serial SPECT imaging in assessing a treatment-related surrogate end point (ischemic burden). Obviously, adequately powered clinical event trials are needed to better define the independent and combined roles of medical and revascularization strategies in suppressing ischemia and improving clinical outcomes, such as death, MI, and recurrent severe angina after ACS.

Closing the Treatment Gap

The current state of risk factor management in the United States is a cause for concern in the medical community. Analysis of National Health and Nutrition Examination Survey (NHANES) data from three separate time periods shows a disturbing trend in hypertension awareness, treatment, and control. In the latest survey, awareness decreased to 68%, treatment to 54%, and control to 27% (296). Extrapolated to 2000 population statistics for the United States, this translates to 32.3 million people with uncontrolled systolic hypertension and 13.2 million with uncontrolled diastolic hypertension (297,298). An estimated 100 million individuals in the United States have total serum cholesterol levels greater than 200 mg/dL. The Lipid Treatment Assessment Project (L-TAP) examined how well cholesterol was controlled according to the old NCEP-ATP II guidelines (299). It showed that only 38% of patients in all categories met their LDL goals; and in the group with established CAD, the LDL goal of 100 mg/dL was achieved in only 18%. The new ATP III guidelines have broadened eligibility criteria and made treatment even more aggressive. Using a subsample of participants in the NHANES study, the impact of these changes on the treatment-eligible population was projected by Fedder and coworkers (300). From an estimated 15 million individuals in the United States eligible for drug treatment to control cholesterol using the ATP II, the number of patients currently eligible for treatment by ATP III is increased to 36 million. These data emphasize the need for cardiologists and other physicians who treat patients at high risk—namely those with atherothrombosis, diabetes, or a high global risk score (301)—to manage risk factors far more aggressively than in the past, and in more patients.

The changing demographics of the U.S. population will contribute to the growth of the population at risk for cardiovascular disease. The age shift that is occurring as the baby boomers join the ranks of the elderly will lead to an estimated more than 50% increase in the prevalence of coronary heart disease from 2000 to 2030 (302,303). In addition, adverse lifestyle trends are leading to an alarming increase in the prevalence and level of major risk factors. For example, it is estimated that the number of adults with diabetes worldwide will explode from 135 million in 1995 to 300 million in 2025 (304). The increasing prevalence of diabetes correlates with the prevalence of obesity, and the increase in obesity is projected to continue driving the diabetes epidemic.

Obesity is defined as a body mass index (BMI; weight/height^2) of 30 kg per square meter or greater, and overweight is defined as a BMI of 25 kg per square meter. Since 1991, the prevalence of obesity has increased by 65%, and currently more than half of the people in the United States are considered overweight (BMI > 25) and 23% are considered obese (305). The epidemic of obesity and the metabolic syndrome in the United States has been featured on the covers of several national news magazines and has been identified as a medical priority by the U.S. Surgeon General (306).

Within the last few years, several U.S. and worldwide surveys of coronary patients, including those recovering from an ACS, have been reported (307–309). These surveys show a high prevalence of unhealthy lifestyles, modifiable risk factors, and inadequate use of drug therapies that have been shown to improve clinical outcomes. Thus, it appears that substantial gaps between knowledge and practice continue to exist and that there is considerable potential for increasing the standard of preventive cardiology in the United States and throughout the world (310).

SUMMARY AND FUTURE DIRECTIONS

The ACSs continue to be an important health care problem, accounting for approximately 2 million hospitalizations annually in the United States. Despite major advances in treatment, the rates of mortality, MI, and readmission for recurrent chest pain and/or decompensated heart failure at 6-month follow-ups remain high. Clinical practice guidelines, if more widely applied, would surely reduce short- and long-term mortality and mitigate the suffering and economic consequences of unnecessary morbidity. In light of our current understanding and new evidence from recently published clinical trials, the following recommendations can be made:

1. *Patients with STEMI require immediate coronary recanalization with PCI or thrombolysis.* PCI is strongly preferred and efforts should be made to effectively change the approach of the emergency medical response system so that all patients with STEMI have timely access to catheter-based reperfusion. On admission, all patients with STEMI are candidates for aspirin; clopidogrel, if PCI is performed; a thrombin inhibitor; a β-blocker, especially if heart rate or blood pressure level is increased, an ACE inhibitor, and a statin class drug.

2. *Patients without persistent STEMI should receive initial baseline treatment with aspirin; clopidogrel; enoxaparin (unless significant renal dysfunction exists); a β-blocker, if heart rate or blood pressure level is increased and there is no contraindication; a nitrate; and a statin class drug.* Risk stratification should be performed at the time of admission, using clinical data, serial ECGs, and biomarkers. Patients judged to be at low risk for an adverse outcome are managed conservatively, whereas those judged to be at intermediate- or high-risk receive additional therapy with a

GPIIb/IIIa receptor inhibitor and undergo prompt coronary angiography and appropriate revascularization.

3. *In patients treated medically and in those who have had a revascularization procedure, it is important to attempt to eliminate all modifiable risk factors that might influence plaque vulnerability and CAD progression.* In particular, every effort should be made to control the adverse effects of oxidized LDL cholesterol by adhering to a low-cholesterol, Mediterranean-type diet and an exercise program appropriate for the individual patient, as well as by the administration of a statin class drug, not only for its LDL reducing properties, but for its many beneficial pleiotropic effects. In addition, control of blood pressure, reduction in weight if BMI is less than 25 kg per square meter, avoidance of smoking, and reduction in the level of stress, if possible, constitute important lifestyle alterations in attempting to prevent progression of CAD. All patients should receive chronic therapy with agents that inhibit platelet aggregation, and the current recommendation is to combine aspirin with clopidogrel for up to 1 year. In light of the published results of the ASPECT and WARIS-2 trials, oral anticoagulant therapy should be strongly considered for all patients at risk for thromboembolic events, those with thrombophilia involving the arterial system, and—pending further investigation of combination antiplatelet therapy in ACS—patients with possible aspirin resistance. A nitrate preparation is added if the patient has exertional angina, such as an ACE inhibitor and a β-blocker if LV function is reduced or blood pressure is increased. Patients should be followed up periodically to evaluate the success of risk-modifying strategies and compliance with medications. If angina limits the lifestyle the patient wishes to lead despite medical therapy, referral for coronary angiography and myocardial revascularization is appropriate.

4. *In the chronic or postdischarge phase, all patients should be followed by a physician knowledgeable in "best medical practice" and skilled in techniques that help patients follow prescribed treatment* (311). Studies have shown that ambulatory care, with these two caveats in mind, is best accomplished by certified cardiologists (312).

In the future, we can expect to see even greater emphasis on prognostication in medical decision-making. Clinicians will begin using more robust risk stratification schemes that incorporate an array of biomarkers, as well as genetic screening techniques, to help guide the selection of appropriate candidates for various medical therapies. The use of revascularization procedures, especially PCI with coated stents, will see increased scrutiny in a health care environment that places considerable emphasis on cost control and managed care. It is no longer adequate to simply show that an interventional procedure has immediate therapeutic value. It is now necessary to demonstrate that PCI or coronary artery bypass graft surgery adds significantly to the therapeutic value of comprehensive, long-term "best medical" care. In an analogous way, it is important to ask what more invasive and expensive strategies add to the value of less expensive risk factor modification and targeted medical therapy.

One also can expect the development of new drugs, such as orally administered direct thrombin inhibitors that may prove to be a "better aspirin," as well as gene therapy strategies that hasten endothelial healing and health. In our search for the "magic bullet," we should not lose sight of what works today, or lose our enthusiasm for closing the treatment gap. The challenge in 2004 and beyond is to translate best practice into common practice. This remains a formidable worldwide task. The power of effective prevention measures and their current low priority emerge as the major message of the 2002 *World Health Report* (313). There are hundreds of millions of individuals with undiagnosed occult atherothrombosis, and these people require treatment for hypertension, high cholesterol, obesity, diabetes, and nicotine dependence. For these patients, who are seen daily by clinicians, advice about diet, tobacco use, and physical exercise can make a difference to their long-term survival. Assessment of blood pressure, glucose, and cholesterol followed by best treatment, especially among patients who have already had a cardiovascular event, could save innumerable lives in the short and long term. A combination of drugs, including antiplatelet agents, a statin, and appropriate antihypertensive therapy can decrease risks for repeated events. These proven effective preventive measures are too infrequently practiced, and when they are practiced, the tendency remains to manage risk separately. In 2002, the *Ottawa Charter* emphasized the need to tackle risks together and within a social, economic, and political context (314). Unless the deeper determinants of health and illness are addressed, single–risk factor approaches will have a limited impact. In addition to selecting the most cost-effective interventions for selected risk factors, we need stronger health systems that have transformed from focusing on acute episodic care to providing new models of chronic care (315–317). Despite our improved drug arsenal and greater access to invasive interventions, the global challenge of cardiac health has yet to be fully met.

One other area of potential future interest is the developing ability to evaluate atherothrombotic plaques in individual patients for their propensity to rupture. One half or more of AMIs occur in patients with a "culprit" lesion that does not reduce luminal diameter by more than 50% (318,319). Indeed, many of these culprit lesions can not be identified by stress imaging studies and some are not visible by x-ray angiography. Studies have suggested that such disruption-prone plaques in the coronary arteries, the so-called vulnerable plaques, are characterized by a thin fibrous cap (cap thickness of 65–150 μm), a large lipid core, and significant inflammatory cell infiltration manifest by temperature and pH heterogeneity (320–323). Clinical studies are underway to determine whether vulnerable plaques may be identified in individual patients using catheter-based methods and noninvasive imaging techniques (324–329) with a goal of identifying patients for more intensive therapy before events occur. If this proves possible, additional therapeutic advances that are preventive of ACS may be expected in the future.

REFERENCES

1. Maseri A, L'Abbate A, Pesola A, et al. Coronary vasospasm in angina pectoris. *Lancet* 1977;1:713–717.
2. DeWood MA, Spores J, Notske R, et al. Prevalence of total coronary occlusion during the early hours of transmural myocardial infarction. *N Engl J Med* 1980;303:897–902.
3. Buja LM, Willerson JT. Clinicopathologic correlates of acute ischemic heart disease syndromes. *Am J Cardiol* 1981;47:343–356.
4. Willerson JT, Campbell WB, Winniford MD, et al. Conversion from chronic to acute coronary artery disease: speculation regarding mechanisms. *Am J Cardiol* 1984;54:1349–1354.
5. Willerson JT, Hillis LD, Winniford MD, et al. Speculations regarding mechanisms responsible for acute ischemic heart disease syndromes. *J Am Coll Cardiol* 1986;8:245–250.
6. Sherman CT, Litvak F, Grundfest W, et al. Coronary angioscopy in patients with unstable angina pectoris. *N Engl J Med* 1986;315:913–919.
7. Falk E. Plaque rupture with severe pre-existing stenosis precipitating coronary thrombosis: characteristics of coronary atherosclerotic plaques underlying fatal occlusive thrombi. *Br Heart J* 1983;50:127–134.
8. Davies MJ, Thomas AC. Plaque fissuring as the cause of acute myocardial infarction, sudden ischemic death, and crescendo angina. *Br Heart J* 1985;53:363–373.
9. Gotoh K, Minamino T, Katoh O, et al. The role of intracoronary thrombus in unstable angina: angiographic assessment and thrombolytic therapy during ongoing anginal attacks. *Circulation* 1988;77:526–534.
10. Hirsh PD, Hillis LD, Campbell WB, et al. Release of prostaglandins and thromboxane into the coronary circulation in patients with ischemic heart disease. *N Engl J Med* 1981;304:685–691.
11. Fitzgerald DJ, Roy L, Catella F, et al. Platelet activation in unstable coronary disease. *N Engl J Med* 1986;315:983–989.
12. Hamm CW, Lorenz R, Bleifeld W, et al. Biochemical evidence of platelet activation in patients with persistent unstable angina. *J Am Coll Cardiol* 1987;9:998–1004.
13. Van den Berg EK, Schmitz JM, Benedict CR, et al. Transcardiac serotonin concentration is increased in selected patients with limiting angina and complex coronary lesion morphology. *Circulation* 1989;79:116–124.
14. Rubanyi GM, Frye RL, Holmes DR, et al. Vasoconstrictor activity of coronary sinus plasma from patients with coronary artery disease. *J Am Coll Cardiol* 1987;9:1243–1249.
15. Gibson RS, Beller GA, Gheorghiade M, et al. The prevalence and clinical significance of residual myocardial ischemia two weeks after uncomplicated non-Q wave infarction: a prospective natural history study. *Circulation* 1986;73:1186–1198.
16. Gibson RS. Non-Q wave myocardial infarction: diagnosis, prognosis and management. *Curr Prob Cardiol* 1988;13:9–72.
17. Gibson RS. Non-Q wave myocardial infarction. In: Fuster V, Ross R, Topol EJ, eds. *Atherosclerosis and coronary artery disease.* New York: Lippincott-Raven Publishers, 1996:1097–1124.
18. Ryan TJ, Antman EM, Califf M, et al. ACC/AHA guidelines for the management of patients with acute myocardial infarction. *Circulation* 1999;100:1016–1030.
19. Braunwald E, Antman EM, Beasley JW, et al. ACC/AHA 2002 guideline update for the management of patients with unstable angina and non-ST-segment elevation myocardial infarction. *J Am Coll Cardiol* 2002;40:1366–1374.
20. Bertrand ME, Simoons ML, Fox KA, et al. Management of acute coronary syndromes in patients presenting without persistent ST-segment elevation. The Task Force on the Management of Acute Coronary Syndromes of the European Society of Cardiology. *Eur Heart J* 2002;23:1809–1840.
21. Mehta RH, Montoye CK, Gallogly M, et al. Improving quality of care for acute myocardial infarction. The Guidelines Applied to Practice (GAP) Initiative. *JAMA* 2002;287:1269–1276.
22. Cannon CP, Hand MH, Bahr R, et al. Critical pathways for management of patients with acute coronary syndromes: an assessment by the National Heart Attack Alert Program. *Am Heart J* 2002;143:777–789.
23. Eagle KA, Gallogly M, Mehta RH, et al. Taking the National Guideline for care of acute myocardial infarction to the bedside: developing the Guideline Applied to Practice (GAP) Initiative in Southeast Michigan. *Jt Comm J Qual Improve* 2002;28:5–19.
24. Mani O, Mehta RH, Tsai T, et al. Assessing performance reports to individual providers in the care of acute coronary syndromes. *Jt Comm J Qual Improve* 2002;28:220–232.
25. Mehta RH, Das S, Tsai TT, et al. Quality improvement initiative and its impact on the management of patients with acute myocardial infarction. *Arch Intern Med* 2000;160:3057–3062.
26. Fonarow GC, Gawlinski A, Moughrabi S, et al. Improved treatment of coronary heart disease by implementation of a Cardiac Hospitalization Atherosclerosis Management Program (CHAMP). *Am J Cardiol* 2001;87:819–822.
27. Grimshaw JM, Russel IT. Effect of clinical guidelines on medical practice: a systematic review of rigorous evaluations. *Lancet* 1993;342:1317–1322.
28. Giugliano RP, Lloyd-Jones DM, Camargo CA Jr, et al. Association of unstable angina guideline care with improved survival. *Arch Intern Med* 2000;160:1775–1780.
29. DeFranco AC, Rivera W, Farrehi P, et al. Implementation of ACC/AHA guidelines results in profound NSTEMI mortality reduction. *Circulation* 2002;106[Suppl]:II-400(abst).
30. Harrington R, Smith S, Brindis R, et al. National Report from the Executive Committee of the CRUSADE National Quality Improvement Initiative. Newsletter. November 2002, pp. 1–4.
31. Peterson ED, Canto JG, Pollack CV, et al. Early use of glycoprotein 2b3a inhibitors and outcomes in non-ST elevation MI: observations from the NRMI-4. *J Am Coll Cardiol* 2002:303A(abst).
32. Califf RM, Peterson ED, Gibbons RJ, et al. Integrating quality into the cycle of therapeutic development. *J Am Coll Cardiol* 2002;40:1895–1901.
33. Hunt SA, Baker DW, Chin MH, et al. ACC/AHA guidelines for the evaluation and management of chronic heart failure in the adult: executive summary. *J Am Coll Cardiol* 2001;38:2101–2113.
34. Rose EA, Gelijns AC, Moskowitz AJ, et al. Long-term use of a left ventricular assist device for end-stage heart failure. *N Engl J Med* 2001;345:1435–1443.
35. Cazeau S, Leclercq C, Lavergne T, et al. Effects of multisite biventricular pacing in patients with heart failure and intraventricular conduction delay. *N Engl J Med* 2001;344:873–880.
36. Moss AJ, Zareba W, Hall J, et al. Prophylactic implantation of a defibrillator in patients with myocardial infarction and reduced ejection fraction. *N Engl J Med* 2002;346:877–883.
37. Abraham WT, Fisher WG, Smith AL, et al. Cardiac resynchronization in chronic heart failure. *N Engl J Med* 2002;346:1845–1853.
38. Grines CL, Westerhausen DR, Grines LL, et al. A randomized trial of transfer for primary angioplasty versus on-site thrombolysis in patients with high-risk myocardial infarction. The Air Primary Angioplasty in Myocardial Infarction Study. Air PAMI Study Group. *J Am Coll Cardiol* 2002;39:1713–1719.
39. Widimsky P, Groch L, Zelizko M, et al. Multicentre randomized trial comparing transport to primary angioplasty vs immediate thrombolysis vs combined strategy for patients with acute myocardial infarction presenting to a community hospital without a catheterization laboratory. The PRAGUE Study. *Eur Heart J* 2000;21:823–831.
40. Moon JC, Kalra PR, Coats AJ. DANAMI-2: is primary angioplasty superior to thrombolysis in acute MI when the patient has to be transferred to an invasive centre? *Int J Cardiol* 2002;85:199–201.
41. Weaver WD, Simes RJ, Betriu A, et al. Comparison of primary coronary angioplasty and intravenous thrombolytic therapy for acute myocardial infarction. A quantitative review. *JAMA* 1997;278:2093–2098.
42. Magid DJ, Calonge BN, Rumsfeld JS, et al. Relation between hospital primary angioplasty volume and mortality for patients with acute MI treated with primary angioplasty vs thrombolytic therapy. *JAMA* 2000;284:3131–3138.
43. Aversano T, Aversano LT, Passamani E, et al. Thrombolytic therapy vs primary percutaneous coronary intervention for myocardial infarction in patients presenting to hospitals without on-site cardiac surgery. A randomized controlled trial. *JAMA* 2002;287:1943–1957.
44. Brodie BR, Stuckey TD, Wall TC, et al. Importance of time to reperfusion for 30-day and late survival and recovery of left ventricular

function after primary angioplasty for acute myocardial infarction. *J Am Coll Cardiol* 1998;32:1312–1319.

45. Kastrati A, Mehilli J, Dirschinger J, et al. Time-to-treatment interval and myocardial salvage after stenting or thrombolysis in patients with acute myocardial infarction. *Circulation* 2002;106[Suppl]:II-333(abst).

46. Kastrati A, Mehilli J, Dirschinger J, et al. Myocardial salvage after coronary stenting plus abciximab versus fibrinolysis plus abciximab in patients with acute myocardial infarction: a randomised trial. *Lancet* 2002;359:920–925.

47. Schomig A, Kastrati A, Dirschinger J, et al. Coronary stenting plus platelet glycoprotein IIb/IIIa blockade compared with tissue plasminogen activator in acute myocardial infarction: Stent versus Thrombolysis for Occluded Coronary Arteries in Patients with Acute Myocardial Infarction Study Investigators. *N Engl J Med* 2000;343:385–391.

48. Limbruno U, Micheli A, Petronio AS, et al. Prevention of no-reflow during primary percutaneous coronary angioplasty with a porous distal embolic protection device. *Circulation* 2002,106.II-446(abst).

49. Cannon CP. Primary percutaneous coronary intervention for all? *JAMA* 2002;287:1987–1988.

50. Cannon CP, Baim DS. Expanding the reach of primary percutaneous coronary intervention for the treatment of acute myocardial infarction. *J Am Coll Cardiol* 2002;39:1720–1722.

51. Schomig A, Kastrati A, Dirschinger J, et al. Coronary stenting plus platelet glycoprotein IIb/IIIa blockade compared with tissue plasminogen activator in acute myocardial infarction: Stent versus Thrombolysis for Occluded Coronary Arteries in Patients with Acute Myocardial Infarction Study Investigators. *N Engl J Med* 2000; 343:385–391.

52. Grines CL. Updated meta-analysis of primary PCI vs thrombolysis. Presented at American College of Cardiology Scientific Sessions; March 19, 2002; Atlanta, GA.

53. Mark DB, Lee TH. Conservative management of acute coronary syndrome: cheaper and better for you? *Circulation* 2002;105:666–668.

54. Yarlagadda RK, Boden WE. Cardioprotective effects of an early invasive strategy for non-ST-segment elevation acute coronary syndromes. *J Am Coll Cardiol* 2002;40:1915–1918.

55. Michalis LK, Stroumbis CS, Pappas K, et al. Treatment of refractory unstable angina in geographically isolated areas without cardiac surgery: invasive versus conservative strategy (TRUCS study). *Eur Heart J* 2000;23:1909–1910.

56. Spacek R, Widimsky P, Straka E, et al. Value of first day angiography/angioplasty in evolving non-ST segment elevation myocardial infarction: an open multicentre randomized trial: the VINO study. *Eur Heart J* 2002;23:230–238.

57. McCulloch PA, O'Neill WW, Graham M, et al. A prospective randomized trial of triage angiography in acute coronary syndromes ineligible for thrombolytic therapy. *J Am Coll Cardiol* 1998;32: 396–405.

58. Effects of tissue plasminogen activator and a comparison of early invasive and conservative strategies in unstable angina and non-Q-wave myocardial infarction. Results of the TIMI IIIB Trial. Thrombolysis in Myocardial Ischemia. *Circulation* 1994;89:1545–1556.

59. Boden WE, O'Rourke RA, Crawford MH, et al. The Veterans Affairs non-Q-wave infarction strategy: outcomes in patients with acute non-Q-wave myocardial infarction randomly assigned to an invasive as compared with a conservative management strategy. *N Engl J Med* 1998;338:1785–1792.

60. Wallentin L, Lagerqvist B, Husted S, et al. Outcome at 1-year after an invasive compared with a non-invasive strategy in unstable coronary-artery disease: the FRISC II invasive randomised trial. *Lancet* 2000;356:9–16.

61. Cannon CP, Weintraub WS, Demopoulos LA, et al. Comparison of early invasive and conservative strategies in patients with unstable coronary syndromes treated with the glycoprotein IIb/IIIa inhibitor tirofiban. *N Engl J Med* 2001;344:1879–1887.

62. Fox KA, Poole-Wilson PA, Henderson RA, et al. Interventional versus conservative treatment for patients with unstable angina or non-ST-elevation myocardial infarction: the British Heart Foundation RITA 3 randomised trial. *Lancet* 2002;360:743–751.

63. Lagerquist S, Safastrom K, Stahle E, et al. Is early invasive treatment of unstable coronary artery disease equally effective for both women and men? *J Am Coll Cardiol* 2001;38:41–48.

64. Morrow DA, Cannon CP, Rifai N, et al. Ability of minor elevations of troponins I and T to predict benefit from an early invasive strategy in patients with unstable angina and non-ST elevation myocardial infarction. *JAMA* 2001;286:2405–2412.

65. Wexler LF, Blaustein AS, Lavori PW, et al. Non-Q-wave myocardial infarction following thrombolytic therapy: a comparison of outcomes in patients randomized to invasive or conservative post-infarct assessment strategies in the Veterans Affairs Non-Q-Wave Infarction Strategies In-Hospital (VANQWISH) Trial. *J Am Coll Cardiol* 2001;37:19–25.

66. Goyal A, Samaha FF, Boden WE, et al. Stress test criteria used in the conservative arm of the FRISC-II trial underdetects surgical coronary artery disease when applied to patients in the VANQWISH Trial. *J Am Coll Cardiol* 2002;39:1601–1607.

67. Solomon DH, Stone PH, Glynn RJ, et al. Use of risk stratification to identify patients with unstable angina likeliest to benefit from an invasive versus conservative management strategy. *J Am Coll Cardiol* 2001;38:969–976.

68. Yao S-S, Rozanski A. Myocardial perfusion scintigraphy in conjunction with exercise and pharmacologic stress: prognostic applications in the clinical management of patients with coronary artery disease. In: DePuey EG, Garcia EV, Berman DS, eds. *Cardiac SPECT imaging,* 2nd ed. Philadelphia: Lippincott Williams & Wilkins, 2001:264–296.

69. Madsen JK, Grande P, Saunamaki K, et al. Danish multicenter randomized study of invasive versus conservative treatment in patients with inducible ischemia after thrombolysis in acute myocardial infarction (DANAMI). DANAMI Study Group. *Circulation* 1997;96:748–755.

70. Use of a monoclonal antibody directed against the platelet glycoprotein IIb/IIIa receptor in high-risk coronary angioplasty. The EPIC Investigators. *N Engl J Med* 1994;330:956–961.

71. Platelet glycoprotein IIb/IIIa blockade and low-dose heparin during percutaneous coronary revascularization. The EPILOG Investigators. *N Engl J Med* 1997;336:1689–1696.

72. Randomized placebo-controlled and balloon-angioplasty-controlled trial to assess safety of coronary glycoprotein IIb/IIIa blockade. EPISTENT Investigators. *Lancet* 1998;352:87–92.

73. Hamm CW, Heeschen C, Goldmann B, et al. Benefit of abciximab in patients with refractory unstable angina in relation to serum troponin T levels. c7E3 Fab Antiplatelet Therapy in Unstable Refractory Angina (CAPTURE) Study Investigators. *N Engl J Med* 1999;340:1623–1629.

74. Randomised placebo-controlled trial of effect of eptifibatide on complications of percutaneous coronary intervention. IMPACT-II investigators. *Lancet* 1997;349:1422–1428.

75. A comparison of aspirin plus tirofiban with aspirin plus heparin for unstable angina. Platelet Receptor Inhibition in Ischemic Syndrome Management (PRISM) Study Investigators. *N Engl J Med* 1998;338: 1498–1505.

76. Inhibition of the platelet glycoprotein IIb/IIIa receptor with tirofiban in unstable angina and non-Q-wave myocardial infarction. Platelet Receptor Inhibition in Ischemic Syndrome Management in Patients Limited by Unstable Signs and Symptoms (PRISM-PLUS) Study Investigators. *N Engl J Med* 1998;338:1488–1497.

77. Inhibition of platelet glycoprotein IIb/IIIa with eptifibatide in patients with acute coronary syndromes: platelet glycoprotein IIb/IIIa in unstable angina: receptor suppression using integrelin therapy. The PURSUIT Trial Investigators. *N Engl J Med* 1998;339:436–443.

78. International, randomized, controlled trial of lamifiban (a platelet glycoprotein IIb/IIIa inhibitor), heparin, or both in unstable angina: platelet IIb/IIIa antagonism for the reduction of acute coronary syndrome events in a global organization network. The PARAGON Investigators. *Circulation* 1998;97:2386–2395.

79. Goodman S. Integrilin and Enoxaparin randomized assessment of acute coronary syndromes treatment (INTERACT) trial. Presented at 51st Annual Scientific Session of American College of Cardiology; March 2002; Atlanta, GA.

80. Bhatt DL, Topol EJ. Need to test the arterial inflammation hypothesis. *Circulation* 2002;106:136–140.

81. Robbins M, Topol EJ. Inflammation in acute coronary syndromes. *Cleveland Clin J Med* 2002;69[Suppl 2]:SII130–SII142.

82. Ross R. Atherosclerosis: an inflammatory disease. *N Engl J Med* 1999;340:115–126.

83. Barnett PG, Chen S, Boden WE, et al. Cost-effectiveness of a conservative, ischemia-guided management strategy after non-Q-wave myocardial infarction. Results of a randomized trial. *Circulation* 2002;105:680–684.

84. Shaw LJ, Hachamovitch R, Berman DS, et al. The economic consequences of available diagnostic and prognostic strategies for the eval-

uation of stable angina patients: an observational assessment of the value of precatheterization ischemia. The Economics of Noninvasive Diagnosis (END) Multicenter Study Group. *J Am Coll Cardiol* 1999;33:661–669.

85. Brown, KA. Cardiac risk defined by stress myocardial perfusion imaging: impact on physician decision-making and cost savings. *J Nucl Cardiol* 2002;9:124–126.

86. Nallamothu N, Pancholy SB, Lee KR, et al. Impact of exercise single-photon emission computed tomographic thallium imaging on patient management and outcome. *J Nucl Cardiol* 1995;2:334–338.

87. Hachamovitch R, Berman DS, Shaw LJ, et al. Incremental prognostic value of myocardial perfusion single photon emission computed tomography for the prediction of cardiac death: differential stratification for risk of cardiac death and myocardial infarction [Erratum in: *Circulation* 1998;98:190]. *Circulation* 1998;97:535–543.

88. Zellweger MJ, Dubois EA, Lai S, et al. Risk stratification in patients with remote prior myocardial infarction using rest-stress myocardial perfusion SPECT: prognostic value and impact on referral to early catheterization. *J Nucl Cardiol* 2002;9:23–32.

89. Morrow DA, Antman EM, Charlesworth A, et al. TIMI risk score for ST-elevation myocardial infarction: a convenient, bedside, clinical score for risk assessment at presentation: an intravenous nPA for treatment of infarcting myocardium early II trial substudy. *Circulation* 2000;102:2031–2037.

90. Morrow DA, Antman EM, Giugliano RP, et al. A simple risk index for rapid initial triage of patients with ST-elevation myocardial infarction: an InTIME II substudy. *Lancet* 2001;358:1571–1575.

91. Tang WH, Gurm HS, Piedmonte M, et al. A simple risk score for prediction of 30-day mortality in patients presenting with acute coronary syndrome without persistent ST-elevation: insights from GUSTO IV. *J Am Coll Cardiol* 2001;39[Suppl A]:197A(abst).

92. Krumholz HM, Chen J, Chen YT, et al. Predicting one-year mortality among elderly survivors of hospitalization for an acute myocardial infarction: results from the Cooperative Cardiovascular Project. *J Am Coll Cardiol* 2001;38:453–459.

93. Singh M, Reeder GS, Jacobsen SJ, et al. Scores for post-myocardial infarction risk stratification in the community. *Circulation* 2002;106:2309–2314.

94. Jacobs DR Jr, Kroenke C, Crow R, et al. PREDICT: a simple risk score for clinical severity and long-term prognosis after hospitalization for acute myocardial infarction or unstable angina: the Minnesota Heart Survey. *Circulation* 1999;100:599–607.

95. Morrow DA, Antman EM, Parsons L, et al. Application of the TIMI risk score for ST-elevation MI in the National Registry of Myocardial Infarction 3. *JAMA* 2001;286:1356–1359.

96. Antman EM, Cohen M, Bernink PJ, et al. The TIMI risk score for unstable angina/non-ST elevation MI: a method for prognostication and therapeutic decision making. *JAMA* 2000;284:835–842.

97. Boersma E, Pieper KS, Steyerberg EW, et al. Predictors of outcome inpatients with acute coronary syndromes without persistent ST-segment elevation: results from an international trial of 9461 patients. The PURSUIT Investigators. *Circulation* 2000;101:2557–2567.

98. Lagerqvist B, Diderholm E, Lindahl B, et al. High risk score predicts bad outcome in patients with unstable coronary artery disease: FRISCII sub-study. *Circulation* 2001;104[Suppl II]:II-648(abst).

99. Antman EM, Tanasijevic MJ, Thompson B, et al. Cardiac-specific troponin I levels to predict the risk of mortality in patients with acute coronary syndromes. *N Engl J Med* 1996;335:1342–1349.

100. Morrow DA, Rifai N, Antman EM, et al. C-reactive protein is a potent predictor of mortality independently and in combination with troponin T in acute coronary syndromes: a TIMI IIA substudy. *J Am Coll Cardiol* 1998;31:1460–1465.

101. Morrow DA, Ridker PM. C-reactive protein, inflammation, and coronary risk. *Med Clin North Am* 2000;84:1491–1461.

102. de Lemos JA, Morrow DA, Bentley JH, et al. The prognostic value of B-type natriuretic peptide in patients with acute coronary syndromes. *N Engl J Med* 2001;345:1014–1021.

103. Sabatine MS, Morrow DA, de Lemos JA, et al. Multimarker approach to risk stratification in non-ST elevation acute coronary syndromes. Simultaneous assessment of troponin I, C-reactive protein, and B-type natriuretic peptide. *Circulation* 2002;105:1760–1763.

104. Smith S, Blair S, Bonow R, et al. AHA/ACC guidelines for preventing heart attack and death in patients with atherosclerotic cardiovascular disease: 2001 update. *Circulation* 2001;104:1577–1579.

105. Cortez D, O'Rourke RA. Current approaches to patients with acute coronary syndromes. *Curr Prob Cardiol* 2002;27:149–177.

106. Waters D. Diagnosis and management of patients with unstable angina. In: Fuster V, Alexander RW, O'Rourke RA, et al., eds. *Hurst's the Heart*, 10th ed. New York: McGraw-Hill, 2001:2129–2142.

107. Balsano F, Rizzon P, Violi F, et al. Antiplatelet treatment with ticlopidine in unstable angina: a controlled multicenter clinical trial. The Studio della Ticlopidinas nell' Angina Instabile Group. *Circulation* 1990;82:17–26.

108. A randomised, blinded trial of clopidogrel versus aspirin in patients at risk of ischemic events (CAPRIE). CAPRIE Steering Committee. *Lancet* 1996;348:1329–1339.

109. Effects of clopidogrel in addition to aspirin in patients with acute coronary syndromes without ST-segment elevation. The Clopidogrel in Unstable Angina to Prevent Recurrent Events Trial Investigators. *N Engl J Med* 2001;345:494–502.

110. Mehta S, Yusuf S, Peters R, et al. Effects of pretreatment with clopidogrel and aspirin followed by long-term therapy in patients undergoing percutaneous coronary intervention: the PCI-CURE study. *Lancet* 2001;358:527–533.

111. Berger PB, Steinhubl S. Clinical implications of Percutaneous Coronary Intervention–Clopidogrel in Unstable Angina to Prevent Recurrent Events (PCI-CURE) Study. A US Perspective. *Circulation* 2002;106:2284–2287.

112. Lau WC, Waskell LA, Watkins PB. Atorvastatin reduces the ability of clopidogrel to inhibit platelet aggregation. A new drug-drug interaction. *Circulation* 2003;107:32–37.

113. Topol EJ, Moliterno DJ, Herrmann HC, et al. Comparison of two platelet glycoprotein IIb/IIIa inhibitors, tirofiban and abciximab, for the prevention of ischemic events with percutaneous coronary revascularization. *N Engl J Med* 2001;344:1888–1894.

114. Steinhubl SR, Berger PB, Mann JT 3rd, et al. Early and sustained dual oral antiplatelet therapy following percutaneous coronary intervention. A randomized controlled trial. *JAMA* 2002;288:2411–2420.

115. Yusuf S, Wittes J, Friedman L. Overview of results of randomized clinical trials in heart disease: unstable angina and heart failure. *JAMA* 1988;260:2259–2263.

116. Yusef S, Peto R, Lewis J, et al. Beta blockade during and after myocardial infarction: an overview of the randomized trials. *Prog Cardiovasc Dis* 1985;27:335.

117. Yusef S, Witles J, Probstfield J. Evaluating effects of treatment in subgroups of patients within a clinical trial: the case on non-Q wave myocardial infarction and beta blockers. *Am J Cardiol* 1990;66:220–222.

118. A randomized trial of propranolol in patients with acute myocardial infarction: I. Mortality results. β-Blocker Heart Attack Trial Research Group. *JAMA* 1982;147:1707.

119. Gheorghiade M, Schultz L, Tilley B, et al. Effects of propranolol in non-Q wave acute myocardial infarction in the beta blocker heart attack trial. *Am J Cardiol* 1990;66:129–133.

120. Mortality results. The MIAMI Trial Research Group. *Am J Cardiol* 1985;56[Suppl G]:12.

121. Timolol-induced reduction in mortality and reinfarction in patients surviving acute myocardial infarction. Norwegian Multicenter Study Group. *N Engl J Med* 1981;304:801.

122. Overskeid K, Abrahamsen AM, Frisvold OI, et al. Letter to the editor. *N Engl J Med* 1981;305:407.

123. Effects of carvedilol on outcome after myocardial infarction in patients with left-ventricular dysfunction: the CAPRICORN randomised trial. The CAPRICORN Investigators. *Lancet* 2001;357:1385–1390.

124. Dargie HJ, Sharpe N, Remme W, et al. Effects of carvedilol on death and major coronary events inpatients with ST elevation and non ST elevation myocardial infarction: the CAPRICORN trial. *Circulation* 2002;106[Suppl II]:II-320(abst).

125. Murrell W. Nitroglycerine as a remedy for angina pectoris. *Lancet* 1879;1:642.

126. Lan JY, Chesebro JH, Fuster V. Platelets, vasoconstriction and nitroglycerin during arterial wall injury: a new antithrombotic role for an old drug. *Circulation* 1988;78:712.

127. Diodati J, Theroux P, Latour JG. Effects of nitroglycerin at therapeutic doses on platelet aggregation in unstable angina pectoris and acute myocardial infarction. *Am J Cardiol* 1990;66:683.

128. Folts JD, Stamler J, Loscalzo J. Intravenous nitroglycerin infusion inhibits cyclic blood flow responses caused by periodic platelet throm-

bus formation in stenosed canine coronary arteries. *Circulation* 1991; 83:2112.

129. Chai AU, Crawford MH. "Traditional" medical therapy for unstable angina. How important? How to use? *Cardiol Clin* 1999;17:359–372.

130. Effect of nicorandil on coronary events in patients with stable angina: the Impact Of Nicorandil in Angina (IONA) randomised trial. The IONA Study Group. *Lancet* 2002;359:1269–1275.

131. Sato T, Sasaki N, O'Rourke B, et al. Nicorandil, a potent cardioprotective agent, acts by opening mitochondrial ATP-dependent potassium channels. *J Am Coll Cardiol* 2000;35:514–518.

132. Gibson RS. Current status of calcium channel-blocking drugs after Q-wave and non-Q wave myocardial infarction. *Circulation* 1989; 80[Suppl 4]:107–119.

133. Gibson RS, Boden WE, Theroux P, et al. Diltiazem and reinfarction in patients with non-Q wave myocardial infarction: results of a double-blind, randomized, multicenter trial. *N Engl J Med* 1986;315:423–429.

134. Gibson RS, Young PM, Boden WE, et al. Prognostic significance and beneficial effect of diltiazem on the incidence of early recurrent ischemia after non-Q wave myocardial infarction: results from the multicenter diltiazem reinfarction study. *Am J Cardiol* 1987;60:203–209.

135. The effect of diltiazem on mortality and reinfarction after myocardial infarction. The Multicenter Diltiazem Postinfarction Trial Research Group. *N Engl J Med* 1988;319:385–392.

136. Gibson RS, Hansen JF, Messerli F, et al. Long-term effects of diltiazem and verapamil on mortality and cardiac events in non-Q-wave acute myocardial infarction without pulmonary congestion: post hoc subset analysis of the Multicenter Diltiazem Postinfarction Trial and the Second Danish Verapamil Infarction Trial Studies. *Am J Cardiol* 2000;86:275–279.

137. Munzel T, Keaney JF Jr. Are ACE inhibitors a "magic bullet" against oxidative stress? *Circulation* 2001;104:1571–1574.

138. Pfeffer MA, Braunwald E, Moye LA, et al. Effect of captopril on morbidity and mortality in patients with left ventricular dysfunction after myocardial infarction: results of the survival and ventricular enlargement trial. The SAVE Investigators. *N Engl J Med* 1992;327:669.

139. ISIS-4: a randomized factorial trial assessing early oral captopril, oral mononitrate, and magnesium sulphate in 58,050 patients with suspected acute myocardial infarction. ISIS-4 Collaborative Group. *Lancet* 1995;345:669.

140. GISSI-3: effects of lisinopril and transdermal glycerol trinitrate singly and together on 6-week mortality and ventricular function after acute myocardial infarction. Gruppo Italiano per lo Studio della Sopravvivenza nell'Infarto Miocardico. *Lancet* 1994;343:1115–1122.

141. Effect of ramipril on mortality and morbidity of survivors of acute myocardial infarction with clinical evidence of heart failure. Acute Infarction Ramipril Efficacy (AIRE) Study Investigators. *Lancet* 1993; 342:821.

142. Kober L, Torp-Pederson C, Carlsen JE, et al. A clinical trial of the angiotensin-converting enzyme inhibitor trandolapril in patients with left ventricular dysfunction after myocardial infarction. Trandolapril Cardiac Evaluation (TRACE) Study Group. *N Engl J Med* 1995;333: 1670.

143. Dzau V. Mechanism of protective effects of ACE inhibition on coronary artery disease. *Eur Heart J* 1998;19[Suppl J]:2–6.

144. Effects of angiotensin-converting enzyme inhibitor ramipril on cardiovascular events in high-risk patients. HOPE Investigators (The Heart Outcomes Prevention Evaluation Study Investigators). *N Engl J Med* 2000;342:145.

145. Dagenais GR, Yusuf S, Bourasa MG, et al. Effects of ramipril on coronary events in high-risk persons: results of the Heart Outcomes Prevention Evaluation Study. *Circulation* 2001;104:522–526.

146. Dickstein K, Kjekshus J; OPTIMAAL Steering Committee for the OPTIMAAL Study Group. Effects of losartan and captopril on mortality and morbidity in high-risk patients after acute myocardial infarction: the OPTIMAAL randomised trial. Optimal Trial in Myocardial Infarction with Angiotensin II Antagonist Losartan. *Lancet* 2002; 360:752–760.

147. Pitt B, Poole-Wilson PA, Segal R, et al. Effect of losartan compared with captopril on mortality in patients with symptomatic heart failure: randomised trial: the Losartan Heart Failure Survival Study ELITE II. *Lancet* 2000;355:1582–1587.

148. Randomized trial of cholesterol lowering in 4444 patients with coronary heart disease: the Scandinavian Simvastatin Survival Study (4S). *Lancet* 1994;344:1383–1389.

149. Shepherd J, Cobbe SM, Ford I, et al. Prevention of coronary heart disease with pravastatin in men with hypercholesterolemia. West of Scotland Coronary Prevention Study Group. *N Engl J Med* 1995; 333:1301–1307.

150. Sacks FM, Pfeffer MA, Moye LA, et al. The effect of pravastatin on coronary events after myocardial infarction in patients with average cholesterol levels. Cholesterol and Recurrent Events Trial Investigators. *N Engl J Med* 1996;335:1001–1009.

151. Prevention of cardiovascular events and death with pravastatin in patients with coronary heart disease and a broad range of initial cholesterol levels. The Long-Term Intervention with Pravastatin in Ischaemic Disease (LIPID) Study Group. *N Engl J Med* 1998;339:1349–1357.

152. Downs JR, Clearfield M, Weis S, et al. Primary prevention of acute coronary events with lovastatin in men and women with average cholesterol levels: results of AFCAPS/TexCAPS. Air Force/Texas Coronary Atherosclerosis Prevention Study. *JAMA* 1998;279:1615–1622.

153. The effect of aggressive lowering of low-density lipoprotein cholesterol levels and low-dose anticoagulation on obstructive changes in saphenous-vein coronary-artery bypass grafts. The Post Coronary Artery Bypass Graft Trial Investigators. *N Engl J Med* 1997;336:153–162.

154. MRC/BHF Heart Protection Study of cholesterol lowering with simvastatin in 20,536 high-risk individuals: a randomised placebo-controlled trial. Heart Protection Study Collaborative Group. *Lancet* 2002;360:7–22.

155. Shepherd J, Blauw GJ, Murphy MB, et al. Pravastatin in elderly individuals at risk of vascular disease (PROSPER): a randomised controlled trial. *Lancet* 2002;360:1623–1630.

156. Serruys PW, de Feyter P, Macaya C, et al. Fluvastatin for prevention of cardiac events following successful first percutaneous coronary intervention. A randomized controlled trial. *JAMA* 2002;287:3215–3222.

157. La Rosa JC, He J, Vupputuri S. Effect of statins on risk of coronary disease: a meta-analysis of randomized controlled trials. *JAMA* 1999; 282:2340–2346.

158. Wood D, De Backer G, Faergeman O, et al. Prevention of coronary heart disease in clinical practice. Recommendations of the Second Joint Task Force of European and Other Societies on coronary prevention. *Eur Heart J* 1998;19:1434–1503.

159. Executive summary of the third report of the National Cholesterol Education Program (NCEP) expert panel on detection, evaluation, and treatment of high blood cholesterol in adults (Adult Treatment Panel III). *JAMA* 2001;285:2486–2497.

160. Chen Z, Peto R, Collins R, et al. Serum cholesterol concentration and coronary heart disease in population with low cholesterol concentrations. *BMJ* 1991;303:276–282.

161. Pitt B, Waters D, Brown WV, et al. Aggressive lipid-lowering therapy compared with angioplasty in stable coronary artery disease. *N Engl J Med* 1999;341:70–76.

162. Smilde TJ, van Wissen S, Wollersheim H, et al. Effect of aggressive versus conventional lipid lowering on atherosclerosis progression in familial hypercholesterolaemia (ASAP): a prospective, randomised, double-blind trial. *Lancet* 2001;357:577–581.

163. Brown BG, Zhao XQ, Chait A, et al. Simvastatin and niacin, antioxidant vitamins, or the combination for the prevention of coronary disease. *N Engl J Med* 2001;345:1583–1592.

164. Taylor AJ, Kent SM, Flaherty PJ, et al. ARBITER: Arterial Biology for the Investigation of the Treatment Effects of Reducing Cholesterol: a randomized trial comparing the effects of atorvastatin and pravastatin on carotid intima medial thickness. *Circulation* 2002;106: 2055–2060.

165. Sever PS, Dahlof B, Poulter NR, et al. Rationale, design, methods and baseline demography of participants of the Anglo-Scandinavian Cardiac Outcomes Trial. ASCOT Investigators. *J Hypertens* 2001;19: 1139–1147.

166. Anglo-Scandinavian Cardiac Outcomes Trial. Atorvastatin shown to decrease heart disease and stroke in patients with hypertension and low cholesterol [press release]. Available at: http://biz.yahoo.com/prnews/021010/lnth011_l.html. Accessed October 10, 2002.

167. Gooszen M, Hoffmeyer MR, Lefar DJ. Simvastatin reduces myocardial ischemia/reperfusion injury in Apo E deficient mice. *Circulation* 2000;II-271(abst).

168. Lacoste I, Lam JY, Hung J, et al. Hyperlipidemia and coronary disease. Correction of the increased thrombogenic potential with cholesterol reduction. *Circulation* 1995;92:3172–3177.

169. Dangas G, Badimon JJ, Smith DA, et al. Pravastatin therapy in hyper-

lipidemia: effects on thrombus formation and the systemic hemostatic profile. *J Am Coll Cardiol* 1999;33:1294–1304.

170. Simpson IA, Lorimer AR, Walker ID, et al. Effect of ciprofibrate on platelet aggregation and fibrinolysis in patients with hypercholesterolemia. *Thromb Haemost* 1985;54:442–444.

171. Szczeklik A, Musial J, Undas A, et al. Inhibition of thrombin generation by simvastatin and lack of additive effects of aspirin in patients with marked hypercholesterolemia. *J Am Coll Cardiol* 1999;33:1286–1293.

172. Notarbartolo A, Davi G, Averna M, et al. Inhibition of thromboxane biosynthesis and platelet function by simvastatin in type IIa hypercholesterolemia. *Arteriascleros Thromb Vasc Biol* 1995;15:247–251.

173. Stroes ES, Koomans HA, de Bruin TW, et al. Vascular function in the forearm of hypercholesterolemic patients off and on lipid-lowering medication. *Lancet* 1995;346:467–471.

174. Dupuis J, Tardif JC, Cernacek P, et al. Cholesterol reduction rapidly improves endothelial function after acute coronary syndromes. The RECIFE (reduction of cholesterol in ischemia and function of the endothelium) trial. *Circulation* 1999;99:3227–3233.

175. Ling M, Ukkonen H, Ruddy T, et al. Early improvement of myocardial perfusion using statin therapy in patients with coronary artery disease. *Circulation* 2002;106:II-477(abst).

176. Mansur AP, Serrano CV, Nicolau JC, et al. Effect of cholesterol lowering treatment on positive exercise tests in patients with hypercholesterolemia and normal coronary angiograms. *Heart* 1999;82:689–693.

177. Ramires JA, Sposito AC, Mansur AP, et al. Cholesterol lowering with statins reduces exercise-induced myocardial ischemia in hypercholesterolemic patients with coronary artery disease. *Am J Cardiol* 2001; 88:1134–1138.

178. Crisby M, Nordin-Fredriksson G, Shah PK, et al. Pravastatin treatment increases collagen content and decreases lipid content, inflammation, metalloproteinases, and cell death in human carotid plaques. *Circulation* 2001;103:926–933.

179. Williams JK, Sukhova GK, Herrington DM, et al. Pravastatin has cholesterol-lowering independent effects on the artery wall of atherosclerotic monkeys. *J Am Coll Cardiol* 1998;31:684–691.

180. Bellosta S, Via D, Canavesi M, et al. HMG-CoA reductase inhibitors reduce MMP-9 secretion by macrophages. *Arterioscler Thromb Vasc Biol* 1998;18:1671–1678.

181. Jialal I, Stein D, Balis D, et al. Effect of hydroxymethyl glutaryl coenzyme A reductase inhibitor therapy on high sensitive C-reactive protein. *Circulation* 2001;103:1933–1935.

182. Plenge JK, Hernandez TL, Weil KM, et al. Simvastatin lower C-reactive protein within 14 days: an effect independent of low-density lipoprotein concentration reduction. *Circulation* 2002;106:1447–1452.

183. Rosenson RS, Tangney CC. Antiatherothrombotic properties of statins: implications for cardiovascular event reduction. *JAMA* 1998;279: 1643–1650.

184. Ridker PM, Cushman M, Stampfer MJ, et al. Inflammation, aspirin and the risk of cardiovascular disease in apparently healthy men. *N Engl J Med* 1997;336:973–979.

185. Ridker PM, Hennekens CH, Buring JE, et al. C-reactive protein and other markers of inflammation in the prediction of cardiovascular disease in women. *N Engl J Med* 2000;342:836–843.

186. Ridker PM, Rafai N, Pfeffer MA, et al. Inflammation, pravastatin, and the risk of coronary events after myocardial infarction in patients with average cholesterol levels: Cholesterol And Recurrent Events (CARE) Investigators. *Circulation* 1998;98:839–844.

187. Chew DP, Bhatt DL, Robbins MA, et al. Incremental prognostic value of elevated baseline C-reactive protein among established markers of risk in percutaneous coronary intervention. *Circulation* 2001;104:992–997.

188. Walter DH, Fichtlscherer S, Britten MB, et al. Statin therapy abrogates the increased risk associated with elevated C-reactive protein levels after coronary stent implantation. *Circulation* 2000;102[Suppl II]:II-390(abst).

189. Schiele R, Gitt AK, Heer T, et al. Early statin use in acute myocardial infarction is associated with a reduced hospital mortality: results of the Mitra-2 Study. *Circulation* 2000;102:II-435(abst).

190. Walter DH, Fichtlscherer S, Britten MB, et al. Initiation of statin therapy immediately after stent implantation: profound benefit in patients with acute coronary syndromes. *Circulation* 2000;102:II-435(abst).

191. Aronow HD, Topol EJ, Roe MT, et al. Effect of lipid-lowering therapy on early mortality after acute coronary syndromes: an observational study. *Lancet* 2001;357:1063–1068.

192. Stenestrand U, Wallentin L, for the Swedish Registry of Cardiac Intensive Care (RIKS-HIA). Early statin treatment following acute myocardial infarction and 1-year survival. *JAMA* 2001;285:430–436.

193. Cannon CP, McCabe CH, Bentley J, et al. Early statin therapy is associated with markedly lower mortality in patients with acute coronary syndromes: observations from OPUS-TIMI 16. *J Am Coll Cardiol* 2001;37:A334.

194. Giugliano RP, Antman EM, Thompson SL, et al. Lipid-lowering drug therapy initiated during hospitalization for acute MI is associated with lower postdischarge 1-year mortality. *J Am Coll Cardiol* 2001; 37:A316.

195. Heeschen C, Hamm CW, Laufs U, et al. Withdrawal of statins increases event rates in patients with acute coronary syndromes. *Circulation* 2002;105:1446–1452.

196. Fonarow GC, Wright RS, Spenser F, et al. Statin use within the first 24 hours of admission for acute MI is associated with reduction in early morbidity and mortality. *Circulation* 2002;106:II-400(abst).

197. Arntz H, Agrawal R, Wunderlich W, et al. Beneficial effects of pravastatin (±cholestyramine/niacin) initiated immediately after a coronary event (The Randomized Lipid-Coronary Artery Disease [L-CAD] Study). *Am J Cardiol* 2000;86:1293–1298.

198. Schwartz GG, Olsson AG, Ezekowitz MD, et al. Effects of atorvastatin on early recurrent ischemic events in acute coronary syndromes. The MIRACL study: a randomized controlled trial. *JAMA* 2001;285: 1711–1718.

199. Muhlestein JB, Horne BD, Bair TL, et al. Usefulness of in-hospital prescription of statin agents after angiographic diagnosis of coronary artery disease in improving continued compliance and reduced mortality. *Am J Cardiol* 2001;87:257–261.

200. Grady D, Rubin SM, Petitti DB, et al. Hormone therapy to prevent disease and prolong life in postmenopausal women. *Ann Intern Med* 1992;117:1016–1037.

201. Grodstein F, Stampfer MJ, Manson JE, et al. Postmenopausal estrogen and progestin use and the risk of cardiovascular disease. *N Engl J Med* 1996;335:453–461.

202. Sullivan JM, El-Zeky F, Vandez Zwaag R, et al. Effect on survival of estrogen replacement therapy after coronary artery bypass grafting. *Am J Cardiol* 1997;79:947–950.

203. Shilpak MG, Angeja BG, Go AS, et al. Hormone therapy and in-hospital survival after myocardial infarction in postmenopausal women. *Circulation* 2001;104:2300–2304.

204. Mendelsohn ME, Karas RH. The protective effect of estrogen on the cardiovascular system. *N Engl J Med* 1999;340:1801–1811.

205. Hulley S, Grady D, Bush T, et al. Randomized trial of estrogen plus progestin for secondary prevention of coronary heart disease in postmenopausal women. Heart and Estrogen/progestin Replacement Study (HERS) Research Group. *JAMA* 1998;280:605–613.

206. Grady D, Herrington D, Bittner V, et al., for the HERS Research Group. Cardiovascular outcomes during 6-8 years of hormone therapy: Heart and Estrogen/progestin Replacement Study follow-up (HERS II). *JAMA* 2002;288:49–57.

207. Herrington DM, Reboussin DM, Brosnihan KB, et al. Effects of estrogen replacement on the progression of coronary-artery atherosclerosis. *N Engl J Med* 2000;343:522–529.

208. Viscoli CM, Brass LM, Kernan WN, et al. A clinical trial of estrogen-replacement therapy after ischemic stroke. *N Engl J Med* 2001;345: 1243–1249.

209. Angerer P, Stork S, Kothny W, et al. Effect of oral postmenopausal hormone replacement on progression of atherosclerosis. A randomized, controlled trial. *Arterioscler Thromb Vasc Biol* 2001;21:262–268.

210. Cherry N, Gilmour K, Hannaford P, et al. Oestrogen therapy for prevention of reinfarction in postmenopausal women: a randomised placebo controlled trial. *Lancet* 2002;360:2001–2008.

211. Waters DD, Alderman ED, Hsia J, et al. Effects of hormone replacement therapy and antioxidant vitamin supplements on coronary atherosclerosis in postmenopausal women. A randomized controlled trial. *JAMA* 2002;288:2432–2440.

212. Wilson PW, Garrison RJ, Castelli WP. Postmenopausal estrogen use, cigarette smoking and cardiovascular risk in women over 50: the Framingham Study. *N Engl J Med* 1985;313:1038–1043.

213. The Coronary Drug Project. Initial findings leading to modifications of its research protocol. *JAMA* 1970;214:1303–1313.

214. The Coronary Drug Project. Initial findings leading to the discontinuation of the 2.5-mg day estrogen group. The coronary Drug Project Research Group. *JAMA* 1973;226:652–657.

215. Alexander KP, Newby LK, Hellkamp AS, et al. Initiation of hormone replacement therapy after acute myocardial infarction is associated with more cardiac events during follow-up. *J Am Coll Cardiol* 2001;38:1–7.

216. Grodstein F, Manson JE, Stampfer MJ. Postmenopausal hormone use and secondary prevention of coronary events in the Nurses' Health Study. A prospective, observational study. *Ann Intern Med* 2001; 135:1–8.

217. Heckbert SR, Kaplan RC, Weiss NS, et al. Risk of recurrent coronary events in relation to use and recent initiation of postmenopausal hormone therapy. *Arch Intern Med* 2001;161:1709–1713.

218. Ferrara A, Quesenberry CP, Karter AJ, et al. Current use of unopposed estrogen and estrogen plus progestin and the risk of acute myocardial infarction among women with diabetes: the Northern California Kaiser Permanente Diabetes Registry, 1995-1998. *Circulation* 2003;107: 43–48.

219. Risks and benefits of estrogen plus progestin in healthy postmenopausal women. Principal results from the Women's Health Initiative Randomized Controlled Trial. Writing Group for the Women's Health Initiative Investigators. *JAMA* 2002;288:321–333.

220. Rossouw JE. Early risk of cardiovascular events after commencing hormone replacement therapy. *Curr Opin Lipidol* 2001;12:371–375.

221. Rabbani LE, Seminario NA, Sciacca RR, et al. Oral conjugated equine estrogen increases plasma von Willebrand Factor in postmenopausal women. *J Am Coll Cardiol* 2002;40:1991–1999.

222. Ridker PM, Hennekens CH, Rifai N, et al. Hormone replacement therapy and increased plasma concentration of C-reactive protein. *Circulation* 1999;100:713–716.

223. Cushman M, Legault C, Barrett-Connor E, et al. Effect of postmenopausal hormones on inflammation-sensitive proteins: the Postmenopausal Estrogen/Progestin Interventions (PEPI) Study. *Circulation* 1999;100:717–722.

224. van Baal WM, Kenemans P, van der Mooren MJ, et al. Increased C-reactive protein levels during short-term hormone replacement therapy in healthy postmenopausal women. *Thromb Haemost* 1999;81:925–928.

225. Mosca L, Collins P, Herrington DM, et al. Hormone replacement therapy and cardiovascular disease: a statement for healthcare professionals from the American Heart Association. *Circulation* 2001;104:499–503.

226. Manson JE, Greenland P, LaCroix AZ. Walking compared with vigorous exercise for the prevention of cardiovascular events in women. *N Engl J Med* 2002;347:716–725.

227. Collaborative overview of randomized trials of antiplatelet therapy—I: prevention of death, myocardial infarction, and stroke by prolonged antiplatelet therapy in various categories of patients. Antiplatelet Trialists' Collaboration. *BMJ* 1994;308:81–106.

228. Teo KK, Yusuf S, Furberg CD. Effects of prophylactic antiarrhythmic drug therapy in acute myocardial infarction: an overview of results from randomized controlled trials. *JAMA* 1993;270:1589–1595.

229. Neal B, MacMahon S, Chapman N. Effect of ACE inhibitors, calcium antagonists and other blood pressure-lowering drugs: results of prospectively designed overviews of randomized trials. *Lancet* 2000; 356:1955–1964.

230. Herbert PR, Gaziano JM, Chan KS, et al. Cholesterol lowering with statin drugs, risk of stroke and total mortality: an overview of randomized trials. *JAMA* 1997;278:313–321.

231. Krauss RM. Individualized hormone-replacement therapy? *N Engl J Med* 2002;346:1017–1018.

232. Psaty BM, Smith NL, Lamaitre RN, et al. Hormone replacement therapy, prothrombotic mutations, and the risk of incident nonfatal myocardial infarction in postmenopausal women. *JAMA* 2001;285:906–913.

233. Glueck CT, Wang P, Fontaine RN, et al. Effect of exogenous estrogen on artherothrombotic vascular disease risk related to the presence or absence of the Factov V Leiden mutation (resistance to activated protein C). *Am J Cardiol* 1999;84:549–554.

234. Herrington DM, Howard TD, Hawkins GA, et al. Estrogen-receptor polymorphisms and effects of estrogen replacement on high-density lipoprotein cholesterol in women with coronary disease. *N Engl J Med* 2002;346:967–975.

235. McGuigan FE, Armbrecht G, Smith R, et al. Prediction of osteoporotic fractures by bone densitometry and COLIA1 genotyping: a prospective, population based study of men and women. *Osteoporos Int* 2001;12:91–96.

236. King MC, Wieand S, Hale K, et al. Tamoxifen and breast cancer incidence among women with inherited mutations in BRCA1 and BRCA2: national surgical adjuvant breast and bowel project (NSABP-P1) breast cancer prevention trial. *JAMA* 2001;286:2251–2256.

237. Ettinger B, Black DM, Mitlak BH, et al. Reduction of vertebral fracture risk in postmenopausal women with osteoporosis treated with raloxifene: results from a 3-year randomized clinical trial. *JAMA* 1999;282:637–645.

238. Cummings SR, Eckert S, Krueger KA, et al. The effect of raloxifene on risk of breast cancer in postmenopausal women. *JAMA* 1999;281: 2189–2197.

239. Barrett-Connor E, Grady D, Sashegyi A, et al. Raloxifene and cardiovascular events in osteoporotic postmenopausal women. Four-year results from the MORE (Multiple Outcomes of Raloxifene Evaluation) randomized trial. *JAMA* 2002;287:847–857.

240. Mosca L, Barrett-Connor E, Wenger NK, et al. Design and methods of the Raloxifene Use for The Heart (RUTH) Study. *Am J Cardiol* 2001;88:392–395.

241. Anand SS, Yusuf S. Oral anticoagulant therapy in patients with coronary artery disease: a meta-analysis *JAMA* 1999;282:2058 2067.

242. van Es RF, Jonker JJC, Verheugt FW, et al. Aspirin and Coumadin after acute coronary syndromes (the ASPECT-2 study): a randomised controlled trial. *Lancet* 2002;360:109–113.

243. Arnesen H. WArfarin Re-Infarction Study (WARIS)-2. Presented at 23rd European Congress of Cardiology; September 2001; Stockholm, Sweden.

244. Randomised double-blind trial of fixed low-dose warfarin with aspirin after myocardial infarction. Coumadin Aspirin Reinfarction Study (CARS) Investigators. *Lancet* 1997;350:389–396.

245. Effects of long-term, moderate-intensity oral anticoagulation in addition to aspirin in unstable angina. The Organization to Assess Strategies for Ischemic Syndromes (OASIS-2) Investigators. *J Am Coll Cardiol* 2001;37:475–484.

246. Fiore LD, Ezekowitz MD, Brophy MT, et al. Department of Veterans Affairs cooperative studies program clinical trial comparing combined warfarin and aspirin with aspirin alone in survivors of acute myocardial infarction: primary results of the CHAMP study. *Circulation* 2002;105:557–563.

247. Daly LE, Mulcahy R, Graham IM, et al. Long term effect on mortality of stopping smoking after unstable angina and myocardial infarction. *Br Med J* (Clin Res Ed) 1983;287:324–326.

248. Smoking cessation. Rockville, MD: Agency for Health Care Policy and Research and the National Heart, Lung, and Blood Institute, US Public Health Service, US Department of Health and Human Services; 1996. AHCPR Publication No. 96-0692.

249. Froelicher ES, Houston NM, Christopherson DJ, et al. Efficacy of smoking cessation intervention in women hospitalized with cardiovascular disease: Women's Initiative for Nonsmoking (WINS). *Circulation* 2002;106[Suppl II]:II-735.

250. Mahmarian JJ, Moye LA, Nasser GA, et al. Nicotine patch therapy in smoking cessation reduces the extent of exercise-induced myocardial ischemia. *J Am Coll Cardiol* 1997;30:125–130.

251. Taylor R, Brown A, Stone JA. The effectiveness of cardiac rehabilitation: systematic review and meta-regression of randomised controlled trials. *Circulation* 2002;106[Suppl II]:II-711(abst).

252. DeSouza CA, Shapiro LF, Clevenger CM, et al. Regular aerobic exercise prevents and restores age-related declines in endothelium-dependent vasodilation in healthy men. *Circulation* 2000;102:1351–1357.

253. Rauramaa R, Vaisanen SB, Lakka TA, et al. Physical exercise retards progression of carotid artery atherosclerosis: a five-year controlled randomized clinical trial. *Circulation* 2002;106[Suppl II]:II-735(abst).

254. Hoff JA, Sevrukov A, Gray H, et al. Subclinical coronary artery disease in women: is exercise protective? *Circulation* 2002;106 [Suppl II]:II-735(abst).

255. Hata T, Okazawa H, Inuzuka Y, et al. Beneficial effects of exercise training on coronary artery flow reserve in patients with recent myocardial infarction. *Circulation* 2002;106[Suppl II]:II-438(abst).

256. Whelton SP, Chin A, Xin X, et al. Effect of aerobic exercise on blood pressure: a meta-analysis of randomized, controlled trials. *Ann Intern Med* 2002;136:493–503.

257. LaMonte MJ, Durstine JL, Yanowitz FG, et al. Cardiorespiratory fitness and C-reactive protein among a tri-ethnic sample of women *Circulation* 2002;106:403–406.

258. Malmberg K, Ryden L, Efendic S, et al. Randomized trial of insulin-glucose infusion followed by subcutaneous insulin treatment in dia-

betic patients with acute myocardial infarction (DIGAMI study): effects on mortality at 1 year. *J Am Coll Cardiol* 1995;26:57–65.

259. American Diabetes Association. Standards of medical care for patients with diabetes mellitus (position statement). *Diabetes Care* 1999;22[Suppl II]:S32–S41.

260. Intensive blood-glucose control with sulphonylureas or insulin compared with conventional treatment and risk of complications in patients with type 2 diabetes (UKPDS 33). UK Prospective Diabetes Study (UKPDS) Group. *Lancet* 1998;352:837–853.

261. Effect of intensive blood-glucose control with metformin on complications in overweight patients with type 2 diabetes (UKPDS 34) [Erratum in: *Lancet* 1998;352:1557]. UK Prospective Diabetes Study (UKPDS) Group. *Lancet* 1998;352:854–865.

262. UK Prospective Diabetes Study Group. Tight blood pressure control and risk of macrovascular and microvascular complications in type 2 diabetes: UKPDS 38. *BMJ* 1998;317:703–713.

263. Stampfer MJ, Malinow MR, Willett WC, et al. A prospective study of plasma homocysteine and risk of myocardial infarction in US physicians. *JAMA* 1992;268:877–881.

264. Ubbink JB, Vermaak WJ, van der Merwe A, et al. Vitamin B-12, vitamin B-6, and folate nutritional status in men with hyperhomocysteinemia. *Am J Clin Nutr* 1993;57:47–53.

265. Schnyder G, Roffi M, Pin R, et al. Decreased rate of coronary restenosis after lowering of plasma homocysteine levels. *N Engl J Med* 2001;345:1593–1600.

266. Baker F, Picton D, Blackwood S, et al. Blinded comparison of folic acid and placebo inpatients with ischemic heart disease: an outcome trial. *Circulation* 2002;106[Suppl II]:II-741(abst).

267. Steinberg D. Low density lipoprotein oxidation and its pathobiological significance. *J Biol Chem* 1997;272:20963–20966.

268. Juliano L, Mauriello A, Sbarigia E, et al. Radiolabeled native low-density lipoprotein injected into patients with carotid stenosis accumulates in macrophages of atherosclerotic plaque: effect of vitamin E supplementation. *Circulation* 2000;101:1249–1254.

269. Fang JC, Kinlay S, Beltrame J, et al. Effect of vitamins C and E on progression of transplant-associated arteriosclerosis: a randomised trial. *Lancet* 2002;359:1108–1113.

270. Vivekananthan DP, Sapp S, Penn MS, et al. Vitamin E does not reduce mortality or cardiovascular morbidity: a pooled analysis of randomized trials. *Circulation* 2002;106[Suppl II]:II-736(abst).

271. Cheung MC, Zhao XQ, Chait A, et al. Antioxidant supplements block the response of HDL to simvastatin-niacin therapy in patients with coronary artery disease and low HDL. *Arterioscler Thromb Vasc Biol* 2001;21:1320–1326.

272. Tardif JC, Cote G, Lesperance J, et al. Probucol and multivitamins in the prevention of restenosis after coronary angioplasty. *N Engl J Med* 1997;337:365–372.

273. Burr ML, Fehily AM, Gilbert JF, et al. Effects of changes in fat, fish, and fibre intakes on death and myocardial reinfarction: diet and reinfarction trial (DART). *Lancet* 1989;2:757–761.

274. Singh RB, Rastogi SS, Verma R, et al. Randomised controlled trial of cardioprotective diet in patients with recent acute myocardial infarction: results of one year follow-up. *BMJ* 1992;304:1015–1019.

275. de Lorgeril M, Renaud S, Mamelle N, et al. Mediterranean alpha-linolenic acid-rich diet in secondary prevention of coronary heart disease. *Lancet* 1994;343:1454–1459.

276. de Lorgeril M, Salen P, Monjaud I, et al. The diet heart hypothesis in secondary prevention of coronary heart disease. *Eur Heart J* 1997;18:14–18.

277. de Lorgeril M, Salen P, Martin JL, et al. Mediterranean diet, traditional risk factors, and the rate of cardiovascular complications after myocardial infarction: final report of the Lyon Diet Heart Study. *Circulation* 1999;99:779–785.

278. Singh RB, Dubnov G, Niaz MA, et al. Effect of an Indo-Mediterranean diet on progression of coronary artery disease in high risk patients (Indo-Mediterranean Diet Heart Study): a randomised single-blind trial. *Lancet* 2002;360:1455–1461.

279. Leaf A. The electrophysiologic basis for the antiarrhythmic actions of polyunsaturated fatty acids. *Eur Heart J* 2001;22:D98–D105.

280. Daviglus ML, Stamler J, Orencia AJ, et al. Fish consumption and the 30-year risk of fatal myocardial infarction. *N Engl J Med* 1997;336:1046–1053.

281. Albert CM, Hennekens CH, O'Donnell CJ, et al. Fish consumption and risk of sudden death. *JAMA* 1998;279:23–28.

282. Marchioli R, Barzi F, Bomba E, et al. Early protection against sudden death by n-3 polyunsaturated fatty acids after myocardial infarction. Time-course analysis of the results of the Gruppo Italiano per lo Studio della Sopravvivenza nell'Infarto Miocardico (GISSI)-Prevenzione. *Circulation* 2002;105:1897–1903.

283. Kris-Etherton PM, Harris WS, Appel LJ, for the Nutrition Committee. Fish consumption, fish oil, omega-3 fatty acids, and cardiovascular disease. *Circulation* 2002;106:2747–2757.

284. Pepine CJ, Cohn PF, Deedwania PC, et al. Effects of treatment on outcome in mildly symptomatic patients with ischemia during daily life: the Atenolol Silent Ischemia Study (ASIST). *Circulation* 1994;90:762–768.

285. Frishman W, Charlap S, Kimmel B, et al. Diltiazem, nifedipine, and their combination in patients with stable angina pectoris: effects on angina, exercise tolerance, and the ambulatory electrocardiographic ST segment. *Circulation* 1988;77:774–786.

286. Subramanian VB, Bowles MJ, Khurmi NS, et al. Rationale for the choice of calcium antagonists in chronic stable angina: an objective double-blind placebo-controlled comparison of nifedipine and verapamil. *Am J Cardiol* 1982;50:1173–1179.

287. Shehata AR, Gillam LD, Mascitelli VA, et al. Impact of acute propranolol administration on dobutamine-induced myocardial ischemia as evaluated by myocardial perfusion imaging and echocardiography. *Am J Cardiol* 1997;80:268–272.

288. Aoki M, Sakai K, Koyanagi S, et al. Effect of nitroglycerin on coronary collateral function during exercise evaluated by quantitative analysis of thallium-201 single photon emission computed tomography. *Am Heart J* 1991;121:1361–1366.

289. Mahmarian JJ, Fenimore NL, Marks GF, et al. Transdermal nitroglycerin patch therapy reduces the extent of exercise-induced myocardial ischemia: results of a double-blind, placebo-controlled trial using quantitative thallium-201 tomography. *J Am Coll Cardiol* 1994;24:25–32.

290. Stegaru B, Loose R, Keller H, et al. Effects of long-term treatment with 120 mg of sustained-release isosorbide dinitrate and 60 mg of sustained-release nifedipine on myocardial perfusion. *Am J Cardiol* 1988;61:74E–77E.

291. O'Rourke RA, Chaudhuri T, Shaw L, et al. Resolution of stress-induced myocardial ischemia during aggressive medical therapy as demonstrated by single photon emission computed tomography imaging. *Circulation* 2001;103:2315.

292. Sdringola S, Nakagawa K, Nakagawa Y, et al. Combined intense lifestyle and pharmacologic lipid treatment further reduce coronary events and myocardial perfusion abnormalities compared with usual-care cholesterol-lowering drugs in coronary artery disease. *J Am Coll Cardiol* 2003;41:263–272.

293. Knatterud GL, Bourassa MG, Pepine CJ, et al.Effects of treatment strategies to suppress ischemia in patients with coronary artery disease: 12-week results of the Asymptomatic Cardiac Ischemia Pilot (ACIP) study. ACIP Investigators. *J Am Coll Cardiol* 1994;24:11–20.

294. Pratt CM, McMahon RP, Goldstein S, et al. Comparison of subgroups assigned to medical regimens used to suppress cardiac ischemia (the Asymptomatic Cardiac Ischemia Pilot [ACIP] study). ACIP Investigators. *Am J Cardiol* 1996;77:1302–1309.

295. Dakik HA, Kleiman NS, Farmer JA, et al. Intensive medical therapy versus coronary angioplasty for suppression of myocardial ischemia in survivors of acute myocardial infarction. A prospective, randomized pilot study. *Circulation* 1998;98:2017–2023.

296. The Sixth Report of the Joint National Committee on Prevention, Detection, Evaluation, and Treatment of High Blood Pressure. Bethesda, MD: National Institutes of Health, National Heart, Lung, and Blood Institute, 1997.

297. L'Italien GL, Lapuerta P. Population blood pressure control in patients with diabetes and congestive heart failure. *Am J Hypertens* 1999;12:92A(abst).

298. Whyte JL, Lapuerta P, L'Italien GJ, et al. The challenge of controlling systolic blood pressure: data from the National Health and Nutrition Examination Survey (NHANES III), 1988-1994. *J Clin Hypertens* 2001;3:211–216.

299. Pearson TA, Laurora I, Chu H, et al. The Lipid Treatment Assessment Project (L-TAP): a multicenter survey to evaluate the percentages of dyslipidemic patients receiving lipid-lowering therapy and achieving low-density lipoprotein cholesterol goals. *Arch Intern Med* 2000;160:459–467.

300. Fedder DO, Koro CE, L'Italien CJ. New National Cholesterol Education Program III guidelines for primary prevention lipid-lowering

drug therapy: projected impact on the size, sex, and age distribution of the treatment-eligible population. *Circulation* 2002;105:152–156.

301. Executive Summary of the Third Report of the National Cholesterol Education Program (NCEP) Expert Panel on Detection, Evaluation, and Treatment of High Blood Cholesterol in Adults (Adult Treatment Panel III). *JAMA* 2001;285:2486–2497.

302. Foot DK, Lewis RP, Pearson TA, et al. Demographics and cardiology, 1950-2050. *J Am Coll Cardiol* 2000;35:1067–1081.

303. Beller GA. Coronary heart disease in the first 30 years of the 21st century; challenges and opportunities: the 33rd Annual James B. Herrick Lecture of the Council on Clinical Cardiology of the American Heart Association. *Circulation* 2001;103:2428–2435.

304. King H, Aubert RE, Herman WH. Global burden of diabetes, 1995-2025. *Diabetes Care* 1998;21:1414–1431.

305. Mokdad AH, Serdula MK, Dietz WH, et al. The spread of the obesity epidemic in the United States, 1991-1998. *JAMA* 1999;282:1519–1522.

306. Overweight and obesity threaten U.S. health gains; communities can help address the problem. Surgeon General says [press release]. Available at: http://www.hhs.gov/news/press/2011213.html. U.S. Department of Health and Human Services; December 13, 2001. Accessed September 20, 2002.

307. O'Connor GT, Quinton HB, Traven ND, et al. Geographic variation in the treatment of acute myocardial infarction. The Cooperative Cardiovascular Project. *JAMA* 1999;281:627–633.

308. Fox KAA, Goodman SG, Klein W, et al. Management of acute coronary syndromes. Variations in practice and outcome. Findings from the Global Registry of Acute Coronary Events (GRACE). GRACE Investigators. *Eur Heart J* 2002;23:1177–1189.

309. Lifestyle and risk factor management and use of drug therapies in coronary patients from 15 countries. Principal results from EUROASPIRE II Euro Heart Survey Programme. EUROASPIRE II Study Group. *Eur Heart J* 2001;22:554–572.

310. Bonow RO, Smaha LA, Smith SC Jr, et al. World Heart Day 2002. The international burden of cardiovascular disease: responding to the emerging global epidemic. *Circulation* 2002;106:1602–1605.

311. Haynes RB, McDonald HP, Garg AX. Helping patients follow prescribed treatment. Clinical applications. *JAMA* 2002;288:2880–2883.

312. Ayanian JZ, Landrum MB, Guadagnoli E, et al. Specialty of ambulatory care physicians and mortality among elderly patients after myocardial infarction. *N Engl J Med* 2002;347:1678–1686.

313. World Health Report 2002. Reducing risks, promoting healthy life. Geneva: World Health Organization; 2002. Available at: www.who.int/whr. Accessed October 30, 2002.

314. Ottawa Charter for Health Promotion. First international conference on health promotion. Geneva: World Health Organization (WHO/HPR/HEP/95.1). November 21, 1986; Ottawa, Canada. Available at: http://www.who.int/hpr/archive/docs/ottawa.html. Accessed October 28, 2002.

315. Innovative care for chronic conditions: building blocks for action. Geneva: World Health Organization (WHO/MNC/CCH/02.01); 2002. Available at: http://www.who.int/ned/chronic_care/innovative_care/iccc_report.pdf. Accessed October 28, 2002.

316. Grumbach K, Bodenheimer T. A primary care home for Americans. Putting the house in order. *JAMA* 2002;288:889–893.

317. Casalino L, Gillies RR, Shortell SM, et al. External incentives, information technology, and organized processes to improve health care quality for patients with chronic diseases. *JAMA* 2003;289:434–441.

318. Falk E, Shah PK, Fuster V. Coronary plaque disruption. *Circulation* 1995;92:657–671.

319. Goldstein JA. Angiographic plaque complexity, the tip of the unstable plaque iceberg. *J Am Coll Cardiol* 2002;39:1464–1467.

320. Davies MJ, Richardson PD, Woolf N, et al. Risk of thrombosis in human atherosclerotic plaques: role of extracellular lipid, macrophage and smooth muscle content. *Br Heart J* 1993;69:377–381.

321. Davies MJ. Stability and instability: two faces of coronary atherosclerosis. The Paul Dudley White Lecture 1995. *Circulation* 1996;94:2013–2020.

322. Casscells W, Hathorn B, Krabach T, et al. Thermal detection of cellular infiltrates in living atherosclerotic plaques: possible implications for plaque rupture and thrombosis. *Lancet* 1996;347:1447–1451.

323. Naghavi M, John R, Naguib S, et al. pH heterogeneity of human and rabbit atherosclerotic plaques: a new insight into detection of vulnerable plaque. *Atherosclerosis* 2002;164:27–35.

324. Hatsukami TS, Ross R, Polissar NL, et al. Visualization of fibrous cap thickness and rupture in human atherosclerotic carotid plaque in vivo with high-resolution magnetic resonance imaging. *Circulation* 2000;102:959–964.

325. Fayad ZA, Fuster V. Clinical imaging of the high-risk or vulnerable atherosclerotic plaque. *Circ Res* 2001;89:305–316.

326. Stefanadis C, Diamantopoulos L, Dernellis J, et al. Thermal heterogeneity within human atherosclerotic coronary arteries detected in vivo: a new method of detection by application of a special thermography catheter. *Circulation* 1999;99:1965–1971.

327. Fayad ZA, Fuster V, Nikolaou K, et al. Computed tomography and magnetic resonance imaging for noninvasive coronary angiography and plaque imaging: current and potential future concepts. *Circulation* 2002;106:2026–2034.

328. Tsimikas S. Noninvasive imaging of oxidized low-density lipoprotein in atherosclerotic plaques with tagged oxidation-specific antibodies. *Am J Cardiol* 2002;90[Suppl]:22L–27L.

329. Madjid M, Naghavi M, Malik BA, et al. Thermal detection of vulnerable plaque. *Am J Cardiol* 2002;90[Suppl]:36L–39L.

CHAPTER 78

Value of Myocardial Perfusion Scintigraphy in Risk Stratification and Clinical Decision-making

Robert S. Gibson and George A. Beller

Key Words: Myocardial perfusion imaging; risk stratification.

INTRODUCTION

Myocardial perfusion imaging (MPI) with thallium-201 (^{201}Tl) or technetium-99m (^{99m}Tc)-sestamibi is an established noninvasive technique that is currently the most widely used nuclear cardiology procedure for assessing nutrient blood flow reserve at the myocapillary level and for measuring left ventricular (LV) function. When performed in conjunction with exercise or pharmacologic stress testing, it offers a unique means of diagnostic evaluation in patients with known or suspected coronary artery disease (CAD). Moreover, the prognostic value of MPI is currently well established. The ability of MPI to distinguish patients at high risk from those at low risk has become a valuable adjunct for determining management of patients across a wide spectrum of clinical settings.

In previous reviews published between 1982–1996 (1–5), Brown and others described the evolution of data that allowed MPI to emerge from a diagnostic to a prognostic tool capable of playing an important role in patient-care decisions. At the time, limitations of the technique and gaps in our knowledge were discussed. Since then, the technology has continued to mature and new data have been reported. Contemporaneously, health care has evolved dramatically,

R. S. Gibson: Department of Medicine, Division of Cardiology, University of Virginia, Charlottesville, Virginia.
G. A. Beller: Department of Medicine, Division of Cardiology, University of Virginia, Charlottesville, Virginia.

placing greater emphasis on cost control and managed care. In this environment, all technology use will see increased scrutiny. Therefore, it is of value to review new developments in the use of MPI for risk stratification that have emerged in the last 5 to 8 years.

BASIC REQUIREMENTS FOR RISK STRATIFICATION STRATEGIES

Although statistically significant risk stratification can be achieved by any of a number of methods, based on prognostic studies performed to date, certain conceptual criteria have emerged as minimal standards for clinically acceptable risk stratification by a noninvasive imaging modality.

- The preferred noninvasive test is one that provides the most quantitatively accurate information about a specific risk predictor (e.g., myocardial ischemia) for which definitive treatment exists (e.g., revascularization) with the fewest complications and the lowest cost to the patient.

- A normal test result should be associated with a low cardiac event rate. As described previously, the criteria generally referred to are those listed in the 2002 Unstable Angina/Non-ST Segment Elevation Myocardial Infarction guideline (6) that categorize "low risk" as one that implies a less than 1% risk for cardiac death during the subsequent year, as well as a low probability of infarction or readmission to the hospital for medically resistant angina pectoris.

- Not only should the cardiac event rate associated with an abnormal scan be statistically significantly greater that that associated with a normal- or low-risk result, but the risk ratio of an abnormal scan relative to a normal scan should greatly exceed 1. The relative risk ratio defines the effectiveness of the stratification method. This takes on greater importance as the cost efficiency of noninvasive testing tends to parallel the effectiveness of stratification achieved. Enhanced stratification results in more patients in the low-risk group (lower cost of care) and less patients in the high-risk group (a greater cost group that will have more resource use over time). In other words, a sufficient number of patients would be reclassified as low-risk by normal studies, thus obviating the need for further testing, for the strategy to be cost-effective.

- Given the recent evolution of health care, it is no longer adequate to demonstrate simply that a procedure such as MPI has prognostic value. It is now necessary to show that such testing adds significantly to the predictive value of data that are less expensive to obtain, such as that derived from the clinical history, risk factors, standard electrocardiography (ECG), or the exercise ECG. In an analogous way, it is important to ask what more invasive and expensive procedures such as coronary angiography add to the value of less expensive testing with MPI.

- Results of noninvasive risk stratification should have a significant influence on clinical decision-making. That is, the method should function as a "gatekeeper" for invasive management strategies (4,5,7) because it effectively identifies low-risk groups who have an excellent prognosis with medical therapy and do not benefit from early revascularization. Conversely, the identification of high-risk patients who would most likely benefit from revascularization on the basis of an expected high cardiac event rate with medical management also would be accomplished. This management approach, in which referral for cardiac catheterization is ischemia driven, also is highly cost-effective.

APPLICATION OF STRESS NUCLEAR TEST RESULTS IN CLINICAL PRACTICE

On the basis of published prognostic literature, the Cedars-Sinai group (8) derived the following four points that can serve as general *rules of thumb* for the use of scintigraphic testing in clinical practice:

1. A normal scintigraphic study at a moderate or high level of stress confers a benign prognosis. For example, Steinberg and coworkers (9) reported the outcomes of 309 patients with normal ^{201}Tl imaging who were followed for 10 years. In this cohort, the annualized cardiac event rate was 0.1% for cardiac death and 0.6% for nonfatal myocardial infarction (MI). Similar findings have been validated in a series of 32 other studies (10–41), using either ^{201}Tl or ^{99m}Tc-sestamibi in more than 11,000 patients (Table 78–1), which evaluated annualized event rates during follow-up of patients who had normal findings during the performance of exercise or pharmacologic stress MPI for suspected CAD. This benign prognosis appears to persist even in patients with positive exercise electrocardiograms or angiographically significant CAD (25–27,42–44).

2. An equivocal scintigraphic study generally also conveys a benign prognosis. For example, Berman and colleagues (34) reported on a cohort of patients referred for exercise ^{99m}Tc-sestamibi single-photon emission computed tomography (SPECT) who were followed for 20 ± 5 months. Among 1,702 patients, no hard events occurred in the 87 patients with an equivocal scan. Similar results have been reported in a study of 505 patients by Yao and coworkers (45) with a mean follow-up of 19 ± 7 months. Equivocal studies were present in 61 (12%) SPECT studies. They were grouped as either small defects according to semiquantitative visual analysis or because of technical problems arising from, most commonly, attenuation artifacts or patient motion. At 1-year follow-up, there was only one confirmed cardiac event (MI) that occurred in the subgroup with technical problems. Thus, despite the lack of diagnostic certainty with

TABLE 78–1. *Annualized cardiac event rates in patients with normal stress thallium-201 and technetium-99m–sestamibi myocardial perfusion imaging results*

Study, year (reference)	Patients, n[a]	Type of stress	Mean follow-up, mo	Annualized cardiac event rate (myocardial infarction/death)
Thallium-201 MPI				
Brown, 1983 (10)	61	Exercise	44	0.8
Pamelia, 1985 (11)	345	Exercise	34	1.1
Wackers, 1985 (12)	95	Exercise	22	1.2
Wahl, 1985 (13)	455	Exercise	14	0.8
Ladenheim, 1986 (14)	851	Exercise	12	1.3
Staniloff, 1986 (15)	374	Exercise	12	0.5
Iskandrian, 1986 (16)	183	Exercise	25	0.2
Gill, 1987 (17)	192	Exercise	58	0.8
Heo, 1987 (18)	519	Exercise	27	0.5
Koss, 1987 (19)	309	Exercise	36	0.5
Koll, 1988 (20)	39	Exercise	64	0.5
Younis, 1989 (21)	36	Dipyridamole	24	0.0
Bairey, 1989 (22)	144	Exercise	12	2.1
Fleg, 1990 (23)	352	Exercise	55	0.9
Hendel, 1990 (24)	172	Dipyridamole	21	1.7
Brown, 1993 (25)	176	Exercise	24	0.9
Steinberg, 1993 (9)	309	Exercise	120	0.7
Schalet, 1993 (26)	164	Exercise	34	0.0
Fattah, 1994 (27)	97	Exercise	32	1.2
Pavin, 1997 (28)	171	Exercise	104	1.7
Total	5,044			
Average			36.1 mos	0.87%
Technetium-99m–sestamibi MPI				
Brown, 1994 (29)	234	Exercise/dipyridamole	10	0.5
Raiker, 1994 (30)	208	Exercise	14	0.4
Stratmann, 1994 (31)	206	Exercise	13	0.5
Stratmann, 1994 (32)	179	Dipyridamole	13	1.6
Zanco, 1995 (33)	58	Exercise	43	0.0
Berman, 1995 (34)	1,131	Exercise	20	0.1
Heller, 1995 (35)	216	Dipyridamole	13	1.2
Gelejinse, 1996 (36)	80	Dobutamine	23	0.0
Hachamovitch, 1996 (37)	2,511	Exercise	20	0.5
Nallamouthu, 1996 (38)	295	Exercise	17	0.2
Boyne, 1997 (39)	155	Exercise	19	0.8
Hachamovitch, 1997 (40)	444	Adenosine	28	1.6
Gibson, 2002 (41)	652	Exercise/dipyridamole	22	0.1
Total	6,369			
Average			19.6 mos	0.58%

[a]Patients with normal myocardial perfusion imaging scan results.

equivocal studies, they are associated with a benign prognosis in patients with a high likelihood of CAD.

3. The cardiac event rate associated with an abnormal scan is substantially greater that that associated with a normal scan. In a review, by Iskander and coworkers (46), of 14 studies comprising more than 12,000 patients, the relative risk ratios ranged from 4.4 to 39. Pooled analysis showed that a normal stress SPECT sestamibi scan was associated with an average annual death and MI rate of 0.6%. In contrast, patients with an abnormal scintiscan had a 12-fold greater event rate (7.4% annually). As demonstrated by Berman and coworkers (4), the effectiveness of stress MPI in risk stratification extends across the full range of pretest probabilities of CAD (Fig. 78–1).

4. Clinical parameters may powerfully modify the assessment of cardiac risk associated with stress myocardial perfusion defects. For example, peak heart rate has a strong influence on the likelihood of cardiac events, independent of the defect size on MPI, as demonstrated by Ladenheim and coworkers (14). When patients were divided into those who did and those who did not achieve an adequate heart rate (i.e., >85% of the maximum predicted heart rate), the cardiac event rate for a given magnitude of myocardial ischemia was approximately threefold greater for patients who could not exercise to more than 85% of their maximum predicted heart rate. Such data illustrate the importance of incorporating clinical data into the as-

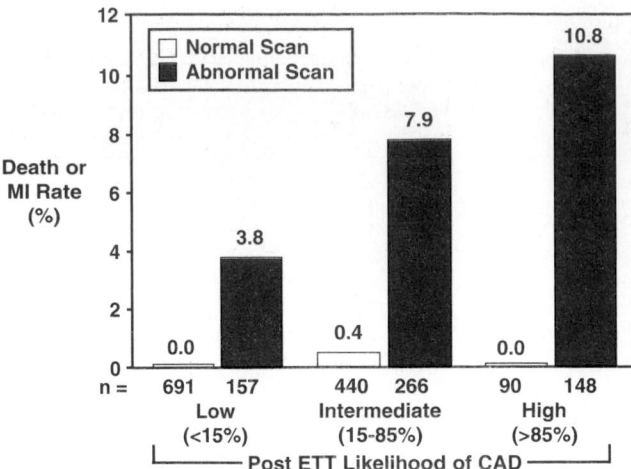

FIG. 78–1. Event rate (cardiac death or myocardial infarction *[MI]* over 20 ± 5 months) as a function of technetium-99m sestamibi and prescan likelihood of coronary artery disease *(CAD)*. ETT, exercise treadmill test. (Adapted from Berman DS, Hachamovitch R. Risk assessment in patients with stable coronary artery disease: incremental value of nuclear imaging. *J Nucl Cardiol* 1996;3:41–49, with permission.)

sessment of cardiac risk when analyzing the results of MPI studies.

SCINTIGRAPHIC PREDICTORS OF CARDIAC EVENTS

The prognostic utility of MPI derives from its ability to reliably detect the presence of reversible ischemia, manifesting as a transient perfusion defect, during exercise or during pharmacologic stress testing with dipyridamole, adenosine, dobutamine, or arbutamine. Numerous studies have shown that the summed defect score, as well as the amount of defect reversibility, are key predictors of future cardiac events. In addition, there are several other scintigraphic variables (Table 78–2) that have been found to provide incremental prognostic information (10,34,37,40,47–58). Each of these variables can be identified qualitatively and quantitatively,

TABLE 78–2. *Scintigraphic predictors of cardiac events*

Perfusion variables
- Numerically significant focal defect
- Defect reversibility
- Quantified magnitude of ischemic jeopardy
- Number of vascular territories with defects

Nonperfusion variables
- Left ventricular dilation (transient or fixed)
- Lung/heart ratios of radioactivity
- Left ventricular ejection fraction from gated single-photon emission computed tomography (rest and exercise)
- Absolute left ventricular volumes
- Poststress wall motion abnormalities

and the prognostic window can be modulated according to the combination of criteria used.

Exponential Relation between Ischemic Burden and Likelihood of Cardiac Events

The relation between the magnitude of inducible myocardial ischemia and the likelihood of subsequent cardiac events is not linear. Rather, previous investigation has shown an exponential relation (14). Accordingly, patients who demonstrate only mild ischemia at peak stress have only a small, relatively flat increase in the likelihood of cardiac events as compared with patients who manifest no scintigraphic evidence of inducible ischemia (Fig. 78–2). This is particularly true if LVEF is normal. By contrast, once ischemia progresses to a moderate magnitude, the likelihood of cardiac events begins to increase sharply. The cutoff point that seems to distinguish mild from moderate defect size is approximately 10% to 20% of the left ventricle (37,51,52,55).

Transient Ischemic Dilation and Increased Lung Uptake

In addition to the aforementioned variables, two other abnormalities should be observed and, when present, described. These include transient ischemic dilation (TID) of the left ventricle (59–62) and abnormalities of lung uptake (17,63–69). TID is considered present when the LV cavity appears to be significantly larger in the poststress images than in the rest images. The degree of enlargement needed depends on the imaging protocol used. For example, with dual-isotope protocols, the greater Compton scatter associated with ^{201}Tl causes the myocardial walls to appear intrin-

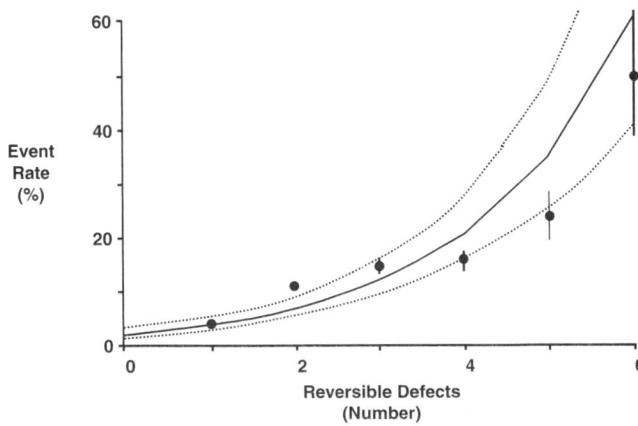

FIG. 78–2. Plot of risk for future cardiac events as a function of number of reversible thallium-201 perfusion defects. Relation is exponential (*r* = 0.97; *p* < 0.001). (Adapted from Ladenheim ML, Pollock BH, Rozanski A, et al. Extent and severity of myocardial hypoperfusion as predictors of prognosis in patients with suspected coronary artery disease. *J Am Coll Cardiol* 1986;7:464–471, with permission.)

sically thicker (and the cavity smaller) in ^{201}Tl rest images compared with poststress ^{99m}Tc-sestamibi images (60). Therefore, a greater degree of transient enlargement must be evident for a dual-isotope study to be considered to show TID. Patients who have TID are more likely to have severe and extensive CAD (i.e., >90% stenosis of the proximal left anterior descending coronary artery [LAD] or of multiple vessels), and it has been shown that TID is more specific than other established markers of severe and extensive CAD (59,60), such as the presence of multiple perfusion defects involving different vascular beds. Also, TID has similar clinical and prognostic implications whether it is observed on exercise or pharmacologic stress studies (61,62). The mechanism of TID is thought to be stress-induced subendocardial ischemia because the total size of the left ventricle is not greater on the poststress compared with the rest images. Only the cavity size of the left ventricle is greater.

The degree of lung uptake of myocardial perfusion tracers should be noted from visual inspection of the raw projection images. Quantitative lung/heart ratios for ^{201}Tl have been shown to have an upper limit of normal of 0.54 (65–67), whereas preliminary data for ^{99m}Tc-sestamibi suggest an upper limit of 0.44 (68). In general, there is a strong linear correlation between the degree of lung uptake and the pulmonary capillary wedge pressure at the time of stress injection (69). Regardless of whether qualitative or quantitative methods of analysis are used, increased lung radioactivity has consistently been found to be a marker of severe underlying CAD, reduced LV contractile reserve, or both. Because an increased lung/heart ratio of radioactivity indicates a high probability of multivessel CAD, even when it is associated with less extensive perfusion defects, it is not surprising that this scintigraphic parameter has been found to have prognostic value.

Quantitative Assessment of Left Ventricular Function and Volumes

The value of LV function and size in risk stratification has been well documented, particularly in identifying patients at increased risk for cardiac death (70–75). With the addition of ECG gating to SPECT imaging, it is now possible to acquire highly accurate and reproducible measurements of left ventricular ejection fraction (LVEF) (76,77). Also, it has been demonstrated that quantitative assessment of absolute LV cavity volumes by gated SPECT is feasible and correlate well with echocardiography (78), thermal dilution cardiac catheterization methods (79), and magnetic resonance imaging (80). Several studies have shown that poststress LVEF and end-systolic volume by gated SPECT have incremental prognostic values over prescan and perfusion information in predicting cardiac death and readmission to the hospital for congestive heart failure (81–84). An example of the relation between LVEF by gated SPECT and survival is shown in

Figure 78–3. In addition to prognostication, both variables can help guide the use of angiotensin-converting enzyme inhibitors (85).

With gated SPECT imaging, it also is possible to identify the development of new wall motion abnormalities by comparing the poststress and rest images. In general, the development of a discrete poststress wall motion or wall thickening abnormality implies the presence of ventricular stunning and is highly specific for severe CAD (>90% narrowing) (86–88). This finding might be missed by perfusion defect assessment alone, particularly in patients with a greater degree of ischemia in a region other than that demonstrating the wall motion abnormality. Assessment of regional thickening or wall motion abnormalities on gated SPECT images obtained after either exercise or pharmacologic stress increases the identification of patients with three-vessel disease compared with evaluation of perfusion images alone.

Assessment of Myocardial Viability

The presence of myocardial viability is implied with the perfusion tracers if the degree of uptake at rest, redistribution, or after a nitrate-augmented rest injection is normal or nearly normal. If a region has severely reduced or no uptake of radioactivity in these settings, it is considered to be nonviable. Areas with a moderate reduction in counts are usually partially viable, and patients in this group have a variable response in terms of postrevascularization improvement (89,90). Although some authors have suggested that a single cutoff point (chosen as a percentage of maximal counts in the myocardium) is predictive of viability in a region in question (89,91,92), others prefer the use of the number of standard deviations below normal, because the latter would take in account the rather marked reduction in counts that occurs in the inferior wall of nonattenuation-corrected myocardial perfusion SPECT images. Another clue of viability is the degree of wall thickening. Demonstration of systolic thickening indicates substantial preservation of myocardial viability.

Assessment of myocardial viability after MI, particularly in patients with severe LV dysfunction, is important for those patients at greatest risk who might benefit from revascularization. As pointed out by DiCarli (93), there is growing and consistent evidence that patients with relatively large areas of dysfunctional but viable myocardium after MI have improved function, symptoms, and survival with prompt revascularization compared with medical management alone. A pooled analysis of 24 viability studies in the literature showed that in patients with viability, revascularization was associated with a 79.6% reduction in annual mortality (16% vs. 3.2%) compared with medical treatment (94). It thus appears that long-term survival with revascularization in these patients may be comparable with that achieved with cardiac transplantation.

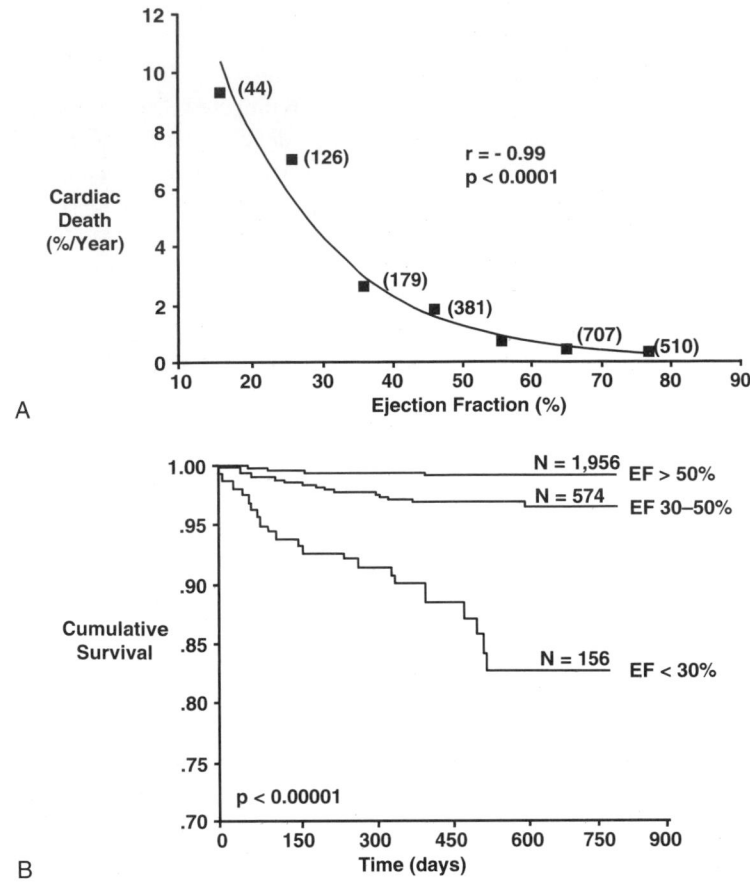

FIG. 78–3. A: Annual cardiac death rate as a function of poststress ejection fraction *(EF)* by gated single-proton emission computed tomography. Number of patients at each 10% interval is indicated in parentheses. **B:** Cumulative survival with stratification by left ventricular EF. (Adapted from Sharir T, Germano G, Kang X, et al. Prediction of myocardial infarction versus cardiac death by gated myocardial perfusion SPECT: risk stratification by the amount of stress-induced ischemia and post-stress ejection fraction. *J Nucl Med* 2001;42:831–837, with permission.)

INCREMENTAL VALUE OF MYOCARDIAL PERFUSION IMAGING

Because stress MPI tests are not inexpensive, for their application to be cost-effective, the data obtained from these tests should contribute incremental information that cannot be derived from the patient's clinical history and risk factors, rest ECG, and exercise ECG findings. An important step to address these issues was taken by Iskandrian and coworkers (49), who determined the additive incremental prognostic value of MPI in patients with angiographically defined CAD.

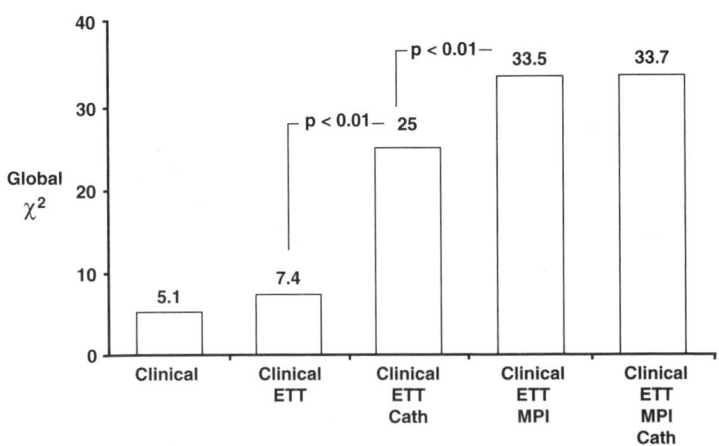

FIG. 78–4. Incremental prognostic information of clinical, exercise treadmill test *(ETT)*, catheterization, and single-photon emission computed tomography thallium variables, shown by global χ^2 value. Cath, catheterization; MPI, myocardial perfusion imaging. (Adapted from Iskandrian AS, Chae SC, Heo J, et al. Independent and incremental prognostic value of exercise single-photon emission computed tomographic (SPECT) thallium imaging in coronary artery disease. *J Am Coll Cardiol* 1993;22:665–670, with permission.)

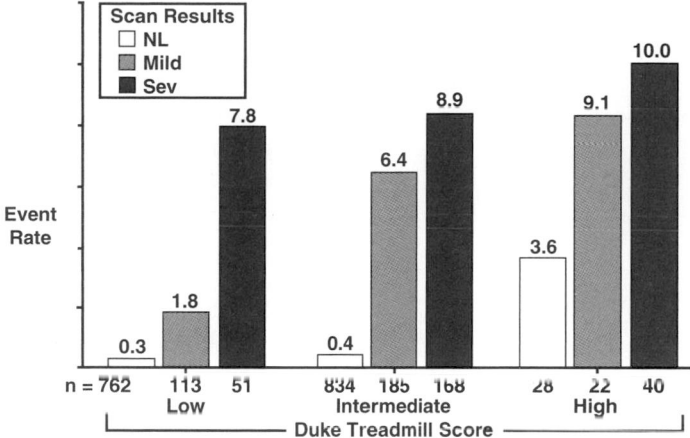

FIG. 78–5. Event rate (cardiac death or myocardial infarction) as a function of Duke Treadmill Score category and scan results. NL, normal; Sev, severe. (Adapted from Hachamovitch R, Berman DS, Kiat H, et al. Exercise myocardial perfusion SPECT in patients without known CAD. Incremental prognostic value and use in risk stratification. *Circulation* 1996;93:905–914, with permission.)

They found that, among all patient variables (including clinical, exercise ECG, MPI, and cardiac catheterization data), MPI had the greatest predictive value. More important, when these variables were evaluated in a hierarchal incremental manner, they found that exercise ECG did not add significant predictive value to clinical variables, but the addition of MPI data improved prognostic value by a factor of greater than 4 (Fig. 78–4). Furthermore, the increment in prognostic value was greater with MPI data than with cardiac catheterization data. Cardiac catheterization data did not add significant prognostic value to thallium scintigraphic data. Thus, MPI greatly improved the prognostic value of the less expensive stress ECG, whereas compared with MPI, the more expensive cardiac catheterization data did not.

The incremental prognostic value of MPI has been shown for patients with suspected and established CAD, with exercise or pharmacologic stress, with both planar and SPECT ^{201}Tl, and with ^{99m}Tc-sestamibi SPECT imaging (10,34,37,40,47–58,81–84,95–100). The Cedars-Sinai group has continued to contribute important new information (81,83,97–100). In a study by Hachamovitch and coworkers (98), nuclear stress testing was found to add significant incremental value to the Duke treadmill score for risk assessment. As shown in Figure 78–5, there were 834 patients classified as having an intermediate risk for subsequent death or infarction on the basis of the Duke treadmill score and normal scan results. The subsequent hard event rate was 0.4% in this group. Multiple logistic regression analysis revealed that scan information contributed 95% of all information regarding referral to catheterization. In another publication by Hachamovitch and coworkers (37), the Cedars-Sinai group reported results from 4,136 patients who underwent dual isotope SPECT imaging and who were followed for 20 ± 5 months. Their data show the incremental prognostic value

of MPI for both men and women (Fig. 78–6). In 1998, this same group demonstrated in a large patient cohort that the results of SPECT imaging can assist in deciding which patients with chronic stable CAD and an abnormal scan might do well with medical therapy compared with early revascularization (99) (Fig. 78–7). They found that the annual cardiac death rate was only 0.8% in patients with a mildly abnormal scan who received medical treatment after testing versus 0.9% for similar patients who had early revascularization after testing. In contrast, patients with moderately or severely abnormal scans (more extensive perfusion defects) benefited from revascularization early after nuclear stress testing.

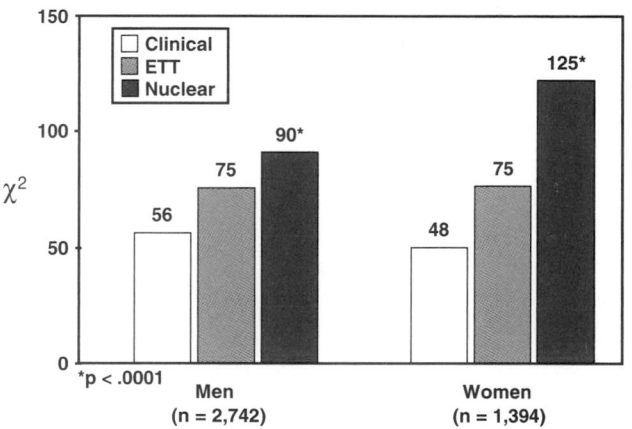

FIG. 78–6. Incremental prognostic information of clinical, exercise treadmill test *(ETT)*, and technetium-99m single-photon emission computed tomography for men and women, shown by global χ^2 values. (Adapted from Hachamovitch R, Berman DS, Kiat H, et al. Effective risk stratification using exercise myocardial perfusion SPECT in women: gender-related differences in prognostic nuclear testing. *J Am Coll Cardiol* 1996;28:34–44, with permission.)

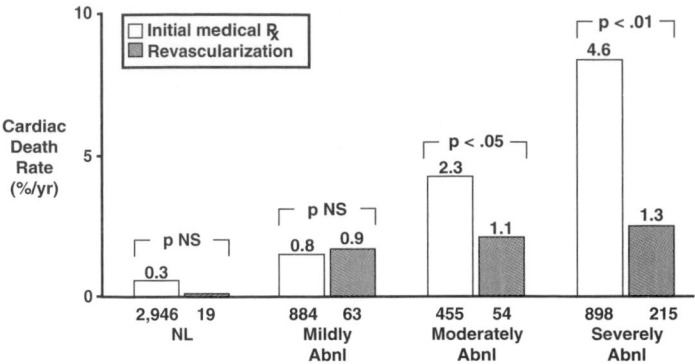

FIG. 78–7. Rates of cardiac death per year as a function of scan result and type of therapy. Abnl, abnormal; NL, normal; NS, not significant; Rx, treatment. (Adapted from Hachamovitch R, Berman DS, Shaw LJ, et al. Incremental prognostic value of myocardial perfusion single photon emission computed tomography for the prediction of cardiac death: differential stratification for risk of cardiac death and myocardial infarction. *Circulation* 1998;97:535–543, with permission.)

EFFECT OF STRESS NUCLEAR MYOCARDIAL PERFUSION IMAGING ON DOWNSTREAM RESOURCE USE

In addition to its ability to provide valuable information regarding risk stratification, stress MPI is increasingly seen as a "gatekeeper" for more costly diagnostic and interventional procedures (4,5,7). In 1991, Steingart and coworkers (101) evaluated 378 patients across a full range of pretest probabilities of CAD and showed that the results of nuclear stress testing significantly reduced referring physicians' likelihood of recommending cardiac catheterization on average by 49%. Bateman and coworkers (102) demonstrated in a large retrospective study of 4,162 patients that the results of SPECT scintigraphy overpowered all other clinical and treadmill variables in determining the likelihood of subsequent coronary angiography. When no reversible defects were present, only 3.5% of patients went on to cardiac catheterization compared with 32% of patients with reversible defects. Among those with reversible defects, 60% of patients with high-risk imaging results (defined as multiregion defects, anterior or anteroseptal defects, or increased lung uptake) went on to angiography compared with only 9% of patients without these findings. Thus, clinicians were clearly acting on the results of MPI, limiting referral for cardiac catheterization principally to the group with significant ischemia. Similar results reported by Nallamothu and coworkers (103) showed that the results of exercise SPECT ^{201}Tl imaging had a substantial impact on patient management and outcome. Coronary angiography, myocardial revascularization procedures, and cardiac events were all found to be rare in patients with normal scintiscans. In a subsequent study by Hachamovitch and coworkers (104), it was shown that the results of stress MPI influenced referral to cardiac catheterization without a sex-related referral bias. Importantly, the decision to perform invasive and interventional procedures was related to the degree of abnormality of imaging results, corresponding to the perceived (and documented) risk for future cardiac events (105). In studies by Mishra and coworkers (106) and Zellweger and coworkers (107), involving more than 8,000 patients with an intermediate to high probability of CAD, it was shown that screening patients by stress SPECT MPI results in lower uti-

lization rates for coronary angiography and coronary revascularization and is economically superior to a strategy based on cardiac catheterization as the initial screening test.

CURRENT EVIDENCE ON COST-EFFECTIVENESS OF STRESS NUCLEAR MYOCARDIAL PERFUSION IMAGING

In an era of cost containment, it also is important to determine whether noninvasive test results can be cost-effective. To this end, Shaw and coworkers (100) evaluated 11,372 consecutive

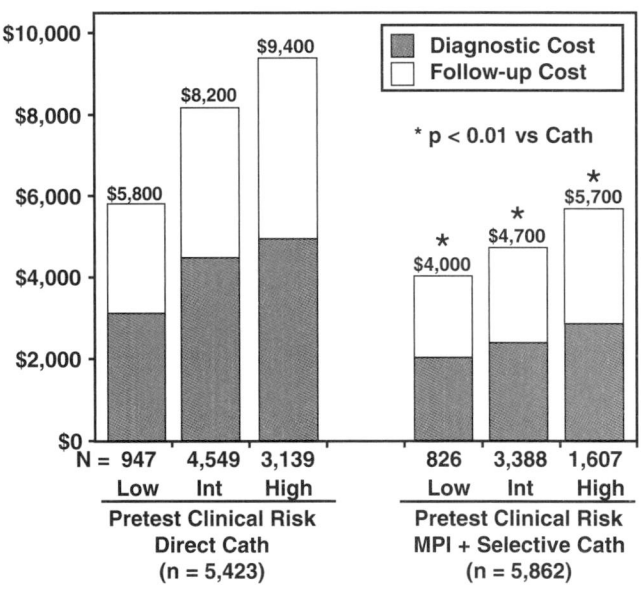

FIG. 78–8. Comparative cost between screening strategies using direct catheterization *(cath)* and myocardial perfusion imaging *(MPI)* with selective catheterization. *Low, Int,* and *High* represent low-, intermediate-, and high-risk subsets of patients with stable angina. (Adapted from Shaw LJ, Hachamovitch R, Berman DS, et al. The economic consequences of available diagnostic and prognostic strategies for the evaluation of stable angina patients: an observational assessment of the value of precatheterization ischemia. The Economics of Noninvasive Diagnosis (END) Multicenter Study Group. *J Am Coll Cardiol* 1999;33:661–669.)

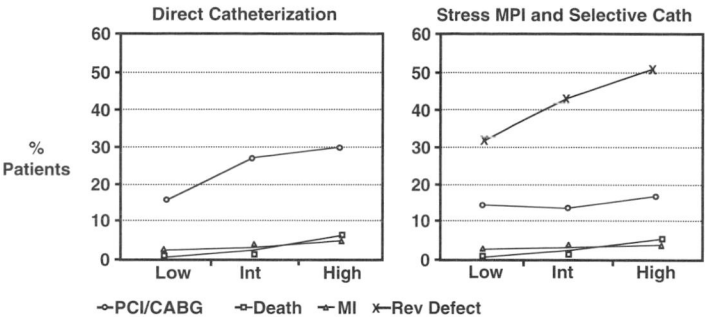

FIG. 78–9. Subsequent event rates in the patient populations illustrated in Figure 78–8. The rates of myocardial infarction and cardiac death were identical between the populations. *Low, Int,* and *High* rep resent low , intermediate-, and high-risk subsets of patients with stable angina; *circles* represent percutaneous coronary intervention; *squares* represent death; *triangles* represent myocardial infarction; *X* represents reversible defect. CABG, coronary artery bypass graft; MI, myocardial infarction; MPI, myocardial perfusion imaging; PCI, percutaneous coronary intervention; Rev Defect, Reversible Defect. (Adapted from Shaw LJ, Hachamovitch R, Berman DS, et al. The economic consequences of available diagnostic and prognostic strategies for the evaluation of stable angina patients: an observational assessment of the value of precatheterization ischemia. The Economics of Noninvasive Diagnosis (END) Multicenter Study Group. *J Am Coll Cardiol* 1999;33:661–669, with permission.)

patients with chronic stable CAD gathered in a large multicenter trial comprising 6 different laboratories from around the United States. In a matched cohort study comparing a direct catheterization approach to initial stress MPI with selective catheterization of high-risk patients (clinically at high risk and those with ischemia on MPI), for all levels of pretest clinical risk, there was a substantial reduction (31–50%) in costs using the MPI plus selective catheterization approach. This cost reduction was seen in both the diagnostic (early) and follow-up (late) costs, which included costs of revascularization (Fig. 78–8). Importantly, the two cohorts had virtually identical rates of subsequent nonfatal MI and cardiac death during 3 years of follow-up. What was significantly different was the rate of revascularization, which was reduced by almost 50% in the MPI with selective catheterization cohort (Fig. 78–9). Thus, these data reveal that patients who undergo a more aggressive diagnostic strategy incur greater costs without a resultant improvement in outcome. The lack of improvement in

3-year outcome decries the aggressive management approach and supports the cost savings yielded by using noninvasive testing for patients with stable CAD.

Other investigators have evaluated the cost-effectiveness of MPI in various clinical settings (106–112). In one study by Patterson and coworkers (109), stress MPI was shown to be more cost efficient that either stress ECG alone or stress ECG combined with echocardiographic imaging across a wide range of pretest disease probabilities (Table 78–3).

RISK STRATIFICATION AFTER AN ACUTE CORONARY SYNDROME

In survivors of acute MI (AMI), many high-risk clinical and laboratory variables have been identified. These variables include recurrent angina, LV failure, malignant arrhythmias, and conduction system abnormalities, to name a few (6,113). In the subset of patients with an uncomplicated MI (asymptomatic and without severely reduced LVEF), 1-year mortality ranges from less than 2% to 7.5% (114). The aim of noninvasive testing before hospital discharge in these patients, therefore, is the identification of those who are at relatively lower or greater risk for subsequent death or recurrent infarction on the basis of residual ischemic myocardium, either adjacent to or remote from the infarct zone.

TABLE 78–3. *Cost savings of stress imaging compared with stress electrocardiography*

	Imaging modality	
Probability of CAD	Echocardiography	SPECT MPI
0.20	−16.4%	−21.1%
0.40	−10.4%	−19.2%
0.60	−6.9%	−18.2%
0.80	−4.4%	−17.5%

CAD, coronary artery disease; MPI, myocardial perfusion imaging; SPECT, single-photon emission computed tomography.

Comparison of cost ($) per quality adjusted life-year for stress echocardiography and MPI versus stress electrocardiography alone.

Advantages of Myocardial Perfusion Imaging versus Stress Electrocardiographic Testing Alone

Whereas exercise ECG may be used in isolation to assess ischemia in patients after MI, there is a decided advantage to using combined MPI and ECG monitoring for assessing such risk. For example, numerous studies published over the last two decades (51,54,55,115–135) have shown that perfusion imag-

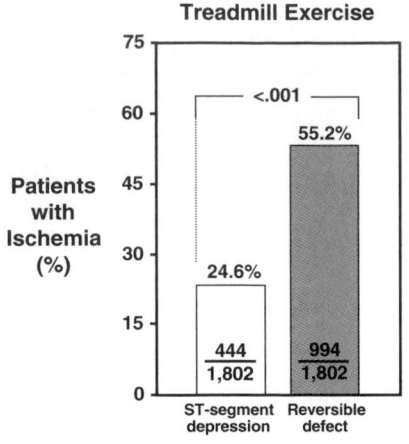
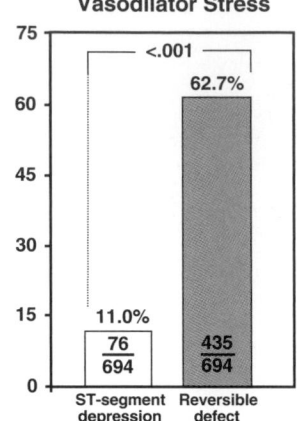

FIG. 78–10. Comparison of stress testing techniques for detecting residual ischemia in medically stabilized patients with acute myocardial infarction.

ing is innately more sensitive for detecting myocardial ischemia (Fig. 78–10) and is more accurate in quantifying its magnitude. Not infrequently, patients after MI with negative predischarge stress tests (defined as no angina or ST-segment depression at > 5 metabolic equivalents [METS]) will have scintigraphic evidence of residual ischemia, either in the infarct zone or in myocardial segments remote from the zone of infarction. Among these patients with negative exercise ECG tests, clinical outcome studies (136) have shown that those with ischemia by MPI have a significantly greater cardiac event rate during long-term follow-up (Fig. 78–11). These results indicate that MPI is a valuable adjunct to stress ECG testing because its use can identify a large group of patients after infarction with prognostically important ischemia who otherwise would not have been detected. Other studies comparing exercise ECG to radionuclide ventriculography (137–139), positron emission tomography (140), and endocardial or intracoronary electrograms (141,142) have all revealed the surface ECG to be relatively insensitive for ischemia detection.

Previously, physicians have assumed that exercise-induced ST-segment depression is a specific marker of residual ischemia in patients recovering from an acute Q-wave MI. This assumption is generally true for patients experiencing angina in conjunction with ST-segment depression. However, in our experience, less than 50% of patients with painless ST-segment depression during predischarge exercise ECG testing show evidence of ischemia by quantitative scintigraphic criteria (143). These false-positive ECG responses are particularly common among patients with large Q-wave infarctions resulting from occlusion of the right or left circumflex coronary arteries.

In contrast to stress ECG testing, segmental analysis of ^{201}Tl or ^{99m}Tc-sestamibi scintiscans allows one to localize ischemia to a particular area or areas subtended by a specific coronary artery. Because of this, it is possible to distinguish periinfarction ischemia from ischemia involving myocardial segments in the distribution of coronary arteries other than those associated with the acute infarction. Many studies have demonstrated that the presence of infarct zone ischemia is highly predictive of adverse outcome, even in patients with single-vessel CAD (122), and that stress MPI can effectively stratify patients with multivessel CAD into high-

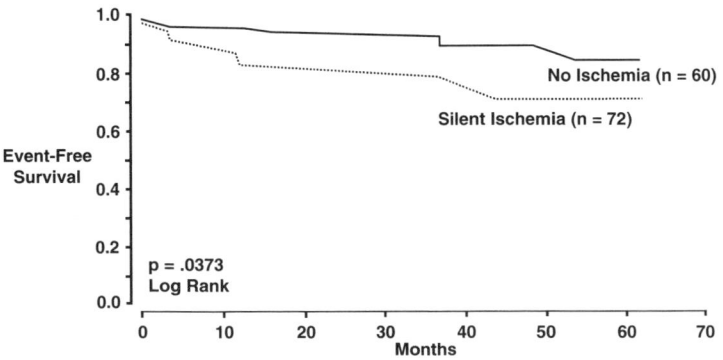

FIG. 78–11. Survival rates with reinfarction for patients with negative predischarge exercise test according to the presence or absence of thallium-201 ischemia. (Adapted from Gibson RS, Watson DD. The value of planar thallium-201 imaging in risk stratification of patients recovering from acute myocardial infarction. *Circulation* 1991;84[Suppl 1]:148–162, with permission.)

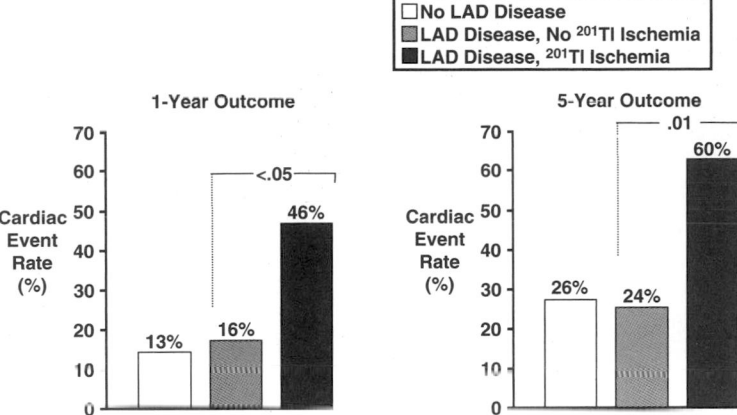

FIG. 78–12. Bar graph showing event rates in 125 patients with inferior wall myocardial infarction according to results of coronary angiography and exercise thallium-201 (^{201}Tl) scintigraphy. *Red bars,* left anterior descending coronary artery disease (LAD) with ^{201}Tl ischemia; *pink bars,* LAD disease without ^{201}Tl ischemia; *open bars,* no LAD disease. (Adapted from Gibson RS, Watson DD. The value of planar thallium-201 imaging in risk stratification of patients recovering from acute myocardial infarction. *Circulation* 1991;84[Suppl 1]:148–162, with permission.)

and low-risk subsets. For example, not all patients with proximal LAD disease, observed in conjunction with an acute inferior MI and occlusion of the right coronary artery, will behave similarly. In some patients, exercise stress will produce marked ischemia of the apical, anterolateral, and septal regions, indicating a large amount of myocardium at risk for subsequent infarction. Other patients with similar anatomy will not demonstrate remote ischemia in the LAD territory and might be expected to do well after recovery from inferior wall infarction (Fig. 78–12).

Prospective Outcome Studies in the Prethrombolytic Era

In 1983, our group compared the prognostic efficiency of exercise ECG, stress-redistribution myocardial perfusion scintigraphy with ^{201}Tl, and cardiac catheterization, all performed before hospital discharge, in 140 consecutive patients with an uncomplicated AMI (116). The patients were followed for a mean of 15 months. The results of the follow-up are shown in Figure 78–13. Test results that were typical of a high risk were associated with the same frequency of cardiac events, whereas strikingly different results were noted among these tests for the prediction of a low risk. Both a negative exercise ECG response and the absence of multivessel CAD were unreliable predictors of low risk. Only a nonischemic ^{201}Tl study (i.e., no reversible defects or abnormal lung uptake) proved to be an accurate predictor of low risk, as summarized in Figure 78–13. Subsequent studies by our group and others have shown that predischarge exercise MPI adds significant prognostic value in medically stabilized patients with either Q-wave or non–Q-wave MI (120, 143–148).

A number of studies have established the prognostic efficiency of pharmacologic stress testing in association with MPI in patients after MI (52,55,96,118,129–135,149). The

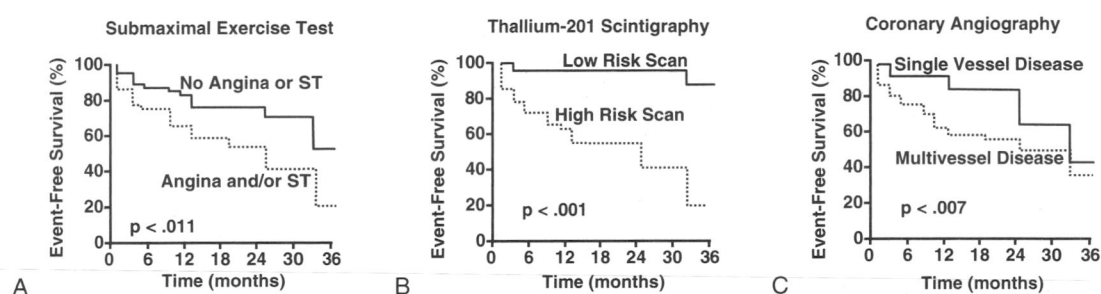

FIG. 78–13. Cumulative probability of event-free survival for six different subgroups of patients after infarction formed by the submaximal exercise test result **(left),** thallium-201 scintigraphic findings **(middle),** and angiographic extent of coronary artery disease **(right).** (Adapted from Gibson RS, Watson DD, Craddock GB, et al. Prediction of cardiac events after uncomplicated myocardial infarction: a prospective study comparing predischarge exercise thallium-201 scintigraphy and coronary angiography. *Circulation* 1983;68:321–336, with permission.)

pattern of results parallels those noted for exercise MPI, including the relatively low risk of cardiac events in patients without evidence of defect reversibility or ischemia, and the marked increased frequency of cardiac events in patients who manifest evidence of defect reversibility within the initial infarct zone, or in myocardial regions remote from the zone of infarction. In a pooled analysis of studies in the literature performed by Shaw and coworkers (150), the mortality rate was 7.1% in postinfarction patients with stress-induced reversible defects on stress imaging compared with 1.6% in those without a reversible defect. Similarly, patients with defects in more than one coronary supply region (a multivessel disease pattern) had a 16.7% combined death or MI rate compared with a 2% event rate in patients without a multivessel disease scan pattern.

Value of Myocardial Perfusion Imaging in the Thrombolytic Era

With the introduction of thrombolytic therapy to the treatment of patients with acute ST-segment elevation MI, attention has been focused on identifying patients who have residual "salvaged" viable myocardium that remains potentially threatened by a high-grade residual stenosis (5). Previously, coronary angiography has been used to define high-risk groups, based on the finding of severe residual stenosis of the infarct-related artery. However, accumulating data from several randomized controlled trials (151–160), registries, and observational studies (161–167) have shown that such "anatomy-driven" care does not usually have an advantage over a more conservative approach, whereby cardiac catheterization and intervention are reserved only for patients who have high-risk clinical features, recurrent angina, or provocable ischemia on predischarge stress testing.

MPI is particularly well suited for risk stratification of patients after MI after thrombolysis because of its aforementioned ability to identify and localize the presence of residual jeopardized viable myocardium. Even when a significant residual stenosis is demonstrated in the infarct vessel angiographically, noninvasive testing can provide valuable information about risk stratification. Ellis and coworkers (156) reported their observations in patients receiving thrombolytic therapy who had high-grade residual angiographic stenosis in the infarct vessel and who were randomized to either PTCA or risk stratification with stress imaging. In the subgroup undergoing noninvasive risk stratification, when provocable ischemia was not present, the subsequent infarct-free survival rate was 98% at 12 months compared with 91% in patients who were randomized to angioplasty at the time of discharge ($p = 0.07$). Thus, noninvasive risk stratification was able to identify low-risk patients for whom further intervention is unnecessary.

Retrospective studies by Tilkemeir and coworkers (124) and Miller and coworkers (127) suggested that stress ^{201}Tl imaging may not be useful in patients with AMI receiving thrombolysis, alone or in conjunction with PCI. More recent studies, however, have shown that stress nuclear MPI retains its prognostic value in such patients (51,52,54,95,128,160, 168). For example, Dakik and coworkers (51) assessed the prognostic efficiency of exercise SPECT MPI in 71 patients receiving thrombolytic therapy for AMI and found that LVEF and the summed ^{201}Tl perfusion defect score were the only significant predictors of future cardiac events by multivariate analysis. The combination of ejection fraction and thallium tomography added significant incremental prognostic information to the clinical data, whereas angiography did not further improve a model that included clinical, ejection fraction, and tomographic variables. In addition, several investigators have demonstrated that MPI was as effective in risk stratification of reperfused patients as it was for patients not receiving reperfusion therapy. In a report by Mahmarian and coworkers (52), it was shown that the quantified extent of scintigraphic ischemia by adenosine SPECT predicted future cardiac events, irrespective of whether patients received acute reperfusion therapy. More than 50% of patients with a greater than 10% ischemic perfusion defect had an event by 1 year compared with less than 10% of patients with smaller perfusion defects. Importantly, none of the latter patients died during follow-up.

In patients treated with thrombolytic therapy, scintigraphic evidence of ischemia is still more prevalent than ST-segment depression (44% vs. 13%), but the prevalence of inducible ischemia is less than that observed in the prethrombolytic era (55% for MPI and 24% for ECG). Therefore, although fewer ischemic responses are found in patients who undergo reperfusion therapy, detection of ischemia is better achieved with stress nuclear MPI than with exercise ECG alone.

Diagnostic and Prognostic Value of Myocardial Perfusion Imaging in Unstable Angina

MPI may also be used to detect residual ischemia and assess the likelihood of cardiac events among patients with unstable angina who have been medically stabilized. No fewer than eight studies (58,169–175) have evaluated such patients and shown that MPI is not only more sensitive than exercise ECG in identifying ischemia (Table 78–4), but it also is capable of providing highly accurate differentiation of high- and low-risk patient subsets. For example, Brown (173) performed a 39-month follow-up study in 52 consecutive patients with unstable angina who responded to medical therapy and then underwent exercise ^{201}Tl MPI. Among the 23 patients (44%) with reversible perfusion defects, the subsequent cardiac death and MI rate was 26% versus only 3% in the 29 patients in whom reversible defects were not induced during stress. In another study, Amanullah and coworkers (175) evaluated 39 patients with unstable angina who had stabilized on medical therapy, despite that 32 of the 39 patients (82%) had transient ST-T wave changes on admission. Patients underwent predischarge stress ECG testing with ^{201}Tl scintigraphy and echocardiography. A total of 23 patients had an event during a mean follow-up of 2.5 years,

TABLE 78–4. *Comparison of stress electrocardiography versus thallium-201 myocardial perfusion imaging in unstable angina*

Study, year	Patients, n	Type of test	Ischemic response	
			ST-segment depression	Reversible defect
Hillert, 1986 (169)	37	Exercise	8 (22%)	19 (51%)
Madsen, 1988 (170)	158	Exercise	16 (10%)	29 (18%)
Brown, 1991 (173)	52	Exercise	11 (21%)	23 (44%)
Zhu, 1991 (174)	170	Dipyridamole	20 (12%)	126 (74%)
Amanallah, 1993 (175)	40	Exercise	18 (45%)	25 (64%)
Summary	457		73 (16%)	222 (49%)

and 91% of these patients with an event had a reversible perfusion defect. In contrast, only 1 of 13 patients (4 5%) with a nonischemic ^{201}Tl scintiscan experienced an event (an event rate of 1.8% per year). Among the 37 patients who had exercise ECG and both imaging studies, the number of myocardial segments with ^{201}Tl redistribution was the only significant predictor of future cardiac events ($p < 0.0005$). The absence of exercise-induced angina or ST-segment depression did not exclude prognostically important ischemia; 39% of patients with a negative exercise ECG had an event. A third study by Stratmann and coworkers (58) examined the prognostic value of exercise SPECT ^{99m}Tc-sestamibi imaging in 121 patients who were followed for 12 ± 7 months. An abnormal ^{99m}Tc-sestamibi study with a reversible defect was a strong predictor of cardiac events by multivariate analysis. The risk for a cardiac event was 25% in patients with a reversible defect as opposed to 2% for those with normal scan results. These data suggest that stress MPI can be safely undertaken for risk stratification among patients with unstable angina who are medically stabilized.

Acute Rest Myocardial Perfusion Imaging in the Emergency Room or Chest Pain Center

The initial evaluation of patients presenting to an emergency department (ED) with chest pain of suspected cardiac origin is critical in determining hospital admission or discharge. It is generally agreed that clinical data alone are inaccurate in the decision process and 30% to 40% of patients with no CAD are hospitalized, and up to 5% of patients with AMI are discharged. This situation is further complicated by the fact that many hospitals, particularly in large metropolitan centers, are above capacity, resulting in closing of hospital admitting and EDs to critically ill patients.

Injection of a MPI agent during or shortly after an episode of chest pain was initially suggested as a potentially useful diagnostic adjunct in the decision-making process for the ED physician. It was first described by Wackers and coworkers (176) more than 20 years ago but did not get much consideration until the advent of managed care with its subsequent pressure to rapidly triage patients and not admit patients at low risk for CAD. As pointed out in a review by Heller (177), a large body of literature now exists that strongly supports the value of acute rest MPI (ARMPI) in patients with chest pain and nondiagnostic electrocardiograms (178–186). ARMPI in this setting is highly sensitive for the detection of AMI, and it appears to provide incremental value over clinical, ECG, and cardiac biomarker testing in the prediction of short-term cardiac events. The consistently high negative predictive value found in many studies, comprising more than 2,000 patients (Table 78–5), indicate that patients with a normal ARMPI scan can be safely discharged from the ED and scheduled for outpatient follow-up at a later time. Not surprisingly, ARMPI-guided management has been shown to be a cost-saving strategy, and physicians who have access to MPI results seem to order fewer cardiac catheterizations without any difference in outcome at 30-day follow-up. In the randomized trial by Udelson and coworkers (185), the hospitalization rate was 52% with usual care and 42% with sestamibi perfusion imaging among patients without acute cardiac ischemia; among patients with AMI, 97% versus 96% were hospitalized. Clearly, if institutions implement a multidisciplinary, protocol-driven ARMPI approach, appropriate patients can

TABLE 78–5. *Value of resting myocardial perfusion imaging in the emergency department*

Study, year	Patients, n	CER with normal MPI		CER with abnormal MPI		
		NPV	Death/MI	Revasc	Death/MI	Revascularization
Varetto, 1993 (178)	64	100%	0%	0%	43%	17%
Hilton, 1994 (179)	102	100%	0%	1%	41%	38%
Kontos, 1997 (181)	532	99.4%	0.6%	3%	15%	27%
Tatum, 1997 (180)	438	100%	0%	3%	7%	32%
Heller, 1998 (182)	357	99.1%	0.9%	5%	12%	16%
Kontos, 1999 (183)	620	98.7%	1.3%	3%	22%	20%

CER, cardiac event rate; NPV, negative predictive value; Revasc, percutaneous coronary intervention or coronary bypass grafting surgery.

be safely discharged from the ED, reserving cardiac beds for those who will benefit most from their use (177).

Thallium-201 versus Technetium-99m–Sestamibi Scintigraphy for Risk Stratification

Since our last review, there have been many technologic advances in MPI. Several new ^{99m}Tc-labeled myocardial perfusion agents have been introduced into clinical practice. ^{99m}Tc-sestamibi and ^{99m}Tc-tetrofosmin are the ones that have been approved in the United States for clinical imaging. Image quality with these radiopharmaceuticals is superior to that obtained with ^{201}Tl because of the more favorable dosimetry and physical characteristics of ^{99m}Tc for imaging with a γ camera. Approximately 10 to 20 times larger doses can be administered than are feasible with ^{201}Tl, yielding a greater count density in both planar and SPECT images. Compared with ^{201}Tl, the ^{99m}Tc tracers produce much less scatter and attenuation and result in improved defect resolution and sensitivity for CAD detection (8,187). ECG gating of SPECT images can be readily accomplished because of the high count rate with ^{99m}Tc tracers, which allows quantitative assessment of LVEF and regional myocardial thickening fractions. This latter point is particularly important because a single-stress SPECT ^{99m}Tc perfusion study can now provide information about exercise capacity, LV function, and stress-induced ischemia to aid in clinical decision-making, obviating the need for separate tests to assess LVEF. This means that a single test can provide the practicing clinician with all the information needed for noninvasive risk stratification.

Exercise, Pharmacologic Stress Myocardial Perfusion Imaging, or Both?

Current practice guidelines (6,113) seem to favor treadmill exercise stress as a more physiologic stimulus. Its safety is well established when applied to medically stabilized patients, and the workload information is helpful in quantifying functional capacity, estimating prognosis, and in prescribing a rational exercise program. Compared with vasodilator stress, exercise does not typically induce dilation of splanchnic vasculature. Exercise promotes a redistribution of blood flow, shunting it to the skeletal musculature and away from intraabdominal organs such as the liver. These effects result in a greater, or more favorable, heart-to-liver activity ratio in images obtained during exercise compared with those obtained during dipyridamole infusion (188,189), which, in turn, greatly diminishes the frequency of artifacts in the inferior and inferoseptal regions of the heart (190,191).

Pharmacologic stress is an acceptable alternative to treadmill exercise (6,113), particularly for patients who are unable to exercise adequately for a variety of noncardiac reasons, such as lower extremity claudication, amputation or disabling arthritis, stroke-related neurologic deficit, chronic pul-

monary disease, and poor motivation to exercise or fear of the treadmill. In these patients, vasodilator stress with either dipyridamole or adenosine is preferred unless there is a history of asthma, in which case β-adrenergic stimulation with dobutamine or arbutamine is recommended. The cardiac safety profile of vasodilator stress testing has been firmly established (192–195). In 1995, Lette and coworkers (193) reported that the combined major adverse events among 73,806 patients who underwent dipyridamole ^{201}Tl MPI included cardiac death (0.95/10,000), nonfatal MI (1.76/10,000), nonfatal sustained ventricular arrhythmias (0.81/10,000), transient cerebral ischemic attacks (1.22/10,000), and severe bronchospasm (1.22/10,000).

Vasodilator stress testing with dipyridamole, unlike exercise or β-adrenergic stimulation with dobutamine or arbutamine, causes only modest changes in hemodynamic determinants of myocardial oxygen demand and can be rapidly reversed with aminophylline. Thus, for risk stratification, vasodilator stress MPI may potentially be safely applied much earlier after AMI than can exercise. Indeed, several prospective studies have now established the safety of early postinfarction (2–4 days) administration of intravenous dipyridamole in conjunction with MPI in patients after uncomplicated AMI (96,129,132,149,195). The performance of MPI in conjunction with vasodilator stress testing, either with dipyridamole or adenosine, has essentially the same sensitivity and specificity for detecting CAD as does symptom-limited (maximal effort) exercise MPI, and it also provides comparable prognostic information (196). Moreover, the multicenter report by Brown and coworkers (96) provides "proof of concept" that dipyridamole ^{99m}Tc-sestamibi SPECT imaging is safe and has powerful prognostic value when performed as early as 2 days after an uncomplicated AMI. Not only was early dipyridamole MPI predictive of in-hospital and postdischarge cardiac events, but it was found to be a more powerful predictor of late events than predischarge submaximal exercise MPI. As pointed out in an accompanying editorial by Wackers and Zaret (197), this option may be of particular interest to smaller hospitals without immediate access to angiography and angioplasty, because vasodilator MPI can be used as a gatekeeper for discriminating between those patients who require transfer to larger centers for revascularization and those who are at low risk and can be managed conservatively in the local hospital. Obviously, if this management strategy of early postinfarction risk stratification is widely adopted, substantial cost savings could be realized in appropriate patient populations.

Recently, there has been a growing interest in combining pharmacologic stress with low-level exercise (198–204). The addition of 4 to 6 minutes of exercise to vasodilator stress (with either dipyridamole or adenosine) improves the heart-to-liver ratio on ^{201}Tl and ^{99m}Tc-sestamibi images, reduces the frequency of image artifacts involving the inferior and inferoseptal regions, decreases some of the side effects attributable to the vasodilator (e.g., hypotension), and increases the sensitivity of the ECG to detect ischemia. It also provides the possibility of obtaining at least an idea of the patient's physical capacity, recovering some of the information lost when a purely pharmacologic test with dipyridamole or adenosine is performed. Currently, however, there have been no prospective randomized trials comparing the prognostic value of pharmacologic testing supplemented with exercise with conventional exercise or pharmacologic stress alone.

Stress Radionuclide Angiography and Echocardiography for Prognostication

Exercise radionuclide angiography has been successfully used for risk stratification of patients recovering from an acute coronary syndrome (205–215). However, this technique is no longer widely performed and most clinicians now favor either stress perfusion imaging with ^{99m}Tc-sestamibi or echocardiography performed in conjunction with upright treadmill testing or dobutamine stress for predischarge risk stratification.

Stress echocardiography and gated SPECT imaging can be used to simultaneously evaluate ischemia and LV function. Until recently, there were only a small amount of prospective data comparing the relative prognostic value of these two imaging modalities after AMI. Candell-Riera and coworkers (168) confirmed the utility of stress nuclear MPI and the shortcomings of stress echocardiography in the post-MI setting. A total of 103 patients with first MI underwent predischarge maximal effort exercise echocardiography and gated SPECT with ^{99m}Tc-tetrofosmin imaging, a mean of 7 days after admission. The cohort included 43 patients who received thrombolytic therapy and 14 patients with non–Q-wave MI. Predischarge imaging yielded a mean LVEF of 55% + 11% by echocardiography and 47% ± 11% by gated SPECT. Only 21 patients (20%) had 1 or more ischemic segments by stress echocardiography versus 51 patients (49%) by gated SPECT. Also, the mean number of ischemic segments per patient was significantly greater with SPECT. During a 12-month follow-up, 2 patients died, 9 had Class III-IV heart failure, and 29 had ischemic complications (4 reinfarctions and 25 patients with Class II-IV angina). Predictive variables for heart failure in multivariate analysis were ejection fraction less than 40% by echocardiography (odds ratio [OR] 8.5; $p = 0.016$) and by gated SPECT (OR, 10.7; $p = 0.009$). Predictive variables for ischemic complications included inability to achieve a 5 MET or greater exercise workload (OR, 5.2; $p = 0.007$) and greater than 15% ischemic burden by SPECT (OR, 3.6; $p = 0.04$). Thus, both exercise echocardiography and SPECT MPI were predictive of heart failure, but only SPECT MPI had predictive power for ischemic complications. That none of the echocardiographic variables, including ischemia (new or worsening regional wall motion), predicted ischemic cardiac events is somewhat discordant with previous studies (135,216–218). However, as pointed out by Brown in an accompanying editorial (219), there are at least 12 other studies detailing the limitations of stress echocardiography imaging (220–231). These latter studies amply illustrate the lower sensitivity of the echocardiographic technique for detecting jeopardized viable myocardium compared with nuclear MPI or positron emission tomography, and they offer several possible explanations for this shortcoming, including: (a) hypoperfusion as detected by MPI precedes the development of regional wall motion abnormalities and may occur in its absence; and (b) the technical difficulty of stress echocardiography in imaging all of the LV myocardium in all patients. In the study by Candell-Riera (168), 21 of the 103 echocardiographic studies were considered suboptimal. Similar findings have been described in previous stress echocardiography studies (226–231). In the most recent of these studies, Hoffman and coworkers (229) found that there was inadequate visualization of at least 2 of 16 segments in 90 of 150 (60%) patients. Furthermore, there is the well recognized problem in detecting new regional wall motion abnormalities when significant resting segmental dysfunction is present. A report by Amanullah and coworkers (225) highlights this limitation. Among 796 segments with resting dysfunction, 518 (65%) had evidence of ischemia with dobutamine SPECT MPI compared with only 265 (33%) with dobutamine echocardiography.

SUMMARY AND FUTURE PERSPECTIVE

Although stress testing with ECG monitoring has been shown to have prognostic value after AMI, exercise or pharmacologic stress perfusion scintigraphy offers several potential advantages, including: (a) increased sensitivity and specificity for detecting residual jeopardized myocardium; (b) the ability to localize ischemia to a specific area or areas subtended by the specific coronary artery; (c) the ability to quantify resting LV function and volumes and to identify stress-induced LV dysfunction that is manifested by transient LV dilatation or an abnormal lung/heart ratio of radioactivity; and (d) more reliable risk stratification of individual patients. The more optimal prognostic efficiency of stress perfusion scintigraphy partially results from the fact that the error rate in falsely classifying patients as low risk is significantly smaller with scintigraphy than with stress electrocardiography. Because of these substantial advantages, there seems to be adequate rationale for recommending perfusion imaging in conjunction with exercise or pharmacologic stress, rather than exercise electrocardiography alone or combined with echocardiography, as the preferred method for evaluating mortality and morbidity rates after an acute coronary syndrome in patients judged to be at low or intermediate risk based on clinical and serum marker variables. Currently, gated SPECT with a ^{99m}Tc-labeled imaging agent is the preferred noninvasive test because it can simultaneously evaluate exercise capacity, resting LV function, infarct size, and ischemic jeopardy, and it has been shown to provide incremental prognostic information in a cost-effective manner.

On the basis of available data, patients who show scintigraphic evidence of prognostically important residual myocardial ischemia are optimal candidates for intensive medical therapy, for cardiac catheterization and revascularization, or for both. Conversely, asymptomatic patients with normal or low-risk test results have little to gain from revascularization because the risk for a future cardiac event is quite low. However, such patients are candidates for intensive risk factor modification, early rehabilitation, and rapid return to productive life styles.

We are currently in an era of health care system reform in which attention must be paid to the cost-effectiveness of diagnostic testing in the risk stratification process after an acute coronary syndrome. There is little justification from randomized controlled clinical trials, registries, and other observational data for routine coronary angiography in all medically stabilized patients. Indeed, these studies indicate that routine cardiac catheterization and "anatomy-driven" revascularization does not reduce mortality or reinfarction rates after an acute coronary syndrome among patients with preserved LV function and no spontaneous or provocable myocardial ischemia. However, it should be remembered that a noninvasive strategy can be used successfully for risk stratification only if the data from nuclear cardiology procedures are of high quality and the interpreters of test results are well trained to accurately distinguish high-risk from low-risk scintigrams.

REFERENCES

1. Gibson RS, Beller GA. Should exercise electrocardiographic testing be replaced by radionuclide methods? In: Rahimtoola SH, Brest AN, eds. *Controversies in coronary artery disease.* Philadelphia: FA Davis, 1982:1–32.
2. Brown KA. Prognostic value of thallium-201 myocardial perfusion imaging: a diagnostic tool comes of age. *Circulation* 1991;83:363–381.
3. Gibson RS, Watson DD. The value of planar thallium-201 imaging in risk stratification of patients recovering from acute myocardial infarction. *Circulation* 1991;84[Suppl 1]:148–162.
4. Berman DS, Hachamovitch R. Risk assessment in patients with stable coronary artery disease: incremental value of nuclear imaging. *J Nucl Cardiol* 1996;3:41–49.
5. Brown KA. Prognostic value of myocardial perfusion imaging: state of the art and new developments. *J Nucl Cardiol* 1996;3:516–537.
6. Braunwald E, Antman EM, Beasley JW, et al. ACC/AHA 2002 guideline update for the management of patients with unstable angina and non-ST-segment elevation myocardial infarction. *J Am Coll Cardiol* 2002;40:1366–1374.
7. Beller GA. Perfusion imaging. *J Am Coll Cardiol* 1999;34:9–11.
8. Yao S, Rozanski A. Myocardial perfusion scintigraphy in conjunction with exercise and pharmacologic stress: prognostic applications in the clinical management of patients with coronary artery disease. In: DePuey EG, Garcia EV, Berman DS, eds. *Cardiac SPECT imaging.* Philadelphia: Lippincott Williams & Williams, 2001:263–296.
9. Steinberg EH, Koss JH, Lee M, et al. Prognostic significance from 10-yr follow-up of a qualitatively normal planar exercise thallium test in suspected coronary artery disease. *Am J Cardiol* 1993;71:1270–1273.
10. Brown KA, Boucher CA, Okada RD, et al. Prognostic value of exercise thallium-201 imaging in patients presenting for evaluation of chest pain. *J Am Coll Cardiol* 1983;1:994–1001.
11. Pamelia FX, Gibson RS, Watson DD, et al. Prognosis with chest pain and normal thallium-201 exercise scintigrams. *Am J Cardiol* 1985;55:920–926.
12. Wackers FJ, Russo DJ, Russo D, et al. Prognostic significance of normal quantitative planar thallium-201 stress scintigraphy in patients with chest pain. *J Am Coll Cardiol* 1985;6:27–30.
13. Wahl JM, Hakki AH, Iskandrian AS. Prognostic implications of normal exercise thallium-201 images. *Arch Intern Med* 1985;145:263–266.
14. Ladenheim ML, Pollock BH, Rozanski A, et al. Extent and severity of myocardial hypoperfusion as predictors of prognosis in patients with suspected coronary artery disease. *J Am Coll Cardiol* 1986;7:464–471.
15. Staniloff HM, Forrester JS, Berman DS, et al. Prediction of death, myocardial infarction, and worsening chest pain using thallium scintigraphy and exercise electrocardiography. *J Nucl Med* 1986;27:1842–1848.
16. Iskandrian AS, Hakki AH, Kane-Marsch S. Exercise thallium-201 scintigraphy in men with nondiagnostic exercise electrocardiograms: prognostic implications. *Arch Intern Med* 1986;146:2189–2193.
17. Gill JB, Ruddy TD, Newell JB, et al. Prognostic importance of thallium uptake by the lungs during exercise in coronary artery disease. *N Engl J Med* 1987;317:1485–1489.
18. Heo J, Thompson WO, Iskandrian AS. Prognostic implications of normal exercise thallium images. *Am J Noninvas Cardiol* 1987;1:209–212.
19. Koss JH, Kobren SM, Grunwald AM, et al. Role of exercise thallium-201 myocardial perfusion scintigraphy in predicting prognosis in suspected coronary artery disease. *Am J Cardiol* 1987;59:531–534.
20. Kaul S, Finkelstein DM, Homma S, et al. Superiority of quantitative exercise thallium-201 variables in determining long-term prognosis in ambulatory patients with chest pain: a comparison with cardiac catheterization. *J Am Coll Cardiol* 1988;12:25–34.
21. Younis LT, Byers S, Shaw L, et al. Prognostic importance of silent myocardial ischemia detected by intravenous dipyridamole-thallium myocardial imaging in asymptomatic patients with coronary artery disease. *J Am Coll Cardiol* 1989;14:1635–1641.
22. Bairey CN, Rozanski A, Maddahi J, et al. Exercise thallium-201 scintigraphy and prognosis in typical angina pectoris and negative exercise electrocardiography. *Am J Cardiol* 1989;64:282–287.
23. Fleg JL, Gerstenblith G, Zonderman AB, et al. Prevalence and prognostic significance of exercise-induced silent myocardial ischemia detected by thallium scintigraphy and electrocardiography in asymptomatic volunteers. *Circulation* 1990;81:428–436.
24. Hendel RC, Layden JJ, Leppo JA. Prognostic value of dipyridamole-thallium scintigraphy for evaluation of ischemic heart disease. *J Am Coll Cardiol* 1990;15:109–116.
25. Brown KA, Rowen M. Prognostic value of a normal exercise myocardial perfusion imaging study in patients with angiographically significant coronary artery disease. *Am J Cardiol* 1993;71:865–867.
26. Schalet BD, Kegel JG, Heo J, et al. Prognostic implications of normal exercise SPECT thallium images in patients with strongly positive exercise electrocardiograms. *Am J Cardiol* 1993;72:1201–1203.
27. Fattah AA, Kamal AM, Pancholy S, et al. Prognostic implications of normal exercise tomographic thallium images in patients with angiographic evidence of significant coronary artery disease. *Am J Cardiol* 1994;74:769–771.
28. Pavin D, Delonca J, Siegenthaler M, et al. Long-term (10 years) prognostic value of a normal thallium-201 myocardial exercise scintigraphy in patients with coronary artery disease documented by angiography. *Eur Heart J* 1997;18:69–77.
29. Brown KA, Altland E, Rowen M. Prognostic value of normal technetium-99m-sestamibi cardiac imaging. *J Nucl Med* 1994;35:554–557.
30. Raiker K, Sinusas AJ, Wackers FJ, et al. One-year prognosis of patients with normal planer or single-photon emission computed tomographic technetium 99m-labeled sestamibi exercise imaging. *J Nucl Cardiol* 1994;1:449–456.
31. Stratmann HG, Williams GA, Wittry MD, et al. Exercise technetium-99m sestamibi tomography for cardiac risk stratification of patients with stable chest pain. *Circulation* 1994;89:615–622.
32. Stratmann HG, Tamesis BR, Younis LT, et al. Prognostic value of dipyridamole technetium-99m sestamibi myocardial tomography in patients with stable chest pain who are unable to exercise. *Am J Cardiol* 1994;73:647–652.
33. Zanco P, Zampiero A, Favero A, et al. Myocardial technetium-99m sestamibi single-photon emission tomography as a prognostic tool in CAD: multivariate analysis in a long-term prospective study. *Eur J Nucl Med* 1995;22:1023–1028.
34. Berman DS, Hachamovitch R, Kiat H, et al. Incremental value of prognostic testing in patient with known or suspected ischemic heart disease: a basis for optimal utilization of exercise technetium-99m

sestamibi myocardial perfusion SPECT. *J Am Coll Cardiol* 1995;26: 639–647.

35. Heller GV, Herman SD, Travin MI, et al. Independent prognostic value of intravenous dipyridamole with technetium-99m sestamibi tomographic imaging in predicting cardiac events and cardiac-related hospital admissions. *J Am Coll Cardiol* 1995;26:1202–1208.

36. Geleijnse MI, Elhendy A, Van Domburg RT, et al. Prognostic value of dobutamine-atropine stress technetium-99m sestamibi perfusion scintigraphy in patients with chest pain. *J Am Coll Cardiol* 1996;28: 447–454.

37. Hachamovitch R, Berman DS, Kiat H, et al. Effective risk stratification using exercise myocardial perfusion SPECT in women: gender-related differences in prognostic nuclear testing. *J Am Coll Cardiol* 1996;28:34–44.

38. Nallamouthu N, Araujo L, Russell J, et al. Prognostic value of simultaneous perfusion and function assessment using technetium-99m sestamibi. *Am J Cardiol* 1996;78:562–564.

39. Boyce TS, Koplan BA, Parsons WJ, et al. Predicting adverse outcome with exercise SPECT Technetium-99m sestamibi imaging in patients with suspected or known CAD. *Am J Cardiol* 1997;79:270–274.

40. Hachamovitch R, Berman DS, Kiat H, et al. Incremental prognostic value of adenosine stress myocardial perfusion SPECT and impact on subsequent management in patients with or suspected of having myocardial ischemia. *Am J Cardiol* 1997;80:426–433.

41. Gibson PB, Demus D, Noto R, et al. Low event rate for stress-only perfusion imaging inpatients evaluated for chest pain. *J Am Coll Cardiol* 2002;39:999–1004.

42. Krishnan R, Lu J, Dae MW, et al. Does myocardial perfusion scintigraphy demonstrate clinical usefulness in patients with markedly positive exercise tests: an assessment of the method in a high-risk subset? *Am Heart J* 1994;127:804–816.

43. Abdel-Farrah A, Kamal AM, Pancholy S, et al. Prognostic implications of normal exercise tomographic thallium images in patients with angiographic evidence of significant coronary artery disease. *Am J Cardiol* 1994;74:769–771.

44. Gibbons RJ, Hodge DO, Berman DS, et al. Long-term outcome of patients with intermediate-risk exercise electrocardiograms who do not have myocardial perfusion defects on radionuclide imaging. *Circulation* 1999;100:2140–2145.

45. Yao S, Chandra P, Dorbala S, et al. Assessment of type, frequency and prognostic value of equivocal test responses during myocardial perfusion SPECT studies. *Circulation* 1998;98:I-653.

46. Iskander S, Iskandrian AE. Risk assessment using single-photon emission computed tomographic technetium-99m sestamibi imaging. *J Am Coll Cardiol* 1998;32:57–62.

47. Pollock SG, Abbott RD, Boucher CA, et al. Independent and incremental prognostic value of tests performed in hierarchical order to evaluate patients with suspected coronary artery disease. *Circulation* 1992;85:237–248.

48. Kaul S, Lilly DR, Gasho JA, et al. Prognostic utility of the exercise thallium-201 test in ambulatory patients with chest pain. *Circulation* 1988;77:745–748.

49. Iskandrian AS, Chae SC, Heo J, et al. Independent and incremental prognostic value of exercise single-photon emission computed tomographic (SPECT) thallium imaging in coronary artery disease. *J Am Coll Cardiol* 1993;22:665–670.

50. Palmas W, Bingham S, Diamond GA, et al. Incremental prognostic value of exercise thallium-201 myocardial single-photon emission computed tomography late after coronary artery bypass surgery. *J Am Coll Cardiol* 1995;25:403–409.

51. Dakik HA, Mahmarian JJ, Kimball KT, et al. Prognostic value of exercise ^{201}Tl tomography in patients treated with thrombolytic therapy during acute myocardial infarction. *Circulation* 1996;94:2735–2742.

52. Mahmarian JJ, Mahmarian AC, Marks CF, et al. Role of adenosine thallium-201 tomography for defining long-term risk in patients after acute myocardial infarction. *J Am Coll Cardiol* 1995;25:1333–1340.

53. Amanullah AM, Berman DS, Erel J, et al. Incremental prognostic value of adenosine myocardial perfusion single photon emission computed tomography in women with suspected coronary artery disease. *Am J Cardiol* 1998;82:725–730.

54. Travin MI, Dessouki A, Cameron T, et al. Use of exercise technetium-99m sestamibi SPECT imaging to detect residual ischemia and for risk stratification after acute myocardial infarction. *Am J Cardiol* 1995;74:665–669.

55. Mahmarian JJ, Pratt CM, Nishimura S, et al. Quantitative adenosine ^{201}Tl single photon computed tomography for the early assessment of patients surviving acute myocardial infarction. *Circulation* 1993;87: 1197–1210.

56. Hachamovitch R, Berman DS, Kiat H, et al. Incremental prognostic value of adenosine stress myocardial perfusion single-photon emission computed tomography and impact on subsequent management in patients with or suspected of having myocardial ischemia. *Am J Cardiol* 1997;80:426–433.

57. Machecort J, Longere P, Fagret D, et al. Prognostic value of thallium-201 SPECT myocardial perfusion imaging according to the extent of the myocardial perfusion defect: a study of 1926 patients with follow-up at 33 months. *J Am Coll Cardiol* 1994;23:1096–1106.

58. Stratmann HG, Younis LT, Wittry MD, et al. Exercise technetium-99m myocardial tomography for the risk stratification of men with medically-treated unstable angina pectoris. *Am J Cardiol* 1995;76:236–240.

59. Weiss AT, Berman DS, Lew AS, et al. Transient ischemic dilation of the left ventricle on stress thallium-201 scintigraphy: a marker of severe and extensive coronary artery disease. *J Nucl Med* 1981,22.585–593.

60. Mazzanti M, Germano G, Kiat H, et al. Identification of severe and extensive coronary artery disease by automatic measurement of transient ischemic dilation of the left ventricle in dual-isotope myocardial perfusion SPECT. *J Am Coll Cardiol* 1996;27:1612–1620.

61. Chouraqui P, Rodrigues EA, Berman DS, et al. Significance of dipyridamole-induced transient dilation of the left ventricle during thallium-201 scintigraphy in suspected coronary artery disease. *Am J Cardiol* 1990;66:689–694.

62. McClellan JR, Travin MI, Herman SO, et al. Prognostic importance of scintigraphic left ventricular cavity dilation during intravenous dipyridamole technetium-99m sestamibi myocardial tomographic imaging in predicting coronary events. *Am J Cardiol* 1997;79:600–605.

63. Gibson RS, Watson DD, Carabello BA, et al. Clinical implications of increased lung uptake of thallium-201 during exercise scintigraphy 2 weeks after myocardial infarction. *Am J Cardiol* 1982;49:1586–1593.

64. Aksut SV, Mallavarapu C, Russell J, et al. Implications of increased lung thallium uptake during exercise single photon emission computed tomography imaging. *Am Heart J* 1995;130:367–373.

65. Jain D, Thompson B, Wackers FJ, et al. Relevance of increased lung thallium uptake on stress imaging in patients with unstable angina and non-Q wave myocardial infarction: results of the thrombolysis in myocardial infarction (TIMI)-IIIB study. *J Am Coll Cardiol* 1997;30: 421–429.

66. Vaccaarino RA, Johnson LL, Antunes ML, et al. Thallium-201 lung uptake and peak treadmill exercise first-pass ejection fraction. *Am Heart J* 1995;129:320–329.

67. Liu P, Kiess M, Okada RD, et al. Increased thallium lung uptake after exercise in isolated left anterior descending coronary artery disease. *Am J Cardiol* 1985;55[13 Pt 1]:1469–1473.

68. Bacher-Stier C, Kavanagh P, Sharir T, et al. Post-exercise tc-99m sestamibi lung uptake determined by a new automatic technique. *J Nucl Med* 1998;39:104P.

69. Martinez EE, Horowitz SF, Castello HJ, et al. Lung and myocardial thallium-201 kinetics in resting patients with congestive heart failure: correlation with pulmonary capillary wedge pressure. *Am Heart J* 1992;123:427–432.

70. Risk stratification and survival after myocardial infarction. Multicenter Postinfarction Research Group. *N Engl J Med* 1983;309:331–339.

71. White HD, Norris RM, Brown MA, et al. Left ventricular end-systolic volume as the major determinant of survival after recovery from myocardial infarction. *Circulation* 1987;76:44–51.

72. Pryor DB, Harrel FE, Lee KL, et al. Prognostic indicators from radionuclide angiography in medically treated patients with coronary artery disease. *Am J Cardiol* 1984;53:18–22.

73. Jones RH, Johnson SH, Bigelow C, et al. Exercise radionuclide angiocardiography predicts cardiac death in patients with coronary artery disease. *Circulation* 1991;84:152–158.

74. Buxton AE, Lee KL, Hafley GE, et al. Relation of ejection fraction and inducible ventricular tachycardia to mode of death in patients with coronary artery disease: an analysis of patients enrolled in the Multicenter Unsustained Tachycardia Trial. *Circulation* 2002;106:2466–2472.

75. Swan G, Castanner A. Determinants of prognosis in survivors of acute myocardial infarction: a prospective clinical angiographic study. *N Engl J Med* 1982;306:1065–1070.

76. Berman D, Germano G, Lewin H, et al. Comparison of post-stress

ejection fraction and relative left ventricular volumes by automatic analysis of gated myocardial perfusion single-photon emission computed tomography acquired in the supine and prone positions. *J Nucl Cardiol* 1998;5:40–47.

77. Germano G, Berman D. On the accuracy and reproducibility of quantitative gated myocardial perfusion SPECT. *J Nucl Med* 1999;40:810–813.

78. Cwajg E, Cwajg J, He Z, et al. Comparison between gated-SPECT and echocardiography for the analysis of global and regional left ventricular function and volumes. *J Am Coll Cardiol* 1998;31[Suppl A]: 440A–441A.

79. Iskandrian A, Germano G, VanDecker W, et al. Validation of left ventricular volume measurements by gated SPECT Tc-99m sestamibi imaging. *J Nucl Cardiol* 1998;5:574–578.

80. He Z, Vick G, Vaduganathan P, et al. Comparison of left ventricular volumes and ejection fraction measured by gated SPECT and by cine magnetic resonance imaging. *J Am Coll Cardiol* 1998;31[Suppl A]:44A.

81. Sharir T, Germano G, Kavangh PB, et al. Incremental prognostic value of post-stress left ventricular ejection fraction and volume by gated myocardial perfusion single photon emission computed tomography. *Circulation* 1999;100:1035–1042.

82. Kroll D, Farah W, McKendall GR, et al. Prognostic value of stress-gated ^{99m}TC-sestamibi SPECT after acute myocardial infarction. *Am J Cardiol* 2001;876:381–386.

83. Sharir T, Germano G, Kang X, et al. Prediction of myocardial infarction versus cardiac death by gated myocardial perfusion SPECT: risk stratification by the amount of stress-induced ischemia and post-stress ejection fraction. *J Nucl Med* 2001;42:831–837.

84. Yamagishi H, Shirai N, Yoshiyama M, et al. Incremental value of left ventricular ejection fraction for detection of multivessel coronary artery disease in exercise ^{201}Tl gated myocardial perfusion imaging. *J Nucl Med* 2002;43:131–139.

85. Pfeffer MA, Braunwald E, Moye LA, et al. Effect of captopril on mortality and morbidity in patients with left ventricular dysfunction after myocardial infarction. Results of the survival and ventricular enlargement trial. The SAVE Investigators. *N Engl J Med* 1992;327:669–677.

86. Johnson LL, Verdesca SA, Aude WY, et al. Postischemic stunning can affect left ventricular ejection fraction and regional wall motion on post-stress gated sestamibi tomograms. *J Am Coll Cardiol* 1997;30: 1641–1648.

87. Sharir T, Bacher-Stier C, Dhar S, et al. Identification of severe and extensive coronary artery disease by post-exercise regional wall motion abnormalities in 99mTc-sestamibi gated single photon emission computed tomography. *Am J Cardiol* 2000;86:1171–1175.

88. Emmett L, Iwanochko RM, Freeman MR, et al. Reversible regional wall motion abnormalities on exercise technetium-99m-gated cardiac single photon emission computed tomography predicts high-grade angiographic stenosis. *J Am Coll Cardiol* 2002;39:991–998.

89. Gibson RS, Watson DD, Taylor GJ, et al. Prospective assessment of regional myocardial perfusion before and after coronary revascularization surgery by quantitative thallium-201 scintigraphy. *J Am Coll Cardiol* 1983;1:804–815.

90. Ragosta M, Beller GA, Watson DD, et al. Quantitative planar rest-redistribution 201Tl imaging in the detection of myocardial viability and prediction of improvement in left ventricular function after coronary bypass surgery in patients with severely depressed left ventricular function. *Circulation* 1993;87:1630–1641.

91. Udelson JE, Coleman PS, Metherall J, et al. Predicting recovery of severe regional ventricular dysfunction. Comparison of resting scintigraphy with 201Tl and 99mTc-sestamibi. *Circulation* 1994;89:2552–2561.

92. Bonow R. Assessment of myocardial viability with thallium-201. In: Zaret BL, Beller G, eds. *Nuclear cardiology: state of the art and future directions,* 2nd ed. St. Louis, MO: Mosby, 1998:503–512.

93. DiCarli MF. Assessment of myocardial viability after myocardial infarction. *J Nucl Cardiol* 2002;9:229–235.

94. Allman KC, Shaw LJ, Hachamovitch R, et al. Myocardial viability testing and impact of revascularization on prognosis in patients with coronary artery disease and left ventricular dysfunction: a meta-analysis. *J Am Coll Cardiol* 2002;39:1151–1158.

95. Pancholy SB, Fattah AA, Kamal AM, et al. Independent and incremental prognostic value of exercise thallium single-photon emission computed tomography in women. *J Nucl Cardiol* 1995;2:110–116.

96. Brown KA, Heller GV, Landin RS, et al. Early dipyridamole ^{99m}Tc-sestamibi single photon emission computed tomographic imaging 2

to 4 days after acute myocardial infarction predicts in-hospital and post-discharge cardiac events: comparison with submaximal exercise imaging. *Circulation* 1999;100:2060–2066.

97. Berman DS, Hachamovitch R, Kiat H, et al. Incremental value of prognostic testing in patients with known or suspected ischemic heart disease: a basis for optimal utilization of exercise technetium-99m sestamibi myocardial perfusion single-photon emission computed tomography. *J Am Coll Cardiol* 1996;27:756.

98. Hachamovitch R, Berman DS, Kiat H, et al. Exercise myocardial perfusion SPECT in patients without known CAD. Incremental prognostic value and use in risk stratification. *Circulation* 1996;93:905–914.

99. Hachamovitch R, Berman DS, Shaw LJ, et al. Incremental prognostic value of myocardial perfusion single photon emission computed tomography for the prediction of cardiac death: differential stratification for risk of cardiac death and myocardial infarction [Erratum in: *Circulation* 1998;98:190]. *Circulation* 1998;97:535–543.

100. Shaw LJ, Hachamovitch R, Berman DS, et al. The economic consequences of available diagnostic and prognostic strategies for the evaluation of stable angina patients: an observational assessment of the value of precatheterization ischemia. The Economics of Noninvasive Diagnosis (END) Multicenter Study Group. *J Am Coll Cardiol* 1999; 33:661–669.

101. Steingart RM, Wassertheil-Smoller S, Tobin JN, et al. Nuclear exercise testing and the management of coronary artery disease. *J Nucl Med* 1991;32:753–758.

102. Bateman TM, O'Keefe JH, Dong VM. Coronary angiographic rates after stress single-photon emission computed tomographic scintigraphy. *J Nucl Cardiol* 1995;2:217–223.

103. Nallamothu N, Pancholy SB, Lee KR, et al. Impact of exercise single-photon emission computed tomographic thallium imaging on patient management and outcome. *J Nucl Cardiol* 1995;2:334–338.

104. Hachamovitch R, Berman DS, Kiat H, et al. Gender-related differences in clinical management after exercise nuclear testing. *J Am Coll Cardiol* 1995;26:1457–1464.

105. Brown KA. Cardiac risk defined by stress myocardial perfusion imaging: impact on physician decision-making and cost savings. *J Nucl Cardiol* 2002;9:124–126.

106. Mishra JP, Acio E, Heo J, et al. Impact of stress single-photon emission computed tomography perfusion imaging on downstream resource utilization. *Am J Cardiol* 1999;83:1401–1403.

107. Zellweger MJ, Dubois EA, Lai S, et al. Risk stratification in patients with remote prior myocardial infarction using rest-stress myocardial perfusion SPECT: prognostic value and impact on referral to early catheterization. *J Nucl Cardiol* 2002;9:23–32.

108. Christian TF, Miller TD, Bailey KR, et al. Exercise tomographic thallium-201 imaging in patients with severe coronary artery disease and normal electrocardiograms. *Ann Intern Med* 1994;121:825–832.

109. Patterson RE, Eisner RL. Cost analysis of noninvasive testing. In: Marwick TH, ed. *Cardiac stress testing and imaging.* New York: Churchill Livingstone, 1996:113–124.

110. Hachamovitch R, Shaw LJ. Cost-effectiveness of myocardial perfusion SPECT. In: DePuey EG, Garcia EV, Berman DS, eds. *Cardiac SPECT imaging.* Philadelphia: Lippincott Williams & Williams, 2001:397–410.

111. Stowers SA, Eisenstein EL, Wackers FJ, et al. An economic analysis of an aggressive diagnostic strategy with SPECT myocardial perfusion imaging and early stress testing in emergency department patients who present with chest pain but nondiagnostic electrocardiograms: results from a randomized trial. *Ann Emergency Med* 2000;35: 17–25.

112. Abbott BG, Abdel-Aziz I, Nagula S, et al. Selective use of single-photon emission computer tomography myocardial perfusion imaging in a chest pain center. *Am J Cardiol* 2001;87:1351–1355.

113. Ryan TJ, Antman EM, Brooks NH, et al. ACC/AHA guideline for the management of patients with acute myocardial infarction. *J Am Coll Cardiol* 1996;28:1328–1428.

114. Epstein S, Palmeri ST, Patterson RE. Evaluation of patients after acute myocardial infarction: indications for cardiac catheterization and surgical intervention. *N Engl J Med* 1982;307:1487–1492.

115. Buda AJ, Dubbin JD, MacDonald IL, et al. Spontaneous changes in thalllium-201 myocardial perfusion imaging after myocardial infarction. *Am J Cardiol* 1982;50:1271–1278.

116. Gibson RS, Watson DD, Craddock GB, et al. Prediction of cardiac events after uncomplicated myocardial infarction: a prospective study

comparing predischarge exercise thallium-201 scintigraphy and coronary angiography. *Circulation* 1983;68:321–336.

117. Hung J, Gordon EP, Houston N, et al. Changes in rest and exercise myocardial perfusion and left ventricular function 3 to 26 weeks after clinically uncomplicated acute myocardial infarction. *Am J Cardiol* 1984;54:943–950.

118. Leppo JA, O'Brien J, Rothendler JA, et al. Dipyridamole-thallium-201 scintigraphy in the prediction of future cardiac events after acute myocardial infarction. *N Engl J Med* 1984;310:1014–1018.

119. Hung J, Goris ML, Nash E, et al. Comparative value of maximal treadmill testing, exercise thallium myocardial perfusion scintigraphy and exercise radionuclide ventriculography for distinguished high- and low-risk patients soon after acute myocardial infarction. *Am J Cardiol* 1984;53:1221–1227.

120. Gibson RS, Beller GA, Gheorghiade M, et al. The prevalence and clinical significance of residual myocardial ischemia two weeks after uncomplicated non-Q wave infarction: a prospective natural history study. *Circulation* 1986;73:1186–1198.

121. Abraham RD, Freedman SB, Dunn RF, et al. Prediction of multivessel coronary artery disease and prognosis early after acute myocardial infarction by exercise electrocardiography and thallium-201 myocardial perfusion scanning. *Am J Cardiol* 1986;58:423–427.

122. Wilson WW, Gibson RS, Nygaard TW, et al. Acute myocardial infarction associated with single vessel coronary artery disease: an analysis of clinical outcome and the prognostic importance of vessel patency and residual ischemic myocardium. *J Am Coll Cardiol* 1988;11:223–234.

123. Touchstone DA, Beller GA, Nygaard TW, et al. Functional significance of predischarge exercise thallium-201 findings following intravenous streptokinase therapy during acute myocardial infarction. *Am Heart J* 1988;116:1500–1507.

124. Tilkemeir PL, Guiney TE, LaRaia PJ, et al. Prognostic value of predischarge low-level exercise thallium testing after thrombolytic treatment of acute myocardial infarction. *Am J Cardiol* 1990;66:1203–1207.

125. Sutton JM, Topol EJ. Significance of a negative exercise thallium test in the presence of a critical residual stenosis after thrombolysis for acute myocardial infarction. *Circulation* 1991;83:1278–1286.

126. Haber HL, Beller GA, Watson DD, et al. Exercise thallium-201 scintigraphy after thrombolytic therapy with or without angioplasty for acute myocardial infarction. *Am J Cardiol* 1993;71:1257–1261.

127. Miller TD, Gersh BJ, Christian TF, et al. Limited prognostic value of thallium-201 exercise treadmill testing early after myocardial infarction in patients treated with thrombolysis. *Am Heart J* 1995;120:259–266.

128. Basu S, Senior R, Dore C, et al. Value of thallium-201 imaging in detecting adverse cardiac events after myocardial infarction and thrombolysis: a follow up of 100 consecutive patients. *Br Med J* 1997;314:225–226.

129. Pirelli S, Inglese E, Suppa M, et al. Dipyridamole-thallium 201 scintigraphy in the early postinfarction period. (Safety and accuracy in predicting the extent of coronary disease and future recurrence of angina in patients suffering from their first myocardial infarction). *Eur Heart J* 1988;9:1324–1331.

130. Younis LT, Byers S, Shaw L, et al. Prognostic value of intravenous dipyridamole thallium scintigraphy after an acute myocardial ischemic event. *Am J Cardiol* 1989;64:161–166.

131. Gimple LW, Hutter AM, Guiney TE, et al. Prognostic utility of predischarge dipyridamole-thallium imaging compared to predischarge submaximal exercise electrocardiography and maximal exercise thallium imaging after uncomplicated acute myocardial infarction. *Am J Cardiol* 1989;64:1243–1248.

132. Brown KA, O'Meara, Chambers CE, et al. Ability of dipyridamole-thallium-201 imaging one to four days after acute myocardial infarction to predict in-hospital and late recurrent myocardial ischemic events. *Am J Cardiol* 1990;65:160–167.

133. Hendel RC, Gore JM, Alpert JS, et al. Prognosis following interventional therapy for acute myocardial infarction: utility of dipyridamole thallium scintigraphy. *Cardiology* 1991;79:73–80.

134. Chiamvimonvat V, Goodman SG, Langer A, et al. Prognostic value of dipyridamole SPECT imaging in low-risk patients after myocardial infarction. *J Nucl Cardiol* 2001;8:136–143.

135. Lancellotti P, Benoit T, Rigo P, et al. Dobutamine stress echocardiography versus quantitative technetium-99m sestamibi SPECT for detecting residual stenosis and multivessel disease after myocardial infarction. *Heart* 2001;86:510–515.

136. Gibson RS. Non-Q-wave myocardial infarction: diagnosis, prognosis and management. *Curr Probl Cardiol* 1988;13:9–72.

137. Corbett JR, Dehmer GJ, Lewis SE, et al. The prognostic value of submaximal exercise testing with radionuclide ventriculography before hospital discharge in patients with recent myocardial infarction. *Circulation* 1981;64:535–544.

138. Upton MT, Palmeri ST, Jones RH, et al. Assessment of left ventricular function by resting and exercise radionuclide angiocardiography following acute myocardial infarction. *Am Heart J* 1982;104:1232–1243.

139. Currie PH, Kelly MJ, Harper RW, et al. Incremental value of clinical assessment, supine exercise electrocardiography and biplane exercise radionuclide ventriculography in the prediction of coronary artery disease in men with chest pain. *Am J Cardiol* 1983;52:927–935.

140. Deanfield JE, Kensett M, Wilson RA, et al. Silent myocardial ischemia due to mental stress. *Lancet* 1984;2:1001–1004.

141. Friedman PL, Shook TL, Kirshenbaum JM, et al. Value of the intracoronary electrocardiogram to monitor ischemia during percutaneous transluminal coronary angioplasty. *Circulation* 1986;74:330–339.

142. Nable EG, Shook TL, Meyerovitz M, et al. Detection of pacing-induced myocardial ischemia by endocardial electrograms recorded during cardiac catheterization. *J Am Coll Cardiol* 1988;11:983–992.

143. Gibson RS, Beller GA, Kaiser DL. Prevalence and clinical significance of painless ST segment depression during early postinfarction exercise testing. *Circulation* 1987;75[Suppl II]:36–39.

144. Gibson RS, Taylor GJ, Watson DD, et al. Predicting the extent and location of coronary artery disease during the early postinfarction period by quantitative thallium-201 scintigraphy. *Am J Cardiol* 1981;47:1010–1019.

145. Legrand V, Rigo P, Kulbertus HE. Complementary role of thallium-201 scintigraphy to predischarge exercise electrocardiography for patient stratification after a first myocardial infarction. *Eur Heart J* 1986;7:644–653.

146. Haines DE, Beller GA, Watson DD, et al. Exercise-induced ST segment elevation 2 weeks after uncomplicated myocardial infarction: contributing factors and prognostic significance. *J Am Coll Cardiol* 1987;9:996–1003.

147. de Cock CC, Visser FC, Van Eenige MJ, et al. Prognostic value of thallium-201 exercise scintigraphy in low-risk patients after Q-wave myocardial infarction: comparison with exercise testing and catheterization. *Cardiology* 1992;81:342–350.

148. Brophy JM, Kerouac M. Risk stratification in patients with non Q-wave myocardial infarction: a role for thallium exercise testing. *Can J Cardiol* 1990;6:435–438.

149. Bosch X, March B, Magrina J, et al. Prediction of in-hospital cardiac events using dipyridamole perfusion scintigraphy early after myocardial infarction. *Circulation* 1989;80[Suppl II]:II-307.

150. Shaw LJ, Peterson ED, Kesler K, et al. A metaanalysis of predischarge risk stratification after acute myocardial infarction with stress electrocardiographic, myocardial perfusion, and ventricular function imaging. *Am J Cardiol* 1996;78:1327–1337.

151. Topol EJ, Califf RM, George BS, et al. A randomized trial of immediate versus delayed elective angioplasty after intravenous tissue plasminogen activator in acute myocardial infarction. *N Engl J Med* 1987;317:581–588.

152. Guerci AD, Gersteinblith G, Brinker JA, et al. A randomized trial of intravenous tissue plasminogen activator for acute myocardial infarction with subsequent randomization to elective coronary angioplasty. *N Engl J Med* 1987;317:1613–1618.

153. Comparison of invasive and conservative strategies after treatment with intravenous tissue plasminogen activator in acute myocardial infarction. The TIMI Study Group. *N Engl J Med* 1989;320:618–627.

154. Barbash GI, Roth A, Hod H, et al. Randomized controlled trial of the late in-hospital angiography and angioplasty versus conservative management after treatment with recombinant tissue-type plasminogen activator in acute myocardial infarction. *Am J Cardiol* 1990;66:538–545.

155. Trial of delayed elective intervention vs conservative treatment after thrombolysis with anistreplase in acute myocardial infarction. SWIFT (Should We Intervene Following Thrombolysis) Trial Study Group. *Br Med J* 1991;302:555–560.

156. Ellis SG, Mooney MR, George BS, et al. Randomized trial of late elective angioplasty versus conservative management for patients with residual stenoses after thrombolytic treatment of myocardial in-

farction. Treatment of Post-Thrombolytic Stenoses (TOPS) Study Group. *Circulation* 1992;86:1400–1406.

157. Effects of tissue plasminogen activator and a comparison of early invasive and conservative strategies in unstable angina and non-Q-wave myocardial infarction: results of the TIMI 3B trial. The TIMI Study Group. *Circulation* 1994;89:1545–1556.

158. McCullough PA, O'Neill WW, Graham M, et al. A prospective randomized trial of triage angiography in acute coronary syndromes ineligible for thrombolytic therapy. Results of the Medicine versus Angiography in Thrombolytic Exclusion (MATE) trial. *J Am Coll Cardiol* 1998;32:596–605.

159. Boden WE, O'Rourke RA, Crawford MH, et al. Outcomes in patients with acute non-Q-wave myocardial infarction randomly assigned to an invasive as compared with a conservative management strategy. *N Engl J Med* 1998;338:1785–1792.

160. Wexler LF, Blaustein AS, Lavori PW, et al. Non-Q-wave myocardial infarction following thrombolytic therapy: a comparison of outcomes in patients randomized to invasive or conservative post-infarct assessment strategies in the VANQWISH trial. *J Am Coll Cardiol* 2001; 37:19–25.

161. Rouleau JL, Moye LA, Pfeffer MA, et al. A comparison of management patterns after acute myocardial infarction in Canada and the United States. *N Engl J Med* 1993;328:779–784.

162. Pilote L, Miller DP, Califf BM, et al. Determinants of the use of coronary angiography and revascularization after thrombolysis for acute myocardial infarction. *N Engl J Med* 1996;335:1198–1205.

163. Every NR, Parson LS, Fihn SD, et al. Long-term outcome in acute myocardial infarction patients admitted to hospitals with and without on-site cardiac catheterization facilities. *Circulation* 1997;96:1770–1775.

164. Marrugat J, Sanz J, Masia R, et al. Six-month outcome in patients with myocardial infarction initially admitted to tertiary and nontertiary hospitals. RESCATE Investigators. *J Am Coll Cardiol* 1997;30:1187–1192.

165. Yusuf S, Flather M, Pogue P, et al. Variations between countries in invasive cardiac procedures and outcomes in patients with suspected unstable angina or myocardial infarction without initial ST elevation. *Lancet* 1998;352:507–514.

166. Ghazzal Z, Chalassani Y, Shen WS. Long-term outcome of patients with non Q-wave myocardial infarction with and without revascularization. *J Am Coll Cardiol* 1998;31:14A.

167. Anderson HV, Gibson RS, Stone PH, et al. Management of unstable angina and acute non-Q-wave myocardial infarction in the United States and Canada. *Am J Cardiol* 1997;79:1441–1446.

168. Candell-Riera J, Llevadot J, Santana C, et al. Prognostic assessment of uncomplicated first myocardial infarction by exercise echocardiography and Tc-99m tetrofosmin gated SPECT. *J Nucl Cardiol* 2001;8:122–128.

169. Hillert MC, Narahara KA, Smitherman TC, et al. Thalliu-201 perfusion imaging after the treatment of unstable angina pectoris—relationship to clinical outcome. *West J Med* 1986;145:335–340.

170. Madsen JK, Stubgaard M, Utne HE, et al. Prognosis and thallium-201 scintigraphy in patients admitted with chest pain without confirmed acute myocardial infarction. *Br Heart J* 1988;59:184–189.

171. Freeman MR, Chisholm RJ, Armstrong PW. Usefulness of exercise electrocardiography and thallium scintigraphy in unstable angina pectoris in predicting the extent and severity of coronary artery disease. *Am J Cardiol* 1988;62:1164–1170.

172. Marmur JD, Freeman MR, Langer A, et al. Prognosis in medically stabilized unstable angina: early Holter ST-segment monitoring compared with predischarge exercise thallium tomography. *Ann Intern Med* 1990;113:575–579.

173. Brown KA. Prognostic value of thallium-201 myocardial perfusion imaging in patients with unstable angina who respond to medical treatment. *J Am Coll Cardiol* 1991;17:1053–1057.

174. Zhu YY, Chung WS, Botvinick EH, et al. Dipyridamole perfusion scintigraphy: the experience with its application in one hundred seventy patients with known or suspected unstable angina. *Am Heart J* 1991;121:33–43.

175. Amanullah AM, Lindvall K, Bevegard S. Prognostic significance of exercise thallium-201 myocardial perfusion imaging compared to stress echocardiography and clinical variables in patients with unstable angina who respond to medical treatment. *Intl J Cardiol* 1993; 39:71–78.

176. Wackers FJ, Lie KI, Liem KL, et al. Thallium-201 scintigraphy in unstable angina pectoris. *Circulation* 1978;57:738–742.

177. Heller GV. Acute rest myocardial perfusion imaging in the emergency department: a technique whose time has come, or gone? *J Nucl Cardiol* 2002;9:350–352.

178. Varetto T, Cantalupi D, Altieri A, et al. Emergency room technetium-99m sestamibi imaging to rule out acute myocardial ischemic events inpatients with nondiagnostic electrocardiograms. *J Am Coll Cardiol* 1993;22:1804–1808.

179. Hilton TC, Thompson RC, Williams HJ, et al. Technetium-99m sestamibi myocardial perfusion imaging in the emergency room evaluation of chest pain. *J Am Coll Cardiol* 1994;23:1016–1022.

180. Tatum JL, Jesse RL, Kontos MC, et al. Comprehensive strategy for the evaluation and triage of the chest pain patient. *Ann Emerg Med* 1997;29:116–123.

181. Kontos MC, Jesse RL, Schmidt KL, et al. Value of acute rest sestamibi perfusion imaging for evaluation of patients admitted to the emergency department with chest pain. *J Am Coll Cardiol* 1997;30:976–982.

182. Heller GV, Stowers SA, Hendel RC, et al. Clinical value of acute rest technetium-99m tetrofosmin tomographic myocardial perfusion imaging inpatients with acute chest pain and nondiagnostic electrocardiograms. *J Am Coll Cardiol* 1998;31:1011–1017.

183. Kontos MC, Jesse RL, Anderson FP, et al. Comparison of myocardial perfusion imaging and cardiac troponin I in patients admitted to the emergency department with chest pain. *Circulation* 1999;99:2073–2078.

184. Bilodeau L, Theroux P, Gregoire J, et al. Technetium-99m sestamibi tomography in patients with spontaneous chest pain, correlations with clinical, electrocardiographic and angiographic findings. *J Am Coll Cardiol* 1991;18:1684–1691.

185. Udelson JE, Beshansky JR, Ballin DS, et al. Myocardial perfusion imaging for evaluation and triage of patients with suspected acute cardiac ischemia: results of the ERASE Chest Pain Trial. *JAMA* 2002; 288:2693–2700.

186. Duca MD, Giri S, Wu AH, et al. Comparison of acute rest myocardial perfusion imaging and serum markers of myocardial injury in patients with chest pain syndromes. *J Nucl Cardiol* 1999;6:570–576.

187. Berman DS, Hayes SW, Germano G. Assessment of myocardial perfusion and viability with technetium-99m, perfusion agents. In: DePuey EG, Garca EV, Berman DS, eds. *Cardiac SPECT imaging.* Philadelphia: Lippincott Williams & Williams, 2001:179–210.

188. Primeau M, Tallifer R, Essiambre R, et al. Technetium 99m sestamibi myocardial perfusion imaging: comparison between treadmill, dipyridamole and transesophageal atrial pacing "stress" tests in normal subjects. *Eur J Nucl Med* 1991;18:247–251.

189. Pennell DJ, Ell PJ. Whole body imaging of thallium-201 after six different stress regimens. *J Nucl Med* 1994;35:425–428.

190. Germano G, Chua T, Kiat H, et al. A quantitative phantom analysis of artifacts due to hepatic activity in technetium-99m myocardial perfusion SPECT studies. *J Nucl Med* 1994;35:356–359.

191. Nuyts J, Dupont P, Maegdenbergh VV, et al. A study of the liver-heart artifact in emission tomography. *J Nucl Med* 1995;36:133–139.

192. Ranhosky A, Kempthorne J. The safety of intravenous dipyridamole thallium perfusion imaging. Intravenous Dipyridamole Thallium Imaging Study Group. *Circulation* 1990;81:1205–1209.

193. Lette J, Tatum JL, Fraser S, et al. Safety of dipyridamole testing in 73,806 patients: the Multicenter Dipyridamole Safety Study. *J Nucl Cardiol* 1995;2:3–17.

194. Cerqueira MD, Verani MS, Schwaiger M, et al. Safety profile of adenosine stress perfusion imaging: results from the Adenoscan Multicenter Trial Registry. *J Am Coll Cardiol* 1994;23:384–389.

195. Heller GV, Brown KA, Landin RJ, et al. Safety of early intravenous dipyridamole technetium 99m sestamibi SPECT myocardial perfusion imaging after uncomplicated first myocardial infarction. *Am Heart J* 1997;134:105–111.

196. Maddahi J, Berman DS. Detection, evaluation and risk stratification of coronary artery disease by thallium-201 myocardial perfusion scintigraphy. In: DePuey EG, Garcia EV, Berman DS, eds. *Cardiac SPECT imaging.* Philadelphia: Lippincott Williams & Williams, 2001:155–177.

197. Wackers FJ, Zaret BL. Risk stratification soon after acute infarction. *Circulation* 1999;100:2040–2042.

198. Stern S, Greenberg D, Corne R. Effect of exercise supplementation on dipyridamole thallium-201 image quality. *J Nucl Med* 1991;32:1559–1564.

199. Kettunen R, Hurikuri HV, Heikkila J, et al. Usefulness of technetium-99m-MIBI and thallium-201 in tomographic imaging combined with high dose dipyridamole and handgrip exercise for detecting coronary artery disease. *Am J Cardiol* 1991;68:575–579.

200. Pennel DJ, Mavrogeni SI, Forbat SM, et al. Adenosine combined with dynamic exercise of myocardial perfusion imaging. *J Am Coll Cardiol* 1995;25:1300–1309.

201. Candell-Riera J, Santana-Boado C, Castell-Conesa J, et al. Simultaneous dipyridamole/maximal subjective exercise with ^{99m}Tc-MIBI SPECT: improved diagnostic yield in coronary artery disease. *J Am Coll Cardiol* 1997;29:531–536.

202. Jamil G, Ahlberg AW, Elliot MD, et al. Impact of limited treadmill exercise on adenosine Tc-99m sestamibi single-photon emission computed tomographic myocardial perfusion imaging in coronary artery disease. *Am J Cardiol* 1999;84:400–403.

203. Vitola JV, Brambatt JC, Caligoris F, et al. Exercise supplementation to dipyridamole prevents hypotension, improves electrocardiogram sensitivity and increases heart-to-liver activity ratio on TC-99m sestamibi imaging. *J Nucl Cardiol* 2001;8:652–659.

204. Samady H, Wackers FJ, Joska TM, et al. Pharmacologic stress perfusion imaging with adenosine: role of simultaneous low-level treadmill exercise. *J Nucl Cardiol* 2002;9:188–196.

205. Corbett JR, Dehmer GJ, Lewis SE, et al. The prognostic value of submaximal exercise testing with radionuclide ventriculography before hospital discharge in patients with recent myocardial infarction. *Circulation* 1981;64:535–544.

206. Wasserman AG, Katz RJ, Cleary P, et al. Noninvasive detection of multivessel disease after myocardial infarction by exercise radionuclide ventriculography. *Am J Cardiol* 1982;50:1242–1247.

207. Morris KG, Palmeri ST, Califf RM, et al. Value of radionuclide angiography for predicting specific cardiac events after acute myocardial infarction. *Am J Cardiol* 1985;55:318–324.

208. Dewhurst NG, Muir AL. Comparative prognostic value of radionuclide ventriculography at rest and during exercise in 100 patients after first myocardial infarction. *Br Heart J* 1983;49:111–121.

209. Abraham RD, Harris PJ, Roubin GS, et al. Usefulness of ejection fraction response to exercise one month after acute myocardial infarction in predicting coronary anatomy and prognosis. *Am J Cardiol* 1987;60:225–230.

210. Zaret BL, Wackers FJ, Terrin ML, et al. Assessment of global and regional left ventricular performance at rest and during exercise after thrombolytic therapy for acute myocardial infarction: results of the Thrombolysis in Myocardial Infarction (TIMI) II Study. *Am J Cardiol* 1992;69:1–9.

211. Rogers WJ, Bourge RC, Papapietro SE, et al. Variables predictive of good functional outcome following thrombolytic therapy in the Thrombolysis in Myocardial Infarction Phase II (TIMI II) pilot study. *Am J Cardiol* 1989;63:503–512.

212. Fioretti P, Brower RW, Simoons ML, et al. Relative value of clinical variables, bicycle ergometry, radionuclide ventriculography and 24-hour ambulatory electrocardiographic monitoring at discharge to predict 1-year survival after myocardial infarction. *J Am Coll Cardiol* 1986;8:40–49.

213. Kuchar DL, Freund J, Yeates M, et al. Enhanced prediction of major cardiac events after myocardial infarction using exercise radionuclide ventriculography. *Aust NZ J Med* 1987;17:228–233.

214. Zhu WX, Gibbons RJ, Bailey KR, et al. Predischarge exercise radionuclide angiography in predicting multivessel coronary artery disease and subsequent cardiac events after thrombolytic therapy for acute myocardial infarction. *Am J Cardiol* 1994;74:554–559.

215. Murray DP, Rafiqi E, Murray RG, et al. Prognostic investigations after myocardial infarction: a comparison of radionuclide angiography and ^{201}Tl scintigraphy. *Eur J Nucl Med* 1986;11:381–385.

216. Jaarsma W, Visser CA, Kupper AJ, et al. Usefulness of two-dimensional exercise echocardiography shortly after myocardial infarction. *Am J Cardiol* 1986;57:86–90.

217. Applegate RJ, Dell'Italia LJ, Crawford MH. Usefulness of two-dimensional echocardiography during low-level exercise testing early after uncomplicated acute myocardial infarction. *Am J Cardiol* 1987;60:10–14.

218. Quintana M, Lindvall K, Ryden L, et al. Prognostic value of predischarge exercise stress echocardiography after acute myocardial infarction. *Am J Cardiol* 1995;76:1115–1121.

219. Brown KA. Post-myocardial infarction risk stratification with stress nuclear myocardial perfusion imaging versus echocardiography: separate but not equal. *J Nucl Cardiol* 2001;8:215–218.

220. Pozzoli MM, Fioretti PM, Salustri A, et al. Exercise echocardiography and technetium-99m MIBI single photon emission computed tomography in the detection of coronary artery disease. *Am J Cardiol* 1991;67:350–355.

221. Quinones MA, Verani MS, Haichin RM, et al. Exercise echocardiography versus thallium-201 single-photon emission computed tomography in evaluation of coronary artery disease: analysis of 292 patients. *Circulation* 1992;85:1026–1031.

222. Forster T, McNeill AJ, Salustri A, et al. Simultaneous dobutamine stress echocardiography and technetium-99m isonitrile single-photon emission computed tomography in patients with suspected coronary artery disease. *J Am Coll Cardiol* 1993;21:1591–1596.

223. Simeck CL, Watson DD, Smith WH, et al. Dipyridamole thallium-201 imaging versus dobutamine echocardiography for the evaluation of coronary artery disease in patients unable to exercise. *Am J Cardiol* 1993;72:1257–1262.

224. Brown KA. Prognostic value of cardiac imaging in patients with known or suspected coronary artery disease: comparison of myocardial perfusion imaging, stress echocardiography, and positron emission tomography. *Am J Cardiol* 1995;75:35D–41D.

225. Amanullah AM, Chaudhry FA, Heo J, et al. Comparison of dobutamine echocardiography, dobutamine sestamibi, and rest-redistribution thallium-201 single-photon emission computed tomography for determining contractile reserve and myocardial ischemia in ischemic cardiomyopathy. *Am J Cardiol* 1999;84:739–741.

226. Marwick TH, Nemec JJ, Pashkow FJ, et al. Accuracy and limitations of exercise echocardiography in a routine clinical practice. *J Am Coll Cardiol* 1992;19:74–81.

227. Panza JA, Laurienzo JM, Quyyumi AA, et al. Transesophageal dobutamine stress echocardiography for evaluation of patients with coronary artery disease. *J Am Coll Cardiol* 1994;24:1260–1267.

228. Tauke JT, Wiet SP, Shelton-Zoiopoulos LY, et al. Simultaneous transthoracic and transesophageal dobutamine stress echocardiography. *J Am Coll Cardiol* 1994;23:360A(abst).

229. Hoffmann R, Lethen H, Marwick T, et al. Analysis of interinstitutional observer agreement in interpretation of dobutamine stress echocardiograms. *J Am Coll Cardiol* 1996;27:330–336.

230. Bonow RO. Diagnosis and risk stratification in coronary artery disease: nuclear cardiology versus stress echocardiography. *J Nucl Cardiol* 1997;4:S172–S178.

231. Maciero-Coelho E, Dionisio I, Garcia-Alves M, et al. Comparison between dobutamine echocardiography and thallium-201 scintigraphy in detecting residual stenosis, ischemia and necrosis inpatients with prior myocardial infarction. *Clin Cardiol* 1997;20:351–356.

CHAPTER 79

Role of Signal Averaging

J. Anthony Gomes

Key Words: Late potentials; myocardial infarction; reperfusion; signal averaging; thrombolysis.

INTRODUCTION

The mortality of patients surviving an acute myocardial infarction (MI) has declined since the use of intravenous and oral β-adrenergic blocker agents and the use of thrombolytic therapy (1–12). It is estimated that, currently, the mortality rate is in the range of 3% to 5% per annum (13). Notably, however, 50% of patients who die after a MI will die suddenly. In addition, mortality remains high in those patients who do not undergo thrombolysis, those with a large anterior wall MI, with a closed coronary artery, with severe left ventricular dysfunction, with the presence of late potentials (LPs), and with ventricular arrhythmias (14).

In the last decade, the technique of signal averaging has been used in electrocardiography as a method for improvement of the signal-to-noise ratio of the surface electrocardiogram (ECG) (15–19). This technique enables identification of low-amplitude cardiac signals, measuring a few microvolts, that otherwise are not readily discernible with standard ECG techniques. The process of signal averaging assumes that the signal of interest (that is, the QRS complex) repeats with every beat in the average, whereas the interfering noise from sources such as skeletal muscle, power line frequency interference, filter noise, and others, is a random event and is therefore canceled in proportion to the square root of the number of beats averaged. The signal-averaging process uses a computer to detect and align the QRS complexes. The average is performed for a specified number of beats, making it possible to decrease the noise level in the range of 0.3 μV or less (20,21).

The signal-averaged ECG (SAECG) was originally used in electrocardiography to record signals from the His-Purkinje system noninvasively (16,17). However, the technique has gained popularity since it was used to detect the presence of LPs that originate from scarred myocardium with inhomogeneous slow conduction. This chapter discusses the value of the SAECG in predicting postinfarction survival.

LATE POTENTIALS AS A MARKER OF THE ARRHYTHMIC SUBSTRATE

The interest in SAECG emanates from the observation that LPs are markers of the arrhythmic substrate. In this regard, it is important to bear in mind that the arrhythmic substrate identified by the SAECG is an anatomic or functional substrate with slow propagation of conduction as a result of factors discussed subsequently. The concept that LPs are markers of the arrhythmic substrate has been supported by the following observations in several independent laboratories (23,24):

1. LPs recorded on the SAECG correspond to fragmented and delayed electrical activity at epicardial and en-

J. A. Gomes: The Zena and Michael A. Wiener Cardiovascular Institute, Mount Sinai Medical Center of NYU, 1-Gustave L. Levy Place, New York, New York 10029.

docardial sites in the animal model after experimental occlusion of the coronary artery and in patients with ventricular arrhythmias after MI.

2. Removal of the arrhythmic substrate by endocardial resection/aneurysmectomy after endocardial mapping can abolish LPs.

3. There is a high correlation between induction of ventricular tachycardia (VT) in patients with previous MI and the presence of LPs.

However, it is important to bear in mind that this concept has important limitations (25–27), including the following:

1. Although slow conduction is an important condition for the occurrence of reentry, other elements that support reentry, such as differential refractoriness, unidirectional block, and recovery of excitability, are likewise of importance to sustain a reentrant tachyarrhythmia.

2. Although reentry is the likely mechanism of most late ventricular tachyarrhythmias after MI, other mechanisms such as triggered activity also could play a role.

3. Although there may be a substrate, which may be anatomic or functional in nature, there may be an exit block from the substrate to the normal myocardium, in which case ventricular tachyarrhythmia will not manifest itself.

Finally, the mechanism of sudden death is likely multifactorial. There could be other factors such as ischemia on top of scarred myocardium, particularly in patients after MI. In addition, the roles of autonomic, metabolic, and chemical factors remain poorly defined at this time; thus, no single test will permit identification of patients for sudden death with a high enough positive predictive accuracy.

MECHANISM OF LATE POTENTIALS

Studies in the intact human heart in patients with VT after MI have confirmed observations reported in the animal model. Endocardial recordings from left ventricular sites have revealed LPs and fragmented activity, as well as bridging in diastole during VT (28). Similarly, LPs have been recorded from epicardial sites and often from the site of reentrant excitation. Recordings from a 56-year-old man with recurrent VT 4 weeks after MI are shown in Figure 79–1. LPs were noted in sinus rhythm at the epicardial border zone of the infarct. During induced VT, the site from which LPs were recorded also was the site of continuous electrical activity and the site of the block around which reentrant excitation circulated. LPs can result from slow conduction velocity and a long conduction pathway. Isochronal maps of activation have shown slow conduction velocity in ischemic and scarred myocardium. Slow conduction velocity is likely a result of anisotropic conduction caused by increased cell coupling resistance in scarred myocardium, which consists anatomically of surviving muscle elements interspersed in dense connective tissue (29). LPs also can be the result of repolarization abnormalities; thus, triggered activity may give rise to signals with morphologic characteristics of LPs. Notably, however, LPs have more often been used to characterize depolarization abnormalities than repolarization abnormalities.

EVOLVING PATHOPHYSIOLOGY OF LATE POTENTIALS AFTER MYOCARDIAL INFARCTION

LPs do not have the same characteristics during the acute, subacute, and chronic phases of MI. This evolving pathophysiology of LPs has been studied primarily in animal ex-

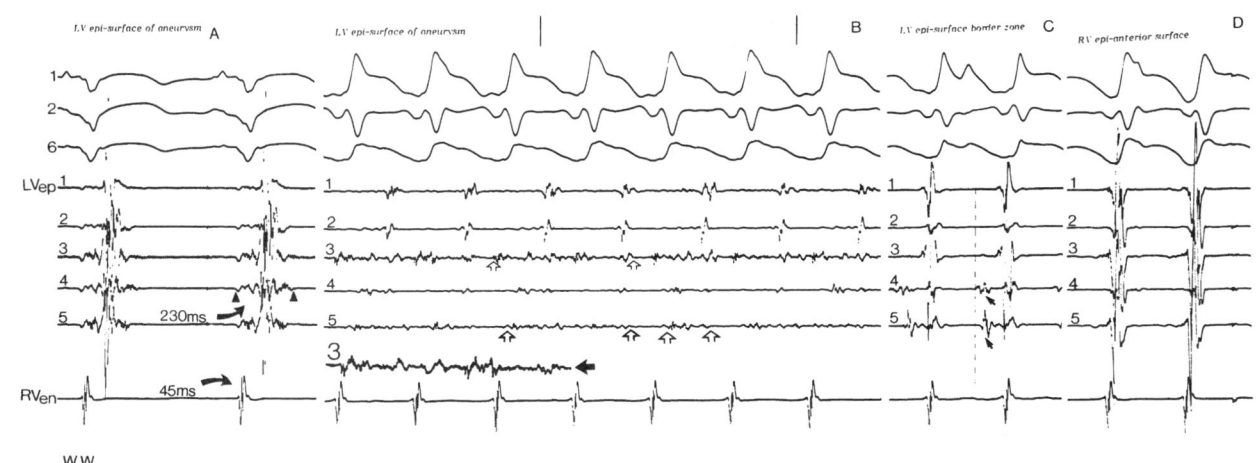

FIG. 79–1. Epicardial bipolar electrocardiograms (ECGs) during sinus rhythm and after induced ventricular tachycardia. From *top* to *bottom* are ECG leads 1, 2, V$_6$, five left ventricular (LV) epicardial, and one right ventricular (RV) endocardial bipolar recordings. **A:** LV epicardial surface of aneurysm during sinus rhythm. **B:** LV epicardial surface of aneurysm during ventricular tachycardia (VT). **C:** LV epicardial surface of border zone. **D:** RV epicardial anterior surface. In **A,** late potentials are seen at epicardial sites 1 through 5. In **B,** during VT, continuous electrical activity is seen at sites 3 and 5, and a block at site 4. In **C,** pre-QRS activity is seen at the LV epicardial border zone, and, in **D,** note that no late potentials are seen in the RV epicardial/endocardial sites.

perimental models. In acute ischemia, the resting membrane potential and maximal transmembrane potential rate of increase is less than in the normal myocardium. The extracellular electrograms from ischemic tissue have lower amplitude and slew rates. Spach and coworkers (30) have shown that in anisotropic tissue, the magnitude of the extracellular potential is decreased because of a reduction in conduction velocity irrespective of the changes in the rate of increase of extracellular action potentials. The longer duration of the upstroke in ischemic tissue results in a longer duration of the extracellular electrogram. The increase in path length secondary to functional and anatomic conduction block may also be responsible for delayed conduction. In the acutely ischemic canine infarction model, delayed activation occurs in the subendocardium and midmyocardium, whereas in infarcts that are 3 to 7 days old, delayed potentials are seen in the epicardial layer overlying the infarct (31,32). It is not uncommon in the human heart to see LPs epicardially (Fig. 79–1), as well as an epicardial site of origin of VT in fresh infarcts.

Unlike the morphology of LPs in the acute and subacute infarction model, the morphology of the extracellular LPs in the chronic infarct model are different in that they are fractionated with multiple high-frequency deflections of low amplitude and longer duration. Gardner and coworkers (31–33) found longer durations in 2-week-old infarcts as compared to 2- to 18-month-old infarcts. The mechanisms of these fractionated electrograms have been shown to be the result of slow conduction (33). In contrast, extracellular potentials recorded from these myocardial sites of fragmentation are similar to normal action potentials (33). Notably, these fragmented electrograms may not necessarily be late in relation to the QRS complex.

CRITERIA FOR IDENTIFICATION OF LATE POTENTIALS

LPs are identified on a SAECG by the quantitative method originally described by Simson (34). Definition of a LP is based on the high-pass filter settings used for analysis (Table 79–1). The most common high-pass filter settings used for analysis are 25 Hz and 40 Hz. Three parameters are identified on the vector magnitude (Fig. 79–2): (a) the

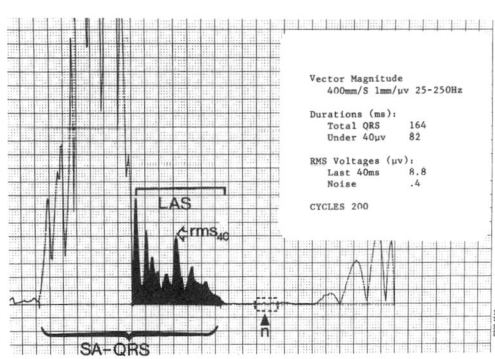

FIG. 79–2. Quantitative measurements of signal-averaged parameters on the vector magnitude. The *brackets* show the quantitative signal-averaged variables; the *stippled box* shows the noise level in the ST segment. (Reprinted with permission from Gomes JA. The vector magnitude, time domain analysis and standards for late potential. In: Gomes JA, ed. *Signal averaged electrocardiography: concepts, methods and applications.* Dordrecht: Kluwer, 1993:69–80.)

entire duration of the filtered signal-averaged QRS complex (SA-QRS); (b) the root mean square voltage of the terminal 40 ms of the QRS complex (RMS40); and (c) the duration of low-amplitude signals of less than 40 μV. It is noteworthy that in the criteria described, 25- and 40-Hz (Table 79–1) filtering is used only for patients without bundle branch block. In addition, criteria for patients with intraventricular conduction defects are not currently well established.

The criteria at 40-Hz high-pass filtering originally described by Gomes and coworkers (35) have been accepted by the Committee of Standards for the SAECG (36). Independent studies have shown that the SA-QRS duration, when used as a continuous variable, is the most significant independent predictor of an arrhythmic event after MI (37). Although identification of LPs in the time domain method with the use of the vector magnitude is the standard method used in clinical practice, other methods are in development, such as the use of the fast Fourier transform analysis to identify the spectral frequencies and the power of LPs in the terminal part of the QRS complex or the entire QRS complex. However, these methods currently remain experimental (38–44).

TABLE 79–1. *Criteria for late potentials*

Author (reference)	High-pass filtering, Hz	RMS40, μV	LAS, ms	SA-QRS, ms
Simson et al. (22)	25	<25	—	>110
Kuchar et al. (47)	40	<20	—	>120
Gomes et al. (35)	25	<25	>32	>114
El-Sherif (25)	40	<20	>38	>114

LAS, low-amplitude signals; RMS40, root mean square voltage of the terminal 40 ms of the QRS complex; SA-QRS, signal-averaged QRS.

From, Gomes JA. The vector magnitude, time domain analysis and standards for late potential. In: Gomes JA, ed. *Signal averaged electrocardiography: concepts, methods and applications.* Dordrecht: Kluwer, 1993:69–80.)

PROGNOSTIC SIGNIFICANCE OF LATE POTENTIALS IN PREDICTING ARRHYTHMIC RISK AFTER MYOCARDIAL INFARCTION

Because LPs are noninvasive markers of the presence of slow and inhomogeneous propagation of conduction in the ventricular myocardium after a MI, it is not surprising that several large-scale studies were directed to determine the role of the LPs as either dependent or independent predictors of arrhythmic events after MI (37,45–50). Furthermore, in many of these studies, the relative value of other predictors such as Holter monitoring, left ventricular function, and heart rate variability also were compared with those of signal averaging. Table 79–2 summarized the results of seven large studies comprising a total of 1,371 patients who had SAECGs, plotted from 6 days to as long as 6 weeks after MI. In these studies, approximately 27% of patients had LPs (range 27–42%), and approximately 70% did not have LPs (range 54–76%). During a mean follow-up of approximately 1 year, the event rate, defined as the occurrence of either sustained VT or sudden cardiac death, was about 16% (range 12–26%) in patients with LPs, whereas in those patients without LPs, the event rate was approximately 3% (range 1–4%). This difference in event rate in patients with or without LPs was highly significant in all studies.

Breithardt and associates (45) studied a total of 152 patients for up to 6 weeks after MI. They did not use quantitative methods in their study but identified LPs qualitatively, which could be subject to interobserver variability. In their study, a high percentage of patients, about 45%, had LPs, and the remaining 55% did not. The patients with LPs had a 12% event rate, whereas in patients without LPs, the event rate was 3% ($p < 0.05$).

An Australian study by Denniss and coworkers (46) assessed the relation of the SAECG results and survival in 306 patients after MI. The presence of LPs was defined as a QRS duration of longer than 120 ms. Using this criteria, they found LPs in 26% of patients. About 19% of patients with LPs had arrhythmic events for a follow-up period of 12 months; in contrast, 4% of patients without LPs had arrhythmic events ($p < 0.00$). In their study, the authors also assessed the efficacy of inducibility of ventricular tachyarrhythmias in the electrophysiology (EP) laboratory and found a good correlation between the presence of LPs after MI and inducibility of ventricular tachyarrhythmia. Another Australian study by Kuchar and coworkers (47) comprised a total of 200 patients after MI. They defined the presence of LPs as a filtered QRS duration of more than 120 ms or an RMS40 of less than 20 μV or low-amplitude signal duration of more than 38 ms. Using these criteria, they noted LPs in 32% of patients. Arrhythmic events occurred in 27% of patients with LPs in contrast to 4% of patients without LPs ($p < 0.001$).

A British study by Cripps and coworkers (48) assessed 159 patients after MI. In their study, LPs were present in 24% of patients and absent in 76% of patients. Arrhythmic events occurred in 26% of patients with LPs and in only 1% of patients without LPs ($p < 0.001$).

El-Sherif and coworkers (49) studied 156 patients by standard quantitative methods. LPs were found in 25% of patients. During a follow-up period of 12 months, arrhythmic events occurred in 23% of patients with LPs and in only 3% of patients without LPs ($p < 0.001$). They also observed that the SAECGs recorded before 5 days did not correlate with arrhythmic events; in contrast, SAECGs recorded 6 to 30 days after MI correlated with arrhythmic events. They recommended that SAECGs should be obtained 6 to 30 days after MI for risk assessment.

Pedretti and coworkers (50) studied 303 patients after MI with signal averaging. A total of 27% of patients had LPs, whereas 73% did not. Over a follow-up period of 15 ± 7 months, 14% of patients with LPs had arrhythmic events, whereas the incidence of arrhythmic events was 3% in patients without LPs ($p < 0.001$).

Several studies also have established the independent prognostic power of LPs relative to clinical variables, results of Holter monitoring, and ejection fraction (EF). Kuchar and associates (47) found that LPs, when defined as an abnormal RMS40 of less than 20 μV or a SA-QRS complex of more than 120 ms at 40-Hz high-pass filtering, and left ventricular EF were independent predictors of the occurrence of arrhythmic events. However, results of Holter monitoring were not predictive of an event. Gomes and coworkers (37), in their study of 115 patients after MI, noted that EF, LPs, and nonsustained VT on 24-hour Holter monitoring were independent predictors of an arrhythmic event. In the Cox regression analysis of 27 clinical and noninvasive variables,

TABLE 79–2. *Prospective studies of the significance of late potentials (LP) after myocardial infarction*

Study	Patients, n	LP$^+$, %	LP$^-$, %	Follow-up, mo	Event rate, % LP$^+$	Event rate, % LP$^-$	p Value
Breidthardt et al. (45)	132	45	55	15 ± 10	12	3	<0.05
Denniss et al. (46)	306	26	74	12	19	4	<0.001
Kuchar et al. (47)	200	39	61	14	17	1	<0.001
Gomes et al. (37)	115	42	58	14 ± 8	27	4	<0.001
Cripps et al. (48)	159	24	76	12 ± 6	26	1	<0.001
El-Sherif et al. (49)	156	25	75	12	23	3	<0.001
Pedretti et al. (50)	303	27	73	15 ± 7	14	3	<0.001
Total	1,371	33	67	13	20	3	

LP, late potentials.

as well as the 3 quantitative SAECG variables, they found that the duration of the SA-QRS complex was the most important variable in predicting arrhythmic events, followed by EF.

These observations have been confirmed in the Cardiac Arrhythmia Suppression Trial (CAST) (51). A total of 1,158 patients without bundle branch block from 10 centers were followed for 10.3 ± 3.2 months. Several clinical variables, ventricular arrhythmias on Holter, six SAECG parameters, and EF were analyzed. There were 45 patients with serious arrhythmic events over the follow-up period. In the Cox repression analysis, a QRS duration at 40-Hz filtering of 120 ms or shorter was the most significant predictor ($p < 0.0001$) of an arrhythmic event. The positive and negative total predictive accuracy and odds ratio for QRS duration of 120 ms or shorter at 40 Hz were 17%, 98%, 88%, and 8.4%, respectively. When combined with an EF of 40% or smaller and complex arrhythmias on Holter, it improved to 32%, 97%, and 16.7%, respectively.

In summary, the presence of LPs is an independent predictor of an arrhythmic event. However, the positive predictive value as seen from Table 79–1 is indeed low, ranging from 12% to 27%, whereas the negative predictive value is extremely high, ranging from 96% to 99%. Thus, it seems that the absence of LPs has more clinical utility because of the high negative predictive value. Nonetheless, it should be kept in mind that the positive predictive value of other noninvasive tests such as left ventricular function assessment, 24-hour monitoring, and heart rate variability is not substantially greater than that of LPs alone.

There are several other important elements that need to be considered when using the SAECG for risk stratification after MI, including time-dependent changes in the SAECG (52). It has been shown that in 16% of patients, the SAECG normalizes in 6 weeks, and in 30% of patients, it normalizes at 1 year. Thus, information gathered in the first few days of MI, or in the first few weeks, may not be applicable beyond 1 year and may yield a lower predictive value even beyond 6 months. The prognostic significance of the SAECG will depend on the site of MI. In one study (53) of 99 patients, 49 of whom had an inferior wall MI and 50 of whom had an anterior wall MI, the site of MI and the presence of LPs relative to the event rate were assessed. Of these 99 patients, 35 had arrhythmic events for a follow-up period of 8 to 24 months

after MI. The remaining 64 patients had no arrhythmic events for a similar follow-up period. These latter patients served as control subjects. LPs in this study were defined as the presence of any one single abnormal criterion (LP_1) or the presence of an abnormal QRS duration and abnormal RMS40 (LP_2). The sensitivity for predicting arrhythmic events was 56% for LP_1, and the specificity was 84% for patients with anterior MI. The sensitivity of LP_1 was 94% and the specificity was 57% for patients with inferior wall MI. For LP_2, the sensitivity was 39% and specificity was 94% for anterior wall MI, whereas it was 82% and 84%, respectively, for patients with inferior wall MI. It is clear from this study that the sensitivity of LPs in inferior MI is greater than that for anterior wall MI.

ROLE OF NONINVASIVE INDEX FOR RISK STRATIFICATION

In view of a low positive predictive value of LPs in predicting arrhythmic events after MI, several investigators have assessed the value of a combined noninvasive index using information obtained from the SAECG, left ventricular function, Holter monitoring, and heart rate variability. The results of six independent studies (47,49,50,51,54,55) are summarized in Table 79–3. A total of 1,859 patients were followed for a total of 10 to 16 months. Multivariate analysis revealed that the SAECG prolonged filtered QRS duration, EF, complex ventricular ectopy (repetitive forms, nonsustained VT), and abnormal heart rate variability were independent predictors of arrhythmic events. The combination of these tests (i.e., two or more) could identify patients with a high positive value. The combination of LP (defined as any single abnormal parameter) and an abnormal EF of 40% or greater had a high sensitivity of 80% to 100% and a specificity of 59% to 89% in these studies. Of patients in whom these two variables were abnormal, the event rate was 34% to 36%. Patients with all three abnormal tests (i.e., LP, EF, and Holter) had an arrhythmic event rate of 28% to 57%. In contrast, only 2% of patients with all three normal tests had an event. Farrell and coworkers (55) combined an abnormal heart rate variability with the presence of LPs and repetitive forms on Holter monitor. The presence of these variables was associated with an event rate of 58% with a negative predictive value of 95%. Pedretti and coworkers (50), in a

TABLE 79–3. *Noninvasive index*

Algorithm	Gomes et al. (54) PPV	Gomes et al. (54) NPV	Kuchar et al. (47) PPV	Kuchar et al. (47) NPV	El-Sherif et al. (49) PPV	El-Sherif et al. (49) NPV	Farrell et al. (55) PPV	Farrell et al. (55) NPV	Pedretti et al. (50) PPV	Pedretti et al. (50) NPV	CAST/El-Sherif et al. (51) PPV	CAST/El-Sherif et al. (51) NPV
LP + EF	36	100	34	100	27	98	19	94				
LP + Holter	35	100	31	100	27	99	19	94				
LP + EF + Holter	50	100	—	—	57	98	28	97	—	—	32	97
LP + HRV + Holter	—	—	—	—	—	—	—	—	—	—	—	—
EF + Holter + (QRS duration > 106)	—	—	—	—	—	—	—	—	44	99		

EF, ejection fraction; HRV, heart rate variability; LP, late potentials; NPV, negative predictor value; PPV, positive predictor value.

more recent study, found the greatest positive predictive value of 44% when using a combination of an abnormal EF (<40%), two or more runs of nonsustained VT, and SA-QRS duration of 106 ms or longer. The negative predictive value of this algorithm was 99%. These authors also tested a hypothesis proposed originally by Gomes and coworkers (54): They used the noninvasive algorithm (LP + Holter + left ventricular EF) to select patients for programmed electrical stimulation. Of 303 patients, 67 of whom (22%) had these abnormalities, 47 consented to undergo programmed ventricular stimulation. A positive EP study (i.e., sustained monomorphic VT at a rate <270 beats/min) was found to be the strongest independent predictor of arrhythmic events in patients preselected by this noninvasive algorithm. Thus, the combined use of noninvasive tests and electrophysiologic study selected a group of patients after MI with a 65% event rate. They suggested that this schema is the most appropriate for selecting patients for invasive strategies after acute MI. What role, if any, thrombolytic therapy could play in this schema was not addressed in this study.

PREDICTION OF LONG-TERM OUTCOMES BY SIGNAL-AVERAGED ELECTROCARDIOGRAPHY IN PATIENTS WITH UNSUSTAINED VENTRICULAR TACHYCARDIA, CORONARY ARTERY DISEASE, PREVIOUS MYOCARDIAL INFARCTION, AND LEFT VENTRICULAR DYSFUNCTION

The long-term predictive value of the SAECG was prospectively assessed in the Multicenter Unsustained Ventricular Tachycardia Trial (MUSST) (56). Of 2,002 patients enrolled at 85 sites in the United States and Canada from November 1, 1990 to October 31, 1996, baseline SAECGs were obtained in 1,925 patients. The SAECG of 1,268 patients (66%) qualified for this analysis. Tracings of 612 patients (32%) with bundle branch block or intraventricular conduction defects (>120 ms), 30 patients (1.6%) with ventricular-paced rhythm, and 15 patients (0.8%) with unreadable trac-

ings were excluded from analysis. Of the 1,268 patients, 364 had inducible sustained VT and were randomized into the trial; 193 patients were randomized to no antiarrhythmic therapy and 171 patients to electrophysiologically guided antiarrhythmic therapy. The remaining 904 patients were followed in a registry. All tracings were obtained with commercially available systems and analyzed at core laboratories without knowledge of treatments or outcomes or whether sustained VT was inducible. In all patients, SAECG quantitative variables were processed at 40 to 250 Hz and included filtered QRS duration, the RMS40, and duration of low-amplitude signals (<40 μV). Variables were measured with computer-derived algorithms.

The primary end point of the trial was cardiac arrest or death from arrhythmia. Secondary end points were cardiac death and total mortality. There were 230 cardiac arrests or deaths from arrhythmia (18%), 341 cardiac deaths (27%), and 457 total deaths (36%) among the 1,268 patients. All patients had coronary artery disease; 90% had had a previous MI. The median EF was 30% (25th and 75th percentiles, 25% and 35%). A filtered QRS duration greater than 114 ms (abnormal SAECG) independently predicted the primary end point and cardiac death, independent of clinical variables, cardioverter-defibrillator implantation, and antiarrhythmic drug therapy. With an abnormal SAECG, the 5-year rates of the primary end point (28% vs. 17%; $p = 0.0001$; Fig. 79–3), cardiac death (37% vs. 25%; $p = 0.0001$; Fig. 79–4), and total mortality (43% vs. 35%; $p = 0.0001$) were significantly greater. The combination of EF less than 30% and abnormal SAECG identified a particularly high-risk subset that constituted 21% of the total population. A total of 36% and 44% of patients with this combination succumbed to arrhythmic and cardiac death, respectively.

The observation that SAECG was not a specific predictor of arrhythmic death but was a more powerful predictor of cardiac death is interesting, inasmuch as the original hypothesis was that the SAECG could predict only arrhythmic events. Although the reason for this observation is unclear, it

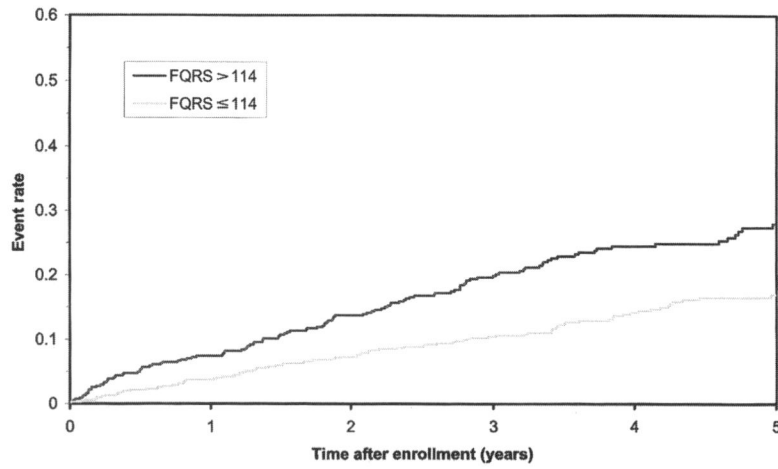

FIG. 79–3. Kaplan-Meier estimates of arrhythmic death or cardiac arrest by signal-averaged electrocardiogram result. $p < 0.001$ between groups. FQRS, filtered QRS duration.

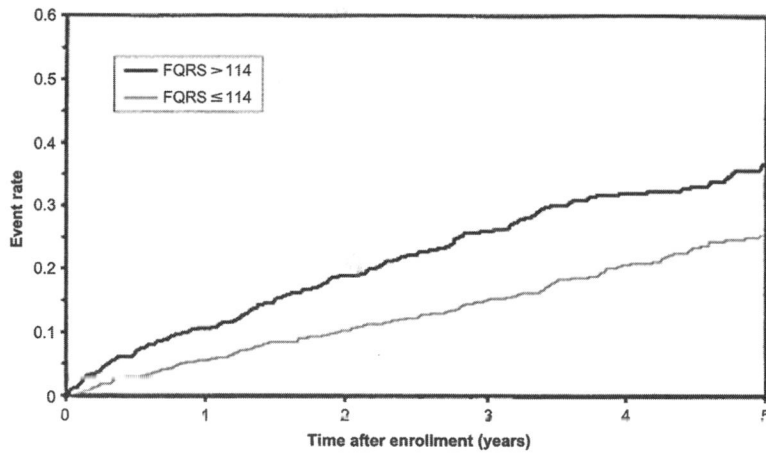

FIG. 79–4. Kaplan-Meier estimates of cardiac death by signal-averaged electrocardiogram result. $p < 0.001$ between groups FQRS, filtered QRS duration.

is tempting to speculate that the longer the filtered QRS, the greater the myocardial scarring, resulting in heterogeneous propagation not only in the terminal depolarization wave front (LPs) but perhaps also in the initial and midportions of the depolarization wave front. Furthermore, a prolonged filtered QRS may reflect an early stage in the development of overt widening of the QRS complex secondary to extensive scar. These abnormalities could, in turn, predispose patients to sudden or nonsudden cardiac death. It may explain the poorer predictive abilities of the other two SAECG variables.

An important new observation from this study was that the SAECG remained a powerful predictor of survival regardless of whether the patients received treatment, were inducible, or received an implantable cardioverter-defibrillator. The obvious implication is that if the SAECG is abnormal, the prognosis for survival from cardiac death and total mortality is worse, irrespective of treatment, including implantable cardioverter-defibrillators. This would suggest that the filtered QRS is valuable in long-term prognostication.

This prospective randomized study indicated that patients who have coronary artery disease, unsustained VT, an EF less than 40%, previous MI, and a prolonged filtered QRS, without bundle branch block or intraventricular conduction defects, have significantly greater rates of arrhythmic deaths or cardiac arrest, cardiac mortality, and all-cause mortality than do patients with a normal SAECG. The greater mortality at 2 and 5 years occurred in patients with an EF less than 30% and filtered QRS greater than 114 ms. This noninvasive algorithm using SAECG and EF may be valuable in the selection of high-risk patient subsets for intervention such as use of the implantable defibrillator and for long-term prognostication.

REFERENCES

1. Norris RM. The changing natural history and prognosis of acute myocardial infarction. In: Gersh BJ, Rahimtoola SH, eds. *Acute myocardial infarction.* New York: Elsevier, 1991:87–97.
2. Timolol-induced reduction in mortality and reinfarction in patients surviving acute myocardial infarction. *N Engl J Med* 1981;304:801–807.
3. A randomized trial of propanolol in patients with acute myocardial infarction. I. Mortality Results. Beta-Blocker Heart Attack Research Group *JAMA* 1982;247:1717–1724.
4. The Beta-Blocker Pooling Project (BBPP): subgroup findings from randomized trials in post infarction patients. The Beta-Blocker Pooling Project Research Group. *Eur Heart J* 1988;9:8–16.
5. Randomized trial of intravenous streptokinase, oral aspirin, both, or neither among 17,187 cases of suspected acute myocardial infarction: ISIS2. ISIS-2 (Second International Study of Infarct Survival) Collaborative Group. *Lancet* 1988;2:349–369.
6. Muller DW, Topol EJ, George BS, et al. Long-term follow-up in the Thrombolysis and Angioplasty in Acute Myocardial Infarction (TAM) trials: comparison of trials with thrombolysis alone. *Circulation* 1989;80[Suppl II]:II-520.
7. Long-term effects of intravenous thrombolysis in acute myocardial infarction: final report of the GISSI study. Gruppo Italiano per lo Studio della Streptochi-nasi nell'Infarto Miocardico (GISSI). *Lancet* 1987;2:871–874.
8. Williams DO, Braunwald E, Knatterud G, et al. The Thrombolysis in Myocardial Infarction (TIMI) trial: outcome at one year of patients randomized to either invasive or conservative management. *Circulation* 1989;80[Suppl II]:II-519.
9. Schroder R, Neuhaus KL, Leizorovicz A, et al. A prospective placebo-controlled double-blind multicenter trial of intravenous streptokinase in acute myocardial infarction (ISAM): long-term mortality and morbidity. *J Am Coll Cardiol* 1987;9:197–203.
10. Simoons ML, Arnold A. One year follow-up of rt-PA without and with immediate PTCA. *Circulation* 1980;80[Suppl II]:II-520.
11. Van De Werf F, Arnold AE. The European Co-operative rt-PA vs Placebo trial: 1 year follow-up *Circulation* 1989;80[Suppl II]:II-520.
12. Dalen JE, Gore JM, Braunwald E, et al. Six- and twelve-month follow-up of the phase I Thrombolysis in Myocardial Infarction (TIMI) trial. *Am J Cardiol* 1988;62:179–185.
13. Taylor GJ, Moses HW, Katholi RE, et al. Six-year survival after coronary thrombolysis and early revascularization for acute myocardial infarction. *Am J Cardiol* 1992;70:26–30.
14. Gomes JA, Winters SL, Ip J. Post infarction high risk of sudden death. In: Akhtar M, Meyerburg RJ, Ruskin JN, eds. *Sudden cardiac death: prevalence, mechanism and approaches to diagnosis.* Baltimore: Williams and Wilkins, 1994:531–538.
15. Berbari EJ. A non-invasive technique for recording the depolarization of the heart's electrical conduction systems. Master's Thesis, University of Miami, 1973.
16. Berbari EJ, Lazarra R, Samet P, et al. Noninvasive technique for detection of electrical activity during the P-R segment. *Circulation* 1973;348:1005.
17. Flowers NC, Hand RC, Orander PC, et al. Surface recording of electrical activity from the region of the bundle of His. *Am J Cadiol* 1974;33:384.
18. Stopczyk MJ, Kopec J, Zochowski RJ, et al. Surface recording of electrical activity during the P-R segment in man by computer averaging technique. *Int Res Comput Syst* 1973;73-78:II-212.
19. Wajszczuk WJ, Sopczyk MJ, Moskowitz MS, et al. Non-invasive

recording of His Purkinje activity in man by QRS-triggered signal averaging. *Circulation* 1978;58:95–102.

20. Steinberg JS, Lender P. Importance of noise reduction for signal-averaged electrocardiography. In: Gomes JA, ed. *Signal-averaged electrocardiography: concepts, method and applications.* Dordrecht: Kluwer, 1992:203–220.

21. Gomes JA, Winters SL, Ip J. Signal averaging of the surface QRS complex: practical applications. *J. Cardiovasc Electrophysiol* 1991;2:316–330.

22. Simson MB, Untereker WJ, Spielman SR, et al. Relations between late potentials on the body surface and directly recorded fragmented electrograms in patients with ventricular tachycardia. *Am J Cardiol* 1993;57:105–112.

23. Marcus NH, Falcone RA, Harken AH, et al. Body surface late potential in patients with ventricular tachycardia. *Circulation* 1984;70:632–637.

24. Kanovsky MS, Falcone RA, Dresden CA, et al. Identification of patients with ventricular tachycardia after myocardial infarction: signal-averaged electrocardiogram, Holter monitoring and cardiac catheterization. *Circulation* 1984;79:264–270.

25. El-Sherif N. Electrophysiologic mechanisms of reentrant ventricular tachyarrhythmias. In: Gomes JA, ed. *Signal-averaged electrocardiography: concepts, methods and applications.* Dordrecht: Kluwer, 1993:28–46.

26. El-Sherif N, Mehra R, Gough WB, et al. Ventricular activation pattern of spontaneous and induced ventricular rhythms in canine one-day-old myocardial infarction. Evidence for focal and reentrant mechanisms. *Circ Res* 1982;68:518–533.

27. El-Sherif N, Gough WB, Restivo M. Electrophysiologic correlates of ventricular late potentials. In: El-Sherif N, Turrito G, eds. *High resolution electrocardiography.* Mount Kisco, NY: Futura, 1992:279–298.

28. Josephson ME, Horrowith LN, Farshidi A. Continuous local electrical activity. A mechanism of recurrent ventricular tachycardia. *Circulation* 1978;57:659–665.

29. Mehra R. Pathophysiology of late potentials. In: Gomes JA, ed. *Signal-averaged electrocardiography: concepts, methods and applications.* Dordrecht: Kluwer, 1993:11–27.

30. Spach MS, Barr RC, Serwer GA, et al. Extracellular potentials related to intracellular action potentials in the dog Purkinje system. *Circ Res* 1972;30:505–519.

31. Ursell PC, Gardner PI, Albala A, et al. Structural and electrophysiological changes on the epicardial border zone of canine myocardial infarcts. *Circ Res* 1988;63:182–206.

32. Gardner PI, Ursell PC, Pham TD, et al. Experimental chronic ventricular tachycardia, anatomic and electrophysiologic substrates. In: Josephson ME, Wellens HJ, eds. *Tachycardias: mechanisms, diagnosis, treatment.* Philadelphia: Lea & Febiger, 1984:29–60.

33. Gardner PI, Ursell PC, Pham TD, et al. Electrophysiologic and anatomic basis for fractionated electrograms recorded from healed myocardial infarcts. *Circulation* 1985;72:596–611.

34. Simson MB. Use of signal in the terminal QRS complex to identify patients with ventricular tachycardia after myocardial infarction. *Circulation* 1982;64:235.

35. Gomes JA, Winters SL, Stewart D, et al. Optimal bandpass filters for time-domain analysis of the signal-averaged electrocardiogram. *Am J Cardiol* 1987;60:1290.

36. Breithardt G, Cain ME, El-Sherif N, et al. Standards for analysis of ventricular late potentials using high resolution or signal-averaged electrocardiography. A statement by a Task Force Committee between the European Society of Cardiology, the American Heart Association and the American College of Cardiology. *Circulation* 1991;83:1481.

37. Gomes JA, Winters SL, Martinson M, et al. The prognostic significance of quantitative signal-averaged variables relative to clinical variables, site, of myocardial infarction, ejection fraction and ventricular premature beats: a prospective study. *J Am Coll Cardiol* 1988;13:337–384.

38. Cain ME, Ambos HD, Witkowski FX, et al. Fast-Fourier transform analysis of signal-averaged electrocardiograms for identification of patients prone to sustained ventricular tachycardia. *Circulation* 1984;69:711–720.

39. Haberl R, Jilge G, Pulter R, et al. Spectral mapping of the electrocardiogram with Fourier transform for identification of patients with sustained ventricular tachycardia and coronary artery disease. *Eur Heart J* 1989;10:316.

40. Kelen GJ, Henkin R, Starr AM, et al. Spectral turbulence analysis of the signal-averaged electrocardiogram and its predictive accuracy for inducible sustained monomorphic ventricular tachycardia. *Am J Cardiol* 1991;7:965.

41. Machac J, Weiss A, Winters SL, et al. A comparative study of frequency domain and time domain analysis of signal-averaged electrocardiograms in patients with ventricular tachycardia. *J Am Coll Cardiol* 1988;11:284.

42. Kelen GJ, Henkin R, Fontaine JM, et al. Effects of analyzed signal duration and phase on the results of fast-Fourier transform analysis of the surface electrocardiogram in subjects with and without late potentials. *Am J Cardiol* 1987;60:1282.

43. Malik M, Kulakowski P, Poloviccki J, et al. Frequency versus time domain analysis of signal-averaged electrocardiogram. I. Reproducibility of the results. *J Am Coll Cardiol* 1992;20:127.

44. Kulakowski P, Malik M, Poloviccki J, et al. Frequency versus time domain analysis of signal-averaged electrocardiograms. II. Identification of patients with ventricular tachycardia after myocardial infarction. *J Am Coll Cardiol* 1992;20:135.

45. Breithardt G, Borgrefe M, Haarten K. Role of programmed ventricular stimulation and non-invasive recording of ventricular late potentials for the identification of patients at risk of ventricular arrhythmias after acute myocardial infarction. In: Zipes DP, Jalife J, eds. *Cardiac electrophysiology and arrhythmias.* Orlando, FL: Grune & Stratton, 1984:553–561.

46. Denniss AR, Richards DA, Cody DV, et al. Prognostic significance of ventricular tachycardia and fibrillation induced at programmed stimulation and delayed potentials detected on the signal-averaged electrocardiograms of survivors of acute myocardial infarction. *Circulation* 1986;74:731–745.

47. Kuchar DL, Thorburn CW, Samuel NL. Late potentials detected after myocardial infarction: natural history and prognostic significance. *Circulation* 1986;74:1280–1289.

48. Cripps T, Bennett ED, Camm AJ, et al. High gain signal averaged electrocardiogram combined with 24 hour monitoring in patients early after myocardial infarction for bedside prediction of arrhythmic events. *Br Heart J* 1988;60:181.

49. El-Sherif N, Ursell SN, Bekheit S, et al. Prognostic significance of the signal averaged electrocardiogram depends on the time of recording in the post-infarction period. *Am Heart J* 1989;118:256–264.

50. Pedretti R, Etro MD, Laporta A, et al. Prediction of late arrhythmic events after acute myocardial infarction from combined use of noninvasive prognostic variables, and inducibility of sustained monomorphic ventricular tachycardia. *Am J Cardiol* 1993;71:1131–1141.

51. el-Sherif N, Denes P, Katz R, et al. Definition of the best prediction criteria of the time domain signal-averaged electrocardiogram for serious arrhythmic events in the postinfarction period. The Cardiac Arrhythmia Suppression Trial/Signal-Averaged Electrocardiogram (CAST/SAECG) Substudy Investigators. *J Am Coll Cardiol* 1995;25:908–914.

52. Kuchar DL. Natural history of late potentials after myocardial infarction. In: Gomes JA, ed. *Signal-averaged electrocardiography: concepts, methods and applications.* Dordrecht: Kluwer, 1993:443–448.

53. Gomes JA, Winters L. The prognostic significance of the signal-averaged electrocardiogram in the infarct survivor. In: Gersh BJ, Rahimtoola SA, eds. *Acute myocardial infarction.* New York: Elsevier, 1991:423–437.

54. Gomes JA, Winters SL, Stewart D, et al. A new noninvasive index to predict sustained ventricular tachycardia and sudden death in the first year after myocardial infarction: based on signal-averaged electrocardiogram, radionuclide ejection fraction and Holter monitoring. *J Am Coll Cardiol* 1987;10:349–357.

55. Farrell TG, Bashier Y, Cripps E, et al. Risk stratification for arrhythmic events in postinfarction patients based on heart rate variability, ambulatory electrocardiographic variables and the signal-averaged electrocardiogram. *J Am Coll Cardiol* 1991;18:687–697.

56. Gomes JA, Cain ME, Buxton AE. Prediction of long-term outcomes by signal-averaged electrocardiography in patients with unsustained ventricular tachycardia, coronary artery disease, and left ventricular dysfunction. *Circulation* 2001;104:436.

CHAPTER **80**

Role of Electrophysiologic Testing Before Hospital Discharge

Eric N. Prystowsky

Key Words: Arrhythmia; atrioventricular block; electrophysiologic testing; myocardial infarction; sudden death; tachycardia.

INTRODUCTION

The use of electrophysiologic testing in patients after acute myocardial infarction (AMI) has changed dramatically over time. Currently, the emphasis is on identifying patients at risk for sustained ventricular tachycardia (VT) or sudden cardiac death. Three randomized controlled trials, two using electrophysiologic testing, have enabled clinicians to identify patients at increased mortality risk that is markedly reduced with an implantable cardioverter-defibrillator (ICD). This chapter reviews the current status of electrophysiologic testing in patients after MI.

BRADYARRHYTHMIAS

Sinus Node Dysfunction

Sinus node dysfunction may occur in up to 4% to 5% of patients during AMI, typically patients with an inferior wall MI (1–3). Although patients may require temporary pacing, most frequently the dysfunction is transient and permanent

E. N. Prystowsky: The Care Group, LLC, 8333 Naab Road, Suite 400, Indianapolis, Indiana 46260.

pacing is not required. Correlation between persistent bradycardia resulting from sinus node dysfunction and patient symptoms will dictate whether a permanent pacemaker is necessary. Electrophysiologic testing is not needed in these patients unless data from the study will affect the type of pacemaker being implanted. Asymptomatic patients are not candidates for sinus node evaluation at electrophysiologic study.

Atrioventricular Block

Two basic patterns of complete atrioventricular (AV) block have been identified with AMI. One type occurs without bundle branch block and typically is associated with an inferior wall MI (Fig. 80–1). The usual course is resumption of reasonable AV conduction without the need for permanent pacing. In some patients, this may take more than 1 week and appropriate times should be allowed before deciding on the need for permanent pacing. Electrophysiologic testing is typically not indicated in these individuals.

The second form of AV block occurs with bundle branch block and is usually associated with anterior wall MI. In-hospital mortality is relatively high in these individuals, who often have substantial myocardial necrosis. The updated American College of Cardiology/American Heart Association/North American Society of Pacing and Electrophysiology (NASPE) Guidelines list transient advanced (second-or

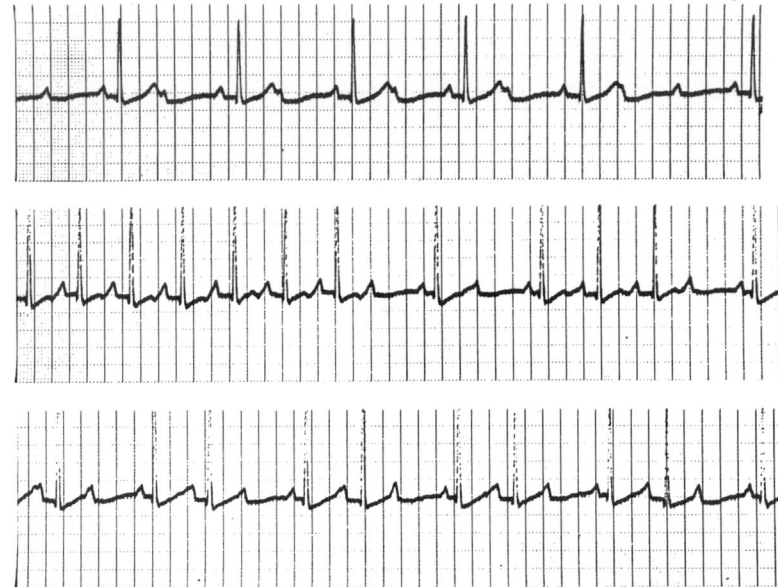

FIG. 80–1. Various electrocardiographic patterns of atrioventricular (AV) conduction in a patient with recent acute inferior wall myocardial infarction. **Top:** Tracing showing 2:1 AV conduction until the end of the recording when 3:1 conduction occurs. **Middle:** Tracing starting with 1:1 AV conduction that proceeds to 2:1 and then Wenckebach conduction patterns. **Bottom:** Tracing demonstrating 3:2 Wenckebach block. The presence of 2:1 and Wenckebach block in a patient with a narrow QRS complex strongly suggests the AV node as the site of bock. This patient regained 1:1 AV conduction before hospital discharge and required no further workup.

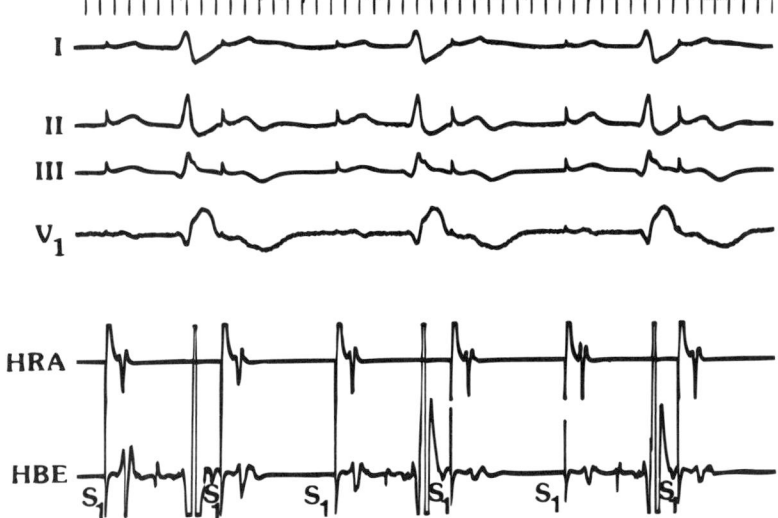

FIG. 80–2. Right bundle branch block with 2:1 atriventricular (AV) conduction during high right atrial (HRA) pacing. Paced atrial complexes 2, 4, and 6 are blocked, and no His bundle activation occurs in the blocked complex. Thus, the AV node is site of block. Simultaneous recordings from electrocardiographic leads I, II, III, and V$_1$ and intracardiac leads from the HRA and His bundle area (HBE).

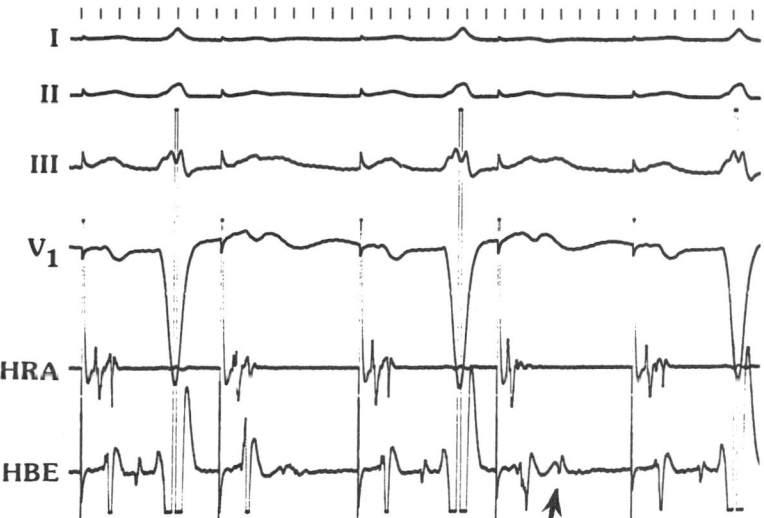

FIG. 80–3. Left bundle branch block with 2:1 atrioventricular conduction during high right atrial (HRA) pacing. The tracings are set up as in Figure 80–2. Paced atrial complexes 2 and 4 are blocked. Note that block occurs below the recorded His depolarization *(arrow).* This patient required permanent pacing. HBE, His bundle area.

third-degree) infranodal AV block associated with bundle branch block after MI as a Class I indication for a permanent pacemaker (4). An electrophysiologic study may be necessary if the site of block is uncertain (Figs. 80–2 and 80–3).

SUPRAVENTRICULAR TACHYCARDIA

Atrial fibrillation and atrial flutter are the most common sustained supraventricular tachycardias that occur with AMI. Rarely, sustained AV nodal–dependent tachycardia may occur during or shortly after AMI (5). Electrophysiologic testing and possible radiofrequency catheter ablation may be indicated in some of these patients with recurrent arrhythmias.

VENTRICULAR ARRHYTHMIAS

Sustained Monomorphic Ventricular Tachycardia

Patients in whom sustained monomorphic ventricular tachycardia (SMVT) develop more than 48 hours after AMI should undergo electrophysiologic testing (6,7). These individuals usually have substantial reduction in left ventricular function, and the SMVT typically is initiated at electrophysiologic testing (Fig. 80–4). Long-term antiarrhythmic therapy is necessary in almost all cases. Few data are available to aid the clinician in the management of patients with SMVT that occurs within 48 hours of AMI. Elder and coworkers (8) reported an incidence of only approximately 0.3%. Furthermore, patients were not prospectively treated by any specific protocol. Our bias is to evaluate these patients with electrophysiologic testing when the patient is in a relatively stable state. An ICD is selected for most of these patients, but some may also re-

quire pharmacologic treatment to suppress recurrences of sustained VT (7,9,10).

Ventricular Fibrillation/Polymorphic Sustained Ventricular Tachycardia

Conventional wisdom holds that ventricular fibrillation (VF) and sustained rapid polymorphic VT that occur within the first 48 hours of an AMI do not require further arrhythmic workup before hospital discharge, assuming that no further sustained ventricular arrhythmias occur (6,11). One should carefully evaluate for recurrent ischemia in these individuals. Electrophysiologic testing is not necessary.

When these same arrhythmias occur after 2 days, there also should be an aggressive workup for recurrent ischemia (6). If no clearcut reversible causes for VF can be found, these individuals should undergo electrophysiologic testing. We recommend long-term antiarrhythmic therapy with an ICD, but some also will require drug therapy (7,9,10).

The dividing line for early (<48 hours) and late (≥48 hours) VF after AMI is arbitrary. Early VF is thought to occur from an ischemic milieu that is unstable but transient. Late VF presumably arises in a more stable electrophysiologic environment, and therefore would portend a much greater chance for recurrence after hospital discharge. Clearly, this dividing "line" should be considered more of a "gray zone" (12). Furthermore, it is unclear whether these data apply to patients who received acute reperfusion during MI. One study seems to support the lack of a clear division between early and late VF, although antiarrhythmic drug therapy was given to more patients with late VF (13). Regardless, these authors noted that although patients with late VF were at greater risk for early death than were those

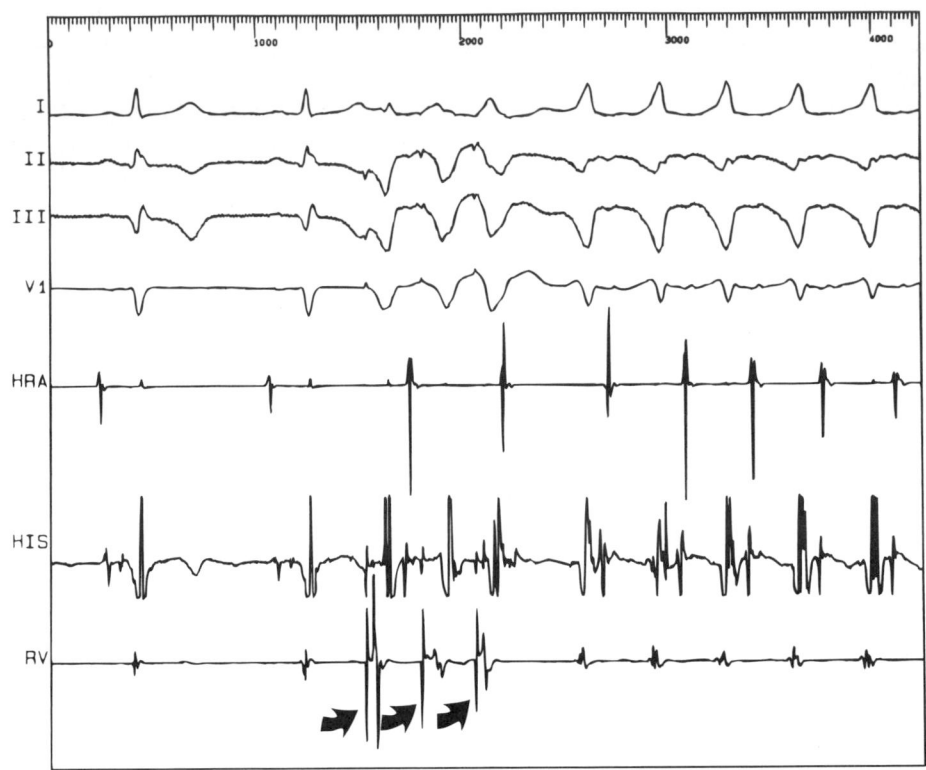

FIG. 80–4. Induction of sustained monomorphic ventricular tachycardia after myocardial infarction. Simultaneous tracings are recorded from electrocardiogram leads I, II, III, and V₁ and from intracardiac leads from the high right atrial (HRA), His bundle area (HBE), and right ventricle (RV). Three extrastimuli *(arrows)* were introduced in sinus rhythm and initiated sustained ventricular tachycardia with 1:1 ventriculoatrial conduction.

with early VF, this was explained by the presence of heart failure (13).

NONSUSTAINED VENTRICULAR ARRHYTHMIAS AND RISK STRATIFICATION

The latest statistics on the epidemic of sudden cardiac death are alarming, and more than 460,000 patients died suddenly in the United States in 1999 (14). It is not surprising that many investigators have evaluated methods to identify patients at high risk and treatment options to prevent sudden death (15,16). Several studies have evaluated the use of programmed ventricular stimulation to induce sustained VT as a means to identify patients at high risk for subsequent overall mortality and arrhythmic death (17–19). More recently, the use of low left ventricular ejection fraction without electrophysiologic testing was studied (20). The results of these randomized trials are reviewed later in this chapter.

Multicenter Automatic Defibrillator Implantation Trial

Moss and coworkers (17) conducted a prospective, randomized, controlled trial in 32 centers (30 were in the United States). Patients were eligible for enrollment if they were 25 to 80 years of age, had a Q-wave or enzyme-positive MI at least 3 weeks before entry, had asymptomatic nonsustained VT greater than 120 beats per minute, had a left ventricular ejection fraction of 0.35 or less, were not New York Heart Association functional Class IV for heart failure, and had no indication for coronary artery bypass grafting or coronary angioplasty. Patients underwent electrophysiologic study, and if sustained VT or VF was induced and not suppressed after intravenous antiarrhythmic therapy (typically procainamide), they qualified for enrollment in the study. Patients were randomized to receive an ICD or "conventional" medical therapy, which was at the discretion of the individual investigator. Notably, most patients in the conventional group received empiric amiodarone treatment that was not guided by electrophysiologic testing.

The 196 randomized patients had a mean left ventricular ejection fraction of 0.26, and New York Heart Association Class II and III congestive heart failure was present in 65% of the patients. Importantly, approximately 75% of the patients were enrolled at least 6 months after their most recent MI. Regarding other medical therapy, there was an imbalance of the use in β-adrenergic blockers with only 8% of the patients in the conventional medical group receiving these drugs compared with 26% in the ICD group.

The primary end point of Multicenter Automatic Defibrillator Implantation Trial (MADIT) was death from all causes.

The trial was prematurely terminated with an average follow-up of 27 months because the ICD group demonstrated a 56% reduction in mortality compared with the conventional group (Fig. 80–5).

Multicenter Unsustained Tachycardia Trial

Buxton and coworkers (18,19) evaluated the hypothesis that antiarrhythmic therapy guided by electrophysiologic testing could reduce the risk for sudden death and cardiac arrest in patients with coronary artery disease, spontaneous nonsustained VT, and a left ventricular ejection fraction of 0.40 or less. There were 85 participating centers in the United States and Canada in the Multicenter Unsustained Tachycardia Trial (MUSTT). Nonsustained VT had to occur at least 4 days after a MI or revascularization procedure but within 6 months of enrollment in MUSTT. Exercise-induced ischemia required therapy before a patient could be enrolled in the trial. Patients were excluded if they were New York Heart Association Class IV for heart failure.

Potential candidates for enrollment in MUSTT underwent electrophysiologic testing and could be included if either SMVT was initiated with three or less extrastimuli or sustained polymorphic VT was induced with one or two extrastimuli. There were two major hypotheses being tested in MUSTT, whether therapy directed by electrophysiology testing could reduce mortality and whether electrophysiologic testing could identify patients at risk for sudden death.

Patients with inducible sustained ventricular tachyarrhythmias were randomized to either no specific antiarrhythmic treatment—that is, a true control group—or they underwent electrophysiologically guided therapy. An antiarrhythmic agent was randomly chosen and tested, and an ICD could be implanted if at least one drug trial proved ineffective. Of 767 eligible patients, 704 agreed to randomization. Patients who were not randomized were followed in a registry. A total of 353 patients were in the control group given no specific antiarrhythmic therapy, and 351 received electrophysiologically guided treatment. The mean time from the most recent MI to enrollment in MUSTT was 39 months, and the mean left ventricular ejection fraction was 0.30. There were 64% of patients who were New York Heart Association Class II or III for congestive heart failure. Notably, patients in the control group had a greater incidence of β-adrenergic blocker use—51% compared with 29% in the electrophysiologically guided treatment group.

The median follow-up duration was 39 months. At 2 and 5 years, respectively, the overall mortality rates were 22% and 40% for patients randomized to electrophysiologically guided therapy compared with 28% and 48% in the control group, which approached but did not achieve statistical significance ($p = 0.06$). The arrhythmic death or cardiac arrest end point at 2 and 5 years was 12% and 25%, respectively, for patients randomized to electrophysiologically guided therapy compared with 18% and 32% for the control group ($p = 0.04$). Further analysis demonstrated that the ICD was responsible for the lower arrhythmic death rate and total mortality. For example, the 5-year rate of cardiac arrest or arrhythmic death was 9% in patients who received an ICD compared with 37% for those treated with antiarrhythmic drugs. The 5-year overall mortality was 24% for the patients who received an ICD compared with 55% for those who received an antiarrhythmic drug (Fig. 80–5). Further analysis showed that there was no difference among the antiarrhythmic drugs and their ability to prolong survival (21).

Because the goal of MUSTT was not specifically to test the advantage of an ICD over antiarrhythmic drugs, a series of further analyses were performed by Lee and coworkers (22). They concluded that the benefit of electrophysiologically guided antiarrhythmic therapy observed in MUSTT

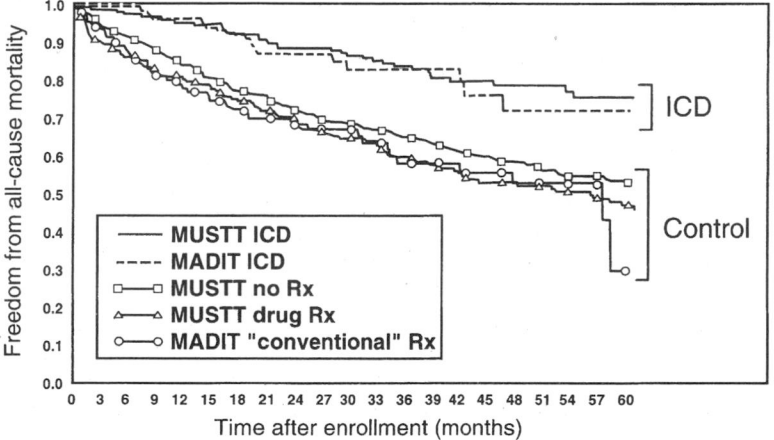

FIG. 80–5. Kaplan-Meier survival curves for all-cause mortality in the Multicenter Unsustained Tachycardia Trial (MUSTT) and Multicenter Automatic Defibrillator Implantation Trial (MADIT) studies. ICD, Implantable cardioverter defibrillator; Rx, treatment. (From Prystowsky EN. Screening and therapy for patients with nonsustained ventricular tachycardia. *Am J Cardiol* 2000;86[Suppl]:34K–39K, with permission.)

was related to the ICD and not to any of the antiarrhythmic drugs.

MUSTT also evaluated whether electrophysiologic testing is useful to predict patients at risk for arrhythmic death after MI (19). A comparison was made between 1,397 patients in the registry and 353 patients who had inducible ventricular tachyarrhythmias and were assigned randomly to receive no specific antiarrhythmic therapy. The 2- and 5-year rates of cardiac arrest or death from an arrhythmia were 12% and 24%, respectively, for the registry patients compared with 18% and 32% in the randomized group ($p <$ 0.001). After 5 years, the overall mortality rate was 44% in the registry patients compared with 48% in the randomized group ($p = 0.005$). Thus, for patients such as those in MUSTT, the inability to induce sustained ventricular tachyarrhythmias imports a lower risk for sudden death or cardiac arrest and lower overall mortality.

Commentary

Evaluation of Figure 80–5, which is a composite of the Kaplan-Meier survival curves for all-cause mortality in the MUSTT and MADIT studies, shows striking similarities in the results of these trials. The overall message is that treatment with an ICD resulted in an approximately 50% lower overall mortality rate than either "conventional" therapy in MADIT or electrophysiologically guided drug treatment or no treatment in MUSTT. These two trials present clear and convincing evidence that patients who meet the MUSTT and MADIT criteria should undergo electrophysiologic testing and have an ICD implanted if a qualifying ventricular tachyarrhythmia is initiated.

Multicenter Automatic Defibrillator Implantation Trial II

Both MUSTT and MADIT I used electrophysiologic testing to stratify risk in patients after a MI. An unanswered question was whether electrophysiologic testing was necessary to stratify risk in all patients with left ventricular ejection fraction of 0.40 or less. That is, could there be a subgroup of patients in whom merely a low enough left ventricular ejection fraction might be useful to stratify risk? A separate analysis of the MUSTT registry addressed this question (23). A comparison was made between patients who had sustained VT initiated but were randomized to no specific antiarrhythmic therapy and various subgroups in the registry. Preliminary data showed that combinations of clinical variables in the nonrandomized group were associated with mortalities that were equal to and in some cases greater than that in patients who had inducible sustained ventricular arrhythmias. Importantly, analysis of the subgroup of patients who had a left ventricular ejection fraction of 0.30 demonstrated no significant difference in the 5-year mortality curves between patients with and without inducible sustained VT.

A prospective randomized controlled trial, MADIT II, was initiated to evaluate the potential survival benefit of an ICD given to patients in the absence of electrophysiologic testing who had a prior MI and left ventricular ejection fraction of 0.30 or less (20). There were 76 enrolling centers (71 were in the United States). Patients were eligible if they were older than 21 years, had an MI 1 month before entry, and had a left ventricular ejection fraction of 0.30 or less obtained within 3 months before entry into the study. Importantly, patients did not have to demonstrate nonsustained VT and did not need to undergo electrophysiologic study for entry into the MADIT II. Patients were excluded if they had New York Heart Association functional Class IV congestive heart failure or if they had undergone coronary revascularization within the preceding 3 months. The 1,232 patients were randomized to receive an ICD or conventional therapy. The average follow-up was 20 months, and the baseline characteristics and various cardiac medications were similar between the groups. The mean left ventricular ejection fraction was 0.23, and 70% of patients received β-adrenergic blockers.

The primary end point of overall mortality demonstrated a clear benefit for patients receiving an ICD. For the average follow-up of 20 months, the mortality rates were 14.2% in the ICD group compared with 19.8% in the conventional therapy group; overall, there was an approximately 31% reduction in the risk for death.

Commentary

The above results suggest that patients with similar clinical characteristics to those enrolled in MADIT II should be seriously considered for ICD therapy. It is quite possible that electrophysiologic testing would enable more precise risk stratification in these patients, and other factors such as QRS duration may also prove useful. However, these require further study. It should be remembered that patients within the first month after MI or within 3 months after coronary revascularization were excluded from MADIT II, and the advantage of an ICD without electrophysiologic testing in these patients is unknown. Because MUSTT enrolled patients 4 days after MI or revascularization and showed a definite benefit of ICD therapy if sustained VT was induced, a reasonable approach would be to perform long-term monitoring on these patients to identify nonsustained VT; electrophysiologic testing would be recommended with ICD therapy if sustained ventricular tachyarrhythmias were induced.

REFERENCES

1. Hatle L, Bathen J, Rokseth R. Sinoatrial disease in acute myocardial infarction: long-term prognosis. *Br Heart J* 1976;38:410–414.
2. Parameswaran R, Ohe T, Goldberg H. Sinus node dysfunction in acute myocardial infarction. *Br Heart J* 1976;38:93–96.
3. Simonsen E, Nielsen BL, Nielsen JS. Sinus node dysfunction in acute myocardial infarction. *Acta Med Scand* 1980;208:463–469.

4. Gregoratos G, Abrams J, Epstein AE, et al. ACC/AHA/NASPE 2002 guideline update for implantation of cardiac pacemakers and antiarrhythmia devices: summary article: a report of the American College of Cardiology/American Heart Association Task Force on Practice Guidelines (ACC/AHA/NASPE Committee to Update the 1998 Pacemaker Guidelines). *Circulation* 2002;106:2145–2161

5. Prystowsky EN, Heger JJ, Jackman WM, et al. Post-myocardial infarction incessant supraventricular tachycardia due to concealed accessory pathway. *Am Heart J* 1982;103:426–430.

6. Hurwitz JL, Prystowsky EN. Ventricular arrhythmias after acute myocardial infarction. In: Califf RM, Mark R, Wagner G, eds. *Acute coronary care,* 2nd ed. St. Louis, MO: Mosby, 1995:617–623.

7. Prystowsky EN, Klein GJ. *Cardiac arrhythmias: an integrated approach for the clinician.* New York: McGraw-Hill, 1995:188–190.

8. Eldar M, Sievner Z, Goldbourt U, et al. Primary ventricular tachycardia in acute myocardial infarction; clinical characteristics and mortality. *Ann Intern Med* 1992;117:31–36.

9. A comparison of antiarrhythmic-drug therapy with implantable defibrillators in patients resuscitated from near-fatal ventricular arrhythmias. The Antiarrhythmics Versus Implantable Defibrillators (AVID) Investigators. *N Engl J Med* 1997;337:1576–1583.

10. Pacifico A, Hohnloser SH, Williams JH, et al. Prevention of implantable-defibrillator shocks by treatment with sotalol. d,l-Sotalol Implantable Cardioverter-Defibrillator Study Group. *N Engl J Med* 1999;340:1855.

11. Birnbaum Y, Sclarovsky S, Ben-Ami R, et al. Polymorphous ventricular tachycardia early after acute myocardial infarction. *Am J Cardiol* 1993;71:745–749.

12. Anderson JL, Hallstrom AP, Epstein AE, et al. Design and results of the antiarrhythmics vs implantable defibrillators (AVID) registry. The AVID Investigators. *Circulation* 1999;99:1692–1699.

13. Jensen GV, Torp-Pedersen C, Kober L, et al. Prognosis of late versus early ventricular fibrillation in acute myocardial infarction. *Am J Cardiol* 1990;66:10–15.

14. State-specific mortality from sudden cardiac death—United States, 1999. *MMWR Morb Mortal Wkly Rep* 2002;51:123–126.

15. Cannom DS, Prystowsky EN. Management of ventricular arrhythmias: detection, drugs, and devices. *JAMA* 1999;281:172–179.

16. Exner DV, Klein GJ, Prystowsky EN. Primary prevention of sudden death with implantable defibrillator therapy in patients with cardiac disease: can we afford to do it? (Can we afford not to?). *Circulation* 2001;104:1564–1570.

17. Moss AJ, Hall WJ, Cannom DS, et al. Improved survival with an implanted defibrillator in patients with coronary disease at high risk for ventricular arrhythmia. Multicenter Automatic Defibrillator Implantation Trial Investigators. *N Engl J Med* 1996;335:1933–1940.

18. Buxton AE, Lee KL, Fisher JD, et al. A randomized study of the prevention of sudden death in patients with coronary artery disease. Multicenter Unsustained Tachycardia Trial Investigators. *N Engl J Med* 1999;341:1882–1890.

19. Buxton AE, Lee KL, DiCarlo L, et al. Electrophysiologic testing to identify patient with coronary artery disease who are at risk for sudden death. Multicenter Unsustained Tachycardia Trial Investigators. *N Engl J Med* 2000;342:1937–1945.

20. Moss AJ, Zareba W, Hall WJ, et al. Prophylactic implantation of a defibrillator in patients with myocardial infarction and reduced ejection fraction. Multicenter Automatic Defibrillator Implantation Trial II Investigators. *N Engl J Med* 2002;346:877–883.

21. Wyse DG, Talajic M, Hafley GE, et al. Antiarrhythmic drug therapy in the Multicenter UnSustained Tachycardia Trial (MUSTT): drug testing and as-treated analysis. *J Am Coll Cardiol* 2001;38:344–351.

22. Lee KL, Hafley G, Fisher JD, et al. Effect of implantable defibrillators on arrhythmic events and mortality in the multicenter unsustained tachycardia trial. Multicenter Unsustained Tachycardia Trial Investigators. *Circulation* 2002;106:233–238.

23. Prystowsky EN, Hafley GE, Buxton AE. Are there subgroups of patients at high risk for sudden death and cardiac arrest without inducible sustained monomorphic ventricular tachycardia—results from Multicenter Unsustained Tachycardia Trial (MUSTT). *Circulation* 1999;100:I-81.

CHAPTER 81

Role of Renin-Angiotensin-Aldosterone System in Cardiovascular Disease

Pathophysiologic Insights and Therapeutic Implications

Gary H. Gibbons and Marc A. Pfeffer

Key Words: Atherosclerosis; endothelial dysfunction; remodeling; vasoactive.

INTRODUCTION

Recent advances in the treatment of cardiovascular disease are based on new insights into the fundamental pathobiologic mechanisms that promote heart disease. In particular, a rapidly emerging body of evidence indicates that the activity of the renin-angiotensin-aldosterone system (RAAS) is an important determinant of cardiovascular function and structure in health and disease. This chapter reviews how these new pathobiologic insights discovered in the experimental laboratory have become translated into the practice of cardiovascular medicine. The development of pharmacologic inhibitors of the renin-angiotensin-aldosterone axis represents a milestone in cardiovascular therapeutics. This chapter describes the results of clinical trials that have established the efficacy

of inhibiting this system as a means of altering the natural history of cardiovascular disease.

CARDIOVASCULAR CONTINUUM: THE PROGRESSION FROM ENDOTHELIAL DYSFUNCTION TO END-STAGE HEART DISEASE

Advances in cardiovascular medicine have improved our capacity to prolong the lives of patients who have had myocardial infarctions (MIs) or congestive heart failure. The traditional therapeutic approach to treating heart disease has focused on the treatment of symptomatic heart disease at the latter stages in the natural history of the disease. However, the current challenge is to develop pharmacotherapies that interrupt the mechanistic underpinnings of disease pathogenesis such that clinicians can prevent the development of end-stage coronary heart disease.

Epidemiologic studies have established that a variety of risk factors such as hypertension, dyslipidemia, obesity, diabetes, and aging are major risk factors for the development of heart disease. Recent advances in vascular biology have provided a unifying framework for understanding how various risk factors activate pathogenic processes that promote cardiovascular injury, pathologic remodel-

G. H. Gibbons: Cardiovascular Research Institute, Morehouse School of Medicine, 720 Westview Drive, Atlanta, Georgia 30310.

M. A. Pfeffer: Cardiovascular Division, Brigham and Women's Hospital, 75 Francis St., Boston, Massachusetts 02115.

ing, and eventual cardiac failure. It is now recognized that each of the classical risk factors is associated with subclinical impairments in vascular function that presage the progression toward clinically evident cardiovascular disease.

The vasculature is now recognized as a complex organ capable of responding to its local milieu and modulating its own function and structure to maintain homeostasis. The ubiquity of the vasculature within each organ provides a platform by which perturbations in vascular biology can induce tissue injury and result in end-stage organ failure. The capacity of the endothelium to regulate tissue blood flow, thrombosis, and the inflammatory response provides the means for the vasculature to be a critical determinant of cardiac function and structure. The normal endothelium has the intrinsic capacity to prevent vascular disease and preserve normal cardiac function. An impairment of endothelial function, manifested as abnormal endothelium-dependent vasorelaxation, reflects a perturbation in this normal homeostatic balance. This state of vascular dysfunction promotes the generation of pathologic mediators that alter cardiac function and structure and eventuates in end-stage cardiac failure. It is therefore not surprising that the characterization of endothelial dysfunction appears to have prognostic value in identifying individuals with subclinical vascular disease at increased risk for cardiovascular complications (1,2).

Endothelial dysfunction is typically characterized on the basis of a physiologic impairment in endothelium-dependent vasorelaxation. The principal factor that mediates this endothelium-dependent vasorelaxation is nitric oxide (NO). Although there are several potential causes of decreased NO bioactivity, several lines of evidence suggest that increased catabolism of NO by reactive oxygen species is the principal factor. Indeed, a recurring theme among cardiovascular risk factors (e.g., smoking, obesity, diabetes, and hypertension) is their association with a state of increased oxidative stress. A growing body of evidence indicates that the RAAS plays an intimate role in this pathogenic process. It is noteworthy that clinical studies of blockade of angiotensin (Ang II) activation by either angiotensin-converting enzyme (ACE) inhibition or angiotensin II receptor type 1 (AT-1R) blockade favorably restores the appropriate Ang II-NO balance in patients with coronary artery disease (3). In addition, these investigators observed that angiotensin blockade was associated with decreased oxidative stress in association with the up-regulation of the endogenous antioxidant, superoxide dismutase. This finding indicates that Ang II promotes oxidative stress in humans by enhancing the generation of reactive oxygen species and that restoration of the redox balance by either ACE inhibition or angiotensin receptor blockade ameliorates vascular function in human atherogenesis. Thus, the local generation of angiotensin and aldosterone within vascular tissues appears to play an important role in accelerating the transition from the early stage of endothelial dysfunction

to the final stages of atherothrombotic complications and heart failure.

THE RENIN-ANGIOTENSIN-ALDOSTERONE SYSTEM AND ATHEROTHROMBOSIS

Advances in our understanding of vascular biology have redefined atherothrombosis as a chronic inflammatory disease. Endothelial dysfunction is one of the earliest discernible signs of the atherothrombotic process and reflects a functional deficiency in one of the major intrinsic antiatherogenic factors within the vasculature: NO. NO preserves normal vascular homeostasis by tonically maintaining vasodilation and normotension, reducing inflammatory cell influx into the vessel wall, attenuating vascular smooth muscle cell growth within lesions, inhibiting thrombus formation, and promoting plaque stability within the extracellular matrix (4). A growing body of evidence indicates that Ang II generated within the vessel wall contributes to the state of endothelial dysfunction and accelerated atherogenesis by promoting increased oxidative stress and stimulating proinflammatory pathways (5).

Studies have documented that human atherothrombotic lesions are characterized by an increased expression of ACE within foamy macrophages that populate the plaque (6). Indeed, ACE expression is further increased within recently ruptured plaques compared with stable atherothrombotic lesions (7). Oxidized low-density lipoprotein (LDL) cholesterol appears to stimulate the expression of ACE within macrophages. Conversely, Ang II appears to promote the oxidation of LDL cholesterol, thereby establishing a vicious cycle. Ang II activates nicotinamide adenine dinucleotide phosphate oxidase to generate reactive oxygen species in both vascular cells and inflammatory cells. This prooxidant signaling pathway stimulates a redox-sensitive, proinflammatory transcriptional cascade mediated by the transcription factors nuclear factor-κB and activator protein-1 (AP-1). These transcription factors, in turn, induce the coordinate up-regulation of cytokines (e.g., tissue necrosis factor and interleukin-6), chemoattractants (e.g., monocyte chemoattractant protein-1), and leukocyte adhesion molecules (e.g., vascular cell adhesion molecule-1) that are necessary for atherothrombotic lesion formation (8–11). In addition to its effects on macrophages, Ang II is generated by lymphocytes and appears to influence the balance of T helper cell 1 (Th1) and Th2 cells such that the "proinflammatory" Th1 cells predominate and further amplify the activation of macrophages (12). Thus, it is apparent that Ang II triggers a cascade of events that result in a vicious cycle of positive feedback loops in which a prooxidant, proinflammatory state promotes vascular injury, accelerates the process of leukocyte infiltration, and augments atherothrombotic plaque formation. In addition, the combination of the prooxidant milieu with the influx of inflammatory cells increases the expression and activation of metalloproteinases, which weaken the integrity of the thin fibrous cap and predispose to plaque rupture (13).

Based on these molecular insights, it is not surprising that studies in animal models of atherogenesis have documented that the infusion of Ang II markedly potentiates the process of atherothrombotic lesion formation (14). Conversely, blockade of angiotensin with either ACE inhibitors or angiotensin receptor blockers (ARBs) significantly reduces vascular oxidative stress, down-regulates the local expression of chemokines, and attenuates atherothrombotic lesion formation in these models (15). It also is intriguing that pharmacologic blockade of the mineralocorticoid receptor with antagonists such as eplerenone also is associated with decreased generation of reactive oxygen species and the inhibition of atherogenesis (16). Thus, a variety of animal model studies of atherogenesis ranging from genetically modified mice to nonhuman primates have documented that the inhibition of the RAAS has efficacy in attenuating the process of atherogenesis. Recently, these animal model studies have been extended to the clinical context. Clinical trials using carotid ultrasound have documented that ACE inhibitor treatment of patients with cardiovascular disease at high risk attenuates the progression of human atherothrombotic lesions (secure).

Although there is a compelling body of evidence that Ang II and aldosterone appear to accelerate atherogenesis, it is recognized that thrombus formation on a ruptured atherothrombotic plaque is a critical pathobiologic mechanism of acute coronary syndromes. A critical determinant of the clinical significance of an acute plaque rupture relates to the local regulatory mechanisms that govern thrombus formation in this context. It is noteworthy that tissue factor is a major mediator of plaque thrombosis and that Ang II is an important inducer of increased tissue factor expression within macrophages and vascular cells within lesions. In addition to promoting fibrin deposition, Ang II also promotes thrombus formation by sensitizing platelets to the effects of other known agonists (17). As a result, angiotensin-treated platelets are more reactive to the aggregating effects of epinephrine, adenosine diphosphate, and collagen. Finally, once the thrombus forms, the vasculature has intrinsic homeostatic mechanisms that are capable of inducing spontaneous thrombolysis by the local generation of urokinase or tissue plasminogen activators (t-PA). Angiotensin is capable of subverting this endogenous defense mechanism against thrombosis by inducing increased levels of the t-PA antagonist, plasminogen activator inhibitor-1 (PAI-1) (18).

These studies in the experimental laboratory indicate that pharmacologic blockade of Ang II may reduce thrombotic cardiovascular complications by modulating the intrinsic fibrinolytic balance governed by influence of t-PA versus PAI-I (19). Indeed, clinical studies have documented an increase in the plasma t-PA:PAI-I ratio in patients with coronary heart disease after treatment with ACE inhibitors. Thus, there are multiple potential mechanisms by which blockade of Ang II may result in the prevention of acute atherothrombotic clinical events.

CARDIOVASCULAR REMODELING: MEDIATOR ROLE OF THE RENIN-ANGIOTENSIN-ALDOSTERONE SYSTEM

A striking pathogenic feature of the progression of cardiovascular disease involves changes in organ architecture in response to tissue injury. The heart has the capacity to remodel itself in response to hemodynamic conditions, acute ischemic events, or both. This process of ventricular remodeling can be adaptive hypertrophy in response to body growth or exercise. In some pathophysiologic circumstances of heightened workload such as hypertension or after a MI, an initial adaptive response may transition to maladaptive structural changes in which altered geometry contributes to further deterioration of cardiac function. Similarly, the process of pathologic vascular remodeling contributes to organ failure by predisposing to tissue ischemia. Structural changes within the microvasculature compromise coronary reserve in hypertrophied hearts, increase the susceptibility to stroke and vascular dementia, and contribute to the progression of glomerular injury toward renal failure. These changes in tissue architecture are fundamental to the progression of cardiovascular disease toward end-organ failure.

The process of cardiovascular remodeling is determined by fundamental cellular processes such as cell growth, cell death, matrix modification, and the response to tissue injury and repair. The cell mass of an organ depends on the balance of cell growth by hypertrophy or hyperplasia versus cell death by either necrosis or apoptosis. Apoptosis is a form of "cell suicide" in which a carefully regulated genetic program deletes a cell from a tissue, thereby compromising tissue function and structure. Studies have documented that apoptosis occurs in contexts of ventricular and vascular remodeling in patients with cardiovascular disease (20–23). An increase in myocardial cell death appears to contribute to the evolution of the dilated cardiomyopathy that occurs after infarction. A series of provocative studies indicates that this process of cell loss in response to tissue injury is mitigated by an intrinsic process of tissue repair involving the replacement of injured cells by undifferentiated progenitor cells that are induced to become new cardiac myocytes. Progenitor cells residing in the bone marrow or resident within the heart, or both, are capable of homing to the site of cardiac injury, replacing the injured cells, and contributing to the preservation of normal cardiac function and structure. Indeed, stem cells may evolve into a promising approach to enhance the process of tissue repair after infarction. Thus, the balance among cell growth, cell death, and cell replacement by progenitor cells is an important determinant of tissue architecture. It is intriguing that a growing body of evidence indicates that the RAAS may play a role in modulating each of these determinants of cardiovascular structure (24). Activation of the AT-1 receptor is coupled to growth-promoting cellular signaling pathways (e.g., mito-gen-activated protein kinase) and also induces cardiovascular cells to synthesize growth factors such as platelet-derived growth factor, basic fibroblast growth factor, and transforming growth factor-β_1 (25). Similarly, the AT-1 receptor is coupled to the regulation of apoptosis by signaling pathways (e.g., Akt) and the induction of growth factors that also modulate cell death (e.g., transforming growth factor-β_1).

In addition to these changes in the cellular compartment, organ structure also is modified by remodeling of the extracellular matrix. An imbalance between matrix protein production and matrix degradation results in maladaptive remodeling and tissue fibrosis. Ang II alters extracellular matrix composition through its effect on the expression of thrombospondin, fibronectin, osteopontin, glycosaminoglycan expression, and plasminogen activator activity (26–28). Similarly, aldosterone has potent profibrotic properties by stimulating collagen synthesis and reducing its degradation. Moreover, an important component of tissue repair after injury involves the process of wound contracture in which the structure of the matrix is remodeled and shaped by contractile forces of myofibroblasts. It is noteworthy that ACE is expressed in myofibroblasts and Ang II appears to stimulate this process of matrix remodeling and contracture (29).

Taken together, the pleiotropic effects of Ang II on matrix degradation, production, contracture, and tissue injury and repair may induce profound influences on cardiac, vascular, or glomerular structure. Indeed, a variety of experimental studies in animal models supports the concept that Ang II is a potent modifier of tissue architecture. These mechanistic insights into the pathogenesis of organ failure have formed the basis of the hypothesis that pharmacologic blockade of Ang II will have particular efficacy in preventing the inexorable progression of heart failure, renal failure, stroke, and dementia. Clinical trials that have tested this hypothesis are reviewed in the next section.

RENIN-ANGIOTENSIN-ALDOSTERONE SYSTEM: BIOCHEMICAL CASCADES

It is important to recognize that the clinical impact of ACE inhibitors, Ang II receptor blockers, and mineralocorticoid receptor antagonists rests on a foundation of experimental studies seeking to understand the physiologic and biochemical mechanisms regulating the RAAS enzymatic cascade. A century has passed since Tigerstedt and Bergman discovered renin as a pressor substance present within the kidney. It is now established that renin initiates the cascade by enzymatic cleavage of the liver-derived substrate angiotensinogen to the decapeptide Ang I (Fig. 81–1). Ang I is then converted to the octapeptide Ang II by the action of ACE, predominately during passage through the lung. Recently, this classical cascade has been further embellished by new discoveries that document a complex interchange between enzymes that result in the generation of multiple vasoactive peptides beyond

Ang II. It is now appreciated that there is a tissue RAAS in addition to the classical endocrine RAAS. Indeed, the tissue RAAS appears to be particularly significant in the context of pathologic states as a determinant of tissue injury, repair, and remodeling. It is well established that the tissue RAAS is up-regulated in the context of the heart after MI (30), the brain after ischemic injury (31), the kidney after renal injury (32), and the myocardium during the progression of heart failure (33). The potential clinical importance of the tissue angiotensin system is implicit in the notion that the therapeutic efficacy of inhibition occurs at doses well beyond that necessary to inhibit the endocrine RAAS.

In addition to the compartmentalization of the RAAS, another feature of its complex regulation involves the dynamic interplay between multiple enzymatic cascades and the resultant generation of many vasoactive peptides. For example, it was recognized quite early that ACE also functions as a kininase that destroys bradykinin in addition to generating Ang II. Similarly, a second ACE enzyme was recently discovered, ACE2, that exhibits a strikingly different pattern of expression, with high levels observed in the heart and kidney. ACE2 also has a distinct biochemical structure that competes with ACE for the substrate Ang I and ++converts it to Ang 1-9. This nonapeptide product of ACE2 product can then be converted by ACE to Ang 1-7. In contrast to Ang II, Ang 1-7 functions as a vasodilator and inhibitor of vascular smooth muscle cell growth. Thus, it has been suggested that the ACE2 axis of the cascade may function to mitigate the vasopressor and remodeling effects of Ang II. Indeed, studies using genetically modified mouse models deficient in ACE2 indicate that integrity of this pathway may play a significant role as a determinant of cardiac function and structure (34). Given that conventional ACE inhibitors fail to influence the activity of ACE2, it is speculated that increased generation of bradykinin and Ang 1-7 observed during ACE inhibition may contribute to the salutary effects of ACE inhibitors beyond the decrease in Ang II levels.

In addition to this interplay between ACE and ACE2, it is well documented that Ang II also can be generated by non–ACE-dependent pathways such as chymase, tonin, and cathepsins. In some species and in certain tissue contexts, these non–ACE-dependent pathways may predominate over the classical ACE cascade as determinants of local Ang II generation within tissues (35). The existence of these non–ACE-dependent pathways for Ang II generation have fostered the hypothesis that blockade of the RAAS at the level of the AT-1 receptor may have greater clinical efficacy than ACE inhibition, may enhance the therapeutic effectiveness of concomitant ACE inhibition in certain clinical contexts, or both. This hypothesis is actively being tested in a series of ongoing clinical trials as detailed next in this chapter.

Ang II alters cellular function by activating one of at least two major classes of Ang II receptors: AT-1 and AT-2. The AT-1 receptor is the main receptor that mediates most of the well characterized actions of Ang II. Ang II induces vaso-

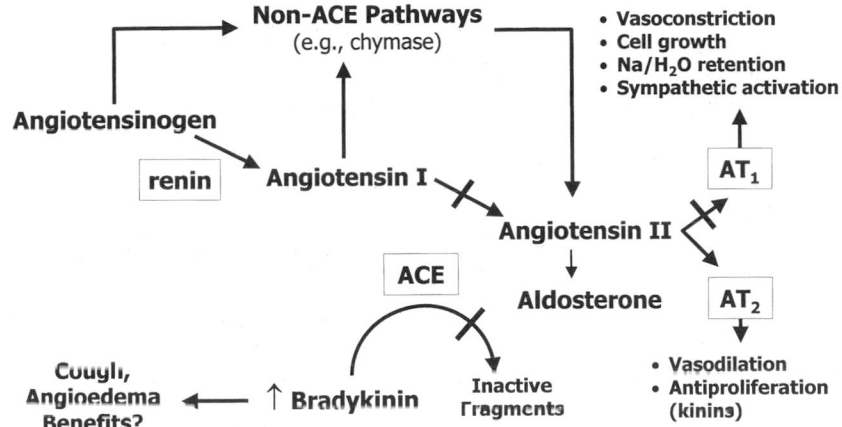

FIG 81–1. Angiotensin-converting enzyme (ACE) and kininase II. Inhibition of converting enzyme and kininase II reduces the vasoconstriction caused by angiotensin II, increases the level of vasodilator prostaglandins, and promotes sodium excretion. AT_1, angiotensin II type 1; AT_2, angiotensin II type 2; H_2O, water; Na, sodium. (Adapted from Williams GH. Converting enzyme inhibitors in the treatment of hypertension. *N Engl J Med* 1988;319:1517, with permission.)

constriction, stimulates aldosterone production, and activates vascular smooth muscle cell growth, migration, and extracellular matrix production through the activation of the AT-1 receptor. In contrast, the AT-2 receptor is much less abundant in adult cardiovascular tissues and appears to play a countervailing role to the AT-1 receptor. The AT-2 receptor appears to induce vasodilation through the generation of bradykinin and NO generation. Similarly, the AT-2 counteracts the trophic effects of the AT-1 receptor on cardiovascular structure by inhibiting cell growth and inducing programmed cell death (36). In the clinical context of AT-1 receptor blockade, it is postulated that the resultant accumulation of Ang II increases the activation of the AT-2 receptor. It is postulated that the salutary effects of AT-1 receptor blockade may involve the combined effects of a decrease in the deleterious effects of the AT-1 receptor–mediated events, as well as an increase in the beneficial influence of the AT-2 receptor on cardiovascular function and structure. These new insights into the complex biochemical pathways involved in Ang II generation have opened the intriguing possibility that combination therapy at more than one site in the RAAS cascade may result in a more optimal balance of vasoactive mediators and greater cardioprotection. As discussed in the next section, emerging clinical trials are testing the relative merits of blocking the RAAS at the level of ACE, the AT-1 receptor, and/or the mineralocorticoid receptor in various patient subsets.

The Clinical Context: Demonstrated Value of Renin-Angiotensin-Aldosterone System Inhibition

High Blood Pressure

Inhibitors of the RAAS were all initially developed as antihypertensive agents. For the most part, these are well toler-

ated and effective blood pressure reducing therapies currently used safely in millions of patients with hypertension. The fundamental importance of blood pressure control for subsequent cardiovascular risk reduction demonstrated in the early Veterans Administration trials remains the central tenet for antihypertensive therapy (37,38). In patients with hypertension, the extent of control of arterial pressure increases is the predominant factor in the reduction of risk for subsequent cardiovascular death, stroke, heart failure, and MIs. More recent attempts to compare antihypertensive agents targeting similar blood pressure reduction have produced a quagmire of apparently conflicting information (39). Currently, in uncomplicated hypertension, although ACE inhibitors are of proven value in a variety of clinical disorders (discussed later), they are not convincingly considered to have unique clinical outcome benefits beyond that achieved by other blood pressure reducing therapies.

The Captopril Prevention Project (CAPPP) was one of the first major outcomes trials in hypertension to compare an ACE inhibitor regimen to a β-blocker. Using a prospective, randomized, open treatment with blinded end point evaluation design (40), CAPPP randomized 10,985 patients to either captopril or a diuretic/β-blocker–based antihypertensive regimen. After 6 years of follow-up, no difference was found between groups in the primary outcome measure of cardiovascular death and nonfatal MI and strokes. In the relatively small (572 patients) subgroup with diabetes, fewer cardiovascular events occurred in those randomized to the ACE inhibitor (40).

The Swedish Trial in Old Patients with Hypertension-2 (STOP-Hypertension-2) used the same type of design in more than 6,000 patients with hypertension older than 70 years. No difference in rates of a combined outcome of fatal and nonfatal cardiovascular events was found comparing blood pressure reduction based on an ACE inhibitor/calcium channel blocker or diuretic/β-blocker regimen (41).

The Antihypertensive and Lipid-Lowering Treatment to Prevent Heart Attack Trial (ALLHAT) (42) and the Second Australian National Blood Pressure Study (ANBP2) (43) underscore the complexity of comparing active antihypertensive agents in the modern era when multiple drug regimens are commonly used to adequately control arterial pressure. ALLHAT randomized more than 40,000 patients with hypertension at high risk to a regimen initially starting with a calcium channel blocker, an α-adrenergic blocker, or an ACE inhibitor or the diuretic chlorthalidone. The Data and Safety Monitoring Board stopped the α-adrenergic blocker arm early because of excess in event rates, principally the development of heart failure compared with the diuretic (44). The other three groups went to completion, and with almost 5 years of follow-up, no difference in the primary end point of fatal coronary heart disease and nonfatal MI was found (42). For secondary end points, a greater frequency of heart failure was reported in the lisinopril group compared with chlorthalidone. In contrast, ANBP2 reported a benefit of an ACE inhibitor–based approach versus the diuretic hydrochlorothiazide in the treatment of elderly individuals with hypertension with a significant 11% reduction in the primary end point incorporating death and multiple major cardiovascular events (43). These apparent discrepancies in trial results have been the subject of several scholarly editorials (44–47). Although there is no consensus, differences in patient populations, ACE inhibitor and diuretics used, blood pressures achieved, second and third agents used for blood pressure control, and specific trial design fea-

tures have all been implicated to various degrees in attempts to explain the discrepancies among trials (44–47). The importance of diuretics and the frequent need of combination therapy to achieve adequate blood pressure control were consistent and important messages. There was general agreement that ACE inhibitors are of proven value in higher risk populations.

More recently developed ARBs also are effective antihypertensive agents with an excellent tolerability profile. The Losartan Intervention For Endpoint reduction in hypertension study (LIFE) randomized more than 9,000 patients with hypertension and electrocardiographic left ventricular hypertrophy to either the ARB losartan or the β-blocker atenolol (48). The primary end point of the study death from any cause, nonfatal MI, or nonfatal stroke was significantly less in the ARB group relative to the β-blocker group. Evaluation of the components of the primary end point indicated that the major difference among the antihypertensive agents was in the risk for stroke that was significantly lower in the ARB group. With minimal differences in blood pressures achieved and similar second line use of other agents such as diuretics, it is fair to conclude that inhibiting the renin-angiotensin system in these patients with an ARB resulted in lower clinical risk that could not be explained solely by blood pressure reduction (Fig. 81–2). The Study on Cognition and Prognosis in the Elderly (SCOPE) compared the primary end point of a decline in cognitive function with blood pressure control on the basis of either the ARB candesartan or a diuretic-based regimen. With approximately 5,000 patients, no differences in mental status decline were observed between the two groups (49). However, a qualitatively similar pattern of

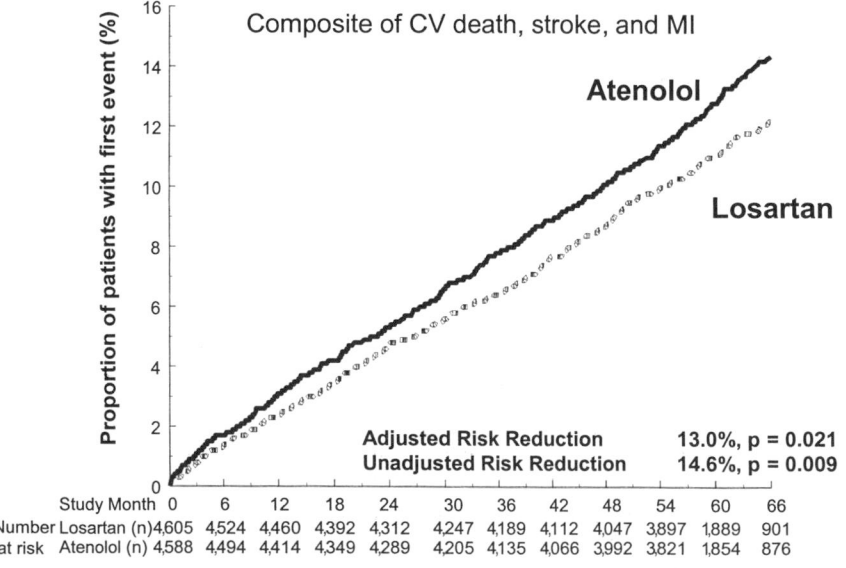

FIG. 81–2. Losartan Intervention For Endpoint reduction in hypertension study (LIFE) Kaplan-Meier curves for primary composite end point. CV, cardiovascular; MI, myocardial infarction. (From Dahlof B, Devereux RB, Kjeldsen SE, et al. Cardiovascular morbidity and mortality in the Losartan Intervention For Endpoint reduction in hypertension study (LIFE): a randomised trial against atenolol. *Lancet* 2002;359:995–1003, with permission.)

trends of reductions in cardiovascular events observed in LIFE was observed in SCOPE. Both studies provided an interesting observation of fewer ARB-treated patients experiencing development of diabetes during the follow-up.

The soon to be completed Valsartan Antihypertensive Long-term Use Evaluation (VALUE) trial comparing clinical outcomes in more than 15,000 patients with hypertension plus an associated risk factor randomized to the ARB valsartan or the calcium channel blocker amlodipine is well poised to address the issue of potential clinical benefits beyond blood pressure reduction (50). However, currently, adequate blood pressure control remains the primary focus of treatment.

Diabetes and Renal Protection

Inhibitors of the renin-angiotensin system have earned their unique place as effective cardiovascular/renal clinical event reducers in more selected patient populations. Animal studies first suggested beneficial roles of inhibiting the renin-angiotensin system in protecting declines in glomerular function and structure that was out of proportion to their blood pressure reducing actions (51). These pioneering studies provided the rationale for definitive clinical outcome trials, which have established the importance of inhibiting the renin-angiotensin system to attenuate progressive renal dysfunction in patients with diabetes and hypertension.

The clinical relevance of these observations was soon confirmed in a placebo-controlled trial demonstrating that captopril reduced the risk for overt deterioration of renal function leading to a doubling of creatinine or need for dialysis in patients with type 1 diabetes (52). The importance of inhibiting the renin angiotensin system and preventing risk for clinically important declines in renal function were extended to non–insulin-dependent diabetics and patients without diabetes with renal insufficiency caused by a variety of glomerulopathies (53–55). As such, ACE inhibitors earned their central role in the treatment of patients at risk for clinically important renal disease.

With the development of ARBs, there was an almost accepted assumption that they would be equally efficacious in reducing clinical events. Two major randomized trials of ARBs did in fact demonstrate important reductions in progression of renal disease in patients with type II diabetes with overt proteinuria (56,57). Notably, the central tenant of blood pressure control was built into the design of both the Irbesartan Diabetic Nephropathy Trial (IDNT) and the Reduction of Endpoints in NIDDM with the Angiotensin II Antagonist Losartan (RENAAL) trial, so that their impressive findings of a reduced need for dialysis and doubling of serum creatinine can be attributed to additional properties of the ARBs (irbesartan and losartan, respectively). It is of interest that a major study directly comparing the clinical efficacy of ACE inhibitors and ARBs has not been conducted in this field (58). Microalbuminuria, an early indication of renal and cardiovascular risk (59), was first observed to be re-

duced by ACE inhibitors and also favorably influenced by ARBs. Several well conducted studies have shown that of the level of proteinuria and the risk for development of proteinuria are reduced with ARBs (60,61). As such, these agents appeared beneficial in the prevention of clinical progression of renal disease. It is important to underscore that these inhibitors of the renin-angiotensin system should be viewed as a component of a multifactorial approach to diabetes care, which includes lifestyle modifications, glycemic control, blood pressure reduction modifications, lipid levels, and aspirin, all coupled with intensive medical care aimed at global risk reductions (62).

Heart Failure

The original Vasodilator-Heart Failure Trial (V-HeFT) provided the first demonstration of a survival benefit with medical therapy in chronic heart failure and ushered in the era of afterload reduction therapy (63). This three-arm trial demonstrated that the combination of hydralazine and nitrates reduced mortality compared with placebo in patients treated with conventional therapy. Of interest, the third arm compared prazosin with placebo and did not show a benefit on survival, although the blood pressure decrease was greatest in the prazosin group (63). ACE inhibitors also were considered as an "afterload reducing therapy" and had initial successes in improving hemodynamic abnormalities short-term in patients with severe heart failure (64,65). The translation of these effects to improved clinical outcomes was first demonstrated in the Cooperative North Scandinavian Enalapril Survival Study (CONSENSUS). The 31% reduction in the risk for death in these exceedingly high-risk patients had a rather pronounced impact on the field (66). The Studies Of Left Ventricular Dysfunction (SOLVD) has provided the most definitive information in this important field (67,68). Conducted as two parallel trials in patients with either symptomatic or relatively asymptomatic heart failure both with reduced ejection fraction (left ventricular ejection fraction [LVEF] ≤35%), a clear reduction in the risk for death and other major cardiovascular events was achieved with the use of the ACE inhibitor enalapril in this broader range of patients with symptomatic heart failure with depressed ejection fraction (67). With more than 2,500 patients and excellent long-term follow-up, the 16% reduction in the risk for death was quite definitive. In the even larger asymptomatic or prevention component, hospitalizations for heart failure were significantly reduced by enalapril, and there was a trend for reduction in mortality (68). With the recent extended follow-up data obtained through national death registries, it was shown that this early reduction in risk for hospitalization was an important indicator of clinical efficacy because long-term (12-year) survival was improved in those patients initially randomized to the ACE inhibitor (69). The consistent benefits of ACE inhibitors in symptomatic heart failure patients has led to their acceptance as a "cornerstone" therapy (70).

The initial expectations for ARBs in heart failure were quite high. Perceived as potentially a more complete inhibitor of the deleterious actions of Ang II and better tolerated, these agents were anticipated to represent a major advance. The initial results of the Evaluation of Losartan in the Elderly (ELITE), an important pilot study that compared renal tolerability of the ARB losartan with the ACE inhibitor captopril, fueled this speculation (71). Although there was no difference in the primary end point of this 722-patient study, the 49 deaths that occurred during the observation period were unevenly distributed. Fewer patients in the losartan group died, and this difference was statistically significant (71). This observation was enough to convince many that ARBs offered a survival advantage over ACE inhibitors in patients with heart failure. However, other investigators and regulatory agencies required a more rigorous test of this observation. ELITE II was designed as a proper mortality trial testing the same therapeutic strategies in a similar patient population but with the prespecified end point of mortality with sufficient statistical power. With ten times as many deaths as in the pilot study, the ARB was not found to be superior and, indeed, the trend was inferior to the ACE inhibitor (72).

The Valsartan Heart Failure Trial (Val-HeFT) investigators adopted another approach to studying the potential merits of an ARB in patients with heart failure. Rather than a direct comparison to an ACE inhibitor, they chose a design in which the ARB, valsartan, was added to optimal conventional therapy, which in most cases included an ACE inhibitor (73). Using coprimary end points, Val-HeFT did not find a survival advantage with the addition of the ARB to conventional therapy. However, a significant reduction in the risk for death combined with several major nonfatal cardiovascular events, predominantly hospitalizations for heart failure, was found (73). The most robust interpretation of Val-HeFT is that the addition of the ARB to conventional therapy reduces morbidity in patients with symptomatic heart failure with depressed ejection fraction. However, subgroup analyses regarding concomitant medical therapies have somewhat "muddied" this overall study interpretation. In the relatively small (7%) proportion of patients that were not receiving an ACE inhibitor at randomization, the use of the ARB was associated with statistically greater benefits than the remainder of the population. Patients treated with a β-blocker appeared to have less benefit and potentially an adverse effect when treated concomitantly with the ARB. In further secondary or even tertiary analyses, a concerning hazard ratio was observed in patients in whom the ARB was added to both an ACE inhibitor and β-blocker baseline therapies. This so-called triple therapy based on subgroup analysis appeared hazardous. Because ACE inhibitors and β-blockers alone and in combination have clear survival benefits in the treatment of patients with symptomatic heart failure with depressed LVEF, it was clear that these are the preferred agents. Currently, ARBs, specifically valsartan, are approved for these patients with heart failure who are not

being treated with an ACE inhibitor or the combination of ACE inhibitor and β-blocker.

The Candesartan in Heart Failure Assessment of Reduction in Mortality and morbidity (CHARM) program addressed many of these issues. This program of research was specifically designed as three parallel, independent, placebo-controlled, randomized trials of candesartan in patients with LVEF less than 40% either on an ACE inhibitor (74) or not receiving an ACE inhibitor because of prior intolerance (75), and the third component, those patients with symptomatic heart failure with an LVEF greater than 40% regardless whether receiving an ACE inhibitor (76). For those with reduced ejection fraction, including those not receiving an ACE inhibitor because of prior intolerance or those currently receiving an ACE inhibitor, randomization to candesartan resulted in significant reductions in the risk for cardiovascular death or hospitalization for heart failure (74,75). Patients with heart failure with an ejection fraction greater than 40% had a strong trend for improved outcomes with significant reductions in hospital admissions for heart failure (76). In the overall program, there was a reduction in cardiovascular deaths and hospital admissions for heart failure (77) (Fig. 81–3). The study reduced prior concerns about "triple therapy" and demonstrated that ARBs can be considered as a clinically effective therapy that produces incremental reductions in cardiovascular mortality and morbidity in the broad population of patients with symptomatic heart failure. An intriguing additional observation of reductions in the new onset of diabetes mellitus with the ARB supports the concept that inhibiting the renin-angiotensin system favorably alters this process (77).

Myocardial Infarction

The rationale to evaluate the effects of ACE inhibitors in patients with acute and chronic MIs was derived from animal studies that demonstrated that the loss of myocardium from an infarct could result in progressive ventricular enlargement (remodeling) that contributes to a further deterioration in cardiac function (78). This process of ventricular remodeling after MI was found to be attenuated by ACE inhibitor therapy with resultant improved ventricular performance and increased survival in the animal model (78,79). Early pilot clinical studies confirm the enlargement process after infarction and did indicate that ACE inhibitors could be effective in reducing this process (80,81). Major international, randomized, placebo-controlled, clinical trials involving more than hundreds of thousands of patients have proven the clinical utility of this use of ACE inhibitors in reducing risk for death, heart failure, and, in some instances, recurrent MI (82).

These trials can be categorically considered as either having broad inclusion criteria with short-term follow-up (83–86) or selecting for patients at greater risk because of left ventricular dysfunction or heart failure and generally providing longer follow-up (87–90). In both instances, there

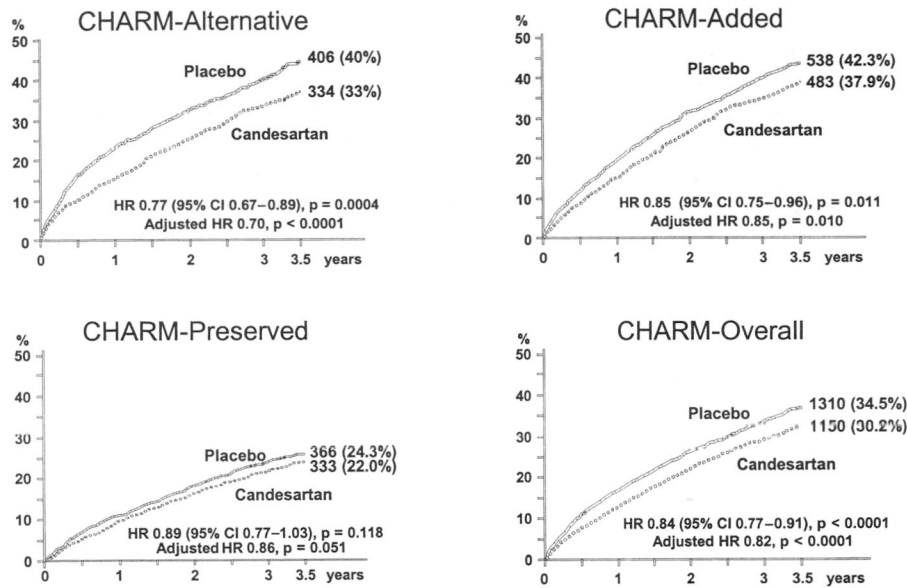

FIG. 81–3. Candesartan in Heart failure—Assessment in Reduction in Morbidity and mortality (CHARM): cardiovascular death or heart failure hospitalization for each of the components and for the CHARM-Overall program. CI, confidence interval; HR, hazard ratio.

was a favorable influence of ACE inhibitor therapy on survival (82,91). Approximately 5 lives per 1,000 treated were saved with broad use in the first 4 to 6 weeks of MI, whereas 40 to 70 lives per 1,000 patients treated were saved treating patients at greater risk for several years. ACE inhibitor therapy also was effective in preventing the development of chronic heart failure in survivors of MIs. Perhaps the most intriguing observations that have stimulated major new clinical trials and intensified basic investigations were the findings from both the Survival And Ventricular Enlargement (SAVE) and SOLVD studies that fewer patients treated with

the ACE inhibitor experienced a MI during the active follow-up phase (87,92,93).

With the demonstrated efficacy of ACE inhibitors in reducing mortality of patients with acute MI, the potential utility of ARBs in these patients had to be determined relative to an ACE inhibitor and not placebo. Two major mortality trials directly compared an ARB to a proven dose of captopril (target dosage 150 mg daily). In Optimal Trial in Myocardial Infarction with Angiotensin II Antagonist Losartan (OPTIMAAL), losartan at a target dose of 50 mg was not as effective as captopril in reducing mortality in high-risk patients with MI (94).

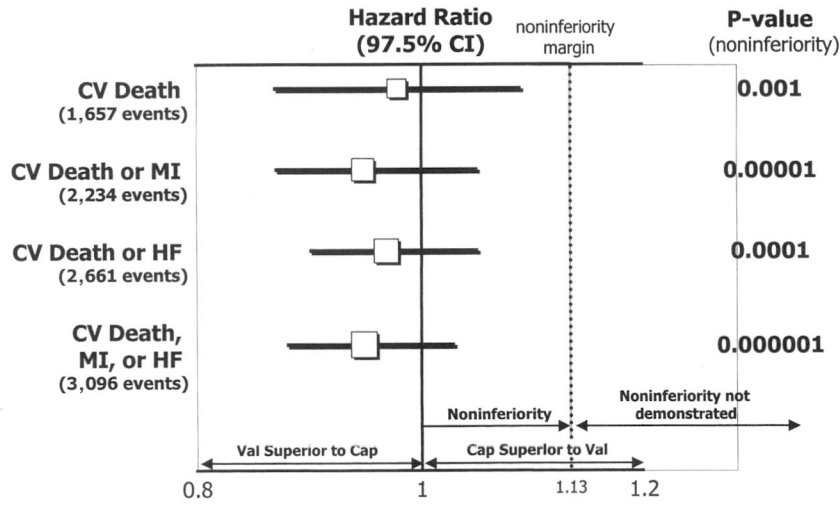

FIG. 81–4. Valsartan in Acute Myocardial Infarction (VALIANT): cardiovascular (CV) mortality and morbidity: valsartan (Val) versus captopril (Cap). CI, confidence interval; HF, heart failure; MI, myocardial infarction.

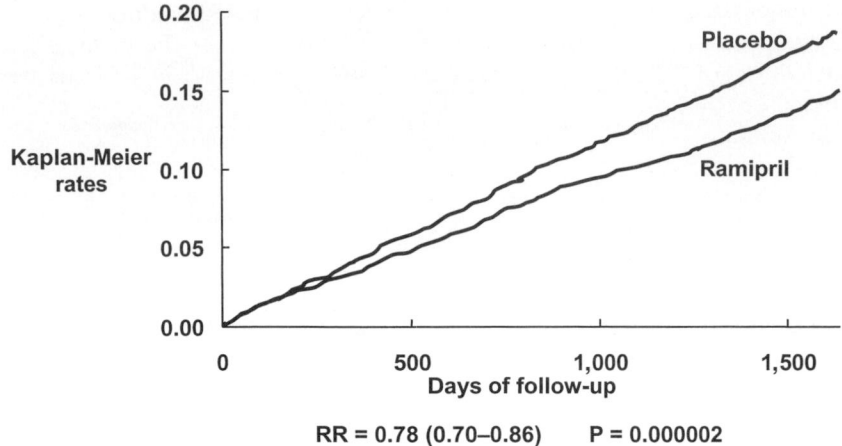

RR = 0.78 (0.70–0.86)   P = 0.000002

FIG. 81–5. Heart Outcomes Prevention Evaluation (HOPE): Kaplan-Meier curves for primary outcome. (The HOPE Study Investigators. Effects of an angiotensin-converting-enzyme inhibitor, ramipril, on cardiovascular events in high-risk patients. RR, relative risk. *N Engl J Med* 2000;342:145–153, with permission.)

Valsartan in Acute Myocardial Infarction (VALIANT), with more than 14,000 patients, demonstrated that valsartan titrated to the target dosage of 160 mg twice daily was as effective as captopril in reducing not only risk for death but also hospitalizations for heart failure and recurrent MIs (Fig. 81–4) (95). As such, this regimen of valsartan can be considered as an alternative to an ACE inhibitor in patients with high-risk MI (96). VALIANT also tested the hypothesis that adding the ARB valsartan to a proven dose of captopril would result in incremental clinical benefits. This hypothesis had to be rejected when the combination was found to be no better than the monotherapy and was associated with more adverse drug-related events. However, the direct comparison of an ARB and an ACE inhibitor in VALIANT does support the conclusion that when given in the appropriate doses, these different inhibitors of the renin-angiotensin system can produce comparable clinical benefits.

Atherothrombotic Vascular Disease

The initial results from both the SAVE and SOLVD trials indicating a reduction in the number of patients with left ventricular dysfunction experiencing a MI when randomized to an ACE inhibitor provided the initial rationale for both the

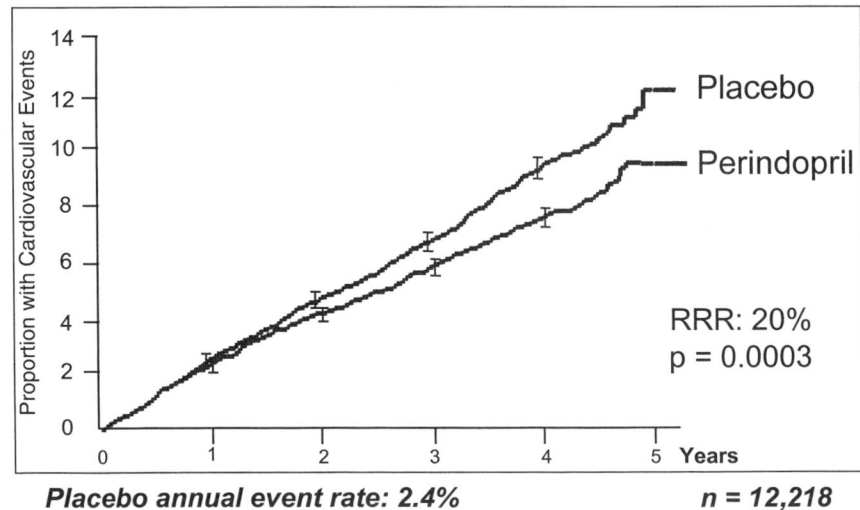

Placebo annual event rate: 2.4%   *n = 12,218*

FIG. 81–6. EUropean trial on Reduction Of cardiac events with Perindopril in patients with stable coronary Artery disease (EUROPA): time to first occurrence of primary end point. RRR, relative risk reduction. (From EUROPA Investigators. Efficacy of perindopril in reduction of cardiovascular events among patients with stable coronary artery disease: randomised, double-blind, placebo-controlled, multicentre trial. *Lancet* 2003;362:782–788, with permission.)

basic investigations discussed in this chapter and three major international, randomized, placebo-controlled, clinical trials. The Heart Outcomes Prevention Evaluation (HOPE) trial definitively demonstrated that use of the ACE inhibitor ramipril would lead to reductions in risk for cardiovascular death, MI, strokes, and other atherothrombotic events in patients with vascular disease excluding those with known left ventricular dysfunction (97) (Fig. 81–5). This was a major advance demonstrating the benefits of ACE inhibitors in preventing manifestations of atherothrombosis. These results were confirmed and expanded in the EUropean trial on Reduction Of cardiac events with Perindopril in patients with stable coronary Artery disease (EUROPA) (98). This trial demonstrated a significant reduction in the risk of the composite of cardiovascular death, MI, or cardiac arrest with the use of the ACE inhibitor in a lower risk, modernly managed, coronary artery disease population (Fig. 81–6). Although the Prevention of Events with ACE inhibition (PEACE) trial is in its final phases of closeout (99), the consistent clinical benefits already achieved with HOPE and EUROPA demonstrate the important value of ACE inhibitors in the treatment of patients with vascular and coronary disease.

Whether an ARB alone or in combination with an ACE inhibitor can achieve or produce a further improvement in clinical outcomes is currently being evaluated in the ongoing Ongoing Telmisartan Alone and in Combination with Ramipril Global Endpoint Trial (ON TARGET), which is randomizing patients with vascular disease to either ramipril, telmisartan, or their combination (100).

SUMMARY AND FUTURE PERSPECTIVES

The current challenge facing clinicians is to develop therapeutic strategies that move beyond the treatment of symptoms toward a new agenda in which interventions actually prevent the onset of cardiovascular disease and interrupt the progression toward the development of end-stage organ failure. The development of new strategies to alter the natural history of cardiovascular disease will be fostered by gaining insights into the fundamental pathobiologic mechanisms that promote the morbidity and mortality of these disorders. An emerging body of evidence indicates that the RAAS is an important determinant of the natural history of vascular disease.

Although there has been a wealth of basic science and clinical investigation on the RAAS, advances in our understanding have raised additional questions that remain to be addressed in future studies, for example:

- Does RAAS blockade reduce cardiovascular morbidity/mortality in high-risk subjects with the metabolic syndrome?
- Can the onset of incident diabetes be prevented by RAAS blockade in obese, insulin-resistant subjects?
- Is RAAS blockade indicated in normotensive patients with diabetes without microalbuminuria or clinically manifest coronary artery disease?

- Will blockade of the RAAS at the level of the AT-1 receptor have similar efficacy to ACE inhibition in preventing atherothrombotic disease progression as demonstrated in HOPE and EUROPA.
- What is the role of risk factor reduction and RAAS blockade in preventing cognitive decline in subjects at risk for vascular dementia?
- Have we identified the full spectrum of high-risk patients with hypertension who would benefit most from combination therapy involving RAAS blockade and diuretics in contrast to other drug combinations?
- Is there particular efficacy for RAAS blockade in the secondary prevention of stroke beyond blood pressure reduction alone?

It is exciting to observe that the horizon of potential indications for RAAS continues to expand, improving our ability to reduce cardiovascular morbidity and mortality.

REFERENCES

1. Suwaidi JA, Hamasaki S, Higano ST, et al. Long-term follow-up of patients with mild coronary artery disease and endothelial dysfunction. *Circulation* 2000;101:948–954.
2. Halcox JP, Schenke WH, Zalos G, et al. Prognostic value of coronary vascular endothelial dysfunction. *Circulation* 2002;106:653–658.
3. Hornig B, Landmesser U, Kohler C, et al. Comparative effect of ACE inhibition and angiotensin II type 1 receptor antagonism on bioavailability of nitric oxide in patients with coronary artery disease: role of superoxide dismutase. *Circulation* 2001;103:799–805.
4. Walford G, Loscalzo J. Nitric oxide in vascular biology. *J Thromb Haemost* 2003;1:2112–2118.
5. Nickenig G, Harrison DG. The AT(1)-type angiotensin receptor in oxidative stress and atherogenesis: part I: oxidative stress and atherogenesis. *Circulation* 2002;105:393–396.
6. Diet F, Pratt RE, Berry GJ, et al. Increased accumulation of tissue ACE in human atherosclerotic coronary artery disease. *Circulation* 1996;94:2756–2767.
7. Cipollone F, Fazia M, Iezzi A, et al. Blockade of the angiotensin II type 1 receptor stabilizes atherosclerotic plaques in humans by inhibiting prostaglandin E2-dependent matrix metalloproteinase activity. *Circulation* 2004;109:1482–1488.
8. Ni W, Kitamoto S, Ishibashi M, et al. Monocyte chemoattractant protein-1 is an essential inflammatory mediator in angiotensin II-induced progression of established atherosclerosis in hypercholesterolemic mice. *Arterioscler Thromb Vasc Biol* 2004;24:534–539.
9. Sun Y, Zhang J, Lu L, et al. Tissue angiotensin II in the regulation of inflammatory and fibrogenic components of repair in the rat heart. *J Lab Clin Med* 2004;143:41–51.
10. Brasier AR, Recinos A 3rd, Eledrisi MS. Vascular inflammation and the renin-angiotensin system. *Arterioscler Thromb Vasc Biol* 2002;22:1257–1266.
11. Shao J, Nangaku M, Miyata T, et al. Imbalance of T-cell subsets in angiotensin II-infused hypertensive rats with kidney injury. *Hypertension* 2003;42:31–38.
12. Hao L, Du M, Lopez-Campistrous A, et al. Agonist-induced activation of matrix metalloproteinase-7 promotes vasoconstriction through the epidermal growth factor-receptor pathway. *Circ Res* 2004;94:68–76.
13. Arenas IA, Xu Y, Lopez-Jaramillo P, et al. Angiotensin II-induced MMP-2 release from endothelial cells is mediated by TNF-alpha. *Am J Physiol (Cell Physiol)* 2004;286:C779–C784.
14. Bruemmer D, Collins AR, Noh G, et al. Angiotensin II-accelerated atherosclerosis and aneurysm formation is attenuated in osteopontin-deficient mice. *J Clin Invest* 2003;112:1318–1331.
15. Hayek T, Pavlotzky E, Hamoud S, et al. Tissue angiotensin-converting-enzyme (ACE) deficiency leads to a reduction in oxidative

stress and in atherosclerosis: studies in ACE-knockout mice type 2. *Arterioscler Thromb Vasc Biol* 2003;23:2090–2096.

16. Rajagopalan S, Duquaine D, King S, et al. Mineralocorticoid receptor antagonism in experimental atherosclerosis. *Circulation* 2002;105:2212–2216.

17. Lonn E, Yusuf S, Dzavik V, et al. Effects of ramipril and vitamin E on atherosclerosis: the study to evaluate carotid ultrasound changes in patients treated with ramipril and vitamin E (SECURE). *Circulation* 2001;103:919–925.

18. Matys T, Kucharewicz I, Pawlak R, et al. Nitric oxide-dependent antiplatelet action of AT1-receptor antagonists in a pulmonary thromboembolism in mice. *J Cardiovasc Pharmacol* 2003;42:710–713.

19. Pretorius M, Murphey LJ, McFarlane JA, et al. Angiotensin-converting enzyme inhibition alters the fibrinolytic response to cardiopulmonary bypass. *Circulation* 2003;108:3079–3083.

20. Oh H, Bradfute SB, Gallardo TD, et al. Cardiac progenitor cells from adult myocardium: homing, differentiation, and fusion after infarction. *Proc Natl Acad Sci USA* 2003;100:12313–12318.

21. Quaini F, Urbanek K, Beltrami AP, et al. Chimerism of the transplanted heart. *N Engl J Med* 2002;346:5–15.

22. Caplice NM, Bunch TJ, Stalboerger PG, et al. Smooth muscle cells in human coronary atherosclerosis can originate from cells administered at marrow transplantation. *Proc Natl Acad Sci USA* 2003;100:4754–4759.

23. Haznedaroglu IC, Ozturk MA. Towards the understanding of the local hematopoietic bone marrow renin-angiotensin system. *Int J Biochem Cell Biol* 2003;35:867–880.

24. Berry C, Touyz R, Dominiczak AF, et al. Angiotensin receptors: signaling, vascular pathophysiology, and interactions with ceramide. *Am J Physiol Heart Circ Physiol* 2001;281:H2337–H2365.

25. Yan C, Kim D, Aizawa T, et al. Functional interplay between angiotensin II and nitric oxide cyclic GMP as a key mediator. *Arterioscler Thromb Vasc Biol* 2003;23:26–36.

26. Gonzalez A, Lopez B, Diez J. Fibrosis in hypertensive heart disease: role of the renin-angiotensin-aldosterone system. *Med Clin North Am* 2004;88:83–97.

27. Sun Y, Zhang J, Lu L, et al. Tissue angiotensin II in the regulation of inflammatory and fibrogenic components of repair in the rat heart. *J Lab Clin Med* 2004;143:41–51.

28. Delcayre C, Swynghedauw B. Molecular mechanisms of myocardial remodeling. The role of aldosterone. *J Mol Cell Cardiol* 2002;34:1577–1584.

29. Shindo T, Manabe I, Fukushima Y, et al. Kruppel-like zinc-finger transcription factor KLF5/BTEB2 is a target for angiotensin II signaling and an essential regulator of cardiovascular remodeling. *Nat Med* 2002;8:856–863.

30. Sakata Y, Yamamoto K, Mano T, et al. Activation of matrix metalloproteinases precedes left ventricular remodeling in hypertensive heart failure rats: its inhibition as a primary effect of angiotensin-converting enzyme inhibitor. *Circulation* 2004;109:2143–2149.

31. Dzau VJ, Bernstein K, Celermajer D, et al., Working Group on Tissue Angiotensin-converting enzyme, International Society of Cardiovascular Pharmacotherapy. The relevance of tissue angiotensin-converting enzyme: manifestations in mechanistic and endpoint data. *Am J Cardiol* 2001;88:1L–20L.

32. Serneri GG, Boddi M, Cecioni I, et al. Cardiac angiotensin II formation in the clinical course of heart failure and its relationship with left ventricular function. *Circ Res* 2001;88:961–968.

33. Crackower MA, Sarao R, Oudit GY, et al. Angiotensin-converting enzyme 2 is an essential regulator of heart function. *Nature* 2002;417:822–828.

34. Boehm M, Nabel EG. Angiotensin-converting enzyme 2--a new cardiac regulator. *N Engl J Med* 2002;347:1795–1797.

35. Carey RM, Siragy HM. Newly recognized components of the renin-angiotensin system: potential roles in cardiovascular and renal regulation. *Endocr Rev* 2003;24:261–271.

36. Henrion D, Kubis N, Levy BI. Physiological and pathophysiological functions of the AT(2) subtype receptor of angiotensin II: from large arteries to the microcirculation. *Hypertension* 2001;38:1150–1157.

37. Effects of treatment on morbidity in hypertension. Results in patients with diastolic blood pressures averaging 115 through 129 mm Hg. *JAMA* 1967;202:1028–1034.

38. Effects of treatment on morbidity in hypertension. II. Results in patients with diastolic blood pressure averaging 90 through 114 mm Hg. *JAMA* 1970;213:1143–1152.

39. Turnbull F; Blood Pressure Lowering Treatment Trialists' Collaboration. Effects of different blood-pressure-lowering regimens on major cardiovascular events: results of prospectively-designed overviews of randomised trials. *Lancet* 2003;362:1527–1535.

40. Hansson L, Lindholm LH, Niskanen L, et al. Effect of angiotensin-converting-enzyme inhibition compared with conventional therapy on cardiovascular morbidity and mortality in hypertension: the Captopril Prevention Project (CAPPP) randomised trial. *Lancet* 1999;353:611–616.

41. Lindholm LH, Hansson L, Dahlof B, et al. The Swedish Trial in old patients with hypertension-2 (STOP-hypertension-2): a progress report. *Blood Press* 1996;5:300–304.

42. Major outcomes in high-risk hypertensive patients randomized to angiotensin-converting enzyme inhibitor or calcium channel blocker vs diuretic: the Antihypertensive and Lipid-Lowering Treatment to Prevent Heart Attack Trial (ALLHAT). *JAMA* 2002;288:2981–2997.

43. Wing LM, Reid CM, Ryan P, et al. A comparison of outcomes with angiotensin-converting enzyme inhibitors and diuretics for hypertension in the elderly. *N Engl J Med* 2003;348:583–592.

44. Major cardiovascular events in hypertensive patients randomized to doxazosin vs chlorthalidone: the antihypertensive and lipid-lowering treatment to prevent heart attack trial (ALLHAT). ALLHAT Collaborative Research Group. *JAMA* 2000;283:1967–1975.

45. Frohlich ED. Treating hypertension—what are we to believe? *N Engl J Med* 2003;348:639–641.

46. Sever P. ALLHAT: definitive answers or continuing uncertainty? *J Renin Angiotensin Aldosterone Syst* 2003;4:3–5.

47. Chalmers J. All hats off to ALLHAT: a massive study with clear messages. *J Hypertens* 2003;21:225–258.

48. Dahlof B, Devereux RB, Kjeldsen SE, et al. Cardiovascular morbidity and mortality in the Losartan Intervention For Endpoint reduction in hypertension study (LIFE): a randomised trial against atenolol. *Lancet* 2002;359:995–1003.

49. Lithell H, Hansson L, Skoog I, et al. The Study on Cognition and Prognosis in the Elderly (SCOPE): principal results of a randomized double-blind intervention trial. *J Hypertens* 2003;21:875–886.

50. Kjeldsen SE, Julius S, Brunner H, et al. Characteristics of 15,314 hypertensive patients at high coronary risk. The VALUE trial. The Valsartan Antihypertensive Long-term Use Evaluation. *Blood Press* 2001;10:83–91.

51. Mackenzie HS, Brenner BM. Current strategies for retarding progression of renal disease. *Am J Kidney Dis* 1998;31:161–170.

52. Lewis EJ, Hunsicker LG, Bain RP, et al. The effect of angiotensin-converting-enzyme inhibition on diabetic nephropathy. The Collaborative Study Group. *N Engl J Med* 1993;329:1456–1462.

53. Ravid M, Lang R, Rachmani R, et al. Long-term renoprotective effect of angiotensin-converting enzyme inhibition in non-insulin-dependent diabetes mellitus. A 7-year follow-up study. *Arch Intern Med* 1996;156:286–289.

54. Maschio G, Alberti D, Janin G, et al. Effect of the angiotensin-converting-enzyme inhibitor benazepril on the progression of chronic renal insufficiency. The Angiotensin-Converting-Enzyme Inhibition in Progressive Renal Insufficiency Study Group. *N Engl J Med* 1996;334:939–945.

55. Randomised placebo-controlled trial of effect of ramipril on decline in glomerular filtration rate and risk of terminal renal failure in proteinuric, non-diabetic nephropathy. The GISEN Group (Gruppo Italiano di Studi Epidemiologici in Nefrologia). *Lancet* 1997;349:1857–1863.

56. Lewis EJ, Hunsicker LG, Clarke WR, et al. Renoprotective effect of the angiotensin-receptor antagonist irbesartan in patients with nephropathy due to type 2 diabetes. *N Engl J Med* 2001;345:851–860.

57. Brenner BM, Cooper ME, de Zeeuw D, et al. Effects of losartan on renal and cardiovascular outcomes in patients with type 2 diabetes and nephropathy. *N Engl J Med* 2001;345:861–869.

58. Hostetter TH, Pfeffer JM, Pfeffer MA, et al. Cardiorenal hemodynamics and sodium excretion in rats with myocardial infarction. *Am J Physiol* 1983;245:H98–H103.

59. Effects of ramipril on cardiovascular and microvascular outcomes in people with diabetes mellitus: results of the HOPE study and MICRO-HOPE substudy. Heart Outcomes Prevention Evaluation Study Investigators. *Lancet* 2000;355:253–259.

60. Parving HH, Lehnert H, Brochner-Mortensen J, et al. The effect of irbesartan on the development of diabetic nephropathy in patients with type 2 diabetes. *N Engl J Med* 2001;345:870–878.

61. Nakao N, Yoshimura A, Morita H, et al. Combination treatment of angiotensin-II receptor blocker and angiotensin-converting-enzyme inhibitor in non-diabetic renal disease (COOPERATE): a randomised controlled trial. *Lancet* 2003;361:117–124.

62. Gaede P, Vedel P, Larsen N, et al. Multifactorial intervention and cardiovascular disease in patients with type 2 diabetes. *N Engl J Med* 2003;348:383–393.

63. Cohn JN, Archibald DG, Ziesche S, et al. Effect of vasodilator therapy on mortality in chronic congestive heart failure. Results of a Veterans Administration Cooperative Study. *N Engl J Med* 1986;314:1547–1552.

64. Dzau VJ, Colucci WS, Williams GH, et al. Sustained effectiveness of converting enzyme inhibition in patients with severe congestive heart failure. *N Engl J Med* 1980;302:1373–1379.

65. Gavras H, Faxon DP, Berkoben J, et al. Angiotensin converting enzyme inhibition in patients with congestive heart failure. *Circulation* 1978;58:770–776.

66. Effects of enalapril on mortality in severe congestive heart failure. Results of the Cooperative North Scandinavian Enalapril Survival Study (CONSENSUS). The CONSENSUS Trial Study Group. *N Engl J Med* 1987;316:1429–1435.

67. Effect of enalapril on survival in patients with reduced left ventricular ejection fractions and congestive heart failure. The SOLVD Investigators. *N Engl J Med* 1991;325:293–302.

68. Effect of enalapril on mortality and the development of heart failure in asymptomatic patients with reduced left ventricular ejection fractions. The SOLVD Investigators. *N Engl J Med* 1992;327:685–691.

69. Jong P, Yusuf S, Rousseau MF, et al. Effect of enalapril on 12-year survival and life expectancy in patients with left ventricular systolic dysfunction: a follow-up study. *Lancet* 2003;361:1843–1848.

70. Braunwald E. ACE inhibitors—a cornerstone of the treatment of heart failure. *N Engl J Med* 1991;325:351–353.

71. Pitt B, Segal R, Martinez FA, et al. Randomised trial of losartan versus captopril in patients over 65 with heart failure (Evaluation of Losartan in the Elderly Study, ELITE). *Lancet* 1997;349:747–752.

72. Pitt B, Poole-Wilson PA, Segal R, et al. Effect of losartan compared with captopril on mortality in patients with symptomatic heart failure: randomised trial—the Losartan Heart Failure Survival Study ELITE II. *Lancet* 2000;355:1582–1587.

73. Cohn JN, Tognoni G. A randomized trial of the angiotensin-receptor blocker valsartan in chronic heart failure. *N Engl J Med* 2001;345:1667–1675.

74. McMurray JJ, Östergren J, Swedberg K, et al. Effects of candesartan in patients with chronic heart failure and reduced left-ventricular systolic function taking angiotensin-converting-enzyme inhibitors: the CHARM-Added trial. *Lancet* 2003;362:767–771.

75. Granger CB, McMurray JJ, Yusuf S, et al. Effects of candesartan in patients with chronic heart failure and reduced left-ventricular systolic function intolerant to angiotensin-converting-enzyme inhibitors: the CHARM-Alternative trial. *Lancet* 2003;362:772–776.

76. Yusuf S, Pfeffer MA, Swedberg K, et al. Effects of candesartan in patients with chronic heart failure and preserved left-ventricular ejection fraction: the CHARM-Preserved trial. *Lancet* 2003;362:777–781.

77. Pfeffer MA, Swedberg K, Granger CB, et al. Effects of candesartan on mortality and morbidity in patients with chronic heart failure: the CHARM-Overall programme. *Lancet* 2003;362:759–766.

78. Pfeffer JM, Pfeffer MA, Fletcher PJ, et al. Progressive ventricular remodeling in rat with myocardial infarction. *Am J Physiol* 1991;260: H1406–H1414.

79. Pfeffer MA, Pfeffer JM, Steinberg C, et al. Survival after an experimental myocardial infarction: beneficial effects of long-term therapy with captopril. *Circulation* 1985;72:406–412.

80. Pfeffer MA, Lamas GA, Vaughan DE, et al. Effect of captopril on progressive ventricular dilatation after anterior myocardial infarction. *N Engl J Med* 1988;319:80–86.

81. Sharpe N, Smith H, Murphy J, et al. Treatment of patients with symptom-less left ventricular dysfunction after myocardial infarction. *Lancet* 1988;1:255–259.

82. Indications for ACE-inhibitors in the early treatment of acute myocardial infarction: systematic overview of individual data from 100,000 patients in randomized trials. ACE Inhibitor Myocardial Infarction Collaborative Group. *Circulation* 1998;97:2202–2212.

83. Swedberg K, Held P, Kjekshus J, et al. Effects of the early administration of enalapril on mortality in patients with acute myocardial infarction. Results of the Cooperative New Scandinavian Enalapril Survival Study II (CONSENSUS II). *N Engl J Med* 1992;327:678–684.

84. ISIS-4: A randomised factorial trial assessing early oral captopril, oral mononitrate, and intravenous magnesium sulphate in 58,050 patients with suspected acute myocardial infarction. ISIS-4 (Fourth International Study of Infarct Survival) Collaborative Group. *Lancet* 1995; 345:669–685.

85. GISSI-3: Effects of lisinopril and transdermal glyceryl trinitrate singly and together on 6-week mortality and ventricular function after acute myocardial infarction. Gruppo Italiano per lo Studio della Sopravvivenza nell'Infarto Miocardico. *Lancet* 1994;343:1115–1122.

86. Oral captopril versus placebo among 13,634 patients with suspected acute myocardial infarction: interim report from the Chinese Cardiac Study (CC-1). *Lancet* 1995;345:686–687.

87. Pfeffer MA, Braunwald E, Moye LA, et al. Effect of captopril on mortality and morbidity in patients with left ventricular dysfunction after myocardial infarction. Results of the survival and ventricular enlargement trial. The SAVE Investigators. *N Engl J Med* 1992;327:669–677.

88. Effect of ramipril on mortality and morbidity of survivors of acute myocardial infarction with clinical evidence of heart failure. Acute Infarction Ramipril Efficacy (AIRE) Study Investigators. *Lancet* 1993;342:821–828.

89. Kober L, Torp-Pedersen C, Carlsen JE, et al. A clinical trial of the angiotensin-converting-enzyme inhibitor trandolapril in patients with left ventricular dysfunction after myocardial infarction. Trandolapril Cardiac Evaluation (TRACE) Study Group. *N Engl J Med* 1995;333:1670–1676.

90. Ambrosioni E, Borghi C, Magnani B. The effect of the angiotensin-converting-enzyme inhibitor zofenopril on mortality and morbidity after anterior myocardial infarction. The Survival of Myocardial Infarction Long-Term Evaluation (SMILE) Study Investigators. *N Engl J Med* 1995;332:80–85.

91. Flather MD, Yusuf S, Kober L, et al. Long-term ACE-inhibitor therapy in patients with heart failure or left-ventricular dysfunction: a systematic overview of data from individual patients. *Lancet* 2000;355: 1575–1581.

92. Yusuf S, Pepine CJ, Garces C, et al. Effect of enalapril on myocardial infarction and unstable angina in patients with low ejection fractions. *Lancet* 1992;340:1173–1178.

93. Rutherford JD, Pfeffer MA, Moy_ LA, et al. Effects of captopril on ischemic events after myocardial infarction. Results of the Survival and Ventricular Enlargement Trial. SAVE Investigators. *Circulation* 1994;90:1731–1738.

94. Dickstein K, Kjekshus J. Effects of losartan and captopril on mortality and morbidity in high-risk patients after acute myocardial infarction: the OPTIMAAL randomised trial. Optimal Trial in Myocardial Infarction with Angiotensin II Antagonist Losartan. *Lancet* 2002;360:752–760.

95. Pfeffer MA, McMurray JJ, Velazquez EJ, et al. Valsartan, captopril, or both in myocardial infarction complicated by heart failure, left ventricular dysfunction, or both. *N Engl J Med* 2003;349:1893–1906.

96. Mann DL, Deswal A. Angiotensin-receptor blockade in acute myocardial infarction—a matter of dose. *N Engl J Med* 2003;349: 1963–1965.

97. Effects of an angiotensin-converting-enzyme inhibitor, ramipril, on cardiovascular events in high-risk patients. The Heart Outcomes Prevention Evaluation Study Investigators. *N Engl J Med* 2000;342:145–153.

98. Fox KM, EURopean trial On reduction of cardiac events with Perindopril in stable coronary Artery disease Investigators. Efficacy of perindopril in reduction of cardiovascular events among patients with stable coronary artery disease: randomised, double-blind, placebo-controlled, multicentre trial (the EUROPA study) *Lancet* 2003;362:782–788.

99. Pfeffer MA, Domanski M, Verter J, et al. The continuation of the Prevention of Events With Angiotensin-Converting Enzyme Inhibition (PEACE) Trial. *Am Heart J* 2001;142:375–377.

100. Yusuf S. From the HOPE to the ONTARGET and the TRANSCEND studies: challenges in improving prognosis. *Am J Cardiol* 2002;89: 18A–26A.

CHAPTER 82

Role of β-Adrenergic Blockade

William H. Frishman

Key Words: β-Blockade; myocardial infarction; risk stratification.

INTRODUCTION

Despite a decline in the incidence of coronary heart disease in the United States, more than 600,000 patients are admitted to hospitals annually with a diagnosis of acute myocardial infarction (AMI) (1). For patients having their first infarction, without pharmacologic intervention there is a 13% in-hospital mortality rate; the figure is greater for patients with recurrent infarctions (2,3). On hospital discharge, patients continue to have an increased risk for cardiovascular morbidity and mortality. Patients younger than 70 years who survive the in-hospital phase of MI have a 10% mortality rate in the first year after discharge, with the greatest proportion of deaths occurring within the first 3 months (2,3). Subsequently, there is a 5% annual mortality rate, which is six times greater than the expected rate in an age-matched population without coronary disease (2). Approximately 85% of deaths that occur after hospital discharge are related to coronary artery disease, and almost half are sudden deaths. Related to recurrent coronary artery thrombosis, both ventricular tachyarrhythmias and bradyarrhythmias appear to be primary causes of sudden death.

Prospective epidemiologic studies have identified subsets of infarct patients with a high, intermediate, or low risk for mortality, related in part to left ventricular (LV) functioning (4,5). Prolonging life in this heterogeneous

group of patients is a major goal of preventive therapy. To reach this goal, a variety of therapeutic approaches have been evaluated, including lifestyle measures (dietary modification, cessation of smoking, physical exercise) and coronary artery reconstructive procedures (6). Specific pharmacologic agents have included lipid-lowering drugs, anticoagulants, thrombolytic drugs, drugs that inhibit platelet aggregation, antiarrhythmic drugs, angiotensin-converting enzyme (ACE) inhibitors, calcium-entry blockers, and β-adrenergic blockers (6). The calcium-entry blockers and β-adrenergic blockers have always appeared to be attractive preventive measures in patients because of their antiischemic, antiarrhythmic, and antihypertensive actions (7), and aspirin is attractive because of its antithrombotic activity (8).

β-ADRENERGIC BLOCKADE

β-Adrenergic blockers have been proven safe and effective for the treatment of patients with various cardiovascular disorders (9). Since 1965, they have been considered as possible therapies for extending life in patients who survived MI (6). On the basis of multiple long-term clinical studies, the efficacy of β-blockers in reducing the risk for mortality and nonfatal reinfarction in survivors of an AMI has been proven (6,10). They also have been shown to reduce the extent of myocardial injury and mortality during the acute phase of MI (6). Finally, β-blockers have been suggested for the primary prevention of MI and death in patients with hypertension, stable angina, and unstable angina; their protective effects in these conditions, however, are less well defined (11,12).

W. H. Frishman: New York Medical College/Westchester Medical Center, Munger Pavillon, Valhalla, New York 10595.

Long-Term Reduction of Cardiovascular Mortality Risk in Survivors of Acute Myocardial Infarction

The presumed major mechanism for increased risk for cardiovascular mortality during the postinfarction period include persistent myocardial ischemia and reinfarction, cardiac arrhythmias, and LV dysfunction (1–6,11). Increases in plasma catecholamine levels or enhanced sympathetic drive can increase both the severity of myocardial ischemia and the frequency of ventricular arrhythmias. After the clinical introduction of propranolol for therapy of angina pectoris and arrhythmias, it was proposed that a β-blocker might favorably influence the natural history of patients with MI by attenuating the undesirable consequences of increased sympathetic nervous system activity (6,11,13). Depression of LV function, the other major risk factor contributing to mortality after infarction, can be caused by β-blockade (9,13). For this reason, β-blockers were initially avoided or used in small doses in patients with MI. Only in the last 25 years have the results of long-term studies demonstrated the benefit of β-blockade in reducing total mortality and nonfatal reinfarction (6,10,11).

Long-Term β-Blocker Prevention Trials

Since 1974, 16 major randomized controlled trials with β-blockers after AMI have been reported, with treatment and mean follow-up extending from 9 months to 6 years (14–36). More than 18,000 survivors of AMI were studied in an attempt to document reductions in total mortality, cardiovascular mortality, coronary mortality, sudden death, and nonfatal reinfarction. Eleven different β-blockers have been evaluated in these studies: acebutolol, alprenolol, atenolol, carvedilol, metoprolol, oxprenolol, pindolol, practolol, propranolol, sotalol, and timolol (Table 82–1) (14–36). The 16 trials met the following criteria for study design: a trial end

TABLE 82–1. *Pharmacologic properties of the β-adrenoceptor blocking drugs tested in long-term trials*

Drug	Relative β-selectivity	Intrinsic sympathomimetic activity	Membrane-stabilizing activity
Acebutolol	+	+	0
Alprenolol[a]	0	+	+
Atenolol	+	0	0
Carvedilol[b]	0	0	0
Metoprolol	+	0	0
Oxprenolol[a]	0	+	+
Pindolol	0	++	0
Practolol[a]	+	+	0
Propranolol	0	0	++
Sotalol	0	0	0
Timolol	0	0	0

[a]Not available for clinical use in the United States.
[b]Has additional α-adrenergic blocking activity.
From Frishman WH, Furberg DC, Friedewald WT. β-Adrenergic blockade for survivors of acute myocardial infarction. *N Engl J Med* 1984;310:830–836, with permission.

point of total mortality or a clearly defined cause-specific mortality, a total sample size of at least 200, and random assignment of patients to either the β-blocker group or a concurrently following control group. The study populations contained from 230 to 3,837 patients (14–36). Fifteen of the 16 trials used a placebo-treated control group and had a double-blind phase. The time between the infarction and the start of β-blocker or placebo treatment ranged from less than 24 hours to 7.5 years. In 12 trials, patients in the low- and intermediate-risk groups were studied predominantly (14–16,18–21,25–32), and in four trials only high-risk patients were evaluated (17,24,33,34).

The results from 13 of the 16 long-term trials showed a lower mortality rate in the β-blocker group than in the placebo group (Table 82–2) (14–17,19,20,24–26,28–34,36). In the four large studies, the reduction in mortality with β-blockade was statistically significant (20,28,29,34,36). In the remaining nine trials, the results were not always conclusive with regard to overall mortality.

With the results of all 16 β-blocker trials combined, mortality was reduced by approximately 21%. Caution is advised in interpreting such results from pooled data because of the inherent differences among the studies in the patient population, type and dosage of β-blocker, and time of initiation and duration of treatment (6,10,11,23).

Eleven of the 12 trials reporting on the incidence of nonfatal reinfarction showed lower rates in the actively treated groups (6,11,33,34). This lower incidence was statistically significant in only two of the trials. A comparison of the effect of treatment on the incidence of nonfatal reinfarction is complicated for many reasons. The diagnostic criteria for infarction differed among the trials, for example, resulting in large differences in incidence. A statistical test for homogeneity, however, indicated that the result of each trial was consistent with those of the others. When all the findings from the 12 placebo-controlled, double-blind trials are pooled, the reduction in nonfatal reinfarction is 22%, a benefit almost identical to that for overall mortality.

It has been suggested that β-blocker treatment should be started on admission to the hospital to reduce the high rate of mortality among inpatients. In general, short-term intravenous treatment trials were designed to provide information about infarct size, arrhythmias, and pain relief, not mortality (10,11,35). In three large studies in which intravenous β-blocker treatment was followed by oral treatment, a true reduction of about 15% was observed in the inpatient mortality compared with placebo or control (36–38).

Possible Mechanisms of Benefit

Antiarrhythmic Effects

An analysis of cause-specific mortality in the β-blocker trials indicates that the reductions in total mortality were caused by a reduction in cardiovascular deaths (Table 82–1) (6,11). Although different definitions of sudden death were

TABLE 82–2. *Results of long-term (more than 9 months) β-blocker trials*

Author/Study (reference)	Number of patients		Mortality		
	Control	Randomized intervention	Control, %	Intervention, %	p Value[a]
Wilhelmsson et al. (32)	116	114	12.1	6.1	0.18
Ahlmark and Saetre (14)[b]	93	69	11.8	7.2	0.48
Barber et al. (19)[c]	147	151	31.3	27.2	0.51
Multicentre International Study (29)	1,520	1,533	8.2	6.3	0.051
Andersen et al. (16)[c]	242	238	26.2	25.2	0.92
Baber et al. (18)	3,654	355	7.4	7.9	0.91
Norwegian Multicenter Study (28)	939	945	16.2	10.4	0.0003
BHAT (20)	1,921	1,916	9.8	7.2	0.005
Hansteen et al. (24)	282	278	13.1	9.0	0.16
Julian et al. (26)	583	873	8.9	7.3	0.32
Taylor et al. (30)	471	632	10.2	9.5	0.78
Pindolol Study Group (17)	266	263	17.7	17.1	0.36
European Infarction Study (21)	880	861	5.1	6.6	0.14
Lopressor Intervention Trial (27)	1,200	1,195	5.2	5.5	0.90
Boissel et al. (33)	309	298	11.0	5.7	0.013
CAPRICORN (34)	984	975	15.0	12.0	0.031

BHAT, Beta-Blocker Heart Attack Trial; CAPRICORN, Carvedilol Post-Infarct Survival Control in Left Ventricular Dysfunction Study.
[a]p Values computed for χ^2 test comparing the proportion of deaths in each.
[b]Incomplete reporting.
[c]Mortality includes all in-hospital deaths.
From Frishman WH. *Clinical pharmacology of the beta-adrenergic blocking drugs,* 2nd ed. Norwalk: Appleton-Century-Croft, 1984:319.

reported in the trials, a large part of the benefit from β-blocker therapy appears to have stemmed from the prevention of these deaths (6,11,22). Nine trials reported on sudden death; the rates of sudden cardiac death were lower in the β-blocker group for all nine trials (22,33). β-Blocker treatment appears to manifest a trend toward a greater overall reduction in sudden cardiac death than in all-cause mortality. The weighted risk ratios for sudden cardiac death vary between 0.15 and 0.84 (mean 0.67), indicating an overall reduction of 33% in sudden cardiac death. Indeed, if sudden cardiac deaths are subtracted from all-cause mortality, the remaining death rate is 3.5% in the intervention group and 4.4% in the control group, which represents an intervention/control risk ratio of nonsudden death of 0.8. Thus, although nonsudden deaths are reduced by 20% in these trials, the sudden cardiac death rate is reduced to a greater extent.

For witnessed instantaneous deaths, an even larger relative benefit from β-blocker therapy was recorded. The reduction was 59% in one study (28), 46% in a second (24), and 37% in a third (19), corresponding to an average reduction in instantaneous death of 46%. For these three trials, the pooled reduction in all-cause mortality was 31%, indicating that the relative reduction in instantaneous deaths is about 50% greater than that in all-cause mortality. When the instantaneous deaths are removed from the all-cause mortality, the pooled reduction in death in the remaining patients becomes 23%, and the relative reduction in instantaneous deaths is twice as great.

Three of the seven trials obtained 24-hour ambulatory electrocardiographic (ECG) records on a subset of their participants, both at trial entry and at a subsequent follow-up visit (20,26,28). The findings of these three trials are similar. In the subgroup of survivors who entered the trial with frequent ventricular premature beats, fewer patients demonstrated this type of arrhythmia at a later follow-up visit than in the placebo groups (26,39,40). Among patients with frequent ventricular premature beats at entry, many continued to have this type of arrhythmia at follow-up, although fewer patients were on β-blockers than on placebo (26,39,40). Although the recorded episodes of ventricular tachycardia were few in all trials at follow-up, this arrhythmia was less common in patients receiving β-blockers than in those on placebo.

In the trials, a greater serum potassium level and a shorter corrected ECG QT interval were noted in patients receiving β-blockers compared with those receiving placebo (26,41). β-Blockers have been observed to attenuate transmembrane potassium fluxes in response to high catecholamine levels (42). Perhaps part of the protective effect of β-blockade comes from its ability to preserve normal serum potassium levels, especially in those patients receiving concurrent diuretic therapy (41). Propranolol also helps to restore heart rate variability after MI, which is associated with increased parasympathetic tone, decreased morning sympathetic tone, and improved clinical outcomes (43).

The Cardiac Arrhythmia Suppression Trial (CAST) showed antiarrhythmic drug suppression of asymptomatic ventricular arrhythmias in survivors of MI to be harmful (44). In contrast, in those patients who received optional β-blocker therapy, there was significantly enhanced survival at 30 days and at 1 to 2 years of follow-up against all-cause and arrhythmic death or nonfatal cardiac arrest. β-Blockers were independently associated with a one-third reduction in arrhythmic death or cardiac arrest. In CAST patients with a history of congestive heart failure, β-blocker therapy was independently associated with a longer time to occurrence of new or worsened congestive heart failure. The study supports the secondary preventive benefit of β-blocker therapy in high-risk patients after MI and provides evidence that β-blockers may counteract the proarrhythmic effects of other antiarrhythmic drugs (45).

Antiischemic Effects

Because the incidence of nonsudden cardiac deaths and nonfatal reinfarction was reduced by β-blockade in the long-term trials, the antiischemic actions of the drugs also may have contributed to their beneficial effects in the postinfarction period (Table 82–3).

Stimulation of cardiac β-adrenergic receptors by endogenous catecholamines increases myocardial oxygen consumption and can thereby aggravate the ischemic process. Drugs that block the β-adrenergic receptor reduce the effects of catecholamines and decrease myocardial oxygen requirements by reducing systemic arterial pressure, heart rate, and myocardial contractility at rest and during exercise (6,9). The effects of these drugs on coronary blood flow are less well defined. β-Blockers may decrease coronary blood flow by allowing the unopposed influence of coronary vasoconstrictor impulses to prevail. Furthermore, these drugs may also augment or maintain overall coronary blood flow by slowing the heart rate and increasing diastolic perfusion time (6,9,46). More controversial are those studies reporting favorable effects of β-blockers on myocardial metabolism, apoptosis, the coronary microvasculature, collateral blood flow, the distribution of myocardial blood flow, and oxygen–hemoglobin affinity. One or several of these antiisch-

---

TABLE 82–3. *Possible mechanisms by which β-blockers protect the ischemic myocardium*

- Reduction in myocardial consumption, heart rate, blood pressure, and myocardial contractility
- Augmentation of coronary blood flow; increase in diastolic perfusion time by reducing heart rate, augmentation of collateral blood flow, and coronary flow reserve; and redistribution of blood flow to ischemic areas
- Prevention of attenuation of atherothrombotic plaque, rupture, and subsequent coronary thrombosis
- Alterations in myocardial substrate utilization
- Decrease in microvascular damage
- Stabilization of cell and lysosomal membranes
- Shift of oxyhemoglobin dissociation curve to the right
- Inhibition of platelet aggregation
- Inhibition of myocardial apoptosis, allowing natural cell regeneration to occur

From Frishman WH. Alpha- and beta-adrenergic blocking drugs. In: Frishman WH, Sonnenblick EH, Sica DA, eds. *Cardiovascular pharmacotherapeutics,* 2nd ed. New York: McGraw-Hill, 2003:67–97, with permission.

---

emic mechanisms may underlie the beneficial effects of β-blocker therapy in survivors of MI.

Prevention of Atherothrombotic Plaque Tears

Coronary thrombi large enough to be detected by angiography often are associated with tears (fissures) in the caps of atherothrombotic plaques (47,48). These tears allow blood to penetrate into the arterial wall, leading to thrombus formation within the intima; this may be followed by propagation of thrombosis into the vessel lumen. This process was described more than 75 years ago (49,50); however, its clinical importance has been realized more recently after the microanatomy of coronary thrombi was established by serial histologic sectioning (51–54). Plaque tears have been recognized in the angiograms of living patients with unstable angina (55), in patients with AMI (56), and in patients resuscitated from sudden cardiac death (57). Angioscopy in living patients with unstable angina also has confirmed the presence of mural thrombi on torn atherothrombotic plaques in the coronary arteries (58,59).

Why a plaque becomes susceptible to rupture is not known. It is presumed to be a dynamic, reversible disorder caused by changes in the constituents of the plaque, its blood supply through the vasa vasorum, the influence of matrix metalloproteinases, or the functional integrity of the overlying endothelium (60,61). Computer modeling of different forms of plaque have shown that the distribution of circumferential tensile stress across the intima can be radically influenced by atherothrombotic plaques. Regions of high circumferential stress correlated closely with the sites of intimal tears found on autopsy.

It has been proposed that sudden increases in blood pressure, myocardial contractility, or both precipitated by physical or mental stress and surges in sympathetic tone could produce hemodynamic changes leading to plaque rupture. These surges in sympathetic nervous activity also could increase platelet aggregability and possibly coronary vascular tone. β-Adrenergic blockade may modulate or attenuate the consequences of these sympathetic nervous system surges by inhibiting the effects of catecholamines on blood pressure, heart rate, and myocardial contractility (62).

β-Blockers are known to protect the aorta from acute dissection and to reduce the incidence of recurrent dissection (9). This is accomplished, in part, by the ability of β-blockers to reduce blood pressure and myocardial contractility. Comparing propranolol with hydralazine, using Doppler ultrasonography, Spence (63) found that propranolol was more likely to reduce the velocity of blood flow and the likelihood of nonlaminar blood flow in the aorta, thereby reducing turbulence and vortex formation (as heart rate blood velocity product is a determinant of arterial blood flow disturbance). It is postulated that this effect of β-blockers also could reduce the risk for endothelial damage and plaque rupture; subsequent coronary thrombosis would be less likely to occur. In addition, some β-blockers also have weak antiplatelet effects that, in addition, might prevent the development or propagation, or both, of clots (8,64).

β-Adrenoceptor Blockade in the Early Phase of Myocardial Infarction

β-Adrenergic blockers have been considered for use as standard therapy in patients with AMI to prevent the undesirable consequences of increased sympathoadrenal discharge, arrhythmogenesis, and extension of myocardial injury (10, 20,37). The drugs can alter those factors that determine increases in myocardial oxygen consumption and may augment coronary blood flow by increasing diastolic perfusion time (46). They also may reduce the incidence of ventricular fibrillation. However, β-adrenergic blockade can have unfavorable consequences in some cases of acute infarction. Cardiac impulse formation may be impaired greatly, and conduction diminished to a degree that causes cardiac arrest (46). Furthermore, exacerbation of congestive heart failure in those patients dependent on the positive inotropic effect of catecholamines is a well recognized sequela of β-blockade (46).

Clinical Recommendations

Intravenous administration of a β-blocker within a few hours after the onset of chest pain markedly reduces pain and the need for narcotic analgesia in patients with MI (35). Pain relief is associated closely with a reduction in the systolic blood pressure and heart rate product. β-Blockade also reduces the number of episodes of ventricular fibrillation compared with placebo treatment in patients with MI (35). On thesis of crude measures of infarct size, such as cumulative creatine phosphokinase (CPK) release and development of Q waves on the ECG, it is clear that β-blockade is associated with less creatine phosphokinase release and better preservation of the R wave on the ECG than placebo (10, 11,35,65–69). β₁-Adrenergic blockade appears to be necessary. Compared with placebo, the pyrexial response that accompanies MI is diminished by β-blockade (35), serum potassium is preserved at a more normal level (41,70), and the number of patients with threatened infarction going on to frank infarction often is reduced (35,69).

It has been suggested that β-blocker treatment should be started on admission to the hospital to reduce the high rate of mortality among inpatients. In general, short-term intravenous treatment trials were designed to provide information about infarct size, arrhythmias, and pain relief, not mortality (10,11,35). In three large studies in which intravenous β-blocker treatment was followed by oral treatment, a true reduction of about 15% was observed in the inpatient mortality rate compared with placebo or control (10,36,37).

The Metoprolol in Acute Myocardial Infarction (MIAMI) study set out to evaluate the effect of metoprolol on mortality in patients entering the hospital within 24 hours of the onset of chest pain (38). Included in the study were 5,778

patients considered to be in a low-risk category, in that patients with bradycardia, hypotension, and LV failure were excluded. Patients received either placebo or intravenous metoprolol (15 mg) followed by oral metoprolol for 15 days. A nonsignificant reduction in mortality of 13% was observed. Retrospective subgroup analysis suggested that an older population of patients with associated risks (previous angina, previous infarction, and diabetes) experienced a 29% reduction in mortality (38).

The First International Study of Infarct Survival (ISIS-I) was a large, simple, open, randomized investigation designed to establish the effect of short-term atenolol treatment on total mortality and cardiovascular mortality at 1 week and 1 year after the onset of chest pain (37). Intravenous atenolol (5–10 mg) was administered, followed by oral atenolol, 100 mg daily for 1 week. As in the MIAMI trial (38), a low-risk population was studied (4.5% mortality at 1 week in the control group) (37). More than 16,000 patients were randomized; 80% were admitted to the study within 8 hours of chest pain. A significant reduction in cardiovascular mortality of 15% was observed with atenolol therapy. The benefit of atenolol was confined to the first 36 hours. The reduction in mortality on Day 0 to Day 1 was 32% (similar to that observed in the MIAMI study). Nonfatal cardiac arrests were not reduced by atenolol treatment, suggesting a reduction in infarct size as a cause for the mortality reduction (35,37), but a subsequent analysis implied a major benefit from atenolol on the frequency of cardiac rupture (37).

Patients in the ISIS were followed for 1 year. The cardiovascular mortality rate was 10.1% in the atenolol group and 11.3% in the control group, representing a 10.6% reduction in mortality (37). The extra lives saved during Days 8 to 365 most likely were related to intravenous β-blockade, because, at hospital discharge, more patients in the atenolol group remained on β-blocker than in the control group (35% vs. 26%) (37). An early intervention study in 1,395 patients with MI randomized to receive intravenous metoprolol followed by 200 mg per day orally or placebo for 3 months (36) showed that the significant early benefit in mortality reduction at 90 days was still present 2 years later. The benefit, however, was not present 5 years later (71).

There is evidence from the Thrombolysis in Myocardial Infarction Trial (TIMI) and the Global Utilization for Streptokinase and tPA for Occluded Coronary Arteries (GUSTO-I) that concomitant β-blockade with thrombolysis during AMI could reduce subsequent ischemic events (72,73).

Use of β-Blockade in Clinical Practice

It has been demonstrated conclusively that β-blockers can prolong life in patients who have had infarction (11). Should all patients receive β-blockers after an MI? There are obvious contraindications to the use of β-blockers, such as pulmonary edema, Raynaud's phenomenon, bronchospastic conditions, significant disorders of atrioventricular and sinus node function, and possibly vasospastic angina (Table 82–4). These conditions restrict the postinfarction population in whom β-blocker therapy can be administered. Moreover, in the major postinfarction β-blocker studies, approximately 50% of the eligible patients (including many high-risk individuals) were excluded (11). Similar patient selection should be used if comparable mortality reduction is to be achieved in standard clinical practice. It is estimated that 80% of infarction survivors who survive the acute phase of MI can be safely started on β-blockers. Why this is not happening in clinical practice probably relates to the ongoing misconception that β-blockers should not be used in patients with LV dysfunction or in patients with chronic obstructive lung disease without bronchospasm (74). It also has been shown that if patients are not discharged from the hospital on β-blockers, they are unlikely to be started on them as outpatients (75).

Use of β-blocker therapy has been shown to be a more common practice among cardiologists than general internists and family practitioners, demonstrating the need to educate practicing physicians about the results of clinical trials (76). It appears from the findings of recent studies that the greatest benefit from β-blocker therapy is achieved in patients who are older than 60 years and in the medium- or high-risk postinfarction group (i.e., patients with LV dysfunction, arrhythmias, or both) (10,11,77). There is a serious question whether the low-risk postinfarction patient (first infarct, no LV dysfunction, normal predischarge exercise test results, and absence of complex ventricular arrhythmias) who has a 1-year posthospital discharge mortality rate of 2% requires prophylactic treatment with β-blockers (76). It also is unknown whether β-blockers should be used as long-term prophylactic therapy in those patients who have undergone successful coronary bypass surgery or angioplasty (11). Certainly, postinfarction patients with angina pectoris, hypertension, supraventricular arrhythmias, or strongly positive graded exercise tests should be considered for treatment with β-blockers as soon as these indications arise (11).

Is one β-adrenergic blocker superior to another in survivors of AMI, or is there a common protective effect seen with all the drugs in this class? Trials investigating 11 different β-blockers found favorable mortality trends, suggesting that the benefit is conferred by the drug class rather than by a specific β-blocker.

TABLE 82–4. *Contraindications to β-adrenergic blockade during acute myocardial infarction*

- Heart failure with pulmonary congestion
- Heart block (disorders of atrioventricular and sinus node function) unless pacemaker in place
- Inferior wall myocardial infarction with suspect right ventricular infarction
- Bronchospastic lung disease
- Hypotension
- Previous problems with β-blocker treatment

When should treatment be initiated with β-blockers, by what route, at which dose, and for how long? It appears from multiple studies that β-adrenergic blockade can be initiated early and safely to hemodynamically stable patients with and without thrombolysis (approximately 50% of patients with MIs) (10). Caution should be given in administering β-blockers to patients with transmural inferior wall MI, where hemodynamic complications of a right ventricular infarction might be unmasked.

Intravenous metoprolol and atenolol are currently approved for use in MI. Timolol was the first orally active β-blocker to be approved by the U.S. Food & Drug Administration as a long-term prophylactic agent in survivors of an AMI, at a fixed daily dose of 20 mg in 2 divided doses. Propranolol also was approved for this use at a range of 180 to 240 mg daily in 2 to 3 divided doses to be started 5 to 21 days after the onset of infarction. Oral metoprolol in doses of 100 mg twice daily and oral atenolol are approved for long-term use. Whether the sustained-release form of propranolol or metoprolol will be effective as a postinfarction treatment needs to be determined. Sustained-release metoprolol and carvedilol were approved for use in patients with LV dysfunction already receiving ACE inhibitors (78,79). It also is not clear whether a fixed-dose regimen of these drugs is preferable to a titration until clinical β-adrenergic blockade is achieved. In patients having MI and LV dysfunction, it is best to titrate the β-blocker dose gradually to avoid decompensation of ventricular function (34,78,80).

No conclusive data are available regarding the effect of β-blocker therapy or mortality if the drugs are started months to years after acute infarction. Nevertheless, it is reasonable to assume that mortality and morbidity would be reduced if treatment were initiated within a few months after hospitalization. Support of this view arose from retrospective subgroup analyses of a long-term prevention study with oxprenolol in coronary heart disease (30). A beneficial effect on survival was noted if treatment was started within 4 months of an AMI, but there was no benefit if therapy was started 4 months or more after the event.

Some studies suggest that the major beneficial effects of β-blockers accrue during the first 12 to 18 months after infarction and that the incremental benefit thereafter is small (81). Limited information from one trial shows more deaths in the placebo treatment groups than in the β-blocker group as far out as 72 months (81), which suggests a sustained benefit from continued therapy.

If one is concerned with the extended use of these drugs in the general postinfarction population, patients in the intermediate- and high-risk subsets, who benefit the most from β-blocker therapy, might be candidates for longer courses of therapy. An argument for stopping β-blocker treatment after a fixed time period stems from the recent observation that some β-blockers can decrease plasma high-density lipoprotein cholesterol levels and triglyceride levels, potentially increasing the risk for atherogenesis (82). Whether this should

TABLE 82–5. *Recommendations for aspirin, β-adrenergic blockade, calcium entry blockade, and angiotensin-converting enzyme inhibition in patients with acute myocardial infarction*

Condition	Recommendations
Hyperacute phase	Thrombolysis, β-adrenergic blockade, aspirin, or their combination; use ACE inhibitors with caution
Long-term treatment of survivors[a]	
Q-wave infarction (good LV function)	β-Adrenergic blockade, ACE inhibitors, aspirin, or their combination; calcium entry blockers (diltiazem or verapamil) in patients who cannot tolerate β-blockade
Q-wave infarction (diminished LV function, EF < 40%)	β-Adrenergic blockade (if tolerated), aspirin, ACE inhibitors; avoid calcium channel blockade
Non–Q-wave infarction (good LV function)	Calcium channel blockade (diltiazem), aspirin, β-adrenergic blockade, or their combination
Non–Q-wave infarction (diminished LV function, EF <40%)	β-Adrenergic blockade (if tolerated), aspirin, ACE inhibitors

ACE, angiotensin-converting enzyme; EF, ejection fraction; LV, left ventricular.

[a]All long-term survivors should have their low-density lipoprotein cholesterol reduced <100 mg/dL with dietary or pharmacologic therapy, or both, and be encouraged to stop tobacco smoking.

Adapted from Skolnick AE, Frishman WH. Calcium channel blockers in myocardial infarction. *Arch Intern Med* 1989; 149:1675, with permission.

be a concern in patients who already have advanced heart disease is debatable.

Finally, in the long-term postinfarction trials, there was no evidence of a β-blocker "withdrawal reaction" in patients who discontinued active treatment (83). Patients who require continued β-blocker treatment for other reasons (angina pectoris, hypertension, migraine, and arrhythmias) should be maintained on this treatment regimen as needed.

How will postinfarction β-blocker therapy affect use of coronary reconstructive procedures in this population? Myocardial revascularization surgery appears to be of benefit in patients with significant angina and angiographically documented severe left main or three-vessel coronary artery disease. Therapy with β-blockers should reduce the frequency and severity of angina and, therefore, may diminish clinical indications for coronary angiography, angioplasty, and bypass surgery. In addition, because there is a documented reduction in 1-year postinfarction mortality with β-blockers, risk–benefit considerations may now favor continued medical therapy rather than surgical intervention in many patients (11,75).

Is there a difference in the postinfarction safety profiles of the different β-blockers? Severe side effects from β-adrenergic blocking drugs were infrequent in the postinfarction trials. Compared with placebo, there appeared to be a greater incidence of symptomatic congestive heart failure, sinus bradycardia, hypotension, bronchial obstruction, fatigue, and mental depression with the β-blockers (84). Caution still should be exercised, however, when using β-blockers in high-risk patients whose myocardial function may be dependent on stimulation from the sympathetic nervous system. However, with the concomitant use of ACE inhibitors and diuretics, β-blockers appear to be well tolerated in most patients with LV dysfunction (85).

SUMMARY

Independent of mechanism, appropriate use of β-blockers in postinfarction patients should improve the outcome of many patients with MI. The addition of β-blockers to acute thrombolysis may improve patient outcome to a greater extent than either drug alone (72). The long-term benefit of combining β-blockers with antiplatelet agents and ACE inhibitors seems to be an ideal approach for reducing mortality and morbidity in survivors of an AMI. An approach to using β-blockers relative to other protective therapies in MI is shown in Table 82–5.

REFERENCES

1. May GS, Furberg CD, Eberlein KA, et al. Secondary prevention after myocardial infarction: a review of short-term acute phase trials. *Prog Cardiovasc Dis* 1983;25:335–359.
2. May GS, Eberlein KA, Furberg CD, et al. Secondary prevention after myocardial infarction: a review of long-term trials. *Prog Cardiovasc Dis* 1982;24:331–352.
3. Law MR, Watt HC, Wald NJ. The underlying risk of death after myocardial infarction in the absence of treatment. *Arch Intern Med* 2002;162: 2405–2410.
4. Davis HT, DeCamilla J, Bayer LW, et al. Survivorship patterns in posthospital phase of myocardial infarction. *Circulation* 1979;60:1252–1258.
5. Risk stratification after myocardial infarction. Multicenter Postinfarction Research Group. *N Engl J Med* 1983;309:331–336.
6. Frishman WH, Furberg DC, Friedewald WT. β-Adrenergic blockade for survivors of acute myocardial infarction. *N Engl J Med* 1984;310: 830–836.
7. Frishman WH, Skolnick AE, Lazar EJ, et al. β-Adrenergic blockade and calcium channel blockade in myocardial infarction. *Med Clin North Am* 1989;73:409–436.
8. Miller KP, Frishman WH. Platelets and antiplatelet therapy in ischemic heart disease. *Med Clin North Am* 1988;72:117–184.
9. Frishman WH. Alpha- and beta-adrenergic blocking drugs. In: Frishman WH, Sonnenblick EH, Sica DA, eds. *Cardiovascular pharmacotherapeutics*, 2nd ed. New York: McGraw Hill, 2003:67–97.
10. Yusuf S, Peto R, Lewis J, et al. β-Blockade during and after myocardial infarction: an overview of the randomized trials. *Prog Cardiovasc Dis* 1985;27:335–371.
11. Frishman WH, Furberg CD, Friedewald WT. The use of β-adrenergic blocking drugs in patients with myocardial infarction. *Curr Prob Cardiol* 1984;9:1–50.
12. Braunwald E, Antman EM, Beasley JW, et al. ACC/AHA 2002 guideline update for the management of patients with unstable angina and non-ST-segment elevation myocardial infarction–summary article: a report of the American College of Cardiology/American Heart Associ-

ation task force on practice guidelines (Committee on the Management of Patients With Unstable Angina). *Circulation* 2002;106:1893–1900.

13. Frishman WH. β-Adrenoceptor antagonists. New drugs and new indications. *N Engl J Med* 1981;305:500–506.

14. Ahlmark G, Saetre H. Long-term treatment with β-blockers after myocardial infarction. *Eur J Clin Pharmacol* 1976;10:77–83.

15. Ahlmark G, Saetre H, Korsgren M. Reduction of sudden deaths after myocardial infarction. *Lancet* 1974;2:1563.

16. Andersen MP, Bechsgaard P, Frederiksen J, et al. Effect of alprenolol on mortality among patients with definite or suspected acute myocardial infarction: preliminary results. *Lancet* 1979;2:865–868.

17. The effect of pindolol on the two years mortality after complicated myocardial infarction. *Eur Heart J* 1983;4:367–375.

18. Baber NS, Wainwright-Evans D, Howitt G, et al. Multicentre postinfarction trial of propranolol in 40 hospitals in the United Kingdom, Italy, and Yugoslavia. *Br Heart J* 1980;44:96–100.

19. Barber JM, Boyle DM, Chaturvedi NC, et al. Practolol in acute myocardial infarction. *Acta Med Scand* 1975;587[Suppl]:213–219.

20. A randomized trial of propranolol in patients with acute myocardial infarction. I. Mortality results. Beta-Blocker Heart Attack Trial Research Group. *JAMA* 1981;247:1707–1714.

21. European Infarction Study (E.I.S.). A secondary prevention study with slow release oxprenolol after myocardial infarction: morbidity and mortality. *Eur Heart J* 1984;5:189–202.

22. Frishman WH, Laifer LI, Furberg CD. β-Adrenergic blockers in the prevention of sudden death. In: Josephson ME, ed. *Sudden cardiac death.* Philadelphia: FA Davis, 1985:249–264.

23. Furberg CD, Bell RL. Effect of β-blocker therapy on recurrent nonfatal myocardial infarction. *Circulation* 1983;67[6 Pt 2]:I-83–I-85.

24. Hansteen V, Moinichen E, Lorentsen E, et al. One year's treatment with propranolol after myocardial infarction: preliminary report of Norwegian multicentre trial. *Br Med J* 1982;284:155–160.

25. Improvement in prognosis of myocardial infarction by long-term β-adrenoceptor blockade using practolol. A multicenter international study. *Br Med J* 1975;3:735–740.

26. Julian DG, Prescott RJ, Jackson FS, et al. A controlled trial of sotalol for 1 year after myocardial infarction. *Lancet* 1982;1:1142–1147.

27. The Lopressor Intervention Trial: multicentre study of metoprolol in survivors of acute myocardial infarction. Lopressor Intervention Trial Research Group. *Eur Heart J* 1987;8:1056–1064.

28. Timolol reduces mortality and reinfarct in patients surviving acute myocardial infarct. *N Engl J Med* 1981;304:801–807.

29. Greene KG, Chamberlain DA, Rulton RM, et al. Reduction in mortality after myocardial infarction with long-term β-adrenoceptor blockade: multicentre international study. Supplementary report. *Br Med J* 1977;2:419–421.

30. Taylor SH, Silke B, Ebbutt A, et al. A long-term prevention study with oxprenolol in coronary heart disease. *N Engl J Med* 1982;307:1293–1301.

31. Vedin A, Wilhelmsson C, Werko L. Chronic alprenolol treatment of patients with acute myocardial infarction after discharge from hospital: effects on mortality and morbidity. *Acta Med Scand* 1975;575[Suppl]:1–40.

32. Wilhelmsson C, Vedin JA, Wilhelmsen L, et al. Reduction of sudden deaths after myocardial infarction by treatment with alprenolol: preliminary results. *Lancet* 1974;2:1157–1160.

33. Boissel JP, Leizorovicz A, Picolet H, et al. Secondary prevention after high-risk acute myocardial infarction with low-dose acebutolol. *Am J Cardiol* 1990;66:251–260.

34. Dargie HJ. Effect of carvedilol on outcome after myocardial infarction in patients with left-ventricular dysfunction: the CAPRICORN randomised trial. *Lancet* 2001;357:1385–1390.

35. Cruickshank JM, Prichard BN. *β-Blockers in clinical practice.* Edinburgh: Churchill Livingstone, 1987:435–504.

36. Hjalmarson A, Elmfeldt D, Herlitz J, et al. Effect on mortality of metoprolol in acute myocardial infarction: a double-blind randomized trial. *Lancet* 1981;2:823–827.

37. Randomised trial of intravenous atenolol among 16,027 cases of suspected acute myocardial infarction. ISIS-I. First International Study of Infarct Survival Collaborative Group. *Lancet* 1986;2:57–66.

38. Metoprolol in acute myocardial infarction (MIAMI). A randomized placebo-controlled international trial. The MIAMI Trial Research Group. *Eur Heart J* 1985;6:199–226.

39. Lichstein E, Morganroth J, Harrist R, et al. Effect of propranolol on ventricular arrhythmias. The Beta-Blocker Heart Attack Trial. *Circulation* 1983;67[Suppl 1]:I-5–I-10.

40. von der Lippe G, Lund-Johansen P, Kjekshus J. Effect of timolol on late ventricular arrhythmias after myocardial infarction. *Acta Med Scand* 1981;651[Suppl]:253–258.

41. Nordrehaug JE, Johannessen KA, von der Lippe G, et al. Effect of timolol on changes in serum potassium concentration during acute myocardial infarction. *Br Heart J* 1985;53:388–393.

42. Brown MJ, Brown DC, Murphy MB. Hypokalemia from β$_2$-receptor stimulation by circulating epinephrine. *N Engl J Med* 1983;309:1414–1419.

43. Lampert R, Ickovics JR, Viscoli CJ, et al. Effects of propranolol on recovery of heart rate variability following acute myocardial infarction and relation to outcome in the beta-blocker heart attack trial. *Am J Cardiol* 2003;91:137–142.

44. Preliminary report: effect of encainide and flecainide on mortality in a randomized trial of arrhythmia suppression after myocardial infarction. The Cardiac Arrhythmia Suppression Trial (CAST) Investigators *N Engl J Med* 1989;321:406–412.

45. Kennedy HL, Brooks MM, Barker AH, et al. Beta-blocker therapy in the Cardiac Arrhythmia Suppression Trial. CAST Investigators. *Am J Cardiol* 1994;74:674–680.

46. Frishman WH. Multifactorial actions of β-adrenergic blocking drugs in ischemic heart disease. Current concepts. *Circulation* 1983;67[6 Pt 2]:I-11–I-18.

47. Richardson PD, Davies MJ, Born GV. Influence of plaque configuration and stress distribution on fissuring of coronary atherosclerotic plaques. *Lancet* 1989;2:941–944.

48. Davies MJ, Thomas AC. Thrombosis and acute coronary artery lesions in sudden cardiac ischemic death. *N Engl J Med* 1984;310:1137–1140.

49. Benson RL. The present status of coronary arterial disease. *Arch Pathol* 1926;2:870–916.

50. Contantinides P. Plaque fissuring in human coronary thrombosis. *J Atheroscler Res* 1966;6:1–17.

51. Fulton WF. *The coronary arteries: arteriography, microanatomy and pathogenesis of obliterative coronary disease.* Springfield, IL: Charles C. Thomas, 1965:230–296.

52. Davies MJ, Thomas AC. The pathological basis and microanatomy of occlusive thrombus formation in human coronary arteries. *Phil Trans R Soc Lond D* 1981;294:225–229.

53. Davies MJ, Thomas AC. Plaque fissuring—the cause of acute myocardial infarction, sudden ischaemic death and crescendo angina. *Br Heart J* 1985;53:363–373.

54. Levin DC, Fallon JT. Significance of the angiographic morphology of localized coronary stenosis: histopathologic correlations. *Circulation* 1982;66:316–320.

55. Ambrose JA, Winters SL, Aora RR. Angiographic evolution of coronary artery morphology in unstable angina. *J Am Coll Cardiol* 1986;7:472–478.

56. Ambrose JA, Tannenbaum MA, Alexopoulos DA, et al. Angiographic progression of coronary artery disease and the development of myocardial infarction. *J Am Coll Cardiol* 1988;12:56–62.

57. Lo YS, Cutler JE, Blake K, et al. Angiographic coronary morphology in survivors of cardiac arrest. *Am Heart J* 1988;115:781–785.

58. Sherman CT, Litvack F, Grundfest W, et al. Coronary angioscopy in patients with unstable angina pectoris. *N Engl J Med* 1986;315:913–919.

59. Forrester JS, Litvack F, Grundfest W, et al. A perspective of coronary disease seen through the arteries of a living man. *Circulation* 1987;75:505–513.

60. Muller JE, Tofler GH, Stone PH. Circadian variation and triggers of onset of acute cardiovascular disease. *Circulation* 1989;79:733–743.

61. Smeglin A, Frishman WH. Elastinolytic matrix metalloproteinases and their inhibitors as therapeutic targets in atherosclerotic plaque instability. *Heart Dis* 2004;12:141–150.

62. Frishman WH, Lazar EJ. Reduction of mortality, sudden death and nonfatal reinfarction with beta-adrenergic blockers in survivors of acute myocardial infarction: a new hypothesis regarding the cardioprotective action of beta-adrenergic blockade. *Am J Cardiol* 1990;66:66G–70G.

63. Spence JD. Effects of hydralazine versus propranolol on blood velocity in patients with carotid stenosis. *Clin Sci* 1983;65:91–93.

64. Weksler BB, Gillich M, Pink J. Effect of propranolol on platelet function. *Blood* 1977;49:185–196.

65. Hjalmarson A, Herlitz J. Limitation of infarct size by β-blockers and its potential role of prognosis. *Circulation* 1983;67[Suppl I]:I68–I71.

66. Reduction of infarct size with the early use of timolol in acute myocar-

dial infarction. International Collaborative Study Group. *N Engl J Med* 1984;310:9–15.

67. Peter T, Norris RM, Clarke ED, et al. Reduction of enzyme levels by propranolol after acute myocardial infarction. *Circulation* 1978;57: 1091–1095.

68. Rogue F, Amuchastegui LM, Lopez-Morillos MA, et al. Beneficial effects of timolol on infarct size and late ventricular tachycardia in patients with acute myocardial infarction. *Circulation* 1987;76:610–617.

69. Yusuf S, Sleight P, Rossi P, et al. Reduction in infarct size, arrhythmias and chest pain by early intravenous β-blockade in suspected myocardial infarction. *Circulation* 1983;67[Suppl I]:I-32–I-41.

70. Jardine RM, Obel IW, Smith AM. Intravenous acebutolol raises serum potassium in acute myocardial infarction. *Eur Heart J* 1986;7:140–145.

71. Herlitz J, Hjalmarson A, Swedberg K, et al. Effects on mortality during 5 years after early intervention with metoprolol in suspected acute myocardial infarction. *Acta Med Scand* 1988;223:227–231.

72. Comparison of invasive and conservative strategies after treatment with intravenous tissue plasminogen activator in acute myocardial infarction: Results of the thrombolysis in myocardial infarction (TIMI) phase II trial. TIMI Study Group. *N Engl J Med* 1989;320:618–627.

73. Pfisterer M, Cox JL, Granger CB, et al. Atenolol use and clinical outcomes after thrombolysis for acute myocardial infarction: the GUSTO-1 experience. Global Utilization of Streptokinase and TPA (alteplase) for Occluded Coronary Arteries *J Am Coll Cardiol* 1998;32:634–640.

74. Sirak TE, Jelic S, LeJemtel TH. Therapeutic update: non-selective beta- and alpha-adrenergic blockade in patients with coexistent chronic obstructive pulmonary disease and chronic heart failure. *J Am Coll Cardiol* 2004;44:497–502.

75. Barron HV, Viskin S. Dispelling the myths surrounding the use of beta blockers in patients with acute myocardial infarction. *Prev Cardiol* 1998;3:13.

76. Gheorghiade M, Goldstein S. β Blockers in the post-myocardial infarction patient. *Circulation* 2002;106:394–398.

77. Gottlieb SS, McCarter RJ, Vogel RA. Effect of beta blockade on mortality among high-risk and low-risk patients after myocardial infarction. *N Engl J Med* 1998;339:489–497.

78. Hjalmarson A, Goldstein S, Fagerberg B, et al. Effects of controlled-release metoprolol on total mortality, hospitalizations, and well-being in patients with heart failure: the Metoprolol CR/XL Randomized Intervention Trial in congestive heart failure (MERIT-HF). MERIT-HF Study Group. *JAMA* 2000;283:1295–1302.

79. Packer M, Fowler MB, Roecker EB, et al. Effect of carvedilol on morbidity of patients with severe chronic heart failure. Results of the Carvedilol Prospective Randomized Cumulative Survival (COPERNICUS) Study Group. *Circulation* 2002;106:2194–2199.

80. Frishman WH. Carvedilol. *N Engl J Med* 1998;339:1759–1765.

81. Pedersen TR. Six-year follow-up of the Norwegian Multicenter Study on Timolol after Acute Myocardial Infarction. *N Engl J Med* 1985; 313:1055–1058.

82. Frishman WH, Clark A, Johnson B. Effects of cardiovascular drugs on plasma lipids and lipoproteins. In: Frishman WH, Sonnenblick EH, eds. *Cardiovascular pharmacotherapeutics*. New York: McGraw-Hill, 1997:1515–1559.

83. Frishman WH. β-Adrenergic blocker withdrawal. *Am J Cardiol* 1987; 59:26F–32F.

84. Friedman LM. How do the various β-blockers compare in type, frequency and severity of their adverse effects? *Circulation* 1983;67[Suppl I]: I-89–I-90.

85. LeJemtel TH, Sonnenblick EH, Frishman WH. Diagnosis and management of heart failure. In: Fuster V, Alexander RW, O'Rourke RA, et al. eds. *Hurst's the heart*, 11th ed. New York: McGraw Hill 2004; 723–762.

CHAPTER 83

Antithrombotic Therapy after Discharge

W. Lane Duvall and David A. Vorchheimer

Key Words: Antiplatelet therapy; antithrombotic therapy; post-myocardial infarction.

INTRODUCTION

Coronary heart disease is the leading cause of death in the United States and the industrialized world. The majority of morbidity and mortality comes from first infarctions, but a substantial portion stems from reinfarction; although there are more than 1.1 million myocardial infarctions (MIs) annually in the United States, 450,000 of these represent reinfarctions (1). Furthermore, there are more than 7.5 million people alive with a history of MI, and they have a 15% to 20% risk for death or having a reinfarction in the 2 to 5 years after their initial infarction (1). Secondary prevention, therefore, is of utmost importance in decreasing the overall morbidity and mortality of patients with coronary heart disease.

Thrombosis and clot formation play an integral role in the pathophysiology of acute myocardial infarction (AMI), both through platelet-mediated processes and the contribution of the coagulation system (2,3). Secondary prevention of MI has thus focused on antithrombotic therapy targeting platelet inhibition and anticoagulation. A substantial body of clinical trial literature has established the efficacy of these two approaches to antithrombotic therapy. In addition, antithrombotic agents also have been used in patients with AMI to prevent left ventricular thrombus formation and systemic embolization.

W. L. Duvall: Mount Sinai Medical Center, The Zena and Michael A. Wiener Cardiovascular Institute, One Gustave L. Levy Place, Box 1030, New York, New York 10029.

D. A. Vorchheimer: Mount Sinai Medical Center, The Zena and Michael A. Wiener Cardiovascular Institute, One Gustave L. Levy Place, Box 1030, New York, New York 10029.

SECONDARY PREVENTION

Antiplatelet Therapy

Aspirin

Multiple clinical trials during the last 15 years have established aspirin as one of the most cost-effective therapies for secondary prevention of MI. Aspirin as antiplatelet therapy has been shown to reduce both reinfarction and mortality during and after MI.

The Second International Study of Infarct Survival (ISIS-2) trial was a landmark study responsible for establishing the efficacy of aspirin in reducing cardiovascular events during and after AMI (4). In the aspirin arm of the trial, more than 17,000 patients were randomized to receive either aspirin (160 mg/d for 1 month) or placebo, and at 5 weeks, vascular mortality was reduced by 23% ($p < 0.0001$) and was maintained over 10 years of follow-up with aspirin therapy (5). There also was a significant reduction in stroke (36%) and reinfarction (44%) in the patients treated with aspirin, and there was no counterbalancing increase in major bleeds or cerebral hemorrhage during treatment. Efficacy did not appear to be dependent on time: Aspirin was effective when given in the first 4 hours after MI (25% mortality reduction), after 12 hours (21% mortality reduction), or after 12 to 24 hours (21% mortality reduction).

In 2002, The Antithrombotic Trialists' Collaboration, which periodically and thoroughly reviews the literature on antiplatelet agents, analyzed data from 12 trials involving 18,788 patients with a history of MI treated with aspirin or other platelet inhibitors (the majority received aspirin) who received therapy for a mean duration of 27 months (6). Treatment resulted in 36 less serious vascular events per 1,000 patients treated, which reflects significant reductions in reinfarction (18/1,000), vascular death (14/1,000), and nonfatal stroke (5/1,000). The collaboration also reviewed 195 trials examining the long-term use of antiplatelet therapy (again mostly aspirin) in 135,640 patients at high risk for development of occlusive arterial disease. Among these patients at high risk, antiplatelet therapy reduced the risks for serious vascular events by 19%, nonfatal MI by 34%, stroke by 25%, and vascular death by 15% ($p < 0.0001$).

Recent data from metaanalyses indicate that high-dose (500–1,500 mg) aspirin is no more effective at reducing cardiovascular events than medium (160–325 mg) or low doses (75–150 mg) during long-term chronic administration (6) (Fig. 83–1). Among trials comparing varying doses of aspirin with placebo, the proportional reduction in vascular events was 19% with 500 to 1,500 mg, 26% with 160 to 325 mg, and 32% with 75 to 160 mg. Higher doses of aspirin have been associated with increased gastrotoxicity (7). Thus, the available evidence supports a daily dosage of 75 to 160 mg for secondary prevention and a loading dose of 160 to 325 mg in acute clinical situations when an immediate effect is required. Very low dosages of aspirin of less than 75 mg daily have been less widely assessed than low-dose aspirin, but the available data suggest that very low doses are less effective (13% reduction in events) (6).

The risks associated with aspirin administration in patients with vascular disease are small but real and include mainly bleeding complications such as gastrointestinal toxicity and hemorrhagic stroke. The American College of Chest Physicians Consensus Conference on Antithrombotic Therapy reports the absolute excess of intracranial hemorrhage with aspirin therapy is less than 1 per 1,000 in high-risk trials (8), and a metaanalysis of 16 trials comprising 55,462 patients demonstrated an increased relative risk of 1.84 (9). Gastrointestinal side effects also have been shown to be increased with aspirin therapy with an incidence of minor gastrointestinal symptoms of 5.2% to 40% in aspirin users compared with 0.7% to 34% of patients taking placebo, peptic ulcers in 0.8% to 2.6% versus 0% to 1.2%, and major gastrointestinal bleeding in less than 1% in both groups (7). A metaanalysis of 24 aspirin therapy trials and almost 66,000 participants found that gastrointestinal bleeding occurred in 2.47% of patients taking aspirin versus 1.42% of those taking placebo, corresponding to an odds ratio of 1.68 (10). Although this metaanalysis did not support a statistically significant reduction in bleeding with reduced aspirin dose (1.5% relative risk reduction [RRR] per 100 mg reduction of aspirin dose), a previous overview found that gastrointestinal toxicity was dose related with daily doses between 30 and 1,300 mg (11). The United Kingdom Transient Ischemic Attack (UK-TIA) trial supported this dose–response relation, finding that gastrointestinal symptoms were significantly more frequent in the high-dose (1,200 mg/d) group than in the low-dose (300 mg/d) group (12). A recent analysis evaluated the risks and benefits of aspirin therapy for secondary prevention of vascular events and found that the number needed to treat for aspirin to prevent 1 death from any cause was 67, whereas 100 patients would need to be treated to detect 1 nonfatal gastrointestinal tract hemorrhage (13).

Although aspirin reduces the risk for cardiovascular events and death by 25%, it appears that aspirin's antiplatelet effect may not be uniform in all patients as 10% to 20% of patients treated with aspirin have recurrent vascular events (14). Clinical aspirin resistance includes patients who, despite being on therapeutic doses of aspirin, experience thrombotic or embolic vascular events. Measurements of platelet aggregation, platelet reactivity, bleeding time, and thromboxane A_2 production have confirmed the variable effect of aspirin on individual patients (15). Previous studies have estimated that between 8% and 45% of the population are resistant to aspirin, (15) and current explanations include that platelet can be activated by pathways not blocked by aspirin, that greater doses of aspirin may be necessary to achieve optimal antithrombotic effect in some patients, and that certain patients can generate thromboxane A_2 despite usual therapeutic doses of aspirin.

Clopidogrel

Clopidogrel versus Aspirin

Clopidogrel is a thienopyridine derivative that blocks the activation of platelets by adenosine diphosphate by selectively and irreversibly inhibiting the binding of this agonist to its receptor on platelets.

Category of trial	No. of trials with data	No. (%) of vascular events		Observed-expected	Variance	Odds ratio (CI) Antiplatelet : control	% Odds reduction (SE)
		Allocated antiplatelet	Adjusted control				
Aspirin alone (mg daily)							
500–1500	34	1,621/11,215 (14.5)	1,930/11,236 (17.2)	−147.1	707.8		19 (3)
160–325	19	1,526/13,240 (11.5)	1,963/13,273 (14.8)	−219.9	742.6		26 (3)
75–150	12	366/3,370 (10.9)	517/3,460 (15.2)	−72.0	183.8		32 (6)
<75	3	316/1,827 (17.3)	354/1,828 (19.4)	−18.9	136.5		13 (8)
Any aspirin*	65	3,829/29,652 (12.9)	4,764/29,743 (16.0)	−452.3	1,717.0		23 (2)

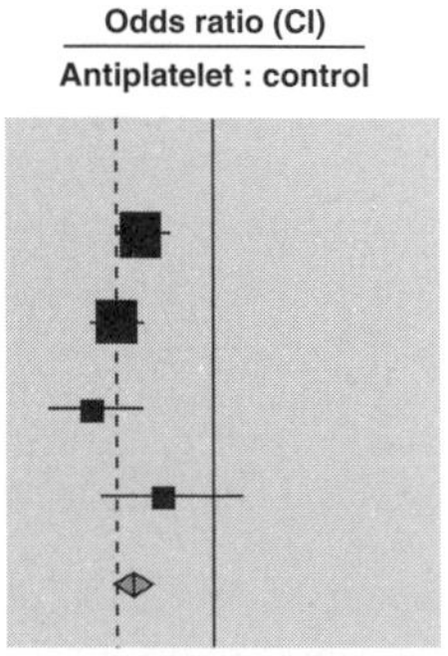

FIG. 83–1. Comparisons of different aspirin doses on vascular events in high risk patients (6). CI, confidence interval; SE, standard error.

The Clopidogrel versus Aspirin in Patients at Risk of Ischaemic Events (CAPRIE) trial was designed to assess the efficacy of clopidogrel compared with aspirin in preventing cardiovascular events in patients with known atherothrombotic vascular disease (16). More than 19,000 patients with either recent ischemic stroke (within last 6 months), recent MI (within last 35 days), or symptomatic peripheral vascular disease were randomized to either clopidogrel (75 mg daily) or aspirin (325 mg daily) and were followed for an average of 1.9 years for the occurrence of the composite end point of ischemic stroke, MI, or vascular death. The intention-to-treat analysis demonstrated a RRR of 8.7% (95% confidence interval [CI], 0.3–16.5%; $p = 0.043$) in favor of clopidogrel with an on-treatment analysis yielding a RRR of 9.4%. The reduction in the composite end point was driven mostly by a 16% reduction in nonfatal MIs and a 22% reduction in fatal MIs. There were no major differences in side effects, with aspirin showing an increase in gastrointestinal hemorrhage (2.66% vs. 1.99%), gastrointestinal intolerance (17.59% vs. 15.01%), and neutropenia (0.17% vs. 0.10%) and clopidogrel having an increase in rash (6.02% vs. 4.61%). Interestingly, there was a nonstatistically significant trend toward lack of benefit of clopidogrel in the MI subgroup (event rate of 5.03% vs. 4.84%; $p = 0.66$). To clarify this issue, all patients with a previous history of MI in the ischemic stroke and peripheral vascular disease group (2,144) were combined with the patients in the MI group (6,302) and found to have a nonsignificant 7.4% (95% CI, −5.2% to 18.6%) RRR in the composite primary end point.

Another secondary analysis of the CAPRIE data was undertaken in the 617 patients in whom AMI developed during the follow-up period (17). The analysis found that clopidogrel imparted a 19.2% RRR in the occurrence of MI, that the risk for infarction was less for clopidogrel in all risk categories, and that the benefit was consistent across all subgroups. The combined event rates for the 1,480 patients with a history of coronary artery bypass graft (CABG) also were reviewed in a secondary analysis (18). There was a 36.3% RRR (95% CI, 13.4–53.1%; $p = 0.004$) in the CAPRIE composite end point of vascular death, MI, and ischemic stroke. As a result of the CAPRIE study, clopidogrel was approved for the reduction of atherothrombotic events in patients with recent strokes, patients with MIs, or patients who have established peripheral vascular disease.

Clopidogrel plus Aspirin

The Clopidogrel in Unstable Angina to Prevent Recurrent Events (CURE) trial examined the use of clopidogrel plus aspirin in acute coronary syndromes and their continued use for secondary prevention of MI (19). The study randomized 12,562 patients who presented within 24 hours of onset of symptoms with electrocardiographic changes or increased cardiac enzymes to either clopidogrel (300-mg load followed by 75 mg daily) or placebo in addition to aspirin (75–325 mg daily). Patients were treated for a mean duration of 9 months and followed for a primary outcome of a composite of cardiovascular death, MI, or stroke. After 1 year of follow-up, there was a 20% RRR with clopidogrel (95% CI, 0.10–0.28; $p < 0.001$). Event reductions were seen during the acute phase in the first 30 days (21% RRR) and also during the chronic phase of prevention from 30 days to the end of the study (18% RRR) (Fig. 83–2 [19]). There were significantly more patients with major (3.7% vs. 2.7%) and minor (5.1% vs. 2.4%) bleeding in the clopidogrel group than the placebo group, but no significant increase in life-threatening bleeding or hemorrhagic stroke. In a retrospective analysis of bleeding events in the CURE study, it was found that the major and life-threatening bleeding risks with the combination of clopidogrel and aspirin were dose dependent, whereas there was no increase in efficacy with increasing aspirin doses (20). Integrating the results of the CURE study into current practice has been limited because the trial was conducted in a mostly European environment of conservative, noninvasive management in which only 5.9% to 7.2% of patients received glycoprotein IIb/IIIa inhibitors and only about 20% underwent a revascularization procedure during their hospitalization. This practice was quite different from the more aggressive, invasive North American style and has limited the applicability of the trial findings. Although not strictly a secondary prevention study, CURE suggests that there is benefit to the chronic addition of clopidogrel to aspirin after MI, but at the cost of increased bleeding.

The Clopidogrel for the Reduction of Events During Observation (CREDO) trial investigated the use of long-term clopidogrel combined with aspirin to prevent cardiovascular events after percutaneous intervention (21). Although CREDO was not specifically designed as a secondary prevention study, as patients were enrolled after elective percutaneous intervention, 13% of subjects had a history of a prior MI and more than 50% were enrolled with unstable angina. However, the second part of the study randomized 2,116 subjects treated with clopidogrel for the standard 28 days to either further clopidogrel (75 mg daily) or placebo with all subjects taking daily aspirin (81–325 mg). At 1 year, there was a 26.9% RRR (95% CI, 3.9–44.4%; $p = 0.02$) in the composite primary end point of death, MI, and stroke. The benefit occurred beyond the standard 28-day period of treatment, as there was a 37.4% (95% CI, 1.8–60.1%; $p = 0.04$) RRR from 4 weeks to 1 year. There was a trend toward an increase in major bleeding in the clopidogrel group (8.8% vs. 6.7%; $p = 0.7$) with approximately two-thirds of all major bleeds occurring in patients undergoing CABG. In the Can Rapid Risk Stratification of Unstable Angina Patients Suppress Adverse Outcomes with Early Implementation of the American of Cardiology/American Heart Association guidelines (CRUSADE) registry, 62% of patients with acute coronary syndrome underwent diagnostic cardiac angiography and 36% underwent percutaneous coronary intervention (22). As the routine invasive approach to patients with acute coronary syndrome continues to emerge as the predominant strategy, combination clopidogrel and aspirin is likely to be adopted

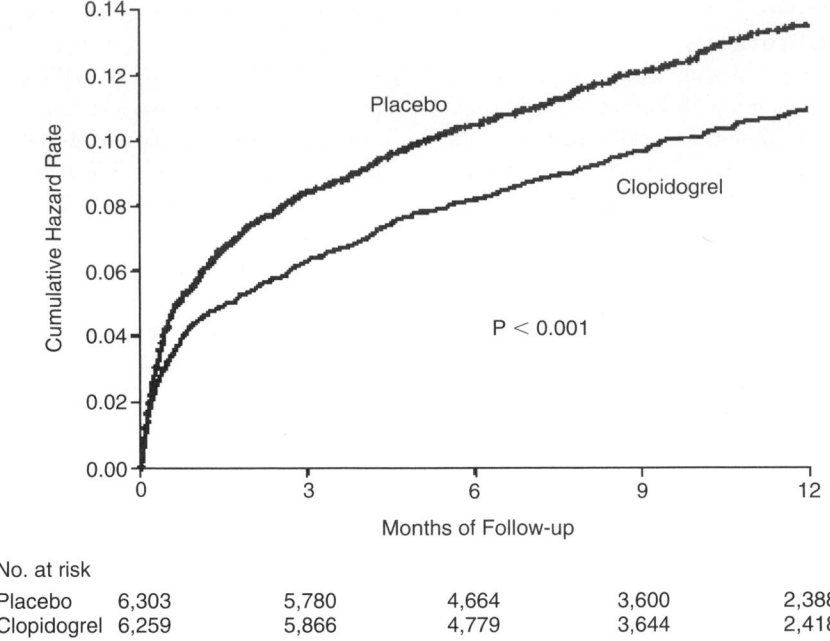

No. at risk

Placebo	6,303	5,780	4,664	3,600	2,388
Clopidogrel	6,259	5,866	4,779	3,644	2,418

FIG. 83–2. Cumulative hazard rates for the occurrence of cardiovascular death, myocardial infarction, or stroke during the Clopidogrel in Unstable Angina to Prevent Recurrent Events (CURE) trial demonstrating the sustained effect of clopidogrel (19).

as standard care for secondary prevention after percutaneous intervention.

Dipyridamole

Dipyridamole alone and in combination with aspirin has been evaluated in a handful of relatively small studies. With regard to monotherapy, no benefit was found in a small study of dipyridamole versus placebo in the month after MI (23). The two Persantine-Aspirin Reinfarction Studies evaluated aspirin, aspirin plus dipyridamole, and placebo in more than 5,000 patients after MI and found reductions of 25% in the composite of coronary death and reinfarction and of 20% to 37% in reinfarction with aspirin plus dipyridamole versus placebo (24,25). Finally, in both European Stroke Prevention Studies, patients with a previous cerebrovascular event had a reduction in MIs when treated with aspirin plus dipyridamole compared with placebo (26,27). However, this reduction only reached statistical significance in the first European Stroke Prevention Study with a RRR of 38.9% (*p* < 0.01).

Antithrombotic Therapy

Oral Anticoagulation (Warfarin)

The role of long-term anticoagulation with warfarin as effective secondary prevention continues to evolve. This therapeutic debate has spanned nearly 50 years as the first studies were performed in the 1950s and large randomized studies have been published in each of the last few years.

Many of the early trials produced conflicting results and are subject to major criticisms on several points, some of which are crucial. Most trials were open- or single-blinded and not properly randomized; they all had a small sample sizes, and historical control subjects often were used. A further criticism is that the intensity of the anticoagulation was not well maintained because of inadequate quality control. Because of these shortcomings, in 1970, an International Review Group (28) reviewed the results of 9 prospective trials in 2,487 men after MI, and adequate levels of anticoagulation were found in only 50% of the trials. On the basis of these pooled data, the mortality rate was reduced by 20% but was restricted to patients with prolonged angina or previous infarction on admission to the trial. Given these equivocal results and the high frequency of bleeding complications, the practice of maintaining patients on long-term anticoagulation was abandoned in many countries despite the observed decrease in death rate. Because of the uncertainties regarding the value of long-term anticoagulant therapy, a new series of well designed clinical studies was started in the mid-1980s in an effort to address this unresolved issue (Table 83–1).

Warfarin versus Placebo

The Norwegian Warfarin Re-Infarction Study (WARIS) trial randomized 1,214 patients within 30 days of a MI to either oral anticoagulation with an International Normalized Ratio (INR) goal of 2.8 to 4.8 or placebo (29). During a mean follow-up of 37 months, risk reduction with coumarin by intention-to-treat analysis in total mortality was 24% (95% CI,

TABLE 83–1. *Comparison of secondary prevention studies of oral anticoagulation*

Study	Date	Patients, n	End point	Follow-Up	Aspirin	Warfarin	Combination
WARIS (29)	1990	1,214	Mortality	4 yr	—	INR 2.8–4.8	—
WARIS-2 (38)	2002	3,630	Death, MI, stroke	4 yr	160 mg	INR 2.8–4.2	75 mg + INR 2.0–2.5
ASPECT (30)	1994	3,404	Mortality	4 yr	—	INR 2.4–4.8	—
ASPECT-2 (37)	2002	999	Death, MI, stroke	1 yr	80 mg	INR 3.0–4.0	80 mg + INR 2.0–2.5
APRICOT (31)	1993	300	Patency	3 mo	325 mg	INR 2.8–4.0	—
APRICOT-2 (36)	2002	308	Patency	3 mo	80 mg	—	80 mg + INR 2.0–3.0
CARS (33)	1997	8,803	Death, MI, stroke	14 mo	160 mg	—	80 mg + 1mg or 3 mg
CHAMP (35)	2002	5,059	Death, MI, stroke	2.7 yr	162 mg	—	81 mg + INR 1.5–2.5
OASIS (34)	2001	3,712	Death, MI, stroke	5 mo	[a]	INR 2.0–2.5	[a]

APRICOT, Antithrombotics in the Prevention of Reocclusion in Coronary Thrombolysis; ASPECT, Anticoagulants in the Secondary Prevention of Events in Coronary Thrombosis; CARS, Coumadin Aspirin Reinfarction Study; CHAMP, Combination Hemotherapy and Mortality Prevention; INR, International Normalized Ratio; MI, myocardial infarction; OASIS, Organization to Assess Strategies for Ischemic Syndromes; WARIS, Norwegian Warfarin Re-Infarction Study.

[a]Patients were randomized to anticoagulation or standard therapy. The majority of subjects in both groups were receiving aspirin.

4–44%; $p < 0.03$), 34% in nonfatal MI (95% CI, 19–54%; $p < 0.001$), and 55% in cerebrovascular accidents (95% CI, 33–77%; $p < 0.002$). The incidence of major bleeding was 0.6% per year, which represented a twofold increase in major hemorrhage. Quality control revealed that two-thirds of the patients were in the preset INR range of between 2.8 and 4.8.

The Dutch trial of Anticoagulants in the Secondary Prevention of Events in Coronary Thrombosis (ASPECT) recruited 3,404 hospital survivors of MI and randomly assigned them to coumarin (INR range between 2.4 and 4.8) or placebo within 8 weeks of hospital admission (30). After a mean follow-up period of 37 months, the all-cause mortality rate was nonsignificantly reduced by 10% (95% CI, −11% to 27%), but statistically significant reductions were seen in recurrent MI (relative risk 53%; 95% CI, 41–62%) and cerebrovascular events (relative risk 40%; 95% CI, 10–60%). Quality control demonstrated that two-thirds of all INR values were in the range of 2.4 to 4.8. The combined end point (vascular death, MI, or cerebral event) was reduced from 17.5% in the control group to 9.5% in the anticoagulated group but at the cost of a 3.87-fold increase in major bleeding with anticoagulation. This translates into the prevention of 3.1 vascular events per 100 patient-years at the cost of one episode of major bleeding.

Warfarin versus Aspirin

The Antithrombotics in the Prevention of Reocclusion in Coronary Thrombolysis (APRICOT) trial enrolled 300 subjects after MI successfully treated with thrombolytics demonstrated at angiography and assigned them to either Coumadin, aspirin, or placebo while still in the hospital (31). At 3 months, 248 subjects had repeat angiography that found no statistically significant difference in vessel patency rates (30%, 25%, and 32%) or mortality. A statistically significant improvement was seen with aspirin in reinfarction,

revascularization, and left ventricular ejection fraction, but not with Coumadin.

Warfarin Plus Aspirin

Considering the importance of both platelets and coagulation in the pathogenesis of AMI, the combination of aspirin and oral anticoagulants would seem to be a logical proposition. In fact, a metaanalysis of the use of anticoagulation in patients with coronary heart disease published in 1999 suggested that both high-dose warfarin alone and moderate-dose warfarin with aspirin were superior to aspirin alone (32).

The Coumadin Aspirin Reinfarction Study (CARS) trial enrolled 8,803 patients after MI and compared aspirin (160 mg) to a combination of either 1 or 3 mg of fixed-dose warfarin in combination with aspirin (80 mg) (33). This study showed no significant benefit of combination therapy in reducing the primary end point of reinfarction, stroke, or cardiovascular death after a median of 14 months of follow-up with event rates of 8.6% with aspirin alone, 8.4% for 3 mg warfarin plus aspirin, and 8.8% with 1 mg warfarin and aspirin. Although the higher-dose warfarin group only achieved a mean INR of 1.3 over the course of the study period, spontaneous major hemorrhage was doubled in this group compared with aspirin alone (1.4% vs. 0.74%).

The Organization to Assess Strategies for Ischemic Syndromes (OASIS) trial evaluated anticoagulation therapy in addition to aspirin in patients with unstable angina (34). Overall, in the 3,712 patients randomized to warfarin (INR goal, 2.0–2.5) or standard therapy, there was a small, nonsignificant trend of reduction in the primary end point of cardiovascular death, MI, and stroke (relative risk, 0.90; 95% CI, 0.72–1.14; $p = 0.40$) in the anticoagulation group at 5 months. When subjects were divided into groups on the basis of location in countries with good or bad compliance, there was a significant reduction in the primary outcome in the anticoagulation group in countries with good compliance (6.1% vs. 8.9%; relative risk, 0.68; 95% CI, 0.48–0.95). Again, there was an excess of major bleeding (2.7% vs. 1.3%) in the warfarin group, which was more dramatic in the countries with good compliance. Over the course of the study, anticoagulated patients had an INR greater than 2.0 approximately 70% of the time.

The Combination Hemotherapy and Mortality Prevention (CHAMP) study also found no significant benefit to combination therapy after randomizing 5,059 patients within 2 weeks of MI and following them for a median of 2.7 years (35). There were no significant differences in end points of mortality, MI, and stroke between the aspirin (162 mg) and aspirin (81 mg) plus warfarin (INR goal 1.5–2.5) groups. Again there was an almost doubling of the major bleeding rate in the combination arm compared with the aspirin only group (1.28 vs. 0.72 events per 100 person-years). The mean INR achieved during the study duration was 1.8, which together with the data from the other negative trials supports the concept of a threshold INR needed to show benefit of antithrombotic therapy or combination therapy over traditional antiplatelet therapy.

The Dutch APRICOT 2 trial randomized subjects treated with thrombolytics to 80 mg aspirin or combination therapy with an INR goal of 2.0 to 3.0 (36). Patients had repeat angiograms at 3 months to reevaluate vessel patency. After achieving a mean INR of 2.6, there was a statistically significant RRR of 45% in flow equal to or less than TIMI 2, with 15% in the combination group versus 28% in the aspirin only arm ($p < 0.02$). There also was a significant reduction in reinfarction and revascularization with survival rates free from events of 66% and 86%, respectively ($p < 0.01$). In this small study, bleeding complications were infrequent with TIMI major and minor bleeding occurring in 5% and 3% of patients (p = not significant).

The ASPECT-2 trial strove to further clarify the issue of a threshold of anticoagulation and the use of combination therapy for secondary prevention of MI (37). A total of 999 patients were randomized to low-dose aspirin (80 mg), high-dose warfarin (INR, 3.0–4.0), or combined low-dose aspirin (80 mg) and moderate-dose warfarin (INR, 2.0–2.5) after MI and were followed for a median of 12 months. Although the trial was terminated prematurely because slow patient recruitment, the composite end point was reduced with borderline statistical significance in both anticoagulation groups. Reinfarction, stroke, or death saw a 9% reduction in subjects treated with aspirin, 5% reduction in subjects treated with high-dose warfarin (hazard ratio [HR], 0.55; 95% CI, 0.30–1.00; p = 0.0479), and 5% reduction in subjects who received combination therapy (HR, 0.50; 95% CI, 0.27–0.92; p = 0.03). All-cause mortality was actually statistically significantly decreased from 4% to 1% in the high-dose warfarin group (HR, 0.2; 95% CI, 0.09–0.82). There were no significant differences in rates of major bleeding among groups, occurring in 1% receiving aspirin, 1% receiving high-dose warfarin, and 2% receiving combination

therapy. The mean INR in the high-dose warfarin group was 3.2 with approximately 50% of the patients within the range of 3.0 to 4.0, whereas the mean INR was 2.4 in the combination group with about 40% of subjects in the target range of 2.0 to 2.5.

The WARIS II trial followed up these results in a larger, randomized, open-label, multicenter trial of 3,630 patients enrolled from 20 Norwegian hospitals (38). Patients hospitalized for an AMI were randomized to either 160 mg aspirin, warfarin adjusted to an INR of 2.8 to 4.2, or 80 mg aspirin and warfarin adjusted to an INR of 2.0 to 2.5 and were followed for an average of 4 years. In an intention-to-treat analysis of the composite end point (death, reinfarction, or ischemic stroke), the study found that there was a statistically significant 29% (95% CI, 17–40%; p = 0.001) reduction in the combination group and a 19% (95% CI, 5–31%; p = 0.03) reduction in the warfarin group compared with aspirin alone. The mean INR achieved was 2.2 in the combination group and 2.8 in patients receiving warfarin alone. The reduction in the composite end point was driven by significant reductions in reinfarction (44% and 26%) and stroke (48% and 48%) in the combination and warfarin only groups. Major bleeding episodes were four times more likely (0.68% per year) in patients receiving warfarin and three times as likely (0.57% per year) in the combination group compared with aspirin alone (0.17% per year), whereas minor bleeding was increased 3-fold and 2.5-fold in the combination and warfarin arms, respectively. Finally, compliance with warfarin therapy proved to be difficult with 40% and 32% of patients discontinuing therapy in the combination and warfarin groups compared with only 16% in the aspirin arm.

As a whole, these trials demonstrate that long-term anticoagulant treatment after MI results in modest reductions in mortality and substantial reductions in the risk for recurrent MIs and cerebrovascular events. However, this benefit is at the cost of increased risk for bleeding (Table 83–2). It appears that there is a threshold level of anticoagulation needed to demonstrate benefit over aspirin alone. The most impressive results were from studies conducted in the medical systems of Scandinavia where national resources for anticoagulation management are available. In the United States, fear of bleeding complications and the complexity of proper medication adjustment continue to make physicians hesitant to adopt routine anticoagulation as first-line secondary prevention when antiplatelet therapy is available as an effective and safe alternative.

Direct Thrombin Inhibitor

Ximelagatran is an oral direct thrombin inhibitor that is rapidly absorbed after oral administration and converted to its active form, Melagatran (39). Ximelagatran has predictable pharmacokinetics, low variability between individuals, and no relevant food interactions allowing for fixed oral dosing without the need for titration or coagulation monitoring. These ad-

TABLE 83–2. *Major bleeding risks in secondary prevention trials of antiplatelet and antithrombotic therapy*

Study	Follow-up	Aspirin	Aspirin + clopidogrel	Warfarin	Warfarin + aspirin	*p* Value
CURE (19)	1 yr	2.7%	3.7%	—	—	0.001
CREDO (21)	1 yr	6.7%	8.8%	—	—	0.07
WARIS-2 (38)	4 yr	0.6%	—	2.7%	2.3%	—
ASPECT-2 (36)	1 yr	1%	—	1%	2%	NS
CARS (33)	14 mo	0.74%	—	—	1.4%	0.014

Note varying length of follow-up and varying definitions of major bleeding.
ASPECT, Anticoagulants in the Secondary Prevention of Events in Coronary Thrombosis; CARS, Coumadin Aspirin Reinfarction Study; CREDO, Clopidogrel for the Reduction of Events During Observation; CURE, Clopidogrel in Unstable Angina to Prevent Recurrent Events; NS, not significant; WARIS, Norwegian Warfarin Re-Infarction Study.

vantages of ximelagatran make it an attractive alternative to oral vitamin K antagonists such as warfarin that have all of these limitations.

Early-phase clinical trials are currently underway evaluating ximelagatran as a potential treatment for post-MI and postacute coronary syndrome therapy. Currently, ximelagatran and Melagatran have mainly been investigated in phase II or III studies of prophylaxis of venous thromboembolic events (40–44). More than 3,000 patients have been studied comparing ximelagatran with or without Melagatran subcutaneously to either warfarin or low–molecular weight heparin, and the direct thrombin inhibitor has been found to be as safe and effective as current therapy in this setting. Although also not in the acute coronary syndrome area, the Stroke Prevention Using an Oral Thrombin Inhibitor in Atrial Fibrillation (SPORTIF) III trial compared ximelagatran with warfarin in the prevention of stroke and systemic embolic events in patients with atrial fibrillation (45). In the 3,407 patients randomized in this open-label study, ximelagatran was found to be as effective as warfarin with a 29% RRR (1.6% vs. 2.3%; *p* = not significant) in the intention-to-treat analysis of the primary end point and to be superior in the on-treatment analysis with a 41% RRR (1.3% vs. 2.2%; *p* = 0.018). No significant differences were found in the rates of intracerebral hemorrhage and major bleeding, but ximelagatran demonstrated a significant reduction in the rate of combined major and minor bleeding (25.5% vs. 29.5%; *p* = 0.007).

PREVENTION OF VENTRICULAR THROMBUS AND ARTERIAL EMBOLI

The major cause of systemic arterial emboli in patients with AMI is left ventricular mural thrombosis usually occurring after an acute anterior wall infarction. Among pooled data from several echocardiographic studies, left ventricular thrombi were found in 4% of inferior infarctions (range 0–15%) and in 30% of anterior MIs (range 20–40%) (46). Large anterior infarctions may be associated with mural thrombosis in up to 60% of cases (47). Two-thirds of left ventricular thrombi occur within 2 days after a MI, and systemic emboli occur on average 2 weeks later. The incidence of systemic emboli appears to be about

10% of the incidence of mural thrombus. One autopsy study found a 50% incidence of systemic embolization after MI, but in patients surviving infarction, the incidence of clinically evident systemic emboli resulting from dislodgment of left ventricular thrombi is much less, ranging from 5% to 26% in patients with echocardiographic evidence of mural thrombus (48–52).

Data from the National Registry of Myocardial Infarction (53) demonstrates that in the current era of MI therapy, there has been an increase in the prevalence of non–Q-wave infarctions (from 45% in 1994 to 63% in 1999; *p* = 0.0001) with a corresponding decrease in patients with ST-segment elevation or left bundle branch block (from 36.4% in 1994 to 27.1% in 1999; *p* ≤ 0.001). The combination of fewer transmural MIs and increased used of antithrombotic and antiplatelet agents has caused the occurrence of left ventricular thrombus to be less common. Anticoagulation with immediate warfarin, unfractionated or low–molecular weight heparin, or treatment with antithrombotic agents (aspirin plus dipyridamole) have been shown to be effective in reducing the formation of left ventricular thrombi (54–59), but aspirin alone does not prevent left ventricular thrombus formation (60). In patients with left ventricular thrombus present by echocardiography at hospital dismissal, oral anticoagulation and aspirin were equally effective, and better than no treatment, in the resolution of left ventricular thrombus and prevention of arterial thromboembolia (61). Currently, the American College of Chest Physicians in their Consensus Conference on Antithrombotic Therapy recommends the use of warfarin therapy for 1 to 3 months in clinical settings of increased embolic risk after MI such as anterior wall MI, severe left ventricular dysfunction, congestive heart failure, previous emboli, echocardiographic evidence of mural thrombosis, or atrial fibrillation (62).

CONCLUSIONS

In light of the many options for antithrombotic therapy in secondary prevention of MI, it often is the initial management of the infarction that guides subsequent therapy. Patients with large, transmural anterior infarctions or those with comorbidities such as atrial fibrillation or prosthetic valves are commonly treated with anticoagulation for secondary prevention because anticoagulation is indicated for the treatment of the concomitant conditions. Patients who receive thrombolysis as the sole form of reperfusion, in contrast, may be treated with the minimum of aspirin monotherapy as no other comorbidity requires additional therapy. Patients managed conservatively for their non–ST-segment elevation MI, who were initially treated with a combination of aspirin and clopidogrel during the acute phase, may be considered for long-term therapy with both agents. And more recently, even those patients whose acute coronary syndrome was treated with percutaneous intervention may be candidates for long-term treatment with not only aspirin, but also clopidogrel. Each antithrombotic therapy then carries with it risks and benefits whose net balance depends on the group in which it is used.

REFERENCES

1. *Morbidity & mortality: 2002 chart book on cardiovascular, lung, and blood diseases.* Bethesda, MD: National Heart, Lung, and Blood Institute, 2002.
2. Fuster V, Badimon L, Badimon JJ, et al. The pathogenesis of coronary artery disease and the acute coronary syndromes (2). *N Engl J Med* 1992;326:310–318.
3. Fuster V, Badimon L, Badimon JJ, et al. The pathogenesis of coronary artery disease and the acute coronary syndromes (1). *N Engl J Med* 1992;326:242–250.
4. Randomised trial of intravenous streptokinase, oral aspirin, both, or neither among 17,187 cases of suspected acute myocardial infarction: ISIS-2. ISIS-2 (Second International Study of Infarct Survival) Collaborative Group. *Lancet* 1988;2:349–360.
5. Baigent C, Collins R, Appleby P, et al. ISIS-2: 10 year survival among patients with suspected acute myocardial infarction in randomised comparison of intravenous streptokinase, oral aspirin, both, or neither. The ISIS-2 (Second International Study of Infarct Survival) Collaborative Group. *BMJ* 1998;316:1337–1343.
6. Collaborative meta-analysis of randomised trials of antiplatelet therapy for prevention of death, myocardial infarction, and stroke in high risk patients. Antithrombotic Trialists' Collaboration *BMJ* 2002;324:71–86.
7. Awtry EH, Loscalzo J. Aspirin. *Circulation* 2000;101:1206–1218.
8. Patrono C, Coller B, Dalen JE, et al. Platelet-active drugs: the relationships among dose, effectiveness, and side effects. *Chest* 2001;119:39S–63S.
9. He J, Whelton PK, Vu B, et al. Aspirin and risk of hemorrhagic stroke: a meta-analysis of randomized controlled trials. *JAMA* 1998;280:1930–1935.
10. Derry S, Loke YK. Risk of gastrointestinal hemorrhage with long term use of aspirin: meta-analysis. *BMJ* 2000;321:1183–1187.
11. Roderick PJ, Wilkes HC, Meade TW. The gastrointestinal toxicity of aspirin: an overview of randomised controlled trials. *Br J Clin Pharmacol* 1993;35:219–226.
12. United Kingdom transient ischaemic attack (UK-TIA) aspirin trial: interim results. UK-TIA Study Group. *Br Med J (Clin Res Ed)* 1988;296:316–320.
13. Weisman SM, Graham DY. Evaluation of the benefits and risks of low-dose aspirin in the secondary prevention of cardiovascular and cerebrovascular events. *Arch Intern Med* 2002;162:2197–2202.
14. Eikelboom JW, Hirsh J, Weitz JI, et al. Aspirin-resistant thromboxane biosynthesis and the risk of myocardial infarction, stroke, or cardiovascular death in patients at high risk for cardiovascular events. *Circulation* 2002;105:1650–1655.
15. Gum PA, Kottke-Marchant K, Poggio ED, et al. Profile and prevalence of aspirin resistance in patients with cardiovascular disease. *Am J Cardiol* 2001;88:230–235.
16. A randomised, blinded, trial of clopidogrel versus aspirin in patients at risk of ischaemic events (CAPRIE). CAPRIE Steering Committee. *Lancet* 1996;348:1329–1339.
17. Cannon CP. Effectiveness of clopidogrel versus aspirin in preventing acute myocardial infarction in patients with symptomatic atherothrombosis (CAPRIE trial). *Am J Cardiol* 2002;90:760–762.
18. Bhatt DL, Chew DP, Hirsch AT, et al. Superiority of clopidogrel versus aspirin in patients with prior cardiac surgery. *Circulation* 2001;103:363–368.
19. Yusuf S, Zhao F, Mehta SR, et al. Effects of clopidogrel in addition to aspirin in patients with acute coronary syndromes without ST-segment elevation. *N Engl J Med* 2001;345:494–502.
20. Peters RJ, Zao F, Lewis BS, et al. Aspirin dose and bleeding events in the CURE study. *Eur Heart J* 2002;23:510.
21. Steinhubl SR, Berger PB, Mann JT 3rd, et al. Early and sustained dual oral antiplatelet therapy following percutaneous coronary intervention: a randomized controlled trial. *JAMA* 2002;288:2411–2420.
22. *The CRUSADE registry.* Berlin: European Society of Cardiology Scientific Sessions, 2002.
23. Gent AE, Brook CG, Foley TH, et al. Dipyridamole: a controlled trial of its effect in acute myocardial infarction. *Br Med J* 1968;4:366–368.
24. Persantine and aspirin in coronary heart disease. The persantine-aspirin reinfarction study research group (PARIS). *Circulation* 1980;62:449–461.
25. Klimt CR, Knatterud GL, Stamler J, et al. Persantine-Aspirin Reinfarction Study. Part II. Secondary coronary prevention with persantine and aspirin. *J Am Coll Cardiol* 1986;7:251–269.
26. European Stroke Prevention Study. ESPS Group. *Stroke* 1990;21:1122–1130.
27. Diener HC, Cunha L, Forbes C, et al. European Stroke Prevention Study. 2. Dipyridamole and acetylsalicylic acid in the secondary prevention of stroke. *J Neurol Sci* 1996;143:1–13.
28. Collaborative analysis of long-term anticoagulant administration after acute myocardial infarction. An international anticoagulant review group. *Lancet* 1970;1:203–209.
29. Smith P, Arnesen H, Holme I. The effect of warfarin on mortality and reinfarction after myocardial infarction. *N Engl J Med* 1990;323:147–152.
30. Effect of long-term oral anticoagulant treatment on mortality and cardiovascular morbidity after myocardial infarction. Anticoagulants in the Secondary Prevention of Events in Coronary Thrombosis (ASPECT) Research Group. *Lancet* 1994;343:499–503.
31. Meijer A, Verheugt FW, Werter CJ, et al. Aspirin versus coumadin in the prevention of reocclusion and recurrent ischemia after successful thrombolysis: a prospective placebo-controlled angiographic study. Results of the APRICOT Study. *Circulation* 1993;87:1524–1530.
32. Anand SS, Yusuf S. Oral anticoagulant therapy in patients with coronary artery disease: a meta-analysis. *JAMA* 1999;282:2058–2067.
33. Randomised double-blind trial of fixed low-dose warfarin with aspirin after myocardial infarction. Coumadin Aspirin Reinfarction Study (CARS) Investigators. *Lancet* 1997;350:389–396.
34. Effects of long-term, moderate-intensity oral anticoagulation in addition to aspirin in unstable angina. The Organization to Assess Strategies for Ischemic Syndromes (OASIS) Investigators. *J Am Coll Cardiol* 2001;37:475–484.
35. Fiore LD, Ezekowitz MD, Brophy MT, et al. Department of Veterans Affairs Cooperative Studies Program Clinical Trial comparing combined warfarin and aspirin with aspirin alone in survivors of acute myocardial infarction: primary results of the CHAMP study. *Circulation* 2002;105:557–563.
36. Brouwer MA, van den Bergh PJ, Aengevaeren WR, et al. Aspirin plus coumarin versus aspirin alone in the prevention of reocclusion after fibrinolysis for acute myocardial infarction: results of the Antithrombotics In the Prevention of Reocclusion In Coronary Thrombolysis (APRICOT)-2 Trial. *Circulation* 2002;106:659–665.
37. van Es RF, Jonker JJ, Verheugt FW, et al. Aspirin and coumadin after acute coronary syndromes (the ASPECT-2 study): a randomised controlled trial. *Lancet* 2002;360:109–113.
38. Hurlen M, Abdelnoor M, Smith P, et al. Warfarin, aspirin, or both after myocardial infarction. *N Engl J Med* 2002;347:969–974.
39. Eriksson UG, Johansson L, Frison L, et al. Single and repeated oral dosing of H 376/95, a prodrug of the direct thrombin inhibitor melagatran, to young healthy male subjects. *Blood* 1999;94[Suppl]:26a.
40. Heit JA, Colwell CW, Francis CW, et al. Comparison of the oral direct thrombin inhibitor ximelagatran with enoxaparin as prophylaxis against venous thromboembolism after total knee replacement: a phase 2 dose-finding study. *Arch Intern Med* 2001;161:2215–2221.
41. Francis CW, Davidson BL, Berkowitz SD, et al. Ximelagatran versus

warfarin for the prevention of venous thromboembolism after total knee arthroplasty. A randomized, double-blind trial. *Ann Intern Med* 2002;137:648–655.

42. Eriksson BI, Arfwidsson AC, Frison L, et al. A dose-ranging study of the oral direct thrombin inhibitor, ximelagatran, and its subcutaneous form, melagatran, compared with dalteparin in the prophylaxis of thromboembolism after hip or knee replacement: METHRO I. MElagatran for THRombin inhibition in Orthopaedic surgery. *Thromb Haemost* 2002;87:231–237.

43. Eriksson BI, Bergqvist D, Kalebo P, et al. Ximelagatran and melagatran compared with dalteparin for prevention of venous thromboembolism after total hip or knee replacement: the METHRO II randomised trial. *Lancet* 2002;360:1441–1447.

44. Eriksson BI, Agnelli G, Cohen AT, et al. Direct thrombin inhibitor melagatran followed by oral ximelagatran in comparison with enoxaparin for prevention of venous thromboembolism after total hip or knee replacement. *Thromb Haemost* 2003;89:288–296.

45. Halperin JL. Stroke Prophylaxis Using an Oral Thrombin Inhibitor in Atrial Fibrillation (SPORTIF III) trial. American College of Cardiology Scientific Session; Chicago, March 30–April 2, 2003.

46. Israel DH, Stein B, Cheseboro JH, et al. Antithrombotic therapy for the prevention of cardiac and arterial thromboembolism. In: Messerli FH, ed. *Cardiovascular drug therapy*. Philadelphia: WB Saunders, 1990.

47. Meltzer RS, Visser CA, Fuster V. Intracardiac thrombi and systemic embolization. *Ann Intern Med* 1986;104:689–698.

48. Haugland JM, Asinger RW, Mikell FL, et al. Embolic potential of left ventricular thrombi detected by two-dimensional echocardiography. *Circulation* 1984;70:588–598.

49. Visser CA, Kan G, Lie KI, et al. Left ventricular thrombus following acute myocardial infarction: a prospective serial echocardiographic study of 96 patients. *Eur Heart J* 1983;4:333–337.

50. Friedman MJ, Carlson K, Marcus FI, et al. Clinical correlations in patients with acute myocardial infarction and left ventricular thrombus detected by two-dimensional echocardiography. *Am J Med* 1982;72:894–898.

51. McEntee CW, Van Reet RE, Winters WL. Incidence and natural history

of mural thrombi in acute myocardial infarction by two-dimensional echocardiography. *Circulation* 1981;64:IV-93.

52. Visser CA, Kan G, Meltzer RS, et al. Embolic potential of left ventricular thrombus after myocardial infarction: a two-dimensional echocardiographic study of 119 patients. *J Am Coll Cardiol* 1985;5:1276–1280.

53. Rogers WJ, Canto JG, Lambrew CT, et al. Temporal trends in the treatment of over 1.5 million patients with myocardial infarction in the US from 1990 through 1999: the National Registry of Myocardial Infarction 1, 2 and 3. *J Am Coll Cardiol* 2000;36:2056–2063.

54. Anticoagulants in acute myocardial infarction: results of a cooperative clinical trial. *JAMA* 1973;225:724–729.

55. Reeder GS, Lengyel M, Tajik AJ, et al. Mural thrombus in left ventricular aneurysm: incidence, role of angiography, and relation between anticoagulation and embolization. *Mayo Clin Proc* 1981;56:77–81.

56. Nordrehaug JE, Johannessen KA, von der Lippe G. Usefulness of high-dose anticoagulants in preventing left ventricular thrombus in acute myocardial infarction. *Am J Cardiol* 1985;55.1491–1493.

57. Johannessen KA, Stratton JR, Taulow E, et al. Usefulness of aspirin plus dipyridamole in reducing left ventricular thrombus formation in anterior wall acute myocardial infarction. *Am J Cardiol* 1989;63:101–102.

58. Iacono A. Mean-term calcium heparin treatment in acute transmural anterior myocardial infarction: effects on left ventricular thrombosis and its complications. *Cardiologia* 1997;42:1251–1255.

59. Kontny F, Dale J, Abildgaard U, et al. Randomized trial of low molecular weight heparin (dalteparin) in prevention of left ventricular thrombus formation and arterial embolism after acute anterior myocardial infarction: the Fragmin in Acute Myocardial Infarction (FRAMI) Study. *J Am Coll Cardiol* 1997;30:962–969.

60. Kupper AJ, Verheugt FW, Peels CH, et al. Effect of low dose acetylsalicylic acid on the frequency and hematologic activity of left ventricular thrombus in anterior wall acute myocardial infarction. *Am J Cardiol* 1989;63:917–920.

61. Kouvaras G, Chronopoulos G, Soufras G, et al. The effects of long-term antithrombotic treatment on left ventricular thrombi in patients after an acute myocardial infarction. *Am Heart J* 1990;119:73–78.

62. Cairns JA, Theroux P, Lewis HD Jr, et al. Antithrombotic agents in coronary artery disease. *Chest* 2001;119:228S–252S.

CHAPTER 84

Cardiac Rehabilitation and Risk Factor Modification

Fredric J. Pashkow and Richard C. Pasternak

Key Words: Cardiac rehabilitation; coronary artery disease risk factors; exercise training; MET; physical conditioning; quality of life; risk stratification.

INTRODUCTION

This chapter examines cardiac rehabilitation as a component of preventive cardiology and a distinct modality in the contemporary therapy of patients with coronary artery disease (CAD). In view of the extensive discussion in other chapters in this textbook of risk stratification and risk factors for coronary atherothrombosis, this chapter focuses particularly on the contribution of cardiac rehabilitation to outcomes, especially survival, after acute coronary syndromes and after

revascularization procedures. Cardiac rehabilitation is currently recognized as a synthesis of exercise training, risk factor modification, psychosocial support, and education for the purpose of facilitating readaptation to normal life through the achievement of improved functional performance and the reduction of coronary heart disease risk factors.

Randomized studies performed mainly between 1975 and 1985 typically suggested a 20% to 30% reduction in cardiovascular mortality and sudden cardiac death but failed to achieve individual statistical significance largely because of insufficient sample size. Beyond traditional cardiac end points, improved quality of life and cost utility also have become important contemporary outcome goals.

Cardiac rehabilitation is rapidly changing with the dynamics of shortened length of hospital stays and a changing patient population. It is provided now by multiple models. Newer findings suggest that those patients stratified at low risk will benefit most by the modification of coronary risk fac-

F. J. Pashkow: John A. Burns School of Medicine, University of Hawaii, Honolulu, Hawaii 96815.
R. C. Pasternak: Cardiology Division, Massachusetts General Hospital, Harvard Medical School, Boston, Massachusetts 02114.

tors and that patients previously thought to be poor candidates for rehabilitation (such as the elderly or those with significant left ventricular [LV] dysfunction and low work capacity) may experience substantial relative functional benefits.

Beyond exercise training, the role of risk factor modification in patients with known coronary disease has become even more established. In addition to the reduction of subsequent acute coronary events and the need for subsequent revascularization, newer data suggest the possibility of arrest, plaque stabilization, and in some cases, actual regression of coronary atherothrombosis.

CARDIAC REHABILITATION AS A MODALITY OF THERAPY IN THE CURRENT TREATMENT OF CORONARY ARTERY DISEASE

Evolution of Cardiac Rehabilitation from Progressive Activity

Up to the early 1950s, activity after acute myocardial infarction (AMI) was thought to be ill advised (1). Levine and others experimented with earlier activities such as chair sitting (2) and progressive ambulation (3). Cardiac rehabilitation had its beginnings as a formalization of progressive earlier activity after AMI (4). It evolved into structured exercise training before or after hospital discharge, or both (5), but more recently it has matured into a multidisciplinary effort serving as a comprehensive preventive cardiac practice encompassing risk stratification, exercise training, secondary risk factor modification, and personal/vocational adjustment (6).

Physiology of Exercise Relevant to Conditioning in Patients with Coronary Artery Disease

Peripheral adaptations, mainly consisting of more efficient oxygen extraction and use of oxygen by skeletal muscle, account for most of the improvement in functional capacity associated with exercise training (7). The reduction in activity-related symptoms experienced by many patients with coronary disease who have received moderate-intensity exercise training is in large part a result of the diminished coronary blood supply required to meet the reduced myocardial oxygen demand needed to perform a given amount of physical work (8). This is especially evident at submaximal workloads, below the anaerobic threshold. The anaerobic threshold is the greatest oxygen uptake that can be maintained without an increase in lactate (9). It effectively delineates routine daily activities from athletic endeavors. Exercise results in a decrease of peripheral vascular resistance, heart rate, and intramyocardial wall tension during physical activity. Although these changes generally produce an improvement in exercise duration, such measures, which often are offered as proof of efficacy for therapeutic interventions, also can be changed by a learning effect, the exercise protocol itself, and patient motivation.

Exercise alone has not been studied in coronary angiographic regression trials. However, an intensive physical training program in association with a moderate diet intervention has been shown to affect favorably the progression of coronary atherothrombotic lesions and stress-induced myocardial ischemia in patients with stable angina pectoris (10). Furthermore, this same group has shown that the extent of improvement (progression, stabilization, and regression) was associated with the weekly amount of physical exercise. Regression was seen only in patients exercising an average of 2,200 kcal per week, whereas angiographically determined slowing of coronary lesion progression was seen in patients averaging approximately 1,500 kcal per week (11). The salutary effect of exercise training on peripheral vascular resistance (12), autonomic nervous system adaptations (13) including heart rate variability (14), blood coagulation, and rheology (15,16), and platelet function (17) will likely be linked both to the process of primary atherogenesis and to the role of plaque rupture leading to initiation of acute coronary events.

The mechanisms involved in mediating the positive effects on myocardial perfusion in patients with CAD have been controversial: Both regression of coronary artery stenosis (18) and improvement of collateralization have been suggested as potential adaptations (19,20). Studies of acetylcholine-induced coronary vasoconstriction have provided evidence of a direct effect of exercise on coronary endothelial function. Exercise training attenuates paradoxic vasoconstriction in CAD and increases coronary blood flow in response to acetylcholine and sensitizes resistance arteries for the vasodilatory effects of adenosine, providing a pathophysiologic framework to explain the improvement of myocardial perfusion in the absence of changes in baseline coronary artery diameter (21).

Ejection fraction is a poor predictor of endurance functional capacity. This appears to be related primarily to the intrinsic capacity of the patient's heart rate to increase appropriately and secondarily to the capability to improve stroke volume by changes in load or contractility (22). A patient with an extremely large heart and an adequate heart rate reserve (through a normal chronotropic response) may have adequate cardiac output to perform moderate endurance exercise despite a very low ejection fraction (23). Kellermann (24) reports that in some selected patients an increased ejection fraction occurred during exercise training. In most cases, it is likely that there is modest improvement in myocardial contractility and stroke volume, the latter as a consequence of adaptive changes in preload and afterload.

Data suggest that greater intensity, long-term exercise training can result in favorable central adaptations to exercise. Central cardiovascular adaptations occurred in patients with CAD after a year-long program of 1 hour of exercise at 70% to 90% of Vo_{2max} 5 days per week using electrocardiographic (ECG), echocardiographic, hemodynamic, and radionuclide evidence (25). These training-induced adaptations are consistent with an improvement in myocardial

TABLE 84–1. *Components of cardiac rehabilitation and associated goals**

Initial evaluation
Take medical history and perform physical examination
Measure risk factors
Obtain electrocardiograms at rest and during exercise
Provide vocational counseling
Determine level of risk
Goal: formulation of prevention plan in collaboration with primary care physician

Management of lipid levels
Assess and modify diet, physical activity, and drug therapy
Primary goal: LDL cholesterol level < 70 mg/dL
Secondary goal: HDL cholesterol level > 45 mg/dL, triglyceride level < 200 mg/dL

Management of hypertension
Measure blood pressure frequently at rest and during exercise
If resting systolic pressure is 130–139 mm Hg or diastolic pressure is 85–89 mm Hg, recommend lifestyle modification, including exercise weight management, sodium restriction, and moderation of alcohol intake; if patient has diabetes or chronic renal or heart failure, consider drug therapy
Monitor effect of intervention in collaboration with primary care physician
Goal: blood pressure < 140/90 mm Hg (or <130/85 mm Hg if patient has diabetes or chronic heart or renal failure)

Cessation of smoking
Document smoking status (never smoked, stopped smoking in remote past, stopped smoking recently, or currently smokes)
Determine patient's readiness to quit; if ready, pick date
Offer nicotine-replacement therapy, bupropion, or both
Offer behavioral advice and group or individual counseling
Goal: long-term abstinence

Weight reduction
Consider for patients with BMI > 25 or waist circumference > 100 cm (in men) or > 90 cm (in women), particularly if associated with hypertension, hyperlipidemia, or insulin resistance or diabetes
Provide behavioral and nutritional counseling with follow-up to monitor progress in achieving goals
Goals: loss of 5–10% of body weight and modification of associated risk factors

Management of diabetes
Identify candidates on the basis of the medical history and baseline glucose test
Develop a regimen of dietary modification, weight control, and exercise combined with oral hypoglycemic agents and insulin therapy
Monitor glucose control before and after exercise sessions and communicate results to primary care physician
For newly detected diabetes, refer patient to primary care physician for evaluation and treatment
Goals: normalization of fasting plasma glucose level (80–110 mg/dL) or glycosylated hemoglobin level (<7.0%) and control of associated obesity, hypertension, and hyperlipidemia

Psychosocial management
Identify psychosocial problems such as depression, anxiety, social isolation, anger, and hostility by means of an interview, standardized questionnaires, or both
Provide individual or group counseling, or both, for patients with clinically significant psychosocial problems
Provide stress reduction class for all patients
Goal: absence of clinically significant psychosocial problems and acquisition of stress management skills

Physical activity counseling and exercise training
Assess current physical activity and exercise tolerance with monitored exercise stress test
Identify barriers to increased physical activity
Provide advice regarding increasing physical activity
Develop an individualized regimen of aerobic and resistance training, specifying frequency, intensity, duration, and types of exercise
Goals: increases in regular physical activity, strength, and physical functioning, expenditure of at least 1,000 kcal per week in physical activity

The body mass index (BMI) is the weight in kilograms divided by the square of the height in meters. To convert the values for low-density lipoprotein (LDL) and high-density lipoprotein (HDL) cholesterol to millimoles per liter, multiply by 0.02586. To convert the value for triglyceride levels to millimoles per liter, multiply by 0.01129. To convert the values for glucose to millimoles per liter, multiply by 0.05551.

oxygenation and concomitantly with enhanced LV function in these patients. The program also resulted in improvements in glucose tolerance, insulin sensitivity, and plasma lipoprotein lipid profile. These beneficial cardiovascular and metabolic adaptations were maintained during 6 years of additional training in these patients. These results do not imply that all patients with CAD should initiate such an intense training program but rather that, in selected patients undergoing a training regimen well in excess of that conventionally prescribed for coronary patients, the training-induced adaptations may be greater than previously believed (25). Furthermore, improved cardiorespiratory fitness is firmly established as having a favorable impact on long-term prognosis in patients with established CAD (26,27).

Exercise influences a wide variety of individual factors associated with CAD risk. A salutary benefit of exercise on factors of the coagulation process has been demonstrated. Exercise training resulted in an alteration of fibrinolytic variables among older individuals 60 to 82 years of age. Fibrinogen and plasminogen activator inhibitor decreased significantly, and tissue plasminogen activity increased (28). Decreased platelet aggregability and a significant inhibition of secondary platelet aggregation from 27% to 36% were observed in the men participating in regular exercise (17). Physical conditioning has improved coagulation indicators after MI as well. Levels of fibrinogen, factor VIII:C, and von Willebrand antigen and activities of angiotensin II receptor type III (AT-III) and plasminogen were significantly decreased in 56 subjects after MI with physical training ($p < 0.05$), whereas values were unchanged in a control group (15). Physical activity may directly mitigate inflammation as inflammatory markers, including C-reactive protein, are less in individuals engaging in regular exercise (29,30). Finally, exercise training appears to lead to at least a modest (16%) decrease in homocysteine levels (31).

Components of Program Design

Cardiac rehabilitation programs have evolved considerably since they first appeared in the 1960s. Key standards and goals are regularly updated. Balady and coworkers (32) has adapted the most recent nationally published guidelines as shown in Table 84–1.

Cardiac rehabilitation programs have traditionally been designated by phases according to the temporal and functional status of the patient relative to an index coronary event. Although no longer applicable with current inpatient lengths of stay, this designation system remains useful for program and patient classification purposes. Phase I rehabilitation is an inpatient therapy. The major goal for the physical activity portion of the phase I program is to condition the patient for the exertional demands required after discharge (33). This has been a reasonably straightforward task because most activities of daily living in the home environment are below the 3 to 4 MET level (1 MET = *metabolic* oxygen requirement for resting conditions). However, short-

ening lengths of stay have essentially eliminated the time available for inpatient exercise training, and the time available is not adequate to acquire the skills required for self-monitoring of exercise activity or for adequately achieving an understanding of the disease process (6). With patients often overwhelmed by the volume of new information to assimilate and remember, it is difficult to do more than begin the process of identifying risk factors and changing lifestyles. Thus, an appropriate trend in phase I programs is to focus more on evaluation of risks and needs and to motivate patients to participate in the appropriate outpatient (phase II or III) rehabilitation program.

Phase II programs are both ECG monitored and supervised; phase III programs are supervised only. Whether phase II or III, current outpatient programs are generally institutionally based group experiences offering ECG monitoring, exercise supervision, education, and risk factor management. The exercise component occurs concurrently with education and psychosocial support for modification of coronary-prone behavior and for satisfactory return to a suitable and active lifestyle (34). By use of a multifactorial approach, all potential risk factors should be addressed (35). In patients of working age, there usually are also vocational and job-specific issues (36). With an increasing emphasis on quality survival (37) and economic valuation of the service (38), the major focus of many programs has gone well beyond the putative impact of exercise training on mortality (39,40). Currently, cardiac rehabilitation is being refashioned as a "soft technology" with great potential to influence outcomes including, but not limited to, long-term postinfarction survival (41). It is likely that in the future the emphasis will be on phase III-like outpatient programs that can provide supervision and guidance to large numbers of patients in relatively low-cost, community-based or at-home programs (42–45).

IMPACT OF CARDIAC REHABILITATION ON SURVIVAL AND SUBSEQUENT MYOCARDIAL INFARCTION

Trials of Exercise Alone or Exercise Plus Additional Interventions

Individual prospective studies performed mainly from the 1970s to the early 1980s showed a trend toward reduced mortality in those participating after an AMI. Insufficient sample size, limited follow-up duration, and dropout rates as high as 50% resulted in insufficient statistical power for any single randomized trial of exercise training to prove its efficacy (46). Most of the studies used life-table analysis for the determination of statistical significance. Had crude death rate (number of deaths/number of patients followed) been used, several of the individual studies would have been significant.

In 1988, Oldridge (47) published a metaanalysis of 10 randomized clinical trials (4,347 patients) that suggested a reduction in the incidence rate of overall and cardiovascular mortality of about 25% in those participating in exercise rehabilitation. Exercise training started between 8 and 36 weeks after infarction, and duration varied between 6 and 48 months. In these pooled data, there was a significant reduction in both all-cause and cardiovascular mortality rates with an odds ratio (OR) of 0.76 (95% confidence interval [CI], 0.63–0.92; $p = 0.004$]. The OR and CI for cardiovascular mortality were nearly identical, which is not surprising because almost all deaths occurring in the patients enrolled in these trials were cardiovascular. The decrease in total and cardiovascular mortality did not depend on when the exercise training was initiated or on whether the program included some risk factor modification or was primarily an exercise-based intervention. The reduction in mortality, however, was more marked in those patients exercising for 52 weeks or more and was only marginally significant among those exercising 12 to 52 weeks. There was no statistically significant effect on mortality observed for those exercising 12 weeks or less. This is especially noteworthy because most contemporary programs deliver (and are only maximally reimbursed for) 8 to 12 weeks of program participation, with variable (and largely unknown) participation thereafter.

O'Connor and associates (48) performed a similar analysis and came to a similar conclusion: Namely, that cardiac rehabilitation reduced overall and cardiovascular mortality by 20% (Fig. 84–1). They further noted that there was a 37% reduction in the incidence of sudden cardiac death (OR, 0.63; 95% CI, 0.41–0.97) within the first year after exercise training. The ORs and 95% CIs at 2 and 3 years were 0.76 (0.54–1.06) and 0.92 (0.69–1.23), respectively, which suggest a benefit, but they are not statistically significant (48). Consistent with this observation, Hämäläinen and coworkers (49), in a single prospective study, noted that the significantly lower sudden death and coronary mortality observed 3 years after MI persisted at 10-year follow-up in the intervention group (35.1% coronary mortality) compared with control groups (47.1% coronary mortality; $p = 0.02$).

The early results reported by Hämäläinen's group (49) were included in both Oldridge's (47) and O'Connor's meta-analysis (48). In a 1979 study, 375 patients were consecutively randomized to a multifactorial intervention program. There was an 18.6% cardiovascular mortality rate in the intervention group and a 29.41% mortality in the control group ($p = 0.02$). This difference was mainly associated with a reduction of sudden deaths in the intervention group (5.8% vs. 14.4%; $p < 0.01$). This was the only "early" study individually achieving such statistical significance (50).

After 10 years of follow-up, the significantly lower sudden death and coronary mortality observed 3 years after MI still persisted in the intervention group (188 patients) compared with the control group (187 patients) (49). The incidence of sudden death in the intervention group was 12.8% compared with 23.0% in the control group ($p = 0.01$). The

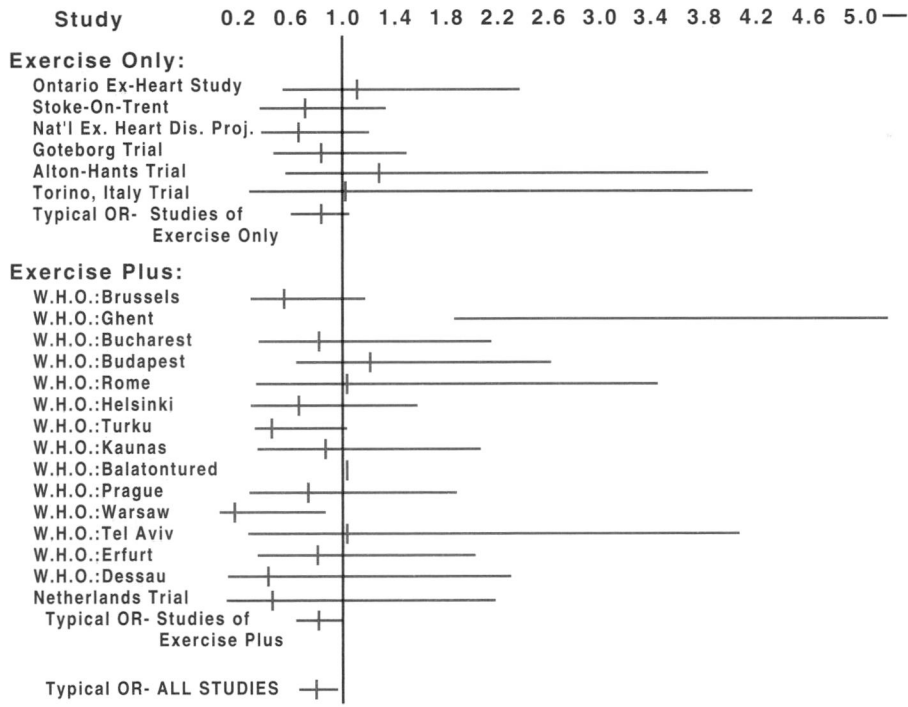

FIG. 84–1. Chart of effects of pooling from randomized trials of cardiac rehabilitation on the estimate of mortality 3 years after randomization. *Short vertical lines* indicate the point estimates; *horizontal lines* depict the 95% confidence intervals. OR, odds ratio; W.H.O., World Health Organization. (Adapted from O'Connor GT, Buring JE, Yusuf S, et al. An overview of randomized trials of rehabilitation with exercise after myocardial infarction. *Circulation* 1989;80:234–244, with permission.)

incidence of coronary mortality was 35.1% and 47.1%, respectively ($p = 0.02$). During the first year, when the mortality difference was most marked, the use of β-blockers was not significantly different between the groups. It is unfortunate that late follow-up is not more uniformly available from other earlier studies. Perhaps similar long-term favorable findings might influence contemporary referral patterns.

Interestingly, the studies discussed above consistently found that the incidence of sudden death is favorably influenced by exercise training (49,50), as did another study regarding regular exercise (51). There are implications for this finding related to the fundamental mechanisms of sudden cardiac death after MI. Exercise may contribute to improved electrical stability of the myocardium by virtue of a number of different mechanisms: decreased regional ischemia at submaximal exercise, decreased ambient catecholamines in myocardial substrate at rest and submaximal exercise, and increased ventricular fibrillation threshold because of a reduction of cyclic adenosine monophosphate (52).

Other explanations for the impact on mortality have been postulated. An alteration of the balance between sympathetic and parasympathetic activity occurs in those undergoing endurance exercise training. This was documented in the modification of heart rate variability observed by spectral analysis indicating an increase in vagal tone with physical training (13). Posel and associates (53) noted that exercise training after experimental MI in an isolated animal heart increases the ventricular fibrillation threshold before and after the onset of reinfarction. Exercise conditioning improved heart rate variability in 20 prospectively studied cardiac patients, particularly in those who achieved a threshold of greater than 1.5 training METs increase over a 12-week period (14). These study results are supportive of the concept that exercise training decreases the risk for sudden cardiac death through increased vagal tone, which likely beneficially alters ventricular fibrillatory and ischemic thresholds.

The increased surveillance present in the rehabilitation environment may in part explain the one-third reduction in the incidence of sudden death (39). The frequent regular contact with knowledgeable and experienced staff provides an opportunity for earlier discovery of potentially destabilizing factors such as ischemia, decompensated heart failure, presyncopal symptoms, and adverse drug reactions. The fact that patients do well when exercising under direct observation in the rehabilitation environment is further suggested by Van Camp's 1986 survey (54) that revealed only 3 deaths among 21 cardiac arrests occurring during more than 2,000,000 patient hours of exercise training. Thus, cardiac rehabilitation may influence both the incidence of sudden death and survival from sudden death.

Both the Oldrich (47) and O'Connor (48) metaanalyses failed to show any decrease in the prevention of nonfatal reinfarction after MI with exercise-based cardiac rehabilitation programs. In addition to the possibility that this lack of effect is real, other factors may explain this observation, including inadequate attention to other risk factors, selection bias leading to lower participation in rehabilitation programs for patients with ongoing symptoms and risk for reinfarction, and finally, statistically insufficient follow-up. Consistent with the latter suggestion is the late follow-up from a comprehensive rehabilitation program in Sweden (55). In this study of more than 300 patients, in the intervention group, recurrent nonfatal MIs were statistically less frequent at both 5 and 10 years after the initial event. Furthermore, at the 10-year follow-up, far more patients continued to be active and at work (51.8 vs. 27.4%; $p < 0.01$) in the intervention group compared with the group receiving standard care. Newer potent lipid-active agents, currently recognized as capable of reducing the incidence of a variety of cardiac events after MI, when added to physical training as part of a comprehensive cardiac rehabilitation approach, would be likely to yield more favorable results with respect to nonfatal recurrent cardiac events. However, as discussed later, it is unlikely that further randomized trials of cardiac rehabilitation will be carried out in the current era.

Bittner and Oberman (52) speculated that the age of prospective randomized trials for cardiac rehabilitation has probably ended. They contended that to document conclusive changes in mortality would require too large a sample size given the difficulties encountered with recruitment and compliance, that low event rates are likely to get even lower with continuing refinements in medical and interventional therapy, and that analysis will be confounded by contemporary changes in lifestyle and risk factor management. All of these predictions have been proven true. Also, recruitment into a post-MI trial of cardiac rehabilitation with a control group is unlikely to be acceptable to most investigators and patients. The trials of the future will likely be multicentered and likely will use substitute surrogates in lieu of a total mortality endpoint—both noninvasive (e.g., carotid intimal thickening) and invasive (e.g., coronary intravascular ultrasound), as well as newer validated tools such as refined quality of life measures and economic evaluation.

Modifications of Other Risk Factors for Coronary Artery Disease

Because of the multifactorial causes of CAD and the multidisciplinary interventions used by contemporary cardiac rehabilitation programs, it is difficult to determine the benefits of individual interventions targeted to specific risk factors. Clearly, implementation of an aggressive secondary preventive approach has had an impact on both the design and the outcomes of cardiac rehabilitation programs. Several lines of evidence point to the benefits of the multifactorial approach. In addition to exercise (discussed earlier) and psychological factors (discussed in the following sections), attention is appropriately directed to control of lipid abnormalities (see Chapter 11), hypertension (see Chapter 16), and diabetes (see Chapter 19). In the context of appropriate risk stratification (see Chapter 78–80), to identify and treat conditions (e.g., recurrent angina, heart failure, and ventricular ectopy), smoking cessation (see Chapter 18) and antithrombotic and antiplatelet therapies (see Chapter 83) also should be addressed. One of the earliest and most successful demonstrations of the benefits of a multifactorial approach is the 1979 study of Kallio and coworkers (50), reported as part of a World Health Organization effort to assess the benefit of comprehensive rehabilitation. This program included emphasis on health education, smoking cessation, diet, stress reduction, and pharmacologic interventions, as well as physical activity. The impact on cardiovascular mortality, particularly sudden cardiac death, is discussed in detail earlier. Results of the Swedish study discussed earlier also confirm the benefit of a "comprehensive" intervention (55).

The individual benefits of various risk factor interventions are well documented and are reviewed in detail in chapters focusing on these specific factors elsewhere in this textbook. In particular, the last decade has witnessed an explosive growth of data supporting the value of lipid-altering therapy in patients with CAD (56,57). Older comprehensive reviews of secondary prevention after MI (46,58,59) suggest that the benefit of antiplatelet drugs, anticoagulants, and β-blockers are roughly equivalent to the benefit from physical training.

Advances in our understanding of the pathogenesis of acute coronary syndromes (60) has led to an evolution of secondary preventive approaches that rationally combine multiple risk factor interventions targeted to an individual's unique combination of risk factors. Understanding of patient-based lifestyle and behavioral factors relevant to modification of appropriate risk factors is ideally managed through the multidisciplinary individualized approach available in comprehensive postinfarct cardiac rehabilitation programs (61). Such programs have been shown to improve both intermediate (e.g., lipids, blood pressure, fitness, and others) and clinical outcomes (62–65).

Psychological Stress and Depression and Their Impact on Cardiac Events and Survival

The relation between the heart and the higher nervous system has been the subject of speculation for perhaps thousands of years, but an understanding of the details of this association and its impact on the prognosis and treatment of CAD is only a relatively recent occurrence. Lown and Verrier (66,67) documented a relation between neural activity and ventricular fibrillation in the mid-1970s and demonstrated that psychological and psychosocial stressors predispose experimental animals to ventricular fibrillation.

In humans, the relation between psychological distress and ventricular ectopy has been investigated extensively. In one study, a correlation between self-reported distress levels and occurrence of ectopic beats in patients after MI was found (68).

Carney and associates (69) have examined the potential relation between psychiatric depression and ventricular arrhythmias in patients with CAD. Among the 103 patients with coronary disease studied, they found 21 (20%) who met the criteria for either major or minor depression. There were no significant differences between patients with or without depression in severity of CAD, age, or use of β-blockers; however, five (23.8%) of the patients with depression exhibited episodes of ventricular tachycardia during ambulatory ECG monitoring compared with only three (3.7%) patients who did not experience depression ($p = 0.008$) (69).

The existence and association of certain specific personality characteristics with CAD has been controversial (70,71). The "type A" personality profile includes such behavioral characteristics as aggressiveness/competitiveness, time urgency, and labile hostility. It has been linked to mortality from CAD (72) and to the extent (73) and progression of coronary atherothrombosis (74). However, other studies have failed to confirm a relation between type A and acute coronary incidents including death (75,76). In a cohort of 257 patients (all men) who died during the 20 years after classification as type A, of 26 subjects who died within 24 hours of a cardiac event, personality type was unrelated to mortality occurrence, and for the remaining subjects who died after the first 24 hours, the likelihood of being type A personality was considerably *lower* than expected (77). An apparent link to atherothrombosis progression also has been suggested for psychological factors including low social support, cynical hostility, and anger. At a 2-year angiographic follow-up, psychological variables were associated with a significantly greater risk for CAD progression (78).

Depression is commonly present in patients with CAD, particularly in the post-MI period. Kavanagh and associates (79) found that one-third of a group of more than 100 patients participating in a cardiac rehabilitation program 16 to 18 months after MI had scores consistent with severe depression. They noted that the severely depressed patients were older and had a greater tendency to have poorly controlled hypertension and active angina. They also noted that those with severe depression have a tendency to accomplish less with exercise training despite an equal intensity of endurance exercise. In a more recent study, depressive symptoms, easily assessed by a simple questionnaire, also was predictive of diminished functional improvement after cardiac rehabilitation (80).

Although the severity of depression may not be associated with the severity of cardiac illness, depression is associated with the presence of comorbid medical conditions (81). Furthermore, depressed patients often do not return to work and only receive psychiatric treatment sporadically (81).

The use of even more stringent diagnostic criteria for major depressive disorder continues to reveal a relatively high incidence (18%) of major depression in patients with coronary disease (82). Increasingly, it is recognized that the presence of major depressive disorder is predictive of future acute cardiac events occurring in patients with CAD, regardless of the severity of the coronary disease, LV ejection fraction, and the presence of smoking (83).

In an extremely important study, Frasure-Smith and coworkers (84) have shown that major depression after MI has a significant independent impact on cardiac mortality over the first 6 months after hospital discharge. In this prospective evaluation of the impact of depression, using a modified version of the National Institute of Mental Health Diagnostic Interview Schedule to detect major depression, Frasure-Smith and her associates (84) evaluated the independent impact of depression after control for significant clinical predictors. A total of 222 patients who met the established criteria for MI during the study period were interviewed up to 15 days after discharge and were followed for 6 months. By 6 months, 12 patients had died; all from cardiac causes. Depression was the most significant predictor of mortality (hazard ratio [HR] 5.74; 95% CI, 4.61–6.87; $p = 0.0006$). The impact of depression remained significant after control for LV dysfunction and previous MI, which also were significant multivariate predictors of mortality (adjusted HR, 4.29; 95% CI, 3.14–5.44; $p = 0.013$). Late (5-year) follow-up demonstrated a continued link between depression and mortality (85). The severity of depression at the time of admission for MI was more closely associated with mortality than was improvement in symptoms at 1 year. Thus, major depression in patients hospitalized after an MI is an independent and powerful risk factor for mortality, at least equivalent to that of LV dysfunction and history of prior infarction.

Roose and Dalack (86) have further connected the phenomenon of sudden cardiac death with the affective disorders such as major depression by observing that parasympathetic activity, measured by analysis of heart rate variability, is decreased in patients with depression in comparison with normal control subjects (86). They note that others have found that, after adjusting for significant cardiac parameters, low heart rate variability also emerged as a significant predictor of mortality in a group of patients after MI. These studies are consistent with Frasure-Smith's finding that patients with affective disorders have a greater than expected rate of morbidity and mortality from cardiovascular disease and suggest that this may be caused by abnormal autonomic nervous system activity (87).

Other manifestations of psychosocial dysfunction are important prognostically as well. Interviews with 2,320 male survivors of AMI revealed two psychological variables strongly associated with an increased 3-year mortality risk: social isolation and a high degree of life stress. Even with other important prognostic factors such as LV function controlled, the patients classified as being socially isolated and having a high degree of life stress had more than four times the risk for death than the subjects with low levels of both stress and isolation (88).

Unfortunately, major affective and stress disorders in patients with coronary heart disease often are unrecognized clinically. Consequently, these disorders usually remain untreated. Rose and Robins (89) have confirmed that the deficiency of treatment is a likely result of a lack of appreciation of the presence and nature of psychological complications by the managing physician, who "in seeking to understand and empathize with the patient's loss, ascribes the patient's emotional state to a 'normal reaction' to illness" (89). This lack of appreciation may account for subsequent mortality that may be as high as 15% to 20% per year, a figure that is comparable to untreated moderate to severe LV dysfunction (71)!

Beneficial Influence of Exercise Training on Neural and Psychological Function

Exercise has been popularly credited with improving psychological well-being. Gentry (90) has observed that on entering cardiac rehabilitation programs, patients typically experience fear of recurrence, death, decreased performance, and damaged self-concept. Anecdotally, patients report significant subjective improvements in mood, anxiety, and self-confidence. The emphasis of studies relevant to this issue has been on specific alterations of psychological measures or personality (91). Hellerstein (92), for example, reported that feelings of depression were significantly reduced in a cohort of 100 patients participating in exercise training. Patients and their spouses observed improvements in sleep, cognitive thinking, fatigue, perception of stress, and well-being in those participating in the exercise program compared with their pretraining condition.

In a small prospective study, Naughton and colleagues (91) reported that patients undergoing exercise training experienced less tension, worry, and anxiety (64% of exercise group vs. 43% of sedentary control group). Exercisers reported improved attitudes and spousal/family relationships and a trend toward improved measures of depression and invalid behavior. Rovario and associates (93) compared patients with coronary disease who participated in a comprehensive cardiac rehabilitation program with nonparticipating patients. The rehabilitation patients reported increased positive self-concept and physical self-esteem, decreased signs of personal maladjustment, improved employment-related stress, and increased participation in leisure time and sexual activity, and they had fewer diagnoses of other psychiatric disorders. There was no difference in total depression scores, however, but certain components of depressed affect such as mood and fatigue improved. Interestingly, the investigators report that patients who had their qualifying event more than 6 months previously derived as much benefit from the program as those entering acutely, and the beneficial effects persisted up to 4 months after completion of the 3-month experience. However, data suggest that changes in major affective psychological disorders are difficult to achieve with exercise training alone (94). Thus, the clinician should not expect that major affective disorders (e.g., severe depression) will be demonstrably influenced by regular exercise per se. Patients with evidence of these disorders need specialized attention.

Specific neurovascular changes occur as a result of strenuous and prolonged endurance training in healthy, previously sedentary, middle-aged and older men (13), and thus are likely to occur in patients with CAD patients. With large increases in maximal exercise capacity, there are small reductions in heart rate at rest, an increase in cardiac vagal tone at rest, and a diminished forearm vasoconstrictor response to reductions in baroreflex sympathoinhibition, but no significant influence on sympathetic neural activation during acute exercise or cold pressor stress (95).

In patients with ischemic heart disease, Cooksey and colleagues (96) have found that a 3-month program of exercise training reduced plasma norepinephrine level during supine rest (320 ± 23 to 191 ± 20 pg/mL; $p < 0.01$), but plasma epinephrine values were unchanged. When these previously sedentary patients exercised on a treadmill to the maximal level attained before exercise training, the mean plasma norepinephrine and plasma epinephrine concentrations were significantly reduced, suggesting that the beneficial adaptations of the cardiovascular system to exercise training are at least partially mediated by changes in the catecholamine response to exercise (96). Clinically, these findings are consistent with the observation that although heavy exercise can "trigger" AMI, increased amounts of habitual physical exercise are associated with decreased relative risk for MI overall (51).

Thus, cardiac rehabilitation produces measurable worthwhile psychological effects in patients with coronary heart disease and provides an adjunct for improving pathologic psychological conditions (97). In those with serious affective disorders who are at greatest risk for experiencing increased mortality as a manifestation of their depression, combination therapy involving psychotropic drugs, psychotherapy, and exercise may prove most appropriate (71). Nevertheless, cardiac rehabilitation, especially when psychological issues are attended to, has been shown to improve certain disorders, including depression and hostility (98–100).

A metaanalysis reviewed psychological treatment with cardiac rehabilitation in 23 randomized controlled trials including 3,180 subjects (101). Treated patients demonstrated a reduction in psychological distress associated with greater improvement in systolic blood pressure, cholesterol level, and trends toward improved mortality and morbidity, compared with patients not receiving psychological treatment. Benefits were continued for 2 years and diminished thereafter. Several more recent small trials suggest that cardiac rehabilitation complemented by psychological interventions result in improved cardiovascular outcomes compared with usual care or with exercise programs alone (102,103). Results of a randomized trial of a selective serotonin reuptake inhibitor, sertraline, in patients with acute coronary syndromes has been reported (104). The principal goals of the trial were to demonstrate safety of the agent in this patient group and to establish antidepressant efficacy. Both goals were accomplished. Furthermore, "severe" cardiovascular events appeared to be less frequent with sertraline (14.5% vs. 22.4%) at 24 weeks.

OTHER GOALS AND END POINTS

Quality of Life: An Alternative End Point

Appropriately, investigators and clinicians have increasingly focused on quality of life as a key outcome in medicine and cardiology (105,106). As measures of quality of life have become better understood and more standardized, these subjective outcomes for cardiac rehabilitation have been more closely assessed (37,107–110). However, valid measures remain an issue (110–112).

Although difficult to consistently demonstrate (113), cardiac rehabilitation does appear to generally improve perceived quality of life (39,114). Oldridge and colleagues (40), for example, have demonstrated that patients at low risk will likely recover normal performance of routine activities of daily living, regardless of whether they participate in an exercise rehabilitation program. Rehabilitation is less likely to affect their perception of quality of life.

Substantial evidence currently supports favorable changes in physical functioning in response to cardiac rehabilitation. Ades and coworkers (8) reported marked improvement in physical functioning assessed by the Medical Outcomes Score Short-Form (SF 36). Others have reported similar improvements (97,115).

Improvement in the Atherothrombotic Process

During recent decades, there has been a heightened focus on secondary prevention of atherothrombosis and CAD events within the context of cardiac rehabilitation programs (41,61). Numerous clinical studies using serial angiography have provided convincing evidence that a slowing or halting of progression or frank regression of coronary atherothrombosis can occur with interventions (10,63,116–118). Most studies have focused on strategies to improve serum lipids through the use of drugs, diet, and exercise. Ornish and colleagues (118) published results from a prospective, randomized, controlled trial suggesting that comprehensive lifestyle changes can affect coronary atherothrombosis after only 1 year. In this study, 28 patients were assigned to an experimental group (low-fat vegetarian diet, smoking cessation, stress management training, and moderate exercise), and 20 to a usual-care control group; 195 coronary artery lesions were analyzed by quantitative coronary angiography. The average percentage diameter stenosis regressed from 40.0% (SD 16.9) to 37.8% (SD 16.5) in the experimental group, but progressed from 42.7% (SD 15.5) to 46.1% (18.5) in the control group.

Significant regression of atherothrombotic lesions after aggressive lipid-lowering treatment without lipid-lowering drugs also has been documented with angiographic studies by Schuler and his associates (10). Treatment comprised intensive physical exercise in group training sessions (minimum 2 h/wk) plus daily home exercise periods (minimum 20 min/d) and a low-fat, low-cholesterol diet (American Heart Association phase 3 diet). After 12 months of participation, repeat coronary angiography was performed. In patients participating in the intervention group, body weight decreased by 5% ($p < 0.001$), total cholesterol by 10% ($p < 0.001$), and triglyceride levels by 24% ($p < 0.001$); high-density lipoprotein levels increased by 3% (not significant). Physical work capacity improved by 23% ($p < 0.0001$), and myocardial oxygen consumption, as estimated from maximal rate–pressure product, by 10% ($p < 0.05$). Stress-induced myocardial ischemia decreased concurrently, indicating improvement of myocardial perfusion. In the intervention group, progression of coronary lesions was noted in 9 patients (23%), no change was noted in 18 patients (45%), and regression occurred in 13 patients (32%). In the control group, metabolic and hemodynamic variables remained essentially unchanged, whereas progression of coronary lesions was noted in 25 patients (48%), no change in 18 patients (35%), and regression in 9 patients (17%). These changes were significantly different from the intervention group ($p < 0.05$).

In a large randomized trial, Haskell and his associates (63) have reported that intensive multiple risk factor reduction delivered through a home-based model, analogous to a comprehensive long-term cardiac rehabilitation program, over an extended period (4 years), significantly reduced the rate of progression of atherothrombosis in the coronary arteries of men and women with CAD and decreased hospitalizations for clinical cardiac events.

Although angiographic "regression" trials allow for increased understanding of the potential efficacy of new and evolving regimens and yield information about the nature of progressive atherothrombotic lesions (119,120), metaanalyses of these trials have consistently demonstrated that the clinical benefit of the intervention (in terms of cardiac event reduction) are of much greater magnitude than expected from the angiographic improvement (120). In view of our current understanding of plaque vulnerability and the plaque-stabilizing effect of preventive efforts, particularly lipid-lowering therapy, the reality that clinical events can be prevented by risk factor interventions should no longer surprise clinicians (60).

CHANGING DEMOGRAPHICS AND INCREASINGLY COMPLEX PATIENTS

Impact of Interventions and Coronary Bypass Surgery on the Cardiac Rehabilitation Population

The patient population admitted to the hospital for acute coronary syndromes is changing; as a result, those referred for cardiac rehabilitation are changing as well. Patients are increasingly older, sicker, and more complex. These patients were formerly thought to pose increased risk and, because of compromise in their circulatory hemodynamics, were thought to be poor candidates for the exercise portion of the rehabilitation (121). Ironically, the current thinking is that formal exercise training may be of relatively little short-term benefit to the completely uncomplicated patient and that the intensive rehabilitative process is now more appropriately directed to-

ward secondary risk factor modification and education (122). Nevertheless, there appears to be a growing population of medically complex cardiac patients who are likely to benefit from cardiac rehabilitation (123).

The principles of risk stratification apply regardless of the intervention. Patients at high risk will potentially benefit most (124).

Percutaneous coronary intervention (PCI) is currently commonly performed after AMI. Improved functional capacity has been demonstrated with cardiac rehabilitation after PCI, but this may represent a simple conditioning effect after relief of ischemic symptoms (125). Ben-Ari and colleagues (126) have reported significant differences in work capacity and favorable changes in low- and high-density lipoproteins in those participating for less than 6 months in a comprehensive rehabilitation program. Participation had no influence on the rate of restenosis (30% vs. 32%), however, or the incidence of subsequent coronary bypass (5% vs. 4.4%) and MI (1.6% vs. 1.4%) (126). Support for cardiac rehabilitation after PCI also comes from the observation that earlier studies had shown a disappointing rate of return to work after PCI although the patients were physically capable (127), possibly related to a lack of self-efficacy and persistence of the "sick role," those who have angina after angioplasty are less likely to return to work (128).

A number of studies have been reported indicating that rehabilitation after coronary bypass surgery has efficacy as well and that results can be long lasting (129,130). Weiner and others (131) reported early on that sustained, measurable improvements in functional capacity occurred in patients who participated in exercise rehabilitation and they continued for 36 to 48 months (131). Oldridge and coworkers (129) have demonstrated a significant functional difference that persists in those who participate in exercise rehabilitation for extended periods. Froelicher (130) has shown increased oxygen uptake and decreased resting and submaximal heart rates in patients after conditioning regardless of whether revascularization appeared complete or incomplete. This finding has implications regarding the efficacy of rehabilitation for incompletely revascularized patients regardless of the technique used. Institution of a simple postrevascularization referral system can dramatically increase the appropriate referral of patients who stand to benefit greatly from cardiac rehabilitation (132).

Among cardiac rehabilitation candidates are increasingly complex patients who have concurrent valvular heart disease, LV dysfunction (133), cardiac transplantation (123), or cardiac devices such as rate-adaptive pacemakers, or automated implantable cardioverter-defibrillators (134).

Exercise Training in Patients with Left Ventricular Dysfunction

Aggressive cardiac care has contributed to the survival of many patients with severe LV dysfunction. This group of patients is one of the fastest growing in the cardiac rehabilitation patient population (135,136). These patients present a different set of problems and expectations and may realize different outcomes from the cardiac rehabilitation process. They are at greater risk for sudden death (137–139) and may be emotionally depressed by the long-standing ordeal of their cardiac disease and their marked limitation (140,141).

The patient with poor LV function shows a varying and inconsistent response to exercise (121). Limitation of exercise capacity is probably the earliest quantifiable finding in heart failure and may actually represent a symptom of functional impairment. The normal central and peripheral effects of exercise may not occur in these patients (142). Exercise can cause an additional reduction in ejection fraction, a decrease in stroke volume, and exertional hypotension. Those with the most severe dysfunction may not increase cardiac output sufficiently to generate a dynamic exercise response (143). Surprisingly, all of these adverse alterations in hemodynamics correlate inconsistently with overall exercise capacity in patients with clinically evident heart failure (144). This occurs because the status of the patient's LV dysfunction is vulnerable to influence by multiple factors (145). The patient may be in atrial fibrillation, for example, or have significant active ischemia. He or she may have forgotten to take prescribed medications, may be salt overloaded, become dehydrated or heat intolerant, or have a concurrent infection. Exercise duration or intensity achieved during a given exercise test or rehabilitation session may be significantly affected.

Exercise intolerance in patients with significant LV dysfunction appears most consistently related to the early onset of anaerobic metabolism in peripheral muscle leading to the development of leg fatigue (121). This is thought to result from both reduced muscle perfusion and reduced aerobic enzyme activity. In the majority of patients, it is not related to greater pulmonary capillary wedge pressures or to increased pulmonary dead space and ventilation in relation to oxygen uptake (121). Despite the observation of inconsistent responses to exercise, there are theoretic, as well as demonstrated, benefits of exercise in patients with heart failure (145,146). Patients with severe LV dysfunction can condition safely by gradually increasing their heart rates above resting level (147). With time, they are able to extract more oxygen from the blood during exercise, thus widening the arteriovenous oxygen difference.

One study raised concern that ventricular remodeling may worsen with exercise in patients with large anterior MIs (148). Subsequent work suggests that beginning moderate exercise training 4 to 8 weeks after an anterior MI in patients with poor LV function neither prevents nor worsens the LV dilation and remodeling that inevitably occurs in such patients (149). This was corroborated in a study by Dubach and colleagues (150) in which a high-intensity cardiac rehabilitation program resulted in substantial increases in exercise capacity among patients with reduced LV function and had no deleterious effects on LV volume, function, or wall thickness regardless of infarct area.

Even patients with profound deconditioning awaiting cardiac transplant who are implanted with an implantable LV assist device (LVAD) are capable of participating in an exercise training program and achieving tangible improvements in exercise capacity (151,152). With the LVAD and a progressive training regimen, all patients achieved New York Heat Association functional Class I-II from Class IV and were walking an average of more than 8,000 feet at the exercise session just before transplant. Another group has reported a similar experience with LVAD therapy and intense exercise training and implied that this observed improvement may have an impact on survival and length of stay after cardiac transplant (151).

The effects of exercise training on mortality for patients with severe LV dysfunction is unknown, but in most, exercise tolerance is improved as illustrated by lower heart rates during submaximal exercise and increased maximal workloads (153). Endurance and fatigue levels must be considered in addition to aerobic capacity. Patients with heart failure may be able to achieve high aerobic workloads but then experience prolonged fatigue for hours or days after an exercise session (143). All of these considerations require careful program design and precautions (133,147).

Wenger (154) noted that the goal of therapy in patients with severe symptomatic heart failure is to improve symptoms and maintain functional abilities and comfort, and that hemodynamic features of heart failure (such as ejection fraction) are generally not well correlated with quality-of-life attributes. For a person who is severely limited, in distinction from the low-risk patient, even modest improvement is likely to have a noticeable impact on functional capacity (155). It is ironic that patients with severely reduced exercise tolerance were formerly excluded from exercise rehabilitation on the assumption that they would derive little tangible benefit (136). The use of β-blockers in patients with heart failure does not eliminate the benefits of such exercise training (156).

Age and Sex Issues Relevant to Cardiac Rehabilitation

Cardiac rehabilitation has increasingly been applied to older populations (157,158). Even in the ninth decade of life exercise training as part of comprehensive cardiac rehabilitation can improve functional capacity and other risk factors (159). With small increments in exercise capacity, the elderly have the capability of maintaining independence and provision of self-care (160). Four to five METs, a work capacity achievable by even some of the very elderly (161), is adequate to perform most activities of daily living such as light housework, shopping, and other domestic functions (123).

Women derive benefits comparable to those achieved by men from cardiac rehabilitation (162), but unfortunately, in part because they are usually older and have other comorbidities, they are not referred as often (163,164). Compared with men, women appear to use cardiac rehabilitation programs less frequently than men, have greater dropout rates, and return to work less frequently and after a longer period (165). However, women completing cardiac rehabilitation can be expected to have similar improvement in risk factors and functional capacity compared with men (166,167). Although the risk factors for coronary disease, other than estrogen, are the same for women as for men, the frequency and relative impact of the risk factors differ (168,169). These findings have important implications for the design of rehabilitation programs.

SUMMARY AND FUTURE DIRECTIONS

Cardiac rehabilitation has evolved into a multifactorial composite therapy of exercise training, risk factor modification, psychosocial support, and education with the two major goals of (a) returning patients to normalcy after acute coronary syndromes or procedures, and (b) reducing the chances of subsequent coronary events. This process especially appears to succeed in patients with significant levels of deconditioning before entering therapy. Survival itself is likely improved, as suggested by metaanalyses of randomized studies performed mainly between 1975 and 1985. A reduction in cardiovascular mortality of 20% to 30% can be anticipated largely through a decrease in the incidence of sudden cardiac death. Improved quality of life and cost utility also have become important contemporary outcomes. Finally, the potential impact of risk factor modification on the fundamental pathologic process of coronary atherothrombosis, thereby mediating the impact of both acute and chronic coronary disease events, may be the most important outcome of cardiac rehabilitation. Future developments in the field of cardiac rehabilitation will be driven by changes in the coronary disease patient population, the rapidly evolving changes in practice and reimbursement including shortening length of hospital stay, increased interest in and confidence in the benefit, and economic pressures. In combination, these factors will continue to drive the development of more diverse models of outpatient rehabilitation services. Home-based rehabilitation will be an attractive option, particularly for lower risk individuals. Reimbursement is currently based primarily on payment for ECG monitoring during exercise, rather than for the personal supervision and often complex clinical management that occurs in comprehensive cardiac rehabilitation programs. This problem is especially relevant in the elderly and in important subsets of patients such as those with severe LV dysfunction. Although these patients were previously thought to be poor candidates for rehabilitation, they potentially can realize the most substantial functional benefits. Likewise, patients who are depressed may realize significant help from group programs that address psychological issues and reduce social isolation. Those patients stratified as low risk will benefit most from lifestyle improvements and management of their coronary risk factors. However, a major problem for all patients is adherence to both lifestyle recommendations and drug therapy. Ongoing efforts and research are needed to make substantial improvements with this important aspect of preventive care delivery.

Considerable clinical trial evidence currently indicates that risk factor modification in patients with known coronary disease should be central to their medical management. Favorable modification of these factors can slow the progression of, stabilize, and in some cases actually reverse, coronary atherothrombosis. These interventions have the potential to greatly reduce the burden of subsequent acute coronary events and the need for future revascularization. Unfortunately, low adherence to preventive care in general, and low referral rates to structured cardiac rehabilitation programs, specifically, have markedly limited this potential. Advanced, comprehensive, cardiac rehabilitation is both a clinically and cost-effective strategy to dramatically improve secondary prevention of coronary heart disease (38,170–174).

REFERENCES

1. Levine SA, Lown B. The "chair" treatment of acute thrombosis. *Trans Assoc Am Physicians* 1951;64:316–327.
2. Levine SA, Lown B. "Armchair" treatment of acute coronary thrombosis. *JAMA* 1952;148:1365–1369.
3. Newman LB, Andrews MF, Koblish MO, et al. Physical medicine and rehabilitation in acute myocardial infarction. *Arch Intern Med* 1952;89:552–561.
4. Brummer P, Linko E, Kasanen A. Myocardial infarction treated by early ambulation. *Am Heart J* 1956;52:269–272.
5. Wenger NK. Early ambulation after myocardial infarction. The inpatient exercise program. *Clin Sports Med* 1984;3:333–348.
6. Wenger NK. Future directions in cardiovascular rehabilitation. *J Cardiopulmonary Rehabil* 1987;7:168–174.
7. Perk J, Veress G. Cardiac rehabilitation: applying exercise physiology in clinical practice. *Eur J Appl Physiol* 2000;83:457–462.
8. Ades PA, Maloney A, Savage P, et al. Determinants of physical functioning in coronary patients: response to cardiac rehabilitation. *Arch Intern Med* 1999;159:2357–2360.
9. Weber KT, Janicki JS, McElroy PA. Determination of aerobic capacity and the severity of chronic cardiac and circulatory failure. *Circulation* 1987;76:V140–V145.
10. Schuler G, Hambrecht R, Schlierf G, et al. Regular physical exercise and low-fat diet. Effects on progression of coronary artery disease. *Circulation* 1992;86:1–11.
11. Hambrecht R, Niebauer J, Marburger C, et al. Various intensities of leisure time physical activity in patients with coronary artery disease: effects on cardiorespiratory fitness and progression of coronary atherosclerotic lesions. *J Am Coll Cardiol* 1993;22:468–477.
12. Aronow WS. Exercise therapy for older persons with cardiovascular disease. *Am J Geriatr Cardiol* 2001;10:245–252.
13. Seals DR, Chase PB. Influence of physical training on heart rate variability and baroreflex circulatory control. *J Appl Physiol* 1989;66:1886–1895.
14. Pardo Y, Merz CN, Velasquez I, et al. Exercise conditioning and heart rate variability: evidence of a threshold effect. *Clin Cardiol* 2000;23:615–620.
15. Suzuki T, Yamauchi K, Yamada Y, et al. Blood coagulability and fibrinolytic activity before and after physical training during the recovery phase of acute myocardial infarction. *Clin Cardiol* 1992;15:358–364.
16. Church TS, Lavie CJ, Milani RV, et al. Improvements in blood rheology after cardiac rehabilitation and exercise training in patients with coronary heart disease. *Am Heart J* 2002;143:349–355.
17. Rauramaa R, Salonen JT, Seppanen K, et al. Inhibition of platelet aggregability by moderate-intensity physical exercise: a randomized clinical trial in overweight men. *Circulation* 1986;74:939–944.
18. Schuler G, Hambrecht R, Schlierf G, et al. Myocardial perfusion and regression of coronary artery disease in patients on a regimen of in-

tensive physical exercise and low fat diet. *J Am Coll Cardiol* 1992;19:
34–42.

19. Ridocci F, Velasco JA, Echanove I, et al. Effects of a 1-year exercise
training program on myocardial ischemia in patients after myocardial
infarction. *Cardiology* 1992;80:406–412.

20. Haskell WL, Sims C, Myll J, et al. Coronary artery size and dilating
capacity in ultradistance runners. *Circulation* 1993;87:1076–1082.

21. Gielen S, Schuler G, Hambrecht R. Exercise training in coronary artery disease and coronary vasomotion. *Circulation* 2001;103:
E1–E6.

22. Szmedra L, Bacharach DW, Buckenmeyer PJ, et al. Response of patients with coronary artery disease stratified by ejection fraction following short-term training. *Int J Cardiol* 1994;46:209–222.

23. Litchfield RL, Kerber RE, Benge JW, et al. Normal exercise capacity
in patients with severe left ventricular dysfunction: compensatory
mechanisms. *Circulation* 1982;66:129–134.

24. Kellermann JJ. The role of exercise therapy in patients with impaired
ventricular function and chronic heart failure. *J Cardiovasc Pharmacol* 1987;10:7.

25. Hagberg JM. Physiologic adaptations to prolonged high-intensity exercise training in patients with coronary artery disease. *Med Sci
Sports Exerc* 1991;23:661–667.

26. Kavanagh T, Mertens DJ, Hamm LF, et al. Prediction of long-term
prognosis in 12,169 men referred for cardiac rehabilitation. *Circulation* 2002;106:666–671.

27. Myers J, Prakash M, Froelicher V, et al. Exercise capacity and mortality
among men referred for exercise testing. *N Engl J Med* 2002;346:
793–801.

28. Stratton JR, Chandler WL, Schwartz RS, et al. Effects of physical
conditioning on fibrinolytic variables and fibrinogen in young and old
healthy adults. *Circulation* 1991;83:1692–1697.

29. Ford ES. Does exercise reduce inflammation? Physical activity and
C-reactive protein among U.S. adults. *Epidemiology* 2002;13:561–568.

30. Geffken D, Cushman M, Burke G, et al. Association between physical
activity and markers of inflammation in a healthy elderly population.
Am J Epidemiol 2001;153:242–250.

31. Ali A, Mehra MR, Lavie CJ, et al. Modulatory impact of cardiac rehabilitation on hyperhomocysteinemia in patients with coronary artery
disease and "normal" lipid levels. *Am J Cardiol* 1998;82:1543–545,A8.

32. Balady GJ, Ades PA, Comoss P, et al. Core components of cardiac re-
habilitation/secondary prevention programs: A statement for healthcare professionals from the American Heart Association and the
American Association of Cardiovascular and Pulmonary Rehabilitation Writing Group. *Circulation* 2000;102:1069–1073.

33. Froelicher V. Cardiac REHABILITATION. In: Parmley W, Chatterjee
K, eds. *Cardiology.* Philadelphia: JB Lippincott Company, 1989:6–9.

34. Fletcher GF. Rehabilitative exercise for the cardiac patient. Early
phase. *Cardiol Clin* 1993;11:267–275.

35. Kellermann JJ. Long-term comprehensive cardiac care—the perspectives and tasks of cardiac rehabilitation. *Eur Heart J* 1993;14:
1441–1444.

36. Dafoe WA, Franklin BA, Cupper L. Vocational issues and disability.
In: Pashkow F, Dafoe W, eds. *Clinical cardiac rehabilitation: a cardiologist's guide.* Baltimore, MD: Williams & Wilkins, 1992:227–242.

37. Katz S. The science of quality of life. *J Chronic Dis* 1987;40:459–463.

38. Oldridge N, Furlong W, Feeny D, et al. Economic evaluation of cardiac rehabilitation soon after acute myocardial infarction. *Am J Cardiol* 1993;72:154–161.

39. Pashkow FJ. Issues in contemporary cardiac rehabilitation: a historical perspective. *J Am Coll Cardiol* 1993;21:822–834.

40. Oldridge N, Guyatt G, Jones N, et al. Effects on quality of life with
comprehensive rehabilitation after acute myocardial infarction. *Am J
Cardiol* 1991;67:1084–1089.

41. Ades PA. Cardiac rehabilitation and secondary prevention of coronary heart disease. *N Engl J Med* 2001;345:892–902.

42. Pashkow FJ, Schafer M, Pashkow P. HeartWatchers-low cost, community centered cardiac rehabilitation in Loveland, Colorado. *J Cardiopulm Rehabil* 1986;6:469–473.

43. DeBusk RF, Haskell WL, Miller NH, et al. Medically directed at-
home rehabilitation soon after clinically uncomplicated acute myocardial infarction: a new model for patient care. *Am J Cardiol*
1985;55:251–257.

44. Carlson JJ, Johnson JA, Franklin BA, et al. Program participation, exercise adherence, cardiovascular outcomes, and program cost of tradi-

tional versus modified cardiac rehabilitation. *Am J Cardiol* 2000;
86:17–23.

45. Gordon NF, English CD, Contractor AS, et al. Effectiveness of three
models for comprehensive cardiovascular disease risk reduction. *Am J
Cardiol* 2002;89:1263–1268.

46. Greenland P, Chu JS. Efficacy of cardiac rehabilitation services: with
emphasis on patients after myocardial infarction. *Ann Intern Med*
1988;109:650–653.

47. Oldridge NB. Cardiac rehabilitation exercise programme, exercise compliance and compliance-enhancing strategies. *Sports Med* 1988;6:
42–55.

48. O'Connor GT, Buring JE, Yusuf S, et al. An overview of randomized
trials of rehabilitation with exercise after myocardial infarction. *Circulation* 1989;80:234–244.

49. Hämäläinen H, Luurila OJ, Kallio V, et al. Long-term reduction in
sudden deaths after multifactorial intervention programme in patients
with myocardial infarction. 10-year results of a controlled investigation. *Eur Heart J* 1989;10:55–62.

50. Kallio V, Hämäläinen H, Hakkila J, et al. Reduction of sudden deaths
by a multifactorial intervention program after acute myocardial infarction. *Lancet* 1979;2:1091–1094.

51. Mittleman MA, Maclure M, Tofler GH, et al. Triggering of acute
myocardial infarction by heavy physical exertion. Protection against
triggering by regular exertion. Determinants of Myocardial Infarction
Onset Study Investigators. *N Engl J Med* 1993;329:1677–1683.

52. Bittner V, Oberman A. Efficacy studies in coronary rehabilitation.
Cardiol Clin 1993;11:333–347.

53. Posel D, Noakes T, Kantor P, et al. Exercise training after experimental myocardial infarction increases the ventricular fibrillation threshold before and after the onset of reinfarction in the isolated rat heart.
Circulation 1989;80:138–145.

54. Van Camp SP, Peterson RA. Cardiovascular complications of outpatient cardiac rehabilitation programs. *JAMA* 1986;256:1160–1163.

55. Hedbäck B, Perk J, Wodlin P. Long-term reduction of cardiac mortality after myocardial infarction: 10-year results of a comprehensive rehabilitation programme. *Eur Heart J* 1993;14:831–835.

56. Kromhout D, Menotti A, Kesteloot H, et al. Prevention of coronary heart
disease by diet and lifestyle: evidence from prospective cross-cultural,
cohort, and intervention studies. *Circulation* 2002;105:893–898.

57. LaRosa JC, He J, Vupputuri S. Effect of statins on risk of coronary disease: a meta-analysis of randomized controlled trials. *JAMA* 1999;282:
2340–2346.

58. May GS, Eberlein KA, Furberg CD, et al. Secondary prevention after
myocardial infarction: a review of long-term trials. *Prog Cardiovasc
Dis* 1982;24:331–352.

59. Yusuf S, Wittes J, Friedman L. Overview of results of randomized
clinical trials in heart disease. II. Unstable angina, heart failure, primary prevention with aspirin, and risk factor modification. *JAMA*
1988;260:2259–2263.

60. Fuster V, Badimon L, Badimon JJ, et al. The pathogenisis of coronary
artery disease and the acute coronary syndromes. Parts I and II. *N
Engl J Med* 1992;326:242–250,310–318.

61. Pashkow F, Dafoe W. Cardiac rehabilitation as a model of integrated
cardiovascular care. In: Pashkow F, Dafoe W, eds. *Clinical cardiac rehabilitation: a cardiologist's guide.* Baltimore, MD: Williams &
Wilkins, 1992:3–24.

62. DeBusk RF, Miller NH, Superko HR, et al. A case-management system for coronary risk factor modification after acute myocardial infarction. *Ann Intern Med* 1994;120:721–729.

63. Haskell WL, Alderman EL, Fair JM, et al. Effects of intensive multiple risk factor reduction on coronary atherosclerosis and clinical cardiac events in men and women with coronary artery disease. The
Stanford Coronary Risk Intervention Project (SCRIP). *Circulation*
1994;89:975–990.

64. Allison TG, Squires RW, Johnson BD, et al. Achieving National Cholesterol Education Program goals for low-density lipoprotein cholesterol in cardiac patients: importance of diet, exercise, weight control,
and drug therapy. *Mayo Clin Proc* 1999;74:466–473.

65. Gordon NF, Salmon RD, Mitchell BS, et al. Innovative approaches
to comprehensive cardiovascular disease risk reduction in clinical
and community-based settings. *Curr Atheroscler Rep* 2001;
3:498–506.

66. Lown B, Verrier RL. Neural activity and ventricular fibrillation. *N
Engl J Med* 1976; 294:1165–1170.

67. Lown B, Verrier RL, Rabinowitz SH. Neural and psychologic mechanisms and the problem of sudden cardiac death. *Am J Cardiol* 1977; 39:890–902.

68. Follick MJ, Gorkin L, Capone RJ, et al. Psychological distress as a predictor of ventricular arrhythmias in a post-myocardial infarction population. *Am Heart J* 1988;116:32–36.

69. Carney RM, Freedland KE, Rich MW, et al. Ventricular tachycardia and psychiatric depression in patients with coronary artery disease. *Am J Med* 1993;95:23–28.

70. Littman AB. Review of psychosomatic aspects of cardiovascular disease. *Psychother Psychosom* 1993;60:148–167.

71. Januzzi JL Jr, Stern TA, Pasternak RC, et al. The influence of anxiety and depression on outcomes of patients with coronary artery disease. *Arch Intern Med* 2000;160:1913–1921.

72. Jenkins C, Zyzanski S, Rosenman R. Risk for new myocardial infarction in middle-aged men with manifest coronary heart disease. *Circulation* 1976;53:342.

73. Blumenthal J, Williams R, Kong Y, et al. Type A behavior pattern and coronary atherosclerosis. *Circulation* 1978;58:634–639.

74. Krantz DS, Sanmarco MI, Selvester RH, et al. Psychological correlates of progression of atherosclerosis in men. *Psychosom Med* 1979; 41:467–475.

75. Case RB, Heller SS, Case NB, et al. Type A behavior and survival after acute myocardial infarction. *N Engl J Med* 1985;312:737–741.

76. Shekelle RB, Hulley SB, Neaton JD, et al. The MRFIT behavior pattern study. II. Type A behavior and incidence of coronary heart disease. *Am J Epidemiol* 1985;122:559–570.

77. Ragland DR, Brand RJ. Type A behavior and mortality from coronary heart disease. *N Engl J Med* 1988;318:65–69.

78. Angerer P, Siebert U, Kothny W, et al. Impact of social support, cynical hostility and anger expression on progression of coronary atherosclerosis. *J Am Coll Cardiol* 2000;36:1781–1788.

79. Kavanagh T, Shephard RJ, Tuck JA. Depression after myocardial infarction. *Can Med Assoc J* 1975;113:23–27.

80. Milani R, Littman A, Lavie C. Depressive symptoms predict functional improvement following cardiac rehabilitation and exercise program. *J Cardiopulm Rehabil* 1993;13:406–411.

81. Schleifer SJ, Macari-Hinson MM, Coyle DA, et al. The nature and course of depression following myocardial infarction. *Arch Intern Med* 1989;149:1785–1789.

82. Carney RM, Rich MW, Tevelde A, et al. Major depressive disorder in coronary artery disease. *Am J Cardiol* 1987;60:1273–1275.

83. Carney RM, Rich MW, Freedland KE, et al. Major depressive disorder predicts cardiac events in patients with coronary artery disease. *Psychosom Med* 1988;50:627–633.

84. Frasure-Smith N, Lesperance F, Talajic M. Depression following myocardial infarction. Impact on 6-month survival. *JAMA* 1993;270: 1819–1825.

85. Lesperance F, Frasure-Smith N, Talajic M, et al. Five-year risk of cardiac mortality in relation to initial severity and one-year changes in depression symptoms after myocardial infarction. *Circulation* 2002; 105:1049–1053.

86. Roose SP, Dalack GW. Perspectives on the relationship between cardiovascular disease and affective disorder. *J Clin Psychiatry* 1990; 51:4–9.

87. Roose SP, Dalack GW, Woodring S. Death, depression, and heart disease. *J Clin Psychiatry* 1991;52:34–39.

88. Ruberman W, Weinblatt E, Goldberg JD, et al. Psychosocial influences on mortality after myocardial infarction. *N Engl J Med* 1984; 311:552–559.

89. Rose M, Robbins B. Psychosocial recovery issues and strategies in cardiac rehabilitation. In: Pashkow F, Dafoe W, eds. *Clinical cardiac rehabilitation: a cardiologist's guide.* Baltimore, MD: Williams & Wilkins, 1992:248–262.

90. Gentry WD. Psychosocial concerns and benefits in cardiac rehabilitation. In: Pollock ML, Schmidt DH, eds. *Heart disease and rehabilitation.* Boston: Houghton Mifflin, 1979.

91. Naughton J, Bruhn JG, Lategola MT. Effects of physical training on physiologic and behavioral characteristics of cardiac patients. *Arch Phys Med Rehabil* 1968;49:131–137.

92. Hellerstein H. Exercise therapy in coronary disease. *Bull NY Acad Med* 1968;44:1028.

93. Rovario S, Holmes DS, Holmsten RD. Influence of a cardiac rehabilitation program on the cardiovascular, psychological, and social functioning of cardiac patients. *Behav Med* 1984;7:61–81.

94. Gentry WD, Stewart MA. Psychologic effects of exercise training in coronary-prone individuals and in patients with symptomatic coronary heart disease. *Cardiol Clin* 1985:255–260.

95. Seals DR. Sympathetic neural adjustments to stress in physically trained and untrained humans. *Hypertension* 1991;17:36–43.

96. Cooksey JD, Reilly P, Brown S, et al. Exercise training and plasma catecholamines in patients with ischemic heart disease. *Am J Cardiol* 1978;42:372–376.

97. Cohen RA, Moser DJ, Clark MM, et al. Neurocognitive functioning and improvement in quality of life following participation in cardiac rehabilitation. *Am J Cardiol* 1999;83:1374–1378.

98. Milani RV, Lavie CJ, Cassidy MM. Effects of cardiac rehabilitation and exercise training programs on depression in patients after major coronary events. *Am Heart J* 1996;132:726–732.

99. Lavie CJ, Milani RV. Effects of cardiac rehabilitation and exercise training programs on coronary patients with high levels of hostility. *Mayo Clin Proc* 1999;74:959–966.

100. Lavie CJ, Milani RV, Cassidy MM, et al. Effects of cardiac rehabilitation and exercise training programs in women with depression. *Am J Cardiol* 1999;83:1480–1483,A7.

101. Linden W, Stossel C, Maurice J. Psychosocial interventions for patients with coronary artery disease: a meta-analysis. *Arch Intern Med* 1996;156:745–752.

102. Blumenthal JA, Babyak M, Wei J, et al. Usefulness of psychosocial treatment of mental stress-induced myocardial ischemia in men. *Am J Cardiol* 2002;89:164–168.

103. Denollet J, Brutsaert DL. Reducing emotional distress improves prognosis in coronary heart disease: 9-year mortality in a clinical trial of rehabilitation. *Circulation* 2001;104:2018–2023.

104. Glassman AH, O'Connor CM, Califf RM, et al. Sertraline treatment of major depression in patients with acute MI or unstable angina. *JAMA* 2002;288:701–709.

105. Wenger NK, Mattson ME, Furberg CD, et al. Assessment of quality of life in clinical trials of cardiovascular therapies. *Am J Cardiol* 1984; 54:908–13.

106. Oldridge NB. Outcome assessment in cardiac rehabilitation. Health-related quality of life and economic evaluation. *J Cardiopulm Rehabil* 1997;17:179–194.

107. Gorkin L, Norvell NK, Rosen RC, et al. Assessment of quality of life as observed from the baseline data of the Studies of Left Ventricular Dysfunction (SOLVD) trial quality-of-life substudy. *Am J Cardiol* 1993;71:1069–1073.

108. Michel T. Outcome assessment in cardiac rehabilitation. *Int J Technol Assess Health Care* 1992;8:76–84.

109. Oldridge N, Gottlieb M, Guyatt G, et al. Predictors of health-related quality of life with cardiac rehabilitation after acute myocardial infarction. *J Cardiopulm Rehabil* 1998;18:95–103.

110. Oldridge N, Perkins A, Marchionni N, et al. Number needed to treat in cardiac rehabilitation. *J Cardiopulm Rehabil* 2002;22:22–30.

111. Shephard RJ, Franklin B. Changes in the quality of life: a major goal of cardiac rehabilitation. *J Cardiopulm Rehabil* 2001;21:189–200.

112. Jamieson M, Wilcox S, Webster W, et al. Factors influencing health-related quality of life in cardiac rehabilitation patients. *Prog Cardiovasc Nurs* 2002;17:124–131.

113. Torrance GW. Utility, decision, and quality of life. *J Chron Dis* 1987;40:593–600.

114. Simchen E, Naveh I, Zitser-Gurevich Y, et al. Is participation in cardiac rehabilitation programs associated with better quality of life and return to work after coronary artery bypass operations? The Israeli CABG Study. *Isr Med Assoc J* 2001;3:399–403.

115. Beniamini Y, Rubenstein JJ, Zaichkowsky LD, et al. Effects of high-intensity strength training on quality-of-life parameters in cardiac rehabilitation patients. *Am J Cardiol* 1997;80:841–846.

116. Blankenhorn DH, Nessim SA, Johnson RL, et al. Beneficial effects of combined colestipol-niacin therapy on coronary atherosclerosis and coronary venous bypass grafts [Erratum in: *JAMA* 1988 May 13;259(18):2698]. *JAMA* 1987;257:3233–3240.

117. Brown G, Albers JJ, Fisher LD, et al. Regression of coronary artery disease as a result of intensive lipid-lowering therapy in men with high levels of apolipoprotein B. *N Engl J Med* 1990;323: 1289–1298.

118. Ornish D, Brown SE, Scherwitz LW, et al. Can lifestyle changes reverse coronary heart disease? The Lifestyle Heart Trial. *Lancet* 1990;336:129–133.
119. Blankenhorn D, Hodis H. Arterial imaging and atherosclerosis reversal. *Arterioscler Thromb* 1994;14:177–192.
120. Brown BG, Zhao XQ, Sacco DE, et al. Lipid lowering and plaque regression. New insights into prevention of plaque disruption and clinical events in coronary disease. *Circulation* 1993;87:1781–1791.
121. Sullivan MJ, Higginbotham MB, Cobb FR. Exercise training in patients with severe left ventricular dysfunction. Hemodynamic and metabolic effects. *Circulation* 1988;78:506–515.
122. Wenger NK, Alpert JS. Rehabilitation of the coronary patient in 1989. *Arch Intern Med* 1989;149:1504–1506.
123. Pashkow FJ. Rehabilitation strategies for the complex cardiac patient. *Cleve Clin J Med* 1991;58:70–75.
124. Hotta S. Cardiac rehabilitation programs: heart transplant, percutaneous transluminal coronary angioplasty, and heart valve surgery patients. Washington, DC: U.S. Department of Health and Human Services, 1991.
125. Okada RD, Lim YL, Boucher CA, et al. Clinical, angiographic, hemodynamic, perfusional and functional changes after one-vessel left anterior descending coronary angioplasty. *Am J Cardiol* 1985;55:347–356.
126. Ben-Ari E, Rothbaum MD, Linnemeir TJ, et al. Benefits of a monitored rehabilitation program versus physician care after emergency percutaneous transluminal coronary angioplasty: follow-up of risk factors and rate of restonosis. *J Cardiopulmonary Rehabil* 1989;7:281–285.
127. Danchin N, Juilliere Y, Selton-Suty C, et al. Return to work after percutaneous transluminal coronary angioplasty: a continuing problem. *Eur Heart J* 1989;10:54–57.
128. McGee HM, Graham T, Crowe B, et al. Return to work following coronary artery bypass surgery or percutaneous transluminal coronary angioplasty. *Eur Heart J* 1993;14:623–628.
129. Oldridge NB, Nagle FJ, Balke B, et al. Aortocoronary bypass surgery: effects of surgery and 32 months of physical conditioning on treadmill performance. *Arch Phys Med Rehabil* 1978;59:268–275.
130. Froelicher V, Jensen D, Sullivan M. A randomized trial of the effects of exercise training after coronary artery bypass surgery. *Arch Intern Med* 1985;145:689–692.
131. Weiner DA, McCabe CH, Roth RL, et al. Serial exercise testing after coronary artery bypass surgery. *Am Heart J* 1981;101:149–154.
132. Pasquali SK, Alexander KP, Lytle BL, et al. Testing an intervention to increase cardiac rehabilitation enrollment after coronary artery bypass grafting. *Am J Cardiol* 2001;88:1415–1416,A6.
133. Pashkow FJ, Pashkow PS, Schafer MN. Complicating conditions. In: *Successful cardiac rehabilitation: the complete guide for building cardiac rehab programs.* Loveland, CO: The HeartWatchers Press, 1988:228–247.
134. Pashkow F. Patients with implanted pacemakers or implanted cardioverter defibrillators. In: Wenger N, Hellerstein H, eds. *Rehabilitation of the coronary patient,* 3rd ed. New York: Churchill Livingston, 1992:431–438.
135. Kokkinos PF, Choucair W, Graves P, et al. Chronic heart failure and exercise. *Am Heart J* 2000;140:21–28.
136. Humphrey R, Bartels MN. Exercise, cardiovascular disease, and chronic heart failure. *Arch Phys Med Rehabil* 2001;82:S76–S81.
137. Packer M. Sudden unexpected death in patients with congestive heart failure: a second frontier. *Circulation* 1985;72:681–685.
138. Kannel WB, Plehn JF, Cupples LA. Cardiac failure and sudden death in the Framingham Study. *Am Heart J* 1988;115:869–875.
139. Cleland JG, Chattopadhyay S, Khand A, et al. Prevalence and incidence of arrhythmias and sudden death in heart failure. *Heart Fail Rev* 2002;7:229–242.
140. MacMahon KM, Lip GY. Psychological factors in heart failure: a review of the literature. *Arch Intern Med* 2002;162:509–516.
141. Rozzini R, Sabatini T, Frisoni GB, et al. Depression and major outcomes in older patients with heart failure. *Arch Intern Med* 2002;162:362–364.
142. Arvan S. Exercise performance of the high risk acute myocardial infarction patient after cardiac rehabilitation [Erratum in: *Am J Cardiol* 1988 Nov 15;62(16):1153]. *Am J Cardiol* 1988;62:197–201.
143. Dubach P, Froelicher VF. Cardiac rehabilitation for heart failure patients. *Cardiology* 1989;76:368–373.
144. McKirnan MD, Sullivan M, Jensen D, et al. Treadmill performance and cardiac function in selected patients with coronary heart disease. *J Am Coll Cardiol* 1984;2:1.
145. Smith LK. Exercise training in patients with impaired left ventricular function. *Med Sci Sports Exerc* 1991;23:654–660.
146. Shabetai R. Beneficial effects of exercise training in compensated heart failure. *Circulation* 1988;78:775–776.
147. Mathes P. Physical training in patients with ventricular dysfunction: choice and dosage of physical exercise in patients with pump dysfunction. *Eur Heart J* 1988;9:67–69.
148. Jugdutt BI, Michorowski BL, Kappagoda CT. Exercise training after anterior Q wave myocardial infarction: importance of regional left ventricular function and topography. *J Am Coll Cardiol* 1988;12:362–372.
149. Giannuzzi P, Tavazzi L, Temporelli PL, et al. Long-term physical training and left ventricular remodeling after anterior myocardial infarction: results of the Exercise in Anterior Myocardial Infarction (EAMI) trial. EAMI Study Group. *J Am Coll Cardiol* 1993;22:1821–1829.
150. Dubach P, Myers J, Dziekan G, et al. Effect of exercise training on myocardial remodeling in patients with reduced left ventricular function after myocardial infarction: application of magnetic resonance imaging. *Circulation* 1997;95:2060–2067.
151. Kormos RL, Murali S, Dew MA, et al. Chronic mechanical circulatory support: rehabilitation, low morbidity, and superior survival. *Ann Thorac Surg* 1994;57:51–57.
152. McCarthy PM, James KB, Savage RM, et al. Implantable left ventricular assist device. Approaching an alternative for end-stage heart failure. Implantable LVAD Study Group. *Circulation* 1994;90:II83–II86.
153. Lee AP, Ice R, Blessey R, et al. Long-term effects of physical training in coronary patients with impaired ventricular function. *Circulation* 1979;60:1519.
154. Wenger NK. Quality of life: can it and should it be assessed in patients with heart failure? *Cardiology* 1989;79:391–398.
155. Sullivan MJ, Higginbotham MB, Cobb FR. Exercise training in patients with chronic heart failure delays ventilatory anaerobic threshold and improves submaximal exercise performance. *Circulation* 1989;79:324–329.
156. Curnier D, Galinier M, Pathak A, et al. Rehabilitation of patients with congestive heart failure with or without beta-blockade therapy. *J Card Fail* 2001;7:241–248.
157. Lavie CJ, Milani RV. Benefits of cardiac rehabilitation and exercise training in elderly women. *Am J Cardiol* 1997;79:664–666.
158. Williams MA, Fleg JL, Ades PA, et al. Secondary prevention of coronary heart disease in the elderly (with emphasis on patients > or =75 years of age): an American Heart Association scientific statement from the Council on Clinical *Cardiology* Subcommittee on Exercise, Cardiac Rehabilitation, and Prevention. *Circulation* 2002;105:1735–1743.
159. Vonder Muhll I, Daub B, Black B, et al. Benefits of cardiac rehabilitation in the ninth decade of life in patients with coronary heart disease. *Am J Cardiol* 2002;90:645–648.
160. Caldwell MA, Dracup K. Team management of heart failure: the emerging role of exercise, and implications for cardiac rehabilitation centers. *J Cardiopulm Rehabil* 2001;21:273–279.
161. Lavie CJ, Milani RV, Littman AB. Benefits of cardiac rehabilitation and exercise training in secondary coronary prevention in the elderly. *J Am Coll Cardiol* 1993;22:678–683.
162. Blumenthal JA, Emery CF, Madden DJ, et al. Effects of exercise training on cardiorespiratory function in men and women older than 60 years of age. *Am J Cardiol* 1991;67:633–639.
163. Haskell WL. Cardiac rehabilitation and secondary prevention: issues of participation and benefit for women. In: Wenger NK, Speroff L, Packard B, eds. *Cardiovascular Health and Disease in Women.* Greenwich, CT: Le Jacq Communications Inc., 1993:123–128.
164. Ades PA, Waldmann ML, Polk DM, et al. Referral patterns and exercise response in the rehabilitation of female coronary patients aged greater than or equal to 62 years. *Am J Cardiol* 1992;69:1422–1425.
165. Hamilton GA. Recovery from acute myocardial infarction in women. *Cardiology* 1990;77:58–70.
166. Cannistra LB, Balady GJ, O'Malley CJ, et al. Comparison of the clinical profile and outcome of women and men in cardiac rehabilitation. *Am J Cardiol* 1992;69:1274–1279.
167. Caras DS, Wenger NK. Exercise rehabilitation of women with coronary heart disease. *J of Myocardial Ischemia* 1993;5:42–52.
168. Corrao JM, Becker RC, Ockene IS, et al. Coronary heart disease risk factors in women. *Cardiology* 1990;77:8–24.

169. Pashkow FJ. The Mona Lisa smiles: impact of risk factors for coronary artery disease in women. *Cleve Clin J Med* 1993;60: 411–414.

170. Levin LA, Perk J, Hedback B. Cardiac rehabilitation—a cost analysis. *J Intern Med* 1991;230:427–434.

171. Ades PA, Pashkow FJ, Nestor JR. Cost-effectiveness of cardiac rehabilitation after myocardial infarction. *J Cardiopulm Rehabil* 1997;17: 222–231.

172. Taylor R, Kirby B. The evidence base for the cost effectiveness of cardiac rehabilitation. *Heart* 1997;78:5–6.

173. Collins L, Scuffham P, Gargett S. Cost-analysis of gym-based versus home-based cardiac rehabilitation programs. *Aust Health Rev* 2001; 24:51–61.

174. Robertson KA, Kayhko K. Cost analysis of an intensive home follow-up program for first-time post-myocardial infarction patients and their families. *Dynamics* 2001;12:25–31.

Other Unstable Conditions

CHAPTER 85

Variant Angina Pectoris

Heidar Arjomand and Marc Cohen

Key Words: Coronary vasospasm; Prinzmetal's angina; variant angina.

INTRODUCTION

In contrast to the average patient with atherothrombotic heart disease presenting with unstable angina, Prinzmetal (1), in 1959, used the term "variant angina" to describe patients whose chest pain occurred at rest, was usually associated with ST-segment elevation on the surface 12-lead electrocardiogram, and who, in general, had normal or near-normal exercise tolerance and no effort-related symptoms of chest discomfort. Variant angina represents only one manifestation of ischemic heart disease in which coronary vasospasm plays the major provocative role (2–4). Acute or chronic ischemic coronary syndromes, or both, triggered by coronary vasospasm include acute myocardial infarction (AMI) (2–4), severe cardiac dysrhythmias, and sudden death (5).

H. Arjomand: Seacoast Cardiology Associates, 750 Central Avenue, Suite U, Dover, New Hampshire 03820.
M. Cohen: Division of Cardiology, Newark Beth Israel Medical Center, 201 Lyons Avenue, Newark, New Jersey 07112.

Coronary artery vasospasm causing a sudden severe reduction in lumen diameter (Fig. 85–1) can occur in patients with either angiographically normal coronary arteries or in patients with atherothrombotic coronary artery disease. Characteristically, the myocardial ischemia resulting in variant angina occurs at rest, in the absence of a stimulus that induces increased oxygen demand such as an increase in blood pressure, or in heart rate (6,7). In general, coronary spasm results from smooth muscle cell contraction in the media of the vessel—that is, an event occurring external to the bloodstream. Nevertheless, it is important to remember that elements within the bloodstream also can precipitate cyclical, severe reduction in blood flow (8). Patients with sudden plaque rupture narrowing the lumen are likely to exhibit platelet aggregation, embolization, and reaggregation, which can result in transient episodes of rest angina. The interrelation between intraluminal events and changes in vessel tone is quite complex and is discussed later.

HISTORICAL AND PATHOPHYSIOLOGIC PERSPECTIVES

Subsequent to the description of Prinzmetal, the concept regarding the mechanism of myocardial ischemia, promul-

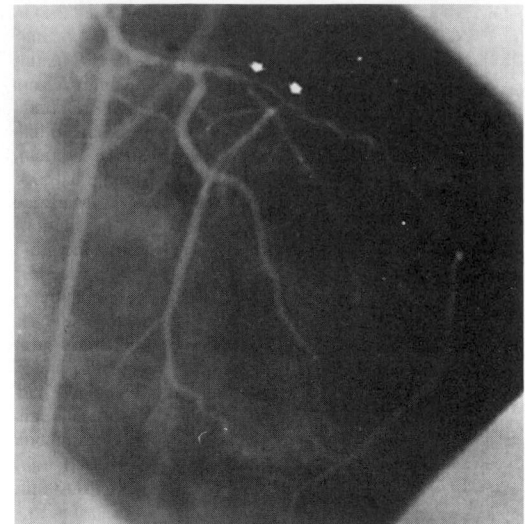

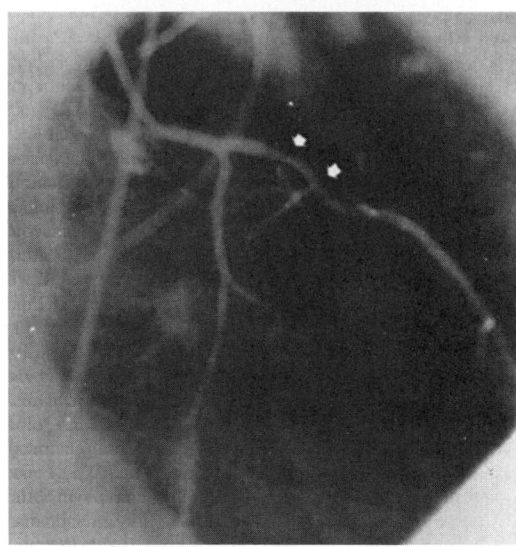

FIG. 85–1. A 41-year-old woman with chest pain and an electrocardiogram showing acute anterior ischemia. **A:** Spasm of the proximal left anterior descending artery and left main. **B:** Reversal of the spasm after intracoronary nitroglycerin. (From Jang IK. Acute myocardial infarction and coronary spasm. *N Engl J Med* 1994;330:1420, with permission.)

gated in the 1960s and early 1970s, was that angina was caused by a severe reduction in coronary flow reserve (caused by a fixed plaque), such that any increase in oxygen demand greater than the basal metabolic needs would result in ischemia. Subsequently, this concept was attacked. In a series of landmark investigations in patients with rest angina using different techniques, Oliva and coworkers (2,3), Maseri and coworkers (4–6), and Figueras and coworkers (7,9) consistently observed a reduction in myocardial blood supply related to the onset of symptoms that was independent of the severity of the fixed coronary atherothrombotic lesion and that was independent of any precipitating increase in the level of the double product (blood pressure X

heart rate) before the onset of angina. Subsequent investigations focused on what triggered the arterial segment to spasm.

RACIAL/ETHNIC VARIATION

A 1999 review of more than 600 original studies of variant angina identified a significant proportion of these studies (30%) had been performed on Japanese patients (10). This has led to the belief that variant angina is more prevalent in Japan and also led to the notion of "Japanese Type Variant Angina." There are clinical and pathophysiologic differences between Japanese and white patients with variant angina. Japanese patients with variant angina appear to have diffusely hyperreactive coronary arteries and multivessel coronary spasm. In contrast, studies in Europe and North America have noted that coronary artery spasm in variant angina is usually focal and rarely involves multiple vessels (10). Clinical differences between Japanese and white patients include a lower prevalence rate of prior MI in Japanese patients (7% vs. 24%; $p < 0.0001$), a lower incidence rate of fixed obstructive coronary disease (41% vs. 66%; $p < 0.0001$), and better survival (97% vs. 89%; $p < 0.0001$) at 3-year follow-up (10). In some Japanese studies, a localized deficiency of coronary nitric oxide production has been implicated to cause coronary spasm in patients with variant angina (10–13). It is, therefore, important to note these racial differences between Japanese and white patients with variant angina because data derived from studies in one population can no longer be automatically extrapolated to another population.

MECHANISMS

Several mechanisms have been proposed to explain the predilection of certain patients to coronary artery spasm. Although one mechanism may be clearly documented in a particular patient, it is likely that different etiologic factors apply to different patients. For example, in patients with variant angina in the setting of significant plaque narrowing, the coronary artery lumen may have different mechanisms triggering coronary spasm than patients with variant angina and no angiographic evidence of plaque. Kaski and coworkers (14) studied 28 patients with Prinzmetal's angina using multiple, different provocative tests in the same patient. Provocative testing was done with ergonovine, hyperventilation, cold pressor test, and histamine infusion. Ergonovine induced coronary spasm in 96% of patients. In 82% of patients, two different provocative tests induced coronary spasm. This suggested that there was a nonspecific reactivity or supersensitivity on the part of these local segments.

Thrombosis

In patients with atherothrombotic coronary artery disease, platelet aggregation, embolization, and reaggregation is the mechanism for cyclic flow reductions to the point of total occlusion in damaged coronary arteries (8). The release of potent vasoconstrictive agents from the activated platelets provides a likely mechanism for some coronary spasm and rest angina in this patient subset. However, in those patients with nonobstructive coronary disease who have variant angina, investigations have suggested that neither thrombosis nor antithrombotic therapy with either heparin or antiplatelet agents such as aspirin, or both, are relevant to patients with recurrent bouts of coronary spasm and variant angina. Robertson and coworkers (15) did not observe an increase in the coronary sinus levels of the platelet metabolite thromboxane A_2 before or early during the episodes of symptomatic ischemia or ST-segment deviations in patients with variant angina. Furthermore, neither inhibition of thromboxane synthesis with low-dose aspirin and/or indomethacin (16) nor intravenous heparin (17) suppressed the variant angina attacks in this population. It is more likely that intracoronary thrombosis is the result of, rather than the cause of, variant anginal attacks (18).

In patients in whom coronary spasm occurs in the setting of an obstructive plaque within a coronary artery, an investigation by Bogaty and coworkers (19) focused attention on the vasoreactivity of the culprit lesion in patients with unstable angina. Using the cold pressor test as a provocation for vasospasm, they observed that patients with stable angina and obstructive plaques had an insignificant change in luminal diameter of the culprit lesion after provocation with cold. In contrast, the culprit lesions in patients with unstable angina demonstrated significant reduction in luminal diameter after provocation with cold suggesting an abnormal vasoreactivity within the culprit lesion.

Endothelial Function and Localized versus Diffuse Hypersensitivity

In white patients with variant angina, coronary spasm occurs in a focal, rather than a diffuse, pattern in the coronary artery tree (11). In patients with atherothrombotic plaques, the site of spasm is usually adjacent to the plaque. In these patients, endothelial function is probably markedly abnormal making them more susceptible to the lack of endothelial-derived relaxing factor. However, although these patients may have less coronary vasodilator reserve, it is still unclear what the positive trigger for transient vasospasm is. Originally, the use of intracoronary acetylcholine as a provocative test for coronary spasm was prompted by the hypothesis that there may be endothelial dysfunction in these patients (20). In fact, intracoronary acetylcholine is a highly specific agent for the identification of patients with coronary spasm. Nevertheless, the mechanism by which acetylcholine induces coronary spasm may not be entirely related to endothelial dysfunction.

In patients with normal coronary arteries or those without angiographic evidence of significant atherothrombotic plaques, several studies have provided insight into coronary tone in patients with variant angina. Hoshio and coworkers (21) observed that ergonovine not only induced significant reduction in luminal diameter at the spastic sites in patients with variant angina, but also induced a greater than normal vasoconstrictor response throughout the entire coronary tree. This suggested that coronary tone in patients with Prinzmetal's angina was heightened. Toyo-oka and coworkers (22) observed that the baseline levels of circulating endothelin in 12 patients with coronary spasm was, on average, more than twice the level of that in the control patients without coronary spasm. Using intracoronary nitroglycerin to measure the degree of coronary tone, Kuga and coworkers (23) observed that there was a greater level of resting coronary tone in patients with coronary spasm who only needed low doses of ergonovine (1–5 μg) to elicit vasospasm. In contrast, those patients with variant angina who needed significantly greater doses of ergonovine to elicit coronary spasm usually had a coronary tone similar to control patients without variant angina. It is likely that the majority of patients with coronary spasm have a heightened resting coronary tone.

The role of endothelial nitric oxide and endothelial dysfunction in patients with variant angina is debatable. In 1996, Kugiyama and coworkers (11) demonstrated a deficiency of nitric oxide bioavailability at the site of coronary artery spasm. In 1997, the same group of investigators showed that flow-dependent, nitric-oxide mediated, coronary dilation was impaired in patients with variant angina (13). Using quantitative coronary angiography to assess coronary dilation in the proximal left anterior descending artery (LAD), after infusing adenosine into the mid/distal LAD, they showed significantly less flow-dependent dilation of the proximal LAD in 10 patients with variant angina as compared with 11 control patients. When L-N^G-monomethyl-arginine (L-NMMA), a competitive inhibitor of nitric oxide production, was infused in the proximal LAD, the flow-dependent (nitric oxide–mediated) dilation was suppressed in control patients but not in patients with variant angina (14). By using high-resolution ultrasound to measure vasodilation, Hamabe and coworkers (24) showed that flow-mediated, endothelium-dependent vasodilation also was impaired in the brachial arteries of patients with variant angina. They postulated that this may be because of increased oxidant stress in the systemic arteries. In 2002, Kawano and coworkers (25) showed a diurnal fluctuation in flow-mediated vasodilation of brachial arteries of patients with variant angina, which was associated with variation in the frequency of ischemic episodes. There was deterioration of flow-mediated vasodilation in the early morning that correlated with the greatest frequency of spontaneous ischemic episodes from midnight to morning. In addition, patients with variant angina were shown to have a normal or exaggerated vasodilator response to nitroglycerin, suggesting that endothelium-independent (not nitric oxide–mediated) vasodilation was intact in these patients (11,12, 14,24).

In contrast to the above studies, other investigators have reported that endothelial nitric oxide production is intact in patients with variant angina (13,26). Okumura and coworkers (26) evaluated 70 patients with and 93 patients without variant angina. Using the endothelium-dependent relaxation factor substance P, patients identified as having coronary spasm using intracoronary acetylcholine were found to have normal coronary vascular relaxation with substance P infusion at the site of acetylcholine-induced spasm. In a parallel investigation also using the endothelium-dependent vasodilator substance P, Egashira and coworkers (27) studied 9 patients and observed normal vasodilation after substance P, both at the site of acetylcholine-induced spasm and in the neighboring normal segments. These two investigations strongly suggested that endothelial function at the site of acetylcholine-induced coronary spasm was normal.

In a subsequent study of 36 patients with variant angina, Okumura and coworkers (28) used quantitative coronary angiography to evaluate coronary artery diameter response to intracoronary acetylcholine at the proximal, mid, and distal segments of major epicardial arteries. They showed that there was a diffuse hyperreactive response to the constrictor effects of acetylcholine. Moreover, multivessel spasm was seen in 15 of 36 (42%) patients. Interestingly, there also was a hyperreactive response to dilator effects of intracoronary nitroglycerin, with epicardial arteries of patients with variant angina showing significantly more vasodilation as compared with control patients (28).

Microvascular Spasm

Variant angina is typically caused by spasm of an epicardial coronary artery. However, in a study of 26 patients with variant angina, Akasaka and coworkers (29) assessed coronary flow reserve by measuring the ratio of hyperemic to baseline time-averaged peak velocity. Patients with diffuse vasospasm had lower coronary flow reserve compared with those with focal vasospasm and control patients, suggesting that microvascular coronary spasm may be responsible. In 2002, Sun and coworkers (30) reported on a group of Japanese patients with variant angina. In their study, the submaximal dose of acetylcholine induced myocardial ischemia (chest pain, ischemic electrocardiographic changes, and increased myocardial lactate production) without epicardial coronary spasm in 14 of 55 (25.5%) patients. This subgroup of patients were typically women who had a history of prolonged chest pain. They postulated that these patients most likely had severe spasm at the level of coronary microcirculation (30).

Neurogenic Factors

Neurogenic factors have been implicated as triggers of coronary spasm. Total cardiac denervation by autotransplantation resulted in cessation of symptoms in several patients with disabling variant angina, suggesting a role for the autonomic nervous system (31,32). It is still unclear how sympathetic or parasympathetic hyperactivity mediate the induction of coronary spasm. However, it has been shown that cardiac sympathetic nerve activity reflects disease activity in variant angina. Sakata and coworkers (33), by performing iodine-123 metaiodobenzylguanidine (MIBG) nuclear imaging, assessed the sympathetic nerve activity in different phases of variant angina. As compared with MIBG washout in the stable and remission phases (no chest pain for >3 months), the washout rate of MIBG from spastic territories was significantly lower in the active phase (recent onset of chest pain), indicating a high sympathetic nerve activity in the active phase of variant angina.

Insulin Resistance

Insulin resistance and metabolic syndrome, a known risk factor for atherothrombotic obstructive coronary disease, also has recently been found in patients with variant angina. Botker and coworkers (34) found that insulin sensitivity (using glucose tolerance) was significantly reduced in 15 patients with variant angina compared with healthy control subjects. In addition, these patients had reduced maximal oxygen uptake. In a more recent study, Hirashima and coworkers (35) also found a greater incidence of impaired glucose tolerance in patients with variant angina than in control patients (41% vs. 10%; $p = 0.02$). In this study, improvement in insulin sensitivity with vitamin C infusion was associated with improvement in flow-mediated vasodilation in brachial artery (35).

Minerals, Vitamins, and Vasoactive Compounds

Several studies have suggested that magnesium may play a role in the pathogenesis of variant angina. There is a correlation between body magnesium status and the frequency of anginal attacks in patients with variant angina; patients with more severe magnesium deficiency have more frequent symptoms (36). Intravenous infusion of magnesium sulfate has been shown to terminate anginal attacks provoked by the cold pressor test, as well as by either hyperventilation or exercise (37–39).

Deficiency of certain antioxidant vitamins has been associated with coronary artery spasm. In a study by Hirashima and coworkers (35), basal vitamin C levels were lower and flow-mediated dilation was reduced in patients with variant angina compared with control subjects. As mentioned earlier, infusion of vitamin C augmented flow-mediated dilation in patients with variant angina but not in the control group (35). Miwa and coworkers (39) showed that patients with active variant angina had lower plasma levels of vitamin E compared with subjects without coronary spasm and patients with inactive variant angina, suggesting that plasma vitamin E status is linked to the activity of coronary artery spasm.

The circulating level of endothelin, a potent vasoconstrictor, is greater than normal baseline level in patients with coronary spasm (22). The description by Schecter and coworkers (40) of the efficacy of cyproheptadine, an antiserotonin agent, in patients with variant angina suggests a role for serotonin (41). However, the use of Ketanserin, an oral serotonin receptor antagonist, has been disappointing (42).

Drug-induced Variant Angina

Several case reports over the last two decades have provided clearcut documentation that several therapeutic drugs can trigger coronary spasm in susceptible individuals. Although these case reports document the role of these agents in individual patients, they do not help provide insight into the larger population of patients with variant angina who are not exposed to these agents. The first such drug-induced variant angina model was described by Lange and coworkers (43), who studied patients with nonatheromatous heart disease and found a high incidence of variant angina occurring after withdrawal from chronic industrial nitroglycerin exposure. The role of the sympathomimetic agent cocaine in inducing coronary artery vasoconstriction (44) is now well established. Most recently, two observations were made in patients receiving the chemotherapeutic agents cyclophosphamide (45) and high-dose 5-fluorouracil (46).

HISTOPATHOLOGY

Several histopathologic observations have been made in patients with variant angina. Forman and coworkers (47) showed that the number of inflammatory and mast cells is increased in the adventitia of coronary arteries excised from a patient with variant angina. Mast cells produce a variety of vasoactive mediators that may cause coronary vasospasm. Umemoto and coworkers (48) found that eosinophil counts were significantly greater in patients with severe variant angina than in the control subjects. Also, phospholipase activity C is greater in the cultured skin fibroblasts of patients with variant angina compared with control subjects (49). This enzyme is involved in the release of Ca^{2+} from the intracellular stores, which then causes contraction of smooth muscle cells. This may also contribute to coronary vasospasm in patients with variant angina, especially because there was a positive correlation between phospholipase C activity and acetylcholine-induced vasoconstriction (49).

In a study using intravascular ultrasound (IVUS), Hong and coworkers (50) analyzed focal spasm sites in 36 patients with variant angina. By IVUS, early atherothrombotic lesions were observed at all coronary spasm sites. The mean plaque burden measured 56% at the spasm sites and 36% at the nonspasm sites. Plaque composition at the spasm sites was mostly hypoechoic and highly eccentric, with no evidence of calcium. These IVUS feature are consistent with mild atherothrombosis at the sites of coronary spasm.

DIAGNOSIS-PROVOCATIVE TESTING

Ergonovine

Several pharmacologic agents, as well as other nondrug-related regimens, have been used for provocative testing in patients being evaluated for variant angina. Of these, the ergonovine test has enjoyed many patient-years of evaluation and has evolved as the most sensitive and useful test (51,52). In the United States, ergonovine is currently becoming more difficult to obtain from manufacturers; therefore, the use of acetylcholine is gaining in popularity.

Given intravenously, ergonovine bathes all of the coronary arteries simultaneously and in susceptible patients produces focal, severe coronary artery narrowing on a background of diffuse mild narrowing of the entire coronary tree. In general, the patients experience some nausea and hypertension as a sign that the ergonovine has in fact been adequate to induce changes in the coronary arteries. In general, a test dose of 0.05 mg is given followed by incremental doses of 0.1 mg every 5 minutes (52). A total dose of 0.4 mg is usually considered adequate to elicit coronary spasm. A true-positive rate of between 93% and 99%, and a false-positive rate of between 0% and 5% has been observed.

Investigators from Duke University published their 10-year retrospective analysis of 3,447 patients without obvious signs and symptoms of variant angina, given ergonovine during cardiac catheterization (53). In this study, the role of ergonovine testing was evaluated specifically in patients who did not have a high clinical suspicion for Prinzmetal's variant angina. Overall, 4% of these patients did have a positive ergonovine test eliciting focal coronary arterial spasm. Complications occurred in about 0.03% of patients. Two independent predictors of a positive ergonovine test were the presence of coronary disease and history of cigarette smoking. The investigators suggested that the presence of these two variables in patients without a clinical history of variant angina is associated with a positive ergonovine test in 10% of cases.

Ergonovine provocation also has been used with echocardiography as a screening test for diagnosis of variant angina before coronary angiography. In a study of 80 patients with chest pain suggestive of variant angina and negative stress tests, Song and coworkers (54) showed that ergonovine echocardiography could diagnose coronary vasospasm with a sensitivity of 91% and specificity of 88%.

Acetylcholine

In 1986, Yasue and coworkers (20) provided a major advance in the field of provocative testing by identifying selective intracoronary acetylcholine injection as being a reliable provocative agent for coronary arterial spasm in patients with variant angina. Subsequent investigations (55,56) identified the value of acetylcholine in larger populations, as well as its inherent ability to identify individual vessels susceptible to spasm. Okumura and coworkers (55) studied 33 patients with variant angina by administering acetylcholine in incremental doses of 20, 50, and 100 μg into the left coronary artery and 20 and 50 μg into the right coronary artery. Thirty-two of the 33 patients had a positive test; the 1 patient with a negative response to acetylcholine had a positive ergonovine provocation. Of these 33 patients, 24 were identified as having multivessel susceptibility to coronary spasm (55). Seventy-six percent of the 33 patients were free of angiographically significant coronary artery disease. These investigators extended their observations to a total population of 70 patients. Acetylcholine provocation was 99% specific, had a positive predictive value of 98%, and had a negative predictive value of 93% (56). Because of its high specificity and ability to be given into individual coronary arteries, acetylcholine will probably become the standard provocative test in the catheterization laboratory.

Hyperventilation and Cold

In 1983, Mortensen and coworkers (57) described nonpharmacologic triggers of coronary vasospasm. He identified hyperventilation as a means of inducing coronary vasospasm in patients with variant angina. Ardissino and coworkers (58) applied hyperventilation as a test to predict restenosis after percutaneous transluminal coronary angioplasty (PTCA). Sudden exposure of extremities to cold should induce an increase in catecholamines and function as a sympathomimetic. The investigation by Bogaty and coworkers (19) used the cold pressor test as a means of identifying vasoreactivity of the culprit lesion in unstable angina. In general, however, hyperventilation and cold pressor are not reliable screens in patients who have only sporadic attacks of variant angina.

DIAGNOSIS-METAIODOBENZYLGUANIDINE IMAGING

There is high sympathetic nerve activity in the active phase of variant angina as shown by a low washout rate of iodine-123 MIBG from myocardial segments supplied by the spastic arteries. In a prospective study of 104 patients suspected of having variant angina, Sakata and coworkers (59) assessed the ability of MIBG nuclear imaging to identify and localize coronary spasm. They showed that regional washout analysis of MIBG imaging has a sensitivity of 76% and specificity of 87% for determining the presence and location of coronary artery spasm. When MIBG imaging is combined with thallium-201 imaging, the sensitivity and specificity of this technique increase to 92% and 88%, respectively.

CLINICAL MANIFESTATIONS

Variant Angina and Exertional Angina

Variant angina, by definition, indicates that patients are experiencing ischemic chest pain at rest or with minimal effort. In general, these patients do not experience exercise-induced chest discomfort or exercise-induced abnormalities during stress testing. During the episode of pain at rest, a wide variety of electrocardiographic changes may be manifest. Classically, variant angina is associated with ST-segment elevations paralleling the discrete severe nature of the coronary vasospasm. However, other transient electrocardiographic changes such as transient Q waves (60), transient hemiblocks, and ST-segment depression (61) also have been seen. In patients whose transient coronary spasm elicits recruitable collateral circulation from the contralateral coronary artery (61,62), the degree of ST-segment elevation may be minimal and ST-segment depression may be the more common presentation.

Alternatively, profound bradycardia or even asystole may be a presenting electrocardiographic correlate to the patient's symptoms. A smaller fraction of patients with variant angina also experience exercise-induced coronary arterial vasospasm (63).

Acute Myocardial Infarction

Some of the earlier investigations in variant angina indicated that coronary arterial vasospasm, the presumed trigger for variant angina, also could be a cause for AMI (3,4). These studies used noninvasive scintigraphy and coronary arteriography to document spasm at the site of the acute total coronary occlusion. The large-scale Gruppo Italiano per lo Studio della Sopravvivenza nell'Infarto Miocardico (GISSI-3) study (64) did not observe any effect on mortality of transdermal glycerol trinitrate in patients receiving thrombolysis for AMI. The lack of evidence in the GISSI-3 trial for a benefit from nitrates diminishes somewhat the enthusiasm regarding antispasm therapy during AMI. It is conceivable that stronger antispasm agents may be more useful, but, currently, none have been established as effective adjuncts to thrombolytics.

The incidence of coronary spasm after MI is greater in Japanese than white patients (10). In a study of Japanese and Italian patients, 80% of the Japanese but only 37% of the white patients had inducible coronary spasm 7 to 10 days after MI (65).

Sudden Cardiac Death and Malignant Ventricular Arrhythmia

As early as 1982, it was observed that some patients with variant angina experienced sudden death suggesting that coronary arterial spasm also could play a role in this acute coronary syndrome. Miller and coworkers (66) identified characteristics in patients with variant angina that were predictive of sudden death: ventricular tachycardia, ventricular fibrillation, or high-degree atrioventricular block during spontaneous episodes of pain. Some investigators (67) observed greater overall levels of ST-segment elevation during variant angina in those patients susceptible to sudden death.

In general, serious arrhythmias (ventricular dysrhythmias, complete atrioventricular block) occur in patients with variant angina who manifest ST-segment elevation, rather than ST-segment depression, during coronary spasm (68). In a study by Suzuki and coworkers (69), patients with variant angina had greater QT dispersion than patients with atypical chest pain. During acetylcholine provocation, 24 of 50 patients with variant angina experienced development of ventricular arrhythmias. At baseline, QT dispersion was significantly greater in patients with than without ventricular arrhythmias. Therefore, measurement of QT dispersion may help predict which patients with variant angina are at high risk for ventricular arrhythmia during ischemia. Moreover, patients with variant angina in whom ventricular tachycardia/fibrillation develops during spasm-induced ischemia are at high risk for recurrent ventricular arrhythmias and sudden death (70).

MacAlpin (71) studied 81 patients with variant angina. Nine of these patients experienced sudden death and 13 had significant cardiac arrhythmia. Overall, he observed that sudden death correlated with arrhythmia and a lack of severe coronary stenosis in the patients prone to sudden cardiac death. Therefore, provocative testing may be warranted in patients with sudden cardiac death to rule out coronary spasm.

Spasm after Coronary Artery Bypass Grafting

The occurrence of coronary artery spasm immediately after uncomplicated coronary artery bypass grafting (CABG) has been observed for more than 14 years. Waters and coworkers in 1980 (72) and Buxton and coworkers in 1981 (73) investigated several patients experiencing either severe chest pain (72) or major cardiovascular collapse and death after coronary surgery (73). The disturbing feature was that several of these patients experienced spasm in vessels that were not severely obstructed and bypassed. The addition of the priming solution used during cardiopulmonary bypass may be effective in preventing perioperative coronary spasm (74). Intravenous calcium channel blocking agents are now routinely administered after surgery in patients receiving free radial artery bypass grafts.

Spasm after Percutaneous Coronary Intervention

Several investigations have focused attention on the role of vasoreactivity at the angioplasty site in patients undergoing PTCA of significant fixed, coronary stenoses (58,75). Bertrand and coworkers (75) observed similar rates of restenosis among patients with and without ergonovine-induced coronary spasm superimposed on their atherothrombotic plaques. Subsequently, Ardissino and coworkers (58) observed that either ST-segment elevation during spontaneous ischemia or a positive hyperventilation test during the early recovery phase after PTCA was associated with a restenosis rate that was twice that of those who had a negative hyperventilation provocation. In the current era of coronary stenting, these findings may not be as relevant.

TREATMENT

Medical Therapy

The treatment of patients with variant angina is to some extent dependent on whether these patients are experiencing coronary spasm superimposed on an atherothrombotic coronary stenosis or whether the patients do not have any angiographic evidence of coronary artery disease. Patients with variant angina in the setting of atherothrombotic coronary artery disease obviously would benefit from therapy with nitrates and calcium channel blockade. However, β-adrenergic receptor blockade, usually beneficial in patients with classical coronary disease, may be somewhat detrimental in patients with both variant angina and significant coronary obstructions.

The main treatment for patients with vasospastic angina in the absence of coronary stenoses is vasodilator therapy with calcium channel blocking agents. The addition of nitrates may be effective for patients breaking through calcium blockers. However, long-term treatment with nitrates is usually associated with tolerance, and the major treatment effect probably would derive from therapy with calcium blockers. It is not recommended for any patient with coronary vasospasm to be treated with nitrates alone. Similar efficacy rates have been reported for nifedipine, diltiazem, and verapamil (76). In addition, it has been suggested that rebound symptoms may occur on withdrawal of calcium channel blockers (77). Amlodipine and related compounds should have a similar efficacy compared with the classical calcium channel blockers described earlier.

Occasionally, patients will be encountered who are refractory to medical therapy with calcium channel blockade. α-Adrenergic receptor blockade with prazosin has been found to be of value in such patients (78). Schecter and coworkers (40) observed that two patients, refractory to medical therapy, benefited from a nonselective serotonin antagonist cyproheptadine. Unfortunately, ketanserin, another serotonin antagonist, failed to prevent recurrent symptoms in six patients hospitalized for variant angina (42).

Several studies have indicated that antioxidant vitamins may be useful in the treatment of patients with variant angina. In one study, oral administration of vitamin E improved endothelium-dependent vasodilation in the brachial arteries of patients with variant angina (79). In another study, vitamin C infusion suppressed acetylcholine-induced constriction in coronary arteries of patients with variant angina (80). These data conflict with the data from the recent HDL-Atherosclerosis Treatment Study (HATS) trial (81), where a combination of antioxidant vitamins, including vitamin C and E, appeared to be detrimental in patients with coronary artery disease.

In a study of patients with diabetes with variant angina (82), administration of troglitazone improved endothelium-dependent vasodilation in brachial arteries and reduced anginal episodes and anginal duration. Reduction of anginal duration correlated with the improvement of endothelium-dependent vasodilation. In postmenopausal women with variant angina, estradiol supplementation prevented hyperventilation-induced anginal attacks and augmented endothelium-dependent vasodilation (83). On the basis of the results of the Heart and Estrogen/progestin Replacement Study (HERS) trial (84) and the recently halted Women's Health Initiative study (85), hormone replacement therapy increased the risk for coronary heart disease, stroke, and pulmonary embolism, in women, especially in smokers.

Surgical Treatment

Patients who do not respond to all drug therapy are candidates for surgical denervation and autotransplantation. This procedure was described by two groups in 1977 (31,32), who surgically excised and retransplanted the patient's heart, thereby denervating all sympathetic input into the coronary circulation.

In those patients who experience variant angina in the setting of significant coronary stenoses, percutaneous coronary intervention or CABG (74) can clearly improve circulation to the heart and improve symptoms. As mentioned earlier, however, patients with variant angina may have a high restenosis rate after PTCA and may also be at greater risk in the perioperative period after CABG. Therefore, any mechanical therapy for fixed coronary obstructions in patients with variant angina needs to be followed with a rigorous antispasm medical regimen.

LONG-TERM PROGNOSIS

In general, the natural history of Prinzmetal's angina is characterized by periods of frequent symptoms of variant angina alternating with periods in which the patient is asympto-

matic (86,87). In the setting of high-dose calcium channel blockade, patients with a shorter duration of symptoms and freedom from fixed coronary obstructions usually go into complete remission (88). Long-term survival at 5 years runs between 89% and 97% (89,90). As is established for patients with stable angina, the extent and severity of coronary artery disease, as well as the adequacy of ventricular function, are preeminent predictors of long-term survival.

Compared with Japanese patients, white patients with variant angina have a worse overall survival rate, which may relate to their more extensive atherothrombotic coronary disease, greater incidence of MI, and more frequent left ventricular dysfunction (10). In a pooled analysis, the survival rate at 3-year follow-up was 97% in Japanese patients versus 89% in white patients (10).

More recently, several investigations have appeared regarding long-term prognosis in patients with variant angina treated with calcium channel blockade. Ozaki at el. (91) followed 322 patients with positive ergonovine provocation testing and nonobstructive coronary disease. They observed a relatively benign prognosis on therapy for several years. However, repeat ergonovine testing, even after long symptom-free intervals, was able to induce the typical focal coronary spasm that the patients had at their onset of symptoms (Fig. 85–2). MacAlpin in 1988 (92) presented a study on 80 patients with variant angina; 28% had significant coronary artery disease. In general, the risk for recurring pain, MI, or death appeared more closely linked to the initial response to vasodilator therapy and *not* to the presence of severe fixed coronary artery disease (Fig. 85–3). The same investigator in 1993 (71) indicated that sudden death was more closely associated to presentation with severe arrhythmias during variant angina and lack of severe coronary stenoses. Although these investigations seem to contradict earlier ones identifying extent of coronary disease and ventricular func-

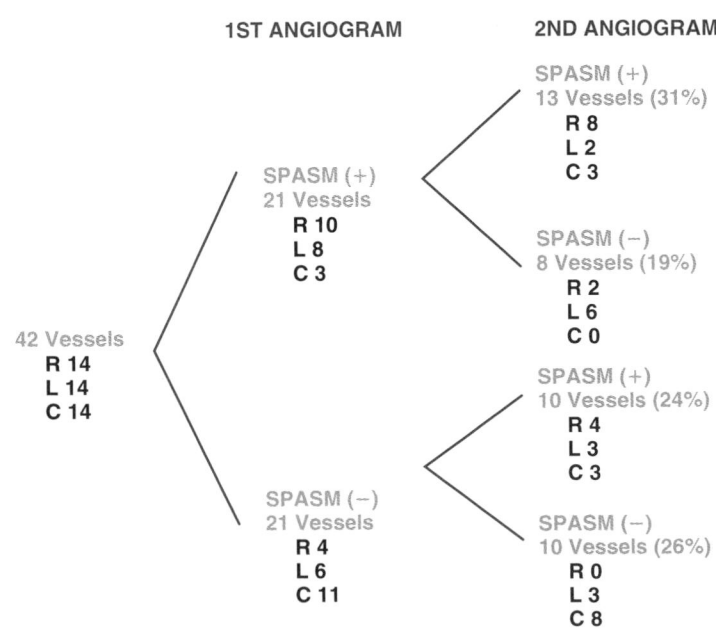

FIG. 85–2. Results of ergonovine testing in 42 vessels during the first and second angiograms. +, spasm; −, no spasm; C, left circumflex; I, left anterior descending; R, right coronary artery. (From Ozaki Y, Takatsu F, Osugi J, et al. Long-term study of recurrent vasospastic angina using coronary angiograms during ergonovine provocation tests. *Am Heart J* 1992;123:1191–1198, with permission.)

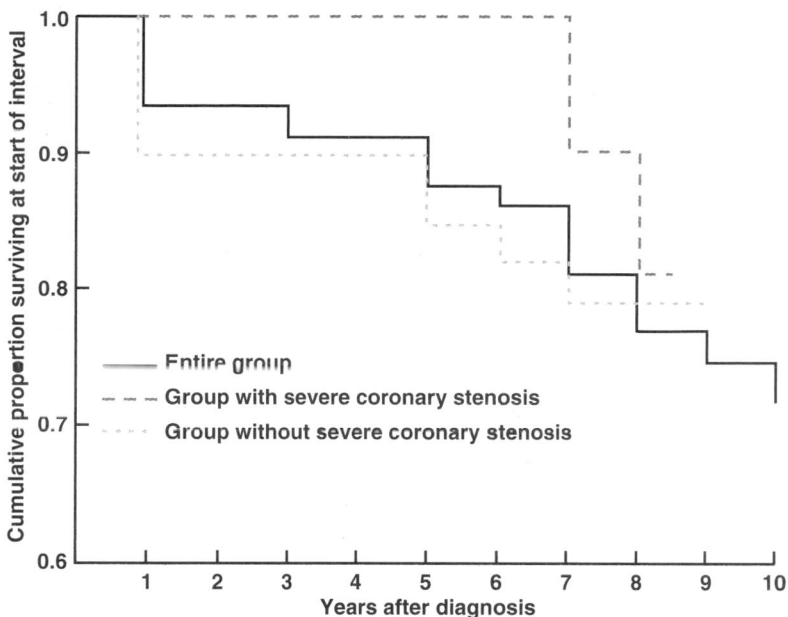

FIG. 85–3. Survival for subjects with and without any coronary artery stenoses greater than 70%. (From MacAlpin RN. Early evolution of symptoms and long-term prognosis in variant angina: importance of the functional component of coronary arterial disease. *Am J Med* 1988;85:19–28, with permission.)

tion as important predictors, they do indicate other variables that are of prognostic value.

FUTURE RESEARCH

For the most part, the cause of coronary spasm triggering variant angina remains a mystery. Techniques such as intravascular coronary ultrasound or angioscopy may help to identify mechanisms of variant angina. Using angioscopy, Etsuda and coworkers (93) observed that 4 of 10 patients with variant angina had angioscopic evidence of intimal injury at the site of focal acetylcholine-induced spasm (Fig. 85–4). Future investigations using these newer technologies may help to determine those factors that are responsible for localized reac-

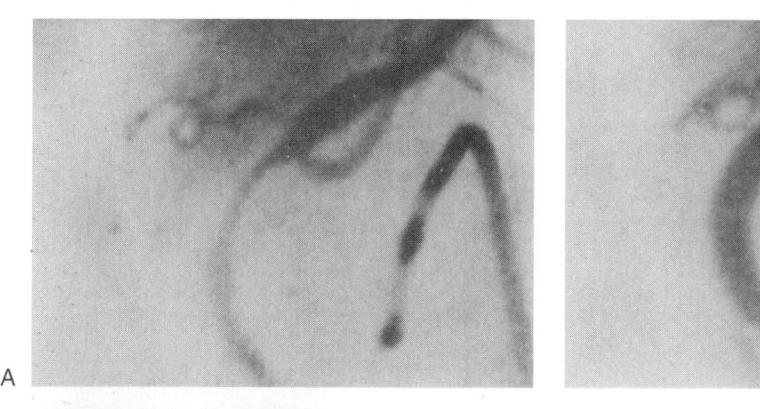
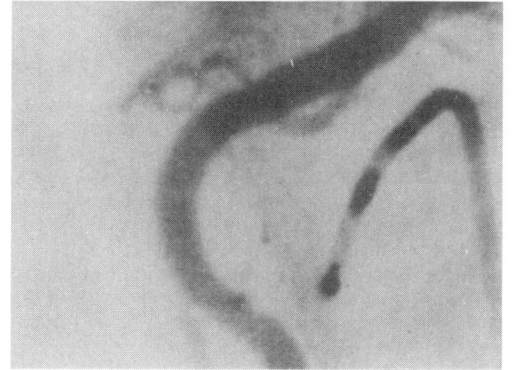
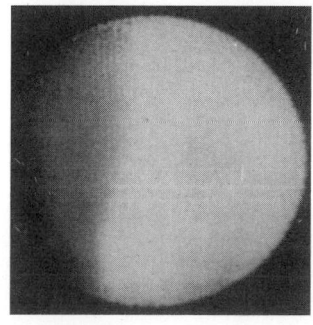

FIG. 85–4. After releasing coronary artery spasm in the proximal left anterior descending artery **(top left).** Intimal hemorrhage at 2 o'clock position **(top right),** and intracoronary thrombus between 5 and 8 o'clock **(bottom).** (From Etsuda H, Mizuno K, Arakawa K, et al. Angioscopy in variant angina: coronary artery spasm and intimal injury. *Lancet* 1993;342:1322–1324, with permission.)

tivity. In addition, emerging data indicate that some genetic abnormalities may contribute to coronary spasm and variant angina (94–96). Nakayama and coworkers (94) reported that T-786→C mutation in endothelial nitric oxide synthase gene reduces nitric oxide synthesis and may predispose the patients with this mutation to coronary spasm. Preliminary data suggest that intracoronary infusion of fasudil, a selective Rho-kinase inhibitor, prevents acetylcholine-induced coronary spasm and resultant myocardial ischemia in patients with variant angina (97). The role of this and similar agents in treating patients with variant angina in everyday clinical practice needs to be further elucidated. In addition, enhanced understanding of endothelial biology and new medical therapies such as endothelin blockers may improve our treatment success.

REFERENCES

1. Prinzmetal M, Kennamer R, Merliss R, et al. Angina pectoris. I. A variant form of angina pectoris; preliminary report. *Am J Med* 1959;27:375–388.
2. Oliva PB, Potts DE, Pluss RG. Coronary arterial spasm in Prinzmetal angina. Documentation by coronary arteriography. *N Engl J Med* 1973;288:745–748.
3. Oliva PB, Breckinridge JC. Arteriographic evidence of coronary arterial spasm in acute myocardial infarction. *Circulation* 1977;56:366–374.
4. Maseri A, L'Abbate A, Baroldi G, et al. Coronary vasospasm as a possible cause of myocardial infarction. A conclusion derived from the study of "preinfarction" angina. *N Engl J Med* 1978;299:1271–1277.
5. Maseri A, Severi S, De Nes M, et al. "Variant" angina: one aspect of a continuous spectrum of vasospastic myocardial ischemia. Pathogenetic mechanisms, estimated incidence and clinical and coronary arteriographic findings in 138 patients. *Am J Cardiol* 1978;42:1019–1035.
6. Maseri A, Parodi O, Severi S, et al. Transient transmural reduction of myocardial blood flow, demonstrated by thallium-201 scintigraphy, as a cause of variant angina. *Circulation* 1976;54:280.
7. Figueras J, Singh BN, Ganz W, et al. Mechanism of rest and nocturnal angina: observations during continuous hemodynamic and electrocardiographic monitoring *Circulation* 1979;59:955–968.
8. Folts JD, Gallagher K, Rowe GG. Blood flow reduction in stenosed coronary arteries: vasospasm or platelet aggregation? *Circulation* 1982;65:248–255.
9. Figueras J, Lidon RM, Seres L. Ischemic threshold and haemodynamic changes during angina at rest in patients with unstable angina. *Eur Heart J* 1993;14:1170–1178.
10. Beltrame JF, Sasayama S, Maseri A. Racial heterogenicity in coronary artery vasomotor reactivity: differences between Japanese and Caucasian patients. *J Am Coll Cardiol* 1999;33:1442–1452.
11. Kugiyama K, Yasue H, Okumura K, et al. Nitric oxide activity is deficient in spasm arteries of patients with coronary spastic angina. *Circulation* 1996;94:266–271.
12. Egashira K, Katsuda Y, Mohri M, et al. Basal release of endothelium-derived nitric oxide at site of spasm in patients with variant angina. *J Am Coll Cardiol* 1996;27:1444–1449.
13. Kugiyama K, Ohgushi M, Motoyama T, et al. Nitric oxide-mediated flow-dependent dilation is impaired in coronary arteries in patients with coronary spastic angina. *J Am Coll Cardiol* 1997;30:920–926.
14. Kaski JC, Crea F, Meran D, et al. Local coronary supersensitivity to diverse vasoconstrictive stimuli in patients with variant angina. *Circulation* 1986;74:1255–1265.
15. Robertson RM, Robertson D, Roberts LJ, et al. Thromboxane A$_2$ and vasotonic angina pectoris: evidence from direct measurements and inhibitor trials. *N Engl J Med* 1981;304:998–1003.
16. Chierchia S, de Caterina R, Crea F, et al. Failure of thromboxane A2 blockade to prevent attacks of vasospastic angina. *Circulation* 1982;66:702–705.
17. Irie T, Imaizumi T, Matuguchi T, et al. Increased fibrinopeptide A during angina attacks in patients with variant angina. *J Am Coll Cardiol* 1989;14:589.
18. Ogawa H, Yasue H, Oshima S, et al. Circadian variation of plasma fibrinopeptide A level in patients with variant angina. *Circulation* 1989;80:1617.
19. Bogaty P, Hackett D, Davies G, et al. Vasoreactivity of the culprit lesion in unstable angina. *Circulation* 1994;90:5–11.
20. Yasue H, Horio Y, Nakamura N, et al. Induction of coronary artery spasm by acetylcholine in patients with variant angina: possible role of the parasympathetic nerve system in the pathogenesis of coronary artery spasm. *Circulation* 1986;74:955.
21. Hoshio A, Kotare H, Mashiba H. Significance of coronary artery tone in patients with vasospastic angina. *J Am Coll Cardiol* 1989;14:604.
22. Toyo-oka T, Aizawa T, Suzuki N, et al. Increased plasma level of endothelin-1 and coronary spasm induction in patients with vasospastic angina pectoris. *Circulation* 1991;83:476–483.
23. Kuga T, Egashira K, Inou T, et al. Correlation of basal coronary artery tone with constrictive response to ergonovine in patients with variant angina. *J Am Coll Cardiol* 1993;22:44–50.
24. Hamabe A, Takase B, Uehata A, et al. Impaired endothelium-dependent vasodilation in the brachial artery in variant angina pectoris and the effect of intravenous administration of vitamin C. *Am J Cardiol* 2001;87:1154–1159.
25. Kawano H, Motoyama T, Yasue H, et al. Endothelial function fluctuates with diurnal variation in the frequency of ischemic episodes in patients with variant angina. *J Am Coll Cardiol* 2002;40:266–270.
26. Okumura K, Yasue H, Ishizaka H, et al. Endothelium-dependent dilator response to substance P in patients with coronary spastic angina. *J Am Coll Cardiol* 1992;20:838–844.
27. Egashira K, Inou T, Yamada A, et al. Preserved endothelium-dependent vasodilation at the vasospastic site in patients with variant angina. *J Clin Invest* 1992;89:1047–1052.
28. Okumura K, Yasue H, Matsuyama K, et al. Diffuse disorder of coronary artery vasomotility in patients with coronary spastic angina. Hyperreactivity to the constrictor effects of acetylcholine and the dilator effects of nitroglycerine. *J Am Coll Cardiol* 1996;27:45–52.
29. Akasaka T, Yoshida K, Hozumi T, et al. Comparison of coronary flow reserve between focal and diffuse vasoconstriction induced by ergonovine in patients with vasospastic angina. *Am J Cardiol* 1997;80:705–710.
30. Sun H, Mohri M, Shimokawa H, et al. Coronary microvascular spasm causes myocardial ischemia in patients with vasospastic angina. *J Am Coll Cardiol* 2002;39:847–851.
31. Clark DA, Quint RA, Mitchell RL, et al. Coronary artery spasm. Medical management, surgical denervation, and autotransplantation. *J Thorac Cardiovasc Surg* 1977;73:332.
32. Grondin CM, Limet R. Sympathetic denervation in association with coronary artery grafting in patients with Prinzmetals' angina. *Ann Thorac Surg* 1977;23:111–117.
33. Sakata K, Yoshida H, Hoshino T, et al. Sympathetic nerve activity in the spasm-induced coronary artery region is associated with disease activity of vasospastic angina. *J Am Coll Cardiol* 1996;28:460–464.
34. Botker HE, Frobert O, Moller N, et al. Insulin resistance in cardiac syndrome X and variant angina: influence of physical capacity and circulating lipids. *Am Heart J* 1997;134:229–237.
35. Hirashima O, Kawano H, Motoyama T, et al. Improvement of endothelial function and insulin resistance with vitamin C in patients with coronary spastic angina. *J Am Coll Cardiol* 2000;35:1860–1866.
36. Satake K, Lee JD, Shimizu H, et al. Relation between severity of magnesium deficiency and frequency of anginal attacks in men with variant angina. *J Am Coll Cardiol* 1996;28:897–902.
37. Cohen L, Kitzes R. Prompt termination and/or prevention of cold-pressor-stimulus-induced vasoconstriction of different vascular beds by magnesium sulfate in patients with Prinzmetal's angina. *Magnesium* 1986;5:144.
38. Miyagi H, Yasue H, Okumura K, et al. Effect of magnesium on anginal attack induced by hyperventilation in patients with variant angina. *Circulation* 1989;79:597.
39. Miwa K, Miyagi Y, Igawa A, et al. Vitamin E deficiency in variant angina. *Circulation* 1996;94:14–18.
40. Schecter AD, Chesebro JH, Fuster V. Refractory Prinzmetal angina treated with Cyproheptadine. *Ann Intern Med* 1994;121:113–114.
41. McFadden EP, Clarke JG, Davies GJ, et al. Effect of intracoronary serotonin on coronary vessels in patients with stable angina and patients with variant angina. *N Engl J Med* 1991;324:648.
42. Mata-Bourcart LE, Waters DD, Bouchard A, et al. Failure of Ke-

tanserin a serotonin inhibitor to prevent spontaneous or ergonovine induced attacks of variant angina. *Can J Cardiol* 1985;1:168–171.

43. Lange RL, Reid MS, Tresch DD, et al. Nonatheromatous ischemic heart disease following withdrawal from chronic industrial nitroglycerin exposure. *Circulation* 1972;46:666–678.

44. Lange RA, Cigarroa RG, Yancy CW, et al. Cocaine induced coronary artery vasoconstriction. *N Engl J Med* 1989;321:1557.

45. Stefenelli T, Zielinski CC, Mayr H, et al. Prinzmetal's angina during cyclophosphamide therapy. *Eur Heart J* 1988;9:1155.

46. Kleiman NS, Lehane DE, Geyer CE Jr, et al. Prinzmetal's angina during 5-fluorouracil chemotherapy. *Am J Med* 1987;82:566–568.

47. Forman MB, Oates JA, Robertson D, et al. Increased adventitial mast cells in a patient with coronary spasm. *N Engl J Med* 1985;313:1138–1141.

48. Umemoto S, Suzuki N, Fujii K, et al. Eosinophil counts and plasma fibrinogen in patients with vasospastic angina pectoris. *Am J Cardiol* 2000;85:715–719.

49. Okumura K, Osanai T, Kosugi T, et al. Enhanced phospholipase C activity in the cultured skin fibroblast obtained from patients with coronary spastic angina: possible role for enhanced vasoconstrictor response. *J Am Coll Cardiol* 2000;36:1847–1852.

50. Hong MK, Park SW, Whan C, et al. Intravascular ultrasound findings of negative arterial remodeling at sites of focal coronary spasm in patients with vasospastic angina. *Am Heart J* 2000;140:395–401.

51. Schroeder JS, Bolen JL, Quint RA, et al. Provocation of coronary spasm with ergonovine maleate. New test with results in 57 patients undergoing coronary arteriography. *Am J Cardiol* 1977;40:487–491.

52. Heupler FA Jr, Proudfit WL, Razavi M, et al. Ergonovine maleate provocative test for coronary arterial spasm. *Am J Cardiol* 1978;41:631–640.

53. Harding MB, Leithe ME, Mark DB, et al. Ergonovine maleate testing during cardiac catheterization: a 10-year perspective in 3,447 patients without significant coronary artery disease or Prinzmetal's variant angina. *J Am Coll Cardiol* 1992;20:107–111.

54. Song JK, Lee SJ, Kang DH, et al. Ergonovine echocardiography as a screening test for diagnosis of vasospastic angina before coronary angiography. *J Am Coll Cardiol* 1996;27:1156–1161.

55. Okumura K, Yasue H, Horio Y, et al. Multivessel coronary spasm in patients with variant angina: a study with intracoronary injection of acetylcholine. *Circulation* 1988;77:535–542.

56. Okumura K, Yasue H, Matsuyama K, et al. Sensitivity and specificity of intracoronary injection of acetylcholine for the induction of coronary artery spasm. *J Am Coll Cardiol* 1988;12:883.

57. Mortensen SA, Vilhelmsen R, Sandoe E. Non-pharmacological provocation of coronary vasospasm. Experience with prolonged hyperventilation in the coronary care unit. *Eur Heart J* 1983;4:391.

58. Ardissino D, Barberis P, De Servi S, et al. Abnormal coronary vasoconstriction as a predictor of restenosis after successful coronary angioplasty in patients with unstable angina pectoris. *N Engl J Med* 1991;325:1053–1057.

59. Sakata K, Shirotani M, Yoshida H, et al. Iodine-123 metaiodobenzylguanidine cardiac imaging to identify and localize vasospastic angina without significant coronary artery narrowing. *J Am Coll Cardiol* 1997;30:370–376.

60. Meller J, Conde CA, Donoso E, et al. Transient Q waves in Prinzmetal's angina. *Am J Cardiol* 1975;35:691.

61. Takeshita A, Koiwaya Y, Nakamura M, et al. Immediate appearance of coronary collaterals during ergonovine induced arterial spasm. *Chest* 1982;82:319.

62. Tada M, Yamagishi M, Kodama K, et al. Transient collateral augmentation during coronary arterial spasm associated with ST-segment depression. *Circulation* 1983;67:693.

63. Boden WE, Bough EW, Core AS, et al. Exercised induced coronary spasm with ST segment depression and normal coronary arteriography. *Am J Cardiol* 1981;48:193–197.

64. GISSI-3: effects of lisinopril and transdermal glyceryl trinitrate singly and together on 6-week mortality and ventricular function after acute myocardial infarction. Gruppo Italiano per lo Studio della Sopravvivenza nell'Infarto Miocardico. *Lancet* 1994;343:1115–1122.

65. Pristipino C, Beltrame JF, Finocchiaro ML, et al. Major racial differences in coronary constrictor response between Japanese and Caucasians with recent myocardial infarction. *Circulation* 2000;101:1102–1108.

66. Miller DD, Waters DD, Szlachcic J, et al. Clinical characteristics associated with sudden death in patients with variant angina. *Circulation* 1982;66:588.

67. Bayes de Luna A, Carreras F, Cladellas M, et al. Holter ECG study of the electrocardiographic phenomena in Prinzmetal angina attacks with emphasis on the study of ventricular arrhythmias. *J Electrocardiol* 1985;18:267.

68. Onaka H, Hirota Y, Shimada S, et al. Clinical observation of spontaneous anginal attacks and multivessel spasm in variant angina pectoris with normal coronary arteries: evaluation by 24-hour 12-lead electrocardiography with compute analysis. *J Am Coll Cardiol* 1996;27:38–44.

69. Suzuki M, Nishizaki M, Arita M, et al. Increased QT dispersion in patients with vasospastic angina. *Circulation* 1998;98:435–440.

70. Meisel SR, Mazur A, Chetboun I, et al. Usefulness of implantable cardioverter-defibrillators in refractory variant angina pectoris complicated by ventricular fibrillation in patients with angiographically normal coronary arteries. *Am J Cardiol* 2002;89:1114–1116.

71. MacAlpin RN. Cardiac arrest and sudden unexpected death in variant angina: complications of coronary spasm that can occur in the absence of severe organic coronary stenosis. *Am Heart J* 1993;125:1011–1107.

72. Waters DD, Theroux P, Crittin J, et al. Previously undiagnosed variant angina as a cause of chest pain after coronary artery bypass surgery. *Circulation* 1980;61:1159.

73. Buxton AE, Goldberg S, Harken A, et al. Coronary artery spasm immediately after myocardial revascularization. *N Engl J Med* 1981;304:1249–1253.

74. Katsumoto K, Niibori T. Prevention of coronary spasms during aortocoronary (A-C) bypass surgery for variant angina and effort angina with ST-elevation. *J Cardiovasc Surg* 1988;29:343.

75. Bertrand ME, LaBlanche JM, Thieuleux FA, et al. Comparative results of percutaneous transluminal coronary angioplasty in patients with dynamic versus fixed coronary stenosis. *J Am Coll Cardiol* 1986;8:504–508.

76. Antman E, Muller J, Goldberg S, et al. Nifedipine therapy for coronary-artery spasm. Experience in 127 patients. *N Engl J Med* 1980;302:12.

77. Passola A, Lauro A, Gallo R, et al. Efficacy of Diltiazem in variant angina: results of a double-blind cross over study in CCU by Holter monitoring: the possible occurrence of a withdrawal syndrome. *G Ital Cardiol* 1987;17:329.

78. Tzivoni D, Keren A, Benhorin J, et al. Prazosin therapy for refractory variant angina. *Am Heart J* 1983;105:262.

79. Motoyama T, Kawano H, Kugiyama K, et al. Vitamin E administration improves impairment of endothelium-dependent vasodilation in patients with coronary spastic angina. *J Am Coll Cardiol* 1998;32:1672–1679.

80. Kugiyama K, Motoyama T, Hirashima O, et al. Vitamin C attenuates abnormal vasomotor reactivity in spasm coronary arteries in patients with coronary spastic angina. *J Am Coll Cardiol* 1998;32:103–109.

81. Brown BG, Zhao XQ, Chait A, et al. Simvastatin and niacin, antioxidant vitamins, or the combination for the prevention of coronary disease. *N Engl J Med* 2001;345:1583–1592.

82. Murakami T, Mizuno S, Ohsato K, et al. Effects of troglitazone on frequency of coronary vasospastic-induced angina pectoris in patients with diabetes mellitus. *Am J Cardiol* 1999;84:92–94.

83. Kawano H, Motoyama T, Hirai N, et al. Estradiol supplementation suppresses hyperventilation-induced attacks in postmenopausal women with variant angina. *J Am Coll Cardiol* 2001;37:735–740.

84. Cardiovascular disease outcomes during 6.8 years of hormone therapy: Heart and Estrogen/progestin Replacement Study follow-up (HERS II). *JAMA* 2002;288:49–57.

85. Rossouw JE, Anderson GL, Prentice RL, et al. Risks and benefits of estrogen plus progestin in healthy postmenopausal women: principal results from the Women's Health Initiative randomized controlled trial. *JAMA* 2002;288:321–323.

86. Waters DD, Miller D, Szlachcic J, et al. Factors influencing the long-term prognosis of treated patients with variant angina. *Circulation* 1983;68:258.

87. Mark DB, Califf RM, Morris KG, et al. Clinical characteristics and long-term survival of patients with variant angina. *Circulation* 1984;69:880.

88. Previtali M, Panciroli C, Ardissino D, et al. Spontaneous remission of variant angina documented by Holter monitoring and ergonovine testing in patients treated with calcium antagonists. *Am J Cardiol* 1987;59:235.

89. Walling A, Waters DD, Miller DD, et al. Long-term prognosis of patients with variant angina. *Circulation* 1987;76:990.

90. Yasue H, Takizawa D, Nagao M, et al. Long-term prognosis for patients with variant angina and influential factors. *Circulation* 1988;78:1.

91. Ozaki Y, Takatsu F, Osugi J, et al. Long-term study of recurrent vasospastic angina using coronary angiograms during ergonovine provocation tests. *Am Heart J* 1992;123:1191–1198.

92. MacAlpin RN. Early evolution of symptoms and long-term prognosis in variant angina: importance of the functional component of coronary arterial disease. *Am J Med* 1988;85:19–28.

93. Etsuda H, Mizuno K, Arakawa K, et al. Angioscopy in variant angina: coronary artery spasm and intimal injury. *Lancet* 1993;342:1322–1324.

94. Nakayama M, Yasue H, Yoshimura M, et al. T-786→C mutation in the 5′-flanking region of the endothelial nitric oxide synthase gene is associated with coronary spasm. *Circulation* 1999;99:2864–2870.

95. Yoshimura M, Yasue H, Nakayama M, et al. A missense Glu298Asp variant in the endothelial nitric oxide synthase gene is associated with coronary spasm in the Japanese. *Hum Genet* 1998;103:65–69.

96. Ito T, Yasue H, Yoshimura M, et al. Paraoxonase gene Gln192Arg (Q192R) polymorphism is associated with coronary artery spasm. *Hum Genet* 2002;110:89–94.

97. Masumoto A, Mohri M, Shimokawa H, et al. Suppression of patients with vasospastic angina. *Circulation* 2002;105:1545–1547.

CHAPTER 86

Silent Ischemia in Unstable Angina

Juan Carlos Kaski and Juan Cosín-Sales

Key Words: Acute coronary syndrome; non-STEMI; silent myocardial ischemia; unstable angina.

INTRODUCTION

The acute coronary syndrome (ACS) encompassing unstable angina (UA) and non–ST-segment elevation myocardial infarction (non-STEMI) affects approximately 1.5 million new individuals annually in the United States and is associated with high morbidity and mortality (1). In recent years the American College of Cardiology/American Heart Association (ACC/AHA) Task Force on Practice Guidelines (1) defined UA and non-STEMI as closely related conditions with similar pathogenesis and clinical presentation, albeit of differing severity. In patients with UA, as recently defined (1), biochemical markers of myocardial necrosis are not increased. In non-STEMI, however, myocardial ischemia is severe enough to cause myocardial damage, which results in the release of detectable quantities of markers of myocardial injury—that is, troponin I (TnI), troponin T (TnT), and creatine phosphokinase-MB isoenzyme. The Joint European Society of Cardiology (ESC)/ACC Committee (2) has defined myocardial infarction (MI) as a typical increase and gradual decrease of troponin (or more rapid increase and decrease of creatine phosphokinase-MB isoenzyme) in the

    J. C. Kaski: Coronary Artery Disease Research Unit, Department of Cardiological Sciences, St George's Hospital Medical School, Cranmer Terrace, London SW17 0RE, UK.
    J. Cosín-Sales: Coronary Artery Disease Research Unit, Department of Cardiological Sciences, St George's Hospital Medical School, Cranmer Terrace, London, SW17 0RE, UK.

presence of at least one of the following: (a) ischemic symptoms; (b) development of pathologic Q waves on the electrocardiogram (ECG); (c) ECG changes indicative of myocardial ischemia (ST-segment elevation or depression); and (d) coronary artery intervention (e.g., coronary angioplasty). The majority of studies discussed in this chapter were carried out before the recently proposed definition of MI. Analysis and interpretation of these studies will be carried out in light of previous definitions of ACS.

Patients with UA represent a heterogeneous population regarding both clinical features and outcome. Patient heterogeneity also results from the diversity of pathogenetic mechanisms responsible for the syndrome. Patients with UA/non-STEMI usually have obstructive coronary artery disease, but the severity of their coronary stenoses varies markedly. The most common pathogenic mechanisms in ACS are atheromatous plaque disruption and endothelial erosion with subsequent acute intraluminal thrombosis (3,4). Occasionally, however, patients with ACS are found to have normal coronary arteriograms. When this occurs, coronary artery spasm, microvascular angina, or a small plaque fissure with spontaneous lysis of a coronary thrombus may be implicated (5).

Before the most recent definition of UA and non-STEMI, several clinical classifications existed for UA on the basis of clinical presentation, severity of symptoms, response to treatment, cardiac troponin levels, and the presence or absence of ECG changes during pain (6,7).

Chest pain is of paramount importance for the diagnosis of ACS as attested by that widely used UA definitions such as that of Braunwald (8) are based on the occurrence of chest pain. However, it has become apparent in recent years that a large proportion of patients with UA/non-STEMI have silent myocardial ischemia, albeit usually in addition to anginal episodes (9,10). Completely silent MIs have been shown to occur frequently, mainly in the elderly and in patients with diabetes mellitus (11). The incidence of completely silent ACS is unknown. Whether the presence of silent ischemic ECG changes in patients with unstable coronary syndromes has prognostic importance has been a matter of speculation for several decades. This chapter reviews the evidence regarding the prognostic value of continuing silent myocardial ischemia in patients who are hospitalized with the syndrome of UA/non-STEMI.

RELATION BETWEEN CLINICAL PRESENTATION AND OUTCOME

It has been suggested that a comprehensive clinical classification of UA may help to identify patients who are at greater risk for infarction and sudden death and may also provide clues as to possible disease mechanisms (6,7). Clinical classifications are useful only if they provide prognostic information or identify subgroups of patients who may benefit from specific therapeutic interventions. Bertolet and coworkers (12) assessed one classification system in 129 consecutive patients with UA discharged from the coronary care unit and observed that subclassification of patients with UA based on clinical characteristics at presentation was not useful to predict subsequent ACS. Other authors have reported that clinical characteristics (i.e., recurrent chest pain) after maximal treatment in patients diagnosed of UA do not correlate with their coronary anatomy (13) or their short- and middle-term outcome (14).

As both myocardial damage (i.e., increased cardiac troponins) (15) and prolonged transient myocardial ischemia (12) correlate with patient outcome, it has been suggested that unrecognized (silent) persistent myocardial ischemia may be responsible for the high incidence of events observed within a few months after discharge from coronary care units in patients with UA.

SILENT MYOCARDIAL ISCHEMIA IN PATIENTS WITH UNSTABLE ANGINA/NON–ST-SEGMENT ELEVATION MYOCARDIAL INFARCTION

Although similar in character, location, and radiation to that observed in chronic stable angina pectoris, chest pain in UA occurs at rest and is usually more severe and longer in duration. As in other forms of coronary artery disease, chest pain in UA is the symptom that most commonly alerts both patient and physician as to the possible serious nature of the chest discomfort. However, when continuous monitoring of the ST segment is carried out, a relatively large proportion of patients with UA have typical ischemic ECG changes that are not associated with chest pain ("silent myocardial ischemia"). Moreover, continuous ST-segment monitoring in individual patients has revealed that from 75% (13) to 90%

(16) of ischemic episodes are not associated with chest pain. It is therefore reasonable to assume that if we rely on chest pain only, we may just see the tip of the iceberg as patients with "completely silent" unstable syndromes will go undetected.

It is important to remember that episodes of silent ischemia do not differ from painful episodes with respect to ECG manifestations, hemodynamic effects, or myocardial perfusion defects. In the 1980s, Gottlieb and coworkers (16) observed a high prevalence of silent ischemic episodes in 70 patients with UA admitted to the coronary care unit. These patients underwent continuous 48-hour monitoring for the assessment of ST-segment changes while treated with conventional antianginal drugs. Thirty-seven (53%) had at least 1 episode of silent myocardial ischemia; of the 37 patients, 8 had both silent and painful episodes and 29 had only silent ST-segment depression. Of all 205 episodes of ST-segment depression detected in the study, 90% were asymptomatic. Similarly, studies by von Arnim and coworkers (17) indicate that more than 40% of patients admitted to the hospital with UA have transient myocardial ischemia on ambulatory monitoring, and more than 80% of the ischemic episodes detected in these patients are silent. A metaanalysis involving 995 patients showed that episodes of silent ischemia were detected in 271 patients (27%) using continuous 24-hour ECG monitoring (14).

Mechanisms of Silent Ischemia

Although previously the symptom of angina was considered to be vital for the diagnosis of myocardial ischemia, it is currently accepted that silent ischemic episodes are probably the most common manifestation of myocardial ischemia. Why some patients have myocardial ischemia without symptoms whereas others have only symptomatic ischemia is unknown. Moreover, the reason within patients some episodes are symptomatic and others asymptomatic despite similar ECG characteristics also is controversial. Mazzone and coworkers (18) observed that patients with silent ischemia had lower CD11b leukocyte adhesion molecule expression and greater concentrations of antiinflammatory cytokines (interleukin [IL]-4, IL-10, and transforming growth factor-β) compared with symptomatic patients. They speculated that in patients with silent ischemia a T helper cell 2 (Th2) type response could induce the production of antiinflammatory cytokines and endogenous opioids, together with a greater expression of peripheral benzodiazepine receptors. It could be speculated that antiinflammatory cytokines may increase the threshold for nerve activation, thus blocking pain transmission pathways. In addition, antiinflammatory cytokines exert a prolonged inhibitory effect on transcription factor nuclear factor-κB leading to a reduction or elimination of pain-mediating substances.

Myocardial ischemia in patients with UA is usually associated with the presence of obstructive coronary artery disease, albeit coronary arteriographic findings vary in different series. Approximately 50% of patients have three-vessel disease, whereas single-vessel disease is found in less than 20% (19). The incidence of single-vessel disease is larger in patients with recent-onsct angina. Angiographically normal coronary arteriograms are seen in less than 15% of patients admitted with UA. Nademanee and coworkers (20) observed that the greater the number of diseased coronary arteries, the longer the cumulative duration of ischemia documented during 24-hour ambulatory monitoring (13).

In a prospective observational study in patients with UA who had been maximally treated medically, Patel and coworkers (13) showed that silent ischemic episodes were a powerful predictor of the presence of complex stenosis and intracoronary thrombus (odds ratio, 7.1). It is established that patients with UA with complex stenoses morphology and intracoronary thrombus, representing atheromatous plaque disruption, have an adverse outcome (21) and show persistent plaque activity (22,23). This association may explain why transient ischaemia is a predictor of poor outcome in patients with UA.

Reduced Heart Rate Variability and Silent Ischemia in Patients with Unstable Angina

Reduced heart rate variability has been demonstrated in patients with MI and appears to be a marker of poor outcome in this setting. Huang and coworkers (24) observed that during 48-hour continuous ECG monitoring, all measures of heart rate variability were markedly reduced in patients with UA, particularly in those with ischemic ST-segment changes. The magnitude of the reduction in heart rate variability in UA was similar to that reported in patients with acute MI. Both patients who remained symptomatic and patients who continued to have silent myocardial ischemia during the last 24 hours of monitoring showed a further reduction of heart rate variability compared with the initial 24-hour period and compared with patients who were clinically improved by treatment. Along the same lines, Lanza and coworkers (25) investigated whether analysis of both time domain and frequency domain heart rate variability could further improve the prognostic yield of Holter monitoring in unstable patients. Although they found that transient ischemia on Holter monitoring was a powerful predictor of cardiac events (odds ratio, 12.2), there were no significant differences between patients with and those without events. An imbalance in cardiac autonomic tone, however, toward increased sympathetic activity (increased low-/high-frequency ratio) was observed in a subgroup of patients with increased risk for serious events.

Myocardial Damage and Silent Ischemia

The presence of myocardial damage, as assessed by cardiac enzyme increase or increases of cardiac troponin, has become an important prognostic marker in the setting of acute chest pain (6). Severe transient silent myocardial ischemia in patients with UA may be associated with myocardial

damage as shown by Botker and coworkers (26). These authors observed that patients with ACS and evidence of myocardial damage, as assessed by serial measurements of creatine kinase MB, also had repetitive ischemic episodes, both painful and silent, during continuous ST-segment monitoring. In the study by Botker and coworkers (26), coronary events during follow-up occurred only in those patients who had increased creatine kinase levels. Similar findings were reported by Hamm and coworkers (27) using TnT to detect myocardial necrosis. The presence of detectable serum levels of TnT during the first 2 days of hospital stay was a sensitive and specific marker for myocardial cell damage and predicted the clinical outcome during hospitalization. Norgaard and coworkers (28) found that among patients with UA, those with at least one silent ischemic episode had a median TnT level greater than or equal to 0.15 μg per liter compared with 0.01 μg per liter in patients without ischemic episodes ($p = 0.0003$). They also found a moderate positive relation between the number of ischemic episodes and TnT levels. Interestingly, when TnT levels and the presence of ischemic episodes were considered together, they provided a more powerful and accurate risk stratification method than either variable alone.

PROGNOSTIC IMPLICATIONS

There is increasing evidence that in patients with UA the presence of continuing silent ischemic episodes of ST-segment depression or elevation has prognostic importance. It has been observed that despite achieving control of symptoms with medical therapy, patients with UA continue to have a high incidence of recurrent angina and MI (16), as well as rapid coronary stenosis progression (29,30). Ambulatory ECG monitoring appears to identify subsets of patients with an increased risk (Figs. 86–1 and 86–2). More than two decades ago, Johnson and coworkers (31) described findings in a subgroup of patients with UA who were at high risk for adverse events. These were hospitalized patients who on continuous monitoring had transient ischemic ST-segment shifts. Transient ST-segment changes were predictors of advanced coronary artery disease and poor prognosis at 3 months. However, although the authors did not analyze results in silent versus painful episodes, their clinical observations were conceptually important and helped to increase awareness among physicians as to the prognostic role of continuing ischemia in UA.

Later, Gottlieb and coworkers (16) and Nademanee and coworkers (20) observed that in patients with UA the persistence of silent ischemic episodes on Holter recordings was associated with severe advanced coronary disease and identified a subset of patients with an increased incidence of recurrent angina, MI, and death, despite marked amelioration of symptoms with conventional therapy during hospital admission. Akkerhuis and coworkers (14) confirmed these initial findings in a metaanalysis involving almost 1,000 patients.

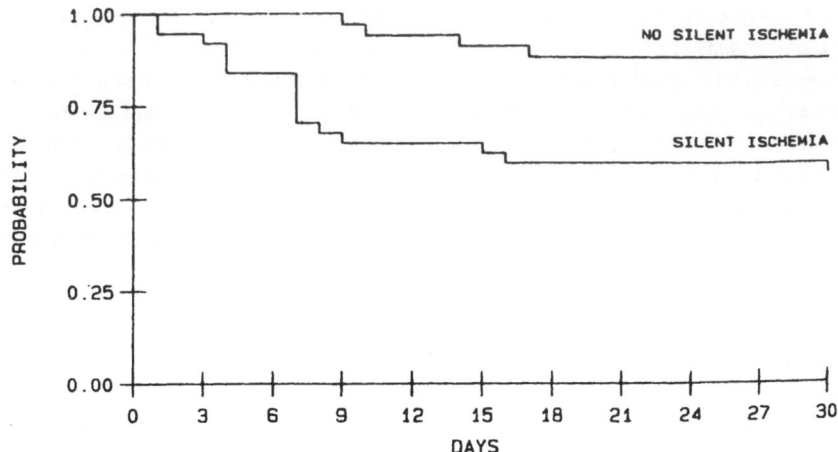

FIG. 86–1. Prognostic value of silent myocardial ischemia in patients with unstable angina 1 month after hospital discharge. Kaplan-Meier curves illustrating the probabilities of not experiencing death or myocardial infarction over 30 days of follow-up. (From Gottlieb et al., ref. 16, with permission.)

In the studies by Gottlieb and coworkers (16,32), 70 patients with UA hospitalized and medically treated were assessed after 1-month follow-up and, subsequently, after 2 years to ascertain the prognostic value of transient myocardial ischemia on 48-hour Holter monitoring. More than 50% of patients with UA had silent ischemic episodes, which correlated significantly with early (1 month) (Fig. 86–1) and late (2 years) (Fig. 86–2) patient outcome. The total duration of silent ST-segment changes also was found to be of prognostic relevance in these studies (16,20). Actuarial Kaplan-Meier analysis at 1-month follow-up showed a significantly greater likelihood of adverse events—that is, recurrence of symptoms requiring revascularization, nonfatal MI, or cardiac death—in patients with more than 60 minutes of silent ischemia than in patients with a shorter total ischemic time. In patients reassessed at 2-year follow-up, multivariate

analysis showed a fivefold greater relative risk for adverse events in the group with silent ischemia compared with the group without silent ischemia (32). In the majority of patients in the study, the adverse clinical outcome occurred within the first few months of follow-up (Fig. 86–2), suggesting that continuing ischemia was related to plaque instability.

Similar findings were reported by Akkerhuis and coworkers (14) in a metaanalysis involving 995 patients who took part in large trials (c7E3 Fab Anti Platelet Therapy in Unstable REfractory angina [CAPTURE], Platelet Glycoprotein IIb-IIIa in Unstable Angina: Receptor Suppression Using Integrilin Therapy [PURSUIT], and Fibrinogen Receptor Occupancy Study [FROST]) evaluating the use of glycoprotein IIb/IIIa blockers in patients with non–ST-elevation ACS. These patients, who may be considered a representative sam-

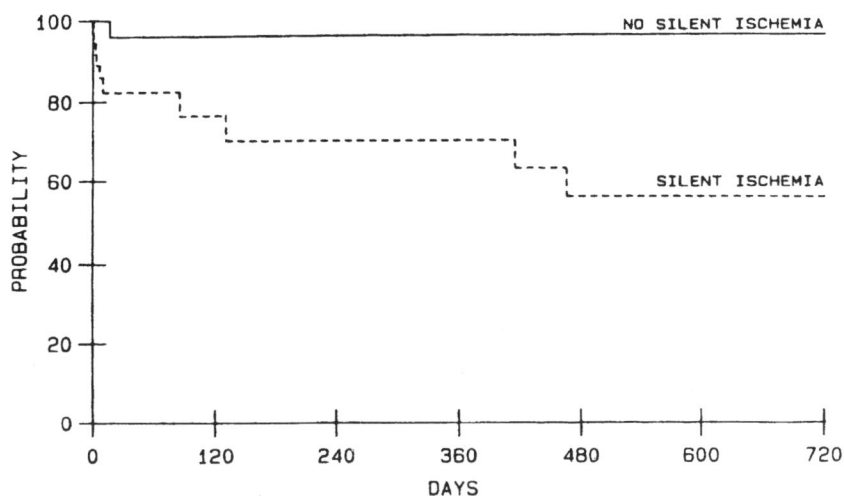

FIG. 86–2. The probabilities of not experiencing serious coronary events (death and myocardial infarction) over the 2-year follow-up period in the study by Gottlieb and coworkers (From Gottlieb et al., ref. 32, with permission.)

ple of receiving management state of art, were continuously monitored for 24 hours after enrollment, using a computer-assisted 12-lead ECG or a vectorcardiographic (VCG) ECG-ischemia monitoring device. Ischemic episodes were detected in 271 (27%) patients, and the authors found a direct relation between the number of ischemic episodes per 24 hours and the probability of cardiac events at 5 and 30 days. The 30-day composite end point of death and MI occurred in 5.7% of patients without episodes and increased to 19.7% in patients with 5 or more episodes. After adjustment for baseline predictors of adverse outcome, the relative risk of death or MI at 5 and 30 days increased by 25% for each additional ischemic episode per 24 hours (Fig. 86 3).

As previously mentioned, the prognostic information derived from continuous ST-segment monitoring can be improved significantly with the use of biochemical markers of myocardial injury such as cardiac troponins. Aguiar and coworkers (33) prospectively studied 183 patients admitted to hospital with chest pain at rest suggestive of ACS. Patients underwent continuous ST-segment monitoring for 24 hours, and TnI levels were measured at admission and every 6 hours for the first 24 hours. Study end points were death or nonfatal MI within 30 days of follow-up. Fifty patients (27%) who had at least one episode of ischemic ST-segment depression showed a worse 30-day outcome (22% event rate) compared with patients without ST segment shifts (7% event rate) ($p = 0.003$). Multivariate analysis showed that the presence of ST-segment depression (hazard ratio, 3.07) and peak TnI levels greater than 0.2 μg per liter (hazard ratio, 2.65) were independent predictors of prognosis. The combined use of both markers allowed the identification of

patients at low, intermediate, and high risk for events at 30 days. In another study involving 232 patients with UA, Norgaard and coworkers (28) assessed whether the addition of 24-hour continuous vectorcardiography ST-segment monitoring (cVST) provides prognostic information in addition to that of TnT. They observed that both early determination of continuous TnT and subsequent cVST for 24 hours offered independent prognostic information. Moreover, patients with a TnT level of 0.20 μg per liter or greater and 1 or more episodes of ST-segment shift were at a particularly high risk for events (25.8%) at 30 days. These findings, however, were not confirmed by Rebuzzi and coworkers (34), who compared four prognostic indicators available on hospital admission—that is, chest pain in the last 24 hours, baseline 12-lead ECG, TnT, and C-reactive protein [CRP])—versus 24-hour Holter monitoring—in 102 patients with Braunwald Class IIIB UA. The Rebuzzi study (34) showed that MI was more frequent in patients with increased TnT levels (50% vs. 9%; $p = 0.001$) and those with increased CRP levels (24%) compared with patients with normal CRP levels (4%; $p = 0.01$). Only 1 of 46 patients with negative TnT and CRP developed MI in their series. Multivariate analysis showed that TnT ($p = 0.02$) and CRP ($p = 0.04$) were independently associated with risk for MI. TnT had the greatest specificity (92%); and CRP had the greatest sensitivity (87%). The presence of myocardial ischemia on Holter monitoring also was associated with the occurrence of MI ($p = 0.003$) but added little to the predictive value of TnT and CRP.

Romeo and coworkers (35), however, did not confirm these findings. They compared the prognostic significance of total

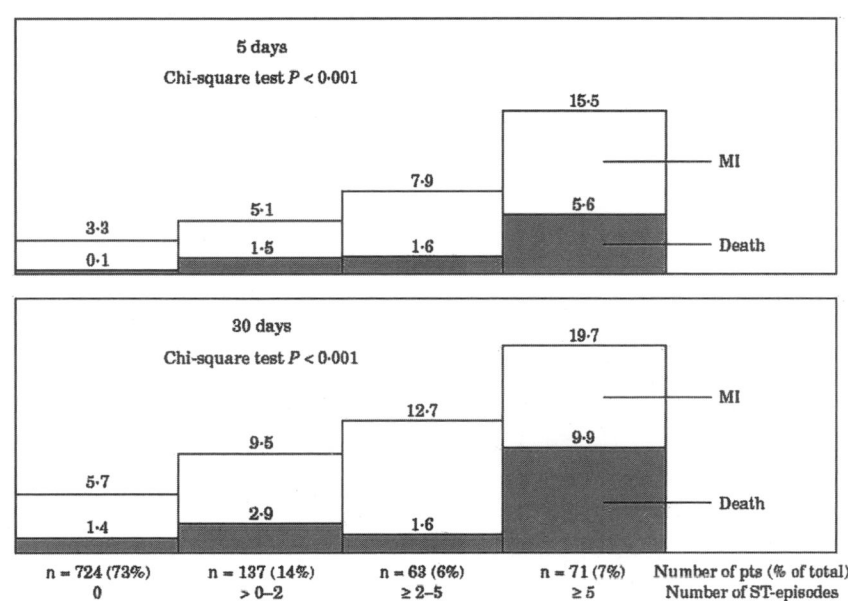

FIG. 86–3. Incidence rate (%) of death and composite of death and myocardial infarction (MI) at Days 5 and 30 in patients with a non–ST-elevation acute coronary syndrome classified according to the number of ischemic episodes per 24 hours as detected by continuous multilead electrocardiogram-ischemia monitoring. (From Akkerhuis et al., ref 14, with permission.)

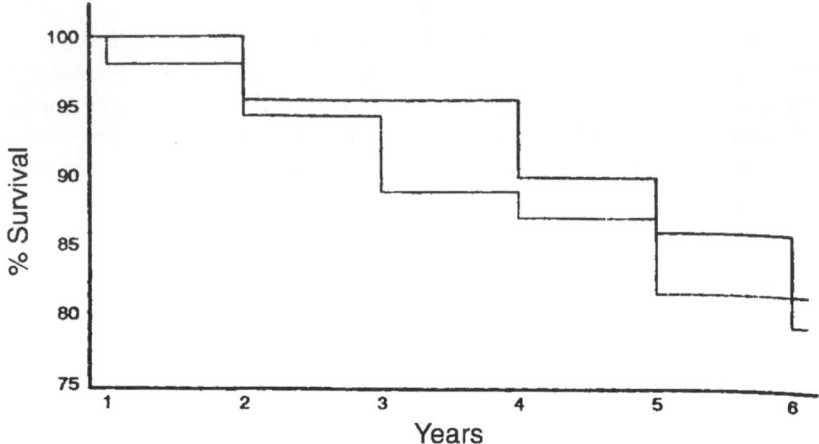

FIG. 86–4. Survival curves of patients with unstable angina who were followed for 6 years. No difference was found in survival at 6 years in patients with silent ischemia *(top line)* compared with patients with symptomatic ischemia *(bottom line)*. (From Romeo et al, ref. 35, with permission.)

ischemic time (silent and painful) versus that of silent ischemia only in 76 patients with UA who stabilized with medical treatment after hospital admission. Multivariate analysis showed that the presence of three-vessel disease was the most important predictor of cardiac mortality and morbidity in their patients. The second most important predictor was *total* ischemic time longer than 60 minutes. Silent ischemia was not found to be an independent predictor of long-term morbidity or mortality (Fig. 86–4). In Romeo's study (35), patients with UA and total ischemic time longer than 60 minutes frequently had silent ischemic episodes on Holter monitoring, a greater extent of coronary disease, and transient myocardial ischemia on the 12-lead ECG. It is not surprising that total ischemic time, and not just the absence of pain during ischemia, is a major determinant of long-term prognosis in patients with UA (Fig. 86–5). Romeo's findings are consistent with previous observations by other authors (17,36,37) and highlight the

fact that prognosis is determined by the duration and severity of myocardial ischemia rather than by chest pain.

DETECTION AND TREATMENT OF SILENT MYOCARDIAL ISCHEMIA

As discussed earlier, regardless of the presence or absence of chest pain, myocardial ischemia carries prognostic value (38). Thus, in our view, the question of whether silent ischemia per se, as opposed to total ischemic burden, is an independent predictor of outcome in patients with UA is probably irrelevant. Current knowledge appears to justify that cardiologists involved in managing patients with UA should aim at identifying and treating myocardial ischemia whatever its presentation may be. Interestingly, perhaps because it is assumed that it may provide redundant information and also because other powerful markers of risk such as cardiac troponins are avail-

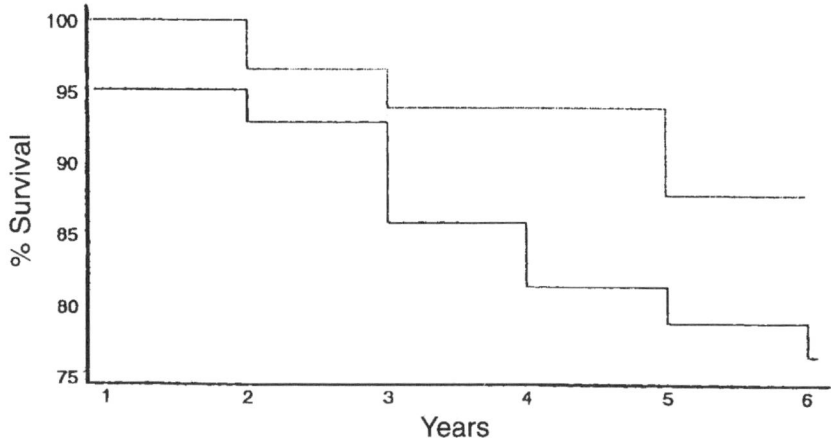

FIG. 86–5. Survival curves of patients with total ischemic time shorter than 60 minutes *(top line)* or 60 minutes or longer *(bottom line)*. Patients with a longer duration of myocardial ischemia during ambulatory electrocardiographic monitoring had a significantly worse prognosis. (From Romeo et al., ref. 35, with permission.)

able, current ACC/AHA guidelines (1,39) do not recommend continuous ECG monitoring for risk assessment in patients with ACS. ESC guidelines (40), however, recommend the routine use of continuous prolonged ECG monitoring.

Accurate tools are currently available for the detection of transient myocardial ischemia including classical continuous Holter monitoring with two, three, or more leads (16) and computer-assisted multilead ECG monitoring, which offers accurate, real-time measurements of QRS complexes and ST-segment shifts (14). Also, 24-hour VCG monitoring is available where ECG signals are collected from body surface electrodes applied to the chest and three orthogonal VCG leads −X, Y, and Z are computed and averaged. In clinical practice, however, these devices are rarely used in non–ST-segment elevation ACS as shown by Euro Heart Survey ACS (41), where 8% of the patients underwent Holter monitoring before hospital discharge. This is a surprising finding if one considers that the assessment of continuing myocardial ischemia, whether painful or silent, may help in risk stratification and provide a useful end point for the evaluation of antianginal therapy. The control of all forms of myocardial ischemia (silent and painful) is certainly a desirable and appropriate objective (42). Indeed, on the basis of the results of the different studies mentioned previously in this chapter, cardiologists should aim at treating myocardial ischemia in patients with UA irrespective of its clinical presentation, with the hope that prognosis would improve accordingly. However, despite the logical intuitive rationale behind this approach, there have been no large-scale trials documenting whether effective treatment of transient asymptomatic myocardial ischemia in UA results in reduction of cardiac mortality, serious coronary events, or both.

Reports from the Asymptomatic Cardiac Ischemia Pilot (ACIP) study have provided important information regarding the feasibility and the effects of suppressing asymptomatic ischemia in patients with chronic forms of coronary artery disease. The ACIP study (43) was designed to assess the feasibility of recruiting patients with documented coronary artery disease and transient myocardial ischemia on both exercise testing and ambulatory ECG monitoring. This information was considered to be of paramount importance for potential large-scale trials on the role of ischemia suppression for patient outcome. Another important goal of the ACIP study was to investigate the efficacy of different treatment strategies in suppressing transient myocardial ischemia during daily life in patients with coronary artery disease. Although the ACIP study enrolled patients with stable angina, some of its findings appear relevant to UA. For example, the prevalence of silent ischemia found in the ACIP study was similar to that reported in previously mentioned UA studies. Also, patients with silent ischemia in the ACIP study had multivessel disease and many additional risk factors that indicate that patients with frequent silent ischemia truly constitute a high-risk group.

Of importance, silent ischemia was frequent in ACIP patients and it was suppressed by treatment (44). Myocardial revascularization suppressed transient myocardial ischemia in more than 50% of patients, and medical treatment did likewise in more than 40% of patients; whereas angina-guided treatment was effective in suppressing ischemia in 39% of patients. Also important are the effects of treatment on patient outcome. Davies and coworkers (45) reported the 2-year follow up results in 558 patients with coronary anatomy suitable for revascularization. Angina-guided drug therapy (n = 183), angina plus ischemia–guided drug therapy (n = 183), and revascularization by angioplasty or bypass surgery (n = 192) were assessed. Two years after randomization, total mortality was 6.6% in the angina-guided strategy, 4.4% in the ischemia-guided strategy, and 1.1% in the revascularization strategy (p < 0.02). The rate of death or MI was 12% in the angina-guided strategy, 8.8% in the ischemia-guided strategy, and 4.7% in the revascularization strategy (p < 0.04) (Fig. 86–6). The rate of death, MI, or re-

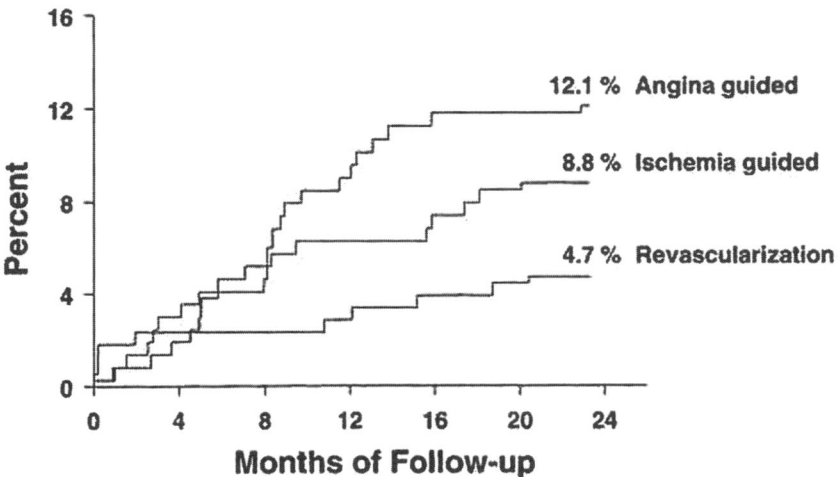

FIG. 86–6. Two-year cumulative rates of death and/or myocardial infarction. Revascularization strategy was significantly different from angina-guided strategy (p < 0.01). (From Davies et al, ref.45, with permission)

current cardiac hospitalization was 41.8% in the angina-guided strategy, 38.5% in the ischemia-guided strategy, and 23.1% in the revascularization strategy ($p < 0.001$). Pairwise testing revealed significant differences between the revascularization and angina-guided strategies for each comparison. When patients undergoing percutaneous transluminal coronary angiography and coronary artery bypass grafting were compared, differences were statistically significant only for death, MI, and hospitalization ($p = 0.005$). Regarding angiographic subgroups, the authors found that patients with proximal left anterior descending coronary artery stenoses and those with three-vessel disease had greater event rates and derived greater benefits from revascularization.

These findings in patients with stable angina pectoris are of practical clinical importance, but whether they can be extrapolated to UA is unknown. Health care cost implications in the detection and treatment of asymptomatic myocardial ischemia should not be ignored. Derived from the ACIP trial, Pepine and coworkers (46) found that although initially medical strategy was cheaper, it could reach or even exceed the costs associated with early revascularization after about 10 years. In view of these results, it seems prudent to recommend an invasive strategy to treat silent ischemia in patients with chronic stable angina. Early invasive approaches have been shown to be more effective than conservative treatment in high- (47) and medium-risk (48,49) patients with ACS.

FUTURE DIRECTIONS

Silent ischemia has prognostic significance in patients with UA. Detection of all forms of myocardial ischemia, including silent ischemia, is desirable and may help in patient risk stratification and management.

Solid data are required to establish whether the presence of silent ischemia offers additional prognostic value over previously increased levels of cardiac troponins and markers of inflammation (CRP), because this may have important clinical implications.

The ACIP trial findings regarding the prognostic role of silent ischemia in patients with stable angina pectoris are of practical importance. They agree with the results of recent studies regarding invasive management of UA/non-STEMI. However, whether these observations can be extrapolated to patients with UA is unknown. Large-scale clinical trials in patients with UA are necessary to prove or disprove whether an association exists between silent ischemia and cardiac mortality and whether silent ischemia has independent prognostic value. Health care cost implications in the detection and treatment of asymptomatic myocardial ischemia are extremely important. The ACIP trial results indicate that in the long term, it may be less costly to treat both symptomatic and asymptomatic ischemia invasively. Monitoring for silent ischemia is likely to be important in patients with normal troponins because the presence of silent ischemia might help to identify a relatively high-risk sub-group of patients who may benefit from an invasive management strategy.

SUMMARY

Evidence has accumulated that continuing transient myocardial ischemia, whether silent or symptomatic, is a marker for poor outcome in patients with UA. Persistence of myocardial ischemia appears to be associated with multivessel disease and may be related to the presence of complex active coronary artery stenoses. Biochemical markers of myocardial injury, such as cardiac troponins, are increased in patients with UA and silent ischemia. Whether silent ischemia provides independent prognostic information over that provided by biochemical markers is unknown.

Despite the availability of useful clinical, angiographic, and biochemical markers of risk, it seems justifiable to evaluate whether treatment of myocardial ischemia (painful or silent) in patients with UA is cost-effective. The question of whether a strategy aimed at suppressing total ischemic burden will reduce cardiac death and rate of MI has been clearly answered for patients with stable angina patients but remains to be investigated in patients with UA.

REFERENCES

1. Braunwald E, Antman EM, Beasley JW, et al. ACC/AHA guidelines for the management of patients with unstable angina and non-ST-segment elevation myocardial infarction. A report of the American College of Cardiology/American Heart Association Task Force on Practice Guidelines (Committee on the Management of Patients With Unstable Angina). *Circulation* 2000;102:1193–1209.
2. Myocardial infarction redefined—a consensus document of The Joint European Society of Cardiology/American College of Cardiology Committee for the redefinition of myocardial infarction. *Eur Heart J* 2000;21:1502–1513.
3. Theroux P, Fuster V. Acute coronary syndromes: unstable angina and non-Q-wave myocardial infarction. *Circulation* 1998;97:1195–1206.
4. Chesebro JH, Fuster V. Thrombosis in unstable angina. *N Engl J Med* 1992;327:192–194.
5. Chierchia S, Brunelli C, Simonetti I, et al. Sequence of events in angina at rest: primary reduction in coronary flow. *Circulation* 1980;61:759–768.
6. Hamm CW, Braunwald E. A classification of unstable angina revisited. *Circulation* 2000;102:118–122.
7. Conti CR. Pathophysiology and management of unstable angina. *Clin Cardiol* 1989;12:616–617.
8. Braunwald E. Unstable angina. A classification. *Circulation* 1989; 80:410–414.
9. Deedwania PC, Carbajal EV. Silent myocardial ischemia. A clinical perspective. *Arch Intern Med* 1991;151:2373–2382.
10. Cohn PF. The value of continuous ST segment monitoring in patients with unstable angina. *Eur Heart J* 2001;22:1972–1973.
11. de Bruyne MC, Mosterd A, Hoes AW, et al. Prevalence, determinants, and misclassification of myocardial infarction in the elderly. *Epidemiology* 1997;8:495–500.
12. Bertolet BD, Dinerman J, Hartke R Jr, et al. Unstable angina: relationship of clinical presentation, coronary artery pathology, and clinical outcome. *Clin Cardiol* 1993;16:116–122.
13. Patel DJ, Gomma AH, Knight CJ, et al. Why is recurrent myocardial ischaemia a predictor of adverse outcome in unstable angina? An observational study of myocardial ischaemia and its relation to coronary anatomy. *Eur Heart J* 2001;22:1991–1996.
14. Akkerhuis KM, Klootwijk PA, Lindeboom W, et al. Recurrent ischaemia during continuous multilead ST-segment monitoring identifies patients with acute coronary syndromes at high risk of adverse cardiac

events; meta-analysis of three studies involving 995 patients. *Eur Heart J* 2001;22:1997–2006.

15. Hamm CW, Ravkilde J, Gerhardt W, et al. The prognostic value of serum troponin T in unstable angina. *N Engl J Med* 1992;327:146–150.

16. Gottlieb SO, Weisfeldt ML, Ouyang P, et al. Silent ischemia as a marker for early unfavorable outcomes in patients with unstable angina. *N Engl J Med* 1986;314:1214–1219.

17. von Arnim T, Gerbig HW, Krawietz W, et al. Prognostic implications of transient—predominantly silent—ischaemia in patients with unstable angina pectoris. *Eur Heart J* 1988;9:435–440.

18. Mazzone A, Cusa C, Mazzucchelli I, et al. Increased production of inflammatory cytokines in patients with silent myocardial ischemia. *J Am Coll Cardiol* 2001;38:1895–1901.

19. Moise A, Theroux P, Taeymans Y, et al. Unstable angina and progression of coronary atherosclerosis. *N Engl J Med* 1983;309:685–689.

20. Nademanee K, Intarachot V, Josephson MA, et al. Prognostic significance of silent myocardial ischemia in patients with unstable angina. *J Am Coll Cardiol* 1987;10:1–9.

21. Bugiardini R, Pozzati A, Borghi A, et al. Angiographic morphology in unstable angina and its relation to transient myocardial ischemia and hospital outcome. *Am J Cardiol* 1991;67:460–464.

22. Chen L, Chester MR, Redwood S, et al. Angiographic stenosis progression and coronary events in patients with 'stabilized' unstable angina. *Circulation* 1995;91:2319–2324.

23. Kaski JC, Chester MR, Chen L, et al. Rapid angiographic progression of coronary artery disease in patients with angina pectoris. The role of complex stenosis morphology. *Circulation* 1995;92:2058–2065.

24. Huang J, Sopher SM, Leatham E, et al. Heart rate variability depression in patients with unstable angina. *Am Heart J* 1995;130:772–779.

25. Lanza GA, Pedrotti P, Rebuzzi AG, et al. Usefulness of the addition of heart rate variability to Holter monitoring in predicting in-hospital cardiac events in patients with unstable angina pectoris. *Am J Cardiol* 1997;80:263–267.

26. Botker HE, Ravkilde J, Sogaard P, et al. Gradation of unstable angina based on a sensitive immunoassay for serum creatine kinase MB. *Br Heart J* 1991;65:72–76.

27. Hamm CW, Ravkilde J, Gerhardt W, et al. The prognostic value of serum troponin T in unstable angina. *N Engl J Med* 1992;327:146–150.

28. Norgaard BL, Andersen K, Dellborg M, et al. Admission risk assessment by cardiac troponin T in unstable coronary artery disease: additional prognostic information from continuous ST segment monitoring. TRIM study group. Thrombin Inhibition in Myocardial Ischemia. *J Am Coll Cardiol* 1999;33:1519–1527.

29. Chen L, Chester MR, Redwood S, et al. Angiographic stenosis progression and coronary events in patients with 'stabilized' unstable angina. *Circulation* 1995;91:2319–2324.

30. Kaski JC, Chester MR, Chen L, et al. Rapid angiographic progression of coronary artery disease in patients with angina pectoris. The role of complex stenosis morphology. *Circulation* 1995;92:2058–2065.

31. Johnson SM, Mauritson DR, Winniford MD, et al. Continuous electrocardiographic monitoring in patients with unstable angina pectoris: identification of high-risk subgroup with severe coronary disease, variant angina, and/or impaired early prognosis. *Am Heart J* 1982;103:4–12.

32. Gottlieb SO, Weisfeldt ML, Ouyang P, et al. Silent ischemia predicts infarction and death during 2 year follow-up of unstable angina. *J Am Coll Cardiol* 1987;10:756–760.

33. Aguiar C, Ferreira J, Seabra-Gomes R. Prognostic value of continuous ST-segment monitoring in patients with non-ST-segment elevation acute coronary syndromes. *Ann Noninvasive Electrocardiol* 2002;7:29–39.

34. Rebuzzi AG, Quaranta G, Liuzzo G, et al. Incremental prognostic value of serum levels of troponin T and C-reactive protein on admission in patients with unstable angina pectoris. *Am J Cardiol* 1998;82:715–719.

35. Romeo F, Rosano GM, Martuscelli E, et al. Unstable angina: role of silent ischemia and total ischemic time (silent plus painful ischemia), a 6-year follow-up. *J Am Coll Cardiol* 1992;19:1173–1179.

36. Johnson SM, Mauritson DR, Winniford MD, et al. Continuous electrocardiographic monitoring in patients with unstable angina pectoris: Identification of high-risk subgroup with severe coronary disease, variant angina, and/or impaired early prognosis. *Am Heart J* 1982;103:4–12.

37. Bugiardini R, Borghi A, Pozzati A, et al. Relation of severity of symptoms to transient myocardial ischemia and prognosis in unstable angina. *J Am Coll Cardiol* 1995;25:597–604.

38. Chatterjee K. Ischemia—silent or manifest: does it matter? *J Am Coll Cardiol* 1989;13:1503–1505.

39. Braunwald E, Antman EM, Beasley JW, et al. ACC/AHA Guideline Update for the Management of Patients With Unstable Angina and Non-ST-Segment Elevation Myocardial Infarction-2002: summary article: a Report of the American College of Cardiology/American Heart Association Task Force on Practice Guidelines (Committee on the Management of Patients With Unstable Angina). *Circulation* 2002;106:1893–1900.

40. Bertrand ME, Simoons ML, Fox KA, et al. Management of acute coronary syndromes: acute coronary syndromes without persistent ST segment elevation; recommendations of the Task Force of the European Society of Cardiology. *Eur Heart J* 2000;21:1406–1432.

41. Hasdai D, Behar S, Wallentin L, et al. A prospective survey of the characteristics, treatments and outcomes of patients with acute coronary syndromes in Europe and the Mediterranean basin; the Euro Heart Survey of Acute Coronary Syndromes (Euro Heart Survey ACS). *Eur Heart J* 2002;23:1190–1201.

42. Deedwania PC. Is there evidence in support of the ischemia suppression hypothesis? *J Am Coll Cardiol* 1994;24:21–24.

43. Pepine CJ, Geller NL, Knatterud GL, et al. The Asymptomatic Cardiac Ischemia Pilot (ACIP) study: design of a randomized clinical trial, baseline data and implications for a long-term outcome trial. *J Am Coll Cardiol* 1994;24:1–10.

44. Knatterud GL, Bourassa MG, Pepine CJ, et al. Effects of treatment strategies to suppress ischemia in patients with coronary artery disease: 12-week results of the Asymptomatic Cardiac Ischemia Pilot (ACIP) study. *J Am Coll Cardiol* 1994;24:11–20.

45. Davies RF, Goldberg AD, Forman S, et al. Asymptomatic Cardiac Ischemia Pilot (ACIP) study two-year follow-up: outcomes of patients randomized to initial strategies of medical therapy versus revascularization. *Circulation* 1997;95:2037–2043.

46. Pepine CJ, Mark DB, Bourassa MG, et al. Cost estimates for treatment of cardiac ischemia (from the Asymptomatic Cardiac Ischemia Pilot [ACIP] study). *Am J Cardiol* 1999;84:1311–1316.

47. Invasive compared with non-invasive treatment in unstable coronary-artery disease: FRISC II prospective randomised multicentre study. FRagmin and Fast Revascularisation during InStability in Coronary artery disease Investigators. *Lancet* 1999;354:708–715.

48. Fox KA, Poole-Wilson PA, Henderson RA, et al. Interventional versus conservative treatment for patients with unstable angina or non-ST-elevation myocardial infarction: the British Heart Foundation RITA 3 randomised trial. Randomized Intervention Trial of unstable Angina. *Lancet* 2002;360:743–751.

49. Cannon CP, Weintraub WS, Demopoulos LA, et al. Comparison of early invasive and conservative strategies in patients with unstable coronary syndromes treated with the glycoprotein IIb/IIIa inhibitor tirofiban. *N Engl J Med* 2001;344:1879–1887.

PART V

Chronic Stable Angina

CHAPTER 87

Pathophysiology of Chronic Stable Angina

Nilesh J. Goswami and Robert A. O'Rourke

Key Words: Coronary autoregulation; effective downstream coronary pressure; myocardial oxygen demand (consumption); myocardial oxygen supply.

INTRODUCTION

William Heberden (1) is credited with the first description of stable angina pectoris in 1772. He described symptoms reproducibly provoked by exertion or meals and relieved by rest as "a painful and most disagreeable sensation in the breast, which seems as if it would extinguish life, if it were to increase or continue."

In the nineteenth century, it became apparent that angina pectoris is associated with obstruction and sometimes with calcification of the coronary arteries (2). However, the pathophysiologic mechanism of anginal pain remained unclear until well into the twentieth century, when the concept that angi-

N. J. Goswami: Department of Internal Medicine, Southern Illinois University School of Medicine, and Coronary Care Unit, Prairie Cardiovascular Consultants, Ltd., Prairie Heart Institute, 619 East Mason Avenue, Springfield, Illinois 62794.

R. A. O'Rourke: Division of Cardiology, University of Texas Health Science Center, 7703 Floyd Curl Drive, San Antonio, Texas 78229.

nal pain resulted from an imbalance of myocardial oxygen supply and demand was identified as the usual feature (3).

This chapter presents the pathophysiologic basis for chest pain in chronic stable angina pectoris. Angina pectoris is the cardinal symptom of myocardial ischemia, which may be defined as a state of tissue perfusion that provides insufficient oxygen delivery to meet metabolic requirements. Accordingly, the chapter discusses the principal determinants of myocardial oxygen supply and demand, the pathophysiologic mechanisms by which the former may be limited and/or the latter augmented, and, finally, the specific mechanisms that apply to the pathophysiology of angina in common clinical conditions (4).

DETERMINANTS OF MYOCARDIAL OXYGEN SUPPLY AND DEMAND

The myocardium has a high metabolic rate that is subject to large and rapid fluctuations, such as during vigorous exercise. Because the myocardium is almost entirely dependent on aerobic metabolism for the synthesis of adenosine triphosphate (ATP), the coronary circulation must adapt to deliver oxygen to the myocardium at widely and rapidly changing rates.

Determinants of Myocardial Oxygen Supply

Myocardial oxygen *delivery* is the product of the coronary flow rate and the coronary arterial oxygen content. Myocardial oxygen *consumption* (MVO_2) is equal to the fraction of delivered oxygen that is extracted across the coronary circulation. The oxygen *supply* to the myocardium is equal to the product of coronary oxygen delivery and maximal myocardial oxygen extraction. Normal values for myocardial blood flow (MBF) and MVO_2 are shown in Table 87–1. Under resting conditions, MBF to left ventricular (LV) myocardium is approximately 0.8 mL per gram^{-1} per minute^{-1} (4). With maximal coronary vasodilation, MBF can increase by five-fold to sixfold. This is the predominant mechanism by which MVO_2 can increase above baseline levels. In contrast, the capacity to increase oxygen extraction above resting levels is quite limited. Approximately 75% of the coronary arterial oxygen content is extracted under resting conditions. During exercise, adrenergic stimulation, or ischemia, *trans*coronary oxygen extraction can increase to approximately 90% (5,6). With maximal exercise, MVO_2 of a healthy subject increases to approximately five times baseline, mainly by increased MBF and less so by increased oxygen extraction.

Determinants of Myocardial Oxygen Demand

The principal determinants of myocardial oxygen demand (or consumption) are mechanical factors—ventricular wall stress, inotropic state, and heart rate. In addition, approximately 25% of resting MVO_2 can be attributed to nonmechanical factors—basal myocardial metabolism and ion pumps (11,12).

The law of Laplace is frequently invoked to explain the determinants of ventricular wall stress or wall tension. This law states that wall tension in a thin-walled shell of well defined shape is directly related to intracavitary pressure and to chamber dimension. Although the mathematic relations applicable to a thick-walled chamber of irregular shape (such as the LV) are more complex (13), the key implication of the law of Laplace still applies to the heart *in vivo*: Generation of a given stroke volume at a given ejection pressure and contractile state requires greater MVO_2 when the end-diastolic volume is increased, because of increased systolic wall stress.

Increased heart rate augments MVO_2 not only by an increase in the number of contractions per unit time, but through the positive staircase, or treppe, effect whereby myocardial contractility increases with the frequency of stimulation (14).

Myocardial contractility is the third principal mechanical determinant of MVO_2. Although quantitative assessment of contractility in the intact heart is difficult, if not elusive, it is clear that qualitative increases in contractility, such as those produced by β-adrenergic agonists or cardiac glycosides (15), are accompanied by increases in MVO_2, even when heart rate and systolic blood pressure are held constant.

Another factor influencing MVO_2 at a given level of mechanical performance is the carbon substrate preference for oxidative metabolism. The principal carbon substrates for myocardial energy metabolism are carbohydrates (e.g., glucose and glycogen), free fatty acids, and lactate. Metabolism of glucose yields ATP from glycolysis and oxidative phosphorylation. Metabolism of lactate or free fatty acids does not yield glycolytic ATP. Accordingly, the molar ratio of ATP synthesized per O_2 consumed is 5.7 for oxidation of palmitate, 6.0 for oxidation of lactate, and 6.3 for oxidation of glucose (16). Alterations in substrate metabolism may play a role in the pathogenesis of angina in diabetes. The rate of myocardial free fatty acid metabolism increases with circulating free fatty acid concentration (17), which is increased in diabetes. Simultaneously, myocardial glucose oxidation is impaired in diabetic hearts (18,19). Enhanced free fatty acid metabolism together with depressed glucose utilization in diabetes may diminish energetic efficiency by increasing MVO_2 for a given rate of ATP synthesis, potentially exacerbating angina in the presence of coronary artery disease.

PATHOPHYSIOLOGIC MECHANISMS OF STABLE ANGINA

Angina Caused by Diminished Myocardial Oxygen Supply

Myocardial oxygen supply may be limited by abnormalities of coronary perfusion pressure, diastolic perfusion time, coronary resistance, blood oxygen content or oxygen exchange, or blood rheology.

TABLE 87–1. *Coronary blood flow and oxygen consumption in the normal heart*

	Rest	Maximum achievable level (condition)
LV blood flow (mL/g · min^{-1})	8–1.0	6.0 (pharmacologic vasodilatation)
LV coronary arteriovenous O_2 extraction (%)	75	90 (ischemia)
LV O_2 consumption (mL/100 g · min^{-1})	8–10	50 (peak exercise)
RV blood flow (mL/g · min^{-1})	0.5–0.7	6.0 (pharmacologic vasodilatation)
RV O_2 consumption (mL/100 g · min^{-1})	5–7	— (undetermined)

Data from References 4 through 10.
LV, left ventricular; RV, right ventricular.

Abnormalities of Coronary Perfusion Pressure

The normal coronary circulation exhibits *autoregulation,* defined as the maintenance of nearly constant perfusion over a range of perfusion pressure when myocardial oxygen demand is held constant (20). In the normal canine LV, the autoregulatory range extends from a mean aortic pressure of approximately 60 mm Hg to approximately 140 mm Hg (Fig. 87–1). Myocardial ischemia may be provoked or exacerbated if coronary perfusion pressure decreases below the autoregulatory range. When perfusion pressure distal to an epicardial coronary stenosis is reduced by the pressure gradient across the stenosis, a portion of the normal autoregulatory capacity is required to maintain perfusion. Further decreases in distal coronary pressure (caused by decreased aortic blood pressure or increased flow and pressure reduction across the epicardial stenosis) have the potential to exhaust autoregulation, resulting in inadequate myocardial perfusion and consequent symptoms of angina.

Perfusion of LV myocardium occurs almost exclusively during diastole. Therefore, myocardial ischemia and angina pectoris are more likely to develop when diastolic aortic pressure declines than when systolic pressure decreases. Of course, changes in diastolic and systolic aortic pressure often occur in parallel. However, conditions that particularly predispose to decreased aortic diastolic pressure, including fever, arteriovenous fistula, and chronic aortic regurgitation, are more likely to compromise myocardial perfusion by this mechanism.

Both upstream (driving) pressure and downstream pressure determine flow through any conduit. In most vascular beds, the downstream pressure is equal to the venous pressure. However, in the coronary circulation, the *effective downstream pressure* is greater than the coronary sinus pressure (by at least 10–15 mm Hg). The effective downstream pressure increases from subepicardium to subendocardium, with increasing coronary vasomotor tone and with increasing LV diastolic pressure. This unusual characteristic of the coronary circulation was determined by studying long diastoles of the canine heart *in situ* (20,21) (Fig. 87–2). Forward coronary flow ceased when the upstream pressure decreased below a critical value, designated $P_{F=0}$, for zero-flow pressure. The dependence of the effective downstream coronary pressure on LV diastolic pressure has potentially important clinical implications: Conditions causing increased LV dias-

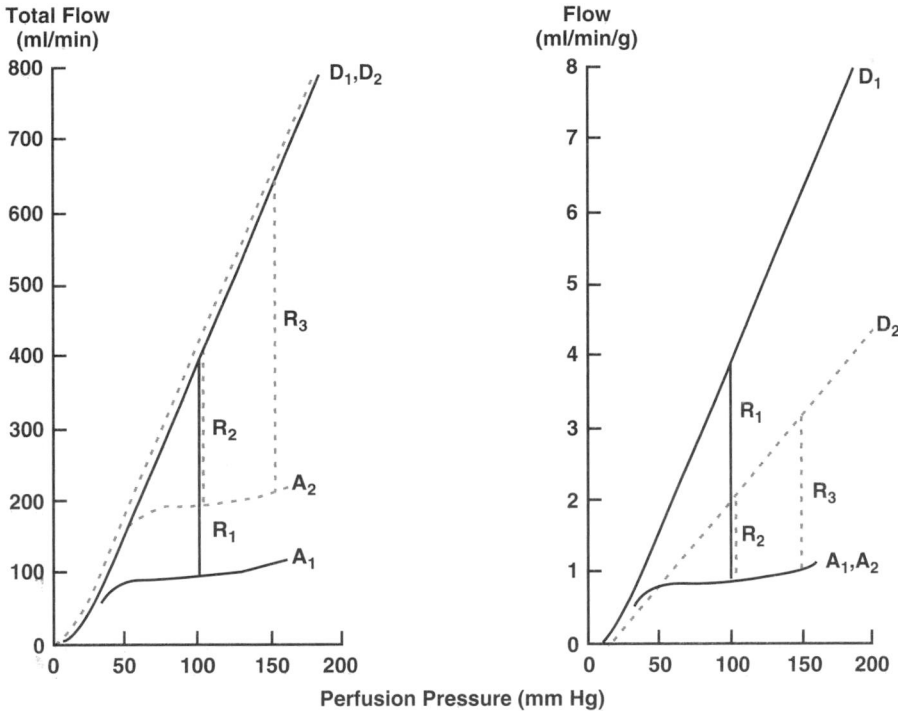

FIG. 87–1. Autoregulation of the coronary circulation. **Left:** Total flow in an epicardial coronary artery. **Right:** Coronary flow per gram of myocardium. Autoregulation maintains nearly constant flow over the physiologic range of perfusion pressure in a healthy heart *(A₁)* and a heart with left ventricular hypertrophy *(A₂)*. During maximal pharmacologic coronary vasodilation, coronary flow per gram is lower in the hypertrophied heart than in the healthy heart (**right;** *D₂* vs. *D₁*). Consequently, coronary reserve (the difference between autoregulated and maximal flows at a given perfusion pressure) is diminished in the hypertrophied heart *(R₂* vs. *R₁)*. However, coronary reserve is augmented at a greater perfusion pressure *(R₃)*. (From Hoffman JIE. A critical view of coronary reserve. *Circulation* 1987;75[Suppl I]:I6–I11, with permission.)

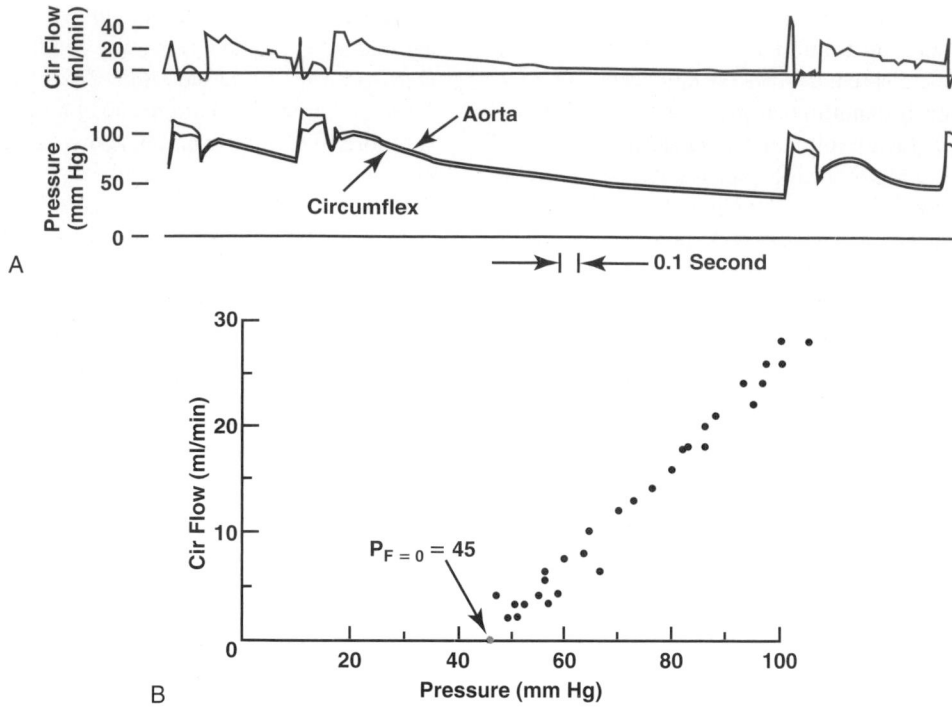

FIG. 87–2. Coronary pressure–flow relations during a single diastole in the conscious dog. Note that by the end of a long diastole, coronary flow has decreased to zero, whereas epicardial coronary artery pressure remains substantially greater than zero **(top).** A plot of instantaneous flow versus pressure indicates a zero-flow pressure of approximately 45 mm Hg **(bottom).** (From Bellamy RF. Diastolic coronary artery pressure-flow relations in the dog. *Circ Res* 1978;43:92–101, with permission.)

tolic volume (e.g., congestive heart failure, aortic or mitral regurgitation) or reduced diastolic compliance (e.g., ischemia, hypertrophy, and aging), or both, may impair coronary perfusion by increasing the effective downstream coronary pressure.

Delayed LV relaxation may also compromise diastolic coronary perfusion and increase the propensity for myocardial ischemia and angina pectoris. The normal isovolumic relaxation time is 10% or less of the cardiac cycle length. However, in conditions such as ischemia, pressure overload hypertrophy, and heart failure, myocardial relaxation may be substantially prolonged (22). Consequently, the effective downstream coronary pressure may remain abnormally high in early diastole, and the pressure gradient for forward coronary flow may be reduced.

Abnormalities of Diastolic Perfusion Time

Coronary perfusion depends not only on upstream and downstream diastolic pressures, but also on the duration of diastole. Tachycardia always results in a relatively greater reduction in the length of diastole compared with systole. Normally, a reduction in diastolic time would be compensated by coronary vasodilation. However, once coronary reserve is exhausted, further decrements in diastolic time have the potential to produce ischemia and angina pectoris (23). Once tachycardia has provoked ischemia, the resultant pro-

longation of LV relaxation may further impede coronary perfusion and exacerbate ischemia. Diastolic perfusion time may also be compromised by delayed relaxation caused by ventricular asynergy in patients with coronary artery disease and previous myocardial infarction (MI) or conduction abnormalities (24).

Abnormalities of Coronary Resistance

In the normal coronary circulation, the pressure decline across the epicardial coronary vessels is only a few millimeters of mercury at low flow rates, but may increase to 10 to 20 mm Hg at peak flow rates (25). However, the principal site of vascular resistance is in coronary arterioles measuring 10 to 150 μm in diameter (4). This resistance is dynamic, responding to changes in perfusion pressure (autoregulation) and myocardial oxygen demand (metabolic vasoregulation). In addition, endothelial-derived relaxing and contracting factors modulate diameter and resistance in both epicardial coronary arteries and small coronary arterioles (26).

Increased coronary resistance may contribute to angina pectoris by stenosis of epicardial coronary arteries, abnormalities of the coronary microvasculature, or abnormalities of coronary endothelial function. The pressure decline across an epicardial coronary stenosis is a function of lesion geometry and flow rate, and involves energy dissipation caused by viscous effects, flow separation in eddies near the vessel wall distal to the stenosis, and turbulence (27). The *trans*stenotic pressure gradient increases as the stenosis diameter decreases or as stenosis length increases; however, there is much stronger dependence on stenosis diameter compared with stenosis length (fourth-order vs. first-order relation). The pressure decrease across a stenosis also varies with stenosis flow. Viscous losses vary linearly with flow rate, whereas losses caused by flow separation depend on the square of the flow. The mechanisms of pressure decline across a stenosis are illustrated in Figure 87–3.

Initially, the pressure decline across an epicardial coronary stenosis is compensated by autoregulation caused by dilation of small resistance vessels. With increasing stenosis severity, increasing flow across the stenosis, and/or decreasing upstream (aortic) blood pressure, the vasodilatory capacity of coronary resistance vessels is outstripped, most readily in the subendocardium, resulting in ischemia and possible angina.

Abnormalities of the coronary microvasculature can occur primarily (as in "syndrome X") or as the result of diseases such as diabetes, vasculitis, or systemic sclerosis. The pathophysiology of these conditions is discussed in more detail elsewhere in Chapters 19, 42, and 47.

Some conditions that cause left ventricular hypertrophy (LVH) (e.g., hypertension and aortic stenosis), but not others (e.g., the athletic heart), are accompanied by an increased propensity for angina pectoris, due in part to abnormal coronary microvascular resistance. Secondary hypertrophy caused by abnormal LV afterload is not matched by a proportional increase in capillary density (28), so that the minimal coronary resistance (during maximal coronary vasodilation) is increased, especially in the subendocardium. In addition, conditions that cause hypertrophy frequently also diminish LV compliance, resulting in greater LV diastolic pressure and increased effective downstream coronary pressure. Consequently, the lower limit of the autoregulatory pressure range is greater in LVH (29). Thus, an epicardial coronary stenosis too mild to compromise perfusion in the nonhypertrophied LV may cause a sufficient transstenotic pressure decrease in the presence of hypertrophy to exhaust autoregulation and provoke ischemia and angina. Even in the absence of any epicardial stenosis, increases in MVO_2 caused by increased LV systolic pressure, diminished capillary density, and increased LV diastolic pressure may produce myocardial ischemia and angina during moderate exercise, tachycardia, and/or sympathetic stimulation in the presence of LVH.

Pathologic increases in coronary resistance in coronary artery disease may also result from abnormal coronary endothelial function. Under normal conditions, numerous circulating and locally produced substances, including acetylcholine, noradrenaline, serotonin, bradykinin, histamine, thrombin, ATP, and adenosine diphosphate, promote vasodilation and increased blood flow that is dependent on the presence of an intact endothelium. A primary increase in blood flow stimulated by endothelium-dependent vasodilation of resistance vessels may be potentiated and prolonged by flow-mediated vasodilation of larger vessels, whereby nitric oxide is released from endothelial cells in response to increased flow-related shear forces on the vessel wall (25). With experimental denudation of endothelium, or with the development of atherothrombosis *in vivo*, the vasomotor response to endothelium-dependent vasodilators or increased blood flow may be blunted or there may even be paradoxic vasoconstriction (30).

Hypercholesterolemia is a frequent contributor to and concomitant of coronary atherothrombosis and is an independent factor leading to abnormal endothelial function and coronary resistance. Endothelium-dependent coronary vasodilation in response to acetylcholine injection is diminished in hypercholesterolemic monkeys (31) and in humans (32,33) even in the absence of atherothrombotic lesions. Endothelial function in humans may be improved by the pharmacologic reduction of serum cholesterol levels (34,35).

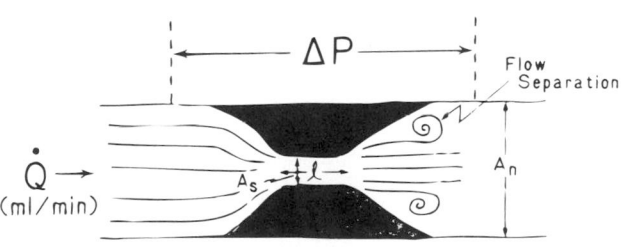

$$\Delta P = \underbrace{f_1\left(\sfrac{1}{A_s^2}, \ell, \dot{Q}\right)}_{\text{VISCOUS}} + \underbrace{f_2\left(\sfrac{1}{A_s^2}, \sfrac{1}{A_n^2}, \dot{Q}^2\right)}_{\text{SEPARATION}}$$

FIG. 87–3. Factors determining the pressure decrease across a coronary stenosis. Viscous (resistive) losses are inversely related to the square of stenosis cross-sectional area (A_s) and directly related to stenosis length *(l)* and flow rate *($\dot{Q}$)*. Flow separation from the downstream vessel wall causes additional losses inversely related to both A_s^2 and the square of the normal vessel cross-sectional area (A_n^2) and directly related to $\dot{Q}^2$. In addition, turbulent flow across the lesion may be responsible for additional pressure decline. (From Klocke FJ. Measurements of coronary blood flow and degree of stenosis: current clinical implications and continuing uncertainties. *J Am Coll Cardiol* 1983;1:31–41, with permission.)

Abnormalities of Blood Oxygen Content

It is a frequent clinical observation that the development of anemia may provoke or exacerbate angina pectoris in patients with coronary artery disease. There is both a reduction in the oxygen-carrying capacity of the blood and an increase in MVO_2 because of increased cardiac output, sympathetic nervous system activity, or both. In this setting, transfusion or stimulation of hematopoiesis may be effective antianginal therapy. Physicians sometimes set an arbitrary therapeutic goal such as a hematocrit of greater than 30% in patients with coronary artery disease. However, because the oxygen-carrying capacity of the blood continues to increase in proportion to hematocrit above this level, the target hematocrit should be individualized based on severity of symptoms versus cost and risk for blood transfusion or hematopoietic therapy.

Abnormalities of Blood Rheology

Angina pectoris, as well as symptoms of peripheral arterial insufficiency, can occur in diseases associated with hyperviscosity (e.g., polycythemia vera), especially when the hematocrit approaches 70%. Angina also occurs frequently in hemoglobinopathies with abnormal red blood cell deformation (e.g., sickle cell anemia).

Angina Caused by Increased Myocardial Oxygen Demand

The role of the MVO_2 in the pathophysiology of angina pectoris is discussed here briefly.

Increased Wall Stress

An increase in systolic pressure, ventricular chamber size, or both will augment wall stress and MVO_2. Increases in systolic pressure occur in the obvious settings of hypertension and obstruction to ventricular outflow caused by discrete subvalvular, valvular, or supravalvular aortic stenosis, hypertrophic cardiomyopathy, or coarctation of the aorta. In addition, systolic pressure frequently increases with advancing age because of diminished compliance of the arterial system. Even when arterial compliance is normal, conditions leading to an increase in stroke volume will augment peak systolic pressure. These include arteriovenous shunts, aortic regurgitation, anemia, and bradycardia. LV chamber size is increased in chronic volume overload states because of aortic or mitral regurgitation, dilated cardiomyopathies, and as a consequence of MI.

Tachycardia

Tachycardia may precipitate or exacerbate angina, either in the setting of a primary arrhythmia or as a secondary effect of exercise, sympathomimetic drugs, fever, pain, emotional excitement, hypoxemia, thyrotoxicosis, anemia, or heart failure. In addition to its direct effects on MVO_2, tachycardia limits diastolic perfusion time (discussed earlier).

Inotropic State

Provocation of angina caused by increased inotropic state most often occurs in the setting of underlying coronary artery disease, with superimposed effects of sympathomimetic drugs or the sympathomimetic effects of the same stimuli responsible for tachycardia. However, some of the increase in MVO_2 caused by inotropic stimulation may be counterbalanced by enhanced chemomechanical efficiency, manifest by a greater ratio of mechanical energy imparted to the blood/MVO_2 (36).

MECHANISMS OF ANGINA IN VARIOUS CLINICAL SETTINGS

In many clinical conditions, angina results from several concomitant pathophysiologic mechanisms that may cause diminished myocardial oxygen supply, increased MVO_2, or both.

Stable Coronary Artery Disease

Epicardial coronary stenoses cause a decrease in downstream coronary artery pressure that limits the potential for further autoregulation of resistance vessels. Myocardial ischemia may be accompanied by reduced LV compliance and delayed and/or asynergic LV relaxation, resulting in increased LV diastolic pressure, a greater effective downstream pressure ($P_{F=0}$) in the coronary circulation, and a shortened diastolic perfusion period. Systolic dysfunction caused by ischemic cardiomyopathy, prior MI, or both may result in a dilated ventricular cavity, thereby increasing wall stress. Hypercholesterolemia and hypertension not only contribute to the development of coronary artery disease, but may independently exacerbate angina in established coronary disease. Hypercholesterolemia impairs endothelial vasodilator function in both angiographically normal and abnormal vascular segments. Hypertension increases LV wall stress, and the secondary development of LVH may limit the minimum achievable coronary resistance, and hence maximum achievable coronary flow.

The susceptibility to myocardial ischemia in coronary artery disease is greatest in the subendocardial region of the LV. This is due in part to greater wall tension and MVO_2 in this region (37). In addition, there is evidence for systolic retrograde coronary blood from subendocardium to subepicardium, simultaneously protecting the subepicardium from ischemia, but also resulting in more compressed vessels in the subendocardium and greater subendocardial resistance to flow at the beginning of the next diastole (38).

The presence of a well developed coronary collateral circulation may mitigate myocardial ischemia and angina pectoris in stable coronary artery disease. Robust coronary collateral flow can attenuate exercise-induced ischemic myocardial dysfunction in the territory of stenotic coronary arteries (39). The adequacy of the coronary collateral circulation varies widely among patients with coronary artery disease of similar severity. However, the perfusion pressure distal to a fully occluded epicardial vessel is less than normal even when robust collateral blood flow is present. Therefore, the coronary collateral circulation often is sufficient to maintain myocardial viability and to prevent resting angina, but not to prevent the development of ischemia and angina with moderate increases in myocardial oxygen demand (40).

Reproducible anginal symptoms may occur with exercise, emotional excitement, or other forms of sympathetic stimulation, postprandially, or nocturnally. In each of these circumstances, several of the above-described mechanisms may be operative. Exercise increases MVO_2 in the healthy heart through increased heart rate and sympathetically mediated increased contractility. In patients with coronary artery disease, the exercise-induced increase in MVO_2 may be amplified by increases in LV end-diastolic volume resulting in increased wall stress. Simultaneously, myocardial oxygen supply may be compromised during exercise in coronary artery disease by an increased transstenotic coronary pressure decrease caused by increased MBF and abnormally increased LV diastolic pressure. In addition, increased sympathetic nervous activity and circulating catecholamines may have paradoxic vasoconstrictive effects in regions with abnormal coronary endothelial function (30). Postprandial angina is most likely related to augmentation of cardiac output by as much as 20%, with resultant increased myocardial oxygen demand (41). Nocturnal angina is thought to be provoked by extravascular-to-intravascular volume shifts, resulting in greater LV end-diastolic volume and wall stress. Circadian alterations in coronary vasomotion may play a role in some cases as well (42). The morning increase in sympathetic activity results in increased heart rates and may cause increased coronary vasoconstriction.

Abnormal Coronary Vasomotion and Microvascular Angina

Although Osler (43) discussed coronary artery spasm in 1910, this explanation of ischemia was disregarded for approximately 70 years. However, there is now abundant evidence that the coronary arteries are not passive conduits for blood, but they exhibit dynamic vasomotion under a variety of stimuli. These include catecholamines, prostaglandins, adenosine, histamine, calcium, serotonin, and cholinergic agonists, as well as endothelium-derived contracting and relaxing factors. Even in the presence of advanced coronary arterial obstruction, coronary vasomotor activity may maintain coronary resistance well above its minimum achievable level.

Under usual circumstances, the coronary vascular tree exhibits the physiologic response of autoregulation as described earlier. However, autoregulation in the presence of fixed obstruction does not entirely explain a number of clinical observations, including a varying anginal threshold throughout the day and the occurrence of rest pain. These phenomena may be partially explained by that a primary decrease in MBF may result from excessive or abnormal coronary vasoconstriction in either large epicardial or smaller resistance vessels (Fig. 87–4). Relatively modest degrees of vasoconstriction may induce ischemic chest pain in the presence of a coronary atherothrombotic lesion; conversely, enhanced coronary vasodilation tends to relieve pain. Quantitative coronary angiography has demonstrated that abnormal vasoconstriction tends to occur in the area of a stenosis, indicating that the obstructed segment is frequently capable of vasomotion (44). In addition, constriction of vessels distal to an obstruction, as well as constriction of collateral vessels, may cause myocardial ischemia in patients with chronic stable angina (45). Thus, in a coronary vessel that has only mild to moderate fixed obstruction, a modest amount of additional constriction produced by coronary vasomotion can lead to critical obstruction. Therapy directed at such vasomotion either can produce dilatation in the area of a critical obstruction or prevent the obstruction from becoming critical.

A third factor also must be considered in the pathogenesis of ischemic chest pain in some patients: Abnormalities of coronary arteriolar or small coronary artery morphology and/or function that cannot be identified by angiography because the vessels are too small. However, such patients will demonstrate reduced coronary flow reserve on the use of intracoronary Doppler techniques in conjunction with coronary vasodilator drugs. This syndrome (syndrome X or microvascular angina; see detailed discussion in Chapter 42) has a good prognosis even when ST-segment depression is produced by exercise. However, some of these patients experience development of constant or rate-dependent left bundle branch block; others manifest significant depression of LV function when followed longitudinally for several years or more (46).

Other associated abnormalities in this apparently heterogeneous subset of patients include abnormal sensitivity to cardiac stimulation (enhanced visceral nociception), esophageal dysmotility, and various types of psychosocial abnormalities, including panic disorder (47).

Left Ventricular Hypertrophy

Angina pectoris may occur in patients with moderate to severe LVH, even in the absence of significant coronary artery disease. LVH usually results from systemic arterial hypertension or aortic valve disease, both of which lead to increases in LV systolic blood pressure and wall stress. Although LVH is probably an adaptive mechanism that tends to blunt the increase in wall stress that would otherwise result from increased systolic pressures, the increase in myocardial mass is not accompanied by a commensurate increase in capillary density (28). Therefore, minimum coronary resistance is increased and maximum MBF per unit myocardial mass is decreased, especially in the subendocardium. LVH is associated with diminished diastolic chamber compliance, resulting in greater LV diastolic pressure, which may diminish the effective pressure gradient for flow through the coronary

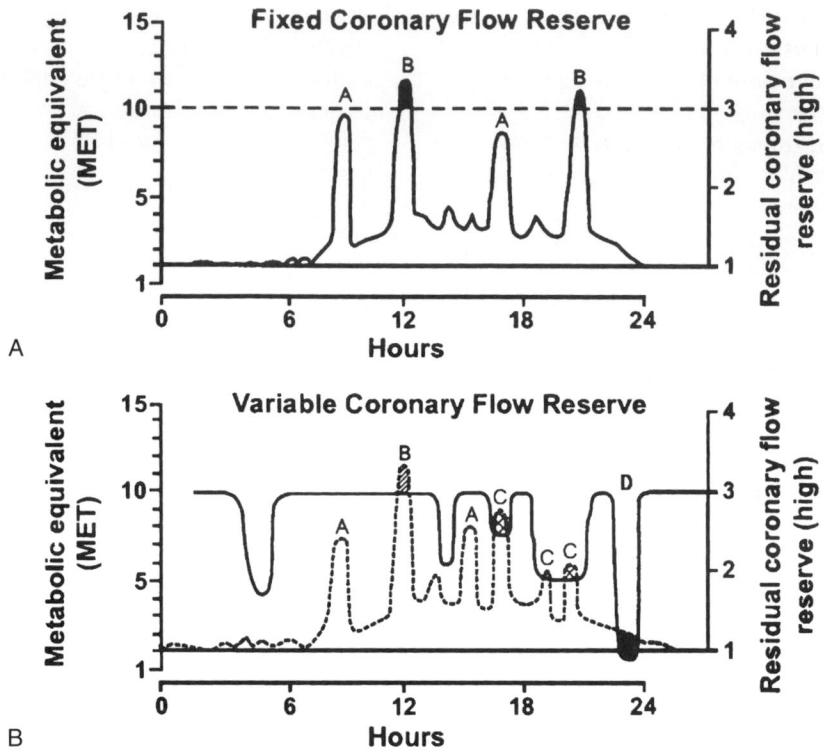

FIG. 87–4. A: Fixed coronary flow reserve in the presences of variable atherothrombotic obstruction. **B:** Variable coronary flow reserve in the presence of variable atherothrombotic obstruction. Episodes not associated with ischemia *(A)*. Ischemic episodes provoked by exercise levels that exceed the threshold of coronary flow reserve *(B)*. Ischemic episodes occurring at lower levels of activity during a period when coronary flow reserve is reduced *(C)*. Ischemic episodes at rest in presence of severe reduction in coronary flow reserve *(D)*. (From Fuster V, Alexander RW, O'Rourke RA. *Hurst's the heart,* 10th ed. New York: McGraw-Hill, 2001:1217, with permission.)

circulation. In patients with LVH, endothelium-dependent coronary vasodilator responses may also be impaired, in the absence of any angiographic evidence of coronary artery disease (48).

Insulin Resistance: Diabetes and the Metabolic Syndrome

There are multiple mechanisms by which diabetes and the metabolic syndrome may cause or exacerbate myocardial ischemia and angina pectoris. The common denominator active in both of these conditions is insulin resistance. Insulin resistance plays a critical role in the development of cardiovascular disease. This resistance to insulin results in two to three times the incidence of atherothrombosis that is commonly accelerated in this patient population (49). The end result often is significant microvascular and epicardial coronary artery stenoses. Diabetes also affects the microvasculature of the heart, with thickening of myocardial capillary basement membranes and development of microaneurysms (50).

Insulin resistance also results in a more atherogenic lipid profile consisting of increased small, dense low-density lipoprotein particles (51). These smaller particles are more susceptible to oxidation that results in inflammatory re-

sponses and plaque formation. Both hyperinsulinemia and hyperlipidemia impair nitric oxide–dependent coronary vasodilation (52). Diabetes appears to be an independent cause of endothelial dysfunction in experimental animal models; however, abnormalities of coronary endothelial function attributable to diabetes has not yet been proven (53).

Hyperinsulinemia also influences the thrombotic potential. In the setting of insulin resistance, the balance between levels of plasminogen activator inhibitor (PAI)-1 and tissue plasminogen activator (t-PA) is altered. Levels of each are increased, which results in impaired fibrinolysis and increased thrombotic potential (54). The relation between PAI-1 and t-PA is being further studied in the Bypass Angioplasty Revascularization Investigation (BARI) 2 Diabetes Trial.

Hypertension is frequently a consequence of insulin resistance. Similarly, diastolic LV function may be abnormal in diabetic hearts, even in the absence of epicardial coronary artery disease, as manifested by delayed ventricular relaxation and diminished compliance (55).

Patients with type II diabetes also have decreased maximal oxygen consumption and slower oxygen uptake (56,57). Myocardial glucose uptake and oxidation are diminished, whereas circulating levels and oxidation of free fatty acids are increased. Because the generation of ATP from oxidation of fatty acids requires more O_2 consumption than glucose oxidation, this shift in substrate preference may have an additional deleterious effect on myocardial O_2 supply–demand imbalance. However, the clinical significance of altered myocardial substrate utilization and its potential treatment remains to be elucidated.

Acquired Aortic and Mitral Valve Disease

Lesions of the aortic and mitral valves are the most common forms of acquired valvular heart disease and may cause or contribute to symptoms of angina pectoris.

Aortic Stenosis

Angina is one of the cardinal symptoms of critical aortic stenosis and may occur without angiographic evidence of coronary artery disease (58). The mechanisms of myocardial ischemia include those generally applicable to LVH. Unlike hypertensive heart disease, however, the aortic blood pressure in aortic stenosis may be normal or low despite markedly increased LV systolic pressure. In addition, the duration of ejection is prolonged in aortic stenosis, so that systolic wall stress is not only increased but more sustained. Therefore, for a given degree of LV systolic pressure increase and LVH, aortic stenosis is associated with a greater propensity for myocardial ischemia and angina than hypertensive heart disease.

Aortic Regurgitation

The increased stroke volume in chronic aortic regurgitation leads to increase of LV systolic blood pressure and stroke work, and chronic volume overload increases LV size. These factors result in augmentation of LV systolic wall stress and MVO_2. Simultaneously, myocardial oxygen supply may be compromised by a wide pulse pressure (reducing diastolic coronary perfusion pressure), high LV diastolic pressure (increasing the effective downstream coronary pressure), and the development of LVH (leading to diminished coronary vasodilator reserve). When both aortic stenosis and regurgitation are present, the pathophysiology of angina may involve a combination of the mechanisms described above.

Mitral Valve Disease

Systolic wall stress and MVO_2 increase with progressive LV dilatation accompanying chronic mitral regurgitation. However, increases in either systolic blood pressure or the duration of ejection are unusual, and a significant reduction in diastolic coronary perfusion pressure does not occur. Therefore, in the absence of coronary artery disease, angina accompanying mitral regurgitation is rare. Because mitral regurgitation may be associated with pulmonary hypertension, angina may occur as a consequence of right ventricular pressure overload and resultant right ventricular ischemia. Chest pain is a prominent symptom in a minority of patients with mitral stenosis. Its cause may be related more to right ventricular ischemia caused by pulmonary hypertension (discussed later) than LV coronary insufficiency.

Dyspnea as an Anginal-equivalent Symptom

Many patients with chronic ischemic heart disease report dyspnea, often without chest pain, with exertion, or even at rest. This symptom may result from several possible mechanisms acting singly or in combination to increase LV diastolic pressure during episodes of myocardial ischemia, including: (a) reduced cardiac output associated with a decline in ejection fraction; (b) decreased LV diastolic compliance; (c) increased venous return during exercise or with assumption of a recumbent position; and (d) decreased diastolic filling period associated with an increased heart rate during exercise. Increased LV diastolic pressure is transmitted in a retrograde manner to the pulmonary capillaries, resulting in the symptom of dyspnea.

It is important to remain cognizant of the differential diagnosis of dyspnea associated with ischemic heart disease. Some disorders that are common in patients with coronary heart disease may cause breathlessness unrelated to myocardial ischemia. These disorders include obesity, chronic obstructive pulmonary disease, or valvular heart disease, among others.

Angina after Revascularization

In many patients, a recurrence of angina that may or may not be considered stable, according to the clinical circumstance, occurs after myocardial revascularization. In patients who have undergone coronary artery bypass surgery, acute closure of vein grafts may occur in the perioperative period, but this likelihood has been reduced by technical advances and the use of antiplatelet drugs, particularly aspirin, immediately after surgery. Because aspirin alone does not prevent graft atherothrombosis, it is recommended that aggressive lipid-lowering and antismoking measures are taken in patients who have had bypass surgery. Recurrent angina in the first 6 to 9 months after coronary artery angioplasty/stenting or atherectomy usually signifies hemodynamically significant restenosis of the affected vessel, which may be prevented by novel stent coatings.

Other Factors

Heritable neuromuscular diseases, such as Duchenne's muscular dystrophy or Friedreich's ataxia, may cause morphologic abnormalities of small coronary arteries, but they are not usually associated with angina. Vascular inflammation or infiltration of the small coronary arteries occurs in diseases such as lupus erythematosus, rheumatoid arthritis, and amyloidosis. Small- and medium-sized coronary arteries may also be involved in polyarteritis nodosa. Small-vessel coronary artery disease in patients with systemic sclerosis is commonly associated with myocardial perfusion abnormalities, but angina pectoris is less frequent. Thrombotic microcirculatory cardiac lesions may occur in thrombotic thrombocytopenic purpura.

A variety of vascular factors may occasionally play a role in the pathogenesis of myocardial ischemia and angina. Among these are myocardial compression, caused by muscle bridges spanning a segment of epicardial coronary artery, and the phenomenon of coronary "steal," in which a low-resistance vessel siphons blood flow from the territory supplied by an obstructed vessel that has a greater resistance to flow; there also is the intriguing observation that coronary vascular reserve is reduced in chronic smokers who have morphologically normal coronary vessels. Coronary ostial narrowing may result from various diseases of the aorta, including atherothrombosis, dissecting and saccular aneurysm, aortitis, calcification of the aorta in proximity to the origin of a coronary artery, and radiation therapy.

Women

Coronary vasoreactivity may differ in men and women. One study evaluated the response to acetylcholine in patients with normal angiographic epicardial coronary arteries and found differences among men and women. In this population, women had more microvascular spasm, whereas men exhibited more large-artery spasm. Microvascular spasm also was associated with greater coronary sinus lactate levels. These data suggest that patterns of ischemia and angina may differ between the two sexes (59).

Drugs and Patient Noncompliance

An important factor to consider in the pathogenesis of angina pectoris is that many patients are noncompliant with medication. Indeed, compliance should be questioned when there is any change in the patient's pattern of previously stable angina. Conversely, many agents may induce or exacerbate angina in previously stable patients. Such drugs are generally agents that increase myocardial oxygen demand by causing an increase in heart rate and contractility. They include β-adrenergic agonists and theophylline-containing compounds used for the treatment of bronchial asthma; direct-acting vasodilators, such as hydralazine and minoxidil, which cause secondary sympathetic nervous system activation; and, paradoxically, agents used to treat angina, such as short-acting dihydropyridine calcium channel blockers (e.g., nifedipine, nicardipine), which may increase heart rate or cause excessive hypotension. An excess of thyroid hormone, either administered exogenously as replacement therapy or occurring endogenously as a result of hyperthyroidism, may lead to angina in susceptible individuals by increasing myocardial metabolic demands beyond the available supply. Other "high-output" states, such as fever, anemia, or arteriovenous fistula, may also provoke angina by a similar mechanism.

Illegal or "recreational" drugs, such as cocaine and amphetamines, may also be responsible for cases of MI and subsequent angina. Cocaine, by blocking uptake of norepinephrine, can cause constriction of epicardial coronary vessels, increase heart rate and blood pressure, and consequently cause myocardial ischemia and chest pain, even in patients without underlying coronary artery atherothrombosis.

As noted earlier, alterations in diastolic filling time significantly influence coronary blood flow. Tachyarrhythmias, either ventricular or supraventricular, may decrease myocardial perfusion by this mechanism, as well as by reducing forward cardiac output and coronary perfusion pressure. Patients with pulmonary hypertension of any cause may also report chest pain that resembles angina pectoris. Experiments in animal models have demonstrated that severe pulmonary hypertension is associated with right ventricular ischemia, especially when coronary perfusion pressure is simultaneously reduced (60). Finally, chronic angina pectoris may be produced by a variety of congenital anomalies of the coronary circulation, including the anomalous origin of a coronary vessel from the pulmonary artery.

MECHANISMS OF ANGINAL PAIN

The pathogenesis of cardiac pain is uncertain, and the precise pathways are not well defined. Afferent fibers running in the cardiac sympathetic nerves are considered to be the major pathways for the transmission of cardiac pain. From the heart these afferent fibers reach the spinal cord through the cardiac nerves, the upper five thoracic sympathetic ganglia, the white rami communicantes, and the upper five thoracic dorsal roots. Impulses mediated by these pathways converge with impulses from somatic thoracic structures into the same ascending spinal neurons. This convergence is thought to account for the projection of cardiac ischemic pain onto various dermatomes and provides the most likely explanation for referred pain. Other possible afferent sensory pathways include the ventral roots and vagal afferents. However, noxious stimuli (presumably hypoxia and acidosis) do not reliably and predictably produce pain. This may, in part, explain the common occurrence of silent ischemia, because pain may be perceived only when a sufficient level of afferent nerve traffic activates ascending neural pathways, thus leading to the conscious perception of discomfort.

There also is evidence that a number of vasoactive factors, including adenosine, are released during myocardial ischemia. These substances may activate cardiac sympathetic afferents to cause reflex sympathoexcitation. Thus adenosine, among other molecules, may be a principal mediator of the sensation of angina pectoris.

FUTURE DIRECTIONS

In the coming years, the key areas in which our understanding of the pathophysiology of chronic angina pectoris is likely to expand include the role of the endothelium in producing abnormal coronary vasoconstriction and increased coronary resistance; the hydraulic, neurohumoral, and/or endothelial mechanisms responsible for increases in the effective downstream coronary pressure; the mechanisms responsible for reduced coronary vasodilator reserve in LVH; and the mechanisms responsible for clinical syndromes of variant angina and angina with angiographically normal coronary arteries.

REFERENCES

1. Heberden W. Some account of a disorder of the breast. *Med Trans Coll Physicians (Lond)* 1772;2:59.
2. Osler W. *The principles and practice of medicine.* New York: Appleton, 1892:655–659.
3. Gorlin R. Pathophysiology of cardiac pain. *Circulation* 1965;32:138–148.
4. Gibbons RJ, Abrams J, Chatterjee K, et al. ACC/AHA 2002 guideline update for the management of patients with chronic stable angina–summary article: a report of the American College of Cardiology/American Heart Association Task Force on practice guidelines (Committee on the Management of Patients with Chronic Stable Angina). 2002. Available at: www.acc.org/clinical/guidelines/stable/stable.pdf (accessed June, 2003).
5. Marcus ML. *The coronary circulation in health and disease.* New York: McGraw-Hill, 1983:65–92.
6. Feigl EO. Coronary physiology. *Physiol Rev* 1983;63:1–205.
7. Weiss HR. Effect of coronary artery occlusion on regional arterial and venous O_2 extraction, blood flow, and O_2 consumption in the dog heart. *Circ Res* 1980;47:400–407.
8. Gibbs CL, Chapman JB. Cardiac energetics. In: Berne RM, ed. *Handbook of physiology, Section 2. The cardiovascular system, vol 1. The heart.* Bethesda, MD: American Physiological Society, 1979:775–804.
9. Weiss HR, Neubauer JA, Sinha AK. Quantitative determination of regional oxygen consumption in the dog heart. *Circ Res* 1978;42:394–401.
10. Gold FL, Horwitz LD, Bache RJ. Adrenergic coronary vasoconstriction in acute right ventricular hypertension. *Cardiovasc Res* 1984;18:447–454.
11. Schwartz GG, Greyson CR, Wisneski JA, et al. Relation among regional O_2 consumption, high-energy phosphates, and substrate uptake in porcine right ventricle. *Am J Physiol* 1994;266:H521–H530.
12. McKeever WP, Gregg DE, Canney PC. Oxygen uptake of the nonworking left ventricle. *Circ Res* 1958;6:612–623.
13. Yaku H, Slinker BK, Mochizuki T, et al. Use of 2,3-butanedione monoxime to estimate nonmechanical VO2 in rabbit hearts. *Am J Physiol* 1993;265:H834–H842.
14. Mirsky I. Elastic properties of the myocardium: a quantitative approach with physiological and clinical applications. In: Berne RM, ed. *Handbook of physiology, Section 2. The cardiovascular system, vol 1. The heart.* Bethesda, MD: American Physiological Society, 1979:497–531.
15. Covell JW, Ross J Jr, Taylor R, et al. Effects of increasing frequency of contraction on force-velocity relation of left ventricle. *Cardiovasc Res* 1967;1:2–8.
16. Covell JW, Braunwald E, Ross J Jr, et al. Studies on digitalis. Effects on myocardial oxygen consumption. *J Clin Invest* 1966;45:1535–1542.
17. White A, Handler P, Smith EL. *Principles of biochemistry,* 5th ed. New York: McGraw-Hill, 1973:437–441,553.
18. Wisneski JA, Gertz EW, Neese RA, et al. Myocardial metabolism of free fatty acids. Studies with 14C-labeled substrates in humans. *J Clin Invest* 1987;79:359–366.
19. Rodrigues B, McNeill JH. The diabetic heart: metabolic causes for the development of a cardiomyopathy. *Cardiovasc Res* 1992;26:913–922.
20. Wall SR, Lopaschuk GD. Glucose oxidation rates in fatty acid-perfused isolated working hearts from diabetic rats. *Biochim Biophys Acta* 1989;1006:97–103.
21. Dole WP. Autoregulation of the coronary circulation. *Prog Cardiovasc Dis* 1987;29:293–323.
22. Klocke FJ, Mates RE, Canty JM, et al. Coronary pressure-flow relationships. Controversial issues and probable implications. *Circ Res* 1985;56:309–323.
23. Harizi RC, Bianco JA, Alpert JS. Diastolic function of the heart in clinical cardiology. *Arch Intern Med* 1988;148:99–109.
24. Canty JM Jr, Giglia J, Kandath D. Effect of tachycardia on regional function and transmural myocardial perfusion during graded coronary pressure reduction in conscious dogs. *Circulation* 1990;82:1815–1825.
25. Yatabe S, Kumada T, Hiro T, et al. The effect of left ventricular wall motion during isovolumetric relaxation period in coronary artery disease. *Jpn Circ J* 1989;53:766–772.
26. Bellamy RF. Diastolic coronary artery pressure-flow relations in the dog. *Circ Res* 1978;43:92–101.
27. Vogel RA. Endothelium-dependent vasoregulation of coronary artery diameter and blood flow. *Circulation* 1993;88:325–327.
28. Brown BG, Bolson EL, Dodge HT. Dynamic mechanisms in human coronary stenosis. *Circulation* 1984;70:917–922.
29. Marcus ML, Harrison DG, Chilian WM, et al. Alterations in the coronary circulation in hypertrophied ventricles. *Circulation* 1987; 75[Suppl I]:I19–I25.
30. Polese A, De Cesare N, Montorsi P, et al. Upward shift of the lower range of coronary flow autoregulation in hypertensive patients with hypertrophy of the left ventricle. *Circulation* 1991;83:845–853.
31. Bassenge E, Busse R. Endothelial modulation of coronary tone. *Prog Cardiovasc Dis* 1988;30:349–380.
32. Selke FW, Armstrong ML, Harrison DG. Endothelium-dependent vascular relaxation is abnormal in the coronary microcirculation of atherosclerotic primates. *Circulation* 1990;81:1586–1593.
33. Zeiher AM, Drexler H, Saurbier B, et al. Endothelium-mediated coronary blood flow modulation in humans. Effects of age, atherosclerosis, hypercholesterolemia, and hypertension. *J Clin Invest* 1993;92:652–662.
34. Egashira K, Inou T, Yamada A, et al. Impaired coronary blood flow response to acetylcholine in patients with coronary risk factors and proximal atherosclerotic lesions. *J Clin Invest* 1993;91:29–37.
35. Egashira K, Hirooka Y, Kai H, et al. Reduction in serum cholesterol with pravastatin improves endothelium-dependent coronary vasomotion in patients with hypercholesterolemia. *Circulation* 1994;89:2519–2524.
36. Leung WH, Lau CP, Wong CK. Beneficial effect of cholesterol-lowering therapy on coronary endothelium-dependent relaxation in hypercholesterolemic patients. *Lancet* 1993;341:1496–1500.
37. Nozawa T, Wada O, Ishizaka S, et al. Dobutamine improves afterload-induced deterioration of mechanical efficiency toward maximal. *Am J Physiol* 1992;263:H1201–H1207.
38. Hoffman JI. Transmural myocardial perfusion. *Prog Cardiovasc Dis* 1987;29:429–464.
39. Flynn AE, Coggins DL, Goto M, et al. Does systolic subepicardial perfusion come from retrograde subendocardial flow? *Am J Physiol* 1992;262:H1759–H1769.
40. Schwarz F, Flameng W, Ensslen R, et al. Effect of collaterals on left ventricular function at rest and during stress. *Am Heart J* 1978;975: 570–577.
41. Figueras J, Singh B, Ganz W, et al. Hemodynamic and electrocardiographic accompaniments of resting postprandial angina. *Br Heart J* 1979;42:402–409.
42. Stern S, Tzivoni D. Dynamic changes in the ST-T segment during sleep in ischemic heart disease. *Am J Cardiol* 1973;32:17–20.
43. Osler W. Lumelian lecture on angina pectoris. In: White PD, ed. The historical background of angina pectoris. *Mod Concepts Cardiovasc Dis* 1974;43:109–112.
44. Gage JE, Hess OM, Murakami T, et al. Vasoconstriction of stenotic coronary arteries during dynamic exercise in patients with classic angina pectoris: reversibility by nitroglycerin. *Circulation* 1986;73:865–876.
45. Pupita G, Maseri A, Kaski JC, et al. Myocardial ischemia caused by distal coronary-artery constriction in stable angina pectoris. *N Engl J Med* 1990;323:514–520.
46. Opherk D, Shuler G, Wetterauer K, et al. Four-year follow-up study in patients with angina pectoris and normal coronary arteriograms ("syndrome X"). *Circulation* 1989;80:1610–1616.
47. Cannon RO 3rd, Quyyumi AA, Schenke WH, et al. Abnormal cardiac sensitivity in patients with chest pain and normal coronary arteries. *J Am Coll Cardiol* 1990;16:1359–1366.
48. Treasure CB, Klein JL, Vita JA, et al. Hypertension and left ventricular hypertrophy are associated with impaired endothelium-mediated relaxation in human coronary resistance vessels. *Circulation* 1993;87: 86–93.
49. Kannel WB, McGhee DL. Diabetes and cardiovascular risk factors: the Framingham study. *Circulation* 1979;59:8–13.
50. Factor SM, Okun EM, Minase T. Capillary microaneurysms in the human diabetic heart. *N Engl J Med* 1980;320:384–388.

51. Reaven GM, Chen YD, Jeppesen J, et al. Insulin resistance and hyperinsulinemia in individuals with small, dense low density lipoprotein particles. *J Clin Invest* 1993;92:141–146.
52. Steinberg HO, Chaker H, Leaming R, et al. Obesity/insulin resistance is associated with endothelial dysfunction: implications for the syndrome of insulin resistance. *J Clin Invest* 1996;97:2601–2610.
53. Vallance P, Calver A, Collier J. The vascular endothelium in diabetes and hypertension. *J Hypertens* 1992;10[Suppl]:S25–S29.
54. Meigs JB, Mittleman MA, Nathan DM, et al. Hyperinsulinemia, hyperglycemia, and impaired hemostasis: the Framingham Offspring Study. *JAMA* 2000;283:221–228.
55. Shapiro LM. Echocardiographic features of impaired ventricular function in diabetes mellitus. *Br Heart J* 1982;47:439–444.
56. Brandenburg SL, Reusch JE, Bauer TA, et al. Effects of exercise training on oxygen uptake kinetic responses in women with type 2 diabetes. *Diabetes Care* 1999;22:1640–1646.
57. Bertrand ME, Lablanche JM, Tilmant PY, et al. Coronary sinus blood flow at rest and during isometric exercise in patients with aortic valve disease: mechanism of angina pectoris in presence of normal coronary arteries. *Am J Cardiol* 1981;47:199–205.
58. Regensteiner JG, Bauer TA, Reusch JE, et al. Abnormal oxygen uptake kinetic responses in women with type II diabetes mellitus. *J Appl Physiol* 1998;85:310–317.
59. Mohri M, Koyanagi M, Egashira K, et al. Angina pectoris caused by microvascular spasm. *Lancet* 1998;351:1165–1169.
60. Vlahakes GJ, Turley K, Hoffman JI. The pathophysiology of failure in acute right ventricular hypertension: hemodynamic and biochemical correlations. *Circulation* 1981;63:87–95.

CHAPTER 88

Clinical Presentation and Diagnostic Techniques

Gordon S. Huggins and Henry Gewirtz

Key Words: Angina; coronary flow reserve; double product; exercise tolerance testing; pharmacologic stress; positron emission tomography; stress echocardiography; stress scintigraphy.

INTRODUCTION

Chronic stable angina is most frequently the result of epicardial stenoses that impair the coronary flow reserve. As the coronary flow reserve is reduced, stress-induced myocardial ischemia can result in angina pectoris. Angina is customarily classified as typical versus atypical angina and is graded according to the amount of effort required to cause angina. A complete evaluation of cardiac risk factors may help to identify patients with chest pain who are at increased risk for having underlying coronary artery disease. There can be variations in the daily anginal pattern if there is a dynamic coronary flow reserve secondary to either epicardial vasomotor tone or ischemic preconditioning. Objective measurements of chronic stable angina rely on subjecting a patient to a myocardial stress (exercise, dobutamine, or adenosine/dipyridamole) and monitoring for the onset of symptomatic angina, ischemic

electrocardiographic changes, altered myocardial perfusion (thallium-201 [^{201}Th] or technetium-99m-methoxyisobutylisonitrile [MIBI] [^{99m}Tc-MIBI]), or left ventricular dyssynergy (echocardiography or magnetic resonance imaging [MRI]). In general, noninvasive markers such as the onset of ischemia at a low level of stress, with a large burden of ischemia and stress-induced left ventricular dysfunction, can help to identify patients with chronic stable angina who are at an increased risk for future adverse outcome. The timely identification of patients at high risk may allow for revascularization with hopes of an improved quality and potentially quantity of life.

PATHOPHYSIOLOGY OF CHRONIC STABLE ANGINA

Chronic stable angina reflects an impaired coronary flow reserve such that myocardial blood flow (MBF) is incapable of increasing sufficiently to meet myocardial oxygen demand, particularly during stress. Coronary arteriolar tone is closely regulated to maintain an adequate resting blood flow over a wide range of perfusion pressures. In response to a stress, under normal conditions, the coronary vascular bed can augment MBF as much as fourfold to fivefold compared with basal levels. However, in the presence of severe coronary artery stenosis, downstream arterioles dilate at rest in an effort to preserve basal flow. In the setting of resting vasodilation,

G. S. Huggins: Cardiology Division, Molecular Cardiology Research Institute, Tufts-New England Medical Center, Boston, Massachusetts 02111.

H. Gewirtz: Cardiac Unit, Massachusetts General Hospital, Boston, Massachusetts 02114.

there is only limited room for additional dilation with stress; thus, the ability of the coronary circulation to increase flow with stress is impaired. When the coronary flow reserve is impaired, the subendocardium develops ischemia before the subepicardium because endocardial flow is impaired to a greater extent than epicardial flow during ventricular systole even under normal conditions. Accordingly, during diastole there is greater endocardial microvascular dilation in comparison with the epicardium with a resultant relative reduction in endocardial flow reserve.

Maximum coronary blood flow is a direct function of coronary perfusion pressure under conditions of full coronary dilation, when microvascular tone is minimal. Ordinarily, epicardial vessels act as conduits, and the microvascular bed is the major source of resistance to flow in the coronary circulation. There is no impairment of coronary flow reserve until a stenosis of any single epicardial artery exceeds 40% of the luminal diameter and the flow reserve becomes significantly impaired with stenoses greater than 70% (1). A single stenosis of 90% to 95% not only is capable of abolishing the coronary

flow reserve, but it often is associated with a reduced resting flow as well (Fig. 88–1). The latter finding is related to Poiseuille's law, according to which the pressure loss across the stenosis is inversely proportional to the vessel luminal radius to the fourth power in the presence of a severe proximal coronary stenosis. The total resistance with two serial stenoses is equal to the sum of the resistance produced by each lesion (2). There is an obligatory loss of pressure (potential energy), at a geometric rate, as blood velocity (kinetic energy) increases across a stenosis of fixed geometry. After the stenosis there is always some pressure recovery with resumption of laminar flow, yet the intraarterial pressure after a significant stenosis is always less than that before the stenosis. These considerations help to explain why exertional angina is frequently seen with a moderate coronary stenosis of approximately 70% luminal diameter reduction and how rest angina may develop with coronary stenoses greater than 90%.

Poiseuille's law also dictates that the length of a stenosis is another factor that can impair coronary flow reserve. For example, there is a greater impairment in coronary flow re-

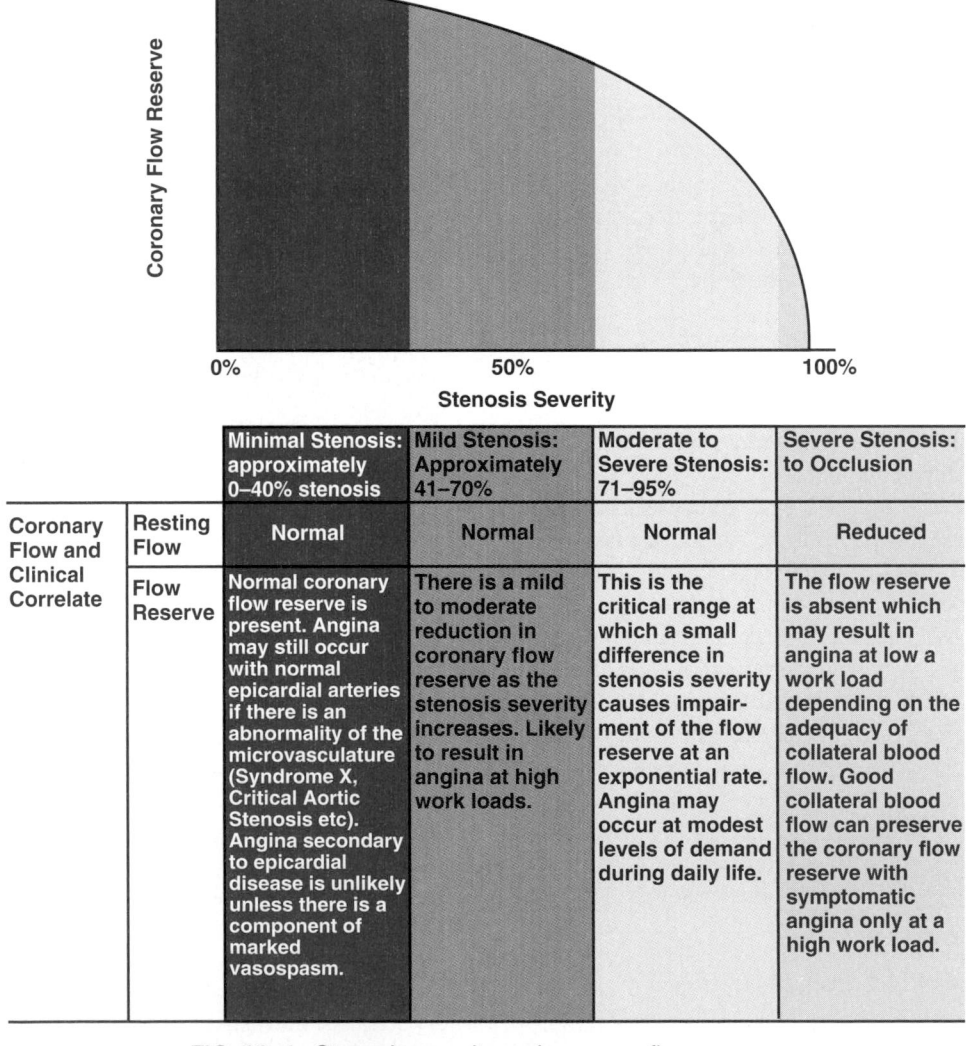

Coronary Flow and Clinical Correlate		Minimal Stenosis: approximately 0–40% stenosis	Mild Stenosis: Approximately 41–70%	Moderate to Severe Stenosis: 71–95%	Severe Stenosis: to Occlusion
	Resting Flow	Normal	Normal	Normal	Reduced
	Flow Reserve	Normal coronary flow reserve is present. Angina may still occur with normal epicardial arteries if there is an abnormality of the microvasculature (Syndrome X, Critical Aortic Stenosis etc). Angina secondary to epicardial disease is unlikely unless there is a component of marked vasospasm.	There is a mild to moderate reduction in coronary flow reserve as the stenosis severity increases. Likely to result in angina at high work loads.	This is the critical range at which a small difference in stenosis severity causes impairment of the flow reserve at an exponential rate. Angina may occur at modest levels of demand during daily life.	The flow reserve is absent which may result in angina at low a work load depending on the adequacy of collateral blood flow. Good collateral blood flow can preserve the coronary flow reserve with symptomatic angina only at a high work load.

FIG. 88–1. Stenosis severity and coronary flow reserve.

serve when a stenosis is 3 mm in length compared with 1 mm in length. In contrast to the additive effects of serial resistances, the lengths of serial lesions have an even greater effect on flow reserve than a single lesion of similar total length. Two serial lesions of 1 mm in length can produce an even greater impairment of coronary blood flow than a single legion of 2 mm in length. This finding can be explained by the loss of kinetic energy in the turbulent flow that occurs in the outlet phase after a stenosis (3). Similarly, complex luminal geometry may impair flow reserve more than simple geometry for a comparable reduction in luminal area (4).

Left ventricular hypertrophy frequently develops in response to the physiologic stress of aortic stenosis or systemic essential hypertension (pressure overload) and aortic insufficiency (pressure and volume overload). An impaired coronary flow reserve with a normal resting coronary blood flow has been found in patients with angina in the setting of normal epicardial arteries and left ventricular hypertrophy secondary to arterial hypertension (5), aortic stenosis (6), and aortic regurgitation (7). In comparison with healthy individuals, there appears to be arteriolar medial hypertrophy, which may impair vasodilation, thereby limiting the coronary flow reserve. In addition to the structural medial hypertrophy, there may be an impairment of dynamic endothelium-dependent vasodilation in patients with essential hypertension (8), although this has been disputed (9). The impaired endothelium-dependent vasodilation may explain the reduced coronary flow reserve found in patients with angina in the setting of arterial hypertension in the absence of left ventricular hypertrophy (10). Finally, the increased resting myocardial oxygen demand with a low coronary flow reserve may contribute to angina in the setting of severe hypertrophic cardiomyopathy with normal epicardial arteries (11,12).

Angina also can result from a reduced coronary perfusion pressure, especially in the setting of impaired coronary flow reserve. Coronary perfusion pressure is related to systemic arterial pressure and left ventricular end-diastolic pressure, both of which can be altered in the setting of left ventricular volume or pressure overload. Volume overload secondary to aortic insufficiency with dilation of the left ventricle can produce both a reduced diastolic arterial pressure and an increased left ventricular end-diastolic pressure as a result of diastolic runoff into the left ventricle. Both factors in association with compensatory left ventricular hypertrophy and a high level of myocardial oxygen demand may be responsible for symptoms of angina with normal coronary arteries in patients with aortic insufficiency (11).

CORONARY ARTERY DISEASE RISK FACTORS

After determining the pattern and characteristics of the chest pain, the estimate of underlying coronary artery disease can be refined by determining if certain risk factors are present. Advancing age is met with an increasing burden of coronary artery disease, with the incidence of coronary artery stenosis increasing from 1.9% in men aged 30 to 39 years to 12.3%

in men aged 60 to 69 years. Women in general are protected from coronary artery disease until after menopause, at which time the incidence of coronary disease increases rapidly reaching that of men. A family history of premature coronary artery disease in first-degree relatives may reflect a genetic predisposition to vascular disease or a familial trend toward hypertension, hyperlipidemia, and tobacco abuse. A family history of premature coronary disease is an independent risk factor for cardiovascular death, especially for men. Hypertension is a prominent risk factor for coronary artery disease, and there is a log-linear relation between diastolic blood pressure and cardiovascular disease as blood pressure increases. Systolic hypertension also is a risk factor for coronary heart disease. Patients with diabetes are more likely to develop peripheral vascular disease, stroke, and premature coronary artery disease than individuals without diabetes. The protective benefit against coronary artery disease enjoyed by women compared with men is lost when diabetes is present. The morbidity and mortality of cardiovascular diseases in diabetic women are actually greater than those in men who do not have diabetes. In men, there is a direct relation between risk for coronary event and the increasing levels of cholesterol and low-density lipoprotein (LDL) cholesterol in patients with and without cardiovascular disease. Correction of hypercholesterolemia by dietary or medical therapy is recommended as an important intervention to reduce the subsequent risk for cardiac events. In the setting of normal LDL levels, increased serum triglyceride levels, reduced high-density lipoprotein (HDL) levels, obesity, insulin resistance, and hypertension comprise a "metabolic syndrome" that is associated with increased risk for vascular disease. Tobacco contributes independently to peripheral and coronary artery disease, and smokers with chronic stable angina have a worse prognosis than nonsmokers.

Patients rarely have only one risk factor when they present with angina. Patients commonly have multiple risk factors, with some factors having greater weight than others. Several prediction models have sought to integrate multiple coronary artery risk factors and to stratify a patient's risk for development of coronary heart disease (13). The Framingham model incorporates age, sex, total cholesterol, HDL level, systolic blood pressure, smoking, diabetes, and left ventricular hypertrophy as diagnosed by an electrocardiogram (14), and it continues to have wide applicability in many ethnic groups (15). Finally, an excellent review of both traditional and emerging risk factors for ischemic heart disease including a practical approach to their integration into clinical practice has been published (16).

CLINICAL PATTERN

Description and Classification

Many patients can recall exactly what they were doing when they first experienced angina. The sensation for some is so unusual and in some cases so alarming for a patient that the character and location of the discomfort are not easily forgotten. In other cases, an anginal discomfort may be so mild and vague that it causes little concern to the patient. Angina is usually described as a substernal chest discomfort that is brought on by exertion and relieved by rest and nitroglycerin. Patients who experience many different types of chest pain may need to be oriented to which pain represents angina as opposed to the discomforts associated with chest wall pain or gastroesophageal reflux. Such patients may mistake a left breast pain for angina because of the mistaken notion that the heart is located under the left breast when their substernal "ache" is actually their angina. Patients with angina will usually deny a "pain," describing a chest "discomfort" instead. The four classical stimulants of angina are: physical exercise, emotional situations, cold weather, and large meals. A patient who has experienced stable angina on a repeated basis can usually describe exactly how much of each of these stimulants is required to provoke the angina, although there may be some variability (17).

There is a considerable difference in the risk for significant coronary artery disease between patients who have typical angina pectoris and patients with atypical angina pectoris. A large autopsy series found that the prevalence of coronary artery disease in men aged 50 to 59 years was 9.7%, whereas patients with atypical angina and typical angina had a prevalence of 58.9% and 92.0%, respectively (18). The Coronary Artery Surgery Study (CASS) registry correlated the presence of significant coronary artery disease defined by angiography with symptoms of chest pain. Patients with "definite" angina were more likely to have a significant coronary luminal stenosis of more than 70% or a left main stenosis of more than 50%, whereas patients with "probable" angina or "nonspecific chest pain" were less likely (19). Patients with symptomatic angina have a worse prognosis than asymptotic patients, even when the coronary anatomy and left ventricular function are similar in both groups (20). The severity of angina in everyday life is commonly gauged using the New York Heart Association classification, which divides anginal severity into four categories depending on the amount of everyday activity required to produce angina. More refined clinometric techniques also have been developed to assess workloads of everyday life and to correlate angina with a patient's functional ability. Although angina has important prognostic value, provided that the symptoms are not unstable, it should be noted that anginal severity has no prognostic significance.

Dynamic Variation

Although it is usually predictable, many patients will describe the phenomenon of "warm-up" or "second-wind" angina in which an activity that initially produces angina will subsequently produce less angina or perhaps no angina later during the same day. Some patients are halted by exertional angina, but after resting they are able to resume the same level of exertion without angina, or with less electro-

cardiographic evidence of ischemia despite a comparable level of stress (21). The warm-up phenomenon likely reflects a component of dynamic epicardial spasm in response to exercise. The administration of nitroglycerin before exercise greatly increases the ischemic threshold of the warm-up patients compared with patients who do not experience the warm-up phenomenon, which may indicate that dynamic variations in coronary tone may contribute to the pathophysiology of the warm-up phenomenon.

In some patients, however, ischemic preconditioning rather than epicardial coronary dilation may be responsible for the "warm-up" phenomenon. Williams and coworkers (22) found that after an initial period of rapid atrial pacing, a lower severity of angina and less electrocardiographic evidence of ischemia in response to a second bout of rapid atrial pacing developed. The major findings were lower myocardial oxygen consumption and an improved lactate extraction in response to the second round of pacing, whereas the great coronary vein blood flow was unaffected by prior rapid atrial pacing. These results were confirmed (23), and increased adenosine was found in the effluent of the great cardiac vein after the second round of exercise. The finding of reduced myocardial oxygen requirements with constant coronary blood flow in the setting of increased adenosine release suggests adenosine-mediated ischemic preconditioning through the adenosine receptor (24) as another potential mechanism underlying the warm-up phenomenon.

The warm-up phenomenon suggests that a patient's anginal history may be variable. Ordinarily, exercise stress tests performed on successive days produce similar results with the development of ischemia at a fixed threshold (25). Some patients, however, with a stable history of exertional angina have marked variability in the threshold for ischemia as determined by exercise testing. Patients with a dynamic ischemic threshold were found to have ergonovine-induced epicardial coronary artery constriction during cardiac catheterization, whereas patients who had a fixed ischemic threshold were found to have no coronary response to ergonovine (26). Thus, patients with a variable threshold for ischemia may have variable coronary flow reserve secondary to epicardial coronary spasm at the site of coronary stenosis or as a result of ischemic preconditioning as discussed earlier.

Associated Silent Ischemia and Diurnal Variations

In the setting of chronic stable angina there is frequently a backdrop of silent ischemia. Alarmingly, Holter monitoring found that only one-fourth of ischemic episodes were accompanied by angina and that ischemia was present at lower heart rate thresholds than found on treadmill exercise testing for each patient (27). Increased blood pressure or altered coronary tone may account for this ischemia, and hourly administration of nitroglycerin greatly reduced the frequency of asymptotic ischemia as measured by Holter monitoring. This observation is compatible either with reduced myocardial oxygen demand with nitroglycerin or increased supply.

Silent ischemia in the setting of stable coronary artery disease frequently follows a bimodal circadian rhythm. The peak incidence of ischemic episodes is in the morning, generally between 7:00 and 11:00 AM, and there also is a smaller evening peak between 5:00 and 9:00 PM. The peak density of silent ischemia occurs immediately on arising in the morning. The ischemic threshold, defined by the heart rate at the time of ischemic changes on an electrocardiogram, also demonstrated a marked circadian rhythm, which can be blunted by the administration of a β-adrenergic receptor antagonist (28). There are several factors such as plasma catecholamine and cortisol levels, blood pressure, and platelet aggregability that seem to follow the daily pattern of the ischemic threshold.

PROGNOSTIC FACTORS OF CHRONIC STABLE ANGINA

Change in Anginal Pattern

There are several prognostic factors that can establish a risk for adverse outcome in patients with chronic stable angina (Table 88–1). Chronic stable angina tends to be predictable with the same limits of exertion evoking angina, albeit with some variability as previously described. Stable angina becomes "unstable" when there is a significant worsening of the frequency or the intensity of angina, or when it presents at a lower than usual workload. An unstable plaque with acute worsening of an epicardial stenosis may cause worsening of anginal symptoms. Alternatively, a condition extrinsic to the heart such as anemia, infection, arrhythmia, or hypoxia may intensify myocardial ischemia. Califf and coworkers (29) devised an angina score formula that incorporates the anginal course (stable, progressive without nocturnal symptoms, progressive with nocturnal symptoms, and unstable or variant angina), the frequency of angina, and the presence of ischemia on a resting electrocardiograph. Patients experiencing crescendo angina had an increased risk for myocardial infarction or death. Patients with unstable symptoms within a 48-hour period not caused by an extra-

TABLE 88–1. *Clinical factors correlated with adverse outcome*

Coronary artery disease
    Left main coronary artery disease
    Three-vessel coronary artery disease
    Two-vessel coronary disease with left ventricular
      dysfunction

Valvular heart disease
    Symptomatic critical aortic stenosis
    Aortic valve insufficiency with marked left ventricular
      dilation

Electrical dysrhythmia
    Sudden death survivor

cardiac condition and associated with dynamic electrocardiographic changes or leakage of the cardiac-specific injury markers troponin I or troponin T have an increased risk for future cardiac events (30). Because of the increase risk for adverse events, these patients are best evaluated by cardiac catheterization rather than noninvasive stress testing, which is contraindicated in high-risk unstable angina.

Multivessel Disease and Ventricular Dysfunction

The presence of multivessel coronary artery disease and resting left ventricular dysfunction are prominent risk factors for future adverse cardiac events. The CASS registry studied 20,088 medically treated patients who had a cardiac catheterization, and 73% of these patients had typical angina (31). The 4-year survival rate for patients with one-, two-, and three-vessel coronary artery stenosis of 70% or more of the coronary luminal diameter was 92%, 84%, and 68%, respectively. Left ventricular dysfunction also was a powerful predictor of survival in this patient population. The 4-year survival rate for patients with a left ventricular ejection fraction (LVEF) greater than 50% was 92%, whereas patients with an ejection fraction between 35% and 49% had a survival of 83%, and patients with an ejection fraction less than 35% had a 58% 4-year survival rate. A study of 1,214 patients performed at Duke University (Durham, NC) also found that multivessel coronary artery disease and left ventricular dysfunction were significant risk factors for death in patients with symptomatic coronary artery disease (32). This study also found that anterior wall asynergy and an increased resting left ventricular end-diastolic pressure were significant risk factors for death over 5 years. Finally, both the CASS and the Duke studies found that a 50% or greater stenosis of the left main coronary artery was an important predictor of an adverse outcome (31,32).

DIAGNOSTIC WORKUP OF CHRONIC STABLE ANGINA

Formulating Diagnostic Strategy

There are no historical points, physical examination findings, or diagnostic tests that can classify patients with chronic stable angina as being at low or high risk for future cardiac events with perfect accuracy. In addition, most of the studies giving prognostic information on clinical evaluations present the data as a relative risk rather than an absolute risk of future event-free survival. Sometimes great pain and effort are put forth to decrease a high relative risk when the underlying absolute risk is low, which makes balancing relative and absolute risks problematic. Often, the evaluation hinges on choosing a test that will refine the probability of potentially dangerous coronary disease rather than provide an absolute answer. Every patient with suspected angina should have an evaluation for the likelihood of coronary artery disease being present and the likelihood of future cardiac events. The cornerstone of this evaluation is a classification of the chest pain as being nonanginal, atypical angina, or typical angina. In addition to coronary risk factors, the pattern of chest pain symptoms, chronic stable, crescendo, or unstable, needs to be elicited from the patient.

Risk stratification begins with the history because as more clues to coronary disease accumulate, there is an increasing need for an objective evaluation of inducible myocardial ischemia. Patients with overt signs of coronary artery disease, such as typical anginal chest pain with marked changes on the electrocardiograph or increased cardiac-specific serum markers, are considered to have a high risk for future coronary event (30) and should be evaluated by cardiac catheterization. Stress testing in such patients is unsafe and should not be performed.

Choosing the optimum method of stress testing entails a number of considerations. The stress modality should be chosen first. Exercise electrocardiography should be reserved for patients with an excellent ability to exercise and a normal resting electrocardiogram. Patients with left bundle branch block, ventricular pacemaker dependency, and the presence of medications that alter the repolarization phase of the electrocardiogram have an absolute need for either stress echocardiography or myocardial perfusion scintigraphy. Patients with known ischemic heart disease generally require an imaging stress test especially if a particular coronary territory needs evaluation. If possible, treadmill exercise should be used to help with risk stratification and to define ischemic threshold. However, if the patient will not be able to exercise adequately, then a pharmacologic stress must be used.

The goal of stress testing should be to identify those patients who are at high risk for development of significant morbidity and, more importantly, mortality from coronary artery disease (Table 88–2). There should be emphasis on screening patients for multivessel coronary artery disease, left main disease, left ventricular dysfunction, and significant valvular heart disease. Timely identification of patients at high risk gives the opportunity for coronary revascularization that may increase the quality of life and

TABLE 88–2. *Noninvasive markers correlated with adverse outcome*

Exercise electrocardiography
    1 mm of horizontal or downsloping ST-segment
        depression before completion of Bruce stage 2 (<6 min
        of the standard protocol)

Stress radionuclide scintigraphy
    Multiple zones of ischemia or infarction
    Exercise-induced increased lung uptake (planar thallium
        scan)
    Exercise-induced left ventricular cavity dilation

Stress echocardiography
    Stress-induced asynergy and reduced wall thickening at a
        low heart rate (dobutamine)
    Multiple regions of stress-induced asynergy

prolong it. Details of stress test procedures are presented in the following section.

Objective Methods of Inducing Myocardial Ischemia

The fundamental basis of cardiovascular stress testing is to apply an intervention (physical or pharmacologic) that drains the coronary flow reserve in the stenosis zone and increases the MBF in the normal zones. Once the flow reserve is surpassed, myocardial ischemia can be detected by monitoring symptoms of angina or by various signs on electrocardiography, radionuclide scintigraphy including positron emission tomography (PET), echocardiography, or MRI.

Exercise

Physical exercise produces the most physiologic stress on the heart. In response to physical exercise, there is an increase in left ventricular contractility, preload, and afterload, which combine to increase myocardial oxygen demand. To avoid myocardial ischemia, there is an increase in MBF through recruitment of the coronary flow reserve. Tachycardia alone markedly consumes the coronary flow reserve, whereas increased blood pressure has a minor effect (33,34). A commonly used index of myocardial oxygen demand, and by extension MBF, in both healthy subjects and patients with ischemic heart disease is the product of the heart rate and the systolic blood pressure, known as the double product (35,36). An exercise stress test is considered adequate if the heart rate increases to more than 85% of the age-adjusted maximum predicted heart rate. Even though coronary flow reserve depends importantly on the heart rate, it is noteworthy that maximal treadmill exercise increases MBF in normally perfused myocardium only two to three times over baseline, whereas pharmacologic stimulation with adenosine or papaverine can increase coronary flow to four or five times baseline. Many patients will not be able to perform an adequate stress test because of claudication, pacemaker dependency, lung disease, or physical deconditioning. Such patients may be candidates for a pharmacologic stress. Because of the important role of an increased heart rate in assessing the coronary flow reserve, medications that can blunt the chronotropic response to exercise should be withheld before stress testing to avoid a false-negative test. Alternatively, antianginal medications can be given before the test to assess the efficacy of these medications at limiting ischemia. Similarly, any patient who cannot easily climb at least one flight of stairs or walk one to two blocks on level ground should not be considered for an exercise test unless the clinical question is to exclude stress-induced myocardial ischemia within the bounds of that patient's capabilities.

Pharmacologic Stress with Adenosine/Dipyridamole

Adenosine is a natural short-acting compound that can produce a dose-dependent myocardial hyperemia secondary to dilation of the coronary microvasculature (37). Coronary pressure distal to an epicardial stenosis declines in response to pharmacologic vasodilation, resulting in an impaired microvascular perfusion pressure. In the setting of a moderate to severe epicardial stenosis, adenosine may cause an intramyocardial "steal" such that endocardial blood flow actually declines, whereas epicardial blood flow is either unchanged or increased (38). The rate–pressure product, which is an index of myocardial oxygen demand, is frequently unchanged or even decreases in response to intravenous adenosine. Accordingly, clinical evidence of myocardial ischemia during adenosine stress in the setting of moderate to severe epicardial stenosis often reflects a decrease in endocardial blood flow in the stenotic zone. In contrast, both endocardial and epicardial blood flow will increase in the nonstenotic zone. Imbalances in coronary blood flow of one zone versus another generally can be most efficiently detected by radionuclide imaging techniques (39,40). Dipyridamole produces myocardial hyperemia by impairing cellular reuptake of adenosine. It differs from adenosine, though, by having a slower onset of action, a longer duration of action, and greater patient-to-patient biologic variation in response and is less potent in terms of coronary dilation at standard clinical dose (41). Methylxanthine compounds such as caffeine and theophylline can block the vasodilating effects of adenosine and dipyridamole because of their ability to compete for the adenosine receptor. Before adenosine or dipyridamole stress testing, all methylxanthines must be held for 24 hours to avoid false-negative stress test results. Patients with obstructive lung disease may experience development of bronchospasm with adenosine or dipyridamole administration, which makes this form of pharmacologic stress testing dangerous in patients with severely reactive airway disease. Dobutamine is preferred in such patients.

Pharmacologic Stress with Dobutamine

Dobutamine is a selective β-adrenergic agonist that produces a positive inotropic and chronotropic effect on the heart. Unlike tests with adenosine, the rate–pressure product with dobutamine can be used as a marker of myocardial oxygen demand, similar to an exercise stress. In addition, dobutamine can directly increase coronary blood flow through β_2 agonist effects. In nonstenosis segments of patients with coronary artery disease, dobutamine increases MBF to levels ~75% of that seen with adenosine (42). The heterogeneity of coronary blood flow in a stenotic zone compared with a nonstenotic zone with dobutamine stress is comparable to an adenosine stress. This finding is particularly true with single-photon emission computed tomography (SPECT) tracers, which are underrepresented in the heart relative to blood flow because they are diffusion limited at hyperemic levels of flow. Transient left ventricular dysfunction as a manifestation of myocardial ischemia may occur with high-dose dobutamine infusion in the setting of coronary artery disease. Accordingly, although dobutamine

stress testing with myocardial perfusion imaging is a useful procedure for patients who cannot safely be given adenosine, it often is used with an imaging modality, such as echocardiography (or MRI), which is designed to detect a transient decline in contractile function as a marker of myocardial ischemia (39). Obviously, effects of dobutamine are blocked by β-adrenergic receptor antagonists, which should be withheld before stress testing with this drug to avoid a false-negative or nondiagnostic response.

Functional Studies of Myocardial Ischemia

Nonimaging Exercise Tolerance Testing

Most laboratories have adopted the standard Bruce protocol, which is a graded exercise test that is run in 3-minute stages with each successive stage requiring a defined amount of work from the patient. The workload required of each of these stages has been correlated to many aspects of everyday life. There are several key prognostic factors that can be determined by exercise testing alone. Patients who were unable to complete the first two stages of the Bruce protocol or who had significant electrocardiogram changes were more likely to have coronary artery disease. Patients who had ischemic electrocardiogram changes and who were unable to complete the first or second stage of the Bruce protocol had a prevalence of significant coronary artery disease that was 98%, and the prevalence of three-vessel coronary artery disease ranged from 51% to 73%. Nearly one-fourth of patients unable to go beyond the second Bruce stage had disease of the left main coronary artery (43). The CASS registry found that the prognosis of any patient with 2 mm or more ST-segment depression in the first stage of the Bruce protocol is poor, with an annual mortality rate of more than 5% (44).

Patients with a normal electrocardiogram at a high workload have a favorable long-term prognosis. The incidence rate of significant coronary artery disease in patients who achieved Bruce stage 4 was 47%, with a 14% incidence rate of three-vessel coronary artery disease; yet, the 1-year survival rate was 99%, and the 4-year survival rate was 95%. These mortality statistics were significantly better than those for patients unable to exercise beyond Bruce stage 1 or 2 (43). The CASS registry also found that patients achieving Bruce stage 3 or greater with less than 1 mm of ST-segment depression have an annual mortality rate of less than 1% (44). Excellent exercise tolerance has a favorable long-term prognosis.

In general, graded exercise tolerance tests are most helpful when the results are markedly positive or negative. Unfortunately, many patients are unable to achieve adequate heart rate and blood pressure goals during an exercise test, which makes risk stratification of a cardiac event with this test alone problematic. In addition, there is a significant incidence of both false-positive and false-negative results with exercise electrocardiography. For this reason, myocardial perfusion scintigraphy and stress echocardiography have been introduced to refine risk stratification.

Myocardial Perfusion Scintigraphy

The essential principles of myocardial perfusion scintigraphy for diagnosis of ischemic heart disease are relatively straightforward and have not changed since introduction of the technology in the 1970s (45). Briefly, the distribution of tracer under resting conditions is compared with that under either exercise or pharmacologic stress. Common pharmacologic stimuli include adenosine, dipyridamole, and dobutamine (40,46). The first two are primary dilators of the coronary circulation, whereas the latter mimics the catecholamine surge associated with physical exertion and also has a component of primary coronary dilation (47). Myocardial regions with relatively normal coronary vessels may increase MBF as much as threefold to fourfold with the coronary dilator adenosine (140 μg/kg/min × 4–6 min) and somewhat less (~75%) with dobutamine at maximal dose (40 μg/kg/min) (42). As reviewed earlier, regions supplied by hemodynamically significant stenosis may increase MBF only modestly with these stimuli or not at all (48). Coronary steal with either adenosine or dobutamine may occur in collateral-dependent segments and is characterized by an absolute decline in MBF compared with baseline (38,49). Conventional SPECT myocardial perfusion images demonstrate relative, not absolute, tracer distribution. Thus, regions perfused by hemodynamically significant stenoses or are collateral dependent typically have substantially less MBF with stress than normally perfused regions of the same heart, and hence appear as defects in SPECT images.

Tracer deposition in the heart is linear up to MBF of 1.5 to 2.0 mL per minute per gram with the two most frequently used myocardial perfusion imaging agents: ^{201}Tl and ^{99m}Tc-MIBI (50,51). However, as MBF increases above these levels, extraction and retention of the tracer lags behind, more so for MIBI versus ^{201}Tl. Accordingly, a plot of tracer activity versus MBF will tend to plateau at MBF greater than ~2 mL per minute per gram with the curve for MIBI being flatter than that for ^{201}Tl (50,51). Because tracer deposition lags behind MBF at higher flows, much of the hyperemia induced by adenosine is wasted in terms of inducing contrast between normal and abnormal regions both for ^{99m}Tc-MIBI and ^{201}Tl. Although the effect is more marked for ^{99m}Tc-MIBI versus ^{201}Tl, the significance is limited for clinical imaging since most published series have reported comparable diagnostic accuracy for the two tracers in detection of ischemic heart disease (52,53). Indeed, a more recent review indicates ^{99m}Tc-MIBI SPECT actually may have a modest edge over ^{201}Tl both in sensitivity and specificity for diagnosis of ischemic heart disease (46). Myocardial segments with normal uptake at rest but definite defects with stress reliably, though not infallibly, indicate ischemia with hemodynamically significant coronary stenosis of the artery supply-

ing the segment (accuracy ~85%) (46,53). Persistent defects, present both at rest and with stress, may reflect either infarct or hibernation, or their combination, provided technical or other artifact can be excluded. The denser the defect the more likely the segment is primarily scar (54,55). Milder fixed defects more often reflect viable, hibernating myocardium (54,55).

The details of various imaging protocols are beyond the scope of this chapter and in many respects reflect local preference. Thus, the following protocols all have their advocates, strengths, and weaknesses, but none has been shown to be clearly superior to any other for assessment of ischemic heart disease in day-to-day use:

1. Thallium stress, redistribution, reinjection imaging (56)
2. Thallium rest, ^{99m}Tc-MIBI stress (57)
3. Same day, low dose (rest); high-dose (stress) ^{99m}Tc-MIBI (53)
4. Two-day protocol (stress one day and rest another) ^{99m}Tc-MIBI (53)

The widespread adoption of SPECT (as opposed to planar) imaging and the use of ^{99m}Tc-MIBI (or tetrofosmin) for gated acquisition represent state of the art, current practice (46). The ability to assess rest (or poststress) ventricular function using gated SPECT imaging adds important information to the myocardial perfusion study. Published data typically report excellent correlation between LVEF measured by gated SPECT and ^{99m}Tc-MIBI compared with other modalities such as echocardiography and MRI (58–60). In addition, assessment of regional contraction also has been reported to be helpful in distinguishing true perfusion abnormality from attenuation artifact (61). Although issues such as evaluation of contractile function in myocardial segments with poor tracer uptake and the validity of LVEF computed in the setting of atrial fibrillation or other irregular cardiac rhythm remain, the technique by and large has proven quite useful and, perhaps best of all, requires little additional effort to obtain.

Stress Echocardiography

Normal myocardial contraction is reflected in vigorous inward systolic wall thickening and wall motion. In response to exercise with a flow-limiting epicardial stenosis, the subendocardial blood flow is compromised before that to the subepicardium, resulting in subendocardial ischemia. Because the subendocardium is responsible for most of the wall thickening during systole, impaired wall thickening is a sensitive indicator of inducible myocardial ischemia. In response to exercise with an epicardial stenosis, there is a direct relation between systolic wall thickening and mean transmural blood flow. Myocardial ischemia also affects ventricular wall motion, resulting in ischemia-induced regional systolic hypokinesis, akinesis, or dyskinesis. Systolic wall thickening is a more sensitive indicator of ischemia than regional wall motion abnormality because abnormal wall thickening can reflect subendocardial ischemia and regional dyssynergy may be affected by motion of the bordering myocardium (62). Because myocardial ischemia reflects the relative balance of myocardial oxygen demand and supply and regional wall motion is sensitive to loading conditions, it is not surprising that there would be considerable variation in the relation between regional blood flow and regional wall motion.

Echocardiography is commonly used to measure systolic wall thickening and wall motion during stress. With the development of digital acquisition techniques, the stress and rest cardiac cycle can be shown simultaneously in a continuous loop format, which improves analysis. Newer techniques of color kinesis and tissue Doppler imaging offer the ability to objectively quantitate left ventricular regions of ischemia. In patients with particularly poor echocardiographic windows, microbubble ultrasound contrast agents can opacify the left ventricular cavity improving endocardial border definition and detection of myocardial perfusion (63). Routine treadmill stress can be used with echocardiography; however, the stress images must be obtained within the first 2 minutes immediately after exercise to identify regions of ischemia. Stress echocardiography is ideally suited for pharmacologic stressors, and most widely used is dobutamine with and without atropine. Dobutamine increases oxygen demand, which in the setting of a flow-limiting epicardial stenosis can produce myocardial ischemia manifest as reduced systolic wall thickening and regional wall motion abnormality. Atropine is occasionally administered at the end of the test to further increase the heart rate if dobutamine alone has failed to achieve the target heart rate goal. The sensitivity of dobutamine stress echocardiography for an epicardial stenosis of 50% or more is 95% with a sensitivity of 85% and an accuracy of 92% (64). This stress modality also is effective in the presence of resting asynergy. Ischemia can be detected in myocardial segments served by all of the major epicardial arteries, and the sensitivity for the detection of coronary disease increases as the burden of coronary disease increases. The development of asynergy with a heart rate less than 125 beats per minute has been associated with an increased likelihood of three-vessel coronary artery disease (65). Dobutamine stress echocardiography can be used to identify patients at high risk for future cardiac events. Mazeika and coworkers (66) found that patients with an abnormal dobutamine stress echocardiograph had a 32-month event rate of myocardial infarction or unstable angina of 32%, whereas patients with negative studies had an event rate of about 8%. The positive predictive value of future events has been estimated at 68% for dobutamine stress echocardiography, and the negative predictive value is 77% (66). The finding of inducible ischemia by dobutamine stress echocardiography in patients with advanced coronary artery disease and left ventricular dysfunction

portends an adverse prognosis, independent of age (67). Finally, an increasing number of myocardial zones found to have inducible ischemia by dobutamine stress echocardiography predicts a worse prognosis and identifies a subset of patients who should undergo intensive management (68–70). Dobutamine stress echocardiography also can detect regions of viable myocardium that benefit from revascularization (71). Improved wall motion of a severely impaired zone with low-dose dobutamine identifies a region of viable myocardium, and revascularization improves left ventricular function (72) and long-term outcomes (73). Dobutamine stress echocardiography compares favorably with other techniques for the detection of viable myocardial segments (74).

Modern digital acquisition techniques have improved *trans*thoracic stress echocardiography. However, in a significant number of patients, the heart cannot be adequately imaged using *trans*thoracic echocardiography. Biplane *trans*esophageal echocardiography is currently performed widely and it offers improved image quality over *trans*thoracic echocardiography. (75). *Trans*esophageal stress echocardiography is a sensitive and specific technique for the detection of coronary artery disease (76,77) that compares favorably with other stress imaging techniques (78). Importantly, though, a negative transesophageal echocardiogram does not offer greater negative predictive value than *trans*thoracic stress echocardiography (79). Widespread application of *trans*esophageal echocardiography is limited by the need for conscious sedation during this minimally invasive procedure.

Positron Emission Tomography

The role of PET myocardial perfusion imaging in the evaluation of patients with chronic stable angina pectoris is still limited by availability, but it has increased in recent years especially after approval of reimbursement for myocardial viability studies with [^{18}F]-fluorodeoxyglucose (FDG) and perfusion studies with rubidium-82. The authors' experience using quantitative PET perfusion imaging with ^{13}N-ammonia indicates that it is superior to conventional nuclear imaging for assessment of both reversible ischemia and myocardial viability in patients with chronic stable ischemic heart disease and prior myocardial infarction. The PET image quality is superior, and more importantly, quantitative information contained in parametric images of myocardial perfusion can provide an objective assessment of regional blood flow and flow reserve that is improved compared with currently available conventional nuclear imaging techniques (54,80–84). Quantitative determination of regional MBF is required for assessment of absolute coronary flow reserve (1,81,85), and it permits improved diagnosis of important pathophysiologic phenomena such as coronary "steal" and myocardial hibernation (49,86). The anatomic detail and quantitative data from PET also are remarkably helpful in assessing, and often predicting, the coronary anatomy, including collaterals, seen on coronary arteriograms (87). Important, although specialized, indications for PET imaging in chronic ischemic heart disease are discussed later.

Quantification of Myocardial Blood Flow in Women

Noninvasive evaluation of chronic chest pain syndromes is problematic in women, especially in the 50 to 60 year age group, which represents a transition period between the premenopausal low risk for coronary artery disease and the postmenopausal (older than 65 years) period when the risk is equal to that of men. Another closely related clinical scenario is that of the woman of any age with known coronary artery disease, particularly when it involves the left anterior descending coronary artery. In some women, it may be all but impossible to confidently evaluate inducible ischemia with conventional nuclear imaging, especially in the setting of prior myocardial infarction. Myocardial perfusion imaging with conventional tracers such as ^{99m}Tc-MIBI SPECT or ^{201}Tl is limited in many women because of photon attenuation by breast tissue. Under these circumstances, one is less able to be confident that an anterior or septal defect is a result of breast artifact, especially if the defect shows some evidence of change on rest or redistribution imaging. Women in this age group who present as diagnostic problems, therefore, ideally would be served best by having quantitative PET myocardial perfusion imaging performed once it is clear that a noninvasive diagnostic test beyond history and physical examination is required. An alternative, and in most circumstances more practical, strategy would be to perform conventional SPECT imaging and refer for PET only those in whom an equivocal result is obtained. The cost-effectiveness of such a strategy, however, will depend on local expertise and the confidence and accuracy with which perfusion images are interpreted.

Myocardial Viability

Patients with an ischemic dilated cardiomyopathy frequently will present with left ventricular dysfunction and heart failure. In this circumstance, the clinical question concerns the suitability of a particular segment(s) for revascularization in the hope of either reversing or at least ameliorating clinical congestive heart failure. In this situation, conventional nuclear imaging is frequently used to determine the viability of a particular myocardial segment so that revascularization can be guided effectively (Table 88–3). The literature is divided on the subject, with some reports suggesting that SPECT ^{201}Tl imaging is as effective as PET FDG imaging for detection of myocardial viability (88), and other reports suggesting that ^{201}Tl SPECT may not detect regions of viable myocardium that are apparent with PET FDG (89,90). More recently, there has been increasing recognition of the superiority of PET technology for myocardial viability assessment (46,91).

TABLE 88–3. *Objective markers for viable myocardium*

Technique	Predictors of viable myocardium
Angiography	Improved wall motion in postextra-systolic beat in a baseline akinetic zone
Radionuclide imaging	Reversible defect or, if fixed, with at least 50% tracer uptake (thallium or 99m-techetium-MIBI) compared with a normal segment
Echocardiography	Dobutamine-induced systolic wall thickening in a baseline akinetic zone
Positron emission tomography	Preserved uptake of fluorodeoxy-glucose, especially if in excess of coronary blood flow

Magnetic Resonance Imaging

MRI is a noninvasive imaging technique that can characterize soft-tissue composition of blood vessel walls, measure luminal blood flow velocity, and identify with great precision peripheral vascular stenoses and determine their functional significance. Currently, MRI is a preferred noninvasive technique for analysis of cerebrovascular, aortic, and peripheral vascular disease; yet, cardiac applications have been slowed by the need to correct for motion during the cardiac and respiratory cycles (92–94). Nonetheless, MRI of the coronary circulation is progressing (95). Stress MRI can be performed with adenosine or dobutamine agents. Similar to echocardiography, MRI can be used to detect the development of regional wall motion abnormalities in response to stress. Using a dobutamine/atropine stimulant, stress MRI compares favorably with stress echocardiography for the detection of coronary artery disease (96). With the combination of ultrafast image techniques and rapid intravenous infusion of a contrast agent, MRI can be used to estimate the coronary flow reserve. This technique has excellent spatial resolution allowing estimation of subepicardial and subendocardial flow reserve (97). Adenosine cardiac MRI underestimates coronary flow reserve compared with PET imaging; yet, MRI represents a promising future semiquantitative method of measuring coronary flow reserve (98). Low-dose dobutamine stress MRI can identify viable myocardium after infarction (99,100). Although MRI has become widely available, cardiac stress MRI is still quite unusual. This technique is sometimes limited by patient claustrophobia. Future development of cardiac stress MRI as a mainstay of noninvasive stress testing will rely on more rapid image acquisition, improved gating, collaboration between MRI specialists and cardiologists, and important financial issues related to reimbursement for the procedure.

A VIEW OF THE FUTURE

The current testing modalities can provide qualitative estimates of myocardial perfusion in the setting of a stress.

Qualitative evaluations, of course, rely on one portion of the myocardium being chosen as the reference point with which the other myocardial segments are compared. Quantitation of blood flow would obviate the need for qualitative comparisons of coronary blood flow, and, in addition, the actual coronary flow reserve could be determined. PET with dynamic parametric imaging is currently capable of making these measurements using ^{13}N-ammonia. PET also is currently capable of providing quantitative assessment of myocardial glucose and fatty acid metabolism, as well as measurement of myocardial oxygen consumption. MRI has the potential in the not too distant future to provide quantitative assessment of MBF, contractile function, and metabolism, as well as delineation of coronary artery anatomy. The challenge will be to bring these expensive and at times cumbersome technologies into the clinical arena in a form in which the information can be acquired quickly and easily. Finally, the data must be made rapidly available to referring clinicians in a manner that is easily understood and that not only facilitates but improves clinical decision-making.

REFERENCES

1. Demer LL, Gould KL, Goldstein RA, et al. Assessment of coronary artery disease severity by positron emission tomography. Comparison with quantitative arteriography in 193 patients. *Circulation* 1989;79: 825–835.
2. Gould KL, Lipscomb K. Effects of coronary stenoses on coronary flow reserve and resistance. *Am J Cardiol* 1974;34:48–55.
3. Feldman RL, Nichols WW, Pepine CJ, et al. Hemodynamic effects of long and multiple coronary arterial narrowings. *Chest* 1978;74:280–285.
4. Fedele FA, Sharaf B, Most AS, et al. Details of coronary stenosis morphology influence its hemodynamic severity and distal flow reserve. *Circulation* 1989;80:636–642.
5. Opherk D, Mall G, Zebe H, et al. Reduction of coronary reserve: a mechanism for angina pectoris in patients with arterial hypertension and normal coronary arteries. *Circulation* 1984;69:1–7.
6. Marcus ML, Doty DB, Hiratzka LF, et al. Decreased coronary reserve: a mechanism for angina pectoris in patients with aortic stenosis and normal coronary arteries. *N Engl J Med* 1982;307:1362–1366.
7. Nitenberg A, Foult JM, Antony I, et al. Coronary flow and resistance reserve in patients with chronic aortic regurgitation, angina pectoris and normal coronary arteries. *J Am Coll Cardiol* 1988;11: 478–486.
8. Panza JA, Quyyumi AA, Brush JE Jr, et al. Abnormal endothelium-dependent vascular relaxation in patients with essential hypertension. *N Engl J Med* 1990;323:22–27.
9. Cockcroft JR, Chowienczyk PJ, Benjamin N, et al. Preserved endothelium-dependent vasodilatation in patients with essential hypertension. *N Engl J Med* 1994;330:1036–1040.
10. Brush JE, Cannon RO, Schenke WH, et al. Angina due to coronary microvascular disease in hypertensive patients without left ventricular hypertrophy. *N Engl J Med* 1988;319:1302–1307.
11. Strauer BE. The significance of coronary reserve in clinical heart disease. *J Am Coll Cardiol* 1990;15:775–783.
12. Lewis EF, Edelman ER. Images in cardiovascular medicine. Acute ST depressions in a patient with idiopathic hypertrophic subaortic stenosis and normal coronary arteries. *Circulation* 2002;106:757–758.
13. Orford JL, Sesso HD, Stedman M, et al. A comparison of the Framingham and European Society of Cardiology coronary heart disease risk prediction models in the normative aging study. *Am Heart J* 2002;144:95–100.
14. Anderson KM, Wilson PW, Odell PM, et al. An updated coronary risk profile. A statement for health professionals. *Circulation* 1991;83: 356–362.
15. D'Agostino RB Sr, Grundy S, Sullivan LM, et al. Validation of the Framingham coronary heart disease prediction scores: results of a multiple ethnic groups investigation. *JAMA* 2001;286:180–187.
16. Grundy SM, Pasternak R, Greenland P, et al. Assessment of cardiovascular risk by use of multiple-risk-factor assessment equations: a statement for healthcare professionals from the American Heart Association and the American College of Cardiology. *Circulation* 1999; 100:1481–1492.
17. Shub C. Stable angina pectoris: 1. Clinical patterns. *Mayo Clin Proc* 1990;65:233–242.
18. Diamond GA, Forrester JS. Analysis of probability as an aid in the clinical diagnosis of coronary-artery disease. *N Engl J Med* 1979; 300:1350–1358.
19. Chaitman BR, Bourassa MG, Davis K, et al. Angiographic prevalence of high-risk coronary artery disease in patient subsets (CASS). *Circulation* 1981;64:360–367.
20. Cohn PF, Harris P, Barry WH, et al. Prognostic importance of anginal symptoms in angiographically defined coronary artery disease. *Am J Cardiol* 1981;47:233–237.
21. Jaffe MD, Quinn NK. Warm-up phenomenon in angina pectoris. *Lancet* 1980;2:934–936.
22. Williams DO, Bass TA, Gewirtz H, et al. Adaptation to the stress of tachycardia in patients with coronary artery disease: insight into the mechanism of the warm-up phenomenon. *Circulation* 1985;71: 687–692.
23. Okazaki Y, Kodama K, Sato H, et al. Attenuation of increased regional myocardial oxygen consumption during exercise as a major cause of warm-up phenomenon. *J Am Coll Cardiol* 1993;21:1597–1604.
24. Schulz R, Cohen MV, Behrends M, et al. Signal transduction of ischemic preconditioning. *Cardiovasc Res* 2001;52:181–198.
25. Waters DD, McCans JL, Crean PA. Serial exercise testing in patients with effort angina: variable tolerance, fixed threshold. *J Am Coll Cardiol* 1985;6:1011–1015.
26. Crea F, Margonato A, Kaski JC, et al. Variability of results during repeat exercise stress testing in patients with stable angina pectoris: role of dynamic coronary flow reserve. *Am Heart J* 1986;112:249–254.
27. Cecchi AC, Dovellini EV, Marchi F, et al. Silent myocardial ischemia during ambulatory electrocardiographic monitoring in patients with effort angina. *J Am Coll Cardiol* 1983;1:934–939.
28. Benhorin J, Banai S, Moriel M, et al. Circadian variations in ischemic threshold and their relation to the occurrence of ischemic episodes. *Circulation* 1993;87:808–814.
29. Califf RM, Mark DB, Harrell FE, et al. Importance of clinical measures of ischemia in the prognosis of patients with documented coronary artery disease. *J Am Coll Cardiol* 1988;11:20–26.
30. Hamm CW, Braunwald E. A classification of unstable angina revisited. *Circulation* 2000;102:118–122.
31. Mock MB, Ringqvist I, Fisher LD, et al. Survival of medically treated patients in the coronary artery surgery study (CASS) registry. *Circulation* 1982;66:562–568.
32. Harris PJ, Harrell FE, Lee KL, et al. Survival in medically treated coronary artery disease. *Circulation* 1979;60:1259–1269.
33. McGinn AL, White CW, Wilson RF. Interstudy variability of coronary flow reserve. Influence of heart rate, arterial pressure, and ventricular preload. *Circulation* 1990;81:1319–1330.
34. Rossen JD, Winniford MD. Effect of increases in heart rate and arterial pressure on coronary flow reserve in humans. *J Am Coll Cardiol* 1993;21:343–348.
35. Gobel FL, Norstrom LA, Nelson RR, et al. The rate-pressure product as an index of myocardial oxygen consumption during exercise in patients with angina pectoris. *Circulation* 1978;57:549–556.
36. Nelson RR, Gobel FL, Jorgensen CR, et al. Hemodynamic predictors of myocardial oxygen consumption during static and dynamic exercise. *Circulation* 1974;50:1179–1189.
37. Wilson RF, Wyche K, Christensen BV, et al. Effects of adenosine on human coronary arterial circulation. *Circulation* 1990;82:1595–1606.
38. Gewirtz H, Gross SL, Williams DO, et al. Contrasting effects of nifedipine and adenosine on regional myocardial flow distribution and metabolism distal to a severe coronary arterial stenosis: observations in sedated, closed-chest, domestic swine. *Circulation* 1984;69:1048–1057.
39. Fung AY, Gallagher KP, Buda AJ. The physiologic basis of dobutamine as compared with dipyridamole stress interventions in the assessment of critical coronary stenosis. *Circulation* 1987;76:943–951.
40. Marwick T, Willemart B, D'Hondt AM, et al. Selection of the optimal nonexercise stress for the evaluation of ischemic regional myocardial

1324 / CHAPTER 88

dysfunction and malperfusion. Comparison of dobutamine and adenosine using echocardiography and 99mTc-MIBI single photon emission computed tomography. *Circulation* 1993;87:345–354.

41. Rossen JD, Quillen JE, Lopez AG, et al. Comparison of coronary vasodilation with intravenous dipyridamole and adenosine. *J Am Coll Cardiol* 1991;18:485–491.

42. Skopicki HA, Abraham SA, Picard MH, et al. Effects of dobutamine at maximally tolerated dose on myocardial blood flow in humans with ischemic heart disease. *Circulation* 1997;96:3346–3352.

43. McNeer JF, Margolis JR, Lee KL, et al. The role of the exercise test in the evaluation of patients for ischemic heart disease. *Circulation* 1978;57:64–70.

44. Weiner DA, Ryan TJ, McCabe CH, et al. Prognostic importance of a clinical profile and exercise test in medically treated patients with coronary artery disease. *J Am Coll Cardiol* 1984;3:772–779.

45. Zaret BL, Strauss HW, Martin ND, et al. Noninvasive regional myocardial perfusion with radioactive potassium. Study of patients at rest, with exercise and during angina pectoris. *N Engl J Med* 1973; 288:809–812.

46. Beller GA, Zaret BL. Contributions of nuclear cardiology to diagnosis and prognosis of patients with coronary artery disease. *Circulation* 2000;101:1465–1478.

47. Vanoverschelde JL, Wijns W, Essamri B, et al. Hemodynamic and mechanical determinants of myocardial O2 consumption in normal human heart: effects of dobutamine. *Am J Physiol* 1993;265:H1884–H1892.

48. Berman M, Fischman AJ, Southern J, et al. Myocardial adaptation during and after sustained, demand-induced ischemia. Observations in closed-chest, domestic swine. *Circulation* 1996;94:755–762.

49. Holmvang G, Fry S, Skopicki HA, et al. Relation between coronary "steal" and contractile function at rest in collateral-dependent myocardium of humans with ischemic heart disease. *Circulation* 1999; 99:2510–2516.

50. Ruiz M, Takehana K, Petruzella FD, et al. Arbutamine stress perfusion imaging in dogs with critical coronary artery stenoses: (99m)Tc-sestamibi versus (201)Tl. *J Nucl Med* 2002;43:664–670.

51. Glover DK, Okada RD. Myocardial kinetics of Tc-MIBI in canine myocardium after dipyridamole. *Circulation* 1990;81:628–636.

52. Sinusas AJ, Beller GA, Smith WH, et al. Quantitative planar imaging with technetium-99m methoxyisobutyl isonitrile: comparison of uptake patterns with thallium-201. *J Nucl Med* 1989;30:1456–1463.

53. Verani M. Thallium-201 and technetium-99m perfusion agents where are we in 1992? In: Zaret BL, Beller GA, eds. *Nuclear cardiology: state of the art and future directions.* St. Louis: Mosby-Year Book, 1993:216–224.

54. Gewirtz H, Fischman AJ, Abraham SA, et al. Positron emission tomographic measurements of absolute regional myocardial blood flow permits identification of nonviable myocardium in patients with chronic myocardial infarction. *J Am Coll Cardiol* 1994;23:851–859.

55. Bax JJ, Wijns W, Cornel JH, et al. Accuracy of currently available techniques for prediction of functional recovery after revascularization in patients with left ventricular dysfunction due to chronic coronary artery disease: comparison of pooled data. *J Am Coll Cardiol* 1997;30:1451–1460.

56. Dilsizian V, Perrone-Filardi P, Arrighi JA, et al. Concordance and discordance between stress-redistribution-reinjection and rest-redistribution thallium imaging for assessing viable myocardium. Comparison with metabolic activity by positron emission tomography. *Circulation* 1993; 88:941–952.

57. Berman DS, Kiat H, Friedman JD, et al. Separate acquisition rest thallium-201/stress technetium-99m sestamibi dual-isotope myocardial perfusion single-photon emission computed tomography: a clinical validation study. *J Am Coll Cardiol* 1993;22:1455–1464.

58. Faber TL, Cooke CD, Folks RD, et al. Left ventricular function and perfusion from gated SPECT perfusion images: an integrated method. *J Nucl Med* 1999;40:650–659.

59. Vallejo E, Dione DP, Bruni WL, et al. Reproducibility and accuracy of gated SPECT for determination of left ventricular volumes and ejection fraction: experimental validation using MRI. *J Nucl Med* 2000; 41:874–882.

60. Vallejo E, Dione DP, Sinusas AJ, et al. Assessment of left ventricular ejection fraction with quantitative gated SPECT: accuracy and correlation with first-pass radionuclide angiography. *J Nucl Cardiol* 2000;7: 461–470.

61. Smanio PE, Watson DD, Segalla DL, et al. Value of gating of technetium-99m sestamibi single-photon emission computed tomographic imaging. *J Am Coll Cardiol* 1997;30:1687–1692.

62. Picano E. Stress echocardiography. From pathophysiological toy to diagnostic tool. *Circulation* 1992;85:1604–1612.

63. Gunda M, Mulvagh SL. Recent advances in myocardial contrast echocardiography. *Curr Opin Cardiol* 2001;16:231–239.

64. Marwick T, D'Hondt AM, Baudhuin T, et al. Optimal use of dobutamine stress for the detection and evaluation of coronary artery disease: combination with echocardiography or scintigraphy, or both? *J Am Coll Cardiol* 1993;22:159–167.

65. Segar DS, Brown SE, Sawada SG, et al. Dobutamine stress echocardiography: correlation with coronary lesion severity as determined by quantitative angiography. *J Am Coll Cardiol* 1992;19:1197–1202.

66. Mazeika PK, Nadazdin A, Oakley CM. Prognostic value of dobutamine echocardiography in patients with high pretest likelihood of coronary artery disease. *Am J Cardiol* 1993;71:33–39.

67. Williams MJ, Odabashian J, Lauer MS, et al. Prognostic value of dobutamine echocardiography in patients with left ventricular dysfunction. *J Am Coll Cardiol* 1996;27:132–139.

68. Senior R, Soman P, Khattar RS, et al. Prognostic value of dobutamine stress echocardiography in patients undergoing diagnostic coronary arteriography. *Am J Cardiol* 1997;79:1610–1614.

69. Poldermans D, Rambaldi R, Fioretti PM, et al. Prognostic value of dobutamine-atropine stress echocardiography for peri-operative and late cardiac events in patients scheduled for vascular surgery. *Eur Heart J* 1997;18[Suppl D]:D86–D96.

70. Poldermans D, Arnese M, Fioretti PM, et al. Sustained prognostic value of dobutamine stress echocardiography for late cardiac events after major noncardiac vascular surgery. *Circulation* 1997;95: 53–58.

71. Singh BK, Chaudhry FA. Echocardiographic assessment of viable myocardium. *Prog Cardiovasc Dis* 2001;43:351–361.

72. Meluzin J, Cigarroa CG, Brickner ME, et al. Dobutamine echocardiography in predicting improvement in global left ventricular systolic function after coronary bypass or angioplasty in patients with healed myocardial infarcts. *Am J Cardiol* 1995;76:877–880.

73. Afridi I, Grayburn PA, Panza JA, et al. Myocardial viability during dobutamine echocardiography predicts survival in patients with coronary artery disease and severe left ventricular systolic dysfunction. *J Am Coll Cardiol* 1998;32:921–926.

74. Nagueh SF, Vaduganathan P, Ali N, et al. Identification of hibernating myocardium: comparative accuracy of myocardial contrast echocardiography, rest-redistribution thallium-201 tomography and dobutamine echocardiography. *J Am Coll Cardiol* 1997;29:985–993.

75. Hoffmann R, Lethen H, Falter F, et al. Dobutamine stress echocardiography after coronary artery bypass grafting. Transthoracic vs biplane transoesophageal imaging. *Eur Heart J* 1996;17:222–229.

76. Panza JA, Laurienzo JM, Curiel RV, et al. Transesophageal dobutamine stress echocardiography for evaluation of patients with coronary artery disease. *J Am Coll Cardiol* 1994;24:1260–1267.

77. Prince CR, Stoddard MF, Morris GT, et al. Dobutamine two-dimensional transesophageal echocardiographic stress testing for detection of coronary artery disease. *Am Heart J* 1994;128:36–41.

78. Laurienzo JM, Cannon RO, Quyyumi AA, et al. Improved specificity of transesophageal dobutamine stress echocardiography compared to standard tests for evaluation of coronary artery disease in women presenting with chest pain. *Am J Cardiol* 1997;80:1402–1407.

79. Kamalesh M, Matorin R, Sawada S. Comparative prognostic significance of transesophageal versus transthoracic stress echocardiography. *Echocardiography* 2002;19:313–318.

80. Choi Y, Huang SC, Hawkins RA, et al. A simplified method for quantification of myocardial blood flow using nitrogen-13-ammonia and dynamic PET. *J Nucl Med* 1993;34:488–497.

81. Gewirtz H, Skopicki HA, Abraham SA, et al. Quantitative PET measurements of regional myocardial blood flow: observations in humans with ischemic heart disease. *Cardiology* 1997;88:62–70.

82. Schelbert HR. PET contributions to understanding normal and abnormal cardiac perfusion and metabolism. *Ann Biomed Eng* 2000;28:922–929.

83. Schelbert HR, Phelps ME, Huang SC, et al. N-13 ammonia as an indicator of myocardial blood flow. *Circulation* 1981;63:1259–1272.

84. Shah A, Schelbert HR, Schwaiger M, et al. Measurement of regional myocardial blood flow with N-13 ammonia and positron-emission tomography in intact dogs. *J Am Coll Cardiol* 1985;5:92–100.

85. Uren NG, Melin JA, De Bruyne B, et al. Relation between myocardial

blood flow and the severity of coronary artery stenosis. *N Engl J Med* 1994;330:1782–1788.

86. Tawakol A, Skopicki HA, Abraham SA, et al. Evidence of reduced resting blood flow in viable myocardial regions with chronic asynergy. *J Am Coll Cardiol* 2000;36:2146–2153.

87. Gould KL. Coronary collateral function assessed by PET. In: Gould KL, ed. *Coronary artery stenosis and reversing atherosclerosis,* 2nd ed. New York: Arnold/Oxford University Press, 1999.

88. Bonow RO, Berman DS, Gibbons RJ, et al. Cardiac positron emission tomography. A report for health professionals from the Committee on Advanced Cardiac Imaging and Technology of the Council on Clinical Cardiology, American Heart Association. *Circulation* 1991;84: 447–454.

89. Brunken R, Schwaiger M, Grover-McKay M, et al. Positron emission tomography detects tissue metabolic activity in myocardial segments with persistent thallium perfusion defects. *J Am Coll Cardiol* 1987; 10:557–567.

90. Tillisch J, Brunken R, Marshall R, et al. Reversibility of cardiac wall-motion abnormalities predicted by positron tomography. *N Engl J Med* 1986;314:884–888.

91. Maddahi J, Schelbert H, Brunken R, et al. Role of thallium-201 and PET imaging in evaluation of myocardial viability and management of patients with coronary artery disease and left ventricular dysfunction. *J Nucl Med* 1994;35:707–715.

92. Blankenship J, Iliadis L. Coronary magnetic resonance angiography. *N Engl J Med* 2002;346:1413–1414.

93. Worthley SG, Helft G, Fayad ZA, et al. Cardiac gated breath-hold black blood MRI of the coronary artery wall: an in vivo and ex vivo comparison. *Int J Cardiovasc Imaging* 2001;17:195–201.

94. Fayad ZA, Fuster V. Clinical imaging of the high-risk or vulnerable atherosclerotic plaque. *Circ Res* 2001;89:305–316.

95. Kim WY, Danias PG, Stuber M, et al. Coronary magnetic resonance angiography for the detection of coronary stenoses. *N Engl J Med* 2001;345:1863–1869.

96. Nagel E, Lehmkuhl HB, Bocksch W, et al. Noninvasive diagnosis of ischemia-induced wall motion abnormalities with the use of high-dose dobutamine stress MRI: comparison with dobutamine stress echocardiography. *Circulation* 1999;99:763–770.

97. Panting JR, Gatehouse PD, Yang GZ, et al. Abnormal subendocardial perfusion in cardiac syndrome X detected by cardiovascular magnetic resonance imaging. *N Engl J Med* 2002;346:1948–1953.

98. Ibrahim T, Nekolla SG, Schreiber K, et al. Assessment of coronary flow reserve: comparison between contrast-enhanced magnetic resonance imaging and positron emission tomography. *J Am Coll Cardiol* 2002;39:864–870.

99. Baer FM, Theissen P, Crnac J, et al. Head to head comparison of dobutamine-transoesophageal echocardiography and dobutamine-magnetic resonance imaging for the prediction of left ventricular functional recovery in patients with chronic coronary artery disease. *Eur Heart J* 2000;21:981–991.

100. Gunning MG, Anagnostopoulos C, Knight CJ, et al. Comparison of 201Tl, 99mTc-tetrofosmin, and dobutamine magnetic resonance imaging for identifying hibernating myocardium. *Circulation* 1998;98:1869–1874.

CHAPTER 89

Medical Management

John D. Rutherford

Key Words: Angiotensin-converting enzyme inhibitors; β-blockers; calcium antagonists; chronic stable angina; high-density lipoprotein cholesterol; low-density lipoprotein cholesterol; myocardial infarction; nitrate.

INTRODUCTION

Traditionally, clinicians have based treatment plans on the symptomatic response of patients with stable angina to therapy. In general, each of the major classes of therapeutic agents (nitrates, β-blockers, and calcium antagonists) have reduced symptoms and improved exercise performance. In addition to providing symptomatic relief and increased freedom to participate in normal daily activities, it has been our hope that various therapies will prevent the occurrence of acute myocardial infarction (AMI) and reduce mortality in patients with chronic stable angina. There is no substantive evidence that any of these therapies mentioned reduces mortality in patients with chronic stable angina. However, there is evidence that aspirin and effective lipid-lowering regimens will reduce both morbidity and mortality (Table 89–1).

In 25% to 50% of patients with chronic stable angina, episodes of asymptomatic ischemia (detected by ambulatory electrocardiographic monitoring) occur (1–3), and this asymptomatic ischemia as a part of the "total ischemic burden" has been linked to adverse events (4–7). Specifically, in patients with stable symptoms of coronary disease, the presence of ischemia on ambulatory monitoring has been a significant predictor of outcome, whereas exercise test charac-

teristics have not (4). Patients with evidence of ischemia recorded on ambulatory monitoring during daily activities have a worse prognosis than patients free from such episodes (5). It is currently believed that ambulatory ischemia may be a powerful and independent predictor of subsequent myocardial infarction (MI) and death (6,7). Interestingly, this type of asymptomatic ischemia can occur at a heart rate threshold 10% to 20% less than the threshold for ischemia during an exercise stress test, suggesting that coronary artery vasoconstriction may play a role, and it has been demonstrated that this can occur about 20% of the time (8). A number of trials suggest that asymptomatic ischemia can be suppressed in patients with coronary artery disease (1,9–11) and that β-blockers administered in relatively modest doses seem more effective than calcium channel antagonists in suppressing this ischemia (1,10,12). Although if the mean heart rate is reduced to a similar degree, diltiazem will reduce the ischemic episodes as effectively as atenolol (13). The Atenolol Silent Ischemia Study of asymptomatic or minimally symptomatic patients with proven coronary disease, exercise-induced ischemia, and evidence of asymptomatic ischemia during a 48-hour ambulatory electrocardiographic monitoring showed that atenolol reduced daily-life ischemia and was associated with reduced risk for adverse outcome (11). The Asymptomatic Cardiac Ischemia Pilot (ACIP) Study in 558 patients with coronary anatomy amenable to revascularization randomized patients to different treatment strategies: medication to suppress angina, medication to suppress angina and to eliminate ambulatory electrocardiographic ischemia, or revascularization of patients by percutaneous coronary intervention (PCI) or bypass surgery. Each strategy reduced cardiac ischemia in 40%

J. D. Rutherford: Division of Cardiology, University of Texas Southwestern, Dallas, Texas 75390-8831.

TABLE 89–1. *Pharmacology of chronic stable angina and patients at high risk*

Drug	Benefits			
	Reduce mortality	Prevent AMI	Reduce angina or improve exercise	Disadvantages
Aspirin	+	+		Bleeding
Lipid-lowering agents	+	+		Liver dysfunction
Nitrates			+	Tolerance, hypotension
β-Blockers			+	Bronchoconstriction, AV block, reduce contractility
Calcium blockers			+	Hypotension, AV block, reduce contractility
ACE inhibitors	+	+		Cough

ACE, angiotensin-converting enzyme; AMI, acute myocardial infarction; AV, atrioventricular.

to 55% of patients (1), but follow-up at 3 months, 6 months, and 1 year demonstrated that revascularization was more likely to completely suppress ischemia (14).

ASPIRIN

In patients with coronary artery disease, disruption of atherothrombotic plaques, with subsequent formation of mural thrombus and fibrotic organization of thrombus, may contribute to the progression of coronary atherothrombosis and the syndromes of unstable angina, AMI, and sudden death (15,16). In all patients with symptomatic coronary artery disease (chronic stable angina) it is likely that aspirin therapy is beneficial. In platelets, aspirin prevents the formation of thromboxane A_2 (a substance that facilitates platelet aggregation) for the lifetime of the platelet (about 10 days). In vascular endothelial cells, aspirin also prevents the synthesis of prostacyclin (a substance that inhibits platelet aggregation), but this effect is probably of a shorter duration because endothelial cells can recover cyclooxygenase synthesis, which is irreversibly inhibited in platelets. Numerous clinical studies suggest that the antithrombotic effects of aspirin probably operate through inhibition of thromboxane A_2 (15–17).

The efficacy of aspirin in reducing fatal and morbid events is established for patients with AMI and unstable angina (18). Aspirin should be used in patients with AMI regardless of whether thrombolytic therapy is given (15). Similarly, three major randomized, placebo-controlled, double-blind studies have shown in patients with unstable angina or non–Q-wave infarction that aspirin therapy reduces the risk for MI or death (19–21). In the Veterans Administration Cooperative Study and the Canadian Multicenter Trial, large doses of aspirin were used; but in the RISC Study, efficacy was seen in men with unstable angina using a dosage of 75 mg aspirin daily (20).

Until recently, the evidence that aspirin may be beneficial in patients with *chronic stable angina* has been less impressive. In the Physicians' Health Study (a primary-prevention trial) (22), low-dose aspirin (325 mg on alternate days) was associated with a highly significant reduction in risk for a first MI. In more than 300 male physicians in this study who had chronic stable angina (with no prior history of MI,

stroke, or a transient ischemic attack), aspirin therapy did not reduce the incidence of symptomatic angina pectoris (23), but it did reduce the risk for MI during 5 years of follow-up by 87% (24). Furthermore, in a study of 2,035 male and female patients with a history of angina for more than 1 month but no history of prior MI, aspirin therapy (75 mg/d) resulted in a 34% risk reduction of the incidence of MI and sudden death during a follow-up period of 50 months (25).

Therefore, as for patients with MI and unstable angina, patients with chronic stable angina should be treated with aspirin. It has been shown that low-dose aspirin therapy (75 mg/d) is clinically effective and can significantly reduce chronic thromboxane synthesis and prevent release of thromboxane into the plasma during acute episodes of myocardial ischemia while preserving endothelial prostacyclin synthesis (26).

LIPID REDUCTION

Both men and women with known coronary artery disease have a substantially increased risk for development of an AMI compared with populations who have no prior clinical manifestations of coronary disease (27–29). In patients with coronary disease, total cholesterol and low-density lipoprotein (LDL) cholesterol are predictors of future MI (27,30, 31), even for patients with relatively low cholesterol levels (30). Analyses of secondary prevention trials suggest that cholesterol-lowering therapy reduces both recurrent coronary events and mortality (32–34). Furthermore, coronary angiographic studies have shown that intensive cholesterol reduction will retard the rate of progression of documented atherothrombosis and, in some patients, will lead to modest regression of atherothrombotic lesions (9,35–40). In major primary-prevention trials, up to 5 years of therapy has been required to show benefit (41,42). Secondary-prevention trials have demonstrated a reduction in total death rate (33) without a significant increase in noncardiovascular deaths, including those from injury, homicide, suicide, or cancer. Finally, there is accumulating evidence that 3-hydroxy-3-methylglutaryl coenzyme A (HMG-CoA) reductase inhibitors have both lipid-lowering and antiinflammatory properties (43,44), which together may play a role in modifying the pathogenesis of acute coronary events.

All patients who have established coronary heart disease or other evidence of clinical atherothrombotic disease should have lipoprotein analysis for LDL cholesterol determination after an overnight fast, on 2 occasions, 1 to 8 weeks apart. In patients who have distinct increases of LDL cholesterol levels, the third report of the Expert Panel on Detection, Evaluation, and Treatment of High Blood Cholesterol in Adults suggested that prompt initiation of drug therapy is acceptable (45). The committee now believes that the target goal for LDL cholesterol reduction should be 70 mg/dL or less for persons with known coronary artery disease and for those with multiple risk factors and increased 10-year risk for coronary heart disease events (e.g., persons with diabetes). A number of patients with coronary heart disease have an "isolated" low high-density lipoprotein (HDL) cholesterol level (46). In this situation, encouragement should be given to cigarette smokers to stop smoking, an effort should be made to get patients to control weight optimally and to exercise, and careful treatment should be undertaken in patients with hypertension and diabetes mellitus. In men and women without clinically evident atherothrombotic cardiovascular disease and average cholesterol and LDL levels but below-average HDL levels who were treated with an HMG-CoA reductase inhibitor, lovastatin, for 5 years, the incidence of first acute major coronary events and coronary revascularization procedures was reduced (47).

NITRATES

Organic nitrates are used chronically as prophylaxis against myocardial ischemia and also acutely to terminate angina. Nitrate therapy in the form of sublingual nitroglycerin, long-acting oral nitrates, and transdermal nitroglycerin preparations reduces ischemia frequency (silent and symptomatic) in patients with angina (48).

Organic nitrates relax vascular smooth muscle. Dilation of veins and arteries occurs when nitric oxide is produced after the interaction of organic nitrates with sulfhydryl groups. Nitric oxide then initiates the conversion of guanosine triphosphate to cyclic guanosine monophosphate by activating the enzyme guanylate cyclase. Thus, nitric oxide stimulates guanylate cyclase resulting in the formation of cyclic guanosine monophosphate, which causes smooth muscle relaxation. It is currently thought that nitric oxide plays a role in maintaining vasodilator tone by activation of endothelial cells by stimuli of shear stress and pulsatile flow (49). In addition, nitric oxide inhibits platelet aggravation responses through activation of guanylate cyclase (50).

Organic nitrates act by causing vasodilating effects on the systemic circulation by causing venodilation and increasing venous capacitance; as a result, cardiac venous return is decreased with a secondary reduction in ventricular volumes and pressures. In addition, and probably to a lesser extent, nitrates reduce arterial and arteriolar vasoconstrictor tone and decrease blood pressure, afterload, and ventricular vol-

umes. These changes in afterload and preload reduce myocardial oxygen needs. Organic nitrates have been shown to dilate both normal and stenotic epicardial coronary arteries (51), prevent exercise-induced constriction of stenotic arteries (52), and, in addition, attenuate the exercise-induced abnormalities in left ventricular end-diastolic pressure and left ventricular volume (53) and reduce the size of perfusion defects in patients with coronary disease (54).

The term "nitrate tolerance" refers to the attenuation or loss of the effects of organic nitrates when administered as frequent doses of long-acting nitrates, by continuous-delivery systems (intravenous infusion or transdermal patches), or as long-acting (sustained-release) preparations where "therapeutic" plasma nitrate concentrations are constantly maintained. Induction of nitrate tolerance is probably contributed to by several mechanisms (55–59). The development of tolerance has been demonstrated with depletion of intracellular sulfhydryl cofactors, which are required in the conversion of organic nitrates to nitric oxide, or S-nitrosothiols. Cysteine acts as a sulfhydryl group donor in the activation of organic nitrates, and, in humans, the administration of N-acetylcysteine and methionine (which are converted into cysteine) have reversed nitrate tolerance in some studies (60). There also is some evidence that a nonspecific interaction exists between nitroglycerin and N-acetylcysteine, because the hemodynamic effects of nitroglycerin can be potentiated (and episodes of hypotension can occur) when both agents are coadministered (60,61). It is possible that neurohormonal responses initiated by the hypotensive actions of organic nitrates may act to attenuate or reverse the effects of nitrates. Continuous administration of organic nitrates in healthy volunteers has been associated with increases in plasma renin activity, plasma norepinephrine, and arginine vasopressin (62). In addition, plasma volume expansion and sodium retention have been observed (57). Finally, prolonged administration of nitroglycerin leads to a decrease in the hematocrit, sodium retention, and plasma volume expansion (62,63). Attenuation of organic nitrate effect also has been thought to be related to an increase in intravascular volume resulting from activation of the renin-angiotensin system and limiting the ability of the drug to decrease cardiac filling pressures. It seems that the plasma volume expansion is caused primarily by a fluid shift from the extravascular compartment to the intravascular space after continuous therapy with organic nitrates, and in healthy volunteers, diuretic therapy does not prevent this plasma volume expansion (64). Also, an angiotensin-converting enzyme inhibitor did not modify the hemodynamic responses to continuous transdermal nitroglycerin therapy in healthy volunteers (63). Therefore, it is likely that plasma volume expansion plays a more important role than neurohormonal responses in the loss of nitrate effects during sustained therapy in healthy volunteers.

In patients with stable angina, attenuation of nitrate effect has been demonstrated both with long-acting oral nitrates (isosorbide dinitrate) and transdermal nitrate patches (57,65). After three doses of isosorbide dinitrate administered at 8 AM, 1 PM, and 6 PM, successive reduction in the mean exercise time to angina has been demonstrated (65). If a nitrate patch is applied for 24 hours, there is an early increase in time to exercise-induced angina, but after continuous therapy for 24 hours, there is no significant increase in exercise duration despite persistent decreases in systolic blood pressure and "therapeutic" blood plasma nitroglycerin levels. In patients randomized to either placebo or intermittent active nitroglycerin patch therapy (0.4 mg/h, 12 hours on and 12 hours off), nitroglycerin reduced the size of exercise-induced thallium-201 perfusion defects compared with patients treated with placebo, confirming the efficacy of organic nitrates in reducing myocardial ischemia (54).

β-BLOCKERS

The β receptor is located on the cell membrane and is linked by the G protein system, when it is in the stimulatory configuration, to the adenylate cyclase system. Activated adenylate cyclase produces adenosine monophosphate from adenosine triphosphate. Cyclic adenosine monophosphate is the messenger within the cell after β receptor stimulation and it acts to open calcium channels and promote a positive inotropic effect, as well as a relaxing or lusitropic effect (by increasing the reuptake of cytosolic calcium into the sarcoplasmic reticulum). β Receptors have been classically divided into β_1 receptors, which are found in myocardium (β_2 receptors also exist there), and β_2 receptors of vascular smooth muscle and bronchial muscle (Table 89–2). The effect of any given β-blocking drug depends on pharmacologic properties, such as absorption, binding to plasma proteins, and lipid solubility, and also on its ability to block or inhibit the β receptor. Most β-blocking drugs have some capacity to activate the receptor (agonist activity), which is also called intrinsic sympathomimetic activity (ISA).

Many β-blockers act on all the β receptors, β_1 and β_2 (e.g., propranolol, timolol, nadolol, sotalol), and therefore are termed nonselective β-blockers. Other agents, given in appropriate dosage, are relatively selective (66) and tend to act on mainly β_1 receptors (e.g., atenolol, metoprolol, and acebutolol). With high doses of these latter agents cardioselectivity is lost or is diminished. It is important for the clinician to understand that this β_1 selectivity does not confer protection for the patient with asthma and that bronchial constriction may still occur in susceptible patients. Newer agents with β-blocking properties may also have the ability to cause vasodilation, for example, labetalol (a β_2 agonist and an α-adrenergic blocking drug).

The lipid solubility (or hydrophilicity) of β-blockers determines their manner of absorption and metabolism. In general, the lipid-soluble agents are readily absorbed from the gastrointestinal tract, are metabolized predominantly by the liver, have a relatively short half-life, are more likely to cross the blood–brain barrier, and usually require administration twice or more daily to achieve adequate pharmacologic effect (e.g., propranolol, metoprolol, pindolol). Lipid-soluble β-blockers are metabolized extensively by the liver (first-pass metabolism) before they reach the systemic circulation, and for this reason, intravenous dosing of such agents has much greater potency than oral dosing (e.g., propranolol and metoprolol) (66). The water-soluble β-blockers are not as readily absorbed from the gastrointestinal tract, are not as extensively metabolized, have relatively long plasma half-lives, and often can be administered once daily. Such agents are preferable in patients with hepatic or renal dysfunction and are less likely to cross the blood–brain barrier (e.g., atenolol, sotalol, and nadolol). The correlation among lipid solubility, crossing the blood–brain barrier, and central nervous system side effects of β-blockers is inconsistent. Side effects attributed to disturbance of the central nervous system, including depression, nightmares, sleep disturbances, fatigue, and weakness, occur to an equal degree with atenolol and metoprolol, despite large differences in lipid solubility (67).

In the clinical setting, β-blocking drugs attenuate the cardiac responses to adrenergic stimuli (mainly increases in heart rate and contractility) and act to reduce myocardial oxygen demand during exercise or times of increased sympathetic activity. They also reduce arterial pressure. The term *potency* refers to the ability of β-blockers to inhibit the tachycardia produced by isoproterenol. The reference drug is propranolol, which is given a value of 1.0; by comparison, timolol and pindolol are the most potent agents (values of 6.0), and acebutolol and labetalol are the least potent (values of 0.3). Agents equivalent in potency to propranolol include atenolol, metoprolol, and nadolol.

Although it is important for the clinician to know the influence of an administered β-blocker on resting heart rate, it is probably more important to observe the influence of the drug during exercise when sympathetic activity is heightened. In general, the goal is to reduce resting heart rate to 50 to 60 beats per minute, and with moderate exercise, an increase of

TABLE 89–2. β-blockers

	Acebutolol	Atenolol	Metoprolol	Nadolol	Pindolol	Propranolol	Sotalol	Timolol
Cardioselective (mainly β_1 receptors)	+	+	+					
Nonselective (β_1 and β_2 receptors)				+	+	+	+	+
Lipid solubility	Low	Low	Moderate	Low	Moderate	High	Low	Low
Intrinsic sympathetic activity	+							

less than 20 to 30 beats per minute in heart rate should occur. To the extent that attenuation of the heart rate responses to increased sympathetic activity is a major mechanism by which β-blocking drugs help patients with angina pectoris, cardioselectivity is not usually a major consideration in the selection of agents, because at the doses required to appropriately alter heart rate, both β₁ and β₂ receptors are blocked.

The author believes that a history of asthma or wheezing constitutes an absolute contraindication to the use of β-blockers, because effective heart rate control can usually be achieved with calcium channel blockers (diltiazem or verapamil). Too little attention is paid by clinicians to the response of the angina patient's heart rate to mild or moderate exercise in formulating the appropriate dosage or agent.

In addition to reducing myocardial oxygen demand, β-blockade may also improve myocardial oxygen supply. During normal daily activities in the patient with chronic stable angina, continuous ambulatory electrocardiographic and intraarterial blood pressure monitoring suggest that many ischemic events may be precipitated by transient impairment of regional myocardial perfusion rather than by increases in myocardial oxygen demand. In such patients, β-blockers have been shown to reduce significantly episodes of transient myocardial ischemia (11). Indeed, in the Atenolol Silent Ischemia Study (ASIST), more than 300 patients with mild or no angina, abnormal exercise tests, and ischemia on ambulatory monitoring were randomized to receive either placebo or atenolol (100 mg/d). After 4 weeks of treatment, the number and average duration of ischemic episodes as recorded on 48-hour ambulatory monitoring decreased in the patients treated with atenolol. Furthermore, atenolol treatment was associated with reduced risk for adverse outcome (11).

Usually these drugs are well tolerated by the majority of patients with angina pectoris; however, their β-blocking properties can lead to adverse effects (severe sinus bradycardia, atrioventricular [AV] block, reduced left ventricular contractility, fatigue, depression, nightmares, sexual dysfunction). In usual therapeutic doses, the membrane-stabilizing activity or "quinidine-like" effect of certain β-blockers (propranolol, acebutolol) is not relevant. However, if a patient taking a lipid-soluble β-blocker exhibits an exaggerated clinical response (e.g., extreme bradycardia), this may be because of slow oxidative metabolism of the drug and prolongation of the elimination half-life (68). It is

possible that the variability of the pharmacokinetics, drug metabolism, and pharmacodynamics of the lipid-soluble β-blockers is in part related to genetically determined rates of hydroxylation or metabolism. Abrupt withdrawal of β-blockers, particularly those with a short half-life (propranolol, pindolol, metoprolol), should be avoided because coronary events may be exacerbated (69).

β-Blocking drugs are known to alter serum lipids (Table 89–3). For example, propranolol can increase plasma triglycerides by up to 50% and reduce HDL cholesterol by approximately 15% (70,71). In general, other agents such as propranolol, which do not have ISA cause no significant changes in total cholesterol or LDL cholesterol, but they can increase triglyceride levels and decrease HDL cholesterol levels. An exception to this is sotalol, a drug without ISA, which increases total cholesterol and LDL cholesterol and triglycerides and also decreases HDL cholesterol. Pindolol and acebutolol, which have ISA, do not significantly change total cholesterol, triglyceride, or LDL cholesterol levels, but pindolol increases serum HDL cholesterol levels. In patient populations with chronic stable angina, the benefits of β-blocking drugs in general will outweigh these effects on cholesterol and triglyceride levels and do not constitute a contraindication to their use. In patients with chronic stable angina, close attention is now being paid to substantially decreasing lipid levels to achieve an LDL cholesterol level of 100 mg/dL or less as part of secondary prevention, and many patients will be taking both a β-blocker and a lipid-lowering agent.

There is some evidence that in the treatment of angina pectoris the use of a β-blocker alone, in maximally tolerated doses, confers as much benefit to a patient as using the combination of a β-blocker and a calcium channel antagonist. However, in patients who remain symptomatic despite maximally tolerated doses of β-blockers, the addition of a calcium channel antagonist has been shown to decrease the frequency of anginal attacks and increase exercise tolerance (72,73).

CALCIUM CHANNEL ANTAGONISTS

Calcium channel antagonists selectively inhibit the inward calcium current through the conventional (L-channel) so that less calcium is available to the contractile apparatus in smooth muscle and myocardium. In the myocardium, cal-

TABLE 89–3. Effect of β-blocking drugs on serum lipids

	Total cholesterol	Triglycerides	LDL cholesterol	HDL cholesterol
Without ISA				
All except sotalol	No change	Increase	No change	Increase
Sotalol	Increase	Increase	Increase	Decrease
With ISA				
Acebutolol	No change	No change	No change	No change
Pindolol	No change	No change	No change	Increase

HDL, high-density lipoprotein; ISA, intrinsic sympathomimetic activity; LDL, low-density lipoprotein.
Data from Lehtonen A. Effect of beta-blockers on blood lipid profile. *Am Heart J* 1985;109:1192–1196.

cium ions and troponin C facilitate actin–myosin interaction. In smooth muscle, calcium ions interact with calmodulin, which then stimulates myosin light-chain kinase to phosphorylate the myosin light chains and allow actin–myosin interaction.

All calcium channel antagonists inhibit the L-channel in arterial smooth muscle, leading to coronary vasodilation and afterload reduction (Table 89–4). In clinical dosages, the dihydropyridine calcium antagonists (nifedipine, nicardipine, amlodipine) cause significant arterial vasodilation and exert negligible influence on AV node conduction, and the arterial vasodilation usually counteracts their direct negative inotropic effect. In addition to arterial dilation, verapamil has a direct negative inotropic effect and has a major effect on AV nodal conduction. It increases AV block and the effective refractory period of the AV node, explaining its efficacy in the therapy of reentrant supraventricular arrhythmias and in reducing the ventricular rate in patients with atrial flutter and fibrillation. It also has a direct negative inotropic effect. Diltiazem appears to affect AV nodal conduction to a lesser degree than verapamil, but it also is active on the sinoatrial node and can reduce heart rate effectively. Diltiazem also has a direct negative inotropic effect.

Nifedipine

Nifedipine is a more potent vasodilator than either diltiazem or verapamil, but in clinical practice the potential negative inotropic effects and effects on AV conduction are rarely a problem. There is a high first-pass hepatic metabolism of nifedipine. Nifedipine is a useful therapeutic agent in patients with chronic stable angina (particularly if they have associated hypertension) and in patients with coronary artery spasm, but it should not be used as a single agent in patients with unstable angina (74). In patients with unstable angina, the addition of nifedipine to β-blocker therapy (75) or to a combination of nitrates and β-blockers (74) is useful in relieving angina (75) and reducing the subsequent short-term risk for death or MI or the need for urgent coronary surgery (76). In patients with chronic stable angina, if symptoms persist despite optimal doses of a β-blocker, then the addition of a calcium antagonist (including nifedipine) is likely to reduce angina and improve exercise performance

(77). Obviously, in patients with AV conduction system disease, a dihydropyridine type of calcium antagonist is preferred. Because it has been found that maximally tolerated doses of nifedipine result in a significant increase in heart rate at rest and at peak exercise, in patients with chronic stable angina, this agent is usually used in combination with a β-blocking agent (78). Provided the appropriate dosage of the drug is used, it is usually safe; however, it can cause hypotension with associated symptoms. The bilateral ankle edema associated with nifedipine use can be troublesome and is to some extent dose dependent. Adverse effects appear to be minimized by use of the extended-release preparations.

Diltiazem

The pharmacologic actions of diltiazem are intermediate between those of verapamil and nifedipine. Diltiazem is a less potent vasodilator than nifedipine and it is less likely to inhibit AV nodal conduction than verapamil, although it will reduce heart rate by its actions on the sinoatrial node. In patients with coronary artery disease, diltiazem has been demonstrated to have a peripheral vasodilator effect; it has a negative inotropic effect, although left ventricular relaxation is improved (79), and it has been demonstrated to prevent exercise-induced coronary vasoconstriction (80). Diltiazem undergoes first-pass hepatic metabolism and is acetylated in the liver, so that whereas 90% of the agent is absorbed after oral administration, approximately 45% is available. Most of the drug is excreted by the gastrointestinal tract, in contrast to verapamil and nifedipine, which are excreted more by the kidneys. Diltiazem is a useful drug in patients with chronic stable angina because it decreases heart rate, does not have a profound effect on AV conduction, and is not associated with severe constipation (as is verapamil), and it is less likely to cause ankle edema than is nifedipine. However, the combination of nifedipine and a β-blocker is less likely to cause problems with significant bradycardia or impaired AV conduction than is the combination of diltiazem and a β-blocker.

Verapamil

Verapamil has been in use for more than 30 years and causes dilation of systemic and coronary arterial vessels, has a significant direct negative inotropic effect, and increases AV block. Accordingly, it has been used in patients with supraventricular arrhythmias, chronic stable angina, and hypertension.

The drug is almost completely absorbed after oral administration, but because of a high first-past liver metabolism (to norverapamil, an active metabolic), most of the drug is excreted by the kidneys and less by the gastrointestinal tract. The most troublesome side effect of the drug is constipation (especially in the elderly), and it causes ankle edema in a similar frequency to diltiazem (but less than nifedipine). Its

TABLE 89–4. *Calcium channel antagonists*

Clinical effect	Nifedipine	Diltiazem	Verapamil
Coronary artery dilation	+++	++	++
Peripheral arterial dilation	+++	++	++
Negative clinical inotropic effects	+	++	+++
Atrioventricular node depression	–	+	+++
Sinus node depression	–	+	++

major action on AV nodal conduction is its strength and its weakness. Because of this property it is particularly useful in treating patients who have chronic stable angina and atrial fibrillation, because it effectively controls the ventricular response. It also is clearly useful in patients with a combination of chronic stable angina and hypertension provided they do not have sick sinus syndrome or preexisting AV nodal disease. In studies of patients with exercise-induced angina, verapamil compares favorably with β-blocker therapy (usually propranolol) in reducing symptoms, and in one study verapamil was more effective than propranolol as an antianginal agent (81). Extreme care should be used if the combination of verapamil and a β-blocker is contemplated. Although some patients will tolerate oral regimens of both drugs, administration of intravenous verapamil to a patient taking oral β-blockers or of intravenous β-blockers to a patient taking oral verapamil should be avoided. If a β-blocker is to be used in combination with verapamil, it is probably wise to choose a water-soluble β-blocker (atenolol or nadolol) that is not extensively metabolized by the liver.

ANGIOTENSIN-CONVERTING ENZYME INHIBITORS

In survivors of AMI (82) and in patients with low ejection fractions (83), treatment with angiotensin-converting enzyme inhibitors has been shown to reduce subsequent ischemic events (recurrent MI [82–84] and subsequent hospitalization with unstable angina [83]). These findings have been now extended to patients at high risk for cardiovascular events (55 years or older, evidence of vascular disease or diabetes and one other cardiovascular risk factor) without overtly impaired cardiac function who were randomized to placebo or ramipril (10 mg daily) for a mean of 5 years (85). It was found that therapy with the angiotensin-converting enzyme inhibitor reduced cardiovascular deaths, MI, and stroke. Thus, the benefits of angiotensin-converting enzyme inhibitors may now be extended to patients at high risk for cardiovascular events.

COMBINATION THERAPY

All patients with chronic stable angina should receive lifelong aspirin (if tolerated), their lipid profile should be assessed, and, if appropriate, they should receive aggressive dietary or pharmacologic lipid-lowering therapy, or both. The recommendation for lifelong aspirin therapy is based on the accumulated evidence of its efficacy in preventing fatal and morbid events in survivors of AMI, patients with unstable angina, and, more recently, patients with chronic stable angina. The accumulating evidence that effective total cholesterol (or LDL cholesterol) reduction will reduce total mortality and cardiovascular mortality in secondary prevention trials is compelling. Furthermore, the importance of aggressive LDL reduction in individuals with diabetes without known coronary artery disease has been emphasized in recent guidelines (45).

Sublingual nitroglycerin remains the treatment of choice for acute anginal episodes, and the prophylactic use of sublingual nitroglycerin (before stressful situations or increased physical activity known to produce angina) is encouraged. Too few clinicians instruct their patients in the prophylactic use of nitroglycerin. Long-acting nitrate therapy as an adjunct to this is useful. Organic nitrates dilate both normal and stenotic epicardial coronary arteries (51), prevent exercise-induced constriction of stenotic arteries (52), and also attenuate exercise-induced abnormalities in left ventricular function. However, nitrate tolerance develops rapidly, and the rapid attenuation of the positive effects of long acting nitrates on exercise performance has been clearly demonstrated (65). Careful dosing regimens need to be formulated to provide a 10- or 12-hour nitrate-free interval within any 24-hour period. This interval should be designed to occur either at the time of minimal activity of the patient (i.e., during sleep) or at the time of maximum action of other antianginal drugs. During such a nitrate-free interval, use of sublingual nitroglycerin, either acutely or prophylactically, is important.

One of the major determinants of myocardial oxygen demand is heart rate, and to control heart rate at rest and during exercise β-blockers, diltiazem, or verapamil provide therapeutic options. It has been pointed out that the optimal use of these agents as monotherapy may be as effective in reducing angina and improving exercise performance as combination therapy (72,73). Nevertheless, it is clear that in patients who continue to have angina despite optimal β-blockade, the addition of a calcium antagonist is likely to reduce symptoms and improve exercise performance (77). Conversely, it is not clear that the addition of a β-blocker to therapy with diltiazem or verapamil improves antianginal efficacy (72), although combination of a β-blocker and nifedipine does. The newer long-acting preparations of the various agents are likely to lead to greater compliance, and in some instances adverse effects appear to be minimized (e.g., long-acting or extended-release nifedipine preparations). In patients with chronic stable angina, other conditions such as hypertension, heart failure, atrial fibrillation, diabetes mellitus, and conduction system disease play a major role in the choice of appropriate therapy. With care, both angina frequency and exercise performance can be improved. Finally, long-term therapy with the angiotensin-converting enzyme inhibitor ramipril has been shown to reduce cardiovascular events in patients at high risk (55 years or older, evidence of vascular disease or diabetes and one other cardiovascular risk factor).

MEDICAL THERAPY VERSUS REVASCULARIZATION

Angina is a diagnosis made by taking a careful history. In patients with a chronic, stable pattern of angina, in addition to historical information, two key pieces of information are required to plan overall management strategy: (a) knowledge of the patient's ventricular function and (b) the response of the patient to some form of stress testing. In patients with angina, significant coronary artery disease, and moderately or severely impaired left ventricular function, there is substantial evidence that if significant three-vessel coronary artery disease or two-vessel coronary artery disease with involvement of the proximal left anterior descending coronary artery exists, then revascularization should be considered, to prolong survival (86,87) (Table 89–5). Obviously, other factors are taken into consideration, such as age of the patient, sex, associated comorbid conditions such as pulmonary or renal disease, and whether the contemplated areas of myocardium for revascularization are viable rather than infarcted. It also is clear that patients with significant left main coronary artery stenoses should be revascularized for survival reasons if they are deemed appropriate candidates.

For these reasons, for patients with chronic stable angina who exhibit moderately or severely impaired left ventricular function (on the basis of myocardial ischemia) or who have a positive stress test at a low workload or at a workload that they would normally exceed during regular daily activities, strong consideration should be given to diagnostic cardiac catheterization. Normally, patients with left main coronary artery disease, severe stenoses of the three major coronary arteries, or a critical proximal stenosis of the left anterior descending coronary artery and one other coronary arteries will be candidates for revascularization. Apart from the efficacy of either angioplasty or bypass grafting surgery in relieving the frequency and severity of angina in patients who have not responded to medical therapy, revascularization

improves survival in patients with left main coronary artery disease and those with multivessel coronary artery disease who have involvement of the proximal left anterior descending artery and left ventricular systolic dysfunction (86). This strategy in part is a consequence of the European Coronary Surgery Study Group emphasizing that the presence of a significant proximal left anterior descending coronary artery stenosis (as a component of two- or three-vessel coronary artery disease) in a population of patients with stable angina pectoris and normal left ventricular ejection fractions was the strongest predictor of a poor prognosis with medical therapy and an improved prognosis with bypass grafting (87). In patients with multivessel coronary disease considered good candidates for either angioplasty or surgery, the rates of procedure-related mortality are similar (88,89). Patients undergoing bypass grafting are more likely to have procedure-related Q-wave MI, but most of these events are well tolerated (90). Subsequently, patients who undergo bypass grafting appear to have less angina and less requirement for antianginal medication and are less likely to need another revascularization procedure (90) than those treated by angioplasty. Although the categories of patients with improved long-term survival after revascularization surgery (compared with medical management) are to a large extent clearly established, similar long-term data for percutaneous transluminal coronary angioplasty are not available. In patients with significant two-vessel coronary artery disease, the options of medical therapy, PCI, and coronary artery bypass graft (CABG) surgery are considered (91,92). As mentioned previously, if a significant stenosis of the proximal left anterior descending coronary artery is a component of two-vessel coronary artery disease, then revascularization will be recommended to improve survival (86). In these patients, PCI represents an intermediate therapy between medical therapy and CABG surgery. PCI is a less traumatic revascularization procedure than CABG associated with a shorter hospital stay and convalescence; however, the relief of angina is less complete, and approximately 33% of patients need to be revascularized within 1 year (92). In other categories of significant two-vessel coronary artery disease, survival outcome is similar in patients who are treated medically or with revascularization, although the latter therapy provides better symptomatic relief. In patients with stable coronary artery disease, the prognosis for patients with preserved ventricular function and single-vessel disease is good, and PCI of a significant stenosis does not reduce the subsequent mortality or MI rate but does provide better symptomatic relief and improved exercise tolerance compared with medical therapy (93). Optimal lipid reduction as a component of medical therapy reduces subsequent myocardial ischemic events at least as effectively as PCI (94) and also reduces the risk for subsequent cardiac events after initial successful PCI (95). There are no current trials comparing morbidity and mortality in patients with stable one- or two-vessel coronary disease treated with optimal medical therapy (including aspirin, LDL reduction, β-blockers, and

TABLE 89–5. *Five-year survival with symptomatic coronary artery disease: medical therapy versus percutaneous transluminal coronary angioplasty versus coronary artery bypass grafting*

Disease type	Survival results
One-vessel disease	Medical equivalent to revascularization therapy
Two-vessel disease	
Without 95% LAD stenosis	Revascularization therapy better (PTCA better)
With 95% LAD stenosis	Revascularization therapy better (CABG better)
Three-vessel disease	Revascularization therapy better (CABG better)

Duke Cardiovascular Disease Databank cohort of patients with angina in 65% to 71%, prior myocardial infarction in 59% to 71%, heart failure in 7% to 17%, left ventricular ejection fractions ~52% (range 39–60%), one-vessel disease in 40%, two-vessel disease in 31%, and three-vessel disease in 29%.

[a]Medical therapy: n = 3,557; percutaneous transluminal coronary angioplasty (PTCA): n = 2,626; coronary artery bypass grafting (CABG): n = 3,080.

Adapted from Mark DB, Nelson CL, Califf RM, et al. Continuing evolution of therapy for coronary artery disease. Initial results from the era of coronary angioplasty. *Circulation* 1994;89:2015–2025.

angiotensin-converting inhibitors in patients at high risk) and PCI with the latest techniques. Nevertheless, the available data do not suggest an advantage of PCI over medical therapy for these patients except for symptomatic relief or in those patients with a proximal left anterior descending coronary artery stenosis (93,96).

SUMMARY

During daily activities many patients with chronic stable angina have asymptomatic ischemia detected by ambulatory electrocardiographic monitoring. This has been linked to adverse events. The ACIP study showed that revascularization and medical therapy used to suppress angina or to suppress angina and ambulatory ischemia reduced cardiac ischemia in 40% to 55% of patients (1), but follow-up at 3 months, 6 months, and 1 year demonstrated that revascularization was more likely to completely suppress ischemia (14).

Although each of the major classes of therapeutic agents (nitrates, β-blockers, and calcium antagonists) will reduce angina and improve exercise performance, only aspirin, effective lipid-lowering regimens, and the use of the angiotensin-converting enzyme inhibitor ramipril in patients at high risk have been clearly demonstrated to reduce both morbidity and mortality in patients with chronic stable angina. In addition to historical information, knowledge of the patient's ventricular function and response to some form of stress testing are essential in deciding whether to manage the patient medically or contemplate revascularization. The goals of revascularization are either to provide better symptom relief or to improve survival of patients compared with medical therapy. (There is no evidence that MI will be prevented by revascularization, although subsequent infarction may be better tolerated after revascularization). The categories of patients with improved long-term survival after revascularization surgery (compared with medical management) are to a large extent clearly established, although similar data for percutaneous transluminal coronary angioplasty are not yet available.

REFERENCES

1. Knatterud GL, Bourassa MG, Pepine CJ, et al. Effects of treatment strategies to suppress ischemia in patients with coronary artery disease: 12-week results of the Asymptomatic Cardiac Ischemia Pilot (ACIP) study. *J Am Coll Cardiol* 1994;24:11–20.
2. Mulcahy D, Keegan J, Crean P, et al. Silent myocardial ischemia in chronic stable angina: a study of its frequency and characteristics in 150 patients. *Br Heart J* 1988;60:417–423.
3. Deedwania PC, Carbajal EV. Prevalence and patterns of silent myocardial ischemia during daily life in stable angina patients receiving conventional antianginal drug therapy. *Am J Cardiol* 1990;65:1090–1096.
4. Rocco MB, Nabel EG, Campbell S, et al. Prognostic importance of myocardial ischemia detected by ambulatory monitoring in patients with stable coronary artery disease. *Circulation* 1988;78:877–884.
5. Tzivoni D, Weisz G, Gavish A, et al. A comparison of mortality and myocardial infarction rates in stable angina pectoris with and without ischemic episodes during daily activities. *Am J Cardiol* 1989;63:273–276.
6. Deedwania P, Carbajal EV. Silent ischemia during daily life is an independent predictor of mortality in stable angina. *Circulation* 1990;81:748–756.
7. Yeung AC, Barry J, Orav J, et al. Effects of asymptomatic ischemia on long-term prognosis in chronic stable coronary disease. *Circulation* 1991;83:1598–1604.
8. Andrews TC, Fenton T, Toyosaki N, et al. Subsets of ambulatory myocardial ischemia based on heart rate activity. Circadian distribution and response to anti-ischemic medication. The Angina and Silent Ischemia Study Group (ASIS). *Circulation* 1993;88:92–100.
9. Kane JP, Malloy MJ, Ports TA, et al. Regression of coronary atherosclerosis during treatment of familial hypercholesterolemia with combined drug regimens. *JAMA* 1990;264:3007–3012.
10. Stone PH, Gibson RS, Glasser SP, et al. Comparison of propranolol, diltiazem, and nifedipine in the treatment of ambulatory ischemia in patients with stable angina. Differential effects on ambulatory ischemia, exercise performance, and anginal symptoms. *Circulation* 1990;82:1962–1972.
11. Pepine CJ, Cohn PF, Deedwania PC, et al. Effects of treatment on outcome in mildly symptomatic patients with ischemia during daily life. The Atenolol Silent Ischemia Study (ASIST). *Circulation* 1994;90:762–768.
12. Pepine CJ. β-Blockers or calcium antagonists in silent ischemia? *Eur Heart J* 1993;14:7–14.
13. Pratt CM, McMahon S, Goldstein S, et al. Comparison of subgroups assigned to medical regimens used to suppress cardiac ischemia (the Asymptomatic Cardiac Ischemia Pilot (ACIP) Study. *J Am Coll Cardiol* 1996;77:1302–1309.
14. Rogers WJ, Bourassa MG, Andrews TC, et al. Asymptomatic Cardiac Ischemia Pilot (ACIP) Study: outcome at 1 year for patients with asymptomatic cardiac ischemia randomized to medical therapy or revascularization. *J Am Coll Cardiol* 1995;26:594–605.
15. Fuster V, Badimon L, Badimon JJ, et al. The pathogenesis of coronary artery disease and the acute coronary syndromes. *N Engl J Med* 1992;326:242–250,310–318.
16. Fuster V, Dyken ML, Vokonas PS, et al. Aspirin as a therapeutic agent in cardiovascular disease. AHA Medical/Scientific Statement. *Circulation* 1993;87:659–675.
17. Hirsh J, Dalen J, Fuster V, et al. Aspirin and other platelet active drugs: the relationship between dose, effectiveness, and side effects. *Chest* 1992;102[Suppl]:327S–336S.
18. Randomised trial of intravenous streptokinase, oral aspirin, both, or neither among 17,187 cases of suspected acute myocardial infarction: ISIS-2. ISIS-2 (Second International Study of Infarct Survival) Collaborative Group. *Lancet* 1988;2:349–360.
19. Lewis HD, Davis JW, Archibald GD, et al. Protective effects of aspirin against acute myocardial infarction and death in men with unstable angina. *N Engl J Med* 1983;309:396–403.
20. Risk of myocardial infarction and death during treatment with low dose aspirin and intravenous heparin in men with unstable coronary artery disease. The RISC Group. *Lancet* 1990;340:1421–1425.
21. Cairns JA, Gent M, Singer J, et al. Aspirin, sulfinpyrazone, or both in unstable angina. Results of a Canadian multicenter trial. *N Engl J Med* 1985;313:1369–1375.
22. Final report on the aspirin component of the ongoing physicians' health study. *N Engl J Med* 1989;321:129–135.
23. Manson JE, Grobbee DE, Stampfer MJ, et al. Aspirin in the primary prevention of angina pectoris in a randomized trial of United States physicians. *Am J Med* 1990;89:772–776.
24. Ridker PM, Manson JE, Gaziano M, et al. Low-dose aspirin therapy for chronic stable angina. *Ann Intern Med* 1991;114:835–839.
25. Juul-Moller S, Edvardsson N, Jahnmatz B, et al. Double-blind trial of aspirin in primary prevention of myocardial infarction in patients with stable chronic angina pectoris. The Sweden Angina Pectoris Aspirin Trial (SAPAT) Group. *Lancet* 1992;340:1421–1425.
26. Montalescot G, Maclouf J, Drobinski G, et al. Eicosanoid biosynthesis in patients with stable angina: beneficial effects of very low dose aspirin. *J Am Coll Cardiol* 1994;24:33–38.
27. Roussouw JE. Clinical trials of lipid-lowering drugs. In: Rifkind BM, ed. *Drug treatment of hyperlipidemia.* New York: Marcel Dekker, Inc., 1991:67–88.
28. Wenger NK. Gender, coronary artery disease, and coronary bypass surgery. *Ann Intern Med* 1990;112:557–558.
29. Second Report of the Expert Panel on Detection, Evaluation, and Treatment of High Blood Cholesterol in Adults. Bethesda, MD: Na-

tional Institutes of Health, National Heart, Lung, and Blood Institute, 1993.

30. Pekkanen J, Linn S, Heiss G, et al. Ten-year mortality from cardiovascular disease in relation to cholesterol level among men with and without preexisting cardiovascular disease. *N Engl J Med* 1990;322:1700–1707.

31. Wong ND, Wilson PW, Kannel WB. Serum cholesterol as a prognostic factor after myocardial infarction: the Framingham Study. *Ann Intern Med* 1991;115:687–693.

32. Prevention of cardiovascular events and death with pravastatin in patients with coronary heart disease and a broad range of initial cholesterol levels. The Long-Term Intervention with Pravastatin in Ischaemic Disease (LIPID) Study Group *N Engl J Med* 1998;339:1349–1357.

33. Randomised trial of cholesterol lowering in 4444 patients with coronary heart disease: the Scandinavian Simvastatin Survival Study (4S). *Lancet* 1994;344:1383–1389.

34. Sacks FM, Pfeffer MA, Moye LA, et al. The effect of pravastatin on coronary events after myocardial infarction in patients with average cholesterol levels. *N Engl J Med* 1996;335:1001–1009.

35. Brown BG, Albers JJ, Fisher LD, et al. Regression of coronary artery disease as a result of intensive lipid-lowering therapy in men with high levels of apolipoprotein B. *N Engl J Med* 1990;323:1289–1298.

36. Buchwald H, Varco RL, Matts JP, et al. Effect of partial ileal bypass surgery on mortality and morbidity from coronary heart disease in patients with hypercholesterolemia: report of the Program on the Surgical Control of Hyperlipidemias. *N Engl J Med* 1990;323:946–955.

37. Blankenhorn DH, Nessim SA, Johnson RL, et al. Beneficial effects of combined colestipol-niacin therapy on coronary atherosclerosis and coronary venous bypass grafts. *JAMA* 1987;257:3233–3240.

38. Ornish D, Scherwitz LW, Billings JH, et al. Intensive lifestyle changes for reversal of coronary heart disease. *JAMA* 1998;280:2001–2007.

39. Watts GF, Lewis B, Brunt JN, et al. Effects on coronary artery disease of lipid-lowering diet, or diet plus cholestyramine, in the St. Thomas' Atherosclerosis Regression Study (STARS). *Lancet* 1992;339:563–569.

40. Waters D, Higginson L, Gladstone P, et al. Effects of monotherapy with an HMG-CoA reductase inhibitor on the progression of coronary atherosclerosis as assessed by serial quantitative arteriography. The Canadian Coronary Atherosclerosis Intervention Trial. *Circulation* 1994;89:959–968.

41. Frick MH, Elo MO, Haapa K, et al. Helsinki Heart Study: primary-prevention trial with gemfibrozil in middle-aged men with dyslipidemia. Safety of treatment, changes in risk factors, and incidence of coronary heart disease. *N Engl J Med* 1987;317:1237–1245.

42. The Lipid Research Clinics Coronary Primary Prevention Trial results. I. Reduction in incidence of coronary heart disease. *JAMA* 1984;251:351–364.

43. Albert MA, Danielson E, Rifai N, et al. Effect of statin therapy on C-reactive protein levels: the pravastatin inflammation/CRP evaluation (PRINCE): a randomized trial and cohort study. *JAMA* 2001;286:64–70.

44. Ridker PM, Rifai N, Clearfield M, et al. Measurement of C-reactive protein for the targeting of statin therapy in the primary prevention of acute coronary events. *N Engl J Med* 2001;344:1959–1965.

45. Executive Summary of the Third Report of the National Cholesterol Education Program (NCEP) Expert Panel on Detection, Evaluation, And Treatment of High Blood Cholesterol In Adults (Adult Treatment Panel III). *JAMA* 2001;285:2486–2497.

46. Sacks FM. The Role of High-Density Lipoprotein (HDL) Cholesterol in the Prevention and Treatment of Coronary Heart Disease: Expert Group Recommendations. *Am J Cardiol* 2002;90:139–143.

47. Downs JR, Clearfield M, Weis S, et al. Primary prevention of acute coronary events with lovastatin in men and women with average cholesterol levels: results of AFCAPS/TexCAPS. Air Force/Texas Coronary Atherosclerosis Prevention Study. *JAMA* 1998;279:1615–1622.

48. Pepine CJ. Daily life ischemia and nitrate therapy. *Am J Cardiol* 1992;70:54B–63B.

49. Moncada S, Higgs A. Mechanisms of disease: the L-arginine nitric oxide pathway. *N Engl J Med* 1993;329:2002–2012.

50. Loscalzo J. Antiplatelet and antithrombotic effects of organic nitrates. *Am J Cardiol* 1992;70:18B–22B.

51. Brown BG, Bolson E, Petersen RB, et al. The mechanisms of nitroglycerin action: stenosis vasodilation as a major component of the drug response. *Circulation* 1981;64:1089–1097.

52. Gage JE, Hess OM, Murakami T, et al. Vasoconstriction of stenotic coronary arteries during dynamic exercise in patients with classic angina pectoris: reversibility by nitroglycerin. *Circulation* 1986;73:865–876.

53. De Coster PM, Chierchia S, Davies GJ, et al. Combined effects of nitrates on the coronary and peripheral circulation in exercise-induced ischemia. *Circulation* 1990;81:1881–1886.

54. Mahmarian JJ, Fenimore NL, Marks GF, et al. Transdermal nitroglycerin patch therapy reduces the extent of exercise-induced myocardial ischemia: results of a double-blind, placebo-controlled trial using quantitative thallium-201 tomography. *J Am Coll Cardiol* 1994;24:25–32.

55. Parker JD, Parker JO. Nitrate tolerance: current concepts concerning mechanisms and implications for therapy. *ACC Curr J Rev* 1993;2:77–79.

56. Packer M. What causes tolerance to nitroglycerin? The 100 year old mystery continues. *J Am Coll Cardiol* 1990;16:932–935.

57. Parker JO. Nitrate tolerance. A problem during continuous nitrate administration. *Eur J Clin Pharmacol* 1990;38[Suppl 1]:S21–S25.

58. Parker JD, Parker JO. Nitrate therapy for stable angina pectoris. *N Engl J Med* 1998;338:520–531.

59. Elkayam U. Tolerance to organic nitrates: evidence, mechanisms, clinical relevance, and strategies for prevention. *Ann Intern Med* 1991;114:667–677.

60. Horowitz JD, Henry CA, Syrjanen ML, et al. Combined use of nitroglycerin and N-acetylcysteine in the management of unstable angina pectoris. *Circulation* 1988;77:787–794.

61. Fung HL, Chong S, Kowaluk E, et al. Mechanisms for the pharmacologic interaction of organic nitrates with thiols. Existence of an extracellular pathway for the reversal of nitrate tolerance by N-acetylcysteine. *J Pharmacol Exp Ther* 1988;245:524–530.

62. Parker J, Farrell B, Fenton T, et al. Counter-regulatory responses to continuous and intermittent therapy with nitroglycerin. *Circulation* 1991;84:2336–2345.

63. Parker JD, Parker JO. Effect of therapy with an angiotensin-converting enzyme inhibitor on hemodynamic and counterregulatory responses during continuous therapy with nitroglycerin. *J Am Coll Cardiol* 1993;21:1445–1453.

64. Dupuis J, Lalonde G, Lemieux R, et al. Tolerance to intravenous nitroglycerin in patients with congestive heart failure: role of increased intravascular volume, neurohumoral activation and lack of prevention with N-acetylcysteine. *J Am Coll Cardiol* 1990;16:923–931.

65. Bassan MM. The daylong pattern of antianginal effect of long-term three times daily administered isosorbide dinitrate. *J Am Coll Cardiol* 1990;16:936–940.

66. Cruickshank JM. The clinical importance of cardioselectivity and lipophilicity in beta blockers. *Am Heart J* 1980;100:160–178.

67. Gengo FM, Huntoon L, McHugh WB. Lipid-soluble and water soluble B-Blockers. Comparison of the central nervous system depressant effect. *Arch Intern Med* 1987;147:39.

68. Lennard MS, Silas JH, Freestone S, et al. Oxidation phenotype: major determinant of metoprolol metabolism and response. *N Engl J Med* 1982;307:1558–1560.

69. Miller RR, Olson HG, Amsterdam EA, et al. Propranolol withdrawal rebound phenomenon. Exacerbation of coronary events after abrupt cessation of antianginal therapy. *N Engl J Med* 1975;293:416.

70. Lehtonen A. Effect of beta-blockers on blood lipid profile. *Am Heart J* 1985;109:1192–1196.

71. Northcote RJ, Todd IC, Ballantyne D. Beta blockers and lipoproteins: a review of current knowledge. *Scott Med J* 1986;31:220–228.

72. Packer M. Combined beta-adrenergic and calcium entry blockade in angina pectoris. *N Engl J Med* 1989;320:709–718.

73. Strauss WE, Parisi AF. Combined use of calcium-channel and beta-adrenergic blockers for the treatment of chronic stable angina. Rationale, efficacy and adverse effects. *Ann Intern Med* 1988;109:570–581.

74. Held PH, Yusuf S. Calcium antagonists in the treatment of ischemic heart disease: myocardial infarction. *Coron Artery Dis* 1994;5:21–26.

75. Muller JE, Turi ZG, Pearle DL, et al. Nifedipine and conventional therapy for unstable angina pectoris. A randomized, double-blind comparison. *Circulation* 1984;69:728.

76. Gerstenblith G, Ouyang P, Achuff SC, et al. Nifedipine in unstable angina. A double-blind, randomized trial. *N Engl J Med* 1982;306:885–889.

77. Nesto RW, White HD, Wynne J, et al. Comparison of nifedipine and isosorbide dinitrate when added to maximal propranolol therapy in stable angina pectoris. *Am J Cardiol* 1987;60:256.

78. Wallace WA, Wellington KL, Murphy GW, et al. Comparison of antianginal efficacies and exercise hemodynamic effects of nifedipine and diltiazem in angina pectoris. *Am J Cardiol* 1989;63:414.

79. Murakami T, Hess OM, Krayenbuehl HP. Left ventricular function be-

fore and after diltiazem in patients with coronary artery disease. *J Am Coll Cardiol* 1985;5:723.

80. Nonogi H, Hess OM, Ritter M, et al. Prevention of coronary vasoconstriction during dynamic exercise in patients with coronary artery disease. *J Am Coll Cardiol* 1988;12:892.

81. Leon MB, Rosing DR, Bonow RO, et al. Clinical efficacy of verapamil alone and combined with propranolol in treating patients with chronic stable angina pectoris. *Am J Cardiol* 1981;131:131-9.

82. Pfeffer MA, Braunwald E, Moye LA, et al. Effect of captopril on mortality and morbidity in patients with left ventricular dysfunction after myocardial infarction. Results of the Survival and Ventricular Enlargement Trial. *N Engl J Med* 1992;327:669–677.

83. Yusuf S, Pepine CJ, Garces C, et al. Effect of enalapril on myocardial infarction and unstable angina in patients with low ejection fractions. *Lancet* 1992;340:1173–1178.

84. Rutherford JD, Pfeffer MA, Moye LA, et al. Effects of captopril on ischemic events after myocardial infarction. Results of the survival and ventricular enlargement Trial. *Circulation* 1994;90:1731–1738.

85. Yusuf S, Sleight P, Pogue J, et al. Effects of an angiotensin converting-enzyme inhibitor, ramipril, on cardiovascular events in high-risk patients. The Heart Outcomes Prevention Evaluation Study Investigators. *N Engl J Med* 2000;342:145–153.

86. Yusuf S, Zucker D, Peduzzi P, et al. Effect of coronary artery bypass graft surgery on survival: overview of 10-year results from randomised trials by the Coronary Artery Bypass Graft Surgery Trialists Collaboration. *Lancet* 1994;344:563–570.

87. Varnauskas E. Twelve-year follow-up of survival in the randomized European Coronary Surgery Study. *N Engl J Med* 1988;319:332–337.

88. King SB, Lembo NJ, Weintraub WS, et al. A randomized trial comparing coronary angioplasty with coronary bypass surgery. *N Engl J Med* 1994;331:1044–1050.

89. Hamm CW, Reimers J, Ischinger T, et al. A randomized study of coronary angioplasty compared with bypass surgery in patients with symptomatic multivessel coronary disease. *N Engl J Med* 1994;331:1037–1043.

90. Hillis LD, Rutherford JD. Coronary angioplasty compared with bypass grafting. *N Engl J Med* 1994;331:1086–1087.

91. Bucher HC, Hengstler P, Schindler C, et al. Percutaneous transluminal coronary angioplasty versus medical treatment for non-acute coronary heart disease: meta-analysis of randomised controlled trials. *BMJ* 2000;321:73–77.

92. Pocock SJ, Anderson RA, Rickards AF, et al. Meta-analysis of randomised trials comparing coronary angioplasty with bypass surgery. *Lancet* 1995;346:1184–1189.

93. Blumenthal RS, Cohn G, Schulman SP. Medical therapy versus coronary angioplasty in stable coronary artery disease: a critical review of the literature. *J Am Coll Cardiol* 2000;36:668–673.

94. Pitt B, Waters D, Brown WV, et al. Aggressive lipid-lowering therapy compared with angioplasty in stable coronary artery disease. *N Engl J Med* 1999;341:70–76.

95. Serruys PW, de Feyter P, Macaya C, et al. Fluvastin for prevention of cardiac events following successful first percutaneous coronary intervention: a randomized controlled trial. *JAMA* 2002;287:3215–3222.

96. Greenbaum AB, Califf RM, Jones RH, et al. Comparison of medicine alone, coronary angioplasty, and left internal mammary artery-coronary artery bypass for one-vessel proximal left anterior descending coronary artery disease. *Am J Cardiol* 2000;86:1322–1326.

Interventional Approach

CHAPTER 90

Role of Coronary Angiography

Stephen G. Ellis

Key Words: Coronary angiography; infarction; left ventricular dysfunction; revascularization; videodensitometry.

INTRODUCTION

Although now slightly tarnished as a diagnostic "gold standard" because of its capacity to visualize only the lumen and not the wall of a potentially diseased coronary artery, coronary angiography still remains the most frequently relied on tool by which clinical cardiologists ascertain the extent and severity of their patients' atherosclerotic coronary disease. It continues to hold this position largely because of the well recognized relation between findings at catheterization and clinical events over spans of more than 5 to 10 years (1), the relative simplicity of its performance, and a level of complications and cost that have been acceptable in relation to its diagnostic utility compared with other techniques. This chapter focuses on the role of coronary angiography in the management of patients with chronic stable coronary disease.

S. G. Ellis: Sones Cardiac Catheterization Laboratories, Department of Cardiovascular Medicine, The Cleveland Clinic Foundation, Cleveland, Ohio 44195.

BRIEF HISTORY

Building on the work of Forssmann, Cournand, Zimmerman, and others (2–4), Mason Sones initiated a program at the Cleveland Clinic in 1958 to study the possibility of selectively opacifying the coronary arteries, largely because there was no suitable benchmark for the diagnosis of coronary artery disease at the time other than the necropsy table. The equipment was extremely primitive by today's standards, and the first selective coronary injection was somewhat inadvertent (a supravalvular aortogram was intended) (5), but the technique led to a revolution in the care of patients with atherothrombotic heart disease. Currently, it is estimated that more than 1,500,000 patients undergo coronary angiography annually in the United States. Without this procedure, of course, coronary revascularization in the forms of bypass surgery (first done in 1967), balloon angioplasty (first done in 1977), coronary stenting (first done in 1986), and others would never have been developed.

CORONARY ANATOMY VIEWED
WITH CONTRAST ANGIOGRAPHY

The technique of coronary angiography has been well described (6,7) and is beyond the scope of this chapter. Vascular access is usually obtained using 4- to 6-F catheters through the femoral, brachial, or radial artery approach.

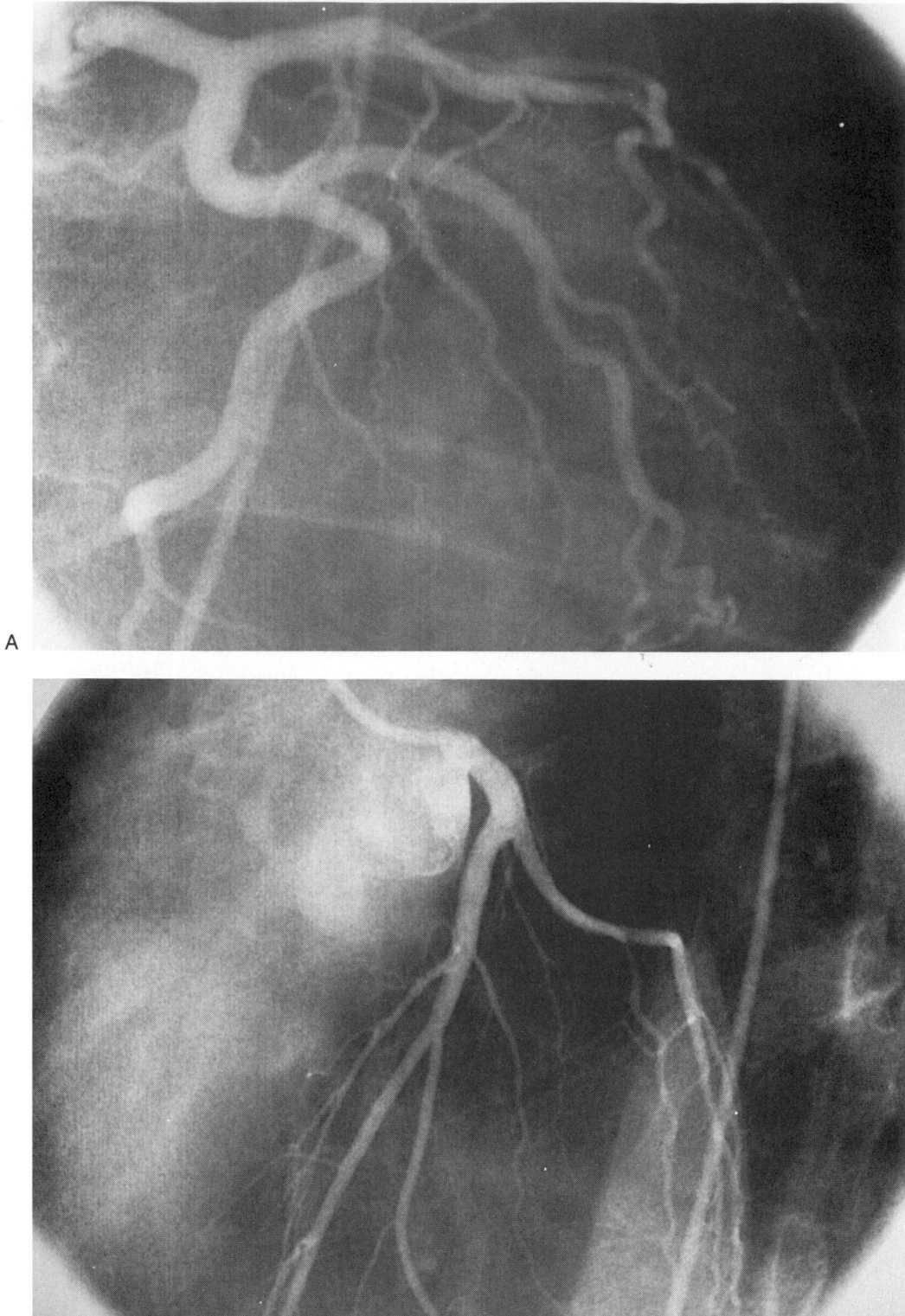

FIG. 90–1. Left coronary artery in the **(A)** right anterior oblique and **(B)** cranially angulated left anterior oblique projections.

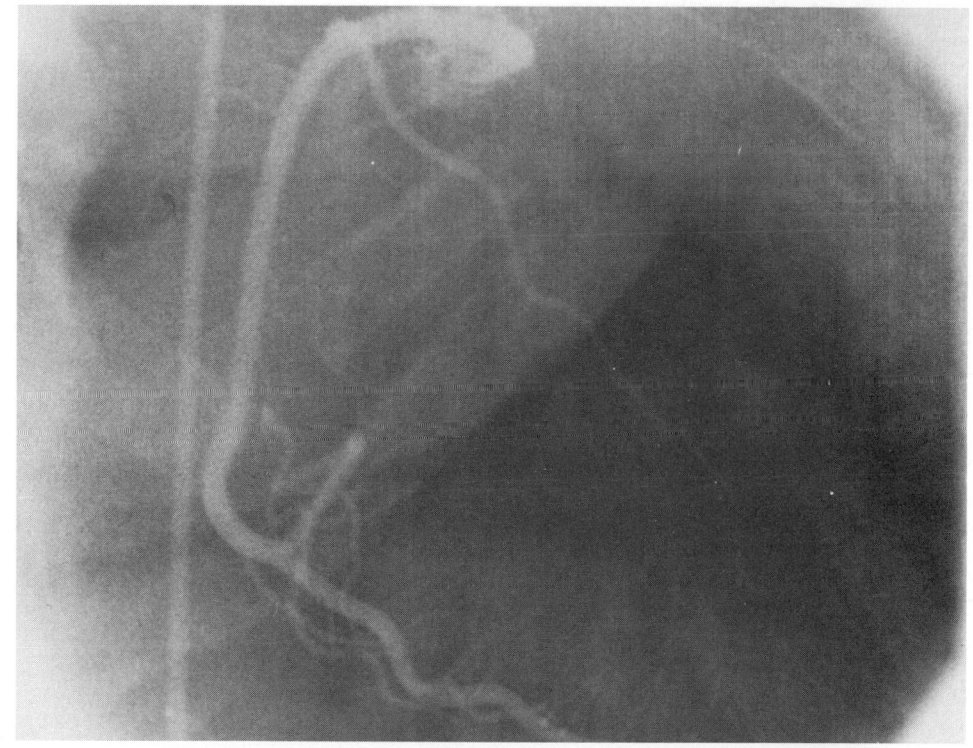

A

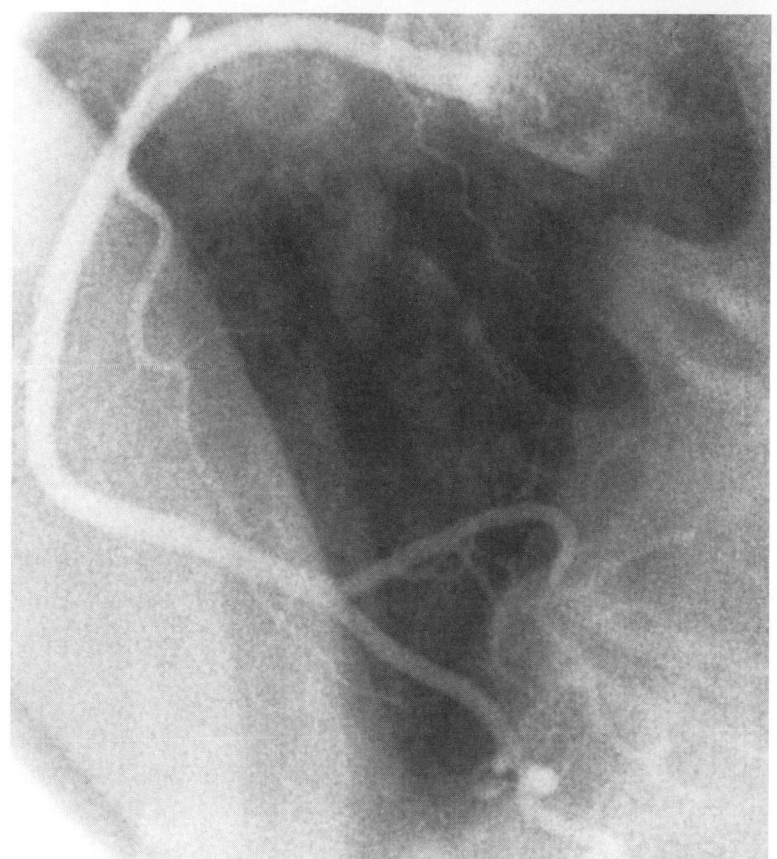

B

FIG. 90–2. Right coronary artery in the **(A)** right anterior oblique and **(B)** left anterior oblique projections.

Representative still frames from left and right anterior oblique angiograms of the left and right coronary arteries are displayed in Figures 90–1 and 90–2.

DIAGNOSIS OF CORONARY ARTERY DISEASE

As atherothrombosis progresses from the fatty streak to the eccentric lipid-filled plaque, luminal encroachment readily detectable by routine angiographic means is a relatively late event because of the compensatory enlargement of the vessel wall (the Glagov effect) (Fig. 90–3) (8). Hence, both necropsy and intravascular ultrasound studies have demonstrated that the extent of plaque mass is grossly underestimated by coronary angiography (9). Furthermore, severe luminal encroachment is not a prerequisite for heightened risk for rapid progression to total coronary occlusion and myocardial infarction (MI). Indeed, Little and colleagues (10), studying patients with diagnostic angiography before infarction, found that 66% of patients had less than 50% maximal narrowing in the infarct vessel before infarction and 17% had less than 30% narrowing, yet all had at least luminal irregularities (10). Furthermore, nearly 10% of all patients with a recent MI, after lysis of the thrombus overlying the causative ruptured plaque, have less than 50% narrowing in the infarct artery at cardiac catheterization (11). Thus, although a greater than 50% diameter narrowing of at least one major epicardial coronary artery has typ-

ically been required "to make the diagnosis" of coronary artery disease, a more functionally meaningful definition would require only detection of enough plaque burden to increase the risk for subsequent coronary events (at least one 20–30% stenosis, and perhaps only luminal irregularities [Fig. 90–4]). Diagnosis and prognosis hence are inexorably intertwined.

The greater than 50% diameter stenosis requirement to make the diagnosis of coronary artery disease is not without rationale, however. First, in the 1960s and 1970s, when the diagnostic role of angiography was in its infancy, and when high-resolution, high-contrast image intensifiers were not available, and the importance of cranially and caudally angulated projections was underappreciated, it often was difficult enough to ascertain whether any lesion was present, let alone distinguish the details of its severity. A loss of half the apparently normal artery size was relatively simple to detect. Second, in 1974, Gould and colleagues published their classic work (12) correlating the degree of stenosis to reduction in blood flow and found that coronary artery flow reserve, or the artery's capacity to increase flow at peak demand, was reduced only by a stenosis greater than 50% (measured by quantitative means) (Fig. 90–5). Finally, a substantial body of knowledge developed linking this definition of coronary disease with a patient's prognosis (vide infra).

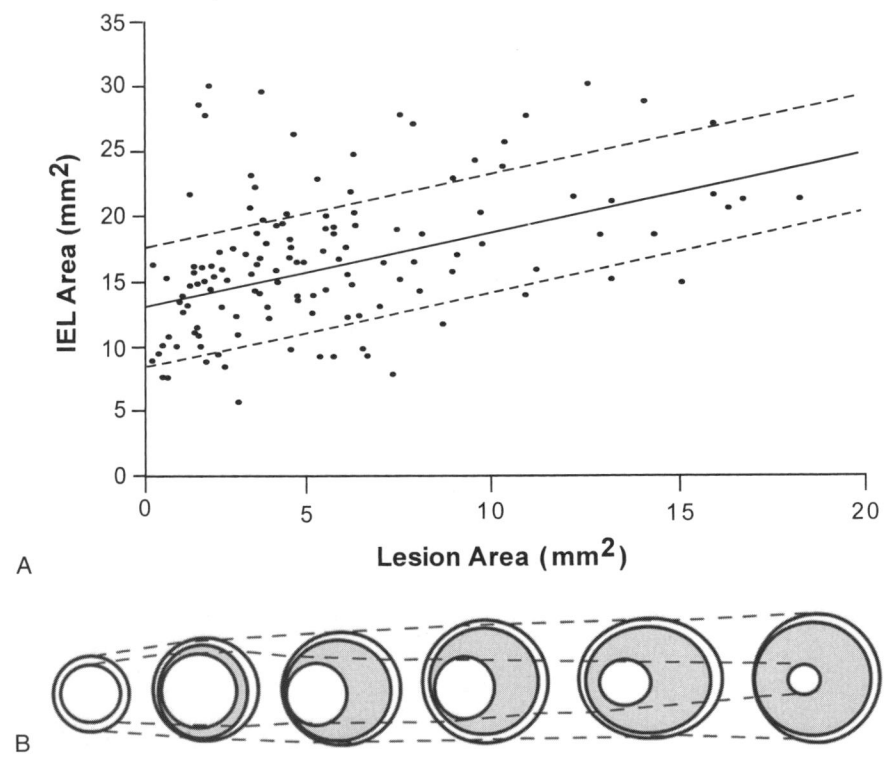

FIG. 90–3. Compensatory arterial dilatation with development of atherothrombosis (the Glagov effect). IEL, internal elastic lamina.

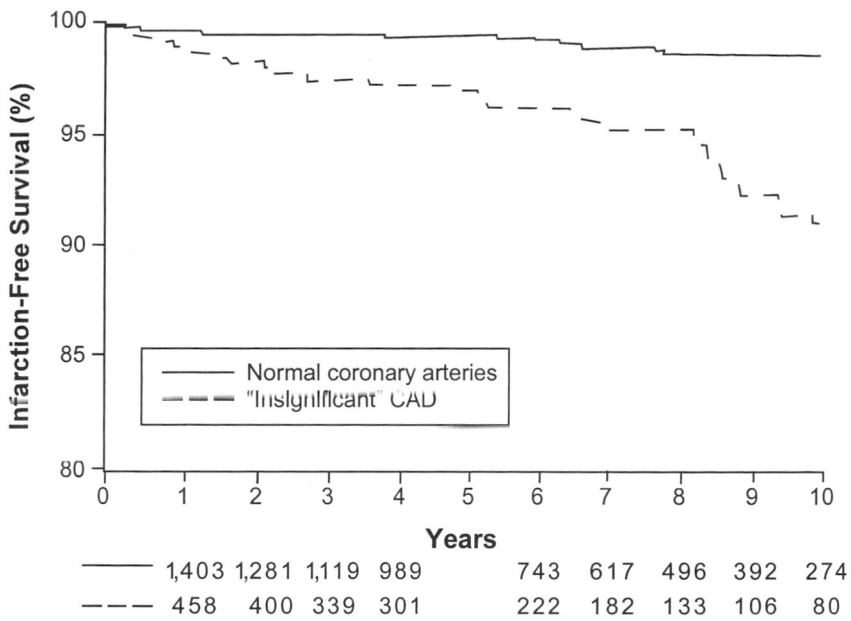

FIG. 90–4. Prognostic importance of risk for myocardial infarction of 25% to 50% ("insignificant") stenoses compared with less than 25% stenoses in patients from the Duke Cardiovascular database. CAD, coronary artery disease.

ASSESSING THE RISK FOR CORONARY ARTERY DISEASE

Cardiac Survival

Although clinical factors such as age, sex, and diabetes contribute to risk in patients with established coronary disease (13–16), risk for death is most closely linked to left ventricular (LV) function (17), the extent and severity of coronary narrowings (18), and the degree of electrical instability (19).

Parameters detected at exercise stress testing such as ST-segment depression or exercise limitation by severe angina or dyspnea at low levels of exercise (e.g., <6 minutes exercise on the Bruce protocol) provide a highly useful estimate of ventricular function and ischemic burden, as well as prognosis (20,21). Coronary angiography and ventriculography add some further prognostic information in patients at moderate to high risk by clinical and noninvasive screening and,

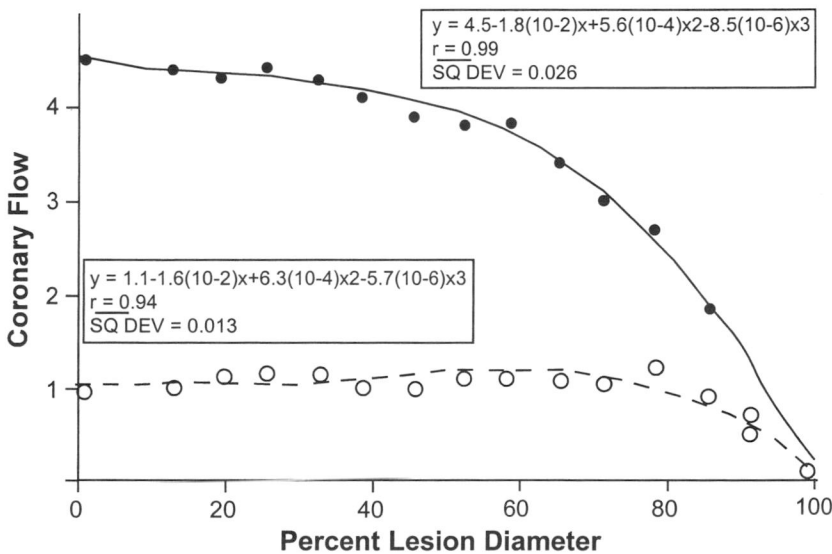

FIG. 90–5. Relation of baseline and hyperemic coronary flow to percentage diameter stenosis in a focal stenosis model.

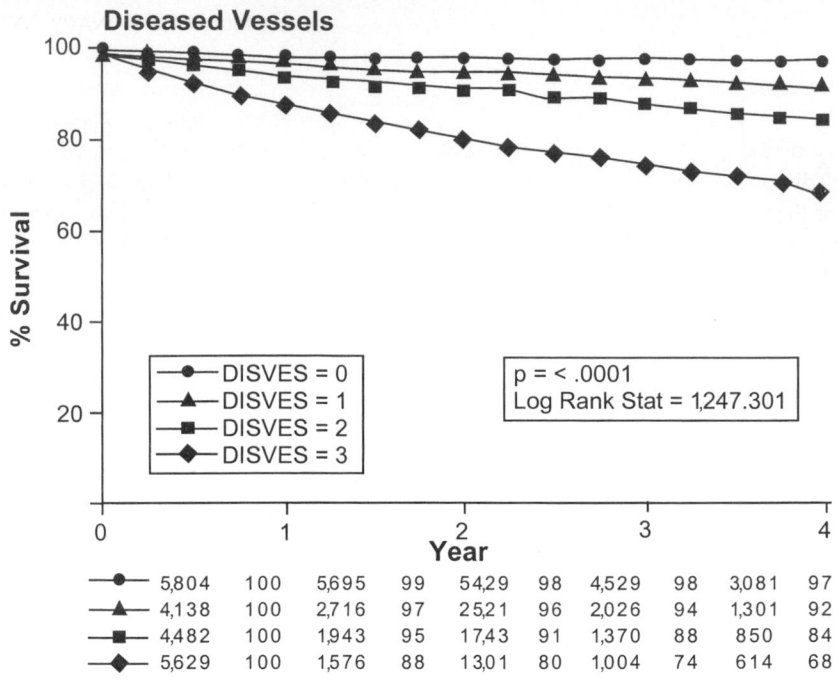

●	5,804	100	5,695	99	54,29	98	4,529	98	3,081	97
▲	4,138	100	2,716	97	25,21	96	2,026	94	1,301	92
■	4,482	100	1,943	95	17,43	91	1,370	88	850	84
◆	5,629	100	1,576	88	13,01	80	1,004	74	614	68

FIG. 90–6. Survival in medically treated patients, subdivided by the number of diseased vessels *(DISVES)* (from the Coronary Artery Surgery Study [CASS] registry experience).

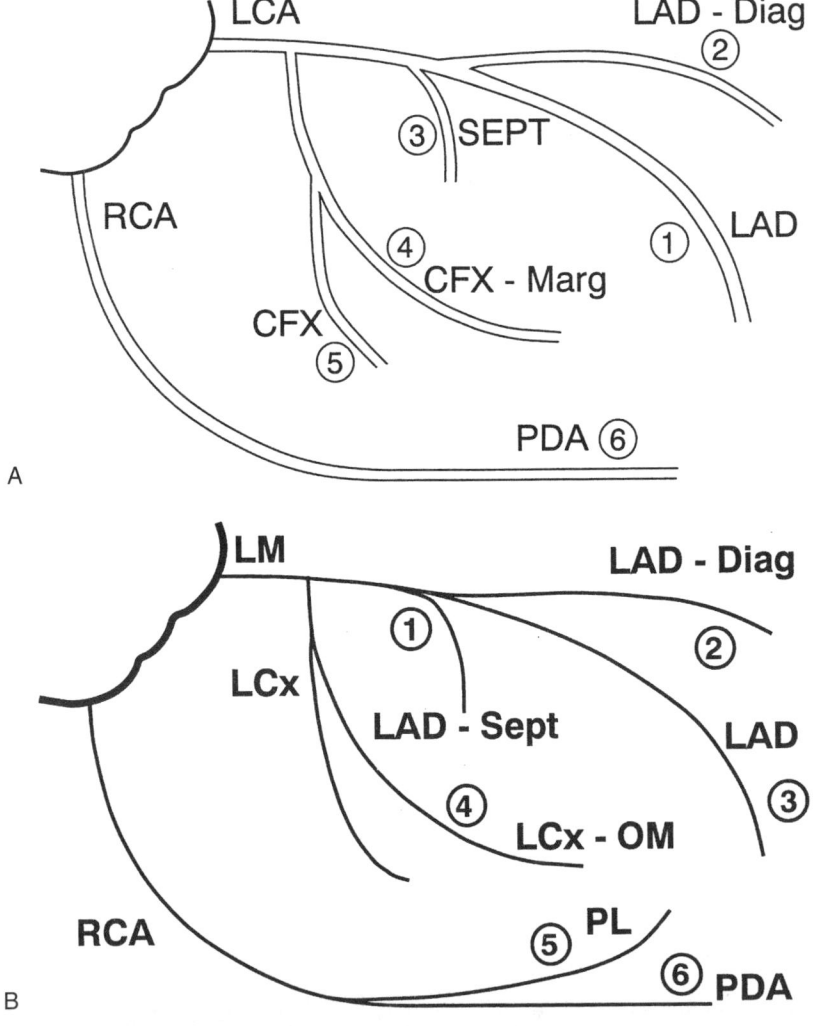

FIG. 90–7. The "jeopardy score" for **(A)** left-dominant and **(B)** right-dominant coronary systems. CFX, circumflex; Cx, circumflex; Diag, diagonal; LAD, left anterior descending; LCA, left coronary artery; LM, left main; Marg, obtuse marginal; OM, obtuse marginal; PDA, posterior descending; PL, posterolateral; RCA, right coronary artery; Sept, septal.

just as important, are requisite for determining suitability for revascularization (22–24).

The extent of coronary disease is traditionally described in terms of the number of diseased vessels (≥50–70% diameter stenosis(es) in any of the three major epicardial vessels or their major branches). Although of considerable prognostic use (Fig. 90–6) (25), this concept is somewhat limited in that a narrowing in a small or moderate branch vessel "counts" as much as one in the proximal segment of a major vessel, which potentially compromises much more myocardium. The concept of the "jeopardy score" (Fig. 90–7) was developed by Califf and colleagues (26) to circumvent this problem and provides further prognostic information (Fig. 90–8). Further prognostic information is available by integrating the number of diseased vessels with the severity and more precise location of the disease location, as in the Duke Risk Score (Table 90–1) (27).

Justification for a 50% to 75% cutoff can be found in the large Duke Cardiovascular Database, wherein cardiac sur-

vival over 10 years in patients with at least 1 greater than 75% coronary narrowing (62%) was markedly reduced compared with that in patients with only 25% to 50% narrowing (97%) or less than 25% narrowing (100%; but note that lesion severity was only visually approximated as <25%, 25%, 50%, 75%, 95%, or 100%) (Fig. 90–9) (28).

Risk for Infarction

Atherothrombotic plaques most likely to fissure or rupture, leading to thrombotic coronary obstruction, tend to be those with a degenerated or lipid-laden core and a thin, macrophage-invaded fibrous cap (29,30). Certainly angiography, only capable of evaluating the lumen and surface of the vessel wall, would not be expected to be highly predictive of the risk for infarction. Nonetheless, by virtue of giving an estimate of plaque burden and of surface characteristics (e.g., roughness and ulceration), angiography has prognostic value in assessing the risk for infarction.

A number of studies have semiquantitatively assessed the degree of coronary involvement and found that markers of the extent of disease do predict risk for infarction. For example, in a study of 313 patients treated medically for an average of 39 months at the Montreal Heart Institute, Moise and coworkers (31) found that a marker of extent of disease (the number of >75% stenoses) and the presence of at least one stenosis greater than 80% correlated with future total occlusion. It should be acknowledged, however, that not all occlusions result in infarction and, furthermore, that previous high-grade stenoses, by inducing collaterals, have a smaller chance of producing Q-wave infarction when they occlude than do less severe stenoses (that do not induce collaterals) (32). Ellis and colleagues (33) from the Coronary Artery Surgery Study (CASS) study found that the risk for anterior wall infarction during 3-year follow-up with medical therapy was 2% for a worst left anterior descending stenosis of 0% to 49%, 6% for stenoses of 50% to 60%, 7% for stenoses

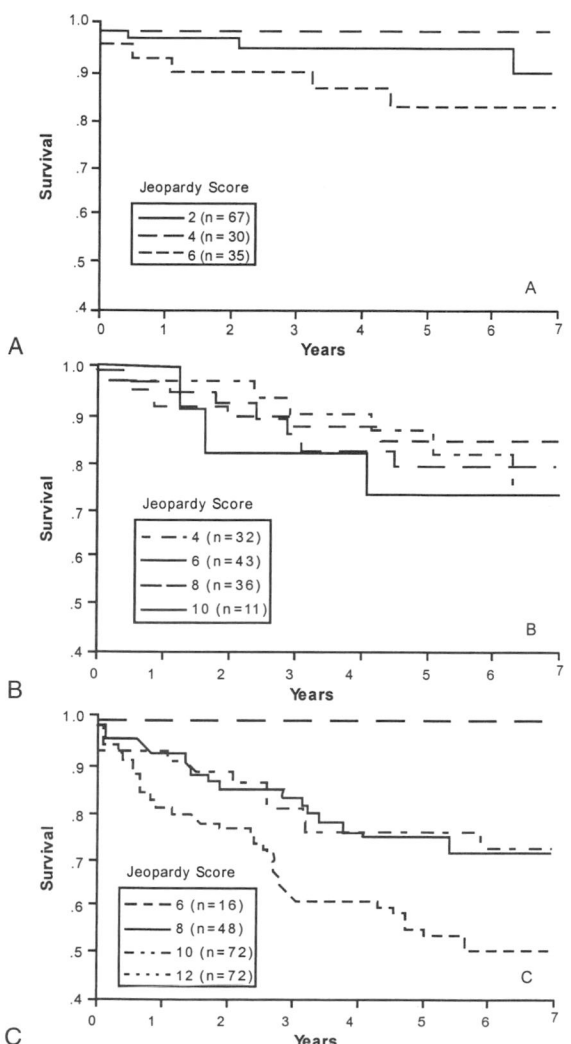

FIG. 90–8. The prognostic impact of the jeopardy score in patients with **(A)** single-vessel, **(B)** double-vessel, and **(C)** triple-vessel disease from the Duke Cardiovascular database.

TABLE 90–1. *Duke index*

Extent of CAD	Prognostic weight (0–100)
No ≥ CAD 50%	0
1 VD 50–74%	19
>1 VD 50–74%	23
1 VD (75%)	23
1 VD (≥95%)	32
2 VD	37
2 VD (both ≥95%)	42
1 VD, ≥95% proximal LAD	48
2 VD, ≥95% LAD	48
2 VD, ≥95% proximal LAD	56
3 VD	56
3 VD, ≥95% in at least one	63
3 VD, 75% proximal LAD	67
3 VD, ≥95% proximal LAD	74
Left main (75%)	82
Left main (≥95%)	100

CAD, coronary artery disease; LAD, left anterior descending coronary artery; VD, vessel disease.

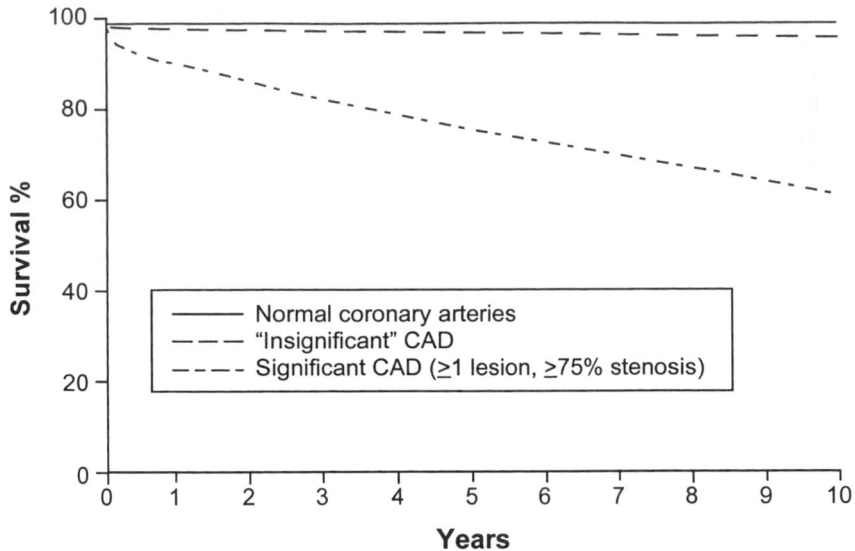

FIG. 90–9. Prognostic importance for survival of at least one greater than 75% diameter stenosis, compared with lesser, no, or inapparent disease in patients from the Duke Cardiovascular database. CAD, coronary artery disease.

of 70% to 89%, 9% for stenoses of 90% to 98%, and 8% for stenoses of 99% to 100%. Multiple stenoses in the same territory further increased the risk. Finally, and importantly, Papanicolaou and coworkers (28) noted in a study of 1,861 patients followed for up to 10 years that patients with worst stenoses of 25% to 50% had a significantly worse 10-year infarct-free survival (89%) than did patients with normal or less than 25% stenoses (99%) (Fig. 90–4).

Despite the correlation of "plaque burden" to risk of infarction, it is well worth recalling that the most severe stenosis in a coronary vessel is not necessarily the one most likely to lead to infarction. In fact, several studies have shown that relatively rapid progression of lesser stenoses is the most common cause of infarction (Table 90–2). Although the literature in this area is scant (34–38), only half of lesions destined to lead to infarction within 12 months reduce their normal vessel diameter by more than 50% when visualized at prior angiography. When the duration between initial and infarction-related angiography is extended to more than 12 months, only about 25% of lesions leading to infarction are narrowed more than 50%.

Somewhat more recently, building on the work of Levin and Fallon (39), who had demonstrated that plaque fissuring could be detected by postmortem angiography, Ambrose and coworkers (40) and Ellis and coworkers (41) separately explored and demonstrated the importance of stenosis morphology in correlation with unstable coronary ischemic syndromes. In their seminal papers in 1985, Ambrose and coworkers (40) demonstrated that eccentric plaques with narrow necks and overhanging edges or scalloped borders (type II plaques) were much more likely to be found in patients with unstable ischemic syndromes than were concentric lesions with smooth borders (type I plaques). In a case–control study of 259 patients followed for 3 years, Ellis and colleagues (41) found that lesion roughness (irregular borders) was the most powerful quantitative (all sites were

measured using edge-detection quantitation) or morphologic correlate of later infarction (relative risk 6.6 compared with smooth-bordered stenoses) (41).

Risk for Disease Progression

Optimal detection of disease progression requires meticulous attention to angiographic technique, quantitative, as opposed to visual, dimensional assessment, and an understand-

TABLE 90–2. *Angiographic precursors of acute ischemic syndromes*

	<50%	50–70%	>70%
All studies			
Unstable angina			
Ambrose (34) (n = 25)	72	16	12
Non–Q-wave MI			
Ambrose (35) (n = 8)	25	12	63
Dacanay (36) (n = 38)	55	21	21
Q-wave or unspecified MI			
Ambrose (35) (n = 15)	60	40	0
Little (10) (n = 29)	66	31	3
Giroud (37) (n = 92)	78	9	13
Nobuyoshi (38) (n = 39)	59	15	26
Dacanay (36) (n = 32)	50	34	16
Total (n = 278)	65	19	16
Angiography within 12 months			
Non–Q-wave MI			
Dacanay (36) (n = 5)	40	0	60
Q-wave or unspecified MI			
Little (10) (n = 14)	71	29	0
Giroud (37) (n = 23)	52	17	30
Dacanay (36) (n = 6)	16	33	50
Total ≤12 mo (n = 48)	52	21	27[a]
Total >12 mo (n = 142)	72	18	9

MI, myocardial infarction.
[a] $p = 0.013$ compared with studies >12 months.

ing of the extent and determinants of interobserver variability (42,43). Properly performed studies suggest that in addition to clinical factors (unstable angina [44], younger patient age [44], high cholesterol levels [45–47], smoking [46,47], treatment with cholesterol-lowering [48,49] treatments), angiographic factors may be important correlates of future disease progression. The risk factors for progression to infarction (discussed earlier) may differ somewhat from those implicated in risk for progression to subtotally occlusive stenoses, because large thrombus formation plays a greater role in the pathogenesis of the former process. The extent of initial disease (measured as the number of coronary segments with 50% to 75% stenosis) (45), large (>3 mm) vessel site (50), proximal stenosis location (50), right coronary artery location (51), and the presence of a patent bypass graft around a coronary segment (52) all increase the rate of progression of coronary narrowing.

Adjuncts to coronary angiography such as fractional flow reverse, intravascular ultrasound, and thermography may provide additional prognostic information.

Risk for Complications with Coronary Revascularization

The likelihood of major periprocedural complications with bypass surgery is directly related to patient age, LV function, need for concomitant cardiac procedures such as mitral valve repair or ventricular aneurysmectomy, and whether the patient has had prior bypass surgery (53).

In contrast, the risk for percutaneous coronary intervention (PCI; stenting, balloon angioplasty, or atherectomy) is most closely related to the nature of the critical stenosis itself and secondarily related to clinical factors and LV function. A number of morphologic features of the stenosis itself—its length, degree of angulation and calcification, and presence of associated thrombus or bifurcation—increase the risk for vessel closure during PCI. Each increases the risk by 1.5- to 2-fold over baseline, and the effects are generally additive. A formal scheme relating lesion morphology to risk was proposed in 1987 by the American College of Cardiology and the American Heart Association (54), and a modification of that classification scheme by Ellis and coworkers (55) has been used widely since 1990. More contemporary risk factor schemes have been proposed (56,57), which improve somewhat on predictive capability. Nonetheless, the capacity to predict major in-hospital complications of PCI (death, unplanned bypass surgery, or MI) remains modest (area under receiver operating curve of 0.70–0.75 at best) (56,57).

COMPLICATIONS

Major complications of diagnostic angiography as it is currently performed are rare. In 58,332 cases in the Society for Cardiac Angiography database for 1990, death occurred in 0.08%, major neurological events in 0.06%, MI in 0.03%,

TABLE 90–3. *Correlates of the major complications of coronary angiography*

Variable	Odds ratio (95% CI)
Moribund	10.2 (3.8–27.8)
NYCA CHF Class	
I	1.0
II	1.1 (0.9–1.4)
III	1.3 (0.9–1.5)
IV	1.5 (1.2–1.7)
Hypertension	1.4 (1.2–1.7)
Shock	6.5 (4.2–10.2)
Aortic valve disease	2.7 (2.0–3.7)
Outpatient	0.6 (0.5–0.8)
Renal insufficiency	3.3 (2.4–4.6)
Unstable angina	1.4 (1.2–1 7)
Mitral valve disease	2.3 (1.8–3.1)
Acute myocardial infarction	4.0 (2.6–6.2)
Cardiomyopathy	3.3 (2.2–49)

CHF, congestive heart failure; CI, confidence interval; NYHA, New York Heart Association.

and major vascular complications occurred in 0.40% of cases (58). Multivariate correlates of major complications in that data set are shown in Table 90–3 and include most prominently moribund status before the procedure, cardiogenic shock, acute myocardial infarction (AMI), cardiomyopathy, and renal insufficiency (58). Complications of lesser severity such as nausea and transient bradycardia are much more common. Their incidence, as well as that of more severe problems, also is in part related to the use of the more expensive, but less toxic, low-osmolar contrast agents (59,60). Because of their cost, such agents are best used only in patients at greater risk (61). A clinically useful algorithm for their use has been developed by Hirshfeld and colleagues from a prospective database of 2,245 procedures. They concluded that only patients in the highest quartile of risk (any two of age >65 years, LV end-diastolic pressure >15 mm Hg, New York Heart Association congestive heart failure Class IV, or prior contrast agent reaction) should receive such low-osmolar contrast agents (61). To this should be added patients with AMI of moderate to large size, with estimated aortic valve area less than or equal to 0.4 cm^2 per square meter or baseline creatinine greater than 2.0 mg/dL, all of whom were underrepresented in the data set. Radiation exposure to patient and physician with appropriate shielding and attention to detail is very low. However, prolonged fluoroscopy or repeated cine runs with the same camera position may cause acute or delayed local [skin] radiation "burns."

PITFALLS AND LIMITATIONS

As a well established procedure with credentialing guidelines for teaching and practice (62), the performance and interpretation of coronary angiography only rarely produces major errors. Occasionally, however, whole vessels or lesions can be missed. Somewhat more commonly, the physiologic importance of a stenosis may be misjudged.

The two most common reasons for failure to visualize all arteries are coronary anomalies and unrecognized bypass grafts. The most common origin anomalies, high right coronary artery takeoff (2%) and origin of the circumflex from the right coronary artery or sinus of Valsalva (1%), are generally readily detected. An anterior and superior origin of the right coronary artery (0.5%) often is more difficult to recognize (63). A high degree of suspicion and use of a multipurpose or Amplatz configuration catheter usually solves this problem. Particularly if the number of bypass grafts is unknown, one may be missed. Usually, adherence to the adage "if a myocardial segment contracts yet seems to have no corresponding antegrade or collateral blood supply, then a conduit has not been visualized" will keep the angiographer from making this mistake. An aortic root injection (40–50 mL over 2 s, depending on the size of the root) often will yield a clue to the "missing" graft's origin.

Lesions are seldom missed if the angiographer requires that all parts of the major epicardial vessels be visualized in at least two, somewhat orthogonal, nonforeshortened projections. The orientation of these projections will depend on the size and orientation of the heart and coronaries; imaging "standard" projections by rote frequently will be inadequate. Because of the prognostic importance of the left main trunk and proximal anterior descending/circumflex arteries, careful visualization of this territory is imperative. Damping (decreased systolic and diastolic pressure with loss of greater frequency elements of the waveform as transmitted from the tip of the diagnostic catheter) or ventricularization of the waveform (transition of the usual waveform to that more closely resembling an LV tracings) also can be clues of an ostial left main narrowing. Steeply angulated caudal left and right anterior oblique projections are frequently useful.

Assessment of the severity of stenoses by visual approximation as is commonly done in clinical practice is difficult and may rather often lead to errors of judgment. Numerous studies have shown that if two experienced angiographers are asked to estimate the degree of narrowing of a given stenosis, their estimate will vary by 14% to 18% (64,65). Discrepancies in the interpretation of the severity of left main trunk stenoses are particularly common (66). Because of the prognostic importance of lesions at this site, consideration of imaging with intravascular ultrasound (with the "guiding catheter" withdrawn into the aorta so as not to mask an ostial narrowing) when there is any question of left main disease is advisable (67). Furthermore, compared with more vigorous methods of quantitative measurement such as edge detection or even caliper measurement, visual assessments tend to overestimate severity in moderately narrowed vessels (50–80% diameter stenosis) by as much as 20% to 30% and to underestimate the severity of stenoses actually narrowed by less than 50% (68). Similarly, most angiographers overestimate the degree of stenosis before PCI, yet underestimate the severity of the lesion after treatment (68). The underestimation of stenosis severity by many angiographers has been confirmed repeatedly by comparisons of angiography to autopsy findings (9) and, more recently, to intravascular ultrasound (69,70).

QUANTITATIVE CORONARY ANGIOGRAPHY

Many, but not all, of the above mentioned problems can be circumvented by the use of quantitative coronary angiography (QCA). A number of techniques have been developed (71). Most rely on image acquisition when the coronary artery has the least movement (generally at end-diastole), digital acquisition or conversion, and optical magnification before analysis. Many increase their signal-to-noise ratio by averaging several video frames before storage. For most, a region of interest about a given stenosis or segment is chosen by the operator. The arterial centerline is then automatically determined using analysis of circular pixel density profiles, and then linear density profiles perpendicular to the centerline are automatically drawn. Vessel edges are then determined by analysis of the rate of grayscale change on the perpendicular approaching the centerline. Most systems find an initial edge by determining a weighted average of the first and second derivatives of density change and then use smoothing algorithms to detect and replace point outliers. Manual editing is possible but should be used judiciously. Dimensions are calibrated, generally by analyzing the coronary catheter (of known dimension) in the same cine frame using the same technique. Maximum and minimum vessel diameter for a given segment, percentage stenosis, and estimates of atheroma mass can be derived (Fig. 90–10). Comparison of diameters found using such techniques to those of phantoms of known dimension have been excellent ($r = 0.992$; standard error of the estimate [SEE] = 0.19 mm) (72). However, they still rely on the angiographer displaying the coronary segment in a nonforeshortened view and the often eccentric stenosis at its most severe aspect.

A number of other factors often diminish accuracy and reproducibility: vessel motion, vasomotor tone, overlapping side branches, inadequate mixing of contrast with blood, the three-dimensional distance between the calibrating object and the coronary segment of interest, finite focal spot size (as the vessel diameter approaches that of the focal spot, 0.5–0.8 mm, the penumbra becomes disproportionate to the vessel diameter; in effect, the edges must physically blur), veiling glare, and pincushion distortion (71). The system's appreciation of scaling objects of apparently known size (coronary catheters) also varies by catheter composition (73) and by whether they are filled with contrast. In practice, variations by 0.22 to 0.36 mm in obstruction diameter and by 0.15 to 0.66 mm in "normal" reference diameter (to calculate percentage diameter stenosis) can be expected, even for the best of analytic laboratories (74). Furthermore, different yet well regarded systems can differ considerably in their estimation of stenosis diameter (75). Many systems now can analyze a coronary segment for quantitative dimensions in less than 1 to 3 minute. Still, for most clinical work, this is slow and labor intensive.

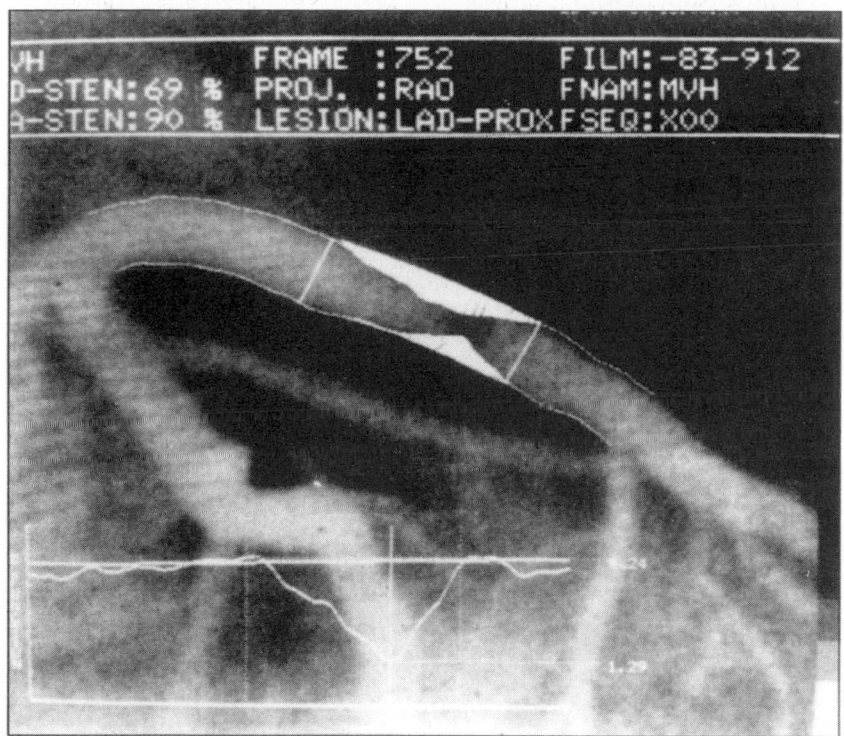

FRAME :752   FILM:-83-912
D-STEN:69 %   PROJ. :RAO   FNAM:MVH
STEN:90 %   LESION:LAD-PROXFSEQ:XOO

FIG. 90–10. Quantitative coronary angiography using the Cardiovascular Angiography Analysis System (CAAS), illustrating edge detection of a proximal left anterior descending lesion with minimum luminal diameter of 1.29 mm.

Electronic digital calipers applied to magnified images can reduce some of the error of visual estimation of stenosis severity and can be performed in a fraction of the time it takes because of true QCA. Controversy exists as to how closely caliper measurement approximates that of QCA (76,77), but it likely represents a compromise adequate for clinical work but too inexact for research application in a situation where precision is required (e.g., studies of coronary progression and regression, vasomotor tone).

Even the determination of percentage stenosis by QCA has major limitations, however. Harrison and colleagues (78) compared QCA-measured percentage stenosis with peak or resting hyperemic responses (using a 20-second occlusion) in the proximal left anterior descending coronary artery of 23 patients. Substantial overlap between those with normal hyperemic responses (peak/resting flow >3.5:1) and those with abnormal response was noted (Fig. 90–11). In contrast, vessels with normal and abnormal hyperemic responses were well categorized by minimum cross-sectional area greater than or less than 3.5 mm^2 (70). These investigators and others concluded that as a result of the often diffuse involvement of the artery with atheromatous plaque (9), as well as early compensatory vessel enlargement (8), determining a true "normal" uninvolved site for reference (required, of course, to determine a percentage stenosis) is nearly impossible.

In clinical practice this should translate into two principles. First, in assessing, and certainly before treating, what appears to be a 50% to 80% diameter stenosis, it is important to ascertain its physiologic importance by correlation with markers of induced ischemia. This may not, however, be easy to do. Recall that a reversible defect on thallium scanning, for instance, only implies a difference in augmented flow between areas of myocardium. Especially in the presence of a totally occluded coronary or an area of infarction, detection of another physiologically important stenosis may be difficult because its flow will still be greater than that beyond the occluded vessel or in the infarcted territory (79). Furthermore, as noted earlier, there is not a one-to-one correlation between the obstructive capacity of a stenosis and its propensity to worsen suddenly and cause an infarction. Second, in a vessel that appears diffusely irregular or smaller than expected for a patient's size and apparent LV mass, or both, use minimum lumen diameter (MLD) of the proximal vessels and percentage stenosis to assess the degree and importance of a narrowing. In general, a MLD less than 1.0 mm of a proximal coronary indicates a flow-limiting narrowing, regardless of the percentage diameter stenosis (80).

INDICATIONS

Referral of a patient for cardiac catheterization and angiography should be based on a thorough understanding of the prognostic implications of potential findings (in relation to clinical and noninvasive test findings) and the limitations

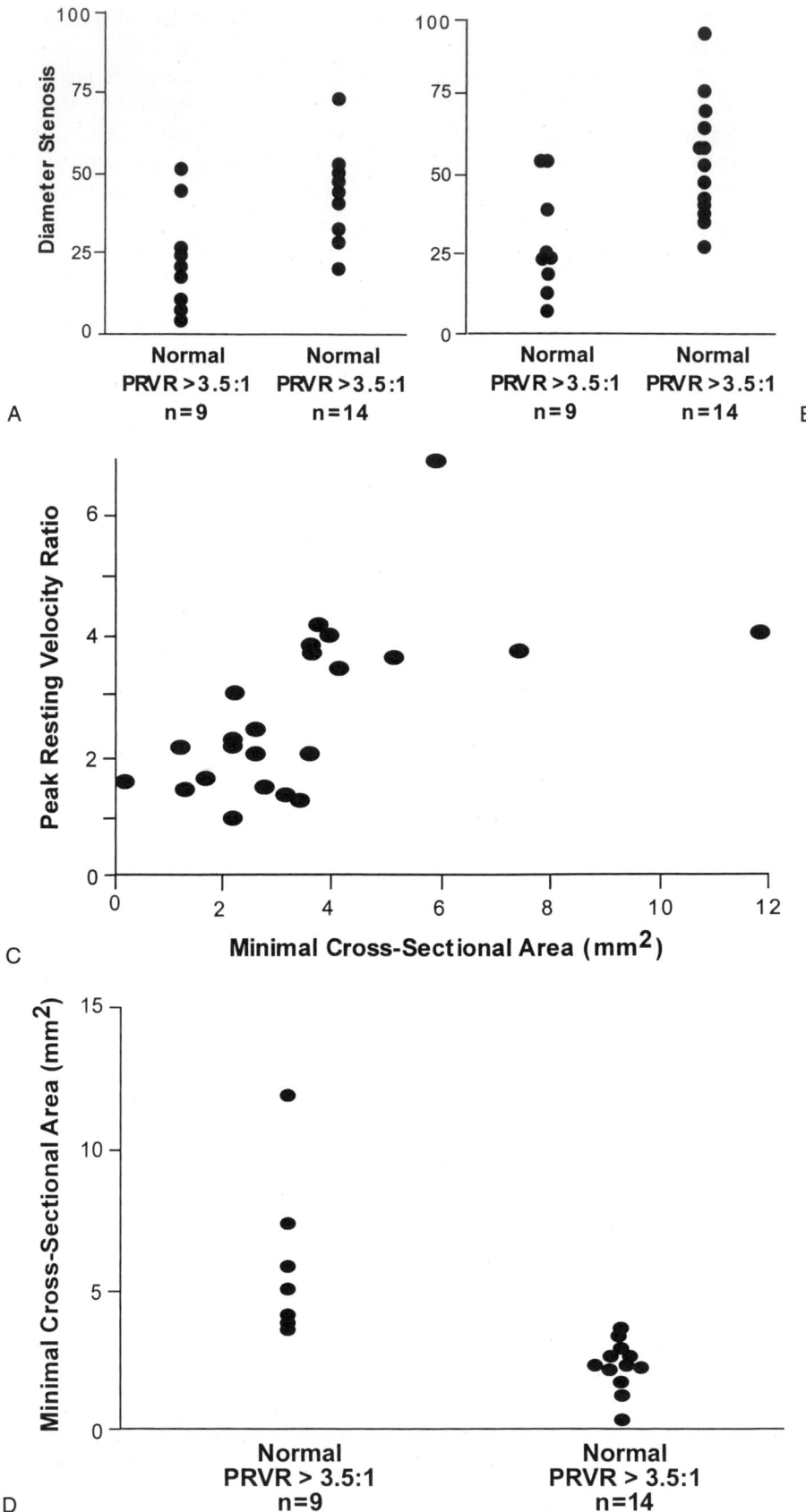

FIG. 90–11. Relation of coronary flow reserve to **(A)** percentage diameter stenosis, **(B)** percentage area stenosis, and **(C** and **D)** minimal cross-sectional lumen area in patients with diffuse coronary artery disease requiring bypass surgery. PRVR, peak resting velocity ratio.

and complications of angiography. Because each patient's situation is different, firm guidelines for the procedure can even be dangerous and should be avoided, yet general guidelines may be helpful.

Such guidelines were developed by the American College of Cardiology and American Heart Association most recently for diagnostic catheterization in 1999 (81). (Guidelines for the procedure itself are provided, with the author's comments, in the Appendix.)

SUMMARY

Like any other diagnostic test, coronary angiography is best applied with clear indications for its performance, an understanding of the prognostic implications of its findings, and a knowledge of its limitations and complications. Because of the proven survival advantage for patients with advanced disease (especially left main stenosis ≥50%, three-vessel disease, and two-vessel disease with proximal left anterior descending coronary involvement [82–85]) when treated with surgery compared with medical therapy, and the reduction of symptoms for patients appropriately treated with bypass surgery or percutaneous revascularization, diagnostic angiography as a prelude to such therapy is invaluable. Furthermore, important psychological relief for patients with troubling symptoms and inconclusive noninvasive test results can be provided by a truly normal study. However, the demonstration of angiographically "mild" disease (stenoses 25–49%) does not provide insurance against MI or suggest that risk factor modification should not be pursued (27). Finally, although the performance of the technique is considered nearly "routine," its rare serious complications and need for appropriate training in its performance should not be underestimated. In the next decade, less invasive imaging modalities such as cine computed tomography may well lessen the clinical need for this time-honored diagnostic tool, especially in patients with relatively low likelihood of disease severe enough to warrant revascularization. Nonetheless, catheter-based angiography will continue to provide the basis for percutaneous revascularization into the foreseeable future.

APPENDIX: AMERICAN COLLEGE OF CARDIOLOGY/AMERICAN HEART ASSOCIATION GUIDELINES FOR CORONARY ANGIOGRAPHY: A REPORT OF THE TASK FORCE ON PRACTICE GUIDELINES (COMMITTEE ON CORONARY ANGIOGRAPHY)

I. CLASSIFICATION OF APPLICATIONS OF CORONARY ANGIOGRAPHY

In considering the use of coronary angiography in specific disease states, the following classification (81) is used throughout this report:

Class I: Conditions for which there is general agreement that coronary angiography is justified. A Class I indication should not be taken to mean that coronary angiography is the only acceptable diagnostic procedure.

Class II: Conditions for which coronary angiography is frequently performed, but there is a divergence of opinion with respect to its justification in terms of value and appropriateness.

Class III: Conditions for which there is general agreement that coronary angiography is not ordinarily justified.

Specific disease states are considered in the following categories: known or suspected coronary heart disease, atypical chest pain, AMI, valvular heart disease, congenital heart disease, and other conditions.

It is recognized that the field of coronary angiography is undergoing considerable change, and as new insights are gained we can anticipate further refinement of the guidelines for coronary angiography set forth in this document.

II. CORONARY ANGIOGRAPHY FOR SPECIFIC CONDITIONS

A. Patients with Known or Suspected Coronary Heart Disease

1. Stable Angina

Recommendations for Coronary Angiography in Patients with Known or Suspected Coronary Artery Disease Who Are Currently Asymptomatic or Have Stable Angina

Class I
1. Canadian Cardiovascular Society (CCS) Class III and IV angina on medical treatment (Level of Evidence: B).
2. High-risk criteria on noninvasive testing regardless of anginal severity* (Level of Evidence: A).
3. Patients who have been successfully resuscitated from sudden cardiac death or have sustained (>30 seconds) monomorphic ventricular tachycardia or nonsustained (<30 seconds) polymorphic ventricular tachycardia (Level of Evidence: B).

Class IIa
1. CCS Class III or IV angina, which improves to Class I or II with medical therapy (Level of Evidence: C).

---

*1. Severe resting left ventricular dysfunction (left ventricular ejection fraction [LVEF] <35%)

2. High-risk Duke treadmill score (score ≤ −11)

3. Severe exercise left ventricular dysfunction (exercise LVEF <35%)

4. Stress-induced large perfusion defect (particularly if anterior)

5. Stress-induced, moderate-sized multiple perfusion defects

6. Large, fixed perfusion defect with left ventricular dilatation or increased lung uptake (201Th)

7. Stress-induced, moderate-sized perfusion defect with left ventricular dilatation or increased lung uptake (201Th)

8. Echocardiographic wall motion abnormally (involving >2 segments) developing at low dose of dobutamine (≤10 mg/kg · min^{-1}) or at a low hear rate (<120 beats/min)

9. Stress echocardiographic evidence of extensive ischemia

2. Serial noninvasive testing with identical testing protocols, at the same level of medical therapy, showing progressively worsening abnormalities (Level of Evidence: C).

3. Patients with angina and suspected coronary disease who, because disability, illness, or physical challenge, cannot be adequately risk stratified by other means (Level of Evidence: C).

4. CCS Class I or II angina with intolerance to adequate medical therapy or with failure to respond, or patients who have recurrence of symptoms during adequate medical therapy as defined earlier (Level of Evidence: C).

5. Individuals whose occupation involves the safety of others (e.g., pilots, bus drivers, and others) who have abnormal but not high-risk stress test results or multiple clinical features that suggest high risk (Level of Evidence: C).

Class IIb

1. CCS Class I or II angina with demonstrable ischemia but no high-risk criteria on noninvasive testing (Level of Evidence: C).

2. Asymptomatic man or postmenopausal woman without known coronary heart disease with two or more major clinical risk factors and abnormal but not high-risk criteria on noninvasive testing (performed for indications stated in the American College of Cardiology/American Heart Association (ACC/AHA) noninvasive testing guidelines) (Level of Evidence: C).

3. Asymptomatic patients with prior MI with normal resting left ventricular function and ischemia on noninvasive testing but without high-risk criteria (Level of Evidence: C).

4. Periodic evaluation after cardiac transplantation (Level of Evidence: C).

5. Candidate for liver, lung, or renal transplant in patients 40 years or older as part of evaluation for transplantation (Level of Evidence: C).

Class III

1. Angina in patients who prefer to avoid revascularization even though it might be appropriate (Level of Evidence: C).

2. Angina in patients who are not candidates for coronary revascularization or in whom revascularization is not likely to improve quality or duration of life (Level of Evidence: C).

3. As a screening test for coronary artery disease (CAD) in asymptomatic patients (Level of Evidence: C).

4. After coronary artery bypass grafting or angioplasty when there is no evidence of ischemia on noninvasive testing, unless there is informed consent for research purposes (Level of Evidence: C).

5. Coronary calcification on fluoroscopy, electron beam computed tomography, or other screening tests without criteria listed earlier (Level of Evidence: C).

2. Treatment of Patients with Nonspecific Chest Pain

Chest pain syndromes that are not characteristic of angina have been previously called noncardiac, atypical, or angiographically negative chest pain, as well as chest pain of undetermined origin. Chest pain of this type is rarely caused by myocardial ischemia, but when it is, less common causes of ischemia, such as variant angina, cocaine abuse, and syndrome X should be suspected. Other cardiac causes of nonspecific chest pain include mitral valve prolapse, myocarditis, pericarditis, and aortic dissection. Noncardiac causes include costochondritis and esophageal disorders. The latter has been implicated as a cause of nonspecific chest pain in 25% of patients. Noninvasive testing should be performed in patients with cardiovascular risk factors and those in whom a noncardiac cause has been excluded or is unlikely.

Recommendations for Coronary Angiography in Patients with Nonspecific Chest Pain

Class I
High-risk findings on noninvasive testing (Level of Evidence: B).
Class IIa
None.
Class IIb
Patients with recurrent hospitalizations for chest pain who have abnormal (but not high-risk) or equivocal findings on noninvasive testing (Level of Evidence: B).
Class III
All other patients with nonspecific chest pain (Level of Evidence: C).

3. Unstable Angina

The guidelines recommended either conservative or invasive management for those judged to be at low risk at presentation. Patients with high-risk criteria for adverse outcome (see footnote in section II.A.1) or who have recurrent ischemia are then candidates for coronary angiography. Patients with unstable angina who are thought to be at intermediate or high risk for death or nonfatal MI at presentation should be admitted to the hospital for intensive medical treatment and early diagnostic angiography. With the early invasive strategy, all in-hospital patients without contraindications receive elective cardiac catheterization within 48 hours (high risk patients are probably best treated even earlier [81a]). With the early conservative strategy, only patients with high-risk indications (prior revascularization, congestive heart failure (CHF), LVEF < 0.05, malignant ventricular arrhythmia, persistent or recurrent ischemic pain, and/or functional study indicating high risk) are referred for cardiac catheterization. Other candidates for elective catheterization include patients with significant mitral regurgitation, aortic stenosis, or hypertrophic cardiomyopathy.

Patients with variant angina may present with unstable chest pain and acute electrocardiographic (ECG) changes. Coronary angiography often is performed in these patients to establish a diagnosis and to exclude fixed obstructive disease that might require revascularization.

Recommendation for Coronary Angiography in Unstable Coronary Syndromes

Class I

1. High or intermediate risk for adverse outcome in patients with unstable angina refractory to initial adequate medical therapy or recurrent symptoms after initial stabilization. Emergent catheterization is recommended (Level of Evidence: B).
2. High risk for adverse outcome in patients with unstable angina. Urgent catheterization is recommended (Level of Evidence: B).
3. High- or intermediate-risk unstable angina that stabilizes after initial treatment (Level of Evidence: A).
4. Initially low short-term risk unstable angina that is subsequently high risk on noninvasive testing (Level of Evidence: B).
5. Suspected Prinzmetal variant angina (Level of Evidence: C).

Class IIa

None.

Class IIb

Low short-term risk unstable angina, without high-risk criteria on noninvasive testing (Level of Evidence: C).

Class III

1. Recurrent chest discomfort suggestive of unstable angina but without objective signs of ischemia and with a normal coronary angiogram during the last 5 years (Level of Evidence: C).
2. Unstable angina in patients who are not candidates for coronary revascularization or in patients for whom coronary revascularization will not improve the quality or duration of life (Level of Evidence: C).

4. Recurrence of Ischemia after Revascularization

Most revascularization procedures are performed when there is likely to be a survival benefit for patients with a high risk for adverse outcome or when there is a large amount of myocardium at risk. Therefore, postrevascularization recurrence of ischemia in these patients is generally managed aggressively.

Acute coronary closure complicates 1% to 5% of percutaneous coronary interventions and is associated with a high incidence of complications. Coronary angiography is generally performed emergently on any patient with suspected abrupt closure with the intent to repeat intervention, if possible.

Recurrence of stenosis after percutaneous transluminal coronary intervention (although much less common in the era of drug-eluting stents [81b]) is still the major limitation to long-term clinical success of the procedure. A distinction should be made between clinical and angiographic restenosis. Clinical (i.e., symptomatic) restenosis should be suspected in patients who present with recurrent angina within 9 months of a catheter-based revascularization procedure. Coronary angiography is generally performed in symptomatic patients with suspected restenosis to reassess anatomy and repeat revascularization as needed. Although coronary angiography may reveal angiographic restenosis in asymptomatic patients after angioplasty who have a positive stress test result, these patients generally have a good outcome, and asymptomatic angiographic restenosis may regress. Therefore, the committee recommends against routine noninvasive evaluation of asymptomatic patients after angioplasty. When noninvasive testing is done in asymptomatic patients and reveals high-risk markers for adverse outcome, coronary angiography is indicated.

Patients with prior coronary artery bypass surgery who experience development of angina after surgery represent an important subset of patients who require aggressive therapy. Graft obstruction within 1 to 2 months of surgery is generally related to a technical problem and often can be treated with percutaneous techniques as can graft disease within the first year. There are no data that compare outcomes in patients with late postoperative angina or ischemia who are treated medically with those treated with revascularization techniques. Most bypass patients who are suitable candidates for further revascularization and who have noninvasive evidence of high risk for adverse outcome are appropriate subjects for coronary angiography. Those who are symptomatic but deemed to be low risk by noninvasive testing can be treated medically before angiography is considered.

Recommendations for Coronary Angiography in Patients with Postrevascularization Ischemia

Class I

1. Suspected abrupt closure or subacute stent thrombosis after percutaneous revascularization (Level of Evidence: B).
2. Recurrent angina or high-risk criteria on noninvasive evaluation (see footnote in section II.A.1) within 9 months of percutaneous revascularization (Level of Evident: C).

Class IIa

1. Recurrent symptomatic ischemia within 12 months of coronary artery bypass graft (Level of Evidence: B).
2. Noninvasive evidence of high-risk criteria at any time after surgery (Level of Evidence: B).
3. Recurrent angina inadequately controlled by medical means after revascularization (Level of Evidence: C).

Class IIb

1. Asymptomatic patients after percutaneous transluminal coronary angioplasty (PTCA) suspected of having restenosis within the first months after angioplasty be-

cause of an abnormal noninvasive test result but without noninvasive high-risk criteria (Level of Evidence: B).

2. Recurrent angina without high-risk criteria on noninvasive testing occurring more than 1 year after surgery (Level of Evidence: C).

3. Asymptomatic patients after bypass in whom a deterioration in serial noninvasive testing has been documented but who is not at high risk on noninvasive testing (Level of Evidence: C).

Class III

1. Symptoms in a patients after bypass who is not a candidate for repeat revascularization (Level of Evidence: C).

2. Routine angiography in asymptomatic patients after PTCA or other surgery, unless as part of an approved research protocol (Level of Evidence: C).

5. Acute Myocardial Infarction

Although coronary angiography may be performed during or after MI solely for diagnostic purposes, most studies are done to evaluate the patient for a percutaneous or surgical revascularization procedure. Therefore, the appropriateness of performing coronary angiography after MI is, by necessity, linked to the efficacy of these revascularization procedures as measured by improved outcome for the patient. Guidelines covering PTCA, coronary artery bypass graft surgery, and management of acute MI have been published by the ACC/AHA Task Force on the Assessment of Diagnostic and Therapeutic Procedures within the last 5 years and include recommendations relevant to the use of coronary angiography.

In practical terms, the use of coronary angiography in patients with acute MI is considered during three separate time periods. The first is related to the use of coronary angiography during recognition and treatment of MI in the emergency department. It is only applicable to patients who present with an acute evolving MI within a time frame when reperfusion therapy will likely be beneficial. It is useful to stratify these patients by the presence or absence of ST-segment elevation on the ECG. Because clinical outcomes, especially with thrombolysis, are similar, the committee included in the group with ST-segment elevation patients with typical ischemic chest pain and a new or presumed new left bundle branch block (BBB) obscuring the ECG diagnosis of MI. In the presence of ongoing ischemic chest pain and ST-segment elevation (or left BBB), the clinician must quickly weigh the risks and benefits of reperfusion therapy and determine whether to use thrombolysis or mechanical techniques, with the latter being performed if available in a timely fashion. Patients with ongoing ischemic chest pain but without ST-segment elevation are a distinct group with different indications for coronary angiography compared with those with ST-segment elevation.

The second time period relates to the use of coronary angiography during the hospital management phase, after completion of reperfusion therapy, if used, or immediately if reperfusion therapy is not used. Throughout the remainder of the hospital management phase, the clinician is mainly concerned with treatment of various complications, such as arrhythmia, heart failure, or recurrent ischemia that may develop.

The final time period is defined not by a specific time but rather by evaluations to determine the risk for future morbid events and the need for additional therapies. In these guidelines, the risk stratification phase refers to testing specifically performed in the patient with MI to determine if high-risk indicators are present.

Recommendations for Coronary Angiography during the Initial Management of Acute Myocardial Infarction (Myocardial Infarction Suspected and ST-Segment Elevation of Bundle Branch Block Present) Coronary Angiography Coupled with the Intent to Perform Primary Percutaneous Transluminal Coronary Angioplasty

Class I

1. As an alternative to thrombolytic therapy in patients who can undergo angioplasty of the infarct artery within 12 hours of the onset of symptoms or beyond 12 hours if ischemic symptoms persist, if performed in a timely fashion (performance standard: within 90 minutes) by individuals skilled in the procedure (individuals who perform >75 PTCA procedures per year) and supported by experienced personnel in an appropriate laboratory environment (centers that perform >200 PCTA procedures per year and have cardiac surgical capability) (Level of Evidence: A).

2. In patients who are within 36 hours of an acute ST-segment elevation/Q-wave or new LBBB MI who experience development of cardiogenic shock, are younger than 75 years, and in whom revascularization can be performed within 18 hours of the onset of shock.

Class IIa

As a reperfusion strategy in patients who are candidates for reperfusion but who have a contraindication to fibrinolytic therapy, if angioplasty can be performed as outline above in Class I (Level of Evidence: C).

Class III

1. In patients who are beyond 12 hours from onset of symptoms and who have no evidence of myocardial ischemia (Level of Evidence: A).

2. In patients who are eligible for thrombolytic therapy and are undergoing primary angioplasty by an unskilled operator in a laboratory that does not have surgical capability (Level of Evidence: B).

Recommendations for Early Coronary Angiography in the Patient with Suspected Myocardial Infarction (ST-Segment Elevation or Bundle Branch Block Present) Who Has Not Undergone Primary Percutaneous Transluminal Coronary Angioplasty

Class I
None.

Class IIa

Cardiogenic shock or persistent hemodynamic instability (Level of Evidence: B).

Class IIb

1. Evolving large or anterior infarction after thrombolytic treatment when it is believed that reperfusion has not occurred and rescue PTCA is planned (Level of Evidence: B).
2. Marginal hemodynamic status but not actual cardiogenic shock when standard management (optimizing filling pressures) does not result in improvement (Level of Evidence: C).

Class III

1. In patients who have received thrombolytic therapy and have no symptoms of ischemia (Level of Evidence: A).
2. Routine use of angiography and subsequent PTCA within 24 hours of administration of thrombolytic agents (Level of Evidence: A).

Recommendations for Early Coronary Angiography in Acute Myocardial Infarction (Myocardial Infarction Suspected but No ST-Segment Elevation)

Class I

1. Persistent or recurrent (stuttering) episodes of symptomatic ischemia, spontaneous or induced, with or without associated ECG changes (Level of Evidence: A).
2. The presence of shock, severe pulmonary congestion, or continuing hypotension (Level of Evidence: B).

Class II

None.

Class III

None.

Recommendations for Coronary Angiography during the Hospital Management Phase (Patients with Q-Wave and Non–Q-Wave Infarction)

Class I

1. Spontaneous myocardial ischemia or myocardial ischemia provoked by minimal exertion, during recovery from infarction (Level of Evidence: C).
2. Before definitive therapy of a mechanical complication of infarction such as acute mitral regurgitation, ventricular septal defect, pseudoaneurysm, or left ventricular aneurysm (Level of Evidence: C).
3. Persistent hemodynamic instability (Level of Evidence: B).

Class IIa

1. When MI is suspected to have occurred by a mechanism other than thrombotic occlusion at an atherothrombotic plaque (e.g., coronary embolism, arteritis, trauma, certain metabolic or hematologic diseases, or coronary spasm) (Level of Evidence: C).

2. Survivors of acute MI with LVEF less than or equal to 0.40, CHF, prior revascularization, or malignant ventricular arrhythmias (Level of Evidence: C).
3. Clinical heart failure during the acute episode, but subsequent demonstration or preserved left ventricular function (LVEF > 0.40) (Level of Evidence: C).

Class IIb

1. Coronary angiography to find a persistently occluded infarct-related artery in an attempt to revascularize that artery (open artery hypothesis) (Level of Evidence: C).
2. Coronary angiography performed without other risk stratification to identify the presence of left main or three-vessel disease (Level of Evidence: C).
3. All patients after a non–Q-wave MI (Level of Evidence: C).
4. Recurrent ventricular tachycardia, fibrillation, or both, despite antiarrhythmic therapy, without evidence of ongoing myocardial ischemia (Level of Evidence: C).

Class III

Patients who are not candidates for or who refuse coronary revascularization (Level of Evidence: C).

Recommendations for Coronary Angiography during the Risk Stratification Phase (Patients with All Types of Myocardial Infarction)

Class I

Ischemia at low levels of exercise with ECG changes (≥1 mm ST-segment depression or other predictors of adverse outcome) (Table 90–3) and/or imaging abnormalities (Level of Evidence: B).

Class IIa

1. Clinically significant CHF during the hospital course (Level of Evidence: C).
2. Inability to perform an exercise test with LVEF of 0.45 or less (Level of Evidence: C).

Class IIb

1. Ischemia occurring at high levels of exercise (Level of Evidence: C).
2. Non–Q-wave MI in a patient who is an appropriate candidate for a revascularization procedure (Level of Evidence: C).
3. Need to return to an unusually active form of employment (Level of Evidence: C).
4. Remote history of MI without evidence of CHF during the current event and without evidence of inducible ischemia (Level of Evidence: C).
5. Recurrent ventricular tachycardia, fibrillation, or both, despite antiarrhythmic therapy, without ongoing myocardial ischemia (Level of Evidence: C).

Class III

Patients who are not candidates for or who refuse coronary revascularization (Level of Evidence: C).

6. Perioperative Coronary Angiography for Patients Undergoing Noncardiac Surgery

The perioperative evaluation of patients undergoing noncardiac surgery was detailed in the "ACC/AHA Guidelines for Perioperative Cardiovascular Evaluation for Noncardiac Surgery." This document outlines a comprehensive approach to perioperative risk assessment that stresses the patient's prior clinical indicators of coronary heart disease, functional status, type of noncardiac surgery, and the role of selected preoperative stress testing in patients thought to be at intermediate or high risk for major perioperative coronary events.

Generally, in patients who are being considered for noncardiac surgery, the indications for coronary angiography should be identical to those outlined in this document. However, the presentation for noncardiac surgery, its potential urgency, the level of cardiovascular stress anticipated, and the patient's general condition all play critical roles in determining the most logical sequence of events for a given patient.

Recommendations for Coronary Angiography in Perioperative Evaluation before (or after) Noncardiac Surgery

Class I: Patients with suspected or known CAD

1. Evidence for high risk for adverse outcome based on noninvasive test results (see footnote) (Level of Evidence: C).
2. Angina unresponsive to adequate medical therapy (Level of Evidence: C).
3. Unstable angina, particularly when facing intermediate* or high-risk* noncardiac surgery (Level of Evidence: C).
4. Equivocal noninvasive test result in a patient with a high clinical risk† undergoing high-risk* surgery (Level of Evidence: C).

Class IIa

1. Multiple intermediate clinical risk markers† and planned vascular surgery (Level of Evidence: B).
2. Ischemia on noninvasive testing but without high-risk criteria (see footnote) (Level of Evidence: B).

3. Equivocal noninvasive test result in a patients with intermediate clinical risk† undergoing high-risk* noncardiac surgery (Level of Evidence: C).
4. Urgent noncardiac surgery while convalescing from acute MI (Level of Evidence: C).

Class IIb

1. Perioperative MI (Level of Evidence: B).
2. Medically stabilized Class III or IV angina and planned low-risk minor* surgery (Level of Evidence: C).

Class III

1. Low-risk* noncardiac surgery, with known CAD and no high-risk results on noninvasive testing (Level of Evidence: B).
2. Asymptomatic after coronary revascularization with excellent exercise capacity (≥7 METs [metabolic equivalent]) (Level of Evidence: C).
3. Mild stable angina with good left ventricular function and no high-risk noninvasive test results (Level of Evidence: B).
4. Noncandidate for coronary revascularization owing to concomitant medical illness, severe left ventricular dysfunction (e.g., LVEF < 0.20), or refusal to consider revascularization (Level of Evidence: C).
5. Candidate for liver, lung, or renal transplant (≥40 years old) as part of evaluation for transplantation, unless noninvasive testing reveals high risk for adverse outcome (Level of Evidence: C).

B. Valvular Heart Disease

In all forms of valvular heart disease, the presence of significant coronary disease worsens prognosis. Most practitioners feel compelled to assess coronary anatomy before valve surgery and to bypass significant obstructions during surgery with the hope of avoiding late reoperation. Although there are no large clinical trials to prove its value, angiography seems to play an important role in the preoperative evaluation of patients with valvular heart disease.

That role continues to evolve. All patients with chest pain or noninvasive evidence of coronary disease should undergo coronary angiography. It still seems prudent to perform coronary angiography in patients who are at increased risk for coronary disease because of age or other risk factors.

Recommendations for Use of Coronary Angiography in Patients with Valvular Heart Disease

Class I

1. Before valve surgery or balloon valvotomy in an adult with chest discomfort, ischemia by noninvasive imaging, or both (Level of Evidence: B).
2. Before valve surgery in an adult free of chest pain but of substantial age and/or with multiple risk factors for coronary disease (Level of Evidence: C).
3. Infective endocarditis with evidence of coronary embolization (Level of Evidence: C).

---

*Cardiac risk according to type of noncardiac surgery. High risk: emergent major operations, aortic and major vascular, peripheral vascular, anticipated prolonged surgical procedures associated with large fluid shifts and/or blood loss; intermediate risk: carotid endarterectomy, major head and neck, intraperitoneal and/or intrathoracic, orthopedic surgery, prostrate surgery; low risk: endoscopic procedures, superficial procedures, cataract surgery, breast surgery.

†Cardiac risk according to clinical predictors of perioperative death, MI, or CHF. High clinical risk: unstable angina, recent MI and evidence of important residual ischemic risk, decompensated CHF, high degree of atrioventricular block, symptomatic ventricular arrhythmias with known structural heart disease, severe symptomatic valvular heart disease, multiple intermediate risk markers such as prior MI, CHF, and diabetes; intermediate clinical risk: CCS Class I or II angina, prior MI by history or ECG, compensated or prior CHF, diabetes mellitus.

Class IIa
None.
Class IIb
During left-heart catheterization performed for hemodynamic evaluation before aortic or mitral valve surgery in patients without preexisting evidence of coronary disease, multiple CAD risk factors, or advanced age (Level of Evidence: C).
Class III
1. Before cardiac surgery for infective endocarditis when there are no risk factors for coronary disease and no evidence for coronary embolization (Level of Evidence: C).
2. In asymptomatic patients when cardiac surgery is not being considered (Level of Evidence: C).
3. Before cardiac surgery when preoperative hemodynamic assessment by catheterization is unnecessary, and there is neither preexisting evidence of coronary disease nor risk factors for CAD (Level of Evidence: C).

C. Congenital Heart Disease

Although there are no large trials to support its use, coronary angiography is performed in congenital heart disease for two broad categorical indications. The first is to assess the hemodynamic impact of congenital coronary lesions. The second is to assess the presence of coronary anomalies, which by themselves may be innocent but whose presence, if unrecognized, may lead to coronary injury during correction of other congenital heart lesions.

In some cases, surgical correction is performed when the patient is older and risk for coronary disease increases. It seems prudent to perform coronary arteriography in patients being considered for repair of congenital heart disease if angina, ischemia on noninvasive testing, or multiple coronary risk factors are present.

Recommendations for Use of Coronary Angiography in Patients with Congenital Heart Disease

Class I
1. Before surgical correction of congenital heart disease when chest discomfort or noninvasive evidence is suggestive of associated CAD (Level of Evidence: C).
2. Before surgical correction of suspected congenital coronary anomalies such as congenital coronary artery stenosis, coronary arteriovenous fistula, and anomalous origin of left coronary artery (Level of Evidence: C).
3. Forms of congenital heart disease frequently associated with coronary artery anomalies that may complicate surgical management (Level of Evidence: C).
4. Unexplained cardiac arrest in a young patient (Level of Evidence: B).
Class IIa
Before corrective open heart surgery for congenital heart disease in an adult whose risk profile increases the likelihood of coexisting coronary disease (Level of Evidence: C).

Class IIb
During left-heart catheterization for hemodynamic assessment of congenital heart disease in an adult in whom the risk for coronary disease is not high (Level of Evidence: C).
Class III
In the routine evaluation of congenital heart disease in asymptomatic patients for whom heart surgery is not planned (Level of Evidence: C).

D. Congestive Heart Failure

Coronary angiography should be strongly considered for patients with systolic left ventricular dysfunction and a strong suspicion of hibernating myocardium based on the findings of noninvasive evaluation. In patients with normal systolic function but otherwise unexplained episodes of acute pulmonary edema, coronary angiography may be necessary to rule out ischemically related systolic and/or diastolic left ventricular dysfunction.

Recommendations for Use of Coronary Angiography in Patients with Congestive Heart Failure

Class I
1. CHF caused by systolic dysfunction with angina or with regional wall motion abnormalities and/or scintigraphic evidence of reversible myocardial ischemia when revascularization is being considered (Level of Evidence: B).
2. Before cardiac transplantation (Level of Evidence: C).
3. CHF secondary to postinfarction ventricular aneurysm or other mechanical complications of MI (Level of Evidence: C).
Class IIa
1. Systolic dysfunction with unexplained cause despite noninvasive testing (Level of Evidence: C).
2. Normal systolic function, but episodic heart failure increases suspicion of ischemically mediated left ventricular dysfunction (Level of Evidence: C).
Class III
CHF with previous coronary angiograms showing normal coronary arteries, with no new evidence to suggest ischemic heart disease (Level of Evidence: C).

E. Other Conditions

Recommendations for Use of Coronary Angiography in Other Conditions

Class I
1. Diseases affecting the aorta when knowledge of the presence or extent of coronary artery involvement is necessary for management (e.g., aortic dissection or aneurysm with known coronary disease) (Level of Evidence: B).
2. Hypertrophic cardiomyopathy with angina despite medical therapy when knowledge of coronary anatomy might affect therapy (Level of Evidence: C).

3. Hypertrophic cardiomyopathy with angina when heart surgery is planned (Level of Evidence: B).

Class IIa

1. High risk for coronary disease when other cardiac surgical procedures are planned (e.g., pericardiectomy or removal of chronic pulmonary emboli) (Level of Evidence: C).

2. Prospective immediate cardiac transplant donors whose risk profile increases the likelihood of coronary disease (Level of Evidence: B).

3. Asymptomatic patients with Kawasaki disease who have coronary artery aneurysms on echocardiography (Level of Evidence: B).

4. Before surgery for aortic aneurysm/dissection in patients without known coronary disease.

5. Recent blunt chest trauma and suspicion of acute MI, without evidence of preexisting CAD (Level of Evidence: C).

REFERENCES

1. Bruschke AV, Proudfit WL, Sones FM Jr. Progress study of 590 consecutive nonsurgical cases of coronary disease followed 5–9 years. I. Arteriographic correlations. *Circulation* 1973;47:1147–1153.
2. Forssmann W. The catheterization of the right side of the heart. *Klin Wochenschr* 1928;8:2085.
3. Cournand A. Cardiac catheterization: development of the technique, its contributions to experimental medicine, and its initial applications in man. *Acta Med Scand (Suppl)* 1975;579:7.
4. Zimmerman HA, Scott RW, Becker NO. Catheterization of the left side of the heart in man. *Circulation* 1950;1:357.
5. Hurst JW. History of cardiac catheterization. In: King SB 3rd, Douglas JS Jr, eds. *Coronary arteriography and angioplasty.* New York: McGraw-Hill, 1985:1–9.
6. Judkins MP. Selective coronary arteriography. I. A percutaneous transfemoral technique. *Radiology* 1976;89:815.
7. King SB 3rd, Douglas JS Jr. Coronary arteriography and left ventriculography: multipurpose technique. In: King SB 3rd, Douglas JS Jr, eds. *Coronary arteriography and angioplasty.* New York: McGraw-Hill, 1985:239.
8. Glagov S, Weisenberg E, Zarins CK, et al. Compensatory enlargement of human atherosclerotic coronary arteries. *N Engl J Med* 1987;316:1371–1375.
9. Arnett EN, Isner JM, Redwood DR, et al. Coronary artery narrowing in coronary heart disease: comparison of cineangiographic and necropsy findings. *Ann Intern Med* 1979;91:350.
10. Little WC, Constantinescu M, Applegate RJ, et al. Can coronary angiography predict the site of a subsequent myocardial infarction in patients with mild-to-moderate coronary artery disease? *Circulation* 1988;78:1157–1166.
11. Kereiakes DJ, Topol EJ, George BS, et al. Myocardial infarction with minimal coronary atherosclerosis in the era of thrombolytic reperfusion. The Thrombolysis and Angioplasty in Myocardial Infarction (TAMI) Study Group. *J Am Coll Cardiol* 1991;17:304–312.
12. Gould KL, Lipscomb K, Hamilton GW. Physiologic basis for assessing critical coronary stenosis: instantaneous flow response and regional distribution during coronary hyperemia as measures of coronary flow reserve. *Am J Cardiol* 1974;33:87–94.
13. Tofler GH, Stone PH, Muller JE, et al. Effects of gender and race on prognosis after myocardial infarction: adverse prognosis for women, particularly black women. *J Am Coll Cardiol* 1987;9:473.
14. DeBusk RF, Kraemer HC, Nash E, et al. Stepwise risk stratification soon after acute myocardial infarction. *Am J Cardiol* 1983;52:1161.
15. Merrilees MA, Scott PJ, Norris RM. Prognosis after myocardial infarction: results of 15-year follow-up. *Br Med J* 1984;288:356.
16. Smith JW, Marcus FI, Serokman R. Prognosis of patients with diabetes mellitus after acute myocardial infarction. *Am J Cardiol* 1984;54:718.
17. Risk stratification and survival after myocardial infarction. *N Engl J Med* 1983;309:331–336.
18. Sanz G, Castañer A, Betriu A, et al. Determinants of prognosis in survivors of myocardial infarction. A prospective clinical angiographic study. *N Engl J Med* 1982;306:1065–1070.
19. Bigger JT Jr, Fleiss JL, Kleiger R, et al. The relationships among ventricular arrhythmias, left ventricular dysfunction, and mortality in the 2 years after myocardial infarction. *Circulation* 1984;69:250.
20. Fioretti P, Brower RW, Simoons ML, et al. Relative value of clinical variables, bicycle ergometry, rest radionuclide ventriculography and 24-hour ambulatory electrocardiographic monitoring at discharge to predict 1-year survival after myocardial infarction. *J Am Coll Cardiol* 1986;8:40.
21. Dagenais GR, Rouleau JR, Christen A, et al. Survival of patients with a strongly positive exercise electrocardiogram. *Circulation* 1982;65:452.
22. Alderman EL, Bourassa MG, Cohen LS, et al. Ten-year follow-up of survival and myocardial infarction in the randomized Coronary Artery Surgery Study. *Circulation* 1990;82:1629–1646.
23. Varnauskas E. Twelve-year follow-up of survival in the randomized European Coronary Surgery Study. *N Engl J Med* 1988;319:332–337.
24. Ellis SG, Roubin GS, King SB, et al. Angiographic and clinical predictors of acute closure after native vessel coronary angioplasty. *Circulation* 1988;77:372–379.
25. Mock MB, Ringqvist I, Fisher LD, et al. Survival of medically treated patients in the coronary artery surgery study (CASS) registry. *Circulation* 1982;66:562–568.
26. Califf RM, Phillips HR 3rd, Hindman MC, et al. Prognostic value of a coronary artery jeopardy score. *J Am Coll Cardiol* 1985;5:1055–1063.
27. Mark DB, Nelson CL, Califf RM, et al. Continuing evolution of therapy for coronary artery disease. Initial results from the era of coronary angioplasty. *Circulation* 1994;89:2015–2025.
28. Papanicolaou MN, Califf RM, Hlatky MA, et al. Prognostic implications of angiographically normal and insignificantly narrowed coronary arteries. *Am J Cardiol* 1986;58:1181–1187.
29. Davies MJ. A macro and micro view of coronary vascular insult in ischemic heart disease. *Circulation* 1990;82:II-38–II-46.
30. Fuster V, Stein B, Ambrose JA, et al. Atherosclerotic plaque rupture and thrombosis. Evolving concepts. *Circulation* 1990;82:II-47–II-59.
31. Moise A, Lesperance J, Theroux P, et al. Clinical and angiographic predictors of new total coronary occlusions in coronary artery disease: analysis of 313 unoperated patients. *Am J Cardiol* 1984;54:1176–1181.
32. Fuster V, Badimon L, Badimon JJ, et al. The pathogenesis of coronary artery disease and the acute coronary syndromes. *N Engl J Med* 1992;326:310–318.
33. Ellis S, Alderman E, Cain K, et al. Prediction of risk of anterior myocardial infarction by lesion severity and measurement method of stenoses in the left anterior descending coronary distribution: a CASS Registry Study. *J Am Coll Cardiol* 1988;11:908–916.
34. Ambrose JA, Winters SL, Arora RR, et al. Angiographic evolution of coronary artery morphology in unstable angina. *J Am Coll Cardiol* 1986;7:472–478.
35. Ambrose JA, Tannenbaum MA, Alexopoulos D, et al. Angiographic progression of coronary artery disease and the development of myocardial infarction. *J Am Coll Cardiol* 1988;12:56–62.
36. Dacanay S, Kennedy HL, Uretz E, et al. Morphological and quantitative angiographic analyses of progression of coronary stenoses. A comparison of Q-wave and non-Q-wave myocardial infarction. *Circulation* 1994;90:1739–1746.
37. Giroud D, Li JM, Urban P, et al. Relation of the site of acute myocardial infarction to the most severe coronary arterial stenosis at prior angiography. *Am J Cardiol* 1992;69:729–732.
38. Nobuyoshi M, Tanaka M, Nosaka H, et al. Progression of coronary atherosclerosis: is coronary spasm related to progression? *J Am Coll Cardiol* 1991;18:904–910.

39. Levin DC, Fallon JT. Significance of the angiographic morphology of localized coronary stenoses: histopathologic correlations. *Circulation* 1982;66:316–320.

40. Ambrose JA, Winters SL, Arora RR, et al. Coronary angiographic morphology in myocardial infarction: a link between the pathogenesis of unstable angina and myocardial infarction. *J Am Coll Cardiol* 1985;6:1233–1238.

41. Ellis S, Alderman EL, Cain K, et al. Morphology of left anterior descending coronary territory lesions as a predictor of anterior myocardial infarction: a CASS registry study. *J Am Coll Cardiol* 1989;13:1481–1491.

42. Brown BG, Bolson EL, Dodge HT. Arteriographic assessment of coronary atherosclerosis. Review of current methods, their limitations and clinical applications. *Arteriosclerosis* 1982;2:2–15.

43. Ellis S, Sanders W, Goulet C, et al. Optimal detection of the progression of coronary artery disease: comparison of methods suitable for risk factor intervention trials. *Circulation* 1986;74:1235–1242.

44. Moise A, Theroux P, Taeymans Y, et al. Clinical and angiographic factors associated with progression of coronary artery disease. *J Am Coll Cardiol* 1984;3:659–667.

45. Arntzenius AC, Kromhout D, Barth JD, et al. Diet, lipoproteins, and the progression of coronary atherosclerosis. The Leiden Intervention Trial. *N Engl J Med* 1985;312:805–811.

46. Raichlen JS, Healy B, Achuff SC, et al. Importance of risk factors in the angiographic progression of coronary artery disease. *Am J Cardiol* 1986;57:66–70.

47. Lichtlen PR, Nikutta P, Jost S, et al. Anatomical progression of coronary artery disease in humans as seen by prospective, repeated, quantitated coronary angiography. Relation to clinical events and risk factors. The INTACT Study Group. *Circulation* 1992;86:828–838.

48. Brown G, Albers JJ, Fisher LD, et al. Regression of coronary artery disease as a result of intensive lipid-lowering therapy in men with high levels of apolipoprotein B. *N Engl J Med* 1990;323:1289–1298.

49. Ornish D, Brown SE, Scherwitz LW, et al. Can lifestyle changes reverse coronary heart disease? *Lancet* 1990;336:129–133.

50. Jost S, Deckers JW, Nikutta P, et al. Progression of coronary artery disease is dependent on anatomic location and diameter. The INTACT investigators. *J Am Coll Cardiol* 1993;21:1339–1346.

51. Alderman EL, Corley SD, Fisher LD, et al. Five-year angiographic follow-up of factors associated with progression of coronary artery disease in the Coronary Artery Surgery Study (CASS). CASS Participating Investigators and Staff. *J Am Coll Cardiol* 1993;22:1141–1154.

52. Bourassa MG, Enjalbert M, Campeau L, et al. Progression of atherosclerosis in coronary arteries and bypass grafts: ten years later. *Am J Cardiol* 1984;53:102C–107C.

53. Kirklin JW, Blackstone EH, Rogers WJ. The plights of the invasive treatment of ischemic heart disease. *J Am Coll Cardiol* 1985;5:158–167.

54. Guidelines for percutaneous transluminal coronary angioplasty. A report of the American College of Cardiology/American Heart Association Task Force on Assessment of Diagnostic and Therapeutic Cardiovascular Procedures (Subcommittee on Percutaneous Transluminal Coronary Angioplasty). *J Am Coll Cardiol* 1988;12:529–545.

55. Ellis SG, Vandormael MG, Cowley MJ, et al. Coronary morphologic and clinical determinants of procedural outcome with angioplasty for multivessel coronary disease. Implications for patient selection. *Circulation* 1990;82:1193–1202.

56. Ellis SG, Guetta V, Miller D, et al. Relation between lesion characteristics and risk with percutaneous intervention in the stent and glycoprotein IIb/IIIa era: an analysis of results from 10,907 lesions and proposal for new classification scheme. *Circulation* 1999;100:1971–1976.

57. Moscucci M, Kline-Rogers E, Share D, et al. Simple bedside additive tool for prediction of in-hospital mortality after percutaneous coronary interventions. *Circulation* 2001;104:263–268.

58. Laskey W, Boyle J, Johnson LW. Multivariable model for prediction of risk of significant complication during diagnostic cardiac catheterization. *Cath Cardiovasc Diagn* 1993;30:185–190.

59. Steinberg EP, Moore RD, Gopalan R, et al. Safety and cost effectiveness of high-osmality as compared with low-osmolality contrast material in patients undergoing cardiac angiography. *N Engl J Med* 1992;326:425–430.

60. Hill JA, Winniford M, Van Fossen DB, et al. Nephrotoxicity following cardiac angiography: a randomized double-blind multicenter trial of ionic and nonionic contrast media in 1194 patients. *Circulation* 1991;84:II 333.

61. Matthai WH, Kussmaul WG 3rd, Krol J, et al. A comparison of low-

with high-osmolality contrast agents in cardiac angiography. Identification of criteria for selective use. *Circulation* 1994;89:291–301.

62. Guidelines for coronary angiography. A report of the American College of Cardiology/American Heart Association Task Force on Assessment of diagnostic and therapeutic cardiovascular procedures (subcommittee on coronary angiography). *J Am Coll Cardiol* 1987;10:935–950.

63. Douglas JS Jr, Franch RH, King SB 3rd. Coronary artery anomalies. In: King SB 3rd, Douglas JS Jr, eds. *Coronary arteriography and angioplasty.* New York: McGraw-Hill, 1985:33–85.

64. DeRouen TA, Murray JA, Owen W. Variability in the analysis of coronary arteriograms. *Circulation* 1977;55:324–328.

65. Sanmarco ME, Brooks SH, Blankenhorn DH. Reproducibility of a consensus panel in the interpretation of coronary angiograms. *Am Heart J* 1978;96:430–437.

66. Fisher LD, Judkins MP, Lesperance J, et al. Reproducibility of coronary arteriographic reading in the Coronary Artery Surgery Study (CASS). *Cath Cardiovasc Diagn* 1982;8:565–575.

67. Elliott J, Tuzcu EM, Guyer S, et al. Relationship of left main coronary dimension to branch vessel size: a new index for detection of LMCA disease. *J Am Coll Cardiol* 1994;210A.

68. Fleming RM, Kirkeeide RL, Smalling RW, et al. Patterns in visual interpretation of coronary arteriograms as detected by quantitative coronary arteriography. *J Am Coll Cardiol* 1991;18:945–951.

69. Painter JA, Mintz GS, Pichard AD, et al. Clinical correlates of atherosclerosis in angiographically normal coronary artery reference segments: an intravascular ultrasound study. *J Am Coll Cardiol* 1994;25:373A.

70. Erbel R, Ge J, Haude M, et al. Intracoronary ultrasound imaging of angiographically unidentified left main coronary artery atherosclerosis. *J Am Coll Cardiol* 1994;6:290A.

71. Mancini GB. Quantitative coronary arteriography: development of methods, limitations, and clinical applications. *Am J Card Imaging* 1988;2:98–109.

72. Mancini GB, Simon SB, McGillem MJ, et al. Automated quantitative coronary arteriography: morphologic and physiologic validation in vivo of a rapid digital angiographic method. *Circulation* 1987;75:452–460.

73. Fortin DF, Spero LA, Cusma JT, et al. Pitfalls in the determination of absolute dimensions using angiographic catheters as calibration devices in quantitative angiography. *Am J Cardiol* 1991;68:1176–1182.

74. Reiber JH, Serruys PW, Kooijman CJ, et al. Assessment of short-, medium-, and long-term variations in arterial dimensions from computer-assisted quantitation of coronary cineangiograms. *Circulation* 1985;71:280–288.

75. Desmet WJ, De Scheerder IK, Piessens JH. Systematic differences between systems routinely used for quantitative coronary analysis. *Circulation* 1994;90:I-487.

76. Kalbfleisch SJ, McGillem MJ, Pinto MF, et al. Comparison of automated quantitative coronary angiography with caliper measurements of percent diameter stenosis. *Am J Cardiol* 1990;65:1181–1184.

77. Uehata A, Matsuguchi T, Bittl JA, et al. Accuracy of electronic digital calipers compared with quantitative angiography in measuring coronary arterial diameter. *Circulation* 1993;88:1724–1729.

78. Harrison DG, White CW, Hiratzka LF, et al. The value of lesion cross-sectional area determined by quantitative coronary angiography in assessing the physiologic significance of proximal left anterior descending coronary arterial stenoses. *Circulation* 1984;69:1111–1119.

79. Haber HL, Beller GA, Watson DD, et al. Exercise thallium-201 scintigraphy after thrombolytic therapy with or without angioplasty for acute myocardial infarction. *Am J Cardiol* 1993;71:1257–1261.

80. McMahon MM, Brown BG, Dukingnan R, et al. Quantitative coronary angiography: measurement of the "critical" stenosis in patients with unstable angina and single-vessel disease without collaterals. *Circulation* 1979;60:106–113.

81. Scanlon PJ, Faxon DP, Audet AM, et al. ACC/AHA Guidelines for Coronary Angiography: Executive Summary and Recommendations. *Circulation* 1999;99:2345–2357.

81a. Neumann FJ, Kastrati A, Pogatsa-Murray G, et al. Evaluation of prolonged antithrombotic pretreatment ("cooling-off" strategy) before intervention in patients with unstable coronary syndromes: a randomized controlled trial. *JAMA* 2003;290:1593–1599.

81b. Moses JW, Leon MB, Popma JJ, et al. Sirolimus-eluting stents versus standard stents in patients with stenosis in a native coronary artery. *N Engl J Med* 2003;349:1315–1323.

82. Chaitman BR, Fisher LD, Bourassa MG, et al. Effect of coronary bypass surgery on survival patterns in subsets of patients with left main coronary artery disease. Report of the Collaborative Study in Coronary Artery Surgery (CASS). *Am J Cardiol* 1981;48:765–777.
83. Long-term results of prospective randomised study of coronary artery bypass surgery in stable angina pectoris. European Coronary Surgery Study Group. *Lancet* 1982;2:1173–1180.
84. Kaiser GC, Davis KB, Fisher LD, et al. Survival following coronary artery bypass grafting in patients with severe angina pectoris (CASS). *J Thorac Cardiovasc Surg* 1985;89:513–524.
85. Parisi AF, Folland ED, Hartigan P. A comparison of angioplasty with medical therapy in the treatment of single-vessel coronary artery disease. Veterans Affairs ACME Investigators. *N Engl J Med* 1992;326:10–16.

CHAPTER 91

Interventional Applications of Coronary Intravascular Ultrasound, Doppler Flow, and Fractional Flow Reserve

Anthony C. De Franco, E. Murat Tuzcu, Steven E. Nissen, and Sorin Brener

Key Words: Coronary stenting; Doppler flow; fractional flow reserve; intravascular ultrasound; percutaneous coronary intervention.

INTRODUCTION

The principal clinical indication for coronary angiography is to determine the presence and extent of hemodynamically significant lesions; however, cardiologists now recognize that the ability of angiography to make this determination has limitations in particular clinical situations. New coronary imaging devices are rapidly altering conventional paradigms in the diagnosis and therapy of coronary artery disease. Technical advances within the last decade have enabled intraluminal evaluation of the coronary arteries using miniaturized ultrasound imaging, Doppler probes, and pressure sensors; these devices are increasingly used to supplement angiographic data. Many studies have documented the clinical situations in which these techniques provide incremental information to angiographic evaluation of the morphologic and physiologic disturbances produced by coronary atherothrombosis.

The application of these procedures during percutaneous coronary interventions (PCIs) can provide important information about the mechanism and extent of lumen enlargement, the presence of complications, and the relative improvement in blood flow. This chapter reviews the status of

A. C. De Franco: McLaren Heart and Vascular Center, Division of Cardiology, McLaren Regional Medical Center; Department of Medicine, Michigan State University, Flint, Michigan.

E. M. Tuzcu: Intravascular Ultrasound Laboratory; Department of Medicine, The Cleveland Clinic Foundation, Cleveland, Ohio.

S. E. Nissen: Division of Cardiology, Cleveland Clinic Foundation; Department of Medicine, The Cleveland Clinic Foundation, Cleveland, Ohio.

S. Brener: Angiographic Core Laboratory, Department of Medicine, The Cleveland Clinic Foundation, Cleveland, Ohio.

these technologies in the interventional laboratory and the implications of these findings for understanding the pathogenesis and optimal management of coronary artery disease.

RATIONALE FOR NEW IMAGING MODALITIES

Although angiography remains a valuable method to assess coronary artery disease severity clinically, cardiologists now recognize its limitations in certain clinical situations (Table 91–1). For the interventionalist, three observations are particularly important. First, angiography is an indirect and relative measure of luminal narrowing. To evaluate the severity of a lesion, the angiographer measures the diameter of a "reference site," which is presumed to be disease-free. However, postmortem studies have consistently demonstrated that coronary atherothrombosis is typically a diffuse, rather than focal, process. Accordingly, no truly normal reference segment exists from which to calculate percentage stenosis. In the most dramatic circumstances, diffuse, concentric, and symmetric coronary disease can affect the entire length of the vessel, resulting in an angiographic appearance of a small artery with minimal luminal irregularities. In the presence of diffuse vessel involvement, determination of percent diameter stenosis will predictably underestimate true disease severity.

Second, angiography often cannot accurately depict irregular lumen shapes, which commonly occur in acute coronary syndromes and after nonstent interventions. The silhouette perspective of angiography usually misrepresents these complex or even bizarrely distorted luminal shapes (see Chapter 50 for examples). Nonstent coronary interventions typically exaggerate the complexity of luminal shape by dissecting, fracturing, or distorting the atheroma (Fig. 91–1). Accordingly, the postintervention lumen may appear significantly larger by angiography, exaggerating the gain in lumen size. The postintervention site is frequently described

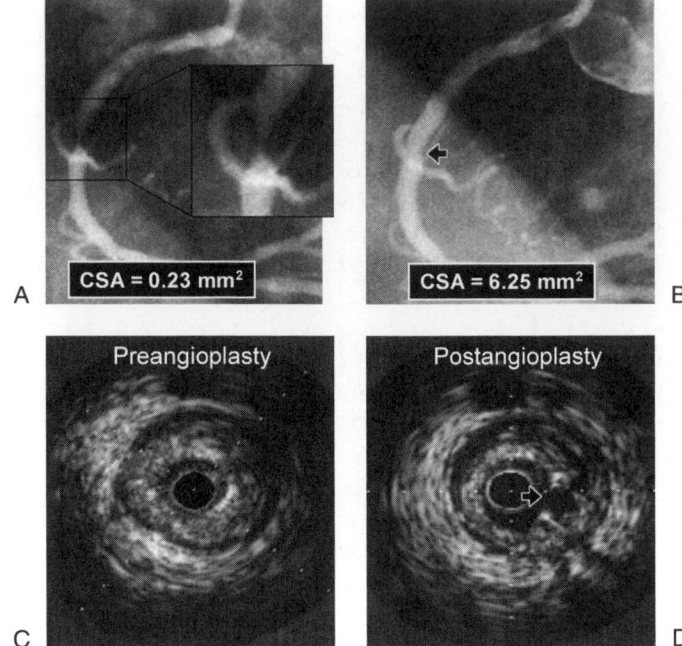

FIG. 91–1. Nonstent coronary interventions frequently exaggerate luminal shapes and make accurate assessment of stenosis severity and luminal size impossible. Balloon angioplasty of this lesion resulted in the angiographic illusion of restoration of near-normal lumen dimensions. **A:** Preprocedure angiogram demonstrates severe stenosis. **B:** After balloon angioplasty, the angiogram demonstrates a minimal residual luminal narrowing. **C:** Preprocedure IVUS. **D:** Postballoon angioplasty IVUS, which demonstrates that although lumen enlargement has occurred, contrast permentes the resulting dissection deep into the plaque (*arrow*, dissection entry site), giving the illusion that the procedure has achieved a gain in lumen size much larger than actual. CSA, cross-sectional area; IVUS, intravascular ultrasound.

TABLE 91–1. *Some limitations of angiographic assessment of coronary atherothrombosis*

- Necropsy cases reveal major differences between the angiographic lesion severity and histologic examination.
- Atherothrombosis is typically diffuse rather than focal, often lacking truly normal reference segments from which to calculate percent stenosis.
- Necropsy studies demonstrate that angiography significantly underestimates atherothrombosis extent.
- The accuracy and reproducibility of coronary arteriography is suboptimal; visual interpretation has clinically significant intraobserver and interobserver variability.
- Quantitative coronary angiography has improved the luminal measurement reproducibility, but it is limited by magnification errors and inability to detect disease reference segment.
- Angiography cannot accurately depict irregular lumen shapes, which commonly occur in acute coronary syndromes and after nonstent interventions.
- Angiography does not assess hemodynamics.

---

as "hazy," which may result from an irregular lumen shape, an intramural dissection, thrombus, or a combination of these mechanisms. Third, angiography does not assess actual coronary flow before or after the intervention. In the absence of data regarding flow reserve, practitioners traditionally have relied on indirect techniques such as exercise testing or nuclear scintigraphy to assess the necessity for and results of percutaneous revascularization. Thus, the rationale for adjunctive imaging is to supplement angiographic data in these particular clinical situations.

CORONARY INTRAVASCULAR ULTRASOUND

Rationale

Intravascular ultrasound (IVUS) has several properties that allow more precise quantification of coronary disease. First, the tomographic orientation enables visualization of the full 360-degree vessel circumference, rather than a two-dimensional silhouette. Lumen dimensions can be directly planimetered on a cross-sectional image. Ultrasound systems contain an internally generated electronic scale that is overlaid on the image. Because the velocity of sound within soft tissues is nearly constant, ultrasound measurements are inherently accurate and do not require additional calibration. Accordingly, many authorities consider IVUS the current "gold standard" for measurement of luminal dimensions.

Second, ultrasound permits direct inspection of the vessel wall, enabling visualization of coronary atheromas *in vivo*. Data are emerging that atheroma morphology is an important factor influencing the natural history and prognosis of coronary disease. For the interventionalist, plaque morphology is a critical determinant of the response of the vessel to mechanical interventions. For example, angiographically occult calcification can significantly prevent adequate expansion of metallic stents, even when high-pressure deployment is used. Ultrasound is exquisitely sensitive for the detection of coronary atherothrombosis, even in vessels that are typically difficult to assess by angiography, such as diffusely diseased segments, ostial and bifurcation sites, and highly eccentric plaques. In such circumstances, foreshortening or overlapping structures may preclude accurate angiographic imaging; however, IVUS is usually unaffected by these factors.

Ultrasound Catheters and Computerized Image Construction

Intracoronary ultrasound equipment consists of two major components: a catheter with a miniature ultrasound transducer and a console with the electronics to reconstruct the image. Transducers operate at relatively high frequencies, typically in the range of 20 to 40 MHz, because wavelength determines the maximum resolution and is inversely proportional to the frequency. Axial resolution approaches 80 μm, whereas lateral resolution is depth-dependent and averages about 150 to 200 μm. Contemporary devices produce remarkably high image quality. There are two different technical approaches to transducer design: mechanically rotated devices and multielement electronic arrays, which have significantly different imaging and catheter-handling characteristics. Mechanical probes use a drive cable running the length of the catheter that rotates a single piezoelectric transducer mounted near the distal catheter tip. A rotation rate of 1,800 g corresponds to 30 full revolutions per second, yielding 30 images per second. Alternatively, fully electronic ultrasound systems have probes with an annular array of multiple piezoelectric transducer elements (currently up to 64) that are activated sequentially to generate the image. The electronic signals are processed by several ultraminiaturized integrated circuits near the catheter tip; thus, only two conductive wires (rather than a drive cable) are required within the catheter. To generate the image, electronic systems use a reconstruction algorithm known as a "synthetic aperture array." Radial scan lines are reconstructed using data derived from multiple transducer elements, using fewer numbers of elements for pixels near the catheter surface and a larger number for pixels in the far field.

Intracoronary ultrasound catheters have an outer diameter between 2.9 and 3.5 French (0.96–1.17 mm in diameter). These small devices are suitable for examination of more distal coronary locations and permit examination of almost all stenotic segments before intervention. The smallest catheters can now be placed through a 6 French guiding catheter. Most ultrasound catheters are monorail designs to facilitate rapid exchanges. Although the mechanical properties and catheter size have vastly improved, handling characteristics remain inferior to angioplasty equipment. Multielement designs generally result in catheters with greater flexibility, whereas mechanical probes have traditionally offered superior image quality. However, these differences have narrowed in recent years.

The second component of all ultrasound systems is the console, which includes the processors to reconstruct the image and an integrated digital recording system for archival storage. Additional processing allows real-time three-dimensional reconstruction, computerized measurement packages, color depictions of coronary flow, and other enhancements. Although these techniques have limitations, each can be useful clinically.

Examination Technique

IVUS examination is performed with standard interventional techniques for catheter delivery. A 6 or 7 French guiding catheter with good support is desirable, because current catheters have less trackability and a larger profile than angioplasty catheters. Heparin (3,000–5,000 U) must be administered before imaging; in addition, intracoronary nitroglycerin (100–200 μg) immediately before each imaging run can prevent coronary spasm and standardizes arterial dimensions under maximal vasodilation. A motorized pullback device to withdraw the catheter at a constant speed is essential for several reasons. By starting every IVUS study at a fiduciary point (such as a side branch) and recording a "pullback" from that point, the imaging run can be systematically reviewed "offline." With experience, motorized pullback substantially shortens the time required to obtain accurate measurements. Motorized pullback offers the only accurate method to measure lesion length, which at times can be vital for stent selection. In addition, motorized pullback allows systematic review after the procedure, without having to guess in which direction the catheter was moving at a particular point. Occasionally, extremely focal lesions (such as at ostia and bifurcations) necessitate supplemental *manual* interrogation *after* a motorized survey.

The safety of IVUS imaging has been well documented. Although the immediate adverse effects are few, the most frequently encountered is focal coronary spasm (5–10%), which usually responds rapidly to intracoronary nitroglycerin. Data from several large series report complication rates in the range of 0.5% to 1.5%, the majority of which are reversible or readily treatable (spasm, vessel dissection, and others) (1). With lower profiles of newer catheters the incidence of vasospasm may be even lower. Even annual three-vessel coronary IVUS imaging in cardiac transplant recipients is safe and does not accelerate transplant coronary artery disease (2).

Normal and Abnormal Morphology

Ultrasound vividly depicts normal and abnormal coronary anatomy. With low-frequency transducers (20 MHz) the lumen is essentially sonolucent. At greater frequencies (>30 MHz), blood appears as faint, finely textured specular echoes that swirl during flow, because of signal return from circulating blood cells. Blood echogenicity can help to identify the lumen–wall interface and any dissection channels. However, when velocities are reduced (such as when the catheter itself occludes the lumen at a severe stenosis), the signal from the slowly flowing blood has an increased echogenicity that can sometimes confound the distinction between lumen and the intima.

IVUS depicts normal arteries as circular lumens surrounded by distinct layers of differing echogenicity (see Fig. 50–3) with two basic patterns. Some sites have a trilaminar appearance, with three discrete layers corresponding to the intima, media, and adventitia. Although there is still some controversy regarding the genesis of these ultrasonic layers, most authorities agree that the innermost band represents reflections from the internal elastic lamina. Many investigators use 0.25 to 0.30 mm as an upper limit of normal. In normal arteries with distinct layers, the middle sonolucent layer is primarily vessel media. The third and deepest layer often has an "onionskin" pattern and represents the adventitia and periadventitial tissues. About 50% of healthy subjects, particularly younger individuals, exhibit a monolayered appearance. At these sites, the internal elastic lamina is exceedingly thin and presumably reflects little of the ultrasound signal. The appearance and thickness of the innermost layer is age dependent, with older subjects exhibiting values at the upper end of this range (3).

Subjects with atherothrombotic vessels have much more varied spectrum of sonographic features that reflect disease severity and plaque composition. At sites with minimal disease, there is thickening of the intimal leading edge, whereas more advanced lesions typically appear as large echogenic masses that may or may not encroach on the lumen. Intravascular ultrasonographers classify atheromas into one of three categories according to their echogenicity: Plaques are described as soft, fibrous, or calcified (see Fig. 50–5). "Soft" plaques are those less echogenic (sonolucent) than the surrounding adventitia; *in vitro* studies demonstrate that these lesions often have high lipid content. "Fibrous" plaques have an echodensity similar to adventitia; whereas "calcified" lesions are segments more echogenic than surrounding adventitia, with acoustic shadowing of the deeper structures. This effect occurs because the calcified areas attenuate the transmission of the ultrasound signal to these deeper layers.

Some caution is necessary in the interpretation of IVUS images, because they represent reconstruction of the acoustic reflections from the wall, rather than *actual* histology. The echogenicity and texture of many different histologic features may appear quite similar by IVUS. For example, a "soft" lesion may represent adherent thrombus, but a nearly identical image from another site may represent atheroma. It is prudent to avoid dogmatic conclusions regarding the tissue content of individual lesions. For example, the genesis of some types of images is controversial. The middle, sonolucent layer becomes relatively thick (0.5–1.5 mm) in some diseased arteries. Some investigators propose that this zone is primarily normal media; however, pathology studies demonstrate that in most diseased vessels, the media thins or is completely absent. Other investigators suggest that differences in instrumentation or attenuation of the ultrasound signal explains this appearance, and still others propose that a high lipid content, the age of the lesion, or the type of artery (muscular versus elastic) affect this appearance. Newer approaches in ultrasound signal processing, such as tissue backscatter analysis may allow more definitive interpretation of the actual histology.

Despite these limitations, the general classification of coronary plaques into the categories of soft, fibrous, or calcified has significant clinical importance to the interventionalist. These three categories often respond quite differently to interventional devices. Densely fibrotic or calcified plaques often resist expansion even with high-pressure stent deployment; in selected cases, pretreatment with either rotational atherectomy or cutting balloon angioplasty (BA) can significantly improve final instent lumen dimensions.

Standardization of Measurements

As with transthoracic echocardiography, all measurements during intravascular ultrasonography are taken "leading edge to leading edge." The American College of Cardiology has recently standardized criteria for IVUS acquisition, nomenclature, and measurements (4); this is essential reading for any cardiologist who performs IVUS. Key measurements are illustrated in Fig. 91–2. Several points of the new guidelines are particularly noteworthy. The official nomenclature discourages the use of the term "vessel area"; this ambiguous term can cause confusion in the catheterization laboratory. Instead, the terms "EEM CSA" (the cross-sectional area bounded by external elastic membrane) and "lumen CSA" are preferred. Second, measurement of vessel and lumen dimensions at a single site cannot be used to calculate "percent stenosis." Because of the phenomenon of coronary remodeling (discussed later), the EEM area at the lesion site may be significantly larger or smaller than at the same site at an earlier, disease-free time point. As discussed later, absolute lumen area and, in some cases, comparison of absolute lumen area at the lesion to absolute lumen area at an appropriate reference site are better predictors of the hemodynamic significance of a diseased segment.

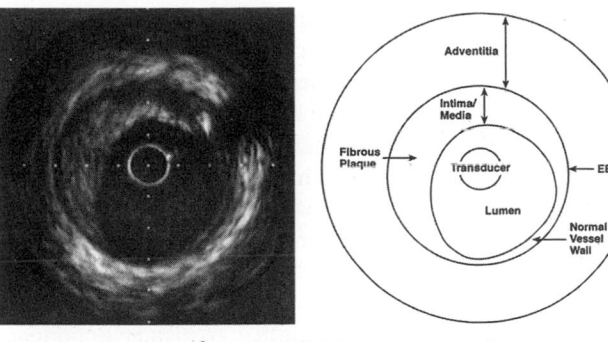

Plaque Area (mm²) = EEM Area–Lumen Area
CSN (%) = Plaque Area/EEM Area

FIG. 91–2. Key intravascular ultrasound measurements for the interventional cardiologist. CSN (%), cross-sectional narrowing (percent); EEM, external elastic membrane.

For longitudinal coronary regression or stabilization studies, other standardized measurements include *intimal thickness,* which is defined as the distance from the intimal leading edge to the external elastic membrane. In very diseased sections, this is called the "intima-media" or "plaque plus media" thickness. By definition, this layer will include the intima, media, and any atheroma (5). The rationale for this convention is twofold. First, the normal media is not always distinguishable as a clear layer because its thickness is only slightly greater than the axial resolution of the imaging systems. Conversely, the external elastic lamina that separates media from adventitia can often be recorded as clear border, and therefore is a reliable boundary for tracing. Second, on many images the media can appear erroneously thin because of an effect known as signal blooming, in which the transition of the ultrasound signal from a region of higher (intima/plaque) to lower (media) reflectivity results in spreading of the signal into the media region. Thus, the intima may appear to be thicker at the expense of media, which appears thinner. The method of delineating the EEM is accurate compared with histology.

Imaging Artifacts

All current IVUS devices generate artifacts that may lessen image quality, reduce measurement accuracy, or alter clinical interpretation (Fig. 91–3). Differential mechanical drag on the drive shaft during the rotational cycle can produce oscillations in rotational speed, called nonuniform rotational distortion (NURD). Common causes include excessive angulation of the catheter shaft adjacent to the motor assembly, overtightening of the hemostatic valve, or examination of a tortuous coronary segment. NURD usually produces "stretching" of a portion of the image with "compression" of the contralateral vessel wall. Transducer "ring-down" is present to some degree in all images. Acoustic oscillations in the piezoelectric transducer material result in high-amplitude signals that obscure the near-field, resulting in an inability to image structures that are immediately adjacent to the transducer.

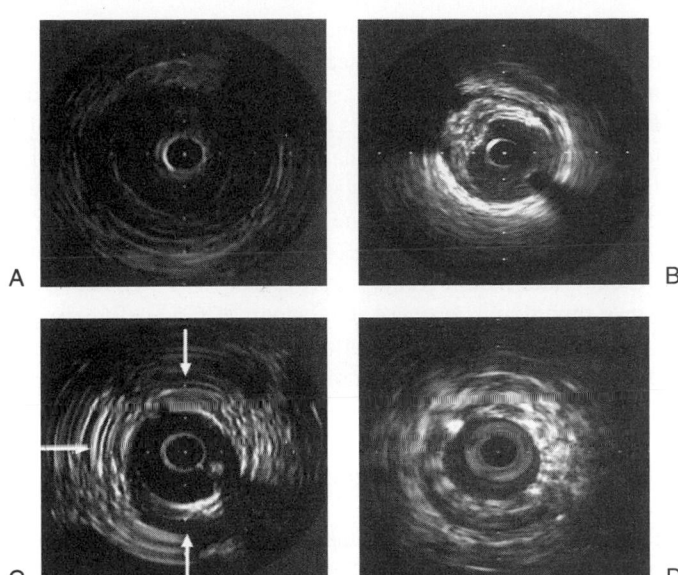

FIG. 91–3. Artifacts on intravascular ultrasound imaging. **A:** Signal dropout. The image is indistinct and lacks signal intensity. This is most often caused by a minute amount of air adjacent to the transducer and is remedied by flushing the catheter. **B:** Guidewire artifact. The shadow at 5 o'clock is caused by the 0.014-inch guidewire, which appears larger than actual size because of wire movement. **C:** Nonuniform rotational distortion, caused by variations in rotation of mechanical transducers. **D:** Ring-down.

Longitudinal reconstruction is currently available in commercial devices and three-dimensional algorithms are in development, both as a means to facilitate understanding of the spatial relation between the structures within different tomographic cross sections. However, the algorithms applied cannot fully account for the vessel curvature, off-axis catheter position, systolic vessel expansion, and "saw tooth" movement of the catheter with each cardiac cycle. Accordingly, the reconstructed L-mode images are not always faithful representations of the vessel and should not be used for quantitation (4).

Impact on Understanding Atherothrombosis and Implications for Revascularization

Disease Severity and Atheroma Distribution

Ultrasound has confirmed necropsy studies from as early as the 1960s that far more atheroma is present than is revealed by angiography and, even more importantly, that extensive disease may be present in young subjects before clinical events and before any angiographic abnormalities are present. In a large number of transplant recipients, Tuzcu (3,6) documented evidence of atherothrombosis in the majority of donors younger than 40 years and early (or more severe) disease in a substantial number of donors before the age of 30 years. Although the majority of these cases may not yet have hemodynamically significant effects from an "obstruction" standpoint, studies using coronary Doppler demonstrate that even the earliest stages of disease can be associated with abnormalities of coronary vasoregulation and endothelial function. By the time patients have obstructive stenoses, ultrasound studies document that most of the coronary tree is involved in the atherothrombotic process. Ultrasound also has revised concepts of plaque distribution. Lesions that appear concentric angiographically are often eccentric by ultrasound and histologically, and vice versa (7). If selective use of directional coronary atherectomy (DCA) before drug-eluting stent (DES) implantation is demonstrated to be useful, operators will likely rely on ultrasound guidance for optimal and safe debulking before stenting.

Plaque Composition

Data are accumulating that the ultrasonic characteristics of plaque composition may predict the probability of subsequent acute coronary syndromes (see Chapter 50) and, for the interventionalist, may predict the probability of acute complications. Plaque burden as assessed by ultrasound is associated with greater postprocedure creatine kinase level increases (8); similarly, positive remodeling is associated with greater in-hospital complications and long-term target vessel revascularization (TVR) rates (9). Extensive dissection after BA is associated with lesions that have soft plaque adjacent to heavy calcification (10). "No-reflow" is associated with plaques that contain a "lipid pool" and a greater overall plaque burden (11). However, these characteristics are not sufficiently established to warrant preprocedure imaging to modify the interventional approach to minimize complications.

Arterial Remodeling

Remodeling is defined as a change in vessel area (i.e., within the external elastic membrane) as the atherothrombosis develops. *Positive remodeling* occurs when the area within the EEM area *increases* as atheroma develops. Glagov and colleagues (12) first described these phenomena in peripheral specimens and then in coronary specimens in necropsy studies; subsequent IVUS studies corroborated these observations *in vivo* (13,14). In positively remodeled segments, Glagov hypothesized that vessel expansion is "compensatory," because *lumen* size was relatively preserved despite considerable amounts of atheroma compared with more normal segments in the same vessel. However, beyond a certain limit, in the range of 30% to 50% cross-sectional narrowing, this "compensatory" mechanism fails, luminal dimensions become progressively compromised, and hemodynamically significant obstruction occurs.

Histopathologic and IVUS studies have demonstrated that in *de novo* coronary lesions remodeling can be *negative,* as well as positive (see Fig. 50–4). At negatively remodeled sites, EEM-CSA is significantly *less* than at the reference site. Thus, at some lesions in the coronaries, the presence of a stenosis is caused by "shrinkage" of the area within the

EEM (negative remodeling) *as well as* atheroma accumulation (15). In some stenoses, the relative contribution of negative remodeling can even exceed that of atheroma accumulation in producing the lesion.

Although the biologic mechanisms responsible for remodeling are unknown, the remodeling phenomenon has several critical implications. Most contemporary studies of regression or stabilization of coronary atherothrombosis use some modality that can accurately measure the effects of the intervention on remodeled segments (see Chapter 50). For the interventionalist, remodeling has particular importance in correct device and stent sizing.

Detection of Coronary Calcification

The presence and extent of coronary calcification is an important determinant of final stent dimensions in both bare-metal and DESs. Clinically, the severity of calcification is quantified by both the angle subtended by the calcified and by the position (whether superficial or deep with respect to the lumen). Whereas modest amounts of calcification, particularly when deep, have little or no effect on transcatheter revascularization, extensive (>180 degrees) and superficial calcification can substantially reduce stent expansion. The most critical aspect of coronary calcification for the interventionalist is that in many cases it is angiographically occult. Many studies document the poor correlation between fluoroscopically and ultrasonically determined calcification (16, 17). Even when fluoroscopy does not suggest calcification at a lesion site, calcification elsewhere in the vessel often predicts extensive lesion calcification that can be ultrasonically. This observation is particularly important for optimal deployment of DESs, because suboptimal expansion in a heavily calcified region leaves no viable options for effective transcatheter re-treatment (Fig. 91–4). Furthermore, as vessel size decreases, the incidence of fluoroscopically occult calcification increases (18). Thus, in small vessels, selective use of IVUS can be clinically important. The optimal deployment of small (<3 mm) DESs may still benefit from pretreatment (either with debulking or balloon predilatation rather than "direct" stenting) because suboptimal deployment because of occult heavy calcification may still result in a hemodynamically significant lesion, even in the absence of subsequent neointimal hyperplasia. Finally, 10% to 20% of lesions are still treated with stand-alone BA, and calcification is a predictor of final lumen dimensions and the probability of extensive dissection and complications (10).

Diagnostic Applications and Implications for Revascularization

Angiographically Intermediate Lesions

Lesions of "moderate" severity (50–75% narrowing) are a common dilemma, yet angiography is often least accurate in this (Fig. 91–5). In such situations IVUS can planimeter lu-

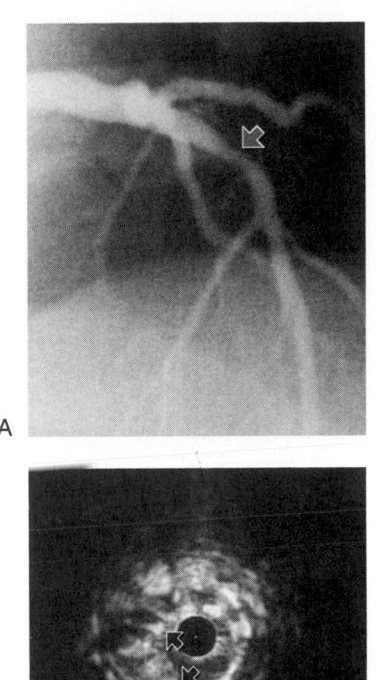

A

B

FIG. 91–4. Extensive calcification may be angiographically occult and may preclude adequate deployment of drug-eluting stents. Intravascular ultrasound was performed when this patient presented with "restenosis." In fact, the predominant mechanism of recurrence was inadequate expansion and the time of deployment, caused by a heavy superficial calcification *(arrows)*, which can still be seen beneath the stent struts.

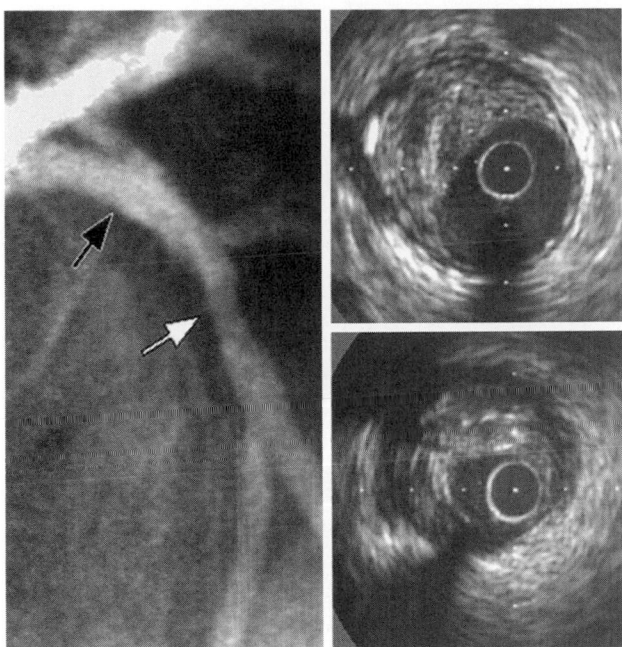

FIG. 91–5. Ultrasound utility in assessing lumen dimensions in an angiographically intermediate lesion. On the angiogram, the quantitative coronary angiography–measured reference diameter *(black arrow)* and the lesion site *(white arrow)* are similar, yet the lesion appears "hazy" or less dense than the reference. Intravascular ultrasound at the reference **(top right)** demonstrates a large, angiographically occult atheroma. The lumen area at the lesion site **(bottom right)** demonstrates a severely compromised lumen (<2 mm^2).

men area directly. Several studies suggest that in a major epicardial coronary artery other than the left main, an absolute lumen area of less than 4 mm^2 has a high probability of ischemia on functional testing (19–21). The decision to defer revascularization in lesions with absolute lumen areas greater than 4 mm^2 also is supported by a study in which intervention was deferred by this criterion (22). However, in many such cases, flow reserve may be a superior method to evaluate these problem lesions (discussed later).

Intermediate Left Main Lesions

The left main has three characteristics that make angiographic estimation of lesion severity potentially problematic: It is short in length, it often is diffusely diseased, and it contains both an ostium and a bifurcation. The short length and diffuse disease may eliminate any true "reference segment"; contrast in the aortic cusp may obscure the ostium, or "streaming" of contrast from the injection vortex can create the false impression of ostial narrowing.

IVUS assessment of angiographically indeterminate or intermediate left main lesions is among the most common clinical indications for the procedure. In our laboratories, IVUS is most useful to exclude significant disease, particularly at the ostium, where angiographic artifacts are not uncommon; in some cases, ultrasound demonstrates an adequate lumen area and minimal atheroma burden and unnecessary revascularization can be deferred (Fig. 91–6). Unfortunately, when plaque volume is greater and residual lumen area is moderately compromised, there are relatively few studies to guide recommending or deferring revascularization (Fig. 91–7). Abizaid and colleagues (23) identified criteria for left main lesions that can safely be followed clinically versus those that should be considered for immediate revascularization. When the residual left main lumen area is less than 6 to 7 mm^2, particularly in the presence of diabetes or a larger than 50% angiographic lesion in another major epicardial vessel, revascularization should be considered (24). Of course, in clinical practice, incorporation of clinical and functional test data into this decision is vital; thus, ultrasound often is most useful when the functional testing indicates either left coronary ischemia but only a "moderate" left main lesion, or when there is no evidence of ischemia in this territory, but a "lesion" (which may be an angiographic artifact) is observed. Until additional data are available, ultrasound is best used in an incremental fashion to supplement information from functional studies.

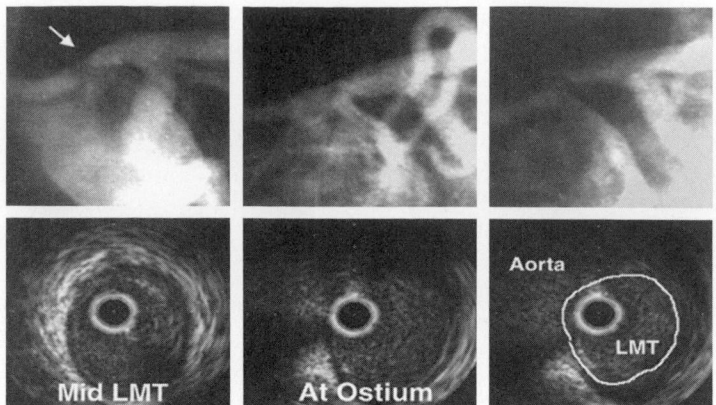

FIG. 91–6. Ostial "lesions" are occasionally angiographic artifacts, presumably caused by streaming of contrast from the catheter into the vessel. LMT, left main trunk.

Ostial and Bifurcation Lesions

Ostial and bifurcation lesions often elude accurate angiographic assessment despite multiple projections (Fig. 91–8). The tomographic orientation of IVUS usually permits accurate measurement of lumen dimensions. In the absence of published data regarding IVUS criteria for revascularization, most operators use similar criteria to those discussed earlier (absolute lumen area ≤ 4.0 mm^2, area stenosis >60–70%), in combination with symptom status and the results of functional testing, to determine the need for revascularization. As with the left main ostium, occasionally an ostial "stenosis" is caused by an angiographic artifact (caused by angulation of the vessel off the aorta) in the absence of a significant stenosis; ultrasound can be useful in obviating the need for intervention (25).

Optimal Coronary Intervention: Intravascular Ultrasound Insights

Most contemporary coronary interventions involve stent implantation, and IVUS has played a critical role in this revolution by revealing the limitations of BA and other nonstent interventions, by identifying the mechanisms of restenosis in these lesions, by defining lesion subsets that may benefit from "debulking," by determining the utility and optimal dose of brachytherapy, and by identifying optimal stent deployment criteria.

Limitations of Nonstent Interventions

Before the widespread use of stents in the mid-1990s, data from ultrasound studies revealed that underlying atheroma morphology strongly influenced final lumen size and morphology after nonstent interventions (26). For example, lesions that contained a moderate to large amount of superficial calcium often were resistant to balloon dilation and at times resulted in extensive dissection. In addition, nonstent interventions often produced irregular or distorted lumen shapes. Angiography often overestimated the size of these irregular lumens, in which the actual gain in lumen area was modest (27). The effectiveness of DCA also was limited by these factors; ultrasound studies revealed that despite a successful angiographic result after atherectomy, 40% to 60% or more of the cross-sectional vessel area at the target site is still occupied by atheroma (28). Several

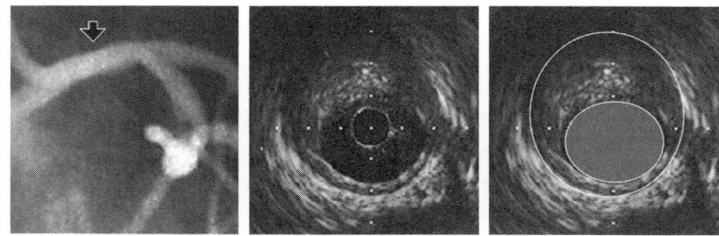

FIG. 91–7. Utility of intravascular ultrasound in accurate diagnosis of left main disease. This left main did not contain a focal stenosis angiographically but appeared somewhat "small" compared with the guiding catheter and the remainder of the left coronary system. Ultrasound confirmed the presence of a substantial atheroma burden distributed throughout the vessel, as well as a small lumen area throughout (<6 mm^2).

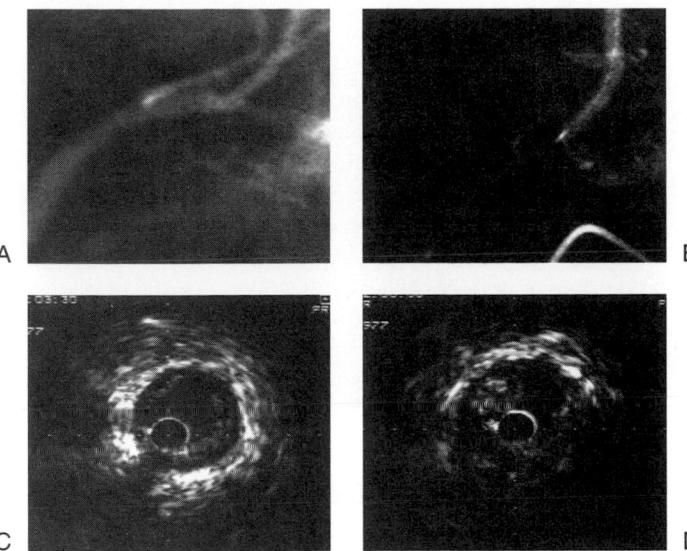

FIG. 91–8. Utility of intravascular ultrasound (IVUS) in ostial disease. **A:** The angiogram suggests the possibility of an ostial lesion right at the catheter tip. **B:** Correct coaxial alignment of the IVUS with the ostium. **C:** Reference site in the proximal right coronary artery, demonstrating a modest amount of atheroma and an adequate lumen. **D:** IVUS precisely at the ostium, demonstrating a large atheroma and a severely compromised lumen (<3 mm²).

studies using angiography as the "gold standard" described the ability of various functional tests to predict the subsequent occurrence of restenosis after apparently successful BA. In retrospect, these studies were probably identifying the subset of patients with an angiographically apparent success but in whom lumen enlargement was suboptimal and in whom subsequent additional negative remodeling occurred.

Restenosis after Nonstent Interventions

In nonstent coronary interventions, ultrasound studies completely revised notions of the restenotic process. Based primarily on animal models and case reports from patients who died soon after angioplasty, the paradigm of human restenosis was predominantly intimal hyperplasia. Instead, ultrasound studies in the mid-1990s demonstrated that the vascular response after nonstent intervention is more complex. In the first month, there is an increase in both plaque-plus-media area and EEM area; however, from Months 2 to 6 there often is a substantial *decrease* in EEM area. Restenotic lesions have a larger degree of EEM reduction; thus, on average, the progressive diminution in lumen area is primarily caused by late vessel constriction or negative remodeling (29–33) with a relatively minor contribution by neointimal hyperplasia (Fig. 91–9). In contrast, coronary stents completely eliminate vessel contraction (34); it is by this mechanism that stents have had such a profound impact on contemporary revascularization.

Lesion Subsets That May Benefit from "Debulking"

Directional Atherectomy

DCA studies of the late 1990s suggested that ultrasound guidance, by defining plaque location and circumferential distribution, could achieve larger lumens and less residual plaque than angiographically guided procedures (7,28,35). Ultrasound allows more aggressive debulking, leading to greater plaque removal and a larger final lumen diameter. Despite these "stent-like" immediate results angiographically, ultrasound revealed a persistent large residual plaque area (approximately 55–60%). Six-month angiographic restenosis rates of approximately 30% and target lesion revascularization rates of 15% to 20% were comparable to bare-metal stenting. However, there are only limited data to suggest that ultrasound-guided DCA versus stenting leads to comparable long-term outcomes. In the randomized STent versus directional coronary Atherectomy Randomized Trial (START) trial, serial ultrasound imaging achieved a residual plaque burden of 52%; restenosis was significantly lower in the group receiving aggressive IVUS-guided atherectomy (16%) compared with stenting (36). With the advent of DESs, atherectomy may have some role before stenting, but few operators are likely to embrace a stand-alone atherectomy strategy.

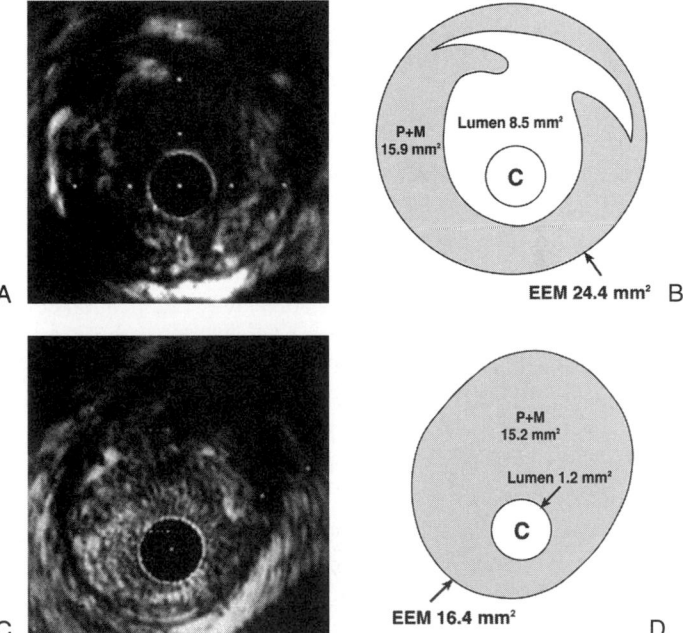

FIG. 91–9. Most of the restenotic process after nonstent interventions is because of negative remodeling. **A:** Lesion before directional atherectomy. **B:** After directional atherectomy. **C:** After adjunctive balloon, at the conclusion of the index procedure. **D:** When the patient returned with restenosis, there has been minimal change in plaque plus media area but substantial negative remodeling, which has caused nearly all of the loss in lumen area. EEM, external elastic membrane.

"Debulking" before Stenting

In 2003, there were two unanswered questions regarding prestent debulking with DCA. First, are the results of bare-metal stenting improved with "debulking"; and, given the added cost of DESs, could this strategy result in comparable outcomes at lower cost? A large plaque burden before bare-metal stenting adversely affects both final instent area (which, for bare-metal stents, is a major determinant of target lesion revascularization) and more aggressive neointimal hyperplasia (37–39). In a nonrandomized series, ultrasound-guided DCA followed by stent implantation resulted in fewer target lesion revascularizations (7% vs. 19%; $p = 0.03$) (40). Nevertheless, the technical challenges of IVUS-guided DCA compared with the relative ease of stenting are likely to limit widespread application. Although prototypes of a combined atherectomy-ultrasound device have been developed, it is unlikely to see commercial development. Second, given the excellent long-term results of DESs, will there be any role for prestent DCA with these devices? Inclusion criteria for nearly all of the DES trials to date have excluded some lesion subsets that might not obtain the same single-digit restenosis rates as the lesions included in these studies. For example, aorto-ostial vein graft lesions have high restenosis rates with or without debulking before bare-metal stenting (41). Target lesion revascularization after DES placement is still unknown; whether debulking will have any role in this subset is unknown.

Rotational Ablation

Rotational ablation is effective in the treatment of heavily calcified coronary lesions and in selected bifurcation stenoses. As discussed earlier, there is a poor correlation between ultrasound and fluoroscopy in assessing the presence and extent of calcification. The greater the arc of superficial calcium, the smaller is the final minimal lumen diameter (42). Accordingly, the ultrasonic demonstration of heavily calcification occasionally leads some operators to "debulk" with prestent rotational ablation. There are insufficient data to recommend precise guidelines for this approach. Nevertheless, some centers perform preinterventional IVUS if there is moderate or extensive calcification anywhere in the target vessel and use rotational ablation if the arc of superficial calcium is greater than 180 degrees in multiple cross sections along the stenotic segment. It often is difficult to determine the "normal" vessel dimensions (and, hence, the optimal stent size) without ultrasound. A series of 75 patients suggested that IVUS-guided rotational ablation before stenting resulted in a restenosis rate of 22.5% (substantially less than historical control subjects), but there was no comparison stenting comparable targets without atherectomy or IVUS (43). Given the incremental cost of DESs, this strategy may remain important in this small but important minority of cases. A randomized trial of this strategy in these lesion subsets might have important clinical implications, but no data are currently available.

Cutting Balloon

Cutting balloon technology uses atherotomes attached to a balloon to exert controlled incision of atheroma. The hypothesis behind the development of this device was that "scoring" the lesion would allow more controlled vessel expansion and less recoil. However, ultrasound data suggest that, in *de novo* lesions, lumen enlargement occurs predominantly by enhanced axial plaque redistribution and, to a lesser degree, vessel expansion; this relation is the reverse of that seen in conventional balloon dilation (44,45).

Coronary Stent Deployment

Ultrasound Contribution to Bare-Metal Stenting

The first generation of slotted-tube stents were deployed using balloon pressures of only 6 to 10 atm, and patients had to receive aggressive anticoagulation during and immediately after the procedure with both antiplatelet and antithrombotic agents to prevent subacute stent thrombosis (46,47). Although these studies proved a reduction in the restenosis rate compared with BA and led to U.S. Food and Drug Administration approval, hemorrhagic complications, long hospital stays, and occasionally fatal subacute thrombosis were obstacles to universal use.

Critical observations from IVUS made possible the contemporary era of coronary stenting, because these studies demonstrated that deployment at only 6 to 10 atm often lead to unexpanded stents, unopposed struts despite excellent angiographic results, or both (48–51). Contrast can flow outside of a partially deployed stent resulting in the angiographic illusion of full deployment (Figs. 91–10 and 91–11). In a large, nonrandomized but nevertheless pivotal study, Columbo and coworkers (50) redefined optimal deployment technique. By using routine ultrasound after conventional, low-pressure angiographically guided stent deployment, his group demonstrated frequent incomplete apposition and a mean residual lumen area stenosis of greater than 50%. Using this IVUS information, when apposition was incomplete or instent area was considered suboptimal, operators per-

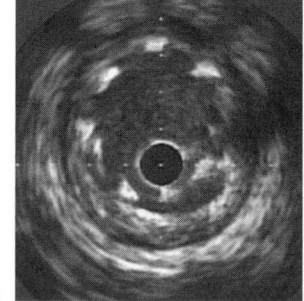
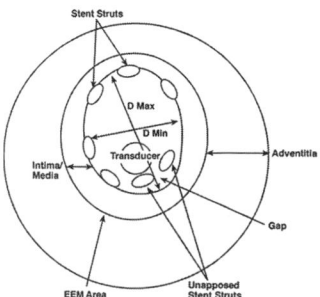

A   B

FIG. 91–10. Malapposition. The stent struts at 5 o'clock are not apposed to the atheroma, creating a gap between the stent struts and the vessel wall. EEM, external elastic membrane.

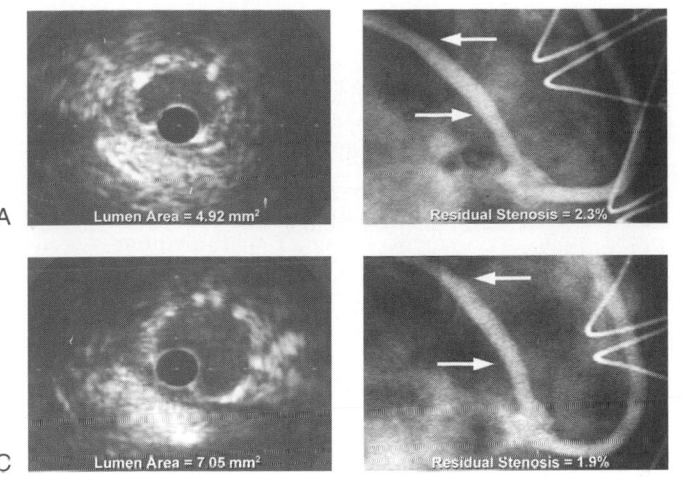

A — Lumen Area = 4.92 mm²
B — Residual Stenosis = 2.3%
C — Lumen Area = 7.05 mm²
D — Residual Stenosis = 1.9%

FIG. 91–11. Malexpansion. Intravascular ultrasound revealed an inadequate minimum instent area **(A)** despite an adequate angiographic appearance **(B)**. Additional inflations led to a substantial increase in final minimum instent area **(C)**. There has been no significant change in the angiographic appearance **(D)**. *Arrows* indicate the stent margins. Although subsequent neointimal hyperplasia in a drug-eluting stent may be negligible, angiographically occult malexpansion may result in persistent ischemia.

formed additional inflations at greater pressures (typically 18–20 atm) or with larger balloons, or both, resulting in larger mean instent lumen areas and more complete apposition. A low subacute thrombosis rate of only 0.3% was achieved using aspirin and ticlopidine without warfarin. This strategy remains the standard technique for stent deployment. Ultrasound also provided insights into the mechanisms of lumen enlargement after stenting, including vessel expansion, plaque compression, and atheroma redistribution from the center of the lesion axially along the vessel (52).

Despite the pivotal role of ultrasound in defining current technique, there are widespread differences in IVUS use in different laboratories and in different countries. In the United States, approximately 7% of interventional procedures use ultrasound, but in Japan (where IVUS reimbursement is adequate) nearly 50% of PCI procedures use ultrasound (53). With current high-pressure deployment, ultrasound-triggered additional dilation is less than initially reported, and routine high-pressure deployment without ultrasound can achieve excellent outcomes and low subacute thrombosis rates (51). However, ultrasound frequently leads to further balloon dilation or alteration of stent length or positioning, with increased instent lumen area and a decrease in residual stenosis at the edges (54). In two large but nonrandomized series that included a large percentage of patients at high risk for restenosis with bare-metal stents (such as diabetics; ostial, long, or restenotic lesions; small vessels; and total occlusions), the angiographic restenosis rates ranged from 10% to 21%, with repeat revascularization required in approximately half (50,55). These results are superior to reports using angiographic guidance alone.

Ultrasound in the Drug-eluting Stent Era

Recently, DESs have been approved for use in the United States; whether these devices will render bare-metal stents obsolete is uncertain because of their substantial incremental cost. Some argue that mass production and market competition will eventually reduce price to the point where bare-metal stents will be obsolete. Conversely, others argue that IVUS-guided bare metal stenting can achieve restenosis rates comparable to DESs, and that if the cost of DES does not decrease substantially, IVUS-guided bare metal stenting could become an alternative to routine DES placement in carefully selected subsets. Because the latter strategy may retain clinical utility, and because many observations of IVUS-guided bare metal stenting have implications for DES deployment, a summary of trials of ultrasound-guided bare metal stenting remains relevant.

With bare-metal stents, ultrasound-measured instent lumen area strongly predicts restenosis. The larger the minimum instent lumen area, the greater is the area to accommodate neointimal hyperplasia, resulting in lower restenosis and revascularization rates. Even after routine high-pressure dilatation, ultrasound-guided additional inflations can increase lumen areas, decreasing restenosis. In the nonrandomized Can Routine Ultrasound Influence Stent Expansion (CRUISE) study, investigators assigned ten centers to angiographic guidance and eight centers to ultrasound guidance (56). In the ultrasound-guided cohort, mean instent lumen area was 0.9 mm larger, and TVR was reduced by 38%, from 14.9 to 8.9%. Three multicenter, randomized trials have tested this hypothesis. The OPTICUS (OPTimization with ICUS to reduce stent restenosis) study randomized 550 patients and did not demonstrate a significant difference in restenosis between ultrasound versus angiographic guidance (57). Although the difference in stent dimensions between the groups was smaller than in other trials. The REStenosis after Ivus guided STenting (RESIST) trial randomized 155 patients to the two strategies and reported a 6.3% absolute reduction in TVR, but this difference did not reach statistical significance because of the small sample size (58). The Antiarrhythmics versus Implantable Defibrillators (AVID) trial randomized 759 patients and demonstrated a trend for improved 12-month TVR with IVUS guidance, but this did not achieve statistical significance (8% vs. 12%; $p = 0.06$). However, this study observed a strong, statistically significant difference in favor of IVUS guidance in vessels with reference diameter less than 3.25 mm, in more severe lesions in saphenous vein grafts (59); subset analysis from other randomized studies and single-center, nonrandomized series also support these data.

There is no consensus on the optimal end points for ultrasound-guided deployment of bare-metal stents. Although complete stent apposition is generally accepted, there are no universally accepted criteria for optimal expansion. Colombo and coworkers (50) initially aimed to achieve 60% or more of the average reference lumen area, but later revised their target to 100% or more of the distal reference vessel area (50).

These more aggressive criteria were revised and tested in the Multicenter Ultrasound Guided Stent Implantation in the Coronaries (MUSIC) trial (60). Using optimal expansion criteria of 100% or more of the distal and 80% or more (for large vessels) or 90% or more of the average proximal and distal reference lumen area, this study reported a subacute thrombosis rate of only 0.6% and a restenosis rate of less than 10%. Other criteria also have been proposed, but from a practical standpoint many are difficult to achieve routinely (59–61). In the Optimal Stent Implantation (OSTI) Trial, investigators serially dilated stents to 12, 15, and 18 atm and quantified the result at each pressure by both QCA and IVUS. Ultrasound quantified a significant increase in stent expansion with successively greater pressures, and these increases (on average) were inapparent angiographically. At an inflation pressure of 15 atm, the predefined target end points of either more than 90% of the average reference or more than 100% of the smaller reference were not achieved in half of the stents; at 18 atm, these end points were achieved in only 60% (62). In the AVID trial, the target end point of 90% or more of the distal reference was not achieved in two-thirds of the patients, and 27% of the patients required further intervention because of inadequate dilatation (59). Taken together, these findings suggest that in different target lesions a given deployment pressure results in markedly different degrees of stent expansion and that intraprocedural IVUS measurements can obviate the need for very high deployment pressures in some stents, as well as indicate the need for additional high-pressure inflations in other stents.

In the search for "optimal" criteria to minimize the risk for restenosis with bare-metal stents, the predictive value of the stent-to-reference ratio also has been studied (63); however, restenosis and TVR rates appear more consistently related (inversely) to the absolute minimum instent lumen area. Most studies indicate that predefined stent-to-reference area ratios are difficult to achieve, are subject to interobserver variability, and correlate only weakly with stent thrombosis and restenosis (63–69).

Many interventionalists conclude from these data that ultrasound is most useful when applied *selectively* to patient and lesion subsets at high risk for restenosis and target lesion revascularization. In bare-metal stents, restenosis is caused by neointimal proliferation (70,71). Because the degree of intimal hyperplasia is independent of the final stent lumen size (72), the larger the in-sent area, the lower is the probability of restenosis. Many studies document the greatest restenosis rates in smaller vessels (<3.25 mm), in diabetics, in long lesions, and in particular anatomic locations, such as ostial and bifurcation lesions (73). In these subsets, an inadequately expanded stent further increases the risk for restenosis by limiting the area available to accommodate the inevitable intrusion of neointimal hyperplasia. Thus, studies suggest that ultrasound is most likely to minimize repeat revascularization in bare-metal stents when it is applied to these high-risk subsets (55,56,59,74). From a practical standpoint, al-

though larger absolute instent lumen area is correlated with lower TVR rates, the extent of stent expansion is limited primarily by the size of the artery itself. Because intimal hyperplasia thickness is independent of vessel size (72), stents in small vessels are more vulnerable to restenosis. Several studies indicate the potential for a substantial reduction in restenosis when ultrasound guidance is used to guide stent deployment in small and medium vessels (56,59,75). As the vessel size increases, the incremental value of ultrasound diminishes (54).

Intravascular Ultrasound and Bare-Metal Stenting: Implications for Drug-eluting Stents

Perhaps the most profound impact of DESs in the studies published to date is the profound reduction in restenosis in subsets at high-risk for restenosis with bare-metal stents. Thus, although the preceding discussion provides an important perspective on the current status of IVUS, to some extent it is academic. DESs appear to have such a profound reduction in restenosis in *high-risk* lesions (such as diabetics, long lesions [>10 mm], and in other subsets) that ultrasound-guided bare-metal stenting seems unlikely to achieve comparable results. Nevertheless, two important questions remain. First, in subsets at *low* risk for restenosis with bare metal stents (such as large-size vessels, vein grafts, and others), can routine or selective IVUS use produce long-term results equivalent to DES implantation, at lower cost and with comparable procedure times? Second, for high-risk lesion subsets that have thus far been *excluded* from the initial randomized trials of DES (such as left main, aortoostial lesions, and heavily calcified lesions, and so on), will angiographic guidance of DES placement result in acceptable restenosis and revascularization rates, or will selective ultrasound guidance improve these end points? Both of these questions are critically important clinically and require further data before any conclusions can be made.

Table 91–2 summarizes the most important indications learned from studies of IVUS-guided bare-metal stenting that are likely to remain relevant in the DES era. Angiogra-

TABLE 91–2. *Clinical applications of intravascular ultrasound in the drug-eluting stent era: lessons from bare-metal stent intravascular ultrasound studies*

- Accurate diagnosis of lesion length
- Accurate diagnosis of vessel size
- Accurate diagnosis of peristent "haziness"
- Optimal treatment of high-risk subsets (left main, complex multivessel disease)
- Assessment of "new" lesions that appear after stent deployment
- Accurate diagnose of instent or peristent recurrence, especially if early
- Assessment of the need for lesion modification before drug-eluting stent
- Assess angiographically intermediate or ambiguous lesions

phy frequently underestimates actual vessel size; a critical potential contribution of ultrasound is to identify which angiographically "small" vessels can actually benefit from a larger deployment balloon or high pressures to maximize instent area and minimize the risk for persistent ischemia or symptoms with DES. Thus, an important indication for ultrasound imaging is to accurately measure vessel size (most often before stenting) in small and medium vessels (angiographic diameter <3–3.25 mm), because many "small" coronary arteries are actually considerably larger than their angiographic silhouette and contain a large plaque burden. In one recent study, 71% of 419 lesions that appeared to be 2.75 mm or smaller by QCA were larger (by ≤1 mm) by IVUS (76). This finding appears to be more common in proximal or mid-left anterior descending (LAD) lesions, in obtuse marginal and circumflex branches (76), in women, and in diabetics (77).

In addition to assessment of final lumen area and strut apposition, IVUS is useful in evaluating vessel anatomy at the edges of the stent, where tissue prolapse, residual or redistributed atheroma (52), dissections (particularly after high-pressure inflations), and intramural hematomas can occur; these lesions can occasionally cause acute or subacute occlusion and can be angiographically occult (50). It is not uncommon to see a "step down" or areas of "haziness" at the stent margins. The differential diagnosis includes all of these phenomena; one study suggests that angiography often is unhelpful in distinguishing among these events (78). One the one hand, the natural history of appears to be benign and does not require further intervention (79,80); on the other hand, persistent dissections that are "obstructive" or that occur with a residual area stenosis of greater than 60%, may benefit from additional stent deployment to prevent complications (81). The appearance of a "new" lesion angiographically after stent deployment may herald an intramural hematoma with a high risk for acute occlusion (82,83) and is a strong indication for ultrasound imaging because accurate diagnosis can both guide or obviate (84) the need for further stent deployment (Fig. 91–12). Similarly, incomplete strut

apposition to the vessel wall occurs in 10% to 15% of stents and when "mild" does not appear to be related to complications (85); however, when ultrasound documents severe malapposition, most operators will perform additional inflations with a larger balloon. Finally, residual plaque burden that is not covered by the stent at its margins has been correlated with the extent of subsequent neointimal hyperplasia (86). As with any diagnostic modality, the incremental value and cost-effectiveness of ultrasound per se is difficult to assess and has not been studied sufficiently.

Ultrasound and Drug-eluting Stents

Although angiography can document an extremely low percent diameter stenosis after DES placement, the ability of ultrasound to examine stent–vessel wall relations and to quantify neointimal volume precisely has made it invaluable in the development of these devices (87–93). For example, quantitative volumetric analysis can discriminate different effects of stents with drug coatings at different concentrations, whereas these differences may not be discernible by QCA (94). Because some brachytherapy patients exhibited unique complications, ultrasound analysis of DES also has focused on whether late stent malapposition, edge effects, and late stent thrombosis occur with these devices. Thus far, IVUS suggests that paclitaxel-coated stents do result in a greater incidence of these late stent malapposition than bare-metal stents in the control arm, but in the short and medium term this observation has not been associated with adverse clinical events (90). Additional data on this point and on optimal dosing regimens, agents, and delivery platforms are required.

The widespread availability of DES may result in some increase in ultrasound use for several reasons. First, DES will open certain high-risk subsets for percutaneous intervention that were most often the domain of the cardiac surgeon, such as multivessel disease and left main revascularization. Actual left main size and plaque distribution (95,96) and, in some cases, the very existence of lesion versus angiographic artifact (25) can be difficult to assess. Several studies have suggested that ultrasound guidance improves the result of unprotected left main stenting (96,97); given the need for a "perfect" result even with an eluting stent, we anticipate that prestent and poststent ultrasound will be routine if selected, and unprotected left main lesions are to be commonly stented. Second, there are many predeployment and postdeployment situations in which IVUS is useful, as summarized in Tables 91–2 and 91–3. Third, as the cost of a stent increases dramatically, and as patients with multi- and three-vessel disease are more commonly treated percutaneously, the relative incremental cost of IVUS will be much less than it is with bare-metal stents in 2003. The futility of placing a DES suboptimally because of angiographically occult calcification, uncertain lesion length, or imprecise vessel sizing will further prompt leading interventionalists to use IVUS when this incremental information is essential.

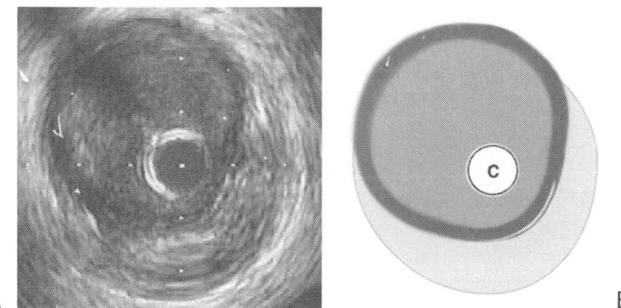

A   B

FIG. 91–12. Intramural hematoma. A new lesion appeared angiographically after a stent was deployed proximally in this vessel. Intravascular ultrasound revealed a large intramural hematoma that extended for more than 15 mm. Such lesions are at high risk for acute closure, which occurred in this case.

TABLE 91–3. *Possible additional intravascular ultrasound applications in the drug-eluting stent era*

Potential clinical applications
- IVUS-guided bare-metal stenting could become an alternative to routine drug-eluting stent placement in carefully selected subsets
- Drug-eluting stents have not been extensively tested in lesions at high risk for recurrence with bare-metal stenting, such as aortoostial lesions and bifurcations
- To obviate high-pressure deployment
- Provisional stenting
- Brachytherapy of bare-metal stents

Research applications
- To evaluate stent coatings with different drug concentrations or different polymer delivery systems
- To assess pharmacologic strategies for disease regression or stabilization (see Chapter 50)
- To assess the effects of new interventional devices or combinations of devices on acute and long-term lumen dimensions and arterial anatomy
- To further understand the natural history of coronary artery disease

In addition to the indications listed in Table 91–3, research is underway to determine these additional potential applications of intravascular ultrasound (IVUS).

Provisional Stenting

Although not widely used, provisional stenting has been advocated as a means of obviating stent placement in patient subsets (98). For example, one study indicates the profound hazards of stent implantation before noncardiac surgery; in such situations, a temporizing strategy of BA may be safer (99) and IVUS guidance may optimize balloon PCI results. In addition, approximately 20% of contemporary coronary interventions in the United States do not involve stent placement. Two early studies suggested that IVUS-guided balloon sizing (which in many cases led to the use of a larger balloon than with angiographic vessel sizing) could improve postprocedure lumen area without increasing short-term complications (100). In two subsequent reports, each reporting on more than 250 patients after the availability of stents, bailout stenting (for suboptimal lumen gain or extensive dissection) was required only approximately half the lesions, and long-term TLR rates also were reduced by approximately half (101,102). Colombo and coworkers (102a) demonstrated that in a consecutive series of 130 long lesions (mean angiographic length, 26.5 mm), a strategy of "spot stenting"—balloon dilation followed by stenting of areas with a residual lumen area of less than 5.5 mm^2 or a greater than 50% reduction in vessel cross-sectional area—resulted in a lower restenosis rate (25% vs. 39%; $p < 0.05$) than stenting of the entire long lesion. These observations were supported by data indicating that nonobstructive dissections after balloon-only procedures are associated with lower restenosis rates than results without dissection (103). No randomized study has yet proven lower long-term event rates with bare-metal stenting in small vessels (<2.75 mm); ultrasound triage has been suggested as a means to better

identify criteria for provisional stenting to decrease TVR rates in these lesions at high risk for restenosis.

Diagnosing the Mechanism of Instent Restenosis

Although brachytherapy has been a major advance in the treatment of bare-metal stent restenosis, many investigators use routine ultrasound imaging to identify the precise mechanism of restenosis, because in a substantial minority, imaging reveals gross malapposition or malexpansion, incorrect placement (the initial deployment may have missed part of the target lesion), or, rarely, stent dislodgement and crush (resulting from slippage off the balloon). In such cases, ultrasound-guided balloon up-sizing, greater pressures, or additional stenting may obviate debulking or brachytherapy. Ultrasound may be particularly important when stent restenosis occurs soon after initial deployment (<1–2 months), or if it was performed with only angiographic guidance, because there is a significant incidence of mechanical problems rather than neointimal hyperplasia as the cause of "restenosis" (104) (Fig. 91–13). DESs are not immune to these types of mechanical problems; thus, the potential use of IVUS in early recurrence is likely to remain clinically important.

Ultrasound and Brachytherapy

The optimal treatment of bare-metal stent restenosis is problematic. Repeat bare-metal stenting is ineffective because of exaggerated neointimal hyperplasia as documented by ultrasound in the absence of brachytherapy or DES placement (105). Debulking with rotational atherectomy followed by adjunctive balloon redilation often leads to excellent immediate outcomes; however, despite a combination of plaque atheroma removal and extrusion, as well as further stent expansion, IVUS studies document tissue reintrusion within 1 hour of this approach, which often is not apparent angiographically (106). Randomized trials of this strategy (which did not include IVUS-guided balloon sizing) failed to show a reduction in repeat revascularization (107), whereas nonrandomized, single-center experiences with IVUS guidance reported persistently high repeat revascularization rates of approximately 50%, although this rate is less than in historical control subjects (108). The cutting balloon appears to allow more efficient extrusion of neointimal through the stent struts in restenotic lesions (109).

Intracoronary brachytherapy is a major advance in treating stent restenosis (110); IVUS has played a critical role in elucidating the effects of brachytherapy. The methodologic issues are complex and have been detailed in a review (111). Ultrasound has confirmed that brachytherapy of instent restenotic lesions reduces late lumen loss mainly by inhibiting neointimal hyperplasia (110,112,113). Ultrasound also has revealed potential causes of brachytherapy failure, such as "geographic miss," in which lesion recurrence is caused by inadequate irradiation at the edge of the stent; the difficulty in achieving adequate doses when treating long

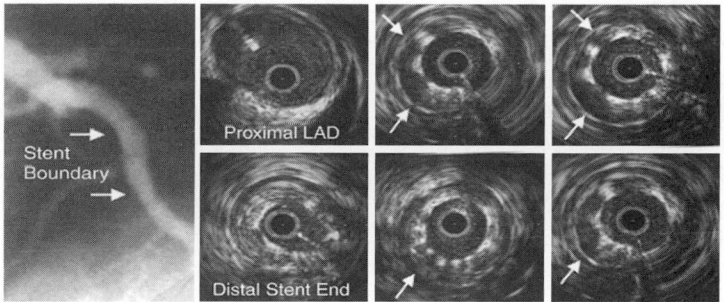

FIG. 91–13. Ultrasound often is useful in rare cases of subacute thrombosis. A stent was placed in the left anterior descending (LAD) during an acute myocardial infarction and appeared adequately deployed at the initial procedure (**left,** *arrows* indicate stent margins). Three days later the stent completely reoccluded; flow was reestablished before any additional inflations. Compared with the proximal reference, the distal stent end is malexpanded, as is the remainder of the stent. In addition, there is gross malapposition throughout the stent *(arrows),* which may be because of the extensive plaque rupture at the time of the initial infarct (predisposing to the angiographic appearance of complete deployment), embolization of atheroma after deployment, or both. All of these factors presumably predispose to acute closure.

restenotic segments explains in part the high recurrence rates in long lesions (114). Ultrasound also has provided several insights into radiation treatment failures. Homogeneity of the delivered dose is an important issue when treating coronary segments with varying curvature, remodeling, plaque extent, and tapering, particularly with β-radiation, which has a rapid-dose drop-off. Dose–volume histograms obtained by ultrasound have been implemented to guide dosimetry; a study of 18 patients demonstrated a wide dose distribution range in the irradiated segments and a lower-than-prescribed dose to the adventitia (115). Compared with conventional stenting, ultrasound reveals that brachytherapy results in an increased incidence of late stent malapposition (because of exaggerated positive remodeling and the absence of neointimal hyperplasia) (115,116), and a greater incidence of echolucent neointimal tissue (called the "black hole" phenomenon) (117). After BA, brachytherapy may result in an increased incidence of unhealed dissections; the frequency of this phenomenon after brachytherapy for stent restenosis is unknown. Whether any of these events increase the risk for late stent thrombosis or other complications remains unclear.

The future role of brachytherapy (and of ultrasound guidance of this procedure) depends on the ultimate market penetration of DESs and whether a subset of DES will have restenosis rates sufficient to retain brachytherapy as a treatment modality. Both of these factors remain to be determined.

Future Developments in Intracoronary Ultrasound

Anticipated technologic advances in IVUS include *guidewire-sized devices* (which may also serve as a stent-delivery wire) (118) and *combination devices* (which incorporate both imaging and a therapeutic device); both may enable simultaneous imaging during the procedure. Other imaging catheters also are under development that incorporate a tip-mounted Doppler flow probe to allow simultaneous cross-

sectional area and flow velocity measurements. To allow uniform radiation to the vessel wall, catheters with capability to image and to selectively shield desired circumference of the vessel wall have been designed. Similarly, stents mounted on the IVUS catheters may also become available. *Tissue characterization* may provide insights into plaque vulnerability and is discussed in Chapter 50. *Higher frequency catheters* may yield significantly improved spatial resolution (100,119–121). There is the potential to derive hemodynamic information from the ultrasound signal, and ultrasound-derived fractional flow reserve (FFR) is in development.

DOPPLER FLOW AND FRACTIONAL FLOW RESERVE

In the last decade, physiologic assessment of coronary flow and endothelial function has become widely used. This resurgence in popularity parallels the development of adequate tools and the recognition that anatomy does not always represent accurately the functional impact of coronary narrowings. The two modalities used in the angiography suite are based on the measurement of coronary flow velocity (Doppler flow probe) or coronary pressure (FFR probe). Invasive physiologic assessment of coronary flow is used mainly in the evaluation of intermediate-grade coronary stenoses and in the assessment of the functional result after PCI. Additional research has focused on the determination of myocardial viability and the response to modifications of endothelial function.

Principles of Invasive Physiologic Assessment of Coronary Flow

Invasive physiologic assessment of coronary flow is performed in the resting condition and after stimulation of coronary flow with a vasodilator drug, simulating an exercise stress test. Typically, the stimulator is adenosine (intra-coronary bolus of 12–48 µg or continuous intravenous infusion at 140 µg/kg/min) (122) because of its ability to dilate preferentially the microcirculation and its short duration of action, which allows repeat measurements. Adenosine has a small effect on the epicardial vessels (~10% change in diameter), thus requiring preceding administration of intra-coronary nitroglycerin (50–200 µg) to ensure maximal epicardial vasodilation. Patients intolerant to adenosine can receive papaverine (7–12 mg bolus), which causes sustained hyperemia for up to 20 minutes (123). Both substances are endothelium-independent vasodilators.

Doppler Velocimetry

The FloWire (JOMED, Helsinborg, Sweden) is a 0.014-inch wire suitable for PCI. It has a 12-MHz piezoelectric transducer located ~3 cm from the proximal tip. The FloWire transducer uses a pulsed-waveform Doppler that samples at 5.2 mm beyond the guidewire tip. It samples a relatively large blood volume by using an ultrasound beam that diverges at an angle of 14 degrees on either side of the centerline of flow. The sample volume approximates 0.65 mm in thickness and 2.25 mm in diameter. In contrast to earlier catheter-mounted probes, the Doppler guidewire uses the fast Fourier transformation method for signal processing, generating approximately 90 spectra per second. An adjustable pulse repetition frequency ranges from 16 to 94 kHz, and the sampling delay is only 0.5 ms, providing satisfactory parameters for spectral analysis. It measures coronary flow velocity rather than flow, but because the epicardial vessel diameter (as well as area) is kept constant during measurement, after nitroglycerin-mediated vasodilatation, changes in flow velocity are directly proportional to changes in volumetric flow. Three parameters can be measured with this technique (124,125):

1. Diastolic/systolic velocity ratio (DSVR): Because of left ventricular systolic contraction, most of the flow (~75% in the left coronary artery and ~50% in the right coronary artery) occurs during diastole. When a significant epicardial obstruction exists, flow can occur preferentially in systole, when systolic ejection force overcomes the lesion resistance. DSVR less than 1.8 (particularly for the left coronary artery) is abnormal.

2. Proximal/distal (P/D) velocity ratio: Because the volume of blood present in the proximal part of an artery must reach its distal end and despite branching of the coronary tree, blood travels at a fairly constant velocity throughout the arterial system. Thus, hemodynamically coronary stenoses will cause an increase in P/D velocity ratio and shunting of blood to unaffected branches. This principle is obviously not applicable to nonbranching arteries or segments. A P/D greater than 1.7 is considered abnormal.

3. Coronary flow reserve (CFR): CFR is the most widely used parameter in clinical practice. It measures the ability of

the microcirculation to dilate in response to physiologic increases in oxygen, such as occurs with exertion or pharmacologic vasodilatation. Normally, coronary blood flow can increase three to five times its basal value, and at least half of this change is because of increased capacitance of the capillary network. The other part is provided by chronotropic response to exercise. As a coronary stenosis progresses, there is compensatory decline in the capillary resistance to maintain adequate basal flow. The use of this reserve at rest diminishes the ability to further increase flow in response to exertion or vasodilatation and is the hallmark of an epicardial coronary narrowing. As elegantly demonstrated by Gould and coworkers (126–129), this reserve is completely exhausted when the stenosis approaches 90%. In clinical use, the assessment of CFR integrates the limitation to flow imposed by the epicardial stenosis and the ability of the microcirculation to respond to an endothelium-independent vasodilator, such as adenosine. As such, it cannot always differentiate between abnormalities in either one of the components. A CFR less than 2.0 is considered abnormal. To circumvent the possibility that abnormal microcirculation is responsible for this defect (such as in patients with diabetes, severe hyperlipidemia, previous infarction, ventricular hypertrophy, and so on), one can measure the relative CFR (rCFR), which is the ratio between CFR in an affected artery and CFR in an angiographically (near) normal artery, supplying a territory without previous infarction. A value greater than 0.8 is considered normal. Thus, if CFR in distal LAD is 1.7 and rCFR is 0.9 (measuring LAD and left circumflex artery, for example), it can be concluded that there is abnormal flow reserve in all arteries and that the epicardial lesion may or may not be hemodynamically significant. In contrast, a CFR of 1.7 in the LAD and rCFR of 0.6 would indicate an important epicardial stenosis.

The main limitations of Doppler velocimetry stem from the dependence on operator ability to properly place the wire and obtain adequate signal, the variability in measured parameters with hemodynamic conditions (arterial blood pressure, heart rate, presence of ischemia, left ventricular end-diastolic pressure) and, most importantly, the lack of perfect discrimination between epicardial and myocardial (microcirculatory) abnormalities (discussed earlier).

Fractional Flow Reserve

FFR is a 0.014-inch angioplasty-suitable wire with a pressure transducer mounted ~3 cm from its proximal tip (Jometrics SmartWire; JOMED, Helsinborg, Sweden; PressureWire; RADI Medical Systems, Uppsala, Sweden). It measures the decrease in pressure across a coronary stenosis (expressed as ratio between aortic pressure and intra-coronary pressure) rest and in response to a vasodilator, such as adenosine. As coronary flow increases with physiologic stress, so does the gradient across the narrowing. Accordingly, each artery serves as its own control, and the previously mentioned limitations of the Doppler FloWire are eliminated. A value less than 0.75 is considered to indicate a hemodynamically significant lesion (130,131). This device is much easier to use than the FloWire, and its measurements are more reproducible (132). In the presence of serial lesions in an epicardial artery, it is possible to measure FFR for each lesion using pressures just proximal and distal to it, but this method introduces a significant overestimation of the true FFR of each lesion. A simpler approach is to intervene on the more severe lesion and reassess FFR of the less severe lesion after PCI (133). FFR measurements also allow the assessment of the burden of moderate coronary disease in an artery. By producing continuous hyperemia with intravenous adenosine and slowly withdrawing the pressure wire from distal to proximal, one can document either a progressive increase in FFR (indicative of moderate diffuse disease that does not require revascularization) or a sharp increase in FFR (corresponding to a severe stenosis within a diseased segment amenable to PCI) (134).

Both FFR and CFR can be measured using 6F diagnostic angiography catheters after adequate anticoagulation. It is important to maintain coaxial alignment of the catheter with the ostium of the artery to allow the hyperemia to occur. The main difference in the information derived from either method is summarized in Figure 91–14.

Clinical Applications of Invasive Physiologic Assessment of Coronary Flow

Lesions of Indeterminate (Moderate) Severity

Although easy to determine the appropriate treatment in patients with clearly minimal or very severe stenoses, an important segment of the patients undergoing angiography have lesions in the 30% to 70% stenosis range without a prior functional test (135). The angiographic appearance of

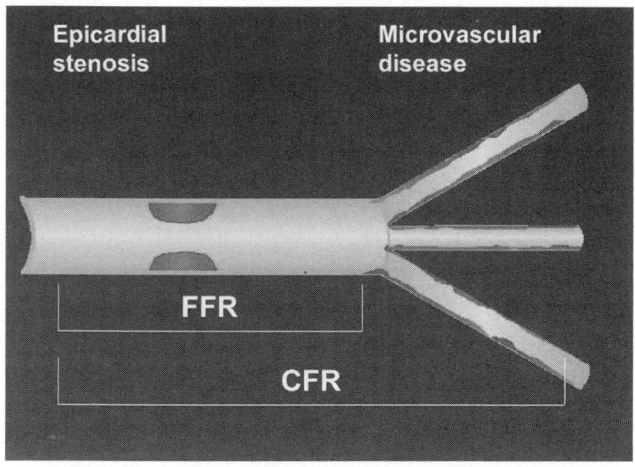

FIG. 91–14. Concepts of physiologic assessment of coronary narrowings. CFR, coronary flow reserve; FFR, fractional flow reserve.

these lesions may be misleading, as outlined in detail earlier in this chapter. Although IVUS may delineate the anatomic and morphologic characteristics of the lesion, physiologic evaluation is essential to prevent both unnecessary revascularization ("oculostenotic" reflex) and underestimation of important lesions. In such cases, invasive assessment of coronary flow may assist in proceeding with or deferring revascularization. In other cases it may change the type of revascularization in accordance with the extent of physiologically significant coronary disease.

Joye and coworkers (136) validated Doppler velocimetry (CFR) in a comparison study using single-photon emission computed tomography (SPECT) thallium to identify ischemia. In 30 patients referred for elective angiography, 16 arteries demonstrated CFR less than 2.0. In 15 of these patients, there was a corresponding defect on thallium scintigraphy. Overall, the predictive accuracy of CFR measurement was 94%. Similar accuracy was obtained in comparison with measurement of translesional gradient (137). CFR measurement correlated better with scintigraphy than either quantitative coronary angiography or IVUS (138). Deferring intervention in patients with normal flow physiology was safe and was associated with a low rate of infarction or need for revascularization (139).

Pijls and coworkers (131) reported on 45 patients studied with noninvasive stress tests and FFR measurements. All 21 patients with abnormal FFR had an abnormal stress test (accuracy 93%, specificity 100%, sensitivity 88%). FFR normalized in all patients after revascularization. In the 24 patients with normal FFR, there was no need for revascularization over a 2-year follow-up. These results were confirmed in another observational series (140). The DEFER trial used FFR to guide the need for revascularization (141). Among 325 patients with moderate coronary stenoses and without objective proof of ischemia, PCI was performed in 144 patients with FFR less than or equal to 0.75. The remaining 181 patients with FFR greater than 0.75 were randomized to PCI (n = 90) or medical therapy (n = 91). At 1 and 2 years there was no significant difference in event-free survival (92% vs. 89% and 89% vs. 83%, respectively) for patients randomized to deferral or PCI. There also was no significant difference between the two groups in the frequency of freedom from angina. The same investigators also evaluated the role of FFR measurement in patients with moderate left main trunk stenosis (142). Among 30 patients with FFR less than or equal to 0.75 who underwent surgical revascularization, the 3-year survival and event-free survival rates were 97% and 83%, not different from 100% and 76%, respectively, among 24 patients with FFR greater than 0.75 who were treated medically.

Guidance of Percutaneous Coronary Intervention Strategy

There has been considerable interest in predicting the risk for restenosis after successful PCI and the need for stent im-

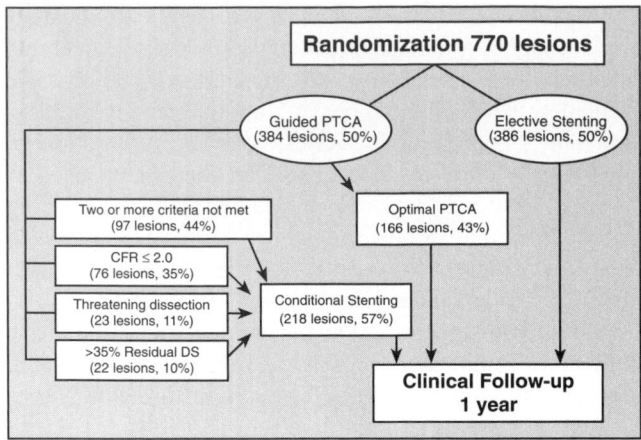

FIG. 91–15. Doppler Endpoint STenting INternational Investigation (DESTINI) study protocol. CFR, coronary flow reserve; PTCA, percutaneous transluminal coronary angiography. (From Di Mario C, Moses JW, Anderson TJ, et al. Randomized comparison of elective stent implantation and coronary balloon angioplasty guided by online quantitative angiography and intracoronary Doppler. DESTINI Study Group (Doppler Endpoint STenting INternational Investigation). *Circulation* 2000;102:2938–2944, with permission.)

plantation, despite a satisfactory BA result. The "stent-like result" concept evolved to describe patients with excellent angiographic outcome after BA alone who may have similar rates of restenosis as patients treated with stents. Naturally, physiologic assessment of coronary flow after PCI became a prime candidate in this quest, recognizing the limitations of angiography in identifying dissections and lumen irregularity after angioplasty.

The ability to predict recurrent ischemia and restenosis was studied in the Doppler Endpoints Balloon Angioplasty Trial Europe (DEBATE) (143). Among 225 patients with successful BA, a residual diameter stenosis less than 35% and CFR of at least 2.5 (achieved in 52%) predicted a low rate of recurrent ischemia at 6 months (23% vs. 47%; $p = 0.005$) and restenosis (16% vs. 41%; $p = 0.002$), compared with patients who did not meet these criteria. Patients with suboptimal CFR after BA had greater baseline flow velocity

before and after BA and a transient reduction in peak velocity after BA, which were associated with increasing age and female sex (144).

In the Doppler Endpoint STenting INternational Investigation (DESTINI) trial, 730 patients were treated with elective stenting or CFR-guided provisional stenting after successful BA (145). The criteria for provisional stenting (any of >35% residual diameter stenosis, threatening dissection or CFR ≤ 2.0) were satisfied in 57% of lesions randomized to guide percutaneous transluminal coronary angiography (PTCA) strategy and provisional stenting was performed (Fig. 91–15). At 1 year, the composite of death, infarction, or TVR occurred in similar proportions of patients assigned elective stenting or guided PTCA (Fig. 91–16) Among patients with guided PTCA, there were no significant differences among those who had provisional stenting or those treated with BA alone. These results led to the conclusion that when angiographic and functional parameters are met (nearly 50% of patients), patients can be treated with BA alone with excellent outcome.

To further explore the role of physiologically guided provisional stenting after BA, the Doppler Endpoints Balloon Angioplasty Trial Europe (DEBATE II) was conducted (146). Its design was similar to DESTINI (Fig. 91–17) except for the further randomization to stent or BA alone after determination of angiographic and physiologic parameters of optimal BA. Forty-eight percent of patients had a residual diameter stenosis of less than 35% without important dissections and CFR of at least 2.5, satisfying the criteria for optimal BA. At 1 year, the composite of death, infarction, or revascularization of the target vessel occurred less frequently in stented patients than in those undergoing BA and also less frequently in those with optimal angiographic and physiologic result than in patients with suboptimal result. Although, overall, there was no significant difference in outcome between patients with primary stenting and those with provisional stenting, there was no economic advantage to the CFR-guided strategy. A low CFR after PCI (regardless of stent implantation) was an independent predictor of adverse outcome at 1 year, particularly related to excess events at 30 days (147).

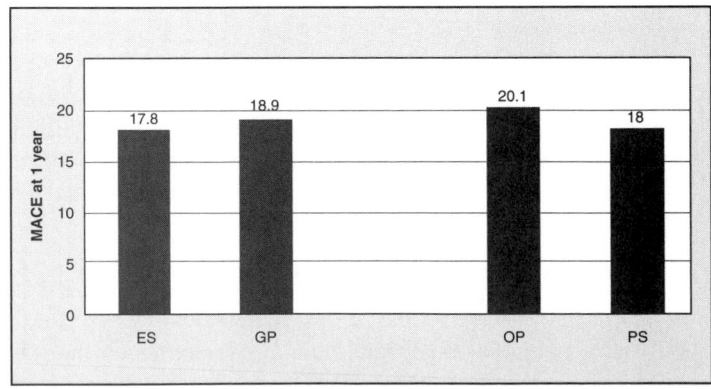

FIG. 91–16. Outcomes in Doppler Endpoint STenting INternational Investigation (DESTINI) at 1 year. ES, elective stenting; GP, guided PTCA; MACE, major adverse cardiac events; OP, optimal PTCA; PS, provisional stenting; PTCA, percutaneous transluminal coronary angiography. (From Di Mario C, Moses JW, Anderson TJ, et al. Randomized comparison of elective stent implantation and coronary balloon angioplasty guided by online quantitative angiography and intracoronary Doppler. DESTINI Study Group (Doppler Endpoint STenting INternational Investigation). *Circulation* 2000; 102:2938–2944, with permission.)

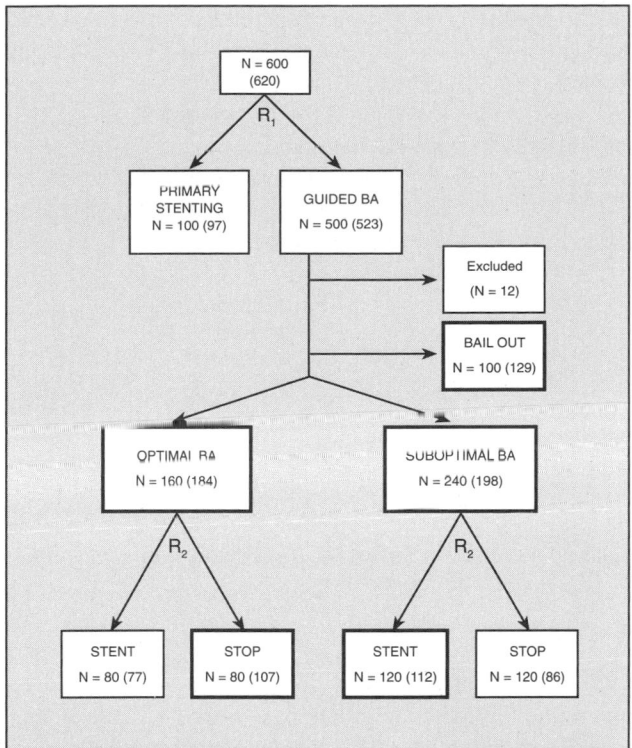

FIG. 91–17. DEBATE II study protocol. BA, balloon angioplasty. (From Serruys PW, de Bruyne B, Carlier S, et al. Randomized comparison of primary stenting and provisional balloon angioplasty guided by flow velocity measurement. Doppler Endpoints Balloon Angioplasty Trial Europe (DEBATE) II Study Group. *Circulation* 2000;102:2930–2937, with permission.)

Outcome after Stenting

Even though stenting improves outcome compared with BA, even in these patients physiologic evaluation provides further risk stratification. In the DESTINI trial, patients with coronary stenting who had CFR less than 2.0 after procedure had a twofold increase in revascularization (22% vs. 11%; $p = 0.01$) compared with those with optimal flow, even after adjustment for all factors known to affect restenosis (148).

Measurement of FFR after stenting is equally effective in predicting outcome (149). As shown in Figure 91–18, the incidence of adverse events (death, infarction, or revascularization) was significantly correlated with poststent FFR, which was the most powerful independent predictor of unfavorable outcome.

When comparing CFR and FFR after stenting, 15% to 20% of patients demonstrate normal FFR and abnormal CFR, as a result of distal microembolization after stenting and stunning of the microcirculation (150).

Assessment of Epicardial Lesions after Myocardial Infarction and Impact on Ventricular Function

After fibrinolytic therapy for acute myocardial infarction, there is frequently a need to predict recovery of left ventricular function and to assess severity of the residual stenosis. In a consecutive series of 57 patients with recent infarction, De Bruyne and coworkers (151) showed that an FFR greater than 0.75 reliably predicts the lack of residual ischemia on SPECT thallium imaging and correlates (inversely) with convalescent ejection fraction. Similar data were observed in 22 patients undergoing acute infarct angioplasty. The CFR after PCI increased from 1.8 ± 0.7 to 2.6 ± 1.0 ($p < 0.0008$) and was an excellent predictor of regional and global ejection fraction at 10 days after procedure (152). Even though CFR may not improve dramatically immediately after PCI in acute infarct angioplasty (because of stunning of the microcirculation), even values of 1.1 to 1.5 are associated with improved recovery compared with patients without any flow reserve after PCI (153).

Endothelial Function

Unlike adenosine and papaverine, acetylcholine (ACh) produces vasodilatation by stimulating a normally reacting endothelium, in doses of 10^{-8} to 10^{-6} M. It can cause paradoxic vasoconstriction in the epicardial arteries in patients with significant endothelial dysfunction (154,155). The serial use of endothelium-dependent and independent vasodilators can differentiate between a reduced CFR caused by

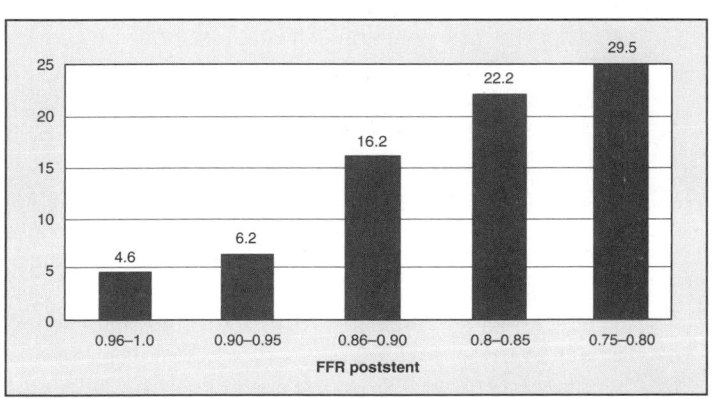

FIG. 91–18. Outcome in 750 patients in a stent registry. FFR, fractional flow reserve. (Adapted from Pijls NH, Klauss V, Siebert U, et al. Coronary pressure measurement after stenting predicts adverse events at follow-up: a multicenter registry. *Circulation* 2002;105: 2950–2954, with permission.)

TABLE 91–4. *Comparison of clinically available imaging and hemodynamic techniques*

Target assessment	Digital angiography	Intravascular ultrasound	Angioscopy	Doppler FloWire	Pressure wire
Vessel lumen detail	+	+ +	+ + + +	−	−
Vessel wall detail	−	+ + + +	−	−	−
Plaque composition	−	+ + +	+ + +	−	−
Vessel dimensions	+.+	+ + + +	−	−	−
Identify disease in "normal" vessel	+	+ + + +	+ +	−	−
Detect diffuse disease	+	+ + + +	+ +	−	±
Evaluate "haziness"	±	+ + +	+ + +	−	±
Arterial remodeling	±	+ + + +	−	−	−
Borderline lesions—morphology	+	+ + + +	−	−	−
Borderline lesions—physiology	−	+	−	+ + + +	+ + + +
Suboptimal results	+	+ + +	+ +	+ + +	+ + + +
Clot vs. dissection	±	+ + +	+ + + +	−	−
Predict complications	+	Possible	Possible	+ + +	Possible
Predict restenosis	+	+ +	−	+ +	Unknown
Diagnose microvascular disease	−	−	−	+ + +	−

−, no value; ±, limited value; + thru + + + +, increasing value.
Modified from DeFranco AC, Safian RD, Ziada KM, et al. Intravascular ultrasound. In: Safian RD, Freed MS, eds. *The manual of interventional cardiology,* 3rd ed. Royal Oak: Physician's Press, 2001:693–733, with permission.

anatomic defects (i.e., lack of response to any agent as seen after myocardial infarction) and that resulting from endothelial dysfunction (i.e., normal response to adenosine and abnormal reaction to ACh), as seen in diffuse atherothrombosis, transplant vasculopathy, or similar conditions.

Evaluation of Collateral and Augmented Flow

The contribution of collateral flow to myocardial perfusion can be measured with Doppler velocimetry distal to balloon occlusion, as demonstrated by Pijls and coworkers (156). Furthermore, physiologic assessment of coronary flow can demonstrate the salutary effect intraaortic balloon counterpulsation has in patients with severe coronary ischemia, particularly in the presence of arterial hypotension (157).

In summary, physiologic assessment of coronary flow is a useful tool in streamlining care of patients with coronary artery disease. Flow and pressure indices are reliable indicators of the need for and results of revascularization and correlate well with clinical and angiographic outcome. Beyond clinical use, these instruments provide invaluable insight into endothelial function and may assist in serial evaluation of interventions geared to alter it.

SUMMARY

Which Adjunctive Modality Is "Best?"

For the research cardiologist, IVUS will continue to be an indispensable tool to evaluate new therapeutic devices; Doppler flow and fractional flow provide invaluable insight into endothelial function and can assess the efficacy of pharmacologic or other interventions prescribed to alter it. For the practitioner, IVUS and FFR will continue to be an indis-

pensable tool for evaluating intermediate lesions, particularly in the left main and in regions where a silhouette technique is suboptimal, such as in plaque rupture, angiographic "haziness," and at the edges of bare-metal or DESs. Physiologic assessment of coronary flow is a useful tool in optimizing patient care. Doppler velocimetry has documented the common finding of endothelial dysfunction as a cause of angina in patients with normal or angiographically mild disease. FFR is likely to gain increasing acceptance to assess intermediate lesions, especially with the increased cost of DESs and the financial and clinical advantages of deferring intervention in lesions without documented hemodynamic significance. Combination devices are in development that will allow pressure and velocity measurements with a single device; such practical advances may speed more widespread acceptance of adjunctive imaging modalities. Flow and pressure indexes are reliable indicators of the need for and results of revascularization and correlate well with clinical and angiographic outcome. Although coronary angiography will not be supplanted by adjunctive modalities, they will provide critical ancillary information in selected patients not only in the research setting, but also in state-of-the-art clinical practice.

Perhaps the most common indication for adjunctive imaging is to assess an intermediate lesion and the adequacy of stenting; the practitioner then needs to choose among these modalities. Available data comparing different techniques in *de novo* lesions and for assessing adequacy of stent deployment suggest that they are comparable (19,158). There are no studies that compare ultrasound with flow reserve in a "head-to-head" comparison in intermediate or angiographically indeterminate lesions. In our experience, when confronted with an intermediate lesion, adjunctive imaging (either with IVUS or flow reserve) is most useful when there is discordance between the patient's symptoms or the results of functional testing and the angiogram. For example, in the patient with angina and a reversible defect nuclear imaging but who has only a "mild" stenosis angiographically, the angiogram may be underestimating the hemodynamic significance of the lesion. Although studies that suggest that IVUS can differentiate "significant" lesions in this situation, overall, the data are stronger for the use of FFR in these situations. Anecdotally, IVUS tends to be most useful when the operator suspects an anatomic reason for angiographic underestimation (such as markedly different stenosis severity in different views of ostial or bifurcation lesion, overlapping vessels, suspected dissection, or angiographic "haze") or when additional anatomic information is necessary to guide intervention. Flow reserve often is more helpful in situations in which these factors are less of a role, in long intermediate lesions, and in assessing sequential stenoses in diffusely diseased vessels. In clinical practice, the modality with which the operator and laboratory are most facile should be chosen to make such important decisions.

Current and Future Status of Adjunctive Imaging

The imaging modalities reviewed in this chapter have been available for more than a decade, and one might rightly ask why they have not been more widely adopted. The slow acceptance of ultrasound, Doppler flow, and FFR is because of several phenomena. First, many cardiologists are reluctant to abandon their dependence on the diagnostic accuracy of coronary angiography. Despite overwhelming evidence of the limitations of angiography, particularly in clinical situations, many practitioners still consider the angiogram to be a "gold standard." Second, the incremental cost of any adjunctive modality adds several hundred dollars to procedural cost; in the current climate of cost-containment, many institutions are unwilling to embrace any new technology without rigorous data on cost-effectiveness. However, many diagnostic imaging modalities have never been subjected to this scrutiny. It is difficult to demonstrate cost-effectiveness for any diagnostic imaging modality, because it is difficult to analyze the subtle and complex decision making that diagnostic imaging influence. There are little or no data "proving" the cost efficacy of echocardiography after myocardial infarction, of chest radiography in suspected pneumonia, or of magnetic resonance imaging in acute joint disorders. Third, as laboratories first begin to adopt these modalities, the inexperience of catheterization laboratory staff may frustrate the physician and lead to the erroneous conclusion that these procedures are time-consuming. But in experienced centers, their selective use adds little or no overall increase in procedural time, in part because the information obtained sometimes obviates additional intervention or more rapidly measures the "correct" size of the device used (102). Finally, adjunctive imaging modalities may reveal to the practitioner information that he or she might not really want to obtain. Deferring angioplasty after IVUS-measured lumen area of more than 4 mm^2, or an FFR greater than 0.75, or Doppler

CFR greater than 2.5 is psychologically (and, perhaps, economically) difficult.

However, all of the adjunctive modalities discussed would benefit from additional, well designed, prospective clinical trials. Unfortunately, cost issues have impeded industry funding for such studies, and few well controlled prospective trials using these new modalities have been completed. Until there are economic and outcome-based rewards for using adjunctive imaging in situations in which they have proven benefit and until additional trials are completed, the full potential of adjunctive imaging modalities may not be realized.

REFERENCES

1. Hausmann D, Erbel R, Alibelli-Chemarin MJ, et al. The safety of intracoronary ultrasound. A multicenter survey of 2207 examinations. *Circulation* 1995;91:623–630.
2. Ramasubbu K, Schoenhagen P, Balghith MA, et al. Repeated intravascular ultrasound imaging in cardiac transplant recipients does not accelerate transplant coronary artery disease. *J Am Coll Cardiol* 2003;41:1739–1743.
3. Tuzcu EM, Hobbs RE, Rincon G, et al. Occult and frequent transmission of atherosclerotic coronary disease with cardiac transplantation. Insights from intravascular ultrasound. *Circulation* 1995;91:1706–1713.
4. Mintz GS, Nissen SE, Anderson WD, et al. American College of Cardiology Clinical Expert Consensus Document on Standards for Acquisition, Measurement and Reporting of Intravascular Ultrasound Studies (IVUS). A report of the American College of Cardiology Task Force on Clinical Expert Consensus Documents. *J Am Coll Cardiol* 2001;37:1478–1492.
5. Metz JA, York PG, Fitzgerald PJ. Intravascular ultrasound: basic interpretation. *Cardiol Clin* 1997;15:1–15.
6. Tuzcu EM, Kapadia SR, Tutar E, et al. High prevalence of coronary atherosclerosis in asymptomatic teenagers and young adults: evidence from intravascular ultrasound. *Circulation* 2001;103:2705–2710.
7. Mintz GS, Popma JJ, Pichard AD, et al. Limitations of angiography in the assessment of plaque distribution in coronary artery disease: a systematic study of target lesion eccentricity in 1446 lesions. *Circulation* 1996;93:924–931.
8. Mehran R, Dangas G, Mintz GS, et al. Atherosclerotic plaque burden and CK-MB enzyme elevation after coronary interventions: intravascular ultrasound study of 2256 patients. *Circulation* 2000;101:604–610.
9. Wexberg P, Gyongyosi M, Sperker W, et al. Pre-existing arterial remodeling is associated with in-hospital and late adverse cardiac events after coronary interventions in patients with stable angina pectoris. *J Am Coll Cardiol* 2000;36:1860–1869.
10. De Franco AC, Nissen S, Tuzcu E, et al. Ultrasound plaque morphology predicts major dissections following stand-alone and adjunctive balloon angioplasty. *Circulation* 1994;90:I–59(abst).
11. Tanaka A, Kawarabayashi T, Nishibori Y, et al. No-reflow phenomenon and lesion morphology in patients with acute myocardial infarction. *Circulation* 2002;105:2148–2152.
12. Glagov S, Weisenberg E, Zarins C, et al. Compensatory enlargement of human atherosclerotic coronary arteries. *N Engl J Med* 1987;316:1371–1375.
13. Schoenhagen P, Ziada KM, Vince DG, et al. Arterial remodeling and coronary artery disease: the concept of "dilated" versus "obstructive" coronary atherosclerosis. *J Am Coll Cardiol* 2001;38:297–306.
14. Schoenhagen P, Ziada KM, Kapadia SR, et al. Extent and direction of arterial remodeling in stable versus unstable coronary syndromes: an intravascular ultrasound study. *Circulation* 2000;101:598–603.
15. Mintz GS, Kent KM, Pichard AD, et al. Contribution of inadequate arterial remodeling to the development of focal coronary artery stenoses. An intravascular ultrasound study. *Circulation* 1997;95:1791–1798.
16. Mintz GS, Douek P, Pichard AD, et al. Target lesion calcification in coronary artery disease: an intravascular ultrasound study. *J Am Coll Cardiol* 1992;20:1149–1155.
17. Tuzcu E, Berkalp B, De Franco A, et al. The dilemma of diagnosing

coronary calcification: angiography vs. intravascular ultrasound. *J Am Coll Cardiol* 1996;27:832–838.

18. Mintz GS, Pichard AD, Kent KM, et al. Interrelation of coronary angiographic reference lumen size and intravascular ultrasound target lesion calcium. *Am J Cardiol* 1998;81:387–391.

19. Briguori C, Anzuini A, Airoldi F, et al. Intravascular ultrasound criteria for the assessment of the functional significance of intermediate coronary artery stenoses and comparison with fractional flow reserve. *Am J Cardiol* 2001;87:136–141.

20. Nishioka T, Amanullah AM, Luo H, et al. Clinical validation of intravascular ultrasound imaging for assessment of coronary stenosis severity: comparison with stress myocardial perfusion imaging. *J Am Coll Cardiol* 1999;33:1870–1878.

21. Abizaid A, Mintz GS, Pichard AD, et al. Clinical, intravascular ultrasound, and quantitative angiographic determinants of the coronary flow reserve before and after percutaneous transluminal coronary angioplasty. *Am J Cardiol* 1998;82:423–428.

22. Abizaid AS, Mintz GS, Mehran R, et al. Long-term follow-up after percutaneous transluminal coronary angioplasty was not performed based on intravascular ultrasound findings: importance of lumen dimensions. *Circulation* 1999;100:256–261.

23. Abizaid AS, Mintz GS, Abizaid A, et al. One-year follow-up after intravascular ultrasound assessment of moderate left main coronary artery disease in patients with ambiguous angiograms. *J Am Coll Cardiol* 1999;34:707–715.

24. Russo RM. Personal communication.

25. Iyisoy A, Ziada K, Schoenhagen P, et al. Intravascular ultrasound evidence of ostial narrowing in nonatherosclerotic left main coronary arteries. *Am J Cardiol* 2002;90:773–775.

26. Mintz GS, Pichard AD, Kovach JA, et al. Impact of preintervention intravascular ultrasound imaging on transcatheter treatment strategies in coronary artery disease. *Am J Cardiol* 1994;73:423–430.

27. Berkalp B, Badak O, Schoenhagen P, et al. Influence of various percutaneous coronary interventional devices on postinterventional luminal shape and plaque surface characteristics as determined by intravascular ultrasound. *Am J Cardiol* 2003;19:1269–1272.

28. Simonton CA, Leon MB, Baim DS, et al. 'Optimal' directional coronary atherectomy: final results of the Optimal Atherectomy Restenosis Study (OARS). *Circulation* 1998;97:332–339.

29. Mintz GS, Popma JJ, Pichard AD, et al. Intravascular ultrasound predictors of restenosis after percutaneous transcatheter coronary revascularization. *J Am Coll Cardiol* 1996;27:1678–1687.

30. Kimura T, Kaburagi S, Tamura T, et al. Remodeling of human coronary arteries undergoing coronary angioplasty or atherectomy. *Circulation* 1997;96:475–483.

31. de Vrey EA, Mintz GS, von Birgelen C, et al. Serial volumetric (three-dimensional) intravascular ultrasound analysis of restenosis after directional coronary atherectomy. *J Am Coll Cardiol* 1998;32:1874–1880.

32. Mintz GS, Kimura T, Nobuyoshi M, et al. Intravascular ultrasound assessment of the relation between early and late changes in arterial area and neointimal hyperplasia after percutaneous transluminal coronary angioplasty and directional coronary atherectomy. *Am J Cardiol* 1999;83:1518–1523.

33. Meine TJ, Bauman RP, Yock PG, et al. Coronary artery restenosis after atherectomy is primarily due to negative remodeling. *Am J Cardiol* 1999;84:141–146.

34. Painter JA, Mintz GS, Wong SC, et al. Serial intravascular ultrasound studies fail to show evidence of chronic Palmaz-Schatz stent recoil. *Am J Cardiol* 1995;75:398–400.

35. Umans VA, Baptista J, di Mario C, et al. Angiographic, ultrasonic, and angioscopic assessment of the coronary artery wall and lumen area configuration after directional atherectomy: the mechanism revisited. *Am Heart J* 1995;130:217–227.

36. Tsuchikane E, Sumitsuji S, Awata N, et al. Final results of the STent versus directional coronary Atherectomy Randomized Trial (START). *J Am Coll Cardiol* 1999;34:1050–1057.

37. Prati F, Di Mario C, Moussa I, et al. In-stent neointimal proliferation correlates with the amount of residual plaque burden outside the stent: an intravascular ultrasound study. *Circulation* 1999;99:1011–1014.

38. Shiran A, Weissman NJ, Leiboff B, et al. Effect of preintervention plaque burden on subsequent intimal hyperplasia in stented coronary artery lesions. *Am J Cardiol* 2000;86:1318–1321.

39. Endo A, Hirayama H, Yoshida O, et al. Arterial remodeling influences

40. Moussa I, Moses J, Di Mario C, et al. Stenting after optimal lesion debulking (sold) registry. Angiographic and clinical outcome. *Circulation* 1998;98:1604–1609.

41. Ahmed JM, Hong MK, Mehran R, et al. Comparison of debulking followed by stenting versus stenting alone for saphenous vein graft aortoostial lesions: immediate and one-year clinical outcomes. *J Am Coll Cardiol* 2000;35:1560–1568.

42. Hoffmann R, Mintz GS, Popma JJ, et al. Treatment of calcified coronary lesions with Palmaz-Schatz stents. An intravascular ultrasound study. *Eur Heart J* 1998;19:1224–1231.

43. Moussa I, Di Mario C, Moses J, et al. Coronary stenting after rotational atherectomy in calcified and complex lesions. Angiographic and clinical follow-up results. *Circulation* 1997;96:128–136.

44. Goicolea J, Martinez D, Alfonso F, et al. Intravascular ultrasound findings after cutting balloon angioplasty. *Circulation* 1996;94[Suppl I]:I-3815–I-3824.

45. Hara H, Nakamura M, Asahara T, et al. Intravascular ultrasonic comparisons of mechanisms of vasodilatation of cutting balloon angioplasty versus conventional balloon angioplasty. *Am J Cardiol* 2002;89:1253–1256.

46. Serruys P, de Jaegere P, Kiemeniej F, et al. A comparison of balloon-expandable-stent implantation with balloon angioplasty in patients with coronary artery disease. *N Engl J Med* 1994;331:489–495.

47. Fischman D, Leon M, Baim D, et al. A randomized comparison of coronary-stent placement and balloon angioplasty in the treatment of coronary artery disease. *N Engl J Med* 1994;331:496–501.

48. Nakamura S, Colombo A, Gaglione A, et al. Intracoronary ultrasound observations during stent implantation. *Circulation* 1994;89:2026–2034.

49. Goldberg SL, Colombo A, Nakamura S, et al. Benefit of intracoronary ultrasound in the deployment of Palmaz-Schatz stents. *J Am Coll Cardiol* 1994;24:996–1003.

50. Colombo A, Hall P, Nakamura S, et al. Intracoronary stenting without anticoagulation accomplished with intravascular ultrasound guidance. *Circulation* 1995;91:1676–1688.

51. Karrillon GJ, Morice MC, Benveniste E, et al. Intracoronary stent implantation without ultrasound guidance and with replacement of conventional anticoagulation by antiplatelet therapy. 30-day clinical outcome of the French Multicenter Registry. *Circulation* 1996;94:1519–1527.

52. Ahmed JM, Mintz GS, Weissman NJ, et al. Mechanism of lumen enlargement during intracoronary stent implantation: an intravascular ultrasound study. *Circulation* 2000;102:7–10.

53. Data on File, Boston Scientific Corporation.

54. Ziada KM, Kapadia SR, Belli G, et al. Prognostic value of absolute versus relative measures of the procedural result after successful coronary stenting: importance of vessel size in predicting long-term freedom from target vessel revascularization. *Am Heart J* 2001;141:823–831.

55. Hong MK, Park SW, Mintz GS, et al. Intravascular ultrasonic predictors of angiographic restenosis after long coronary stenting. *Am J Cardiol* 2000;85:441–445.

56. Fitzgerald PJ, Oshima A, Hayase M, et al. Final results of the Can Routine Ultrasound Influence Stent Expansion (CRUISE) study. *Circulation* 2000;102:523–530.

57. Mudra H, di Mario C, de Jaegere P, et al. Randomized comparison of coronary stent implantation under ultrasound or angiographic guidance to reduce stent restenosis (OPTICUS Study). *Circulation* 2001;104:1343–1349.

58. Schiele F, Meneveau N, Vuillemenot A, et al. Impact of intravascular ultrasound guidance in stent deployment on 6-month restenosis rate: a multicenter, randomized study comparing two strategies—with and without intravascular ultrasound guidance. RESIST Study Group. REStenosis after Ivus guided STenting. *J Am Coll Cardiol* 1998;32:320–328.

59. Russo RJ, Nicosia A, Teirstein PS, et al. Angiography versus intravascular ultrasound-directed stent placement. *J Am Coll Cardiol* 1997;29:369A(abst).

60. de Jaegere P, Mudra H, Figulla H, et al. Intravascular ultrasound-guided optimized stent deployment. Immediate and 6 months clinical and angiographic results from the Multicenter Ultrasound Stenting in Coronaries Study (MUSIC Study). *Eur Heart J* 1998;19:1214–1223.

61. Bermejo J, Botas J, Garcia E, et al. Mechanisms of residual lumen stenosis after high-pressure stent implantation: a quantitative coronary angiography and intravascular ultrasound study. *Circulation* 1998;98:112–118.

the development of intimal hyperplasia after stent implantation. *J Am Coll Cardiol* 2001;37:70–75.

62. Stone GW, St Goar FG, Hodgson JM, et al. Analysis of the relation between stent implantation pressure and expansion. Optimal Stent Implantation (OSTI) Investigators. *Am J Cardiol* 1999;83:1397–1400,A8.
63. Moussa I, Moses J, Di Mario C, et al. Does the specific intravascular ultrasound criterion used to optimize stent expansion have an impact on the probability of stent restenosis? *Am J Cardiol* 1999;83:1012–1017.
64. Blessing E, Hausmann D, Sturm M, et al. Intravascular ultrasound and stent implantation: intraobserver and interobserver variability. *Am Heart J* 1999;137:368–371.
65. Ziada KM, Tuzcu EM, De Franco AC, et al. Absolute, not relative, post-stent lumen area is a better predictor of clinical events. *Circulation* 1996;94:I-453(abst).
66. Hoffmann R, Mintz GS, Mehran R, et al. Intravascular ultrasound predictors of angiographic restenosis in lesions treated with Palmaz-Schatz stents. *J Am Coll Cardiol* 1998;31:43–49.
67. de Feyter PJ, Kay P, Disco C, et al. Reference chart derived from post-stent-implantation intravascular ultrasound predictors of 6-month expected restenosis on quantitative coronary angiography. *Circulation* 1999;100:1777–1783.
68. Hong MK, Mintz GS, Hong MK, et al. Intravascular ultrasound predictors of target lesion revascularization after stenting of protected left main coronary artery stenoses. *Am J Cardiol* 1999;83:175–179.
69. Schiele F, Meneveau N, Seronde MF, et al. Predictors of event-free survival after repeat intracoronary procedure for in-stent restenosis; study with angiographic and intravascular ultrasound imaging. *Eur Heart J* 2000;21:754–762.
70. Hoffmann R, Mintz GS, Dussaillant GR, et al. Patterns and mechanisms of in-stent restenosis. A serial intravascular ultrasound study. *Circulation* 1996;94:1247–1254.
71. Mehran R, Mintz GS, Hong MK, et al. Validation of the in vivo intravascular ultrasound measurement of in-stent neointimal hyperplasia volumes. *J Am Coll Cardiol* 1998;32:794–799.
72. Hoffmann R, Mintz GS, Pichard AD, et al. Intimal hyperplasia thickness at follow-up is independent of stent size: a serial intravascular ultrasound study. *Am J Cardiol* 1998;82:1168–1172.
73. Kastrati A, Schomig A, Elezi S, et al. Predictive factors of restenosis after coronary stent placement. *J Am Coll Cardiol* 1997;30:1428–1436.
74. Oemrawsingh PV, Mintz GS, Schalij MJ, et al. Intravascular ultrasound guidance improves angiographic and clinical outcome of stent implantation for long coronary artery stenoses: final results of a randomized comparison with angiographic guidance (TULIP Study). *Circulation* 2003;107:62–77.
75. Okabe T, Asakura Y, Ishikawa S, et al. Determining appropriate small vessels for stenting by intravascular ultrasound. *J Invasive Cardiol* 2000;12:625–630.
76. Briguori C, Tobis J, Nishida T, et al. Discrepancy between angiography and intravascular ultrasound when analysing small coronary arteries. *Eur Heart J* 2002;23:247–254.
77. Moussa I, Kobayashi Y, Adamian M, et al. Characteristics of patients with a large discrepancy in coronary artery diameter between quantitative angiography and intravascular ultrasound. *Am J Cardiol* 2001;88:294–296.
78. Ziada KM, Tuzcu EM, De Franco AC, et al. Intravascular ultrasound assessment of the prevalence and causes of angiographic "haziness" following high-pressure coronary stenting. *Am J Cardiol* 1997;80:116–121.
79. Sheris SJ, Canos MR, Weissman NJ. Natural history of intravascular ultrasound-detected edge dissections from coronary stent deployment. *Am Heart J* 2000;139[1 Pt 1]:59–63.
80. Hong MK, Park SW, Lee NH, et al. Long-term outcomes of minor dissection at the edge of stents detected with intravascular ultrasound. *Am J Cardiol* 2000;86:791–795,A9.
81. Nishida T, Colombo A, Briguori C, et al. Outcome of nonobstructive residual dissections detected by intravascular ultrasound following percutaneous coronary intervention. *Am J Cardiol* 2002;89:1257–1262.
82. Maehara A, Mintz GS, Bui AB, et al. Incidence, morphology, angiographic findings, and outcomes of intramural hematomas after percutaneous coronary interventions: an intravascular ultrasound study. *Circulation* 2002;105:2037–2042.
83. Ziada KM, Roffi M, Crowe TD, et al. Adventitial hematoma triggering coronary spasm during percutaneous coronary intervention. *J Invasive Cardiol* 2001;13:464–466.
84. Grewal J, Ganz P, Selwyn A, et al. Usefulness of intravascular ultra-

85. Kasaoka S, Tobis JM, Akiyama T, et al. Angiographic and intravascular ultrasound predictors of in-stent restenosis. *J Am Coll Cardiol* 1998;32:1630–1635.
86. Hoffmann R, Mintz GS, Kent KM, et al. Serial intravascular ultrasound predictors of restenosis at the margins of Palmaz-Schatz stents. *Am J Cardiol* 1997;79:915–953.
87. Rensing BJ, Vos J, Smits PC, et al. Coronary restenosis elimination with a sirolimus eluting stent: first European human experience with 6-month angiographic and intravascular ultrasonic follow-up. *Eur Heart J* 2001;22:2125–2130.
88. Sousa JE, Costa MA, Abizaid AC, et al. Sustained suppression of neointimal proliferation by sirolimus-eluting stents: one-year angiographic and intravascular ultrasound follow-up. *Circulation* 2001;104:2007–2011.
89. Degertekin M, Serruys PW, Foley DP, et al. Persistent inhibition of neointimal hyperplasia after sirolimus-eluting stent implantation: long-term (up to 2 years) clinical, angiographic, and intravascular ultrasound follow-up. *Circulation* 2002;106:1610–1613.
90. Serruys PW, Degertekin M, Tanabe K, et al. Intravascular ultrasound findings in the multicenter, randomized, double-blind RAVEL (RAndomized study with the sirolimus-eluting VElocity balloon-expandable stent in the treatment of patients with de novo native coronary artery Lesions) trial. *Circulation* 2002;106:798–803.
91. Grube E, Silber S, Hauptmann KE, et al. TAXUS I: six- and twelve-month results from a randomized, double-blind trial on a slow-release paclitaxel-eluting stent for de novo coronary lesions. *Circulation* 2003;107:38–42.
92. Sousa JE, Costa MA, Abizaid A, et al. Sirolimus-eluting stent for the treatment of in-stent restenosis: a quantitative coronary angiography and three-dimensional intravascular ultrasound study. *Circulation* 2003;107:24–27.
93. Tanabe K, Serruys PW, Grube E, et al. TAXUS III Trial: in-stent restenosis treated with stent-based delivery of paclitaxel incorporated in a slow-release polymer formulation. *Circulation* 2003;107:559–564.
94. Hong MK, Mintz GS, Lee CW, et al. Paclitaxel coating reduces in-stent intimal hyperplasia in human coronary arteries: a serial volumetric intravascular ultrasound analysis from the ASian Paclitaxel-Eluting Stent Clinical Trial (ASPECT). *Circulation* 2003;107:517–520.
95. Hermiller JB, Buller CE, Tenaglia AN, et al. Unrecognized left main coronary artery disease in patients undergoing interventional procedures. *Am J Cardiol* 1993;71:173–176.
96. Park SJ, Hong MK, Lee CW, et al. Elective stenting of unprotected left main coronary artery stenosis: effect of debulking before stenting and intravascular ultrasound guidance. *J Am Coll Cardiol* 2001;38:1054–1060.
97. Hong MK, Park SW, Lee CW, et al. Intravascular ultrasound findings in stenting of unprotected left main coronary artery stenosis. *Am J Cardiol* 1998;82:670–673,A8.
98. Cantor WJ, Peterson ED, Popma JJ, et al. Provisional stenting strategies: systematic overview and implications for clinical decision-making. *J Am Coll Cardiol* 2000;36:1142–1151.
99. Wilson SH, Fasseas P, Orford JL, et al. Clinical outcome of patients undergoing non-cardiac surgery in the two months following coronary stenting. *J Am Coll Cardiol* 2003;42:234–240.
100. Stone GW, Hodgson JM, St Goar FG, et al. Improved procedural results of coronary angioplasty with intravascular ultrasound-guided balloon sizing: the CLOUT Pilot Trial. Clinical Outcomes With Ultrasound Trial (CLOUT) Investigators. *Circulation* 1997;95:2044–2052.
101. Abizaid A, Pichard AD, Mintz GS, et al. Acute and long-term results of an intravascular ultrasound-guided percutaneous transluminal coronary angioplasty/provisional stent implantation strategy. *Am J Cardiol* 1999;84:1298–1303.
102. Frey AW, Hodgson JM, Muller C, et al. Ultrasound-guided strategy for provisional stenting with focal balloon combination catheter: results from the randomized Strategy for Intracoronary Ultrasound-guided PTCA and Stenting (SIPS) trial. *Circulation* 2000;102:2497–2502.
102a. Colombo A, De Gregorio J, Moussa I, et al. Intravascular ultrasound-guided percutaneous transluminal coronary angioplasty with provisional spot stenting for treatment of long coronary lesions. *J Am Coll Cardiol* 2001;38:1427–1433.
103. Schroeder S, Baumbach A, Mahrholdt H, et al. The impact of un-

treated coronary dissections on acute and long-term outcome after intravascular ultrasound guided PTCA. *Eur Heart J* 2000;21:137–145.

104. Mintz GS, Hoffmann R, Mehran R, et al. In-stent restenosis: the Washington Hospital Center experience. *Am J Cardiol* 1998;81(7A):7E–13E.

105. Morino Y, Limpijankit T, Honda Y, et al. Late vascular response to repeat stenting for in-stent restenosis with and without radiation: an intravascular ultrasound volumetric analysis. *Circulation* 2002;105:2465–2468.

106. Shiran A, Mintz GS, Waksman R, et al. Early lumen loss after treatment of in-stent restenosis: an intravascular ultrasound study. *Circulation* 1998;98:200–203.

107. vom Dahl J, Dietz U, Haager PK, et al. Rotational atherectomy does not reduce recurrent in-stent restenosis: results of the angioplasty versus rotational atherectomy for treatment of diffuse in-stent restenosis trial (ARTIST). *Circulation* 2002;105:583–588.

108. Radke PW, Klues HG, Haager PK, et al. Mechanisms of acute lumen gain and recurrent restenosis after rotational atherectomy of diffuse in-stent restenosis: a quantitative angiographic and intravascular ultrasound study. *J Am Coll Cardiol* 1999;34:33–39.

109. Ahmed JM, Mintz GS, Castagna M, et al. Intravascular ultrasound assessment of the mechanism of lumen enlargement during cutting balloon angioplasty treatment of in-stent restenosis. *Am J Cardiol* 2001;88:1032–1034.

110. Teirstein PS, Massullo V, Jani S, et al. Catheter-based radiotherapy to inhibit restenosis after coronary stenting. *N Engl J Med* 1997;336:1697–1703.

111. Mintz GS, Weissman NJ, Fitzgerald PJ. Intravascular ultrasound assessment of the mechanisms and results of brachytherapy. *Circulation* 2001;104:1320–1325.

112. Waksman R, White RL, Chan RC, et al. Intracoronary gamma-radiation therapy after angioplasty inhibits recurrence in patients with in-stent restenosis. *Circulation* 2000;101:2165–2171.

113. Mintz GS, Weissman NJ, Teirstein PS, et al. Effect of intracoronary gamma-radiation therapy on in-stent restenosis: an intravascular ultrasound analysis from the gamma-1 study. *Circulation* 2000;102:2915–2918.

114. Ahmed JM, Mintz GS, Waksman R, et al. Serial intravascular ultrasound analysis of edge recurrence after intracoronary gamma radiation treatment of native artery in-stent restenosis lesions. *Am J Cardiol* 2001;87:1145–1149.

115. Sabate M, Marijnissen JP, Carlier SG, et al. Residual plaque burden, delivered dose, and tissue composition predict 6-month outcome after balloon angioplasty and beta-radiation therapy. *Circulation* 2000;101:2472–2477.

116. Kozuma K, Costa MA, Sabate M, et al. Late stent malapposition occurring after intracoronary beta-irradiation detected by intravascular ultrasound. *J Invasive Cardiol* 1999;11:651–655.

117. Castagna MT, Mintz GS, Weissman N, et al. "Black hole": echolucent restenotic tissue after brachytherapy. *Circulation* 2001;103:778.

118. TenHoff H, Hamm MA, Lowe GE, et al. Technical aspects of ultrasound imaging guidewires. *Semin Interv Cardiol* 1997;2:63–68.

119. Lockwood GR, Ryan LK, Foster FS. A 45 to 55 MHz needle-based ultrasound system for invasive imaging. *Ultrason Imaging* 1993;15:1–13.

120. Foster FS, Knapik DA, Machado JC, et al. High-frequency intracoronary ultrasound imaging. *Semin Interv Cardiol* 1997;2:33–41.

121. Brezinski ME, Tearney GJ, Weissman NJ, et al. Assessing atherosclerotic plaque morphology: comparison of optical coherence tomography and high frequency intravascular ultrasound. *Heart* 1997;77:397–403.

122. Jeremias A, Whitbourn RJ, Filardo SD, et al. Adequacy of intracoronary versus intravenous adenosine-induced maximal coronary hyperemia for fractional flow reserve measurements. *Am Heart J* 2000;140:651–657.

123. Wilson RF, White CW. Intracoronary papaverine: an ideal coronary vasodilator for studies of the coronary circulation in conscious humans. *Circulation* 1986;73:444–451.

124. Ofili EO, Kern MJ, St Vrain JA, et al. Differential characterization of blood flow, velocity, and vascular resistance between proximal and distal normal epicardial human coronary arteries: analysis by intracoronary Doppler spectral flow velocity. *Am Heart J* 1995;130:37–46.

125. Kern MJ. A simplified method to measure coronary blood flow velocity in patients: validation and application of a Judkins-style Doppler-tipped angiographic catheter. *Am Heart J* 1990;120:1202–1212.

126. Gould KL, Lipscomb K. Effects of coronary stenoses on coronary flow reserve and resistance. *Am J Cardiol* 1974;34:48–55.

127. Gould KL, Lipscomb K, Hamilton GW. Physiologic basis for assessing critical coronary stenosis. Instantaneous flow response and re-gional distribution during coronary hyperemia as measures of coronary flow reserve. *Am J Cardiol* 1974;33:87–94.

128. Lipscomb K, Gould KL. Mechanism of the effect of coronary artery stenosis on coronary flow in the dog. *Am Heart J* 1975;89:60–67.

129. Gould KL, Lipscomb K, Calvert C. Compensatory changes of the distal coronary vascular bed during progressive coronary constriction. *Circulation* 1975;51:1085–1094.

130. Pijls NH, Van Gelder B, Van der Voort P, et al. Fractional flow reserve. A useful index to evaluate the influence of an epicardial coronary stenosis on myocardial blood flow. *Circulation* 1995;92:3183–3193.

131. Pijls NH, De Bruyne B, Peels K, et al. Measurement of fractional flow reserve to assess the functional severity of coronary-artery stenoses. *N Engl J Med* 1996;334:1703–1708.

132. De Bruyne B, Baudhuin T, Melin JA, et al. Coronary flow reserve calculated from pressure measurements in humans. Validation with positron emission tomography. *Circulation* 1994;89:1013–1022.

133. De Bruyne B, Pijls NH, Heyndrickx GR, et al. Pressure-derived fractional flow reserve to assess serial epicardial stenoses: theoretical basis and animal validation. *Circulation* 2000;101:1840–1847.

134. De Bruyne B, Hersbach F, Pijls NH, et al. Abnormal epicardial coronary resistance in patients with diffuse atherosclerosis but "normal" coronary angiography. *Circulation* 2001;104:2401–2406.

135. Topol EJ, Ellis SG, Cosgrove DM, et al. Analysis of coronary angioplasty practice in the United States with an insurance-claims data base. *Circulation* 1993;87:1489–1497.

136. Joye JD, Schulman DS, Lasorda D, et al. Intracoronary Doppler guide wire versus stress single-photon emission computed tomographic thallium-201 imaging in assessment of intermediate coronary stenoses. *J Am Coll Cardiol* 1994;24:940–947.

137. Donohue TJ, Kern MJ, Aguirre FV, et al. Assessing the hemodynamic significance of coronary artery stenoses: analysis of translesional pressure-flow velocity relations in patients. *J Am Coll Cardiol* 1993;22:449–458.

138. Moses JW, Undermir C, Strain JE, et al. Relation between single tomographic intravascular ultrasound image parameters and intracoronary Doppler flow velocity in patients with intermediately severe coronary stenoses. *Am Heart J* 1998;135[6 Pt 1]:988–994.

139. Kern MJ, de Bruyne B, Pijls NH. From research to clinical practice: current role of intracoronary physiologically based decision making in the cardiac catheterization laboratory. *J Am Coll Cardiol* 1997;30:613–620.

140. Bech GJ, De Bruyne B, Bonnier HJ, et al. Long-term follow-up after deferral of percutaneous transluminal coronary angioplasty of intermediate stenosis on the basis of coronary pressure measurement. *J Am Coll Cardiol* 1998;31:841–847.

141. Bech GJ, De Bruyne B, Pijls NH, et al. Fractional flow reserve to determine the appropriateness of angioplasty in moderate coronary stenosis: a randomized trial. *Circulation* 2001;103:2928–2934.

142. Bech GJ, Droste H, Pijls NH, et al. Value of fractional flow reserve in making decisions about bypass surgery for equivocal left main coronary artery disease. *Heart* 2001;86:547–552.

143. Serruys PW, di Mario C, Piek J, et al. Prognostic value of intracoronary flow velocity and diameter stenosis in assessing the short- and long-term outcomes of coronary balloon angioplasty: the DEBATE Study (Doppler Endpoints Balloon Angioplasty Trial Europe). *Circulation* 1997;96:3369–77.

144. Albertal M, Regar E, Van Langenhove G, et al. Flow velocity and predictors of a suboptimal coronary flow velocity reserve after coronary balloon angioplasty. *Eur Heart J* 2002;23:133–138.

145. Di Mario C, Moses JW, Anderson TJ, et al. Randomized comparison of elective stent implantation and coronary balloon angioplasty guided by online quantitative angiography and intracoronary Doppler. DESTINI Study Group (Doppler Endpoint STenting INternational Investigation). *Circulation* 2000;102:2938–2944.

146. Serruys PW, de Bruyne B, Carlier S, et al. Randomized comparison of primary stenting and provisional balloon angioplasty guided by flow velocity measurement. Doppler Endpoints Balloon Angioplasty Trial Europe (DEBATE) II Study Group. *Circulation* 2000;102:2930–2937.

147. Albertal M, Voskuil M, Piek JJ, et al. Coronary flow velocity reserve after percutaneous interventions is predictive of periprocedural outcome. *Circulation* 2002;105:1573–1578.

148. Nishida T, Di Mario C, Kern MJ, et al. Impact of final coronary flow velocity reserve on late outcome following stent implantation. *Eur Heart J* 2002;23:331–340.

149. Pijls NH, Klauss V, Siebert U, et al. Coronary pressure measurement after stenting predicts adverse events at follow-up: a multicenter registry. *Circulation* 2002;105:2950–2954.
150. Kern MJ, Puri S, Bach RG, et al. Abnormal coronary flow velocity reserve after coronary artery stenting in patients: role of relative coronary reserve to assess potential mechanisms. *Circulation* 1999;100:2491–2498.
151. De Bruyne B, Pijls NH, Bartunek J, et al. Fractional flow reserve in patients with prior myocardial infarction. *Circulation* 2001;104:157–162.
152. Suryapranata H, Zijlstra F, MacLeod DC, et al. Predictive value of reactive hyperemic response on reperfusion on recovery of regional myocardial function after coronary angioplasty in acute myocardial infarction. *Circulation* 1994;89:1109–1117.
153. Mazur W, Bitar JN, Lechin M, et al. Coronary flow reserve may predict myocardial recovery after myocardial infarction in patients with TIMI grade 3 flow. *Am Heart J* 1998;136:335–344.
154. Hodgson JM, Marshall JJ. Direct vasoconstriction and endothelium-dependent vasodilation. Mechanisms of acetylcholine effects on coronary flow and arterial diameter in patients with nonstenotic coronary arteries. *Circulation* 1989;79:1043–1051.
155. Werns SW, Walton JA, Hsia HH, et al. Evidence of endothelial dysfunction in angiographically normal coronary arteries of patients with coronary artery disease. *Circulation* 1989;79:287–291.
156. Pijls NH, van Son JA, Kirkeeide RL, et al. Experimental basis of determining maximum coronary, myocardial, and collateral blood flow by pressure measurements for assessing functional stenosis severity before and after percutaneous transluminal coronary angioplasty. *Circulation* 1993;87:1354–1367.
157. Kern MJ, Aguirre FV, Tatineni S, et al. Enhanced coronary blood flow velocity during intraaortic balloon counterpulsation in critically ill patients. *J Am Coll Cardiol* 1993;21:359–368.
158. Hanekamp CE, Koolen JJ, Pijls NH, et al. Comparison of quantitative coronary angiography, intravascular ultrasound, and coronary pressure measurement to assess optimum stent deployment. *Circulation* 1999;99:1015–1021.

CHAPTER 92

Percutaneous Coronary Revascularization for Chronic Coronary Artery Disease

David R. Holmes, Jr. and Spencer B. King III

Key Words: Elastic recoil; percutaneous coronary intervention; percutaneous transluminal coronary angiography; remodeling; restenosis; stent placement.

INTRODUCTION

The introduction and widespread use of percutaneous revascularization techniques has revolutionized the treatment of patients with coronary artery disease. Before the initial description of this technique in 1977, only medical and surgical options were available. The widespread acceptance of these techniques has been the result of several factors including technical advances, increasing operator experience, and expanded patient and angiographic selection criteria. Advances continue with the development of new modalities aimed at addressing the problems of conventional percutaneous transluminal coronary angioplasty (PTCA). Resolution of these problems of adverse lesion characteristics, acute closure, and restenosis should continue to encourage growth of the field and its wider application for the treatment of patients with acute and chronic coronary artery disease.

D. R. Holmes, Jr.: Division of Cardiovascular Diseases, Mayo Clinic, Rochester, Minnesota 55905.

S. B. King III: The Fuqua Heart Center, Piedmont Hospital, Atlanta, Georgia 30309.

BACKGROUND

The advent of interventional cardiology can be dated to October 1958 (1,2). At that time, during performance of aortic root angiography, Mason Sones noted that the catheter had selectively engaged the coronary artery. Drs. Sones and Sheldon have summarized the experience (1,2). When Dr. Sones realized that selective opacification of the dominant right coronary artery had occurred, he also realized that asystole had resulted. The patient remained conscious and responded to the urgent demands for ongoing coughing until sinus rhythm was restored. This event led to the development of invasive cardiology. The second event occurred during performance of a femoral arterial procedure by Charles Dotter (3,4). During this procedure, a catheter was inadvertently passed retrogradely through an occluded iliac artery, thus restoring patency. Both of these seminal events set the stage for the eventual development of PTCA by Andreas Gruntzig, which has revolutionized modern cardiology (5,6).

In addition to these two seminal observations, we have learned a great deal about vascular biology including response to arterial injury and atherosclerosis. The whole concept of changes in arterial geometry over time has been developed and substantiated. These changes have been characterized by the "bigger is better theory" (7–9), which was developed to explain phenomena that were documented after percutaneous coronary intervention (PCI). Changes in external vascular dimensions also have been described during the development of atherosclerosis and affect not only the coronary arteries, but the peripheral vessels as well (10–13). Elastic recoil of the vessel occurs after PTCA, but there often is also constriction or negative remodeling of the lumen in response to chronic injury. Serial intravascular ultrasound studies have documented that there is either lack of arterial enlargement or constriction in patients in whom restenosis develops (14). This may be a dominant mechanism in some patients after dilatation or treatment with new devices. Stents may act by mechanically remodeling the vessel (15–21). They do not prevent neointimal hyperplasia; in fact, they stimulate it. Such constriction may account for as much as 50% of the loss of lumen diameter after conventional dilatation.

The initial PTCA performed in 1977 relied on equipment that by current standards looks not only formidable but potentially dangerous, being large, stiff, and neither very steerable nor trackable. Despite this, the procedure was a success. It also was long lasting at the time of follow-up angiography in 1987–10 years later, the initially treated left anterior descending artery remained widely patent (Fig. 92–1). Even later angiographic follow-up in 2000 documented continued patency. Given the early prototype equipment, additional lesion and patient selection criteria were stringent. Since that time the field has changed dramatically with increased operator experience, broadening of patient and lesion selection criteria, and improved equipment; new generations of therapeutic devices have been introduced and evaluated including a variety of debulking devices—for example, directional coronary atherectomy (DCA) and rotational atherectomy and stents. Many of these devices were received with great acclaim; not all have become main line procedures and some have virtually disappeared. Even the name of the procedure has changed from PTCA, which relied on balloon dilatation alone, to now PCI, which currently, in most cases, is stent based. The number of procedures has increased dramatically, and PCI has now surpassed the frequency of coronary artery bypass graft (CABG) surgery as a means of revascularization for ischemic heart disease.

There have been dramatic changes in patient and lesion selection criteria since the early years of PTCA. The initial patient selection criteria included those with symptomatic but stable myocardial ischemia and well preserved left ventricular function who were candidates for surgical revascularization (22–25). The initial lesion selection criteria were significantly more limited and included proximal, subtotal, concentric, noncalcified, discrete stenoses in large vessels without significant tortuosity and a single culprit lesion; many of the patients only had single-vessel disease. These patients were chosen for two reasons: They had clear documentation of the source of ischemia so that the results of the PTCA procedure could be easily measured by the relief of symptoms and by objective testing. More importantly, the anatomic lesions could be accessed by the early equipment,

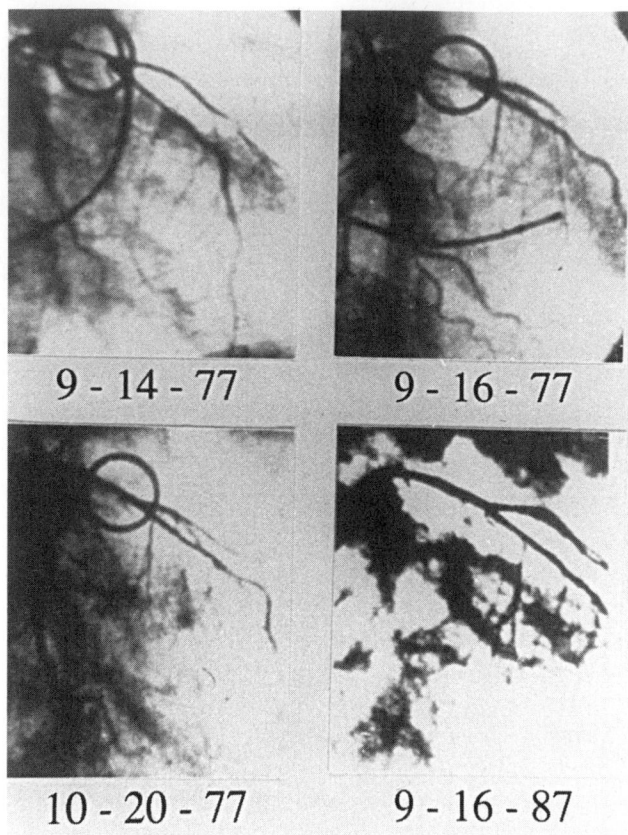

FIG. 92–1. Angiography from the first patient undergoing percutaneous transluminal coronary angioplasty by Andreas Gruntzig. Diagnostic angiography on September 14, 1977 (9-14-77) documenting severe proximal left anterior descending stenosis. The successful dilatation results after this initial dilatation procedure can be seen on October 20, 1977 (10-20-77) and are continued throughout September 16, 1987 (9-16-87), 10 years later.

and the risk for dilatation was believed to be relatively low. From historical interest, despite these strict lesion criteria, in early series, success rates of only 60% to 65% were relatively common. Of the initial consecutive 169 patients treated by Andreas Gruntzig, 133 (79%) were successfully dilated (26, 27). Relief of angina and objective measures of exercise performance were improved, although approximately 25% had a positive exercise test. Ten-year follow-up of this initial cohort of patients documented 95% survival in patients with single-vessel disease and 81% survival with multivessel disease (27). The explosive growth of percutaneous revascularization has been dependent on changes in patient and lesion selection criteria.

LESION SELECTION CRITERIA

Initial lesion selection criteria were aimed at identifying lesions with the greatest success rate and fewest complications. These criteria were based on that the equipment was often the rate-limiting factor; in many patients, the lesion could not be accessed or dilatation resulted in vessel compromise. The major early complication was acute closure, the incidence of which was relatively constant from 4% to 8%; even though relatively uncommon, acute closure accounted for the majority of myocardial infarctions (MIs), emergent or urgent surgical procedures, and mortality during and immediately after intervention (28–33). The other impediment to long-term outcome was restenosis; in one of the earliest publications from the National Heart, Lung and Blood Institute (NHLBI) PTCA registry, this was evaluated in 665 patients who had undergone successful PTCA from 1979 to 1981 (34). A total of 557 of these patients had follow-up angiography at a mean of 188 days. Restenosis, usually associated with recurrent angina, was documented in 33.6% of patients.

In an attempt to optimize outcome, a series of lesion classifications were developed that were intended to be a guide for case selection. Although these classification schemes are still currently used, they are considerably less relevant since the introduction of new technology aimed at making the procedure safer and more successful, namely stent implantation.

DEVICE SELECTION

Multiple new devices and new categories of devices have been developed in an attempt to improve outcome and in response to the problems of conventional PTCA (Fig. 92–2). All of these devices went through the steps of early single-center and multicenter registries, randomized clinical trials, device U.S. Food and Drug Administration (FDA) approval, and then clinical use. Some of these devices have since been virtually abandoned clinically, such as DCA or laser angioplasty, whereas others have been relegated to niche status, such as rotational atherectomy, and still others have achieved dominant roles, such as stents.

Atherectomy

Several atherectomy devices are available and have been relatively widely tested. The first was DCA (Fig. 92–3), which has been extensively studied in multiple randomized trials (35–37). It was originally developed to make PCI safer and more reliable; but then it was most widely tested as a means to decrease restenosis and to improve clinical outcome. Early trials were not convincing in terms of the clinically utility of DCA, and issues of safety were even raised because of increased cardiac enzymes periprocedurally compared with PTCA. The most recent study (Atherectomy before Multi-Link improves luminal gain and clinical outcome [AMIGO]) (38) was aimed at comparing debulking and stent implantation versus stent implantation alone and documented no clearcut advantage for the combined approach versus stent implantation alone. Directional atherectomy remains a demanding discipline. The device is difficult to position optimally and monitoring of the amount of tissue re-

moved can be problematic. Currently, DCA is used infrequently and in some centers not at all; it still may be useful to debulk large proximal bulky or excentric lesions or to treat selected bifurcation lesions.

The second atherectomy device is rotational atherectomy (Fig. 92–4), which consists of an olive-shaped burr that is coated with 5-μm diamond chips and rotates at 150,000 to 200,000 g in the coronary artery, polishing the internal lumen of the vessel wall (39–45). This device uses the principle of differential cutting to selectively ablate atheromatous tissue, which is embolized as small microparticles less than 5 μm, which are then cleared by the reticuloendothelial system. More normal arterial wall is spared in this differential cutting process. Although attractive conceptually, there are specific complication patterns associated with the device, namely slow-flow or no-reflow, which may be difficult to treat and can result in adverse hemodynamic and clinical outcomes. In addition, perforation from wire bias is a significant concern for angulated lesions. Rotational atherectomy has been tested in multicenter randomized trials (43,44) and has not been found to improve restenosis even in high-risk lesions. Because of the complication patterns, the complexity of the device, and lack of restenosis benefit, it has been used recently only as a niche device (46). It is still useful to treat hard fibrocalcific lesions that cannot be dilated with conventional high-pressure balloons, some patients with diffuse instent restenosis, and some ostial lesions that tend to be poorly treated with conventional PTCA.

Lasers

A second group of nonballoon devices are intracoronary lasers, developed with the intent to ablate plaque (47–55). Although several forms of laser energy have been used, only two were used clinically: the excimer laser with a wavelength of 308 nm and a holmium YAG laser with a wavelength of 2 μm (Fig. 92–5). Both lasers are over-the-wire systems with the energy being delivered through a fiberoptic bundle. Tissue ablation is achieved by a combination of photoablation and mechanical disruption. Excimer lasers have been compared with conventional PTCA in two randomized trials—Amsterdam-Rotterdam (AMRO) (54) and Excimer Laser, Rotational Atherectomy, and Balloon Angioplasty Comparison (ERBAC) (44)—and were not found to be dramatically effective. Accordingly, lasers have been relegated to a very small niche and many centers have no experience with them. They may still be useful for treatment of instent restenosis but even this application is uncommon.

Stents

Stents have revolutionized interventional cardiology and are currently the backbone of the field, being used in approximally 90% of all interventional cases (55–61). They have been subjected to multiple randomized clinical trials: initially, stents versus conventional PTCA, and then later stents

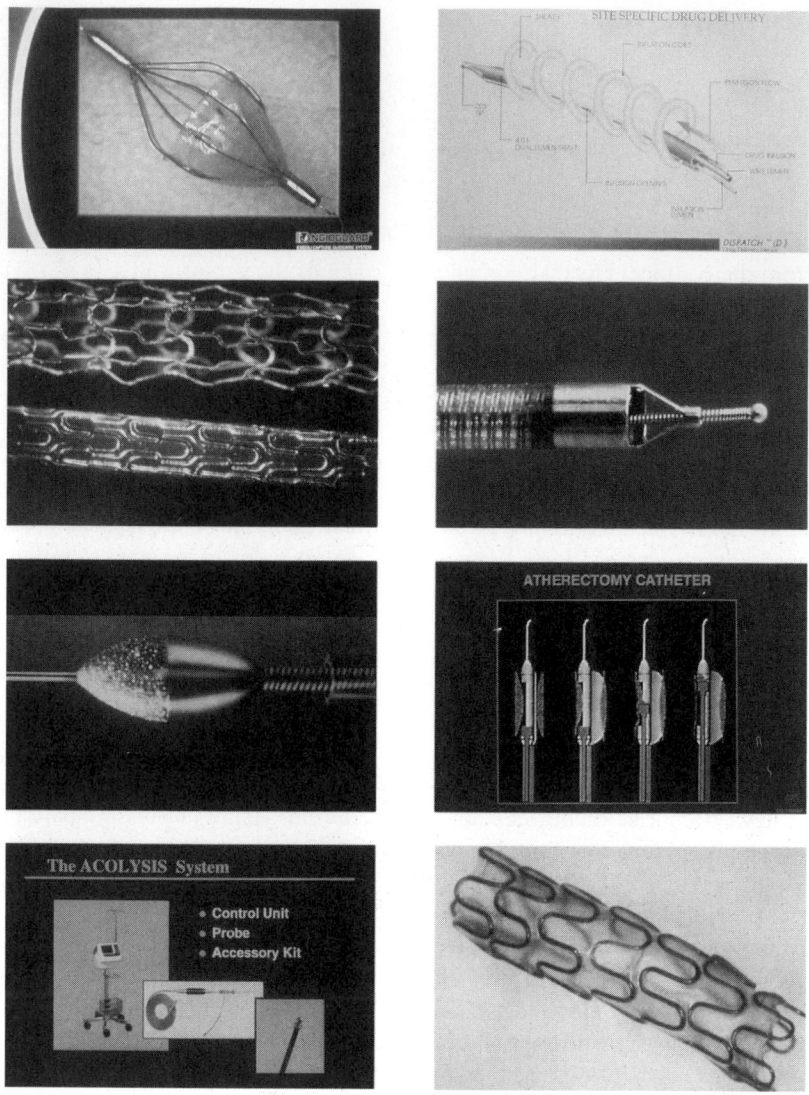

FIG. 92–2. Collage of directional coronary atherectomy, transluminal extraction atherectomy catheter (TEC), rotational atherectomy, laser, rheolytic thrombectomy, and stent.

of different design and configurations with each other. They also have been the focus of two expert consensus American College of Cardiology documents. This widespread use has been the result of several factors: (a) the typical, predictable, and optimal stable angiographic appearance of lesions treated with stent implantation largely irrespective of baseline lesion complexity compared with conventional PTCA; (b) deliverability and ease of use of the newer generation devices that allow stents to be placed relatively easily to all coronary arterial segments; (c) documented decrease in restenosis rates compared with conventional PTCA; (d) ability to treat or prevent subacute closure. With current stent-based approaches, the need for urgent or emergent surgery as a complication of intervention is approximately 0.5%.

There are still issues that are not completely resolved with stenting. First, subacute closure was a relatively infrequent but a prominent clinical problem in the early days of stent experience that resulted in infarction and even mortality.

With dual antiplatelet therapy and high-pressure dilatation, even in unselected patient series, subacute closure rates are now less than 1%. When it does occur, however, it is still associated with major adverse events and a striking increased incidence of death and/or MI (62–68). Second, instent restenosis is a substantial problem even though it occurs less frequently than restenosis after conventional dilatation. Different patterns of instent restenosis have been described (69) that have significant prognostic implications and may require different approaches (*vide infra*). Third, specific lesion characteristics also are problematic for stents including: (a) bifurcation lesions (70–72), which currently appear to be best treated with stent placement in only the main vessel with conventional dilatation or debulking of the side branch; (b) small diffusely diseased vessels that may limit placement of the stent and treatment of which is associated with increased restenosis; (c) severe calcification that limits the ability to fully deploy the stent. Solutions to these problems

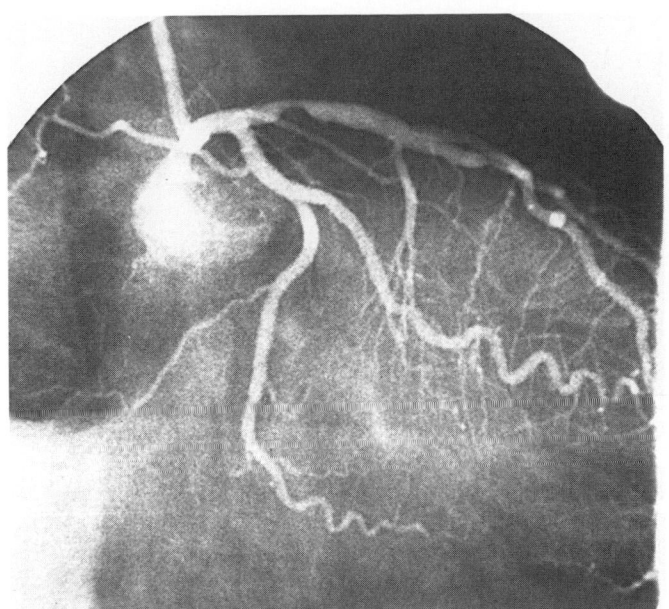
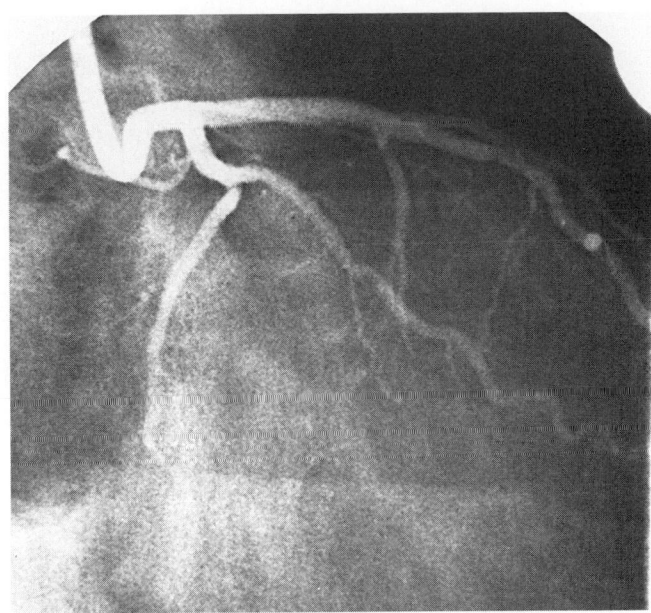

FIG. 92–3. Right anterior oblique view of proximal left anterior descending artery with a lesion ideal for atherectomy. **A:** Before atherectomy. **B:** After atherectomy.

and introduction of new stent modifications such as drug-eluting or coated stents will make this type of therapy even more ubiquitous.

Newer Devices/Distal Protection Devices

Early on in the field of interventional cardiology, distal embolization during the course of an interventional procedure was believed to be uncommon and not a clinically important problem (73,74). Subsequent to these perceptions, there has been more attention paid to the issue (75,76). In postmortem specimens, multiple small emboli have been documented in the watershed distribution downstream from treated lesions (73,74,76). These findings have led to the development of a variety of distal protection devices—some of these are based on balloon occlusion and subsequent aspiration, whereas others are based on a filter design, which allows flow during treatment with subsequent removal of the filter. Although

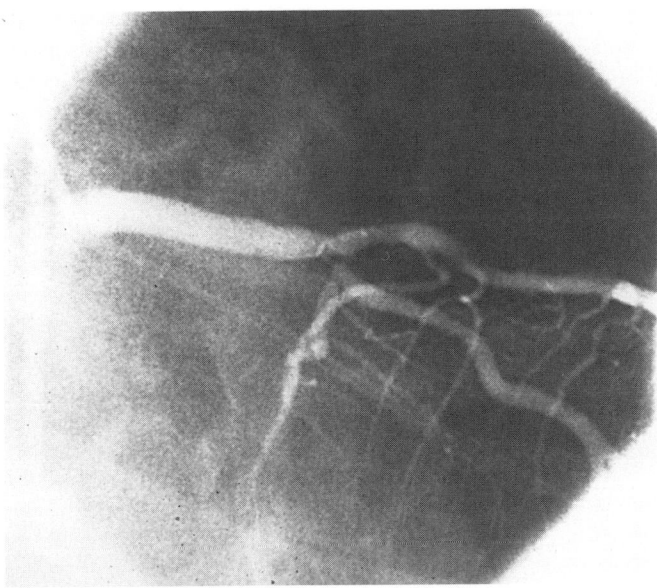
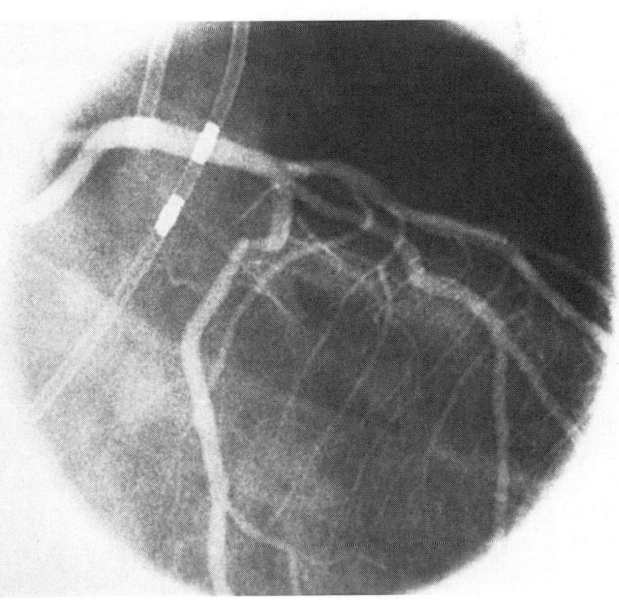

FIG. 92–4. Right anterior oblique view of ostial circumflex lesion (baseline **A**). Rotablator burr is used to treat lesion, followed by adjunctive percutaneous transluminal coronary angiography to give final result **(B)**.

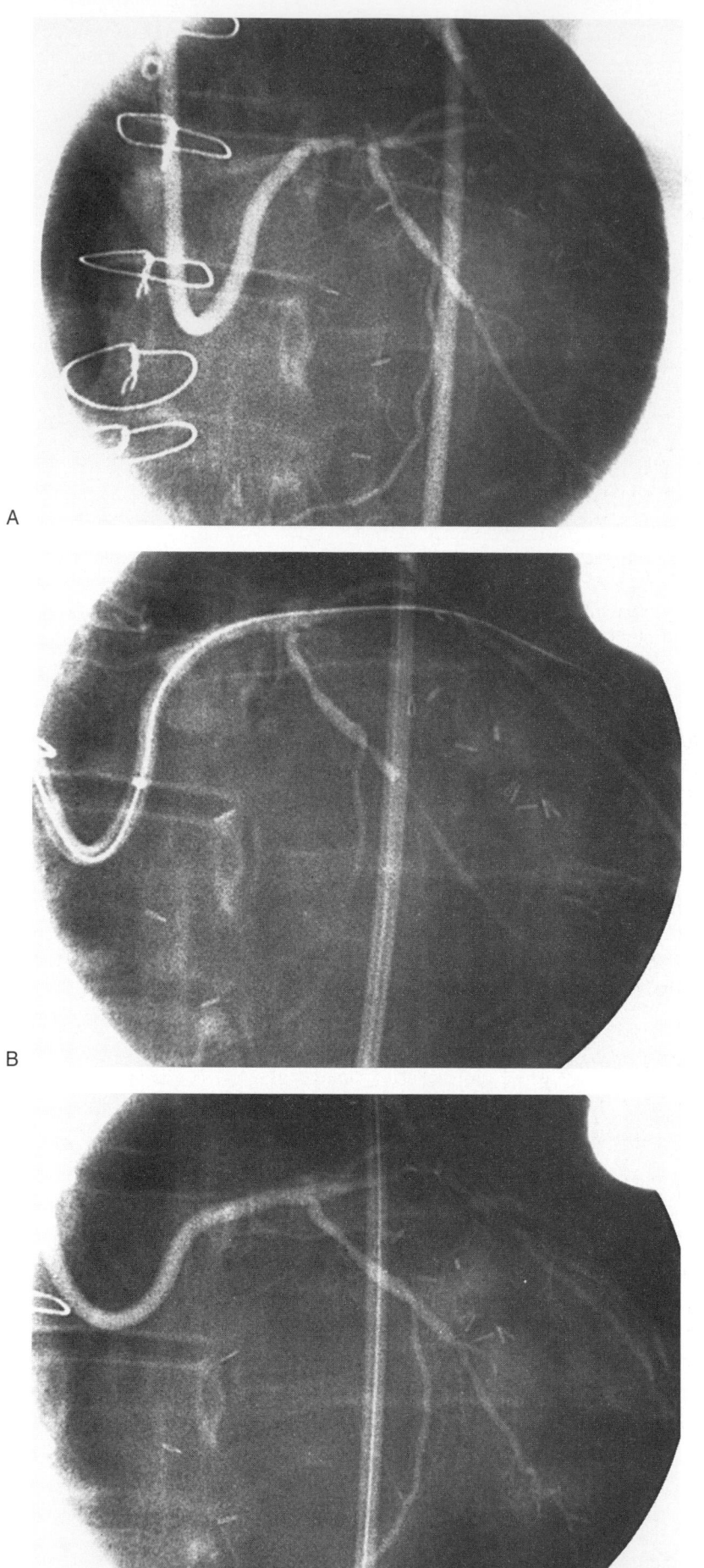

FIG. 92–5. Directional laser fibers have been developed to treat eccentric and branch lesions. **A:** Eccentric lesion in left main coronary artery in a patient who had previously undergone bypass surgery. **B:** The eccentric laser catheter is advanced through the lesion, directing the energy into the eccentric plaque. **C:** After ablation there is excellent improvement in the eccentric stenosis.

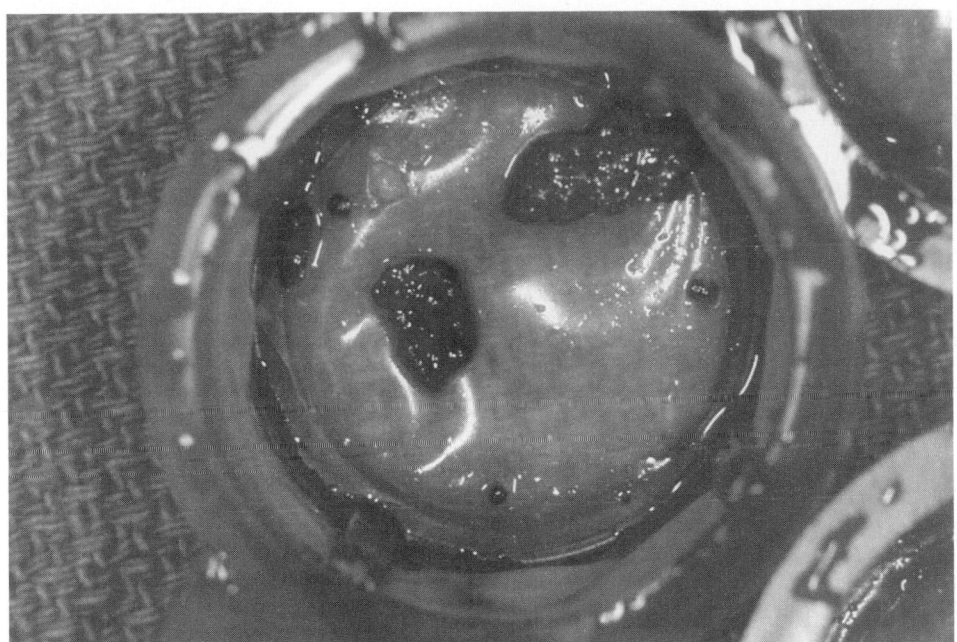

FIG. 92–6. Particulate debris and thrombus retrieved from a diffusely diseased vein graft undergoing stent implantation.

only one device (77) has been approved and has become a predicate device, it is anticipated that multiple other devices will become available for clinical use.

It has become apparent that particulate debris is common (Fig. 92–6); Webb and coworkers (78) evaluated a distal embolic occlusion device in 27 percutaneous interventional vein graft procedures. With this device, the vein graft distal to the lesion is occluded, the stenosis is treated, then the graft is aspirated before restoring flow. The graft age in this study was 8.7 ± 5 years. Occlusion times varied but averaged 150 ± 54 seconds. Particulate material was retrieved from 21 of 23 procedures and consisted of necrotic core with cholesterol clefts, lipid-rich macrophages, and fibrin strands. This device was subsequently tested in a multicenter, multinational trial of 103 consecutive patients undergoing planned stenting of 105 vein graft patients. In this experience, the distal occlusion balloon was inflated for 5.4 ± 3.7 minutes; macroscopic debris was retrieved in 91% of the patients. The pivotal U.S. trial, Saphenous vein graft Angioplasty Free of Emboli Randomized (SAFER), randomized 551 patients to either conventional therapy or distal embolic protection (77). This trial was stopped prematurely with documentation that there was an approximate 50% reduction in major adverse cardiac event rates at 30 days from 19.8% in the control arm to 9.6% in the distal protection group. This distal protection device was subsequently approved for use by the FDA and has become the predicate device for treatment of saphenous vein graft disease. Other approaches such as filters that do not occlude flow are currently being tested for treatment of vein graft disease and acute MI (79,80). As these devices become more streamlined and user friendly, they may be used in the majority of

interventions to prevent distal embolization and to potentially decrease periprocedural enzyme level increase.

Thrombectomy Devices

Thrombus continues to be a problem for interventional cardiology *(vide infra)* (Fig. 92–7). Two different devices are being used with increasing frequency in this setting. Rheolytic thrombectomy is the most prominently used. The AngioJet (Possis Medical, Minneapolis, MN) device has three separate

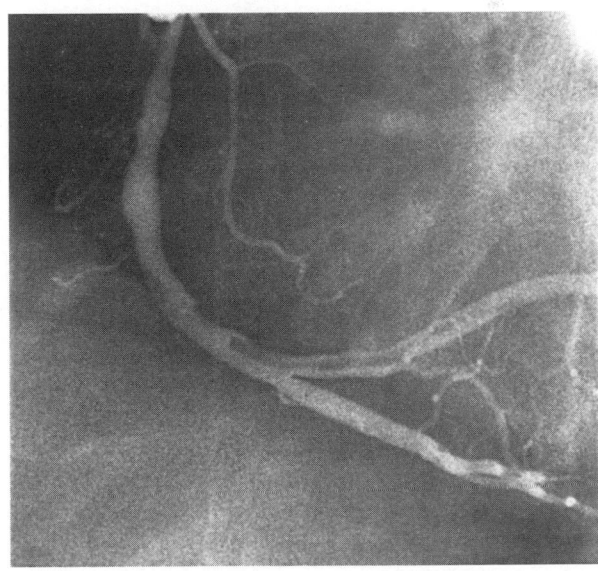

FIG. 92–7. Left anterior oblique of the distal right coronary artery with a larger filling defect consistent with thrombus.

components: a drive unit, a pulsatile pump, and the catheter. High-pressure saline jets are produced by applying pressure and forcing the saline through the catheter. This results in a vortex that causes fragmentation of thrombus and then allows removal of debris. Current device iterations can be used with a 6-French guiding catheter. The safety and efficacy of this system have been documented in single-center experiences of vein graft disease and native coronary arteries with complex thrombus-containing lesions (81–83). This device also has been studied in a randomized multicenter trial (Vein Graft AngioJet Study [VEGAS-2]) of 346 patients (81). This trial randomized patients with angiographically visible thrombus to either rheolytic thrombectomy or urokinase before PTCA or stenting and documented improved procedural success and improved 1-year, major, adverse, cardiac event-free survival in the thrombectomy group. There are some specific complication patterns that may be seen with this device, specifically AV block. Accordingly, in treating a dominant

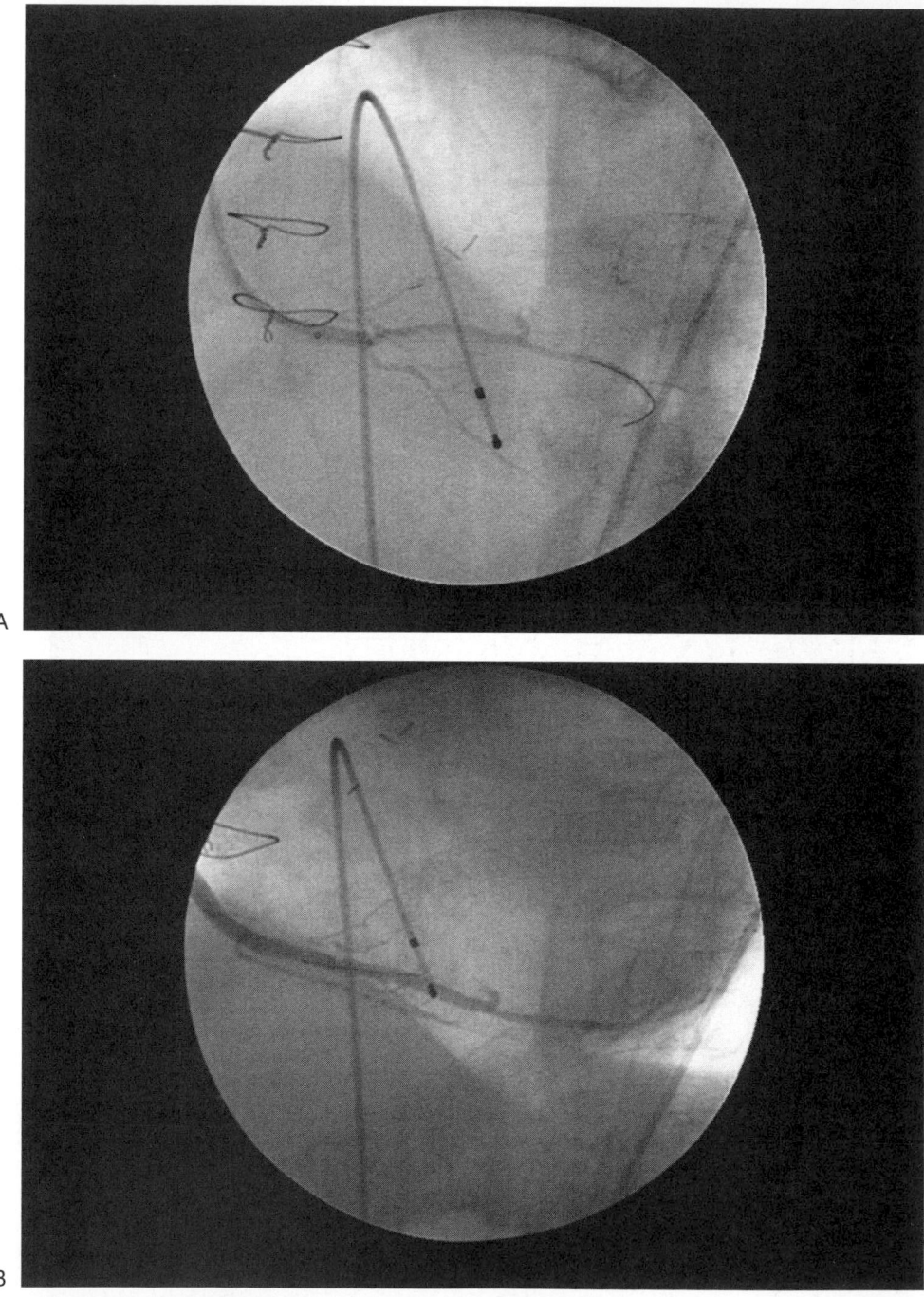

FIG. 92–8. Left anterior oblique view of distal right coronary artery. **A:** A large filling defect is present before rheolytic thrombectomy **(B).** After rheolytic thrombectomy, there has been resolution with full flow although a branch remains occluded.

right coronary artery or a left dominant circumflex coronary artery, a temporary pacemaker should be placed. For the treatment of left anterior descending distribution lesions, not all patients will require a temporary pacemaker; instead, a venous sheath may be placed prophylactically. Currently, this device is helpful in treating thrombotic lesions in either the native coronary arteries or vein grafts (Fig. 92–8).

The other device currently being tested is the X sizer (ev3, Plymouth, MN) (84), which acts on the principle of the Archimedes screw. The Endicor X sizer catheter system is designed for selective removal of thrombus and occlusion tissue. The inner lumen of the catheter contains a hollow torque cable that houses a helical cutter at the tip. It has been tested in both native coronary vessels and vein graft disease. In an initial pilot study of 50 patients (85), acute technical success rate was 86% and preexisting thrombus was effectively removed. This device has been tested in an 800-patient multicenter trial (84) of target lesions in a native coronary artery with definite or presumed thrombus or a saphenous vein graft. The primary end points included 30-day major adverse cardiac event (cardiac death, MI, target vessel revascularization). The 30-day major adverse cardiac event rate was similar in both groups— 17% of the X-sizer group and 17.4% of the control group. Although Q-wave MI occurred with a similar incidence in both groups, a large MI was less frequent in the X-sizer group.

SINGLE-VESSEL DISEASE

PCI is the treatment of choice for patients with single-vessel disease who require revascularization. In these patients, the primary goals of therapy are to improve symptoms or reduce ischemia. In patients with single-vessel disease and well preserved left ventricular function, there are no data to suggest that any type of revascularization will improve longevity. In those patients with acute coronary syndromes and single-vessel disease, PCI may be used to prevent infarction or reinfarction or minimize any ongoing ischemic insult.

The importance of lesion complexity in patients with single-vessel disease is currently less critical than previously because of the widespread use of stent implantation. There are still occasional circumstances in which patients with single-vessel disease with ischemia who require revascularization may be considered for surgical as compared with PCI revascularization, including. (a) projected inability to deliver a stent; (b) involvement of a major bifurcation lesion such as a large diagonal branch that cannot be treated percutaneously because of local arterial geometry or anatomy; (c) absolute contraindication to any antiplatelet therapy that would preclude placement of a stent. An additional group of patients that may be considered for surgical revascularization are those in whom stent placement could be predicted to have an increased likelihood of compromising a major side branch. The typical example of this situation would include an isolated *ostial* left anterior descending lesion (Fig. 92–9), which if treated percutaneously would result in an increased chance of compromising the ostium of the circumflex. In this particular setting, a left internal thoracic artery bypass surgical approach may be preferred. In addition, in this particular setting, with a percutaneous approach, restenosis rates have been found to be increased. A final group of pa-

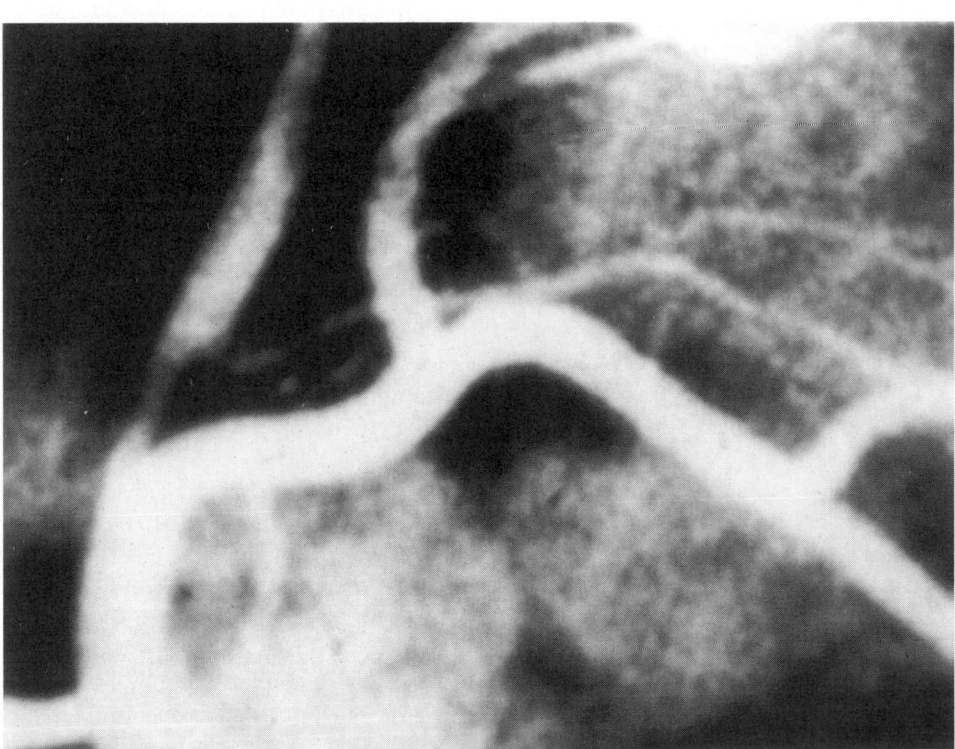

FIG. 92–9. Right anterior oblique view of the left coronary artery. There is an ostial left anterior descending stenosis. Treatment of this may result in compromise of the circumflex.

TABLE 92–1. *Six-month major adverse cardiac events*

MACE	Stent group (n = 108)	Surgical group (n = 108)	*p* Value	RR (95% CI)
Cardiac death	0	2 (2%)	0.99	
Acute infarction	3 (3%)	5 (5%)	0.68	1.77 (0.41–7.58)
<30 days	2 (2%)	4 (4%)		
30–180 days	1 (1%)	1 (1%)		
Acute infarction or cardiac death	3 (3%)	7 (6%)	0.50	2.33 (0.34–43.73)
Target vessel revascularization	31 (29%)	9 (8%)	0.003	0.29 (0.09–0.65)
<30 days	2 (2%)	4 (4%)		
30–180 days	29 (27%)	5 (5%)		
Any MACE	34 (31%)	16 (15%)	0.02	0.47 (0.21–0.89)

CI, confidence interval; MACE, major adverse cardiac event; RR, risk ratio.

tients might be those in the small group who have had recurrent instent restenosis even after subsequent treatment with vascular brachytherapy.

A randomized comparison of stenting versus minimally invasive bypass surgery for stenosis of the left anterior descending coronary artery has been reported (86). In this study, 220 symptomatic patients with high-grade lesions in the proximal left anterior descending (proximal to the first major septal branch) were randomized to surgery (n = 110) or stenting (n = 110). The primary end point for this trial was the combined end point of freedom from major adverse cardiac events including death from cardiac causes, MI, and the need for repeat revascularization of the target lesion within 6 months. Ejection fraction was well preserved at approximately 63%, although 45% of patients had a prior MI. Secondary end points of the trial included composite end point of clinical status and need for antianginal drugs at 6 months. This study was carried out between 1997 and 2001 and represents a reasonably concurrent practice. Stenting was successful in all patients and there were no complications. On average, 1.2 stents were implanted, and the mean stent length was 15.1 mm. There were two episodes of stent thrombosis that resulted in acute MI. Both of these were treated with a catheter-based approach. In the surgical group, minimally invasive surgery was successfully performed in 95% of the patients; however, in five patients, conversion to a full sternotomy was necessary. Three patients underwent reoperation during hospitalization for the first surgery because of anastomotic stenoses or occlusion; two of these patients had a perioperative MI. Two additional patients also had a perioperative MI, and one patient had an ischemic stroke 5 days after a procedure. The major adverse cardiac events during 6 months of follow-up can be seen in Table 92–1. As can be seen, there was no difference in death from cardiac causes, acute MI, or a combined end point of MI or death from cardiac causes. Despite the use of stents, revascularization of the target vessel was required from 1 to 6 months in 27% of the stent group and only 5% in the surgical group. Any major adverse cardiac event rate also was more frequent in the stent group at 31% versus 15% in the surgical group, again driven by the need for repeat revascularization.

The authors concluded that stenting resulted in excellent short-term outcome with fewer periprocedural adverse events, but surgery was superior with regard to the need for repeated intervention and also freedom from angina at 6 months. It is anticipated that drug-coated stents (*vide infra*) will dramatically affect the practice particularly in these high-risk patients.

PERCUTANEOUS CORONARY INTERVENTION VERSUS MEDICAL THERAPY

In many centers, PCI also is offered as an alternative to medical therapy. There are relatively limited controlled data on this approach. In addition, it is limited by that medical therapy has changed dramatically, and even more importantly, that medical therapy should be used in all patients with coronary artery disease, particularly a statin, an angiotensin-converting enzyme (ACE) inhibitor, aspirin, and a β-blocker. Many of the randomized trials of PCI versus medical therapy included patients with multivessel disease. A recent metaanalysis (87) has been performed which included six randomized controlled trials, three of which included patients with multivessel disease. A total of 1,904 patients were included in this analysis. In these trials, stent implantation was infrequent. Also, these patients included relatively stable patients in whom the ejection fraction was well preserved and the majority of whom had stable angina. Success rates for PCI ranged from 80% to 100% with the earlier series having lower success rates. Complication rates varied; periprocedural infarction ranged from 0.01% to 2.8% and emergency CABG surgery from 1.5% to 2.8%. The mean follow-up ranged from 6 to 57 months. The pooled risk ratios of different events can be seen in Figure 92–10 (87). There was no significant difference in death or the combined end point of death and MI. Patients treated with initial PTCA required more frequent subsequent surgical procedures; however, patients treated with PTCA had less angina. This metaanalysis illustrates some important points: (a) in patients with stable angina, PCI will not reduce the already low incidence of death alone or death and MI; (b) angina relief is better with PCI than medical therapy; (c) PCI may result in

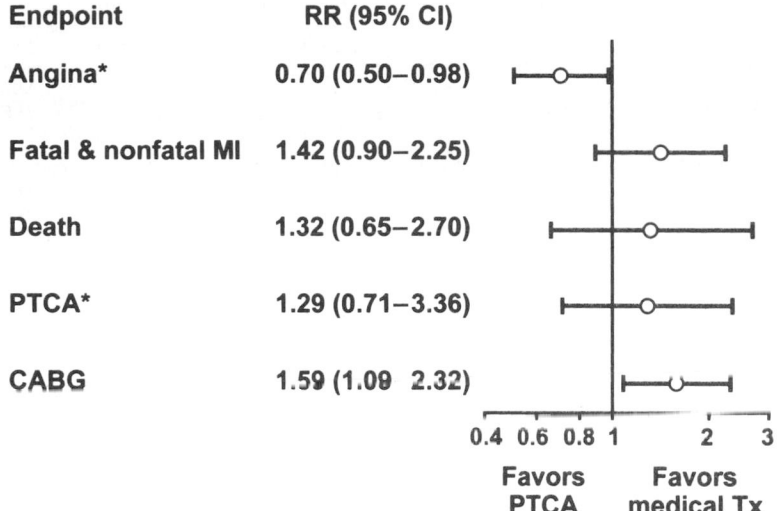

Endpoint	RR (95% CI)
Angina*	0.70 (0.50–0.98)
Fatal & nonfatal MI	1.42 (0.90–2.25)
Death	1.32 (0.65–2.70)
PTCA*	1.29 (0.71–3.36)
CABG	1.59 (1.09 2.32)

Favors PTCA   Favors medical Tx

FIG. 92–10. Pooled risk ratios. *Test of heterogeneity: $p < 0.001$. CABG, coronary artery bypass graft; CI, confidence interval; MI, myocardial infarction; PTCA, percutaneous transluminal coronary angiography; RR, relative risk; Tx, treatment. (From Bucher HC, Hengstler P, Schindler C, et al. Percutaneous transluminal coronary angioplasty versus medical treatment for non acute coronary heart disease: meta-analysis of randomized controlled trials. *BMJ* 2000;321:73–77, with permission.)

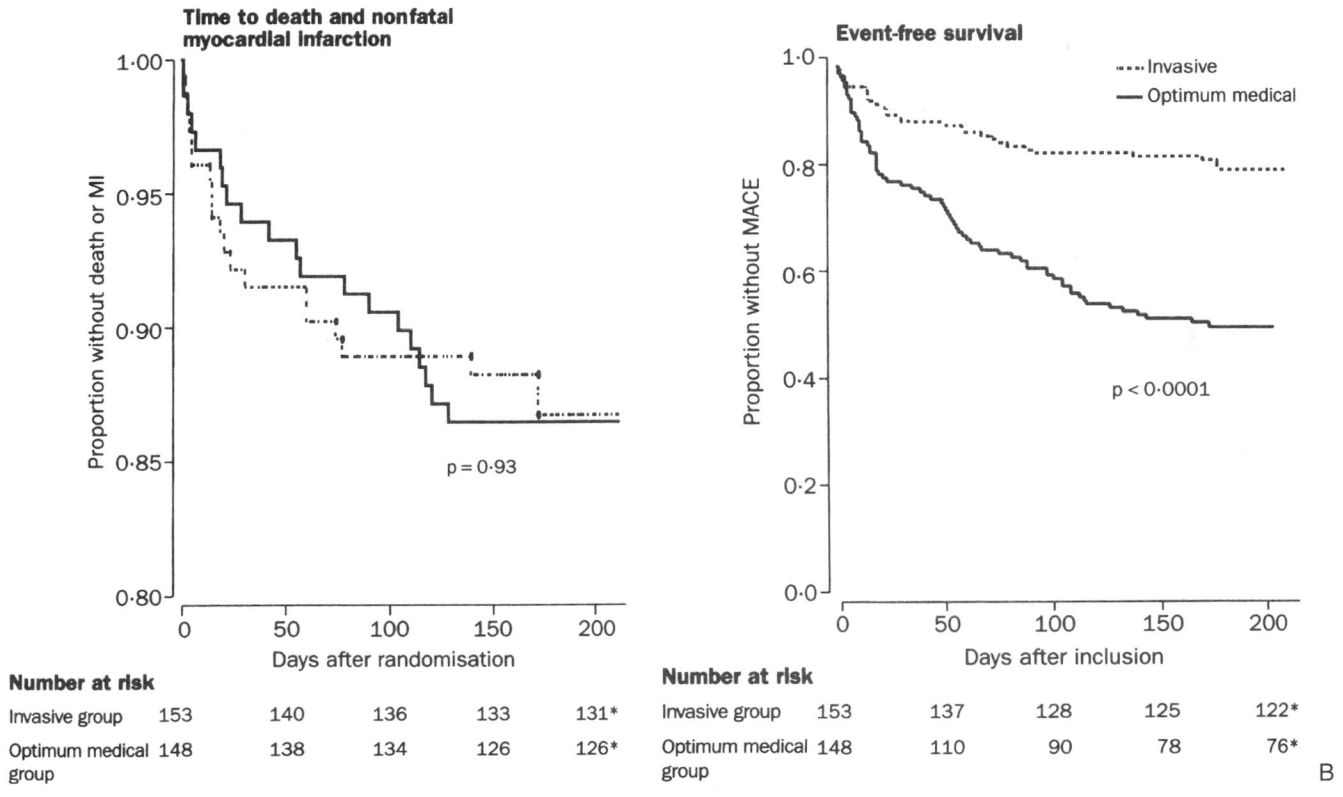

FIG. 92–11. A: Freedom from death or myocardial infarction in the TIME trial (89). **B:** Freedom from major adverse cardiac event (MACE). MI, myocardial infarction. (From The TIME Investigators. Trial of invasive versus medical therapy in elderly patients with chronic symptomatic coronary artery disease (TIME): a randomized trial. *Lancet* 2001;358:951–957, with permission.)

the need for more subsequent procedures because of restenosis.

An additional trial has been subsequently reported in 303 patients aged 75 years or older (88). These patients had more severe symptoms, with angina pectoris, Canadian Cardiovascular Society Class 2 or greater, and were treated with two or more antianginal drugs. Patients were randomized to either PCI or to a conservative approach. The primary end points were quality of life after 6 months including major adverse cardiac events (death, MI, and admission for acute coronary syndromes). There was no difference in death or nonfatal MI (Fig. 92–11); but again in those patients treated by an invasive strategy, the angina severity, quality of life, and need for repeat hospitalizations for acute coronary syndromes were improved in the invasive strategy group compared with the group treated with more intensive medical therapy.

NEW TECHNOLOGY OPPORTUNITIES

The development of these new devices and continued development of balloon technology will continue to allow more lesions and more patients to be treated with percutaneous interventions. A prominent thrust will be the integration of new technology and balloons to optimize the initial result. Intravascular ultrasound is being evaluated as a potential means to match the specific lesion with the optimal device for that lesion. Randomized trials are currently being performed to test the effect of this match on outcome. Currently, broad groups of lesions can be matched with specific technical approaches.

Specific lesion subsets remain problematic (Tables 92–2 and 92–3). Chronic total occlusions often remain unsuitable for treatment with percutaneous techniques (Fig. 92–12). The presence of a chronic total occlusion in a patient with viable myocardium is still the most common reason to choose coronary surgery in preference to PCI. Although large series of chronic total occlusions have been reported, these are in selected patients. Patients with unfavorable anatomy often are not even offered interventional proce-

TABLE 92–2. *Lesion characteristics that can affect procedural outcome*

Decreased success rates
    Chronic coronary occlusion
    Branch lesions
    Ostial lesions
    Severe calcification

Increased incidence of complications
    Preexisting thrombus
    Diffuse disease
    Severe lesion angulation
    Lesion eccentricity
    Lesion calcification
    Friable vein graft disease
    Tandem lesions

dures. Even in those selected series that have been reported, success rates of 60% to 70% are common (89–98). New technology as yet has not been a great help. Excimer laser was used in the past; unfortunately, it required crossing the chronic total occlusion with a guidewire that is in itself the most difficult part of the procedure. A whole new series of guidewires of variable stiffness has been developed, some of which are hydrophilic, which can be used to penetrate and make a small pilot channel. More recently, two new devices have been tested. The first involves blunt dissection with a reverse bioptome action to gain access to the distal vessels. The other device involves the use of optical coherence reflectometry, which allows interrogation of the chronic total occlusion in an attempt to differentiate plaque from more normal arterial wall. Once that differentiation is made, more forceful probing may be effective in crossing the occlusion. If these systems are found to be effective, they would greatly increase the number of patients who could benefit from a percutaneous approach.

Long diffuse disease also remains a problem (Fig. 92–13). These lesions often are calcified. Although PTCA can be performed with long balloons, the results are sometimes suboptimal; unfortunately, this is unpredictable. If there is a large distal vascular bed, then rotational atherectomy can be helpful, although distal embolization and noreflow is a problem; laser may also be used, although the incidence of dissection continues to be increased compared with cohorts of patients treated with PTCA. After conventional PTCA, stent deployment should be considered. If the lesion is calcified, it may not be improved with stent placement. Other problems include (a) that stent length and number of stents placed are both variable and associated with increased subacute closure; (b) stent length is directly related to the development of subsequent restenosis; (c) longer lesions more often involve side branches, which may be compromised resulting in periprocedural enzyme elevation; and (d) that if the stent is too long, it may prevent performance of subsequent surgical revascularization of that vessel. This is particularly true for the left anterior descending. If too long a stent is placed, it may compromise the ability of cardiovascular surgery to place a left internal mammary artery graft in the future if it becomes necessary.

A third lesion that remains problematic is one that is occluded and contains thrombus (Fig. 92–14) (99–105). These lesions were initially identified as having a strikingly increased risk for acute closure with conventional PTCA. With improvements in technique and equipment, the risk of treating these lesions appears to have decreased. However, Reeder and coworkers (104) evaluated whether thrombus remains a risk factor for angioplasty failure by analyzing outcome of procedures in three time periods from 1984 to 1991. In this analysis, they found that of all clinical and angiographic factors, only three were independently associated with angioplasty failure: coronary thrombus, history of congestive heart failure, and multivessel disease. Over the entire 7-year period, multivariate analysis documented that the ef-

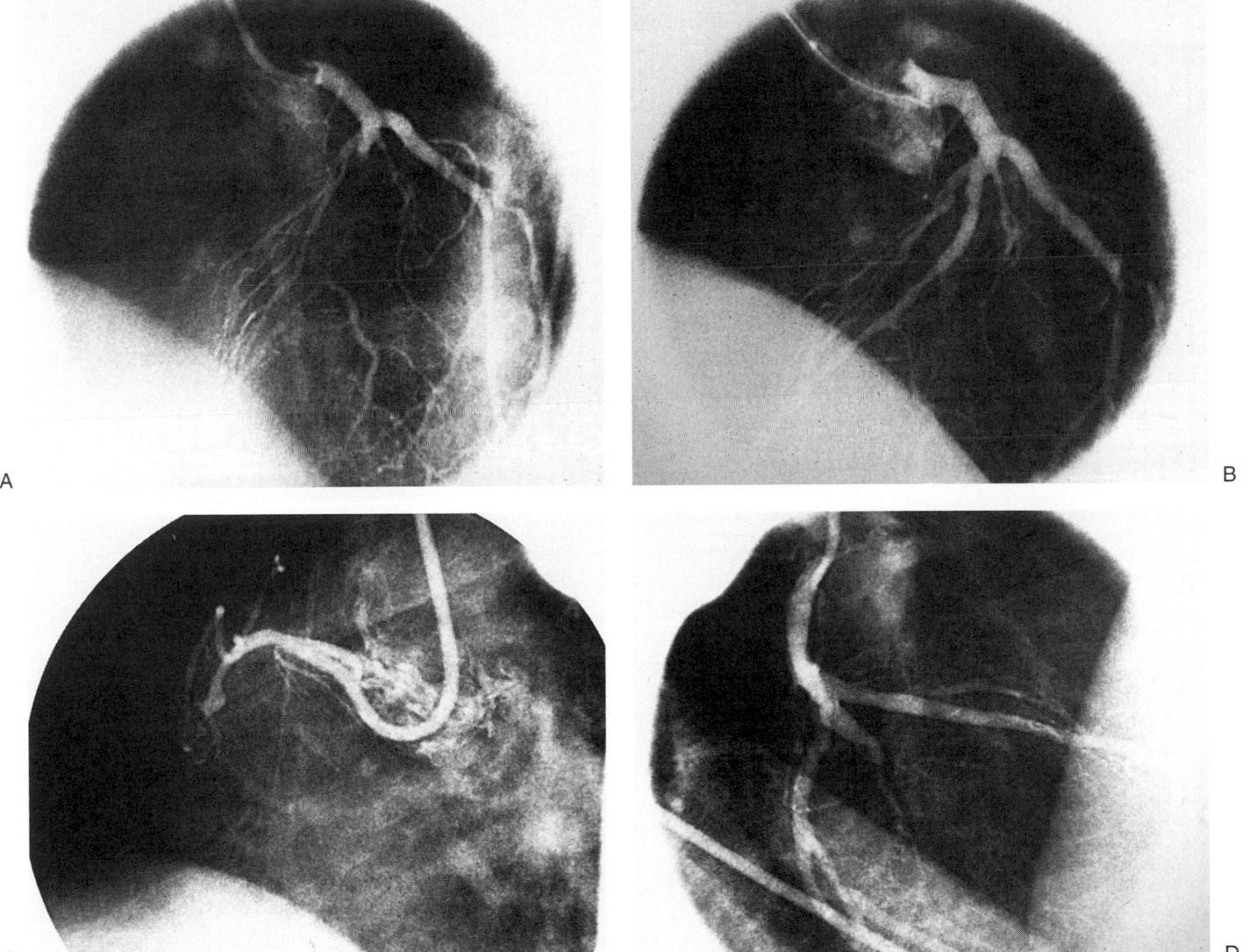

FIG. 92–12. A, B: Left anterior oblique view of occluded left coronary artery with features to suggest good potential success rate including tapered tip, straight vessel course, and visualization of the distal vessel, before and after percutaneous transluminal coronary angiography. **C:** Left anterior oblique view of right coronary artery with an occluded segment with adverse features, most prominently adventitial collaterals. Adverse lesion morphology in a left coronary branch occlusion. At the site of occlusion is a large side branch **(D).**

fect of thrombus on angioplasty failure had not changed in magnitude. Singh and coworkers (106) reviewed a data set from 6 prospective randomized trials including 7,917 patients. Angiographic evidence of thrombus was seen in 2,752 patients (35%). Although inhospital mortality rates were low in groups with (0.8%) and without thrombus (0.6%), several adverse outcomes were greater in patients with thrombus. These included death, MI (8.4% vs. 5.5%; $p < 0.001$), abrupt closure (5.9% vs. 3.9%; $p \leq 0.001$), and the inhospital composite of death, MI, and a repeat revascularization (15.4% vs. 11.2%; $p \leq 0.001$). The introduction and widespread use of new antithrombotic and antiplatelet drugs such as bivalirudin and IIb/IIIa receptor blockers may potentially improve outcome in these patients.

A fourth problematic lesion is the hard calcific plaque that opens inadequately or not at all with balloons. Rotablator has

a unique role to play in these lesions because it preferentially ablates hard unyielding tissue. Rotablator may also, by debulking the lesion, result in a lower acute dissection rate in such lesions. The cutting balloon also has been useful in this setting. This balloon has stainless steel microtome blades on the surface of the balloon. Inflation of the balloon presses these blades against the atherosclerotic plaque at the restenotic lesion. It has the advantage that balloon movement is minimal, and it can create predefined stress lines in the plaque so that subsequent inflation and stent deployment are more optional. They do have the disadvantage of relative inflexibility and inability to deliver the device in tortuous vessels. These devices have been studied in registry experiences and in small randomized trials. A randomized trial (107) enrolled 1,238 patients—617 to cutting balloon and 621 to PTCA. The primary end point was angiographic restenosis

TABLE 92–3. *Characteristics of type A, B, and C lesions influencing successful percutaneous transluminal coronary angioplasty*

Type A lesions (high success; low risk)
    Discrete (<10 mm in length)   Little or no calcification
    Concentric   Less than totally occlusive
    Readily accessible   Not ostial in location
    Nonangulated segment (<45 degrees)   No major branch involvement
    Smooth contour   Absence of thrombus
Type B lesions (moderate success; moderate risk)[a]
    Tubular (10–20 mm in length)   Moderate to heavy calcification
    Eccentric   Total occlusion <3 mo old
    Moderate tortuosity of proximal segment   Ostial location
    Moderately angulated segment (>45 degrees but <90 degrees)   Bifurcation lesions requiring double guidewires
    Irregular contour   Some thrombus present
        B_1 lesions, one characteristic
        B_2 lesions, one characteristic
Type C lesions (low success; high risk)
    Diffuse (>20 mm in length)   Total occlusion >3 mo old
    Excessive tortuosity of proximal segment   Inability to protect major side branches
    Extremely angulated segments (>90 degrees)   Degenerated vein grafts with friable lesions

[a]Although the risk for abrupt vessel closure is moderate, in certain instances the likelihood of a major complication may be low, such as in dilation to total occlusions less than 3 months old or when abundant collateral channels supply the distal vessel.

and was 31.4% for cutting balloon and 30.4% for PTCA ($p = 0.75$). The authors concluded that cutting balloon should be reserved for difficult lesions in which the results with PTCA could be predicted to be suboptimal. These might include ostial lesions, focal fibrocalcific lesions, and instent restenosis.

A final group of lesions that remain very problematic are diffuse vein graft stenoses (77–80,108–115). The treatment of vein graft disease is associated with poor initial results, a high chance of distal embolism, and the long-term effect of high restenosis rates and increased mortality. This is particularly true if the vein graft is occluded (Fig. 92–14). Previously used strategies of transluminal extraction atherectomy catheter (TEC) laser, and prolonged urokinase infusions have been abandoned. As previously mentioned, distal protection devices and rheolytic thrombectomy have been documented in multicenter randomized clinical trials to result in

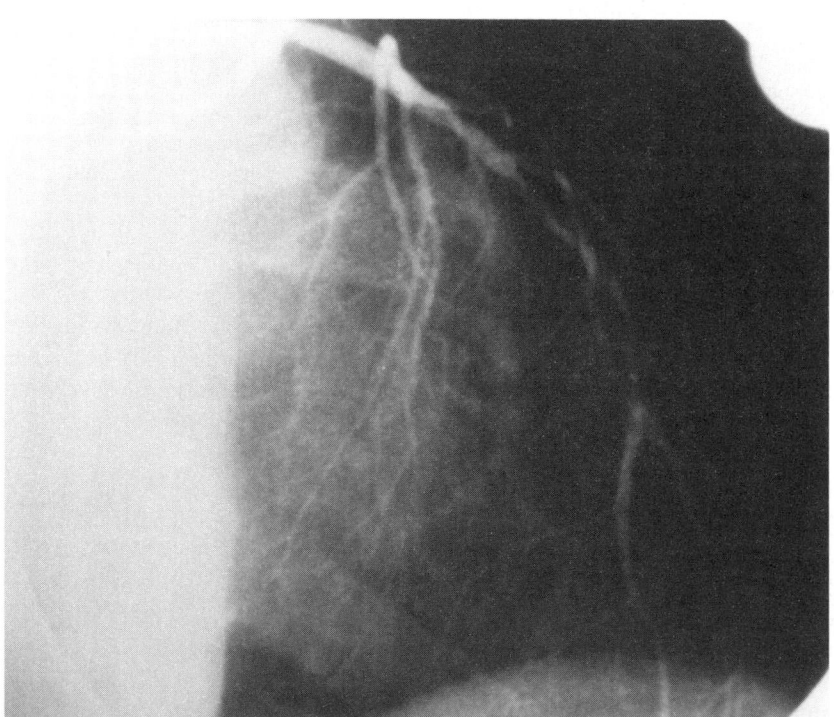

FIG. 92–13. Right anterior oblique cranial view of the left coronary artery documenting a long diffuse severe stenosis in the mid left anterior descending artery.

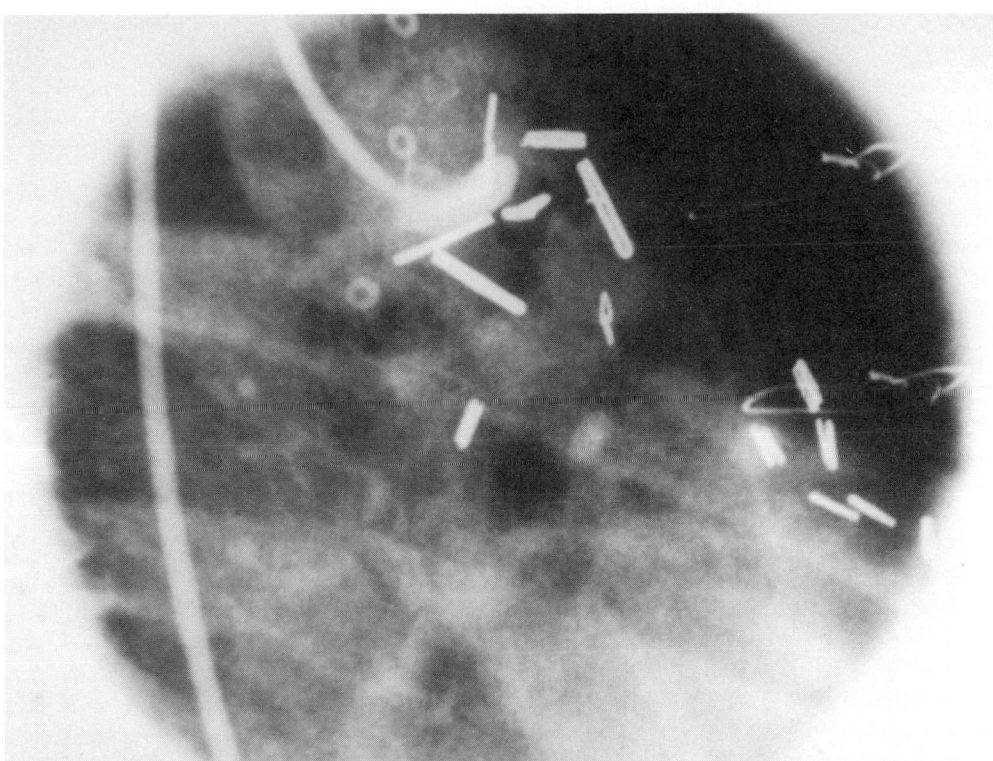

FIG. 92–14. Right anterior oblique of an occluded vein graft.

improved outcome compared with conventional treatment (77). A controversial area has been the need for adjunctive therapy with a IIb/IIIa agent (116–118). Available data would indicate that these agents do not improve outcome in these patients at high risk; this probably relates to the atheroembolic debris that is not affected by IIb/IIIa receptor blockage. Covered stents may be helpful in this regard to prevent distal embolization and are currently being tested in registries and randomized clinical trials.

MULTIVESSEL DISEASE

Application of PCI in multivessel disease has been the major reason for the striking increase in the number of procedures (119–125). It is used as an alternative to either medical therapy or surgical revascularization.

There are multiple important issues in evaluation of dilatation for multivessel disease. The risk/benefit ratio of each lesion must be evaluated. This must be considered in light of the concept of completeness of revascularization. This concept was initially developed in surgical series in which patients with a graft placed to each ischemic bed or territory had improved outcome compared with patients in whom some lesions were not grafted. This concept has important implications for dilatation practice. The frequency with which complete revascularization can be achieved depends in part on the number of diseased vessels (126,127). In patients with three-vessel disease, the ability to achieve complete revascularization with PTCA is less than with two-

vessel disease. Inability to achieve complete revascularization has been studied in the most recent NHLBI PTCA Registry. Bourassa and coworkers (126) noted that complete revascularization was achieved in only 19% of patients (Table 92–4). In this series, the presence of lesions not amenable to PTCA, including an undilatable chronic total occlusion, was the reason for inability to completely revascularize 24% of patients. More frequently, the operator identified lesions that could be dilated but were not attempted as the most frequent cause for not achieving complete revascularization. This was seen in 42% of patients. Such a strategy is the result of attempts to identify the angina-producing or culprit lesion and has the advantage that the risk for dilating angiographically significant but functionally unimportant lesions can be avoided. Identification of the "culprit" lesion is sometimes easy and straightforward, based either on the re-

TABLE 92–4. *National Heart, Lung and Blood Institute Percutaneous Transluminal Coronary Angiography Registry 1985–1986: dilatation strategy*

	Percentage
All lesions amenable and intended but not all attempted	6
All lesions amenable, intended, and attempted—not all successful	9
Complete revascularization	19
Not all lesions amenable	24
All lesions amenable, but not all intended	42

sults of angiography, the results of functional testing, or a combination. More often, however, it is difficult.

The importance of complete revascularization is still the subject of considerable debate (127–132). Intuitively, it makes sense that fewer severe residual stenoses should translate into an improved outcome. However, not all studies have documented this. Some reports have indicated that patients in whom complete revascularization cannot be achieved have more adverse baseline characteristics—for example, more diffuse disease or more chronic total occlusions—so they will not have as optimal an outcome for that reason alone. It appears that there is a significant interrelation, however, among left ventricular function, anginal severity, and number of diseased vessels. In patients with left ventricular dysfunction, unstable angina, and three-vessel disease, it is more important to achieve complete revascularization to optimize the long-term outcome. This has important implications for patients with one or more chronic total occlusions that cannot be dilated.

Since the Bypass Angioplasty Revascularization Investigation (BARI) and other trials have documented increased mortality in patients with diabetes at 5 to 7 years in the angioplasty group, there has been a concerted effort to provide more complete revascularization by PCI or CABG (133–135). The ongoing BARI 2D trial compares patients treated with revascularization or medical therapy only. Because of the ability to choose PCI or surgery, complete revascularization can be offered in that trial. Among the first 293 patients randomized to revascularization, 92 had CABG and 201 had PCI. PCI was chosen for 34% with one-vessel disease, 35% with two-vessel disease, 29% with three-vessel disease, and CABG was chosen for 5% with one-vessel disease, 23% with two-vessel disease, and 72% with three-vessel disease. Although revascularization by strict criteria of including every vessel was 97% with CABG and 58% with PCI, a definition of functionally complete revascularization that included all major branches was achieved in 100% of patients with CABG and 89% of patients with PCI (K. M. Detre, Pittsburgh School of Public Health BARI Data Coordinating Center, Pittsburgh, PA).

The goal of achieving complete revascularization must be balanced by the risks for dilating multiple lesions. In general, the most important functional lesion should be treated first. If that is not successful, then other lesions should not be approached. A potential exception to this is the patient with a chronic total occlusion that supplies collaterals to the target lesion. This chronic total occlusion may be attempted first to improve the safety of dilating the target lesion. Resource consumption must be kept in mind in approaching these chronic total occlusions. The amount of contrast used is not inconsequential; in a patient with abnormal renal function, treatment of the nonessential chronic total occlusion may use enough contrast to increase the potential for renal toxicity even before the true target lesion is approached.

The risk for dilating multiple lesions during the same procedure is difficult to quantitate. In the PTCA Registry of 1985–1986, dilatation was successful in 86% of patients with two-vessel disease and 88% of patients with three-vessel disease. Mortality rates increased as the number of vessels diseased increased: 0.2% in single-vessel disease, 0.9% in two-vessel disease, and 2.8% in three-vessel disease. The concern has been that if a complication occurs during dilatation of a second lesion that results in hypotension, the first lesion also will occlude. This has been less a problem since stenting became the primary intervention. However, when excess contrast media has been used or the patient becomes unstable, it may be preferable to stage subsequent lesions.

An important consideration in multivessel disease in addition to lesion type is left ventricular function. Patients with depressed left ventricular function may tolerate complications of the procedure less well than patients with normal left ventricular function. This has been assessed in multiple series (136–139). The risks of treating patients with decreased left ventricular function do appear to be increased, but not prohibitively so. The most important consideration is the long-term follow-up of these patients. Event-free survival continues to be affected adversely in these patients. The need to achieve complete revascularization may be of more importance in this group.

ANGIOPLASTY VERSUS SURGERY FOR MULTIVESSEL DISEASE

There have been multiple observational studies of angioplasty that have been compared with surgical series (Fig. 92–15) (140–143). In general, in these series, patients treated with angioplasty had more two-vessel disease and better left ventricular function compared with surgical patients, who had more three-vessel disease and worse left ventricular function. The observational trials showed that the risks of the procedure in terms of mortality and procedural infarction were similar, but initial hospitalization was shorter with PTCA. During follow-up, mortality and infarction rates also were similar, but because of restenosis, patients undergoing PTCA had an increased need for repeat revascularization procedures compared with patients initially treated surgically. Given the competing nature of these two strategies in patient care, in the latter part of the 1980s, randomized trials were initiated.

Two trials, sponsored by the NHLBI, were performed in the United States. The first was the Emory Angioplasty vs. Surgery Trial (EAST). The primary composite end point at 3 years was not different, but repeat revascularization was much more common in the angioplasty group. A completed 8-year follow-up showed 82.7% survival in the surgery group and 79.3% survival in the PTCA group, which was not different (134). The larger BARI was the first trial to show a difference between the treated patients with and without diabetes. Among patients without diabetes fol-

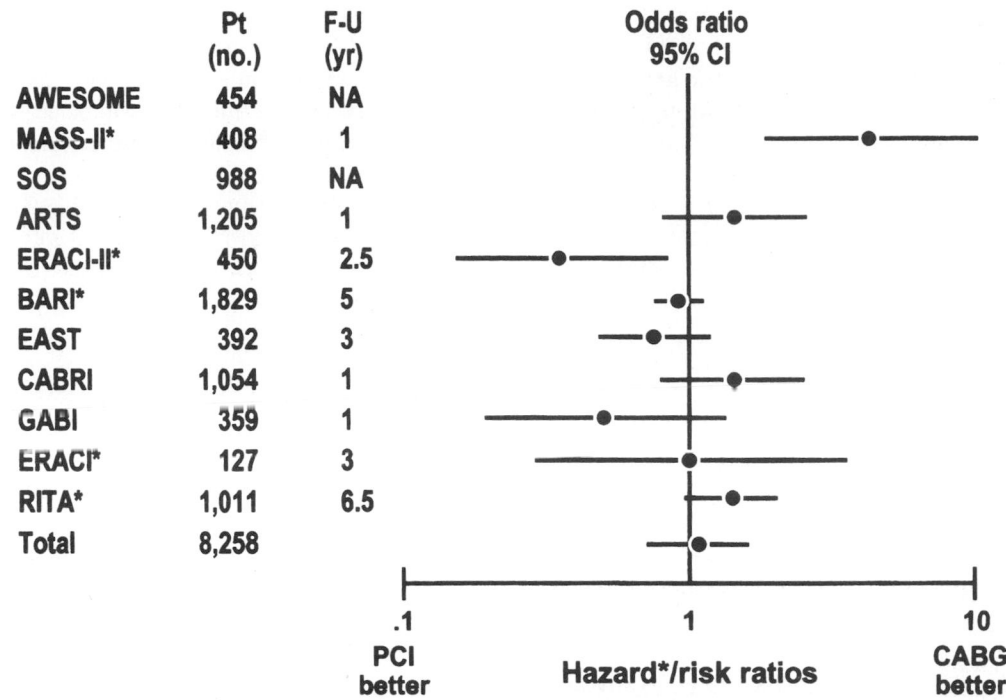

	Pt (no.)	F-U (yr)
AWESOME	454	NA
MASS-II*	408	1
SOS	988	NA
ARTS	1,205	1
ERACI-II*	450	2.5
BARI*	1,829	5
EAST	392	3
CABRI	1,054	1
GABI	359	1
ERACI*	127	3
RITA*	1,011	6.5
Total	8,258	

FIG. 92–15. Odds ratio for outcome of surgery in percutaneous coronary intervention (PCI). ARTS, Arterial Revascularization Therapy Study; AWESOME, Angina With Extremely Serious Operative Mortality Evaluation; BARI, Bypass Angioplasty Revascularization Investigation; CABG, coronary artery bypass graft; CABRI, Coronary Angioplasty Versus Bypass Revascularization Investigation; CI, confidence interval; EAST, Emory Angioplasty vs. Surgery Trial; ERACI, Coronary Angioplasty with Stenting Versus Coronary Bypass Surgery in Patients with Multiple-Vessel Disease; GABI, German Angioplasty Bypass Surgery Investigation; MASS, Medicine-Antibody-Surgery Study; RITA, Randomized Intervention Treatment of Angina; SOS, Stent or Surgery. (From Holmes D, Berger P. Complex intervention. In: Topol EJ, ed. *Textbook of interventional cardiology*, 4th ed. 2003:201–222, with permission.)

lowed to 7 years, the survival rate was almost identical at 86.5%. The patients with diabetes, however, fared much better with surgery with a survival rate of 76.4% compared with 55.7% in the angioplasty group. These patients with diabetes have become the focus of newly initiated trials (133). Despite that poor outcome in the randomized diabetic cohort undergoing PTCA, the registry patients in BARI who underwent PTCA had a better outcome (144). These two techniques also have been studied in the context of multiple randomized trials (145–148). A meta-analysis of randomized trials comparing PTCA and CABG and including Randomized Intervention Treatment of Angina (RITA), Coronary Angioplasty Versus Bypass Revascularization Investigation (CABRI), German Angioplasty Bypass surgery Investigation, Coronary Angioplasty with Stenting Versus Coronary Bypass Surgery in Patients with Multiple-Vessel Disease (ERACI), and Medicine-Antibody-Surgery Study (MASS), as well as EAST and BARI, reported no difference in mortality or MI at 1 year but close to 30% to 40% of patients treated with conventional PTCA required an additional procedure, be it surgery or angioplasty, within that first year; in those patients treated with stent implantation, the risk difference was reduced to 15% at 1 and 3 years (148).

Speculation as to why overall survival was similar but the diabetic populations did better with bypass surgery have included greater restenosis rates, more progression of disease, and greater noncardiac mortality in the patients with diabetes.

With the advent of stenting, two trials were initiated in Europe to compare angioplasty and bypass surgery. These are the Arterial Revascularization Therapy Study (ARTS) trial and the Stent or Surgery (SOS) trial. ARTS has reported 1-year follow-up (149). That trial of 1,205 patients with multivessel disease required that lesions be suitable for stenting for bypass surgery. Bypass grafting resulted in 2.7 grafts per patient, and there were 2.7 stents placed per patient. The results at 1 year showed no difference in mortality or MI (stent 7.8% and surgery 6.8%). The need for additional surgery or angioplasty was approximately one half of that seen in the previous balloon angioplasty trials. The much watched diabetic population had a lower mortality than seen in the previous BARI trial but still favored surgery with a stenting mortality rate at 1 year of 6.4% and a surgical mortality rate of 3.1%.

The SOS trial (150) enrolled 998 patients with multivessel disease with a strategy of applying stenting or bypass surgery. Once again in this trial, the repeat interventions were reduced by use of stenting with 20.7% of patients in the PCI group requiring additional revascularization compared with 6% of the surgery group. Death or Q-wave MI was similar at 9.4% in the PCI group and 9.8% in the CABG group. Mortality with surgery was exceptionally good with a 1-year mortality rate of 1.6% compared with 4.5% in the PCI group.

The NHLBI Dynamic Registry is another source for understanding recent practice results with stenting compared with older randomized balloon angioplasty trials. Patients with characteristics similar to the BARI patients treated in 1997 to 1999 had similar survival rates at approximately 95%, but the requirement for repeat intervention at 1 year was reduced from approximately 40% in the BARI trial to less than 20% in the current NHLBI registry.

A smaller study, ERACI-II (151), carried out in Argentina randomized 450 patients to stenting or surgery. The surgical mortality rate in this trial was greater at 5.7%, and the survival rate at 18 months was 92.5% in the surgery group compared with 96.9% in the PCI group. Subsequent revascularization was performed in 16.8% of the PCI patients versus 4.8% of the surgical group.

In summary, therefore, the newer stent trials seem to show somewhat better overall survival than the earlier studies using balloon angioplasty but also better survival in the surgical cohort. The major difference in the stent trials is a reduction in the need for repeat intervention by approximately one half compared with previous trials that included only conventional balloon angioplasty.

The next development in interventional cardiology, namely the stents that elute antirestenotic drugs, will be tested against surgery as well. This will be carried out in the diabetic population in the Future Revascularization Evaluation on Patients with Diabetes Mellitus: Optimal Management of Multivessel Disease (FREEDOM) study, which is supported by the NHLBI but which has not yet begun enrolling patients. It would be expected that this approach should reduce further the reintervention rate, and as followup continues, it will be important to understand whether this will narrow the gap in survival between the patients with diabetes having surgery and those undergoing percutaneous intervention. It must be remembered that much of the mortality in this diabetic population is likely because of progression of disease and noncardiac causes that will not be influenced by improvements in stenting alone.

Recognition of the progressive nature of multivessel disease in patients with diabetes has led to the initiation of two trials to test patients who are less severely symptomatic and to understand whether intervention is effective in prolonging survival. These trials use recently recognized measures to improve survival of both patients with and without diabetes, such as tight blood pressure control, increased lipid management, vigorous control of hyperglycemia, and liberal use of β-blockers, ACE inhibitors, and antithrombotic drugs. These studies are Clinical Outcomes Utilizing Revascularization and Aggressive Drug Evaluation (COURAGE), which is a trial that will contain approximately 30% patients with dia-

betes and the BARI 2D trial, which will be composed entirely of patients with diabetes. These trials will go a long way toward establishing whether the most modern percutaneous interventional methods combined with well established secondary prevention measures can be superior to this excellent medical therapy alone.

It is difficult to select care for individual patients based on protocols. Patient and physician expectations must be kept in mind. For some patients, the primary concern is symptom relief without undergoing CABG, whereas in other patients, the primary concern is to avoid repeat procedures. Selection of the treatment for these two groups of patients will be quite different even if their anatomy is very similar.

Of patients who were eligible for randomization in the BARI trial at Mayo Clinic but declined to be randomized, approximately 50% chose PTCA and 50% chose surgery. The most common reason for choosing PTCA was to avoid the need for initial thoracotomy, whereas the most common reason for choosing CABG was to avoid the need for repeat procedures to treat restenosis. As mentioned earlier, a solution to the problem of restenosis will have a major impact on revascularization strategy in the future.

The American College of Cardiology and American Heart Association (ACC/AHA) Task Force on new technology assessment has published revised guidelines for PTCA. In this report, new devices and conventional PTCA are considered together (152). These revised guidelines reflect the dominance of coronary stenting in the field of interventional cardiology, both for single-vessel and multivessel disease. Since the 1993 guidelines (153), the definition of success has changed. Improvement in artery diameter so there is less than 50% stenosis has been revised to suggest that a 20% residual stenosis should be the benchmark of success. The improvements in stenting and other devices and adjunctive therapies, such as glycoprotein IIb/IIIa, platelet receptor antagonists, and thienopyridines, are emphasized.

The guidelines discuss optimal features for success with interventional procedures, bypass surgery, or medical therapy and emphasize three special categories—that is, women, the elderly, and individuals with diabetes. The benefit of interventional procedures in women and the older age group seems comparable to other groups. The challenge of managing patients with diabetes with percutaneous techniques remains as alluded to earlier. For symptomatic patients, Class 1 and 2 indications include lesions amenable to angioplasty with a moderate or high chance of success and a low to moderate risk for mortality or morbidity in the setting of angina unresponsive to medical therapy. For patients who are asymptomatic or only mildly symptomatic, more severe ischemia on functional testing or documentation of severe prior ischemia is required, and the lesion or lesions to be treated should have a high likelihood of success and only a low risk for mortality and morbidity.

The practice of interventional cardiology is changing rapidly. There are several areas that will have great impact on the continued role of this approach, such as restenosis, new adjunctive medications, brachytherapy, chronic total occlusions, and device- and lesion-specific therapy.

RESTENOSIS

Restenosis has been documented since the initial days of dilatation (Fig. 92–16) (154–157). It was observed by Gruntzig in 31% of his initial cohort of successful PTCA patients (26,27). The frequency has varied depending on patient subsets studied and definitions used. Although there has been substantial progress in understanding the pathophysiology in animal models, knowledge of the human situation remains somewhat limited (15–21). Although numerous clinical and angiographic factors are known to be associated with the occurrence of restenosis, their predictive value is limited for any one specific patient. The process is complex and ubiquitous, is seen with all new devices, and is in part a response to arterial injury. There are, however, multiple factors involved, including neointimal hyperplasia, vascular remodeling, matrix formation, thrombus formation, and elastic recoil. In any one given patient, it may be difficult to identify the specific cause.

A controversy has developed around the principle that has been widely termed "bigger is better." On the one hand, in animal models, the more arterial damage to the arterial wall, the greater the neointimal hyperplasia (Fig. 92–17); but on the other hand, there was the observation that the most important determinant of restenosis was maximal luminal diameter after treatment. This controversy has been largely resolved by taking into account the differences between neointimal hyperplasia and restenosis. The concept of acute gain, late loss, net gain, and loss index have been widely accepted (7,8,158). In response to arterial damage, there is always neointimal hyperplasia; this occurs with conventional PTCA and with new devices, and the more the damage, the more the hyperplasia. However, the key finding is that the neointimal hyperplasia is well tolerated and does not produce clinical restenosis if the initial acute gain is large enough.

A variety of animal models have been developed in different species, in different arterial beds, and using different stimuli (15,158–161). These models have been used to study the pathophysiology of the phenomena and then to screen strategies for prevention. The most commonly used model in the past to screen preventive strategies is the rat carotid model (162–164). Several approaches have been found to be successful in inhibiting neointimal hyperplasia in this model, for example, ACE inhibitors. However, in the human situation, few have been successful. This may be because of the difference in arterial structure, for example, an elastic versus a muscular artery, the lack of atherosclerosis, or the exuberant smooth muscle cell hyperplasia in the rat, which is not necessarily the dominant problem in patients. None of the other models is ideal. The porcine coronary (16–18) model is perhaps the closest to the human coronary artery. With this model, arterial damage can be performed with overinflation, stent implantation, heat, or radiofrequency energy. The degree of neointimal hyperplasia is directly related to the extent and depth of arterial damage (Fig. 92–17). It remains uncertain whether approaches shown to work in this model will be translatable to the human atherosclerotic coronary artery. Recently, two approaches have been documented to be successful: One is low tech and the other is high tech. A small pilot trial of folic acid (1 mg), vitamin B_{12} (400 mg), and pyridoxine (10 mg) has been performed in 205 patients (165). The primary end point was restenosis assessed by quantitation coronary angiography. At 6 months, the rate of restenosis was significantly lower in patients given folate (19.6% vs. 37.6%; $p = 0.01$). In addition, target lesion revascularization also was decreased (10.0% vs. 22.3%; $p = 0.47$). A larger trial has confirmed these initial results and found decreased clinical and angiographic restenosis (166).

The high-tech approach has involved drug-coated or drug-eluting stents. This is a complex field because it requires careful selection of drug, the polymer for delivery, and the time course of drug administration. In the past, biocompatible polymers were not found to be blood compatible and resulted in severe local tissue damage. Several drugs have been tested, most prominently, sirolimus, an agent approved for use in the setting of renal transplantation and a Taxol derivative. The most complete data set currently is with sirolimus (167–169). In the initial clinical study of 30 patients, there was no restenosis and only minimal late loss

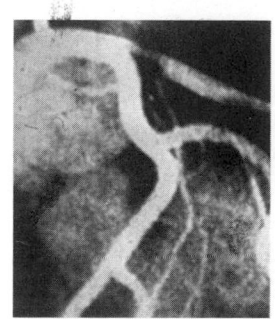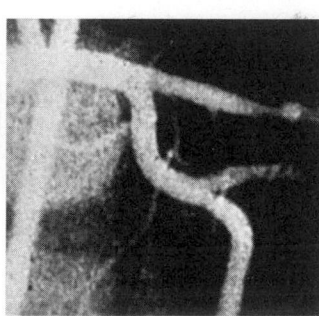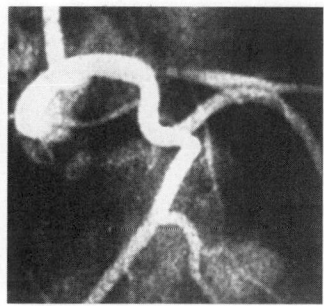

FIG. 92–16. Angiographic stenosis before percutaneous transluminal coronary angiography (PTCA; **left**), immediately after PTCA **(middle)**, and at 6 months **(right)**.

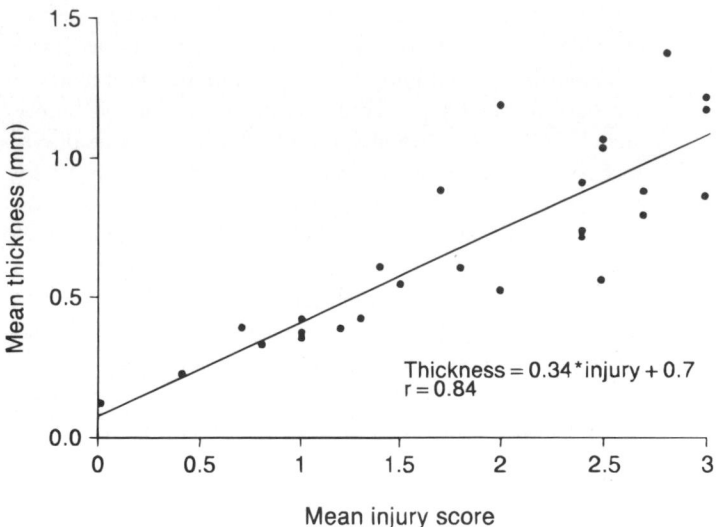

FIG. 92–17. In the porcine model, there is a definite relation between the depth and severity of arterial injury and the mean neointimal thickness. This relation has been validated in the human experience (106–108).

(0.09 mm). This drug-eluting stent was then tested in a multicenter European trial, Randomized Comparison of a Sirolimus Eluting Stent with a Standard Stent For Coronary Revascularization (RAVEL) (169). The primary end point was instent late lumen loss measured by intravascular ultrasound. At 6 months, late lumen loss was markedly less in the sirolimus limb (-0.01 ± 0.33 mm) versus the control stent (0.80 ± 0.53 mm) ($p < 0.001$). None of the sirolimus patients developed restenosis versus 26.6% in the standard bare stent. The larger U.S. trial, Prospective, Randomized Evaluation of the Sirolimus-eluting Stent in Patients with De Novo Coronary Lesions (SIRIUS), has been completed but not yet published. Preliminary data in the first 400 patients documented a restenosis rate of approximately 2% in the stent; there was some evidence of edge effect, but still there was a dramatic reduction compared with the control arm, which had a restenosis rate of 27%. Preliminary data with Paclitaxel also looks promising. Current studies are aimed at greater risk results of patients—left main coronary artery, instent restenosis, and bifurcations.

Other approaches have not been as successful. There was initial great enthusiasm for tranilast on the basis of experimental animal models and small randomized clinical trials. This led to the largest interventional restenosis trial (170), Prevention of Restenosis with Tranilast and Its Outcomes (PRESTO), which randomized approximately 11,500 patients with successful PCI to either placebo or 1 of 2 doses of tranilast delivered for 2 different time periods. There was no significant difference in restenosis in any of the four treatment arms or the placebo group. Restenosis ranged from 33% to 35%, and there was no reduction in the composite of major adverse cardiac events.

Other approaches have been developed, tested, and approved. Vascular brachytherapy has been studied in multiple randomized clinical trials (171–177). Both γ and β systems have been tested, and the devices have been tested in both *de*

novo lesions for prevention of restenosis and in restenosis lesions for prevention of recurrent restenosis. Experimental animal studies documented a consistent reduction in restenosis or recurrent restenosis irrespective of whether γ and β sources were used. These data led to clinical evaluation with multiple randomized clinical trials (171–178) (Fig. 92–18), which have documented a 36% to 39% reduction in recurrent restenosis in patients with instent restenosis. This improvement was not seen in the Beta Cath study of 1,455 patients with native lesions in which the 8-month primary end point was not different between placebo and patients treated with β-radiation. Some specific issues have come up with radiation (179–181). First, delayed subacute closure has been documented in up to 8% to 10% of patients and results in increased mortality and morbidity. This phenomenon is mitigated if placement of a new stent is avoided and if dual antiplatelet therapy is continued for an extended period. Second, geographic miss describes the phenomenon in which the radiation source does not fully cover the injured arterial segment. When there is geographic miss, restenosis is increased at that site; this may reflect a prostimulatory effect of low-dose radiation. Currently, vascular brachytherapy is performed using an approved γ and β source and is restricted to treatment of instent stenosis.

New adjunctive medications will play an increasingly important role. In the past, heparin and aspirin were the mainstays of treatment to prevent acute complications. Although the former is undoubtedly important and the latter has been proven to result in decreased acute complications, more powerful adjunctive medications are Currently available. Intravenous IIb/IIIa platelet receptor inhibitors that improve the initial outcome of procedure have been subjected to intense study and are widely used. Hirudin also has been used, as well as other direct antithrombins, and may replace heparin, although again the incidence of bleeding may be increased.

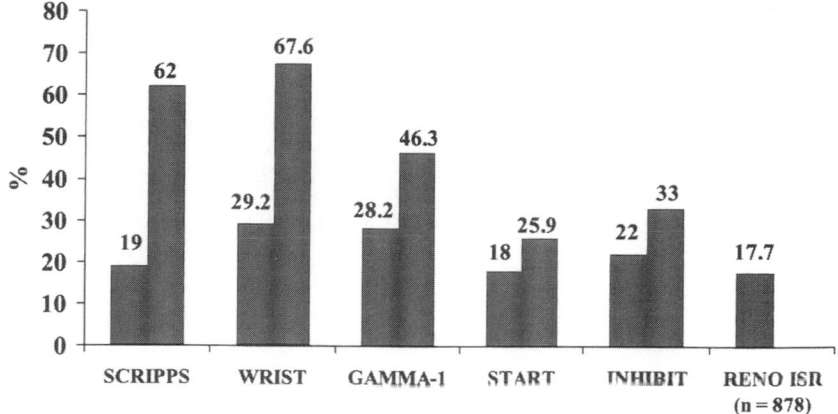

FIG. 92–18. Composite figure of reduction in subsequent recurrent restenosis with vascular brachytherapy. GAMMA-1, gamma radiation; INHIBIT, INtimal Hyperplasia Inhibition with Beta In-stent Trial; RENO ISR, Restenosis Novoste; SCRIPPS, Scripps Coronary Radiation to Inhibit Proliferation Post Stenting; START, Stent versus Angioplasty Restenosis Trial; WRIST, Washington Radiation for In-Stent restenosis Trial. (From Waksman R. Radiation for restenosis. In: Topol EJ. *Textbook of interventional cardiology,* 4th ed. 2003:725–745, with permission.)

FUTURE DIRECTIONS

Since 1977, percutaneous revascularization procedures have revolutionized the treatment of coronary artery disease. These techniques have grown from a procedure with crude equipment used in a small number of patients to a procedure that is currently used more frequently than CABG. When it is successful and leads to long-term good outcome, there is no question that it is preferred over CABG, which requires a thoracotomy and a long recovery time. Resolution of all the problems with percutaneous techniques would go far toward making percutaneous procedures the treatment of choice for coronary artery disease. Even if restenosis is almost completely eliminated, not all problems will be completely alleviated. Technical problems dealing with specific lesion subsets, particularly chronic occlusion, and diffuse disease will remain. For the foreseeable future, CABG remains a reasonable alternative option to PCI in some patients. Selection of the ideal means for revascularization will depend on several factors, including the following:

1. The results of the randomized trials: Results are now accumulating and confirm the observations of prior studies, which indicate that in carefully selected patients, the risks for mortality and MI during the initial procedure and follow-up up to 2 to 3 years are similar between PCI and CABG. Improvement in symptoms is noted in the majority of patients irrespective of the treatment selected, but more patients initially treated with PCI have required repeat revascularization, and more patients initially treated with CABG are asymptomatic.

2. The extent and severity of coronary artery disease and amount of viable myocardium in jeopardy: The more severe the extent of disease, the greater is the chance of achieving only incomplete revascularization with PCI and of leaving

behind unrevascularized ischemic myocardium. The more severe the ischemia, the more important complete revascularization becomes, which may mandate surgery. Alternatively, if single-vessel disease or two-vessel disease with both lesions amenable to PCI is present, strong consideration should be given to the use of a percutaneous approach. The lesion subtype must be kept in mind with the use of a variety of technologies to optimize the outcome. If the risk outweighs the benefit, it should not be performed, and instead an alternative means of revascularization should be selected.

3. The presence and severity of left ventricular dysfunction: There is increasing information that the more severe the left ventricular dysfunction, the more important is complete revascularization for the long term. In addition, the degree of left ventricular dysfunction may necessitate a different initial interventional strategy.

4. Resolution of the problem of restenosis: This has been the greatest impediment to long-term success and is a negative trial end point in all of the trials. The development and testing of some of the drug-eluting stents appears to be associated with dramatically decreased restenosis rates and markedly less need for repeat procedures. Widespread use of these specific stents will expand the number of patients who will be treated with a percutaneous approach.

5. Patient and physician expectations: These are crucial issues. Patients are increasingly sophisticated and often wish to have significant input into their medical care. An open and full discussion of the risks and benefits—both short- and long-term outcome—must be carried out so that an informed decision can be made. For the physician, the charge is to select the optimal treatment strategy, deciding whether revascularization is needed and, if so, then what type, again considering the totality of the patient, the degree and sever-

ity of coronary artery disease and left ventricular function, and the specific technique available to achieve optimal intervention.

SUMMARY

The field of interventional cardiology is changing rapidly. Restenosis rates are dramatically improved with drug-eluting stents. However, problems remain and include technical problems dealing with specific lesion subsets including chronic occlusion and diffuse disease. In addition, acute coronary syndromes result in increased morbidity and even mortality, even with all of the new techniques available. The future will depend in part on resolution of these problems. It can be anticipated that there will be increased emphasis on matching the specific device with the specific lesion to optimize the initial and long-term outcome.

REFERENCES

1. Sheldon WC. F. Mason Sones, Jr.—stormy petrel of cardiology. *Clin Cardiol* 1994;17:405–407.
2. Hurst JW. History of cardiac catheterization. In: King SB 3rd, Douglas JS Jr, eds. *Coronary arteriography and angiography.* New York: McGraw-Hill, 1985;1–9.
3. Dotter CT. Transluminal angioplasty: background and rationale. *Proceedings of the workshop on percutaneous transluminal coronary angioplasty.* Bethesda, MD: U.S. Department of Health, Education and Welfare. NIH Publication No. 80-2030; 1980:5.
4. Dotter CT, Judkins MP. Transluminal treatment of arteriosclerotic obstruction: description of a new technique and a preliminary report of its application. *Circulation* 1964;30:654–670.
5. Gruntzig A. Transluminal dilation of coronary-artery stenosis [letter]. *Lancet* 1978;1:263.
6. Gruntzig AR, Senning A, Siegenthaler WE. Nonoperative dilatation of coronary-artery stenosis: percutaneous transluminal coronary angioplasty. *N Engl J Med* 1979;301:61–68.
7. Kuntz RE, Safian RD, Levine MJ, et al. Novel approach to the analysis of restenosis after the use of three new coronary devices. *J Am Coll Cardiol* 1992;19:1493–1499.
8. Kuntz RE, Gibson CM, Nobuyoshi M, et al. A generalized model of restenosis following conventional balloon angioplasty, stenting, and directional atherectomy. *J Am Coll Cardiol* 1993;21:15–25.
9. Beatt JK, Serruys PW, Luitjten HE, et al. Restenosis after coronary angioplasty: the paradox of increased lumen diameter and restenosis. *J Am Coll Cardiol* 1992;19:258–266.
10. Haude M, Erbel R, Issa H, et al. Quantitative analysis of elastic recoil after balloon angioplasty and after intracoronary implantation of balloon-expandable Palmaz-Schatz stents. *J Am Coll Cardiol* 1993;21:26–34.
11. Isner JM. Vascular remodeling: honey, I think I shrunk the artery. *Circulation* 1994;89:2937–2942.
12. Kakuta T, Currier JW, Haudenscheld CC. Differences in compensatory vessel enlargement, not intimal formation, account for restenosis after angioplasty in the hypercholesterolemic rabbit model. *Circulation* 1994;89:2809–2816.
13. Post MJ, Borst C, Keintz RE. The relative importance of arterial remodeling compared with intimal hyperplasia on lumen narrowing after balloon angioplasty: a study in the normal rabbit and the hypercholesterolemic Yucatan micropig. *Circulation* 1994;89:2816–2822.
14. Mintz GS, Popma JJ, Hong MK, et al. Intravascular ultrasound to discern device specific effects and mechanisms of restenosis. *Am J Cardiol* 1996;78:18–22.
15. Schwartz RS, Holmes DR. Pigs, dogs, baboons and man: lessons for stenting from animal studies. *J Interv Cardiol* 1994;7:355–368.
16. Schwartz R, Huber K, Murphy J, et al. Restenosis and the proportional neointimal response to coronary artery injury: results in a porcine model. *J Am Coll Cardiol* 1992;19:267–274.
17. Schwartz RS, Edwards WD, Huber KC, et al. Coronary restenosis: prospects for solution and new perspectives from a porcine model. *Mayo Clin Proc* 1993;68:54–62.
18. Schwartz R, Holmes D Jr, Topol E. The restenosis paradigm revisited: an alternative proposal for cellular mechanisms. *J Am Coll Cardiol* 1992;20:1284–1293.
19. Schwartz RS, Murphy JG, Edwards WD, et al. Restenosis after balloon angioplasty: a practical proliferative model in porcine coronary arteries. *Circulation* 1990;82:2190–2200.
20. Farb A, Sangiorgi G, Carter AJ, et al. Pathology of acute and chronic coronary stenting in humans. *Circulation* 1999;99:44–52.
21. Virmani R, Farb A. Pathology of in-stent restenosis. *Curr Opin Lipidol* 1999;10:499–506.
22. Detre K, Holubkov R, Kelsey S, et al. Percutaneous transluminal coronary angioplasty in 1985–1986 and 1977–1981. The National Heart, Lung, and Blood Institute Registry. *N Engl J Med* 1988;318:265–270.
23. Vlietstra RE, Holmes DR Jr. PTCA in acute ischemic syndromes. *Curr Probl Cardiol* 1987;12:699.
24. Holmes DR Jr, Vlietstra RE. Balloon angioplasty in acute and chronic coronary artery disease. *JAMA* 1989;261:2109.
25. Holmes DR Jr, Cohen HA, Vlietstra RE. Optimizing the results of balloon coronary angioplasty of "nonideal" lesions. *Prog Cardiovasc Dis* 1989;32:149–170.
26. Gruntzig AR, King SB, Schlumpf M, et al. Long-term follow-up after percutaneous transluminal coronary angioplasty: the early Zurich experience. *N Engl J Med* 1987;316:1127–1132.
27. King SB 3rd, Schlumpf M. Ten-year completed follow-up after percutaneous transluminal coronary angioplasty: the early Zurich experience. *J Am Coll Cardiol* 1993;22:353–360.
28. Detre KM, Holmes DR, Holubkov R, et al. Incidence and consequences of periprocedural occlusion: The 1985-1986 National Heart, Lung, and Blood Institute Percutaneous Transluminal Coronary Angioplasty Registry. *Circulation* 1990;82:739–750.
29. de Feyter PJ, van den Brand M, Laarman GJ, et al. Acute coronary artery occlusion during and after percutaneous transluminal coronary angioplasty. Frequency, prediction, clinical course, management, and follow-up. *Circulation* 1991;83:927–936.
30. Holmes DR, Holubkov R, Vlietstra RE, et al. Comparison of complications during percutaneous transluminal coronary angioplasty from 1977–1981 and from 1985–1986: the National Heart, Lung, and Blood Institute Percutaneous Transluminal Coronary Angioplasty Registry. *J Am Coll Cardiol* 1988;12:1149–1155.
31. Sinclair IN, McCabe CH, Sipperly ME, et al. Predictors, therapeutic options and long-term outcome of abrupt reclosure. *Am J Cardiol* 1988;61:61G–66G.
32. Simpfendorfer C, Belardi J, Bellamy G, et al. Frequency, management and follow-up of patients with acute coronary occlusions after percutaneous transluminal coronary angiography. *Am J Cardiol* 1987;59:267–269.
33. Kuntz RE, Piana R, Pomerantz RM, et al. Changing incidence and management of abrupt closure following coronary intervention in the new devices era. *Cathet Cardiovasc Diagn* 1992;27:183–190.
34. Holmes DR, Vlietstra RE, Smith HC, et al. Restenosis after percutaneous transluminal coronary angioplasty (PTCA): a report from the PTCA Registry of the National Heart, Lung, and Blood Institute. *Am J Cardiol* 1984;53:77C–81C.
35. Holmes DR, Topol EJ, Adelman AG, et al. Randomized trials of directional coronary atherectomy: implications for clinical practice and future investigation. *J Am Coll Cardiol* 1994;24:431–440.
36. Baim DS, Cutlip DE, Sharma SK, et al. Final results of the Balloon vs Optimal Atherectomy Trial (BOAT). *Circulation* 1998;97:322–331.
37. Lefkovits J, Holmes DR, Califf RM, et al. Predictors and sequelae of distal embolization during saphenous vein graft intervention from the CAVEAT-II trial. *Circulation* 1995;92:734–740.
38. Stankovic G, Colombo A, Bersin R., et al; AMIGO Investigators. Comparison of directional coronary atherectomy and stenting versus stenting alone for the treatment of de novo and restenotic coronary artery narrowing. *Am J Cardiol* 2004;93:953–958.
39. Reisman M, Harms V, Whitlow P, et al. Comparison of early and recent results with rotational atherectomy. *J Am Coll Cardiol* 1997;29:353–357.
40. Reisman M. Technique and strategy of rotational atherectomy. *Cathet Cardiovasc Diagn* 1996;[Suppl 3]:2–14.
41. Ellis SG, Popma JJ, Buchbinder M, et al. Relation of clinical presenta-

tion, stenosis morphology, and operator technique to the procedural results of rotational atherectomy and rotational atherectomy-facilitated angioplasty. *Circulation* 1994;89:882–892.

42. Whitlow PL, Bass TA, Kipperman RM, et al. Results of the study to determine rotablator and transluminal angioplasty strategy (STRATAS). *Am J Cardiol* 2001;87:699–705.

43. Safian RD, Feldman T, Muller DW, et al. Coronary angioplasty and Rotablator atherectomy trial (CARAT): immediate and late results of a prospective multicenter randomized trial. *Catheter Cardiovasc Interv* 2001;53:213–220.

44. Reifart N, Vandormael M, Krajcar M, et al. Randomized comparison of angioplasty of complex coronary lesions at a single center: Excimer Laser, Rotational Atherectomy, and Balloon Angioplasty Comparison (ERBAC) study. *Circulation* 1997;96:91–98.

45. Warth D, Leon M, O'Neill W. Rotational atherectomy multicenter registry: acute results, complications and 6-month angiographic follow-up in 709 patients. *J Am Coll Cardiol* 1994;24:641–648.

46. Laskey W, Kimmel S, Krone R. Contemporary trends in coronary intervention: a report from the Registry of the Society for Cardiac Angiography and Interventions. *Catheter Cardiovasc Interv* 2000;49: 19–22.

47. Litvack F, Eigler N, Margolis J, et al. Percutaneous excimer laser coronary angioplasty: results in the first consecutive 3000 patients. *J Am Coll Cardiol* 1994;23:323–330.

48. Reference deleted in proofs.

49. Bittl JA, Sanborn TA. Excimer laser-facilitated coronary angioplasty. Relative risk analysis of acute and follow-up results in 200 patients. *Circulation* 1992;86:71–80.

50. Koster R, Kahler J, Terres W, et al. Six-month clinical and angiographic outcome after successful excimer laser angioplasty for in-stent restenosis. *J Am Coll Cardiol* 2000;36:69–74.

51. Hamburger JN, Foley DP, de Feyter PJ, et al. Six-month outcome after excimer laser coronary angioplasty for diffuse in-stent restenosis in native coronary arteries. *Am J Cardiol* 2000;86:390–394.

52. Dahm JB. Excimer laser coronary angioplasty for diffuse instent restenosis: beneficial long-term results after sufficient debulking with a lesion-specific approach using various laser catheters. *Lasers Med Sci* 2001;16:84–89.

53. Holmes DR Jr, Forrester JS, Litvack F, et al. Chronic total obstruction and short-term outcome: the excimer laser angioplasty registry experience. *Mayo Clin Proc* 1993;68:5–10.

54. Appelman YE, Piek JJ, Strikwerda S, et al. Randomized trial of excimer laser versus balloon angioplasty for treatment of obstructive coronary artery disease. *Lancet* 1996;346:79–84.

55. Holmes DR, Hirshfeld J, Faxan D, et al. ACC consensus document on coronary artery stents. *J Am Coll Cardiol* 1998;32:1471–1482.

56. Al Suwaidi J, Berger PB, Holmes DR Jr, et al. Coronary artery stents. *JAMA* 2000;284:1828–1836.

57. Rankin JM, Spinelli JJ, Carere RG, et al. Improved clinical outcome after widespread use of coronary-artery stenting in Canada. *N Engl J Med* 1999;341:1957–1965.

58. Kimmel SE, Localio AR, Krone RJ, et al. The effects of contemporary use of coronary stents on in-hospital mortality. *J Am Coll Cardiol* 2001;37:499–504.

59. Fischman DL, Leon MB, Baim DS, et al. Stent Restenosis Study Investigators. A randomized comparison of coronary-stent placement and balloon angioplasty in the treatment of coronary artery disease. Stent Restenosis Study Investigators. *N Engl J Med* 1994;331: 496–501.

60. Serruys PW, de Jaegere P, Kiemeneij F, et al. A comparison of balloon-expandable-stent implantation with balloon angioplasty in patients with coronary artery disease. Benestent Study Group. *N Engl J Med* 1994;331:489–495.

61. George BS, Voorhees WD 3rd, Roubin GS, et al. Multicenter investigation of coronary stenting to treat acute or threatened closure after percutaneous transluminal coronary angioplasty: clinical and angiographic outcomes. *J Am Coll Cardiol* 1993;22:135–143.

62. Schomig A, Neumann FJ, Kastrati A, et al. A randomized comparison of antiplatelet and anticoagulant therapy after the placement of coronary-artery stents. *N Engl J Med* 1996;334:1084–1089.

63. Leon MB, Baim DS, Popma JJ, et al. A clinical trial comparing three antithrombotic regimens after coronary artery stenting. *N Engl J Med* 1998;339:1665–1671.

64. Cutlip DE, Baim DS, Hok KL, et al. Stent thrombosis in the modern era: a pooled analysis of multicenter coronary stent clinical trials. *Circulation* 2001;103:1967–1971.

65. Colombo A, Hall P, Nakamura S, et al. Intracoronary stenting without anticoagulation accomplished with ultrasound guidance. *Circulation* 1995;91:1676–1688.

66. Bertrand ME, Rupprecht HJ, Urban P, et al. Double blind study of the safety of clopidogrel with and without a loading dose in combination with aspirin compared with ticlopidine in combination with aspirin after coronary stenting: the clopidogrel aspirin stent international cooperative study (CLASSICS). *Circulation* 2000;102:624–629.

67. Berger PB, Bell MR, Rihal CS, et al. Clopidogrel versus ticlopidine after intracoronary stent placement. *J Am Coll Cardiol* 1999;34:1891–1894.

68. Moussa I, Oetgen M, Roulin G, et al. Effectiveness of clopidogrel and aspirin versus ticlopidine and aspirin in preventing stent thrombosis after coronary stent placement. *Circulation* 1999;99:2364–2366.

69. Mehran R, Dangas G, Abizaid AS, et al. Angiographic patterns of in-stent restenosis: classification and implication for long-term outcome. *Circulation* 1999;100:1872–1878.

70. Carrie D, Karouny E, Chauairi S, et al. "T"-shaped stent placement: a technique for the treatment of dissected bifurcation lesions. *Cathet Cardiovasc Diagn* 1996;37:311–313.

71. Al Suwaidi J, Berger PB, Rihal CS, et al. Immediate and long-term outcome of intracoronary stent implantation for true bifurcation lesions. *J Am Coll Cardiol* 2000;35:929–936.

72. Yamashita T, Nishida T, Adamian MG, et al. Bifurcation lesions: two stents vs. one stent immediate and follow-up results. *J Am Coll Cardiol* 2000;35:1145–1151.

73. Saber RS, Edwards WD, Holmes DR, et al. Balloon angioplasty of aortocoronary saphenous vein bypass grafts: a histopathologic study of six grafts from five patients with emphasis on restenosis and embolic complications. *J Am Coll Cardiol* 1988;12:1501–1510.

74. Saber RS, Edwards WD, Bailey KR, et al. Coronary embolization after balloon angioplasty and thrombolytic therapy: an autopsy study of 32 cases. *J Am Coll Cardiol* 1993;22:1283–1288.

75. Topol EJ, Yadav JS. Recognition of the importance of embolization in atherosclerotic vascular disease. *Circulation* 2000;101:570–580.

76. Frink RJ, Ostrach LH, Rooney PA, et al. Coronary thrombosis, ulcerated atherosclerotic plaques and platelet/fibrin microemboli in patients dying with acute coronary disease: a large autopsy study. *J Clin Invest* 1990;2:199–210.

77. Baim DS, Wahr D, George B, et al. Randomized trial of a distal embolic protection device during percutaneous intervention of saphenous vein aorto-coronary bypass grafts. *Circulation* 2002;105:1285–1290.

78. Webb JG, Carere RG, Virmani R, et al. Retrieval and analysis of particulate debris after saphenous vein graft intervention. *J Am Coll Cardiol* 1999;34:468–475.

79. Steve GW, Rogers C, Ramee S, et al. Distal filter protection during saphenous vein graft stenting: technical and clinical correlation of effusion. *J Am Coll Cardiol* 2002;40:1882–1888.

80. Grube E, Gerckens U, Young A, et al. Prevention of distal embolization during coronary angioplasty in saphenous vein grafts and native vessels using porous filter protection. *Circulation* 2001;104:2436–2441.

81. Kuntz RE, Baim DS, Cohen DJ, et al. A trial comparing rheolytic thrombectomy with intracoronary urokinase for coronary and vein graft thrombus (The Vein Graft Angiojet Study (VEGAS-2). *Am J Cardiol* 2002;89:326–330.

82. Singh M, Tiede DJ, Mathew V, et al. Rheolytic thrombectomy with Angiojet in thrombus containing lesions. *Cath Cardiovasc Interv* 2002;56:1–7.

83. Rinfret S, Katsiyiannis PT, Ho KK, et al. Effectiveness of rheolytic coronary thrombectomy with the AngioJet catheter. *Am J Cardiol* 2002;89:470–476.

84. Stone GW, Cox DA, Babb J, et al. Prospective, randomized evaluation of thrombectomy prior to percutaneous intervention in diseased saphenous vein grafts and thrombus containing coronary arteries. *J Am Coll Cardiol* 2003;42:2007–2013.

85. Stone GW, Cox DA, Low R, et al. Safety and efficacy of a novel device for treatment of thrombotic and atherosclerotic lesions in native coronary arteries and saphenous vein grafts. *Catheter Cardiovasc Interv* 2003;58:419–427.

86. Diegeler A, Thiele H, Falk V, et al. Comparison of stenting with minimally invasive bypass surgery for stenosis of the left anterior descending coronary artery. *N Engl J Med* 2002;347:561–566.

87. Bucher HC, Hengstler P, Schindler C, et al. Percutaneous translumi-

nal coronary angioplasty versus medical treatment for non-acute coronary heart disease: meta-analysis of randomized controlled trials. *BMJ* 2000;321:73–77.

88. TIME Investigators. Trial of invasive versus medical therapy in elderly patients with chronic symptomatic coronary artery disease (TIME): a randomised trial. *Lancet* 2001;358:951–957.

89. Holmes DR Jr, Vlietstra RE, Reeder GS, et al. Angioplasty in total coronary artery occlusion. *J Am Coll Cardiol* 1984;3:845–849.

90. Holmes DR Jr, Vlietstra RE. Angioplasty in total coronary arterial occlusion. *Herz* 1985;10:292–297.

91. Safian RD, McCabe CH, Siperly ME, et al. Initial success and long-term follow-up of percutaneous transluminal coronary angioplasty in chronic total occlusions versus conventional stenoses. *Am J Cardiol* 1988;61:23G–28G.

92. Bell MR, Berger PB, Bresnahan JF, et al. Initial and long term outcome of 354 patients following coronary balloon angioplasty of total coronary artery occlusions. *Circulation* 1992;85:1003–1011.

93. Stone GW, Rutherford BD, McConahay DR, et al. Procedural outcome of angioplasty for total coronary artery occlusion: an analysis of 971 lesions in 905 patients. *J Am Coll Cardiol* 1990;15:849–856.

94. Jost S, Nolte CW, Simon R, et al. Angioplasty of subacute and chronic total coronary occlusions: success, recurrence rate, and clinical follow-up. *Am Heart J* 1991;122:1509–1514.

95. Ivanhoe RJ, Weintraub WS, Douglas JS, et al. Percutaneous transluminal coronary angioplasty of chronic total occlusions. Primary success, restenosis and long term clinical follow-up. *Circulation* 1992;85:106–115.

96. Holmes DR, Faxon D, Serruys PW, et al. Restenosis with chronic total occlusion: the MARCATOR randomized trial experience. *J Am Coll Cardiol* 1994;1A:472A.

97. Holmes DR, Forrester JS, Litvack F, et al. Chronic total obstruction and short-term outcome: The Excimer Laser Coronary Angioplasty Registry experience. *Mayo Clin Proc* 1993;68:54–62.

98. Suero JA, Marso SP, Jones PG. Procedural outcomes and long term survival among patients undergoing percutaneous coronary intervention of a chronic total occlusion in native coronary arteries: a 20 year experience. *J Am Coll Cardiol* 2001;38:404–414.

99. Mabin TA, Holmes DR Jr, Smith HC, et al. Intracoronary thrombus: role in coronary occlusion complicating percutaneous transluminal coronary angioplasty. *J Am Coll Cardiol* 1985;5:198–202.

100. Surgrue D, Holmes D Jr, Smith H, et al. Coronary artery thrombus as a risk factor for acute vessel occlusion during percutaneous transluminal coronary angioplasty: improving results. *Br Heart J* 1986;56:62–66.

101. Vaitkus P, Herrmann H, Laskey W. Management and immediate outcome of patients with intracoronary thrombus during percutaneous transluminal coronary angioplasty. *Am Heart J* 1992;124:1–8.

102. Buchalter M, Been M, Williams D, et al. The occurrence of early sudden coronary artery occlusion following angioplasty may be predicted from the clinical characteristics of the patients and their coronary lesion morphology. *Jpn Heart J* 1992;33:295–302.

103. Mooney MR, Mooney JF, Goldenberg IF, et al. Percutaneous transluminal coronary angioplasty in the setting of large intracoronary thrombi. *Am J Cardiol* 1990;65:427–431.

104. Reeder GS, Bryant SL, Suman VJ, et al. Intracoronary thrombus: still a risk factor for PTCA failure. *Cath Cardiovasc Diagn* 1995;34:191–195.

105. Singh M, Berger PB, Ting HH, et al. Influence of coronary thrombus in outcome of percutaneous coronary angioplasty in the current era (Mayo Clinic). *Am J Cardiol* 2001;88:1091–1096.

106. Singh M, Reeder GS, Ohman EM, et al. Does the presence of thrombus seen on a coronary angiogram affect the outcome after percutaneous coronary angioplasty? An Angiographic Trials Pool data experience. *J Am Coll Cardiol* 2001;38:624–630.

107. Mauri L, Bonan R, Weiner BH, et al. Cutting balloon angioplasty for the prevention of restenosis: results of the cutting balloon global randomized trial. *Am J Cardiol* 2002;90:1079–1083.

108. Wong SC, Popma JJ, Hong MK, et al. Procedural results and long term clinical outcome in aorto-ostial saphenous vein graft lesions after new device angioplasty. *J Am Coll Cardiol* 1995;25[Suppl A]:394A.

109. Bittl JA, Sanborn TA, Yardley DE, et al. Predictors of outcome of percutaneous excimer laser coronary angioplasty of saphenous vein bypass graft lesions. *Am J Cardiol* 1994;74:144–148.

110. Barness GW, Buller C, Ohman EM, et al. Reduced thrombus burden with abciximab delivered locally before percutaneous intervention in saphenous vein grafts. *Am Heart J* 2000;139:824–829.

111. Piana RN, Paik GY, Moscucci M, et al. Incidence and treatment of "no-reflow" after percutaneous coronary intervention. *Circulation* 1994;89:2514–2518.

112. Hong MK, Mehran R, Dangas G, et al. Are we making progress with percutaneous saphenous vein graft treatment? *J Am Coll Cardiol* 2001;38:150–154.

113. Mathew V, Berger PB, Lennon RJ, et al. Comparison of percutaneous interventions for unstable angina pectoris in patients with and without previous coronary artery bypass grafting. *Am J Cardiol* 2000;86:931–937.

114. Hartmann JR, McKeever LS, Stamato NJ, et al. Recanalization of chronically occluded aortocoronary saphenous vein bypass grafts by extended infusion of urokinase: initial results and short-term clinical follow-up. *J Am Coll Cardiol* 1991;18:1517–1523.

115. Rosenschein U, Gaul G, Erbel R, et al. Percutaneous transluminal therapy of occluded saphenous vein grafts: can the challenge be met with ultrasound thrombolysis? *Circulation* 1999;99:26–29.

116. Ellis SG, Lincoff AM, Miller D, et al. Reduction in complications of angioplasty with abciximab occurs largely independently of baseline lesion morphology. EPIC and EPILOG Investigators. Evaluation of 7E3 for the Prevention of Ischemic Complications. Evaluation of PTCA To Improve Long-term Outcome with abciximab GPIIb/IIIa Receptor Blockade. *J Am Coll Cardiol* 1998;32:1619–1623.

117. Mathew V, Grill DE, Scott CG, et al. The influence of abciximab use on clinical outcome after aortocoronary vein graft interventions. *J Am Coll Cardiol* 1999;34:1163–1169.

118. Roffi M, Mukherjee D, Chen DP, et al. Lack of benefit from intravenous platelet glycoprotein IIb/IIIa receptor inhibitors as adjunctive treatment for percutaneous intervention aortocoronary bypass grafts: a pooled analysis of five randomized clinical trials. *Circulation* 2002;106:3063–3067.

119. Landau C, Lange RA, Hillis LD. Percutaneous transluminal coronary angioplasty. *N Engl J Med* 1994;330:981–993.

120. Talley JD, Hurst JW, King SB, et al. Clinical outcome 5 years after attempted percutaneous transluminal coronary angioplasty in 427 patients. *Circulation* 1988;77:820–829.

121. Cowley MJ, Vetrovec GW, DiSciasio G, et al. Coronary angioplasty of multiple vessels: short-term outcome and long-term results. *Circulation* 1985;72:1314–1320.

122. O'Keefe JH Jr, Rutherford BD, McConahay DR, et al. Multivessel coronary angioplasty from 1980–1989: procedural results and long-term outcome. *J Am Coll Cardiol* 1990;16:1079–1102.

123. Myler RK, Topol EJ, Shaw RE, et al. Multiple vessel coronary angioplasty: classification, results, and patterns of restenosis in 494 consecutive patients. *Cath Cardiovasc Diagn* 1987;13:1–15.

124. DiSciascio G, Cowley MJ, Vetrovec GW, et al. Triple vessel coronary angioplasty: acute outcome and long-term results. *J Am Coll Cardiol* 1988;12:42–48.

125. Vandormael MG, Deligonul U, Kern MJ, et al. Multilesion coronary angioplasty: clinical and angiographic follow-up. *J Am Coll Cardiol* 1987;10:246–252.

126. Bourassa MG, Holubkov R, Yeh W, et al. Strategy of complete revascularization in patients with multivessel coronary artery disease. (A report from the 1985–86 NHLBI PTCA Registry.) *Am J Cardiol* 1992;70:174–178.

127. Reeder GS, Holmes DR Jr, Detre K, et al. Degree of revascularization in patients with multivessel coronary disease: a report from the National Heart, Lung, and Blood Institute Percutaneous Transluminal Coronary Angioplasty Registry. *Circulation* 1988;77:638–644.

128. Bell MR, Bailey KR, Reeder GS, et al. Percutaneous transluminal angioplasty in patients with multivessel coronary disease: How important is complete revascularization for cardiac event-free survival? *J Am Coll Cardiol* 1990;16:553–562.

129. Vandormael MG, Chaitman BR, Ischinger T, et al. Immediate and short-term benefit of multilesion coronary angioplasty: influence of degree of revascularization. *J Am Coll Cardiol* 1985;6:983–991.

130. Mabin TA, Holmes DR Jr, Smith HC, et al. Follow-up clinical results in patients undergoing percutaneous transluminal coronary angioplasty. *Circulation* 1985;71:754.

131. Vacek JL, Rosamond TL, Stites HW, et al. Comparison of percutaneous transluminal coronary angioplasty versus coronary bypass grafting for multivessel coronary artery disease. *Am J Cardiol* 1992;69:592–597.

132. Faxon DP, Ghalilli K, Jacobs AK. The degree of revascularization and outcome after multivessel coronary angioplasty. *Am Heart J* 1992; 123:854.

133. Seven-year outcome in the Bypass Angioplasty Revascularization Investigation (BARI) by treatment and diabetes status. *J Am Coll Cardiol* 2000;35:1122–1129.

134. King SB 3rd, Kosinski AS, Guyton RA, et al. Eight-year mortality in the Emory Angioplasty versus Surgery Trial (EAST). *J Am Coll Cardiol* 2000;35:1116–1121.

135. Kurbaan AS, Bowker TJ, Ilsley CD, et al. Difference in the mortality of the CABRI diabetic and nondiabetic populations and its relation to coronary artery disease and the revascularization mode. *Am J Cardiol* 2001;87:947–950.

136. Holmes DR, Detre K, Williams DO, et al. Long-term outcome of patients with depressed left ventricular function undergoing percutaneous transluminal coronary angioplasty: the NHLBI PTCA Registry. *Circulation* 1993;87:21–29.

137. Stevens T, Kahn JK, McCallister BD, et al. Safety and efficacy of percutaneous transluminal coronary angioplasty in patients with left ventricular dysfunction. *Am J Cardiol* 1991;68:313.

138. Kohli RS, DiSciascio G, Cowley MJ, et al. Coronary angioplasty in patients with severe left ventricular dysfunction. *J Am Coll Cardiol* 1990;16:807–811.

139. Keelan PC, Johnston JM, Koru-Sengul T, et al. Comparison of in-hospital and one-year outcomes in patients with left ventricular ejection fractions < or = 40%, 41 to 49%, and > or = 50% having percutaneous coronary revascularization. *Am J Cardiol* 2003;91:1168–1172.

140. Mark DB, Nelson CL, Califf RM, et al. Continuing education of therapy for coronary artery disease. Initial results from the era of coronary angioplasty. *Circulation* 1994;89:2015–2025.

141. Hartz AJ, Kuhn EM, Pryer DB, et al. Mortality after coronary angioplasty and coronary artery bypass surgery (The National Medicare Experience). *Am J Cardiol* 1992;70:179–185.

142. Weintraub WS, Jones EL, King SB 3rd, et al. Changing use of coronary angioplasty and coronary bypass surgery in the treatment of chronic coronary artery disease. *Am J Cardiol* 1990;65:183–188.

143. O'Keefe JH Jr, Allan JJ, McCallister BD, et al. Angioplasty versus bypass surgery for multivessel coronary artery disease with left ventricular ejection fraction ≤40 percent. *Am J Cardiol* 1993;71:897–901.

144. Detre KM, Guo P, Holubkor R, et al. Coronary revascularization in diabetic patients. A comparison of the randomized and observational component of the Bypass Angioplasty Revascularization Investigation. *Circulation* 1999;99:633–640.

145. King SB 3rd, Lembo NJ, Weintraub WS, et al. A randomized trial comparing coronary angioplasty to coronary bypass surgery. Emory Angioplasty versus Surgery Trial (EAST) *N Engl J Med* 1994;331:1044–1050.

146. Coronary angioplasty versus coronary artery bypass surgery: the Randomized Intervention Treatment of Angina (RITA) trial. *Lancet* 1993;341:573–580.

147. Rodriquez A, Boullon F, Perez-Balino N, et al. Argentine randomized trial of percutaneous transluminal coronary angioplasty versus coronary artery bypass surgery in multivessel disease (ERACI): in hospital results and 1 year follow-up. *J Am Coll Cardiol* 1993;22:1060–1067.

148. Hoffman SN, TenBrook JA, Wolf MP, et al. A meta-analysis of randomized controlled trials comparing coronary artery bypass graft with percutaneous transluminal coronary angioplasty: one to eight year outcomes. *J Am Coll Cardiol* 2003;41:1293–1304.

149. Serruys PW, Unger F, Sousa JE, et al. Comparison of coronary artery bypass surgery and stenting for the treatment of multivessel disease. *N Engl J Med* 2001;344:1117–1124.

150. SoS Investigators. Coronary artery bypass surgery versus percutaneous coronary intervention with stent implantation in patients with multivessel coronary artery disease (the Stent or Surgery Trial): a randomized controlled trial. *Lancet* 2002;360:965–970.

151. Rodriguez A, Bernardi V, Navia J, et al. Argentine Randomized Study: Coronary Angioplasty with Stenting versus Coronary Bypass Surgery in patients with Multiple-Vessel Disease (ERACI II): 30-day and one-year follow-up results. ERACI II Investigators. *J Am Coll Cardiol* 2001;37;51–58.

152. Smith SC Jr, Dove JT, Jacobs AK, et al. ACC/AHA guidelines of percutaneous coronary interventions (revisions of the 1993 PTCA guidelines)—executive summary. A report of the American College of Cardiology/American Heart Association Task Force on Practice Guidelines (committee to revise the 1993 guidelines for percutaneous transluminal coronary angioplasty). *J Am Coll Cardiol* 2001;37:2215–2239.

153. Ryan TJ, Bauman WB, Kennedy WJ, et al. Guidelines for percutaneous transluminal coronary angioplasty. A report of the American Heart Association/American College of Cardiology Task Force on Assessment of Diagnostic and Therapeutic Cardiovascular Procedures (Committee on Percutaneous Transluminal Coronary Angioplasty). *Circulation* 1993;88:2987–3007.

154. Holmes DR, Vlietstra RE, Smith HC, et al. Restenosis after PTCA: a report from the PTCA Registry of the National Heart, Lung and Blood Institute. *Am J Cardiol* 1984;53[Suppl C]:77.

155. Serruys PW, Luijten HE, Beatt KJ, et al. Incidence of restenosis after successful coronary angioplasty: a time-related phenomenon. A quantitative angiographic study in 342 consecutive patients at 1, 2, 3, and 4 months. *Circulation* 1988;77:361–371.

156. Nobuyoshi M, Kimura T, Nosaka H, et al. Restenosis after successful percutaneous transluminal coronary angioplasty. serial angiographic follow-up of 229 patients. *J Am Coll Cardiol* 1988;12:616–623.

157. Rensing BJ, Hermans WR, Deckers JW, et al. Lumen narrowing after percutaneous transluminal coronary angioplasty follows a near Gaussian distribution: a quantitative angiographic study in 1,445 successfully dilated lesions. *J Am Coll Cardiol* 1992;19:939–945.

158. Hirshfeld JW, Schwartz JS, Jugo R, et al. Restenosis after coronary angioplasty: a multivariate statistical model to relate lesion and procedural variables to restenosis. *J Am Coll Cardiol* 1991;18:647–656.

159. Muller DW, Ellis SG, Topol EJ. Experimental models of coronary artery restenosis. *J Am Coll Cardiol* 1992;19:418–432.

160. Karas SP, Gravanis MB, Santoian EC, et al. Coronary intimal proliferation after balloon injury and stenting in swine: an animal model of restenosis. *J Am Coll Cardiol* 1992;20:467–474.

161. Gravanis MB, Robinson K, Santoian EC, et al. The reparative phenomena at the site of balloon angioplasty in humans and experimental models. *Cardiovasc Pathol* 1993;2:263–273.

162. Fishman JA, Ryan GB, Karnovsky MJ. Endothelial regeneration in the rat carotid artery and the significance of endothelial denudation in the pathogenesis of myointimal thickening. *Lab Invest* 1975;32:339–351.

163. Clowes AW, Reidy MA, Clowes MM. Kinetics of cellular proliferation after arterial injury. 1. Smooth muscle cell growth in the absence of endothelium. *Lab Invest* 1983;49:337.

164. Fingerle J, Au YP, Clowes AW, et al. Intimal lesion formation in rat carotid arteries after endothelial denudation in the absence of medial injury. *Arteriosclerosis* 1990;10:1082–1087.

165. Schnyder G, Roffi M, Pin R, et al. Decreased rate of coronary restenosis after lowering of plasma homocysteine levels. *N Engl J Med* 2001; 345:1593–1600.

166. Schnyder G, Roffi M, Flammer Y. Effect of homocysteine lowering therapy with folic acid, vitamin B_{12} and vitamin B_6 on clinical outcome after percutaneous coronary intervention: the SWISS Heart Study. *JAMA* 2002;288:973–979.

167. Serruys PW, Degertekin M, Tanabe K, et al. Intravascular ultrasound findings in the multicenter randomized double blind RAVEL (RAndomized study with the sirolimus-eluting Velocity balloon-expandable stent in the treatment of patients with de novo native coronary artery Lesions) trial. *Circulation* 2002;106:798–803.

168. Regar E, Serruys PW, Bode C, et al. Angiographic Findings of the Multicenter Randomized Study with the Sirolimus-Eluting Bx Velocity Balloon Expandable Stent (RAVEL): sirolimus-eluting stents inhibit restenosis irrespective of the vessel size. *Circulation* 2002;106:1949–1956.

169. Morice MC, Serruys PW, Sousa JE, et al. Randomized Study with the Sirolimus-Coated Bx Velocity Balloon Expandable Stent in the Treatment of Patients with de Novo Native Coronary Artery Lesions. RAVEL Study Group. *N Engl J Med* 2002;346:1773–1780.

170. Holmes DR, Savage M, LaBlanche JM, et al. Results of Prevention of Restenosis with Tranilast and Its Outcomes (PRESTO) Trial. *Circulation* 2002;106:1243–1250.

171. King SB 3rd, Williams DO, Chaugule P, et al. Endovascular beta-radiation to reduce restenosis after coronary balloon angioplasty: results of the Beta Energy Restenosis Trial (BERT). *Circulation* 1998; 97:2025–2030.

172. Raizner AE, Osterle SN, Waksman R, et al. Inhibition of restenosis with β-emitting radiotherapy: Report of the Proliferation Reduction with Vascular Energy Trial (PREVENT). *Circulation* 2000;102:951–958.

173. Verin V, Popowski Y, de Bruyne B, et al. Endoluminal beta-radiation

therapy for the prevention of coronary restenosis after balloon angioplasty. *N Engl J Med* 2001;344:243–249.

174. Popma J. Late clinical and angiographic outcomes after use of ^{90}Sr/^{90}Y beta radiation for the treatment of in-stent restenosis: results from the ^{90}Sr Treatment of Angiographic Restenosis (START) trial. *J Am Coll Cardiol* 2000;36:311–312.

175. Condado JA, Waksman R, Gurdiel O, et al. Long-term angiographic and clinical outcome after percutaneous transluminal coronary angioplasty and intracoronary radiation therapy in humans. *Circulation* 1997;96:727–732.

176. Teirstein PS, Massullo V, Jani S, et al. Catheter-based radio-therapy to inhibit restenosis after coronary stenting. *N Engl J Med* 1997;336: 1697–1703.

177. Leon MB, Teirstein PS, Moses JW, et al. Localized intracoronary gamma-radiation therapy to inhibit the recurrence of restenosis after stenting. *N Engl J Med* 2001;344:250–256.

178. Popma JJ, Suntharalingam M, Lansky AJ, et al. Randomized trial of 90Sr/90Y beta radiation versus placebo control for treatment of in-stent restenosis. *Circulation* 2002;106:1090–1096.

179. Waksman R, Bhargava B, Mintz GS, et al. Late total occlusion after intracoronary brachytherapy for patients with in-stent restenosis. *J Am Coll Cardiol* 2000;36:65–68.

180. Costa MA, Sabat M, van der Giessen WJ, et al. Late coronary occlusion after intracoronary brachytherapy. *Circulation* 1999;100:789–792.

181. Sabate M, Serruys PW, van der Giessen WJ, et al. Geometric vascular remodeling after balloon angioplasty and beta-radiation therapy: a three-dimensional intravascular ultrasound study. *Circulation* 1999; 100:1182–1188.

CHAPTER 93

Clinical Evaluation of Restenosis

Albert W. Chan and David J. Moliterno

Key Words: Angioplasty; coronary artherosclerosis; evaluation; restenosis; stent.

INTRODUCTION

Since the introduction of percutaneous transluminal coronary angioplasty (PTCA) more than a quarter of a century ago (1), procedural techniques and equipment have continuously evolved. With the vast variety of interventional devices including stents, the safety and efficacy of interventional procedures have steadily improved, and favorable outcomes have been sustained over long-term follow-up. Percutaneous coronary interventions (PCIs) have become the dominant revascularization modality for obstructive coronary artery disease (2). Between 1986 and 2000, the number of PCIs performed each year has increased by six-fold in the United States (Fig. 93–1). However, restenosis remains as the Achilles heel of PCI. Out of 1.5 million PCIs performed annually worldwide, clinically important restenosis occurs at a rate of 10% to 15%, although the incidence may be yet decreased with the introductions of

A. W. Chan: Department of Cardiology, Royal Columbian Hospital, 206-301 E. Columbia St., New Westminster, British Columbia, V3L 3W5, Canada.

D. J. Moliterno: Department of Cardiovascular Medicine, University of Kentucky, 900 S. Limestone Avenue, 317 Health Sciences Building, Lexington, Kentucky 40536-0200.

brachytherapy and drug-eluting stents. From both the individual and societal perspectives, the health care cost for diagnosing and treating restenosis is large, mounting to more than $1 billion annually. Drug-eluting stents, which will decrease restenosis rates, is estimated to cost three times as much as the conventional stents and is not expected to relieve the overall financial burden.

Given the complexity of the restenotic process, the rapid technology evolution, and the inherent limitations of many clinical studies in restenosis, the literature has wide-ranging observations and recommendations. The scope of this chapter is to review the clinical issues and the clinical trials in restenosis with specific attention to the evaluation of patients in whom restenosis is suspected.

PATHOGENESIS OF RESTENOSIS

Restenosis is the response to vascular injury associated with coronary intervention. All PCI causes a degree of restenosis, but this "reparative process" becomes excessive in some cases, causing significant angiographic or clinical effects. Renarrowing after PCI develops over weeks to months, in contrast to *de novo* coronary narrowings that develop over years, likely reflecting the difference in the degree of inflammation between these lesion types. The process of restenosis can be broadly categorized into four interrelated facets—*vessel recoil, thrombus formation and organization, vascular remodeling, and*

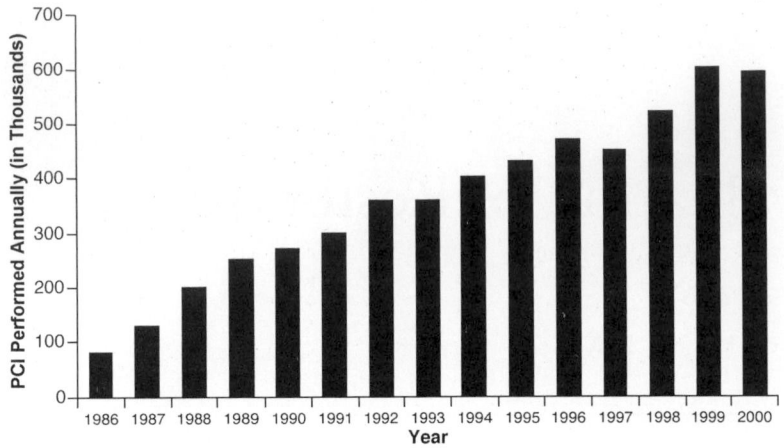

FIG. 93–1. Number of percutaneous coronary interventions (PCIs) performed in the United States from 1986 to 2000. (Data adapted from the Centers of Disease Control and Prevention. Atlanta, GA. Available at: http://www.cdc.gov.)

neointimal growth—that begin immediately after the procedure and continue during the next 6 to 9 months (Fig. 93–2).

Early Phase

The acute reduction of the arterial lumen is related to the combination of elastic recoil and thrombus formation. Vascular recoil is related to "springlike" rebound of the arterial segment, or may simply reflect persistence of the temporarily displaced atherothrombotic plaque. Within minutes of balloon deflation, the vessel may approximate its predilation shape, thereby negating much of the original gain. Small or distal segments are more prone to recoil as the reference diameter may be overestimated. The process of vasoconstriction is fueled by thrombus formation after the cascade of plaque disruption, platelet adhesion, activation, and aggre-

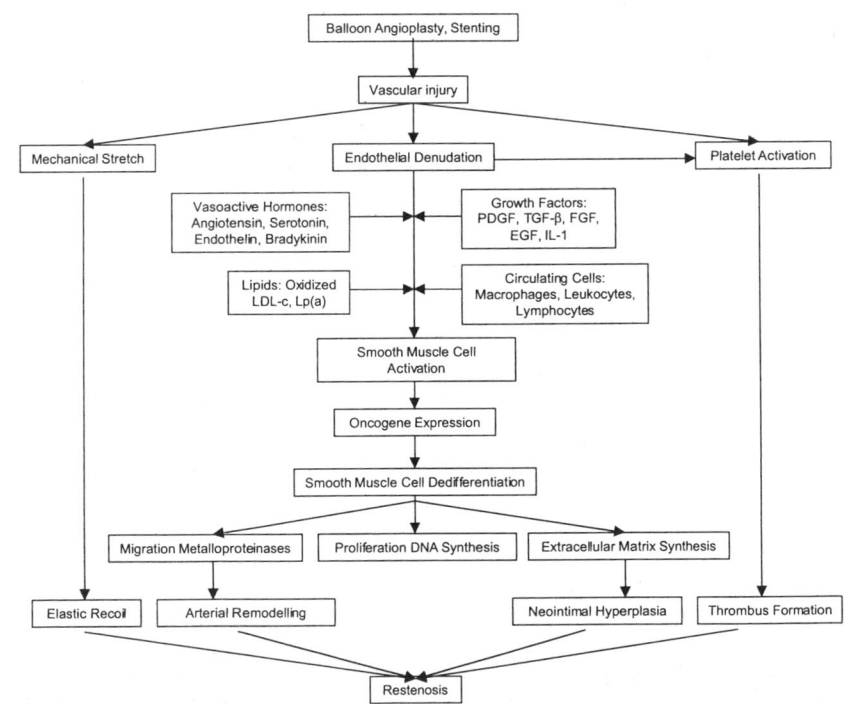

FIG. 93–2. Pathophysiology of restenosis after percutaneous coronary intervention. After balloon injury, elastic recoil and thrombus formation take place almost immediately, whereas arterial remodeling and neointimal hyperplasia occur during the subsequent months. Arterial remodeling is the predominant factor of restenosis after balloon angioplasty, and neointimal hyperplasia has a major role in restenosis after stenting. EGF, endothelial growth factor; FGF, fibroblast growth factor; IL-1, interleukin-1; LDL-c, low-density lipoprotein cholesterol; Lp(a), lipoprotein(a); PDGF, platelet-derived growth factor; TGF, transforming growth factor.

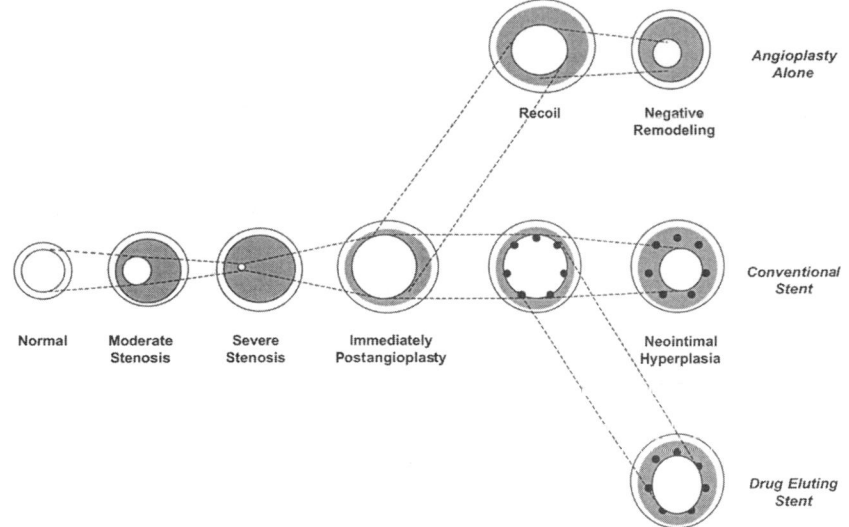

FIG. 93–3. The Glagov Phenomenon. By serial ultrasound studies, the cross-sectional area of the external elastic membrane enlarges as the plaque volume increases. The increase in plaque volume, compensated by the enlargement of the arterial diameter, results in modest reduction of luminal area until advanced atherothrombosis. The angiographic appearance differs after various modality of revascularization.

gation. The presence of thrombus either before or after angioplasty is associated with immediate vessel renarrowing or its extreme presentation—abrupt vessel closure. Beyond the acute phase, platelets also release a host of growth factors and chemokines (platelet-derived growth factor, tissue growth factor-β, basic fibroblast growth factor, epidermal growth factor, and interleukin-1), which can further stimulate smooth muscle cell proliferation and migration, thereby promoting fibromuscular growth during the next several months (3–5).

Late Phase

Neointimal hyperplasia predominates the luminal narrowing beyond the acute phase after balloon angioplasty. After medial wall injury, the reparative process is orchestrated by thrombosis, inflammation, smooth muscle cell proliferation, and extracellular matrix formation (6–9). The arterial wall may remodel in response to PTCA, resulting in an increase, decrease, or no change in the cross-sectional area (CSA) of the artery. This so-called Glagov phenomenon (10), combined with extracellular matrix formation and smooth muscle cell proliferation, represents the final wave of the restenotic process, and it usually extends up to 6 to 9 months (Fig. 93–3). Histologic examination of human atherectomy tissue from restenotic stents suggested cell-depleted myxoid tissue is a major component of instent restenosis (9).

TYPE OF RESTENOSIS

Depending on the circumstances, whether it is in the context of clinical care or research, restenosis has been defined in different ways, namely angiographic, clinical, and silent. Each definition has different relevance.

Angiographic Restenosis

Among the studies evaluating the efficacy of PCI strategies or devices over the last two decades, many definitions for angiographic restenosis have evolved (Table 93–1). The extent of angiographic restenosis follows a normal distribution after either angioplasty or stent placement. The rates of restenosis can be reported as a frequency distribution (Fig. 93–4) or as a cumulative distribution (Fig. 93–5) of either

TABLE 93–1. *Restenosis criteria for follow-up angiography*

1. Diameter stenosis ≥50%
2. Reduction ≥30% in diameter stenosis (NHLBI 1)
3. An immediate post-PTCA <50% diameter stenosis that increases to ≥70% at follow-up (NHLBI 2)
4. Return to within 10% of pre-PTCA diameter stenosis (NHLBI 3)
5. Loss of at least 50% of the initial gain (NHLBI 4)
6. Diameter stenosis ≥70%
7. Area stenosis ≥85%
8. An immediate post-PTCA <50% diameter stenosis that increases to ≥50% at follow-up
9. Reduction ≥20% in diameter stenosis
10. Loss of ≥1 mm² in stenosis area
11. Loss of ≥0.50 mm in minimal lumen diameter
12. Loss of ≥0.72 mm in minimal lumen diameter

NHLBI, National Heart, Lung and Blood Institute; PTCA, percutaneous transluminal coronary angiography.
From Serruys PW, Foley DP, Kirkeeide RL, et al. Restenosis revisited: insights provided by quantitative coronary angiography. *Am Heart J* 1993;126:1243–1267, with permission.

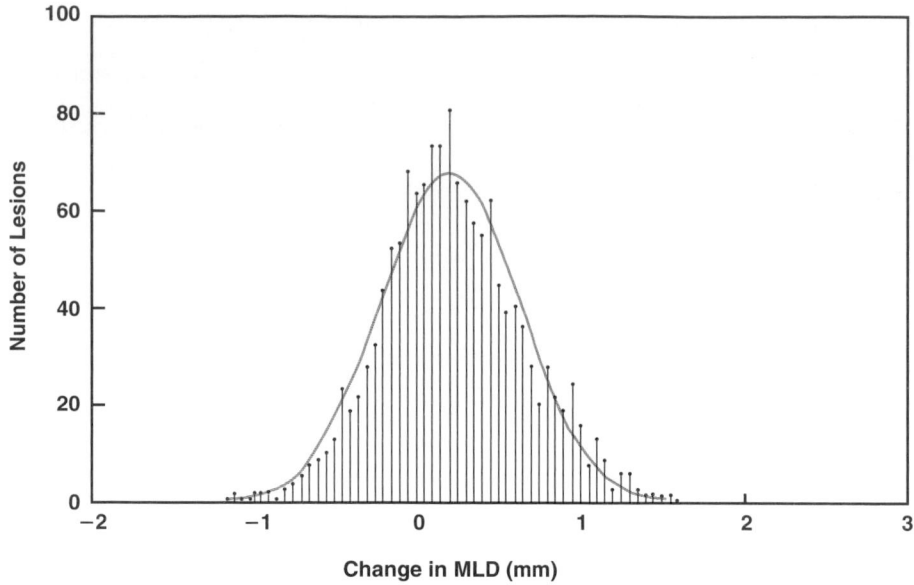

FIG. 93–4. Histogram of the individual changes in minimum lumen diameter (MLD) between the immediate postprocedure angiogram and that at 6 month follow-up in 1,375 lesions. Lesions that progressed to total occlusion were not included. A positive value corresponds to a decrease in MLD. The curve superimposed on the distribution depicts the theoretic Gaussian distribution. (From van der Giessen WJ, Hermans WR, Rensing BJ, et al. Clinical and angiographic definitions of restenosis: Recommendations for clinical trials. In: Schwartz RS, ed. *Coronary restenosis.* Boston: Blackwell Scientific, 1993:169–191, with permission.)

the degree of stenosis or luminal diameter. Although there is no consensus among interventional cardiologists as to which definition is the best, 50% or greater diameter stenosis (dichotomous) at follow-up angiography is the most commonly used criterion in clinical trials. Depending on the definition used, the same angiographic result can lead to different interpretations of the rate of restenosis (Fig. 93–6).

Alternatively, reporting of the target lesion minimum luminal diameter (MLD) may avoid variation in the interpretation of angiographic restenosis. The difference between the immediate postprocedural MLD and the preprocedural MLD is defined as acute gain, and the difference between the MLD at follow-up and the postprocedural MLD is equal to late loss (Fig. 93–7). Acute gain is the lowest with balloon

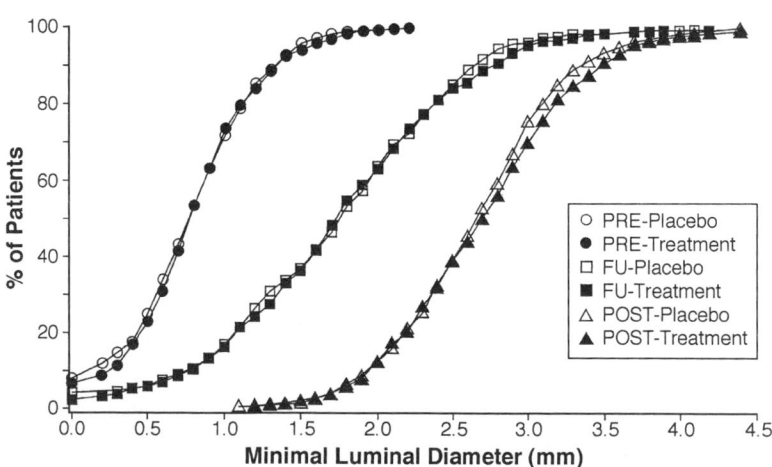

FIG. 93–5. Cumulative distribution curve of the continuous change in minimum luminal diameter from immediately after percutaneous coronary intervention to follow-up in the tranilast group and the control group of the PRESTO study. (From Holmes DR Jr, Savage M, LaBlanche JM. Results of Prevention of REStenosis with Tranilast and its Outcomes (PRESTO) trial. *Circulation* 2002;106:1243–1250, with permission.)

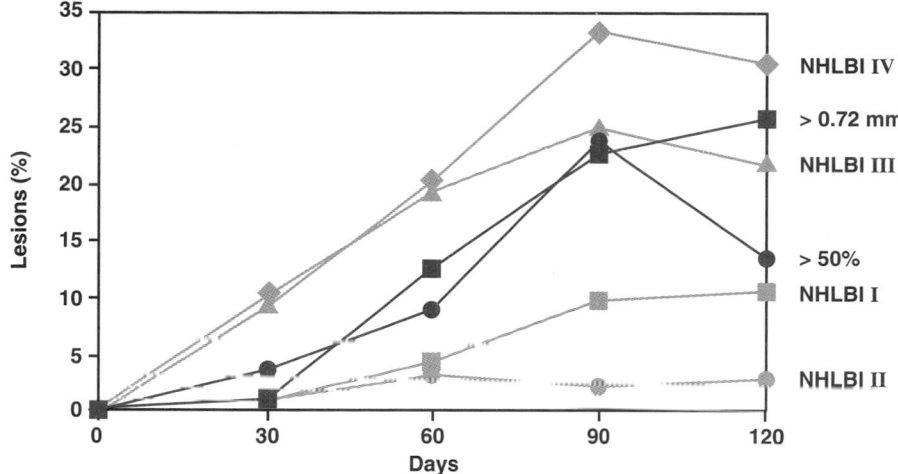

FIG. 93–6. Restenosis rate per lesion according to various restenosis definitions at 30, 60, 90, and 120 days. Variability among definitions is wide throughout the entire time range, but by most criteria restenosis is complete by 3 months after angioplasty. NHLBI, National Heart, Lung and Blood Institute. (Adapted from Serruys PW, Luijten HE, Beatt KJ, et al. Incidence of restenosis after successful coronary angioplasty: a time-related phenomenon. A quantitative angiographic study in 342 consecutive patients at 1, 2, 3, and 4 months. *Circulation* 1988;77:361–371, with permission.) NHLBI, National Heart, Lung and Blood Institute.

angioplasty, which is followed by atherectomy; whereas stents usually achieve the greatest acute gain.

Moreover, visual methods of assessing angiographic stenosis severity are prone to interobserver and intraobserver variability and bias, especially in the midrange (30–70%) of stenosis estimates. It is generally found that simple visual assessment overestimates lesion severity by 15% to 20% when compared with more accurate quantitative methods. Quantitative coronary angiography using either digital calipers or computer-assisted edge-detection system is highly reproducible and is the standard technique used in most contemporary research trials. However, quantitative coronary angiography is not so accurate for the assessment of bifurcation lesions, or in the absence of disease-free reference segments.

Using a simple angiographic definition of restenosis of greater than 50% lumen diameter stenosis, several large, clinical trials with standardized follow-up demonstrated an angiographic restenosis rate of approximately 30% to 50% at 6 months after balloon angioplasty (PTCA) (11–25) and 10% to 30% after stent implantation (22,23,26–36); these values may be greater in clinical practice because the lesions selected for clinical trials were "ideal" lesions. A report from the National Heart, Lung and Blood Institute (NHLBI) PTCA Registry containing follow-up angiography in 84% of 665 patients from 1979 to 1982 cited an angiographic

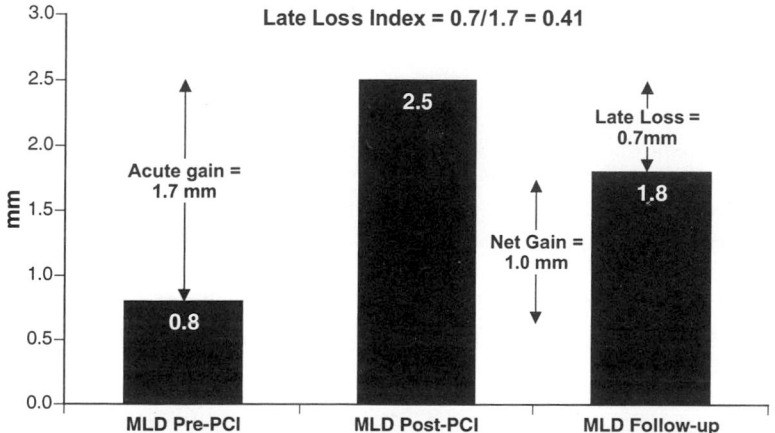

FIG. 93–7. The relation between various indexes of minimum lumen diameter (MLD) (acute gain, late loss, net gain, and late loss index). PCI, percutaneous coronary intervention.

restenosis rate of 34% (37). In the Coronary Angioplasty Versus Excisional Atherectomy Trial (CAVEAT), 53% had angiographic restenosis at 6-month follow-up (16).

Notably, the reported rate is largely dependent on the method and definition adopted by the angiographic core laboratory. For instance, in the CAVEAT trial, the "worst view" method, which reported the angiographic view demonstrating the most severe stenosis was used. When the "average view" was used, the restenosis rate was decreased from 53% to 45%. Although it is uncertain which analysis method is more clinically relevant, these findings have important implications for comparing results among different angiographic trials of restenosis.

Clinical Restenosis

Because all angiographic definitions for restenosis are arbitrary, the importance of restenosis becomes clinically relevant only if it is linked to symptoms or some functional parameters. Coronary artery restenosis may present as angina, exertional dyspnea, a positive stress test, or rarely with myocardial infarction (MI) or sudden cardiac death. Because the process of restenosis is usually gradual, and the newly formed lesion is "stabilized" with fibrous tissue and smooth muscle cells, recurrent angina is the most common presenting feature, whereas MI and sudden death are infrequent (38). The proportion of patients with recurrent chest pain who have angiographically demonstrable restenosis ranges from 48% to 92% (38,39). Hence, the positive predictive value (PPV) of symptoms alone is only moderate. Other difficulties in evaluating restenosis relate to the use of noninvasive modalities (e.g., exercise electrocardiography, nuclear scintigraphy, and stress echocardiography). It is important to understand that to use a noninvasive modality to convincingly demonstrate restenosis, one has to perform the test serially and to demonstrate normalization of the test after index procedure and becoming abnormal during the following months.

Finally, clinical restenosis is roughly correlated with the need of repeat revascularization (either by repeat PCI or bypass surgery). Traditionally, target lesion revascularization has been used in many of the interventional trials designed to test various pharmacologic therapies, whereas target vessel revascularization (TVR) has been used among device trials (e.g., brachytherapy, radioactive stents, and drug-eluting stents) in which the effect of the device on the vessel segment adjacent to the target lesions also needs to be taken consideration for adverse events. More recently, the term *target vessel failure* has become popular, and it refers to repeat vessel revascularization plus death or MI caused by restenosis or reocclusion of the target coronary vessel. In view of the low event rates at follow-up, many clinical trials use a composite of death, MI, and TVR as the primary end point.

Interpretation regarding clinical restenosis rates using this composite end point should be cautious. Early complications including cardiac death or MI may be related to periprocedural complications rather than restenosis. For example, in the Evaluation of Platelet IIb/IIIa Inhibition and Stenting

(EPISTENT) trial, the composite event of death, MI, and TVR was significantly different between stent plus abciximab and stent alone (13.0% vs. 18.3%); however, the rates of repeat revascularization were similar (8.7% and 11.6%, respectively) (40). Likewise, in the Enhanced Suppression of the Platelet IIb/IIIa Receptor with Integrilin Therapy (ESPRIT) (41) trial and the Do Tirofiban and ReoPro Give Similar Efficacy Trial (TARGET) (42,43), the extent of reduction in primary composite death, MI, and revascularization within 30 days and at 6 months did not correlate with the TVR rates at 6 months with "active" treatments. Thus, with different ways to estimate clinical restenosis, reported rates may be as low as 5% to 10% for only major late adverse events or as high as 20% to 30% for all clinical presentation including symptoms.

Silent Restenosis

Because the definition of angiographic restenosis is arbitrary, the incidence of silent restenosis, which is defined by angiographic restenosis without ischemic symptoms, also is variable. Using 50% diameter stenosis as the angiographic restenosis definition, half of the patients with restenosis after PTCA would present with angina, whereas the rest would be defined as having silent restenosis (37,44–49). Besides the arbitrariness of defining angiographic restenosis, absence of symptoms or ischemia on stress test may be caused by less severe coronary obstructions (45,46), vessels supplying nonviable myocardium, presence of diabetes mellitus, or abundant collaterizations (45,47). The long-term prognosis of silent restenosis is uncertain. In one report, Popma and coworkers (45) suggested about half of asymptomatic patients with angiographic restenosis at 6 months would experience symptoms in later months. On the contrary, two studies reported by Kovac and coworkers (50) and Laarman and coworkers (51), respectively, concluded that the majority of patients with documented silent restenosis were event-free over a 3-year period. In summary, the importance of silent restenosis in clinical practice remains controversial.

CLINICAL PRESENTATION OF RESTENOSIS

Timing

Irrespective of the treatment modality of PCI, three events can occur after coronary intervention that may result in ischemic events. First, elastic recoil, which takes place within seconds to hours after PTCA, produces suboptimal angiographic result rather than acute symptoms. Elastic recoil has been largely eliminated in the era of routine stenting. On the other hand, abrupt vessel closure often results in acute MI. Acute stent thrombosis occurs at a rate of about 1% and is present when there is stent malapposition, residual dissection, or hypercoagulable state, despite conventional dual antiplatelet regimen after stenting (52). Stent thrombosis after brachytherapy could occur in months especially with new stent placement, but this appears to be largely resolved with prolongation of antiplatelet therapy (53–55). Strictly speaking, elastic recoil and abrupt vessel closure are not considered to be restenosis. Finally, over the weeks to months after PCI, substantial neointimal growth occurs in 10% to 30% of patients, producing luminal renarrowing and typical angina. This final process is what is generally considered restenosis and, in most cases, is complete within 3 to 4 months after angioplasty (Fig. 93–8).

Serial angiographic studies performed on patients after PTCA by Nobuyoshi and coworkers (56) shed some light on the relative contribution of each step in the restenotic process. Within 24 hours after PTCA, an appreciable loss (>0.5 mm) in lumen diameter was detected in 15% of patients, consistent with lesion recoil or thrombus formation. Of these, approximately half proceeded to restenosis. Within the first month, most lesions remained unchanged or regressed with a mean improvement in lumen diameter. During this period, few (12%) patients were classified as having restenosis. The actuarial patient rate of restenosis increased markedly (from 12% to 43%) between 1 and 3 months and increased only modestly thereafter. From this and other studies using serial angiography (57), it is evident that the majority of restenosis occurs within the first 3 months after balloon angioplasty, and occurrence after 3 to 6 months is infrequent. Joelson and coworkers (58) showed that symptom recurrence more than 6 months after angioplasty usually represented progression of disease in another vessel rather than restenosis. With coronary stents, the time course for restenosis is delayed by 1 to 3 months. Hence, patients who are free of restenosis at 6 to 8 months after coronary stenting are likely to enjoy long-term patency within the index lesion.

Symptoms

Regardless of the device used, the majority of patients who have restenosis experience the gradual return of symptom similar in nature to that occurring before the revascularization procedure. In pooling data of 1,475 patients who presented with recurrent chest pain and underwent angiography, the best correlation of symptom and angiographic restenosis occurred among those presenting within the first 4 months after intervention. Patients (a) with atypical chest pain, (b) with pain different from that before PCI, or (c) early (e.g., within a month) after PCI are unlikely to have restenosis. They may represent cases of incomplete revascularization (37,48,58). Patients presenting beyond 6 to 9 months may have other lesions. Reporting on a portion of the NHLBI PTCA Registry with an 84% angiographic follow-up rate, Holmes and coworkers (37) found that only 56% of patients with definite or probable angina had angiographic restenosis; whereas among patients without chest pain, 14% had restenosis. Thus, the predictive value of recurrent symptoms is modest for restenosis, because of incomplete revascularization, asymptomatic restenosis, and withdrawal bias.

PREDICTORS FOR RESTENOSIS

Evaluation plans after a coronary interventional procedure can be guided by assessing the likelihood of restenosis. However, identification of the risk factors for restenosis in clinical trials has been limited by small sample size in some studies, selection bias from incomplete follow-up, inconsistently

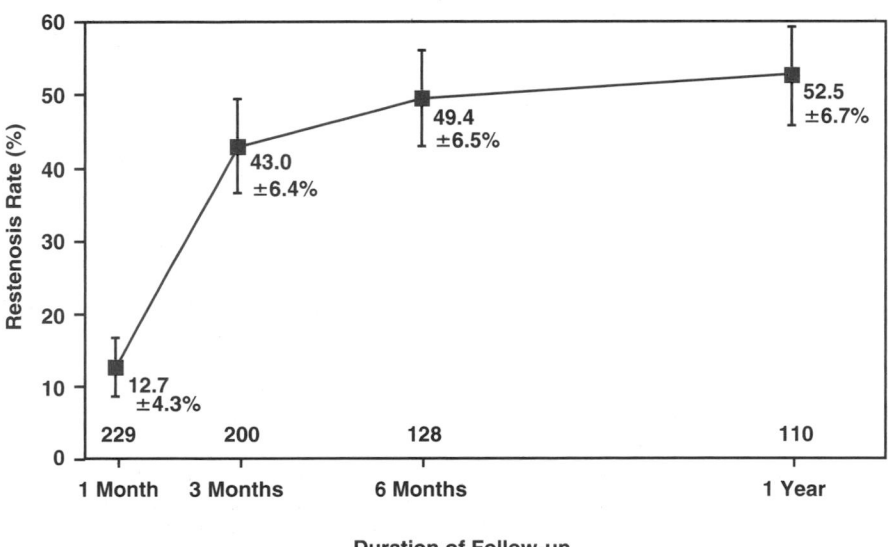

FIG. 93–8. Occurrence of restenosis in 229 patients undergoing serial angiography after coronary angioplasty. Restenosis is expressed as the mean ± 1.96 standard error (95% confidence limits). The numbers above the horizontal line represent the patients at risk at the end of each interval. (Adapted from Nobuyoshi M, Kimura T, Nosaka H, et al. Restenosis after successful percutaneous transluminal coronary angioplasty: serial angiographic follow-up of 229 patients. *J Am Coll Cardiol* 1988;12:616–623, with permission by the American College of Cardiology.)

defined angiographic end points, and retrospective analysis; thus, conclusions have been rather varied among clinical trials. Predictors for restenosis after PTCA, stenting, and brachytherapy also differ. Table 93–2 summarizes the risk factors for restenosis, which can be categorized as those related to the patients, the lesions, and the procedures.

Patient-related Factors

In contrast to the *de novo* coronary lesions, the traditional cardiovascular risk factors (i.e., smoking, hypertension, and hypercholesterolemia) are not associated with a risk for restenosis, except for diabetes mellitus. Patients who have a history of coronary restenosis are more likely to have restenosis. This emphasizes the importance of some patient-

related factors for restenosis (59). However, only diabetes mellitus and presentation of unstable angina are the patient characteristics that have been consistently shown to be predictive for restenosis (37,40,60–72).

Diabetes Mellitus

It is well known that diabetes, especially insulin-dependent diabetes, is a strong risk factor for atherothrombotic heart disease, and it is generally held that diabetes is an important risk factor for restenosis (40,69,70,73–78). Table 93–3 depicts the possible mechanisms for hyperglycemia in causing greater restenosis rates. The risk for restenosis among individuals with diabetes was approximately 1.3 times that of individuals without diabetes after PTCA in the NHLBI data-

TABLE 93–2 *Predictors for restenosis*

Balloon Angioplasty[a]	Bare Metal Stents	Brachytherapy	Drug-Eluting Stents
Clinical factors			
ACE-D genotype	ACE-D genotype	Diabetes mellitus	Diabetes mellitus[b]
Acute coronary syndrome	Acute coronary syndrome	History of restenosis	
Age	Arterial hypertension		
Diabetes mellitus[b]	Diabetes mellitus[b]		
End-staged renal disease	Elevated hsCRP		
History of restenosis	Glycoprotein PI[A] polymorphism		
Hypercholesterolemia	History of restenosis		
Elevated hsCRP	Tobacco use		
Male sex			
Multisite angioplasty			
Prior myocardial infarction			
Variant angina			
Lesion morphology			
Angulated lesion (>45 degrees)	Chronic total occlusion	Long lesion[b]	Long lesion (stent) length[b]
Bifurcation lesion	Left anterior descending	Small vessel diameter	Small vessel diameter[b]
Calcification	Long lesion (stent) length[b]		
Chronic total occlusion[b]	Saphenous vein grafts (especially in proximal segment or degenerated grafts)		
Collateral vessels	Severe preprocedural stenosis or small MLD[b]		
Early restenosis (< 3 months)	Small vessel diameter[b]		
Left anterior descending			
Long lesion[b]			
Ostial location			
Proximal location			
Saphenous vein grafts[b]			
Small vessel diameter			
Severe preprocedural stenosis or small MLD[b]			
Thrombus			
Procedural characteristics			
Abrupt closure	Final MLD by angiography[b]	Geographic miss	
Dissection	Final CSA by IVUS	Restenting	
Duration of balloon inflation	Stent design		
Final MLD[b]	Stent length		
CFR < 2.0–2.5 or FFR < 0.9	Stent material (gold-coated)		

Data from References 37, 40, 59, 61, 64, 66, 67, 70, 73, 75, 77, 83, 85, 111, 112, 119, 120, 146, 147, 150, 151, 166, 167, 170, 174, 180, 193, 195, 202, 204, 207, 211, 221, 226, 228, 230, 231, 292–307.
[a]Include nonstented cases that have undergone atherectomy, excimer laser angioplasty.
[b]Factors that have been consistently demonstrated to be associated with restenosis.
ACE-D, angiotensin-converting enzyme deletion; CSA, cross-sectional area; CFR, coronary flow velocity reserve; FFR, fractional flow reserve; hsCRP, high-sensitivity C-reactive protein; IVUS, intravascular ultrasound; MLD, minimal luminal diameter.

TABLE 93–3 *Pathophysiology of hyperglycemia in causing restenosis*

Endothelial dysfunction	↓ Endothelial-derived relaxation factor ↓ Prostaglandin production ↓ Endothelial cell replication ↓ Platelet-derived relaxation factor ↑ Insulin-like growth factor ↑ Endothelin-1 ↑ Fibroblast growth factor ↑ Transforming growth factor-β
Platelet hyperaggregability and thrombogenicity	Platelet activation ↑ Platelet adhesiveness (↑ thromboxane A_2 synthesis, ↑ fibrinogen) ↑ Macrophage concentration in vessel wall

base. Among the patients with diabetes enrolled in the Bypass Angioplasty Revascularization Investigation (BARI) trial, the 5-year survival rates were 66% after PTCA and 81% after bypass surgery; and the repeat revascularization rate for the PTCA group reached almost 60% at 7 years (Fig. 93–9) (79). In the stent era, diabetes remains an important predictor for restenosis (40,73,75,80), particularly a diffuse-type in-stent restenosis (76). In the EPISTENT, patients with diabetes had almost twice the TVR rate at follow-up after stenting relative to those without diabetes (16.6% vs. 8.8%) (Fig. 93–10) (40). Interestingly, among the patients with diabetes treated with stents, those who were treated with abciximab had a similar TVR rate to those patients without diabetes in the same study. In the largest contemporary coronary stent trial, TARGET, patients with diabetes whose anatomy was considered suitable for PCI still had a greater incidence of TVR at 6 months as compared with the patients without diabetes (10.3% vs. 7.8%) (43,81). Pooling the data of 6,186 patients who were enrolled in multicenter trials also confirmed diabetes as an independent predictor for restenosis after coronary stenting (82). In the Prospective, Randomized Evaluation of the Sirolimus-eluting Stent in Patients with De Novo Coronary Lesions (SIRIUS) trial, diabetes remains an independent predictor for angiographic restenosis (83); however, compared with the bare-metal stent arm, the angiographic restenosis was reduced from 49% to ~8%. Optimal glycemic control (HgbA_1c < 7%) has been associated with a 33% reduction in restenosis rate after coronary stenting among patients with diabetes (84).

Acute Coronary Syndromes

Coronary artery plaque rupture results in exposure of subendothelial tissue and is associated with thrombus formation, platelet activation, and vasoconstriction. This leads to the release and local enrichment of a number of mitogens and cytokines. Vascular injury during balloon angioplasty further increases the number of inflammatory cells in the local tissue, promoting further release of cytokines, growth factors, and metalloproteinases, leading to further neointimal growth and constrictive scarring of the adventitia.

Early studies using balloon angioplasty as the primary revascularization modality reveal that acute coronary syndromes (ACSs) are associated with a 1.2- to 1.7-fold increase in the risk for restenosis, as compared with patients with chronic stable angina (37,66,67,85). Pooling the results of more than 6,000 patients enrolled in coronary stent trials, unstable angina remains as an independent predictor for TVR (82). Among the 4,809 patients enrolled in TARGET (72), ACS was associated with a significantly greater TVR

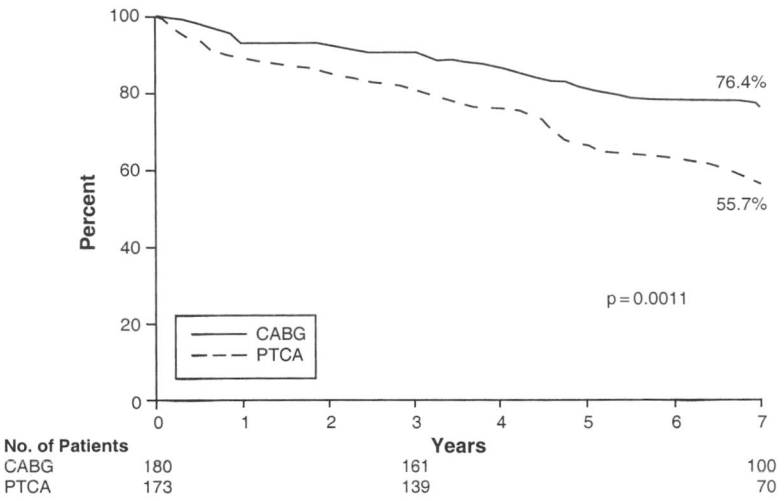

No. of Patients			
CABG	180	161	100
PTCA	173	139	70

FIG. 93–9. Kaplan-Meier curves of the mortality over 7 years of follow-up in the BARI trial. CABG, coronary artery bypass graft; PTCA, percutaneous transluminal coronary angiography. (Adapted from Seven-year outcome in Bypass Angioplasty Revascularization Investigation (BARI) by treatment and diabetic status. *J Am Coll Cardiol* 2000;35:1122–1129, with permission by the American College of Cardiology.)

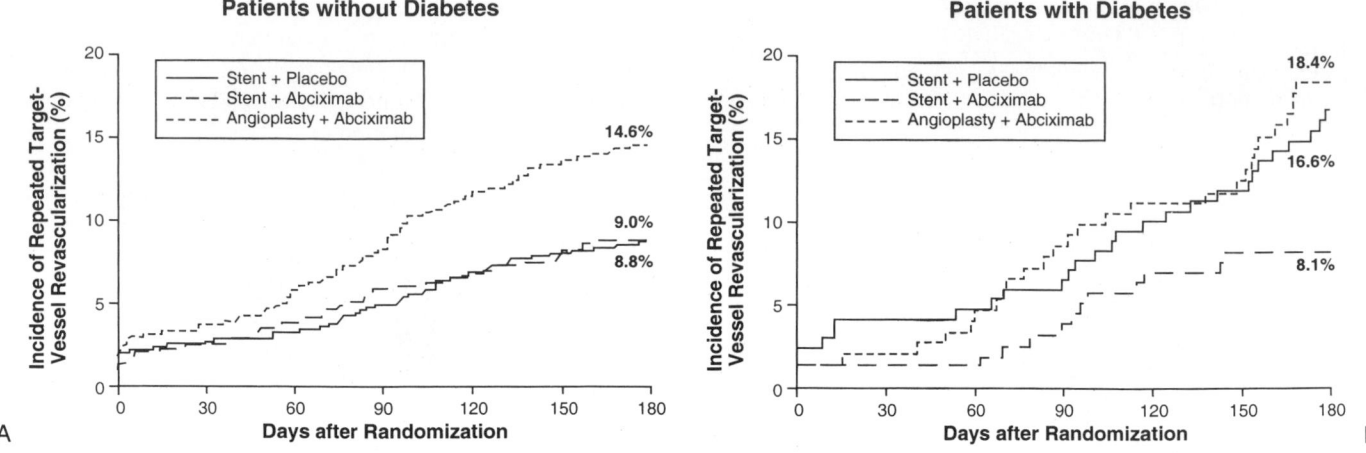

FIG. 93–10. Kaplan-Meier estimates of the target vessel revascularization (TVR) rates within 6 months after randomization in the Evaluation of Platelet IIb/IIIa Inhibition and Stenting (EPISTENT) study among patients with **(A)** and without diabetes **(B)**. Similar to many other studies, diabetes was associated with increased TVR after angioplasty and stenting. However, in this study, patients with diabetes who received abciximab at the time of stenting had a similar rate of TVR as in the patients without diabetes, suggesting profound benefit of abciximab among patients with diabetes undergoing coronary stenting. (From Lincoff AM, Califf AM, Moliterno DJ, et al. Complementary clinical benefits of coronary-artery stenting and blockade of platelet glycoprotein IIb/IIIa receptors. Evaluation of Platelet IIb/IIIa Inhibition in Stenting Investigators. *N Engl J Med* 1999;341:319–327, with permission. Copyright 1999 Massachusetts Medical Society.)

rate at 6 months than patients without ACS (9.7% vs. 7.1%; $p = 0.003$).

Lipoprotein

An association between hypercholesterolemia and restenosis has not been well established. Although various lipoproteins including triglycerides (86), total cholesterol (87), low-density lipoprotein cholesterol, high-density lipoprotein cholesterol (87), and lipoprotein(a) (88–91) have been linked to the risk for restenosis in early studies, these associations were not confirmed in large clinical trials (92–94). Medications used in decreasing low-density lipoprotein cholesterol levels were unsuccessful in decreasing the subsequent risk for restenosis, as evident in three large trials that used angiographic restenosis as the primary end point (17,21,95). Among 1,677 patients randomized in the Lovastatin Intervention Prevention Study (LIPS), a trend toward lower revascularization rate (either bypass surgery or coronary intervention) was reported among patients randomized to statin therapy by 6 months after coronary stenting as compared with placebo (19.8% vs. 23.3%) (96). In summary, whereas lipoprotein levels are related to progression of *de novo* atherothrombotic lesions, any effect of lipoproteins on the process of restenosis is uncertain.

Inflammatory Status

Inflammation plays a pivotal role in the pathogenesis of coronary atherothrombosis and acute coronary events (97–99). C-reactive protein (CRP) reduces nitric oxide production and increases expression of adhesion molecules by endothelial cells (100,101). It also plays a crucial role in chemotaxis of monocytes and foam cell formation in atherothrombotic plaques (102,103). Apart from its direct role in plaque formation, CRP also enhances vasoreactivity of unstable plaques (100,104,105).

Increased baseline high-sensitivity C-reactive protein (hs-CRP) as a measure of the degree of vascular inflammation has been suggested to correlate with recurrent events after PCI, especially in the absence of statin therapy (106–113). Sustained increase of hs-CRP after stent implantation was suggested to correlate with prolonged vascular inflammation, and hence restenosis (108). Although statins have been shown to have no direct effect on decreasing restenosis through its lipid-lowering effect (17,21, 95,96), in two large consecutive series of patients who underwent PCI, patients who received statin and had an increased baseline hs-CRP did have a lower revascularization rate at 1 year compared with those who were not receiving statins (rate of revascularization among statin group vs. nonstatin group in first to third hs-CRP quartiles: 19.0% vs. 18.9%; hs-CRP in fourth quartile: 11.3% vs. 16.7%) (Fig. 93–11). This suggests an interaction of statins and inflammation in attenuating the atherothrombotic process because of inflammation (109,110). Because widespread inflammation and multifocal ulcerative plaques often are present in patients with ACS (97,114), systemic therapy with statins not only has positive impact on the target lesions but also throughout the coronary, and noncoronary, circulation (110). Infective pathogens such as cytomegalovirus or *Chla-*

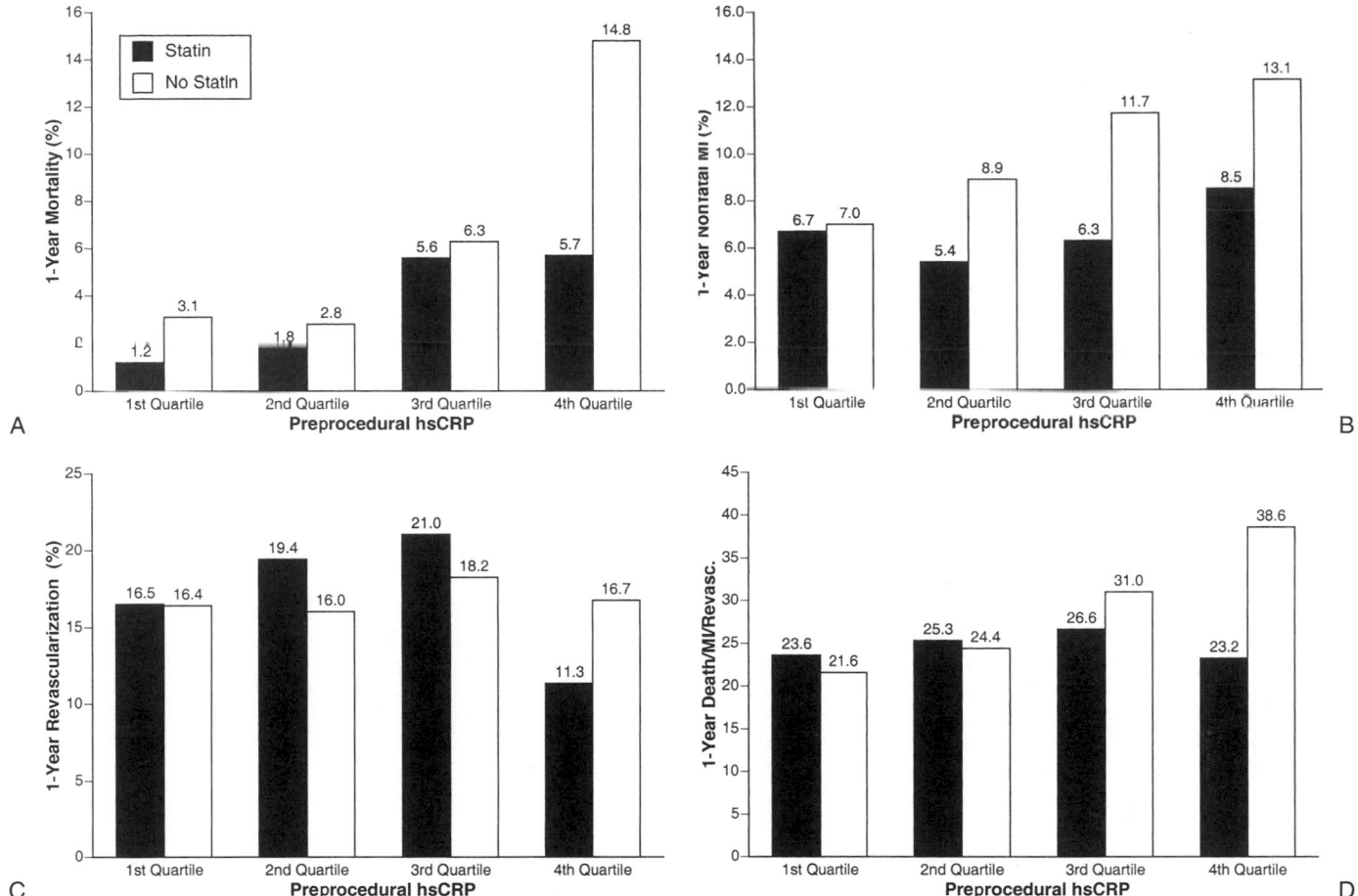

FIG. 93–11. Direct association of the baseline high-sensitivity C-reactive protein (hsCRP) levels with major cardiac adverse events after percutaneous coronary intervention (PCI). HsCRP is a strong predictor for death and myocardial infarction (MI) after PCI. Among patients receiving statins, this association was blunted, and revascularization rate was decreased significantly in high hsCRP levels, suggesting statin effect on reducing the detrimental effect of inflammation on subsequent cardiac events. (Adapted from Chan et al. Relation of inflammatory status and effect of statins following percutaneous coronary interventions. *Circulation* 2003 *(In press)*.)

mydia pneumoniae may be associated with restenosis or accelerated bypass graft closure, but this remains inconclusive (113,115–117).

Genetics

Evidence supports that genetic predisposition may partly explain the increased risk for restenosis (118). Patients with a history of restenosis within a segment of the coronary circulation have a greater propensity of restenosis at another site during subsequent PCI (59,119). Using quantitative analysis of 6-month follow-up angiography among 1,244 patients who underwent coronary stenting, Kastrati and coworkers reported that the presence of a restenotic lesion independently increases likelihood of restenosis of a companion lesion by 2.5-fold after multilesion intervention (120). This suggests there are unidentified factors in each individual other than the conventional clinical and angiographic characteristics that can predict restenosis.

Table 93–4 lists the potential genes that have been reported to be associated with coronary restenosis. Genetic epidemiology studies have shed light on the significance of gene polymorphism in association with restenosis. One of the more frequently studied genes is the insertion/deletion polymorphism of the 287–base pair Alu element in intron 16 of the angiotensin-converting enzyme *(ACE)* gene (121–133). The renin-angiotensin system plays an important role in cell growth and arterial wall repair, and *ACE deletion (D)* allele is associated with atherothrombosis and MI (121,134). Whether *ACE-D* allele is related to restenosis after balloon angioplasty remains controversial, at least partly related to the small size of these studies and publication bias (123,124,135). Although *lipolipoprotein E* genotype itself does not predict restenosis (136), one report observed the presence of both *apolipoprotein E4* genotype and *ACE-D* allele to be associated with a 16-fold increase in the likelihood of restenosis, suggesting an interdependence of polygenic predisposition in restenosis (124). Considering coronary

TABLE 93–4 *Potential genes associated with coronary restenosis*

Candidate genes	Allele	References
Angiotensin-converting enzyme gene polymorphism	*Insertion/Deletion* allele	121–133, 137, 138
	M235T	308
Platelet glycoprotein IIIa polymorphism	*Pl^A* polymorphism	143, 144, 309–311
Human leukocyte antigen-C locus	*Cw1*	312
Apolipoprotein	*Eε4* genotype	88, 124, 136, 313
Endothelial nitric oxide synthase (eNOS) polymorphism	*298Asp* allele of the eNOS Glu298Asp, *786C* allele of the eNOS-786T > C	314

stent implantation, the association *ACE* genotype with restenosis also is inconclusive (126,127,137,138). A meta-analysis reported by Agema and coworkers (139) concluded that no definitive association was present between clinical restenosis and *ACE D/D* homozygous gene (odds ratio [odds ratio], 1.15; 95% confidence interval [CI], 0.98–1.32) (139). It appears that this polymorphism has moderate impact on the cardiovascular response to ACE inhibitors, but there is no consensus as to which allele confers a greater effect. Although ACE inhibition can reduce neointimal hyperplasia in animal models (140), it has not been shown to reduce angiographic restenosis in clinical trials (24,124,129,137,141).

Pl^A polymorphism of glycoprotein IIIa has been linked with both coronary thrombosis and restenosis (142). Among 1,150 patients with angiographic follow-up after coronary stenting, *Pl^A* allele carrier was independently factor associated with restenosis (OR, 1.35; 95% CI, 1.07–1.70), with 53.1% of homozygous *Pl^A* patients having angiographic restenosis (143). Pooled data from six studies confirmed similar findings (144). In summary, it is likely that the

process of restenosis is influenced by multiple genes, which emphasizes the importance of the role of genomic epidemiology studies in further enhancing our understanding and targeting of genetic therapy for restenosis.

Lesion-related Factors

Vessel Diameter

Since the late loss indexes are similar across various revascularization modalities (Fig. 93–8), the greater the reference diameter of the vessel implies a greater luminal diameter at the end of the healing process (145). The inverse relation between vessel size and restenosis has been confirmed in many clinical trials (64,82,146–148). Despite some studies reporting a superior result with stenting as compared with PTCA in large vessels (>2.9mm diameter) and also in small vessels in some studies (≤2.9mm) (22,23), coronary stenting in relatively small vessels has a worse outcome than in large vessels (Fig. 93–12) (148). Metaanalysis of several multicenter random-

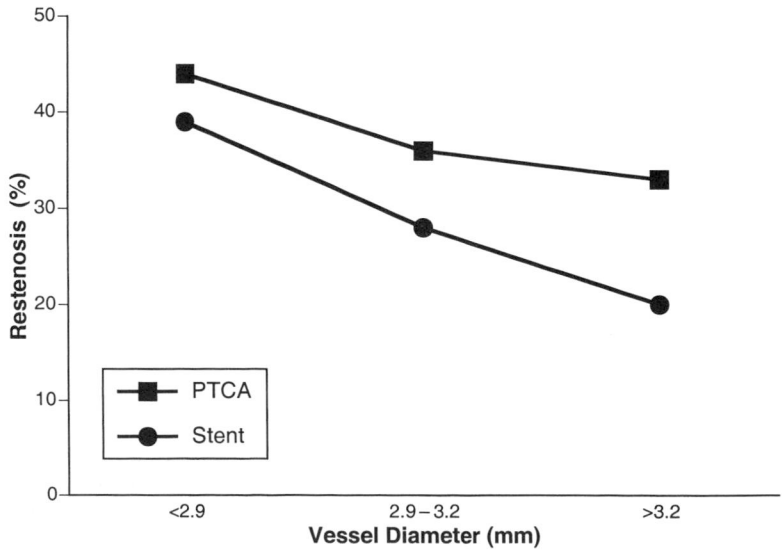

FIG. 93–12. The relation of reference vessel diameter and rate of restenosis after balloon angioplasty or stenting. (Adapted from Hirshfeld JW Jr, Schwartz JS, Jugo R, et al. Restenosis after coronary angioplasty: a multivariate statistical model to relate lesion and procedure variables to restenosis. The M-HEART Investigators. *J Am Coll Cardiol* 1991;18:647–656; and Elezi S, Kastrati A, Neumann FJ, et al. Vessel size and long-term outcome after coronary stent placement. *Circulation* 1998;98:1875–1880, with permission.) PTCA, percutaneous transluminal coronary angiography.

ized clinical trials confirmed reference diameter as a leading independent factor for restenosis (82). Additional risk factors such as diabetes or complex lesion morphology increase the risk for restenosis within small vessels from 30% to more than 50% (148). Vessel diameter also is an independent predictor for re-restenosis among patients randomized in the brachytherapy trials (149,150). Furthermore, vessel diameter is correlated even with restenosis in drug-eluting stents. In the SIRIUS study, the angiographic restenosis rate of the small vessels was 5.3% as compared with 1.9% in large vessel, although the gradient of the differences was much smaller than that observed with the bare stents (83,151).

Recurrent Restenosis

A history of restenosis within the target lesion or elsewhere in the coronary circulation is a predictor of recurrent restenosis (59,119,120,152). Indeed, restenosis rates after the first repeat PTCA range from 25% to 47%, and it ranges between 34% and 69% for a third and fourth PTCA (153–162). The occurrence of restenosis did increase dramatically in patients who underwent the third angioplasty within 3 months of the previous procedure (157,161), and it was greater than 50% after a fourth PTCA (158,163). For instent restenosis, the risk for recurrence of restenosis treated with balloon angioplasty alone also is related to the number of prior interventions within the stent (164,165). Although the risk for recurrent restenosis is halved with the use of adjunctive brachytherapy while treating instent restenosis (166–173), history of multiple episodes of prior instent restenosis is a risk factor for TVR and subacute thrombosis even after γ brachytherapy (174). More recently, drug-eluting stents also show promise as treatment of restenosis after stenting (175–177), and data are continuing to emerge.

Vein Graft

Saphenous vein grafts have a markedly greater rate of restenosis compared with native coronary arteries after balloon angioplasties (146,178–181) (Fig. 93–13). Pooled analysis of 5 interventional trials (EPIC, Evaluation in PTCA to Improve Long-term Outcome with Abcimixab GP IIb/IIIa blockage [EPILOG], EPISTENT, Integrilin to Manage Platelet Aggregation to Prevent Coronary Thrombosis [IMPACT] II, and Platelet Glycoprotein IIb/IIIa in Unstable Angina: Receptor Suppression Using Integrilin Therapy [PURSUIT]) revealed a greater 6-month composite event (death, MI, or TVR; 37.1% vs 25.4%; $p < 0.001$), and TVR (24.5% vs 19.1%; $p = 0.003$) was significantly greater after vein graft intervention (n = 627) as compared with those of native coronary arteries (n = 13,158) (181). Early observational studies suggested some benefits with stents in bypass graft intervention (182–184). In a randomized trial, although stents achieved a significantly greater angiographic success (92% vs. 69%; $p < 0.001$), this initial success did not translate to reduction of angiographic restenosis (37% in stent group vs. 46% in PTCA group at 6

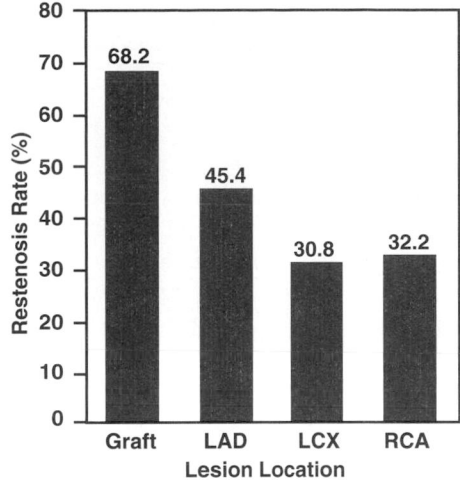

A

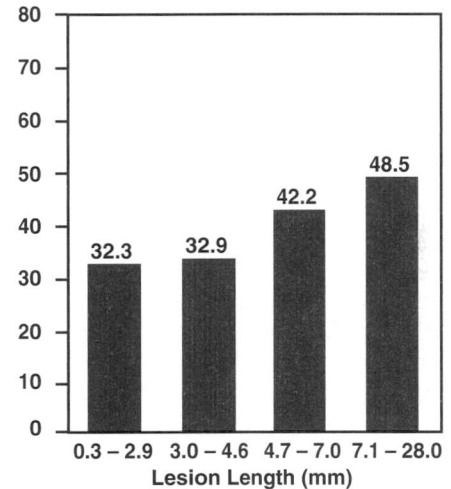

B

FIG. 93–13. Relations of lesion-related variables associated with restenosis among 598 treated sites: lesion location **(A)** and lesion length **(B).** In both panels the height of each column represents the restenosis rate for each group of segregated lesions. In **A,** lesion location, saphenous vein graft conduit *(Graft),* left anterior descending artery *(LAD),* left circumflex artery *(LCX),* right coronary artery *(RCA)* yielded a $\chi^2 p = 0.003$. In **B,** lesion length segregated by quartiles was found to be associated significantly with restenosis, $\chi^2 p = 0.013$, with the rate of stenosis recurrence increasing for lesions greater than 4.6 mm. (Adapted from Hirshfeld JW Jr, Schwartz JS, Jugo R, et al. Restenosis after coronary angioplasty: a multivariate statistical model to relate lesion and procedure variables to restenosis. The M-HEART Investigators. *J Am Coll Cardiol* 1991;18:647–656, with permission.)

months; $p = 0.24$) (185). Age of the vein graft is an important predictor for restenosis, and this is independent of the modality of revascularization (183,186).

Location

The left anterior descending artery (LAD) was associated with about a 30% increase in risk for restenosis after balloon angioplasty (64,146,147) (Fig. 93–13), possibly related to the presence of interventricular muscular septum surrounding the vessel or undersizing of balloon catheter in this large epicardial artery. Because LAD provides major blood supply to the left ventricle, coronary bypass surgery was frequently a consideration if a proximal LAD obstructive lesion was present.

When revascularization other than balloon angioplasty is performed, the association between LAD and restenosis risk becomes more controversial. LAD location was not shown to be associated with restenosis in any of the major coronary atherectomy studies (16,19,145,187–190). Pooling the data from the pivotal U.S. stent approval trials—Stent Restenosis Study (STRESS), Belgian Netherlands Stent (BENE-STENT)-I, BENESTENT-II—vessel diameter rather than LAD location was an independent predictor for restenosis after coronary stenting (23,191,192). In the largest stent trial to date, TARGET, which enrolled 4,809 patients, LAD was an independent predictor for composite of death, MI, or TVR at 6 months among patients with ACS (hazard ratio, 1.55; 95% CI, 1.29–1.86; $p < 0.001$) (72), but not within the non-ACS group. With the use of the newly introduced sirolimus-coated stents, the restenosis risk is essentially ameliorated, and target vessel (LAD vs. non-LAD) is not a consideration for risk for restenosis (83).

Aortoostial lesions are more likely to be associated with a lower immediate angiographic success and greater restenosis risk after balloon angioplasty, probably related to the greater muscular recoil, plaque volume, and fibrotic characteristics of these plaques (193–195). This location becomes a less important consideration when a stent is placed in these lesions. Although some studies have shown that angulated lesions are associated with restenosis (65,196), no data have consistently shown that atherectomy, stenting, or balloon angioplasty alone could provide superior long-term results in these complex lesions relative to one other.

Lesion Length

Prospective clinical trials have consistently demonstrated the association between lesion length and restenosis after balloon angioplasty (Fig. 93–13) (66,146,197). With stents, restenosis risk increased by ~50% among lesions 15 mm or greater in length relative to those less than 15 mm (198). When pooling the data of coronary stent trials, lesion length remains as an independent predictor for restenosis after adjusting for diabetic status, vessel size, stent length, and smoking history (82). Long lesion length may also predict reduced efficacy of radiation in decreasing recurrence rate of instent restenosis (149,199), and even with the use of drug-eluting stents. In the SIRIUS study, instent restenosis rate was increased by 1.6% for every additional 10 mm of implanted stent length (83).

Preprocedural Minimum Luminal Diameter

Compared with lesions with moderate severity, severe lesions contain greater plaque burden and inflammatory cell density,

which, in turn, is associated with thrombogenesis, greater lumen loss, negative remodeling, and neointimal growth (200). Indeed, many studies have consistently shown that the restenosis rate increases with the severity of the stenosis after angioplasty (37,62,63,67,146,197,201). In the Multi-Hospital Eastern Atlantic Restenosis Trial (M-HEART) study, restenosis rate increased from 25% to 44% when comparing lesions 74% or greater in severity with those less than 74% in severity (Fig. 93–14) (146). Two analyses using multivariate predictive models also demonstrated preprocedural MLD was corre-

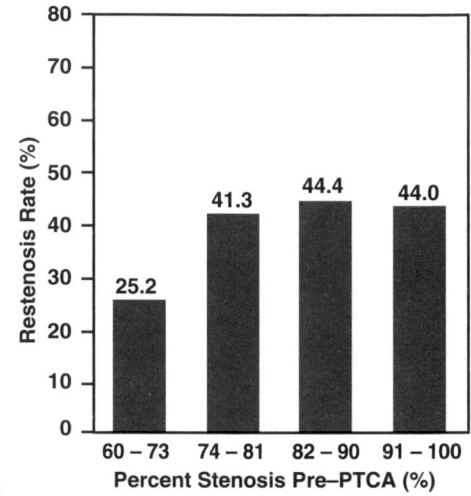

A

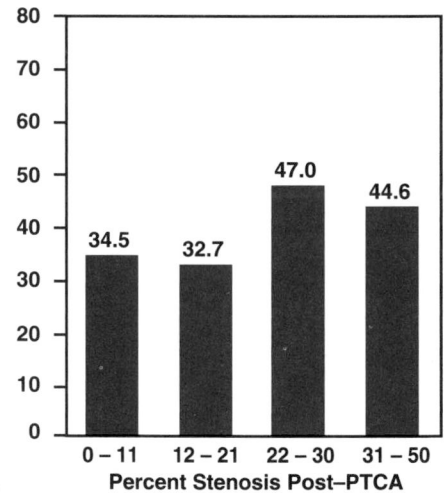

B

FIG. 93–14. Relations of preprocedural **(A)** and postprocedural **(B)** stenosis severity on restenosis among 598 treated sites. In both panels the height of each column represents the restenosis rate for each group of segregated lesions. In **A**, preprocedural stenosis severity was observed to be associated with restenosis (χ^2 $p = 0.004$), with greater restenosis rates among lesions with greater than 73% in lumen diameter narrowing. Similarly, the postprocedural stenosis severity **(B)** was associated with restenosis (χ^2 $p = 0.022$), with a greater incidence of restenosis among lesions with a residual narrowing greater than 21%. (Adapted from Hirshfeld JW Jr, Schwartz JS, Jugo R, et al. Restenosis after coronary angioplasty: a multivariate statistical model to relate lesion and procedure variables to restenosis. The M-HEART Investigators. *J Am Coll Cardiol* 1991;18:647–656, with permission.)

lated with better acute gain but a more significant late loss at follow-up after angioplasty (62,147). Interestingly, in studies involving coronary stents, preprocedural MLD was less consistently associated with restenosis (77,82,156,191,202). In some of these studies, preprocedural lesion severity loses ground as an independent predictor after adjusting for other characteristics.

Chronic total occlusion has been considered as a continuum of this angiographic characteristic in the prediction of restenosis (62). In fact, it has been unequivocally demonstrated as a predictor for restenosis and reocclusion, especially for those that have been occluded for a long period (e.g., >3 months) (203–206). With angioplasty alone, about 40% of patients had recurrence of anginal symptoms after an apparently successful revascularization (206–211), whereas an additional 20% could have silent reocclusion (204,207, 208,210–214). With stents, angiographic restenosis was reduced by ~50% (212,213,215–220).

Procedure-related Factors

Postprocedural Minimum Luminal Diameter

Severity of residual stenosis remains an important predictor for restenosis (66,77,146,191). Kuntz and coworkers (145) proposed "bigger is better" as the main factor that determined the long-term patency with various interventional devices. In the balloon angioplasty era, final residual stenosis was an independent predictor for restenosis in two large registry reports (Fig. 93–14) (66,146). Pooling the results of four MultiLink stent trials, Kereiakes and coworkers (221)

reported postprocedural MLD as the strongest independent predictor for restenosis at 6 to 9 months of follow-up (221). Other investigators also reported the same conclusions using multivariate analyses (77). One remaining issue is whether routine high-pressure inflation with the intention to "oversizing" stents would ensure adequate stent apposition and avoid stent thrombosis. However, with dual antiplatelet protection after stenting, stent thrombosis is infrequent, and oversizing of stents paradoxically may increase restenosis rate, perhaps because of more severe vascular injury (222). More recent studies suggested that residual luminal diameter is irrelevant for predicting restenosis after the use of brachytherapy or drug eluting stents (83,223,224)

Fractional Flow Reserve

Fractional flow reserve (FFR) is calculated as the ratio of distal mean coronary pressure divided by the simultaneous mean aortic pressure during maximal hyperemia. It has been found useful as a "point-of-care" invasive physiologic assessment for restenosis. An FFR greater than 0.90 immediately after angioplasty combining with a diameter stenosis less than 35% was noted to correspond to a lower restenosis rate during follow-up (Fig. 93–15) (225). Among 750 patients undergoing stent implantation, postprocedural FFR is an independent predictor for TVR at 6 months (Fig. 93–15) (226). A FFR greater than 0.94 had a 91% concordance with IVUS for optimal stent apposition and deployment (227). Several studies have illustrated the predictive value of FFR in predicting restenosis after balloon angioplasty and stent,

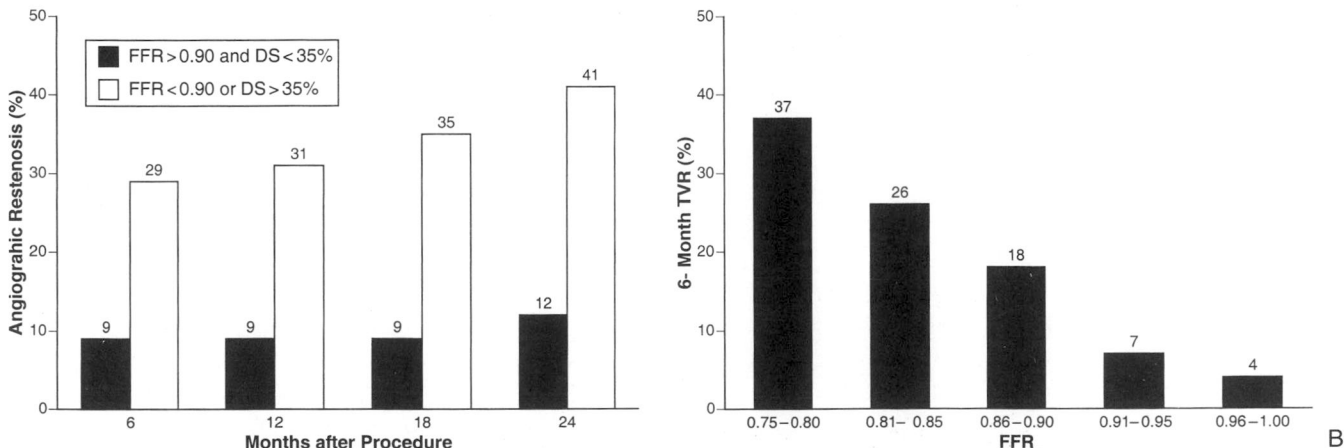

FIG. 93–15. Event-free survival after balloon angioplasty **(left)** and stenting **(right)** according to fractional flow reserve (FFR) parameters. **Left:** Out of 58 patients, 26 patients achieved FFR greater than 0.90 and diameter stenosis (DS) less than 35% after balloon angioplasty. When compared with the 32 patients who did not achieve either one of these two criteria, these 26 patients had a better event-free survival during follow-up. **Right:** Out of a series of 750 patients, FFR was a strong predictor for target vessel revascularization (TVR) at 6 months. When poststent FFR was greater than 0.90, TVR was less than 7%. However, when it was reduced to less than 0.85, TVR was increased to greater than 26%. (Adapted from Bech GJ, Pijls NH, De Bruyne B, et al. Usefulness of fractional flow reserve to predict clinical outcome after balloon angioplasty. *Circulation* 1999;99:883–888; and Pijls NH. Fractional flow reserve after stenting to predict need for repeated target vessel revascularization during follow-up. *J Am Coll Cardiol* 2002;39:34A, with permission.)

although the utilization has been limited because of physicians' preference and improvement in stent design (225, 227,228).

Ultrasound-guided Percutaneous Coronary Intervention

Intravascular ultrasound (IVUS) provides both guidance for optimal stent placement and prediction of restenosis (229–231). Postprocedural CSA was the strongest predictor for restenosis after coronary angioplasty (229) and coronary stenting (230,232–235). Among 425 patients who underwent IVUS-guided stent implantation, Moussa and coworkers (231) reported that the combination of final minimal lumen CSA greater than or equal to 55% of average reference vessel CSA and an absolute CSA of 9 mm² or greater was a strong independent predictor for freedom of restenosis. Although long stent length correlates with restenosis, a CSA greater than or equal to 7 mm² even with long stent length is associated with low restenosis rate (Fig. 93–16) (230). The Restenosis after IVUS-guided Stenting (RESIST) study, the Multicenter Ultrasound Stenting in Coronaries Study (MUSIC), and the Strategy for Intracoronary Ultrasound-guided PTCA and Stenting (SIPS) trial all demonstrated favorable outcome in restenosis with IVUS guidance stent implantation (35,236,237). The amount of plaque burden behind the stent after stent deployment was associated with increased neointimal hyperplasia in one study (238). Nevertheless, in daily practice, routine high-pressure inflation to ensure stent apposition vastly has eliminated IVUS-facilitated stent implantation (239).

Stent Type and Strut Thickness

Stent implantation has become an integral part of contemporary PCI practice, based on the results of the STRESS and BENESTENT trials (22,23). The reported restenosis rates vary among various types of stents, suggesting the importance of stent design in relation to restenosis risk (156, 240–242). During a follow-up of 4,510 consecutive patients after stenting, Kastrati and coworkers (156) reported coronary stent design was the second most important factor in determining restenosis risk.

Several features of the stents may determine restenosis, namely stent type, strut thickness, and covering material. Coiled stent has been found to be inferior to slotted-tube design in maintaining long-term patency (29). The markedly increased restenosis rate at 1 year after gold-coated NIR (Boston Scientific Scimed Inc., Maple Grove, MN) stent placement outweighs the benefits derived from the enhanced radiopacification of the stent (243–245). Furthermore, strut thickness also is an independent factor to determine restenosis, particularly among patients with small coronary vessels (reference diameter <3.0 mm). Out of 821 patients with angiographic follow-up, the restenosis rate was 28.5% in the thin group (<0.1mm) and 36.6% in the thick group (≥0.1mm; $p = 0.009$), and thick strut independently predicted restenosis (OR, 1.68; $p = 0.001$) (246).

Drug-eluting stents (e.g., with sirolimus or paclitaxel coatings, with or without controlled release) provide all the advantages of the bare stents and also reduce intimal proliferation. They bring the TVR rates to less than 5% within the first year after the procedure (83,177,247–258).

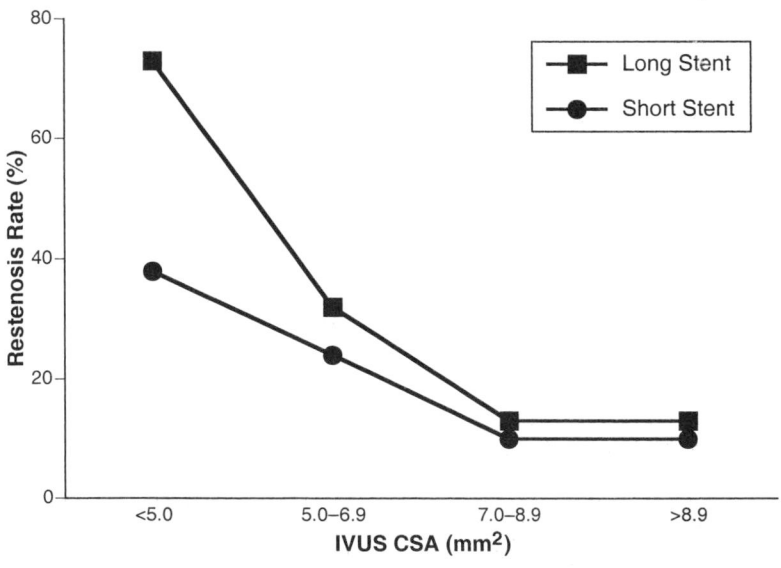

FIG. 93–16. The relation of postprocedural luminal cross-sectional area (CSA) measured by intravascular ultrasound (IVUS) and angiographic restenosis. As the CSA increases, the restenosis rate decreases. This graph also indicates that short stent length (<20 mm; mean, 16 mm) provides more impact than long stent (≥20 mm; mean, 30 mm) in decreasing restenosis rate if the CSA is small. FFR, fractional flow reserve; TVR, target vessel revascularization. (Data from Hong MK, Park SW, Mintz GS, et al. Intravascular ultrasonic predictors of angiographic restenosis after long coronary stenting. *Am J Cardiol* 2000;85:441–445.)

NONINVASIVE EVALUATION OF RESTENOSIS

Invasive versus Noninvasive

Recurrent angina within 9 months of percutaneous coronary revascularization has been adopted by the American College of Cardiology and American Heart Association as a Class 1 indication for repeat coronary angiography (259). As previously mentioned, coronary angiography is the mainstay of definitive diagnosis of restenosis and is the essential tool for evaluating investigational devices. Intravascular ultrasonography and assessment of coronary flow reserve could be used as adjunctive modalities for assessment of intermediate lesions. However, the routine angiography to detect silent restenosis has not been shown beneficial to patients and is not practically or economically feasible for most parts of the world (260). Furthermore, it may lead to many unnecessary interventions. Noninvasive tests hence play an important role among patients with atypical symptoms or asymptomatic patients, because they carry relatively less risk, cost, and time, as compared with coronary angiography. The advantages of an accurate and readily available noninvasive test for restenosis are obvious. The Asymptomatic Cardiac Ischemia Pilot (ACIP) study suggested that revascularization might improve survival among patients with silent ischemia found in exercise or pharmacologic stress testing compared with medical therapy alone, although this study excluded patients with restenosis (261,262). The noninvasive tests that are commercially available for restenosis evaluation include exercise treadmill testing (ETT), exercise or pharmacologic nuclear scintigraphy, stress echocardiography, and positron emission tomography (PET), whereas magnetic resonance angiography or ultrafast computed tomography scanning has not yet been proven valuable for this purpose.

Exercise Treadmill Testing

Myocardial stress testing with exercise electrocardiography is widely available and has moderate sensitivity for detecting myocardial ischemia. Testing in the early PCI setting can be performed relatively safely within days of procedure (263–266), although most clinicians have focused on the 3- to 6-month postprocedure interval, because this is when restenosis typically becomes manifest and predictive accuracy is greater. Factors that limit the sensitivity and specificity of ETT for restenosis include baseline electrocardiographic abnormalities, the extent of atherothrombosis at untreated sites, and an inability to obtain an adequate rate–pressure product. Compounding the issues of reporting the accuracy of noninvasive tests was that there were no well defined criteria for angiographic restenosis. Although the sensitivity of ETT increases with the number of diseased vessels, the sensitivity of detecting restenosis of a single coronary artery is only modest (267). In the Glaxo Restenosis and Symptoms Project (GRASP) trial in which angiography follow-up was used, the sensitivity of patient-reported angina or ST-segment changes on ETT was only 44%, and the specificity was 72% (264). Summarizing 15 treadmill studies totaling 2,249 patients with angiographic follow-up, the PPV ranges from 15% to 89% (mean 50%), and the negative predictive values (NPVs) were 48% to 95% (mean 76%) (Table 93–5) (48,51,264,268–278).

Nuclear Scintigraphy

Nuclear scintigraphy improves predictive values relative to electrocardiography alone for noninvasively assessing restenosis. The radionuclide modalities used in evaluating restenosis include planar thallium-201 myocardial perfusion

TABLE 93–5 *Exercise treadmill testing in the evaluation of restenosis*

First author (reference)	Year	Single-vessel CAD, %	n	Interval from PTCA to ETT, mo	Angiographic restenosis, %	Positive predictive value, %	Negative predictive value, %
Scholl (272)	1982	83	30	6	31	63	83
Ernst (279)	1984	100	25	4–8	16	50	95
Wijns (268)	1985	96	89	6	39	50	65
O'Keefe	1988	56	48	4–8	27	29	73
Honan (269)	1989	57	144	6	40	57	64
Korzick (273)	1990	46	218	7 d to 6 mo	46	40	48
Laarman (51)	1990	100	141	3	12	15	87
Bengston (48)	1990	67	205	6	25	39	84
El-Tamimi (271)	1990	100	31	6	45	93	94
Pirelli (274)	1991	91	75	6	15	29	90
Hillegass (264)	1992	NA	703	6	37	65	79
Roth (275)	1994	100	78	6	28	37	77
Desmet (276)	1995	NA	191	6	33	52	70
Azpitarte (277)	1995	NA	213	6	39	60	72
Pooled			2,249		34	50	76

CAD, coronary artery disease; ETT, exercise treadmill test; NA, not available; PTCA percutaneous transluminal coronary angiography.
References (48,51,264,268–277).

imaging, single-photon emission computed tomography (SPECT) thallium-201 and technetium-99 imaging, and PET.

Pooling the data from 4 studies involving a total of 221 patients, the PPV and NPV of thallium-201 scintigraphy were 63% and 84%, respectively (Table 93–6) (268,272, 279,280). SPECT thallium-201 imaging more effectively localizes the coronary vascular territory of ischemia than planar imaging techniques and may be advantageous in patients with known multivessel coronary artery disease or incomplete revascularization after PCI. Four studies concluded that it had an improved PPV (83%) and NPV (93%) as compared with planar imaging (235,281–284). For patients who could not achieve target heart rate or could not exercise, dobutamine SPECT thallium-201 scanning was found to have similar predictive values as exercise stress nuclear scanning (285). Because of the high accuracy, SPECT imaging is considered the diagnostic tool of choice for detecting restenosis.

PET and isonitrile imaging also are sensitive tools for detecting restenosis. Apart from assessing myocardial perfusion, PET scanning using Rb-82 and nitrogen-13 ammonia uptake may also provide precise information on regional myocardial metabolism (286). Although the technology has superior accuracy in assessing myocardial perfusion and viability, its availability is limited to some selected centers.

Stress Echocardiography

The relatively low cost and easy availability are the main advantages of stress echocardiography in clinical practice for assessment of myocardial ischemia, including coronary restenosis. However, the accuracy of stress echocardiography relies on interpreters' experience. Several studies have been completed on exercise and pharmacologic stress echocardiography (Table 93–6) (287–290). In a study from Duke University (Durham, NC) (289), the sensitivity and specificity of dobutamine echocardiography in detecting restenosis were 38% and 79%, respectively. The restenosis rate and the high prevalence in the single-vessel disease cohort may explain the low predictive value. In another study by Hecht and coworkers (288), using supine bicycle stress echocardiography to detect restenosis among 129 treated sites in 80 patients, the sensitivity and specificity were 87% and 95%, respectively.

CONCLUSIONS AND FUTURE PERSPECTIVES

With the refinement in the interventional technology and improvement in pharmacology over the last quarter century, the number of patients undergoing PCI has been increasing and the types of lesions receiving treatment are becoming more complex (long lesions, small vessels, ostial lesions, bifurca-

TABLE 93–6 *Nuclear scintigraphy and echocardiographic stress test in evaluation of restenosis*

First author (reference)	Year	n	Interval from PCI to stress test	Angiographic restenosis, %	Sensitivity, %	Specificity, %	PPV, %	NPV, %
Planar thallium-201								
Scholl (272)	1982	36	1 mo	31	77	100	100	82
Wijns (268)	1985	89	1mo	39	74	83	74	83
Ernst (279)	1985	25	4–8 mo	16	100	81	50	100
Hardoff (280)	1990	71	1 d	32	77	67	53	86
Total		221		33	76	77	63	84
SPECT thallium-201								
Jain (315)	1988	22	3 d	33	77	88	77	88
Breisblatt (281)	1988	121	3–13 mo	33	98	96	93	93
Hecht (282)	1990	116	3–9 mo	46	93	74	80	92
Marie (283)	1993	62	5–7 mo	26	94	84	68	98
Total		321		36	91	87	83	93
SPECT technetium-201								
Milan (316)	1996	37	NA	53	75	74	81	86
Georgoulias (278)	1998	41	6 mo	39	81	88	77	90
Total		78		46	78	81	79	88
Echocardiography								
Aboul-Enein (287)[a]	1991	101	6 mo	47	67	83	78	73
Hecht (288)[a]	1993	80	3–9 mo	56	87	95	95	85
Heinle (289)[b]	1993	103	6 mo	44	38	79	59	62
Takeuchi (290)[b]	1995	53	5 mo	43	78	93	87	85
Total		337		47	66	86	81	74
Pooled		957		40	77	84	76	84

NA, not applicable; NPV, negative predictive value; PCI, percutaneous coronary intervention; PPV, positive predictive value; SPECT, single-photon emission computed tomography.

[a]Exercise stress echocardiography.
[b]Dobutamine stress echocardiography.

tions, left main coronary lesions). Several different types of restenosis exist—angiographic, clinical, and silent—and each of these has several different definitions. In general, the process of restenosis is complete within 4 to 6 months after angioplasty or atherectomy alone, 6 to 9 months after stenting, and may be up to 3 years after brachytherapy. The model of restenosis in drug-eluting stents needs to be defined. With about 80% of patients receiving stents, angiographic restenosis occurs in 30% of patients, clinical restenosis in 10% to 20%, and silent restenosis in about 10%. The introduction of drug-eluting stents markedly reduces each of these values to less than 5%, and this is becoming the new reference standard for comparison of new interventional devices.

The majority of the patients having restenosis have recurrent angina, and those with MI represents a minority. Limitations of studying restenosis clinically stem from the modest predictive value of symptoms alone and significant selection and withdrawal bias in angiographic studies. The list of pharmacologic and mechanical therapies studied in an attempt to reduce the occurrence of restenosis is extensive and, unfortunately, nearly all have failed. The number of patients with restenosis has been increasing with the diversity of lesions attempted. Brachytherapy successfully halves the recurrence of instent restenosis, and subsequently decreases the number of patients returning to the catheterization laboratory. The introduction of drug-eluting stents proves to be a major step forward to eliminate restenosis and may possibly be beneficial for treatment of instent restenosis. These stents target the key mechanisms of restenosis—early elastic recoil, thrombus organization, negative remodeling, and neointimal hyperplasia.

The evaluation of patients in whom restenosis is suspected can begin with a consideration of patient-, lesion-, and procedure-related factors that have been associated with an increased risk for restenosis. The four major predictive factors that have consistently been identified for restenosis include diabetes mellitus, vessel diameter, postprocedural diameter, and lesion length. Although ACS and increased inflammatory status were observed in many studies as a predictor for restenosis after stents, target lesion in LAD has lost the importance with stent placement. Large-scale genomic sequencing and genetic epidemiology studies are underway to identify genes correlating with restenosis.

Recurrence of symptoms and exercise electrocardiography test are only modestly reliable for detecting restenosis. SPECT sestamibi imaging and stress echocardiography improve the PPVs of the assessment. Despite these tests, alone or in combination, the greatest PPVs on average reach only 80%. New imaging techniques such as magnetic resonance angiography may have a role in the future but will remain investigational within the next few years. For now, invasive assessment with contrast angiography remains the gold standard.

Although general recommendations for evaluating patients after interventional cardiology procedures can be made, our approach is to individualize follow-up care. For patients who have a relatively low risk for restenosis—that is, no or one associated risk and a small area of myocardium of risk—simple clinical follow-up for symptom recurrence is acceptable providing the patient has had symptoms of ischemia before revascularization procedure. On the other hand, patients who have several known factors associated with an increased risk restenosis or who have a substantial area of myocardium at risk should undergo stress perfusion imaging 4 to 6 months after coronary intervention. In cases where these tests are positive and repeat revascularization is appropriate, coronary angiography should be performed. Although moving into the era of routine "drug-eluting stenting," this strategy may become less important. New approaches for follow-up evaluation of restenosis may need to be established as the incidence of restenosis diminishes.

REFERENCES

1. Gruentzig A. Transluminal dilatation of coronary-artery stenosis. *Lancet* 1978;1:263.
2. American Heart Association. *2001 heart and stroke statistical update.* Dallas, Texas: American Heart Association. Available at: http://www.americanheart.org/statistics/index.html.
3. Le Breton H, Plow EF, Topol EJ. Role of platelets in restenosis after percutaneous coronary revascularization. *J Am Coll Cardiol* 1996;28: 1643–1651.
4. Lindner V, Reidy MA. Expression of basic fibroblast growth factor and its receptor by smooth muscle cells and endothelium in injured rat arteries. An en face study. *Circ Res* 1993;73:589–595.
5. Shimokawa H, Ito A, Fukumoto Y, et al. Chronic treatment with interleukin-1 beta induces coronary intimal lesions and vasospastic responses in pigs in vivo. The role of platelet- derived growth factor. *J Clin Invest* 1996;97:769–776.
6. Clowes AW, Reidy MA, Clowes MM. Kinetics of cellular proliferation after arterial injury. I. Smooth muscle growth in the absence of endothelium. *Lab Invest* 1983;49:327–333.
7. Schwartz RS, Huber KC, Murphy JG, et al. Restenosis and the proportional neointimal response to coronary artery injury: results in a porcine model. *J Am Coll Cardiol* 1992;19:267–274.
8. Forrester JS, Fishbein M, Helfant R, et al. A paradigm for restenosis based on cell biology: clues for the development of new preventive therapies. *J Am Coll Cardiol* 1991;17:758–769.
9. Chung I, Gold HK, Schwartz SM, et al. Enhanced extracellular matrix accumulation in restenosis of coronary arteries after stent deployment. *J Am Coll Cardiol* 2002;40:2072–2081.
10. Glagov S, Weisenberg E, Zarins CK, et al. Compensatory enlargement of human atherosclerotic coronary arteries. *N Engl J Med* 1987;316:1371–1375.
11. Schwartz L, Bourassa MG, Lesperance J, et al. Aspirin and dipyridamole in the prevention of restenosis after percutaneous transluminal coronary angioplasty. *N Engl J Med* 1988;318:1714–1719.
12. Ellis SG, Roubin GS, Wilentz J, et al. Effect of 18- to 24-hour heparin administration for prevention of restenosis after uncomplicated coronary angioplasty. *Am Heart J* 1989;117:777–782.
13. Pepine CJ, Hirshfeld JW, Macdonald RG, et al. A controlled trial of corticosteroids to prevent restenosis after coronary angioplasty. M-HEART Group. *Circulation* 1990;81:1753–1761.
14. Knudtson ML, Flintoft VF, Roth DL, et al. Effect of short-term prostacyclin administration on restenosis after percutaneous transluminal coronary angioplasty. *J Am Coll Cardiol* 1990;15:691–697.
15. Adelman AG, Cohen EA, Kimball BP, et al. A comparison of directional atherectomy with balloon angioplasty for lesions of the left anterior descending coronary artery. *N Engl J Med* 1993;329:228–233.
16. Topol EJ, Leya F, Pinkerton CA, et al. A comparison of directional atherectomy with coronary angioplasty in patients with coronary artery disease. The CAVEAT Study Group. *N Engl J Med* 1993;329:221–227.
17. Weintraub WS, Boccuzzi SJ, Klein JL, et al. Lack of effect of lovastatin on restenosis after coronary angioplasty. Lovastatin Restenosis Trial Study Group. *N Engl J Med* 1994;331:1331–1337.

18. Savage MP, Goldberg S, Bove AA, et al. Effect of thromboxane A2 blockade on clinical outcome and restenosis after successful coronary angioplasty. Multi-Hospital Eastern Atlantic Restenosis Trial (M-HEART II). *Circulation* 1995;92:3194–3200.

19. Baim DS, Cutlip DE, Sharma SK, et al. Final results of the Balloon vs Optimal Atherectomy Trial (BOAT). *Circulation* 1998;97:322–331.

20. Gibson CM, Goel M, Cohen DJ, et al. Six-month angiographic and clinical follow-up of patients prospectively randomized to receive either tirofiban or placebo during angioplasty in the RESTORE trial. Randomized Efficacy Study of Tirofiban for Outcomes and Restenosis. *J Am Coll Cardiol* 1998;32:28–34.

21. Serruys PW, Foley DP, Jackson G, et al. A randomized placebo-controlled trial of fluvastatin for prevention of restenosis after successful coronary balloon angioplasty; final results of the fluvastatin angiographic restenosis (FLARE) trial. *Eur Heart J* 1999;20:58–69.

22. Serruys PW, de Jaegere P, Kiemeneij F, et al. A comparison of balloon-expandable-stent implantation with balloon angioplasty in patients with coronary artery disease. Benestent Study Group. *N Engl J Med* 1994;331:489–495.

23. Fischman DL, Leon MB, Baim DS, et al. A randomized comparison of coronary-stent placement and balloon angioplasty in the treatment of coronary artery disease. Stent Restenosis Study Investigators. *N Engl J Med* 1994;331:496–501.

24. Faxon DP. Effect of high dose angiotensin-converting enzyme inhibition on restenosis: final results of the MARCATOR Study, a multicenter, double-blind, placebo-controlled trial of cilazapril. The Multicenter American Research Trial With Cilazapril After Angioplasty to Prevent Transluminal Coronary Obstruction and Restenosis (MARCATOR) Study Group. *J Am Coll Cardiol* 1995;25:362–369.

25. Franzen D, Schannwell M, Oette K, et al. A prospective, randomized, and double-blind trial on the effect of fish oil on the incidence of restenosis following PTCA. *Cathet Cardiovasc Diagn* 1993;28:301–310.

26. Serruys PW, van Hout B, Bonnier H, et al. Randomised comparison of implantation of heparin-coated stents with balloon angioplasty in selected patients with coronary artery disease (Benestent II). *Lancet* 1998;352:673–681.

27. Baim DS, Cutlip DE, Midei M, et al. Final results of a randomized trial comparing the MULTI-LINK stent with the Palmaz-Schatz stent for narrowings in native coronary arteries. *Am J Cardiol* 2001;87:157–162.

28. Baim DS, Cutlip DE, O'Shaughnessy CD, et al. Final results of a randomized trial comparing the NIR stent to the Palmaz-Schatz stent for narrowings in native coronary arteries. *Am J Cardiol* 2001;87:152–156.

29. Lansky AJ, Roubin GS, O'Shaughnessy CD, et al. Randomized comparison of GR-II stent and Palmaz-Schatz stent for elective treatment of coronary stenoses. *Circulation* 2000;102:1364–1368.

30. Neumann FJ, Kastrati A, Schmitt C, et al. Effect of glycoprotein IIb/IIIa receptor blockade with abciximab on clinical and angiographic restenosis rate after the placement of coronary stents following acute myocardial infarction. *J Am Coll Cardiol* 2000;35:915–921.

31. Acute platelet inhibition with abciximab does not reduce in-stent restenosis (ERASER study). The ERASER Investigators. *Circulation* 1999;100:799–806.

32. Meneveau N, Schiele F, Grollier G, et al. Local delivery of nadroparin for the prevention of neointimal hyperplasia following stent implantation: results of the IMPRESS Trial. A multicentre, randomized, clinical, angiographic and intravascular ultrasound study. *Eur Heart J* 2000;21:1767–1775.

33. Kiesz RS, Buszman P, Martin JL, et al. Local delivery of enoxaparin to decrease restenosis after stenting: results of initial multicenter trial: Polish-American Local Lovenox NIR Assessment Study (The POLONIA Study). *Circulation* 2001;103:26–31.

34. Heuser R, Lopez A, Kuntz R, et al. SMART: The microstent's ability to limit restenosis trial. *Catheter Cardiovasc Interv* 2001;52:269–277.

35. Frey AW, Hodgson JM, Muller C, et al. Ultrasound-guided strategy for provisional stenting with focal balloon combination catheter: results from the randomized Strategy for Intracoronary Ultrasound-guided PTCA and Stenting (SIPS) trial. *Circulation* 2000;102:2497–2502.

36. Serruys PW, Foley DP, Hofling B, et al. Carvedilol for prevention of restenosis after directional coronary atherectomy: final results of the European carvedilol atherectomy restenosis (EUROCARE) trial. *Circulation* 2000;101:1512–1518.

37. Holmes DR, Vlietstra RE, Smith HC, et al. Restenosis after percutaneous transluminal coronary angioplasty (PTCA): a report from the PTCA registry of the National Heart, Lung, and Blood Institute. *Am J Cardiol* 1984;53:77C–81C.

38. Piessens JH, Stammen F, Desmet W, et al. Immediate and 6-month follow-up results of coronary angioplasty for restenosis: analysis of factors predicting recurrent clinical restenosis. *Am Heart J* 1993;126:565–570.

39. Simonton CA, Mark DB, Hinohara T, et al. Late restenosis after emergent coronary angioplasty for acute myocardial infarction: comparison with elective coronary angioplasty. *J Am Coll Cardiol* 1988;11:698–705.

40. Lincoff AM, Califf RM, Moliterno DJ, et al. Complementary clinical benefits of coronary-artery stenting and blockade of platelet glycoprotein IIb/IIIa receptors. Evaluation of Platelet IIb/IIIa Inhibition in Stenting Investigators. *N Engl J Med* 1999;341:319–327.

41. O'Shea JC, Hafley GE, Greenberg S, et al. Platelet glycoprotein IIb/IIIa integrin blockade with eptifibatide in coronary stent intervention: the ESPRIT trial: a randomized controlled trial. *JAMA* 2001;285:2468–2473.

42. Topol EJ, Moliterno DJ, Herrmann HC, et al. Comparison of two platelet glycoprotein IIb/IIIa inhibitors, tirofiban and abciximab, for the prevention of ischemic events with percutaneous coronary revascularization. *N Engl J Med* 2001;344:1888–1894.

43. Moliterno DJ, Yakubov SJ, DiBattiste PM, et al. Outcomes at 6 months for the direct comparison of tirofiban and abciximab during percutaneous coronary revascularisation with stent placement: the TARGET follow-up study. *Lancet* 2002;360:355–360.

44. Levine S, Ewels CJ, Rosing DR, et al. Coronary angioplasty: clinical and angiographic follow-up. *Am J Cardiol* 1985;55:673–676.

45. Popma JJ, van den Berg EK, Dehmer GJ. Long-term outcome of patients with asymptomatic restenosis after percutaneous transluminal coronary angioplasty. *Am J Cardiol* 1988;62:1298–1299.

46. Vetrovec GW, DiSciascio G, Hugo R. Comparative clinical and angiographic findings in patients with symptomatic and asymptomatic restenosis following angioplasty. *J Am Coll Cardiol* 1990;15:59A(abst).

47. Hernandez RA, Macaya C, Iniguez A, et al. Midterm outcome of patients with asymptomatic restenosis after coronary balloon angioplasty. *J Am Coll Cardiol* 1992;19:1402–1409.

48. Bengtson JR, Mark DB, Honan MB, et al. Detection of restenosis after elective percutaneous transluminal coronary angioplasty using the exercise treadmill test. *Am J Cardiol* 1990;65:28–34.

49. Mata LA, Bosch X, David PR, et al. Clinical and angiographic assessment 6 months after double vessel percutaneous coronary angioplasty. *J Am Coll Cardiol* 1985;6:1239–1244.

50. Kovac JD, Brack MJ, Harley A, et al. Longer-term clinical outcome in patients presenting with asymptomatic restenosis at 4 month trial angiography (abstract). *Circulation* 1995;92:I-347.

51. Laarman G, Luijten HE, van Zeyl LG, et al. Assessment of "silent" restenosis and long-term follow-up after successful angioplasty in single vessel coronary artery disease: the value of quantitative exercise electrocardiography and quantitative coronary angiography. *J Am Coll Cardiol* 1990;16:578–585.

52. Cutlip DE, Baim DS, Ho KK, et al. Stent thrombosis in the modern era: a pooled analysis of multicenter coronary stent clinical trials. *Circulation* 2001;103:1967–1971.

53. Waksman R, Ajani AE, Kim HS, et al. Is 6 months of plavix enough to prevent late total occlusion after gamma radiation for in-stent restenosis? *J Am Coll Cardiol* 2001;37:14A.

54. Waksman R, Ajani AE, Pinnow E, et al. Twelve versus six months of clopidogrel to reduce major cardiac events in patients undergoing gamma-radiation therapy for in-stent restenosis: Washington Radiation for In-Stent restenosis Trial (WRIST) 12 versus WRIST PLUS. *Circulation* 2002;106:776–778.

55. Waksman R, Ajani AE, White RL, et al. Prolonged antiplatelet therapy to prevent late thrombosis after intracoronary gamma-radiation in patients with in-stent restenosis: Washington Radiation for In-Stent Restenosis Trial Plus 6 Months of Clopidogrel (WRIST PLUS). *Circulation* 2001;103:2332–2335.

56. Nobuyoshi M, Kimura T, Ohishi H, et al. Restenosis after percutaneous transluminal coronary angioplasty: pathologic observations in 20 patients. *J Am Coll Cardiol* 1991;17:433–439.

57. Serruys PW, Luijten HE, Beatt KJ, et al. Incidence of restenosis after successful coronary angioplasty: a time-related phenomenon. A quantitative angiographic study in 342 consecutive patients at 1, 2, 3, and 4 months. *Circulation* 1988;77:361–371.

58. Joelson JM, Most AS, Williams DO. Angiographic findings when

chest pain recurs after successful percutaneous transluminal coronary angioplasty. *Am J Cardiol* 1987;60:792–795.

59. Weintraub WS, Brown CL, Liberman HA, et al. Effect of restenosis at one previously dilated coronary site on the probability of restenosis at another previously dilated coronary site. *Am J Cardiol* 1993;72:1107–1113.
60. Myler RK, Topol EJ, Shaw RE, et al. Multiple vessel coronary angioplasty: classification, results, and patterns of restenosis in 494 consecutive patients. *Cathet Cardiovasc Diagn* 1987;13:1–15.
61. Weintraub WS, Kosinski AS, Brown CL 3rd, et al. Can restenosis after coronary angioplasty be predicted from clinical variables? *J Am Coll Cardiol* 1993;21:6–14.
62. Rensing BJ, Hermans WR, Deckers JW, et al. Which angiographic variable best describes functional status 6 months after successful single-vessel coronary balloon angioplasty? *J Am Coll Cardiol* 1993;21:317–324.
63. Lambert M, Bonan R, Cote G, et al. Multiple coronary angioplasty: a model to discriminate systemic and procedural factors related to restenosis. *J Am Coll Cardiol* 1988;12:310–314.
64. Weintraub WS, Douglas JS Jr, Ghazzal Z, et al. Evaluation and prediction of clinical restenosis. *Circulation* 1996;94:I-90(abst).
65. Hermans WR, Foley DP, Rensing BJ, et al. Usefulness of quantitative and qualitative angiographic lesion morphology, and clinical characteristics in predicting major adverse cardiac events during and after native coronary balloon angioplasty. CARPORT and MERCATOR Study Groups. *Am J Cardiol* 1993;72:14–20.
66. Bourassa MG, Lesperance J, Eastwood C, et al. Clinical, physiologic, anatomic and procedural factors predictive of restenosis after percutaneous transluminal coronary angioplasty. *J Am Coll Cardiol* 1991;18:368–376.
67. Leimgruber PP, Roubin GS, Hollman J, et al. Restenosis after successful coronary angioplasty in patients with single-vessel disease. *Circulation* 1986;73:710–717.
68. Maresta A, Balducelli M, Cantini L, et al. Trapidil (triazolopyrimidine), a platelet-derived growth factor antagonist, reduces restenosis after percutaneous transluminal coronary angioplasty. Results of the randomized, double-blind STARC study. Studio Trapidil versus Aspirin nella Restenosi Coronarica. *Circulation* 1994;90:2710–2715.
69. Carrozza JP Jr, Kuntz RE, Fishman RF, et al. Restenosis after arterial injury caused by coronary stenting in patients with diabetes mellitus. *Ann Intern Med* 1993;118:344–349.
70. Abizaid A, Mehran R, Bucher TA, et al. Does diabetes influence clinical recurrence after coronary stent implantation? *J Am Coll Cardiol* 1996;27:528–535.
71. Moustapha A, Assali AR, Sdringola S, et al. Percutaneous and surgical interventions for in-stent restenosis: long-term outcomes and effect of diabetes mellitus. *J Am Coll Cardiol* 2001;37:1877–1882.
72. Stone GW, Moliterno DJ, Bertrand M, et al. Impact of clinical syndrome acuity on the differential response to 2 glycoprotein IIb/IIIa inhibitors in patients undergoing coronary stenting: The TARGET Trial. *Circulation* 2002;105:2347–2354.
73. Abizaid A, Kornowski R, Mintz GS, et al. The influence of diabetes mellitus on acute and late clinical outcomes following coronary stent implantation. *J Am Coll Cardiol* 1998;32:584–589.
74. Aronson D, Bloomgarden Z, Rayfield EJ. Potential mechanisms promoting restenosis in diabetic patients. *J Am Coll Cardiol* 1996;27:528–535.
75. Elezi S, Kastrati A, Pache J, et al. Diabetes mellitus and the clinical and angiographic outcome after coronary stent placement. *J Am Coll Cardiol* 1998;32:1866–1873.
76. Lee SG, Lee CW, Hong MK, et al. Predictors of diffuse-type in-stent restenosis after coronary stent implantation. *Catheter Cardiovasc Interv* 1999;47:406–409.
77. Kastrati A, Schomig A, Elezi S, et al. Predictive factors of restenosis after coronary stent placement. *J Am Coll Cardiol* 1997;30:1428–1436.
78. Klugherz BD, Meneveau NF, Kolansky DM, et al. Predictors of clinical outcome following percutaneous intervention for in-stent restenosis. *Am J Cardiol* 2000;85:1427–1431.
79. Seven-year outcome in the Bypass Angioplasty Revascularization Investigation (BARI) by treatment and diabetic status. *J Am Coll Cardiol* 2000;35:1122–1129.
80. Serruys PW, Unger F, Sousa JE, et al. Comparison of coronary-artery bypass surgery and stenting for the treatment of multivessel disease. *N Engl J Med* 2001;344:1117–1124.

81. Roffi M, Moliterno DJ, Meier B, et al. Impact of different platelet glycoprotein IIb/IIIa receptor inhibitors among diabetic patients undergoing percutaneous coronary intervention: Do Tirofiban and ReoPro Give Similar Efficacy Outcomes Trial (TARGET) 1-year follow-up. *Circulation* 2002;105:2730–2736.
82. Cutlip DE, Chauhan MS, Baim DS, et al. Clinical restenosis after coronary stenting: perspectives from multicenter clinical trials. *J Am Coll Cardiol* 2002;40:2082–2089.
83. Leon MB. SIRIUS study. Presented at the Transcatheter Cardiovascular Therapeutics. Washington DC; September 2002. Available at: http://www.theheart.org.
84. Miyoshi H, Kamihata H, Sutani Y, et al. Glycemic control and in-stent restenosis in patients with diabetes mellitus. *J Am Coll Cardiol* 2002;39:74A.
85. Rupprecht HJ, Brennecke R, Bernhard G, et al. Analysis of risk factors for restenosis after PTCA. *Cathet Cardiovasc Diagn* 1990;19:151–159.
86. Reis GJ, Kuntz RE, Silverman DI, et al. Effects of serum lipid levels on restenosis after coronary angioplasty. *Am J Cardiol* 1991;68:1431–1435.
87. Arora RR, Konrad K, Badhwar K, et al. Restenosis after transluminal coronary angioplasty: a risk factor analysis. *Cathet Cardiovasc Diagn* 1990;19:17–22.
88. Desmarais RL, Sarembock IJ, Ayers CR, et al. Elevated serum lipoprotein(a) is a risk factor for clinical recurrence after coronary balloon angioplasty. *Circulation* 1995;91:1403–1409.
89. Yamamoto H, Imazu M, Yamabe T, et al. Risk factors for restenosis after percutaneous transluminal coronary angioplasty: role of lipoprotein (a). *Am Heart J* 1995;130:1168–1173.
90. Miyata M, Biro S, Arima S, et al. High serum concentration of lipoprotein(a) is a risk factor for restenosis after percutaneous transluminal coronary angioplasty in Japanese patients with single-vessel disease. *Am Heart J* 1996;132:269–273.
91. Chiarugi L, Prisco D, Antonucci E, et al. Lipoprotein (a) and anticardiolipin antibodies are risk factors for clinically relevant restenosis after elective balloon percutaneous transluminal coronary angioplasty. *Atherosclerosis* 2001;154:129–135.
92. Rozenman Y, Gilon D, Welber S, et al. Plasma lipoproteins are not related to restenosis after successful coronary angioplasty. *Am J Cardiol* 1993;72:1206–1207.
93. Ribichini F, Steffenino G, Dellavalle A, et al. Plasma lipoprotein(a) is not a predictor for restenosis after elective high-pressure coronary stenting. *Circulation* 1998;98:1172–1177.
94. Violaris AG, Melkert R, Serruys PW. Influence of serum cholesterol and cholesterol subfractions on restenosis after successful coronary angioplasty. A quantitative angiographic analysis of 3336 lesions. *Circulation* 1994;90:2267–2279.
95. Bertrand ME, McFadden EP, Fruchart JC, et al. Effect of pravastatin on angiographic restenosis after coronary balloon angioplasty. The PREDICT Trial Investigators. Prevention of Restenosis by Elisor after Transluminal Coronary Angioplasty. *J Am Coll Cardiol* 1997;30:863–869.
96. Serruys PW, De Feyter P, Macaya C, et al. Fluvastatin for prevention of cardiac events following successful first percutaneous coronary intervention: a randomized controlled trial. *JAMA* 2002;287:3215–3222.
97. Buffon A, Biasucci LM, Liuzzo G, et al. Widespread coronary inflammation in unstable angina. *N Engl J Med* 2002;347:5–12.
98. Ross R. Atherosclerosis—an inflammatory disease. *N Engl J Med* 1999;340:115–126.
99. Yeh ET, Anderson HV, Pasceri V, et al. C-reactive protein: linking inflammation to cardiovascular complications. *Circulation* 2001;104:974–975.
100. Verma S, Wang CH, Li SH, et al. A self-fulfilling prophecy: C-reactive protein attenuates nitric oxide production and inhibits angiogenesis. *Circulation* 2002;106:913–919.
101. Pasceri V, Willerson JT, Yeh ET. Direct proinflammatory effect of C-reactive protein on human endothelial cells. *Circulation* 2000;102:2165–2168.
102. Torzewski M, Rist C, Mortensen RF, et al. C-reactive protein in the arterial intima: role of C-reactive protein receptor-dependent monocyte recruitment in atherogenesis. *Arterioscler Thromb Vasc Biol* 2000;20:2094–2099.
103. Zwaka TP, Hombach V, Torzewski J. C-reactive protein-mediated low density lipoprotein uptake by macrophages: implications for atherosclerosis. *Circulation* 2001;103:1194–1197.
104. Fichtlscherer S, Rosenberger G, Walter DH, et al. Elevated C-reactive

protein levels and impaired endothelial vasoreactivity in patients with coronary artery disease. *Circulation* 2000;102:1000–1006.

105. Tomai F, Crea F, Gaspardone A, et al. Unstable angina and elevated C-reactive protein levels predict enhanced vasoreactivity of the culprit lesion. *Circulation* 2001;104:1471–1476.

106. Buffon A, Liuzzo G, Biasucci LM, et al. Preprocedural serum levels of C-reactive protein predict early complications and late restenosis after coronary angioplasty. *J Am Coll Cardiol* 1999;34:1512–1521.

107. Biasucci LM, Liuzzo G, Buffon A, et al. The variable role of inflammation in acute coronary syndromes and in restenosis. *Semin Interv Cardiol* 1999;4:105–110.

108. Gottsauner-Wolf M, Zasmeta G, Hornykewycz S, et al. Plasma levels of C-reactive protein after coronary stent implantation. *Eur Heart J* 2000;21:1152–1158.

109. Walter DH, Fichtlscherer S, Sellwig M, et al. Preprocedural C-reactive protein levels and cardiovascular events after coronary stent implantation. *J Am Coll Cardiol* 2001;37:839–846.

110. Chan AW, Bhatt DL, Chew DP, et al. Early and sustained survival benefit associated with statin therapy at the time of percutaneous coronary intervention. *Circulation* 2002;105:691–696.

111. Beygui F, Laporte M, Le Feuvre C, et al. In-hospital C-reactive protein is a predictor of in-stent restenosis after primary stenting for acute myocardial infarction. *Circulation* 2002;106:II-583.

112. Croitoru M, Holmes DR, Bamlet WE, et al. Elevated serum C-reactive protein predict clinical outcomes after percutaneous revascularization. *Circulation* 2002;106:II-589.

113. Rahel BM, Diepersloot RJ, de Jongh BM, et al. Role of acute phase reactants and infection as predictors for major adverse clinical events and angina pectoris after percutaneous coronary intervention. *J Am Coll Cardiol* 2002;39:273A.

114. Rioufol G, Finet G, Ginon I, et al. Multiple atherosclerotic plaque rupture in acute coronary syndrome: a three-vessel intravascular ultrasound study. *Circulation* 2002;106:804–808.

115. Bartels C, Maass M, Bein G, et al. Detection of Chlamydia pneumoniae but not cytomegalovirus in occluded saphenous vein coronary artery bypass grafts. *Circulation* 1999;99:879–882.

116. Muhlestein JB, Horne BD, Carlquist JF, et al. Cytomegalovirus seropositivity and C-reactive protein have independent and combined predictive value for mortality in patients with angiographically demonstrated coronary artery disease. *Circulation* 2000;102:1917–1923.

117. Maier W, Corti M, Orsucci T, et al. Role of chlamydia pneumoniae after percutaneous coronary intervention: the SWICA (Swiss Cardiovascular Center Chlamydia) trial. *J Am Coll Cardiol* 2002;39:31A.

118. Kastrati A, Dirschinger J, Schomig A. Genetic risk factors and restenosis after percutaneous coronary interventions. *Herz* 2000;25:34–46.

119. Bresee SJ, Jacobs AK, Garber GR, et al. Prior restenosis predicts restenosis after coronary angioplasty of a new significant narrowing. *Am J Cardiol* 1991;68:1158–1162.

120. Kastrati A, Schomig A, Elezi S, et al. Interlesion dependence of the risk for restenosis in patients with coronary stent placement in multiple lesions. *Circulation* 1998;97:2396–2401.

121. Cambien F, Poirier O, Lecerf L, et al. Deletion polymorphism in the gene for angiotensin-converting enzyme is a potent risk factor for myocardial infarction. *Nature* 1992;359:641–644.

122. Hamon M, Bauters C, Amant C, et al. Relation between the deletion polymorphism of the angiotensin-converting enzyme gene and late luminal narrowing after coronary angioplasty. *Circulation* 1995;92:296–299.

123. Samani NJ, Martin DS, Brack M, et al. Insertion/deletion polymorphism in the angiotensin-converting enzyme gene and risk of restenosis after coronary angioplasty. *Lancet* 1995;345:1013–1016.

124. van Bockxmeer FM, Mamotte CD, Gibbons FA, et al. Angiotensin-converting enzyme and apolipoprotein E genotypes and restenosis after coronary angioplasty. *Circulation* 1995;92:2066–2071.

125. Amant C, Bauters C, Bodart JC, et al. D allele of the angiotensin I-converting enzyme is a major risk factor for restenosis after coronary stenting. *Circulation* 1997;96:56–60.

126. Ribichini F, Steffenino G, Dellavalle A, et al. Plasma activity and insertion/deletion polymorphism of angiotensin I-converting enzyme: a major risk factor and a marker of risk for coronary stent restenosis. *Circulation* 1998;97:147–154.

127. Koch W, Kastrati A, Mehilli J, et al. Insertion/deletion polymorphism of the angiotensin I-converting enzyme gene is not associated with restenosis after coronary stent placement. *Circulation* 2000;102:197–202.

128. Gurlek A, Gulec S, Karabulut H, et al. Relation between the insertion/deletion polymorphism of the angiotensin I converting enzyme gene and restenosis after coronary stenting. *J Cardiovasc Risk* 2000;7:403–407.

129. Meurice T, Bauters C, Hermant X, et al. Effect of ACE inhibitors on angiographic restenosis after coronary stenting (PARIS): a randomised, double-blind, placebo-controlled trial. *Lancet* 2001;357:1321–1324.

130. Bauters C, Amouyel P, Bertrand ME. ACE gene polymorphism and coronary restenosis. *Semin Interv Cardiol* 1999;4:145–149.

131. Okamura A, Ohishi M, Rakugi H, et al. Pharmacogenetic analysis of the effect of angiotensin-converting enzyme inhibitor on restenosis after percutaneous transluminal coronary angioplasty. *Angiology* 1999;50:811–822.

132. Beohar N, Damaraju S, Prather A, et al. Angiotensin-I converting enzyme genotype DD is a risk factor for coronary artery disease. *J Investig Med* 1995;43:275–280.

133. Kasi JC, Zhang Y, Calvino R, et al. Angiotensin-converting enzyme insertion/deletion polymorphism and restenosis after coronary angioplasty in unstable angina pectoris. *Am J Cardiol* 1996;77:875–877.

134. Lindpaintner K, Pfeffer MA, Kreutz R, et al. A prospective evaluation of an angiotensin-converting-enzyme gene polymorphism and the risk of ischemic heart disease. *N Engl J Med* 1995;332:706–711.

135. Ohishi M, Fujii K, Minamino T, et al. A potent genetic risk factor for restenosis. *Nat Genet* 1993;5:324–325.

136. Samani NJ, Martin DS, Brack M, et al. Apolipoprotein E polymorphism does not predict risk of restenosis after coronary angioplasty. *Atherosclerosis* 1996;125:209–216.

137. Jorgensen E, Kelbaek H, Helqvist S, et al. Predictors of coronary in-stent restenosis: importance of angiotensin-converting enzyme gene polymorphism and treatment with angiotensin-converting enzyme inhibitors. *J Am Coll Cardiol* 2001;38:1434–1439.

138. Ferrari M, Mudra H, Grip L, et al. Angiotensin-converting enzyme insertion/deletion polymorphism does not influence the restenosis rate after coronary stent implantation. *Cardiology* 2002;97:29–36.

139. Agema WR, Jukema JW, Zwinderman AH, et al. A meta-analysis of the angiotensin-converting enzyme gene polymorphism and restenosis after percutaneous transluminal coronary revascularization: evidence for publication bias. *Am Heart J* 2002;144:760–768.

140. Huber KC, Schwartz RS, Edwards WD, et al. Effects of angiotensin converting enzyme inhibition on neointimal proliferation in a porcine coronary injury model. *Am Heart J* 1993;125:695–701.

141. Desmet W, Vrolix M, De Scheerder I, et al. Angiotensin-converting enzyme inhibition with fosinopril sodium in the prevention of restenosis after coronary angioplasty. *Circulation* 1994;89:385–392.

142. Weiss EJ, Bray PF, Tayback M, et al. A polymorphism of a platelet glycoprotein receptor as an inherited risk factor for coronary thrombosis. *N Engl J Med* 1996;334:1090–1094.

143. Kastrati A, Schomig A, Seyfarth M, et al. PlA polymorphism of platelet glycoprotein IIIa and risk of restenosis after coronary stent placement. *Circulation* 1999;99:1005–1010.

144. Di Castelnuovo A, de Gaetano G, Donati MB, et al. Platelet glycoprotein receptor IIIa polymorphism PIA1/PIA2 and coronary risk: a meta-analysis. *Thromb Haemost* 2001;85:626–633.

145. Kuntz RE, Gibson CM, Nobuyoshi M, et al. Generalized model of restenosis after conventional balloon angioplasty, stenting and directional atherectomy. *J Am Coll Cardiol* 1993;21:15–25.

146. Hirshfeld JW Jr, Schwartz JS, Jugo R, et al. Restenosis after coronary angioplasty: a multivariate statistical model to relate lesion and procedure variables to restenosis. The M-HEART Investigators. *J Am Coll Cardiol* 1991;18:647–656.

147. Foley DP, Melkert R, Serruys PW. Influence of coronary vessel size on renarrowing process and late angiographic outcome after successful balloon angioplasty. *Circulation* 1994;90:1239–1251.

148. Elezi S, Kastrati A, Neumann FJ, et al. Vessel size and long-term outcome after coronary stent placement. *Circulation* 1998;98:1875–1880.

149. Ajani AE, Waksman R, Cha DH, et al. The impact of lesion length and reference vessel diameter on angiographic restenosis and target vessel revascularization in treating in-stent restenosis with radiation. *J Am Coll Cardiol* 2002;39:1290–1296.

150. Costantini CO, Lansky AJ, Mehran R, et al. Impact of vessel size after coronary vascular brachytherapy: a report of 990 patients. *J Am Coll Cardiol* 2002;39:14A.

151. Popma JJ, Cox NR, Moses JW, et al. Effect of vessel size on angiographic restenosis in a randomized comparison of bare metal and sirolimus-eluting Bx Velocity stents: a SIRIUS trial substudy. *Circulation* 2002;106:II-520.

152. Berger PB, Bell MR, Holmes DR Jr, et al. Effect of restenosis after an earlier angioplasty at another coronary site on the frequency of restenosis after a subsequent coronary angioplasty. *Am J Cardiol* 1992;69:1086–1089.

153. Kitazume H, Ichiro K, Iwama T, et al. Repeat coronary angioplasty as the treatment of choice for restenosis. *Am Heart J* 1996;132:711–715.

154. Glazier JJ, Varricchione TR, Ryan TJ, et al. Outcome in patients with recurrent restenosis after percutaneous transluminal balloon angioplasty. *Br Heart J* 1989;61:485–488.

155. Colombo A, Ferraro M, Itoh A, et al. Results of coronary stenting for restenosis. *J Am Coll Cardiol* 1996;28:830–836.

156. Kastrati A, Mehilli J, Dirschinger J, et al. Restenosis after coronary placement of various stent types. *Am J Cardiol* 2001;87:34–39.

157. Tan KH, Sulke N, Taub N, et al. Efficacy of a third coronary angioplasty for a second restenosis: short-term results, long-term follow up, and correlates of a third restenosis. *Br Heart J* 1995;73:327–333.

158. Teirstein PS, Hoover CA, Ligon RW, et al. Repeat coronary angioplasty: efficacy of a third angioplasty for a second restenosis. *J Am Coll Cardiol* 1989;13:291–296.

159. Joly P, Bonan R, Palisaitis D, et al. Treatment of recurrent restenosis with repeat percutaneous transluminal coronary angioplasty. *Am J Cardiol* 1988;61:906–908.

160. Dimas AP, Grigera F, Arora RR, et al. Repeat coronary angioplasty as treatment for restenosis. *J Am Coll Cardiol* 1992;19:1310–1314.

161. Bauters C, Mc Fadden EP, Lablanche JM, et al. Restenosis rate after multiple percutaneous transluminal coronary angioplasty procedures at the same site. A quantitative angiographic study in consecutive patients undergoing a third angioplasty procedure for a second restenosis. *Circulation* 1993;88:969–974.

162. Williams DO, Guruntzig AR, Kent KM, et al. Efficacy of repeat percutaneous transluminal coronary angioplasty for coronary restenosis. *Am J Cardiol* 1984;53:32C–35C.

163. Quigley PJ, Hlatky MA, Hinohara T, et al. Repeat percutaneous transluminal coronary angioplasty and predictors of recurrent restenosis. *Am J Cardiol* 1989;63:409–413.

164. Williams DO, Selzer F, Johnston JM, et al. Repeat revascularization in the stent era: a report from the NHLBI dynamic registry. *Circulation* 2001;104:II-387.

165. Galassi AR, Foti R, Azzarelli S, et al. Long-term angiographic follow-up after successful repeat balloon angioplasty for in-stent restenosis. *Clin Cardiol* 2001;24:334–340.

166. Teirstein PS, Massullo V, Jani S, et al. Catheter-based radiotherapy to inhibit restenosis after coronary stenting. *N Engl J Med* 1997;336:1697–1703.

167. Teirstein PS, Massullo V, Jani S, et al. Three-year clinical and angiographic follow-up after intracoronary radiation: results of a randomized clinical trial. *Circulation* 2000;101:360–365.

168. Grise MA, Jani S, Russo RJ, et al. Five-year clinical follow-up after intracoronary radiation: results of a randomized trial. *Circulation* 2001;104:II-348.

169. Waksman R, White RL, Chan RC, et al. Intracoronary gamma-radiation therapy after angioplasty inhibits recurrence in patients with in-stent restenosis. *Circulation* 2000;101:2165–2171.

170. Waksman R, Ajani AE, Kim HS, et al. Three-year follow-up after intracoronary gamma radiation therapy for in-stent restenosis: results from a randomized clinical trial. *Circulation* 2001;104:II-348.

171. Leon MB, Teirstein PS, Moses J, et al. Localized intracoronary gamma-radiation therapy to inhibit the recurrence of restenosis after stenting. *N Engl J Med* 2001;344:250–256.

172. Stone GW, Mehran R, Midei M, et al. Beta radiation for de novo and in-stent restenotic lesions in saphenous vein grafts: the SVG BRITE trial. *Circulation* 2002;106:II-335.

173. Waksman R, Ajani AE, White RL, et al. Four-year follow-up after intracoronary gamma radiation therapy for in-stent restenosis: results from a randomized clinical trial. *J Am Coll Cardiol* 2002;39:64A.

174. Ashby DT, Dangas G, Mehran R, et al. Do multiple prior interventions for in-stent restenosis impact the success of gamma brachytherapy? *J Am Coll Cardiol* 2002;39:58A.

175. Grube E, Serruys PW. Safety and performance of a paclitaxel-eluting stent for the treatment of in-stent restenosis: preliminary results of the TAXUS III trial. *J Am Coll Cardiol* 2002;39:58A.

176. Serruys PW, Abizaid AA, Foley D, et al. Sirolimus-eluting stents abolish neointimal hyperplasia in patients with in-stent restenosis: late angiographic and intravascular ultrasound results. *J Am Coll Cardiol* 2002;39:37A.

177. Sousa JE, Costa MA, Abizaid A, et al. Sirolimus-eluting stent for the treatment of in-stent restenosis: a quantitative coronary angiography and three-dimensional intravascular ultrasound study. *Circulation* 2003;107:24–27.

178. Webb JG, Myler RK, Shaw RE, et al. Coronary angioplasty after coronary bypass surgery: initial results and late outcome in 422 patients. *J Am Coll Cardiol* 1990;16:812–820.

179. de Feyter PJ, van Suylen RJ, de Jaegere PP, et al. Balloon angioplasty for the treatment of lesions in saphenous vein bypass grafts. *J Am Coll Cardiol* 1993;21:1539–1549.

180. Platko WP, Hollman J, Whitlow PL, et al. Percutaneous transluminal angioplasty of saphenous vein graft stenosis: long term follow up. *J Am Coll Cardiol* 1989;14:1645–1650.

181. Roffi M, Mukherjee D, Chew DP, et al. Lack of benefit from intravenous platelet glycoprotein IIb/IIIa receptor inhibition as adjunctive treatment for percutaneous interventions of aortocoronary bypass grafts: a pooled analysis of five randomized clinical trials. *Circulation* 2002;106:3063–3067.

182. Wong SC, Baim DS, Schatz RA, et al. Immediate results and late outcomes after stent implantation in saphenous vein graft lesions: the multicenter U.S. Palmaz-Schatz stent experience. The Palmaz-Schatz Stent Study Group. *J Am Coll Cardiol* 1995;26:704–712.

183. Brener SJ, Ellis SG, Apperson-Hansen C, et al. Comparison of stenting and balloon angioplasty for narrowings in aortocoronary saphenous vein conduits in place for more than five years. *Am J Cardiol* 1997;79:13–18.

184. Bhargava B, Kornowski R, Mehran R, et al. Procedural results and intermediate clinical outcomes after multiple saphenous vein graft stenting. *J Am Coll Cardiol* 2000;35:389–397.

185. Savage MP, Douglas JS Jr, Fischman DL, et al. Stent placement compared with balloon angioplasty for obstructed coronary bypass grafts. Saphenous Vein De Novo Trial Investigators. *N Engl J Med* 1997;337:740–747.

186. Ribeiro PA, Scavetta K, Oh C, et al. Long-term clinical results after stent implantation in old obstructed saphenous vein grafts. *Chest* 2000;118:750–755.

187. Boehrer JD, Ellis SG, Pieper K, et al. Directional atherectomy versus balloon angioplasty for coronary ostial and nonstial left anterior descending coronary artery lesions: results from a randomized multicenter trial. The CAVEAT-I investigators. Coronary Angioplasty Versus Excisional Atherectomy Trial. *J Am Coll Cardiol* 1995;25:1380–1386.

188. Foley DP, Melkert R, Umans VA, et al. Differences in restenosis propensity of devices for transluminal coronary intervention. A quantitative angiographic comparison of balloon angioplasty, directional atherectomy, stent implantation and excimer laser angioplasty. CARPORT, MERCATOR, MARCATOR, PARK, and BENESTENT Trial Groups. *Eur Heart J* 1995;16:1331–1346.

189. Mehran R, Dangas G, Mintz GS, et al. Treatment of in-stent restenosis with excimer laser coronary angioplasty versus rotational atherectomy: comparative mechanisms and results. *Circulation* 2000;101:2484–2489.

190. Simonton CA, Leon MB, Baim DS, et al. 'Optimal' directional coronary atherectomy: final results of the Optimal Atherectomy Restenosis Study (OARS). *Circulation* 1998;97:332–339.

191. Serruys PW, Kay IP, Disco C, et al. Periprocedural quantitative coronary angiography after Palmaz-Schatz stent implantation predicts the restenosis rate at six months: results of a meta-analysis of the BElgian NEtherlands Stent study (BENESTENT) I, BENESTENT II Pilot, BENESTENT II and MUSIC trials. Multicenter Ultrasound Stent In Coronaries. *J Am Coll Cardiol* 1999;34:1067–1074.

192. Schomig A, Kastrati A, Elezi S, et al. Bimodal distribution of angiographic measures of restenosis six months after coronary stent placement. *Circulation* 1997;96:3880–3887.

193. Topol EJ, Ellis SG, Fishman J, et al. Multicenter study of percutaneous transluminal angioplasty for right coronary artery ostial stenosis. *J Am Coll Cardiol* 1987;9:1214–1218.

194. Whitworth HB, Pilcher GS, Roubin GS, et al. Do proximal lesions involving the origin of the left anterior descending artery (LAD) have a

higher restenosis rate after coronary angioplasty (PTCA)? *Circulation* 1985;72:III-398(abst).

195. Mathias DW, Mooney JF, Lange HW, et al. Frequency of success and complications of coronary angioplasty of a stenosis at the ostium of a branch vessel. *Am J Cardiol* 1991;67:491–495.

196. Ellis SG, Roubin GS, King SB 3rd, et al. Importance of stenosis morphology in the estimation of restenosis risk after elective percutaneous transluminal coronary angioplasty. *Am J Cardiol* 1989;63:30–34.

197. Rensing BJ, Hermans WR, Deckers JW, et al. Lumen narrowing after percutaneous transluminal coronary balloon angioplasty follows a near gaussian distribution: a quantitative angiographic study in 1,445 successfully dilated lesions. *J Am Coll Cardiol* 1992;19:939–945.

198. Hamasaki N, Nosaka H, Kimura T, et al. Influence of lesion length on late angiographic outcome and restenotic process after successful stent implantation. *J Am Coll Cardiol* 1997;29:239A.

199. Ahmed JM, Mintz GS, Waksman R, et al. Serial intravascular ultrasound analysis of the impact of lesion length on the efficacy of intracoronary gamma-irradiation for preventing recurrent in-stent restenosis. *Circulation* 2001;103:188–191.

200. Farb A, Weber DK, Kolodgie FD, et al. Morphological predictors of restenosis after coronary stenting in humans. *Circulation* 2002;105:2974–2980.

201. Macdonald RG, Henderson MA, Hirshfeld JW Jr, et al. Patient-related variables and restenosis after percutaneous transluminal coronary angioplasty—a report from the M-HEART Group. *Am J Cardiol* 1990;66:926–931.

202. Schofer J, Schluter M, Rau T, et al. Influence of treatment modality on angiographic outcome after coronary stenting in diabetic patients: a controlled study. *J Am Coll Cardiol* 2000;35:1554–1559.

203. Ellis SG, Guetta V, Miller D, et al. Relation between lesion characteristics and risk with percutaneous intervention in the stent and glycoprotein IIb/IIIa era: an analysis of results from 10,907 lesions and proposal for new classification scheme. *Circulation* 1999;100:1971–1976.

204. Meier B. Total coronary occlusion: a different animal? *J Am Coll Cardiol* 1991;17:50B–57B.

205. Bell MR, Berger PB, Bresnahan JF, et al. Initial and long-term outcome of 354 patients after coronary balloon angioplasty of total coronary artery occlusions. *Circulation* 1992;85:1003–1011.

206. Safian RD, McCabe CH, Sipperly ME, et al. Initial success and long-term follow-up of percutaneous transluminal coronary angioplasty in chronic total occlusions versus conventional stenoses. *Am J Cardiol* 1988;61:23G–28G.

207. DiSciascio G, Vetrovec GW, Cowley MJ, et al. Early and late outcome of percutaneous transluminal coronary angioplasty for subacute and chronic total coronary occlusion. *Am Heart J* 1986;111:833–839.

208. Berger PB, Holmes DR Jr, Ohman EM, et al. Restenosis, reocclusion and adverse cardiovascular events after successful balloon angioplasty of occluded versus nonoccluded coronary arteries. Results from the Multicenter American Research Trial With Cilazapril After Angioplasty to Prevent Transluminal Coronary Obstruction and Restenosis (MARCATOR). *J Am Coll Cardiol* 1996;27:1–7.

209. Kereiakes DJ, Selmon MR, McAuley BJ, et al. Angioplasty in total coronary artery occlusion: experience in 76 consecutive patients. *J Am Coll Cardiol* 1985;6:526–533.

210. Clark DA, Wexman M, Murphy MC, et al. Factors predicting recurrence in patients who have had angioplasty of total occluded vessels. *J Am Coll Cardiol* 1986;7:20A.

211. Melchior JP, Meier B, Urban P, et al. Percutaneous transluminal coronary angioplasty for chronic total coronary arterial occlusion. *Am J Cardiol* 1987;59:535–538.

212. Nienaber C, Fratz S, Lund G, et al. Primary stent placement or balloon angioplasty for chronic coronary occlusions: a matched pair analysis of 100 patients. *Circulation* 1996;94:I-686.

213. Etsuo T, Osamu K, Masanobu F, et al. Impact of coronary stenting on PTCA of chronic coronary total occlusions. *Circulation* 1996;94:I-249.

214. Cerisier A, Isaaz K, Dacosta A, et al. Prevention of reocclusion after successful balloon PTCA of totally occluded coronary arteries: a prospective randomized pilot-study comparing ticlopidine-aspirin association with aspirin alone. *J Am Coll Cardiol* 1997;29:395A.

215. Sirnes PA, Golf S, Myreng Y, et al. Stenting in Chronic Coronary Occlusion (SICCO): a randomized, controlled trial of adding stent implantation after successful angioplasty. *J Am Coll Cardiol* 1996;28:1444–1451.

216. Sirnes PA, Golf S, Myreng Y, et al. Sustained benefit of stenting chronic coronary occlusion: long-term clinical follow-up of the Stenting in Chronic Coronary Occlusion (SICCO) study. *J Am Coll Cardiol* 1998;32:305–310.

217. Werner GS, Gastmann O, Ferrari M, et al. Determinants of stent restenosis in chronic coronary occlusions assessed by intracoronary ultrasound. *Am J Cardiol* 1999;83:1164–1169.

218. Buller CE, Dzavik V, Carere RG, et al. Primary stenting versus balloon angioplasty in occluded coronary arteries: the Total Occlusion Study of Canada (TOSCA). *Circulation* 1999;100:236–242.

219. Sallam M, Spanos V, Briguori C, et al. Predictors of re-occlusion after successful recanalization of chronic total occlusion. *J Invasive Cardiol* 2001;13:511–515.

220. Lotan C, Rozenman Y, Hendler A, et al. Stents in total occlusion for restenosis prevention. The multicentre randomized STOP study. The Israeli Working Group for Interventional Cardiology. *Eur Heart J* 2000;21:1960–1966.

221. Kereiakes D, Linnemeier TJ, Baim DS, et al. Usefulness of stent length in predicting in-stent restenosis (the MULTI- LINK stent trials). *Am J Cardiol* 2000;86:336–341.

222. Sick P, Huttl T, Niebauer J, et al. Influence of residual stenosis after percutaneous coronary intervention with stent implantation on development of restenosis and stent thrombosis. *Am J Cardiol* 2003;91:148–153.

223. Cheneau E, Ajani AE, Leborgne L, et al. Relation of residual stenosis after angioplasty to long-term outcome of patients treated for in-stent restenosis with intravascular radiation therapy. *Am J Cardiol* 2002;89:1426–1428.

224. Costantini CO, Lansky AJ, Mehran R, et al. Is bigger better with vascular brachytherapy (VBT) for in-stent restenosis? Impact of optimal final angiographic results and predictors of restenosis in 990 VBT patients. *J Am Coll Cardiol* 2002;39:20A.

225. Bech GJ, Pijls NH, De Bruyne B, et al. Usefulness of fractional flow reserve to predict clinical outcome after balloon angioplasty. *Circulation* 1999;99:883–888.

226. Pijls NH. Fractional flow reserve after stenting to predict need for repeated target vessel revascularization during follow-up. *J Am Coll Cardiol* 2002;39:34A.

227. Hanekamp CE, Koolen JJ, Pijls NH, et al. Comparison of quantitative coronary angiography, intravascular ultrasound, and coronary pressure measurement to assess optimum stent deployment. *Circulation* 1999;99:1015–1021.

228. Serruys PW, di Mario C, Piek J, et al. Prognostic value of intracoronary flow velocity and diameter stenosis in assessing the short- and long-term outcomes of coronary balloon angioplasty: the DEBATE Study (Doppler Endpoints Balloon Angioplasty Trial Europe). *Circulation* 1997;96:3369–3377.

229. Mintz GS, Popma JJ, Pichard AD, et al. Intravascular ultrasound predictors of restenosis after percutaneous transcatheter coronary revascularization. *J Am Coll Cardiol* 1996;27:1678–1687.

230. Hong MK, Park SW, Mintz GS, et al. Intravascular ultrasonic predictors of angiographic restenosis after long coronary stenting. *Am J Cardiol* 2000;85:441–445.

231. Moussa I, Moses J, Di Mario C, et al. Does the specific intravascular ultrasound criterion used to optimize stent expansion have an impact on the probability of stent restenosis? *Am J Cardiol* 1999;83:1012–1017.

232. Kasaoka S, Tobis JM, Akiyama T, et al. Angiographic and intravascular ultrasound predictors of in-stent restenosis. *J Am Coll Cardiol* 1998;32:1630–1635.

233. Hong MK, Lee CW, Kim JH, et al. Impact of various intravascular ultrasound criteria for stent optimization on the six-month angiographic restenosis. *Catheter Cardiovasc Interv* 2002;56:178–183.

234. Hong MK, Park SW, Lee CW, et al. Relation between residual plaque burden after stenting and six-month angiographic restenosis. *Am J Cardiol* 2002;89:368–371.

235. Jain SP, Jain A, Collins TJ, et al. Predictors of restenosis: a morphometric and quantitative evaluation by intravascular ultrasound. *Am Heart J* 1994;128:664–673.

236. Schiele F, Meneveau N, Vuillemenot A, et al. Impact of intravascular ultrasound guidance in stent deployment on 6-month restenosis rate: a multicenter, randomized study comparing two strategies—with and without intravascular ultrasound guidance. RESIST Study Group. REStenosis after Ivus guided STenting. *J Am Coll Cardiol* 1998;32:320–328.

237. de Jaegere P, Mudra H, Figulla H, et al. Intravascular ultrasound-

guided optimized stent deployment. Immediate and 6 months clinical and angiographic results from the Multicenter Ultrasound Stenting in Coronaries Study (MUSIC Study). *Eur Heart J* 1998;19:1214–1223.

238. Prati F, Di Mario C, Moussa I, et al. In-stent neointimal proliferation correlates with the amount of residual plaque burden outside the stent: an intravascular ultrasound study. *Circulation* 1999;99:1011–1014.

239. Nakamura S, Hall P, Gaglione A, et al. High pressure assisted coronary stent implantation accomplished without intravascular ultrasound guidance and subsequent anticoagulation. *J Am Coll Cardiol* 1997;29:21–27.

240. Colombo A, Stankovic G, Moses JW. Selection of coronary stents. *J Am Coll Cardiol* 2002;40:1021–1033.

241. Escaned J, Goicolea J, Alfonso F, et al. Propensity and mechanisms of restenosis in different coronary stent designs: complementary value of the analysis of the luminal gain-loss relationship. *J Am Coll Cardiol* 1999;34:1490–1497.

242. Hoffmann R, Mintz GS, Haager PK, et al. Relation of stent design and stent surface material to subsequent in-stent intimal hyperplasia in coronary arteries determined by intravascular ultrasound. *Am J Cardiol* 2002;89:1360–1364.

243. Silber S, Reifart N, Morice MC, et al. The NUGGET trial (NIR Ultimate Gold-Gilded Equivalency Trial): 6 months post procedure safety and efficacy results. *Circulation* 2001;104:II-623.

244. Kastrati A, Schomig A, Dirschinger J, et al. Increased risk of restenosis after placement of gold-coated stents: results of a randomized trial comparing gold-coated with uncoated steel stents in patients with coronary artery disease. *Circulation* 2000;101:2478–2483.

245. Park SJ, Lee CW, Hong MK, et al. Comparison of gold-coated NIR stents with uncoated NIR stents in patients with coronary artery disease. *Am J Cardiol* 2002;89:872–875.

246. Briguori C, Sarais C, Pagnotta P, et al. In-stent restenosis in small coronary arteries: impact of strut thickness. *J Am Coll Cardiol* 2002;40:403–409.

247. Sousa E, Abizaid A, Abizaid A, et al. First human experience with sirolimus coated BX velocity stent: clinical, angiographic and ultrasound late results. *Circulation* 2000;102:II-815.

248. Sousa JE, Costa MA, Abizaid A, et al. Lack of neointimal proliferation after implantation of sirolimus-coated stents in human coronary arteries: a quantitative coronary angiography and three-dimensional intravascular ultrasound study. *Circulation* 2001;103:192–195.

249. Park SJ, H SW, Ho DS, et al. The clinical effectiveness of paclitaxel-coated coronary stents for the reduction of restenosis in the ASPECT trial. *Circulation* 2001;104:II-464.

250. Grube E, Silber SM, Hauptmann KE. Taxus I: prospective, randomized, double-blind comparison of NIRx™ stents coated with paclitaxel in a polymer carrier in de novo coronary lesions compared with uncoated controls. *Circulation* 2001;104:II-463.

251. Sousa JE, Morice MC, Serruys PW, et al. The RAVEL study: a randomized study with the sirolimus coated BX Velocity balloon-expandable stent in the treatment of patients with de novo native coronary artery lesions. *Circulation* 2001;104:II-463.

252. Abizaid AS, Costa MA, Abizaid AA, et al. Lack of edge effect after implantation of sirolimus-eluting BX-Velocity stent. *Circulation* 2001;104:II-771.

253. Abizaid AA, Sousa A, Abizaid AS, et al. Sustained suppression of neointimal preoliferation late (1 year) after implantation of Sirolimus-eluting Bx-Velocity stent. *Circulation* 2001;104:II-464.

254. Gershlick AH, Chevalier B, Camenzind E, et al. Local drug delivery to inhibit coronary artery restenosis. Data from the ELUTES (EvaLUation of PacliTaxel Eluting Stent) clinical trial. *Circulation* 2001;104:II-417.

255. Serruys PW, Degertekin M, Tanabe K, et al. Intravascular ultrasound findings in the multicenter, randomized, double-blind RAVEL (RANdomized study with the sirolimus-eluting VElocity balloon-expandable stent in the treatment of patients with de novo native coronary artery Lesions) trial. *Circulation* 2002;106:798–803.

256. Grube E, Bullesfeld L. Initial experience with paclitaxel-coated stents. *J Interv Cardiol* 2002;15:471–475.

257. Morice MC, Serruys PW, Sousa JE, et al. A randomized comparison of a sirolimus-eluting stent with a standard stent for coronary revascularization. *N Engl J Med* 2002;346:1773–1780.

258. Grube E, Silber S, Hauptmann KE, et al. TAXUS I: six- and twelve-month results from a randomized, double-blind trial on a slow-release

paclitaxel-eluting stent for de novo coronary lesions. *Circulation* 2003;107:38–42.

259. Ryan TJ, Antman EM, Brooks NH, et al. 1999 update: ACC/AHA Guidelines for the Management of Patients with Acute Myocardial Infarction: Executive Summary and Recommendations: A report of the American College of Cardiology/American Heart Association Task Force on Practice Guidelines (Committee on Management of Acute Myocardial Infarction). *Circulation* 1999;100:1016–1030.

260. Friedrich SP, Kuntz RE, Gordon PC, et al. "Moderate" restenosis has a favorable natural history. *J Am Coll Cardiol* 1993;21:321A(abst).

261. Davies RF, Goldberg AD, Forman S, et al. Asymptomatic Cardiac Ischemia Pilot (ACIP) study two-year follow-up: outcomes of patients randomized to initial strategies of medical therapy versus revascularization. *Circulation* 1997;95:2037–2043.

262. Pepine CJ, Mark DB, Bourassa MG, et al. Cost estimates for treatment of cardiac ischemia (from the Asymptomatic Cardiac Ischemia Pilot [ACIP] study). *Am J Cardiol* 1999;84:1311–1316.

263. Balady GJ, Leitschuh ML, Jacobs AK, et al. Safety and clinical use of exercise testing one to three days after percutaneous transluminal coronary angioplasty. *Am J Cardiol* 1992;69:1259–1264.

264. Hillegass WB, Ancukiewicz M, Bengtson JR, et al. Does follow-up exercise testing predict restenosis after successful angioplasty? *Circulation* 1992;86:I-137(abst).

265. Hillegass WB, Bengtson JR, Ancukiewicz M, et al. Pre-discharge exercise testing does not predict clinical events or restenosis after successful angioplasty. *Circulation* 1992;86:I-137(abst).

266. Deligonul U, Vandormael MG, Younis LT, et al. Prognostic significance of silent myocardial ischemia detected by early treadmill exercise after coronary angioplasty. *Am J Cardiol* 1989;64:1–5.

267. Hlatky MA, Mark DB. *Overview of diagnostic test assessment.* In: Califf RM, Mark DB, Wagner GS, eds. *Acute coronary care in the thrombolytic era.* Chicago: Year–Book Medical Publishers, 1988:91–99.

268. Wijns W, Serruys PW, Simoons ML, et al. Predictive value of early maximal exercise test and thallium scintigraphy after successful percutaneous transluminal coronary angioplasty. *Br Heart J* 1985;53:194–200.

269. Honan MB, Bengtson JR, Pryor DB, et al. Exercise treadmill testing is a poor predictor of anatomic restenosis after angioplasty for acute myocardial infarction. *Circulation* 1989;80:1585–1594.

270. Coma-Canella I, Daza NS, Orbe LC. Detection of restenosis with dobutamine stress test after coronary angioplasty. *Am Heart J* 1992;124:1196–1204.

271. El-Tamimi H, Davies GJ, Hackett D, et al. Very early prediction of restenosis after successful coronary angioplasty: anatomic and functional assessment. *J Am Coll Cardiol* 1990;15:259–264.

272. Scholl JM, Chaitman BR, David PR, et al. Exercise electrocardiography and myocardial scintigraphy in the serial evaluation of the results of percutaneous transluminal coronary angioplasty. *Circulation* 1982;66:380–390.

273. Korzick DH, Underwood DA, Simpfendorfer CC. Early exercise testing following percutaneous transluminal coronary angioplasty. *Cleve Clin J Med* 1990;57:53–56.

274. Pirelli S, Danzi GB, Alberti A, et al. Comparison of usefulness of high-dose dipyridamole echocardiography and exercise electrocardiography for detection of asymptomatic restenosis after coronary angioplasty. *Am J Cardiol* 1991;67:1335–1338.

275. Roth A, Miller HI, Keren G, et al. Detection of restenosis following percutaneous coronary angioplasty in single-vessel coronary artery disease: the value of clinical assessment and exercise tolerance testing. *Cardiology* 1994;84:106–113.

276. Desmet W, De Scheerder I, Piessens J. Limited value of exercise testing in the detection of silent restenosis after successful coronary angioplasty. *Am Heart J* 1995;129:452–459.

277. Azpitarte J, Tercedor L, Melgares R, et al. The value of exercise electrocardiography testing in the identification of coronary restenosis: a probability analysis. *Int J Cardiol* 1995;48:239–247.

278. Georgoulias P, Demakopoulos N, Kontos A, et al. Tc-99m tetrofosmin myocardial perfusion imaging before and six months after percutaneous transluminal coronary angioplasty. *Clin Nucl Med* 1998;23:678–682.

279. Ernst SM, Hillebrand FA, Klein B, et al. The value of exercise tests in the follow-up of patients who underwent transluminal coronary angioplasty. *Int J Cardiol* 1985;7:267–279.

280. Hardoff R, Shefer A, Gips S, et al. Predicting late restenosis after coronary angioplasty by very early (12 to 24 h) thallium-201 scintig-

raphy: implications with regard to mechanisms of late coronary restenosis. *J Am Coll Cardiol* 1990;15:1486–1492.

281. Breisblatt WM, Barnes JV, Weiland F, et al. Incomplete revascularization in multivessel percutaneous transluminal coronary angioplasty: the role for stress thallium-201 imaging. *J Am Coll Cardiol* 1988;11: 1183–1190.

282. Hecht HS, Shaw RE, Bruce TR, et al. Usefulness of tomographic thallium-201 imaging for detection of restenosis after percutaneous transluminal coronary angioplasty. *Am J Cardiol* 1990;66:1314–1318.

283. Marie PY, Danchin N, Karcher G, et al. Usefulness of exercise SPECT-thallium to detect asymptomatic restenosis in patients who had angina before coronary angioplasty. *Am Heart J* 1993;126:571–577.

284. Lefkowitz CA, Ross BL, Schwartz L, et al. Superiority of tomographic thallium imaging for the detection of restenosis after percutaneous transluminal coronary angioplasty. *J Am Coll Cardiol* 1989;13:161A(abst).

285. Caner B, Oto A, Ovunc K, et al. Prediction of restenosis after successful percutaneous coronary angioplasty by dobutamine thallium-201 scintigraphy. *Int J Cardiol* 1998;66:175–181.

286. vom Dahl J, Altehoefer C, Sheehan FH, et al. Recovery of regional left ventricular dysfunction after coronary revascularization. Impact of myocardial viability assessed by nuclear imaging and vessel patency at follow-up angiography. *J Am Coll Cardiol* 1996;28:948–958.

287. Aboul-Enein H, Bengston JR, Adams DB, et al. Effect of the degree of effort on exercise echocardiography for the detection of restenosis after coronary artery angioplasty. *Am Heart J* 1991;122:430–437.

288. Hecht HS, DeBord L, Shaw R, et al. Usefulness of supine bicycle stress echocardiography for detection of restenosis after percutaneous transluminal coronary angioplasty. *Am J Cardiol* 1993;71:293–296.

289. Heinle SK, Lieberman EB, Ancukiewicz M, et al. Usefulness of dobutamine echocardiography for detecting restenosis after percutaneous transluminal coronary angioplasty. *Am J Cardiol* 1993;72:1220–1225.

290. Takeuchi M, Miura Y, Toyokawa T, et al. The comparative diagnostic value of dobutamine stress echocardiography and thallium stress tomography for detecting restenosis after coronary angioplasty. *J Am Soc Echocardiogr* 1995;8:696–702.

291. Serruys PW, Foley DP, Kirkeeide RL, et al. Restenosis revisited: insights provided by quantitative coronary angiography. *Am Heart J* 1993;126:1243–1267.

292. Topol EJ, Califf RM, Weisman HF, et al. Randomised trial of coronary intervention with antibody against platelet IIb/IIIa integrin for reduction of clinical restenosis: results at six months. The EPIC Investigators. *Lancet* 1994;343:881–886.

293. Genuth S. Exogenous insulin administration and cardiovascular risk in non-insulin- dependent and insulin-dependent diabetes mellitus. *Ann Intern Med* 1996;124:104–109.

294. Tenaglia AN, Fortin DF, Frid DJ, et al. Long-term outcome following successful reopening of abrupt closure after coronary angioplasty. *Am J Cardiol* 1993;72:21–25.

295. Kastrati A, Schomig A, Dirschinger J, et al. A randomized trial comparing stenting with balloon angioplasty in small vessels in patients with symptomatic coronary artery disease. *Circulation* 2000;102:2593–2598.

296. Doucet S, Schalij MJ, Hilton D, et al. The SISA study: a randomized comparison of balloon angioplasty and stent to prevent restenosis in small arteries. Presented at the Canadian Cardiovascular Congress; Vancouver, British Columbia, Canada; 2000.

297. Goldberg SL, Loussararian A, De Gregorio J, et al. Predictors of diffuse and aggressive intra-stent restenosis. *J Am Coll Cardiol* 2001; 37:1019–1025.

298. Di Mario C, Moses JW, Anderson TJ, et al. Randomized comparison of elective stent implantation and coronary balloon angioplasty guided by online quantitative angiography and intracoronary Doppler. DESTINI Study Group (Doppler Endpoint STenting INternational Investigation). *Circulation* 2000;102:2938–2944.

299. Serruys PW, de Bruyne B, Carlier S, et al. Randomized comparison of primary stenting and provisional balloon angioplasty guided by flow velocity measurement. Doppler Endpoints Balloon Angioplasty Trial Europe (DEBATE) II Study Group. *Circulation* 2000;102:2930–2937.

300. Briguori C, Sarais C, Spanos V, et al. Impact of strut's thickness on restenosis after stent implantation in small coronary vessels. *Circulation* 2001;104:II-665.

301. Stankovic G, Ferraro M, Takagi T, et al. Effect of strut thickness on angiographic restenosis rate after coronary stenting. *Circulation* 2001;104:II-665.

302. Silber S, Reifart N, Morice MC, et al. The Nugget trial (NIR Ultimate Gold-gilded Equivalency Trial): 6 months post-procedure safety and efficacy results. *Circulation* 2001;104:II-623.

303. Waksman R. Use of localised intracoronary b radiation in treatment of in-stent restenosis: the INHIBIT randomised controlled trial. *Lancet* 2002;359:551–557.

304. Waksman R, Ajani AE, White RL, et al. Intravascular gamma radiation for in-stent restenosis in saphenous-vein bypass grafts. *N Engl J Med* 2002;346:1194–1199.

305. Ajani AE, Canos DA, Gevorkian N, et al. Correlates of radiation failure for in-stent restenosis. *Circulation* 2002;106:II-392.

306. Toutouzas K, Stankovic G, Takagi T, et al. Impact of stent length on restenosis rate in small vessels. *J Am Coll Cardiol* 2002;39:53A.

307. Syeda B, Schmid R, Wexberg P, et al. Effects of geographic miss during intracoronary brachytherapy on edge stenosis at follow-up. *J Am Coll Cardiol* 2002;39:23A.

308. Hertwig S, Volzke H, Robinson DM, et al. Angiotensinogen M235T gene polymorphism and recurrent restenosis after repeated percutaneous transluminal coronary angioplasty. *Clin Sci (Lond)* 2002;103:101–106.

309. von Beckerath N, Koch W, Mehilli J, et al. Glycoprotein Ia C807T polymorphism and risk of restenosis following coronary stenting. *Atherosclerosis* 2001;156:463–468.

310. Bottiger C, Kastrati A, Koch W, et al. Polymorphism of platelet glycoprotein IIb and risk of thrombosis and restenosis after coronary stent placement. *Am J Cardiol* 1999;84:987–991.

311. Abbate R, Marcucci R, Camacho-Vanegas O, et al. Role of platelet glycoprotein PL(A1/A2) polymorphism in restenosis after percutaneous transluminal coronary angioplasty. *Am J Cardiol* 1998;82:524–525.

312. Watanabe Y, Yamada N, Yokoi H, et al. Relationship between HLA-C locus and restenosis after coronary artery balloon angioplasty. *JAMA* 1997;277:983–984.

313. Cooke T, Sheahan R, Foley D, et al. Lipoprotein(a) in restenosis after percutaneous transluminal coronary angioplasty and coronary artery disease. *Circulation* 1994;89:1593–1598.

314. Gomma AH, Elrayess MA, Knight CJ, et al. The endothelial nitric oxide synthase (Glu298Asp and -786T>C) gene polymorphisms are associated with coronary in-stent restenosis. *Eur Heart J* 2002;23:1955–1962.

315. Jain A, Mahmarian JJ, Borges-Neto S, et al. Clinical significance of perfusion defects by thallium-201 single photon emission tomography following oral dipyridamole early after coronary angioplasty. *J Am Coll Cardiol* 1988;11:970–976.

316. Milan E, Zoccarato O, Terzi A, et al. Technetium-99m-sestamibi SPECT to detect restenosis after successful percutaneous coronary angioplasty. *J Nucl Med* 1996;37:1300–1305.

CHAPTER 94

Use of New Angioplasty Devices for the Treatment of Stable Angina

Martin B. Leon and Donald S. Baim

INTRODUCTION

Despite its humble beginnings, as percutaneous coronary intervention (PCI) passes its twenty-fifth anniversary (September 1977 to September 2002) it currently stands as the dominant form of coronary revascularization. Annual volumes of procedures currently exceed 1 million, more than doubling the annual volume of coronary bypass surgery (1). Much of the growth of this procedure has been the result of technologic improvements that have increased the range of treatable lesion types, the predictability of acute success, procedural safety, and durability of an initially successful result (2). This technologic improvement has included the introduction of a range of new devices that are the subject of this chapter. Including coronary stents, introduced into clinical use in the United States in 1993–1994, the new devices discussed in this chapter account for 90% of coronary intervention, whereas the original stand-alone balloon angioplasty procedure introduced by Gruntzig has been almost completely supplanted (3).

ATHERECTOMY

The goal of the atherectomy class of device is to remove (rather than simply displace or scaffold in place) the ob-

structing atherothrombotic lesion. A variety of strategies have been used to achieve this goal.

Directional Coronary Atherectomy

Directional coronary atherectomy (DCA; Guidant vascular intervention), approved by the Food and Drug Administration in 1990, was the first new angioplasty device to enter clinical practice (Fig. 94–1A). The device consists of a windowed steel cylinder that contains a spinning, cup-shaped blade. A low-pressure positioning balloon attached to the back of the cylinder (opposite the window) is inflated to press the window against the obstructing plaque. Advancement of the blade across the window cuts off any plaque that protrudes into the window and traps it in the flexible nose cone of the device. This procedure is repeated with different orientations of the window within the lesion until a large lumen result is achieved. Early devices were available with housing sizes of 5, 6, and 7 French (F) to treat different vessel sizes; more recent realizations of this device use a common 6-F housing with different size balloons to accommodate for the reference vessel diameter. This has allowed reduction in the size of the guiding catheter needed, from 10 to 8 F. Other improvements such as an improved nose cone and shorter rigid length have added to device deliverability, and a hardened cutter has allowed more efficient cutting of fibrous or even moderately calcified plaque. A newer DCA variant (Fox Hollow Technology) uses a different strategy wherein a smaller (4-F) catheter is positioned just proximal

M. B. Leon: Department of Medicine, Cardiovascular Interventional Therapy, Columbia University College of Physicians and Surgeons, New York, New York.

D. S. Baim: Department of Medicine, Harvard Medical School; and Center for Integration of Medicine and Innovative Technology, Brigham and Women's Hospital, Boston, Massachusetts.

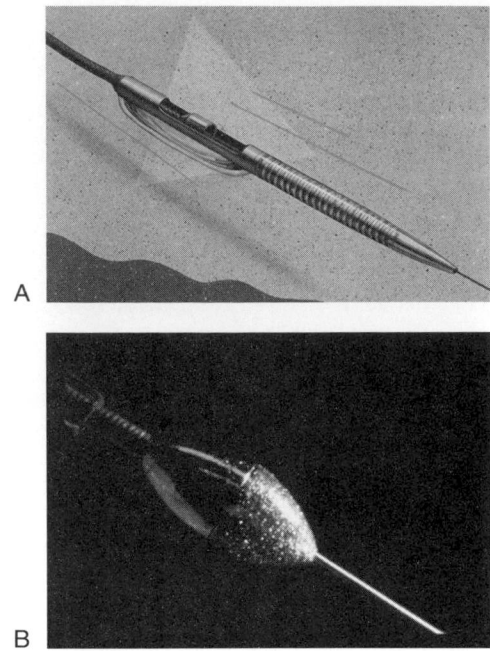

FIG. 94–1. Coronary atherectomy catheters (**A:** directional atherectomy; **B:** rotational atherectomy).

to the target lesion over a guidewire, and its tip is deflected to expose a spinning blade and press it against the lesion, as the entire catheter is advanced across the lesion (4). Excised plaque strips are deflected into a nose cone, and the procedure is repeated with different device orientations until the desired degree of debulking is obtained.

An average of 13 to 18 mg tissue is removed during the average DCA procedure, which accounts for only about half of the observed lumen improvement. The remainder of lumen improvement results from mechanical dilation, and the post-DCA result therefore can be further improved by balloon angioplasty or stent placement. Intravascular ultrasound has shown, however, that the amount of tissue removal is important to the long-term result of DCA (5). Aggressive debulking to a residual plaque area (as a percentage of the overall vessel or external elastic laminar area) less than 50% provides a larger acute lumen and requires correspondingly less mechanical dilation, with an improved resistance to subsequent restenosis.

Much of the variability in reported DCA results seem to stem from the extent of debulking achieved with the device. In the early Coronary Angioplasty Versus Excisional Atherectomy Trial (CAVEAT) trial, 1,000 patients were randomized to DCA or conventional balloon angioplasty (6). Relatively conservative debulking using the 6-F device in 3-mm arteries and a limited use of balloon after dilation left an average 30% residual restenosis and gave a nearly 50% angiographic restenosis rate, which was not significantly better than the 57% restenosis rate observed with balloon angioplasty (6,7). With this lack of benefit, the slightly greater complication rate with DCA led to limited

clinical use in many centers (8). Subsequent trials such as Optimal Atherectomy Restenosis Study (OARS), Balloon vs Optimal Atherectomy Trial (BOAT), and Adjunctive Balloon Angioplasty After Coronary Atherectomy Study (ABACAS) have used more aggressive debulking and more common balloon after dilation to achieve lower residual restenosis (10–15%), a lower angiographic restenosis rate (15–20%), and a lower angiographic restenosis rate (15–20%), with no increase in acute major complications (death, Q-wave myocardial infarction [MI], emergency bypass surgery) compared with balloon angioplasty, although the incidence of postprocedure creatine kinase (CK)-MB level increase is twice as great with DCA (9–12). Although histology shows that recovery of deep vessel wall elements (media and even adventitia) are commonly recovered in DCA specimens, the incidence of frank vessel perforation is less than 1% (13,14).

In the wake of stent availability after 1994, the use of DCA has decreased to well less than 1% of coronary interventions. Its current use is restricted to origin left anterior descending (LAD) coronary artery lesions where plaque shifting into the origin circumflex by stenting would be problematic, certain large and noncalcified bifurcation lesions, debulking of instent restenosis, and debulking before stent placement (15–20). Even these indications are controversial, however. In bifurcations, DCA of the parent vessel and the involved side branch followed by kissing-balloon dilation gives a superior acute result to balloon alone, and registry data suggest reduced recurrence rates. Conversely, new stenting strategies (culottes stenting, crushing of the side branch stent) may give equivalent short- and long-term results, particularly with the advent of the drug-eluting stents (21). Instent restenosis is a pure case of excessive neointimal hyperplasia, and initial treatment focused on reexpanding the lumen by balloon (or cutting balloon) dilation (22). DCA offered the option of removing the obstructing tissue to provide a larger acute lumen and less tendency for tissue reintrusion, and also suggested reduced clinical restenosis in some series. Conversely, the cutting balloon (equipped with three or four microscopic blades on its surface) provides effective dilation because of its resistance to slippage out of the restenotic lesion, and when coupled with intracoronary (β or γ) brachytherapy, it reduces the recurrence rate of instent restenosis markedly (from roughly 60% to roughly 20%) (23–25). The concept that debulking before stent placement would allow better initial stent expansion and reduce the amount of instent hyperplasia was asserted by the Stenting after Optimal Lesion Debulking (SOLD) registry (5), but it failed to be confirmed (except in a subset with more aggressive debulking) in the randomized Atherectomy before Multilink Improves lumen Gain and clinical Outcomes (AMIGO) trial. In any event, the hoped for benefit can now be achieved with greater simplicity using drug-eluting stents.

In summary, although DCA does provide a safe and effective alternative means of enlarging a stenotic coronary lumen and appears to offer benefit in certain clinical and anatomic niches, the availability of simpler and technically less demanding alternatives has reduced its current impact on coronary intervention.

Rotational Atherectomy

The concept of rotational atherectomy (Boston Scientific, Natick, MA) uses microscopic diamond chips attached to a football-shaped burr that spins at 150,000 g to abrade plaque from obstructing lesions (Fig. 94–1B). By the principle of differential cutting, harder plaque elements are abraded, whereas softer vessel wall is spared. Abraded plaque is reduced to particles that generally are small enough (≤10 micron) to pass through the distal microcirculation without sequela. Burrs are available in sizes ranging from 1.25 mm to a maximum of 2.5 mm. For improving the compliance of calcified lesions ("lesion modification"), only a single 1.5- or 1.75-mm burr may be used, whereas "complete" debulking would involve use of a series of burrs starting at 1.5 mm and increasing in 0.5-mm steps to a maximum of 70% to 75% of the reference vessel diameter. Only the smallest burrs can be advanced through 6-F guiding catheters, whereas the largest burr requires a 9-F guiding catheter. The desired burrs are advanced over a special purpose 0.009-inch guidewire whose tip is placed in the vessel beyond the target lesion. Forward pressure on the device is modulated carefully by the operator to avoid excessive slowing of the rotational speed, which can cause heating of the vessel, dissection, and creation of larger debris particles. Similarly, the duration of a rotational atherectomy "run" is usually limited to 30 seconds before the burr is pulled back away from the lesion to allow initial debris clearance before proceeding with further ablation. Great care must be taken as the end of the lesion is approached to avoid abrupt exit of the burr into the distal vessel, which can cause dissection or even perforation. The final result can be improved further by balloon dilation (typically at pressures as low as 4–6 atm) or stent implantation.

Initial data suggested a procedural success rate of roughly 95%, even in calcified or diffuse lesions that were poorly suited to conventional balloon angioplasty (26–28). Major complications were seen in 3% of cases (including death in 0.8%, Q-wave MI in 0.9%, and emergency surgery in 1.7%). Dissections (10%), diffuse coronary spasm, vessel perforation (1%), slow flow in the distal vessel because of embolization, and postprocedural CK level increase, were other common complications of rotational atherectomy. When rotational atherectomy is performed in right coronary lesions, burr activation can trigger profound bradycardia, making use of atropine or temporary right ventricular pacing a requirement. This complication profile has decreased progressively with greater understanding of optimal technique, including burr sizing, lower rotational speeds (140,000 rather than 180,000–200,000 g), allowance of intermittent distal perfusion, and avoidance of speed decreases more than 10,000 g during lesion ablation.

Although it was hoped that less traumatic removal of plaque by rotational atherectomy would reduce the incidence of complications compared with balloon angioplasty, randomized data from the Study To determine Rotablator and Transluminal Angioplasty Strategy (STRATAS) (29) and Dilatation vs Ablation Revascularization Trial Targeting Restenosis (DART) (30) trials show that there is no benefit of rotational atherectomy whether a conservative (smaller maximal burr size) or aggressive (larger final burr/artery ratio) is used. The main uses of rotational atherectomy are thus treatment of heavily calcified or resistant lesions, treatment of ostial or diffuse disease, debulking or instent restenosis, and debulking before stent implantation. Whereas the treatment of *calcified or resistant lesions* remains a useful application, challenged only partially by the cutting balloon or force-focused angioplasty balloon (FX-MiniRail [Guidant, VI, Santa Clara, CA]; X Technology) (31); this accounts for no more than 5% to 10% of interventions. Debulking of instent restenosis is possible, but it usually requires two burrs and (despite positive registry data) failed to show benefit over balloon angioplasty in the Angioplasty versus Rotational Atherectomy for Treatment of Diffuse In-stent Restenosis Trial (ARTIST) trial (32). The availability of cutting balloon, brachytherapy, and drug-eluting stents all challenge this role. Although rotablator of a resistant lesion before stent placement is beneficial in allowing complete stent expansion, the Stent Implantation Post Rotational Atherectomy Trial (SPORT) trial showed no benefit of routine rotational atherectomy debulking before stent placement (33).

Laser Atherectomy

Transmission of excimer (308 micron; Spectranetics [Colorado Springs, CO]) or HoYAG (>1000 micron) laser light through multifiber optical catheters can produce ablation of plaque from coronary atherothrombotic lesions. Laser catheter diameters from 0.9 to 2.5 mm are available and are placed over a standard 0.014-inch angioplasty guidewire. The excimer laser was originally felt to vaporize plaque by direct photochemical ablation, but it is now accepted that all lasers invoke a combination of photothermal and photoacoustic (shock wave) plaque disruption. Although eccentric catheters have been introduced in an effort to cut a vessel lumen larger than the catheter dimension, laser atherectomy procedures must generally be completed by balloon angioplasty and stent placement.

Data on this technology come almost exclusively from registries that contain up to 3,000 patients (34–36). Although lesion success in these registries is generally greater than 90%, major in-hospital complications occur in up to 6.4% of patients, including death in 0.5%, Q-wave MI in 2.1%, and urgent bypass surgery in 3.8%. The incidence of coronary perforation was as high as 1.4%, but has decreased to roughly 0.3% with technical enhancements including saline flush to remove blood and contrast from the laser path to minimize photoacoustic vessel disruption. Long-term follow-up has shown no improvement in angiographic or clinical restenosis rates compared with conventional balloon angioplasty (37).

With these clinical trial findings, the role of laser angioplasty as a primary interventional modality has almost vanished. Some aficionados still favor excimer laser angioplasty for treatment of resistant lesions, degenerated vein grafts, debulking of instent restenosis, or to facilitate crossing of total occlusions after guidewire recanalization (0.9-mm-diameter catheter) (38,39).

THROMBECTOMY DEVICES

When large thrombi are present, the risk for coronary intervention increases. Older strategies, such as prolonged anticoagulation or overnight intracoronary infusion of streptokinase, have now been supplanted by newer mechanical devices for thrombus removal. Although some claims for thrombectomy had been made by the earlier transluminal extraction catheter, this device has been designed predominantly as an atherectomy device with leading cutting blades that produced high levels of vessel trauma, and with relatively weak evacuation capacity by the application of external suction through the small-caliber central lumen. More recently, devices targeting thrombus removal more specifically have been developed, including the Possis AngioJet rheolytic thrombectomy catheter (Possis Medical, Minneapolis, MN) (40–44).

The AngioJet catheter in its current 4F XMI embodiment uses high-pressure (10,000 psi) infusion of saline through a small hypotube, and directed retrograde down the catheter lumen, to create intense local suction by the Bernoulli principle (pressure decreases adjacent to areas of rapid fluid flow). This local suction creates a vortex-like flow near the tip of the catheter that pulls soft fresh thrombus into the catheter openings, macerates it, and propels it through the catheter central lumen to an external collection bag. Early studies in saphenous vein grafts (SVGs; Vein Graft AngioJet Study [VeGAS I] and II) showed that it was highly effective in removing large "rat-tail" filling defects in SVGs and native coronary arteries, and it did so with fewer acute complications than the alternative treatment (overnight selective infusion of a thrombolytic agent into the affected vessel) (43). Experience in native vessels has concentrated on patients with unstable angina or acute myocardial infarction (AMI) in whom angiographic thrombus is present. Other devices include an Archimedes screw–assisted aspiration (X-sizer [eV3, Plymouth, MN]) and various ultrasonically active devices (OmniSonics [Wilmington, MA]) that break up thrombus by local cavitation (45–47).

The use of thrombectomy devices is generally confined to cases where a large thrombus burden is present on angiography. It is currently unclear whether routine use of a thrombectomy device would improve the procedural outcome of AMI. This is currently being evaluated in the AngioJet In Myocardial Infarction (AIMI) Trial.

DISTAL EMBOLIC PROTECTION

Although the early clinical and animal studies with balloon angioplasty suggested that distal embolization of atherothrombotic debris was distinctly uncommon, work with distal embolic protection devices in diseased SVGs has now established that distal atheroembolization is seen in more than 95% of cases (Fig. 94–2). Histologic examination shows that these emboli consist of cholesterol crystals, foam cells, and fibrous tissue—in short, the constituents of the underlying plaque (48–50). Moreover, trials comparing stenting over a conventional guidewire to stenting over distal occlusion device (PercuSurge GuardWire [Medtronic, Minneapolis, MN]) that allows aspiration of the debris containing stagnant column of blood before the occlusion device is deflated and flow restored have established the role of such emboli in producing clinical complications (51). In the Saphenous vein graft Angioplasty Free of Emboli Randomized (SAFER) trial of 801 patients, the use of this distal protection device thus reduced the incidence of major adverse clinical events (death, MI defined as CK-MB greater than three times the upper limit of normal, urgent target vessel revascularization) within 30 days of SVG PCI by 42% (51). This was largely because of reduction in the incidence of CK-MB level increase (across the range from three to ten times normal), but there were parallel reductions in mortality and the incidence of the "no-reflow" phenomenon (from 8% to 3%). Although the transient reduction of antegrade flow and associated ischemia in the absence of identifiable epicardial obstruction (stenosis, spasm, dissection, macroembolus) had previously been seen as a consequence of inappropriate distal arteriolar vasospasm requiring treatment with intracoronary infusion of arteriolar vasodilators (calcium channel blockers, nitroprusside, or adenosine) or platelet aggregation (requiring use of platelet glycoprotein IIb/IIIa receptor blockers), neither of these treatment modalities has shown the ability to reduce significantly the incidence of either no-reflow or major adverse clinical events in SVG intervention (52). The nearly ubiquitous recovery of distal emboli and the unprecedented ability of distal embolic protection to reduce these adverse events thus established the role of distal emboli (and the benefit of embolic protection) in this lesion type.

Although the distal occlusion system provides effective embolic protection, it has disadvantages including the need for several minutes of arterial occlusion with resulting ischemia and user complexity relating to sealing and unsealing the proximal end of the occlusion guidewire. In response, alternative devices using self-expanding basket or umbrella-like filters mounted on self-expanding nitinol armatures have been developed. These devices seem to provide a similar level of clinical benefit, although their 100-micron pore size does not allow them to block the smallest embolic particles or humoral mediators of distal microvascular spasm. Data from the recent FilterWire EX Randomized Evaluation (FIRE) trial of 650 patients showed that the Boston Scientific EPI FilterWire was equivalent to the PercuSurge GuardWire in preventing major adverse clinical events during SVG intervention (53).

Newer proximal occlusion devices, which reverse graft flow and allow debris aspiration through the guiding

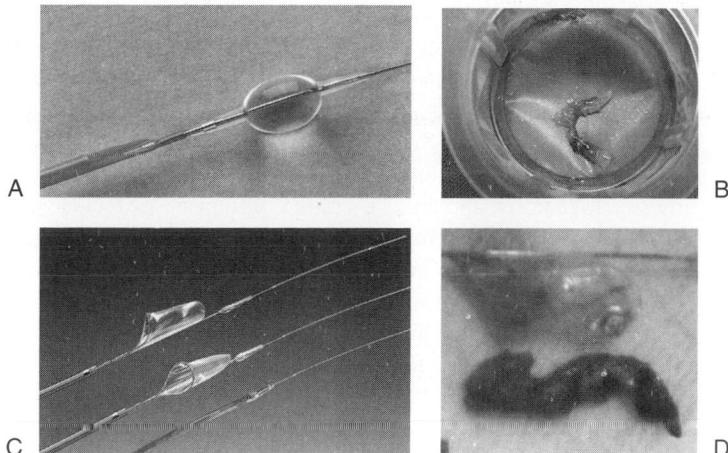

FIG. 94-2. Distal embolic protection devices (**A** and **C**) and associated debris retrieval during angioplasty of saphenous vein grafts (**B** and **D**).

catheter, are currently entering clinical trials. They offer the prospect of protection before the lesion is crossed with the guidewire and the possibility of "pressure-washing" the stented segment to remove any plaque material protruding through the stent struts, before antegrade flow is restored.

The findings regarding the benefit of distal embolic protection in SVG may well extend to other vessels. Small series of stents in carotid and renal arteries do show similar high frequencies of distal embolic recovery and suggest that intervention with distal embolic protection decreases the frequency of end-organ damage during the procedure (54–56). The definitive randomized trials, however, have not yet been performed. Similarly, provocative data have been obtained in native coronary arteries treated in the context of primary stenting of AMI. These data show a high frequency of recovery of both thrombotic and atherothrombotic debris and suggest better postintervention myocardial perfusion as measured by TIMI flow, myocardial blush score, and ST-segment resolution. A randomized trial known as Enhanced Myocardial Efficacy and Removal by Aspiration of Liberated Debris (EMERALD), however, has failed to show a clinical benefit of distal embolic protection with the GuardWire, using radionuclide-measured myocardial infarct size as the primary endpoint.

TOTAL OCCLUSION CROSSING DEVICES

The advances in PCI described earlier have concerned culprit lesions that are subtotally stenosed and can be crossed with angioplasty guidewires. Patients with one or more chronic total occlusions, or diffuse disease, present unmet clinical challenges (57–62). There are data suggesting that revascularization of chronic total occlusions is beneficial, but the success rate for conventional polymerase chain reaction attempts remains only 60% to 70%. Earlier attempts to use guidewires associated with energy sources (e.g., lasers) often have resulted in vessel dissection or perforation. Newer approaches include blunt microdissection with the Lumend FrontRunner

(Lumend, Redwood City, CA), or the combination of optical coherence reflectometry with pulses of radiofrequency energy in the IntraLuminal Therapeutics SafeCross device (IntraLuminal Therapeutics, Carlsbad, CA) (63,64).

When the vessels are still not suitable for revascularization, attempts have been made to provide other sources of collateral blood flow. One such approach is to arterialize the coronary venous system by connecting it to an adjacent coronary artery (TransVascular [Medtronic, Minneapolis, MN]) or the left ventricle (Percardia [Merrimack, NH]) (65). Ventricular sourcing directly to the myocardium also has been attempted through the use of laser-drilled channels, with some improvement in anginal frequency and exercise time compared with open-label medical therapy. But such channels seem to close spontaneously within several weeks, and randomized double-blinded studies have shown similar benefits in laser- and medically-treated patients, suggesting a potent "placebo" effect (66,67).

Another approach (discussed in Chapter 23) is angiogenesis—stimulated collateral growth through the systemic, intracoronary, pericardial, or myocardial injection of growth factors (or genes coding for such factors) (68). Results in patients with severe angina but no conventional revascularization options have been mixed. Given the profound placebo effect demonstrated for percutaneous laser myocardial revascularization, such trials will need to be analyzed carefully before the therapies are accepted as effective alternative forms of revascularization.

BRACHYTHERAPY

Recent experience with both β and γ catheter–based brachytherapy has been proven a successful way to prevent this neointimal regrowth after mechanical treatment of in-stent restenosis (69–71). Catheter-based sources can deliver the required 13- to 20-Gray radiation dose to the vessel wall in dwell times from 3 (β sources) to 20 minutes (γ sources). Care should be taken to cover the stent and generous proximal and distal margins (including all points of balloon injury) to minimize the risk for late failure caused by "geographic miss" (72). With effective brachytherapy, the chance of diffuse instent restenosis is reduced from roughly 50% to 20% (69–71). Because brachytherapy also inhibits beneficial endothelial coverage of the stent, new stent implantation should be avoided when performing brachytherapy, and antiplatelet drugs (aspirin and Plavix) should be continued for at least 9 months after treatment (73,74). It also should be appreciated that the effects of radiation on the arterial wall are cumulative, and brachytherapy can be used only once on a given lesion or vessel segment. A promising alternative to brachytherapy for the treatment of instent restenosis may be the implantation of a drug-eluting stent within the restenotic lumen.

STENTS

The concept of implanting a permanent endoluminal scaffold to maintain arterial patency was first proposed by Charles Dotter in 1969 (75). Practical devices for coronary use, however, were not introduced into clinical practice until 1985 in the form of a self-expanding wire mesh stent: the Wallstent (76–78). The rationale for stent implantation was based on the commonly accepted notion that unpredictable vessel wall disruption after balloon dilation results in deep vessel wall injury, as well as both microdissections and macrodissections, leading to abrupt vessel closure or restenosis. A rigid metallic endoluminal scaffold serves to "seal" dissections, creates a uniform circular lumen that improves flow characteristics, and provides a larger initial lumen cross-sectional area to accommodate postprocedural neointimal hyperplasia (Fig. 94–3). In the mid-1990s, on the basis of extensive serial intravascular ultrasound assessments, it became clear that vascular "remodeling," or late vessel wall constriction, rather than neointimal hyperplasia was the major contributor to late lumen cross-sectional area reduction after angioplasty. Importantly, placement of a stent not only prevents early mechanical recoil but also eliminates vascular remodeling as a restenosis mechanism.

Several years of clinical study were required to mature both stent designs and operator techniques, such that stents

could be used as a primary interventional therapy. The subsequent explosive growth of stents as the "default" therapy in coronary intervention is due to the following reasons: (a) stent delivery systems became sufficiently flexible to negotiate distal and tortuous regions of the coronary tree; (b) stents were associated with a dramatic reduction in postangioplasty abrupt vessel closure; (c) optimal stent technique combined with appropriate adjunctive pharmacology (aspirin plus thienopyridines) markedly reduced the frequency of subacute stent thrombosis (Intracoronary Stenting and Antithrombotic Regimen [ISAR] and STent Antithrombotic Regimens Study [STARS] trials) (79,80); and (d) stents were shown to reduce restenosis (vs. balloon angioplasty) by 30% (Belgium Netherlands stent [BENESTENT] and Stent Restenosis Study [STRESS] trials) (81,82). By the end of 2002, in the United States, balloon-expandable stents were being implanted in more than 90% of all interventional coronary procedures, attesting to the generalized acceptance of this breakthrough technology.

Bare-Metal Stents

Stent Designs

Most coronary stents are constructed from common biocompatible metals (usually 316L stainless steel) and are delivered through a balloon-expandable delivery system; that is, the stent is securely crimped or compressed over a balloon catheter and is deployed on balloon inflation after delivery to the lesion site. Stent designs are loosely categorized in three general groups: wire coils, slotted tubes, and modular rings. The earliest version of the Gianturco-Roubin stent was a wire coiled in a serpiginous pattern of reversing loops. This stent was successful as a device to scaffold dissections and prevent abrupt vessel closure (83). However, excessive plaque prolapse through the coils and inadequate radial support resulted in greater than expected restenosis. Several alternative versions and iterations of wire-coiled designs have been proposed and tested over the last decade, but none has demonstrated competitive antirestenosis efficacy, and this design configuration is currently no longer used for coronary applications.

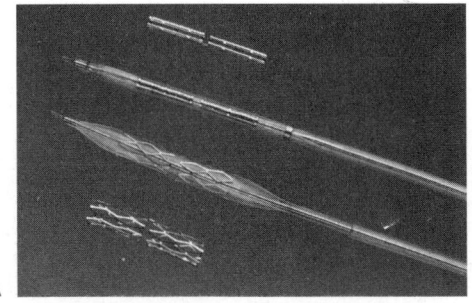
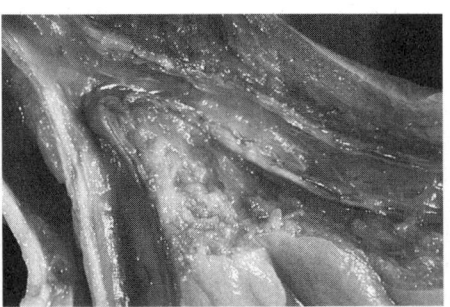

FIG. 94–3. The first-generation Palmaz-Schatz coronary stent **(A)** and necropsy section of coronary stent in place demonstrating scaffolding properties **(B).**

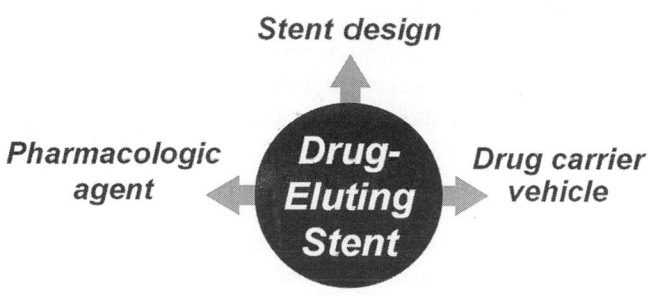

FIG. 94–4. The three components of a drug-eluting stent system.

The slotted tube design concept was embodied in the original Palmaz-Schatz stent, which was introduced as an investigational device in 1987 (Fig. 94–4) (84). The unexpanded offset rows of rectangular slots became plastically deformed into supporting diamonds with high radial strength after balloon inflation. A central articulating "bridge" was added to improve axial flexibility, and an overriding sheath was used to ensure stent retention before deployment. Although this stent design produced homogeneous scaffolding and provided favorable antirestenosis efficacy, the inherent rigidity of a continuous slotted tube design rendered delivery of the Palmaz-Schatz stent into challenging coronary anatomy problematic. This led to a variety of next-generation devices based on the slotted tube concept, including the Multilink stent (Guidant, Vl, and Santa Clara, CA) and the NIR stent (Boston Scientific, Natick, MA), wherein flexible connectors were added to continuous closed or open cell designs. These more flexible stents allowed distribution of stent bending throughout the stent length while maintaining requisite scaffolding properties. Third-generation stent designs within this category have incorporated lower overall profiles (<1 mm in diameter), further improvements in system flexibility, and thinner struts. Most recently, stent material changes have been emphasized, including cobalt-chromium alloys, which improve radial strength and radiopacity, despite thinner struts and lower profile designs.

Modular stent designs were developed to emphasize deliverability and radial support. The earliest designs (AVE Microstent [Medtronic, Minneapolis, MN]), consisting of discontinuous repeating zigzag rings, however, were unsuccessful in that the modules telescoped or separated on deployment, and the separation between rings encouraged excessive plaque prolapse. Current versions of modular stent designs have now incorporated laser welded connections between rings, shorter distances between modules (to reduce plaque prolapse and improve scaffolding), and thinner struts to reduce overall stent profile (including cobalt-chromium alloys).

A final category of stent designs are the self-expanding stents. This genre of stent consists of either woven strands of stainless steel in the form of a compressed meshlike tube or restrained modular geometries with struts composed of superelastic shape memory alloys such as nickel-titanium (nitinol) (85). Self-expanding stents are always held firmly in a compressed state onto the delivery catheter by a sheath or membrane, which is unfolded or withdrawn to allow expansion and deployment at the lesion site. Generally, these stents are intentionally "oversized," which ensures optimal vessel wall contact and expansile force. Although self-expanding stents may be very deliverable within the coronary tree, accuracy of positioning to lesion sites has been troublesome and antirestenosis of some designs has been suboptimal. Currently, self-expanding stents have been largely relegated to extracoronary applications in appropriate anatomies, such as carotid bifurcation disease and femoropopliteal lesions.

Clinical Indications

The clinical indications for bare-metal stents can be divided into urgent (or emergent) and elective applications. Most importantly, stents have dramatically improved the safety of coronary angioplasty procedures by virtue of reversing or preventing acute and "threatened" closure syndromes. Several registry studies involving multiple stent designs were shown to significantly reduce the need for emergency coronary bypass surgery after successful stent treatment of severe dissections and closure due to balloon angioplasty. Perhaps more important is the prevention of acute closure associated with the widespread use of elective stents (rather than balloon angioplasty) in clinical practice. Thus, a vital contribution of stent technology to PCI procedures has been the improvement in patient safety and the predictability of excellent angiographic outcomes, thereby eliminating the need for standby surgical backup (to manage complications or emergencies) and increasing the operator confidence to treat complex lesion morphologies.

During the decade of the 1990s, much investigator effort was directed toward the evidence-based medicine demonstration of superiority in safety and efficacy of coronary stent implantation versus balloon angioplasty (or coronary atherectomy) in a variety of clinical and anatomic situations. The principle justification for elective stenting has been both the prevention of acute closure and a 30% to 50% reduction in subsequent restenosis. Studies have been completed in *de novo* in patients with native coronary lesions, restenosis native coronary lesions, long lesions (diffuse disease), lesions in small vessels, aortoostial lesions, bifurcation lesions, SVG lesions, total occlusions, AMI lesions, and multivessel disease. There is an overriding consensus that elective stenting provides safer and more predictable periprocedural outcomes compared with alternative procedures. There also is agreement that stent implantation reduces subsequent restenosis, although the magnitude of restenosis reduction is somewhat dependent on lesion subtype (e.g., marked reduction in total occlusions, whereas modest reduction in small vessels). There is still an ongoing debate over whether elective stents are indicated in situations where the antirestenosis benefits are small versus a strategy of "provisional" stenting, which advocates initial balloon angioplasty and stent placement only if suboptimal angiographic results are achieved (usually about 50% of cases). Another technique that has become popular among interventional operators is so-called direct stenting—that is, stent implantation without antecedent predilation using a balloon catheter. This technique emphasizes the modern-day simplicity of coronary stenting procedures—easy deliverability of flexible low-profile stent systems to complex lesion morphologies, often without predilation, producing excellent angiographic results with rare complications and reduced restenosis.

Complications

Complications after stent procedures should be viewed in the context of frequency and importance. Stent embolization (dislodgement from the balloon delivery catheter) is extremely uncommon in the current era of stent implantation. Vessel perforation and side branch occlusion also are uncommon and occur with similar frequency during alternative interventional modalities. The two most important stent-related complications are stent thrombosis and late instent restenosis.

Stent thrombosis can occur within 24 hours of the index procedure (acute), within 30 days (subacute), or within the first 9 months (late). Both acute and late stent thrombosis are uncommon (combined <1%) and are usually associated with identified procedural technical difficulties (acute), endogenous patient-related thrombogenic milieu (hypercoaguable states or thrombocytosis), concomitant procedures (including general surgery after stent placement or vascular brachytherapy for instent restenosis), or withdrawal of appropriate antiplatelet medications. Subacute stent thrombosis (between 1 and 30 days after the stent procedure) occurs more frequently, and most disturbingly, and it can occur without warning or identifiable causation. All stents should be considered foreign body implants that elicit thrombogenic and inflammatory reactions. Until a biocompatible neointima is formed with overlying functioning endothelium, stents require meticulous treatment with advanced antiplatelet agents. Initially (late 1980s), the subacute stent thrombosis frequency was 15% to 20% because of improper implantation techniques combined with frustrating trial and error use of exotic cocktails of antithrombotic and antiplatelet agents. The application of aggressive long-term systemic anticoagulation (intravenous heparin with inhospital crossover to oral warfarin) reduced subacute stent thrombosis to 3%, but also resulted in markedly increased hemorrhagic complications and prolonged (and costly) hospital stays. A crucial breakthrough was pioneered by Colombo and coworkers (86) in the early 1990s: The combination of improved stent implantation techniques and additional antiplatelet therapy reduced subacute stent thrombosis to less than 1%. Thus, flush apposition of the stent struts to the vessel wall, using high-pressure balloon inflation that often was guided using intravascular ultrasound, rendered stents less thrombogenic, and the addition of oral thienopyridines (first ticlopidine and more recently clopidogrel) to aspirin eliminated the need for long-term antithrombotic agents. Despite these improvements, the syndrome of stent thrombosis continues to be a serious complication, because it often occurs suddenly when patients are out of the hospital and is generally associated with AMI and even sudden death (about 20% of cases).

Instent restenosis, or excessive necintima formation within or around the implanted stent, is observed in approximately 15% to 35% of cases depending on the stent design, the lesion morphology, and the clinical scenario. In approximately 60% of instent restenosis cases, the lesions are diffuse (>10 mm in length) and are more difficult to treat without secondary recurrence. A series of stent versus stent studies were performed in the mid and late 1990s to determine if stent design impacts the frequency and pattern of instent restenosis. In general, thinner strut balloon-expandable stents with optimized scaffolding features tend to have lower subsequent instent restenosis. Longer lesions in small vessels (especially in patients with diabetes) are associated with the greatest in-stent restenosis rates. The severity of the instent restenosis lesion predicts subsequent treatment success; thus, proliferative diffuse lesions or total occlusions after stent implantation will have as high as a 60% to 80% likelihood of recurrence after PCI reestablishment of optimal lumen dimensions. These poor results in the management of diffuse instent restenosis led to the application of intracoronary radiation as a new modality to prevent recurrence. Using catheter-based β- and γ-radiation sources that were exposed to the diseased stented vessel segment for up to 20 minutes, subsequent restenosis was reduced by as much as 50% compared with conventional therapies (69–71). Importantly, vascular brachytherapy has deleterious effects on vessel wall healing responses, which result in more frequent late stent thrombosis (after 30 days) and require prolonged dual antiplatelet therapy (from the standard 1 month for up to 1 year).

Clearly, the iterative development of improved stent systems, improved operator technique, and advanced adjunctive pharmacology heralded the era of "stent frenzy," which rapidly captured the imagination of interventional operators around the world. Nevertheless, even under the best circumstances, instent restenosis remained problematic and provoked the continued investigation of other biotechnology platforms.

"Covered" Stents

Overlapping the era of bare-metal "stent frenzy," several creative modifications of stent designs were proposed and evaluated in clinical investigations. One of the more innovative concepts was to use the bare-metal stent as a scaffold for a covering or graft material to create a flexible solid endovascular tube. These devices became known as "covered" stents or stent grafts, perhaps borrowing somewhat from the larger stent graft devices that were being developed to treat expanding abdominal aortic aneurysms. The clinical applications of coronary "covered" stents include the following treatment scenarios: (a) treatment of acute (and often life-threatening) procedure-related coronary perforations; (b) treatment of coronary aneurysms, pseudoaneurysms, and arteriovenous communications; (c) treatment of degenerative SVG disease; and (d) as an antirestenosis therapy (either alone or combined with embedded pharmacotherapy) in either native coronaries or SVGs (87). The graft coverings included biologic and prosthetic materials such as autologous vein (or artery), bovine pericardium, and polytetrafluoroethylene (PTFE).

The earliest (and most primitive) stent graft devices consisted of autologous vein, which was sewn onto a bare-metal stent immediately after harvesting and subsequently implanted by conventional balloon expansion techniques. Although initial success in treating coronary perforations and excluding coronary aneurysms was observed, this technique was too laborious and required too much time to be of practical value to the majority of practicing interventionalists. These "homemade" devices were rapidly replaced by commercial versions consisting of thin microporous PTFE graft materials that could be elastically stretched by either balloon expansion or on a self-expanding nitinol stent platform. Because the consequences of PCI-induced severe coronary perforations can be catastrophic (death in 19%, Q-wave MI in 15%, and emergency coronary reparative surgery in 63%), the availability of a covered stent device for urgent placement to seal the perforation site can be life-saving. In the first consecutive case registry evaluating the clinical efficacy of a balloon-expandable, PTFE-covered stent for severe coronary perforations, deployment success was achieved in all patients, and there were no adverse clinical events (death, Q-wave MI, or emergency coronary surgery).

Although the importance of stent grafts to treat severe coronary perforations has been established, the value of these devices as an anti-restenosis therapy in either native coronaries or SVGs has been disappointing. In two randomized clinical trials completed in Europe (Randomized Evaluation of polytetrafluoroethylene-COVERed stent in Saphenous vein grafts [RECOVERS] and STents IN Grafts [STING]) (88,89) comparing balloon-expandable covered stents versus bare-metal stents in SVG lesions, there was no indication of reduced restenosis frequency in patient treated with the covered stents. Additional studies in the United States are ongoing comparing a novel self-expanding encapsulated PTFE-covered stent design to determine if this newer version of a covered stent will reduce distal embolization, will improve restenosis frequency compared with conventional therapy, or both.

Drug-eluting Stents

Underlying Concepts

The application of bare-metal stents to reduce restenosis provides the dual benefits of blocking early recoil and late remodeling and providing an initially larger lumen area after angioplasty. However, stents do not prevent intimal hyperplasia,

and, in fact, the volume of neointima formation is four times greater in a stented artery compared with an artery treated using balloon angioplasty. A drug-eluting stent represents an elegant solution to the Achilles heel of angioplasty—restenosis—by incorporating a stent backbone and potent therapeutic agents that elute from the implanted stent surface into the vessel wall and can abolish subsequent intimal hyperplasia (90–93). A successful drug-eluting stent system represents an advanced biotechnology challenge that requires the synchronous integration of a stent, a carrier vehicle, and a drug (Fig. 94–3). A critical feature of the stent design is to provide optimized geometry with uniform interstrut distances on expansion, even within vessel bends (94). The carrier vehicle is probably the most undervalued and least understood component of a drug-eluting stent system. Many different synthetic and natural substances have been used as drug carriers for medical applications. Remarkably diverse carrier vehicle technologies have been studied in experimental models and have already been subjected to early clinical testing in patients (95–99). The most carefully examined drug carrier vehicles are thin layers (<20 microns in thickness) of elastomeric biostable polymers, which fully encapsulate the entire stent surface. The pharmaceutical agent selected for a drug-eluting stent is usually the most readily identified feature. The four general classes of drug compounds being investigated for drug-eluting stent clinical applications are antiinflammatory agents, antiproliferative agents, migration inhibitors and extracellular matrix modulators, and agents that promote healing usually by accelerating reendothelialization of the denuded vascular surface. Currently, the lead drug candidates for an ideal drug-eluting stent system have multiple modes of action, emphasizing antiinflammatory and antiproliferative properties. Among the important features of a successful pharmaceutical agent in a drug-eluting stent are the following: (a) known and targeted mechanism of action at the prescribed doses; (b) acceptable pharmacokinetic release profiles of the formulated compounds; (c) favorable therapeutic dosing "window" (broad dose range between optimal therapeutic and toxic doses); (d) no systemic toxicity and vascular biocompatibility at the prescribed and "real-world" doses; and (e) acceptable logistical factors, such as no alteration of drug activity after sterilization and drug stability over time.

Sirolimus-eluting Stents

The Cypher stent (Cordis Corporation, Warren, NJ) is the first U.S. Food and Drug Administration (FDA)–approved drug-eluting stent in the United States. Over the subsequent 6 months since FDA approval on April 24, 2003, there have been more than 250,000 Cypher stents implanted in patients in the United States. The three components of the Cypher stent include the Bx VELOCITY closed-cell stent platform, a biostable polymer for drug delivery, and the drug sirolimus. The Bx VELOCITY stent is a third-generation, flexible, closed-cell geometry stainless steel stent, which is mounted on a low-profile, semicompliant balloon delivery system. The closed-cell geometry favors homogeneous drug distribution into the vascular tissue on elution from the stent strut surfaces. The drug carrier vehicle selected for Cypher is a combination of biostable polymers (poly ethylene-co-vinyl acetate [PEVA] and poly n-butyl methacrylate [PBMA]) used for decades in biomedical applications and proven to be both safe and durable. Animal studies have demonstrated that the polymer combination does not erode over time and is neither proinflammatory nor thrombogenic. The drug is mixed with the polymers and the mixture forms a thin coat (5–10 microns) over the stent surface (Fig. 94–5). Drug release from the polymer-encapsulated stent is governed by simple principles of diffusion. This usually results in an early burst release followed by a secondary slower release, both of which depend on the drug/polymer weight ratios, the polymer thickness, the molecular weight of the drug, and the water solubility—characteristics of the drug and the polymer. This so-called matrix release pattern from biostable polymers is currently the most commonly used drug carrier vehicle for drug-eluting stent systems. To further delay the initial burst release, a drug-free, polymer-only "topcoat" can be added to the formulation. The topcoat serves as a diffusion barrier that importantly alters the elution kinetic profiles. The Cypher drug carrier system consists of the polymer drug base coat covered by a thin drug-free polymer topcoat tailored to elute approximately 50% of the drug (sirolimus) in the first week, 80% in the first month, and 100% in the first 3 months after stent implantation. Because sirolimus is very water-insoluble (i.e., lipophilic), almost no drug is released into the bloodstream during stent advancement to the lesion site, and after stent implantation, the diffusion gradient favors elution into tissue, again limiting the amounts of circulating free sirolimus.

Sirolimus (originally known as rapamycin) is a macrocyclic lactone fermentation product that was discovered by scientists from Wyeth Laboratories in the 1970s from soil

samples on the remote island of Rapa Nui. Originally thought to be an antifungal agent, this low–molecular weight, highly lipophilic compound was soon found to possess potent immunosuppressant properties. Sirolimus, in an oral formulation, under the trade name Rapamune, is an FDA-approved drug for the clinical indication of immunosuppression to prevent rejection after renal transplantation. More recently, vascular biologists learned that sirolimus also has potent cytostatic antiproliferative properties, thereby reducing intimal hyperplasia formation in animal models of balloon injury and stent implantation. Sirolimus interferes with the cell cycle before the critical G1 checkpoint, thereby allowing cells to remain viable and to return to a resting (nonproliferating) state. The sequential mechanisms of action of sirolimus as a cytostatic antiproliferative agent are as follows: (a) the highly lipophilic sirolimus molecule rapidly crosses smooth muscle cell membranes; (b) sirolimus binds avidly to an intracellular protein, called FKBP, which is up-regulated after vascular injury (during stent implantation); (c) sirolimus-FKBP now binds to a critical signal transduction protein, called mTOR (mammalian target of rapamycin); and (d) the sirolimus-FKBP-mTOR complex interferes with cell cycle events such as blocking proteins that activate the cell cycle, stimulating natural cell cycle inhibitors (especially p27), and turning off the cell cycle at the G1-S phase. Sirolimus also has well described and specific antiinflammatory effects including reduced T-cell proliferation and macrophage function, as well as interfering with cell surface, cytokine-mediated stimulation of inflammation (Fig. 94–6).

The pivotal clinical trials with the Cypher sirolimus-eluting stent should serve as a model for the evidence-based medicine introduction of future drug-eluting stent systems. Every patient was captured in the context of carefully planned and meticulously analyzed clinical trials. The clinical trials that form the basis for assessing the safety and efficacy of the Cypher sirolimus-eluting stent include a "first-in-man" experience at two centers, a multicenter blinded randomized trial outside the United States in simple coronary lesions (RAndomized study with the sirolimus-eluting VElocity balloon-expandable stent in the treatment of patients with de novo native coronary artery Lesions [RAVEL]), and a multicenter blinded randomized trial in the United States in more complex coronary lesions (Prospective, Randomized Evaluation of the SIRolImUS-eluting stent in de novo native coronary arteries [SIRIUS]). The first-in-man studies, performed in Sao Paulo, Brazil, and in Rotterdam, The Netherlands, were designed to assess the safety and preliminary efficacy of fast and slow release formulations in 45 carefully selected patients with simple *de novo* coronary lesions. Important lessons from these first-in-man cases can be summarized as follows: (a) Cypher was safe without evidence of stent thrombosis or other untoward clinical events; (b) angiography and intravascular ultrasound indicated a striking efficacy with marked reduction in binary restenosis, late loss, and percent volume obstruction; (c) clinical outcomes

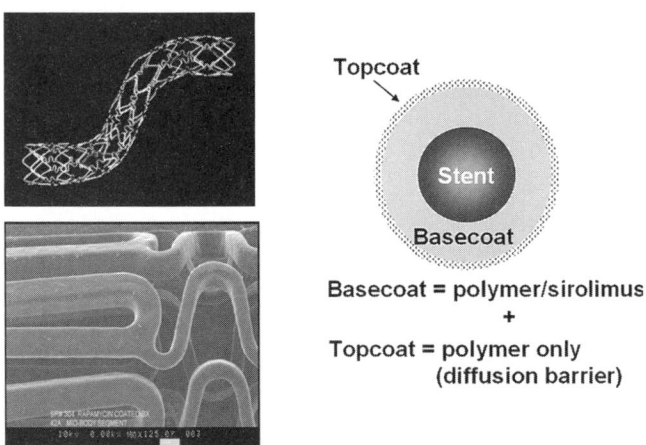

FIG. 94–5. The Cypher sirolimus drug-eluting stent system, demonstrating the stent geometry **(top left),** scanning electron micrograph of the stent surface **(bottom left),** and the multilayer polymer delivery system with topcoat (drug free) and base coat (containing sirolimus).

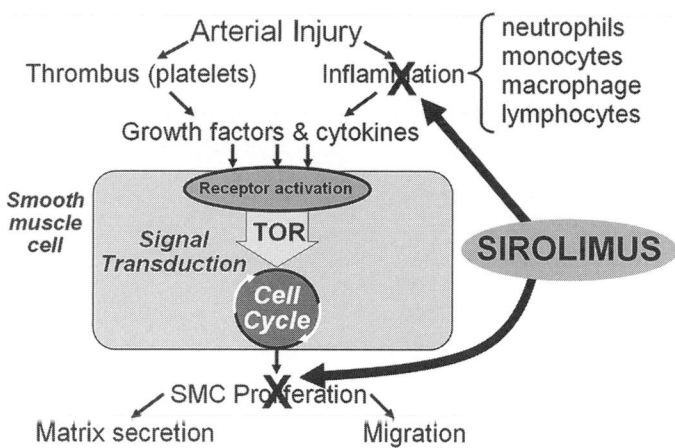

FIG. 94–6. Pictorial schematic showing the sites of action of sirolimus on the restenosis process. SMC, smooth muscle cell; TOC, target of rapamycin.

showed a similar striking reduction in target lesion and target vessel revascularization; (d) there were no differences between the fast- and slow-release formulations; and (e) the angiographic and clinical results were durable with maintained efficacy (current assessments at 4 years) (100–104) (Fig. 94–7).

The RAVEL trial was a double-blind, randomized trial of 238 patients with simple *de novo* coronary lesions in 19 clinical centers from Europe and Latin America. The slow-release Cypher formulation was used, and all lesions were required to be covered by a single 18-mm-long stent (either Bx VELOCITY or Cypher). Once again, the results were striking and corroborated the earlier first-in-man findings. RAVEL has been whimsically called the "zero study"; angiographic binary restenosis, late loss, target lesion and target vessel revascularization, and stent thrombosis were all zero in the 120 patients randomized to the Cypher stent (105–107).

SIRIUS was the pivotal Cypher clinical trial in the United States involving 52 clinical centers and 1,101 patients (108). Compared with first-in-man studies and RAVEL, this double-blinded, randomized trial included more complex patients (more patients with diabetes) and longer lesions, often requiring overlapping stents. In SIRIUS, the Cypher stent was safe with an overall stent thrombosis frequency of 0.4%. In these more complex patients and lesions, Cypher was still associated with a striking greater than 90% reduction of neointimal hyperplasia within the stent (assessed by quantitative intravascular ultrasound methodologies) (Fig. 94–8), and angiographic outcomes also were markedly improved, with 70% to 80% reductions in late loss and restenosis (overall restenosis reduced to 8.9% and target lesion revascularization reduced to 4.1%). Importantly, the subgroup analyses from SIRIUS indicate that the safety and effectiveness of Cypher sirolimus-eluting stents extend to a broad cross section of patients and lesions, including small

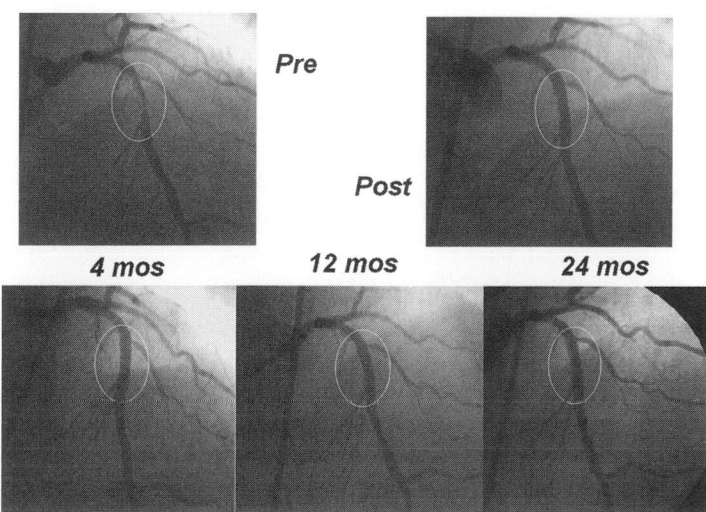

FIG. 94–7. Angiogram from the first-in-man experience showing widely patent stent site at four months, one year, and two years after the index procedure.

Neointimal Hyperplasia (NIH)

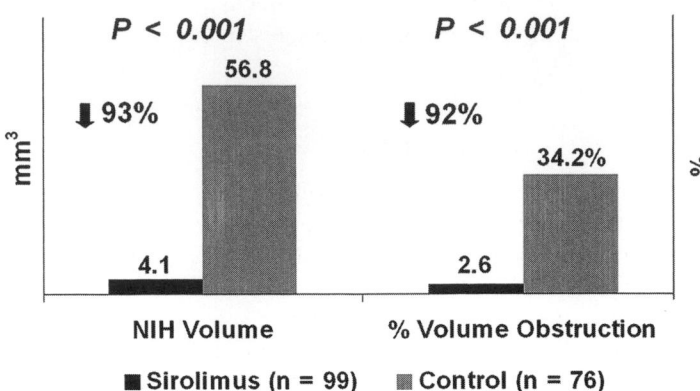

FIG. 94–8. Data from the Prospective, Randomized Evaluation of the Sirolimus-eluting Stent in Patients with De Novo Coronary Lesions (SIRIUS) clinical trial showing dramatic reduction in intimal hyperplasia (intravascular ultrasound assessments) within the stent compared with bare-metal control stents 8 months after stent placement.

and large vessels, short and long lesions, diabetes, lesions involving the LAD, and lesions treated with single or overlapping stents (Fig. 94–9).

From these pivotal trials, it is justified to conclude the following: (a) Cypher stents are safe without known untoward complications (such as increased stent thrombosis or aneurysms); (b) Cypher stents have shown consistent dramatic reduction in poststent implantation neointimal hyperplasia assessed by quantitative angiographic and intravascular ultrasound techniques (far greater effects than were anticipated on the basis of earlier animal studies); (c) Cypher stents have consistently demonstrated improved clinical outcomes, especially the need for repeat revascularization of the target lesions; (d) the effects of Cypher stents appear durable with 3-year data from first-in-man, 2-year data from RAVEL, and 1-year data from SIRIUS, all indicating maintained efficacy at late follow-up intervals;

(e) Cypher stents are an effective antirestenosis therapy in both simple and complex lesions (although additional data would be important in several lesion subsets) (109); and (f) precise implantation techniques for Cypher stents (such as longer stent/lesion length ratios) are required to obtain optimal follow-up results.

Paclitaxel-eluting Stents

The TAXUS drug-eluting stent platform (Boston Scientific) is the next important biotechnology antirestenosis therapy that will be available in the United States. This device consists of a highly deliverable bare-metal stent system (the Express^2), encapsulated by a thin layer of a biostable elastomeric polymer that contains the drug paclitaxel. As with many antiproliferative agents used in drug-eluting stent systems to treat restenosis, paclitaxel, which is the active com-

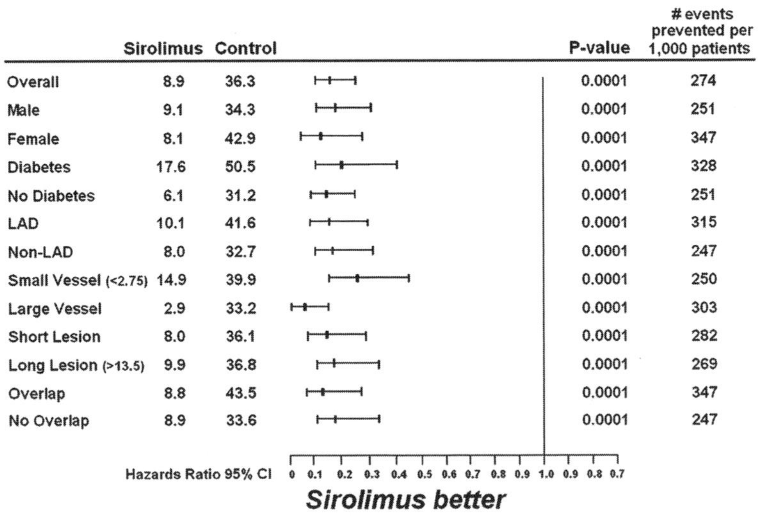

	Sirolimus	Control	Hazards Ratio 95% CI	P-value	# events prevented per 1,000 patients
Overall	8.9	36.3		0.0001	274
Male	9.1	34.3		0.0001	251
Female	8.1	42.9		0.0001	347
Diabetes	17.6	50.5		0.0001	328
No Diabetes	6.1	31.2		0.0001	251
LAD	10.1	41.6		0.0001	315
Non-LAD	8.0	32.7		0.0001	247
Small Vessel (<2.75)	14.9	39.9		0.0001	250
Large Vessel	2.9	33.2		0.0001	303
Short Lesion	8.0	36.1		0.0001	282
Long Lesion (>13.5)	9.9	36.8		0.0001	269
Overlap	8.8	43.5		0.0001	347
No Overlap	8.9	33.6		0.0001	247

Hazards Ratio 95% CI   0 0.1 0.2 0.3 0.4 0.5 0.6 0.7 0.8 0.9 1.0 0.9 0.8 0.7

Sirolimus better

FIG. 94–9. Data from the Prospective, Randomized Evaluation of the SIRolImUS-eluting stent in de novo native coronary arteries (SIRIUS) clinical trial showing odds ratio results of restenosis in various patient and lesion subgroups. CI, confidence interval; LAD, left anterior descending.

ponent of Taxol, is a commonly used chemotherapy agent. Paclitaxel is an extremely hydrophobic compound that is extracted from the Pacific Yew tree, Taxus Brevifolia, found in the Northwest United States and Canada. Paclitaxel has multifunctional activities with dose-dependent cellular effects including antiproliferative and antiinflammatory actions and inhibition of smooth muscle cell migration. At high doses, paclitaxel promotes apoptosis, but at doses in the therapeutic range, the effects on the cell cycle appear to be cytostatic. The predominant mechanism of action that has been associated with paclitaxel has been the suppression of microtubule dynamics involved in cell division. Paclitaxel binds to microtubules, which causes stabilization of microtubule deconstruction, the formation bundles and multiple asters, and cell cycle mitotic arrest, thereby inhibiting cell proliferation and migration.

The clinical trials performed with the Taxus drug-eluting stent have again followed a deliberate pathway, starting with first-in-man experiences (TAXUS 1) (110), advancing to blinded randomized clinical trials using different release formulations in simple coronary lesions (ASian Paclitaxel-Eluting Stent Clinical Trial [ASPECT] and TAXUS 2) (111–113), and concluding with a blinded randomized trial in the United States (the FDA pivotal study) using the slow-release formulation in more complex coronary lesions (TAXUS IV) (114). In TAXUS I, the slow-release paclitaxel-eluting stent resulted in a reduced late lumen loss (0.36 mm) and no episodes of angiographic restenosis or target lesion revascularization at follow-up in 31 patients with simple coronary lesions. TAXUS II studied both the slow- and moderate-release paclitaxel-eluting stent formulations in sequential blinded randomized clinical trials versus control bare-metal stents (total n = 536 patients). The results indicated (a) infrequent stent thrombosis, comparable to bare-metal stents and similar with both slow- and moderate-release formulations; (b) marked reduction in angiographic late loss and restenosis (for slow release from 20.1% to 5.5% and for moderate release from 23.8% to 8.6%); (c) marked improvement in target lesion revascularization at follow-up (for slow release from 14.3% to 7.3% and for moderate release from 17.7% to 6.2%). Because there was no incremental efficacy between the slow- and moderate-release paclitaxel formulations, the subsequent U.S. clinical trial, TAXUS IV, involved only the use of slow-release paclitaxel-eluting stents. TAXUS IV was a double-blind, randomized study of 1,314 patients conducted at 73 U.S. sites comparing the slow-release paclitaxel-eluting stent versus a bare-metal stent in patients with moderately complex coronary lesions. Stent thrombosis was low (<1%) in both groups, attesting to the safety of the drug-eluting stent in this study. At 9-month follow-up angiographic study, in patients treated with the paclitaxel-eluting stent, the late lumen loss was reduced from 0.61 to 0.23 mm and restenosis was reduced from 26.6% to 7.9%. Similarly, clinical end points, such as target lesion revascularization, were dramatically reduced to 3% at 9-month follow-up assessments. Because the patient and lesion demo-

graphics of SIRIUS and TAXUS IV were similar, it would be reasonable to suggest that a preliminary cross-study comparison indicates that these two drug-eluting stent systems are "essentially comparable" from the standpoint of safety and efficacy.

Drug-eluting Stents in the Future

The rapid proliferation of drug-eluting stent use in the United States since mid-2003 represents the most radical shift in interventional therapeutics over the past 25 years. Most assuredly, considerable additional clinical trial data are required before a blanket recommendation can be made to implant drug-eluting stents in all patients who are appropriate candidates for interventional therapy of obstructive coronary disease. Many lesion subsets, including SVG lesions, left main lesions, bifurcation disease, instent restenosis lesions, AMI lesions, and chronic total occlusions have not been fully evaluated, and clinical trial results in the next 2 years will indicate whether treatment should be extended to these more complex lesion morphologies. Finally, the durability (both safety and efficacy) of the early favorable data must be carefully scrutinized, because true long-term data (>3 years of follow-up) exist for only a handful of patients.

Clearly, there will be several additional innovative biotechnology devices in the future involving improved stent design and delivery platforms, novel and precise drug carrier vehicles without early or late inflammatory changes, and alternative pharmaceutical agents, alone and in combination, which can address problematic patient subsets, such as patients with severe diabetes. Moreover, the concept of site-specific stent-based drug delivery may have other interesting clinical applications including treatment of vulnerable plaque, angiogenesis or myogenesis, and myocardial preservation AMI.

REFERENCES

1. Topol EJ, Ellis SG, Cosgrove DM, et al. Analysis of coronary angioplasty practice in the United States with an insurance-claims data base. *Circulation* 1993;87:1489–1497.
2. Popma JJ, Wang JC. Advances in percutaneous coronary intervention. *Adv Intern Med* 2001;46:307–358.
3. Gruntzig AR, Senning A, Siegenthaler WE. Nonoperative dilatation of coronary-artery stenosis: percutaneous transluminal coronary angioplasty. *N Engl J Med* 1979;301:61–68.
4. Orlic D, Reimers B, Stankovic G, et al. Initial experience with a new 8 French-compatible directional atherectomy catheter: immediate and mid-term results. *Catheter Cardiovasc Interv* 2003;60:159–166.
5. Moussa I, Moses J, Di Mario C, et al. Stenting after optimal lesion debulking (sold) registry. Angiographic and clinical outcome. *Circulation* 1998;98:1604–1609.
6. Topol EJ, Leya F, Pinkerton CA, et al. A comparison of directional atherectomy with coronary angioplasty in patients with coronary artery disease. The CAVEAT Study Group. *N Engl J Med* 1993;329:221–227.
7. Elliott JM, Berdan LG, Holmes DR, et al. One-year follow-up in the Coronary Angioplasty Versus Excisional Atherectomy Trial (CAVEAT I). *Circulation* 1995;91:2158–2166.
8. Omoigui NA, Califf RM, Pieper K, et al. Peripheral vascular complications in the Coronary Angioplasty Versus Excisional Atherectomy Trial (CAVEAT-I). *J Am Coll Cardiol* 1995;26:922–930.

9. Simonton CA, Leon MB, Baim DS, et al. 'Optimal' directional coronary atherectomy: final results of the Optimal Atherectomy Restenosis Study (OARS). *Circulation* 1998;97:332–339.

10. Baim DS, Cutlip DE, Sharma SK, et al. Final results of the Balloon vs Optimal Atherectomy Trial (BOAT). *Circulation* 1998;97:322–331.

11. Lansky AJ, Popma JJ, Cutlip D, et al. Comparative analysis of early and late angiographic outcomes using two quantitative algorithms in the Balloon versus Optimal Atherectomy Trial (BOAT). *Am J Cardiol* 1999;83:1611–1616.

12. Suzuki T, Hosokawa H, Katoh O, et al. Effects of adjunctive balloon angioplasty after intravascular ultrasound-guided optimal directional coronary atherectomy: the result of Adjunctive Balloon Angioplasty After Coronary Atherectomy Study (ABACAS). *J Am Coll Cardiol* 1999;34:1028–1035.

13. Gruberg L, Pinnow E, Flood R, et al. Incidence, management, and outcome of coronary artery perforation during percutaneous coronary intervention. *Am J Cardiol* 2000;86:680–682,A8.

14. Von Sohsten R, Kopistansky C, Cohen M, et al. Cardiac tamponade in the "new device" era: evaluation of 6999 consecutive percutaneous coronary interventions. *Am Heart J* 2000;140:279–283.

15. Adelman AG, Cohen EA, Kimball BP, et al. A comparison of directional atherectomy with balloon angioplasty for lesions of the left anterior descending coronary artery. *N Engl J Med* 1993;329:228–233.

16. Airoldi F, Di Mario C, Stankovic G, et al. Clinical and angiographic outcome of directional atherectomy followed by stent implantation in de novo lesions located at the ostium of the left anterior descending coronary artery. *Heart* 2003;89:1050–1054.

17. Cohen EA, Sykora K, Kimball BP, et al. Clinical outcomes of patients more than one year following randomization in the Canadian Coronary Atherectomy Trial (CCAT). *Can J Cardiol* 1997;13:825–830.

18. Brener SJ, Leya FS, Apperson-Hansen C, et al. A comparison of debulking versus dilatation of bifurcation coronary arterial narrowings (from the CAVEAT I Trial). Coronary Angioplasty Versus Excisional Atherectomy Trial-I. *Am J Cardiol* 1996;78:1039–1041.

19. Karvouni E, Di Mario C, Nishida T, et al. Directional atherectomy prior to stenting in bifurcation lesions: a matched comparison study with stenting alone. *Catheter Cardiovasc Interv* 2001;53:12–20.

20. Mahdi NA, Pathan AZ, Harrell L, et al. Directional coronary atherectomy for the treatment of Palmaz-Schatz in-stent restenosis. *Am J Cardiol* 1998;82:1345–1351.

21. Robinson NM, Balcon R, Layton CA, et al. Intravascular ultrasound assessment of culotte stent deployment for the treatment of stenoses at major coronary bifurcations. *Int J Cardiovasc Interv* 2001;4: 21–27.

22. Airoldi F, Di Mario C, Stankovic G, et al. Effectiveness of treatment of in-stent restenosis with an 8-French compatible atherectomy catheter. *Am J Cardiol* 2003;92:725–728.

23. Adamian M, Colombo A, Briguori C, et al. Cutting balloon angioplasty for the treatment of in-stent restenosis: a matched comparison with rotational atherectomy, additional stent implantation and balloon angioplasty. *J Am Coll Cardiol* 2001;38:672–679.

24. Kobayashi Y, Mehran R, Mintz GS, et al. Acute and long-term outcomes of cutting balloon angioplasty followed by gamma brachytherapy for in-stent restenosis. *Am J Cardiol* 2003;92:1329–1331.

25. Roguelov C, Eeckhout E, De Benedetti E, et al. Clinical outcome following combination of cutting balloon angioplasty and coronary beta-radiation for in-stent restenosis: a report from the RENO Registry. *J Invasive Cardiol* 2003;15:706–709.

26. Kobayashi Y, De Gregorio J, Kobayashi N, et al. Lower restenosis rate with stenting following aggressive versus less aggressive rotational atherectomy. *Catheter Cardiovasc Interv* 1999;46:406–414.

27. Dietz U, Rupprecht HJ, Ekinci O, et al. Angiographic analysis of immediate and long-term results of PTCR vs. PTCA in complex lesions (COBRA study). *Catheter Cardiovasc Interv* 2001;53:359–367.

28. Safian RD, Feldman T, Muller DW, et al. Coronary angioplasty and Rotablator atherectomy trial (CARAT): immediate and late results of a prospective multicenter randomized trial. *Catheter Cardiovasc Interv* 2001;53:213–220.

29. Whitlow PL, Bass TA, Kipperman RM, et al. Results of the study to determine rotablator and transluminal angioplasty strategy (STRATAS). *Am J Cardiol* 2001;87:699–705.

30. Mauri L, Reisman M, Buchbinder M, et al. Comparison of rotational atherectomy with conventional balloon angioplasty in the prevention of restenosis of small coronary arteries: results of the Dilatation vs Ablation Revascularization Trial Targeting Restenosis (DART). *Am Heart J* 2003;145:847–854.

31. Ischinger TA, Solar RJ, Hitzke E. Improved outcome with novel device for low-pressure PTCA in de novo and in-stent lesions. *Cardiovasc Radiat Med* 2003;4:2–6.

32. vom Dahl J, Dietz U, Haager PK, et al. Rotational atherectomy does not reduce recurrent in-stent restenosis: results of the angioplasty versus rotational atherectomy for treatment of diffuse in-stent restenosis trial (ARTIST). *Circulation* 2002;105:583–588.

33. Buchbinder M, Fortuna R, Sharma SK, et al. Debulking prior to stenting: long term clinical and angiographic results from the SPORT trial. *Circulation* 2000;102:II,663 (abst).

34. Safian RD, Freed M, Reddy V, et al. Do excimer laser angioplasty and rotational atherectomy facilitate balloon angioplasty? Implications for lesion-specific coronary intervention. *J Am Coll Cardiol* 1996; 27:552–559.

35. Hong MK, Popma JJ, Baim DS, et al. Frequency and predictors of major in-hospital ischemic complications after planned and unplanned new-device angioplasty from the New Approaches to Coronary Intervention (NACI) registry. *Am J Cardiol* 1997;80:40K–49K.

36. Mehran R, Dangas G, Mintz GS, et al. Treatment of in-stent restenosis with excimer laser coronary angioplasty versus rotational atherectomy: comparative mechanisms and results. *Circulation* 2000;101:2484–2489.

37. Reifart N, Vandormael M, Krajcar M, et al. Randomized comparison of angioplasty of complex coronary lesions at a single center. Excimer Laser, Rotational Atherectomy, and Balloon Angioplasty Comparison (ERBAC) Study. *Circulation* 1997;96:91–98.

38. Strauss BH, Natarajan MK, Batchelor WB, et al. Early and late quantitative angiographic results of vein graft lesions treated by excimer laser with adjunctive balloon angioplasty. *Circulation* 1995;92:348–356.

39. Almeida M, Cavaco DM, Ribeiro MA, et al. The angioplasty of chronic coronary occlusions with the excimer laser for debulking followed by stent implantation. *Rev Port Cardiol* 2000;19:67–71.

40. Topaz O, Bernardo N, Desai P, et al. Acute thrombotic-ischemic coronary syndromes: the usefulness of TEC. *Catheter Cardiovasc Interv* 1999;48:406–420.

41. Nakagawa Y, Matsuo S, Kimura T, et al. Thrombectomy with Angio-Jet catheter in native coronary arteries for patients with acute or recent myocardial infarction. *Am J Cardiol* 1999;83:994–999.

42. Rinfret S, Katsiyiannis PT, Ho KK, et al. Effectiveness of rheolytic coronary thrombectomy with the AngioJet catheter. *Am J Cardiol* 2002;90:470–476.

43. Kuntz RE, Baim DS, Cohen DJ, et al. A trial comparing rheolytic thrombectomy with intracoronary urokinase for coronary and vein graft thrombus (the Vein Graft AngioJet Study [VeGAS 2]). *Am J Cardiol* 2002;89:326–330.

44. Singh M, Tiede DJ, Mathew V, et al. Rheolytic thrombectomy with Angiojet in thrombus-containing lesions. *Catheter Cardiovasc Interv* 2002;56:1–7.

45. Kwok OH, Prpic R, Gaspar J, et al. Angiographic outcome after intracoronary X-Sizer helical atherectomy and thrombectomy: first use in humans. *Catheter Cardiovasc Interv* 2002;55:133–139.

46. Stone GW, Cox DA, Low R, et al. X-TRACT Investigators. Safety and efficacy of a novel device for treatment of thrombotic and atherosclerotic lesions in native coronary arteries and saphenous vein grafts: results from the multicenter X-Sizer for treatment of thrombus and atherosclerosis in coronary applications trial (X-TRACT) study. *Catheter Cardiovasc Interv* 2003;58:419–427.

47. Rosenschein U, Brosh D, Halkin A. Coronary ultrasound thrombolysis: from acute myocardial infarction to saphenous vein grafts and beyond. *Curr Interv Cardiol Rep* 2001;3:5–9.

48. Grube E, Gerckens U, Yeung AC, et al. Prevention of distal embolization during coronary angioplasty in saphenous vein grafts and native vessels using porous filter protection. *Circulation* 2001;104:2436–2441.

49. Lowe HC, Houser SL, Aretz T, et al. Significant atheromatous debris following uncomplicated vein graft direct stenting: evidence supporting routine use of distal protection devices. *J Invasive Cardiol* 2002; 14:636–639.

50. Moreno PR, Lodder RA, Purushothaman KR, et al. Detection of lipid pool, thin fibrous cap, and inflammatory cells in human aortic atherosclerotic plaques by near-infrared spectroscopy. *Circulation* 2002;105: 923–927.

51. Baim DS, Wahr D, George B, et al. Saphenous vein graft Angioplasty Free of Emboli Randomized (SAFER) Trial Investigators. Random-

ized trial of a distal embolic protection device during percutaneous intervention of saphenous vein aorto-coronary bypass grafts. *Circulation* 2002;105:1285–1290.

52. Eeckhout E, Kern MJ. The coronary no-reflow phenomenon: a review of mechanisms and therapies. *Eur Heart J* 2001;22:729–739.

53. Stone GW, Rogers C, Hermiller J, et al. FilterWire EX Randomized Evaluation Investigators. Randomized comparison of distal protection with a filter-based catheter and a balloon occlusion and aspiration system during percutaneous intervention of diseased saphenous vein aorto-coronary bypass grafts. *Circulation* 2003;108: 548–553.

54. Grube E, Colombo A, Hauptmann E, et al. Initial multicenter experience with a novel distal protection filter during carotid artery stent implantation. *Catheter Cardiovasc Interv* 2003;58:139–146.

55. Al-Mubarak N, Roubin GS, Vitek JJ, et al. Microembolization during carotid stenting with the distal-balloon antiemboli system. *Int Angiol* 2002;21:344–348.

56. Henry M, Klonaris C, Henry I, et al. Protected renal stenting with the PercuSurge GuardWire device: a pilot study. *J Endovasc Ther* 2001; 8:227–237.

57. Finci L, Meier B, Favre J, et al. Long-term results of successful and failed angioplasty for chronic total coronary arterial occlusion. *Am J Cardiol* 1990;66:660–662.

58. Ruocco NA Jr, Ring ME, Holubkov R, et al. Results of coronary angioplasty of chronic total occlusions (the National Heart, Lung, and Blood Institute 1985-1986 Percutaneous Transluminal Angioplasty Registry). *Am J Cardiol* 1992;69:69–76.

59. Kinoshita I, Katoh O, Nariyama J, et al. Coronary angioplasty of chronic total occlusions with bridging collateral vessels: immediate and follow-up outcome from a large single-center experience. *J Am Coll Cardiol* 1995;26:409–415.

60. Puma JA, Sketch MH Jr, Tcheng JE, et al. Percutaneous revascularization of chronic coronary occlusions: an overview. *J Am Coll Cardiol* 1995;26:1–11.

61. Suero JA, Marso SP, Jones PG, et al. Procedural outcomes and long-term survival among patients undergoing percutaneous coronary intervention of a chronic total occlusion in native coronary arteries: a 20-year experience. *J Am Coll Cardiol* 2001;38:409–414.

62. Ivanhoe RJ, Weintraub WS, Douglas JS Jr, et al. Percutaneous transluminal coronary angioplasty of chronic total occlusions. Primary success, restenosis, and long-term clinical follow-up. *Circulation* 1992; 85:106–115.

63. Morales PA, Heuser RR. Chronic total occlusions: experience with fiber-optic guidance technology—optical coherence reflectometry. *J Interv Cardiol* 2001;14:611–616.

64. Tadros P. Successful revascularization of a long chronic total occlusion of the right coronary artery utilizing the frontrunner X39 CTO catheter system. *J Invasive Cardiol* 2003;15:3.

65. Boeksteegers P, Raake P, Al Ghobainy R, et al. Stent-based approach for ventricle-to-coronary artery bypass. *Circulation* 2002;106:1000–1006.

66. Laham RJ, Simons M, Pearlman JD, et al. Magnetic resonance imaging demonstrates improved regional systolic wall motion and thickening and myocardial perfusion of myocardial territories treated by laser myocardial revascularization. *J Am Coll Cardiol* 2002;39:1–8.

67. Stone GW, Teirstein PS, Rubenstein R, et al. A prospective, multicenter, randomized trial of percutaneous transmyocardial laser revascularization in patients with nonrecanalizable chronic total occlusions. *J Am Coll Cardiol* 2002;39:1581.

68. Patterson C, Runge MS. Therapeutic myocardial angiogenesis via vascular endothelial growth factor gene therapy: moving on down the road. *Circulation* 2000;102:940–942.

69. Teirstein PS, Massulo V, Jani S, et al. Catheter-based radiotherapy to inhibit restenosis after coronary stenting. *N Engl J Med* 1997;336: 1697–1703.

70. Waksman R, Bhargava B, White L, et al. Intracoronary beta-radiation therapy inhibits recurrence of in-stent restenosis. *Circulation* 2000; 101:1895–1898.

71. Leon MB, Teirstein PS, Moses JW, et al. Localized intracoronary gamma-radiation therapy to inhibit the recurrence of restenosis after stenting. *N Engl J Med* 2001;344:250–256.

72. Sabate M, Costa MA, Kozuma K, et al. Geographic miss: a cause of treatment failure in radio-oncology applied to intracoronary radiation therapy. *Circulation* 2000;101:2467–2471.

73. Waksman R, Bhargava B, Mintz GS, et al. Late total occlusion after

74. Waksman R, Ajani A, Pinnow E, et al. Twelve versus six months of clopidogrel to reduce major cardiac events in patients undergoing gamma-radiation therapy for in-stent restenosis: Washington radiation for In-Stent restenosis Trial (WRIST) 12 versus WRIST PLUS. *Circulation* 2002;106:776–778.

75. Dotter CT. Transluminally placed coil spring arterial tube grafts: long-term patency in canine popliteal artery. *Invest Radiol* 1969;4: 329–334.

76. Sigwart U, Puel J, Mirkovitch V, et al. Intravascular stent to prevent occlusion and restenosis after transluminal angioplasty. *N Engl J Med* 1987;316:701–707.

77. Roubin GS, Robinson KA, King SB 3rd, et al. Early and late results of intracoronary arterial stenting after coronary angioplasty in dogs. *Circulation* 1987;76:891–899.

78. Palmaz JC, Sibbitt RR, Reuter SR, et al. Expandable intraluminal graft: preliminary study. *Radiology* 1985;156:73–81.

79. Schomig A, Neumann FJ, Kastrati A, et al. A randomized comparison of anti-platelet therapy and anticoagulation therapy after placement of coronary artery stents. *N Engl J Med* 1996;334:1084–1092.

80. Leon MB, Baim DS, Popma JJ, et al. A clinical trial comparing three anti-thrombotic drug regimens after coronary artery stenting. *N Engl J Med* 1998;339:1665–1674.

81. Serruys PW, de Jaegere P, Kiemeneij F, et al. A comparison of balloon-expandable stent implantation with balloon angioplasty in patients with coronary artery disease. *N Engl J Med* 1994;331:489–497.

82. Fischman DL, Leon MB, Baim DS, et al. A randomized comparison of coronary stent placement and balloon angioplasty in the treatment of coronary artery disease. *N Engl J Med* 1994;331:497–506.

83. George BS, Voohees WD 3rd, Roubin GS, et al. Multicenter investigation of coronary stenting to treat acute or threatened closure after percutaneous transluminal coronary angioplasty: clinical and angiographic outcomes. *J Am Coll Cardiol* 1993;22:135–144.

84. Schatz RA, Baim DS, Leon MB, et al. Clinical experience with the Palmaz-Schatz coronary stent: Initial results of a multicenter study. *Circulation* 1991;83:148–157.

85. Serruys PW, Strauss BH, Beatt KJ, et al. Angiographic follow-up after placement of a self-expanding coronary stent. *N Engl J Med* 1991; 324:13–19.

86. Colombo A, Hall P, Nakamura S, et al. Intracoronary stenting without anticoagulation accomplished with intravascular ultrasound guidance. *Circulation* 1995;91:676–684.

87. Gercken U, Lansky AJ, Buellesfeld L, et al. Results of the Josent coronary stent graft implantation in various clinical settings: procedural and follow-up results. *Catheter Cardiovasc Interv* 2002;56:353–360.

88. Stankovic G, Colombo A, Presbitero P, et al. Randomized evaluation of polytetrafluoroethylene-covered stent in saphenous vein grafts: the Randomized Evaluation of polytetrafluoroethylene-COVERed stent in Saphenous vein grafts (RECOVERS) trial. *Circulation* 2003;108:37–42.

89. Schachinger V, Hamm CW, Munze, T, et al. A randomized trial of polytetrafluoroethylene-membrane covered stents compared with conventional stents in aortocoronary saphenous vein grafts. *J Am Coll Cardiol* 2003;42:1360–1369.

90. Sousa JE, Serruys PW, Costa MA. New frontiers in cardiology. Drug-eluting stents: Part I. *Circulation* 2003;107:2274–2279.

91. Sousa JE, Costa MA, Sousa AG. What is "the matter" with restenosis in 2002? *Circulation* 2002;105:2932–2933.

92. Sousa JE, Serruys PW, Costa MA. New frontiers in cardiology: drug-eluting stents: Part II. *Circulation* 2003;107:2383–2389.

93. Teirstein PS. Living the dream of no restenosis. *Circulation* 2001; 104:1996–1998.

94. Rogers CD. Drug-eluting stents: role of stent design, delivery vehicle, and drug selection. *Rev Cardiovasc Med* 2002;3[Suppl 5]:S10–S15.

95. Suzuki T, Kopia G, Hayashi S, et al. Stent-based delivery of sirolimus reduces neointimal formation in a porcine coronary model. *Circulation* 2001;104:1188–1193.

96. Drachman DE, Edelman ER, Seifert P, et al. Neointimal thickening after stent delivery of paclitaxel: change in composition and arrest of growth over 6 months. *J Am Coll Cardiol* 2000;36:2325–2332.

97. Heldman AW, Cheng L, Jenkins GM, et al. Paclitaxel stent coating inhibits neointimal hyperplasia at 4 weeks in a porcine model of coronary restenosis. *Circulation* 2001;103:2289–2295.

98. Hong MK, Kornowski R, Bramwell O, et al. Paclitaxel-coated

Gianturco-Roubin II (GR II) stents reduce neointimal hyperplasia in a porcine coronary in-stent restenosis model. *Coron Artery Dis* 2001; 12:513–515.

99. Schwartz RS, Edelman ER, Carter A, et al. Drug-eluting stents in preclinical studies: recommended evaluation from a consensus group. *Circulation* 2002;106:1867–1873.

100. Sousa JE, Costa MA, Abizaid A, et al. Lack of neointimal proliferation after implantation of sirolimus-coated stents in human coronary arteries: a quantitative coronary angiography and 3-dimensional intravascular ultrasound study. *Circulation* 2001;103:192–195.

101. Sousa JE, Costa MA, Abizaid AC, et al. Sustained suppression of neointimal proliferation by sirolimus-eluting stents: one-year angiographic and intravascular ultrasound follow-up. *Circulation* 2001;104:2007–2011.

102. Sousa JE, Costa MA, Abizaid A, et al. Sirolimus-eluting stent for the treatment of in-stent restenosis: a quantitative coronary angiography and 3-dimensional intravascular ultrasound study. *Circulation* 2003; 107:24–27.

103. Sousa JE, Costa MA, Sousa AG, et al. Two-year angiographic and intravascular ultrasound follow-up after implantation of sirolimus-eluting stents in human coronary arteries. *Circulation* 2003;107:381–383.

104. Degertekin M, Serruys PW, Foley DP, et al. Persistent inhibition of neointimal hyperplasia after sirolimus-eluting stent implantation: long-term (up to 2 years) clinical, angiographic, and intravascular ultrasound follow-up. *Circulation* 2002;106:1610–1613.

105. Morice MC, Serruys PW, Sousa JE, et al. A randomized comparison of a sirolimus-eluting stent with a standard stent for coronary revascularization. *N Engl J Med* 2002;346:1773–1780.

106. Serruys PW. ARTS I—the rapamycin-eluting stent; ARTS II—the rosy prophecy. *Eur Heart J* 2002;23:757–759.

107. Serruys PW, Degertekin M, Tanabe K, et al. Intravascular ultrasound findings in the multicenter, randomized, double-blind RAVEL (RAndomized study with the sirolimus-eluting VElocity balloon-expandable stent in the treatment of patients with de novo native coronary artery Lesions) trial. *Circulation* 2002;106:798–803.

108. Moses JW, Leon MB, Popma JJ, at al. Sirolimus-eluting stents versus standard stents in patients with stenosis in a native coronary artery. *N Engl Med* 2003;349:315–323.

109. Degertekin M, Regar E, Tanabe K, et al. Sirolimus-eluting stent for treatment of complex in-stent restenosis: the first clinical experience. *J Am Coll Cardiol* 2003;41:184–189.

110. Grube E, Bullesfeld L. Initial experience with paclitaxel-coated stents. *J Interv Cardiol* 2002;15:471–475.

111. Hong MK, Mintz GS, Lee CW, et al. Paclitaxel coating reduces instent intimal hyperplasia in human coronary arteries. A serial volumetric intravascular ultrasound analysis from the ASian Paclitaxel-Eluting Stent Clinical Trial (ASPECT). *Circulation* 2003;107:517–520.

112. Park SJ, Shim WH, Ho DS, et al. A paclitaxel-eluting stent for the prevention of coronary restenosis. *N Engl J Med* 2003;348:1537–1545.

113. Colombo A, Drzewiecki J, Banning A, et al. Randomized study to assess the effectiveness of slow- and moderate-release polymer-based paclitaxel-eluting stents for coronary artery lesions. *Circulation* 2003; 108:788–794.

114. Stone GW, Ellis SE, Cox DA, et al. A polymer-based, paclitaxel-eluting stent in patients with coronary artery disease. *N Engl J Med* 2004;350:221–231.

CHAPTER 95

Role of Bypass Surgery

William L. Holman, David C. McGiffin, and James K. Kirklin

Key Words: Angioplasty; clinical trials; platelet inhibitors; restenosis; stents; stress testing.

INTRODUCTION

Coronary artery bypass grafting (CABG) surgery has benefited many patients through its capacity to relieve the symptoms of angina pectoris and, in certain situations, to prolong life. The maturation process of CABG required not only the development of contemporary operations but, of equal importance, the distillation of information from numerous clinical studies to determine the place of CABG along with other invasive and noninvasive therapies.

HISTORICAL OVERVIEW

The earliest attempts to relieve the symptoms of angina involved indirect procedures such as division of neural connections to the heart or thyroidectomy to reduce

W. L. Holman: Department of Surgery, Division of Cardiothoracic Surgery, University of Alabama at Birmingham, 719 Zeigler Research Building, Birmingham, Alabama 35294.

D. C. McGiffin, Department of Surgery, Division of Cardiothoracic Surgery, University of Alabama at Birmingham, 780 Lyons-Harrison Research Building, Birmingham, Alabama 35294.

J. K. Kirklin, Department of Surgery, Division of Cardiothoracic Surgery, University of Alabama at Birmingham, 739 Zeigler Research Building, Birmingham, Alabama 35294.

myocardial energy requirements. Sympathectomy appears to have been first used by Charles Mayo sometime during 1913 (1). The sympathectomy by Jonnesco (2) for the treatment of angina was reported in 1920. Thyroidectomy in euthyroid patients for relief of angina arose from the observation that symptoms of heart failure and angina in hyperthyroid states were relieved by thyroidectomy (3).

A number of indirect approaches to increasing myocardial blood flow were investigated both experimentally and clinically, commencing in the early 1930s. These procedures included the induction of pericardial to myocardial adhesions (4) and the use of pedicled muscle (5) or pedicled omental grafting (6) to the myocardium. Great cardiac vein ligation (7) and even coronary sinus ligation (8) were explored. The Vineberg operation (9) is the one procedure from that era that persisted because it did have at least the suggestion of some therapeutic efficacy.

The notion of directly increasing coronary blood flow by means of a bypass graft can be attributed to Carrel in 1910 (10). Murray in 1954 (11) alluded to the possible clinical application of interposing grafts in the coronary arterial tree, which he performed experimentally. The first clinical application of CABG appears to be the unsuccessful carotid-coronary artery graft by Mustard in 1953 (10). The earliest attempts at coronary endarterectomy were performed in 1956 and 1957 by Longmire and Bailey (10), working independently.

Important clinical contributions were made by a number of surgeons. In the early 1960s, Sabiston (12) and DeBakey (13) independently performed interposition saphenous vein grafts between the aorta and a coronary artery. The clinical experience of Favaloro (14) during this era did much to open the way for the wide application of reversed saphenous vein bypass grafting. Work by Effler and coworkers (15) (coronary endarterectomy with patch grafting) and Green and coworkers (16) (internal mammary artery–coronary artery anastomosis using microsurgical techniques) also contributed to the popularization of surgical procedures for coronary artery disease.

PRINCIPLES OF CORONARY ARTERY SURGERY

Coronary artery surgery for most cardiac surgeons is a reproducible and technically precise procedure. The primary goal is to achieve complete revascularization of the ventricles, because incomplete revascularization has an adverse effect on survival. This is true even when the left anterior coronary artery is the target vessel and an internal mammary artery is used as the graft conduit (17).

Minimization of Perioperative Myocardial Ischemia

More than any other patient undergoing cardiac surgery, patients with coronary artery disease are vulnerable to myocardial oxygen supply/demand imbalance before the initiation of cardiopulmonary bypass. In the face of a relatively fixed coronary blood supply to areas of myocardium supplied by stenotic coronary arteries, blunting the release of catecholamines, avoidance of pharmacologic agents that increase heart rate and contractility, and prevention of left atrial hypertension are important in preventing myocardial ischemia. Additional maneuvers to minimize perioperative myocardial ischemia include continuance of β-blocking drugs (except in large doses) (18), calcium channel–blocking drugs, and nitrates up until the time of the surgery. Placement of an intraaortic balloon pump before incision may be beneficial in patients with severe unstable angina, very poor ventricular function, or other important risk factors for perioperative morbidity (19–21).

Myocardial Management

Protection of the myocardium during the period of aortic cross-clamping and metabolic resuscitation of ischemic myocardium are of special importance in patients undergoing coronary artery surgery. Numerous strategies for myocardial management are in use, but as Buckberg (22) has quite correctly pointed out, adversarial positions tend to be taken (crystalloid vs. blood cardioplegia, anterograde vs. retrograde administration of cardioplegia). Numerous strategies are available, many of which can be integrated or applied flexibly to particular situations. Coronary artery surgery using hypothermia and ventricular fibrillation can be performed with results comparable to that achieved with cardioplegic techniques (23–25). Novel methods, such as pharmacologically mimicking ischemic preconditioning (26), are actively being developed.

Conduits for Coronary Artery Surgery

Several autogenous conduits are available for coronary artery surgery. The most widely used conduit is the long saphenous vein. If the long saphenous vein has been previously stripped for varicose vein disease or is unsuitable because of small caliber or varicosities, the short saphenous vein may be used. The thin-walled cephalic vein should be used only when no other conduit is available because of its poor patency (27). Cryopreserved allograft vein has been used as a conduit with poor patency (28).

Arterial grafts for coronary artery surgery are the preferred conduit because their patency is superior to that of venous conduits (29,30). The left internal thoracic artery currently is incorporated in most coronary bypass procedures. Use of both internal mammary arteries provides superior long-term patency (31–33), although this advantage is eroded somewhat by advancing age or death caused by comorbid conditions (34). Bilateral internal mammary artery dissection markedly decreases the blood supply to the sternum for a period of weeks. This is the reason for the greater incidence of poor healing, sternal osteomyelitis, and mediastinitis in patients, especially those with diabetes, who undergo bilateral internal mammary artery grafting.

Other arterial conduits that are used include the radial artery (35), the inferior epigastric artery (36,37), and the right gastroepiploic artery (38–40) as a pedicled or free graft. Over the last several years, there has been renewed interest in the radial artery. Radial arteries are readily available with little if any morbidity in properly selected patients (41–43). The radial artery may not be suitable because of atherothrombosis in some patients (e.g., patients with chronic diabetes or severe generalized peripheral vascular disease), but this is relatively uncommon. Nonrandomized studies suggest that the patency rate for radial artery grafts is at least intermediate between saphenous vein and internal mammary artery grafts and may be equivalent to *in situ* internal mammary artery grafts (44–47). A prospective, randomized, multicenter trial sponsored by the Veterans Administration is underway that will compare radial artery with saphenous vein patency rates.

Analysis of large collective experiences provides useful information to guide the choice of conduits. For example, analysis of the Society of Thoracic Surgeons national database for cardiac surgery argues compellingly for increased use of at least one internal mammary artery graft in elderly patients (48). Information from future analyses is expected to further refine the accuracy of judgments regarding conduit use for individual patients.

Other Procedures for Relieving Coronary Stenosis

Endarterectomy is a procedure used to relieve coronary stenosis, but it is primarily reserved for vessels with distal disease that precludes satisfactory distal grafts. Most commonly, endarterectomy is applied to the right coronary artery at and beyond the bifurcation, although the diffusely diseased left anterior descending coronary artery may also be dealt with by endarterectomy. Although there is no uniform agreement, there is evidence to suggest that the use of coronary endarterectomy is associated with a greater operative mortality rate (49), greater incidence of perioperative myocardial infarction (49), and lower long-term graft patency rates (when a graft is anastomosed to an endarterectomized vessel) compared with coronary revascularization without the use of endarterectomy (50). Also, patency of the endarterectomized arteries is unpredictable, perhaps because of progressive cicatrization (51). However, extensive coronary endarterectomy has been performed with good results (52).

Conduct of the Coronary Bypass Surgery

CABG is a straightforward and reproducible procedure, and clearly there are many technical variations to the conduct of the operation. The most recent are the procedures that are performed through small incisions or without cardiopulmonary bypass. The indications for these newer approaches are evolving and remain somewhat controversial (53–57). However, there is increasing use of off-pump CABG procedures based on personal experience and from studies primarily showing advantages in recovery time from CABG surgery and improved outcomes for patients with comorbid conditions (e.g., pulmonary dysfunction).

The surgery is most commonly performed through a median sternotomy. The long saphenous vein is removed, and arterial conduits, which may include one or both internal mammary arteries, one or both radial arteries, the right gastroepiploic artery, and the inferior epigastric artery, are mobilized. If cardiopulmonary bypass is used, heparin is given, then hypothermic cardiopulmonary bypass is commenced followed by cardioplegic myocardial arrest.

The distal and proximal vein graft and free arterial graft anastomoses are performed, as well as the distal anastomoses of the pedicled arterial grafts. The order in which the anastomoses are performed varies from surgeon to surgeon and is almost certainly not important. However, the end result should be complete revascularization by bypassing all arteries with stenosis resulting in at least a 50% reduction in diameter, except for vessels 1 mm in diameter or less.

Controversy exists as to any potential benefits of sequential anastomoses in terms of long-term patency. Because of this uncertainty, one strategy is to use one or more arterial grafts and three segments of saphenous vein for the remaining coronary arteries before using sequential grafts (58). The internal mammary artery (as well as other arterial grafts) has been used for sequential grafts with good results (59), including triple sequential grafts (60), indicating that these vessels appear to have adequate flow reserve in the multivessel configuration. Bilateral internal mammary artery grafting can be used with low mortality (61), but the use of this

technique is an independent and important risk factor for postoperative sternal infection (62–64), presumably related to impairment of sternal blood flow after internal mammary artery mobilization (65,66).

To extend the use of arterial conduits, the internal mammary artery has been used as T grafts, where segments of free internal mammary artery are anastomosed end to side to the other internal mammary artery, which is used as a pedicled graft (67,68). Internal mammary artery graft patency, when it is used in this configuration, appears identical to that achieved with a single pedicled internal mammary artery graft (68).

Secondary Prevention in Patients Having Coronary Artery Bypass Surgery

During the last decade there has been an increasing appreciation for the importance of secondary prevention measures that are undertaken during hospitalization for CABG. Regional quality improvement initiatives are one method for disseminating best practice guidelines and promoting their uniform application (69,70). The focus of these efforts has been on improving processes of care that are likely to improve outcome for patients. These processes include the use of at least one internal mammary artery graft; prescription of aspirin at discharge; use of β-blocking drugs before, during, and after the CABG procedure; and appropriate lipid management (including medication to decrease lipid levels if necessary). The importance of some of these measures is well established, whereas the evidence supporting other measures (e.g., perioperative β-blocker use [71] and appropriate lipid management [72–74]) is evolving with ongoing studies of large data sets.

Reoperative Coronary Artery Bypass Surgery

Coronary reoperation may be required as treatment for progression of native vessel coronary artery disease or the development of vein graft atherothrombosis, or both. A number of technical problems must be dealt with during reoperative coronary artery surgery. Reopening of the sternum must be performed without damage to underlying structures such as the aorta, right ventricle, or patent grafts. Patent but atherothrombotic vein grafts, on handling, can readily embolize atherothrombotic material. The approach to angiographically unobstructed vein grafts is not uniform. Lytle and Cosgrove (75) advise replacement of all vein grafts that are older than 5 years, even if angiographically free of disease. However, others (58) have advised replacing only grafts that have angiographic or palpable disease.

Novel approaches for reoperative surgery such as the use of a left thoracotomy with or without femorofemoral cardiopulmonary bypass for access to the lateral aspect of the left ventricle have been used with good results (76,77). A right thoracotomy approach has been used successfully for revascularization of the right coronary system (78).

THE BASIS FOR DECISION-MAKING
IN CORONARY ARTERY DISEASE

The exponential growth in the number of patients undergoing CABG from its earliest days resulted in part from the clear efficacy of the surgery in relieving angina. However, with the improvements in pharmacologic therapy for angina and the development of percutaneous coronary interventions (PCIs) came the responsibility to compare outcomes after each of these therapies. However, this process is fraught with a number of complexities.

The results of randomized trials comparing survival of patients undergoing medical versus surgical therapy for coronary artery disease, most notably the Coronary Artery Surgery Study (CASS) and Veterans Administration Coronary Artery Bypass Surgery Cooperative study group, have found their way into the daily decision-making process for patients with coronary artery disease. Unfortunately, the shortcomings of the analytic approach used in these studies are not widely appreciated, and the results are frequently unhesitatingly applied to individual patients.

Randomized trials provide secure evidence of differences among therapies applied to randomized patients, but randomized patients do not necessarily reflect the entire spectrum of patients with coronary artery disease. For example, the CASS study excluded patients with left main coronary artery disease. There are many risk factors that have been identified that adversely impact on survival (and other unfavorable events) after treatment for coronary artery disease. Randomized trials cannot hope to account for all of these risk factors; therefore, a trial of this nature must necessarily restrict patient selection for randomization to a subset of the full spectrum of patients with coronary artery disease or ignore important risk factors, although the inferences of the study may subsequently be applied to all patients with coronary artery disease. The usual presentation of the differences in survival between patients randomized to medical or surgical therapy is by actuarial depiction. The difference between the curves is indicated by a global p value. For example, Figure 95–1 is taken from a CASS report (79) that depicts the survival of patients with three-vessel coronary disease, mild angina, and left ventricular dysfunction (left ventricular ejection fraction between 0.35 and 0.50). The global p value by log-rank test is 0.0094, and the usual interpretation is that surgical therapy is advisable in patients with three-vessel disease and left ventricular dysfunction because of a demonstrated surgical survival advantage. However, what does this global p value mean, and what is the magnitude of this surgical survival advantage? The global p value indicates that there is a difference between the two curves, but it does not specify where that difference may be. By a reanalysis of these CASS data, Kirklin and colleagues (80) brought the magnitude of the difference between these curves into sharp focus. Figure 95–2 represents a reanalysis of the CASS information using parametric methods. The difference in survival between the two groups is only 1% at 1 year and 10% at 5 years. The 70% confidence limits around the estimates overlap for the first 5 years, indicating that at 5 years, the better survival in surgically treated patients could result from chance. A time-related p-value depiction (Fig. 95–3) demonstrates that the difference in survival may possibly represent something other than chance ($p < 0.05$) only at 7 years.

Parametric survival analysis (81) offers particular advantages over other statistical methods of studying the results of therapy for coronary artery disease. As outlined by Naftel (82), this system allows the application of parametric equations to a variety of possible survival distributions, for example, death after CABG. Because the distribution of death after CABG is not constant across time, the method incorporates a mixture of up to three distributions or phases (such as an early phase reflecting operative mortality, a constant phase, followed by a rising phase reflecting increasing risk for death from graft closure and coronary artery disease progression). Once the distribution of death (or other events such as return of angina or reoperation) has been estimated, risk factors that increase the probability of the event can be identified during each of these phases. Then, risk-adjusted comparisons can be made between therapies (e.g., medical vs. surgical therapy) or certain aspects

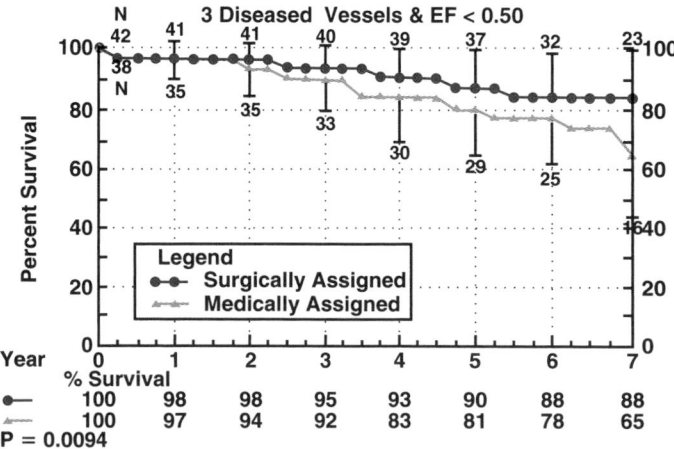

FIG. 95–1. Actuarial survival of patients with three-vessel coronary artery disease, left ventricular dysfunction (left ventricular ejection fraction [EF], 0.35–0.50), and mild angina, randomized to medical or surgical therapy. The global p value for the difference is 0.0094 (log-rank test). (From Killip T, Passamani E, Davis K, CASS Principal Investigators and their associates. Coronary artery surgery study [CASS]: a randomized trial of coronary bypass surgery. Eight years follow-up and survival in patients with reduced ejection fraction. *Circulation* 1985;72[Suppl V]: V-102–V-109, by permission of the American Heart Association.)

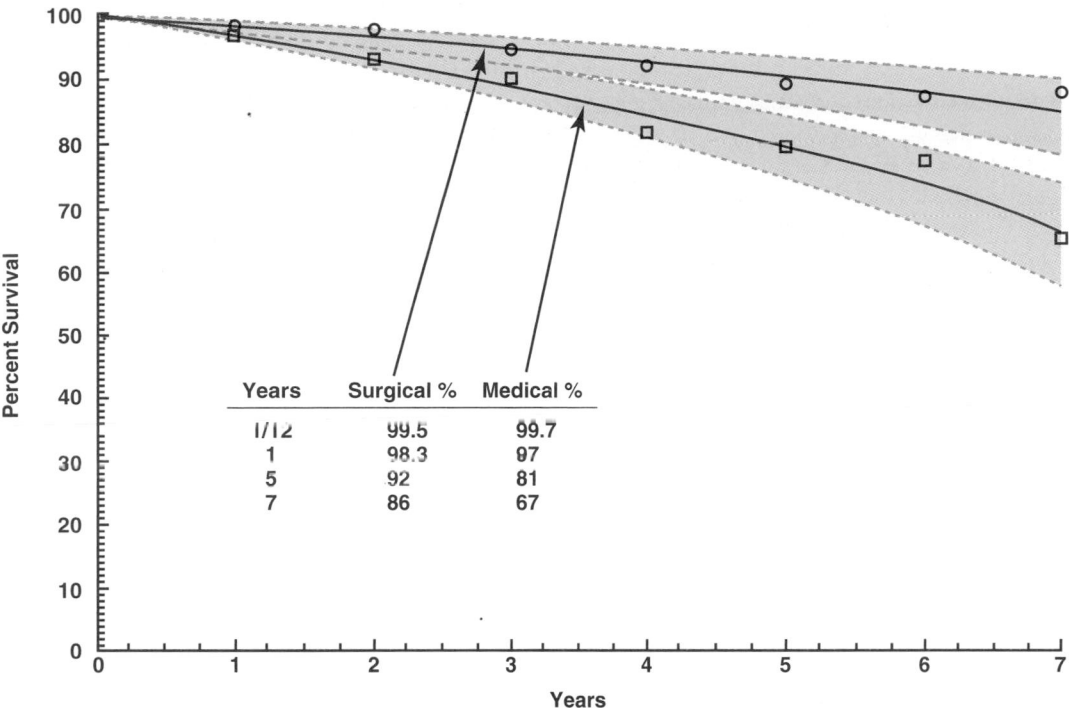

Years	Surgical %	Medical %
1/12	99.5	99.7
1	98.3	97
5	92	81
7	86	67

FIG. 95–2. Parametric estimates of survival for patients depicted in Figure 95–4. The *solid lines* are the parametric estimates, and the *dotted* and *dashed lines* are the 70% confidence limits. The *circles* and *squares* are the actuarial estimates from the original data. (From Kirklin JW, Frye RL, Blackstone EH, et al. Some comments on the indications for the coronary artery bypass graft operation. *Int J Cardiol* 1991;31:23–30, with permission.)

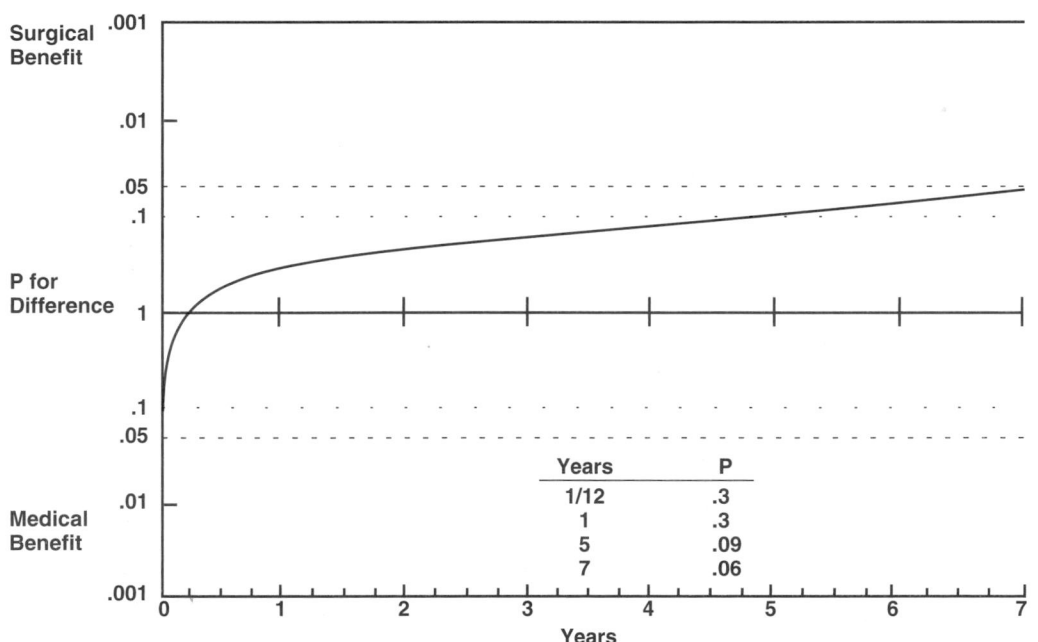

Years	P
1/12	.3
1	.3
5	.09
7	.06

FIG. 95–3. Time-related *p* value for the difference in percentage survival between the medical and surgical groups in Figure 95–5. The *dashed* and *dotted lines* at 0.05 and 0.1 are there to assist with interpretation of the figure. (From Kirklin JW, Frye RL, Blackstone EH, et al. Some comments on the indications for the coronary artery bypass graft operation. *Int J Cardiol* 1991;31:23–30, with permission.)

of the same treatment such as hospitals, surgeons, or eras. Furthermore, it is possible to make patient-specific predictions of the time-related probability of death. This feature of the parametric methodology has allowed the development of software to assist clinicians in making recommendations to individual patients as to the most appropriate therapy for their coronary artery disease, on the basis of the patient's specific risk factors (83). These prediction equations are not meant to replace clinical judgment on the part of the physician, but rather to provide useful information to guide the decision for a therapeutic pathway for an individual patient.

INDICATIONS FOR CORONARY BYPASS SURGERY

The decision regarding a therapeutic course for an individual patient among CABG, medical treatment, and PCI is complicated by the lack of comparisons among therapies with adjustment for the risk factors. Clearly, CABG is effective in relieving angina, but perhaps of most interest (especially to the patient) is the benefit of one therapy over another in terms of survival. The American College of Cardiology/American Heart Association Guidelines and Indications for Coronary Artery Bypass Graft Surgery (84) represents the most reliable and rational distillation of available data into a series of indications for CABG. The authors of this report have devised three treatment classes reflecting the believed benefit (in terms of survival) of CABG over other therapies. However, until patient-specific predictions of death (and other unfavorable events) after CABG and patient-specific comparisons between CABG and alternative therapies become widely available and in general use, only oversimplified and imprecise generalizations can be made.

The roles for CABG and PCIs for the treatment of coronary artery disease continue to evolve as new information is generated from large clinical trials and as the techniques for both methods of revascularization improve. The recently reported Stent or Surgery (SoS) Trial (85) compared patients with multivessel coronary artery disease treated with either CABG or PCI that included stents. The results of this trial were similar to previous comparisons (e.g., the Bypass Angioplasty Revascularization Investigation [BARI] trial) in that the reintervention rate was greater for patients receiving PCI as compared with patients receiving CABG. However, the use of stents appears to have reduced the rate of reintervention for the PCI group as compared with reintervention rates from the era of balloon angioplasty without stents. Interestingly, there was a survival benefit for patients with CABG in the SoS trial, although it was not clear whether this benefit was because of the population that was studied or because of a somewhat greater number of cancer deaths in the PCI group as compared with the CABG group.

The Arterial Revascularization Therapy Study (ARTS) found similar survival in patients with multivessel coronary artery disease who were randomly assigned to either CABG

or PCI. However, the subgroup of patients with diabetes had superior survival after CABG (86), which mirrored findings from the earlier BARI Trial. A separate *post hoc* analysis of the ARTS data found that an abnormal increase of creatine kinase (CK)-MB isoenzymes (i.e., 61.9% of patients) was not uncommon after CABG for multivessel coronary artery disease. Moreover, CK-MB isoenzyme increase was an independent risk factor for late adverse events and death (87), highlighting the continuing need for attention to myocardial protection during CABG surgery.

The Bypass Angioplasty Revascularization Investigation 2 Diabetes (BARI 2D) Trial is currently underway. This study has a relatively complex experimental design that is examining questions of diabetic management together with questions regarding optimal timing for revascularization therapy (PCI or CABG) in this complex patient population (88). It is expected that the results of this trial will have a major impact on evidence-based treatment guidelines for patients with diabetes and concomitant coronary artery disease.

RESULTS OF CORONARY ARTERY BYPASS SURGERY

Survival

The risk profile of patients undergoing CABG has increased over the last decade, yet the risk-adjusted mortality of patients with CABG has decreased (89). This is probably because of the cumulative mortality benefit of many advances. Scrutiny of other well validated data sets has yielded information describing the impact of CABG on the clinical course of patients with coronary atherothrombosis. After CABG in one large group of patients (90), survival was 95% at 1 year and 60% at 15 years (Fig. 95–4A). The hazard function for death (90) demonstrates an early and rapidly declining risk for death (corresponding to operative mortality) merging with a constant risk at approximately 3 months after surgery and an increasing risk commencing 6 years after surgery (see Fig. 95–4B). This increasing phase of risk is probably associated with graft closure or progression of native vessel disease, or both. A number of multivariable analyses have been performed to identify risk factors for death after CABG, and, generally speaking, the important findings of most analyses are similar and intuitive. One particular study by Sergeant and colleagues (91) found that some of the important risk factors were lower pre-CABG left ventricular ejection fraction, incomplete revascularization, nonuse of the internal mammary artery, older age at operation, and presence of insulin-dependent diabetes. The strength of risk factors may be portrayed using nomograms that predict the probability of death (or other events) in a risk-adjusted manner. For example, Figure 95–5 depicts the nomogram of the solution to a multivariable equation illustrating the risk-adjusted effect of increasing left ventricular dysfunction on the risk for death after CABG. Figure 95–6 indicates, in a risk-adjusted way, the survival benefit of the

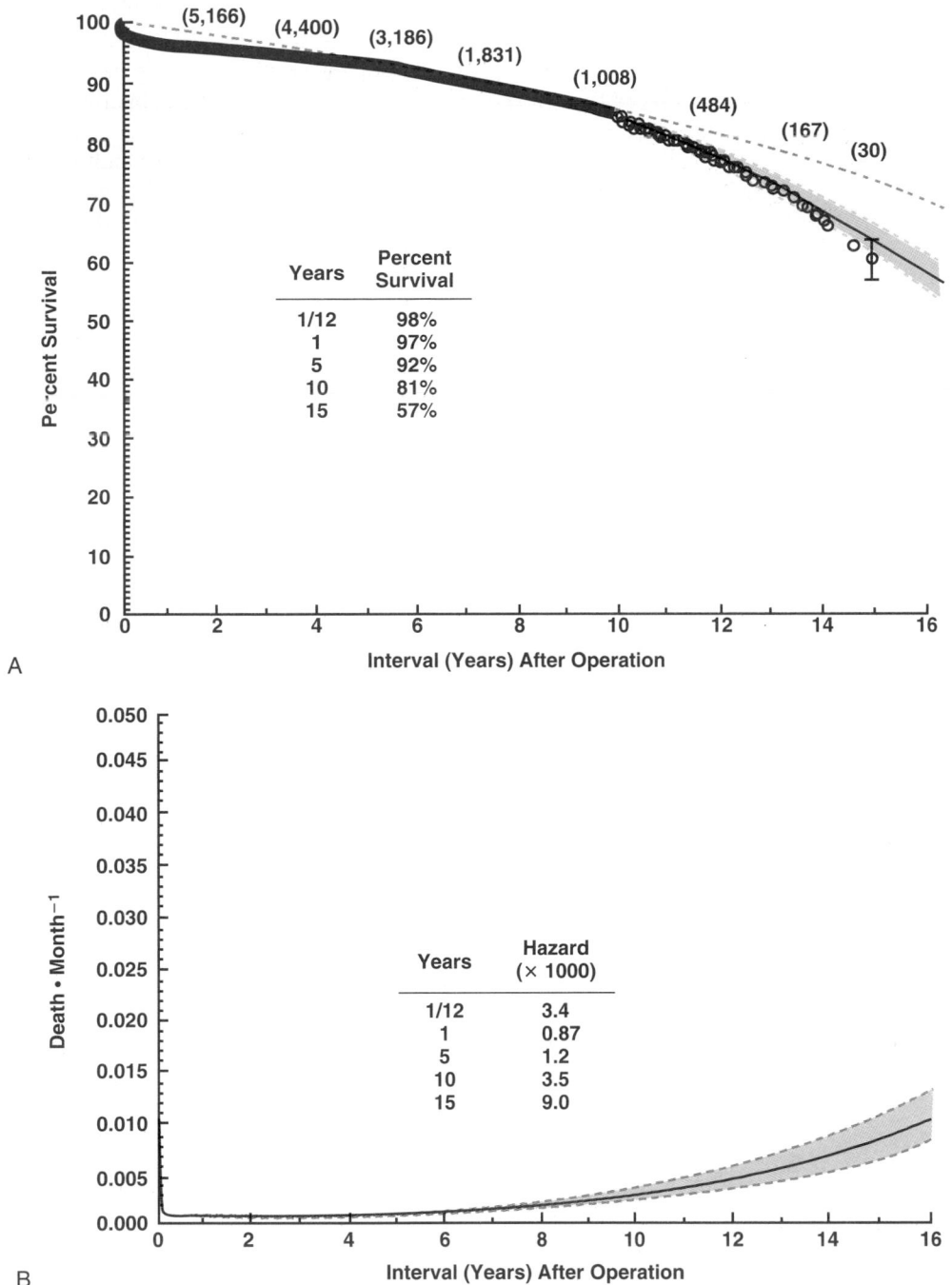

FIG. 95–4. A: Probability of survival after coronary artery bypass grafting (CABG) in a heterogeneous group of patients. The *solid line* is the parametric estimate, the *dashed lines* are the 70% confidence limits around the parametric estimate, and the *dotted-dashed line* is the survivorship of an age-, sex-, and race-matched general population. The *circles* represent individual deaths. The numbers in parentheses indicate the number of patients being traced at each time. **B:** Hazard function (or instantaneous risk) for death in the group of patients in **A.** There is a rapidly declining phase of risk merging with a constant phase at approximately 3 months after CABG, followed by an increasing late phase of risk commencing approximately 6 years after surgery. (From ACC/AHA guidelines and indications for the coronary artery bypass graft operation. A report of the American College of Cardiology/American Heart Association Task Force on Assessment of Diagnostic and Therapeutic Cardiovascular Procedures [Subcommittee on Coronary Artery Bypass Graft Surgery]. *J Am Coll Cardiol* 1991;17:543–589; and *Circulation* 1991;83:1125–1173, with permission.)

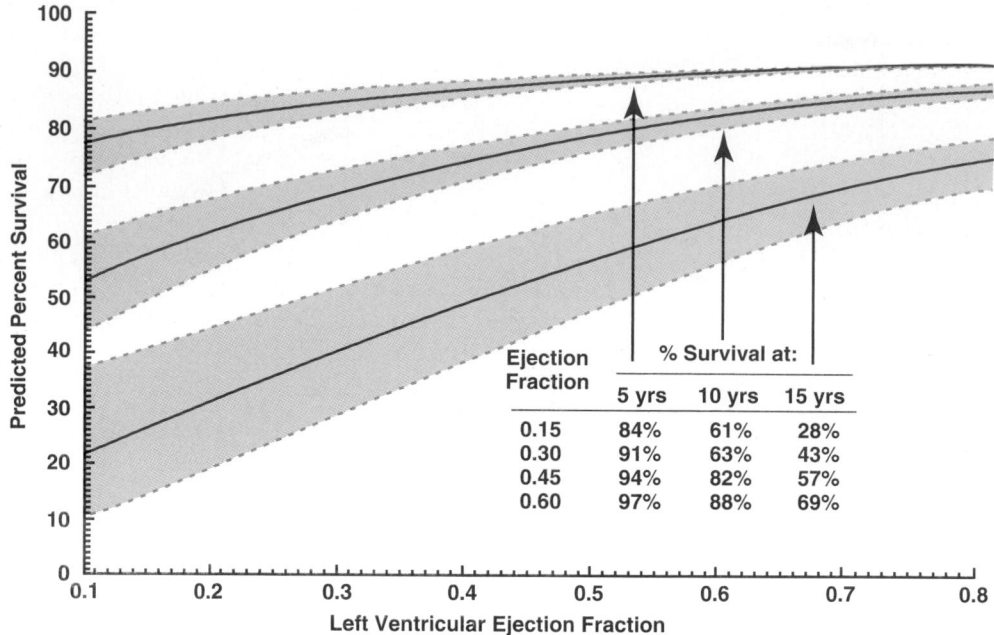

Ejection Fraction	% Survival at:		
	5 yrs	10 yrs	15 yrs
0.15	84%	61%	28%
0.30	91%	63%	43%
0.45	94%	82%	57%
0.60	97%	88%	69%

FIG. 95–5. Nomogram of the risk-adjusted effect of left ventricular ejection fraction on survival at 5, 10, and 15 years after surgery. (From Sergeant PT, Blackstone EH, Lasaffre E, et al. Unpublished study cited in: Kirklin JW, Barratt-Boyes BG, eds. *Cardiac Surgery, Vol 1,* 2nd ed. New York: Churchill Livingstone, 1993, with permission.)

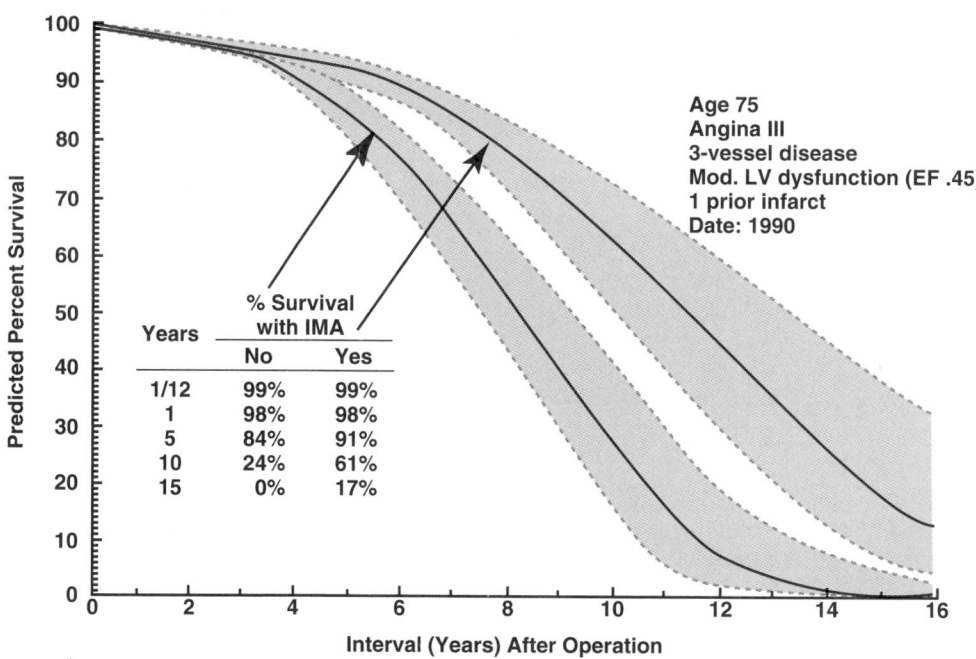

Age 75
Angina III
3-vessel disease
Mod. LV dysfunction (EF .45)
1 prior infarct
Date: 1990

Years	% Survival with IMA	
	No	Yes
1/12	99%	99%
1	98%	98%
5	84%	91%
10	24%	61%
15	0%	17%

FIG. 95–6. Nomogram illustrating the survival advantage of the use of the internal mammary artery in the coronary artery bypass grafting surgery in an elderly patient. EF, ejection fraction; IMA, internal mammary artery; LV, left ventricular. (From ACC/AHA guidelines and indications for the coronary artery bypass graft operation. A report of the American College of Cardiology/American Heart Association Task Force on Assessment of Diagnostic and Therapeutic Cardiovascular Procedures [Subcommittee on Coronary Artery Bypass Graft Surgery]. *J Am Coll Cardiol* 1991;17:543–589; and *Circulation* 1991;83:1125–1173, with permission.)

use of an internal mammary artery in the CABG procedure, even in the elderly patient. Notably, this benefit does not become apparent until approximately 4 years after CABG.

Return of Angina

The most frequent ischemic event after CABG is return of angina (other ischemic events include sudden death and myocardial infarction). After CABG, 95%, 83%, and 63% of patients are free of angina after 1, 5, and 10 years (92). Of particular importance is the time course of return of angina, which is illustrated by the hazard function curve from the study by Sergeant and colleagues (92) (Fig. 95–7). The early peak phase may represent early graft closure and incomplete revascularization, whereas the late increasing phase likely represents progression of native vessel disease or development of graft atherothrombosis, or both.

Myocardial Infarction

On the basis of the development of new Q waves on the electrocardiogram, the incidence rate of perioperative acute myocardial infarction is approximately 4.6%. Perioperative Q-wave infarction reduces long- (93,94) and short-term survival.

Reintervention after Coronary Artery Bypass Graft

Reintervention after CABG may be required for, most frequently, vein graft atherothrombosis, progression of native vessel coronary artery disease, or both (95). The form of re-intervention may be by percutaneous transluminal coronary angioplasty (PTCA) or atherectomy device or by reoperation CABG. By 5, 10, and 15 years after CABG, approximately 97%, 91%, and 66% of patients, respectively, will be free of reintervention either by reoperation CABG or, less frequently in this study, by PTCA (96). The hazard function curve, which depicts how time to reintervention is distributed across time, has a shape similar to that of return of angina and acute myocardial infarction after CABG. The probability of requiring reintervention after CABG appears to have been reduced by the use of the internal mammary artery (97,98).

BIOLOGY OF CONDUITS FOR CORONARY ARTERY BYPASS GRAFT

After implantation as coronary bypass conduits, arterial and venous grafts do not necessarily behave as passive tubes. The tone of normal blood vessels can be viewed as a balance between vasodilating and vasoconstricting responses of neurogenic and humorally mediated influences. Bypass grafts, both arterial and venous, have the capacity for relaxation and contraction. The mechanisms involved in the modulation of vascular tone by interaction of vasoactive substances with vascular endothelium and vascular smooth muscle are complex. However, a useful framework for considering those interactions is to view the vasodilatation and vasoconstriction as either endothelium dependent or independent (99). Endothelium-dependent vasodilatation is mediated through the release of endothelium-derived relaxing factor (EDRF), which is now known to be nitric oxide, and prostacyclin. Endothe-

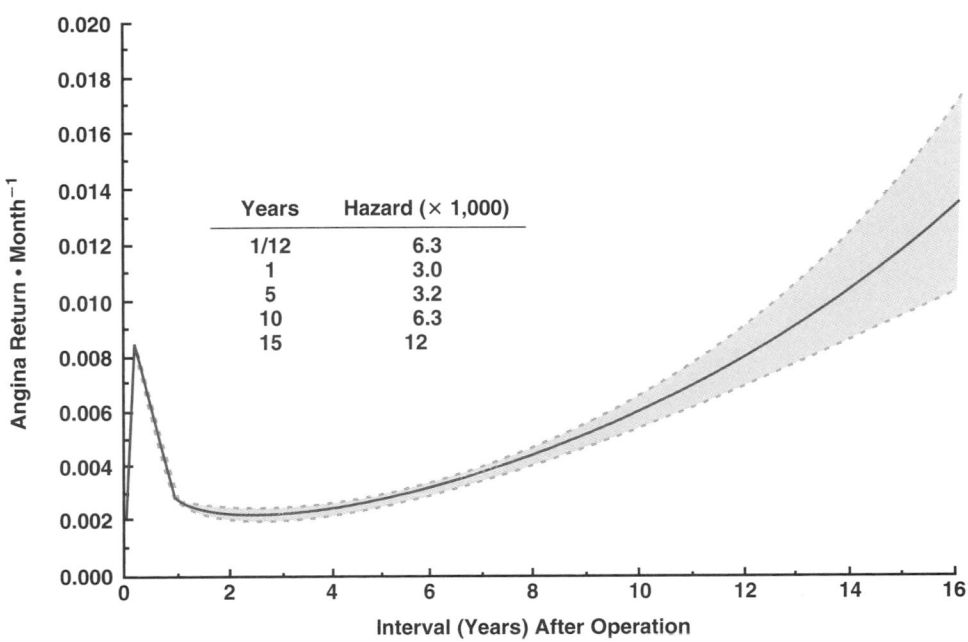

FIG. 95–7. Hazard function for return of angina after coronary artery bypass grafting. (From Sergeant P, Lesaffre E, Flameng W, et al. The return of clinically evident ischemia after coronary artery bypass grafting. *Eur J Cardiothorac Surg* 1991;5:447–457, with permission.)

lium also releases a vasoconstrictor substance, endothelin (100), although the vasodilatory influences predominate. Vasodilator and vasoconstrictor substances also can act directly on vascular smooth muscle without the need for an intact endothelium.

Reduction in EDRF release from arterial and venous graft endothelium after CABG may impact on graft function in at least two major ways. In the immediate postoperative period, impairment of the constant basal release of EDRF may expose the smooth muscle of the graft to unbalanced vasoconstrictor influences, which may result in graft spasm, producing myocardial ischemia and its fatal and nonfatal consequences. This is probably more likely to occur in arterial than venous grafts. A simplification of a complex interplay is illustrated in Figure 95–8.

The other major impact that impairment of EDRF release may have on arterial and venous grafts is the development of graft closure by thrombosis and atherothrombosis. More than 90% of internal mammary artery grafts anastomosed to the left anterior descending coronary artery are patent 10 years after CABG (101). This may in part be related to the protective effect of a functional endothelium. Moreover, the endothelium of arterial grafts appears to be a crucial sensor and effector in chronic remodeling of the artery after CABG (102). In contrast, saphenous vein grafts have a less satisfactory patency. It should be noted that grafts (arterial and venous) may close for a variety of reasons not predominantly related to endothelial responses, such as poor coronary vessel runoff, anastomotic problems, and other technical factors, some of which are related to surgical expertise. Although the patency rate of vein grafts is quite variable, at least 10% have closed in the first few postoperative weeks (103,104) from thrombosis as a result of endothelial damage and technical factors. A process of intimal hyperplasia resulting in a reduction in diameter of the vein graft is the usual appearance after 1 month (105–107) and should probably be regarded as an adaptation process of the conduit to flow.

By 3 years after CABG, some 60% to 70% of vein grafts have evidence of atherothrombotic change (108,109). Vein graft atherothrombosis is a diffuse, soft, and friable lesion compared with native coronary artery disease, which tends to be proximal and eccentric. The role of an intact vein graft endothelium in reducing the probability of early vein graft closure and the late development of atherothrombosis is still uncertain. However, the use of strategies to reduce endothelial injury in conduits for CABG seems prudent.

The internal mammary artery only rarely develops atherothrombosis. Part of the explanation for this phenomenon is the much higher level of EDRF seen in internal mammary artery grafts compared with saphenous vein grafts. Furthermore, the lack of discontinuities in the internal elastic lamina of the internal mammary artery (110) may prevent the earliest lesion of the atherothrombotic process. This lesion is the migration of smooth muscle cells of the media through fenestrations in the internal elastic lamina to the intima (111), a feature seen in muscular arteries other than the internal mammary artery.

During the last decade, gene-based therapies have been developed to suppress intimal proliferation, and hence re-

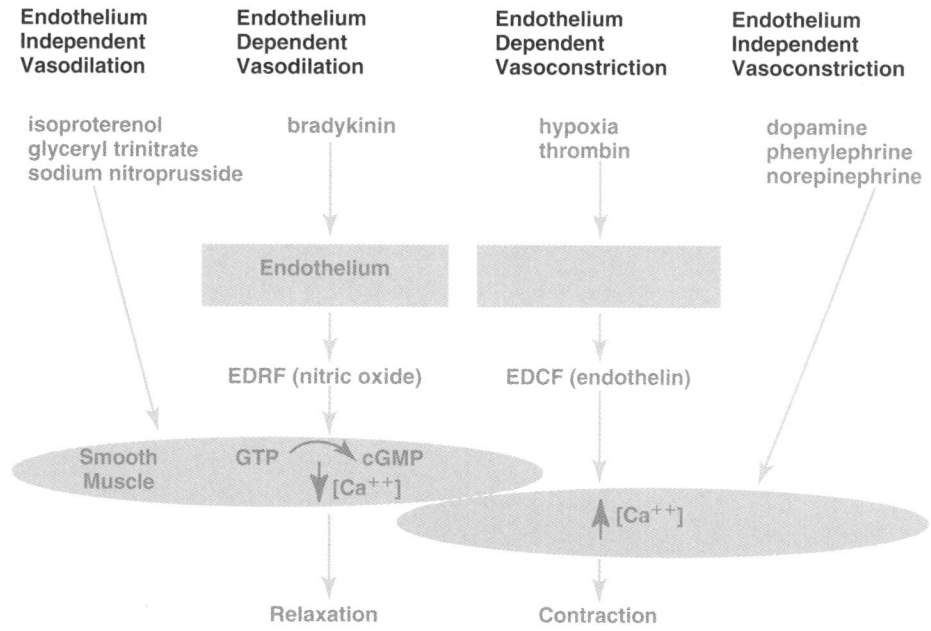

FIG. 95–8. Schematic diagram of some of the possible influences on vasomotor tone in the early postoperative period after coronary artery bypass grafting. cGMP, cyclic guanosine monophosphate; Ca^{++}, cytosolic calcium; EDCF (EDRF), endothelial cell-derived constricting (relaxing) factor; GTP, guanosine triphosphate.

duce the incidence of saphenous vein obstruction and the development of accelerated atherothrombosis. A number of approaches have been used (112,113), but studies with E2F-decoy oligodeoxynucleotide (ODN) have progressed the furthest. For this therapy, saphenous vein segments are treated with E2F-decoy ODN (or other similar decoy ODN) after procurement and before placement as an aortocoronary bypass graft. On the basis of studies in nonprimate species (114), it appears that suppression of early smooth muscle responses to arterial pressure confers long-lasting protection against intimal hyperplasia in the grafted segment of vein. Initial trials in humans that studied saphenous vein grafts in the infrainguinal region have shown safety and inhibition of regulatory genes for cell cycling (115). On the basis of these encouraging early results, trials are planned using the E2F-decoy ODN in humans undergoing CABG.

SUMMARY

The methods for CABG continue to evolve toward providing an even more durable procedure that can be applied safely to patients with an enlarging spectrum of important comorbid conditions. An important challenge for the future is the widespread application of patient-specific prediction equations so that recommendations regarding the most appropriate therapy for an individual patient can be made with some security.

REFERENCES

1. Mayo CH. Discussion: Lilienthal, Howard, cervical sympathectomy in angina pectoris. A report of three cases. *Arch Surg* 1925;10:531–543.
2. Jonnesco T. Angine de poitrine gu_rie par le r_section due sympathique cervicothoracic. *Bull Acad Med* 1920;84:93–102.
3. Rosenblum HH, Levine SA. What happens eventually to patients with hyperthyroidism and significant heart disease following subtotal thyroidectomy? *Am J Med Sci* 1933;185:219–233.
4. Shrager JB. The Vineberg procedure: the immediate forerunner of coronary artery bypass grafting. *Ann Thorac Surg* 1994;57:1354–1364.
5. Beck CS. Further data on the establishment of a new blood supply to the heart by operation. *J Thorac Surg* 1936;5:605–611.
6. O'Shaughnessy L. The surgery of the heart. *Practitioner* 1938;140:603–618.
7. Fauteux M. Surgical treatment of angina pectoris. Experiences with ligation of the great cardiac vein and pericoronary neurectomy. *Ann Surg* 1946;124:1041–1046.
8. Gross L, Blum L, Silverman G. Experimental attempts to increase the blood supply to the dog's heart by means of coronary sinus occlusion. *J Exp Med* 1937;65:91–108.
9. Vineberg AM, Miller G. Internal mammary coronary anastomosis in the surgical treatment of coronary artery insufficiency. *Can Med Assoc J* 1951;64:204–210.
10. Shumaker HB Jr. *The evolution of cardiac surgery.* Bloomington, IN: Indiana University Press, 1992.
11. Murray G, Porcheron R, Hilario J, et al. Anastomosis of a systemic artery to the coronary. *Can Med Assoc J* 1954;71:594–597.
12. Sabiston DC Jr. The William F. Rienhoff, Jr. lecture. The coronary circulation. *Johns Hopkins Med J* 1974;134:314–329.
13. Garrett HE, Dennis EW, DeBakey ME. Aortocoronary bypass with saphenous vein graft. Seven-year follow-up. *JAMA* 1973;223:792–794.
14. Favaloro RG, Effler DB, Groves LK, et al. Direct myocardial revascularization with saphenous vein autograft. Clinical experience in 100 cases. *Dis Chest* 1969;56:279–283.
15. Effler DB, Groves LK, Sones FM, et al. Endarterectomy in the treatment of coronary artery disease. *J Thorac Cardiovasc Surg* 1964;47:98–108.
16. Green GE, Stertzer SH, Reppert EH. Coronary arterial bypass grafts. *Ann Thorac Surg* 1968;5:443–450.
17. Scott R, Blackstone EH, McCarthy PM, et al. Isolated bypass grafting of the left internal thoracic artery to the left anterior descending coronary artery: late consequences of incomplete revascularization. *J Thorac Cardiovasc Surg* 2000;120:173–184.
18. Wechsler AS. Assessment of prospectively randomized patients receiving propranolol therapy before coronary bypass operation. *Ann Thorac Surg* 1980;30:128–136.
19. Christenson JT. Preoperative intraaortic balloon therapy. *Ann Thorac Surg* 1999;68:1438–1439.
20. Dietl CA, Berkheimer MD, Woods EL, et al. Efficacy and cost-effectiveness of preoperative IABP in patients with ejection fraction of 0.25 or less. *Ann Thorac Surg* 1996;62:401–409.
21. Holman WL, Li Q, Kiefe CI, et al. Prophylactic value of preincision intra-aortic balloon pump: analysis of a statewide experience. *J Thorac Cardiovasc Surg* 2000;120:1112–1119.
22. Buckberg GD. Warm versus cold blood cardioplegia: a self-imposed and counterproductive dilemma. *Ann Thorac Surg* 1993;56:1007–1010.
23. Akins CW. Noncardioplegic myocardial preservation for coronary revascularization. *J Thorac Cardiovasc Surg* 1984;88:174–181.
24. Akins CW, Carroll DL. Event-free survival following nonemergency myocardial revascularization during hypothermic fibrillatory arrest. *Ann Thorac Surg* 1987;43:628–633.
25. Bonchek LI, Burlingame MW, Vazales BE, et al. Applicability of noncardioplegic coronary bypass to high-risk patients. *J Thorac Cardiovasc Surg* 1992;103:230–237.
26. Stadler B, Phillips J, Toyoda Y, et al. Adenosine-enhanced ischemic preconditioning modulates necrosis and apoptosis: effects of stunning and ischemia-reperfusion. *Ann Thorac Surg* 2001;72:555–564.
27. Wijnberg DS, Boeve WJ, Ebels T, et al. Patency of arm vein grafts used in aorto-coronary bypass surgery. *Eur J Cardiothorac Surg* 1990;4:510–513.
28. Laub GW, Muralidharan S, Clancy R, et al. Cryopreserved allograft veins as alternative coronary artery bypass conduits: early phase results. *Ann Thorac Surg* 1992;54:826–831.
29. Boylan MJ, Lytle BW, Loop FD, et al. Surgical treatment of isolated left anterior descending coronary stenosis. Comparison of left internal mammary artery and venous autograft at 18 to 20 years of follow-up. *J Thorac Cardiovasc Surg* 1994;107:657–662.
30. Cohn LH. Use of the internal mammary artery graft and in-hospital mortality and other adverse outcomes associated with coronary artery bypass surgery. *Circulation* 2001;103:483–484.
31. Lytle BW, Loop FD. Superiority of bilateral internal thoracic artery grafting: it's been a long time comin'. *Circulation* 2001;104:2152–2154.
32. Endo M, Nishida H, Tomizawa Y, et al. Benefit of bilateral over single internal mammary artery grafts for multiple coronary artery bypass grafting. *Ann Thorac Surg* 2001;104:2164–2170.
33. Lytle BW, Blackstone EH, Loop FD, et al. Two internal thoracic artery grafts are better than one. *J Thorac Cardiovasc Surg* 1999;117:855–872.
34. Blackstone EH, Lytle BW. Competing risks after coronary bypass surgery: the influence of death on reintervention. *J Thorac Cardiovasc Surg* 2000;119:1221–1230.
35. Acar C, Jebara VA, Portoghese M, et al. Revival of the radial artery for coronary artery bypass grafting. *Ann Thorac Surg* 1992;54:652–660.
36. Buche M, Scheovaerdts JC, Louagie Y, et al. Use of the inferior epigastric artery for coronary bypass. *J Thorac Cardiovasc Surg* 1992;103:665–670.
37. Milgalter E, Pearl JM, Laks H, et al. The inferior epigastric arteries as coronary bypass conduits. *J Thorac Cardiovasc Surg* 1992;103:463–465.
38. Suma H, Wanibuchi Y, Furuta S, et al. Does use of gastroepiploic artery graft increase the surgical risk? *J Thorac Cardiovasc Surg* 1991;101:121–125.
39. Perrault LP, Carrier M, Hebert Y, et al. Clinical experience with the right gastroepiploic artery in coronary artery bypass grafting. *Ann Thorac Surg* 1993;56:1082–1084.
40. Newman MA. Arterial grafts for coronary artery bypass: experience with the right gastroepiploic artery and internal mammary artery. *Australas J Cardiac Thorac Surg* 1993;2:77–79.
41. Denton TA, Trento L, Cohen M, et al. Radial artery harvesting for

coronary bypass operations: neurologic complications and their potential mechanisms. *J Thorac Cardiovasc Surg* 2001;121:951–956.

42. Brodman RF, Hirsh LE, Frame R. Effect of radial artery harvest on collateral forearm blood flow and digital perfusion. *J Thorac Cardiovasc Surg* 2002;123:512–516.

43. Anyanwu AC, Saeed I, Bustami M, et al. Does routine use of the radial artery increase complexity or morbidity of coronary bypass surgery? *Ann Thorac Surg* 2001;71:555–559.

44. Tatoulis J, Royse AG, Buxton BF, et al. The radial artery in coronary surgery: a 5-year experience—clinical and angiographic results. *Ann Thorac Surg* 2002;73:143–147.

45. Cohen G, Tamariz MG, Sever JY, et al. The radial artery versus the saphenous vein graft in contemporary CABG: a case-matched study. *Ann Thorac Surg* 2001;71:180–185.

46. Weinschelbaum EE, Macchia A, Caramutti VM, et al. Myocardial revascularization with radial and mammary arteries: initial and mid-term results. *Ann Thorac Surg* 2000;70:1378–1383.

47. Iaco AL, Teodori G, Di Giammarco G, et al. Radial artery for myocardial revascularization: long-term clinical and angiographic results. *Ann Thorac Surg* 2001;72:464–468.

48. Ferguson TB Jr, Coombs LP, Peterson ED. Internal thoracic artery grafting in the elderly patient undergoing coronary artery bypass grafting: room for process improvement? *J Thorac Cardiovasc Surg* 2002;123:869–880.

49. Livesay JJ, Cooley DA, Hallman GL, et al. Early and late results of coronary endarterectomy. *J Thorac Cardiovasc Surg* 1986;92:649–660.

50. Yeh TJ, Heidary D, Shelton L. Y-grafts and sequential grafts in coronary bypass surgery: a critical evaluation of patency rates. *Ann Thorac Surg* 1979;27:409–412.

51. Goldstein J, Cooper E, Saltups A, et al. Angiographic assessment of graft patency after coronary endarterectomy. *J Thorac Cardiovasc Surg* 1991;102:539–545.

52. Brenowitz JB, Kayser KL, Johnson WD. Triple vessel coronary artery endarterectomy and reconstruction: results in 144 patients. *J Am Coll Cardiol* 1988;11:706–711.

53. Bonchek LI, Ullyot DJ. Minimally invasive coronary bypass: a dissenting opinion. *Circulation* 1998;98:495–497.

54. Van Dijk D, de Jaegere PP. Neuropsychological outcome after off-pump versus on-pump coronary bypass surgery: the octopus randomized trial. *Circulation* 2002;105:E179.

55. Van Dijk D, Nierich AP, Jansen EW, et al. Early outcome after off-pump versus on-pump coronary bypass surgery: results from a randomized study. *Circulation* 2001;104:1761–1766.

56. Yacoub M. Off-pump coronary bypass surgery: in search of an identity. *Circulation* 2001;104:1743–1745.

57. Puskas JD, Thourani VH, Marshall JJ, et al. Clinical outcomes, angiographic patency, and resource utilization in 200 consecutive off-pump coronary bypass patients. *Ann Thorac Surg* 2001;71:1477–1483.

58. Kirklin JW, Barratt-Boyes BG. *Cardiac surgery, Vol 1,* 2nd ed. New York: Churchill Livingstone, 1993.

59. McBride LR, Barner HB. The left internal mammary artery as a sequential graft to the left anterior descending system. *J Thorac Cardiovasc Surg* 1983;86:703–705.

60. van Sterkenburg SM, Ernst SM, de la Riviere A, et al. Triple sequential grafts using the internal mammary artery. An angiographic and short-term follow-up study. *J Thorac Cardiovasc Surg* 1992;104:60–65.

61. Galbut DL, Traad EA, Dorman MJ, et al. Seventeen-year experience with bilateral internal mammary artery grafts. *Ann Thorac Surg* 1990;49:195–201.

62. Kouchoukos NT, Wareing TH, Murphy SF, et al. Risks of bilateral internal mammary artery bypass grafting. *Ann Thorac Surg* 1990;49:210–219.

63. Grover FL, Johnson RR, Marshall G, et al. Impact of mammary grafts on coronary bypass operative mortality and morbidity. Department of Veterans Affairs Cardiac Surgeons. *Ann Thorac Surg* 1994;57:559–569.

64. Grossi EA, Esposito R, Harris LJ, et al. Sternal wound infections and use of internal mammary artery grafts. *J Thorac Cardiovasc Surg* 1991;102:342–347.

65. Carrier M, Gregoire J, Tronc F, et al. Effects of internal mammary artery dissection on sternal vascularization. *Ann Thorac Surg* 1992;53:115–119.

66. Seyfer AE, Shriver CD, Miller TR, et al. Sternal blood flow after median sternotomy and mobilization of the internal mammary arteries. *Surgery* 1988;104:899–904.

67. Slater AD, Gott JP, Gray LA. Extended use of bilateral internal mammary arteries for coronary artery disease. *Ann Thorac Surg* 1990;49:1014–1015.

68. Tector AJ, Amundsen S, Schmahl TM, et al. Total revascularization with T grafts. *Ann Thorac Surg* 1994;57:33–39.

69. O'Connor GT, Plume SK, Olmstead EM, et al. A regional intervention to improve the hospital mortality associated with coronary artery bypass graft surgery. The Northern New England Cardiovascular Disease Study Group. *JAMA* 1996;275:841–846.

70. Holman WL, Allman RM, Sansom M, et al. Alabama coronary artery bypass grafting project: results of a statewide quality improvement initiative. *JAMA* 2001;285:3003–3010.

71. Mangano DT, Layug EL, Wallace A, et al. Effect of atenolol on mortality and cardiovascular morbidity after noncardiac surgery. *N Engl J Med* 1996;335:1713–1720.

72. The effect of aggressive lowering of low-density lipoprotein cholesterol levels and low-dose anticoagulation on obstructive changes in saphenous vein coronary artery bypass grafts. The Post Coronary Artery Bypass Graft Trial Investigators. *N Engl J Med* 1997;336:153–162.

73. White CW, Gobel FL, Campeau L, et al. Effect of an aggressive lipid lowering strategy on progression of atherosclerosis in the left main coronary artery from patients in the post coronary artery bypass graft trial. *Circulation* 2001;104:2660–2665.

74. Hunninghake DB. Is aggressive cholesterol control justified? Review of the post-coronary artery bypass graft trial. *Am J Cardiol* 1998;82[Suppl T]:45T–48T.

75. Lytle BW, Cosgrove DM. Coronary artery bypass surgery. *Curr Probl Surg* 1992;29:742–807.

76. Knight JL, Cohn LH. Left thoracotomy and femoro-femoral bypass for reoperative revascularization of the posterior coronary circulation. *J Card Surg* 1987;2:343–349.

77. Gandjbakhch I, Acar C, Cabrol C. Left thoracotomy approach for coronary artery bypass grafting in patients with pericardial adhesions. *Ann Thorac Surg* 1989;48:871–873.

78. Uppal R, Wolfe WG, Lowe JE, et al. Right thoracotomy for reoperative right coronary artery bypass procedures. *Ann Thorac Surg* 1994;57:123–125.

79. Killip T, Passamani E, Davis K. Coronary artery surgery study (CASS): a randomized trial of coronary bypass surgery. Eight years follow-up and survival in patients with reduced ejection fraction. *Circulation* 1985;72[Suppl V]:V-102–V-109.

80. Kirklin JW, Frye RL, Blackstone EH, et al. Some comments on the indications for the coronary artery bypass graft operation. *Int J Cardiol* 1991;31:23–30.

81. Blackstone EH, Naftel DC, Turner ME Jr. The decomposition of time-varying hazard into phases, each incorporating a separate stream of concomitant information. *J Am Stat Assoc* 1986;81:615–624.

82. Naftel DC. Survival analysis methods for medical treatment effectiveness research. *Medical Effectiveness Research Data Methods.* US Department of Health and Human Services, Agency for Health Care Policy and Research. 1992;92-0056:137–150.

83. Naftel DC, Blackstone EH, Kirklin JW. Patient-specific predictions and comparisons for patients with coronary artery disease [software]. UA Health Services Foundation 1993.

84. Eagle KA, Guyton RA, Davidoff R, et al. ACC/AHA guidelines for coronary artery bypass graft surgery: executive summary and recommendations: a report of the American College of Cardiology/American Heart Association Task Force on Practice Guidelines (Committee to revise the 1991 guidelines for coronary artery bypass graft surgery). *Circulation* 1999;100:1464–1480.

85. SoS Investigators. Coronary artery bypass surgery versus percutaneous coronary intervention with stent implantation in patients with multivessel coronary artery disease (the Stent or Surgery trial): a randomized controlled trial. *Lancet* 2002;360:965–970.

86. Abizaid A, Costa MA, Centermero M, et al. Clinical and economic impact of diabetes mellitus on percutaneous and surgical treatment of multivessel coronary disease patients: insights from the Arterial Revascularization Therapy Study (ARTS) Trial. *Circulation* 2001;104:533–538.

87. Costa MA, Carere RG, Lichtenstein SV, et al. Incidence, predictors, and significance of abnormal cardiac enzyme rise in patients treated with bypass surgery in the Arterial Revascularization Therapies Study (ARTS). *Circulation* 2001;104:2689–2693.

88. Sobel BE, Frye R, Detre KM. Burgeoning dilemmas in the manage-

ment of diabetes and cardiovascular disease: rationale for the Bypass Angioplasty Revascularization Investigation 2 Diabetes (BARI 2D) Trial. *Circulation* 2003;107:636–642.

89. Ferguson TB Jr, Hammill BG, Peterson ED, et al. A decade of change—risk profiles and outcomes for isolated coronary artery bypass grafting procedures, 1990-1999: a report from the STS National Database Committee and the Duke Clinical Research Institute. Society of Thoracic Surgeons. *Ann Thorac Surg* 2002;73:480–489.

90. ACC/AHA guidelines and indications for the coronary artery bypass graft operation. A report of the American College of Cardiology/American Heart Association Task Force on Assessment of Diagnostic and Therapeutic Cardiovascular Procedures (Subcommittee on Coronary Artery Bypass Graft Surgery). *J Am Coll Cardiol* 1991;17:543–589; and *Circulation* 1991;83:1125–1173.

91. Sergeant PT, Blackstone EH, Lasaffre E, et al. Unpublished study cited in: Kirklin JW, Barratt-Boyes BG, eds. *Cardiac Surgery, Vol 1,* 2nd ed. New York: Churchill Livingstone, 1993.

92. Sergeant P, Lesaffre E, Flameng W, et al. The return of clinically evident ischemia after coronary artery bypass grafting. *Eur J Cardiothorac Surg* 1991;5:447–457.

93. Fremes SE, Tamariz MG, Abramov D, et al. Late results of the Warm Heart Trial: the influence of nonfatal cardiac events on late survival. *Circulation* 2000;102[10 Suppl 3]:III339–III345.

94. Chaitman BR, Alderman EL, Sheffield LT, et al. Use of survival analysis to determine the clinical significance of new Q waves after coronary bypass surgery. *Circulation* 1983;67:302–309.

95. Janardhan T, Ross JK, Shore DF, et al. Reoperation for recurrent angina after aortocoronary bypass surgery. *Eur J Cardiothorac Surg* 1990;4:29–32.

96. Kirklin JW, Naftel DC, Blackstone EH, et al. Summary of a consensus concerning death and ischemic events after coronary artery bypass grafting. *Circulation* 1989;79[Suppl I]:I81–91.

97. Cameron A, Kemp HG Jr, Green GE. Bypass surgery with the internal mammary artery graft: 15 year follow-up. *Circulation* 1986; 74[Suppl III]:30–36.

98. Salomon NW, Page US, Bigelow JC, et al. Reoperative coronary surgery: comparative analysis of 6591 patients undergoing primary bypass and 508 patients undergoing reoperative coronary artery bypass. *J Thorac Cardiovasc Surg* 1990;100:250–260.

99. Zilla P, von Oppell U, Deutsch M. The endothelium: a key to the future. *J Card Surg* 1993;8:32–60.

100. Yanagisawa M, Kurihara H, Kimura S, et al. A novel potent vasoconstrictor peptide produced by vascular endothelial cells. *Nature* 1988;332:411–415.

101. Loop FD, Lytle BW, Cosgrove DM, et al. Influence of the internal mammary artery graft on 10-year survival and other cardiac events. *N Engl J Med* 1986;314:1–6.

102. Barner HB. Remodeling of arterial conduits in coronary grafting. *Ann Thorac Surg* 2002;73:1341–1345.

103. Bourassa MG, Fisher LD, Campeau L, et al. Long-term fate of bypass grafts. The Coronary Artery Surgery Study (CASS) and Montreal Heart Institute experiences. *Circulation* 1985;72:V71–V78.

104. Bourassa MG, Campeau L, Lesperance J. Changes in grafts and coronary arteries after coronary bypass surgery. *Cardiovasc Clin* 1991;21: 83–100.

105. Barboriak JJ, Van Horn DL, Pintar K, et al. Scanning electron microscope study of human veins and aorta-coronary vein grafts. *J Thorac Cardiovasc Surg* 1976;71:673–679.

106. Kern WH, Dermer GB, Lindesmith GG. The intimal proliferation in aortic-coronary saphenous vein grafts: light and electron microscopic studies. *Am Heart J* 1972;84:771–777.

107. Smith SH, Geer JC. Morphology of saphenous vein coronary artery bypass grafts: 7-116 months postoperative. *Arch Pathol Lab Med* 1983; 107:13–18.

108. Lie JT, Lawrie GM, Morris GC. Aortocoronary bypass graft atherosclerosis. Anatomic study of 99 vein grafts from normal and hyperlipoproteinemic patients up to 75 months postoperatively. *Am J Cardiol* 1977;40:906–914.

109. Neitzel GF, Barboriak JJ, Pintar K, et al. Atherosclerosis in aortocoronary bypass grafts. Morphologic study and risk factor analysis 6 to 12 years after surgery. *Arteriosclerosis* 1986;6:594–600.

110. Sims FH. Discontinuities in the internal elastic lamina: a comparison of coronary and internal mammary arteries. *Artery* 1985;13:127–143.

111. Ross R. The pathogenesis of atherosclerosis: an update. *N Engl J Med* 1986;314:488–500.

112. White SJ, Newby AC. Gene therapy for all aspects of vein-graft disease. *J Card Surg* 2002;17:549–555.

113. Mannion JD, Ormont ML, Magno MG, et al. Sustained reduction of neointima with *c-myc* antisense oligonucleotides in saphenous vein grafts. *Ann Thorac Surg* 1998;66:1948–1952.

114. Ehsan A, Mann MJ, Dell'Acqua G, et al. Long-term stabilization of vein graft wall architecture and prolonged resistance to experimental atherosclerosis after E2F decoy oligonucleotide gene therapy. *J Thorac Cardiovasc Surg* 2001;121:714–722.

115. Mann MJ, Whittemore AD, Donaldson MC, et al. Ex-vivo gene therapy of human vascular bypass grafts with E2F decoy: the PREVENT single-centre, randomized, controlled trial. *Lancet* 1999;354:1493–1498.

Other Stable Conditions

CHAPTER 96

Silent Ischemia

Peter F. Cohn

Key Words: Antiischemic agents; coronary angioplasty; coronary artery surgery; exercise testing; Holter monitoring; silent ischemia.

INTRODUCTION

Silent ischemia—that is, objective documentation of myocardial ischemia in the absence of angina or anginal equivalents—is currently recognized as an important part of the ischemic spectrum, with solid evidence linking its occurrence (by whatever means of detection) to an adverse prognosis. This review addresses the pathophysiology, detection, prognosis, and therapy of silent ischemia in totally asymptomatic patients, patients after infarction, and patients with chronic angina.

PATHOPHYSIOLOGY

Pain Studies

The exact nature of the cardiac pain mechanism remains uncertain, but important data from Maseri's laboratory has identified adenosine as the chemical mediator for this process (1). A variety of clinical studies have shed light on the clinical relevance of cardiac pain. In particular, the pio-

P. F. Cohn: Department of Medicine, Cardiology Division, State University of New York Health Sciences Center, Stony Brook, New York 11794.

neering somatic pain threshold studies of Droste and Roskamm (2) suggested differences between coronary patients with and without angina. These differences were subsequently confirmed by other authors.

A possible role for endorphin mechanisms in the pain responses also has been extensively studied. Normally, varying concentrations of these opioid-like substances exist in plasma and cerebrospinal fluid and may be important in mediating pain sensitivity. Several articles from different laboratories have dealt directly with this issue through measurements of plasma endorphin levels. Sheps and coworkers (3) reported greater levels in silent ischemia. Data from Falcone and coworkers (4) during coronary angioplasty procedures (Fig. 96–1) also suggested a link between endorphin levels and symptoms. By contrast, Marchant and coworkers (5) reported that endorphin levels were similar in patients with painful and silent ischemia, suggesting that "endogenous opiates do not play an important role in modulating symptoms in myocardial ischemia." In summary, the evidence linking endorphins to silent myocardial ischemia is suggestive but not conclusive. Whether more recent data relating inflammatory cytokines to silent ischemia (6) can be confirmed remains unclear, especially in diabetes. Patients with diabetes often have overt neuropathy as a cause for their silent ischemia, but in many instances, the neuropathy is subclinical and can only be detected when autonomic impairment is demonstrated (7).

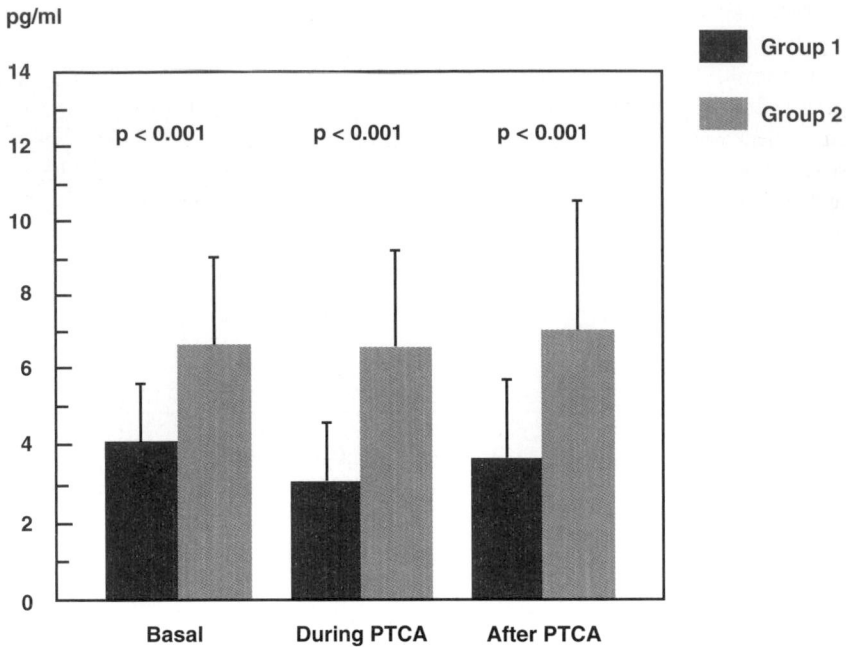

FIG. 96–1. β-Endorphin plasma levels in symptomatic (Group 1) and asymptomatic (Group 2) patients before, during, and after coronary angioplasty (PTCA). The asymptomatic patients showed greater opiate levels during basal conditions, during balloon occlusion, and after the procedure, as compared with patients in Group 1. (From Falcone C, Guasti L, Ochan M, et al. Beta-endorphins during coronary angioplasty in patients with silent or symptomatic myocardial ischemia. *J Am Coll Cardiol* 1993;22: 1614–1620, with permission.)

Hemodynamic Abnormalities

Coronary angioplasty (percutaneous transluminal coronary angioplasty [PTCA]) has allowed the sequence of ischemic events to be precisely defined in a controlled setting. During the first 30 seconds after occlusion, Sigwart and coworkers (8) found that relaxation parameters were the most sensitive of all variables measured. This confirmed earlier reports in experimental animals and other PTCA studies in humans. Angina, when it occurred, was later than 25 seconds after balloon occlusion and was usually preceded by electrocardiographic (ECG) changes. This transition to a symptomatic stage does not necessarily occur, however, as demonstrated by Hauser and coworkers (9), who studied 18 patients with echocardiography during PTCA. Thus, on the basis of exercise studies, hemodynamic monitoring, and, most importantly, transient coronary artery obstruction during PTCA as described earlier, it is apparent that pain is the final event in the sequence of events that characterizes an ischemic episode.

The amount of myocardium rendered ischemic is difficult to quantitate in humans, but comparisons between symptomatic and silent ischemia have been attempted using a variety of techniques. For example, Hirzel and colleagues (10) reported on both wall motion disorders and hemodynamic changes in their series of 36 patients with exercise-induced silent ischemia and 36 matched patients with exercise-induced angina. Under similar exercise conditions, comparable hemodynamic and wall motion abnormalities indicative of ischemia were ob-

served in both groups of patients. Results from our laboratory (11) using exercise radionuclide ventriculography in 40 patients agreed with these findings, whereas Iskandrian and Hakki (12), using similar techniques, disagreed.

When evaluating myocardial perfusion with the exercise thallium-201 scintigram, Travin and coworkers (13) found less ischemia in those patients who experienced silent exercise-induced thallium defects. By contrast, Gasperetti and coworkers (14) reported similar degrees of thallium perfusion defects in their patient groups, as did Mahmarian and coworkers (15), with the latter using the single-photon emission computed tomography technique. Another type of myocardial perfusion technique uses an intravenous infusion of rubidium-82. In a frequently quoted study, Deanfield and coworkers (16) obtained positron tomograms of rubidium uptake from five regions of interest during 24-hour ambulatory monitoring, exercise tests, and cold pressor tests in 34 patients with histories of angina. No significant difference in the change in uptake of rubidium-82 in the abnormal segment of myocardium was observed in episodes accompanied by angina compared with those without pain. The rubidium studies (and to a lesser degree the thallium studies) tend to refute the hypothesis that lesser amounts of myocardium are injured during painless ischemia.

Holter monitoring also has proven useful in clarifying pathophysiologic mechanisms during silent ischemia. Deanfield and coworkers (16) noted approximately 75% of total ischemic episodes were silent. As more and more studies using the Holter monitor have been published, it is apparent that there is circadian variation in ischemic episodes, with most coming after arousal in the morning, or waking and rising at night. In recent studies, silent ST-segment depression on Holter recordings has been related to more severe disease, as defined by angiography and exercise scintigraphy (17).

Ischemia on the Holter monitor also has been linked with enhanced platelet aggregation or variations in vascular tone, or both. Physical exertion, anger, smoking, and mental stress are well documented as "triggers" (18). The latter has received special attention. For example, Kop and coworkers (19) measured heart rate variability using Holter monitoring 60 minutes before and after each of 68 ischemic events triggered by mental stress and found that autonomic change (consistent with vagal withdrawal) may be contributing to silent ischemia.

One of the most intriguing physiologic observations during Holter monitoring has been the steady increase in heart rate preceding the ischemic episode. Even when not frankly tachycardic, this increased heart rate suggests more of a "demand" than "supply" imbalance as a basis for many of the episodes that were once thought to be vasospastic in origin.

DETECTION

In discussing detection of silent ischemia, we consider three separate populations (18): totally asymptomatic individuals, those who are asymptomatic postinfarction, and those with both symptomatic and asymptomatic ischemic episodes.

Asymptomatic Populations

One approach to estimating the prevalence of asymptomatic disease is through pathologic surveys of atherothrombotic heart disease in adult populations who were apparently free of clinical coronary artery disease at time of death and who died of trauma or noncardiac causes. In the nearly 24,000 autopsies reported by Diamond and Forrester (20), the mean prevalence of coronary artery disease was 4.5%.

Another approach to estimating the prevalence of coronary artery disease in asymptomatic individuals is by screening large numbers of asymptomatic individuals and then subjecting positive responders to coronary angiography. This screening can be done with various noninvasive techniques. Currently, ultrafast (electron-beam) computed tomography is attracting interest in detecting coronary calcification. The severity of coronary artery calcification predicted silent ischemia on subsequent radionuclide exercise test in one recent study (Fig. 96–2) (21). Using exercise tests alone, pioneering U.S. Air Force studies in 1,390 men (22) revealed 111 cases with positive exercise tests in a single lead, of whom 34 (about 2.5%) had lesions of at least 50% stenosis. In their landmark study, Erikssen and Thaulow (23) studied 2,014 male office workers in Norway who were 40

to 59 years old. A total of 69 had at least 50% stenosis in one coronary artery, and 50 of these (2.8% of the total) were completely asymptomatic. This percentage is similar to that in the U.S. Air Force study but greater than that reported in 1993 in a multicenter Italian investigation (24).

Because of the problem of false-positive responses in an asymptomatic population, stress tests should be considered as screening procedures for coronary artery disease only in those individuals with multiple risk factors, family histories of premature coronary artery disease, or both. Despite the impressive results of exercise testing in predicting future cardiac events, its limitations in regard to "false-negative" responders must also be noted. In large-scale surveys, the *absolute* number of persons experiencing subsequent cardiac events is larger in the negative-responder group than in the positive-responder group, even though the event *rate* is greater in the latter group. This is, in part, explained by the larger number of individuals in the negative response group, some of whom may have noncritical stenoses at the time of exercise testing that will be acutely transformed (by plaque disruption and other factors) into total or subtotal occlusions.

One of the ways to enhance the diagnostic yield of exercise testing is to combine it with other procedures. For example, Uhl and coworkers (25) studied 191 airmen with abnormal exercise ECGs. Using coronary angiography, the predictive value of the ECG alone was 21% compared with 75% with scintigraphy. Fleg and coworkers (26), using thallium scan and ECG findings, reported a progressive increase in the prevalence of exercise-induced silent ischemia in apparently healthy individuals from one age decade to the next.

Within the asymptomatic population, individuals with diabetes show an especially high prevalence of exercise-induced silent ischemia (27). This is true not only for ECG findings but also for thallium defects. Hypertensive populations also have increased evidence of silent ischemia (28), as do asymptomatic siblings of patients with coronary artery disease (29).

Patients after Infarction

Prevalence statistics also are available in patients who have had myocardial infarctions (MIs) but now are asymptomatic. For example, on the basis of exercise test data, about 50,000 asymptomatic patients per year have silent myocardial ischemia in the initial 30-day postinfarction period (18). In patients who are unable to exercise because of peripheral vascular disease or other problems, Holter monitoring has been used with increasing frequency to document the occurrence of silent ischemia. The intravenous administration of dipyridamole, adenosine, or dobutamine also has been used in place of exercise. For example, stress echocardiography with dipyridamole was used by Bolognese and coworkers (30) to induce wall motion abnormalities in patients after infarction. They were able to induce such abnormalities in 189 of 217 patients; in 94 of those 189 (41%), the abnormalities were unaccompanied by angina. By whatever technique, the

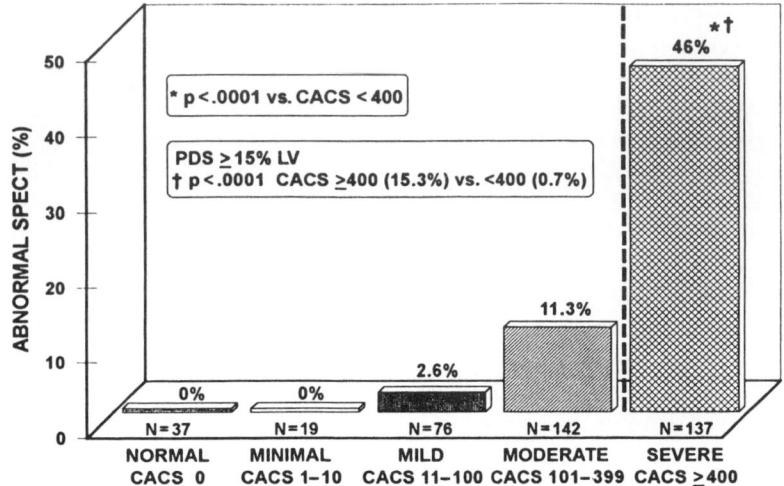

FIG. 96–2. Single-photon emission computed tomography (SPECT) results based on total coronary artery calcium scores (CACS). Few subjects with CACS less than 400 had abnormal SPECT (6.6%), and most (99.3%) had only small (<15%) perfusion defect size (PDS). LV, left ventricle. (From He ZX, Hedrick TD, Pratt CM, et al. Severity of coronary artery calcification by electron beam computed tomography predicts silent myocardial ischemia. *Circulation* 2000;101:244–251, with permission)

reported frequency of silent ischemia in patients after infarction varies from 30% to 42% (18).

Patients with Chronic Angina

The first Holter study to specifically evaluate the significance of asymptomatic episodes in patients with chronic angina was that of Schang and Pepine (31). They indirectly "proved" that the silent ST-segment episodes were truly ischemic by markedly reducing their occurrence with the frequent prophylactic use of nitrate preparations.

Deanfield and coworkers (16) combined Holter monitoring with rubidium perfusion studies to validate ST-segment changes. Of the 1,934 episodes of horizontal or downsloping ST-segment depression that they reported, only 470 (or 24%) were accompanied by angina, a figure almost identical to that of Schang and Pepine (25%) (31).

The number of patients with angina who also have asymptomatic episodes of myocardial ischemia is large, but the exact percentage is unknown. In general, about half of the patients with angina (stable or unstable) have silent ischemia on Holter monitoring, with some series reporting much greater frequencies in their study populations (18). In medically treated patients with minimal residual angina, the figure decreases to about one-fourth to one-third. (See Chapter 86 for a detailed discussion of unstable angina by Kaski.)

PROGNOSIS

Asymptomatic Populations

It has been well established that abnormal exercise tests in asymptomatic individuals help to predict future cardiac

events. Two of the largest epidemiologic studies are the Multiple Risk Factor Intervention Trial (MRFIT) (Fig. 96–3) (32) and the Lipid Research Clinics Mortality Follow-Up Study (33). More recently, the Kuopio study of asymptomatic middle-aged Finnish men found exercise-induced silent ischemia to be a strong predictor of coronary mortality when at least one conventional risk factor also was present (34).

The importance of serial exercise testing has been demonstrated by Josephson and coworkers (35) in their asymptomatic cohort from the Baltimore Longitudinal Aging Study. In this study, conversion from a normal to an abnormal ST-segment response carried the same risk for future cardiac events as an initially abnormal response did.

In the series performed in Norway by Erikssen and colleagues (23), after an 8- to 10-year period of following the 50 asymptomatic men (15 of whom had one-vessel disease, 18 had two-vessel disease, and 17 had three-vessel disease), the authors found that 3 died of cardiac disease and 7 had a MI (5 of which were silent). In addition, angina pectoris developed in 16 other men. Clinical events were observed mostly in men with multivessel disease. At the 15-year mark (36) there were 14 deaths overall (Fig. 96–4), including 8 deaths in the three-vessel disease group. Warning signs, such as typical angina, often were absent before death or nonfatal MI. Thus, the yearly mortality rate in the three-vessel disease group was 3% compared with approximately 1% in the patients with one- and two-vessel disease combined. Asymptomatic diabetics with exercise-induced silent ischemia and microalbuminuria have been shown to have a worse prognosis than patients with diabetes without microalbuminuria (29).

In addition to exercise studies, there are reports of Holter monitoring studies in asymptomatic populations. In 1989,

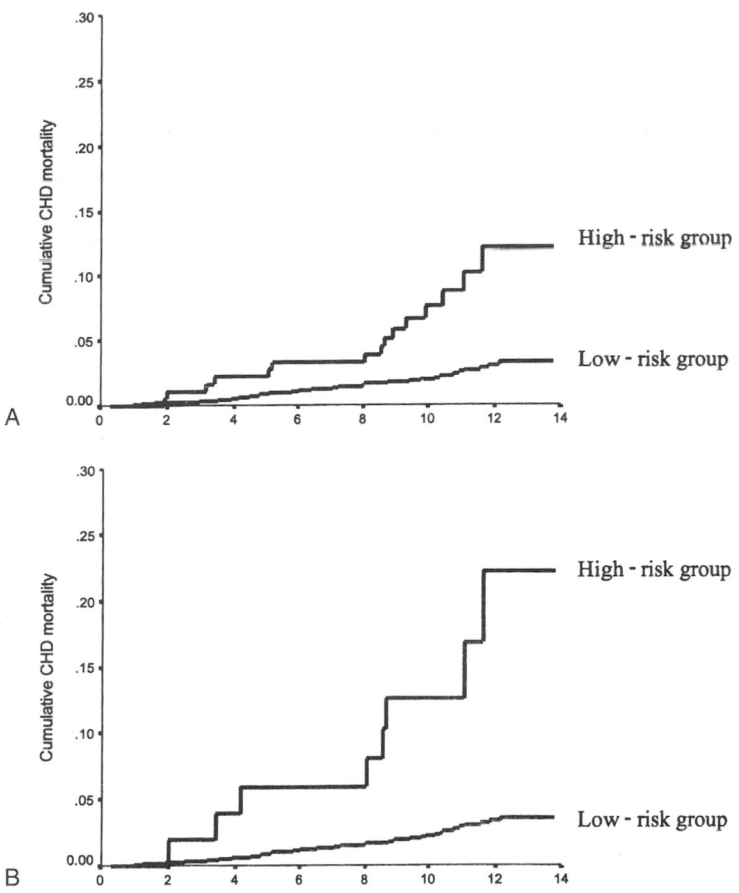

FIG. 96–3. Cumulative hazards of coronary mortality in men with silent myocardial ischemia (high-risk group) during exercise (high-risk group) **(A)** or in the recovery period after exercise **(B)** versus all others (low-risk group). CHD, coronary heart disease. (From Laukkanen JA, Kurl S, Lakka TA, et al. Exercise-induced silent myocardial ischemia and coronary morbidity and mortality in middle-aged men. *J Am Coll Cardiol* 2001;38:72–79, with permission.)

Hedblad and coworkers (37) reported the results of their "Men born in 1914" study from Sweden. Of the 394 men who had ST-segment analysis after 24 hours of Holter monitoring, 341 had no prior history of coronary artery disease. Of these 341 men, 70 had at least 1 episode of ST-segment depression, and 12 (14%) died over the course of the 43-month follow-up period. This incidence rate was twice as high as that observed in the 262 men without ST-segment depression (19 deaths or 7%; $p < 0.005$). Despite this study, the use of ambulatory monitoring for detecting silent ischemia in asymptomatic persons without coronary arteriographic evidence of coronary artery disease is not recommended as a valid "screening" test when compared with exercise testing.

A discussion of prognosis would not be complete without consideration of the initial presentation of coronary artery disease in previously asymptomatic individuals, some of whom presumably had silent ischemia. On the basis of data from the Framingham study and other surveys of apparently healthy individuals, it is apparent that angina is the initial presentation in only about half of these individuals. MI and sudden death are the other common presentations. Similar data have been reported by Thaulow and coworkers (36) (Fig. 96–4) in angiographically documented coronary artery disease and by Fleg and Kennedy (38), but not by Droste and coworkers (39).

Few studies have addressed the issue of whether the population with asymptomatic coronary artery disease forms the pool from which a certain number of persons will surface each year as victims of sudden death or nonfatal MIs. Evidence from a study performed at the Hennepin County Medical Center in Minnesota (40) provides some tentative conclusions in this regard. These investigators studied 15 individuals who were successfully resuscitated from ventricular fibrillation that took place outside the hospital. Nine of the 15 had no prior history of heart disease. Nearly all the patients showed silent myocardial ischemia on their ECGs and left ventriculograms during exercise testing. Norris and coworkers (41) found that 25% of 43 out-of-hospital survivors of ventricular fibrillation had silent ischemia on subsequent Holter monitoring. Thus, one could speculate that episodes of silent ischemia may occur before ventricular fi-

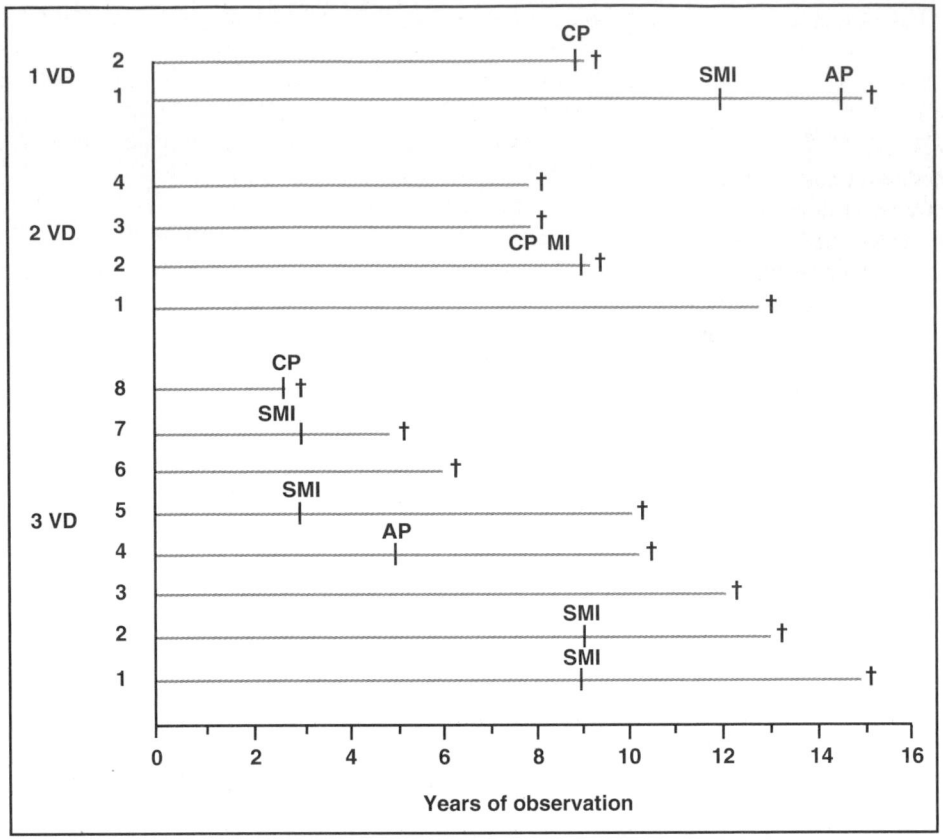

FIG. 96–4. Lifetime curves after first identification of a significant exercise-induced ST-segment depression in 14 asymptomatic men with angiographically proven coronary artery disease who died during the first 15 years of follow-up. AP, clinical angina pectoris; CP, atypical chest pain; MI, clinically evident myocardial infarction; SMI, silent myocardial infarction; 1 VD, one-vessel disease; 2 VD, two-vessel disease; 3 VD, three-vessel disease; *dagger,* death. (From Thaulow E, Erikssen J, Sandik L, et al. Initial clinical presentation of cardiac disease in asymptomatic men with silent myocardial ischemia and angiographically documented coronary artery disease [the Oslo Ischemia Study]. *Am J Cardiol* 1993;72: 629–633, with permission.)

brillation and may play a role in the genesis of sudden death in some individuals.

Patients after Infarction

Data are also available in patients who are asymptomatic after an MI. The Coronary Artery Surgery Study (CASS) registry consists largely of asymptomatic or mildly symptomatic patients after infarction. In a 1987 report, Weiner and coworkers (42) found painless exercise-induced ischemia to carry the same prognosis as painful ischemia. The subgroup of patients with three-vessel disease had a 6% annual mortality rate.

In addition to these studies, there are numerous reports describing prognosis in patients who had sustained an acute MI. Short-term survival statistics based on the postinfarction exercise studies indicate that exercise-induced ST-segment depression markedly increases the 1-year mortality rate. For example, in the study by Theroux and coworkers (43), the 1-year mortality rate was 2.1% (3 of 146) in patients without

ischemic ST-segment changes during exercise and 27% (17 of 64) in those with such changes ($p < 0.001$). The authors reported that angina in the presence of ST-segment depression had no effect on these statistics. deBelder and coworkers (44) studied 262 patients 7 days after infarction; 104 had a positive exercise test, and 67 had silent ischemia. In the first year after the infarction, these latter patients had 12 times as high a cardiac mortality rate as the negative responders (and twice as high a rate as patients with angina and ST-segment depression). These figures are similar to those reported by Theroux and coworkers (43).

Data also are available from Holter studies in patients after infarction. Gottlieb and coworkers (45) reported that in patients after infarction who were not suitable for exercise testing, silent ischemia on Holter monitoring was a significant predictor of 1-year mortality rates. Tzivoni and coworkers (46) compared the value of Holter monitoring versus exercise testing as risk prognosticators. The subsequent cardiac event rate was significantly greater in those patients with both abnormal Holter reports and abnormal exercise tests; these results have been confirmed by Jereczek and coworkers (47).

Patients with Chronic Angina

Several studies have investigated the prognosis of patients with chronic angina who have a positive exercise test without pain. Presumably, these individuals have both symptomatic and silent ischemic episodes during daily activities. Falcone and coworkers (48) followed 269 patients with painful ischemia during exercise and 204 patients with painless ischemia. Survival curves were similar regardless of the presence or absence of pain during the test. By contrast, Mark and coworkers (49) found ST-segment depression without angina to have the same prognostic importance as a negative exercise test. Studies using radionuclide techniques have not supported the results of Mark and coworkers (49). For example, Assay and coworkers (50) found a worse prognosis in silent than in painful ischemia in their series of 55 patients studied with exercise thallium tests. Other reports citing exercise thallium scintigraphy or exercise radionuclide ventriculography also have shown silent ischemia to carry the same adverse prognosis as painful ischemia.

There is currently a considerable amount of data concerning prognosis in stable angina patients who have undergone long-term ambulatory ECG monitoring. In general, these reports show that Holter evidence of ischemia adds potentially important incremental data to those obtained from the clinical history, exercise testing, or both. For example, Deedwania and Carbajal (51) found that silent ischemia occurs frequently (even in apparently adequately medically treated patients) and identifies a subset of patients at high risk for cardiac death. This has been confirmed in a 1994 study by deMarchena and coworkers (52) but questioned by Gandhi and coworkers (53) in another report that year and by Mulcahy and coworkers in 1997 (54). The issue is not resolved and research in this area is still active. Data from the Asymptomatic Cardiac Ischemic Pilot (ACIP) study are important in this regard and is considered in detail later in this chapter in the section on effect of treatment on prognosis. Additional Holter data also are available in patients with unstable angina (see Chapter 86 by Kaski).

The prognostic importance of silent ischemia has now been demonstrated in an entirely new setting. For example, it is becoming increasing clear that not only exercise testing (with or without radionuclide scintigraphy) but also Holter monitoring can be used to assess the perioperative risk for cardiovascular morbidity and mortality in patients undergoing a variety of noncardiac surgical procedures. Even in patients with histories of angina, most of the ischemia found by these tests is silent. Eagle and coworkers (55) have reviewed the value of preoperative chemical radionuclide imaging, which continues to be popular in patients who cannot exercise because of peripheral vascular disease. Studies comparing dipyridamole scintigraphy with Holter monitoring find each to be helpful. The latter procedure has grown in popularity with both cardiologists and anesthesiologists. Mangano and coworkers (56) have published several studies attesting to its utility. For example, they found that postoperative myocardial ischemia occurred in 41% of their Holter-monitored patients and was associated with a significant increase in the risk for an adverse cardiovascular event. Landesberg and coworkers (57) correlated prolonged silent ischemia on Holter monitoring perioperatively to postoperative infarcts.

MANAGEMENT

Medical Treatment

Perhaps no single area concerning coronary artery disease is as controversial as management of individuals who are totally asymptomatic. Because the prognosis in individuals in this category is generally favorable, the simplest approach is to modify risk factors when they are present and reduce physical activities so that myocardial ischemia does not develop. It is the patients who demonstrate extensive ischemia that merit special concern. These individuals are more likely to have multivessel disease with its correspondingly worse prognosis. As opposed to asymptomatic persons with single-vessel disease, who may be in a "presymptomatic" stage and go on to angina or nonfatal infarction, asymptomatic individuals with triple-vessel or left main disease appear to be at greater risk for sudden death or massive infarctions. One end point of therapy could be improved exercise tolerance—that is, prolonging the time at which ischemia develops. Another end point could be improved wall motion in ischemic zones.

The use of pharmacologic agents and PTCA is discussed in more detail in connection with silent ischemia in patients with known coronary artery disease because there is a greater consensus concerning treatment of these patients. For example, medical treatment with β-blockers is recommended for patients after infarction to reduce short-term mortality and reinfarction. Furthermore, initial data have appeared that suggest, but do not prove, that the β-blockers improve prognosis in patients after infarction by reducing ischemia. Ruberman and coworkers (58) conducted a large case–control study using data from the Beta Blocker Heart Attack Trial (BHAT). The investigators found that ST-segment depression on Holter monitoring was associated with increased mortality and that the more ischemic time on Holter monitoring, the greater the risk for subsequent death. Most importantly, in terms of medical management, the relative risk in the propranolol-treated group was significantly less than in the placebo-treated group.

Patients who have both symptomatic and asymptomatic myocardial ischemia are the most commonly encountered patients by practitioners. Previously, there has been a tendency to discount the importance of the asymptomatic episodes and to treat "symptoms." With the report of several groups that asymptomatic episodes often greatly outnumber symptomatic episodes (as determined by Holter monitoring), there is a growing trend toward considering the asymptomatic episodes to be of equal importance to the symptomatic ones. Physicians have a full range of therapeutic options to choose from, including long-acting nitrates, either as ointment, isosorbide dinitrate, or isosorbide mononitrate preparations, and also calcium antagonists and β-blockers. The combination of nifedipine and β-blockers was used in the Nifedipine-Total Ischemia Awareness Program (TIAP) (59). The beneficial effects of combination therapy were especially marked in the patients with the most total ischemic activity. A third generation calcium antagonist (amlodipine) was subsequently introduced and tested in another large multicenter study (60). The results were impressive, especially in combination with a β-blocker (61).

Choice of medications depends on whether the ischemia is caused by increased work of the heart or by a vasospastic component, or both. In the former case, myocardial oxygen requirements are raised, usually because of increases in heart rate and blood pressure, two of the major factors regulating myocardial oxygen consumption. For these episodes, β-blockers would appear to be reasonable agents. Although early studies of silent myocardial ischemia on Holter monitoring suggested that many of the episodes did not appear to be associated with increased work of the heart, this has not been borne out by subsequent studies, as noted earlier in this review. Thus, despite observations concerning relatively low heart rates at the onset of most episodes of out-of-hospital ischemia and the lack of association with strenuous exercising, the sum of the data concerning treatment of ambulatory ischemia indicates that the β-blockers are still the most efficacious agents (62). The key to this seeming paradox is in the small but significant increase in heart rate preceding the ischemic event. By preventing this increase, β-blockers can be a highly effective form of therapy, more so even than calcium blockers, as demonstrated by several comparative studies (63–66). The possibility that the effect of β-blocking drugs on platelet aggregability was responsible for their abolition of the circadian variation in ischemic events has been proposed, but currently no conclusive results have been reported (67).

In a large Swedish study (68), investigators found aspirin to be a protective agent against future infarctions (Fig. 96–5). This study is important in light of increased data concerning the role of enhanced platelet aggregability (which can be blocked by aspirin) in precipitating ischemic events. Statins also can reduce ischemic events (69), presumably by favorable effects on endothelial function.

PTCA represents a great advance in the treatment of myocardial ischemia, whether painful or silent. Documentation of persistent but silent ischemia after the procedures offers physicians an opportunity to diagnose restenosis before dangerous events occur. Documentation of such ischemia carries an unfavorable prognosis (18).

Whether any therapies short of revascularization surgery favorably affect the prognosis of patients with chronic myocardial ischemia is still unclear. In selected patients, both β-blockers and aspirin improve prognosis (e.g., in patients after infarction), but it is still unproven that abolition of ischemic episodes per se has the same effect. Lim and cowork-

ers (70) reported that patients who had their exercise-induced painless wall motion abnormalities abolished by medications did better at 9-month follow-up than patients in whom the abnormalities persisted. Other evidence is less direct. In the BHAT study (58), patients on placebo had a much greater frequency of abnormal Holter recordings and a worse prognosis than those patients receiving propranolol.

Data on the effect of treatment on prognosis has come from the results of multicenter trials in which patients are randomized to different treatment regimens (with ischemic episodes documented by exercise testing and Holter monitoring) and followed for subsequent development of cardiovascular events. The largest of these trials, ACIP, was sponsored by the National Institutes of Health (NIH) and directed by Conti (71). Patients were randomized to angina-guided medical therapy, ischemia-guided (Holter-driven) medical therapy, or revascularization. The primary goals were (a) to compare the 12-week efficacy of the three treatment strategies in suppressing cardiac ischemia and (b) to assess the feasibility for a larger prognosis trial in patients with asymptomatic ischemia. A total of 618 patients were enrolled in the pilot study with cardiac ischemia suppressed in 40% to 55% of patients at 12 weeks, using either low or moderate doses of a multidrug medical regimen or revascularization. After 1 year of follow-up, revascularization was superior to both angina-guided and ischemia-guided medical strategies in suppressing ischemia and also was associated with a better clinical outcome (Fig. 96–6) (72). Within the revascularization arm, bypass surgery was superior to angioplasty in suppressing cardiac ischemia (73). At 2 years, the benefits of revascularization were still present (74).

Other trials of prognostic importance also have been completed albeit with mixed results. In the Atenolol Silent Ischemic Trial (ASIST) (75), atenolol-treated patients with coronary disease and mild or no ischemia had fewer adverse events, fewer ischemic episodes, and shorter duration ischemia compared with placebo. At 1-year follow-up, the patients treated with atenolol also had fewer cardiac events. The Total Ischemic Burden European Trial (TIBET) (76) had a different protocol in that there was no placebo arm but rather treatment with atenolol, slow-release nifedipine, and a combination of the two drugs. That study showed no evidence of an association between ischemic events or hard and soft end points after 2 years of follow-up. The Angina Pectoris Study in Stockholm (APSIS) (77) also did not show a reduction in cardiac events on combined treatment, but the Total Ischemic Burden Bisoprolol Study (TIBBS) did (78). In another example of the value of β-blockers, the use of atenolol to prevent perioperative ischemia in noncardiac surgical cases and to improve the adverse prognosis cited earlier has been reported by Mangano and coworkers (79).

Surgical Treatment

Coronary bypass surgery in small numbers of asymptomatic patients are usually reported as part of a mixed series that in-

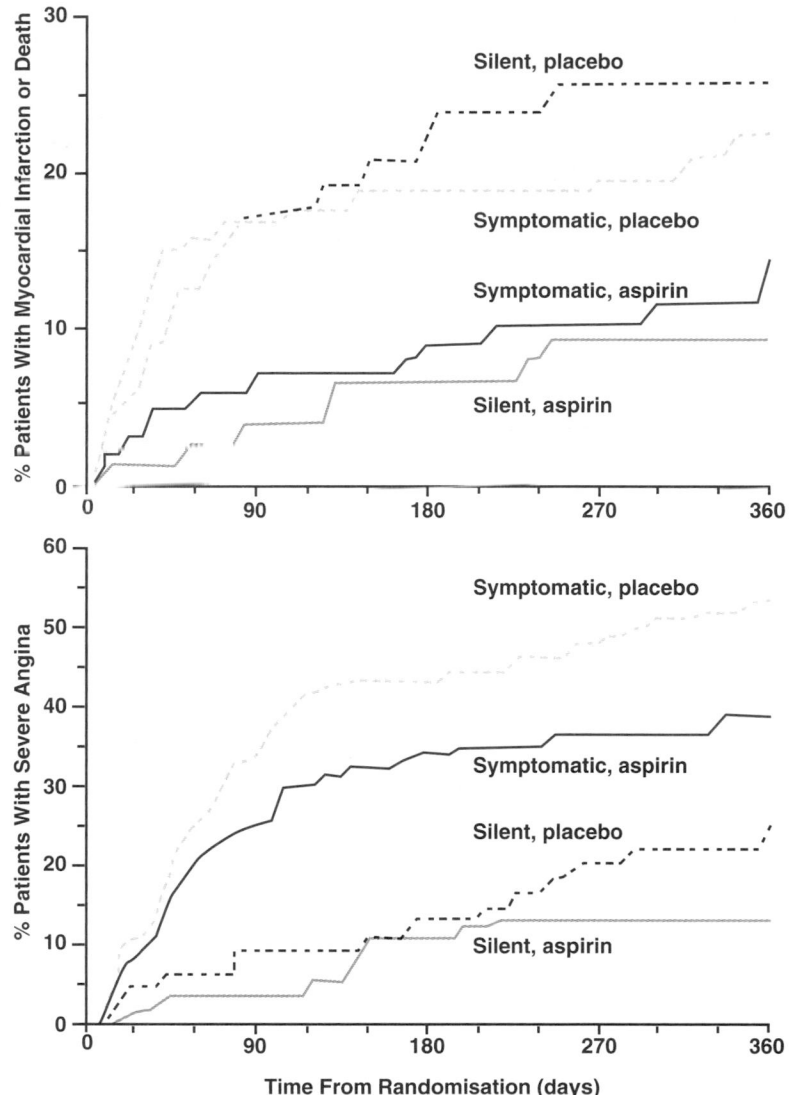

FIG. 96–5. Life-table analysis of rates of death, myocardial infarction, and severe angina in patients with silent and symptomatic ischemia on exercise tests. A comparison of aspirin versus placebo therapy. (From Nyman I, Larsson H, Wallentin L. Prevention of serious cardiac events by low-dose aspirin in patients with silent myocardial ischemia. The Research Group on Instability in Coronary Artery Disease in Southeast Sweden. *Lancet* 1992;340:497–501, with permission.)

cludes asymptomatic and mildly symptomatic patients. The results involving the asymptomatic patients must then be dissected out from the main body of data. The study from the Seattle Heart Watch conducted by the University of Washington School of Medicine is one such study (80). Even though the study was nonrandomized, it provides important data because the medically and surgically treated patients had similar baseline variables. The surgically treated patients had a lower mortality rate (via life-table analysis) than their medical counterparts, with the largest difference in survival seen in patients with triple-vessel disease and ejection fractions between 31% and 50%. This is the only nonrandomized study with control patients; it suggests a beneficial effect of surgery on mortality in asymptomatic patients.

In addition to this retrospective "matched" study from the University of Washington, there also have been several reports of surgical series without attempts to have control groups. The Peter Bent Brigham Hospital (now Brigham and Women's Hospital, Boston, MA) is a good example (81). Twenty patients were studied, 14 of whom were totally asymptomatic. Six of these had sustained a prior MI. This series was unique in that 16 patients had preoperative exercise tests, of which 14 demonstrated silent ischemia. The only death in this series occurred 5 years after surgery. There were 12 patients with both preoperative and postoperative exercise tests; in 8 of these patients the test became completely normal, and in the other 4, less of an ischemic response was observed than in the preoperative test.

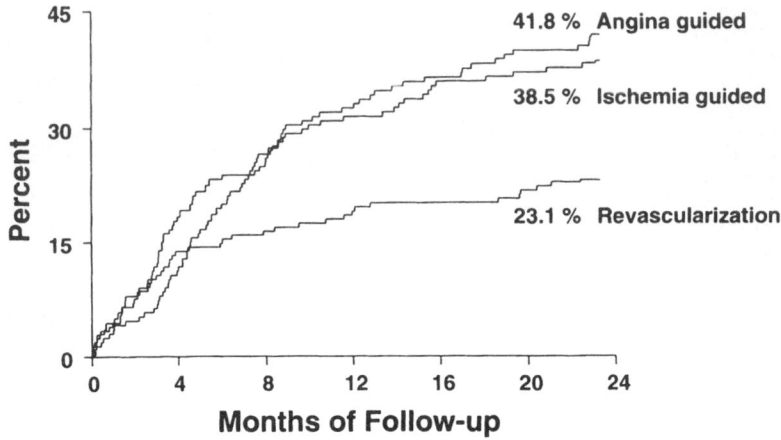

FIG. 96–6. Two-year cumulative rates of death, myocardial infarction, or cardiac hospitalization in the Asymptomatic Cardiac Ischemic Pilot (ACIP) trial. Differences were significant between revascularization strategy and both angina-guided and ischemia-guided strategies ($p < 0.003$). The latter were not significantly different from each other ($p = 48$). (From Davies RF, Goldberg D, Forman S, et al. Asymptomatic cardiac ischemia pilot [ACIP] study two-year follow-up. *Circulation* 1997;95:2037–2043, with permission.)

The multicenter CASS (82,83) has provided additional data both for and against surgical intervention. Unlike the Seattle report, this was a randomized study, but one with certain qualifying features. First, many patients had sustained MIs. Second, they all had undergone coronary arteriography before randomization. Third, patients with left main lesions or ejection fractions less than 35% were excluded. Fourth, although only patients with no angina or mild angina (New York Heart Association Class I and II) were included, many patients required medication to attain this pain-free or mild-pain classification. With only one exception, there were no statistically significant differences in survival in patients receiving medical versus surgical therapy. The exception was the triple-vessel disease subgroup with ejection fraction less than 50%. The existence of patients at high risk within the three-vessel disease subgroup with normal left ventricular function can best be demonstrated when the exercise test is used. The CASS Registry also included 53 asymptomatic patients with left main disease. Their outlook was significantly better when treated with bypass surgery compared with medical therapy (84). Others have reported similar findings (85). The ACIP study, with its impressive surgical results, has been discussed earlier in this chapter (71–74).

SUMMARY

Since the first edition of this book appeared, and despite important new data, certain questions still remain unanswered, especially concerning the pathophysiology of silent ischemic episodes. Why do they occur in some patients and not others? Why do they occur in some instances in a given individual but not at other times? Of more importance to the clinician is the issue of whether antiisch-

emic therapy with drugs or revascularization procedures can improve morbidity and mortality. Results of clinical trials concluded since 1996 have provided more information for the latter area.

To summarize the most important aspects of this chapter: (a) the pathophysiology of silent ischemia remains unclear, but it is extremely prevalent in patients with coronary artery disease; (b) stress testing is the preferred method of detection, but Holter monitoring is reliable in recording ischemia during daily life and in evaluating therapy; (c) prognosis is adversely affected by silent ischemia whether the patient is symptomatic or asymptomatic, especially during stress testing; and (d) a variety of pharmacologic agents can reduce the ischemic burden, but currently there are only limited data suggesting that such therapy improves prognosis. By contrast, revascularization, especially coronary artery surgery, does appear to improve longevity.

REFERENCES

1. Crea F, Pupita G, Galassi AR, et al. Role of adenosine in the pathogenesis of anginal pain *Circulation* 1990;81:164–172.
2. Droste C, Roskamm H. Experimental pain measurement in patients with asymptomatic myocardial ischemia. *J Am Coll Cardiol* 1983;81:164–172.
3. Sheps DS, Adams KF, Hinderliter A, et al. Endorphins are related to pain perception in coronary artery disease. *Am J Cardiol* 1987;59:523–527.
4. Falcone C, Guasti L, Ochan M, et al. Beta-endorphins during coronary angioplasty in patients with silent or symptomatic myocardial ischemia. *J Am Coll Cardiol* 1993;22:1614–1620.
5. Marchant B, Umachandran V, Wilkinson P, et al. Reexamination of the role of endogenous opiates in silent myocardial ischemia. *J Am Coll Cardiol* 1994:23:645–651.
6. Mazzone A, Cusa C, Mazzucchelli I, et al. Increased production of inflammatory cytokines in patients with silent myocardial ischemia. *J Am Coll Cardiol* 2001;38:1895–1901.
7. Marchant B, Umachandran V, Stevenson R, et al. Silent myocardial

ischemia: role of subclinical neuropathy in patients with and without diabetes. *J Am Coll Cardiol* 1993;22:1433–1437.

8. Sigwart U, Gerbic M, Payot M, et al. Ischemic events during coronary artery balloon occlusion. In: Rutishauswer W, Roskamm H, eds. *Silent myocardial ischemia.* Berlin: Springer-Verlag, 1984:29–36.

9. Hauser AM, Gangadharan V, Ramos RG, et al. Sequence of mechanical, electrocardiographic and clinical effects of repeated coronary occlusion in human beings: echocardiographic observations during coronary angioplasty. *J Am Coll Cardiol* 1985;5:193–197.

10. Hirzel HO, Leutwyler R, Krayenbuehl HP. Silent myocardial ischemia: hemodynamic changes during dynamic exercise in patients with proved coronary artery disease despite absence of angina pectoris. *J Am Coll Cardiol* 1985;6:275–284.

11. Cohn PF, Brown EJ, Wynne J, et al. Global and regional left ventricular ejection fraction abnormalities during exercise in patients with silent myocardial ischemia. *J Am Coll Cardiol* 1983;1:931–933.

12. Iskandrian AS, Hakki AH. Left ventricular function in patients with coronary heart disease in the presence or absence of angina pectoris during exercise radionuclide ventriculography. *Am J Cardiol* 1984;53:1239–1243.

13. Travin MI, Fores AR, Boucher CA, et al. Silent versus symptomatic ischemia during a thallium-201 exercise test. *Am J Cardiol* 1991;68:1600–1608.

14. Gasperetti CM, Burwell LR, Beller GA. Prevalence of and variables associated with silent myocardial ischemia on exercise thallium-201 stress testing. *J Am Coll Cardiol* 1990;16:115–123.

15. Mahmarian JJ, Pratt CM, Cocanougher MK, et al. Altered myocardial perfusion in patients with angina pectoris or silent ischemia during exercise as assessed by quantitative thallium-201 single-photon emission computed tomography. *Circulation* 1990;82:1305–1315.

16. Deanfield JE, Shea M, Ribiero P, et al. Transient ST-segment depression as a marker of myocardial ischemia during daily life. *Am J Cardiol* 1984;54:1195–1200.

17. Baszko A, Ochotny R, Blaszyk K. Correlation of ST-segment depression during ambulatory electrocardiographic monitoring with myocardial perfusion and left ventricular function. *Am J Cardiol* 2001;87:959–963.

18. Cohn PF. *Silent myocardial ischemia and infarction, 4th ed.* New York: Marcel Dekker, 2000.

19. Kop WJ, Verdino RJ, Gottdiener JS. Changes in heart rate and heart rate variability before ambulatory ischemic events. *J Am Coll Cardiol* 2001;38:742–749.

20. Diamond GA, Forrester JS. Analysis of probability as an aid in the clinical diagnosis of coronary artery disease. *N Engl J Med* 1979;300:1350–1358.

21. He ZX, Hedrick TD, Pratt CM, et al. Severity of coronary artery calcification by electron beam computed tomography predicts silent myocardial ischemia. *Circulation* 2000;101:244–251.

22. Froehlicher VF, Thompson AJ, Longo MR Jr, et al. Value of exercise testing for screening symptomatic men for latent coronary artery disease. *Prog Cardiovasc Dis* 1976;16:265–276.

23. Erikssen J, Thaulow E. Follow-up of patients with asymptomatic myocardial ischemia. In: Rutishauser W, Roskamm H, eds. *Silent myocardial ischemia.* Berlin: Springer-Verlag, 1984:156–164.

24. Fazzini PF, Prati PL, Rovelli F, et al. Epidemiology of silent myocardial ischemia in asymptomatic middle-aged men (the ECCIS Project). *Am J Cardiol* 1993;72:1383–1388.

25. Uhl GS, Kay TN, Hickman JR Jr. Comparison of exercise radionuclide angiography and thallium perfusion imaging in detecting coronary artery disease in asymptomatic men. *J Cardiac Rehabil* 1983;2:118–124.

26. Fleg JL, Gerstenblith G, Zonderman AB, et al. Prevalence and prognostic significance of exercise-induced silent myocardial ischemia detected by thallium scintigraphy and electrocardiography in asymptomatic volunteers. *Circulation* 1990;81:428–436.

27. Rutter MK, Wahid ST, McComb JM, et al. Significance of silent ischemia and microalbuminuria in predicting coronary events in asymptomatic patients with type 2 diabetes. *J Am Coll Cardiol* 2002;40:56–61.

28. Massie BM, Szlachcic Y, Tubau JF, et al. Scintigraphic and electrocardiographic evidence of silent coronary artery disease in asymptomatic hypertension: a case-control study. *J Am Coll Cardiol* 1993;22:1598–1606.

29. Blumenthal RS, Becker DM, Yanek LR, et al. Detecting occult coronary disease in a high-risk asymptomatic population. *Circulation* 2003;107:702–707.

30. Bolognese L, Rossi L, Sarasso G, et al. Silent versus symptomatic dipyridamole-induced ischemia after myocardial infarction: clinical and prognostic significance. *J Am Coll Cardiol* 1992;19:953–959.

31. Schang SJ, Pepine CJ. Transient asymptomatic ST-segment depression during daily activity. *Am J Cardiol* 1977;39:396–402.

32. Rautaharju PM, Prineas RJ, Eifler WJ, et al. Prognostic value of exercise electrocardiogram in men at high risk of future coronary heart disease: Multiple Risk Factor Intervention Trial experience. *J Am Coll Cardiol* 1986;8:1–10.

33. Gordon DJ, Elelund LG, Karon JM, et al. Predictive value of the exercise tolerance test for mortality in North American men: the Lipid Research Clinics Mortality Follow-Up study. *Circulation* 1986;2:252–226.

34. Laukkanen JA, Kurl S, Lakka TA, et al. Exercise-induced silent myocardial ischemia and coronary morbidity and mortality in middle-aged men. *J Am Coll Cardiol* 2001;38:72–79.

35. Josephson RA, Shefrin E, Lakatta EG, et al. Can serial exercise testing improve the prediction of coronary events in asymptomatic individuals? *Circulation* 1990;81:20–24.

36. Thaulow E, Erikssen J, Sandik L, et al. Initial clinical presentation of cardiac disease in asymptomatic men with silent myocardial ischemia and angiographically documented coronary artery disease (the Oslo Ischemia Study). *Am J Cardiol* 1993;72:629–633.

37. Hedblad B, Juell-Moller S, Svensson K, et al. Increased mortality in men with ST segment depression during 24 h ambulatory long-term ECG recording. Results from prospective population study "Men born in 1914," from Malmo, Sweden. *Eur Heart J* 1989;10:149–158.

38. Fleg JL, Kennedy HL. Prognostic significance of Holter monitoring in apparently healthy older subjects. *J Am Coll Cardiol* 1991;17:330A(abst).

39. Droste C, Ruf G, Greenlee MW, et al. Development of angina pectoris pain and cardiac events in asymptomatic patients with myocardial ischemia. *Am J Cardiol* 1993;72:121–127.

40. Sharma B, Asinger R, Francis GS, et al. Demonstration of exercise-induced painless myocardial ischemia in survivors of out-of-hospital ventricular fibrillation. *Am J Cardiol* 1987;59:740–745.

41. Norris B, Callahan DB, Emery M, et al. Silent ischemia in survivors of out-of-hospital ventricular fibrillation. *J Am Coll Cardiol* 1988;11:96A(abst).

42. Weiner DA, Ryan TJ, McCabe CH, et al. Significance of silent myocardial ischemia during exercise testing in patients with coronary artery disease. *Am J Cardiol* 1987;59:725–729.

43. Theroux P, Waters DD, Halphen C, et al. Prognostic value of exercise testing soon after myocardial infarction. *N Engl J Med* 1979;301:341–345.

44. de Belder M, Skehan D, Pumphrey C, et al. Identification of a high risk subgroup of patients with silent ischaemia after myocardial infarction: a group for early therapeutic revascularisation? *Br Heart J* 1990;63:145–150.

45. Gottlieb SO, Gottlieb SH, Ashuff SC, et al. Silent ischemia on Holter monitoring predicts mortality in high-risk post infarction patients. *JAMA* 1988;259:1030–1035.

46. Tzivoni D, Gavish A, Zin D, et al. Prognostic significance of ischemic episodes in patients with previous myocardial infarction. *Am J Cardiol* 1988;62:661–664.

47. Jereczek M, Andresen D, Schroder J, et al. Prognostic value of ischemia during Holter monitoring and exercise testing after acute myocardial infarction. *Am J Cardiol* 1993;72:8–13.

48. Falcone C, de Servi S, Poma E, et al. Clinical significance of exercise-induced silent myocardial ischemia in patients with coronary artery disease. *J Am Coll Cardiol* 1989;14:1175–1180.

49. Mark DB, Hlatky MA, Califf RM, et al. Painless exercise ST deviation on the treadmill: long-term prognosis. *J Am Coll Cardiol* 1989;14:885–892.

50. Assay ME, Walters GL, Hendrix GH, et al. Incidence of acute myocardial infarction in patients with exercise-induced silent myocardial ischemia. *Am J Cardiol* 1987;59:497–500.

51. Deedwania PC, Carbajal EV. Silent ischemia during daily life is an independent predictor of mortality in stable angina. *Circulation* 1990;81:748–756.

52. de Marchena E, Asch J, Martinez J, et al. Usefulness of persistent silent myocardial ischemia in predicting a high cardiac event rate in men with medically controlled, stable angina pectoris. *Am J Cardiol* 1994;73:390–392.

53. Gandhi MM, Wood DA, Lampe FC. Characteristics and clinical significance of ambulatory myocardial ischemia in men and women in the general population presenting with angina pectoris. *J Am Coll Cardiol* 1994;23:74–81.

54. Mulcahy D, Husain S, Zalos G, et al. Ischemia during ambulatory monitoring as a prognostic indicator in patients with stable coronary artery disease. *JAMA* 1997;277:318–324.

55. Eagle KA, Coley CM, Newell JB, et al. Combining clinical and thallium data optimizes preoperative assessment of cardiac risk before major vascular surgery. *Ann Intern Med* 1989;110:859–865.

56. Mangano DT, Browner WS, Hollenberg M, et al. Association of perioperative myocardial ischemia with cardiac morbidity and mortality in men undergoing noncardiac surgery. The Study of Perioperative Ischemia Research Group. *N Engl J Med* 1990;323:1781–1788.

57. Landesberg G, Mosseri M, Zahger D, et al. Myocardial infarction after vascular surgery: the role of prolonged stress-induced, ST depression-type ischemia. *J Am Coll Cardiol* 2001;37:1839–1845.

58. Ruberman W, Crow R, Rosenberg CR, et al. Intermittent ST depression and mortality after myocardial infarction. *Circulation* 1992;85:1440–1446.

59. Cohn PF, Vetrovec GW, Nesto R, et al. The Nifedipine–Total Ischemia Awareness Program: a national survey of painful and painless myocardial ischemia including results of antiischemic therapy. *Am J Cardiol* 1989;63:534–539.

60. Deedwania PC. Anti-ischemic effects of amlodipine in patients with stable angina pectoris and myocardial ischemia during daily life. Amlodipine Study Group *Am J Cardiol* 1999;83:1117–1119.

61. Davies RF, Habibi H, Klinke WP, et al. Effect of amlodipine, atenolol and their combination on myocardial ischaemia during treadmill exercise and ambulatory monitoring. Canadian Amlodipine/Atenolol in Silent Ischemia Study (CASIS) Investigators. *J Am Coll Cardiol* 1995;25:619–625.

62. Parker JD, Testa MA, Jimenez AH, et al. Morning increase in ambulatory ischemia in patients with stable coronary artery disease: importance of physical activity and increased cardiac demand. *Circulation* 1994;89:604–614.

63. Stone PH, Gibson RS, Glasser SP, et al. Comparison of propranolol, diltiazem, and nifedipine in the treatment of ambulatory ischemia in patients with stable angina: differential effects on ambulatory ischemia, exercise performance, and anginal symptoms. *Circulation* 1990;82:1962–1972.

64. Frishman WH, Glasser S, Stone P, et al. Comparison of controlled-onset, extended-release verapamil with amlodipine and amlodipine plus atenolol on exercise performance and ambulatory ischemia in patients with chronic stable angina pectoris. *Am J Cardiol* 1999;83:507–514.

65. Hill JA, Gonzalez JI, Kolb R, et al. Effects of atenolol alone, nifedipine alone and their combination on ambulant myocardial ischemia. *Am J Cardiol* 1991;67:671–675.

66. Deedwania PC, Carbajal EV, Nelson JR, et al. Anti-ischemic effects of atenolol versus nifedipine in patients with coronary artery disease and ambulatory silent ischemia. *J Am Coll Cardiol* 1991;17:963–969.

67. Willich SN, Pohjola-Sintonen S, Bhatia SJ, et al. Suppression of silent ischemia by metoprolol without alteration of platelet aggregability in patients with coronary artery disease. *Circulation* 1989;79:557–565.

68. Nyman I, Larsson H, Wallentin L. Prevention of serious cardiac events by low-dose aspirin in patients with silent myocardial ischemia. The Research Group on Instability in Coronary Artery Disease in Southeast Sweden. *Lancet* 1992;340:497–501.

69. Andrews TC, Raby K, Naimi BJ, et al. Effect of cholesterol reduction on myocardial ischemia in patients with coronary disease. *Circulation* 1997;95:324–328.

70. Lim R, Dyke L, Dymond DS. Effect on prognosis of abolition of exercise-induced painless myocardial ischemia by medical therapy. *Am J Cardiol* 1992;69:733–735.

71. Knatterud GL, Bourassa MG, Pepine CJ, et al. Effects of treatment strategies to suppress ischemia in patients with coronary artery disease: 12-week results of the Asymptomatic Cardiac Ischemia Pilot (ACIP) Study. *J Am Coll Cardiol* 1994;24:11–20.

72. Forslund L, Hjemdahl P, Held C, et al. Prognostic implications of ambulatory electrocardiography, exercise treadmill testing and electrocardiogram at rest to predict cardiac events by one year. The asymptomatic cardiac ischemia pilot (ACIP) Study. *Am J Cardiol* 1997;80:1395–1401.

73. Bourassa MG, Pepine CJ, Forman SA, et al. Asymptomatic cardiac ischemia pilot (ACIP) study: effects of coronary angioplasty and coronary artery bypass graft surgery on recurrent angina and ischemia. *J Am Coll Cardiol* 1995;26:606–614.

74. Davies RF, Goldberg D, Forman S, et al. Asymptomatic cardiac ischemia pilot (ACIP) study two-year follow-up. *Circulation* 1997;95:2037–2043.

75. Pepine CJ, Cohn PF, Deedwania PC, et al. Effects of treatment on outcome in mildly symptomatic patients with ischemia during daily life. The Atenolol Silent Ischemia Study (ASIST). *Circulation* 1994;90:762–768.

76. Dargie HJ, Ford I, Fox K. Effects of ischaemia and treatment with atenolol, nifedipine SR and their combination on outcome in patients with chronic stable angina. The TIBET Study Group. *Eur Heart J* 1996;17:104–112.

77. Forslund L, Hjemdahl P, Held C, et al. Prognostic implications of ambulatory myocardial ischemia and arrhythmias and relations to ischaemia on exercise in chronic stable angina pectoris (The Angina Prognosis Study in Stockholm [APSIS]). *AM J Cardiol* 1988;62:661–664.

78. Von Arnim T. Prognostic significance of transient ischaemic episodes: response to treatment shows improved prognosis. Results of the Total Ischaemic Burden Bisoprolol Study (TIBBs) follow-up. *J Am Coll Cardiol* 1996;28:20–24.

79. Mangano DT, Layug EL, Wallace A, et al. Effect of atenolol on mortality and cardiovascular morbidity after noncardiac surgery. *N Engl J Med* 1996;335:1713–1762.

80. Hammermeister KE, DeRouen TA, Dodge HT. Effect of coronary surgery on survival in asymptomatic and minimally symptomatic patients. *Circulation* 1980;62:98–105.

81. Wynne J, Cohn LH, Collins JJ Jr, et al. Myocardial revascularization in patients with multivessel coronary artery disease and minimal angina pectoris. *Circulation* 1978;58[Suppl]:I-92–I-95.

82. Weiner DA, Ryan TJ, McCabe CH, et al. Comparison of coronary artery bypass surgery and medical therapy in patients with exercise-induced silent myocardial ischemia. *J Am Coll Cardiol* 1988;12:595–599.

83. Weiner DA, Ryan TJ, McCabe CH, et al. The role of exercise-induced silent myocardial ischemia in patients with abnormal left ventricular function: a report from the Coronary Artery Surgery Study (CASS) Registry. *Am Heart J* 1989;118:649–655.

84. Taylor HA, Deumite J, Chaitman BR, et al. Asymptomatic left main coronary artery disease in the Coronary Artery Surgery Study (CASS) Registry. *Circulation* 1989;79:1171–1179.

85. Shawl FA, Chun PK, Mutter ML, et al. Asymptomatic left main coronary artery disease and silent myocardial ischemia. *Am Heart J* 1989;117:537–541.

CHAPTER 97

Chest Pain with Normal Coronary Angiograms

Richard O. Cannon III

Key Words: Angina pectoris; coronary microcirculation; endothelium; myocardial ischemia; pain; syndrome X.

INTRODUCTION

Patients with angina-like chest pain whose coronary angiograms show no evidence of obstructive coronary artery disease and who have no evidence of organic heart disease are a common and frustrating problem for physicians. Several published series, including the National Institutes of Health (NIH)–sponsored Coronary Artery Surgery Study and the Women's Ischemia Syndrome Evaluation, have indicated that from 10% to 30% of patients undergoing coronary angiography are found to have normal or near-normal epicardial coronary arteries (1–3). Many features of this patient population have been identified for more than four decades: a female predominance, onset of symptoms commonly between 40 and 50 years of age, chest pain generally "atypical" for ischemic heart disease, pain that is particularly severe and disabling, and inconsistent responses to conventional antiischemic therapy. Because many patients are found to have abnormal noninvasive test results (such as an ischemic-appearing electrocardiogram during exercise testing) that prompted the performance of cardiac catheterization, studies have sought to demonstrate an association with myocardial ischemia. Indeed, abnormalities in coronary flow and metabolic responses to stress have been demonstrated by several groups, findings consistent with a microvascular cause for ischemia and symptoms. However, other studies have questioned an ischemic cause for symptoms, even in patients se-

lected for abnormal noninvasive testing. For several groups, attention has focused on abnormal cardiac pain perception as being a fundamental abnormality in this patient population, with recent evidence that approaches useful in the management of chronic pain syndromes may also be of benefit to this population.

HISTORICAL BACKGROUND

Soon after the advent of coronary angiography, it became clear that not all patients with a clinical diagnosis of coronary artery disease had evidence of significant atherothrombotic obstruction of their epicardial coronary arteries. In 1967, Likoff and coworkers (4) reported 15 women ranging in age from 30 to 53 years with normal coronary angiograms but with electrocardiographic (ECG) abnormalities at rest (ST-segment depression or T-wave inversion) that were accentuated by exercise. Despite the ECG changes during exercise, the hemodynamic response, as assessed by pulmonary artery pressure, cardiac output, and oxygen consumption, were reported as normal in the eight patients in whom these measurements were made. The authors stated that "usual therapy of coronary artery disease was ineffective and unwarranted" in this setting.

That same year, Kemp and coworkers (5) reported studies performed in 50 patients (62% women) with angina-like chest pain and normal coronary angiograms, commenting that, as a group, "these patients may frequently have the most severe pain syndromes, often proving refractory to conventional forms of therapy." Of the 41 patients who underwent metabolic study during isoproterenol, 11 (27%) demonstrated myocardial lactate production supportive of myocardial ischemia. Four of these 11 patients had ischemic-appearing ECGs during exercise stress; however, five additional patients with ischemic-appearing ECGs dur-

R. O. Cannon III: Cardiovascular Branch, National Heart, Lung and Blood Institute, National Institutes of Health, Building 10, Room 7B-15, 10 Center Drive, MSC 1650, Bethesda, Maryland 20892-1650.

ing exercise stress did not demonstrate myocardial lactate production during isoproterenol infusion. In a 1973 editorial, Kemp (6) noted the heterogeneity of patients included in studies of patients with chest pain despite normal coronary angiogram results, thereby increasing the difficulty of drawing general conclusions about this syndrome. The term "syndrome X" was used in Kemp's editorial to denote the uncertainty of the cause of chest pain in these patients; this term subsequently has been used by other investigators, but often with different criteria for its definition.

Despite differences in opinion regarding cardiac versus noncardiac mechanisms of chest pain in this population, there has been virtually universal agreement that the long-term survival of patients with chest pain syndromes associated with normal coronary angiograms is probably no different than the general population (7–11). Although reassurance helps many patients, most continue to have episodic chest pain resulting in visits to the emergency room, admission to the coronary care unit, and even repeat cardiac catheterization (12–14). Thus, an apparently benign condition may have considerable adverse effects on the quality of life, employment, and use of health care resources, with their attendant expenses.

THE CASE FOR MYOCARDIAL ISCHEMIA

Over the last two decades, several groups have examined the possibility of abnormal coronary flow responsiveness as a mechanism for ischemia responsible for chest pain symptoms and ST-segment depression during exercise in patients designated as having syndrome X, reporting limited coronary flow responses to pacing stress or to microvascular dilators such as papaverine, dipyridamole, and adenosine (15). A coronary microvascular cause for symptoms has certain appeal because small arteries (especially arterioles) within the myocardium regulate the coronary blood flow response to stress so that the metabolic needs of the myocardium are closely matched by appropriate perfusion and oxygen delivery to permit augmented cardiac work. A growing list of abnormalities have been described in series of patients with syndrome X to account for coronary microvascular dysfunction, including altered autonomic tone (16,17), insulin resistance (18–20), enhanced ion transport across cell membranes (21), increased endothelin-1 release (22, 23), estrogen deficiency (24), and endothelial dysfunction (25–27). Maseri and coworkers (28) have proposed that patchy or diffuse microvascular constriction (or absence of appropriate vasodilation) may produce myocardial ischemia during stress that does not affect myocardial contractility because of compensatory vasodilation of adjacent arterioles. Maseri's group (29) measured lipid hydroperoxides and conjugated dienes—molecules generated on reoxygenation of ischemic tissue—as metabolic markers of ischemia in arterial and great cardiac vein blood. Samples were drawn before and after rapid atrial pacing in nine patients with chest pain and normal coronary angiograms, seven of whom had ischemic-appearing ST-segment depression during exercise stress and five of whom had reversible perfusion defects on exercise thallium scintigraphy. These measurements were compared with those of five patients with mitral valve disease who underwent this study and served as control subjects. Curiously, levels of these molecules were greater in great cardiac vein blood than arterial blood before pacing in patients, whereas the reverse was true in control subjects. In patients, but not control subjects, great cardiac venous levels of these molecules increased after pacing (160 beats/min or heart rate at development of ST-segment depression for 3 minutes), which induced ST-segment depression and chest pain in all but one patient.

Buchthal and coworkers (30) from the Women's Ischemia Syndrome Evaluation group reported that 7 of 35 women with chest pain and normal coronary angiograms who underwent nuclear magnetic resonance spectroscopy had findings compatible with myocardial ischemia during hand-grip exercise. This conclusion was based on reduction in spectral signals from the phosphate of creatine phosphate relative to the phosphate of adenosine triphosphate that was similar to the decline in the ratio of these high-energy phosphate spectra recorded in patients with coronary artery disease. Results of treadmill exercise testing to identify who in this group had syndrome X were not reported. However, the frequency of exercise-induced thallium perfusion defects and abnormal brachial artery endothelial testing (flow-mediated dilation) was similar for the 7 women with reduction in the ratio of high-energy phosphate spectra and the 28 women with smaller reduction (or actual increases) in these spectra.

Panting and coworkers (31) performed myocardial perfusion magnetic resonance imaging in 20 patients (16 women and 4 men) with syndrome X and in 10 age- and sex-matched control subjects. Fourteen of the patients had undergone single-photon emission computed tomography thallium imaging studies. None showed reversible perfusion abnormalities after stress to suggest inducible myocardial ischemia. Using gadopentetate dimeglumine as the contrast agent, magnetic resonance images were obtained at baseline and during adenosine infusion to dilate the coronary microcirculation and maximally increase coronary blood flow. In control subjects, adenosine increased perfusion in the endocardium and the epicardium by analysis of short-axis slices of the left ventricle. In contrast, patients with syndrome X showed less increase in endocardial perfusion, but preserved increase in epicardial perfusion in response to adenosine was shown. During the adenosine infusion, 19 of 20 patients with syndrome X experienced chest pain, often intense in severity, whereas 4 of 10 control subjects experienced chest pain, generally mild in severity. The investigators concluded that coronary microvascular dysfunction in syndrome X may limit appropriate increases in endocardial blood flow. Why ischemic chest pain should have occurred when endocardial perfusion was not actually reduced by adenosine in this study was not explained.

THE CASE AGAINST MYOCARDIAL ISCHEMIA

Although many of the studies cited earlier in this chapter support the paradigm that abnormal coronary microvascular dilator responsiveness to stress may precipitate myocardial ischemia, other studies beginning with the report from the Montreal Heart Institute (32) that prompted Kemp's 1973 editorial (6) have questioned the existence of myocardial ischemia in patients with chest pain despite normal coronary angiogram results, including the subset with syndrome X on the basis of their ischemic-appearing exercise test. Thus, Camici and coworkers (33) found no metabolic evidence of myocardial ischemia by analysis of coronary sinus metabolites of carbohydrates and fatty acids in 12 women with syndrome X during rapid atrial pacing. Nihoyannopoulos and coworkers (34) reported normal left ventricular systolic function by echocardiography immediately after exercise and during rapid atrial pacing in 18 patients with syndrome X, despite experiencing chest pain with ischemic-appearing ST-segment depression during these stresses. Rosano and coworkers (35) performed pH monitoring of coronary sinus blood before and during rapid atrial pacing in 14 patients with chest pain and normal coronary angiograms, 11 of whom had ischemic-appearing ST-segment depression during exercise and 6 of whom had reversible perfusion defects on exercise thallium scintigraphy. During pacing, despite chest pain provoked in 11 of the 14 patients, only 3 showed declines in coronary sinus pH that approached the magnitude of reduction in pH measured in patients with coronary artery disease subjected to pacing stress.

We evaluated 70 consecutive patients with angina-like chest pain and normal coronary angiograms, 22 of whom had syndrome X by virtue of ischemic-appearing ST-segment depression during exercise (36). Thirteen patients had reversible perfusion defects during exercise by thallium scintigraphy, abnormalities consistent with myocardial ischemia. However, the findings of thallium scintigraphy did not correlate with the presence of ST-segment depression during exercise testing. The results of exercise testing and dobutamine stress echocardiography from these 70 patients were compared with those of 26 healthy volunteers. We used the transesophageal route for imaging to maximize the number of ventricular segments visualized and the quality of images for assessment of contractility. Dobutamine infused in stepwise increments to 40 μg per kilogram per minute induced chest pain in 59 patients, but in none of the control subjects. Ischemic-appearing ST-segment depression developed in 22 patients (19 with syndrome X) and in 2 control subjects. Wall motion abnormalities occurred in none of the patients or the control subjects. Importantly, no differences were observed in transmural contractile response to dobutamine between patients and control subjects. Indeed, of the 70 patients with chest pain despite normal coronary angiogram results, the quantitative myocardial contractile response to dobutamine was virtually identical in the 22 patients with syndrome X and the 48 patients without ischemic-appearing ST-segment depression during infusion. Thus, despite the frequent provocation of characteristic chest pain and, in the syndrome X subset, ischemic-appearing ST-segment depression, patients with chest pain and normal coronary angiograms do not demonstrate concomitant regional wall motion abnormalities and, in fact, show a quantitatively normal myocardial contractile response to dobutamine.

Thus, the debate continues. However, the studies cited above suggest that conventional noninvasive testing (e.g., stress ECG, echocardiographic, or nuclear perfusion testing) may not reliably identify the subset of patients who have stress-induced myocardial ischemia as a cause of chest pain symptoms, and that specialized testing (endothelial function, nuclear magnetic resonance spectroscopy, magnetic resonance imaging) may be required. However, for such specialized—and not widely available—testing to be clinically useful, investigators must show that patients identified as having abnormalities by their test of choice respond to specific therapies or have a different natural history to their disorder than patients who do not have abnormalities.

ABNORMAL CARDIAC PAIN PERCEPTION: THE SENSITIVE HEART

The observation that patients with chest pain and normal coronary angiograms, regardless of whether they are defined as having syndrome X on the basis of their exercise electrocardiogram results, commonly experience their characteristic chest pain during the performance of diagnostic cardiac catheterization has led several groups to consider abnormal cardiac pain perception as a fundamental abnormality in this patient population (37–41). We found that in 36 patients with chest pain and normal coronary angiogram results, characteristic chest pain could be provoked in 86% by electrical stimulation (right ventricular pacing) at a heart rate 5 beats faster than their resting heart rate, with the pain worsened by increasing the stimulus intensity (38). In more than half of these same patients, pain also could be provoked by simply injecting contrast media into the left coronary artery. In contrast, pain responses to right ventricular pacing or contrast media injection were seen in only 2 of 42 patients with coronary artery disease and in none of the 10 patients with valvular heart disease asymptomatic for chest pain. Other potent stimuli for pain provocation in patients with syndrome X are dipyridamole and adenosine infusion (39,40).

It is unknown whether heightened intracardiac pain sensitivity demonstrated in patients with chest pain and normal coronary angiograms represents one extreme of the normal "bell curve" distribution of visceral sensory function or is indicative of a true abnormality in visceral sensory function. These patients may represent the opposite end of the cardiac pain spectrum from the subgroup of patients with coronary artery disease who have "silent ischemia." Similar observations of exaggerated visceral pain sensitivity had been made within the esophagus of patients with chest pain and normal or near-normal coronary angiogram results and may explain why increased esophageal pressures and acid reflux, generally unrecognized by healthy subjects, cause chest pain in some patients (42). In addition, exaggerated visceral pain sensitivity has been demonstrated within the rectum, sigmoid colon, and small intestines of patients with irritable bowel syndrome (43). Thus, patients with "sensitive hearts" may represent one manifestation of chronic pain associated with heightened visceral pain sensitivity. In addition, the mechanism of exaggerated visceral pain sensitivity may be neurophysiologically linked to whatever is responsible for anxiety and panic disorders commonly noted with patients with chest pain and normal coronary angiogram results (44,45).

Rosen and coworkers (46) have considered the possibility that central neural processing of sensory input from viscera might be important in understanding symptoms in this patient population. They measured regional cerebral blood flow (positron emission tomography) as an index of neuronal activity at rest and during dobutamine stress in eight patients with syndrome X (six women) and eight control subjects (five women). Dobutamine precipitated severe chest pain and ST-segment depression in all patients with syndrome X, although echocardiography showed increased left ventricular contractility. Patients with syndrome X and control subjects showed similar increases in blood flow in the hypothalamus, thalami, right orbitofrontal cortex, and anterior temporal lobes. In patients, but not control subjects, increased blood flow also was noted in the right anterior insula/frontal operculum junction. In a previous study of identical design but with patients with coronary artery disease, dobutamine infusion provoked chest pain and echocardiographic evidence of myocardial ischemia; no increased blood flow in the right insula was noted in these patients with ischemia-provoked chest pain (47). Thus, patients with syndrome X have an altered pattern of cortical activation by visceral afferent signals, which may contribute to abnormal pain perception during cardiac stress even in the absence of ischemia.

TREATMENT TRIALS

Perhaps the most frustrating aspect of the syndrome of chest pain despite normal coronary angiogram results, including the syndrome X subset, is the management of chest pain symptoms, as was recognized in the earliest reports in the literature. Numerous therapies have been reported to be successful in clinical trials generally including small numbers of patients, including nitrates (48,49), β-blockers (49,50), calcium channel blockers (49,50), angiotensin-converting enzyme inhibitors (51), tricyclic antidepressants (52), aminophylline (53), estrogen replacement therapy (54), and L-arginine (55). However, the clinical experience often has been that pain relief with medical therapy is not sustained over time, and patients are commonly prescribed a large number of drugs, with associated side effects. Of interest, nonpharmacologic approaches may be of symptom benefit in this patient population. In this regard, Eriksson and cowork-

ers (56) randomized 26 women with syndrome X to 2 exercise training groups (cycle ergometry for 30 minutes at 50% peak workload 3 times a week for 8 weeks) or to no exercise training. In the exercise groups, peak capacity improved by 34% and onset of chest pain was delayed by 100% from pretraining values. Cunningham and coworkers (57) reported that 3-month training in transcendental meditation reduced chest pain frequency and severity and improved quality of life assessed by questionnaires in nine postmenopausal women with syndrome X. Of interest, this treatment also improved the time to ST-segment depression and maximum ST-segment depression during treadmill exercise testing compared with baseline values. Cognitive behavioral therapy with clinical psychologists has been reported to be of value in reducing symptoms and improving quality of life (58). For those patients resistant to these pharmacologic and nonpharmacologic approaches described earlier, transcutaneous electrical nerve stimulation or spinal cord stimulation may be of symptom benefit (59–62).

APPROACH TO PATIENT MANAGEMENT

The management recommendations that follow are predicated on determination of normal cardiac pressures and angiograms during cardiac catheterization, a normal echocardiogram showing absence of myocardial or valvular disease, no evidence of coronary artery spasm (absence of characteristic ST-segment changes during spontaneous episodes of chest pain or negative ergonovine challenge), and no gastroesophageal source of symptoms. Given this constellation of findings, the patient should be reassured that he or she has a chest pain syndrome that poses no increased cardiovascular morbidity or mortality risk over that of the general population. Patients with luminal irregularities on coronary angiography or "nonsignificant" coronary artery disease should undergo aggressive risk factor management and begin daily aspirin therapy.

All patients should be started on a regular exercise program to improve their stamina (many are severely deconditioned) and to encourage a positive attitude regarding their state of health. Efforts should be made to discontinue all unnecessary medications. In some, this approach will sufficiently alleviate symptoms, and thus no further evaluation is necessary. Should symptoms persist, empiric trials of antiischemic therapy, angiotensin-converting enzyme inhibitors, L-arginine, estrogen replacement therapy, or tricyclic antidepressants (coupled with a β-blocker to block anticholinergic effects of this therapy) may be required.

Currently, there is no widely available or accepted test to determine whether the patient has an ischemic cause for symptoms. However, greater experience with stress nuclear magnetic resonance spectroscopy or cardiovascular magnetic resonance imaging at specialized centers, with confirmation of findings reported thus far in small numbers of patients, may resolve this dilemma in the future. Should exercise and therapeutic trials fail to control chest pain symptoms, referral to a pain clinic may be necessary for a multidisciplinary approach to pain management.

REFERENCES

1. Proudfit WL, Shirey EK, Sones FM. Selective cine coronary arteriography. Correlation with clinical findings in 1,000 patients. *Circulation* 1966;33:901–910.
2. Kemp HG, Kronmal RA, Vliestra RE, et al. Seven year survival of patients with normal or near normal coronary arteriograms: a CASS registry study. *J Am Coll Cardiol* 1986;7:479–483.
3. Sharaf BL, Pepine CJ, Kerensky RA, et al. Detailed angiographic analysis of women with suspected ischemic chest pain (pilot phase data from the NHLBI-sponsored Women's Ischemia Syndrome Evaluation [WISE] Study Angiographic Core Laboratory). *Am J Cardiol* 2001;87:937–941.
4. Likoff W, Segal BL, Kasparian H. Paradox of normal selective coronary arteriograms in patients considered to have unmistakable coronary heart disease. *N Engl J Med* 1967;276:1063–1066.
5. Kemp HG, Elliott WC, Gorlin R. The anginal syndrome with normal coronary arteriography. *Trans Assoc Am Physicians* 1967;80:59–70.
6. Kemp HG. Left ventricular function in patients with the anginal syndrome and normal coronary arteriograms. *Am J Cardiol* 1973;32:375–376.
7. Kemp HG Jr, Vokonas PS, Cohn PF, et al. The anginal syndrome associated with normal coronary angiograms. Report of a six year experience. *Am J Med* 1973;54:735–742.
8. Pasternak RC, Thibault GE, DeSanctis RW, et al. Chest pain with angiographically insignificant coronary arterial obstruction: clinical presentation and long-term follow-up. *Am J Med* 1980;68:813–817.
9. Dart AM, Davies HA, Dalal J, et al. "Angina" and normal coronary arteriograms: a follow-up study. *Eur Heart J* 1980;1:97–100.
10. Wielgosz AT, Fletcher RH, McCants CB, et al. Unimproved chest pain in patients with minimal or no coronary disease: a behavioral phenomenon. *Am Heart J* 1984;108:67–72.
11. Papaniculaou MN, Califf RM, Hlatky MA, et al. Prognostic implications of angiographically normal and insignificantly narrowed coronary arteries. *Am J Cardiol* 1986;58:1181–1187.
12. Day LJ, Sowton E. Clinical features and follow-up of patients with angina and normal coronary arteries. *Lancet* 1976;2:334–337.
13. Ockene IS, Shay MJ, Alpert JS, et al. Unexplained chest pain in patients with normal coronary arteriograms: a follow-up study of functional status. *N Engl J Med* 1980;303:1249–1252.
14. Isner JM, Salem DN, Banas JS, et al. Long-term clinical course of patients with normal coronary arteriography: follow-up study of 121 patients with normal or nearly normal coronary arteriograms. *Am Heart J* 1981;102:645–653.
15. Cannon RO, Camici PG, Epstein SE. Pathophysiological dilemma of syndrome X. *Circulation* 1992;85:883–892.
16. Rosano GM, Ponikowski P, Adamopoulos S, et al. Abnormal autonomic control of the cardiovascular system in syndrome X. *Am J Cardiol* 1994;73:1174–1179.
17. Frobert O, Molgaard H, Botker HE, et al. Autonomic balance in patients with angina and a normal coronary angiogram. *Eur Heart J* 1995;16:1356–1360.
18. Chauhan A, Foote J, Petch MC, et al. Hyperinsulinemia, coronary artery disease and syndrome X. *J Am Coll Cardiol* 1994;23:364–368.
19. Swan JW, Walton C, Godsland IF, et al. Insulin resistance syndrome as a feature of cardiological syndrome X in non-obese men. *Br Heart J* 1994;71:41–44.
20. Botker HE, Moller N, Schmitz O, et al. Myocardial insulin resistance in patients with syndrome X. *J Clin Invest* 1997;100:1919–1927.
21. Gaspardone A, Ferri C, Crea F, et al. Enhanced activity of sodium-lithium countertransport in patients with cardiac syndrome X. A potential link between cardiac and metabolic syndrome X. *J Am Coll Cardiol* 1998;32:2031–2034.
22. Kaski JC, Elliott PM, Salomone O, et al. Concentration of circulating plasma endothelin in patients with angina and normal coronary angiograms. *Br Heart J* 1995;74:620–624.
23. Lanza GA, Luscher TF, Pasceri V, et al. Effects of atrial pacing on arterial and coronary sinus endothelin-1 levels in syndrome X. *Am J Cardiol* 1999;84:1187–1191.
24. Rosano GM, Collins P, Kaski JC, et al. Syndrome X in women is associated with oestrogen deficiency. *Eur Heart J* 1995;16:610–614.
25. Egashira K, Inou T, Hirooka Y, et al. Evidence of impaired endothelium-dependent coronary vasodilation in patients with angina pectoris and normal coronary angiograms. *N Engl J Med* 1993;328:1659–1664.
26. Zeiher AM, Krause T, Schachinger V, et al. Impaired endothelium-dependent vasodilation of coronary resistance vessels is associated with exercise-induced myocardial ischemia. *Circulation* 1995;91:2345–2352.
27. Hasdai D, Gibbons RJ, Holmes DR Jr, et al. Coronary endothelial dysfunction in humans is associated with myocardial perfusion defects. *Circulation* 1997;96:3390–3395.
28. Maseri A, Crea F, Kaski JC, et al. Mechanisms of angina pectoris in syndrome X. *J Am Coll Cardiol* 1991;17:499–506.
29. Buffon A, Rigattieri S, Santini SA, et al. Myocardial ischemia-reperfusion damage after pacing-induced tachycardia in patients with cardiac syndrome X. *Am J Physiol Heart Circ Physiol* 2000;279:H2627–H2633.
30. Buchthal SD, den Hollander JA, Merz CN, et al. Abnormal myocardial phosphorous 31 nuclear magnetic resonance spectroscopy in women with chest pain but normal coronary angiograms. *N Engl J Med* 2000;342:829–835.
31. Panting JR, Gatehouse PD, Yang GZ, et al. Abnormal subendocardial perfusion in cardiac syndrome X detected by cardiovascular magnetic resonance imaging. *N Engl J Med* 2002;346:1948–1953.
32. Arbogast R, Bourassa MG. Myocardial function during atrial pacing in patients with angina pectoris and normal coronary arteriograms: comparison with patients having significant coronary artery disease. *Am J Cardiol* 1973;32:257–263.
33. Camici PG, Marraccini P, Lorenzoni R, et al. Coronary hemodynamics and myocardial metabolism in patients with syndrome X: response to pacing stress. *J Am Coll Cardiol* 1991;17:1461–1470.
34. Nihoyannopoulos P, Kaski JC, Crake T, et al. Absence of myocardial dysfunction during stress in patients with syndrome X. *J Am Coll Cardiol* 1991;18:1463–1470.
35. Rosano GM, Kaski JC, Arie S, et al. Failure to demonstrate myocardial ischaemia in patients with angina and normal coronary arteries. Evaluation by continuous coronary sinus pH monitoring. *Eur Heart J* 1997;17:1175–1180.
36. Panza JA, Laurienzo JM, Curiel RV, et al. Investigation of the mechanism of chest pain in patients with angiographically normal coronary arteries using transesophageal dobutamine stress echocardiography. *J Am Coll Cardiol* 1997;29:293–301.
37. Shapiro LM, Crake T, Poole-Wilson PA. Is altered cardiac sensation responsible for chest pain in patients with normal coronary arteries? Clinical observation during cardiac catheterization. *BMJ* 1988;296:170–171.
38. Cannon RO 3rd, Quyyumi AA, Schenke WH, et al. Abnormal cardiac pain sensitivity in patients with chest pain and normal coronary arteries. *J Am Coll Cardiol* 1990;16:1359–1366.
39. Lagerqvist B, Sylven C, Waldenstrom A. Lower threshold for adenosine-induced chest pain in patients with angina and normal coronary angiograms. *Br Heart J* 1992;68:282–285.
40. Rosen SD, Uren NG, Kaski JC, et al. Coronary vasodilator reserve, pain perception, and sex in patients with syndrome X. *Circulation* 1994;90:50–60.
41. Pasceri V, Lanza GA, Buffon A, et al. Role of abnormal pain sensitivity and behavioral factors in determining chest pain in syndrome X. *J Am Coll Cardiol* 1998;31:62–66.
42. Richter JE, Barish CF, Castell DO. Abnormal sensory perception in patients with esophageal chest pain. *Gastroenterology* 1986;91:845–852.
43. Lynn RB, Friedman LS. Irritable bowel syndrome. *N Engl J Med* 1993;329:1940–1945.
44. Bass C, Wade C, Hand D, et al. Patients with angina with normal and near normal coronary arteries: clinical and psychosocial state 12 months after angiography. *Br Med J* 1983;287:1505–1508.
45. Beitman BD, Mukerji V, Lamberti JW, et al. Panic disorder in patients with chest pain and angiographically normal coronary arteries. *Am J Cardiol* 1989;63:1399–1403.
46. Rosen SD, Paulesu E, Wise RJ, et al. Central neural contribution to the perception of chest pain in cardiac syndrome X. *Heart* 2002;87:513–519.
47. Rosen SD, Paulesu E, Frith CD, et al. Central neural correlates of angina pectoris as a model of visceral pain. *Lancet* 1994;344:147–150.

48. Lanza GA, Manzoli A, Bia E, et al. Acute effects of nitrates on exercise testing in patients with syndrome X: clinical and pathophysiological implications. *Circulation* 1994;90:2695–2700.

49. Lanza GA, Colonna G, Pasceri V, et al. Atenolol versus amlodipine versus isosorbide-5-mononitrate on anginal symptoms in syndrome X. *Am J Cardiol* 1999;84:854–856.

50. Bugiardini R, Borghi A, Biagetti L, et al. Comparison of verapamil versus propanolol therapy in syndrome X. *Am J Cardiol* 1989;63:286–290.

51. Kaski JC, Rosano GM, Gavrielides S, et al. Effects of angiotensin-converting enzyme inhibition on exercise-induced angina and ST segment depression in patients with microvascular angina. *J Am Coll Cardiol* 1994;23:652–657.

52. Cannon RO 3rd, Quyyumi AA, Mincemoyer R, et al. Imipramine in patients with chest pain despite normal coronary angiograms. *N Engl J Med* 1994;330:1411–1417.

53. Elliott PM, Krzyzowska-Dickinson K, Calvino R, et al. Effect of oral aminophylline in patients with angina and normal coronary arteriograms (cardiac syndrome X). *Heart* 1997;77:523–526.

54. Rosano GM, Peters NS, Lefroy D, et al. 17-beta-Estradiol therapy lessens angina in postmenopausal women with syndrome X. *J Am Coll Cardiol* 1996;27:1500–1505.

55. Lerman A, Burnett JC Jr, Higano ST, et al. Long-term L-arginine supplementation improves small-vessel coronary endothelial function in humans. *Circulation* 1998;97:2123–2128.

56. Eriksson BE, Tyni-Lenne R, Svedenhag J, et al. Physical training in syndrome X: physical training counteracts deconditioning and pain in syndrome X. *J Am Coll Cardiol* 2000;36:1619–1625.

57. Cunningham C, Brown S, Kaski JC. Effects of transcendental meditation on symptoms and electrocardiographic changes in patients with cardiac syndrome X. *Am J Cardiol* 2000;85:653–655.

58. Mayou RA, Bryant BM, Sanders C, et al. A controlled trial of cognitive behavioural therapy for non-cardiac chest pain. *Psychol Med* 1997;27: 1021–1031.

59. Sanderson JE, Woo KS, Chung HK, et al. The effect of transcutaneous electrical nerve stimulation on coronary and systemic hemodynamics in syndrome X. *Coron Artery Dis* 1996;7:547–552.

60. Anderson C, Hole P, Oxhoj H. Spinal cord stimulation as a pain treatment for angina pectoris. *Pain Clin* 1995;8:333–339.

61. Eliasson T, Albertsson P, Hardhammar P, et al. Spinal cord stimulation in angina pectoris with normal coronary arteriograms. *Coron Artery Dis* 1993;4:819–827.

62. Lanza GA, Sestito A, Sandric S, et al. Spinal cord stimulation in patients with refractory anginal pain and normal coronary arteries. *Ital Heart J* 2001;2:25–30.

PART VI

Noncoronary Atherothrombosis

CHAPTER 98

Epidemiologic Relation of Cardiovascular Disease among Different Vascular Territories

William B. Kannel

Introduction
Cardiovascular Events after Peripheral Arterial Disease
Atherothrombotic Events after Coronary Disease
Atherothrombotic Events after Cardiac Failure
Atherothrombotic Events after Stroke

Impact of Risk Factors
Implications
Acknowledgments
References

Key Words: Vascular disease in different territories.

INTRODUCTION

Atherothrombotic cardiovascular disease is a diffuse condition involving the arterial circulation to the heart, brain, and periphery. The underlying atherothrombotic disease is common to clinical events in all these areas, and most of the risk factors that apply to one arterial bed also apply to the others (1). It is to be expected that having one atherothrombotic cardiovascular event increases the risk for development of the others. This is mainly because of shared predisposing risk factors, but also because one cardiovascular disease may directly predispose to another. For example, cardiac failure and coronary disease may predispose to a stroke by producing a source for emboli or compromising the circulation to the brain.

The Framingham Study, which has been following a cohort of 5,209 individuals for more than three decades for development of initial and recurrent cardiovascular events, provides data on the concordance of disease in the different arterial vascular beds (1). It also provides data on the impact of cardiovascular risk factors on development of atherothrombotic cardiovascular events in the different vascular territories.

W. B. Kannel: Boston University School of Medicine and National Heart, Lung and Blood Institute's Framingham Heart Study, National Institutes of Health, 73 Mt. Wayte Avenue, Framingham, Massachusetts 01702-5827.

CARDIOVASCULAR EVENTS AFTER PERIPHERAL ARTERIAL DISEASE

More than half of individuals with intermittent claudication already have coexistent overt atherothrombotic cardiovascular disease when initially diagnosed (2). This suggests that it may also be a marker for predisposition to other cardiovascular disease. This proved to be the case when risk for other atherothrombotic events over decades of follow-up in individuals with intermittent claudication as their first manifestation of atherothrombotic cardiovascular disease was determined in the Framingham Study cohort (2). This indicated a twofold to fourfold excess risk for development of overt coronary disease, stroke/transient ischemic attack (TIA), or cardiac failure compared with individuals of the same age without the complaint. Over a 10-year period, the incidence rate of coronary heart disease (CHD) in those with the condition was 40% in women and 47% in men, respectively, a twofold to threefold greater risk than that of the general population of comparable age (Table 98–1). The absolute risk was comparable between the two sexes, but the relative risk was greater in women.

Stroke risk also was increased twofold to threefold with a greater relative risk in men. The absolute risk was similar at about 20% over 10 years in each sex for all ages combined (Table 98–1), but in patients younger than 65 years, the risk for stroke associated with claudication in men (19%) was twice that in women (8%). Heart failure occurred in 22% to 27% of patients with intermittent claudication, primarily because of hypertension or coronary disease (Table 98–1), a 3.5-fold to 4.5-fold increased risk, with a substantially

TABLE 98–1. *Risk for specified atherothrombotic cardiovascular events after occurrence of coronary, stroke, peripheral artery, and heart failure: Framingham Study subjects aged 35 to 94 years old*

	Age-adjusted 10-year percent probability					
	Coronary disease		Stroke or TIA		Heart failure	
Initial event	Men	Women	Men	Women	Men	Women
Peripheral artery disease	46%	40%	22%	20%	22%	27%
Myocardial infarction	—	—	16%	24%	27%	31%
Heart failure	50%	42%	42%	34%	—	—
Stroke	44%	25%	—	—	16%	15%

TIA, transient ischemia attack.

greater relative risk for patients who had claudication who were younger than versus older than age 65 years. Risk ratios were greater in women than men.

Vascular bruits often signify diseased vessels; hence, it is not surprising that femoral bruits are associated with a high prevalence (20–30%) of intermittent claudication (Table 98–2). It is interesting, however, that these femoral bruits also are associated with a significantly increased prevalence of atherothrombotic cardiovascular problems in other vascular territories such as the coronary arteries (2). Femoral vascular bruits also are associated with cardiac failure. Thus, peripheral arterial disease is clearly part of a problem of widespread atherothrombotic disease (2). Because the peripheral vessels are more accessible to noninvasive assessment of obstructed flow than the coronary arteries, there is merit in early detection of presymptomatic peripheral arterial disease so that timely preventive measures to protect against more lethal clinical manifestations of accelerated atherogenesis can be vigorously instituted.

ATHEROTHROMBOTIC EVENTS AFTER CORONARY DISEASE

Patients with initial myocardial infarctions (MIs) often have preexisting cardiovascular conditions such as strokes, heart failure, and intermittent claudication, suggesting the likelihood of further occurrence of concordant cardiovascular events (Table 98–3). After an initial MI, other atherothrombotic events, such as stroke and cardiac failure, occur at a threefold to sixfold excess rate, with risk ratios greater in women than men at all ages. The 10-year rate of stroke after MI is 16% in men and 24% in women for all ages combined

(Table 98–1). Cardiac failure rates were greater at all ages than stroke rates, presumably because of a more direct adverse effect of the MI on cardiac function. About 30% of MI victims experienced development of heart failure over 10 years, a rate four to six times that of the general population of the same age (Table 98–1). Coronary disease increases stroke risk in the absence of hypertension and cardiac failure, suggesting a direct relation (3).

ATHEROTHROMBOTIC EVENTS AFTER CARDIAC FAILURE

After cardiac failure, new coronary events and strokes occur at two to five times the general population rates (Table 98–1). Risk ratios are greater in women than men except for strokes in the elderly. Coronary events occur within 10 years after onset of failure in 42% to 50% of patients, presumably because of shared risk factors or the presence of occult coronary disease underlying the failure (Table 98–1). Strokes also are distressingly common after onset of heart failure, occurring within 10 years in 42% of men and 34% of women (Table 98–1).

ATHEROTHROMBOTIC EVENTS AFTER STROKE

Atherothrombotic brain infarctions are associated with about a twofold excess risk for cardiac failure and coronary disease, presumably on the basis of diffuse atherothrombosis. Cardiac failure occurs in about 15% of stroke patients over 10 years with rates in men and women virtually identical at all ages (Table 98–1). Coronary events occur in 44% of men and 25% of women presumably because of shared

TABLE 98–2. *Prevalence of heart failure, coronary disease, and intermittent claudication by femoral bruit status: Framingham Study age-adjusted prevalence per 1,000 subjects*

	Cardiac failure		Coronary disease		Intermittent claudication	
	Absent	Present	Absent	Present	Absent	Present
Men	22	39[a]	165	291[b]	44	300[b]
Women	24	67[b]	104	140[a]	26	199[b]

[a]$p < 0.05$; [b]$p < 0.001$.
From Kannel WB, McGee DL. Update on some epidemiologic features of intermittent claudication. *J Am Geriatric Soc* 1985;33:13–18, with permission.

TABLE 98–3. *Preexisting conditions in patients with initial myocardial infarction: 34-year follow-up Framingham Study*

Prior condition	Men n	Men %	Women n	Women %
Total MI	532	—	296	—
Angina	111	20.9	73	24.7
Intermittent claudication	50	9.4	35	10.5
Stroke/TIA	28	5.3	24	8.1
Heart failure	18	3.4	29	9.8
None	365	68.6	179	60.5

MI, myocardial infarction; TIA, transient ischemic attack.
Cupples LA, Gagnon DR, Wong ND, et al. Preexisting cardiovascular conditions and long-term prognosis after initial myocardial infarction: the Framingham Study. *Am Heart J* 1993,125:863–872.

predisposing hypertension and diabetes. Carotid bruits indicate vascular disease in the cerebral circulation and, as expected, are associated with a twofold to threefold increase in the risk for stroke. However, these bruits also signify widespread atherothrombotic disease as indicated by their association with twofold or threefold increased risk for coronary disease, heart failure, and peripheral artery disease (Table 98–4).

IMPACT OF RISK FACTORS

The major cardiovascular risk factors influence clinical events in all vascular territories in one age and sex subgroup or another, but with some noteworthy differences in their impact (Table 98–5). Hypertension is a prominent risk factor for all the atherothrombotic cardiovascular outcomes, with a greater impact of the systolic and pulse pressures than diastolic blood pressure (4). Risk ratios are greatest for stroke and cardiac failure, but the absolute risk is greatest for CHD. The risk imposed by hypertension persists into old age with a lower risk ratio for all atherothrombotic cardiovascular outcomes (Table 98–5), which is, however, offset by a greater absolute risk in the elderly.

TABLE 98–4. *Risk for cardiovascular events in subjects with carotid bruits: Framingham Study*

CV event	Biennial age-adjusted rate per 1,000 subjects with carotid bruit Men Absent	Men Present	Women Absent	Women Present
Stroke	13.6	25.1	10.3	29.8[c]
CHD	39.9	49.6	23.7	45.4[b]
CHF	13.3	30.5[a]	9.9	24.7[c]
I.C.	10.7	20.3[a]	6.1	17.7[a]

Persons free of specified conditions placed at risk.
CHD, coronary heart disease; CHF, congestive heart failure; CV, cardiovascular; I.C., intermittent claudication.
[a]p < 0.05; [b]p < 0.01; [c]p < 0.001.

Increased serum total cholesterol level appears to have little impact on stroke and heart failure (Table 98–5). However, the total/high-density lipoprotein cholesterol level ratio, which is the best lipid profile for prediction of atherothrombotic cardiovascular events, predicts coronary disease and peripheral artery disease at all ages in both men and women (5). Although total and low-density lipoprotein (LDL) cholesterol levels appear unrelated to occurrence of brain infarction, blood lipids have been found to be related to carotid disease (6). Also, statin treatment of dyslipidemia has been shown to prevent strokes (7).

Diabetes and glucose intolerance increase risk for all atherothrombotic cardiovascular events at all ages in both sexes (Table 98–5). The risk ratios diminish with age, but this is offset by a greater absolute risk in advanced age. The impact of diabetes is greater in women than men and tends to eliminate their cardiovascular disease advantage over men.

Cigarette smoking is a reversible risk factor for cardiovascular events with a greater absolute and relative impact in men than women younger than 65 years (Table 98–5). In women older than 65 years, smoking has a significant impact on the rate of development of brain infarction and stroke. For both sexes, its strongest impact, in terms of relative risk, is for peripheral artery disease.

Obesity is an important correctable predisposing condition for coronary disease, heart failure, and brain infarction. Visceral adiposity in particular is a hazard because of its propensity to induce insulin resistance and an accumulation of atherogenic risk factors including dyslipidemia, hypertension, and diabetes (8).

IMPLICATIONS

The foregoing epidemiologic data indicate that development of a clinical atherothrombotic event in one arterial vascular territory is usually a hallmark of diffuse atherothrombosis and a heightened risk for clinical atherothrombotic events in other areas. The impact of the major cardiovascular risk factors on all arterial vascular territories probably explains why persons who experience development of one clinical manifestation of atherothrombosis have increased vulnerability to another. This suggests a common cause or pathogenesis underlying the disease, but other influences also are operative.

The presence of cardiovascular risk factors common to all of the atherothrombotic cardiovascular disease outcomes suggests a pathogenesis universal to atherothrombosis in all vascular territories. However, some nontrivial differences exist. Serum cholesterol and its LDL cholesterol fraction are unrelated to the rate of development of atherothrombotic brain infarction. Diabetes has a much greater pathogenetic impact on peripheral arterial disease and cardiac failure than on coronary disease or stroke. The greater impact of diabetes in women than men also is noteworthy. A better understanding of the reason for these differences is needed. How-

TABLE 98–5. *Impact of cardiovascular risk factors in different vascular territories: 36-year follow-up Framingham Study cohort*

| | Age-adjusted risk ratio | | | | | | | |
| | Coronary disease | | Brain infarction | | Heart failure | | Peripheral artery disease | |
Risk factor	Men	Women	Men	Women	Men	Women	Men	Women
Hypertension								
Age 35–64 yr	2.0^c	2.2^c	5.7^c	4.0^c	4.0^c	4.2^c	2.0^c	3.7^c
65–94 yr	1.6^c	1.9^c	2.0^c	2.6^c	1.9^c	1.9^c	1.6^a	2.0^b
Cholesterol								
Age 35–64 yr	1.9^b	1.8^c	1.0	1.1	1.2	0.7	2.0^b	1.9
65–94 yr	1.2	2.0^c	0.7	0.6	1.0	0.8	1.4	0.8
Diabetes								
Age 35–64 yr	1.5^c	3.7^c	3.0^c	2.4^a	4.4^c	7.8^c	3.4^c	6.4^c
65–94 yr	1.6^c	2.1^c	1.6	2.9^c	2.0^c	3.6^c	1.9^c	2.6^b
Cigarettes								
Age 35–64 yr	1.5^c	1.1	2.5^b	0.7	1.4^c	1.1	2.5^c	2.0^b
65–94 yr	1.0	1.2	1.4	1.9^c	1.0	1.3^a	1.8^b	1.8^a

$^aP < 0.05$; $^bP < 0.01$; $^cP < 0.001$.

ever, it seems clear that measures taken to prevent one atherothrombotic disease (e.g., coronary disease) should carry a substantial bonus in preventing atherothrombotic events in other vascular territories. Each of the risk factors considered has been shown to independently contribute to the occurrence of the atherothrombotic cardiovascular events, but the risk each imposes varies widely depending on the associated burden of other risk factors. This necessitates global risk evaluation using multivariable risk formulations (9).

It also is important to recognize that the ultimate morbidity and mortality associated with any particular atherothrombotic cardiovascular event may be profoundly influenced by coexistent overt or silent cardiovascular disease soon to make its appearance (2). For example, mortality is increased in persons with intermittent claudication, femoral bruits, or other evidence of peripheral arterial disease, but this occurs chiefly from stroke, cardiac failure, and coronary disease (2). Not only do carotid bruits predict strokes, they also presage coronary disease, heart failure, and peripheral artery disease as well.

That coronary disease is associated with an increased stroke risk in the absence of hypertension or cardiac failure, and that angina carries half the stroke risk of a MI, suggests a direct effect by embolization or inadequate maintenance of cerebral blood flow as a result of rhythm disturbances or cardiac failure. Coronary disease can provide a source for embolism in akinetic segments of the myocardium or in a fibrillating atrium. Coronary disease places a patient in jeopardy not only of recurrent infarction, angina, cardiac failure, and

sudden death, but also from atherothrombosis in other vascular territories in the form of strokes, TIAs, and intermittent claudication.

ACKNOWLEDGMENTS

Framingham Heart Study research is supported by National Institutes of Health/National Heart, Lung and Blood Institute Contract No. 01-HC-25195 and the Visiting Scientist Program, which is supported by Astra-Zeneca.

REFERENCES

1. Cupples LA, D'Agostino RB. Survival following initial cardiovascular events. The Framingham Study. 30-year follow-up. Section 35. National Institutes of Health Publication no. 88-2909; 1988.
2. Kannel WB, McGee DL. Update on some epidemiologic features of intermittent claudication. *J Am Geriatric Soc* 1985;33:13–18.
3. Kannel WB, Wolf PA, Verter J. Manifestations of coronary disease predisposing to stroke. *JAMA* 1983;250:2942–2946.
4. Franklin SS, Kahn SA, Wong ND, et al. Is pulse pressure useful in predicting risk for coronary heart disease? *Circulation* 1999;100:354–360.
5. Kannel WB. Risk factors for atherosclerotic cardiovascular outcomes in different vascular territories. *J Cardiovasc Risk* 1994;1:1–7.
6. O'Leary DH, Anderson KM, Wolf PA, et al. Cholesterol and carotid atherosclerosis: the Framingham Study. *Ann Epidemiol* 1992;2:147–153.
7. Sacks FM, Pfeffer MA, Moye LA, et al. The effect of pravastatin on coronary events after myocardial infarction in patients with average cholesterol levels: Cholesterol and Recurrent Events Trial investigators. *N Engl J Med* 1996;335:1001–1009.
8. Reaven GM. Syndrome X: 6 years later. *J Intern Med* 1994;736:13–22.
9. Wilson PW, D'Agostino RB, Levy D, et al. Prediction of coronary heart disease using risk factor categories. *Circulation* 1998;97:1837–1847.

CHAPTER 99

Diagnosis and Treatment of Atherothrombotic Diseases of the Aorta

Jonathan L. Halperin and Jeffrey W. Olin

Key Words: Aneurysms; aorta; aortic dissection; aortoiliac disease; atheroembolism.

ATHEROTHROMBOSIS OF THE AORTA

Pathologic evidence of atherothrombosis arises earlier in the aorta than in any other vascular tissue, and the usual risk factors (tobacco smoking, diabetes mellitus, hypertension, hypercholesterolemia, obesity, and sedentary lifestyle) and novel risk factors (e.g., increased plasma levels of homocysteine and C-reactive protein) are related to progression and complications. In the infrarenal aorta, atherothrombosis may be asymptomatic or produce intermittent claudication, critical limb ischemia, or atheromatous embolism. Atherothrombosis less commonly affects the supraceliac portion of the abdominal aorta and the descending thoracic aorta (1), but involvement of the origins of the brachiocephalic, carotid, and subclavian vessels and the aortic arch has well characterized

   J. L. Halperin: The Zena and Michael A. Wiener Cardiovascular Institute, Mount Sinai School of Medicine, Fifth Avenue at 100th Street, New York, New York 10029.
   J. W. Olin: The Zena and Michael A. Wiener Cardiovascular Institute, Mount Sinai School of Medicine, Fifth Avenue at 100th Street, New York, New York 10029.

clinical manifestations (2). Atherothrombosis of the thoracic aorta is a strong predictor of initial and recurrent stroke, coronary events, and death (3–5), reflecting either an embolic mechanism or associated vascular pathology.

AORTOILIAC OBSTRUCTIVE DISEASE

Isolated aortoiliac atherothrombosis typically occurs in younger individuals who smoke cigarettes. Almost half of the cases are women, who may exhibit the "hypoplastic aortic syndrome," characterized by small-caliber aortic, iliac, and femoropopliteal arteries, and atherothrombosis confined to the aortic bifurcation (6). Men generally present older and with more diffuse disease (type II involving the aorta, common and external iliac arteries, and type III widespread disease both above and below the inguinal ligament) (7,8). Disease localized to the distal aorta and common iliac arteries (type I) rarely produces limb-threatening ischemia because of extensive collateral vessels. The classical presentation is the Leriche syndrome—a clinical triad of intermittent claudication involving the low back, buttocks, hip, or thigh, often mistaken for degenerative joint disease of the low back or hips; impotency (which occurs in 30–50% of male individuals with aortoiliac occlusive disease); and so-called global atrophy of the lower extremities, reflecting the chronicity of low-grade ischemia (9). The femoral pulses often are weak or absent, but the ankle–brachial index may be normal at rest. A decline in ankle systolic pressure after exercise confirms hemodynamically significant stenosis.

Treatment

Treatment of patients with occlusive atherothrombosis of the aorta is directed at improving symptoms or claudication or limb ischemia, and thus quality of life, as well as reduction of overall cardiovascular risk. The latter involves measures comparable to those for other manifestations of systemic atherothrombosis or peripheral arterial disease. Patients with symptomatic aortoiliac occlusive disease may not respond as well to exercise or medications such as pentoxifylline or cilostazol as those patients with infrainguinal peripheral arterial disease. Catheter-based intervention to relieve aortic obstruction may be useful for those patients with critical limb ischemia or severe claudication. Percutaneous catheter-based interventions under local anesthesia have largely replaced surgical revascularization (e.g., endarterectomy, aortoiliac or aortobifemoral bypass) because they avoid abdominal incision, abbreviate hospital stay, reduce cost, accelerate recovery, and are associated with lower short-term morbidity and mortality rates (10).

The Transatlantic Inter-societal Consensus group classified patients with aortoiliac occlusive disease in four categories: types A, B, C, and D. Endovascular therapy was favored for patients with type A lesions; surgery was preferred for those with type D lesions (11). Although the available evidence did not support firm recommendations for type B or C aortoiliac lesions, subsequent advances currently justify angioplasty and stenting for most cases meeting clinical criteria for revascularization, unless obstructive disease extends into the common femoral artery. Surgical revascularization of aortoiliac lesions is associated with 74% to 95% patency rates at 5 years (12), which is similar but not superior to results with catheter-based interventions (13). A multicenter trial of primary iliac stenting in 486 patients demonstrated clinical benefit in 91% at 1 year, 84% at 2 years, and 63% at 43-month follow-up; the angiographic patency rate was 92% (14).

ACUTE OCCLUSIVE SYNDROMES

Sudden occlusion of the terminal aorta may result from "saddle" embolism at the iliac bifurcation (15), trauma, dissection, or *in situ* thrombosis. Most saddle emboli originate in the heart in patients with mitral stenosis, atrial fibrillation, acute anterior myocardial infarction (MI), or infective endocarditis, or involve paradoxic embolism through a right-to-left intracardiac shunt from a peripheral venous source. When thrombotic occlusion of the aorta develops at a point of atherothrombotic narrowing, collateral perfusion is usu-

ally sufficient to prevent acute limb ischemia. Acute aortic occlusion related to thrombosis of an abdominal aortic aneurysm is considerably less common than thrombosis of popliteal aneurysms.

Unlike gradually progressive obstruction, abrupt interruption of flow through the terminal aorta or common iliac arteries poses an immediate threat to life and limb. Although the clinical picture varies depending on collaterals, presentation may be characterized by severe pain in the back, buttocks, perineum, abdomen, and legs with diffuse cyanosis from the umbilicus to the feet, and the lower limbs may be pale, cold, and pulseless with numbness, paresthesiae, or paralysis. Unless circulation is restored promptly, muscle necrosis may produce myoglobinuria, renal failure, acidosis, hyperkalemia, and death.

Treatment

Acute aortic occlusion calls for immediate revascularization. The optimum procedure depends on etiologic factors and the strategy for prevention of recurrent embolism. Transfemoral catheter-based embolectomy can extract even large amounts of embolic material from the distal aorta. Even after circulation has been restored, however, mortality related to the underlying disease is high (16).

ATHEROMATOUS EMBOLISM

Embolism of cholesterol-laden material and thrombus from the surface of the aorta occurs commonly in patients with severe aortic atherothrombosis (17). Atheroembolism may be spontaneous, although it occurs more frequently after surgical or arteriographic manipulation, such as catheter-based coronary or peripheral interventions. The most important predictive factor is the severity of aortic atherothrombosis, but whether anticoagulant and thrombolytic drugs exacerbate atheroembolism is controversial (18,19). Among 71 autopsied cases, cholesterol embolism was detected in 27% of patients who had undergone arteriography before death, compared with 4.3% of age- and disease-matched control subjects who had not undergone angiography (20). The incidence rate of clinical atheroembolism was 0.002% in a series of 4,587 cardiac catheterization procedures (21), and in another of 3,733 cardiac catheterization, angioplasty, and intraaortic balloon pump procedures (22), and none was observed when access was obtained through the brachial artery. In another study of 7,621 cardiac catheterization cases, histologic evidence of atheroembolism was found in 0.54% without clinically apparent ischemic complications (23).

Patients with atheromatous embolism typically have a history of angina pectoris, MI, transient ischemic attack, stroke, intermittent claudication, or peripheral gangrene. Clinical signs and symptoms vary depending on the amount, size, and site of origin of the atheromatous material, as well as on the tissue affected. Macroembolism may present catastrophically as an acute ischemic limb, whereas patients with microembolism may have milder localized signs or a clinical picture suggesting systemic illness, including fever, weight loss, anorexia, myalgia, headache, nausea, vomiting, or diarrhea. Occasionally, the presentation may suggest vasculitis, infective endocarditis, or malignancy (24). Cutaneous manifestations are the most frequent findings (25) and include cyanotic toes, gangrenous digits, livedo reticularis, or nodules (Fig. 99–1) (26). When atheroembolism affects both lower extremities, the source is generally the aorta, but when only one extremity is involved, it may be difficult to determine whether the origin is a diseased ipsilateral artery or a more proximal site.

Atheromatous embolism arising from the aortic arch or the carotid and vertebral arteries may cause stroke, transient ischemic attack, amaurosis fugax, blindness, headache, confusion, organic brain syndromes, dizziness, or spinal cord infarction. Retinal artery occlusion may be identified by Hollenhorst plaque on ophthalmoscopic examination as yellow, highly refractile atheromatous material at an arteriolar bifurcation. The risk for ischemic events in the central nervous system appears related to specific morphologic features of atheromatous aortic plaque defined by transesophageal echocardiography (TEE), including thickness, ulceration, or the presence of mobile elements (Figs. 99–2 and 99–3) (4,27,28).

Atheroembolism originating from the suprarenal aorta may involve the kidneys, producing small-vessel occlusive disease with accelerated hypertension, microscopic hematuria, or seg-mental ischemic atrophy. Various patterns of renal insufficiency may progress over weeks or months to irreversible renal failure requiring dialysis (29). To distinguish this syndrome from renal artery stenosis, renal artery thrombosis, infective endocarditis, vasculitis, and other causes of acute renal failure no single laboratory test is diagnostic, because acceleration of the erythrocyte sedimentation rate, leukocytosis with eosinophilia and anemia, azotemia, and abnormalities of the urinary sediment are common to many of these conditions (30). Increased serum levels of amylase, hepatic transaminase levels, creatine kinase, or aldolase arise from atheroembolic involvement of the liver, pancreas, or skeletal muscle. Renal biopsy may reveal pathognomonic needle-shaped cholesterol clefts within small vessels. Atheroembolic renal disease carries a poor prognosis, with a mortality rate of 81% in one series, the most common causes were cardiac, renal, or multiorgan failure (25).

Treatment

Treatment seldom reverses damage, therefore emphasis is on prevention of subsequent ischemic events. Treatment also should involve symptomatic care of the affected ischemic tissue and risk factor modification to prevent progression of atheromatous disease and to promote plaque stabilization. When lower extremity ischemia is present, local care of ulceration is appropriate, and amputation may be required when gangrene is present. Although controversial, sympathectomy may help to control intractable pain. In cases of renal atheroembolism, dialysis is used to control

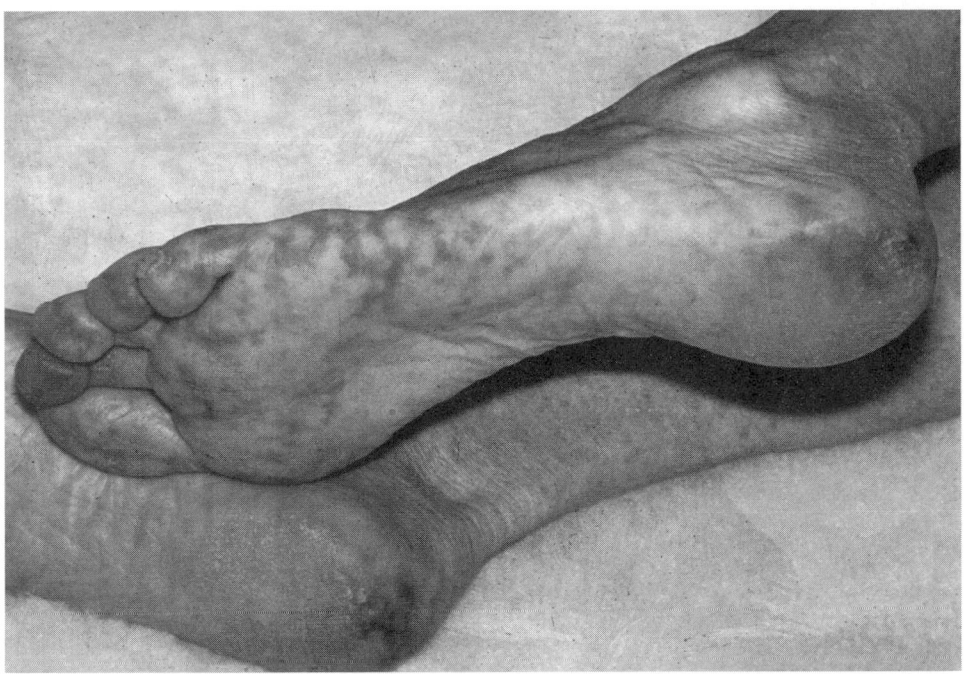

FIG. 99–1. Atheroembolism (cholesterol embolism) involving the feet in a patient with aortic atherothrombotic disease.

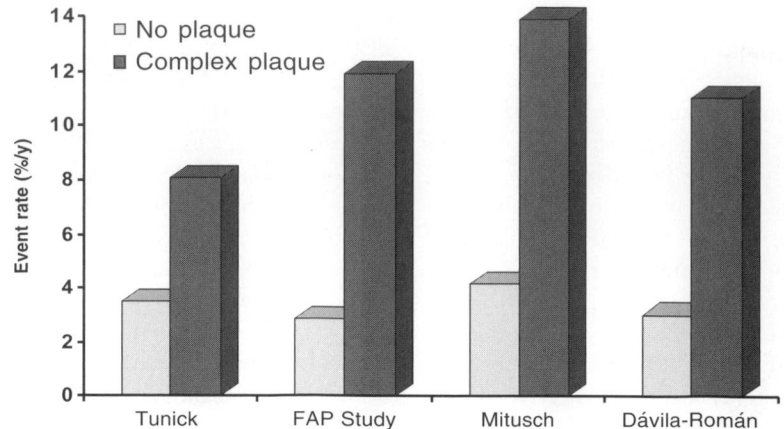

FIG. 99–2. Incidence of ischemic events in observational series of patients (Tunick [215], French Study of Aortic Plaques *[FAP]* [4], Mitusch [216], and Dávila-Román [217]) with morphologically complex atheromatous disease of the aortic arch compared with patients without plaque identified by transesophageal echocardiography.

uremic manifestations and hypertension is managed pharmacologically.

Optimum antithrombotic therapy (anticoagulants, platelet inhibitors, or a combination of both) has not been defined for atheromatous embolism, but the agents involved decrease the long-term risk for cardiovascular ischemic events. 3-hydroxy-3-methylglutaryl coenzyme A (HMG CoA) reductase inhibitor ("statin") drugs improve plaque stabilization in patients with coronary disease (31), and case reports (32) and nonrandomized series (33) support their use in patients with atheroembolism (Fig. 99–4).

When the source of embolism can be localized, it may be possible to isolate or replace a segment of the aorta by surgery, angioplasty, or stent-graft insertion. Surgical or endovascular therapy has been advocated when the source of embolism is localized in the aortoiliac segment. Aortobiiliac or aortobifemoral bypass is indicated when atheromatous disease is infrarenal (the most common location). Because considerable perioperative morbidity and mortality is involved, replacement of the suprarenal aorta is reserved for patients in life-threatening situations (34). In poor candidates for aortic replacement, ligation of the common femoral arteries together with extraanatomic bypass may prevent recurrent lower limb ischemia, but intestinal and renal ischemia is not avoided (35). Aortic stent grafting to overlay the atheromatous material and to prevent future em-

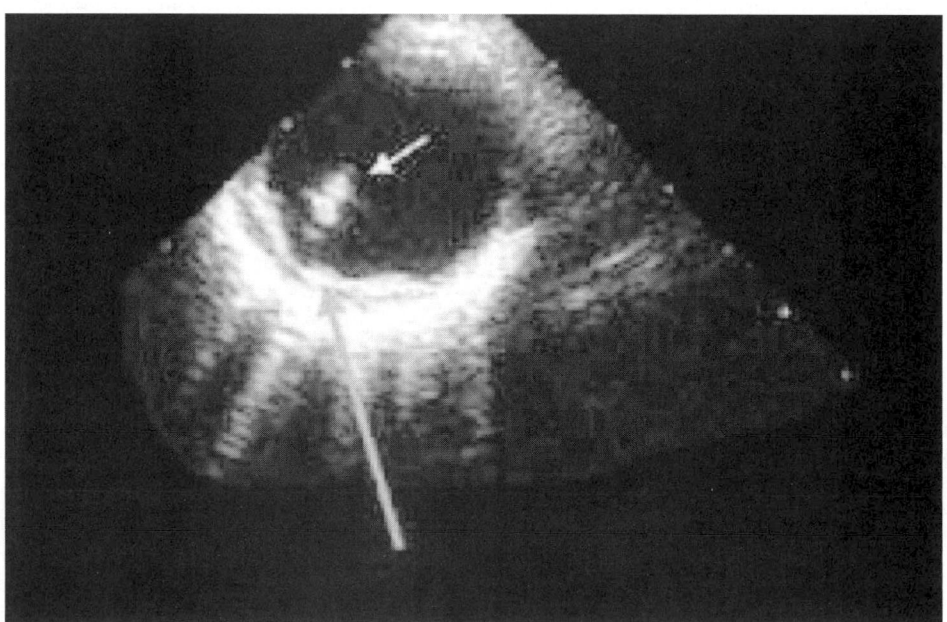

FIG. 99–3. Complex atherothrombotic plaque in the aortic arch with protruding, mobile elements *(arrows)* imaged by transesophageal echocardiography.

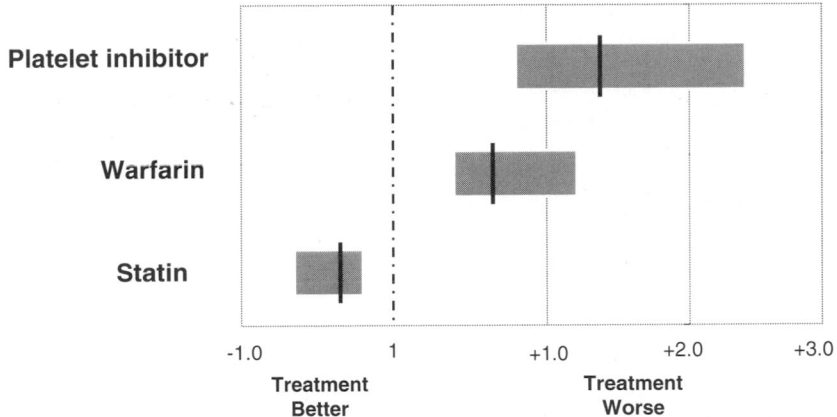

FIG. 99–4. Comparison of estimated odds ratios for stroke and systemic embolism during treatment of patients with aortic atherothrombosis with platelet inhibitor, oral anticoagulant, and 3-hydroxy-3-methylglutaryl coenzyme A reductase inhibitor ("statin") agents in a retrospective analysis of 519 cases. (From Tunick PA, Nayar AC, Goodkin GM, et al. Effect of treatment on the incidence of stroke and other emboli in 519 patients with severe thoracic aortic plaque. *Am J Cardiol* 2002;90:1320–1325, with permission.)

bolism also has been described. It may be difficult to localize the source of embolism when atherothrombosis is diffusely distributed, and no well designed trials have compared nonsurgical with surgical therapy for patients with atheroembolism (36).

ANEURYSMAL DISEASE

Aneurysm formation is considerably more widespread along the length of the aorta than obstructive atherothrombotic disease, potentially affecting almost the entire vessel, whereas obstruction tends to involve only the abdominal portion of the aorta, when the iliac arteries are commonly affected as well. Dilatation of the aorta may occur as a consequence of atherothrombosis alone, as well as of aging, infection, inflammation, trauma, congenital anomalies, and medial degeneration or in combinations of pathologic states. The pathologic changes that accompany these conditions cause the aorta to thicken, thin, bulge, tear, rupture, narrow, dissect, or be altered by combinations of these conditions.

The principal histologic feature of aortic aneurysms is destruction of the media and elastic tissue. Excessive proteolytic enzyme activity may promote deterioration of structural matrix proteins, such as elastin and collagen, in the aortic wall (37). Smooth muscle cells derived from patients with aortic aneurysms display invasive properties compared with those from normal aortas. This increased migration, which appears to be caused by overproduction of the matrix metalloproteinase-2, may lead to extracellular matrix remodeling and subsequent medial disruption in the aneurysmal aorta (38). Abnormal biochemical elastolytic and active proteolytic activity also have been identified in tissue from aneurysmal aortas (39). An abnormal presence of macrophages (40) and increased levels of cytokines (41) in

aneurysmal aortic tissue likewise indicate that an active inflammatory process may contribute to the pathogenesis of aortic aneurysms. Cultured smooth muscle cells from aneurysmal aortas produce increased levels of plasminogen activators compared with cells from normal aortas (42). This could increase the amount of plasmin available for zymogen activation of matrix metalloproteinases, which would favor proteolysis in the absence of a reciprocal increase in plasmin activator inhibitor. Matrix metalloproteinases thus may play a major role in the aortic wall degeneration that leads to aneurysm formation.

The pathophysiologic processes that underlie aneurysm expansion have not been clearly defined, but appear to involve elastolysis and collagenolysis promoted by inflammatory changes within the aortic wall and by hypertension (43). An increased level of C-reactive protein (a marker of inflammation) correlates with poor prognosis in patients with symptomatic aortic aneurysms or dissection (44). A relation between inflammatory processes and atherothrombotic aortic aneurysmal disease is supported by an abnormal accumulation of macrophages and increased levels of cytokines in aneurysmal aortic tissue (40,41). Despite the greater risk for rupture with large aneurysms, it has been difficult to establish a clear correlation between the rate of aneurysm expansion and the risk for rupture. The problem may be one of observational methodology, however, and there is little reason to doubt that rapid expansion is a harbinger of rupture (45). It is widely believed, but difficult to prove, that symptomatic aneurysms or those that generate a local or systemic inflammatory response show an earlier propensity to rupture. The prevalence of abdominal aortic aneurysm increases with age, occurring more frequently in patients aged 60 to 70 years than in younger individuals, although affected individuals range from age 30 to older than 90 years (46,47). Coronary artery disease, peripheral arterial disease, and other manifestations of systemic atherothrombosis occur frequently in patients with abdominal aortic aneurysms, and hypertension often coexists (48). Whether hypertension correlates with the risk for rupture is controversial (49).

Atherothrombotic Thoracic Aortic Aneurysm

The most common cause of ascending aortic aneurysm, cystic medial necrosis, usually affects the ascending aorta and may involve the sinuses of Valsalva (50), whereas atherothrombosis of the aorta, the topic of this chapter, is an unusual cause of ascending aortic aneurysms, and when it is the cause, there is usually extensive atherothrombosis elsewhere. Proximal atherothrombotic aneurysms are typically fusiform and extend into the arch. Aneurysms of the aortic arch therefore often are contiguous with aneurysms in the ascending aorta, and occur more frequently in men than in women (51). More frequently, atherothrombotic aneurysms affect the distal aspect of the arch and descending thoracic aorta (52). Proximal aortic aneurysms caused by atherothrombosis are usually part of a more diffuse atherothrombotic process and must be distinguished from cystic medial necrosis, syphilitic aneurysms, and other aneurysms of infectious or inflammatory causes in this location. In contrast, the majority of aneurysms of the descending thoracic aorta are associated with atherothrombosis (53–55). These are typically fusiform, often begin distal to the origin of the left subclavian artery, and may extend to the level of the abdominal aorta (56).

Aneurysms of the thoracic aorta typically produce no symptoms, but a variety of symptom complexes may arise related to the size of the aneurysm and its location within the thorax. Chest pain, typically positional, may occur when the aneurysm compresses surrounding structures or erodes into adjacent bone, such as the ribs or sternum. Aneurysms of the aortic arch may produce symptoms by compression of contiguous structures, but most are asymptomatic. Dyspnea or cough may be caused by compression of the trachea or mainstem bronchi, dysphagia by compression of the esophagus, or hoarseness secondary to left vocal cord paralysis related to compression of the left recurrent laryngeal nerve (53,55,57,58). Rupture may occur into the left pleural space, mediastinum, pericardium, pulmonary artery, superior vena cava, tracheobronchial tree (causing hemoptysis), or esophagus (causing hematemesis) (50,59,60). Symptoms frequently are a harbinger of rupture or death in patients with thoracic aortic aneurysm, which call for a more aggressive approach. In asymptomatic patients, prophylactic surgery is indicated for atherothrombotic aneurysms a maximum of 6 cm diameter.

Thoracoabdominal Aortic Aneurysm

As suggested by the nomenclature, thoracoabdominal aortic aneurysms have features of both thoracic and abdominal

aortic aneurysms. Although they constitute only about 3% of all aortic aneurysms, thoracoabdominal aneurysms are considered a separate class because of the diffuse and extensive aortic involvement and special considerations for surgical repair, which may entail reimplantation of the origins of visceral arteries (61). Among the various proposed classification schemes, Crawford (62) delineated four types of thoracoabdominal aortic aneurysms according to the segment and extent of aorta involved. In keeping with the notion that thoracoabdominal aortic aneurysms represent a diffusely atherothrombotic and ectatic aorta with one or more aneurysmal segments of variable length, two types that are essentially confined to the abdominal aorta are included. The principal clinical implication is that surgical repair may require reimplantation or reconstruction of the origins of major branch arteries, which entails risks for ischemic tissue injury greater than those associated with aneurysmectomy alone.

Because they occur less frequently than discrete aneurysms of the aorta, relatively little information is available regarding the natural history of thoracoabdominal aneurysms. The etiologic factors and clinical presentation are more comparable to aneurysms of the abdominal than the thoracic aorta; thus, it has been speculated that the risk for rupture is similar to abdominal aortic aneurysms of equivalent diameter.

Although most patients with thoracoabdominal aortic aneurysms are asymptomatic, discomfort occasionally develops in the epigastrium or left upper quadrant of the abdomen. Back or flank pain may occur when the patient lies in the left lateral decubitus position. Erosion of the anterior surfaces of the vertebral bodies may occur, leading to radiculopathy (63–65). Visceral artery occlusion may occur, but frank ischemia and infarction are infrequent (65). Patients who report claudication also may have occlusive atherothrombotic disease of the aorta, iliac, or more distal arteries. Mural thrombosis is common in atherothrombotic aneurysms, and may be the source of peripheral atheroembolism, causing occlusion of distal vessels (66,67). Rupture of the thoracic component of these aneurysms generally occurs into the left pleural space, producing hemothorax; the abdominal component may rupture into the retroperitoneum, inferior vena cava, or duodenum.

Abdominal Aortic Aneurysm

Aneurysms of the abdominal aorta account for approximately 15,000 deaths annually in the United States. The incidence rate of abdominal aortic aneurysms in autopsy series has ranged from 1.8% to 6.6% of cases, leading to an estimated occurrence rate of 15 to 37 cases per 100,000 patient-years (68–78). The incidence increases with age, ranging from less than 2.1 per 100,000 patient-years between the ages of 40 and 49 years to more than 280 per 100,000 patient-years among individuals older than 80 years (76,77). Abdominal aortic aneurysms occur two to five times more frequently in male than female individuals, and more often in white than black individuals (76,77). One autopsy series reported an incidence rate of 4.2% among white male individuals compared with 1.5% among black male individuals (71). The prevalence of abdominal aortic aneurysms is greater in patients with clinical evidence of atherothrombosis. In patients with coronary artery disease, for instance, the prevalence of abdominal aneurysms is approximately 5%, and nearly 10% of patients with atherothrombotic peripheral arterial obstructive disease have associated abdominal aortic aneurysms (70,79–81).

In more than 90% of cases, the superior margins of abdominal aortic aneurysms are below the level of the renal arteries (82–87). Several reports of familial clustering of abdominal aortic aneurysm have appeared, and decreased type 3 collagen and elastin content of the aortic wall and increased collagenase activity have been identified in some familial cases (88–93). Whether atherothrombosis is the inciting cause of these aneurysms or a cofactor in otherwise predisposed individuals remains uncertain (94,95).

Survival is limited in patients with abdominal aortic aneurysms because of the potential for aortic rupture and the prevalence of coronary artery disease. In 1950, the survival rates of 102 patients with abdominal aortic aneurysms identified on physical examination or radiography, most of which were atherothrombotic (96), were 67% at 1 year, 49% at 3 years, and 19% at 5 years. Of the fatalities, 63% were related to rupture. Others have subsequently reported similar statistics (97–100). The survival rate for patients with aneurysms smaller than 6 cm in one series was 75% after 1 year, 68% after 3 years, and 48% after 5 years. For those with aneurysms larger than 6 cm, the survival rate was 48% at 1 year, 12% at 3 years, and 6% at 5 years. Follow-up after up to 20 years of 127 patients initially deemed medically unfit for surgery (predominantly because of severe coexisting coronary artery disease) reported a mortality rate of 71%, with 28% on the basis of rupture (101). In other series, rupture was reported in 20% of patients over a 30-year period, most with aneurysms greater than 5 cm in diameter (77), and the following survival rates have been described in patients with untreated abdominal aortic aneurysms: 62% after 1 year, 32% after 3 years, and 19% after 5 years (102). About 38% of the patients died as a consequence of rupture; 55% of those with aneurysms larger than 6 cm died of rupture compared with 16% of those with aneurysms smaller than 6 cm in diameter. In a group of patients with aneurysms initially 3 to 6 cm in diameter, the mean expansion rate was 0.4 cm per year (103).

Most patients with abdominal aortic aneurysms are asymptomatic; others experience abdominal discomfort, back pain, or abdominal pulsation (104,105). Less frequently, pain may occur in the legs, chest, or groin; anorexia, nausea, vomiting, constipation, or dyspnea may develop. Compression of the left iliac vein may cause left leg swelling, just as compression of the left ureter may cause hydronephrosis, or compression of testicular veins may cause varicocele. As the aneurysm expands and compresses

vertebrae and lumbar nerve roots, pain may develop in the lower back and radiate to the posterior aspects of the legs. Flank pain radiating to the anterior left thigh or scrotum may reflect compression of the left genitofemoral nerve. Nausea and vomiting may occur as the aneurysm compresses the duodenum. Bladder compression may cause urinary frequency or urgency.

The key physical finding is a pulsatile abdominal mass. Typically, aneurysms larger than 4 cm in diameter are palpable except in obese individuals or when examination is impeded by guarding. A pulsatile epigastric or periumbilical mass may be visible as well as palpable, expanding laterally with systole (106). Abdominal bruits are not specific for aneurysm formation, and only about 40% of such aneurysms are associated with bruits. The finding of a pulsatile mass in the groin (suggesting iliac artery aneurysm) or in the popliteal fossa (suggesting popliteal artery aneurysm) should raise suspicion that an abdominal aortic aneurysm may be present, because multiple aneurysms often coexist. Carotid bruits or diminished arterial pulses in the lower extremities may reflect atherothrombosis of other vessels.

The triad of chronic abdominal pain, weight loss, and an accelerated sedimentation rate in a patient with an abdominal aortic aneurysm is highly suggestive of an inflammatory aneurysm. Inflammatory aortic or iliac aneurysms were present in 4.5% of the 2,816 patients who underwent elective abdominal aortic aneurysm repair at the Mayo Clinic from 1955 to 1985 (107). Compared with patients with noninflammatory atherothrombotic aneurysms, those with inflammatory aneurysms were more likely to have symptoms, weight loss, a greater sedimentation rate, larger diameter, more intense retroperitoneal inflammatory reaction, and greater operative mortality (107,108).

Ultrasound Screening

Accurate, cost-effective screening for abdominal aortic aneurysm is an important health economic issue, considering the prevalence of and mortality associated with this disease. In a population-based investigation of 67,800 men aged 65 to 74 years initiated in the United Kingdom in 1997, 33,839 were randomly invited to undergo abdominal ultrasound scanning and be compared with 33,961 subjects in a control group in whom scans were not performed (109). Men with aortic aneurysms measuring at least 3 cm in diameter were followed with repeat scans for a mean of 4.1 years, and surgical treatment was considered when the diameter reached 5.5 cm, when expansion occurred at a rate of more than 1 cm per year, or when symptoms occurred. More than 27,000 (80%) of the men invited agreed to screening, and 1,333 aneurysms were detected. There were 65 aneurysm-related deaths (absolute risk, 0.19%) in this group, compared with 113 (0.33%) in the control group (relative risk reduction, 42%; $p = 0.0002$), including a 53% reduction of risk among those who actually underwent screening. The 30-day mortality rate was 6% after elective aneurysm repair, compared with 37% after emergency surgeries. Over 4 years, 47 less deaths related to abdominal aortic aneurysms occurred in the screened group than in the control group, but the additional costs incurred were £2.2 million (approximately $3.5 million). After adjustment for censoring and a discount of 6%, the mean additional cost of screening was £63.4 ($98) per patient. Over four years, the mean incremental cost-effectiveness ratio for screening was £28,400 ($45,000) per life-year gained, corresponding to approximately £36,000 ($57,000) per quality-adjusted life-year. After 10 years, this figure declined to approximately £8,000 ($12,500) per life-year gained (110).

Aneurysm Rupture

Rupture of an abdominal aortic aneurysm usually presents clinically as an abdominal catastrophe. Patients frequently have severe abdominal or back pain, but the pattern of pain varies considerably. The aneurysm may rupture into the retroperitoneum or into the peritoneal or pleural cavities, leading to hypotension, tachycardia, pallor, diaphoresis, or deep shock, depending on the extent of rupture and associated blood loss into the extravascular space. On occasion, rupture occurs directly into the duodenum, causing an aorto-duodenal fistula and acute gastrointestinal bleeding. This possibility should be considered when gastrointestinal bleeding is evident together with signs of an aneurysm on physical examination. Rupture may also occur into the inferior vena cava or iliac veins, producing an arteriovenous fistula; this is suggested by rapid development of leg swelling or high-output congestive heart failure in the presence of an abdominal aortic aneurysm. Despite surgical advances, mor-

tality is still the most frequent outcome because abrupt circulatory collapse usually prevents timely intervention.

Elective Surgical and Endograft Repair to Prevent Rupture

During the last decade, randomized trials comparing early intervention versus expectant management of infrarenal abdominal aortic aneurysms measuring 4.0 to 5.4 cm in diameter have been conducted in the United Kingdom and by the Veterans Administration (VA) in the United States (111, 112). By protocol, elective surgical treatment was not offered to patients allocated to the nonoperative cohort in each trial until aneurysms exceeded 5.4 cm in size on serial imaging studies. Women comprised 17% of the patients in the U.K. study but only 0.8% of the VA population. Thirty-day operative mortality rates (U.K.: 5.4%; VA: 2.1%) were competitive with those from other multicenter studies. Endografts were used in 27 patients in the surgical arm of the U.K. trial (4.8%) but in just 2 patients in the VA trial.

After a mean follow-up of 4.9 years, early aneurysm repair produced no significant benefits with respect to the incidence of either aneurysm-related deaths or deaths from all causes in the VA trial. The same conclusions were reached at a mean follow-up of 4.6 years in the U.K. trial in 1998 (Fig. 99–5). Although the U.K. surgical cohort had a lower overall mortality rate than the nonoperative cohort at 8 years ($p = 0.03$), this finding has been attributed in part to a greater rate of smoking cessation in the early-surgery group (113). The annual rupture rate was negligible (0.6%) for observed aneurysms in the VA trial and was 3.2% in the U.K. trial. Rupture in the U.K. trial was more likely to occur in women (odds ratio, 4.0; $p < 0.001$), accounting for 14% of all

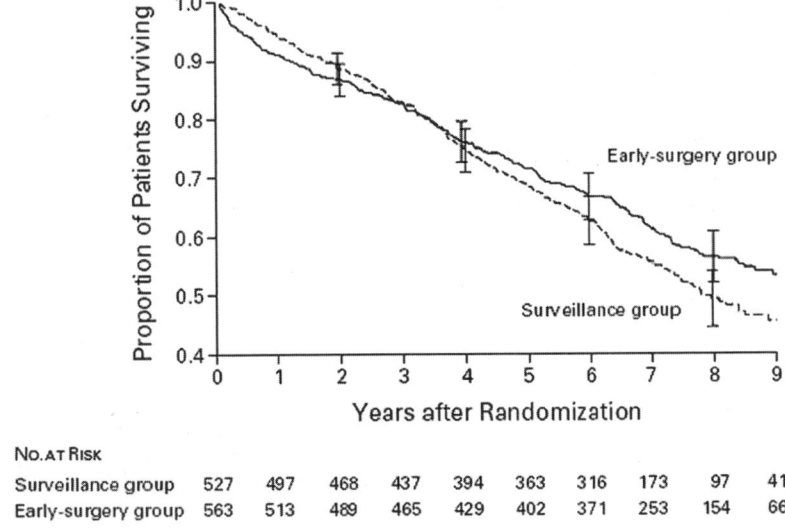

No. at Risk									
Surveillance group	527	497	468	437	394	363	316	173	97	41
Early-surgery group	563	513	489	465	429	402	371	253	154	66

FIG. 99–5. Overall survival according to treatment group in the U.K. Small Aneurysm Trial. (From United Kingdom Small Aneurysm Trial Participants. Long-term outcomes of immediate repair compared with surveillance of small abdominal aortic aneurysms. *N Engl J Med* 2002;346:1445–1452, with permission.)

deaths in women compared with 4.6% of all deaths in men ($p < 0.001$). Aneurysm size at the time of randomization did not influence the risk for rupture in the U.K. trial or the long-term mortality rate in either trial, which may reflect the promptness with which intervention was performed when aneurysms reached a diameter of 5.5 cm or larger. More than 60% of the patients in the nonoperative arm of each of these trials have undergone aneurysm repair because of documented enlargement, including 81% of the patients in the VA trial whose aneurysms were 5.0 to 5.4 cm in diameter when recruited.

Endovascular Repair

Parodi and coworkers (114) first reported the technique of transfemoral catheter-based repair of infrarenal abdominal aortic aneurysms in 1991 as an alternative for management of patients at high risk for complications with conventional surgical treatment. Over the following decade, a variety of stent grafts and delivery systems have been introduced, all of which require open exposure of the common femoral arteries for sheath insertion. In addition, extraperitoneal incisions may be necessary to establish temporary access conduits to the iliac arteries when the size or tortuosity of the external iliac arteries precludes transfemoral cannulation. By avoiding major abdominal/retroperitoneal surgery, however, endovascular repair under regional or local anesthesia has become a valuable alternative for patients in whom severe cardiopulmonary disease, advanced age, morbid obesity, or a previously instrumented abdomen present obstacles to safe, direct, surgical reconstruction.

Most stent-graft devices have a modular construction consisting of a metallic exoskeleton surrounding an intimal fabric graft to maintain linear stability and to avoid kinking (Fig. 99–6). The aortic stem and one contiguous iliac limb are inserted through one femoral artery and the other iliac limb is then positioned using a separate delivery system through the contralateral femoral artery. The conventional technique required an adequate aortic segment of relatively normal caliber below the renal arteries, but newer devices incorporate barbed hooks to secure the stent graft to the aorta above the renal arteries. To avoid obstructing the origins of the renal arteries by the fabric component of the endograft, at least a 1- to 1.5-cm relatively straight aortic segment measuring no more than 28 mm in diameter should be available below the renal arteries. This poses a particular challenge in female patients, in whom the aortoiliac arteries are generally smaller and more angulated than in men (115–118).

Continued blood flow into the excluded sac of an aneurysm, termed an *endoleak,* represents an important complication of endograft repair (Fig. 99–7) (119). *Type I* endoleaks are caused by incompetent proximal or distal attachments, produce high intrasac pressure that can lead to rupture, and should be repaired using intraluminal extension cuffs or conversion to an open procedure as soon as they are

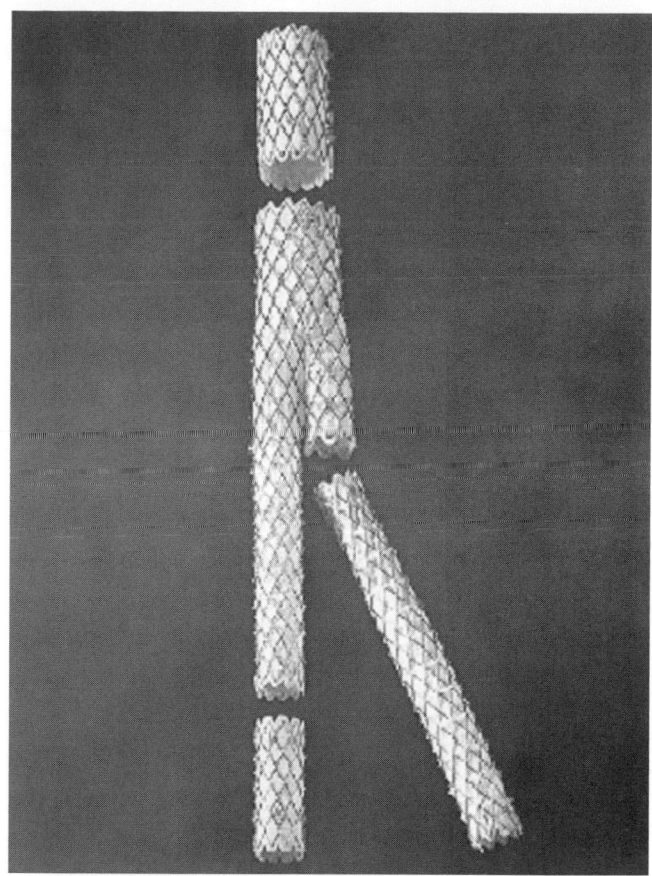

FIG. 99–6. Modular aortic stent-graft system.

discovered. *Type II* endoleaks result from retrograde flow from branch vessels (e.g., the lumbar or inferior mesenteric arteries) and occur in as many as 40% of patients after endograft implantation. These may be corrected by selective arterial embolization, but more than half seal spontaneously, and when persistent do not appear to increase the risk for rupture over 18 to 36 months (120–123). *Type III* endoleaks are caused by fabric defects or tears or disruption of modular graft components. These carry the same potential for delayed aneurysm rupture as type I endoleaks and should, therefore, be promptly repaired. *Type IV* endoleaks, the least common, result from high graft porosity and diffuse leakage through interstices and usually occur within 30 days of implantation. Because of the potential for endoleaks, follow-up imaging every 6 to 12 months is recommended after endovascular stent-graft repair (119,124).

Other complications of endovascular stent-graft repair of abdominal aortic aneurysms include occlusion of the iliac limbs of bifurcation endografts (125,126), migration from the proximal attachment related to progressive aortic expansion (127,128), which can be detected by serial imaging studies in 13% of patients at 1 year after endovascular aneurysm repair, in 21% at 2 years, and in 19% at 3 years (129). These and other complications may become increasingly apparent as the follow-up of patients undergoing endograft repair grows longer.

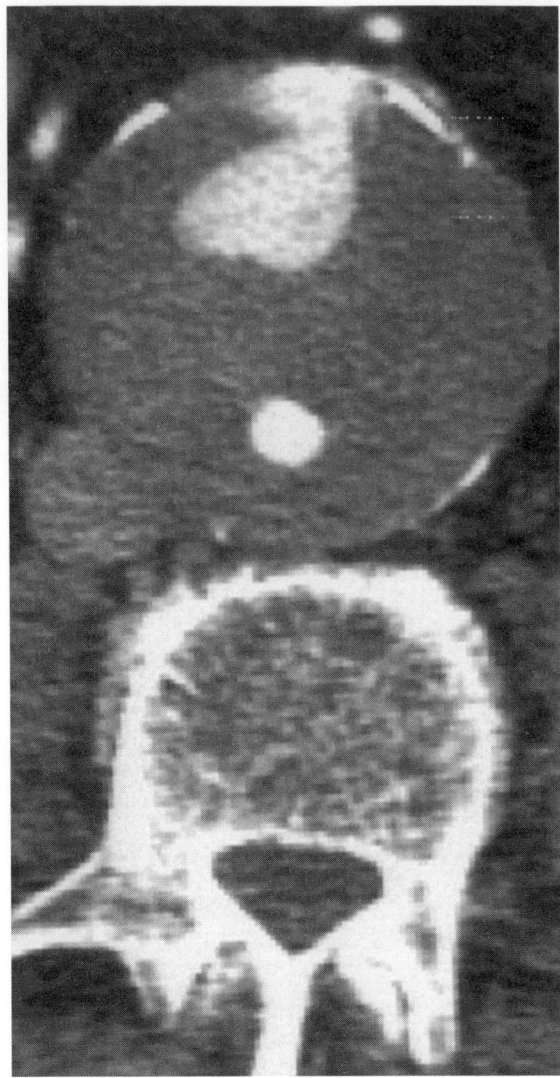

FIG. 99–7. Contrast-enhanced computed tomography scan demonstrating aortic stent-graft endoleak in the sagittal plane. (Courtesy of Dr. Michael L. Marin, Division of Vascular Surgery, Mount Sinai Medical Center, New York, NY.)

Concomitant Coronary Artery Disease

Coronary artery disease is the most important risk factor for cardiac events and death in patients undergoing aneurysm surgery (130–133). Because operative mortality is related mainly to myocardial ischemia, it has been suggested that coronary revascularization be performed in certain patients before abdominal aortic aneurysm resection (134–137). No well designed studies are available that compare the outcome of serial myocardial revascularization and abdominal aortic aneurysm repair with aneurysm surgery alone. Even so, an effort should be made to identify those patients at greatest cardiac risk before surgery using noninvasive diagnostic methods (133,138,139). Abnormal findings indicative of extensive myocardial ischemia may prompt angiography to determine the nature of coronary artery disease and left ventricular function. Thereafter, decisions regarding coronary revasculariza-

tion must be based on symptoms, angiographic findings, and other elements of risk. It is reasonable to consider coronary revascularization before aneurysm surgery in patients with left main coronary artery disease, stenosis greater than 70% in each of the three major coronary arteries in the presence of impaired left ventricular function, and active angina pectoris.

AORTIC DISSECTION

Without early diagnosis and aggressive treatment, aortic dissection often is fatal. The presenting symptoms and signs are so myriad and nonspecific that dissection may be overlooked initially in up to 40% of cases and the diagnosis in a substantial proportion of cases is only established after death (140). Few other conditions demand such prompt diagnosis and treatment, because the mortality rate of untreated dissection approaches 1% per hour during the first 48 hours, 80% at 14 days and 90% at 3 months (141).

Dissection is considered acute when identified within 2 weeks of onset and is chronic when symptoms have been present longer. Several schemes for classification of aortic dissections have been proposed, but the simplest is based on distinguishing those originating proximal or distal to the left subclavian artery. For the former, early surgical intervention is generally recommended, whereas the latter may be managed medically or by endovascular therapy.

The inciting event is usually an intimal tear that propels blood from the true lumen into the middle or outer layer of aortic media, forming a second or false lumen separated by an intimal flap (142,143). In some cases, however, intramural hematoma precedes perforation of the intima (144). The dissection may propagate proximally (retrograde), distally (antegrade), or both, and may narrow or occlude the origin of any branch artery arising from the aorta; the antegrade type is most common. Spiral dissection may leave some aortic branches supplied by the true lumen and others supplied by the false lumen, or pressure from one lumen may compress portions of the other.

The intimal tear originates in the ascending aorta in 65% of cases, the transverse arch in 10%, the upper descending aorta (just beyond the origin of the left subclavian artery) in 20%, and more distally in 5% of cases (142). The false lumen may terminate at any point along the length of the aorta, iliac, or femoral arteries, and there are sometimes multiple flaps and levels of reentry. The false lumen can undergo retrograde dissection, thrombotic occlusion, pseudoaneurysm formation, compression, or rupture. Associated with these are obstruction of the coronary ostia, incompetence of the aortic valve, or pericardial tamponade (145).

Left untreated, less than 10% of patients with proximal aortic dissection survive the first year; most succumb within the first 3 months (146), usually of acute aortic insufficiency, major branch vessel occlusion, or rupture into the pericardium, mediastinum, or left hemithorax. In 20 years of follow-up of 527 patients with aortic dissection, nearly 30% of late deaths were caused by ruptured aortic aneurysm (147).

Aortic dissection occurs more often in male than female individuals, with a 2:1 to 5:1 preponderance (148), usually in the sixth and seventh decades of life. Systemic hypertension is the major predisposing risk factor. In the International Registry of Acute Aortic Dissection, 194 of 289 patients (69%) with proximal dissections and 132 of 175 (77%) with distal dissections had a history of hypertension (149); similar ratios were reported at the Mayo Clinic (Rochester, MN) (148). Other predisposing conditions are the Marfan syndrome, bicuspid aortic valve, Ehlers-Danlos syndrome, Turner's syndrome, Noonan's syndrome, aortic aneurysm, and annuloaortic ectasia, many of which are associated with cystic medial necrosis. The most common causes of aortic dissection in patients younger than 40 years are Marfan's syndrome and pregnancy. Iatrogenic trauma resulting from catheter manipulation is the culprit in approximately 5% of cases, usually involving the descending thoracic or abdominal aorta. Cocaine abuse is another predisposing factor (150).

The most common symptom is chest or upper back pain of sudden onset classically described as ripping, tearing, or shearing in quality (143). In the International Registry, chest pain was present in more than 95% of all patients, 79% of patients with type A dissections, and 63% of those with type B dissections (149). In one large series, painless dissection occurred in only 15% of patients (148). Impending aortic rupture should be considered when pain subsides and later recurs (146).

Aortic insufficiency occurs in 18% to 55% of patients with proximal aortic dissection. In the International Registry, a diastolic murmur of aortic insufficiency was identified in 44% of patients with proximal aortic dissection compared with 12% of those with distal aortic dissection (149). After aortic rupture, the second most common cause of death in patients with aortic dissection is acute, severe aortic insufficiency caused by dilatation of the aortic root, annulus, and valve cusps. Most patients with aortic dissection are hypertensive, but 3% to 18% present in shock, sometimes secondary to extension of dissection into the coronary arteries, acute MI, left ventricular dysfunction, acute severe aortic insufficiency, cardiac tamponade, or aortic rupture. Coronary perfusion may be compromised by retrograde dissection, compression by the false lumen, or hypotension (151). Differential pulse volume and blood pressure between the right and left upper extremities was detected in 38% of patients with proximal aortic dissection in one series (152). An abrupt loss of pulse can affect the carotid, subclavian, axillary, radial, ulnar, or femoral arteries, and acute limb ischemia has been reported in 20% of patients (153–155).

A neurologic deficit develops in approximately 15% to 20% of patients with aortic dissection, with transient cerebral ischemia or stroke in up to 10% of cases as a result of extension of dissection into the carotid or vertebral arteries (156). In the International Registry, syncope was a presenting symptom in 13% of patients with proximal dissection and 4% of those with distal dissection (149). Interruption of circulation to the spinal cord can lead to paraplegia (157). Less common neurologic abnormalities include Horner's syndrome, hoarseness, and ischemic neuropathy.

Diagnosis

A high index of suspicion is required to establish the diagnosis promptly, because the presentations of aortic dissection are so myriad and mimic a wide array of other diseases. Accordingly, simple diagnostic tests are used to exclude other causes of the symptoms. An electrocardiogram should be performed to exclude acute MI, because administration of thrombolytic drugs in patients with acute aortic dissection is associated with a high mortality rate (158). Chest radiography results were normal in 12.4% of 427 patients in the International Registry (149), but may help exclude other causes of chest pain, such as pneumothorax. The most common findings in patients with dissection include widening of the mediastinal shadow, pleural effusion, or greater than 10 mm separation of aortic intimal calcification (159).

The most frequently used modalities to identify dissection and to define the sites of origin and termination are computerized tomography (CT), TEE, and magnetic resonance (MR) imaging. The primary diagnostic criterion for diagnosis of aortic dissection by CT is demonstration of two contrast-filled lumens separated by an intimal flap (160). The sensitivity of this method ranges from 93% to 100% and specificity from 87% to 100% (161–163). Inaccuracy may result from inadequate contrast opacification, nonvisualization of the intimal flap, artifacts extending across the aortic lumen that simulate an intimal flap, misinterpretation of adjacent vessels or prominent sinus of Valsalva as the flap, atelectasis, pleural thickening, or thrombosis of the false lumen. Multidetector-row CT scanners offer more rapid image acquisition, variable section thickness, three-dimensional rendering, diminished helical artifacts, and smaller contrast requirements, overcoming many of these pitfalls (164).

The sensitivity and specificity of MR imaging for diagnosis of aortic dissection has been reported to be between 95% and 100% (165–167). The technique enables identification of the entry tear and the extent of dissection; defines the anatomy of the vessels arising from the aortic arch, visceral vessels, and the iliac and common femoral arteries (168–170); and measures blood flow velocities in both the true and false lumens (171,172). When the false lumen is occluded by thrombus, the dissection may be missed and give the appearance of an intact aneurysm (160). Other shortcomings are inaccessibility of the patient for 30 to 60 minutes during image acquisition and unsuitability of the method for those with implanted electronic devices or ferro-magnetic materials. However, a promising potential future application is the use of MR to guide endovascular interventional therapeutic procedures (i.e., fenestration, stenting, and stent grafting) (173,174).

TEE provides rapid multiplane imaging of the aorta and assessment of flow dynamics. The examination can be performed in the emergency department soon after patient presentation (175,176) with sensitivity near 98% and specificity of 63% to 96% (177–180). Limitations are that the coronary arteries and the arch vessels may not be adequately visualized, extension into the visceral or iliac arteries may go undetected, there is a blind spot in the proximal aortic arch (179), and the quality of the study is operator dependent.

Contrast aortography, once the standard method, can accurately identify the site of intimal tear, distinguish the two lumens, define the degree of aortic valve insufficiency, and clearly delineate the branches of the aorta (181). Comparative studies found 88% sensitivity of aortography and 94% specificity for aortic dissection (178). Inaccuracy may arise when there is thrombosis of the false lumen or circumferential dissection. The need for injection of contrast material, the invasive nature of the examination, and delays inherent in preparing the angiography suite have made catheter aortography a secondary diagnostic modality (140).

Intravascular ultrasonography using high-frequency transducers is a promising tool for accurate determination of the location and extent of dissection and assessment of branch vessels. This method may be particularly helpful to differentiate aortic dissection from a penetrating atherothrombotic ulcer, but it has not been widely used (182).

Among the conditions that may initially resemble acute or chronic aortic dissection are MI, thoracic aortic aneurysm without dissection, musculoskeletal chest pain, mediastinal tumors, pericarditis, pleuritis, pneumothorax, pulmonary thromboembolism, cholecystitis, ureteral colic, appendicitis, mesenteric ischemia, pyelonephritis, stroke, transient ischemic attack, and limb ischemia. Given the extensive differential diagnosis, objective diagnostic testing is necessary when the diagnosis of dissection is considered. The diagnosis is most strongly suggested when migratory chest and back pain of less than 24 hours in duration arises in a patient with a history of hypertension.

Treatment

Management of patients with aortic dissection involves decreasing blood pressure and the rate of increase in aortic pressure during ventricular systole (dP/dt), analgesia, and selection of patients who benefit from surgical or endovascular intervention. Both blood pressure and heart rate contribute to the shear force exerted on the aortic wall, which is the major factor responsible for progression of dissection (183). Reduction in the velocity of ventricular contraction retards expansion of the dissection (184). β-Adrenergic antagonists such as intravenous esmolol, propranolol, or metoprolol are the first line of therapy, and they may be given concurrently with sodium nitroprusside to rapidly reduce these hemodynamic forces. Another approach is administration of the α- and β-adrenergic antagonist, labetalol, by intravenous infusion (185). The goal is to decrease systolic blood pressure to the lowest tolerated level without compromising perfusion of vital organs, usually 90 to 110 mm Hg. In patients with reactive airway disease, the calcium channel

antagonists, diltiazem or verapamil, represent potential alternatives to treatment with β-blocker drugs.

Once the diagnosis is established and pain and hemodynamic forces have been controlled, surgical or endovascular intervention may be warranted. In a European cooperative study, continued medical management for patients with type B (distal) aortic dissection was associated with a survival rate no lower that that with surgical therapy (186,187). Survival rates for patients with proximal (type A; DeBakey type I or II) aortic dissection treated medically are poor—43%, 34%, and 28% at 2 weeks, 5 years, and 10 years, respectively (188). A direct comparison of surgical versus medical therapy for type III aortic dissection found comparable survival rates at 1, 5, and 10 years (187). Unless an associated illness precludes surgery, repair is indicated for patients with proximal dissection (189). The usual procedure—replacement of the aortic segment affected by the intimal tear and aneurysmal dilatation with a tubular interposition graft (190)—is associated with a mortality rate between 5% and 32% (191,192).

When insufficiency or other pathology of the aortic valve is present, emergent composite reconstruction carries an 8-year survival rate of 40% to 50% (193). Perioperative complications and mortality increase when dissection extends beyond the ascending aorta into the arch, but operative techniques for reimplantation of the great vessels and coronary arteries have improved. In an international registry of 550 patients with type A aortic dissection, ascending aortic replacement was performed in 91%, root replacement in 32%, and complete arch replacement in 12.6% of patients undergoing surgical repair (194). The overall mortality rate was 27% (23% for patients younger than 70 years and 38% for those older than 70 years; $p = 0.003$).

For survivors of aortic dissection, long-term management should involve β-adrenergic blockade (when not contraindicated) and meticulous blood pressure control. Regardless of the initial management strategy, patients should undergo periodic surveillance imaging by MR imaging or CT scanning every 6 to 12 months to monitor the diameter of the aorta, the extent of dissection, and the status of the repair that might require additional intervention. Clinical events or significant radiographic changes in the extent of dissection or diameter of the aorta warrant consideration of surgical repair, because enlargement of the false channel and late rupture is the most common cause of death after the initial event. Leakage, rupture, arterial compromise producing tissue ischemia because of the dissection, enlargement of aortic diameter beyond 5.0 cm, and extension of dissection despite therapy, persistent pain, or poorly controlled hypertension constitute potential indications for repair (143).

Endovascular stent-graft devices may be placed over the entry tear to control distal thoracic aortic dissection by thrombosis of the false lumen, but there is less experience with this technology in patients with type A than with type B dissections (195). Patency of branch vessels is achieved by supplementary stenting. In one series of 23 patients, the 30-day mortality rate was 16%, but there were no late deaths over a follow-up period of 13 months (196). The procedures may be combined with septal fenestration to equalize pressure in the true and false channels (197,198). As endovascular techniques improve, their role is expected to increase (199,200).

PENETRATING AORTIC ULCER

A penetrating aortic ulcer is an ulcerated atheromatous lesion that disrupts the internal elastic lamina and erodes into the media, which in some cases may mimic or initiate aortic dissection pseudoaneurysm formation, intramural hematoma, or rupture (201). Among 684 aortograms in cases of suspected aortic dissection, the incidence of penetrating ulcer was 2.3% (202). Penetrating ulcers typically cause sudden back or chest pain in elderly patients with hypertension. Intramural hematoma develops without an intimal flap. The extensive atheromatous disease at the site of the ulcer is uncommon in the region of the intimal flap of a dissection. Accurate diagnosis of this condition is critical, because medical management with blood pressure and heart rate control in patients with uncomplicated ulceration is associated with a good outcome (203,204). Surgical intervention is required when hemodynamic instability, pseudoaneurysm, or rupture occurs, but endovascular stent-graft repair has been successfully used in patients (205–207).

INTRAMURAL HEMATOMA

Intramural hematoma constitutes a variant of aortic dissection in which no entry point or intimal flap can be identified. Optimum therapy for this condition is unknown, and complications such as aortic dissection and aortic rupture occur unpredictably (208). Whether the intramural hematoma arises from a small intimal tear or rupture of vasa vasorum within the aortic wall remains controversial (209). On CT scan, intramural hematoma may appear as a crescent-shaped or circumferential thickening of the aortic wall with no flow in the space containing the hematoma. Up to 17% of patients with aortic dissection actually have intramural hematoma, but only CT or MR imaging currently makes the distinction. The clinical course is variable: The hematoma may persist, reabsorb returning the aorta to a normal appearance, lead to aneurysm with the possibility of rupture, or convert to dissection (210).

Among 124 patients with intramural hematoma in one series, in-hospital mortality was 7% for 41 patients with proximal aortic hematomas and 1% for 83 patients with distal hematomas (211), which was substantially better than the 47% mortality rate reported with proximal intramural hematomas and the 13% rate in patients with distal hematomas in another series of medically managed patients (212). In a recent report, hematoma progressed to aortic dissection in 45% of 66 patients and the mortality rate was 20% at 30 days. Late progression occurred in 21% and death occurred in 17% of patients, yielding 1-, 2-, and 5-year survival rates of 76%, 73%, and 43%, respectively. Regardless of aortic diameter, type A intramural hematoma is more likely to progress, and early surgical intervention is recommended for such cases (213). In a metaanalysis of 143 patients, the mortality rate for patients with type A hematomas undergoing surgery was 14% versus 36% for those treated medically, with a relative risk reduction of 75% (95% CI, 57–98%) with surgery ($p < 0.02$). The mortality rate for patients with type B hematomas treated medically was 14%, similar to the outcome in the surgical group (214).

REFERENCES

1. Khoury Z, Gottlieb S, Stern S, et al. Frequency and distribution of atherosclerotic plaques in the thoracic aorta as determined by transesophageal echocardiography in patients with coronary artery disease. *Am J Cardiol* 1997;79:23–27.
2. Davila-Roman VG, Murphy SF, Nickerson NJ, et al. Atherosclerosis of the ascending aorta is an independent predictor of long-term neurologic events and mortality. *J Am Coll Cardiol* 1999;33:1308–1316.
3. Amarenco P, Cohen A, Tzourio C, et al. Atherosclerotic disease of the aortic arch and risk of ischemic stroke. *N Engl J Med* 1994;331:1474–1479.
4. Atherosclerotic disease of the aortic arch as a risk factor for recurrent ischemic stroke. The French Study of Aortic Plaques in Stroke Group. *N Engl J Med* 1996;334:1216–1221.
5. Fazio GP, Redberg RF, Winslow T, et al. Transesophageal echocardiographically detected atherosclerotic aortic plaque is a marker for coronary artery disease. *J Am Coll Cardiol* 1993;21:144–150.
6. DeLaurentis DA, Friedmann P, Wolferth CC Jr, et al. Atherosclerosis and hypoplastic aortoiliac system. *Surgery* 1978;83:27–37.
7. Brewster DC. Clinical and anatomical considerations for surgery in aortoiliac disease and results of surgical treatment. *Circulation* 1991;83[Suppl I]:I-42–I-52.
8. Debakey ME, Lawrie GM, Glaeser DH. Patterns of atherosclerosis and their surgical significance. *Ann Surg* 1985;201:115–131.
9. Leriche R, Morel A. The syndrome of thrombotic obliteration of the aortic bifurcation. *Ann Surg* 1948;127:193–204.
10. Diethrich EB. Endovascular treatment of abdominal aortic occlusive disease: the impact of stents and intravascular ultrasound imaging. *Eur J Vasc Surg* 1993;7:228–236.
11. Management of peripheral arterial disease (CAD). Transatlantic Intersocietal Consensus (TASC). *J Vasc Surg* 2000;31[Suppl]:S1–S296.
12. Johnston KW. Balloon angioplasty: predictive factors for long-term success. *Semin Vasc Surg* 1989;3:117–122.
13. Sullivan TM, Childs MB, Bacharach JM, et al. Percutaneous transluminal angioplasty and primary stenting of the iliac arteries in 288 patients. *J Vasc Surg* 1997;25:829–839.
14. Palmaz JC, Laborde JC, Rivera FJ, et al. Stenting of the iliac arteries with the Palmaz stent: experience from a multicenter trial. *Cardiovasc Intervent Radiol* 1992;15:291–297.
15. Busuttil RW, Keehn G, Milliken J, et al. Aortic saddle embolus: a twenty-year experience. *Ann Surg* 1983;197:698–706.
16. Fogarty T, Daily P, Shumway N, et al. Experience with balloon catheter technique for arterial embolectomy. *Am J Surg* 1971;122:231–237.
17. Khatibzadeh M, Mitusch R, Stierle U, et al. Aortic atherosclerotic plaques as a source of systemic embolism. *J Am Coll Cardiol* 1996;27:664–669.
18. Hyman BT, Landas SK, Ashman RF. Warfarin-related purple toes syndrome and cholesterol microembolization. *Am J Med* 1987;82:1233–1237.
19. Bruns FJ, Segel DP, Adler S. Control of cholesterol embolization by discontinuation of anticoagulant therapy. *Am J Med Sci* 1978;275:105–108.
20. Ramirez G, O'Neill WM Jr, Lambert R, et al. Cholesterol embolization: a complication of angiography. *Arch Intern Med* 1978;138:1430–1432.
21. Drost H, Buis B, Haan D, et al. Cholesterol embolism as a complication of left heart catheterization. Report of seven cases. *Br Heart J* 1984;52:339–342.
22. Colt HG, Begg RJ, Saporito JJ. Cholesterol emboli after cardiac

catheterization: eight cases and a review of the literature. *Medicine* 1988;67:389–400.

23. Eggebrecht H, Oldenbureg O, Dirsch O, et al. Potential embolization by atherosclerotic debris dislodged from aortic wall during cardiac catheterization: histologic and clinical findings in 7621 patients. *Cathet Cardiovasc Interv* 2000;49:389–394.

24. Olin JW. Syndromes that mimic vasculitis. *Curr Opin Cardiol* 1991;6:768–774.

25. Fine MJ, Kapoor WN, Falanga V. Cholesterol crystal embolization: a review of 221 cases in the English language. *Angiology* 1987;38:769–784.

26. Pennington M, Yeager J, Skelton J, et al. Cholesterol embolization syndrome: cutaneous histopathological features and the variable onset of symptoms in patients with different risk factors. *Br J Derm* 2002;146:511–517.

27. Cohen A, Tzourio C, Bertrand B, et al. Aortic plaque morphology and vascular events: a follow-up study in patients with ischemic stroke: FAPS Investigators. French Study of Aortic Plaques in Stroke. *Circulation* 1997;96:3828–3841.

28. Cohen A, Amarenco P. Atherosclerosis of the thoracic aorta: from risk stratification to treatment. *Am J Cardiol* 2002;90:1333–1335.

29. Scolari F, Tardanico R, Zani R, et al. Cholesterol crystal embolism: a recognizable cause of renal disease. *Am J Kidney Dis* 2000;36:1089–1109.

30. Kasinath BS, Lewis EJ. Eosinophilia as a clue to the diagnosis of atheroembolic renal disease. *Arch Intern Med* 1987;147:1384–1385.

31. Pitt B, Waters D, Brown WV, et al. Aggressive lipid-lowering therapy compared with angioplasty in stable coronary artery disease. *N Engl J Med* 1999;341:70–76.

32. Woolfson RG, Lachmann H. Improvement in renal cholesterol emboli syndrome after simvastatin. *Lancet* 1998;351:1331–1332.

33. Tunick PA, Nayar AC, Goodkin GM, et al. Effect of treatment on the incidence of stroke and other emboli in 519 patients with severe thoracic aortic plaque. *Am J Cardiol* 2002;90:1320–1325.

34. Belenfant X, Meyrier A, Jacquot C. Supportive treatment improves survival in multivessel cholesterol crystal embolization. *Am J Kidney Dis* 1999;33:840–850.

35. Keen RR, McCarthy WJ, Shireman PK, et al. Surgical management of atheroembolization. *J Vasc Surg* 1995;21:773–781.

36. Fisher DF Jr, Clagett GP, Brigham RA, et al. Dilemmas in dealing with the blue toe syndrome: aortic versus peripheral source. *Am J Surg* 1984;148:836–839.

37. Davies MJ. Aortic aneurysm formation: lessons from human studies and experimental models. *Circulation* 1998;98:193–195.

38. Goodall S, Porter KE, Bell PR, et al. Enhanced invasive properties exhibited by smooth muscle cells are associated with elevated production of MMP-2 in patients with aortic aneurysms. *Eur J Vasc Endovasc Surg* 2002;24:72–80.

39. Reilly JM, Brophy CM, Tilson MD. Characterization of an elastase from aneurysmal aorta which degrades intact aortic elastin. *Ann Vasc Surg* 1992;6:499–502.

40. Anidjar S, Dobrin PB, Eichorst M, et al. Correlation of inflammatory infiltrate with the enlargement of experimental aortic aneurysms. *J Vasc Surg* 1992;16:139–147.

41. Pearce WH, Koch AE. Cellular components and features of immune response in abdominal aortic aneurysms. *Ann NY Acad Sci* 1996;800:175–185.

42. Louwrens HD, Kwaan HC, Pearce WH, et al. Plasminogen activator and plasminogen activator inhibitor expression by normal and aneurysmal human aortic smooth muscle cells in culture. *Eur J Vasc Endovasc Surg* 1995;10:289–293.

43. Anidjar S, Dobrin PB, Chejfec G, et al. Experimental study of determinants of aneurysmal expansion of the abdominal aorta. *Ann Vasc Surg* 1994;8:127–136.

44. Schillinger M, Domanovits H, Bayegan K, et al. C-reactive protein and mortality in patients with acute aortic disease. *Intensive Care Med* 2002;28:740–745.

45. Cronenwett JL, Murphy TF, Zelenock GB, et al. Actuarial analysis of variables associated with rupture of small abdominal aortic aneurysms. *Surgery* 1985;98:472–483.

46. Gore I, Hirst AE. Arteriosclerotic aneurysms of the abdominal aorta: a review. *Prog Cardiovasc Dis* 1973;17:113–149.

47. Stokes J, Butcher HR Jr. Abdominal aortic aneurysms: factors influencing operative mortality and criteria of operability. *Arch Surg* 1973;107:297–302.

48. Hall AD, Zubrin JR, Moore WS, et al. Surgical treatment of aortic aneurysm in the aged. *Arch Surg* 1970;100:455–460.

49. Hammond EC, Garfinkel L. Coronary heart disease, stroke, and aortic aneurysm. *Arch Environ Health* 1969;19:167–182.

50. Hahn RT, Roman MJ, Mogtader AH, et al. Association of aortic dilation with regurgitant, stenotic and functionally normal bicuspid aortic valves. *J Am Coll Cardiol* 1992;19:283–288.

51. Noon GP. Aneurysms of the aortic arch. In: Campbell AD, ed. *Aortic aneurysms: surgical therapy*. Mount Kisco, NY: Futura Publishing, 1981;79–100.

52. Morse DE. Embryology, anatomy and histology of the aorta. In: Lindsay J, Hurst JW, eds. *The aorta*. New York: Grune & Stratton, 1979:15–37.

53. Dillon ML, Young WG, Sealy WC. Aneurysms of the descending thoracic aorta. *Ann Thorac Surg* 1967;3:430–438.

54. DeBakey ME, Noon GP. Aneurysms of the thoracic aorta. *Mod Concepts Cardiovasc Dis* 1975;44:53–58.

55. Joyce JW, Fairbairn JF 2nd, Kincaid OW, et al. Aneurysms of the thoracic aorta: a clinical study with special reference to prognosis. *Circulation* 1964;29:176–181.

56. Lindsay J Jr. Thoracic aneurysms. In: Lindsay J, Hurst JW, eds. *The aorta*. New York: Grune & Stratton, 1979:121–130.

57. Varkey B, Tristani FE. Compression of pulmonary artery and bronchus by descending thoracic aortic aneurysm. *Am J Cardiol* 1974;34:610–614.

58. Birnholz JC, Ferrucci JT, Wyman SM. Roentgen features of dysphagia aortica. *Radiology* 1974;111:93–96.

59. Finkbohner R, Johnston D, Crawford ES, et al. Marfan syndrome. Long-term survival and complications after aortic aneurysm repair. *Circulation* 1995;91:728–733.

60. Cranley JJ, Herrmann LG, Preuninger RM. Natural history of aneurysms of the aorta. *Arch Surg* 1954;69:185–197.

61. Fomon JJ, Kurzweg FT, Broadaway RK. Aneurysms of the aorta: a review. *Ann Surg* 1967;165:557–563.

62. Crawford ES, Snyder DM, Cho GC, et al. Progress in treatment of thoracoabdominal and abdominal aortic aneurysms involving celiac, superior mesenteric and renal arteries. *Ann Surg* 1978;188:404–421.

63. Creech O Jr, DeBakey ME, Morris GC Jr. Aneurysm of thoracoabdominal aorta involving the celiac, superior mesenteric and renal arteries. Report of four cases treated by resection and homograft replacement. *Ann Surg* 1956;144:549–573.

64. Etheredge SN, Yee J, Smith JV, et al. Successful resection of a large aneurysm of the upper abdominal aorta and replacement with homograft. *Surgery* 1955;38:1071–1081.

65. Hardy JD, Timmis HH, Saleh SS, et al. Thoracoabdominal aortic aneurysm: simplified surgical management with case report. *Ann Surg* 1967;166:1008–1011.

66. Heyde MN, van der Zwaveling A. Resection of an abdominal aortic aneurysm in a patient with Marfan's syndrome. *J Cardiovasc Surg* 1961;2:359–366.

67. DeBakey ME. Surgical considerations in the treatment of aneurysms of the thoracoabdominal aorta. *Ann Surg* 1965;162:650–662.

68. Auerbach O, Garfinkel L. Atherosclerosis and aneurysm of the aorta in relation to smoking habits and age. *Chest* 1980;78:805–809.

69. Carlsson J, Sternby NH. Aortic aneurysms. *Acta Chir Scand* 1964;127:466–473.

70. Cole C, Barber GG, Bouchard AG, et al. Abdominal aortic aneurysm: consequences of a positive family history. *Can J Surg* 1989;32:117–120.

71. Allardice JT, Allwright GJ, Wafula JM, et al. High prevalence of abdominal aortic aneurysm in men with peripheral vascular disease: screening by ultrasonography. *Br J Surg* 1988;75:240–242.

72. Darling RC, Messina CR, Brewster DC, et al. Autopsy study of unoperated abdominal aortic aneurysms: the case for early resection. *Circulation* 1977;56[Suppl 2]:161.

73. Johansen K, Koepsell T. Familial tendency for abdominal aortic aneurysm. *JAMA* 1986;256:1934–1936.

74. Johnson G Jr, Avery A, McDougal EG, et al. Aneurysms of the abdominal aorta. Incidence in blacks and whites in North Carolina. *Arch Surg* 1985;120:1138–1140.

75. Leopold GR, Goldberger LE, Bernstein EF. Ultrasonic detection and evaluation of abdominal aortic aneurysms. *Surgery* 1972;72:939–945.

76. Scott RA. Ultrasound screening in the management of abdominal aortic aneurysms. *Int Angiol* 1986;5:263–267.

77. Bickerstaff LK, Hollier LH, Van Peenan HJ, et al. Abdominal aortic aneurysms: the changing natural history. *J Vasc Surg* 1984;1:6–12.
78. Bowers D, Cave WS. Aneurysms of the abdominal aorta: a twenty-year study. *J R Soc Med* 1985;78:812–820.
79. Cabellon S Jr, Moncrief CL, Pierre DR, et al. Incidence of abdominal aortic aneurysms in patients with atheromatous arterial disease. *Am J Surg* 1983;146:575–576.
80. Graham M, Chan A. Ultrasound screening for clinically occult abdominal aortic aneurysm. *Can Med Assoc J* 1988;138:627–629.
81. Thurmond AS, Semler HJ. Abdominal aortic aneurysm: incidence in a population at risk. *J Cardiovasc Surg* 1986;27:457–460.
82. Sommerville RL, Allen EV, Edwards JE. Bland and infected arteriosclerotic abdominal aortic aneurysms: a clinicopathologic study. *Medicine* 1959;38:207–221.
83. Friedman SA, Hufnagel CA, Conrad PW, et al. Abdominal aortic aneurysms: clinical status and results of surgery in 100 consecutive cases. *JAMA* 1967;200:1147–1151.
84. Gliedman ML, Ayers WB, Vestal BL. Aneurysms of the abdominal aorta and its branches: a study of untreated patients. *Ann Surg* 1957;146:207–214.
85. Schatz IJ, Fairbairn JR 2nd, Juergens JL. Abdominal aortic aneurysms: a reappraisal. *Circulation* 1962;26:200–205.
86. DeBakey ME, Crawford ES, Cooley DA, et al. Aneurysm of abdominal aorta: analysis of graft replacement therapy 1 to 11 years after operation. *Ann Surg* 1964;160:622–639.
87. Reilly JM, Tilson MD. Incidence and etiology of abdominal aortic aneurysms. *Surg Clin North Am* 1989;69:705–711.
88. Norrgard O, Rais O, Anguist K. Familial occurrence of abdominal aortic aneurysms. *Surgery* 1984;95:650–656.
89. Tilson MD, Seashore M. Human genetics of the abdominal aortic aneurysm. *Surg Gynecol Obstet* 1984;158:129–132.
90. Tilson MD, Seashore M. Fifty families with abdominal aortic aneurysms in two or more first-order relatives. *Am J Surg* 1984;147:551–553.
91. Busuttil RW, Abou-Zamzam AM, Machleder HI. Collagenase activity of the human aorta. A comparison of patients with and without abdominal aortic aneurysms. *Arch Surg* 1980;115:1373–1378.
92. Menashi S, Campa JS, Greenhalgh RM, et al. Collagen in abdominal aortic aneurysm: typing, content, and degradation. *J Vasc Surg* 1987;6:578–582.
93. Sumner D, Hokanson D, Strandness D. Stress-strain characteristics and collagen-elastin content of abdominal aortic aneurysms. *Surg Gynecol Obstet* 1970;130:459–466.
94. Kuivanieri H, Tromp G, Prockup DJ. Genetic causes of aortic aneurysms. *J Clin Invest* 1991;88:1441–144.
95. Ernst CB. Abdominal aortic aneurysm. *N Engl J Med* 1993;328:1167–1172.
96. Estes JE Jr. Abdominal aortic aneurysm: a study of one hundred and two cases. *Circulation* 1950;2:258.
97. Wright B, Urdaneta E, Wright IS. Re-opening the case of the abdominal aortic aneurysm. *Circulation* 1956;13:754–768.
98. Blakemore AH, Voorhees AB Jr. Aneurysm of the aorta: a review of 365 cases. *Angiology* 1954;5:209–231.
99. Kampmeier RH. Aneurysm of the abdominal aorta: a study of 73 cases. *Am J Med Sci* 1936;192:97–109.
100. Szilagyi DE, Smith RF, DeRusso FJ, et al. Contribution of abdominal aortic aneurysmectomy to prolongation of life. *Ann Surg* 1966;164:678–699.
101. Szilagyi DE, Elliott JP, Smith RF. Clinical fate of the patient with asymptomatic abdominal aortic aneurysm and unfit for surgical treatment. *Arch Surg* 1972;104:600–606.
102. Foster JH, Bolasny BL, Gobbel WG Jr. Comparative study of elective resection and expectant treatment of abdominal aortic aneurysm. *Surg Gynecol Obstet* 1969;129:1–9.
103. Bernstein EF, Chan EL. Abdominal aortic aneurysm in high-risk patients: outcome of selective management based on size and expansion rate. *Ann Surg* 1984;200:255–263.
104. Barrat-Boyes BG. Symptomatology and prognosis of abdominal aortic aneurysm. *Lancet* 1957;2:716–720.
105. Tallgren LG, von Bonsdorff CH. Symptomatology and prognosis of abdominal aortic aneurysm. *Acta Med Scand* 1964;175[Suppl 412]:287.
106. Brewster DC, Darling RC, Raines JK, et al. Assessment of abdominal aortic aneurysm size. *Circulation* 1977;56[Suppl 2]:II-164–II-169.
107. Pennell RC, Hollier LH, Lie JT, et al. Inflammatory abdominal aortic aneurysms: a thirty-year review. *J Vasc Surg* 1985;2:859–869.
108. Bonamigo TP, Bianco C, Becker M, et al. Inflammatory aneurysms of infra-renal abdominal aorta. A case-control study. *Minerva Cardioangiol* 2002;50:253–258.
109. Ashton HA, Buxton MJ, Day NE, et al.. The Multicentre Aneurysm Screening Study (MASS) into the effect of abdominal aortic aneurysm screening on mortality in men: a randomised controlled trial. *Lancet* 2002;360:1531–1539.
110. Multicentre Aneurysm Screening Study Group. Multicentre aneurysm screening study (MASS): cost effectiveness analysis of screening for abdominal aortic aneurysms based on four year results from randomised controlled trial. *BMJ* 2002;325:1135–1142.
111. Powell JT, Greenhalgh RM, Ruckley CV, et al. The UK Small Aneurysm Trial. *Ann NY Acad Sci* 1996;800:249–251.
112. Lederle FA, Wilson SE, Johnson GR, et al. Immediate repair compared with surveillance of small abdominal aortic aneurysms. *N Engl J Med* 2002;346:1437–1444.
113. Brady A, Fowkes F, Greenhalgh R, et al. Risk factors for postoperative death following elective surgical repair of abdominal aortic aneurysm: results from the UK Small Aneurysm Trial. *Br J Surg* 2000;87:742–749.
114. Parodi JC, Palamz JC, Barone HD. Transfemoral intraluminal graft implantation for abdominal aortic aneurysms. *Ann Vasc Surg* 1991;5:491–499.
115. Carpenter JP, Baum RA, Barker CF, et al. Impact of exclusion criteria on patient selection for endovascular abdominal aortic aneurysm repair. *J Vasc Surg* 2001;34:1050–1054.
116. Becker GJ, Kovacs M, Mathison MN, et al. Risk stratification and outcomes of transluminal endografting for abdominal aortic aneurysm: 7-year experience and long-term follow-up. *J Vasc Interv Radiol* 2001;12:1033–1046.
117. Mathison M, Becker GJ, Katzen BT, et al. The influence of female gender on the outcome of endovascular abdominal aortic aneurysm repair. *J Vasc Interv Radiol* 2001;12:1047–1051.
118. Wolf YG, Tillich M, Lee WA, et al. Impact of aortoiliac tortuosity on endovascular repair of abdominal aortic aneurysms: evaluation of 3D computer-based assessment. *J Vasc Surg* 2001;34:594–599.
119. Veith FJ, Johnston KW. Endovascular treatment of abdominal aortic aneurysms: an innovation in evolution and under evaluation. *J Vasc Surg* 2002;35:183.
120. White RA, Donayre C, Walot I, et al. Abdominal aortic aneurysm rupture following endoluminal graft deployment: report of a predictable event. *J Endovasc Ther* 2000;7:257–262.
121. Abraham CZ, Chuter TA, Reilly LM, et al. Abdominal aortic aneurysm repair with the Zenith stent graft: short to midterm results. *J Vasc Surg* 2002;36:217–225.
122. Zarins CK, White RA, Hodgson KJ, et al. Endoleak as a predictor of outcome after endovascular aneurysm repair: AneuRx multicenter clinical trial. *J Vasc Surg* 2000;32:90–107.
123. Zarins CK, White RA, Moll FL, et al. The AneuRx stent graft: four-year results and worldwide experience 2000. *J Vasc Surg* 2001;33:S135–S145.
124. Sapirstein W, Chandeysson P, Wentz C. The Food and Drug Administration approval of endovascular grafts for abdominal aortic aneurysm: an 18-month retrospective. *J Vasc Surg* 2001;34:180–183.
125. Stelter W, Umscheid T, Ziegler P. Three-year experience with modular stent-graft devices for endovascular AAA treatment. *J Endovasc Surg* 1997;4:362–369.
126. Amesur NB, Zajko AB, Orons PD, et al. Endovascular treatment of iliac limb stenoses or occlusions in 31 patients treated with the ancure endograft. *J Vasc Interv Radiol* 2000;11:421–428.
127. Greenberg RK, Lawrence-Brown M, Bhandari G, et al. An update of the Zenith endovascular graft for abdominal aortic aneurysms: initial implantation and mid-term follow-up data. *J Vasc Surg* 2001;33:S157–S164.
128. Broeders IA, Blankensteijn JD, Wever JJ, et al. Mid-term fixation stability of the EndoVascular Technologies endograft. EVT Investigators. *Eur J Vasc Endovasc Surg* 1999;18:300–307.
129. Makaroun MS, Deaton DH. Is proximal aortic neck dilatation after endovascular aneurysm exclusion a cause for concern? *J Vasc Surg* 2001;33:S39–S45.
130. Boucher CA, Brewster DC, Darling RC, et al. Determination of car-

diac risk by dipyridamole-thallium imaging before peripheral vascular surgery. *N Engl J Med* 1985;312:389–394.

131. Leppo J, Plaja J, Gionet M, et al. Noninvasive evaluation of cardiac risk before elective vascular surgery. *J Am Coll Cardiol* 1987;9: 269–276.

132. Raby KE, Goldman L, Creager MA, et al. Correlation between preoperative ischemia and major cardiac events after peripheral vascular surgery. *N Engl J Med* 1989;321:1296–1300.

133. Eagle KA, Coley CM, Newell JB, et al. Combining clinical and thallium data optimizes preoperative assessment of cardiac risk before major vascular surgery. *Ann Intern Med* 1989;110:859–866.

134. Hertzer NR, Beven EG, Young JR, et al. Coronary artery disease in peripheral vascular patients. A classification of 1000 coronary angiograms and results of surgical management. *Ann Surg* 1984;199: 223–233.

135. Jamieson WR, Janusz MT, Miyagishima RT, et al. Influence of ischemic heart disease on early and late mortality after surgery for peripheral occlusive vascular disease. *Circulation* 1982;66: I92–I97.

136. Tomatis LA, Fierens EE, Verbrugge GP. Evaluation of surgical risk in peripheral vascular disease by coronary arteriography: a series of 100 cases. *Surgery* 1972;71:429–435.

137. McCollum CH, Garcia-Rinaldi R, Graham JM, et al. Myocardial revascularization prior to subsequent major surgery in patients with coronary artery disease. *Surgery* 1977;81:302–304.

138. Fleisher LA, Rosenbaum SH, Barash PG. Preoperative silent ischemia is a predictor of postoperative cardiac events in patients undergoing elective noncardiac surgery. *Soc Cardiovasc Anesthes* 1990;12:98.

139. McCabe CJ, Reidy NC, Abbott WM, et al. The value of electrocardiogram monitoring during treadmill testing for peripheral vascular disease. *Surgery* 1981;89:183–186.

140. Khan IA, Nair CK. Clinical, diagnostic and management perspectives of aortic dissection. *Chest* 2002;122:311–328.

141. Hirst AE Jr, Johns VJ Jr, Kime SW Jr. Dissecting aneurysms of the aorta: a review of 505 cases. *Medicine* 1958;37:217–279.

142. Crawford ES. The diagnosis and management of aortic dissection. *JAMA* 1990;264:2537–2541.

143. DeSanctis RW, Doroghazi RM, Austen WG, et al. Aortic dissection. *N Engl J Med* 1990;317:1060–1067.

144. Wilson SK, Hutchins GM. Aortic dissecting aneurysms: causative factors in 204 subjects. *Arch Pathol Lab Med* 1982;106:175–180.

145. Coplan NL, Goldman B, Mechanic G, et al. Sudden hemodynamic collapse following relief of cardiac tamponade in a patient with aortic dissection. *Am Heart J* 1986;111:405–406.

146. Meszaros I, Morocz J, Szlavi J, et al. Epidemiology and clinicopathology of aortic dissection. *Chest* 2000;117:1271–1278.

147. DeBakey ME, McCollum CH, Crawford ES, et al. Dissection and dissecting aneurysms of the aorta: twenty-year follow-up of five hundred twenty-seven patients treated surgically. *Surgery* 1982;92:1118–1134.

148. Spittell PC, Spittell JA Jr, Joyce JW, et al. Clinical features and differential diagnosis of aortic dissection: experience with 236 cases (1980 through 1990). *Mayo Clin Proc* 1993;68:642–651.

149. Hagan PG, Nienaber CA, Isselbacher EM, et al. The International Registry of acute Aortic Dissection (IRAD). New Insights into an old disease. *JAMA* 2000;283:897–903.

150. Perron AD, Gibbs M. Thoracic aortic dissection secondary to crack cocaine ingestion. *Am J Emerg Med* 1997;12:507–509.

151. Eisenberg MJ, Rice SA, Paraschos A. The clinical spectrum of patients with aneurysms of the ascending aorta. *Am Heart J* 1993;125: 1380–1385.

152. von Kodolitsch Y, Schwartz AG, Nienaber CA. Clinical prediction of acute aortic dissection. *Arch Intern Med* 2000;160:2977–2982.

153. Fann JI, Sarris GE, Mitchell RS, et al. Treatment of patients with aortic dissection presenting with peripheral vascular complications. *Ann Surg* 1990;212:705–713.

154. Cambria RP, Brewster DC, Gertler J, et al. Vascular complications associated with spontaneous aortic dissection. *J Vasc Surg* 1988;7:199–209.

155. Giles S, Walters H. Aortic dissection presenting as acute leg ischaemia. *Clin Radiol* 1990;42:116–117.

156. Gerber O, Heyer EJ, Vieux U. Painless dissections of the aorta presenting as acute neurologic syndromes. *Stroke* 1986;17:644–647.

157. Strouse PJ, Shea MJ, Guy GE, et al. Aortic dissection presenting as spinal cord ischemia with a false negative aortogram. *Cardiovasc Intervent Radiol* 1990;13:77–82.

158. Butler J, Davies AH, Westaby S. Streptokinase in acute aortic dissection. *BMJ* 1990;300:517–519.

159. Petasnick JP. Radiologic evaluation of aortic dissection. *Radiology* 1991;180:297–305.

160. Cigarroa JE, Isselbacher EM, DeSanctis RW, et al. Diagnostic imaging in the evaluation of suspected aortic dissection-old standards and new directions. *N Engl J Med* 1993;128:35–43.

161. Thorsen MK, San Dretto MA, Lawson TL, et al. Dissecting aortic aneurysms: accuracy of computed tomographic diagnosis. *Radiology* 1983;148:773–777.

162. Nienaber CA, Kodolitsch Y, Nicolas V, et al. The diagnosis of thoracic aortic dissection by noninvasive imaging procedures. *N Engl J Med* 1993;328:1–9.

163. Sommer T, Fehske W, Holzknecht N, et al. Aortic dissection: a comparative study of diagnosis with spiral CT, multiplanar transesophageal echocardiography, and MR imaging. *Radiology* 1996;199:347–352.

164. Rubin GD. MDCT imaging of the aorta and peripheral vessels. *Eur J Radiol* 2003;45[Suppl]:S42–S49.

165. Tomiguchi S, Morishita S, Nakashima R, et al. Usefulness of turbo-FLASH dynamic MR imaging of dissecting aneurysms of the thoracic aorta. *Cardiovasc Intervent Radiol* 1994;17:17–21.

166. Mendelson DS, Apter S, Mitty HA, et al. Residual dissection of the thoracic aorta after repair: MRI-angiographic correlation. *Comput Med Imaging Graph* 1991;15:31–35.

167. White R, Ullyot D, Higgins CB. MR imaging of the aorta after surgery for aortic dissection. *Am J Roentgenol* 1988;150:87–92.

168. Prince MR, Narasimham DL, Stanley JC, et al. Breath-hold gadolinium-enhanced MR angiography of the abdominal aorta and its major branches. *Radiology* 1995;197:785–792.

169. Wolff KA, Herold CJ, Tempany CM, et al. Aortic dissection: atypical patterns seen at MR imaging. *Radiology* 1991;181:489–495.

170. Earls JP, DeSena S, Bluemke DA. Gadolinium-enhanced three-dimensional MR angiography of the entire aorta and iliac arteries with dynamic manual table translation. *Radiology* 1998;209:844–849.

171. Chang JM, Friese K, Caputo GR, et al. MR measurement of blood flow in the true and false channel in chronic aortic dissection. *J Comp Assist Tomogr* 1991;15:418–423.

172. Mitchell L, Jenkins JP, Brownlee WC, et al. Aortic dissection: morphology and differential flow velocity patterns demonstrated by magnetic resonance imaging. *Clin Radiol* 1988;39:458–461.

173. Adam G, Neuerburg J, Bucker A, et al. Interventional magnetic resonance. Initial clinical experience with a 1.5-tesla magnetic resonance system combined with c-arm fluoroscopy. *Invest Radiol* 1997;32: 191–197.

174. Yang X, Bolster BD Jr, Kraitchman DL, et al. Intravascular MR-monitored balloon angioplasty: an in vivo feasibility study. *J Vasc Interv Radiol* 1998;9:953–959.

175. Omoto R, Kyo S, Matsumura M. Evaluation of biplane color Doppler transesophageal echocardiography in 200 consecutive patients. *Circulation* 1992;85:1237–1247.

176. Pearson AC, Castello R, Lebovitz AJ. Safety and utility of transesophageal echocardiography in the critically ill patient. *Am Heart J* 1990;119:1083–1089.

177. Hashimoto S, Kumada T, Osakada G, et al. Assessment of transesophageal Doppler echocardiography in dissecting aortic aneurysm. *J Am Coll Cardiol* 1989;14:1253–1262.

178. Erbel R, Daniel W, Visser C, et al. Echocardiography in diagnosis of aortic dissection. *Lancet* 1989;330:457–460.

179. Keren A, Kim CB, Hu BS, et al. Accuracy of biplane and multiplane transesophageal echocardiography in diagnosis of typical acute aortic dissection and intramural hematoma. *J Am Coll Cardiol* 1996;28: 627–636.

180. Balla RJ, Nanda NC, Gatewood R, et al. Usefulness of transesophageal echocardiography in assessment of aortic dissection. *Circulation* 1991;84:1903–1914.

181. Soto B, Harman MA, Ceballos R, et al. Angiographic diagnosis of dissecting aneurysm of the aorta. *Am J Roentgenol Radium Ther Nucl Med* 1972;116:146–154.

182. Weintraub AR, Erbel R, Gorge G, et al. Intravascular ultrasound imaging in acute aortic dissection. *J Am Coll Cardiol* 1994;24: 495–503.

183. Prokop EK, Palmer RF, Wheat MW. Hydrodynamic forces in dissecting aneurysms: in-vitro studies in a tygon model and in dog aortas. *Circ Res* 1970;27:121–127.

184. Wheat MW Jr, Palmer RF. Treatment of dissecting aneurysms of the aorta without surgery. *Prog Cardiovasc Dis* 1968;11:198–210.
185. Grubb BP, Sirio C, Zelis R. Intravenous labetolol in acute aortic dissection. *JAMA* 1987;258:78–79.
186. Chirillo F, Marchiori MC, Andriolo L. Outcome of 290 patients with aortic dissection: a 12-year multicentre experience. *Eur Heart J* 1990;11:311–319.
187. Glower DD, Fann JI, Speier RH, et al. Comparison of medical and surgical therapy for uncomplicated descending aortic dissections. *Circulation* 1990;82[Suppl IV]:IV-39–IV-46.
188. Masuda Y, Yamada Z, Morooka N, et al. Prognosis of patients with medically treated aortic dissections. *Circulation* 1991;84[Suppl III]:III-7–III-13.
189. Borst HG, Laass J. Surgical treatment of thoracic aortic aneurysms. *Adv Card Surg* 1993;4:47–87.
190. Crawford ES, Svensson LG, Coselli JS, et al. Surgical treatment of aneurysm and/or dissection of the ascending aorta, transverse aortic arch and ascending aorta and transverse aortic arch. *J Thorac Cardiovasc Surg* 1989;98:659–673.
191. Ikonomidis JS, Weisel RD, Mouradian MS, et al. Thoracic aortic surgery. *Circulation* 1991;84[Suppl III].III1-6.
192. Svensson LG, Crawford ES, Hess KR, et al. Dissection of the aorta and dissecting aortic aneurysm. Improving early and long-term surgical results. *Circulation* 1990;82[Suppl IV]:IV2438.
193. Taniguchi K, Nakano S, Matsuda H, et al. Long-term survival and complications after composite graft replacement for ascending aortic aneurysm associated with aortic regurgitation. *Circulation* 1991;84[Suppl III]:III31-9.
194. Mehta RH, O'Gara PT, Bossone E, et al. Acute type A aortic dissection in the elderly: clinical characteristics, management and outcomes in the current era. *J Am Coll Cardiol* 2002;40:685–692.
195. Walker PJ, Dake MD, Mitchell RS, et al. The use of endovascular techniques for the treatment of complications of aortic dissection. *J Vasc Surg* 1993;18:1042–1051.
196. Dake MD, Kato N, Mitchell RS, et al. Endovascular stent-graft placement for the treatment of acute aortic dissection. *N Engl J Med* 1999;340:1546–1552.
197. Slonim SM, Miller DC, Mitchell RS, et al. Percutaneous balloon fenestration and stenting for life-threatening ischemic complications in patients with acute aortic dissection. *Thorac Cardiovasc Surg* 1999;117:1118–1126.
198. Williams DM, Lee DY, Hamilton BH, et al. The dissected aorta: percutaneous treatment of ischemic complications-principles and results. *J Vasc Interv Radiol* 1997;8:605–625.
199. Vedantham S, Picus D, Sanchez LA, et al. Percutaneous management of ischemic complications in patients with type-B aortic dissection. *J Vasc Interv Radiol* 2003;12:181–193.
200. Lopera J, Patino JH, Urbina C, et al. Endovascular treatment of complicated type-B aortic dissection with stent-grafts: midterm results. *J Vasc Interv Radiol* 2003;14:195–203.
201. Cooke JP, Kazmier FJ, Orszulak TA. The penetrating aortic ulcer: pathologic manifestations, diagnosis, and management. *Mayo Clin Proc* 1988;63:718–725.
202. Stanson AW, Kazmier FJ, Hollier LH. Penetrating atherosclerotic ulcers of the thoracic aorta: natural history and clinicopathologic correlations. *Ann Vasc Surg* 1986;1:15–23.
203. Hussain S, Glover JL, Bree R, et al. Penetrating atherosclerotic ulcers of the thoracic aorta. *J Vasc Surg* 1989;9:710–717.
204. Movsowitz HD, Lampert C, Jacobs LE, et al. Penetrating atherosclerotic aortic ulcers. *Am Heart J* 1994;28:1210–1217.
205. Faries PL, Lang E, Ramdev P, et al. Endovascular stent-graft treatment of a ruptured thoracic aortic ulcer. *J Endovasc Ther* 2002;9:II-20–II-24.
206. Kos X, Bouchard L, Otal P, et al. Stent-graft treatment of penetrating thoracic aortic ulcers. *J Endovasc Ther* 2002;9:II-25–II-31.
207. Crane JS, Cowling M, Cheshire NJ. Endovascular stent grafting of a penetrating ulcer in the descending thoracic aorta. *Eur J Vasc Endovasc Surg* 2003;25:178–179.
208. von Kodolitsch Y, Csosz SK, Koschyk DH, et al. Intramural hematoma of the aorta: predictors of progression to dissection and rupture. *Circulation* 2003;107:1158–1163.
209. Cambria RP. Regarding "analysis of predictive factors for progression of type B aortic intramural hematoma with computed tomography." *J Vasc Surg* 2002;35:1295–1296.
210. Isselbacher EM. Intramural hematoma of the aorta: should we let down our guard? *Am J Med* 2002;113:244–246.
211. Song JK, Kim HS, Song JM. Outcomes of medically treated patients with aortic intramural hematoma. *Am J Med* 2002;113:181–187.
212. Sawhney NS, DeMaria AN, Blanchard DG. Aortic intramural hematoma: an increasingly recognized and potentially fatal entity. *Chest* 2001;120:1340–1346.
213. von Kodolitsch Y, Csosz SK, Koschyk DH, et al. Intramural hematoma of the aorta: predictors of progression to dissection and rupture. *Circulation* 2003;107:1158–1163.
214. Maraj R, Rerkpattanapipat P, Jacobs LE, et al. Meta-analysis of 143 reported cases of aortic intramural hematoma. *Am J Cardiol* 2000;86:664–648.
215. Tunick PA, Rosenzweig BP, Katz ES, et al. High risk for vascular events in patients with protruding aortic atheromas: a prospective study. *J Am Coll Cardiol* 1994;23:1085–1090.
216. Mitusch R, Doherty C, Wucherpfennig H, et al. Vascular events during follow-up in patients with aortic arch atherosclerosis. *Stroke* 1997;28:36–39.
217. Dávila-Román VG, Barzilai B, Wareing TH, et al. Atherosclerosis of the ascending aorta: prevalence and role as an independent predictor of cerebrovascular events in cardiac patients. *Stroke* 1994;25:2010–2016.

CHAPTER 100

Cerebrovascular Disease and Neurologic Manifestations of Heart Disease

Joao A. Gomes and Louis R. Caplan

Key Words: Aortic origin embolism; brain embolism; brain infarction; cardiac encephalopathy.

CEREBROVASCULAR DISEASE

Stroke is the third most common cause of death and the leading cause of long-term disability. There are about 4.5 million stroke survivors in the United States alone (1). Stroke is anything but a homogenous entity. Stroke refers to any damage to the brain or spinal cord related to an abnormality in blood supply. Approximately 80% of all strokes are ischemic; the remaining 20% of strokes are hemorrhagic, which can be further subdivided in two subtypes: intracerebral and subarachnoid (2).

Cardiogenic Brain Embolism

Cardiogenic embolism is estimated to account for 15% to 25% of all ischemic strokes (3–6). However, the absence of sensitive and specific criteria for the diagnosis of cardioembolic stroke has precluded an accurate estimation of its true frequency (7), and earlier series using more restrictive criteria and antedating widespread availability of echocardiogra-

J. A. Gomes: Department of Neurology, Stroke Division, Beth Israel Deaconess Medical Center, Harvard Medical School, 330 Brookline Ave., Boston, Massachusetts 02215.
L. R. Caplan: Department of Neurology, Stroke Division, Beth Israel Deaconess Medical Center, Harvard Medical School, 330 Brookline Ave., Boston, Massachusetts 02215.

phy underestimated the role of cardioembolism in stroke patients (8–10).

Maximal deficit at stroke onset, presence of an embolic source, evidence of peripheral emboli, and hemorrhagic transformation on computed tomography (CT) scan are among the features that suggest brain infarction caused by cardioembolism. These criteria, however, are unreliable because 10% to 20% of these patients have a progressive or stuttering course (3,11,12), only 2% have clinically recognized peripheral emboli (13,14), and the presence of an embolic source does not necessarily establish the diagnosis. CT scan evidence of hemorrhagic transformation is found only in about 15% to 30% of embolic strokes (15,16), and atherothrombotic disease in large arteries within the cerebral vasculature can be identified in up to one-third of patients with a potential cardioembolic source (17–19). The growing number of cardiac sources of embolic material can be divided as presented in the following sections (Table 100–1).

Arrhythmias

Atrial Fibrillation

One of every six strokes occurs in patients with atrial fibrillation (AF), and it is estimated that 10% of all ischemic strokes are caused by embolism of left atrial thrombi (20). Various studies have shown that AF is associated with a six-fold increase in the risk for stroke (21–24). However, most patients with AF develop an ischemic event, and the stroke

TABLE 100–1. *Common cardiac sources of emboli*

Arrhythmias
    Atrial fibrillation
    Sick sinus syndrome

Septal abnormalities
    Atrial septal defect
    Patent foramen ovale
    Atrial septal aneurysm

Cardiomyopathies
    Alcohol
    Cocaine
    Myocarditis
    Ischemia
    Sarcoidosis
    Amyloidosis
    Fabry's disease
    Chagas disease

Cardiac chambers lesions
    Myxoma
    Fibroelastoma
    Metastatic tumors
    Ventricular aneurysms
    Hypokinetic/akinetic zones

Valvular disease
    Rheumatic valvular disease (mitral and/or aortic)
    Mitral annulus calcification
    Calcific aortic stenosis
    Bicuspid aortic valve
    Mitral valve prolapse
    Bacterial endocarditis
    Marantic endocarditis
    Libman-Sacks endocarditis
    Behçet's disease

rate varies from 0.5% per year for young patients with "lone AF" (25) to 12% per year for patients with previous strokes (26,27).

Clearly, the cause of AF and associated cardiac and medical factors influence the risk for stroke, for example, being increased 17.6 times in patients with rheumatic heart disease (28). Identification of risk factors in patients with nonvalvular AF allows risk assessment and individualization of therapy. Age older than 75 years, hypertension, history of stroke or transient ischemic attack (TIA), and left ventricular dysfunction predict ischemic stroke in patients with nonvalvular AF (29–31). The presence of diabetes mellitus, sex (women), regular alcohol use, moderate to severe mitral regurgitation, coronary artery disease, or previous myocardial infarction (MI) and postmenopausal hormone replacement therapy are weaker predictors of stroke risk (29,30,32).

Sick Sinus Syndrome

Cardioembolic stroke occurs in approximately 14% to 18% of patients with the sick sinus syndrome (33), and patients with tachyarrhythmias are more likely to embolize than those with only bradyarrhythmias. The use of pacemakers does not reduce the risk for stroke (34,35), and age (>65

years), left atrial size, the presence of spontaneous echo contrast, and atrial ejection force are proposed predictors of embolic stroke in paced patients with sick sinus syndrome (36). Many of these patients have associated AF or atrial flutter with slow ventricular response (34).

Myocardial Wall and Cardiac Chamber Lesions

Paradoxic Embolism and Septal Lesions

Once considered rare, paradoxic embolism and septal lesions are currently being increasingly recognized as potential causes of ischemic stroke, particularly in young adults. The most common intracardiac right-to-left shunt is a patent foramen ovale (PFO); however, the high prevalence of PFOs in the general population (estimated at 25–30%) (37–39), has made it difficult to establish with certainty whether PFOs are more than just an incidental finding in a given patient.

Several studies have shown that PFOs are more often found in stroke patients than in control subjects, particularly in those younger than 55 years without traditional risk factors and with an undetermined cause of stroke (38,40). The annual recurrence of stroke, TIA, or both in patients with PFOs ranges from 2.5% to 5.5% (39,41,42). The association with an atrial septal aneurysm significantly increases this risk (43).

The stroke mechanisms postulated in patients with PFOs include paradoxic embolism from a venous source (deep leg or pelvic), thrombus formation within the PFO itself, or an associated atrial septal aneurysm or atrial arrhythmias (44–48). The presence of a hypercoagulable state, a situation that favors leg or pelvic vein thrombosis, pulmonary embolism temporally related to the stroke, and stroke onset during a Valsalva maneuver (sexual intercourse, straining, physical exertion) are criteria that implicate a PFO as an etiologic factor (49).

Cardiac Myxomas and Other Tumors

Although rare, cardiac tumors represent an important cause of cardioembolism in selected patients. Myxomas originate most often in the left atrium and are usually found in patients between the ages of 30 and 60 years; women seem to be slightly more commonly affected than men (50). Embolism occurs in about 30% to 50% of patients with cardiac myxomas (51), and although the cerebral hemispheres are usually more commonly affected, instances of spinal cord embolism, visual loss, and mycotic aneurysm formation with subsequent bleeding have been reported (52,53).

Cardiac Valve Disease

Mitral Valve Prolapse

Mitral valve prolapse (MVP) continues to be a controversial source of embolism. In the 1980s it was reported that up to 40% of patients younger than 45 years with an acute ischemic stroke had MVP (54). This view, however, has been challenged recently because the diagnostic criteria previously used overestimated the true prevalence of MVP; a clinical study in patients with similar characteristics, but using more reliable two-dimensional echocardiographic criteria, found a 2.8% prevalence of MVP in patients with cryptogenic stroke. This rate does not differ from the 2.7% prevalence found in control subjects (55,56) and the 2.4% reported prevalence among members of the offspring of the Framingham Heart Study with a mean age of 55 years (57).

Mitral Annulus Calcification

Mitral annulus calcification is an uncommonly recognized cause of embolism. Emboli particles composed of calcium have been documented in surgical embolectomies (58), extrusion of calcium through overlapping cusps has been found at necropsy (58), and several series have shown a relation between mitral annulus calcification and stroke (59–61). Despite this evidence, a study from the Netherlands suggested that mitral annulus calcification is not an independent risk factor for stroke. Instead, it is the presence of carotid atheroma and cardiovascular risk factors for stroke commonly found in patients with mitral annulus calcification that account for the high stroke incidence in previous studies (62).

Clinical Syndromes

Approximately 80% of all emboli arising from the heart go into the anterior circulation, whereas the remaining 20% affect the vertebrobasilar system (3,5). Embolic particles have predilection sites within the anterior and posterior circulations. A large embolus would tend to lodge in the common carotid or internal carotid arteries (ICA), whereas if it is small enough to go through, it would most likely lodge in the ICA bifurcation in anterior cerebral (ACA) and middle cerebral (MCA) arteries. Most emboli that pass through the ICA bifurcation go into either the mainstem MCA (M1 segment) or the superior or inferior division of the MCA.

In the posterior circulation, emboli, if large enough, can block the vertebral arteries in the neck or intracranially. However, if they are able to pass through the intracranial vertebral arteries, they reach the distal basilar artery bifurcation (top of the basilar). Table 100–2 summarizes the common clinical findings associated with ischemia in different vascular territories.

Atherothrombotic Carotid Artery Disease

Carotid atherothrombosis accounts for 10% to 20% of cases of brain infarction (63). In the 1950s, Fisher (64) first called attention to extracranial carotid atherothrombosis as an important cause of TIAs and stroke and suggested surgery as a possible therapy.

Inflammation, lipid deposition, endothelial injury, plaque formation, thrombin, platelets, and fibrin all contribute to the pathogenesis of the lesion. After reaching a critical size, plaques can affect the flow of blood creating turbulence, which, in turn, causes complications to develop within the plaque. Plaque ulceration and mural thrombi can develop, and loosely adherent, fresh thrombi rapidly propagate and embolize distally (65).

There are significant race and sex differences in the distribution of cerebral atherothrombosis (66–68). White men have an increased prevalence of atherothrombotic lesions at the origin of the carotid arteries, usually associated with

TABLE 100–2. *Clinical manifestations of ischemic stroke in different vascular territories*

Artery involved	Left hemisphere	Right hemisphere
Anterior cerebral	Contralateral paralysis of the leg with sensory loss. If the lesion is proximal and the recurrent artery of Heubner is involved, weakness of face and arm is usually present.	Same. If bilateral involvement, a state of akinetic-mutism and urinary incontinence usually is added.
Middle cerebral: superior division	Contralateral weakness and sensory loss; Broca's aphasia	Neglect of the left side of space, lack of awareness of deficit and motor impersistence
Middle cerebral: inferior division	Fluent aphasia (Wernicke), superior quadrantanopia, agitation	Agitation, left neglect, hyperactivity, visuospatial impairments
Posterior cerebral	Combination of a homonymous hemianopia with or without sensory loss contralateral to the side involved. Inability to read or name colors.	Left-sided neglect is associated with right-sided lesions.
Top of the basilar	Abnormalities in vertical gaze, hallucinations, apathy, sleepiness and other behavioral abnormalities. Bilateral posterior cerebral artery infarction can result in cortical blindness, severe agitation, and amnesia.	
Posterior–inferior cerebellar artery	Branch of the vertebral artery; usually supplies the inferior aspect of the cerebellum and the posterolateral aspect of the medulla. Ataxia, vomiting, occipital headache, paresis of the palate, and Horner's syndrome are common signs.	

coronary artery disease, hypercholesterolemia, and peripheral vascular disease. Black, Chinese, and Japanese individuals have a high frequency of intracranial occlusive disease and a relatively low frequency of extracranial stenosis. Women and patients with diabetes also have an increased prevalence of intracranial disease.

Ischemic stroke in patients with extracranial stenosis is caused by two different mechanisms: artery-to-artery embolism and hypoperfusion (2). The latter only develops when a critical degree of stenosis is reached, and it is more prominent when the progression is relatively rapid, not allowing the recruitment of collateral circulation. Embolism likely plays a more prominent role in these patients, and microembolic signals can be detected in this setting by means of transcranial Doppler monitoring (69,70).

The two main approaches for the management of carotid stenosis include plaque stabilization (through risk factor modification and medication) and reduction or elimination of the plaque by surgical or endovascular means. This decision is usually based on the degree of stenosis, age, sex, comorbid conditions, overall perceived surgical risk, and the presence of concomitant vascular disease (71). Angioplasty and stenting can be entertained in patients who are believed to be poor surgical candidates.

NEUROLOGIC MANIFESTATIONS OF HEART DISEASE

Ischemic Stroke during Coronary Artery Bypass Surgery

Each year, an estimated 650,000 coronary artery bypass graft (CABG) surgeries are performed in the United States (72). CABG is associated with a 1% to 5% incidence of symptomatic ischemic brain infarcts, and more than a third of patients who have a stroke during CABG die, making it the single most important cause of iatrogenic stroke (73). The occurrence of postoperative stroke increases the length of stays in hospitals and intensive care units (74) and is associated with a fivefold to tenfold increase of in-hospital mortality (75,76). A number of factors associated with stroke after CABG have been identified, including chronic renal failure, recent MI, previous stroke, carotid artery disease, hemodilution, hypertension, diabetes, age older than 75 years, left ventricular dysfunction, atherothrombosis of the ascending aorta, cardiopulmonary bypass (CPB) equipment, postoperative low cardiac output syndrome, and the development of postoperative AF (75,77). Abnormal cardiac function and severe aortic atheromatous disease are likely especially important.

Hemodynamically Mediated Brain Infarcts

Given the circulatory and hemodynamic stress related to heart surgery, there has always been concern that areas supplied by stenosed or occluded arteries may be underperfused during CABG, possibly leading to brain infarction. In this regard, carotid artery stenosis is particularly relevant, not only because of its frequency, but also because it is accessible to surgical treatment, and some investigators support the notion of prophylactic carotid endarterectomy in patients with greater than 75% stenosis who are being considered for nonemergent CABG (76). The prevalence of carotid artery disease in patients undergoing cardiovascular surgery ranges from 6% to 31% (78), and the degree of stenosis seems to be an independent predictor of postoperative stroke as patients with greater than 75% stenosis have a rate of stroke that is five times that of patients with less than 50% disease (76, 79). Cerebral blood flow monitoring has been obtained in a limited number of studies, and several technologies have been used (80,81). Substantial fluctuations in cerebral blood flow occur during different stages of the surgery, with relatively low flow usually occurring during CPB and pH-stat acid-base management stages (80,82). The effect of severe carotid stenosis or occlusion on cerebral blood flow during CABG has been assessed in a limited number of studies, but the data are inconclusive (82). Available data suggest that a short period of hemodynamic instability follows the initiation of CPB, but severe decreases in flow occur only infrequently. The role of hemodynamic changes in the pathogenesis of brain infarction in patients with carotid stenosis undergoing CABG is likely minor, and embolism (either from the carotid or from other sources) is probably more common and a greater concern. Management of combined coronary and cerebral artery disease awaits the outcome of clinical trials.

Embolism-related Brain Infarcts

That most CABG-related strokes do not occur in the immediate postoperative period (i.e., on awakening from anesthesia), as one would expect if the cause were a hemodynamic mechanism, strongly favors embolism as the most likely cause of post-CABG strokes. In two separate studies, the incidence rate of stroke in the immediate postoperative period was only 16% and 17%, respectively (83,84). Furthermore, another study found that the majority of post-CABG strokes were related to macroemboli, as evidenced by the territorial distribution of stroke in CT scan or autopsies (85); in another study using diffusion-weighted imaging, 26% of patients undergoing cardiovascular surgery had asymptomatic lesions compatible with acute stroke in a pattern suggestive of embolization (86).

Although potential sources of emboli in these patients are varied (i.e., left ventricular dysfunction, atrial dilatation, arrhythmias, and atherothrombotic disease of the carotid arteries), there are increasing data suggesting that aortic arch atherothrombosis plays a major role in post-CABG stroke. High prevalence rates of aortic arch atheroma have been documented among patients undergoing cardiovascular surgery (85,87). It also is an area of prominent surgical manipulation where cross-clamping and cannulation take place (85). Finally, the topography of the atheroma within the aortic arch may also be of relevance because the distal anterior segment is usually the most commonly affected by atheroma and is typically the place where most surgeons place the aortic canula (88). Transcranial doppler (TCD) monitoring during CABG surgery has shown that more than one-third of the microembolic signals are detected as the cross-clamps are removed and another one-fourth are detected as aortic partial occlusion clamps are removed (89). Autopsy of patients who underwent cardiac surgery and died demonstrated cholesterol crystal emboli in the small arteries of the brain and other viscera (90).

Encephalopathy and Cognitive Abnormalities after Coronary Artery Bypass Grafting Surgery

The incidence rate of encephalopathy after CABG surgery is estimated at about 7% (91). It has been associated with increased length of hospital stay and up to five times greater mortality (92). CPB time is strongly associated with the development of postoperative encephalopathy, and the probability increases 30% to 50% for every 30 minutes of CPB (92). Likely, it is multifactorial and related to medications, fever, sepsis, hypoxia, hypotension, and metabolic abnormalities, as well as to multiple small brain emboli. Age, history of previous stroke, diabetes, hypertension, and carotid bruit have been used to develop a predictive model for the development of delirium (92).

Impairment in neuropsychological performance often is found in patients undergoing CABG surgery and ranges from 30% (93) to 88% (94), depending on the timing and kind of neuropsychological assessment. The most common cognitive abnormalities are disturbances of memory, concentration, attention, and rapidity of response to stimuli (94). In a prospective study, the early postoperative incidence of cognitive decline was 50%, with improvement at 6 months and a later decline at 5 years in up to 42% of patients (95). In this same study, the level of long-term cognitive function was predicted by age, educational, level and perioperative cognitive decline (95).

Hypoperfusion, hypothermia, and microemboli have been suggested as causative factors of neuropsychological impairment. Recent data obtained using magnetic resonance spectroscopy technology suggest a transient metabolic dysfunction of the frontal lobes in a significant proportion of these patients (86).

Other Neurologic Complications of Coronary Artery Bypass Grafting Surgery

The peripheral nervous system is involved in up to 13% of patients undergoing CABG surgery (96). The brachial plexus is the most common and potentially serious site of involvement. Typically, the lower trunk (C8-T1 roots) is affected resulting in pain, sensory changes, and weakness of the hand. In one study, injury to the brachial plexus correlated with internal jugular vein cannulation (97). Another potential mechanism of injury is plexus stretching from chest wall retraction. Other sites involved include the common peroneal nerve with resultant foot drop, saphenous nerve, phrenic nerve, ulnar nerve, and facial nerve.

Other rare causes of neurologic complications after CABG surgery include intracranial hemorrhage (98), pituitary apoplexy (99), and unilateral hearing loss (100).

Cardiac Encephalopathy

Some patients with acute or chronic heart failure can experience development of an encephalopathy in the absence of any toxic/metabolic abnormality or liver, renal, or pulmonary failure. These patients are usually inattentive, drowsy, unable to interact with the examiner, and at times even wrongly considered to be experiencing development of a dementing process. Two clinical syndromes have been recognized in patients with cardiac encephalopathy (49).

Nonabulic Encephalopathy

Nonabulic encephalopathy resembles in every aspect the encephalopathy seen in patients with metabolic disturbances or organ failure. Inattention is a prominent aspect in these patients, and some may even have an agitated state.

In patients who have congestive heart failure (CHF), systemic venous pressure is increased, resulting in increased venous dural sinus pressure. If a lumbar puncture is performed, the cerebrospinal fluid (CSF) pressure may be increased. Brain edema may result as a consequence of the increased venous pressure.

A gradient between arterial and intracranial pressure is required to maintain adequate cerebral perfusion. If the arteriovenous pressure difference is decreased as a consequence of venous hypertension, arterial pressure and blood flow will have to be augmented. This can be limited in patients with suboptimal heart function. Hypoxia, electrolyte, blood volume, and acid-base abnormalities can compound the cardiac encephalopathy (49).

Abulic Encephalopathy

Abulic encephalopathy is a clinical syndrome similar to that of patients with hydrocephalus. The major feature is abulia, a clinical state in which the patient has severely reduced spontaneous behavior; they just sit or lie about and show little interest in any activity. Spontaneous speech is markedly reduced, and responses are usually short and terse.

This syndrome can be seen not only during exacerbation of CHF, but also even after cardiac compensation has occurred and the patient is recovering from heart failure. Increased venous and intracranial pressure decreases absorption of CSF with resultant fluid accumulation in the cisterns around the brain, in the subarachnoid space, and within the ventricles. CSF is retained intracranially, and on brain imaging this finding can be confused with brain atrophy as CSF accumulates between gyri (external hydrocephalus) and within the ventricular system (internal hydrocephalus). Just as pericardial, peritoneal, and pleural effusions are common in patients with CHF and may persist even after adequate medical treatment sometimes requiring drainage, accumulation of CSF probably has the same mechanism. The meninges are connective tissue membranes that share structural and functional similarities with the pleura, pericardium, and peritoneum.

It is well known that correction of CHF does not necessarily result in complete resolution of pleural and pericardial effusions and ascites, and a similar situation likely occurs in the subarachnoid space. In some of these patients with the abulic syndrome, performance of lumbar puncture and drainage of CSF is associated with marked clinical improvement and reversal of "brain atrophy" on brain imaging (49).

Toxic/Metabolic Encephalopathies in Cardiac Patients

There are a large number of potential causes of encephalopathy in acutely ill cardiac patients. Most often, it is the result of toxic substances or metabolic derangements that interfere with normal brain function.

It is usually helpful to group them into exogenous and endogenous causes. *Endogenous etiologic factors* include liver, renal, and pulmonary failure, electrolyte disturbances, thyroid and adrenal dysfunction, alterations in blood sugar, acid-base abnormalities, changes in blood osmolarity and viscosity, intravascular volume depletion, fever and sepsis, and presence of ketone bodies. Alcohol, psychotropic drugs (i.e., haloperidol, benzodiazepines, barbiturates), pain medications (i.e., morphine), vitamin B_{12}, thiamine, and pyridoxine deficiency are among the most common *exogenous causes* (49).

Nontoxic/Nonmetabolic Encephalopathies

Certain conditions that involve the brain diffusely or multifocally, or involve the meninges, can present with a clinical picture indistinguishable from toxic/metabolic disorders.

Bacterial endocarditis, particularly if caused by *Staphylococcus aureus,* can present with an encephalopathy. It is thought to be caused by the combination of sepsis, single or multiple brain infarcts, and microabscesses (101–103). *Hypercoagulable states* (i.e., cancer, disseminated intravascular coagulation [DIC], and thrombotic thrombocytopenic purpura [TTP]) are associated with scattered small regions of brain infarction, edema and hemorrhage, and an acute encephalopathy (104). *Increased blood viscosity* results in reduced brain and retinal blood flow with diffuse cerebral dysfunction. It is commonly associated with Waldenström's macroglobulinemia, multiple myeloma, hyperlipidemia, and intravascular lymphoma. Dural sinus thrombosis, infectious processes such as viral encephalitis, carcinomatous menin-

gitis, and arteritis also should be considered in the differential diagnosis of these patients (105,106).

Hypoxic Ischemic Encephalopathy and Cardiac Arrest

Within the brain there are regions of "selective vulnerability" to hypoxic–ischemic insults depending on energy requirements, anatomy of arterial circulation, and individual cell susceptibility. This explains why a systemic insult can damage certain cells or regions more than others. The most vulnerable cells are those located in the cerebral cortex, hippocampus, cerebellar cortex (i.e., Purkinje cells), amygdaloid nucleus, basal ganglia, and some brainstem nuclei (107).

Brain regions between arterial territories (so-called border zone or watershed) are more susceptible to ischemia than those located in the center of a major feeding artery in patients with hypotension and global hypoperfusion (2). Damage tends to be more severe in the posterior parieto-temporo-occipital (between MCA and posterior cerebral artery) and in the frontal (between ACA and MCA) areas. Similar border zones exist internally in the cerebral hemispheres, the brainstem between the medial and lateral perforating arteries, the cerebellum, and the spinal cord (2).

Anoxic injuries can be classified as *hypoxic hypoxia* (decreased partial pressure of oxygen as seen in drowning), *histotoxic hypoxia* (inability of the tissues to use oxygen, usually related to a mitochondrial disorder or carbon monoxide intoxication), *anemic hypoxia* (decreased hemoglobin concentration), and *hypoxic ischemic encephalopathy* (as seen after cardiac arrest) (108). The distribution of lesions in diffusion-weighted magnetic resonance imaging correlates well with the distinct neuropathologic features of these entities, and thus may aid in prognosis (109).

If hypoxia is severe, but some degree of circulation is preserved (as in hanging, strangulation, drowning, carbon monoxide poisoning), the basal ganglia and thalamus are usually the main sites of involvement (110). When circulatory arrest is sudden and complete in children and young adults, the brainstem nuclei are severely affected (111), and if the degree of hypoxia is particularly severe, the spinal cord may also be damaged (112).

Clinical Syndromes

The clinical findings in patients who have experienced a hypoxic–ischemic event depend on the duration, severity, and type of insult. Table 100–3 summarizes the clinical syndromes frequently encountered in patients with hypoxic–ischemic injuries.

Prognosis

Predicting outcome is one of the most important issues in patients with hypoxic–ischemic insults. In the initial min-

TABLE 100–3. *Clinical findings in patients with hypoxic–ischemic encephalopathies*

Syndrome	Clinical findings	Pathologic correlate
Brainstem–hemispheral coma	Patients lack so-called brainstem reflexes (i.e., pupillary, corneal, and oculocephalic reflexes), exhibit no movement, and are unable to control respiration. Severe damage results in irreversible coma and death.	Diffuse cortical and brainstem injury
Persistent vegetative state	Certain automatic movements such as blinking and yawning with preservation of brainstem reflexes, but lack of a meaningful response to the environment	Damage to the cerebral cortex with relative sparing of the brainstem centers
Posterior border zone infarct	Usually visual. Patients exhibit poor eye–hand coordination (optic ataxia), difficulty with gaze (optic apraxia), and difficulty integrating all the features of a scene (asimultagnosia). These are features of Balint's syndrome.	Ischemia in the posterior border zone regions
Anterior border zone infarct	Proximal arm and leg weakness with normal strength distally and in the face (man in a barrel syndrome)	Ischemia in the anterior border zone regions

utes and hours after cardiac arrest, the depth and duration of coma and the response to pain are powerful predictors of neurologic outcome (113). The size and reaction of pupils also are useful prognostic indicators. In a case series of cardiopulmonary arrest, all those patients with absent pupillary response by 3 hours after the event died (114). In another series, pupillary dilatation throughout resuscitation carried a poor prognosis (115).

The presence of frequent jerks (myoclonic movements) also aids in prognostication. These movements can involve the face, eyelids, limbs, and jaw and have been associated with poor outcome, particularly if very common (myoclonic status) (116,117).

More recently, the use of neurophysiologic evaluation and biochemical markers has been investigated as a mean of more reliably predicting neurologic outcome after cardiac arrest (118,119). The diagnosis of brain death, however, is still based on clinical evaluation, and the proposed criteria are summarized in Table 100–4.

The use of mild hypothermia in patients successfully resuscitated after cardiac arrest correlated with a favorable neurologic outcome and reduced mortality in two randomized trials (120,121). Although encouraging, further studies of the efficacy and safety of therapeutic hypothermia are needed to validate these results.

TABLE 100–4. *Clinical criteria for the diagnosis of brain death*

Coma
Absence of motor responses
Absence of pupillary responses to light and pupils at midposition with respect to dilatation (4–6 mm)
Absence of corneal reflexes
Absence of caloric responses
Absence of gag reflex
Absence of coughing in response to tracheal suctioning
Absence of sucking and rooting reflexes
Absence of respiratory drive at a partial pressure of arterial carbon dioxide that is 60 or 20 mm Hg above normal baseline values

Modified from Wijdicks EF. The diagnosis of brain death. *N Engl J Med* 2001;344:1215–1221, with permission.

REFERENCES

1. American Heart Association. *2001 heart and stroke statistical update.* Dallas, TX: American Heart Association, 2000. Available at: www.americanheart.org/statistics.
2. Caplan LR. *Caplan's stroke: a clinical approach,* 3rd ed. Boston: Butterworth-Heinemann, 2000.
3. Mohr JP, Caplan LR, Melski JW, et al. The Harvard Cooperative Stroke Registry: a prospective registry. *Neurology* 1978;28:754–762.
4. Wolf PA, Kannel W, McGee DL, et al. Duration of atrial fibrillation and imminence of stroke: the Framingham Study. *Stroke* 1983;14:664–667.
5. Caplan LR, Hier D, D'Cruz I. Cerebral embolism in the Michael Reese Stroke registry. *Stroke* 1983;14:530–537.
6. Grau AJ, Weimar C, Buggle F, et al. Risk factors, outcome, and treatment in subtypes of ischemic stroke. The German Stroke Databank. *Stroke* 2001;32:2559–2566.
7. Cardiogenic brain embolism. Cerebral Embolism Task Force. *Arch Neurol* 1986;43:71–84.
8. Aring CD, Merritt HH. Differential diagnosis between cerebral hemorrhage and cerebral thrombosis. *Arch Intern Med* 1935;56:435–456.
9. Whisnant JP, Fitzgibbons JP, Kurland LT, et al. Natural history of stroke in Rochester, Minnesota, 1945 through 1954. *Stroke* 1971;2:11–22.
10. Matsumoto N, Whisnant JP, Kurland LT, et al. Natural history of stroke in Rochester, Minnesota, 1955 through 1969: an extension of previous study 1945 through 1954. *Stroke* 1973;4:20–29.
11. Fisher CM, Pearlman A. Nonsudden onset of cerebral embolism. *Neurology* 1967;17:1025–1032.
12. Chambers BR, Donnan GA, Bladen PF. An analysis of the first 700 consecutive admissions to the Austin Hospital Stroke Unit. *Aust NZ J Med* 1983;13:57–64.
13. Foulkes MA, Wolf PA, Price TR, et al. The Stroke Data Bank: design, methods, and baseline characteristics. *Stroke* 1988;19:547–554.
14. Bogousslavsky J, van Melle G, Regli F. The Lausanne Stroke Registry: analysis of 1000 consecutive patients with first stroke. *Stroke* 1988;19:1083–1092.
15. Okada Y, Yamaguchi T, Minematsu K, et al. Hemorrhagic transformation in cerebral embolism. *Stroke* 1989;20:598–603.
16. Molina CA, Montaner J, Abilleira S, et al. Timing of spontaneous recanalization and risk of hemorrhagic transformation in acute cardioembolic stroke. *Stroke* 2001;32:1079–1084.
17. Bogousslavsky J, Hachinski VC, Boughner DR, et al. Cardiac and arterial lesions in carotid transient ischemic attacks. *Arch Neurol* 1986;43:223–228.
18. Olsen TS, Skiver EB, Herning M. Cause of cerebral infarction in the carotid territory: its relation to the size and the location of the infarct and to the underlying vascular lesion. *Stroke* 1985;16:459–466.
19. Gagliardi R, Benvenuti L, Frosini F, et al. Frequency of echocardio-

graphic abnormalities in patients with ischemia of the carotid terri-tory—a preliminary report. *Stroke* 1985;16:118–120.

20. Hart RG, Halperin JL. Atrial fibrillation and thromboembolism: a decade of progress in stroke prevention. *Ann Intern Med* 1999;131: 688–695.

21. Wolf PA, Dawber TR, Thomas HE Jr, et al. Epidemiologic assessment of chronic atrial fibrillation and risk of stroke. *Neurology* 1978;28: 973–977.

22. Tanaka H, Hayashi M, Date C, et al. Epidemiologic studies of stroke in Shibata, a Japanese provincial city: preliminary report on risk factors for cerebral infarction. *Stroke* 1985;16:773–780.

23. Onundarsen PT, Thorgeirson G, Jonmundson E, et al. Chronic atrial fibrillation-epidemiologic features and 14 year follow-up: a case control study. *Eur Heart J* 1987;8:521–527.

24. Flegel KM, Shipley MJ, Rose G. Risk of stroke in nonrheumatic atrial fibrillation. *Lancet* 1987;1:526–529.

25. Kopecky SL, Gersh BJ, McGoon MD, et al. The natural history of lone atrial fibrillation. A population-based study over three decades. *N Engl J Med* 1987;317:669–674.

26. Secondary prevention in non-rheumatic atrial fibrillation after transient ischemic attack or minor stroke. EAFT (European Atrial Fibrillation Trial) Study Group. *Lancet* 1993;342:1255–1262.

27. Adjusted-dose warfarin versus low-intensity, fixed-dose warfarin plus aspirin for high-risk patients with atrial fibrillation. Stroke Prevention in Atrial Fibrillation III randomized clinical trial. *Lancet* 1996;348: 633–638.

28. Wolf PA, Abbot RD, Kannel WB. Atrial fibrillation: a major contributor to stroke in the elderly: the Framingham Study. *Arch Intern Med* 1987;147:1561–1564.

29. Hart RG, Pearcy LA, McBride R, et al. Factors associated with ischemic stroke during aspirin therapy in atrial fibrillation: analysis of 2012 participants in the SPAF I-III clinical trials. *Stroke* 1999;30:1223–1229.

30. Predictors of thromboembolism in atrial fibrillation: I. Clinical features of patients at risk. The Stroke Prevention in Atrial Fibrillation Investigators. *Ann Intern Med* 1992;116:1–5.

31. Patients with nonvalvular atrial fibrillation at low risk of stroke during treatment with aspirin: Stroke Prevention in Atrial Fibrillation III Study. The SPAF III Writing Committee for the Stroke Prevention in Atrial Fibrillation Investigators. *JAMA* 1998;279:1273–1277.

32. Nakagami H, Yamamoto K, Ikeda U, et al. Mitral regurgitation reduces the risk of stroke in patients with nonrheumatic atrial fibrillation. *Am Heart J* 1998;136:528–532.

33. Rosenqvist M, Vallin H, Edhag O. Clinical and electrophysiologic course of sinus node disease: five year follow-up study. *Am Heart J* 1985;109:513–522.

34. Orencia AJ, Hammill SC, Whisnant JP. Sinus node dysfunction and ischemic stroke. *Heart Dis Stroke* 1994;3:91–94.

35. Rosenqvist M, Brandt J, Schuller H. Long-term pacing in sinus node disease: effects of stimulation mode on cardiovascular morbidity and mortality. *Am Heart J* 1988;116:16–22.

36. Mattioli AV, Castellani ET, Matiolli G. Stroke in paced patients with sick sinus syndrome: influence of left atrial function and size. *Cardiology* 1999;91:150–155.

37. Hagen PT, Scholz D, Edwards WD. Incidence and size of patent foramen ovale during the first 10 decades of life: an autopsy study of 965 normal hearts. *Mayo Clin Proc* 1984;59:17–20.

38. Lechat PH, Mas JL, Lascault G, et al. Prevalence of patent foramen ovale in patients with stroke. *N Engl J Med* 1988;318:1148–1152.

39. Nedeltchev K, Arnold M, Wahl A, et al. Outcome of patients with cryptogenic stroke and patent foramen ovale. *J Neurol Neurosurg Psychiatry* 2002;72:347–350.

40. Lamy C, Giannesine C, Zuber M, et al. Clinical and imaging findings in cryptogenic stroke patients with and without patent foramen ovale. The PFO-ASA study. *Stroke* 2002;33:706–711.

41. Mas JL, Zuber M. Recurrent cerebrovascular events in patients with patent foramen ovale, atrial septal aneurysm, or both and cryptogenic stroke or transient ischemic attack. *Am Heart J* 1995;130: 1083–1088.

42. Bogousslavsky J, Garazi S, Jeanrenaud X, et al. Stroke recurrence in patients with patent foramen ovale: the Lausanne study. *Neurology* 1996;46:1301–1305.

43. Mas JL, Arquizan C, Lamy C, et al. Recurrent cerebrovascular events associated with patent foramen ovale, atrial septal aneurysm, or both. *N Engl J Med* 2001;345:1740–1746.

44. Mas JL. Patent foramen ovale, atrial septal aneurysm and ischaemic stroke in young adults. *Eur Heart J* 1994;15:446–449.

45. Ranoux D, Cohen A, Cabanes L, et al. Patent foramen ovale: is stroke due to paradoxical embolism? *Stroke* 1993;24:31–34.

46. Silver MD, Dorsey JS. Aneurysms of the septum primum in adults. *Arch Pathol Lab Med* 1978;102:62–65.

47. Mugge A, Daniel WG, Angermann C, et al. Atrial septal aneurysm in adult patients. A multicenter study using transthoracic and transesophageal echocardiography. *Circulation* 1995;91:2785–2792.

48. Berthet K, Lavergne T, Cohen A, et al. Significant association of atrial vulnerability with atrial septal abnormalities in young patients with ischemic stroke of unknown cause. *Stroke* 2000;31:398–403.

49. Caplan LR, Hurst JW, Chimowitz MI. *Clinical neurocardiology*. New York: Marcel Dekker, 1999.

50. Reynen K. Cardiac myxomas. *N Engl J Med* 1995;333:1610–1617.

51. Blondaeu P. Primary cardiac tumors—French studies of 533 cases. *Thorac Cardiovasc Surg* 1990;38[Suppl 2]:192–195.

52. Sandok BA, von Estorff I, Giuliani ER. CNS embolism due to atrial myxoma: clinical features and diagnosis. *Arch Neurol* 1980;37: 485–488.

53. Damasio H, Seabra-Gomes R, daSilva JP, et al. Multiple cerebral aneurysms and cardiac myxomas. *Arch Neurol* 1975;32:269–270.

54. Barnett HJ, Boughner DR, Taylor DW, et al. Further evidence relating mitral valve prolapse to cerebral ischemic events. *N Engl J Med* 1980; 302:139–144.

55. Boughner DR, Barnett HJ. The enigma of the risk of stroke in mitral valve prolapse. *Stroke* 1985;16:175–177.

56. Gilon D, Ferdinando SB, Marshall MJ, et al. Lack of evidence of an association between mitral-valve prolapse and stroke in young patients. *N Engl J Med* 1999;341:8–13.

57. Freed LA, Levy D, Levine RA, et al. Prevalence and clinical outcome of mitral-valve prolapse. *N Engl J Med* 1999;341:1–7.

58. Pomerance A. Pathological and clinical study of calcification of the mitral valve ring. *J Clin Pathol* 1970;23:354–361.

59. DeBono D, Warlow C. Mitral annulus calcification and cerebral or retinal ischemia. *Lancet* 1979;2:383–385.

60. Benjamin EJ, Plehn JF, D'Agostino RB, et al. Mitral annular calcification and the risk of stroke in an elderly cohort. *N Engl J Med* 1992; 327:374–379.

61. Aronow WS. Mitral annular calcification: significant and worth acting upon. *Geriatrics* 1991;46:73–75.

62. Boon A, Lodder J, Cheriex E. Mitral annulus calcification is not an independent risk factor for stroke: a cohort study of 657 patients. *J Neurol* 1997;244:535–541.

63. Sacco RL, Ellenberg JH, Mohr JP, et al. Infarcts of undetermined cause: the NINCDS Stroke Data Bank. *Ann Neurol* 1989;25: 382–390.

64. Fisher CM, Gore I, Okabe N, et al. Atherosclerosis of the carotid and vertebral arteries-extracranial and intracranial. *J Neuropathol Exp Neurol* 1965;24:455–476.

65. Fisher CM, Ojemann RG. A clinico-pathologic study of carotid endarterectomy plaques. *Rev Neurol (Paris)* 1986;142:573–589.

66. Caplan LR, Gorelick PB, Hier DB. Race, sex, and occlusive vascular disease: a review. *Stroke* 1986;17:648–655.

67. Gorelick PB, Caplan LR, Hier DB, et al. Racial differences in the distribution of posterior circulation occlusive disease. *Stroke* 1985;16: 785–790.

68. Feldman E, Daneault N, Kwan E, et al. Chinese-white differences in the distribution of occlusive cerebrovascular disease. *Neurology* 1990; 40:1541–1545.

69. Spencer MP, Thomas GI, Nicholls SC, et al. Detection of middle cerebral artery emboli during carotid endarterectomy using transcranial Doppler ultrasonography. *Stroke* 1990;21:415–423.

70. Markus HS, Brown MM. Differentiation between different pathological cerebral embolic materials using transcranial Doppler in an in vitro model. *Stroke* 1993;24:1–5.

71. Sacco RL. Extracranial carotid stenosis. *N Engl J Med* 2001;345: 1113–1118.

72. Selnes OA, Goldsborough MA, Borowicz LM, et al. Neurobehavioral sequelae of cardiopulmonary bypass. *Lancet* 1999;353:1601–1606.

73. Silver B. Editorial comment. *Stroke* 2001;32:1512–1513.

74. Wolman RL, Nussmeir NA, Aggarawal A, et al. Cerebral injury after cardiac surgery: identification of a group at extraordinary risk. Multicenter Study of Perioperative Ischemia Research Group (McSPI) and

the Ischemia Research Education Foundation (IREF) Investigators *Stroke* 1999;30:514–522.

75. Stamou S, Hill P, Dangas G, et al. Stroke after coronary artery bypass. Incidence, predictors, and clinical outcomes. *Stroke* 2001;32:1508–1513.

76. Hirotami T, Kameda T, Kumamoto T, et al. Stroke after coronary artery bypass grafting in patients with cerebrovascular disease. *Ann Thorac Surg* 2000;70:1571–1576.

77. Goto T, Baba T, Yoshitake A, et al. Craniocervical and aortic atherosclerosis as neurologic risk factors in coronary surgery. *Ann Thorac Surg* 2000;69:834–840.

78. Furlan AJ, Craciun AR. Risk of stroke during coronary artery bypass graft surgery in patients with internal carotid artery disease documented by angiography. *Stroke* 1985;16:797–799.

79. Dashe JF, Pessin MS, Murphy RE, et al. Carotid occlusive disease and stroke risk in coronary artery bypass graft surgery. *Neurology* 1997;49:678–686.

80. Triverdi UH, Patel R, Turtle MR, et al. Relative changes in cerebral blood flow during cardiac operations using xenon-133 clearance versus transcranial Doppler sonography. *Ann Thorac Surg* 1997;63:167–174.

81. Von Reutern GM, Hetzel A, Birnbaum D, et al. Transcranial Doppler ultrasonography during cardiopulmonary bypass in patients with severe carotid stenosis or occlusion. *Stroke* 1988;19:674–680.

82. Wijman CA, Schauble B, Vakili K, et al. Cerebral hemodynamic changes during coronary artery bypass surgery. *Ann Neurol* 1998;44:494(abst).

83. Wijdicks EF, Jack CR. Coronary artery bypass grafting-associated ischemic stroke. *J Neuroimaging* 1996;6:20–22.

84. Tettenborn B, Caplan LR, Sloan MA, et al. Postoperative brainstem cerebellar infarcts. *Neurology* 1993;43:471–477.

85. Borger MA, Ivanov J, Weisel RD, et al. Stroke during coronary bypass surgery: principal role of cerebral macroemboli. *Eur J Cardiothoracic Surg* 2001;19:627–632.

86. Bendszus M, Reents W, Franke D, et al. Brain damage after coronary artery bypass grafting. *Arch Neurol* 2002;59:1090–1095.

87. Blauth CI, Cosgrove DM, Webb BW, et al. Atheroembolism from the ascending aorta: an emerging problem in cardiac surgery. *J Thorac Cardiovasc Surg* 1992;103:1104–1112.

88. van der Linder J, Hadjinikolaou L, Bergman P, et al. Postoperative stroke in cardiac surgery is related to the location and extent of atherosclerotic disease in the ascending aorta. *J Am Coll Cardiol* 2001;38:131–135.

89. Barbut D, Hinton RB, Szatrowski TP, et al. Cerebral emboli detected during bypass surgery are associated with clamp removal. *Stroke* 1994;25:2398–2402.

90. Price DL, Harris J. Cholesterol emboli in cerebral arteries as a complication of retrograde aortic perfusion during cardiac surgery. *Neurology* 1970;20:1207–1214.

91. Calabrese J, Skwerer R, Gulledge A, et al. Incidence of postoperative delirium following myocardial revascularization. *Cleve Clin J Med* 1987;54:29–32.

92. McKhann GM, Grega MA, Borowicz LM, et al. Encephalopathy and stroke after coronary artery bypass grafting. Incidence, consequences, and prediction. *Arch Neurol* 2002;59:1422–1428.

93. Sotaniemi KA, Mononen H, Hokkanen TE. Long-term cerebral outcome after open-heart surgery: a five-year neuropsychological follow-up study. *Stroke;* 1986:17:410–416.

94. McKhann GM, Borowicz L, Goldsborough M, et al. Depression and cognitive decline after coronary artery bypass grafting. *Lancet* 1997;349:1282–1284.

95. Newman MF, Kirchner JL, Phillips-Bute B, et al. Longitudinal assessment of neurocognitive function after coronary-artery bypass surgery. *N Engl J Med* 2001;344:395–402.

96. Lederman R, Breuer A, Hanson M, et al. Peripheral nervous system complications of coronary artery bypass graft surgery. *Ann Neurol* 1982;12:297–301.

97. Hanson MR, Breuer AC, Furlan AJ, et al. Mechanism and frequency of brachial plexus injury in open-heart surgery: a prospective analysis. *Ann Thorac Surg* 1983;36:675–679.

98. Humphreys R, Hoffman H, Mustard W, et al. Cerebral hemorrhage following heart surgery. *J Neurosurg* 1975;43:671–675.

99. Cooper D, Bazaral M, Furlan A, et al. Pituitary apoplexy: a complication of cardiac surgery. *Ann Thorac Surg* 1986;41:547–550.

100. Plasse H, Mittleman M, Frost J. Unilateral sudden hearing loss after open heart surgery: a detailed study of seven cases. *Laryngoscope* 1981;91:101–109.

101. Kanter MC, Hart RG. Neurologic complications of infective endocarditis. *Neurology* 1991;41:1015–1020.

102. Bertorini TE, Laster RE, Thompson BF, et al. Magnetic resonance imaging of the brain in bacterial endocarditis. *Arch Intern Med* 1989;149:815–817.

103. Gransden WR, Eykyn SJ, Leach RM. Neurological presentation of native valve endocarditis. *Q J Med* 1989;73:1135–1142.

104. Ridolfi RL, Bell WR. Thrombotic thrombocytopenic purpura: report of 25 cases and review of the literature. *Medicine* 1981;60:413–427.

105. Bousser MG, Ross RR. *Cerebral venous thrombosis.* London: WB Saunders, 1997.

106. Hankey GJ. Isolated angiitis/angiopathy of the central nervous system. *Cerebrovasc Dis* 1991;1:2–15.

107. Ellison D, Love S, Chimelli L, et al. *Neuropathology: a reference text of CNS pathology.* St. Louis: Mosby.

108. Brierley JB, Graham DI. Hypoxia and vascular disorders of the central nervous system. In: Adams JH, Corsellis JA, Duchen LW, eds. *Greenfield's neuropathology,* 4th ed. London: Edward Arnold, 1984:125–207.

109. Singhal AB, Topcuoglu MA, Koroshetz WJ. Diffusion MRI in three types of anoxic encephalopathy. *J Neurol Sci* 2002;196:37–40.

110. Dooling E, Richardson EP. Delayed encephalopathy after strangling. *Arch Neurol* 1976;33:196–199.

111. Gilles F. Hypotensive brainstem necrosis. *Arch Pathol* 1969;88:32–41.

112. Caronna JJ, Finkelstein S. Neurological syndromes after cardiac arrest. *Stroke* 1978;9:517–520.

113. Levy DE, Caronna JJ, Singer BH, et al. Predicting outcome from hypoxic-ischemic coma. *JAMA* 1985;253:1420–1426.

114. Snyder BD, Gumnit RJ, Leppik IE, et al. Neurologic prognosis after cardiopulmonary arrest: IV. Brainstem reflexes. *Neurology* 1981;31:1092–1097.

115. Steen-Hansen JE, Hansen NN, Vaagenes P, et al. Pupil size and light reactivity during cardiopulmonary resuscitation. A clinical study. *Crit Care Med* 1988;16:69–70.

116. Young GB, Gilbert JJ, Zochodne D. The significance of myoclonic status epilepticus in postanoxic coma. *Neurology* 1990;40:1843–1848.

117. Wijdicks EF, Parisi JE, Sharbrough FW. Prognostic value of myoclonic status in comatose survivors of cardiac arrest. *Ann Neurol* 1994;35:239–243.

118. Nakabayashi M, Kurokawa A, Yamamoto Y. Immediate prediction of recovery of consciousness after cardiac arrest. *Intensive Care Med* 2001;27:1210–1214.

119. Bottiger BW, Mobes S, Glatzer R. Astroglial protein S-100 is an early and sensitive marker of hypoxic brain damage and outcome after cardiac arrest in humans. *Circulation* 2001;103:2694–2698.

120. Hypothermia after Cardiac Arrest Study Group. Mild therapeutic hypothermia to improve the neurologic outcome after cardiac arrest. *N Engl J Med* 2002;346:549–556.

121. Bernard SA, Gray TW, Buist MD, et al. Treatment of comatose survivors of out-of-hospital cardiac arrest with induced hypothermia. *N Engl J Med* 2002;346:557–563.

CHAPTER 101

Diagnosis and Management of Diseases of the Peripheral Arteries and Veins

Paul Wade Wennberg and Thom W. Rooke

Arterial Disease	Venous Disease
Assessment of Arterial Disease	Laboratory Assessment: Venous Disease
Laboratory Assessment	Venous Syndromes
Arterial Syndromes	**References**

Key Words: Deep vein thrombosis; peripheral arterial diseases; venous insufficiency.

ARTERIAL DISEASE

Assessment of Arterial Disease

History

General information including age, sex, associated medical problems (including prior trauma, vascular and orthopedic procedures, and past or current medication use) and risk factors for atherothrombosis should be obtained when taking a patient's history. Symptoms including onset, progression, and aggravating or alleviating factors should be clarified. Claudication, ischemic rest pain, or skin ulceration are the usual presenting complaints of occlusive arterial disease. The description of symptoms may be quite different from patient to patient.

Claudication ("limping") is reproducible discomfort in single or multiple muscle groups brought on by exercise and relieved by rest. Discomfort is typically described as cramping, but it may also be described as numbness, weakness, giving way, aching, burning, or pain. Onset is usually predictable. It is important to remember that claudication from ischemic sources occurs in muscle groups, not in joints. Relief with rest is independent of position. If relief of pain is dependent on po-

P. W. Wennberg: Department of Medicine, Division of Cardiovascular Diseases, Gonda Vascular Center, Mayo Clinic, Rochester, Minnesota.

T. W. Rooke: Department of Medicine, Gonda Vascular Center, Division of Cardiovascular Diseases, Mayo Clinic, Rochester, Minnesota.

sition or is specifically localized to a joint, musculoskeletal or neurologic disorders should be suspected.

Quantization of disease severity by history alone is unreliable. Patient estimates of pace, workload, and distance are unreliable. Standardized treadmill testing with ankle–brachial indices (ABIs) provides objective measurement required for prognostication and long-term follow-up.

Ischemic Rest Pain

When perfusion deficit is severe, patients can experience persistent pain at rest. Pain may be either ischemic *muscular* pain (sensation of cramps) or present as an ischemic *neuropathic* pain (burning or dysthetic in quality). Pain may be confined to digits, a foot, a hand, ulcerated areas, or, less commonly, an entire limb. A local area of trauma in a poorly perfused limb is a frequent cause of such pain (1).

Nocturnal rest pain is common. It is relieved by dependency such as hanging the limb off the bed, sleeping in a chair, or walking. Dependency can lead to edema, further complicating the ischemia. In more severe stages pain may become constant, preventing sleep and causing anorexia and weight loss. Large doses of analgesics may be required and depression often is present.

Examination

Inspection

A red or purplish color of the forefoot that is present during dependency (dependent rubor) is common with severe ischemia. True dependent rubor will give way to pallor with elevation. ABIs will differentiate occlusive disease from these vasomotor changes. Pallor during dependency may be present in chronic ischemia, but it is seen more often in acute ischemia.

Palpation

The aorta, radial, ulnar, subclavian, carotid, temporal, occipital, femoral, popliteal, posterior tibial, and dorsalis pedis arteries are accessible (although the dorsalis pedis artery is congenitally absent in a small minority). Pulses are graded on many scales, the authors use a scale of 0 (absent) to 4 (normal). If a pulse is not palpable, Doppler examination should be performed to establish whether the pulse is absent or below the level of detection by palpation. Temperature is reduced when perfusion is compromised.

Auscultation

Blood pressure should be taken in both arms. If a large difference is noted between arms (>16 mm Hg), blood pressures should be rechecked. If the difference is real, simultaneous pressures (two examiners) should be used to confirm the finding. The femoral, iliac, aortic, carotid, and subclavian arteries should be auscultated routinely. Simultaneous palpation of a radial artery will improve appreciation of subtle bruits and also allows timing of bruits into diastole. As a rule, the further a bruit extends into diastole, the greater is the degree of stenosis. Abdominal bruits are difficult to differentiate, especially if bowel sounds are vigorous. A renal artery source may be suspected if the bruit lateralizes to a flank.

Laboratory Assessment

Vascular testing are traditionally considered as invasive or noninvasive. However, a better classification scheme may be one based on the type of information provided—anatomic, hemodynamic, or functional.

Anatomic Studies

Arteriography is the standard by which all other imaging techniques are judged. It provides reproducible information with high resolution not yet matched by other readily available modalities. Assessment of distal vessels, fine structural detail, and shunting with early venous filling are still best determined by this means. Drawbacks include an arterial catheterization and the risks inherent to arterial puncture. Iodinated contrast also is used, posing a small risk for anaphylactoid reactions and contrast nephropathy.

Computed tomography (CT) and the emerging technique of *computerized tomographic angiography* (CTA) provide detailed anatomic information without need of arterial access. Iodinated contrast is required. CTA also has become the standard for assessing and planning endograft repair of infrarenal

aortic aneurysm since accurate measurement of the "landing zone" (distance between the renal arteries and the neck of the aneurysm) can be made. Magnetic resonance imaging (MRI) and *magnetic resonance angiography* (MRA) provide information similar to CT and CTA, but iodinated contrast is not required (Fig. 101–1). Gadolinium-based contrast agents often are needed, but risk for nephropathy is minimal (2,3). This technique should be considered for patients with renal insufficiency in place of conventional angiography, and if detail is not sufficient, it serves as a screen to limit iodinated contrast during more targeted conventional angiography. MRA, like CTA, provides a three-dimensional image and is able to include or exclude structures of interest. Patients with implantable devices such as pacemakers, automated defibrillators, recently placed arterial stents, and intracranial clips cannot be safely placed into the magnetic field.

Two-dimensional ultrasound provides safe and reliable data of not only anatomy, but also hemodynamic effect of stenosis if and when Doppler analysis of flow is incorporated. Contrast is not required and no ionizing radiation is required. Ultrasound is portable, allowing bedside data acquisition. However, data acquisition may be limited by overlying structures such as bowel gas and other tissues that interfere with imaging.

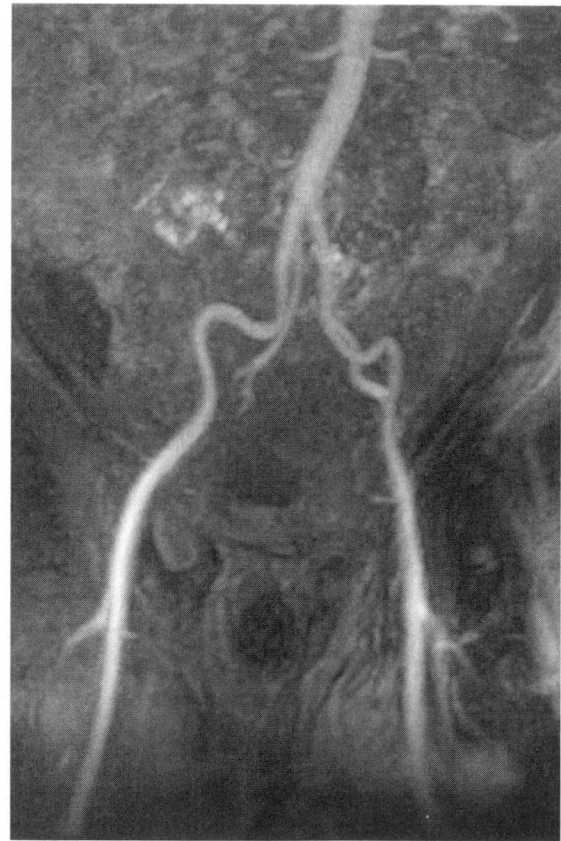

FIG. 101–1. Magnetic resonance angiography of the aorta and iliac system obtained in an obese patient at risk for contrast nephropathy.

Hemodynamic Studies

The hemodynamic significance of a stenosis may be assessed by multiple methods. Invasive measurement of a pressure decrease or gradient across a stenosis is the "gold standard" for hemodynamic assessment. The pressure waveform is valuable information as well, with the normal triphasic waveform changing to monophasic waveform in the presence of severe stenosis. Noninvasive evaluation is available by measuring externally applied pressure at multiple levels (segmental pressures, discussed later in chapter) or by Doppler-derived flow velocities and waveforms.

Functional Studies

When the information obtained by anatomic or hemodynamic testing is insufficient to explain the symptoms or degree of impairment described by the patient, a functional assessment is appropriate. Functional studies involve some form of applied stress, such as treadmill testing, to assess claudication.

Continuous wave Doppler (CWD) detects blood motion and may be used alone as a means of screening for vascular disease (4,5), or it may be an integral part of other tests such as segmental pressure determination (described later).

In a normal artery, the waveform is triphasic. A hemodynamically significant stenosis changes the normal triphasic wave to a biphasic waveform, then monophasic, and then absent as the artery is occluded. Location of a stenosis may be estimated by assessing the Doppler signal at multiple sites along the limb. CWD is inexpensive and may be performed at the bedside as an extension of the vascular examination. Handheld devices often are available on nursing units or may be purchased for personal use. Use of a handheld Doppler requires training and practice to be effective, and the information obtained is limited by that it is a "blind" technique. Duplicated vessels, anatomic variations, and obesity may reduce its accuracy.

Segmental pressures provide a simple, reproducible, inexpensive, and accurate method of determining whether arterial obstruction is present, the severity of the obstruction, and the approximate location of the obstruction(s). Pneumatic cuffs are placed around the thigh, calf, ankle, upper or lower arm, or digits. A CWD probe (discussed earlier) is positioned over the artery at a site distal to the pressure cuff(s) and is used to determine the systolic pressure at which arterial flow resumes as the cuff is deflated. The limb pressures are divided by a reference arterial pressure (i.e., brachial artery systolic pressure) to create an index. The most commonly reported segmental pressure is the ABI. Severity of disease is graded by individual laboratories. Normal is usually defined as an ABI of 1.0 (0.90 is used in some laboratories), with severe disease indicated by an ABI less than 0.50.

There are patients, particularly those with diabetes and those on dialysis, who deposit calcium in the media of conduit arteries (Mönckeberg's calcification) (6). The biggest disadvantage of segmental pressure measurement is that it cannot be reliably used in patients with noncompressible or poorly compressible vessels (7). This occurs most commonly in patients with diabetes. When vessels are stiff, the cuff cannot produce sufficient pressure to obliterate blood flow, and the arterial pressure cannot be determined. Even when the large vessels of the limb are noncompressible, the digital vessels in the toes and fingers often remain noncalcified and can be used to estimate pressure with an appropriate-sized cuff. Many groups use the great toe index in such situations. Pulse volume recording, laser–Doppler studies, and transcutaneous oximetry can be effectively used in these patients as well.

After exercise, ABIs are able to identify arterial lesions that are too minor to produce pressure changes at rest. A decrease in ABI or a change in Doppler signal can be detected after exercise. The subject is placed on a treadmill and exercise is performed under a standardized protocol (8). Elements of the lower extremity study (i.e., ABI or CWD analysis) are performed before and after exercise. With exercise the systolic blood pressure increases as peripheral resistance decreases, resulting in a larger pressure gradient.

Exercise studies also provide ancillary data such as the walking distance to onset of symptoms, absolute walking distance, and blood pressure response during exercise (9). These parameters can be useful for assessing medical and procedural outcomes. They also correlate symptoms, which may be vague, with the data generated, providing objective evidence of the patient's symptoms (10).

Transcutaneous oxygen measurement ($Tcpo_2$) is used to evaluate skin blood flow (11). Oxygen-sensing electrodes are attached with an airtight seal to the skin by means of adhesive rings. The surface temperature of the electrode is maintained at 43°C to 45°C so that the small vessels underlying the electrode are maximally dilated. The amount of oxygen that diffuses out of the skin depends on numerous factors including the arterial partial pressure of oxygen (Pao_2), cutaneous blood flow, and the rate of oxygen consumption by the skin. When cutaneous blood flow is high (relative to the metabolic rate of the skin), $Tcpo_2$ approaches Pao_2. In contrast, when the cutaneous blood flow is low, $Tcpo_2$ is reduced (12). $Tcpo_2$ is not so much a measurement of skin blood flow as it is a measurement of the adequacy of cutaneous oxygen delivery, and it has been shown to be useful in a number of situations including evaluation of critical ischemia. $Tcpo_2$ can be used to predict whether the cutaneous perfusion is adequate for healing at a given amputation site. Values greater than 40 mm Hg are typically sufficient for healing, whereas those less than 20 mm Hg are not likely to heal (13). Certain disease states may affect the small vessels or microcirculation without involving larger arteries. When this occurs, techniques such as CWD, segmental pressures, and pulse volume recording (PVR) will not detect a significant abnormality. In contrast, $Tcpo_2$ measurements will demonstrate the inadequacy of circulation when it is caused by small, nutritive vessel occlusive disease. $Tcpo_2$ determination is valuable in the assessment of patients with diabetes (when noncompressible or poorly compressible vessels are present), small-vessel disease, or both. Although $TcpO_2$ measurement is an accurate way to assess the severity of cutaneous ischemia, it has several limitations including the inability to localize the disease to a particular segment or vessel (14,15).

Arterial Syndromes

Claudication

Peripheral arterial disease (PAD) caused by atherothrombosis is the most common cause of lower extremity ischemic syndromes in Western societies, regardless of age (16,17). Symptoms of PAD are variable. On one extreme, acute onset of ischemic limb pain can occur in the setting of embolic events or thrombosis in situ. On the other extreme, symptoms may go unnoticed as subtle, progressive adaptation of lifestyle compensates for the disease process.

Prevalence and Natural History

The prevalence of PAD is high and increases with age (18). Framingham Study data estimate the annual incidence rate of symptomatic disease at 0.3% and 0.1% for men and women, respectively (19,20). Prevalence of intermittent claudication increases with age: 1.8% for individuals younger than 60 years, 3.7 % for those 60 to 70 years old, and just greater than 5% for those 70 years and older. Risk factors for peripheral arterial disease (PAD) reflect those of coronary disease (21). Diabetes increases the risk for ASO threefold (more so if asymptomatic ASO is included) (22). In a hypertensive elderly population, the incidence of ASO as defined by an ABI less than 0.90 was slightly greater than 25%. The PARTNERS study elegantly demonstrated the high incidence of PAD, especially in the setting of coronary artery disease (CAD) (23). The risk for death, usually because of a cardiovascular event, increases dramatically as the ABI decreases (24). The 5-year mortality rate of a patient with an ABI less than 0.85 is 10%. At an ABI of less than 0.40, the 5-year mortality rate approaches 50% (Fig. 101–2) (25). Mortality is caused by concomitant coronary and cerebrovascular disease. Death primarily caused by PAD complication is rare. The relative risk of death for all-cause mortality is 3.1 in patients with PAD versus the general population (26). The relative risk for coronary heart disease death is 6.9, accounting for more than two-thirds of death in cohorts studied (27).

Although the long-term prognosis of patients with PAD is sobering, the rate of progression and need for revascularization is low (28). Symptoms worsen at 5 years in approximately 20% of patients (29). Requirement for revascularization because of imminent tissue or limb loss or rest pain is around 5% per year. Amputation rates are similarly low, at about 1% per year (30). However, up to 15% of those who continue smoking undergo amputation within 5 years. Patients with diabetes have an amputation rate of 25% over 10 years, which has changed little over time (31–33). Although overall amputation rates for PAD have declined, the increase in the diabetic population has increased, leaving the total number of amputations unchanged. Current practice demonstrates a shift toward distal amputation (below knee), however (34). When PAD is present in a young patient, in the fourth or fifth decade, progression of disease resulting in multiple interventions occurs in approximately 40% of these patients (35). Aggressive medical therapy and close follow-up are indicated. This "premature atherothrombosis" group justifies ongoing intense research efforts.

Treatment

Aggressive risk factor modification is the cornerstone of therapy in all patients. The slow rate of progression and high incidence of cardiovascular comorbidities creates the optimal situation for modifying the underlying atherothrombotic process. Unfortunately, secondary prevention has been disappointing in this group (36). The PARTNERS study found that in patients with PAD, there is a markedly lower rate of treatment for risk factors and antiplatelet medications than in those with coronary disease. This was found in both established and newly diagnosed PAD. The one exception was in smoking cessation where PAD had a greater rate of intervention than CAD. Smoking cessation in PAD is mandatory. The rate of progression and amputation in those who continue to smoke is more than twofold greater than in those who quit smoking (37). It also is the most cost-effective measure available (38). Patients with diabetes have a substantially increased risk for amputation. Tight control of blood sugar reduces complications. Hyperlipidemia and hyperhomocystinemia should be treated.

A walking program should be initiated in all patients with claudication. The effectiveness of a structured walking program has been well demonstrated (39–41). Twenty to 30 minutes, 4 to 5 days per week improves functional capacity, exercise capacity, and increases total and absolute walking distance from 50% to 300% (39). The mechanism of this improvement is not clear, but increased collateral formation or recruitment, muscle training, improved oxygen uptake, or improved mechanics of walking are all plausible (41,42). Diligent foot care and protection must be emphasized, particularly in patients with diabetes and those with severe reductions in ABI or $TcpO_2$ values. Footwear must be supportive and protective, and nail care should be performed regularly by professionals (43). Routine foot care in patients with diabetes with PAD may reduce amputation rates up to four times (44).

Medical therapy for PAD has been slow to develop. Pentoxifylline has been proven effective for increasing claudication distance in some patients with ASO (45). Cilostazol has been approved for use for patients with claudication. It is ef-

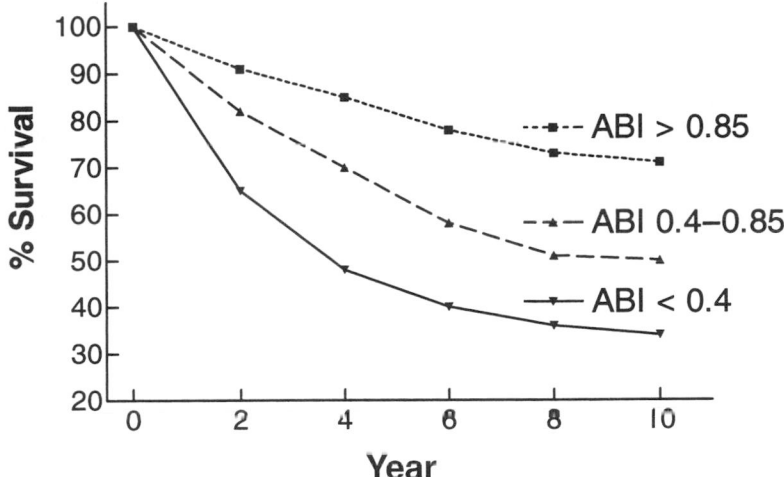

FIG. 101–2. Percent survival over time stratified by ankle–brachial index (ABI). (Adapted from McKenna M, Wolfson S, Kuller L. The ratio of ankle and arm blood pressure as an independent risk factor of mortality. *Atherosclerosis* 1991;87:199–228, with permission.)

fective in increasing walking distance, but the effect is lost when the drug is stopped (46,47). The group shown to benefit includes those with diabetes (48). Direct vasodilators have proven ineffective with the exception of verapamil. In a double-blind, dose-adjusted, placebo-controlled study, verapamil increased pain free walking distance 29% and maximal walking distance 49% (49). β-Blockade has long been believed to be contraindicated for patients with ASO, but studies have refuted this idea (50,51). Given the beneficial effects of β-blockade in patients with CAD, these agents should not be withheld in patients with peripheral ASO.

Antiplatelet agents including aspirin and clopidogrel should be considered first-line agents for patient with PAD. Aspirin therapy has shown benefit after surgical revascularization of the periphery (52). However, in patients with PAD, up to 40% may not respond to aspirin at either low (100 mg daily) or high (300 mg daily) doses (53). The Clopidogrel versus Aspirin in Patients at Risk of Ischaemic Events (CAPRIE) trial showed a benefit of clopidogrel over aspirin in all-cause cardiovascular mortality (54). Patients with PAD had the most significant improvement and should be strongly considered for antiplatelet therapy (55).

Lipid reduction has a beneficial role in patients with PAD. Goals for cholesterol are identical to those for patients with CAD (56). Lipid reduction in CAD has been shown to decrease rates of cerebrovascular events and rate of new claudication symptoms (57). Hypertension has long been associated with PAD. Control should be optimized; recognizing that pressure reduction in the setting of severe stenosis may worsen symptoms in the short term (58). Homocystinemia plays an independent role in development of PAD. The mechanism is at least in part related to an inborn genetic mutation affecting methylene tetrahydrofolate reductase, result-

ing in accelerated intimal damage and early atherothrombosis (59,60). Treatment with folic acid and vitamins B_{12} and B_6 is appropriate when levels are increased (61).

L-carnitine has been studied and shown to improve mitochondrial metabolism in patients with PAD (62–64). Work has been promising, with suggestions that patients with diabetes may benefit greater than patients without diabetes. Prostacyclins, such as beraprost and iloprost, are direct vasodilators that have shown promise in PAD (65,66). Iloprost infusion is effective in acute large and small arterial syndromes in the setting of critical ischemia (67–69). Indication and duration parameters remain to be defined. Orally available prostacyclins such as beraprost have shown mixed results in treatment of claudication. Although promising initially, a recent study in claudication was disappointing (70). Therefore, further study is needed.

Revascularization should be considered in patients with rest pain, impending tissue loss, or significant limitation of lifestyle. Surgical revascularization has been available for years. Large-vessel bypass surgery with vein or synthetic graft material is well established and durable. Percutaneous transluminal angioplasty (PTA), with or without stent placement, is useful for lesions or the renal, iliac, and proximal superficial femoral arteries. Cost-effectiveness of PTA and surgical revascularization compared with walking and medical therapy alone show a benefit at a cost of $38,000 for PTA and $311,000 for surgical revascularization per quality-adjusted life-years over medical therapy alone (71). Despite the advantages of PTA over surgical revascularization, it is important to point out the decreasing long-term effectiveness of PTA in distal vessels and long stenosis. This likely is a reflection of decreasing arterial size limiting rate of flow. However, for patients at high risk for limb loss (deemed poor surgical candidates or technically unfeasible for revascularization), it is reasonable to consider distal angioplasty for limb salvage (72).

Acute Arterial Occlusion

Acute arterial occlusion presents suddenly as a clinical pentad of pain, pallor, paresthesia, paralysis, and pulselessness. The limb may also be cold (polar). Limb survival is at risk if flow is not restored quickly. Distal changes of livedo caused by microembolization may also be seen. Severe ischemia is suggested by pallor at rest, profound coolness, tender or hard muscles, and loss of motor and or sensory functions.

The cause of acute arterial occlusions can be classified into three groups: trauma and dissection, thrombosis *in situ,* and embolism. Attention to arterial integrity is of prime importance in injuries caused by penetration (including medical interventions), crush or fracture, and deceleration injuries. *In situ* thrombosis occurs with both occlusive and aneurysmal disease. Aneurysms, clotting disorders, atherothrombosis, and recent arterial manipulation may precipitate acute occlusion.

Arterial emboli may come from any proximal source, occlusive or aneurysmal, but the majority of emboli originate from the heart. Both the left ventricle and atrium may harbor thrombus (73). Emboli tend to be multiple and recurrent and to distribute randomly, primary to the legs, but with a significant incidence of cerebral, renal, visceral, and arm events (74). Venous thrombi from the right heart or limbs can pass across cardiac septal defects or patent foramen ovale and cause arterial events (75). Echocardiography is useful to determine source (76).

Immediate measures are needed to protect the limb and to restore blood flow. Heparin is given to prevent clot propagation and to stabilize the embolic source(s). Angiography may be required to plan repair when there is preexisting occlusive or aneurysmal disease, or when the cause is unclear. Embolectomy without angiography may be performed when an embolic source is certain and the vessel is considered acceptable to pass a catheter. Ideally, all acute occlusions should be considered for repair, but urgency is governed by the degree of ischemia. When severe ischemia is present, repair must occur within hours to salvage the limb. Additional time may be taken to address ancillary problems in lesser degrees of ischemia, and, at times, no repair is elected when the occlusion has minimal impact on the patient's symptoms or lifestyle. When indicated, thrombolysis of acute occlusion can be effective (77–79) (Fig. 101–3). Bleeding risk and stroke risk must be considered, particularly in the elderly.

Arteriopathies and Other Arterial Syndromes

Buerger's Disease

Thromboangiitis obliterans (TAO) (Buerger's disease), described by Buerger in the late nineteenth century, is an inflammatory vasculopathy with a characteristic, highly cellu-

lar, intraluminal thrombus that affects small- and medium-sized arteries and veins. TAO is always associated with tobacco use, and there may be an autoimmune response to it. Historically, TAO was seen predominantly in male individuals in the second through fifth decades of life, although the incidence in women is increase (80,81). This likely reflects the demographics of tobacco use. Clinically, TAO differs from atherothrombosis in that concurrent involvement of the upper extremity is common. The initial involvement is in digital, pedal, and hand vessels; progression to the calf, thigh, and forearm is brisk and occurs over a few months or years. One-third of patients report Raynaud's phenomenon (82). Recurrent episodes of superficial phlebitis of the calves or forearms are frequently seen. Biopsy of acute lesions, particularly accessible veins, is diagnostic, and angiographic features are characteristic. Rare manifestations include coronary, cerebral, or visceral artery lesions. Stability or improvement is variable and possible only after all exposure to tobacco ceases (83). Cannabis, either on its own or because of contamination with tobacco, may cause a similar entity, and its use also should be addressed (84). Sympathectomy and intravenous prostacyclin analogs can accelerate healing of ischemic lesions, but amputation of damaged digits and limbs often is required (85). Angiogenesis by protein or gene therapy is likely to prove the best hope for this otherwise difficult disease (86).

Popliteal Entrapment and Adventitial Cystic Disease

Popliteal entrapment syndrome occurs when the popliteal artery is trapped by the medial gastrocnemius or various muscular and ligamentous bands during passive dorsiflexion or active plantar flexion (87). Entrapment may cause claudication (and late occlusion) usually in relatively young, healthy individuals. Surgical repair is the treatment of choice. Although uncommon, entrapment syndromes also can be seen at other sites (88,89). Adventitial cystic disease is analogous in structure and content to a ganglion or mucoid cyst. It slowly grows into the popliteal space (or occasionally common femoral artery, or rarely a venous structure), causing claudication or occlusion. Surgical repair is the preferred treatment (90).

Takayasu's and Giant Cell Arteritis

Takayasu's arteritis and giant cell (temporal) arteritis (GCA) are similar in pathologic process but affect different age groups. Differing criteria for age may be argued, but in general Takayasu's arteritis affects individuals younger than 40 years, with GCA usually affecting those older than 60 years. Either may be seen in the fifth and sixth decades of life (91). Also a generality, Takayasu's arteritis involves arteries below the neck, and GCA involves arteries above the neck (92). However, involvement of the aorta, subclavian, axillary, renal, iliac, femoral, and superficial femoral arteries has been described in both. Disease is usually bilateral and

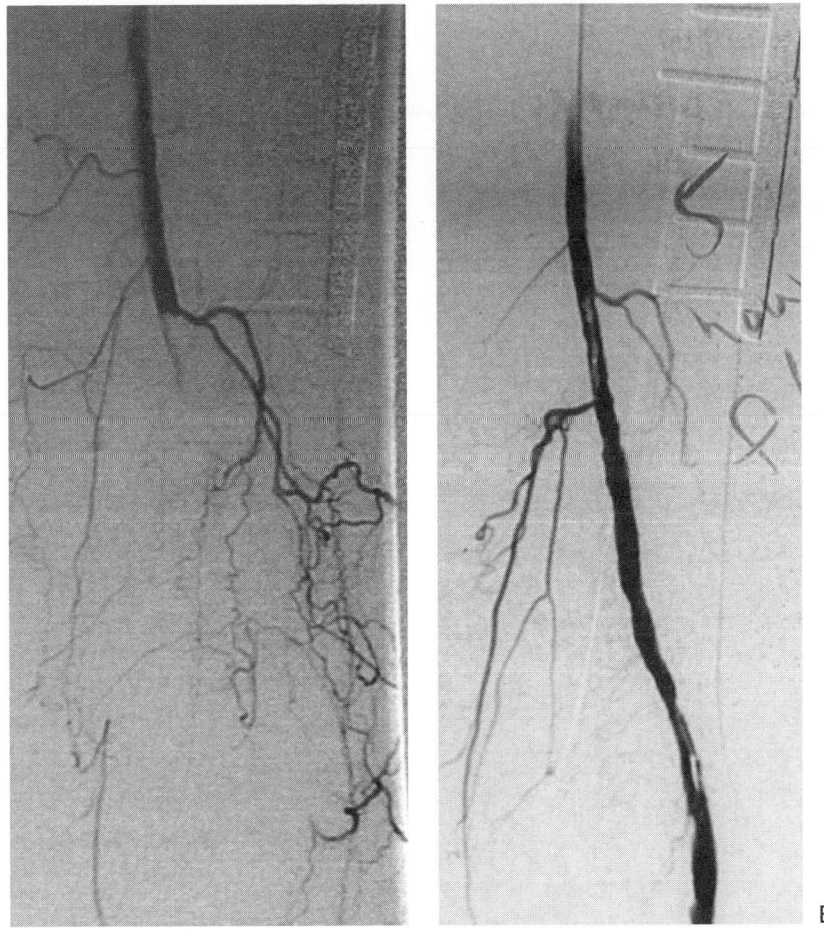

FIG. 101–3. A: Acute occlusion caused by embolic event in the superficial femoral artery. **B:** Repeat angiography after 5 hours of catheter-directed lytic therapy demonstrating preexisting atherothrombosis.

results in rapidly progressive claudication. Ischemia is rare. Both have characteristic clinical and laboratory findings including an increased sedimentation rate (most common, but not in all) and typical arteriographic features. For GCA, confirmatory biopsy of the temporal artery within 3 days of starting steroids is the gold standard (93). These diseases are unique among arteriopathies in that the acutely stenotic lesions improve rapidly with steroid therapy (94–96). Revascularization, when required, is best performed when the inflammatory process is quiet or "burned out" and steroids have been discontinued or requirements tapered to a low maintenance dose (97,98).

Ergot

Ergot compounds can induce Raynaud's phenomenon, claudication, acute ischemia, or tissue infarction. Problems are usually seen in those patients using ergot for treatment migraine headaches. Intravenous nitroprusside infusion may help acute ischemia (99). The incidence of ergot toxicity is decreasing as alternatives for migraine treatment become available, but it should be considered in patients with ischemia and few, if any, risk factors (100).

Fibromuscular Dysplasia

Fibromuscular dysplasia has been described in almost all named arteries. It most commonly affects middle-aged women. Renal artery disease is most common, affecting 4% to 5% of the population. Cut carotid, mesenteric, and both upper and lower extremity diseases may be seen. Bilateral disease is present in about 10% of cases (101). Arterial dissection is associated with fibromuscular dysplasia, causing about 10% of total spontaneous dissections; more than 20% of carotid dissections in women (102).

Aneurysms

Arterial aneurysms are a major cause of death and disability. Early detection allows definitive repair. The three most common aneurysms are accessible to examination including 40% to 60% of abdominal aortic aneurysms and almost all popliteal and femoral aneurysms (103). Several general characteristics of aneurysmal disease are useful in clinical decision making. Aneurysms caused by degenerative etiologic factors enlarge over years to decades. Aneurysms caused by infectious or traumatic etiologic factors expand over days to months. It should be noted that aneurysms tend to occur concurrently at multiple sites. About 5% to 10% of patients with an aortic aneurysm and 50% of those with peripheral aneurysms will have aneurysms elsewhere (104). Therefore, when a popliteal aneurysm is found, a careful search for iliac, femoral, and aortic aneurysms should be performed. Aortic aneurysms are discussed elsewhere in this textbook.

Treatment of aneurysm is undergoing a radical change. Effective and durable treatment by surgical resection of abdominal aortic aneurysm and synthetic graft placement is well established. Over the last decade, advances in endovascular repair have occurred. However, minor complications including endograft leak require increased surveillance after the procedure. A type II endoleak, from a side vessel into the aneurysm sack, is the most common (105).

Vasospastic Disorders

Color and warmth of the acral parts vary considerably from person to person in a normal population, reflecting individual vasomotor tone. Livedo reticularis, acrocyanosis, and Raynaud's phenomenon are distinctive clinical syndromes manifest by abnormal color and temperature changes of the skin. These syndromes are induced or intensified as a result of stimuli from cold, emotion, or drugs. They cause spasm in digital arteries, arterioles, and venules. These disorders are usually benign, lifelong, primary processes, but all three syndromes can have important secondary causes. Careful clinical examination and selective testing will usually confirm the specific cause and define prognosis and the direction of therapy.

Livedo

Livedo reticularis is characterized by a persistent, symmetric, bluish, lacy pattern on the extremities and sometimes the trunk with variable extent and intensity. It is most apparent after stimulation by cold or emotion and fades with warmth and exercise. It is first seen in childhood or at puberty and is more common in women and fair-skinned individuals. It is so frequent in its milder form that it often is overlooked or considered a variant of normal skin. It is postulated that spasm of the cutaneous arterioles (with secondary dilation of the capillaries and venules) causes slow flow, increased oxygen uptake, and reduced oxyhemoglobin, producing color change. Primary livedo reticularis often is seen with acrocyanosis and primary Raynaud's disease. Treatment rarely is needed. Secondary livedo reticularis is patchy, focal, or asymmetric in distribution, relatively late in onset, and may be complicated by local infarction or ulceration. The lesions may be elevated or tender when caused by vasculitis. Therapy is directed at the underlying cause. Severe livedo reticularis in the setting of multiple cerebrovascular events may suggest Sneddon's syndrome. In this group, antiphospholipid antibodies are common (106).

Acrocyanosis

Acrocyanosis is a benign, persistent, cyanotic discoloration and coolness of the hands (or fingers, sometimes the feet) more commonly seen in women. Cold and emotion intensify—whereas warmth and exercise ameliorate—the findings. Mild local edema is not uncommon and bothersome; associated hyperhidrosis may require treatment. Acrocyanosis is painless and does not ulcerate, but it is a bothersome cosmetic problem for some. Calcium entry blockers or α_1 antagonists often will reduce the symptoms. A modest degree of acrocyanosis is sometimes seen in limbs immobilized by neurogenic deficits. Rarely, β-blockade will induce the syndrome. It may also present as a paraneoplastic phenomenon (107,108).

Raynaud's Phenomenon

Raynaud's phenomenon is diagnosed from history alone. It is difficult to demonstrate, even with ice immersion, as whole body cooling may be needed to induce findings. The syndrome is defined as episodes of blue or white color changes of the digits induced by cold or emotional stimuli followed by reactive hyperemia during recovery. Most patients describe the white phase and the red of the hyperemic phase, but few will spontaneously describe blue changing to white or blue only. A dead, numb feeling (but rarely pain) accompanies the ischemic phase, and a dysthetic, throbbing, or painful sensation is common in recovery. Fingers are involved more often than toes—initially the distal digits and later the entire digit, but rarely the palm. The thumbs often are spared. Recovery time is 3 to 10 minutes but can exceed 1 hour in advanced cases, usually of secondary origin (109). Allen and Brown (110) defined primary Raynaud's phenomenon as episodes of bilateral color changes induced by cold or emotion without evidence of ischemia or other disease for 2 years. Later development of secondary disease was noted in 2% to 5% of patients (111). A prospective study confirms that patients without laboratory evidence of digital occlusive, clotting, or serologic abnormalities have a benign course, with only 2% showing secondary causes in the subsequent decade (112).

Unilateral Raynaud's phenomenon, trophic skin changes, and ischemic lesions suggest a secondary process and often accompanying occlusion (113). Causes of secondary Raynaud's phenomenon are diverse. Most can be defined by history and examination, knowledge of their natural behavior, vascular laboratory measurements of digital obstruction, and clotting or serologic tests. Vibratory tools such as chain saws, grinders, and jackhammers can induce hand dysesthesias and Raynaud's phenomenon when used for several years. Symptoms initially occur during use, but they may become chronic in later stages. Ischemia is a rare and late occurrence (114,115).

Most patients with primary Raynaud's phenomenon require no therapy and quickly learn to keep not only their hands but their whole body warm. Arteriography (from the arch through the digits, bilaterally) is useful in difficult cases or when surgical intervention is considered. Treatment of secondary forms is directed at the underlying cause when feasible. Calcium channel blockers and α-blockade, alone or in combination, can suppress the episodes in some patients, but they may have little impact on ischemic complications. These are best treated as conservatively as possible with local debridement and control of infection and pain.

Thoracic Outlet Syndrome

Thoracic outlet syndrome is difficult to diagnose and to treat. This difficulty reflects the anatomy, in that the artery, vein, and nervous bundle all pass through a small, dynamic space as they leave the thorax. The usual mechanism of damage is from the clavicle and a cervical rib (or the first rib) impinging on the subclavian artery like scissors. The result is stenosis and possible poststenotic aneurysm of the subclavian artery. Hypertrophy of the scalene musculature may add to the osseous cause or may be present independently (116). Aneurysmal dilatation is prone to thrombus formation, leading to thromboembolism and distal arterial occlusion (Fig. 101–4). Raynaud's phenomenon is common. Venous occlusion or "effort thrombosis" in the subclavian artery (Paget-Schroetter syndrome) may be the presenting complaint. This is most frequently seen in active individuals—such as construction workers and athletes—with repetitive motion closing the venous outflow (117). Neurogenic complaints may be present and difficult to isolate. In cases with pure neurologic findings, long-term resolution after intervention is less reliable (118).

It is important to point out that *the presence of positive thoracic outlet maneuvers does not equal the diagnosis of thoracic outlet syndrome.* Imaging for the presence of an aneurysm or a stenosis, dynamic or static, with Duplex ultrasound or arteriography is needed when the diagnosis is entertained. Clinical correlation is required for the diagnosis. Initial treatment for uncomplicated cases—that is, no distal embolization or arterial damage—should include thoracic outlet opening exercises (119). If arterial damage or distal embolization has occurred, resection of a cervical rib or first rib, or both, frequently is required (120). However, improvement of symptoms is variable (121). For venous occlusion, initial treatment should be aimed at opening the subclavian vein, most frequently with thrombolysis. The optimal timing of further surgical intervention, immediate or delayed with several weeks to months of anticoagulation, is not yet established (122).

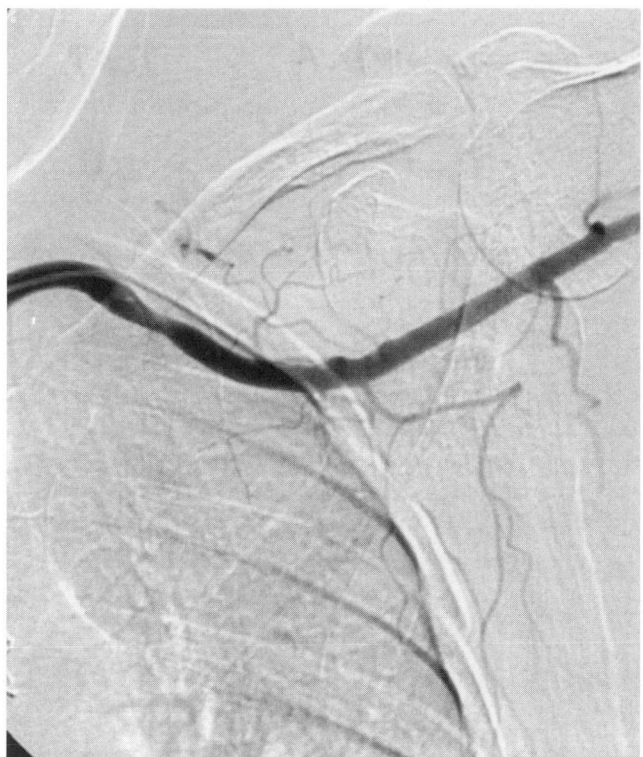
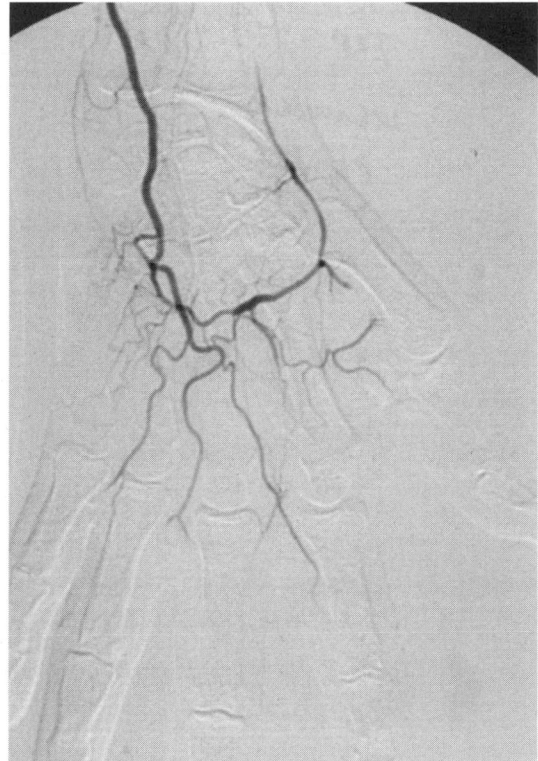

FIG. 101–4. A: Stenosis of the left subclavian artery caused by impingement between the first rib and the clavicle. **B:** Distal emboli of the left radial artery and in multiple digital arteries. Film is taken in early phase demonstrating collateralization through the palmar arch.

VENOUS DISEASE

Laboratory Assessment: Venous Disease

Venous tests may be invasive (i.e., venography) or noninvasive. The information provided may be classified as anatomic, hemodynamic, or functional. Indications for venous testing include objective documentation supporting the diagnosis of venous disease, assessment of severity, and monitoring of progression or regression of disease.

Anatomic Studies

Duplex ultrasound, CT, MRI, and venography are anatomic methods available for evaluation of the venous system. Venography is considered the "gold standard" for determination of deep vein thrombosis (DVT). However, venous *duplex ultrasound* is the most commonly used technique. Duplex has the advantage of differentiating acute from old thrombus based on the presence of venous distension (common in acute clot) and increased echogenicity (common in chronic clot). Compared with venography, duplex ultrasound is less sensitive both above the groin and below the knee. *CT venography* is widely used as a rapid and reliable screen for pulmonary embolism (Fig. 101–5). *MR venography* is emerging. In addition to providing accurate information above the groin in the iliac veins, despite body habitus, they may be performed concurrently with pulmonary embolism studies and dovetail nicely with duplex ultrasound.

Physiologic Studies

CWD provides qualitative (but not quantitative) information about blood movement, and thus the presence of reflux or obstruction. There are five general features of venous CWD addressed at each level examined. Venous flow should be *spontaneous, phasic* with respiratory variation, *competent* to proximal compression, *augment* with distal compression, and be free of *pulsatility.* Deep vein obstruction is likely to be present if spontaneity, phasicity, or augmentation is lost. Deep vein incompetence is present if compression of a proximal segment results in flow reversal. A pulsatile signal suggests increased central venous pressure or arterial venous fistula. These data may be obtained with duplex evaluation as part of a full venous assessment.

By examining multiple levels, localization of incompetence or obstruction can be made (specificity 88%, sensitivity 85%) (123). However, CWD alone is a poor technique for evaluating partially obstructing thrombus or confirming acute DVT. And, although it is sensitive for detecting hemodynamically significant valvular incompetence, it cannot determine the functional significance of venous incompetence. In contrast to the triphasic arterial signal, the venous signal is much more complex.

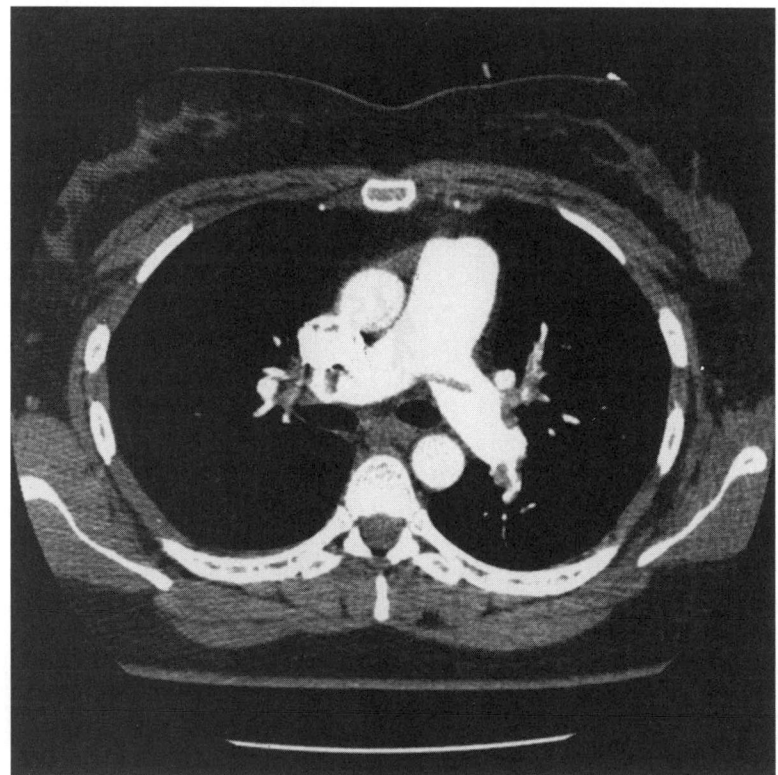

FIG. 101–5. Computed tomography scan of the pulmonary vasculature demonstrating multiple, bilateral pulmonary emboli seen as filling defects in the contrast-enhanced pulmonary vasculature. In this patient, filling defects were present in fourth-order vessels.

Plethysmography

Plethysmography measurement records the change in limb volume caused by arterial inflow, venous outflow, or venous reflux over time. The rate of change is increased with venous incompetence or is decreased when venous outflow is impeded. The most common plethysmographic techniques are strain gauge plethysmography, air plethysmography, and impedance plethysmography (IPG). Photo plethysmography is not truly a plethysmographic technique, but instead estimates the amount of blood in the limb by reflecting infrared light off red blood cells flowing through the cutaneous vasculature (124).

Plethysmography for Venous Incompetence

Passive drainage can be assessed by raising the legs and reaching a low volume steady state. The patient is then tipped forward and blood refills the venous system. If incompetent, blood fall from the proximal veins (retrograde) and calf volume increases rapidly. If competent, refilling time is slower, relying on arterial inflow to fill the venous structure (antegrade). Once the blood has been emptied, the patient is returned to the upright position and the veins refill (125). The next question is whether the incompetence is located in the superficial or deep venous elements, or both. If the incompetence is primarily superficial, placing light tourniquets around the leg or directly compressing an incompetent superficial vein with a finger, or both, will normalize refilling time (126).

Outflow Plethysmography

Plethysmography is useful in screening limbs for venous outflow obstruction. IPG is the best studied technique (127–129). Unlike anatomic tests such as venography or ultrasound scanning (i.e., tests that directly image the thrombus), IPG identifies the presence of functional venous obstruction.

To test for the presence of venous outflow obstruction, the patient lies supine with the legs elevated and slightly flexed. A pneumatic cuff placed around the thigh is inflated to greater than venous pressure but below arterial pressure (typically 40–50 mm Hg), blood becomes trapped beyond the cuff and the volume of the lower leg increases. After equilibrium is reached (1–2 minutes typically), the cuff is rapidly deflated, blood drains from the limb, and volume decreases rapidly. The rate of outflow against is plotted against the increase in volume during venous occlusion on a standard curve. If outflow rate is brisk, the venous system is considered patent. If outflow rate is slow, obstruction may be present. The role of IPG for screening is giving way to Duplex ultrasound in most centers. Because IPG relies on indirect evidence of venous obstruction, it may be subject to more false-positive and negative results than the imaging tests (130–132). Nevertheless, the ease of performance, low cost, and reasonable overall accuracy of IPG make it a useful screening tool.

Developing Techniques

CT and MR venography are proving to be accurate and applicable in clinical practice (133–136). A negative D-dimer profile has been shown to be an excellent predictor for no acute thrombosis (137–139).

Venous Syndromes

Varicose Veins

Varicosities of the superficial veins may be classified as primary or secondary. *Primary varicosities* often are familial, first appearing during the teen years or during pregnancy. Burning, bursting, bruising, or aching are just some of the sensations reported by patients. Elevation or walking/exercise will relieve symptoms. Symptoms are exacerbated by prolonged standing or dependency, obesity, and pregnancy. *Secondary varicosities* reflect underlying deep venous obstruction and/or incompetence, or perforator vein incompetence. Any of these anomalies shifts venous from the deep venous structures to the superficial veins. Common secondary causes of varicosities include extrinsic venous compression, prior DVT, congenital lesions, arteriovenous fistulas, and right heart disease. Edema and venous stasis changes rarely are caused by primary varicosities and usually signal the presence of an underlying secondary process. The history, examination, and (when necessary) laboratory evaluation of the deep venous system usually will allow the physician to differentiate primary from secondary varicosities.

Varicose veins are common (140). The varicosities may ache or burn with standing or prolonged sitting with the legs in a dependent position. Episodes of superficial thrombophlebitis may occur, and if repetitive. ablation of the veins is appropriate. Rarely, veins may bleed; this bleeding often is brisk despite the venous because venous pressure is increased when the limb is dependent. Control of bleeding must therefore include pressure and limb elevation. Symptoms can be improved by graduated compression hose of 20 to 30 mm Hg or more. Ablation of the vein should be considered if complications or discomfort interfere with occupation or lifestyle. Sclerotherapy is effective for certain varicosities and cutaneous "spiders." Laser therapy is effective for small "spider veins" and telangiectasias (141). Surgical removal is indicated for longer segments of proximal varicosities, especially if perforator or saphenofemoral incompetence is present (142). Recently, endovascular techniques have become available (143).

Superficial Thrombophlebitis

Superficial thrombophlebitis presents as a warm, tender, erythematous, and indurated linear lesion in the anatomic course of a superficial vein. Ultrasound can differentiate thrombophlebitis from lymphangitic streaks, erythema nodosum, and other lesions. Thrombophlebitis often occurs in a varicose vein or at sites of indwelling catheters or intravenous injections. Active infection may be associated with the latter and, in such cases, antibiotics should be considered. Evaluation for underlying diseases that can predispose to clotting or a clotting abnormality should be considered. One study suggested one-third of patients with a primary DVT have an underlying clotting abnormality (144). Superficial thrombophlebitis is usually self-limited. Recovery can be accelerated by rest, topical warmth, and antiinflammatory agents. Systemic anticoagulation is appropriate for lesions that progress with conservative care or are located proximally in the lesser or greater saphenous veins such that minimal extension would enter the deep system. There is a high incidence of concurrent DVT in superficial thrombophlebitis (145). Duplex ultrasound should be used to screen for DVT because management with chronic anticoagulation would then be indicated.

Deep Vein Thrombosis

The morbidity and mortality of DVT remain high. Risk factors for DVT and pulmonary embolism have been well defined in several studies (146). The signs and symptoms of DVT are not specific (often findings are absent or subtle), but they include prominent superficial venous pattern, edema, discomfort at rest, and pain with compression. Objective testing to confirm and define the extent of DVT should be obtained whenever one is suspected. Confirmed diagnosis strengthens the decision to treat when anticoagulation is relatively contraindicated. Less than half of patients considered to have DVT have the diagnosis confirmed when tested objectively (147,148). If the diagnosis is disproved, the cost of treatment and the risks for hemorrhage, heparin-induced thrombocytopenia, and warfarin necrosis are avoided.

When DVT or thromboembolic events occur without a recognized risk factor, a search for venous compression, inherited or acquired clotting abnormalities, systemic disease, and age-appropriate cancer screening is appropriate (138, 149,150). Such screening is valuable, even when the results are negative, in establishing prognosis and planning duration of anticoagulation therapy (151). Evaluation for known thrombophilia is indicated when there is a strong family history of thrombosis or when the precipitating event seems mild. As good techniques become more readily available and at a lower cost, the indications should expand.

Treatment with heparin acutely followed by warfarin chronically is highly effective in preventing clot propagation and pulmonary embolism. Duration of treatment for optimal risk–benefit ratio is unknown. Recent literature suggests treatment for a minimum of 6 to 12 months in patients with spontaneous DVT (152,153). Low–molecular weight heparins (adjusted for weight) have shown promise in treating DVT and can be used for outpatient management in uncomplicated cases (154,155). It also serves as an excellent bridge for short-term anticoagulation while Coumadin effect is increasing (or decreasing before a procedure). The risk for major hemorrhage from anticoagulation is 1% to 3% per year when control is strict and attention is paid to drugs that alter warfarin effect (156,157). The risk for bleeding increases markedly when the international normalized ratio (INR) is greater than 4.0 (158). The INR should be followed to ensure consistency among laboratories. Patients should be encouraged to know and record their INR for potential emergencies. The most common mistake in treatment of DVT is failure to use adequate compression. The result is swelling that often is mistaken for failure of Coumadin therapy. Elastic wrapping initially followed by several months of use of 20- to 30-mm Hg or, if tolerated, 30- to 40-mm Hg compression stockings is appropriate.

Thrombolytic therapy, given early, accelerates recovery and may reduce incidence and severity of postphlebitic syndrome (159,160). It appears to be most effective in ileo-femoral DVT (161). Mechanical thrombectomy also is promising and may be combined with thrombolysis (162). However, well defined indications for thrombolytic therapy in DVT have not yet been established. Long-term use of compression stockings to the knee (or above, if tolerated) drastically reduces the incidence of postphlebitic syndrome, venous stasis changes, and venous ulceration (163–165).

DVT isolated to the calf is thought to be less dangerous than DVT of the thigh, but, in fact, upward of 20% of such thrombi extend proximally and 10% embolize (166). Ultrasound surveillance is required if anticoagulants are withheld. Patients with isolated calf DVT also are prone to persistent symptoms and postphlebitic syndrome (167).

Prophylactic anticoagulation is warranted in all patients in the setting of trauma, medical or surgical illness, or prolonged bed rest (168–172). If anticoagulation must be interrupted for a surgical procedure, a baseline duplex ultrasound and postoperative surveillance ultrasound (on or about Day 2 after surgery) may be obtained. With this approach acute clot in the presence of chronic clot is more easily detected. In patients with absolute contraindication for anticoagulation and at high risk for pulmonary embolism, an inferior vena cava filter should be considered. This does not decrease the risk for DVT, and anticoagulation should begin as soon as possible.

Complications

Heparin-induced thrombocytopenia is detected by daily monitoring of platelets. If there is known heparin-induced thrombocytopenia or it is suspected, all heparin exposure must stop immediately (173,174). Hirudin or danaparoid may be used in place of heparin until Coumadin effect is therapeutic (175,176). Warfarin-induced necrosis, although rare, may be avoided by overlapping heparin with warfarin for 4 to 5 days (177,178).

Phlegmasia cerulea dolens is a rare complication of DVT characterized by rapid, massive edema, severe pain, and cyanosis. This most commonly occurs in the setting of extensive iliofemoral thrombosis. One-third of patients die of pulmonary embolism, and distal gangrene develops in half of patients. It is seen most commonly with advanced malignancy or severe infections but can follow surgery, fractures, and other common precipitants of thrombosis. Urgent treatment including placement of a caval filter, heparinization, and often physical removal of the clot by thrombectomy (surgical or endovascular) and thrombolysis is essential to minimize loss of life or limb (179).

Thrombosis in Central Veins

Superior vena cava syndrome is rare. Etiologic factors include radiation, central lines, tumor, adenopathy, or fibrosing mediastinitis (180–182). Symptoms and signs include head fullness or headache and neck, face, and arm swelling. The presence of superficial collateral veins across the chest is best appreciated with the patient upright. *Inferior vena cava* syndrome may be an acute event or may occur gradually from extrinsic compression (Fig. 101–6) or extension of ileofemoral thrombosis. The acute syndrome produces massive

lower extremity swelling and discomfort. Venous collaterals across the abdomen and pelvis are prominent in chronic occlusion. Bilateral severe leg swelling and pain is the most common symptom (183). Both inferior and superior vena cava syndromes may be the initial manifestation of a primary clotting abnormality. Thrombolytic therapy may clear thrombosis when given early. Endovascular stenting or bypass surgery is effective in selected instances of either syndrome, but frequently may only be offered for temporary relief.

Acute and chronic *hepatic vein thrombosis* (Budd-Chiari syndrome) presents with varying degrees of hepatic failure and ascites; clotting disorders, tumors, and congenital venous anomalies are the most common causes (184,185). Axillo-subclavian thrombosis (Paget-Schroetter syndrome) often is attributed to unusual effort or positioning. There often is evidence of thoracic outlet obstruction. Catheter-related thrombus, central or peripheral, is treated by removing the line and treating with heparin if possible. Thrombolytic therapy can be effective when given early and followed by chronic anticoagulation.

Postphlebitic Syndrome

Chronic *deep venous incompetence,* with or without venous obstruction, causes venous hypertension. This is characterized by leg edema, venous dilation, and intradermal deposition of proteins and hemosiderin. Cutaneous changes of fibrosis, lichenification, cellulitis, and ulceration may follow. Edema of the foot (with sparing of the toes) differentiates edema of chronic venous insufficiency from lymphedema. Postphlebitic syndrome occurs months to years after DVT and onset of deep venous incompetence (186). Symptoms include heavy, congested limbs, venous claudication, pruritus, and skin ulceration that often is painless. Increased ambulatory pressure can be confirmed by direct measurement or plethysmography. Both incompetence and obstruction can be documented by bidirectional Doppler, ultrasound, duplex ultrasound, or venography (187).

Venous ulceration is usually perimalleolar and is medial more often than lateral. This area receives the greatest venous pressure, often in excess of perfusion pressure, resulting in chronic hypoxic skin prone to injury. Once ulceration has occurred, successful management is staged. Reduction of the edema and debridement of the ulcer must occur first, followed by healing of the ulcer, and finally lifelong control of venous hypertension using elastic support at 30 to 40 mm Hg of compression (more if required). If venous ulceration occurs on the setting of moderate to severe PAD, treatment may be difficult. Compression must still be applied, but with a low stretch rap to avoid further reduction of arterial inflow.

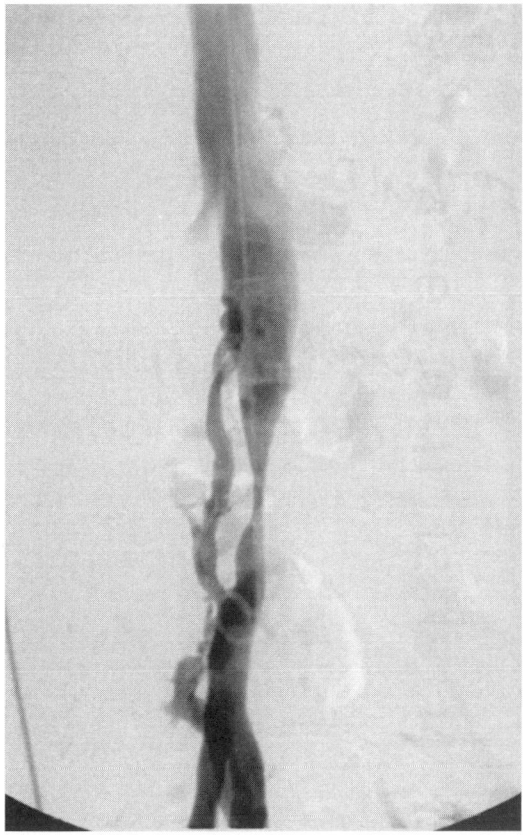

FIG. 101–6. Inferior cavogram demonstrating extrinsic compression of the inferior vena cava because of retroperitoneal fibrosis. Note the collateral vessel.

REFERENCES

1. Burns SL, Leese GP, McMurdo ME. Older people and ill fitting shoes. *Postgrad Med J* 2002;78:344–346.
2. Tombach B, Bremer C, Reimer P, et al. Using highly concentrated

gadobutrol as an MR contrast agent in patients also requiring hemodialysis: safety and dialysability. *AJR Am J Roentgenol* 2002;178:105–109.

3. Bellin MF, Deray G, Assogba U, et al. Gd-DOTA: evaluation of its renal tolerance in patients with chronic renal failure. *Magn Reson Imaging* 1992;10:115–118.

4. Strandness DJ, Schultz R, Sumner D, et al. Ultrasound flow detection: a useful technic in the evaluation of peripheral vascular disease. *Am J Surg* 1967;113:311–320.

5. Strandness DJ, McCutcheon E, Rushmer R. Application of transcutaneous Doppler flowmeter in evaluation of occlusive arterial disease. *Surg Gynecol Obstet* 1966;122:1039–1045.

6. Lanzer P. Topographic distribution of peripheral arteriopathy in non-diabetics and type 2 diabetics. *Z Kardiol* 2001;90:99–103.

7. Hobbs J, Yao J, Lewis J, et al. A limitation of the Doppler ultrasound method of measuring ankle systolic pressure. *Vasa* 1974;160–164.

8. Regensteiner JG, Gardner A, Hiatt WR. Exercise testing and exercise rehabilitation for patients with peripheral arterial disease: status in 1997. *Vasc Med* 1997;2:147–155.

9. Regensteiner JG, Hiatt WR. Medical management of peripheral arterial disease. *J Vasc Interv Radiol* 1994;5:669–677.

10. McDermott MM, Mehta S, Liu K, et al. Leg symptoms, the ankle-brachial index, and walking ability in patients with peripheral arterial disease. *J Gen Intern Med* 1999;14:173–181.

11. Rooke T. The use of transcutaneous oximetry in the noninvasive vascular laboratory. *Int Angiol* 1992;36–40.

12. Rooke T, Hollier L, Osmundson P. The influence of sympathetic nerves on transcutaneous oxygen tension in normal and ischemic lower extremities. *Angiology* 1987;38:400–410.

13. Bacharach J, Rooke T, Osmundson P, et al. Predictive value of transcutaneous oxygen pressure and amputation success by use of supine and elevation measurements. *J Vasc Surg* 1992;558–563.

14. Rooke T, Osmundson P. The influence of age, sex, smoking, and diabetes on lower limb transcutaneous oxygen tension in patients with arterial occlusive disease. *Arch Intern Med* 1990;150:129–132.

15. Rooke TW, Osmundson PJ. Variability and reproducibility of transcutaneous oxygen tension measurements in the assessment of peripheral vascular disease. *Angiology* 1989;40:695–699.

16. Criqui MH, Denenberg JO, Langer RD, et al. The epidemiology of peripheral arterial disease: importance of identifying the population at risk. *Vasc Med* 1997;2:221–226.

17. Criqui MH, Fronek A, Barrett-Connor E, et al. The prevalence of peripheral arterial disease in a defined population. *Circulation* 1985;71:510–515.

18. Criqui MH. Peripheral arterial disease—epidemiological aspects. *Vasc Med* 2001;6:3–7.

19. Kannel WB, Vokonas PS. Demographics of the prevalence, incidence, and management of coronary heart disease in the elderly and in women. *Ann Epidemiol* 1992;2:5–14.

20. Kannel W, McGee D. Update on some epidemiologic features of intermittent claudication: the Framingham Study. *J Am Geriatr Soc* 1985;33:13.

21. Hooi JD, Kester AD, Stoffers HE, et al. Incidence of and risk factors for asymptomatic peripheral arterial occlusive disease: a longitudinal study. *Am J Epidemiol* 2001;153:666–672.

22. Hooi J, Stoffers H, Kester A, et al. Risk factors and cardiovascular diseases associated with asymptomatic peripheral arterial occlusive disease. The Limburg PAOD Study. Peripheral Arterial Occlusive Disease. *Scand J Prim Health Care* 1998;16:177–182.

23. Hirsch AT, Criqui MH, Treat-Jacobson D, et al. Peripheral arterial disease detection, awareness, and treatment in primary care. *JAMA* 2001;286:1317–1324.

24. Hooi JD, Stoffers HE, Knottnerus JA, et al. The prognosis of non-critical limb ischaemia: a systematic review of population-based evidence. *Br J Gen Pract* 1999;49:49–55.

25. McKenna M, Wolfson S, Kuller L. The ratio of ankle and arm blood pressure as an independent risk factor of mortality. *Atherosclerosis* 1991;87:199–228.

26. Criqui M, Langer R, Fronek A, et al. Mortality over a period of 10 years in patients with peripheral arterial disease. *N Engl J Med* 1992;326:381–386.

27. Lassila R, Lepantalo M, Lindfors O. Peripheral arterial disease—natural outcome. *Acta Med Scand* 1986;220:295–301.

28. McDaniel M, Cronenwett J. Basic data related to the natural history of intermittent claudication. *Ann Vasc Surg* 1989;3:273.

29. Imparato A, Kim G, Davidson T, et al. Intermittent claudication: its natural course. *Surgery* 1975;78:795–799.

30. Feinglass J, Brown J, LoSasso A, et al. Rates of lower extremity amputation and arterial reconstruction in the United States, 1979 to 1996. *Am J Public Health* 1999;89:1222–1227.

31. Moss SE, Klein R, Klein BE. The 14-year incidence of lower-extremity amputation in a diabetic population. The Wisconsin Epidemiologic Study of Diabetic Retinopathy. *Diabetes Care* 1999;22:951–959.

32. Juergens J, Barker N, Hines EJ. Arteriosclerosis obliterans: review of 520 cases with special reference to pathogenic and prognostic factors. *Circulation* 1960;21:188–195.

33. Schadt D, Hines AJ, Juergens J, et al. Chronic atherosclerotic occlusion of the femoral artery. *JAMA* 1961;175:937–940.

34. Fletcher DD, Andrews KL, Hallett JW Jr, et al. Trends in rehabilitation after amputation for geriatric patients with vascular disease: implications for future health resource allocation. *Arch Phys Med Rehabil* 2002;83:1389–1393.

35. Valentine RJ, Jackson MR, Modrall JG, et al. The progressive nature of peripheral arterial disease in young adults: a prospective analysis of white men referred to a vascular surgery service. *J Vasc Surg* 1999;30:436–444.

36. McDermott M, Mehta S, Ahn H, et al. Atherosclerotic risk factors are less intensively treated in patients with peripheral arterial disease than in patients with coronary artery disease. *J Gen Intern Med* 1997;12:209–215.

37. Dormandy J, Heeck L, Vig S. Predicting which patients will develop chronic critical leg ischemia. *Semin Vasc Surg* 1999;12:138–141.

38. West JA. Cost-effective strategies for the management of vascular disease. *Vasc Med* 1997;2:25–29.

39. Regensteiner JG, Steiner JF, Hiatt WR. Exercise training improves functional status in patients with peripheral arterial disease. *J Vasc Surg* 1996;23:104–115.

40. McDermott MM, Greenland P, Liu K, et al. The ankle brachial index is associated with leg function and physical activity: the Walking and Leg Circulation Study. *Ann Intern Med* 2002;136:873–883.

41. Gardner AW, Katzel LI, Sorkin JD, et al. Effects of long-term exercise rehabilitation on claudication distances in patients with peripheral arterial disease: a randomized controlled trial. *J Cardiopulm Rehabil* 2002;22:192–198.

42. Hiatt WR, Regensteiner JG, Wolfel EE, et al. Effect of exercise training on skeletal muscle histology and metabolism in peripheral arterial disease. *J Appl Physiol* 1996;81:780–788.

43. Rith-Najarian SJ, Reiber GE. Prevention of foot problems in persons with diabetes. *J Fam Pract* 2000;49:S30–S39.

44. Sowell RD, Mangel WB, Kilczewski CJ, et al. Effect of podiatric medical care on rates of lower-extremity amputation in a Medicare population. *J Am Podiatr Med Assoc* 1999;89:312–317.

45. Hood S, Moher D, Barber G. Management of intermittent claudication with pentoxifylline: meta-analysis of randomized controlled trials. *Can Med Assoc J* 1996;155:1053–1058.

46. Strandness DE Jr, Dalman RL, Panian S, et al. Effect of cilostazol in patients with intermittent claudication: a randomized, double-blind, placebo-controlled study. *Vasc Endovascular Surg* 2002;36:83–91.

47. Reilly MP, Mohler ER 3rd. Cilostazol: treatment of intermittent claudication. *Ann Pharmacother* 2001;35:48–56.

48. Uchikawa T, Murakami T, Furukawa H. Effects of the anti-platelet agent cilostazol on peripheral vascular disease in patients with diabetes mellitus. *Arzneimittelforschung* 1992;42:322–324.

49. Bagger J, Helligose P, Randsbaek F, et al. Effect of verapamil in intermittent claudication: a randomized, double-blind, placebo-controlled, cross-over study after individual dose response assessment. *Circulation* 1997;95:422–424.

50. Hiatt W, Stoll S, Nies A. Effect of beta-adrenergic blockers in the peripheral circulation in patients with peripheral arterial disease. *Circulation* 1985;72:1226–1231.

51. Radack K, Deck C. Beta-adrenergic blocker therapy does not worsen intermittent claudication in subjects with peripheral arterial disease. A meta-analysis of randomized controlled trials. *Arch Intern Med* 1991;151:1769–1776.

52. Girolami B, Bernardi E, Prins MH, et al. Antiplatelet therapy and other interventions after revascularisation procedures in patients with peripheral arterial disease: a meta-analysis. *Eur J Vasc Endovasc Surg* 2000;19:370–380.

53. Roller RE, Dorr A, Ulrich S, et al. Effect of aspirin treatment in pa-

tients with peripheral arterial disease monitored with the platelet function analyzer PFA-100. *Blood Coagul Fibrinolysis* 2002;13:277–281.

54. A randomised, blinded, trial of clopidogrel versus aspirin in patients at risk of ischaemic events (CAPRIE). CAPRIE Steering Committee. *Lancet* 1996;348:1329–1339.

55. Hiatt WR. Preventing atherothrombotic events in peripheral arterial disease: the use of antiplatelet therapy. *J Intern Med* 2002;251:193–206.

56. Barndt R, Blankenhorn D, Crawford D, et al. Regression and progression of early femoral atherosclerosis in treated hyperlipoproteinemic patients. *Ann Intern Med* 1977;86:139–146.

57. Pedersen TR, Kjekshus J, Pyorala K, et al. Effect of simvastatin on ischemic signs and symptoms in the Scandinavian simvastatin survival study (4S). *Am J Cardiol* 1998;81:333–335.

58. Leng GC, Price JF, Jepson RG. Lipid-lowering for lower limb atherosclerosis. *Cochrane Database Syst Rev* 2000(3):000123.

59. Kuan YM, E Dear A, Grigg MJ. Homocysteine: an aetiological contributor to peripheral vascular arterial disease. *ANZ J Surg* 2002;72:668–671.

60. Hansrani M, Gillespie JI, Stansby G. Homocysteine in myointimal hyperplasia. *Eur J Vasc Endovasc Surg* 2002;23:3–10.

61. Weiss N, Feussner A, Hailer S, et al. Influence of folic acid, pyridoxal phosphate and cobalamin on plasma homocyst(e)ine levels and the susceptibility of low-density lipoprotein to ex-vivo oxidation. *Eur J Med Res* 1999;4:425–432.

62. Hou XY, Green S, Askew CD, et al. Skeletal muscle mitochondrial ATP production rate and walking performance in peripheral arterial disease. *Clin Physiol Funct Imaging* 2002;22:226–232.

63. Barker GA, Green S, Askew CD, et al. Effect of propionyl-L-carnitine on exercise performance in peripheral arterial disease. *Med Sci Sports Exerc* 2001;33:1415–1422.

64. Brass EP, Hiatt WR. The role of carnitine and carnitine supplementation during exercise in man and in individuals with special needs. *J Am Coll Nutr* 1998;17:207–215.

65. Melian EB, Goa KL. Beraprost: a review of its pharmacology and therapeutic efficacy in the treatment of peripheral arterial disease and pulmonary arterial hypertension. *Drugs* 2002;62:107–133.

66. Mohler ER 3rd, Klugherz B, Goldman R, et al. Trial of a novel prostacyclin analog, UT-15, in patients with severe intermittent claudication. *Vasc Med* 2000;5:231–237.

67. Loosemore TM, Chalmers TC, Dormandy JA. A meta-analysis of randomized placebo control trials in Fontaine stages III and IV peripheral occlusive arterial disease. *Int Angiol* 1994;13:133–142.

68. Cozzolino D, Coppola L, Masi S, et al. Short- and long-term treatments with iloprost in diabetic patients with peripheral vascular disease: effects on the cardiovascular risk factor plasminogen activator inhibitor type-1. *Eur J Clin Pharmacol* 1999;55:491–497.

69. Melillo E, Iabichella L, Berchiolli R, et al. Transcutaneous oxygen and carbon dioxide during treatment of critical limb ischemia with iloprost, a prostacyclin derivative. *Int J Microcirc Clin Exp* 1995;15:60–64.

70. Moller ER 3rd, Klugherz B, Goldman R, et al. Trial of a novel prostacyclin analog, UT-15, in patients with severe intermittent claudication. *Vasc Med* 2000;5:231–237.

71. de Vries SO, Visser K, de Vries JA, et al. Intermittent claudication: cost-effectiveness of revascularization versus exercise therapy. *Radiology* 2002;222:25–36.

72. Faglia E, Mantero M, Caminiti M, et al. Extensive use of peripheral angioplasty, particularly infrapopliteal, in the treatment of ischaemic diabetic foot ulcers: clinical results of a multicentric study of 221 consecutive diabetic subjects. *J Intern Med* 2002;252:225–232.

73. Hight D, Tilney N, Couch N. Changing clinical trends in patients with peripheral arterial emboli. *Surgery* 1976;79:172–176.

74. Darling R, Austen W, Linton R. Arterial embolism. *Surg Gynecol Obstet* 1967;106–114.

75. Meister S, Grossman W, Dexter L, et al. Paradoxical embolism: diagnosis during life. *Am J Med* 1972;53:292–298.

76. Mariano MC, Gutierrez CJ, Alexander J, et al. The utility of transesophageal echocardiography in determining the source of arterial embolization. *Am Surg* 2000;66:901–904.

77. Ouriel K, Veith FJ, Sasahara AA. Thrombolysis or peripheral arterial surgery: phase I results. TOPAS Investigators. *J Vasc Surg* 1996;23:64–75.

78. Laird JR. The management of acute limb ischemia: techniques for dealing with thrombus. *J Interv Cardiol* 2001;14:539–546.

79. Semba CP, Murphy TP, Bakal CW, et al. Thrombolytic therapy with use of alteplase (rt-PA) in peripheral arterial occlusive disease: review of the clinical literature. The Advisory Panel. *J Vasc Interv Radiol* 2000;11:149–161.

80. Wysokinski WE, Kwiatkowska W, Sapian-Raczkowska B, et al. Sustained classic clinical spectrum of thromboangiitis obliterans (Buerger's disease). *Angiology* 2000;51:141–150.

81. Wysokinski WE, Kwiatkowska W, Maslowski L, et al. Buerger's disease in two brothers: iliac artery occlusion by thromboangiitis obliterans—case reports. *Angiology* 1998;49:409–414.

82. Shionoya S. Diagnostic criteria of Buerger's disease. *Int J Cardiol* 1998;66[Suppl 1]:S243–S247.

83. Olin JW, Young JR, Graor RA, et al. The changing clinical spectrum of thromboangiitis obliterans (Buerger's disease). *Circulation* 1990;82:IV3–IV8.

84. Disdier P, Granel B, Serratrice J, et al. Cannabis arteritis revisited—ten new case reports. *Angiology* 2001;52:1–5.

85. Ishibashi H, Hayakawa N, Yamamoto H, et al. Thoracoscopic sympathectomy for Buerger's disease: a report on the successful treatment of four patients. *Surg Today* 1995;25:180–183.

86. Isner JM, Baumgartner I, Rauh G, et al. Treatment of thromboangiitis obliterans (Buerger's disease) by intramuscular gene transfer of vascular endothelial growth factor: preliminary clinical results. *J Vasc Surg* 1998;28:964–975.

87. Ring DH Jr, Haines GA, Miller DL. Popliteal artery entrapment syndrome: arteriographic findings and thrombolytic therapy. *J Vasc Interv Radiol* 1999;10:713–721.

88. Ohara N, Miyata T, Oshiro H, et al. Surgical treatment for popliteal artery entrapment syndrome. *Cardiovasc Surg* 2001;9:141–144.

89. Lambert AW, Wilkins DC. Popliteal artery entrapment syndrome. *Br J Surg* 1999;86:1365–1370.

90. Tsolakis IA, Walvatne CS, Caldwell MD. Cystic adventitial disease of the popliteal artery: diagnosis and treatment. *Eur J Vasc Endovasc Surg* 1998;15:188–194.

91. Singh S, Dass R. Clinical approach to vasculitides. *Indian J Pediatr* 2002;69:881–888.

92. Layne RD, Lerfald NM. Diagnosing temporal arteritis [letter]. *JAMA* 2002;288:1352–1353.

93. Achkar AA, Hunder GG, Gabriel SE. Effect of previous corticosteroid treatment on temporal artery biopsy results. *Ann Intern Med* 1998;128:410.

94. Hoffman GS, Cid MC, Hellmann DB, et al. A multicenter, randomized, double-blind, placebo-controlled trial of adjuvant methotrexate treatment for giant cell arteritis. *Arthritis Rheum* 2002;46:1309–1318.

95. Evans JM, O'Fallon WM, Hunder GG. Increased incidence of aortic aneurysm and dissection in giant cell (temporal) arteritis. A population-based study. *Ann Intern Med* 1995;122:502–507.

96. Hall S, Hunder GG. Treatment of Takayasu's arteritis. *Ann Intern Med* 1986;104:288.

97. Salvarani C, Hunder GG. Giant cell arteritis with low erythrocyte sedimentation rate: frequency of occurrence in a population-based study. *Arthritis Rheum* 2001;45:140–145.

98. Stone JH, Calabrese LH, Hoffman GS, et al. Vasculitis. A collection of pearls and myths. *Rheum Dis Clin North Am* 2001;27:677–728,v.

99. Shepherd R. Ergotism. In: White RA, Hollier LH, eds. *Vascular surgery: basic science and clinical correlations.* Philadelphia: JB Lippincott, 1994:177–191.

100. Tay JC, Chee YC. Ergotism and vascular insufficiency: a case report and review of literature. *Ann Acad Med Singapore* 1998;27:285–288.

101. Andreoni KA, Weeks SM, Gerber DA, et al. Incidence of donor renal fibromuscular dysplasia: does it justify routine angiography? *Transplantation* 2002;73:1112–1116.

102. Muller BT, Luther B, Hort W, et al. Surgical treatment of 50 carotid dissections: indications and results. *J Vasc Surg* 2000;31:980–988.

103. Lederle F, Walker J, Reinke D. Selective screening for abdominal aortic aneurysms with physical examination and ultrasound. *Arch Intern Med* 1988;1753–1756.

104. Joyce J, Fairbairn JI, Kincaid O, et al. Aneurysms of the thoracic aorta: a clinical study with special reference to prognosis. *Circulation* 1964;29:176–181.

105. Hoffer EK, Sclafani SJ, Herskowitz MM, et al. Natural history of arterial injuries diagnosed with arteriography. *J Vasc Interv Radiol* 1997;8:43–53.

106. Frances C, Papo T, Wechsler B, et al. Sneddon syndrome with or

without antiphospholipid antibodies. A comparative study in 46 patients. *Medicine (Baltimore)* 1999;78:209–219.

107. Poszepczynska-Guigne E, Viguier M, Chosidow O, et al. Paraneoplastic acral vascular syndrome: epidemiologic features, clinical manifestations, and disease sequelae. *J Am Acad Dermatol* 2002;47: 47–52.

108. Lauchli S, Widmer L, Lautenschlager S. Cold agglutinin disease—the importance of cutaneous signs. *Dermatology* 2001;202:356–358.

109. Weil JS, Maurel A, Van Frenkel R, et al. [Cutaneous pulpar temperature and cold test. Predictive specificity and sensitivity in pharmacoclinical studies]. *J Mal Vasc* 1995;20:38–44.

110. Allen E, Brown G. Raynaud's disease: a critical review of minimal requisites for diagnosis. *Am J Med Sci* 1932;187–200.

111. Priollet P, Vayssairat M, Housset E. How to classify Raynaud's phenomenon. Long-term follow-up study of 73 cases. *Am J Med* 1987; 83:494–498.

112. Landry G, Edwards J, McLafferty R, et al. Long-term outcome of Raynaud's syndrome in a prospectively analyzed patient cohort. *J Vasc Surg* 1996;23:76–86.

113. Coffman J. *Raynaud's phenomenon.* New York: Oxford University Press, 1989.

114. Bovenzi M. Vibration-induced white finger and cold response of digital arterial vessels in occupational groups with various patterns of exposure to hand-transmitted vibration. *Scand J Work Environ Health* 1998;24:138–144.

115. Chetter IC, Kent PJ, Kester RC. The hand arm vibration syndrome: a review. *Cardiovasc Surg* 1998;6:1–9.

116. Jordan SE, Ahn SS, Freischlag JA, et al. Selective botulinum chemodenervation of the scalene muscles for treatment of neurogenic thoracic outlet syndrome. *Ann Vasc Surg* 2000;14:365–369.

117. Zell L, Scheffler P, Heger M, et al. [Paget-von Schroetter syndrome as an occupational accident]. *Dtsch Med Wochenschr* 2001;126: 326–328.

118. Landry GJ, Moneta GL, Taylor LM Jr, et al. Long-term functional outcome of neurogenic thoracic outlet syndrome in surgically and conservatively treated patients. *J Vasc Surg* 2001;33:312–319.

119. Lindgren KA. Conservative treatment of thoracic outlet syndrome: a 2-year follow-up. *Arch Phys Med Rehabil* 1997;78:373–378.

120. Kieffer E, Vasseur MA. [Surgery of thoracic outlet syndromes]. *Rev Med Interne* 1999;20[Suppl 5]:506S–514S.

121. Le Forestier N, Moulonguet A, Maisonobe T, et al. True neurogenic thoracic outlet syndrome: electrophysiological diagnosis in six cases. *Muscle Nerve* 1998;21:1129–1134.

122. Rutherford RB, Hurlbert SN. Primary subclavian-axillary vein thrombosis: consensus and commentary. *Cardiovasc Surg* 1996;4: 420–423.

123. Wheeler HB, Anderson FJ Jr, Cardullo PA, et al. Suspected deep vein thrombosis. Management by impedance plethysmography. *Arch Surg* 1982;1296–1309.

124. Abramowitz H, Queral L, Flinn W, et al. The use of photoplethysmography in the assessment of venous insufficiency: a comparison to venous pressure measurements. *Surgery* 1979;86:434–441.

125. Bygdeman S, Aschberg S, Hindmarsh T. Venous plethysmography in the diagnosis of chronic venous insufficiency. *Acta Chir Scand* 1971; 137:423–428.

126. Holm JS. A simple plethysmographic method for differentiating primary from secondary varicose veins. *Surg Gynecol Obstet* 1976;143: 609–612.

127. Huisman MV, Buller HR, ten Cate JW, et al. Serial impedance plethysmography for suspected deep venous thrombosis in outpatients. The Amsterdam General Practitioner Study. *N Engl J Med* 1986;314:823–828.

128. Brown J, Ward P, Wilkinson A, et al. Impedance plethysmography: a screening procedure to detect deep vein thrombosis. *J Bone Joint Surg* 1987;69:264–267.

129. Kahn SR, Joseph L, Grover SA, et al. A randomized management study of impedance plethysmography vs. contrast venography in patients with a first episode of clinically suspected deep vein thrombosis. *Thromb Res* 2001;102:15–24.

130. Chong D. IPG screening for asymptomatic DVT. *Arch Phys Med Rehabil* 1996;77:211.

131. Katz RT, McCulla MM. Impedance plethysmography as a screening procedure for asymptomatic deep venous thrombosis in a rehabilitation hospital. *Arch Phys Med Rehabil* 1995;76:833–839.

132. Kahn CE Jr, Haddawy P. Optimizing, diagnostic, and therapeutic strategies using decision- theoretic planning: principles and applications. *Medinfo* 1995;8[Pt 2]:894–898.

133. Washington L, Goodman LR, Gonyo MB. CT for thromboembolic disease. *Radiol Clin North Am* 2002;40:751–771.

134. Ciccotosto C, Goodman LR, Washington L, et al. Indirect CT venography following CT pulmonary angiography: spectrum of CT findings. *J Thorac Imaging* 2002;17:18–27.

135. Kroencke TJ, Taupitz M, Arnold R, et al. Three-dimensional gadolinium-enhanced magnetic resonance venography in suspected thrombo-occlusive disease of the central chest veins. *Chest* 2001;120:1570–1576.

136. Montgomery KD, Potter HG, Helfet DL. The detection and management of proximal deep venous thrombosis in patients with acute acetabular fractures: a follow-up report. *J Orthop Trauma* 1997;11:330–336.

137. Schutgens RE, Esseboom EU, Haas FJ, et al. Usefulness of a semiquantitative D-dimer test for the exclusion of deep venous thrombosis in outpatients. *Am J Med* 2002;112:617–621.

138. Hirsh J, Lee AY. How we diagnose and treat deep vein thrombosis. *Blood* 2002;99:3102–3110.

139. Palareti G, Legnani C, Cosmi B, et al. Risk of venous thromboembolism recurrence: high negative predictive value of D-dimer performed after oral anticoagulation is stopped. *Thromb Haemost* 2002;87:7–12.

140. Franks PJ, Wright DD, Moffatt CJ, et al. Prevalence of venous disease: a community study in west London. *Eur J Surg* 1992;158:143–147.

141. Flordal PA, Berggvist D, Burmark US, et al. Risk factors for major thromboembolism and bleeding tendency after elective general surgical operations. The Fragmin Multicentre Study Group. *Eur J Surg* 1996;162:783–789.

142. Harris EJ Jr. Endovascular obliteration of saphenous vein reflux: a perspective. *J Vasc Surg* 2002;35:1292–1294.

143. Jeanneret C, Fischer R, Chandler JG, et al. Great saphenous vein stripping with liberal use of subfascial endoscopic perforator vein surgery (SEPS). *Ann Vasc Surg* 2003;17:539–549.

144. Hanson JN, Ascher E, DePippo P, et al. Saphenous vein thrombophlebitis (SVT): a deceptively benign disease. *J Vasc Surg* 1998; 27:677–680.

145. Guex JJ. Thrombotic complications of varicose veins. A literature review of the role of superficial venous thrombosis. *Dermatol Surg* 1996;22:378–382.

146. O'Fallon W, Heit J, Mohr D, et al. Predictors of recurrence after deep vein thrombosis and pulmonary embolism: a population-based cohort study. *Blood* 1998;10:560a–561a.

147. Ouriel K, Whitehouse WJ, Zarins C. Combined use of Doppler ultrasound and phleborheography in suspected deep venous thrombosis. *Surg Gynecol Obstet* 1984;242–246.

148. Haeger K. Problems of acute deep vein thrombosis: the interpretation of signs and symptoms. *Angiology* 1969;20:219–223.

149. Tripodi A, Mannucci PM. Laboratory investigation of thrombophilia. *Clin Chem* 2001;47:1597–1606.

150. Freedman MD, Young M. Venous thrombosis: diagnosis and treatment; new methods and strategies for management. *Compr Ther* 1999;25: 13–19.

151. Piccioli A, Prandoni P. Idiopathic venous thromboembolism as a first manifestation of cancer. *Haemostasis* 2001;31[Suppl 1]:37–39.

152. Kearon C, Gent M, Hirsh J, et al. A comparison of three months of anticoagulation with extended anticoagulation for a first episode of idiopathic venous thromboembolism. *N Engl J Med* 1999;340: 901–907.

153. Agnelli G, Prandoni P, Santamaria MG, et al. Three months versus one year of oral anticoagulant therapy for idiopathic deep venous thrombosis. Warfarin Optimal Duration Italian Trial Investigators. *N Engl J Med* 2001;345:165–169.

154. Rymes NL, Lester W, Connor C, et al. Outpatient management of DVT using low molecular weight heparin and a hospital outreach service. *Clin Lab Haematol* 2002;24:165–170.

155. Litin SC, Heit JA, Mees KA. Use of low-molecular-weight heparin in the treatment of venous thromboembolic disease: answers to frequently asked questions. The Thrombophilia Center Investigators. *Mayo Clin Proc* 1998;73:545–551.

156. Anand SS. Comparison of 3 and 6 months of oral anticoagulant therapy after a first episode of proximal deep vein thrombosis or pulmonary embolism and comparison of 6 and 12 weeks of therapy after isolated calf deep vein thrombosis. Pinede L, Ninet J, Duhaut P, et al for the Investigators of the 'Duree Optimale du Traitement Antivita-

mines K' (DOTAVK) study. *Vasc Med* 2001;6:269–270; and *Circulation* 2001;103:2453–2460.

157. Robitaille P, Le Clerc JR, Brave G. Treatment of venous thromboembolism. In: Le Clerc JR, ed. *Venous thromboembolic disorders.* Philadelphia: Lea & Febiger, 1991:267–302.

158. Palareti G, Legnani C, Lee A, et al. A comparison of the safety and efficacy of oral anticoagulation for the treatment of venous thromboembolic disease in patients with or without malignancy. *Thromb Haemost* 2000;84:805–810.

159. Comerota A. Venous thromboembolism. In: Rutherford RB, ed. *Vascular surgery,* 4th ed. Philadelphia: WB Saunders, 1995:1785–1814.

160. Rhodes JM, Cho JS, Gloviczki P, et al. Thrombolysis for experimental deep venous thrombosis maintains valvular competence and vasoreactivity. *J Vasc Surg* 2000;31:1193–1205.

161. Elsharawy M, Elzayat E. Early results of thrombolysis vs anticoagulation in iliofemoral venous thrombosis. A randomised clinical trial. *Eur J Vasc Endovasc Surg* 2002;24:209–214.

162. Mewissen MW, Seabrook GR, Meissner MH, et al. Catheter-directed thrombolysis for lower extremity deep venous thrombosis: report of a national multicenter registry. *Radiology* 1999;211:39–49.

163. Ginsberg JS, Hirsh J, Julian J, et al. Prevention and treatment of postphlebitic syndrome: results of a 3-part study. *Arch Intern Med* 2001;161:2105–2109.

164. Owens LV, Farber MA, Young ML, et al. The value of air plethysmography in predicting clinical outcome after surgical treatment of chronic venous insufficiency. *J Vasc Surg* 2000;32:961–968.

165. Prandoni P, Lensing A, Cogo A, et al. The long-term clinical course of acute deep venous thrombosis. *Ann Intern Med* 1996;125:1–7.

166. Harris M, Grange J. Management of calf deep venous thrombosis. *Ann Emerg Med* 2000;35:629.

167. Meissner MH, Caps MT, Bergelin RO, et al. Early outcome after isolated calf vein thrombosis. *J Vasc Surg* 1997;26:749–756.

168. Ryan MG, Westrich GH, Potter HG, et al. Effect of mechanical compression on the prevalence of proximal deep venous thrombosis as assessed by magnetic resonance venography. *J Bone Joint Surg Am* 2002;84-A:1998–2004.

169. Ahmad HA, Geissler A, MacLellan DG. Deep venous thrombosis prophylaxis: are guidelines being followed? *ANZ J Surg* 2002;72:331–334.

170. Arnold DM, Kahn SR, Shrier I. Missed opportunities for prevention of venous thromboembolism: an evaluation of the use of thromboprophylaxis guidelines. *Chest* 2001;120:1964–1971.

171. Pierson JL, Tavel ME. Thromboembolic prophylaxis in total joint replacement. *Chest* 2001;120:302–304.

172. Hull RD, Pineo GF. Prophylaxis of deep venous thrombosis and pulmonary embolism. Current recommendations. *Med Clin North Am* 1998;82:477–493.

173. Lindhoff-Last E, Nakov R, Misselwitz F, et al. Incidence and clinical relevance of heparin-induced antibodies in patients with deep vein thrombosis treated with unfractionated or low- molecular-weight heparin. *Br J Haematol* 2002;118:1137–1142.

174. Warkentin TE. Heparin-induced thrombocytopenia: a ten-year retrospective. *Annu Rev Med* 1999;50:129–147.

175. Ibbotson T, Perry CM. Danaparoid: a review of its use in thromboembolic and coagulation disorders. *Drugs* 2002;62:2283–2314.

176. Acostamadiedo JM, Iyer UG, Owen J. Danaparoid sodium. *Exp Opin Pharmacother* 2000;1:803–814.

177. Miura Y, Ardenghy M, Ramasastry S, et al. Coumadin necrosis of the skin: report of four patients. *Ann Plast Surg* 1996;37:332–337.

178. Anderson DR, Brill-Edwards P, Walker I. Warfarin-induced skin necrosis in 2 patients with protein S deficiency: successful reinstatement of warfarin therapy. *Haemostasis* 1992;22:124–128.

179. Wood KE, Reedy JS, Pozniak MA, et al. Phlegmasia cerulea dolens with compartment syndrome: a complication of femoral vein catheterization. *Crit Care Med* 2000;28:1626–1630.

180. Wudel LJ Jr, Nesbitt JC. Superior vena cava syndrome. *Curr Treat Options Oncol* 2001;2:77–91.

181. Barakat K, Robinson NM, Spurrell RA. Transvenous pacing lead-induced thrombosis: a series of cases with a review of the literature. *Cardiology* 2000;93:142–148.

182. Mahajan V, Strimlan V, Ordstrand HS, et al. Benign superior vena cava syndrome. *Chest* 1975;68:32–35.

183. Hausler M, Hubner D, Delhaas T, et al. Long term complications of inferior vena cava thrombosis. *Arch Dis Child* 2001;85:228–233.

184. Espinosa G, Font J, Garcia-Pagan JC, et al. Budd-Chiari syndrome secondary to antiphospholipid syndrome: clinical and immunologic characteristics of 43 patients. *Medicine (Baltimore)* 2001;80:345–354.

185. Emre A, Ozden I, Poyanli A, et al. Vena cava stenting and portorenal shunt in Budd-Chiari syndrome: combination of the 'modern' and the 'classical.' *Dig Surg* 2001;18:223–225.

186. Haenen JH, Janssen MC, Wollersheim H, et al. The development of postthrombotic syndrome in relationship to venous reflux and calf muscle pump dysfunction at 2 years after the onset of deep venous thrombosis. *J Vasc Surg* 2002;35:1184–1189.

187. Nicolaides A, Christopoulos D, Vasdekis S. Progress in the investigation of chronic venous insufficiency. *Ann Vasc Surg* 1989;3:278–292.

CHAPTER 102

Surgical Treatment of Peripheral Vascular Disease

Victor J. Weiss, Thomas F. Dodson, and Robert B. Smith III

Introduction	**Surgical Options for Aortoiliac Disease**
Symptoms of Peripheral Vascular Disease and	**Femoropopliteal Disease**
Indications for Intervention	**Surgical Options for Infrainguinal Disease**
Differential Diagnosis	**Results of Bypass for Infrainguinal Disease**
Angioplasty/Stent or Surgical Intervention?	**References**

Key Words: Bypass; iliac femoropopliteal; peripheral; vascular.

INTRODUCTION

Atherothrombosis involving the infrarenal aorta and more distal vessels of the lower extremities may produce characteristic symptoms if the degree of stenosis is sufficient to produce hemodynamic compromise. The diagnosis of chronic arterial insufficiency, the differentiation from acute embolic disease, and the minimally invasive methods of treatment are presented elsewhere in this textbook. The focus of this chapter is to discuss chronic arterial insufficiency and the surgical treatment options designed to improve distal perfusion.

SYMPTOMS OF PERIPHERAL VASCULAR DISEASE AND INDICATIONS FOR INTERVENTION

Chronic lower extremity arterial insufficiency may take one of several different symptom patterns. A hemodynamically significant stenosis of the lower extremities may only be noted by the patient if the demands of oxygen delivery to the leg muscles can not be met during the period of activity.

V. J. Weiss: University of Mississippi School of Medicine, Cardiovascular Surgical Clinic, 501 Marshall Street, Suite 100, Jackson, Mississippi 39202.

T. F. Dodson: Division of Vascular Surgery, Emory University School of Medicine, 1364 Clifton Road, NE, Atlanta, Georgia 30322.

R. B. Smith III: Division of Vascular Surgery, Emory University School of Medicine, 1364 Clifton Road, NE, Atlanta, Georgia 30322.

Therefore, the earliest stages of this disease are usually asymptomatic, particularly if an individual is sedentary. The most common early sign of arterial insufficiency is pain in the involved extremity with walking, termed claudication. The location of the discomfort depends on the level of disease, with aortoiliac disease typically causing hip, thigh, and buttock claudication. This may be associated at times with vasculogenic impotence, collectively termed Leriche syndrome. Disease of the femoropopliteal segment causes symptoms in the calf. The characteristic history is that this pain or discomfort is not present at rest or when the patient first begins to walk. Once a certain distance has been reached, the discomfort begins in the involved extremity (or both extremities) in the characteristic location. Resting reliably alleviates this pain after a minute or so, and the patient can then continue walking. Activities that increase oxygen demand (such as climbing stairs or walking on an incline) would be expected to produce these symptoms after a shorter distance. If the patient's history does not fit well with this description, other causes of leg pain must be entertained. An ankle–brachial index in such a patient might measure anywhere from 0.9 to 0.4, depending on the severity of claudication symptoms. It must be kept in mind that the reserve of the arterial system is tremendous. This is the reason patients who present with disabling claudication typically have already developed occlusion of the superficial femoral artery for a variable length. With more severe symptoms, the location of disease would be expected to be located at multiple levels.

Rest pain indicates an increasing severity of vascular insufficiency. When the patient assumes a recumbent position and gravity is no longer able to assist in perfusion of the legs, ischemic pain is produced. The pain is typically noted during the night and occurs in the foot. The patient may discover that placing the limb in a dependent position or standing and walking a short distance improves the pain. Rest pain is of severe intensity, and it typically prevents the patient from sleeping. Ankle–brachial indices in a patient with rest pain often are in a range from 0.4 to 0.1. Intervention is usually indicated for these patients, but in those with more mild symptoms and severely diseased runoff vessels, close observation may be prudent. Ulcerations or gangrene can develop in an ischemic extremity and can represent a more urgent indication for intervention for limb preservation.

Patients with severe rest pain, gangrene, or ischemic ulcerations typically require timely evaluation and treatment, because these symptoms indicate a threatened limb. Patients with claudication may or may not have a justifiable indication for intervention, and in these patients experienced judgment is crucial. In keeping with the dictum *primum non nocere,* it is imperative to recognize that within 5 years of the onset of claudication approximately 5% to 7% of patients will require amputation (1,2). Without treatment, 10% to 15% of patients with intermittent claudication will improve, whereas 60% to 70% will remain stable (1,2). This is in distinct contrast to those patients with ischemic ulceration or rest pain, with approximately 20% requiring immediate amputation (3). Not uncommonly, a failed bypass performed for claudication can place a limb at risk that would have had a benign course if no treatment had been undertaken initially. Therefore, indications for surgical intervention for claudication should be quite compelling. A history of very short distance claudication or claudication in a patient with an occupation requiring significant ambulation are two such conditions.

DIFFERENTIAL DIAGNOSIS

Lower extremity pain can have numerous cause, only some of which are related to arterial insufficiency. Claudication has very characteristic features, including an onset of symptoms only after a period of exertion when the oxygen demand has exceeded the supply. Thus, the symptoms of claudication do not begin immediately with walking and they do not occur at rest. The description of symptoms that the patient describes can be quite variable and may include heaviness, weakness, burning, or a "charley horse." Musculoskeletal pain often can be distinguished from that of arterial insufficiency because musculoskeletal pain typically is present when first walking and may not be precipitated by walking. Neurogenic pain may be caused by compression of the lower spinal cord or cauda equina. Often, these patients may have a peripheral vascular examination that does not correlate with the degree of symptoms, leading the physician to search for other causes of leg pain.

Lower extremity ulceration may be of either arterial or venous etiology. Typically, the patient with venous ulceration has a history of chronic venous insufficiency, with characteristic hyperpigmentation and stasis changes, and most commonly ulceration involving the lateral malleolus. These patients often have lower extremity swelling, which makes assessment of pedal pulses difficult. Ankle–brachial indices should be preserved in the patient with ulceration of purely venous etiology. Ulcerations of the lower extremity as a result of arterial insufficiency often are more painful than venous ulcers. The location of these arterial ulcers is variable, but may frequently be located overlying bony prominences (i.e., malleoli or the plantar aspect of the metatarsal heads). These patients will typically have risk factors associated with peripheral vascular disease, such as a history of smoking, diabetes, and/or chronic renal insufficiency. Other findings on physical examination often will be identified, such as dependent rubor, atrophic nail growth, and abnormal pulse examination results on the contralateral extremity. Ankle–brachial indices are characteristically in the range of 0.4 and less.

When evaluating the patient with reports of lower extremity chronic arterial insufficiency, the systemic nature of the atherothrombotic process should be kept in mind. Attention to risk factor modification must focus on treating hypercholesterolemia and cessation of tobacco use. If operative intervention is planned, cardiac evaluation may be performed for risk stratification and to identify correctable coronary artery disease (4).

ANGIOPLASTY/STENT OR SURGICAL INTERVENTION?

Once the decision has been made to intervene on a patient, the next question to be answered is how best to treat the patient and his/her lesion(s). What type of imaging study should be performed? Should a minimally invasive intervention be attempted? Are the lesions amenable to angioplasty and stent, and would this intervention be likely to give a durable result? Is an open surgical approach more likely to provide the patient with a lasting result? Is the patient's general medical condition favorable enough to tolerate an open surgical procedure? These questions are crucial in the decision about intervention, and often are best addressed either by individuals with expertise in both methods of vascular intervention or by a multidisciplinary approach.

The most commonly used techniques of vascular imaging include contrast arteriography, magnetic resonance angiography, computed angiographic tomography, and duplex ultrasonography. Each modality has particular advantages and shortcomings. The appropriate use and limitations of each study, however, is beyond the scope of this chapter.

If the patient's history suggests a recent, acute deterioration of symptoms, or if there is an angiographic suggestion of an embolic process, the use of mechanical or pharmacologic thrombolysis, or both, may be warranted. Lesion morphology and anatomic location play a significant role in determining the optimal treatment modality. Surgical treatment is most often reserved for longer occlusive lesions rather than for short stenoses, which might be effectively treated with angioplasty/stent. Similarly, multisegment infrainguinal disease is more commonly treated with bypass, although percutaneous interventions are receiving increasing attention in this location (5). Stenotic lesions of the iliac system, including some completely occlusive lesions, may be optimally treated by percutaneous means (6).

There are specific locations where surgical intervention may be initially favored over percutaneous intervention for fear that a failed angioplasty might limit remedial surgical options. Angioplasty/stent of a common iliac artery that places an internal iliac artery orifice at risk for occlusion, particularly if the contralateral internal iliac artery is occluded, might best be avoided as pelvic ischemia with bilateral internal iliac artery occlusion often is difficult or impossible to improve on. Occlusive disease of the distal external iliac or common femoral arteries often is easily treated with endarterectomy or bypass; thus, surgical options are typically favored in this location. Angioplasty/stent is appropriately avoided in this region for several reasons. The inguinal ligament is rarely a site of stent placement because the repetitive motion at the hip joint is likely to induce metal fatigue and stent fracture. Furthermore, stents placed at the unprotected area of the groin are susceptible to extrinsic compression. The femoral bifurcation also is frequently avoided as a site for angioplasty/stent, because preservation of the orifice of the profunda femoris is of supreme importance in maintaining adequate pedal perfusion. Any procedure that may jeopardize perfusion through this critical vessel should be avoided. Lesions involving the popliteal artery at the level of the knee are usually treated surgically, because there is concern about the durability and integrity of stent placement at this region where a great deal of motion occurs.

The appropriate intervention after a failed angioplasty with or without stent is complex. Many factors, including the duration of patency after the initial angioplasty, lesion morphology, anatomic location, and patient comorbidity are all considered when planning remedial therapy after a failed attempt at angioplasty/stent.

SURGICAL OPTIONS FOR AORTOILIAC DISEASE

The patient with isolated aortoiliac occlusive disease typically presents with hip, thigh, and/or buttock claudication and occasionally with reports of impotence if there is limited blood flow to both internal iliac arteries. Physical examination reveals diminished or absent femoral pulse(s), although with sufficient collateralization pedal pulses may be present. An arteriogram demonstrating iliac occlusion or diffuse severe stenosis throughout the distal aorta and/or iliac system might best be treated by surgical means. Focal aortoiliac disease may be appropriately treated with endarterectomy, which typically requires open exposure of the involved vessel and removal of the inciting plaque down to the level of the media. Endarterectomy in this location is as-

sociated with a 95% 5-year patency (6,7). Suitable candidates for aortoiliac endarterectomy must have disease localized to the distal aorta and common iliac arteries. This is rarely the case, however, because posterior plaque commonly extends into the external iliac artery. Therefore, aortoiliac endarterectomy is an infrequently performed procedure, with more diffuse disease often treated with bypass.

Bypass for aortoiliac disease may take the form of an anatomic (aortobiiliac or bifemoral bypass) or extraanatomic bypass (axillary bifemoral, axillary unifemoral, or femorofemoral bypass). Each procedure has specific advantages and disadvantages. Typically, direct aortic reconstruction (aortobifemoral or aortobiiliac bypass) is favored for its superior durability, despite a greater physiologic stress to the patient and slightly greater morbidity and mortality. In certain patients, an extraanatomic bypass may be chosen for its reduced morbidity and mortality, despite the inferior long-term results.

Aortobiiliac or aortobifemoral bypass involves a laparotomy incision (either a transperitoneal or retroperitoneal approach) and a proximal anastomosis arising from the infrarenal aorta. This anastomosis may be performed in an end-to-end or end-to-side configuration. Most often, if the aorta is occluded, an end-to-end anastomosis is performed. If antegrade flow is required to perfuse the inferior mesenteric or internal iliac arteries, an end-to-side anastomosis is performed.

The results of aortobifemoral bypass are excellent, with many centers reporting 85% to 90% graft patency at 5 years, and 70% to 75% patency at 10 years (6,8,9). The procedure is associated with a morbidity of well less than 3%. The most frequent late complication after aortobifemoral bypass is graft occlusion, occurring in 5% to 10% of patients at 5 years, and 15% to 30% at and beyond 10 years (10,11). Graft infection, late anastomotic pseudoaneurysm formation, and aortoduodenal fistula formation are rare complications from aortobiiliac or bifemoral bypass. Although the results for aortic bypass are quite good, subgroups have been identified with predictably inferior results. Younger patients have been noted to have increased late graft thrombosis, with a 50% 5-year patency in patients younger than 50 years (12). These same investigators found a 6-year patency rate of 20% in patients with aortic diameters less than 1.8 cm, compared with a 6-year patency rate of 60% with aortas greater than 1.8 cm.

Extraanatomic bypass is typically reserved for patients with severe comorbidities, which make laparotomy and direct aortic reconstruction prohibitively risky. The most common extraanatomic bypass for aortoiliac disease is the axillobifemoral bypass (Fig. 102–1). This allows for the perfusion of the lower extremities from a donor axillary artery, accessed under the clavicle. The graft (Dacron or polytetrafluoroethylene [PTFE]) is tunneled from an infraclavicular incision in a subcutaneous plane, along the chest wall and medial to the anterior superior iliac spine to the groin. A side limb is attached to the graft and tunneled in a cross pu-

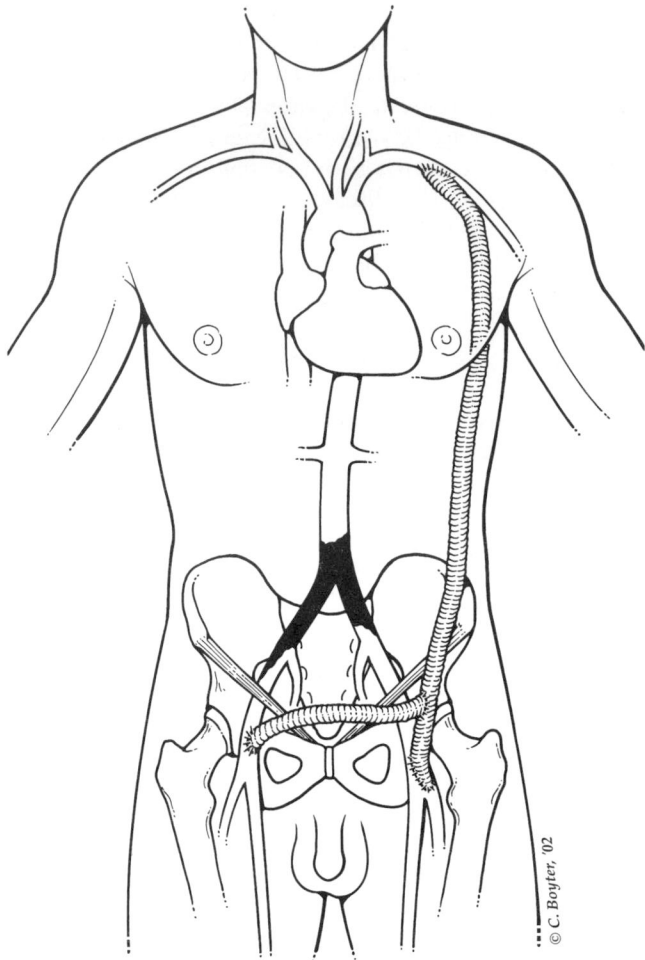

FIG. 102–1. An axillobifemoral bypass.

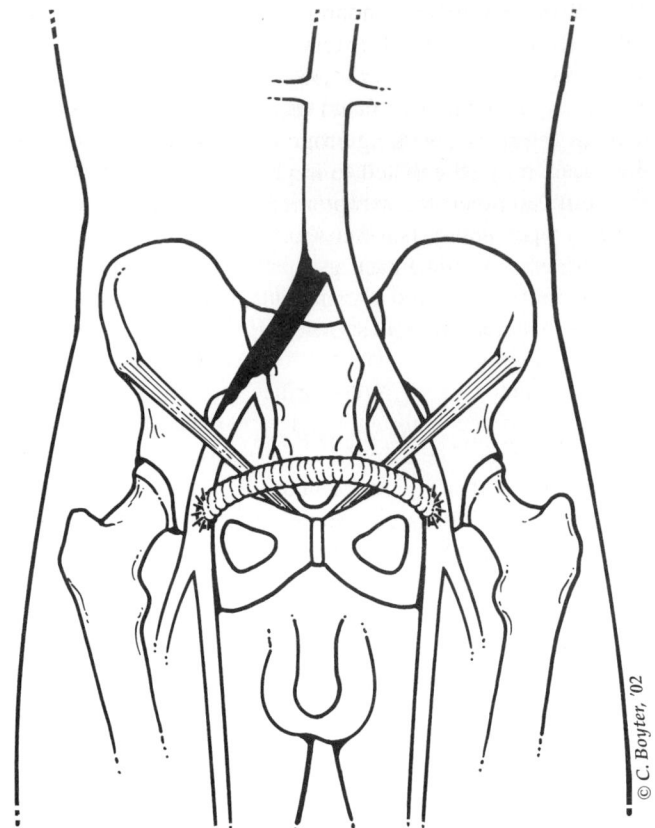

FIG. 101–2. A femorofemoral bypass.

bic location toward the contralateral groin. Because neither the thoracic nor peritoneal cavity is opened, the procedure is less stressful, particularly in the patient with multiple medical comorbidities. Axillobifemoral bypass is associated with a 5-year cumulative patency rate of approximately 70% to 75% (13–15), which has been demonstrated to be statistically inferior to the results of direct aortic reconstruction. Therefore, this procedure is typically reserved for patients at increased risk for direct aortic bypass who are at risk for limb loss or severe disability by chronic arterial insufficiency.

Patients with occlusive disease isolated to one iliac artery, with the aorta and contralateral iliac system free of disease, may be suitable for femorofemoral bypass grafting (Fig. 102–2). When evaluating a patient for this procedure, one must be certain that the donor iliac and femoral system is free of hemodynamically significant disease. Biplanar angiography is the preferred imaging modality, but physiologic testing also should be assessed. A normal femoral pulse, a normal thigh–brachial index, a thigh plethysmographic tracing with a brisk upstroke, and triphasic wave-

form on Doppler tracing all indicate a suitable donor iliofemoral segment. Femorofemoral bypass is well suited to the patient with multiple comorbidities, as the bypass can be constructed under spinal, epidural, or even local anesthesia with conscious sedation. In this procedure, both femoral arteries are exposed, and a graft is tunneled in a subcutaneous plane across the pubis. Femorofemoral bypass is associated with a 5-year patency rate of 60% to 85% (16,17). The patency of this bypass is significantly reduced if the recipient superficial femoral artery is occluded, and in this setting the likelihood of symptomatic relief or limb salvage also is reduced.

FEMOROPOPLITEAL DISEASE

Patients with arterial insufficiency of the lower extremities frequently have atherothrombotic disease of the superficial femoral artery. If localized to the femoropopliteal segment, symptoms most often will involve calf claudication. When the patient with such symptoms is initially evaluated, a detailed history and physical examination is obtained, including an evaluation of the ankle–brachial index. The decision regarding further imaging studies is based on whether the patient has symptoms deemed severe enough to warrant intervention. As previously discussed, claudication (particularly in the nondiabetic, nonrenal failure population) has a relatively benign natural history, with ultimate limb loss of approximately 1% per year (1,18). Most often, these patients are best treated with risk factor modification and are encouraged to begin on a walking program. Occasionally, pharmacotherapy may be enlisted to improve the claudication distance. If, however, the symptoms appear severe enough to warrant intervention (severe, short distance claudication or limb-threatening ischemia), an arteriogram is most often obtained. Other imaging options exist, but this discussion is beyond the scope of this chapter.

SURGICAL OPTIONS
FOR INFRAINGUINAL DISEASE

Intervention for infrainguinal atherothrombotic disease has most commonly centered around surgical options, because angioplasty and stent have traditionally had less durable results in the occluded femoropopliteal segment (19,20). The prime modality for surgical revascularization of the infrainguinal segment has been bypass. Bypass may be accomplished with a variety of conduits, including autogenous vein (most commonly greater saphenous, lesser saphenous, and/or cephalic vein), prosthetic material (expanded PTFE, Dacron), or biomaterials (human umbilical vein, cryopreserved human vessels).

The most durable results for infrainguinal bypass are achieved with autogenous vein as the bypass conduit (Table 102–1). The most commonly used vein is the greater saphenous, although the lesser saphenous and cephalic veins often are suitable if the greater saphenous veins have previously been harvested, or if they are diseased. Autogenous veins may be placed in a reversed fashion to permit for the flow of blood across the valves, or in a nonreversed fashion with the valves manually lysed. Although autogenous vein harvest requires additional incisions, this often is the preferred conduit because of its proven durability and freedom from infectious complications (21). Expanded PTFE is the most common prosthetic graft chosen for lower extremity bypass, although Dacron fabric also can be used. Operative times are shorter because the vein is not harvested, and incision length is kept to a minimum compared with autogenous vein bypass. The prosthetic grafts are obviously more costly than using the patient's own vein, and as described later, long-term patency is generally significantly less with the prosthetic grafts compared with vein bypass. The biomaterial grafts also introduce additional cost but make for a shorter operative time.

RESULTS OF BYPASS
FOR INFRAINGUINAL DISEASE

The results of bypass for infrainguinal disease are dependent on several different factors, including the indication for the procedure, the type of conduit used, the location of the distal anastomosis, and the status of the inflow and outflow vessels. Quinones-Baldrich and coworkers (22) demonstrated 5-year primary patency rates using PTFE of 69% when claudication was the indication for surgery, but this figure decreased to 49% when the bypass was performed for critical limb ischemia. Similarly, both the choice of conduit and the location of the distal anastomosis can influence long-term results. Comparing PTFE and reversed saphenous vein grafts (RSVGs) in both the above knee and below knee popliteal arteries, Plecha reported 4-year patency rates of 100% for above knee RSVGs and 57% for above knee PTFE grafts (22a). In the below knee position, he reported a 72% patency rate for RSVGs and a 47% rate for PTFE. These findings are in keeping with those of most other reports: In general, patency is best using autogenous vein and having a distal anastomosis at the above knee location. Human umbilical vein grafts have been noted to give results either equal to or superior to those obtained with PTFE (23). More recently, experience has been reported with cadaveric cryopreserved saphenous vein used as a conduit for infrainguinal bypass. Results are variable, however, with a postoperative antiplatelet and anticoagulation regimen; 1-year primary patency rates of 82% and limb salvage rates of 80% have been reported (24,25).

As operative techniques have improved over the last 20 years, more distal bypasses have been performed in patients with occlusive disease involving the tibial vessels. With

TABLE 102–1. *Infrainguinal bypass with autogenous vein*

Study	Limbs, n	Operative mortality rate, %	Primary patency	Secondary patency	Limb salvage	Patient survival
Taylor et al., 1990 (30)	516	1	75	80	90	28
Bergamini et al., 1991 (31)	361	3	63	81	86	57
Donaldson et al., 1991 (32)	440	2	72	83	84	66
Leather et al., 1992 (33)	1688	3	70	81	92	58
Total/weighted average	3005	2	70	81	90	54

Graft patency, limb salvage, and survival are based on 5-year cumulative rates (%).
From Whittemore AD, Belkin M. Infrainguinal bypass. In: Rutherford RB, ed. *Vascular surgery,* 5th ed. Philadelphia: WB Saunders, 2000:1012, with permission.

TABLE 102–2. *Paramalleolar infrapopliteal reconstruction with autogenous vein*

Study	Limbs, n	2- to 3-Year primary patency rates, %	4- to 5-Year primary patency rates, %	4- to 5-Year limb salvage rate, %
Andros et al., 1988 (34)	224	62	40	71
Klamer et al., 1990 (35)	68	81	81	95
Pomposelli et al., 1990 (36)	97	80	—	—
Shah et al., 1992 (37)	270	74	61	89
Harrington et al., 1992 (38)	73	59	50	74
Total/weighted average	732	70	55	82

From Whittemore AD, Belkin M. Infrainguinal bypass. In: Rutherford RB, ed. *Vascular surgery,* 5th ed. Philadelphia: WB Saunders, 2000:1012, with permission.

proper patient selection, the results of tibial bypass are quite good (Table 102–2). Reviewing an experience extending over 10 years and including more than 2,000 patients, Shah and coworkers (26) reported 10-year cumulative secondary patency rates of 91%, 81%, and 70% at 1, 5, and 10 years, with limb salvage rates of 97%, 95%, and 90% at 1, 5, and 10 years.

Arterial endarterectomy, that is, manually removing the atheromatous plaque from the diseased vessel, has experienced a resurgence. This procedure had previously been performed through long incisions to completely expose the diseased vessel. The artery is opened longitudinally, the plaque removed, and the artery closed. With proper patient selection, results with this method were acceptable, with a patency rate of 75% at 1 year, 66% at 3 years, and 57% at 7 years (27). More recently, experiences with remote endarterectomy have been detailed. Using a plaque stripping device on a long handle, and working through an open femoral artery exposure, plaque in the superficial femoral artery can be removed remotely. Once an end point has been identified, a plaque-cutting stripper can then be advanced over the plaque to divide it. The end point may then be tacked down with an intraluminal stent. Results of this technique have been variable, with a reported patency rate at 1 year of 26% to 61% (28,29). Much of the enthusiasm about this procedure revolves not necessarily around the current results but around the potential of placing drug-eluting stents after remote endarterectomy to minimize restenosis. If the early success of these drug-coated stents in the coronary circulation translates to the lower extremity, this might represent another method for providing improved flow to the lower extremity, with a result perhaps more durable than the current minimally invasive methods.

REFERENCES

1. Imparato AM, Kim GE, Davidson T, et al. Intermittent claudication: its natural course. *Surgery* 1975;78:795–797.
2. Boyd AM. Natural course of arteriosclerosis of lower extremities. *Proc R Soc Med* 1962;53:591–593.
3. Juergens JL, Barker NW, Hines EA Jr. Arteriosclerosis obliterans: review of 520 cases with special reference to pathogenic and prognostic factors. *Circulation* 1960;21:188–193.
4. Hertzer NR, Beven EG, Young JR, et al. Coronary artery disease in peripheral vascular patients: a classification of 1000 coronary angiograms and results of surgical management. *Ann Surg* 1984;199: 223–233.
5. Vraux H, Hammer F, Verhelst R, et al. Subintimal angioplasty of tibial vessel occlusions in the treatment of critical limb ischaemia: mid-term results. *Eur J Vasc Endovasc Surg* 2000;20:441–446.
6. Brewster DC, Darling RC. Optimal methods of aortoiliac reconstruction. *Surgery* 1978;84:739–748.
7. Stoney EJ, Reilly LM. Endarterectomy for aortoiliac occlusive disease. In: Ernst CB, Stanley JC, eds. *Current therapy in vascular surgery.* Philadelphia: BC Decker, 1987:157.
8. Martinez BD, Hertzer NR, Beven EG. Influence of distal arterial occlusive disease on prognosis following aortobifemoral bypass. *Surgery* 1980;88:795–805.
9. Crawford ES, Bomberger RA, Glaeser DH, et al. Aortoiliac occlusive disease: factors influencing survival and function following reconstructive operation over a twenty five year period. *Surgery* 1981;90: 1555–1567.
10. Brewster DC, Meier GH, Darling RC, et al. Reoperation for aortofemoral graft limb occlusion: optimal methods and long term results. *J Vasc Surg* 1987;5:363–374.
11. Nevelsteen A, Suy R. Graft occlusion following aortofemoral Dacron bypass. *Ann Vasc Surg* 1991;5:32–37.
12. Valentine RJ, Hansen ME, Myers SI, et al. The influence of sex and aortic size on late patency after aortofemoral revascularization in young adults. *J Vasc Surg* 1995;21:296–306.
13. Harris EJ Jr, Taylor LM Jr, McConnell DB, et al. Clinical results of axillobifemoral bypass using externally supported polytetrafluoroethylene. *J Vasc Surg* 1990;12:416–421.
14. el-Massry S, Saad E, Sauvage LR, et al. Axillofemoral bypass with externally supported, knitted Dacron grafts: a follow-up through twelve years. *J Vasc Surg* 1993;17:107–114.
15. Passman MA, Taylor LM, Moneta GL, et al. Comparison of axillofemoral and aortofemoral bypass for aortoiliac occlusive disease. *J Vasc Surg* 1996;23:263–269.
16. Criado E, Burnham SJ, Tinsley EA Jr, et al. Femoralfemoral bypass graft: analysis of patency and factors influencing long term outcome. *J Vasc Surg* 1993;18:495–504.
17. Farber MA, Hollier LH, Eubanks R, et al. Femoralfemoral bypass: a profile of graft failure. *South Med J* 1990;83:1437–1443.
18. McAllister FF. The fate of patients with intermittent claudication managed non-operatively. *Am J Surg* 1976;132:593–595.
19. Krepel VM, van Andel GJ, van Erp WF, et al. Percutaneous transluminal angioplasty of the femoropopliteal artery: initial and long-term results. *Radiology* 1985;156:325–328.
20. Capek P, MacLean GK, Berkowitz HD. Femoral angioplasty: factors influencing long term success. *Circulation* 1991;183:767–771.
21. Taylor LM, Edwards JM, Porter JM. Present status of reversed vein bypass grafting: five-year results of a modern series. *J Vasc Surg* 1990;11:193–205.
22. Quinones-Baldrich WJ, Busittil RW, Baker JD, et al. Is the preferential use of polytetrafluoroethylene grafts for femoropopliteal bypass justified? *J Vasc Surg* 1988;8:219–228.
22a. Plecha EJ, Freischlag JA, Seabrook GR, et al. Femoropopliteal bypass revisited: an analysis of 138 cases. *CV Surg* 1996;4:195–199.
23. McCollum C, Kenchington G, Alexander C, et al. PTFE or HUV for

femoro-popliteal bypass: a multi-center trial. *Eur J Vasc Surg* 1991;5:435–443.

24. Buckley CJ, Abernathy S, Lee SD, et al. Suggested treatment protocol for improving patency of femoral-infrapopliteal cryopreserved saphenous vein allografts. *J Vasc Surg* 2000;32:731–738.

25. Harris L, O'Brien-Irr M, Ricotta JJ. Long-term assessment of cryopreserved vein bypass grafting success. *J Vasc Surg* 2001;33:528–532.

26. Shah D, Darling R, Chang B, et al. Long-term results of in situ saphenous vein bypass: analysis of 2058 cases. *Ann Surg* 1995;222:438–446.

27. Ouriel K, Smith CR, DeWeese JA. Endarterectomy for localized lesions of the superficial femoral artery at the adductor canal. *J Vasc Surg* 1986;3:531–534.

28. Nelson PR, Powell RJ, Proia RR, et al. Results of endovascular superficial femoral endarterectomy. *J Vasc Surg* 2001;34:526–531.

29. Rosenthal D, Schubart PJ, Kinney EV, et al. Remote superficial femoral artery endarterectomy: multicenter medium-term results. *J Vasc Surg* 2001;34:428–433.

30. Taylor LM, Edwards JM, Porter JM. Present status of reversed vein bypass grafting: five-year results of a modern series. *J Vasc Surg* 1990;11:193–205.

31. Bergamini TM, Towne JB, Bandyk DF, et al. Experience with in-situ saphenous vein bypasses during 1981 to 1989: determinant factors of long-term patency. *J Vasc Surg* 1991;13:137–147.

32. Donaldson MC, Mannick JA, Whittemore AD. Femoral-distal bypass with in-situ greater saphenous vein: long-term results using the Mills valvulotome. *Ann Surg* 1991;213:457–464.

33. Leather RP, Fitzgerald K. From: Vascular Data Registry, Department of Surgery, Albany Medical College, October 19, 1992.

34. Andros G, Harris RW, Salles-Cunha SX, et al. Bypass grafts to the ankle and foot. *J Vasc Surg* 1988;7:785–794.

35. Klamer TW, Lambert GE, Richardson JD, et al. Utility of inframalleolar arterial bypass grafting. *J Vasc Surg* 1990;11:164–169.

36. Pomposelli FB, Jespen SJ, Gibbons GW, et al. Efficacy of the dorsal pedal bypass for limb salvage in diabetic patients: short-term observations. *J Vasc Surg* 1990;11:745–751.

37. Shah DM, Darling RC, Change BB, et al. Is long vein bypass from groin to ankle a durable procedure? An analysis of a ten-year experience. *J Vasc Surg* 1992;15:402–407.

38. Harrington ED, Harrington ME, Schanzer H, et al. The dorsalis pedis bypass: moderate success in difficult situations. *J Vasc Surg* 1992;15:409–414.

CHAPTER 103

Nonsurgical Management of Carotid Disease

Samir R. Kapadia and Jay S. Yadav

Key Words: Carotid endarterectomy; carotid stenosis; carotid stenting; cerebrovascular disease; stroke.

Carotid artery stenosis has emerged as an important and potentially modifiable cause for ischemic strokes since the first implication of carotid disease in genesis of stroke by C. Miller Fisher in 1951 (1). Carotid artery disease, both symptomatic and asymptomatic, increases the risk for ischemic strokes and the risk increases with worsening severity of stenosis (2). Considering that ischemic strokes account for more than 80% of all strokes and that stroke is the third most common cause of death in the United States, the public health implication of carotid disease is substantial. Various treatments including medical management, surgery in the form of carotid endarterectomy (CEA), and percutaneous therapy with balloon angioplasty and stenting have been successfully used to decrease the risk for ischemic stroke in patients with carotid artery disease (3–9). This chapter reviews the epidemiology, clinical presentations, diagnosis, and nonsurgical management of carotid disease.

S. R. Kapadia: The Cleveland Clinic Foundation, 9500 Euclid Ave., F25, Cleveland, Ohio 44195.

J. S. Yadav: The Cleveland Clinic Foundation, 9500 Euclid Ave., F25, Cleveland, Ohio 44195.

EPIDEMIOLOGY

Prevalence

Stroke is the third leading cause of death in the United States after cardiovascular disease and cancer, causing 163,601 deaths in 2001 (10). Overall, approximately 730,000 people experience either an initial or recurrent stroke each year, with approximately 40,000 more women than men having a stroke each year (11). In 2000, more than $51 billion dollars was spent on the diagnosis and treatment of stroke in the United States. In addition to the acute clinical and financial consequences, there are significant long-term effects related to stroke. Stroke is the most common cause of long-term disability, with 20% of victims needing institutional care 3 months after the event. Furthermore, almost one-fourth of all stroke patients will die within 1 year after the event, and this number is even greater for those who are older than 65 years.

The predominant cause (>80%) of stroke is the abrupt interruption of cerebral blood flow described as ischemic stroke. Almost one-third (15–40%) of ischemic strokes result from plaque rupture and local thrombosis of atherothrombotic lesions in the aortic arch, carotid bifurcation, or intracranial vessels, resulting in distal embolism of the clot with total occlusion of the smaller distal vessels. Cardiac sources of embolism (20–30%) and lacunar infarctions (15–30%) from *in situ* thrombosis are other important causes (12).

Several population-based epidemiologic studies using duplex scanning have shown that the prevalence rate of asymptomatic carotid stenosis of 50% or greater is between 4% and 8% in adults (13–17) and that of less than 50% is between 28% and 54% in adults (18,19). Presence and severity of carotid atherothrombosis correlates with the presence and severity of coronary atherothrombosis and peripheral vascular disease (20–23). Patients with severe peripheral vascular disease (e.g., ankle–brachial index < 0.4, aortic aneurysms) have been reported to have high prevalence of carotid disease (24,25). About 5% to 10% of patients with coronary artery disease also will have severe carotid atherothrombosis, but the prevalence of significant carotid stenosis is greater in patients with left main disease or severe three-vessel coronary disease. On the other hand, approximately one-third of patients with carotid disease have severe coronary stenosis (26).

Risk Factors

The risk factors for coronary atherothrombosis also are associated with carotid atherothrombosis (27–30). The incidence of severe carotid disease increases with age in men and women. Half of men older than 75 years have some carotid atherothrombosis by ultrasonography, but more than 50% stenosis is present only in 5% (18,31). There may be substantial racial differences in the severity and distribution of carotid atherothrombosis. White patients have predominantly extracranial carotid artery atherothrombosis, whereas black, Japanese, and Chinese patients have predominantly intracranial vascular lesions (32,33). Smoking is the most important risk factor for prediction of carotid atherothrombotic disease, followed by hypertension, diabetes, male sex, and increased systolic blood pressure (34). Association of hypercholesterolemia with stroke has been clouded by that many epidemiologic studies failed to separate ischemic and hemorrhagic strokes for analysis. Therefore, hypercholesterolemia did not always pan out to be a risk factor for "stroke" (35). Ischemic stroke, however, has been associated with greater serum cholesterol levels (36). Multiple studies have now associated increased total cholesterol, increased low-density lipoprotein (LDL) cholesterol, increased triglycerides, and decreased high-density lipoprotein (HDL) cholesterol levels with carotid atherothrombosis (30,37–39). Even low level of HDL cholesterol without elevated levels of LDL or total cholesterol in patients with coronary disease has been associated with carotid disease (40). Metaanalyses with clinical trials of 3-hydroxy-3-methylglutaryl coenzyme A (HMG-CoA) inhibitors have further added support to the association between hypercholesterolemia and ischemic stroke (41–44). Two recent trials, the Myocardial Ischemia Reduction with Aggressive Cholesterol Lowering (MIRACL) and the Heart Protection Study (HPS), provide strong prospective evidence that statin therapy effectively reduces stroke (45,46). Stroke was reduced by 51% in the MIRACL study and 25% in the HPS study. Furthermore, the HPS study helps to refute the prior concerns that cholesterol therapy increases the risk for hemorrhagic stroke, because the hemorrhagic stroke rate was similar in simvastatin and placebo arms. The roles of various lipid reducing therapies on carotid atherothrombosis will become more clear as many prospective clinical trials are using carotid intima-media thickness to monitor atherothrombosis progression or regression (47,48).

Natural History

Once carotid atheromatous lesions have formed, the severity of stenosis and associated symptoms are predictive of the risk for stroke (49,50). In asymptomatic carotid stenosis of 60% or greater, the annual risk for stroke has been found to be 2.1% (3). The addition of symptoms such as transient ischemic attack (TIA) significantly increases the risk for stroke in patients with even moderate stenosis, and this risk increases in a stepwise fashion with increasing severity of stenosis. The risk for stroke after a TIA was 40% in the Framingham study, and two-thirds of these strokes occurred within the first 6 months (34). The North American Symptomatic Carotid Endarterectomy Trial (NASCET) demonstrated the risk for ipsilateral stroke to be 18.7% over 5 years in medically treated patients with greater than 50% symptomatic stenosis and 22.2% in those with 50% to 69% symptomatic stenosis (51). Mortality also increases with worsening severity of stenosis. The adjusted relative risk for death is 1.32 for stenoses less than 45%, 2.22 for stenoses 45% to 74%, and 3.24 for stenoses 75% to 99% (52).

CLINICAL PRESENTATION

Carotid bruits can be auscultated over one or both carotid arteries and typically have a harsh blowing quality. Evidence of a carotid bruit on physical examination is the most common finding leading to the diagnosis of asymptomatic carotid stenosis. Although carotid bruits are poor predictors of the severity of atherothrombosis, they have been associated with an increased risk for stroke, myocardial infarction (MI), and death (53).

A TIA is the most common presentation of symptomatic carotid stenosis. By definition, a TIA lasts for less than 24 hours and typically resolves within 30 minutes. Symptoms from a TIA are related to the distribution affected by the area of ischemia. Importantly, TIAs caused by vertebrobasilar insufficiency must be differentiated from those secondary to carotid origin by careful history taking and physical examination. Carotid-related symptoms include aphasia and contralateral sensory and motor deficits. Visual disturbances such as ipsilateral amaurosis fugax or contralateral homonymous hemianopia also can be present. Conversely, symptoms related to vertebrobasilar insufficiency include transient cranial nerve findings, diplopia, and dysarthria. Motor deficits are ipsilateral, and visual losses are frequently bilateral.

DIAGNOSIS

Ultrasonography

The standard noninvasive method for the evaluation of carotid artery stenosis is duplex ultrasonography. Several studies encouraged the diagnosis of carotid artery stenosis severity on the basis of ultrasound alone, without the need for angiography (54–58). Results concerning the diagnostic accuracy of carotid ultrasound in the centers participating in the NASCET study, however, cast some doubt on the validity of ultrasound because the sensitivity and specificity of carotid ultrasound were only 68% and 67%, respectively (59). This poor performance has been attributed to many factors, including variations in patient selection, imaging device performance, and the imaging protocols used. Ultrasound evaluation faired better in the Asymptomatic Carotid Atherosclerosis Study (ACAS). In this study, centers had to show evidence of Doppler measurements and carotid arteriography correlation, and a standard protocol was adopted. This helped to increase the specificity of carotid ultrasound to 95% (60). Properly trained sonographers and a routine quality assurance program are critical to the better sensitivity and specificity of ultrasound examination. Many experienced laboratories report sensitivity greater than 80% and specificity greater than 90% in identifying severe carotid stenosis (61).

Magnetic Resonance Angiography

Magnetic resonance angiography (MRA) has been used to evaluate the carotid bifurcation, because this segment of the carotid artery is relatively motionless, superficial, and large enough for visualization. Newer methods of MRA have addressed some of the shortcomings associated with initial techniques and have made better visualization possible with reliable imaging of the carotids from their origin to the intracranial branches.

Three-dimensional (3D) contrast-enhanced MRA of the carotid and thoracic aorta has made significant advancements for noninvasive examination of the extracranial carotid and the aortic arch. Before the evolution of 3D gadolinium-contrasted MRA as a standard part of MRA, it was routine to use two-dimensional (2D) time of flight (TOF) and 3D multislab TOF MRA alone. These techniques are complementary, making it important to use them together to accurately diagnose stenoses. They are limited by their flow dependence and their susceptibility to motion artifacts. Advantages of gadolinium-enhanced MRA for carotid angiography include the ability to image plaque ulcerations (which often are not seen on TOF), lack of flow-related artifacts, which can degrade tortuous vessels by inplane saturation, short imaging times with excellent signal-to-noise ratio, and the ability to image from the aortic arch to circle of Willis in approximately 30 seconds. Contrast-enhanced magnetic resonance imaging (MRI) is limited by interference from contrast in the jugular vein, which may impair visualization of the carotid artery, thereby decreasing the sensitivity for measuring stenoses when a long scan time is used. Conversely, using the shorter scan time decreases the spatial resolution. A study comparing the sensitivity and specificity of noninvasive imaging with angiography on 569 patients demonstrated that MRA was associated with a sensitivity of 75% and specificity of 88%. However, concordant noninvasive testing with Doppler ultrasound and MRA resulted in an improved sensitivity of 96% and specificity of 85%, suggesting that surgical decisions should be made cautiously if based solely on the results of individual noninvasive studies (62). Concordant Doppler ultrasound and MRA may result in better sensitivity and specificity, possibly reducing the need for invasive diagnostic angiography.

Digital Subtraction Angiography

Angiography remains the gold standard of assessing the severity of carotid stenosis severity. There are several factors that make angiography unique and attractive in its detection of atherothrombotic plaque. It provides high-resolution images of the stenosis and plaque surface and is able to distinguish easily between a high-grade stenosis and occlusion. It allows the simultaneous study of the origin of the neck vessels and intracranial circulation. This is important for the detection of tandem stenoses, which pose diagnostic problems for Doppler ultrasound. The ability to assess collateral circulation, intracranial lesions, and adequacy of anterior and posterior communicating vessels can be useful in determining the safety of temporary carotid occlusion associated with either CEA or carotid artery stenting. The risks associated with angiography include embolization and dissection, but these risks have been shown to be relatively low, particularly when performed in the cardiac catheterization laboratory (63).

NONSURGICAL MANAGEMENT

Medical Management

Antiplatelet Agents

The long-standing foundation of antiplatelet therapy in atherothrombotic disease management has been aspirin. Aspirin exerts its antiplatelet effect by acetylating platelet cyclooxygenase, thereby irreversibly inhibiting platelet-dependent thromboxane formation. The Antithrombotic Trialists' Collaboration has documented in its most recent metaanalysis of more than 200,000 patients from 287 randomized trials the powerful effect of antiplatelet agents, primarily aspirin, in reducing both fatal and nonfatal strokes compared with control subjects. Aspirin was found to be effective in dosages ranging from less than 75mg to 1,500 mg without a dose-associated difference in effect. There are substantially less data for doses less than 75 mg, however, which leaves uncertain the effectiveness of this small dose. This trial also reported the results from six trials that specifically evaluated the use of antiplatelet agents in patients with carotid stenosis. This subanalysis of five CEA trials and one asymptomatic carotid disease trial demonstrated a 19% reduction in vascular events, which, although it did not reach statistical significance, demonstrated a consistent trend with that seen in other high-risk patient populations in the metaanalysis (64).

Clopidogrel and ticlopidine are thienopyridine inhibitors. They inhibit adenosine diphosphate (ADP)–induced platelet aggregation by direct inhibition of ADP binding to its receptor and the subsequent activation of the glycoprotein IIb/IIIa complex. The Ticlopidine Aspirin Stroke Study compared the use of ticlopidine and aspirin in patients with a history of TIA, reversible ischemic neurologic deficit, or minor stroke. Ticlopidine significantly reduced the risk for fatal and nonfatal stroke by 24% ($p = 0.011$) compared with aspirin. This effect was even greater during the first year, with a 48% reduction in the risk for stroke (65). In The Canadian American Ticlopidine Study, patients with a history of previous atherothrombotic stroke were treated with ticlopidine or placebo for up to 3 years. Ticlopidine significantly reduced the relative risk for stroke by 24% over 3 years ($p = 0.017$) (66). However, secondary to complications associated with ticlopidine, such as neutropenia and thrombotic thrombocytopenic purpura, the use of a newer thienopyridine inhibitor, clopidogrel, has become standard.

The Clopidogrel vs. Aspirin in Patients at Risk of Ischemic Events trial (CAPRIE) was a randomized, double-blind trial that compared clopidogrel and aspirin in patients with a history of recent MI, ischemic stroke, or peripheral vascular disease. Clopidogrel demonstrated an 8.7% relative risk reducing for the primary outcome of stroke, MI, or vascular death ($p = 0.04$). In a subgroup analysis of patients with a history of a previous stroke, there was a trend toward decreasing the risk for adverse events with a relative risk reduction of 7.3% in favor of clopidogrel ($p = 0.26$) (67).

The Clopidogrel in Unstable Angina to Reduce Ischemic Events study (CURE) included patients with acute coronary syndrome without ST-segment elevation (68). Patients were randomized to receive clopidogrel or placebo and were treated for up to 1 year. All patients also were treated with aspirin. There was a 20% relative risk reduction in the occurrence of cardiovascular death, MI, or stroke for the group treated with clopidogrel. There was a small and statistically insignificant reduction of ischemic stroke favoring clopidogrel (1.2% clopidogrel vs. 1.4% placebo; $p =$ not significant).

The ongoing Management of Atherothrombosis with Clopidogrel in High-risk Patients with Recent Transient Ischaemic Attack or Ischaemic Stroke (MATCH) trial will evaluate the efficacy and safety of clopidogrel plus aspirin versus clopidogrel alone in patients with recent TIA or ischemic stroke. The Clopidogrel for High Atherothrombotic Risk and Ischemic Stabilization, Management and Avoidance (CHARISMA) trial also is designed to investigate the role of adding clopidogrel to aspirin therapy in pa-

tients with vascular disease including coronary or cerebrovascular disease.

Dipyridamole is an antiplatelet agent that inhibits cyclic adenosine monophosphate (cAMP)–dependent phosphodiesterase, which, in turn, increases intraplatelet cAMP. It also effectively inhibits the cellular uptake of adenosine. The effect of dipyridamole in patients with stroke and TIA has been investigated in five studies (69–73). The most recent study compared the efficacy of aspirin and an extended-release formulation of dipyridamole with aspirin alone for prevention of stroke or death (73). The study included 6,602 patients with stroke (76.3%) or TIA (23.7%) within 3 months of enrollment. Compared with placebo, 25 mg aspirin twice a day reduced stroke risk by 18%, dipyridamole alone reduced stroke risk by 16%, and the combination of aspirin and dipyridamole reduced stroke by 37%. Although individual prior studies did not prove benefit of dipyridamole, the aggregate data from these four trials do show 15% stroke reduction by adding dipyridamole to aspirin therapy.

Anticoagulants

Although there is evidence that warfarin reduces the risk for stroke in specific subsets of patients, such as those with atrial fibrillation, there is no convincing evidence that it is superior to aspirin in patients with a history of ischemic stroke from a noncardioembolic source (74). The Stroke Prevention in Reversible Ischemia Trial evaluated the use of warfarin with a target International Normalized Ratio (INR) of 3.0 to 4.5 compared with aspirin for the prevention of adverse events in patients with a history of noncardioembolic TIA or stroke. Warfarin was associated with twice the risk for vascular death, stroke, MI, or major bleeding complications compared with aspirin (12.4% vs. 5.4%; $p < 0.05$). This poor outcome was mainly attributable to excess bleeding complications, including 27 intracranial bleeds associated with warfarin (75). The Warfarin Aspirin Recurrent Stroke Study compared warfarin with a lower target INR of 1.4 to 2.8 and aspirin in 2,206 patients with a history of ischemic, noncardioembolic stroke. The rates of complications including major hemorrhage were not statistically different between the two treatment groups with the more conservative dosing of warfarin, and there was no difference between aspirin and warfarin for the prevention of recurrent ischemic stroke or death (17% vs. 16%; $p = 0.25$) (76). Thus, current data do not support the use of warfarin over aspirin for the prevention of strokes.

Antihyperlipidemics

The treatment of hyperlipidemia has been confirmed in multiple studies to confer a cardiovascular and mortality benefit (43,45,46,77–79). More specifically, the use of HMG-CoA reductase inhibitors (statins) also has been shown to be of benefit in reducing stroke and treating carotid atherothrombosis. Three separate metaanalyses have demonstrated a reduction in stoke with the use of statins. Bucher and coworkers (43) analyzed the results from more than 100,000 patients treated with statins, fibrates, resins, or dietary intervention. Only statins were associated with a reduction in the risk for stoke ($p < 0.05$). Blauw and coworkers (42) evaluated the effect of statins compared with placebo in more than 20,000 patients. Statins were associated with a 31% risk reduction of stroke compared with placebo ($p < 0.05$). Hebert and coworkers (44) evaluated the results from more than 29,000 patients. Those assigned to statin drugs experienced a 29% risk reduction of stroke (95% confidence interval, 14–41%).

There also is evidence that statin therapy has a positive effect on carotid atherothrombotic lesions. Thirty-five aortic and 25 carotid artery plaques were monitored by serial MRIs of the aorta and carotid at baseline and 6 and 12 months after initiation on simvastatin. Statin therapy was found to be associated with significant reductions in vessel wall thickness and vessel wall area over 12 months of follow-up in both aortic and carotid arteries ($p < 0.001$) (80). Further work by Corti and coworkers (81) on 44 aortic and 32 carotid artery plaques detected by MRI in 21 patients with asymptomatic hypercholesterolemia demonstrated not only a decrease in vessel wall thickness and vessel wall area after treatment with simvastatin, but also an increase in lumen area, ranging from 4% to 6% at 18 and 24 months in both carotid and aortic lesions (81). The largest study to evaluate the effect of statins on carotid stenoses is The Carotid Atherosclerosis Italian Ultrasound Study (CAIUS). It was performed to test the effect of lipid reduction on the progression of carotid intima-media thickness in 305 asymptomatic patients. Progression intimal-medial thickness was less in the group treated with pravastatin compared with control ($p < 0.0007$) (82).

CAROTID STENTING

Evolution of Technique

Surgical treatment of carotid stenosis was first attempted in 1951 at the Institute of Experimental Medicine in Buenos Aires by a neurosurgeon named Raúl Carrea. He reconstructed the internal carotid by anastomosing the normal distal internal carotid with the normal proximal external carotid artery. In 1954, at St. Mary's Hospital in London, Eastcott resected the diseased portion of internal carotid and reanastomosed it to the common carotid artery. In 1953, Dr. Kenneth Strully attempted endarterectomy at Montefiore Hospital (Montefiore, NY), but the antegrade flow could not be established. The first successful endarterectomy was performed by Drs. DeBakey and Crawford at the Methodist Hospital in Houston in 1953, but it was not reported until 1975 (83).

The most significant attempt to study the results of CEA was the "Joint Study," which reported its results in series of publications. However, there were many criticisms of this

early effort. Subsequent well planned and executed studies, including NASCET, the European Carotid Surgery Trialists' Collaboration (ECST), and the Veterans Administration (VA) Cooperative trial demonstrated a decrease in the risk for stroke for patients with severe, symptomatic carotid stenosis treated with CEA compared with medical management (6,9,46). The ACAS study showed that asymptomatic patients with greater than 60% stenosis treated with CEA had a decreased risk for stroke at 5 years compared with those treated with medical management (3). Surgery, however, is not without limitations. The risk for stroke associated with CEA ranged from 2.9% to 10.7% in these trials (3,6,9,46). In addition, there are several groups of patients that are considered to be at high risk for CEA including severe coronary atherothrombotic disease, a history of head or neck radiation, previous ipsilateral CEA, or contralateral carotid occlusion. Therefore, there was need for a less invasive strategy for revascularization.

The first percutaneous transluminal angioplasty of the carotid artery in humans was reported by both Mullan and coworkers (84) and Kerber and coworkers (85) in 1980. This was followed by widespread controversy associated with the investigation of carotid angioplasty. In Kachel's 1996 review (86), the results of more than 500 carotid angioplasties are presented demonstrating a low event rate comparable to CEA. Acute closure, vascular recoil, and dissection during angioplasty compelled many investigators to use stents. Initially, only balloon-expandable stents were available. Because of the superficial nature of the carotid artery and constant external forces resulting from neck movements and swallowing, stent deformation was encountered in some patients (87). This led to the development and use of self-expanding alloy stents (Wallstent, Boston Scientific Vascular, Minneapolis, MN) or nitinol stents (Precise, Cordis Endovascular, Warren, NJ; Memotherm, Angiomed Barol, Murray Hill, NJ; Acculink, Guidant, Indianapolis, IN) that continue to exert outward forces for carotid stenting. With widespread availability of deliverable, durable, and self-expanding stents, stand-alone carotid artery angioplasty quickly fell out of favor.

The modern era of percutaneous carotid artery intervention was heralded by the development of the distal emboli prevention device. Numerous studies have demonstrated the occurrence of microemboli as detected by transcranial Doppler during carotid artery stenting and CEA (88–90). There is correlation between the number of emboli and neurologic events after CEA (91–93). Accordingly, numerous mechanical devices have been developed to prevent the distal embolization of debris during carotid artery stenting. There are three major types of emboli prevention devices (EPD): the distal occlusive balloon, the proximal occlusive balloon, and the filter wire (Fig. 103–1) (see color insert).

The PercuSurge GuardWire (Medtronic, Santa Rosa, CA) is the prototypical distal occlusive EPD. A low-pressure balloon is located at the distal tip of a hollow wire. This balloon is inflated after the lesion is crossed and traps any debris released during the percutaneous procedure in the internal carotid artery, which is then aspirated before deflation of the balloon. The advantages of this system include a low crossing profile and superior wire flexibility. Disadvantages include the occlusive nature of this device, which is not well tolerated in patients without good collateral flow, and potential damage to the distal internal carotid artery by the device. In addition, after inflation of the balloon, angiography to localize balloon or stent placement is difficult.

Proximal occlusion balloon systems create retrograde flow in the internal carotid artery, which prevents emboli from traveling to the cerebral circulation. Like the Guard-Wire (Medtronic Corp., Minneapolis, MN) device, this requires occlusive balloon inflation and can cause vessel damage. Good collateral circulation also is critical. Examples of these devices include the Parodi (Arteria Medical Science, San Francisco, CA) and MOMA (Invatec, Italy) devices.

The AngioGuard Emboli Capture Guidewire (Cordis, Miami, FL) was the first distal filtration wire system designed to conform to the artery and trap microemboli while maintaining distal flow through a filter umbrella with multiple perfusion pores. The major advantage of filters is the preservation of flow during the intervention and the ability to visualize the vessel with contrast material throughout the procedure. Disadvantages of filters include a larger crossing profile, which may necessitate predilatation before placement of the filter distal to the lesion. Many other filter devices, such as Accunet (Guidant), FilterWire EX (Boston Scientific), Sulzer-IntraGuard (IntraTherapeutics, St. Paul, MN), MDT-Filter (Medtronic), SpideRX (EV3, Plymouth, MN), and Mednova (Mednova Inc., Galway, Ireland) (Abbott/Mednova), have been under investigation.

Current Carotid Stenting Procedure

Carotid stenting typically requires an overnight hospital stay, although ambulatory stenting also appears to be safe (94). The procedure is commonly performed using a 6- to 8-French femoral sheath. Heparin is used to achieve an activated clotting time (ACT) of 250 to 300 seconds. A guiding catheter or a sheath is advanced to the common carotid artery, and the lesion is crossed with an EPD. The device is deployed in the in-ternal carotid artery, and the lesion is predilated with a small coronary balloon. The lesion is then stented with a self-expanding stent, and the stent is postdilated to the appropriate diameter. The EPD is captured and removed at the end of the procedure. Routine use of a temporary pacing wire is not necessary. Intracardiac filling pressure monitoring is helpful in patients with severe left ventricular dysfunction, in patients with severe aortic stenosis, or in hemodynamically unstable patients. Adjunctive treatment with glycoprotein IIb/IIIa inhibitors has been evaluated in small studies and may be beneficial, but it has been largely supplanted by EPDs (95–98). Aspirin is continued permanently, and clopidogrel is continued for at least 1 month after the procedure.

Outcome

The initial experience of carotid stenting, before the routine use of EPD, was reported by several investigators as consecutive patient series. The 30-day outcome of the larger series ($\geq$100 patients) is summarized in Table 103–1. The majority of patients included in these reports were at high surgical risk for CEA. There also is a significant learning curve effect as this procedure was evolving in that era. Despite these, the safety and durability of carotid stenting in these patients at high risk was remarkable. This generated appropriate enthusiasm and interest in the procedure worldwide. This was evident in the Multi-Center Carotid World Registry where 6,734 patients from 42 centers in the United States, Europe, and South America were enrolled. The study reported a total stroke and mortality rate at 30 days of 5.8%, of which 1.02% were nonprocedure-related deaths. The technical success rate of the study was 98.5%, with a reported major stroke rate of 1.3% and minor stroke rate of 2.7% (99).

With availability of various EPDs, the carotid stenting procedure has become safer. Various investigators have reported their experience with these devices in the form of consecutive case series (Table 103–2). These results are encouraging and convincing regarding the efficacy of the devices in reducing procedural stroke compared with retrospective cohorts where these devices were not available. Most recently, the preliminary data from the ARCHeR (Acculink for Revascu-

TABLE 103–1. *Carotid stenting without emboli prevention devices*

Study	Year	30-Day outcomes						
		Arteries, n	Minor stroke	Major stroke	Death	All	Follow-up, mo	Restenosis
Cremonesi (114)	2000	119	3	0	0	3	6–12	6
Criado (115)	2002	135	2	1	0	3	16	4
Dangas (116)	2000	140	8	1	0	9	10	1
Diethrich (117)	1996	129	10	2	1	14	7.6	2
Gupta (118)	2000	100	0	1	0	1	12.1	1
Kapadia (96)	2001	151	2	1	1	4	1	0
Roubin (119)	2001	604	29	6	8	43	17	16
Shawl (120)	2000	192	4	1	0	5	19	3
All		1,570	58 (3.6%)	13 (0.8%)	10 (0.6%)	82 (5.2%)		33 (2.1%)

TABLE 103–2. *Emboli prevention device experience*

Study	Year	Procedures, n	Device	30-Day events (includes procedural)			
				Minor stroke	Major stroke	Death	All
Al-Mubarak (121)	2002	164	NeuroShield	2	0	2	4
Guimaraens (122)	2002	194	Multiple	2	0	3	5
Henry (123)	1999	184	GuardWire	0	2	1	3
Reimers (124)	2001	88	Filters	1	0	1	2
Tubler (125)	2001	58	GuardWire	0	1	0	1
Whitlow (126)	2002	75	GuardWire	0	0	0	0
All		763		5 (0.6%)	3 (0.4%)	7 (0.9)%	15 (1.96%)

larization of Carotids in High-Risk Patients) registry were presented at the American College of Cardiology meeting in 2003 (Chicago, March 30–April 2) by Wholey and coworkers. Patients with high surgical risk were enrolled in this registry. A total of 437 patients from 41 centers underwent carotid stenting where EPD (Accunet) was used in 278 (64%) patients in latter phase of the trial. In all patients enrolled in the study, the 30-day major adverse event rate— defined as all-cause stroke (5.3%), death (2.3%), and MI (2.1%)—was 7.8%. The event rates from subgroup of patients treated with EPDs were not presented. All currently ongoing randomized trials comparing carotid stenting with CEA use EPDs (Table 103–3). Furthermore, EPDs have become the standard of care for carotid stenting procedure in clinical practice. Currently, there are no studies comparing safety and efficacy of different EPDs.

Complications

There are several important issues, some unique to carotid artery stenting and some similar to those seen in percutaneous coronary intervention, that the physician must be mindful of to avert an adverse and potentially catastrophic outcome. The major periprocedural complications of carotid artery stenting are stroke, MI, and death. Other associated adverse events are intracranial hemorrhage, bradycardia, hypotension, seizures, contrast nephrotoxicities, and access site complications.

Although the majority of ischemic complications occur during the procedure, they can occur several hours later. Careful neurologic examination is essential to identify these complications. Routine use of cerebral angiography before and after stenting can help to identify occluded intracranial vessels. Intraarterial thrombolytic therapy has been used to

TABLE 103–3. *Carotid stent trials*

Trial acronym	Trial name	Comment
ARCHeR	ACCULINK for Revascularization of Carotids in High-Risk Patients	Registry, high-risk patients treated with ACCULINK stent and now with ACCUNET (endoscopic papillary balloon dilation). PI: L. Nelson Hopkins and Mark H. Wholey
CREST	Carotid Revascularization Endarterectomy vs. Stent Trial	Randomized American Trial, National Institutes of Health funded, endarterectomy vs. stenting in symptomatic patients, n = 2500. PI: Robert W. Hobson II
EVA-3S	Endarterectomy Versus Angioplasty in patients with Severe Symptomatic carotid Stenosis	Randomized French trial, endarterectomy vs. angioplasty and stenting in symptomatic patients, n = 1900. PI: Jean-Louis Mas and Gilles Chatellier
ICSS (CAVATAS-2)	International Carotid Stenting Study	Randomized English trial, endarterectomy vs. stenting in symptomatic patients, n = 2000. PI: Martin M. Brown
MAVErIC	Evaluation of the Medtronic AVE Self-Expanding Carotid Stent System With Distal Protection In the Treatment of Carotid Stenosis	Registry, high-risk patients for endarterectomy
PASCAL	Performance And Safety of the Medtronic AVE Self-Expandable Stent in Treatment of Carotid Artery Lesions	Registry, carotid stenting in patients with coronary artery disease
SHELTER	Stenting of High risk patients Extracranial Lesions Trial with Emboli Removal	Registry, high-risk patients for endarterectomy. PI: Sriram Iyer
SPACE	Stent-protected Percutaneous Angioplasty of the Carotid vs. Endarterectomy	Randomized German trial, endarterectomy vs. stenting in symptomatic patients, n = 1900, PI: Werner Hacke

treat this complication, but with limited success, reflecting that embolic materials are commonly plaque fragments and not thrombus (100). Furthermore, the risk for intracranial hemorrhage with this approach is substantial. Mechanical dislodgement of the embolic debris with soft wire may be the best approach to minimize the size of cerebral infraction.

The carotid sinus reflex is most often responsible for the bradycardia and hypotension associated with carotid sinus manipulation. In anticipation of this effect, antihypertensives are typically held the morning of the procedure, and depending on the response to stenting, may also be held until the following morning. Adequate volume expansion is the cornerstone of effective treatment. Atropine is helpful in cases of severe bradycardia. Vasopressors may be required for severe and persistent hypotension. The carotid sinus reflex is typically transient, but it may continue to be a concern for up to 24 hours after the procedure.

On the other side of the spectrum, brisk return of blood flow distal to a chronically ischemic cerebral hemisphere with disordered cerebral autoregulation can lead to problems. Hyperperfusion syndrome is a potentially deadly complication from carotid artery stenting or CEA. Severe hypertension, critical carotid stenosis, and contralateral carotid occlusion appear to be predisposing factors. Strict monitoring of blood pressure with appropriate treatment is crucial to preventing this. All patients undergoing carotid artery stenting should be instructed on the importance of medication compliance and home blood pressure monitoring. They should be instructed to keep their systolic blood pressure less than 140 mmHg. Furthermore, patients must be instructed to monitor for headaches localized to one side associated with nausea, vomiting, and photophobia. Treatment of hyperperfusion syndrome includes strict blood pressure control with the reduction of systolic blood pressure to approximately 100 mm Hg.

Comparisons with Carotid Endarterectomy

Although carotid artery stenting is a less invasive method of treating carotid artery stenosis compared with CEA, extensive evidence of the safety and feasibility of CEA have made it difficult to establish carotid artery stenting as a viable alternative. Two major studies comparing these procedures have been completed, however, and many more are currently enrolling subjects.

The Carotid and Vertebral Artery Transluminal Angioplasty study (CAVATAS) compared the outcomes of percutaneous angioplasty and stenting to surgical CEA in 504 patients with carotid stenosis (101). Stents were used only in 55 patients (26%) treated by percutaneous approach. The rates of any stroke or death at 30 days were similar between endovascular treatment and surgery (10% vs. 9.9%). Cranial neuropathy was reported in 22 surgical patients (8.7%), but not after endovascular treatment. Major groin or neck hematoma occurred less often after endovascular treatment than after surgery (1.2% vs. 6.7%; $p < 0.0015$). Restenosis

at 1 year was more common after endovascular treatment (14% vs. 4%; $p < 0.001$); however, there was no difference in ipsilateral stroke rate. This trial has been criticized for having greater than expected complication rates with CEA. However, the percutaneous method used would not be considered state of the art by current standards because only 25% of the patients undergoing percutaneous revascularization received stents and EPDs were not used in this study.

More recently, results from the Stenting and Angioplasty with Protection in Patients at High Risk for Endarterectomy (SAPPHIRE) trial were reported at the American Heart Association Scientific Sessions in Chicago (November 2002) (102). This trial randomized 307 patients to either carotid angioplasty or stenting with emboli protection or CEA. Patients were either asymptomatic with 80% or greater stenosis by ultrasound or symptomatic with 50% or greater stenosis. All patients enrolled had a comorbid condition, which increased the risk for CEA. The inclusion criteria included previous CEA, congestive heart failure, severe coronary artery disease, previous radical neck surgery or radiation therapy, and chronic obstructive pulmonary disease. Patients who in the opinion of a vascular surgeon were not eligible for surgery were enrolled in a stent registry (409 patients). Patients considered too high risk for percutaneous management were likewise enrolled in a surgical registry (17 patients). The primary end point was major adverse cardiovascular events (MACE), including death, stroke, or MI within 30 days of the procedure. The 30-day MACE rate was markedly reduced in the percutaneous treatment group compared with the CEA group (5.8% vs. 12.6%; $p = 0.047$). In the registry data, the 30-day MACE rate was 7.8% for stenting (32/409) and 14.3% (1/7) for CEA. There were no significant differences between the two groups with regard to either major bleeding (8.3% vs. 10.6%; $p = 0.56$) or TIA (3.85 vs. 2.0%; $p = 0.5$), but carotid stenting did have an advantage over CEA with regard to cranial nerve injury (0% vs. 5.3%; $p < 0.01$). Restenosis rates were not presented. This trial clearly demonstrated a reduction in risk for MACE for patients at high risk treated with carotid stenting compared with conventional CEA.

Use in Specific Situations

There are several patient subgroups that have posed special challenges for the vascular surgeon contemplating a surgical approach to treatment of their carotid artery stenosis. Existing data support the treatment of these patients with carotid artery stenting instead of CEA.

Concomitant Carotid Stenosis and Coronary Artery Disease

An important issue surrounding the treatment of carotid artery atherothrombosis is the optimal treatment strategy used to treat those with both significant carotid artery disease and coronary atherothrombosis. Approaches using CEA followed by open heart surgery (OHS), OHS followed by CEA, or combined OHS and CEA have been studied. Whether to use staged approach where CEA is preformed before CABG or simultaneous CEA and CABG during the same anesthesia (CEA is typically performed before CABG) is dependent on institutional preference. There are conflicting data whether one approach is better than the other (103,104). However, it is clear that the risk for stroke, MI, and death are significantly high (combined events >15%) with all of these strategies. Furthermore, recent analysis would suggest that the outcome in community might even be worse than reported in the literature (105).

Considering these limitations of current therapy, carotid stenting has been explored as a treatment option for these patients. Ziada and coworkers (106) evaluated the outcomes of 64 patients with both severe carotid stenosis and coronary atherothrombosis who were treated with carotid stenting followed by coronary artery bypass surgery and compared them to 112 patients who underwent combined CEA and OHS. The stent group had a much greater prevalence of unstable angina, poor left ventricular function, critical aortic valve stenosis, TIA or stroke, and history of previous OHS. Although there was no difference in mortality, the stent patients had significantly lower incidence rates of stroke (2% vs. 9%; $p = 0.05$) and strokes or MI (6% vs. 19%; $p = 0.02$) compared with those who received concomitant CEA and OHS (106). This is consistent with the recent data from the SAPPHIRE trial where carotid stenting was associated with a lower rate of MI compared with CEA (2.6% vs. 7.3%) (102). However, carotid stenting also is not a perfect solution for this situation, because antiplatelet therapy poses a challenge for patients scheduled for immediate surgery. It is preferable if patients can wait 2 to 4 weeks after stenting and be kept on aspirin and clopidogrel during this time. Anecdotal use of short-acting glycoprotein IIb/IIIa inhibitors until the cardiac surgery, and immediate loading with clopidogrel and aspirin after the surgery, has been reported with success. The availability of heparin-coated stents may reduce the need for dual antiplatelet therapy and make this an even better option in patients requiring OHS.

Radical Neck Surgery and Radiation Therapy

Extracranial carotid stenosis frequently occurs in patients who have had surgery and head and neck irradiation for cancer therapy. Tissue dissection is complicated by the extensive fibrosis of the arterial wall and normal tissue planes, and the difficult locations of the lesions because of extensive involvement of long segments of the carotid artery above and below the carotid bifurcation make access difficult (107). Carotid stenting has been reported as safe and effective in the treatment of this problem (108–112). The procedural risks are not increased compared with stenting for conventional atherothrombotic carotid disease treatment. Therefore, carotid stenting can be considered the treatment of choice for severe carotid stenosis requiring revascularization after cervical radiation or radical neck surgery.

Restenosis after Endarterectomy

There is a greater surgical risk for patients with restenotic lesions after CEA compared with those undergoing CEA for the first time. Occasionally, the lesion also is in an anatomically unfavorable location for surgery. These lesions can be successfully treated with percutaneous stenting with no increased risk. Data from a multicenter registry of 14 centers in the United States included 338 patients undergoing carotid stenting of 358 arteries for restenosis after CEA revealed an overall 30-day stroke and death rate of 3.7% (113). There was one fatal (0.3%) and one nonfatal (0.3%) stroke during the follow-up period. The overall 3-year rate of freedom from all fatal and nonfatal strokes was 96%. These results suggest that carotid artery stenting is an excellent treatment alternative for restenosis after CEA.

FUTURE

Several trials to evaluate the percutaneous treatment of carotid artery atherothrombosis are ongoing (the updated information on these trials is available online at: www. strokecenter.org). The Carotid Revascularization Endarterectomy versus Stent Trial (CREST) is a multicenter randomized trial comparing CEA with carotid artery stenting using EPD. Unlike SAPPHIRE, the patients studied in this trial are at low risk; therefore, this trial will add insight into the use of this treatment strategy in additional patient populations. Furthermore, there are several ongoing registries for carotid artery stenting patients who are not eligible for randomized trials. With increasing understanding of the procedure and the technologic advances, carotid stenting will become an even safer and more widely used therapy for carotid stenosis.

REFERENCES

1. Fisher M. Occlusion of internal carotid artery. *Arch Neurol Psychol* 1951;65:364–377.
2. Wilterdink JL, Easton JD. Vascular event rates in patients with atherosclerotic cerebrovascular disease. *Arch Neurol* 1992;49:857–863.
3. Endarterectomy for asymptomatic carotid artery stenosis. Executive Committee for the Asymptomatic Carotid Atherosclerosis Study. *JAMA* 1995;273:1421–1428.
4. Hobson RW 2nd, Weiss DG, Fields WS, et al. Efficacy of carotid endarterectomy for asymptomatic carotid stenosis. The Veterans Affairs Cooperative Study Group. *N Engl J Med* 1993;328:221–227.
5. Carotid surgery versus medical therapy in asymptomatic carotid stenosis. The CASANOVA Study Group. *Stroke* 1991;22:1229–1235.
6. Beneficial effect of carotid endarterectomy in symptomatic patients with high-grade carotid stenosis. North American Symptomatic Carotid Endarterectomy Trial Collaborators. *N Engl J Med* 1991;325:445–453.
7. Randomised trial of endarterectomy for recently symptomatic carotid stenosis: final results of the MRC European Carotid Surgery Trial (ECST). *Lancet* 1998;351:1379–1387.
8. Rothwell PM, Gutnikov SA, Warlow CP. Reanalysis of the final results of the European Carotid Surgery Trial. *Stroke* 2003;34:514–523.
9. Mayberg MR, Wilson SE, Yatsu F, et al. Carotid endarterectomy and

prevention of cerebral ischemia in symptomatic carotid stenosis. Veterans Affairs Cooperative Studies Program 309 Trialist Group. *JAMA* 1991;266:3289–3294.

10. Arias E, Smith BL. Deaths: Preliminary data for 2001. *Natl Vital Stat Rep* 2003;51:1–44.

11. Broderick J, Brott T, Kothari R, et al. The Greater Cincinnati/Northern Kentucky Stroke Study: preliminary first-ever and total incidence rates of stroke among blacks. *Stroke* 1998;29:415–421.

12. Baumgartner RW, Sidler C, Mosso M, et al. Ischemic lacunar stroke in patients with and without potential mechanism other than small-artery disease. *Stroke* 2003;34:653–659.

13. Ricci S, Flamini FO, Marini M, et al. [The prevalence of stenosis of the internal carotid in subjects over 49: a population study]. *Epidemiol Prev* 1991;13:173–176.

14. O'Leary DH, Anderson KM, Wolf PA, et al. Cholesterol and carotid atherosclerosis in older persons: the Framingham Study. *Ann Epidemiol* 1992;2:147–153.

15. Pujia A, Rubba P, Spencer MP. Prevalence of extracranial carotid artery disease detectable by echo-Doppler in an elderly population. *Stroke* 1992;23:818–822.

16. Mannami T, Konishi M, Baba S, et al. Prevalence of asymptomatic carotid atherosclerotic lesions detected by high-resolution ultrasonography and its relation to cardiovascular risk factors in the general population of a Japanese city: the Suita study. *Stroke* 1997;28: 518–525.

17. Mineva PP, Manchev IC, Hadjiev DI. Prevalence and outcome of asymptomatic carotid stenosis: a population-based ultrasonographic study. *Eur J Neurol* 2002;9:383–388.

18. Colgan MP, Strode GR, Sommer JD, et al. Prevalence of asymptomatic carotid disease: results of duplex scanning in 348 unselected volunteers. *J Vasc Surg* 1988;8:674–678.

19. Fine-Edelstein JS, Wolf PA, O'Leary DH, et al. Precursors of extracranial carotid atherosclerosis in the Framingham Study. *Neurology* 1994;44:1046–1050.

20. Hertzer NR, Beven EG, Young JR, et al. Coronary artery disease in peripheral vascular patients. A classification of 1000 coronary angiograms and results of surgical management. *Ann Surg* 1984;199:223–233.

21. Chambers BR, Norris JW. Outcome in patients with asymptomatic neck bruits. *N Engl J Med* 1986;315:860–865.

22. Dormandy J, Heeck L, Vig S. Lower-extremity arteriosclerosis as a reflection of a systemic process: implications for concomitant coronary and carotid disease. *Semin Vasc Surg* 1999;12:118–122.

23. Simons PC, Algra A, Eikelboom BC, et al. Carotid artery stenosis in patients with peripheral arterial disease: the SMART study. SMART study group. *J Vasc Surg* 1999;30:519–525.

24. Cina CS, Safar HA, Maggisano R, et al. Prevalence and progression of internal carotid artery stenosis in patients with peripheral arterial occlusive disease. *J Vasc Surg* 2002;36:75–82.

25. Kang SS, Littooy FN, Gupta SR, et al. Higher prevalence of abdominal aortic aneurysms in patients with carotid stenosis but without diabetes. *Surgery* 1999;126:687–692.

26. Hertzer NR, Young JR, Beven EG, et al. Coronary angiography in 506 patients with extracranial cerebrovascular disease. *Arch Intern Med* 1985;145:849–852.

27. Crouse JR, Toole JF, McKinney WM, et al. Risk factors for extracranial carotid artery atherosclerosis. *Stroke* 1987;18:990–996.

28. Howard G, Wagenknecht LE, Burke GL, et al. Cigarette smoking and progression of atherosclerosis: the Atherosclerosis Risk in Communities (ARIC) Study. *JAMA* 1998;279:119–124.

29. Kallikazaros I, Tsioufis C, Sideris S, et al. Carotid artery disease as a marker for the presence of severe coronary artery disease in patients evaluated for chest pain. *Stroke* 1999;30:1002–1007.

30. Salonen JT, Seppanen K, Rauramaa R, et al. Risk factors for carotid atherosclerosis: the Kuopio Ischaemic Heart Disease Risk Factor Study. *Ann Med* 1989;21:227–229.

31. Josse MO, Touboul PJ, Mas JL, et al. Prevalence of asymptomatic internal carotid artery stenosis. *Neuroepidemiology* 1987;6:150–152.

32. Heyman A, Fields WS, Keating RD. Joint study of extracranial arterial occlusion. VI. Racial differences in hospitalized patients with ischemic stroke. *JAMA* 1972;222:285–289.

33. Leung SY, Ng TH, Yuen ST, et al. Pattern of cerebral atherosclerosis in Hong Kong Chinese. Severity in intracranial and extracranial vessels. *Stroke* 1993;24:779–786.

34. Whisnant JP, Homer D, Ingall TJ, et al. Duration of cigarette smoking

is the strongest predictor of severe extracranial carotid artery atherosclerosis. *Stroke* 1990;21:707–714.

35. Cholesterol, diastolic blood pressure, and stroke: 13,000 strokes in 450,000 people in 45 prospective cohorts. Prospective studies collaboration. *Lancet* 1995;346:1647–1653.

36. Iso H, Jacobs DR Jr, Wentworth D, et al. Serum cholesterol levels and six-year mortality from stroke in 350,977 men screened for the multiple risk factor intervention trial. *N Engl J Med* 1989;320:904–910.

37. Bonithon-Kopp C, Scarabin PY, Taquet A, et al. Risk factors for early carotid atherosclerosis in middle-aged French women. *Arterioscler Thromb* 1991;11:966–972.

38. Bonithon-Kopp C, Touboul PJ, Berr C, et al. Relation of intima-media thickness to atherosclerotic plaques in carotid arteries. The Vascular Aging (EVA) Study. *Arterioscler Thromb Vasc Biol* 1996;16:310–316.

39. Salonen R, Seppanen K, Rauramaa R, et al. Prevalence of carotid atherosclerosis and serum cholesterol levels in eastern Finland. *Arteriosclerosis* 1988;8:788–792.

40. Wilt TJ, Rubins HB, Robins SJ, et al. Carotid atherosclerosis in men with low levels of HDL cholesterol. *Stroke* 1997;28:1919–1925.

41. Babatasi G, Theron J, Massetti M, et al. [Associated carotid and coronary lesions: carotid endoluminal angioplasty before coronary surgery]. *Presse Med* 1996;25:1623–1626.

42. Blauw GJ, Lagaay AM, Westendorp RG. Statins for prevention of stroke. *Lancet* 1998;352:144.

43. Bucher HC, Griffith LE, Guyatt GH. Effect of HMGcoA reductase inhibitors on stroke. A meta-analysis of randomized, controlled trials. *Ann Intern Med* 1998;128:89–95.

44. Hebert PR, Gaziano JM, Chan KS, et al. Cholesterol lowering with statin drugs, risk of stroke, and total mortality. An overview of randomized trials. *JAMA* 1997;278:313–321.

45. Waters DD, Schwartz GG, Olsson AG, et al. Effects of atorvastatin on stroke in patients with unstable angina or non-Q-wave myocardial infarction: a Myocardial Ischemia Reduction with Aggressive Cholesterol Lowering (MIRACL) substudy. *Circulation* 2002;106:1690–1695.

46. Heart Protection Study Collaborative Group. MRC/BHF Heart Protection Study of cholesterol lowering with simvastatin in 20,536 high-risk individuals: a randomised placebo-controlled trial. *Lancet* 2002; 360:7–22.

47. O'Leary DH, Polak JF, Kronmal RA, et al. Carotid-artery intima and media thickness as a risk factor for myocardial infarction and stroke in older adults. Cardiovascular Health Study Collaborative Research Group. *N Engl J Med* 1999;340:14–22.

48. O'Leary DH, Polak JF. Intima-media thickness: a tool for atherosclerosis imaging and event prediction. *Am J Cardiol* 2002;90:18L–21L.

49. Taylor LM Jr, Loboa L, Porter JM. The clinical course of carotid bifurcation stenosis as determined by duplex scanning. *J Vasc Surg* 1988;8:255–261.

50. Fabris F, Poli L, Zanocchi M, et al. A four year clinical and echographic follow-up of asymptomatic carotid plaque. *Angiology* 1992; 43:590–598.

51. Barnett HJ, Taylor DW, Eliasziw M, et al. Benefit of carotid endarterectomy in patients with symptomatic moderate or severe stenosis. North American Symptomatic Carotid Endarterectomy Trial Collaborators. *N Engl J Med* 1998;339:1415–1425.

52. Joakimsen O, Bonaa KH, Mathiesen EB, et al. Prediction of mortality by ultrasound screening of a general population for carotid stenosis: the Tromso Study. *Stroke* 2000;31:1871–1876.

53. Norris JW, Zhu CZ, Bornstein NM, et al. Vascular risks of asymptomatic carotid stenosis. *Stroke* 1991;22:1485–1490.

54. Erdoes LS, Marek JM, Mills JL, et al. The relative contributions of carotid duplex scanning, magnetic resonance angiography, and cerebral arteriography to clinical decision making: a prospective study in patients with carotid occlusive disease. *J Vasc Surg* 1996;23:950–956.

55. Chervu A, Moore WS. Carotid endarterectomy without arteriography. *Ann Vasc Surg* 1994;8:296–302.

56. Dawson DL, Zierler RE, Strandness DE Jr, et al. The role of duplex scanning and arteriography before carotid endarterectomy: a prospective study. *J Vasc Surg* 1993;18:673–683.

57. Horn M, Michelini M, Greisler HP, et al. Carotid endarterectomy without arteriography: the preeminent role of the vascular laboratory. *Ann Vasc Surg* 1994;8:221–224.

58. Mattos MA, Hodgson KJ, Faught WE, et al. Carotid endarterectomy without angiography: is color-flow duplex scanning sufficient? *Surgery* 1994;116:776–783.

59. Eliasziw M, Rankin RN, Fox AJ, et al. Accuracy and prognostic consequences of ultrasonography in identifying severe carotid artery stenosis. North American Symptomatic Carotid Endarterectomy Trial (NASCET) Group. *Stroke* 1995;26:1747–1752.
60. Howard G, Baker WH, Chambless LE, et al. An approach for the use of Doppler ultrasound as a screening tool for hemodynamically significant stenosis (despite heterogeneity of Doppler performance). A multicenter experience. Asymptomatic Carotid Atherosclerosis Study Investigators. *Stroke* 1996;27:1951–1957.
61. Hood DB, Mattos MA, Mansour A, et al. Prospective evaluation of new duplex criteria to identify 70% internal carotid artery stenosis. *J Vasc Surg* 1996;23:254–262.
62. Johnston DC, Goldstein LB. Clinical carotid endarterectomy decision making: noninvasive vascular imaging versus angiography. *Neurology* 2001;56:1009–1015.
63. Fayed AM, White CJ, Ramee SR, et al. Carotid and cerebral angiography performed by cardiologists: cerebrovascular complications. *Catheter Cardiovasc Interv* 2002;55:277–280.
64. Collaborative meta-analysis of randomised trials of antiplatelet therapy for prevention of death, myocardial infarction, and stroke in high risk patients. *BMJ* 2002;324:71–86.
65. Hass WK, Easton JD, Adams HP Jr, et al. A randomized trial comparing ticlopidine hydrochloride with aspirin for the prevention of stroke in high-risk patients. Ticlopidine Aspirin Stroke Study Group. *N Engl J Med* 1989;321:501–507.
66. Gent M, Blakely JA, Easton JD, et al. The Canadian American Ticlopidine Study (CATS) in thromboembolic stroke. *Lancet* 1989;1:1215–1220.
67. A randomised, blinded, trial of clopidogrel versus aspirin in patients at risk of ischaemic events (CAPRIE). CAPRIE Steering Committee. *Lancet* 1996;348:1329–1339.
68. Yusuf S, Zhao F, Mehta SR, et al. Effects of clopidogrel in addition to aspirin in patients with acute coronary syndromes without ST-segment elevation. *N Engl J Med* 2001;345:494–502.
69. Diener HC, Cunha L, Forbes C, et al. European Stroke Prevention Study. 2. Dipyridamole and acetylsalicylic acid in the secondary prevention of stroke. *J Neurol Sci* 1996;143:1–13.
70. Guiraud-Chaumeil B, Rascol A, David J, et al. [Prevention of recurrences of cerebral ischemic vascular accidents by platelet antiaggregants. Results of a 3-year controlled therapeutic trial]. *Rev Neurol* 1982;138:367–385.
71. Bousser MG, Eschwege E, Haguenau M, et al. 'AICLA' controlled trial of aspirin and dipyridamole in the secondary prevention of atherothrombotic cerebral ischemia. *Stroke* 1983;14:5–14.
72. Persantine Aspirin Trial in cerebral ischemia. Part II: Endpoint results. The American-Canadian Co-Operative Study group. *Stroke* 1985;16:406–415.
73. The European Stroke Prevention Study (ESPS). Principal end-points. The ESPS Group. *Lancet* 1987;2:1351–1354.
74. Risk factors for stroke and efficacy of antithrombotic therapy in atrial fibrillation. Analysis of pooled data from five randomized controlled trials. *Arch Intern Med* 1994;154:1449–1457.
75. A randomized trial of anticoagulants versus aspirin after cerebral ischemia of presumed arterial origin. The Stroke Prevention in Reversible Ischemia Trial (SPIRIT) Study Group. *Ann Neurol* 1997;42:857–865.
76. Mohr JP, Thompson JL, Lazar RM, et al. A comparison of warfarin and aspirin for the prevention of recurrent ischemic stroke. *N Engl J Med* 2001;345:1444–1451.
77. Randomised trial of cholesterol lowering in 4444 patients with coronary heart disease: the Scandinavian Simvastatin Survival Study (4S). *Lancet* 1994;344:1383–1389.
78. Prevention of cardiovascular events and death with pravastatin in patients with coronary heart disease and a broad range of initial cholesterol levels. The Long-Term Intervention with Pravastatin in Ischaemic Disease (LIPID) Study Group. *N Engl J Med* 1998;339:1349–1357.
79. Sacks FM, Pfeffer MA, Moye LA, et al. The effect of pravastatin on coronary events after myocardial infarction in patients with average cholesterol levels. Cholesterol and Recurrent Events Trial investigators. *N Engl J Med* 1996;335:1001–1009.
80. Corti R, Fayad ZA, Fuster V, et al. Effects of lipid-lowering by simvastatin on human atherosclerotic lesions: a longitudinal study by high-resolution, noninvasive magnetic resonance imaging. *Circulation* 2001;104:249–252.
81. Corti R, Fuster V, Fayad ZA, et al. Lipid lowering by simvastatin induces regression of human atherosclerotic lesions: two years' follow-up by high-resolution noninvasive magnetic resonance imaging. *Circulation* 2002;106:2884–2887.
82. Mercuri M, Bond MG, Sirtori CR, et al. Pravastatin reduces carotid intima-media thickness progression in an asymptomatic hypercholesterolemic Mediterranean population: the Carotid Atherosclerosis Italian Ultrasound Study. *Am J Med* 1996;101:627–634.
83. Friedman SG. Carotid endarterectomy: a champion turns fifty. *J Vasc Surg* 2001;34:569–571.
84. Mullan S, Duda EE, Patronas NJ. Some examples of balloon technology in neurosurgery. *J Neurosurg* 1980;52:321–329.
85. Kerber CW, Cromwell LD, Loehden OL. Catheter dilatation of proximal carotid stenosis during distal bifurcation endarterectomy. *AJNR Am J Neuroradiol* 1980;1:348–349.
86. Kachel R. Results of balloon angioplasty in the carotid arteries. *J Endovasc Surg* 1996;3:22–30.
87. Mathur A, Dorros G, Iyer SS, et al. Palmaz stent compression in patients following carotid artery stenting. *Cathet Cardiovasc Diagn* 1997;41:137–140.
88. McCleary AJ, Nelson M, Dearden NM, et al. Cerebral haemodynamics and embolization during carotid angioplasty in high-risk patients. *Br J Surg* 1998;85:771–774.
89. Topol EJ, Yadav JS. Recognition of the importance of embolization in atherosclerotic vascular disease. *Circulation* 2000;101:570–580.
90. Markus HS, Clifton A, Buckenham T, et al. Carotid angioplasty. Detection of embolic signals during and after the procedure. *Stroke* 1994;25:2403–2406.
91. Ackerstaff RG, Jansen C, Moll FL, et al. The significance of microemboli detection by means of transcranial Doppler ultrasonography monitoring in carotid endarterectomy. *J Vasc Surg* 1995;21:963–969.
92. Gaunt ME, Martin PJ, Smith JL, et al. Clinical relevance of intraoperative embolization detected by transcranial Doppler ultrasonography during carotid endarterectomy: a prospective study of 100 patients. *Br J Surg* 1994;81:1435–1439.
93. Jansen C, Ramos LM, van Heesewijk JP, et al. Impact of microembolism and hemodynamic changes in the brain during carotid endarterectomy. *Stroke* 1994;25:992–997.
94. Al-Mubarak N, Roubin GS, Vitek JJ, et al. Procedural safety and short-term outcome of ambulatory carotid stenting. *Stroke* 2001;32:2305–2309.
95. Hofmann R, Kerschner K, Steinwender C, et al. Abciximab bolus injection does not reduce cerebral ischemic complications of elective carotid artery stenting: a randomized study. *Stroke* 2002;33:725–727.
96. Kapadia SR, Bajzer CT, Ziada KM, et al. Initial experience of platelet glycoprotein IIb/IIIa inhibition with abciximab during carotid stenting: a safe and effective adjunctive therapy. *Stroke* 2001;32:2328–2332.
97. Qureshi AI, Ali Z, Suri MF, et al. Open-label phase I clinical study to assess the safety of intravenous eptifibatide in patients undergoing internal carotid artery angioplasty and stent placement. *Neurosurgery* 2001;48:998–1005.
98. Qureshi AI, Suri MF, Ali Z, et al. Carotid angioplasty and stent placement: a prospective analysis of perioperative complications and impact of intravenously administered abciximab. *Neurosurgery* 2002;50:466–475.
99. Wholey MH, Wholey M, Mathias K, et al. Global experience in cervical carotid artery stent placement. *Catheter Cardiovasc Interv* 2000;50:160–167.
100. Wholey MH, Tan WA, Toursarkissian B, et al. Management of neurological complications of carotid artery stenting. *J Endovasc Ther* 2001;8:341–353.
101. Endovascular versus surgical treatment in patients with carotid stenosis in the Carotid and Vertebral Artery Transluminal Angioplasty Study (CAVATAS): a randomised trial. *Lancet* 2001;357:1729–1737.
102. Investigators YJfS. Stenting and angioplasty with protection in patients at high risk for endarterectomy. *American Heart Association Scientific Sessions*, Chicago, IL; November 2002.
103. Moore WS, Barnett HJ, Beebe HG, et al. Guidelines for carotid endarterectomy. A multidisciplinary consensus statement from the Ad Hoc Committee, American Heart Association. *Circulation* 1995;91:566–579.
104. Borger MA, Fremes SE, Weisel RD, et al. Coronary bypass and carotid endarterectomy: does a combined approach increase risk? A metaanalysis. *Ann Thorac Surg* 1999;68:14–21.
105. Brown KR, Kresowik TF, Chin MH, et al. Multistate population-

based outcomes of combined carotid endarterectomy and coronary artery bypass. *J Vasc Surg* 2003;37:32–39.

106. Ziada KM, Kapadia SR, Bhatt DL, et al. Approach to carotid stenosis in patients undergoing open heart surgery: stenting or endarterectomy? *J Am Coll Cardiol* 2001;37:648A.

107. Friedell ML, Joseph BP, Cohen MJ, et al. Surgery for carotid artery stenosis following neck irradiation. *Ann Vasc Surg* 2001;15:13–18.

108. Houdart E, Mounayer C, Chapot R, et al. Carotid stenting for radiation-induced stenoses: a report of 7 cases. *Stroke* 2001;32:118–121.

109. Paniagua D, Howell M, Strickman N, et al. Outcomes following extracranial carotid artery stenting in high-risk patients. *J Invasive Cardiol* 2001;13:375–381.

110. Dangas G, Laird JR Jr, Mehran R, et al. Carotid artery stenting in patients with high-risk anatomy for carotid endarterectomy. *J Endovasc Ther* 2001;8:39–43.

111. Alric P, Branchereau P, Berthet JP, et al. Carotid artery stenting for stenosis following revascularization or cervical irradiation. *J Endovasc Ther* 2002;9:14–19.

112. Al-Mubarak N, Roubin GS, Iyer SS, et al. Carotid stenting for severe radiation-induced extracranial carotid artery occlusive disease. *J Endovasc Ther* 2000;7:36–40.

113. New G, Roubin GS, Iyer SS, et al. Safety, efficacy, and durability of carotid artery stenting for restenosis following carotid endarterectomy: a multicenter study. *J Endovasc Ther* 2000;7:345–352.

114. Cremonesi A, Castriota F, Manetti R, et al. Endovascular treatment of carotid atherosclerotic disease: early and late outcome in a nonselected population. *Ital Heart J* 2000;1:801–809.

115. Criado FJ, Lingelbach JM, Ledesma DF, et al. Carotid artery stenting in a vascular surgery practice. *J Vasc Surg* 2002;35:430–434.

116. Dangas G, Laird JR Jr, Satler LF, et al. Postprocedural hypotension after carotid artery stent placement: predictors and short- and long-term clinical outcomes. *Radiology* 2000;215:677–683.

117. Diethrich EB, Ndiaye M, Reid DB. Stenting in the carotid artery: initial experience in 110 patients. *J Endovasc Surg* 1996;3:42–62.

118. Gupta A, Bhatia A, Ahuja A, et al. Carotid stenting in patients older than 65 years with inoperable carotid artery disease: a single-center experience. *Catheter Cardiovasc Interv* 2000;50:1–9.

119. Roubin GS, New G, Iyer SS, et al. Immediate and late clinical outcomes of carotid artery stenting in patients with symptomatic and asymptomatic carotid artery stenosis: a 5-year prospective analysis. *Circulation* 2001;103:532–537.

120. Shawl F, Kadro W, Domanski MJ, et al. Safety and efficacy of elective carotid artery stenting in high-risk patients. *J Am Coll Cardiol* 2000; 35:1721–1728.

121. Al-Mubarak N, Colombo A, Gaines PA, et al. Multicenter evaluation of carotid artery stenting with a filter protection system. *J Am Coll Cardiol* 2002;39:841–846.

122. Guimaraens L, Sola MT, Matali A, et al. Carotid angioplasty with cerebral protection and stenting: report of 164 patients (194 carotid percutaneous transluminal angioplasties). *Cerebrovasc Dis* 2002;13:114–119.

123. Henry M, Henry I, Klonaris C, et al. Benefits of cerebral protection during carotid stenting with the PercuSurge GuardWire system: midterm results. *J Endovasc Ther* 2002;9:1–13.

124. Reimers B, Corvaja N, Moshiri S, et al. Cerebral protection with filter devices during carotid artery stenting. *Circulation* 2001;104:12–15.

125. Tubler T, Schluter M, Dirsch O, et al. Balloon-protected carotid artery stenting: relationship of periprocedural neurological complications with the size of particulate debris. *Circulation* 2001;104:2791–2796.

126. Whitlow PL, Lylyk P, Londero H, et al. Carotid artery stenting protected with an emboli containment system. *Stroke* 2002;33:1308–1314.

CHAPTER 104

Minimally Invasive Treatment of Peripheral Vascular Disease

Alfio Carroccio, Sharif H. Ellozy, Robert A. Lookstein, Larry H. Hollier, and Michael L. Marin

Key Words: Aneurysm; angioplasty; arterial; endovascular; graft; occlusive; percutaneous; stent.

INTRODUCTION

Since the first report of transluminal angioplasty by Charles Dotter in 1964, minimally invasive treatment of peripheral vascular disease has gained growing popularity. The patient with peripheral arterial occlusive disease often has diffuse atherothrombosis of his or her vascular system, as well as multiple medical comorbidities, which has further prompted a search for a less morbid therapy, thus avoiding conventional open surgery. This chapter reviews currently accepted therapies of occlusive and aneurysmal disease of peripheral

A. Carroccio: Department of Surgery, Division of Vascular and Endovascular Surgery, The Mount Sinai Medical Center, 5 East 98th Street, New York, New York 10029.

S. H. Ellozy: Department of Surgery, Division of Vascular and Endovascular Surgery, The Mount Sinai Medical Center, 5 East 98th Street, New York, New York 10029.

R. A. Lookstein: Department of Interventional Radiology, Division of Vascular and Endovascular Surgery, The Mount Sinai Medical Center, 5 East 98th Street, New York, New York 10029.

L. H. Hollier: Department of Surgery, Division of Vascular and Endovascular Surgery, The Mount Sinai Medical Center, 5 East 98th Street, New York, New York 10029.

M. L. Marin: Department of Surgery, Division of Vascular and Endovascular Surgery, The Mount Sinai Medical Center, 5 East 98th Street, New York, New York 10029.

arteries, results of these therapies, and potential future developments in minimally invasive therapies.

PERIPHERAL ARTERY OCCLUSIVE DISEASES

Peripheral artery occlusive disease includes atherothrombosis affecting all vascular beds except the coronary and intracerebral circulation. Endovascular therapy has been attempted in all of these beds, with varying results. Minimally invasive therapeutic options for treatment of arterial occlusive disease include balloon angioplasty with or without stenting, thrombolysis, atherectomy, and stented grafts. The experience with drug-eluting stents in the coronary circulation recently has been extended to the periphery, with benefits soon to be determined.

OCCLUSIVE DISEASE OF THE AORTIC ARCH VESSELS

Symptomatic occlusive disease of the brachiocephalic arteries is a rare but debilitating entity. Patients may present with cerebral neurologic deficit, upper extremity weakness, claudication, rest pain, or distal ulcerations. The presenting signs and symptoms can result from high-grade stenosis impeding adequate flow, embolic debris from ulcerated plaques, or thrombus lining a poststenotic dilatated segment of artery. Occasionally, a proximal subclavian stenosis may present with no arm symptomatology; however, a resulting steel

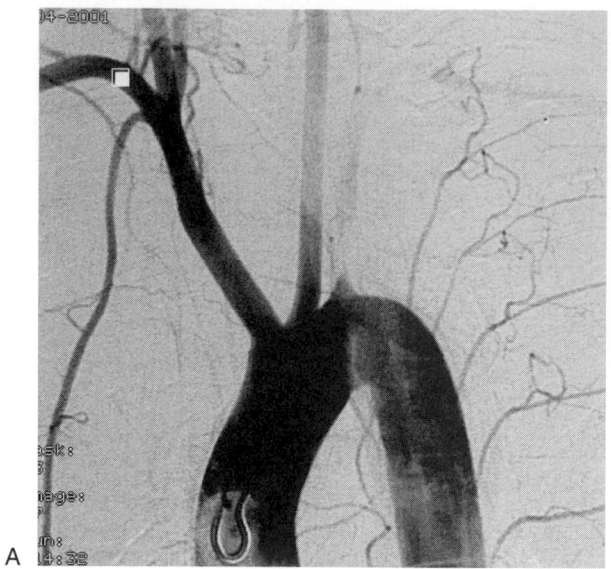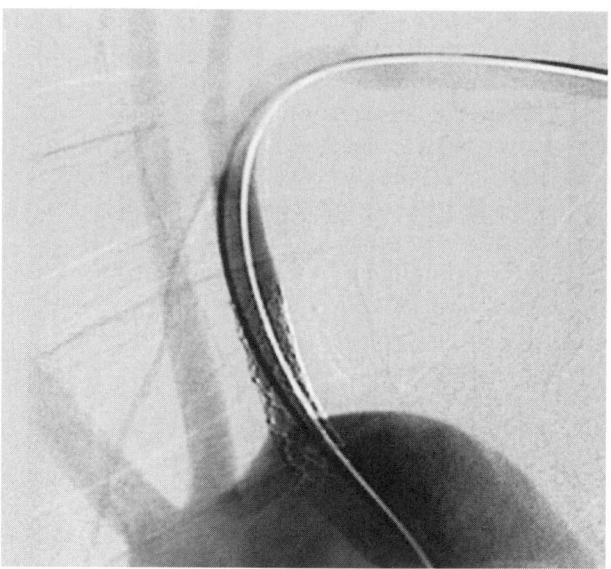

FIG. 104–1. A: Angiogram demonstrating near-occlusion of the left subclavian artery. **B:** Completion angiography showing a good result after angioplasty and stenting.

from a vertebral artery or internal mammary artery used in bypass surgery can present with vertebrobasilar symptoms or myocardial ischemic symptoms, respectively. With these anatomic or lesion characteristics in mind, the appropriate treatment can be planned. Given the anatomic location of

these vessels, one can appreciate the benefit of catheter-based therapy as apposed to the conventional endarterectomy or surgical bypass, which often require intrathoracic surgery.

Single-center case series have reported initial technical success rates of 92% to 100% for arterial occlusive lesions

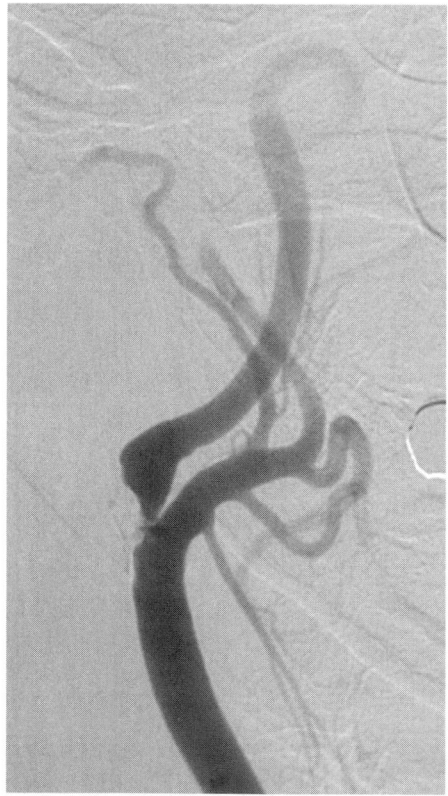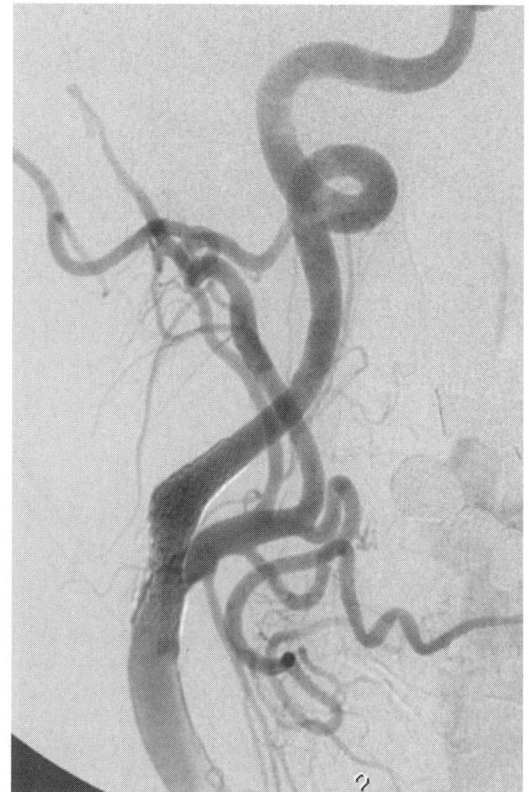

FIG. 104–2. A: Angiogram demonstrating 95% stenosis of the right internal carotid artery. **B:** Completion angiogram after angioplasty and stenting.

in this area (1–3). Primary patency rates greater than 90% on long-term follow-up have been reported. In addition, either relief or improvement in symptoms can be expected in most patients. Although the presence of these lesions is not uncommon, associated symptoms are rare. This must be kept in mind, because treatment is not without consequences. Aside from access-related complications, embolization or dissection into the cerebral circulation can have devastating consequences. With this in mind, anatomically favorable lesions may be better treated with endovascular therapy as the first-line treatment (Fig. 104–1).

Occlusive disease affecting the carotid bifurcation is, by comparison, a much more significant public health problem. Indications for therapy include symptomatic carotid stenosis greater than 70% or asymptomatic carotid stenosis greater than 60%. Carotid endarterectomy, the traditional gold standard therapy, is a well studied and safe approach to stroke prevention. However, several large, single-center series have reported good results with carotid bifurcation angioplasty

and stenting, with minimal morbidity (4,5) (Fig. 104–2). As such, there is much controversy surrounding the debate between surgical and endovascular therapy for carotid stenosis. Most experts agree that angioplasty and stenting should play a role in the treatment of patients at high risk with symptoms, recurrent carotid stenosis, postirradiation stenosis, and surgically inaccessible lesions such as the high-carotid bifurcation (6). The advent of cerebral protection devices holds the promise of minimizing the potential for embolic complications. Currently, there are a number of prospective, randomized, multicenter clinical trials aimed at resolving the debate between endarterectomy and carotid stenting (7).

Interestingly, although the debate over angioplasty/stenting versus carotid endarterectomy ensues, the perceived benefit of procedural intervention over medical management should be readdressed. In previous years, medical management in stroke prevention and death used aspirin therapy, but significant progress has ensued in the various antiplatelet

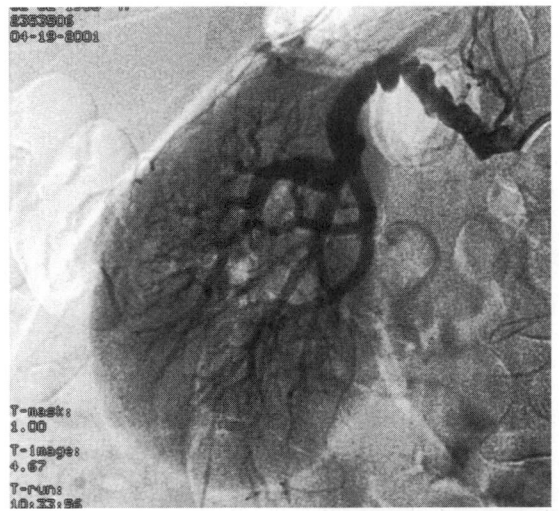

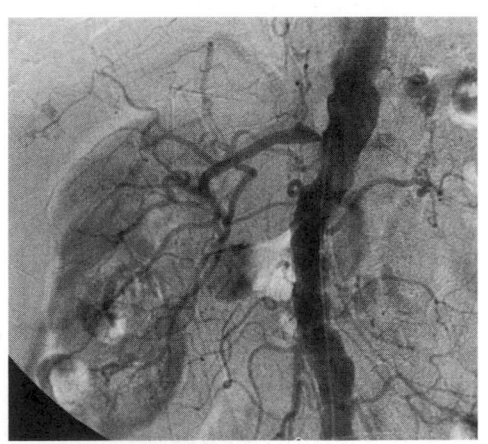

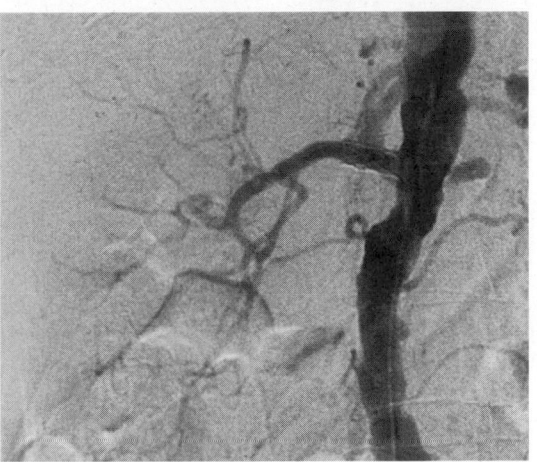

FIG. 104–3. A: Renal angiogram showing the characteristic "string-of-beads" appearance associated with fibromuscular dysplasia. **B:** High-grade renal artery stenosis in a patient with a single kidney. **C:** Completion angiography showing a good result after angioplasty and stenting.

therapies, as well as lipid reduction therapies and cardioprotective antihypertensives.

OCCLUSIVE DISEASE OF THE RENAL ARTERIES

Renal artery angioplasty and stenting have received increasing attention over the last decade. Significant improvements in catheter and stent technology have increased the safety and rates of procedural success. Incidental renal artery stenosis is fairly common, yet true renovascular hypertension accounts for only 1% to 5% of all cases of hypertension (8). The two most common causes of renal artery stenosis are fibromuscular dysplasia, typically seen in young women, and atherothrombosis, seen in older individuals (Fig. 104–3). Patients with hypertension secondary to fibromuscular dysplasia respond well to angioplasty alone. However, controversy regarding the indications for therapy of atherothrombotic renal artery stenosis exists because of a relative lack of controlled clinical trials. Patients with atherothrombotic renal artery stenosis of at least 70% of one or both renal arteries may be considered for revascularization. Generally accepted indications include hypertension not responsive to multiple medications, chronic renal failure that is not attributable to another cause (disease should be bilateral), and recurrent congestive heart failure or flash pulmonary edema that is not caused by coronary ischemia. Technical success rates in most large, recent series range from 90% to 100%; however, in 15% to 20% of patients, renal function does not improve and may worsen, and blood pressure is not improved in 20% to 50% of patients (8,9). Improving on these results will require two things: advances in preoperative evaluation to determine who will respond to angioplasty and stenting, and technical adjuncts such as distal protection devices and therapy aimed at reducing recurrent stenosis.

OCCLUSIVE DISEASE OF THE MESENTERIC ARTERIES

Chronic intestinal ischemia is a rare disease that presents significant diagnostic and therapeutic challenges. In its classic presentation, patients present with significant weight loss and postprandial abdominal pain. Exclusion of other more likely diagnoses and the presence of occlusion or high-grade stenosis of two visceral vessels suggest a compromised blood supply to the abdominal organs (Fig. 104–4). Results of minimally invasive treatment of patients with this pathology has been acquired in the last decade; however, given the time frame and the paucity of patients with this condition, there are limitations. Reported results include a variety of experi-

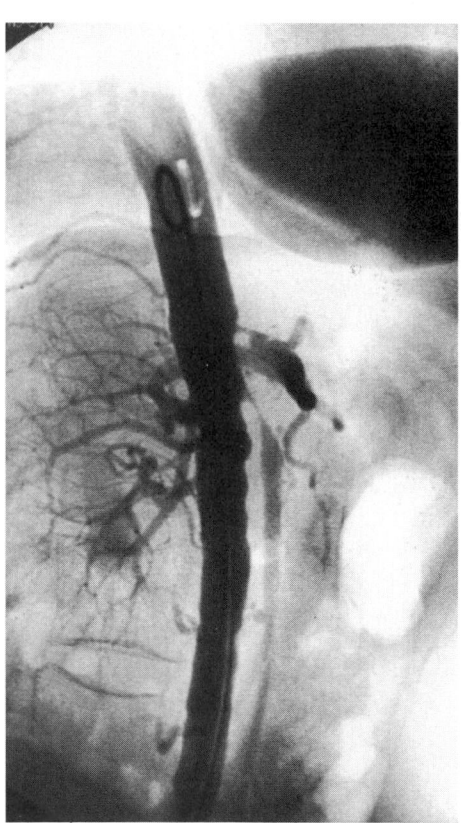
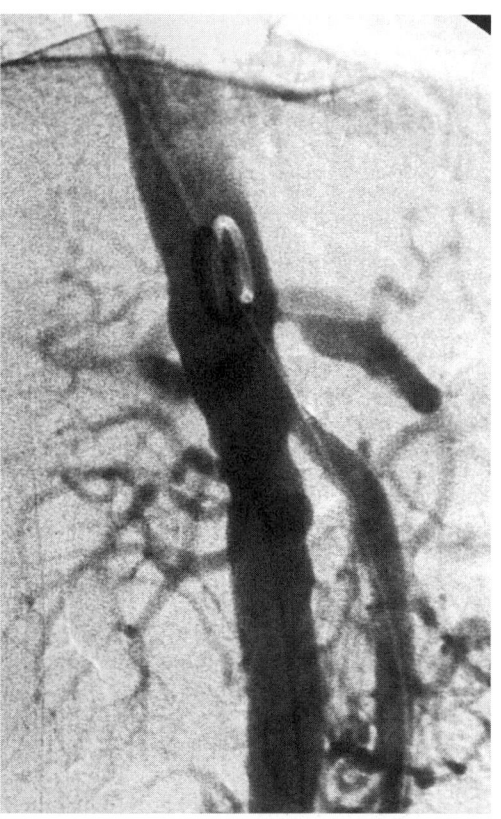

A

B

FIG. 104–4. A: Lateral aortogram demonstrating high-grade stenosis of the celiac and superior mesenteric artery origins in a patient with chronic mesenteric ischemia. **B:** Completion angiography after angioplasty and stenting of the superior mesenteric artery.

ences including different lesion characteristics (stenosis and/or occlusion), number of vessels treated, method of treatment (angioplasty with or without stenting), duration, modality, and volume of patient at follow-up. Technical success can be achieved in 80% to 100% of patients, with complete alleviation of symptoms in more than 80% of patients. In patients with clinically successful procedures, long-term clinical success has been reported in more than 80%. The majority of patients with recurrent symptoms often are successfully retreated with endovascular therapy, yielding primary, assisted, long-term clinical success rates of greater than 90% (9,10).

OCCLUSIVE DISEASE OF THE ILIAC, FEMORAL, POPLITEAL, AND TIBIAL ARTERIES

Treatment of occlusive disease affecting the lower extremities is performed to improve on patient mobility and to avoid placing a patient at risk for limb loss. Currently accepted indications for intervention include rest pain, infection in the setting of vascular insufficiency, nonhealing ulcer, and gangrene. Relative indications include disabling claudication.

Endovascular therapy has emerged as the mainstay of therapy for aortoiliac occlusive disease. Stenosis less than 10 cm in length or occlusions less than 5 cm in length are believed to be better treated with angioplasty and stenting than with surgery (Fig. 104–5). Good long-term patency with relief of symptoms has been achieved in this setting (11). Suitability of this therapy for occlusive disease in the superficial femoral artery is being evaluated. Although feasible, the data regarding the preferred treatment in this area is not clearcut and may not be so simple as patency rates in the long term. Despite less favorable patency rates, endovascular therapy is less invasive and often preferable in situations where the more desirable autogenous vein graft conduits are not available, or when the life expectancy of the patient is minimal and a temporizing measure is the best option. Infrainguinal occlusive disease tends to be more diffuse at presentation, rendering it less amenable to endovascular therapy. Unlike in the aortoiliac segment, definitive data regarding primary stenting of superficial femoral artery lesions are not available, whereas overall the tendency appears to favor stenting. The lack of clear benefit over angioplasty alone possibly is because of high rates of instent restenosis

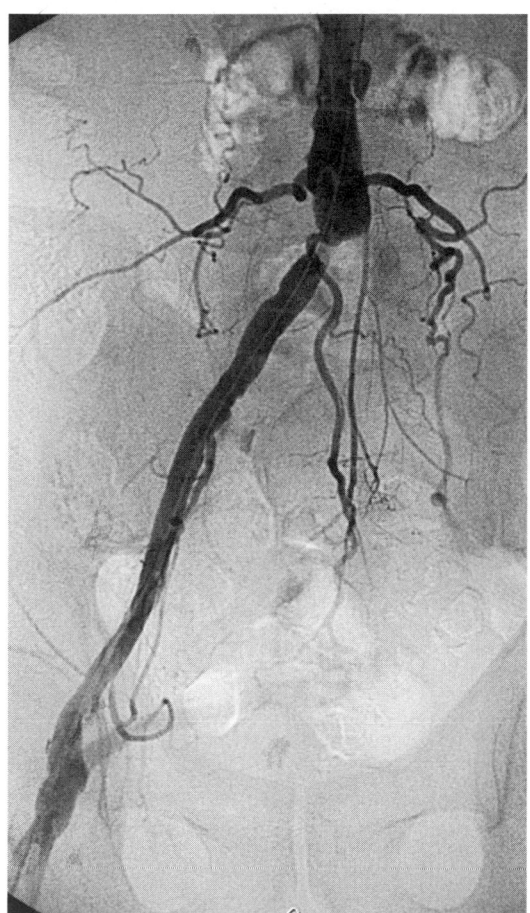 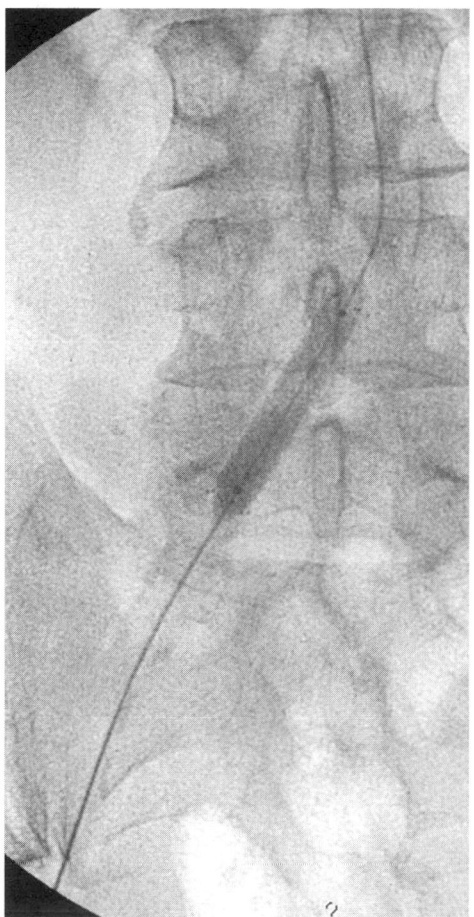

FIG. 104–5. A: Tight stenosis of the origin of the right common iliac artery in a patient with a femoro-femoral bypass. **B:** Angioplasty and stenting of the right common iliac artery. **C:** Completion angiogram.

continued

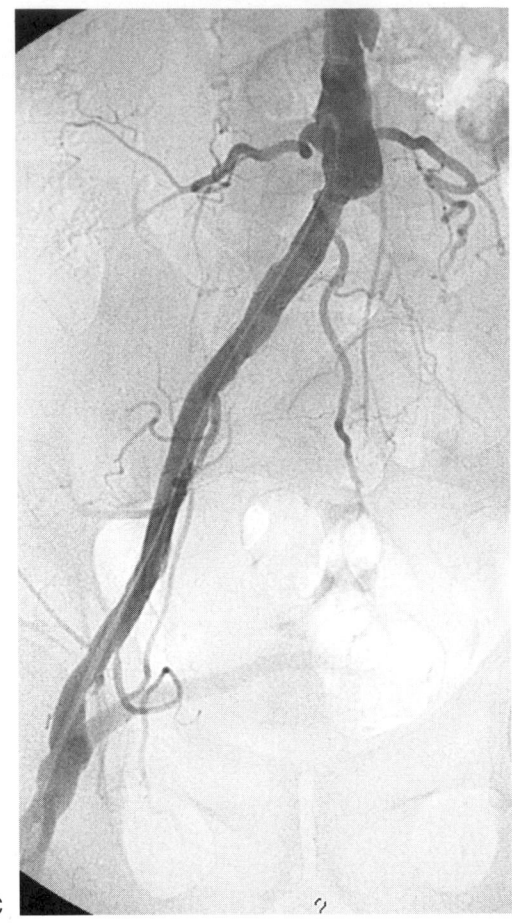

C

FIG. 104–5. *Continued.*

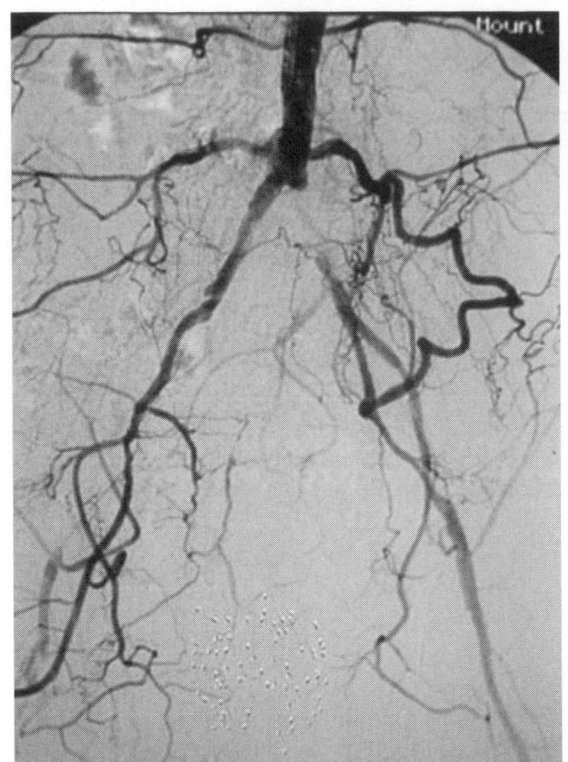

A

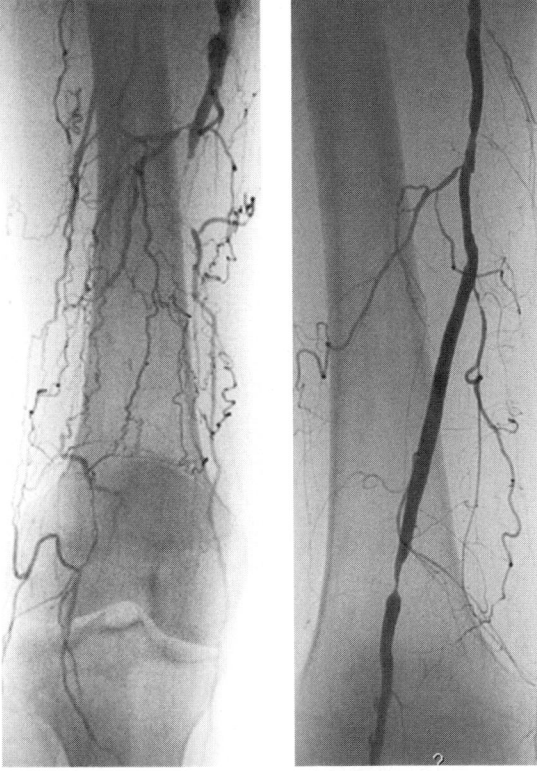

B   C

(11). Early data with the use of drug-eluting stents in the treatment of these lesions show some promise (12).

Minimally invasive therapy for infrapopliteal disease has not been widely embraced. Single centers have reported acceptable patency rates with percutaneous transluminal angioplasty of the crural vessels (13); however, these results have not been widely duplicated, and surgical bypass should still be the first-line therapy in acceptable patients.

The more reasonable current status is to decide on a treatment plan on the basis of the overall medical condition of the patient and the various available conduits for bypass in the need for distal revascularizations. Often, the best treatment option may involve a combination of endovascular therapy with surgical revascularization to optimize the available vein conduits.

ENDOVASCULAR STENT GRAFTS FOR THE TREATMENT OF OCCLUSIVE DISEASE

When the nature of occlusive disease is extensive or multifocal (Fig. 104–6), results of endoluminal therapy are less favorable in terms of long-term durability compared with short focal lesions (14,15). Efforts to improve on long-term success have combined vascular grafts with stent technol-

FIG. 104–6. Angiogram demonstrating the more challenging long-segment occlusion of the iliac **(A)** and superficial femoral artery **(B)**. Alternatively **(C)**, the short focal high-grade stenosis of the superficial femoral artery may be more facile to manage.

ogy. The potential benefit of endovascular stent grafts in this setting is the ability of synthetic graft material to reline the luminal surface of various lengths of occlusive vasculature after angioplasty. A long segment of treated vessel may then have a new luminal surface that is uniform (Fig. 104–7). Treatment of occlusive disease in the aortoiliac segment with self-expanding stent grafts (Wallgraft, Boston Scientific, Boston, MA; and Viabahn, W. L. Gore, Flagstaff, AZ) (Fig. 104–8) reported a 12-month primary patency rate of 70% and primary assisted patency rate of 88% in a study of 34 patients with rest pain or tissue loss (16). Durability of treatment in the femoropopliteal segment as demonstrated by Matsi and coworkers (17) is similarly related to the length of area being treated. Two studies of self-expanding stent graft in the femoropopliteal segment report primary and secondary patency rates of 73% to 78% and 82% to 93%, respectively, at 1 year (18,19). Two-year experience with primary and secondary patency rates of 74.1% and 83.2%, respectively, have subsequently been reported (20).

Less favorable results of 40% and 67% for 1-year primary and secondary patency rates, respectively, have been reported by Fischer and coworkers (21). The authors believed that the results were attributable to poor runoff, calcifications, and multiple-vessel lesions (Fig. 104–9). Patients with more favorable proximal or distal vascular beds displayed more favorable results, with 1-year primary and secondary patency rates of 80% and 100%, respectively. Clearly, success is not strictly dependent on lesion length or endoluminal device; multiple factors play a role, such as inflow, outflow, and optimal medical management. Optimization of all of these variables is of critical importance when choosing this therapeutic option.

ANEURYSMAL DISEASE OF THE AORTA AND PERIPHERAL ARTERIES

Aneurysmal disease of the aorta and peripheral vessels has been progressing over the last decade. Since the first de-

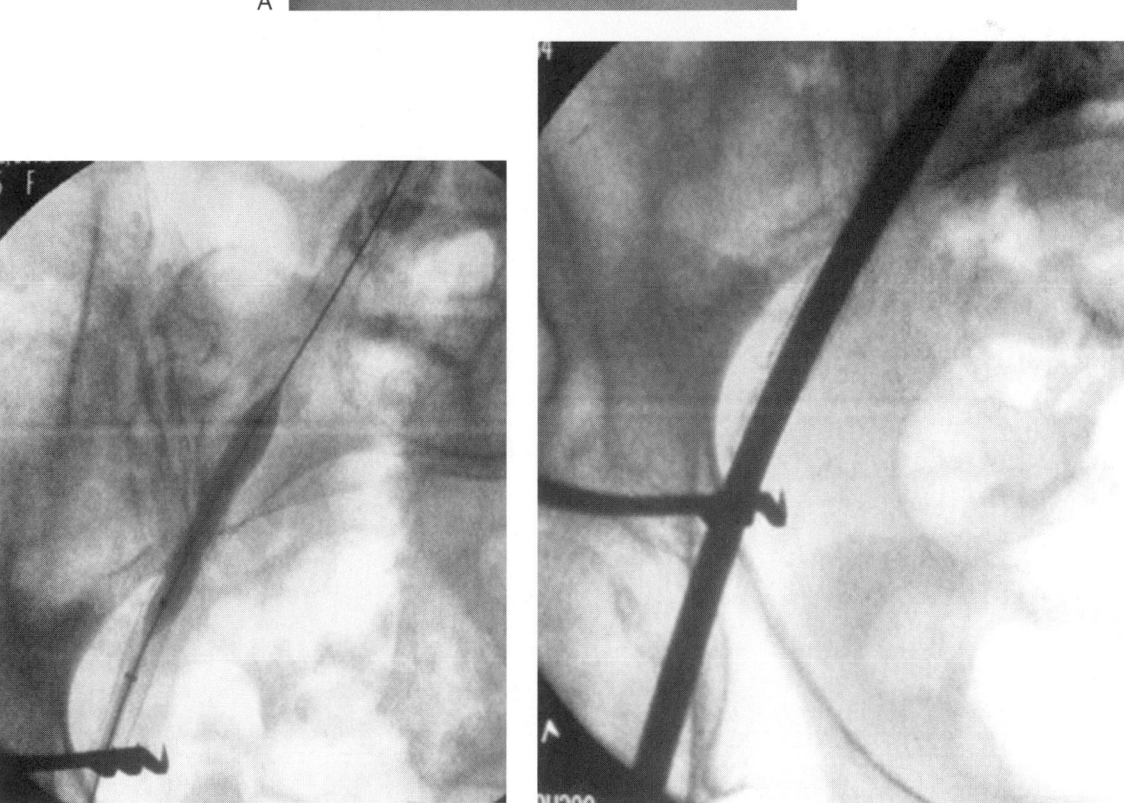

FIG. 104–7. A: Photo of a balloon-expandable stent fixed within a length of polytetrafluoroethylene (PTFE) graft. **B:** Intraoperative imaging of balloon angioplasty after deployment of the stent in the common iliac artery with extension of the PTFE through the iliac artery to terminate in the external iliac artery. **C:** Completion angiography after the relining of the iliac arteries with a PTFE conduit.

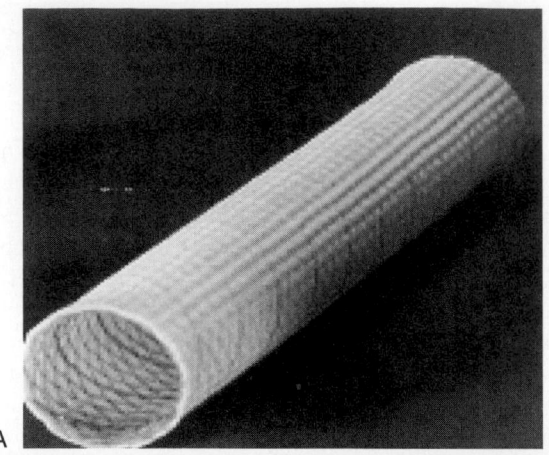

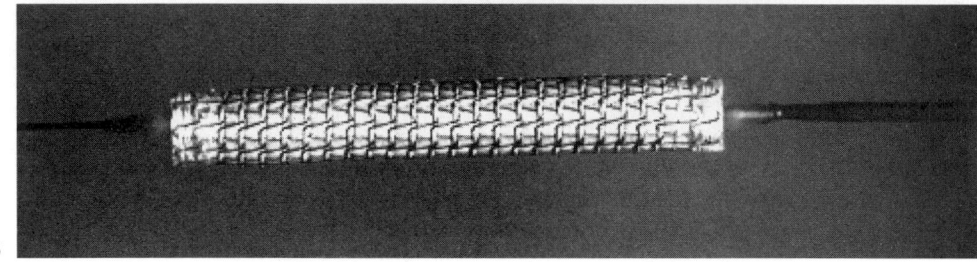

FIG. 104–8. Photograph of graft-covered stents.

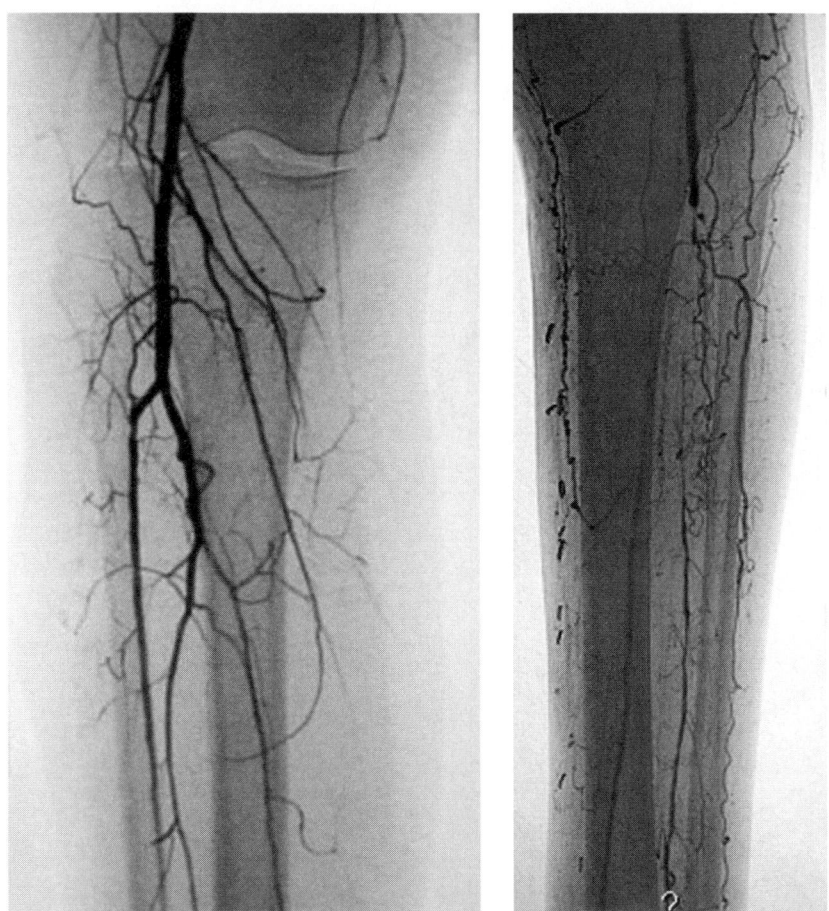

FIG. 104–9. A: Angiogram demonstrating a more favorable runoff vascular bed below the popliteal artery. **B:** In contrast, a high-resistance minimal runoff is visualized in this angiogram of the below knee popliteal artery segment.

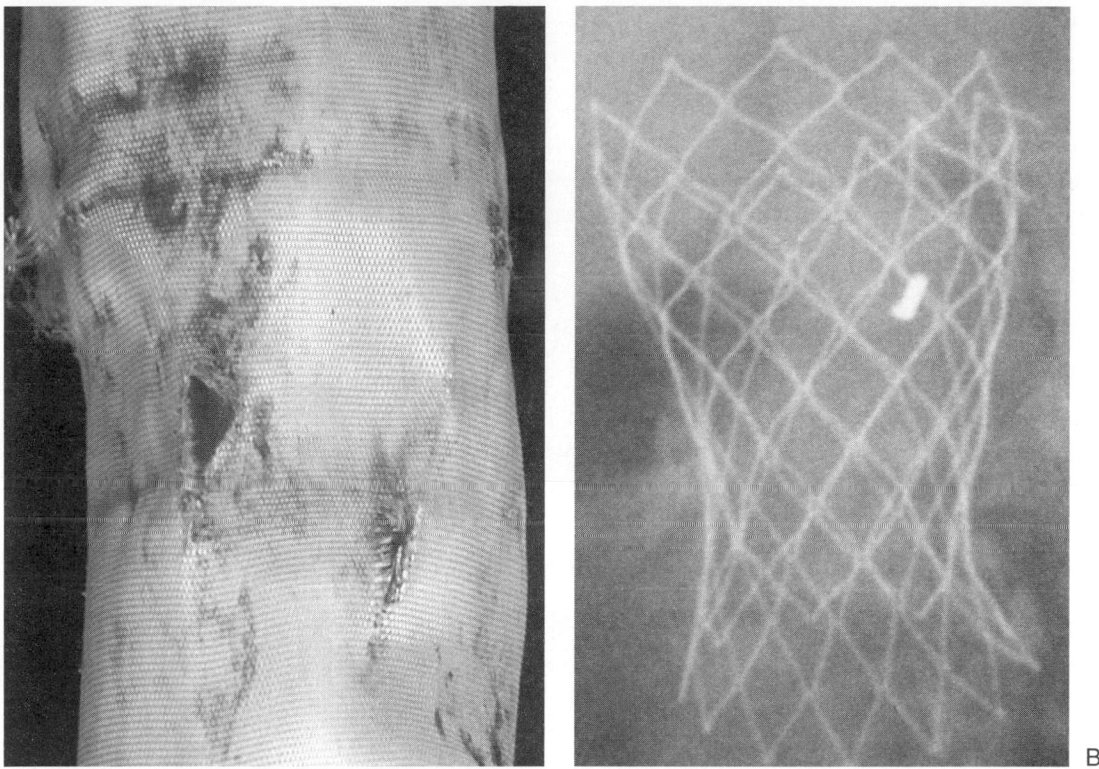

FIG. 104–10. Photographs of aortic stent graft device breakdown. **A:** Tear within the fabric of the device. **B:** Metallic stint fracture.

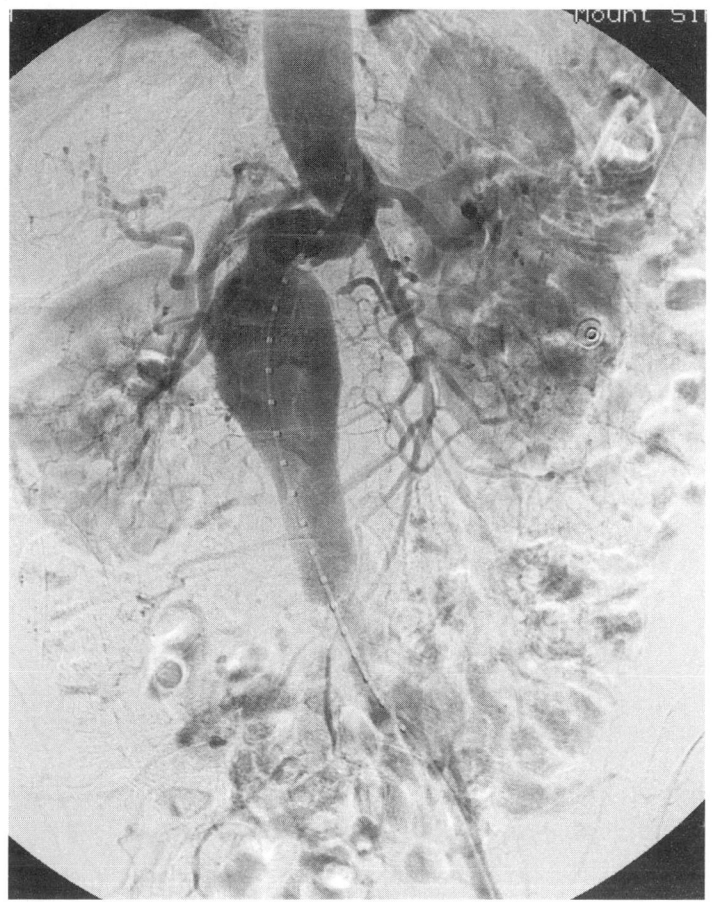

FIG. 104–11. Angiogram of an infrarenal aortic aneurysm with an acutely angled neck immediately below the renal arteries. This demonstrates a difficult angle in which to position an endograft.

scription in 1991 by Parodi and associates (22), the endoluminal approach to aneurysm repair requires three essential elements. Successful exclusion depends on adequate proximal and distal fixation sites, a durable conduit (endograft) to bridge the aneurysm, and access vessels that permit the passage of a device. More than a decade has passed since its introduction, and improvements in these basic elements have revealed that it is an alternative treatment option that is feasible, durable, and associated with less morbidity as determined in the intermediate follow-up (23–27). An area of great concern is the need for reintervention that often is required on follow-up, particularly when considering the treatment of thoracic and abdominal aortic aneurysms. Despite the need for reintervention, endovascular techniques allow treatment in most cases. Stent-graft modification and use of more refined microcatheters allow for a greater ability to treat than was previously possible.

Although this treatment modality has been applied to the thoracic and abdominal aorta, it also has been extended to aneurysms in the periphery (28–30). Despite progress in this area, device fatigue (Fig. 104–10) and anatomic restrictions (Fig. 104–11) allow for further improvement to extend the applicability of this modality.

ENDOVASCULAR GRAFTS FOR TRAUMATIC VASCULAR INJURIES

Injury to an artery whether from traumatic events in the community or iatrogenic result in hemorrhage, pseudoaneurysm formation, or an arteriovenous fistula. Relining the injured segment with a stent graft delivered from a remote access site can exclude the aneurysm or fistula from the circulation while avoiding surgical dissection in a traumatized field. Experience with endovascular treatment of arterial trauma extends from the acute thoracic aortic disruption after blunt trauma to endograft exclusion of injuries to the more peripheral vessels (31–33) (Fig. 104–12). Acute thoracic aortic disruption is an example of the huge benefit endovascular therapy can provide. As is often the case, rapid deceleration injuries can cause, in addition to aortic disruption, a multitude of concomitant injuries. Quick control of a potentially lethal problem under regional anesthesia with avoidance of a thoracotomy can allow for close observation of other injuries in an awake communicating patient. As the physician becomes more facile with these procedures, larger experience can accumulate.

SUMMARY

Endovascular treatment of peripheral vascular disease is a growing area of interest, with constantly evolving technology and equipment contributing to advances in this treatment. An understanding of the pathology of vascular disease and limitations of the minimally invasive approach are required to optimize the benefits. Both physician and patient

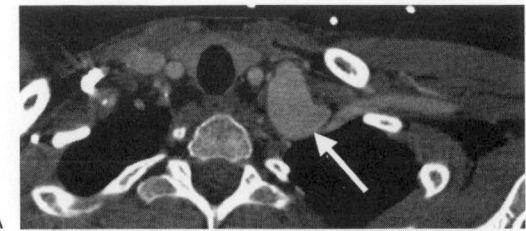
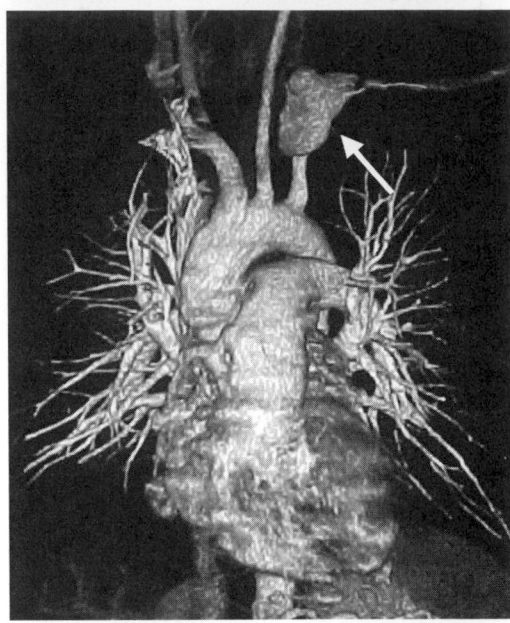
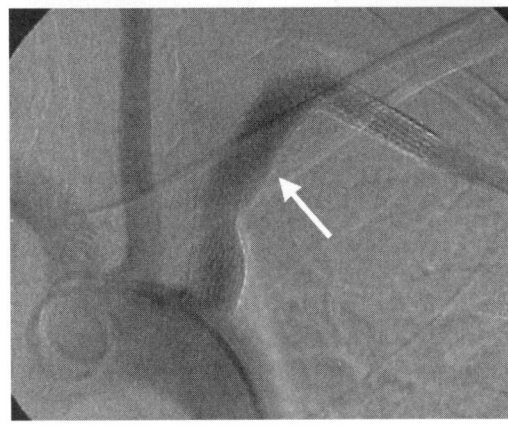

FIG. 104–12. Computed tomography angiogram of a left subclavian artery pseudoaneurysm seen in both **(A)** axial and **(B)** three-dimensional reconstruction before treatment. **C:** Intraoperative angiogram after stint graft exclusion of the aneurysm.

seek the appeal of a less invasive option; however, the long-term results must be evaluated to select the best therapy for each individual patient.

REFERENCES

1. Diethrich EB. Endovascular management of brachiocephalic arterial occlusive disease. *Ann Vasc Surg* 2000;14:189–192.
2. Kandarpa K, Becker GJ, Hunink MG, et al. Transcatheter interventions

for the treatment of peripheral atherosclerotic lesions: part I. *J Vasc Interv Radiol* 2001;12:683–695.

3. Huttl K, Nemes B, Simonffy A, et al. Angioplasty of the innominate artery in 89 patients: experience over 19 years. *Cardiovasc Intervent Radiol* 2002;25:109–114.

4. Roubin GS, New G, Iyer SS, et al. Immediate and late clinical outcomes of carotid artery stenting in patients with symptomatic and asymptomatic carotid artery stenosis: a 5-year prospective analysis. *Circulation* 2001;103:532–537.

5. Wholey MH, Wholey MH, Tan WA, et al. A comparison of balloon-mounted and self-expanding stents in the carotid arteries: immediate and long-term results of more than 500 patients. *J Endovasc Ther* 2003;10:171–181.

6. Veith FJ, Amor M, Ohki T, et al. Current status of carotid bifurcation angioplasty and stenting based on a consensus of opinion leaders. *J Vasc Surg* 2001;33[2 Suppl]:S111–S116.

7. Roubin GS, Hobson RE 2nd, White R, et al. CREST and CARESS to evaluate carotid stenting: time to get to work! *J Endovasc Ther* 2001;0. 107–110,

8. Olin JW. Atherosclerotic renal artery disease. *Cardiol Clin* 2002;20: 547–562.

9. Sharafuddin MJ, Olson CH, Sun S, et al. Endovascular treatment of celiac and mesenteric arteries stenoses: applications and results. *J Vasc Surg* 2003;38:692–698.

10. Matsumoto AH, Angle JF, Spinosa DJ, et al. Percutaneous transluminal angioplasty and stenting in the treatment of chronic mesenteric ischemia: results and longterm followup. *J Am Coll Surg* 2002; 194[1 Suppl]:S22–S31.

11. Kandarpa K, Becker GJ, Hunink MG, et al. Transcatheter interventions for the treatment of peripheral atherosclerotic lesions: part I. *J Vasc Interv Radiol* 2001;12:683–695.

12. Duda SH, Pusich B, Richter G, et al. Sirolimus-eluting stents for the treatment of obstructive superficial femoral artery disease: six-month results. *Circulation* 2002;106:1505–1509.

13. Ingle H, Nasim A, Bolia A, et al. Subintimal angioplasty of isolated infragenicular vessels in lower limb ischemia: long-term results. *J Endovasc Ther* 2002;9:411–416.

14. Powell RJ, Fillinger M, Bettmann M, et al. The durability of endovascular treatment of multisegment iliac occlusive disease. *J Vasc Surg* 2000;31:1178–1184.

15. Powell RJ, Fillinger M, Walsh DB, et al. Predicting outcomes of angioplasty and selective stenting of multisegment iliac artery occlusive disease. *J Vasc Surg* 2000;32:564–569.

16. Rzucidlo EM, Powell RJ, Zwolak RM, et al. Early results of stent-grafting to treat diffuse aortoiliac occlusive disease. *J Vasc Surg* 2003; 37:1175–1180.

17. Matsi PJ, Manninen HI, Vanninen RL, et al. Femoropopliteal angioplasty in patients with claudication: primary and secondary patency in 140 limbs with 1–3-year follow-up. *Radiology* 1994;191:727–733.

18. Bauermeister G. Endovascular stent-grafting in the treatment of superficial femoral artery occlusive disease. *J Endovasc Ther* 2001;8:315–320.

19. Lammer J, Dake MD, Bleyn J, et al. Peripheral arterial obstruction: prospective study of treatment with a transluminally placed self-expanding stent-graft. International Trial Study Group. *Radiology* 2000;217:95–104.

20. Jahnke T, Andresen R, MŸller-HŸlsbeck S, et al. Hemobahn stent-grafts for treatment of femoropopliteal arterial obstructions: midterm results of a prospective trial. *J Vasc Interv Radiol* 2003;14:41–51.

21. Fischer M, Sakriss U, Stalke J, et al. Hemobahn endoprosthesis: experience with percutaneous placing in the arteria femoralis superficialis. *Zentralbl Chir* 2001;126:138–143.

22. Parodi JC, Palmaz JC, Barone HD. Transfemoral intraluminal graft implantation for abdominal aortic aneurysms. *Ann Vasc Surg* 1991;5: 491–499.

23. Ouriel K, Greenberg RK, Clair DG, et al. Endovascular aneurysm repair: gender-specific results. *J Vasc Surg* 2003;38:93–98.

24. Alric P, Hinchliffe RJ, MacSweeney ST, et al. The Zenith aortic stent-graft: a 5-year single-center experience. *J Endovasc Ther* 2002;9: 719–728.

25. Abraham CZ, Chuter TA, Reilly LM, et al. Abdominal aortic aneurysm repair with the Zenith stent graft: short to midterm results. *J Vasc Surg* 2002;36:217–225.

26. Chaikof EL, Lin PH, Brinkman WT, et al. Endovascular repair of abdominal aortic aneurysms: risk stratified outcomes. *Ann Surg* 2002; 235:833–841.

27. Thompson CS, Gaxotte VD, Rodriguez JA, et al. Endoluminal stent grafting of the thoracic aorta: initial experience with the Gore Excluder. *J Vasc Surg* 2002;35:1163–1170.

28. Kasirajan K, Greenberg RK, Clair D, et al. Endovascular management of visceral artery aneurysm. *J Endovasc Ther* 2001;8:150–155.

29. Tielliu IF, Verhoeven EL, Prins TR, et al. Treatment of popliteal artery aneurysms with the Hemobahn stent-graft. *J Endovasc Ther* 2003;10: 111–116.

30. Sanada J, Matsui O, Terayama N, et al. Stent-graft repair of a mycotic left subclavian artery pseudoaneurysm. *J Endovasc Ther* 2003; 10:66–70.

31. Ohki T, Veith FJ, Marin ML, et al. Endovascular approaches for traumatic arterial lesions. *Semin Vasc Surg* 1997;10:272–285.

32. Kato N, Dake MD, Miller DC, et al. Traumatic thoracic aortic aneurysm: treatment with endovascular stent-grafts. *Radiology* 1997; 205:657–662.

33. Criado E, Marston WA, Ligush J, et al. Endovascular repair of peripheral aneurysms, pseudoaneurysms, and arteriovenous fistulas. *Ann Vasc Surg* 1997;11:256–263.

CHAPTER 105

Behavioral and Alternative Medicine in the Treatment of Atherothrombosis

Thomas G. Pickering, Karina W. Davidson, Lynn P. Clemow, and William Gerin

Key Words: Anxiety; depression; exercise; obesity; smoking; stress.

INTRODUCTION

It has been estimated that approximately 50% of deaths in the United States in 1993 (the majority of which were caused by heart disease) were attributable to behavioral or lifestyle factors, including smoking, poor diet, physical inactivity, and alcohol (1). Although genetic factors contribute to susceptibility to these factors, a prime ingredient is the in-

T. G. Pickering: Behavioral Cardiovascular Health and Hypertension Program, Columbia University Medical College, 622 W 168th Street, New York, New York 10032.

K. W. Davidson: Behavioral Cardiovascular Health and Hypertension Program, Columbia University Medical College, 622 W 168th Street, New York, New York 10032.

L. P. Clemow: Behavioral Cardiovascular Health and Hypertension Program, Columbia University Medical College, 622 W 168th Street, New York, New York 10032.

W. Gerin: Behavioral Cardiovascular Health and Hypertension Program, Columbia University Medical College, 622 W 168th Street, New York, New York 10032.

dividual's behavior. The costs of treating heart disease are escalating at an increasingly rapid pace, because of the widespread use of sophisticated and expensive treatments such as coated coronary artery stents and implantable defibrillators. Most efforts to contain the increase in health care costs have focused on limiting supply and imposing some sort of rationing. However, Fries and coworkers (2) pointed out that reducing demand could achieve the same objective. These authors identified six factors, four of which are directly relevant to this chapter: (a) much disease is preventable; (b) risky behavior costs money; (c) self-management can result in savings; and (d) health behavior promotion at work has successfully reduced costs.

This chapter focuses on the major behavioral and psychological factors that influence the course of atherothrombosis and how they can be treated. The behavioral factors are smoking, diet, and physical inactivity; and the psychological factors are hostility, depression, and anxiety.

Psychosocial factors can influence the course of chronic disease by two main pathways: first, by inducing behavioral or lifestyle patterns such as smoking, which are themselves injurious; and second, by a direct effect of social and environmental factors such as socioeconomic status and stress on the disease process. Personality and emotional characteristics such as hostility and depression interact with both pathways—they influence how people choose their lifestyles and how they react to stress. For example, hostility may be a risk factor for atherothrombosis; hostile persons show an exaggerated cardiovascular reactivity to stress, which may contribute to the development of atherothrombosis or may trigger an acute event. Hostile individuals also are more likely to smoke and less likely to quit (3).

An example of the importance of psychological factors was seen in a study that evaluated 381 patients after hospitalization for an acute coronary event (4). Patients were evaluated for traditional risk factors and for psychological distress (including depression). Over a 6-month period it was found that individuals high in psychological distress were three times more likely to be hospitalized for recurrent coronary events; other less powerful predictive factors included no previous bypass procedure (odds ratio [OR], 2.73), diabetes (OR, 2.65), and ejection fraction less than 40% (OR, 1.98). A second example comes from a study of patients undergoing coronary angioplasty, which found that after controlling for standard risk factors, men who scored high on anger had a threefold increase in the rate of recurrent events compared with men with lower scores (5).

BARRIERS TO BEHAVIORAL INTERVENTIONS AND THE ROLE OF COLLABORATIVE MANAGEMENT OF PATIENTS WITH ATHEROTHROMBOSIS

Atherothrombosis is chronic, and its successful management requires an active collaboration between patient and health care provider. Patients often lack the knowledge and motivation to make behavioral changes, and the training of cardiologists rarely includes anything related to behavioral intervention. Physicians generally have a low perception of the effectiveness of behavioral interventions and no particular incentive to implement them, let alone the time; and because neither patients nor physicians have pressured the health care system to recognize the importance of making these changes, behavioral interventions rarely have been reimbursed. Recent (2002) changes in Medicare policy have for the first time introduced the possibility of reimbursing providers such as health psychologists for assessment and treatment of health behaviors related to medical diagnoses.

Despite these limitations, physicians can use behavioral techniques to improve self-care techniques. These include contracting with the patient to reach specific goals, evaluating the patient's readiness for self-care, breaking self-care tasks into small, manageable steps, providing personalized feedback to the patient, self-monitoring health-related behaviors, enlisting social support, checking patient commitment to key tasks, and providing structure through follow-up appointments. One of the first tasks is to define the behav-

ioral problem clearly. Physicians are usually concerned with items such as poor compliance and unhealthy lifestyle behavior, whereas patients often are more concerned about symptoms and emotional distress. Few physicians ask patients to identify the biggest problems faced in managing their illness.

Given the lack of training in behavioral techniques and the time limitations of cardiologists, a team approach ideally should be used. Behavioral interventions tend to require relatively large amounts of time, but nurses, psychologists, dietitians, and social workers can contribute this time. The end of this chapter discusses specific strategies that can be easily used by the physician to help patients make necessary changes in their behavior.

SMOKING CESSATION

The cardiovascular health risks associated with smoking are almost completely reversible after quitting (6,7), and smoking cessation has been shown to be one of the most cost-effective interventions in the field of medicine (8). Considerable evidence suggests that patients who have had acute coronary syndromes can cut their risk for a recurrent event in half by quitting smoking (9). (See Chapter 18 for a more indepth treatment of smoking cessation issues.) A brief overview of physician-delivered approaches to smoking cessation is outlined below and serves as one of the best-developed models for health behavior counseling.

Agency for Healthcare Research and Quality Guidelines

The effectiveness of smoking cessation programs has been reviewed by the Agency for Healthcare Research and Quality (AHRQ; formerly the Agency for Health Care Policy and Research [AHCPR]) who issued guidelines in 1996 (10) and provided an update in 2000 (11). These guidelines state that healthcare clinics such as cardiology practices are ideal settings for the promotion of such treatments. The guidelines emphasize that a variety of effective strategies can be adopted, some very simple, others more complex. Five steps are recommended. First, identify the smokers. Although this seems obvious, recent data show that only about 50% of smokers report ever having been asked by a physician if they smoked (12). There is evidence that adding smoking status to the vital sign stamp on clinical records increases the likelihood that the physician will discuss smoking with the patient (11). Second, advise the smoker to quit. Although this may seem trivial, an analysis of several studies has shown that the quit rate will increase from 7.9% to 10.2%, an increment that again may seem insubstantial, except that each smoker who quits will add up to 15 years to his or her life expectancy (10). Moreover, this number will increase with each succeeding examination in which the physician advises the patient to quit. Third, assess the smoker's willingness to quit and to provide informational support appropriate to their readiness to quit (e.g., personalized information on why they should quit for people who are not thinking of quitting, or reviewing treatment options for those ready to act). The fourth step deals with the smoker who is unwilling to attempt to quit. This involves promoting the patient's readiness to quit and emphasizes four Rs: personal Relevance to the patient's medical and social situation, the Risks associated with smoking, the Rewards of quitting, and the Repetition of a stop-smoking message. Fifth, develop the strategy that is chosen for the patient who is willing to quit. A general rule is that "more is better," or that the quit rate is proportional to the amount of effort that is put in. For example, a 5- to 7-minute brief counseling intervention using the counseling model suggested above increased cessation rates to 20% compared the 7% to 10% cessation rates with advice alone (13). The options, which are not mutually exclusive, include counseling, which has two basic components: providing social support and boosting skills in problem-solving. A state-funded telephone quit line to provide brief counseling services also has been proven to be effective (14). Other components include the use of nicotine replacement therapy, which can be delivered in a variety of ways, including gum, skin patches, and nasal sprays. A number of clinical trials have shown that the nicotine patches can double the quit rates (15). Finally, the use of the antidepressant drug bupropion (Zyban or Wellbutrin) is generally well tolerated by patients and also has been found to be effective in approximately doubling quit rates (16).

Barriers to Physician Intervention in Smokers

Why do so few physicians pay attention to smoking cessation? First, many physicians are not trained in behavioral techniques such as counseling, even though this is an activity to which they devote substantial time. They believe that their patients already know that smoking is harmful and are not interested in hearing about smoking, and that counseling is unlikely to have any significant effect. Second, that they are pressed for time and counseling is poorly reimbursed by health insurance gives it a low priority (17). However, the reason most often cited in recent surveys is that physicians do not think their patients will follow through (18). This is particularly unfortunate in that even a low rate of success in encouraging smoking cessation would yield substantial health benefits in a population of patients. It has been established that brief (approximately 3 minutes) counseling from a physician can double the spontaneous quit rate of smokers, which is about 2.5% per year. If a physician counsels 100 patients per year, 95% will continue to smoke, a despairingly large number. But of the 2.5 smokers who quit—above the further 2.5 smokers who will quit spontaneously—1 ex-smoker will avoid a premature smoking-related death, and another ex-smoker will gain up to 15 years of life expectancy. The cost of this benefit will have been 3 hours and 20 minutes of the physician's time.

DIETARY INTERVENTIONS

Dietary factors have a substantial impact on the development of cardiovascular disease (CVD). Many studies show that saturated fat and lipids intake are associated with rates of CVD-related death and all-cause mortality (19,20). On the basis of epidemiologic and observational studies in men, women, black, and elderly individuals, as well as postmortem angiographic studies in young persons, the National Institutes of Health (NIH) and the European Atherosclerosis Society have concluded that the intake of fats is a causal factor in coronary artery disease (20–22).

Low-density lipoprotein cholesterol (LDL-C) levels and other components of the lipid profile are affected by dietary intervention (23). This has led to strong recommendations by the National Cholesterol Education Program (NCEP) that dietary counseling should form the basis of lipid-regulating regimens for both the prevention and clinical management of CVD (24,25). Reductions in lipid levels are readily achievable through careful adherence to dietary changes.

Compared with pharmacologic intervention, dietary intervention has produced less net reduction in total cholesterol and LDL-C levels in randomized trials (26). However, two recent secondary intervention trials comparing a Mediterranean, α-linolenic–rich diet, one conducted in France (27–29) and the other in India (30), reported remarkably similar reductions in cardiac deaths over 2 to 5 years, which approached 50%. However, only a small proportion of these patients were taking statins.

Comprehensive reviews of dietary intervention studies (20,31,32) lead to the conclusion that aggressive treatment with a diet low in total and saturated fat produce decreased serum lipid levels and positive angiographic changes, as well as potentially helping to improve angina and other nonlipid related symptoms. Reducing fat intake alone only goes so far, however. A review by Hu and Willett (33) proposed that at least three strategies are effective in preventing coronary heart disease (CHD): substituting nonhydrogenated unsaturated fats for saturated and trans-fats, increasing consumption of ω3 fatty acids, and consuming a diet high in fruits, vegetables, and grains. However, achieving and maintaining dietary adherence on a long-term basis remains a major challenge.

There is evidence that physicians can successfully counsel patients regarding dietary changes to reduce lipids, but the counseling is effective in significantly changing patient outcomes only when there are office systems in place that assist and prompt the intervention (34). Individual and group nutrition interventions also can be effective, although, as noted earlier, long-term adherence can be difficult.

For patients with hypertension, the Dietary Approaches to Stop Hypertension (DASH) diet has been shown to be highly effective at reducing blood pressure (35), particularly when combined with salt restriction (36). This is basically a Mediterranean type of diet with the addition of low-fat dairy products to provide extra calcium. It also decreases total and LDL cholesterol levels (37), but in common with some other diets such as the Ornish diet, high-density lipoprotein cholesterol may also be reduced (38).

National Cholesterol Education Program Guidelines

On the basis of the cumulative scientific evidence from epidemiologic and controlled clinical trials, the NCEP advocated diet as the cornerstone of treatment in its reports of the Adult Treatment Panel, as well as the Population Based Panel and Pediatric Panel reports (24,25,39). In 1989, both the NCEP and the American Heart Association announced population-wide recommendations for the Step I and Step II diets as the primary strategies for the prevention and treatment of high blood lipid levels (24,40). The most recent report, published in 2001 (25), introduced stricter guidelines than previously, and it emphasized the importance of four behavioral interventions: reduced intake of saturated fats and cholesterol, increased intake of plant sterols and fiber, weight reduction, and exercise. These interventions are generally similar to the recommendations of Hu and Willett summarized earlier (33).

The last two decades have seen improvement in some aspects of the U.S. diet and corresponding declines in blood lipid levels (31,32). Although most U.S. adults still eat more than the recommended 30% of total calories as fat, the country as a whole has had a major downward shift in total fat intake.

Obesity and weight are increasing at epidemic rates, however, especially among young women and children (22). This is because of other factors, such as levels of inactivity, and other aspects of the U.S. diet such as energy sources. Thus, childhood obesity has been related both to watching television (41) and to the intake of sweetened drinks (42). It has been estimated that 52 million individuals in the United States are candidates for diet therapy to reduce high blood lipid levels; however, according to recent surveys, less than 10% have been prescribed such diets (43,44).

Other Nutrients, Antioxidants, and Homocysteine

Other nutrients also have been explored regarding their impact on blood lipids. Antioxidant vitamins E, C, and β-carotene delay and reduce the oxidation of LDL-C *in vitro* and may be especially important among smokers (45–48). Observational studies in female nurses and male health professionals have reported favorable reductions in CHD risk among those who took vitamin E supplements. For example, use of vitamin E supplements was associated with a 35% reduction in CHD after adjustment for other risk factors, multiple vitamins, β-carotene, and vitamin C (46). However, intervention trials have shown no benefits of vitamin E supplementation (47), even when given in combination with vitamin C and β-carotene (49). Conversely, iron has been suggested to serve as a prooxidant in the arterial wall, thereby potentially contributing to LDL oxidation, endothelial injury, and myocardial injury (50). Studies on iron and risk for CHD are currently inconclusive.

Increased levels of homocysteine damage endothelial cells and promote arterial occlusion (51). Homocysteine is produced by the demethylation of methionine, an amino acid found mainly in animal protein foods. This conversion is dependent on folic acid, with vitamins B_6- and B_{12}-dependent enzymes playing a role as well. If these factors are reduced or inactivated, increases in homocysteine can result. Diets rich in dark green and yellow fruits and vegetables and whole grains that provide an optimal amount of 400 mg per day of folate are adequate to produce serum folate levels of 15 μmol per liter. As the therapeutic level is in the usual recommended dietary allowance range, supplementation is thought to be extremely safe, although the efficacy supplementation remains unclear. Two metaanalyses have reviewed the evidence relating homocysteine to CVD and estimated that a reduction of serum homocysteine (achievable with folic acid supplementation) would result in a reduction of risk for cardiovascular events of between 11% and 16% (52,53).

Herbal Remedies

Most physicians, including cardiologists, have little knowledge of the potential harms and benefits of herbal supplements, although they are increasingly being used by the general public (54). In 2001, $17.8 billion was spent on dietary supplements in the United States, of which $4.2 billion was for herbal remedies (55). These products can be marketed without proof of either efficacy or safety, and it is virtually impossible for the consumer to know how much of the supposed active ingredient is present, or whether they are adulterated with additives such as heavy metals and pharmaceuticals, both of which are commonly present (55). These remedies are marketed as treatment for a variety of CVDs, including hypertension, hyperlipidemia, and heart failure. Examples are garlic (used for hypertension and hyperlipidemia), hawthorn (heart failure), ginseng (hypertension and heart failure), and ginkgo (cerebrovascular disease). These and others have been reviewed by Valli and Giardina (56). Clinical trials with these agents are few and rarely placebo-controlled, although at least one randomized, double-blind trial of hawthorn (crataegus extract) is currently being conducted in patients with heart failure (57). The possibility that these agents may have adverse effects also should be borne in mind; ginseng has been reported in an open-label trial to decrease 24-hour blood pressure (58), whereas a ginseng-abuse syndrome has been reported to be associated with increased blood pressure (59). Thus, when taking a patient's history, it is important to ask about the use of herbal remedies and supplements.

OBESITY

Independent of the qualitative objectives of dietary adherence, obesity both directly and indirectly plays a major causal role in CHD and stroke (60). It contributes to dyslipidemia, diabetes, and hypertension, and its strong association with reduced physical activity further exacerbates CVD (61–63). The prevalence of obesity has increased markedly in the United States and other countries in the last 20 years; in 1978, one-fourth of individuals in the United States were overweight (defined by a body mass index [BMI] between 25 and 30 kg/m^2), and in 1990, one-third of the U.S. population was overweight—a 33% increase. The latest figures from the Centers for Disease Control show that 60% of the U.S. population is currently overweight. Similarly, the prevalence of obesity (defined as a BMI > 30 kg/m^2) has increased from 12% in 1991 to 19% in 1999 (64), and by a staggering 5.6% between 2000 and 2001 (65). It has been estimated that 300,000 deaths per year are attributable to obesity, and that it accounts for nearly 10% of national health costs (64).

Excess body weight has been causally linked with deleterious changes in the lipoprotein profile (61). Several studies document that lipoprotein abnormalities are induced with weight gain and reversed with weight loss (66,67). Particularly in obese children, even small amounts of weight loss can result in dramatic normalization of the lipid profile (67).

In summary, the research suggests that a diet reduced in total and saturated fat, lipids, *trans*-fatty acids, homocysteine, sodium, and excess calories and increased in dietary fiber (especially soluble fiber), folate, vitamin B$_6$, and ω3 fatty acids will decrease cardiovascular risk for most individuals. The resulting dietary pattern is rich in fruits and vegetables, whole grains and cereals, low-fat and skim dairy products, and fish, lean meats, and/or soy protein foods. Foods should be cooked without added saturated fat and, when necessary, cooked in a small amount of liquid vegetable oil, preferably olive, canola, or other monounsaturated nonhydrogenated liquid oil.

Prevention and Treatment of Obesity

An NIH conference on Voluntary Methods for Weight Loss and Control concluded that most existing adult obesity interventions are ineffective, with one-third to two-thirds of the weight loss being regained in 1 year and almost all of the weight being regained within 5 years (68). Training and calorie restrictions and use of packaged diet food are not effective long term. The greatest success in treating obese adults has occurred with combined dietary fat restriction, behavioral skill development, and regular exercise (69,70). The importance of exercise has been well demonstrated in a study of postmenopausal women, for whom a year-long program of modest exercise (mostly walking) resulted in a small but significant loss of weight and a more marked reduction of intraabdominal fat (71). Other effective strategies include family-oriented interventions and booster sessions (72). A number of diets such as the Atkins high-protein diet have become popular, but their role remains uncertain (73). Pharmacologic appetite suppressants and gene therapy may offer promising options in the future for some patients, but inevitably diet and energy balance must be addressed.

Factors Related to Good Dietary Adherence

In a review of 30 studies reporting changes in fat intake, Barnard and coworkers (74) summarized the factors that were commonly associated with increased adherence. These factors include:

- Stricter Limits on Fat Intake: Somewhat surprisingly, studies that set a lower limit of fat intake achieved better results.
- Frequent Monitoring: At least monthly monitoring is recommended.
- Vegetarian Diets: Adherence to a vegetarian diet more often achieved recommended fat intake than nonvegetarian approaches.
- Initial Residential Treatment: Attending a spa or similar facility that provides intensive training, monitoring, provision of food, and group support may result in better adherence to self-selected diets over the long term. However, this option may be impractical in many cases.
- Family Involvement: Involvement by family members results in improved adherence.
- Group Support: This is not mandatory, but can be helpful.
- Providing Food: Entire meals are not required, but some provision of acceptable products is important.
- Symptomatic Patients: Symptomatic patients appear to be more motivated to comply with dietary regimens; healthy patients at high risk appear to be similarly motivated.

Relevant sources of total and saturated fat and lipids should be identified before attempting to prescribe a new dietary pattern for any patient. Two large-scale, controlled, clinical trials reported that meats, fats and oils, dairy, and baked goods contributed more total and saturated fat to the diets of adults than any other food groups (75,76). Fortunately, there are now many acceptable alternatives to these high-fat foods. Substitution of lower-fat or fat-free versions for the high-fat foods (e.g., skim milk for whole milk, fat-free salad dressing for full-fat salad dressing) and adding more servings of fruits, vegetables, and grains to compensate for fewer servings of high-fat meats, dairy, and baked goods are essential components. The food industry has aggressively responded to the request for lower-fat or no-fat products. The greater challenge is achieving the desired shift to greater intake of complex carbohydrate foods.

Changing Dietary Behavior, One Patient at a Time

Van Horn and Kavey (22) have made the following suggestions, which can help to promote successful dietary adherence:

- Start with dietary assessment, then individualize the dietary intervention. Assessing baseline intake is the only way to identify the foods that are contributing the most saturated fat, lipids, and calories to a patient's diet. In adults, these are often meats, fats, and sweets. In children, it is often whole milk dairy products and sodas. In children who consume the recommended four servings of dairy foods per day, it may be possible to achieve adherence to the Step I diet (≤10% saturated fatty acid) simply by switching to skim milk and low-fat dairy products at school and at home.

- Provide clear goals. For example, the current food labels make it possible to establish a fixed "Fat Gram Goal" rather than the less precise recommendations to eat less than 30% calories from total fat. It provides each person with an objective target they can self-monitor. Similarly, establishing the goal number of servings of fruits, vegetables, and grains can further assist the individual in achieving increased fiber, folate, and antioxidant intake.

- Assess the patient's level of confidence in achieving a self-determined adherence goal. Reassess the patient's status at each subsequent visit.

- Encourage self-monitoring through the use of food records or other simplified fat/fiber goal-counting records, or both. Likewise, encourage nonfood self-rewards when goals are met.

- Promote the benefit of adopting other health-oriented behaviors. These behaviors include exercise, relaxation techniques, stress reduction, and others.

- Prevent relapse through ongoing follow-up, reassessment, and establishment of new goals.

- Patients who are referred to trained nutrition counselors may require relatively little follow-up. Comprehensive feedback on dietary adherence can be provided to the referring physician by these other health professionals for consideration in determining future treatment plans.

EXERCISE

Physical inactivity is recognized as a major risk factor for CVD, and numerous studies have shown that even mild exercise can reduce the probability of morbid events and can improve longevity. Only 22% of adults engage in 30 minutes or more of light to moderate exercise 5 or more times a week (the recommended amount for cardiovascular benefit) (77). Despite that patients with cardiac disease are seen regularly by both cardiologists and primary care physicians, most physicians do not counsel their patients about physical activity (78,79). In 2000, one of the goals of the national Health Promotion Objectives was to increase to at least 50% the number of primary care physicians who assess and advise their patients about exercise. The benefits of regular exercise are substantial and can be seen with several different types. Thus, men who run for an hour or more per week have a 42% reduction of cardiovascular risk, those who train with weights for 30 minutes have a 23% reduction, and 30 minutes per day of brisk walking is associated with an 18% reduction (80).

Two studies have investigated the efficacy of exercise counseling by physicians. The Physician-based Assessment and Counseling for Exercise (PACE) study (81) gave patients a questionnaire to assess their readiness to engage in an exercise program and spent about 5 minutes describing the program. There also was a follow-up call from a health educator. This simple intervention resulted in almost double the number of minutes of walking per week in the intervention group (average increase = 37 minutes) without any significant change in the control subjects. However, follow-up duration was only 6 weeks. A second trial, Physically Active for Life (PAL) (82), used a similar design and demonstrated a marginally significant positive effect at 6 weeks, but the effect had disappeared when assessed at 8 months. One reason for the more disappointing results in PAL may have been that the participants were older (average age, 65 years).

There are a number of methods that help to improve adherence to exercise regimens. The first method is to educate and motivate patients on the benefits of exercise. The second method is to set reasonable goals, which can be gradually increased over time. It may be helpful for the patient and the interventionist to agree on a "behavioral contract" with a date set for achieving a particular goal. Self-monitoring also is helpful (keeping a log of daily activities, for example), as well as feedback and reinforcement provided regularly to the participant. It also is important to identify barriers that may hinder progress and to find ways to overcome these. For example, if a patient has no easy means of getting to a gym, a home exercise program can be recommended.

MULTIPLE RISK FACTORS

It is clear that the behavioral and psychosocial risk factors for CVD are not distributed evenly across the population (83). Many patients have a cluster of behavioral risk factors that interact to multiply their risk for atherothrombosis. The most prominent example of this is the metabolic syndrome, which might be termed "the American Disease," which has been estimated to be present in 57 million individuals in the United States (84) and has been associated with a nearly threefold increase of cardiovascular mortality, even after adjusting for risk factors such as smoking and LDL cholesterol levels (85). The clinical management of these patients is a daunting challenge. It often is difficult to know where to start, and there is little guidance in this process from randomized controlled trials (86). Many clinicians would suggest that if the patient is a smoker, the risk reduction gained from changing that behavior is the quickest and of greatest magnitude. However, clinical experience suggests that this is not always a successful strategy. One study in a work site population of middle-aged adults suggests that exercise may be an excellent "gateway" behavioral change that may facilitate other subsequent changes in smoking and diet (87), and there is support from the weight management literature on the value of exercise as a starting point (88). The best clinical rule of thumb is to conduct a thorough assessment of the patient's behavioral and psychosocial issues and engage in a conversation with the patient regarding the prioritizing of risk behavior change and devising a strategy and a follow-up plan. Although such a comprehensive assessment is beyond the scope of traditional cardiology practice, with a team approach including psychologists, nurses, exercise specialists, and nutritionists, such a program can form the basis for cardiac rehabilitation after a cardiac event or for services in the secondary prevention setting.

PSYCHOSOCIAL RISK FACTORS

Stress, depression, anger/hostility, Type A behavior pattern, and anxiety have each been proposed as possible CVD risk factors. Each construct is theoretically and operationally distinct from the other, and the empirical support for each as a CVD risk factor varies. Furthermore, recent technology and animal experiments suggest that some of these psychosocial factors contribute to the pathogenesis of CVD, whereas others do not (89).

Stress

Stress to the lay person typically encompasses, among other issues, work and family stress, social isolation, and the occurrence of recent acute and chronic life events. Work stress, defined as a combination of having low control over the way in which work is done, but high work demands, has been implicated as a reliable and consistent predictor of progression of hypertension (in men, but not in women) (90), carotid atherothrombosis (91), cardiac events, and death (92,93). Other theorists in this area have argued that work stress is better assessed as low job control, and this index of work stress also has been found to predict future cardiac events (94,95). Marital stress (but not work stress) has been reported to worsen the prognosis of women with CHD, whereas the opposite may be true of men (96).

Social isolation (having few friends, family, or close others) and perceived lack of social support have consistently been found to predict acute myocardial infarction (MI) and cardiac death. The relative risks in the 15 most recent studies indicate a threefold mortality risk for patients with CVD who are socially isolated or perceive poor social support, or both (97). Acute mental stress (such as the sudden loss of a loved one, or an earthquake) has consistently been shown to provoke silent myocardial ischemia and to predict increased CVD incidence and death in epidemiologic studies (98,99).

Depression

Depressive symptoms and depressive disorders predict cardiac recurrence and mortality with relative risks ranging from 2.6 to 7.8 in cardiac patients (100,101). These risk ratios remain when controlling for all other known predictors of MI recurrence, and depressive symptoms predict MI recurrence in a dose–response fashion. Thus, there is consider-

able evidence that a cardiac patient who is depressed is at substantially greater risk for a future event. There is extensive evidence that depression, both clinical and subclinical, predicts the initial development of CHD (102), the recurrence of cardiac events in patients who have experienced a MI (103,104), unstable angina (105), or coronary bypass surgery (106). Currently, it is unclear whether treatment of depression will reduce the risk for recurrent events (107).

Anxiety

There have been fewer investigations of the relation of anxiety to cardiac disease and recurrence (100,101,108,109). Most studies of anxiety disorders have examined the increased occurrence of CVD mortality in psychiatric patients known to have some type of anxiety disorder (110–112), although some studies have found a relation between anxiety and sudden cardiac death in patients with CVD (97,101, 108,109,112). However, anxiety symptoms are not associated with MI recurrence in these studies. Rozanski and coworkers (97) and others (113,114) hypothesize that anxiety disorders and the associated symptoms may cause an alteration in cardiac autonomic tone through impaired vagal control or reduced heart rate variability, or both, to cause increased risk for sudden cardiac death in cardiac patients. Apart from the direct impact of anxiety on morbidity and mortality, the clinician should be alert to the presence of panic disorder in patients with CVD because of the effect on quality of life. Because many of the symptoms of panic disorder can mimic symptoms of CVD, patients with CVD can develop a particularly heightened sense of vigilance and distress in response to anxiety symptoms (115).

Type A Behavior Pattern

Friedman and Rosenman (116) first proposed that a constellation of competitive, hostile, time-pressured behaviors comprised a personality trait ("Type A") that predisposed patients to CVD. Although the Western Collaborative Group study found a twofold risk for CVD and a fivefold risk for MI recurrence by the Types A and B categorization, several more recent studies have failed to find such a difference (117). Many investigators have suggested that hostility, or the tendency to view others with suspicion and skepticism, may be the toxic component of the Type A behavior pattern, and that this component should be evaluated independently for its prediction of increased risk in cardiac patients. Four small studies of patients with CVD have found that the presence of high hostility is associated with more rapid progression of atherothrombosis, more ischemia, a faster rate of restenosis after angioplasty, and a greater probability of recurrent MI (118–120).

Psychosocial Interventions

Given the emphasis that patients with CVD place on stress and psychosocial factors contributing to their disease, and some of the recent evidence suggesting that psychosocial factors predict CVD recurrence and death, offering psychosocial interventions for patients with CVD seems reasonable. However, there are many different types of interventions aimed at different psychosocial factors and different outcomes.

Linden and coworkers (121) conducted a metaanalysis of 23 controlled psychosocial intervention studies. All patients were receiving standard medical and surgical care, and most were additionally receiving standard cardiac rehabilitation interventions. For follow-up periods of less than 2 years, there was a 41% reduction in mortality and a 46% reduction in MI recurrence as a result of psychosocial interventions. There also were significant and clinically meaningful reductions in measures of psychosocial distress (such as depression and anxiety) and in cardiovascular risk factors such as blood pressure and lipid levels. There were only three randomized trials that reported results for more than 2 years of follow-up, and in none of these trials did the effects of psychosocial intervention on mortality or MI recurrence remain significant.

There are two large, published studies of psychosocial interventions that deserve special comment. In 1997, Frasure-Smith and coworkers (122) reported favorable survival results for patients after MI (n = 229) who received a home- and telephone-based stress monitoring nursing intervention. As a result of this outcome, a larger randomized trial of a similar intervention was conducted (n = 1376). In this trial, there was no overall survival impact of the program, and in elderly women, there was a paradoxically increased cardiac and all-cause mortality rate. In the second study, Jones and West (123) conducted a randomized controlled psychological intervention trial in 2,328 patients after MI. They also found no difference in cardiac event recurrence and mortality at 12 months of follow-up. There are two important features of these two studies that may explain their negative results: Neither one actually achieved the objective of significantly reducing stress, and neither study screened patients to determine if they, in fact, exhibited any symptoms of stress or of the psychological factor that was being targeted by the intervention. Frasure-Smith (124) conducted a reanalysis of her original nursing intervention and reported that only those patients who reported distress during hospitalization benefited from the psychosocial intervention, which is consistent with our speculation that those not at risk for psychosocial difficulties will not benefit from a psychosocial intervention. However, a firm conclusion about the efficacy of psychosocial interventions in cardiac patients awaits larger, randomized trials that target those at risk. Such a trial has been conducted by the NIH (called Enhancing Recovery in Coronary Heart Disease Patients [ENRICHD]), and it examined the efficacy of cognitive–behavioral interventions on cardiac, psychosocial, and CVD risk factor outcomes in socially isolated and/or depressed patients after MI (125). The intervention did not in fact reduce recurrent events, which may be because it was relatively ineffective in improving depression scores. However, a more encouraging result was obtained with a trial

of an antidepressant drug (sertraline) in patients after an acute coronary syndrome, which showed a generally favorable outcome, although the study was not powered to detect differences in morbidity (107).

Clinical Implications

Because of the dearth of large, randomly assigned psychosocial interventions, there is not yet sufficient evidence to either recommend or caution against psychosocial interventions for altering cardiac outcomes in patients with atherothrombosis. There is, however, ample evidence that improvement in psychosocial functioning can be obtained by standardized, empirically supported therapy protocols administered by mental health professionals to patients who are at psychosocial risk. Improving the quality of life, and decreasing the psychological distress of cardiac patients, may also have other benefits. First, many of the mechanisms proposed to account for the association between psychosocial factors and CVD are behavioral. Thus, decreasing depressive symptoms is hypothesized to decrease smoking rates, increase engagement in physical activity, and improve dietary habits (126). Second, decreasing psychosocial distress is thought to increase patient compliance with physicians' recommendations, but testing these behavioral mechanisms, as well as the pathophysiologic mechanisms addressed elsewhere, again awaits larger controlled trials.

COMPLIANCE: THE KEY TO SUCCESSFUL INTERVENTIONS

The evidence for the intervention strategies reviewed in this chapter points to the inescapable conclusion that changing lifestyle habits will significantly reduce risk for CVD. No matter how efficacious the intervention strategy, however, it is doomed to failure unless the patient complies with the requirements of the intervention. Nonadherence crosses treatment regimens, age and sex groups, and socioeconomic strata, and, moreover, varies across the treatment course (127,128).

Thus, patients are asked to change their diets, eat less, exercise more, quit smoking, and reduce the amount of stress they experience and the ways in which they express their anger. These changes, however, are difficult. Knowledge of the risks is clearly insufficient to produce changes; most individuals know by now that smoking is bad for them, that their diet could be improved, and so on. These behaviors, however, are reinforcing in their own right. Smoking is pleasurable, as is the avoidance of nicotine withdrawal; high-fat foods taste good; exercise is time-consuming, and may be boring and even painful for many individuals. Coping with stress and anger means having to examine our lives in ways that may be unpleasant and even traumatic for many of us. Thus, patients with poor health habits, which may have been reinforced over the course of a lifetime, are very resistant to change. Clearly, it is vitally important to begin establishing healthy behavior habits early in life; however, parents and teachers themselves may provide poor models for these behaviors, having been acculturated in a time during which such concerns were virtually nonexistent.

Much of the adherence problem occurs early in treatment. It is estimated that 50% of patients discontinue participation in cardiac rehabilitation programs within the first year (129). The smoking cessation literature reports that 70% of post-treatment relapse occurred within the first 4 months (130). Early adherence rates are predictive of longer term adherence (130,131).

The primary care physician and the cardiologist can play a major role in helping patients to alter poor health habits and to establish healthy behaviors. The physician is regarded by many patients as a source of authority, and can have a large impact on behavior change (132). In addition, the physician can refer patients to other health professionals such as nutrition and exercise counselors and stress- and anger-reduction therapists. This often does not occur, however, for a number of reasons. First, physicians may be convinced that patients will simply not engage in healthy behaviors, or they may not be aware of how to suggest such changes, or to whom to refer these patients. Second, given the current reimbursement climate, many physicians have only a few minutes to spend with each patient.

The fact is a great deal is now known about how to maximize the likelihood that patients will adhere to healthy behavior regimens. An excellent review by Burke and colleagues (133) provides a great amount of detail concerning these regimens; a brief summary is provided below that briefly describes strategies that have been demonstrated to be successful in improving compliance to CVD behavioral intervention strategies.

Signed agreements: A written contract is drawn up between the patient and the physician or other health professional, in which a specific set of behaviors to be followed by the patient are agreed on. These should be as specific as possible (e.g., number of calories per day, number of servings of fruits and vegetables per day, number of minutes of cardiovascular-strengthening exercise, number of hours of stress-reduction therapy). The patient should maintain behavior logs.

Behavioral skill training: Patients can attend classes that teach healthy cooking, proper stretching techniques before and after exercise, or how to respond to an anger-provoking situation. Patients may have the desire to engage in healthy behaviors, but without the skills, they tend to fall back on previous behaviors.

Self-monitoring: Many patients are truly unaware of the extent to which they engage in certain unhealthy behaviors. It is useful to have patients monitor the number of cigarettes they smoke, their daily intake of fat (current packaging requirements make this relatively easy), and so on. The first step in changing behavior is to establish a baseline, so that the patient can see improvement.

Self-efficacy enhancement: A patient's confidence in his or her ability to engage in a particular behavior, such as eating in more healthy ways or exercising with a specified frequency, has been shown to be an important factor in their motivation to engage in these behaviors. Self-monitoring (discussed earlier) provides a baseline level and can then document improvement. Even small changes will increase the patient's self-efficacy for a given behavior, so that he or she is motivated to continue, which will produce additional positive changes, which then enhance self-efficacy even more, and so on. The physician, or other health professional, can focus on such improvement as a means of further enhancing the patient's self-efficacy for behavior change.

Telephone/mail contact: Reminders have been shown to have a positive effect on compliance.

Spouse/Social support: A great deal of research shows that others in the patient's social environment can have a dramatic impact on compliance. When discussing behavior change with the patient, it is helpful for such a support person to be present as well. If an exercise or diet regimen, or both, is agreed on (possibly using a contract, as described earlier), having a support person participate will significantly enhance the likelihood that the patient will adhere to the program. Having a close friend or relation, such as a spouse, continue in her or his own unhealthy behavior patterns, such as continuing to smoke or to express anger in an abusive or unhealthy manner, will hinder the possibility for change on the part of the patient.

Stages of change: Different patients may be in a different stage of readiness to change behavior (134). Thus, one patient may be ready only to begin discussing the need to stop smoking, whereas another may be ready to begin the actual quitting. Research shows that it is helpful to tailor advice to the patient's current stage of readiness. The techniques described earlier are clearly additive, more than one may be usefully combined to help the patient comply. It also is clear that, in trying, many patients will not succeed. However, it is worth noting that a patient cannot quit smoking until he or she first *tries* to quit; therefore, efforts to produce this behavior are a good investment of the physician's time.

Professional support: We strongly recommend that cardiologists develop a network of health care professionals who can support their efforts, that is, to whom patients can be referred for help with specific intervention strategies.

We are a long way from eliminating the need for medication and surgical intervention for CVD. However, we are not as far as we were only a relatively short time ago. By advocating such strategies, prescribing them, discussing them with patients, and referring patients to other health professionals, a substantial proportion of the need for more traditional interventions can be eliminated.

CONCLUSIONS

The potential applications of behavioral techniques in cardiology are enormous and largely unrealized. In principle, they can help to prevent the onset of disease, to treat it once established, and to be used in conjunction with virtually any other kind of treatment. In practice, few cardiologists have either the time or the interest to pay much attention to them, despite the demonstrated efficacy of many programs. Future success depends on better education of physicians, incorporation of a team approach, and the wider recognition of the value of behavioral interventions by third-party payers.

ACKNOWLEDGMENTS

Preparation of this review was supported by American Heart Association grant 9750544N and National Institutes of Health/National Heart, Lung and Blood Institute grants HL47540, HL67677, and HL04458.

REFERENCES.

1. McGinnis JM, Foege WH. Actual causes of death in the United States. *JAMA* 1993;270:2207–2212.
2. Fries JF, Koop CE, Beadle CE, et al. Reducing health care costs by reducing the need and demand for medical services. The Health Project Consortium. *N Engl J Med* 1993;329:321–325.
3. Lipkus IM, Barefoot JC, Williams RB, et al. Personality measures as predictors of smoking initiation and cessation in the UNC Alumni Heart Study. *Health Psychol* 1994;13:149–155.
4. Allison TG, Williams DE, Miller TD, et al. Medical and economic costs of psychologic distress in patients with coronary artery disease. *Mayo Clin Proc* 1995;70:734–742.
5. Mendes de Leon CF, Kop WJ, de Swart HB, et al. Psychosocial characteristics and recurrent events after percutaneous transluminal coronary angioplasty. *Am J Cardiol* 1996;77:252–255.
6. Rosenberg L, Kaufman DW, Helmrich SP, et al. The risk of myocardial infarction after quitting smoking in men under 55 years of age. *N Engl J Med* 1985;313:1511–1514.
7. Gordon T, Kannel WB, McGee D, et al. Death and coronary attacks in men after giving up cigarette smoking. A report from the Framingham study. *Lancet* 1974;2:1345–1348.
8. Warner KE. Smoking out the incentives for tobacco control in managed care settings. *Tob Control* 1998;7[Suppl]:S50–S54.
9. Wilhelmsen L. Effects of cessation of smoking after myocardial infarction. *J Cardiovasc Risk* 1998;5:173–176.
10. Fiore MC, Jorenby DE, Baker TB. Smoking cessation: principles and practice based upon the AHCPR Guideline, 1996. Agency for Health Care Policy and Research. *Ann Behav Med* 1997;19:213–219.
11. Fiore MC. US public health service clinical practice guideline: treating tobacco use and dependence. *Respir Care* 2000;45:1200–1262.
12. Anda RF, Remington PL, Sienko DG, et al. Are physicians advising smokers to quit? The patient's perspective. *JAMA* 1987;257:1916–1919.
13. Ockene JK. Smoking among women across the life span: prevalence, interventions, and implications for cessation research. *Ann Behav Med* 1993;15:135–148.
14. McDonald HP, Garg AX, Haynes RB. Interventions to enhance patient adherence to medication prescriptions: scientific review. *JAMA* 2002;288:2868–2879.
15. Silagy C, Mant D, Fowler G, et al. Meta-analysis on efficacy of nicotine replacement therapies in smoking cessation. *Lancet* 1994;343:139–142.
16. Jorenby DE, Leischow SJ, Nides MA, et al. A controlled trial of sustained-release bupropion, a nicotine patch, or both for smoking cessation. *N Engl J Med* 1999;340:685–691.
17. Saywell RM, Jay SJ, Lukas PJ, et al. Indiana family physician attitudes and practices concerning smoking cessation. *Indiana Med* 1996;89:149–156.
18. Goldstein MG, Niaura R, Willey-Lessne C, et al. Physicians counseling smokers. A population-based survey of patients' perceptions of health care provider-delivered smoking cessation interventions. *Arch Intern Med* 1997;157:1313–1319.
19. Keys A. *Seven countries: a multivariate analysis of death and coronary heart disease.* Cambridge, MA: Harvard University Press, 1980.
20. Levine G, Keaney J, Vita J. Cholesterol reduction in cardiovascular disease. *N Engl J Med* 1995;332:512–521.
21. The Lipid Research Clinics Coronary Primary Prevention Trial re-

22. Van Horn L, Kavey RE. Diet and cardiovascular disease prevention: what works? *Ann Behav Med* 1997;19:197–212.
23. Greenland P, Hayman L. Making cardiovascular disease prevention a reality. *Ann Behav Med* 1997;19:193–196.
24. National Cholesterol Education Program. Report of the Expert Panel on Population Strategies for Blood Cholesterol Reduction. Besthesda, MD: U.S. Department of Health and Human Services, Public Health Service, National Institutes of Health, National Heart, Lung and Blood Institute. DHHS Publication No. (NIH) 90-30-46; 1990.
25. Executive Summary of The Third Report of The National Cholesterol Education Program (NCEP) Expert Panel on Detection, Evaluation, And Treatment of High Blood Cholesterol In Adults (Adult Treatment Panel III). *JAMA* 2001;285:2486–2497.
26. Holme I. An analysis of randomized trials evaluating the effect of cholesterol reduction on total mortality and coronary heart disease incidence. *Circulation* 1990;82:1916–1924.
27. Renaud S, de Lorgeril M, Delaye J, et al. Cretan Mediterranean diet for prevention of coronary heart disease. *Am J Clin Nutr* 1995; 61[Suppl]:1360S–1367S.
28. de Lorgeril M, Renaud S, Mamelle N, et al. Mediterranean alpha-linolenic acid-rich diet in secondary prevention of coronary heart disease. *Lancet* 1994;343:1454–1459.
29. de Lorgeril M, Salen P. Alpha-linolenic acid and coronary heart disease. *Nutr Metab Cardiovasc Dis* 2004;14:162–169.
30. Singh RB, Dubnov G, Niaz MA, et al. Effect of an Indo-Mediterranean diet on progression of coronary artery disease in high risk patients (Indo-Mediterranean Diet Heart Study): a randomised single-blind trial. *Lancet* 2002;360:1455–1461.
31. Buefel RR. Assessment of the U.S diet in national nutrition surveys: national collaborative efforts and NHANES. *Am J Clin Nutr* 1994; 59[Suppl]:1645–1675.
32. Nationwide Food Consumption Survey, Continuing Survey of Food Intake by Individuals: Women 19-50 Years and Children 1-5 Years, 4 Days. Washington, DC: U.S. Department of Agriculture, Human Nutrition Information Service, 1996.
33. Hu FB, Willett WC. Optimal diets for prevention of coronary heart disease. *JAMA* 2002;288:2569–2578.
34. Ockene IS, Hebert JR, Ockene JK, et al. Effect of physician-delivered nutrition counseling training and an office-support program on saturated fat intake, weight, and serum lipid measurements in a hyperlipidemic population: Worcester Area Trial for Counseling in Hyperlipidemia (WATCH). *Arch Intern Med* 1999;159:725–731.
35. Appel LJ, Moore TJ, Obarzanek E, et al. A clinical trial of the effects of dietary patterns on blood pressure. DASH Collaborative Research Group. *N Engl J Med* 1997;336:1117–1124.
36. Sacks FM, Svetkey LP, Vollmer WM, et al. Effects on blood pressure of reduced dietary sodium and the Dietary Approches to Stop Hypertension (DASH) diet. DASH-Sodium Collaborative Research Group. *N Engl J Med* 2001;344:3–10.
37. Obarzanek E, Sacks FM, Vollmer WM, et al. Effects on blood lipids of a blood pressure-lowering diet: the Dietary Approaches to Stop Hypertension (DASH) Trial. *Am J Clin Nutr* 2001;74:80–89.
38. Ornish D, Brown SE, Scherwitz LW, et al. Lifestyle changes and heart disease. *Lancet* 1990;336:741–742.
39. Summary of the Second Report of the National Cholesterol Education Program (NCEP) Expert Panel on Detection, Evaluation, and Treatment of High Blood Cholesterol in Adults (Adult Treatment Panel II). *JAMA* 1993;269:3015–3023.
40. LaRosa JC, Hunninghake D, Bush D, et al. The cholesterol facts: a summary of the evidence relating dietary facts, serum cholesterol, and coronary heart disease: a joint statement by the American Heart Association and the National Heart, Lung, and Blood Institute. *Circulation* 1990;81:1721–1733.
41. Gortmaker SL, Must A, Sobol AM, et al. Television viewing as a cause of increasing obesity among children in the United States, 1986-1990. *Arch Pediatr Adolesc Med* 1996;150:356–362.
42. Ludwig DS, Peterson KE, Gortmaker SL. Relation between consumption of sugar-sweetened drinks and childhood obesity: a prospective, observational analysis. *Lancet* 2001;357:505–508.
43. Sempos C, Cleeman J, Carroll M, et al. Prevalence of high blood cholesterol among U.S. adults. *JAMA* 1993;269:3009–3014.
44. Schucker B, Wittes JT, Santanello NC, et al. Change in cholesterol

sults. I. Reduction in incidence of coronary heart disease. *JAMA* 1984;251:351–364.

awareness and action: results from national physician and public surveys. *Arch Intern Med* 1991;151:666–673.

45. Stone NJ. Diet, blood cholesterol levels, and coronary heart disease. *Coron Artery Dis* 1993;4:871–881.

46. Princen HM, van Poppel G, Vogelezang C, et al. Supplementation with vitamin E but not beta-carotene in vivo protects low density lipoprotein from lipid peroxidation in vitro. Effect of cigarette smoking. *Arterioscler Thromb* 1992;12:554–562.

47. Stamler MJ, Hennekens CH, Manson JE, et al. Vitamin E consumption and the risk of coronary disease in women. *N Engl J Med* 1993;328:1444–1449.

48. Steinberg D, Parthasarathy S, Carew TE, et al. Beyond cholesterol: modifications of low-density lipoprotein that increase its atherogenicity. *N Engl J Med* 1989;320:915–924.

49. MRC/BHF Heart Protection Study of antioxidant vitamin supplementation in 20,536 high-risk individuals: a randomised placebo-controlled trial. *Lancet* 2002;360:23–33.

50. Hoffman RM, Garewal HS. Antioxidants and the prevention of coronary heart disease. *Arch Intern Med* 1995;155:241–246.

51. Boushey CJ, Beresford SA, Omenn GS, et al. A quantitative assessment of plasma homocysteine as a risk factor for vascular disease. Probable benefits of increasing folic acid intakes. *JAMA* 1995; 274:1049–1057.

52. Wald DS, Law M, Morris JK. Homocysteine and cardiovascular disease: evidence on causality from a meta-analysis. *BMJ* 2002;325:1202.

53. Homocysteine and risk of ischemic heart disease and stroke: a meta-analysis. *JAMA* 2002;288:2015–2022.

54. De Smet PA. Herbal remedies. *N Engl J Med* 2002;347:2046–2056.

55. Marcus DM, Grollman AP. Botanical medicines—the need for new regulations. *N Engl J Med* 2002;347:2073–2076.

56. Valli G, Giardina EG. Benefits, adverse effects and drug interactions of herbal therapies with cardiovascular effects. *J Am Coll Cardiol* 2002;39:1083–1095.

57. Holubarsch CJ, Colucci WS, Meinertz T, et al. Survival and prognosis: investigation of Crataegus extract WS 1442 in congestive heart failure (SPICE)—rationale, study design and study protocol. *Eur J Heart Fail* 2000;2:431–437.

58. Han KH, Choe SC, Kim HS, et al. Effect of red ginseng on blood pressure in patients with essential hypertension and white coat hypertension. *Am J Chin Med* 1998;26:199–209.

59. Siegel RK. Ginseng abuse syndrome. Problems with the panacea. *JAMA* 1979;241:1614–1615.

60. Hubert HB, Feinleib M, McNamara PM, et al. Obesity as an independent risk factor for cardiovascular disease: a 26-year follow-up of participants in the Framingham Heart Study. *Circulation* 1983;67: 968–977.

61. Denke MA, Sempos CT, Grundy SM. Excess body weight: an underrecognized contributor to high blood cholesterol levels. *Arch Intern Med* 1993;153:1093–1103.

62. Medalie JH, Papier CM, Goldbourt U, et al. Major factors in the development of diabetes mellitus in 10,000 men. *Arch Intern Med* 1975; 135:811–817.

63. Tobian L. Hypertension and obesity. *N Engl J Med* 1978;298:46–60.

64. Mokdad AH, Serdula MK, Dietz WH, et al. The continuing epidemic of obesity in the United States. *JAMA* 2000;284:1650–1651.

65. Mokdad AH, Ford ES, Bowman BA, et al. Prevalence of obesity, diabetes, and obesity-related health risk factors, 2001. *JAMA* 2003;289: 76–79.

66. Wood PD, Stefanick ML, Williams PT, et al. Changes in plasma lipids and lipoproteins in overweight men during weight loss through dieting as compared with exercise. *N Engl J Med* 1988;319:1173–1179.

67. Becque MD, Katch VL, Rocchini AP, et al. Coronary risk incidence of obese adolescents: reduction by exercise plus diet intervention. *Pediatrics* 1988;81:605–612.

68. Health implications of obesity. National Institutes of Health Consensus Development Conference Statement. *Ann Intern Med* 1985; 103[Pt 2]:1073–1077.

69. O'Leary KD, Wilson GT. *Behavior therapy: application and outcome.* Englewood Cliffs, NJ: Prentice Hall, 1975.

70. Brownell KD, Heckerman C, Westlake R. The behavior control: a descriptive analysis of a large scale program. *J Clin Psychol* 1979;35:864.

71. Irwin ML, Yasui Y, Ulrich CM, et al. Effect of exercise on total and intra-abdominal body fat in postmenopausal women: a randomized controlled trial. *JAMA* 2003;289:323–330.

72. Garner D, Wooley S. Confronting the failure of behavior and dietary treatments for obesity. *Clin Psychol Rev* 1991;11:729–780.

73. Pickering TG. Diet wars: from Atkins to the Zone. Who is right? *J Clin Hypertens (Greenwich)* 2002;4:130–133.

74. Barnard N, Akhtar A, Nicholson A. Factors that facilitate compliance to lower fat intake. *Arch Fam Med* 1995;4:153–158.

75. Tinker L, Burrows E, Henry H, et al. The Women's Health Initiative: overview of the nutrition components. In: Krummel D, Kris-Etherton P, ed. *Nutrition in women's health.* Gaithersberg, MD: Aspen Publications, 1996:510–542.

76. Dolecek TA, Milas NC, Van Horn LV, et al. A long-term nutrition intervention experience: lipid responses and dietary adherence patterns in the Multiple Risk Factor Intervention Trial (MRFIT). *J Am Diet Assoc* 1986;86:752–758.

77. U.S. Department of Health and Human Services. Healthy people 2000: national health promotion and disease prevention objectives. Washington, DC: U.S. Department of Health and Human Services. DHHS Publication No. (PHS) 91 50212; 1990.

78. Wells KB, Lewis CE, Leake B, et al. The practices of general and subspecialty internists in counseling about smoking and exercise. *Am J Public Health* 1986;76:1009–1013.

79. Orleans CT, George LK, Houpt JL, et al. Health promotion in primary care: a survey of U.S. family practitioners. *Prev Med* 1985;14:636–647.

80. Tanasescu M, Leitzmann MF, Rimm EB, et al. Exercise type and intensity in relation to coronary heart disease in men. *JAMA* 2002; 288:1994–2000.

81. Calfas KJ, Long BJ, Sallis JF, et al. A controlled trial of physician counseling to promote the adoption of physical activity. *Prev Med* 1996;25:225–233.

82. Goldstein MG, Pinto BM, Lynn H, et al. Physician-based physical activity counseling for middle-aged and older adults: a randomized trial. *Ann Behav Med* 1999;21:40–47.

83. Patterson RE, Haines PS, Popkin BM. Health lifestyle patterns of U.S. adults. *Prev Med* 1994;23:453–460.

84. Ford ES, Giles WH, Dietz WH. Prevalence of the metabolic syndrome among US adults: findings from the third National Health and Nutrition Examination Survey. *JAMA* 2002;287:356–359.

85. Lakka HM, Laaksonen DE, Lakka TA, et al. The metabolic syndrome and total and cardiovascular disease mortality in middle-aged men. *JAMA* 2002;288:2709–2716.

86. Strecher V, Wang C, Derry H, et al. Tailored interventions for multiple risk behaviors. *Health Educ Res* 2002;17:619–626.

87. Emmons KM, Marcus BH, Linnan L, et al. Mechanisms in multiple risk factor interventions: smoking, physical activity, and dietary fat intake among manufacturing workers. Working Well Research Group. *Prev Med* 1994;23:481–489.

88. Foreyt JP, Goodrick GK. Factors common to successful therapy for the obese patient. *Med Sci Sports Exerc* 1991;23:292–297.

89. Rozanski A, Blumenthal JA, Kaplan J. Impact of psychological factors on the pathogenesis of cardiovascular disease and implications for therapy. *Circulation* 1999;99:2192–2217.

90. Schnall PL, Schwartz JE, Landsbergis PA, et al. A longitudinal study of job strain and ambulatory blood pressure: results from a three-year follow-up. *Psychosom Med* 1998;60:697–706.

91. Lynch J, Krause N, Kaplan GA, et al. Work place demands, economic reward, and progression of carotid atherosclerosis. *Circulation* 1997;96:302–307.

92. Theorell T, Tsutsumi A, Hallqist J, et al. Decision latitude, job strain, and myocardial infarction: a study of working men in Stockholm. The SHEEP Study Group. *Am J Public Health* 1998;88:382–388.

93. Karasek RA, Theorell T, Schwartz JE, et al. Job characteristics in relation to the prevalence of myocardial infarction in the U.S. Health Examination Survey (HESS) and the Health and Nutrition Examination Survey (HAINES). *Am J Public Health* 1988;78:910–918.

94. Johnson JV, Stewart W, Hall EM, et al. Long-term psychosocial work environment and cardiovascular mortality among Swedish men. *Am J Public Health* 1996;86:324–331.

95. Marmot MG, Bosma H, Hemingway H, et al. Contribution of job control and other risk factors to social variations in coronary heart disease incidence. *Lancet* 1997;350:235–239.

96. Orth-Gomer K, Wamala SP, Horsten M, et al. Marital stress worsens prognosis in women with coronary heart disease: the Stockholm Female Coronary Risk Study. *JAMA* 2000;284:3008–3014.

97. Rozanski A, Blumenthal JA, Kaplan J. Impact of psychological fac-

tors on the pathogenesis of cardiovascular disease and implications for therapy. *Circulation* 1999;99:2192–2217.

98. Kario K, Matsuo T, Kobayashi H, et al. Earthquake-induced potentiation of acute risk factors in hypertensive elderly patients: possible triggering of cardiovascular events after a major earthquake. *J Am Coll Cardiol* 1997;29:926–933.

99. Gabbay FH, Krantz DS, Kop WJ, et al. Triggers of myocardial ischemia during daily life in patients with coronary artery disease: physical and mental activities, anger and smoking. *J Am Coll Cardiol* 1996;27:585–592.

100. Denollet J, Brutsaert DL. Personality, disease severity, and the risk of long-term cardiac events in patients with a decreased ejection fraction after myocardial infarction. *Circulation* 1998;97:167–173.

101. Hermann C, Brand-Driehorst S, Kaminsky B, et al. Diagnosis groups and depressed mood as predictors of 22-month mortality in medical patients. *Psychosom Med* 1998;60:570–577.

102. Ferketich AK, Schwartzbaum JA, Frid DJ, et al. Depression as an antecedent to heart disease among women and men in the NHANES I study. National Health and Nutrition Examination Survey. *Arch Intern Med* 2000;160:1261–1268.

103. Barefoot JC, Helms MJ, Mark DB, et al. Depression and long-term mortality risk in patients with coronary artery disease. *Am J Cardiol* 1996;78:613–617.

104. Frasure-Smith N, Lesperance F, Talajic M. Depression and 18-month prognosis after myocardial infarction. *Circulation* 1995;91:999–1005.

105. Lesperance F, Frasure-Smith N, Juneau M, et al. Depression and 1-year prognosis in unstable angina. *Arch Intern Med* 2000;160:1354–1360.

106. Connerney I, Shapiro PA, McLaughlin JS, et al. Relation between depression after coronary artery bypass surgery and 12-month outcome: a prospective study. *Lancet* 2001;358:1766–1771.

107. Glassman AH, O'Connor CM, Califf RM, et al. Sertraline treatment of major depression in patients with acute MI or unstable angina. *JAMA* 2002;288:701–709.

108. Frasure-Smith N, Lesperance F, Talajic M. The impact of negative emotions on prognosis following myocardial infarction: is it more than depression? *Health Psychol* 1995;14:388–398.

109. Moser DK, Dracup K. Is anxiety early after myocardial infarction associated with subsequent ischemic and arrhythmic events? *Psychosom Med* 1996;58:395–401.

110. Kawachi I, Colditz GA, Ascherio A, et al. Prospective study of phobic anxiety and risk of coronary heart disease in men. *Circulation* 1994;89:1992–1997.

111. Kawachi I, Sparrow D, Vokonas PS, et al. Symptoms of anxiety and risk of coronary heart disease. The Normative Aging Study. *Circulation* 1994;90:2225–2229.

112. Kubzansky LD, Kawachi I, Weiss ST, et al. Anxiety and coronary heart disease: a synthesis of epidemiological, psychological, and experimental evidence. *Ann Behav Med* 1998;20:47–58.

113. Watkins LL, Grossman P, Krishnan R, et al. Anxiety and vagal control of heart risk. *Psychosom Med* 1998;60:498–502.

114. Kawachi I, Sparrow D, Vokonas PS, et al. Decreased heart rate variability in men with phobic anxiety (data from the Normative Aging Study). *Am J Cardiol* 1995;75:882–885.

115. Bovasso G, Eaton W. Types of panic attacks and their association with psychiatric disorder and physical illness. *Compr Psychiatry* 1999; 40:469–477.

116. Friedman M, Rosenman RH. Association of specific overt behavior pattern with blood and cardiovascular findings: blood cholesterol level, blood clotting time, incidence of arcus senilis, and clinical coronary artery disease. *JAMA* 1959;169:1286–1296.

117. Miller TQ, Turner CW, Tindale RS, et al. Reasons for the trend toward null findings in research on Type A behavior. *Psychol Bull* 1991; 110:469–485.

118. Koskenvuo M, Kaprio J, Rose RJ, et al. Hostility as a risk factor for mortality and ischemic heart disease in men. *Psychosom Med* 1988;50:330–340.

119. Hecker MH, Chesney MA, Blacks GW, et al. Coronary-prone behaviors in the Western Collaborative Group Study. *Psychosom Med* 1988;50:153–164.

120. Dembroski TM, MacDougall JM, Costa PT, et al. Components of hostility as predictors of sudden death and myocardial infarction in the Multiple Risk Factor Intervention Trial. *Psychosom Med* 1989;51: 514–522.

121. Linden W, Stossel C, Maurice J. Psychosocial interventions for patients with coronary artery disease: a meta-analysis. *Arch Intern Med* 1996;156:745–752.

122. Frasure-Smith N, Lesperance F, Prince RH, et al. Randomised trial of home-based psychosocial nursing intervention for patients recovering from myocardial infarction. *Lancet* 1997;350:473–479.

123. Jones DA, West RR. Psychological rehabilitation after myocardial infarction: multicentre randomised controlled trial. *BMJ* 1996;313: 1517–1521.

124. Frasure-Smith N. In-hospital symptoms of psychological stress as predictors of long-term outcome after acute myocardial infarction in men. *Am J Cardiol* 1991;67:121–127.

125. Berkman, LF, Blumenthal J, Burg M, et al. Effects of treating depression and low perceived social support on clinical events after myocardial infarction: the Enhancing Recovery in Coronary Heart Disease Patients (ENRICHD) Randomized Trial. *JAMA* 2003;289:3106–3116.

126. Glassman, AH, Helzer JE, Covey LS, et al. Smoking, smoking cessation, and major depression. *JAMA* 1990;264:1546–1549.

127. Stewart RB, Caranasos GJ. Medication compliance in the elderly. *Med Clin North Am* 1989;73:1551–1563.

128. Dunbar-Jacob J, Mortimer-Stephens MK. Treatment adherence in chronic disease. *J Clin Epidemiol* 2001;54[Suppl 1]:S57–S60.

129. Ades PA. Cardiac rehabilitation and secondary prevention of coronary heart disease. *N Engl J Med* 2001;345:892–902.

130. Brandon TH, Tiffany ST, Obremski KM, et al. Postcessation cigarette use: the process of relapse. *Addict Behav* 1990;15:105–114.

131. Westman EC, Behm FM, Simel DL, et al. Smoking behavior on the first day of a quit attempt predicts long-term abstinence. *Arch Intern Med* 1997;157:335–340.

132. Caggiula A, Watson J, Kuller L, et al. Cholesterol-lowering intervention program: effect of the Step I diet in community office practices. *Arch Intern Med* 1996;156:1205–1213.

133. Burke LE, Dunbar-Jacob JM, Hill MN. Compliance with cardiovascular disease prevention strategies: a review of the research. *Ann Behav Med* 1997;19:239–263.

134. Prochaska JO, DiClemente CC, Norcross JC. In search of how people change. Applications to addictive behaviors. *Am Psychol* 1992;47: 1102–1114.

Subject Index

Page numbers followed by "f" denote figures; those followed by "t" denote tables

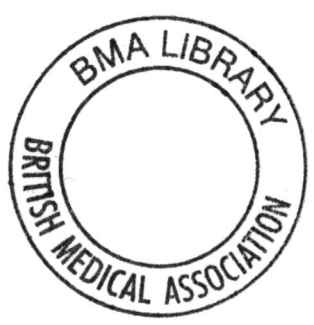